PSYCHOPHARMACOLOGY

The Third Generation of Progress

In association with the
American College of Neuropsychopharmacology

PSYCHOPHARMACOLOGY
The Third Generation of Progress

In association with the
American College of Neuropsychopharmacology

Editor

Herbert Y. Meltzer, M.D.
Director, Laboratory of Biological Psychiatry
Douglas Danford Bond Professor of Psychiatry
Case Western Reserve University
Cleveland, Ohio

Associate Editors

Basic Neurobiology

Joseph T. Coyle, M.D.
Johns Hopkins School of Medicine
Baltimore, Maryland

Irwin J. Kopin, M.D.
Intramural Research Program, National Institute of
Neurological and Communicative Disorders and Stroke
Bethesda, Maryland

Biological Psychiatry

William E. Bunney, Jr., M.D.
University of California, Irvine
Irvine, California

Kenneth L. Davis, M.D.
Bronx Veterans Administration Medical Center
Bronx, New York

Clinical Psychopharmacology

Charles R. Schuster, Ph.D.
National Institute of Drug Abuse
Bethesda, Maryland

Richard I. Shader, M.D.
Tufts University School of Medicine
Boston, Massachusetts

George M. Simpson, M.D.
Medical College of Pennsylvania
Philadelphia, Pennsylvania

Raven Press New York

Raven Press, 1185 Avenue of the Americas, New York, New York 10036

Made in the United States of America

Library of Congress Cataloging-in-Publication Data

Psychopharmacology: the third generation of
progress.

Includes bibliographies and index.
1. Psychopharmacology—Congresses. 2. Neurobiology—
Congresses. 3. Biological psychiatry—Congresses.
I. Meltzer, Herbert Y. [DNLM: 1. Psychopharmacology—
history. 2. Psychotropic Drugs.   QV 11.1 P974]
RC483.P7784 1987   615′.78   85-43136
ISBN 0-88167-273-4

9 8 7 6 5 4 3 2 1

Preface

Psychopharmacology: The Third Generation of Progress is similar to the two preceding editions, in that it provides a definition of and treatise about the domain of psychopharmacology as understood by the American College of Neuropsychopharmacology (ACNP): to utilize drugs and other chemical agents to understand neural function, to prevent and treat mental illness, drug abuse, and alcoholism; and to understand how nontherapeutic psychoactive drugs and natural substances alter human mood, mentation, motor activity, endocrine, and other centrally mediated functions. A comparison of this edition with its predecessors reveals the remarkable developments in psychopharmacology, and why publication of a new volume is both desirable and timely. The explosion of information—a consequence of the huge increase in the number of neuroscientists and a more modest but nonetheless significant increase in the number of clinical investigators—has made some changes in format desirable. The book is divided into three major sections: Basic Neurobiology, Biological Psychiatry, and Clinical Psychopharmacology. The authors have, for the most part, eschewed textbook-type presentations in favor of critical evaluation of the most worthy research findings of the past nine years, often concluding with suggestions for future research.

This edition will help to educate scientists and clinicians who are encountering psychopharmacology for the first time, to broaden the knowledge of those already in the field, and to stimulate further research through an emphasis on the crucial areas of psychopharmacology where the opportunity for advancement is greatest.

Herbert Y. Meltzer

Acknowledgments

The Editor would like to take this opportunity to thank the ACNP council for the trust placed in him with regard to this project, to the Associate Editors whose tremendous efforts made it possible to organize and edit this book, and to Mrs. Diane Mack, his secretary, whose good spirits, organizational skills, and tireless energies provided the means to actually get the job done.

American College of Neuropsychopharmacology and the History of This Edition

The American College of Neuropsychopharmacology (ACNP) has grown in its 25 years of existence from a membership of about 50 to approximately 400. From inception, its members recognized that psychopharmacology was a dynamic field that would need to incorporate as well as catalyze developments in diverse areas of clinical and basic neuroscience were it to fulfill its inherent mission.

The common bond of the pioneering, as well as subsequent ACNP members, is an active research or administrative interest in understanding the structure and function of the central nervous system and its behavioral output in health and illness. Publication of symposia from its annual meeting as well as periodic review volumes has been a key function of the ACNP.

This edition is a product of the college membership. The Editor and Associate Editors identified the major areas of psychopharmacology and chose Section Editors to oversee the writing of chapters by contributing authors who were agreed on by all three editorial levels. Most, but not all, first authors are ACNP members.

The first edition of *Psychopharmacology, A Review of Progress 1957–1967* was published in 1968 by the U.S. Government Printing Office. The 116 papers included in it constituted the proceedings of the sixth annual meeting of the ACNP. Eight sessions were held at that meeting, and in each of these, either original work or reviews of a significant area of psychopharmacology, were addressed. The second edition, entitled *Psychopharmacology: A Generation of Progress* was prepared in 1976 to mark the twentieth year of the National Institute of Mental Health's Psychopharmacology Research Branch and the fifteenth year of the ACNP. The book was 1,731 pages long and contained 149 chapters prepared by 241 contributing authors, most of whom were members or guests of the ACNP. This, the third edition contains 184 chapters prepared by 271 contributors and is 1,840 pages long. The explosion of information, reflected in the exponential growth of original and review publications in refereed journals, is evidence that this edition could have been much longer. Its length has been restricted by the editorial decision to limit the contents to a single volume.

Comparison of the two preceding editions with the present one reveals that the major concerns of both basic and clinical psychopharmacology have not changed, but the sophistication of the methods with which these problems are addressed has been enhanced in many areas. The basic neuroscience addressed in the first edition described the key outlines of the chemical neuroanatomy and biochemical pharmacology of the central nervous system, electrophysiological indicators of drug action, the biology of memory and learning and central nervous system toxicology. Clinical sections were devoted to the anxiolytic agents, the antidepressants, antipsychotic agents, and psychotomimetics. A section was devoted to alcohol and drug addiction. In still other sections, considerable attention was paid to research methodology in human psychopharmacology and to ethical and legal considerations of research in the area of brain and behavior.

The Second Edition updated newer research findings in these areas and added the emerging areas of research with receptors, the neuropeptides, neuroendocrinology, and animal models. Clinical sections dealing with the psychopharmacology of neurological, pediatric, and geriatric disorders were introduced. The major outlines of some of the current theories of the etiology of schizophrenia and depression were described.

This edition will help to prepare the current generation of psychopharmacologists to understand the contributions of molecular biology.

Introduction

The first section of *Psychopharmacology: The Third Generation of Progress,* Basic Neurobiology, provides extensive consideration of the anatomy, biochemistry, and physiology of monoaminergic systems, including excitatory amino acids. Key findings in receptors of monoamines and other neurotransmitters as well as ion channels are thoroughly reviewed. This area has made enormous progress in the past decade, influencing psychotropic drug development and contributing greatly to the understanding of the mechanism of action of psychotropic drugs and the role of neurotransmitters in neuropsychiatric disorders. Neurotoxins, which have emerged as potential etiological agents in Parkinson's disease and schizophrenia as well as research tools are emphasized.

Molecular biology, like neuroscience, at the cutting edge of modern medicine, is systematically considered for the first time in the section on Neuropeptides. The focus is on the biosynthesis of peptides from prohormone precursors. Molecular biology has already provided important information about receptor structure and the identification of the genes involved in Huntington's chorea and Alzheimer's disease. The search for the genes that cause mental illnesses is well underway. Success in this endeavor will clarify the crucial nosological questions that continue to elude definitive resolution. Identification of the genes that predispose to mental illness is likely to eventually transform the professional lives of psychopharmacologists even more profoundly than the discovery of the currently available psychotropic drugs, by assisting in diagnosis and, possibly, by permitting novel approaches to prevention and treatment by manipulation of genes. Molecular biology has enabled us to begin to understand how genes, acting in concert, lead to the development of the brain we so indelicately perturb with drugs, how genes, when required, guide the remodeling of the brain, and how genes ultimately orchestrate the complex sequence of biochemical events that underlie our thoughts and feelings.

The emphasis of this volume on the Biological Psychiatry section reflects the value placed by modern psychopharmacology on the pathophysiology of mental illness as well as normal brain functioning, in order to understand and monitor drug action, to identify predictors of drug response, and to help in the search for clues as to new strategies for drug development. This section provides overviews of the biological theories of the etiology of affective disorders (and aggression), schizophrenia, childhood behavioral disorders (including mental retardation), dementia and anxiety, and the somatic treatments that have proven to be most effective, including mood-altering therapies, such as carbamazepine and light therapy. A molecular biological approach to mental retardation is also described. For now, the genetic, biochemical, neuroendocrine, electrophysiologic, neuroanatomic, and brain imaging studies appear best organized along disease lines. This is true even though many of the biological markers thus far identified appear to be nonspecific vulnerability factors, and that key neurotransmitters, such as dopamine, serotonin, norepinephrine, and γ-aminobutyric acid (GABA), appear to have crucial roles in a wide range of neuropsychiatric disorders.

The chapters in this section reveal steady progress in translating the new knowledge of basic science (described in the first part of this edition) into clinical studies. Thus, the relevance of receptor subtypes, neurotransmitter interactions, neuropeptides, and new information about the structural organization of the brain for biological hypotheses have begun to be tested by clinical neuroscientists in both pre- and postmortem studies. Clinical tools, such as ligand binding procedures, receptor assays, high-pressure liquid chromatography, and positron emission tomography that have emerged from the basic scientist's laboratory have been developed rapidly. Advances in the techniques of PET scanning will no doubt provide knowledge about normal and abnormal brain functioning not possible through other means. When coupled with other brain imaging techniques, such as magnetic resonance imaging and, perhaps, brain electrical activity mapping, it may be possible to discern the abnormal interactions of regions of the brain that lead to pathological behaviors.

The section on Clinical Psychopharmacology is the largest component of the triad that comprises psychopharmacology. The state of the art of developing new psychopharmacologic means to treat the affective disorders, schizophrenia, geriatric psychiatric disorders, anxiety, childhood psychiatric disorders, and eating disorders is considered. Subsections consider pharmacokinetics, major drug side effects, the effects of psychotropic drugs on various functions in normal humans and infrahuman species, alcohol and drug abuse, and the development of new drugs from the viewpoint of industry and federal regulators. The importance of assessment methods using standardized interviewing schedules and explicit diagnostic criteria is highlighted throughout the clinical psychopharmacology section.

Thirty years ago, psychiatric theory and practice were dominated by psychodynamic psychoanalytic thinking. Psychopharmacology emerged empirically, and its demonstrable results quickly made it competitive. Early debates between the advocates of the two schools of thought were often acrimonious. Psychoanalytic practitioners called psychotropic drugs "chemical straight jackets," and some psychopharmacologists predicted the demise of psychological approaches. Over the past 30 years, both extremes have been proven to be wrong. This edition demonstrates much of the change in psychopharmacology. Less evident (in this edition) are the changes in psychosocial treatments, which now include group, family, and social modalities, as well as cognitive therapy, desensitization, and behavioral shaping. Although some degree of competitiveness will continue to be inevitable, it becomes increasingly clear that both modalities will continue to be necessary: psychotropic drugs to reduce vulnerability and psychological treatments to enhance coping skills. Currently, both have limitations. Fortunately, the therapeutic armamentaria of both types of treatment modalities are constantly increasing. It seems likely that the future will bring more precise and powerful drugs. It is equally likely that improving clinical and laboratory skills will permit the development of biological and behavioral markers that will permit early detection and intervention. Biological and psychological approaches should no longer be competitive but, rather, cooperative in the interest of the mentally ill. The issue for the future should no longer be one of pharmacotherapy versus psychotherapy but rather, which of the large number of available drugs should be employed for what conditions and with which of the increasing number of psychosocial interventions to enhance prevention and treatment.

The Psychopharmacology section presents the steady progress that has been made in developing new drug strategies in many conditions, even though truly novel approaches that are of dramatic therapeutic advantage have not yet been developed. Alprazolam and buspirone for the treatment of anxiety, carbamazepine for the treatment of affective disorders, clonidine for the treatment of opioid withdrawal states and perhaps other addictions are examples of novel drugs that were not present a decade ago, but have since gained some measure of acceptance in clinical practice. The use of lithium to potentiate antidepressant action in nonresponders is an excellent example of the application of basic neuroscience knowledge to a therapeutic problem. Progress in treating schizophrenia has been least impressive. Some of the reasons for this are discussed by Hollister and Klerman in the introductory and final subsections. The novel approaches to drug treatment of schizophrenia described by Tamminga and Gerlach in Chapter 116 are not without benefit for some patients. Atypical neuroleptic drugs, such as clozapine and the benzamides, may yet find their way into broader clinical use for schizophrenia. This decade has been one of fine tuning our ability to use already-available drugs discovered in affective disorders, anxiety disorders, childhood disorders, schizophrenia, eating disorders, and sleep disturbances. The chapters concerning these topics describe the results of important studies that target predictors of response, duration of treatment, dosage schedule, side effects, withdrawal effects, etc., that are of great importance for safe and optimal drug utilization.

The tremendous importance the ACNP attaches to the understanding of all aspects of substance abuse for the well-being of our society is evidenced by the attention given in this edition to biological and psychopharmacologic studies of ethanol, cocaine, opioids, marijuana, phencyclidine, tobacco, and the phenylisopropylamines. There has been a vast increase in our knowledge of opioid mechanisms and how phencyclidine acts at a basic level. Clinical studies of alcohol, cocaine, and tobacco abuse as documented here have become much more sophisticated and have produced important data on risk factors and reward mechanisms.

This edition includes a chapter on teaching psychopharmacology. The ACNP has developed a model curriculum to facilitate educating medical students, residents, and mental health professionals of all disciplines in psychopharmacology. The philosophy behind this curriculum and its major elements are described.

Psychopharmacology began as an empirical science that quickly demonstrated clinical utility. Ultimately, its progress will be judged on the basis of its capacity to prevent and to treat neurological and psychiatric illnesses effectively. Both the prospects for and the impediments to rapid progress are impressive. We have much reason to believe that insights offered by the new technologies of neuroscience and molecular biology will lead to better and more specific diagnosis and treatment. New discoveries about multiple receptors for the monoamine neurotransmitters and the mechanisms involved in the regulation of their sensitivity and number will likely lead to new drugs with greater specificity and fewer adverse side effects. Methods probably will be developed for introducing neuropeptides or smaller molecules, which possess their activity, into the brain. Linkage studies and the methods of the molecular biologist may well permit the identification of absent or aberrant genes that predispose people to genetic vulnerability to the major mental illnesses. Environmental factors that convert the genotype to the phenotype will likely be better understood. Scientifically, prospects for the future are rosy.

Yet, impediments are formidable. Clearly, the major mental illnesses differ from the simple illnesses that are caused by the toxic or deficiency states in which medicine has had its greatest successes. Rather, they resemble those illnesses, like hypertension and some forms of diabetes or cancer, in which appropriate regulation of physiological processes is either inadequate or overwhelmed by environmental events. Animal models for the major human mental illnesses are still inadequate, and even these are threatened by political movements that oppose animal experimentation. Uncertain economic forecasts and fragile international relationships make for an unstable economy and national priorities that compete with those of health-related research. Even in the health research area, there is competition between mental health research and the physical illnesses that are still a burden to society. Along with the brilliant advances in science, there is emerging an antiscience manifested by a resurgence of creationism, fundamentalism, and intense nationalism.

Given these opposing forces and the intense competition among them, it is hazardous to predict where we will be a decade from now. On the optimistic assumption that all will go well in the basic and clinical neurosciences, we may confidently predict that in the next decade there will be very many surprises.

Herbert Y. Meltzer
Morris A. Lipton

Contents

BASIC NEUROBIOLOGY

Ethical Precepts and Research Strategies in Psychopharmacology

Neuroanatomic and Neurochemical Mechanisms

Amino Acids and Acetylcholine

Receptors

Neurotoxins

Neuropeptides

BIOLOGICAL PSYCHIATRY

Biology of Affective Disorders and Aggression

Biology of Schizophrenia

Biology of Psychiatric Disorders of Childhood

Biology of Dementia

CLINICAL PSYCHOPHARMACOLOGY

Clinical Psychopharmacology of Schizophrenia

Geriatric Psychopharmacology: Treatment Update

Treatment of Anxiety

Treatment of Childhood Disorders

Treatment of Eating Disorders

General Topics

Effects of Psychotropic Drugs on Major Functions in Normal Humans and Infrahuman Species

Alcohol and Drug Abuse

Development of New Drugs

Future Directions

Contributors

Sigurd Ackerman   *Cornell University Medical College, New York Hospital/Westchester Division, 21 Bloomingdale Road, White Plains, New York 10605*

Joshua E. Adler   *Department of Neurology, Division of Developmental Neurology, Cornell University Medical College, 515 East 71st Street, New York, New York 10021*

G. K. Aghajanian   *Department of Psychiatry, Yale University School of Medicine, 34 Park Street, New Haven, Connecticut 06508*

Bernard W. Agranoff   *Neuroscience Laboratory, 1103 East Huron, Ann Arbor, Michigan 48109*

Huda Akil   *Department of Psychiatry, Mental Health Research Institute, University of Michigan, Ann Arbor, Michigan 48109-0720*

Paul Ambrosini   *University Hospitals of Cleveland, Hanna Pavilion, 2040 Abington Road, Cleveland, Ohio 44106*

Nancy Andreasen   *Department of Psychiatry, The University of Iowa, 500 Newton Road, Iowa City, Iowa 52242*

George W. Arana   *Department of Psychiatry and Behavioral Sciences, University of South Carolina, 171 Ashley Avenue, Charleston, South Carolina 29425-0742*

Marie Åsberg   *Departments of Psychiatry and Psychology, Karolinska Hospital, S-104 01 Stockholm, Sweden*

Charanjit S. Aulakh   *Laboratory of Clinical Science, National Institute of Mental Health, National Institutes of Health Clinical Center, 10/3D41, Bethesda, Maryland 20892*

Efrain Azmitia   *Department of Biology, 1009 Main Building, New York University, 100 Washington Square East, New York, New York 10003*

Ross J. Baldessarini   *Mailman Research Center, McLean Hospital, 115 Mill Street, Belmont, Massachusetts 02178*

Robert L. Balster   *Department of Pharmacology and Toxicology, Medical College of Virginia, Virginia Commonwealth University, Richmond, Virginia 23298-0001*

Thomas A. Ban   *Division of Psychopharmacology, Vanderbilt University, Medical Arts Building, Room 242, Nashville, Tennessee 37212*

Jack David Barchas   *Department of Psychiatry and Behavioral Sciences, Stanford University Medical Center, Room R-321, Stanford, California 94305*

James E. Barrett   *Department of Psychiatry, Uniformed Service University Health Science, 4301 Jones Bridge Road, Bethesda, Maryland 20814*

Raymond T. Bartus   *Department of CNS Research, Lederle Laboratories of American Cyanamid, Pearl River, New York 10965*

Michel Baudry   *Center for the Neurobiology of Learning and Memory, University of California, Irvine, Irvine, California 92717*

Reina Bendayan   *University of Toronto, 33 Russell Street, Toronto, Ontario, Canada M5S 2S1*

Philip A. Berger   *Department of Psychiatry and Behavioral Sciences, TD-114, Stanford University School of Medicine, Stanford, California 94305*

Wade H. Berrettini   *National Institute of Mental Health, National Institutes of Health, 9000 Rockville Pike, 10/3N218, Bethesda, Maryland 20892*

J. Thomas Bigger, Jr.   *Departments of Medicine and Pharmacology, College of Physicians and Surgeons, 630 West 168th Street, New York, New York 10032*

Garth Bissette   *Assistant Professor of Psychiatry, Duke University Medical Center, Box 3859, Durham, North Carolina 27710*

Ira B. Black   *Department of Neurology, Cornell University Medical College, 515 East 71st Street, New York, New York 10021*

Barry Blackwell   *Department of Psychiatry, University of Wisconsin Medical School, Milwaukee Clinical Campus, 950 North Twelfth Street, Milwaukee, Wisconsin 53233*

Floyd E. Bloom   *10666 North Torrey Pines Road, La Jolla, California 92037*

Malcolm B. Bowers, Jr.   *Department of Psychiatry, Yale University School of Medicine, 25 Park Street, New Haven, Connecticut 06519*

George R. Breese   *Biological Sciences Research Center, University of North Carolina at Chapel Hill, Chapel Hill, North Carolina 27514*

John C. S. Breitner   *Department of Psychiatry, Duke University Medical Center, Durham, North Carolina 27710*

Andrew W. Brotman   *ACC 707, Massachusetts General Hospital, 32 Fruit Street, Boston, Massachusetts 02114*

Monte S. Buchsbaum   *Department of Psychiatry and Human Behavior, University of California, Irvine, Medical Sciences I, Room D-404, Irvine, California 92717*

Benjamin S. Bunney   *Departments of Psychiatry and Pharmacology, Yale University School of Medicine, New Haven, Connecticut 06510*

William E. Bunney, Jr.   *California College of Medicine, University of California, Irvine, Medical Science I Building, Room D-440, Irvine, California 92717*

Nelson Butters   *Department of Psychiatry, M-003, University of California, San Diego, La Jolla, California 92093*

Magda Campbell   *Department of Psychiatry, New York University Medical Center, 550 First Avenue, New York, New York 10016*

Arvid Carlsson   *Department of Pharmacology, University of Göteborg, P.O. Box 33031, S-400 33, Göteborg, Sweden*

William T. Carpenter, Jr.   *Maryland Psychiatric Research Center, Box 3235, Baltimore, Maryland 21228*

Daniel E. Casey   *Psychiatry Service (116A), Veterans Administration Medical Center, P.O. Box 1034, Portland, Oregon 97207*

Dennis S. Charney   *Connecticut Mental Health Center, 34 Park Street, New Haven, Connecticut 06508*

Roland D. Ciaranello   *Department of Psychiatry and Behavioral Science, Stanford University School of Medicine, Stanford, California 94305*

Paula J. Clayton   *Department of Psychiatry, University of Minnesota, 393 Mayo, 420 Delaware Street, Southeast Minneapolis, Minnesota 55455*

C. Robert Cloninger   *Departments of Psychiatry and Genetics, Washington University School of Medicine and Jewish Hospital, 216 South Kingshighway Boulevard, St. Louis, Missouri 63110*

Donald J. Cohen   *Child Study Center, Yale University School of Medicine, P.O. Box 3333, New Haven, Connecticut 06510*

Robert Cohen   *Laboratory of Cerebral Metabolism, National Institute of Mental Health, National Institutes of Health, Bethesda, Maryland 20892*

Michael Comb   *Department of Molecular Biology, Massachusetts General Hospital, 32 Fruit Street, Boston, Massachusetts 02114*

P. Jeffrey Conn   *Department of Pharmacology, Yale University School of Medicine, Sterling Hall of Medicine, New Haven, Connecticut 06510-8066*

Thomas B. Cooper   *Analytical Psychopharmacy, New York State Psychiatric Institute, Orangeburg, New York 10962*

Erminio Costa   *FIDIA-Georgetown Institute for the Neurosciences, Georgetown Medical School, Washington, D.C. 20007*

Carl W. Cotman   *Department of Psychobiology, University of California, Irvine, California 92717*

Joseph T. Coyle   *The Johns Hopkins University School of Medicine, Meyer 4-163, 600 North Wolfe Street, Baltimore, Maryland 21205*

Ian Creese   *Department of Neuroscience M-008, University of California, San Diego, La Jolla, California 92093*

Thomas H. Crook   *Western Psychiatric Institute and Clinic, 3811 O'Hara Street, Pittsburgh, Pennsylvania 15213*

Christine Cross   *3317 Shadyside Lane, Chesapeake, Virginia 23321*

George Cuff   *Lilly Research Laboratories, Lilly Corporate Center, Indianapolis, Indiana 46285*

Edward I. Cullen   *Department of Neuroscience, The Johns Hopkins University School of Medicine, 725 North Wolfe Street, Baltimore, Maryland 21205*

Neal R. Cutler   *Center for Aging and Alzheimer's, 8500 Wilshire Boulevard, Lobby Suite, Beverly Hills, California 90211*

Michael Davidson   *Department of Psychiatry, Bronx Veterans Administration Medical Center, 130 West Kingsbridge Road, Bronx, New York 10468*

Kenneth L. Davis   *Psychiatry Service (116A), Bronx Veterans Administration Medical Center, 130 West Kingsbridge Road, Bronx, New York 10468*

Reginald Dean   *Department of CNS Research, Lederle Laboratories of American Cyanamid, Pearl River, New York 01965*

Lynn DeLisi *Clinical Neurogenetics Branch, National Institute of Mental Health, National Institutes of Health, Room 3N/220, Building 10, Bethesda, Maryland 20892*

William C. Dement *Association of Sleep Disorders Centers, Stanford University School of Medicine, Sleep Disorders Center TD-114, Stanford, California 94305*

Ariel Y. Deutch *Departments of Pharmacology and Psychiatry, Yale University School of Medicine, 333 Cedar Street, New Haven, Connecticut 06510*

David De Wied *Rudolf Magnus Institute for Pharmacology, Vondellaan 6, 3521 GD Utrecht, The Netherlands*

Cheryl F. Dreyfus *Department of Neurology, Division of Developmental Neurology, Cornell University Medical College, 515 East 71st Street, New York, New York 10021*

Bernard Dubnick *Cardiovascular—CNS Research Section, American Cyanamid Company, Lederle Laboratories, Pearl River, New York 10965*

David L. Dunner *Department of Psychiatry and Behavioral Sciences, Harborview Medical Center, 325 Ninth Avenue, Seattle, Washington 98104*

James H. Eberwine *Nancy Pritzker Laboratory of Behavioral Chemistry, Department of Psychiatry and Behavioral Sciences, Stanford University School of Medicine, Stanford, California 94305*

Burr Eichelman *Department of Psychiatry, University of Wisconsin Medical School, 600 Highland Avenue, Madison, Wisconsin 53792*

Betty A. Eipper *Department of Neuroscience, The Johns Hopkins University School of Medicine, 725 North Wolfe Street, Baltimore, Maryland 21205*

Everett H. Ellinwood, Jr. *Department of Psychiatry, Duke University Medical Center, Box 3870, Durham, North Carolina 27710*

Jean Endicott *Research Assessment and Training Unit, New York State Psychiatric Institute, 722 West 168th Street, New York, New York 10032*

S. J. Enna *Departments of Pharmacology, Neurobiology, and Anatomy, University of Texas Medical School/Houston, P.O. Box 20708, Houston, Texas 77025*

Christopher J. Evans *Nancy Pritzker Laboratory of Behavioral Chemistry, Department of Psychiatry and Behavioral Sciences, Stanford University School of Medicine, Stanford University Medical Center, Stanford, California 94305*

Kym F. Faull *Nancy Pritzker Laboratory of Behavioral Chemistry, Department of Psychiatry and Behavioral Sciences, Stanford University School of Medicine, Stanford University Medical Center, Stanford, California 94305*

John L. Falk *Department of Psychology, Rutgers University, New Brunswick, New Jersey 08903*

William E. Falk *Department of Psychiatry, Massachusetts General Hospital, 32 Fruit Street, Boston, Massachusetts 02114*

David A. Feingold *Institute for Study of Human Issues, 210 South 13th Street, Philadelphia, Pennsylvania 19107*

Hans C. Fibiger *Department of Psychiatry, University of British Columbia, Vancouver, British Columbia, Canada, V6T 1W5*

Max Fink *Department of Psychiatry and Behavioral Sciences, School of Medicine, State University of New York at Stony Brook, Long Island, New York 11794*

Marian W. Fischman *Department of Psychiatry and Behavioral Sciences, The Johns Hopkins University School of Medicine, 600 North Wolfe Street, Baltimore, Maryland 21205*

Abraham Fisher *Department of Organic Chemistry, Israel Institute for Biological Research, P.O. Box 19, Ness Ziona 70450, Israel*

Seymour Fisher *Department of Psychiatry and Behavioral Sciences, University of Texas, Medical Branch, 219 Administration Annex D-41, Galveston, Texas 77550*

Stephen K. Fisher *Neuroscience Laboratory, 1103 East Huron, Ann Arbor, Michigan 48109*

Charles Flicker *Department of CNS Research, Lederle Laboratories of American Cyanamid, Pearl River, New York 10965*

Frode Fonnum *Norwegian Defince Research Establishment, Division for Environmental Toxicology, P.O. Box 25, N-2007 Kjeller, Norway*

William J. Freed *Preclinical Neuroscience Section, Neuropsychiatry Branch, National Institute of Mental Health, National Institutes of Health, St. Elizabeth's Hospital, Washington, D.C. 20032*

Daniel X. Freedman *Department of Psychiatry and Behavioral Sciences, NPI/UCLA, 760 Westwood Plaza, Los Angeles, California 90024*

Wilma J. Friedman *Department of Neurology, Division of Developmental Neurology, Cornell University Medical College, 515 East 71st Street, New York, New York 10021*

Abby J. Fyer *Department of Psychiatry, College of Physicians and Surgeons, Columbia University, 722 West 168th Street, New York, New York 10032*

Minna Fyer *The New York Hospital, 525 East 68th Street, New York, New York 10021*

Donald M. Gallant *Department of Psychiatry, Tulane Medical School, 1430 Tulane Avenue, New Orleans, Louisiana 70112*

James C. Garbutt *Clinical Research Unit, Dorthea Dix Hospital, Raleigh, North Carolina 27611*

Blynn L. Garland-Bunney *Department of Psychiatry, Medical Sciences I D440, University of California, Irvine, Irvine, California 92717*

Nancy A. Garrick *Laboratory of Clinical Science, National Institute of Mental Health, National Institutes of Health Clinical Center, 10/3D41, Bethesda, Maryland 20892*

Alan J. Gelenberg *The Arbour Hospital, 49 Robinwood, Jamaica Plain, Massachusetts 02138*

Joel Gelernter *National Institutes of Health, Building 10, Room 3N216, Bethesda, Maryland 20892*

Jes Gerlach *SCT Hans Hospital, Department H, DK-4000, Roskilde, Denmark*

Nino-Murcia German *Stanford Sleep Disorders Clinic, 211 Quarry Road, Stanford, California 94305*

Elliot S. Gershon *Clinical Neurogenetics, Intramural Research Program—National Institute of Mental Health, National Institutes of Health, 9000 Rockville Pike, 10/3N218, Bethesda, Maryland 20892*

Sylvia C. Gerson *812 Cape View Drive, Fort Meyers, Florida 33907*

Elsa-Grace Giardina *Department of Medicine, College of Physicians and Surgeons, Columbia University, 630 West 168th Street, New York, New York 10032*

James Gibbs *Cornell University Medical College, New York Hospital/Westchester Division, 21 Bloomingdale Road, White Plains, New York 10605*

J. Christian Gillin *Department of Psychiatry 116A, University of California, San Diego, San Diego Veterans Administration Medical Center, 3350 LaJolla Village Drive, San Diego, California 92161*

Alexander H. Glassman *New York State Psychiatric Institute, 722 West 168th Street, New York, New York 10032*

Richard A. Glennon *Department of Medical Chemistry, School of Pharmacy, Medical College of Virginia, Virginia Commonwealth University, Richmond, Virginia 23298*

Ira Glick *Payne Whitney Clinic, New York Hospital-Cornell Medical Center, 525 East 68th Street, New York, New York 10021*

Nick E. Goeders *Department of Pharmacology, Louisiana State University, Medical Center, P.O. Box 33932, Shreveport, Louisiana 71130*

Philip W. Gold *Biological Psychiatry Branch, National Institute of Mental Health, National Institutes of Health, Building 10, Room 3S239, 9000 Rockville Pike, Bethesda, Maryland 20892*

Morton E. Goldberg *Biomedical Research, Stuart Pharmaceuticals, ICI Americas, Concord Pike and Murphy Road, Wilmington, Delaware 19897*

Solomon C. Goldberg *Department of Psychiatry Medical College of Virginia, MCV Box 710, Richmond, Virginia 23298*

Lynn R. Goldin *National Institute of Mental Health, National Institutes of Health, 10/3N218, 9000 Rockville Pike, Bethesda, Maryland 20892*

Menek Goldstein *New York University Medical Center, 550 First Avenue, New York, New York 10016*

Frederick K. Goodwin *Mental Health Intramural Research Program, National Institute of Mental Health, National Institutes of Health, Building 10, Room 4N-224, 9000 Rockville Pike, Bethesda, Maryland 20205*

Jack M. Gorman *Department of Psychiatry, New York State Psychiatric Institute, College of Physicians and Surgeons, 722 West 168th Street, New York, New York 10032*

Jack Peter Green *Department of Pharmacology, Mount Sinai School of Medicine, One Gustave L. Levy Place, New York, New York 10029*

David J. Greenblatt *Department of Psychiatry, Tufts University School of Medicine, Box 1007, 171 Harrison Avenue, Boston, Massachusetts 02111*

Lloyd A. Greene *Department of Pharmacology, New York University Medical Center, Room M493, 550 First Avenue, New York, New York 10016*

Roland R. Griffiths *Departments of Psychiatry and Behavioral Sciences, and Neuroscience, The Johns Hopkins School of Medicine, 720 Rutland Avenue, Baltimore, Maryland 21205*

C. Thomas Gualtieri *Department of Psychiatry, School of Medicine, University of North Carolina, Chapel Hill, North Carolina 27514*

Alessandro Guidotti *FGIN, 3900 Reservoir Road, Room SE 402, Washington, D.C. 20007*

Sally Guthrie *Laboratory of Clinical Studies, DICBR, National Institute on Alcohol Abuse and Alcoholism, National Institutes of Health, 9000 Rockville Pike, Bethesda, Maryland 20205*

Katherine A. Halmi *Department of Psychiatry, Cornell University Medical College, New York Hospital/Westchester Division, 21 Bloomingdale Road, White Plains, New York 10605*

Israel Hanin *Departments of Pharmacology and Experimental Therapeutics, Loyola University Stritch School of Medicine, 2160 South First Avenue, Maywood, Illinois 60153*

John A. Harvey *Departments of Psychology and Pharmacology, The University of Iowa, Iowa City, Iowa 52242*

Edward M. Hawes *College of Pharmacy, University of Saskatchewan, Saskatoon, Saskatchewan, Canada S7N 0W0*

George R. Heninger *Yale University, 34 Park Street, New Haven, Connecticut 06508*

Fritz A. Henn *Department of Psychiatry and Behavioral Sciences, Health Science Center, State University, New York, New York 11794-8101*

Edward Herbert *(Deceased)*

Barrie Hesp *Stuart Pharmaceuticals, Division of ICI Americas Inc., Concord Pike and Murphy Road, Wilmington, Delaware 19897*

Robert M. A. Hirschfeld *Division of Clinical Research, National Institute of Mental Health, National Institutes of Health, Parklawn Building, Room 10-C-24, 5600 Fishers Lane, Rockville, Maryland 20857*

Carolyn C. Hoch *Western Psychiatric Institute and Clinic, 3811 O'Hara Street, Pittsburgh, Pennsylvania 15213*

Paula L. Hoffman *Section on Receptor Mechanisms, Laboratory of Physiologic and Pharmacologic Studies, National Institute on Alcohol Abuse and Alcoholism, 12501 Washington Avenue, Rockville, Maryland 20852*

Gerard E. Hogarty *Western Psychiatric Institute and Clinic, 3811 O'Hara Street, Pittsburgh, Pennsylvania 15213*

Tomas Hökfelt *Department of Histology, Karolinska Institutet, P.O. Box 60400, S-104 01 Stockholm, Sweden*

Vicky Holets *Department of Neurological Surgery, Research Laboratories, University of Miami, 1600 Northwest 10th Avenue, Miami, Florida 33136*

Leo Hollister *Senior Medical Investigator, Veterans Administration Center (151-H), 3801 Miranda Avenue, Palo Alto, California 94304*

Daniel W. Hommer *Clinical Neuroscience Branch, National Institute of Mental Health, National Institutes of Health, Building 10, Room 4N214, Bethesda, Maryland 20892*

Heide Hörtnagl *Institute of Biochemical Pharmacology, Borschkeg 8a, A-1090 Vienna, Austria*

John W. Hubbard *College of Pharmacy, University of Saskatchewan, Saskatoon, Saskatchewan, Canada S7N 0W0*

Thomas R. Insel *P.O. Box 289, Building 110, Poolesville, Maryland 20837*

Barry L. Jacobs *Department of Psychology, Princeton University, Princeton, New Jersey 08544*

Jerome H. Jaffe   *NIDA Research Addiction Center, 4940 Eastern Avenue, Baltimore, Maryland 21224*

Aaron Janowsky   *Department of Psychiatry, Vanderbilt University School of Medicine, Nashville, Tennessee 37232*

David S. Janowsky   *Department of Psychiatry, School of Medicine, University of North Carolina, Chapel Hill, North Carolina 27514*

Robin B. Jarrett   *The University of Texas, Health Science Center at Dallas, 5323 Harry Hines Boulevard, Dallas, Texas 75235*

Murray E. Jarvik   *Psychopharmacology Unit, Veterans Administration Medical Center, West Los Angeles, California 90074*

Lissy F. Jarvik   *Neuropsychiatric Institute and Hospital, Center for the Health Sciences, 760 Westwood Plaza, Los Angeles, California 90024*

Donald J. Jenden   *Department of Pharmacology and Brain Research, University of California, Center for Health Science, Los Angeles, California 90024*

David C. Jimerson   *Laboratory of Clinical Science, Intramural Research Program, National Institute of Mental Health, National Institutes of Health, Building 10, Room 3S231, Bethesda, Maryland 20892*

Chris-Ellyn Johanson   *Office of Scientific Affairs, American Psychological Association, 1200 Seventeenth Street, Northwest, Washington, D.C. 20036*

Olle Johansson   *Department of Histology, Karolinska Institute, Box 60400, S-104 01 Stockholm, Sweden*

Kenneth M. Johnson, Jr.   *Department of Pharmacology and Toxicology, University of Texas Medical Branch, Galveston, Texas 77550*

Reese T. Jones   *Drug Dependence Clinical Research Center, Langley Porter Psychiatric Institute, University of California, San Francisco, San Francisco, California 94145*

Lewis L. Judd   *Department of Psychiatry, M-003 University of California, San Diego, La Jolla, California 92093*

John M. Kane   *Department of Psychiatric Research, Hillside Hospital, 75-59 263rd Street, Glen Oaks, New York 11004*

Charles Kaufmann   *New York State Psychiatric Institute, 722 West 168th Street, New York, New York 10032*

Kenneth S. Kendler   *Departments of Psychiatry and Human Genetics, Medical College of Virginia, MCV P.O. Box 710, Richmond, Virginia 23298*

John S. Kennedy   *Valleview Provincial Hospital, 500 Lougheed Highway, Port Coquitlam, British Columbia, Canada*

Donald F. Klein   *College of Physicians and Surgeons, Columbia University, 722 West 168th Street, New York, New York 10032*

Rachel Gittelman Klein   *New York State Psychiatric Institute, Columbia University, 722 West 168th Street, New York, New York 10032*

Gerald L. Klerman   *Payne Whitney Clinic, New York Hospital-Cornell Medical Center, 525 East 68th Street, New York, New York 10021*

Peter J. Knott   *Box 1230, Mount Sinai School of Medicine, Fifth Avenue at 99th Street, New York, New York 10029*

B. Kenneth Koe *Department of Pharmacology, Pfizer Inc., Groton, Connecticut 06340*

Irwin J. Kopin *National Institute of Neurological and Communicative Disorders and Stroke, National Institute of Mental Health, Building 10, Room 5N214, Bethesda, Maryland 20205*

Elarien D. Korchinski *Department of Family Medicine, University Hospital, Saskatoon, Saskatchewan, Canada S7N 0W0*

Mary Jeanne Kreek *The Rockefeller University, 1230 York Avenue, New York, New York 10021*

Michael J. Kuhar *Department of Neuroscience, National Institute on Drug Abuse, 4940 Eastern Avenue, Baltimore, Maryland 21224*

David J. Kupfer *Western Psychiatric Institute and Clinic, 3811 O'Hara Street, Pittsburgh, Pennsylvania 15213*

Neil M. Kurtz *Bristol-Myers Company, P.O. Box 5100, 5 Research Parkway, Wallingford, Connecticut 06492*

Edmund F. LaGamma *Department of Pediatrics, School of Medicine, State University of New York at Stony Brook, Stony Brook, New York 11794-8111*

S. Lal *Department of Psychiatry, Montreal General Hospital, 1650 Cedar Avenue, Montreal, Quebec, Canada H3G 1A4*

Barrie Lancaster *Department of Pharmacology, University of California, San Francisco, California 94143*

Elizabeth A. Lane *National Institute on Alcohol Abuse and Alcoholism, 9000 Rockville Pike, Building 10, Bethesda, Maryland 20892*

Salomon Z. Langer *Department of Biology, Laboratoires d'Etudes et de Recherches Synthélabo, 58 Rue de la Glacière, 75013 Paris, France*

Louis Lasagna *Sackler School of Graduate Biomedical Sciences, Tufts University, 136 Harrison Avenue, Boston, Massachusetts 02111*

Paul Leber *Division of Neuropharmacological Drug Products, National Center of Drugs and Biologics, HFN-120 FDA, Rockville, Maryland 20857*

James F. Leckman *I-269 Sterling Hall of Medicine, Child Study Center, Yale University School of Medicine, P.O. Box 3333, New Haven, Connecticut 06510*

Louis Lemberger *Departments of Pharmacology and Psychiatry, Lilly Laboratory for Clinical Research, Wishard Memorial Hospital, Indianapolis, Indiana 46202*

Bernard Lerer *Director of Research, Jerusalem Mental Health Center, Ezrath Nashim, Jerusalem, Israel*

Leonard I. Leven *Box 1230, Mount Sinai School of Medicine, Fifth Avenue at 99th Street, New York, New York 10029*

Steven M. Leventer *Departments of Pharmacology and Experimental Therapeutics, Loyola University of Chicago, Stritch School of Medicine, 2160 South First Avenue, Maywood, Illinois 60153*

Jerome Levine *Maryland Psychiatric Research Center, School of Medicine, University of Maryland, P.O. Box 21247, Baltimore, Maryland 21228*

Douglas F. Levinson *Medical College of Pennsylvania, Eastern Pennsylvania Psychiatric Institute, 3200 Henry Street, Philadelphia, Pennsylvania 19129*

Jeffrey A. Lieberman *Long Island Jewish Medical Center, Hillside Hospital, 75-59 263rd Street, Glen Oaks, New York 11004*

Michael R. Liebowitz *722 West 168th Street, New York, New York 10032*

Markku Linnoila *National Institute on Alcohol Abuse and Alcoholism, National Institutes of Health, 9000 Rockville Pike, Building 10, Room 3B19, Bethesda, Maryland 20892*

K. G. Lloyd *Laboratoires d'Etudes et de Recherches, Synthélabo, 31, Avenue Paul Vaillant Couturier, 92220 Bagneux, France*

Peter T. Loosen *Veterans Administration Medical Center, Room 116-A, 1310 24th Avenue South, Nashville, Tennessee 37203*

Miklos F. Losonczy *Department of Psychiatry, Bronx Veterans Administration Medical Center, 130 West Kingsbridge Road, Bronx, New York 10468*

Martin T. Lowy *Department of Psychiatry, Case Western Reserve University, 2040 Abington Road, Cleveland, Ohio 44106*

Gary S. Lynch *Department of Psychobiology, University of California, Irvine, Irvine, California 92717*

Daniel V. Madison *Department of Physiology, Yale University, School of Medicine, New Haven, Connecticut 06510*

Richard E. Mains *Department of Neuroscience, The Johns Hopkins University School of Medicine, 725 North Wolfe Street WBSB 914, Baltimore, Maryland 21205*

Sal Mannuzza *Department of Psychiatry, College of Physicians and Surgeons, Columbia University, 722 West 168th Street, New York, New York 10032*

Victor May *Department of Neuroscience, The Johns Hopkins University School of Medicine, 725 North Wolfe Street, WBSB 914, Baltimore, Maryland 21205*

Bjorn Meister *Department of Histology, Karolinska Institute, Box 60400, S-104 01, Stockholm, Sweden*

Tor Melander *Department of Histology, Karolinska Institute, Box 60400, S-104 01, Stockholm, Sweden*

Erling Mellerup *Psychochemistry Institute, Rigshospitalet, 9 Blegdamsvej, DK-2100 Copenhagen Ø, Denmark*

Nancy K. Mello *Alcohol and Drug Abuse Research Center, Harvard Medical School— McLean Hospital, 115 Mill Street, Belmont, Massachusetts 02178*

Herbert Y. Meltzer *Case Western Reserve University School of Medicine, Hanna Pavilion, 2040 Abington Road, Cleveland, Ohio 44106*

Jack H. Mendelson *Alcohol and Drug Abuse Research Center, Harvard Medical School— McLean Hospital, 115 Mill Street, Belmont, Massachusetts 02178*

Wallace B. Mendelson *Section on Sleep Studies, National Institute of Mental Health, National Institutes of Health, Parklawn Building, 5600 Fishers Lane, Rockville, Maryland 20857*

Kamal K. Midha *Colleges of Pharmacology and Medicine, University of Saskatchewan, Saskatoon, Saskatchewan, Canada S7N 0W0*

Teresa A. Milner *Department of Neurology, Cornell University Medical College, New York, New York 10021*

James E. Mitchell   *Department of Psychiatry, University of Minnesota Medical School, Box 393 Mayo, 420 Delaware Street, Southeast, Minneapolis, Minnesota 55455*

Hans Mohler   *Medical Research Department, F. Hoffmann-La Roche, Basel, Switzerland*

Richard C. Mohs   *Psychiatry Service (116A), Bronx Veterans Administration Medical Center, 130 West Kingsbridge Road, Bronx, New York 10468*

Daniel T. Monaghan   *Department of Psychobiology, University of California, Irvine, Irvine, California 92717*

Kenneth E. Moore   *Departments of Pharmacology and Toxicology, Michigan State University, East Lansing, Michigan 48824*

John E. Morley   *Department of Medicine, Geriatric Research Education and Clinical Center, University of California, Sepulveda Veterans Administration Medical Center, 16111 Plummer Street, Sepulveda, California 91343*

Paolo L. Morselli   *Laboratoires d'Etudes et de Recherches Synthélabo, 58 Rue de la Glacière, 75013 Paris, France*

Robert A. Mueller   *Department of Anesthesiology, School of Medicine, University of North Carolina, Chapel Hill, North Carolina 27514*

Dennis L. Murphy   *Laboratory of Clinical Science, National Institute of Mental Health, National Institutes of Health, Clinical Center, Room 3D41, 9000 Rockville Pike, Bethesda, Maryland 20892*

Adavi S. N. Murthy   *(Deceased)*

Gordon McKay   *College of Pharmacy, University of Saskatchewan, Saskatoon, Saskatchewan, Canada S7N 0W0*

William T. McKinney   *Department of Psychiatry, University of Wisconsin Medical School, Clinical Science Center, 600 Highland Avenue, Madison, Wisconsin 53792*

Charles B. Nemeroff   *Department of Psychiatry, Pharmacology and Center for Aging and Human Development, Duke University Medical Center, Durham, North Carolina 27710*

Jeffrey H. Newcorn   *Box 1229, Mount Sinai School of Medicine, Fifth Avenue at 99th Street, New York, New York 10029*

Karl M. Newell   *Department of Physical Education, University of Illinois, 117 Freer Hall, Urbana, Illinois 61801*

Paul Newhouse   *Department of Behavioral Biology, Walter Reed Army Institute of Research, Building 189 Neuropsychiatry Division, Washington, D.C. 20307*

Roger A. Nicoll   *Department of Pharmacology, S-1210, University of California, San Francisco, California 94143*

Arlene M. Nikaido   *Department of Psychiatry, Duke University Medical Center, Box 3870, Durham, North Carolina 27710*

G. Nino-Murcia   *Stanford Sleep Disorders Clinic, 211 Quarry Road, Stanford, California 94305*

John Nurnberger, Jr.   *Indiana University Medical Center, Institute of Psychiatric Research, 791 Union Drive, Indianapolis, Indiana 46223*

David S. Olton   *Department of Psychology, The Johns Hopkins University, Baltimore, Maryland 21218*

John E. Overall   *Department of Psychiatry and Behavioral Sciences, University of Texas Medical School, P.O. Box 20708, Houston, Texas 77225*

Ken A. Paller   *San Diego Veterans Administration Medical Center, La Jolla, California 92093*

Steven M. Paul   *National Institutes of Health, Room 4N214, Bethesda, Maryland 20892*

Barry S. Pallotta   *Department of Pharmacology, University of North Carolina School of Medicine, Chapel Hill, North Carolina 27514*

Barbara L. Parry   *University of San Diego T-004, La Jolla, California 92093*

Gavril W. Pasternak   *The Cotias Laboratory of Neuro-Oncology, Memorial Sloan-Kettering Cancer Center, 1275 York Avenue, New York, New York 10021*

Kennerly S. Patrick   *Department of Medicinal Chemistry, College of Pharmacy, University of Tennessee, Memphis, Tennessee 38163*

Cort A. Pedersen   *Department of Psychiatry, University of North Carolina, School of Medicine, Chapel Hill, North Carolina 27514*

William Pendlebury   *Department of Pathology, The University of Vermont, Burlington, Vermont 05405*

Daniel P. Perl   *Division of Neuropathology, Mount Sinai Medical Center, Annenberg 15-76, One Gustave L. Levy Place, New York, New York 10029*

Stephen J. Peroutka   *Departments of Neurology and Pharmacology, Stanford University Medical Center, Stanford, California 94305*

Elaine K. Perry   *Department of Neuropathology, Regional Neurological Centre, Newcastle General Hospital, Newcastle Upon Tyne NE4 6BE, England*

Virginia Pickel   *Cornell University Medical College, 411 East 69th Street, New York, New York 10021*

Per Plenge   *Psychochemistry Institute, Rigshospitalet, 9, Blegdamsvej, DK-2100, Copenhagen Ø, Denmark*

D. A. Plotkin   *Department of Psychiatry, University of California, Los Angeles, Los Angeles, California 90024*

Robert M. Post   *Biological Psychiatry Branch, National Institute of Mental Health, National Institutes of Health, Building 10, Room 3N212, 9000 Rockville Pike, Bethesda, Maryland 20892*

Pamela Potter   *Departments of Pharmacology and Experimental Therapeutics, Loyola University of Chicago, Stritch School of Medicine, 2160 South First Avenue, Maywood, Illinois 60153*

William Z. Potter   *Section of Clinical Pharmacology, Laboratory of Clinical Science, National Institute of Mental Health, National Institutes of Health, Building 10, Room 2D46, Bethesda, Maryland 20892*

Arthur J. Prange, Jr.   *Department of Psychiatry, University of North Carolina, School of Medicine, Chapel Hill, North Carolina 27514*

Robert F. Prien   *Psychopharmacology Research Branch, National Institute of Mental Health, National Institutes of Health, Parklawn Building 10C 06, 5600 Fishers Lane, Rockville, Maryland 20857*

Joaquim Puig-Antich *Department of Psychiatry, University of Pittsburgh, Pittsburgh, Pennsylvania 15213*

Ole J. Rafaelsen *Psychochemistry Institute, Rigshospitalet, 9, Blegdamsvej, DK-2100, Copenhagen Ø, Denmark*

Judith L. Rapoport *Unit on Childhood Psychiatry, National Institute of Mental Health, National Institutes of Health, Building 10, Room 3N-204, Bethesda, Maryland 20205*

K. Rasmussen *Department of Psychiatry, Yale University School of Medicine, 34 Park Street, New Haven, Connecticut 06508*

D. E. Redmond, Jr. *Neurobehavioral Laboratory and Department of Psychiatry, Yale University School of Medicine, P.O. Box 3333, New Haven, Connecticut 06510*

James F. Resch *ICI Pharmaceuticals Group, Division of ICI Americas Inc., Concord Pike and Murphy Road, Wilmington, Delaware 19879*

Charles F. Reynolds, III *Department of Psychiatry, University of Pittsburgh School of Medicine, Pittsburgh, Pennsylvania 15213*

Howard M. Rhoades *Department of Psychiatry and Behavioral Sciences, University of Texas Medical School, P.O. Box 20708, Houston, Texas 77225*

George A. Ricaurte *Department of Neurology C338, Stanford University, Stanford, California 94305*

Karl Rickels *Department of Psychiatry, University of Pennsylvania, University Hospital, 203 Piersol Building, 3400 Spruce Street, Philadelphia, Pennsylvania 19104*

Mark A. Riddle *Child Study Center, Yale University School of Medicine, P.O. Box 3333, New Haven, Connecticut 06510*

Arthur Rifkin *Mount Sinai Services, 79-01 Broadway, Elmhurst, New York 11373*

Samuel Craig Risch *University of California, San Diego, School of Medicine, La Jolla, California 92093*

Arthus H. Roach *% J.-M. Matthieu, Laboratoire de Neurochimie, Service de Pediatrie, Centre Hospitalier Universitaire Vaudois, CH-1011 Lausanne, Switzerland*

Donald S. Robinson *Bristol-Myers Company, Pharmaceutical, Research and Development Division, Wallingford, Connecticut 06492*

William R. Roeske *Departments of Internal Medicine and Pharmacology, University of Arizona, College of Medicine, Tucson, Arizona 85724*

Steven P. Roose *Department of Psychiatry, New York State Psychiatric Institute, 722 West 168th Street, New York, New York 10032*

Norman E. Rosenthal *National Institutes of Health, Building 10, Room 4S 239, Bethesda, Maryland 20502*

Robert H. Roth *Department of Pharmacology and Psychiatry, Yale University School of Medicine, New Haven, Connecticut 06510*

Walton J. Roth *Psychiatry Service (116A3), Veterans Administration Medical Center, Palo Alto, California 94304*

John Rotrosen *Psychiatry Service, New York Veterans Administration Medical Center, 408 First Avenue, New York, New York 10010*

Peter P. Roy-Byrne   *University of Washington, School of Medicine, Department of Psychiatry, RP #10, Seattle, Washington 98195*

Robert T. Rubin   *Department of Psychiatry, Harbor UCLA Medical Center, Torrance, California 90509*

David R. Rubinow   *Unit of Peptide Studies, BPB, National Institute of Mental Health, National Institutes of Health, Room 4C418, 9000 Rockville Pike, Bethesda, Maryland 20892*

Matthew V. Rudorfer   *Laboratory of Clinical Science, National Institutes of Health, Building 10, Room 2D46, 9000 Rockville Pike, Bethesda, Maryland 20892*

John A. Rush   *Affective Disorders Unit, Department of Psychiatry, The University of Texas, Health Science Center at Dallas, 5323 Harry Hines Boulevard, Dallas, Texas 75235*

David A. Sack   *National Institutes of Health, Building 10, Room 4S 239, Bethesda, Maryland 20502*

David P. Salmon   *Department of Psychiatry, University of California, San Diego, La Jolla, California 92093*

Carl Salzman   *Massachusetts Mental Health Center, Harvard Medical School, 74 Fenwood Road, Boston, Massachusetts 02115*

Elaine Sanders-Bush   *Departments of Pharmacology and Psychiatry, Vanderbilt University School of Medicine, Nashville, Tennessee 37232*

Christine A. Sannerud   *Department of Psychiatry and Behavioral Sciences, The Johns Hopkins University, School of Medicine, 720 Rutland Avenue, Baltimore, Maryland 21205*

Sheryl Sato   *Department of Health and Human Services, Public Health Services, National Institutes of Health, Building 6, Room 339, Bethesda, Maryland 20892*

Daisy Schalling   *Department of Psychiatry, Karolinska Hospital, S-104 01 Stockholm, Sweden*

Sigmund Schildcrout   *Lilly Research Laboratories, Lilly Corporate Center, Indianapolis, Indiana 46285*

Nina R. Schooler   *National Institute of Mental Health, National Institutes of Health, Room 10C06, 5600 Fishers Lane, Rockville, Maryland 20857*

Marc A. Schukit   *San Diego Veterans Administration Medical Center, 3350 La Jolla Village Drive, San Diego, California 92161*

Charles R. Schuster   *National Institute on Drug Abuse, Parklawn Building, Room 10-03, 5600 Fishers Lane, Rockville, Maryland 20857*

Edward Schweizer   *University of Pennsylvania, Psychopharmacology Research and Treatment Clinic, 133 South 36th Street, Suite 402, Philadelphia, Pennsylvania 19104*

Audrey Seasholtz   *The Oregon Health Science University, Vollum Institute for Advanced Biomedical Research, 3181 Southwest Sam Jackson Park Road, Portland, Oregon 97201*

Lewis S. Seiden   *Department of Pharmacological and Physiological Sciences, The University of Chicago, 947 East 58th Street, Chicago, Illinois 60637*

E. M. Sellers   *Departments of Pharmacology and Medicine, University of Toronto, 33 Russell Street, Toronto, Ontario, Canada M5S 2S1*

Susan R. Sesack *Department of Pharmacology, Yale University School of Medicine, 333 Cedar Street, New Haven, Connecticut 06510*

Richard Shader *Department of Psychiatry, Tufts University School of Medicine, New England Medical Center Hospital, 171 Harrison Avenue, Boston, Massachusetts 02111*

Richard C. Shelton *Department of Psychiatry, Vanderbilt University Medical Center, Medical Center North, Room A-2215, Nashville, Tennessee 37232*

Larry J. Siever *Department of Psychiatry-116A, Bronx Veterans Administration Medical Center, 130 West Kingsbridge Road, Bronx, New York 10468*

Carolyn R. Sikes *Payne Whitney Clinic, New York Hospital-Cornell Medical Center, 525 East 68th Street, New York, New York 10021*

Nancy L. Silva *Laboratory of Neurophysiology, National Institutes of Health, NINCDS, Building 36, Room 2C02, Bethesda, Maryland 20892*

George M. Simpson *Medical College of Pennsylvania, 3200 Henry Avenue, Philadelphia, Pennsylvania 19129*

Samuel G. Siris *Department of Psychiatry, Mount Sinai Medical Center, One Gustave L. Levy Place, New York, New York 10029*

Phil Skolnick *National Institutes of Health, Building 8, Room 103, Bethesda, Maryland 20892*

Gerard Smith *Eating Disorders Institute, New York Hospital, Cornell Medical Center, 21 Bloomingdale Road, White Plains, New York 10605*

R. Michael Snider *Neuroscience Laboratory, Departments of Biological Chemistry and Pharmacology, University of Michigan, Ann Arbor, Michigan 48104–1687*

Solomon H. Snyder *Department of Neuroscience, The Johns Hopkins University School of Medicine, 725 North Wolfe Street, Baltimore, Maryland 21205*

Bert Spilker *Burroughs Welcome Company, 3030 Cornwallis Road, Research Triangle Park, North Carolina 27709*

Robert L. Sprague *Institute for Child Behavior and Development, University of Illinois, 51 Getty Drive, Champaign, Illinois 61820*

J. S. Sprouse *Department of Psychiatry, Yale University School of Medicine, 34 Park Street, New Haven, Connecticut 06508*

Larry R. Squire *Department of Psychiatry, San Diego Veterans Administration Medical Center, La Jolla, California 92093*

Peter E. Stokes *Payne Whitney Clinic, New York Hospital-Cornell Medical Center, 525 East 68th Street, New York, New York 10021*

Fridolin Sulser *Departments of Pharmacology and Psychiatry, Vanderbilt University School of Medicine, Nashville, Tennessee 37232*

Trey Sunderland *Laboratory of Clinical Science, National Institute of Mental Health, NIH Clinical Center, 10/3D41, Bethesda, Maryland 20892*

Boris Tabakoff *Laboratory of Physiologic and Pharmacologic Studies, National Institute on Alcohol Abuse and Alcoholism, National Institutes of Health Clinical Center, Building 10, Room 3C103, Bethesda, Maryland 20892*

Carol A. Tamminga *Maryland Psychiatric Research Center, P.O. Box 21247, Baltimore, Maryland 21228*

Pierre Tariot   *Monroe Community Hospital, 435 East Henrietta Road, Rochester, New York 14603*

Kazuhiko Tatemoto   *Nancy Pritzker Laboratory of Behavioral Chemistry, Department of Psychiatry and Behavioral Sciences, Stanford University School of Medicine, Stanford University Medical Center, Stanford, California 94305*

Joy L. Taylor   *Veterans Administration Medical Center, 116A3, 3801 Miranda, Palo Alto, California 94304*

Gary Thomas   *The Oregon Health Science University, Vollum Institute for Advanced Biomedical Research, 3181 Southwest Sam Jackson Park Road, Portland, Oregon 97201*

Karen Thompson   *Unit of Cognitive Studies, National Institute of Mental Health, National Institutes of Health, Bethesda, Maryland 20892*

Barbara Thorne   *The Oregon Health Science University, Vollum Institute for Advanced Biomedical Research, 3181 Southwest Sam Jackson Park Road, Portland, Oregon 97201*

Jared R. Tinklenberg   *Veterans Administration Medical Center, 116A, 3801 Miranda Avenue, Palo Alto, California 94304*

Kenneth E. Towbin   *Child Study Center, Yale University School of Medicine, P.O. Box 3333, New Haven, Connecticut 06510*

Lil Träskman-Bendz   *Department of Psychiatry, Karolinska Hospital, S-104 01 Stockholm, Sweden*

E. H. Uhlenhuth   *Department of Psychiatry, University of New Mexico, 2400 Tucker, Northeast, Albuquerque, New Mexico 87131*

Karen L. Valentino   *Nancy Pritzker Laboratory of Behavioral Chemistry, Department of Psychiatry and Behavioral Sciences, Stanford University School of Medicine, Stanford University Medical Center, Stanford, California 94305*

Daniel P. van Kammen   *Psychiatry Service, Veterans Administration Medical Center (11), Highland Drive, Pittsburgh, Pennsylvania 15206*

Jan M. Van Ree   *Rudolf Magnus Institute of Pharmacology, Medical Faculty, University of Utrecht, Vondellaan 6, 3521 GD Utrecht, The Netherlands*

Steven R. Vincent   *Division of Neurological Sciences, Department of Psychiatry, University of British Columbia, 2255 Westbrook Mall, Vancouver, B.C. Canada V6T 2A1*

Anna Wägner   *Department of Psychiatry and Psychology, Karolinska Hospital, 104 01 Stockholm, Sweden*

John T. Walkup   *Child Study Center, Yale University School of Medicine, P.O. Box 3333, New Haven, Connecticut 06510*

Thomas J. Walsh   *Department of Psychiatry, Rutgers University, Busch Campus, New Brunswick, New Jersey 08903*

Timothy B. Walsh   *College of Physicians and Surgeons, Columbia University, 722 West 168th Street, New York, New York 10032*

Mark Watson   *Department of Pharmacology, New Jersey Medical School, University of Medicine and Dentistry, 100 Bergen Street, Newark, New Jersey 07103*

Stanley J. Watson   *Mental Health Research Institute, University of Michigan, 205 Washtenaw Place, Ann Arbor, Michigan 48109-0720*

Thomas A. Wehr   *National Institutes of Health, Building 10, Room 4S 239, Bethesda, Maryland 20502*

Daniel R. Weinberger   *Section on Clinical Neuropsychiatry, NIMH-Intramural Research Program, Saint Elizabeth's Hospital, William A. White Building, Room 500, Washington, D.C. 20032*

Herbert Weingartner   *Department of Psychology, George Washington University, Washington, D.C. 20052*

Albert Weissman   *Department of Pharmacology, Pfizer Central Research, Pfizer Inc., Groton, Connecticut 06340*

Myrna M. Weissman   *Department of Psychiatry, College of Physicians and Surgeons, Columbia University, 722 West 168th Street, Box 14, New York, New York 10032*

Gary L. Wenk   *Department of Psychology, The Johns Hopkins University, Baltimore, Maryland 21218*

Michael Williams   *J-206A CIBA-Geigy, 556 Morris Avenue, Summit, New Jersey 07901*

Gail Winger   *Department of Pharmacology, M6322 Medical Science I, University of Michigan Medical School, Ann Arbor, Michigan 48109*

Marina E. Wolf   *Laboratory of Neurochemistry, Center for Cell Biology, Sinai Hospital of Detroit, 6767 West Outer Drive, Detroit, Michigan 48235*

Adam Wolkin   *New York Veterans Administration Medical Center/116A, 408 First Avenue, New York, New York 10010*

Dona L. Wong   *Department of Psychiatry and Behavioral Sciences, Stanford University School of Medicine, Stanford, California 94305*

James H. Woods   *Departments of Pharmacology and Psychology, University of Michigan Medical School, Ann Arbor, Michigan 48109*

William L. Woolverton   *Department of Pharmacological and Physiological Science, University of Chicago, 947 East 58th Street, Chicago, Illinois 60637*

Richard J. Wyatt   *St. Elizabeth's Hospital, William A. White Building, Room 536, Washington, D.C. 20032*

Henry I. Yamamura   *Departments of Pharmacology, Internal Medicine, and Biochemistry, University of Arizona, College of Medicine, Tucson, Arizona 85724*

J. Gerald Young   *Department of Psychiatry, Mount Sinai School of Medicine, One Gustave L. Levy Place, New York, New York, 10029*

Alan J. Zametkin   *Child Psychiatry Branch, Building 10, Room 6N-240, National Institute of Mental Health, National Institutes of Health, 9000 Rockville Pike, Bethesda, Maryland 20892*

Joseph Zohar   *National Institute of Mental Health, National Institutes of Health, Building 10, Room 3D/41, Bethesda, Maryland 20892*

Psychopharmacology:
The Third Generation of Progress,
edited by Herbert Y. Meltzer.
Raven Press, New York © 1987.

CHAPTER 1

Ethical Dilemmas in Neuropsychopharmacologic Research

Donald M. Gallant and Burr Eichelman

Over the past decade and a half there has been a renewed awareness of ethical issues in neuropsychopharmacologic research. The biomedical community has been particularly concerned with the rights of human subjects in research. For example, congressional committees have reviewed experimental treatments (behavior modification) (1), and the National Commission for the Protection of Human Subjects has produced monographs on the use of prisoners as research subjects (2) and the use of children or others for whom informed consent is an issue (3). The recommendations from the Commission became United States governmental research policy as implemented through the Federal Register (4–6), which has included the establishment of active Institutional Review Boards (IRBs).

An awareness of ethical issues has been reflected in the activities of the American College of Neuropsychopharmacology (ACNP). In 1974, at the request of the President of the ACNP, the Ethics Committee began to develop "A Statement of Principles of Ethical Conduct for Neuropsychopharmacologic Research in Human Subjects" (7). It was recognized at that time that there was a need for a Statement of Principles that would exist independently of standards contained in law, since governmental regulations would vary over time, and some universal standards were necessary for the conduct of neuropsychopharmacologic research in human subjects. The first and second drafts of this statement were reviewed by the members of the ACNP council, the members of the Ethics Committee, and many other individuals whose diverse professional experiences made their suggestions particularly helpful. The majority of the suggestions were incorporated into a third draft which was sent to the entire voting membership in September 1975; the open meeting on this draft was conducted in December 1975. The fourth and fifth (final) drafts were formulated from the suggestions and advice offered at this meeting. The final draft of the Statement was approved by the membership of the ACNP in a mail ballot in June 1976. A revised Statement was ratified by the ACNP in 1985 (Appendix 1).

Programmatically in 1976, the ACNP sponsored a symposium on ethical issues in psychopharmacologic treatment and research. The papers from the symposium, which were published as a book (7), review such complex issues in research (8) and treatment (9) as consent, the balancing of risks and benefits, and issues of deception. Such analyses have also been published by the ACNP membership on an individual basis (10).

The Statement of Principles was designed to serve as an ethical guide for neuropsychopharmacologic research with human subjects. The document states specifically that it was "neither to be used as a legal statement nor as a binding legal document, either in a court of law or within the ACNP." It was the intention of the ACNP that the Statement of Principles would serve as a framework for meeting existing as well as evolving concepts for ethical neuropsychopharmacologic research and thus pass the test of time as new ethical problems arose.

Designing and conducting neuropsychopharmacologic research that is responsive to ethical issues would be enhanced by a review of research practices focusing on ethical principles. The ACNP's Statement of Principles was created in this way. A statement of principles, however, is of little use in stimulating investigator thought regarding the ethical issues of research protocols unless it is applied and discussed in the context of real-life situations.

Six case descriptions with appended commentary are presented to illustrate the application of the Statement of Principles to the problem of ethically sensitive neuropsychopharmacologic research.

CASE 1: INVESTIGATIONAL DRUGS IN SCHIZOPHRENIA

Case Description

A 37-year-old male patient is diagnosed as schizophrenic disorder–disorganized type by DSM-III criteria. Among his presenting symptoms are a flat affect, apathy, and frequent episodes of incoherence. His past history reveals a mental illness of at least 15 years with numerous lengthy hospitalizations and a premorbid schizoid adjustment with an insidious onset of psychotic symptoms. Family members abandoned the patient years ago and their addresses are unknown. Numerous trials of FDA-approved neuroleptics, singly and in combination with other compounds in attempts to potentiate the antipsychotic activity, have resulted in only temporary reduction of psychotic symptomatology. However, no significant improvement occurred and the patient has never been able to function adequately in the social and economic areas outside the institutional setting. When the patient is not receiving psychiatric drugs, he is totally unmanageable and unable to care for himself. At present, he is receiving large doses of a standard neuroleptic, which enables him to integrate his thought processes enough to cooperate within the ward milieu but thought dissociations are still frequent. He is developing symptoms of tardive dyskinesia and it appears that this drug-related problem will increase if the present medication regimen is continued.

Drug X is a new investigational antipsychotic agent that has undergone early drug testing in Europe. The extrapyramidal side effects are minimal and the drug appears to have activating as well as antipsychotic activity. Of the first 100 patients receiving this drug in therapeutic doses for 12 months or longer, only one potential case of tardive dyskinesia has been reported. However, of several thousand patients receiving the drug, four cases of granulocytopenia have been described in the literature. The patient's psychiatrist believes that the patient may profit from the investigational new drug, but the patient is quite negative about any new drugs, stating that he is "tired of all of these medications." This is the only coherent statement that the patient is able to make about the proposed drug study.

Commentary

Principle 5 of the Statement, "Considerations in Determining Who May Be a Proper Subject in a Research Study," is satisfied in this case because an anticipated therapeutic effect is a major (but not necessarily the exclusive) goal of this drug trial. The requirement of Principle 7, "Ethical Considerations in Evaluating Potential Research Study Benefits and Risks," is also met because there is an apparent "reasonable belief that the research may ultimately produce beneficial changes in the patient's clinical condition." Principle 8, "Informed Consent," poses the obvious dilemma since the patient lacks the capacity to give informed consent and does object to the investigation. The section reads, "Where a subject lacks capacity to consent, the scientific investigator shall obtain the consent from a person authorized to give consent on behalf of the subject or shall take other legally appropriate actions." This wording in the Statement, "other legally appropriate actions," does allow for a "court of competent jurisdiction" to play a decisive role in the final decision for consent to research. The Federal Register states that research may be conducted in subjects "who are institutionalized as mentally infirm" where there is more than minimal risk, even if the subject objects to participation, only if the "subject's participation is specifically authorized by a court of competent jurisdiction," providing that the requirements of methodology and benefits versus risks have been approved by the Institutional Review Board (4). In this particular case, there is no apparent conflict between the Statement of Principles and federal regulations.

The court would probably make its decision based on the stated facts that (a) the subject appears to lack the capacity to give informed consent; (b) there is no authorized person to give consent; and (c) the requirements of methodology and benefit versus risk have been approved by an IRB. The court would further consider the patient-subject's background and whether or not the patient would have consented if he were competent at the present time. Considering the moral tradition of "the overall good of the patient" and the realistic assessment that this new medication may benefit the mental illness while it reduces the severity of the side effects, it would be our hope that the courts would decide that the research drug would be quite appropriate for this particular patient (11). In this case, the ethical dilemma of informed consent in the incompetent schizophrenic patient who rejects a new research treatment modality is apparently resolved by appropriate use of the Statement of Principles. The Statement does not offer a final decision but does provide a guideline for ethical conduct in neuropsychopharmacologic research in schizophrenic patients.

CASE 2: BASIC RESEARCH IN SCHIZOPHRENIA

Case Description

A 42-year-old female patient had been diagnosed as schizophrenic disorder–paranoid type by several different psychiatrists during separate admissions to the inpatient service. Her premorbid history revealed a good adjustment in high school, where she had been a member of several extracurricular groups such as the school choral and girls' basketball team. During her first year of college away from home, the patient had several painful experiences, which involved rejection by a desired sorority and by her first serious boyfriend. She gradually withdrew from other social activities, began to display episodes of accusatory behavior, and was frequently seen mumbling to herself. Her school grades deteriorated over a period of 3 to 4 months. These symptoms of disorganized behavior finally culminated in the patient's first overt psychotic episode, with persecutory delusions that her roommates were poisoning her. She had auditory hallucinations, hearing voices of the college president and her dormitory advisor accusing her of having sexual relations with the entire basketball team.

During the following 13 years, the patient had six similar psychotic paranoid episodes; each remission was accompanied by progressive social and economic deterioration. However, her affect during remissions was not considered to be flat or too restricted. The patient had always shown a good response to neuroleptics but would discontinue them after several months and subsequently have a rapid relapse. Family history was negative for schizophrenic disorder except that her father was described as an emotionally isolated individual with some eccentricity. However, he always functioned well at his job and was seen as someone who loved his family but had difficulty expressing his feelings.

Present physical and psychiatric evaluation showed a patient who fit all of the criteria for the diagnosis of schizophrenic disorder–paranoid type. Present paranoid delusions were directed toward the hospital staff and the patient's legal representative, a lawyer appointed by the hospital to protect patients' rights. She accused him and the staff of having planned to kill her. Her anger was explosive, and assaultive behavior was a frequent problem. Naturally, the patient adamantly refused any new research endeavors. Laboratory workup, including EEG and CT scan, was within normal limits. Despite the duration of the patient's mental illness, it was the opinion of the staff that she was a "good prognosis" schizophrenic if her compliance with neuroleptic medication could be sustained.

Drug Y, a new oral, long-acting neuroleptic, is being considered for this patient. Theoretically, this investigational new drug has a duration of antipsychotic activity of 1 to 2 weeks after one administration. The extrapyramidal side effects are minimal and it appears to have a large differential between its therapeutic and toxic activity. The clinical advantage of this drug is that it can easily be administered at home by visiting human service workers without the need for subcutaneous injection by a trained individual. As part of the research protocol for the controlled evaluation of drug Y, the investigator at one of the medical schools has added cerebrospinal fluid (CSF) assays for N,N-dimethyltryptamine (DMT), 5-methoxy-N,N-dimethyltryptamine (5-MeO-DMT), and homovanillic acid (HVA), along with urine assays for 3,4-dimethoxyphenethylamine (DMPEA) at baseline, midway, and termination of the study. The investigator has the opinion that "good prognosis" schizophrenics who more readily respond to neuroleptics are more likely to display significant elevations in CSF HVA with antipsychotic drug administration as compared with "poor prognosis" patients who may have some atrophy on CAT scan. In addition, the presence of DMPEA in a "good prognosis" subgroup of unmedicated and medicated patients as well as in "poor prognosis" patients can be more adequately compared. CSF assays for DMT and 5-MeO-DMT will be performed in order to investigate previous conflicting reports in the literature about the transmethylation hypothesis and presence or absence of methylated toxins in schizophrenic patients.

Commentary

Principle 5, Section 1, is met because the major goal of the study is an "anticipated therapeutic effect." It appears that Section 2 of Principle 5 is also satisfied. This section states, "Patients who are mentally incompetent should not be subjects in neuropsychopharmacologic research studies which have no diagnostic, therapeutic, or prophylactic goals for the subject except in those cases where there are no 'realistic risks' involving long-term side effects or toxicity." In addition to the therapeutic goals of using drug Y, it may be argued that spinal taps for CSF assays, if performed by experienced clinicians, offer no "realistic risks" to the patients.

As in the previous case, Principle 8 (Informed Consent) is complied with by the requirement that "legally appropriate action" is necessary for subjects who lack capacity to consent. However, Principle 3 states the need for review and approval of human research studies by an IRB or an appropriate, qualified reviewing body. This board has the obligation to review the risks of the spinal tap versus the possible future benefits to patients with similar psychiatric illnesses. This type of subjective evaluation could result in different decisions by various IRBs, with approval for the entire protocol by some IRBs and recommendations for approval, but only if the CSF assays are eliminated, by other IRBs.

The federal regulations are more specific for this particular case. On page 11332 of the Federal Register of March 17, 1978, a spinal tap would be considered more than minimal risk (4). "Minimal risk" is defined as "the risk (probability and magnitude of physical or psychological harm or discomfort) that is normally encountered in the daily lives, or in the *routine* [italics added] medical or psychological examination, of normal persons." This section infers that mentally incompetent patients may react even more severely than normal persons to certain routine procedures; thus, the intrusive spinal tap procedure could possibly be viewed as even more of a psychologic risk to the "mentally infirm" than to the "normal person." Later in this same issue of the Federal Register, Recommendation 4 further addresses this problem of basic research in schizophrenia. It states, "Research in which *more than minimal risk* [italics added] to subjects who are institutionalized as mentally infirm is present by an intervention that does not hold out the prospect of direct benefit for the individual subjects, or by a monitoring procedure that is not required for well-being of the subjects, may be conducted or supported provided an Institutional Review Board has determined that: if the subject is incapable of assenting, a guardian of the person gives permission (if a guardian of the person has not been appointed, such appointment should be requested at a court of competent jurisdiction)." However, "A subject's *objection* [italics added] to research that is reviewed under Recommendation 4 should be *binding* [italics added]" (4). Here, we see a more well-defined limitation on certain technical procedures required for basic research and a potential conflict between one interpretation of the Statement of Principles and the federal regulations.

CASE 3: CONSENT FOR CHILDREN IN NEUROPSYCHOPHARMACOLOGIC RESEARCH

Case Description

A 12-year-old male had been previously diagnosed as having Tourette's disorder with a history of recurrent involuntary, rapid movements of the head, torso, and upper and lower limbs starting at the age of 7 years. These movements were accompanied by multiple focal tics, occasionally consisting of scatological words or grunts. These symptoms had progressed to the point that the patient was unable to function in the school environment by the time he was 9 years old. Various neuroleptics had been tried; haloperidol produced the best therapeutic response, although a relatively high dosage of 18 mg per day was required. At this dosage, the patient had problems with akinesia, which apparently were alleviated by an antiparkinsonian medication. His overall improvement allowed him to return to school and once again function adequately in the school environment. The main concern of the family at this time was the potential risk of later development of tardive dyskinesia. They asked the child's neurologist if there were any new medications that were just as efficacious and had less of a risk of tardive dyskinesia. The neurologist informed them that an investigational new drug, drug A, was being evaluated at that time and that the patient could be included in a drug study that was scheduled to begin the following month.

Clinical psychopharmacologic data from Europe indicate a low incidence of extrapyramidal side effects associated with drug A and a possible low occurrence of tardive dyskinesia. Significant benefits have been reported with use of this compound in reducing the symptoms of Tourette's disorder. The methodology described in the research protocol for drug A utilizes a randomized double-blind design with a placebo group as a control. The duration of this drug-placebo evaluation period is 12 weeks. At that time, the patients will resume their former medications or be allowed to continue on drug A if the therapeutic response has been significant and if side effects have been considerably less than those produced by the previous medication. The patient, with his parents' approval, agreed to enter the drug study.

Commentary

Under Principle 2, "Design and Methodology of Research Studies," the Commentary states, "In research designs of studies in patients, randomization of assignment for treatment should be employed only when the scientific question requires such a procedure and when increased risk is considered to be minimal." Since Tourette's disorder can vary in the intensity of the symptoms over weeks or months, the use of randomization and the double-blind procedure with a control group is indicated. However, since the patient may be assigned to a placebo group, the risk may be more than minimal. Discontinuing the haloperidol and administering placebo for 12 weeks could result in a clinical relapse with a resultant deterioration and failure in school performance with attendant psychologic consequences. Therefore, this particular patient may not be appropriate for the specific study that has been proposed, although the study would be quite suitable for this patient if the control group received haloperidol. On the other hand, if the patient had not been functioning in school and had not shown any significant therapeutic gains with previous psychopharmacologic agents, then the possibility of being administered placebo would offer no more than minimal risk. In this type of research patient evaluation, using the Statement of Principles, the final ethical decision may vary according to the baseline functioning of the patient or with the specific type of substance used for the control group.

In the Federal Register of March 8, 1983, *Children Involved as Subjects in Research,* in the subsection, "Research involving greater than minimal risk but presenting the prospect of direct benefit to the individual subjects," the Department of Health and Human Services' (DHHS) position is that "research studies involving placebo may be conducted . . . depending upon the individual activity" (5). The discretion allowed the IRBs in this section is reflected by the statement, "The Department believes that it is an appropriate responsibility of the IRBs to determine when the research would involve a minor increase over minimal risk." Here again, we can find no conflict between the Statement of Principles and the federal regulations.

CASE 4: NEUROPSYCHOPHARMACOLOGIC RESEARCH IN PRISONERS

Case Description

A 32-year-old inmate of a state penitentiary presented a history of episodes of violence against people that had begun when he was 11 or 12 years old. Pertinent data in the history revealed an alcoholic father who had been extremely brutal to the patient. At times, the mother would try to intervene, but she died when the patient was 11 years old. Until her death, the patient's performance in school had been above average; afterwards, he developed progressive difficulty with his anger. His aggressive explosive behavior was vented on his schoolmates until he was finally expelled from school at the age of 14 after numerous suspensions for fighting. The remainder of his adolescent and adult years were divided between jail for arrests on charges of assault or destruction of property and working as a heavy equipment operator in the community. His alcohol intake increased, and he became even more dangerous when he was intoxicated, particularly during alcohol-induced blackouts. Even when sober, he reacted with violence that was out of proportion to the environmental stress. Between the violent episodes, there were no overt signs of impulsivity and there was no evidence of a psychotic disorder. He had had two marriages, both of them disrupted by his violence during drinking episodes. Feelings of guilt would occur after most of these episodes. His alcohol intake had progressed until his "binges" occurred every weekend, and he began to show "morning shakes" the day after each of these binges. Despite these significant problems with alcohol and anger, the patient was considered to be a very conscientious, reliable worker and was not known to exhibit any other type of antisocial behavior.

During the intervals between outbursts of anger, the patient complained about a chronic feeling of tension and simmering anger, recognizing that he could lose control at any time. The current incarceration was a 5- to 10-year sentence for injury to a fellow worker by causing a fracture of the skull with subsequent subdural hematoma and a residual hemiparesis. The victim had teased him about his weight while they were drinking in a bar. During the interview session, he sat with one leg crossed over the other, continuously swinging it back and forth. The interviewer could feel the tension that was conveyed by the patient's body movements and staccato speech. There was no evidence of a psychotic disorder and the early childhood history revealed no history of attention deficit disorder. The patient's diagnoses are alcohol dependence (alcoholism) and intermittent explosive disorder. He has volunteered for the following research study.

A research team from a nearby university is studying the association between aggressive behavior and alcohol-associated neurophysiologic changes. The initial protocol outlines the methodology for administering alcohol intravenously to those patients incarcerated for aggressive acts following alcohol ingestion. A question and answer (q + a) session will be conducted one evening during the period of alcohol administration, and the same q + a session will be conducted the following morning. Among the neurophysiologic and biochemical evaluations planned are serial EEGs and evoked potentials during the time of alcohol administration and the following morning. A comparison group of nonalcoholics with no history of unusual violent behavior will undergo the same procedure. If the results of this study reveal that certain patients have low thresholds for explosive behavior associated with neurophysiologic-related abnormalities that can be activated by alcohol (alcohol-aggressive patient), a second study will be undertaken. The latter study will evaluate the antiaggressive efficacy of a new compound in the alcohol-aggressive patients during abstinent states and alcohol-induced conditions. This compound has already been shown to display antiaggressive properties in animals, and early uncontrolled trials in human volunteers have been impressive.

Commentary

Before reviewing the Statement of Principles for research pertaining to prisoners, the investigators should be aware of their state legislation and departmental prison policies. Less than half of the states permit biomedical and behavioral research in prisons (6).

The problem of consent in prisoners is one of the main reasons for the additional protection for prisoners in the federal regulations (12). The inherently coercive nature of imprisonment and the relative isolation of the prisoner from society impose additional responsibilities, as mentioned in the Statement of Principles, to "ascertain that the patient is truly a volunteer, that the prisoner understands he is under no obligation to participate, and that the prisoner has full information about the study and its possible effects on him" (7). In Principle 8, "Informed Consent," the section on prison inmates recognizes the difficult problem in evaluating the ability of the prisoner to give informed consent and places the major responsibility for this judgment on the shoulders of the IRB or other reviewing body: "When an investigator proposes to select as volunteer subjects individuals who are involuntarily institutionalized or subject to some legal restraint or whose personal circumstances are such that their need for volunteer compensation . . . may cloud their caution or judgment, the final approval concerning such a research study shall reside with the appropriate, qualified reviewing body." The reviewing body for the prisoner cited in this section will have to determine if the risk of reexposure to alcohol will outweigh the potential benefits of the first research protocol. One of the major goals of this research is to find possible neurophysiologic predictors of violence for a particular group of patients. The second protocol, which relates more specifically to the patient's treatment, should not be considered since the patient may be found unsuitable for that drug study.

The Federal Register is more specific about permitted research involving prisoners. The November 16, 1978, issue states, "Biomedical or behavioral research conducted or supported by DHEW may involve prisoners as subjects only if . . . [the study involves] possible causes, effects, and processes of incarceration and of criminal behavior, provided that the study presents no more than minimal risk and no more than inconvenience to the subjects" (12). Using the definition of minimal risk by DHHS, which was earlier described, the procedure of intravenous administration of alcohol to the alcohol-aggressive patient can be considered more than minimal risk. However, in Subsection C of this section in the Federal Register, which pertains to research on "social and psychologic problems such as alcoholism," the particular research project may be allowed if the Secretary, after consultation with experts, approves and publishes notice of this intent in the Federal Register. Of course, approval by the appropriate IRB is also necessary. This particular section on prisoner research seems to be ambivalent since some research projects in prisoners can contain goals which evaluate the possible causes of incarceration as well as the psychological problems of alcoholism or other substances of abuse. It appears that if the investigator changes the main thrust of his study of alcohol-related violence to research on psychological problems rather than on possible causes of incarceration, the project could be approved. However, it would have been disapproved if the latter goal was the major emphasis of the project. Either using the Statement of Principles or following the guidelines of the Federal Register, the final decision concerning approval for the study is based on the estimation of the degree of risk when exposing an alcoholic patient to the administration of alcohol. In prison settings, the necessary additional caution may result in rejection of this research proposal while it may be entirely appropriate to conduct this research project in volunteer-patients who are not incarcerated.

CASE 5: CONSENT FOR PRIMARY DEGENERATIVE DEMENTIA PATIENTS

Case Description

A 64-year-old woman presented at a medical institution with a 4-year history of slowly progressive memory difficulties, impairment of judgment with serious mistakes in financial decisions, concretization of thought processes, recent difficulty in recognizing the names of people as well as of objects, and recent personality changes with occasional explosive outbursts of anger which precipitated the present admission. Psychologic testing showed moderate problems in spoken and comprehensive language ability, impaired

recall of test instructions and commands, some evidence of nominal aphasia, and sporadic disorientation for time and person. Constructional apraxia was not significant. Presence of severe paranoid delusions was noted. The family history revealed that the patient's mother had been diagnosed as having Alzheimer's disease when she was 66 years old. The patient's physical examination and laboratory workup showed cortical atrophy and no focal neurologic signs. There was no evidence of generalized atherosclerosis and no history of alcoholism, two other relatively frequent causes of dementia.

Two years before the current admission, the patient had been diagnosed as having senile dementia of the Alzheimer's type (SDAT). At that time, she was still oriented, had not yet developed delusions, and was considered mentally competent. Having been informed of the diagnosis and nature of this disease, she had decided to use a durable-power-of-attorney, which she assigned to her nephew with whom she had a close relationship. The patient had never married and the nephew was her closest living relative as well as her heir. This durable-power-of-attorney permitted her nephew to assume legal responsibility for her at some time in the future if and when she was adjudged to be incompetent. It was understood at that time that the nephew would be a proxy decision maker and give instructions regarding her case.

Drug Q had been found to have cholinergic facilitating properties in rats as well as very potent dopaminergic and serotonergic properties. Initial studies in 400 human volunteers indicated that the drug may have some antidepressant properties, but several drug-related convulsions were reported. In view of the enhanced central cholinergic activity produced by drug Q, it was proposed that the drug be evaluated in patients with SDAT. The initial phase of the research protocol required each patient to have an intravenous physostigmine test to determine which patients showed temporary improvement on the psychologic test measurements, which included the Alzheimer's Disease Assessment Scale, the Memory-Information Test, and the Stuard Hospital Geriatric Rating Scale. One of the hypotheses of the research study design was that there may exist an SDAT subgroup of patients who have definite diminished central cholinergic function, respond temporarily to intravenous physostigmine, and show a more significant response to cholinergic enhancing agents such as drug Q than do physostigmine nonresponders. Each of the physostigmine responders and nonresponders was then to be randomly assigned to either the active drug Q group or to a placebo group in order to provide adequate controls for the study.

The patient, who had now been declared mentally incompetent as a result of her psychiatrist's testimony in court, refused to participate in the study because she thought that it was a plot by her nephew to kill her and inherit her estate. However, the nephew, using his durable-power-of-attorney, gave permission for this study. It had been explained to the nephew that the anticipated benefits for the patient would probably be no more than mild at best. The potential side effects of drug Q and physostigmine were adequately reviewed for him before he signed the consent.

Commentary

In Principle 5 of the Statement of Principles, "Considerations in Determining Who May Be a Proper Subject in a Research Study," Section 2 states, "Patients who are mentally incompetent should not be subjects in neuropsychopharmacologic research studies which have no diagnostic, therapeutic, or prophylactic goals for the subject except in those cases where there are no 'realistic risks' involving long-term side effects or toxicity." With the inclusion of a placebo group that would be exposed to intravenous physostigmine, an agent capable of producing such side effects as convulsions and bradycardia, without the potential benefits of drug Q, interpretation of this Principle would negate the study unless the placebo group was excluded from the protocol. In Section 2 of Principle 7, "Ethical Considerations in Evaluating Potential Research Study Benefits and Risks," the inclusion of a placebo group would also be negated by the statement, "The scientific investigator shall not use a research procedure . . . if the reasonably anticipated benefits to a patient are outweighed by reasonably forseeable disadvantages." (Since the Statement of Principles is not intended to be a legal document, the subject of durable-power-of-attorney is not addressed.)

As previously noted in the case that was concerned with basic research in schizophrenia, the Federal Register states that in those research studies in the mentally infirm in which more than minimal risk is present with an intervention that does not hold out the prospect of direct benefit for the patient, a subject's objection to research is binding (4). Therefore, the placebo group would have to be excluded under the federal regulations as well as the Statement of Principles. If this placebo group were eliminated from the study, then the protocol would be acceptable according to the guidelines in the Statement of Principles and the Federal Register.

However, the ACNP Statement of Principles does not address the durable-power-of-attorney and the Federal Register does not outline policy directions for assessing the validity of the durable-power-of-attorney.

As of March 1983, 42 states had statutes on the durable-power-of-attorney, but not all of these statutes specifically mention medical decision making (13,14). Therefore, it is incumbent on the research investigator to be familiar with the state law, since a "general" durable-power-of-attorney may not support medical decision making. A court ruling in the state may be necessary to determine whether or not a "general" durable-power-of-attorney includes medical decision making. In those states that expressly authorize a proxy to make medical decisions, there would be no question of the authority.

CASE 6: COVERT INFLUENCES ON NONINSTITUTIONALIZED NONPATIENT RESEARCH VOLUNTEERS

Case Description

Twenty students had enrolled in a postgraduate course titled "Physiologic Psychology." One of the goals of the course was to show the pharmacologic effects of some psychoactive agents on behavior. Midway through the course, the professor asked for volunteers to demonstrate the effects of alcohol on emotion and cognition and the possible enhancement of these effects by the addition of a minor tranquilizer. The subjects were to be randomly assigned to either an ethanol plus diazepam (e + d) group or an ethanol plus placebo (e + p) group. Standardized identical testing sessions were to be administered at baseline, after ethanol, and again the next day at baseline and after either e + d or e + p. They would complete a preethanol test battery before receiving a dose of 1.5 ml/kg of 95% ethanol in orange juice. Blood alcohol measurements would be obtained 15 min after consumption of the ethanol; the subjects would then be asked to complete the first post-ethanol test battery. On the next day, the same procedure would be followed with the blind addition of diazepam, 0.20 mg/kg, to the e + d group and placebo for the e + p subjects. The self-rating test battery included the Profile of Mood States and a line analog scale for estimation of intoxication. The cognitive test battery consisted of the Standardized Serial Seven Test, Porteus Maze, Speed of Closure Test, Digit Symbol Substitution Test, Minnesota Clerical Test, and Trail Making Tests A and B with equivalent but different forms used during each of the four experimental sessions. The students were informed that those who volunteered would be given additional credit toward their final grade. This protocol was submitted to the IRB.

Commentary

As stated in Principle 8, "Informed Consent," "When an investigator proposes to select as volunteer subjects, individuals . . . whose personal circumstances are such that their need for volunteer compensation or course accreditation (students) may cloud their caution or judgment, the final approval concerning such a research study shall reside with the appropriate, qualified reviewing body." In this particular case, the IRB may determine that the investigator has not made any special efforts to eliminate or decrease the covert pressure. In fact, the investigator in this case has increased the covert pressure since additional credit for grades could skew the grade curve and actually penalize those students who do not volunteer. The last sentence of the final paragraph in Principle 8 states, "The investigator should make special efforts to eliminate or decrease external pressures or reject volunteers who have been subjected to substantial external pressures."

Although the Federal Register does not specifically address the facts in the above case, it should be noted that the National Commission for the Protection of Human Subjects of Biomedical and Behavioral Research (NCPHSBBR) did publish recommendations in the Federal Register about student volunteers who may be coerced or unduly influenced (15). The Commission recommended that protective steps for students who are asked to be research subjects should include a descriptive statement at the onset of the course that such a request will be made and that "reasonable alternatives are offered." If the IRB follows this suggestion, then the protocol would be rejected.

DISCUSSION

The authors selected some typical and atypical cases in hopes of providing thought-provoking problems for the clinical investigator. The cases discussed illustrate some of the technical issues that must be addressed in neuropsycho-pharmacologic research. The moral solution to these problems is a process, not adherence to fixed legislative mandates, but an evolving fluid awareness of the need to conduct both basic and therapeutic research with ethical insight.

Medical research, although traditionally subject to a self-imposed conformance to ethical principles, has now become the object of significant legal constraints, including litigation, legislation, and administrative regulation. When the question of "rights" in medical research is considered from the perspective of the patient or subject, a complex balancing of factors is involved. Conducting research is not necessarily an issue of an ethically sound approach contrasted with an unsound one; it often involves the balancing of two ethically sound arguments. For example, the obtaining of informed consent from a research subject acknowledges the ethically sound principle of Respect for Persons. However, the difficulty in obtaining "pure" informed consent from psychotic, retarded, or demented patients can have a social effect of reducing the research effort related to their specific disorders. This, in turn, could produce a diminished allocation of research effort for these populations given their potentially increased social need. The resultant potential unjust distribution may be unethical in accordance with the principles of Distributive Justice. Consent issues in research also contrast respect for the rights of the individual versus the desire to reduce harm caused by ineffective or dangerous treatments.

In summary, ethical research should begin with an awareness by the researcher of general principles provided in the ACNP Statement of Principles. From these principles and a discussion of the application of these principles to research problems, more ethically responsive research will be generated.

REFERENCES

1. Individual Rights and the Federal Role in Behavioral Modification (1974): U.S. Government Printing Office, Washington.
2. Research Involving Prisoners. Appendix to Report and Recommendations (1976): National Commission for the Protection of Human Subjects of Biomedical and Behavioral Research. U.S. Government Printing Office, Washington.
3. Research Involving Children. Report and Recommendations (1977): The National Commission for the Protection of Human Subjects of Biomedical and Behavioral Research. U.S. Government Printing Office, Washington.
4. Federal Register—DHEW (1978): Research involving those who are mentally infirm. Vol. 43 (No. 53), March 17, 1978.
5. Federal Register—DHHS (1983): Children involved as subjects in research; additional protection. Vol. 48 (No. 46), March 8, 1983.
6. Federal Register—DHEW (1977): Research involving prisoners. Vol. 43 (No. 10), January 14, 1977.
7. Gallant, D. M., and Force, R. (1978): *Legal and Ethical Issues in Human Research and Treatment. Psychopharmacologic Considerations.* Spectrum Publications, New York.
8. Lebacqz, K. (1978): In: *Legal and Ethical Issues in Human Research and Treatment,* edited by D. M. Gallant and R. Force, pp. 113–142. Spectrum Publications, New York.
9. Jonsen, A. R., and Eichelman, B. (1978): In: *Legal and Ethical Issues in Human Research and Treatment: Psychopharmacologic Considerations,* edited by D. M. Gallant and R. Force, pp. 143–175. Spectrum Publications, New York.
10. Eichelman, B., Wikler, D., and Hartwig, A. (1984): *Am. J. Psychiatry,* 141:400–405.
11. McCormick, R. A. (1978): In: *Legal and Ethical Issues in Human Research and Treatment: Psychopharmacologic Considerations,* edited by D. M. Gallant and R. Force, pp. 158–166. Spectrum Publications, New York.
12. Federal Register—DHEW (1978): Additional protections pertaining to biomedical and behavioral research involving prisoners as subjects. Vol. 43 (No. 222), November 16, 1978.
13. Lynn, J. (1985): *N. Engl. J. Med.,* 312:248.
14. Fish, D. G. (1985): *N. Engl. J. Med.,* 312:248.
15. Federal Register—DHEW (1978): Protection of human subjects. Institutional Review Board; Report and Recommendations of National Commission for the Protection of Human Subjects of Biomedical and Behavioral Research. Vol. 43 (No. 231), November 30, 1978.

APPENDIX: A Statement of Principles of Ethical Conduct for Neuropsychopharmacologic Research in Human Subjects

The request to develop the Statement of Principles was made by Dr. Philip R. May, President of the ACNP, to Dr. Donald M. Gallant, Chairman of the Ethics Committee, in December 1974. The final draft of the Statement was approved by the membership of the ACNP in a mail ballot in June 1976. In 1985, a revised Statement of Principles was ratified by the ACNP membership.

INTRODUCTION

This Statement of Principles is intended to serve as an ethical guide to apply specifically to neuropsychopharmacologic research with human subjects performed by the members of the ACNP. Neuropsychopharmacologic research is here defined as the evaluation of the effects of synthetic compounds or natural products employed as investigational agents that affect the brain, and/or the peripheral nervous system, and behavior. While the Principles formulated herein may be relevant to other areas of research with human subjects, this Statement of Principles was not designed with that broad goal in mind. This Statement of Principles is neither to be used as a legal statement nor as a binding legal document, either in a court of law or within the ACNP. It is not intended to be the ultimate statement of ethical principles, but rather a framework for meeting existing as well as evolving concepts. It should not be used retrospectively to judge research conducted prior to its adoption by the ACNP.

To distinguish and clarify various ethical obligations which may be applicable in some research studies and not in others, this Statement of Principles employs the following terms to describe various types of subjects and the distinction between therapeutic and nontherapeutic research:

1. Patient—a person who has entered into a doctor-patient relationship with the scientific investigator or another

physician in the facility and who is a subject in a research study primarily intended to bring about beneficial changes in the condition being treated.

2. Patient-Volunteer—a patient who is a subject in a research study not primarily intended to bring about beneficial changes in the condition being treated, but which may add to the knowledge about emotional and mental disorders.

3. Nonpatient-Volunteer—a person who is a subject in a research study primarily intended to benefit society, not the subject; however, in certain studies, this person may also benefit.

4. Subject—an encompassing term which refers to all persons described in the three previous categories.

Neuropsychopharmacologic research has made significant contributions to human welfare. For example, as a result of the discovery and development of new drugs, patients with severe psychiatric and neurological illnesses, who were once considered untreatable and relegated to overcrowded institutions, have been able to return to their families and communities, often as productive persons. Others have been able to avoid institutionalization or to reduce its duration substantially as a result of drug therapy administered in outpatient treatment programs. However, the imperfections of existing treatment methods require increased scientific efforts to decrease the pain and suffering of patients and their families.

Scientific research does not exist in a vacuum. It should be emphasized that all persons living in society have a moral responsibility to participate in efforts to promote and contribute to the present and future welfare of that society. Research is one of these obligations. Notwithstanding the substantial benefits to society derived from neuropsychopharmacologic research, another societal interest must be considered—the welfare of each research subject. These Principles are designed to reconcile society's need for both advancing knowledge and for maintaining the dignity and rights of research subjects. It should also be recognized that advancement in medical research with subsequent benefit to society is impossible without some risks.

This Statement of Principles *exists independently of standards currently contained in law or proposed governmental regulations.* This independence has significant implications: (1) While law and ethics interrelate, they are by no means identical in that ethical requirements may affect behavior not within legal control. (2) This Statement of Principles applies to all neuropsychopharmacologic research in human subjects. (3) Standards of governmental regulations may vary, and there is no assurance that present standards will prevail in the future. (4) Finally, the existence of a Statement of Principles provides a reference point for the conduct of neuropsychopharmacologic research in human subjects.

One of the moral obligations and responsibilities of biomedical scientists is the acquisition of knowledge to preserve and enrich life. In accordance with scientific tradition, there are certain identifiable ethical values that should be supported for the maintenance and improvement of society. However, these underlying values are not described specifically in the Statement of Principles; instead,

it addresses itself to what the scientific investigator must or may do. Implicit in the Principles are the recognition and acceptance of these cardinal ethical values, as exemplified by voluntary consent, consideration of risks versus benefits, avoidance of unnecessary pain or disabling long-term effects, and benefits to both the individual and society.

The Principles are phrased in general terms without enumerating every possible ethical problem. A Statement of Principles of such specificity would require volumes, yet would inevitably be incomplete. The general principles expressed in this Statement should provide clear standards for resolving specific ethical questions which may arise in the course of neuropsychopharmacologic research and the use of data resulting from such studies.

Important distinctions are made in this Statement among various types of human subjects, especially such vulnerable groups as institutionalized people and children. Notwithstanding the premise that in all research unnecessary harm to the subject should be avoided and that any possible disadvantages which may result should be disclosed to the subject, ethical propriety of neuropsychopharmacologic research in any given case also depends on the subject's status as a patient, a patient-volunteer, or a nonpatient-volunteer.

The scientific investigator has certain ethical obligations to a "patient" which are inherently different from those of the researcher to the "patient-volunteer" or the "nonpatient-volunteer" (as these terms are defined above). In studies with patients, the individual patient should reasonably be expected to benefit from the research results. Research studies with volunteers, both patients and nonpatients, should reasonably be expected to produce benefits for society.

Procedures for securing subjects' consent to participate may depend on whether the subject is incompetent or competent, a child or an adult, or a member of a group particularly vulnerable to undue influence, or whether the research is therapeutic or nontherapeutic. The resolution of many ethical problems may well depend on the awareness and intelligent application of these distinctions.

The Statement of Principles, generally, is phrased in terms of what the scientific investigator may do in order to assure ethical requirements. In addition, this Statement addresses itself to the qualifications of the scientific investigator and takes the position that any clinical research undertaken by an unqualified investigator is, of itself, unethical behavior.

PRINCIPLE 1: QUALIFICATIONS OF THE SCIENTIFIC INVESTIGATOR

A scientific investigator, before assuming full responsibility for conducting neuropsychopharmacologic research studies with human subjects, shall have had adequate training and experience to conduct the research study proposed.

Commentary

The scientific investigator's prior experience as an assistant in neuropsychopharmacologic studies with human subjects shall be given weight in assessing competence. The adequacy of the investigator's experience should be a concern of the Institutional Review Board or its equivalent.

PRINCIPLE 2: DESIGN AND METHODOLOGY OF RESEARCH STUDIES

A neuropsychopharmacologic research study with human subjects shall be designed and carried out in accordance with generally accepted scientific principles.

Commentary

Experimentation with human subjects without reasonable anticipation of patient benefit or without reasonable anticipation of adding to the body of scientific knowledge is ethically unacceptable. Therefore, no risks can be justified when the experimental design is poor. The scientific investigator has the general obligation to extract the greatest amount of useful information from the smallest number of subjects with minimal risk or discomfort.

The following examples are some of the considerations that should be taken into account in the preparation of research protocols: (1) Subjects should be selected only if they appear suitable to test the specific hypotheses proposed in the research. (2) Whenever feasible, studies should be planned so that the number of subjects in the study is consistent with the statistical requirements necessary to assure that the data obtained or the conclusions drawn are likely to be valid. (3) When appropriate, provision should be made for control or comparison groups, or for subjects who serve as their own controls, to assure that information gathered has potential utility. (4) The investigator should have access to appropriate statistical expertise to assure that the results of the experiment will be meaningful to the scientific community. (5) In research designs of studies in patients, randomization of assignment to treatment should be employed only when the scientific question requires such a procedure and when increased risk is considered to be minimal.

It is recommended that a letter including a clear statement that Institutional Review Board approval for the protocol was obtained accompany research papers submitted for publication.

PRINCIPLE 3: REVIEW AND APPROVAL OF HUMAN RESEARCH STUDIES

A scientific investigator shall not undertake a neuropsychopharmacologic research study involving human subjects without the approval of an appropriate, qualified reviewing body. The investigator shall ascertain that the reviewing body has specific guidelines for the submission, initial approval, and periodic review of all protocols for research studies with human subjects. Once having secured initial approval, the investigator should obtain subsequent approval for any substantial deviation from the protocol.

Commentary

The organization of Institution Review Boards for approval and review of research studies with human subjects

has been advocated by scientific investigators and required by the United States Department of Health, Education and Welfare (DHEW), as described in the Federal Register (1–5).

The law requiring Institutional Review Boards was passed and enacted in 1974, and guidelines necessary for appropriate operation of Institutional Review Boards as recommended by the National Commission for the Protection of Human Subjects of Biomedical and Behavioral Research (NCPHSBBR) were published in the Federal Register in 1978 (3,4). In 1981, standards for Institutional Review Boards for clinical investigation and the list of research activities which the Boards may review through expedited review procedures set forth in FDA regulations for the protection of human subjects were published in the Federal Register (5). In accordance with these guidelines, this committee of the institution sponsoring investigation with human subjects serves to protect the rights and welfare of the participants.

No individual investigator, regardless of qualifications and competency, is infallible. Thus, both the scientific investigator and the subject benefit from the establishment of review committees, the very existence of which stimulates thoughtfulness and encourages responsibility on the part of the scientific investigator.

A scientific investigator who is not affiliated with an institution which has an Institutional Review Board shall not undertake a neuropsychopharmacologic research study unless it is initially approved and periodically reviewed by an independent review body that is substantially the equivalent of an Institutional Board.

In the event that HHS should ultimately abandon or substantially restrict its requirements for Institutional Review Boards, review and approval of research studies by appropriate review bodies would continue to be required by this Statement of Principles. The intent of this Principle is that all human research, regardless of the source of funds, should be subject to review.

The scientific investigator has the responsibility to serve on an Institutional Review Board or its equivalent, when requested, in order to maintain the necessary principle of review of research by one's peers. If the scientific investigator is a member of an Institutional Review Board which is considering the investigator's own project, the investigator should not participate in the vote relative to that research project.

Reviewing bodies have an obligation to establish a fair procedure for approval and independent review of their decisions.

PRINCIPLE 4: RESPONSIBILITIES OF THE SCIENTIFIC INVESTIGATOR AND THE APPLICATION OF THIS STATEMENT OF PRINCIPLES

Individual Responsibility

Each scientific investigator shall ascertain and consider the current ethical standards applicable to neuropsychopharmacologic research studies with human subjects.

Application of This Statement of Principles

1. The scientific investigator shall conduct studies in neuropsychopharmacologic research with human subjects in substantial accordance with the ethical principles contained in this Statement of Principles—with respect for subjects and with concern for their dignity, welfare, and rights. This responsibility, in addition, is imposed on all associates, employees, or students who assist the scientific investigator.

2. The scientific investigator shall take reasonable precaution to assure that the Principles contained in this Statement are observed by all persons who assist in the research study.

3. The ethical responsibilities imposed by this Statement of Principles shall become applicable when the scientific investigator makes the initial decision to undertake a neuropsychopharmacologic research study with human subjects and shall continue through the conclusion of the research study, including all necessary steps to protect any privileged or confidential material pertaining to subjects in the study.

4. The scientific investigator shall take reasonable precautions to become acquainted with regulations which are relevant to the research study proposed.

PRINCIPLE 5: CONSIDERATIONS IN DETERMINING WHO MAY BE A PROPER SUBJECT IN A RESEARCH STUDY: GOAL OF RESEARCH STUDY DETERMINES TYPE OF SUBJECT

General Responsibilities

The scientific investigator engaged in neuropsychopharmacologic research with human subjects shall take all reasonable precautions for preserving the dignity, rights, and safety of all subjects.

Studies with Patients

1. In neuropsychopharmacologic research involving patients, an anticipated therapeutic effect should be the primary but not necessarily the exclusive goal. The scientific investigator should evaluate the research regimen with a view toward doing no harm to the patient by withholding treatment which has a very high degree of probability of significantly improving the patient's condition. Some research might be designed primarily to make an accurate diagnosis prior to definitive treatment or to develop prognostic indicators for selection of optimal treatment of the patient's disease.

2. Patients who are mentally incompetent should not be subjects in neuropsychopharmacologic research studies which have no diagnostic, therapeutic, or prophylactic goals for the subject except in those cases where there are no "realistic risks" involving long-term side effects or toxicity. Some examples of relatively minor safe procedures are comparisons of physical measurements, psychological test surveys, and the taking of small samples of biologic fluids for qualitative or quantitative analyses.

Studies with Patient-Volunteers

1. A patient may be included as a volunteer in a research study unrelated to the disease or condition being treated if the study is not reasonably expected to interfere with the welfare of the patient or the treatment regimen, and the patient otherwise satisfies the prerequisites of a volunteer.

2. When performing research with patient-volunteers, the investigator should obtain from the patient's physician an opinion that the patient may justifiably be included in the research project.

Studies with Nonpatient-Volunteers

In neuropsychopharmacologic research with volunteers, the attainment of scientific knowledge may be regarded as a primary goal. Research with volunteer subjects, i.e., mentally competent, fully informed adults, nevertheless imposes ethical responsibilities for the safety, dignity, and rights of these subjects.

Commentary

Many of the ethical problems dealt with in this Principle and in other Principles have been given thoughtful, detailed consideration in Ethical Principles in the Conduct of Research with Human Participants and in Ethical Principles of Psychologists, both published by the American Psychological Association (6,7)

PRINCIPLE 6: ETHICAL RESPONSIBILITY—PHYSICAL AND MENTAL DISCOMFORT

The scientific investigator has the obligation to minimize, to the extent possible, all undue physical and mental discomfort of the subject. When it appears that a research study may have resulted in undesirable consequences for the subject, the investigator shall make every reasonable attempt to detect them and to provide adequate follow-up treatment to remove, correct, or relieve those consequences.

Commentary

In scientific investigations of subjects involving physical and/or mental discomfort, the nature of the anticipated physical and/or mental discomfort should be explained to the subject in advance. Furthermore, the investigator should be reasonably certain, on the basis of existing knowledge, that the anticipated physical and/or mental discomfort will not have long-term adverse consequences for the nonpatient-volunteer.

PRINCIPLE 7: ETHICAL CONSIDERATIONS IN EVALUATING POTENTIAL RESEARCH STUDY BENEFITS AND RISK; RESEARCH PROCEDURES

Patients

Research studies with patients shall be conducted only when the expectation of anticipated results will justify the experiment. At the time the research study is undertaken and throughout its performance, there should exist a scientific basis for a reasonable belief that the research may ultimately produce beneficial changes in the patient's clinical condition.

Patient-Volunteers and Nonpatient-Volunteers

1. Scientific gains expected from research studies with volunteers shall be weighed against the reasonably anticipated risks involved. At the time the research study is undertaken and throughout its performance, there should exist a scientific basis for a reasonable belief that the research study will ultimately produce scientific knowledge which will benefit patients in the future.

2. The scientific investigator shall not use a research procedure if it is likely to cause disabling or lasting harm to subjects or if the reasonably anticipated benefits to a patient are outweighed by reasonably foreseeable disadvantages.

Subjects of Limited Mental Capacity

1. Children may be subjects in a neuropsychopharmacologic research study when they need treatment and are reasonably expected to benefit from their participation in the study. They may also be included as "normal control" subjects in comparison studies. In general, research studies of drugs in children shall not be undertaken unless similar studies in adults have proved reasonably safe.

A drug that has been proved to be safe but ineffective in adults may be evaluated in children if there is a reasonable basis for expecting it to be effective in children. In some specific disorders which are unique to children, such as childhood autism, prior demonstration of drug efficacy in adults may be irrelevant. Research studies in these uniquely pediatric disorders are not foreclosed under this Principle because of the lack of such a disease process in adults.

2. A research study with subjects who are mentally incompetent or with children involves additional considerations because of the limitations of the subjects or their inability to understand fully the procedures and implications of the research study and to communicate their feelings and responses to the investigator.

Inert Substances

The scientific investigator who proposes to use an "inert" substance (placebo) as part of the methodological requirement of a study shall examine carefully both the necessity and ethical considerations of the procedure as it relates to the specific illness or particular research problem. This approach shall be reviewed carefully by the Institutional Review Board or qualified review body.

The scientific investigator who proposes to use an "inert" substance as part of the research study shall carefully differentiate among patient groups in evaluating expected improvement against possible deterioration (8).

Commentary

Prior to the introduction of a neuropsychopharmacologic agent in man, studies of the agent in several different animal species shall have indicated the probability that a substantial risk of organ system injury will not result from its administration in humans. However, in experimentation, it is impossible to predetermine the exact scope of the risks or benefits. This lack of precise foreknowledge of risks and benefits should be specified in the protocol and should be communicated to the subject, or in cases where informed consent cannot be obtained, to the person authorized to give consent. The existence of this uncertainty and honest realization of the limits of knowledge concerning the experiment should not itself be the cause for abandoning the research.

The use of a placebo in severely ill patients, such as very disturbed and/or severely deteriorated chronic schizophrenic patients who present gross thought disorders and hallucinations, should be carefully reviewed by the investigator. It may be quite appropriate to use a placebo control group in evaluating treatment in conditions with a tendency toward spontaneous remission. Thirty to forty percent of patients diagnosed as acute schizophrenics may show moderate to marked improvement with placebo (8), while such improvement in very disturbed or severely deteriorated chronic schizophrenics is rare. In nonpsychotic conditions, such as anxiety and depression, the "superiority of standard existing drugs over placebo is of sufficiently modest extent to make the administration of placebo to some patients in a study justifiable, particularly if there are explicit provisions for removing from the study patients whose clinical condition worsened" (9).

Patients in any study, including those in which a placebo is being used, even under "blind" conditions, should be removed from the study at any clearly discernible sign of substantial worsening of their conditions and treated as expeditiously as possible.

The report and recommendations by the NCPHSBBR on research involving children were published in the Federal Register of January 13, 1978 (10). In 1983, additional protections for children involved as subjects in research as well as requirements for permission by parents or guardians were prescribed in the Federal Register (11).

PRINCIPLE 8: INFORMED CONSENT

The Requirements of Informed Consent

Research studies with human subjects require informed consent of the subjects. Where a subject lacks capacity to consent, the scientific investigator shall obtain the consent from a person authorized to give consent on behalf of the subject or shall take other legally appropriate action.

Informed consent as used in the context of these Principles is the agreement obtained from a subject (or from an authorized representative) to participate in a neuropsychopharmacologic research study. The basic elements of informed consent are:

1. An explanation of the procedures to be followed, including an identification of those that are experimental.

2. A description of the reasonably foreseeable attendant discomforts and risks and a statement of the uncertainty of the anticipated risks due to the inherent nature of the research process.

3. A description of the benefits that may be expected.

4. A disclosure of appropriate and available alternate procedures that might be advantageous for the subject.

5. An offer to answer any inquiries concerning the procedures.

6. A statement that information may be withheld from the subject in certain cases when the investigator believes that full disclosure may be detrimental to the subject or fatal to the study design (providing, however, that the Institutional Review Board has given prior approval to such withholding of information).

7. A disclosure of the probability that the subject may be given a placebo at some time during the course of the research study if placebo is to be utilized in the study.

8. An explanation of the probability that the subject may be placed in one or another treatment group and a definition of this probability in lay terms if randomization is a necessary part of the study design.

9. An instruction that consent may be withdrawn and participation in the study may be discontinued at any time.

10. An explanation that there is no penalty for not participating in or withdrawing from the study once the project has been initiated.

11. A statement that the investigator will inform the patient of any significant new information arising from the experiment or other ongoing experiments which bear on the patient's choice to remain in the study (12).

12. A statement that the investigator shall provide a review of the nature and results of the study to those subjects who request such information.

The Federal Register of January 27, 1981, contains the Food and Drug Administration (FDA) requirements for informed consent, including the requirement that the subject be informed that FDA may inspect the records. Thus, the subject should be informed about the extent to which confidentiality of the records identifying the subject will be maintained (5).

Subjects Who Lack the Capacity to Consent

1. When a patient is mentally incompetent or too young to comprehend, informed consent must be obtained from one who is legally authorized to consent on behalf of the proposed subject. As the study progresses, the investigator also shall keep the person who consents on behalf of the subjects informed of any major changes in the research protocol or significant side effects.

2. If a mentally incompetent or incapacitated subject is capable of exercising some judgment concerning the nature of the research study and participation in it, the investigator shall obtain the informed consent of the subject in addition to the person legally authorized to consent. Supplemental guidelines for research involving those institutionalized as mentally infirm were published in the Federal Register in 1978 (13).

3. When the subject is a child who has reached the age of some discretion, and the subject is otherwise mentally competent, the scientific researcher shall obtain the subject's informed consent in addition to the person legally authorized to consent (10).

Patients unable to give informed consent pose special problems (14,15). The scientific investigator assumes additional ethical responsibilities to the patient, who because of lack of capacity, may not be able to make rational judgments concerning participation or withdrawal from the research study (14).

Consent of Prison Inmates and Other Especially Vulnerable Groups

1. With nonpatient-volunteers who are involuntarily institutionalized or subject to some legal restraint, investigators should take special precautions to assure the subjects the opportunity to obtain full information about the research study, including the right to refuse to participate or to withdraw from the study at any time without penalty. Guidelines for conditions under which research involving prisoners is permitted were published in the Federal Register of November 16, 1978 (16).

2. When an investigator proposes to select as volunteer subjects individuals who are involuntarily institutionalized or subject to some legal restraint or whose personal circumstances are such that their need for volunteer compensation or course accreditation (students) may cloud their caution or judgment, the final approval concerning such a research study shall reside with the appropriate, qualified reviewing body.

Commentary

Consent of the subject is an ethical prerequisite. This Statement of Principles establishes the ethical requirements of consent, but takes no position on the legal sufficiency of the Principles.

The authority of a person to provide informed consent on behalf of one who lacks capacity may vary from state to state. Parental consent is usually required when children comprise the subject group in well-designed neuropsycho-pharmacologic experiments. However, the parent or court-appointed proxy has no moral right to give consent for the child to participate in an experiment which has no specific etiologic, diagnostic, or therapeutic goals for the disease presented by the child, except in those cases where there are no reasonably foreseeable risks. With regard to persons who are mentally incompetent, some states may require informed consent from the closest living relative; some states may require consent by a legal guardian; and finally, some states may insist on approval from a court. The scientific investigator should make further inquiries to resolve any doubts as to the appropriate person to give consent. This Principle does not contend that persons who may be vulnerable to undue influence must be automatically excluded as potential volunteers. Such decisions should be made by an appropriate Institutional Review Board on a protocol-by-protocol basis.

These Principles recognize the great difficulty that has surrounded the issue of informed consent. A further problem exists in subsequently proving, years later, that one did in fact secure informed consent. The use of forms detailing risks and benefits is presently the dominant means of dealing with this problem. An alternative procedure may involve the utilization of an individual not involved in the research study who would be present at the time consent is secured. Such an individual would assist the subject by explaining the risks and benefits to the subject and could certify for the purpose of documentation that informed consent had in fact been obtained. Utilization of such an individual would facilitate the explanation of risks and benefits in a manner appropriate for the subject, or person giving consent on his behalf, as well as providing subsequent proof of the occurrence of this procedure.

A person who is incarcerated as a result of a criminal conviction should not be disqualified from being a volunteer in a neuropsychopharmacologic research study merely because he is a prisoner. Furthermore, a nonpatient-volunteer who is a prisoner should not be denied the opportunity to be exposed to a research study that undertakes an evaluation of an illness that may have been directly or indirectly associated with the prisoner's incarceration. For example, a prisoner with a history of heroin addiction that resulted in illegal activity and subsequent incarceration should have the opportunity to participate voluntarily in research studies of treatment with narcotic-blocking agents. If such a research endeavor were successful, the prisoner would then have gained a definite benefit from the particular experiment. However, the relative isolation of the prisoner from society and the inherently coercive environment of the prison imposes on the scientific investigator the additional obligation to take all practical measures to ascertain that the prisoner is truly a volunteer, that the prisoner understands that he is under no obligation to participate, and that the prisoner has full information about the study and its possible effects on him.

Careful consideration should be given to studies with residents of a poverty area whose need for paid volunteer fees may outweigh their caution or with college students who may participate in a drug research study if it is perceived as a requirement to a course or because of faculty pressure. Every volunteer is responding to some pressures; however, there is a difference between gross external pressures brought about, for example, by prison officials or teachers and internal pressures which are complex and vary among individuals. It may be difficult or impossible for the scientific investigator to be aware of and to evaluate complex internal pressures in a potential volunteer. The investigator should make special efforts to eliminate or decrease external pressures or reject volunteers who have been subjected to substantial external pressures.

PRINCIPLE 9: SUBJECT'S RIGHT TO DECLINE OR WITHDRAW

Right to Decline Participation and Right to Withdraw

The investigator shall respect the freedom of the individual subject or, in the case of those who lack capacity to consent, the person legally authorized to act on the patient's behalf to decline to participate in a research study or to discontinue participation at any time without penalty.

Reviewing Body

The obligation to insure that the project protocol protects the subject's freedom to participate and withdraw is the responsibility of the reviewing body as well as of the individual investigator. The reviewing body shall determine whether or not the research procedures protect the subject from deceit or any type of undue influence.

Commentary

In studies with mentally competent individuals, the subject may withdraw from the research project at any time. However, patients unable to give informed consent pose particular problems (14). The scientific investigator assumes additional ethical responsibilities to the patient who, because of lack of capacity, may not be able to make rational judgments concerning withdrawal from the research study. These additional responsibilities require exceptionally careful attention to a patient's attempted rejection of a particular treatment.

Regardless of the research subject's mental competency, the investigator may be uniquely able to anticipate adverse consequences from the continuation of an experiment. It is his responsibility to withdraw the patient from the study if such a situation appears imminent; this responsibility includes patients receiving either active drugs or placebo.

PRINCIPLE 10: INFORMATION

Confidentiality

The scientific investigator shall have responsibility for not improperly releasing information pertaining to subjects in the study. This responsibility includes not only information protected by law, which often does not apply to all subjects, but also information that affects the privacy and dignity of subjects. When there is a likelihood that others may obtain access to such information derived from the research, the investigator, in obtaining informed consent, shall explain this possibility and the plans for maintaining confidentiality to the subject or, in the case of those lacking mental capacity, to the person who provides consent on behalf of the patient.

Explanation to Subjects

1. Information about foreseeable side effects should be given to the subject and/or the person who consented to the patient's treatment.

2. After the data are collected, the investigator shall provide a review of the nature and results of the study to those subjects who request such information. When scientific or humane values justify delaying or withholding information, the investigator incurs a special responsibility to

take reasonable precautions that this action would not be expected to result in damaging consequences for the subject.

3. After termination of studies involving those who lack the capacity to consent, such as mentally incompetent persons and young children, the investigator shall reveal on request important and pertinent results to the person who provided consent for the patient.

PRINCIPLE 11: ETHICAL OBLIGATIONS OF INVESTIGATOR FOR FOLLOW-UP TREATMENT OF THE PATIENT

Responsibility of the Investigator to Communicate Research Results

The scientific investigator has the responsibility to inform the patient or the consenting person whether the research treatment has been effective or ineffective if the investigator believes that this information would be beneficial.

Responsibility for Follow-Up Treatment for the Patient

The scientific investigator shall take reasonable steps to see that the patient is treated in the most appropriate manner. These steps may include the continuation of a research program if such a procedure is possible: if not, the best alternative should be sought.

REFERENCES

1. Federal Register—DHEW-PHS (1974): Protection of human subjects: Policies and procedures. Vol. 39 (No. 105), May 30, 1974.

2. The Institutional Guide to DHEW Policy on Protection of Human Subjects (1971): DHEW Pub. No. 72–102, December 1, 1971.
3. Pub. L. 93–348, 1974.
4. Federal Register—DHEW (1978): Protection of human subjects, Institutional Review Board. Report and recommendations of National Commission for the protection of human subjects of biomedical and behavioral research. Vol. 43 (No. 231), November 30, 1978.
5. Federal Register—DHHS (1981): Protection of human subjects; Informed consent; Standards for Institutional Review Board for clinical investigations; and clinical investigations which may be reviewed through expedited review procedures. Vol. 46 (No. 17), January 27, 1981.
6. Ad Hoc Committee on Ethical Standards in Psychological Research (1973): Ethical Principles in the Conduct of Research with Human Participants. American Psychological Association, 1973.
7. Ethical Principles of Psychologists (1981): *Am. Psychologist,* 36: 633–638.
8. Bishop, M. P., and Gallant, D. M. (1966): *Arch. Gen. Psychiatry,* 14:497–503.
9. FDA Guidelines for Psychotropic Drugs (1975): *Psychopharmacol. Bull.,* 4:7–28.
10. Federal Register—DHEW (1978): Research involving children. Report and recommendations of the National Commission for the Protection of human subjects of biomedical and behavioral research. Vol. 43 (No. 9), January 13, 1978.
11. Federal Register—DHHS (1983): Children involved as subjects in research; Additional protections. Vol. 48 (No. 46), March 8, 1983.
12. Fried, C. (1974): *Medical Experimentation: Personal Integrity and Social Policy.* American Elsevier Publishing Co., New York.
13. Federal Register—DHEW (1978): Research involving those who are mentally infirm. Vol. 43 (No. 53), March 17, 1978.
14. Gallant, D. M. (1970): *Psychopharmacol. Bull.,* 6:4–12.
15. Gallant, D. M., and Force, R. (1978): *Legal and Ethical Issues in Human Research and Treatment.* Spectrum Press, New York.
16. Federal Register—DHEW (1978): Additional protections pertaining to biomedical and behavioral research involving prisoners as subjects. Vol. 43 (No. 222), November 16, 1978.

Psychopharmacology:
The Third Generation of Progress,
edited by Herbert Y. Meltzer.
Raven Press, New York © 1987.

CHAPTER 2

Molecular Strategies in Neuropsychopharmacology: Old and New

Solomon H. Snyder

Psychiatry and neurology have often been regarded as the scientific weak sisters of the medical disciplines. In contrast to the substantial understanding of molecular mechanisms in "conventional" diseases, too many disorders in psychiatry and neurology are "idiopathic." However, in one area psychiatrists and neurologists can be proud. In these disciplines more is known of the mechanism of action of therapeutic drugs than in most fields of medicine. Moreover, psychotropic drugs have provided virtually the most powerful probes permitting the modern explosion in the neurosciences. Basic research in psychopharmacology has been important in two ways. Understanding molecular mechanisms of drug action provides means for designing new, more potent and selective therapeutic agents with fewer side effects. With selective ligands it has been possible to sort out the nuances of neurotransmitter receptors and enzymes involved in processing neurotransmitters, thereby enhancing greatly our understanding of the molecular mechanisms of nervous function.

Almost all drugs that affect the brain do so by influences on synaptic transmission. Hence this essay will focus largely on molecular aspects of neurotransmission. Drugs can affect the storage of a neurotransmitter, its release, its inactivation by enzymatic or uptake mechanisms, its metabolism, or its action on receptors. The first generation of basic research into psychoactive drug mechanisms dealt largely with influences on neurotransmitter storage, release, and inactivation. The discovery that reserpine interrupts storage of biogenic amines, depleting them and causing attendant depression, stands as one of the cornerstones of psychopharmacology. At about the same time it became apparent that monoamine oxidase is responsible for the degradation of biogenic amines and that the antidepressant monoamine oxidase inhibitors owe their therapeutic effects to actions on this enzyme. The subsequent

discovery that tricyclic antidepressants inhibit the reuptake in activation of amines and the evidence that the euphoric effects of amphetamines were due to amine release filled out an elegant, if somewhat simplistic, view of the ways in which mood can be titrated up or down by manipulating amines.

Many of these advances were made possible by techniques developed by Sidney Udenfriend to measure amines chemically by fluorescent emissions and the pioneering work of Bernard Brodie utilizing these techniques to demonstrate drug-induced changes in amine content. Of particular importance was the development by Julius Axelrod of ways to monitor amine disposition with radiolabeled neurotransmitters, permitting the first direct evidence that antidepressants block catecholamine uptake. Radiolabeled catecholamines and their precursor amino acids provided tools to monitor the turnover of norepinephrine and dopamine, a biochemical means to assess the overall firing rate of amine-containing neurons in the periphery and in the brain. The work of Udenfriend identifying and characterizing tyrosine hydroxylase resulted in the discovery of inhibitors of this rate-limiting enzyme in catecholamine biosynthesis, permitting another elegant way of assessing amine turnover. Similar studies of tryptophan hydroxylase afforded insights into serotonin turnover.

This biochemical work on amine neurotransmitters took place in the 1950s and the 1960s. In the late 1960s it was increasingly appreciated that amino acids such as glycine and glutamic acid are also neurotransmitters and γ-aminobutyric acid (GABA) was accepted as the major inhibitory neurotransmitter in the brain. The demonstration of specific, high-affinity, sodium-requiring uptake systems for neurotransmitter amino acids into nerve terminals permitted a discrimination of the neurotransmitter pools of these amino acids from the general metabolic pool.

RECEPTORS

Until 1970 very little if anything had been done to identify the sites where neurotransmitters are recognized to influence adjacent neurons, namely, synaptic receptors. In 1970 several laboratories used potent snake neurotoxins to label nicotinic acetylcholine receptors in the electric organs of certain fish. The very success of this work implied that it would be impossible to do the same for the major neurotransmitters in mammalian brain, since the cholinergic receptor in these electric organs comprises 20% of total membrane protein, and the snake toxin ligands are extraordinarily potent and almost irreversible. By contrast, neurotransmitter receptors in the brain are only about one millionth of total brain weight, and no unique toxins exist for such receptors. Thus, it was something of a surprise when, in 1973, reversibly acting, common drugs successfully labeled opiate receptors in crude brain homogenates. Strategic elements contributing to this success were radiolabeled drugs of high specific activity and high affinity for receptors, as well as extensive and rapid washing to remove nonspecific interactions of drug with membranes while preserving receptor binding. The techniques that made possible identification of opiate receptors could be readily applied to receptors for the major neurotransmitters in the brain. Within 5 years several dozen neurotransmitter receptors were characterized.

Measuring receptor recognition sites by simple binding techniques has had many implications for psychopharmacology. First of all, it became possible to clarify mechanisms for therapeutic actions of drugs. For instance, the hypothesis that neuroleptics act by blocking dopamine receptors was established unequivocally by showing that the relative potencies of an extensive series of neuroleptics in blocking dopamine receptors closely parallel their therapeutic potencies, whereas the effects of these drugs on serotonin, histamine, and norepinephrine receptors show no correlation with therapeutic effects. The increasing subtlety with which one could biochemically dissect receptors with radioligands permitted the identification of receptor subtypes. In the case of dopamine, binding studies, in conjunction with influences on adenylate cyclase, discriminated two major subtypes of dopamine receptors, D1 and D2. The antischizophrenic actions of neuroleptics could be ascribed to blockade of D2 and not D1 receptors.

Receptor research made possible an understanding of drug side effects. For instance, the sedative and hypotensive effects of neuroleptics correlate with their potencies in blocking α_1-adrenergic receptors, whereas muscarinic anticholinergic actions are inversely correlated with extrapyramidal side effects. Anticholinergic drugs, of course, are therapeutic in Parkinson's disease and neuroleptics have varying anticholinergic potencies. Thus, neuroleptics that are more potent anticholinergics alleviate the extrapyramidal side effects which they themselves provoke by blocking dopamine receptors.

Technically, receptor binding techniques are sufficiently straightforward that a worker can readily assay a thousand test tubes in a day. Since one can secure specific molar potencies of drugs and receptors, it becomes possible to conduct sophisticated structure-activity analysis for developing drugs of increased potency. Such techniques, now routinely employed in the drug industry, permit the sculpting of drugs to secure receptor selectivity. Because of the lag of many years between the identification of a test chemical with a potentially therapeutic action and the commercialization of the resultant drug, new, more selective agents with fewer side effects are just reaching clinical trial. It is likely that a new generation of such agents will influence clinical psychopharmacology in coming decades.

SECOND MESSENGERS

Receptor binding identifies only the recognition site of the neurotransmitter receptor. After recognition, second messenger events alter cellular function. There are two major classes of second messengers, the adenylate cyclase and the phosphoinositide systems. Both of these act through third messengers, the phosphorylation of various protein and nonprotein substrates. The great diversity of protein kinase systems has been elucidated largely through the efforts of Paul Greengard. He and his students have characterized a series of different protein kinase enzymes and also isolated their specific protein substrates.

The phosphoinositide (PI) cycle has been appreciated as a major second messenger system only in the last few years, based in large part on the contributions of Bernard Agranoff, Yasutomi Nishizuka, Robert Michell, Michael Berridge, and their colleagues. Interestingly, Lowell and Mabel Hokin first demonstrated phosphoinositide turnover enhancement by acetylcholine in 1953. In this system, receptor recognition triggers the hydrolysis of phosphatidyl-inositol-bis-phosphate to form inositol triphosphate and diacylglycerol. Diacylglycerol stimulates the activity of protein kinase C, which can phosphorylate a number of substrates to alter cellular function. Inositol triphosphate liberates calcium from the endoplasmic reticulum. The released calcium synergizes with diacylglycerol in stimulating protein kinase C activity. As many transmitters act through the PI cycle as via adenylate cyclase. The PI cycle mediates α-adrenergic, serotonin S_2, bradykinin, muscarinic cholinergic M_1, and histamine H_1 synaptic actions, as well as effects of numerous hormones.

The PI cycle is more sensitive to feedback influences than almost any other metabolic cycle. Phorbol esters, inflammatory and tumor-promoting substances, potently mimic diacylglycerol to augment protein kinase C activity. In some synaptic systems they produce effects reflecting enhanced PI cycle activity, whereas in other systems they have opposite actions.

The cyclic AMP system and PI cycle can be imaged on a microscopic level (Fig. 1). Their reciprocal localizations may reflect reciprocal functions, a "ying-yang" phenomenon. Conceivably these two major counterbalanced systems will provide insight into the "big picture" of emotional regulation, a picture presently obscured by the literally hundreds of discrete neurotransmitters.

At therapeutic blood levels lithium inhibits phosphatases, which degrade inositol phosphates to permit the reformation of inositol, thus slowing the PI cycle and potentially dam-

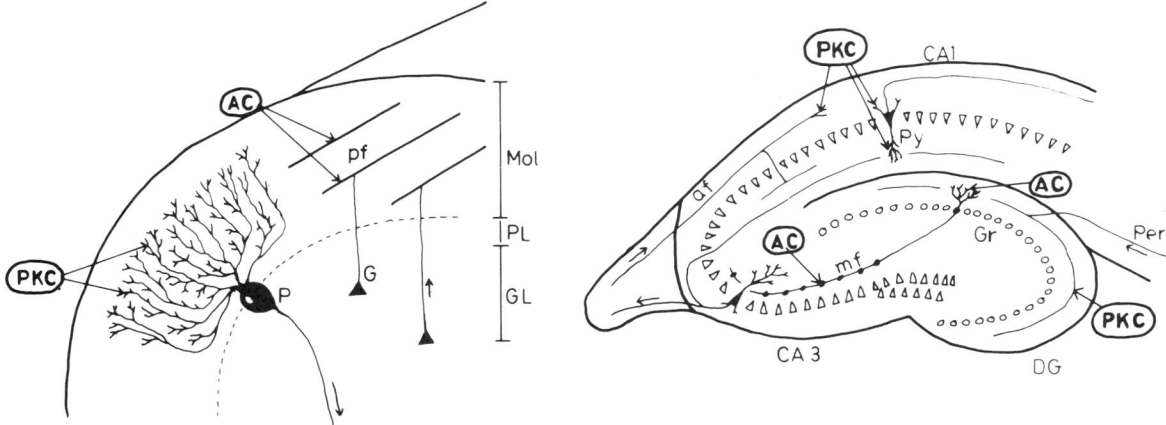

FIG. 1. Postulated localizations of adenylate cyclase and protein kinase C in the cerebellum and hippocampus. Diagrammatic presentation of cerebellum (**left**) and hippocampus (**right**) shows proposed predominant localizations of adenylate cyclase (AC) and protein kinase C (PKC) based on autoradiographic studies with [3H]forskolin and [3H]phorbol-12,13-dibutyrate ([3H]PBt2). In the cerebellum both ligands selectively label the molecular layer (Mol), which contains both Purkinje cell (P) dendrites and parallel fibers (pf), while both the Purkinje cell layer (PL) and granule cell layer (GL) have lower grain densities. Within the molecular layer adenylate cyclase is localized to parallel fiber axons and terminals, which are processes of the granule cells (G). In contrast, protein kinase C appears to be predominantly localized within Purkinje cell dendrites. In the hippocampus adenylate cyclase is concentrated in the molecular layer of the dentate gyrus (DG), where it is present in granule cell (Gr) dendrites. In addition, the mossy fiber (mf) projection of the granule cells which extends to the CA3 division of the hippocampus is also enriched with [3H]forskolin binding. Protein kinase C has a wider distribution in the hippocampal formation. In the dentate, it is located in afferents to the molecular layer, here represented as part of the perforant pathway (Perf). In CA1 and CA3, protein kinase C is thought to be present in both apical and basal dendrites of pyramidal neurons (Py) as well as hippocampal afferent (af). (Adapted from ref. 2.)

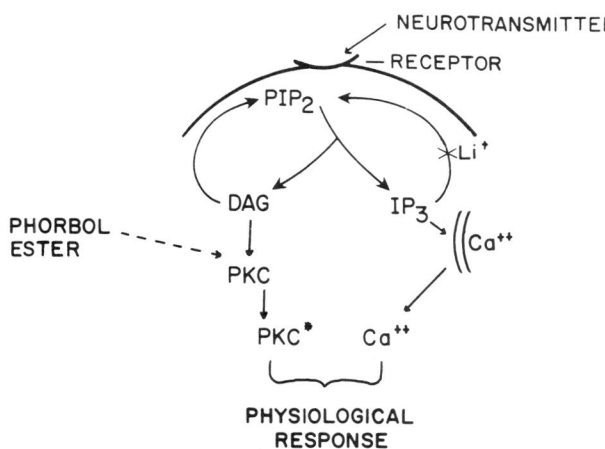

FIG. 2. Schematic diagram of phosphoinositide (PI) cycle and effect of lithium. Receptor stimulation by agonist triggers hydrolysis of phosphatidyl-inositol-bis-phosphate (PIP2) to diacylglycerol (DAG) and inositol trisphosphate (IP3). Diacylglycerol activates protein kinase C (PKC), an action mimicked by phorbol esters. Inositol trisphosphate releases calcium from intracellular stores. Activated protein kinase C (PKC*) and elevated levels of intracellular calcium act together in mediating physiological responses to receptor stimulation. Inositol phosphates and diacylglycerol are recycled to replenish PIP2 stores. Reutilization of inositol phosphate is blocked by lithium so that lithium may alter PI-mediated responses. (Adapted from ref. 1.)

pening related synaptic events (Fig. 2). Such an effect may explain the perplexing ability of lithium to relieve both depressive and manic symptoms and to afford prophylaxis against the two poles of affective illness. Let us assume that different transmitters that influence the PI cycle are respectively hyperactive in mania and depression. A dampening effect will be most pronounced on that system which is most overactive. Thus lithium will "slow down" whatever excess activity accounts for mania or depression. For its prophylactic effects, we speculate that lithium prevents both the manic and depressive synaptic systems from "overheating."

Up to the present time no major therapeutic drugs have been introduced that act via second messenger systems. The paucity of drug development in this area may reflect a prejudice that substances that influence something so universal as a second messenger system would grossly disrupt brain function. Such a conclusion may be premature. One might similarly conclude that drugs that influence GABA, a neurotransmitter at up to 40% of all brain synapses, would be similarly disruptive. However, we now know that benzodiazepines act by markedly facilitating synaptic actions of GABA throughout the brain.

MULTIPLE NEUROTRANSMITTERS

Until the mid-1970s the major neurotransmitters known were the handful of biogenic amines, amino acids, and a few neuropeptides such as substance P. The remarkable properties of opiate receptors suggested that there might exist an endogenous opiate-like neurotransmitter. The subsequent identification of the enkephalins and the endorphins greatly stimulated what had been a slowly growing interest in neurotransmitter peptides. Within a few years as many as 50 distinct neurotransmitter peptides were isolated and characterized. Most of these have been discovered by indirect ways. There have been few systematic attempts to identify "all" the potential neuropeptides in the brain. Thus, what we presently know of neuropeptides may only be the tip of the iceberg. It would not be surprising if there existed as many as 200 distinct neuropeptides. Immuno-histochemical techniques have permitted the mapping of almost all the major neuropeptides. Each resides in a distinctive set of neuronal pathways just as interesting as neuronal systems for the enkephalins and the catecholamines. Accordingly, each of these peptides provides a target for the development of psychotropic agents with therapeutic potential which, in principle, would be just as important as any of the presently available psychoactive agents. The means whereby one could discover novel drugs acting through peptides are readily available. Most peptide receptors have been identified by binding techniques, so that one could readily screen chemical structures for active agents.

The biosynthesis and degradation of neuropeptides constitutes a rapidly developing area of research. Virtually all biologically active peptides are synthesized by being cleaved from large protein precursors. Within these precursors the active peptide is flanked on both sides by pairs of basic amino acids. The liberation of the transmitter peptide from the precursor usually requires the action of two sequential enzymes. First a trypsin-like enzyme cleaves to the right-hand side (carboxyl terminus) of all the basic amino acids. This liberates the active peptide with one basic amino acid attached on the carboxyl terminus. Then, a carboxypeptidase-B-like enzyme removes the basic amino acid. This pattern of metabolism was elucidated by Donald Steiner in the mid-1960s for the processing of insulin and subsequently shown to be universal for biologically active peptides. Despite the many years of investigation of this biosynthetic pathway, until recently it was not clear whether specific enzymes process individual peptides or whether generalized enzymes exert these actions for all peptides.

Recently a carboxypeptidase that synthesizes enkephalin has been isolated and designated enkephalin convertase or carboxypeptidase E. Autoradiography with the potent inhibitor [3H]GEMSA (guanidinoethylmercaptosuccinic acid) reveals a relatively selective localization to enkephalin-containing neuronal pathways. Since enkephalin convertase is localized also to some other areas that are not enriched in enkephalin, this enzyme probably acts as well on a few other neuropeptides. Such a pattern is reminiscent of angiotensin converting enzyme, which is also highly localized in the brain to areas, such as the subfornical organ, that contain angiotensin and to other areas, such as the striatonigral pathway, that are devoid of angiotensin. Here the enzyme must have some other endogenous substrate, perhaps substance P or substance K. Whether there are

selective trypsin-like enzymes for the processing of each neuropeptide is unclear.

How are neuropeptides inactivated after synaptic release in receptor action? Peptides do not appear to be inactivated via reuptake systems. Instead, peptidases seem to degrade them. Again, one might ask whether selective peptidases are involved. Recently several laboratories have characterized an enkephalin-degrading enzyme known as enkephalinase or endopeptidase 24.11. The enzyme has been imaged microscopically by immunohistochemistry, by autoradiography with a potent inhibitor of the enzyme, and by a colorimetric histochemical technique. With all three procedures the enzyme is highly localized to areas enriched in enkephalin terminals and opiate receptors. Thus, this enzyme, whose catalytic properties are those of a neutral endopeptidase, is selective for enkephalin. One would anticipate that inhibitors of the enzyme should exert opiate agonist-like properties. The limited work that has been done with a few inhibitors of the enzyme accords with this prediction. The successful work with enkephalin convertase and enkephalinase suggests that potent and selective inhibitors of biosynthetic and degrading enzymes for neuropeptides will afford novel psychoactive drugs.

FUTURE DIRECTIONS

Exploiting the advances already made will likely occupy the pharmaceutical industry for many years to come. With the rapidly escalating developments in molecular neuroscience, it is likely that there will be yet other fundamental opportunities.

Molecular biological techniques have permitted the cloning of genes for the acetylcholine receptor and a fairly detailed characterization of the three-dimensional structure of this receptor and the sodium ion channel contained within this macromolecule. Similar successes are likely within a few years for the β-adrenergic and benzodiazepine-GABA receptors. Drugs may be designed systematically to "fit" the pocket in a receptor that recognizes the transmitter. Gene delivery via retroviruses may someday correct the molecular abnormalities in genetically determined conditions ranging from Huntington's disease and hemophilia to schizophrenia and affective disorders. Peptides and proteins synthesized by cDNA techniques may find therapeutic application, but only after means have been devised to facilitate their absorption into the circulation and penetration of the blood-brain barrier.

Before concluding that pharmacologists and biochemists are obsolete as gene cloners can take care of everything, one should remember that clinically useful drugs will always derive largely from small organic molecules. The difficulties inherent in the use of macromolecules as drugs suggest that the link between present "old-fashioned" pharmaceuticals and the new molecular biology will come with small organic molecules that mimic or block effects of proteins and genes. Not only genes that code for specific enzymes, receptors, and structural proteins, but also promoters, enhancers, and other regulatory genes determine the rate at which other genes will be transcribed. Drugs in psychopharmacology as well as general medicine may interact with proteins that bind to regulatory genes. Examples already exist. Glucocorticoids act by binding to protein receptors, which in turn attach to promoter elements in the genome. Conceivably, drugs in the future will bind to gene regulators turning on or off the synthesis of neuropeptides or receptors.

Whether or not gene-selective drugs emerge, we can be confident that new psychotropic agents will emerge with extraordinary potency and selectivity for one or another neuropeptide or second messenger. These drugs will permit us to modulate selectively emotional nuances which today are so subtle that they reside in the vocabulary of poets, not psychiatrists.

ACKNOWLEDGMENTS

This research was supported by USPHS grants DA-00266, MH-18501, NS-16375, and RSA Award DA-00074 and a grant from the Laboratories for Therapeutic Research. Experimental studies of the localization of protein kinase C and adenylate cyclase and actions of lithium were conducted in collaboration with Jay Baraban, Paul Worley, and Harold Menkes.

REFERENCES

1. Menkes, H. A., Baraban, J. M., Freed, A. N., and Snyder, S. H. (1986). *Proc. Natl. Acad. Sci. USA*, 83:5727–5730.
2. Worley, P. F., Baraban, J. M., De Souza, E. B., and Snyder, S. H. (1986): *Proc. Natl. Acad. Sci. USA*, 83:4053–4057.

Psychopharmacology:
The Third Generation of Progress,
edited by Herbert Y. Meltzer.
Raven Press, New York © 1987.

CHAPTER 3

Strategies for Research in Biological Psychiatry

Daniel X. Freedman

NEUROPSYCHOPHARMACOLOGY AND CLINICAL DISORDER

The broadly open-ended activities of the American College of Neuropsychopharmacology are not centered on diseases but spring from varied interests in behavior and CNS pharmacology of both the clinical and nonclinical disciplines. Yet, with drugs to change or to probe biobehavioral processes or to discern neuronal, molecular, and biophysical mechanisms, we do have "points of leverage"—frameworks of facts and concepts to be subsequently tested in basic or clinical research. This interplay, in part, provides the context in which to place the role and relevance of the striking momentum of research in biological psychiatry. New mechanisms of drug actions and refined treatment strategies are in hand. Clinical research has defined "markers" and patterns of changed brain physiology and has delineated biologically or descriptively based subtypes for each of the major disorders as detailed throughout these volumes. New uses of old drugs (carbamazapine for mania, clonidine for Tourette's, or phenelzine for panic disorder) and new antidepressants and neuroleptics have been tested. In brief, a large corpus of reliable information along a number of fronts now guides the search for definitive causal and remedial mechanisms in the study of disease.

The serendipitous observations of drug effects on psychiatric disorders in the early 1950s had two major consequences. In clinical science, strategies to define and assess the selective use of the novel therapeutic agents in objectively classified patients had to be developed. Secondly, neurochemistry was drastically redefined. By tracing drug effects on the CNS, we gained our initial grip on a functionally relevant brain chemistry and a world of new mechanisms by which drugs act. This has not directly led to the causal effects of the initial disequilibria and the cascade of consequences we recognize as symptomatic disease. It has provided mechanisms and processes to test and, thus, transformed the focus, range, and zest of clinical investigations.

Historical reconstructions of these developments are requisite (and tempting to document), but beyond our scope. We can, however, be sensitive to the intrinsic snobbery of the present looking at the past (this will be the privilege of the future assessing us!). Looking briefly back, we should at least recognize the long history of systematic attempts to link brain and behavior. By 1950, just before chlorpromazine's neuroleptic effects were tested, this research had finally provided a brain that worked! We now deal with "wires" and "juices," but before World War II we had a switchboard ("off" or "on") model of neural function. This could not tell us *how* hormones (e.g., thyroid excess or deficiency), drugs, or anesthetics could affect function nor even how neuronal operations could possibly accomplish what introspection and observations of the brain's dissociations and disinhibitions required. Neural operations (graded potentials) and systems for graded states of consciousness, linking internal and external signals and simultaneously "alerting" or recruiting cognitive, as well as affective and bodily processes, were then discovered. The role of an intrinsic brain chemistry as a signaling system influencing behavior, one differentially altered not only by different classes of drugs (10) but by environmental signals (3), and the observation of membrane and structural changes responsive to experience and to maturation (6) were yet to come.

Even in the immediate "predrug" era, it was evident that to internal or external signals perceived as stress a number of synchronized behavioral and bodily systems responded. "Logic" required mediation by both neural and hormonal signals regulated through feedback loops—"molecules talking to molecules." By 1950, the basic search for hypothalamic events had just begun and finally eventuated in the prohormones that are now central for clinical investigations. Vast uncharted territories separated the few measurable substances out of which one could deduce the logic of neurohormonal regulations and behavioral adaptations. It was evident—as it should now be—that while "go for broke" hypotheses abounded, absent good fortune, painstakingly detailed physiology to link relevant processes was required.

The overriding strategy was that mental disorder should be reflected in some sign of dysregulation, lack of synchrony, or imbalance in these signals and adaptive processes. If substances relevant to the signaling processes were different at steady state or with challenge, then the deviation should provide an investigatory or therapeutic lead, whether it represented cause or consequences. Many measures, such as of autonomic function, adrenal hormones, psychotoxic indoles, or methoxylated phenylethylamines, or differences in energy metabolism, were attempted in psychiatric disorders. For all of our contemporary power to understand fundamental synaptic regulations (and with molecular biology probing the determinants of gene expression), we are still calibrating exactly where and how these substances, processes, and mechanisms are relevant to the manifestations of disease that clinical science identifies. We now continue to find both differences and overlaps of biological processes in different disorders, search for therapeutic mechanisms (such as for electroconvulsive therapy), and seek to sort these out. Essentially, we examine the unity, diversity, and variability of clinical phenomena to see what they reveal about the significance of biological measures and *vice versa* (8). Thus, the basic strategies of bench and bedside have shifted in their focus but still fundamentally persist.

Bench and Bedside

It is an absolute requisite that clinical disorders be reliably classified and subsequently reclassified with the advent of new findings. Yet to understand the neurobiological relevance of a clinical finding or to apply a neurobiological finding to clinical disorder is not a trivial task. Quite different knowledge structures (each rightly pursuing its own agenda) have to be translated. Only in the past decade have clinical observations of the rate of change following a therapeutic drug regimen set the agenda for the laboratory in determining chronic as well as acute drug effects. Drugs induce "periods of neurochemical change" (13), and correlations with such temporal dimensions are now a part of strategies for both clinical and basic research, as are other temporal parameters (e.g., the study of intrinsic biorhythms in clinical, neuroendocrine, and sleep research).

Bench and bedside are neatly linked when the binding of neuroleptics at a dopamine receptor subtype can be correlated with their clinical antipsychotic potency (estab-

lished by the assessment tools developed in clinical psychopharmacology). It is rarely that neat! Clinical investigations in depression and schizophrenia now use peripheral measures of amine turnover. Not definitively diagnostic, they do help to define subtypes, predict clinical response, or define correlations with symptom severity, etc. However, we do not speak of unequivocal "abnormal" values, but rather establish correlations with components of clinical dysfunction. Neither the physiological "meaning" nor the central and/or peripheral sources of variations in these measures are instantly apparent. Indeed this becomes, *per se,* a new research topic.

The obvious strategies derive from neuropharmacology's focus on brain neurotransmission, receptors, and interdependent transmitter systems. From the clinical vantage, the focus is too exclusive. Most studies are in rodents where brain biochemistry and "receptorology" have but recently begun to be coupled with concomitant blood and urine measures. Yet the linkages are a central methodologic and conceptual problem for clinical research. For the full physiology of the multiple compartmental fluxes and disposition of amine precursors and metabolites neither physiology nor clinical pathology texts provide the maps. The relevant information has to be built as the clinical research develops. We know something of "upstairs" and "downstairs" regulatory processes (12); we must still explicate their autonomy, their linkages, and their feedback loops in different psychobiological states (21). This is equally true for neuroendocrines studied.

We also have to decide what is logical to require of these measures. A reliable "marker"—biological or genetic—has obvious utility for "next steps" in the study of disease, but a direct consequence on brain function is not a requisite for useful leads. Whether a measure reflects cause, consequence, a compensatory or incidental process, or a correlation can rarely be inferred but has to be systematically established whether we study life events, parental loss, or β-receptor down-regulation with antidepressants.

Quite similarly, the psychobiology of arousal, perception, attention, anxiety, or information processing was developed in animals usually independently from clinical data and *vice versa.* New linkages in these areas have been generated as clinical studies gain in focus. Disease mechanisms sought in animal models must ultimately be tested in the clinic, as is done in current "challenge" studies of panic disorder. Bench and bedside have, thus, been strikingly joined as mental, autonomic, and biochemical components of "anxiety" are "dissected" in both animals and the human. Both the locus ceruleus and γ-aminobutyric acid (GABA) receptors (and possible endogenous ligands) are probed. Linked or dissociated responses [e.g., elevated 3-methoxy-4-hydroxyphenylglycol (MHPG) with yohimbine but diminished symptoms with the concomitant use of diazepam, etc.] can be based on the internal "logic" of these different limbic and brainstem systems.

There is, however, an uncanny ease with which we can take assertions too literally from either the bench or clinic. We have endured "eras" of hypotheses readily degraded to dogma rather than the sheerly pragmatic working tools they are. Notions of "one juice, one disease" for schizophrenia or depression are of little service. Nor are drug actions as simple as our classificatory conveniences connote;

further, the therapeutic mode of action of the same drug in different disorders may (or may not) be different. Today we use far more rigorous and objectifiable clinical criteria and specified variants of statements that initially served as a hopeful (and, in some senses, useful) guiding beacon.

Old legends die hard, but practical spinoffs eventually ensue. Thus, amphetamine, once an antidepressant, became a "model" for "schizophrenia." Yet, all are true: amphetamine, a dopamine agonist antagonized by neuroleptics, produces schizophrenia-like states; a given dose is *not* reliably psychotogenic; the drug exacerbates schizophrenic psychosis; very often, it clearly does *not*. In fact, stimulant-induced "schizophrenias" are paranoid and delusional states. These clinically can occur alone and in disorders *other* than schizophrenia. Further, stimulants—within given dosage ranges—*enhance* focused attention and skilled motor performance. But these very processes are *diminished* in chronic schizophrenia and most clearly improved by dopamine-blocking agents (27). Finally, there are multiple actions of the drug and different ones for different stimulants.

What I once called "metapharmacology" (13)—explanatory "stories" about plausible but unobserved events—can facilely reconcile apparently contradictory statements. Today experts reasonably propose pre- or postsynaptic down- or up-receptor regulation, or a GABA-mediated destabilization of dopamine subsystems to account for the varied amphetamine effects. The range and control of attentional states (shifting from scattered to paranoid rigidity) may be explored for differentiating clues. More critically, we can now rapidly test the verity and revise the utility of hypotheses. The strategy of testing CNS "prior state" (13)—however it is ultimately defined—may be a practical technique in schizophrenia to predict vulnerability to relapse or to tardive dyskinesia. A hormonal rather than behavioral response to the stimulant probe may prove useful (as it has with various probes of CNS status in depression). But, *diagnostically* specific biological "definitions" of prior state in untreated patients remain the ultimate goal yet to be satisfactorily achieved.

We have moved far from the notion that a simple excess of dopamine is directly schizophrenogenic. We do not know where the story will end but pathophysiological sequences involving dopamine or receptors in schizophrenia are appropriately sought at autopsy, in positron emission tomography (PET) scans, or in peripheral measures of homovanillic acid (HVA), and useful next steps (a focus on dopamine function in mesolimbic systems and frontal lobe) have ensued. Similarly, we have moved from concepts of simple deficits of norepinephrine as causal in major depression to a more usefully formulated "dysregulation" in these systems. To paraphrase Judson (17), one should not be surprised that in every once-absorbing problem there are small or more precise problems struggling to get out of the perplexities in which they are enmeshed.

CALIBRATING EXPECTATIONS OF CURRENT STRATEGIES

The "Ways" of Science

Problems posed by clinical disorders transcend questions of drug actions and effects. Powerful and consequential strategies lie in the domains of epidemiologic, nosologic, family history, neurobehavioral, and genetic research. Both categories and dimensions of behavior—both diagnoses and processes cutting across them (such as "reactivity" or impulsivity correlated with low brain serotonin)—are relevant research parameters. Nevertheless, the task is to understand how a "fact," in actuality, is generated and the particularities of the problem for which a "fact" is deemed to be germane. We must further calibrate our expectations as we piece together these elements of a "story" and where they fit. In all of medicine we usually have partial stories. And so it is—and has been—if we bother to gain some perspective of discovery and solution in the clinical sciences. It is a long trajectory involving oscillations between clinical observation, basic science, accidents of nature, and serendipitous occasions as well. We need not require of each effort the eureka-like leap from the unknown to the definitive final answer. Many promising starts in biological psychiatry still await completion (8). In this, we should appreciate the "helpless opportunism" (17) of all science, awaiting the right tools, discovery, or concepts with which to pursue, "frame," and tell a completed story.

With scientific inquiry, we lose breadth but gain specificity with the limitations of method, as in the quest for answers we search for the sources of error. We gain in relevance reviewing the "problem," carefully scanning present and past inquiry (too rarely done), and noting untested assumptions and discrepancies. Generally, through laborious bits and pieces, through convergent as well as linear pursuits, we are in the incessant business of knowledge construction, generating new questions—but only occasionally new paradigms.

Useful discovery can be impeded by knowing too much! An absorption in detail can impede the effort even to try; yet, many useful findings were undertaken for what turned out to be the wrong reasons. In fact, "theory" has rarely predicted either the behavioral or biochemical advances we currently have in hand (11). More critically, prevailing "rules" and logic may blind one to opportunity, to what has been overlooked or what is not quite right with the wisdom of the day. The exceptions to or flaws in current knowledge structures have provided powerful leverage for useful new insights (19). Thus, although discovery does not require that working hypotheses be accurately based or that the exceptions be noted, the test of discovery and a critically articulated knowledge base surely do!

Interdisciplinary Work: Complexities, Pieties, and Purpose

We now have salient tools and cogent questions to be tested in designed clinical investigations. The sheer consumption of time and effort simply to recruit patient samples and manage the ethical execution of protocols—even for a simple study—is, however, worth noting. Further, even small-scale inquiries now also require multiple and highly specialized talents. Complex analyses of computerized data bases distance investigators from their observational sources and increase the task of differentiating chance from "meaningful" correlations. The consequences of all this for the funding and conduct of science, for the meaning of accountable "authorship," or for the development and test of ideas will surely affect research strategy and policy.

The power of collaborative studies to verify hypotheses and maximize the needed numbers of subjects has long been clear [and virtually pioneered in psychopharmacology (24)], and the unique potential of prospective studies to define critical disease parameters is obvious. But large projects also may lose essential information and, if lengthy, enshrine the state of yesterday's art! On the other hand, selection of the right pedigree or of the extremes on a distribution may maximize the chance for salient discovery. So, we require different arrangements shrewdly selected because they are appropriate to the phase of the science problems pursued.

However these complexities unfold, there is no pietistic virtue simply in assembling different disciplines without clarity about what is to be solved. The extended time and resources required for exploration or for even "narrow" pursuit of conclusive information (for completing the unfinished "stories") can conflict with the needs of granting agencies. Some prefer requisitioning the few experts hard at work for a novel interdisciplinary agenda. There often is a lofty assumption that the "answers" to difficult clinical problems readily lie secreted in the treasure houses of disciplines that logically "sound" as if they *ought* to be relevant! It is quite different when the involved investigators themselves perceive a need to be enabled to reach beyond their current methodologies for new perspectives and tools or colloquy on strategies.

Technology's triumphs (e.g., automated biochemical analyses) may replace technical expertise with a seemingly simple routine. Even so, for the responsible pursuit of articulated scientific questions there can be no escape from critically appraising where and when other disciplines and expertise are needed and why. We also require sustained fundamental inquiry unfettered by the moment's agenda precisely because we cannot know the unknown until we come upon it. With perhaps half of human DNA devoted to brain—what has yet to be mined!

THE STUDY OF DISEASES

Progress in Investigating All Diseases

The astonishing progress in both biology and therapeutics since World War II has affected research strategies for psychiatric disorders as profoundly as for most other medical diseases. Yet one still encounters denigration of the status of psychiatry and neurology in biomedicine. The sources for this misperception are many, including enchantment with putative or proven prizes currently in hand (the moment's hot tools or leads). In fact, the full infrastructure or "architecture" (7) of clinical biomedical research, as an organized topic, is relatively new and its applicability to all disorders is not widely grasped. Nor is the relative state of the art with respect to biomedical disorders.

Thus, unequivocally established sets of definitive causes, their precise treatment and prevention are few beyond some infectious and deficiency diseases (two psychiatric disorders, paresis due to syphilis and pellagra due to niacin

deficiency, are examples). Rather, we have so-called "halfway technologies." The "logic of nature" should increasingly provide the leads to attain precision in untangling the nexus of causal sequences *and* an understanding of the *intrinsic* sources of variability—and unpredictability—in them. Etiopathology, however, is still less developed than is our growing grasp of pathophysiological sequences or (more frequently) therapeutic mechanisms and the refinement of steps toward specific efficient remedies. This is essentially true for psychiatric as well as other disorders, but less confidently appreciated.

Similar Strategies for Psychiatric and Medical Disorders

We do know more about readily accessible and less complex organ systems than brain, and hence about measures of their operations. These, while rarely pathognomonic, are aids for arriving at a diagnosis or, more often, "signals" for considering one or another intervention. Objective evidence of bodily and brain dysfunction in different psychiatric disorders (and of typical patterns of disturbed mentation and behavior) is solid and growing. Although laboratory "definitions" of diagnosis, other than for exclusion, are few [also true for many medical disorders (15)], there are salient strategies to search for pathophysiologic processes.

Any medical text reveals that, even with our measurements, processes related to causes and phases of disorders still require search. Only since the 1970s have the different mechanisms begun to be identified that lead to elevated blood sugar (and even the risks of mildly elevated levels determined). Yet, insulin had been in hand for well over 50 years! For even longer (as is the *clear* case for schizophrenia, affective, and anxiety disorders) a distinct familial clustering was evident, but only recently clarified for type I and type II diabetes.

This research now focuses on disease subtypes, on subsensitive insulin receptors, and on autoimmune mechanisms affecting receptors or substrate (5). Current work seeks to detect the symptomatically silent long prodromal phases or the determinants for disease expression and the genetic, environmental, and molecular mechanisms influencing both. Animal models and twin studies are used to find predictors and define "necessary but not sufficient" factors, i.e., vulnerabilities. Interactions with the environment—restored receptor sensitivity with weight loss, or the vulnerability to viral instigation of type I diabetes—is under study. So too the management and etiopathology of the unexplained late phase chronic effects on cardiovascular and neurological systems. All these efforts—if retranslated—reflect the same fundamental parameters used in research on schizophrenia or the major depressions.

Failure to readily grasp these commonalities of approach may also derive from distracting ideologies about "the mentally ill" (as if we globally could usefully discuss "the febrile"). This obscures perspective on the tasks, accomplishments, and ways of proceeding of psychiatry as one of medicine's scientific disciplines. So we should briefly examine the function of clinical sciences; the confusion about whether psychiatric disorders are medically relevant; and, apart from the term's convenience in emphasizing currently "hot" strategies, query the utility of further specifying "Biological Psychiatry."

THE STUDY OF PSYCHIATRIC DISORDERS

Can "Medical" Research Strategies Be Relevant?

Past definitional detours concerned the "medical model." Essentially, the "model" is rooted in an ethic of professional accountability that employs a systematic mode of proceeding—the "clinical process" (11). More than simple trial and error, this entails a commitment to a logical investigation of the evidence that both the patient and scientific data provide. Mastery of the scientific knowledge base and tutored clinical judgment then guide the steps for diagnosis, treatment, and reassessment as the individual's response is monitored and the optimal possible function is achieved. This is how physicians proceed, whether psychiatrists or internists. The *source* of data, the *type* of intervention—*or* medicines—do not make a medical model. Instead, the way they are assessed and used in the management of a disorder is subsumed *in* the model. One may use the patient's report, the family history, or the laboratory in diagnosis; and one may manipulate diet or environment or prescribe exercise, medicines, or the acquisition of new skills or attitudes to compensate for impairment—whether we deal with diabetes, heart disease, arthritis, aphasia, asthma, depression, or agoraphobia.

Psychiatric disorder was also declared out of medical bounds when the secondary consequences of initially being ill, "labeling" and stigma, were construed to be the primary illness. There was no disease—only socially conditioned deviant behaviors—a view fueled by a diffuse agenda concerning the quality of public treatment facilities, the "civil right to be crazy" (rather than a functional incapacity to *not* be), and the arrogation of "power" by psychiatrists presuming to intervene in a purely social problem. Hardly illuminating the tasks of clinical or basic science research, these scholastic forays have been saliently critiqued (25).

A focus in modern biomedicine is now on the signaling and recognition systems of physiological regulatory mechanisms so that we no longer sharply distinguish the "organic" and the "functional" (and never should have). The implication was that the one can be seen and its cause thereby can be established, whereas the other was only imagined or groundlessly inferred—as if function could not be mediated by demonstrable processes. With the advent of psychometric assessment and diagnostic techniques, and of imaging and laboratory measures, structure and function, lesion and consequence are no longer alien domains but rather dynamically related. The autopsy may have a say (recently, even in schizophrenia) but no longer contains the final word about disease whether it is hypertension, migraine, gout, viral hepatitis, epilepsy, or fatal cardiac arrhythmia.

A century ago, the "father" of pathology, Virchow, noted that diseases are not intrusive "entities" but represent "only the course of physiological phenomena under altered conditions." There is dysfunction without lesions, and not all lesions produce symptoms. Probing these issues, Guze (15) concluded that the dictionary definition of disease can do for all: "An impairment of the normal state of the living animal or plant body that affects the performance of vital functions." Thus, the central issue is comprehending how to investigate characteristic clusters of symptoms and signs of dysfunctions (and their underlying processes) that in their origins, course, intensity, resolution, or response to treatment, are most usefully studied as diseases.

The Clinical Sciences and Their Function

Unlike the broader functions of the College, the narrowed task of the clinical sciences—and, paradoxically, the broad choice of strategies—is directed by an ineluctably pragmatic focus on disease. Thus, psychiatry, as does internal medicine, probes for predisposing causes, precipitants, courses, outcomes, and prognoses; etiopathological and pathophysiological processes; risks, vulnerabilities, modifying factors and resistance; treatments, their indications, efficacy, efficient delivery, and mechanisms of action; and means of prevention. Each specialty extracts and calibrates information from all sciences, and will use technological and methodological developments for the problem at hand. Clinical sciences also have a unique scholarly role. Dependent on many sources of knowledge, they must aggregate all data to assess the state of the art for the disorders in their purview. This is not the prime agenda of the essential contributory disciplines.

Overview of Clinical Research Strategy in Psychiatry

Analysis of the performances, characteristics, vulnerabilities, and responses to treatment or to biological or psychobiological (28) probes of defined clinical populations is a key clinical research activity. Clinical science investigations use anthropological (23) or epidemiological (2,7,20) tools to detect risk factors and disease variations not encountered in the clinic or correlations for which mechanisms must then be sought. Studies range from careful observational information to systematic inquiry in descriptively or biologically defined subgroups of patients. The question may be treatment response and side effects, therapeutic or disease mechanisms, or descriptive characteristics for subtypes (such as age of onset, severity, or prognostic profiles). Familial patterns of disorders may identify subtypes of depressive disorders or aid in differential diagnoses of schizophrenia and bipolar disease (18,29).

Disease "state" or enduring trait markers—behavioral, molecular, neuromuscular, etc.—may be sought. Signs of HPA axis overactivity are measured (as with the DST) to reflect state and diagnostic subtype status in depression, or decreased platelet serotonin uptake is seen as a trait marking "vulnerability" to delusional depression (22). Similar correlations of state, subtype, and amine receptor status are studied with various probes of neurohormonal response. "Sporadic" and "familial" schizophrenia may be differentiated based on brain morphological changes and symptomatic criteria ("positive" or "negative" symptoms) or perinatal history; lateralization of brain functions, information processing changes, or deviant eye tracking (as a trait) are also current topics of pursuit (1). Medical morbidity and mortality risks are assessed (and found to be elevated in schizophrenia, anxiety, and affective disorders).

Populations are thus studied cross-sectionally or over time using psychometric, biochemical, neuropsychological, electrophysiological, neurophysiological, brain imaging, molecular, genetic, pharmacologic, or epidemiological tools. Many psychiatric disorders and their subtypes "breed true." Populations may be selected as in family studies for prospective or retrospective inquiry for clues to transmission. Family studies may be designed to find useful pedigrees or to otherwise maximize the detection of mechanisms and markers or of predispositional traits, phases of disease, or prodromal signs, or of subgroups with distinct coexisting disorders [such as anxiety and depression (29)]. The continuities and discontinuities of childhood, adult, and geriatric disorders may be sought.

The clinical scientist may search in tissue cultures or, as noted, invent animal models further to elucidate mechanisms exposed in descriptive and correlational disease research. Research strategies seeking signs of the role of genetics range from the search for "markers" to familial, twin, and cross-fostering studies to mathematical models to linkage analyses using the tools of molecular genetics. These will increasingly be central across all disease research and be refining our current strategies. All are used in current research in schizophrenia, depression, obsessive or anxiety disorders, alcoholism, or somatoform disorder and more. We can search for neurobehavioral mechanisms mediating genetic factors prior to precise molecular definitions (26) and already know that with postnatal genetic rearrangements we can no longer directly infer an environmental component in the simple lack of full concordance in monozygotic twins (5).

As critical to psychiatric disease research as any known biological measure has been the development of instruments for structured interviews and use of explicit diagnostic criteria, a sustained focus on ascertainment bias, and unrelenting search for the sources of information and criterion variance when subgroups are described. The key aim is to clarify the question of diagnostic heterogeneity and homogeneity—of subtypes in disorders where phenotypes may be only apparently similar.

"Mechanisms of access" to the limited number of final common pathways have to be studied. Various broad conceptions of disease are in question: some view the depressions, or indeed all psychoses, as one disorder distinguished by degrees of severity. At bottom the question is when "more" is more—or different; are vigilance, anxiety, panic, terror, and confusion on a continuum or do they represent distinct organizations of biobehavioral mechanisms, or both? Whether there is one etiopathology for several outcomes or there are multiple etiologies for one phenotype are lively questions. Primary psychopathology and secondary and tertiary factors [e.g., stress of illness (14)] have to be sorted out as we attempt descriptive precision for biological subtyping. In broad brush, these systematic approaches (and their now intricate methodologies) reflect some of the panoply of strategies disease research entails in psychiatry as in all of medicine.

PSYCHIATRY AND BIOLOGY

Biological Psychiatry

Surveying strategies, what do we intend by "Biological Psychiatry?" The term today is a redundancy, but it arose in reaction to once-dominant interests in intrapsychic contents and mechanisms (9). For some, it refers to a highly restrictive set of measures or interventions—one side of a bad coin vainly separating mind from body or nature from nurture. Currently, it often connotes a special mode of practice, rather than a growing body of special knowledge. Thus, "neuropsychiatry" is rediscovered simply because it is now more relevant than it *recently* was to learn about function from brain lesions (as was commonly done by Freud, Kraepelin, Schilder, or students of lobotomy or limbic function and experimental psychobiology in "predrug" eras). We should not confuse special inquiry (neuropsychological correlations) or domains of knowledge (psychopharmacology)—or the use of laboratory tests, drug challenges, and endocrine or electrophysiological measures and pharmacokinetics to aid in clinical decisions—with a brand "new" clinical discipline. Practice generally adapts—as it ought—to new tools and applications of new knowledge.

Pragmatically, most of us have in mind merely an emphasis on biochemical or physiological processes and the tools to analyze them whether the "signals" are symbols, environmental cues, or internal "codes." Even if, as a working hypothesis (not an ideological position), we are in hot pursuit of an endogenous psychotogenic molecular mechanism effecting the genetic diathesis of schizophrenia, such "biological" investigation has as its ultimate reference specific patterns of "behavings." Human biology has to be concerned with the experience and operations of the mind and the events of behavior as they effect or express organismic adaptations. For psychiatry, these events symptomatically express and—for the moment—conclusively identify the presence of psychiatric disorder. Systematic language analysis currently "objectively" differentiates mania and schizophrenia better than any direct biological measure (16). Admixture and discriminant statistical analyses of symptoms can identify those differentiating schizophrenia from other disorders (4). So a biological psychiatry without a behavioral science and systematic psychological observations is as useless as a hammer without an anvil, and, perhaps, as dangerous. Such generalities aside, we can, in brief conclusory sweep, note what is intrinsically "biological" about the study of brain function and behavior, and essentially what our inferences and strategies must probe.

What Is Biological About Psychiatry?

Fundamentally, psychiatry and medicine as a part of the "life sciences" will ultimately have to discern the arrangements and subsequent operations of what is prepared in the human genome. We should come to understand the range of mechanisms, both endogenous *and* exogenous to nuclear DNA, by which apparently similar phenotypes can be observed. This intrinsic genetic design "expects" an environment with which to transact; the structure of DNA itself provides for order, error, and chance from conception throughout the life cycle. Whether we deal with the simplest of organisms or the human, the instructional and expressive design entails a ceaseless interplay of the "seeking and the sought" through molecular, cellular, and behavioral communications. We see this in embryology, with a nerve seeking the target that signals an "interest" or in the developed human seeking its sources of emotional nurturance. At bottom, then, we are built to behave.

This choreography of signaled events underlies the study of stability and change in living organisms. Their sustained identity but openness toward flexibility for adaptations was clearly expressed in nineteenth-century physiology by Claude Bernard. The organism is tending always toward equilibrium and, with perturbation, regulating itself to cope. With feedbacks, new governing "setpoints" for equilibria are constructed, providing an internally regulated organism that can optimally transact with and utilize the milieu it is built to seek. Fundamentally, this was Freud's approach when he elaborated how ongoing neuronal activity begins to acquire new secondary functions—i.e., how the cue of the parental intervener becomes a part of the organizing regulatory "memory structures" and control systems through and with which bodily and environmental needs are transacted.

Studying hormones or amines, we catch a snapshot of system with regulated equilibria and with compensatory processes. We attempt to discern the range over which any one system can fluctuate, but the prior state of any ongoing active system, simple or complex, will change the impact and meaning of a signal impinging upon it. The brain also is a dynamic organ built to behave, and one with "blank spaces." Through changes in its microstructure to the organization of limbic and frontal cortex, it is built to acquire information, memory, and a history to serve organismic needs in an expectable fashion. In so doing, it constructs an identity, style, or unique thumbprint. We know that learned familial rules and signals and personal memories structure the individual's interpretation not only of stressors but of options for goal setting and problem solving. The "psychosocial" is, thus, biologically rooted and a part of the regulatory operations we must study *and* use.

That fundamental neurobehavioral processes—sensitization, habituation, selection, inhibition—might be key in understanding how environmental signals are amplified or dampened or how behaviors become entrenched or too readily elicited, forecasts the profound clinically relevant work yet to be done in psychobiology. The challenge is great, entailing analyses from the molecular to organ system functions. Thus, even if we imagine the power to engineer it, exactly *how* the neuronal operation of differentiated but coordinated brain systems *should* be "set right" in schizophrenia would still elude us! For that goal, we have but

glimpses of what is going wrong (e.g., 1,27,28) and of the functions that neural systems and specialized brain areas do or don't accomplish. Loss of considerable brain tissue—even a hemisphere—does not abolish drug-responsive bipolar disease or the vegetative symptoms of melancholia. We will aim, then, to conceive of disease in terms of a useful grasp at the level both of brain neurobehavioral systems and of their underlying basic processes.

Clinically, we are searching for compensatory or regulatory processes that are excessive or inadequate in amount, in kind, or in their temporal or their articulated arrangements. Drugs in their effects on attention, perception, cognitive operations, or arousal and affective mechanisms are, in fact, influencing stop and start mechanisms and thresholds which, in turn, change the rate and range of signals through which a nervous system operates. To understand these operations in their simpler forms will bring a better grasp of the molecular mechanisms and functional brain systems necessary for the more complex expressions of human behavior which we study in their own right. In all this, to understand "the way things are"—rather than what we wish them to be—positions us to know what really may be possible. In this sense, both medicine and psychiatry will become increasingly unified in what is essentially a dynamic physiology, understanding the operations of the varied organ and molecular systems to be coordinated for optimal function. This is the broadly "biological" agenda that is at the heart of psychiatry's foreseeable future.

REFERENCES

1. Andreasen, N. C., ed. (1986): *Can Schizophrenia Be Localized in the Brain?* American Psychiatric Press, Washington, DC.
2. *Arch. Gen. Psychiatry* (1984): 41:921–1012.
3. Barchas, J. D., and Freedman, D. X. (1963): *Biochem. Pharmacol.,* 12:1225–1238.
4. Cloninger, C. R., Martin, R. L., Guze, S. B., and Clayton, P. J. (1985): *Arch. Gen. Psychiatry,* 42:15–25.
5. Eisenbarth, G. S. (1986): *N. Engl. J. Med.,* 314:1360–1368.
6. Feinberg, I. (1982/83): *J. Psychiatr. Res.,* 17:319–334.
7. Feinstein, A. R. (1985): *Clinical Epidemiology: The Architecture of Clinical Research.* W. B. Saunders Co., Philadelphia.
8. Freedman, D. X., ed. (1975): *Biology of the Major Psychoses: A Comparative Analysis.* Raven Press, New York.
9. Freedman, D. X. (1978): *Yale J. Biol. Med.,* 51:117–131.
10. Freedman, D. X. (1981): In: *Handbook of Biological Psychiatry, Vol. II, Part IV,* edited by H. M. van Praag, M. H. Lader, O. R. Rafaelsen, and E. J. Sachar, pp. 859–884. Marcel Dekker, New York.
11. Freedman, D. X. (1982): *Am. J. Psychiatry,* 139:1087–1095.
12. Freedman, D. X., Belendiuk, K., Belendiuk, G. W., and Crayton, J. W. (1981): *Arch. Gen. Psychiatry,* 38:655–659.
13. Freedman, D. X., and Giarman, N. J. (1963): In: *EEG and Behavior,* edited by G. H. Glaser, pp. 198–243. Basic Books, New York.
14. Gardner, R., Jr. (1982): *Arch. Gen. Psychiatry,* 39:1436–1441.
15. Guze, S. B. (1978): *Compr. Psychiatry,* 19:295–307.
16. Hoffman, R. E., Stopek, S., and Andreasen, N. C. (1986): *Arch. Gen. Psychiatry,* 43:831–838.
17. Judson, H. F. (1980): *The Eighth Day of Creation.* Simon & Schuster, New York.
18. Kendler, K. S., Gruenberg, A. M., and Tsuang, M. T. (1985): *Arch. Gen. Psychiatry,* 42:770–779.
19. Klein, D. S. (1981): In: *Anxiety: New Research and Changing*

Concepts, edited by D. S. Klein and J. G. Rabkin, pp. 235–262. Raven Press, New York.

20. Klerman, G. L., and Weissman, M. M. (1984): In: *Normality and the Life Cycle: A Critical Integration,* edited by D. Offer and M. Sabshin, pp. 315–344. Basic Books, New York.

21. Maas, J. W., and Leckman, J. F. (1983): In: *MHPG: Basic Mechanisms and Psychopathology,* edited by J. W. Maas, pp. 33–43. Academic Press, New York.

22. Meltzer, H. Y., Arora, R. C., Tricou, B. J., and Fang, V. S. (1983): *Psychiatry Res.,* 8:41–47.

23. Murphy, J. M. (1976): *Science,* 191:1019–1028.

24. NIMH-PSC Collaborative Study Group (1964): *Arch. Gen. Psychiatry,* 10:246.

25. Pies, R. (1979): *Arch. Gen. Psychiatry,* 36:139–144.

26. Schuckit, M. A. (1985): *Arch. Gen. Psychiatry,* 42:375–379.

27. Spohn, H. E., Lacoursiere, R. B., Thompson, K., and Coyne, L. (1977): *Arch. Gen. Psychiatry,* 34:633–644.

28. Weinberger, D. R., Berman, K. F., and Zec, R. F. (1986): *Arch. Gen. Psychiatry,* 43:114–124.

29. Weissman, M. M., Merikangas, K. R., Wickramaratne, P., Kidd, K. K., Prusoff, B. A., Leckman, J. F., and Pauls, D. L. (1986): *Arch. Gen. Psychiatry,* 43:430–434.

Psychopharmacology:
The Third Generation of Progress,
edited by Herbert Y. Meltzer.
Raven Press, New York © 1987.

CHAPTER **4**

Strategies for Research in Clinical Psychopharmacology

Leo E. Hollister

I should like to address several somewhat unrelated issues in clinical psychopharmacology that are important now and that will probably remain important for the next several years. Not all of these issues are solely the province of the clinical psychopharmacologist, but they do impinge on what we do.

NEED FOR DEVELOPMENT OF NEW DRUGS

For whatever reasons, the development of new psychotherapeutic drugs has slowed perceptibly. If one considers only the new chemical entities that have reached the marketplace, things don't look so bad. If one considers the novelty of these as drugs, they do. Many reasons account for this dearth of new drugs, despite the fact that a new drug with any clear advantage over existing drugs would be an enormous commercial success. In fact, some drugs have become so in the absence of convincing evidence of superiority. Let us now consider the four major classes of psychotherapeutic drugs, pointing out the deficiencies and problems associated with present drugs and the tentative searches for new ones.

Antipsychotic Drugs

Present Antipsychotics

It is most discouraging that more effective pharmacotherapy for schizophrenia has not been developed in the more than three decades since the introduction of the first effective drugs. The present large array of antipsychotic drugs have many deficiencies: they are not curative; their ameliorative effects are often limited; many patients remain totally unresponsive; they are unpleasant to take, so that many patients are less than fully compliant; and they produce major side effects, such as tardive dyskinesia and tardive psychosis, whose full implications are still uncertain.

Development of highly potent agents, or depot preparations that permit better compliance, or drugs with more specific actions on dopamine receptors has advanced the art of treatment. However, no presently available drug has been proved conclusively to be more effective, overall, than chlorpromazine, and therapeutic advantages have not been impressive. Having a good battery of predictive animal tests for typical antipsychotics, it has been possible to discover many chemicals with similar properties, but few really new drugs. No new antipsychotic drug has been introduced to the U.S. market for at least 10 years.

Many unsolved or controversial issues still surround the use of present drugs. Extensive studies aimed at determining the characteristics of patients who might respond selectively to antipsychotics are generally unrewarding (16). Differences in response may be mediated more by individual differences among patients than by differences between the drugs. Choice of drug for individual patients is made either on the basis of past experience of that patient or empirically.

Even the proper dose of antipsychotic is uncertain. Customary doses have increased during the past two decades. This trend may be in part attributable to the desire to obtain a quicker and more complete response or to increased needs of patients who become "tolerant" to the drug after long exposure. Another consideration is the fact that the availability of high-potency drugs permits use of much larger therapeutic doses than was possible with low-potency drugs.

The practice of using very large initial doses of drug in an attempt to gain a more rapid or more complete remission no longer seems to be justified. On the other hand, the question of whether larger than usual doses may salvage refractory patients is still not fully answered. Some preliminary studies suggest that some patients may require supranormal doses (19).

The duration of treatment and the best form of maintenance treatment are controversial. As it is impossible to be sure which patients will do well without drugs following remission of an initial episode of schizophrenia, the usual practice has been to withdraw antipsychotics in all patients. The rapidity and severity of relapse will determine the future course of maintenance treatment. The goal in maintenance treatment has been to keep the total exposure of the patient to the drug as low as is consistent with good control of symptoms. Whether these aims are best realized by treating intermittently ("drug holidays") or continually is still argued (2).

Although it is technically possible to measure plasma concentrations of several antipsychotic drugs, it has not yet been established that routine monitoring of such concentrations enhances drug therapy (20). In fact, with only a few drugs has it been possible to suggest a therapeutic range of plasma concentrations. The most secure data have emerged for haloperidol, but even with this drug, different therapeutic ranges may be defined for different types of patients. A range of 8 to 18 ng/ml is reasonable for newly admitted patients, whereas a range of 18 to 42 ng/ml is reasonable for previously refractory patients. Thus, although the laboratories can produce numbers, their clinical meaning is uncertain.

The late consequences of treatment with antipsychotics now include tardive dyskinesia, chronic akathisia, supersensitivity psychosis, and tardive dysmentia. The clinical implications of these developments for individual patients are uncertain and the proper management of such complications is controversial. These late complications have promoted a generally more conservative approach to use of antipsychotic drugs than that which prevailed a few years ago.

Atypical Neuroleptics

The earliest atypical neuroleptic was thioridazine, which lacked the antiemetic action of the others and tended to produce few extrapyramidal syndromes. Clozapine was the first true atypical drug and was of interest mainly because it had little tendency to evoke tardive dyskinesia. However, the threat of agranulocytosis has limited use of this compound. A related drug, fluperlapine, has suffered the same fate.

Recognition of two dopamine receptors, one linked to adenylate cyclase (D-1) and the other not (D-2), suggested that a drug acting specifically on D-2 receptors might have

less tendency to produce tardive dyskinesia. The benzamide, sulpiride, is such a drug and does seem to have minimal likelihood of producing tardive dyskinesia. It is also somewhat less effective as an antipsychotic (12).

Many other drugs are being investigated to determine if it is possible to separate the antipsychotic action from that which produces extrapyramidal effects. Zetidolone, setoperone, and BW-234U are examples of such drugs, but even early in their clinical testing, the latter two drugs have been withdrawn. Although such a separation would be valuable in that potentially disabling side effects might be reduced, no evidence suggests that any of these compounds developed thus far are more effective than traditional drugs.

Benzodiazepines

Interest in using benzodiazepines to treat schizophrenics has revived during the past few years. Diazepam, clonazepam, estazolam, and alprazolam have been used in much larger doses than customary for treating anxiety with initially favorable reports (21). Although it is conceivable that benzodiazepines, like the barbiturates which preceded them, may be useful for controlling agitated behavior and thus be considered as "sparing" antipsychotics, it seems unlikely that they would have specific antipsychotic actions in their own right.

Propranolol

After almost two decades of use as an antipsychotic, it is difficult to determine how effective propranolol is. Rather than being used as a sole treatment for schizophrenia, as originally proposed, it is now used as an adjunctive treatment in patients in whom traditional antipsychotics have failed (25). Propranolol has also gained a reputation as being an effective adjunct for patients who are aggressive. Despite the high dose used, the drug appears to be safe. Whether the mechanism of improvement is due to β-receptor blockade, a membrane-stabilizing action, or simply additional sedation, is not clear.

Clonidine

Clonidine, an α_2-adrenoreceptor agonist, was first tried in schizophrenics soon after its development due to its obvious sedating action. Six schizophrenic patients were treated, with negative results (27). Recently interest in this drug has revived, based on its ability to diminish noradrenergic activity.

Lithium and Carbamazepine

Many clinicians add lithium to the treatment of schizophrenics who have not responded to antipsychotics. Whether lithium simply has a nonspecific effect on excitement and aggression, or whether it specifically affects schizophrenic symptoms is uncertain. In any case, the effects of lithium become apparent rapidly, the majority of patients showing either a positive or negative effect after 1 week of treatment (31).

Carbamazepine has emerged as an alternative to lithium for a number of indications, including the adjunctive treatment of schizophrenia. As with lithium, the drug curbed violent behavior in some patients (1).

Dopamine Receptor Agonists

The concept of presynaptic receptors for dopamine that monitor its release by feedback inhibition offered an appealing method for reducing dopaminergic activity. Apomorphine has long been recognized as a dopamine receptor agonist, and it was thought to act selectively as a presynaptic receptor agonist in low doses. After some initial trials that looked promising, interest in this drug has waned. A drug that appeared to be highly selective for presynaptic dopamine receptor (3PPP) has been dropped from clinical investigation due to toxicity.

Proponents of the presynaptic approach forget that this method of treatment has been widely tried before. Reserpine, which acted by depleting aminergic neurotransmitters presynaptically, was an effective antipsychotic drug but was not considered to be as effective as the phenothiazines and became obsolete. It is difficult to imagine any presynaptic approach that could surpass the effect of reserpine.

Levodopa, in small doses, and bromocriptine, in substantial doses, have been used to treat schizophrenia with unimpressive results.

Naloxone and Opioid Peptides

It may seem somewhat illogical to link naloxone, an opiate antagonist, with endogenous or synthetic opioid peptides, yet similar claims have been made for both. A review of all the studies of naloxone in schizophrenia concluded that such "positive" effects as were mentioned were really quite small and that many trials were negative (28). Most studies were done with single doses. More chronic studies have been negative (30).

The initial glowing report on the efficacy of β-endorphin in schizophrenia led to many subsequent trials, most of which were not confirmatory. A synthetic homolog, des-tyrosine-γ-endorphin (DTE), has been most often used recently. It seems to work only in the Netherlands, where it originated.

Cholecystokinin Peptides

It is likely that every peptide hormone found in the brain will ultimately be tried in schizophrenia. Thyrotropin-releasing hormone (TRH) was the first one to be tried; it made schizophrenics worse (5). Recently, the major brain peptide of interest has been the gut hormone cholecystokinin (CCK). Most studies have used the decapeptide homolog of CCK ceruletide (or cerulein, as both names are used). Most studies have been negative (17). Problems with peptides are great: only very small ones are effective orally; penetration of the larger ones into brain is questionable,

even when given parenterally; most have half-lives measured in minutes. It will take a while to sort things out.

Other Possible New Treatment

Prostaglandin E_1 had prolonged antipsychotic effects following a single infusion (18). This remarkable report awaits confirmation.

Although no clinical studies have been done to date, one can confidently predict that calcium channel blockers will be tried in schizophrenia. The rationale stems from observations that trifluoperazine, as well as some of the diphenylbutylpiperidine antipsychotics, is a calcium channel blocker (11). Already some calcium channel blockers have been used to treat mania. The penetration of available calcium channel blockers into the brain is not high, but newer ones may prove to be better.

On the whole, development of new antipsychotics has followed a circular course. Pharmacological screening tests can be devised that characterize most clinically effective drugs. These tests can be used to discover a new chemical that shares many actions of existing drugs. Thus, we have new chemicals but old drugs.

Another factor that has slowed development of new antipsychotics has been the fact that the "dopamine" hypothesis, despite the lack of direct proof, still prevails. Although some drugs currently being tested involve primarily other neurotransmitters (setoperone, serotonin; clonidine, norepinephrine), a strong case cannot yet be made for neurotransmitters or neuropeptides other than dopamine. Until new hypotheses are proposed, the circular trap may continue to operate.

Antidepressants

Older Antidepressants

Tricyclic antidepressants and monoamine oxidase (MAO) inhibitors have been used clinically for almost 30 years. The numbers of both types of drugs have leveled off. For practical purposes, about seven or eight tricyclics and three MAO inhibitors are available in the United States. The advent of these drugs has ameliorated the treatment of depressed patients. Few patients now endure the chronic depressions of the past that resulted in years of continual hospitalization or multiple electroconvulsive treatments (ECT). On the other hand, relegating ECT to a place as a last-choice treatment has diminished the appropriate use of this highly effective treatment. The main disadvantage of these older drugs is that they fail to alleviate depression in 30 to 40% of patients, and in many others symptoms are not fully controlled. Further, they have many noxious side effects that make them unpleasant for patients to take. Thus, many failures of treatment may be due to the patients' not being able to take a full therapeutic dose or being noncompliant.

Another problem with tricyclics is that they affect multiple receptors. By blocking the uptake of neurotransmitters released into the synapse they produce a "down-regulation" of postsynaptic receptors, either for norepinephrine or serotonin. This action is believed to explain their antidepressant efficacy. However, they affect as well muscarinic-acetylcholine receptors, α_1 and α_2-adrenoreceptors, and histamine-1 and histamine-2 receptors (26). These latter actions produce side effects characterized by sedation, anticholinergic effects, orthostatic hypotension, and sympathomimetic effects. Clearly, a great fault with tricyclics is their lack of specificity of action.

The selection of an antidepressant for an individual patient is largely empirical. MAO inhibitors were thought to be primarily useful for "atypical" depressions characterized by anxiety, somatic complaints, and obsessive-compulsive-phobic features. Recent studies indicate that they are probably equally effective in "endogenous" depressions. Tricyclic antidepressants have their most specific effect in "endogenous" depressions. Biological correlates of such depression, such as nonsuppression of cortisol by dexamethasone, blunting of thyrotropin responses to thyrotropin-releasing hormone, and shortened latency of rapid eye-movement sleep, are said to augur a good response to tricyclics. That is, the more "endogenous" a depression, the better the response.

The selection of drug for individual patients has been less clear. Attempts to classify depressions as "noradrenergic" or "serotonergic" based on excretion patterns of neurotransmitter metabolites, particularly 3-methoxy-4-hydroxy-phenylglycol (MHPG), have not proven to be clinically useful.

Failure to respond to tricyclics has been alleged to be due to inadequate treatment. In many patients, the dose of drug does not relate well with plasma concentrations. Accordingly, monitoring plasma concentrations of these drugs is considered to eliminate the possibility of under-treatment or, in the case of some drugs, such as nortriptyline, overtreatment. Whether routine monitoring should be employed is controversial. The main difficulty is that one has little confidence in the ranges proposed for therapeutic concentrations. Even in the case of nortriptyline, about which there is most agreement, the contribution of a much more abundant active metabolite, 10-hydroxy-nortriptyline, has been overlooked. In the case of MAO inhibitors, it has been possible to gain some idea of their effect by measuring platelet MAO activity (although this measurement is not easy) or by simply testing for orthostatic hypotension, but correlations with clinical responses have been lacking.

Newer Antidepressants

As a result of the defects of older antidepressants, considerable current activity is directed at discovering new antidepressants. Five new antidepressants have entered the market during the past 6 years and more are expected soon. Major claims made for them are (a) faster onset of action, (b) fewer anticholinergic side effects, and (c) less cardiotoxicity. No claim of greater therapeutic efficacy has ever been validated. These drugs, and the others to follow, have been called "second- (or third-) generation" drugs, "atypical antidepressants," or "heterocyclic antidepressants." Experience to date with these new antidepressants has

not been encouraging (4). Amoxepine has no clinically significant faster onset of action, its side effect profile has been enlarged to include some side effects associated with antipsychotics, and its neurotoxicity in overdose may be greater than the cardiotoxicity of tricyclics. The combination of antipsychotic action and antidepressant effect may make it the drug of choice for psychotic depressions. Maprotiline seems to act specifically by blocking uptake of norepinephrine, similar to desipramine. As desipramine has the least sedative and anticholinergic actions of any tricyclic, assertions for fewer of these actions for maprotiline would be valid were the drug compared directly with desipramine, which has not yet been done. A faster onset of action is dubious, as is any advantage of greater safety when the drug is taken in overdose. Dose-related seizures are more common with this drug than with tricyclics.

Trazodone still remains something of a puzzle. Although it is thought to work primarily through an action on serotonin, the precise mechanism is unknown. Clinical responses have been spotty: either excellent results or very poor results; either marked sedation or scarcely any. Side effects, other than sedation, are minimal and overdoses are handled easily. Its efficacy relative to tricyclics has been questioned.

Nomifensine was of interest in that it acted by blocking uptake of both dopamine and norepinephrine. It had no sedative or anticholinergic actions. Its major problems were that it can act as an immunogen, and immunologic side effects led to its withdrawal. Buproprion also acted through dopaminergic mechanisms, by ways still poorly understood. It, too, was withdrawn due to dose-related seizures. These two drugs, both of which were effective antidepressants, raise the question of the role of dopamine in depression.

Greatest interest in developing new antidepressants has focused on selective inhibitors of serotonin uptake. The first of these, zimelidine, was most encouraging except for neurotoxicity, which caused the drug to be abandoned. A host of other selective inhibitors of serotonin uptake are in clinical trial: fluoxetine, paroxetine, femoxetine, fluvoxamine, clovoxamine, alaproclate, citalprolam, and indalpine. It remains to be seen whether any of these drugs can achieve the success of zimelidine with less danger.

Selective inhibition of MAO isozymes, A and B, could result in safer treatment. Clorgyline and deprenyl have been under investigation. A number of selective drugs that are also short-lived are also in trial.

Down-regulation of β-adrenoreceptors can be accomplished by direct β-adrenoreceptor agonists. Salbutamol and clenbuterol are the drugs of most interest. If such down-regulation is the final common pathway of action of antidepressants, this approach could achieve this end with much more specificity.

The role of alprazolam as an antidepressant is unclear (7). Should this atypical benzodiazepine have true antidepressant properties, it could represent a new and perhaps safer class of drug for treating depression.

Development of new antidepressants is limited in a way similar to antipsychotics. So much emphasis has been placed on the "amine hypothesis" that few drugs are considered as potential antidepressants unless they have some action on enhancing aminergic neurotransmitters at the synapse or mimicking their actions at the receptor. Until some new approaches are postulated, it is unlikely that we shall have new antidepressants that are more efficacious than the present ones, but we may obtain drugs with greater specificity of action.

Mood Stabilizers

Lithium and, more recently, carbamazepine, have been the drugs most often used to stabilize mood in patients with manic-depressive disorder. Although it is likely that an acute manic attack can be ameliorated in about 80% of patients by one or the other of these drugs, it is less likely that maintenance therapy with either drug will do as well in preventing future episodes. The recent expansion of mood stabilizers to other anticonvulsants, such as valproate sodium or clonazepam, cannot be interpreted as indicating that the anticonvulsant action itself is important. Phenytoin is ineffective. In fact, very little is known about the presumed mode of action of either of the two proven drugs. As many patients will be refractory to all these drugs, clearly better ones are needed. However, without a clear idea of both the pathogenesis of the disorder and the mechanism by which mood swings can be controlled by these drugs, problems in developing new ones are formidable.

The adjunctive role of antidepressants during the depressed phase and of antipsychotics during the manic phase is well established. Still uncertain is the extent to which their use may predispose to rapid cycling with an apparent worsening of the condition. Nor are there any data regarding which antidepressants or antipsychotics, if any, may be optimal for such use.

Antianxiety Agents

The era of the benzodiazepines may be coming to a close. The exact role of the triazolobenzodiazepines is still uncertain. Despite extensive investigation, it is still uncertain how they may differ from conventional benzodiazepines. The 1,5-benzodiazepines also do not differ materially in their spectrum of pharmacological actions; differences in pharmacokinetics may make certain members of this class more suitable for clinical indications other than anxiety.

The great contribution of the benzodiazepine era, besides providing drugs with advantages over barbiturates, has been the delineation of the benzodiazepine-γ-aminobutyric acid macromolecular complex (29). Several consequences of this discovery have already evolved. First, antagonists to benzodiazepines not only provide pharmacological tools but may be useful for expanding some clinical indications of these drugs and for managing overdoses. Second, the discovery of "inverse agonists," which bind to the receptor but which have actions opposite to the benzodiazepines, revives the issue of the pathogenesis of pathological anxiety. It is highly probable that the vulnerability to such anxiety may be mediated by biological mechanisms. Third, nonbenzodiazepine structures that bind to these receptors may suggest novel agents, especially if different benzodiazepine receptors are found to mediate different pharmacological

effects. The goal of separating sedative from antianxiety actions might be realized finally, either by developing mixed agonist-antagonist drugs, such as has been done for opiates, or by developing compounds specific for different types of receptors.

However, the most promising new lead has come from a drug that is neither a benzodiazepine nor one that binds to the receptor. Whether buspirone is as effective an antianxiety drug as the benzodiazepines and by what mechanisms its antianxiety action is mediated are important clinical and theoretical questions (10). Interactions between benzodiazepine receptors and adenosine receptors or β-adrenereceptors obviously require much more study.

BARRIERS TO NOVELTY IN DRUG DEVELOPMENT

The present system of investigational new drug (IND) applications may hinder some clinical pharmacological investigations testing a new hypothesis or new approaches to treatment. Each drug trial requires virtually the same formalities as though the drug were sponsored by a drug company and were likely to enter commerce. Yet many drug trials might use drugs as tools to test a hypothesis or as probes for new treatments. Only single doses or short-term treatment may be intended.

Recently, I cleaned out an old file relating to a study of melatonin in humans. One would think that a study of a naturally occurring substance, a relatively simple chemical, and one given in single doses, might be very uncomplicated. I could not believe the amount of correspondence involved in getting an IND for that study. Maybe I am getting old, but I should not have pursued the investigation today. Furthermore, as often happens with such studies, nothing publishable ensued.

It has been proposed that local Institutional Review Boards (IRBs) be given the authority to pass on all clinical trials of drugs. This responsibility would be too much to expect of most of these IRBs, whose membership cannot possibly include all the areas of expertise needed for making such a decision. Further, there is little reason to change the IND system as it applies to drugs sponsored by a drug company. This system works reasonably well. It is only when these formalities are extended to clinical trials of a truly investigational nature that progress seems to be impeded. The labor of obtaining certifications of purity of manufacture and extensive toxicological studies for compounds that might be used only a few times in humans deters all but the most obsessive investigator.

An abbreviated process might be developed for nonsponsored drugs or those which are to be used as tools to test a hypothesis. Investigators doing such trials should be able to send to the FDA a letter of notification of a proposed trial, along with available supporting data regarding the source of the chemical, its toxicological studies, and a copy of the protocol for the clinical study. Unless asked for additional information by the FDA within 60 days of submission, they should be able then to proceed with the proposed study.

The present system may be too cumbersome to permit much novelty. Drug companies that have a primary commercial interest in a compound will be able and willing to meet the requirements. Someone starting with a compound that cannot be patented and that may simply test a hypothesis should be covered under some separate "orphan drug" procedure. One wonders whether John Cade would ever have tried lithium had he had to meet the current requirements for an IND.

CLINICAL PHARMACOLOGICAL ISSUES

Clinical Trials

The present methodology of clinical trials is such that it is impossible to conceive of an adequate study that would miss an effective drug or ascribe efficacy to an ineffective drug. The largest remaining problems are defining selected efficacy of new drugs, that is, those patients for whom the drug may have the most to offer. Comparative efficacy is often inadequately studied by using sample sizes that are too small to reject the null hypothesis. This error leads to the "no different from therefore equal to" fallacy. It can be corrected by using ample sample sizes.

Bioavailability

During phase 1 studies of drugs with clear-cut subjective or objective effects, bioavailability is not a problem. Discernible clinical effects that are dose-related virtually assure that effective amounts of drug have entered the systemic circulation. When such effects are absent or equivocal, one cannot be sure whether adequate amounts of drug are available or whether the drug truly lacks these properties. Such determinations might be important, for instance, in the case of a presumed anxiolytic with no sedating effects. It is also obvious that before a drug is abandoned as being less than adequately effective in clinical trials, one should determine that adequate amounts of the drug have been made available to test the presumed therapeutic action.

The comparative bioavailability of different dosage forms of a drug could be of clinical importance (15). Many physicians (and their patients) have learned the hard way that 200 mg of chlorpromazine given intramuscularly is three or four times as potent as the same dose given orally. The ratio with the high-potency drugs is usually less; parenteral doses are usually not more than twice as potent.

Metabolism in Humans

The importance of determining early on the metabolic fate of a new drug is that a very large number of psychotherapeutic drugs have active metabolites that account for all, or a major portion, of their clinical effects (6). Such drugs include thioridazine, amitriptyline, imipramine, chlordiazepoxide, and diazepam. An active metabolite of each of these drugs has been marketed as a separate entity. Other psychotherapeutic drugs in which the role of active metabolites seems to be important, though less clear, include nortriptyline, desipramine, doxepin, amoxepine, and alprazolam. Active metabolites have been suspected to be important in the clinical actions of buproprion, nomifensine, maprotiline, and trazodone.

Early identification of metabolites of a new drug may allow for testing them for pharmacologic activity and a better appreciation of their role in its clinical action. It may also lead, as it has done repeatedly in the past, to the introduction of the active metabolite as a drug in its own right. Another consideration is that one can scarcely make an accurate appraisal of the relationship between clinical response and plasma concentrations unless active metabolites are also taken into account.

Clinical Pharmacokinetics

Pharmacokinetic studies have universally shown that different patients display widely varying plasma concentrations of drug, either after single doses or at steady-state conditions. The implication is clear that not all patients are best treated with the same dosage schedule. Rather, doses should be titrated to the needs of individual patients. Most clinical protocols now allow for some degree of flexibility of doses. The extent of such flexibility might best be determined by earlier studies indicating the degree of variation in plasma concentrations among a sample of potential patients.

Pharmacokinetic studies, and the use of these parameters in clinical trials, should always be accompanied by clinical observations of the pharmacodynamic actions of the new drug. Long ago it became obvious that the duration of action of antipsychotics was much longer than the plasma half-life indicated. On the other hand, good clinical observations may anticipate the half-lives of the drug being studied. The classification of duration of action of various barbiturates was determined both by clinical observations and a few studies of sleeping time in animals, long before accurate measurements of the concentrations of these drugs in bodily fluids could verify these estimates.

Therapeutic Ranges of Plasma Concentrations

Establishing relationships between steady-state plasma concentrations of psychotherapeutic drugs and clinical response has usually been done, if at all, long after the drug has been marketed. Despite a great amount of work during the past two decades, one still cannot speak with much assurance about a therapeutic range of plasma concentrations for any psychotherapeutic drug other than lithium. This question is fraught with difficulties. Yet, if a suitable method for measuring plasma concentrations of a drug is available, it would seem a pity not to take advantage of the unique situation in late phase 3 clinical trials in which doses of drug are tightly controlled and careful and frequent measurements of clinical response are made.

Another possible reason for measuring plasma concentrations of drugs early in the course of their development is to check on compliance. Very little attention has been paid to this aspect of drug trials. Clinical experience with monitoring plasma concentrations of antidepressants among outpatients suggests a rate of 20% noncompliance (13). Monitoring of plasma concentrations of diazepam among outpatients indicated that about 35% of patients had lower levels than would have been expected had they taken the drug as prescribed (14). A number of techniques have been used in the past to monitor compliance (pill counts, riboflavin excretion in urine, qualitative tests for drug in urine), but determination of plasma concentrations of drug would provide the most useful information. At present, we have no idea of how noncompliance with scheduled drug taking affects the results of clinical trials.

Potential Drug Interactions

Each member of the four major classes of psychotherapeutic drugs may be combined with one or more of the others. Therefore, it makes sense to explore systematically the consequences of such combinations.

Many pharmacodynamic interactions can be predicted on the basis of known pharmacological effects of the drugs in question. For instance, if two drugs both have sedative or anticholinergic or adrenoreceptor-blocking actions, these will become additive when the drugs are combined. Such interactions are by far the most common and most important clinically. Systematic exposure of patients to a new drug in combination with other drugs that may also be used simultaneously should detect any major interactions, the mechanisms of which can be worked out later on.

Patients often take drugs in the presence of other disease states than those for which the drug is given. The usual mode of testing new drugs prior to marketing virtually completely eliminates the possibility of detecting any interactions between the new drugs and a disease state. Subjects for study are deliberately chosen on the basis of their not taking other drugs or having other illnesses. It is not surprising that major problems associated with the use of new drugs often do not appear until the drug has already been marketed. It would seem desirable that during some part of the development of a new drug, it be used in patients with concurrent liver, heart, lung, or kidney disease. Probably such observations would best be made during the late stage 3 phase of drug development. These observations need not use any blind controls but should be made systematically, using commonly available techniques for ascertaining any adverse effects on the function of these various organ systems.

Overdoses

Psychotherapeutic drugs are used in patients who have a high risk for suicide. Frequently, patients use the drugs prescribed for their emotional disorder to attempt to end their lives. It would be nice to know in advance of the actual clinical situation what sort of problems might be encountered with overdoses of various new drugs and what measures might be taken to mitigate them.

Obviously, such studies cannot be done in humans. Probably dogs would be the best animals for such overdose studies. It might not be difficult to detect in overdosed dogs whether a new drug might create life-threatening ventricular arrhythmias or seizures. If such were the case, one might also study the best methods for managing such complications, in the choice of either antiarrhythmics or anticonvulsants. The severe and uncontrollable convulsions that follow overdoses of amoxepine might have come as less of a surprise had animal studies of the effects of overdoses been done prior to its release (22).

Studies in humans might be directed at determining ways in which absorption of large therapeutic doses of the drug may be impaired, or, conversely, its elimination enhanced. Presumably any methods that would work in this situation should be equally effective in the overdose situation.

Special Problems

Most clinical trials of new drugs during the developmental stages place an age limit on the subjects. Usually, this limit is considerably below that of many potential patients who might receive the drug in practice. Such age limits should be abandoned, provided no other contraindications to the use of the drug exist. Systematic observation of the effects of the drug in the elderly, along with pharmacokinetic data, could afford the basis for more accurate labeling of the new drug in regard to its use in elderly patients.

Increasing evidence indicates that virtually any centrally active drug (as well as many that are not) may be associated with withdrawal phenomena when the drug is suddenly stopped. Tests for such withdrawal effects might very well be done in animals, as even rodents provide adequate models (8). If the withdrawal effects of the drug are not too severe in animal models, then it might be feasible to do clinical studies of various modes of withdrawal of the drug, ranging from abrupt to phased withdrawal. The mere fact that a drug produced such a syndrome would not, in itself, be cause for abandoning it. The main purpose would be to alert clinicians who prescribe the drug to the possibility and to promote guidelines for avoiding or for managing the problem.

NEW AREAS OF DRUG DEVELOPMENT

Some areas of interest to clinical psychopharmacologists have not seen the development of effective drugs at all. These areas might lead to a "wish list" of drugs of great interest and great commercial value. Here are some likely candidates.

Drugs to Facilitate Learning and Memory

Mental retardation is a major psychiatric problem for which no drug therapy exists. Although it is likely that the causes of mental retardation are multiple, a drug that might nonspecifically improve attention, alertness, and memory would be of great value. Amphetamines and other sympathomimetic stimulants have many drawbacks. The newer peptides, such as corticotropin (ACTH) fragments and vasopressin analogs, seem to work much better in animals than in humans. Thus, the field is wide open. Such drugs might also be useful in the elderly who find some difficulty in retrieval of information. In fact, they might be generally applicable, for who would spurn a "smartness drug"?

Drugs That Would Alter the Pathology of Alzheimer's Disease

This disease, formerly considered to be rather uncommon, now looms as a major problem due to the increasing age of our population. Drug treatment has generally been without much effect. The symptomatic control of behavioral disturbances has been most fruitful. Depending upon which hypothesis for the pathogenesis of Alzheimer's disease one would embrace, drugs of this type might be antivirals, immunosuppressives, chelating agents, or products of genetic engineering. Unfortunately, the uncertain pathogenesis of this disorder prevents any rational development of drugs to treat it. The current line being followed, that of augmenting cholinergic neurotransmission, is analogous to the augmentation of dopamine in Parkinson's disease (23). Even a successful approach using this limited hypothesis would be valuable and may be the most one can expect over the near term.

Drugs That Would Decrease the Reward from Alcohol or Other Dependence-Producing Drugs

Between them, alcohol abuse and nicotine dependence contribute more premature deaths by far than any other cause. No amethystic agent (that is, an antidote to alcohol's effects) has ever been developed. The recent reports suggesting that specific serotonin uptake inhibitors limit alcohol consumption requires verification (24). Current attempts to treat nicotine dependence by administering the drug in a different form require more time for evaluation. If the observation that clonidine may actually decrease craving for nicotine is confirmed, this approach might also be promising (9). One would like to think that some drug that would block access of dependence-producing substances to the sites in the brain that lead to reinforcement of drug-taking behavior might be generally applicable to many problems with dependence-producing drugs. Maybe that is too naive a hope.

Drugs That Would Augment Sexual Interest and Performance

The search for an aphrodisiac is ancient and is no closer to fruition now than it was many years ago. The news about drugs and sex is that whatever effects drugs may have are usually all bad. With 10% of adult males bothered by partial or total impotence, and with a steadily aging population, one would predict that any drug that offered hope would be highly successful commercially. Even the old and formerly discredited drug, yohimbine, is making a comeback (3). The hope engendered by the discovery of releasing hormones has proven to be elusive. But the effort to develop such drugs would be worth making.

EPILOGUE

When the late Kenneth Clark undertook to write about a broad topic, *Civilization*, he added a subtitle to the book: *A Personal View*. Such a limiting statement was not mere modesty but an acceptance of reality. As the topic of this essay is similarly broad, I am sure that my coverage of it also represents a personal view. Many of my colleagues, given the same chore, might have turned out pieces greatly different. Indeed, I hope that this chapter will be as provocative as it is informative. As we think in broad terms of the problems that face us, we can better devise strategies for their solution. Defining the problem is the first step.

REFERENCES

1. Ballenger, J. C., and Post, R. M. (1984): *Psychopharmacol. Bull.,* 20:572–584.
2. Carpenter, W., Jr. (1986): *J. Clin. Psychiatry,* 47(*Suppl*):23–29.
3. Clark, J. T., Smith, E. R., and Davidson, J. M. (1984): *Science,* 225:847–848.
4. Coccaro, E. F., and Siever, L. J. (1985): *J. Clin. Psychopharmacol.,* 25:241–260.
5. Davis, K. L., Hollister, L. E., and Berger, P. A. (1975): *Am. J. Psychiatry,* 132:951–953.
6. Drayer, D. E. (1982): *Drugs,* 24:519–542.
7. Feighner, J. P., Aden, G. C., Fabvre, L. F., Rickels, K., and Smith, W. T. (1983): *JAMA,* 249:3057–3064.
8. Gallaher, E. J., Henauer, S. A., Jacques, C. J., and Hollister, L. E. (1986): *J. Pharmacol. Exp. Ther.,* 237:462–467.
9. Glassman, A. H., Jackson, W. K., Walsh, B. T., Roose, S. P., and Rosenfeld, B. (1984): *Science,* 226:864–866.
10. Goa, K. L., and Ward, A. (1986): *Drugs,* 32:114–129.
11. Gould, R. J., Murphy, K. M. M., Reynolds, I. J., and Snyder, S. H. (1983): *Proc. Natl. Acad. Sci. USA,* 80:5122–5123.
12. Harnryd, C., Bjerkenstedt, L., Bjork, K., Gullberg, B., Oxenstein, G., Sedvall, G., Wiesel, F.-A., Wik, G., and Aberg-Wistedt, A. (1984): *Acta Psychiatr. Scand.,* 69(*Suppl* 311):7–30.
13. Hollister, L. E. (1982): *J. Clin. Psychiatry,* 42:66–69.
14. Hollister, L. E., Conley, F. K., Britt, R. H., and Shuer, L. (1981): *JAMA,* 246:1568–1570.
15. Hollister, L. E., Curry, S. F., Derr, J., and Kanter, S. (1970): *Clin. Pharmacol. Ther.,* 11:49–59.
16. Hollister, L. E., Overall, J. E., Kimbell, I., Jr., Pokorny, A. (1974): *Arch. Gen. Psychol.,* 30:94–99.
17. Itoh, E., and Study Group for CLN. (1986): *Clin. Eval.,* 14:175–216.
18. Kaiya, H. (1984): *Biol. Psychiatry,* 19:457–463.
19. Kim, D. Y., and Hollister, L. E. (1984): *J. Clin. Psychopharmacol.,* 4:32–35.
20. Kucharski, L. T., Alexander, P., Tune, L., and Coyle, J. (1984): *Psychopharmacology,* 82:194–198.
21. Lingjaerde, O. (1982): *Acta Psychiatr. Scand.,* 65:339–354.
22. Litovitz, T. L., and Troutman, W. G. (1983): *JAMA,* 250:1069–1071.
23. Mohs, R. C., Davis, B. M., Greenwald, B. S., Mathe, A. A., Johns, C., Horvath, T. B., and Davis, K. L. (1985): *J. Am. Geriatr. Soc.,* 33:749–757.
24. Naranjo, C. A., Sellers, E. M., and Lawrin, M. O. (1986): *J. Clin. Psychiatry,* 47(*Suppl*):16–22.
25. Pugh, C. R., Steinert, J., and Priest, R. G. (1983): *Br. J. Psychiatry,* 143:151–155.
26. Richelson, E. (1979): *Psychiatr. Ann.,* 9:195–196.
27. Simpson, G. M., Dunz-Bartholini, E., and Watts, T. P. S. (1967): *J. Clin. Pharmacol.,* 7:221–225.
28. Skrabanek, P. (1982): *Lancet,* 2:1270.
29. Tallman, J. F. (1985): *Prog. Neuropsychopharmacol. Biol. Psychiatry,* 9:545–549.
30. Verhoeven, W. M. A., Van Praag, H. M., and Van Ree, J. M. (1984): *Psychiatry Res.,* 12:297–312.
31. Zemian, F. P., Hirschowitz, J., Saulter, F. J., and Garver, D. L. (1984): *Br. J. Psychiatry,* 144:64–69.

Psychopharmacology:
The Third Generation of Progress,
edited by Herbert Y. Meltzer.
Raven Press, New York © 1987.

CHAPTER 5

Monoamines of the Central Nervous System: A Historical Perspective

Arvid Carlsson

The concept of chemical neurotransmission goes back to the beginning of this century, but its relevance for the central nervous system became evident much later. In 1963 McLennan (92) concluded: "In the vertebrate central nervous system there is only one synapse identified whose operation can, with assurance, be ascribed to acetylcholine." The synapse referred to was located to the Renshaw cells in the spinal cord receiving innervation from collaterals of the motoneurons. Obviously no generalizations could be made from this very special case. Regarding the monoamines and other putative neurotransmitters, McLennan found himself unable to identify a single case where any of them could be ascribed a role as a neurotransmitter in the vertebrate central nervous system. Yet at this time a development was already in progress that was to change this picture dramatically.

The new development was triggered by a number of parallel events in the 1950s: the discovery of "sympathin" (a mixture of norepinephrine and epinephrine, ref. 111) and 5-hydroxytryptamine (5-HT, serotonin, refs. 3, 106) in the brain, the introduction of the modern psychotropic drugs, and the development of sensitive and specific biochemical and histochemical methods for the detection of the monoamines and their precursors and metabolites in tissues and body fluids.

The blockade of peripheral 5-HT receptors by the hallucinogen LSD led to some intriguing speculations concerning a role for 5-HT in mental functions (67,113), and this in turn prompted Brodie and Shore (101) to investigate the interactions between 5-HT, LSD, and the newly discovered antipsychotic agent reserpine. They speculated that reserpine might act by releasing 5-HT. Moreover, they were in an excellent position to examine their hypothesis, thanks

to an important methodological innovation being developed in Brodie's laboratory at the National Heart Institute in Bethesda, Maryland. Together with Dr. Udenfriend, Dr. Brodie had persuaded Dr. Bowman, an M.D. with exceptional talents, to construct the first prototype of a spectrophotofluorimeter. This instrument was soon to revolutionize the analysis of biogenic amines and numerous other important body constituents. Using this instrument Brodie and his colleagues now made a great discovery: following treatment with reserpine the stores of 5-HT in the brain and other tissues were almost completely depleted, with a concomitant increase in the urinary excretion of the 5-HT metabolite 5-hydroxyindoleacetic acid (99,101).

Thus, for the first time, a psychotropic agent had been shown to exert a dramatic action on an endogenous putative agonist in the brain. I was fortunate enough to arrive in Dr. Brodie's laboratory only a few months later and to spend a very stimulating 6-month period with Drs. Brodie and Shore. Together with them I had the opportunity to demonstrate in *in vitro* experiments on platelets that reserpine acts directly on the storage mechanism for 5-HT (45).

After returning from Bethesda to my hometown of Lund in Sweden I found myself in another fortunate circumstance: Dr. Hillarp, working in the Department of Histology, had recently discovered the organelles, so-called granules, storing the catecholamines in the adrenal medulla (75) together with stoichiometric amounts of ATP (74). In Bethesda I had found fairly large amounts of ATP in platelets, as shortly afterwards reported by Born (18), and thus a link between the storage of 5-HT and catecholamines was suggested. Hillarp and I joined forces, and we discovered the virtually complete disappearance of catecholamines from the adrenal medulla following reserpine treatment

(33). Shortly afterward, together with my graduate students Bertler and Rosengren, I demonstrated the depletion of norepinephrine in the heart and brain by reserpine and the failure of noradrenergic nerves to function following this depletion (11,44). Similar observations were made by Vogt and her colleagues (80,94).

Much to our regret we had to disagree with my tutors and friends Drs. Brodie and Shore concerning the mode of action of reserpine. They had suggested that the behavioral action of this agent was due to the continuous release of 5-HT onto receptors following depletion of the stores. This interpretation was logical in view of their interaction experiments referred to above, indicating that 5-HT and reserpine acted similarly as LSD antagonists in sleeping time experiments in mice. However, their interpretation was open to the criticism that 5-HT, given systemically, does not penetrate readily into the brain. On the basis of our own observations we felt that not only 5-HT but also the catecholamines should be considered in attempts to explain the action of reserpine. Moreover, the functional failure of the adrenergic nerves suggested that lack of monoamines at receptor sites, rather than continuous stimulation of the receptors, might be the crucial functional result of reserpine's action. To test this hypothesis we administered dopa and 5-hydroxytryptophan (5-HTP) to reserpine-treated animals and discovered the remarkable stimulating action of dopa, leading to the virtually complete reversal of reserpine's sedative action (40).

DISCOVERY OF DOPAMINE IN THE BRAIN: AN ENDOGENOUS BEHAVIORAL STIMULANT

Following the discovery of dopa decarboxylase in 1938 (79) and the formulation of the synthetic pathway for catecholamines (17), dopamine was recognized as an intermediate in the synthesis of the two important catecholamines, norepinephrine and epinephrine. The weak sympathomimetic activity of dopamine argued against a role for this amine in its own right. In 1957 Montagu (93) reported the presence in brain extracts of a compound, called "X," which on a paper chromatogram behaved as dopamine.

In the further analysis of our reserpine-dopa experiment we found that norepinephrine remained at a very low level in the brain despite the dramatic reversal of the action of reserpine by dopa. We were thus forced to turn our attention to dopamine. After developing a method for its detection (46), which could be adapted to our previous method for the measurement of epinephrine and norepinephrine (12), we found that the stimulating action of dopa was closely correlated to the appearance of dopamine in the brain. Moreover, we observed that dopamine occurs normally in the brain in amounts comparable to those of norepinephrine and that it was made to disappear, like norepinephrine, after treatment with reserpine. This led us to propose that dopamine is not merely a precursor but also serves as an agonist in its own right in the brain (42). Shortly afterwards we discovered the peculiar distribution of dopamine, with by far the highest amounts in the striatum. Given the recently discovered extrapyramidal effects of reserpine, we suggested that dopamine is involved in extrapyramidal functions, excess and deficiency of this agonist leading to Parkinsonism and chorea, respectively (14,24).

My colleagues and I were excited by these observations. We felt that the opposite behavioral actions of a monoamine-depleting agent and a catecholamine precursor made a strong case for the catecholamines as agonists in the central nervous system. However, we were disappointed by meeting a lot of scepticism against our views. This is evident, for example, from the proceedings of the Ciba Foundation Symposium on Adrenergic Mechanisms (110), where our ideas were not well received. Thus, Sir John Gaddum, in his final remarks, concluded (p. 594): "The meeting was in a critical mood, and no-one ventured to speculate on the relation between catecholamines and the function of the brain." My attempts in this direction were simply ignored. This negative attitude was the more remarkable, as our most salient observations had actually been confirmed or independently demonstrated by others.

Shortly afterward, Ehringer and Hornykiewicz (56) reported their discovery of low levels of dopamine in the basal ganglia of Parkinson patients, and a therapeutic effect of L-dopa was demonstrated in this disorder (10,15). No doubt these important discoveries contributed to bring the central monoamines into focus. Incidentally, they supported our deficiency theory for the action of reserpine. However, the real breakthrough came with the histochemical techniques permitting the visualization of the monoamines in the fluorescence microscope.

VISUALIZATION OF THE MONOAMINES IN THE FLUORESCENCE MICROSCOPE

The fascinating story of the development of a histochemical technique for the visualization of monoamines in the fluorescence microscope is closely linked to the late Dr. Nils-Åke Hillarp, a highly talented histologist who died at the untimely age of 48 in 1965 (for a detailed review, see ref. 54). Hillarp had already in the 1940s and 1950s made several important discoveries in the area of the autonomic nervous system, partly referred to above. Our collaboration was not confined to the mechanism of storage of catecholamines; we also engaged in attempts to visualize the catecholamines under the microscope. At that time such visualization was possible only in the chromaffin cells of, e.g., the adrenal medulla, using the so-called chromaffin reaction or, as shown by Eränkö (59), by the green fluorescence occurring in sections of the adrenal medulla following formalin fixation (see also ref. 62).

When I was appointed to the chair of pharmacology at the University of Göteborg in 1959, I was delighted to learn that Hillarp wanted to join me. This was made possible through a grant from the Swedish Medical Research Council, which enabled Hillarp to take leave from his associate professorship at the University of Lund. In 1960 we moved into the newly built Department of Pharmacology in Göteborg. The university had allowed fairly generous funding for the equipment of the new institution, and

Hillarp and I could start our research in Göteborg without delay.

Our first attempt to visualize catecholamines in the fluorescence microscope utilized the principle of the so-called trihydroxyindole method for quantitative analysis of catecholamines, i.e., the principle used, for example, by Bertler et al. (12). Tissue sections were in a first step exposed to iodine to oxidize the catecholamines to adrenochromes, and in a second step to ammonia to rearrange the adrenochromes to fluorescent adrenolutines. Our efforts were very successful in so far as the adrenal medulla was concerned: a highly intensive fluorescence developed; it was reduced, though still clearly visible, after removing more than 95% of the catecholamines by reserpine treatment (31). However, for some unknown reason, perhaps diffusion of the amines out of the tissue, the adrenergic transmitter could not be visualized in nerve terminals or cell bodies. Nevertheless, the results were considered encouraging, and Hillarp was now convinced that the project would ultimately prove successful.

Hillarp decided to try another principle for the development of fluorescence from monoamines, based on the method of Hess and Udenfriend (71) for measurement of, e.g., tryptamine. In this method tryptamine is condensed with formaldehyde to form a highly fluorescent product. Together with his skillful research engineer Georg Thieme, Hillarp started to investigate systematically this reaction in histochemical model experiments. Amines were dissolved in solutions of serum albumin, sucrose, gelatin, or gliadin, spotted on glass slides, and air dried. Upon treatment with formaldehyde vapor, generated from a 35% solution of formaldehyde, a very strong fluorescence developed in spots of, e.g., norepinephrine or dopamine. Protein catalyzed the reaction. The fluorescence products were identified as tetrahydroisoquinolines, later verified by Corrodi and Hillarp (51).

The paper reporting these fundamental model experiments, all of which were performed by Hillarp and Thieme in the Department of Pharmacology at the University of Göteborg, was authored by Falck, Hillarp, Thieme, and Torp (63), one of the 100 most cited publications from 1961 to 1982. After Hillarp's move to Göteborg, Falck remained at the Department of Histology, University of Lund. After the model experiments were completed, a considerable part of the experiments on tissue specimens was performed in collaboration with Falck in Lund, since a histology department was of course better equipped for this purpose. Various attempts were made, though without any clear-cut success, until one day in late August 1961, when Hillarp visited Falck and his old department, and Hillarp proposed that they try air-dried stretch preparations of thin tissue specimens, such as rat iris and mesentery. Hillarp was familiar with these preparations from his previous work (72,73), classical treatises on the functional organization of the autonomic ground plexus. Such preparations were now exposed to dry formaldehyde gas generated from paraformaldehyde powder. The outcome was dramatic: in the fluorescence microscope Hillarp and Falck saw the same nerve-plexus pattern as previously observed by Hillarp following staining with methylene blue. But this time it was the adrenergic transmitter that showed up as

green fluorescence as a consequence of treatment with formaldehyde. In addition, yellow fluorescence derived from mast-cell 5-HT could be seen in the mesentery preparations. In principle, a great discovery had thus been made, but needless to say, a lot of work remained. For example, the technique had to be adapted to embedded tissue specimens. This work was first performed in Lund and later, after Hillarp's move to take over the chair of histology at the Karolinska Institute in Stockholm in 1962, also by a rapidly growing group of young, enthusiastic students in Hillarp's new working place. For a detailed account of the further development of the histofluorescence techniques, see refs. 16 and 54. Evidently the new technique was a powerful tool, which helped to solve a large number of important problems in the monoamine field.

CELLULAR LOCALIZATION AND MAPPING OF THE MONOAMINES

A major initial step was the demonstration of the monoamines in nerve cell bodies and nerve terminals of the central nervous system (30). The neuronal localization of the central monoamines was confirmed by lesion experiments. The first lesion experiments, which demonstrated the virtually complete disappearance of monoamines from the spinal cord below a transection, utilized biochemical techniques only (43,90), shortly before the demonstration of the descending bulbospinal monoaminergic pathways by means of the histofluorescence technique (29). The first lesion experiments to confirm the neuronal localization of a monoamine in the brain demonstrated the disappearance of dopamine, measured biochemically, and of green-fluorescent nerve terminals from the rat neostriatum following a lesion of the substantia nigra (5). Moreover, removal of the striatum was followed by an accumulation of fluorescent material in the cell bodies of the substantia nigra and in axons proximal to the lesion, thus demonstrating the existence of a nigrostriatal dopamine pathway. Independent work in Lund (13) gave similar results.

But these were only beginnings. An enormous amount of work remained to map out all the monoaminergic pathways in the central nervous system. A large number of workers became engaged in this important mapping, starting with Dahlström and Fuxe (55) and Fuxe (66), and followed by Ungerstedt (107) and many others (see refs. 16, 87). Needless to say, the detailed knowledge of the central monoaminergic pathways has been of fundamental importance for the further development of this research field. For example, it enabled Andén and his colleagues (see ref. 6) to develop simple and useful functional models for the individual monoamines, and Aghajanian and his colleagues (see ref. 2 and chapters by Aghajanian and Bunney, *this volume*) to embark on their pioneer studies of the electrophysiological activity of monoaminergic neurons.

EMERGING SYNAPTOLOGY

The impact of the histochemical visualization of the monoamines goes of course far beyond the mapping of monoamine-carrying neuronal pathways. After the introduction of the new technique, previous doubts expressed about the transmitter function of the monoamines gradually changed into a debate on the complex issue of neurotransmitter versus neuromodulator function. Today nobody appears to question the neurotransmitter function of the monoamines in the central nervous system, at least in a broad sense of this term. Rather, the monoamines have become "spearheads" in neurotransmission research, especially in the central nervous system. In particular, the monoaminergic synapse has become a very useful model. Fitting together the various pieces of the "synapse puzzle" has been a cumbersome process; a few early recollections will be briefly reviewed below.

In 1960 Axelrod et al. (see ref. 9) discovered the uptake of circulating catecholamines by adrenergic nerves. This uptake proved to be an important inactivation mechanism. According to Axelrod it could be blocked by a large number of drugs, for example, reserpine, chlorpromazine, cocaine, and imipramine, leading to supersensitivity to catecholamines and acceleration of their metabolism. This interpretation was not entirely in line with ours, especially in so far as reserpine was concerned; we considered the action of reserpine on the adrenergic transmitter to be a strictly intraneuronal event (see below). The discrepancy could be resolved by combined biochemical (35,84) and histochemical studies (91). Two different amine-concentrating mechanisms could be distinguished, i.e., uptake at the level of the cell membrane, sensitive, e.g., to cocaine and imipramine, and uptake by the storage granules or synaptic vesicles, sensitive, e.g., to reserpine. Blockade of the former, but not the latter, mechanism leads to catecholamine supersensitivity directly (although secondary receptor supersensitivity may develop after blockade of the latter). In the presence of reserpine, extracellular amine is still pumped into the cytoplasm with unabated efficiency. However, it cannot be stored but is deaminated by intraneuronal monoamine oxidase (MAO) (see also ref. 27).

Interesting perspectives emerged after the discovery by Axelrod and his colleagues of catechol-O-methyltransferase (COMT). Axelrod (8) proposed that COMT was mainly responsible for the metabolism of catecholamines, whereas MAO was thought to be primarily involved in the metabolism of the O-methylated metabolites of the catecholamines. Axelrod referred to the intracellular geography: since COMT occurs in the cell sap, newly released catecholamines will be primarily exposed to this enzyme and only secondarily to the mitochondrially located MAO. However, our reserpine data (44), as well as our observations on the accumulation of catecholamines and their metabolites following treatment with L-dopa (41), suggested to us that intraneuronally released catecholamines would primarily be metabolized by MAO; only after release into the extracellular space would they be exposed to COMT (25,34). This concept was later substantiated by numerous experiments and is now generally accepted (see refs. 9, 81, 112).

In the mid-1960s opinions still differed considerably concerning the subcellular distribution of the monoaminergic transmitters. In the fluorescence microscope the accumulation of monoamines in the so-called varicosities of nerve terminals was obvious. This corresponded to the distribution of synaptic vesicles, as observed in the electron microscope. In fact, Hökfelt (78) was able to demonstrate the localization of central as well as peripheral monoamines to synaptic vesicles in the electron microscope. However, there was controversy about the nature and size of the extravesicular (or extragranular) pool of neurotransmitter. This is evident from the recorded discussions of the symposium "Mechanisms of Release of Biogenic Amines," held in Stockholm in 1965 (61). For example, Drs. Axelrod and von Euler maintained that a considerable part of the transmitter was located outside the granules, mainly in a bound form. This fraction was proposed to be more important than the granular fraction, since it was thought to be more readily available for release. Indeed, the granules were facetiously referred to as "garbage cans." Our group had arrived at a different view, based on a variety of biochemical, histochemical, and pharmacological data. We felt that the granules were essential in transmission, and that the transmitter had to be taken up by them in order to become available for release by the nerve impulse. In favor of this contention was our finding, mentioned above, that reserpine's site of action is the amine uptake mechanism of the granules. The failure of adrenergic transmission as well as the behavioral actions of reserpine were correlated to the blockade of granular uptake induced by the drug, rather than to the size of the transmitter stores (89). Moreover, extragranular norepinephrine (accumulated in adrenergic nerves by pretreatment with reserpine, followed by an inhibitor of MAO and systemically administered norepinephrine), was unavailable for release by the nerve impulse, as observed histochemically (91). We proposed that under normal conditions the extragranular fraction of monoaminergic transmitters was very small, owing to the presence of MAO intracellularly. Subsequent work in numerous laboratories has lent support to these views. Already at the Symposium, Douglas presented evidence suggesting a Ca^{2+}-triggered fusion between the granule and cell membranes, preceding the release. The release is now generally assumed to take place as "exocytosis," even though the complete extrusion of the granule content may still be debatable.

The regulation of monoamine synthesis attracted considerable interest. The above-mentioned rapid conversion of administered dopa to dopamine indicated that the first step in the pathway was rate limiting, i.e., the conversion of tyrosine to dopa. Perhaps the first evidence for a regulation of catecholamine synthesis came from the observation that the accumulation of catecholamines and their O-methylated basic metabolites in mouse brain following inhibition of MAO leveled off within a few hours, suggesting that the synthesis was brought to a standstill when the stores had been filled (41). Subsequent, more sophisticated work in a large number of laboratories has revealed that catecholamine synthesis is regulated by several independent mechanisms. After the isolation of tyrosine hydroxylase Udenfriend and his colleagues discovered an inhibitory action of catechols on this enzyme (95), leading to reduced affinity for the tetrahydropteridine coenzyme. End-product inhibition was thus demonstrated, and was for several years believed to be the only mechanism of short-term control of catecholamine synthesis. For the long-term control, variation in the number of enzyme molecules via enzyme induction was shown to be responsible (104). However, short-term activation of tyrosine hydroxylase can take place in dopamine neurons *in vivo* despite an increase in dopamine levels, indicating the existence of an additional, rapid control mechanism (36,37). Phosphorylation of the enzyme seems to be involved in this regulation (88).

Several *in vitro* and *in vivo* approaches have been used to demonstrate and measure the release of amine transmitters and its dependence on the nerve impulses. Release *in vivo* has been shown using, e.g., push-pull cannulas (48), semipermeable tubes (108), and voltammetry (1). Indirect, but nontraumatic, biochemical approaches to the quantitation of transmitter synthesis, turnover, and release have also proven useful, such as measurements of the rate of transmitter disappearance following inhibition of its synthesis (see refs. 6, 20), the rate of accumulation of dopa and 5-HTP, induced by inhibition of the aromatic L-amino acid decarboxylase (37), or the accumulation of monoamines (20) or of *O*-methylated basic catecholamine metabolites following inhibition of MAO (82). The data thus obtained demonstrate that dopamine, norepinephrine, and serotonin are released from nerve terminals by the nerve impulses. However, in the somatodendritic region of the nigral dopamine neurons, a rapid release and turnover of dopamine appears to occur more or less independently of the nerve impulses and beyond the reach of receptor-mediated control (see refs. 48, 98). The physiological significance of this observation is not known, but the implications are intriguing.

THE FALSE-TRANSMITTER CONCEPT

Alpha-methyl-meta-tyrosine was reported to deplete central norepinephrine stores, while leaving the 5-HT stores intact (70). Since no sedation occurred after treatment with this agent despite the virtually complete depletion of norepinephrine stores, it was suggested that the central action of reserpine was unrelated to catecholamine deficiency but was rather induced by 5-HT release (ref. 53; dopamine was ignored in this context, which was not unusual at that time). At the First International Catecholamine Symposium in Stockholm in 1961, we challenged this interpretation (26). We had found that alpha-methyl-meta-tyrosine and alpha-methyl-dopa yield decarboxylation products that displace the catecholamines from their storage sites stoichiometrically. To explain the lack of sedation by alpha-methyl-meta-tyrosine and the fact that only very mild sedation was induced by alpha-methyl-dopa, we pointed out that these agents, unlike reserpine, do not appear to block the storage mechanism. We proposed that the amines formed from these amino acids are able to take over the functions of the displaced endogenous amines (38). The "false-transmitter" concept thus formulated was then thoroughly investigated in numerous laboratories (for review, see ref. 86). Not only the mentioned decarboxylation products but several other amines were found to be taken up in monoamine stores, thereby displacing the endogenous transmitters, and to be released by the nerve impulses, causing postsynaptic effects.

The false-transmitter concept, as it is nowadays often understood, assumes that the false transmitter is less active than the endogenous transmitter. Thus the displacement of the latter by the former amine should lead to a deficient transmission mechanism. It seems doubtful, however, to what extent this actually occurs. To account for the lack of sedative action of alpha-methyl-meta-tyrosine, the possibility should be considered that despite the pronounced displacement of the endogenous catecholamines by the alpha-methylated decarboxylation products, newly synthesized endogenous transmitter may still be available for release in sufficient amounts to keep the function intact. The reduction of blood pressure by alpha-methyl-dopa, an action not shared by alpha-methyl-meta-tyrosine, appears to be induced by a complex mechanism. It is central in origin: the effect persists after pretreatment with a peripheral decarboxylase inhibitor but is prevented by a centrally acting inhibitor (69). The hypotensive action may be analogous to that of clonidine, i.e., it may be due to preferential activation of alpha-2 receptors by alpha-methyl-norepinephrine (4). Not only differences in potency but also in pharmacological profile between the endogenous and the false transmitter should thus be taken into account.

RECEPTOR RESEARCH

For a long time the synthesis, storage, release, and metabolism of the monoamines attracted most attention. During the last ten to fifteen years, however, the monoaminergic receptors have attracted an ever-increasing interest. These studies have utilized, for example, the biochemical changes induced by receptor manipulation *in vivo,* the electrophysiological changes caused by such manipulations in both pre- and postsynaptic neurons, and receptor binding studies *in vitro* as well as *in vivo*. Much progress has also been made in elucidating the events occurring beyond the receptors (see ref. 97).

The discovery of the dopamine-receptor blocking action of the major neuroleptic (antipsychotic) agents has attracted a lot of interest. Our first study in this area (39) was undertaken in the hope that our recently improved fluorimetric methods for the determination of basic catecholamine metabolites would enable us to solve the riddle, why the major antipsychotic agents, such as chlorpromazine and haloperidol, have a reserpine-like pharmacological and clinical profile and yet lack the monoamine-depleting properties of the latter drug. We found that chlorpromazine and haloperidol accelerated the formation of the dopamine metabolite 3-methoxytyramine and of the norepinephrine metabolite normetanephrine, while leaving the neurotransmitter levels unchanged. In support of the specificity, promethazine, a sedative phenothiazine lacking antipsychotic and neuroleptic properties, did not change the turnover of the catecholamines. It did not seem far-fetched, then, to propose that rather than reducing the availability of monoamines, as does reserpine, the major antipsychotic drugs block the receptors involved in dopamine and norepinephrine neurotransmission. This would explain their reserpine-like pharmacological profile. To account for the enhanced catecholamine turnover we proposed that neurons can increase their physiological activity in response to receptor blockade. This, I believe, was the first time that a receptor-mediated feedback control of neuronal activity was proposed. These findings and interpretations have been amply confirmed and extended by numerous workers, using a variety of techniques. In the following year three of my students discovered the neuroleptic-induced increase in the concentrations of deaminated dopamine metabolites (7). Despite confirmatory work by others, our findings did not receive much attention until several years later. A possible explanation for this was that, as mentioned, most workers in this field were focusing on other aspects of neurotransmission in the 1960s. In the 1970s the picture changed; the ability of catecholaminergic, especially dopaminergic, agonists and antagonists to induce and alleviate, respectively, psychotic symptoms, started to attract a lot of interest and led to the much-debated "dopamine hypothesis of schizophrenia." For a review of the historical background and recent developments in this area, see ref. 28.

The further analysis of receptor-mediated feedback control of neuronal activity, which, incidentally, soon proved to occur also in noradrenergic and serotonergic systems (see refs. 2, 6, and Aghajanian, *this volume*) and in other systems as well, revealed that this control was largely, if not entirely, mediated by a special population of receptors, apparently located on the monoaminergic neuron itself. These receptors have been called presynaptic receptors or, perhaps preferably, autoreceptors, since they have various locations on the neuron but share the property of being sensitive to the neuron's own neurotransmitter. The first suggestion of the existence of such receptors came from studies on brain tissue slices (64, see also Langer, *this volume*), demonstrating inhibition and stimulation of nerve-impulse-induced dopamine release by dopamine agonists and antagonists, respectively. Subsequent *in vivo* studies demonstrated inhibition of striatal dopamine synthesis by the dopamine-receptor agonist apomorphine and blockade of this action by the neuroleptic agent haloperidol; moreover, this effect persisted after cutting the dopaminergic axons, thus demonstrating that this feedback control was not loop mediated but was restricted to the nerve-terminal area (83). Finally, Aghajanian and Bunney (see Bunney, *this volume*) demonstrated a similar control in the somatodendritic part of dopamine neurons, leading to a decreased firing by dopamine-receptor agonists and a blockade of this action by dopamine-receptor antagonists. Further work along this line has led to the discovery of selective dopamine-autoreceptor agonists and antagonists with interesting pharmacological properties and potential clinical utility (see refs. 49, 50, 103).

FUNCTIONAL AND CLINICAL PERSPECTIVES

Various aspects of monoaminergic brain function and dysfunction are discussed in a specific manner in other chapters of this volume. Some general reflections are given below.

The majority of monoaminergic neurons are located in the lower brain stem. From a narrow area they project to all parts of the central nervous system. Indeed, it will probably prove difficult to identify any region or function of the brain or spinal cord that is not under some kind of monoaminergic influence. It is not surprising, then, that our present knowledge of the physiology and pathophysiology of the monoaminergic systems is fragmentary. It seems evident, however, that these systems play a modulating rather than an executive role. An impressive illustration is afforded by the reserpine-treated animal, in which the monoaminergic systems can be assumed to be largely out of function. In this animal the most elementary functions of the central nervous system seem to be preserved, but some of them appear to operate at an extremely low level. From this it may be inferred that the monoaminergic systems play a facilitating role on a variety of central nervous functions. The reserpine syndrome appears to be grossly dominated by dopamine deficiency, as suggested by its dramatic reversal of L-dopa and other dopamine-receptor agonists. However, after the elimination of the deficiency in dopamine, abnormalities caused by lack of the other monoamines become evident. An instructive example is the aggressiveness displayed by animals made deficient in 5-HT preferentially (22).

The functions of the central monoaminergic neurons and their role in neurological and psychiatric disorders are more poorly understood than the morphology and synaptology of these systems. Perhaps the part played by dopamine is least obscure. That the nigrostriatal dopamine system is involved in extrapyramidal functions and disorders, especially Parkinson's disease, is clearly established. The role of the tuberoinfundibular dopamine pathway in the control of prolactin secretion is also obvious, and even though the pathogenetic role of dopamine in clinical hyperprolactinemia is doubtful, the use of dopamine agonists in such cases is a significant advance. That dopamine plays a role in important mental functions is evident from the therapeutic actions of dopamine antagonists, as well as from the psychotomimetic effects of dopamine agonists. However, no disturbance in dopamine function has as yet been demonstrated beyond doubt in schizophrenia or any other psychotic condition (see ref. 28).

The side effects of the antipsychotic agents are a matter for serious concern. Especially the tardive dyskinesia should restrict the use of these agents to psychotic conditions and a limited number of additional indications. Experience with clozapine and to some extent also with other agents such as thioridazine strongly suggests that antipsychotic efficacy can be achieved without any serious extrapyramidal side effects. We can thus expect that much better antipsychotic drugs will be developed in the not too distant future. Whether they will be directly based on the clozapine lead is difficult to predict, however. In animal models selective dopamine autoreceptor agonists have shown an interesting profile, and clinical trials with such agents are eagerly awaited.

Paradoxically, selective dopamine autoreceptor agonists appear to be active anti-Parkinson agents (21,52). This was predicted from animal data, showing that selective dopamine autoreceptor agonists in general possess affinity for the postsynaptic dopamine receptors, too. However, their intrinsic activity on these receptors is very low. In contrast, when postsynaptic dopamine receptors become supersensitive following denervation, the intrinsic activity of these agonists increases considerably. Thus, the dopamine auto-receptor agonists are capable of stimulating postsynaptic supersensitive receptors selectively: normosensitive post-synaptic dopamine receptors are not stimulated but can actually be influenced in the opposite direction, owing to competition with the endogenous transmitter, dopamine. This opens up new therapeutic perspectives in Parkinson's disease and may lead to more satisfactory responses with fewer side effects. The theoretical implications of the relation between receptor sensitivity and intrinsic activity are also intriguing (see ref. 50).

We probably do not fully appreciate how profound the influence of the monoaminergic systems is and how it extends to all aspects of brain function. A recent observation may be quoted to illustrate this. In spontaneously hypertensive rats the development of hypertension can be prevented by treating the animals at an early stage with 6-hydroxydopamine, leading to destruction of central catecholaminergic pathways. A closer examination revealed that this prevention was linked to the destruction of dopaminergic cell bodies in the A9 region; noradrenergic pathways seemed to be unimportant in this respect. Along with the prevention of hypertension the signs of apparent hyperarousal of these spontaneously hypertensive rats (SHR) were reduced (23). If these observations can be confirmed, they open up new perspectives on the biology of the nigrostriatal system. It may extend far beyond the functions that we generally connect with this pathway.

Our knowledge of the physiology and pathology of central norepinephrine, not to speak of epinephrine, is also very fragmentary. Like dopamine, norepinephrine seems to be somehow involved in arousal, and locus ceruleus seems to respond very vividly to incoming stimuli, especially when they signify novelty. Stimulation of norepinephrine neurons, e.g., by electrical stimulation of locus ceruleus or by yohimbine-induced blockade of alpha-2-adrenergic autoreceptors, seems to cause strong arousal accompanied by severe anxiety. Conversely, stimulation of alpha-2-adrenergic receptors by clonidine causes—in addition to a decrease in blood pressure—sedation and anxiolysis. Bilateral destruction of locus ceruleus has a similar effect. Both dopamine and norepinephrine appear to be somehow involved in the positive reinforcing action of dependence-producing drugs, and especially clonidine appears to be capable of alleviating certain withdrawal reactions (for review, see refs. 57, 58).

The fairly marked age dependence of central catecholamine neurons (discussed in several chapters of ref. 68) is possibly related to the formation of toxic metabolites and oxygen species in the autoxidation of these amines. The discovery of 5-S-cysteinyldopamine and related metabolites in dopamine-rich brain regions (65,100) lends some support to this hypothesis.

The functions and pathophysiological significance of 5-HT are also poorly comprehended. As already referred to, animal data support the contention that serotonergic systems exert an inhibitory function on aggressive behavior (109). The serotonergic system appears to be more strongly developed in female than in male rats (47), which may at least partly account for the well-known sex difference in aggressive behavior among vertebrates. The serotonergic systems seem to control the mating behavior of both sexes,

but here the situation may be more complex, with notable species differences. That 5-HT also plays a part in the control of motor functions is suggested by the "5-HT motor syndrome," but the physiological implications of this phenomenon are obscure. Similarly, the role of 5-HT and the other monoamines in various aspects of sleep seems to be established, although the available data are contradictory in certain respects.

Evidence for a role of 5-HT, norepinephrine, and dopamine in the control of mood and psychomotor activity and in affective disorders and anxiety has also been presented, and some impressive observations relating 5-HT to suicidal behavior have been published (105). Moreover, all the three major monoamines appear to play a role in various central neuroendocrinological and autonomic nervous functions.

The tricyclic antidepressant agents, although clinically effective, have some disturbing side effects that limit their use, especially in geriatric practice. The most important lead in this area is the fact that practically all antipsychotic drugs have been shown to promote monoaminergic transmission in various ways. Doubt has been cast on this mechanism, mainly because the action on monoaminergic transmission is followed by an antidepressant response only after some delay. However, this does not exclude a causal relationship, given the well-known fact that neurotransmission not only involves immediate neurophysiological responses but also various long-term, "trophic" influences, leading, for example to changes in receptor responsiveness. Various delayed receptor changes have, in fact, been described following subchronic treatment with antidepressants, and some workers have suggested that one or a few of these changes can be identified as crucial component(s) underlying the therapeutic response. Although such possibilities are not excluded, it is equally probable that the whole cascade of secondary events following on the initial change in monoaminergic neurotransmission is responsible for the therapeutic action. In any event, the best lead available today is the ability of antidepressant agents to promote monoaminergic transmission, and thus the logical step should be to develop more selective drugs possessing this property. Such agents are now underway, and some of them appear to be promising. For example, the selective 5-HT uptake inhibitor zimelidine proved to be an efficient antidepressant devoid of the classical side effects of the tricyclics (32); unfortunately the drug had to be withdrawn owing to a rare side effect, appearing as Guillain-Barré syndrome. Nevertheless, it seems obvious that effective antidepressants can be developed, lacking the bothersome classical side effects of the tricyclics.

Experimental and clinical observations using zimelidine suggest that 5-HT plays a role as inhibitor of ethanol-seeking behavior (discussed in several chapters in ref. 96).

The discovery of the therapeutic efficacy of tricyclic antidepressants in "panic disorders" deserves mentioning in this context (85). The mechanism of this action is not clear but will hopefully be elucidated, leading to the development of more specific drugs and a better understanding of these disorders.

On the whole, anxiety disorders are mainly treated with benzodiazepines, in so far as drugs are concerned. These are of course excellent drugs, not least because of their low toxicity, and their dependence liability does not seem to be a matter for major concern. Nevertheless, alternatives would be welcome. Among possible candidates, buspirone has attracted some interest in recent years. The mode of action of this compound is not clear. Originally it was thought to be a selective dopamine autoreceptor agonist, but the selectivity for autoreceptors could not be substantiated. Today the ability of this agent to stimulate 5-HT receptors (76), while at the same time blocking dopamine receptors, looks like a plausible mode of action. If this proves to be the basis for the anxiolytic action, we can foresee the development of other 5-HT receptor agonists with or without an additional dopamine-receptor blocking action. Possibly an important therapeutic application of 5-HT receptor agonists will thus be opened up. The newly discovered 5-HT agonist 8-hydroxy-2-(dipropylamine) tetralin (8-OH-DPAT) (77) may serve as a prototype.

As mentioned, animal data strongly implicate 5-HT as an important endogenous inhibitor of aggressiveness. In one clinical study aggressiveness could be correlated to a low ratio of tryptophan to competing large neutral amino acids in plasma (19). Directly or indirectly acting 5-HT agonists might thus prove useful in aggressiveness. Alternatively, the entry of tryptophan (and its competitors) through the blood-brain barrier could be promoted. This transport mechanism appears to be controlled by adrenergic beta receptors (60), and thus beta-receptor agonists might not only alleviate depression (102) but also aggressiveness.

The possibility may be considered that the apparent antidepressant, anti-ethanol-seeking, anxiolytic, and antiaggressive functions of 5-HT are interrelated; maybe a basic function of central 5-HT neurons is to regulate the threshold for a variety of stressful and noxious stimuli.

CONCLUDING REMARKS

The rise of neuropsychopharmacology in the 1950s is closely linked to the discovery of the antipsychotic and antidepressant drugs and the subsequent elucidation of their mode of action. The impact of these discoveries on basic as well as clinical brain research is obvious. In light of the tremendous progress made in basic knowledge, it is remarkable, however, how modest the development in pharmacotherapy has been since the 1950s. The first generation of antipsychotic and antidepressant agents still plays a dominating role, despite the fact that they are far from ideal as regards efficacy or side effects. The only really striking therapeutic spinoff from basic research is the introduction of L-dopa in the treatment of Parkinson's disease. Enormous efforts are obviously required to obtain a comprehensive picture of the biological and clinical significance of the monoaminergic systems. More sophisticated animal models and human studies using, for example, modern imaging techniques, will be needed. Although pharmacological tools have contributed much, better ones are wanted. Especially, more selective monoaminergic agonists and antagonists, applicable also to humans, would prove useful. Hopefully, at least some of the many fascinating leads that are presently pursued in numerous laboratories and clinics, aiming to improve the therapy of neuropsychiatric disorders, will be successful.

REFERENCES

1. Adams, R. N., and Marsden, C. A. (1982): In: *Handbook of Psychopharmacology, Vol. 15,* edited by L. L. Iversen, S. D. Iversen, and S. H. Snyder, pp. 1–74. Plenum Press, New York.
2. Aghajanian, G. K. (1984): In: *Catecholamines. Part B: Neuropharmacology and Central Nervous System—Theoretical Aspects,* edited by E. Usdin, A. Carlsson, A. Dahlström, and J. Engel, pp. 85–92. Alan R. Liss, New York.
3. Amin, A. H., Crawford, T. B. B., and Gaddum, J. H. (1954): *J. Physiol. (Lond.),* 126:596–618.
4. Andén, N.-E. (1979): *Naunyn Schmiedeberg's Arch. Pharmacol,* 306:263–266.
5. Andén, N.-E., Carlsson, A., Dahlström, A., Fuxe, K., Hillarp, N.-Å., and Larsson, K. (1964): *Life Sci.,* 3:523–530.
6. Andén, N.-E., Carlsson, A., and Häggendal, J. (1969): *Annu. Rev. Pharmacol.,* 9:119–134.
7. Andén, N.-E., Roos, B.-E., and Werdinius, B. (1964): *Life Sci.,* 3:149–158.
8. Axelrod, J. (1960): In: *Ciba Foundation Symposium on Adrenergic Mechanisms,* edited by J. R. Vane, G. E. W. Wolstenholme, and M. O'Connor, pp. 558–559. J & A Churchill, London.
9. Axelrod, J. (1964): In: *Progress in Brain Research, Vol. 8: Biogenic Amines,* edited by H. E. Himwich and W. A. Himwich, pp. 81–89. Elsevier, Amsterdam.
10. Barbeau, A., Sourkes, T. L., and Murphy, G. F. (1962): In: *Monoamines et Systeme Nerveux Central,* edited by J. de Ajuriaguerra, pp. 247–262. Georg Masson, Geneva.
11. Bertler, Å., Carlsson, A., and Rosengren, E. (1956): *Naturwissenschaften,* 22:521.
12. Bertler, Å., Carlsson, A., and Rosengren, E. (1958): *Acta Physiol. Scand.,* 44:273–292.
13. Bertler, Å., Falck, B., Gottfries, C. G., Ljunggren, L., and Rosengren, E. (1964): *Acta Pharmacol.,* 21:283–289.
14. Bertler, Å., and Rosengren, E. (1959): *Experientia,* 15:10.
15. Birkmayer, W., and Hornykiewicz, O. (1962): *Arch. Psychiatr. Nervenkr.,* 203:560–574.
16. Björklund, A., and Hökfelt, T., editors (1984): *Handbook of Chemical Neuroanatomy, Vol. 2: Classical Transmitters in the CNS, Part I.* Elsevier, Amsterdam.
17. Blaschko, H. (1939): *J. Physiol. (Lond.),* 96:50P–51P.
18. Born, G. V. R. (1956): *Biochem. J.,* 62:33P.
19. Branchey, L., Branchey, M., Shaw, S., and Lieber, C. S. (1984): *Psychiatry Res.,* 12:219–226.
20. Brodie, B. B., Costa, E., Dlabac, A., Neff, N. H., and Smokler, H. H. (1966): *J. Pharmacol. Exp. Ther.,* 154:493–498.
21. Brücke, T., Danielczyk, W., Simanyi, M., Sofic, E., and Riederer, P. (1985): *Proc. VIIIth Int. Symp. on Parkinson's Disease.* New York, p. 109.
22. Butcher, L. L., and Dietrich, A. P. (1973): *Naunyn Schmiedebergs Arch. Pharmacol.,* 277:61–70.
23. Buuse, M. van den (1985): Brain Catecholamines and the Development of Hypertension in the Spontaneously Hypertensive Rat. Thesis, University of Utrecht, pp. 1–156.
24. Carlsson, A. (1959): *Pharmacol. Rev.,* 11:490–493.
25. Carlsson, A. (1960): In: *Ciba Foundation Symposium on Adrenergic Mechanisms,* edited by J. R. Vane, G. E. W. Wolstenholme, and M. O'Connor, pp. 558–559. J & A Churchill, London.
26. Carlsson, A. (1962): In: *Pharmacological Analysis of Central Nervous Action,* edited by W. D. M. Paton and P. Lindgren, pp. 71–74. Pergamon Press, Oxford.
27. Carlsson, A. (1966): In: *Mechanisms of Release of Biogenic Amines,* edited by U. S. von Euler, S. Rosell, and B. Uvnäs, pp. 331–346. Pergamon Press, Oxford.
28. Carlsson, A. (1983): In: *Discoveries in Pharmacology, Vol. 1: Psycho- and Neuro-Pharmacology,* edited by M. J. Parnham and J. Bruinvels, pp. 197–206. Elsevier, Amsterdam.

29. Carlsson, A., Falck, B., Fuxe, K., and Hillarp, N.-Å. (1964): *Acta Physiol. Scand.,* 60:112–119.
30. Carlsson, A., Falck, B., and Hillarp, N.-Ä. (1962): *Acta Physiol. Scand.,* 56(*Suppl.* 196):1–27.
31. Carlsson, A., Falck, B., Hillarp, N.-Å., Thieme, G., and Torp, A. (1961): *Med. Exper.,* 4:123–125.
32. Carlsson, A., Gottfries, C.-G., Holmberg, G., Modigh, K., Svensson, T., and Ögren, S.-O., editors (1981): *Recent Advances in the Treatment of Depression. Acta Psychiat. Scand.,* 63(*Suppl.* 290).
33. Carlsson, A., and Hillarp, N.-Å. (1956): *Kgl. Fysiogr. Sällsk. Förhandl.,* 26(8).
34. Carlsson, A., and Hillarp, N.-Å. (1962): *Acta Physiol. Scand.,* 55: 95–100.
35. Carlsson, A., Hillarp, N.-Å., and Waldeck, B. (1963): *Acta Physiol. Scand.,* 59(*Suppl.* 215):1–38.
36. Carlsson, A., Kehr, W., and Lindqvist, M. (1976): *J. Neural Transm.,* 39:1–19.
37. Carlsson, A., Kehr, W., Lindqvist, M., Magnusson, T., and Atack, C. V. (1972): *Pharmacol. Rev.,* 24:371–384.
38. Carlsson, A., and Lindqvist, M. (1962): *Acta Physiol. Scand.,* 54: 87–94.
39. Carlsson, A., and Lindqvist, M. (1963): *Acta Pharmacol.,* 20: 140–144.
40. Carlsson, A., Lindqvist, M., and Magnusson, T. (1957): *Nature,* 180:1200.
41. Carlsson, A., Lindqvist, M., and Magnusson, T. (1960): In: *Ciba Foundation Symposium on Adrenergic Mechanisms,* edited by J. R. Vane, G. E. W. Wolstenholme, and M. O'Connor, pp. 432–439. J & A Churchill, London.
42. Carlsson, A., Lindqvist, M., Magnusson, T., and Waldeck, B. (1958): *Science,* 127:471.
43. Carlsson, A., Magnusson, T., and Rosengren, E. (1963): *Experientia,* 19:359.
44. Carlsson, A., Rosengren, E., Bertler, Å., and Nilsson, J. (1957): In: *Psychotropic Drugs,* edited by S. Garattini and V. Ghetti, pp. 363–372. Elsevier, Amsterdam.
45. Carlsson, A., Shore, P. A., and Brodie, B. B. (1957): *J. Pharmacol. Exp. Ther.,* 120:334–339.
46. Carlsson, A., and Waldeck, B. (1958): *Acta Physiol. Scand.,* 44: 293–298.
47. Carlsson, M., Svensson, K., Eriksson, E., and Carlsson, A. (1985): *J. Neural Transm.,* 63:297–313.
48. Cheramy, A., Leviel, V., and Glowinski, J. (1981): *Nature,* 289: 537–542.
49. Clark, D., Carlsson, A., and Hjorth, S. (1985): *J. Neural Transm.,* 62:1–52.
50. Clark, D., Hjorth, S., and Carlsson, A. (1985): *J. Neural Transm.,* 62:171–207.
51. Corrodi, H., and Hillarp, N.-Å. (1964): *Helv. Chim. Acta,* 47: 911–918.
52. Corsini, G. U., Horowski, R., Rainer, R., and Del Zompo, M. (1984): *Clin. Neuropharmacol.,* 7(*Suppl.* 1):950–951.
53. Costa, E., Gessa, G. L., Kuntzman, R., and Brodie, B. B. (1962): In: *Pharmacological Analysis of Central Nervous Action,* edited by W. D. M. Paton and P. Lindgren, pp. 43–71. Pergamon Press, Oxford.
54. Dahlström, A., and Carlsson, A. (1986): In: *Discoveries in Pharmacology, Vol. 3: Chemical Pharmacology and Chemotherapy,* edited by M. J. Parnham and J. Bruinvels, pp. 97–125. Elsevier, Amsterdam.
55. Dahlström, A., and Fuxe, K. (1964): *Acta Physiol. Scand.,* 62(*Suppl.* 232):1–55.
56. Ehringer, H., and Hornykiewicz, O. (1960): *Klin. Wochenschr.,* 38:1236–1239.
57. Elam, M. (1985): On the Physiological Regulation of Brain Norepinephrine Neurons in Rat Locus Ceruleus, pp. 1–43. Thesis, University of Göteborg.
58. Engel, J., and Carlsson, A. (1977): In: *Current Developments in Psychopharmacology, Vol. 4,* edited by W. B. Essman and L. Valzelli, pp. 3–32. Spectrum Publications, New York.
59. Eränkö, O. (1955): *Acta Endocrinol.,* 18:180–188.
60. Eriksson, T. (1985): Regulation of Monoamine-Precursor Transport into the Brain. Thesis, University of Göteborg.
61. Euler, U. S. von, Rosell, S., and Uvnäs, B., editors (1966): *Mechanisms of Release of Biogenic Amines,* discussion, pp. 469–477. Pergamon Press, Oxford.
62. Falck, B., and Hillarp, N.-Å. (1959): *Acta Anat.,* 38:277–279.
63. Falck, B., Hillarp, N.-Å., Thieme, G., and Torp, A. (1962): *J. Histochem. Cytochem.,* 10:348–354.
64. Farnebo, L.-O., and Hamberger, B. (1971): *Acta Physiol. Scand.* (*Suppl.* 371), pp. 35–44.
65. Fornstedt, B., Rosengren, E., and Carlsson, A. (1986): *Neuropharmacology,* 25:451–454.
66. Fuxe, K. (1965): *Acta Physiol. Scand.* (*Suppl.* 247), 64:37–84.
67. Gaddum, J. H. (1954): In: *Ciba Foundation Symposium on Hypertension: Humoral and Neurogenic Factors,* edited by J. H. Gaddum, pp. 75–77. Little, Brown, Boston.
68. Gaitz, C. M., and Samorajski, T., editors (1985): *Aging 2000: Our Health Care Destiny. Vol. I: Biomedical Issues.* Springer Verlag, New York.
69. Henning, M. (1969): *Acta Physiol. Scand.,* 76(*Suppl.* 322), pp. 1–37.
70. Hess, S. M., Connamacher, R. H., Ozaki, M., and Udenfriend, S. (1961): *J. Pharmacol. Exp. Ther.,* 134:129–138.
71. Hess, S. M., and Udenfriend, S. (1959): *J. Pharmacol. Exp. Ther.,* 127:175–177.
72. Hillarp, N.-Å. (1946): *Acta Anat.* (*Suppl.* 4):1–153.
73. Hillarp, N.-Å. (1959): *Acta Physiol. Scand.,* 46(*Suppl.* 157):1–38.
74. Hillarp, N.-Å., Högberg, B., and Nilsson, B. (1955): *Nature,* 176: 1032–1033.
75. Hillarp, N.-Å., Lagerstedt, S., and Nilsson, B. (1953): *Acta Physiol. Scand.,* 28:251–263.
76. Hjorth, S., and Carlsson, A. (1982): *Eur. J. Pharmacol.,* 83:131–134.
77. Hjorth, S., Carlsson, A., Lindberg, P., Sanchez, D., Wikström, H., Arvidsson, L.-E., Hacksell, U., and Nilsson, J. L. G. (1982): *J. Neural Transm.,* 55:169–188.
78. Hökfelt, T. (1968): Electron Microscopic Studies on Peripheral and Central Monoamine Neurons, pp. 1–30. Thesis, Stockholm.
79. Holtz, P., Heise, R., and Ludtke, K. (1938): *Arch. Exp. Pathol. Pharmakol.,* 191:87–118.
80. Holzbauer, M., and Vogt, M. (1956): *J. Neurochem.,* 1:8–11.
81. Jonason, J., and Rutledge, C. O. (1968): *Acta Physiol. Scand.,* 73:411–417.
82. Kehr, W. (1976): *Naunyn Schmiedebergs Arch. Pharmacol.,* 293: 209–215.
83. Kehr, W., Carlsson, A., Lindqvist, M., Magnusson, T., and Atack, C. (1972): *J. Pharm. Pharmacol.,* 24:744–747.
84. Kirshner, N. (1962): *J. Biol. Chem.,* 237:2311–2317.
85. Klein, D. F. (1964): *Psychopharmacologia,* 5:397–408.
86. Kopin, I. J. (1968): *Annu. Rev. Pharmacol.,* 8:377–394.
87. Lindvall, O. (1974): The Glyoxylic Acid Fluorescence Histochemical Method for Monoamines. Chemistry, Methodology and Neuroanatomical Application. Thesis, University of Lund.
88. Lovenberg, W., Bruckwick, E. A., and Hanbauer, I. (1975): *Proc. Natl. Acad. Sci. USA,* 72:2955–2958.
89. Lundborg, P. (1963): *Experientia,* 19:479–480.
90. Magnusson, T., and Rosengren, E. (1963): *Experientia,* 19:229.
91. Malmfors, T. (1965): *Acta Physiol. Scand.,* 64(*Suppl.* 248):1–93.
92. McLennan, H. (1963): *Synaptic Transmission,* pp. 1–134. WB Saunders Co., Philadelphia.
93. Montagu, K. R. (1957): *Nature,* 180:244–245.
94. Muscholl, E., and Vogt, M. (1958): *J. Physiol. (Lond.),* 141:132–155.
95. Nagatsu, T., Levitt, B. G., and Udenfriend, S. (1964): *J. Biol. Chem.,* 238:2910–2917.
96. Naranjo, C. A., and Sellers, E. M., editors (1985): *Research Advances in New Psychopharmacological Treatments for Alcoholism.* Excerpta Medica, Amsterdam.
97. Nestler, E. J., and Greengard, P. (1984): In: *Catecholamines, Part A: Basic and Peripheral Mechanisms,* edited by E. Usdin, A. Carlsson, A. Dahlström, and J. Engel, pp. 9–22. Alan R. Liss, New York.
98. Nissbrandt, H., Pileblad, E., and Carlsson, A. (1985): *J. Pharm. Pharmacol.,* 37:884–889.
99. Pletscher, A., Shore, P. A., and Brodie, B. B. (1955): *Science,* 122:374–375.

100. Rosengren, E., Linder-Eliasson, E., and Carlsson, A. (1985): *J. Neural Transm.*, 63:247–253.
101. Shore, P. A., Silver, S. L., and Brodie, B. B. (1955): *Science*, 122: 284–285.
102. Simon, P., Lecrubier, Y., Jouvent, R., Puech, A. J., Allilaire, J. F., and Widlocher, D. (1978): *Psychol. Med.*, 8:335–338.
103. Svensson, K., Carlsson, A., Johansson, A. M., Arvidsson, L.-E., and Nilsson, J. L. G. (1986): *J. Neural Transm.*, 65:29–38.
104. Thoenen, H., Otten, U., and Oesch, F. (1973): In: *Frontiers in Catecholamine Research*, edited by E. Usdin and S. Snyder, pp. 179–185. Pergamon Press, Oxford.
105. Träskman, L., Åsberg, M., Bertilsson, L., and Sjöstrand, L. (1981): *Arch. Gen. Psychiatry*, 38:631–636.
106. Twarog, B. M., and Page, I. H. (1954): *Am. J. Physiol.*, 175:157–161.
107. Ungerstedt, U. (1971): On the Anatomy, Pharmacology and Function of the Nigrostriatal Dopamine System. Thesis, Karolinska Institutet, Stockholm.
108. Ungerstedt, U., Herrera-Marschitz, M., Ståhle, L., Tossman, U., and Zetterström, T. (1983): In: *Dopamine Receptor Agonists 1*, edited by A. Carlsson and J. L. G. Nilsson, pp. 165–181. Swedish Pharmaceutical Press, Stockholm.
109. Valzelli, L. (1974): *Adv. Biochem. Psychopharmacol.*, 11:255–264.
110. Vane, J. R., Wolstenholme, G. E. W., and O'Connor, M., editors (1960): *Ciba Foundation Symposium on Adrenergic Mechanisms*. J & A Churchill, London.
111. Vogt, M. (1954): *J. Physiol. (Lond.)*, 123:451–481.
112. Westerink, B. H. C., and Spaan, S. J. (1982): *J. Neurochem.*, 38: 680–686.
113. Woolley, D. W., and Shaw, E. (1954): *Science*, 119:587–588.

Psychopharmacology:
The Third Generation of Progress,
edited by Herbert Y. Meltzer.
Raven Press, New York © 1987.

CHAPTER 6

Electron Microscopy of Central Catecholamine Systems

Virginia M. Pickel and Teresa A. Milner

During the last decade use of immunocytochemistry for the electron microscopic localization of catecholamine-synthesizing enzymes has considerably broadened our knowledge of the morphology and synaptic associations of catecholaminergic neurons (5,6,11,38,41,43–50). The most extensively studied enzymes include (a) tyrosine hydroxylase (TH; EC 1.14.16.2), which catalyzes the first step in the biosynthesis of catecholamines and thus is a specific marker common to dopaminergic, noradrenergic, and adrenergic neurons (29); (b) dopamine-beta-hydroxylase (DBH; EC 1.14.17.1), which converts dopamine to norepinephrine and hence is a marker of noradrenergic and adrenergic neurons (24); and (c) phenylethanolamine *N*-methyltransferase (PNMT; EC 2.1.1.28), which converts norepinephrine to epinephrine and thus is a marker for adrenergic neurons (26,28,40). This review is focused principally on the ultrastructural localization of TH in dopaminergic neurons of the nigrostriatal system and in pathways from the medial nuclei of the solitary tracts (m-NTS) to the parabrachial region (PBR), DBH in the ceruleocortical noradrenergic pathways, and PNMT in adrenergic cell groups in the rostral ventrolateral medulla and m-NTS. The features of the catecholaminergic neurons determined by immunocytochemistry will be compared to the results with other histochemical (83) and autoradiographic (2,4) methods.

NIGROSTRIATAL DOPAMINERGIC SYSTEM

The nigrostriatal dopaminergic system includes perikarya located in the pars compacta of the substantia nigra, dendrites from these neurons that radiate ventrally into the pars reticulata, and axons that traverse the lateral hypothalamus to innervate the neostriatum (3). The dopaminergic *perikarya* in the substantia nigra are medium-sized and have multiple processes. The nucleus is large and eccentrically located within the perikaryon, has a relatively smooth contour, and contains a prominent nucleolus. In conventionally stained electron micrographs, the cells have a semidark appearance attributed largely to peripheral masses of Nissl bodies, clusters of polyribosomes, and stacks of rough endoplasmic reticulum (17).

Other notable cytoplasmic organelles that may be associated with the synthesis and packaging of dopamine include the numerous Golgi saccules, granular and agranular vesicles, mitochondria, and tubular profiles of smooth endoplasmic reticulum (49). The abundant dopamine seen by fluorescence histochemistry (3) and the relative sparsity of dense core or clear vesicles found in the soma and dendrites of perikarya in the substantia nigra (17) may be interpreted in at least three ways with regard to the storage of the biogenic amine: (a) The dopamine in perikarya may be labile and not associated with vesicles as suggested by the recent demonstration that dopamine is found in massive Cr-positive areas in the cytoplasm as seen by X-ray microanalysis (69). (b) The dopamine may be associated with smooth endoplasmic reticulum, as suggested by the dense labeling in saccules of smooth reticulum following uptake of the catecholamine congener 5-hydroxydopamine (5-OHDA) (33,68). Thus, the storage and transport of dopamine in dendrites might be similar to certain types of axonal transport involving smooth endoplasmic reticulum

(18). (c) Dopamine could be stored in vesicles that are undetected in conventionally stained material. Using uptake of 5-OHDA, Wilson et al. (68) showed many small densely labeled vesicles throughout the cytoplasm of neurons within the substantia nigra.

The *dendrites* from perikarya in the pars compacta of the substantia nigra extend unbranched for some distance into the pars reticulata. The dendrites are often seen in clusters and are found near blood vessels (57). The dendrites sometimes form dendrodendritic junctions and contain aggregates of small vesicles that are selectively labeled following uptake of 5-OHDA (68). Dendrites of the substantia nigra also contain immunoreactivity for TH (49) and release dopamine by calcium-dependent mechanisms (9,20). Self-modulation through dendritic or axonic interactions has been suggested from pharmacological studies showing that norepinephrine and dopamine are inhibited by local administration of their own transmitters (8,62). However, except for the dendrodendritic synapses described above, there is little morphological evidence for direct feedback of dopaminergic neurons on other similar neurons in the substantia nigra. In addition to possible self-regulation, through interaction with other dopaminergic dendrites, the released dopamine also may influence other nondopaminergic neurons.

Dopaminergic axons and axon terminals in the striatum have been extensively examined by immunocytochemistry for TH (6,43) and autoradiographic localization of incorporated [3H]dopamine (15). As seen by both methods, the majority of the dopaminergic axons in the rat neostriatum are thin (0.1–0.3 μm) and unmyelinated. The terminals are 0.5 to 1.0 μm in diameter and have closely packed vesicles. In striatal sections labeled with TH by the peroxidase-antiperoxidase (PAP) immunocytochemical method of Sternberger (60), large dense core vesicles are rarely detected. The large dense core vesicles in axon terminals of the caudate nucleus are also rarely seen following 5-OHDA uptake, which produces a dense central core in virtually all smaller vesicles (1).

In contrast to the nigrostriatal afferents, the terminals of the more medial dopaminergic neurons in the nucleus accumbens contain many large dense core vesicles (5). The difference in content of large dense core vesicles between the caudate nucleus and the nucleus accumbens may be related to the fact that the ventral tegmental neurons that supply the dopaminergic innervation to the nucleus accumbens contain cholecystokinin, whereas the dopaminergic neurons projecting to the neostriatum do not contain this peptide (27). The presence of large dense core vesicles is a common feature of many peptidergic neurons (42) and may represent one of the primary storage sites for the peptides that are costored with catecholamines or other classical transmitters (32).

The synaptic specializations of dopaminergic terminals have been described as either symmetric (15,43), asymmetric (1), or without membrane densities (67). The occurrence of symmetric and asymmetric synapses is compatible with physiological evidence that dopamine may have both inhibitory and excitatory properties in the striatum (12,31,37). There is also evidence that one of the dopamine-sensitive

receptors may be on dendrites or postsynaptic sites whereas others may be presynaptically located on axon terminals (36). Appositions without observed specializations of the membranes have been reported between adjacent TH-labeled terminals (43) and between TH-labeled axon terminals and degenerating afferents seen after removal of the cerebral cortex (6). The "non-synaptic" interactions could provide an anatomical substrate for the presynaptic release of dopamine by L-glutamate and a variety of other transmitters (21,22).

NORADRENERGIC NEURONS OF THE CERULEOCORTICAL PROJECTION

Several groups of perikarya in the medulla and pons exhibit fluorescent properties of noradrenergic neurons (14) and contain immunocytochemically detectable levels of TH and DBH, but not PNMT (11,48). The locus ceruleus or A6 group of noradrenergic neurons and noradrenergic terminals in the cerebral cortex, many of which belong to the ceruleocortical system (65), have been most extensively investigated.

Perikarya of the noradrenergic neurons in the locus ceruleus of the rat are closely packed, medium-sized, and multipolar or fusiform (63). Conventional electron microscopic staining demonstrates an abundance of cytoplasmic organelles including cisterns of rough-surfaced endoplasmic reticulum, Golgi saccules, mitochondria, dense bodies, and a few granular vesicles (52). As seen for the perikaryon in the adjacent parabrachial region (Fig. 1), many of these organelles are obscured by peroxidase reaction product following immunocytochemical labeling for TH by the PAP method. The noradrenergic neurons in the locus ceruleus are also characterized by spines and synapses on both soma and dendrites. The numerous spines, which have large amounts of actin (13), may account for the well-known capacity of noradrenergic neurons for regeneration and sprouting (59).

Few small or large dense vesicles are seen in noradrenergic neurons even after uptake of 5-OHDA and KMnO₄ fixation (25,58). Thus, the storage of norepinephrine may be accounted for by mechanisms similar to those described for dopamine in the substantia nigra. The storage of norepinephrine in central neurons may differ from those in peripheral systems such as the superior cervical ganglia where Richards and Tranzer (53,54) showed that uptake of 5-OHDA was found in large (85 nm) and small (50 nm) vesicles and in a tubular (15 nm) reticulum which occurred in isolated saccules or in clusters. Alternatively, the storage organelles may be more rapidly transported into axons and dendrites within the central neurons. Figure 2 shows the localization of TH by radioimmunocytochemistry (45) in a presumably noradrenergic neuron of the m-NTS 24 hr after intraventricular injection of colchicine (75 μg in 10 μl saline). The accumulation of small clear and large dense core vesicles more closely resembles that reported by Richards and Tranzer (54) in peripheral sympathetic neurons. The identification of vesicles is also greatly facilitated by

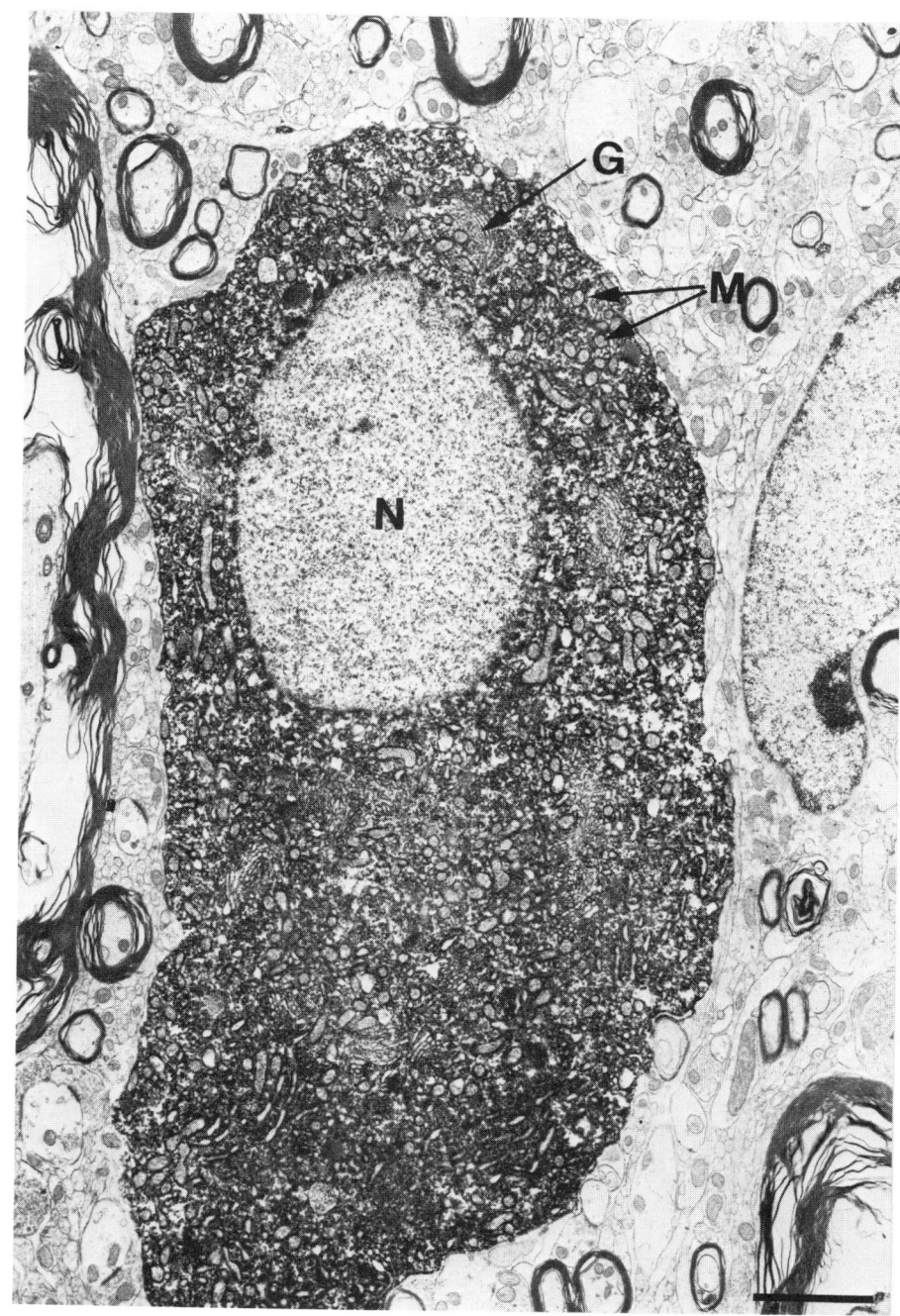

FIG. 1. Immunocytochemical localization of TH within a neuronal perikaryon in the lateral parabrachial region using PAP method. The labeling is diffusely distributed throughout the cytoplasm, whereas the nucleus (N) and surrounding neuropil are devoid of immunoreactivity. Numerous mitochondria (M) and Golgi saccules (G) are seen in the cytoplasm. Bar = 2.0 μm.

the use of ^{125}I-labeled secondary immunoglobulins rather than PAP for detection of TH-antiserum.

Fluorescence histochemistry has shown that *dendrites* of the neurons of the locus ceruleus extend for some distance outside the confines of the nucleus (63). The dendrites of the locus ceruleus show TH-immunoreactivity by the PAP method (48). The diffuse peroxidase labeling for TH in dendrites is analogous to that seen in other catecholaminergic processes (34) (Fig. 3). The dendrites contain a few vesicles, polyribosomes, smooth reticulum, mitochondria, microtubules, and multivestibular bodies. The dendrites

are principally innervated by unlabeled (noncatecholaminergic) terminals. Both the dendrites and perikarya are usually ensheathed in thin laminar glial processes except at the location of synaptic contacts (Fig. 3A).

Nonadrenergic *terminals* identified by uptake of [3H]norepinephrine (16) or by immunocytochemistry for DBH (38) are characterized by a mixed population of many small (30–50 nm) clear and usually five or more large (100 nm) dense core vesicles. As many as 95% (2,16) or possibly as few as 40% (38) of the noradrenergic terminals in the frontal cortex lack synaptic specializations. These

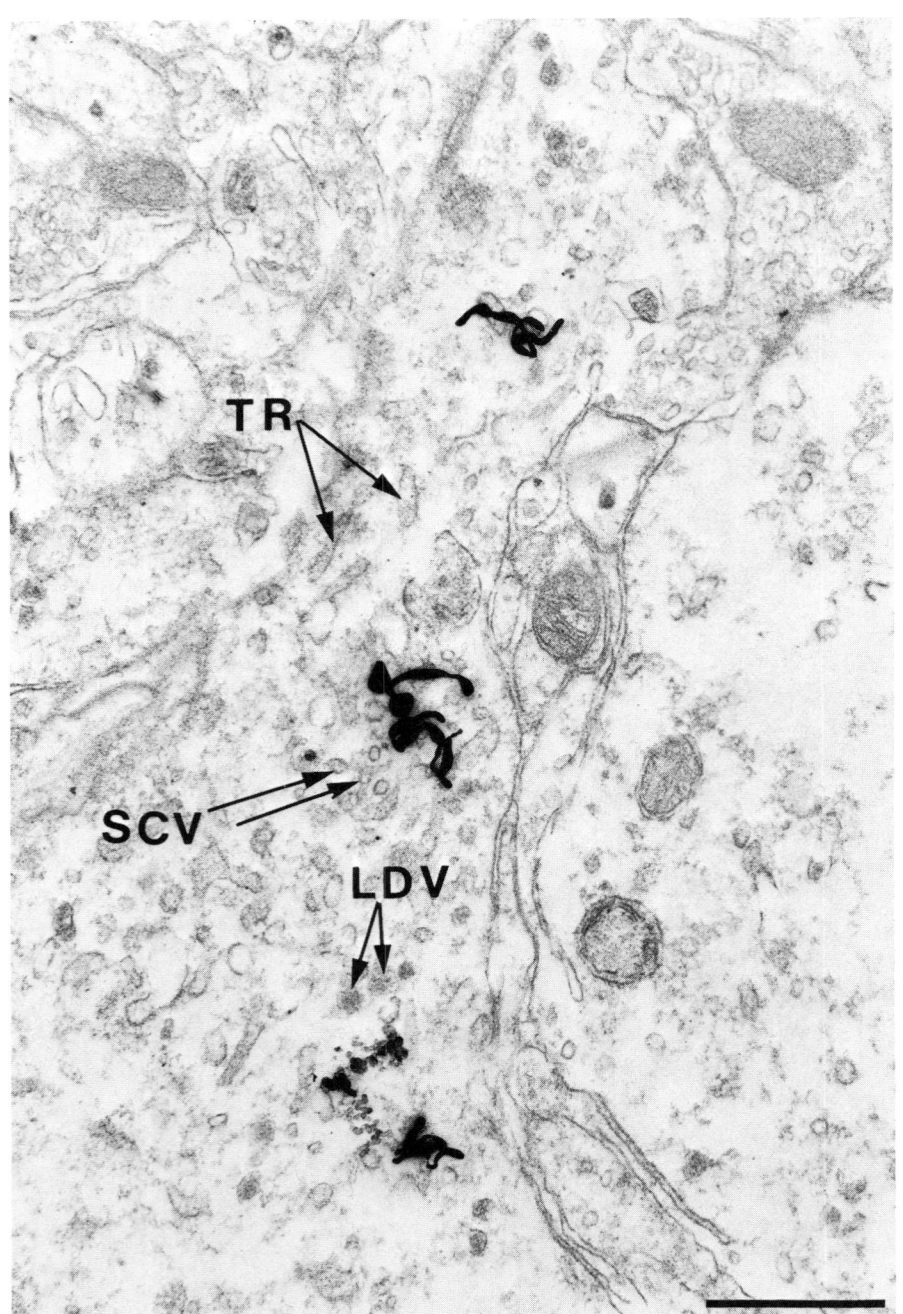

FIG. 2. Autoradiographic immunocytochemical localization of TH using ^{125}I-secondary immunoglobulin. Silver grains are exclusively seen over the neuronal perikaryon and proximal dendrite. Numerous large dense vesicles (LDV), small clear vesicles (SCV), and tubular reticulum (TR) are evident. Bar = 0.5 μm.

observations led to the hypothesis that central noradrenergic terminals may be comparable to peripheral sympathetic axons, which also lack synaptic specializations (2,56). Several lines of evidence support the possibility that at least some central noradrenergic terminals may have a wide range of effects on other neurons as well as on neighboring glia or blood vessels (51). First, beta-adrenergic receptors have been demonstrated on glia and on preterminal axons where there is no morphological evidence of synaptic associations (39). Second, centrally derived axon terminals showing uptake of 5-OHDA have been demonstrated in direct apposition to the basal laminae of blood vessels in the paraventricular nuclei of the hypothalamus (64). Third, many of the noradrenergic and adrenergic neurons in brain contain a recently discovered peptide, neuropeptide Y, which is found also in peripheral sympathetic neurons and which acts synergistically with norepinephrine (19). In addition to the observed "nonsynaptic" associations, immunocytochemical labeling with DBH revealed that at least 58% of the noradrenergic terminals in the cerebral cortex make conventional axodendritic synapses usually with an asymmetric density (38). The possible multiple types of

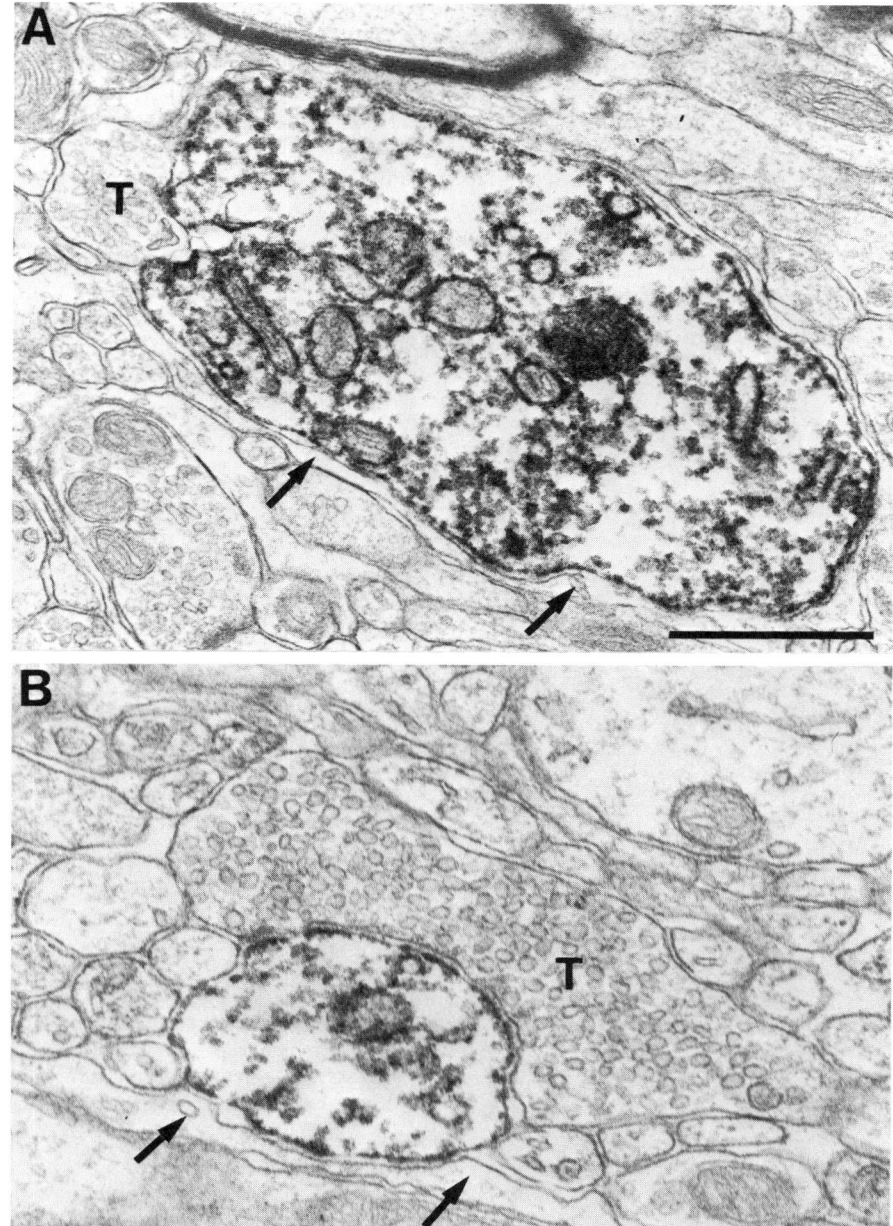

FIG. 3. Peroxidase immunocytochemistry for TH in proximal (**A**) and more distal (**B**) dendrite in the lateral parabrachial region. The labeled dendrites are postsynaptic to unlabeled terminals (T) and are invested in a thin lamina of glial processes (*arrows*). Bar = 0.5 µm.

terminations for noradrenergic axons labeled with immunocytochemical or autoradiographic methods may indicate multiple types of receptor-mediated interactions.

CATECHOLAMINERGIC PATHWAY FROM THE SOLITARY NUCLEI TO THE PARABRACHIAL REGION

The catecholaminergic neurons of the caudal m-NTS include principally the noradrenergic neurons of the A2

group (14). However, recently Kalia et al. (30) and Ruggiero et al. (55) have used immunocytochemistry for the respective synthesizing enzymes to demonstrate that the caudal m-NTS also contains both dopaminergic and adrenergic neurons. Immunoreactivity for TH is found in all three types of catecholaminergic neurons. Thus the described ultrastructural features and afferent and efferent connections of TH-labeled neurons cannot exclusively be ascribed to the noradrenergic neurons in the m-NTS.

The cytological features of TH-labeled perikarya and dendrites in the m-NTS are similar to those described in the locus ceruleus and thus will not be given in detail. The somatic and dendritic spines are numerous on labeled neurons in the m-NTS. Cytoplasmic organelles such as the tubular endoplasmic reticulum and both small clear and large dense core vesicles are readily evident with autoradiographic immunolabeling of TH (Fig. 2).

Unlabeled (presumably noncatecholaminergic) and TH-labeled terminals form synapses with perikarya and dendrites showing immunoreactivity for the enzyme. At least some of the unlabeled afferents to the catecholaminergic neurons in the m-NTS are derived from sensory neurons located in the nodose ganglia (61). Serotonergic (47), GABAergic (44), and peptidergic (50) neurons also directly terminate on

TH-labeled dendrites in the m-NTS. The TH-labeled terminals within the m-NTS are relatively sparse as compared with the density of catecholaminergic terminals identified by uptake of 5-OHDA (10,66), presumably reflecting the difficulty in localizing TH in noradrenergic axon terminals by electron microscopy (48). Thus the examples of TH-labeled terminals on similarly labeled dendrites most likely demonstrate interactions between two different types of catecholaminergic neurons.

The projections of TH-labeled neurons from the m-NTS to the lateral PBR have been extensively studied by combined light microscopic tracing and by electron microscopy (34). The terminals with TH-immunoreactivity in the PBR

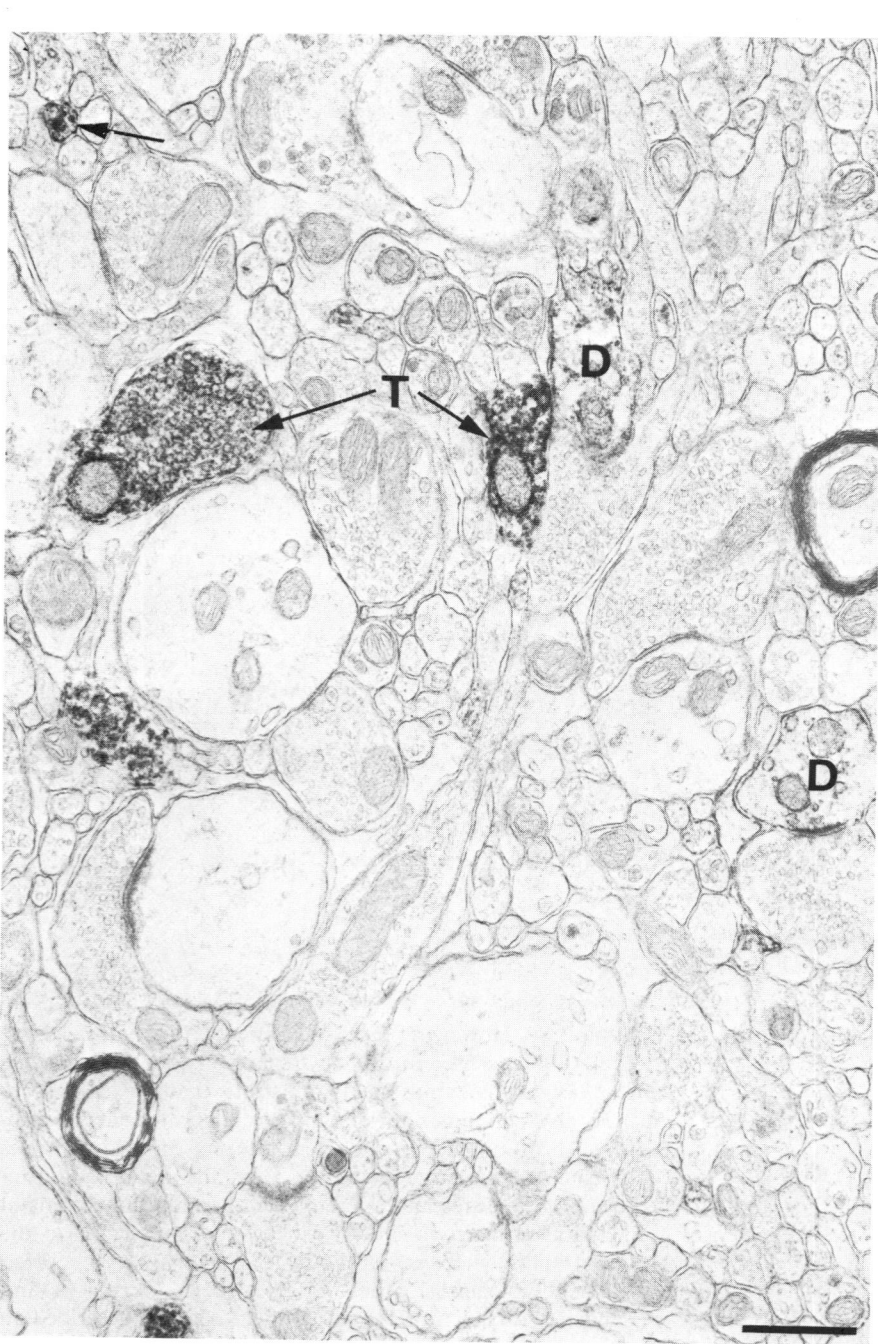

FIG. 4. Peroxidase labeling for TH in the lateral parabrachial region. Immunoreactivity is seen in a small unmyelinated axon (arrows), axon terminals (T), and dendrites (D). Bar = 0.5 μm.

(Fig. 4) are similar to dopaminergic terminals both in ease of detection and in morphological characteristics. In tissues prepared for electron microscopy, areas containing predominantly dopaminergic terminals are readily labeled with TH in the absence of detergents or other agents to enhance penetration of the antisera (43). In contrast, regions containing primarily noradrenergic terminals such as the cerebellum and portions of the cerebral cortex exhibit few, if any, TH-labeled axons in similarly prepared tissues. This difference is believed to be largely attributable to lower quantities or less accessibility of TH within noradrenergic axons (48). In the PBR, TH-immunoreactivity is readily detected with glutaraldehyde or acrolein fixation and thus appears more similar to dopaminergic terminals (34). The labeled terminals of the PBR also share several common morphological characteristics with the dopaminergic terminals of the caudate and accumbens nuclei. These include multiple types of synaptic vesicles and the formation of symmetric, asymmetric, and nonsynaptic junctions.

The catecholaminergic terminals in the PBR form synapses principally with neurons that lack immunoreactivity for TH. However, a few perikarya and dendrites in the lateral PBR contain TH-immunoreactivity and receive synapses from other labeled terminals (34). These observations provide additional support for a direct modulatory interaction between catecholaminergic neurons.

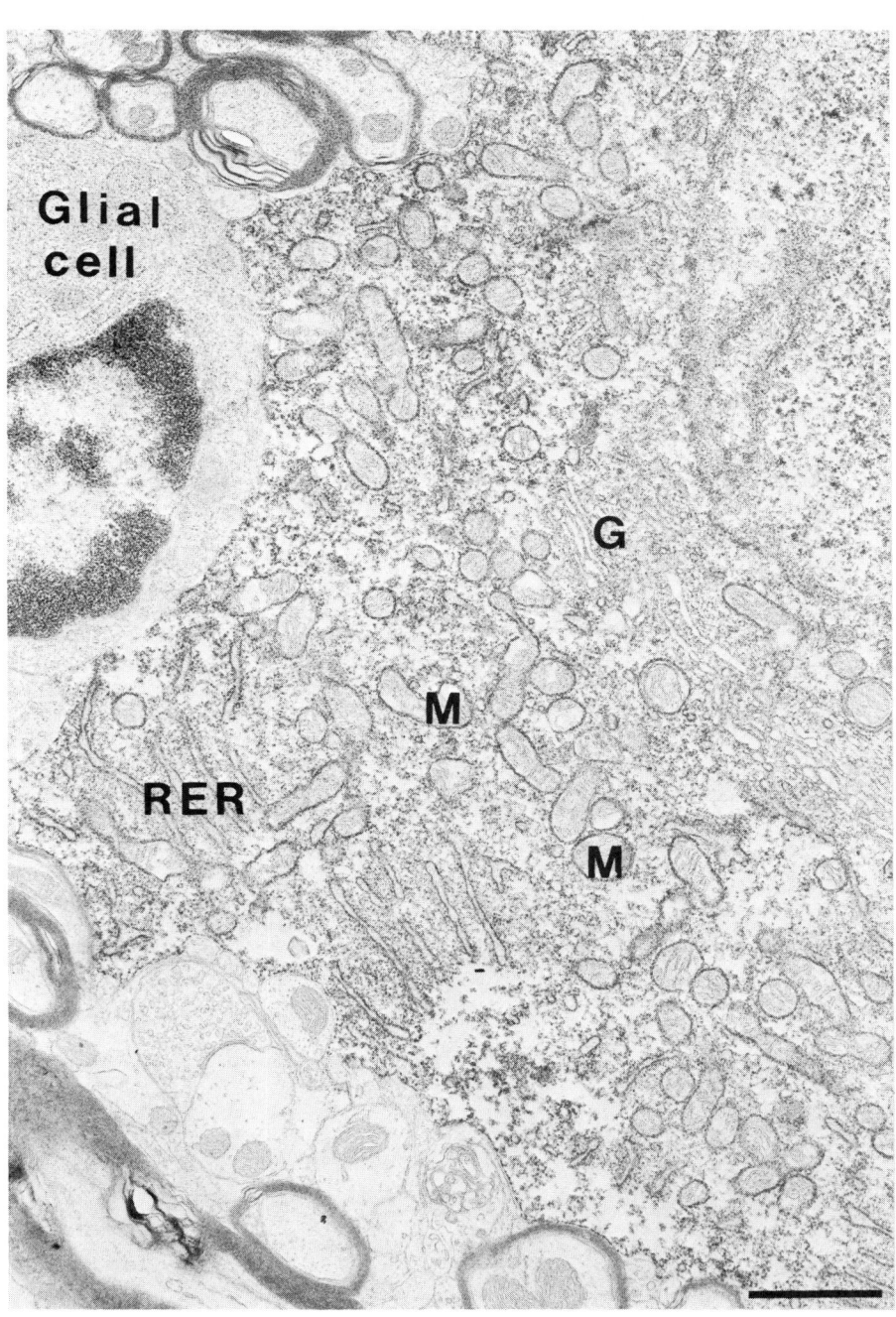

FIG. 5. Peroxidase immunoreactivity for PNMT in cytoplasm of a perikaryon in the rostral ventrolateral medulla. The cytoplasm of the labeled neuron is characterized by Golgi apparatus (G), mitochondria (M), and rough endoplasmic reticulum (RER). The labeled neuronal perikaryon is in direct apposition to an unlabeled supporting glial cell. Bar = 0.1 μm.

ADRENERGIC NEURONS OF THE ROSTRAL VENTROLATERAL MEDULLA AND SOLITARY NUCLEI

Until extremely recently (35,46) there were no ultrastructural studies of adrenergic neurons. This deficiency was accounted for largely by nonselectivity of [³H]epinephrine as an uptake marker for adrenergic neurons (4). Furthermore, PNMT had exclusively been used for light microscopy (26). We have now examined the ultrastructural localization of PNMT within the C1 group of adrenergic neurons in the rostral ventrolateral medulla (RVL) (35) and in the caudal m-NTS and dorsal motor nuclei of the vagus (46).

In the RVL, peroxidase immunoreactivity for PNMT is diffusely distributed throughout the cytoplasm of select perikarya. The most outstanding ultrastructural feature of the PNMT-containing perikarya in the RVL is their high density of mitochondria (Fig. 5). The cells are also heavily invested in glial processes and are found in close proximity to neighboring blood vessels (35). These ultrastructural characteristics are consistent with a high metabolic activity and possible chemosensory function for adrenergic neurons in the RVL (23). Similar ultrastructural features were

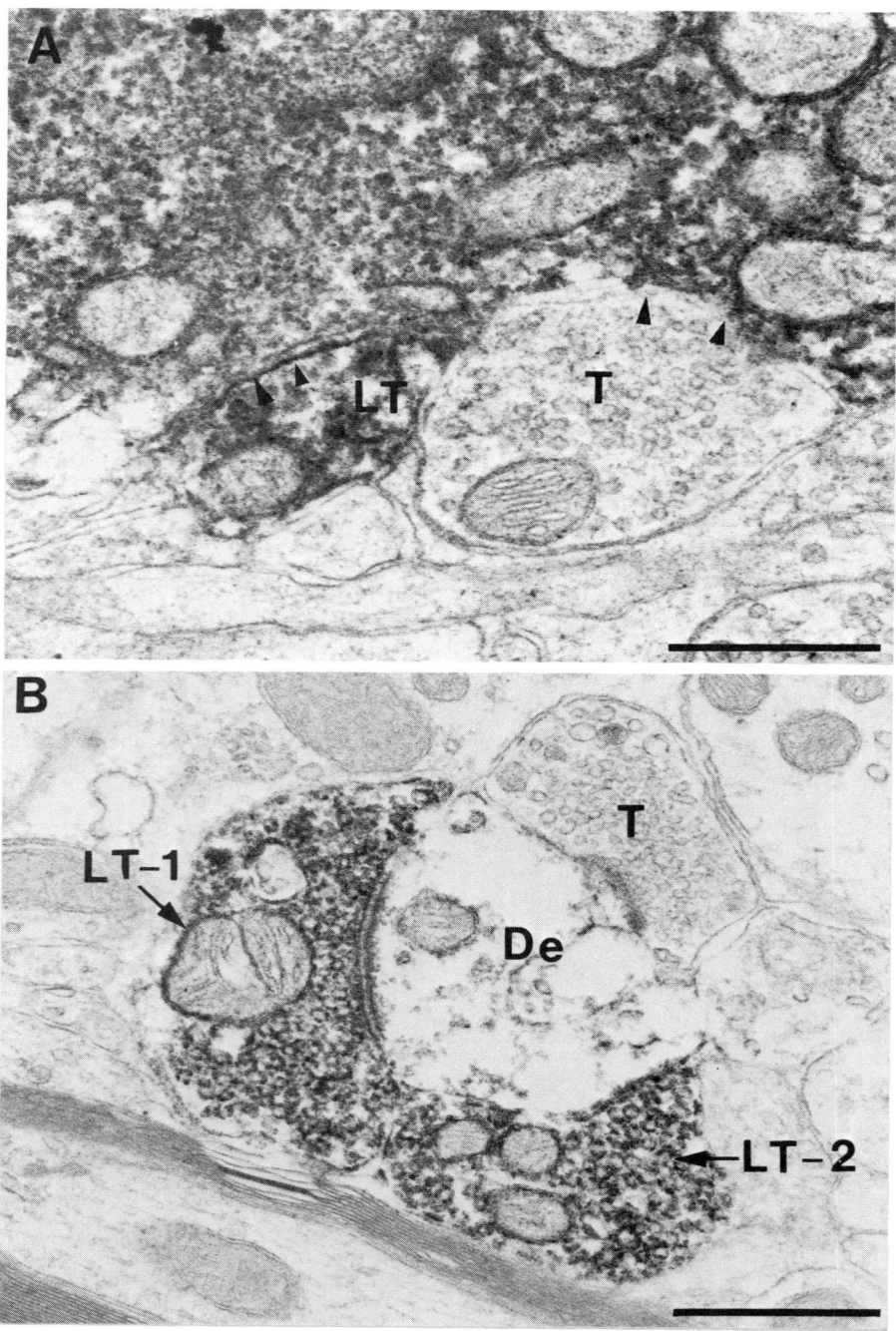

FIG. 6. Synaptic interaction between PNMT-labeled profiles in the rostral ventrolateral medulla. **A:** Electron micrograph shows appositions (*arrowheads*) between a peroxidase-immunoreactive neuronal perikaryon and a labeled terminal (LT) and an unlabeled terminal (T). **B:** Electron micrograph shows two labeled terminals (LT-1 and LT-2) and an unlabeled terminal (T) which converge on a dendrite (De). The dendrite also contains a small accumulation of peroxidase immunoreactivity for PNMT. Bar = 0.5.

described by Zhigadlo and Belova (70) for presumed epinephrine-synthesizing neurons in the ventrolateral medulla, but without confirmatory labeling with PNMT.

The PNMT-containing perikarya in the RVL received synaptic contacts from unlabeled as well as PNMT-containing terminals (Fig. 6A). The somatic junctions usually are not characterized by synaptic densities, which are recognizable due to the dense peroxidase immunoreactivity at the postsynaptic site. Dendrites with immunoreactivity for PNMT also receive synaptic input from both labeled and unlabeled axon terminals (Fig. 6B).

The *axons* with PNMT immunoreactivity in the RVL are principally small and unmyelinated. However, a few larger axons also exhibit several layers of myelin. The thin unmyelinated and myelinated axons could provide a basis for differences in conduction velocity in bulbospinal autonomic pathways (7).

The PNMT-containing perikarya in *the caudal portion of the m-NTS* have only recently been described by light (30,35) and electron microscopy (46). Failure to detect these perikarya in initial studies by Hökfelt et al. (26) is probably attributable to lower quantities of the enzyme or

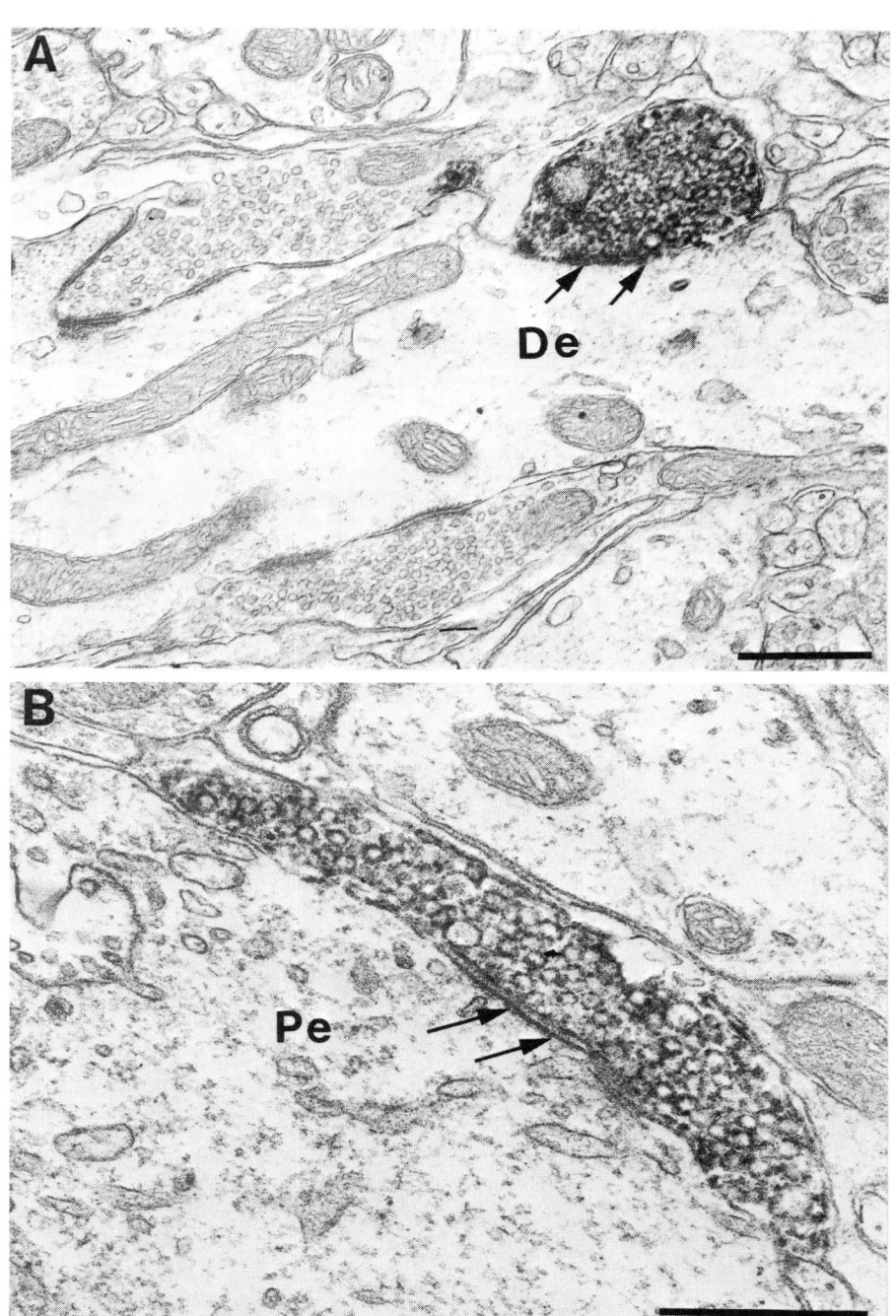

FIG. 7. PNMT-containing terminals in the dorsal motor nucleus of the vagus. Immunoreactive terminals form symmetric synapses (*arrows*) with unlabeled (**A**) dendrite (De) and (**B**) perikaryon (Pe). Bar = 0.5 μm.

different sensitivities to aldehyde fixatives. The majority of the PNMT-labeled perikarya in m-NTS are small (10–15 μm), contain only a thin rim of cytoplasm, and are located in the dorsomedial subdivision near the ventrolateral boundaries of the area postrema. Most of the labeled perikarya in the m-NTS differ from those in the RVL by their smaller size, less dense PNMT-immunoreactivity, and fewer mitochondria (46).

Axons and axon terminals labeled for PNMT are far more numerous in the m-NTS and in the dorsal motor nuclei of the vagus than in the RVL. The PNMT-containing terminals form synapses primarily with unlabeled soma and dendrites in both the sensory (m-NTS) and motor nuclei of the vagus (Fig. 7). In the m-NTS a small portion of the PNMT-containing terminals also form synapses with labeled dendrites, thus again supporting a functional interaction between the adrenergic neurons.

SUMMARY

The ultrastructural features of a few of the histologically and functionally more well-characterized central catecholaminergic systems have been reviewed. The described morphological characteristics are not sufficiently unique to allow identification of catecholaminergic neurons without additional labels such as immunoreactivity for the synthesizing enzymes, uptake of catecholamine congeners like 5-OHDA, or autoradiographic detection of incorporated [3H]dopamine or [3H]norepinephrine. However, the structural studies provide a morphological substrate for direct synaptic interactions between catecholaminergic and non-catecholaminergic neurons and suggest a possibly nonsynaptic relationship between central catecholaminergic neurons and other axons, neighboring glia, and blood vessels. The morphological studies also provide a structural basis for the increasing body of physiological evidence that the activity of central catecholaminergic, particularly adrenergic, neurons is influenced by synaptic input from other neurons containing the same or a different catecholamine.

ACKNOWLEDGMENTS

We gratefully acknowledge the support of grants from NSF (BNS 80-23914), NIH (HL 18974), and NIMH (MH 00078 and MH 40342).

REFERENCES

1. Arluison, M., Agid, Y., and Javoy, F. (1978): *Neuroscience, 3:* 657–673.
2. Beaudet, A., and Descarries, L. (1978): *Neuroscience,* 3:851–860.
3. Björklund, A., and Lindvall, O. (1975): *Brain Res.,* 83:531–537.
4. Bosler, O., and Calas, A. (1982): *Brain Res. Bull.,* 9:151–169.
5. Bouyer, J. J., Joh, T. H., and Pickel, V. M. (1984): *J. Comp. Neurol.,* 227:92–103.
6. Bouyer, J. J., Park, D. H., Joh, T. H., and Pickel, V. M. (1984): *Brain Res.,* 302:267–275.
7. Brown, D. L., and Guyenet, P. G. (1984): *Am. J. Physiol.,* 247: R1009–R1016.
8. Bunney, B. S., Walters, J. R., Roth, R. H., and Aghajanian, G. K. (1973): *J. Pharmacol. Exp. Ther.,* 185:560–571.
9. Cheramy, A., Leviel, V., and Glowinski, J. (1981): *Nature,* 289: 537–542.
10. Chiba, T., and Kato, M. (1978): *Brain Res.,* 151:323–338.
11. Cimarusti, D. L., Saito, K., Vaughn, J. E., Barber, R., Roberts, R., and Thomas, P. E. (1979): *Brain Res.,* 162:55–67.
12. Cohen, R. S., Carlin, R. K., Grab, D. J., and Siekevitz, P. (1982): *Prog. Brain Res.,* 56:49–76.
13. Crick, F. (1982): *Trends Neurosci.,* 5:44–46.
14. Dahlström, A., and Fuxe, K. (1964): *Acta. Physiol. Scand.,* 62(Suppl. 232):1–55.
15. Descarries, L., Bosler, O., Berthelet, F., and Des Rosiers, M. H. (1980): *Nature,* 284:620–622.
16. Descarries, L., Watkins, K. C., and Lapierre, Y. (1977): *Brain Res.,* 133:197–222.
17. Domesick, V. B., Stinus, L., and Paskevich, P. A. (1983): *Neuroscience,* 8:743–765.
18. Droz, B., Rambourg, A., and Koenig, H. L. (1975): *Brain Res.,* 93:1–13.
19. Everitt, B. J., Hökfelt, T., and Terenius, L. (1984): *Neuroscience,* 11:443–462.
20. Geffen, L. B., Jessell, T. M., Cuello, A. C., and Iversen, L. L. (1976): *Nature,* 260:258–260.
21. Giorguieff, M. F., Kemel, M. L., and Glowinski, J. (1977): *Neurosci. Lett.,* 6:73–77.
22. Giorguieff, M. F., LeFloch, M. L., Westfall, T. C., Glowinski, J., and Bensson, M. J. (1976): *Brain Res.,* 106:117–131.
23. Granata, A. R., Ruggiero, D. A., Park, D. H., Joh, T. H., and Reis, D. J. (1985): *Heart Circ. Phys.,* 17:H547–567.
24. Grzanna, R., and Coyle, J. T. (1976): *J. Neurochem.,* 27:1091–1096.
25. Hökfelt, T. (1967): *Z. Zellforsch. Mikrosk. Anat.,* 79:110–117.
26. Hökfelt, T., Fuxe, K., Goldstein, M., and Johnsson, O. (1974): *Brain Res.,* 66:235–251.
27. Hökfelt, T., Skirboll, L., Rehfeld, J. F., Goldstein, M., Markey, K., and Dann, O. (1980): *Neuroscience,* 5:2093–2124.
28. Howe, P. R. C., Costa, M., Furness, J. B., and Chalmers, J. P. (1980): *Neuroscience,* 5:2229–2238.
29. Joh, T. H., Gegham, C., and Reis, D. J. (1973): *Proc. Natl. Acad. Sci. USA,* 70:2767–2771.
30. Kalia, M., Fuxe, K., and Goldstein, M. (1985): *J. Comp. Neurol.,* 233:308–332.
31. Kitai, S. T., Sugimori, M., and Kocis, J. (1976): *Exp. Brain Res.,* 24:351–363.
32. Lundberg, J. M., Hedlund, B., Anggard, A., Fahrenkrug, J., Hökfelt, T., Tatemoto, K., and Bartfait, T. (1982): In: *Systemic Role of Regulatory Peptides,* edited by S. R. Bloom, J. M. Polak, and E. Lindlaub, pp. 93–119. Schottauer and Stuttgard Publishers, New York.
33. Mercer, L., Del Fiacoo, M., and Cuello, A. C. (1979): *Experientia,* 35:101–103.
34. Milner, T. A., Joh, T. H., and Pickel, V. M. (1986): *J. Neurosci.,* 6:2585–2603.
35. Milner, T. A., Pickel, V. M., Park, D. H., Joh, T. H., and Reis, D. J. (1987): *Brain Res.,* 6–77.
36. Nagy, J. I., Lee, T., Seeman, P., and Fibiger, H. C. (1978): *Nature,* 274:278–281.
37. Norcross, K., and Spehlmann, R. (1978): *Brain Res.,* 156:168–174.
38. Olschowka, J. A., Molliver, M. E., Grzanna, R., Rice, R. L., and Coyle, J. T. (1981): *J. Histochem. Cytochem.,* 29:271–280.
39. Palmer, G. C. (1980): *Neuropharmacology,* 19:17–23.
40. Park, D. H., Baetge, E. E., Kaplan, B., Albert, V. R., Reis, D. J., and Joh, T. H. (1982): *J. Neurochem.,* 38:410–414.
41. Pickel, V. M. (1981): In: *Neuroanatomical Tract-Tracing Methods,* edited by L. Heimer and M. J. Robards, pp. 483–509. Plenum Press, New York.
42. Pickel, V. M. (1984): In: *Handbook of Chemical Neuroanatomy, Vol. III,* edited by A. Björklund and T. Hökfelt. Elsevier, Amsterdam.
43. Pickel, V. M., Beckley, S. C., Joh, T. H., and Reis, D. J. (1981): *Brain Res.,* 225:373–385.
44. Pickel, V. M., Chan, J., Joh, T. H., and Massari, J. V. (1984): *Soc. Neurosci. Abst.,* 10:537.

45. Pickel, V. M., Chan, J., and Milner, T. A. (1986): *J. Histochem. Cytochem.,* 34:707–718.
46. Pickel, V. M., Chan, J., Park, D. H., Joh, T. H., and Milner, T. A. (1986): *J. Neurosci. Res.,* 15:436–456.
47. Pickel, V. M., Joh, T. H., Chan, J., and Beaudet, A. (1984): *J. Comp. Neurol.,* 225:291–302.
48. Pickel, V. M., Joh, T. H., and Reis, D. J. (1976): *J. Histochem. Cytochem.,* 24:792–806.
50. Pickel, V. M., Joh, T. H., Reis, D. J., Leeman, S. E., and Miller, R. J. (1979): *Brain Res.,* 160:387–400.
51. Raichle, M. E., Hartman, B. K., Eichling, J. O., and Sharpe, L. G. (1975): *Proc. Natl. Acad. Sci. USA,* 72:3726–3730.
52. Ramon-Moliner, E. (1974): *Cell Tissue Res.,* 149:205–221.
53. Richards, J. G. (1983): In: *Handbook of Chemical Neuroanatomy, Volume I: Methods in Chemical Neuroanatomy,* edited by A. Björklund and T. Hökfelt, pp. 122–146. Elsevier, Amsterdam.
54. Richards, J. G., and Tranzer, J. P. (1975): *J. Ultrastruct. Res.,* 53:204–216.
55. Ruggiero, D. A., Ross, C. A., Anwar, M., Park, D. H., Joh, T. H., and Reis, D. J. (1985): *J. Comp. Neurol.,* 239:127–154.
56. Santer, R. M., Lever, J. D., and Davies, T. W. (1981): *Histochemistry,* 71:155–160.
57. Scheibel, A. B., and Tomiyasu, U. (1980): *Exp. Neurol.,* 70:717–720.
58. Shimizu, N., and Imamoto, K. (1970): *Arch. Histol. Jpn.,* 31:229–246.
59. Stenevi, U., Björklund, A., and Moore, R. Y. (1972): *Exp. Neurol.,* 35:290–299.
60. Sternberger, L. A. (1979): In: *Immunocytochemistry,* pp. 436–440. John Wiley and Sons, New York.
61. Sumal, K. K., Blessing, W. W., Joh, T. H., Reis, D. J., and Pickel, V. M. (1983): *Brain Res.,* 277:31–40.
62. Svensson, T. H., Bunney, B. S., and Aghajanian, G. K. (1975): *Brain Res.,* 92:291–306.
63. Swanson, L. W. (1976): *Brain Res.,* 110:39–56.
64. Swanson, L. W., Connelly, M. A., and Hartman, B. K. (1977): *Brain Res.,* 136:166–173.
65. Swanson, L. W., and Hartman, B. K. (1975): *J. Comp. Neurol.,* 163:467–505.
66. Takahashi, Y., Tohyama, M., Satoh, K., Sakumoto, T., Kashiba, A., and Shimizu, N. (1980): *J. Comp. Neurol.,* 189:525–535.
67. Tenneyson, V. M., Heikkila, R., Mytilineou, C., Cote, L., and Cohen, G. (1974): *Brain Res.,* 82:341–348.
68. Wilson, C. J., Groves, P. M., and Fifkova, E. (1977): *Exp. Brain Res.,* 30:161–174.
69. Wood, J. G. (1982): *Brain Res. Bull.,* 9:178–188.
70. Zhigadlo, B. A., and Belova, T. I. (1983): *Neurosci. Behav. Physiol.,* 12:407–415.

Psychopharmacology:
The Third Generation of Progress,
edited by Herbert Y. Meltzer.
Raven Press, New York © 1987.

CHAPTER 7

The CNS Serotonergic System: Progression Toward a Collaborative Organization

Efrain C. Azmitia

Serotonergic cells are phylogenetically ancient and have been identified in nearly every nervous system studied from coelenterates (review 36) to human (7). Ontogenetically, detectable levels of serotonin (5-HT) and tryptophan hydroxylase activity are present in the fertilized egg (30). Nearly every cell has 5-HT until the gastrula stage is complete. The distribution of this important monoamine becomes increasingly restricted to a small proportion of cells in the CNS, peripheral nervous system, and some nonnervous tissues (e.g., lung, pineal). The CNS cells develop mainly in the brainstem ventricular zone at days 12 to 14 (38). The cells form just lateral to the midline and migrate toward the raphe after day 18 of gestation in the rat (39). The cells begin to develop homotypic collaterals among themselves before they establish long target projections (29,54). These interconnections play a major role in synchronizing the firing rate of the 5-HT cells.

Electrophysiological studies by Jacobs (*this volume*) indicate that 5-HT identified cells in the same vicinity have remarkable similar firing characteristics. Thus, the close apposition of the neurons has the benefit of allowing many cells to function as closely knit groups. Mesencephalic cultures treated with the serotonergic agonist 5-methoxy-tryptamine produce cells whose transmitter maturation is inhibited and whose processes can actually encircle the soma (55). So 5-HT itself might act as a neurotropic agent in directing the initial outgrowth of serotonergic cells. In *Helisoma* (a snail), application of 5-HT to the growth cone of an axon can change its migration rate (31).

Later, the cells grow out in fasciculus anteriorly toward the cortex, and caudally extend into the spinal cord. Groups of 5-HT cells innervate interconnecting terminal areas. When these terminal regions are activated in concert, their coordinated activity will be facilitated. Thus, the collaborative organization developed during early ontogeny permits clusters of raphe cells to function as a coordinated group in controlling complex neuronal circuits. The collaborative arrangement of the 5-HT cells allows more closely knit cells to have a more powerful combined effect. Lower species such as the rat have more tightly clustered cells than do cat or monkey, where few of the cells have migrated toward the actual midline. *The implications of this increased independence of 5-HT neuronal functioning may actually correspond with the greater complexity of human thought.*

This chapter provides morphological data on the anatomical distribution of the serotonergic system in the primate, cat, and rat brain and will emphasize the main differences occurring among them. We shall discuss the CNS cell groups lying outside the brainstem: the 5-HT-IR (5-HT-immunoreactive) cells in the hypothalamic dorsomedial nucleus in the rat, and in the cervical spinal cord of the monkey. A nomenclature based on Olszewski and Baxter (45) will be presented that differs significantly from previous reports.

FINDINGS

Cell Bodies

The 5-HT-IR cell bodies in the brain can be divided into rostral and caudal brainstem groups. The rostral group essentially consists of four main nuclei: the nucleus centralis superior (B5, B7, and B8), the nucleus raphe dorsalis (B6 and B7), the nucleus prosupralemniscus (B9), and the hypothalamic dorsomedial nucleus. The caudal group consists of five main nuclei: the nucleus raphe obscurus (B2), the nucleus raphe pallidus (B1), the nucleus raphe magnus (B3), the nucleus raphe ventricularis (B4), and the fifth group of 5-HT-IR cells in the nucleus reticularis lateralis

(LRN) and the nucleus paragigantocellularis lateralis (NPGL).

With regard to the rostral group, one of the main features of our classification is that the nucleus annularis (23,52) or the nucleus interfascicularis (5,57), located between the medial longitudinal fasciculi (MLF), is combined with the nucleus centralis superior (NCS) as proposed by Olszewski and Baxter (45) instead of the nucleus raphe dorsalis (NRD) as suggested by Dahlstrom and Fuxe (19). There is both historical and anatomical justification for including this group with NCS. First, these cells are spindle shaped and perpendicularly oriented as distinct from the cells seen dorsally in the central gray. Second, the ascending projections of the NCS dorsalis closely overlie the cells of NCS medialis. In the rat both groups project to the dorsal hippocampus (5,57) whereas in the monkey they both project to the cingulate and prefrontal cortex (47). Third, in the caudal midbrain, behind the superior cerebellar decussation, the cells of NCS dorsalis merge caudally with B5 and ventrally with B8 (NCS ventralis). The cells of NRD, on the other hand, merge caudally with B6. Another interesting observation is the group of small 5-HR-IR cells in the dorsomedial nucleus of the hypothalamus. The cells have only been seen in the rat brain. Their position in the hypothalamus, their small size and round soma, and their short projections make this a unique collection of serotonergic cells.

With regard to the caudal group, several points should be emphasized. The 5-HT-IR cells in nucleus raphe obscurus (NRO) extend into the spinal cord in the monkey, where they are associated with the descending MLF, the central canal (lamina X), and the motor neurons (lamina IX). This group merges rostrally with NRO. A second point is the existence of a large cluster of neurons on the ventrolateral floor of the medulla oblongata. These cells are located in the LRN and more rostrally in the NPGL and extend from the emergence of nerve VI to that of nerve XII. In this ventral position, the cells are often associated with blood vessels entering the brain at this level. This nucleus may be a major afferent of the nucleus locus ceruleus (2). The final point is the existence of small 5-HT-IR cells in the area postrema of monkey, cat, and rat.

Rostral Brainstem Group

Nucleus centralis superior (B8, B5, part of B7). Nucleus centralis superior (NCS), using the division proposed by Olszewski and Baxter (45), can be divided into three components in the monkey brain: dorsalis, medialis, and lateralis (see Fig. 1). The dorsal component lies between the MLF. This group is continuous with B5 nucleus raphe pontis (NRPo) in the pons, and extends as far rostrally as the oculomotor nuclei remaining superior to the superior cerebellar decussation.

The medialis component is generally considered to be B8. It is a paramedian and median cluster of cells. The group has a rostrocaudal oblique orientation as previously described in the rat (5,40). The cells of the medialis component remain ventral to the decussation of the superior cerebellar peduncle. Rostrally, the cells from this group end

around and within the interpeduncular nucleus. Caudally, the ventral border of this group is the trapezoid body.

The final cluster of cells of NCS is the lateralis group, which is seen ventrolateral to the MLF. A large number of cells extend from this group into the midbrain reticular formation. These cells in the monkey and cat are widely scattered and seem to form a ring around the nucleus reticularis pontis oralis. In the cat the NCS begins as a single cluster of cells at the level of the dorsal tegmental nucleus of the cat (34). The cluster lies in paramedian columns (approximately 60–70 cells per section) extending ventrally from the fourth ventricle. The dorsalis group (approximately 20 5-HT cells per section at this level) separates rostrally and lies between the MLF and is bordered ventrally by the superior cerebellar descussation (SCD). The main medialis division extends ventrally from the SCD to an area just dorsal to the medial lemniscus (ML). The nucleus has two paramedian columns separated by as much as 400 μm and has about 100 5-HT cells, which increase to about 200 cells rostrally.

Nucleus raphe pontis (B5). A small paramedian cluster of 5-HT-IR cells with a few cells lying directly on the midline forms the caudal border of the nucleus centralis superior dorsalis (B8). The cells are located just medial and ventral to the MLF and extend caudally to the level of the abducens nucleus. Some of the cells and many dendrites are situated within the MLF. At the very caudal portion of this group, the cells are situated dorsal to the raphe magnus cells. In the cat and monkey, these cells are not aggregated closely enough to be described as a separate nucleus. In the rat, this group was described as being continuous with the median raphe nucleus (40).

Nucleus raphe dorsalis. The NRD is divided into a medial and lateral component. The medial component is in the central gray just below the cerebral aqueduct. These cells extend caudally to merge with B6 in the pons. The cells extend rostrally to the caudal border of the oculomotor nuclei. This group is clearly visible in all three species. In the cat it contains a maximum of about 100 cells per section.

The lateral component (the wings) forms the larger division of NRD and extends as far rostrally as the oculomotor nuclei. The wings are best developed at the level of the rostral pole of the trochlear nucleus. In the cat, the number of cells is approximately 180 cells per section. This pair of laterally situated 5-HT-IR cells (Fig. 9) extends caudally and can be seen in the central gray of the pons just ventral to the fourth ventricle. The cells lie between the MLF and the locus ceruleus and some of the cells penetrate into the boundaries of these two areas. The serotonergic cells in the nucleus of locus ceruleus were first described by Sladek and Walker (51) in the brains of stump-tailed macaques. The cells comprising the B6 groups are first seen at the level of the motor nucleus of V and become continuous rostrally with the lateral wings of NRD. This continuity was also seen in the developing rat brain (40).

Nucleus prosupralemniscus (B9). This group is located along the dorsal surface of the medial lemniscus from the rostral border of the inferior olive to the level of the red nucleus. These cells are occasionally continuous with the

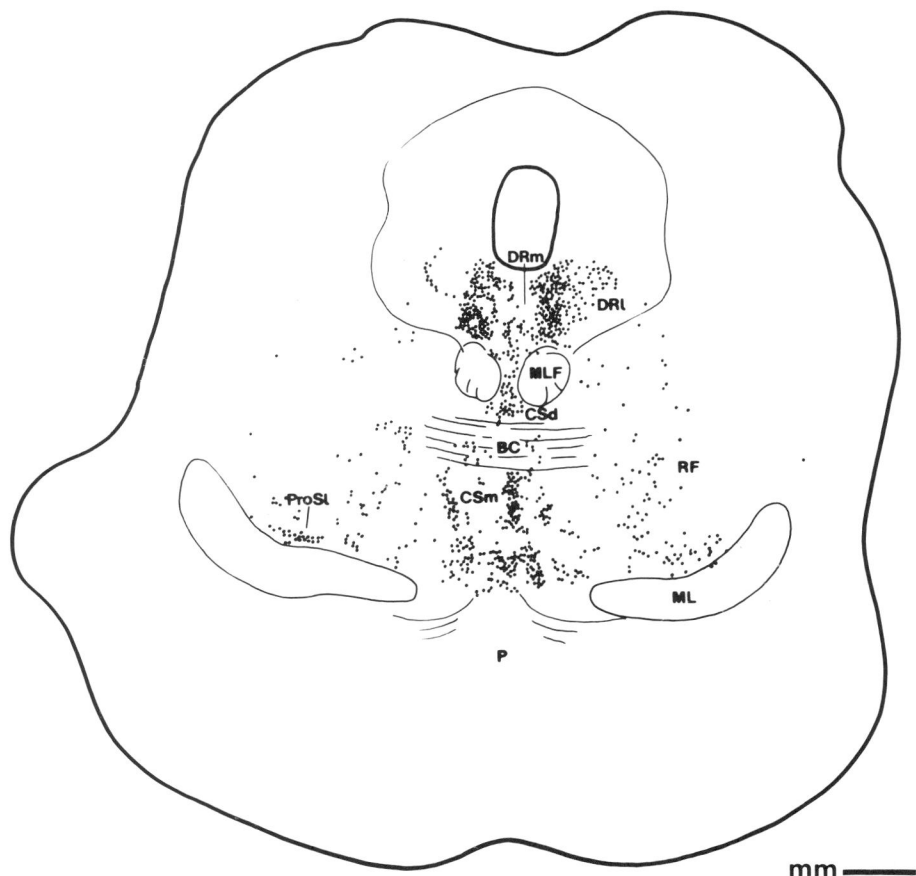

FIG. 1. Representative section from the brainstem of *M. fascicularis* coronally sectioned at 100 μm and reacted with an antibody raised against serotonin. ●, 5-HT-immunoreactive (5-HT-IR) cells. The major divisions of the nucleus centralis superior are dorsalis (CSd), medialis (CSm), and lateralis (not labeled but cells seen in the reticular formation, RF). The nucleus raphe dorsalis contains the medialis (DRm) and the lateral wings (DRl). The 5-HT-IR cells in nucleus prosupralemniscus (ProSl) are shown. MLF, Medial longitudinal fasciculus; BC, decussation of the brachium conjunctivum; P, pons; ML, medial lemniscus. (From ref. 7.)

paramedian cells of the medial component of the NCS. The similar cytological and fluorescent characteristics of the cells in NCS and nucleus prosupralemnscus (ProSL) were first noted in the brainstem of the squirrel monkey by Hubbard and DiCarlo (33). In the cat, these cells can be seen to be continuous with NCS, medialis, and form the ventral part of the ring of cells that surrounds the reticular nucleus. These findings confirm the similarity between these two nuclei shown in the rat by Dahlstrom and Fuxe (19).

Nucleus dorsalis medialis of the hypothalamus. Using fluorescence histochemistry following intraventricular infusion of 5-HT in nialamide-pretreated rats, Fuxe and Ungerstedt (27) identified an additional group of 5-HT cells located in the dorsomedial nucleus (DMN) of the hypothalamus. This provided the first evidence that the hypothalamus contains an endogenous source of 5-HT. Biochemical support for the hypothalamus containing 5-HT-producing cells comes from the high concentrations of 5-HT and tryptophan hydroxylase present in the surgically isolated mediobasal hypothalamus (12). Beaudet and Descarries (10) using [³H]5-HT *in vivo* uptake radioautography,

found a single cluster of labeled cells in the ventral part of the DMN. We observed a group of small round "immature" 5-HT-IR cells in the same area described previously only if the animal was pretreated with tryptophan and pargyline (25,26) (Fig. 2).

Further evidence for the serotonergic nature of the 5-HT-IR cells in the ventromedial DMN of the hypothalamus was their apparent destruction by 5,7-DHT but not by hydroxydopamine dense concentration of fine fibers (6-OHDA). However, preliminary studies done in collaboration with Alain Beaudet (Montreal) showed that the 5-HT cells are still alive and capable of concentrating [³H]5-HT after 5,7-dihydroxytryptamine (5,7-DHT) injection. Thus the cells exposed to 5,7-DHT can lose their capacity to synthesize and/or store 5-HT, but still maintain an active "high-affinity" uptake mechanism. Cells with only a 5-HT high-affinity uptake mechanism have been shown in the anterior pituitary (35) and in the retina (21). It may be pertinent that in certain neurons it has been shown that the high-affinity uptake mechanism develops before the neuron is able to synthesize and store its own transmitter.

Should the 5-HT-IR cells in the DMN be designated

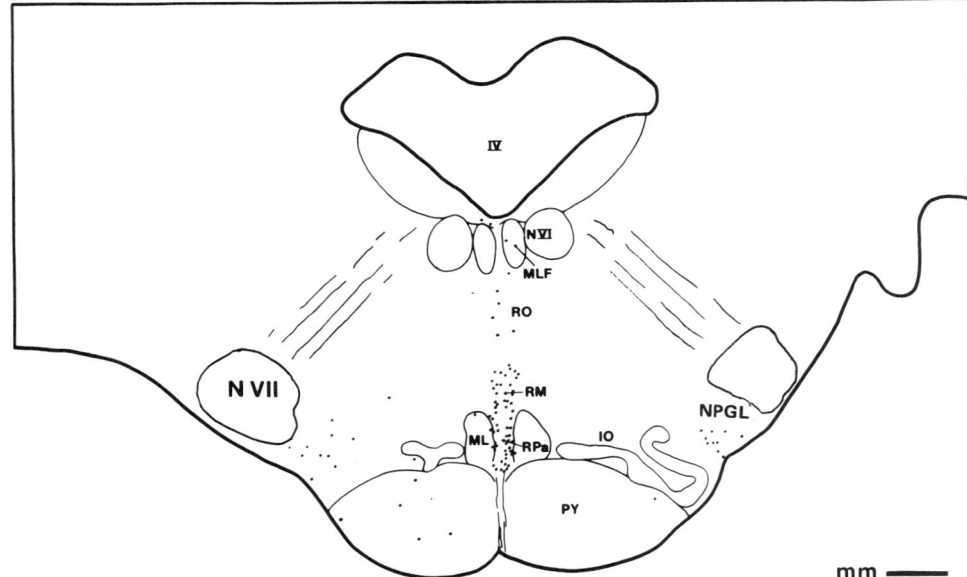

FIG. 2. Brainstem section caudal to that shown in Fig. 1 illustrating the position of the nuclei of the raphe obscurus (RO), raphe magnus (RM), raphe pallidus (RPa), and lateral paragigantocellularis (NPGL). A few cells seen under the fourth ventricle are part of nucleus ventricularis. IO, Inferior olive; PY, pyramidal tract. (From ref. 7.)

B10? There are several criteria for establishing the presence of a putative transmitter in a given cell group. These are, briefly, that the neurons possess the ability to synthesize, store, release, inactivate, and mimic the postsynaptic effect of the putative transmitter. At present three of these criteria have been met. The cells can synthesize 5-HT, they can store 5-HT, and they possess both the major mechanism of inactivation, reuptake, and the major degradative enzyme for 5-HT, monoamine oxidase (MAO). Thus, two additional criteria remain to be established: the release of 5-HT from these cells and a comparison of the postsynaptic effects after stimulation of the cells with the effects of 5-HT itself. These cells have not been observed in either the monkey or the cat hypothalamus.

Caudal Brainstem Group

Nucleus raphe obscurus (B2). The largest collection of 5-HT-IR neurons lies in a symmetrical paramedian cluster that extends caudally from the border of the pons to the cervical spinal cord. In the spinal cord, the cells are scattered in the central gray area just ventral to the central canal of the spinal cord and on the medial border of the ventral horn. The majority of these neurons are associated with the fibers of the MLF and the tectospinal tract as these tracts move from their superior position in the medulla to an inferior position in the spinal cord. The cells in the spinal cord lying below the central canal have been previously described by LaMotte et al. (37). In the cat at the level of the decussation of the pyramidal tract, 5-HT cells are seen off the midline along the border between the MLF and the pyramidal decussations just ventral to the central canal. These cells in the cat and monkey become continuous rostrally with NRO. In the rat, Dahlstrom and

Fuxe considered the few cells in the caudal medulla to be a part of nucleus raphe pallidus (B1).

NRO extends rostrally up to the level of the exit of nerve VI (see Fig. 3). In the cat, this nucleus reaches its greatest extent at the caudal end of the fourth ventricle (40–50 cells per section) where it appears as two tightly packed and closely spaced paramedian columns. In the rat, this nucleus (as well as nucleus raphe pallidus) is completely fused in a midline group by postnatal day 6 (39). At these anterior levels a smaller number of 5-HT-IR cells have split dorsally from the main cluster and are designated nucleus raphe ventricularis (NRV).

Raphe pallidus (B1). A midline cluster extends from nerve XII to the rostral pole of the inferior olive. The cells lie mainly between the pyramidal tracts both dorsally and ventrally. The dorsal border is continuous with the raphe magnus rostrally. The dorsal group forms two paramedian clusters and some cells are actually located directly on the midline. Cells extend caudally along the medial border of the ML. The majority of the 5-HT cells are found in the ventral aspect of the nucleus and stretch laterally into the LRN along fibers in the mediolateral plane. In the cat, nucleus raphe pallidus contains approximately 50 cells per section at its densest. In this species the cells form paramedian columns whereas in the rat the cells are fused.

Nucleus raphe magnus (B3). This group of large cells is more random and extends much more laterally into the nucleus reticularis gigantocellularis. The group extends rostrocaudally from the emergence of the nerve XII roots to the rostral inferior olive. Its location overlaps the trapezoid body and the dorsal border of the ML. It is continuous at certain points with both B1 and B2. In the cat, at the level of the rostral half of the facial nucleus, nucleus raphe magnus is located on the midline between the ML. The cells of this nucleus remain on the midline and scattered

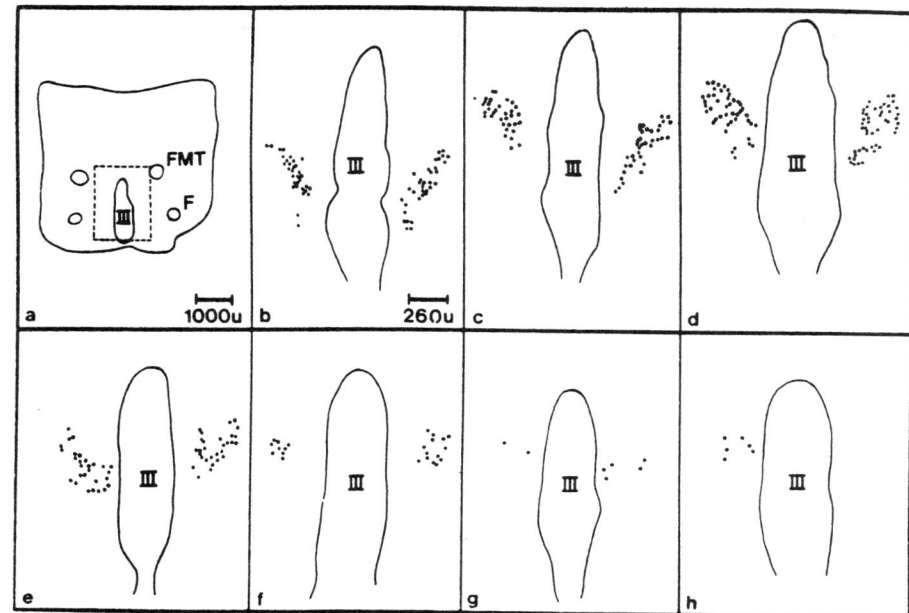

FIG. 3. Diagram of a hypothalamic section midway between the suprachiasmatic nuclei and the interthalamic adhesion. Rectangular area is enlarged in **b-h:** 50-μm coronal sections through the medial hypothalamus (100 μm apart) showing the rostrocaudal extent of the 5-HT-IR cells. III, Third ventricle; FMT, fasciculus mammillothalamicus; F, fornix. (From ref. 26.)

cells can be seen above the ML and superior olivary complex and within the trapezoid body. At its greatest density it contains approximately 25 to 40 5-HT cells per section.

Nucleus reticularis-paragigantocellularis lateralis. Neurons from this group extend laterally along the trapezoid, ML, and pyramidal fibers. These 5-HT-IR cells are located in the reticular formation of the ventrolateral medulla. Rostrally they appear to be in the NPGL and caudally in the ventral part of the LRN. This substantial group of cells extends from the emergence of the roots of nerve XII to the rostral part of the inferior olivary nucleus. This lateral group was described by Schofield and Dixon (49) in the common marmoset and called the nucleus reticularis paragigantocellularis lateralis (1,15). In the developing rat brain, this group was attributed to a lateral wing of B1 by Lidov and Molliver (40). The original classification proposed by Dahlstrom and Fuxe (19) in the adult rat assigned the cells to both B1 and B3. In the cat, these cells were described as reaching the floor of the medulla (56). In our preparations, the cells in the monkey and cat also reached the ventral pia and in certain cases were associated with the large blood vessels entering the medulla. The 5-HT cells are surrounded by a dense plexus of 5-HT fibers in this area (the LRN). At its greatest extent in the cat, as many as 25 cells per section are found in this nucleus. At the rostral end of the inferior olive, the 5-HT cells move medially and become continuous with the nucleus raphe magnus and the nucleus raphe pallidus.

Nucleus raphe ventricularis (B4). A group of 5-HT-IR cells was seen in the monkey just ventral to the fourth ventricle at the level of the genu of nerve VII and extended caudally to join the NRO. The cells were small and located on the midline. This group was not previously described in the primate brain and may have been visible in our preparation because the animals were pretreated with pargyline and tryptophan. In the rat, B4 has been described

as being continuous with B7 (the superior medial component) (40). In the monkey preparation, the ventricular raphe group appears distinct from B7, but is continuous with B3. In the cat, this group has a similar position but rostrally appears to be continuous with B6/7 as described in the rat.

Summary of Cellular Organization

5-HT-IR neurons are closely associated with major motor and sensory pathways. The cells of NCS, NRD, and NRO are located near or within the MLF, which interconnects the oculomotor nuclei, the spinal motor neurons, and the vestibular nuclei. The cells of ProSL and nucleus raphe magnus (NRM) lie adjacent to the ML tract which conveys proprioceptive information from the spinal cord. The cells of NRM are associated with the trapezoid body which transmits auditory signals to the midbrain. The cells of nucleus raphe pallidus (NRPa) are around, and within, the pyramidal tract. Finally, the lateral 5-HT-IR cells in the LRN and NPGL are associated with the tractus spinal olivaris and tractus spinal thalamicus, which transmits sensory input from the spinal cord to the brainstem.

5-HT cells are also associated with brainstem nuclei involved in integrating higher and lower centers. The NCS surrounds the interpeduncular nucleus, which receives descending information from the habenula. Cells from this serotonergic nucleus also extend laterally into the reticular formation of the brainstem. Cells from NRM and NRPa extend into the inferior olive and into the medullary reticular formation. The cells in the ventrolateral medulla are associated with the lateral reticular and lateral paragigantocellular nuclei. Finally, the cells of NRD and NRO lie within the central gray from the midbrain to the cervical spinal cord.

Associations are also seen with nonneuronal cell types. Neurons in the NRD and NCS are in apposition to oligodendrocytes (3,20). 5-HT-IR cells from the NRD and the ventricular nucleus are associated with the ependymal cells of the cerebral aqueduct and the fourth ventricle. We have also seen the rare ependymal cells that were immunoreactive to our 5-HT antibody (*unpublished observation*). Bundles of 5-HT dendrites and ventricular tanocytes have been reported (24). Finally, 5-HT cells are commonly associated with large blood vessels. This is most evident in the NCS medialis and the NPGL. The final point to be mentioned is the very small 5-HT cells in the area postrema visible in pretreated monkey and rats. Serotonin probably serves a unique function in this nucleus.

The strategic location of the 5-HT cells among important brainstem nuclei and fiber pathways provides a means for direct 5-HT modulation of both sensory and motor functions. The numerous and varied contacts with nonneuronal cells suggest that generalized mental states (e.g., anxiety, depression, euphoria), possibly hormonal in nature, should be strongly influenced by serotonergic neurons.

Pathways

Descending Projection to Spinal Cord and Brainstem

Pathways and terminals. There is good evidence that serotonin modulates both motor and sensory processing at the level of the brainstem and spinal cord. In the brainstem, the distribution of 5-HT-IR fibers in the trigeminal nuclear complex of the rat was studied (18). Dense innervation was noted in the sensory nuclei primarily associated with nociceptive afferent activity, and sparse in the sensory nuclei related to nonnociceptive afferent activity. Specifically, the marginal and gelatinosa layers of the spinal subnucleus caudalis had a dense number of fine fibers. The motor nucleus contained as many immunoreactive fibers as the subnucleus caudalis but the fibers here were thicker and

varicosities more irregularly spaced than in caudalis. In the monkey, NRO could be seen to contribute fibers to the hypoglossal nucleus and the dorsal motor nucleus of the vagus (24).

In the spinal cord, a dense plexus of 5-HT-IR fibers is present in the substantia gelatinosa and around the motor neurons in the ventral horn. Serotonergic endings have been shown to make direct contact with the neurons in the dorsal horn that give rise to the spinothalamic tract. This projection is believed to be important in the transmission of nociceptive information in humans and monkeys (28) and is believed to originate in the raphe magnus. Serotonergic endings have also been seen directly on motor neurons and these excitatory contacts probably originate in the raphe obscurus. Large injections of horseradish peroxidase (HRP) into the lumbar spinal cord in *Macaca fascicularis* label cells in NRO, NRM, and the nucleus gigantocellularis (11). A few cells have also been seen in the medial and lateral division of the NRD in squirrel monkeys and a baboon (41).

Nobin and Bjorklund (43) described a single ventral descending tract in the human fetal brain. Felten and Sladek (24) report a dorsal descending pathway from B2 and a ventral descending one from B1 and B3. However, we have observed no dorsal route but a medioventral and a lateral descending pathway. It appears from our material that the fibers of B2 (NRO) project to the motor neurons of the ventral horn using the descending MLF as a guide. Thus, the fibers in the ventral descending tract moved into this inferior position at the level of the decussation of the pyramidal tract along with the fibers comprising the MLF. This innervation of the motor neurons of the ventral horn is consistent with the other projections from NRO to the motor neurons of the brainstem nuclei of nerves X and XII (24). We have termed this ventral descending tract the Raphe Obscurus Spinal Tract (ROST) (Fig. 4). The cells of

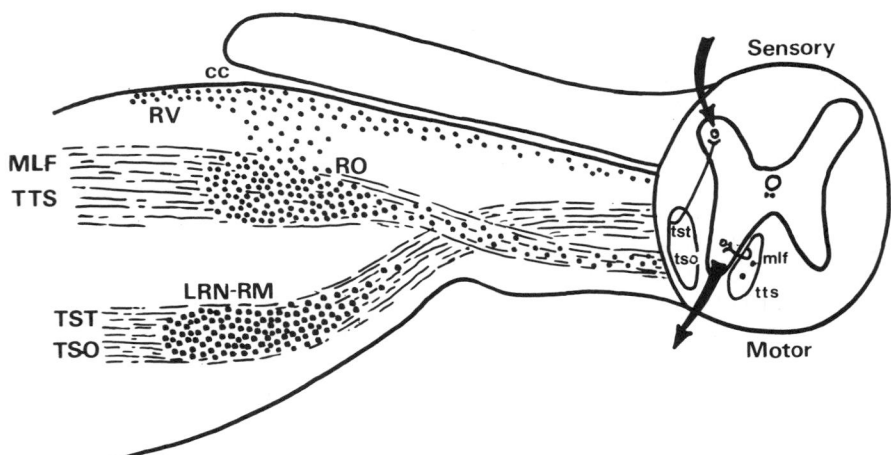

FIG. 4. Sagittal section modified from Ramon y Cajal's (13) Fig. 409 showing the descending projections of the medial longitudinal fasciculus (MLF). The serotonergic cells in nucleus raphe magnus (RM) and lateral reticular nucleus (LRN) and in obscurus (RO) are shown giving rise to two descending projections. It should be noted that the LRN and RM project along the tracti spinal thalamicus (TST) and spinal olivaris (TSO) whereas the NRO projects ventrally along the MLF. The raphe magnus spinal tract (RMST) projects via a lateral descending route to innervate the substantia gelatinosa whereas the raphe obscurus spinal tract (ROST) projects via a ventromedial descending route to innervate the motor neurons of the anterior horn. TTS, tractus tectospinalis; cc, central canal; RV, raphe ventricularis. (From ref. 7.)

the B3 complex (NRM, NPGL, and LRN) descend in the same position but in the opposite direction as the ascending sensory fibers in tractus spinal olivaris and tractus spinal thalamicus. In the cervical levels of the spinal cord, the 5-HT-IR fibers appear to extend dorsally to innervate the substantia gelatinosa. We have termed this lateral descending tract the Raphe Magnus Spinal Tract. There is evidence that some of these fibers may be myelinated. Ruda and Gobel (48) showed a few examples of myelinated fibers in the rat labeled after incubation with [³H]5-HT and pro-

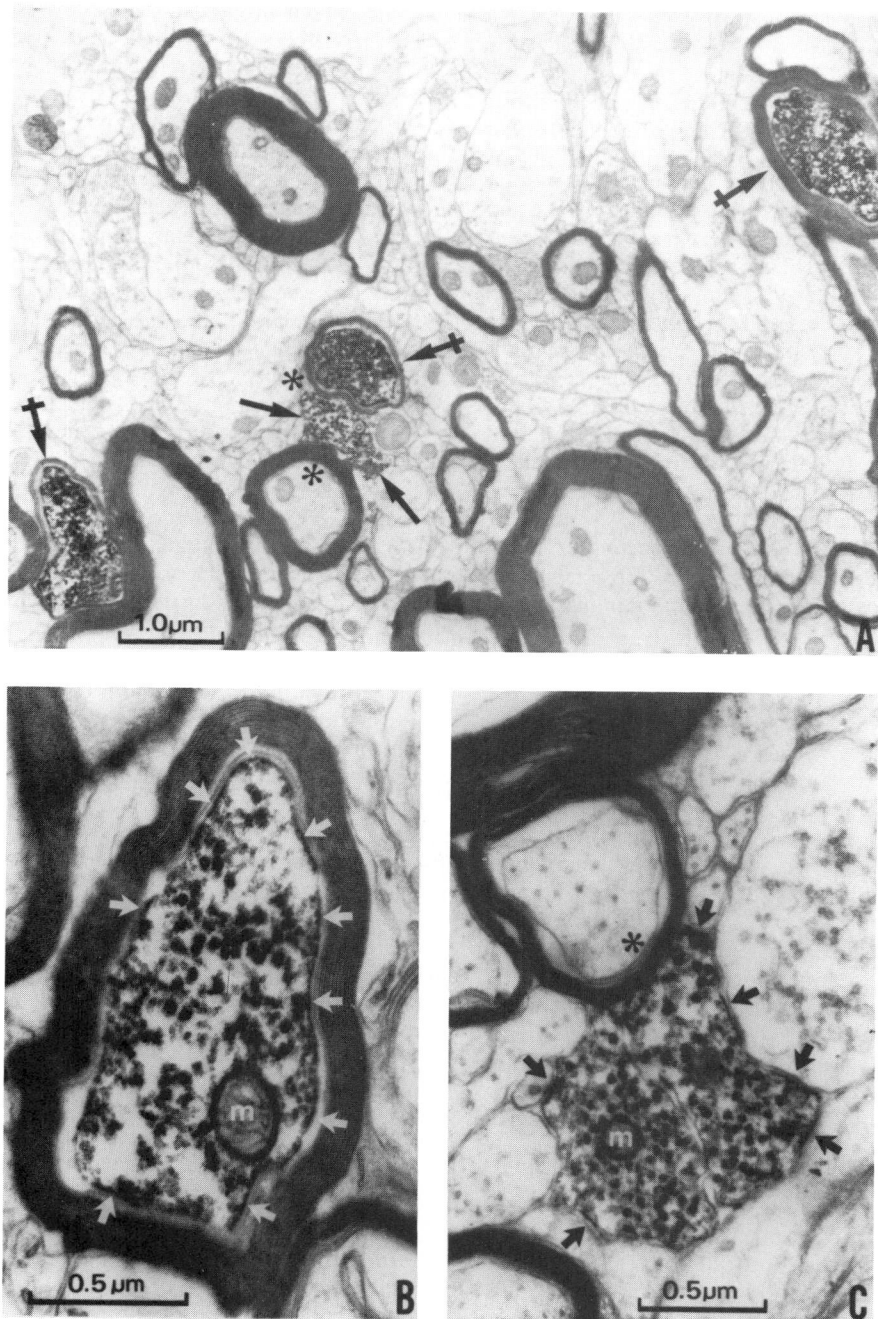

FIG. 5. Electron photomicrographs of the rat MFB showing 5-HT-immunoreactive axons in cross-section. **A:** A low power view showing six unmyelinated axons (*arrows*) and a single myelinated axon (*arrow with bar*) immunoreactive to a specific 5-HT antibody. All immunoreactive axons shown are in close apposition to unreactive myelinated axons (*asterisk*). **B:** High power electron micrograph of myelinated axon stained with the 5-HT antibody. The staining is mainly restricted to vesicles and patches along the cytoplasmic leaf of the axonal membrane (*arrow*). **C:** unmyelinated axon shown in close apposition to unreactive myelinated axon (*asterisk*). The cytoplasmic distribution of the reaction product is as described above in B. In addition, the outer mitochondrial membrane is stained. Note the densities between the immunoreactive axon and the unreactive myelinated and unmyelinated fibers (*arrows*). (Modified from ref. 6.)

cessing the tissue for electron microscopic radioautography. Chan Palay (15,16) also reported a few cases of myelinated fibers labeled by [³H]5-HT in the lower brainstem of the monkey. The frequency and distribution of these fibers remain to be determined.

Ascending Projections to Forebrain

Pathways and terminals. Ascending 5-HT-containing fibers, first visualized with histochemical fluorescence methods, were classically described as being unmyelinated (19). We observed myelinated and unmyelinated serotonin-containing axons in the medial forebrain bundle of rats and monkeys with an antibody against serotonin (5-HT) conjugated to hemocyanin (6). 5-HT-IR was seen predominantly in unmyelinated axons (0.2–1.25 μm in diameter) surrounded by unlabeled processes. More than half of these 5-HT-IR fibers were in apposition with unreactive myelinated axons in the hypothalamus of both the rat (55%) and the monkey (54%). In addition to the unmyelinated fibers, intensely labeled myelinated axons (1.0–2.1 μm) were seen in the medial forebrain bundle of both rats and monkeys (Fig. 5). The percentage of 5-HT-IR myelinated axons was greater in the monkey than in the rat (25.4% versus 0.7% of the total number of 5-HT-IR fibers, respectively).

The serotonergic fibers projecting to the forebrain originate mainly in the rostral nuclei. Two main ascending

bundles have been described in the primate brain (43,49,50). In the human fetus, 5-HT fibers were seen (a) in the central gray near the ependyma of the fourth ventricle and the aqueduct and (b) in a position between the medial raphe cells and the lateral cell system (43).

In juvenile macaques, two main ascending bundles were described. A dorsal bundle was seen just ventral to the MLF, which originated at the level of locus ceruleus and received fibers from NRD and nucleus annularis (NCS dorsalis). These fibers appear to turn ventrally at the level of the red nucleus. A second bundle of ventrally flowing serotonergic fibers lateral to NCS originated at the level of the trochlear nucleus and received fibers from the midline NRD and NCS. These fibers appear to turn rostrally just dorsal to nucleus interpeduncularis (50).

In our monkey preparations, dense staining was present in the two areas described by Schofield and Everitt (50). In addition, we also saw fibers near the cerebral aqueduct in the hypothalamus and projecting lateroventrally from the NRD. Thus, all of the 5-HT fiber bundles observed in the rat (8) can be observed in the primate brainstem. In addition, in the monkey the main ascending bundle through the hypothalamus may not be the medial forebrain bundle (MFB) as it is in the rat. Examination of the caudal hypothalamic area (Fig. 6) shows two main ascending bundles previously described in the rat (the MFB and the dorsal raphe cortical tract, DRCT). However, in the primate, the latter tract, which ascends to the cerebral cortex via the internal capsule, is larger than the MFB. The DRCT thus

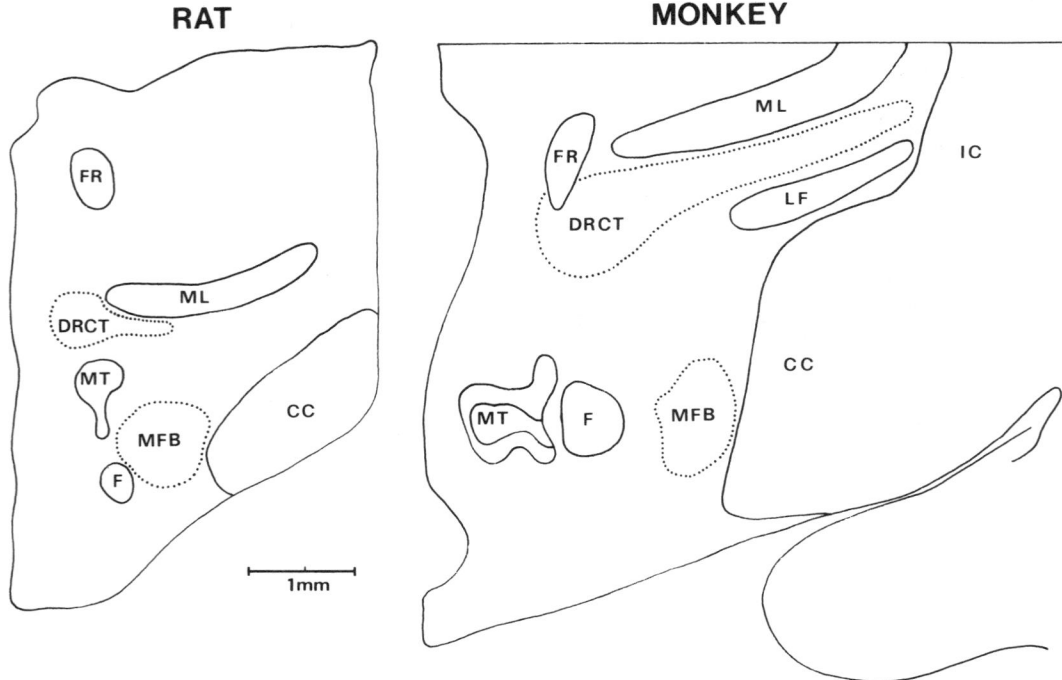

FIG. 6. Schematic drawing of coronal sections at the level of the posterior hypothalamus in the rat and monkey brain. The two main ascending pathways are the medial forebrain bundle (MFB) and the dorsal raphe cortical tract (DRCT) and these are outlined with dashed lines. The relative size and position of the MFB are similar in these two species. However, the

DRCT is much larger in the monkey than in the rat brain, although it does occupy a similar relative position in both species. CC, Crus cerebri; F, fornix; FR, fasciculus retroflexus; IC, internal capsule; ML, medial lemniscus; MT, mammillo-thalamic tract. (Modified from ref. 6.)

appears to have undergone a significant increase in absolute size when compared to the homologous pathway in the rat. This probably represents an increase in the projection from the NRD and the NCS dorsalis to the primate cerebral cortex.

Subcortical distribution of 5-HT fibers. Several studies have used immunocytochemical methods to study 5-HT fibers. In the rat, an exhaustive study of the development of the ascending projection was done by Lidov and Mollier (40). We studied the distribution in the thalamus and found a marked regional distribution (17). Innervation was greatest in those thalamic nuclei associated with limbic functions (e.g., nucleus reuniens and nucleus anterior dorsalis) and with sensory transmission, either nociceptive (e.g., posterior complex) or visual (e.g., nucleus dorsalis corporis geniculati lateralis). In the monkey, 5-HT-IR axons were seen in both regions of the substantia nigra, although mainly in the pars reticularis (32). In the neostriatum of the same species, 5-HT-IR fibers were particularly abundant in the ventromedial region of the caudate head bordering the nucleus accumbens where the plexus was heavier (46). The number of fibers in the caudate was reduced in more dorsal and lateral areas. The fibers were uniformly distributed in the putamen. Fibers were fine and had irregularly spaced fusiform varicosities.

A comparative study in monkey, cat, and rat of the olfactory bulb was performed with a 5-HT antibody. Serotonergic fibers were seen in all layers except for the olfactory nerve layer in *Macaca fuscata* (53). The fibers were observed to form a chain of large varicosities in the periglomerular region. The 5-HT distribution was predominantly in the internal plexiform layer. In some portions, a dense plexus of 5-HT fibers extended to the external plexiform layer. The number of 5-HT-IR fibers was also numerous in the inner portions of the granular cell layer. Finally, and in contrast to both rat and cat, the distribution of 5-HT-IR fibers was scanty and partial in the glomerular layer. In this area, only a few of the glomeruli (no more than 5%) possessed 5-HT-IR axons.

The distribution of [³H]5-HT accumulation in monkey shows high levels are seen in amygdala, the rectus gyrus of the frontal lobe, and the inferior and superior gyri of the temporal lobe (Fig. 7). The lowest levels are seen in the occipital lobe and the precentral (motor) cortex of the frontal lobe. The differences within the major cortical lobes are pronounced. The rectus gyrus of the frontal lobe has four times as much uptake of [³H]5-HT as the precentral motor cortex of the same lobe. In the occipital lobe, the calcarine region has double the uptake of the surrounding cortex. Finally, the variation within the hippocampal complex is striking. The entorhinal cortex and the dentate gyrus are high in uptake whereas the subiculum and the cornu ammonis (CA) are low.

These results demonstrate the heterogeneous distribution of serotonergic fibers in the primate brain. Highest levels are seen in limbic centers (temporal lobe, amygdaloid nuclei, and cingulate gyrus) and with sensory centers (visual—calcarine, auditory—superior temporal gyrus, somatosensory—postcentral cortex, and olfaction—amygdaloid nuclei and entorhinal cortex). The lowest levels are found in the frontal lobe (with the exception of the rectus

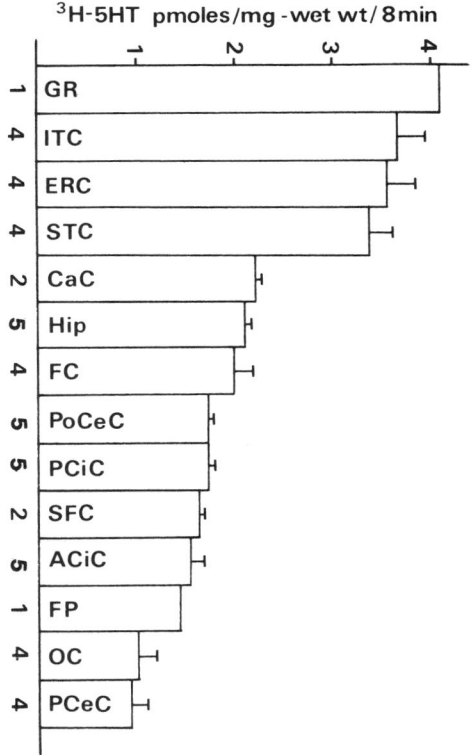

FIG. 7. Synaptosomal specific uptake of serotonin in different cortical brain regions of *M. fascicularis*. The numbers of animals sampled are beneath each column and the brain regions are labeled within each column. The ordinate shows the amount of specific uptake of serotonin after incubating synaptosomal fractions in 5×10^{-8} M [³H]5-HT for 8 min at 37°C. The bars at the top of each column are the standard deviations of the mean. ACiC, Anterior cingulate cortex; CaC, calcarine cortex; ERC, entorhinal cortex; FC, frontal cortex; GR, rectus gyrus; Hip, hippocampus; ITC, inferior temporal cortex; OC, occipital cortex; PCeC, precentral cortex; PCiC, posterior cingulate cortex; PoCeC, postcentral cortex; SFC, superior frontal cortex; STC, superior temporal cortex; FP, frontal pole. (From ref. 7.)

gyrus). The distribution is quite varied even within the subregions of the hippocampal complex. As a general rule it may be proposed that serotonin levels are highest in those regions of cortex having more granule cells, since these cells are associated with sensory receiving areas.

Laminar distribution in the cortex. Little is known of the serotonin distribution in the cerebral cortex of the rat (see ref. 22 for review). Chan-Palay (14) reported highest density of 5-HT fibers after intraventricular administration of [³H]5-HT in the cingulate cortex whereas other parts contain only low densities. Beaudet and Descarries (9) using radioautography with [³H]5-HT reported that the intralaminar density increased progressively from layer V to layer I.

Our results showed a clear laminar pattern in several layers of cerebral cortex. In all regions examined, a clear lamination was observed with the highest densities in layer I and in layer IV (7). The density in layer IV again indicates a preferential innervation of granule cells by 5-HT fibers.

Studies in the hippocampal formation showed that the granule cells of the dentate gyrus were very heavily innervated whereas the innervation of the CA was much weaker. It is interesting that the pattern seen in the monkey dentate gyrus is similar to that observed in the rat, whereas the density in monkey CA is much less (4). This difference between rat and monkey may represent an increased specialization in the primate brain.

Morrison et al. (42) found in the squirrel monkey primary visual cortex a very dense serotonergic projection to layer IV. These workers conclude: "The 5-HT projection is in a position to modulate neuronal activity at the initial stage of signal processing in cortex. Layer IV cells are closely linked to the thalamic input" (p. 2405). Our finding in *M. fascicularis* that 5-HT fibers heavily innervate layer IV in a number of cortical areas, that the innervation of the

dentate gyrus remains constant from rat to monkey, and that 5-HT reuptake is highest in those regions of cortex having a significant layer IV (e.g., sensory cortex), all indicate a special relationship between serotonergic fibers and granule cells.

CONCLUSION

The serotonergic system in the primate brain has remained relatively stable throughout evolution (Fig. 8). The main cellular nuclei in the brainstem first described in the rat and cat are still present in the monkey brain. The ascending nuclei (NCS, NRD, and ProSL) use multiple ascending tracts to innervate most of the subcortical and cortical areas of the forebrain with a distribution pattern

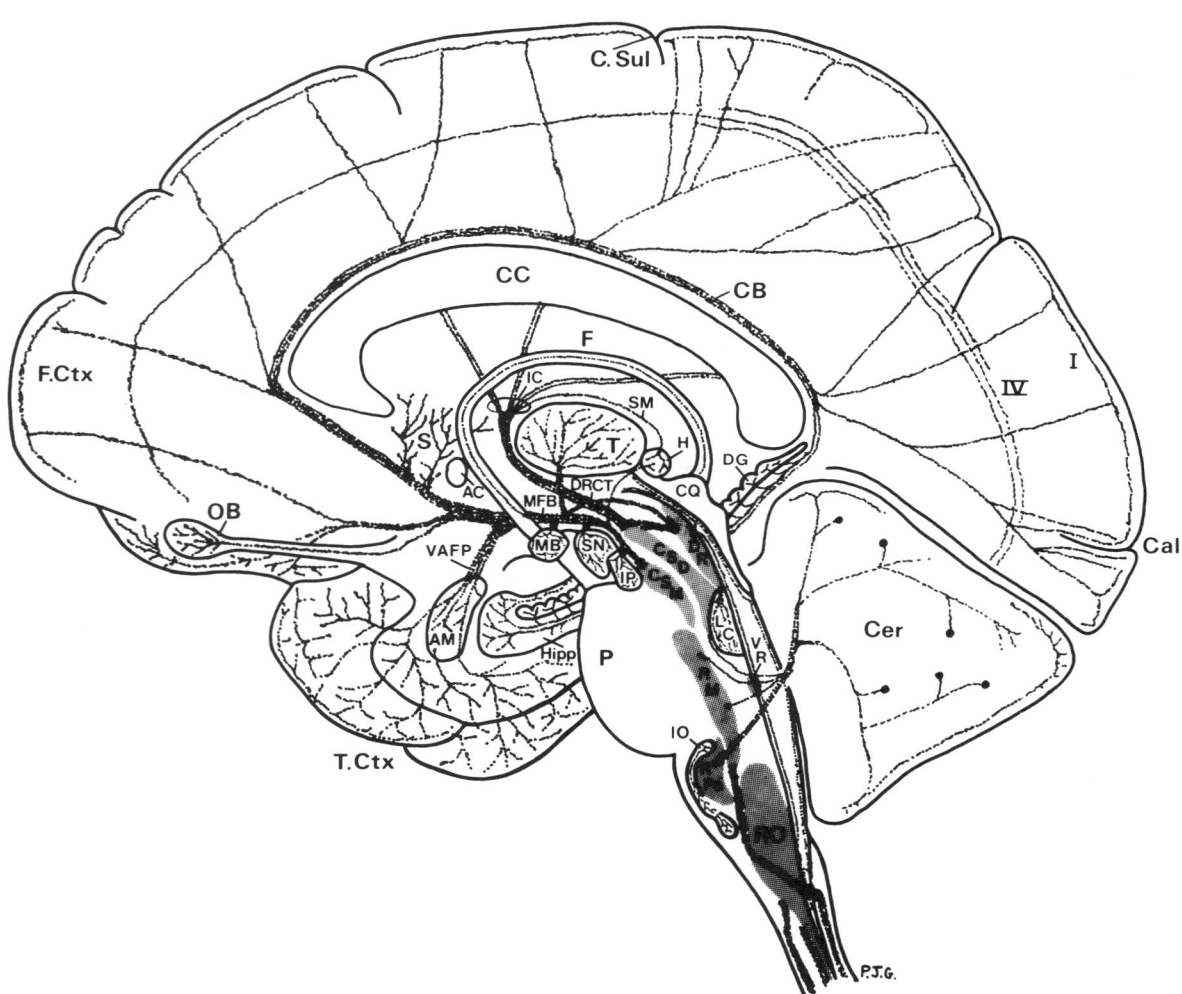

FIG. 8. Summary diagram of the primate serotonergic system. The main nuclei are *shaded*. The fiber pathways are shown as *broken lines*. Abbreviations are as follows: AC, anterior commissure; Am, amygdaloid nuclei; CC, corpus callosum; Cer, cerebellum; CQ, corpus quadrigimini; CSd, centralis superior nucleus, pars dorsalis; CSM, centralis superior nucleus, pars medialis; Csul, central sulcus; DG, dentate gyrus; DR, dorsal raphe nucleus; DRCT, dorsal raphe cortical tract; F, fornix; FCII, frontal cortex; Hipp, hippocampus; IC, interna capsule; IO, inferior olivary nuclei; IP, interpeduncular; LC, locus ceruleus; MB, mammillary body; MFB, medial forebrain bundle; OB, olfactory bulb; P, pons; RM, raphe magnus; RO, raphe obscurus; RPa, raphe pallidus; S, septum; SM, stria medullaris; SN, substantia nigra; STC, superior temporal cortex; T, thalamus; TCtx, temporal cortex; VAFP, ventro amygdaloid fugal pathway; VR, raphe ventriculus. (From ref. 7.)

consistent in part with that reported in the rat. Many of the minor and unusual groups seen in the rat and cat were present in our monkey material (7). The B4 group has not been described in any primate brain previously, yet a number of neurons were seen as part of the nucleus raphe ventricularis. Furthermore, the small serotonin cells noted in the area postrema by Dahlstrom and Fuxe (19) were seen in the pretreated primate brain. Finally, the termination patterns seen are fairly similar to those in subprimates. The serotonergic fibers enter the various target structures through similar pathways and appear to innervate the appropriate neurons. For instance, the labeling patterns seen in the dentate gyrus of monkey are almost indistinguishable from those seen in the rodent (4).

However, the concept of an evolutionarily stable system does not appear justified when all the comparative evidence is closely scrutinized. The nuclear organization in the primate brain does differ from that of the rodent in several important aspects. First, in the rat brain the majority of the serotonergic nuclear groups are indeed raphe nuclei, that is, the cells are tightly clustered on the midline seam and extend laterally from this line (39). In the primate, few cells lie on the midline and most have at best a paramedian organization. Second, the nucleus centralis superior is larger and more varied in the monkey. The inclusion of the dorsalis portion of this nucleus as proposed by Olszewski and Baxter (45) makes this the major ascending group rather than the NRD as proposed for the rat. Third, the serotonergic cells from NRO extend far more caudally in the primate brain and reach the cervical levels of the spinal cord. The location of these cells in laminae X and IX indicates a more important relationship between serotonergic cells and motor neurons in the primate brain. Finally, the hypothalamic serotonin-concentrating cells described by several groups in the rat (10,19,25) were not seen in the primate hypothalamus.

Differences are noted in the projection pathways. The descending fibers to the ventral horn motor neurons in the rat originate from NRM and NRPa, but appear to originate only from NRM in the primate (11). The ascending fibers to the forebrain in the rat use mainly the MFB (3), but in the monkey the DRCT may be quantitatively larger (6). Finally, the fibers in the primate brain have been noted by several workers to be myelinated (6,14–16,37). Although myelinated serotonin fibers have been noted in rodents (48), we have found the occurrence in rat (0.7%) to be much lower than in the monkey (25%) (6).

The termination patterns in certain areas of the cortex and subcortical regions are also different between primates and subprimates. We have reported that the innervation density of the CA region of the primate is markedly less than in the rat and mouse, although the innervation of the dentate gyrus is similar (4). The pattern of 5-HT-IR fibers in the olfactory bulb of the monkey is also different from that of the rat or cat because of an almost total absence of serotonergic fibers innervating the glomeruli in the monkey, in sharp contrast to subprimates (53). Biochemical studies have revealed marked variations in the cortical distribution of the serotonin system whereas studies in the rodent indicated a more uniform distribution (22). These studies indicate that the termination of 5-HT fibers is becoming more restricted in the primate brain compared to rat and cat.

It would appear, therefore, that although the primate and subprimate serotonergic systems have many similarities, there are important differences in cellular organization, projecting pathways, and innervation patterns. The studies on the rodent serotonergic system led to the conclusion that the axons, being fine and unmyelinated, possess a slow rate of conduction and have a scarcity of postsynaptic membrane specialization and are thus not a part of the "hard wiring" involved in the rapid stimulus-response organization of the brain (3). This view must be modified because of the studies performed on the primate brain. A number of concepts regarding serotonergic functions should be retained. It remains a very expansive chemical network, a part of the reticular formation, and organized in tightly clustered groups with extensive homotypic interconnections and long projections to interacting target areas.

These traits can best be understood by studying how the collaborative organization arises during early development. The initial axonal elongation from 5-HT-IR cells begins very early in the rat (day 13–16 of gestation) (40). The serotonergic axons extend along the entire floor of the diencephalon (44). These fibers are thus in a key position of the forebrain during the development of diencephalic and telencephalic interconnections. The 5-HT-IR cells appear to possess the ability to be guided by developing nonserotonergic tracts in growing into selected target areas. This process, which we have termed epiphytic guidance (3), encourages appropriate 5-HT axons to utilize many "classical" pathways such as the MLF and the fornix. This epiphytic guidance not only selects a single terminal zone, but provides a mechanism for innervation of interconnected areas (e.g., septum and hippocampus, interpenduncular nucleus and habenula, oculomotor nuclei, and the motor neurons of the cranial nuclei and the ventral horn of the spinal cord). Thus, groups of cells whose axons travel in the same fascicles would innervate similar termination areas by having access to the same routes of entry (Fig. 9).

The fact that these systems are predominantly unmyelinated also allows the interaction occurring between the 5-HT soma to extend along the length of the axon. The observation that 5-HT cells have sensitive autoreceptors would allow the fibers to respond to the firing of nearby homotypic axons. The 5-HT neurons would thus maintain a high degree of collaboration from the soma to the terminal. The implication that a large number of 5-HT fibers in the primate brain are myelinated may have profound implications beyond the obvious fact that the conduction velocity is dramatically increased. However, it appears that this primitive system has evolved certain properties in the cat and primate brain to adapt to the enlargement of the cerebral cortex and the corresponding changes in the regulation of sensory, motor, endocrine, and cognitive processes. The trend appears directed toward increased independence in the grouping and projections of the 5-HT cells but at the expense of a loss of overall influence in directing the behavioral patterns of the animals.

In most of the 5-HT cells occurring in the vertebrate brains, the collaborative arrangement suggests that the more closely-knit and the larger the number of cells in the

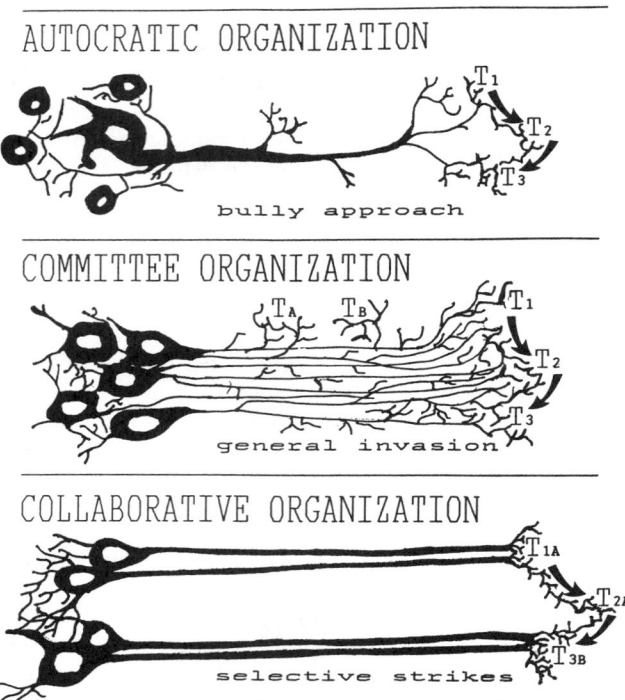

AUTOCRATIC ORGANIZATION

bully approach

COMMITTEE ORGANIZATION

general invasion

COLLABORATIVE ORGANIZATION

selective strikes

FIG. 9. The three types of serotonergic neuronal organization seen in the brain. The *Autocratic Organization* is seen in invertebrate cerebral ganglion, where there are a few "giant" serotonergic neurons. These cells develop very early and have strong effects on the motor behavior of the organism. The action of these cells can be described as a "bully approach" because they are so much larger than the neighboring cells. The second approach, the *Committee Organization,* has been described in the rat (3). The cells form a large cluster comprising almost the entire nucleus which probably involves the coordinated action of hundreds of neurons. This tight cluster innervates similar areas as large fasciculus of unmyelinated axons (general invasion). The action of the cluster may modulate many of the stereotyped behaviors. The final type of organization is most evident in the monkey. Here the clusters are smaller but much more numerous within a given nucleus. A large proportion of the axons are myelinated so there is rapid transmission to selected targets. The innervation pattern in these higher vertebrates has now become more restricted to a particular type of target. The *Collaborative Organization* permits more precise control over a larger number of interacting circuits (selective strikes). In all examples, there is a significant interaction between the serotonergic cell bodies and their terminals in the primary target areas. T_1, T_2, and T_3 are interacting target areas. T_{1A}, T_{2A}, and T_{3B} are subdivisions within these areas. T_A and T_B are brain structures near fibers of passage but whose function is not related to the interacting primary targets.

functional clusters, the more powerful their combined effect would be in controlling the behavior of the animal (Fig. 8). In lower invertebrates, a single giant serotonergic neuron will have extensive connections to motor and sensory ganglia. The single giant cell in the snail is surrounded by many smaller 5-HT cells (J. Goldberg and S. Kater, *in preparation*). In rodents, large tight clusters of medium-sized 5-HT cells have dense projections to appropriate interconnecting target areas (3). Thus, the group of 5-HT neurons, extensively interconnected, projects and functions as a large collection of cells. The situation in cats has changed. The 5-HT cells are more scattered and tightly clustered into smaller units than seen in the rat. The greater number of 5-HT clusterings would enable more independent biasing of interacting target connections. In the monkey, the cells have the same general distributions as seen in the cat, but now a significant proportion of the cells are myelinated. The insulation of the fibers prevents influences from reaching the cells along their route to the target area. Furthermore, the termination patterns have become more restricted to certain cell populations. The 5-HT system now is sensitive to collaborative influences only in their soma and their restricted terminal fields. The 5-HT neurons have evolved a more rapid, independent, and precise form of communication, but have retained the clustering organization that has characterized this group of neurons since they were first utilized in the brains of invertebrates.

ACKNOWLEDGMENT

The research for this chapter was supported by the National Science Foundation with a grant from the Behavioral Neuroscience Program 83-04704.

REFERENCES

1. Andrezik, J. A., Chan-Palay, V., and Palay, S. L. (1981): *Anat. Embryol.,* 151:355–371.
2. Aston-Jones, G., Ennis, M., Pieribone, U., Nickell, W. T., and Shipley, M. T. (1986): *Science,* 234:734–737.
3. Azmitia, E. C. (1978): In: *Handbook of Psychopharmacology, Vol. 9,* edited by L. L. Iversen, S. D. Iversen, and S. H. Snyder, pp. 233–314. Plenum Press, New York.
4. Azmitia, E. C. (1981): *J. Physiol. (Paris),* 77:175–182.
5. Azmitia, E. C. (1981): *J. Comp. Neurol.,* 203:737–743.
6. Azmitia, E. C., and Gannon, P. J. (1983): *J. Neurosci.,* 3:2083–2090.
7. Azmitia, E. C., and Gannon, P. J. (1986): In: *Advances in Neurology, Vol. 43: Myoclonus,* edited by S. Fahn et al. Raven Press, New York, pp. 407–468.
8. Azmitia, E. C., and Segal, M. (1978): *J. Comp. Neurol.,* 179:641–659.
9. Beaudet, A., and Descarries, L. (1976): *Brain Res.,* 111:301–309.
10. Beaudet, A., and Descarries, L. (1979): *Brain Res.,* 160:231–243.
11. Bowker, R. M., Westlund, K. N., and Coulter, J. D. (1982): *Brain Res. Bull.,* 9:271–278.
12. Brownstein, M. J., Palkovits, M., Tappaz, M. L., Saavedra, J. M., and Kizer, J. S. (1976): *Brain Res.,* 117:287–295.
13. Cajal, S. R. (1909): *Histologie du Systeme Nerveux de L'Homme and des Vertebres,* transl. L. Azoulay, *Vol. I,* p. 913. A. Maloine, Paris.
14. Chan-Palay, V. (1976): *Brain Res.,* 102:103–130.
15. Chan-Palay, V. (1978): In: *Amino Acids as Chemical Transmitter,* NATO Advanced Study Symposium, pp. 1–30. Plenum Press, New York.
16. Chan-Palay, V. (1978): *J. Neurocytol.,* 7:419–442.
17. Cropper, E. C., Eisenman, J. S., and Azmitia, E. C. (1984): *J. Comp. Neurol.,* 224:38–50.
18. Cropper, E. C., Eisenman, J. S., and Azmitia, E. C. (1984): *Exp. Brain Res.,* 55:515–522.
19. Dahlstrom, A., and Fuxe, K. (1964): *Acta Physiol. Scand. (Suppl. 62),* 232:1–55.

20. Descarries, L., Watkins, K. C., Garcia, S., and Beaudet, A. (1982): *J. Comp. Neurol.*, 207:239–254.
21. Ehinger, B., and Floren, I. (1980): *Neurochemistry,* 1:209–229.
22. Emson, P. C., and Lindvall, O. (1979): *Neuroscience,* 4:1–30.
23. Felten, D. L., Laties, A. M., and Carpenter, M. B. (1974): *Am. J. Anat.,* 139:153–166.
24. Felten, D. L., and Sladek, J. R. (1983): *Brain Res. Bull.,* 10:171–284.
25. Frankfurt, M., and Azmitia, E. C. (1983): *Brain Res.,* 261:91–99.
26. Frankfurt, M., Lauder, J. M., and Azmitia, E. C. (1981): *Neurosci. Lett.,* 24:277.
27. Fuxe, K., and Ungerstedt, U. (1968): *Histochemie,* 13:16–28.
28. Giesler, G. J., Gerhart, K. D., Yezierski, R. P., Wilcox, T. K., and Willis, W. D. (1981): *Brain Res.,* 204:184–188.
29. Golden, G. S. (1973): *Dev. Biol.* 33:300–311.
30. Harris, W. A. (1981): *Annu. Rev. Physiol.,* 43:689–710.
31. Haydon, P. G., McCobb, D. P., and Kater, S. B. (1984): *Science,* 226:561–564.
32. Holstein, G., Pasik, T., and Pasik, P. (1983): *Soc. Neurosci. Abst.,* 9:661.
33. Hubbard, J. E., and Di Carlo, V. (1974): *J. Comp. Neurol.,* 153:385–398.
34. Jacobs, B., Gannon, P. J., and Azmitia, E. C. (1984): *Brain Res. Bull.,* 13:1–31.
35. Johns, M. A., Azmitia, E. C., and Krieger, D. T. (1982): *Endocrinology,* 110:754–760.
36. Klemm, N. (1985): In: *Neurobiology,* edited by R. Gillies and J. Balthazart, pp. 280–296. Springer-Verlag, Berlin, Heidelberg.
37. LaMotte, C. C., Johns, D. R., and De Lanerolle, N. C. (1982): *J. Comp. Neurol.,* 206:359–370.
38. Lauder, J. M., and Bloom, F. E. (1974): *J. Comp. Neurol.* 155:469–481.
39. Levitt, P., and Moore, R. Y. (1978): *Anat. Embryol.,* 154:241–251.
40. Lidov, H. G. W., and Molliver, M. E. (1982): *Brain Res. Bull.,* 9:559–604.
41. Mantyh, P. W., and Peschanski, M. (1982): *Neuroscience,* 11:2769–2776.
42. Morrison, J. H., Foote, S. L., Molliver, M. E., Bloom, F. E., and Lidov, G. W. (1982): *Proc. Natl. Acad. Sci. USA,* 79:2401–2405.
43. Nobin, A., and Bjorklund, A. (1973): *Acta Physiol. Scand. (Suppl.* 388):1–40.
44. Olson, L., and Seiger, A. (1972): *Z. Anat. Entw. Gesch.,* 137:301–316.
45. Olszewski, J., and Baxter, D. (1954): *Cytoarchitecture of the Human Brain Stem.* J. B. Lippincott, Philadelphia.
46. Pasik, T., and Pasik, P. (1982): *Acta Biol. Acad. Sci. Hung.,* 33:277–288.
47. Porrino, L. J., and Goldman-Rakic, P. S. (1982): *J. Comp. Neurol.,* 205:63–76.
48. Ruda, M. A., and Gobel, S. (1980): *Brain Res.,* 184:57–83.
49. Schofield, S. P. M., and Dixon, A. F. (1982): *J. Anat.,* 134:315–338.
50. Schofield, S. P. M., and Everitt, B. J. (1981): *J. Comp. Neurol.,* 197:369–383.
51. Sladek, J. R., and Walker, P. (1977): *Brain Res.,* 134:359–366.
52. Taber, E., Brodal, A., and Walberg, F. (1960): *J. Comp. Neurol.,* 114:161–187.
53. Takeuchi, Y., Kimura, H., and Sano, Y. (1982): *Histochemistry,* 75:461–471.
54. Wallace, J. A., and Lauder, J. M. (1983): *Brain Res. Bull.,* 10:459–479.
55. Whitaker-Azmitia, P. M., and Azmitia, E. C. (1984): In: *Developmental Neuroscience: Physiological, Pharmacological and Clinical Aspects,* edited by F. Caciagli, E. Giacobini, and R. Paoletti, pp. 251–257. Elsevier Science Publishers B. V., Amsterdam, New York, Oxford.
56. Wiklund, L., Leger, L., and Persson, M. (1981): *J. Comp. Neurol.,* 203:613–647.
57. Zhou, F. C., and Azmitia, E. C. (1983): *Brain Res. Bull.,* 10:445–451.

Psychopharmacology:
The Third Generation of Progress,
edited by Herbert Y. Meltzer.
Raven Press, New York © 1987.

CHAPTER 8

Activation of Tyrosine Hydroxylase by Phosphorylation

Menek Goldstein and Lloyd A. Greene

The first step in the biosynthesis of dopamine (DA) is catalyzed by tyrosine hydroxylase (TH), which utilizes tetra-hydropteridine ($DMPH_4$) as a cofactor in the enzymatic hydroxylation reaction. The activity of TH in the peripheral and central nervous system is subject to short- and long-term regulation by extra- and intracellular signals. This provides mechanisms by which the amount of DA synthesized and available for secretion can be modulated in response to physiological requirements.

Conditions that yield increased secretion of catecholamine *in vivo* and *in vitro* from adrenergically innervated tissues are associated with accelerated catecholamine biosynthesis. It has been postulated that enhanced secretion of endogenous catecholamines causes a decrease in tonic end-product inhibition of TH by catecholamine and thereby results in an acceleration of synthesis. However, the findings that catecholamines inhibit *in vitro* TH activity only at relatively high concentrations, and that accelerated catecholamine biosynthesis induced by nerve stimulation is not completely surmountable by exogenous catecholamines (6), suggest that end-product inhibition is not the major regulatory pathway. This consideration has led to a search for additional regulatory mechanisms. Evidence has accumulated that cyclic AMP-dependent phosphorylation of proteins plays a role in neuronal functions. The stimulation of DA synthesis in striatal slices (2) and synaptosomes (8,13,18) by dibutyryl cyclic AMP (dB cyclic AMP) provided the first clue that phosphorylation of TH might be involved in short-term regulation of catecholamine biosynthesis. This idea was further substantiated by a number of studies that have shown that cyclic AMP-dependent protein kinase (kinase A) phosphorylates and activates TH *in vitro*

(24,29,35) and that activation of the enzyme by nerve stimulation produces similar changes in its kinetic constants as those produced *in vitro* following phosphorylation by kinase A (39). We and others have subsequently shown that a number of extracellular signals produce activation and phosphorylation of TH and do so via at least several different protein kinases. The purpose of this presentation is to describe the activation and phosphorylation of TH by various extracellular signals and to compare the kinetic properties of the enzyme phosphorylated *in vitro* by different protein kinases. The effects of phosphorylation of TH on its regulation by DA autoreceptors will also be discussed.

ACTIVATION AND PHOSPHORYLATION OF TH *IN SITU* BY EXTRACELLULAR SIGNALS

The finding that dB cyclic AMP stimulates DA biosynthesis and TH activity in striatal slices and synaptosomes (2,8,13) has led to a number of studies on the activation and phosphorylation of TH *in vitro* and *in vivo*. TH, like some other neuronal proteins, is activated and phosphorylated *in situ* in response to external signals that elevate intracellular cyclic AMP and/or Ca^{2+} levels. It is evident from the results summarized in Table 1 that cyclic AMP analogs and agents that increase cyclic AMP levels activate TH in striatal slices (2), synaptosomes (8,13,18), and cultured cells (20,26,42,45). In many instances it was found that the activation of TH by cyclic AMP is associated with an increased synthesis of catecholamines. The increased incorporation of ^{32}P into TH was also demonstrated in cultured cells preincubated with [^{32}P]orthophosphate and

TABLE 1. *Stimulation of TH activity* in situ *by extracellular and intracellular signals*

Extracellular signal	Intracellular signal (second messenger)	Response
Forskolin, cholera toxin Adenosine derivatives Peptides, VIP, secretin	Cyclic AMP	Phosphorylation and activation by protein kinase A
Cyclic AMP analogs Depolarizing agents (K$^+$, AcCh)	Mimics cyclic AMP Ca^{2+}	Phosphorylation and activation by a Ca^{2+}-CaM-dependent protein kinase
Muscarinic agonists	Ca^{2+}/phospholipids, diacylglycerol (mimicked by phorbol ester)	Phosphorylation and activation by protein kinase C
Growth factors (NGF, EGF, etc.)		Phosphorylation and activation by kinases activated by growth factors

exposed to cyclic AMP analogs (29,31). Interestingly, an adenosine kinase-deficient mutant of cultured PC12 pheochromocytoma cells is resistant to (R)N^6-phenylisopropyladenosine (PIA)-induced activation of TH because the response of adenylate cyclase to PIA is defective in this mutant (12). This provides genetic evidence that adenosine-dependent activation of TH is mediated by an acute activation of adenylate cyclase. In additional experiments among a number of peptides tested, it was found that secretin and vasoactive intestinal peptide (VIP) increase TH activity by increasing ganglionic cyclic AMP levels (21,23). It can therefore be assumed that these peptides activate the enzyme by a protein kinase A-mediated phosphorylation.

Within intact cells, TH also appears to be a substrate for the widely distributed Ca^{2+}/phospholipid-dependent protein kinase (kinase C). This is suggested by the observation that exposure of PC12 cells to phorbol ester (PMA), a potent activator of kinase C, leads to enhanced TH phosphorylation (30).

TH activity is also increased *in situ* by exposure of striatal slices, synaptosomes, or cultured PC12 cells to depolarizing concentrations of K$^+$ (2,26,42) (Table 1). The activation of TH by elevated K$^+$ is additive with the activation by cyclic AMP analogs, suggesting that depolarization and cyclic AMP activate the enzyme by different mechanisms (2,17,26). The enzyme extracted from striatal slices exposed to dB cyclic AMP or forskolin (an activator of adenylate cyclase activity) is further activated by Ca^{2+}-dependent phosphorylation, whereas the enzyme extracted from slices exposed to high K$^+$ is not further activated under Ca^{2+}-dependent phosphorylation conditions (9,11). These results provide further evidence that depolarization by high K$^+$ elicits activation of TH by a different mechanism than cyclic AMP and suggest a role for a Ca^{2+}-dependent kinase in this event.

In addition to depolarization, TH activity is also increased in response to other agents that might elevate free intracel-

lular Ca^{2+}. Thus acetylcholine (AcCh) and other nicotinic agonists increase TH activity and catecholamine synthesis in intact preparations (20,21). The effects of AcCh on TH activity, like those of elevated K$^+$, are dependent on extracellular Ca^{2+} and are suppressed by known Ca^{2+}/calmodulin (CaM) inhibitors.

The time course of stimulation of TH activity by elevated K$^+$ in cultured PC12 cells does not strictly correlate with degree of phosphorylation of the enzyme (26,42). The effects of K$^+$ on enhanced incorporation of ^{32}P into TH show a biphasic time course with one maximum at approximately 30 sec of exposure and a second after 10 min (26). Activation of the enzyme, in contrast, occurs within about 30 sec. The full significance of these observations is not clear.

TH is also activated and phosphorylated *in situ* in response to nerve growth factor (NGF) (17,26,30) and epidermal growth factor (EGF) (30). Increased phosphorylation of TH was detected with 0.1 nM NGF and reached maximal levels at 0.3 to 1 nM of NGF (26). The time course of enhancement of TH activity by NGF did not strictly correlate with the increased phosphorylation. The increased phosphorylation elicited by NGF showed an initial lag of several minutes followed by a monophasic increase in phosphorylation to reach a plateau within about 10 min. Maximal activation of TH occurred within 10 min. The increased TH phosphorylation by NGF does not require extracellular Ca^{2+} and is not suppressed by known CaM activity inhibitors (26).

KINETIC CORRELATES OF ACTIVATION IN CELLULAR PREPARATIONS

Kinetic studies in intact and lysed striatal synaptosomes reveal that activation of TH by cyclic AMP analogs results in a decreased K_M for pteridine cofactor, an increased K_i for DA, no change in the V_{max}, and an increase in pH optimum toward the physiological range (10,11,13). In contrast, activated enzyme from depolarized tissues exhibits no change in the K_M for pteridine cofactor, an increase in V_{max}, and no shift in pH optimum (10,11). Activation of TH in PC12 cells by NGF also reflects an increase in V_{max}, with no shift in apparent K_M for tyrosine.

PHOSPHORYLATION AND ACTIVATION OF TH BY VARIOUS PROTEIN KINASES IN PURIFIED ENZYME PREPARATIONS

It is now well documented that TH is a substrate for at least three protein kinases: kinase A, CaM multiple protein kinase (CaM protein kinase II), and kinase C. The phosphorylation and activation of TH mediated by kinase A have been most extensively studied. Initially, it was questionable whether TH itself is a substrate for kinase A (28), but subsequently it was demonstrated that kinase A mediates phosphorylation of TH and that the phosphorylation correlates with increased TH catalytic activity (13,24,31,35). In purified TH preparations from cultured PC12 cells, purified exogenous kinase A increases ^{32}P incorporation from γ-[^{32}P]ATP and the radioactivity is associated with the 62-kDa subunit of the enzyme (15,20).

Phosphorylation of TH is also catalyzed by CaM-dependent protein kinase II (40,41,44) and Ca^{2+}-phospholipid-dependent protein kinase C (1,37). The activation of TH by CaM-dependent protein kinase II appears to require the presence of an activating protein and the phosphorylated enzyme shows a pH profile similar to that of the nonphosphorylated enzyme (44). The mechanism by which the activating protein stimulates TH activity is not yet known. CaM-dependent protein kinase I apparently does not phosphorylate or activate TH. TH phosphorylated by protein kinase C has kinetic properties that are similar to those of TH phosphorylated by protein kinase A (Table 2) (1). Thus, the enzyme phosphorylated either by protein kinase A or C has a higher affinity for pteridine cofactor and lower affinities for catechol end-products. It was also found that TH in striatal homogenates exists in two kinetically different forms, one with a low K_M and the other with a high K_M value for pteridine cofactor (34,37). Exposure of striatal homogenates to phosphorylating conditions in the presence of protein kinase A causes TH to be almost entirely converted to the phosphorylated form with the low K_M value for pteridine cofactor. These kinetic changes suggest

that phosphorylation of TH by kinases A and C may be involved in the control of TH activity in physiological and pathological states and that the nonphosphorylated form of the enzyme may represent an inactive or less active reservoir. Furthermore, the finding that phosphorylation-dephosphorylation of TH is a reversible process associated with activation and deactivation of the enzyme (43) also supports the idea that these mechanisms have a regulatory function in the synthesis of catecholamines.

ANALYSIS OF PHOSPHOPEPTIDES OF TH

A comparison of two-dimensional maps of phosphopeptides generated by tryptic-chymotryptic digestion of TH reveals a single major species when phosphorylation is catalyzed by protein kinases A or C (1), and two phosphopeptides (A and B) when phosphorylation is catalyzed by CaM protein kinase II (40,41).

Exposure of ^{32}P-phosphate-labeled adrenal medullary cells to AcCh stimulates the incorporation of ^{32}P into TH peptides (A and C), whereas exposure to cyclic AMP analogs stimulates the incorporation of ^{32}P into only one TH peptide (19). Peptide [sodium dodecyl sulfate-polyacrylamide gel electrophoresis (SDS-PAGE)] analysis after digestion of TH-labeled PC12 cells with protease *Staphylococcus aureus* V8 reveals several phosphopeptides. Exposure of PC12 cells to elevated K$^+$ stimulates incorporation of ^{32}P into three of these peptides, whereas exposure to NGF stimulates incorporation of ^{32}P into only one peptide (Fig. 1). Thus, enhanced phosphorylation by elevated K$^+$

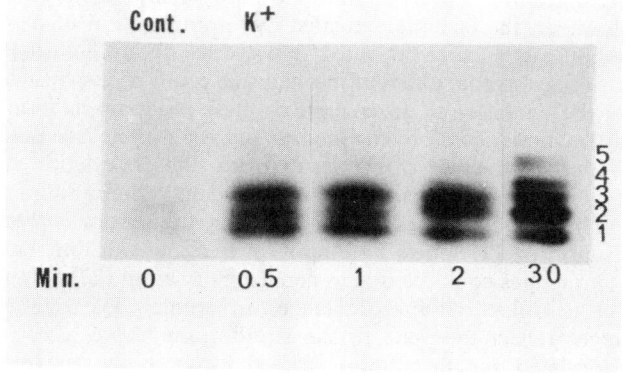

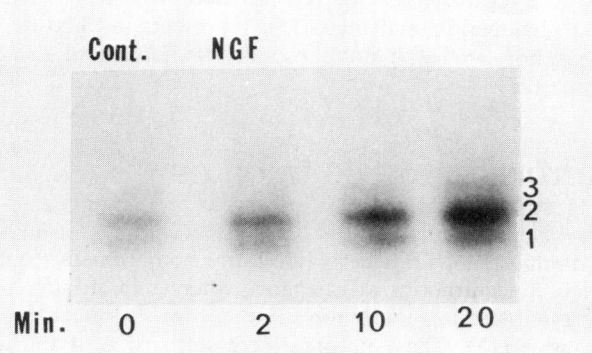

FIG. 1. Patterns of phosphorylated peptides of PC12 cell TH at various time intervals of exposure of the cells to elevated K$^+$ or NGF. (For experimental procedure, see ref. 26.)

TABLE 2. *Effect of phosphorylation on kinetic parameters of soluble TH*

Source of TH	Treatment	K_M for DMPH$_4$ (μM)	K_i for DA (μM)
Striatum	None	170.0	60.0
	Kinase A	80.0	200.0
Purified from cultured PC12 cells	None	200.0	10.0
	Kinase A	90.0	78.0
Purified from PC12 cells	None	450.0	4.5
	Kinase C	110.0	47.5

K_M and K_i values are as taken from the literature (1,13,29).

differs from the enhanced phosphorylation by NGF (26). The enhanced phosphorylation of TH by NGF appears to be mediated by a kinase that is distinct from other characterized kinases and studies are in progress to characterize this enzyme. However, in work from a different laboratory, it was reported that the site phosphorylated in response to NGF is also phosphorylated in response to dB cyclic AMP and cholera toxin (30). It was also found that in response to EGF, another site in TH is phosphorylated which differs from that affected by NGF, whereas a third site is phosphorylated in response to K^+ and a fourth site in response to PMA (30). Clearly, more work is in order to consolidate these various observations.

The relevance of phosphorylation at each site to the activity of TH is not yet known. It will be of interest to determine the effect of TH activity produced by sequential phosphorylation with various kinases.

ACTIVATION OF TH BY NEUROLEPTICS

Acute administration of neuroleptics causes an increase in the firing rate of DA neurons and an increase of turnover and synthesis of DA (46). Several lines of evidence suggest that activation of TH following neuroleptic administration might be due to phosphorylation of the enzyme. First, phosphorylation of TH by kinase A or C or by acute administration of neuroleptics produces similar changes in the affinity of the enzyme for pterine cofactor (27). Second, the activation of striatal TH by neuroleptics and by phosphorylation is higher at physiological pH values than at the pH optimum, 6.0, of the nonphosphorylated enzyme (14). However, the enzyme activated by administration of neuroleptics is further activated in vitro by dB cyclic AMP. This suggests that different mechanisms could be responsible for the activation of the enzyme by these two manipulations (14). One is therefore tempted to suggest that neuroleptic-induced activation might result from phosphorylation of the enzyme by a cyclic AMP-independent protein kinase.

The above findings also suggest that the reported deactivation of TH following long-term treatment of rats with neuroleptics could be due to dephosphorylation (27). Thus, the neuroleptic-induced changes in striatal TH activity might reflect the state of the equilibrium between phosphorylated and nonphosphorylated forms of the enzyme. In this regard, based on kinetic data, it was postulated that haloperidol-activated TH represents a mixture of phosphorylated and nonphosphorylated forms of the enzyme (25).

AUTORECEPTOR CONTROL OF TH ACTIVITY

Inhibition of TH activity in cell-free homogenates requires high concentrations of catechols, whereas in striatal slices or synaptosomes inhibition occurs at much lower concentrations (15). These findings were supportive of the idea that inhibition of TH by DA and by DA agonists might be due to stimulation of presynaptic DA receptors (autoreceptors). Indeed, Apo inhibits striatal and mesolimbic synaptosomal TH activity at low concentrations, and this inhibition is partially reversed by DA antagonists such as haloperidol, fluphenazine, (+)butaclamol, etc. (4,13). It has been postulated that Apo exerts a dual inhibitory action on TH activity, one related to its direct inhibitory property as a catechol derivative, and the other related to its DA agonist activity at presynaptic DA receptors (13).

The dual inhibitory action of Apo on synaptosomal TH activity was confirmed by measuring the enzyme activity extracted from synaptosomes incubated with DA agonists (10). Some noncatechol DA agonists such as the partial ergoline LY 171555 or 3-PPP also inhibit TH activity, and this effect appears to be dependent on the stimulation of presynaptic DA autoreceptors (10). However, some noncatechol D_2-DA agonists (e.g., lergotrile, lisuride, bromocriptine) do not inhibit, or only slightly inhibit, synaptosomal TH activity (16). It was suggested that the lack of synaptosomal TH inhibition by ergot derivatives might be due to the thermolability of presynaptic DA receptors in synaptosomal preparations (38).

We have investigated the possible relationships between stimulation of DA autoreceptors and phosphorylation of TH. Stimulation of synaptosomal DA autoreceptors by Apo does not seem to affect activation of the enzyme by cyclic AMP analogs (13). However, stimulation of DA autoreceptors by DA agonists may influence DA-sensitive adenylate cyclase activity, and thereby might affect phosphorylation of the enzyme by protein kinase A. Since DA autoreceptors have characteristics similar to D_2-DA receptors, it is conceivable that stimulation of these receptors leads to a decreased formation of cyclic AMP and to a decreased phosphorylation of TH. Indeed, it was reported that the stimulation of DA-sensitive adenylate cyclase by forskolin is inhibited by D_2-DA agonists (3). Based on some recent findings with rat striatal slices and synaptosomes, it was concluded that DA autoreceptors control the activation of TH in depolarized striatal dopaminergic terminals (10).

It is noteworthy that inhibition of synaptosomal TH by Apo is significantly reduced in presence of dB cyclic AMP (13). The reduced efficacy of Apo to inhibit synaptosomal TH in presence of dB cyclic AMP is probably due to the decreased affinity of catechol end-products for the phosphorylated enzyme (see Table 2). Since haloperidol almost completely reverses Apo-induced inhibition of the dB cyclic AMP-activated enzyme, it can be assumed that inhibition by Apo of the phosphorylated enzyme is due solely to stimulation of presynaptic DA receptors.

A number of hypotheses have been postulated to explain the selective ability of some DA agonists to inhibit DOPA synthesis via presynaptic DA receptors. Based on studies with the selective presynaptic DA agonist 3-PPP, it was suggested that the intrinsic activity of this compound correlates with previous agonist occupancy of the receptor and is dependent on conformational changes of the receptor complex (5). We have recently obtained data that might provide an alternative explanation for the selective activation of presynaptic receptors by some DA agonists. The results of our studies show that a large reserve exists of striatal presynaptic DA receptors that are capable of regulating DA synthesis (32,33). A large receptor reserve might produce an increase in the maximal response to partial DA agonists and explain the ability of these compounds to regulate DA synthesis via presynaptic DA receptors. Studies are now in progress to determine whether selective presynaptic DA agonists affect the *in situ* phosphorylation of TH in response to various external stimuli.

DISCUSSION

It is now well established that protein phosphorylation is involved in regulation of neuronal function. At least three distinct classes of well-characterized protein kinases, namely kinase A, kinase C, and CaM kinase II, have been found to catalyze the phosphorylation of a large number of neuronal proteins. Interestingly, TH is a substrate for all three of these kinases as well as perhaps for others, and one may therefore speculate whether phosphorylation of TH by each of these kinases is of physiological importance or whether there is some redundancy in the system.

The phosphorylation and activation of TH by various protein kinases that are controlled by different second messengers (e.g., cyclic AMP, Ca^{2+}, phospholipids, and/or diacylglycerol) raise the question of how these kinases interact in the cell to achieve a coordinated regulation of catecholamine biosynthesis. It is possible that various protein kinases are distributed differently in specific DA and nor-ephinephrine neuronal systems and that in each of these systems a different type of kinase plays a predominant role.

The possibility must also be considered that TH may be a substrate for multiple kinases within the same neuron. This appears to be the case at least in sympathetic neurons. Sustained firing of these neurons, as mediated by nicotinic cholinergic receptors, may cause an increased influx of Ca^{2+} and consequently enhance TH phosphorylation via activation of CaM-dependent kinases. Peptidergic input into these neurons may further regulate TH phosphorylation and activity by increasing cyclic AMP levels and thereby activating kinase A (21,23). There is also evidence (22) that stimulation of muscarinic cholinergic receptors on sympathetic neurons may stimulate TH activity via activation of kinase C. Finally, sympathetic neurons bear receptors for NGF, and this may lead to activation of yet another kinase that can phosphorylate and regulate TH. It must be further kept in mind that multiple TH-regulating kinases may be present within the same CNS neuron. For instance, in rat cerebral cortex, VIP coexists in some neurons with AcCh. Since this peptide has the ability to increase cyclic AMP levels, it is possible that corelease of AcCh and VIP yields activation of both CaM-dependent and cyclic AMP-dependent kinases in the same TH-containing target neurons.

The roles of kinases A and C in the activation of TH deserve some comment. The phosphorylation of TH by either kinase results in activation of the enzyme via similar kinetic changes. Thus, the activation by these two kinases might produce synergistic effects; alternatively, each effect may have a different duration of action. Diacylglycerides and Ca^{2+} are the signals that activate kinase C, and the rapid breakdown of diacylglycerol in cells suggests that kinase C might be involved in acute regulation of TH activity. On the other hand, the equilibrium between soluble and membrane-bound protein kinase C shifts in favor of the membrane form in the presence of Ca^{2+} and phospholipid. Therefore, this kinase may play a specific role in the activation of membrane-bound TH. Although it was shown that TH phosphorylated *in vitro* by kinases A and C contains ^{32}P in the same tryptic peptide, it is possible that *in vivo* these two kinases may phosphorylate TH at distinct sites and thereby modify the enzyme function differently. It is noteworthy that phosphorylation of proteins by kinases A and C can result in synergistic as well as antagonistic effects. For example, in the bag cells of *Aplysia*, activation of protein kinases A and C transforms the electrical properties of these neurons in the same direction by increasing excitability (7), whereas in platelets the activation of protein kinases A and C produces an antagonistic effect (36). Future studies should elucidate whether phosphorylation of TH *in vivo* by these two kinases results in additive, nonadditive, synergistic, or antagonistic effects.

Several proteins whose phosphorylations are stimulated by depolarization were also more heavily phosphorylated by CaM protein kinase in lysed synaptosomes. The increased phosphorylation and activation of TH by depolarizing agents seem not to be mediated by protein kinase A, and the dependence on extracellular Ca^{2+} suggests that CaM protein kinase and/or protein kinase C is involved in this activation. On the basis of kinetic studies of TH in lysed synaptosomes, it seems likely that phosphorylation mediated by CaM protein kinase is responsible for activation of the enzyme in depolarized DA terminals. In several studies it was shown that the influx of Ca^{2+} into synaptosomes activates protein phosphorylation, but that at higher intra-synaptosomal Ca^{2+} levels, dephosphorylation occurs.

Although phosphorylation of TH by different protein kinases has been intensively studied, the mechanisms involved in dephosphorylation of TH have not yet been elucidated. The return of neuronal catecholamine synthetic activity from an activated to a resting state probably depends on the rate of dephosphorylation of TH. Furthermore, it was suggested that the phosphorylation-dephosphorylation reaction may play a role in the activation-deactivation of TH following neuroleptic treatment (27,36).

ACKNOWLEDGMENTS

We wish to thank Ms. Judith Scheer for her excellent editorial assistance. These studies were supported in part by National Institute of Mental Health grant MH 02717 (M.G.), National Institute of Neurological and Communicative Disorders and Stroke (NINCDS) grants 06801 (M.G.) and 16036 (L.A.G.), and grants to M.G. and L.A.G. from the American Parkinson's Disease Foundation.

REFERENCES

1. Albert, K. A., Helmer-Matyjek, E., Nairn, A. C., Muller, T. H., Haycock, J. W., Greene, L. A., Goldstein, M., and Greengard, P. (1984): *Proc. Natl. Acad. Sci. USA*, 81:7713–7717.
2. Anagnoste, B., Shirron, C., Friedman, E., and Goldstein, M. (1974): *J. Pharmacol. Exp. Ther.*, 101:370–376.
3. Battaglia, G., Norman, A. B., Hess, E. J., and Creese, I. (1985): *Neurosci. Lett.*, 59:177–182.

4. Christiansen, J., and Squire, R. F. (1974): *J. Pharm. Pharmacol.,* 26:742–743.
5. Clark, D., Hjorth, S., and Carlsson, A. (1985): *J. Neural Transm.,* 62:171–207.
6. Cloutier, G., and Weiner, N. (1973): *J. Pharmacol. Exp. Ther.,* 186:75–85.
7. DeRiemer, S. A., Greengard, P., and Kacmarek, L. K. (1985): *J. Neurosci.,* 5:2672–2676.
8. Ebstein, B., Roberge, C., Tabachnick, J., and Goldstein, M. (1974): *J. Pharm. Pharmacol.,* 26:975–977.
9. El Mestikawy, S., Glowinski, J., and Hamon, M. (1983): *Nature,* 302:830–832.
10. El Mestikawy, S., Glowinski, J., and Hamon, M. (1986): *J. Neurochem.,* 46:12–22.
11. El Mestikawy, S., Gozlan, H., Glowinski, J., and Hamon, M. (1985): *J. Neurochem.,* 45:173–184.
12. Erny, R., and Wagner, J. A. (1984): *Proc. Natl. Acad. Sci. USA,* 81:4974–4978.
13. Goldstein, M., Bronaugh, R. L., Ebstein, B., and Roberge, C. (1976): *Brain Res.,* 109:563–574.
14. Goldstein, M., Ebstein, B., Bronaugh, R. L., and Roberge, C. (1975): In: *Chemical Tools in Catecholamine Research, Vol. II,* edited by O. Almgren, A. Carlsson, and J. Engel, pp. 257–264. North Holland, Elsevier, New York.
15. Goldstein, M., Freedman, L. S., and Backstrom, T. (1970): *J. Pharm. Pharmacol.,* 22:715–716.
16. Goldstein, M., Lew, J. Y., Nakamura, S., Battista, A. F., Lieberman, A., and Fuxe, K. (1978): *Fed. Proc.,* 37:2202–2206.
17. Greene, L. A., and Rein, G. (1978): *J. Neurochem.,* 30:549–555.
18. Harris, J. E., Morgenroth, V. H., III., Roth, R. H., and Baldessarini, R. J. (1974): *Nature,* 252:156–158.
19. Haycock, J. W., Bennett, W. F., George, R. J., and Waymire, J. C. (1982): *J. Biol. Chem.,* 257:13699–13703.
20. Haycock, J. W., Meligeni, J. A., Bennett, W. F., and Waymire, J. C. (1982): *J. Biol. Chem.,* 257:12641–12648.
21. Horwitz, J., and Perlman, R. L. (1984): *J. Neurochem.,* 43:546–552.
22. Horwitz, J., Tsymbalov, S., and Perlman, R. L. (1984): *J. Pharmacol. Exp. Ther.,* 229:577–582.
23. Ip, N. Y., Baldwin, C., and Zigmond, R. E. (1985): *J. Neurosci.,* 5:1947–1954.
24. Joh, T. H., Park, D. H., and Reis, D. J. (1978): *Proc. Natl. Acad. Sci. USA,* 75:4744–4748.
25. Lazar, M., Mefford, I. N., and Barchas, J. D. (1982): *Biochem. Pharmacol.,* 31:2599–2607.
26. Lee, K. Y., Seeley, P. J., Muller, T. H., Helmer-Matyjek, E.,

Sabban, E., Goldstein, M., and Greene, L. A. (1985): *Mol. Pharmacol.,* 28:220–228.
27. Lerner, P., Nose, P., Gordon, E. K., and Lovenberg, W. (1977): *Science,* 197:181–183.
28. Lloyd, T., and Kaufman, S. (1975): *Biochem. Biophys. Res. Commun.,* 66:907–913.
29. Markey, K. A., Kondo, S., Shenkman, L., and Goldstein, M. (1979): *Mol. Pharmacol.,* 17:79–85.
30. McTigue, M., Cremins, J., and Halegoua, S. (1985): *J. Biol. Chem.,* 260:9047–9056.
31. Meligeni, J. A., Haycock, J. W., Bennett, W. F., and Waymire, J. C. (1982): *J. Biol. Chem.,* 257:12632–12640.
32. Meller, E., Helmer-Matyjek, E., Bohmaker, K., Adler, C. H., Friedhoff, A. J., and Goldstein, M. (1986): *Eur. J. Pharmacol.,* 123:311–314.
33. Meller, E., Matyjek, E., Adler, C. H., Bohmaker, K., Friedhoff, A. J., and Goldstein, M. (1985): *Soc. Neurosci.,* 11:Abstr.3396.
34. Miller, L. P., and Lovenberg, W. (1985): *Neurochem. Int.,* 7:689–697.
35. Morgenroth, V. H., III, Hegstrand, L. R., Roth, R. H., and Greengard, P. (1975): *J. Biol. Chem.,* 250:1946–1948.
36. Nishizuka, Y. (1984): *Science,* 225:1365–1370.
37. Raese, J. D., Edelman, A. M., Makk, G., Bruckwick, E. A., Lovenberg, W., and Barchas, J. D. (1979): *Commun. Psychopharmacol.,* 3:295–301.
38. Tissari, A. H., and Gessa, G. (1983): In: *Lisuride and Other Dopamine Agonists,* edited by D. B. Calne, R. Horowski, R. J. McDonald, and W. Wuttke, pp. 33–43. Raven Press, New York.
39. Vulliet, P. R., Langan, T. A., and Weiner, N. (1980): *Proc. Natl. Acad. Sci.,* 77:92–96.
40. Vulliet, P. R., Woodgett, J. R., and Cohen, P. (1984): *J. Biol. Chem.,* 259:13680–13683.
41. Vulliet, P. R., Woodgett, J. R., Ferrari, S., and Hardie, D. G. (1982): *FEBS Lett.,* 182:335–339.
42. Weiner, N., Yanagihara, N., Tank, A. W., Baizer, L., and Langan, T. A. (1984): In: *Catecholamines: Part A: Basic and Peripheral Mechanisms,* edited by E. Usdin, A. Carlsson, A. Dahlstrom, and J. Engel, pp. 173–181. Alan R. Liss, New York.
43. Yamauchi, T., and Fujisawa, H. (1979): *J. Biol. Chem.,* 254:6408–6413.
44. Yamauchi, T., and Fujisawa, H. (1981): *Biochem. Biophys. Res. Commun.,* 100:807–813.
45. Yanagihara, N., Tank, A. W., and Weiner, N. (1984): *Mol. Pharmacol.,* 26:141–147.
46. Zivkovic, B., Guidotti, A., and Costa, E. (1974): *Mol. Pharmacol.,* 10:727–735.

Psychopharmacology:
The Third Generation of Progress,
edited by Herbert Y. Meltzer.
Raven Press, New York © 1987.

CHAPTER 9

Neurochemistry of Midbrain Dopamine Systems

Robert H. Roth, Marina E. Wolf, and Ariel Y. Deutch

ANATOMICAL CONSIDERATIONS

The dopamine (DA) cells of the ventral midbrain have, over the past quarter century, been among the most intensively studied of neuronal groups. At first believed to be two rather homogeneous groups localized to the substantia nigra and ventral tegmental area, midbrain DA neurons have turned out to be heterogeneous populations consisting of neurons projecting to a variety of overlapping areas in the telencephalon. Since the original histochemical descriptions of the monoaminergic neurons of the brain, anatomical studies have focused on the delineation of the telencephalic projections of the midbrain DA neurons. Over the past decade, advances in neuroanatomical methodologies have led to an appreciation of the striking heterogeneity of the mesencephalic DA neurons, both in terms of their connectivity and in reference to the transmitters and proteins localized to these neurons. Biochemical, pharmacological, and electrophysiological investigations have revealed corresponding heterogeneities in midbrain DA neurons, and have led to an understanding of the diversity of both intrinsic and extrinsic control mechanisms that regulate DA neurons. A conceptual approach that utilizes these anatomical and biochemical heterogeneities to define functional subpopulations of DA cells seems most likely to yield information that may enable the rational pharmacological manipulation of dopaminergic function.

The dopamine neurons of the ventral mesencephalon have been designated the A8, A9, and A10 cell groups (57). There are no clear anatomical boundaries between the neurons of the different cell groups, and the DA neurons forming these populations appear at the same time during development (168). These facts, coupled with the overlap in projection fields of the A8, A9, and A10 cell groups (122,144,145), have led to the suggestion that these neurons be collectively designated the mesotelencephalic DA system (155). However, the ability to functionally and biochemically differentiate both the cell body areas and the DA terminal fields suggests that there may be some utility in the original nomenclature of Dahlstrom and Fuxe.

The A10 DA neurons are located in the ventral tegmental area (VTA), whereas the more lateral DA cells of the substantia nigra (SN) have been designated the A9 cell group; the A8 neurons occupy a more caudal position in the retrorubral field (RRF) of the midbrain. The A9 neurons ascend to provide the majority of the dopaminergic innervation of the striatum, whereas the A10 neurons of the VTA innervate mesolimbic areas (e.g., the nucleus accumbens, olfactory tubercles, amygdala) and mesocortical sites such as the prefrontal cortex (35,122,144,145). The A8 neurons contribute to the DA innervation of striatal and mesolimbic, but not neocortical, sites (61,141). The pattern of innervation of the midbrain DA neurons onto the telencephalon forms a broad topography (77–79,155). However, the topographic scheme is not absolute, and there is overlap in the efferent projections of the midbrain DA neurons such that certain telencephalic areas receive convergent inputs (see Fig. 1). Furthermore, certain subpopulations of midbrain DA neurons have axons that collateralize to innervate two or more terminal field regions (76,147).

Such anatomical overlap in the innervation pattern of DA neurons onto terminal field targets suggests that there may exist a considerable degree of heterogeneity within a

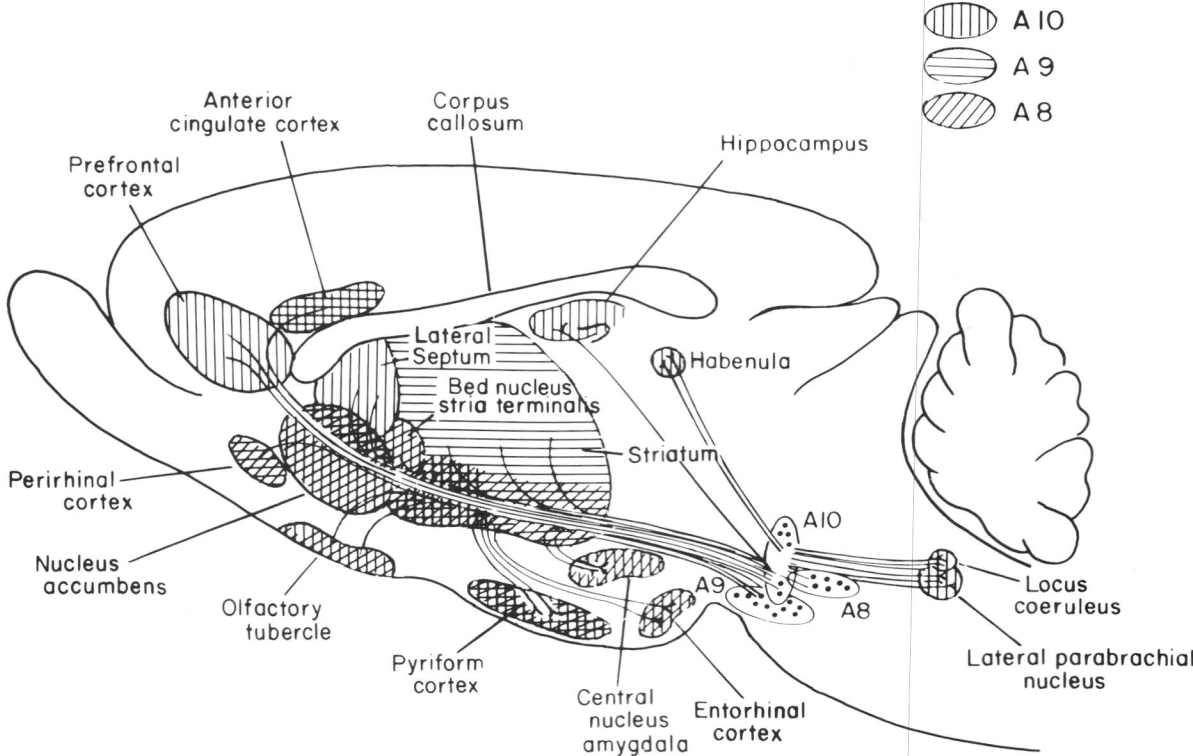

A 10
A 9
A 8

FIG. 1. Schematic representation of the efferent projections of the A8, A9, and A10 dopamine cell groups. The various nondopaminergic projections that originate from neurons in the RRF, SN, and VTA are not shown. The projection fields of the A10 neurons are designated by *vertical* hatching, those of the A9 cells by *horizontal* hatching, and the targets of the A8 DA neurons by *diagonal* hatching. Hatching is not intended to indicate the density of the various projections. A number of regions receive convergent inputs from different cell body regions.

given terminal field. Such heterogeneities are apparent in the striatum, in which there are two distinct nerve terminal DA systems, termed the islandic and diffuse systems (169). These two types of DA innervations originate from different populations of neurons within the midbrain DA cell groups (8,81,127) and exhibit both different basal DA turnover rates and different responsiveness to DA agonists and antagonists (81,82). Such heterogeneities in DA innervation, coupled with histochemically distinct compartments in the striatum with which the different DA systems are in register (101–103), suggest that there may be multiple levels of input-output organization that may be reflected in the functional characteristics of these pathways.

Midbrain DA neurons project extensively to cortical sites, including the prefrontal cortices, cingulate cortex, and certain allocortical sites (144,145). Moreover, recent data indicate that dopaminergic fibers innervate neocortical sites that were previously thought to be devoid of DA input, such as the visual and association cortices (23,24,220,221). Although it is not clear to what degree dopaminergic innervation patterns differ between species, the neocortical DA system appears to be more extensive in primates and felines than in the rat (143,178,220,221). Other relatively minor DA projections that have been uncovered over the past decade indicate that the midbrain DA neurons innervate pontine and diencephalic structures as well as telencephalon sites. These systems include the DA efferents to the locus ceruleus (22,63,195,204), medial parabrachial region (22,112,204), habenula (173,197,204), hippocampus (192,222), and diagonal band of Broca (22,132).

There appear to be extensive connections among the DA terminal field regions, and also efferents from the terminal field regions onto the midbrain cell body areas forming feedback loops. It appears likely that such pathways will be the focus of considerable attention over the next decade, since such interconnections may function in the integration of dopaminergic activity within the telencephalon. The degree of interconnection between the A8, A9, and A10 neurons of the midbrain is not clear, but preliminary data from our laboratory indicate that such interconnections may exist in the rat.

The DA neurons of the midbrain exhibit differences in transmitter and enzyme composition as well as differences in connectivity. Thus, certain of the neurons of the VTA, SN, and RRF contain the peptide transmitter cholecystokinin as well as DA (123,203). Similarly, other subpopulations of midbrain DA cells contain the peptide neurotensin (121); a third group of ventral mesencephalic neurons contain DA, cholecystokinin, and neurotensin (194). There are also patterns of colocalization of DA with certain nontransmitter proteins. Thus, the enzymes protein-*O*-carboxylmethyltransferase (PCM) (30) and acetylcholinesterase (AChE) (104) appear to be present in the DA neurons of the midbrain; cytochrome P450 reductase (107) and a vitamin D-dependent calcium-binding protein (CaBP) (11,88) have also been observed in some, but not all, midbrain DA neurons. Although the functional significance of such colocalization at this time is unclear, these patterns may provide an empirically useful way of identifying subpopulations of DA cells for further study.

SIMILARITIES AND GENERAL BIOCHEMICAL CHARACTERISTICS OF MIDBRAIN DOPAMINE SYSTEMS

It is apparent that considerable biochemical heterogeneity exists among various DA cell groups. Heterogeneity can reflect differences in extrinsic (e.g., afferent inputs) as well as intrinsic (e.g., autoreceptors) regulatory mechanisms. However, the functional output of all DA neurons to a large degree reflects neurochemical features of transmitter synthesis and release that are shared by all DA neurons. It is therefore useful to first consider general characteristics of DA neurochemistry that have been revealed by studies of the "prototypic" nigrostriatal DA projection.

Regulation of Impulse Flow

Action potentials in DA neurons appear to be triggered by slow depolarizing pacemaker-like potentials in the somatodendritic region (97). The likelihood that these potentials will generate an action potential is influenced by many factors, including effects on membrane potential exerted by transmitters released from nondopaminergic neurons in the SN or VTA. Impulse flow also appears to be modulated by DA autoreceptors located on the cell body and/or dendrites of DA neurons. Intracellular recording studies have shown that autoreceptor-selective doses of apomorphine produce a hyperpolarization of A9 DA neurons that is associated with inhibition of the slow depolarizing potential that precedes spontaneously occurring action potentials (99,100). Autoreceptor activation also appears to reduce the occurrence of small, spontaneous fast potentials that apparently arise as a result of electrical coupling between neighboring DA cells. These potentials may trigger action potentials in DA neurons when the membrane potential is close to firing threshold (98).

Several lines of evidence support a role for somatodendritic autoreceptors in regulating DA impulse flow under physiological conditions. First of all, dendrites of both A9 and A10 DA cells have the capacity for high-affinity uptake, storage, and synthesis of DA, and have been found to release both previously taken up radiolabeled DA and endogenous DA in a Ca^{2+}-dependent manner in response to depolarizing stimuli (19–21,34,56,87). Some characteristics of the dendritic release process appear to differ from the release mechanism operative in axon terminals. For example, DA is stored in the smooth endoplasmic reticulum of nigral dendrites rather than in vesicles (56,153,199), and dendritic release of DA is not inhibited by tetrodotoxin (161) or gamma-butyrolactone (113), suggesting that release of DA from dendrites is not impulse dependent. Immunocytochemical studies have shown that dendrodendritic

synaptic contacts are rare in the SN, leading to the suggestion that dendritically released DA exerts a tonic modulatory influence on target sites distributed over a relatively large area (56,231). However, both push-pull cannulation techniques and other in vivo techniques that allow temporal correlation, such as voltammetry and dialysis, have demonstrated that changes in the nigral release of DA are accompanied by oppositely directed changes in DA release from nigrostriatal and mesolimbic DA terminals (42,43, 135,142,150,162). These results are consistent with a model in which activation of somatodendritic autoreceptors by dendritically released DA results in depression of impulse flow in DA neurons, thereby decreasing the impulse-dependent release of DA from nerve terminals in the projection field.

Dopamine Release

Release of DA from nigrostriatal DA terminals appears to be a function of the rate and pattern of impulse flow. For example, recent voltammetric studies have suggested that burst firing in nigrostriatal neurons is associated with a dramatic facilitation of DA release (96). In addition, presynaptic autoreceptors have been shown to regulate the electrically or K^+-evoked release of DA from striatal slices and synaptosomes (53–55,80,120,126,172,179,200,233,234). These release-modulating autoreceptors can be pharmacologically characterized as D-2-type dopamine receptors (114,140,202), develop supersensitivity following chronic exposure to neuroleptics (164), and desensitize rapidly to endogenous DA (6).

In general, DA agonists inhibit while DA antagonists enhance the evoked release of DA, although the extent of these effects has been shown to be critically dependent on experimental conditions that alter synaptic levels of released DA. For example, antagonists are most effective at facilitating DA release evoked by high-frequency, short-duration depolarizing stimuli. This suggests that autoreceptor activation by endogenous DA is greatest under these conditions and may serve to reduce the amount of DA liberated per pulse during high rates of neuronal firing (53,55,120). Release-modulating autoreceptors may therefore be of particular importance under conditions of burst firing. By flattening the frequency-response curve, autoreceptor activation could partially compensate for the marked facilitation of release associated with burst firing. Recent studies have suggested that activation of nerve terminal autoreceptors on striatal terminals results in a decrease in terminal excitability that may reflect hyperpolarization of nerve terminal membranes. Terminal excitability appears to be sensitive to changes in the level of released transmitter that occur over a physiological range of firing frequencies (105,212–214). Autoreceptors may regulate terminal excitability and transmitter release by diminishing a voltage-dependent Ca^{2+} conductance involved in stimulus-secretion coupling or by influencing a coupling step that occurs after the initial influx of Ca^{2+}. Either possibility is consistent with the observation that Ca^{2+}-independent DA release (basal efflux or release evoked by amphetamine or tyramine) is not modulated by autoreceptors (134,200). Alternatively, hyperpolarization of nigrostriatal terminals may reduce the probability that an action potential arriving at the nerve terminal will successfully invade potential sites of DA release.

Although most studies of release-modulating autoreceptors have utilized striatal slices, similar receptors appear to modulate the evoked release of DA from slices of prefrontal cortex (184,241) and entorhinal cortex (174). Since *in vivo* studies employing the gamma-butyrolactone model have shown that mesoprefrontal and mesoentorhinal DA neurons lack synthesis-modulating autoreceptors (14,86,184), this suggests that the autoreceptor-dependent pathway for regulation of DA release can exist independently of the autoreceptor-dependent pathway for the regulation of DA synthesis (86,237,240). Release-modulating autoreceptors may constitute a general feature of dopaminergic nerve terminals in the CNS.

Dopamine Metabolism

DA nerve terminals possess a high-affinity uptake mechanism for DA that is important in terminating transmitter action. Released DA appears to be converted to dihydrophenylacetic acid (DOPAC) by intraneuronal monoamine oxidase following reuptake. Released DA is also converted to homovanillic acid (HVA), probably at an extraneuronal site, either by initial methylation followed by deamination or by methylation after deamination by monoamine oxidase. In most cases, levels of DOPAC and HVA are reliable indicators of dopaminergic activity, i.e., they provide a reasonable combined measure of DA synthesis and metabolism and therefore of impulse flow in DA neurons. However, the minor metabolite 3-methoxytyramine appears to provide a better index of DA release *per se*. Whereas DOPAC is the major metabolite in rat brain, HVA predominates in primates. Sulfate conjugation of DOPAC and HVA occurs to a significant extent in rat but not in primate brain. Pathways of DA metabolism in brain have been reviewed recently (50,232).

Dopamine Synthesis

The rate-limiting step in DA biosynthesis is the conversion of tyrosine to dihydroxyphenylalanine (DOPA) by tyrosine hydroxylase (TH). DOPA is subsequently converted to dopamine by *l*-aromatic amino acid decarboxylase. A number of autoregulatory mechanisms can influence the rate of DA synthesis.

Role of Dopamine, Substrate, and Cofactor Levels

DA itself functions as an end-product inhibitor of TH. Since DA levels in nerve terminals are estimated to be well above the K_i for inhibition of TH by DA, this mechanism should be operative under physiological conditions. In support of this idea, administration of monoamine oxidase inhibitors has been shown to increase DA levels in nigrostriatal, mesolimbic, and mesocortical DA nerve terminals, leading to greatly attenuated rates of DA synthesis in these regions (14,58).

Recent studies suggest that TH activity may be influenced under some experimental circumstances by availability of precursor tyrosine (92,154,209,243). Tyrosine levels may in turn be influenced by dietary intake of tyrosine or other amino acids that compete with tyrosine for transport into the brain. TH activity is also dependent on adequate concentrations of tetrahydrobiopterin cofactor. Estimates of endogenous tetrahydrobiopterin levels have suggested that TH is normally unsaturated with respect to cofactor. Under certain conditions changes in TH activity may reflect alterations in tetrahydrobiopterin availability. Dihydropteridine reductase, which catalyzes the reduction of the quinonoid dihydropterin that has been oxidized during the tyrosine hydroxylation reaction, may represent a potential site for drug intervention in catecholamine biosynthesis.

Role of Impulse Flow

During periods of increased impulse flow in central dopaminergic neurons, the kinetic properties of TH are altered. For example, the enzyme obtained from rat striatum after electrical stimulation of the nigrostriatal tract or acute administration of neuroleptic drugs exhibits an increased affinity for pterin cofactor and a decreased affinity for the normal end-product inhibitor, DA (160,185,188,251). A similar activation of TH can be produced *in vitro* by incubation of striatal slices or homogenates under conditions that promote terminal depolarization (39,181). This post-stimulation activation of TH presumably represents one of the mechanisms by which DA neurons meet the increased demand for DA during periods of enhanced impulse flow and transmitter release.

Phosphorylation of TH *in vitro* has been found to produce a similar kinetic activation of the enzyme. Although it is well established that cyclic AMP-dependent protein kinase can phosphorylate and activate TH (95,108,148, 223,247), recent studies have shown that the Ca^{2+}-phospholipid-dependent protein kinase known as protein kinase C can also phosphorylate and activate TH *in vitro* (3,177). Protein kinase C phosphorylates TH obtained from PC12 cells on the same site as cyclic AMP-dependent protein kinase, resulting in a decreased K_m for 6-methyltetrahydropterine cofactor and an increased K_i for DA (3). Phosphorylation of rat brain TH by Ca^{2+}-calmodulin-dependent kinase II has also been demonstrated, although in this case phosphorylation appears to be accompanied by a kinetic activation only in the presence of an endogenous protein (244–246) which may serve to activate or stabilize the phosphorylated enzyme. Studies using TH purified from rat pheochromocytoma indicate that the secondary site phosphorylated by Ca^{2+}-calmodulin-dependent kinase is apparently the same as that phosphorylated by cyclic AMP-dependent kinase and protein kinase C, although the primary site appears to be unique (224). The interpretation of all of these results is complicated by the possibility that TH may be regulated differently in different systems. For example, phorbol esters (which activate protein kinase C) increase TH activity in adrenal chromaffin cells (175) and superior cervical ganglion (230) but not in striatal slices (138).

It seems most reasonable to speculate that multiple kinases are involved in regulating TH activity in brain. It is possible, for example, that different kinases are involved in maintaining basal as opposed to stimulated TH activity (119). However, considerable evidence suggests that Ca^{2+}-dependent phosphorylation processes (mediated by Ca^{2+}-calmodulin-dependent kinase and/or protein kinase C) are primarily responsible for the *in vivo* and *in situ* activation of TH produced by electrical stimulation of the nigrostriatal tract, acute neuroleptic administration, or K^+-depolarization of striatal slices (40,71,72,95,119,125,138,176,177,196). Ca^{2+}-calmodulin-dependent events also seem to be involved in maintaining basal TH activity in striatal slices (119,138). Recent studies in our laboratory on the mechanism of the depolarization-induced activation of TH in striatal slices suggest that a two-step mechanism may be involved. The K_m for cofactor appears to be decreased via a mechanism involving protein kinase C. However, this kinetic change in itself does not appear to be sufficient for eliciting increased DOPA formation *in situ* unless accompanied by a calmodulin-dependent activational step (238). It is important to note that the available data do not exclude a role for cyclic AMP-dependent phosphorylation in regulating TH activity in response to other types of stimulation or maintaining TH activity under basal conditions.

DA neurons resemble other monoaminergic neurons in their ability to respond to increases in impulse flow by increasing transmitter synthesis. However, if impulse flow is interrupted in DA neurons, either mechanically or pharmacologically by administration of gamma-butyrolactone (GBL), the neurons respond in a unique fashion by increasing the rate of DA synthesis and increasing DA levels in the terminals (1,4,89,90,186,187,228,229). The increase in DA synthesis appears to reflect the fact that inhibition of impulse flow in DA cells also shuts off impulse-dependent DA release from nerve terminals. The resulting decrease in synaptic levels of DA leads to a disinhibition of those events normally under the tonic control of nerve-terminal synthesis-modulating autoreceptors (226,229; see next section). It is not entirely clear how DA synthesis can proceed supranormally in the presence of elevated intraneuronal DA levels, since DA is the natural end-product inhibitor of TH. This may reflect the fact that TH prepared from GBL-treated rats or rats with electrothermic lesions of the nigrostriatal pathway has an increased affinity for pterin cofactor and decreased affinity for DA, rendering it less susceptible to feedback inhibition (158,227).

It has been speculated that the increase in tyrosine hydroxylation produced by GBL or axotomy may result from the decreased Ca^{++} influx that would be expected to accompany a cessation of impulse flow (185,187). This is consistent with the observation that incubation of striatal slices in Ca^{++}-free medium results in enhanced tyrosine hydroxylation (38,94,109,111,138) and a kinetic activation of TH (33,38). However, as noted above, TH is also activated by mechanisms that depend on the presence of extracellular Ca^{2+}, such as K^+-depolarization of striatal slices (39,181) or mechanisms that involve *increases* in intracellular levels of free Ca^{2+}, such as incubation in Na^+-free medium (40). These observations suggest that the dependency of TH activity on intracellular Ca^{2+} levels is extremely complex, since the enzyme can apparently be activated by both decreases and increases in intracellular Ca^{2+}.

Role of Presynaptic Autoreceptors

The rate of tyrosine hydroxylation is under the control of nerve-terminal synthesis-modulating autoreceptors. These receptors modulate DA synthesis independent of changes in intraneuronal DA levels or DA release (86,237), can be classified as D-2-type dopamine receptors (47,218), and have been found to develop supersensitivity following chronic neuroleptic administration (91,165) or prolonged decreases in DA release (7). The question of whether the inhibition of TH activity by autoreceptor activation depends on changes in the kinetic properties of the enzyme has been controversial. Autoreceptor stimulation *in vivo* appears to attenuate the activation of TH produced by GBL administration (158) or electrical stimulation of the medial forebrain bundle (185,188). For example, TH isolated from rat striatum after GBL administration has an increased affinity for pterin cofactor and a decreased affinity for DA. However, if DA agonists are administered in conjunction with GBL, these kinetic changes are reversed, i.e., the isolated enzyme exhibits properties similar to those observed for the enzyme prepared from untreated rats (158,227). Recent studies using striatal slices also suggest that presynaptic autoreceptors modulate the change in the kinetic properties (181) and activity (70,181) of TH produced by K^+-depolarization of striatal slices. We have found that the enhancement of *in situ* DOPA formation produced by K^+-depolarization of striatal slices is accompanied by a substantial decrease in the K_m for pterin cofactor (39,181). When slices are depolarized in the presence of *l*-sulpiride, both the magnitude of the increase in DOPA levels and the magnitude of the decrease in the K_m for cofactor are greater than in the absence of the DA antagonist (181). This suggests that autoreceptor activation by endogenous DA is normally exerting a dampening effect on the depolarization-induced kinetic activation of TH.

However, a number of indirect findings appear to argue against this concept. For example, antipsychotic drugs are known to stimulate DA synthesis in nigrostriatal DA terminals and to produce a kinetic activation of TH characterized by increased affinity for the pterin cofactor (248,251). It has been reported that GBL administration, transection of nigrostriatal fibers, or kainic acid lesions of the striatum prevent the ability of neuroleptics to produce a kinetic activation of TH but not their ability to stimulate DA synthesis and metabolism *in vivo* (66,249,250). On the basis of these observations it was proposed that antipsychotic drugs such as haloperidol produce a kinetic activation of TH as a result of blockade of postsynaptic receptors and subsequent feedback-mediated increases in impulse flow in the nigrostriatal pathway, whereas blockade of presynaptic receptors was proposed to increase DA synthesis through a mechanism that does not depend on kinetic changes in TH (66,219). However, recent studies have shown that SCH 23390 (a D-1-selective DA antagonist) increases the firing rate of nigrostriatal DA neurons to the same extent as the nonselective antagonist haloperidol or the D-2-selective antagonist sulpiride, but does not elicit a kinetic activation of TH (170). D-1-selective antagonists would be expected to block postsynaptic striatal DA receptors but not presynaptic autoreceptors, whereas haloperidol and sulpiride would block both types of receptors. This may suggest that in the case of SCH 23390 the kinetic activation of TH normally associated with increased impulse flow is being masked as a result of activation of synthesis-modulating autoreceptors by DA released from striatal terminals (170). These findings indicate that presynaptic autoreceptors exercise control over the ability of changes in impulse flow to alter the kinetic properties of TH.

What mechanisms might be involved in coupling the occupation of synthesis-modulating autoreceptors to changes in the kinetic properties of TH? It has been suggested that autoreceptors function by gating Ca^{2+} entry into the nerve terminal (166). This would be consistent with the ability of autoreceptors to attenuate the Ca^{2+}-dependent increase in TH activity produced by K^+-depolarization of striatal slices (237). However, autoreceptor stimulation also attenuates the activation of DA synthesis produced by incubating striatal slices in Ca^{2+}-free medium, suggesting that autoreceptor-mediated inhibition of DA synthesis is not dependent on the presence of extracellular Ca^{2+} and does not necessarily involve regulating Ca^{2+} entry into the nerve terminal (33). Furthermore, the mechanism by which autoreceptors inhibit TH activity appears to be sensitive to high levels of intracellular Ca^{2+}, since autoreceptor-mediated inhibition of DA synthesis in striatal slices is impaired by conditions associated with increases in intracellular Ca^{2+}, such as incubation in sodium-free medium or ouabain (33). In addition to attenuating the stimulation of DA synthesis in striatal slices produced by K^+-depolarization or incubation in low-Ca^{2+} medium, it appears that autoreceptors also modulate the unstimulated rate of DA synthesis that occurs in striatal slices (70,237) or synaptosomes (33,110,189,225). However, it should be noted that the "basal" rate of tyrosine hydroxylation in brain slices may be greater than the basal rate that occurs in vivo, suggesting that TH may already be activated to some degree in the slice preparation (119,237).

It seems likely that the kinetic activation of TH produced by GBL, electrical stimulation, Ca^{2+}-free conditions, or K^+-depolarization ultimately results from stimulation of its phosphorylation. Autoreceptors may attenuate TH activity by promoting dephosphorylation. If multiple kinases are involved in regulating TH activity, it is conceivable that autoreceptors regulate tyrosine hydroxylation by altering the activity of kinase(s) that are different from those involved in stimulating TH activity. Some evidence suggests that autoreceptors may inhibit DA synthesis by modulating cyclic AMP-dependent events (70). Alternatively, autoreceptor stimulation may interfere with an activational or stabilizing step rather than with phosphorylation per se.

Dopamine Autoreceptors

The available data suggest that nerve-terminal and somatodendritic autoreceptors have similar pharmacological properties. Both are relatively more sensitive to DA agonists than postsynaptic DA receptors and exhibit similar pharmacological profiles (114). It is conceivable that a single receptor protein might be responsible for modulating such diverse functions as transmitter release, tyrosine hydroxylation, and action potential generation. For example, all of these functions may share a common sensitivity to the initial signaling event (hyperpolarization?) triggered by autoreceptor occupation. However, it is likely that different second messenger systems are ultimately responsible for transducing the signal of autoreceptor occupation into changes in DA synthesis, release, and impulse generation. A schematic model for the modulation of striatal DA synthesis and release by nerve terminal autoreceptors is shown in Fig. 2.

Role of Protein Carboxylmethylation in Autoreceptor Function

Our laboratory has investigated the possible role of protein carboxylmethylation in DA autoreceptor function. Protein-O-carboxylmethyltransferase (PCM; EC 2.1.1.24) catalyzes the transfer of methyl groups from S-adenosylmethionine to free carboxylic acid groups on substrate methyl-acceptor proteins. PCM has been implicated in stimulus-secretion coupling in a number of biological systems (67). PCM has also been suggested to play a role in the repair and/or recognition of damaged proteins (9,128,159). The enzyme exhibits a unique neuron-specific distribution in rat brain, with relatively high levels of immunoreactivity found in catecholamine-containing cell body regions, such as SN, VTA, and locus cerulus, as well as catecholamine projection fields including the striatum, cortex, thalamus, hippocampus, and amygdala (25,27). Recent immunocytochemical studies have suggested that PCM and TH may be colocalized in nigral cells and processes (26), providing an anatomical basis for the hypothesis that PCM modulates dopaminergic function. It has been speculated that one role of PCM in brain may be to regulate the activity of Ca^{2+}-calmodulin-stimulated enzymes, based on the observation that carboxylmethylation of calmodulin-dependent protein kinase, phosphodiesterase, or calcineurin results in a significant attenuation of their calmodulin-stimulated activity (28–30,32,83,84). This raises the interesting possibility that PCM may regulate Ca^{2+}-calmodulin-dependent synaptic events such as transmitter synthesis and release.

We have demonstrated that protein carboxylmethylester formation is increased as a result of DA autoreceptor stimulation in striatal synaptosomes (31) and slices (239). In order to test the possible involvement of PCM in autoreceptor-mediated events, we have attempted to correlate changes in DA release, DA synthesis, and protein carboxylmethylester formation in striatal slices. Our findings suggest that methyltransferase inhibitors interfere with the autoreceptor-mediated regulation of DA release from striatal slices but not with the ability of DA agonists and antagonists to modulate DA synthesis (240,242). This indicates that a methyltransferase-dependent signal transduction step may be involved in the function of release-modulating autore-

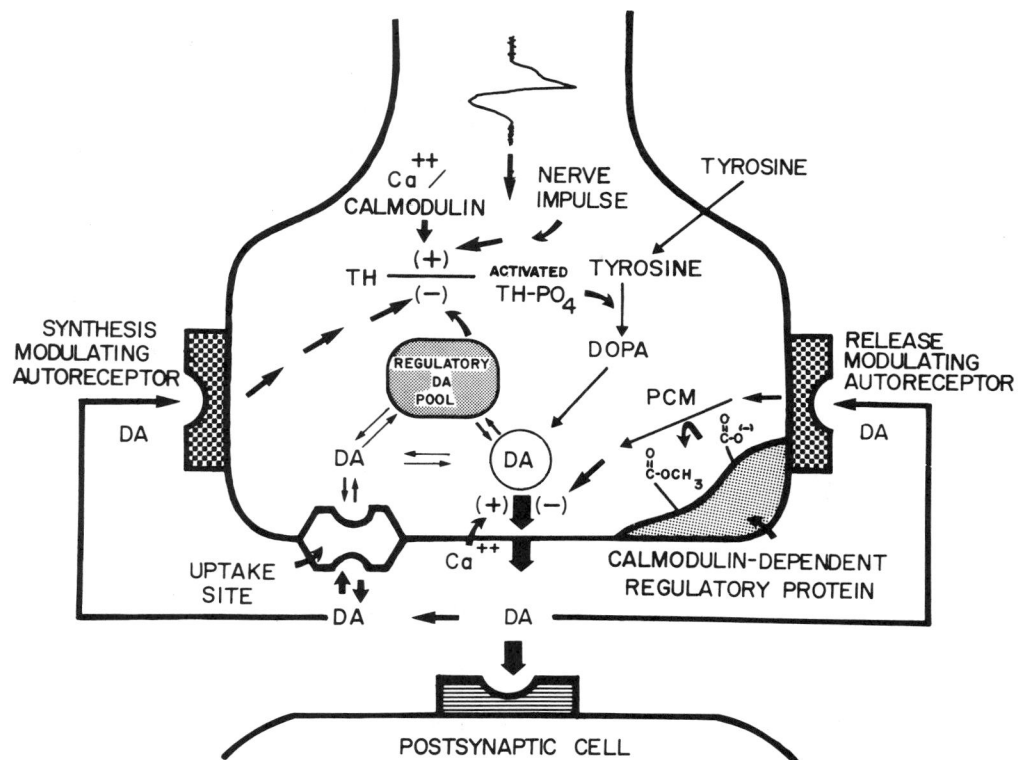

FIG. 2. Schematic model for the modulation of striatal DA synthesis and release by nerve terminal autoreceptors. Invasion of the nerve terminal by an action potential results in Ca^{2+}-dependent release of DA. DA release is attenuated by release-modulating autoreceptors via a coupling mechanism that may involve protein carboxylmethylation; the relevant substrate may be calmodulin or a calmodulin-dependent enzyme. Impulse flow also increases the rate of tyrosine hydroxylation. This may involve the Ca^{2+}-dependent phosphorylation of TH, resulting in conversion to an activated form that exhibits greater affinity for tetrahydrobiopterin cofactor. TH activity is attenuated by end-product inhibition by intraneuronal DA, and by activation of synthesis-modulating autoreceptors. Autoreceptor-mediated inhibition of DA synthesis does not appear to involve a methylation-dependent step and may involve kinetic changes in TH. Release- and synthesis-modulating autoreceptors may represent distinct receptive sites. Alternatively, one site may regulate both functions through distinct transduction mechanisms.

ceptors but not synthesis-modulating autoreceptors and provides additional support for the distinction between autoreceptor-mediated pathways for the regulation of release and synthesis (240). Similar results have been obtained in striatal synaptosomes (189). In addition, these investigators have found that inhibition of methyltransferase activity in brain interferes with the ability of apomorphine to decrease striatal DOPAC levels *in vivo* (190). Since depression of DA metabolite levels by apomorphine may reflect activation of release-modulating autoreceptors and subsequent reductions in DA turnover, these findings are consistent with a role for PCM in the function of release-modulating DA autoreceptors.

Autoreceptors Versus Postsynaptic Dopamine Receptors

The possibility that autoreceptor stimulation might be of therapeutic benefit in patients suffering from diseases thought to involve excessive dopaminergic activity has provided the impetus for the search for DA agonists that would act selectively at autoreceptors. Autoreceptor-selective agonists synthesized in recent years include racemic 3-PPP, the indolylbutylamine EMD 23 448, transdihydrolisuride (TDHL), HW 165, and B-HT 920. These agonists have been demonstrated to inhibit DA release, synthesis, and impulse flow in DA neurons, as well as elicit behavioral responses associated with diminished dopaminergic function (see 48, 49). Studies of these agonists have also yielded considerable insight into what features confer autoreceptor selectivity on a drug. Carlsson (41) has suggested that DA autoreceptors and postsynaptic receptors exist in different adaptational states (i.e., different conformational states) as a result of different degrees of previous occupancy by endogenous transmitter. According to this hypothesis, agents like (−)-3-PPP show high intrinsic activity at receptors that are adapted to low endogenous DA levels, either as a result of denervation (e.g., "autoreceptor-selective" agonists show activity at denervated postsynaptic receptors) or because they are "nonsynaptic" and therefore located at some distance from the release of transmitter (e.g., DA receptors on lactotrophs in the pituitary). This may suggest that central DA autoreceptors, which show high agonist responsiveness, are also located "nonsynaptically" (41,74).

The use of autoreceptor-selective DA agonists to inhibit dopaminergic activity may have therapeutic applications (152). For example, autoreceptor-selective doses of DA agonists have been shown to have beneficial effects in some subtypes of schizophrenic patients (52,210). There is reason to think that autoreceptor-selective agonists might be free of many of the side effects associated with chronic antipsychotic drug administration, possibly because autoreceptor stimulation merely diminishes dopaminergic tone whereas blockade of postsynaptic receptors by neuroleptics presumably results in a complete and abrupt shut-off of dopaminergic output. Autoreceptor stimulation may also be of value in motor disorders believed to be associated with excessive dopaminergic activity, such as tardive dyskinesia and Huntington's chorea. Although clinical trials have been limited, low doses of apomorphine or bromocriptine have proven therapeutic in patients suffering from a variety of movement disorders, whereas preliminary findings suggest that 3-PPP may reduce dyskinetic movements induced by long-term haloperidol administration in monkeys (106). Finally, the fact that autoreceptor-selective agonists are inactive at normosensitive postsynaptic DA receptors but active at supersensitive postsynaptic receptors suggests that these drugs may be useful in the treatment of Parkinson's disease. Autoreceptor agonists could theoretically substitute for depleted DA at supersensitive receptors in striatum without activating normosensitive DA receptors elsewhere in brain. In fact, a recent clinical trial suggests that TDHL is effective in the treatment of Parkinson's disease (51).

HETEROGENEITY OF NIGROSTRIATAL DOPAMINE NEURONS

A number of recent findings have indicated that the nigrostriatal DA system exhibits anatomical, biochemical, electrophysiological, and pharmacological heterogeneity. In addition to overlap in the terminal projection fields of nigral DA neurons (144,155), certain subpopulations of these DA neurons have axons that collateralize and innervate several terminal field regions (76,147). In the striatum there are two distinct nerve-terminal DA systems, referred to as the islandic and diffuse systems (169). These two systems appear to exhibit different basal rates of transmitter turnover and to respond in a quantitatively different fashion to DA agonists and antagonists. For example, certain ergolene derivatives selectively reduce DA turnover rates in the islandic but not diffuse systems of the striatum (80), whereas other DA agonists rather selectively interact with the diffuse DA innervation of the striatum (81).

Heterogeneities in the striatum are also apparent in that there are regional variations in striatal response to DA antagonists such as haloperidol (62). Thus, the magnitudes of both the antipsychotic drug-induced increase in DA metabolite accumulation and the neuroleptic-elicited increase in DA synthesis exhibit a twofold regional variability in the striatum. The greatest increase in turnover and synthesis is observed in the rostral dorsomedial sector of the striatum, whereas the ventrolateral tail of the striatum exhibits the least responsiveness to antipsychotic drugs. Furthermore, the precise mesencephalic source of the DA innervation of the striatum subfields and the biochemical

responsiveness of these regions are highly correlated. Areas of the striatum exhibiting the greatest degree of change in metabolites or synthesis receive their DA innervation from the medial and central regions of the A9 cell group; areas exhibiting low responsiveness are predominantly innervated by A10 and A8 neurons. Those areas intermediate in responsiveness receive mixed A9/A10 inputs.

These data suggest that there might be regional variability in the biochemical responsiveness of different subsets of the mesencephalic cell body regions that project to different striatal sectors. Examination of micropunched samples from different regions of the A8, A9, and A10 cell body areas has revealed that there are significant regional differences within the SN in terms of responsiveness to acute neuroleptic challenge (60,62). Acute treatment with haloperidol produces a significant increase in DA synthesis (as reflected by DOPA accumulation) in the medial and central SN, whereas DOPA accumulation in the lateral SN is unaffected. Within the VTA, only the lateral area (primary source of the mesolimbic efferents) exhibits a significant increase in synthesis in response to haloperidol. The medial sector (source of the mesocortical innervation) of the VTA exhibits no increase in DA synthesis following neuroleptic challenge, probably because the mesoprefrontal cortical neurons lack both synthesis-modulating and somatodendritic autoreceptors (see Heterogeneity of Ventral Tegmental Dopamine Neurons). It is conceivable that the nonresponsive lateral sector of the SN and the A8 regions fail to exhibit an increase in DOPA accumulation in response to haloperidol because these regions share with the medial VTA a lack of synthesis-modulating autoreceptors.

Heterogeneities within the SN are also apparent in an animal model of Parkinson's disease. Administration of 1-methyl-4-phenyl-1,2,3,6-tetrahydropyridine (MPTP) to primate species results in a Parkinsonian-like syndrome and is marked by a selective decrease in striatal, but not mesolimbic, DA levels (73). DA neurons within the lateral A8 cell group and the central SN appear to be preferentially vulnerable to MPTP-induced neurotoxicity (59,73), whereas DA neurons within the medial SN are somewhat less susceptible to MPTP. The DA neurons of the lateral SN do not appear to be damaged by MPTP.

These data indicate that subpopulations of nigral DA neurons can be defined on the basis of anatomical, biochemical, and pharmacological criteria, and suggest that such heterogeneities may be apparent in neurological and psychiatric disorders. Given the degree of nigral heterogeneity, it would appear reasonable to expect corresponding differences in subpopulations of DA neurons within the ventral tegmental area.

HETEROGENEITY OF VENTRAL TEGMENTAL DOPAMINE NEURONS

Differences Related to the Absence of Autoreceptors

Although the majority of ventral tegmental DA neurons appear to possess somatodendritic and synthesis-modulating autoreceptors, the DA cells that project to the prefrontal and cingulate cortices appear either to have a greatly diminished number of these receptors or to lack them entirely (17,44,205,235). The absence of these important modulatory receptors on certain subsets of VTA DA neurons appears in part to be responsible for some of the unique characteristics of these neurons when compared to mesotelencephalic DA neurons that possess autoreceptors [nigrostriatal, mesolimbic, and mesopyriform systems (182,184)]. These properties are summarized in Table 1. Electrophysiological studies have revealed that midbrain DA neurons lacking somatodendritic autoreceptors possess a higher basal rate of physiological activity and exhibit a different pattern of activity, which is characterized by a greater degree of burst firing (44). These electrophysiological studies complement biochemical studies which demonstrate that the turnover rate of DA in the mesoprefrontal and mesocingulate cortices is greater than that observed in the pyriform cortex, or in the projection fields of other midbrain DA neurons that possess autoreceptors (12,16). For example, the $t_{1/2}$ for DA turnover in the prefrontal cortex is about 15 min compared to a $t_{1/2}$ of over 2 hr in the striatum. The interaction of DA agonists and antagonists with DA autoreceptors apparently plays a prominent role in determining the output of the various DA systems in response to acute and chronic treatment with these drugs, since DA neurons that lack autoreceptors show little response [as is the case with the mesoprefrontal or mesocingulate cortical systems (15,16)] or no response [e.g., the tuberoinfundibular system (58)] to acute DA antagonist or agonist challenge. In contrast, dopamine systems that possess autoreceptors (nigrostriatal, mesolimbic, mesopyriform, and tuberohypophyseal systems) exhibit a dramatic response to the administration of DA agonists and antagonists (16,58,182).

A number of independent studies conducted in rodents have demonstrated that DA neurons projecting to the prefrontal and cingulate cortices appear to be resistant to the development of biochemical tolerance following the chronic administration of therapeutically relevant doses of antipsychotic drugs (15,85,130,151,191). This is in contrast to the nigrostriatal, mesolimbic, and mesopyriform DA neurons, which readily develop tolerance during chronic administration of antipsychotic drugs. Furthermore, the time course for the development of tolerance to the biochemical changes elicited by a challenge dose of a DA antagonist parallels the development of autoreceptor supersensitivity (165,166). These studies in rodents have been

extended to nonhuman primates, where tolerance development is observed in the caudate, putamen, and olfactory tubercle, but not in the DA systems projecting to the frontal and cingulate cortices (10,183). Thus it seems likely that autoreceptors may be involved in the development of biochemical tolerance to antipsychotic drugs after longterm administration. The absence of autoreceptors may explain in part why those DA neurons projecting to the prefrontal cortex do not go into depolarization block following chronic treatment with antipsychotic drugs, in contrast to the nigrostriatal and mesolimbic DA neurons (45). However, numerous other mechanisms may also be operative.

The enhanced susceptibility of mesoprefrontal and mesocingulate DA neurons to precursor control of transmitter synthesis may also be related to the absence of DA autoreceptors. These DA neurons selectively increase their synthesis rate following administration of physiologically relevant doses of the precursor tyrosine (209). Precursor dependency has been suggested to be closely related to the physiological firing rate of catecholamine neurons (92,243). The mesoprefrontal and mesocingulate DA neurons exhibit the highest firing frequency and the most bursting of the mesencephalic DA neurons examined (44), probably because they lack impulse-modulating somatodendritic autoreceptors. Thus, it is not surprising that this subset of DA neurons is more susceptible to precursor regulation of transmitter synthesis.

Others

Enhanced Responsiveness of Mesoprefrontal DA Neurons to Stress

It is now well documented that the mesoprefrontal cortical DA system is activated by mild footshock stress or conditioned fear, conditions that do not appreciably activate either other mesotelencephalic (nigrostriatal, mesolimbic, or other mesocortical) DA systems or central noradrenergic systems (36,65,75,115,139,180,216,217). The stress-induced activation of mesoprefrontal DA neurons is antagonized by anxiolytic agents such as diazepam or lorazepam (139,180). The anxiolytic properties of these agents are reversed by benzodiazepine antagonists (171), implicating the involvement of benzodiazepine/γ-aminobutyric acid (GABA) receptors in the stress-induced alterations in mesoprefrontal cortical DA function. The observation that mesoprefrontal neurons differ from nigrostriatal and mesolimbic DA neurons in that they lack impulse-modulating and synthesis-modulating autoreceptors prompted the speculation that lack of autoreceptors might account in part for the unique responsiveness of this system to mild stress (182). However, evidence to date is not entirely consistent with a correlation between lack of autoreceptors and enhanced responsiveness to stress. Although some reports indicate that mesocingulate DA neurons, which also lack autoreceptors, respond to mild stress in a manner similar to mesoprefrontal DA cells (139), other studies have found that the mesocingulate DA system is not activated by mild stress (13,65,115,207). However, stress exposure has been reported to cause small increases in DOPAC or in the ratio

TABLE 1. *Unique characteristics of mesoprefrontal DA neurons compared to nigrostriatal and mesolimbic DA neurons*

1. Higher rate of physiological activity (firing) and a different pattern of activity (more bursting) (44,235)
2. Higher turnover rate of transmitter (2,12,16)
3. Greatly diminished biochemical and electrophysiological responsiveness to DA agonists and antagonists (16,44,235)
4. Lack of tolerance development following chronic antipsychotic drug administration (15,182,191)
5. Resistance to the development of depolarization-induced inactivation following chronic treatment with antipsychotic drugs (46,236)
6. Transmitter synthesis more readily influenced by altered availability of precursor tyrosine (209)

DOPAC/DA in the pyriform cortex, a DA innervation system that possesses autoreceptors (13,17).

It has recently been demonstrated that infusion into the VTA of monoclonal antibodies directed against substance P (SP) prevents the footshock-induced increase in prefrontal cortical DOPAC (13). It therefore seems likely that distinct afferents to different areas within the VTA and SN may, in part, account for the selective responses of various DA systems to stress, rather than solely the presence or absence of somatodendritic and synthesis-modulating nerve terminal DA autoreceptors. The lack of effect of SP antibody infusion on basal mesolimbic or mesocortical DA metabolite levels may argue against a tonic excitatory effect of SP on A10 DA neurons. The precise identity of the VTA neurons innervated by SP afferents remains undetermined, although biochemical studies suggest that only the medial subset of VTA DA neurons show an increase in DA metabolite levels following stress.

Selective Activation of Mesoprefrontal DA Neurons by the Anxiogenic Beta-Carbolines

It is now generally accepted that the pharmacological effects of the anxiolytic benzodiazepines are mediated through specific receptors in the CNS. Beta-Carboline carboxylate esters are specific benzodiazepine receptor ligands that antagonize the various central effects of benzodiazepines (37,198). Some of the beta-carbolines have been found to be anxiogenic in animals and humans (68,163). One of these anxiogenic beta-carbolines, FG 7142 (methyl-beta-carboline-3-carboxamide), produces a dose-dependent increase in DA metabolism in the prefrontal cortex of the rat without causing any significant increase in DA metabolism in other mesocortical, mesolimbic, or nigrostriatal sites (208). This selective increase in DA metabolism induced in the mesoprefrontal DA neurons by FG 7142 is prevented by pretreatment with anxiolytic benzodiazepines (i.e., diazepam, lorazepam) or benzodiazepine antagonists, such as RO 15-1788 (206). These data are consistent with a benzodiazepine-GABA receptor modulation of the mesoprefrontal cortical subset of VTA neurons.

Differential Afferent Control of Ventral Tegmental Neurons

Differential modulation of mesolimbic and mesocortical systems by substance K and substance P. Substance P is a member of a family of peptides known as the tachykinins, which possess the conserved carboxyl terminal sequence -Phe-X-Gly-Leu-Met-NH$_2$. Two other tachykinins, known as substance K (SK; X = Val) and neuromedin K, are also present in mammalian brain (149). The aromatic tachykinin SP (X = Phe) and the aliphatic tachykinin SK are derived from a common prohormone.

SP has been shown to modulate the activity of the mesotelencephalic DA systems (69,93). Thus, unilateral infusion of SP into the region of the A9 DA cells of the SN results in rotational behavior (136), whereas bilateral administration of SP to the A10 DA neurons of the VTA elicits locomotor hyperactivity (133,137). Electrophysiolog-

ical data also suggest that the tachykinins may modulate the activity of dopaminergic neurons in the ventral midbrain (124).

Furthermore, the tachykinins appear to be intricately involved in the response of the prefrontal cortical DA system to stress. Exposure to mild footshock stress selectively activates the prefrontal cortical dopaminergic system arising from VTA neurons (65,216), and results in a concomitant decrease in levels of SP in the VTA (146). This peptidergic involvement in the DA stress response appears to be critical, since immunoneutralization of VTA SP prevents stress-induced mesocortical dopamine activation (13).

Although SP levels decline in the VTA following mild footshock stress (146), recent data indicate that levels of the aliphatic tachykinin SP do not correspondingly decrease (64). Furthermore, VTA injections of SP, but not SK, activate DA metabolism in the prefrontal cortex, whereas SK injections alter DA metabolism in the nucleus accumbens but not the cortical site (64). SK is at least 10 times more potent than SP in inducing locomotor hyperactivity (a mesolimbic phenomena) when injected into the VTA (64,131). These data suggest that SK and SP may differentially modulate subsets of VTA dopaminergic neurons that innervate mesolimbic and mesocortical sites, such that the aromatic tachykinin regulates mesocortical activity, whereas SK represents the physiologically relevant tachykinin that regulates the mesolimbic DA system (64).

Differential modulation of mesolimbic and mesoprefrontal systems by serotonergic and noradrenergic neurons. The VTA receives both serotonergic and noradrenergic afferents from brainstem monoamine neurons (22, 129,156,167,195,201). A number of reports suggest that these monoaminergic inputs to the VTA may be of functional significance in regulating dopaminergic neurons (5,116–118,211). For example, DA utilization is selectively enhanced in the nucleus accumbens but decreased in the prefrontal cortex following electrolytic lesions of the median raphe (117). Lesions of the dorsal raphe reduce dopaminergic utilization in the prefrontal cortex but do not alter DA parameters in the nucleus accumbens (118). Furthermore, DA utilization is decreased in the prefrontal cortex but remains unaltered in the nucleus accumbens following 6-hydroxydopamine-induced degeneration of the noradrenergic fibers projecting to the VTA (116). These results are consistent with the selective modulation of activity of mesolimbic and mesocortical DA neurons by serotonergic and noradrenergic afferents to the VTA. However, it is not clear if such regulation occurs at the level of the cell bodies of origin of these dopaminergic pathways, or alternatively at the terminal field level. Such conclusions will require both the specific delineation of the precise origin of the chemically defined afferents innervating the VTA, and the ruling out of interactive effects occurring either through other afferent inputs or occurring at the level of the terminal fields.

CONCLUSIONS

On the basis of biochemical, anatomical, and electrophysiological studies, there is now compelling evidence that the organization of ascending DA neurons arising from the SN, VTA, and RRF is much more complex than originally suspected. The initial classification scheme indicating the existence of three major systems, namely the nigrostriatal, mesolimbic, and mesocortical systems, no longer seems fully appropriate. It is now recognized that distinct DA subsystems are responsible for the DA innervations of well-defined cortical areas as well as mesolimbic structures. It is also clear that the SN contains DA cells that project not only to the striatum, but to certain cortical and mesolimbic sites as well; furthermore, certain VTA neurons contribute to the striatal dopaminergic innervation. These interdigitating DA subsystems can be distinguished not only on the basis of their origin within the midbrain DA cell groups, but may also be distinguished by virtue of the type of DA neurons they comprise (e.g., shape of the cell body and nature of the dendritic arborization, characteristic axonal morphology, presence of axon collaterals, coexistence of identified peptides or enzymes, existence of autoreceptors), by their physiological profile (e.g., firing rate, degree of bursting, transmitter turnover), by their respective specific afferents, and by their specific reactivity to pharmacological treatments or environmental stimuli. In mesocortical DA systems, such distinctions have been examined extensively in relation to the prefrontal cortical dopaminergic innervation of the rat. Much remains to be done to characterize in a similar way the properties of DA neurons innervating other cortical regions.

The recognition of these important differences in mesotelencephalic DA systems makes it essential for the basic researcher to carefully identify the specific DA subsystem being studied, and to realize that the different subsystems possess different anatomical, biochemical, pharmacological, and physiological characteristics. However, the observed heterogeneity of these mesotelencephalic DA systems portends the development of pharmacological tools that will selectively manipulate various DA subpopulations. The possibility of targeting specific DA systems offers the hope of improved treatments for the neurological and psychiatric disorders believed to be (at least in part) related to a malfunction within these dopaminergic systems.

ACKNOWLEDGMENTS

We thank Amy M. Knorr for helpful discussions. Much of the work cited in this review was supported in part by MH-14092 (R.H.R.), the National Science Foundation (M.E.W.), the Pharmaceutical Manufacturers Association Foundation, Inc. (M.E.W.), MH-09156 (A.Y.D.), the American Parkinson's Disease Association (A.Y.D. and R.H.R.), and the State of Connecticut (R.H.R.).

REFERENCES

1. Aghajanian, G. K., and Roth, R. H. (1970): *J. Pharmacol. Exp. Ther.,* 175:131–137.
2. Agnati, L. F., Fuxe, K., Andersson, K., Benfenati, F., Cortelli, P., and D'Alessandro, R. (1980): *Neurosci. Lett.,* 18:45–51.
3. Albert, K. A., Helmer-Matyjiek, E., Nairn, A. C., Muller, T. H., Haycock, J. W., Greene, L. A., Goldstein, M., and Greengard, P. (1984): *Proc. Natl. Acad. Sci. USA,* 81:7713–7717.
4. Anden, N.-E., Bedard, P., Fuxe, K., and Ungerstedt, U. (1972): *Experientia,* 28:300–302.
5. Antelman, S. M., and Caggiula, A. R. (1977): *Science,* 195:646–653.
6. Arbilla, S., Nowak, J. Z., and Langer, S. Z. (1985): *Brain Res.,* 337:11–17.
7. Argiolas, A., Fadda, F., Melis, M. R., Marcou, M., Porceddu, M. L., and Gessa, G. L. (1982): *Eur. J. Pharmacol.,* 85:23–27.
8. Arluison, M., Javoy-Agid, F., Feuerstein, C., Tauc, M., Verrier, M., and Mailly, P. (1982): *Brain Res. Bull.,* 9:355–366.
9. Aswad, D. W. (1984): *J. Biol. Chem.,* 259:10714–10721.
10. Bacopoulos, N. G., Bustos, G., Redmond, D. E., Baulu, J., and Roth, R. H. (1978): *Brain Res.,* 157:396–401.
11. Baimbridge, K. G., Miller, J. J., and Parks, C. O. (1982): *Brain Res.,* 239:519–525.
12. Bannon, M. J., Bunney, E. B., and Roth, R. H. (1981): *Brain Res.,* 218:376–382.
13. Bannon, M. J., Elliot, P. J., Alpert, J. E., Goedert, M., Iversen, S. D., and Iversen, L. L. (1983): *Nature,* 306:791–792.
14. Bannon, M. J., Michaud, R. L., and Roth, R. H. (1981): *Mol. Pharmacol.,* 19:270–275.
15. Bannon, M. J., Reinhard, J. F., Jr., Bunney, E. B., and Roth, R. H. (1982): *Nature,* 296:444–446.
16. Bannon, M. J., and Roth, R. H. (1983): *Pharmacol. Rev.,* 35:53–68.
17. Bannon, M. J., Wolf, M. E., and Roth, R. H. (1983): *Eur. J. Pharmacol.,* 91:119–125.
18. Beal, M. F., and Martin, J. B. (1985): *Brain Res.,* 358:10–15.
19. Beart, P. M., and Gundlach, A. L. (1980): *Br. J. Pharmacol.,* 69:241–247.
20. Beart, P. M., and McDonald, D. (1980): *J. Neurochem.,* 34:1622–1629.
21. Beart, P. M., McDonald, D., and Gundlach, A. L. (1979): *Neurosci. Lett.,* 15:165–170.
22. Beckstead, R. M., Domesick, V. B., and Nauta, W. J. H. (1979): *Brain Res.,* 175:191–217.
23. Berger, B., and Verney, C. (1984): In: *Monoamine Innervation of Cerebral Cortex,* edited by L. Descarnies, T. R. Reader, and H. H. Jasper, pp. 95–124, Alan R. Liss, New York.
24. Berger, B., Verney, C., Alvarez, C., Vigny, A., and Helle, K. B. (1985): *Neuroscience,* 15:983–998.
25. Billingsley, M. L., and Balaban, C. D. (1985): *Brain Res.,* 358:96–103.
26. Billingsley, M. L., Balaban, C. D., Berresheim, U., and Kuhn, D. M. (1986): *Neurochem. Int.,* 8:255–265.
27. Billingsley, M. L., Kim, S., and Kuhn, D. M. (1985): *Neuroscience,* 15:159–171.
28. Billingsley, M. L., Kincaid, R. L., and Lovenberg, W. (1985): *Proc. Natl. Acad. Sci. USA,* 82:5612–5616.
29. Billingsley, M. L., Kuhn, D., Velletri, P. A., Kincaid, R., and Lovenberg, W. (1984): *J. Biol. Chem.,* 259:6630–6635.
30. Billingsley, M. L., and Lovenberg, W. (1985): *Neurochem. Int.,* 7:575–587.
31. Billingsley, M. L., and Roth, R. H. (1982): *J. Pharmacol. Exp. Ther.,* 223:681–688.
32. Billingsley, M. L., Velletri, P. A., Lovenberg, W., Kuhn, D., Goldenring, J. R., and DeLorenzo, R. J. (1985): *J. Neurochem.,* 44:1442–1450.
33. Bitran, M., and Bustos, G. (1982): *Biochem. Pharmacol.,* 31:2851–2860.
34. Bjorklund, A., and Lindvall, O. (1975): *Brain Res.,* 83:531–537.
35. Bjorklund, A., and Lindvall, O. (1984): In: *Chemical Neuroanatomy: Classical Transmitters in the CNS, Part I,* edited by A. Bjorklund and T. Hokfelt, pp. 55–122. Elsevier, Amsterdam.
36. Blanc, G., Herve, D., Simon, H., Lisoprawski, A., Glowinski, J., and Tassin, J. P. (1980): *Nature,* 284:265–267.
37. Braestrup, C., Schmiechen, R., Neef, G., Nielsen, M., and Petersen, E. N. (1982): *Science,* 216:1241–1243.
38. Bustos, G., and Roth, R. H. (1979): *Biochem. Pharmacol.,* 28:1923–1931.
39. Bustos, G., Roth, R. H., and Morgenroth, V. H., III (1976): *Biochem. Pharmacol.,* 25:2493–2497.
40. Bustos, G., Simon, J., and Roth, R. H. (1980): *J. Neurochem.,* 35:47–57.

41. Carlsson, A. (1983): *J. Neural Transm.*, 57:309–315.
42. Cheramy, A., Leviel, V., and Glowinski, J. (1981): *Nature*, 289: 537–542.
43. Cheramy, A., Nieoullon, A., Michelot, R., and Glowinski, J. (1977): *Neurosci. Lett.*, 4:105–109.
44. Chiodo, L. A., Bannon, M. J., Grace, A. A., Roth, R. H., and Bunney, B. S. (1984): *Neuroscience*, 12:1–16.
45. Chiodo, L. A., and Bunney, B. S. (1983): *J. Neurosci.*, 3:1607–1619.
46. Chiodo, L. A., and Bunney, B. S. (1983): *Neuropharmacology*, 22:1087–1093.
47. Clark, D., and Galloway, M. P. (1985): *Soc. Neurosci. Abstr.*, 11: 1208.
48. Clark, D., Hjorth, S., and Carlsson, A. (1985): *J. Neural Transm.*, 62:1–52.
49. Clark, D., Hjorth, S., and Carlsson, A. (1985): *J. Neural Transm.*, 62:171–207.
50. Cooper, J., Bloom, F., and Roth, R. H. (1986): *The Biochemical Basis of Neuropharmacology.* Oxford University Press, New York.
51. Corsini, G. U., Bonuccelli, U., Rainer, E., and Del Zompo, M. (1985): *J. Neural Transm.*, 64:105–111.
52. Corsini, G. U., Pitzalis, G. F., Bernardi, F., Bocchetta, A., and Del Zompo, M. (1981): *Neuropharmacology*, 20:1309–1313.
53. Cubeddu, L. X., and Hoffmann, I. S. (1982): *J. Pharmacol. Exp. Ther.*, 223:497–501.
54. Cubeddu, L. X., and Hoffmann, I. S. (1983): *J. Neurochem.*, 41: 94–101.
55. Cubeddu, L. X., Hoffmann, I. S., and James, M. K. (1983): *J. Pharmacol. Exp. Ther.*, 226:88–94.
56. Cuello, A. C., and Iversen, L. L. (1978): In: *Interactions Between Putative Neurotransmitters in the Brain*, edited by S. Garattini, J. F. Pujol, and R. Samanin, pp. 127–149, Raven Press, New York.
57. Dahlstrom, A., and Fuxe, K. (1964): *Acta Physiol. Scand.*, 62(*Suppl.* 232):1–64.
58. Demarest, K. T., and Moore, K. E. (1979): *J. Neural Transm.*, 46:263–277.
59. Deutch, A. Y., Elsworth, J. D., Goldstein, M., Fuxe, K., Redmond, D. E., Jr., Sladek, J. R., Jr., and Roth, R. H. (1986): *Neurosci. Lett.*, 68:51–56.
60. Deutch, A. Y., Elsworth, J. D., and Roth, R. H. (1987): *J. Neurochem.* (*submitted*).
61. Deutch, A. Y., Goldstein, M., Bunney, B. S., and Roth, R. H. (1984): *Soc. Neurosci. Abstr.*, 10:9.
62. Deutch, A. Y., Goldstein, M., and Roth, R. H. (1985): *Soc. Neurosci. Abstr.*, 11:208.
63. Deutch, A. Y., Goldstein, M., and Roth, R. H. (1986): *Brain Res.*, 363:307–314.
64. Deutch, A. Y., Maggio, J. E., Bannon, M. J., Kalivas, P. W., Tam, S.-Y., Goldstein, M., and Roth, R. H. (1985): *Peptides*, 6(*Suppl.* 2):113–122.
65. Deutch, A. Y., Tam, S.-Y., and Roth, R. H. (1985): *Brain Res.*, 333:143–146.
66. Di Chiara, G., Onali, P. L., Tissari, A. H., Porceddu, M. L., Morelli, M., and Gessa, G. L. (1978): *Life Sci.*, 23:691–696.
67. Diliberto, E. J., Jr. (1982): In: *Cellular Regulation of Secretion and Release*, edited by M. P. Conn, pp. 147–192, Academic Press, New York.
68. Dorow, R., Horowski, R., Paschelke, G., Amin, M., and Braestrup, C. (1983): *Lancet*, 1:98–99.
69. Elliott, P. J., Alpert, J. E., Bannon, M. J., and Iversen, S. D. (1986): *Brain Res.*, 363:145–147.
70. El Mestikaway, S., Glowinski, J., and Hamon, A. (1986): *J. Neurochem.*, 46:12–22.
71. El Mestikaway, S., Glowinski, J., and Hamon, A. (1983): *Nature*, 302:830–832.
72. El Mestikaway, S., Gozlan, H., Glowinski, J., and Hamon, M. (1985): *J. Neurochem.*, 45:173–184.
73. Elsworth, J. D., Deutch, A. Y., Redmond, D. E., Jr., Sladek, J. R., Jr., and Roth, R. H. (1987): *Life Sci.*, 40:193–202.
74. Eriksson, E., Modigh, K., Carlsson, A., and Wikstrom, H. (1983): *Eur. J. Pharmacol.*, 96:29–36.
75. Fadda, F., Argiolas, A., Melis, M. R., Tissari, A., Onali, P., and Gessa, G. L. (1978): *Life Sci.*, 23:2219–2224.
76. Fallon, J. H. (1981): *J. Neurosci.*, 1:1361–1368.
77. Fallon, J. H., and Moore, R. Y. (1976): *Anat. Rec.*, 185:485.
78. Fallon, J. H., and Moore, R. Y. (1978): *J. Comp. Neurol.*, 180: 545–580.
79. Fallon, J. H., Riley, J. R., and Moore, R. Y. (1978): *Neurosci. Lett.*, 7:157–162.
80. Farnebo, L.-O., and Hamberger, B. (1971): *Acta Physiol. Scand.* (*Suppl.*), 371:35–44.
81. Fuxe, K., Agnati, L. F., Ogren, S.-O., Kohler, C., Calzu, L., Benfenati, F., Goldstein, M., Anderson, K., and Neroth, P. (1983): *Acta Pharm. Suec.* (*Suppl.* 1):60–79.
82. Fuxe, K., Fredholm, B. B., Agnati, L. F., and Corrodi, H. (1978): *Brain Res.*, 146:295–311.
83. Gagnon, C. (1983): *Can. J. Biochem. Cell Biol.*, 61:921–926.
84. Gagnon, C., Kelly, S., Manganiello, V., Vaughn, M., Odya, C., Strittmatter, W., Hoffman, A., and Hirata, F. (1981): *Nature*, 291:515–516.
85. Galloway, M. P., and Roth, R. H. (1983): *Soc. Neurosci. Abstr.*, 9:1003.
86. Galloway, M. P., Wolf, M. E., and Roth, R. H. (1986): *J. Pharmacol. Exp. Ther.*, 236:689–698.
87. Geffen, L. B., Jessell, T. M., Cuello, A. C., and Iversen, L. L. (1976): *Nature*, 260:258–260.
88. Gerfen, C. R., Baimbridge, K. G., and Miller, J. J. (1985): *Proc. Natl. Acad. Sci. USA*, 82:8780–8784.
89. Gessa, G. L., Crabai, F., Vargui, L., and Spano, F. (1968): *J. Neurochem.*, 15:377–381.
90. Gessa, G. L., Vargiu, L., Crabai, F., Boero, C. C., Caboni, R., and Camba, R. (1966): *Life Sci.*, 5:1921–1930.
91. Gianutsos, G., Hynes, M. D., and Lal, H. (1975): *Biochem. Pharmacol.*, 24:581–582.
92. Gibson, C. J. (1985): In: *Handbook of Neurochemistry, Vol. 2*, edited by A. Lajtha, pp. 309–324, Plenum Press, New York.
93. Glowinski, J., Michelot, R., and Cheramy, A. (1980): In: *Neural Peptides and Neural Communication*, edited by E. Costa and M. Trebucchi, pp. 51–61. Raven Press, New York.
94. Goldstein, M., Backstrom, T., Ohi, Y., and Frenkel, R. (1970): *Life Sci.*, 9:919–924.
95. Goldstein, M., Bronaugh, R. L., Ebstein, B., and Roberg, C. (1976): *Brain Res.*, 109:563–574.
96. Gonon, F. G., and Buda, M. J. (1985): *Neuroscience*, 14:765–774.
97. Grace, A. A., and Bunney, B. S. (1983): *Neuroscience*, 10:317–331.
98. Grace, A. A., and Bunney, B. S. (1983): *Neuroscience*, 10:333–348.
99. Grace, A. A., and Bunney, B. S. (1984): In: *Catecholamines: Neuropharmacology and Central Nervous System—Theoretical Aspects*, edited by E. Usdin, A. Carlsson, A. Dahlstrom, and J. Engel, pp. 323–332. Alan R. Liss, New York.
100. Grace, A. A., and Bunney, B. S. (1985): *Brain Res.*, 333:285–298.
101. Graybiel, A. M. (1984): *Neuroscience*, 13:1157–1187.
102. Graybiel, A. M. (1984): In: *Functions of the Basal Ganglia* (Ciba Foundation Symposium 107), pp. 114–149. Pitman, London.
103. Graybiel, A. M., and Ragsddale, C. W., Jr. (1983): In: *Chemical Neuroanatomy*, edited by P. C. Emson, pp. 427–504. Raven Press, New York.
104. Greenfield, S. A. (1985): *Neurochem. Int.*, 7:887–901.
105. Groves, P. M., Fenster, G. A., Tepper, J. M., Nakamura, S., and Young, S. J. (1981): *Brain Res.*, 221:425–431.
106. Haggstrom, J.-E., Gunne, L. M., Carlsson, A., and Wikstrom, H. (1983): *J. Neural Transm.*, 58:135–142.
107. Haglund, L., Kohler, C., Haaparanta, T., Goldstein, M., and Gustafsson, J.-A. (1984): *Nature*, 307:259–262.
108. Harris, J. E., Morgenroth, V. H., III, Roth, R. H., and Baldessarini, R. J. (1974): *Nature*, 252:156–158.
109. Harris, J. E., and Roth, R. H. (1970): *Fed. Proc.*, 29:941.
110. Haubrich, D. R., and Pflueger, A. B. (1982): *Mol. Pharmacol.*, 21:114–120.
111. Haycock, D. A., Greenblatt, S. E., Askins, H. L., and Patrick, R. L. (1984): *Brain Res.*, 299:15–23.
112. Hedreen, J. (1980): *Brain Res. Bull.*, 5:425–436.
113. Hefti, R., Lienhart, R., and Lichtensteiger, W. (1976): *Nature*, 263:341–342.
114. Helmreich, I., Reimann, W., Hertting, G., and Starke, K. (1982): *Neuroscience*, 7:1559–1566.

115. Herman, J. P., Guillonneau, D., Dantzer, R., Scatton, B., Semerdjan-Rouquier, L., and LeMoal, M. (1982): *Life Sci.,* 30: 2207–2214.
116. Herve, D., Blanc, G., Glowinski, J., and Tassin, J. P. (1982): *Brain Res.,* 237:510–516.
117. Herve, D., Simon, H., Blanc, G., LeMoal, M., Glowinski, J., and Tassin, J. P. (1981): *Brain Res.,* 216:422–428.
118. Herve, D., Simon, H., Blanc, G., Lisoprawski, A., LeMoal, M., Glowinski, J., and Tassin, J. P. (1979): *Neurosci. Lett.,* 15:127–133.
119. Hirata, Y., and Nagatsu, T. (1985): *Biochem. Pharmacol.,* 34: 2637–2643.
120. Hoffmann, I. S., and Cubeddu, L. X. (1982): *J. Neurochem.,* 39: 585–588.
121. Hokfelt, T., Everitt, B. J., Theodorsson-Norheim, E., and Goldstein, M. (1984): *J. Comp. Neurol.,* 222:543–559.
122. Hokfelt, T., Martensson, R., Bjorklund, A., Kleinau, S., and Goldstein, M. (1984): In: *Handbook of Chemical Neuroanatomy: Classical Transmitters in the CNS, Part I,* edited by A. Bjorklund and T. Hokfelt, pp. 277–379. Elsevier, Amsterdam.
123. Hokfelt, T., Skirboll, L., Rehfeld, J. F., Goldstein, M., Markey, K., and Dann, O. (1980): *Neuroscience,* 5:2093–2124.
124. Innis, R. B., Andrade, R., and Aghajanian, G. K. (1984): *Brain Res.,* 335:381–383.
125. Iuvone, M. P. (1984): *J. Neurochem.,* 43:1359–1368.
126. Jackisch, R., Zumstein, A., Hertting, G., and Starke, K. (1980): *Naunyn Schmiedebergs Arch. Pharmacol.,* 314:129–133.
127. Jimenez-Castellanos, J., and Graybiel, A. M. (1985): *Soc. Neurosci. Abstr.,* 11:1249.
128. Johnson, B. A., and Aswad, D. W. (1985): *Biochemistry,* 24: 2581–2586.
129. Jones, B. E., and Yang, T.-Z. (1985): *J. Comp. Neurol.,* 242:56–92.
130. Julou, L., Scatton, B., and Glowinski, J. (1977): In: *Advances in Biochemical Psychopharmacology, Vol. 16,* edited by E. Costa and G. L. Gessa, pp. 617–624. Raven Press, New York.
131. Kalivas, P. W., Deutch, A. Y., Maggio, J. E., Mantyh, P. W., and Roth, R. H. (1985): *Neurosci. Lett.,* 57:241–246.
132. Kalivas, P. W., Jennes, L., and Miller, J. S. (1985): *Brain Res.,* 326:229–238.
133. Kalivas, P. W., and Miller, J. S. (1984): *Neurosci. Lett.,* 48:55–59.
134. Kamal, L. A., Arbilla, S., and Langer, S. Z. (1981): *J. Pharmacol. Exp. Ther.,* 216:592–598.
135. Kato, T., Ishii, K., and Ikeda, M. (1984): Voltammetry in unanesthetized rat. *Neurosci. Lett.,* 50:263–267.
136. Kelly, A. E., and Iversen, S. D. (1978): *Brain Res.,* 158:474–478.
137. Kelly, A. E., Stinus, L., and Iversen, S. D. (1979): *Neurosci. Lett.,* 11:335–339.
138. Knorr, A. K., Wolf, M. E., and Roth, R. H. (1986): *Biochem. Pharmacol.,* 35:1929–1932.
139. Lavielle, S., Tassin, J. P., Thierry, A.-M., Blanc, G., Herve, D., Bathelemy, C., and Glowinski, J. (1978): *Brain Res.,* 168:585–594.
140. Lehmann, J., Briley, M., and Langer, S. Z. (1983): *Eur. J. Pharmacol.,* 88:11–26.
141. Lenard, L., and Nauta, W. J. H. (1979): *Neurosci. Lett. (Suppl. 3):570.
142. Leviel, V., Cheramy, A., and Glowinski, J. (1979): *Nature,* 280: 236–239.
143. Levitt, P., Rakic, P., and Goldman-Rakic, P. S. (1984): In: *Monoamine Innervation of Cerebral Cortex,* edited by L. Descarries, T. R. Reader, and H. H. Jasper, pp. 41–59. Alan R. Liss, New York.
144. Lindvall, O., and Bjorklund, A. (1983): In: *Chemical Neuroanatomy,* edited by P. C. Emson, pp. 229–255. Raven Press, New York.
145. Lindvall, O., and Bjorklund, A. (1984): In: *Monoamine Innervation of Cerebral Cortex,* edited by L. Descarries, T. R. Reader, and H. H. Jasper, pp. 9–40. Alan R. Liss, New York.
146. Lisoprawski, A., Blanc, G., and Glowinski, J. (1981): *Neurosci. Lett.,* 25:47–51.
147. Loughlin, S. E., and Fallon, J. H. (1984): *J. Neurosci.,* 11:425–435.
148. Lovenberg, W., Bruckwick, E. A., and Hanbauer, I. (1975): *Proc. Natl. Acad. Sci. USA,* 72:2955–2958.
149. Maggio, J. E., Sandberg, B. E. B., Bradley, C. V., Iversen, L. L., Santikarn, S., Williams, D. H., Hunter, J. C., and Hanley, M. R. (1983): In: *Substance P,* edited by P. Skrabanek and D. Powell, pp. 20–21. Boole Press, Dublin.
150. Maidment, N. J., and Marsden, C. A. (1985): *Brain Res.,* 338: 317–325.
151. Matsumoto, T., Uchimura, H., Hirano, M., Kim, J. S., Yokoo, H., Shimomura, M., Nakahara, T., Inoue, K., and Oomagari, K. (1983): *Eur. J. Pharmacol.,* 89:27–33.
152. Meltzer, H. Y. (1980): *Schizophrenia Bull.,* 6:456–475.
153. Mercer, L., Del Fiacco, M., and Cuello, A. C. (1979): *Experientia,* 35:101–103.
154. Milner, J. D., and Wurtman, R. J. (1986): *Biochem. Pharmacol.,* 35:875–882.
155. Moore, R. Y., and Bloom, F. (1978): *Annu. Rev. Neurosci.,* 1: 129–170.
156. Moore, R. Y., Halaris, A. E., and Jones, B. E. (1978): *J. Comp. Neurol.,* 180:417–438.
157. Morgenroth, V. H., III, Boadle-Biber, M. C., and Roth, R. H. (1976): *Mol. Pharmacol.,* 12:41–48.
158. Morgenroth, V. H., III, Walters, J. R., and Roth, R. H. (1976): *Biochem. Pharmacol.,* 25:655–661.
159. Murray, E. D., Jr., and Clarke, S. (1984): *J. Biol. Chem.,* 259: 10722–10732.
160. Murrin, L. C., Morgenroth, V. H., III, and Roth, R. H. (1976): *Mol. Pharmacol.,* 12:1070–1081.
161. Nieoullon, A., Cheramy, A., and Glowinski, J. (1977): *Nature,* 266:375–377.
162. Nieoullon, A., Cheramy, A., Leviel, A., and Glowinski, J. (1979): *Eur. J. Pharmacol.,* 53:289–296.
163. Ninan, P. T., Insel, T. M., Cohen, R. M., Cook, J. M., Skilnick, P., and Paul, S. M. (1982): *Science,* 218:1332–1334.
164. Nowak, J. Z., Arbilla, S., Galzin, A. M., and Langer, S. Z. (1983): *J. Pharmacol. Exp. Ther.,* 226:558–564.
165. Nowycky, M., and Roth, R. H. (1977): *Naunyn Schmiedebergs Arch. Pharmacol.,* 300:247–254.
166. Nowycky, M., and Roth, R. H. (1978): *Prog. Neuropsychopharmacol.,* 2:139–158.
167. O'Donohue, T. L., Crowley, W. R., and Jacobowitz, D. M. (1979): *Brain Res.,* 172:87–100.
168. Olson, L., and Seiger, A. (1972): *Z. Anat. Entwicklungs.,* 137: 301–346.
169. Olson, L., Seiger, A., and Fuxe, K. (1972): *Brain Res.,* 44:283–288.
170. Onali, P., Mereu, G., Olianas, M. C., Bunse, B., Rossetti, Z., and Gessa, G. L. (1985): *Brain Res.,* 340:1–7.
171. Onel, S., Tam, S.-Y., and Roth, R. H. (1984): *Soc. Neurosci. Abstr.,* 10:881.
172. Parker, E. M., and Cubeddu, L. X. (1985): *J. Pharmacol. Exp. Ther.,* 232:492–500.
173. Phillipson, O. T., and Griffith, A. C. (1980): *Brain Res.,* 197: 213–218.
174. Plantje, J. F., Dijcks, F. A., Verheijden, P. F. H. M., and Stoof, J. C. (1985): *Eur. J. Pharmacol.,* 114:401–402.
175. Pocotte, S. L., and Holz, R. W. (1986): *J. Biol. Chem.,* 261: 1873–1877.
176. Pradhan, S., Alphs, L., and Lovenberg, W. (1981): *Neuropharmacology,* 20:149–154.
177. Raese, J. D., Edelman, A. M., Makk, G., Bruckwick, E. A., Lovenberg, W., and Barchas, J. D. (1979): *Commun. Psychopharmacol.,* 3:295–301.
178. Reader, T. A., Masse, P., and DeChamplain, J. (1979): *Brain Res.,* 177:499–513.
179. Reimann, W., Zumstein, A., Jackisch, R., Starke, K., and Hertting, G. (1979): *Naunyn Schmiedebergs Arch. Pharmacol.,* 306:53–60.
180. Reinhard, J. R., Jr., Bannon, M. J., and Roth, R. H. (1982): *Naunyn Schmiedebergs Arch. Pharmacol.,* 318:374–377.
181. Rosin, D., Wolf, M. E., and Roth, R. H. (1986): *Fed Proc.,* 45: 432.
182. Roth, R. H. (1984): *Ann. NY Acad. Sci.,* 430:27–53.
183. Roth, R. H., Bacapoulos, N. G., Bustos, G., and Redmond, D. E. (1980): *Adv. Biochem. Psychopharmacol.,* 24:513–520.
184. Roth, R. H., Galloway, M. P., Tam, S.-Y., Ono, N., and Wolf, M. E. (1986): In: *Dopamine 84,* edited by G. N. Woodruff, J. A. Poat, and P. J. Roberts, pp. 45–61. Macmillan, London.
185. Roth, R. H., Morgenroth, V. H., III, and Murrin, L. C. (1975):

In: *Antipsychotic Drugs, Pharmacodynamics and Pharmacokinetics,* edited by G. Sedvall, pp. 133–145. Pergamon Press, Oxford and New York.

186. Roth, R. H., and Suhr, Y. (1970): *Biochem. Pharmacol.,* 19: 3001–3012.
187. Roth, R. H., Walters, J. R., and Morgenroth, V. H., III (1974): In: *Neuropsychopharmacology of Monoamines and Their Regulatory Enzymes,* edited by E. Usdin, pp. 369–384. Raven Press, New York.
188. Roth, R. H., Walters, J. R., Murrin, L. C., and Morgenroth, V. H., III (1975): In: *Pre- and Postsynaptic Receptors,* edited by E. Usdin and W. E. Bunney, Jr., pp. 5–46. Marcel Dekker, New York.
189. Saller, C. F., and Salama, A. I. (1984): *J. Neurochem.,* 43:675–688.
190. Saller, C. F., and Salama, A. I. (1985): *Eur. J. Pharmacol.,* 111: 17–22.
191. Scatton, B. (1977): *Eur. J. Pharmacol.,* 46:363–369.
192. Scatton, B., Glowinski, J., and Julou, L. (1976): *Brain Res.,* 109: 184–189.
193. Scatton, B., Simon, H., LeMoal, M., and Bischoff, S. (1980): *Neurosci. Lett.,* 18:125–133.
194. Seroogy, K. B., Mehta, A., and Fallon, J. H. (1987): *Exp. Brain Res. (in press).*
195. Simon, H., LeMoal, M., Stinus, L., and Calas, A. (1979): *J. Neural Transm.,* 44:77–81.
196. Simon, J. R., and Roth, R. H. (1979): *Mol. Pharmacol.,* 16:224–233.
197. Skagerberg, G., Lindvall, O., and Bjorklund, A. (1984): *Brain Res.,* 307:99–108.
198. Skolnick, P., Schweri, M. M., Williams, E. F., Moncada, V. Y., and Paul, S. M. (1982): *Eur. J. Pharmacol.,* 78:133–136.
199. Sotelo, C. (1971): *J. Ultrastruct. Res.,* 36:824–841.
200. Starke, K., Reimann, W., Zumstein, A., and Hertting, G. (1978): *Naunyn Schmiedebergs Arch. Pharmacol.,* 305:27–36.
201. Steinbusch, H. W. M., and Nieuwenhuys, R. (1983): In: *Chemical Neuroanatomy,* edited by P. C. Emson, pp. 131–207. Raven Press, New York.
202. Stoof, J. C., De Boer, T., Sminia, P., and Mulder, A. H. (1982): *Eur. J. Pharmacol.,* 84:211–214.
203. Studler, J. M., Simon, H., Cesselin, F., Legrand, J. C., Glowinski, J., and Tassin, J. P. (1981): *Neuropeptides,* 2:131–139.
204. Swanson, L. W. (1982): *Brain Res. Bull.,* 9:321–353.
205. Tam, S.-Y., Bannon, M. J., and Roth, R. H. (1983): *Soc. Neurosci. Abstr.,* 9:1004.
206. Tam, S.-Y., Deutch, A. Y., Yang, J.-X., Bannon, M. J., and Roth, R. H. (1985): *Soc. Neurosci. Abstr.,* 11:1206.
207. Tam, S.-Y., and Roth, R. H. (1984): *Soc. Neurosci. Abstr.,* 10: 259.11.
208. Tam, S.-Y., and Roth, R. H. (1985): *Biochem. Pharmacol.,* 34: 1595–1598.
209. Tam, S.-Y., and Roth, R. H. (1987): *Life Sci. (in press).*
210. Tamminga, C. A., Gotts, M. D., and Miller, M. R. (1983): *Acta Pharm. Suec. (Suppl. 2)*:153–158.
211. Tassin, J. P., Lavielle, S., Herve, D., Blanc, G., Thierry, A. M., Alvarez, C., Berger, B., and Glowinski, J. (1979): *Neuroscience,* 4:1569–1582.
212. Tepper, J. M., Groves, P. M., and Young, S. J. (1985): *Trends Pharmacol. Sci.,* 6:251–256.
213. Tepper, J. M., Nakamura, S., Young, S. J., and Groves, P. M. (1984): *Brain Res.,* 309:317–333.
214. Tepper, J. M., Young, S. J., and Groves, P. M. (1984): *Brain Res.,* 309:309–316.
215. Thierry, A. M., Chevalier, G., Ferron, A., and Glowinski, J. (1983): *Exp. Brain Res.,* 50:275–282.
216. Thierry, A. M., Tassin, J. P., Blanc, G., and Glowinski, J. (1976): *Nature,* 263:242–244.
217. Thierry, A. M., Tassin, J. P., and Glowinski, J. (1984): In: *Monoamine Innervation of the Cerebral Cortex,* edited by L. Descarries, T. R. Reader, and H. Jasper, pp. 233–262. Alan R. Liss, New York.

218. Tissari, A. H., Atzori, L., and Galdieri, M. T. (1983): *Naunyn Schmiedebergs Arch. Pharmacol.,* 322:89–91.
219. Tissari, H. A., Porceddu, M. L., Argiolas, G., DiChiara, G., and Gessa, G. L. (1978): *Life Sci.,* 23:653–658.
220. Tork, I., Halliday, G., Scheibner, T., and Turner, S. (1984): In: *Modulation of Sensorimotor Activity During Alterations in Behavioral States,* edited by L. Descarries, T. R. Reader, and H. H. Jasper, pp. 39–73. Alan R. Liss, New York.
221. Tork, I., and Turner, S. (1981): *Neurosci. Lett.,* 24:215–219.
222. Verney, C., Baulac, M., Berger, B., Alvarez, C., Vigny, A., and Helle, K. B. (1985): *Neurosci. Lett.,* 14:1039–1051.
223. Vulliet, P. R., Langan, T. A., and Weiner, N. (1980): *Proc. Natl. Acad. Sci. USA,* 77:92–96.
224. Vulliet, P. R., Woodgett, J. R., Ferrari, S., and Hardie, D. G. (1985): *FEBS Lett.,* 182:335–339.
225. Waggoner, W. G., McDermed, J., and Leighton, H. J. (1980): *Mol. Pharmacol.,* 18:91–99.
226. Walters, J. R., and Roth, R. H. (1976): *Naunyn Schmiedebergs Arch. Pharmacol.,* 296:5–14.
227. Walters, J. R., and Roth, R. H. (1976): *Biochem. Pharmacol.,* 25:649–654.
228. Walters, J. R., and Roth, R. H. (1972): *Biochem. Pharmacol.,* 21:2111–2121.
229. Walters, J. R., and Roth, R. H. (1974): *J. Pharmacol. Exp. Ther.,* 191:82–91.
230. Wang, M., Kahill, A. L., and Perlman, R. L. (1986): *J. Neurochem.,* 46:388–393.
231. Wassef, M., Berod, A., and Sotelo, C. (1981): *Neuroscience,* 6: 2125–2139.
232. Westerink, B. H. C. (1985): *Neurochem. Int.,* 7:221–227.
233. Westfall, T. C., Besson, M.-J., Giorguieff, M.-F., and Glowinski, J. (1976): *Naunyn Schmiedebergs Arch. Pharmacol.,* 292:279–287.
234. Westfall, T. C., Perkins, N. A., and Paul, C. (1978): In: *Advances in the Biosciences, Vol. 18: Presynaptic Receptors,* edited by S. Z. Langer, K. Starke, and M. L. Dubocovich, pp. 243–248. Pergamon, Oxford.
235. White, F. J., and Wang, R. Y. (1984): *Life Sci.,* 34:1161–1170.
236. White, F. J., and Wang, R. Y. (1983): *Science,* 221:1054–1057.
237. Wolf, M. E., Galloway, M. P., and Roth, R. H. (1986): *J. Pharmacol. Exp. Ther.,* 236:699–707.
238. Wolf, M. E., Knorr, A. K., Rosin, D., and Roth, R. H. (1987): *(in preparation).*
239. Wolf, M. E., and Roth, R. H. (1985): *J. Neurochem.,* 44:291–298.
240. Wolf, M. E., and Roth, R. H. (1987): In: *Structure and Function of Dopamine Receptors—Receptor Biochemistry and Methodology, Vol. 9,* edited by I. Creese and C. M. Fraser. Alan R. Liss, New York *(in press).*
241. Wolf, M. E., and Roth, R. H. (1987): *Neuropharmacol (in press).*
242. Wolf, M. E., Roth, R. H., Billingsley, M. L., and Lovenberg, W. (1985): In: *S-Adenosylmethionine Interfers With Dopamine AutoReceptor-Mediated Modulation of Dopamine Release But Not Synthesis in Striatal Slices.* Paper presented at The Biochemistry of S-Adenosylmethionine as a Basis for Drug Action—An International Symposium, Bergen, Norway.
243. Wurtman, R. J., Hefti, F., and Melamed, E. (1981): *Pharmacol. Rev.,* 32:315–335.
244. Yamauchi, T., and Fujisawa, H. (1980): *Biochem. Int.,* 1:98–104.
245. Yamauchi, T., and Fujisawa, H. (1981): *Biochem. Biophys. Res. Commun.,* 100:807–813.
246. Yamauchi, T., Nakata, H., and Fujisawa, H. (1981): *J. Biol. Chem.,* 256:5404–5409.
247. Yanagihara, M., Pank, A. W., Langen, T. A., and Weiner, N. (1986): *J. Neurochem.,* 46:562–568.
248. Zivkovic, B., Guidotti, A., and Costa, E. (1974): *Mol. Pharmacol.,* 10:727–735.
249. Zivkovic, B., Guidotti, A., and Costa, E. (1975): *Naunyn Schmiedebergs Arch. Pharmacol.,* 291:193–200.
250. Zivkovic, B., Guidotti, A., and Costa, E. (1975): *Brain Res.,* 92: 516–521.
251. Zivkovic, B., Guidotti, A., Revuelta, A., and Costa, E. (1975): *J. Pharmacol. Exp. Ther.,* 194:37–46.

Psychopharmacology:
The Third Generation of Progress,
edited by Herbert Y. Meltzer.
Raven Press, New York © 1987.

CHAPTER 10

Neurochemistry of Serotonin Neuronal Systems: Consequences of Serotonin Receptor Activation

Elaine Sanders-Bush and P. Jeffrey Conn

During the past decade, emphasis has shifted from the neurochemistry of presynaptic events, such as synthesis and metabolism of the neurotransmitters, to receptor-mediated changes in synaptic neurochemistry. This review reflects that changing emphasis and focuses on the neurochemical consequences of 5HT receptor activation, with particular emphasis on the biochemical transducing systems that are linked to 5HT receptors.

Central serotonin (5HT) receptors have been classified into two major subtypes (5HT-1 and 5HT-2) based on radioligand binding studies (69). The 5HT-1 site has been further subdivided into 5HT-1a, 5HT-1b (67), and 5HT-1c sites (66,84). The classification of the 5HT binding sites is based on the ability of drugs to compete selectively for one or another subsite. However, unless the affinity differences span several orders of magnitude, the "selective" drugs are of limited value in functional studies because of the difficulty in relating doses in a whole-tissue preparation or in the whole animal to the concentrations in membrane-binding assays. Several drugs are selective for the 5HT-2 site versus the 5HT-1a and 5HT-1b sites, including ketanserin (48), mianserin (46,79), LY 53857 (18), and the recently described ritanserin (47), but the selectivity may be lost with the recent discovery of yet another 5HT-1 subtype, the so-called 5HT-1c site (65,66,84). This new site actually has a pharmacology that resembles the 5HT-2 site, but the name 5HT-1c was chosen because, in common with other 5HT-1 sites, it has a high affinity for 5HT.

Whether or not the four 5HT recognition sites defined in binding assays actually function as 5HT receptors remains to be determined. This chapter will review the biochemical studies directed at defining functional correlates of activation of the various 5HT "receptor" subtypes defined in binding assays. Identification of the biochemical transducing systems that are linked to these sites is one important way to evaluate their role. Two major transducing systems that mediate signal transmission for neurotransmitters are the adenylate cyclase/cyclic AMP signal cascade and phospholipase C-mediated hydrolysis of membrane phosphoinositides. Only recently has it been possible to examine the mechanism of signal transduction in central 5HT receptor systems, and evidence is emerging that the two major transducing systems are linked to different 5HT receptors in mammalian brain. These studies will be reviewed. In addition, the biochemical studies of autoreceptor regulation of 5HT release will be examined, with emphasis on the receptor subtype that mediates this response. An obvious limitation of binding assays is the inability to ascertain definitively whether a drug binds to a site as an agonist or as an antagonist. Such classifications depend on functional studies. However, frequently the action of a drug is defined in functional models reflecting a specific site and then generalized to all 5HT receptor sites, when in fact the same drug may have opposite effects at different 5HT receptors. Such examples are pointed out in this article.

HYDROLYSIS OF MEMBRANE PHOSPHOINOSITIDES

The phospholipase C/phosphoinositide hydrolysis mechanism utilizes inositol lipids [phosphatidylinositol (PI), phosphatidylinositol-4-phosphate (PIP), and phosphatidylinositol-4,5-bisphosphate (PIP_2)] in the membrane as a first step in the transducing mechanism (Fig. 1). The interaction of an agonist with its membrane receptor leads to activation of phospholipase C, which catalyzes the hydrolysis of membrane phosphoinositides. It is generally thought that PIP_2 is the primary substrate for the activated enzyme and that both products of PIP_2 hydrolysis, inositol-1,4,5-tris-phosphate (IP_3) and diacylglycerol, act as second messengers to elicit cellular responses. The sugar product, IP_3, elevates cytosol calcium levels by releasing intracellular storage pools. Calcium ions then serve as a "third messenger" to evoke responses such as muscle contraction and neurotransmitter release by activating specific enzymes, e.g., calcium/calmodulin-dependent protein kinases. The second product formed by the hydrolysis of PIP_2 is diacylglycerol. Diacylglycerol stimulates protein kinase C, an enzyme that regulates cellular events by phosphorylating key proteins. The physiological consequences of protein kinase C activation have not been completely worked out, but evidence is emerging that this enzyme is involved in a number of processes, including heterologous receptor desensitization and the control of cell division and differentiation. Another important consequence of the rise in diacylglycerol is the release of arachidonic acid, which leads to the formation of prostaglandins and leukotrienes. These "icosanoids" have numerous cellular effects. Progress in understanding the phospholipase C/phosphoinositide hydrolysis signal-transducing system has recently exploded. Interested readers are referred to reviews by leading authorities for additional details (7,41).

Recent evidence suggests that the phosphoinositide signaling pathway is involved in 5HT transmission. 5HT-stimulated phosphoinositide hydrolysis was first characterized in insect salivary gland, where it was demonstrated that this second messenger system is involved in the regulation of saliva secretion (11). Limited studies by Berridge et al. (10) suggested that 5HT activates phosphoinositide hydrolysis in mammalian brain. We have recently extended these studies with the aim of determining which receptor(s) mediates the 5HT/phosphoinositide effect in rat brain (20,21). For these studies, slices of cerebral cortex were prelabeled with [³H]inositol and the method of Berridge et al. (10) was used to measure the accumulation of [³H]inositol-1-phosphate (IP) as an index of the hydrolysis of radiolabeled phosphoinositides. IP is formed by the sequential dephosphorylation of IP_3 to IP_2 and then to IP (Fig. 1). Further metabolism of IP is prevented by the addition of lithium, which amplifies the response and makes it possible to study 5HT-stimulated phosphoinositide hydrolysis in brain, where the signal is relatively weak.

The addition of increasing concentrations of 5HT to prelabeled cortical slices results in the accumulation of increasing amounts of IP (Fig. 2). The response is maximum at 10 μM and has an EC_{50} value of 1 μM. A number of 5HT agonists, including quipazine, MK212, and 5-fluoro-tryptamine, stimulate phosphoinositide hydrolysis, but the selective 5HT-1 agonist, 8-hydroxy-2-(di-*N*-propyl-amino)tetralin, is inactive. Concentration-effect studies of several 5HT agonists showed that the EC_{50} values and the rank order of potencies at stimulating phosphoinositide hydrolysis in cerebral cortex agree with their potencies at the 5HT-2 binding site (21). Furthermore, a number of 5HT-2 antagonists, including spiperone, ketanserin, LY 53857, pizotifen, pipamperone, and cinanserin, block 5HT activation of phosphoinositide hydrolysis in cortical slices (20,21,44). In order to obtain an estimate of the absolute affinity (K_d) of antagonists for the phosphoinositide-hydrolysis-linked receptor, concentration-response curves of the effect of 5HT were measured in the presence of increasing

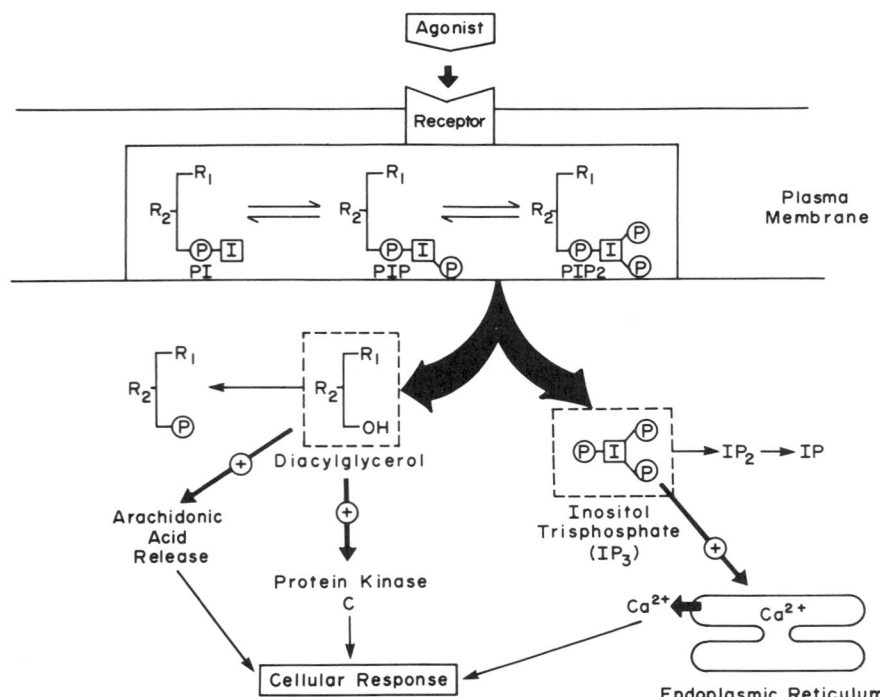

FIG. 1. Schematic illustration of the phospholipase C/phosphoinositide hydrolysis signal cascade. Phosphatidylinositol (PI) is sequentially phosphorylated to phosphatidylinositol-4-phosphate (PIP) and then to phosphatidylinositol-4,5-bisphosphate (PIP_2) by specific kinases. Agonist interaction with membrane receptors leads to the activation of phospholipase C, which catalyzes the hydrolysis of PIP_2 to form inositol-1,4,5-trisphosphate (IP_3) and diacylglycerol. The pathways of inactivation and the second messenger functions are shown.

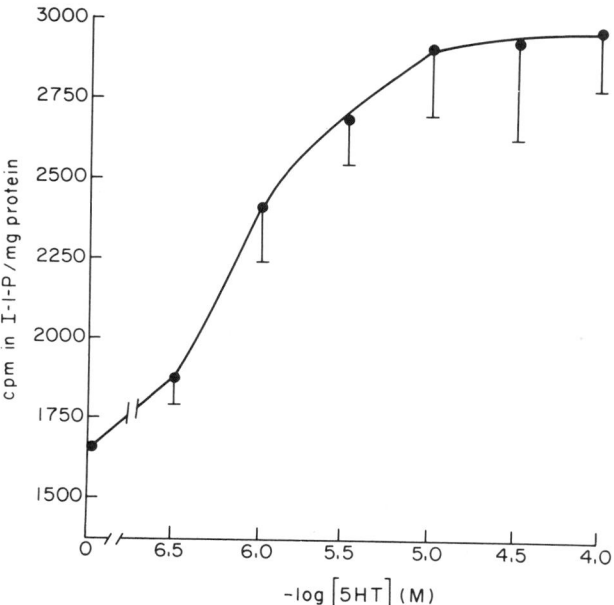

FIG. 2. 5HT-stimulated phosphoinositide hydrolysis in rat cerebral cortex. Cortical slices were prelabeled by incubating with [³H]inositol. Increasing concentrations of 5HT were added and the release of [³H]inositol phosphate was measured as described in Conn and Sanders-Bush (21). The values plotted are the means ±SEM for three determinations.

concentrations of antagonist, as illustrated in Fig. 3 for ketanserin. Dose ratios were determined and analyzed by the method of Arunlakshana and Schild (4). The slope of the Schild plot (inset, Fig. 3) is not different from unity, which suggests that ketanserin is a simple competitive antagonist of the phosphoinositide-hydrolysis-linked receptor. The pA_2 value of ketanserin is −7.93, corresponding to an estimated K_d of 12 nM, which agrees with the K_d value (3 nM) of [³H]ketanserin for the 5HT-2 binding site when measured in the presence of physiological salts. A number of other antagonists were analyzed in this manner, and for those that gave results consistent with competitive antagonism, K_d values were determined (Table 1). A plot of the K_d values determined by Schild analyses versus K_i values at the 5HT-2 binding site is linear (Fig. 4). Regression analysis showed a significant correlation between the potencies of these drugs at inhibiting 5HT-stimulated phosphoinositide hydrolysis and at inhibiting the binding of [³H]ketanserin to the 5HT-2 site (correlation coefficient, 0.99; $p < 0.001$). Furthermore, antagonists of H-1 histaminergic, alpha-1 adrenergic, and muscarinic cholinergic receptors do not block the effect of 5HT, which suggests that these receptors are not involved in this response. Based on these data, we have hypothesized that 5HT-stimulated phosphoinositide hydrolysis in rat cerebral cortex is linked to the 5HT-2 binding site. However, the finding that activation of a given receptor stimulates phosphoinositide hydrolysis does not necessarily mean that the receptor is

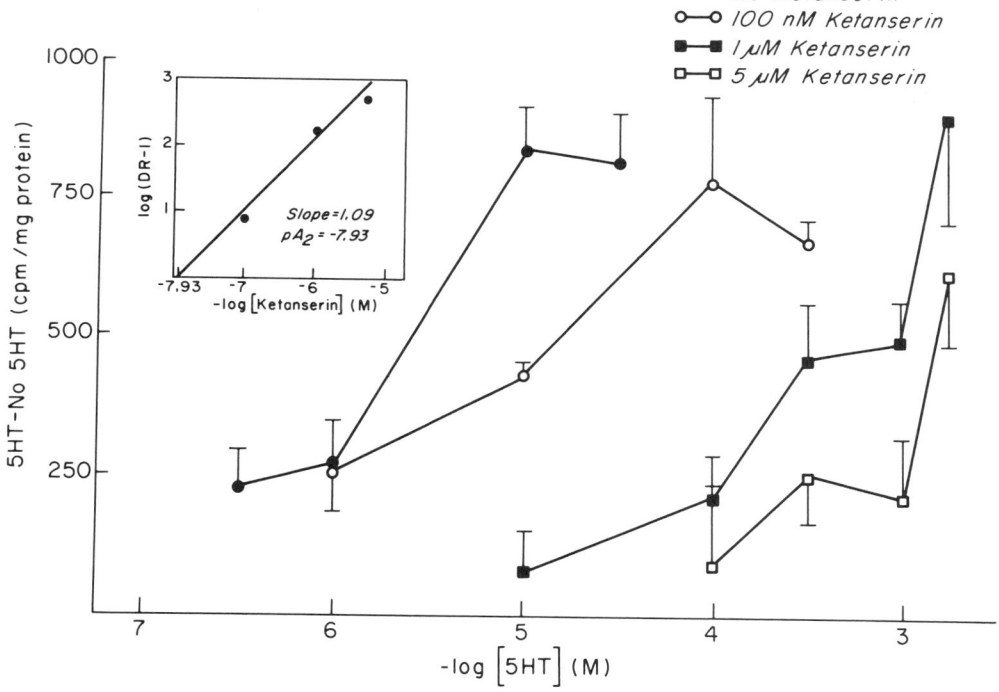

FIG. 3. Schild analysis of ketanserin's antagonism of 5HT-stimulated phosphoinositide hydrolysis in cortical slices. 5HT concentration-response curves were generated in the presence of increasing concentrations of ketanserin. **Inset** shows the Schild plot of the same data. The dose ratio (DR) was calculated by dividing the concentration of 5HT needed to elicit a response of 600 cpm/mg of protein in the presence of ketanserin by the concentration of 5HT needed to elicit the same response in the absence of ketanserin. The pA_2 (−log K_d) value was obtained by extrapolation of the line to the x-axis. Each point represents the mean of two separate experiments, each done in triplicate. Vertical bars represent the SEM. (From ref. 21.)

TABLE 1. K_d values (nM) at cerebral cortex phosphoinositide-hydrolysis-linked receptor and at the 5HT-2 binding site

Antagonist	Response[a]	5HT-2 binding[b]
Spiperone	2	2
Ketanserin	12	3
Pizotifen	12	4
Mianserin	14	7
Cinanserin	148	21
Trazadone	240	24
Promethazine	500	63

[a] K_d values for inhibition of 5HT-stimulated phosphoinositide hydrolysis in rat cerebral cortex were determined by Schild analyses as described in the legend to Fig. 3.

[b] K_d values for the 5HT-2 site were determined by competition with [³H]ketanserin binding in rat frontal cortex membrane preparations.

directly linked to this transducing system. The phosphoinositide hydrolysis response to certain agonists is secondary to receptor-mediated neurotransmitter release (15) or to arachidonate metabolism (72,81). We have shown, however, that the 5HT-2-mediated phosphoinositide hydrolysis response in cerebral cortex is not dependent on either of these indirect mechanisms (22). Taken together, our studies in brain suggest that the 5HT-2-binding site is a functional receptor that utilizes phosphoinositide hydrolysis as its transducing mechanism. Studies of 5HT-stimulated phosphoinositide hydrolysis in platelets (27) and in aorta (73,74) are consistent with this conclusion. The hypothesis that the 5HT-2-binding site employs the phosphoinositide transducing system is supported by several other recent findings. 5HT evokes calcium fluxes in human platelets and this response is blocked by selective 5HT-2 antagonists (2). Furthermore, 5HT stimulates and ketanserin blocks the

phosphorylation of a 40-kDa and 20-kDa protein in human platelets (28). Since these proteins have been shown to be phosphorylated by protein kinase C (63,75), this finding suggests that 5HT may activate the phosphoinositide hydrolysis signal cascade via a 5HT-2 receptor. Lastly, 5HT increases prostacyclin synthesis in cultured cells from bovine aortic smooth muscle and the pharmacology of this response is similar to the pharmacology of the 5HT-2 binding site (24,25).

Studies of the actions of trifluoromethylphenylpiperazine (TFMPP) and *m*-chlorophenylpiperazine (MCPP) on the 5HT-2-linked phosphoinositide hydrolysis system in the cerebral cortex have yielded some surprising findings. These compounds are generally thought to be agonists at all central 5HT receptors with which they interact. However, the efficacy at the various 5HT receptor subtypes has not been rigorously tested. Using the cortical phosphoinositide hydrolysis system, we have characterized the actions of these and other piperazines at central 5HT-2 receptors. Quipazine and MK-212 function as partial agonists at these receptors. In contrast, TFMPP and MCPP fail to stimulate phosphoinositide hydrolysis at concentrations that completely inhibit the response to 5HT (Fig. 5). These drugs shift the 5HT concentration-effect curve to the right without changing the maximum response. Thus, TFMPP and MCPP act as pure antagonists of the 5HT-2 receptors in brain. This finding is consistent with the report that these drugs antagonize the contractile effects of 5HT in vascular smooth muscle (17), a response that is clearly mediated by the 5HT-2 site (19). Since it is unlikely that responses to 5HT that are mimicked by MCPP and TFMPP are mediated by

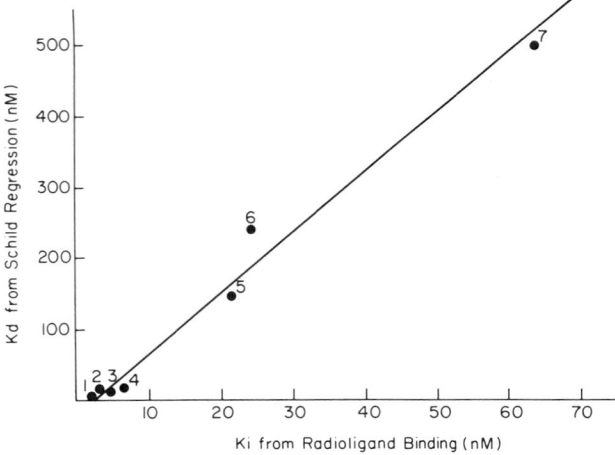

FIG. 4. Correlation between inhibition of 5HT-stimulated phosphoinositide hydrolysis and inhibition of [³H]ketanserin binding to the 5HT-2 site. The values were obtained from Table 1. Symbols: 1, spiperone; 2, ketanserin; 3, pizotifen; 4, mianserin; 5, cinanserin; 6, trazadone; 7, promethazine.

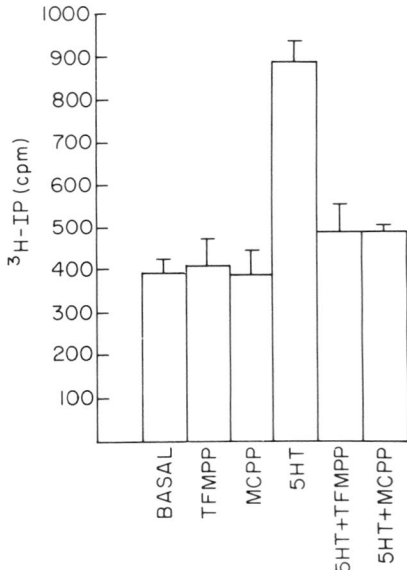

FIG. 5. Antagonism of 5HT-stimulated phosphoinositide hydrolysis by piperazines. Prelabeled rat cerebral cortical slices were incubated with 25-μM concentrations of trifluoromethylphenylpiperazine (TFMPP) or *m*-chlorophenylpiperazine (MCPP) in the presence or absence of 5 μM 5HT. Values plotted are means of three to six determinations ±SEM. The piperazines had no effect on the basal release of [³H]IP, but blocked the stimulatory effect of 5HT.

the 5HT-2 binding site, these compounds will be useful in future studies aimed at determining which 5HT receptor subtype mediates different central effects of 5HT.

The phospholipid substrates and the second messenger products of 5HT-2-initiated phosphoinositide hydrolysis have not yet been characterized in brain. Phospholipase C-type phosphodiesterases catalyze the hydrolysis of all three of the membrane phosphoinositides. With most phosphoinositide-linked receptors, including 5HT-stimulated phosphoinositide hydrolysis in insect salivary gland (6,8,9), the primary substrate for the activated phospholipase C is PIP_2 leading to the formation of two second messengers, IP_3 and diacylglycerol. However, we have been unable to demonstrate 5HT-stimulated formation of IP_3 in cerebral cortex, probably because the signal is too weak. Alternatively, perhaps one of the other phosphoinositides is the substrate for the 5HT-activated phospholipase C in cerebral cortex. This question has more than theoretical interest, since it would determine whether one or two second messengers were formed.

5-HT-stimulated phosphoinositide hydrolysis in subcortical regions of rat brain is apparently mediated by mechanisms other than activation of the 5HT-2 receptor (21,42), but the pharmacology of these effects has not been worked out. We have recently identified a unique 5HT receptor in the choroid plexus that is coupled to phosphoinositide hydrolysis (23). The effect of 5HT on IP formation is much more robust in choroid plexus (fivefold stimulation, Fig. 6) than in cerebral cortex (twofold stimulation, Fig. 2). Furthermore, the potency of 5HT is about 10-fold higher in the choroid plexus. With such a robust signal in choroid plexus, it was possible to follow the time course of the formation of all three inositol sugars (Fig. 7). Both IP_3 and

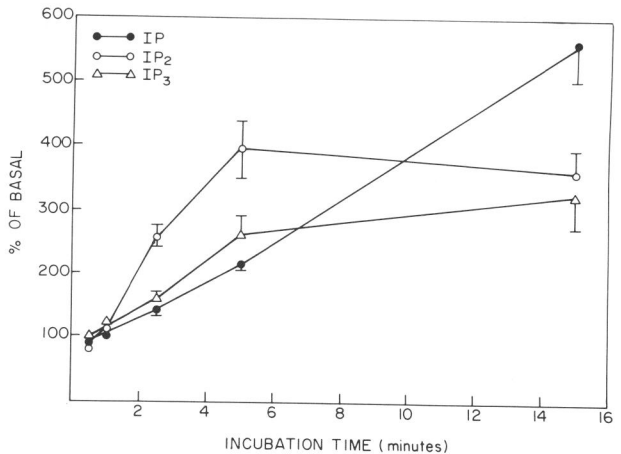

FIG. 7. Time course of the formation of inositol sugars after the addition of 5HT. Individual choroid plexuses were prelabeled with [³H]inositol. 5HT (10 μM) was added at time zero and the incubation was continued for the indicated times. The levels of radioactive IP, IP_2, and IP_3 were measured after purification by anion-exchange chromatography (10). The values are presented as percent of the basal levels and are the mean ±SEM of five or six determinations.

inositol bisphosphate (IP_2) increase early and peak at about 5 min. The levels of IP, on the other hand, continue to rise linearly, reflecting the inhibition of its further metabolism by lithium. These results demonstrate, for the first time, that PIP_2 hydrolysis in brain is activated by 5HT receptors, but they do not exclude the possibility that hydrolysis of the other phosphoinositides is also increased. The finding that 5HT is more potent (EC_{50} 46 nM) in the choroid plexus than it is at the cerebral cortical 5HT-2 receptor (EC_{50} 1,000 nM) suggests that different receptors may mediate these effects. Therefore, the pharmacology of the response in choroid plexus was compared with that in the cerebral cortex, and with the pharmacology of the 5HT-2 binding site. Furthermore, the properties of 5HT-stimulated phosphoinositide hydrolysis in choroid plexus were compared with the recently described 5HT-1c binding site, which is highly localized in this tissue (66,84). The K_i value of 5HT at competing for the 5HT-1C binding site (94 nM) is similar to its EC_{50} value at the phosphoinositide-linked receptor in choroid plexus, but not in cerebral cortex. Furthermore, the rank order and absolute potencies of antagonists in blocking phosphoinositide hydrolysis and 5HT-1C binding are in excellent agreement (Table 2). Consistent with its low potency at the 5HT-1C binding site, spiperone is a very weak antagonist of 5HT-stimulated phosphoinositide hydrolysis in choroid plexus (Table 2), whereas it is the most potent antagonist of the response in cerebral cortex (Table 1). Based on the pharmacological similarity of the phosphoinositide hydrolysis response and the 5HT-1C binding site, we have concluded that the 5HT-1C binding site on choroid plexus epithelial cells is a functional receptor that is linked to phosphoinositide hydrolysis. It remains to be determined if this receptor mediates any of the known physiological effects of 5HT, such as inhibition of cerebrospinal fluid production (51).

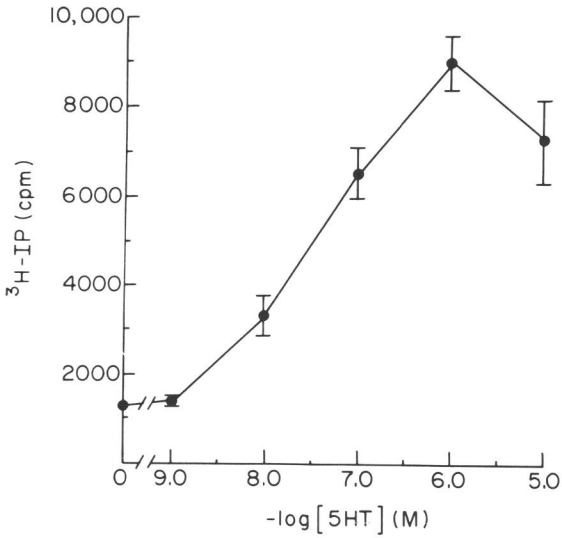

FIG. 6. 5HT-stimulated phosphoinositide hydrolysis in rat choroid plexus. Individual whole choroid plexuses were prelabeled by incubating with [³H]inositol. Increasing concentrations of 5HT were added and the release of [³H]inositol phosphate (IP) was measured as described in Conn et al. (23). Values plotted are means ±SEM for three determinations.

TABLE 2. K_d values (nM) at choroid plexus phosphoinositide-hydrolysis-linked receptor and at 5HT-1c and 5HT-2 binding sites

Antagonist	Response[a]	Radioligand binding	
		5HT-2[b]	5HT-1c[c]
Mianserin	12	7	5
Ketanserin	130	3	195
Spiperone	6,200	2	4,600

[a] Adapted from ref. 23.
[b] Competition with [^{3}H]ketanserin, from ref. 21.
[c] Competition with [^{125}I]LSD, from ref. 23.

The "selective" 5HT-2 antagonist ketanserin has a moderately high affinity for the 5HT-1C receptor (Table 2). Frequently, the finding that a single dose of ketanserin blocks a response to 5HT is taken as evidence that that response is mediated by the 5HT-2 binding site. However, caution should be taken in making such a conclusion since the 5HT-1C receptor is also blocked by ketanserin. Mianserin, another antagonist with selectivity for the 5HT-2 versus the 5HT-1a and 5HT-1b sites, has equal affinity for the 5HT-1c receptor (Table 2) and the 5HT-2 sites (Table 1). Spiperone, on the other hand, distinguishes between 5HT-1c and 5HT-2 sites, with more than three orders of magnitude difference in its affinities for the two sites. It remains to be determined if other "selective" 5HT-2 antagonists remain selective when evaluated at this new receptor site.

The choroid plexus is a relatively simple tissue containing a monolayer of epithelial cells (56), which can readily be dissociated and grown in culture (26). This fact, coupled with the high 5HT-1C receptor density (84) and the robust phosphoinositide response in this tissue, could make it a useful model system for studying the molecular mechanisms underlying the coupling of phosphoinositide-linked receptors to phospholipase C.

ADENYLATE CYCLASE/CYCLIC AMP SIGNAL CASCADE

The second major signaling pathway, adenylate cyclase activation, leads to the formation of cyclic AMP, a second messenger that affects numerous cellular processes by activation of specific protein kinases. 5HT-induced cyclic AMP formation was first demonstrated in tissue particles of the liver fluke *Fasciola hepatica* (53), where cyclic AMP apparently mediates the effects of 5HT on carbohydrate metabolism and on motility (52,80). Since then, 5HT-sensitive adenylate cyclase systems have been described in a number of invertebrate tissues where they are responsible for modulation of functions as diverse as neurotransmitter release (45), muscle contraction (39,45), saliva secretion (11), and permeability of various ion channels (1,71,78). Compared with the invertebrate systems, relatively little is known about the role of cyclic AMP in mediating responses to 5HT in mammalian tissues. In facial motor nucleus of rat brain, 5HT stimulates phosphorylation of protein I by

an apparently cyclic AMP-dependent mechanism (30). Protein I is localized in presynaptic terminals where it may modulate neurotransmitter release. This suggestion is consistent with the cyclic AMP-mediated effect of 5HT on neurotransmitter release at the crustacean neuromuscular junction (45). A role for cyclic AMP in rat adrenal glomerulosa cells is suggested by the finding that in this tissue 5HT stimulates aldosterone and cyclic AMP production with a similar time course (3). Furthermore, nonhydrolyzable analogs of cyclic AMP mimic the effect of 5HT on aldosterone production (38).

The first demonstration that 5HT stimulates adenylate cyclase in a vertebrate tissue was by Kakiuchi and Rall (43), who showed that 5HT elicits a three- to fourfold increase in cyclic AMP levels in slices of rabbit cerebellum. Subsequently, micromolar concentrations of 5HT were found to stimulate adenylate cyclase in a cell-free preparation from immature rat brain (82,83). This adenylate cyclase system is distributed in several cortical and subcortical regions, with the largest response in superior and inferior colliculi. The increase in cyclic AMP, which is maximum (50–80% above basal) in 1- to 3-day-old rats, progressively diminishes with age so that it is barely detectable in 42-day-old rats. Although this may reflect a role of 5HT-stimulated adenylate cyclase in development, it should be noted that basal adenylate cyclase activity increases with age, and when expressed as nanomoles of cyclic AMP formed per milligram of protein per hour, the effect of 5HT is constant during development (33,82). This finding suggests that the number of adenylate-cyclase-coupled 5HT receptors present in the colliculi at birth remains constant during development, while the activity of adenylate cyclase systems that are sensitive to other neurotransmitters increases with age. It is likely that 5HT-sensitive adenylate cyclase in colliculi of immature rats is coupled to a 5HT receptor, since it is stimulated by a variety of 5HT agonists and inhibited by classical 5HT antagonists (34,83). Furthermore, the regional distribution of 5HT-sensitive adenylate cyclase activity is closely related to the distribution of 5HT nerve terminals (33). However, this receptor is apparently distinct from the 5HT binding sites defined in radioligand studies. Nelson et al. (64) showed that the pharmacology of the [^{3}H]5HT binding site is clearly distinct from that of 5HT-stimulated adenylate cyclase. For example, cyproheptadine, clozapine, and thioproperazine are more potent than metergoline at inhibiting 5HT-sensitive adenylate cyclase, but are less potent at competing for the 5HT-1 binding site. Other compounds (e.g., the piperazines) that bind to the 5HT-1 site with relatively high affinity have no effect on collicular 5HT-stimulated adenylate cyclase. Furthermore, 5HT has a nanomolar affinity for the 5HT-1 binding site, whereas the EC_{50} value for stimulating collicular adenylate cyclase is 1 μM. Given the possibility of spare receptors, the EC_{50} value of 5HT at stimulating adenylate cyclase should be equal to or less than its K_i value for the receptor mediating that response. Although it is possible that these differences could be reconciled if the specific 5HT-1 subtypes were taken into account, this seems unlikely. Furthermore, the pharmacological profile of the collicular adenylate-cyclase-linked receptor is clearly distinct from the profiles of the 5HT-2 and 5HT-1c binding sites.

5HT stimulates cyclic AMP production in a striatal crude membrane preparation with two apparent affinities (37). The EC_{50} values are 1 nM and 1 μM. Only the high-affinity system is present in an enriched synaptosomal preparation, whereas both the high- and low-affinity systems are found in a mitochondrial fraction. Since the nanomolar potency of 5HT at the high-affinity adenylate cyclase system is consistent with its K_i at the 5HT-1 binding sites, it is tempting to speculate that this response is mediated by one of these sites. Indeed, cinanserin, methysergide, and cyproheptadine inhibit the effect of 5HT in striatal synaptosomes with potencies that resemble their potencies for [³H]5HT binding. Furthermore, kainic acid lesions of striatal neurons cause a complete loss of [³H]5HT binding and of the high-affinity, but not the low-affinity, 5HT-sensitive adenylate cyclase (36). Further studies are needed to investigate the possibility that a 5HT-1 site is linked to the high-affinity adenylate cyclase system. Unfortunately, only one group has reported detection of the high-affinity system.

A 5HT-activated adenylate cyclase is found in adult rat (5) and guinea pig (76) hippocampus. Pretreatment with reserpine (76) or with para-chlorophenylalanine (5) markedly potentiates this response. Metergoline, spiperone, and pizotifen antagonize 5HT activation of adenylate cyclase in hippocampus, but the selective 5HT-2 antagonists ketanserin and mianserin are inactive. Kainic acid lesions cause a complete loss of 5HT-sensitive adenylate cyclase activity, but only a 40% reduction in the binding of [³H]5HT. Furthermore, 5,7-dihydroxytryptamine lesions cause a smaller increase in [³H]5HT binding than in 5HT-stimulated adenylate cyclase activity. Based on these findings, Barbaccia et al. (5) suggested that the hippocampal response is mediated by a subpopulation of 5HT-1 recognition sites. Shenker et al. (77) found that 5-carboxyamidotryptamine stimulates adenylate cyclase in hippocampus with a biphasic concentration-response curve and suggested that two separate 5HT receptors mediate this response. Spiperone inhibits the response to low concentrations of 5-carboxyamidotryptamine with an apparent K_i value consistent with its K_i value at the 5HT-1a binding site. Furthermore, the selective 5HT-1a ligand 8-hydroxy-2-(di-n-propylamine)tretraline (8-OH-DPAT) is a partial agonist in hippocampal membranes. Although these data are consistent with the argument that the 5HT-1a site is linked to adenylate cyclase, the evidence is not compelling. Potencies of a wide range of antagonists should be compared before making a conclusion about the receptor subtype mediating the hippocampal adenylate cyclase response. Recently, Devivo and Maayani (29) reported that 5HT inhibits forskolin-activated adenylate cyclase in the same hippocampal preparation that was used for the studies of 5HT-stimulated adenylate cyclase. This inhibitory response has the same pharmacological properties as those of 5HT-stimulated adenylate cyclase, leading these authors to conclude that the 5HT-1a site is linked to both stimulation and inhibition of adenylate cyclase. Before accepting such a conclusion, additional studies are needed.

5HT stimulates adenylate cyclase activity in NCB-20 neuroblastoma $\times$ brain cell hybrids (12,50). The relative potencies of four agonists and three antagonists at competing for [³H]5HT binding in these cells closely resemble their relative potencies at the 5HT-sensitive adenylate cyclase. Furthermore, 5HT has a K_d value at the [³H]5HT binding site that is similar to its K_d at the adenylate-cyclase-linked receptor. The addition of gangliosides increases the affinity of 5HT for this binding site and causes a parallel increase in the potency of 5HT in stimulating adenylate cyclase activity (13). Unfortunately, comparison of the antagonist profile suggests that the [³H]5HT binding site on NCB-20 cells may not be identical with the 5HT-1 sites found in brain homogenates.

It warrants mention that Peroutka et al. (68) demonstrated that [³H]5HT binding in brain is modulated by guanine nucleotides, a finding that has since been confirmed by many other laboratories. Based on this finding, Peroutka et al. (68) suggested that the 5HT-1 binding site is linked to adenylate cyclase. However, since then, it has become clear that receptors that are not linked to adenylate cyclase can be modulated by guanine nucleotides (14,35,49).

In summary, although a number of investigators have suggested that 5HT-1 sites are linked to adenylate cyclase, the evidence that this is the case is not compelling. It is clear that the low-affinity 5HT-sensitive adenylate cyclase characterized in immature rat colliculi is not mediated by a 5HT-1 site. Furthermore, it is clear that none of the characterized 5HT-stimulated adenylate cyclase responses are mediated by the 5HT-2 or the 5HT-1c binding sites, both of which are linked to phosphoinositide hydrolysis (see Hydrolysis of Membrane Phosphoinositides). More data must be gathered before definitive conclusions can be made concerning the 5HT-sensitive adenylate cyclase systems in hippocampus, striatum, or NCB-20 cells. In gathering these data, particular attention should be paid to discriminating between 5HT-1a and 5HT-1b binding sites.

RECEPTOR-MEDIATED CHANGES IN 5HT RELEASE

Inhibition of 5HT release is a biochemical measure of 5HT autoreceptor activation. Autoreceptor-mediated inhibition of 5HT release has been demonstrated in vitro using superfusion systems and [³H]5HT or [³H]tryptophan to label the synaptic stores of 5HT. This control mechanism is found in numerous terminal areas, including hippocampus, cerebral cortex, hypothalamus, striatum, cerebellum, and spinal cord. More recently, sensitive high-pressure-liquid chromatography/electrochemical detection (hplc/ec) methodology has made it possible to demonstrate autoreceptor regulation of the release of endogenous 5HT in superfused synaptosomes (70). The properties and role of the terminal 5HT autoreceptors have been extensively reviewed (61). The current article focuses on the more recent work directed at the relation between the autoreceptors and specific 5HT binding sites.

The early studies of Martin and Sanders-Bush (55) in hypothalamic synaptosomes and of Engel et al. (32) in cortical slices demonstrated that the autoreceptor has pharmacological properties in common with the 5HT-1 binding site labeled with [³H]5HT. Both groups found a significant correlation between potencies of agonists at competing for [³H]5HT binding and at inhibiting 5HT release, as illustrated in Fig. 8. Furthermore, the potencies of antagonists for [³H]5HT binding agreed roughly with their ability to block the autoreceptor (32). On the other hand, the potencies of agonists and antagonists at the autoreceptor do not agree

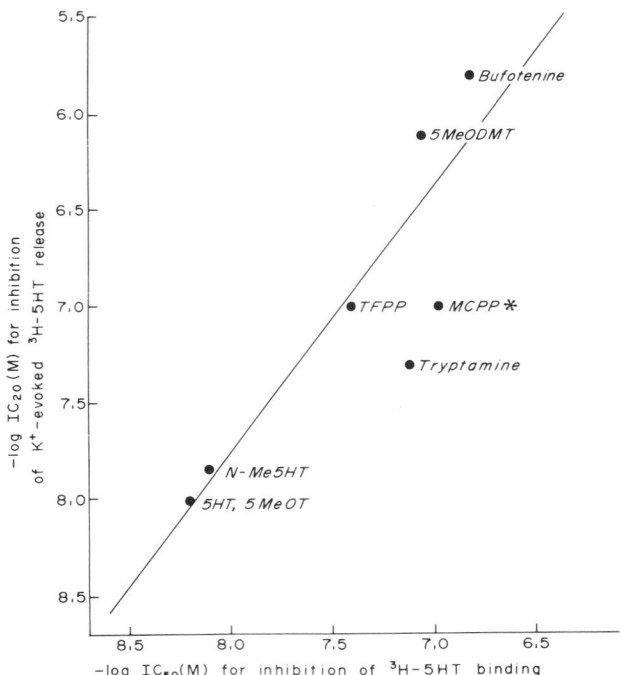

FIG. 8. Correlation between activation of the 5HT autoreceptor and competition for [³H]5HT binding. Inhibition of the release of [³H]5HT was determined in hypothalamic slices; the values plotted are the concentrations required to inhibit K⁺-evoked [³H]5HT release by 20% (IC₂₀ values). IC₅₀ values were determined in competition experiments using [³H]5HT to label the 5HT-1 site(s) in hypothalamic membranes. (From ref. 55.)

with their potencies at the 5HT-2 binding site (55). These studies were performed prior to the recent recognition of multiple subtypes of [³H]5HT binding. With the development of methods to assay each subtype separately, it should be possible to determine the specific receptor subtype of the 5HT-release-inhibiting autoreceptor. Studies to date are not definitive but, for the most part, they are consistent with a 5HT-1b classification. Nonselective 5HT agonists inhibit 5HT release, but the selective 5HT-1a agonist 8OH-DPAT does not (58), except at high, nonspecific concentrations (40). Conversely, RU-24969, which has been proposed to be a selective 5HT-1b agonist (31), interacts with the autoreceptor to block 5HT release (16). However, others have not confirmed that RU-24969 is selective for the 5HT-1b subtype (59). Studies with antagonists have been of limited value in evaluating subtype classification, since most are nonselective, binding to both the 5HT-1a and 5HT-1b sites. However, antagonist studies have ruled out a 5HT-1c classification, since mianserin, a potent 5HT-1c antagonist, does not block the 5HT autoreceptor (54). (−)Propranolol, but not the (+) isomer, antagonizes the effect of 5HT at the autoreceptor with a potency similar to its potency for the 5HT-1b site (57). However, apparently this drug also binds to the 5HT-1a subsite. Spiperone, a potent 5HT-1a antagonist with low affinity for the 5HT1b site, does not block the release-inhibiting effects of 5HT (60). Although consistent with a 5HT-1b classification, these studies are not conclusive, since it was not clear that

the 5HT-1a site was blocked by the concentrations of spiperone that were tested.

SUMMARY AND CONCLUSIONS

Two major transducing systems that carry the extracellular signal of receptor activation across the plasma membrane are phospholipase C/phosphoinositide hydrolysis and the adenylate cyclase/cyclic AMP cascade. These signals modify cellular systems largely via the common mechanism of protein phosphorylation. Studies have demonstrated that at least two 5HT receptor subtypes, the 5HT-2 site and the 5HT-1c site, are linked to phosphoinositide hydrolysis. This multifunctional transducing mechanism has numerous cellular effects, and it is the challenge of the next decade to relate specific cellular responses to specific actions of 5HT. 5HT activation of adenylate cyclase, on the other hand, has been more difficult to characterize, probably because the cyclic AMP signal is small and variable. An increase in cyclic AMP is clearly not related to 5HT-2 or 5HT-1c activation and may instead be mediated by a receptor(s) with properties akin to the other two 5HT-1 sites. Biochemical studies of the terminal autoreceptor that regulates 5HT release suggest that it is also related to a 5HT-1-like site, but additional studies are required before a more precise classification is possible. The second messenger system that mediates the autoreceptor effects is not yet known, but extensive studies have suggested that phosphorylation is involved in neurotransmitter release and this is an obvious point of regulation via an autoreceptor. All three specific protein kinases—cyclic AMP-dependent protein kinase, calcium/calmodulin-dependent protein kinase, and protein kinase C—are found in nerve terminals (62). Each kinase has been implicated in the release process but it is not yet possible to assign a specific or an exclusive role to any one of them or to relate them directly to autoreceptor function.

ACKNOWLEDGMENTS

The original investigations of the authors are supported in part by research grants MH 26463 and MH 34007 from the National Institute of Mental Health and by a fellowship from Lilly Research Laboratories to P.J.C.

REFERENCES

1. Adams, W. B., and Levitan, I. B. (1982): *Proc. Natl. Acad. Sci. USA,* 79:3877–3880.
2. Affolter, H., Erne, P., Burgisser, E., and Pletscher, A. (1984): *Naunyn Schmiedebergs Arch. Pharmacol.,* 325:337–342.
3. Albano, J. D. M., Brown, B. L., Ekins, R. P., Tait, S. A. S., and Tait, J. F. (1974): *Biochem. J.,* 142:391–400.
4. Arunlakshana, O., and Schild, H. O. (1959): *Br. J. Pharmacol.,* 14:48–58.
5. Barbaccia, M. L., Brunello, N., Chuang, D. M., and Costa, E. (1983): *J. Neurochem.,* 40:1671–1679.
6. Berridge, M. J. (1983): *Biochem. J.,* 212:849–858.
7. Berridge, M. J. (1984): *Biochem. J.,* 220:345–360.
8. Berridge, M. J., Buchan, P. B., and Heslop, J. P. (1984): *Mol. Cell. Endocrinol.,* 36:37–42.
9. Berridge, M. J., Dawson, C., Downes, C. P., Heslop, J. P., and Irvine, R. (1983): *Biochem. J.,* 212:473–482.
10. Berridge, M. J., Downes, P. C., and Hanley, M. R. (1982): *Biochem. J.,* 206:587–595.

11. Berridge, M. J., and Heslop, J. P. (1981): *Br. J. Pharmacol.*, 73: 729–738.

12. Berry-Kravis, E., and Dawson, G. (1983): *J. Neurochem.*, 40:977–985.

13. Berry-Kravis, E., and Dawson, G. (1985): *J. Neurochem.*, 45: 1739–1747.

14. Blackmore, P. F., Bocckino, S. B., Waynick, L. E., and Exton, J. H. (1985): *J. Biol. Chem.*, 260:14477–14483.

15. Bone, E. A., and Michell, R. H. (1985): *Biochem. J.*, 227:263–269.

16. Brazell, M. P., Marsden, C. A., Nisbet, A. P., and Routledge, C. (1985): *Br. J. Pharmacol.*, 86:209–216.

17. Cohen, M. L., and Fuller, R. W. (1983): *Life Sci.*, 32:711–718.

18. Cohen, M. L., Fuller, R. W., and Kurz, K. D. (1983): *J. Pharmacol. Exp. Ther.*, 227:327–332.

19. Cohen, M. L., Fuller, R. W., and Wiley, K. S. (1981): *J. Pharmacol. Exp. Ther.*, 218:421–425.

20. Conn, P. J., and Sanders-Bush, E. (1984): *Neuropharmacology*, 23:993–996.

21. Conn, P. J., and Sanders-Bush, E. (1985): *J. Pharmacol. Exp. Ther.*, 234:195–203.

22. Conn, P. J., and Sanders-Bush, E. (1986): *Life Sci.*, 38:663–669.

23. Conn, P. J., Sanders-Bush, E., Hoffman, B. J., and Hartig, P. R. (1986): *Proc. Natl. Acad. Sci. USA*, 83:4086–4088.

24. Coughlin, S. R., Moskowitz, M. A., Antoniades, H. N., and Levine, L. (1981): *Proc. Natl. Acad. Sci. USA*, 78:7134–7138.

25. Coughlin, S. R., Moskowitz, M. A., and Levine, L. (1984): *Biochem. Pharmacol.*, 33:692–695.

26. Crook, R. B., Kasagami, H., and Prusiner, S. B. (1981): *J. Neurochem.*, 37:845–854.

27. de Chaffoy de Courcelles, D., Leysen, J. E., De Clerck, F., Van Belle, H., and Janssen P. A. J. (1985): *J. Biol. Chem.*, 260:7603–7608.

28. de Chaffoy de Courcelles, D., Roevens, P., and Van Belle, H. (1984): *FEBS Lett.*, 171:289–292.

29. Devivo, M., and Maayani, S. (1985): *Eur. J. Pharmacol.*, 119: 231–234.

30. Dolphin, A. C., and Greengard, P. (1981): *Nature*, 289:76–79.

31. Doods, H. N., Kalkman, H. O., DeJonge, A., Thoolen, M. J. M. C., Wilffert, B., Timmerman, P. B. W. M., and Van Zwieten, P. A. (1985): *Eur. J. Pharmacol.*, 112:363–370.

32. Engel, G., Gothert, M., Muller-Schweinitzer, E., Schlicker, E., Sistonen, L., and Stadler, P. A. (1983): *Naunyn Schmiedebergs Arch. Pharmacol.*, 324:116–124.

33. Enjalbert, A., Bourgoin, S., Hamon, M., Adrien, J., and Bockaert, J. (1978): *Mol. Pharmacol.*, 14:2–10.

34. Enjalbert, A., Hamon, M., Bourgoin, S., and Bockaert, J. (1978): *Mol. Pharmacol.*, 14:11–23.

35. Evans, T., Hepler, J. R., Masters, S. B., Brown, J. H., and Harden, T. K. (1985): *Biochem. J.*, 232:751–757.

36. Fillion, G., Beaudoin, D., Rousselle, J. C., Deniau, J. M., Fillion, M. P., Dray, F., and Jacob, J. (1979): *J. Neurochem.*, 33:567–570.

37. Fillion, G., Rousselle, J. C., Beaudoin, D., Pradelles, P., Goiny, M., Dray, F., and Jacob, J. (1979): *Life Sci.*, 24:1813–1822.

38. Fujita, K., Aguilera, G., and Catt, K. J. (1979): *J. Biol. Chem.*, 254:8567–8574.

39. Goy, M. F., Schwarz, T. L., and Kravitz, E. A. (1984): *J. Neurosci.*, 4:611–626.

40. Hamon, M., Bourgoin, S., Gozlan, H., Hall, M. D., Goetz, C., Artaud, F., and Horn, A. S. (1984): *Eur. J. Pharmacol.*, 100:263–276.

41. Hirasawa, K., and Nishizuka, Y. (1985): *Annu. Rev. Pharmacol. Toxicol.*, 25:147–170.

42. Janowsky, A., Labarca, R., and Paul, S. M. (1984): *Life Sci.*, 35: 1953–1961.

43. Kakiuchi, S., and Rall, T. W. (1968): *Mol. Pharmacol.*, 4:367–378.

44. Kendall, D. A., and Nahorski, S. R. (1985): *J. Pharmacol. Exp. Ther.*, 233:473–479.

45. Kravitz, E. A., Beltz, B., Glusman, S., Goy, M., Harris-Warrick, R., Johnston, M., Livingstone, M., Schwarz, T., and Siwicki, K. K. (1985): In: *Model Neural Networks and Behavior*, edited by A. I. Selverston, pp. 339–360. Plenum Publishing Corp., New York.

46. Leysen, J. E., Awouters, F., Kennis, L., Laduron, P. M., Vandenberk, J., and Janssen, P. A. J. (1981): *Life Sci.*, 28:1015–1022.

47. Leysen, J. E., Gommeren, W., Van Gompel, P., Wynants, J., Janssen, P. F. M., and Laduron, P. M. (1985): *Mol. Pharmacol.*, 27:600–611.

48. Leysen, J. E., Niemegeers, C. J. E., Van Nueten, J. M., and Laduron, P. M. (1982): *Mol. Pharmacol.*, 21:6301–6314.

49. Litosch, I., Wallis, C., and Fain, J. N. (1985): *J. Biol. Chem.*, 260: 5464–5471.

50. MacDermot, J., Higashida, H., Wilson, S. P., Matsuzawa, H., Minna, J., and Nirenberg, M. (1979): *Proc. Natl. Acad. Sci. USA*, 76:1135–1139.

51. Maeda, K. (1983): *Nihon Univ. J. Med.*, 25:155–174.

52. Mansour, T. E. (1959): *J. Pharmacol. Exp. Ther.*, 126:212–216.

53. Mansour, T. E., Sutherland, E. W., Rall, T. W., and Bueding, E. (1960): *J. Biol. Chem.*, 235:466–470.

54. Martin, L. L., and Sanders-Bush, E. (1982): *Neuropharmacology*, 21:445–450.

55. Martin, L. L., and Sanders-Bush, E. (1982): *Naunyn Schmiedebergs Arch. Pharmacol.*, 321:165–170.

56. McComb, J. G. (1983): *J. Neurosurg.*, 59:369–383.

57. Middlemiss, D. N. (1984): *Eur. J. Pharmacol.*, 101:289–293.

58. Middlemiss, D. N. (1984): *Naunyn Schmiedebergs Arch. Pharmacol.*, 327:18–22.

59. Middlemiss, D. N. (1985): *J. Pharm. Pharmacol.*, 37:434–437.

60. Monroe, P. J., and Smith, D. J. (1985): *J. Neurochem.*, 45:1886–1894.

61. Moret, C. (1985): In: *Neuropharmacology of Serotonin*, edited by A. R. Green, pp. 21–49. Oxford University Press, Oxford.

62. Nairn, A. C., Hemmings, H. C., Jr., and Greengard, P. (1985): *Annu. Rev. Biochem.*, 54:931–976.

63. Naka, M., Nishikawa, M., Adelstein, R. S., and Hiroyoshi, H. (1983): *Nature*, 306:490–492.

64. Nelson, D. L., Herbet, A., Enjalbert, A., Bockaert, J., and Hamon, M. (1980): *Biochem. Pharmacol.*, 29:2445–2453.

65. Pazos, A., Hoyer, D., and Palacios, J. M. (1984): *Eur. J. Pharmacol.*, 106:531–538.

66. Pazos, A., Hoyer, D., and Palacios, J. M. (1984): *Eur. J. Pharmacol.*, 106:539–546.

67. Pedigo, N. W., Yamamura, H. I., and Nelson, D. L. (1981): *J. Neurochem.*, 36:220–226.

68. Peroutka, S. J., Lebovitz, R. M., and Snyder, S. H. (1979): *Mol. Pharmacol.*, 16:700–708.

69. Peroutka, S. J., and Snyder, S. H. (1979): *Mol. Pharmacol.*, 16: 687–699.

70. Pettibone, D. J., and Pflueger, A. B. (1984): *J. Neurochem.*, 43: 83–90.

71. Pollock, J. D., Bernier, L., and Camardo, J. S. (1985): *J. Neurosci.*, 5:1862–1871.

72. Rittenhouse, S. E. (1984): *Biochem. J.*, 222:103–110.

73. Roth, B. L., Nakaki, T., Chuang, D. M., and Costa, E. (1984): *Neuropharmacology*, 23:1223–1225.

74. Roth, B. L., Nakaki, T., Chuang, D. M., Chernow, B., and Costa, E. (1985): *Fed. Proc.*, 44:1244.

75. Sano, K., Takai, Y., Yamanishi, J., and Nishizuka, Y. (1983): *J. Biol. Chem.*, 258:2010–2013.

76. Shenker, A., Maayani, S., Weinstein, H., and Green, J. P. (1983): *Life Sci.*, 32:2335–2342.

77. Shenker, A., Maayani, S., Weinstein, H., and Green, J. P. (1985): *Eur. J. Pharmacol.*, 109:427–429.

78. Siegelbaum, S. A., Camardo, J. S., and Kandel, E. R. (1982): *Nature*, 299:413–415.

79. Sills, M. A., Wolfe, B. B., and Frazer, A. (1984): *J. Pharmacol. Exp. Ther.*, 231:480–487.

80. Stone, D. B., and Mansour, T. E. (1967): *Mol. Pharmacol.*, 3:161–169.

81. Watson, S. P., Wolf, M., and Lapetina, E. G. (1985): *Biochem. Biophys. Res. Commun.*, 132:555–562.

82. Von Hungen, K., Roberts, S., and Hill, D. F. (1974): *J. Neurochem.*, 22:811–819.

83. Von Hungen, K., Roberts, S., and Hill, D. F. (1975): *Brain Res.*, 84:257–267.

84. Yagaloff, K. A., and Hartig, P. R. (1985): *J. Neurosci.*, 5:3178–3183.

Psychopharmacology:
The Third Generation of Progress,
edited by Herbert Y. Meltzer.
Raven Press, New York © 1987.

CHAPTER **11**

Noradrenergic Modulation of Neuronal Excitability in Mammalian Hippocampus

Roger A. Nicoll, Daniel V. Madison, and Barrie Lancaster

In the past dozen or so years there has been a revolution in the understanding of the cellular mechanisms of norepinephrine (NE) action in the CNS. Early findings that NE could cause small hyperpolarizations of neuronal membrane potentials in several brain regions led to the general idea that NE acted as a more-or-less standard inhibitory neurotransmitter (9,17,18,39,41); that is, that it moved the membrane potential of cells farther from action potential threshold by hyperpolarizing them. But with the advent of the *in vitro* brain slice technique, used in conjunction with intracellular recording, a different and more interesting idea of how NE functions in the CNS has emerged. Based on evidence from several areas of the brain, including that shown in detail in this article, it now appears that NE serves in many systems to modulate the responsiveness of neuronal excitability to other excitatory and inhibitory neurotransmitters.

The idea that NE may be having some modulatory action in the CNS first arose from the observation that the actions of NE in the cerebellum were very slow, and the hyperpolarizations caused by NE application often appeared to occur without any changes in membrane resistance (10). Later observations in the cerebellar cortex (42) and in the hippocampus (40) showed that application of NE could enhance the actions of other transmitters such as glutamate and γ-aminobutyric acid (GABA). In the cerebellar cortex, in particular, NE caused an enhancement of synaptic inhibition and also increased the response of Purkinje neurons to iontophoretically applied GABA (42). The action of the putative excitatory neurotransmitter glutamate is also enhanced by NE in the dorsal lateral geniculate nucleus (37). This enhancement of glutamate action may actually result from a disinhibitory action of NE (22,34). By decreasing tonic inhibitory transmission, NE may indi-

rectly allow excitatory influences, such as those mediated by glutamate, to be more effective. Such a disinhibitory action of NE has been observed in several brain regions, including the hippocampus (24,28), and has been characterized in the olfactory bulb. The principal cell of the olfactory bulb, the mitral cell, receives inhibitory input from the dendrites of interneurons within the bulb. These interneurons are synaptically activated in turn by depolarization of the mitral cell dendrites, so that in effect, activation of the mitral cells results in a reciprocal inhibitory feedback (20). Application of NE to the olfactory bulb results in a reduction of these inhibitory postsynaptic potentials (IPSPs), presumably by an action on the interneuron, since there is no concomitant decrease in the sensitivity of the mitral cell to the inhibitory neurotransmitter GABA (21). The result of this disinhibitory action is that the excitability of the mitral cell is enhanced, since the cell is released from the control of the inhibitory circuits.

We have recently described another type of modulatory action of NE in the hippocampus. Using the *in vitro* hippocampal slice preparation, intracellular recording, and single-electrode voltage-clamp techniques, we have described how a combination of noradrenergic action on pyramidal cells of the rat hippocampus can result in an increase in the signal-to-noise ratio of these neurons. These results have appeared in previous published reports (26,29,30).

ENHANCEMENT OF GLUTAMATE ACTION IN THE HIPPOCAMPUS BY NE

Previous reports in the cerebellar cortex (42) and the hippocampus (40) indicated that excitatory responses of

Purkinje and pyramidal cells to iontophoretic application of glutamate could be enhanced by NE application. Glutamate is the putative excitatory neurotransmitter for many of the synapses onto pyramidal cells. Intracellular recordings from the somata of pyramidal cells show that when glutamate is applied by iontophoresis onto the dendrites of these cells, the cell depolarizes and fires spikes (Fig. 1A₁). During a glutamate application of 1-sec duration, the action potential output of the cell is clustered at the beginning of the glutamate depolarization. Even though the level of depolarization caused by glutamate remains constant or increases throughout the application, the last several hundred milliseconds of depolarization elicit few, if any, action potentials. In addition, the rate of action potential discharge during

the initial spike train declines or accommodates before discharge ceases. Addition of NE to the preparation, either in the bathing medium or by iontophoresis, causes a dramatic change in this glutamate response. In the presence of NE, the glutamate depolarization now elicits action potentials throughout its entire duration, even though the actual size of the depolarization is unchanged (Fig. 1A₁).

NE could cause an enhancement of glutamate responses either by interacting specifically with the glutamate neurotransmission pathway in some manner, or more generally, by altering some aspect of pyramidal cell physiology such that the cell becomes more responsive to any excitatory stimulus. To test for this second possibility, we have simulated the glutamate-induced depolarization by passing

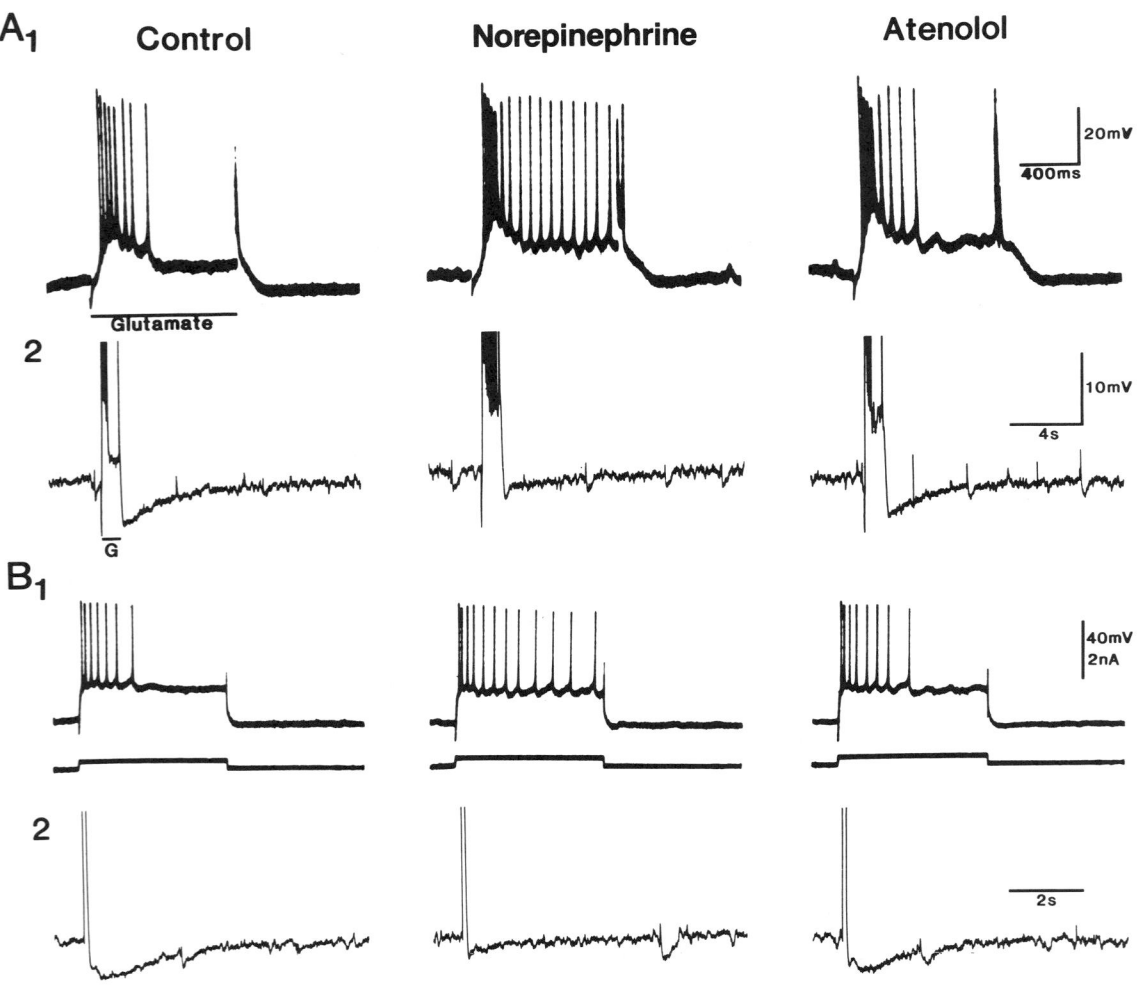

FIG. 1. NE blocks calcium-activated potassium AHPs and accommodation in hippocampal CA1 pyramidal neurons. All records in this figure are from the same pyramidal cell. **A₁:** Glutamate application by iontophoresis onto the apical dendritic region of a pyramidal cell causes a depolarization and elicits action potentials that cluster at the beginning of the stimulus. NE (10 μM) added to the superfusing medium of the slice causes a change in the cell's response to glutamate such that spikes are elicited during the entire duration of the depolarization. **A₂:** Same responses as in A at a slower sweep speed showing the AHP that follows glutamate application. This AHP is nearly abolished by NE. **B₁:** Same cell depolarized with current passed through the recording electrode gives a response pattern similar to that with glutamate, with the action potential discharge clustered near the beginning of the stimulus. As with the glutamate response, addition of NE causes more action potentials to be elicited by the same stimulus such that the cell fires for the entire duration of the stimulus. **B₂:** Short-duration current activation of the cell elicits an AHP that is reduced by NE. All effects of NE illustrated in this figure were reversed by application of the specific beta₁-receptor antagonist, atenolol (3 μM) (with NE still present). (From ref. 29.)

current through the recording electrode to excite the cell in a manner similar to glutamate (Fig. 1B₁). As with glutamate depolarizations, current-induced depolarizations elicit action potentials only during the initial portion of the stimulus, and this initial discharge slows, or accommodates. Also similar to glutamate, application of NE dramatically alters this response pattern to one in which the depolarization generates spikes throughout its duration. Thus, it seems likely that the enhancement of the cell's responsiveness to depolarizing stimuli reflects the action of NE on some general cellular property rather than any specific interaction with glutamate.

Depolarizing responses to glutamate or to current are followed by an afterhyperpolarization (AHP). This AHP has been shown by several laboratories to be due to a calcium-dependent potassium conductance that is turned on by calcium that enters the cell during action potential discharge (5,15,19,27,38). Evidence that this AHP is due to an increase in potassium conductance is summarized in

Fig. 2. First, the AHP is associated with an increase in membrane conductance. This can be seen as a decrease in cell responses to short-duration hyperpolarizing pulses applied through the recording electrode (Fig. 2A₁). This decrease can be seen more clearly when the cell is held near resting potential during the AHP (Fig. 2A₂). Second, the reversal potential of the AHP occurs at a membrane potential consistent with its being mediated by potassium ions (Fig. 2B), and the reversal potential shifts approximately 20 mV to a more depolarized level when the extracellular potassium is doubled (Fig. 2C). These data are consistent with the conclusion that the AHP is a potassium-mediated potential. Evidence that the AHP is activated by calcium entry into the cell can be seen in Fig. 3. Addition of the calcium-channel blocker cadmium reduces the slow phase of the AHP and also increases the number of action potentials that are elicited by depolarizing stimuli. As can be seen in the graph in Fig. 3B, the decrease in the AHP and the increase in the excitability of the cell occur

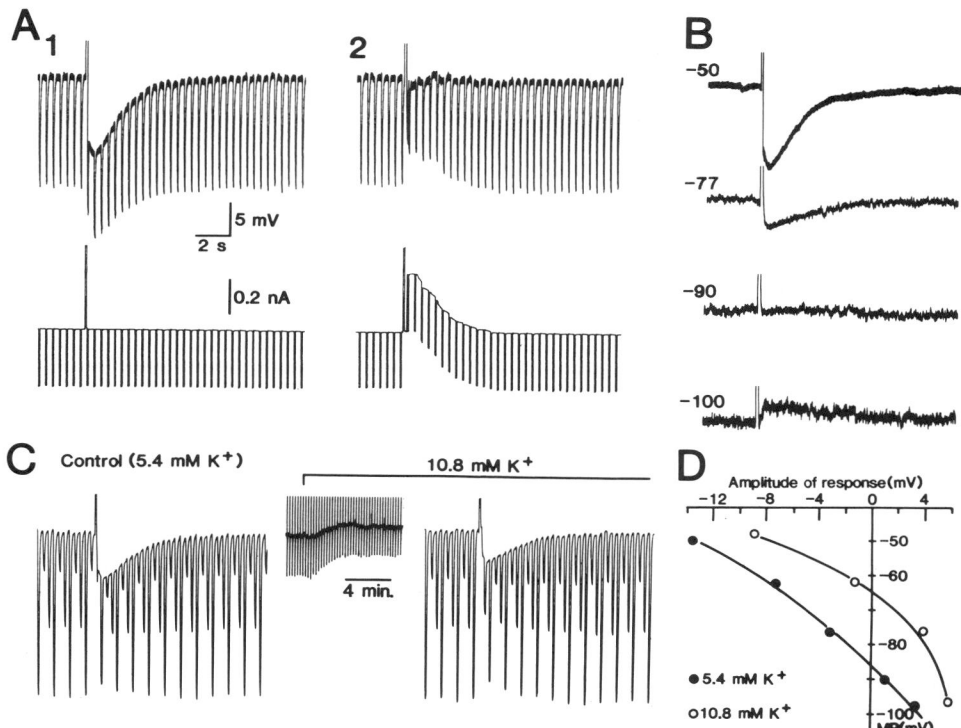

FIG. 2. The AHP is caused by an increase in membrane potassium conductance. Records shown in **A** and **B** are from the same pyramidal cell, and in **C** and **D** are from another cell. **A₁**: AHP elicited by a short-duration depolarizing current pulse. The cell in this figure is bathed in TTX and TEA and the AHP shown follows a single calcium action potential. **A₂**: AHP elicited by an identical stimulus, but with the membrane potential held near rest for the duration of the AHP with current injected into the cell under manual control. In part **A**, the current monitor trace is below the membrane voltage record. The downward deflections are constant-current hyperpolarizing pulses to measure membrane resistance. As can be seen clearly in A₂, the AHP is accompanied by an increase in membrane conductance. **B**: AHPs elicited at various membrane potentials at and on either side of the AHP reversal potential. Note that the AHP reverses at approximately −90

mV, a value consistent with a potassium-mediated potential. **C**: Hyperpolarizing current pulses of three different sizes, the largest of which hyperpolarizes the cell beyond the AHP reversal potential, were applied during the AHP. This allowed us to sample the membrane potential at four points (see ref. 35 for method). This was done in a solution containing our normal potassium concentration (5.4 mM) and with the potassium concentration doubled to 10.8 mM. The voltage gain in **C** is half that in **A**. **D**: Graph of the amplitude of the AHP vs membrane potential plotted from the data in **C**. The point plotted at −90 mV in control is from another trace not shown in this figure. Note that doubling the extracellular potassium concentration shifts the reversal potential of the AHP from approximately −85 to −65 mV. These data indicate that the AHP is due to an increase in potassium conductance.

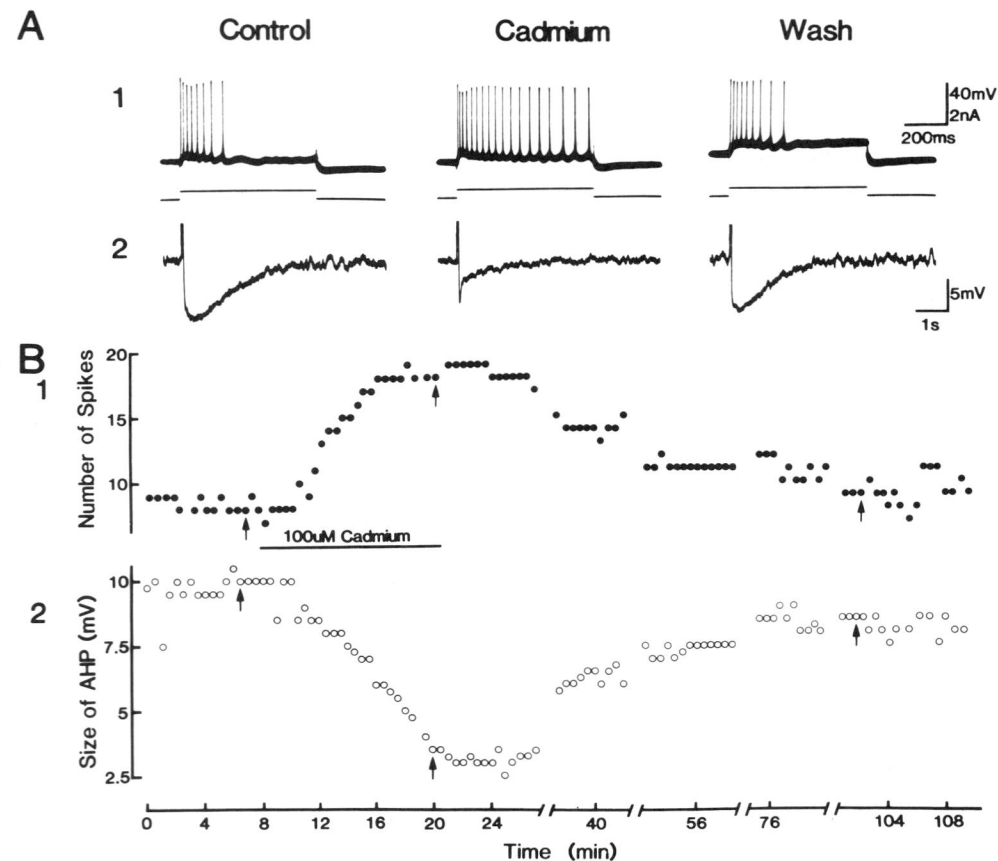

FIG. 3. Cadmium blocks calcium-activated potassium AHPs and accommodation simultaneously. All records in this figure are from the same pyramidal cell. **A$_1$:** Response of the pyramidal cell to a long-duration current pulse. **A$_2$:** AHP caused by a short-duration current pulse. Note that application of cadmium (100 μM) reduces the slow phase of the AHP and increases the excitability of the cell in a manner indistinguishable from NE. **B:** Plot of the number of spikes elicited by the long-duration depolarization (**B$_1$**) and of the amplitude of the AHP (**B$_2$**) during the course of the experiment. Records in **A** were taken at the time indicated by the *arrows*. (Part of this figure is reprinted from ref. 27.)

simultaneously. Similar blockade of the AHP also occurs when applying low-calcium solutions (27), and when cells are injected with the calcium chelator ethyleneglycol bis(aminoethylether)tetraacetate (EGTA) (27,38). All of these treatments that block the AHP also reduce accommodation of the cell's discharge in a manner identical to NE (27).

The calcium-dependent potassium AHP is sensitive to NE (16,26,29). When applied to the preparation in low concentrations, the slow phase of the AHP is abolished by NE (Fig. 1A$_2$ and B$_2$). This occurs simultaneously with the NE-induced increase in excitability of the cell to depolarizing stimuli. The blockade of the AHP by NE is related in a causal way to the increase in firing because any experimental manipulation that blocks the AHP, such as cadmium application or EGTA injection, also causes an identical increase in excitability (27). The calcium-dependent potassium conductance that is turned on during action potential discharge in turn acts in an inhibitory manner to brake the further discharge of the cell within a few hundred milliseconds. Blockade of this conductance by NE allows the cell to fire more freely during depolarizing stimuli. The mechanism of the noradrenergic blockade of the AHP is not

fully elucidated, but it is known that it is not due to a reduction in calcium current across the membrane, since during NE blockade of the AHP both calcium action potentials and calcium currents are undiminished (29).

ON WHAT MEMBRANE CURRENT DOES NE ACT?

It was expected that under voltage clamp NE would block a calcium-dependent potassium current, and this was indeed the case. However, the current observed to be blocked by NE could not unambiguously be identified as the same calcium-dependent current that had been previously described in other preparations. This previously described current (I_c) has a pronounced voltage sensitivity such that at membrane potentials of −60 to −70 mV, this current turns off quite rapidly, i.e., within a few tens of milliseconds (1,7). How then could these channels stay open long enough to underlie the slow AHP, which has a duration of hundreds of milliseconds or even seconds? A second problem is presented by the pharmacology of I_c, which can be blocked by low concentrations of tetraethylammonium (TEA) (1–2 mM) which do not affect the slow AHP (1,36). These difficulties were resolved when it was found that a second calcium-dependent potassium current exists in neuronal membranes. This current, which underlies the AHP, is known as I_{AHP} (36).

Although activation of both I_c and I_{AHP} depends on calcium entry, activation of I_c is additionally favored by membrane depolarization, although this current is rapidly deactivated when the membrane potential returns to rest. On the other hand, I_{AHP} is not rapidly deactivated at rest because this current displays no intrinsic voltage sensitivity (23,36). As described above, the prolonged time course of this current following a burst of action potentials accounts for the slowing down or cessation of action potential firing, which is sensitive to application of NE.

A simple method used to observe I_{AHP} is to make large, short-duration depolarizing steps that elicit a reproducible slow tail current upon return to the holding potential near rest (Fig. 4A). This procedure is similar to the hybrid (current/voltage) clamp method (23,36), in which a train of action potentials is followed by a rapid transition to voltage clamp so as to bring the membrane potential to rest. This procedure demonstrates the outward current that is responsible for the slow AHP. This AHP current is sensitive to application of NE (Fig. 4A). Following longer

(approximately 1 sec) step depolarizing voltage commands from potentials near rest, slow outward current tails can be observed after repolarization to the holding potential. These tail currents show the same time course as I_{AHP} evoked by a short step, and can be blocked by cadmium or NE (Fig. 4B) (23). Simultaneously, much of the outward current that develops during the voltage command is also abolished by these agents (23). Thus under voltage clamp, I_{AHP} is seen to be generated by depolarizing commands to −50 mV or more positive levels and appears to develop rather slowly during a 1-sec command. This contrasts with the generation of an AHP by five or six action potentials covering approximately 60 msec. This presumably reflects the behavior of the underlying calcium current. Inward calcium currents can be activated within 2 msec of depolarization and show a maximum inward current at approximately +10 mV (3,14). A burst of action potentials is therefore an ideal stimulus for rapid calcium entry and can generate an I_{AHP} of comparable amplitude to 1-sec voltage commands to lesser potentials.

In the presence of NE, cadmium-sensitive outward tail currents remain, i.e., there is another calcium-dependent outward current. These tail currents comprise a faster initial decay phase of the total outward tail and are also sensitive to low TEA concentrations (1 mM) (23). This observation

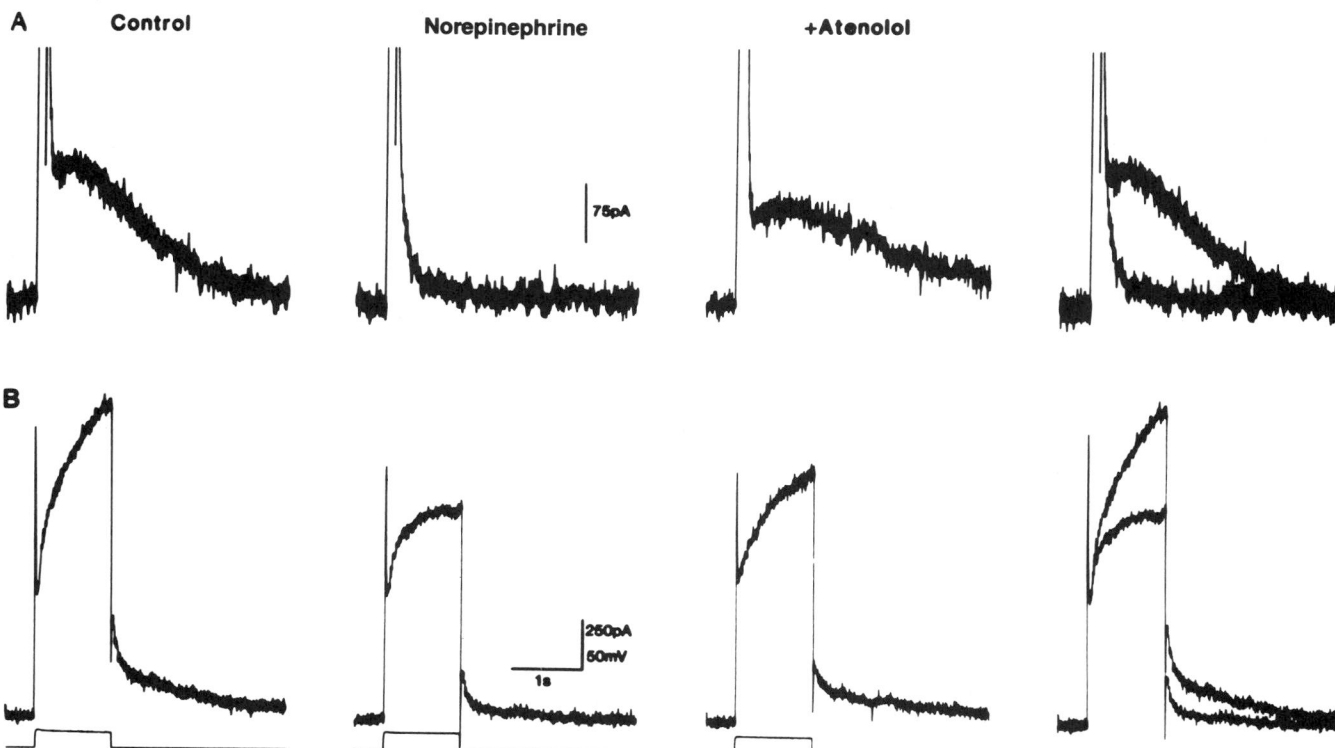

FIG. 4. The current underlying the afterhyperpolarization (I_{AHP}) is reduced by application of NE. All records in this figure are from the same pyramidal cell recorded with a single-electrode voltage clamp. **A:** Tail current following a short depolarizing voltage command, which results from I_{AHP} activated by calcium entry during the depolarizing step, is reduced by application of NE (10 μM). The outward current resulting from a 1-sec duration depolarizing command, and the outward tail current following this current step, both of which are due primarily to I_{AHP}, are reduced by NE. All actions of NE on I_{AHP} were partially reversed by application of 3 μM of the beta$_1$-antagonist, atenolol. This cell was bathed in the sodium channel blocker, TTX, throughout the experiment.

is compatible with a previous report of a voltage- and cadmium-sensitive current that can be recorded to the presence of muscarinic agonists (11) that are known block the AHP (8,12). This additional calcium dependent outward current probably represents I_c.

PHARMACOLOGY AND MECHANISM OF THE ACTION OF NE

The noradrenergic blockade of the AHP and its underlying current is mediated by a beta$_1$-receptor subtype (29). This is known because beta-antagonists, such as propranolol, and specific beta$_1$-antagonists, such as atenolol, block the effect of NA on the AHP, whereas alpha-antagonists and beta$_2$-antagonists have no such effect. Additionally, beta-agonists such as isoproterenol, and dobutamine (a specific beta$_1$-agonist) also cause reductions in the AHP (29).

As is expected for a beta-receptor-mediated response, the noradrenergic blockade of the AHP is mediated by the intracellular second messenger cyclic AMP (30). The evidence for this is summarized as follows. First, application of exogenous membrane-permeant analogs of cyclic AMP, such as 8-bromo-cyclic AMP, exactly mimic the effects of NE, not only in blocking the AHP, but also in producing the increase in excitability to other excitatory stimuli such as injected current (Fig. 5). This blockade of the AHP, similar to the noradrenergic blockade, occurs without any reduction in calcium entry (30). Second, activation of the cell's endogenous adenylate cyclase by forskolin also mimics the effects of NE (30). Third, blockade of the cell's phosphodiesterase, using Ro-20-1724 or IBMX, enhances the action of NE (30). Finally, reduction in adenylate cyclase activity during application of SQ22,536 [9-(tetrahydro-2-furyl)adenine] reduces the effect of NE on the AHP (30).

FUNCTIONAL SIGNIFICANCE OF NORADRENERGIC ACTIONS

In some parts of the CNS, such as in the locus ceruleus (2,13), NE causes large and reproducible hyperpolarizations of neuronal membrane potentials and clearly acts as an inhibitory neurotransmitter. These actions result from NE acting on alpha$_2$-receptors. Comparing these types of nor-adrenergic responses to the very small and slow hyperpolarizations that NE causes in the hippocampus, we were led to conclude that these hyperpolarizations were not the major transmitter action of NE in the hippocampus. Indeed, a much more robust and reproducible action of NE in the hippocampus is the blockade of I_{AHP}. This blockade of the slow calcium-dependent potassium current makes the cell more excitable in response to glutamate action, and indeed, as discussed earlier, to any excitatory stimulus. This action is unlike that of classical neurotransmitters, which simply hyperpolarize or depolarize neurons, in that by blocking I_{AHP} NE does not have much of an effect on the resting state of the neuron when it is activated, but instead, markedly alters the response of the neuron when it is activated.

Although the hyperpolarizing action of NE in the hippocampus is quite small, nonetheless, we find that it may play some role in pyramidal cell physiology in that these hyperpolarizations can interact with the blockade of the AHP to increase the signal-to-noise ratio of these neurons. This interaction is demonstrated in Fig. 6. In this experiment, pyramidal cells, recorded intracellularly, were stimulated with a small ramp of depolarizing current that was adjusted to a level just above threshold for a single action potential. This ramp stimulus was followed by a large, long-duration, square-current pulse, which elicited several action potentials in the familiar accommodating pattern. Application of NE to the preparation reduced the AHP and allowed the cell to discharge action potentials throughout the long-current pulse. At the same time, the small hyperpolarizing action of NE was of sufficient magnitude to inhibit the ability of the near-threshold ramp stimulus to elicit a spike. Thus, the interaction between the membrane potential hyperpolarization and the beta-receptor-mediated decrease in calcium-dependent potassium current is capable of causing an increase in the signal-to-noise ratio of the pyramidal cell such that the cell's response to stimuli near action potential threshold are inhibited, whereas the responses to larger stimuli are enhanced. Some examples of similar increases in signal-to-noise ratios in neuronal responses to sensory stimuli have been described (25,32). The noradrenergic blockade of the AHP may also participate in producing the proconvulsant effects that have been described in hippocampus for beta-receptor agonists (33).

It now appears from several published reports that NE is not the only putative neurotransmitter substance that

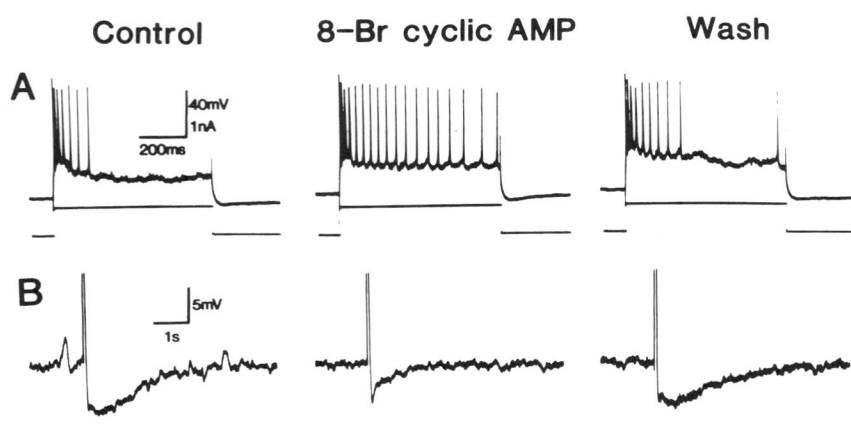

Control   **8-Br cyclic AMP**   **Wash**

A
40mV
1nA
200ms

B
5mV
1s

FIG. 5. Exogenous cyclic AMP analogs application mimics the effects of NE. All records in this figure are from the same pyramidal cell. **A:** Application of the membrane-permeant analog of cyclic AMP, 8-bromo cyclic AMP, causes a decrease in accommodation identical to NE. **B:** Amplitude of the slow AHP is also reduced by 8-bromo cyclic AMP. (From ref. 29.)

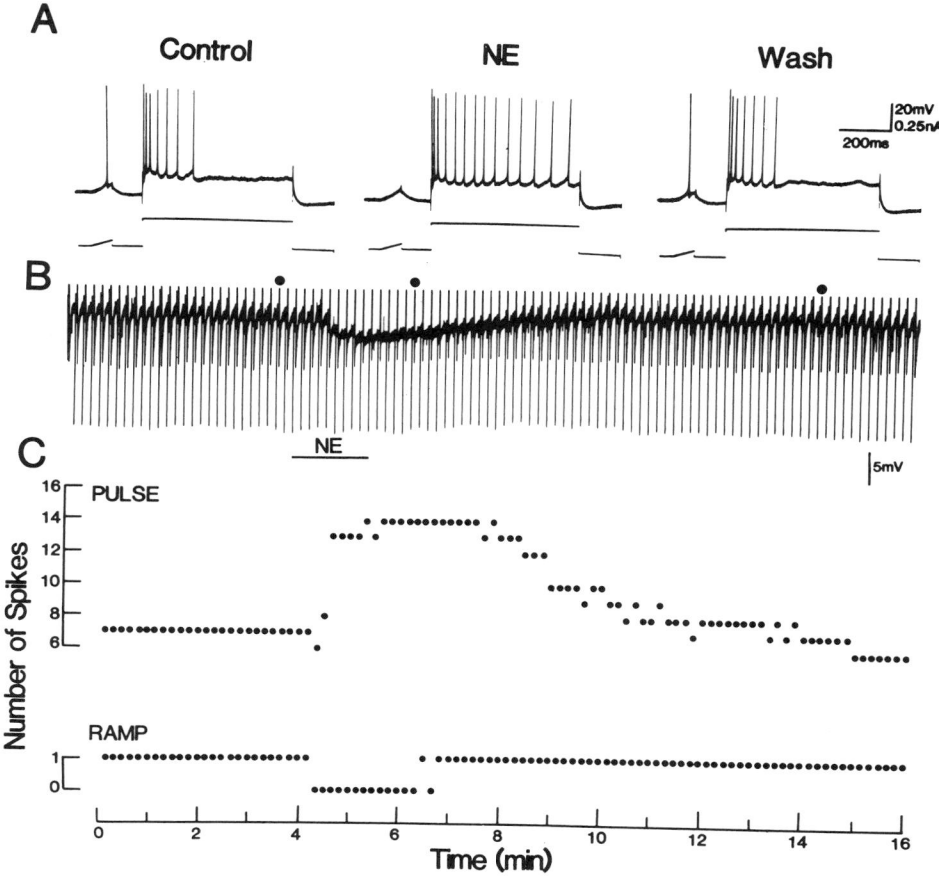

FIG. 6. NE decreases the signal-to-noise ratio of pyramidal neurons. All records in this figure are from the same pyramidal cell. **A:** Pyramidal cells were stimulated with a short ramp of depolarizing current, just threshold for a single action potential, followed by a large, long-duration current pulse. **B:** Continuous record of the pyramidal cell's membrane potential. The longest downward deflections are constant-current hyperpolarizing pulses to measure membrane resistance. The medium-length hyperpolarizing deflections are the AHPs following each depolarizing stimulus. **C:** Note that the small hyperpolarizing action of NE on the resting membrane potential is of sufficient magnitude to inhibit the response of the cell to the near-threshold ramp stimulus, whereas the blockade of the AHP allows the cell to fire more vigorously to the large current pulse. (From ref. 29.)

can cause blockade of calcium-dependent potassium currents. Acetylcholine (8,12), histamine (16), and corticotropin-releasing factor (4) have also been shown to reduce the AHP in the hippocampus. In addition, activation of protein kinase C by phorbol ester application also reduces the AHP in the hippocampus (6,31). The phospholipid-protein kinase C pathway has been proposed to act as a second messenger system for a variety of neurotransmitters including acetylcholine. Thus it appears likely that blockade of calcium-dependent potassium currents may play a key role in the regulation of neuronal excitability and that the calcium-dependent potassium current may be a final common path for the actions of several neurotransmitters.

ACKNOWLEDGMENTS

This work was supported by a Bank of America-Giannini Foundation Fellowship to D.V.M. and NIH grants MH-38256 and MH-00437 (RSDA) and the Klingenstein Fund to R.A.N. B.L. acknowledges the support of the Wellcome Trust.

REFERENCES

1. Adams, P. R., Constanti, A., Brown, D. A., and Clark, R. B. (1982): *Nature,* 296:746–749.
2. Aghajanian, G. K., and VanderMaelen, C. P. (1982): *Science,* 215:1394–1396.
3. Akaike, N., Lee, K. S., and Brown, A. M. (1978): *J. Gen. Physiol.,* 71:509–531.
4. Aldenhoff, J. B., Gruol, D. L., Rivier, J., Vale, W., and Siggins, G. R. (1983): *Science,* 221:875–877.
5. Alger, B. E., and Nicoll, R. A. (1980): *Science,* 210:1122–1124.
6. Baraban, J. M., Snyder, S. H., and Alger, B. E. (1985): *Proc. Natl. Acad. Sci. USA,* 82:2538–2542.
7. Barrett, J. N., Magleby, K. L., and Pallotta, B. S. (1982): *J. Physiol. (Lond.),* 331:211–230.
8. Benardo, L. S., and Prince, D. A. (1982): *Brain Res.,* 249:333–344.
9. Biscoe, T. J., and Straughan, D. W. (1966): *J. Physiol. (Lond.),* 183:341–359.
10. Bloom, F. E. (1973): *Brain Res.,* 62:299–305.
11. Brown, D. A., and Griffith, W. H. (1983): *J. Physiol. (Lond.),* 337:287–301.
12. Cole, A. E., and Nicoll, R. A. (1984): *J. Physiol. (Lond.),* 352:173–188.
13. Egan, T. M., Henderson, G., North, R. A., and Williams, J. T. (1983): *J. Physiol. (Lond.),* 345:477–488.

14. Fenwick, E. M., Marty, A., and Neher, E. (1982): *J. Physiol. (Lond.)*, 331:599–635.
15. Gustafsson, B., and Wigstrom, H. (1981): *Brain Res.*, 206:462–468.
16. Haas, H. L., and Konnerth, A. (1983): *Nature*, 302:432–434.
17. Hoffer, B. J., Siggins, G. R., and Bloom, F. E. (1971): *Brain Res.*, 25:523–534.
18. Hoffer, B. J., Siggins, G. R., Oliver, A. P., and Bloom, F. E. (1973): *J. Pharmacol. Exp. Ther.*, 184:553–569.
19. Hotson, J. R., and Prince, D. A. (1980): *J. Neurophysiol.*, 43:409–419.
20. Jahr, C. E., and Nicoll, R. A. (1982): *J. Physiol. (Lond.)*, 326:213–234.
21. Jahr, C. E., and Nicoll, R. A. (1982): *Nature*, 297:227–229.
22. Kayama, Y., Negi, T., Sugitani, M., and Iwama, K. (1982): *Neuroscience*, 7:655–666.
23. Lancaster, B., and Adams, P. R. (1986): *J. Neurophysiol.*, 55:1268–1282.
24. Langmoen, I. A., Segal, M., and Andersen, P. (1981): *Brain Res.*, 208:349–362.
25. Livingstone, M. S., and Hubel, D. H. (1981): *Nature*, 291:554–561.
26. Madison, D. V., and Nicoll, R. A. (1982): *Nature*, 299:636–638.
27. Madison, D. V., and Nicoll, R. A. (1984): *J. Physiol. (Lond.)*, 354:319–331.
28. Madison, D. V., and Nicoll, R. A. (1984): *Soc. Neurosci. Abstr.*, 10:660.
29. Madison, D. V., and Nicoll, R. A. (1986): *J. Physiol. (Lond.)*, 372:221–244.
30. Madison, D. V., and Nicoll, R. A. (1986): *J. Physiol. (Lond.)*, 372:245–259.
31. Malenka, R. C., Madison, D. V., Andrade, R., and Nicoll, R. A. (1987): *J. Neurosci. (in press)*.
32. Mountcastle, V. B., Andersen, R. A., and Motter, B. C. (1981): *J. Neurosci.*, 1:1218–1235.
33. Mueller, A. L., and Dunwiddie, T. V. (1983): *Epilepsia*, 24:57–64.
34. Nakai, Y., and Takaori, S. (1974): *Brain Res.*, 71:47–60.
35. Newberry, N. R., and Nicoll, R. A. (1985): *J. Physiol. (Lond.)*, 360:161–185.
36. Pennefather, P., Lancaster, B., Adams, P. R., and Nicoll, R. A. (1985): *Proc. Natl. Acad. Sci. USA*, 82:3040–3044.
37. Rogawski, M. A., and Aghajanian, G. K. (1980): *Nature*, 287:731–734.
38. Schwartzkroin, P. A., and Stafstrom, C. E. (1980): *Science*, 210:1125–1126.
39. Segal, M. (1981): *Brain Res.*, 206:107–128.
40. Segal, M. (1982): *Exp. Neurol.*, 77:86–93.
41. Segal, M., and Bloom, F. E. (1974): *Brain Res.*, 72:79–97.
42. Woodward, D. J., Moises, H. C., Waterhouse, B. D., Hoffer, B. J., and Freedman, R. (1979): *Fed. Proc.*, 38:2109–2116.

Psychopharmacology:
The Third Generation of Progress,
edited by Herbert Y. Meltzer.
Raven Press, New York © 1987.

CHAPTER **12**

Midbrain Dopaminergic Systems: Neurophysiology and Electrophysiological Pharmacology

Benjamin S. Bunney, Susan R. Sesack, and Nancy L. Silva

Midbrain dopaminergic (DA) neurons were identified electrophysiologically for the first time in 1973 (25). Five years later their neurophysiological characteristics and electrophysiological pharmacology were reviewed in the last publication of this volume (19). Nine years have now elapsed since that chapter was written and during that time there has been an exponential growth in publications relevant to this area. Discoveries in a variety of related basic science areas as well as the development of entirely new techniques have contributed significantly to this growth. For example, in addition to the discovery that a number of different peptides interact with midbrain DA neurons to modulate their activity, it was found that a subpopulation of these DA cells contain the peptide cholecystokinin (CCK) (63). The discovery that DA and CCK could coexist in the same cell not only started a whole new field of research endeavor (CCK-DA interactions) but served to emphasize a fact already recognized by many, that DA neurons form a very heterogeneous population. Thus, these cells differ not only in terms of their projection areas but also in terms of the types of feedback pathways they receive, the types of afferents that modulate their activity, the presence or absence of coexisting chemical messengers, their responsivity to acutely and chronically administered drugs and the types of receptors present on their terminals, cell bodies, and dendrites. New techniques, not available or at least not applied to this particular system nine years ago, include *in vivo* intracellular recording, extra- and intracellular recording from midbrain DA neurons in slices, and recording from DA neurons in freely moving animals.

Given the mass of new data on the physiology and electrophysiological pharmacology of DA neurons, and the space available in this volume, it would be impossible to do an in depth review of all areas. For this reason, we have arbitrarily chosen some areas to emphasize and some to mention, while totally omitting others. We apologize in advance to the reader who does not find his or her own work covered or a topic reviewed in which he or she is interested.

MIDBRAIN DA NEURONS

In Vivo Studies

Identification

Extracellular. Midbrain DA neurons were first identified electrophysiologically in 1973 (25) using a variety of indirect extracellular methods. Subsequently, a number of studies have added significant further evidence supporting the DA identity of these cells. Guyenet and Aghajanian (60) activated neurons in the zona compacta of the substantia nigra (A9) antidromically from the striatum. Two types of neurons were observed, one of which had identical electrophysiological characteristics to those previously attributed to DA neurons. This latter set of neurons had a conduction velocity of 0.58 m/sec, suggesting that they were unmyelinated, a finding that was compatible with histochemical data describing the axons of DA cells as fine and lacking myelination (64).

Several extracellular studies have contributed further evidence for the DA identity of neurons in the midbrain ventral tegmental area (A10). Deniau et al. (42) activated A10 neurons antidromically from a variety of projection areas. One subpopulation of activated cells possessed many of the electrophysiological characteristics of DA neurons and was found to have slow conduction velocities. In another study, animals were pretreated with the catecholamine (CA) specific neurotoxin 6-hydroxy-dopamine (6-OHDA) (111). In these animals, the number of slow-conducting neurons was greatly diminished. Wang (116) published an elegant set of experiments in which he demonstrated, as had been done previously in the A9 area, that A10 cells could be divided essentially into two groups: those with electrophysiological characteristics (including conduction velocities of approximately 0.5 m/sec) similar to other neurons in the A9/A10 area which had been previously identified as DA, and a heterogeneous group that, when compared to the DA cells, had a higher discharge rate, faster conduction velocity, and shorter spike duration. A10 cells were characterized further in terms of their projection areas by the concomitant use of a fluorescent retrograde tracer and the glyoxylic acid fluorescence histochemical method, which is specific for CA.

Combined, the efforts of the above investigators clearly demonstrate the feasibility of electrophysiologically identifying DA neurons in vivo. However, although sufficient for identification when taken together, the above-mentioned methods provide only indirect proof. One therefore would like a direct confirmation of the DA identity of these cells.

Intracellular. Direct *in vivo* electrophysiological identification of DA neurons depends on the absolute identification of the specific neuron recorded combined with the establishment of that neuron's neurochemical identity. Extracellular recording is not adequate in this regard, as it is impossible to ascertain the exact cell recorded. Intracellular recording, on the other hand, by its very nature allows one to identify the cell studied. One is then left with the problem of establishing the neurochemical identity of the intracellularly recorded cell. This can be accomplished in a variety of ways, but in each case the end result is dependent on a chemical reaction that specifically identifies the neurotransmitter used by the neuron. For the identification of midbrain DA neurons, the specific chemical process consists of the reaction of DA with glyoxylic acid to form a fluorescent product. As glyoxylic acid will also react with other CA to produce fluorescent compounds, the specificity in this case is dependent on the fact that the only CA contained by neurons in the area under study is DA.

Using the above principles, midbrain DA neurons were directly identified electrophysiologically in 1980 (49). This initial identification has subsequently been extended using modifications of the original technique and has been broadened to include A10 DA neurons (30) as well as A9 DA cells (50).

Characterization

Extracellular. DA neurons have now been characterized extracellularly in four *in vivo* animal preparations: (a)

anesthetized (usually using chloral hydrate), (b) gallamine paralyzed, (c) low cerveau isole, (d) unanesthetized freely moving. All four preparations have yielded similar results. DA cells were found to be either nonfiring or firing spontaneously. The nonfiring DA cells made up approximately 20% of the total population and could be activated by intravenous haloperidol administration or by iontophoresis of the excitatory substance glutamic acid. DA cells activated in the latter manner cease firing when glutamate ejection is terminated and are inhibited by coiontophoresis of DA. Intracellular recording from these inactive DA cells demonstrated a higher resting potential (−65 to −75 mV) compared to those firing spontaneously.

Spontaneously active DA cells fire in one or a combination of two modes—single spike and bursting (53,54). Single-spiking DA cells typically fire in a slow irregular pattern with an average rate of 4.5 ± 1.5 spikes/sec. The interspike interval of these cells forms a near normal distribution around 200 to 250 msec. The action potentials are usually biphasic (often with an inflection in the initial positive-going segment) and exhibit a long time-course (2.75 ± 0.5 msec, mean ± SD; range 1.8–4.2 msec).

DA cells can also fire in bursts of 3 to 12 spikes. Spike amplitude progressively decreases and duration increases within each burst. Bursts begin with the first pair of spikes having an interspike interval of 80 msec or less. The termination of these bursts is followed by a long period of silence that averages 343 ± 112 msec in duration. For a given cell, bursting tends to increase as the rate of the cell increases. However, between cells there is a very poor correlation between firing rate and degree of bursting (54).

Both modes of activity, single spiking and bursting, have been observed in freely moving, drug-free rats (83), and cats (110), and DA cells have been seen to spontaneously switch between one mode and the other. These findings suggest that shifting back and forth between modes may be important for the functioning of DA systems (45).

Intracellular. Intracellularly, DA cell action potentials are observed to contain four subcomponents (51): (a) a slow depolarization, approximately 80 msec in duration and of 10 to 15 mV in amplitude; (b) an initial segment (IS) spike; (c) a somatodendritic (SD) spike; and (d) a calcium-dependent after-hyperpolarization (AHP). The slow depolarization brings the DA cell from its resting potential (−55 to −58 mV) to an atypically high spike threshold (−45 mV).

The slow depolarization demonstrates voltage dependency and can be inhibited by systemic administration of autoreceptor doses (106) of apomorphine (APO) (50,53,56). At spike threshold the slow depolarization triggers the lower threshold IS spike. This IS spike can in turn trigger the SD action potential (51).

SD action potentials are of comparatively long duration and small amplitude in a spontaneously firing neuron (e.g., 2.5 msec and 55–65 mV, respectively) and are most likely associated with a significant calcium component. The low amplitude may be due to the presence of a high baseline level of calcium current inactivation, since intracellular injection of ethyleneglycol bis(aminoethylether)tetraacetate (EGTA) will increase the spike amplitude by 20 mV or more above this level (53). An increased calcium entry associated with increased firing rate may be responsible for the rate-dependent decrease in spike amplitude observed during extracellular and intracellular recording (53). The AHP is probably a calcium-activated potassium current ($IK_{(Ca)}$) (82), since it can be specifically blocked by intracellular injection of the calcium chelator EGTA or long-term (30 min or more) intracellular injection of the potassium channel blocker tetraethylammonium (TEA). This $IK_{(Ca)}$ is most likely responsible for the long interspike interval and irregular firing pattern observed in spontaneously discharging DA neurons. *In vivo* intracellular recording has shown that DA cell bursts ride on a depolarizing wave (5–15 mV in amplitude) (49). These bursts are different from those observed in other vertebrate neurons. Due to their long interspike interval within the burst (73 ± 13 msec), DA cell bursts probably do not arise as a result of rebound calcium spikes, which are believed to mediate burst generation in other brain regions (78,132). Burst firing can be triggered by increases in firing rate, as observed with iontophoresis of excitatory compounds or long periods (greater than 3 min) of depolarizing current injection. Initiation of burst firing most likely occurs as a result of an increased spike-dependent calcium event since (a) burst firing is highly correlated with increases in firing rates; (b) the ability of depolarization to induce burst firing is prevented by intracellular EGTA injection; and (c) intracellular injection of calcium will initiate burst firing without concomitant increases in firing rate (54). The ability of calcium to trigger burst firing may depend on its ability to inactivate a voltage-dependent potassium current ($IK_{(v)}$). Thus, depolarization initially decreases DA cell input resistance during periods of firing rate accommodation, but the input resistance typically increases again at the onset of bursting. Furthermore, extracellular iontophoresis of the potassium blocker barium, as well as intracellular injection of the potassium blocker TEA, will trigger burst firing. These potassium blockers also cause an increase in the duration of the action potential. DA cell action potentials occurring in bursts typically show a progressive increase in spike duration as the burst progresses (25,50,54). The increase in spike duration during burst firing in other preparations is believed to occur through an inactivation of the $IK_{(v)}$, lending support for this burst firing model. DA neuron bursts are usually terminated by an $IK_{(Ca)}$ typically occurring 20 msec or more after the last spike of the burst.

One totally unexpected finding resulting from intracellular recording in midbrain DA neurons was electrotonic coupling (52). Spontaneously occurring small (3–15 mV) fast potentials were observed in spontaneously firing DA cells, especially those that were bursting. These fast potentials often triggered action potentials in DA cells when the membrane potential was close to firing threshold. The fast potentials had a rate and pattern similar to DA cell action potentials and could be activated antidromically from the caudate nucleus with a similar constant latency. They also followed high-frequency stimulation at a constant latency and collided with spontaneously occurring fast potentials.

On the other hand, directly elicited action potentials did not collide reliably with antidromically activated fast potentials. Intracellular injection of depolarizing or hyperpolarizing current changed the rate of occurrence of these fast

potentials and their firing rate could be manipulated by i.v. administration of DA agonists and antagonists. Anatomical support for belief that the fast potentials represent electrotonic coupling between DA cells came from intracellular injections of Lucifer Yellow at the end of experiments in which these potentials were observed. Subsequent examination of midbrain slices with a fluorescence microscope revealed one to five cells labeled even though in each case only one DA cell had been injected. Extracellular evidence for electrotonic coupling has been observed in the form of nearly simultaneous, synchronized groups of action potentials (either two or three together). These were observed in all preparations studied including freely moving animals (45) and were recorded in both the A9 and A10 region.

Finally, another state in which DA neurons can be found is characterized by inactivity. However, in this case inactivity results from tonic depolarization block. Such a condition can be induced by the acute administration of CCK or by the repeated administration of antipsychotic drugs (see below).

Modulation

Autoreceptors. In 1972 Kehr et al. (73) published the first biochemical evidence suggesting that there were receptors for DA on DA terminals in the striatum that modulated DA synthesis and release (Fig. 1). Carlsson (27) later termed these receptors "DA autoreceptors." The following year, using electrophysiological techniques, somatodendritic autoreceptors were found on both A9 and A10 DA neurons (1) (Fig. 1). Since that time these findings have been greatly extended. The sensitivity of somatodendritic A9 DA cell autoreceptors was compared to postsynaptic DA receptors in the striatum (106). DA cells were found to be 6 to 10 times more sensitive to the inhibitory effects of iontophoretically applied DA and intravenously administered apomorphine than were the postsynaptic striatal cells tested. Using relatively specific D1 and D2 agonists and antagonists, White and Wang (126) demonstrated that DA autoreceptors in the A10 area were of the D2 type. In addition, a variety of studies using antidromic activation from the nucleus accumbens or the olfactory tubercles has suggested that autoreceptors on A10 DA cells may participate in self-inhibition by DA neurons (47,116,117,118).

The discovery of autoreceptors and the fact that they are more sensitive to directly acting dopamine agonists than are DA postsynaptic receptors have provided the impetus for an intensive search for a *selective* autoreceptor agonist in the hope that such a compound would provide a new treatment for those disorders thought to be due to hyperfunctioning of DA systems. Several such compounds have been studied electrophysiologically, including 3-PPP and EMD 23 448 (39,34, respectively). Of these two compounds, EMD 23 448 was found to be the more selective.

The search for a selective autoreceptor agonist recently took on new meaning when it was discovered that not all midbrain DA neurons possess autoreceptors. The first evidence that this was the case came from biochemical studies in which it was demonstrated that DA terminals in

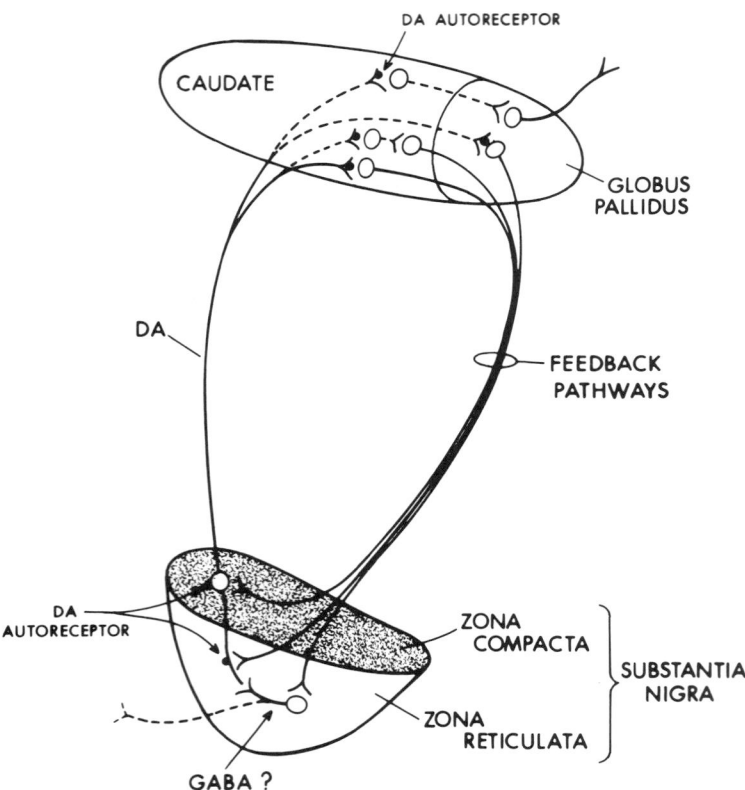

DA AUTORECEPTOR

CAUDATE

GLOBUS PALLIDUS

DA

FEEDBACK PATHWAYS

DA AUTORECEPTOR

ZONA COMPACTA

SUBSTANTIA NIGRA

ZONA RETICULATA

GABA ?

FIG. 1. Schematic representation of mechanisms for the control of DA activity: somatodendritic autoreceptors and feedback pathways. The exact interconnections in the caudate and globus pallidus are unknown and only some of the possibilities are illustrated. It *is* known that at least one feedback pathway uses GABA as its chemical messenger and is inhibitory to both DA neurons and ZR (GABA?) cells. The latter also inhibit DA neurons and are significantly more sensitive to the inhibitory effects of GABA than are the DA cells themselves. Thus, activation of the GABAergic feedback pathway can lead to disinhibition of DA cells (see text).

the prefrontal and cingulate cortices lack synthesis-regulating autoreceptors (7).

Subsequent studies using electrophysiological techniques have demonstrated that antidromically identified DA neurons projecting to the prefrontal and cingulate cortices lack or have a significantly decreased number of somatodendritic autoreceptors (30,102,125). A comparison of the electrophysiological properties of DA neurons projecting to the prefrontal and cingulate cortices with DA cells projecting to the caudate nucleus and accumbens nucleus demonstrated that the former had a higher baseline firing rate and a greater degree of bursting. These findings correlate well with biochemical data demonstrating that mesocortical DA neurons have a higher turnover rate compared to other brain CA systems (30). The discovery that some midbrain DA neurons lack autoreceptors increases the importance of finding selective autoreceptor agonists, as it holds out the possibility that such a pharmacological agent would be selective for some DA systems but not others and thus provide a tool for beginning to discriminate differences in function among the various DA systems.

Peptides. A variety of peptides and their receptors have been reported to be present in both the substantia nigra and the ventral tegmental area. In addition, a subpopulation of midbrain DA neurons has been demonstrated to contain the peptide CCK (63) as well as neurotensin (62).

Perhaps because of its coexistence with DA, CCK has been studied electrophysiologically in by far the greatest detail. CCK was found to be one of the most powerful

excitants of DA neurons studied to date (107). Administered either intravenously in doses as low as 1 mg/kg or applied directly to DA cells by means of microiontophoresis, CCK has a variety of effects, including the ability to (a) activate nonfiring hyperpolarized DA neurons; (b) increase activity and switch to bursting mode all DA neurons in areas where DA and CCK coexist; (c) induce a tonic state of depolarization inactivation in some DA neurons; (d) potentiate the inhibition of DA neurons induced by low doses of apomorphine, which are presumably acting selectively at somatodendritic autoreceptors (67). All of these effects are blocked by the glutaramic acid derivative proglumide, a putative selective CCK antagonist in the CNS (33,38). Studies in freely moving rats have now confirmed both the excitatory and DA potentiating effects of i.v. CCK as well as the ability of proglumide to block its activating effects (44).

Recent evidence suggests that the intravenous effects of the CCK used (in these studies the sulfated form of either CCK 7 or 8) have both a peripheral and a central component (66). Thus, lesions of either the vagal fibers in the medulla or the efferent pathways from the nucleus tractus solitarius significantly decreased the effects of systemically administered CCK on DA cells. On the other hand, neither lesion completely blocked CCK's effect. Thus, CCK has profound effects on DA cell activity; however, the exact role of CCK in the control of that activity has not been discovered.

Although not yet studied in any detail, a variety of other peptides have been found to have excitatory effects on either A9 or A10 DA neurons. These peptides include neurotensin (70), substance P (70,95), substance K (70), and dynorphin (114).

Feedback pathways. Over the years more and more anatomical evidence has accumulated suggesting that many midbrain DA cell projection areas have output neurons that project back to the midbrain (Fig. 1). Electrophysiological studies suggest that many of these neurons form single or multisynaptic pathways that provide feedback control of their DA innervation. Evidence available to date suggests that the most common chemical messenger for these pathways is γ-amino butyric acid (GABA). Most of the electrophysiological experiments carried out to study these feedback pathways have concentrated on the nigrostriatal DA system.

A9 neurons. Evidence for the involvement of feedback pathways in the modulation of A9 DA neurons takes several forms. Stimulation in the caudate nucleus has been found to produce both excitatory and inhibitory effects on A9 DA neurons and on non-DA zona reticulata cells (40,55). In other studies, output neurons from the striatum were destroyed by local injection of a neurotoxin such as kainic acid, electrolytic lesions, or selective knife cuts of the striatonigral feedback pathway and the effects of these lesions on A9 DA cell functioning determined. Such lesions were found to decrease the ability of striatal stimulation to inhibit neurons in the substantia nigra (84) and greatly diminish the effects of indirectly acting DA agonists (e.g., *d*-amphetamine) on A9 DA cells (20). The acute effects of intrastriatal injections of kainic acid itself on A9 DA neurons have also been studied. It was demonstrated that 1 hr after injection, DA cell firing rates were significantly increased, whereas 12 hr after kainic acid injection, although cell firing rate had returned to control levels, the number of spontaneously firing DA cells had significantly decreased. Indirect evidence suggested that the "silent" DA cells were in a state of depolarization inactivation. By 48 hr after kainic acid injection, the number of spontaneously active DA cells was significantly increased, indicating that a subpopulation of DA cells normally not firing had become spontaneously active after destruction of striatonigral feedback pathways (15).

The response of DA cells to the striatal injection of an excitatory substance not only demonstrated the progressive effects of kainic acid on striatal neurons but also the complexity of the interactions between output neurons and DA cells. This complexity is further highlighted by a series of experiments in which it was demonstrated that a systemically administered GABA agonist, muscimol, increased the activity of A9 DA cells (48,79,115,119). At the same time, many of these studies demonstrated that non-DA cells in the zona reticulata (ZR) were inhibited by intravenous muscimol and that ZR neurons were more sensitive to the inhibitory effects of GABA and/or muscimol than were DA cells when these substances were iontophoretically applied. These findings thus formed a paradox—both DA and non-DA ZR cells could be inhibited by local application of GABA or muscimol and yet intravenous muscimol excited DA neurons. The identification of a ZR neuron that was inhibitory to DA cells and was 20 times more

sensitive to iontophoretically applied GABA than DA cells provided an explanation for the paradox (48). Thus, the data suggest that although both cells receive a GABAergic input, and therefore possess GABA receptors, at low doses directly acting GABA agonists will preferentially inhibit the more sensitive ZR interneuron. Since this interneuron is inhibitory on DA cells, the result would be a disinhibition of DA cells and consequently an increase in activity. Further support for this explanation comes from unpublished work by Waszczak (see ref. 119) demonstrating that the excitatory action of systemic muscimol on A9 DA cells is unaffected by kainic acid-induced destruction of striatonigral feedback pathways.

Recently, striatonigral feedback pathway control of A9 DA cells has been studied in great detail using combined *in vivo* extracellular and intracellular techniques (55,56). It was found that stimulation of the striatum resulted in an inhibitory postsynaptic potential (IPSP) and a rebound depolarization in DA cells. A variety of lines of evidence suggest that the IPSP is due to a short-latency conductance increase to chloride ions, suggesting that a GABAergic pathway is involved. Striatal stimulation was also found to elicit IPSPs in a subclass of substantia nigra ZR neurons at the same latency as the IPSPs triggered in DA cells, although their amplitude and duration were longer and there was no depolarizing rebound. These IPSPs were also found to be due to increases in chloride conductance and are therefore assumed to be mediated by a GABAergic input. It was determined that the late component of the IPSP in the ZR neurons corresponded temporally to the rebound depolarization seen in DA cells in response to striatal stimulation. When recorded extracellularly, striatal stimulation was found to inhibit the firing of this class of ZR neurons while exciting DA cells. Combined, the data suggest that striatal cells may send branched fast-conducting GABAergic projections both to ZR and DA neurons. They also add further support to previous work (see above) suggesting that low levels of striatal stimulation can excite DA cells by preferentially inhibiting interneurons in the ZR that are more sensitive to the inhibitory effects of GABA than are DA neurons.

In summary, we now have a detailed understanding of some of the components that make up one of the striatonigral feedback systems responsible for modulating DA cell activity (i.e., those components that reside within the substantia nigra). The parts of the pathway that are located within the striatum and/or globus pallidus remain poorly delineated. Thus, we do not know whether the GABAergic input to the substantia nigra described above receives a direct DA innervation or whether there are one or more neurons intervening between DA innervation to the striatum and the GABAergic feedback pathways. Nevertheless, the fact that activation of GABAergic neurons in the striatum leads to disinhibition of DA cells and that ZR neurons, which are inhibitory to DA neurons, are 20 times more sensitive to the inhibitory effects of GABA than are DA cells themselves adds several layers of complexity to an already complex series of interactions.

How might these complex modulatory systems (i.e., autoreceptor and feedback pathway) function to govern

DA cell activity under more physiological conditions where exogenous administration of pharmacological agents is not involved? Can we develop a model to study how these two modulatory systems interact with each other? One such model system may be available (65). A9 DA cells have been shown to respond to a variety of sensory stimuli (28,29,37,48,65). In an attempt to obtain quantitative information about the effects of peripheral stimulation on DA cell activity, stimulation of the sciatic nerve was used. Stimulation at frequencies of 0.5 Hz or less produced an initial inhibition of DA cell activity followed by oscillations between excitation and inhibition which slowly diminished in amplitude until a return to baseline activity was reached 500 to 1,000 msec after the single stimulus. A reciprocal pattern of the initial activity change was seen in a subpopulation of ZR neurons. Selective knife cuts of the striatonigral feedback pathway totally eliminated the rebound excitation and oscillations recorded in DA cells in response to sciatic nerve stimulation while increasing the initial inhibitory period. Thus it would appear that stimulation in the periphery, through as yet unknown pathways, results in an initial inhibition of DA cell activity. The inhibitory period, however, is cut short due to a rebound excitation mediated through striatonigral feedback pathways that involve a substantia nigra interneuron inhibitory to DA cells. The oscillations in activity thus would seem to be due to feedback pathway responses to intermittent release of DA from terminals in the striatum.

In another series of experiments, the DA receptor blocker haloperidol was administered systemically and its effects on DA cell rate changes induced by sciatic nerve stimulation were studied. Haloperidol attenuated the oscillatory response of DA cells but also decreased the duration of the initial inhibition (65). Preliminary unpublished studies suggest that iontophoretic administration of another DA receptor blocker, trifluoperazine, onto DA cells also decreases the initial inhibition of these neurons induced by sciatic nerve stimulation. Combined, these results would suggest that part of the initial inhibitory period after sciatic nerve stimulation is mediated through dopamine acting on DA autoreceptors. Why DA should be released under these conditions is not clear, although Glowinsky and co-workers (85) have presented evidence suggesting that DA release from dendrites can occur in the absence of impulse flow. In any event, sciatic nerve stimulation-induced changes in DA cell activity may provide a model for studying both feedback pathway and autoreceptor control of DA cell activity.

A10 neurons. Very few studies have been carried out examining the effects of feedback pathways on identified A10 DA cell activity. One study demonstrated that stimulation of the nucleus accumbens would inhibit unidentified neurons within the ventral tegmental area (VTA) and that this inhibition could be blocked by the GABA antagonist bicuculline (131). In another study two GABA agonists, muscimol and 4,5,6,7-tetra hydroisoxazolo-(5,4,-c)-pyridin-3-ol (THIP), administered intravenously, caused a dose-dependent increase in extracellular DA cell activity (120). These results suggest that like A9 DA cells, A10 DA cells may be regulated by feedback pathways involving an inhib-

itory neuron that is inhibited by GABA, thus leading to disinhibition. Much more work needs to be done in this area, however, before we will know for sure that this is the case.

Pharmacology

Since the original electrophysiological identification of midbrain DA neurons (25), a number of studies have been carried out examining the acute and chronic effects of a wide variety of pharmacological agents on DA cell activity. In some cases drugs were used as tools to discover which neurotransmitter systems influence DA cell functioning. In other experiments, drug studies were performed in an attempt to further understand their site and mechanism of action. The former type of experiments has been described, where appropriate, in the above sections. The latter type of studies will be discussed in this section but because of space limitations will be limited solely to the effects of DA antagonists on midbrain DA system functioning.

Most pharmacological agents that fall into the category of DA antagonists have antipsychotic activity and, in addition, produce unwanted neurological side effects. From the time of their initial discovery in 1953, behavioral and biochemical techniques had been used to try to discover the underlying mechanisms and sites of action responsible for these two sets of clinical effects. Electrophysiological techniques, on the other hand, were not extensively used prior to 1973. However, in the ensuing 5 years, the acute effects of a variety of antipsychotic drugs (ADs) were studied in some detail. Since the last publication of this book, researchers' attention has been primarily focused on the effects of repeated AD administration on neurochemically defined systems.

Acute effects. Acutely, ADs change the functioning of midbrain DA neurons in a variety of ways. With the exception of ADs lacking Parkinson-like side effects (e.g., clozapine), all ADs increase the activity of both A9 and A10 neurons. The degree to which they do this is dependent on both the baseline rate of the individual cell being studied (i.e., the faster the baseline activity, the less increase in rate induced by an AD) and on the preparation used (e.g., anesthetics can have a marked effect on the responsivity of DA neurons to a wide variety of pharmacological agents). The increased activity induced by ADs in A9 DA cells has been demonstrated to be, at least in part, dependent on intact striatonigral feedback pathways (65,75).

Another site at which ADs could act to affect the activity of DA cells is at the somatodendritic autoreceptor. The inhibition of these cells by microiontophoretic application of DA has been shown to be blocked by a variety of ADs including i.v. haloperidol (1,28), i.v. chlorpromazine (1), and iontophoretically applied trifluoperazine (2,28,34). On the other hand, trifluoperazine alone has no effect on DA cell discharge rate when administered locally to the cell recorded (2,28,34). In contrast, the local infusion of haloperidol into the substantia nigra was reported to increase the firing rate of A9 cells (58). The reason for the divergent results obtained with these two techniques remains unknown.

DA antagonist blockade of DA autoreceptors can also affect the general responsiveness of DA neurons. For example, the postdischarge inhibitory period observed in the autocorrelation histograms of A9 DA neurons, thought by some to be due to self-inhibitory somatodendritic feedback mechanisms (57,130), is dramatically shortened by the systemic administration of haloperidol (129). Similarly, the inhibition observed in A9 cells after the invasion of the cell body region by a stimulus-elicited antidromic action potential [which is presumably releasing DA from the dendrites of DA neurons (76) and thereby stimulating local inhibitory autoreceptors] is shortened by both systemic haloperidol administration and microiontophoretically applied trifluoperazine (84). In addition, antidromic activation of A10 neurons from the nucleus accumbens has been shown to inhibit the activity of these cells, presumably via similar inhibitory DA somatodendritic mechanisms (116). This inhibitory effect is attenuated by the systemic administration of haloperidol. The fact that this effect is only moderately attenuated by ibotenic acid lesions of the nucleus accumbens further supports the notion that dendritic mechanisms may be important in regulating A10 DA neuronal activity (116,117).

Activation of midbrain DA neurons by ADs is characterized not only by an increase in firing rate but by a change in firing pattern—from a predominantly single-spiking mode to the bursting mode. *In vivo* intracellular recording has demonstrated that i.v. haloperidol depolarizes the membrane of DA cells by 2 to 5 mV and increases their membrane input resistance 20 to 50%. This excitatory action of haloperidol may be due to the removal of an inhibitory GABAergic feedback input to DA cells as the reversal potential of this haloperidol effect was similar to the GABA reversal potential (24). Intravenous haloperidol also increases the rate of occurrence of fast potentials [thought to be due to electrotonic coupling between DA cells (52)] and causes these potentials to be observed where none had been present before. A similar phenomenon has been observed extracellularly. Last, acute AD administration appears to activate a population of "silent" hyperpolarized DA cells, which have been found in every preparation studied to date (23,32). When combined, the above results suggest that the effect of acute AD administration is a marked activation of midbrain DA systems.

Chronic effects. When ADs are administered repeatedly (e.g., once a day for 21 days), their effect differs markedly from that observed after acute administration. The first studies (involving A9 DA cells exclusively) found that the great majority of midbrain DA neurons had become "silent" due to the induction of a tonic state of depolarization inactivation (23). These findings were later confirmed and extended to A10 DA cells (32,123,124). *In vivo* intracellular recording has recently verified that the inactivity is due to depolarization block (24). Feedback pathways would appear to play a role in the development of AD-induced depolarization inactivation of both A9 and A10 neurons, as destruction of the striatonigral and pallidonigral feedback pathways, prior to initiation of repeated haloperidol admin-

istration, totally prevented the development of depolarization inactivation of A9 cells (23) and prior lesioning of the nucleus accumbens produced similar results with A10 cells (123). However, in accordance with the mounting evidence suggesting that autoreceptors play a more important role in regulating A10 DA cell activity than they do for A9 DA cells, acute knife cuts, which transected the midbrain, immediately reversed the depolarization inactivation of A9 but not A10 DA neurons induced by 21 days of repeated chlorpromazine treatment (32). Further support for the possible importance of A10 DA cell autoreceptors in mediating AD-induced depolarization inactivation comes from the finding that there are two sets of midbrain DA cells that do not become inactivated by repeated AD administration—those DA neurons innervating the prefrontal and cingulate cortices (32), both of which lack somatodendritic DA autoreceptors (30).

Time-course studies have demonstrated that 2 weeks of repeated AD administration are necessary to obtain maximal depolarization inactivation (123) and that once obtained, it is still present after 7 months of repeated treatment (36). However, no permanent changes appear to have occurred, since after a 2-week wash-out period (e.g., 2 weeks after discontinuing treatment), the number of DA cells firing in both the A9 and A10 areas has returned to control levels.

Not all ADs induce depolarization inactivation of A9 and A10 neurons. Those drugs that lack or have a markedly decreased incidence of Parkinson-like side effects and tardive dyskinesia (e.g., clozapine) induce depolarization inactivation only in A10 DA neurons (32,124). On the other hand, drugs that possess extrapyramidal side effects but lack or have a low level of antipsychotic efficacy (e.g., metoclopramide) induce depolarization inactivation in A9 cells but not in A10 DA neurons (124). Combined, these findings suggest that depolarization inactivation of DA neurons may be one of the mechanisms underlying both the time-dependent therapeutic and neurological side effects of these drugs.

What makes a drug like clozapine incapable of inducing depolarization inactivation of A9 neurons? In addition to its effects on DA systems, clozapine has at least two other actions in the brain—anticholinergic activity (108) and alpha noradrenergic receptor-blocking properties (26,81,109). In an attempt to determine whether one or the other of these properties might be important in this regard, the number of spontaneously firing DA cells in the A9 and A10 areas was determined after 21 days of pretreatment with haloperidol and the anticholinergic drug trihexyphenidyl, haloperidol and the alpha-1 antagonist prazosin, or haloperidol and the alpha-2 antagonist idazoxan. The results were compared with clozapine or haloperidol treatment alone (35). It was found that concomitant treatment with either trihexyphenidyl or prazosin, but not idazoxan, gave haloperidol a clozapine-like profile in terms of its effect on spontaneous A9 and A10 activity. Thus, when combined with an anticholinergic drug or an alpha-1 blocker, haloperidol no longer induced depolarization inactivation of A9 DA cells. The fact that the alpha-2 blocker did not have this effect ruled out the possibility that these were nonspecific results due to polypharmacy.

In another set of studies, 21 days of treatment with i.p. haloperidol was found to result in A9 DA cell autoreceptor supersensitivity 7 days after cessation of treatment. Furthermore, in a separate group of animals, concurrent administration of lithium carbonate was found to prevent this change in receptor sensitivity (46).

In summary, the above data suggest that the primary effect of repeated AD administration on most midbrain DA neurons is inactivation. This depolarization-induced cessation of spontaneous activity would appear to have a marked effect on both basal and stimulated DA release from nerve terminals in that several studies, using voltametric techniques, have now demonstrated DA release to be diminished under these conditions (12,22,99). These findings stand in marked contrast to the acute effects of ADs where biochemical techniques have been used to demonstrate a marked increase in the release of DA into projection areas (12,68,69). The combined effects of acute and chronic AD administration on midbrain DA cell activity may explain the delay in onset of both their therapeutic and neurological side effects (16,23).

In Vitro Studies

The recently developed midbrain tissue slice preparation offers investigators a new approach to the study of neuronal function. Within the past 5 years a number of laboratories have adopted this preparation to study the electrophysiological and pharmacological properties of midbrain DA systems.

Characterization

In vitro single-unit extracellular recording studies have demonstrated that A9 and A10 DA-sensitive neurons have slow firing rates (1–9 spikes/sec) and long-duration action potentials (>2 msec) (90,98,103,112). These characteristics are identical to those which have been recorded from identified DA neurons in vivo (25,50). Some debate as to whether baseline DA cell firing rates are slower or faster in vitro has arisen. However, this may be due either to the different animals that were used (e.g., rat vs. mouse) or, more probably, to differing ionic constituents that were used in the perfusion medium (especially K^+ concentration). One distinct difference between DA neurons in vivo and DA-sensitive cells in vitro is that, whereas they display an irregular and/or burst firing pattern in vivo, DA-sensitive neurons have a very regular firing pattern with no bursting in vitro. One study did report burst firing; however, in this same study a more regular firing pattern was encountered when synaptic input was eliminated by perfusing the slices with a high-Mg^{2+}, low-Ca^{2+} solution (98). The regular firing pattern is presumed to be due to the loss of afferent input that occurs in the slice preparation.

One intracellular study, thus far, has optimized the use of the nigral slice to investigate the electrophysiological properties of unidentified neurons within the zona compacta (77). Two types of firing patterns, repetitive firing and burst firing, were demonstrated. Depolarization of neurons from

resting membrane potential evoked repetitive firing, whereas depolarization of neurons from a hyperpolarized state evoked burst firing. During perfusions of specific ionic channel blockers, two types of calcium conductances were observed. One was associated with depolarizing pulse injection at resting membrane potentials (high-threshold spike, HTS) and the other was associated with membrane depolarization from a hyperpolarized level (low-threshold spike, LTS). Further, synaptic activation of cells or manipulation of cells' length constant suggested that the sites of generation of the LTS and HTS were located at a distance from the cell body (possibly in the dendrites). In some instances both types of calcium conductances were elicited. As calcium conductances can be associated with both depolarizing and hyperpolarizing events, it was proposed that the above results might help to explain why calcium-dependent dendritic DA release is not so easily correlated with firing rate in vivo. Preliminary intracellular studies of A9 DA-sensitive neurons in our laboratory have shown that spontaneously firing DA neurons in vitro have a spontaneous slow depolarizing potential that initiates the action potential, which, in turn, is followed by an afterhyperpolarization (N. L. Silva and B. S. Bunney, unpublished observations). These findings are identical to those obtained in vivo (53,54). The extremely regular firing pattern exhibited by these cells is most likely due to the intrinsic pacemaker activity and would be predicted from the previously described regulation of DA cell firing pattern observed in vivo (53,54). In accordance with others (74,94), the resting membrane potential of these cells appears to be approximately −60 mV and the 55- to 65-mV action potential occurs following a 12- to 15-mV spontaneous depolarization. These cells maintain a resting input resistance of 100 to 200 MΩ.

Autoreceptors

DA autoreceptors have also been studied in vitro. A reduction of DA cell firing rate was seen following the administration of DA in the perfusion bath (89,90,98,103). This inhibition was dose dependent and was apparently due to an action at somatic or dendritic autoreceptors, as it persisted during perfusion of medium, which blocked synaptic activity. We have carried out a quantitative study combining simultaneous electrophysiological recording and voltametric DA concentration measurements to investigate the effect of known concentrations of DA on A9 DA cell activity (103,104). Dose-response curves revealed that two subpopulations of DA neurons (with respect to their sensitivity to DA) exist within the zona compacta of the substantia nigra. These two populations have parallel dose-response curves, but the concentration of DA that inhibits their firing rates by 50% is separated by approximately an order of magnitude. [Further support for the existence of two populations of DA cells characterized by autoreceptor sensitivity was recently demonstrated in freely moving animal experiments in which the sensitivity to i.v. apomorphine also differed by approximately an order of magnitude between cell groups (44).] Analysis of these two curves suggests that, in both cell populations, the relationship of DA concentration and the percent inhibition of cell firing evoked by DA follows a simple equilibrium model having a stoichiometric relationship of 1:1. Thus, in each population, one unit of DA concentration is associated with one unit of change in physiological response (e.g., inhibition of DA cell firing rate). The specificity of this response has also been examined. DA-evoked inhibition of all cells could be reversed by 1-sulpiride, a selective D_2 antagonist, but not by bicuculline, a GABA antagonist that antagonizes GABA-evoked inhibition of DA cells *in vitro*. These data add further support to *in vivo* studies suggesting that DA autoreceptors are of the D_2 type (41,100,126) and the hypothesis that DA is acting directly on DA cells and not through GABAergic terminals or interneurons (2,20). Only one investigator has used intracellular recording in slices to examine the effects of DA on A9 neurons. This study reported that DA administration was associated with a hyperpolarization and a decrease in input resistance of the cell (94). *In vivo* studies (56) have described a hyperpolarization and slight increase in input resistance following the administration of DA agonists. The reason for this discrepancy is unclear.

Afferent Effects

The deafferented nature of the slice is important because it allows for the investigation of the actions of physiologically significant substances (e.g., neurotransmitters, modulators, hormones) on DA cell activity in a less complex environment than is encountered *in vivo*. Several studies have begun to evaluate the effects of putative neurotransmitters on A9 and A10 neurons. It has been shown that A9 and A10 DA-sensitive neurons are differentially sensitive to β-endorphin and morphine but have similar sensitivities to enkephalin (113). All responses were excitatory, antagonized by naloxone, and persisted during synaptic blockade. DA-sensitive cells within the A9 area are inhibited by norepinephrine, but this response could not be antagonized by propranolol or phentolamine, and it is therefore unlikely that alpha or beta adrenergic receptors are involved (90). The existence of two types of GABA receptors on DA-sensitive neurons in the A9 area has been postulated based on the finding that the GABA-A agonist, muscimol, depolarized these cells, whereas the GABA-B agonist, baclofen, hyperpolarized them and GABA itself could produce both effects (93). Finally, the excitatory effects of neurotensin were reported to be maintained during synaptic blockade, and associated with a depolarization and an increase in input resistance in approximately 60% of the DA-sensitive cells tested (94). Future intracellular recording studies in which the ionic components of the perfusion bath are manipulated will more clearly elucidate the molecular mechanisms underlying these neurotransmitter-evoked events.

Drug Effects

Extracellular recording experiments have studied the actions of several DA agonists and antagonists on DA cell activity in the slice preparation. The primary goal of these studies was to determine if the nigral slice could be utilized as a CNS bioassay system to examine and compare the activity of DA agonists and the potency of DA antagonists with data from biochemical, binding, and clinical studies. In agreement with invertebrate and kidney studies, it was determined that rigid DA analogs such as apomorphine, 2-amino-6,7-dihydroxy-1,2,3,4-tetrahydronaphthalene (ADTN), 6,7-dihydroxy-2-dimethyl aminotetralin (TL-99), and 2-di-*n*-propylamino-4,7-dimethoxyindane (RDS-127) are at least 100 times more potent at inhibiting DA cell firing rate than is DA (90,91). In contrast, the removal or rearrangement of the hydroxyl groups on the catechol ring [e.g., octopamine, *p*-tyramine, norphenephrine, *N*-*n*-propyl-3-(3-hydroxyphenyl)-piperidine (3-PPP), 2-amino-5,6-dihydroxy-1,2,3,4-tetrahydronaphthalene (5,6-ATN)] is associated with decreased potency of DA agonists. All DA agonist activity could be blocked by DA antagonists (e.g., (−)-sulpiride, haloperidol, flupenthixol). Further, when comparing the effects of apomorphine, 5,6-ATN, and ADTN, it was suggested that the potency of apomorphine and ADTN appears to be determined by the active conformation of DA which is contained in apomorphine and ADTN and not by the hydroxyl group position, which is similar in apomorphine and 5,6-ATN.

The mechanism of action of DA antagonists has been quantitatively evaluated by simultaneously perfusing slices with DA and antipsychotic drugs. In one study by Pinnock (92), the effects of (−)-sulpiride, haloperidol, and cis-flupenthixol on DA dose-response curves were studied. The potencies of haloperidol and sulpiride were quite similar to those which have been described in binding studies. However, the potency of cis-flupenthixol was 100 times less than that found with binding and clinical efficacy studies. The reason for this discrepancy is unknown. In the presence of DA antagonists the dose-response curves for DA were shifted in parallel to the right. Schild plot analysis of these data suggests that because the slopes of the plots deviated from unity the antagonism is not competitive. This author cautioned that these experiments are tedious, requiring long recording periods and many perfusion medium changes, risking the stability of the recording. Further, he suggested that Schild plot slopes might deviate from unity for reasons that were not addressed in these experiments. These technical problems need to be worked out to clarify the interpretation of future experiments. Overall, this work suggests that the nigral slice has potential as a CNS preparation that may be used to directly test the actions of experimental drugs on DA cell activity.

The use of the midbrain slice preparation for studying DA cell physiology and pharmacology has just begun. With a few exceptions, most studies, to date, have found that DA neurons *in vitro* behave in a manner quite similar to that observed *in vivo*. However, as experiments become more sophisticated this preparation will allow us to begin to understand DA cell function at a level that would be impossible to obtain *in vivo*.

DA-INNERVATED NEURONS

During the past decade studies aimed at investigating the effects of DA on postsynaptic neurons have improved our understanding of the function of this transmitter within the CNS. While the controversy continues over whether DA is primarily excitatory or inhibitory to its follower cells (see Table 1), attention is turning to perhaps the more relevant issue of neuromodulation. Inspired by demonstrations of a modulatory role for norepinephrine (133), investigators have begun to realize that the obvious changes of spontaneous activity that one sees when DA is applied iontophoretically or released by stimulation of the midbrain may not reflect its most vital postsynaptic functions. Evidence for DA-induced neuromodulation has now been obtained in several of the brain regions innervated by the mesotelencephalic system. Due to limitations of space, only those *in vivo* studies examining the effects of DA on single-unit activity in these regions will be discussed.

Extracellular Studies

Accumbens Nucleus

In the nucleus accumbens the suggestion of a neuromodulatory role for DA comes from the observation that iontophoretic DA inhibits the activity evoked by stimulation of excitatory accumbens afferents (5,134). This inhibition can be blocked by DA receptor antagonists and occurs at iontophoretic currents that produce less suppression of baseline firing rate (134). That the demonstrated neuromodulation may be relevant to DA's physiological role in the accumbens is suggested by evidence that stimulation of the A10 area mimics the effect of DA on evoked activity and that this action is readily antagonized by DA receptor blockers (5,134) or lost in rats with DA specific lesions of the A10 area induced by 6-OHDA (134). Furthermore, there is evidence to suggest that DA's modulatory action in the accumbens may serve to alter the output of this nucleus to other structures (135).

Lateral Septal Nucleus

A recent iontophoretic study in the lateral septal nucleus suggests a modulatory action for DA in this structure similar to that recorded in the accumbens (80). The majority of neurons in the lateral septum respond to DA application with a decrease in the number of evoked spikes produced by stimulation of the fimbria. Facilitatory effects are also noted, however, as well as biphasic responses consisting of an initial facilitation followed by profound inhibition of evoked activity (80). Fluphenazine, a DA receptor antagonist, has been shown to block most of the inhibitory effects of DA on evoked activity as well as a few of the facilitations (80).

Caudate Nucleus

In the caudate nucleus there is still no general agreement regarding the effect of DA on spontaneous activity (see Table 1). Johnson et al. (71), however, suggest that neuromodulation may be a more important function of DA in the caudate than its effect on spontaneous firing rate. Their experiment demonstrates that locally applied DA inhibits spontaneous activity more than the activity evoked by stimulation of cortical afferents, and in some cases DA actually facilitates evoked activity (71). Thus, DA may increase the "signal-to-noise ratio" in the caudate much like the neuromodulatory effect reported for norepinephrine in other brain regions (133). A similar finding was reported by Norcross and Spehlmann (86,87), who demonstrated that iontophoretic application of DA could facilitate evoked responses of caudate neurons. This same group also reported DA attenuation of evoked activity in some instances and showed that both types of modulatory response could be blocked by DA receptor antagonists (86,87).

Cerebral Cortex

One study that suggests a modulatory function for the mesocortical DA system reports the effects of A10 area stimulation on the activity of prefrontal cortex neurons (43). A10 stimulation inhibits spontaneous activity and blocks the excitatory response of prefrontal neurons to thalamic stimulation (43). Evidence that these effects may be DA mediated comes from the demonstration that depletion of DA by systemic alpha-methyl-paratyrosine, a DA synthesis inhibitor, or lesion of the DA innervation by 6-OHDA, significantly reduces the ability of A10 stimulation to inhibit both spontaneous and evoked activity (43). Similar lesion of the noradrenergic cortical innervation does not alter the effects of A10 stimulation, and although this is supportive of a proposed DA neuromodulation in the cortex (43), it will be necessary to examine the action of DA antagonists on these responses before this hypothesis can be substantiated.

Whereas evidence is accumulating for DA neuromodulation of stimulus-evoked activity in several brain regions, studies examining the possible modulatory interactions of DA with other transmitters are also being conducted. In the prefrontal cortex, Palmer and Hoffer (88) have convincingly demonstrated that DA facilitates the expression of inhibitory responses to iontophoretically applied enkephalin. Enkephalin inhibitions can be blocked stereospecifically by DA receptor antagonists and reduced in animals with 6-OHDA lesions of the ascending DA bundle (88). In another investigation, DA was found to attenuate the excitatory response of frontal cortex cells to iontophoretic acetylcholine (96). This modulatory response may not have been specific for DA, however, since other inhibitory transmitters produced similar reductions of acetylcholine-induced activity.

Globus Pallidus

Consistent evidence has been provided for a modulatory role of DA in the globus pallidus. The most striking effect of iontophoretic DA in this structure is its ability to attenuate the inhibition of pallidal neurons by GABA (8). The modulation of GABA inhibitions by DA appears to be independent of its effects on firing rate and, in addition, appears to be specific for DA (8).

TABLE 1. *Effects of DA on single-unit activity recorded in DA-innervated areas*

DA-innervated region	Preparation	Method of DA administration	Effect on baseline activity	Modulatory actions observed	Blocked by DA antagonists	Refs.
Accumbens nucleus	Rat, anesthetized	Iontophoresis	Inhibit[a]	—	Yes	17,128
			Inhibit[b]	—	Yes	128,134
	Rat, paralyzed	Iontophoresis	Inhibit[b]	—	Yes	4
			—	Inhibit evoked activity	Yes	5
	Rat, paralyzed	Stimulate A10 area	Inhibit[a]	—	NT	3
	Rat, anesthetized	Iontophoresis and stimulate A10 area	—	Inhibit evoked activity	Yes	134
	Rat, anesthetized	Iontophoresis	Inhibit[a,b]	Reverse CCK excitation	NT	127
Caudate nucleus	Rat, paralyzed	Iontophoresis	Inhibit[a]	—	NT	72,106
			Inhibit[a]	—	No	105
	Cat, decerebrate	Stimulate A9 area	Excite[a]	—	Yes	86
	Cat, decerebrate	Iontophoresis	Excite[a,b,c] Inhibit[a,b]	—	NT	87
	Cat, decerebrate	Iontophoresis	—	Facilitate or inhibit evoked activity	Yes	86,87
	Rat, anesthetized	Pressure ejection	Inhibit[a,c] Excite[a]	Facilitate evoked activity	NT	71
	Rat, paralyzed	Iontophoresis	Inhibit[a]	Facilitate GABA inhibition; facilitate or attenuate GLU excitation	NT	31
	Rat, paralyzed[d]	Iontophoresis	Inhibit[a]	—	NT	10
	Cat, paralyzed[d]	Iontophoresis	Inhibit[a]	—	No	61
			—	Inhibit evoked activity	Yes	61
Frontal cortex	Rat, anesthetized	Iontophoresis	Excite[a] Inhibit[a]	—	Yes	11,13,14
	Rat, anesthetized	Iontophoresis	Inhibit[a]	Attenuate ACH excitation	NT	96
	Rat, paralyzed[d]	Iontophoresis	Inhibit[a]	Attenuate GLU excitation; inhibit evoked activity	NT	9
Globus pallidus	Rat, anesthetized	Iontophoresis	Excite[a,c] Inhibit[a]	Attenuate GABA inhibition	NT	8
Lateral septal nucleus	Rat, anesthetized	Stimulate A10 area	Excite[a]	—	Yes	6
	Rat, anesthetized	Iontophoresis	Inhibit[a]	Facilitate and/or inhibit evoked activity	Yes	80
Olfactory tubercles	Rat, anesthetized	Iontophoresis	Inhibit[a,c] Excite[a]	—	NT	59
Prefrontal cortex	Rat, decerebrate	Iontophoresis	Inhibit[a]	—	Yes	18,21
			Inhibit[a]	—	NT	101
	Rat, anesthetized	Iontophoresis	Inhibit[a]	—	NT	88
		Endogenous DA	—	Facilitate ENK inhibition	Yes	88
	Rat, anesthetized	Stimulate A10 area	Inhibit[a]	Inhibit evoked activity	NT	43
Substantia nigra, zona reticulata	Rat, anesthetized	Iontophoresis	Excite[a,c] Inhibit[a]	—	Yes	97
	Rat, anesthetized	Iontophoresis	Excite[a,c] Inhibit[a]	Attenuate GABA inhibition	NT	121
	Rat, anesthetized	Iontophoresis	—	Attenuate evoked inhibition	NT	122

[a] Effect on spontaneous activity.
[b] Effect on glutamate-stimulated activity.
[c] Most frequent response listed first.
[d] Intracellular recording.
— Indicates effect listed separately or not reported.
NT, Not tested.
Abbreviations: acetylcholine (ACH), cholecystokinin (CCK), enkephalin (ENK), γ-aminobutyric acid (GABA), glutamate (GLU).

Substantia Nigra Zona Reticulata

The demonstrated neuromodulatory effect of DA in the globus pallidus is reminiscent of an earlier study reporting similar findings in the ZR of the substantia nigra (121). DA iontophoresis onto ZR neurons attenuates the inhibitory response of these cells to GABA, and again this effect of DA appears to be independent of changes in spontaneous activity and to be specific for the two transmitters involved (121). Evidence suggesting a physiological role for this modulatory interaction of DA and GABA has recently been reported (122).

Intracellular Studies

In addition to extracellular investigations of modulatory functions for DA, recent intracellular recordings have begun to examine the responses of DA-innervated neurons in an attempt to study the mechanisms underlying DA's complex actions. The predominant effect of iontophoretic DA recorded so far has been a slow depolarization of membrane potential in both frontal cortex (9) and striatal neurons (10,61). Hyperpolarizing responses in the caudate have also been observed (61). Regardless of the direction of the effect on membrane potential, DA application has consistently produced an inhibition of spontaneous activity (9,10,61). In the frontal cortex DA has been further shown to block the spikes produced by direct current injection and to attenuate the ability of glutamate to stimulate firing (9). DA antagonists have not been used, however, to strengthen the argument for specificity of the cortical DA effect. In the caudate DA has been reported to attenuate cortically evoked excitatory postsynaptic potential (EPSP)/IPSP sequences, and although this effect and the slow depolarization of membrane potential can be blocked by DA receptor antagonists, the inhibition of spontaneous activity does not appear to be antagonized (61). Perhaps more troublesome is the demonstration that compounds unrelated to DA have also been shown to produce nearly identical intracellular responses in caudate neurons (61). Until the action of DA antagonists on these effects is investigated, the specificity of the recorded response to DA in this structure must remain in question.

In summary, investigations of the responses of DA-innervated neurons reveal what may be a general concept regarding DA physiology, namely, that the commonly observed inhibitory or excitatory effects of locally applied DA in terminal regions may not reflect its functional role in these structures. Instead, DA's primary role may be one of neuromodulation. In as much as DA has been shown to alter responses to afferent activity in several terminal fields, the observed effects of DA on firing rate may also depend on the tonic activity of inputs to these regions. Future studies will continue to investigate neuromodulatory actions of DA and, it is hoped, will clarify the intracellular mechanisms that mediate such effects.

EPILOGUE

It is obvious from the above review that over the last 9 years we have greatly expanded our knowledge of the physiology and electrophysiological pharmacology of midbrain DA systems. Given the number of laboratories now working on these systems, the next decade promises to be even more exciting than this one has been. To date, the presynaptic side of midbrain DA systems has continued to receive the most attention. Neurophysiologically, we have begun to make inroads into understanding the ways in which these systems function within the brain, the ways in which they differ, and the incredibly complex ways in which their activity is controlled. Pharmacologically, we have learned that the way that they function in the brain is very much affected by acutely and chronically administered DA agonists and antagonists, and that their remarkable propensity to transiently become inactivated due to depolarization is probably responsible for the unusual effects observed when antipsychotic drugs are administered repeatedly.

The postsynaptic side of these DA systems still remains understudied relative to the DA cells themselves. Very little work has been done to try to electrophysiologically identify those neurons receiving a DA input, and in areas other than the caudate, very little intracellular work has been carried out examining the actions of DA on postsynaptic DA receptors. Perhaps the most exciting information to come out of studies on postsynaptic DA-innervated neurons over the last decade is the finding that DA can act as a neuromodulator. It can be anticipated that this discovery will help us rethink the function that DA neurons have in the central nervous system.

ACKNOWLEDGMENTS

We would like to thank Chen-Lun Pun for laboratory assistance and Stephanie Arrell for manuscript preparation. This work was supported by United States Public Health Service grants MH-28849, MH-25642, MH-14276, and GM-07527, the Robert Alwin Hay Fund for Schizophrenia Research, a James Hudson Brown-Alexander B. Coxe Fellowship, a research grant from the American Parkinson's Disease Association, the Abraham Ribicoff Research Facilities, and the State of Connecticut.

REFERENCES

1. Aghajanian, G. K., and Bunney, B. S. (1974): In: *Frontiers in Neurology and Neuroscience Research,* edited by P. Seeman and G. M. Brown, pp. 4–11. University of Toronto Press, Toronto.
2. Aghajanian, G. K., and Bunney, B. S. (1977): *Naunyn Schmiedebergs Arch. Pharmacol.,* 297:1–7.
3. Akaike, A., Sasa, M., and Takaori, S. (1981): *Brain Res.,* 225: 189–194.
4. Akaike, A., Sasa, M., and Takaori, S. (1983): *Life Sci.,* 32:2649–2653.
5. Akaike, A., Sasa, M., and Takaori, S. (1984): *J. Pharmacol. Exp. Ther.,* 229:859–864.
6. Assaf, S. Y., and Miller, J. J. (1977): *Brain Res.,* 129:353–360.
7. Bannon, M. J., Michaud, R. L., and Roth, R. H. (1981): *Mol. Pharmacol.,* 19:270–275.
8. Bergstrom, D. A., and Walters, J. R. (1984): *Brain Res.,* 310:23–33.
9. Bernardi, G., Cherubini, E., Marciani, M. G., Mercuri, N., and Stanzione, P. (1982): *Brain Res.,* 245:267–274.
10. Bernardi, G., Marciani, M. G., Pavone, F., and Stanzione, P. (1978): *Neurosci. Lett.,* 8:235–240.

11. Bevan, P., Bradshaw, C. M., Pun, R. Y. K., Slater, N. T., and Szabadi, E. (1978): *Neuropharmacology,* 17:611–617.
12. Blaha, C. D., and Lane, R. F. (1984): *Eur. J. Pharmacol.,* 98:113–117.
13. Bradshaw, C. M., Pun, R. Y. K., Slater, N. T., Stoker, M. J., and Szabadi, E. (1983): *Neuropharmacology,* 22:945–952.
14. Bradshaw, C. M., Sheridan, R. D., and Szabadi, E. (1985): *Br. J. Pharmacol.,* 86:483–490.
15. Braszko, J. J., Bannon, M. J., Bunney, B. S., and Roth, R. H. (1981): *J. Pharmacol. Exp. Ther.,* 216:289–293.
16. Bunney, B. S. (1984): *Trends Neurosci.,* 7:212–215.
17. Bunney, B. S., and Aghajanian, G. K. (1975): In: *Antipsychotic Drugs, Pharmacodynamics and Pharmacokinetics,* pp. 305–318. Wenner-Gren Center International Symposium Series. Pergamon Press, New York.
18. Bunney, B. S., and Aghajanian, G. K. (1976): *Life Sci.,* 19:1783–1792.
19. Bunney, B. S., and Aghajanian, G. K. (1978): In: *Psychopharmacology: A Generation of Progress,* edited by M. A. Lipton and A. DiMascio, pp. 159–171. Raven Press, New York.
20. Bunney, B. S., and Aghajanian, G. K. (1978): *Naunyn Schmiedebergs Arch. Pharmacol.,* 304:255–261.
21. Bunney, B. S., and Chiodo, L. A. (1984): In: *Monoamine Innervation of the Cerebral Cortex,* edited by L. Descarries, T. R. Reader, and M. H. Jasper, pp. 263–277. Alan R. Liss, New York.
22. Bunney, B. S., Chiodo, L. A., Grace, A. A., and Schenk, J. O. (1984): In: *Behavioral Pharmacology: Current Status,* edited by L. S. Seiden and R. L. Balsten, pp. 205–210. Alan R. Liss, New York.
23. Bunney, B. S., and Grace, A. A. (1978): *Life Sci.,* 23:1715–1728.
24. Bunney, B. S., and Grace, A. A. (1985): *Neurosci. Abstr.,* 311.15:1076.
25. Bunney, B. S., Walters, J. R., Roth, R. H., and Aghajanian, G. K. (1973): *J. Pharmacol. Exp. Ther.,* 185:560–571.
26. Burki, H. R., Ruch, W., Aspen, H., Beggiolini, M., and Stille, G. (1974): *Eur. J. Pharmacol.,* 27:180–190.
27. Carlsson, A. (1975): In: *Chemical Tools in Catecholamine Research II,* edited by O. Almgren, A. Carlsson, and J. Engel, pp. 219–225. North Holland Publishing Co., Amsterdam.
28. Chiodo, L. A. (1981): Doctoral Dissertation, University of Pittsburgh.
29. Chiodo, L. A., Antelman, S. M., Caggiula, A. R., and Lineberry, C. G. (1980): *Brain Res.,* 189:544–549.
30. Chiodo, L. A., Bannon, M. J., Grace, A. A., Roth, R. H., and Bunney, B. S. (1984): *Neuroscience,* 12:1–16.
31. Chiodo, L. A., and Berger, T. W. (1986): *Brain Res.,* 375:198–203.
32. Chiodo, L. A., and Bunney, B. S. (1983): *J. Neurosci.,* 3:1607–1619.
33. Chiodo, L. A., and Bunney, B. S. (1983): *Science,* 219:1449–1451.
34. Chiodo, L. A., and Bunney, B. S. (1983): *Neuropharmacology,* 22:1087–1093.
35. Chiodo, L. A., and Bunney, B. S. (1985): *J. Neurosci.,* 5:2539–2544.
36. Chiodo, L. A., and Bunney, B. S. (1987): *J. Neurosci. (in press).*
37. Chiodo, L. A., Caggiula, A. R., Antelman, S. M., and Lineberry, C. G. (1979): *Brain Res.,* 176:385–390.
38. Chiodo, L. A., Freeman, A. S., and Bunney, B. S. (1984): *Neurosci. Abstr.,* 24.16:72.
39. Clark, D., Engberg, G., Pileblad, E., Svensson, T. H., Carlsson, A., Freeman, A. S., and Bunney, B. S. (1985): *Naunyn Schmiedebergs Arch. Pharmacol.,* 329:344–354.
40. Collingridge, G. L., and Davies, J. (1981): *Brain Res.,* 212:345–359.
41. Creese, I. (1982): *Trends Neurosci.,* 2:40–43.
42. Deniau, J. M., Thierry, A. M., and Feger, J. (1980): *Brain Res.,* 189:315–326.
43. Ferron, A., Thierry, A. M., Le Douarin, C., and Glowinski, J. (1984): *Brain Res.,* 302:257–265.
44. Freeman, A. S., and Bunney, B. S. (1987): *J. Neurosci. (in press).*
45. Freeman, A. S., Meltzer, L. T., and Bunney, B. S. (1985): *Life Sci.,* 36:1983–1994.
46. Gallager, D. W., Pert, A., and Bunney, W. E., Jr. (1978): *Nature,* 273:309–312.
47. German, D. C., Dalsass, M., and Kiser, R. S. (1980): *Brain Res.,* 181:191–197.
48. Grace, A. A., and Bunney, B. S. (1979): *Eur. J. Pharmacol.,* 59:211–218.
49. Grace, A. A., and Bunney, B. S. (1980): *Science,* 210:654–656.
50. Grace, A. A., and Bunney, B. S. (1983): *Neuroscience,* 10:301–315.
51. Grace, A. A., and Bunney, B. S. (1983): *Neuroscience,* 10:317–331.
52. Grace, A. A., and Bunney, B. S. (1983): *Neuroscience,* 10:333–348.
53. Grace, A. A., and Bunney, B. S. (1984): *J. Neurosci.,* 4:2866–2876.
54. Grace, A. A., and Bunney, B. S. (1984): *J. Neurosci.,* 4:2877–2890.
55. Grace, A. A., and Bunney, B. S. (1985): *Brain Res.,* 333:271–284.
56. Grace, A. A., and Bunney, B. S. (1985): *Brain Res.,* 333:285–298.
57. Groves, P. M., Wilson, C. J., and MacGregor, R. J. (1977): In: *Interactions Among Putative Neurotransmitters in the Brain,* edited by S. Garattini, J. F. Pujol, and R. Samanin, pp. 191–215. Raven Press, New York.
58. Groves, P. M., Wilson, C. J., Young, S. J., and Rebec, G. C. (1975): *Science,* 190:522–529.
59. Guevara-Aguilar, R., Solano-Flores, L. P., Garcia-Diaz, D. E., and Aguilar-Baturoni, H. U. (1985): *Brain Res. Bull.,* 15:665–668.
60. Guyenet, P. G., and Aghajanian, G. K. (1978): *Brain Res.,* 150:69–84.
61. Herrling, P. L., and Hull, C. D. (1980): *Brain Res.,* 192:441–462.
62. Hokfelt, T., Everitt, B. J., Theodorsson-Norheim, E., and Goldstein, M. (1984): *J. Comp. Neurol.,* 222:543–559.
63. Hokfelt, T., Skirboll, L., Rehfeld, J. F., Goldstein, M., Markey, K., and Dann, O. (1980): *Neuroscience,* 5:2093–2124.
64. Hokfelt, T., and Ungerstedt, U. (1973): *Brain Res.,* 60:269–297.
65. Hommer, D. W., and Bunney, B. S. (1980): *Life Sci.,* 27:377–386.
66. Hommer, D. W., Polkovits, M., Paul, S. M., and Skirboll, L. R. (1985): *J. Neurosci.,* 5:1387–1392.
67. Hommer, D. W., and Skirboll, L. R. (1983): *Eur. J. Pharmacol.,* 91:151–152.
68. Huff, R. M., and Adams, R. N. (1980): *Neuropharmacology,* 19:587–590.
69. Imperato, A., and DiChiara, G. (1984): *J. Neurosci.,* 5:297–306.
70. Innis, R. B., Andrade, R., and Aghajanian, G. K. (1984): *Neurosci. Abstr.,* 241.9:812.
71. Johnson, S. W., Palmer, M. R., and Freedman, R. (1983): *Neuropharmacology,* 22:843–851.
72. Kamata, K., and Robec, G. V. (1985): *Eur. J. Pharmacol.,* 106:393–397.
73. Kehr, W., Carlsson, A., Lindqvist, M., Magnusson, T., and Atack, C. V. (1972): *J. Pharm. Pharmacol.,* 24:744–747.
74. Kitai, H., Kita, T., and Kitai, S. T. (1984): *Neurosci. Abstr.,* 10:704.
75. Kondo, Y., and Iwatsubo, K. (1980): *Brain Res.,* 181:237–240.
76. Korf, J., Fieleman, M., and Westernik, B. H. C. (1976): *Nature,* 260:257–258.
77. Llinas, R., Greenfield, S. A., and Jahnsen, M. (1984): *Brain Res.,* 294:127–132.
78. Llinas, R., and Yarom, Y. (1981): *J. Physiol. (Lond.),* 315:560–584.
79. MacNeil, D., Gauer, M., and Szymanska, I. (1978): *Brain Res.,* 154:401–403.
80. Marchand, J. E., and Hagino, N. (1983): *Exp. Neurol.,* 82:683–697.
81. McMillen, B. A., and Shore, P. A. (1978): *Eur. J. Pharmacol.,* 52:225–230.
82. Meech, R. W. (1978): *Annu. Rev. Biophys. Bioeng.,* 7:1–18.
83. Meltzer, L. T., and Bunney, B. S. (1981): *Neurosci. Abstr.,* 7:341.
84. Nakamura, S., Iwatsubo, K., Tsai, C. T., and Iwama, K. (1979): *Exp. Neurol.,* 66:682–691.

85. Nieoullon, A., Cheramy, A., and Glowinski, J. (1977): *Nature,* 266:375–377.
86. Norcross, K., and Spehlmann, R. (1977): *Neurosci. Lett.,* 6:323–328k.
87. Norcross, K., and Spehlmann, R. (1978): *Brain Res.,* 156:168–174.
88. Palmer, M. R., and Hoffer, B. J. (1980): *J. Pharm. Exp. Therap.,* 213:205–215.
89. Pinnock, R. D. (1983): *J. Neurophysiol. (Lond.),* 334:88.
90. Pinnock, R. D. (1983): *Eur. J. Pharmacol.,* 96:269–276.
91. Pinnock, R. D. (1984): *Brain Res.,* 292:190–193.
92. Pinnock, R. D. (1984): *Br. J. Pharmacol.,* 81:631–635.
93. Pinnock, R. D. (1984): *Brain Res.,* 322:337–340.
94. Pinnock, R. D. (1985): *Brain Res.,* 338:151–154.
95. Pinnock, R. D., and Dray, A. (1982): *Neurosci. Lett.,* 29:153–158.
96. Reader, T. A., Ferron, A., Descarries, L., and Jasper, H. H. (1979): *Brain Res.,* 160:217–229.
97. Ruffieux, A., and Schultz, W. (1980): *Nature,* 285:240–241.
98. Sanghera, M. D., Trulson, M. E., and German, D. E. (1984): *Neuroscience,* 12:793–801.
99. Schenk, J. O., and Bunney, B. S. (1983): *Neurosci. Abstr.,* 292:5.
100. Seeman, P. (1981): *Pharmacol. Rev.,* 32:229–331.
101. Sesack, S. R., and Bunney, B. S. (1985): *Neurosci. Abstr.,* 11:1079.
102. Shepard, P. D., and German, D. C. (1984): *Eur. J. Pharmacol.,* 98:455–456.
103. Silva, N. L., Schenk, J. O., and Bunney, B. S. (1985): *Neurosci. Abstr.,* 11:1075.
104. Silva, N. L., Schenk, J. O., and Bunney, B. S. (1986): *J. Neurosci.* (submitted).
105. Skirboll, L. R., and Bunney, B. S. (1979): *Life Sci.,* 25:1419–1434.
106. Skirboll, L. R., Grace, A. A., and Bunney, B. S. (1979): *Science,* 206:80–82.
107. Skirboll, L. R., Grace, A. A., Hommer, D. W., Rehfeld, J., Goldstein, M., Hokfelt, T., and Bunney, B. S. (1981): *Neuroscience,* 6:2111–2124.
108. Snyder, S. H., Banerjee, S. P., Yamamura, H. I., and Greenberg, D. (1974): *Science,* 184:1243–1253.
109. Souto, M., Monti, J. M., and Altier, H. (1979): *Pharmacol. Biochem. Behav.,* 10:5–9.
110. Steinfels, G. F., Heym, J., and Jacobs, B. L. (1981): *Life Sci.,* 29:1435–1442.
111. Thierry, A. M., Deniau, J. M., Herve, D., and Chevalier, G. (1980): *Brain Res.,* 201:210–214.
112. Thomson, A. M. (1982): *J. Neurophysiol. (Lond.),* 338:41.
113. Trulson, M. E., and Arasteh, K. (1985): *Eur. J. Pharmacol.,* 114:105–109.
114. Walker, J. M., and Friederich, M. W. (1985): *Neurosci. Abstr.,* 340.14:1163.
115. Walters, J. R., and Lakoski, J. M. (1978): *Eur. J. Pharmacol.,* 47:469–471.
116. Wang, R. Y. (1981): *Brain Res. Rev.,* 3:123–140.
117. Wang, R. Y. (1981): *Brain Res. Rev.,* 3:141–151.
118. Wang, R. Y. (1981): *Brain Res. Rev.,* 3:153–165.
119. Waszczak, B. L., Eng, N., and Walters, J. R. (1980): *Brain Res.,* 188:185–197.
120. Waszczak, B. L., and Walters, J. R. (1980): *Eur. J. Pharmacol.,* 66:141–144.
121. Waszczak, B. L., and Walters, J. R. (1983): *Science,* 220:218–221.
122. Waszczak, B. L., and Walters, J. R. (1986): *J. Neurosci.,* 6:120–126.
123. White, F. J., and Wang, R. Y. (1982): *Life Sci.,* 32:983–993.
124. White, F. J., and Wang, R. Y. (1983): *Science,* 221:1054–1057.
125. White, F. J., and Wang, R. Y. (1984): *Life Sci.,* 34:1161–1170.
126. White, F. J., and Wang, R. Y. (1984): *J. Pharmacol. Exp. Ther.,* 231:275–280.
127. White, F. J., and Wang, R. Y. (1984): *Brain Res.,* 300:161–166.
128. White, F. J., and Wang, R. Y. (1986): *J. Neurosci.,* 6:274–280.
129. Wilson, C. J., Fenster, G. A., Young, S. J., and Groves, P. M. (1979): *Brain Res.,* 179:165–170.
130. Wilson, C. J., Young, S. J., and Groves, P. M. (1977): *Brain Res.,* 136:243–260.
131. Wolf, P., Olpe, H.-R., Avrith, D., and Haas, H. L. (1978): *Experientia,* 34:73.
132. Wong, R. K. S., and Prince, D. A. (1978): *Brain Res.,* 159:385–390.
133. Woodward, D. J., Moises, H. C., Waterhouse, B. D., Hoffer, B. J., and Freedman, R. (1979): *Fed. Proc.,* 38:2109–2116.
134. Yim, C. Y., and Mogenson, G. J. (1982): *Brain Res.,* 239:401–415.
135. Yim, C. Y., and Mogenson, G. J. (1983): *J. Neurophysiol.,* 50:148–161.

Psychopharmacology:
The Third Generation of Progress,
edited by Herbert Y. Meltzer.
Raven Press, New York © 1987.

CHAPTER **13**

Hypothalamic Dopaminergic Neuronal Systems

Kenneth E. Moore

There are a number of different dopamine (DA)-containing neuronal systems in the brain. Most of what is known about these neurons has been learned from studies on the nigrostriatal system, which is the largest and consequently the most convenient group of DA neurons to study. It is, however, misleading to consider a nigrostriatal DA neuron as a "model" of other DA neurons. Results of studies conducted during the past 10 years reveal that various groups of DA neurons have different functions and characteristics. Indeed, different DA neurons appear to have evolved distinctive properties that are suited to the unique requirements of their specialized functions. This is most apparent when the neurochemical properties and the responses to pharmacological and endocrinological manipulations of the different DA neurons are compared. There are differences among the pharmacological responses of the various subdivisions of the major ascending mesotelencephalic DA neurons (89); this is particularly apparent when the properties of neurons projecting to the cerebral cortex are compared with those projecting to subcortical regions (e.g., 9). These differences probably relate to differences in circuitry of neuronal feedback loops, afferent neuronal connections, and the sensitivity of DA autoreceptors. Even greater differences are noted between DA neurons that comprise the mesotelencephalic system and those DA neurons that are located within the hypothalamus (e.g., 87,88,95). This chapter focuses on the latter neurons; it

reviews the anatomy, the neurochemical characteristics, the methods of regulation, and the possible functions of the different groups of hypothalamic DA neurons.

ANATOMY OF DA NEURONS

Using the Falck-Hillarp paraformaldehyde fluorescence procedure on freeze-dried brain regions and subsequently the more sensitive glyoxylic acid histofluorescent technique on Vibratome sections, neuroanatomists have identified catecholamine-containing perikarya, fibers, and terminals throughout the brain and spinal cord (see reviews 13, 74, 96). Because of similarities in the spectral characteristics of DA, norepinephrine (NE), and epinephrine (EPI), fluorophors, it is difficult to distinguish neurons containing different catecholamines using histofluorescent methods unless the studies are done in conjunction with pharmacological manipulations or following selective lesions. On the other hand, by using immunological procedures to localize catecholamine-synthesizing enzymes, it has been possible to identify EPI-, NE-, and DA-containing neurons (55).

Prior to the advent of immunohistological techniques, Dahlström and Fuxe (22) had suggested a numbering system to identify various groups of catecholamine-containing perikarya (see Fig. 1). The more caudal cells in the

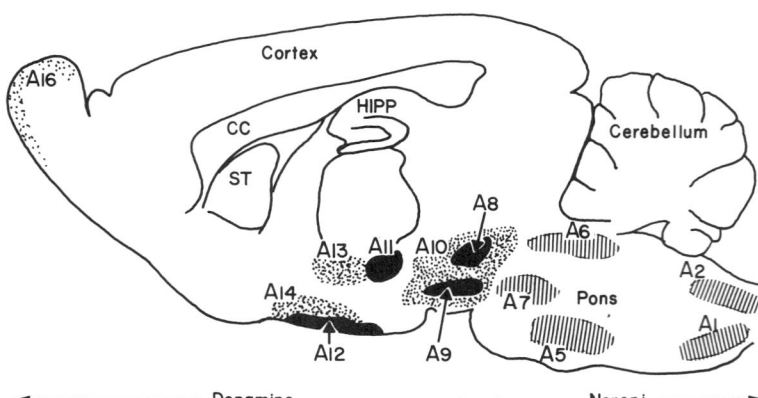

FIG. 1. Sagittal section of the rat brain schematically depicting the location of NE (A_1–A_7) and DA (A_8–A_{16}) perikarya. (Modified from ref. 67.)

pons-medulla (A_1–A_7) represent NE neurons. EPI neurons have also been identified in the medulla. Catecholaminergic perikarya in the mid and rostral parts of the brain are exclusively dopaminergic; they extend from the mesencephalon (A_8–A_{10}) to the olfactory bulb (A_{16}). The large number of DA perikarya that are located in the pars compacta of substantia nigra (A_8–A_9) and in the more medial regions of the ventromedial mesencephalon (A_{10}) give rise to the major ascending DA neurons that have been classified as the "mesotelencephalic" system (13). These neurons have been subdivided into the "mesostriatal" (neurons projecting to the caudate, putamen, and nucleus accumbens) and the "mesocortical" systems (neurons projecting to limbic forebrain regions and several regions of the cerebral cortex). Although this is a logical anatomical classification, most neurochemists and neuropharmacologists employ the original terms "nigrostriatal" (neurons projecting primarily from A_8 and A_9 to the caudate-putamen), "mesolimbic" (neurons projecting from A_{10} to a variety of subcortical regions, e.g., nucleus accumbens, olfactory tubercle, septum), and "mesocortical" (neurons projecting to cingulate, entorhinal, prefrontal, and pyriform cerebral cortices) when referring to these ascending DA neurons.

DA perikarya have also been identified in the more rostral regions of the brain, in the olfactory bulb (A_{16}, ref. 65) and in four regions of the hypothalamus (A_{11}–A_{14}). With the exception of cells in the A_{12} group, the axonal projections from these perikarya are not as well defined as they are for the mesotelencephalic DA neurons. Within the hypothalamus, DA neurons have been divided into two major groups, those comprising the incertohypothalamic dopaminergic (IHDA) system, with cells identified as A_{11},

A_{13}, and A_{14} (14), and those that were originally referred to as the tuberohypophysial system (119), which have perikarya (A_{12}) located within the mediobasal hypothalamus in the arcuate nucleus and in the periventricular nucleus lying just dorsal to the former nucleus. These latter neurons have now been subdivided on the basis of their anatomical distribution: tuberoinfundibular dopaminergic (TIDA) neurons project to the median eminence, and tuberohypophysial dopaminergic neurons (THDA) project to the neural and intermediate lobes of the pituitary (see Fig. 2).

Tuberoinfundibular and Tuberohypophysial DA Neurons

Cell bodies of THDA neurons are located primarily in the rostral regions of the arcuate nucleus. Their axons project ventrally through the median eminence and down the infundibular stalk to terminate in the neurointermediate lobe of the pituitary (NIL). In the intermediate lobe these neurons terminate near endocrine cells where they appear to exert an inhibitory action on the release of α-melanocyte-stimulating hormone (αMSH) and β-endorphin (see review 69). DA terminals throughout the parenchyma of the neural lobe appear to make contact with terminals of neurosecretory axons and pituicyte processes. There is some evidence to suggest that THDA neurons modulate the release of oxytocin and vasopressin (68,114). Some THDA neurons also terminate close to pericapillary spaces, and DA released from these neurons may be transported in the blood to the anterior pituitary where it inhibits the release of prolactin (10). Most of the DA arriving at the anterior pituitary, however, originates from terminals of TIDA neurons.

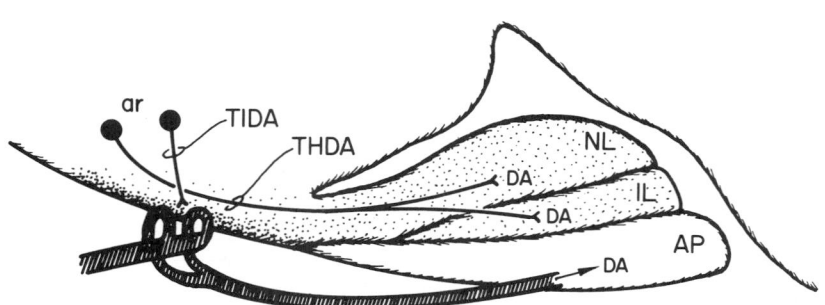

FIG. 2. Schematic depiction of projections of A_{12} DA neurons in the rat brain. TIDA, tuberoinfundibular DA neurons; THDA, tuberohypophysial DA neurons; NL, neural lobe; IL, intermediate lobe; AP, anterior lobe of the pituitary; ar, arcuate nucleus.

TIDA neurons originate in rostral and caudal portions of the arcuate nucleus. Their short axons project ventrally to terminate in the external layer of the median eminence where they are densely packed in a palisade-like manner close to the primary capillary loops of the hypothalamic-hypophysial portal system. The DA-rich regions of the median eminence have been divided into the medial and lateral palisade zones. DA is released into the hypophysial portal blood from both regions, but in the lateral palisade zone DA neurons also appear to terminate in close proximity to luteinizing hormone-releasing hormone (LHRH) neurons and they may modulate the release of this hormone (52). DA released into the portal blood is transported to the anterior pituitary where it activates receptors on lactotrophs (prolactin-secreting cells), resulting in the inhibition of prolactin release (84).

The relatively high concentration of DA in the mediobasal hypothalamus, including the median eminence and NIL, represents only a small percentage of the total hypothalamic content of this amine. Similarly, TIDA and THDA perikarya in the arcuate and periventricular nuclei represent only a small percentage of the total number of DA cells in the whole hypothalamus (120). A relatively large number of DA cells, which constitute IHDA neurons, are scattered throughout the hypothalamus; they contain most of the DA in this brain region.

Incertohypothalamic DA Neurons

DA perikarya located at the mesencephalic-hypothalamic junction (A_{11}), in medial zona incerta (A_{13}), and in the periventricular region of the anterior hypothalamus (A_{14}) are collectively referred to as the IHDA neurons (14; see Fig. 3). The projections and functions of these neurons are largely unknown but they are generally believed to be short

intradiencephalic neurons. On the other hand, some DA neurons originating in A_{11} project to the spinal cord (15) and some of the anterior A_{14} neurons appear to innervate the preoptic-anterior hypothalamic regions (14), suggesting an involvement in neuroendocrine mechanisms. Björklund et al. (14) have divided the incertohypothalamic system into a caudal group of neurons originating in A_{11} and A_{13} and projecting to anterior and dorsal hypothalamic areas (e.g., dorsomedial nucleus, zona incerta) and a rostral group of neurons in A_{14} that possibly project to periventricular, preoptic, and septal regions. One of the difficulties in studying the distribution of axons of the IHDA neurons is that they intermingle with dense plexuses of NE neurons. Following lesions of NE neurons, DA terminals have been identified in a variety of hypothalamic regions (e.g., medial preoptic regions, anterior hypothalamic nucleus, medial zona incerta, dorsomedial nucleus, paraventricular nucleus, suprachiasmatic nucleus, periventricular nucleus; ref. 75). Biochemical evidence suggests that these terminals are of IHDA neurons and not of ascending mesotelencephalic neurons (see below and ref. 80).

BIOCHEMISTRY OF DA NEURONS

Currently held concepts of DA synthesis, storage, release, and metabolism have been derived primarily from studies on nigrostriatal DA neurons; a schematic diagram of the neurochemical events occurring at terminals of these neurons is depicted in Fig. 4 (top). Tyrosine is transported into the nerve terminal where it is converted to L-dihydroxyphenylalanine (DOPA) by tyrosine hydroxylase, the enzyme that regulates this rate-limiting step in DA synthesis. DOPA, in turn, is decarboxylated by aromatic L-amino acid decarboxylase to DA. The newly synthesized DA can be stored in synaptic vesicles or be released in response to the arrival

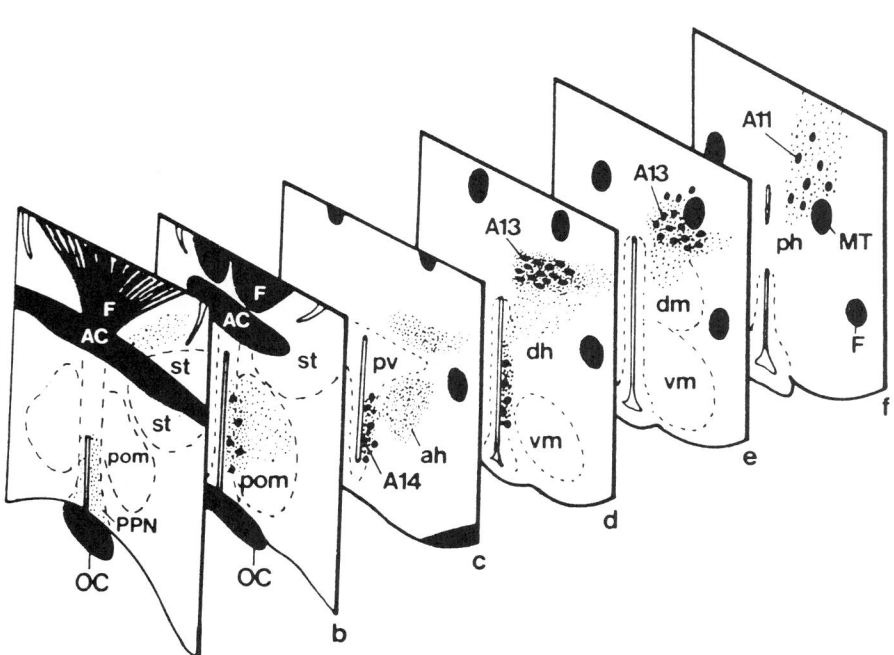

FIG. 3. Sites of incertohypothalamic DA cell bodies and terminals are schematically depicted on frontal sections through the diencephalon of the rat brain. Abbreviations: AC, anterior commissure; ah, anterior hypothalamic area; $A_{11,13,14}$, DA cell groups; dh, dorsal hypothalamic area; dm, dorsomedial nucleus; F, fornix; MT, mammilothalamic tract; OC, optic chiasm; ph, posterior hypothalamus; pom, medial preoptic area; PPN, preoptic periventricular nucleus; pv, paraventricular nucleus; st, bed nucleus of stria terminalis. (From ref. 14.)

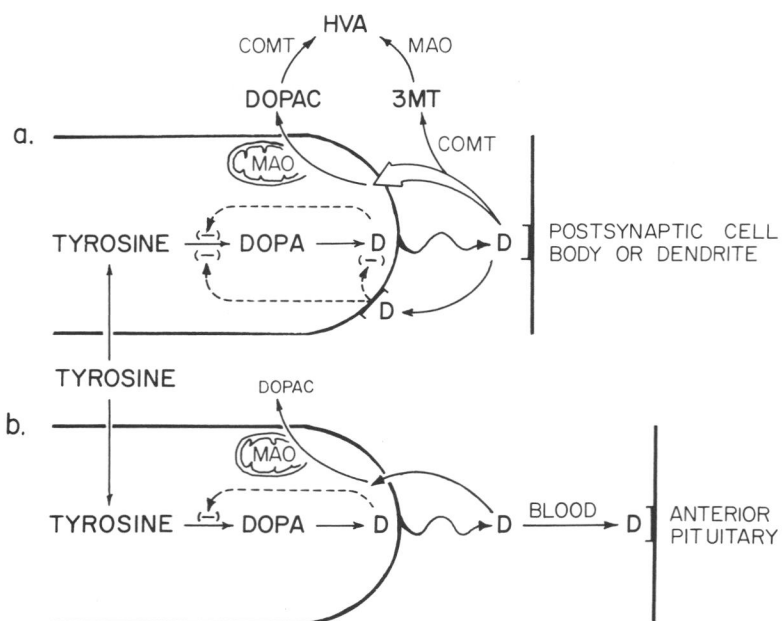

FIG. 4. Schematic diagram of (**a**) nigrostriatal and (**b**) tuberoinfundibular DA neurons. Abbreviations: COMT, catechol-*O*-methyltransferase; D, dopamine; DOPAC, dihydroxyphenylacetic acid; HVA, homovanillic acid; MAO, monoamine oxidase; 3MT, 3-methoxytyramine.

of nerve action potentials. Concentrations of DA in the striatum remain fairly constant despite alterations in the amount of DA released. This is due, in part, to regulation of tyrosine hydroxylase by end-product inhibition and by the activation of DA autoreceptors (schematically represented by dotted lines).

Once DA is released from the nerve terminal it can diffuse across the synaptic cleft and activate receptors located on membranes of dendrites or soma of postsynaptic neurons. Released DA can also activate putative presynaptic receptors (autoreceptors) which inhibit synthesis and possibly release of DA (short-loop feedback). DA is removed from the synaptic cleft by a high-affinity transport system that carries the amine back into the presynaptic nerve terminal where it can reenter the synaptic vesicle and be subsequently released, or it can be converted by intraneuronal monoamine oxidase (MAO) to dihydroxyphenylacetic acid (DOPAC). This metabolite then diffuses from the neuron where it can be converted to homovanillic acid (HVA) by catechol-*O*-methyltransferase (COMT). A small amount of DA that is not recaptured by the presynaptic nerve terminal can be converted by COMT to 3-methoxytyramine (3MT). Changes in the concentrations of DA metabolites (DOPAC, HVA, 3MT) in the striatum or in cerebrospinal fluid have been used in indices of nigrostriatal DA neuronal activity (90,106,125).

Many of the synthetic and metabolic processes described above for the nigrostriatal DA neurons also occur in the terminals of hypothalamic DA neurons. For example, DA synthesis in TIDA and THDA neurons is regulated by end-product inhibition just as it is in nigrostriatal neurons. This is evidenced by the fact that inhibitors of MAO A, but not of MAO B, increase DA concentrations and decrease the rate of DA synthesis in the striatum, median eminence, and NIL (32). Conversely, reserpine reduces DA concentrations and increases DA synthesis in the same brain regions (30).

There are, however, a number of important differences in the neurochemical characteristics of the nigrostriatal and hypothalamic DA neurons. These differences are most apparent when nigrostriatal and TIDA neuronal systems are compared (see Fig. 4). First, most TIDA neurons do not form synapses, but release DA directly into perivascular spaces in the median eminence and thence into the blood of the hypophysial portal system. Second, the concentration of DOPAC, when compared to that of DA, is much lower in the median eminence than it is in other brain regions that contain DA nerve terminals (48,118). This may be due, in part, to the fact that DA is quickly transported away from the TIDA nerve terminal by the blood. In addition, the DA uptake system in terminals of TIDA and THDA neurons has a lower affinity for DA than do nigrostriatal DA terminals (6,29,57). The lower-affinity uptake system for DA in TIDA neurons probably accounts for the resistance of these neurons to destruction by 6-hydroxydopamine, a catecholaminergic neurotoxin that owes its specificity to being selectively accumulated in these neurons (38,115).

Another unusual feature of TIDA neurons is that their activity is not controlled by DA receptor-mediated mechanisms; they lack autoreceptors. Acute lesions of nigrostriatal DA fibers or the administration of drugs [γ-butyrolactone (GBL), baclofen] that block impulse flow in these neurons impairs the release of DA and consequently the activation of autoreceptors at the terminals of these neurons. A decrease in DA autoreceptor activation disinhibits tyrosine hydroxylase so that DA synthesis increases. Since DA continues to be synthesized at an increased rate but is not released, the concentration of the amine in the terminals increases. This biochemical technique has been employed as a test for DA autoreceptor activity since both the increased concentration and the rate of synthesis of DA in the striatum of GBL- or baclofen-treated animals can be reversed by the administration of DA agonists (e.g., apomorphine). Similar events do not occur at terminals of TIDA neurons. That is, following administration of GBL or baclofen the concentration and rate of synthesis of DA in the median eminence do not increase (30). On the other hand, IHDA neurons appear to be regulated by autoreceptors in that the administration of GBL increases the DA content in hypothalamic regions that contain these neurons, and this effect is reversed by the administration of apomorphine (80). In this respect IHDA neurons resemble the nigrostriatal DA neurons rather than the anatomically related TIDA neurons. Not all mesotelencephalic DA neurons are regulated by autoreceptors. DA neurons projecting to the prefrontal and cingulate cortices are also reported to lack autoreceptors (9). Since these receptors are believed to play an important role in neuronal regulation, it is of interest to determine how DA neurons that lack autoreceptors are regulated. Before answering this question, one must consider how the activity of hypothalamic DA neurons can be quantified.

METHODS OF ESTIMATING DA NEURONAL ACTIVITY

The activity (impulse traffic) in DA neurons has been estimated using both electrophysiological and biochemical techniques; most of these studies have been performed on mesotelencephalic DA neurons. The perikarya of these neurons are tightly packed within the A_8–A_{10} regions of the ventral mesencephalon so that it has been possible to record their electrical activity (17). Unfortunately, DA perikarya in the more rostral brain regions are diffusely distributed among non-DA neurons, and to date it has not been possible to record unit activity from confirmed DA cell bodies in these regions. Instead, investigators have had to rely on biochemical techniques to estimate impulse traffic in hypothalamic DA neurons.

Neurochemical estimates of DA neuronal activity are based on coupled relationships among DA synthesis, release, and metabolism. Several *in vivo* biochemical techniques have been employed to estimate the activity of mesotelencephalic DA neurons; these involve measuring the rates of synthesis, turnover, and/or metabolism of DA in brain regions containing terminals of these neurons. Concurrent biochemical and electrophysiological measurements of mesotelencephalic neurons have provided qualitatively similar results. A brief description of these methods and a critical evaluation of their use in estimating the activities of hypothalamic DA neurons are discussed in the next sections.

Concentrations of DA Metabolites

The concentration of DOPAC in the striatum, which presumably reflects DA that has been released and subsequently recaptured by nigrostriatal neurons and then oxidatively deaminated by intraneuronal MAO, increases and decreases in association with increases and decreases in the impulse traffic in these neurons (106). Concentrations of other metabolites of DA (e.g., HVA and 3MT) have also been employed as biochemical estimates of mesotelencephalic DA neuronal activity (125).

One advantage of using DA metabolites to estimate DA neuronal activity is that it requires no pharmacological manipulations that can complicate interpretation of the results (see sections below on measuring rates of DA synthesis and turnover). There are, however, several limitations and disadvantages of using DA metabolites to estimate the activity of hypothalamic DA neurons. In median eminence and NIL, which contain terminals of TIDA and THDA neurons, the concentrations of DOPAC are unusually low (48,118), and in early studies in which this metabolite was measured by radioenzymatic assay, it was found that the concentrations did not reflect impulse traffic in these neurons (118). The lack of effect was postulated to be due to rapid removal of released DA from the terminal regions of TIDA neurons by the blood and to the inefficient uptake systems in the terminals of these neurons. It was initially suggested, therefore, that DOPAC concentrations in the median eminence and NIL could not serve as indices of TIDA and THDA neuronal activity (94). This conclusion may be incorrect because measurements were made near the limits of the sensitivity of the assay. More sensitive methods involving the use of high-performance liquid chromatography (HPLC) coupled to amperometric detectors have recently been employed to quantify the picogram quantities of DOPAC that are present in the median eminence and NIL. Preliminary evidence (K. J. Lookingland and K. E. Moore, *unpublished*) suggests that changes in the concentrations of DOPAC in the median eminence of animals subjected to pharmacological or endocrinological manipulations known to alter the activity of TIDA neurons are consistent with previously reported changes in the rates of DA synthesis and turnover in this region. If these preliminary results can be confirmed, estimations of TIDA neurons can be greatly simplified by measuring DOPAC concentrations in the median eminence.

There is a problem in using changes in DOPAC concentrations to estimate IHDA neuronal activity because brain regions containing cell bodies and terminals of these neurons also contain dense innervations of NE neurons. It has been reported that DOPAC in some hypothalamic regions originates from NE neurons (111), although other reports indicate that concentrations of DA and DOPAC in selected brain regions do not change when NE neurons to these regions are lesioned (123).

Rates of DA Synthesis

DA synthesis is generally coupled to release, and, since the rate of synthesis of this amine is regulated at the step catalyzed by tyrosine hydroxylase, estimates of DA neuronal activity (release) have been made on the basis of the activity of this enzyme. Electrical stimulation of nigrostriatal DA neurons causes an allosteric activation of tyrosine hydroxylase that can be measured *in vitro* (107). The activity of tyrosine hydroxylase in homogenates of the median eminence has also been measured following a variety of endocrinological manipulations (71,72), but because of limitations in the sensitivity of this assay, measurements of the kinetic properties of the enzyme have required pooling of median eminences from several animals.

Radioactive tracer techniques are not sensitive enough to quantify the small amounts of DA that are synthesized *in vivo* in the median eminence or NIL, but a nonradioactive tracer technique developed by Carlsson et al. (19) has been employed successfully to estimate the activity of tyrosine hydroxylase in these regions. This procedure involves measuring the rate of accumulation of DOPA following systemic administration of centrally active inhibitors of aromatic L-amino acid decarboxylase (e.g., NSD 1015; Ro4-4602). In the absence of a decarboxylase inhibitor the concentration of DOPA in the brain is essentially zero, but following the administration of a decarboxylase inhibitor the concentration of this amino acid in the striatum increases linearly with time at a rate that is proportional to impulse traffic in nigrostriatal neurons (97). With the development of sensitive radioenzymatic and HPLC techniques for quantifying picogram quantities of DOPA (31,122), it has been possible to employ this technique to estimate the rate of DA synthesis in terminals of TIDA and THDA neurons in the median eminence and NIL.

One shortcoming of the DOPA accumulation technique is that following inhibition of decarboxylase, DOPA accumulates in both NE and DA neurons. This does not pose a problem in brain regions that contain few NE neurons (e.g., striatum) or where the concentration and rate of turnover of DA far exceed that of NE (e.g., median eminence, NIL). In the latter regions DOPA accumulation has been shown to represent DA synthesis (24). In brain regions containing IHDA neurons the rate of turnover of DA exceeds that of NE (80), but the density of NE terminals is much greater than that of DA so that the rate of DOPA accumulation in most hypothalamic regions represents tyrosine hydroxylase activity in both DA and NE neurons and hence it cannot be used to estimate the activity of either group of neurons.

Rate of Decline of DA After Inhibition of Tyrosine Hydroxylase

Under steady-state conditions the rate of synthesis of DA equals the rate of release so that the concentration of this amine in nerve terminals does not change despite marked changes in impulse traffic. Following the administration of α-methyltyrosine (αMT), an inhibitor of tyrosine hydroxylase, the concentrations of all catecholamines in the brain fall in an exponential manner at a rate that is proportional to the activity of the neurons containing the amine (16). One advantage of this technique is that it permits a concurrent estimate of turnover of all catecholamines, so it can be employed in discrete hypothalamic regions where both NE and DA neurons are present (e.g., 80). Furthermore, the decline of DA following the administration of αMT can be followed using histofluorescent procedures. Fuxe and his collaborators carried out a number of pioneering studies on TIDA neurons, first using semiquantitative measurements (56) and subsequently more quantitative microfluorometric techniques (78) to estimate the decline of DA in the median eminence after the administration of αMT.

Release of DA

The release of DA has been measured *in vitro* from both the median eminence (5,50,100) and the NIL (68,69). The release of DA from terminals of TIDA neurons has also been measured *in vivo* using voltammetric electrodes implanted into the median eminence (103) and by quantifying the concentration of DA in portal blood (12,58). The latter procedure provides a direct measure of DA released from TIDA neurons and thus an index of impulse traffic in these neurons. One shortcoming of this technique is that it must be carried out in anesthetized animals and some anesthetics alter TIDA neuronal activity (102).

There are small amounts of DA in the anterior pituitary, yet this gland does not contain DA nerve terminals and is unable to synthesize this amine. Accordingly, it has been suggested that the concentration of DA within this gland represents the amine that has been released from TIDA neurons, transported in the hypophysial portal blood, and then internalized within cells of the pituitary (8). Subsequent studies, however, have revealed that changes in TIDA neuronal activity do not correlate with the anterior pituitary DA content, indicating that the latter measure is not a reliable index of impulse traffic in TIDA neurons (40,41).

Since each of the neurochemical methods described above has some limitations, it is advisable to compare results of at least "key" experiments with more than one method. Despite the shortcomings of these methods, the results of studies on the various hypothalamic DA neurons by investigators in different laboratories throughout the world are remarkably consistent. In the next sections the mechanisms of regulation of TIDA, THDA, and IHDA neurons and the responses of these neurons to pharmacological, endocrinological, and environmental manipulations are described. Because of space limitations only studies employing biochemical techniques are described in depth. Results from histochemical studies can be found in the references (senior authors: Fuxe, Löfström, Hökfelt).

RESPONSE OF HYPOTHALAMIC DA NEURONS TO PHARMACOLOGICAL MANIPULATIONS

DA Agonists and Antagonists

The first recognized neurochemical effect of antipsychotic drugs (neuroleptics) was the ability of these drugs to increase the concentration of DA metabolites in the striatum (20). This was subsequently found to result from the ability of these drugs to increase the activity of nigrostriatal DA neurons, as evidenced by increased activity of units in the pars compacta substantia nigra and increased rates of synthesis, turnover, and metabolism of DA in the striatum and substantia nigra (see review 95). Similar electrophysiological and biochemical effects were noted in brain regions that contain cell bodies and terminals of other DA ascending neurons that comprise the mesotelencephalic system (89). The compensatory increase in mesotelencephalic DA neuronal activity following the administration of antipsychotic drugs appears to result from the ability of these drugs to block DA autoreceptors and/or postsynaptic DA receptors on neurons that participate in neuronal feedback loops.

TIDA neurons are markedly different from mesotelencephalic DA neurons in that they do not respond to the acute administration of antipsychotic drugs. For up to 2 hr after the administration of neuroleptics the rate of αMT-induced decline of DA, measured histochemically (53) or biochemically (59,60), increased in the striatum and olfactory tubercle but not in the median eminence. Similarly, neuroleptics caused an acute increase in the rate of DOPA accumulation in brain regions containing terminals of mesotelencephalic DA neurons but not in the median eminence (30). Conversely, for up to 2 hr after the administration of DA agonists (e.g., apomorphine, piribedil) the rates of synthesis and turnover of DA decreased in brain regions containing terminals of mesotelencephalic DA neurons, but were unchanged in the median eminence (30,59). Collectively, these results indicate that nigrostriatal but not TIDA neurons are acutely regulated by DA receptor-mediated mechanisms. Furthermore, studies on the actions of GBL and baclofen reveal that TIDA neurons are not modulated by autoreceptors. That is, these drugs increase the concentration and rate of synthesis of DA in brain regions containing terminals of mesotelencephalic DA neurons but not in the median eminence (30).

The lack of response of TIDA neurons to the acute administration of DA agonists and antagonists is not shared by other hypothalamic DA neurons. The rates of turnover of DA in brain regions containing terminals and cell bodies of IHDA neurons increase and decrease following the administration of DA antagonists and agonists, respectively (80). Furthermore, GBL increases the concentrations of DA in various hypothalamic regions just as it does in regions that contain terminals of mesotelencephalic DA neurons (80). Thus, in their response to these drugs, IHDA neurons resemble those DA neurons that comprise the mesotelencephalic system rather than those in the anatomically related TIDA system.

DA agonists decrease and DA antagonists increase the rates of synthesis and turnover of DA in the NIL, but the magnitude of these responses is small when compared to those in the striatum and limbic forebrain regions (30). The reason for the small responses became evident when neurochemical measurements were made in the neural and intermediate lobes separately. Only in the intermediate lobe did the rate of DA turnover change following the administration of DA agonists or antagonists (79). Thus, only those THDA neurons terminating in the intermediate lobe are regulated by DA receptor-mediated mechanisms. On the other hand, THDA neurons terminating in the neural lobe are unresponsive to the direct actions of DA agonists and antagonists, and in this regard they resemble the TIDA neurons that terminate in the median eminence.

As discussed above, DA antagonists have no "acute" effect on TIDA neurons but cause a rapid compensatory increase in the activity of mesotelencephalic DA neurons. Although TIDA neurons are not immediately responsive to DA antagonists, they do exhibit a delayed increase in activity. This is shown in Fig. 5. Between 2 and 12 hr after the injection of a large dose of haloperidol the rate of DA synthesis (DOPA accumulation) increases in the striatum but not in the median eminence. At later times (12–30 hr) the rate of DA synthesis in the median eminence is increased (see also 39). A similar time course was seen when the effects of DA antagonists on the αMT-induced decline of DA were measured in the striatum and median eminence (60). When injected into hypophysectomized rats, DA antagonists still activated mesotelencephalic DA neurons, but the activation of TIDA neurons was blocked (31,60), indicating that DA antagonists influence the activity of these two groups of DA neurons by different mechanisms. These are depicted schematically in Fig. 6. In nigrostriatal DA neurons, pictured on the left, DA antagonists block

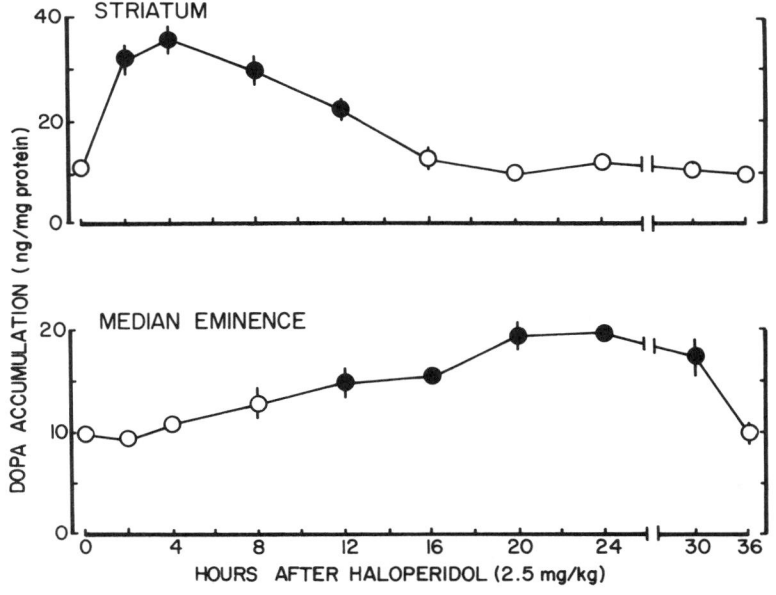

FIG. 5. Effect of haloperidol on the rate of DA synthesis (DOPA accumulation following a decarboxylase inhibitor). Male rats were decapitated at various times after a single injection of haloperidol (2.5 mg/kg, s.c.). Each animal was injected with NSD 1015 (100 mg/kg, i.p.) 30 min prior to sacrifice. Symbols represent means and vertical lines ±1 S.E. (N = 8). Solid symbols indicate those values that are significantly different ($p < 0.05$) from zero time controls.

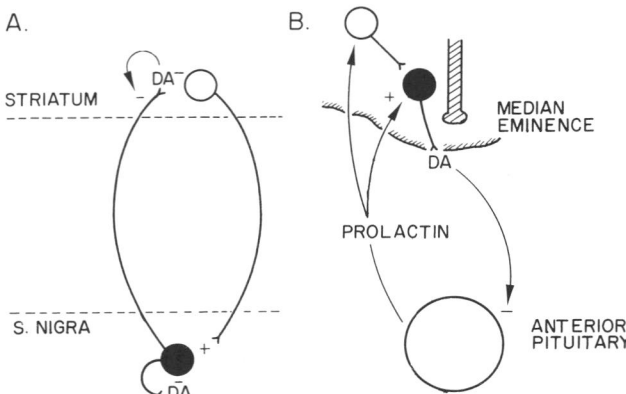

FIG. 6. Schematic representation of the regulation of (**A**) nigrostriatal and (**B**) tuberoinfundibular DA neurons.

DA autoreceptors located on cell bodies and terminals of these neurons, and also block DA receptors on striatonigral feedback loops; the result of this blockade is a prompt compensatory increase in the activity of these neurons. TIDA neurons, on the other hand, are not directly regulated by DA receptor-mediated mechanisms. DA antagonists block DA receptors on prolactin-secreting cells in the anterior pituitary, thereby removing the tonic inhibitory effect of DA on prolactin release. As a result the circulating levels of prolactin increase and feedback to activate TIDA neurons, either by acting directly on these neurons or on neurons that project to the TIDA neurons. In this way, prolactin regulates its own release via a sluggish hormonal-neuronal feedback loop.

A differential response of mesotelencephalic and TIDA neurons to DA antagonists is also apparent when these drugs are administered chronically. Tolerance develops to the actions of these drugs on mesotelencephalic DA neurons (18,110). In animals injected daily with haloperidol for up to 22 days there was a marked reduction in the stimulation of the rate of DA synthesis in striatum and olfactory tubercle, while the serum prolactin concentrations and the rate of DA synthesis in the median eminence remained elevated (91,92). Thus, tolerance develops to the actions of DA antagonists on mesotelencephalic but not to the prolactin-mediated activation of TIDA neurons.

Prolactin

The feedback scheme depicted in Fig. 6 indicates that prolactin stimulates TIDA neurons. This was initially demonstrated by Hökfelt and Fuxe (66), who showed that systemic administration of this hormone increased the αMT-induced decline of DA histofluorescence selectively in the median eminence. Subsequently, using biochemical techniques it was shown that multiple systemic (63,112) and single intracerebroventricular (icv) injections (7,70) of prolactin increased TIDA neuronal activity. This effect is specific for TIDA neurons since prolactin-induced changes in the rates of synthesis and turnover of DA are consistently seen in the median eminence but not in regions containing terminals of mesotelencephalic and THDA neurons.

The prolactin-induced activation of TIDA neurons in intact male and female rats was noted only after a delay of 12 to 16 hr (39,63). The mechanisms of this delayed stimulatory effect are not understood, but as it is markedly reduced by treatment with cycloheximide, it appears to involve protein synthesis (39,70). The delayed *in vivo* action of prolactin on TIDA neurons conflicts with the reported prompt ability of this hormone to release DA from the median eminence *in vitro* (50,100). This difference may be related to the fact that with *in vivo* but not *in vitro* experiments TIDA neurons are tonically activated by endogenous prolactin so that in the former situation the response of these neurons to the administration of exogenous hormone may be masked. This problem is exacerbated by the fact that pharmacological manipulations needed to make biochemical measurements of TIDA neuronal activity (i.e., administration of αMT or NSD 1015) inhibit DA synthesis and thereby increase prolactin secretion. Thus, "control" rates of synthesis and turnover of DA in the median eminence are actually values obtained in the presence of high circulating levels of prolactin that tonically activate TIDA neurons. When this complication is avoided by conducting experiments in hypophysectomized or bromocriptine-treated animals, so as to lower circulating prolactin concentrations and "basal" rates of TIDA neuronal activity, the administration of exogenous prolactin, either by i.p., i.v., or icv routes, increases the rate of DA synthesis and turnover in the median eminence by 2 to 4 hr (rapid "tonic" component) and then causes a further increase by 12 hr (delayed "induction" component; refs. 39,44). Only the latter effect is blocked by cycloheximide. It appears, therefore, that the activity of TIDA neurons at any point in time is dependent on the circulating levels of prolactin at the time of measurement ("tonic" component) and the past history of prolactin concentrations ("induction" component). Thus, subjects treated chronically with a DA antagonist (haloperidol) would have a history of high circulating levels of prolactin; TIDA neurons in these subjects respond to exogenously administered prolactin in an exaggerated manner (44). On the other hand, subjects treated chronically with a DA agonist (bromocriptine) would have a history of low blood levels of prolactin; their TIDA neurons exhibit a reduced response to prolactin (43). Details of the responses of TIDA neurons to prolactin under a variety of situations can be found in recent reviews (92,93).

Estrogens

There are conflicting reports on the effects of estrogens on mesotelencephalic DA neurons and on the characteristics of DA receptors in forebrain regions innervated by these neurons. Results of studies on the effects of estrogens on hypothalamic DA neurons are in general agreement, and they reveal that the responses of these neurons to estrogens are largely the result of increased circulating levels of prolactin. Repeated injections of estrogens into ovariectomized rats increase serum prolactin levels and the αMT-induced decline of histofluorescence in the median eminence (77). Biochemical studies have generally confirmed the results of these histochemical studies. Two or three daily injections of estrogens increase the rate of synthesis and turnover of DA in the median eminence (31,47) and the DA concentration in hypophysial portal blood (61). Since the former effects were not observed in hypophysectomized rats, it was postulated that the estrogen-induced activation of TIDA neurons is not due to a direct action of the hormone *per se,* but rather to its ability to increase circulating concentrations of prolactin.

The acute administration of estrogens to ovariectomized rats is reported to increase DA turnover in both neural and intermediate lobes of the pituitary (108). Estrogen had a differential effect on IHDA neurons in male rats. Following three daily injections of estradiol, DA turnover was increased in caudal regions of the hypothalamus and decreased in rostral regions (81). These effects are mimicked by icv administration of prolactin. The effects of estradiol on IHDA neurons were not seen in hypophysectomized rats, suggesting that these actions are mediated by prolactin.

A complex pattern of effects on TIDA neurons is observed if rats are exposed to estrogens for longer periods (i.e., more than 2 weeks). These include a decrease in the concentration, synthesis, and turnover of DA in the median eminence and a reduced responsiveness of TIDA neurons to prolactin (21,42,117). These effects of estrogens may be due to the direct effect of the hormone, indirectly to the increased circulating levels of prolactin, or to the enlargement and possible tumor development in the anterior pituitary, which can compress the TIDA neurons (105). Most of the effects of chronic estrogen treatment on TIDA neurons are reversible (42), but there are some reports that long-term exposure to this hormone damages TIDA neurons (109).

Opiates

Systemic administration of morphine increases impulse traffic in mesotelencephalic DA neurons, as evidenced by results of electrophysiological recordings of unit activity in the ventral mesencephalon (85,98) and by the results of a variety of neurochemical studies. For example, morphine increases the rate of synthesis (1,101), turnover (51,99), and metabolism (1,124) of DA in striatum and limbic forebrain regions innervated by these DA neurons. Conversely, morphine inhibits TIDA neuronal activity as evidenced by the fact that morphine reduces the rate of synthesis and turnover of DA in the median eminence (1,45) and reduces the content of DA in hypophysial portal blood (62,104). The increase in serum levels of prolactin by morphine appears to be due, at least in part, to the ability of this drug to inhibit TIDA neurons. The stimulatory effects of morphine on mesotelencephalic DA neurons, the inhibitory effects on TIDA neurons, and the stimulatory effects on prolactin secretion are blocked by opiate antagonists. Tolerance develops to inhibitory actions of morphine on TIDA neurons and to the prolactin-releasing effects of this drug (46). Naturally occurring and synthetic opiate peptides mimic the actions of morphine on TIDA neurons (49,54,62,121). The inhibitory actions of morphine on TIDA neurons and on the increase in serum prolactin levels appear to be mediated by serotonin (5HT) neurons since these effects are attenuated in animals in which 5HT neuronal influences are disrupted by 5,7-dihydroxytryptamine-induced lesions of these neurons or by pretreatment with 5HT receptor antagonists (33,73).

The initial report on the effect of morphine on THDA neurons indicated this drug did not alter the rate of synthesis and turnover of DA in the NIL (1). In a more recent study, however, morphine was found to reduce the rate of DA turnover in the neural but not in the intermediate lobe of the pituitary (82). Thus, with respect to their response to morphine, THDA neurons projecting to the neural lobe resemble those of the TIDA system projecting to the median eminence. Finally, morphine increases the concentration of DOPAC and the αMT-induced decline of DA in brain regions that contain cell bodies and terminals of IHDA neurons; these effects are blocked by naltrexone

TABLE 1. *Summary of responses of different DA neurons to pharmacological manipulations*

Neuronal system	Nigrostriatal	TIDA	THDA	IHDA	Refs.
DA antagonists					
Acute (<2 hr)	++	0	+	+	30,59,79,80
Repeated (or >2 hr)	+(T)	+(P)	+	?	39,53,60,92
DA agonists					
Acute (<2 hr)	−	0	−	−	30,59,79,80
Repeated (or >2 hr)	−	−(P)	−	?	34,40,43
GBL or Baclofen	++	0	+	+	30
Prolactin	0	+	0	+, −	7,56,63,70,112
Estrogens	0	+(P)	0	+, −	31,61,76,81,108
Morphine					
Acute	++	−	−	+	1,45,51,62,82
Repeated	+(T)	−(T)	?	?	46

Symbols represent changes in the rates of DA synthesis or turnover: +, Increase; −, decrease; 0, no change; ?, not determined. T, Indicates that the tolerance develops to the response; P, indicates that the response is mediated by changes in circulating levels of prolactin.

(83). Thus, IHDA neurons are stimulated by the acute administration of morphine, and in this respect they resemble extrahypothalamic mesotelencephalic DA neurons rather than the hypothalamic TIDA and THDA neurons.

A summary of the effects of a variety of pharmacological treatments on neurochemical estimates of different DA neuronal systems in the rat brain is compiled in Table 1.

ACTIVITY OF HYPOTHALAMIC DA NEURONS IN DIFFERENT PHYSIOLOGICAL STATES

The following sections briefly summarize recent reports on neurochemical estimates of the activities of TIDA and THDA neuronal systems during various physiological states; additional details can be found in several reviews (87,92,93). At present, little is known about the functions of IHDA neurons and changes in their activity during different physiological states.

TIDA Neurons

Male-Female Differences

To avoid possible confounding variables that might arise as a result of changing hormonal states associated with the estrous cycle, most early neurochemical studies on TIDA neurons were conducted in male rats. In retrospect this was unfortunate because the interactions between prolactin and TIDA neurons are more pronounced and, from a physiological standpoint, more interesting in the female. Indeed, the "basal" rates of synthesis and turnover of DA in the median eminence are two to three times greater in the female (34). Since there is no sexual difference in the steady-state concentrations of DA in the median eminence, it would appear that TIDA neuronal activity (and DA release into the hypophysial portal blood; ref. 12) is greater in the female. There are no major sexual differences in DA neurons that terminate in any other brain region, and the turnover of NE in the median eminence is the same in male and female rats. The sexual differences in TIDA neuronal activity appear to result from neonatal exposure to androgens (27). The neonatal androgen-induced differences in TIDA neuronal activity may be responsible, at least in part, for sexual differences in the hypothalamic regulation of prolactin release. Castration of adult rats results in a differential response in males and females; neurochemical estimates of TIDA neuronal activity are increased in the male but decreased in the female following castration (37,64).

The sexual difference in TIDA neuronal activity results from a greater sensitivity of these neurons in the female to the stimulatory actions of prolactin (34). Hypophysectomy and the administration of bromocriptine, both of which markedly lower circulating concentrations of prolactin, cause a greater decline in TIDA neuronal activity in the female than in the male. Furthermore, although prolactin activates TIDA with a similar time delay in male and female rats, the magnitude of the stimulation of TIDA

neurons is much greater and the dose of prolactin needed to produce this stimulatory effect is much lower in the female (34).

The increase in serum concentrations of prolactin and LH that occur in the late afternoon and early evening of proestrus in the rat are accompanied by small changes in the activities of TIDA neurons. On the morning and early afternoon of proestrus, prior to the time of the prolactin and LH surges, the αMT-induced decline of DA in the median eminence is decreased (26). The results of this biochemical study are in general agreement with the results of earlier studies obtained by histofluorescent techniques (76) and by measuring the concentration of DA in hypophysial portal blood (12).

Pregnancy and Lactation

The daily nocturnal and diurnal surges of prolactin that occur during the first half of pregnancy appear to be necessary for the initiation and maintenance of luteal function in the rat (116). These cyclical changes in prolactin secretion are related to changes in TIDA neuronal activity (86). Up to days 11–13 of pregnancy there are two daily surges of prolactin and biphasic changes in the rate of DOPA accumulation in the median eminence, with the increased serum concentrations of prolactin occurring at the times when TIDA neuronal activity is low. A similar pattern of TIDA neuronal activity and serum levels of prolactin is also seen in rats made pseudopregnant by electrical stimulation of the uterine cervix. The changes in DA synthesis are specific for the median eminence; there are no cyclical changes in the rate of DOPA accumulation in any other brain region. By day 13 of pregnancy and continuing until term the cyclical patterns are lost; serum prolactin levels remain low and the rate of DOPA accumulation in the median eminence high throughout the daily 24-hr periods. Thus, during the first half of pregnancy the two daily surges of prolactin appear to be temporally related to changes in the activity of TIDA neurons. The cyclical patterns of serum prolactin levels and TIDA neuronal activity cease at midpregnancy; this is the result of the actions of placental lactogen, which is released from the uterine-placental unit starting at midpregnancy (35). Placental lactogen stimulates TIDA neurons in a manner similar to that of prolactin (25).

In the lactating rat, suckling causes a marked increase in the serum concentrations of prolactin, due in part to the reduced release of DA into the hypophysial portal blood (11). This appears to be due to the activation of a neuronal circuit that inhibits TIDA neuronal activity and thereby removes inhibitory control over prolactin secretion. Suckling causes an immediate reduction in the rate of synthesis and turnover of DA in the median eminence, but not in other brain regions (28,113). If left undisturbed, lactating rats suckle intermittently throughout the 24-hr period. The rate of synthesis and turnover of DA in the median eminence of these animals is very low despite the fact that circulating levels of prolactin, which normally stimulate TIDA neurons, are very high. This is due to the fact that TIDA neurons in the lactating rat, in contrast to the nonlactating rat, are not stimulated by prolactin (28). This may be the reason that these animals are able to maintain constantly high serum concentrations of prolactin while they are suckling.

Stress

Various types of stressful manipulations increase serum prolactin concentrations, at least in part, as a result of decreased DA inhibitory tone on the secretion of this hormone from the anterior pituitary. Acute stress (e.g., immobilization) causes a prompt reduction in the rates of synthesis and turnover of DA in the median eminence; similar changes do not occur in the striatum or NIL (36). This stress-induced inhibition of TIDA neurons is more pronounced in the female (37) and appears to be due to the activation of an inhibitory neuronal pathway that projects to the mediobasal hypothalamus. The stress-induced increase in serum prolactin levels and the decrease in the activity of TIDA neurons are blocked by pretreatment with 5HT and muscarinic cholinergic antagonists, but not by opiate antagonists. This suggests that 5HT and cholinergic neuronal systems play a role in stress-induced changes in TIDA neuronal activity.

In summary, increases in prolactin secretion that occur in early pregnancy, during suckling, and following restraint stress are accompanied by a decrease in the rate of synthesis and turnover of DA in the median eminence but not in other DA-rich regions of the brain. These results indicate that TIDA neurons are influenced both by prolactin and afferent neuronal circuits.

THDA Neurons

Despite the fact that THDA and TIDA neuronal systems are related anatomically, they differ in their responses to pharmacological, endocrinological, and environmental manipulations. THDA are unresponsive to prolactin, to suckling and to stressful stimuli. On the other hand, THDA neurons are regulated, in part, by the activation of sodium or osmoreceptors. The concentration and the rate of synthesis of DA in the NIL are selectively increased by 3 to 5 days of water deprivation, drinking 2% NaCl (2,3,69), injections of saline or mannitol (4), and hemorrhage (23).

SUMMARY

There are several distinct DA neuronal systems within the mammalian brain that are involved with various functions and are regulated by different mechanisms. Because of these differences it is inappropriate to extrapolate information obtained from one DA neuronal system to another. There are minor differences among the properties of major ascending mesotelencephalic DA neurons that project to various regions of the forebrain, and there are even greater differences between these DA neurons and those that are located within the hypothalamus. These latter neurons have been divided into three major groups:

1. TIDA neurons, which tonically inhibit the release of prolactin from the anterior pituitary, are regulated, in part, by this hormone.

2. THDA neurons, which project to the neural and intermediate lobes of the pituitary, appear to modulate the release of hormones from these structures; their activity is regulated in part by changes in the osmolarity of the blood.

3. IHDA neurons, which share some properties with both mesotelencephalic and the other hypothalamic DA neurons, have functions that currently are not well-defined.

ACKNOWLEDGMENTS

The author's studies cited in this review were supported by USPHS grants NS09174 and NS15911. The assistance of Diane Hummel in the preparation of this manuscript is gratefully acknowledged.

REFERENCES

1. Alper, R. H., Demarest, K. T., and Moore, K. E. (1980): *J. Neural Transm.,* 48:157–165.
2. Alper, R. H., Demarest, K. T., and Moore, K. E. (1980): *Neuroendocrinology,* 31:112–115.
3. Alper, R. H., Demarest, K. T., and Moore, K. E. (1982): *Neuroendocrinology,* 34:252–257.
4. Alper, R. H., and Moore, K. E. (1982): *Neuroendocrinology,* 35: 469–474.
5. Annunziato, L., Cerrito, F., and Raiteri, M. (1981): *Neuropharmacology,* 20:727–731.
6. Annunziato, L., Leblanc, P., Kordon, C., and Weiner, R. I. (1980): *Neuroendocrinology,* 31:316–320.
7. Annunziato, L., and Moore, K. E. (1978): *Life Sci.,* 22:2037–2042.
8. Apud, J., Cocchi, D., Iuliano, E., Casanueva, F., Müller, E. E., and Racagni, G. (1980): *Brain Res.,* 186:226–231.
9. Bannon, M. J., Chiodo, L. A., Bunney, E. B., Wolf, M. E., Grace, A. A., Bunney, B. S., and Roth, R. H. (1984): In: *Catecholamines: Neuropharmacology and Central Nervous System,* edited by E. Usdin, A. Carlsson, A. Dahlström, and J. Engel, pp. 25–36. Alan R. Liss, New York.
10. Ben-Jonathan, N., and Froehlich, J. C. (1985): In: *Catecholamines as Hormone Regulators,* edited by N. Ben-Jonathan, J. M. Bahr, and R. I. Weiner, pp. 145–160. Academic Press, New York.
11. Ben-Jonathan, N., Neill, M. A., Arbogst, L. A., Peters, L. L., and Hoefer, M. T. (1980): *Endocrinology,* 106:690–697.
12. Ben-Jonathan, N., Oliver, C., Weiner, H. J., Mical, R. S., and Porter, J. C. (1977): *Endocrinology,* 100:452–458.
13. Björklund, A., and Lindvall, O. (1978): In: *Limbic Mechanisms,* edited by K. E. Livingston and O. Hornykiewicz, pp. 307–331. Plenum, New York.
14. Björklund, A., Lindvall, O., and Nobin, A. (1975): *Brain Res.,* 89:29–41.
15. Björklund, A., and Skagerberg, G. (1979): *Brain Res.,* 177:170–175.
16. Brodie, B. B., Costa, E., Dlabac, A., Neff, N., and Smookler, H. H. (1966): *J. Pharmacol. Exp. Ther.,* 154:493–498.
17. Bunney, B. S. (1979): In: *The Neurobiology of Dopamine,* edited by A. S. Horn, J. Korf, and B. H. S. Westerink, pp. 417–452. Academic Press, New York.
18. Bunney, B. S., and Grace, A. A. (1978): *Life Sci.,* 23:1715–1728.
19. Carlsson, A., Davis, J. N., Kehr, W., Lindqvist, M., and Atack, C. V. (1972): *Naunyn Schmiedebergs Arch. Pharmacol.,* 275: 153–168.
20. Carlsson, A., and Lindqvist, M. (1963): *Acta Pharmacol. Toxicol.,* 20:140–144.
21. Casanueva, F., Cocchi, D., Locatelli, V., Flauto, C., Zambotti,

F., Bestelli, G., Rossi, G. L., and Müller, E. (1982): *Endocrinology,* 110:590–599.

22. Dahlström, A., and Fuxe, K. (1964): *Acta Physiol. Scand.,* 232(*Suppl.* 62).
23. Demarest, K. T. (1985): *Soc. Neurosci. Abstr.,* 11:1207.
24. Demarest, K. T., Alper, R. A., and Moore, K. E. (1979): *J. Neural Transm.,* 46:183–193.
25. Demarest, K. T., Duda, N. J., Riegle, G. D., and Moore, K. E. (1983): *Brain Res.,* 272:175–178.
26. Demarest, K. T., Johnston, C. A., and Moore, K. E. (1981): *Neuroendocrinology,* 32:24–27.
27. Demarest, K. T., McKay, D. W., Riegle, G. D., and Moore, K. E. (1981): *Neuroendocrinology,* 32:108–113.
28. Demarest, K. T., McKay, D. W., Riegle, G. D., and Moore, K. E. (1983): *Neuroendocrinology,* 36:130–137.
29. Demarest, K. T., and Moore, K. E. (1979): *Brain Res.,* 171:545–551.
30. Demarest, K. T., and Moore, K. E. (1979): *J. Neural Transm.,* 46:263–277.
31. Demarest, K. T., and Moore, K. E. (1980): *Endocrinology,* 106:463–468.
32. Demarest, K. T., and Moore, K. E. (1981): *J. Neural Transm.,* 52:175–187.
33. Demarest, K. T., and Moore, K. E. (1981): *Life Sci.,* 28:1345–1351.
34. Demarest, K. T., and Moore, K. E. (1981): *Neuroendocrinology,* 33:230–234.
35. Demarest, K. T., Moore, K. E., and Riegle, G. D. (1983): *Neuroendocrinology,* 36:409–414.
36. Demarest, K. T., Moore, K. E., and Riegle, G. D. (1985): *Neuroendocrinology,* 41:437–444.
37. Demarest, K. T., Moore, K. E., and Riegle, G. D. (1985): *Neuroendocrinology,* 41:504–510.
38. Demarest, K. T., Riegle, G. D., and Moore, K. E. (1980): *Neuroendocrinology,* 31:222–227.
39. Demarest, K. T., Riegle, G. D., and Moore, K. E. (1984): *Neuroendocrinology,* 38:467–475.
40. Demarest, K. T., Riegle, G. D., and Moore, K. E. (1984): *Endocrinology,* 115:2091–2097.
41. Demarest, K. T., Riegle, G. D., and Moore, K. E. (1984): *Endocrinology,* 115:493–500.
42. Demarest, K. T., Riegle, G. D., and Moore, K. E. (1984): *Neuroendocrinology,* 39:193–200.
43. Demarest, K. T., Riegle, G. D., and Moore, K. E. (1985): *Neuroendocrinology,* 40:369–376.
44. Demarest, K. T., Riegle, G. D., and Moore, K. E. (1986): *Neuroendocrinology,* 44:291–299.
45. Deyo, S. N., Swift, R. M., and Miller, R. J. (1979): *Proc. Natl. Acad. Sci. USA,* 76:3006–3009.
46. Deyo, S. N., Swift, R. H., Miller, R. J., and Fang, V. S. (1980): *Endocrinology,* 106:1469–1474.
47. Eikenburg, D., Ravitz, A. J., Gudelsky, G. A., and Moore, K. E. (1977): *J. Neural Transm.,* 40:235–244.
48. Fekete, M. I. K., Herman, J. P., Kanyicska, B., and Palkovits, M. (1979): *J. Neural Transm.,* 45:207–218.
49. Ferland, L., Fuxe, K., Eneroth, P., Gustafsson, J. A., and Skett, P. (1977): *Eur. J. Pharmacol.,* 43:89–90.
50. Forman, M. M., and Porter, J. C. (1981): *Endocrinology,* 107:800–804.
51. Fuxe, K., Agnati, L., Bolme, P., Everitt, B., Hökfelt, T., Jonsson, G., Ljungdall, A., and Löfström, A. (1975): *Neuropharmacology,* 14:903–912.
52. Fuxe, K., Agnati, L. F., Calza, L., Andersson, K., Giardino, L., Benfenati, F., Camurri, M., and Goldstein, M. (1984): In: *Catecholamines: Neuropharmacology and Central Nervous System,* pp. 441–449. Alan R. Liss, New York.
53. Fuxe, K., Agnati, L. F., Hökfelt, T., Jonsson, G., Lidbrink, P., Ljungdahl, A., Löfström, A., and Ungerstedt, U. (1975): *J. Pharmacol. (Paris),* 6:117–129.
54. Fuxe, K., Andersson, K., Hökfelt, T., Mutt, V., Ferland, L., Agnati, L. F., Ganten, D., Said, S., Eneroth, P., and Gustafson, J. A. (1979): *Fed. Proc.,* 38:2333–2340.
55. Fuxe, K., Hökfelt, T., Agnati, L. F., Johansson, O., Goldstein, M., Perz de la Mora, M., Possani, L., Tapia, R., Teran, L., and Palacios, R. (1978): In: *Psychopharmacology: A Generation of*

Progress, edited by M. A. Lipton, A. DiMascio, and K. F. Killam, pp. 67–94. Raven Press, New York.
56. Fuxe, K., Hökfelt, T., and Nilsson, O. (1969): *Neuroendocrinology,* 5:107–120.
57. George, S. R., and van Loon, G. R. (1982): *Brain Res.,* 234:339–355.
58. Gibbs, D. M., and Neill, J. B. (1978): *Endocrinology,* 102:1895–1900.
59. Gudelsky, G. A., and Moore, K. E. (1976): *J. Neural Transm.,* 38:95–105.
60. Gudelsky, G. A., and Moore, K. E. (1977): *J. Pharmacol. Exp. Ther.,* 202:149–156.
61. Gudelsky, G. A., Nansel, D. D., and Porter, J. C. (1981): *Endocrinology,* 108:440–444.
62. Gudelsky, G. A., and Porter, J. C. (1979): *Life Sci.,* 25:1697–1702.
63. Gudelsky, G. A., Simpkins, J., Mueller, G. P., Meites, J., and Moore, K. E. (1976): *Neuroendocrinology,* 22:206–215.
64. Gunnet, J. W., Lookingland, K. J., and Moore, K. E. (1985): *Soc. Neurosci. Abstr.,* 11:1206.
65. Halasz, N., Ljungdahl, A., Hökfelt, T., Johansson, O., Goldstein, M., Park, D., and Biberfeld, P. (1977): *Brain Res.,* 126:445–474.
66. Hökfelt, T., and Fuxe, K. (1972): *Neuroendocrinology,* 9:100–122.
67. Hökfelt, T., Johansson, O., and Goldstein, M. (1984): *Science,* 225:1326–1334.
68. Holzbauer, M., Muscholl, E., Racke, K., and Sharman, D. F. (1983): In: *The Neurohypophysis: Structure, Function, and Control (Prog. Brain Res.,* 60), edited by B. A. Cross, and G. Long, pp. 357–364. Elsevier, Amsterdam.
69. Holzbauer, M., and Racke, K. (1985): *Med. Biol.,* 63:97–116.
70. Johnston, C. A., Demarest, K. T., and Moore, K. E. (1980): *Brain Res.,* 195:236–240.
71. Kizer, J. S., Humm, J., Nicholson, G., Greeley, G., and Youngblood, W. (1978): *Brain Res.,* 146:95–108.
72. Kizer, J. S., Palkovits, M., Kopin, I. J., Saavedra, J. M., and Brownstein, M. J. (1976): *Endocrinology,* 98:743–747.
73. Koenig, J., Mayfield, M. A., McCann, S. M., and Krulich, L. (1979): *Life Sci.,* 25:853–864.
74. Lindvall, O., and Björklund, A. (1983): In: *Chemical Neuroanatomy,* edited by P. C. Emson, pp. 229–255. Raven Press, New York.
75. Lindvall, O., Björklund, A., and Skagerberg, G. (1984): *Brain Res.,* 306:19–30.
76. Löfström, A. (1977): *Brain Res.,* 120:113–132.
77. Löfström, A., Eneroth, P., Gustafsson, J. A., and Skett, P. (1977): *Endocrinology,* 101:1559–1569.
78. Löfström, A., Jonsson, G., Wiesel, F. A., and Fuxe, K. (1976): *J. Histochem. Cytochem.,* 24:430–442.
79. Lookingland, K. J., Farah, J. M., Lovell, K. L., and Moore, K. E. (1985): *Neuroendocrinology,* 40:145–151.
80. Lookingland, K. J., and Moore, K. E. (1984): *Brain Res.,* 304:329–338.
81. Lookingland, K. J., and Moore, K. E. (1984): *Brain Res.,* 323:83–91.
82. Lookingland, K. J., and Moore, K. E. (1985): *Life Sci.,* 37:1225–1229.
83. Lookingland, K. J., and Moore, K. E. (1985): *Brain Res.,* 348:205–212.
84. MacLeod, R. M. (1976): In: *Frontiers in Neuroendocrinology, Vol. 4,* edited by W. F. Ganong and L. Martini, pp. 169–194. Raven Press, New York.
85. Mathews, R. T., and German, D. C. (1984): *Neuroscience,* 11:617–625.
86. McKay, D. W., Pasieka, C. A., Moore, K. E., Riegle, G. D., and Demarest, K. T. (1982): *Neuroendocrinology,* 34:229–235.
87. Moore, K. E., and Demarest, K. T. (1982): In: *Frontiers in Neuroendocrinology, Vol. 7,* edited by W. F. Ganong and L. Martini, pp. 161–190. Raven Press, New York.
88. Moore, K. E., and Johnston, C. A. (1982): In: *Neuroendocrine Perspectives, Vol. 1,* edited by E. E. Müller and R. M. MacLeod, pp. 23–68. Elsevier, Amsterdam.
89. Moore, K. E., and Kelly, P. H. (1978): In: *Psychopharmacology: A Generation of Progress,* edited by M. A. Lipton, A. DiMascio, and K. F. Killam, pp. 221–234. Raven Press, New York.

90. Moore, K. E., and Nielsen, J. A. (1985): In: *In Vivo Perfusion and the Release of Neuroactive Substances,* edited by A. Bayón and R. Drucker-Collin, pp. 177–199. Academic Press, New York.

91. Moore, K. E., Riegle, G. D., and Demarest, K. T. (1982): *Pharmacologist,* 24:198.

92. Moore, K. E., Riegle, G. D., and Demarest, K. T. (1985): In: *Prolactin: Basic and Clinical Correlates,* edited by R. M. MacLeod, M. O. Thorner, and U. Scapagnini, pp. 543–549. Liviana Press, Padova.

93. Moore, K. E., Riegle, G. D., and Demarest, K. T. (1985): In: *Catecholamines as Hormone Regulators,* edited by N. Ben-Jonathan, J. M. Bahr, and R. I. Weiner, pp. 31–49. Raven Press, New York.

94. Moore, K. E., Umezu, K., and Demarest, K. T. (1979): In: *Catecholamines: Basic and Clinical Frontiers,* edited by E. Usdin, I. J. Kopin, and J. Barchas, pp. 1230–1232. Pergamon Press, New York.

95. Moore, K. E., and Wuerthele, S. M. (1979): In: *Progress in Neurobiology, Vol. 13,* edited by G. A. Kerkut and J. W. Phillis, pp. 325–359. Pergamon Press, New York.

96. Moore, R. Y., and Bloom, F. E. (1978): *Annu. Rev. Neurosci.,* 1: 129–169.

97. Murrin, L. C., and Roth, R. H. (1976): *Mol. Pharmacol.,* 12: 463–475.

98. Nowycky, M. C., Walters, J. R., and Roth, R. H. (1978): *J. Neural Transm.,* 42:99–116.

99. Paalzow, G., and Paalzow, L. (1975): *Psychopharmacology,* 45: 9–20.

100. Perkins, N. A., and Westfall, T. C. (1978): *Neuroscience,* 3:59–63.

101. Persson, S. A. (1979): *Eur. J. Pharmacol.,* 55:121–128.

102. Pilotte, N. S., Gudelsky, G. A., and Porter, J. C. (1980): *Brain Res.,* 193:284–288.

103. Plotsky, P. M., and Neill, J. D. (1982): *Endocrinology,* 110:691–696.

104. Reymond, M. I., Kaur, C., and Porter, J. C. (1983): *Brain Res.,* 262:253–258.

105. Riegle, G. D., Moore, K. E., Lovell, K. L., and Demarest, K. T. (1985): *Soc. Neurosci. Abstr.,* 11:1207.

106. Roth, R. H., Murrin, L. C., and Walters, J. R. (1976): *Eur. J. Pharmacol.,* 36:163–171.

107. Roth, R. H., Walters, J. R., Murrin, L. C., and Morgenroth, V. H. (1975): In: *Pre- and Postsynaptic Receptors,* edited by E. Usdin and W. E. Bunney, pp. 5–46. Dekker, New York.

108. Saavedra, J. M., Chevillard, C., Bisserbe, J. C., and Borden, N. (1984): *Cell. Mol. Neurobiol.,* 4:397–402.

109. Sarkar, D. K., Gottschall, P. E., and Meites, J. (1982): *Science,* 218:684–686.

110. Scatton, B. (1977): *Eur. J. Pharmacol.,* 46:363–369.

111. Scatton, B., Dennis, T., and Curet, O. (1984): *Brain Res.,* 298: 193–196.

112. Selmanoff, M. (1981): *Endocrinology,* 108:1716–1722.

113. Selmanoff, M., and Wise, P. M. (1981): *Brain Res.,* 212:101–116.

114. Share, L. (1983): In: *The Neurohypophysis: Structure, Function and Control (Prog. Brain Res.,* 60), edited by B. A. Cross and G. Long, pp. 425–435. Elsevier, Amsterdam.

115. Smith, G. C., and Helme, R. D. (1974): *Cell Tissue Res.,* 152: 493–512.

116. Smith, M. S., Freeman, M. E., and Neill, J. D. (1975): *Endocrinology,* 96:219–226.

117. Terry, L. C., Craig, R., Hughes, T., Schatzle, J., Zora, M., Ortolano, G. A., and Willoughby, J. O. (1985): *Neuroendocrinology,* 41:269–275.

118. Umezu, K., and Moore, K. E. (1979): *J. Pharmacol. Exp. Ther.,* 208:49–56.

119. Ungerstedt, U. (1971): *Acta Physiol. Scand. (Suppl.* 367):1–48.

120. van de Pol, A. N., Herlist, R., and Powell, J. F. (1984): *Neuroscience,* 13:1117–1152.

121. van Loon, G. R., Ho, D., and Kim, C. (1980): *Endocrinology,* 106:76–80.

122. Wagner, J., Palfreyman, M., and Zraika, M. (1979): *J. Chromatogr.,* 164:41–54.

123. Westerink, B. H. C., and DeVries, J. B. (1985): *Brain Res.,* 330: 164–166.

124. Wood, P. L. (1983): *Peptides,* 4:595–601.

125. Wood, P. L., Nair, N. P. V., and Bozarth, M. (1982): *Neurosci. Lett.,* 32:291–294.

Psychopharmacology:
The Third Generation of Progress,
edited by Herbert Y. Meltzer.
Raven Press, New York © 1987.

CHAPTER 14

Physiology of the Midbrain Serotonin System

G. K. Aghajanian, J. S. Sprouse, and K. Rasmussen

In the mid-1960s, by means of the newly developed Falck-Hillarp histochemical method, neurons containing serotonin (5-hydroxytryptamine, 5-HT) were first found and mapped in the central nervous system (10,22,31,39). This discovery laid the foundation for physiological and biochemical investigations into the status of 5-HT as a central neurotransmitter. Studies conducted in a number of laboratories soon provided evidence that 5-HT met most if not all the classical criteria for a neurotransmitter or neuromodulator (9). This body of work may be summarized as follows: (a) serotonergic neurons possess the biochemical machinery for the synthesis and storage of 5-HT; (b) stimulation of the brainstem raphe nuclei, where most of the cell bodies of serotonergic neurons are located, causes a release of 5-HT in postsynaptic regions; (c) the effects of stimulating 5-HT pathways are mimicked by the direct iontophoretic application of 5-HT onto various postsynaptic neurons in the brain; and (d) blockade of reuptake, the principal mechanism for removal of 5-HT from sites of action, potentiates the physiological effects of stimulating 5-HT pathways. Attempts to block the physiological effects of 5-HT with putative antagonists have yielded less consistent results. Nevertheless, the preponderance of evidence supports the view that 5-HT functions as a neurotransmitter or neuromodulator in the central nervous system. These data, taken together with the fact that the serotonergic neurons of the raphe nuclei have extensive projections to nearly all parts of the neuraxis, point to an important role for this monoamine in brain function as well as in mediating the actions of various psychoactive drugs.

Recent research on the physiology and pharmacology of the midbrain 5-HT system is taking a number of exciting new directions. First, intracellular recording techniques are being introduced to investigate the intrinsic membrane properties of serotonergic neurons. Second, new information is coming to light about afferents to serotonergic neurons as well as the ionic basis for the inhibitory or excitatory effects of such inputs. Last, radiolabeled ligand binding methods have revealed the existence of multiple 5-HT binding sites, stimulating investigations into the physiological correlates of putative 5-HT receptor subtypes. This review will focus on recent developments in these three major areas.

BASIC PROPERTIES OF SEROTONERGIC NEURONS

Identification

In the past, serotonergic neurons had been identified on the basis of relatively indirect methods (e.g., firing pattern, antidromic activation, histological location, destruction by selective neurotoxins, etc.). Recently, by means of a new intracellular double-labeling method, it has been possible to colocalize intracellular injections of an intensely red-fluorescing dye (ethidium bromide) with the yellow, formaldehyde-induced fluorescence of 5-HT; an example of such an experiment is illustrated in Fig. 1 (7). By this method, it can be shown definitively that the slow, rhythmically firing neurons of the dorsal raphe nucleus are in fact the neurons that contain 5-HT.

Pacemaker Activity: Intrinsic Ionic Mechanisms and the Role of Noradrenergic Inputs

To investigate the membrane events underlying their distinctive pacemaker firing pattern, intracellular recordings

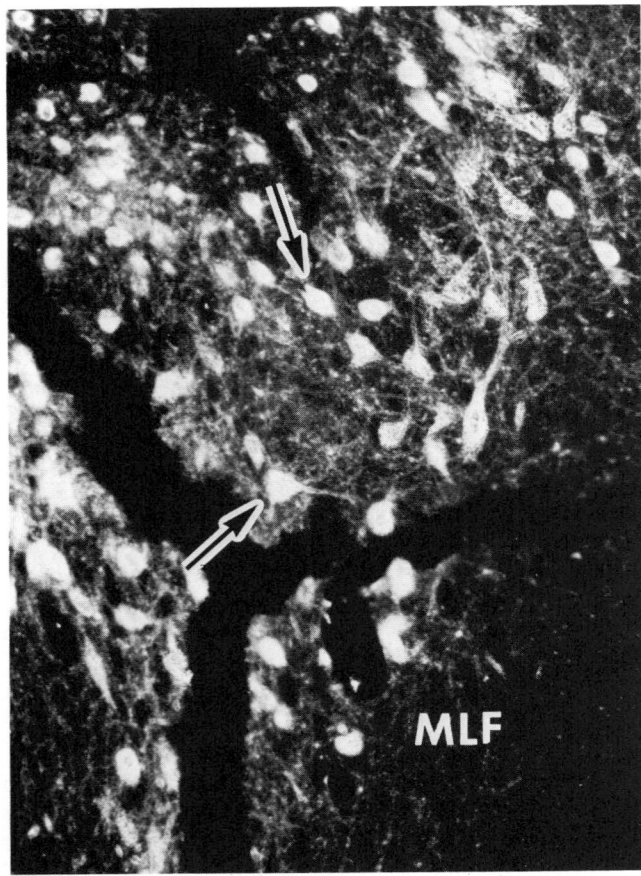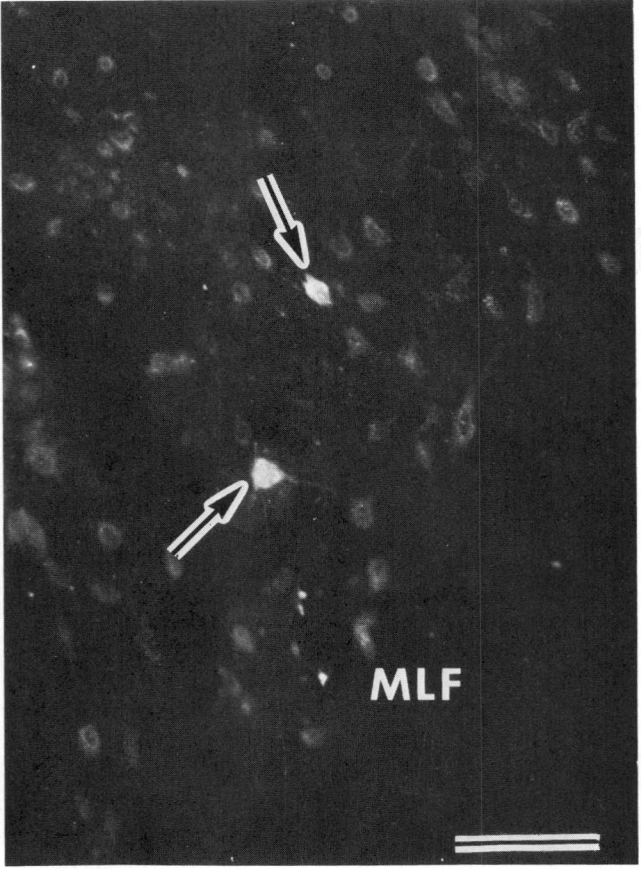

FIG. 1. Fluorescence micrographs of ethidium bromide-labeled cells in the dorsal raphe nucleus. **Left:** With the monoamine filter combination (500 nm peak transmission, 650 nm cutoff), clusters of (yellow) fluorescent serotonergic neurons can be seen; ethidium bromide-labeled cells (*arrows*) cannot be discerned because of their bright (yellow) serotonin-derived fluorescence. **Right:** Micrograph of the same field taken with a red pass barrier filter (590 nm peak transmission); two serotonergic neurons labeled with ethidium bromide can be visualized readily. MLF, Medial longitudinal fasciculus. Scale bar, 0.1 mm. (From ref. 7.)

have been made from serotonergic dorsal raphe neurons both *in vivo* and *in vitro* (from brain slices). These studies show that the typical rhythmic dorsal raphe cells exhibit a large afterhyperpolarization (AHP), which decays slowly during the interspike interval (6,29,112); as illustrated in Fig. 2, spikes arise from such depolarizing ramps (pacemaker potentials) rather than from excitatory postsynaptic potentials (EPSPs). Input resistance is reduced during the AHP, indicating an underlying increase in membrane conductance. Studies in brain slices on the ionic basis for this increased conductance indicate that it is produced by a calcium-activated potassium current (2,111). Thus, the slow, regular firing pattern of serotonergic neurons can be explained, at least in part, by the large amplitude and slow decay of a spike-dependent, calcium-activated outward current.

In addition to such intrinsic ionic mechanisms, there is evidence for noradrenergic modulation of the pacemaker cycle of serotonergic neurons. By electron microscopic autoradiography, identified serotonergic neurons of the dorsal raphe have been shown to receive a direct noradrenergic synaptic input (16). In the anesthetized rat, blockade

of the noradrenergic input to serotonergic neurons results in a cessation of spontaneous activity (14,15). *In vitro,* the majority of dorsal raphe cells are silent, but can be activated by introducing norepinephrine or the α_1-agonist phenylephrine into the medium; this activation can be blocked by specific α_1-antagonists (112). Since the activity of serotonergic neurons, at least in the anesthetized rat, depends on their noradrenergic input, it is possible that the relative lack of spontaneous activity in the dorsal raphe slice is caused by a disfacilitation due to an interruption of a tonic noradrenergic input. Investigations into the ionic basis for the noradrenergic enhancement of serotonergic pacemaker activity reveal that α_1-adrenoceptor stimulation (a) suppresses a resting outward potassium current to produce a steady depolarizing effect, and (b) suppresses a voltage-dependent transient outward potassium current (2), the so-called A-current (25), which normally slows the rate of depolarization during the latter phase of the interspike interval. A suppression of these outward potassium currents leads more rapidly to an activation of a voltage-dependent, low-threshold inward calcium current that triggers the spike toward the end of the pacemaker cycle (21).

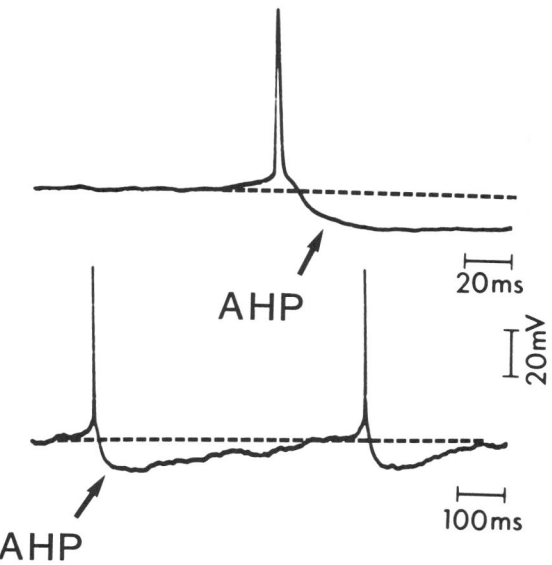

FIG. 2. Oscilloscope tracings showing intracellular recordings from a serotonergic dorsal raphe neuron *in vivo*. **Upper** trace shows a single spike at a relatively fast sweep speed. Note the long-duration spike (∼4 msec) and prominent afterhyperpolarization (AHP), which are characteristic of serotonergic neurons in the dorsal raphe nucleus. **Lower** trace (at a slower sweep speed) shows the gradual interspike depolarization (i.e., pacemaker potential) leading to spike threshold. *Dotted lines* indicate approach to spike threshold. (Provided by G. K. Aghajanian.)

The following sequence of events can now be proposed to account for the pacemaker cycle of serotonergic neurons: (a) calcium enters the cell during a spike through voltage-dependent calcium channels; this leads to a large AHP due to the calcium-activated potassium conductance; (b) the hyperpolarization not only serves to suppress firing but it removes the low-threshold calcium and A-channels from inactivation; (c) the cell gradually depolarizes during the interspike interval as the AHP diminishes (secondary to the sequestration and extrusion of calcium); (d) when the cell's membrane potential enters the appropriate voltage range (i.e., −60 to −58 mV) the low-threshold calcium current triggers a spike; (e) calcium, which enters during the spike, once again induces a large AHP to reinitiate the pacemaker cycle. This scheme is quite similar to that developed for invertebrate neurons and demonstrates the general importance of various calcium and potassium conductances in regulating tonic pacemaker activity (24,46).

Autoreceptors and Collateral Inhibition

It has been shown that serotonergic dorsal raphe neurons can be inhibited via a 5-HT autoreceptor (i.e., a receptor for a neuron's own transmitter). This receptor, which is located in the somatodendritic region of the cell, may function to mediate collateral inhibition within the raphe nuclei (116,119). Similar receptors may also serve to depress the excitability of serotonergic nerve terminals (97). From a pharmacological standpoint, this receptor seems to have a 5-HT$_{1A}$ agonist profile (see below). Lysergic acid diethylamide (LSD) and other indoleamine hallucinogens are powerful agonists at the somatodendritic 5-HT autoreceptor (4,32); phenethylamine hallucinogens (e.g., mescaline) do not share this action (48). Intracellular recordings *in vivo* have shown that the inhibition of dorsal raphe neurons by LSD is caused by a hyperpolarization accompanied by an increase in ionic conductance (6). Studies in the brain slice preparation have revealed that the ionic basis for the effects of 5-HT autoreceptor stimulation is an opening of potassium channels (5).

One physiological role for the 5-HT autoreceptor would be to mediate collateral inhibition in the raphe nuclei. When serotonergic neurons are activated antidromically they exhibit a period of suppressed firing proportional to the strength of the stimulus, a phenomenon suggestive of collateral or recurrent inhibition (116). Furthermore, cross-correlation analysis in the dorsal raphe nucleus has demonstrated mutually inhibitory interactions between adjacent serotonergic neurons (120). Theoretically, these inhibitions could be mediated via recurrent axon collaterals and/or dendrodendritic junctions. Anatomical studies have indicated close approximations between dendrite bundles in the dorsal raphe nucleus (38). In contrast, electron microscopic autoradiographic studies in the dorsal raphe nucleus have failed to reveal [³H]5-HT-labeled axon terminals at junctional sites (16,34). These anatomical observations, although not definitive, seem to favor the view that dendrodendritic rather than axon-collateral interactions may occur between serotonergic neurons.

AFFERENTS TO SEROTONERGIC NEURONS

Excitatory

The dorsal raphe nucleus receives afferents from a number of brain regions; among these are the lateral habenula, the lateral hypothalamic area, and the substantia nigra (8,27,54,81,82,96). Electrical stimulation of the lateral habenula and substantia nigra produces primarily inhibitory responses in the dorsal raphe (see below). In contrast, intracellular recording from dorsal raphe neurons has shown that electrical stimulation of the lateral hypothalamus produces a robust excitatory (depolarizing) response followed by an AHP (80). The depolarization is graded, is associated with an increase in ionic conductance, and can be reversed by the injection of depolarizing current and enhanced with hyperpolarization; thus, it has all the usual properties of an EPSP. The EPSP latency does not change with increasing stimulus strength, indicating that the response is mediated through a monosynaptic pathway. Conversely, the amplitude of the AHP increases with depolarization and can be reversed with hyperpolarization; this would suggest a conductance increase to potassium since the latter has a reversal potential in the hyperpolarizing direction. This ionic mechanism for the AHP would be consistent with a recurrent inhibitory circuit in the dorsal raphe nucleus and/or a calcium-activated potassium conductance.

The above studies show that the lateral hypothalamus gives rise to a major, monosynaptic excitatory forebrain input to the dorsal raphe nucleus. To date, the only other well-characterized excitatory input to the dorsal raphe nucleus is noradrenergic (see above), most likely emanating from sites within the brainstem itself (16). Chronic unit recordings in unanesthetized rats (59) and cats (51,92,93; B. L. Jacobs, *these volumes*) have demonstrated that phasic auditory and/or visual stimuli can activate dorsal or median (central superior) raphe neurons. The anatomical pathways and transmitters involved in the mediation of these effects have not as yet been determined. The central superior raphe nucleus of the cat has been reported to receive afferents from the interpeduncular nucleus as well as the lateral habenula and dorsal tegmental area (67). Central superior neurons are excited by electrical stimulation of the interpeduncular nucleus (66), but it is not yet known whether the affected neurons are serotonergic in identity.

Inhibitory

The habenular-raphe and nigral-raphe pathways have been studied as possible inhibitory inputs to the dorsal raphe nucleus (105,106,117). Electrical stimulation of the lateral habenula or substantia nigra results in a suppression of the spontaneous firing of serotonergic dorsal raphe neurons. The inhibitory effects of habenular stimulation resemble the effects produced by direct iontophoresis of γ-aminobutyric acid (GABA), as both can be blocked by intravenous injections of the GABA antagonist picrotoxin but not the glycine antagonist strychnine. Based on these experiments, GABA was originally proposed as the transmitter in the habenular-raphe pathway (117). This conclusion is supported by intracellular recordings that show that habenular stimulation elicits monosynaptic inhibitory responses in presumed serotonergic neurons of the dorsal raphe nucleus (79). However, biochemical studies do not detect a decrease in the levels of GABA and its synthetic enzyme, glutamic acid decarboxylase, after habenular lesions (47,77). On this basis, it has been hypothesized that excitatory habenular efferents may project to GABA interneurons in the dorsal raphe nucleus, and that these interneurons then terminate on serotonergic cells as part of a polysynaptic pathway (77). Two sets of anatomical data are consistent with this view: (a) immunocytochemical methods have revealed large numbers of GABAergic neurons in the dorsal raphe nucleus (76), and (b) retrograde tracing studies with [³H]aspartate indicate the existence of an excitatory amino acid projection from the lateral habenula to the dorsal raphe nucleus (54). To confirm this polysynaptic model, it will be necessary to show that electrical stimulation of the habenula excites raphe GABA interneurons in the dorsal raphe nucleus and that this, in turn, is responsible for the subsequent inhibition of serotonergic neurons. At this time, however, the precise synaptic mechanisms mediating habenular-raphe interactions remain unresolved.

PHYSIOLOGICAL CORRELATES OF SEROTONIN RECEPTOR SUBTYPES

Basis for Classification

In brain, the existence of multiple 5-HT receptors was first suggested by microiontophoretic studies in the cerebral cortex (95) and subcortical regions (49). In these experiments, putative 5-HT antagonists such as methysergide and cinanserin blocked the excitatory but not the inhibitory effects of 5-HT, suggesting two types of 5-HT receptors in brain, one for excitation and one for inhibition. Radioligand binding techniques also indicate the presence of multiple 5-HT receptors in brain. This conclusion derives from the finding that the neuroleptic agent [³H]spiperone labels 5-HT binding sites in frontal cortex (28,62,63) that exhibit features distinct from those sites labeled by [³H]5-HT itself (88). At the [³H]spiperone-labeled site, putative 5-HT antagonists display nanomolar affinities, whereas 5-HT and 5-HT agonists bind in the micromolar concentration range (90). Conversely, 5-HT and 5-HT agonists display more potent binding affinities than antagonists at the [³H]5-HT-labeled site. LSD binds to [³H]5-HT- and [³H]spiperone-labeled sites with similar affinity. These findings suggested the existence of distinct populations of 5-HT receptor sites, termed 5-HT$_1$ (S$_1$) for the 5-HT-labeled site and 5-HT$_2$ (S$_2$) for the spiperone-labeled site (88). These subtypes display marked regional variations in binding densities, again suggesting that they represent distinct molecular entities (89).

Recent studies have suggested heterogeneity within the 5-HT$_1$ subtype itself based on the finding that spiperone inhibits [³H]5-HT binding in a biphasic manner (86). Binding sites displaying high or low affinity for [³H]spiperone were designated 5-HT$_{1A}$ and 5-HT$_{1B}$, respectively. Subsequently, compounds selective for the 5-HT$_{1A}$ subtype (e.g., 8-OH-2-di-*n*-propyl-aminotetralin or 8-OH-DPAT) and the 5-HT$_{1B}$ subtype (e.g., RU 24969) were identified (74,100). Competition experiments, in which these compounds were tested for their capacity to displace [³H]5-HT binding, revealed high concentrations of 5-HT$_{1A}$ sites in the septal nucleus, hippocampus (CA1–CA4), dentate gyrus, and dorsal raphe nucleus, and high concentrations of 5-HT$_{1B}$ sites in the dorsal subiculum, globus pallidus, and substantia nigra (35,68,85). An additional subtype (5-HT$_{1C}$) has been proposed to account for labeling by mesulergine, 5-HT, and LSD, not similarly observed with 8-OH-DPAT or RU 24969 (26,84).

Because spiperone binds to dopamine-D2 (63) and 5-HT$_{1A}$ sites in addition to 5-HT$_2$ sites, the search began in the early 1980s for a selective 5-HT$_2$ ligand. The discovery of ketanserin (64) and later ritanserin (61), which label preferentially the 5-HT$_2$ site, has permitted further investigation of this binding site subtype (see below).

In summary, there is growing evidence for the existence of distinct 5-HT$_1$ and 5-HT$_2$ binding sites. However, it remains to be established that these binding sites are true functional receptors in brain. The remainder of this section will be devoted to examining correlations between radioligand binding studies and physiological studies.

Physiology of 5-HT$_1$ Receptors

Physiological studies aimed at assigning functional correlates to the 5-HT$_1$ binding site take advantage of the availability of 5-HT$_{1A}$ and 5-HT$_{1B}$ subtype-selective ligands and the heterogeneous distribution of subtype binding sites. Studies in the dorsal raphe nucleus and the hippocampal pyramidal cell layer, two areas containing dense concentrations of 5-HT_{1A} sites, will be considered in the following sections.

Dorsal Raphe Nucleus

A novel agonist with 5-HT-like actions but devoid of an indole or arylpiperazine nucleus, 8-hydroxy-2-(di-*n*-propylamino)tetralin (8-OH-DPAT; ref. 12), possesses an almost 1000-fold selectivity for the 5-HT_{1A} binding site (74). A marked reduction in the binding of 8-OH-DPAT in the dorsal raphe nucleus occurs following 5,7-dihydroxytryptamine-induced degeneration of serotonergic cell bodies (115). As a result, it was proposed that the somatic autoreceptor of neurons in the dorsal raphe is of the 5-HT_{1A} subtype. Consistent with this proposal, small intravenous doses of 8-OH-DPAT were found to inhibit the firing rate of 5-HT neurons in the dorsal raphe of chloral-hydrate-anesthetized rats (37). This observation was confirmed in microiontophoretic studies in which 8-OH-DPAT exerted a depressant effect comparable to LSD (33). Furthermore, buspirone, a purported nonbenzodiazepine anxiolytic that displays 5-HT_{1A} binding properties (87), also has been shown in extracellular recordings to potently inhibit the firing of 5-HT dorsal raphe neurons when administered systemically, microiontophoretically (113), or added to media bathing brain slices (114).

A direct comparison of the effects of 5-HT_{1A}- and 5-HT_{1B}-selective compounds on the spontaneous firing rate of dorsal raphe neurons has disclosed striking differences between the two ligand subtypes (102). The intravenous administration of TVX Q 7821 (ipsapirone) or LY 165163 (*p*-aminophenylethyl-*m*-trifluoromethylphenylpiperazine or PAPP), two long-chain substituted piperazines chosen for their 5-HT_{1A}-binding affinities (13,36,40,91), potently inhibits raphe cell firing in a dose-dependent manner. In contrast, trifluoromethylphenylpiperazine (TFMPP) and *m*-chlorophenylpiperazine (mCPP), two short-chain substituted piperazines chosen for their 5-HT_{1B}-binding affinities (100), display weak or irregular actions. Raphe cell firing is also suppressed by the microiontophoretic application of ipsapirone and PAPP, indicating a direct action on 5-HT neurons. Dose-response curves for these two 5-HT_{1A}-selective compounds are indistinguishable from that of 5-HT. However, the two 5-HT_{1B}-selective compounds, TFMPP and mCPP, when applied by microiontophoresis again appear to be only weak autoreceptor agonists. A representative rate histogram illustrating these differences is presented in Fig. 3.

The efficacy of 5-HT_{1A} ligands in slowing 5-HT cell firing has been further demonstrated by intracellular recordings of dorsal raphe neurons in coronal brain slices maintained *in vitro*. Ipsapirone and PAPP mimic the effects of 5-HT in hyperpolarizing the cell membrane and decreasing input resistance (102).

Direct evidence for the activation of 5-HT somatic autoreceptors by ipsapirone or PAPP ideally should include the demonstration that its effect on spontaneous cell firing can be blocked by autoreceptor antagonists. To date, the classical 5-HT antagonists have proven ineffective in blocking the effect of 5-HT at the autoreceptor, or for that matter, at inhibitory postsynaptic sites (49). However,

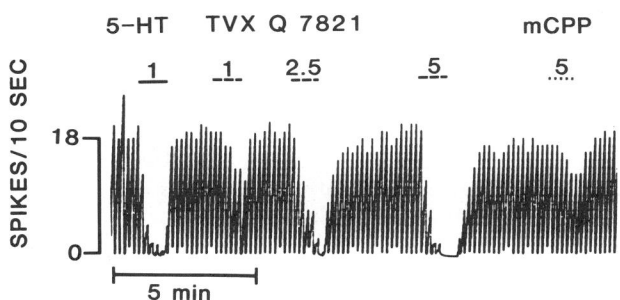

FIG. 3. Effects of microiontophoretic application of 5-HT, TVX Q 7821 (ipsapirone), and *m*-chlorophenylpiperazine (mCPP) on a spontaneously firing neuron in the dorsal raphe nucleus of a chloral-hydrate-anesthetized rat. The duration of each drug ejection is 1 min as indicated by the bars above the record; the numbers directly above each bar refer to the iontophoretic current in nanoamperes used for ejection. 5-HT (*solid bar*) and TVX Q 7821 (*dashed bar*), a 5-HT_{1A}-selective compound, potently suppress firing. In contrast, mCPP (*dotted bar*), a 5-HT_{1B}-selective compound, produces only a minimal suppresion. (Provided by J. S. Sprouse.)

recent behavioral studies have suggested that certain β-adrenoceptor antagonists including (−)-propranolol may possess 5-HT_{1A}-antagonistic properties (45,107,108), and studies in our laboratory indicate that low microiontophoretic currents of (−)- but not (+)-propranolol effectively block the suppressant effects of ipsapirone on raphe cell firing (103).

Hippocampal Pyramidal Cell Layer

Intracellular recordings from hippocampal pyramidal cells (CA1) in rat brain slices have shown that 5-HT produces a membrane hyperpolarization and reduction in the input resistance due to an opening of potassium channels (99). The receptors mediating these events appear to be of the 5-HT_{1A} subtype, as 8-OH-DPAT elicits similar changes in membrane potential and input resistance (11). This latter finding is consistent with radioligand data showing that 8-OH-DPAT potently displaces [^{3}H]5-HT binding in hippocampus (85). Buspirone, a selective 5-HT_{1A} ligand (87) and displacer of 5-HT binding in hippocampal preparations (41), produces only small hyperpolarizations; in addition, it reduces maximal 5-HT responses, which is in accord with a weak partial agonist action at these postsynaptic sites (11).

In rat dorsal hippocampal slices, the predominant effect of 5-HT on population spikes elicited from the pyramidal cell layer (CA1) is a dose-dependent decrease in amplitude, often preceded by a smaller transient increase (17). 8-OH-DPAT and 5-carboxyamidotryptamine, a potent but nonselective 5-HT_1 ligand, also produce a decrease in population spike amplitude, which can be antagonized by spiperone (18). Likewise, application of buspirone or isapirone results in a dose-dependent and reversible reduction of the population spike (69). Together, these data suggest that the decrease in population spike amplitude is mediated by a 5-HT_{1A} receptor.

Although the microiontophoretic application of 5-HT slows the spontaneous firing of hippocampal pyramidal cells in a dose-related fashion, we have found that the 5-HT$_{1A}$ agonists, ipsapirone and PAPP, only weakly suppress spontaneous cell firing (J. S. Sprouse and G. K. Aghajanian, *unpublished observations*). This result is consistent with the proposed agonist role assigned to another 5-HT$_{1A}$ agonist, buspirone (11). The 5-HT$_{1B}$-selective compounds, TFMPP and mCPP, also exhibit only weak effects. To reconcile these findings with the dense labeling of ipsapirone observed in the hippocampus (40,42), a modulatory role for ipsapirone has been sought. Recent experiments in our laboratory indicate that low microiontophoretic currents of ipsapirone, which do not affect spontaneous firing, attenuate glutamate excitation of pyramidal cells (J. S. Sprouse and G. K. Aghajanian, *unpublished observations*). Similar modulatory effects of 5-HT on glutamate excitation have been observed in the cerebral cortex (55), substantia nigra (3), and on cerebellar Purkinje cells (58). However, it has not been demonstrated that these apparent modulatory effects are specifically mediated by 5-HT$_{1A}$ receptors.

Physiology of 5-HT$_2$ Receptors

Initial studies on 5-HT$_2$ binding sites in rat brain indicated a high density in the frontal cortex, striatum, and nucleus accumbens (56,101). Later, a quantitative autoradiographic study confirmed the existence of 5-HT$_2$ binding in these brain areas, and went further to show high concentrations of 5-HT$_2$ sites in the claustrum, olfactory tubercle, layers I and IV of the neocortex, anterior olfactory nucleus, and pyriform cortex, and moderate concentrations in the caudate-putamen, nucleus accumbens, layer V of the neocortex, ventral dentate gyrus, and mammillary bodies (83). Studies in human brain have also shown a high concentration of 5-HT$_2$ sites throughout the cerebral cortex, with the exception of pre- and postcentral gyri (98). This pattern contrasts with rat brain, which displays the highest concentration of 5-HT$_2$ sites in the frontal cortex with a progressively decreasing anterior-posterior gradient (83). Preliminary single-cell studies aimed at examining the physiological role of 5-HT$_2$ binding sites are discussed in the following sections.

Facial Motor Nucleus

Although there generally are very few 5-HT$_2$ binding sites in the brainstem, one exception is the facial motor nucleus (83). In this nucleus the microiontophoretic application of 5-HT or norepinephrine does not by itself excite facial motoneurons but does facilitate the subthreshold and threshold excitatory effects of iontophoretically applied glutamate (70). A similar effect of 5-HT and norepinephrine on glutamate excitation of spinal motoneurons has also been documented (121). Activation of the 5-HT receptor on facial motoneurons has since been shown to cause a slow depolarization, increased input resistance, and increased excitability, probably through a decrease in resting membrane conductance to potassium (109,110).

The facilitation of glutamate excitation by the activation of 5-HT receptors on facial motoneurons appears to be physiologically relevant, since (a) the facial nucleus receives a dense and uniform 5-HT input (31,78); (b) the release of

endogenous 5-HT following iontophoresis of the 5-HT-releasing agent *p*-chloroamphetamine mimics the effects of iontophoretic 5-HT (70); (c) the destruction of the 5-HT terminals with 5,7-dihydroxytryptamine significantly decreases the ejecting current of 5-HT required to excite facial motoneurons (71); (d) the activation of facial motoneurons produced by electrical stimulation of the motor cortex or red nucleus is potentiated by the microiontophoretic application of 5-HT (70). This marked facilitation of excitatory inputs to brainstem and spinal cord motor nuclei may explain the excitatory 5-HT motor syndrome produced by pharmacological treatments that enhance stimulation of postsynaptic 5-HT receptors (53).

An action of 5-HT on 5-HT$_1$ receptors would appear to be mainly responsible for producing the 5-HT motor syndrome (12,65). The action of iontophoretically applied 5-HT in the facial nucleus can be blocked by the classical 5-HT antagonists metergoline, methysergide, cyproheptadine, and cinanserin (72). However, as all of these antagonists have been shown to interact with both the 5-HT$_1$ and 5-HT$_2$ receptors, with greater affinity for 5-HT$_2$ receptors (60), it is conceivable that the action of 5-HT in the facial motor nucleus involves both 5-HT$_1$ and 5-HT$_2$ receptors. Recently, a large number of studies, using behavioral as well as binding techniques, have shown that indoleamine and phenethylamine hallucinogens share the property of interacting with 5-HT$_2$ receptors (20,23,43,44,50,75). Therefore, one would expect members of both classes of hallucinogens to have direct effects in the facial motor nucleus. Thus, it is of interest that the iontophoretic administration of LSD, mescaline, or psilocin, although having little discernible effect by themselves, markedly enhance the facilitation of facial motoneuron excitation produced by iontophoretically applied 5-HT and norepinephrine (73). In essence, the hallucinogens facilitate the facilitation produced by 5-HT and norepinephrine. Two nonhallucinogenic ergot derivatives, lisuride and methysergide, do not enhance the facilitatory effects of 5-HT and norepinephrine, suggesting that the phenomenon is specific to hallucinogens.

Thus, the action of 5-HT in the facial motor nucleus may be a complex one involving a cooperative interaction between 5-HT$_1$ and 5-HT$_2$ receptors. Determination of the exact nature of this interaction awaits experiments employing more selective 5-HT$_2$ and 5-HT$_1$ antagonists.

Prefrontal Cortex

Consistent with the above notion that 5-HT$_2$ receptors can function to modulate physiological effects of 5-HT is the response of prefrontal cortex neurons in the rat to iontophoretic administration of the 5-HT$_2$ antagonist ketanserin (57). In the prefrontal cortex the iontophoretic application of 5-HT almost invariably produces inhibitory responses (57,94). The administration of ketanserin, iontophoretically or systemically, not only fails to antagonize this inhibitory action but, in 60% of the cells examined, potentiates the 5-HT-induced inhibition (57). If this effect of ketanserin is due to the block of a tonic 5-HT$_2$ influence, then this implies that 5-HT$_2$ receptor activation down-modulates the inhibitory action of 5-HT. Methysergide has

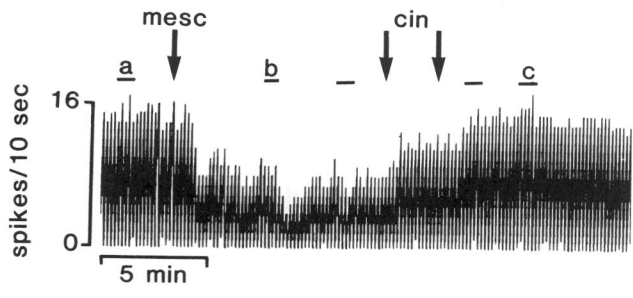

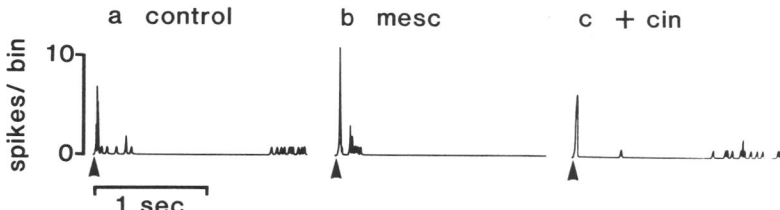

FIG. 4. Effect of mescaline followed by cinanserin on the firing rate (**top**) and response to sciatic nerve stimulation (**bottom**) of a rat locus coeruleus neuron. **Top:** Drugs were given by slow i.v. infusion (*arrows*). The sciatic nerve was stimulated (*bars*) by means of a bipolar electrode inserted into the nerve (0.1–0.2 mA, 0.25 Hz). The results of sciatic nerve stimulation occurring at the bars marked *a, b,* and *c* are displayed in the bottom half of the figure. **Bottom:** Poststimulus time histograms of the response of a locus ceruleus neuron to sciatic nerve stimulation before (*a*) and after (*b*) the administration of mescaline (mesc; 1 mg/kg), and (*c*) after the subsequent administration of cinanserin (cin; 0.5 mg/kg × 2). Each histogram was generated from 10 sweeps initiated by sciatic nerve stimulus (*arrows*). Note the decrease in background firing rate and increase in evoked responses after the administration of mescaline and the reversal of each of these trends after the administration of cinanserin. (Provided by G. K. Aghajanian.)

also been reported to potentiate the depressant effects of 5-HT recorded in the somatosensory cortex (19). Similarly, 5-HT antagonists (e.g., cinanserin, cyproheptadine) not only failed to antagonize the depressant effects of 5-HT in the dorsal (30) and ventral lateral geniculate (49,118), but actually tended to potentiate these inhibitory effects (49).

It appears that in areas of the brain where both 5-HT$_1$ and 5-HT$_2$ receptors exist, the 5-HT$_2$ receptor opposes inhibitory and enhances excitatory effects produced by activation of the 5-HT$_1$ receptor. Thus, in the prefrontal cortex, 5-HT$_2$ receptor activation works in opposition to the depressant effect of 5-HT on cell firing, whereas in the facial motor nucleus, 5-HT$_2$ receptors enhance a facilitatory action of 5-HT on cell firing.

Locus Coeruleus

Another example of a facilitatory effect mediated by 5-HT$_2$ receptors can be observed in the locus coeruleus (LC). In anesthetized rats, systemically administered mescaline or LSD induces a decrease in the spontaneous activity of noradrenergic cells in the LC but, paradoxically, facilitates the activation of these cells by tactile stimuli (1). That the effects of LSD and mescaline on LC neurons are mediated

by 5-HT$_2$ receptors is suggested by the fact that they can be reversed not only by the classical 5-HT antagonists such as cinanserin (Fig. 4; G. K. Aghajanian, *unpublished observations*) but also by the newer, more selective 5-HT$_2$ antagonists such as ritanserin and LY-53857 (92). In addition, 1-(2,5-dimethoxy-4-methylphenyl)-2-aminopropane (DOM) has an extremely potent mescaline-like action on LC neurons (Fig. 5). Thus, the relative potencies of LSD, DOM, and mescaline in their action on LC neurons correlate with their affinity for 5-HT$_2$ receptors (43). However, this action of hallucinogens is not a direct one, as the effects of these drugs given systemically are not mimicked by their iontophoretic application onto LC cell bodies (G. K. Aghajanian, *unpublished observations*). Moreover, the systemic administration of mescaline or LSD does not enhance the excitation of LC neurons evoked by microiontophoretically applied acetylcholine, glutamate, or substance P (1). These results imply that the hallucinogens are acting on afferents to the LC, afferents that are affected directly, or indirectly, by 5-HT$_2$ receptors. When these 5-HT$_2$ receptors are activated, they facilitate the response of the LC to peripheral stimuli. Presumably, the relevant afferents to the LC arise from various sensory relay nuclei in the spinal cord and lower brainstem. However, since 5-HT$_2$ receptors are not located in high densities in these nuclei (83), it is possible that other areas of the brain that are rich in 5-HT$_2$

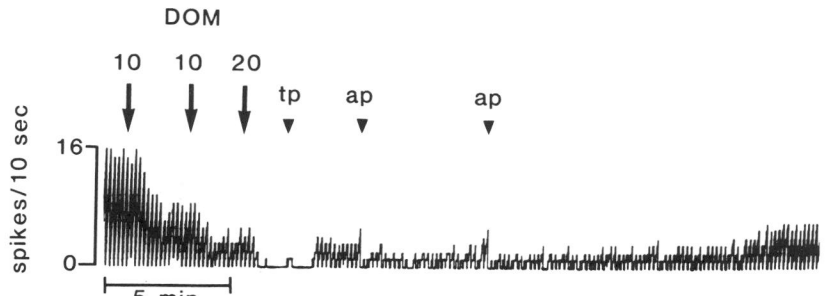

FIG. 5. Effects of DOM on the firing rate and reactivity to peripheral stimuli of a rat locus coeruleus neuron. DOM was administered by slow i.v. infusion (*large arrows*—numbers refer to dose in micrograms per kilogram). Note the dramatic decrease in spontaneous activity following the administration of DOM. A very mild contralateral toe pinch (tp) and air puffs to the animal's back (ap) are indicated. The response to mild toe pinch served to indicate that the cell being recorded was still present. Note the increase in activity caused by air puffs; air puffs would not normally elicit such large increases in activity in anesthetized rats. (Provided by G. K. Aghajanian.)

receptors, e.g., prefrontal cortex, send efferents to these sensory relay nuclei and/or directly to the LC.

SUMMARY AND CONCLUSIONS

This review has emphasized developments in three major areas: (a) the intrinsic membrane properties of serotonergic neurons; (b) the physiology of afferents to the dorsal and median raphe nuclei; and (c) physiological correlates of 5-HT receptor subtypes. Some of the key findings and conclusions are summarized as follows:

1. The firing of serotonergic neurons is tightly regulated by intrinsic ionic mechanisms (e.g., a calcium-activated potassium conductance), accounting for the well-known tonic pacemaker pattern of activity of these cells. The intrinsic pacemaker is modulated by at least two neurotransmitters: (a) norepinephrine, acting through α_1-adrenoceptors, accelerates the pacemaker; and (b) 5-HT, acting through somatodendritic 5-HT autoreceptors, slows the pacemaker.

2. Several excitatory and inhibitory pathways impinge upon midbrain serotonergic neurons; the physiological effects of extrinsic inputs become superimposed upon the intrinsic ionic mechanisms. For example, following excitation there is a prolonged inhibitory period; this postactivation inhibition can be explained by intrinsic ionic mechanisms (e.g., the calcium-activated potassium conductance) and/or autoreceptor-mediated collateral inhibition.

3. The 5-HT_1 receptor subtypes, as identified by radioligand binding techniques, can be differentiated physiologically: (a) 5-HT_{1A} but not 5-HT_{1B} ligands mimic the inhibitory action of 5-HT at somatodendritic autoreceptors; (b) 5-HT_{1A} ligands, although they do not mimic the direct inhibitory action of 5-HT in the hippocampus, share with 5-HT the ability to suppress excitatory responses to glutamate.

4. Complex modulatory interactions appear to exist between 5-HT_2 and 5-HT_1 receptors. Indoleamine hallucinogens have agonist activity at both 5-HT_1 and 5-HT_2 receptors, but phenethylamine hallucinogens are active only at 5-HT_2 receptors. Therefore, it is proposed that an action at 5-HT_2 receptors—not 5-HT_1 receptors—could account for the behavioral and psychological effects that these two major classes of hallucinogens have in common. Finally, because the 5-HT_2 site has a hybrid agonist profile, with both indoleamine and phenethylamine features, the possibility must be considered that there may be an endogenous ligand for this site in addition to 5-HT itself.

ACKNOWLEDGMENTS

This work was supported by PHS Grants MH-17871, MH-14276, and the State of Connecticut.

REFERENCES

1. Aghajanian, G. K. (1980): *Brain Res.*, 186:492–498.
2. Aghajanian, G. K. (1985): *Nature*, 315:501–503.
3. Aghajanian, G. K., and Bunney, B. S. (1974): *Excerpta Med. Int. Cong.*, 359:444–452.
4. Aghajanian, G. K., and Haigler, H. J. (1975): *Psychopharmacol. Commun.*, 1:619–629.
5. Aghajanian, G. K., and Lakoski, J. M. (1984): *Brain Res.*, 305: 181–185.
6. Aghajanian, G. K., and VanderMaelen, C. P. (1982): *Brain Res.*, 238:463–469.
7. Aghajanian, G. K., and VanderMaelen, C. P. (1982): *J. Neurosci.*, 2:1786–1792.
8. Aghajanian, G. K., and Wang, R. Y. (1977): *Brain Res.*, 122: 229–242.
9. Aghajanian, G. K., and Wang, R. Y. (1978): In: *Psychopharmacology: A Generation of Progress*, edited by M. A. Lipton, A. DiMascio, and K. F. Killam, pp. 171–183. Raven Press, New York.
10. Andén, N. E., Dahlström, A., Fuxe, K., Larsson, K., Olson, L., and Ungerstedt, U. (1966): *Acta Physiol. Scand.*, 67:313–326.
11. Andrade, R., and Nicoll, R. A. (1985): *Soc. Neurosci. Abstr.*, 11: 597.
12. Arvidsson, L., Hacksell, U., Nilsson, J. L. G., Hjorth, S., Carlsson, A., Lindberg, P., Sanchez, D., and Wikstrom, H. (1981): *J. Med. Chem.*, 24:921–923.
13. Asarch, K. B., Ransom, R. W., and Shih, J. C. (1985): *Life Sci.*, 36:1265–1273.
14. Baraban, J. M., and Aghajanian, G. K. (1980): *Neuropharmacology*, 19:355–363.
15. Baraban, J. M., and Aghajanian, G. K. (1980): *Eur. J. Pharmacol.*, 66:287–294.
16. Baraban, J. M., and Aghajanian, G. K. (1981): *Brain Res.*, 204: 1–11.
17. Beck, S. G., Clarke, W. P., and Goldfarb, J. (1985): *Eur. J. Pharmacol.*, 116:195–197.
18. Beck, S. G., and Goldfarb, J. (1985): *Life Sci.*, 36:557–563.
19. Bradshaw, C. M., Stoker, M. J., and Szabadi, E. (1983): *Neuropharmacology*, 22:677–683.
20. Buckholtz, N. S., Freedman, D. X., and Middaugh, L. D. (1985): *Eur. J. Pharmacol.*, 109:421–425.
21. Burlhis, T. M., and Aghajanian, G. K. (1986): *Soc. Neurosci. Abstr.*, 12:175.
22. Carlsson, A., Falck, B., and Hillarp, N.-Å. (1962): *Acta Physiol. Scand.*, 196:1–28.
23. Colpaert, F. C., Meert, T. F., Niemegeers, C. J. E., and Janssen, P. A. J. (1985): *Psychopharmacology*, 86:45–54.
24. Connor, J. A. (1978): *Fed. Proc.*, 37:2139–2144.
25. Connor, J. A., and Stevens, C. F. (1971): *J. Physiol. (Lond.)*, 213:21–30.
26. Cortes, R., Palacios, J. M., and Pazos, A. (1984): *Br. J. Pharmacol.*, 82:202P.
27. Cowan, R. L., and Park, M. R. (1985): *Soc. Neurosci. Abstr.*, 2: 1277.
28. Creese, I., and Snyder, S. H. (1978): *Eur. J. Pharmacol.*, 49:201–202.
29. Crunelli, V., Forda, S., Brooks, P. A., Wilson, K. C. P., Wise, J. C. M., and Kelly, J. S. (1983): *Neurosci. Lett.*, 40:263–268.
30. Curtis, D. R., and Davis, R. (1962): *Br. J. Pharmacol.*, 18:217–246.
31. Dahlström, A., and Fuxe, K. (1965): *Acta Physiol. Scand.*, 232: 1–55.
32. deMontigny, C., and Aghajanian, G. K. (1977): *Neuropharmacology*, 16:811–818.
33. deMontigny, C., Blier, P., and Chaput, Y. (1984): *Neuropharmacology*, 23:1511–1520.
34. Descarries, L., Watkins, K. C., Garcia, S., and Beaudet, A. (1982): *J. Comp. Neurol.*, 207:239–254.
35. Deshmukh, P. P., Yamamura, H. I., Woods, L., and Nelson, D. L. (1983): *Brain Res.*, 288:338–343.
36. Dompert, W. U., Glaser, T., and Traber, J. (1985): *Naunyn Schmiedebergs Arch. Pharmacol.*, 328:462–465.
37. Fallon, S. L., Kim, H. S., and Welch, J. J. (1983): *Soc. Neurosci. Abstr.*, 9:716.
38. Felten, D. L., and Harrigan, P. (1980): *Neurosci. Lett.*, 16:275–280.
39. Fuxe, K. (1965): *Acta Physiol. Scand.*, 247:37–85.
40. Glaser, T., Rath, M., Traber, J., Zilles, K., and Schleicher, A. (1985): *Brain Res.*, 358:129–136.
41. Glaser, T., and Traber, J. (1983): *Eur. J. Pharmacol.*, 88:137–138.

42. Glaser, T., and Traber, J. (1985): *Naunyn Schmiedebergs Arch. Pharmacol.*, 329:211–215.
43. Glennon, R. A., Titeler, M., and McKenney, J. D. (1984): *Life Sci.*, 35:2505–2511.
44. Glennon, R. A., Young, R., and Rosecrans, J. A. (1983): *Eur. J. Pharmacol.*, 91:189–196.
45. Goodwin, G. M., and Green, A. R. (1985): *Br. J. Pharmacol.*, 84:743–753.
46. Gorman, A. L. F., Hermann, A., and Thomas, M. V. (1981): *Fed. Proc.*, 40:2233–2239.
47. Gottesfeld, Z., Hoover, D. B., Muth, E. A., and Jacobowitz, D. M. (1978): *Brain Res.*, 141:353–356.
48. Haigler, H. J., and Aghajanian, G. K. (1973): *Eur. J. Pharmacol.*, 21:53–60.
49. Haigler, H. J., and Aghajanian, G. K. (1974): *J. Neural Transm.*, 35:257–273.
50. Heym, J., Rasmussen, K., and Jacobs, B. L. (1984): *Eur. J. Pharmacol.*, 101:57–68.
51. Heym, J., Steinfels, G. F., and Jacobs, B. L. (1984): *Brain Res.*, 291:63–72.
52. Heym, J., Trulson, M. E., and Jacobs, B. L. (1982): *Brain Res.*, 232:29–39.
53. Jacobs, B. L. (1976): *Life Sci.*, 19:777–786.
54. Kalen, P., Karlson, M., and Wiklund, L. (1985): *Brain Res.*, 360:285–297.
55. Krnjevic, K., and Phillis, J. W. (1963): *Br. J. Pharmacol.*, 20:471–490.
56. Laduron, P. M., Janssen, P. F. M., and Leysen, J. E. (1982): *Eur. J. Pharmacol.*, 81:43–48.
57. Lakoski, J. M., and Aghajanian, G. K. (1985): *Neuropharmacology*, 24:265–273.
58. Lee, M., Strahlendorf, J. C., and Strahlendorf, H. K. (1986): *Brain Res.*, 361:107–113.
59. LeMoal, M., and Olds, M. E. (1979): *Physiol. Behav.*, 22:11–15.
60. Leysen, J. E., Awouters, F., Kennis, L., Laduron, P. M., Vandenberk, J., and Janssen, P. A. J. (1981): *Life Sci.*, 28:1015–1022.
61. Leysen, J. E., Gommereu, W., Van Gompel, P., Wynants, J., Janssen, P. F. M., and Laduron, P. M. (1985): *Mol. Pharmacol.*, 27:600–611.
62. Leysen, J. E., and Laduron, P. M. (1977): *Arch. Int. Pharmacodyn. Ther.*, 230:337–339.
63. Leysen, J. E., Niemegeers, C. J. E., Tollenaere, J. P., and Laduron, P. M. (1978): *Nature*, 272:168–171.
64. Leysen, J. E., Niemegeers, C. J. E., Van Nueten, J. M., and Laduron, P. (1982): *Mol. Pharmacol.*, 21:301–314.
65. Lucki, I., Nobler, M. S., and Frazer, A. (1984): *J. Pharmacol. Exp. Ther.*, 228:133–139.
66. Maciewicz, R., Foote, W. E., and Bry, J. (1981): *Brain Res.*, 225:179–183.
67. Maciewicz, R., Taber-Pierce, E., Ronner, S., and Foote, W. E. (1981): *Brain Res.*, 216:414–421.
68. Marcinkiewicz, M., Verge, D., Gozlan, H., Pichat, L., and Hamon, M. (1984): *Brain Res.*, 291:159–163.
69. Mauk, M. D., Peroutka, P. J., and Kocsis, J. D. (1985): *Soc. Neurosci. Abstr.*, 11:135.
70. McCall, R. B., and Aghajanian, G. K. (1979): *Brain Res.*, 169:11–27.
71. McCall, R. B., and Aghajanian, G. K. (1979): *Neuroscience*, 4:1501–1510.
72. McCall, R. B., and Aghajanian, G. K. (1980): *Eur. J. Pharmacol.*, 65:175–183.
73. McCall, R. B., and Aghajanian, G. K. (1980): *Life Sci.*, 26:1149–1156.
74. Middlemiss, D. N., and Fozard, J. R. (1983): *Eur. J. Pharmacol.*, 90:151–153.
75. Mokler, D. J., Stoudt, K. W., and Rech, R. H. (1985): *Pharmacol. Biochem. Behav.*, 22:677–682.
76. Nanopoulos, D., Belin, M. F., Maitre, M., Vincendon, G., and Pujol, J. F. (1982): *Brain Res.*, 232:375–389.
77. Neckers, L. M., Schwartz, J. P., Wyatt, R. J., and Speciale, S. G. (1979): *Exp. Brain Res.*, 37:619–623.
78. Palkovits, M., Brownstein, M., and Saavedra, J. M. (1974): *Brain Res.*, 80:237–249.
79. Park, M. R. (1982): *Soc. Neurosci. Abstr.*, 8:781.
80. Park, M. R. (1985): *Soc. Neurosci. Abstr.*, 11:1227.
81. Pasquier, D. A., Anderson, C., Forbes, W. B., and Morgane, P. J. (1976): *Brain Res. Bull.*, 1:443–451.
82. Pasquier, D. A., Kemper, T. L., Forbes, W. B., and Morgane, P. J. (1977): *Brain Res. Bull.*, 2:323–339.
83. Pazos, A., Cortes, R., and Palacios, J. M. (1985): *Brain Res.*, 346:231–249.
84. Pazos, A., Hoyer, D., and Palacios, J. M. (1985): *Eur. J. Pharmacol.*, 106:539–546.
85. Pazos, A., and Palacios, J. M. (1985): *Brain Res.*, 346:205–230.
86. Pedigo, N. W., Yamamura, H. I., and Nelson, D. L. (1981): *J. Neurochem.*, 36:220–226.
87. Peroutka, S. J. (1985): *Biol. Psychiatry*, 20:971–979.
88. Peroutka, S. J., and Snyder, S. H. (1979): *Mol. Pharmacol.*, 16:687–699.
89. Peroutka, S. J., and Snyder, S. H. (1981): *Brain Res.*, 208:339–347.
90. Peroutka, S. J., and Snyder, S. H. (1983): *Fed. Proc.*, 42:213–217.
91. Ransom, R. W., Asarch, K. B., and Shih, J. C. (1986): *J. Neurochem.*, 46:68–75.
92. Rasmussen, K., and Aghajanian, G. K. (1986): *Brain Res.*, 385:395–400.
93. Rasmussen, K., Heym, J., and Jacobs, B. L. (1984): *Exp. Neurol.*, 83:302–317.
94. Reader, T. A., Ferron, A., Descarries, L., and Jasper, H. H. (1979): *Brain Res.*, 160:217–229.
95. Roberts, M. H. T., and Straughan, D. W. (1967): *J. Physiol. (Lond.)*, 193:269–294.
96. Sakai, K., Salvert, D., Touret, M., and Jouvet, M. (1977): *Brain Res.*, 137:11–35.
97. Sawyer, S. F., Tepper, J. M., Young, S. J., and Groves, P. M. (1985): *Brain Res.*, 332:15–28.
98. Schotte, A., Maloteaux, J. M., and Laduron, P. M. (1983): *Brain Res.*, 276:231–235.
99. Segal, M. (1980): *J. Physiol. (Lond.)*, 303:423–439.
100. Sills, M. A., Wolfe, B. B., and Frazer, A. (1984): *J. Pharmacol. Exp. Ther.*, 231:480–487.
101. Slater, P., and Patel, S. (1983): *Eur. J. Pharmacol.*, 92:297–298.
102. Sprouse, J. S., and Aghajanian, G. K. (1985): *Synapse*, 1:3–9.
103. Sprouse, J. S., and Aghajanian, G. K. (1986): *Eur. J. Pharmacol.*, 128:295–298.
104. Stern, W. C., Johnson, A., Bronzino, J. D., and Morgane, P. J. (1979): *Exp. Neurol.*, 65:326–342.
105. Stern, W. C., Johnson, A., Bronzino, J. D., and Morgane, P. J. (1979): *Brain Res. Bull.*, 4:561–565.
106. Stern, W. C., Johnson, A., Bronzino, J. D., and Morgane, P. J. (1981): *Neuropharmacology*, 20:979–989.
107. Tricklebank, M. D. (1984): *Br. J. Pharmacol.*, 81:26P.
108. Tricklebank, M. D. (1984): *Br. J. Pharmacol.*, 82:204P.
109. VanderMaelen, C. P., and Aghajanian, G. K. (1982): *Brain Res.*, 239:139–152.
110. VanderMaelen, C. P., and Aghajanian, G. K. (1982): *Eur. J. Pharmacol.*, 78:233–236.
111. VanderMaelen, C. P., and Aghajanian, G. K. (1983): *Soc. Neurosci. Abstr.*, 9:500.
112. VanderMaelen, C. P., and Aghajanian, G. K. (1983): *Brain Res.*, 289:109–119.
113. VanderMaelen, C. P., and Wilderman, R. C. (1984): *Fed. Proc.*, 43:947.
114. VanderMaelen, C. P., and Wilderman, R. C. (1984): *Soc. Neurosci. Abstr.*, 11:259.
115. Verge, D., Daval, G., Patey, A., Gozlan, H., El Mestikawy, S., and Hamon, M. (1985): *Eur. J. Pharmacol.*, 113:463–464.
116. Wang, R. Y., and Aghajanian, G. K. (1977): *Brain Res.*, 132:186–193.
117. Wang, R. Y., and Aghajanian, G. K. (1977): *Science*, 197:89–91.
118. Wang, R. Y., and Aghajanian, G. K. (1977): *Brain Res.*, 120:85–102.
119. Wang, R. Y., and Aghajanian, G. K. (1978): *Neuropharmacology*, 17:819–825.
120. Wang, R. Y., and Aghajanian, G. K. (1982): *J. Neurosci.*, 2:11–16.
121. White, S. R., and Neumann, R. S. (1980): *Brain Res.*, 188:119–127.

Psychopharmacology:
The Third Generation of Progress,
edited by Herbert Y. Meltzer.
Raven Press, New York © 1987.

CHAPTER **15**

Presynaptic Regulation of Monoaminergic Neurons

S. Z. Langer

The evidence accumulated during the last 15 years supports the view that presynaptic receptors modulate the release of several neurotransmitters from nerve terminals in the periphery and in the central nervous system (for reviews, see refs. 41, 43, 44). Presynaptic autoreceptors are involved in negative feedback mechanisms for the release of several neurotransmitters of which norepinephrine, serotonin, acetylcholine, and dopamine are examples of well-documented autoreceptor modulation.

The general view that transmitters can regulate their own release through an action on presynaptic inhibitory autoreceptors represents a new concept in the field of neurotransmission. In addition to presynaptic autoreceptors, many nerve terminals possess presynaptic receptors sensitive to endogenous compounds other than the neuron's own transmitter. This second group of presynaptic receptors are referred to as presynaptic heteroreceptors and are acted upon by cotransmitter neuropeptides, by transmitters released from adjacent terminals, or by locally produced or blood-borne substances that either facilitate or inhibit the calcium-dependent release of the neurotransmitter.

In addition to the presynaptic receptors involved in the modulation of transmitter release, presynaptic recognition sites for the transporter that is associated with the neuronal uptake mechanism were characterized in noradrenergic, serotonergic, and dopaminergic neurons. The neuronal uptake system for 5-hydroxytryptamine (5-HT) can be labeled with [³H]imipramine or [³H]paroxetine (31,56), whereas the noradrenergic transporter can be labeled with [³H]desipramine (59,82) and the dopaminergic transporter with [³H]cocaine or [³H]nomifensine (84). More recently the epinephrine transporter has been characterized in the frog heart using [³H]desipramine as a ligand (57). These presynaptic sites associated with the transporter system differ pharmacologically from the presynaptic autoreceptors that modulate the release of serotonin, norepinephrine, or dopamine.

The aim of this chapter is to review the pharmacological and clinical relevance of presynaptic receptors in noradrenergic, dopaminergic, and serotonergic neurons.

PRESYNAPTIC AUTORECEPTORS AND NORADRENERGIC NEUROTRANSMISSION

In support of the view that presynaptic α-adrenoceptors regulate the release of norepinephrine through a negative feedback mechanism, it has been demonstrated under *in vitro* as well as *in vivo* conditions that α-adrenoceptor agonists inhibit, whereas α-adrenoceptor antagonists enhance the release of norepinephrine elicited by nerve stimulation. The effects of α-adrenoceptor agonists and antagonists on noradrenergic neurotransmission are observed regardless of the α or β type of the postsynaptic adrenoceptor that mediates the response of the effector organ.

Before the discovery of presynaptic, release-modulating α-adrenoceptors, it was generally accepted that the α-adrenoceptors represented a single homogeneous class of receptors. Experimental evidence suggesting differences between pre- and postsynaptic α-adrenoceptors was first obtained in the perfused cat spleen (40). Subsequently, it was shown that phenoxybenzamine is nearly 100 times more potent in blocking the postsynaptic α-adrenoceptors than it is in blocking the presynaptic α-adrenoceptors (18,19). These results led to the proposal that the α-adrenoceptors should be subclassified into α_1- and α_2-subtypes (41). Subsequent studies provided the additional pharmacological evidence in terms of differences in the relative order of potencies of α-adrenoceptor agonists and antagonists that is essential for the classification of α-adrenoceptors into α_1- and α_2-subtypes (for reviews, see refs. 44, 51, 88). Among the α-adrenoceptor blocking agents, idazoxan, yohimbine, and rauwolscine are preferential antagonists for the α_2-subtype whereas prazosin, corynanthine, and alfusozin are selective α_1-adrenoceptor antagonists. Among the agonists, UK 14304, guanabenz, clonidine, BHT 933, and the aminotetralins M7 and TL 99 stimulate preferentially the α_2-adrenoceptor. On the other hand, the agonists that stimulate preferentially the α_1-adrenoceptor include phenylephrine, methoxamine, cirazoline, and amidephrine. The neurotransmitter norepinephrine, as well as epinephrine, activates both α_1- and α_2-adrenoceptors. Therefore, the α_1-adrenoceptor can be defined as that stimulated preferentially by cirazoline or phenylephrine and blocked by prazosin, whereas the α_2-adrenoceptor is stimulated by UK 14304 or clonidine and blocked by idazoxan.

Table 1 shows the location as well as the physiological effects linked to the activation of α_1- and α_2-adrenoceptors in the periphery and in the central nervous system. The presynaptic α-adrenoceptors associated with the inhibition of transmitter release in the peripheral and in the central nervous system have the pharmacological characteristics of the α_2-adrenoceptor subtype.

As shown in Table 1, both α_1- and α_2-adrenoceptors mediate contraction in vascular smooth muscle. In most vascular beds the α_1-adrenoceptor is preferentially innervated and is the target of released norepinephrine, whereas the α_2-adrenoceptors are mainly extrasynaptic (probably near the intima) and may be the target for circulating catecholamines rather than endogenously released norepinephrine (61).

The proportion of α_1- and α_2-adrenoceptors in vascular smooth muscle varies with the vascular bed under consideration. For instance, the α_1-adrenoceptor subtype predominates in the renal vascular bed, whereas both α_1- and α_2-adrenoceptors mediate vasoconstriction in the femoral and mesenteric vascular beds (23,51). In the cerebral blood vessels of several species like the dog and the cat, the predominant α-adrenoceptor mediating constriction corresponds to the α_2-subtype (73). There are also species differences in the predominating α-adrenoceptor subtype in the various vascular beds.

POTENTIAL THERAPEUTIC USES OF DRUGS ACTING AT α-ADRENOCEPTOR SUBTYPES

An important consequence of receptor subclassification is the development of selective agents which, acting as agonists or antagonists at these receptor subtypes, can subserve the function of useful therapeutic drugs. Table 2 lists a number of such well-established examples and also potential therapeutic uses of selective agonists or antagonists acting at α_1- or α_2-adrenoceptors.

Local activation of α_1-adrenoceptors produces vasoconstriction in most vascular beds, particularly the nasal mucosa. Systemic administration of α_1-adrenoceptor agonists can be used for the treatment of severe hypotension and shock.

Drugs that selectively block peripheral α_1-adrenoceptors, such as prazosin and alfuzosin, are used successfully in the treatment of essential hypertension. This represents a ra-

TABLE 1. *Location and function of α-adrenoceptor subtypes*

Receptor	Location	Effect
α_1-Adrenoceptors	Postsynaptic in vascular smooth muscle	Contraction
	Postsynaptic in cardiac muscle	Positive inotropism
	Postsynaptic in liver	Activation of glycogen phosphorylase
	Postsynaptic in CNS	Stimulation
Neuronal α_2-adrenoceptors	Postsynaptic in CNS	Hypotension, bradycardia
	Presynaptic in peripheral and central noradrenergic neurons	Inhibition of norepinephrine release
	Presynaptic in peripheral cholinergic neurons	Inhibition of acetylcholine release
	Presynaptic in 5-HT neurons (CNS)	Inhibition of 5-HT release
	Somatodendritic autoreceptors in CNS	Inhibition of firing of noradrenergic neurons
	Sympathetic ganglia	Hyperpolarization
Nonneuronal α_2-adrenoceptors	Platelets	Aggregation
	Pancreatic islets	Inhibition of insulin release
	Human fat cells	Inhibition of lipolysis
	Smooth muscle: Vascular	Contraction
	Bronchial	Contraction

TABLE 2. *Potential therapeutic uses of drugs acting at α-adrenoceptor subtypes*

α_1-Adrenoceptor agonists

Nasal vasoconstrictors
Treatment of hypotension

α_1-Adrenoceptor antagonists

Antihypertensive agents (periphery)
Congestive heart failure
Antiarrhythmics?
Treatment of urinary disorders

α_2-Adrenoceptor agonists

Antihypertensive agents (CNS)
Bradycardic agents (CNS and periphery)
Treatment of glaucoma
Opiate withdrawal syndrome

α_2-Adrenoceptor antagonists

Antidepressant action
Treatment of diabetes
Antiasthmatic drugs
Treatment of obesity

tional therapeutic approach in hypertension as the vascular α_1-adrenoceptor is the preferentially innervated subtype (44,62). α_1-Adrenoceptor antagonists possess vasodilating properties and they can be useful in the treatment of congestive heart failure by reducing venous return. The possibility that peripheral α_1-adrenoceptor antagonists may have antiarrhythmic properties, related to the blockade of α_1-adrenoceptors in the heart, is still an open question, although these effects can be demonstrated in some animal models of arrhythmias. Among the α_1-adrenoceptor antagonists, drugs like alfuzosin are useful in the treatment of the benign hypertrophy of the prostate and other functional urinary disorders. The reason for this beneficial effect of α_1-blockade is the fact that smooth muscle α-adrenoceptors in the urinary tract are of the α_1-subtype.

As indicated in Table 2, stimulation of central α_2-adrenoceptors by drugs like clonidine, guanfacine, and guanabenz produces bradycardia and hypotension, providing a desirable profile for a drug in the treatment of hypertension. The bradycardic action of α_2-adrenoceptor agonists can be of both central and peripheral origin. The peripheral effect is due to the inhibition of the release of norepinephrine at the level of the cardiac pacemaker (49).

Local application of α_2-adrenoceptor agonists was shown to be useful in the treatment of glaucoma because these drugs reduce intraocular pressure. Finally, centrally acting α_2-adrenoceptor agonists like clonidine have been shown to be effective in the treatment of the opiate withdrawal syndrome. The effectiveness of clonidine is most likely due to the ability of α_2-adrenoceptor agonists to reduce the firing and the release of the transmitter from central and peripheral noradrenergic neurons.

The therapeutic potential of drugs that block selectively α_2-adrenoceptors remains a speculative issue, because such agents are in the process of clinical testing for several indications. As shown in Table 2, it is possible that centrally acting α_2-adrenoceptor antagonists by increasing presynaptically the release of norepinephrine may possess antidepressant properties. It is also possible that the association of a centrally acting α_2-adrenoceptor antagonist and a classical tricyclic antidepressant drug may accelerate the onset of antidepressant action and reduce the latency period in antidepressant therapy, which is usually 2 to 3 weeks.

A peripherally acting α_2-adrenoceptor antagonist may be useful in the treatment of diabetes by blocking the α_2-adrenoceptor-mediated inhibition of insulin release. It is not yet clear whether the inhibitory α_2-adrenoceptor in the β-cells of the pancreas is under tonic control of norepinephrine released from sympathetic nerves. Another potential indication involves the treatment of asthma by blocking α_2-adrenoceptors involved in constriction at the level of bronchiolar smooth muscle, although this field is still controversial. Finally, as shown in Table 2, an α_2-adrenoceptor antagonist may be useful in the treatment of obesity because of the blockade of α_2-adrenoceptors that inhibit lipolysis and insulin release.

PRESYNAPTIC RECEPTORS INVOLVED IN THE MODULATION OF THE RELEASE OF NOREPINEPHRINE

As already discussed, the autoreceptor control of the release of norepinephrine is mediated by presynaptic α_2-adrenoceptors that are part of a negative feedback mechanism whereby the synaptic concentration of released norepinephrine can modulate further release of the neurotransmitter.

Several other receptor-mediated inhibitory mechanisms exist at the level of the release of norepinephrine. The inhibition of peripheral noradrenergic neurotransmission by presynaptic muscarinic receptors was mainly studied at the level of the heart (27,68), where it is likely to play a physiological role, since both cholinergic and noradrenergic pathways innervate cardiac muscle (75). The close proximity of cholinergic and noradrenergic terminals in the heart is compatible with the view that the muscarinic receptors on the sympathetic terminals in atria can be activated by acetylcholine released from the parasympathetic nerves.

The presence of presynaptic inhibitory dopamine receptors modulating noradrenergic transmission was first reported in the perfused cat spleen (40) and cat nictitating membrane (25), and these observations have been extended to several isolated blood vessels *in vitro* (33,77). It was also shown that dopamine receptor agonists reduce end-organ responses *in vivo* during sympathetic nerve stimulation (69,72). The presynaptic inhibitory dopamine receptors do not seem to play a physiological role in noradrenergic transmission, because blockade of these receptors by specific antagonists like *S*-sulpiride does not enhance the release of norepinephrine during nerve stimulation (21).

Nevertheless, it is possible that presynaptic inhibitory dopamine-2 (DA$_2$) receptors might be involved in the antihypertensive effects of monoamine oxidase inhibitors.

Following chronic administration of monoamine oxidase inhibitors, enough dopamine may accumulate in noradrenergic nerve terminals and it could be released concomitantly with norepinephrine by nerve impulses. Under these conditions released dopamine could reduce noradrenergic transmission through the activation of presynaptic inhibitory DA_2 receptors (S. Z. Langer and M. J. Vidal, *unpublished observations*). The presynaptic dopamine receptors are of the DA_2 subtype, sensitive to blockade by *S*-sulpiride, and can be differentiated clearly from the peripheral DA_1 receptor subtype, which mediates vasodilatation in certain vascular beds (11,30) and is blocked selectively by the DA_1 antagonist SCH 23390. The reduction in noradrenergic neurotransmission produced by dopamine receptor agonists like *N,N*-di-*n*-propyldopamine and pergolide produces hypotensive and bradycardic effects under *in vivo* conditions (14,72). The peripheral presynaptic inhibitory DA_2 receptors can be considered as potential targets for the development of selective agonists that may be useful antihypertensive agents. However, one potential side effect of this type of drug is likely to be the emetic action.

Among the other types of presynaptic receptors that can modify the release of norepinephrine, two transsynaptic mechanisms involve the formation at the level of the effector organ of substances that can act presynaptically to inhibit the release of norepinephrine. The inhibition of peripheral noradrenergic transmission by prostaglandins of the E series is well documented (6,20,32). The stimulus that triggers the local release of prostaglandins is probably related to the activation by norepinephrine of the postsynaptic adrenoceptor. A similar mechanism may involve the inhibition of the release of norepinephrine through the activation of adenosine receptors (43,70,71). A possible cotransmitter role for ATP in noradrenergic neurons (12,24,87,92) may be relevant to the presynaptic inhibitory effects of adenosine on the release of norepinephrine.

Two receptor-mediated mechanisms that facilitate the release of norepinephrine are both relevant to the cardiovascular system, although it appears that they are also present in the central nervous system. The presence of presynaptic facilitatory β-adrenoceptors was first reported by Adler-Graschinsky and Langer (1,2). Originally, the facilitation of the release of norepinephrine was reported using isoprenaline as an agonist (2); subsequently it was reported that epinephrine can preferentially activate these presynaptic β-receptors (83). The latter may be relevant to the pathogenesis of hypertension and to the influence of stress. It is likely that circulating epinephrine is taken up by sympathetic nerve terminals and stored as a cotransmitter, to be subsequently released to activate presynaptic facilitatory β-receptors. It is generally accepted that the presynaptic β-adrenoceptors are of the $β_2$-subtype (50). The question of whether the clinical efficacy of β-adrenoceptor-blocking drugs in hypertension is related to blockade of presynaptic facilitatory β-adrenoceptors is still open (42,74).

A second facilitatory mechanism in sympathetic nerve endings involves angiotensin. The existence of presynaptic angiotensin II receptors which enhance the release of norepinephrine is well documented (13,29,90,93). It is of interest that angiotensin converting enzyme inhibitors like captopril possess antihypertensive properties and prevent the angiotensin II-mediated facilitation of norepinephrine release (4,16).

PRESYNAPTIC 5-HT AUTORECEPTORS AND THE MODULATION OF THE RELEASE OF SEROTONIN

In analogy with the noradrenergic and dopaminergic system, the experimental evidence available supports the view that presynaptic inhibitory 5-HT autoreceptors are involved in the modulation of the release of serotonin through a negative feedback mechanism. Lysergic acid diethylamide (LSD) and 5-methoxytryptamine are agonists at the level of the 5-HT autoreceptor, whereas methiothepin is the antagonist that shows clear selectivity for the presynaptic autoreceptor (15,28,55). As shown for the release of dopamine, the inhibition by LSD and the increase by methiothepin in the release of [³H]5-HT is observed for the calcium-dependent electrically evoked release, but these drugs do not modify the calcium-independent release of [³H]5-HT induced by fenfluramine (55).

Pharmacologically the 5-HT autoreceptor clearly differs from the $5-HT_2$ receptor and possesses the characteristics of one of the $5-HT_1$ receptor subtypes.

When neuronal uptake of 5-HT is inhibited by drugs like citalopram or paroxetine, the 5-HT autoreceptor agonists like LSD or 5-methoxytryptamine fail to inhibit the electrically evoked release of [³H]5-HT (28,55). This interaction between 5-HT uptake inhibitors and 5-HT autoreceptor agonists does not seem to be due to increased levels of released 5-HT in the synaptic cleft, because a similar interaction is observed following pretreatment with *p*-chlorophenylalanine to deplete the endogenous stores of 5-HT (28). These results suggest that there may exist an interaction between the presynaptic 5-HT autoreceptor and the serotonin transporter responsible for the neuronal uptake of 5-HT (28) (Fig. 1). This interaction may be relevant to the effects of antidepressants that are inhibitors of serotonin uptake and that can enhance serotonergic neurotransmission by producing subsensitivity of the inhibitory 5-HT autoreceptors (Fig 1). In slices of the rat hypothalamus, tricyclic or nontricyclic inhibitors of neuronal uptake of 5-HT do not enhance the electrically evoked release of [³H]5-HT (28,55). Yet, after pretreatment with parachlorophenylalanine (PCPA), both the tricyclic and nontricyclic inhibitors of serotonin uptake produce a marked increase in the stimulation-evoked release of [³H]5-HT (28). It is not clear which mechanism is involved in this interaction between PCPA and 5-HT uptake inhibitors (28), but it is tempting to speculate that it may be related to the observation that PCPA can reverse the clinical improvement in depressed patients during treatment with monoamine oxidase inhibitors or with imipramine (86).

In view of the fact that methiothepin is not a very specific antagonist at the level of the 5-HT autoreceptor because it also blocks dopamine receptors, there is a special interest in the development of new drugs with specific affinity as antagonists of the 5-HT autoreceptor. Such drugs would enhance serotonergic neurotransmission and could be potentially useful in the treatment of depression.

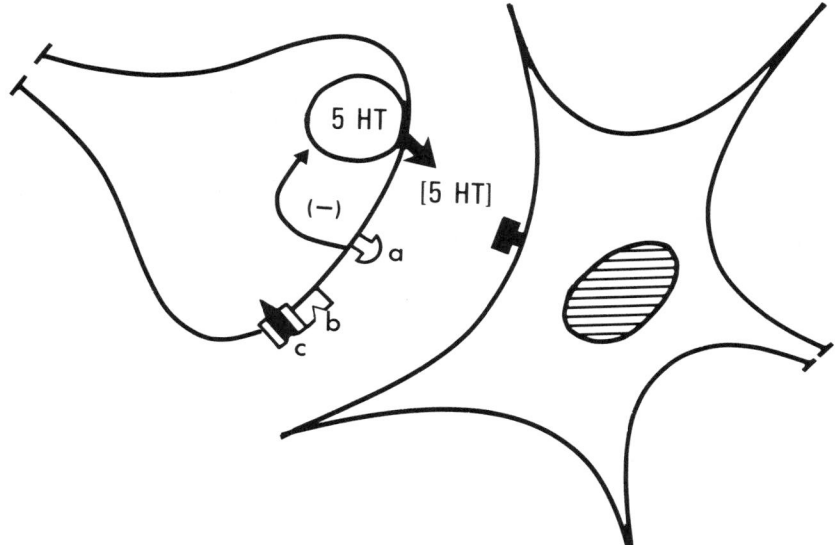

FIG. 1. Schematic representation of a central serotonergic synapse. The following are shown at the presynaptic level: (a) serotonin autoreceptor, mediating a negative feedback mechanism that modulates transmitter release; (b) serotonin transporter complex: modulatory site that can be labeled with [³H]imipramine or [³H]paroxetine; (c) substrate recognition site of the carrier involved in serotonin uptake. The modulatory site of the serotonin transporter appears to be allosterically linked to the substrate recognition site for 5-HT. The recognition site labeled with [³H]imipramine or [³H]paroxetine may be the target of action of an endocoid, different from 5-HT, which subserves the function of modulating neuronal uptake of the transmitter. The figure also shows schematically a single postsynaptic receptor, although it is now well established that several subtypes of postsynaptic 5-HT receptors exist in the central nervous system.

MODULATION OF DOPAMINERGIC NEUROTRANSMISSION THROUGH PRESYNAPTIC DOPAMINE AUTORECEPTORS

In analogy with the negative feedback hypothesis for noradrenergic transmission, the concept of a dopamine autoreceptor on the dopaminergic terminal, sensing the amount of dopamine released and modulating transmitter release, was a predictable possibility. The experimental evidence supports the existence of presynaptic inhibitory dopamine autoreceptors (26,46,89).

Whereas dopamine receptor agonists decrease and antagonists increase the calcium-dependent release of [³H]dopamine evoked by electrical stimulation (36) or elevated potassium (34), the calcium-independent release of [³H]dopamine evoked by amphetamine or tyramine is not subject to this modulation (36). The dopamine autoreceptor possesses the pharmacological properties of the D_2 subtype (5,54,66). It is of interest to note that presynaptic dopamine autoreceptors appear to be also involved in the inhibition of the synthesis of dopamine at the level of tyrosine hydroxylase activity.

Neuroleptics are extensively used in the treatment of schizophrenia, and to the extent of our present knowledge all neuroleptic dopamine receptor antagonists have approximately equal affinity for pre- and postsynaptic D_2 receptors. It should be noted that neuroleptics have to be administered for 2 to 3 weeks before they are fully effective in a patient with an acute psychotic attack. Whereas drug-specific clinical improvement occurs in 2 to 3 weeks following daily neuroleptic administration, the increase in serum prolactin levels caused by the neuroleptic occurs rapidly (17,78), indicating immediate blockade of D_2 receptors. It is possible that initially neuroleptics increase dopamine release (by blocking the autoreceptor) in addition to their antagonist action at the level of the postsynaptic dopamine receptors. This presynaptic effect of neuroleptics by increasing dopamine release may tend to diminish the effectiveness of their

postsynaptic dopamine blockade. Yet as a function of time, neuroleptics produce supersensitivity of presynaptic inhibitory dopamine autoreceptors (76), which would result in decreased dopamine release (65). In support of this mechanism of action, it was shown that low doses of dopamine receptor agonists improve psychotic symptoms without the 2- to 3-week latency described for neuroleptics (91). These results indicate that there is a potential for the clinical use of selective dopamine autoreceptor agonists as therapeutic agents in schizophrenia because they might be effective on acute administration.

HIGH-AFFINITY LABELING OF MONOAMINE TRANSPORTER SYSTEMS: PRESYNAPTIC MODULATION OF NEURONAL UPTAKE

The termination of action for the three transmitters discussed in the previous sections—norepinephrine, dopamine, and serotonin—involves the process of neuronal uptake, namely, the active sodium-dependent transport of the neurotransmitter across the membrane of the nerve terminal.

In analogy with presynaptic receptors that modulate the release of neurotransmitters, it was recently suggested that presynaptic sites may exist that are involved in the modulation of neuronal uptake of these transmitters (45,58).

Both [³H]imipramine and [³H]paroxetine bind with high affinity to a recognition site that is associated with the neuronal uptake of serotonin and that is present in the brain as well as in platelets of different species, including humans (31,48,56,64). There is a good correlation between the potencies of drugs at inhibiting [³H]5-HT uptake and at inhibiting [³H]imipramine binding (56) or [³H]paroxetine binding (31).

Dissociation kinetic experiments indicate that the site labeled by [³H]imipramine is not identical with the substrate recognition site of the serotonin transporter (85). It therefore appears that [³H]imipramine labels a presynaptic modulatory site for the 5-HT transporter system, and it is possible that an endocoid different from serotonin may be the endogenous ligand acting on the [^{3}H]imipramine recognition site to modulate 5-HT uptake (8–10,47,52,53,58,60).

While investigating the structure-activity relationships among known indoleamines that are thought to occur endogenously (3), it was found that substituted tryptolines inhibited both the binding of [^{3}H]imipramine and the uptake of [^{3}H]5-HT (53,60,85). These studies led to the proposal that 5-methoxytryptoline (6-methoxy-tetrahydrobetacarboline) or a close analog may be an endogenous modulator acting on the [^{3}H]imipramine recognition site (53,60). There is evidence in the literature for the presence of 5-methoxytryptoline in the retina and the pineal gland of several species (37,38), although a recent study revealed only trace amounts of 5-methoxytryptoline in the pineal glands of several species (52).

It is still an open question whether 5-methoxytryptoline or a close analog plays a physiological role in the modulation of 5-HT uptake through an action at the level of the [^{3}H]imipramine recognition site. Although the neurochemical and endocrinological profile of 5-methoxytryptoline represents an attractive model to characterize the pharmacological properties of this compound (52), it should be noted that 5-methoxytryptoline appears to be present only in trace amounts in some tissues.

The B_{max} of [^{3}H]imipramine binding in platelets is reduced in untreated severely depressed patients (64,67,79,80,81), and it appears to be a useful biological marker in depression.

In analogy with the labeling by [^{3}H]imipramine or [^{3}H]paroxetine of a high-affinity recognition site associated with the serotonin transporter complex, there are now tritiated ligands that label presynaptic sites associated with the transporter for norepinephrine and dopamine. [^{3}H]Desipramine labels with high affinity a recognition site associated with the transporter for norepinephrine in the peripheral as well as the central nervous system (59,63,82). The dopamine transporter in the central nervous system has been labeled with [^{3}H]cocaine (39,84), [^{3}H]mazindol (35), or [^{3}H]nomifensine (22). It is still an open question whether the high-affinity sites associated with the norepinephrine and dopamine transporters represent modulatory sites for the neuronal uptake of these monoamines, as suggested for [^{3}H]imipramine binding and the neuronal uptake of serotonin.

More recently a high-affinity recognition site associated with the epinephrine transporter has been labeled with [^{3}H]desipramine in the frog heart (57). It is of interest to note that epinephrine and not norepinephrine is the transmitter in the frog heart (7). The pharmacological profile of inhibition by drugs of [^{3}H]desipramine binding to the epinephrine transporter suggests pharmacological differences between the epinephrine and the norepinephrine transporters (57).

CONCLUSIONS

A significant advance in the field of neurotransmission was made with the discovery of presynaptic α_2-adrenoceptors on noradrenergic nerves, because it developed the concept that transmitters can regulate their own release through an action of presynaptic inhibitory autoreceptors. In addition,

this finding developed in parallel with the pharmacological evidence for the presence of two α-adrenoceptor subtypes, the α_1- and α_2-adrenoceptor subtypes, which are defined by a different profile of affinity and relative order of potencies for agonists and for antagonists.

Presynaptic autoreceptors are involved in negative feedback mechanisms for the regulation of the release of several neurotransmitters. In addition to norepinephrine, dopamine, serotonin, and acetylcholine represent well-established examples of modulation of release mediated by presynaptic autoreceptor systems.

In addition to the presynaptic autoreceptors involved in the modulation of transmitter release, it was recently reported that a separate receptor-mediated process modulates the presynaptic transporters for serotonin, norepinephrine, and dopamine. The presynaptic modulation of the neuronal uptake of serotonin, norepinephrine, and dopamine involves a site with many of the properties of a pharmacological receptor that is different from the corresponding autoreceptor involved in modulating transmitter release.

REFERENCES

1. Adler-Graschinsky, E., and Langer, S. Z. (1974): *Acta Physiol. Lat. Am.*, 24, 185P.
2. Adler-Graschinsky, E., and Langer, S. Z. (1975): *Br. J. Pharmacol.*, 53:43–50.
3. Airaksinen, M. M., and Kari, I. (1981): *Med. Biol.*, 59:190–211.
4. Antonaccio, M. J., and Kerwin, L. (1981): *Hypertension*, 3:154–162.
5. Arbilla, S., and Langer, S. Z. (1981): *Eur. J. Pharmacol.*, 76:345–351.
6. Armstrong, J. M. (1982): In: *Cardiovascular Pharmacology of Prostaglandins*, edited by A. G. Herman, P. M. Vanhoutte, H. Denolin, and A. Goosens, pp. 51–64. Raven Press, New York.
7. Azuma, T., et al. (1965): *Am. J. Physiol.*, 209:1287–1294.
8. Barbaccia, M. L., and Costa, E. (1984): *Ann. NY Acad. Sci.*, 430:103–114.
9. Barbaccia, M. L., Gandolfi, O., Chuang, D. M., and Costa, E. (1983): *Proc. Natl. Acad. Sci. USA*, 80:5134–5138.
10. Barbaccia, M. L., et al. (1986): *Eur. J. Pharmacol.*, 123:45–52.
11. Brodde, O. E. (1982): *Life Sci.*, 31:289–306.
12. Burnstock, G., Sneddon, P. (1985): *Clin. Sci.*, 68:89S–92S.
13. Campbell, W. B., and Jackson, E. K. (1979): *Am. J. Physiol.*, 236:211–217.
14. Cavero, I., Massingham, R., and Lefevre-Borg, F. (1982): *Life Sci.*, 31:1059–1069.
15. Cerrito, F., and Raiteri, M. (1979): *Eur. J. Pharmacol.*, 57:427–430.
16. Clough, D. P., Hatton, R., Keddie, J. R., and Collis, M. G. (1982): *Hypertension*, 4:764–772.
17. Crow, T. J., Cross, A. J., Johnstone, E. C., Longden, A., Owen, F., and Ridley, R. M. (1980): In: *Long-Term Effects of Neuroleptics*, edited by Cattabeni et al., pp. 495–503. Raven Press, New York.
18. Cubeddu, L. X., Barnes, E. M., Langer, S. Z., and Weiner, N. (1974): *J. Pharmacol. Exp. Ther.*, 190:431–450.
19. Dubocovich, M. L., and Langer, S. Z. (1974): *J. Physiol. (Lond.)*, 237:505–519.
20. Dubocovich, M. L., and Langer, S. Z. (1975): *J. Physiol. (Lond.)*, 251:737–762.
21. Dubocovich, M. L., and Langer, S. Z. (1980): *J. Pharmacol. Exp. Ther.*, 212:144–152.
22. Dubocovich, M. L., and Zahniser, N. K. (1983): *Soc. Neurosci. Abstr.*, 9:564P.
23. Duval, N., Hicks, P. E., and Langer, S. Z. (1985): *Eur. J. Pharmacol.*, 108:265–272.
24. Duval, N., Hicks, P. E., and Langer, S. Z. (1985): *Eur. J. Pharmacol.*, 110:373–377.
25. Enero, M. A., and Langer, S. Z. (1975): *Naunyn Schmiedebergs Arch. Pharmacol.*, 289:179–203.

26. Farnebo, L.-O., and Hamberger, B. (1973): In: *Frontiers in Catecholamine Research,* edited by E. Usdin and S. H. Snyder, pp. 589–593. Pergamon Press, Oxford.

27. Fozard, J. R., and Muscholl, E. (1972): *Br. J. Pharmacol.,* 45: 616–629.

28. Galzin, A.-M., Moret, C., Verzier, B., and Langer, S. Z. (1985): *J. Pharmacol. Exp. Ther.,* 235:200–211.

29. Garcia-Sevilla, J. A., Dubocovich, M. L., and Langer, S. Z. (1985): *Naunyn Schmiedebergs Arch. Pharmacol.,* 330:9–15.

30. Goldberg, L. I., Volkman, P. H., and Kohli, J. D. (1978): *Annu. Rev. Pharmacol. Toxicol.,* 18:57–79.

31. Habert, E., Graham, D., Tahraoui, L., Claustre, Y., and Langer, S. Z. (1985): *Eur. J. Pharmacol.,* 118:107–114.

32. Hedqvist, P. (1974): In: *Prostaglandin Synthesis Inhibitors,* edited by H. J. Robinson and J. R. Vane, pp. 303–309. Raven Press, New York.

33. Hope, W., McCulloch, M. W., Story, D. F., and Rand, M. J. (1977): *Eur. J. Pharmacol.,* 46:101–111.

34. Jackisch, R., Zumstein, A., Hertting, G., and Starke, K. (1980): *Naunyn Schmiedebergs Arch. Pharmacol.,* 314:129–133.

35. Javitch, J. A., Blaustein, R. O., and Snyder, S. H. (1983): *Eur. J. Pharmacol.,* 90:461–462.

36. Kamal, L. A., Arbilla, S., and Langer, S. Z. (1981): *J. Pharmacol. Exp. Ther.,* 216:592–598.

37. Kari, I. (1981) *FEBS Lett.,* 127:277–280.

38. Kari, I., Airaksinen, M. M., Gynther, J., and Huhtikangas, A. (1983): In: *Recent Developments in Biochemistry, Medicine and Environmental Research, Vol. 8,* edited by A. Frigerio, pp. 19–24. Elsevier, Amsterdam.

39. Kennedy, L. T., and Hanbauer, I. (1983): *J. Neurochem.,* 41:172–178.

40. Langer, S. Z. (1973): In: *Frontiers in Catecholamine Research,* edited by E. Usdin and S. H. Snyder, pp. 543–549. Pergamon Press, Oxford.

41. Langer, S. Z. (1974): *Biochem. Pharmacol.,* 23:1793–1800.

42. Langer, S. Z. (1976): *Clin. Sci. Mol. Med.,* 51:423s–426s.

43. Langer, S. Z. (1977): *Br. J. Pharmacol.,* 60:481–497.

44. Langer, S. Z. (1981): *Pharmacol. Rev.,* 32:337–362.

45. Langer, S. Z. (1984): *Trends Pharmacol. Sci.,* 5:51–52.

46. Langer, S. Z., Arbilla, S., and Kamal, L. A. (1980): In: *Neurotransmitters and Their Receptors,* edited by U. Z. Littauer, Y. Dudai, I. Silman, V. I. Teichberg, and Z. Vogel, pp. 7–21. J. Wiley & Sons. Chichester, England.

47. Langer, S. Z., Arbilla, S., Tahraoui, L., and Lee, C. R. (1984): *Clin. Neuropharmacol.,* 7:868–869.

48. Langer, S. Z., Briley, M. S., Raisman, R., Henry, J.-F., and Morselli, P. L. (1980): *Naunyn Schmiedebergs Arch. Pharmacol.,* 313:189–194.

49. Langer, S. Z., Cavero, I., and Massingham, R. (1980): *Hypertension,* 2:372–382.

50. Langer, S. Z., and Galzin, A.-M. (1983): In: *L.E.R.S. Monograph Series, Vol. 1. Betaxolol: A New Beta₁-adrenoceptor Antagonist,* edited by P. L. Morselli, J. R. Kilborn, I. Cavero, D. C. Harrison, and S. Z. Langer, pp. 21–30. Raven Press, New York.

51. Langer, S. Z., and Hicks, P. E. (1984): *J. Cardiovasc. Pharmacol.,* 6:S547–S558.

52. Langer, S. Z., Lee, C. R., Schoemaker, H., Segonzac, A., and Esnaud, H. (1985): In: *Endocoids,* edited by H. Lal, F. LaBella, and J. Lane, pp. 441–455. Alan R. Liss, New York.

53. Langer, S. Z., Lee, C. R., Segonzac, A., Tateishi, T., Esnaud, H., Schoemaker, H., and Winblad, B. (1984): *Eur. J. Pharmacol.,* 102: 379–380.

54. Langer, S. Z., and Lehmann, J. (1987): In: *Catecholamine II,* edited by U. Trendelenburg and N. Weiner. Springer-Verlag, Heidelberg (*in press*).

55. Langer, S. Z., and Moret, C. (1982): *J. Pharmacol. Exp. Ther.,* 222:220–226.

56. Langer, S. Z., Moret, C., Raisman, R., Dubocovich, M. L., and Briley, M. S. (1980): *Science,* 210:1133–1135.

57. Langer, S. Z., Pimoule, C., and Schoemaker, H. (1987): *Br. J. Pharmacol.,* 90:285P.

58. Langer, S. Z., and Raisman, R. (1983): *Neuropharmacology,* 22: 407–413.

59. Langer, S. Z., Raisman, R., and Briley, M. S. (1981): *Eur. J. Pharmacol.,* 72:423–424.

60. Langer, S. Z., Raisman, R., Tahraoui, L., Scatton, B., Niddam,

R., Lee, C. R., and Claustre, Y. (1984): *Eur. J. Pharmacol.,* 98: 153–154.

61. Langer, S. Z., and Shepperson, N. B. (1982): *Trends Pharmacol. Sci.,* 3:440–444.

62. Langer, S. Z., Shepperson, N. B., and Massingham R. (1981): *Hypertension,* 3:I112–I118.

63. Langer, S. Z., Tahraoui, L., Raisman, R., Arbilla, S., Najar, M., and Dedek, J. (1984): In: *Neuronal and Extraneuronal Events in Autonomic Pharmacology,* edited by W. Fleming et al., pp. 37–49. Raven Press, New York.

64. Langer, S. Z., Zarifian, E., Briley, M. S., Raisman, R., and Sechter, D. (1981): *Life Sci.,* 29:211–220.

65. Lehmann, J., and Langer, S. Z. (1982): In: *Advances in the Biosciences, Vol. 37 (Advances in Dopamine Research),* edited by M. Kohsaka, T. Shohmori, Y. Tsukuda, and G. N. Woodruff, pp. 25–39. Pergamon Press, Oxford.

66. Lehmann, J., Briley, M. S., and Langer, S. Z. (1983): *Eur. J. Pharmacol.,* 88:11–26.

67. Lewis, D. A., and McChesney, C. (1985): *Arch. Gen. Psychiatry,* 42:485–488.

68. Löffelholz, K., and Muscholl, E. (1970): *Naunyn Schmiedebergs Arch. Pharmacol.,* 267:181–184.

69. Long, J. P., Heintz, S., Cannon, J. G., and Kim, J. (1975): *J. Pharmacol. Exp. Ther.,* 192:336–342.

70. Luchelli-Fortis, M. A., Fredholm, B. B., and Langer, S. Z. (1979): *Eur. J. Pharmacol.,* 58:389–397.

71. Luchelli-Fortis, M. A., Fredholm, B. B., and Langer, S. Z. (1981): *J. Pharmacol. Exp. Ther.,* 219:235–242.

72. Massingham, R., Dubocovich, M. L., and Langer, S. Z. (1980): *Naunyn Schmiedebergs Arch. Pharmacol.,* 314:17–28.

73. Medgett, I. C., and Langer, S. Z. (1983): *Naunyn Schmiedebergs Arch. Pharmacol.,* 323:24–32.

74. Misu, Y., and Kubo, T. (1983): *Trends Pharmacol. Sci.,* 4:506–508.

75. Muscholl, E. (1979): In: *The Release of Catecholamines from Adrenergic Neurones,* edited by D. M. Paton, pp. 87–110. Pergamon Press, Oxford.

76. Nowak, J. Z., Arbilla, S., Galzin, A.-M., and Langer, S. Z. (1983): *J. Pharmacol. Exp. Ther.,* 226:558–564.

77. O'Connor, S. E., and Brown, R. A. (1982): *Gen. Pharmacol.,* 13: 185–193.

78. Ohman, R., Larsson, M., Nilsson, I. M., Engel, J., and Carlsson, A. (1977): *Naunyn Schmiedebergs Arch. Pharmacol.,* 299:105–114.

79. Paul, S. M., Rehavi, M., Skolnick, P., Ballenger, J., and Goodwin, F. (1981): *Arch. Gen. Psychiatry,* 38:1315–1317.

80. Raisman, R., Briley, M. S., Bouchami, F., Sechter, D., Zarifian, E., and Langer, S. Z. (1982): *Psychopharmacology,* 77:332–335.

81. Raisman, R., Sechter, D., Briley, M. S., Zarifian, E., and Langer, S. Z. (1981): *Psychopharmacology,* 75:368–371.

82. Raisman, R., Sette, M., Pimoule, C., Briley, M. S., and Langer, S. Z. (1982): *Eur. J. Pharmacol.,* 78:345–351.

83. Rand, M. J., Majewski, H., McCulloch, M. W., and Story, D. F. (1979): In: *Presynaptic Receptors,* edited by S. Z. Langer, K. Starke, and M. L. Dubocovich, pp. 263–269. Pergamon Press, Oxford.

84. Schoemaker, H., Pimoule, C., Arbilla, S., Scatton, B., Javoy-Agid, F., and Langer, S. Z. (1985): *Naunyn Schmiedebergs Arch. Pharmacol.,* 329:227–235.

85. Segonzac, A., Schoemaker, H., Tateishi, T., and Langer, S. Z. (1985): *J. Neurochem.,* 45:249–256.

86. Shopsin, et al. (1976): *Arch. Gen. Psychiatry,* 33:811–819.

87. Sneddon, P., and Burnstock, G. (1984): *Eur. J. Pharmacol.,* 100: 85–90.

88. Starke, K., and Langer, S. Z. (1979): In: *Presynaptic Receptors,* edited by S. Z. Langer, K. Starke, and M. L. Dubocovich, pp. 1–4. Pergamon Press, Oxford.

89. Starke, K., Reimann, W., Zumstein, A., and Hertting, G. (1978): *Naunyn Schmiedebergs Arch. Pharmacol.,* 305:27–36.

90. Starke, K., Werner, U., Hellerforth, R., and Schümann, H. J. (1970): *Eur. J. Pharmacol.,* 9:136–140.

91. Tamminga, C. A., Schaffer, M. H., Smith, R. C., and Davis, J. M. (1978): *Science,* 200:567–568.

92. Vidal, M., Hicks, P. E., and Langer, S. Z. (1986): *Naunyn Schmiedebergs Arch. Pharmacol.,* 332:384–390.

93. Zimmerman, B. G., and Whitmore, L. (1967): *Int. J. Neuropharmacol.,* 6:27–38.

Psychopharmacology:
The Third Generation of Progress,
edited by Herbert Y. Meltzer.
Raven Press, New York © 1987.

CHAPTER 16

Central Monoaminergic Neurons: Single-Unit Studies in Behaving Animals

Barry L. Jacobs

Central monoaminergic neurons exert a modulatory influence over virtually all mammalian psychological, behavioral, and physiological processes. Data presented in a number of chapters in this volume are testimony to this almost ubiquitous functional involvement. Monoaminergic neurons are also the primary site of action of many psychoactive drugs (this follows almost necessarily from the first statement). Nonetheless, the exact nature of the interrelationship among these central neurochemical systems, drug action, and physiology and behavior has remained obscure. This is due, in part, to the fact that most of the studies in this field have employed somewhat imprecise or general methods: lesions, gross neurochemical analyses, brain stimulation, or systemic pharmacology.

In order to understand the specific roles of serotonin (5HT), dopamine (DA), and norepinephrine (NE)[1] in psychoactive drug action and in physiology and behavior, a more precise methodology is needed. Single-unit recording of monoaminergic neurons is an approach that combines the desirable characteristics of neurochemical specificity, precision of localization, minimal perturbation of the system under study, and close temporal contiguity between measurements of the neurochemical system and of the functional variable under investigation.

The fundamental single-unit analyses of these systems began nearly 20 years ago with studies carried out in anesthetized animals (7,18,38). These pioneering investigations laid the foundation for this field and are a continuing source of important information. In recent years, significant progress in these studies has come from the technical advancements of microiontophoresis, recording *in vitro* from tissue slices, and intracellular recordings, both *in vivo* and *in vitro*. These studies have provided an understanding of the basic physiological and pharmacological properties of central monoaminergic neurons. Since these basic studies are described in other chapters in this volume, only brief overviews will be presented here.

It goes without saying that if one is interested in studying the behavioral or physiological roles of monoaminergic neurons, such studies must be carried out in unanesthetized and unrestrained animals. Even the conclusions of pharmacological studies may be compromised by the presence of anesthesia. A few examples will suffice to make these points clearly. 5HT neurons in the dorsal raphe nucleus of the unanesthetized cat are highly responsive to repetitively presented phasic sensory stimuli (click or flash). This responsiveness to sensory inputs is totally blocked when the experiments are repeated while the cat is anesthetized with

---

[1] A fourth monoamine, epinephrine, is also a CNS neurotransmitter, but since it has received relatively little experimental attention, and because there have been no single-unit studies of these neurons in behaving animals, no further reference to epinephrine will be made in this chapter.

chloral hydrate (48). The same study reported that electrical stimulation of the pontine reticular formation strongly excited 5HT neurons, while, once again, chloral hydrate anesthesia completely blocked this response. Another study reported that the systemic administration of morphine produced a small, but significant, *increase* in the activity of NE neurons in the area of the locus ceruleus in behaving cats; however, when this experiment was repeated while the cat was anesthetized with chloral hydrate, morphine now produced a substantial *decrease* in unit activity (75). Both the increase and the decrease in unit activity were naloxone reversible. Thus, these two studies demonstrate that anesthesia can influence dramatically the response of the nervous system to sensory stimuli, electrical brain stimulation, and pharmacological agents. Furthermore, these alterations are not simply modest changes in response magnitude; sometimes they produce complete blockades or even response reversals (it is particularly confounding that the direction of changes induced by anesthesia is not uniform).

For these reasons, and because of growing interest in brain monoaminergic neurons specifically in relationship to behavior and to "physiologically relevant" stimuli, approximately 10 years ago investigators began to study the single-unit activity of these neurons in behaving animals. To date, these studies have been carried out exclusively in rats, cats, and several monkey species. Various methods have been employed to record single-unit activity, but recently an increasing number of studies have used bundles of flexible, low-impedance microwires that can be advanced through the brain by means of an attached mechanical microdrive (44,56). This technique permits stable single-unit recordings over long periods of time (the same cell often can be studied for days) and in spite of gross movements on the part of the animal. Its usefulness may be somewhat restricted to neurons with large somata; however, all, or most, brain monoaminergic neurons have large cell bodies. Finally, the issue of neurochemical identification of the neurons should be mentioned. Since in most cases brain 5HT, DA, and NE neurons are interspersed among nonmonoaminergic neurons, and since these single-unit recording techniques do not allow intracellular marking of the neurons, the cells under study cannot be identified directly. Fortunately, however, neurons in each neurochemical group display a distinctive constellation of characteristics that closely parallels the characteristics of neurons that have been identified directly as 5HT, DA, or NE in acute electrophysiological experiments utilizing intracellular staining. Thus, in most cases, 5HT, DA, or NE neurons can be identified unambiguously by means of indirect criteria (this issue is discussed more fully in refs. 54,56,91).

This chapter provides an overview of the current state of knowledge regarding the behavioral and physiological correlates of monoaminergic unit activity in behaving animals. Although in most cases the data are limited, pharmacological studies of these neurons in behaving animals are also reviewed. A separate section is devoted to each of the three groups of neurons. The final section of this chapter compares and contrasts the data from the three groups, discusses species differences in the data, examines limitations of this approach, and, finally, takes a look into the future.

SEROTONERGIC (5HT) NEURONS

Overview of Basic Characteristics

Cell bodies of 5HT neurons are localized almost exclusively in the brainstem, mostly in several midline clusters that lie within or in close proximity to the classically defined raphe nuclei. When examined in both freely moving cats and anesthetized rats, 5HT neurons display a slow (2–5 spikes/sec) and highly regular discharge pattern (7,103), which is so clocklike in nature that it led us to speculate that these cells might be autoactive. This hypothesis is supported by single-cell recordings of 5HT neurons in tissue slabs maintained *in vitro* (69), and from intracellular analyses of 5HT unit activity both *in vivo* and *in vitro* (8,24,108). Another important neurophysiological variable that controls 5HT unit activity is a local negative feedback mechanism exerted by two separate means: axon collateral inhibition and axosomatic/dendritic or dendrodendritic connections between neighboring 5HT neurons (70,109). We have proposed that the density of these 5HT receptors (sometimes referred to as cell body autoreceptors) in the somadendritic area may determine both the level of spontaneous activity of 5HT neurons and the degree to which they respond to 5HT agonist drugs (47,55).

To date, all of the single-unit studies of brain 5HT neurons in unrestrained and unanesthetized animals have been conducted in cats, in the four nuclei containing the densest aggregations of these cells. Two nuclei lie within the pons/mesencephalon—nucleus raphe dorsalis (DRN) and nucleus centralis superior (NCS)—and the other two lie within the medulla—nucleus raphe magnus (NRM) and nucleus raphe pallidus (NRP). Since most of the studies examining the behavioral or physiological correlates of 5HT unit activity in freely moving cats have focused on the DRN, I shall first describe these results and then compare and contrast them, when possible, with the results from the other groups of 5HT neurons.

Circadian Variation

One of the most basic physiological parameters of a neuron's activity is whether it varies in a circadian manner. Because brain 5HT metabolism is strongly influenced by the light-dark cycle (true circadian rhythmicity has not been closely examined), we decided to see whether the light-dark cycle would influence the activity of DRN neurons (104). When state was held constant, i.e., when the activity of a given neuron was studied during REM sleep (or slow wave sleep or quiet waking) at various times during the light-dark cycle, we found the activity to be completely invariant. Why, then, does 5HT metabolism vary as a function of the light-dark cycle? There are two nonmutually exclusive possibilities. First, since neurotransmitter metabolism occurs predominantly at the axon terminal, local conditions at these sites may modulate metabolism somewhat independently of constant spike discharge at the cell body. Second, the variation in 5HT metabolism across the light-dark cycle may simply be secondary to the well-known distribution of sleep and waking across this cycle.

Sleep-Wake Arousal Cycle

Historically, brain 5HT function was most strongly associated with the initiation and maintenance of sleep (see ref. 57 for an excellent review). Because of the difficulties involved in drawing clear conclusions about much of the lesion and pharmacological data that comprised this field, we decided to examine this issue at the single-unit level. These data also constituted the basic characterization of the activity of these cells across the sleep-wake cycle. The initial study was of the DRN, but these analyses have since been extended to 5HT neurons in the NCS, NRM, and NRP.

DRN unit activity is slow and regular when the cat is in a quiet waking state; however, this activity shows dramatic changes across the sleep-waking cycle (63,103). From a quiet waking rate of approximately 3 spikes/sec, the activity of these neurons will often reach 6 spikes/sec in response to the presentation of a phasically arousing stimulus. Reciprocally, the activity of DRN neurons shows a gradual decline as the cat becomes drowsy and enters slow wave sleep. The culmination of this state-dependent decrease in DRN unit activity occurs during REM sleep when the activity of these neurons typically becomes completely quiescent. At the end of a REM sleep epoch, DRN unit activity returns to levels seen during active or quiet waking. Interestingly, this return of DRN unit activity to waking levels often *precedes* behavioral or polygraphic evidence of waking by several seconds. The activity of DRN neurons also displays a strong inverse relationship with two of the electrophysiological events associated with slow wave sleep and REM sleep, namely, sleep spindles and ponto-geniculo-occipital (PGO) waves, respectively. A somewhat similar pattern of activity across the sleep-wake-arousal cycle is seen with neighboring 5HT neurons in the NCS (74).

5HT neurons in the medulla, however, display a slightly different pattern of activity than DRN and NCS neurons. Although they discharge at an overall higher rate, 5HT neurons in the NRM also display a strong state dependency, but they show no change in activity in relation to sleep spindles or PGO waves (29,84). Similarly, the activity of neurons in the caudal medullary group, NRP, shows no relationship to sleep spindles or PGO waves, and displays less variation across behavioral state (46,84). NRP neurons are generally unresponsive to behaviorally arousing stimuli, and display a more gradual rate of decline in activity from quiet waking, to drowsy, to slow wave sleep. Their activity does, however, precipitously decrease with the onset of REM sleep, although not to as great a degree as 5HT neurons in the other three areas.

These data indicate that brain 5HT neurons do not play an active role in the generation and maintenance of the states of sleep. Rather than *increasing* their activity preceding or coincident with the onset of sleep states, 5HT neurons display a monotonic *decrease* in activity from arousal through waking, drowsy, slow wave sleep, and REM sleep. This type of activity is consistent with 5HT neurons modulating, rather than mediating, a variety of behavioral and physiological processes during waking and sleep. It is clear, for example, from previous pharmacological data and from the single-unit studies described above, that both sleep spindles and PGO waves are modulated by a tonic inhibition exerted by 5HT neurons localized in the pons/mesencephalon.

Sensory Stimulation

Repetitive presentations (once every 2 sec) of phasic auditory (click) or visual stimuli (flash) both produce a similar effect on DRN unit activity, consisting of excitation followed by inhibition (50). We have hypothesized that this response may represent simply a resetting of these highly regular discharging neurons (50). A similar pattern of excitation and inhibition is observed with NCS neurons (74). No evidence of habituation of these responses of DRN and NCS neurons is seen (76). In contrast to the response of DRN and NCS units to phasic auditory and visual stimuli, NRP neurons display little or no response to these same stimuli (46). The response of 5HT neurons in the NRM is intermediate between the strong excitation-inhibition of DRN and NCS neurons and the virtual lack of response of NRP cells (29). Thus, a rostral to caudal gradient of responsiveness of 5HT neurons may exist in the brainstem.

Perhaps of greater importance than the moderate response of these cells to simple phasic sensory stimuli is our failure to observe any specific response of NRM neurons to various types of noxious stimuli: radiant heat applied to the tail, electrical stimulation of the inferior alveolar nerve, pinches applied to the body surface, and the subcutaneous injection of a dilute formalin solution (16). None of these stimuli produced an increase in NRM unit activity that was greater than that observed in response to nonnoxious but arousing stimuli. Furthermore, the increases in NRM unit activity produced by noxious stimuli were not affected by systemic administration of morphine in analgesic doses. The morphine injections also failed to influence significantly the spontaneous activity of NRM neurons. These data do not support hypotheses that implicate changes in neuronal discharge of NRM 5HT neurons in either nociception or analgesia. They are, however, consistent with our general conception of 5HT neurons *modulating* a wide range of sensory and motor processes, including nociception and analgesia.

Behavior and Physiology

One of the initial clues for discovering the behavioral/physiological variables that exert tonic control over 5HT unit activity was the finding that these neurons become totally inactive during REM sleep. Since it is well known that a primary feature of REM sleep is centrally induced atonia, we hypothesized that this might be importantly related to the decrease in DRN unit activity.

This hypothesis has now been tested in several different ways, but only for the DRN group of 5HT neurons. In the first series of studies, we ablated a small area of the pons whose destruction in cats was known to result in REM sleep without atonia (43). An animal with such a lesion has epochs which, by all criteria, look like REM sleep, except that antigravity muscle tonus is present and the animals are therefore capable of engaging in complex behaviors, including locomotion. Consistent with our initial hypothesis, we found that the activity of DRN neurons was significantly increased during REM sleep epochs in these animals (105). In fact, the level of neuronal activity was directly related to the level of restored motor activity during REM sleep. A second series of experiments examined this issue in a somewhat reciprocal manner (92). When the cholinomimetic agent carbachol is injected directly into specific areas of the pons, it can produce atonia in an otherwise awake cat. When the carbachol injection induced atonia, we observed a complete suppression of DRN unit activity, whereas injections in nearby areas, which failed to induce atonia, had no effect on DRN unit activity. Several additional experiments in this series led us to conclude that the critical variable was centrally induced atonia, rather than muscle paralysis *per se*. Administration of dantrolene, a peripherally acting muscle relaxant, or succinylcholine, an antagonist at the neuromuscular junction, produced no change in DRN unit activity in spite of a profound loss of muscle tonus. However, when we administered mephenesin, a centrally acting muscle relaxant, we once again observed a large decrease in DRN unit activity. It should be noted, however, that even if a functional relationship exists between the activity of 5HT neurons and activity in central motor systems, it is not a simple linear one (61). It may be one that is engaged only under specific or extreme conditions.

We are currently attempting to determine whether this relationship perhaps is attributable to a variable that is strongly, and possibly inextricably, linked to central motor activity. A prime candidate for such a concomitant of motor activity is sympathetic tone, or its central representation. It is well known that activity of the autonomic nervous system is often closely tied to somatic motor activity (71). For example, it is known that the somatomotor and cardiovascular systems are coactivated by commands descending from motor cortex (51). Furthermore, and perhaps more importantly, many autonomic reflexes are suppressed during REM sleep (72), and Parmeggiani has suggested that this state is one of suspended homeostasis (73). Therefore, we are examining the issue of whether 5HT neuronal activity is related to changes in sympathetic activity by exposing animals to a variety of environmental and physiological challenges. Thus far, our results are negative. We find that many challenges that elicit sympathetic activation, such as exposure to 100-db white noise, restraint, environmental heating, pyrogen administration, insulin-induced hypoglycemia, and drug-induced hypotension, produce little or no change in DRN unit activity (30, 3a,112b). Perhaps more importantly, these data bear on

fundamental issues such as the role of 5HT neurons in cardiovascular control or thermoregulation. Once again, these negative data indicate that if the hypothesized involvement of 5HT in these processes is valid, it may be due to modulation of axon terminal release of 5HT, rather than to changes in 5HT neuronal discharge.

Pharmacology

Drug studies of 5HT neurons in behaving animals are few in number. Many are based on the findings, in anesthetized rats, that any drug that either acts as a direct 5HT agonist or that increases synaptic levels of 5HT will depress 5HT neuronal activity (2,25,100,102). It is assumed that these compounds do so by acting at the aforementioned 5HT cell body autoreceptors (5). Hallucinogenic drugs that have a structural similarity to 5HT (i.e., those containing an indole nucleus) also depress the activity of 5HT neurons, but this is probably not the critical neuropharmacological action subserving hallucinogenesis (see refs. 50 and 53 for a complete discussion of this issue). No known 5HT antagonist drug is capable of consistently blocking the depression of 5HT neuronal activity produced by either directly or indirectly acting 5HT agonists (42,45). Thus, the 5HT cell body autoreceptor probably represents a different 5HT receptor subtype than those found in other areas of the CNS (5,25).

Diazepam, an anxiolytic drug of the benzodiazepine class, produces no significant effect on DRN unit activity in behaving cats when administered in low doses known to be anxiolytic (107; L. O. Wilkinson et al., *unpublished observations*). However, at higher doses, when sedation and ataxia are seen, diazepam does depress DRN unit activity. By contrast, buspirone, an anxiospecific drug of the azaspirodecanedione class, strongly suppresses DRN unit activity at dose levels that produce no obvious side effects (112a).

Finally, we find that systemic administration of adrenergic agonist and antagonist drugs exerts modest excitatory and suppressant effects, respectively, on DRN unit activity in behaving cats (49,101). This is somewhat at variance with the results from similar studies of DRN neurons examined in chloral-hydrate-anesthetized rats, where adrenergic drugs are found to exert strong effects on DRN neurons (17).

Many other clinically interesting drugs, such as various classes of antidepressants, have yet to be examined for their chronic, or even acute, effects on 5HT neuronal activity in behaving animals.

Conclusions

Brain 5HT neurons discharge with an extraordinary tonic regularity, suggesting that little neuronal information is conveyed by this activity. This is consistent with the concept that the function of these neurons is to modulate a wide variety of behavioral and physiological processes rather than to mediate any one of them. The general lack of perturbability of these neurons, even by strong environmental or physiological stimuli, is in agreement with this concept. (Also consistent is a large body of neurochemical evidence indicating that 5HT turnover is unresponsive to a variety of stressors that are known to influence other central neurochemical systems; refs. 13,60,82.) Furthermore, these data suggest consideration of one of the following two possibilities. First, that much of the function of 5HT neurons is carried out by changes in release, reuptake, etc. at the axon terminal, rather than by changes in neuronal discharge rate. There is ample evidence in the literature supporting the existence of such local influences (e.g., 20,59). Second, and more radically, these single-unit data suggest that hypotheses specifically implicating brain 5HT neurons in processes such as thermoregulation, analgesia, etc. may be incorrect. This does not seem so heretical when we recall that it was data from single-unit studies in behaving animals that provided one of the major arguments in opposition to a strong body of evidence implicating brain 5HT as the active agent in the initiation and maintenance of sleep.

DOPAMINERGIC NEURONS

Overview of Basic Characteristics

Most of the dopaminergic (DA) neurons in the mammalian CNS are found in the ventral mesencephalon (pars compacta of the substantia nigra and the ventral tegmental area). Although a number of different groups of DA neurons have been identified in the CNS, most of the neurophysiological studies have been carried out on these two groups. Under chloral hydrate anesthesia, the activity of these neurons in both rat and cat displays a characteristically slow (2–7 spikes/sec) and fairly regular discharge pattern, with occasional bursts containing spikes of decreasing amplitude (19,90). DA neurons in the substantia nigra are influenced by two different types of negative feedback: long-loop, via the corpus striatum (18), and local, via dendritic release of DA (41). The existence of negative feedback for ventral tegmental DA neurons is not nearly as clear as it is for the substantia nigra. As with 5HT neurons, there is evidence that the discharge rate of DA neurons may be inversely related to the density of autoreceptors in the somadendritic area (21,112). Finally, DA neurons, at least in the substantia nigra, appear to be autoactive (36,88) and also appear to be electrotonically coupled to each other (37).

Several years ago, we reported that DA neurons in freely moving cats display a rate and pattern of neuronal activity similar to that seen under anesthesia (90). Since that time, several reports on DA unit activity in freely moving rats (65) and awake monkeys (89) have described results generally similar to that which we observed in cats. Studies of DA neurons in freely moving animals have focused primarily on those in the substantia nigra. To the degree that DA neurons in the ventral tegmental area of freely moving animals have been examined, their activity conforms closely to that found in the substantia nigra, with one exception noted below.

Sleep-Wake-Arousal Cycle

The rate and pattern of firing of DA neurons displays a remarkable stability across quiet waking, slow wave sleep, and REM sleep (91). The mean discharge rate for DA neurons in the pars compacta of the substantia nigra of the cat is approximately 3 spikes/sec across these three states. This constancy of activity is unique among the various groups of brain neurons that have been examined under similar conditions. A slight overall increase (20%) in the activity of these neurons was observed, however, during active waking, a period associated with gross movement and/or behavioral arousal. A very similar pattern of activity across state is seen for DA neurons in the substantia nigra in rats (65). Although studied less extensively, the rate and pattern of activity for DA neurons in the ventral tegmental area of rats and cats is virtually identical to that for DA neurons in the substantia nigra (65,106).

Sensory Stimulation

Presentation (once every 2 sec) of clicks or flashes elicited a similar pattern of excitation followed by inhibition in most DA neurons in the substantia nigra (91). Interestingly, the response to clicks showed no evidence of habituation, whereas the response to flashes decreased over the course of 64 repetitions (76). DA units in the substantia nigra of monkeys were unaffected by presentation of tones or colored lights, stimuli of lesser intensity and substantially longer duration than the aforementioned clicks and flashes (89). In a recent study, we found that the response of DA neurons in cats to clicks or flashes could be totally blocked by simultaneously presenting any of a variety of arousing and/or distracting stimuli (tail pinch, immersion of feet in ice water, inaccessible food, feeding, grooming, inaccessible rats, and somatosensory stimuli) (94). Interestingly, these sensory evoked unit responses were not blocked by white noise (perhaps because it is a full field stimulus that does not elicit orientation to a particular part of the environment). No data are available for the response characteristics of DA neurons in the ventral tegmental area to these simple sensory stimuli.

Behavior and Physiology

When the aforementioned arousing and/or distracting stimuli were examined for their effect on DA unit activity in the substantia nigra of cats, *none* of them were found to exert a significant effect on the tonic discharge rate of DA neurons, in spite of the fact that the cats often reacted quite strongly to the stimuli (94). A recent study reported that the activity of DA neurons in the ventral tegmental area of the cat was significantly increased above a quiet waking baseline by the presentation of a tone that was paired with a noxious airpuff (106). However, it would seem more appropriate to compare this condition to active waking rather than a quiet waking baseline. When this is done, only 26% of the neurons showed an increase in activity. These data are somewhat at variance with the neurochemical data showing dramatic increases in DA metabolism in forebrain areas in response to stressful stimuli in rats (e.g., 99). This difference may be attributable to that fact that the DA neurons that project to these forebrain areas are localized on or near the midline, whereas all of the neurons sampled in the single-unit study were at least 1 mm off the midline.

Activity of DA neurons in the substantia nigra does not appear to be temporally correlated with the execution of general spontaneous movements. There is only a small increase in activity during periods when the cat is moving as compared to when it is immobile. Furthermore, as discussed above, there is no increase in the activity of these neurons in association with gross movements *per se* (91). This was somewhat surprising to us, since the substantia nigra has long been considered a key structure within the extrapyramidal motor system. More detailed and specific analyses do, however, reveal that the activity of these neurons is related to particular types of motor acts. It appears that DA unit activity may be related to rapidly executed purposive responses involving a large body mass. For example, in monkeys trained to make reaching responses, DA neurons generally displayed increased activity following the initiation of the movement (25% of the cells showed decreases in activity) (89). There was no relationship to smaller movements, such as those of the hand or the eyes, or postural adjustments. The typical pattern of DA unit activity observed in the majority of neurons examined in cats during orientation to a novel or significant stimulus was a short-latency excitation followed by long-lasting depression of unit activity (91). The depression appears to correspond to the period of fixation (possibly response suppression) and focused attention. As orientation to these stimuli habituates, usually within two to four trials, so does the associated suppression of DA unit activity.

The activity of substantia nigra DA neurons in cats was uninfluenced either by feeding to satiation or by systemic glucose administration (95). This is at variance with data from chloral-hydrate-anesthetized rats showing that glucose administration dramatically suppressed substantia nigra DA neuronal activity (85). No explanation for this discrepancy is available. At present, this study of satiation and glucose administration represents the only examination of the influence of a direct physiological manipulation on DA unit activity in an unrestrained and unanesthetized animals.

Pharmacology

There have been very few studies of drug effects on DA unit activity in behaving animals. As with 5HT neurons, DA unit activity in behaving animals is increased by systemic administration of DA antagonist drugs (e.g., haloperidol) and decreased by DA agonist drugs (e.g., apomorphine). This has been reported for DA neurons in both groups in the mesencephalon, and in rats, cats, and monkeys (1,31,90,106).

Conclusions

Any conclusions regarding DA unit activity in behaving animals must be considered tentative since so few studies have been conducted. The constancy of activity across the sleep-wake-arousal cycle and the overall lack of relationship between movement and DA unit activity are somewhat surprising, considering the widely hypothesized involvement of brain DA in behavior, and especially because of the role of the substantia nigra in basal ganglia motor function. However, these data are consistent with evidence indicating that DA's role in brain may be permissive and somewhat neurohumoral rather than neurotransmitter-like. This would explain the capability of nonspecific manipulations such as systemic administration of the DA precursor, L-dopa, and transplantation of DA neurons into the corpus striatum, to restore motor function in Parkinsonian patients and DA-denervated rats, respectively. The available data suggest that the activity of DA neurons may be similar across several mammalian species, but once again the evidence is too limited to permit any firm conclusion to be drawn.

NORADRENERGIC NEURONS

Overview of Basic Characteristics

Cell bodies of noradrenergic (NE) neurons in the mammalian CNS are localized almost exclusively within the brainstem and hypothalamus, mostly in discrete clusters lying off of the midline, and frequently within classically defined nuclei. More than half of all brain NE neurons are localized in the locus ceruleus in the dorsolateral pons. In anesthetized rats, NE neurons in several brain regions, including the locus ceruleus, discharge with a slow (0.5–5.0 spikes/sec) and somewhat regular pattern of activity (11,38,66). Intracellular studies of NE neurons in the rat locus ceruleus, examined *in vivo* and *in vitro,* indicate that these neurons are autoactive (9,113). This autoactivity appears to be controlled by a local negative feedback mechanism mediated by axon collaterals and possibly connections between neighboring NE neurons (6,9). Perhaps even more important is a calcium-activated potassium conductance that produces autoinhibition (9,12).

To date, the only NE neurons that have been studied in unanesthetized rats, cats, and monkeys are those in the area of the locus ceruleus (14,15,28,52,77–79). The spontaneous activity of locus ceruleus NE neurons in these unanesthetized animals displays characteristics similar to those described above for the anesthetized rat. The following sections review the behavioral, environmental, and physiological correlates of locus ceruleus NE single-unit activity examined in behaving animals.

Sleep-Wake-Arousal Cycle

The activity of NE locus ceruleus neurons in rat (14), cat (52,78,79), and monkey (28) is slow (typically below 5 spikes/sec) and fairly regular (less so than when recorded under anesthesia). This activity, however, changes dramatically across the sleep-wake cycle. A number of investigators have studied the activity of locus ceruleus neurons across these state changes in cats (22,52,78,79). Their activity is highest during the active waking state (~2 spikes/sec), decreases during quiet waking (~1 spike/sec), decreases still further during slow wave sleep (~0.5 spikes/sec), and finally, becomes virtually quiescent during REM sleep. (In cats, locus ceruleus unit activity is also inversely related to the emergence of PGO waves in REM sleep; refs. 64,83.) The same state-related pattern of locus ceruleus unit activity observed in cats has also been reported to occur in locus ceruleus neurons examined across the sleep-wake cycle in the albino rat (14). The latter authors also noted that in rats these neurons significantly increased their activity in association with the occurrence of EEG spindles in slow wave sleep, whereas a study in cats failed to observe such a relationship (78). Finally, studies in squirrel monkeys reported a similar magnitude of decrease in activity in going from waking to slow wave sleep (no data were gathered during REM sleep) (28). Thus, the same pattern of locus ceruleus unit activity is observed across the sleep-wake-arousal cycle in the three species that have been studied to date.

Sensory Stimulation

In rat, cat, and monkey, locus ceruleus neurons display dramatic phasic increases in activity in response to any of a variety of arousing stimuli (15,28,40,78). Neuronal activity during these phasic bursts sometimes reaches levels as high as 10 to 20 spikes/sec (see details below).

More systematic analyses have been carried out on the response of locus ceruleus neurons to the repetitive presentation of phasic auditory (tone pips or clicks) or phasic visual (flash) stimuli. In general, the response to both the auditory and visual stimuli is similar in rats, cats, and monkeys (15,28,76,78). Typically, it consists of an excitatory response of relatively short duration, containing 1 to 4 spikes, followed by a longer-lasting inhibitory period.

A more interesting issue than the simple response of locus ceruleus neurons to the repetitive presentation of auditory or visual stimuli is the dynamic nature of this response. Studies in rat, cat, and monkey all report some form of response decrement with stimulus repetition. In the monkey, when the stimulus no longer elicited EEG arousal or orienting responses, it no longer evoked unit activity (28). In rats, large decreases in responsiveness to sensory stimuli were seen in association with decreasing levels of vigilance, but no evidence of habituation was observed when behavioral state was held constant (15). A slightly different pattern is observed in cats (76). The first few presentations of clicks or flashes may elicit several spikes, but this rapidly habituates, presumably in association with a decrease in the stimulus-elicited arousal or orientation response. Thereafter, the number of elicited spikes and/or the probability of eliciting a spike gradually decrease over the next 50 to 60 presentations, in the absence of any concomitant shifts in behavioral state. Thus, response of locus ceruleus neurons to the repeated presentation of simple sensory stimuli can be characterized generally as a dynamic or labile one (cf. the stable response of 5HT neurons; ref. 76).

Behavior and Physiology

Locus ceruleus neuronal activity in rats, cats, and monkeys shows no relationship to movement *per se* (14,28,78).

In addition, the activity of these neurons is unrelated to the performance of simple operant responses in monkeys (32).

These neurons have also been studied during complex naturalistic behaviors. No change in locus ceruleus unit activity was seen during feeding in rhesus monkeys (32), but a decrease in unit activity was reported during feeding in stump-tailed monkeys (40). During feeding in cats, the activity of these neurons is slightly lower than that observed during active waking, but above the activity level observed during quiet waking (78). During the repetitive and often long-lasting motor sequences of grooming, which many mammalian species engage in, locus ceruleus unit activity is also reported to decrease in rats and monkeys (14,40). In cat, much the same type of relationship described above for feeding was seen during grooming, i.e., the level of unit activity was above that observed during a quiet waking state without movement, but slightly below that seen during an active waking state with approximately equivalent level of spontaneous or random motor activity (78). Thus, when animals engage in repetitive, unlearned naturalistic behaviors, especially those that are vegetative in nature, locus ceruleus unit activity may decrease somewhat from a level seen when the animal is generally more attentive to its external environment (15). Locus ceruleus unit activity in cats is also decreased slightly during the vegetative behaviors of defecation and micturition (K. Rasmussen, E. D. Abercrombie, D. A. Morilak, and B. L. Jacobs, *unpublished observations*).

Locus ceruleus unit activity in cats has also been examined during a variety of other complex behaviors (or in response to complex stimuli). Somewhat surprisingly, very little change in unit activity, from that observed during active waking, is observed during these conditions, in spite of the fact that several of them appear to be quite arousing to the animals: presence and mutual sniffing of another cat of the same sex; scratching about the head and neck by the experimenter; exposure to highly preferred, but inaccessible, food; and exposure to inaccessible rats (78).

A great deal of evidence indicates that the activity of locus ceruleus neurons is positively correlated with increases in the animal's level of behavioral arousal. As mentioned above, any of a diverse group of stimuli that phasically elicit behavioral arousal will evoke a concomitant phasic increase in locus ceruleus unit activity. In squirrel monkeys, the sight of a preferred food or an unfamiliar person entering the recording room greatly increases the activity of these neurons (28). A study utilizing stump-tailed monkeys examined the issue of behavioral arousal and locus ceruleus unit activity more extensively (40). The results were similar to those described above for squirrel monkeys. The most impressive increases in activity, often three- to tenfold, were seen in response to human imitations of primate agonistic social signals. Interestingly, these strong responses showed no evidence of habituation (cf. the previous discussion of habituation of response to simple sensory stimuli). A number of other stimuli also elicited locus ceruleus unit responses in stump-tailed monkeys: light pin pricks to the foot; holding the monkey's foot; entrance or exit of the experimenter from the recording room; sight of a mechanism used to present noxious stimuli to the animal;

and sight of desirable foods. The response of locus ceruleus neurons in cats is increased by pinches applied to the tail or paw (78). This typically produced a burst of unit activity lasting for about 1 sec, with an approximately 10-fold increase in discharge rate. A "threat" stimulus (movement of the experimenter's hand rapidly toward the animal's face) also elicited a locus ceruleus unit response in cats that was of short duration and a high level of activity (78). These responses are similar to the characteristic burst-pause response to pinches of locus ceruleus neurons in anesthetized animals (38).

In order to examine further the relationship between locus ceruleus unit activity and behavioral activation, several studies have employed manipulations that unambiguously could be considered challenges to the integrity of the organism. Studies in anesthetized rats have shown that locus ceruleus unit activity is increased by blood volume depletion, hypercapnia, and hypoxia (27,97). This group of investigators also reported that noxious mechanical sensory stimulation, as well as nonnoxious and noxious thermal sensory stimulation, produced parallel and virtually identical increases in locus ceruleus unit activity and peripheral sympathetic nerve discharge (26). These latter results are consistent with the authors' previous data since blood volume depletion, hypoxia, and hypercapnia are all known to produce sympathetic activation. They summarize their findings by suggesting that only imperative stimuli continue to elicit robust locus ceruleus discharge (26).

Experiments in behaving cats have come to a similar conclusion. Spontaneous changes in locus ceruleus activity across the sleep-wake cycle were found to be correlated with the level of activity in the cervical sympathetic trunk (79). Other studies have begun to explore related issues in behaving cats. At the most basic level, the probability of locus ceruleus discharge was found to be temporally related to the cardiac cycle in cats. The excitability of these neurons is at its nadir at the time of occurrence of the r-wave (during systole) and reaches the peak of its excitability approximately 120 msec later (during diastole) (67,68). Further analyses in behaving cats indicated that the activity of locus ceruleus neurons is moderately increased in response to administration of the hypotensive agent hydralazine (68b). This finding is significant because hydralazine elicits sympathetic activation in the absence of an effect on behavioral arousal. Consistent with these results is the finding that the elicitation of thermoregulatory responses in cats, through environmental heating or pyrogen administration, and insulin-induced glucoprivation, all of which evoke sympathetic activation in the absence of behavioral arousal, produce a moderate elevation of locus ceruleus unit activity (68a,68c). In conclusion, studies in anesthetized rats and unanesthetized cats imply that locus ceruleus unit activity often may be correlated with sympathetic activity, but there may be an additional powerful influence of behavioral arousal.

This issue has also been explored, to a limited extent, through the use of behavioral or environmental manipulations. Perhaps the most impressive stimulus for producing a tonic increase in locus ceruleus unit activity is the induction of emesis. Over a 1-min period culminating in emesis, locus ceruleus neurons in cats manifest as much as a 10-fold increase in unit activity (78,79). The effects on locus ceruleus unit activity of two other environmental challenges have also been examined in cats. Fifteen minutes of restraint or exposure to 100-db white noise both produce substantial increases in locus ceruleus unit activity, which peak within the first 5 min at three to four times the baseline level, and then decrease somewhat, leveling off at about twice the baseline level of activity. These changes in unit activity induced by restraint and white noise were accompanied by large increases in plasma catecholamines, and were closely correlated with increases in heart rate (1a).

One of the hallmarks of mammalian behavior is its diversity and the attendant capacity for change as a function of environmental contingencies, i.e., learning. Many theories have implicated brain NE, especially in locus ceruleus neurons, as being important in learning or in the subprocesses, such as attention, that contribute to it (e.g., 23,62,81). Only recently, however, have single-unit studies in behaving animals attempted to assess the role of locus ceruleus neurons in learning. The activity of these neurons was examined in cats during two conditioning paradigms: conditioned emotional response (CER) and conditioned food reward (CFR) training (77). During CER training, locus ceruleus units displayed a severalfold increase in activity in response to a previously neutral stimulus that was paired with a noxious stimulus (airpuff to the face), whereas no increase in unit activity was seen in response to a stimulus that was not paired with the airpuff. By contrast, during CFR training, a previously neutral stimulus paired with a rewarding stimulus (food delivery) did not elicit a significant increase in locus ceruleus unit activity. These data suggest that locus ceruleus neurons are not necessarily implicated in all types of learning, but that they may be preferentially involved in learning contingencies regarding challenging or noxious events (81). These results are consistent with neurochemical studies in rats and brain stimulation studies in pigeons indicating that locus ceruleus neurons play an active role in aversive, but not appetitive, conditioning (33,111).

More generally, since learning is the epitome of adaptation, these data are consistent with the concept that locus ceruleus neurons are mobilized by various challenges to the organism in order to integrate adaptive responses to them by the CNS.

Pharmacology

As with 5HT and DA neurons, the activity of NE neurons is decreased by systemic administration of adrenergic agonist drugs and is increased by adrenergic antagonist drugs. This has been reported in both anesthetized rats (11,66,96,98) and behaving cats (78,80). These effects appear to be mediated by an action at an α_2 cell body autoreceptor.

A number of studies have reported that the systemic administration of morphine, in analgesic doses, produces a substantial decrease in locus ceruleus unit activity in anesthetized rats (3,58). In contrast, when morphine was administered to unanesthetized cats (0.5, 2.0, or 4.0 mg/kg i.p.) it produced a significant *increase* in unit activity that was naloxone reversible (75). The discrepancy between these studies may be attributable to anesthesia, since administration of the same doses of morphine to chloral-hydrate-anesthetized cats resulted in a significant decrease in locus ceruleus NE unit activity, which was also naloxone reversible (75).

In chloral-hydrate-anesthetized rats, diazepam in doses of 0.5 and 1.0 mg/kg i.v. produced 30 to 40% and 60 to 80% reductions in locus ceruleus unit activity, respectively (39,86). In contrast to these results, when diazepam (0.25 or 2.0 mg/kg i.p.) was administered to behaving cats, it produced no significant decrease in locus ceruleus unit activity (77). In this latter study, the lower dose of diazepam was also tested for its efficacy in influencing the sensory responsiveness of locus ceruleus NE neurons to repetitive presentations of clicks or flashes. In spite of the fact that diazepam did not significantly influence the baseline firing rate of these neurons, it markedly suppressed (80–90% reduction) the sensory evoked single-unit responses, suggesting a preferential effect of diazepam on the excitability of these cells (77). Studies of systemically administered buspirone indicate that it suppresses neither spontaneous nor sensory evoked locus ceruleus unit activity in cats (112a), but produces a small increase in locus ceruleus unit activity somewhat similar to that reported in anesthetized rats (87).

Finally, in chloral-hydrate-anesthetized rats, hallucinogens such as mescaline and lysergic acid diethylamide (LSD) are reported to decrease locus ceruleus unit activity while simultaneously increasing their response to somatosensory stimuli (4). These opposite effects would, of course, greatly increase the signal-to-noise ratio (sensory evoked unit activity/spontaneous activity of locus ceruleus unit activity). Initial results in behaving cats indicate that neither LSD nor mescaline nor DOM (2,5-dimethoxy-4-methylamphetamine) significantly affects either spontaneous or sensory evoked locus ceruleus unit activity (K. Rasmussen, E. D. Abercrombie, and B. L. Jacobs, *unpublished observations*).

In general, data from these various pharmacological studies suggest that anesthesia may dramatically change the magnitude and/or direction of response of locus ceruleus neurons to drugs.

Conclusions

These results are consistent with the concept that locus ceruleus neurons play an important role in the integration and orchestration of the adaptive CNS response of mammalian organisms to various stressors or challenges. In behaving animals, locus ceruleus neurons respond to novel neutral phasic stimuli with a moderate increase in unit activity (as these stimuli lose their novelty and/or potential importance to the animal, this response may diminish greatly or even completely); respond to noxious and/or imperative phasic stimuli with a dramatic, but also brief, increase in activity; and respond to tonically challenging or stressful stimuli with a long-lasting elevation in activity. The activity of these neurons manifests little or no change in response to arousing, but nonchallenging, stimuli, and may even decrease somewhat during both active and passive vegetative behaviors. There is evidence to indicate that the activity of locus ceruleus NE neurons generally increases in association with sympathetic activation.

This concept is consistent with an extensive body of neurochemical studies indicating that brain NE neurons, including those in the locus ceruleus, are strongly activated by a variety of stressors (for reviews see 13,35,93). Although widely scattered through the experimental literature, there are also a number of reports that suppression of NE function, including that deriving from the locus ceruleus, impairs the ability of mammalian organisms to respond effectively to challenging situations (e.g., 34,110). These functional data are consonant with the anatomical data indicating that brain NE neurons, and particularly those in the locus ceruleus, have a widespread, almost ubiquitous, projection domain. This is a characteristic that would be critical for a system hypothesized to integrate the activity of CNS structures responsible for sensory, motor, hormonal, autonomic, and cognitive responses to imperative environmental, behavioral, or physiological challenges. It also has been noted that brain NE neurons bear a resemblance, both morphologically and in terms of its modulatory action on its target sites, to the peripheral NE neurons that comprise the sympathetic ganglia of the autonomic nervous system (e.g., 10,114).

GENERAL DISCUSSION

A sufficient amount of information has been accumulated on these three systems, both from single-unit studies in behaving animals and from other approaches, to formulate hypotheses regarding their function. Fortunately, comparisons across single-unit studies employing rats, cats, and monkeys indicate that these data have cross-species generality. Not only does this increase confidence in the significance of data derived from any given species, but it provides a basis for assuming that these results may generalize to humans. Furthermore, any differences noted in the data between species, such as some of those for NE neurons, may be more apparent than real. It must be kept in mind that although the rat, cat, and monkey are all mammals, they belong to different *orders* and thus are markedly different both genotypically and phenotypically. Additionally, these three species exist in extremely different ecological niches and thus would be expected to solve similar environmental and physiological problems by means of different behavioral and physiological mechanisms. One might also expect the cat, a domesticated species, to react to the laboratory setting and handling by experimenters in quite a different way than the nondomesticated rat and monkey. In comparison with the cat, the latter two species may be chronically anxious or vigilant in the laboratory, which could be manifested as differences between them in the spontaneous activity or responsiveness of neurons such as these in the locus ceruleus. Such factors must be recognized when comparing data from different species of animals.

As might be expected from groups of neurons with their cell bodies localized exclusively within the brainstem, monoaminergic neurons appear to subserve basic roles in physiology and behavior. Furthermore, it is hypothesized that these basic functions are invariant across various mammalian species. DA neurons in the substantia nigra appear to play a permissive role with respect to motor activity. Their activity is invariant across state changes and a variety of environmental and physiological challenges. This probably represents evidence that the activity of these neurons is unlikely to be related to changes in major physiological systems (e.g., cardiovascular). The activity of these neurons does, however, change dramatically during rapidly executed purposive or targeted movements, such as orientation and fixation, which involve large body masses. Although the activity of DA neurons in the ventral tegmental area appears similar to that of DA neurons in the substantia nigra, the data on the former group are too limited to allow any conclusions to be drawn. Given the variety of behavioral and physiological processes in which 5HT neurons have been implicated (e.g., thermoregulation, sleep, nociception, hormone release, etc.), the failure to find strong correlations between these variables and 5HT unit activity is surprising. A possible explanation for this is that many of these variables exert their effect directly on axon terminal function of 5HT neurons rather than on 5HT cell discharge activity. Finally, the activity of NE neurons in the area of the locus ceruleus manifests a dynamic relationship to a variety of behavioral and physiological variables. This activity is often correlated with activation of the sympathetic nervous system. Current evidence indicates that these neurons may be preferentially activated by challenges to the integrity of the organism. It is hypothesized that locus ceruleus NE neurons may coordinate diverse sensory, motor, hormonal, and physiological functions to act in a concerted manner as part of the organism's adaptive response to these challenges.

In the future, one obvious direction for studies in this area will be an extension of these analyses to other groups of monoaminergic neurons, including those utilizing epinephrine for neurotransmission. A major limitation of single-unit studies is the fact that they provide evidence only on activity at the cell body level. Therefore, recently developed methods for measuring axon terminal release of monoamines, utilizing either voltammetry or dialysis, represent an important additional technique for studying neurotransmitter function. Finally, the study of the effects of psychoactive drugs on single-unit activity in behaving animals will be exploited in coming years. Since some of the methods employed in these single-unit studies often permit the same neuron to be examined for several days or more, the important area of chronic drug treatment also will soon be explored.

ACKNOWLEDGMENTS

The research from the author's laboratory described in this review was generously supported by grants from the National Institute of Mental Health (MH 23433), the National Science Foundation (BNS 81-19840), and the United States Air Force (AFOSR 85-0034).

REFERENCES

1. Aebischer, P., and Schultz, W. (1984): *Neurosci. Lett.*, 50:25–29.
1a. Abercrombie, E. D., Wilkinson, L. O., and Jacobs, B. L. (1986): *Soc. Neurosci. Abstr.*, 12:1134.
2. Aghajanian, G. K. (1972): *Ann. NY Acad. Sci.*, 193:86–94.
3. Aghajanian, G. K. (1978): *Nature*, 276:186–188.
4. Aghajanian, G. K. (1980): *Brain Res.*, 186:492–498.
5. Aghajanian, G. K. (1981): In: *Serotonin Neurotransmission and Behavior*, edited by B. L. Jacobs and A. Gelperin, pp. 156–185. MIT Press, Cambridge.
6. Aghajanian, G. K., Cedarbaum, J. M., and Wang, R. Y. (1977): *Brain Res.*, 136:570–577.
7. Aghajanian, G. K., Foote, W. E., and Sheard, M. H. (1968): *Science*, 161:706–708.
8. Aghajanian, G. K., and VanderMaelen, C. P. (1982): *Brain Res.*, 238:463–469.
9. Aghajanian, G. K., VanderMaelen, C. P., and Andrade, R. (1983): *Brain Res.*, 273:237–243.
10. Amaral, D. G., and Sinnamon, H. M. (1977): *Prog. Neurobiol.*, 9:147–196.
11. Andrade, R., and Aghajanian, G. K. (1982): *Brain Res.*, 242:125–135.
12. Andrade, R., and Aghajanian, G. K. (1984): *J. Neurosci.*, 4:161–170.
13. Anisman, H., Kokkinidis, L., and Sklar, L. S. (1984): In: *Psychological and Physiological Interaction in Response to Stress*, edited by S. Burchfield, pp. 67–98. Hemisphere, New York.
14. Aston-Jones, G., and Bloom, F. E. (1981): *J. Neurosci.*, 1:876–886.
15. Aston-Jones, G., and Bloom, F. E. (1981): *J. Neurosci.*, 1:887–900.
16. Auerbach, S., Fornal, C., and Jacobs, B. L. (1985): *Exp. Neurol.*, 88:609–628.
17. Baraban, J. M., and Aghajanian, G. K. (1980): *Neuropharmacology*, 19:355–363.
18. Bunney, B. S., and Aghajanian, G. K. (1978): *Naunyn Schmiedebergs Arch. Pharmacol*, 304:255–261.
19. Bunney, B. S., Walters, J. R., Roth, R. H., and Aghajanian, G. K. (1973): *J. Pharmacol. Exp. Ther.*, 185:560–571.
20. Chesselet, M. F. (1984): *Neuroscience*, 12:347–375.
21. Chiodo, L. A., Bannon, M. J., Grace, A. A., Roth, R. H., and Bunney, B. S. (1984): *Neuroscience*, 12:1–16.
22. Chu, N. S., and Bloom, F. E. (1974): *J. Neurobiol.*, 5:527–544.
23. Crow, T. J., and Arbuthnott, G. W. (1972): *Nature*, 238:245–246.
24. Crunelli, V., Forda, S., Brooks, P. A., Wilson, K. C. P., Wise, J. C. M., and Kelly, J. S. (1983): *Neurosci. Lett.*, 40:263–268.
25. de Montigny, C., Blier, P., and Chaput, Y. (1984): *Neuropharmacology*, 23:1511–1520.
26. Elam, M., Svensson, T. H., and Thoren, P. (1986): *Brain Res.*, 366:254–261.
27. Elam, M., Yao, T., Thoren, P., and Svensson, T. H. (1981): *Brain Res.*, 222:373–381.
28. Foote, S. L., Aston-Jones, G., and Bloom, F. E. (1980): *Proc. Natl. Acad. Sci. USA*, 77:3033–3037.
29. Fornal, C., Auerbach, S., and Jacobs, B. L. (1985): *Exp. Neurol.*, 88:590–608.
30. Fornal, C., Morilak, D., Auerbach, S., and Jacobs, B. L. (1985): *Soc. Neurosci. Abstr.*, 11:769.
30a. Fornal, C., Morilak, D. A., and Jacobs, B. L. (1986): *Soc. Neurosci. Abstr.*, 12:1134.
31. Freeman, A. S., Meltzer, L. T., and Bunney, B. S. (1985): *Life Sci.*, 36:1983–1994.
32. German, D. C., and Fetz, E. E. (1976): *Brain Res.*, 109:497–514.
33. Gibbs, C. M., Broyles, J. L., and Cohen, D. H. (1983): *Soc. Neurosci. Abstr.*, 9:641.
34. Glavin, G. B. (1985): *Life Sci.*, 37:461–465.
35. Glavin, G. B. (1985): *Neurosci. Biobehav. Rev.*, 9:233–243.
36. Grace, A. A., and Bunney, B. S. (1983): *Neuroscience*, 10:301–315.
37. Grace, A. A., and Bunney, B. S. (1983): *Neuroscience*, 10:333–348.
38. Graham, A. W., and Aghajanian, G. K. (1971): *Nature*, 234:100–102.
39. Grant, S. J., Huang, Y. H., and Redmond, D. E. (1980): *Life Sci.*, 27:2231–2236.
40. Grant, S. J., and Redmond, D. E. (1984): *Exp. Neurol.*, 84:701–708.
41. Groves, P. M., Wilson, C. J., Young, S. J., and Rebec, G. V. (1975): *Science*, 190:522–529.

42. Haigler, H. J., and Aghajanian, G. K. (1977): *Fed. Proc.*, 36:2159–2164.
43. Henley, K., and Morrison, A. R. (1974): *Acta Neurobiol. Exp.*, 34:215–232.
44. Heym, J., and Jacobs, B. L. (1986): In: *Modern Methods in Pharmacology: Electrophysiological Techniques*, edited by H. M. Geller, pp. 18–34. Alan R. Liss, New York (*in press*).
45. Heym, J., Rasmussen, K., and Jacobs, B. L. (1984): *Eur. J. Pharmacol.*, 101:57–68.
46. Heym, J., Steinfels, G. F., and Jacobs, B. L. (1982): *Brain Res.*, 251:259–276.
47. Heym, J., Steinfels, G. F., and Jacobs, B. L. (1982): *Eur. J. Pharmacol.*, 81:677–680.
48. Heym, J., Steinfels, G. F., and Jacobs, B. L. (1984): *Brain Res.*, 291:63–72.
49. Heym, J., Trulson, M. E., and Jacobs, B. L. (1981): *Eur. J. Pharmacol.*, 74:117–125.
50. Heym, J., Trulson, M. E., and Jacobs, B. L. (1982): *Brain Res.*, 232:29–39.
51. Hobbs, S. F. (1982): In: *Circulation, Neurobiology and Behavior*, edited by O. A. Smith et al., pp. 216–231. Elsevier, Amsterdam.
52. Hobson, J. A., McCarley, R. W., and Wyzinski, P. W. (1975): *Science*, 189:55–58.
53. Jacobs, B. L. (1984): In: *Hallucinogens: Neurochemical, Behavioral, and Clinical Perspectives*, edited by B. L. Jacobs, pp. 183–202. Raven Press, New York.
54. Jacobs, B. L. (1986): *Prog. Neurobiol.*, 27:183–194.
55. Jacobs, B. L., Heym, J., and Rasmussen, K. (1983): *Eur. J. Pharmacol.*, 90:275–278.
56. Jacobs, B. L., Heym, J., and Steinfels, G. F. (1984): In: *Handbook of Psychopharmacology*, edited by L. L. Iversen et al., pp. 343–395. Plenum Press, New York.
57. Jouvet, M. (1972): *Ergeb. Physiol.*, 64:166–307.
58. Korf, J., Roth, R. H., and Aghajanian, G. K. (1974): *Eur. J. Pharmacol.*, 25:165–169.
59. Langer, S. Z. (1981): *Pharmacol. Rev.*, 32:337–362.
60. Lehnert, H., Reinstein, D. K., Strowbridge, B. W., and Wurtman, R. J. (1981): *Brain Res.*, 303:215–223.
61. Lydic, R., McCarley, R. W., and Hobson, J. A. (1983): *Brain Res.*, 274:365–370.
62. Mason, S. T. (1984): *Catecholamines and Behavior.* Cambridge University Press, Cambridge.
63. McGinty, D. J., and Harper, R. M. (1976): *Brain Res.*, 101:569–575.
64. McGinty, D. J., Harper, R. M., and Fairbanks, M. K. (1974): *Adv. Sleep Res.*, 1:173–216.
65. Miller, J. D., Farber, J., Gatz, P., Roffwarg, H., and German, D. C. (1983): *Brain Res.*, 273:133–141.
66. Moore, S. D., and Guyenet, P. G. (1983): *Brain Res.*, 263:211–222.
67. Morilak, D. A., Fornal, C., Auerbach, S., and Jacobs, B. L. (1985): *Soc. Neurosci. Abstr.*, 11:769.
68. Morilak, D. A., Fornal, C., and Jacobs, B. L. (1986): *Brain Res.* 399:262–270.
68a. Morilak, D. A., Fornal, C. A., and Jacobs, B. L. (1987): *Brain Res. (in press)*.
68b. Morilak, D. A., Fornal, C. A., and Jacobs, B. L. (1987): *Brain Res. (in press)*.
68c. Morilak, D. A., Fornal, C. A., and Jacobs, B. L. (1987): *Brain Res. (in press)*.
69. Mosko, S. S., and Jacobs, B. L. (1976): *Neurosci. Lett.*, 2:195–200.
70. Mosko, S. S., and Jacobs, B. L. (1977): *Brain Res.*, 119:291–303.
71. Obrist, P. A. (1976): *Psychophysiology*, 13:95–107.
72. Orem, J., and Barnes, C. D. (1980): In: *Physiology in Sleep.* Academic Press, New York.
73. Parmeggiani, P. L. (1980): In: *Physiology in Sleep*, edited by J. Orem and C. D. Barnes, pp. 97–143. Academic Press, New York.
74. Rasmussen, K., Heym, J., and Jacobs, B. L. (1984): *Exp. Neurol.*, 83:302–317.
75. Rasmussen, K., and Jacobs, B. L. (1985): *Brain Res.*, 344:240–248.
76. Rasmussen, K., Strecker, R. E., and Jacobs, B. L. (1986): *Brain Res.*, 369:336–340.
77. Rasmussen, K., and Jacobs, B. L. (1986): *Brain Res.*, 371:335–344.
78. Rasmussen, K., Morilak, D. A., and Jacobs, B. L. (1986): *Brain Res.*, 371:324–334.
79. Reiner, P. B. (1984): Doctoral dissertation, University of Pennsylvania.
80. Reiner, P. B. (1985): *Eur. J. Pharmacol.*, 115:249–257.
81. Roberts, D. C. S. (1981): In: *Theory in Psychopharmacology*, edited by S. J. Cooper, pp. 123–148. Academic Press, New York.
82. Roth, K. A., Mefford, I. M., and Barchas, J. D. (1982): *Brain Res.*, 239:417–424.
83. Sakai, K. (1980): In: *The Reticular Formation Revisited*, edited by J. A. Hobson and M. A. B. Brazier, pp. 427–447. Raven Press, New York.
84. Sakai, K., Vanni-Mercier, G., and Jouvet, M. (1983): *Exp. Brain Res.*, 49:311–314.
85. Saller, C. F., and Chiodo, L. A. (1980): *Science*, 210:1269–1271.
86. Sanghera, M. K., and German, D. C. (1983): *J. Neural Transm.*, 57:267–279.
87. Sanghera, M. K., McMillen, B. A., and German, D. C. (1983): *Eur. J. Pharmacol.*, 86:107–110.
88. Sanghera, M. K., Trulson, M. E., and German, D. C. (1984): *Neuroscience*, 12:793–801.
89. Schultz, W., Ruffieux, A., and Aebischer, P. (1983): *Exp. Brain Res.*, 51:377–387.
90. Steinfels, G. F., Heym, J., and Jacobs, B. L. (1981): *Life Sci.*, 29:1435–1442.
91. Steinfels, G. F., Heym, J., Strecker, R. E., and Jacobs, B. L. (1983): *Brain Res.*, 258:217–228.
92. Steinfels, G. F., Heym, J., Strecker, R. E., and Jacobs, B. L. (1983): *Brain Res.*, 279:77–84.
93. Stone, E. A. (1975): In: *Catecholamines and Behavior*, edited by A. J. Friedhoff, pp. 31–72. Plenum, New York.
94. Strecker, R. E., and Jacobs, B. L. (1985): *Brain Res.*, 361:339–350.
95. Strecker, R. E., Steinfels, G. F., and Jacobs, B. L. (1983): *Brain Res.*, 260:317–321.
96. Svensson, T. H., Bunney, B. S., and Aghajanian, G. K. (1975): *Brain Res.*, 92:291–306.
97. Svensson, T. H., and Thoren, P. (1979): *Brain Res.*, 172:174–178.
98. Svensson, T. H., and Usdin, T. (1978): *Science*, 202:1084–1091.
99. Thierry, A. M., Tassin, J. P., Blanc, G., and Glowinski, J. (1976): *Nature*, 263:242–244.
100. Trulson, M. E., Crisp, T., and Howell, G. A. (1982): *Neuropharmacology*, 21:681–686.
101. Trulson, M. E., Heym, J., and Jacobs, B. L. (1981): *Brain Res.*, 215:275–293.
102. Trulson, M. E., and Jacobs, B. L. (1976): *Neuropharmacology*, 15:339–344.
103. Trulson, M. E., and Jacobs, B. L. (1979): *Brain Res.*, 163:135–150.
104. Trulson, M. E., and Jacobs, B. L. (1983): *Neurosci. Lett.*, 36:285–290.
105. Trulson, M. E., Jacobs, B. L., and Morrison, A. R. (1981): *Brain Res.*, 226:75–91.
106. Trulson, M. E., and Preussler, D. W. (1984): *Exp. Neurol.*, 83:367–377.
107. Trulson, M. E., Preussler, D. W., Howell, G. A., and Frederickson, C. J. (1982): *Neuropharmacology*, 21:1045–1050.
108. VanderMaelen, C. P., and Aghajanian, G. K. (1983): *Brain Res.*, 289:109–119.
109. Wang, R. Y., and Aghajanian, G. K. (1977): *Brain Res.*, 132:186–193.
110. Weiss, J. M., and Simson, P. G. (1985): *Psychopharmacol. Bull.*, 21:447–457.
111. Welsh, K. A., and Gold, P. E. (1985): *Behav. Neural Biol.*, 43:119–131.
112. White, F. J., and Wang, R. Y. (1984): *Life Sci.*, 34:1161–1170.
112a. Wilkinson, L. O., Abercrombie, E. D., Rasmussen, K., and Jacobs, B. L. (1987). *Eur. J. Pharmacol. (in press)*.
112b. Wilkinson, L. O., Abercrombie, E. D., and Jacobs, B. L. (1986): *Soc. Neurosci. Abstr.*, 12:1134.
113. Williams, J. T., North, R. A., Shefner, S. A., Nishi, S., and Egan, T. M. (1984): *Neuroscience*, 13:137–156.
114. Woodward, D. J., Moises, H. C., Waterhouse, B. D., Hoffer, B. J., and Freedman, R. (1979): *Fed. Proc.*, 38:2109–2116.

Psychopharmacology:
The Third Generation of Progress,
edited by Herbert Y. Meltzer.
Raven Press, New York © 1987.

CHAPTER 17

Amino Acids and Acetylcholine

Hans C. Fibiger

The past 10 years have generated an explosion in knowledge concerning the anatomy, chemistry, pharmacology and function of neurons that use acetylcholine, γ-aminobutyric acid (GABA), or excitatory amino acids as their neurotransmitters. In fact, on reviewing the chapters in this section, it can be argued that during this decade research on these systems has far outpaced most other facets of modern neuropsychopharmacology. The basic and clinical advances on these transmitter-specific systems are such that they have opened entirely new fields of enquiry.

Research on central cholinergic systems offers perhaps the most dramatic example. Because acetylcholine was the first neurotransmitter to be discovered, it is ironic that information concerning the anatomy of cholinergic neurons lagged far behind other, more recently identified neurotransmitter-specific systems. The development of antibodies to choline acetyltransferase, an enzyme that exists in appreciable amounts only in cholinergic neurons, has dramatically changed this state of affairs, and we now possess rather detailed information about the organization of these neurons. These important anatomical advances have occurred in parallel with major neurochemical and neuropathological discoveries showing that degeneration of cholinergic neurons in the basal forebrain is reliably associated with Alzheimer's disease. This in turn has led to many trials with cholinergic agonists and precursors as potential treatments for Alzheimer's disease, and although to date the results of these trials have been disappointing, there is no question that the information that has been garnered on cholinergic systems during this period will figure prominently in the eventual cure or prevention of this disease.

Major advances have also been made concerning neuronal systems that use amino acids such as glutamate and aspartate as their neurotransmitters. Although it has long been known that these molecules can increase the firing rates of most neurons, not until the last decade has the anatomy of glutamate- and aspartate-releasing neurons begun to be appreciated. During the same period, it has been discovered that the action of glutamate may be mediated by at least four different types of receptors. This has created major

new opportunities to develop agonists and antagonists that are selective for each receptor. The clinical applications of such compounds in psychiatry and neurology are potentially great and will offer many new research opportunities in the coming decade. In addition, these advances have generated new research tools, such as the neurotoxins kainic acid and ibotenic acid, which are enjoying widespread use in basic neurobiological research.

Although GABA is no newcomer to neuropsychopharmacology, research on GABAergic neurons and receptors has generated many important new insights during the past decade. Until 7 or 8 years ago, nearly all that was known about the anatomy of GABAergic systems was based on the effects of lesions on glutamic acid decarboxylase (GAD) activity in various brain nuclei thought to be innervated by the lesioned area. The development of specific antibodies to GAD in the mid-1970s and their subsequent use in immunocytochemical studies have generated information about the anatomy of GABAergic neurons that is substantially more detailed than what could be obtained with the earlier approaches. As a result, today our appreciation of the complex anatomy of the major GABAergic systems in the central nervous system is quite advanced. Knowledge concerning the pharmacology of GABA receptors has also experienced important gains in the past decade. Not only have receptor subtypes been identified, but the interactions between GABA and benzodiazepine receptors have been elucidated in considerable detail. This research has led to the development of new pharmacological tools that are proving useful both in the laboratory and in the clinic. Given the widespread distribution of GABAergic neurons and GABA receptors in the central nervous system, it is perhaps not surprising that abnormalities in the function of GABAergic systems have been implicated in the pathophysiology of a broad variety of diseases, including epilepsy, movement disorders, and affective illness. Although it is too early for consensus to have been reached concerning the degree to which newly developed GABAergic agents are useful in the treatment of these conditions, with the rapidly growing interest in "GABAmimetics," it seems certain that this will be achieved during the next decade.

Psychopharmacology:
The Third Generation of Progress,
edited by Herbert Y. Meltzer.
Raven Press, New York © 1987.

CHAPTER **18**

Biochemistry, Anatomy, and Pharmacology of GABA Neurons

Frode Fonnum

Amino acids are quantitatively probably the most important group of neurotransmitters in mammalian brain. The two best established inhibitory transmitter amino acids are γ-aminobutyric acid (GABA) and glycine. GABA seems to be an important inhibitory transmitter in all parts of the CNS, whereas the inhibitory function of glycine is mainly limited to the medulla and the spinal cord (45). Autoradiography after high-affinity uptake of GABA indicates that as much as 10 to 40% of all terminals in cerebral cortex, hippocampus, and substantia nigra may be GABAergic (79,170). Previously GABA was thought to occur exclusively in the CNS but in recent years small amounts of GABA have also been found in several peripheral tissues.

During the last 10 years the main emphasis on GABA research has been to identify and characterize GABAergic structures in CNS using immunocytochemical methods, to characterize the GABA receptors, and to develop GABAergic drugs (receptor agonists, uptake inhibitors, and GABA-T inhibitors). The use of GABAergic drugs has unveiled several unexpected physiological functions involving GABA. GABA has strong sedative and anticonvulsant effects. In addition it has antinociceptive action, has hypothermic effects, reduces food intake, is involved in antidepression, and has effects on the cardiovascular system. In recent years GABAergic drugs have shown promise as antiepileptic, antispastic, and antidepressive drugs. Furthermore, the anxiolytic properties of benzodiazepines are ascribed to their involvement in the modification of the GABA receptor.

SYNTHESIS, STORAGE, AND RELEASE OF GABA

GABA is synthesized from glutamate by the enzyme glutamate decarboxylase (GAD). This enzyme is concentrated in the nerve terminals, most probably in the cytoplasm (44,165). Immunohistochemical methods have never demonstrated GAD within the synaptic vesicle, although association with membranes can never be disregarded. GABA has never been found concentrated in the synaptosome fraction. It is an open question whether this is due to the redistribution of GABA during homogenization of the tissue or whether this reflects the true situation. Recent experiments have at least detected changes in its subcellular localization during the influence of drugs (60). The concentration of GABA in the GABAergic terminals has been estimated to be 50 to 150 mM (54). A large part of this is probably bound to synaptic vesicles, although satisfactory evidence for this has never been obtained (46). The glutamate concentration in the GABAergic terminal is low since they appear negative in immunohistochemistry with glutamate-like immunoactivity (144,145) and since degeneration of GABAergic terminals results in only small losses of glutamate (46,87,119). The glutamate used for synthesis of GABA is mainly derived from glucose or glutamine (46,189). A significant reduction of glutamine under hypoglycemia does not affect the GABA level to the same extent as it affects the glutamate level (38). This indicates that the levels of both glucose and glutamine required to sustain GABA synthesis are low. After release GABA is taken up into its own nerve terminals or into glial cells by high-affinity uptake systems (50). There are some indications that the release of GABA is autoregulated.

The extracellular level of GABA, as reflected in cerebrospinal fluid (CSF) or in ventricular fluids, is low, probably because of the efficient high-affinity uptake systems (39,65). In the CSF the main part of GABA is found in a conjugated form such as homocarnosine. An artificially high level of GABA is often reported from CSF due to spontaneous formation during handling of the samples (43). An increase of GABA in the brain due to the treatment with GABA-T inhibitors is often reflected as increase of GABA in the CSF (17).

PROPERTIES OF GABA ENZYMES

GAD was first extensively purified and studied by Wu (224). In recent years several different molecular forms of the enzyme have been isolated from different species. In mouse brain high- and low-molecular weight fractions have been identified (225). From porcine brain three forms with slightly different K_m values for glutamate have been separated by isoelectric focusing, phenyl-Sepharose chromatography, or polyacrylamide electrophoresis (181). In rats three forms and in humans two forms have been separated by phenyl-Sepharose chromatography (180).

Several studies have indicated that GAD exists in an apoform and in a holoform with strong binding to pyridoxal phosphate. The holoform of GAD is distributed evenly throughout the CNS regions, whereas the apoform varies considerably, having a high level in GABA-rich regions and a low level in GABA-poor regions (11,136).

In agreement with this concept (36), two forms of GAD differing in their binding to pyridoxal phosphate, temperature sensitivity, and electrophoretic mobility have been separated. Several studies have indicated a regulation of GAD through pyridoxal phosphate binding *in vivo*. Adenosine nucleotides and phosphate ions have been implicated in the regulation (113,115,118,175,178). Recently, in the presence of low pyridoxal phosphate concentration, it has also been shown that 5 to 15 mM GABA will substantially inhibit GAD (152). Such a cytoplasmic concentration may not be unphysiological.

GABA is first metabolized by GABA-T to succinic semialdehyde and then subsequently by succinic semialdehyde dehydrogenase to succinic acid. GABA-T, like all aminotransferases, binds pyridoxal phosphate strongly. Biochemical studies have shown that there is not a clear correlation between GAD and GABA-T levels in different brain regions (41). Likewise, subcellular fractionation has shown that the enzyme is linked to the free mitochondrial fraction and not so markedly to the synaptosomal mitochondria (155,165). Lesions of a major GABAergic tract, i.e., the striatal nigral projection, were accompanied by only small losses of GABA-T in substantia nigra. In contrast, histochemical visualization of GABA-T, 24 hr after treatment with an irreversible GABA-T inhibitor, has proved

very efficient in demonstrating GABAergic structures (209,211). It is difficult to reconcile the biochemical and histochemical localization if GABA-T in GABAergic neurons is not rapidly resynthesized. GABA-T is not specifically localized in GABA-receiving neurons (129).

LOCALIZATION OF GABAERGIC STRUCTURES

Methods for Localization of GABAergic Structures in CNS

In 1970 we succeeded by lesion studies in demonstrating the first specific localization of GAD in inhibitory terminals from mammalian tissue, i.e., Purkinje cells in cerebellum (49). Since then, several GABAergic pathways have been identified by studying the loss of GABAergic parameters accompanying the degeneration of inhibitory terminals in well-defined brain regions. The loss can be studied either biochemically (51), by autoradiography after high-affinity GABA uptake (170), by the immunohistochemical localization of GAD (112), or by the pharmacohistochemical demonstration of GABA-T (211,212). Recently the immunohistochemical localization of GABA has also been made possible (69,187). The immunohistochemical methods have proved very important for the description of GABAergic cells at the light microscopic level and for the description of terminals at the electron microscopic level.

Localization in CNS

Neocortex

There are small variations of GAD or GABA in the different cortical layers (68,77). It is generally agreed that GABA content in neocortex is due almost exclusively to local neurons, since undercutting of the cortex does not reduce GABA parameters (154). Recent immunohistochemical studies have, however, indicated a GABAergic projection from hypothalamus to neocortex (209).

Immunohistocytochemical studies of the morphology of GABAergic cells in neocortex have revealed an abundant variety of stained cells distributed throughout all layers. Most of the cells were aspinous or sparsely spinous stellate cells (144,156). Subsequent Golgi studies indicated basket cells (74) and chandelier cells (158) as GAD immunopositive. In monkey striate cortex all cells in layer I were GABA positive, in other layers only a minority of the cells were GABAergic (178). All GAD-stained boutons are symmetrical and they contain pleomorphic vesicles (179). Recently it has been shown that in several neurons from rat, cat, and monkey cortex GAD coexists with somatostatin (168).

Hippocampus

Biochemical studies have shown a bimodal distribution of GAD with a peak in the pyramidal/granular layer and in the molecular layer of the hippocampal formation (186).

Subsequent lesion studies indicated that almost all GAD activity was due to local neurons (52,185). These findings correlate well with the subsequent immunocytochemical localization of GAD (7,160) or GABA (143), and of [³H]GABA high-affinity uptake (199). The high density of GAD/GABA boutons around the pyramidal/granular cells has been considered evidence for basket cell axon terminals. In addition, Somogyi et al. (178) have also found a type of interneurons distinct from the basket cell, which are responsible for the high density of GABAergic boutons exclusively on the initial segments of the pyramidal cell axons. In hippocampus there is evidence that GAD in some neurons is colocalized with cholecystokinin (206) in the molecular layer and with somatostatin in some cells in subcortical white matter (168).

Basal Ganglia

A lot of attention has been focused on the localization and function of GABA in the basal ganglia due to their involvement in several neurological diseases. The levels of GABA parameters were intermediate in caudate-putamen and high in globus pallidus, entopeduncularis, and substantia nigra (47,49). In caudate-putamen GAD has been shown to be present almost exclusively in local neurons from lesion studies and from the effect of kainic acid (31). The neurons have been identified by immunocytochemical methods for GAD to be fusiform or round in shape with somata of 10 to 20 μm (160). Recently it has been suggested that in half of the GAD cells it coexists with leu- or met-enkephalin (6). In this respect one should remember the immunological overlap between leu-enkephalin and dynorphin. Cells with GABA-like immunoreactivity were found to amount to 10 to 15% of the total cell population and were distributed relatively evenly along the rostrocaudal axis (144,145) in agreement with the distribution of GAD activity (47).

In globus pallidus GAD activity was mainly present as terminals that surround the somata and dendrites. Most of the terminals are of the symmetrical type (157). Lesion studies have shown that GAD activity in globus pallidus arises from the cells in caudate-putamen (47,49,130). Following injection of [³H]GABA in globus pallidus, labeling was observed in subthalamic nucleus, indicating also a GABAergic input from the subthalamic nuclei (131). A lesion in globus pallidus also led to a loss of GAD activity or GABA-T staining in subthalamus, indicating that the pallidal-subthalamic pathways are also GABAergic (48,213).

In entopeduncularis GAD is also mainly derived from cells in neostriatum (47). A lesion in entopeduncularis leads to a loss of GAD in the lateral habenulae (29,61,213), indicating that this pathway is GABAergic.

Most of the GABAergic activity in substantia nigra is derived from the neurons in neostriatum, a minor part from neurons in globus pallidus, and a small amount is due to the local GABAergic cells in substantia nigra reticulata (47,130). Approximately 80% of the terminals in substantia nigra pars compacta are GABAergic, and virtually every soma and dendrite in substantia nigra is associated with GABAergic terminals (161). The GABAergic cells in substantia nigra project to superior colliculus, certain thalamic nuclei, and the tegmental area (see below).

Nucleus accumbens and olfactory tubercle have higher GAD and GABA contents than caudate-putamen. From surgical lesions and kainic acid studies it is concluded that the GABAergic neurons are local interneurons (217). A very high level of GAD was found in "ventral globus pallidus" (53) and this has been confirmed by GABAlike and GADlike immunohistochemical staining (144,148). This activity is mainly due to a GABAergic input from nucleus accumbens and olfactory tubercle (216). Electrolytic destruction of nucleus accumbens was further accompanied by a reduction in GAD activity in the rostromedial substantia nigra (218) and a small reduction in the rostral ventral tegmental area. The latter is in agreement with electrophysiological studies (223) and neurochemical studies (214). In contrast to these authors, Walaas and Fonnum (218) stress that only a small part of the ventral tegmental area receives such a projection from nucleus accumbens.

Thalamus

Thalamus is not particularly rich in GABAergic parameters. In thalamus the nucleus reticularis seems to constitute a major source for GABAergic cells which project fibers to several other thalamic regions (26,73,145). These projections may be important in modulating the thalamic releasing cells. There are also intrinsic GABAergic neurons in the dorsal and ventral lateral nuclei and in the pulvinar (28). This picture has been confirmed by GABA-like immunocytochemistry (144). In the thalamic reticular nucleus GAD seems to coexist with somatostatin (137).

The thalamic region also receives a GABAergic input from neurons in substantia nigra pars reticulata. Lesion studies have shown a decrease of GAD and GABA in the ventromedial and the parafascicular nuclei (37,85,183). It has also been claimed, based on kainic acid injection into entopeduncularis, that the entopeduncular/thalamic fibers are GABAergic (147). The entopeduncular-habenulae fibers have already been dealt with.

Hypothalamus

The hypothalamus is a region rich in GABAergic parameters. The highest levels were found in the preoptic and anterior hypothalamic areas (196). On the basis of deafferentation studies (195) it was concluded that GAD was localized to intrinsic fibers, but other studies (116), on the basis of surgical lesions, have suggested a GABAergic input from nucleus accumbens to the supraoptic nucleus. There are, however, few intrahypothalamic centers of GAD or GABA-T containing neurons. One center includes neurons ventral to the posterior hypothalamus, and a few other smaller cell groups exist in other hypothalamic regions (210), including cells in the nucleus arcuatus and ventral periventricular regions (197). Glutamate treatment (215) suggested that GABAergic arcuate neurons projected to infundibulum. Immunohistochemistry showed GABAergic axon terminals on the dopaminergic tubero in fundibular neurons and therefore suggested GABAergic control of dopaminergic cells in the arcuate-periventricular complex (194). The tuberoinfundibular GAD activity was increased by treatment with estradiol benzoate (132). GABA has been suggested to alter the secretion of many adenohypophysical hormones or hypothalamic hypophysiotropic hormones: adrenocorticophin hormones (21), growth hormones (190), luteinizing hormone (207), and prolactin (99,207,208).

Amygdala

In amygdala GABA is more concentrated in the phylogenetically older nuclei (medial, cortical, and ventral) than the more recently evolved nuclei (lateral and basolateral) (15). Most of the activity belongs to local neurons.

Cerebellum

The Purkinje, stellate, basket, and Golgi cells have been identified as GABAergic from topographical studies, lesion studies, autoradiography of the high-affinity uptake studies, and immunocytochemical studies (51,112,144). In several species the Purkinje cells also were found to contain motilin-like immunoreactivity (23,56,133). In rat Purkinje cells, cystein sulphinic acid decarboxylase has also been found by an immunohistochemical method (24). The enzyme product taurine is also present in a high concentration (103). It is interesting that the content of GABA seems to be higher in the Golgi cell bodies than in the Purkinje cell bodies (143,178).

Medulla

Raphe nuclei contain a relatively high level of GABAergic parameters. The GABAergic activity has been suggested to arise from both interneurons and serotonin (5HT) neurons. A GABAergic input from the lateral habenulae seems to be controversial (13,211). The coexistence of GABA and 5HT in 5HT neurons was concluded from the double immunohistochemical localization of 5HT and GAD in some raphe neurons (14). In addition, several GAD-containing neurons were sensitive to 5,7-dihydroxytryptamine treatment. GABA agonists in the raphe nuclei reduce 5HT turnover in all regions with 5HT nerve terminals (134). This effect is believed to be due to an action of GABAergic interneurons on the serotonergic cells in the raphe nuclei.

The information about GABAergic fibers in other mesencephalic regions is scanty. The periaqueductal gray has a high GAD content, which is decreased after medial hypothalamic lesions (166). The eye motor nuclei were found possibly to receive a GABAergic input from the superior vestibular nuclei (163).

A considerable amount of work has been done with neurotransmitter distribution in the cochlear nucleus. Recent work (128) on the immunocytochemistry of GAD shows that the cartwheel, the stellate, and possibly the Golgi cells are GABAergic. In layer 1 the displayed Purkinje cells are also GABAergic (128).

The cardiopulmonary afferents terminate in nucleus tractus solitarius. This region heavily innervates neurons in the rostral ventral medulla (rVL), including the adrenergic cell group, and in the caudal ventrolateral medulla (cVL), overlapping the noradrenergic Al group. In rVL GABA or muscimol reduced the arterial pressure whereas bicuculline elevated it. In cVL the effects were opposite (83,222,228). In nucleus tractus solitarius the distribution of GABA and GAD has been described in detail (106,219). In cVL the GAD neurons were found to be intrinsic (164).

Spinal Cord

GAD-immunoreactive terminals are concentrated in laminae I–III and a moderate number are distributed in other areas of gray matter (59,111). It is generally assumed that these terminals are supplied by short axon intraspinal neurons because GABA was not reduced by dorsal rhizotomy (191) or by transection of the spinal cord (198). It is therefore believed that GABAergic terminals mediate presynaptic inhibition of primary afferent terminals (8), and that GABA interneurons are involved in postsynaptic inhibition of interneurons.

Localization of GABA in Peripheral Tissue

Low levels of GABA were detected in the kidney and other peripheral organs by Zackerman et al. (226). In high concentrations GAD and GABA were first detected in flounder erythrocytes where they may be involved in osmotic regulation (58). Mammalian peripheral organs with high levels of GABA or GAD are the β cells of the pancreatic islets (138), the pituitary gland (12,137), and the fallopian tube (5,40,108). The simultaneous loss of immunohistochemically stained GAD and insulin after treatment with alloxan and the β-cell toxin streptozotogin provided evidence for their coexistence in the β cells (213). The functions of GABA in these tissues are, however, not understood. Low concentrations of GABA were found in the gut, where it was concentrated in Auerbach's plexus (80,117,193), and in the ovary (109). Except in the fallopian tube, the GAD in peripheral tissue did not cross-react immunologically with the brain GAD enzyme (5).

In most peripheral organs GAD cannot be assayed from $^{14}CO_2$ produced from 1-[^{14}C]glutamate. This is due to the decarboxylation of glutamate through other metabolic pathways. The use of a high-speed supernatant of an extract may reduce the alternative metabolic pathways.

Differentiation Between GABA Uptake and Receptor Sites

GABA is a flexible molecule that can occur in several different conformational forms and thereby bind to different target molecules such as uptake sites or receptor sites. There are at least two different high-affinity uptake sites and two different GABAergic receptor sites: one postsynaptic, responsible for the inhibitory effect of GABA (GABA$_A$ receptor), and one presynaptic, regulating the release of other transmitters such as glutamate and monoamines (GABA_B receptor). By synthesizing molecules with restricted conformation it has been possible to obtain molecules with specific affinity for each of the four sites. Flexible molecules such as homo-β-proline and 3-hydroxy GABA have an affinity for all four sites (91). Restricted molecules such as isonipecotic acid, isoguavacine, P-4S, and 4,5,6,7-tetra-hydroiso-xazolo[5,4-C]pyridin-3-ol (THIP) have only ago-nistic properties towards the GABA_A receptor. Extensive structure-activity studies indicated that at this receptor GABA interacts in a partially extended and almost planar form (92). A slightly different position of the nitrogen molecule in the ring of the related nipecotic acids and guavacine made these compounds uptake inhibitors for both glial and neuron cell uptake (89). It is in this context interesting to note that of the two stereoisomers of 4-(Me)-trans-4-amino-pent-2-enoic acid (ACA) one is a GABA agonist whereas the other is an uptake inhibitor (91). β-Alanine and diaminobutyric acid are substrates for the glial and neuronal uptake, respectively, indicating that the two uptake sites react with GABA in a short and extended conformation, respectively (78). 4-Hydroxynipecotic acid and 4,5,6,7-tetrahydroiso-xazolo[4,5-C]pyridin-3-ol (THPO) have been found to be specific glial uptake inhibitors (90). The GABA_B receptor is bicuculline insensitive and the most potent and selective agonist is R-(−)-baclophen (19). This receptor does not bind isoguavacine, P4S, and THIP, whereas the GABA_A receptor does not bind baclophen (66).

GABA Receptor

Virtually all neurons are sensitive to GABA, and GABA receptors are distributed all over the brain. If all neurons in the CNS contain the same type of GABA receptor, administration of GABA agonists or antagonists would affect the entire CNS, and any therapy based on their action would therefore be impossible due to the widespread effects. Fortunately, there is increasing evidence for at least a small degree of heterogeneity among GABA receptors. As discussed above, the receptors can first be separated into bicuculline-sensitive (GABA_A) (33,34) and bicuculline-insensitive (GABA_B) receptors. The GABA_A receptor may be subdivided into synaptic and extrasynaptic receptors, which hyperpolarize and depolarize neurons, respectively (1,4). The two receptors differ in their affinity for different agonists. THIP, which acts preferentially at the synaptic receptors, has therefore a more efficient hyperpolarizing action at the pyramidal cell layer of hippocampus and cells at the spinal cord than a depolarizing action at the spinal roots (1,3). There are also examples of GABA receptors in neurohypophysis and spinal cord that have different speci-ficities toward different agonists (110).

Binding studies have also revealed multiple GABA re-ceptors with various affinities for GABA in the brain. High-, low-, and perhaps intermediate-affinity receptor sites have been suggested from Scatchard plots, polyphasic as-sociation, or disassociation studies, as well as from thermal inactivation (42,139,140,141). According to a model by Olsen and Snowman (142) the three binding sites are linked to the opening of the chloride channel and are intercon-vertible by the action of different drugs. It is interesting that a chemical modification of the GABA receptors with p-diazobenzenesulphonic acid and tetramethionine selec-tively eliminates the low-affinity sites (22,105) and that the chaotrophic anion thiocyanate eliminates the high-affinity GABA sites (20,105). The low-affinity GABA receptor has been suggested to have a hydrophobic accessory site that is critical for the binding of antagonist. In agreement, Triton-X-100 converts the low-affinity GABA binding site to a high-affinity site (94). Cl⁻, on the other hand, is said to mask the high-affinity binding site (104).

The affinity of GABA to membrane fractions is highly dependent on the preparation of the fraction. A variety of possible endogenous inhibitors, of which the best known is GABA-modulin (204), appear to exist. It may well be that these endogenous inhibitors can modulate the receptor interactions *in vivo*.

The GABA_A receptor is closely associated with the chlo-ride ionophore. The ionophore has several different sites, which include a binding site for the convulsive agents picrotoxin, dihydropicrotoxin, or t-butylbicyclophosphoro-thionates (93,139), a group of potential insecticides (93). Barbiturates inhibit the binding of dihydropicrotoxin (182,201,202) and increase the binding of GABA and benzodiazepine agonists (139,201). The interaction of bar-biturates with the picrotoxin sites seems to prolong the duration of the channel opening for chloride (188).

The anticonvulsive effect of pentobarbitals can be blocked by bicuculline, whereas the hypnotic effect is not (153). In the same way it is possible to differentiate between the different physiological effects of optically active isomers of barbiturates. As an example (S+) and (R−) isomers of 1-methyl-5-phenylbarbituric acid display convulsive and de-pressing effects, respectively. The different effects could be due to the fact that the (S+) isomer interacted directly with the picrotoxin site whereas (R−) interacted allosterically (203) with this site.

Avermectin B_{1a}, a powerful antihelmintic and insecticide, also enhances the binding of GABA and benzodiazepine receptor agonists (151). Its site of action and binding to the picrotoxin site appears to be different from that of barbi-turates (142,221). It causes an irreversible and prolonged opening of the chloride channels (57).

Benzodiazepines bind to a receptor site different from the picrotoxin site. Benzodiazepines also increase the binding of GABA to the low-affinity GABA binding site (177). Benzodiazepines act by increasing the frequency of the opening of the chloride channel with little effect on the open-channel lifetime (188).

The GABA_B receptor agonists depress the firing frequency of neurons in most areas of the brain. They modulate monoamine release in the CNS and at the autonomic nerve terminals at the periphery (18). There is some evidence that the GABA_B receptor may be involved in neurodepres-sion (97) and in spasticity.

GABA Dysfunction

From the wide distribution of GABAergic terminals in the brain, one would expect that dysfunction in the GABA system may cause several different physiological effects or symptoms. There are numerous examples where specific localized changes in the GABA system are associated with pathology. In Huntington's chorea there is a significant and well-established reduction of the GABA level in the basal ganglia (16,150). Another violent chorea is hemiballismus, which involves a deficiency in the GABAergic system in subthalamic nuclei and globus pallidus (48). There are several reports of a decrease in GABAergic parameters in the basal ganglia or in the lumbar CSF of untreated patients with Parkinson's disease. During L-dopa therapy the levels are reported to return to normal (71,95,107,200). The neurobiology of epilepsy is complicated, but GABA and acidic amino acids are most certainly involved in the pathology. It may well be that epilepsy is a symptom arising from different origins. In some cases the causative agent is a decrease in GABA, in other cases there is an increase of the excitatory amino acids. Several animal models for epilepsy show a decrease in GABA or GAD at the epileptic foci (159) (for review see 220). Some human samples from around the foci also show a decrease (205) of GABA.

GABAergic agonists (see below) are often effective in treatment of spasticity. This may be explained by an effect on presynaptic inhibition of the monosynaptic reflex in the spinal cord. This could be due to a reduction of the release of the excitatory amino acids from the primary afferents.

Several studies have shown that GABA-T inhibitors can induce a dose-related and long-lasting decrease in food intake (30,75). It is difficult, however, to differentiate between the effect of sedation and food intake. The antinociceptive effect of GABA, GABA agonist, and GABA-T inhibitors is naloxone and bicuculline insensitive (27,67). It may be due to an interaction between GABA and acetylcholine since the effect is atropine sensitive and potentiated by physostigmine (63).

The monoamines occupy a central position in the study of the mechanism and treatment of depression. GABA has, however, been found to be low in the CSF (four of six studies) and in the plasma (six of six studies) of depressed patients (summary in ref. 96). Recently it has also been shown that several antidepressive drugs increase the number of GABA_B receptors (97). Evidence is therefore accumulating that GABA is involved in depression (126).

GABAergic Drugs

GABA Agonists

Progabide (SL 76002) and other SL-analogs. The phenyl groups and the amide form of progabide enhance the passage through the blood-brain barrier. The compound is slowly metabolized in the brain by amidation or by cleavage of the imine group. Progabide has a short onset of action and therefore probably acts in the progabide form and not as a metabolite. The compound acts as a GABA agonist probably at both the GABA_A and GABA_B receptors. It displaces GABA and muscimol from brain membrane fractions and depresses the firing of the cells on the dorsal Deiters' nucleus. The action of progabide is blocked by picrotoxin and bicuculline (9,10).

Progabide is said to be effective as an anticonvulsant in several animal models of convulsion (227). There are also several studies showing it to be beneficial in certain forms of epilepsy (124,127). In other cases the results are negative (35,169). Progabide has been found to be effective in several clinical trials for spastic patients (122). In particular, progabide had a significant effect on many of the symptoms in patients suffering spasticity from multiple sclerosis.

More surprising has been the suggestion that progabide, in a bicuculline-dependent manner, displays a profile simulating tricyclic antidepressant in behavior tests. In an open pilot study (125) and later in a multicentric double-blind study of patients with major depressive disorders, progabide behaved as effectively as imipramine (126). Progabide in this case probably acts by increasing norepinephrine (NE) turnover and decreasing 5HT transmission (96–98).

Progabide has been shown to have at least three different actions in the basal ganglia: reduction in dopamine (DA) release, antagonism of the neuroleptic-induced increase of DA receptor density, and an action beyond the DA synapse (9,10). Repeated administration of progabide together with neuroleptics has been claimed to reduce the enhancement of DA receptor density, the supersensitivity to dopaminomimetics, and the tolerance to catalepsy (9,10,98). In two open studies with patients progabide was claimed to give good results in about 70% of neuroleptic-induced tardive dyskinesia (176). The results of progabide with L-dopa-induced dyskinesia in Parkinson's patients appear controversial (9).

Progabide did not have anxiolytic properties and had little effect in patients with Huntington's disease (125).

THIP and muscimol-like compounds. THIP is a specific GABA agonist with little effect on GABA uptake or other GABAergic parameters such as enzymes (90). Although it is less active than muscimol as a GABA agonist *in vitro*, it is not metabolized by GABA-T and is present in brain in much higher concentration than muscimol after administration of equal doses (123).

The anticonvulsant effect of THIP is well established through several animal models (101,114,120). So far little effect of THIP has been found in trials with epileptic patients (146). In spastic patients THIP reduced the flexor reflex threshold significantly (121). THIP has been found ineffective in a clinical trial with four patients with classical Huntington's chorea (55).

THIP has also been found to induce analgesic effects in different animal models. For this purpose THIP has been applied to postoperative patients and patients with malignant pain (86). THIP has also been used to reduce anxiety in several patients (70). The side effects—sedation and ataxia—have so far limited the use of THIP in clinical testing (70).

GABA-T Inhibitors

γ-Vinyl GABA. γ-Vinyl GABA seems to be one of the most attractive GABA-T inhibitors since it can be used orally and since it has a fairly specific action (81).

It is an anticonvulsant agent in some animal models (64). There have been several trials with epileptic patients where γ-vinyl GABA has had a positive effect

(19,62,162,167). There were no effects on six patients with Huntington's chorea (171).

γ-Vinyl GABA has been found to reduce dyskinesia in three studies. In one study the patients were drug free for 4 weeks prior to the study and no adverse effects were reported (192). In the other two studies γ-vinyl GABA was given together with the patients' neuroleptic regime, and adverse effects were reported in patients with Parkinson's disease or with senile dementia (72,88).

Isoniazide. Isoniazide is metabolized in the liver to hydrazine, an inhibitor of GABA-T. Since hydrazine reacts with pyridoxal phosphate, the compound is administered together with pyridoxine. It has been shown that isoniazide treatment (900 mg/day + pyridoxine 100 mg/day for 4 weeks) increased both the free GABA and the conjugated GABA in the CSF in Huntington's patients (107). One patient treated with isoniazide for 13 months died of suicide with barbiturate. The GABA levels, and particularly homocarnosine, were found to be high in all brain regions in this patient (150). Isoniazide for 4 months or more did not improve the voluntary movements in Huntington's patients, but was claimed to improve the psychiatric situation in some patients (184).

GABA Uptake Inhibitors

A way of enhancing the GABAergic action is to prevent its uptake from the synaptic cleft. Uptake inhibitors have been shown to enhance the depressant action of GABA on spinal neurons, cerebellar, and cerebral cortex neurons (34). A glial uptake inhibitor would increase the reuptake into the nerve terminals and it would therefore be expected to be a better anticonvulsant than a nerve terminal uptake inhibitor (32). THPO, which is a weak blood-brain barrier penetrant, is a specific glial uptake blocker and seems to protect rodents against convulsions. In addition, other modified uptake inhibitors, esters of nipecotic acid, produced similar results (32). When THPO was administered with glycine it protected mice against mercaptopropionic-acid-induced convulsions (174). This is very surprising since mercaptopropionic acid is a specific inhibitor of GAD and should only affect the GABA level (82). This synergistic anticonvulsant effect of glycine and GABAergic compounds has previously been observed with both GABA-T inhibitors and muscimol (172,173).

A group of lipophilic GABA uptake inhibitors has recently been synthesized by introduction of a bulky 4,4-diphenyl-3-butenyl group to the classical GABA uptake inhibitors such as nipecotic acid (2). These compounds were 10 times more efficient than the parent nipecotic acid *in vitro* and much better *in vivo* (100,229). The compounds have both anticonvulsant and antinociceptic effects.

Valproic acid. Valproic acid (VPA) is known as an antiepileptic agent. Its action has for many years been believed to be due to an increase of GABA due to an inhibition of succinic semialdehyde dehydrogenase (76). Valproate also potentiates the depression of neuronal firing by GABA and muscimol (84). In anticonvulsive doses VPA has a rapid onset that cannot easily be explained by an elevation in total brain GABA. It has, however, been shown that the synaptosomal increase of GABA by valproate occurs at a dose and time course in accordance with its anticonvulsive action (102). There is also a marked increase of CSF GABA in epileptic patients in response to valproate treatment (101). Other studies are interpreted to show that valproate has a primary effect on receptors and secondary effects on amino acid metabolism (25). Interestingly, valproate decreases aspartate with a time course similar to that of its anticonvulsant action.

CONCLUDING REMARKS

During the last 5 years we have seen a rapid proliferation of drugs designed to have an action on the GABA system. Several of these show great promise in treatment of epilepsy, spasticity, anxiety, and depression. Due to the widespread action of the GABA system, adverse effects such as sedation are a problem. We already have a good description of the localization of the GABA system in the brain. More and more we are seeing examples of coexistence between GABA and peptides in one neuron. Future work should try to take advantage of these findings to study the possible interaction between peptides and GABA. This may be a way of obtaining GABAergic drugs with more specific action within one brain region or brain system and therefore with fewer adverse effects.

REFERENCES

1. Alger, B. E., and Nicholl, R. A. (1982): *J. Physiol. (Lond.),* 328: 125–141.
2. Ali, F. E., Bondinell, W. E., Dandridge, P. A., Frazee, J. S., Garvey, E., Gerard, G. R., Kaiser, C., Ku, T. W., Lafferty, J. J., Moonsammy, G. I., Oh, H.-Y., Rush, J. A., Seller, P. E., Stringer, O. D., Venslawsky, J. W., Volpe, B. W., and Yunger, L. M. (1985): *J. Med. Chem.,* 28:653–660.
3. Allan, R. D., Evans, R. H., and Johnston, G. A. R. (1980): *Br. J. Pharmacol.,* 70:609–618.
4. Andersen, P., Dingledine, R., Gjerstad, L., Langmoen, I. A., and Mosfeldt Laursen, A. M. (1980): *J. Physiol. (Lond.),* 305:279–296.
5. Apud, J. A., Tappaz, M. L., and Celotti, F., Negri-Cesi, P., Masotto, C., and Racagni, G. (1984): *J. Neurochem.,* 43:120–125.
6. Aronin, N., DiFiglia, M., Graveland, G. A. A., Schwartz, W. J., and Wu, J.-Y. (1984): *Brain Res.,* 300:376–380.
7. Barber, R. P., and Saito, K. C. (1976): In: *GABA in Nervous System Function,* edited by E. Roberts, T. N. Chase, and D. B. Tower, pp. 113–132. Raven Press, New York.
8. Barber, R. P., Vaughn, J. E., Saitio, K., McLaughlin, B., and Roberts, E. (1978): *Brain Res.,* 141:35–55.
9. Bartholini, F. (1984): *Neurosci. Lett.,* 47:351–355.
10. Bartholini, G., Scatton, B., Zirkov, B., Lloyd, K. G., Deportene, H., Langer, S. Z., and Morselli, P. L. (1985): In: *L.E.R.S., Vol. 3,* edited by G. Bartholini, H. Langer, and K. G. Lloyd, pp. 1–30. Raven Press, New York.
11. Bayón, A., Possani, L. D., Tapia, M., and Tapia, R. (1977): *J. Neurochem.,* 29:519–525.
12. Beart, P. M., Kelly, J. D., and Schon, F. (1974): *Biochem. Soc. Trans.,* 2:266–268.
13. Belin, M. F., Aguera, M., Tappaz, M., McRae-Deguerre, A., Babilier, P., and Peyot, J. F. (1979): *Brain Res.,* 170:279–297.
14. Belin, M. F., Nanopoulos, D., Didier, M., Aguera, M., Steinbusch, H., Verkofstad, A., Maitre, M., and Peyot, J. E. (1983): *Brain Res.,* 275:329–341.
15. Ben-Ari, Y., Kanazawa, I., and Zigmond, R. E. (1976): *J. Neurochem.,* 26:1279–1283.

16. Bird, E. D., and Iversen, L. L. (1974): *Brain,* 97:457–472.
17. Böhlen, P., Huot, D., and Palfreyman, M. G. (1979): *Brain Res.,* 167:297–305.
18. Bowry, N. G., Hill, D. R., Hudson, A. L., Dodd, D. S., Middlemiss, D. N., Shaw, J., and Turnbull, M. (1980): *Nature,* 283:92–94.
19. Browne, T. R., Mattson, R. H., Napoliello, M. J., Penry, J. K., Smith, D. B., Treiman, D. M., and Wilder, B. J. (1984): *Neurology,* 33:434–448.
20. Browner, M., Ferkany, J. W., and Enna, S. J. (1981): *J. Neurosci.,* 1:514–518.
21. Buckingham and Hodges (1979): *J. Physiol. (Lond.),* 290:421–431.
22. Burch, T. P., Thyagarajan, R., and Ticker, M. L. (1983): *Mol. Pharmacol.,* 23:52–59.
23. Chan-Palay, V., Lin, C.-T., Palay, S., Yamamoto, M., and Wu, J.-Y. (1982): *Proc. Natl. Acad. Sci. USA,* 79:2695–2699.
24. Chan-Palay, V., Nilaver, G., Palay, S., Beinfeld, M. C., Zimmermann, E. A., Wu, J.-Y., and Donohue, T. L. (1981): *Proc. Natl. Acad. Sci. USA,* 78:7787–7791.
25. Chapman, A. G., Riley, K., Evans, M. C., and Meldrum, B. S. (1982): *Neurochem. Res.,* 7:1087–1105.
26. Chara, P. T., Lieberman, A. R., Hurt, S. P., and Wu, J.-Y. (1983): *Neuroscience,* 8:189–211.
27. Christensen, A. V., and Larsen, J. J. (1982): *Pol. J. Pharmacol. Pharm.,* 34:127–134.
28. Cohen et al. (1987): *(to be published).*
29. Contestabile, A., and Fonnum, F. (1983): *Brain Res.,* 275:287–297.
30. Cooper, B. R., Howard, J. L., White, H. L., Scroka, F., Ingold, K., and Maxwell, R. A. (1980): *Life Sci.,* 26:1997–2002.
31. Coyle, J. T., McGeer, E. G., McGeer, P. L., and Schwarcz, R. (1978): In: *Kainic Acid as a Tool in Neurobiology,* edited by E. G. McGeer, J. W. Olney, and P. L. McGeer, pp. 139–161. Raven Press, New York.
32. Croucher, M. J., Meldrum, B. S., and Krogsgaard-Larsen, P. (1983): *Eur. J. Pharmacol.,* 89:217–228.
33. Curtis, D. R., Duggan, A. W., Felix, D., Johnston, G. A. R., and McLennan, H. (1971): *Brain Res.,* 70:493–499.
34. Curtis, D. R., Game, C. J. A., and Lodge, D. (1976): *Exp. Brain. Res.,* 25:413–428.
35. Dam, M., Gram, L., Philbert, A., Hansen, B. S., Blatt Lyon, B., Christensen, J. M., and Angelo, H. R. (1983): *Epilepsia,* 24:127–134.
36. Denner, L. A., and Wu, J.-Y. (1985): *J. Neurochem.,* 44:957–965.
37. DiChiara, G., Porceddu, M. L., Morelli, M., Mulas, M. S., and Gessa, G. L. (1979): *Brain Res.,* 176:273–284.
38. Engelsen, B. A., and Fonnum, F. (1984): *Neurosci. Lett.,* 42:317–322.
39. Engelsen, B. A., Fosse, V. M., Myrseth, E., and Fonnum, F. (1985): *Neurosci. Lett.,* 62:97–102.
40. Erdö, S. L., Rosdy, B., and Szporny, L. (1982): *J. Neurochem.,* 38:1174–1176.
41. Fahn, S. (1976): In: *GABA in Nervous System Function,* edited by E. Roberts, T. N. Chase, and T. B. Tower, pp. 169–186. Raven Press, New York.
42. Falch, E., and Krogsgaard-Larsen, P. (1982): *J. Neurochem.,* 38:1123–1129.
43. Ferraro, T. N., Maniyama, B. N., and Hare, T. A. (1983): *J. Neurochem.,* 41:1057–1066.
44. Fonnum, F. (1968): *Biochem. J.,* 106:401–412.
45. Fonnum, F. (1978): *Amino Acids as Chemical Transmitters.* Plenum Press, New York.
46. Fonnum, F. (1986): In: *Neurochemical Methods, Vol. 2,* edited by A. Boulton and J. D. Wood, pp. 201–237.
47. Fonnum, F., Grofova, I., and Gottesfeld, Z. (1978): *Brain Res.,* 143:125–138.
48. Fonnum, F., Grofova, I., and Rinvik, E. (1978): *Brain Res.,* 153:370–374.
49. Fonnum, F., Grofova, I., Rinvik, E., Storm-Mathisen, J., and Walberg, F. (1974): *Brain Res.,* 71:77–92.
50. Fonnum, F., Lund Karlsen, R., Malthe-Sørenssen, D., Sterri, S., and Walaas, I. (1980): In: *The Cell Surface and Neuronal Function,* edited by C. W. Cotman, F. Poste, and G. L. Nickolson, pp. 455–504. Elsevier, Amsterdam.
51. Fonnum, F., Storm-Mathisen, J., and Walberg, F. (1970): *Brain Res.,* 20:259–275.
52. Fonnum, F., and Walaas, I. (1978): *J. Neurochem.,* 31:1173–1181.
53. Fonnum, F., Walaas, I., and Iversen, E. (1977): *J. Neurochem.,* 29:221–230.
54. Fonnum, F., and Walberg, F. (1973): *Brain Res.,* 54:115–127.
55. Foster, N. L., Chase, T. N., Denaro, A., Hare, T. A., and Tamminga, C. A. (1983): *Neurology,* 33:637–639.
56. Fratta, W., Panula, P., Yang, H.-Y. T., and Costa, E. (1985): *Brain Res.,* 171–175.
57. Fritz, L. C., Wang, C. C., and Gorio, A. (1979): *Proc. Natl. Acad. Sci. USA,* 76:2062–2066.
58. Fugelli, F., Storm-Mathisen, J., and Fonnum, F. (1970): *Nature,* 228:1001.
59. Fuji, K., Senba, E., Fujui, S., Nømura, I., Wu, J.-Y., Ileda, Y., and Tohyama, M. (1985): *Neuroscience,* 14:881–894.
60. Geddes, J. W., and Wood, J. B. (1984): *J. Neurochem.,* 42:16–24.
61. Gottesfeld, Z., Massari, V. J., Mutt, E. A., and Jakobowitz, D. M. (1977): *Brain Res.,* 130:184–189.
62. Gram, L., Klosterskov, P., and Dam, M. (1985): *Ann. Neurol.,* 17:262–266.
63. Grognet, A., Hertz, F., and DeFeudis, F. V. (1983): *Gen. Pharmacol.,* 14:585–589.
64. Hammond, E. J., and Wilder, B. J. (1983): *Clin. Neuropharmacol.,* 8:1–12.
65. Hare, T. A., and Wood, J. H. (1985): In: *Handbook of Neurochemistry, Vol. 4,* 2nd ed., edited by A. Lajhta, pp. 421–448. Plenum Press, New York.
66. Hill, D. R., and Bowry, N. G. (1981): *Nature,* 290:149–152.
67. Hill, R. C., Maurer, R., Buescher, H.-H., and Roemer, D. (1981): *Eur. J. Pharmacol.,* 69:221–224.
68. Hirsch, H. E., and Robins, E. (1962): *J. Neurochem.,* 9:63–70.
69. Hodgson, A. J., Penke, B., Erdei, A., Chubb, I. W., and Somogyi, P. (1985): *J. Histochem. Cytochem.,* 33:229–239.
70. Hoehn-Saric, R. (1983): *Psychopharmacology,* 80:338–341.
71. Hornykiewicz, O., Lloyd, K. G., and Davidson, L. (1976): In: *GABA System Function,* edited by E. Roberts, T. N. Chase, and D. B. Tower, pp. 479–485. Raven Press, New York.
72. Hosoya, R., Muva, M., Nishamura, K., and Yamamoto, T. (1981): *N. Engl. J. Med.,* 305:381–382.
73. Houser, C. R., Hendry, S. H. C., Jones, E. G., and Vaughn, J. E. (1983): *J. Neurocytol.,* 12:617–638.
74. Houser, C. R., Vaughn, J. E., Barber, R. P., and Roberts, E. (1980): *Brain Res.,* 200:341–354.
75. Howard, J. L., Cooper, B. R., Whitt, H. L., Soroka, F. E., and Maxwell, R. A. (1980): *Brain Res.,* 5:52–56.
76. Iadarola, M. J., Raines, A., and Gale, K. (1979): *J. Neurochem.,* 33:1119–1125.
77. Ishikawa, K., Watabe, S., and Goto, N. (1983): *Brain Res.,* 277:361–364.
78. Iversen, L. L. (1978): In: *Psychopharmacology: A Generation of Progress,* edited by M. A. Lipton, A. DiMascio, and K. F. Killam, pp. 25–37. Raven Press, New York.
79. Iversen, L. L., and Bloom, F. E. (1972): *Brain Res.,* 41:131–143.
80. Jessen, K. R., Mirsky, R., Dennison, M. E., and Burnstock, G. (1979): *Nature,* 281:71–74.
81. Jung, M. J., Lippert, B., Metcalf, B. W., Böhlen, P., and Schechter, P. J. (1977): *J. Neurochem.,* 29:787–802.
82. Karlsson, A., Fonnum, F., Malthe-Sørenssen, D., and Storm-Mathisen, J. (1975): *Biochem. Pharmacol.,* 23:3053–3061.
83. Keeler, J. R., Schultz, C. W., Chase, T. N., and Hilke, C. J. (1984): *Brain Res.,* 197:217–224.
84. Kerwin, R. W., Olpe, H.-R., and Schmutz, M. (1980): *Br. J. Pharmacol.,* 71:545–550.
85. Kilpatrick, I. C., Starr, M. S., Fletcher, A., James, T. A., and McLeod, N. K. (1980): *Exp. Brain Res.,* 40:45–54.
86. Kjaer, M., and Nielsen, H. (1983): *Br. J. Clin. Pharmacol.,* 16:477–485.
87. Korf, J., and Venema, K. (1983): *J. Neurochem.,* 40:1171–1173.

88. Korsgaard, S., Casey, D. E., and Gerlach, J. (1983): *Psychiatric Res.*, 8:261–271.
89. Krogsgaard-Larsen, G. A. R., Curtis, D. R., Game, C. J. A., and McCulloch, R. M. (1975): *J. Neurochem.*, 35:803–809.
90. Krogsgaard-Larsen, P. (1981): *J. Med. Chem.*, 24:1377–1383.
91. Krogsgaard-Larsen, P., Falch, E., Schousboe, A., and Curtis, D. R. (1986): In: *Neurotransmitters, Seizures, and Epilepsy III*, edited by G. Nustrico, J. Engel, R. G. Farello, K. G. Lloyd, and P. L. Morselli, pp. 135–150. Raven Press, New York.
92. Krogsgaard-Larsen, P., Johnston, G. A. R., Lodge, D., and Curtis, D. R. (1977): *Nature*, 268:53–55.
93. Lawrence, L. J., and Casida, J. E. (1983): *Science*, 221:1399–1401.
94. Lloyd, K. G., and Davidson, L. (1979): *Science*, 205:1147–1149.
95. Lloyd, K. G., and Hornykiewitcz, O. (1975): *Nature*, 243:521–523.
96. Lloyd, K. G., and Pichat, P. (1987): In: *New Academic Psychotherapy Drug Research*, edited by S. Dahl, S. M. Paul, and W. Bradley (*in press*).
97. Lloyd, K. G., Thuret, F., and Pilc, A. (1985): *J. Pharmacol. Ther.*, 235:191–199.
98. Lloyd, K. G., and Worms, P. (1980): In: *Long-Term Effects of Neuroleptics*, edited by F. Cattabeni, G. Racagni, P. F. Spano, and E. Costa, pp. 253–258. Raven Press, New York.
99. Locatelli, D., Cocchi, D., Cattabeni, F., Maggi, A., Krogsgaard-Larsen, P., and Müller, E. E. (1978): *Brain Res.*, 145:173–179.
100. Löscher, W. (1985): *Eur. J. Pharmacol.*, 110:103–105.
101. Löscher, W., Frey, H.-H., Reiche, R., and Schultz, D. (1983): *J. Pharmacol. Exp. Ther.*, 226:839–844.
102. Löscher, W., and Vetter, M. (1985): *Biochem. Pharmacol.*, 34:1747–1756.
103. Madsen, S., Ottersen, O. P., and Storm-Mathisen, J. (1985): *Neurosci. Lett.*, 60:255–260.
104. Madthes, A., Jr. (1984): *J. Neurochem.*, 43:1434–1437.
105. Maksay, G., and Tichu, M. K. (1984): *J. Neurochem.*, 43:261–269.
106. Maley, B. E., and Newton, B. W. (1985): *Brain Res.*, 330:364–368.
107. Manyam, B. V. (1982): *Arch. Neurol.*, 39:391–392.
108. Martin del Rio, R. (1981): *J. Biol. Chem.*, 193:265–278.
109. Martin del Rio, R., and Latorre Caballero, A. (1980): *J. Neurochem.*, 34:1584–1586.
110. Mathison, R. D., and Dreifuss, J. J. (1980): *Brain Res.*, 187:476–480.
111. McLaughlin, B. J., Barber, R., Saito, K., Roberts, E., and Wu, J.-Y. (1975): *J. Comp. Neurobiol.*, 169:305–322.
112. McLaughlin, B. J., Wood, J. G., Saito, K., Barber, R., Vaughn, J. E., Roberts, E., and Wu, J.-Y. (1974): *Brain Res.*, 76:377–395.
113. Meley, M. P., and Martin, D. L. (1983): *Cell. Mol. Neurobiol.*, 3:39–56.
114. Meldrum, B., and Horton, R. (1980): *Eur. J. Pharmacol.*, 61:231–237.
115. Meley, M. P., and Martin, D. L. (1983): *Cell. Mol. Neurobiol.*, 3:58–68.
116. Meyer, D. K., Oertel, W. H., and Brownstein, M. J. (1980): *Brain Res.*, 200:165–168.
117. Miki, Y., Taniyama, K., Tanaka, C., and Tobe, T. (1983): *J. Neurochem.*, 40:861–865.
118. Miller, L. P., Martin, D. L., Mazumder, A., and Walters, J. R. (1978): *J. Neurochem.*, 30:361–370.
119. Minchin, M. C. W., and Fonnum, F. (1979): *J. Neurochem.*, 32:203–209.
120. Minchin, M. C. W., and Nutt, D. J. (1983): *Br. J. Pharmacol. Soc.*, 78:10.
121. Mondrup, K., and Pedersen, E. (1983): *Acta Neurol. Scand.*, 67:48–54.
122. Mondrup, K., and Pedersen, E. (1984): *Acta Neurol. Scand.*, 69:200–206.
123. Moroni, F., Forchetti, M. C., Krogsgaard-Larsen, P., and Guidotti, A. (1982): *J. Pharm. Pharmacol.*, 34:676–678.
124. Morselli, P. L. (1985): In: *L.E.R.S., Vol. 3*, edited by G. Bartholini, H. Langer, and K. G. Lloyd, pp. 441–442. Raven Press, New York.
125. Morselli, P. L., Bosse, L., Henry, J. F., Zarifian, E., and Bartholini, G. (1980): *Brain Res. (Suppl. 2)*, 5:411–414.
126. Morselli, P. L., Henry, J. F., Macher, J. P., Bottin, P., Huber, J. P., and van Landeghem, V. H. (1981): In: *Biological Psychiatry*, edited by C. Perris, G. Struwe, and B. Jansson, pp. 440–443. Elsevier, Amsterdam.
127. Morselli, P. L., Lloyd, K. G., Löscher, W., Meldrum, B., and Reynolds, E. H., eds. (1981): *Neurotransmitters, Seizures and Epilepsy*. Raven Press, New York.
128. Mugnaini, E. (1985): *J. Comp. Neurol.*, 235:61–81.
129. Nagai, T., McGeer, P. L., and McGeer, E. G. (1983): *J. Comp. Neurol.*, 218:220–238.
130. Nagy, J. L., Carter, B. A., and Fibiger, H. C. (1978): *Brain Res.*, 158:15–29.
131. Nauta, H. J. W., and Cuenod, M. (1982): *Neuroscience*, 7:2725–2734.
132. Nicoletti, F., Grandison, L., and Meek, J. L. (1985): *J. Neurochem.*, 44:1217–1220.
133. Nilava, G., Defendeni, R., Zimmermann, E. A., Beinfeld, M. C., and Donohue, T. L. (1982): *Nature*, 295:597–598.
134. Nishikawa, T., and Scatton, B. (1985): *Brain Res.*, 331:81–90.
135. Nitsch, C. (1980): *J. Neurochem.*, 34:822–830.
136. Oertel, W. H., Graybiel, A. M., Mugnaini, E., Elde, R. P., Schmechel, D. E., and Kopin, J. Y. (1983): *J. Neurosci.*, 3:1322–1332.
137. Oertel, W. H., Mugnaini, E., Tappaz, M. L., Weise, V. K., Dahl, A. L., Schmechel, D. E., and Kopin, I. J. (1982): *Proc. Natl. Acad. Sci. USA*, 79:675–679.
138. Okada, Y., Taniguchi, H., and Shimada, C. (1976): *Science*, 194:620–622.
139. Olsen, R. W. (1981): *J. Neurochem.*, 37:1–13.
140. Olsen, R. W., Bergmann, M. O., van Ness, P. C., Lummis, S. C., Napias, C., and Greenlee, D. W. (1981): *Mol. Pharmacol.*, 19:217–227.
141. Olsen, R. W., and Snowman, J. N. (1982): *Neuroscience*, 2:1817–1823.
142. Olsen, R. W., and Snowman, J. N. (1985): *J. Neurochem.*, 44:1074–1082.
143. Ottersen, O. P., and Storm-Mathisen, J. (1984): In: *Handbook of Chemical Neuroanatomy, Vol. 3*, edited by A. Björklund, T. Hökfelt, and M. J. Kuhar, pp. 141–246. Elsevier, Amsterdam.
144. Ottersen, O. P., and Storm-Mathisen, J. (1984): *J. Comp. Neurol.*, 229:374–392.
145. Ottersen, O. P., and Storm-Mathisen, J. (1984): *Anat. Embryol.*, 170:197–207.
146. Pedersen, H. R., Jensen, I., and Dam, M. (1983): *Acta Neurol. Scand.*, 67:114–117.
147. Penney, J. B., and Young, A. B. (1981): *Brain Res.*, 207:195–198.
148. Perez de la Mora, M., Possani, L. A., Tapia, R., Teran, L., Palacios, R., Fuxe, K., Hökfelt, T., and Ljungdahl, Å. (1981): *Neuroscience*, 6:875–895.
149. Perry, T. L. (1985): *Neurology*, 35:755–758.
150. Perry, T. L., Hansen, S., and Kloster, S. (1973): *N. Engl. J. Med.*, 288:337–342.
151. Pong, S.-S., and Wang, C. C. (1982): *J. Neurochem.*, 38:375–379.
152. Porter, T. G., and Martin, D. L. (1984): *J. Neurochem.*, 43:1464–1467.
153. Rastogi, S. L., and Tichey, M. K. (1985): *Pharmacol. Biochem. Behav.*, 22:141–148.
154. Reiffenstein, R. J., and Neil, M. J. (1974): *Can. J. Physiol. Pharmacol.*, 52:286–290.
155. Reijnierse, G. L. A., Veldstra, H., and van den Berg, C. J. (1975): *Biochem. J.*, 152:469–475.
156. Ribak, C. E. (1978): *J. Neurocytol.*, 7:461–478.
157. Ribak, C. E. (1981): *Acta Biochem. Psychopharmacol.*, 30:23–37.
158. Ribak, C. E. (1985): *Brain Res.*, 326:251–260.
159. Ribak, C. E., Bradbourne, R. H., and Harris, A. B. (1982): *J. Neurosci.*, 2:461–478.
160. Ribak, C. E., Vaughn, J. E., and Roberts, E. (1979): *J. Comp. Neurol.*, 187:261–283.

161. Ribak, C. E., Vaughn, J. E., and Roberts, E. (1980): *Brain Res.,* 192:413–420.
162. Rimmer, E. M., and Richen, A. (1984): *Lancet,* 1:189–190.
163. Roffler-Tarlov, S., and Tarlov, E. (1975): *Brain Res.,* 91:326–330.
164. Ruggiero, D. A., Meeley, M. P., Anwar, M., and Reis, D. J. (1985): *Brain Res.,* 339:171–172.
165. Salganicoff, L., and De Robertis, E. (1965): *J. Neurochem.,* 12:287–298.
166. Sandner, G., Dessert, D., Schmitt, P., and Karli, P. (1981): *Brain Res.,* 224:279–290.
167. Schechter, P. J., Lewis, P. J., and Newberne, J. W. (1984): *Lancet,* 1:737–738.
168. Schmechel, D. E., Vickeroy, B. G., Fitzpatrick, D., and Elde, R. P. (1984): *Neurosci. Lett.,* 47:227–232.
169. Schmidt, D. (1984): *Neurosci. Lett.,* 47:357–360.
170. Schon, F., and Iversen, L. L. (1974): *Life Sci.,* 15:157–175.
171. Scigliano, G., Giovanni, P., Girotti, F., Grassi, M. P., Caraceni, T., and Schechter, P. J. (1984): *Neurology,* 34:94–96.
172. Seiler, N., and Sarhan, S. (1984): *Naunyn Schmiedebergs Arch. Pharmacol.,* 326:49–57.
173. Seiler, N., and Sarhan, S. (1984): *Gen. Pharmacol.,* 15:367–369.
174. Seiler, N., Sarhan, S., Krogsgaard-Larsen, P., Hjeds, H., and Schousboe, A. (1985): *Gen. Pharmacol.,* 16:509–511.
175. Seligmann, B., Miller, L. P., Brockmann, D. E., and Martin, D. L. (1978): *J. Neurochem.,* 30:371–376.
176. Sevestre, P., Rondot, P., Bathien, N., Morselli, P. L., and van Landeghem, V. M. (1982): *Abstracts 13 C.I.N. P. Congress, Vol. 2,* Jerusalem, p. 663.
177. Skerritt, J. A., Willow, M., and Johnston, G. A. R. (1982): *Neurosci. Lett.,* 38:315–320.
178. Somogyi, P., Hodgson, A. J., Chubb, I. W., Penke, B., and Erdei, A. (1985): *J. Histochem. Cytochem.,* 33:240–248.
179. Somogyi, P., Nemzi, M. G., Gorio, A., and Smith, A. D. (1983): *Brain Res.,* 259:137–142.
180. Spink, D. C., and Martin, D. L. (1983): In: *Glutamine, Glutamate and GABA in the CNS,* edited by L. Hertz, E. Kvamme, E. McGeer, and A. Schousboe, pp. 129–143. Alan R. Liss, New York.
181. Spink, D. C., Wu, S. J., and Martin, D. L. (1983): *J. Neurochem.,* 40:1113–1199.
182. Squires, R. F., Casida, J. E., Richardson, M., and Saedrup, E. (1983): *Mol. Pharmacol.,* 23:326–338.
183. Starr, M. S., and Kilpatrick, I. C., (1981): *Neuroscience,* 6:1098–1104.
184. Stober, T., Schimrigh, K., and Holzer, G., (1983): *J. Neurol.,* 229:237–245.
185. Storm-Mathisen, J. (1972): *Brain Res.,* 40:215–235.
186. Storm-Mathisen, J., and Fonnum, F. (1971): *J. Neurochem.,* 18:1105–1111.
187. Storm-Mathisen, J., Leknes, A. K., Bore, A. T., Vaaland, J. L., Edmundsen, P., Haug, F. M. S., and Ottersen, P. (1983): *Nature,* 301:517–520.
188. Study, R. E., and Barker, J. L. (1981): *Proc. Natl. Acad. Sci. USA,* 78:7180–7184.
189. Szerb, J. C. (1984): *Brain Res.,* 293:293–303.
190. Takahara, Y., Yunoki, S., Hosogi, H., Yakushigi, W., Kageryama, Y., and Osuji, T. (1980): *Endocrinology,* 106:343–347.
191. Takahashi, T., and Otsuka, M. (1975): *Brain Res.,* 87:1–11.
192. Tamminya, C. A., Thaker, G. K., Ferraro, T. N., and Hare, T. A. (1983): *Lancet,* 2:97–98.
193. Taniyama, K., Miki, Y., and Tanaka, C. (1982): *Neurosci. Lett.,* 29:53–56.
194. Tappaz, M. L., Bader, O., Paul, L., and Bered, A. (1985): *Neuroscience,* 16:111–122.
195. Tappaz, M. L., and Brownstein, M. J. (1977): *Brain Res.,* 132:95–107.
196. Tappaz, M. L., Brownstein, M. J., and Kopin, J. Y. (1977): *Brain Res.,* 125:109–121.
197. Tappaz, M. L., Wassef, M., Oertel, W. A., Paul, L., and Peyot, J. F. (1983): *Neuroscience,* 9:271–287.
198. Tappaz, M. L., Zivin, J. A., and Kopin, W. (1976): *Brain Res.,* 111:220–225.
199. Taxt, T., and Storm-Mathisen, J. (1984): *Neuroscience,* 11:79–100.
200. Techenne, P. F., Ziegler, M. G., Lake, C. R., and Enna, C. (1982): *J. Am. Neurol.,* 11:76–79.
201. Tichu, M. K., and Maksay, G. (1983): *Life Sci.,* 33:236.
202. Tichu, M. K., and Olsen, R. W. (1978): *Life Sci.,* 22:1643–1653.
203. Tichu, M. K., Rastogi, S. L., and Thygarjan, R. (1985): *Eur. J. Pharmacol.,* 112:1–9.
204. Vaccarino, F., Conti Tranconi, B. M., Panula, P., Guidotti, A., and Costa, E. (1985): *J. Neurochem.,* 44:278–290.
205. van Gelder, N. M., Sherwin, A., and Rasmusen, T. (1972): *Brain Res.,* 40:385–393.
206. Vickeroy, V. (1983): *Soc. Neurosci. Abstr.,* 9:408.
207. Vijargan, E., and McCann, S. M. (1978): *Brain Res.,* 155:38–43.
208. Vijargan, E., and McCann, S. M. (1978): *Endocrinology,* 103:1888–1893.
209. Vincent, S. R., Hökfelt, T., Skirbole, L. R., and Wu, J.-Y. (1983): *Science,* 200:1309–1311.
210. Vincent, S. R., Hökfelt, T., and Wu, J.-Y. (1982): *Neuroendocrinology,* 36:97–106.
211. Vincent, S. R., Kimura, H., and McGeer, E. G. (1980): *Neurosci. Lett.,* 16:345.
212. Vincent, S. R., Kimura, H., and McGeer, E. G. (1981): *Brain Res.,* 222:198–203.
213. Vincent, S. R., Kimura, H., and McGeer, E. G. (1982): *Brain Res.,* 241:162–165.
214. Waddington, J. L., and Cross, A. J. (1978): *Life Sci.,* 22:1011–1014.
215. Walaas, I., and Fonnum, F. (1978): *Brain Res.,* 153:549–562.
216. Walaas, I., and Fonnum, F. (1979): *Brain Res.,* 177:325–336.
217. Walaas, I., and Fonnum, F. (1979): *Neuroscience,* 4:209–216.
218. Walaas, I., and Fonnum, F. (1980): *Neuroscience,* 5:63–72.
219. Wang, B. H., and Wu, J.-Y. (1984): *Brain Res.,* 302:57–67.
220. Wasterlain, C. G., Moren, A. M., and Dwyer, B. E. (1985): *Handbook of Neurochemistry, Vol. 10,* 2nd ed., edited by A. Lahjta, pp. 386–387. Plenum Press, New York.
221. Williams, M., and Yarbrough, G. G. (1979): *Eur. J. Pharmacol.,* 56:273–276.
222. Williford, D. J., Hamilton, B. L., Souza, J. D., Williams, T. P., DiMicco, J. A., and Gillis, R. A. (1980): *Circ. Res.,* 47:80–88.
223. Wolf, P., Olpe, H. R., Avrith, D., and Haas, H. L. (1978): *Experientia,* 34:73–74.
224. Wu, J.-Y., Matsuda, T., and Roberts, E. (1973): *J. Biol. Chem.,* 248:3029–3036.
225. Wu, J.-Y., Matsuda, E., Saito, K., Roberts, E., and Schousboe, A. (1976): *J. Neurochem.,* 27:653–662.
226. Zackerman, M., Tocci, P., and Nyhan, W. L. (1966): *J. Biol. Chem.,* 241:1355–1360.
227. Zivkovic, B., Lloyd, K. G., and Bartholini, G. (1984): *L.E.R.S., Vol. 3,* edited by G. Bartholini, H. Langer, and K. G. Lloyd, pp. 101–109. Raven Press, New York.
228. Yamada, K. A., McAllen, R. M., and Lowry, A. D. (1984): *Brain Res.,* 292:175–180.
229. Yunger, L. M., Fowler, P. J., Zarevics, P., and Setler, P. E. (1984): *J. Pharmacol. Exp. Ther.,* 228:109–119.

Psychopharmacology:
The Third Generation of Progress,
edited by Herbert Y. Meltzer.
Raven Press, New York © 1987.

CHAPTER 19

Psychopharmacology of GABAergic Drugs

K. G. Lloyd and P. L. Morselli

The understanding of γ-aminobutyric acid (GABA) synapses has greatly evolved since the description of the psychopharmacology of GABA by Iversen in the first edition of this compendium (75). Knowledge of a $GABA_B$ receptor not regulating chloride ion flux (69) has changed certain concepts of GABA synapses, and has opened the door to a new generation of GABAergic mechanisms and drugs. Additionally, GABA has lost its crown as "the" central neurotransmitter with the demonstration that all of the neuronal and synaptic mechanisms necessary for GABAergic transmission exist in the periphery in such organs as the pancreas, kidney, and female reproductive system (cf. ref. 45). In certain species the highest concentrations of GABA exist not in the brain but in peripheral organs. Even within the classical GABA synapse (now termed $GABA_A$) regulating a chloride ionophore, the understanding of the GABA benzodiazepine-chloride ionophore macromolecular complex has greatly increased with the knowledge of different recognition sites for GABA agonists (the $GABA_A$ receptor), benzodiazepines and benzodiazepine displacing agents (BZ_1 and BZ_2 sites), barbiturates (picrotoxinin and other compounds acting at the picrotoxinin-barbiturate site), and modulatory proteins (e.g., gabamodulins, diazepam binding inhibitor (DBI), and related substances) (cf. ref. 13).

In parallel, the pharmacology of GABA synapses has become increasingly complex and the number of compounds modulating GABA function has risen exponentially. The present review will limit itself to the central aspects of GABAergic transmission (for a review of peripheral mechanisms see ref. 45). Furthermore, only the psychopharmacology of agents acting at GABA receptors will be considered, i.e., compounds with a direct action (agonists or

antagonists) or that alter the availability of GABA within the synapse [GABA uptake inhibitors, glutamate decarboxylase (GAD) inhibitors, inhibitors of GABA metabolism, GABA prodrugs].

Advances in the knowledge and understanding of GABA synaptic function will receive priority, as the historically well-known facts of GABAergic transmission are to be found in the review by Iversen (75) in the first edition. One of the most marked of these advances is the availability of GABAergic drugs suitable for use in humans, allowing a real understanding of GABAergic function in neuropsychiatric disorders and providing a validation or refutation of the animal models for these diseases.

NEW ASPECTS OF THE BIOCHEMICAL PSYCHOPHARMACOLOGY OF GABA SYNAPSES

As indicated above, major advances in the biochemical pharmacology of GABA synapses relate to the understanding of the $GABA_A$-benzodiazepine-chloride ionophore complex and the demonstration of a second $GABA_B$ receptor not linked to a chloride ionophore. As the interactions within the $GABA_A$-benzodiazepine receptor complex are treated in detail by others in this volume, and a recent book is dedicated to this subject (13), this will not be considered in detail.

The description of a second major GABA receptor insensitive to bicuculline (e.g., refs. 13, 15, 39, 96, 157) has greatly enlarged our understanding of the function and role of GABA synapses and the mechanism of action of certain drugs. The $GABA_B$ receptor is found both in the periphery (e.g., heart, C fibers) and in the CNS (35,45,69). This recognition site is associated with a distribution and physiological, biochemical, and neuropharmacological activities that differentiate it from GABA$_A$ receptors. GABA$_B$ receptors have their highest density in the interpeduncular nucleus, which apparently does not contain GABA$_A$ receptors. Within the cerebellum GABA$_B$ sites occur at the molecular layer, whereas GABA$_A$ receptors are present in the granule cell layer (16,17,96,155). GABA$_B$ activation results in a decrease in calcium conductance (34,40) and increase in potassium conductance (74,137), whereas GABA$_A$ receptor stimulation alters chloride ion flux (83). GABA$_B$ activation potentiates cyclic AMP formation by norepinephrine, dopamine, and isoproterenol, whereas GABA$_A$ site stimulation is inactive in this respect but diminishes cerebellar cyclic GMP levels (68,80,122).

The differential pharmacological profiles of GABA$_A$ and GABA$_B$ sites are summarized in Table 1. Compounds exerting a full GABAergic action (i.e., acting equally at both sites) include GABA itself, SL 75.102 (see also ref. 16), and β-OH GABA. (−)Baclofen is a specific agonist for the GABA$_B$ site, whereas isoguvacine, 4,5,6,7-tetrahydroisoxazolo-5,4C-pyridin-3-ol (THIP), and piperidine-4-sulfonic acid are specific for the GABA$_A$ site. Muscimol has the highest affinity for the GABA$_A$ site with a weak activity at GABA$_B$ receptors (cf. 12,69,96). Bicuculline is a highly specific antagonist for the GABA$_A$ site (69,77), whereas no specific antagonists are available for the GABA$_B$ site. Two compounds (5-aminovaleric acid and homotaurine) have been described as GABA$_B$ antagonists (56,133,136), but both are GABA$_A$ agonists. GTP decreases the sensitivity of GABA$_B$ sites (14), whereas GABA$_A$ receptor sites are up-regulated by barbiturates and benzodiazepines (13,63,141,176).

This description of two different GABA receptors has eliminated certain apparent discrepancies in the pharmacological profiles of GABAergic agents (e.g., between muscimol, THIP, and SL 75.102). It has provided the psychopharmacologist with a more useful armamentarium for the investigation of GABA synaptic function: (a) those agents with a full GABAergic role—compounds that act at both receptors (progabide, SL 75.102, muscimol), or that increase GABA levels within the synapse (GABA uptake inhibitors, GABA transaminase inhibitors); (b) compounds specific for GABA$_A$ receptors (isoguvacine, THIP); (c) compounds specific for GABA$_B$ receptors (baclofen).

The other major advance in the psychopharmacology of GABAergic agents is the availability of compounds suitable for clinical investigation. Previously, the only useful GABAergic agent was sodium valproate, an inhibitor of GABA transaminase, for which the specificity of effects on GABAergic transmission has been debated. Recently, the highly specific mixed GABA$_{A+B}$ agonist progabide has received extensive clinical trials, the specific GABA$_A$ agonist THIP has been examined less extensively, and a specific GABA-transaminase inhibitor (γ-vinyl GABA) is under investigation (see below). These findings, together with those from the earlier studies on muscimol, have allowed the confirmation of certain GABAergic hypotheses (e.g., of epilepsy, dyskinesia, spasticity) while seemingly refuting some (schizophrenia) and questioning others (anxiety, chorea). A noninclusive list of GABAergic agents useful for *in vivo* psychopharmacological investigation is provided in Table 2. Those in italics have undergone clinical investigation.

PSYCHONEUROPHARMACOLOGY OF GABAERGIC AGENTS IN DIFFERENT ANIMAL MODELS AND CLINICAL CONDITIONS: NEUROLOGICAL ASPECTS

Convulsant Threshold, Seizures, and Epilepsy: The GABAergic Hypothesis of Epilepsy

A physiological parameter closely related to GABA$_A$ synaptic function would appear to be the maintenance of a normal ratio of excitation-inhibition and thus cerebral excitability. When excess excitation or insufficient inhibition arises, especially in certain cortical areas and hippocampus, then convulsions occur. The GABA hypothesis of epilepsy states that one of the major factors in epileptogenesis is a decreased function of GABA$_A$ synapses. A corollary of this hypothesis is that agents that increase GABA$_A$ synaptic function and have a good clinical tolerance should be effective antiepileptic drugs (cf. ref. 97).

Any agent that reduces GABA$_A$ synaptic function provokes convulsions (Table 3). An inhibition of GABA synthesis (by GAD inhibitors) of approximately 40% is sufficient to provoke seizures in rats, mice, baboons, and other species. These seizures may occur even in the presence of increased GABA levels (for example, with compounds such as aminooxyacetic acid or γ-acetylenic GABA, which inhibit both GABA transaminase and GAD activities), indicating that it is the GABA newly synthesized and released from nerve terminals that is essential for the maintenance of sufficient cerebral inhibition (97,183,194,195).

TABLE 1. *Pharmacological profile of [³H]GABA binding to GABA$_A$ and GABA$_B$ receptor recognition sites*

Displacer	GABA$_A$ site[a] (IC$_{50}$, nM)	GABA$_B$ site (IC$_{50}$, nM)
GABA	200	80
Muscimol	24	5,400
3-aminopropane sulfonic acid	70	10,000
Piperidine-4-sulfonic acid	90	>10⁵
Isoguvacine	150	>10⁵
THIP	630	>10⁵
β-OH GABA	700[b]	1,100
SL 75.102	860[b]	500
Bicuculline	2,000	>10⁵
5-Amino valeric Acid	5,000	30,000
(−)Baclofen	>10⁶	130
GTP	No effect	Decrease affinity
Benzodiazepines	Enhance binding	No effect
Barbiturates	Enhance binding	No effect

[a] No Triton-x-100 treatment.
[b] With Triton-x-100.
From refs. 17 and 96.

TABLE 2. *GABAergic agents useful for* in vivo *psychopharmacology*

Enhanced GABA receptor activation

GABA-transaminase inhibitors	*Sodium valproate; γ-vinyl GABA; γ-acetylenic GABA;* ethanolamine-*O*-sulfate; aminooxyacetic acid; various pyridoxal phosphate hydrazides
GABA uptake inhibitors	Various esters of nipecotic acid and isoguvacine; THPO
GABA agonists: GABA$_{A+B}$	*Progabide;* SL 75.102; Kojic amine
GABA$_A$	*Muscimol; THIP;* isoguvacine; 3-aminopropane sulfonic acid
GABA$_B$	*Baclofen*

Diminished GABA receptor activation

Inhibition of GABA synthesis (GAD)	Allylglycine; isonicotinic-acid hydrazide; *cycloserine;* higher doses of aminooxyacetic acid and γ-*acetylenic GABA;* diverse pyridoxal phosphate hydrazides; pyridoxal-5-sulfate
GABA$_A$ receptor antagonists	Bicuculline; Ru 5135
Reduced chloride ionophore opening	Picrotoxinin; convulsant barbiturates

For references, see text and refs. 43, 96, 97.
Compounds in italics have undergone clinical trials.

This maintenance of a physiological level of inhibition by GABA neurons also occurs in humans, as shown by the proconvulsant state and occurrence of tonic-clonic seizures in nonepileptic tuberculosis patients treated with cycloserine (90).

A convulsive state is also induced by the direct blockade of GABA$_A$ receptors (e.g., by bicuculline) or a reduction in the GABA-mediated opening of the chloride ion channel (by picrotoxinin or convulsant barbiturates) (77,140,142,159,179,189). It appears that some brain regions are extremely sensitive to GABA$_A$ receptor blockade with regard to convulsant threshold. Thus, injection of nanomolar amounts of bicuculline into the rat deep prepyriform cortex induces convulsions (51,153).

These data suggest that disinhibition by means of a specific reduction in GABA synaptic activity is sufficient to provoke seizures. There are indications that dysfunctional GABA synaptic activity may be fundamental to at least certain forms of human epilepsy, as decreased GAD activity and GABA$_A$ sites have been demonstrated in epileptogenic

TABLE 3. *Psychopharmacology of GABA synapses and seizures*

Action within GABA synapses	Activity in animal models	Clinical activity
Agents that diminish GABA synaptic activity		
L-Glutamic acid decarboxylase inhibitors	Convulsant	Proconvulsant/convulsant (cycloserine)
GABA$_A$ antagonists	Convulsant	Untested
Reduced chloride ion entry	Convulsant	Untested
Agents that enhance GABA synaptic activity		
GABA-transaminase inhibitors	Broad anticonvulsant spectrum	Antiepileptic (valproate, γ-vinyl GABA)
GABA uptake inhibitors	Anticonvulsant	Untested
GABA agonists: GABA$_{A+B}$	Broad anticonvulsant spectrum	Antiepileptic (progabide)
GABA$_A$	Wide anticonvulsant spectrum (inactive strychnine, electroshock, *Papio papio*)	Limited activity (THIP)
GABA$_B$	Limited anticonvulsant spectrum (pentetrazole, strychnine, audiogenic DBA$_2$ mice)	Not useful as an epileptic (baclofen)

For references, see text and ref. 97.

regions of human brain (4,98,105), but the overall neurochemical pathology of human epilepsy is far from clear (cf. ref. 30).

More importantly for practical purposes, the converse is also true, i.e., increasing GABA synaptic function has an anticonvulsant effect in animals and an antiepileptic activity in humans (Table 3). It appears that GABA$_A$ receptors play a predominant role, as GABA$_A$ agonists (e.g., muscimol, THIP, isoguvacine) have a wide spectrum of anticonvulsant activity (although virtually inactive against electroshock or strychnine convulsions or in the photosensitive *Papio papio*), and the GABA$_B$ agonist baclofen has a very limited anticonvulsant profile (against pentetrazole and strychnine and in audiogenic DBA$_2$ mice) (cf. refs. 97, 106, 115, 124, 196). However, the most marked anticonvulsant effect is obtained with simultaneous stimulation of all GABA receptors, either directly by agonists (e.g., progabide, SL 75.102) or by increasing synaptic GABA levels by inhibition of GABA transaminase or GABA uptake. In this case virtually all seizure models respond to increased GABA receptor activation, including the *Papio papio*, kindling, and models due to hyperexcitability (22,27,79,97,106,115,196).

This broad-spectrum anticonvulsant profile of GABA$_{A+B}$ receptor activation is paralleled by a clinically useful antiepileptic activity. The therapeutic activity of sodium valproate is well known; its mechanism of action involves not only an inhibition of the degradation of GABA (117), but probably also an increase in synthesis and release (114). A more specific GABA-transaminase inhibitor, γ-vinyl GABA, has shown promising activity in early trials (67).

The most direct evidence for the antiepileptic activity of enhanced GABAergic transmission is the therapeutic effect of the GABA$_{A+B}$ agonist progabide. In trials involving over 700 severely or therapy-resistant epileptic patients, progabide was active (>50% reduction of seizures) in primary generalized epilepsy, secondary generalized epilepsy, and partial epilepsy (130) with a very low incidence of adverse reactions (25). In contrast, the trials with a specific GABA$_A$ agonist (THIP) were limited due to the emergence of undesirable secondary effects (150).

GABAergic Agents and Spasticity

Although GABAergic mechanisms regulate (*inter alia*) spinal reflexes and modulate proprioceptive reflexes relevant for spasticity (26,138,154,164), and a decreased GABA release is reported in paraplegic cats (135), few GABAergic agents have been examined in models for spasticity. In contrast, benzodiazepines, which modulate GABAergic transmission at the GABA$_A$ synapse, have received considerable attention (cf. ref. 28).

From the available results it would appear that activation of either GABA$_A$ or GABA$_B$ receptors exerts an action on spinal reflexes that is consistent with an antispastic effect. In cats *l*-baclofen inhibits the patellar, flexor, and linguomandibular reflexes and *d-l* baclofen antagonizes the H-reflex, whereas *d*-baclofen is inactive in these tests (139). This parallels the stereospecificity for baclofen enantiomers at the GABA$_B$ site (10). Baclofen depresses monosynaptic and polysynaptic inhibition of spinal cord neurons in a manner similar to GABA, but this is not reversed by bicuculline (cf. ref. 28).

As baclofen (the most commonly used antispastic agent; ref. 123) exhibits an antispastic action in patients with either a partial or complete lesion of the spinal cord (3,143) and has a therapeutic action after local (intrathecal) administration (144), it can be suggested that the antispastic effect of baclofen is due to an interaction with GABA$_B$ receptors in the spinal cord.

Specific activation of GABA$_A$ synapses apparently also can evoke a partial antispastic activity, as in spastic patients THIP reduces the monosynaptic T-reflex, reinforces vibratory inhibition of the I$_A$ monosynaptic pathway, and is without significant effect on flexor reflexes, resistance to passive movement, or clonus (127).

Simultaneous activation of GABA$_A$ and GABA$_B$ receptors leads to marked antispastic effects in both animal models and spastic patients. Thus, progabide reduces the hypertonia of the gastrocnemius-soleus muscle in the spastic mutant Han-Wistar rat (171). As this effect is partially reduced by bicuculline and picrotoxin, GABA$_A$ receptors that likely play a contributing role. In baboons rendered spastic by either hemispinal or cortical lesions, both progabide and gabaculine (a GABA transaminase inhibitor) reduce both the hyperactive phasic and tonic stretch responses of the soleus muscle, whereas the physiological reflexes in unoperated monkeys are unaltered (M. Hugon, *unpublished results*). Progabide has been shown to be an effective clinical antispastic agent in both open (131) and double-blind (11,128,129) trials, significantly reducing monosynaptic T-reflexes, the duration of clonus, and the latency of the flexor-reflex threshold. Dynamic power was improved and a reduction of spasms was evident. No alteration of vibratory inhibition of the T- and H-reflexes was observed.

GABAergic Agents and Movement Disorders

Basal Ganglia Movement Disorders

The movement disorders associated with basal ganglia dysfunction include Parkinson's disease, Huntington's chorea, and tardive dyskinesia. An altered balance between dopamine and GABA neuron function within the nigro-striato-nigral loop appears to be a common factor. The physiological role of GABA neurons within this circuit is apparently to modulate (decrease) dopamine neuron activity by reducing cell firing, dopamine release, and the postsynaptic consequences of dopamine receptor stimulation or blockade. Both GABA$_A$ and GABA$_B$ receptors are implicated, as GABA$_A$ (muscimol), GABA$_B$ (baclofen), and GABA$_{A+B}$ (progabide, SL 75.102, GABA-transaminase inhibitors) mimetics reduce indices of nigrostriatal dopamine neuron activity (dopamine release, tyrosine hydroxylase activity, dopamine turnover, etc.) under either resting conditions or after dopamine neuron activation (by neuroleptics) (cf. refs. 93, 96, 113, 166, 167). The behavioral correlates of this GABAergic inhibition of nigrostriatal dopamine neuron function include an increase in neuroleptic-induced catalepsy in rats and a decrease in dopamine-mimetic (e.g., apomorphine)-induced activities—stereotypies in mice, rotation in rats with unilateral nigral lesions, abnormal involuntary movements in cats or monkeys (100,104,106,111). Furthermore, coadministration of a GABA agonist (progabide, muscimol) together with a neuroleptic (haloperidol, 14 days) greatly reduces the dopamine receptor supersensitivity observed after the neuroleptic alone, as evidenced by a suppression of the tolerance to the cataleptic action of the neuroleptic, diminished supersensitivity to dopamine agonists, and a prevention of the up-regulation of dopamine receptors (86,100,104,111,112).

It should be noted that under specific circumstances, a biphasic action of GABA agonists can be observed: potentiation of behavior related to nigrostriatal dopamine neuron activity at very low doses of muscimol or progabide (23,111,167,196) in contrast to the inhibition of dopamine neuron activity and receptor-mediated behavior at somewhat higher doses (see above). Furthermore, the effects of local intracerebral injection of GABA agonists (muscimol, THIP) are site specific (167,168) and may differ markedly from the actions seen after their systemic administration.

These modulatory actions of GABA mimetics on nigrostriatal dopamine neuron activity and associated behavior predict that such GABAergic agents might (a) in Parkinson's disease, diminish L-dopa stereotypies but, if anything, exaggerate the underlying Parkinsonism; (b) reduce neuroleptic-induced tardive dyskinesia; (c) reduce the dyskinetic movements in Huntington's chorea. There are now sufficient data available to make a preliminary assessment of GABAergic agents in these clinical conditions.

Parkinson's Disease. The prominent neurochemical deficit in Parkinson's disease is a loss of nigrostriatal dopamine neurons (72,101), although other neurochemical deficits also occur, including a decrease in GAD activity and GABA$_A$ recognition sites in the substantia nigra and striatum (cf. ref. 95).

In parkinsonian patients, specific GABA$_B$ receptor activation by baclofen is without benefit on L-dopa-induced dyskinesia and is reputed to exacerbate rigidity (88).

Activation of both GABA$_{A+B}$ receptors by progabide has led to mixed results: a marked reduction in dyskinetic movements and an exacerbation of parkinsonism at high doses (7); a beneficial increase in the L-dopa "on" time for patients with "on-off" responses to L-dopa, with no change in L-dopa dyskinesia (which was minimal) (8); and a lack of effect on either the parkinsonism or the dyskinetic syndrome (121).

Of these, the most promising response may be the enhancement of the effect of L-dopa during GABA agonist therapy (ref. 8 and also M. Ziegler et al., *unpublished*). This action may be related to the observations that CSF GABA levels are significantly lower in poorly responding and "on-off" parkinsonian patients treated with L-dopa (185), and that successful L-dopa therapy elevates CSF GABA levels in Parkinson's disease (118) [however, this latter finding has not been reproduced (1)].

Thus, the clinical psychopharmacology of progabide in Parkinson's disease is apparently at odds with the predictions from animal models of basal ganglia dysfunction. Plausible explanations for this include the following: (a) the doses used in the clinic (approximately 10–25 mg/kg, p.o.) are similar to those low doses which potentiate rather than

antagonize dopaminergic function in animal models (see above); and (b) the major neuropathology of Parkinson's disease occurs in the substantia nigra (72) and GABA mimetics applied locally within this region both antagonize and enhance dopamine neuron function (168). In contrast to these findings in idiopathic Parkinson's disease, an increase in neuroleptic-induced parkinsonism by muscimol has been reported (181), which is in agreement with the animal models.

Huntington's Chorea. In contrast to the dopamine neuron loss in the substantia nigra in Parkinson's disease, the neurochemical pathology of Huntington's chorea is associated with a disappearance of GABA synapses in the corpus striatum, with evidence for at least a functional dopaminergic hyperactivity (75,94,95). Models of Huntington's chorea (intrastriatal administration of kainic acid) demonstrate similar losses of GABA synaptic function that can be diminished or prevented by pretreatment with GABAergic agents such as GABA-transaminase inhibitors and benzodiazepines (170).

The decrease in GABA levels and GAD activity in Huntington's chorea (44,75,95) can be considered to be a reflection of GABA neuron loss, in a manner parallel to which the low dopamine and DOPA decarboxylase levels reflect dopamine neuron loss in Parkinson's disease (101). It is thus logical to consider GABA replacement therapy for Huntington's chorea, as L-dopa or dopaminomimetic therapy alleviates Parkinson's disease.

Three GABA agonists (progabide, THIP, muscimol) and four GABA-transaminase inhibitors (valproate, isoniazid, aminooxyacetic acid, γ-acetylenic GABA) (48,116, 120,121,131,142,147–149,174,178,184) have been used in clinical trials for Huntington's chorea. Only in one trial was there a notable effect, and then only in recently diagnosed patients (131). In total, only 11 of 101 Huntington patients appeared to have benefited from GABAergic agents, in spite of a demonstrated (threefold) increase in CSF (119,147,184) and brain (146) GABA levels during therapy with GABA-transaminase inhibitors.

A probable contributing factor to the failure of GABA agonist therapy in Huntington's disease is the large decrease of GABA$_A$ receptors in the striatum of these patients (102,191,197), and the large loss of striatal tissue in general. As the site of action for the GABA mimetics is thus greatly reduced, the action of the compounds would necessarily be limited.

In contrast to this lack of effect in Huntington's chorea, Sydenham's chorea has been reported to respond to valproate (36) and hemiballismus to progabide (two neuroleptic-resistant cases) (60).

Tardive Dyskinesia. The dyskinetic syndrome induced by chronic neuroleptic administration is an iatrogenic disorder that can be replicated in animal models. From these studies a picture emerges of striatal dopamine receptor up-regulation and supersensitivity (58) combined with a decrease of nigral GAD activity and GABA$_A$ receptor binding (64,65,111). From such data a GABA hypothesis of tardive dyskinesia has been proposed (47). *A priori* this biochemical model of movement disorders (with behavioral components in primates) should be the closest and most predictive for human movement disorders, as this drug-induced syndrome is apparently not associated with a primary genetic defect or unknown pathogen.

As reviewed above, the basis for the prediction that GABAergic agents may control tardive dyskinesia includes the following: the tonic inhibitory GABAergic control of nigrostriatal dopamine neuron activity; the regulation of postsynaptic DA receptor-mediated events by GABA receptors (e.g., the reversal of apomorphine-induced rotation in rats with unilateral lesions of the nigrostriatal path); the reduction by GABA agonists of dopamine receptor supersensitivity and up-regulation observed after withdrawal from prolonged neuroleptic administration (see above and refs. 20 and 159).

The clinical psychopharmacology of tardive dyskinesia indicates that GABA$_{A+B}$ receptor activation is a potential means of controlling these abnormal involuntary movements. Thus, of 58 patients receiving either progabide (N = 29) (132), γ-vinyl GABA (N = 11) (182,186), γ-acetylenic GABA (N = 10) (21), or muscimol (N = 8) (180), 44 showed a marked improvement during GABAergic drug administration. In contrast, specific GABA$_B$ receptor activation (by baclofen) resulted in improvement in only 37 of 110 patients (cf. ref. 57), and the specific GABA$_A$ agent THIP was without effect in 18 cases (84). In contrast to the marked improvement obtained with the more potent GABA-transaminase inhibitors, sodium valproate did not alter dyskinesia in a series of 24 patients (55).

Other Movement Disorders

Increased GABA receptor activation has been utilized in a variety of movement disorders other than those usually associated with basal ganglia dysfunction. Increasing synaptic GABA levels by valproate (46) or GABA receptor activation by progabide or THIP (125) is reported to improve posthypoxic intention myoclonus. In contrast, patients with benign essential tremor did not respond to progabide (N = 18) (126). Single-patient studies indicate a possible positive effect of GABA$_B$ receptor activation (e.g., baclofen) in hemifacial spasm (161) and stiff-man syndrome (192).

PSYCHOPHARMACOLOGY OF GABAERGIC AGENTS: PSYCHIATRIC ASPECTS

Studies over the past decade have indicated that GABA neuron function is not limited to control and/or modulation of cerebral excitability and involuntary movements, but that GABA synapses play an important role in the cognitive, emotional, and psychological aspects of cerebral function. Studies with GABAergic agents in animal models would predict an efficacy of GABA mimetics in schizophrenia, anxiety, and mood disorders. As for the different neurological correlates of GABA synaptic function, sufficient data now exist to assess the activity of GABAergic agents in these psychiatric disorders.

Anxiety

The hypothetical role of GABAergic agents as potential anxiolytics is based on observations that benzodiazepines (the primary treatment for anxiety) potentiate the neurophysiological actions of GABA at the chloride ion channel (5,66), that they increase the binding of GABA to GABA$_A$ receptors (63,78), and that some membrane recognition sites for benzodiazepines are an integral part of the GABA$_A$-chloride ionophore macromolecular complex (cf. ref. 13). These studies imply that the GABA$_A$ receptor is involved in anxiety and that its direct activation would have an anxiolytic effect.

However appealing this biochemical hypothesis may be, the experimental evidence with GABAergic agents in models of anxiety is rather controversial (162). In punished drinking (Vogel test) and other antipunishment models, GABA agonists such as muscimol (52,61,73,172,187) or progabide (163) do not exert anxiolytic-like effects, although muscimol, THIP, and GABA are active when administered intracerebrally (19,169,188). GABA receptor antagonists and GAD inhibitors block the action of benzodiazepines in models of punished behavior, although not in a dose-dependent manner (61,92,177,198). In contrast to the GABA agonists, GABA transaminase inhibitors exhibit modest antipunishment activity, but not in parallel with elevated GABA levels (52,158,160).

In an aversive model (stimulation of the periaqueductal gray matter in the rat), sodium valproate and progabide increase the escape latency and threshold (10). Progabide is synergistic with diazepam and both drugs are antagonized by bicuculline. The effect of diazepam, but not progabide, is blocked by the benzodiazepine antagonist Ro 15-1788 (10,99).

Similar conflicting data occur for the comparison of actions of GABAergic agents and benzodiazepines on discriminatory stimuli, food and water intake, and other behavioral properties (162).

In therapeutic use the anxiolytic activity of GABAergic agents is not remarkable. Thus, in trials in anxious patients, progabide (104) or THIP (71) produces at most a weak beneficial effect, much less than that observed with benzodiazepines. Furthermore, valproate is not known for anxiolytic effects after several years of use as an antiepileptic. However, in schizophrenic patients muscimol is noted to have an anxiolytic effect, although aggravating the psychosis at higher doses (181). Thus, the clinical results to date do not support a major anxiolytic effect of GABAergic agents.

Schizophrenia

Appealing evidence exists that implies a dysfunction of GABA synapses in schizophrenia, or at least suggests that GABAergic agents could exert an intrinsic antipsychotic action, or potentiate neuroleptics. The biochemical evidence is similar to that reviewed for the antidyskinetic potential of GABAergic agents: the tonic inhibitory control of dopamine neurons by GABA synapses; the inhibition of the feedback activation of dopamine neurons following neuroleptics; the decrease in dopamine receptor up-regulation following chronic dopamine receptor blockade. Behaviorally, GABAergic agents (agonists such as progabide and muscimol, GABA-transaminase inhibitors) potentiate the cataleptogenic and antiapomorphine (stereotypies) action of neuroleptics, and exert some intrinsic antidopamine acti-

TABLE 4. *Clinical psychopharmacology of GABAergic agents in schizophrenia*

Class	No. of patients treated	Improved	Worsened	Refs.
GABA$_A$ agonist				
THIP	18	0	0	84
GABA$_B$ agonist				
Baclofen	132	14	19	49,57,175
GABA$_{A+B}$ agonists				
Progabide	26	0	3	131
Muscimol	6	0	At high doses	180
GABA-transaminase inhibitors				
Valproate	8	0	6	87
γ-Acetylenic acid	10	0	0	21
γ-Vinyl GABA	4	0	0	186

vity such as inhibition of apomorphine stereotypies or decreased amphetamine hyperactivity (see above and refs. 38, 93–95).

These arguments are enhanced by the observation that a direct inhibition of dopamine synthesis potentiates the clinical effect of neuroleptics (18,93–95) and that neurochemical alterations of GABA synaptic activity have been observed in cerebral material from schizophrenic patients (cf. refs. 75 and 190); however, the latter findings are controversial (76). Furthermore, upon both acute and chronic administration, neuroleptics alter indices of GABA synaptic activity (synthesis, levels, and GABA$_A$ receptor binding) (103,109).

Based on these findings, several GABAergic compounds have been tested in schizophrenic patients. As shown in Table 4, GABAergic therapy in schizophrenia has proven to be a total failure; only one (49) of 15 studies with different compounds reports a therapeutic benefit. Overall, more patients have had symptoms exacerbated than ameliorated. This includes agonists specific for GABA$_A$ (THIP) or GABA$_B$ (baclofen) receptors and also agonists with activity at both receptor subtypes (progabide, muscimol) and GABA-transaminase inhibitors (valproate, γ-vinyl GABA, γ-acetylenic GABA).

It is useful to look for a logical explanation for such a discrepancy between the prediction made from animal models and the actual clinical results. It is unlikely that the explanation is an insufficient GABAergic inhibition of striatal dopamine neuron activity, as in several of these trials dyskinetic movements were noticeably decreased (21,131,181,182). It is more probable that separate dopaminergic systems are involved in tardive dyskinesia (nigrostriatal dopamine neurons) and in schizophrenia (mesolimbic and mesocortical dopamine neurons). The GABAergic inhibition of limbic dopamine neurons is less effective than the tonic inhibition of nigrostriatal dopamine neurons as shown by a less marked effect of GABAergic agents (progabide, muscimol) on both basal and neuroleptic-activated mesolimbic dopamine neuron function (113,166). In parallel, GABA agonists (e.g., progabide, muscimol) antagonize apomorphine-induced stereotypies (proposed to

be related to striatal function) but do not reduce apomorphine-induced climbing activity (a limbic event) in the mouse (K. G. Lloyd, *unpublished data*). Furthermore, the locomotor effect of amphetamine is reduced by progabide, whereas the conditioned place preference is unaltered (38). These findings suggest that it is the interpretation of the animal models that has been erroneous.

Mood Disorders

One of the more surprising developments in the psychopharmacology of GABAergic agents has arisen from the study of mood disorders, at biochemical, behavioral, and clinical levels. From these results it would appear that both GABA$_A$ and GABA$_B$ receptor activation participates in the modulation of mood.

In behavioral models of depression (Table 5), GABA mimetics exert an activity similar to that of therapeutically useful antidepressant drugs. In the learned helplessness model, GABAergic agents such as progabide and fengabine, or GABA itself (intracerebrally), antagonize the behavioral

TABLE 5. *Activity of GABAergic compounds in behavioral models for antidepressant drug action*

Model	Active compounds	Refs.
Learned helplessness (rat)	GABA (intracerebral)	151
	Progabide	104
	Fengabine	163
Olfactory bulbectomy (rat)		
Passive avoidance deficit	Progabide	104
	Fengabine	199
	Muscimol	104
Muricidal behavior	Baclofen	31
Open-field activation	Baclofen	89
	γ-vinyl GABA	89
Paradoxical sleep (rat, cat)	Progabide	104
	Fengabine	33

deficits (Table 5). Furthermore, a decrease in GABA release in the hippocampus parallels the onset of the behavioral deficit; both alterations are reversed by imipramine (151). Blockade of GABA$_A$ receptors by bicuculline provokes a learned-helplessness-like state (151,173) and reverses the action of tricyclic antidepressants in this model (199).

In the olfactory bulbectomized rat, GABAergic agents also demonstrate an antidepressant-like activity. Activation of both GABA$_A$ and GABA$_B$ receptors (progabide, fengabine, muscimol) reverses both the passive avoidance deficit (in a bicuculline-sensitive manner) (89,104,163,199) and the open-field activation (γ-vinyl GABA) (89). Specific GABA$_B$ receptor activation by baclofen reverses both the muricidal behavior (32) and the open-field activation (89). Furthermore, GABA$_B$ receptors are decreased in the frontal cortex after olfactory bulbectomy (107). Antidepressant treatment reverses both the GABA$_B$ and the passive avoidance behavior deficits in a parallel manner (K. G. Lloyd and P. Pichat, *unpublished*).

A common action of clinically useful antidepressants is a decrease in paradoxical sleep phases in the rat. GABA receptor activation by either progabide (104) or fengabine (33) reduces the paradoxical sleep content in a manner similar to that of tricyclic antidepressants.

In animal models for antidepressant drug action that depend on an activation of monoaminergic neurons (e.g., reserpine ptosis, 5-hydroxytryptophan head twitches), GABAergic agents are at most weakly active (104).

This antidepressant profile of GABAergic agents is reproduced in clinical trials in which progabide has been shown to be at least as active as tricyclic antidepressants (imipramine, nortryptyline) (6,104,131). Of 71 patients, 46 exhibited an excellent to good response to progabide, with a much lower incidence of undesirable effects as compared to the tricyclics. Similar results have been obtained with fengabine (134). Again, 46 of 71 patients exhibited an excellent to good therapeutic response with a lower incidence of side effects and a possible faster onset of action than tricyclics.

Clinical data with other GABAergic agents support these observations: valproate (but not the specific GABA$_A$ agonist THIP) is reported to have an antimanic activity (41,42), and manic symptomatology has been reported after withdrawal from chronic baclofen (2,193). Furthermore, cycloserine, a glutamic acid decarboxylase inhibitor, is associated with mood changes and depression (even resulting in suicide) that remit upon withdrawal (90).

As the psychopharmacological profiles of GABAergic agents are parallel in both animal models and mood disorders, the possibility should be considered that a deficit in GABAergic mechanisms is fundamental to depression and that the clinical action of antidepressant drugs may be related to GABAergic function rather than to the plethora of different monoaminergic mechanisms that have been proposed.

There is evidence that a deficit in central GABA neuron function exists in depression. Low levels of GAD activity in the frontal cortex (145), and GABA in the CSF (53,54,59,81) and plasma (9,151) have been reported for depressed patients. In a study where different biochemical parameters in the CSF were evaluated by means of a covariant analysis [including homovanillic acid (HVA), 3-methoxy-4-hydroxyphenylethyleneglycol (MO-

PEG), 5-hydroxyindoleacetic acid (5-HIAA), and GABA levels], only GABA was found to be correlated with the changes in depressive symptoms (53,54).

Clinically effective antidepressants and electroshock have a consistent effect on GABA synapses, up-regulating GABA$_B$ receptors in the rat frontal cortex on repeated administration (Table 6). Such alterations are not observed for GABA$_A$ receptors, GABA levels, or GABA synthesis (152). Psychotherapeutic agents that are not antidepressant (neuroleptics, barbiturates, anxiolytics, amphetamine) do not increase GABA$_B$ binding (108,110). Furthermore, some tricyclics (desmethylimipramine, iprindole, amitryptyline, nortryptyline) inhibit GABA uptake at clinically relevant concentrations (108).

It is very probable that GABA neurons and noradrenergic neurons are both involved in the action of antidepressant drugs. Thus, GABA$_B$ up-regulation and β-adrenoceptor down-regulation are the two most consistent biochemical results of repeated antidepressant drug administration (108). GABA synapses modulate noradrenergic synaptic activity as shown by the increase in norepinephrine turnover induced by progabide, fengabine, and other GABA agonists (165,166) and the GABA$_B$ enhancement of the maximal response of β-receptor-induced cyclic AMP formation (68,80).

TABLE 6. *Effect of repeated administration of antidepressant drugs, or electroshock, on GABA$_B$ binding to rat frontal cortex membranes*

Compound (mg/kg/d)	Duration and route	% Control
Uptake inhibitors		
Nonspecific		
Amitryptyline (10)	18d, s.c.	154
Amphetamine (2)	18d, s.c.	119
Norepinephrine		
Desipramine (5)	18d, s.c.	151
Maprotiline (10)	18d, s.c.	135
Viloxazine (10)	18d, s.c.	188
Dopamine		
Nomifensine (5)	18d, s.c.	146
Buproprion (5)	18d, s.c.	154
Serotonin		
Citalopram (10)	18d, s.c.	172
Fluoxetine (10)	6d, i.p.	183
Zimelidine (10)	18d, s.c.	165
Monoamine oxidase inhibitor		
Pargyline (20)	18d, s.c.	142
Electroshock		
150 mA, 0.5 sec/48 hr	10d	177
GABA mimetics		
Progabide (100)	18d, i.p.	127
Fengabine (50)	6d, i.p.	159
Sodium valproate (100)	18d, i.p.	120
Miscellaneous compounds		
Trazodone (10)	18d, s.c.	155
Iprindole (5)	18d, s.c.	129
Mianserine (10)	18d, s.c.	133
Idazoxan (5)	18d, s.c.	207

Data from refs. 108 and 110.
The concentration of [^{3}H]GABA was 10 nM in the presence of 40 μM isoguvacine.

ANALGESIC ACTIVITY

Several GABA agonists with either pure GABA$_A$ (THIP), GABA$_B$ (baclofen), or mixed GABA$_{A+B}$ (muscimol) profiles have been tested for analgesic activity, and all have been shown to be effective in writhing, hot plate, tail flick, arthritic pain, and paw pressure tests (24,29,62,70,82). This action is apparently independent of GABA$_A$ receptors (bicuculline insensitive) and opiate receptors (naloxone insensitive) (70) (cf. also ref. 85). The analgesia related to GABA$_B$ receptors may be at least partially due to a reduction in C fiber transmission at the level of the nerve fibers themselves, or at the dorsal horn of the spinal cord (35,37,156).

In clinical studies baclofen has been reported to be efficacious in trigeminal neuralgia (50). However, in this syndrome the analgesic activity may be due to a direct action at the level of the spinal trigeminal nucleus (50). THIP has been reported to have analgesic activities in humans (91).

SUMMARY AND CONCLUSIONS

In the last decade the psychopharmacology of GABAergic agents has made considerable advances, due mainly to the understanding of the different subtypes of GABA receptors (GABA$_A$ and GABA$_B$) and to the availability of compounds

TABLE 7. *Psychopharmacology of GABAergic agents: correlation between prediction from animal models and clinical responses*

Prediction from animal models	Pathological state	Clinical response
	Epilepsy	
A broad spectrum of antiepileptic action for GABA$_{A+B}$ receptor activation		Positive response to GABA$_{A+B}$ agonists and GABA transaminase inhibitors. GABA$_A$ agonist less effective (progabide, valproate, γ-vinyl GABA, THIP)
	Spasticity	
Antispastic action of GABA receptor activation (GABA$_A$ and/or $_B$)		Positive response to GABA$_A$, GABA$_B$, and GABA$_{A+B}$ agonists (THIP, baclofen, progabide)
	Parkinson's disease	
Exacerbation of parkinsonism Reduction of L-dopa dyskinesia (GABA$_A$)		Little marked effect of parkinsonism. Increased on-time for L-dopa response. Exacerbation of neuroleptic-induced parkinsonism (progabide)
	Huntington's chorea	
Improvement of chorea (GABA$_A$)		No dramatic effect (progabide, THIP, muscimol, γ-vinyl GABA, valproate, γ-acetylenic GABA)
	Tardive dyskinesia	
Improvement of dyskinesia		Positive response to GABA$_A$ and GABA$_{A+B}$ activation (progabide, THIP, muscimol, γ-vinyl GABA). No effect of GABA$_B$ activation (baclofen)
	Schizophrenia	
Decrease in psychosis or increased efficacy of neuroleptics (GABA$_A$ or $_B$)		No reproducible effect with GABA$_A$, GABA$_B$, or GABA$_{A+B}$ mimetics (progabide, muscimol, THIP, baclofen, γ-vinyl GABA, valproate)
	Anxiety	
Anxiolytic action (GABA$_A$)		At most a mild anxiolytic effect (muscimol, THIP, progabide)
	Depression	
Antidepressant activity (GABA$_{A+B}$)		Positive antidepressant effect (progabide, fengabine)

(e.g., progabide, THIP, γ-vinyl GABA) suitable for clinical testing of the hypotheses arising from animal experimentation. As a result a new category of psychopharmacological agents has been conceived: the GABA mimetics. Diseases responsive to this therapeutic category include epilepsy, spasticity, tardive dyskinesia, and depression (Table 7).

To date epilepsy has shown the most promising response, with a high percentage of previously refractory or uncontrolled patients responding to GABA mimetic therapy. These positive results are likely correlated with an underlying deficit in GABA-mediated inhibition in at least some cases of epilepsy. Epilepsy is the only clinical condition for which GABAergic compounds are marketed (valproate, progabide).

Other clinical states exhibiting a positive response to GABA mimetics in parallel with their preclinical activity include spasticity and depression. As for epilepsy, it is highly probable that an underlying pathology of GABA neuron function exists in these conditions. Either GABA$_A$ or GABA$_B$ receptor activation results in an antispastic effect, whereas the antidepressant action of GABAergic agents appears to require both GABA receptor subtypes.

In addition to these neuropsychiatric disorders, GABA mimetics also show a promising activity in the iatrogenic syndrome of tardive dyskinesia. In this condition GABA receptor activation reinstates the physiological balance between striatal dopamine and GABA synaptic transmission that is perturbed by the neuroleptics.

Equally interesting are those states in which the activity of GABA mimetics in animal models apparently erroneously predicted a positive clinical response. Of these, the apparently paradoxical increase in "on-time" for L-dopa in Parkinson's disease corresponds to the potentiation of dopamine mimetics seen with low doses of GABA agonists in animal models. The fact that neuroleptic-induced Parkinsonism is exacerbated at the same doses of GABA mimetics is puzzling, but may reflect a difference in the neurochemistry of Parkinson's disease versus drug-induced Parkinsonism. In contrast, the failure of GABA mimetics to act in Huntington's chorea is not surprising in light of the widespread neuroanatomical destruction occurring in these patients. Prophylactic treatment with GABA agonists might have a greater chance of success.

The apparent paradoxical resistance of schizophrenia and anxiety to GABA mimetic therapy is probably due to the use of animal models that do not reflect the human condition, resulting in a misinterpretation of the biochemical and neuropharmacological data. Perhaps GABA mimetics with a preferential inhibition of mesolimbic dopamine neurons would have positive effects in schizophrenia. In anxiety the profile of GABA mimetics does not resemble that of the benzodiazepines either at the clinical or preclinical levels.

REFERENCES

1. Abbott, R. J., Pye, I. F., and Nahorski, S. R. (1982): *J. Neurol. Neurosurg. Psychiatry,* 45:253–256.
2. Arnold, E. S., Rudd, S., and Kirshner, H. (1980): *Am. J. Psychiatry,* 137:1466–1467.
3. Ashby, P., White, C. J., and Knowles, L. (1973): *J. Neurol. Sci.,* 20:329–338.
4. Bakay, R. A. E., and Harris, A. B. (1984): *Soc. Neurosci. Abstr.,* 10:188.
5. Barker, J. L., Gratz, E., Owen, D. G., and Study, R. E. (1984): In: *Actions and Interactions of GABA and Benzodiazepines,* edited by N. G. Bowery, pp. 203–216. Raven Press, New York.
6. Bartholini, G., Lloyd, K. G., and Morselli, P. L., eds. (1986): *GABA and Mood Disorders.* Raven Press, New York.
7. Bartholini, G., Lloyd, K. G., Worms, P., Costantinidis, J., and Tissot, R. (1979): In: *Advances in Neurology, Vol. 24,* edited by L. J. Poirier, T. L. Sourkes, and P. J. Bedard, pp. 253–257. Raven Press, New York.
8. Bergman, K. J., Limongi, J. C. P., Lowe, Y. H., Mendoza, M. R., and Yahr, M. D. (1984): *Lancet,* 1:559.
9. Berrettini, W. H., Nurnberger, J. I., Hare, T., Gershon, E. S., and Post, R. M. (1982): *Br. J. Psychiatry,* 14:483–487.
10. Bovier, P., Broekkamp, C. L. E., and Lloyd, K. G. (1982): *Brain Res.,* 248:313–320.
11. Bovier, P., Cambier, J., and Morselli, P. L. (1985): *Therapie,* 40:181–185.
12. Bowery, N. G. (1982): *TIPS*(October):400–403.
13. Bowery, N. G., ed. (1984): *Actions and Interactions of GABA and Benzodiazepines.* Raven Press, New York.
14. Bowery, N. G., Hill, D. R., and Hudson, A. L. (1982): *Br. J. Pharmacol.,* 75:86P.
15. Bowery, N. G., Hill, D. R., and Hudson, A. L. (1983): *Br. J. Pharmacol.,* 78:191–206.
16. Bowery, N. G., Hill, D. R., Hudson, A. L., and Price, G. W. (1985): In: *Epilepsy and GABA Receptor Agonists,* edited by G. Bartholini, L. Bossi, K. G. Lloyd, and P. L. Morselli, pp. 63–80. Raven Press, New York.
17. Bowery, N. G., Price, G. W., Hudson, A. L., Hill, P. R., Wilkin, G. P., and Turnbull, M. J. (1984): *Neuropharmacology,* 23:219–231.
18. Brogden, R. N., Heed, R. C., Speight, T. M., and Avery, G. S. (1981): *Drugs,* 21:81–89.
19. Carranzi, A. R., Costa, E., and Guidotti, A. (1980): *Brain Res.,* 196:447–453.
20. Casey, D. E., Chase, T. N., Christensen, A. V., and Gerlach, J., eds. (1985): *Dyskinesia Research and Treatment.* Springer-Verlag, Berlin.
21. Casey, D. E., Gerlach, J., Magelund, G., and Christensen, T. R. (1980): *Arch. Gen. Psychiatry,* 37:1376–1379.
22. Cepeda, C., Worms, P., Lloyd, K. G., and Naquet, R. (1982): *Epilepsia,* 24:463–470.
23. Christensen, A. V., Arnt, J., and Scheel-Kruger, J. (1980): *Brain Res. Bull.,* 5(Suppl. 2):885–890.
24. Christensen, A. V., and Larsen, J. J. (1982): *Pol. J. Pharmacol.,* 34:127–134.
25. Coquelin, J. P., Krall, R., Bossi, L., Musch, B., and Morselli, P. L. (1985): In: *Epilepsy and GABA Receptor Agonists,* edited by G. Bartholini, L. Bossi, K. G. Lloyd, and P. L. Morselli, pp. 431–440. Raven Press, New York.
26. Curtis, D. R., and Malik, R. (1985): *Exp. Brain Res.,* 58:333–337.
27. Czuczar, S. J., Frey, H. H., and Löscher, W. (1986): In: *Workshop on Neurotransmitters in Epilepsy III,* edited by G. Nistiko, P. L. Morselli, K. G. Lloyd, J. Engel, Jr., and R. G. Fariello, pp. 235–245. Raven Press, New York.
28. Davidoff, R. A. (1985): *Ann. Neurol.,* 17:107–116.
29. DeFeudis, F. V. (1982): *Trends Pharmacol. Sci.,* 3:444–446.
30. Delgado-Escueta, A. V., Ward, A. A., Jr., Woodbury, D. M., and Porter, R. J., eds. (1986): *Basic Mechanisms of the Epilepsies.* Raven Press, New York.
31. Delini-Stula, A. (1979): In: *GABA-Neurotransmitters,* edited by P. Krogsgaard-Larsen, J. Scheel-Kruger, and H. Kofod, pp. 482–499. Munksgaard, Copenhagen.
32. Delini-Stula, A., and Vassout, A. (1978): *Arzneim. Forsch.,* 28:1508–1509.
33. Depoortere, H., and Riou-Merle, F. (1986): In: *GABA and Mood Disorders,* edited by G. Bartholini, K. G. Lloyd, and P. L. Morselli, pp. 97–100. Raven Press, New York.
34. Desarmenien, M., Feltz, P., Occhipinti, G., Santangelo, F., and Schlichter, R. (1984): *Br. J. Pharmacol.,* 81:327–333.
35. Desarmenien, M., Santangelo, F., Loeffler, J. P., and Feltz, P. (1984): *Exp. Brain Res.,* 54:521–528.

36. Dhanaraj, M., Radhakrishnan, A. R., Srinivas, K., and Sayeed, Z. A. (1985): *Neurology*, 35:114–115.
37. Dickenson, A. H., Breuer, C. M., and Hayes, N. A. (1985): *Neurosciences*, 4:557–562.
38. Di Scala, G., Martin-Iversen, M. I., Phillips, A. G., and Fibiger, H. C. (1985): *Eur. J. Pharmacol.*, 107:271–274.
39. Drew, C. A., Johnston, G. A. R., and Weatherby, R. P. (1984): *Neurosci. Lett.*, 52:317–321.
40. Dunlap, K. (1981): *Br. J. Pharmacol.*, 74:579–585.
41. Emrich, H. M., Altman, H., Dose, M., and Von Zersen, D. (1985): *Pharmacol. Biochem. Behav.*, 19:369–372.
42. Emrich, H. M., Dose, M., and Von Zerssen, D. (1985): *J. Affective Disord.*, 8:243–250.
43. Enna, S. J., ed. (1983): *The GABA Receptors*. Humana Press, Clifton.
44. Enna, S. J., Stern, L., Wastek, G., and Yamamura, H. I. (1977): *Life Sci.*, 20:205–212.
45. Erdo, S. L., and Bowery, N. G., eds. (1986): *GABAergic Mechanisms in the Mammalian Periphery*. Raven Press, New York.
46. Fahn, S. (1979): *Adv. Neurol.*, 26:49–84.
47. Fibiger, H. C., and Lloyd, K. G. (1984): *Trends Neurosci.*, 7: 462–464.
48. Foster, N. L., Chase, T. N., Denaro, A., Hare, T. A., and Tamminga, C. A. (1983): *Neurology*, 33:637–639.
49. Frederiksen, P. K. (1975): *Lancet*, 1:702.
50. Fromm, G. H., Terrence, C. F., and Chattha, A. S. (1984): *Ann. Neurol.*, 15:240–244.
51. Gale, K. (1986): In: *Workshop on Neurotransmitters in Epilepsy III*, edited by G. Nistico, P. L. Morselli, K. G. Lloyd, J. Engel, Jr., and R. G. Fariello, pp. 205–217. Raven Press, New York.
52. Gardner, C. R., and Piper, C. D. (1982): *Eur. J. Pharmacol.*, 83: 25–33.
53. Gerner, R. H., and Fairbanks, L. (1985): *IV World Congress of Biological Psychiatry*, Abstract 500.1.
54. Gerner, R. H., Fairbanks, L., Andersen, G. E., Young, J. G., Scheinini, M., Lennoila, M., Hare, T. A., Shaywitz, B. A., and Chen, D. J. (1984): *Am. J. Psychiatry*, 141:1533–1540.
55. Gibson, A. C. (1978): *Br. J. Psychiatry*, 133:82–86.
56. Giotti, A., Luzzi, S., Spagnesi, S., and Ziletti, L. (1983): *Br. J. Pharmacol.*, 79:855–862.
57. Glaser, W. M., Moore, D. C., Bowers, M. B., Bunney, B. S., and Roffman, M. (1985): *Psychopharmacology*, 87:480–483.
58. Goetz, C. G., and Klawans, H. L. (1982): In: *Butterworths International Medical Reviews, Neurology 2: Movement Disorders*, edited by C. D. Marsden and S. Fahn, pp. 263–276. Butterworth Scientific, London.
59. Gold, B. I., Bowers, M. B., Roth, R. H., and Sweeney, D. W. (1980): *Am. J. Psychiatry*, 137:362–364.
60. Gonce, M., Schoenen, J., Charlier, M., and Delwaide, P. J. (1983): *J. Neurol.*, 229:121–124.
61. Gray, J. A., Quinters, S., Mellandbry, J., Buckland, C., Fillenz, M., and Fung, S. C. (1984): In: *Actions and Interactions of GABA and Benzodiazepines*, edited by N. G. Bowery, pp. 239–262. Raven Press, New York.
62. Grognet, A., Hertz, F., and De Feudis, F. V. (1983): *Gen. Pharmacol.*, 14:585–589.
63. Guidotti, A., Toffano, G., Grandison, L., and Costa, E. (1978): In: *Amino Acids as Chemical Transmitters*, edited by F. Fonnum, pp. 517–530. Plenum Press, New York.
64. Gunne, L. M., and Haggstrom, J. E. (1983): *Psychopharmacology*, 81:191–194.
65. Gunne, L. M., Haggstrom, J. E., and Sjoqvist, B. (1984): *Nature*, 309:347–349.
66. Haefely, W., Pieri, L., Polc, P., and Schaffner, R. (1981): In: *Handbook of Experimental Pharmacology, 55/II*, edited by F. Hoffmeister and G. Stille, pp. 13–262. Springer-Verlag, Berlin.
67. Hammond, E. J., and Wilder, B. J. (1985): *Clin. Neuropharmacol.*, 8:1–12.
68. Hill, D. R. (1985): *Br. J. Pharmacol.*, 84:249–257.
69. Hill, D. R., and Bowery, N. G. (1981): *Nature*, 290:149–152.
70. Hill, R. C., Maurer, R., Buescher, H. H., and Roemer, D. (1981): *Eur. J. Pharmacol.*, 69:221–224.
71. Hoehn-Saric, R. (1983): *Psychopharmacology*, 80:338–341.
72. Hornykiewicz, O. (1966): *Pharmacol. Revs.*, 18:925–964.
73. Huot, S., Robin, M., and Palfreymann, M. G. (1981): In: *Amino Acid Neurotransmitters*, edited by F. V. De Feudis and P. Mandel, pp. 45–52. Raven Press, New York.
74. Inowe, M., Mabuo, T., and Ogata, N. (1985): *Br. J. Pharmacol.*, 84:843–852.
75. Iversen, L. L. (1978): In: *Psychopharmacology: A Generation of Progress*, edited by M. A. Lipton, A. Di Mascio, and K. F. Killam, pp. 25–38. Raven Press, New York.
76. Iversen, L. L., Bird, E., Spokes, E., Nicholson, S. H., and Suckling, C. J. (1979): In: *GABA Neurotransmitters*, edited by P. Krogsgaard-Larsen, J. Scheel-Kruger, and H. Kofod, pp. 179–190. Munksgaard, Copenhagen.
77. Johnston, G. A. R. (1976): In: *GABA in Nervous System Function*, edited by E. Roberts, T. N. Chase, and D. B. Tower, pp. 395–413. Raven Press, New York.
78. Johnston, G. A. R., and Skerritt, J. H. (1984): In: *Actions and Interactions of GABA and Benzodiazepines*, edited by N. G. Bowery, pp. 179–190. Raven Press, New York.
79. Joy, R. M., Albertson, T. E., and Stark, L. G. (1984): *Exp. Neurol.*, 83:144–154.
80. Karbon, E. W., Duman, R. S., and Enna, S. J. (1984): *Brain Res.*, 306:327–332.
81. Kasa, K., Otsuki, S., Yamamoto, M., Sato, M., Kuroda, H., and Ogawa, N. (1982): *Biol. Psychiatry*, 17:877–883.
82. Kendall, D. A., Browner, M., and Enna, S. J. (1982): *J. Pharmacol. Exp. Ther.*, 220:482–497.
83. Krjnevic, K. (1976): In: *GABA in Nervous System Function*, edited by E. Roberts, T. N. Chase, and D. B. Tower, pp. 395–413. Raven Press, New York.
84. Korsgaard, S., Casey, D. E., Gerlach, J., Hetmar, O., Kaldan, H., and Mikkelsen, L. B. (1982): *Arch. Gen. Psychiatry*, 39:1017–1021.
85. Krogsgaard-Larsen, P., Falch, E., and Christensen, A. V. (1984): *Drugs Fut.*, 9:597–618.
86. Langer, S. Z., Arbilla, S., Scatton, B., Zivkovic, B., Galzin, A. M., Lloyd, K. G., and Bartholini, G. (1985): In: *Epilepsy and GABA Receptor Agonists*, edited by G. Bartholini, L. Bossi, K. G. Lloyd, and P. L. Morselli, pp. 81–90. Raven Press, New York.
87. Lautin, A., Angrist, B., Stanley, M., Gershon, S., Heckl, K., and Karobath, M. (1980): *Br. J. Psychiatry*, 137:240–244.
88. Lees, A. J., Shaw, K. M., and Stern, G. M. (1978): *J. Neurol. Neurosurg. Psychiatry*, 41:707–708.
89. Leonard, B. E. (1984): *Pol. J. Pharmacol.*, 36:561–569.
90. Lewis, W. C., Calden, G., Thurston, J. R., and Gilson, W. E. (1957): *Dis. Chest*, 32:172–182.
91. Lindeburg, T., Foelsgaard, S., Sillesen, H., Jacobsen, E., and Kehlet, H. (1983): *Acta Anaesth. Scand.*, 27:10–12.
92. Lippa, A. S., Nash, P. A., and Greenblatt, E. N. (1979): In: *Anxiolytics*, edited by S. Fielding and H. Lal, pp. 41–81. Futura, New York.
93. Lloyd, K. G. (1977): In: *Essays in Neurochemistry and Neuropharmacology, Vol. 3*, edited by M. B. H. Youdim, W. Lovenberg, D. F. Sharman, and J. R. Lagnado, pp. 129–208. Wiley, New York.
94. Lloyd, K. G. (1978): In: *Cholinergic Monoaminergic Interactions in the Brain*, edited by L. L. Butcher, pp. 363–392. Raven Press, New York.
95. Lloyd, K. G. (1980): In: *Enzymes and Neurotransmitters in Mental Disease*, edited by F. Usdin, T. L. Sourkes, and M. B. H. Youdim, pp. 329–344. Wiley, New York.
96. Lloyd, K. G. (1986): In: *Neuromethods, Vol. IV*, edited by G. Baker and A. A. Boulton, pp. 217–249. Humana Press, Clifton.
97. Lloyd, K. G. (1986): *Rev. Pract. (Paris)*, 36:243–254.
98. Lloyd, K. G., Bossi, L., Morselli, P. L., Munari, C., Rougier, M., and Loiseau, P. (1986): In: *Basic Mechanisms of the Epilepsies*, edited by A. V. Delgado-Escueta, A. A. Ward, Jr., D. M. Woodbury, and R. J. Porter, pp. 1033–1044. Raven Press, New York.
99. Lloyd, K. G., Bovier, P., Broekkamp, C. L. E., and Worms, P. (1981): *Eur. J. Pharmacol.*, 75:77–78.
100. Lloyd, K. G., Broekkamp, C. L. E., and Worms, P. (1983): In: *Application of Behavioral Pharmacology in Toxicology*, edited by G. Zbinden, V. Cuomo, G. Racagni, and B. Weiss, pp. 203–215. Raven Press, New York.

101. Lloyd, K. G., Davidson, L., and Hornykiewicz, O. (1975): *J. Pharmacol. Exp. Ther.*, 195:453–464.
102. Lloyd, K. G., Dreksler, S., and Bird, E. D. (1977): *Life Sci.*, 21:747–749.
103. Lloyd, K. G., and Hornykiewicz, O. (1977): *Life Sci.*, 21:1489–1496.
104. Lloyd, K. G., Morselli, P. L., Depoortere, H., Fournier, V., Zivkovic, B., Scatton, B., Broekkamp, C. L. E., Worms, P., and Bartholini, G. (1983): *Pharmacol. Biochem. Behav.*, 18:957–966.
105. Lloyd, K. G., Munari, C., Bossi, L., and Morselli, P. L. (1983): In: *Workshop on Neurotransmitters in Epilepsy II*, edited by R. G. Fariello, P. L. Morselli, K. G. Lloyd, L. F. Quesney, and J. Engel, pp. 285–293. Raven Press, New York.
106. Lloyd, K. G., Perrault, G., and Zivkovic, B. (1985): *J. Pharmacol. (Paris)*, 16:5–27.
107. Lloyd, K. G., and Pichat, P. (1986): *Br. J. Pharmacol.*, 87:36.
108. Lloyd, K. G., and Pichat, P. (1987): In: *New Advances in Psychotropic Drug Research*, edited by S. Dahl, S. M. Paul, and W. Bradley. Raven Press, New York (*in press*).
109. Lloyd, K. G., Shibuya, M., Davidson, L., and Hornykiewicz, O. (1977): In: *Non-Striatal Dopaminergic Neurons*, edited by E. Costa and G. L. Gessa, pp. 409–416. Raven Press, New York.
110. Lloyd, K. G., Thuret, F., and Pilc, A. (1985): *J. Pharmacol. Exp. Ther.*, 235:191–199.
111. Lloyd, K. G., Willigens, M. T., and Goldstein, M. (1985): In: *Dyskinesia: Research and Treatment*, edited by D. Casey, T. N. Chase, A. V. Christensen, and J. Gerlach, pp. 200–210. Springer-Verlag, Berlin.
112. Lloyd, K. G., and Worms, P. (1980): In: *Long Term Effects of Neuroleptics*, edited by F. Cattabeni, G. Racagni, and P. F. Spano, pp. 253–258. Raven Press, New York.
113. Lloyd, K. G., Worms, P., Zivkovic, B., Scatton, B., and Bartholini, G. (1980): *Brain Res. Bull.* 5(Suppl. 2):439–445.
114. Löscher, W. (1981): *Biochem. Pharmacol.*, 30:1364–1366.
115. Löscher, W. (1982): *Neuropharmacology*, 21:803–810.
116. MacLean, D. R. (1982): *Neurology*, 32:1189–1191.
117. Maitre, M., Csieski, L., and Mandel, P. (1974): *Biochem. Pharmacol.*, 23:2363–2368.
118. Manyam, B. V. (1982): *Arch. Neurol.*, 39:391–392.
119. Manyam, B. V., Hare, T. A., and Katz, L. (1980): *Life Sci.*, 26:1303–1308.
120. Manyam, B. V., Katz, L., Hare, T. A., Kaniefski, K., and Tremblay, R. D. (1981): *Ann. Neurol.*, 10:35–37.
121. Marsden, C. D., and Sheehy, M. P. (1981): In: *GABA and the Basal Ganglia*, edited by G. DiChiara and G. L. Gessa, pp. 225–234. Raven Press, New York.
122. Mao, C. C., Guidotti, A. M., and Costa, E. (1975): *Mol. Pharmacol.*, 10:736–745.
123. McLellan, D. L. (1984): *Int. Rehab. Med.*, 5:141–142.
124. Meldrum, B., Peddley, T., Hanton, R., Horlezark, G., and Franks, A. (1980): *Brain Res. Bull.*, 5(Suppl. 2):685–690.
125. Mondrup, K., Dupont, E., and Braendgaard, H. (1983): *Lancet*, 2:1490.
126. Mondrup, K., Dupont, E., and Pedersen, E. (1983): *Acta Neurol. Scand.*, 68:248–252.
127. Mondrup, K., and Pedersen, E. (1983): *Acta Neurol. Scand.*, 67:48–54.
128. Mondrup, K., and Pedersen, E. (1984): *Acta Neurol. Scand.*, 69:191–199.
129. Mondrup, K., and Pedersen, E. (1984): *Acta Neurol. Scand.*, 69:200–206.
130. Morselli, P. L. (1985): In: *Epilepsy and GABA Receptor Agonists*, edited by G. Bartholini, L. Bossi, K. G. Lloyd, and P. L. Morselli, pp. 441–448. Raven Press, New York.
131. Morselli, P. L., Bossi, L., Henry, J. F., Zarifian, E., and Bartholini, G. (1980): *Brain Res. Bull.*, 5(Suppl. 2):411–414.
132. Morselli, P. L., Fournier, V., Bossi, L., and Musch, B. (1985): In: *Dyskinesia: Research and Treatment*, edited by D. E. Casey, T. N. Chase, A. V. Christensen, and J. Gerlach, pp. 128–136. Springer-Verlag, Berlin.
133. Muhyadden, M., Roberts, P. J., and Woodruff, G. N. (1982): *Br. J. Pharmacol.*, 77:163–168.
134. Musch, B. (1986): In: *GABA and Mood Disorders*, edited by G. Bartholini, K. G. Lloyd, and P. L. Morselli, pp. 171–178. Raven Press, New York.
135. Naftchi, N. E., Schlosser, W., and Horst, W. D. (1979): *Adv. Exp. Biol. Med.*, 123:431–450.
136. Nakahiro, M., Saito, K., Yamada, I., and Yoshida, H. (1985): *Neurosci. Lett.*, 57:263–266.
137. Newberry, N. R., and Nicoll, R. A. (1985): *J. Physiol. (Lond.)*, 348:239–254.
138. Nistri, A. (1983): In: *Handbook of the Spinal Cord, Vol. 1*, edited by R. A. Davidoff, pp. 45–104. Marcel Dekker, New York.
139. Olpe, H. R., Demieville, H., Baltzer, V., Beneze, W. L., Koella, W. P., Wolf, P., and Haas, H. L. (1978): *Eur. J. Pharmacol.*, 52:133–136.
140. Olsen, R. W. (1981): *Mol. Cell. Biochem.*, 39:261–279.
141. Olsen, R. W. (1982): *Annu. Rev. Pharmacol. Toxicol.*, 22:245–277.
142. Pearce, I., Heathfield, K. W. G., and Pearce, J. M. S. (1977): *Arch Neurol.*, 34:308–309.
143. Pedersen, E., Arlien-Soeborg, P., and Maj, J. (1974): *Acta Neurol. Scand.*, 50:665–680.
144. Penn, R. D., and Kroin, J. S. (1985): *Lancet*, 2:125–127.
145. Perry, E. K., Gibson, P. H., Blessed, G., Perry, R. H., and Tomlinsin, B. E. (1977): *J. Neurol. Sci.*, 34:247–265.
146. Perry, T. L., Wall, R. A., and Hansen, S. (1985): *Neurology*, 35:755–758.
147. Perry, T. L., Wright, J. M., Hansen, B. A., Thomas, S. M. B., Allan, B. M., Baird, P. A., and Diewold, P. A. (1982): *Neurology*, 32:354–358.
148. Perry, T. L., Wright, J. M., Hansen, S., Allan, B. M., Baird, P. A., and MacLeod, P. M. (1980): *Neurology*, 30:772–775.
149. Perry, T. L., Wright, J. M., Hansen, S., and MacLeod, P. (1979): *Neurology*, 29:370–375.
150. Petersen, H. R., Jensen, I., and Dam, M. (1983): *Acta Neurol. Scand.*, 67:114–117.
151. Petty, F. (1986): In: *GABA and Mood Disorders*, edited by G. Bartholini, K. G. Lloyd, and P. L. Morselli, pp. 61–66. Raven Press, New York.
152. Pilc, A., and Lloyd, K. G. (1984): *Life Sci.*, 35:2149–2154.
153. Pirreda, S., Lim, C. R., and Gale, K. (1985): *Life Sci.*, 36:1295–1298.
154. Polc, P. (1979): *Neuropsychopharmacology*, 3:345–352.
155. Price, G. W., Blackburn, T. P., Hudson, A. L., and Bowery, N. G. (1984): *Neuropharmacology*, 23(7B):861–862.
156. Price, G. W., Wilkin, G. P., Turnbull, M. J., and Bowery, N. G. (1984): *Nature*, 307:71–73.
157. Rago, L. K., and Zarkovsky, A. M. (1983): *Naunyn Schmiedebergs Arch. Pharmacol.*, 322:166–169.
158. Rasmussen, K. J., Schneider, H. H., and Petersen, E. N. (1981): *Life Sci.*, 29:2163–2170.
159. Rastogi, S. K., Rastogi, R. B., Lapierre, Y. D., and Singhal, R. L. (1982): *Gen. Pharmacol.*, 13:499–504.
160. Rayevsky, K. S., and Kharlamov, A. N. (1983): *Pharmacol. Res. Commun.*, 15:85–96.
161. Sandyk, R. (1984): *Eur. Neurol.*, 23:163–165.
162. Sanger, D. J. (1985): *Life Sci.*, 36:1503–1513.
163. Sanger, D. J., Joly, D., Depoortere, H., Zivkovic, B., and Lloyd, K. G. (1986): In: *GABA and Mood Disorders*, edited by G. Bartholini, K. G. Lloyd, and P. L. Morselli, pp. 77–84. Raven Press, New York.
164. Sastry, B. R. (1979): *Can. J. Physiol. Pharmacol.*, 57:1157–1167.
165. Scatton, B., Nishikawa, T., Dennis, T., Dedek, J., Curet, O., Zivkovic, B., and Bartholini, G. (1986): In: *GABA and Mood Disorders*, edited by G. Bartholini, K. G. Lloyd, and P. L. Morselli, pp. 67–76. Raven Press, New York.
166. Scatton, B., Zivkovic, B., Dedek, J., Lloyd, K. G., Constantinidis, J., Tissot, R., and Bartholini, G. (1982): *J. Pharmacol. Exp. Ther.*, 220:678–688.
167. Scheel-Krüger, J., and Arnt, J. (1985): *Dyskinesia Research and Treatment*, edited by D. E. Casey, T. N. Chase, A. V. Christensen, and J. Gerlach, pp. 46–57. Springer-Verlag, Berlin.
168. Scheel-Krüger, J., Arnt, J., Braestrup, C., Christensen, A. V., and Magelund, G. (1979): In: *GABA-Neurotransmitters*, edited by P. Krogsgaard-Larsen, J. Scheel-Krüger, and H. Kofod, pp. 447–464. Munksgaard, Copenhagen.
169. Scheel-Krüger, J., and Petersen, E. N. (1982): *Eur. J. Pharmacol.*, 82:115–116.

170. Schwarcz, R., Bennet, J. P., Jr., and Coyle, J. T. (1977): *Ann. Neurol.,* 2:299–303.
171. Schwarz, M., Turski, L., and Sontag, K. H. (1983): *Eur. J. Pharmacol.,* 90:139–142.
172. Seppinwall, J., and Cook, L. (1980): *Brain Res. Bull.,* 5(*Suppl.* 2):839–848.
173. Sherman, A. D., and Petty, F. (1982): *Behav. Neurol. Biol.,* 35:344–353.
174. Shoulscn, I., Goldblatt, D., Charlton, M., and Joynt, R. J. (1978): *Ann. Neurol.,* 4:279–284.
175. Simpson, G. M., Branchey, M. H., and Shrivastava, R. K. (1976): *Lancet,* 1:966–967.
176. Skerritt, J. H., Willow, M., and Johnston, G. A. R. (1982): *Neurosci. Lett.,* 29:63–66.
177. Stein, L. (1980): *Drug Res.,* 30:868–873.
178. Symington, G. R., Leonard, O. P., Shannon, P. J., and Vajda, F. J. E. (1978): *Am. J. Psychiatry,* 135:352–354.
179. Takeuchi, A., and Takeuchi, N. (1967): *J. Physiol. (Lond.),* 191:575–590.
180. Tamminga, C. A., Crayton, J. W., and Chase, T. N. (1978): *Am. J. Psychiatry,* 135:746–747.
181. Tamminga, C. A., Crayton, J. W., and Chase, T. W. (1979): *Arch. Gen. Psychiatry,* 36:595–598.
182. Tamminga, C. A., Thaker, G. K., Ferraro, T. N., and Hare, T. A. (1983): *Lancet,* 2:97–98.
183. Tapia, R. (1974): In: *Neurohumoral Coding of Brain Function,* edited by R. D. Meyers and R. R. Drucker-Colin, pp. 3–26. Plenum Press, New York.
184. Tell, G., Böhlen, P., Schechter, P. J., Koch-Weser, J., Agid, Y., Bonnet, A. M., Coquillat, G., Chazot, G., and Fischer, C. (1981): *Neurology,* 31:207–211.
185. Teychenné, P. F., Ziegler, M. G., Lake, C. R., and Enna, S. J. (1982): *Ann. Neurol.,* 11:76–79.
186. Thaker, G. K., Hare, T. A., and Tamminga, C. A. (1983): *Mod. Problems Pharmacopsychiatry,* 21:155–167.
187. Thiebot, M. H., Jobert, A., and Soubrie, R. (1979): *Psychopharmacology,* 61:85–89.
188. Thiebot, M. H., Jobert, A., and Soubrie, P. (1980): *Neurosci. Lett.,* 16:213–217.
189. Ticku, M. J., and Rastogi, S. K. (1986): In: *Workshop on Neurotransmitters in Epilepsy III,* edited by G. Nistico, P. L. Morselli, K. G. Lloyd, J. Engels, Jr., and R. G. Fariello, pp. 163–176. Raven Press, New York.
190. Van Kammen, D. P., Sternberg, D. E., Hare, T. A., Waters, R. N., and Bunney, W. E., Jr. (1982): *Arch. Gen. Psychiatry,* 39:91–97.
191. Van Ness, P. C., Watkins, A. E., Bergman, M. O., Tourtellotte, W. W., and Olsen, R. W. (1982): *Neurology,* 32:63–68.
192. Whelan, J. L. (1980): *Arch. Neurol.,* 37:600–601.
193. Wolf, M. E., Almy, G., Toll, M., and Mosnaim, A. D. (1982): *Biol. Psychiatry,* 17:757–759.
194. Wood, J. D., Kuryls, E., and Peesker, S. J. (1978): In: *Amino Acids as Chemical Neurotransmitters,* edited by F. Fonnum, pp. 439–444. Plenum Press, New York.
195. Wood, J. D., and Peesker, S. J. (1973): *J. Neurochem.,* 20:379–387.
196. Worms, P., Depoortere, H., Durand, A., Morselli, P. L., Lloyd, K. G., and Bartholini, G. (1982): *J. Pharmacol. Exp. Ther.,* 220:660–671.
197. Yamamura, H. I., Reisine, T. D., and Beaumont, K. (1980): *Brain Res. Bull.* 5(*Suppl.* 2):773–775.
198. Zakusov, V. V., Ostroskaya, R. U., Kozhechkin, S. N., Markovich, V. V., Molodavkin, G. M., and Voronina, T. A. (1977): *Arch. Int. Pharmacodyn.,* 229:313–326.
199. Zivkovic, B., Lloyd, K. G., Scatton, B., Sanger, D. J., Depoortere, H., Dedek, J., Arbilla, S., Langer, S. Z., and Bartholini, G. (1986): In: *GABA and Mood Disorders,* edited by G. Bartholini, K. G. Lloyd, and P. L. Morselli, pp. 85–96. Raven Press, New York.

Psychopharmacology:
The Third Generation of Progress,
edited by Herbert Y. Meltzer.
Raven Press, New York © 1987.

CHAPTER 20

Chemistry and Anatomy of Excitatory Amino Acid Systems

Carl W. Cotman and Daniel T. Monaghan

The identification and study of neurons that use catecholamines, acetylcholine, γ-aminobutyric acid (GABA), and peptides as their neurotransmitters has greatly increased our understanding of brain function and brain disorders. However, the majority of the brain does not use these neurotransmitters. Since the excitatory amino acids probably represent the major excitatory neurotransmitter class of mammalian CNS neurons, the identification of neurons that use an excitatory amino acid as a neurotransmitter is one of the major missing links in the understanding of CNS neurotransmitters, and is necessary for understanding much of brain function. In this review we will summarize current progress on the identification of neurons that use excitatory amino acids as neurotransmitters.

Excitatory amino acids usually refer to L-glutamate or L-aspartate. To date, most research has focused on L-glutamate. However, other naturally occurring acidic amino acids and related derivatives also elicit neuronal depolarizations, and these may also be neurotransmitters. These include L-homocysteate, L-cysteate, quinolinate, and *N*-acetylaspartylglutamate (30,50,147,159). Oftentimes, the actual molecule acting at the postsynaptic receptors has not been definitively identified even though pharmacological analysis indicates that the synaptic response is mediated by a particular excitatory amino acid receptor. Thus, it is often more accurate to refer to the transmitter as an excitatory amino acid rather than as L-glutamate.

We will focus this review on recent advances in the identification of excitatory amino acid pathways and receptor systems in the CNS. The availability and use of antagonists that block synaptic transmission at specific pathways has led to important new information on the transmitters at CNS pathways. This information is now being extended by recently developed autoradiographic techniques for localizing receptors and their subtypes. Additionally, by using recently available immunohistochemical and radiohistochemical approaches it is possible to study a variety of transmitter properties with much greater anatomical resolution. These results can now be compared with those obtained with other approaches such as the measurement of (a) free amino acid levels, (b) Ca^{2+}-dependent release of endogenous or exogenously loaded radiolabeled acidic amino acids, and (c) high-affinity amino acid uptake. Presently, data from all these approaches are beginning to converge toward a more comprehensive view of excitatory amino acid systems in the CNS.

EXCITATORY AMINO ACID RECEPTORS

Classification of Receptor Subtypes

A critical link in establishing the neurotransmitter role of an excitatory amino acid at a specific pathway is the demonstration that an excitatory amino acid receptor mediates synaptic transmission at that synapse. Following the identification of the receptor classes that control acidic amino acid depolarizations, it was soon discovered that these receptors are also responsible for mediating synaptic transmission in a variety of CNS pathways.

Currently, there is considerable evidence that indicates that the action of glutamate is mediated by at least four distinct receptors (12,24,47,61,88,146,147). Three of these receptors have been identified by the selective agonist action of the glutamate analogs: N-methyl-D-aspartate (NMDA), kainate (KA), and quisqualate (QA) (or amino-3-hydroxy-5-methyl-4-isoxazolepropionic acid, AMPA). NMDA-induced depolarizations are potently and selectively antagonized by D-2-amino-5-phosphonopentanoate (AP5) and D-2-amino-7-phosphonoheptanoate (AP7), whereas the related analogs, 2-amino-4-phosphonobutyrate (AP4) and 2-amino-6-phosphonohexanoate, are relatively ineffective (see Table 1). AMPA and QA depolarizations are selectively antagonized by glutamate diethylester (GDEE) (47,79,88). In contrast, KA-induced depolarizations are relatively unaffected by both the NMDA antagonists and by GDEE. More potent antagonists of KA and QA responses are now available [kynurenic acid (54,115), N-(p-chlorobenzoyl)piperazine-2,3-dicarboxylic acid (33,53), and others listed in Table 1]. These antagonists do not readily differentiate between the excitatory amino acid receptors, but they are useful for identifying synaptic responses mediated by excitatory amino acids (32,146). Various physiological studies have provided examples of differential localizations of these receptor classes, further indicating that these receptors are distinct entities (27,31,115,117,121). Additionally, studies of ion fluxes, receptor desensitization, the effects of divalent cations, and patch-clamp recordings confirm this classification scheme of the receptor classes (7,82,86,108).

The fourth receptor with which L-glutamate is thought to interact has been characterized by the antagonism of synaptic responses by the glutamate analog L-2-amino-4-phosphonobutyrate (L-AP4) in pathways thought to use glutamate as a neurotransmitter. Synaptic responses in the lateral perforant pathway of the dentate gyrus (75), in the mossy fiber pathway of the guinea pig (80,155), and in the lateral olfactory tract (71) are selectively blocked by micromolar concentrations of L-AP4. In the retina this receptor appears to mediate the hyperpolarizing responses at the ON-bipolar cell (132). Evidence from quantal analysis indicates that L-AP4 action in the mossy fiber pathway may be presynaptic (55). This action would account for the observation that L-AP4 is not a potent antagonist of L-glutamate- or L-aspartate-induced depolarizations yet appears to block synaptic transmission at certain pathways thought to use glutamate as a transmitter (52,71).

Mediation of Synaptic Activity by Excitatory Amino Acid Receptors

Pharmacological analysis has demonstrated that various excitatory synaptic responses are mediated by excitatory amino acid receptors (146). Using the moderately potent, broad-spectrum excitatory amino acid antagonists, synaptic responses are inhibited at antagonist concentrations that inhibit excitatory amino acid depolarizations. Thus the following pathways appear to use an excitatory amino acid as their neurotransmitter: projections from cerebral cortex to striatum (67) and hippocampus (29,54,75); the intrahippocampal mossy fiber system (54,80,155) and the Schaffer collaterals (20,54,76); the dorsal root evoked-monosynaptic response (32,35); the lateral olfactory tract (21); and the primary afferents to the trigeminal nucleus (126). Each of these synaptic responses is insensitive to the potent and selective NMDA antagonists. Therefore, the synaptic receptor mediating the fast excitatory postsynaptic potential (EPSP) appears to be a KA receptor and/or a QA receptor (or possibly another, yet undiscovered, excitatory amino acid receptor). A fast synaptic action of KA or QA receptors is consistent with the observation that these receptors activate voltage-independent Na^+/K^+ channels whereas the NMDA receptor activates a voltage-dependent cation channel that has a low conductance at resting potential (43,86,108).

TABLE 1. *Pharmacology of excitatory amino acid receptors*

	NMDA	KA	QA
Agonists	NMDA L-Glutamate L-Aspartate Ibotenate Quinolinate	KA L-Glutamate Domoate	QA L-Glutamate AMPA
Antagonists	D-AP5 AP7 D-α-Aminoadipate		GDEE?
General antagonists and synaptic antagonists: cis-2,3-piperidine dicarboxylic acid, γ-D-glutamyl-glycine, γ-D-glutamylaminomethyl sulfonate, kynurenic acid, 1-(p-chlorobenzoyl)-piperazine-2,3-dicarboxylic acid			
Radioligands	D-[³H]AP5 L-[³H]Glutamate	[³H]KA L-[³H]Glutamate	[³H]AMPA L-[³H]Glutamate

Synapses that are thought to use the KA and/or QA receptor correspond to pathways presumed to use glutamate or aspartate based on other criteria discussed below.

NMDA receptors appear to play a more interesting and complex role in mediating synaptic transmission. In an initial report it was observed that the NMDA antagonist D-AP5, when iontophoretically applied, would block the formation of long-term potentiation (LTP, a long-lasting increase in synaptic efficacy following high-frequency stimulation) in the hippocampus while not reducing the evoked response (20). Upon analysis of the pharmacological specificity and the potency of this antagonism, it was found that blockade of the formation of LTP showed an exact correspondence to the antagonism of NMDA receptors in the same preparation (65). As described above, the synaptic response appears to be mediated by a KA/QA receptor, whereas the NMDA receptor appears to mediate the formation of LTP (20,65,152).

The voltage-dependent conductance regulated by NMDA receptors appears to involve Mg^{2+} ions (86,108,146). In the presence of Mg^{2+}, NMDA opens a channel more permeable to cations (Na^+, K^+, and Ca^{2+}) at depolarized potentials. When Mg^{2+} is removed, the channel appears to be unblocked and behaves in a voltage-independent manner. As a result of these findings, the effects of NMDA antagonists have been reevaluated in low concentrations of Mg^{2+} at excitatory amino acid synapses (19,137). Accordingly, in low Mg^{2+}, NMDA antagonists block a component of synaptic activity at both intracortical and Schaffer collateral synapses. These results are consistent with previous findings that a late-occurring synaptic response in the spinal cord (dorsal root-evoked, ventral root polysynaptic response) is blocked by NMDA antagonists and by Mg^{2+} ions (147). Consistent with the voltage dependency of this receptor, NMDA receptor activity can be shown in the presence of Mg^{2+} if the resting membrane is partially depolarized (74).

Together these findings indicate that NMDA receptors do not mediate the normal fast EPSP response, but are activated under special conditions and can lead to an altered physiological response. The possibility that a major neurotransmitter can behave in such a modulatory fashion opens up many exciting questions regarding the regulation of synaptic activity in the CNS.

Clinical Applications Involving Excitatory Amino Acid Receptors

With the availability of selective NMDA antagonists, it has become possible to evaluate the role of NMDA and related receptors in pathological brain function. [A detailed critique of this exciting new direction is beyond the scope of the present review, and the reader is referred to other reviews for details (90,123,146,150,151).] These studies have led to several highly significant findings. In brief, NMDA antagonists can protect brain tissue in hypoglycemia, hypoxia, and seizures. The role of these receptors in spatial learning (5) and LTP has also opened up areas of research that may ultimately relate to new therapeutic approaches. With the availability of autoradiographic methods for the study of excitatory amino acid receptors, it is now possible

to study their potential involvement in a variety of neuropathologies.

ANATOMICAL ORGANIZATION OF EXCITATORY AMINO ACID RECEPTORS

Distribution of NMDA Binding Sites

Since NMDA receptors appear to be necessary for LTP (in at least one pathway) and for the formation of a spatial memory, it is possible that the distribution of these sites corresponds to regions that are capable of generating LTP and forming a synaptic component of memory. Additionally, as this system appears to have significant clinical applications, the distribution of these sites suggests brain regions affected by this receptor. There has been considerable progress in the identification of radioligand binding sites that appear to correspond to NMDA receptors. NMDA receptors appear to be labeled in autoradiographic preparations by both L-[^{3}H]glutamate (58,95,97,101) and D-[^{3}H]AP5 (103). The distribution of NMDA receptors has been determined quantitatively by measuring NMDA displacement of L-[^{3}H]glutamate binding under conditions where the majority of the specific binding is NMDA specific (95). Due to the very rapid dissociation of D-[^{3}H]AP5 from the NMDA site, it has not been possible to present a similar detailed analysis with this ligand (103); however, the general distribution obtained with both ligands appears to be similar, particularly within the hippocampus.

NMDA-displaceable L-[^{3}H]glutamate binding sites are found throughout the brain with a predominance in the telencephalon (Fig. 1a) (95). In cerebral cortex there exist both regional and laminar variations. Among regions, NMDA sites are found in higher densities in frontal, anterior cingulate, and pyriform corticies. Lower concentrations are found in the parietal, posterior cingulate, and entorhinal corticies. In neocortex there is a dense band of binding sites corresponding to layers I–III and an additional band in layer Va. Layer IV binding appears to be lowest in regions receiving specific thalamic innervation. Within the basal ganglia, NMDA sites have high concentrations in the nucleus accumbens, slightly lower concentrations in the striatum, and strikingly low levels in the globus pallidus.

In the olfactory bulb the external plexiform layer and the accessory bulb have higher concentrations than the other adjacent regions. More posteriorly, the anterior olfactory nuclei, olfactory tubercles, and the nucleus of the lateral olfactory tract show high levels of binding. Within the amygdala there is a distinct pattern that is also observed with the AMPA sites. Basolateral, lateral, posterior cortical, and the hippocampal-amygdaloid transition area all exhibit higher receptor densities than do the central, medial, and anterior cortical regions. Septum shows higher levels in the lateral nucleus than in the medial component. Ventrally, the bed nucleus of the stria terminalis displays intermediate levels of binding that are higher than the adjacent globus pallidus, ventral pallidum, and preoptic area.

The hippocampus displays a distinctive distribution of NMDA sites. The highest levels of binding in the entire brain are found over the stratum oriens and stratum

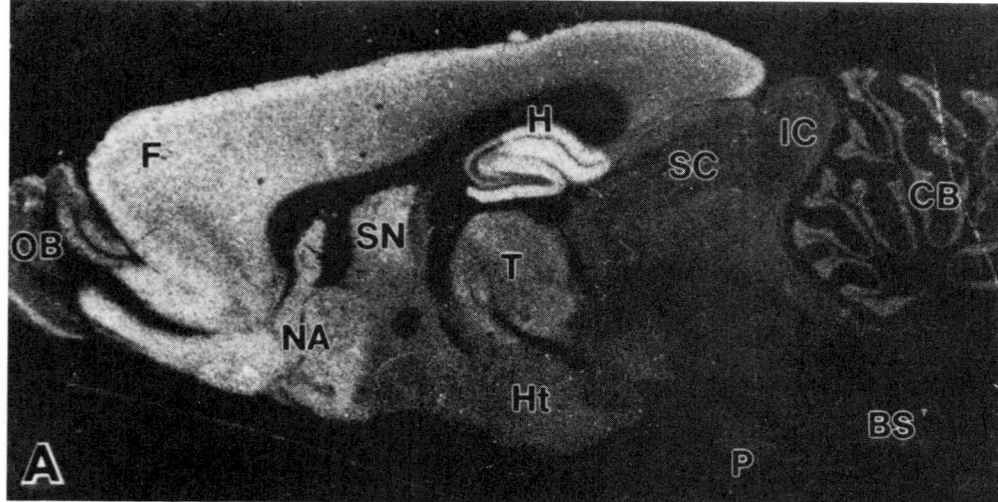

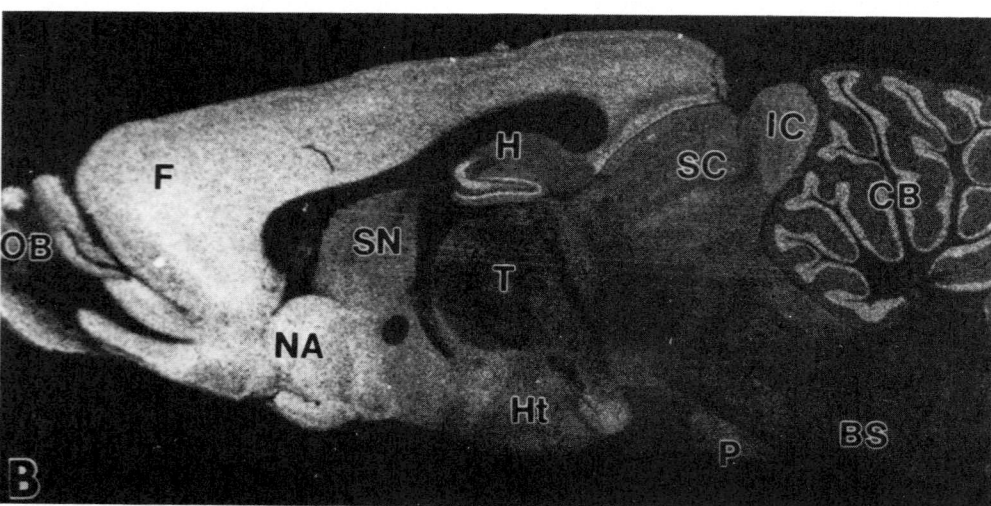

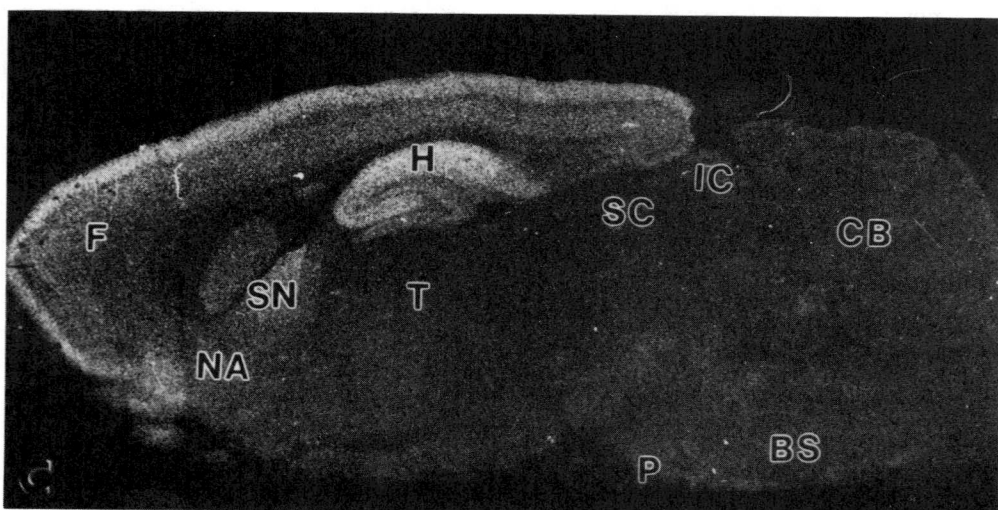

FIG. 1. Receptor autoradiography. Sagittal sections of rodent brain displaying the distribution of various excitatory amino acid receptors. **A:** NMDA receptors labeled with L-[³H]glutamate in the presence of QA to displace binding to the KA and AMPA receptors. **B:** KA receptors labeled with [³H]KA. **C:** QA receptors labeled with [³H]AMPA. Abbreviations used: OB, olfactory bulb; F, frontal cortex; NA, nucleus accumbens; SN, septal nucleus; H, hippocampus; T, thalamus; Ht, hypothalamus; SC, superior colliculus; IC, inferior colliculus; CB, cerebellum; P, pontine nuclei; BS, brainstem.

radiatum of the CA1 field of the hippocampus. In CA3 these layers display moderately high levels whereas the stratum lucidum and stratum pyramidale have distinctly low levels of binding. In the dentate gyrus, the outer molecular layer shows slightly lower levels of binding than does the inner molecular layer, whereas the infragranule and granule cell layers have quite low levels of binding.

Thalamic regions in general have higher levels of NMDA sites than do the hypothalamic regions. Relatively low levels are found in the reticular nucleus and the zona incerta. Using D-[³H]AP5 as a ligand for NMDA receptors, the ventroposterior nucleus was distinctly labeled (103). In both the lateral and medial geniculate, the dorsal subdivisions have higher levels of NMDA sites than the ventral subdivisions. Midbrain and brainstem regions display an overall low density of NMDA sites with certain nuclei showing relatively higher levels of binding sites. These include the superficial and intermediate gray layers of the superior colliculus, dorsal medial inferior colliculus, medial vestibular nucleus, cuneiform nucleus, granule cell layer of the cochlear nucleus, parabrachial nucleus, nucleus of the solitary tract, central gray, the inferior olive, and the substantia gelatinosa of the spinal cord. In general, all along the floor of the fourth ventricle, medially located structures displayed moderate levels of NMDA sites, whereas ventrally located motor structures displayed no selective enrichment of binding sites. The cerebellum displayed overall low levels, with greater levels of binding in the granule cell layer than in the molecular layer. In view of other evidence presented below, it is noteworthy that there was only a slight or no enrichment of NMDA sites found over the substantia nigra, the pontine nuclei, the red nucleus, the trigeminal nucleus, and the cerebellar molecular layer.

Distribution of AMPA Binding Sites

QA receptors appear to be labeled by [³H]AMPA. In isolated membrane preparations (69) and autoradiographic preparations (100,118), [³H]AMPA binds to a distinct class of binding sites that display the same ligand specificity for QA agonists as does the quisqualate receptor. As with the other two receptors, this binding site may also be labeled by L-[³H]glutamate (97,101).

In general, QA sites, as labeled by [³H]AMPA, display a pattern similar to that of NMDA sites (Fig. 1c) (100). Again, outer layers of the cerebral cortex (I–III) have higher levels of binding than do the middle and deep layers. Layer IV has lower levels than do the deeper layers. Regional cortical variations are not large, but they exhibit a similar pattern of variation as displayed by NMDA sites. AMPA sites are enriched in the anterior olfactory nuclei, the olfactory tubercles, the nucleus accumbens, the caudate/putamen, and, especially, the lateral septum. Globus pallidus, ventral pallidum, and substantia innominata exhibit low levels of binding. Unlike NMDA receptors, AMPA sites are low in the external plexiform layer of the olfactory bulb and there is a dense band of AMPA binding in layer Vb of visual cortex (the latter finding may relate to the

relatively greater density of AMPA sites found in the intermediate gray layer of the superior colliculus).

Of the entire brain, the hippocampal pyramidal cell body layer and the induseum griseum display the highest levels of binding. Additionally, the pyramidal cell dendritic fields display high levels of binding, with the CA1 region having higher levels than CA3. Likewise, the dentate gyrus exhibited moderately high levels of binding. As found for NMDA-sensitive L-[³H]glutamate binding sites, the basolateral, lateral, and posteriocortical amygdala are relatively enriched in AMPA sites compared to the other regions of the amygdala. This distribution of sites in the amygdala is similar to that reported for excitatory amino acid uptake sites (discussed below).

Other regions of the brain display relatively low levels of binding. The molecular layer of the cerebellum displays higher binding levels than does the granule cell layer; however, the molecular layer binding is still about one-fifth that found in the hippocampus stratum radiatum. Detailed description of lower brain regions will therefore require further experiments using much longer film exposure times with higher levels of bound radioactivity. Preliminary studies under these conditions indicate that AMPA sites in the thalamus and hypothalamus display a distribution similar to that found for NMDA sites, with higher levels of binding in the thalamus (D. T. Monaghan and C. W. Cotman, *unpublished observations*).

We have also identified the AMPA binding site population by using L-[³H]glutamate as a ligand (97,101). Although the lower levels of binding to this site (due to the lower affinity for glutamate) make the anatomical localization more difficult, these sites were found to exhibit a similar distribution within the CNS. Highest levels were found in the hippocampal pyramidal cell layer. Other regions of high binding were the lateral septum, outer cerebral cortical layers, the dendritic fields of the hippocampal pyramidal cells, and the dentate gyrus.

In summary, the largely overlapping distribution of the NMDA and AMPA binding site populations is consistent with the idea that both of these receptors can be functional in the same synaptic field and may mediate different aspects of synaptic transmission.

Distribution of Kainate Binding Sites

KA receptors can be selectively labeled in both autoradiographic and isolated membrane preparations by [³H]KA (48,81,94,130,138). In addition L-[³H]glutamate can also be shown to label KA sites in autoradiographic preparations (97).

As found for NMDA and AMPA binding sites, [³H]KA binding sites are found predominantly in the telencephalon (Fig. 1b) (94,138). However, within various regions, KA sites display a largely complementary distribution to that found for the other binding sites. In neocortex KA sites are located predominantly in the superficial-most layer and in layers V and VI, with layer VI having a slightly higher density than layer V. Among the various cortical regions, frontal, temporal, insular, and anterior cingulate cortices have generally higher levels of binding than the parietal, pyriform, and entorhinal regions. Caudate/putamen, nucleus accumbens, olfactory tubercles, anterior olfactory nuclei, and the olfactory bulbs display high levels of KA sites; the globus pallidus and septum display low levels. Within the amygdala and ventral pallidum the density of KA sites is moderate with a relatively uniform distribution.

The hippocampus displays a very distinct pattern of KA binding sites. The highest density of KA binding sites in the rat brain corresponds to the stratum lucidum, and moderate concentrations are found in the inner portion of the dentate gyrus molecular layer. With the exception of the hilus and a portion of the stratum lacunosum-molecu-lare, the remainder of the hippocampus displays low levels of KA binding. Thalamic midline nuclei, reticular nucleus, zona incerta, and hypothalamus have moderate levels of binding, whereas the remainder of the thalamus has low levels.

Lower brain regions with moderate levels of binding are the mesencephalic central gray, the granule cell layer of the cerebellum, and the substantia gelatinosa of the spinal cord. To further characterize lower brain regions, again longer film exposures and/or higher radiolabeling of receptors is required. Using [3H]KA of higher specific activity we have recently observed that lower brain regions display a distribution of KA binding sites similar to that found for NMDA sites, with the exception that additional ventrally located structures are also labeled. For example, the pontine nucleus, portions of the red nucleus, hypothalamus, and the substantia nigra contain higher levels of KA sites than their surrounding tissue.

Clearly, NMDA and KA receptors are differentially distributed, and this may provide some clue as to their function. One possibility is that the distribution of NMDA receptors may correspond to regions that are capable of expressing long-term potentiation. In the hippocampus, NMDA receptors have been shown to be necessary for the formation of long-term potentiation—the enhanced synaptic efficacy that follows high-frequency stimulation. Another possibility is that NMDA receptors and KA receptors may correspond to synaptic activity mediated by differing neurotransmitters. Since L-aspartate and L-glutamate recognize NMDA receptors whereas L-glutamate is the preferred ligand for KA sites, it is possible that KA receptors reflect regions that use predominantly L-glutamate (or a related derivative) as a neurotransmitter. Interestingly, in the hippocampus, the highest KA receptor density is found in the stratum lucidum. This dendritic field is also readily labeled by antibodies to L-glutamate and glutaminase, but not by L-aspartate antibodies. In contrast, the stratum radiatum contains L-glutamate- and L-aspartate-like immunoreactivity as well as a high concentration of NMDA receptors (2,114,135).

In summary, the differing excitatory amino acid receptors display a partially nonoverlapping distribution. Added together, their distribution corresponds to that expected for excitatory amino acid terminal fields. One possible exception is the relatively low receptor levels found in the cerebellum molecular layer. This may suggest either that a lower receptor density is adequate in the cerebellum or that a different receptor type is involved at the parallel fiber synapse (see ref. 96 for a detailed discussion of other possible receptor types).

Properties of Excitatory Amino Acid Receptors in Isolated Membranes

Studies of receptors in isolated membranes are valuable for examining the biochemical and regulatory properties of receptors as well as their subcellular distribution (49). Until recently, however, the physiologically defined receptor classes did not correspond to the binding sites for L-[3H]glutamate. It now appears that one of the critical parameters in resolving this mismatch was the predominance of a particular glutamate-binding population in the presence of Cl⁻ ions (47,92). With roughly 80% of the binding representing this site, it was initially thought that this site was homogeneous, and it has been termed the Na^+-independent glutamate binding site (47,60,62). On removal of Cl⁻ ions from the incubation buffer, binding is greatly reduced and the pharmacological character changes, becoming partially sensitive to displacement by NMDA and no longer sensitive to L-AP4. Indeed, results obtained by autoradiography indicate that L-[3H]glutamate binds to NMDA, QA, and KA sites. In agreement with results obtained in autoradiography using L-[3H]glutamate, radioligand binding studies with ligands selective for the three agonist-defined receptors also indicate that L-glutamate has a similar high affinity for each of these sites (69,96,109,130).

[3H]KA binding to membrane fragments displays a ligand specificity indicative of the KA receptor (81,130). On Scatchard analysis of KA binding, both a high- and a low-affinity site is observed. KA binding that appears as high affinity when determined by Scatchard analysis does not appear in the presence of cations (Ca^{2+} ions in particular) (99).

[3H]AMPA appears to be a selective ligand for QA receptors (69). This conclusion is based on the parallel potencies of several AMPA analogs at the displacement of [3H]AMPA binding and at evoking GDEE-sensitive depolarizations. Radioligand binding studies indicate that AMPA has greater selectivity than does QA, and therefore the notation for this receptor may need to be revised in the future. Thus, AMPA may be more selective in physiological studies. Relatively little is known regarding this binding site. It has been difficult to obtain an adequate signal-to-noise ratio with this radioligand; however, it has been recently shown that KSCN increases AMPA affinity without changing other characteristics of the binding site (70). Thus, a more extensive characterization of [3H]AMPA binding sites should now be possible.

NMDA receptors have only recently been described in isolated membrane fractions. Using D-[3H]AP5, Olverman et al. (109) have described a binding site that appears to correspond to the NMDA receptor and to the NMDA-sensitive L-[3H]glutamate binding site observed by autoradiography. The highest levels of this binding site are found in the hippocampus, striatum, and cerebral cortex. Using L-[3H]glutamate a binding site of similar ligand specificity has been described in purified postsynaptic densities (42). More recently, we have found that this binding site may also be characterized in isolated synaptic membrane fractions, thereby permitting a detailed analysis of this binding site (102). Again, the ligand specificity of this binding site corresponds well to that of the NMDA receptor, with NMDA agonists and antagonists displaying affinities for the binding site that correspond to their potencies observed in physiological preparations.

So far, it has not been possible to identify clearly the L-AP4 receptor using radioligand binding techniques. Initial experiments demonstrated the presence of an L-[^{3}H]-glutamate binding site that selectively interacts with L-AP4 with the appropriate affinity and stereoselectivity (17,40,98). However, we have further characterized the pharmacological profile of the L-AP4 receptor and compared this with the displacement potency of various glutamate analogs against L-[^{3}H]AP4 binding and L-AP4-sensitive L-[^{3}H]glutamate binding and find that significant differences exist (15,122). Furthermore, evidence from a variety of experiments indicates that this binding site may actually represent Cl$^-$-dependent uptake (93,116,144).

The value of the receptor autoradiography method as an indicator of glutamate terminal fields depends on the extent that the receptors are preferentially localized in synaptic structures. It has been noted in other transmitter-receptor systems that there is sometimes a mismatch between receptor localization and transmitter localization (66). Are excitatory amino acid receptors junctional or extrajunctional? It is significant that each of the three binding sites corresponding to the three well-described glutamate receptors has been found to be greatly enriched in synaptic structures. The glutamate receptor labeled by KA is enriched in detergent-treated synaptic junctions (48). The receptor that recognizes NMDA is also highly enriched in synaptic junctions (156) and is also found in purified postsynaptic densities (42). The QA receptor likewise appears to be localized in postsynaptic densities (42). Thus these data are consistent with the hypothesis that these binding sites represent markers for the corresponding excitatory amino acid-using synapses and that these sites are involved in synaptic transmission. Nonetheless, light microscopic autoradiography cannot provide definite data on the selective abundance of junctional versus extrajunctional receptors.

L-GLUTAMATE AS A MARKER FOR GLUTAMATE-USING NEURONS

Initial studies on the anatomical distribution of glutamate as a transmitter measured the regional distribution of glutamate levels (11,22,44,57,72,78,113). Glutamate exhibits a two- to threefold range in concentration, with greater levels found in gray matter and higher brain structures. Such a distribution is consistent with glutamate's being a major transmitter with a wide distribution, but it is also consistent with metabolic glutamate being predominant over transmitter glutamate and having a moderate regional variation. The determination of glutamate levels in discrete terminal fields before and after afferent removal has similarly failed to provide clear data. For example, lesions of the entorhinal cortex, which projects to the dentate gyrus, do not result in a significant loss of L-glutamate, whereas

glutamate levels in synaptosomes are reduced (105,107). Thus the failure to measure L-glutamate changes in whole tissue in a relatively large, high innervation density pathway suggests that this method is not very reliable.

A more sensitive approach to the localization of transmitter L-glutamate has been the recent application of immunohistochemical techniques (112–114,135). Storm-Mathisen and colleagues have prepared polyclonal antibodies to L-glutamate linked by glutaraldehyde to bovine serum albumin. This approach has demonstrated a reasonable correlation to other markers of glutamate neurotransmission.

Glutamate-like immunoreactivity shows a distribution similar to, but more uniform than, that found for the glutamate receptors. This correlation appears most noticeable in the olfactory bulb (higher staining in the external plexiform layer and accessory bulb), in basal ganglia (greater staining in the nucleus accumbens and caudate/putamen than in the globus pallidus), in the septum (with lateral septum having higher levels), in the thalamus (midline, reticular, and dorsal lateral geniculate nuclei), and in the brainstem and spinal cord (periventricular gray and substantia gelatinosa).

The finding of a variation in regional glutamate immunoreactivity is somewhat unexpected, but is perhaps explainable in terms of the properties of different glutamate compartments. In studies of both high-affinity glutamate uptake and glutamate content, the preparation of synaptosomes from whole brain tissue is thought to result in a selective retention of an intact transmitter compartment, whereas glial and cell body glutamate and uptake capacity are preferentially lost (41,105). In a similar manner, it has been argued that sectioning of brain tissue prior to fixation preserves the transmitter (or nerve terminal) compartment, whereas nerve and glial cell body glutamate compartments are lost from the cut surface. When hippocampal tissue is first sectioned, then fixed, immunohistochemical localization of L-glutamate shows a very distinct pattern of staining (135). This pattern is strikingly reminiscent of the high-affinity uptake system (see below), and corresponds well to the pathways thought to use L-glutamate as a neurotransmitter. In the hippocampus the stratum radiatum and stratum oriens show higher staining than the stratum lacunosum-moleculare. In the dentate gyrus, the molecular layer has a trilaminar appearance with higher levels of staining in the inner and outer one-third of this layer. The mossy fiber terminal zone, the stratum lucidum, also has selective staining. Consistent with the loss of glutamate from larger structures, cell bodies and dendrites did not exhibit significant labeling. On electron microscopic analysis of the tissue, immunoreactivity was found in synaptic terminals and apparently associated with synaptic vesicles (135).

Two potential problems with this approach are the regionally selective loss of glutamate from fragile nerve terminals (e.g., the large mossy fiber boutons of the hippocampus) and the reuptake of lost glutamate into other tissues during tissue preparation. However, the results of this approach in other brain regions will be very interesting in light of the anatomically distinct results obtained in the hippocampus. The immunohistochemical identification of L-glutamate in tissue also permits the use of lesion experiments that have a much greater level of anatomical resolution and sensitivity. The demonstration of Ca^{2+}-dependent evoked release of L-glutamate from this preparation supports the hypothesis that the remaining glutamate is transmitter glutamate and means that this more stringent criterion of transmitter activity can now be applied at a histochemical level (51,110).

Recently, the localization of L-aspartate by immunocytochemistry has been reported (114). In the hippocampus, this antibody exhibits a pattern of staining similar to that found for the glutamate antibody; however, the mossy fiber terminal zone (stratum lucidum) is not significantly labeled. Another antibody recently developed is that against L-homocysteate (30). With this antibody, staining is seen in the superficial cortical layers and in the striatum. Beitz and colleagues have recently developed a monoclonal antibody raised against γ-L-glutamyl-L-glutamic acid conjugated to keyhole limpet hemocyanin (84). Immunoreactive cells have been found in pyramidal neurons of the cerebral cortex (especially layers V and VI) and in the nucleus accumbens, ventral lateral striatum, cochlear nucleus, cerebellar deep nuclei, pontine nuclei, and cerebellar granule cells (9,84,104).

ENZYMES AS MARKERS FOR EXCITATORY AMINO ACID NEURONS

As expected for a compound that plays a major role in energy and amino acid metabolism, multiple synthetic and degradative enzymes metabolize L-glutamate and other excitatory amino acids. In the specific case of L-glutamate, the synthetic enzymes proposed to generate transmitter glutamate are glutaminase, aspartate transaminase, and ornithine transaminase, corresponding to the putative glutamate precursors glutamine, aspartate and α-ketoglutarate, and ornithine (68). Biochemical studies have demonstrated that glutamine appears to be the preferred precursor to the releasable pool of glutamate. Addition of glutamine to tissue sections in the continued presence of glucose led to a substantial increase in the releasable pool of glutamate. Furthermore, as much as 60 to 80% of released glutamate can be derived from radiolabeled exogenous glutamine (14,63,64). These results are consistent with the "glutamine-glutamate cycle," in which neuronally released glutamate is thought to enter astrocytes where glutamine synthetase is located. Following synthesis, nonexcitatory glutamine can then be transferred back to the neuronal terminal for synthesis into glutamate.

Lesion studies, however, have failed to clarify which of the synthetic enzymes for glutamate is the most important, if indeed one enzyme is primarily responsible. Denervation of the cochlear nucleus results in a significant loss of glutaminase and aspartate transaminase (148); however, elimination of the corticostriatal tract (68,127) and the perforant path to the dentate gyrus (107) results in either a very small or a negligible decrease in glutaminase and aspartate transaminase. Interpretive problems that arise are the extent to which a metabolic enzyme may be preferentially localized in metabolically active nerve terminals in general, the extent that these enzymes may be providing

glutamate as a precursor to GABA, and the possible plastic responses to denervation.

Antibodies to glutaminase and aspartate transaminase appear to label some terminal fields and a greater number of cell bodies, but do not serve as a general marker for glutamate or aspartate terminal fields (38,149). Terminals in the cochlear nucleus contain immunoreactivity to both antibodies, whereas hippocampal mossy fibers appear to contain only the glutaminase immunoreactivity (2–4). Other studies with these antibodies have identified cell bodies with glutaminase-like immunoreactivity in neocortical (layers V and VI) and hippocampal pyramidal cells and granule cells of the cerebellum (38,149). Aspartate transaminase immunoreactivity has also been found in the cerebral cortex (layers II and III) and in the cerebellar granule cells. Although both glutaminase and aspartate transaminase have been suggested to be used by GABAergic neurons, their localization in these neurons by immunocytochemical techniques does not appear to be highly significant, except perhaps GABAergic neurons of the cerebellum, which appear to be labeled by antibodies to aspartate transaminase.

In summary, it appears that currently the immunocytochemical identification of acidic amino acid enzymes is more useful as a means of elucidating the differing biochemical pools than in the identification of excitatory amino acid-using neurons.

RELEASE OF EXCITATORY AMINO ACIDS

A critical proof of the neurotransmitter function of excitatory amino acids is the demonstration that endogenous acidic amino acids are released from nerve terminals in a Ca^{2+}-dependent fashion on stimulation. In the dentate gyrus, electrical and high-potassium stimulation results in a Ca^{2+}-dependent release of L-glutamate (25). The releasable glutamate is reduced by removal of the entorhinal projection to the dentate gyrus. Furthermore, releasable glutamate is enriched in synaptosomal fractions relative to whole homogenates. Results similar to these have now been obtained in a number of systems using both endogenous L-glutamate and/or L-aspartate and exogenously loaded L-glutamate or D-aspartate. Release elicited by either electrical stimulation, high potassium, or veratridine is largely Ca^{2+} dependent and reduced by lesions that remove the presumed glutamate projection. More recently, L-glutamate release has been demonstrated *in vivo* in the perforant path (37).

In addition to L-glutamate, L-aspartate release has been demonstrated in the hippocampal commissural and associational projections (106), the olfactory bulb to olfactory cortex projection (23), and the cerebellar climbing fibers (154). In each of these systems, removal of these synaptic afferents reduces the stimulated efflux of L-aspartate. Recently, it has also been demonstrated that sulfur-containing acidic amino acids also display Ca^{2+}-dependent release (cysteine sulfinic acid, homocysteine sulfinic acid, and especially homocysteic acid) (30). These amino acids, along with quinolinic acid, are candidates for the endogenous NMDA molecule (see refs. 30, 54, 115). The peptide *N*-acetyl-aspartyl-glutamate has been proposed to act on the AP4 receptor (77), although its release has not yet been demonstrated.

Currently, analysis of the release properties of excitatory amino acids is very important for proving that a specific compound is the neurotransmitter for a given pathway. However, current methods are somewhat limited to the study of relatively major projecting pathways. Perhaps as discussed in the previous section, antibodies to specific acidic amino acids can be used for identifying terminal fields that display Ca^{2+}-dependent release. For further discussion of release studies see refs. 13, 24, 25, 39, 41, 119.

HIGH-AFFINITY UPTAKE OF ACIDIC AMINO ACIDS

Since uptake appears to be the means of L-glutamate transmitter inactivation, it is a reasonable hypothesis that a high-affinity uptake system would be uniquely associated with neurons that use glutamate as a transmitter (6,10). The uptake systems located in glial cells may also be associated with the transmitter function of glutamate, since glial cells appear to play a major role in providing transmitter precursor to glutamate nerve terminals.

The majority of information regarding the distribution of L-glutamate-using pathways is derived from studies that use the high-affinity uptake of a radiolabeled acidic amino acid. For high-affinity uptake to be an adequate marker of excitatory amino acid neurons, this uptake system should be present only in these neurons. However, many studies have demonstrated that glial cells can transport L-glutamate with a high affinity (e.g., 120,129). In spite of this problem, neuronal labeling can be discriminated by (a) performing pathway-specific ablations to determine if terminal field uptake is localized to a given pathway; (b) performing transport in thin, fresh tissue sections which are less likely to have an intact glial compartment; and (c) allowing for retrograde transport of the radiolabel in the neuron.

Certain populations of neurons exhibit high-affinity glutamate uptake. Purified GABAergic neurons and regions rich in GABA have lower levels of glutamate uptake (45,158). Furthermore, kainate injections into the striatum reduce both GABA and cholinergic markers, but do not significantly reduce high-affinity glutamate uptake (139). More recent evidence that uptake is selective among neurons has come from studies that permit the retrograde transport of D-[³H]aspartate following uptake. Thus, only certain projections demonstrate retrograde transport of aspartate, whereas many more projections will retrogradely transport horseradish peroxidase (136).

Uptake Labeling of Terminal Fields

Many studies have assessed radiolabeled acidic amino acid uptake before and after ablation of presumed glutamate-using pathways (44,112). A remarkable observation is that often large reductions (60–80%) can be observed in some pathways. The major pathways that exhibit high-affinity acidic amino acid transport that is reduced by afferent ablation are the cortical projections to hippocampus, contralateral cortex, caudate/putamen, nucleus accumbens, amygdala, thalamus, dorsal lateral geniculate body, superior colliculus, pons, red nucleus, substantia nigra, and spinal cord (Fig. 2a). The major intrinsic hippocampal pathways and the hippocampal and subicular efferents (to nucleus accumbens, lateral septum, mammilary bodies, and amygdala) also readily exhibit uptake capacity (Fig. 2b). In addition, the dorsal root and vagal primary afferents likewise display glutamate uptake capacity. As mentioned above, a limitation of this approach is that it is somewhat limited to large and homogeneous pathways, thus making analysis difficult in many subcortical pathways.

Nevertheless, these results have been confirmed and extended by the use of uptake autoradiography. Fonnum, Storm-Mathisen, and colleagues have demonstrated that tissue slices incubated with tritiated L-glutamate or tritiated D-aspartate will take up label into pools that are lost on ablation of the presynaptic component (44,133). Generally, D-[³H]aspartate is used because this label recognizes the transport system and is metabolically inert.

Recently, Ottersen and Storm-Mathisen have provided a detailed description of the distribution of high-affinity uptake autoradiography in mouse brain (112). In neocortex the outer layers I, II, and III have higher levels of activity than the deep layers whereas layer IV is particularly low, especially in the somatosensory barrel fields. It also appears that there is a band of greater activity within layer V. The hippocampal pattern is also quite distinctive with higher levels in stratum radiatum and stratum oriens. Additionally, the molecular layer of the dentate gyrus and the stratum lucidum of CA3 display significant levels of uptake. Within the amygdala region, the lateral, basolateral, and lateral olfactory tract nuclei show greater activity than the central and medial nuclei. In septum, activity was higher in the lateral nucleus than in the medial nucleus. Caudate/putamen, nucleus accumbens, and olfactory tubercles showed much higher uptake levels than the globus pallidus and ventral pallidum. The bed nucleus of the stria terminalis displayed levels higher than in the latter two structures. Thalamus displays higher levels of uptake than the hypothalamus, with distinct nuclei in the thalamus exhibiting uptake. In the lateral geniculate, uptake is confined to the dorsal subdivision. Autoradiographic analysis in conjunction with electron microscopic analysis (134) and lesion studies (133) indicates that the D-[³H]aspartate uptake in the hippocampus is localized to presynaptic terminals.

Low to moderate levels of D-[³H]aspartate uptake are found in the mammilary bodies and substantia nigra, with higher levels in the pars compacta than in the middle and lateral pars reticulata. Within the superior colliculus, the superficial gray layer shows greater uptake capacity. Other notable midbrain structures that take up D-[³H]aspartate are the periaqueductal gray and the dorsal raphe nuclei. These results confirm the description of uptake autoradiography reported by Fonnum and colleagues (45).

Retrograde Transport of D-[³H]Aspartate

The most powerful biochemical approach in mapping excitatory amino acid pathways at present makes use of the retrograde transport of D-[³H]aspartate. Since the initial studies by Streit (136), various studies have confirmed that injections of D-[³H]aspartate in vivo result in its retrograde transport to the cell bodies of only select populations of

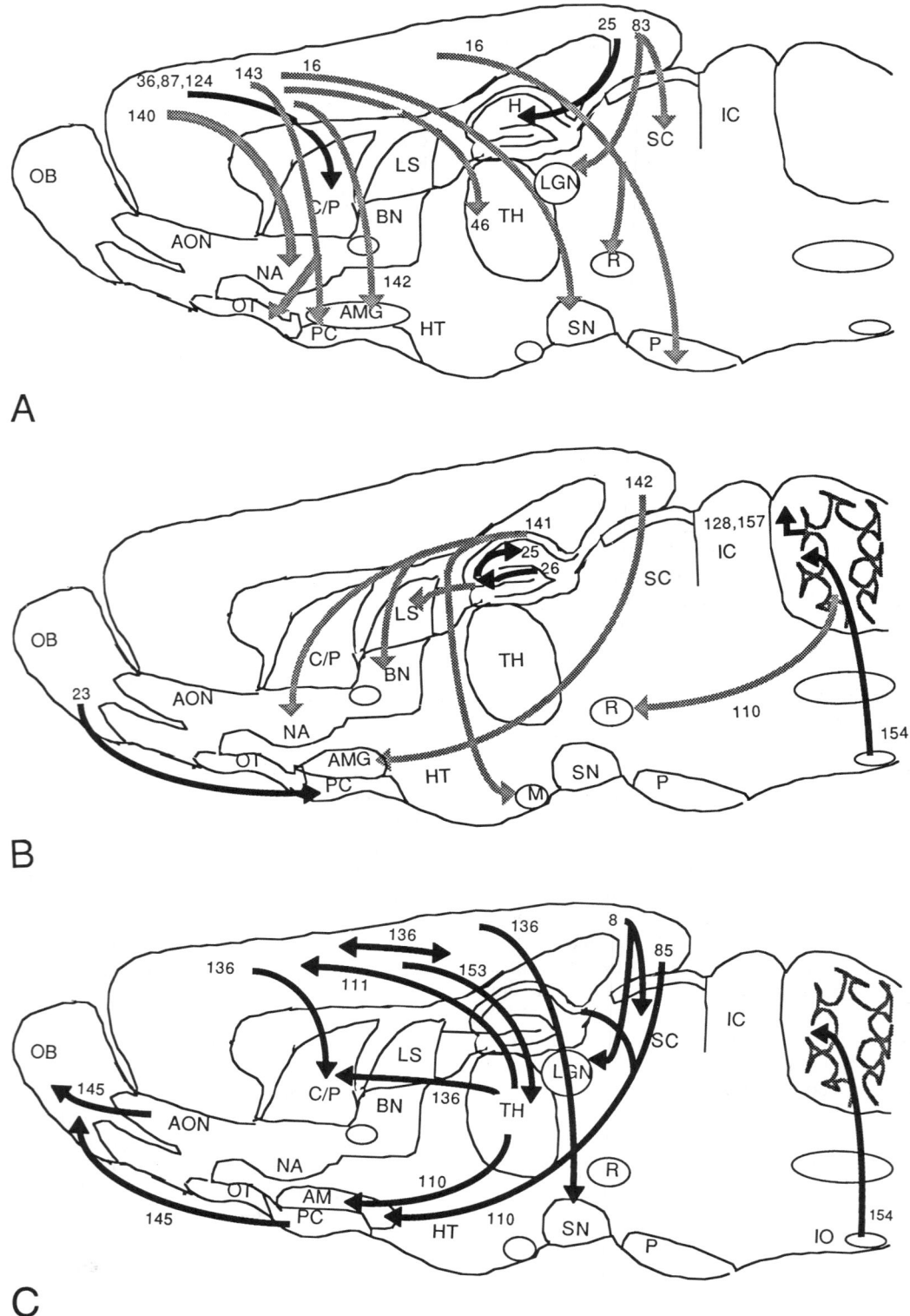

FIG. 2. Summary of CNS pathways that appear to use an excitatory amino acid as a neurotransmitter. **A, B:** Pathways demonstrated on the basis of high-affinity uptake or release of acidic amino acids: those demonstrated by both release and uptake have been marked with *black arrows;* those where only uptake has been described are shown in *gray.* **C:** Pathways demonstrated by retrograde transport of D-[³H]aspartate. Abbreviations used: OB, olfactory bulb; NA, nucleus accumbens; H, hippocampus; TH, thalamus; HT, hypothalamus; SC, superior colliculus; IC, inferior colliculus; CB, cerebellum; P, pontine nuclei; AON, anterior olfactory nucleus; OT, olfactory tubercle; C/P, caudate/putamen; LS, lateral septum; BN, bed nucleus; AMG, amygdala; PC, pyriform cortex; LGN, lateral geniculate nucleus; SN, substantia nigra; R, red nucleus; M, mammillary body; ID, inferior dive.

neurons that project into the injected region. Notably, cells that are known to use a different neurotransmitter (e.g., GABA, serotonin, norepinephrine, and dopamine) do not retrogradely transport D-[³H]aspartate whereas they do transport the protein retrograde tracers and the cell's corresponding radiolabeled transmitters. Thus, D-[³H]aspartate and radiolabeled serotonin injected into the caudate nucleus result in selective D-[³H]aspartate transport to the cerebral cortex and [³H]serotonin transport to the dorsal raphe nucleus.

Interpretive problems with this technique are that fibers of passage may be labeled by the D-[³H]aspartate injections, and it is necessary to differentiate between retrograde transport and anterograde transport (the latter being less substantial and less transmitter specific). It is significant that the relatively dense ventrobasal thalamus to somatosensory cortex projection does not retrogradely transport D-[³H]aspartate, whereas the adjacent agranular cortex readily transports label to the thalamic intralaminar nuclei (111). Thus, innervation density does not seem to affect the ability to observe D-[³H]aspartate transport.

Retrograde transport of D-[³H]aspartate has already confirmed the presence of excitatory amino acid projections from cerebral cortex to the caudate/putamen (125), superior colliculi, thalamus, substantia nigra, and cuneate nucleus (Fig. 2c). Additionally, excitatory amino acid-using pathways having cell bodies in the medial hypothalamus, intralaminar and ventromedial thalamic nuclei, periaqueductal gray, and inferior olive have now been tentatively identified (73).

In summary, the use of this technique should greatly add to the list of proposed excitatory amino acid pathways. Of particular value is the anatomical resolution and sensitivity that this method allows. Thus, this method should be valuable for the analysis of various subcortical pathways that are not amenable to biochemical approaches combined with lesions.

CONCLUSIONS

In this chapter we have summarized the various pathways in the CNS that appear to use an excitatory amino acid as a neurotransmitter and described the characteristics of these systems. The strategies and approaches available to address this issue have greatly increased in recent years. These include the existence of better and more specific antagonists (Table 1), glutamate-specific antibodies to localize terminals that store and secrete this molecule, D-[³H]aspartate as a selective retrograde tracer, and high-resolution light microscopic autoradiography to analyze the organization of the various receptor types.

Each of the currently used markers for excitatory amino acid neurons indicates that the cerebral cortex and hippocampus are major sources of neurons that use acidic amino acids as excitatory neurotransmitters. Many neurons in neocortical and allocortical regions take up and release these transmitters in their commissural, associational, and corticofugal projections. These studies are reinforced by the findings that excitatory amino acid receptors are present in the terminal fields of these pathways. Indeed, in regions

such as amygdala, hippocampus, and cortex there is almost an exact correspondence between the localization of receptors, particularly the NMDA and AMPA sites, and the uptake of D-[³H]aspartate.

The properties of other major excitatory amino acid pathways can now be resolved, for example, the thalamocortical projections. It is noteworthy that cortical regions receiving specific thalamic input, e.g., layer IV of parietal cortex, are relatively low in receptor density. In contrast, cortical regions receiving nonspecific thalamic input, e.g., agranular cortical regions, have a high binding site density. These results are consistent with transport experiments that indicate that the nonspecific thalamic region, the intralaminar nuclei, will transport D-[³H]aspartate whereas the specific thalamic region, the ventrobasal complex, will not retrogradely transport D-[³H]aspartate injected into its terminal field (111).

Overall the evidence continues to grow that excitatory amino acids are the major excitatory transmitters in the CNS. The detailed evidence is best for the perforant path, mossy fiber, and Schaffer collateral systems of the hippocampus where most of the classical criteria have been evaluated and the results shown to be consistent with an excitatory amino acid neurotransmitter. In no case, however, are the data as compelling as those for the peripheral nervous system and the neuromuscular junction. Several issues are in need of resolution. In many cases the action of glutamate and/or aspartate is sufficient to account for the action on receptors; however, other candidate molecules may indeed be used or coexist with these two amino acids. The localization of putative neurotransmitters using selective antibodies to these molecules plus release experiments will help further resolve the issue of which actual product(s) are secreted. Procedures are needed that allow the localization of receptors to specific synapses at the electron microscopic level and the study of specific second messenger systems for each receptor subtype. The availability of antagonists, particularly for NMDA, has greatly increased in recent years; however, antagonists are needed that better discriminate between QA- and KA-type receptors.

It is now possible to evaluate in more detail the involvement of excitatory amino acid pathways in normal brain function and in neuropathological conditions. The participation of NMDA receptors in long-term potentiation provides a strong link between these systems and the mechanisms of learning and memory. NMDA and other excitatory amino acid receptors also appear to play a role in excitotoxic-mediated cell damage caused by seizures, hypoglycemia, and other disturbances associated with excess excitatory amino acids. Excitatory amino acids may be involved in neuropathological disorders to a greater extent than appreciated at the present time. In Alzheimer's disease, for example, recent evidence suggests a vulnerability of NMDA receptors in cerebral cortex (59) and enhancement of KA receptors in hippocampus probably associated with axon sprouting (56). The study of excitatory amino acid-mediated neurotransmission has now reached the point where, particularly for the NMDA system, nearly all aspects of their involvement in various aspects of neurotransmission can be studied.

ACKNOWLEDGMENTS

This work was supported by grants DAMD 17-83-C-3189 and DAAG-29-82-K-0194.

REFERENCES

1. Abarca, J., and Bustos, G. (1985): *Neurochem. Int.,* 7:229.
2. Altschuler, R. A., Monaghan, D. T., Haser, W. G., Wenthold, R. J., Curthoys, N. P., and Cotman, C. W. (1985): *Brain Res.,* 330:225–233.
3. Altschuler, R. A., Neises, G. R., Harmison, G. C., Wenthold, R. J., and Fex, J. (1981): *Proc. Natl. Acad. Sci. USA,* 78:6553–6557.
4. Altschuler, R. A., Wenthold, R. J., Schwartz, A. M., Haser, W. G., Curthoys, N. P., Parakkal, M., and Fex, J. (1984): *Brain Res.,* 291:173–178.
5. Anderson, E., Baudry, M., and Morris, R. G. M. (1985): *Neurosci. Lett. (Suppl.),* 21:552.
6. Balcar, V. J., and Johnston, G. A. R. (1972): *J. Neurochem.,* 19:2657–2666.
7. Baudry, M., Kramer, K., Fagni, L., Recasens, M., and Lynch, G. (1983): *Mol. Pharmacol.,* 24:222–228.
8. Baughman, R. W., and Gilbert, C. D. (1981): *J. Neurosci.,* 1:427.
9. Beitz, A. J., Larson, A. A., Monaghan, P., Altschuler, R. A., Mullett, M. M., and Madl, J. E. (1986): *Neuroscience,* 17:741–753.
10. Bennett, J. P., Logan, W. J., and Snyder, S. H. (1972): *Science,* 178:997–999.
11. Berger, S. J., Carter, J. G., and Lowry, O. H. (1977): *J. Neurochem.,* 28:149–158.
12. Biscoe, T. J., Evans, R. H., Francis, A. A., Martin, M. R., Watkins, J. C., Davies, J., and Dray, A. (1977): *Nature,* 270:743–745.
13. Bradford, H. F., and Richards, C. D. (1976): *Brain Res.,* 105:168–172.
14. Bradford, H. F., Ward, H. K., and Tomas, A. J. (1978): *J. Neurochem.,* 30:1453–1459.
15. Bridges, R., Hearn, T., Monaghan, D. T., and Cotman, C. W. (1986): *Brain Res.,* 375:204–209.
16. Bromberg, M. B., Penney, J. B., Jr., Stephenson, B. S., and Young, A. B. (1981): *Brain Res.,* 215:369–374.
17. Butcher, S. P., Collins, J. F., and Roberts, P. J. (1983): *Br. J. Pharmacol.,* 80:355–364.
18. Carter, C. J. (1982): *Neuropharmacology,* 21:379–383.
19. Coan, E. J., and Collingridge, G. L. (1985): *Neurosci. Lett.,* 53:21–26.
20. Collingridge, G. L., Kehl, S. J., and McLennan, H. (1983): *J. Physiol. (Lond.),* 334:33–46.
21. Collins, G. G. S. (1982): *Brain Res.,* 244:311–318.
22. Collins, G. G. S. (1984): *Brain Res.,* 296:145–147.
23. Collins, G. G. S., Anson, J., and Probett, G. A. (1981): *Brain Res.,* 204:103–120.
24. Cotman, C. W., Foster, A. C., and Lanthorn, T. H. (1981): *Adv. Biochem. Pharmacol.,* 27:1–27.
25. Cotman, C. W., and Nadler, J. V. (1981): In: *Glutamate: Transmitter in the Central Nervous System,* edited by P. J. Roberts, J. Storm-Mathisen, and G. A. R. Johnston, pp. 117–154. John Wiley and Sons, London.
26. Crawford, I. L., and Connor, J. D. (1973): *Nature,* 244:442–443.
27. Crepel, F., Ahanjal, S. S., and Sears, T. A. (1982): *J. Physiol. (Lond.),* 329:297–317.
28. Croucher, M. J., Collins, J. F., Meldrum, B. S. (1982): *Science,* 216:899–901.
29. Crunelli, V., Forda, S., and Kelly, J. S. (1983): *J. Physiol. (Lond.),* 341:627–640.
30. Cuenod, M., Kim, Q. D., Herrling, P. L., Turski, W. A., Matute, C., and Streit, P. (1987): In: *Excitatory Amino Acids and Seizure Disorders,* edited by R. Schwarcz and Y. Ben-Ari. Plenum, New York (*in press*).
31. Davies, J., Evans, R. H., Francis, A. A., and Watkins, J. C. (1979): *J. Physiol. (Paris),* 75:641–645.
32. Davies, J., Evans, R. H., Jones, A. W., Smith, D. A. S., and Watkins, J. C. (1982): *Comp. Biochem. Physiol.,* 72:211–224.
33. Davies, J., Jones, A. W., Sheardown, M. J., Smith, D. A. S., and Watkins, J. C. (1984): *Neurosci. Lett.,* 52:79–84.
34. Davies, J., and Watkins, J. C. (1979): *J. Physiol. (Lond.),* 297:621–635.
35. Davies, J., and Watkins, J. C. (1983): *Exp. Brain Res.,* 49:280–290.
36. Divac, I., Fonnum, F., and Storm-Mathisen, J. (1977): *Nature,* 266:377–378.
37. Dolphin, A. C., Errington, M. L., and Bliss, T. V. P. (1982): *Nature,* 297:496–498.
38. Donoghue, J. P., Wenthold, R. J., and Altschuler, R. A. (1985): *J. Neurosci.,* 5:2597–2608.
39. Fagg, G. E., and Foster, A. C. (1983): *Neuroscience,* 9:701–719.
40. Fagg, G. E., Foster, A. C., Mena, E. E., and Cotman, C. W. (1982): *J. Neurosci.,* 2:958–965.
41. Fagg, G. E., and Lane, J. D. (1979): *Neuroscience,* 4:1015–1036.
42. Fagg, G. E., and Matus, A. (1984): *Proc. Natl. Acad. Sci. USA,* 81:6876–6880.
43. Flatman, J. A., Schwindt, P. C., Crill, W. E., and Stafstrom, C. E. (1983): *Brain Res.,* 266:169–173.
44. Fonnum, F. (1984): *J. Neurochem.,* 42:1–11.
45. Fonnum, F., Soreide, A., Kvale, I., Walker, J., and Walaas, I. (1981): In: *Glutamate as a Neurotransmitter,* edited by G. DiChiara and G. L. Gessa, pp. 29–41. Raven Press, New York.
46. Fonnum, F., Storm-Mathisen, J., and Divac, I. (1981): *Neuroscience,* 6:863–875.
47. Foster, A. C., and Fagg, G. E. (1984): *Brain Res. Rev.,* 7:103–164.
48. Foster, A. C., Mena, E. E., Monaghan, D. T., and Cotman, C. W. (1981): *Nature,* 289:73–75.
49. Foster, A. C., and Roberts, P. J. (1978): *J. Neurochem.,* 31:1467–1477.
50. Foster, A. C., Vezzamo, A., French, E. D., and Schwarcz, R. (1984): *Neurosci. Lett.,* 48:273–278.
51. Fu-long, T., Ottersen, O. P., and Storm-Mathisen, J. (1984): *Neurosci. Lett. (Suppl.),* 18:S196.
52. Ganong, A. H., and Cotman, C. W. (1982): *Neurosci. Lett.,* 34:195–200.
53. Ganong, A. H., Jones, A. W., Watkins, J. C., and Cotman, C. W. (1986): *J. Neurosci.,* 6:930–937.
54. Ganong, A. H., Lanthorn, T. H., and Cotman, C. W. (1983): *Brain Res.,* 273:170–174.
55. Ganong, A. H., Perkins, M., Flatman, J., and Cotman, C. W. (1985): *Soc. Neurosci. Abstr.,* 11:1003.
56. Geddes, J. W., Monaghan, D. T., Cotman, C. W., Lott, I. T., Kim, R. C., and Chiu, H. C. (1985): *Science,* 230:1179–1181.
57. Graham, L. T., Shank, R. P., Werman, R., and Aprison, M. H. (1967): *J. Neurochem.,* 14:465–472.
58. Greenamyre, J. T., Olson, J. M., Penney, J. B., and Young, A. B. (1985): *J. Pharmacol. Exp. Ther.,* 233:254–263.
59. Greenamyre, J. T., Penney, J. B., Young, A. B., D'Amato, C. J., Hicks, S. P., and Shoulson, I. (1985): *Science,* 227:1496–1499.
60. Greenamyre, J. T., Young, A. B., and Penny, J. B. (1983): *Neurosci. Lett.,* 37:155–160.
61. Haldeman, S., and McLennan, H. (1972): *Brain Res.,* 45:393–400.
62. Halpain, S., Wieczorek, C. M., and Rainbow, T. C. (1984): *J. Neurosci.,* 4:2247–2258.
63. Hamberger, A., Chiang, G. H., Nylen, E. S., Scheff, S. W., and Cotman, C. W. (1978): *Brain Res.,* 143:549–555.
64. Hamberger, A., Chiang, G. H., Nylen, E. S., Scheff, S. W., and Cotman, C. W. (1979): *Brain Res.,* 168:513–530.
65. Harris, E. W., Ganong, A. H., and Cotman, C. W. (1984): *Brain Res.,* 323:132–137.
66. Herkenham, M., and McLean, S. (1985): In *Quantitative Receptor Autoradiography,* edited by C. Boast, E. W. Snowhill, and C. A. Alter. Alan Liss, New York.
67. Herrling, P. L., Morris, R., and Salt, T. E. (1983): *J. Physiol. (Lond.),* 339:207–222.
68. Hertz, L., Kvamme, E., McGeer, E. G., and Schousboe, A.

(1983): In: *Glutamine, Glutamate and GABA in the Central Nervous System*, edited by L. Hertz, E. Kvamme, E. G. McGeer, and A. Schousboe, Alan R. Liss, New York.

69. Honore, T., Lauridsen, J., and Krogsgaard-Larsen, P. (1982): *J. Neurochem.*, 38:173–178.

70. Honore, T., and Nielsen, M. (1985): *Neurosci. Lett.*, 54:27–32.

71. Hori, N., Auker, C. R., Braitman, D. J., and Carpenter, D. O. (1981): *Cell. Mol. Neurobiol.*, 1:115–120.

72. Johnson, J. L., and Aprison, M. H. (1970): *Brain Res.*, 24:285–292.

73. Kalen, P., Karlson, M., and Wiklund, L. (1984): *Neurosci. Lett. (Suppl.)*, 18:S190.

74. King, G. L., and Dingledine, R. (1986): In: *Excitatory Amino Acids and Seizure Disorders*, edited by R. Schwarcz and Y. Ben-Ari, pp. 465–474. Plenum, New York.

75. Koerner, J. F., and Cotman, C. W. (1981): *Brain Res.*, 216:192–198.

76. Koerner, J. F., and Cotman, C. W. (1982): *Brain Res.*, 251:105–115.

77. Koller, K. J., and Coyle, J. T. (1985): *J. Neurosci.*, 5:2882–2888.

78. Korf, J., and Venema, K. (1983): *J. Neurochem.*, 40:1171–1173.

79. Krogsgaard-Larsen, P., Honore, T., Hansen, J. J., Curtis, D. R., and Lodge, D. (1980): *Nature*, 284:64–66.

80. Lanthorn, T. H., Ganong, A. H., and Cotman, C. W. (1984): *Brain Res.*, 290:174–178.

81. London, E. D., and Coyle, J. T. (1979): *Mol. Pharmacol.*, 15:492–505.

82. Luini, A., Goldberg, O., and Teichberg, V. I. (1981): *Proc. Natl. Acad. Sci. USA*, 78:3250–3254.

83. Lund-Carlsen, R., and Fonnum, F. (1978): *Brain Res.*, 151:457–467.

84. Madl, J. E., Larson, A. A., and Beitz, A. J. (1986): *J. Histochem. Cytochem.*, 34:317–326.

85. Matute, C., and Streit, P. (1985): *J. Comp. Neurol.*, 241:34–49.

86. Mayer, M. L., Westbrook, G. L., and Guthrie, P. B. (1984): *Nature*, 309:261–263.

87. McGeer, P. L., McGeer, E. G., Scherer, U., and Singh, K. (1977): *Brain Res.*, 128:369–373.

88. McLennan, H. (1981): In: *Glutamate as a Neurotransmitter*, edited by G. DiChiara and G. L. Gessa, pp. 253–264. Raven Press, New York.

89. McLennan, H., and Lodge, D. (1979): *Brain Res.*, 169:83–90.

90. Meldrum, B. S. (1985): *Clin. Sci.*, 68:113–122.

91. Meldrum, B. S., Wardley-Smith, B., Halsey, M., and Rostein, J. C. (1983) *Eur. J. Pharmacol.*, 87:501–502.

92. Mena, E. E., Fagg, G. E., and Cotman, C. W. (1982): *Brain Res.*, 243:378–381.

93. Mena, E. E., Whittemore, S. R., Monaghan, D. T., and Cotman, C. W. (1984) *Life Sci.*, 35:2427–2433.

94. Monaghan, D. T., and Cotman, C. W. (1982): *Brain Res.*, 252:91–100.

95. Monaghan, D. T., and Cotman, C. W. (1985): *J. Neurosci.*, 5:2909–2919.

96. Monaghan, D. T., and Cotman, C. W. (1987): In: *Excitatory Amino Acids*, edited by P. J. Roberts, J. Storm-Mathison, and H. Bradford. Macmillan Press, London (*in press*).

97. Monaghan, D. T., Holets, V. R., Toy, D. W., and Cotman, C. W. (1983): *Nature*, 306:176–179.

98. Monaghan, D. T., McMills, M. C., Chamberlin, A. R., and Cotman, C. W. (1983): *Brain Res.*, 278:137–144.

99. Monaghan, D. T., Nguyen, L., and Cotman, C. W. (1986): *Neurochem. Res.*, 11:1073–1082.

100. Monaghan, D. T., Yao, D., and Cotman, C. W. (1984): *Brain Res.*, 324:160–164.

101. Monaghan, D. T., Yao, D., and Cotman, C. W. (1985): *Brain Res.*, 340:378–383.

102. Monaghan, D. T., Yao, D., Nguyen, L., and Cotman, C. W. (1985): *Soc. Neurosci. Abstr.*, 11:110.

103. Monaghan, D. T., Yao, D., Olverman, H. J., Watkins, J. C., and Cotman, C. W. (1984): *Neurosci. Lett.*, 52:253–258.

104. Monaghan, P. L., Beitz, A. J., Larson, A. A., Altschuler, R. A., Madl, J. E., and Mullett, M. A. (1986): *Brain Res.*, 363:364–370.

105. Nadler, J. V., and Smith, E. M. (1981): *Neurosci. Lett.*, 25:275–280.

106. Nadler, J. V., Vaca, K. W., White, W. F., Lynch, G. S., and Cotman, C. W. (1976): *Nature*, 260:538–540.

107. Nadler, J. V., White, W. F., Vaca, K. W., Perry, B. W., and Cotman, C. W. (1978): *J. Neurochem.*, 31:147–155.

108. Nowak, L., Bregestovski, P., Ascher, P., Herbet, A., and Prochiantz, A. (1984): *Nature*, 307:462–465.

109. Olverman, H. J., Jones, A. W., and Watkins, J. C. (1984): *Nature*, 306:176–179.

110. Ottersen, O. P., Fischer, B. O., Rinvik, E., and Storm-Mathisen, J. (1986): In: *Excitatory Amino Acids and Seizure Disorders*, edited by Y. Ben-Ari and R. Schwarcz, pp. 263–284. Plenum Press, London.

111. Ottersen, O. P., Fischer, B. O., and Storm-Mathisen, J. (1983): *Neurosci. Lett.*, 42:19–24.

112. Ottersen, O. P., and Storm-Mathisen, J. (1984): In: *Handbook of Chemical Neuroanatomy*, edited by A. Bjorklund, T. Hokfelt, and M. J. Kuhar, pp. 141–246. Elsevier/North Holland, Amsterdam.

113. Ottersen, O. P., and Storm-Mathisen, J. (1984): *J. Comp. Neurol.*, 229:374–392.

114. Ottersen, O. P., and Storm-Mathisen, J. (1985): *Neuroscience*, 16:589–606.

115. Perkins, M., and Stone, T. W. (1983): *J. Pharmacol. Exp. Ther.*, 226:551–557.

116. Pin, J.-P., Bockaert, J., and Recasens, M. (1984): *FEBS Lett.*, 175:31–36.

117. Pumain, R., Kurcewicz, L., Louvel, J., and Heinemann, U. (1984): *Neurosci. Lett. (Suppl.)*, 18:S433.

118. Rainbow, T. C., Wieczorek, C. M., and Halpain, S. (1984): *Brain Res.*, 309:173–177.

119. Reubi, J. C., and Cuenod, M. (1979): *Brain Res.*, 176:185–188.

120. Roberts, P. J., and Keen, P. (1974): *Brain Res.*, 74:333–337.

121. Robinson, J. H., and Deadwyler, S. A. (1981): *Brain Res.*, 221:117–127.

122. Robinson, M. B., Crooks, S. L., Johnson, R. L., and Koerner, J. F. (1985): *Biochemistry*, 24:2401–2405.

123. Rothman, S. M., and Olney, J. W. (1986): *Ann. Neurol.*, 19:105–111.

124. Rowlands, G. J., and Roberts, P. J. (1980): *Exp. Brain Res.*, 39:239–240.

125. Rustioni, A., and Cuenod, M. (1982): *Brain Res.*, 236:143.

126. Salt, T. E., and Hill, R. G. (1981): *Neurosci. Lett.*, 22:183–187.

127. Sandberg, M., Ward, K., and Bradford, H. F. (1985): *J. Neurochem.*, 44:42–47.

128. Sandoval, M. E., and Cotman, C. W. (1978): *Neuroscience*, 3:199–206.

129. Schon, F., and Kelly, J. S. (1974): *Brain Res.*, 66:275–288.

130. Simon, J. R., Contrera, J. F., and Kuhar, M. J. (1976): *J. Neurochem.*, 26:141–147.

131. Simon, R. P., Swan, J. H., Griffiths, T., and Meldrum, B. S. (1984): *Science*, 226:850–852.

132. Slaughter, M. M., and Miller, R. F. (1985): *J. Neurosci.*, 5:224–233.

133. Storm-Mathisen, J. (1981): In: *Glutamate: Transmitter in the Central Nervous System*, edited by P. J. Roberts, J. Storm-Mathisen, and G. A. R. Johnston, pp. 43–55. John Wiley and Sons, Chichester.

134. Storm-Mathisen, J., and Iversen, L. L. (1979): *Neuroscience*, 4:1237–1253.

135. Storm-Mathisen, J., Leknes, A. K., Bore, A. T., Vaaland, J. L., Edminson, P., Haug, F. M. S., and Ottersen, O. P. (1983): *Nature*, 301:517–520.

136. Streit, P. (1980): *J. Comp. Neurol.*, 191:429–463.

137. Thomson, A. M., West, D. C., and Lodge, D. (1985): *Nature*, 313:479–481.

138. Unnerstall, J. R., and Wamsley, J. K. (1983): *Eur. J. Pharmacol.*, 86:361–371.

139. Vincent, S. R., and McGeer, E. G. (1980): *Brain Res.*, 184:99–108.

140. Walaas, I. (1981): *Neuroscience*, 6:399–406.

141. Walaas, I., and Fonnum, F. (1980): *Neuroscience*, 5:1691–1698.

142. Walker, J. E., and Fonnum, F. (1983): *Brain Res.*, 267:371–374.

143. Walker, J. E., and Fonnum, F. (1983): *Brain Res.*, 278:283–286.

144. Waniewski, R. A., and Martin, D. L. (1984): *J. Neurosci.,* 4: 2237–2246.
145. Watanabe, K., and Kawana, E. (1984): *Brain Res.,* 296:148–151.
146. Watkins, J. C. (1984): *Trends Pharmacol. Sci.,* 84:373–376.
147. Watkins, J. C., and Evans, R. H. (1981): *Annu. Rev. Pharmacol. Toxicol.,* 21:165–204.
148. Wenthold, R. J. (1980): *Brain Res.,* 190:293–297.
149. Wenthold, R. J., and Altschuler, R. A. (1983): In: *Glutamine, Glutamate, and GABA in the Central Nervous System,* edited by L. Hertz, E. Kvamme, E. G. McGeer, and A. Schousboe. Alan R. Liss, New York.
150. Wieloch, T. (1985): *Science,* 230:681–683.
151. Wieloch, T. (1985): *Prog. Brain Res.,* 63:69–85.
152. Wigström, H., and Gustafson, B. (1984): *Neurosci. Lett.,* 44:327–332.
153. Wiklund, L., and Cuenod, M. (1984): *Neurosci. Lett.,* 46:275.
154. Wiklund, L., Toggenburger, G., and Cuenod, M. (1982): *Science,* 216:78.
155. Yamamoto, C., Sawada, S., and Takada, S. (1983): *Exp. Brain Res.,* 51:128–134.
156. Yao, D., Monaghan, D. T., Ganong, A. H., Harris, E. W., and Cotman, C. W. (1984): *Soc. Neurosci. Abstr.,* 10:419.
157. Young, A. B., Oster-Granite, M. L., Herndon, R. M., and Snyder, S. H. (1974): *Brain Res.,* 73:1–13.
158. Yu, A., and Hertz, L. (1982): *J. Neurosci. Res.,* 7:23–30.
159. Zaczek, R., Koller, K., Cotter, R., Heller, D., and Coyle, J. T. (1983): *Proc. Natl. Acad. Sci. USA,* 80:1116–1119.

Psychopharmacology:
The Third Generation of Progress,
edited by Herbert Y. Meltzer.
Raven Press, New York © 1987.

CHAPTER 21

Anatomy of Central Cholinergic Neurons

Hans C. Fibiger and Steven R. Vincent

The anatomical organization of central cholinergic systems has been under study for many years. Originally, acetylcholinesterase (AChE) histochemical techniques were applied to the brain, culminating in the classic studies of Shute and Lewis (58,94–97). These studies were supplemented by biochemical studies on the distribution of AChE and choline acetyltransferase (ChAT), the enzyme that catalyzes the synthesis of acetylcholine (ACh) (24,47). Later, the pharmacohistochemical technique involving pretreatment with the irreversible AChE inhibitor diisopropylfluorophosphate (DFP) was introduced (11,60) and provided new insights into the distribution of perikarya that are potentially cholinergic (25).

Over the past decade, knowledge concerning the anatomy of central cholinergic neurons has increased dramatically. This has been made possible by the development of antisera and monoclonal antibodies to ChAT (15,16,22,36,37,54, 55,77). The use of these antibodies in immunohistochemical studies has provided a reliable means for visualizing cholinergic cell groups. Using this technique Kimura et al. (46) provided the first detailed atlas of cholinergic neurons in the brain. These findings have since been confirmed and extended by various groups (3,5,23,34,35,53,56,57,61,66–68,72,78,87–89,99,112,113). Others have combined immunohistochemistry or AChE histochemistry with tracing techniques to examine the projections of central cholinergic neurons (1,4,6,12,28,69,71,83,84,92,100,110,113,116–119). This chapter will review the current areas of consensus with regard to the localization of central cholinergic neurons, and examine areas where controversy still exists.

STRIATUM

The presence of cholinergic interneurons in the striatum was first proposed on the basis of lesion studies (62). The pharmacohistochemical AChE technique shows a population of large aspiny neurons in the striatum that stains intensely

for AChE. This led to the suggestion of Lehmann et al. (50) that some large aspiny neurons in the striatum are cholinergic. Subsequent immunohistochemical techniques using antibodies to ChAT have provided overwhelming support for this hypothesis (3,21,34,37,45,46,53,56,67,87–89,99,111). The cells are present in rat (3,21,34,37,45, 53,56,87,99) (see Fig. 1a), cat (46,76,80), monkey (67, 88,89,98), and human (44) caudate-putamen. Similar cells are also found in the nucleus accumbens and olfactory tubercle. In terms of the evolution of this system, it is of interest that such cells have not been detected in the reptilian striatum (70).

The intrinsic nature of the striatal cholinergic neurons has been confirmed with retrograde tracing studies (76,115), whereas the ultrastructure of these cells has been examined using both AChE histochemistry (8,91) and ChAT immunohistochemistry (9,79). These studies have characterized the cholinergic neurons as being large, with eccentric, heavily indented nuclei and possessing aspiny processes. The cholinergic interneurons are distinct from the smaller striatal aspiny interneurons that contain somatostatin, neuropeptide Y, and NADPH-diaphorase activity (108). Cholinergic neurons in dopamine-rich regions of the forebrain (striatum, nucleus accumbens, and olfactory tubercle) are considered to be local circuit neurons because in contrast to those in the basal forebrain, their axons extend for only short distances from the cell body (i.e., on the order of 750 μm in the rat). The dopaminergic afferents to these regions are thought to exert a powerful inhibitory control over the activity of these cholinergic interneurons (51).

ROSTRAL CHOLINERGIC COLUMN OF THE BASAL FOREBRAIN

Shute and Lewis (94,97) first suggested that there are cholinergic neurons in the basal forebrain that project to the cerebral cortex. The effects of lesions of the basal

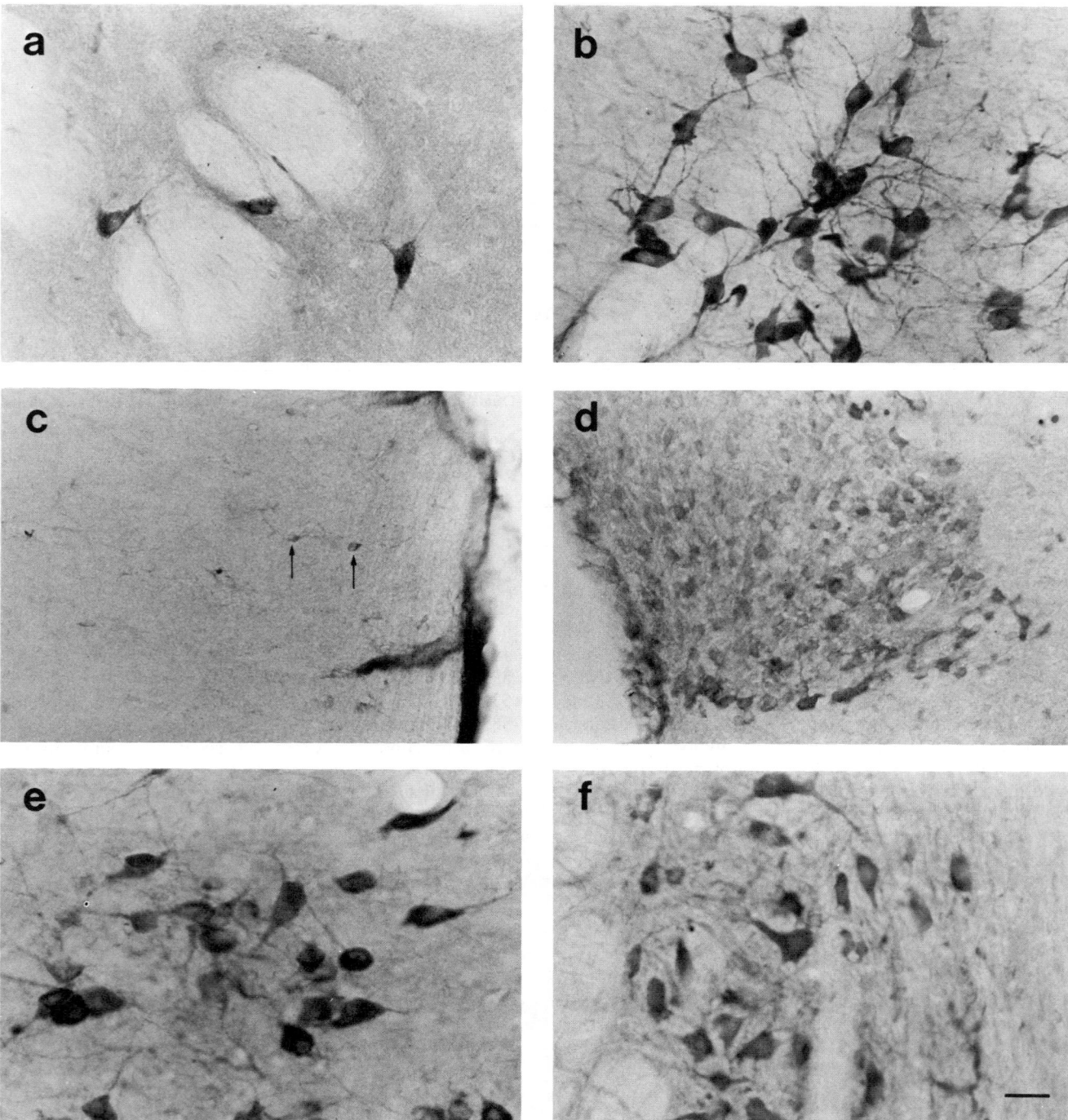

FIG. 1. Examples of the different types of ChAT-immunoreactive neurons in rat brain. **a:** Striatum. **b:** Nucleus of the diagonal band of Broca. **c:** Cerebral cortex. **d:** Medial habenula. **e:** Laterodorsal tegmental nucleus. **f:** Oculomotor nucleus. Scale bar indicates 25 μm for all figures.

forebrain subsequently provided biochemical support for this hypothesis (38,42,52,114). The basal forebrain cholinergic system has since been mapped using AChE histochemistry (25,75,80,86,98,99) and ChAT immunohistochemistry in rat (68,87,99), cat (46), monkey (66,67,88,89), and human (72,86) brain. Although there are species differences in the extent and distribution of this system, the columnar arrangement of cholinergic neurons in the basal forebrain is evident in all species examined to date. The cholinergic cells extend from the medial septum rostrally into the vertical and horizontal limbs of the nucleus of the diagonal band of Broca. Further caudally they occupy the region that has been variously termed the ventral pallidum, substantia innominata, lateral preoptic region, and the basal nucleus of Meynert (87). Although in recent years researchers have been preoccupied with the role of the nucleus basalis in Alzheimer's disease, it should be emphasized that the entire rostral cholinergic column is vulnerable and appears to degenerate in this condition (7,31,85).

Retrograde tracing has been used to examine the projections of this system (4,6,28,64,66,68,69,73,81,83,84,110, 113). The horizontal limb of the nucleus of the diagonal band of Broca (see Fig. 1b) provides the major cholinergic innervation to the olfactory bulb (25,66,68,84). The medial septum and the vertical limb of the nucleus of the diagonal band of Broca provide the input to the hippocampus (66,68,84), whereas the nucleus basalis provides the predominant cholinergic innervation to the cerebral cortex and amygdala (12,66,68,71,84,116). Figure 2 summarizes in schematic form some of the projections of the rostral cholinergic column.

By combining neurophysiological measures with an intracellular horseradish peroxidase technique, Semba et al. (93) have obtained detailed morphological information about basal forebrain neurons that project to the cerebral cortex. The soma of these multipolar cells are large (30–50 μm in the longest dimension) and have extensive dendritic trees that extend between 600 and 900 μm from the soma. The cells have between three and eight primary dendrites that ramify into third to fifth order dendrites. Although the density varies, all of these cells have dendritic spines. An example of such a neuron is seen in Fig. 3. The direct afferent connections of the cholinergic neurons in the basal forebrain remain largely unknown and are an important priority for future research.

Melander et al. (65) have recently found that the peptide galanin is colocalized with ChAT in a subpopulation of neurons in the rostral cholinergic column. Specifically, between 50 and 70% of the cholinergic neurons in the medial septal nucleus and in the vertical and horizontal limbs of the diagonal band were shown to contain galanin-like immunoreactivity. Retrograde tracing experiments indicated that some of these neurons project to the hippocampus. Galanin was not detected in the other components of the rostral cholinergic column (i.e., magnocellular preoptic area and nucleus basalis). At present, no other neuropeptides have been detected in neurons of the rostral cholinergic column.

CEREBRAL CORTEX

The organization of the cholinergic system in the cerebral cortex has been the subject of much research and debate. Biochemical measurements of ChAT and AChE after cortical undercutting point to both intrinsic and extrinsic sources for these cortical cholinergic markers (27,30,103). Conflicting results have been obtained following kainic acid lesions of cortex (39,50). The presence of cholinergic perikarya in cortex is supported by the observation that cultures of rat cerebral cortex can accumulate choline and synthesize ACh (102). Although AChE-positive cells are present in the cortex, there are none that meet the criterion of being intensely stained for AChE 4 to 8 hr after DFP (25). Initial immunohistochemical studies indicated that ChAT-positive cells were present in the rat (63), but the specificity of the antiserum in that study has been questioned. Other immunohistochemical studies failed to demonstrate any cho-

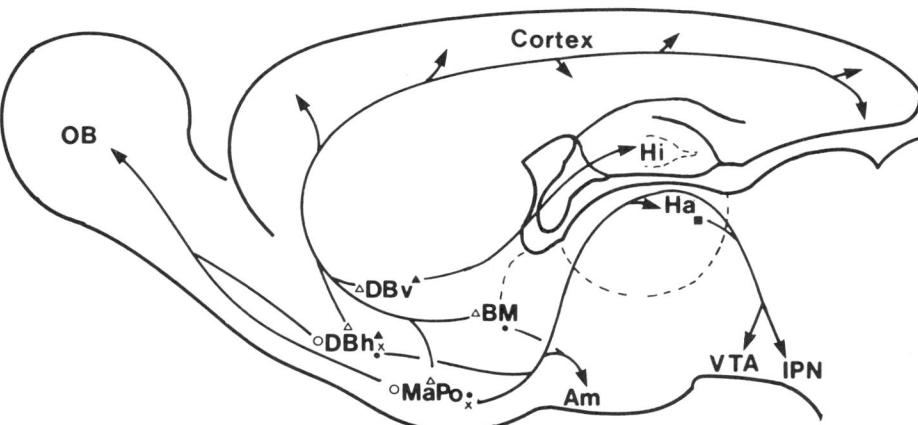

○ OLFACTORY BULB
● AMYGDALA
△ CORTEX
▲ HIPPOCAMPUS
× VTA–IPN

FIG. 2. Sagittal view of some projections of the rostral cholinergic column in the rat. The symbols (○, ●, △, ▲, ×) refer to the origin within the rostral cholinergic column of afferents to the olfactory bulb, amygdala, etc. Abbreviations: Am, amygdala; BM, nucleus basalis; DBh, horizontal limb of diagonal band; DBv, vertical limb of diagonal band; Ha, habenula; Hi, hippocampus; IPN, interpeduncular nucleus; MaPo, magnocellular preoptic area; OB, olfactory bulb; VTA, ventral tegmental area.

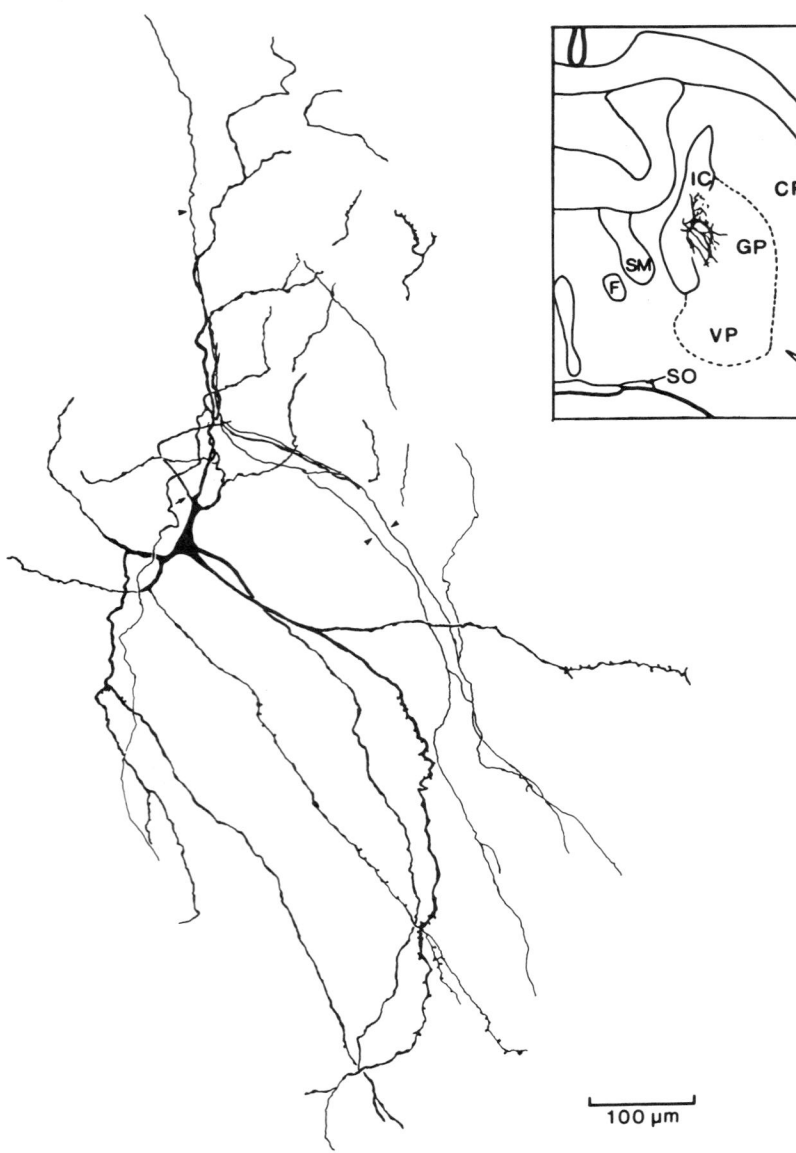

FIG. 3. Cortically projecting neuron in the rostral cholinergic column that was filled intracellularly with horseradish peroxidase by iontophoresis (93). The cell was reconstructed from camera lucida drawings of seven consecutive 100-μm sections. *Arrows* indicate presumptive axons. **Insert** shows the location of the cell on the medial border of the globus pallidus. Abbreviations: CP, caudate putamen; F, fornix; GP, globus pallidus; IC, internal capsule; SM, stria medullaris; SO, supraoptic nucleus; VP, ventral pallidum.

linergic cells (3,45,46,67,68,87–89,99), and cholinergic activity in the cortex was thus considered to arise only from extrinsic sources.

Recently, however, with the application of more sensitive immunohistochemical techniques for detecting ChAT, various groups have now reported the presence of ChAT in neurons in the rat cortex (20,21,34,35,57). This has been demonstrated with a polyclonal antibody and four different monoclonal antibodies recognizing different epitopes on ChAT. This suggests that true ChAT immunoreactivity is being detected in these cells. These cortical neurons are small, bipolar, and, though present in all cortical layers, appear to be concentrated in laminae II–III (Fig. 1c). The morphology of these cells is similar to neurons containing vasoactive intestinal peptide (VIP) in the cortex, and Eckenstein and Baughman (20) have in fact been able to demonstrate that VIP and ChAT coexist in many bipolar cortical neurons. At present these cortical cells have only been detected in the rat.

HABENULA

The habenula is another region about which there has been debate about the presence of cholinergic neurons. It has been suggested (17) that the lateral habenula provides a cholinergic input to the interpeduncular nucleus (IP) in the rat. However, lesions of the lateral habenula do not reduce ChAT in the IP (109). The medial habenula has also been suggested as a possible source of cholinergic input to the IP. However, intensely staining AChE-positive cells cannot be detected in the habenula by the pharmacohistochemical procedure (25,50), and early immunohistochemical studies could not consistently reveal ChAT-positive cells in this region (3,45,46,67,68,87–89). This led to the suggestion that the cholinergic input to the IP arose from cholinergic cells in the basal forebrain that send projections through the habenula and into the fasciculus retroflexus (25). This indeed appears to account for some of the cholinergic input to the IP (1,117).

Subsequent immunohistochemical studies with monoclonal antibodies to ChAT have demonstrated that ChAT-immunoreactive cells are indeed present in the habenula (Fig. 1d). These have been illustrated by Houser et al. (34) in the rat to form a compact cluster in the ventral portion of the medial habenula. Cuello and Sofroniew (18) have since confirmed this, while Keller et al. (41) have demonstrated similar cells in slice cultures of rat habenula. Vincent and Reiner (104) have also noted such cells in the feline medial habenula with a few additional scattered cells in the lateral habenula. These cells seem distinct from the substance P cells of the habenula, which also appear to project to the IP, but are present in a cluster in the dorsal portion of the medial habenula (59).

HYPOTHALAMUS

Many studies have indicated that cholinergic mechanisms may be involved in hypothalamic regulation. Although the activities of ACh, ChAT, and AChE are comparatively low in the hypothalamus (10,24,33,47), intensely staining cells are seen in the hypothalamus with AChE pharmacohistochemistry (25,74). Intense AChE-positive cells are present in the lateral hypothalamus, the dorsomedial nucleus, and around the fornix in the posterior hypothalamus. Some of these cells appear to project to the spinal cord, hippocampus, and cerebral cortex (29,48) and contain α-melanocyte-stimulating-hormone (α-MSH)-like immunoreactivity (48). Studies comparing the distribution of AChE-intense neurons with ChAT-immunoreactive cells indicate that in the rat (21,56,87) and primate (67,89) the AChE-intense cells in the hypothalamus are probably not cholinergic. Kimura et al. (46) also failed to detect cholinergic perikarya in the hypothalamus of the cat. However, a more recent study in the cat using a monoclonal antibody detected many cells in the lateral hypothalamus that are weakly positive for ChAT (104). It remains to be determined whether these cells correspond to the AChE-intense cells reported by others. The presence of cholinergic cells in the basal hypothalamus would be compatible with biochemical studies utilizing selective lesions that indicated the presence of

cholinergic cell bodies in this region (14). At present, however, the existence of such hypothalamic cholinergic neurons awaits confirmation, and deserves further study. The hypothalamus may also receive a cholinergic input from the caudal cholinergic column (see below).

CAUDAL CHOLINERGIC COLUMN OF THE MESENCEPHALIC AND PONTINE RETICULAR FORMATION

Using lesion techniques combined with AChE histochemistry, Shute and Lewis (94,95,97) provided evidence for an ascending cholinergic system arising in the mesencephalic and pontine tegmentum. Lesions of these areas were subsequently found to decrease ChAT activity in various forebrain areas (32). The cholinergic cells responsible for this projection have now been identified immunohistochemically (Fig. 1e) (3,43,46,67,68,87–89,100,101,106, 111). They appear to form a continuous column of cells similar to that in the basal forebrain. The caudal extension of this column of cholinergic cells is the laterodorsal tegmental nucleus in the floor of the fourth ventricle. From this nucleus the column moves rostrally and ventrolaterally around the superior cerebellar peduncle to include the pedunculopontine tegmental nucleus. In the rat the rostral extension of this column is located at the caudal tip of the substantia nigra (87). The cells stain intensely for AChE after DFP (87,88) and also can be selectively stained using NADPH-diaphorase histochemistry (105). Ultrastructurally, these neurons are similar to the large cholinergic neurons of the forebrain (101).

The projections of this system are being studied in detail by combining immunohistochemistry with various tracing techniques. To date, these studies have demonstrated projections to the interpeduncular nucleus (90,117), tectum (90), hypothalamus (90), thalamus (90,100), basal forebrain (90), and medial prefrontal cortex (67,106,119). A summary of the ascending projections of the laterodorsal tegmental nucleus, the caudal component of the caudal cholinergic column, is presented schematically in Fig. 4. Detailed

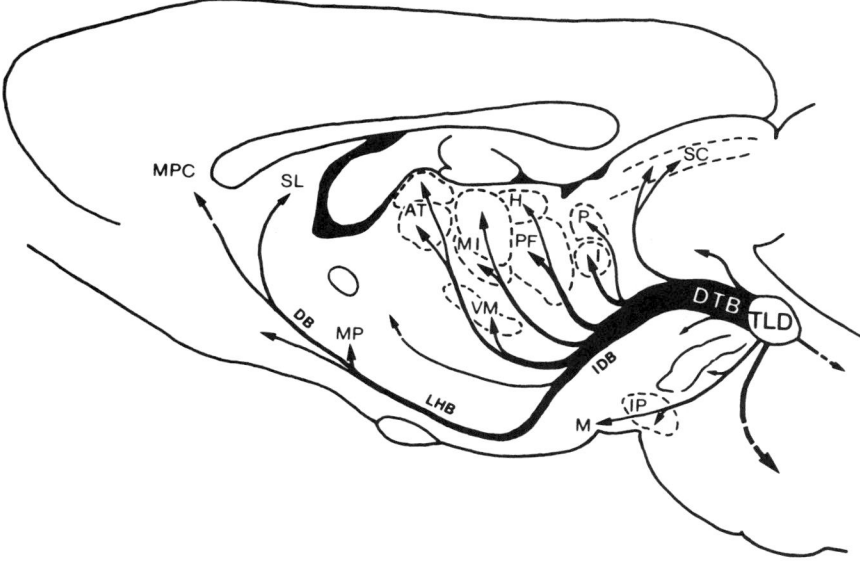

FIG. 4. Sagittal view of some projections of the laterodorsal tegmental nucleus (TLD), the caudal component of the caudal cholinergic column in the rat. Abbreviations: DTB, dorsal tegmental bundle; IDB, intermediate diencephalic bundle; LHB, lateral hypothalamic bundle; DB, diagonal band of Broca; AT, anterior thalamic nuclei; H, lateral habenular nucleus; I, interstitial magnocellular nucleus of the posterior commissure; IP, interpeduncular nucleus; M, lateral mammillary nucleus; MI, mediodorsal (lateral part) and intralaminar thalamic nuclei; MP, magnocellular preoptic nucleus; MPC, medial prefrontal cortex; P, anterior pretectal area; PF, parafascicular thalamic nucleus; SC, superior colliculus; SL, lateral septum; VM, ventromedial thalamic nucleus.

information concerning the projections of the remainder of this group of cells is not presently available.

A number of neuropeptides have been found in the neurons of the caudal cholinergic column. At least a third of these neurons contain substance P immunoreactivity, and these cells innervate the forebrain (106). More recent studies have indicated that other neuropeptides, including bombesin/gastrin-releasing peptide and corticotropin-releasing factor, are also present in some of these cholinergic cells (107). Caudal cholinergic column neurons also contain the enzyme NADPH-diaphorase (105). Although the functional significance of this observation remains unknown, NADPH-diaphorase histochemistry can be used to demonstrate the morphology of these cells in considerable detail and has proven useful in anatomical studies of this cell group (107). At present, it is not known if the caudal cholinergic column degenerates in Alzheimer's disease or whether only cholinergic neurons in the basal forebrain are vulnerable in this condition.

MOTONEURONS AND THE SPINAL CORD

Viscero- and somatomotor perikarya (III, V, VI, VII, IX, X, XI, XII) stain intensely for AChE and are also labeled by ChAT immunohistochemistry (Fig. 1f) (3,5,34,45, 46,78,87–89). In addition, a number of similar neurons can be identified by both techniques outside the boundaries of the cranial nerve nuclei. It appears that these cells, which are scattered in the gigantocellular reticular formation, are displaced motoneurons of the fifth, sixth, and seventh nerve nuclei (87,89).

Some of the vestibular efferents arising from group E medial and lateral to the facial genu display intense AChE activity after DFP challenge as well as ChAT immunoreactivity (92). However, in the rat, cochlear efferents from the lateral superior olive have not been shown to contain ChAT immunoreactivity (92). In the guinea pig (2) and cat (104) ChAT-immunoreactive cells have been observed in the superior olivary complex. Some of these cholinergic cochlear efferents also appear to contain enkephalin-like immunoreactivity (2).

Somatic motoneurons and preganglionic autonomic neurons in the spinal cord have been thought to be cholinergic for half a century. However, only recently have studies demonstrated ChAT in these cell populations using immunohistochemical techniques (5,34,46,63). The postnatal development of ChAT in these cells has now been examined (78) and their detailed morphology determined (5). The most striking finding with regard to the latter is the presence of extensive longitudinal and transverse ChAT-positive dendritic bundles extending from these cells (5). The role these might play in motor coordination remains to be ascertained.

Evidence has been presented for the presence of enkephalin-like immunoreactivity in sympathetic preganglionic neurons (19), and recent double-labeling studies have indeed shown that enkephalin-like and ChAT-like immunoreactivities coexist in some sympathetic preganglionic neurons in the rat spinal cord (49).

Barber et al. (5) have also reported the presence of previously unsuspected cholinergic neurons in the spinal cord. These include what they have termed partition cells in the intermediate gray matter and a population of small cells about the central canal. Barber et al. (5) also found ChAT-positive cell bodies in the dorsal horn in laminae III–V.

CONCLUSIONS

Although much has been learned about the anatomy of central cholinergic systems, many questions remain. Various ChAT-immunoreactive cell groups have been found in areas where other evidence for cholinergic neurons is equivocal. These include the rat cortex, the cat hypothalamus, and the rat spinal cord dorsal horn. These areas warrant further study. The precise input and output relationships of the rostral and caudal cholinergic columns have yet to be determined. Also, with a few exceptions, cholinergic terminal fields have not been successfully visualized with the current techniques. Perhaps with further technical refinements, together with the use of new techniques such as antibodies to cholinergic vesicles (13) or to ACh itself (26), these remaining puzzles will be answered.

The majority of cholinergic neurons in the central nervous system have large perikarya and contain high AChE activity as visualized by the pharmacohistochemical method. This includes the local circuit neurons in dopamine-rich regions of the forebrain, the long-axon neurons that form the rostral and caudal cholinergic columns, and the motoneurons of the cranial motor nuclei and spinal cord. The development of new antibodies to ChAT and the development of more sensitive immunohistochemical procedures have led to the discovery of a new class of ChAT-containing neuron that has substantially different morphological and biochemical characteristics. These cells, which have been observed in the cerebral cortex (Fig. 1c), hippocampus, and medial habenula (Fig. 1d), are small, stain weakly for ChAT, and have little AChE activity as indicated by the pharmacohistochemical procedure. The discovery of these ChAT-containing neurons raises a number of interesting questions. Why, for example, do the ChAT-immunoreactive cells in the cerebral cortex and hippocampus appear to be present only in the rat? Attempts to demonstrate their existence in other species (cat and primate) with the same antibodies have not been successful. Second, although these cells contain small amounts of ChAT-like immunoreactivity, are they "cholinergic" in the sense that they synthesize and release acetylcholine? Immunohistochemical studies on the distribution of tyrosine hydroxylase-immunoreactive neurons may be informative in this regard. Recently, for example, a group of tyrosine hydroxylase-containing neurons have been demonstrated in the area postrema of the rat (40) and cat (82), which do not contain either dopamine-β-hydroxylase or phenethanolamine-N-methyltransferase and might therefore be considered to be dopaminergic. However, fluorescence histochemical studies have consistently failed to demonstrate catecholamine-containing neurons in this part of the brain. It appears, therefore, that although these neurons may contain tyrosine hydroxylase, they do not synthesize detectable amounts of catecholamines. The implications of these observations for cholinergic neuroanatomy are self-evident. It will be important to determine by other methods if all the ChAT-containing neurons identified immunohistochemically are indeed cholinergic.

REFERENCES

1. Albanese, A., Castagna, M., and Altavista, M. C. (1985): *Brain Res.*, 329:334–339.
2. Altschuler, R. A., Fex, J., Parakkal, M. H., and Eckenstein, F. (1984): *J. Histochem. Cytochem.*, 32:839–843.
3. Armstrong, D. M., Saper, C. B., Levey, A. I., Wainer, B. H., and Terry, R. D. (1983): *J. Comp. Neurol.*, 216:53–68.
4. Baisden, R. H., Woodruff, M. L., and Hoover, D. B. (1984): *Brain Res.*, 290:146–151.
5. Barber, R. P., Phelps, P. E., Houser, C. R., Crawford, G. D., Salvaterra, P. M., and Vaughn, J. E. (1984): *J. Comp. Neurol.*, 229:329–346.
6. Bigl, V., Woolf, N. J., and Butcher, L. L. (1982): *Brain Res. Bull.*, 8:727–749.
7. Bird, T. D., Stranahan, S., Sumi, S. M., and Raskind, M. (1983): *Ann. Neurol.*, 14:284–293.
8. Bolam, J. P., Ingham, C. A., and Smith, A. D. (1984): *Neuroscience*, 12:687–709.
9. Bolam, J. P., Wainer, B. H., and Smith, A. D. (1984): *Neuroscience*, 12:711–718.
10. Brownstein, M., Kobayashi, R., Palkovits, M., and Saavedra, J. M. (1975): *J. Neurochem.*, 24:35–38.
11. Butcher, L. L., Talbot, K., and Bilezikjian, L. (1975): *J. Neural Transm.*, 37:127–153.
12. Carlsen, J., Zaborszky, L., and Heimer, L. (1985): *J. Comp. Neurol.*, 234:155–167.
13. Carlson, S. S., and Kelly, R. B. (1980): *J. Cell. Biol.*, 87:98–103.
14. Carson, K. A., Nemeroff, C. B., Rone, M. S., Youngblood, W. W., Prange, A. J., Jr., Hanker, J. S., and Kizer, J. S. (1977): *Brain Res.*, 129:169–173.
15. Cozzari, C., and Hartman, B. K. (1980): *Proc. Natl. Acad. Sci. USA*, 77:7453–7457.
16. Crawford, G. D., Correa, L., and Salvaterra, P. M. (1982): *Proc. Natl. Acad. Sci. USA*, 79:7031–7035.
17. Cuello, A. C., Emson, P. C., Paxinos, G., and Jessell, T. (1978): *Brain Res.*, 149:413–429.
18. Cuello, A. C., and Sofroniew, M. V. (1984): *TINS*, 7:74–78.
19. Dalsgaard, C.-J., Hökfelt, T., Elfvin, L.-G., and Terenius, L. (1982): *Neuroscience*, 7:2039–2050.
20. Eckenstein, F., and Baughman, R. W. (1984): *Nature*, 309:153–155.
21. Eckenstein, F., and Sofroniew, M. V. (1983): *J. Neurosci.*, 3:2286–2291.
22. Eckenstein, F., and Thoenen, H. (1982): *EMBO J.*, 1:363–368.
23. Eckenstein, F., and Thoenen, H. (1983): *Neurosci. Lett.*, 36:211–215.
24. Fahn, S., and Cote, L. J. (1968): *Brain Res.*, 7:323–325.
25. Fibiger, H. C. (1982): *Brain Res. Rev.*, 4:327–388.
26. Geffard, M., McRae-Degueurce, A., and Souan, M. L. (1985): *Science*, 229:77–79.
27. Green, J. R., Halpern, L. M., and Van Niel, S. (1970): *Life Sci.*, 9:481–488.
28. Hardy, H., Heimer, L., Switzer, R., and Watkins, D. (1976): *Neurosci. Lett.*, 3:1–5.
29. Haring, J. H., and Davis, J. N. (1983): *Brain Res.*, 268:275–283.
30. Hebb, C. O., and Silver, A. (1956): *Nature*, 198:692.
31. Henke, H., and Lange, W. (1983): *Brain Res.*, 267:281–291.
32. Hoover, D. B., and Jacobowitz, D. M. (1979): *Brain Res.*, 170:113–122.
33. Hoover, D. B., Muth, E. A., and Jacobowitz, D. M. (1978): *Brain Res.*, 153:295–306.
34. Houser, C. R., Crawford, G. D., Barber, R. P., Salvaterra, P. M., and Vaughn, J. E. (1983): *Brain Res.*, 266:97–119.
35. Houser, C. R., Crawford, G. D., Salvaterra, P. M., and Vaughn, J. E. (1985): *J. Comp. Neurol.*, 234:17–34.
36. Ichikawa, T., Ishida, I., and Deguchi, T. (1983): *FEBS Lett.*, 155:306–310.
37. Ishida, I., Ichikawa, T., and Deguchi, T. (1983): *Neurosci. Lett.*, 42:267–271.
38. Johnston, M. V., McKinney, M., and Coyle, J. T. (1979): *Proc. Natl. Acad. Sci. USA*, 76:5392–5396.
39. Johnston, M. V., McKinney, M., and Coyle, J. T. (1981): *Brain Res.*, 43:159–172.
40. Kalia, M., Fuxe, K., and Goldstein, M. (1985): *J. Comp. Neurol.*, 233:308–332.
41. Keller, F., Rimvall, K., and Waser, P. G. (1984): *Neurosci. Lett.*, 52:299–304.
42. Kelly, P. H., and Moore, K. E. (1978): *Exp. Neurol.*, 61:479–484.
43. Kimura, H., and Maeda, T. (1982): *Brain Res. Bull.*, 9:493–499.
44. Kimura, H., McGeer, E. G., McGeer, P. L., and Peng, J. H. (1979): *Soc. Neurosci. Abstr.*, 5:240.
45. Kimura, H., McGeer, P. L., Peng, J. H., and McGeer, E. G. (1980): *Science*, 208:1057–1059.
46. Kimura, H., McGeer, P. L., Peng, J. H., and McGeer, E. G. (1981): *J. Comp. Neurol.*, 200:151–201.
47. Kobayashi, R. M., Brownstein, M., Saavedra, J. M., and Palkovits, M. (1975): *J. Neurochem.*, 24:637–640.
48. Köhler, C., and Swanson, L. W. (1984): *Neurosci. Lett.*, 49:39–43.
49. Kondo, H., Kuramotot, H., Wainer, B. H., and Yanaihara, N. (1985): *Brain Res.*, 335:309–314.
50. Lehmann, J., and Fibiger, H. C. (1979): *Life Sci.*, 25:1939–1947.
51. Lehmann, J., and Langer, S. Z. (1983): *Neuroscience*, 10:1105–1120.
52. Lehmann, J., Nagy, J. I., Atmadja, S., and Fibiger, H. C. (1980): *Neuroscience*, 5:1161–1174.
53. Levey, A. I., Armstrong, D. M., Atweh, S. F., Terry, R. D., and Wainer, B. H. (1983a): *J. Neurosci.*, 3:1–9.
54. Levey, A. I., Rye, D. B., and Wainer, B. H. (1982): *J. Neurochem.*, 39:1652–1659.
55. Levey, A. I., and Wainer, B. H. (1982): *Brain Res.*, 234:469–473.
56. Levey, A. I., Wainer, B. H., Mufson, E. J., and Mesulam, M.-M. (1983b): *Neuroscience*, 9:9–22.
57. Levey, A. I., Wainer, B. H., Rye, D. B., Mufson, E. J., and Mesulam, M.-M. (1984): *Neuroscience*, 13:341–353.
58. Lewis, P. R., and Shute, C. C. D. (1967): *Brain*, 90:521–540.
59. Ljungdahl, A., Hökfelt, T., and Nilsson, G. (1978): *Neuroscience*, 3:861–943.
60. Lynch, G. S., Lucas, P. A., and Deadwyler, S. A. (1972): *Brain Res.*, 45:617–621.
61. Mason, W. T., Ho, Y. W., Eckenstein, F., and Hatton, G. I. (1983): *Brain Res. Bull.*, 11:617–626.
62. McGeer, P. L., McGeer, E. G., Fibiger, H. C., and Wickson, V. (1971): *Brain Res.*, 135:308–314.
63. McGeer, P. L., McGeer, E. G., Singh, V. K., and Chase, W. H. (1974): *Brain Res.*, 81:373–379.
64. McKinney, M., Coyle, J. T., and Hedreen, J. C. (1983): *J. Comp. Neurol.*, 217:103–121.
65. Melander, T., Staines, W. A., Hökfelt, T., Rökhaeus, A., Eckenstein, F., Salvaterra, P. M., and Wainer, B. H. (1985): *Brain Res.*, 360:130–138.
66. Mesulam, M.-M., Mufson, E. J., Levey, A. I., and Wainer, B. H. (1983a): *J. Comp. Neurol.*, 214:170–197.
67. Mesulam, M.-M., Mufson, E. J., Levey, A. I., and Wainer, B. H. (1984): *Neuroscience*, 12:669–686.
68. Mesulam, M.-M., Mufson, E. J., Wainer, B. H., and Levey, A. I. (1983b): *Neuroscience*, 10:1185–1201.
69. Mesulam, M.-M., and Van Hoesen, G. W. (1976): *Brain Res.*, 109:152–157.
70. Mufson, E. J., Desan, P. H., Mesulam, M. M., Wainer, B. H., and Levey, A. I. (1984): *Brain Res.*, 323:103–108.
71. Nagai, T., Kimura, H., Maeda, T., McGeer, P. L., Peng, F., and McGeer, E. G. (1982): *Neuroscience*, 2:513–520.
72. Nagai, T., McGeer, P. L., Peng, J. H., McGeer, E. G., and Dolman, C. E. (1983): *Neurosci. Lett.*, 36:195–199.
73. Parent, A., Boucher, R., and O'Reilly-Fromentin, J. (1981): *Brain Res.*, 230:356–361.
74. Parent, A., and Butcher, L. L. (1976): *J. Comp. Neurol.*, 170:205–226.

75. Parent, A., and O'Reilly-Fromentin, J. (1982): *Brain Res. Bull.,* 8:183–196.
76. Parent, A., O'Reilly-Fromentin, J., and Boucher, R. (1980): *Neurosci. Lett.,* 20:271–276.
77. Peng, J. H., Kimura, H., McGeer, P. L., and McGeer, E. G. (1981): *Neurosci. Lett.,* 21:281–285.
78. Phelps, P. E., Barber, R. P., Houser, C. R., Crawford, G. D., Salvaterra, P. M., and Vaughn, J. E. (1984): *J. Comp. Neurol.,* 229:347–361.
79. Phelps, P. E., Houser, C. R., and Vaughn, J. E. (1985): *J. Comp. Neurol.,* 238:286–307.
80. Poirier, L. J., Parent, A., Marchand, R., and Butcher, L. L. (1977): *J. Neurol. Sci.,* 31:181–198.
81. Price, J. L., and Stern, R. (1983): *Brain Res.,* 269:352–356.
82. Reiner, P. B., and Vincent, S. R. (1986): *J. Comp. Neurol.,* 248:518–531.
83. Ribak, C. E., and Kramer, W. G., III (1982): *Exp. Neurol.,* 75:453–465.
84. Rye, D. B., Wainer, B. H., Mesulam, M.-M., Mufson, E. J., and Saper, C. B. (1984): *Neuroscience,* 13:627–643.
85. Rylett, R. J., Ball, M. J., and Colhoun, E. H. (1983): *Brain Res.,* 289:169–175.
86. Saper, C. B., and Chelimsky, T. C. (1984): *Neuroscience,* 13:1023–1037.
87. Satoh, K., Armstrong, D. M., and Fibiger, H. C. (1983): *Brain Res. Bull.,* 11:693–720.
88. Satoh, K., and Fibiger, H. C. (1985): *J. Comp. Neurol.,* 236:197–214.
89. Satoh, K., and Fibiger, H. C. (1985): *J. Comp. Neurol.,* 236:215–233.
90. Satoh, K., and Fibiger, H. C. (1986): *J. Comp. Neurol.,* 253:277–302.
91. Satoh, K., Staines, W. A., Atmadja, S., and Fibiger, H. C. (1986): *Neuroscience,* 10:1121–1136.
92. Schwarz, D. W. F., Satoh, K., Schwarz, I. E., Hu, K., and Fibiger, H. C. (1986): *Exper. Brain Res.,* 64:19–26.
93. Semba, K., Reiner, P. B., McGeer, E. G., and Fibiger, H. C. (1985): *Soc. Neurosci. Abstr.,* 11:1238.
94. Shute, C. C. D., and Lewis, P. R. (1963): *Nature,* 199:1160–1164.
95. Shute, C. C. D., and Lewis, P. R. (1965): *Nature,* 205:242–246.
96. Shute, C. C. D., and Lewis, P. R. (1966): *Br. Med. Bull.,* 22:221–226.
97. Shute, C. C. D., and Lewis, P. R. (1967): *Brain,* 90:497–521.
98. Smith, Y., and Parent, A. (1984): *Brain Res. Bull.,* 12:95–104.
99. Sofroniew, M. V., Eckenstein, F., Thoenen, H., and Cuello, A. C. (1982): *Neurosci. Lett.,* 33:7–12.
100. Sofroniew, M. V., Priestley, J. V., Consolazione, A., Eckenstein, F., and Cuello, A. C. (1985): *Brain Res.,* 329:213–223.
101. Sugimoto, T., Mizukawa, K., Hattori, T., Konishi, A., Kaneko, T., and Mizuno, N. (1984): *Neurosci. Lett.,* 51:113–117.
102. Thomas, W. E. (1985): *Brain Res.,* 332:79–89.
103. Ulmar, G., Ljungdahl, A., and Hökfelt, T. (1975): *Exp. Neurol.,* 46:199–208.
104. Vincent, S. R., and Reiner, P. B. (1985): *Soc. Neurosci. Abstr.,* 11:372.
105. Vincent, S. R., Satoh, K., Armstrong, D. M., and Fibiger, H. C. (1983a): *Neurosci. Lett.,* 43:31–36.
106. Vincent, S. R., Satoh, K., Armstrong, D. M., and Fibiger, H. C. (1983b): *Nature,* 306:688–691.
107. Vincent, S. R., Satoh, K., Armstrong, D. M., Panula, P., Vale, W., and Fibiger, H. C. (1986): *Neuroscience,* 17:167–182.
108. Vincent, S. R., Staines, W. A., and Fibiger, H. C. (1982): *Neurosci. Lett.,* 35:111–114.
109. Vincent, S. R., Staines, W. A., McGeer, E. G., and Fibiger, H. C. (1980): *Brain Res.,* 195:479–484.
110. Wahle, P., Sanides-Buchholtz, C., Eckenstein, F., and Albus, K. (1984): *Neurosci. Lett.,* 44:223–228.
111. Wainer, B. H., Bolam, J. P., Freund, T. F., Henderson, Z., Totterdell, S., and Smith, A. D. (1984): *Brain Res.,* 308:69–76.
112. Wainer, B. H., Levey, A. I., Mufson, E. J., and Mesulam, M.-M. (1984b): *Neurochem. Int.,* 6:163–182.
113. Wainer, B. H., and Rye, D. B. (1984): *J. Histochem. Cytochem.,* 32:439–443.
114. Wenk, H., Bigl, V., and Meyer, U. (1980): *Brain Res. Rev.,* 2:295–316.
115. Woolf, N. J., and Butcher, L. L. (1981): *Brain Res. Bull.,* 7:487–507.
116. Woolf, N. J., and Butcher, L. L. (1982): *Brain Res. Bull.,* 8:751–763.
117. Woolf, N. J., and Butcher, L. L. (1985): *Brain Res. Bull.,* 14:63–83.
118. Woolf, N. J., Eckenstein, F., and Butcher, L. L. (1983): *Neurosci. Lett.,* 40:93–98.
119. Woolf, N. J., Eckenstein, F., and Butcher, L. L. (1984): *Brain Res. Bull.,* 13:751–784.

Psychopharmacology:
The Third Generation of Progress,
edited by Herbert Y. Meltzer.
Raven Press, New York © 1987.

CHAPTER 22

Cholinergic Psychopharmacology: An Integration of Human and Animal Research on Memory

Raymond T. Bartus, Reginald L. Dean, and Charles Flicker

Research on the cholinergic system has had a truly rich history. Not only was acetylcholine the first neurotransmitter identified (10,115,157), but subsequent research on the cholinergic system served to help establish many of the basic principles of synaptic function and neurotransmission (52,83,84). Later work, spanning subsequent decades, revealed the ubiquitousness of this neurochemical, demonstrating that its neurons are widely distributed throughout the peripheral and central nervous system, and are involved in a multitude of physiological and behavioral functions (e.g., see 56,107,123,182,222 for earlier reviews). In humans, acetylcholine serves as the neurotransmitter of all voluntary movement. In the parasympathetic and sympathetic nervous systems, it is utilized as the ultimate and penultimate mediator, respectively, of transsynaptic activation. Paradoxically, the essential role played by acetylcholine in the peripheral nervous system has tended to obscure our understanding of its psychopharmacological roles, and has impeded efforts to treat psychopathological changes through the pharmacological manipulation of this chemical in the central nervous system.

Nevertheless, during the past decade, research into the psychopharmacology of the cholinergic system has continued to expand the long list of behaviors in which acetylcholine seems to be involved. For example, the cholinergic system has been implicated in a wide variety of behaviors, including numerous motor-related behaviors (11,46,80,112, 126,131–133,152,170), as well as others including visual acuity (94), self stimulation (105), nociception (231), water intake (199), and temperature regulation (43). Still other investigators have suggested a cholinergic role in more species-specific behaviors, such as grooming (82), aggression

(195), social play (181), exploration (217), odor aversion (33), response to novelty (40,197), lordosis (13,129,223) and other sexual behaviors (2,192). Finally, research of the last decade has also implicated the cholinergic system in more complex behavioral constructs, such as depression (121,122,150,178,202), delirium (187), the response to stress (102,121,203), arousal (116), sleep and dreaming (201,202). It is thus readily apparent that the cholinergic system is involved in a wide variety of behavioral functions and that its role in neural activities is complex and widespread.

Basic neuroscience research of the last decade has also produced a greater awareness of the important interactions that exist among various neurotransmitter systems, and the cholinergic system is certainly no exception. For example, functional interactions have been suggested to exist between cholinergic activity and many of the more classically defined neurotransmitter systems such as dopamine (57,69,87,132, 139,145,146,176,186,194,195,200,209,211), serotonin (87,186,189,220), epinephrine (53,187), norepinephrine (85,118,142,156,168,219), γ-aminobutyric acid (GABA) (86,150,198,217), and glutamate (175). Similar interactions have also been suggested with more recently recognized transmitters or neuropeptides, such as somatostatin (218), the opioids (35,39,49,138,217,233), vasopressin (204), corticotropin (ACTH) and its fragments (82), growth hormone (37,39,97), thyroid-stimulating hormone (TSH) (97), angiotensin II (167,173), and histamine (185).

The widespread localization of cholinergic neurons in the nervous system, coupled with the complexity and diversity of their function, makes any attempt at a complete review of psychopharmacological research of the last decade impossible. Rather, it would seem more practical and instructive to focus our attention on current thinking and experimentation with regard to the involvement of cholinergic neurons in one of the most complex behavioral functions: memory. One area of neuropsychopharmacological investigation, in particular, has fostered intense efforts to integrate the extant literature of the last decade into a conceptual framework that might permit further developments in our knowledge of the role of acetylcholine in learning and memory. This has been the study of the changes in memory function associated with advanced age. The history of the study of the cholinergic role in memory has been incorporated with more contemporary findings into what has come to be called the "cholinergic hypothesis of geriatric memory dysfunction." At the present time, it seems apparent that future studies concerned with the cholinergic role in learning and memory will require interpretation in light of this hypothesis. It is therefore a most useful perspective from which to view our current understanding of this problem.

Stated in its most simple terms, the cholinergic hypothesis asserts that (a) significant, functional disturbances in cholinergic activity occur in the brains of aged and, especially, demented patients; (b) these disturbances play an important role in the memory loss and related cognitive problems associated with old age and dementia; and (c) proper enhancement or restoration of cholinergic function may significantly reduce the severity of the cognitive loss.

Although the relationship between age-related CNS dysfunction and cognitive loss will ultimately prove to be complex and multidimensional, the cholinergic hypothesis has attracted considerable attention and generated a broad range of support, including evidence from pharmacological, biochemical, and electrophysiological studies. Because several detailed reviews of work in this area have been recently published (24,28,51,54,75,76), a comprehensive review of this research will not be repeated here. Rather, this paper will use the cholinergic hypothesis as a point of orientation to review research of the past decade related to several interdependent areas of cholinergic psychopharmacology. The areas selected have all, directly or indirectly, been stimulated by the interest and controversy associated with the cholinergic hypothesis. Further, all have benefited from an exemplary exchange of ideas and information between animal laboratory work and human clinical observations.

PHARMACOLOGICAL STUDIES CONTRIBUTING TO THE CHOLINERGIC HYPOTHESIS

The initial empirical foundation for the cholinergic hypothesis can be traced historically to at least four distinct areas of study: (a) clinical pharmacological observations; (b) animal psychopharmacological studies; (c) basic neuroscience research; and (d) biochemical determinations of brain tissue, particularly from Alzheimer's patients (for detailed review, see 25). Although studies of biochemical changes in Alzheimer's brains (especially the reductions in choline acetyltransferase activity) provided a major catalyst for much of the contemporary thinking and research, drug studies of the cholinergic system provided an equally important empirical foundation for thinking in this area, and continue to provide an important means of empirically testing ideas.

Early animal psychopharmacology research in the 1960s characterizing the behavioral effects of centrally acting drugs began to generate support for an important role of cholinergic activity in learning and memory (70,71,151,227). Most notably, Herz (113) and Meyers and Domino (164,165) suggested specifically that one effect of blocking cholinergic function in the CNS may include an impairment of recent memory. The subsequent systematic studies of Deutsch (70,71) helped demonstrate a clear role for cholinergic-sensitive neurons in mediating learning and memory. Although these early studies were not concerned with age-related changes in memory and are only indirectly related to the specific types of memory problems addressed by the cholinergic hypothesis, they nevertheless played a key role in establishing general acceptance of the idea that cholinergic mechanisms are directly involved in mediating certain learning and memory phenomena.

Similarly, the basic neuroscience research of the same era began to demonstrate that brain regions (now known to be) rich in cholinergic neuronal elements (e.g., hippocampus, septum, amygdala, and frontal cortex) seem to play important roles in learning and memory phenomena (73,119,120,210,221). Indeed, it is interesting to note that in one of the earlier studies of the effects of anticholinergics, it was speculated (on the basis of the nature of the behavioral results) that a hippocampal site of action may mediate the anticholinergic memory deficits observed (165). The existence of dense fields of muscarinic receptors in the hippocampus was not confirmed neurochemically for another decade (137,238–240).

Even before systematic studies with animals began to establish an important role of cholinergic activity in learning and memory, early predescendent clinical records noted that drugs blocking central cholinergic activity produced a dementia-like syndrome, with concomitant memory loss (81,114,151). In fact, this knowledge was employed in the 1950s and 1960s when central anticholinergics were commonly combined with sedative/hypnotics during childbirth to produce an altered state of consciousness in the mother called "twilight sleep." This condition was characterized by an amnesia in which the mothers displayed a marked reduction in their ability to remember events occurring just prior to and during delivery (143,180). Interestingly, this phenomenon, and its therapeutic application, was initially described very early in this century (98) coincidentally close in time to when Alzheimer first published his now-classic case study (4).

To some extent, the initial thinking behind the idea that the specific cognitive deficits associated with advanced age may be similar to those associated with anticholinergic drug treatment (in young subjects) can be traced to these earlier clinical observations. Drachman and Leavitt (77) first formally suggested this possibility. They demonstrated that young subjects given an acute dose of the cholinergic antagonist scopolamine performed various tasks of a cognitive test battery in a manner similar to normal elderly subjects. They concluded that the selective performance failures on certain memory tests that are observed in elderly subjects may therefore be related to a cholinergic deficiency in aged brains. Others have since drawn similar parallels between the memory loss of Alzheimer's patients and the effects of anticholinergic drugs in young subjects (60,205). Finally, more recent studies imply an even greater sensitivity to anticholinergic challenge in nondemented elderly (191) and Alzheimer's patients (213).

Soon after the initial Drachman study, a series of papers was published showing similarly parallel memory deficits in aged monkeys and scopolamine-treated young monkeys (19,29,31). Specifically, aged nonhuman primates tested on a number of different behavioral tasks suffer a very consistent and severe deficit on tasks requiring memory for recent sensory events (21,29,154,159,160,193), with greatest deficits under those conditions requiring longest retention of recent information. This deficit shares many conceptual and operational similarities with that suffered by elderly and demented humans (36,93,190). One of the most consistent and robust pharmacological phenomena observed on these memory tasks is that young monkeys injected with the central cholinergic receptor blocker scopolamine (but not the peripheral blocker methylscopolamine) exhibit a deficit strikingly similar to that occurring naturally in the aged monkeys (31,66). Subsequent studies demonstrated that the deficit produced by scopolamine can be partially, but reliably, reduced by the anticholinesterase physostigmine in both humans (75,163) and monkeys (3,16). Similar beneficial effects were not observed with the CNS stimulants methylphenidate (16) or amphetamine (75). It is therefore unlikely that the retention deficit induced by scopolamine in either human or nonhuman primates can be related to its more general effects on arousal and attention, or to other nonspecific sedative-like effects.

In addition, scopolamine's age-mimicking effects on memory were shown to be at least somewhat specific to its effects on central muscarinic receptors, since similar age-like effects on memory were not obtained with a number of other drug treatments, including dopaminergic or adren-

ergic blockers (15,19), several nonspecific and catecholaminergic stimulants (17), nicotinic receptor blockers (67), and peripheral anticholinergics (67) (see Table 1). Although most researchers readily acknowledge that other neurochemical systems must also be involved in the mediation of recent memory, few noncholinergic pharmacological agents have yet been identified that also produce specific, age-related deficits in memory performance. The two most notable exceptions, observed in both human and nonhuman primates, are diazepam and tetrahydrocannabinol (67,99,155,158,196,212). Interestingly, both drugs show evidence of interacting directly or indirectly with cholinergic neurons (9,72,127,140). However, more recent studies are beginning to suggest that adrenergic mechanisms may also play a similar role in behavior of this type (7,8,241). Further work is required to characterize more clearly this role, as well as the possible interactions that may exist with the cholinergic system.

There is little doubt that, in the final analysis, other neurotransmitter systems will be identified that contribute to the loss of cognitive function in aged or demented patients. However, the establishment of such relationships is not likely to undermine the importance of the role of the cholinergic system. Rather, they will provide a more detailed description of the relationships presumed to exist between the memory disturbance, changes in cholinergic function, and changes in other noncholinergic systems. In this way, a more complete understanding of these relationships may indeed develop.

PRECURSOR MANIPULATION OF CHOLINERGIC FUNCTION

Another area that has been the focus of much attention and controversy during the past decade involves the idea that cholinergic function might be enhanced by the availability of increased quantities of the precursor, choline (or

TABLE 1. *Amnestic effects of drugs in recent memory paradigms*

Drug	Class	Amnestic effect in humans?	Amnestic effect in monkeys?	Monkey dose (mg/kg)
Scopolamine	Centrally acting muscarinic antagonist	Yes	Yes	0.01–0.04
Methylscopolamine	Peripherally acting muscarinic antagonist	No	No	0.01–0.64
Atropine	Centrally acting muscarinic antagonist	Yes	Yes	0.15–0.6
Mecamylamine	Centrally acting nicotinic antagonist	No	No	0.25–12
Haloperidol	Centrally acting dopaminergic antagonist	No	No	0.0125–0.25
Amitriptyline	Tricyclic antidepressant (with strong anticholinergic properties)	Yes	Yes	0.5–4
Desipramine	Tricyclic antidepressant (with weak anticholinergic properties)	No	No	2–32
Diazepam	Anxiolytic (with affinity for all benzodiazepine receptors)	Yes	Yes	3–16
CL 218,872	Anxiolytic (with preferential affinity for type 1 benzodiazepine receptor)	Unknown	Weak	6–72
Δ^9Tetrahydrocannabinol (THC)	Psychoactive cannabinoid	Yes	Yes	0.03–1
Pentobarbital	Sedative hypnotic	Weak	No	2.5–10
Methylphenidate	CNS stimulant	No	No	0.1–0.8
Propranolol	β-Adrenergic antagonist	No	No	0.5–2.0

a primary dietary source of choline, phosphatidylcholine) (12,47,124,125,236). Conceptually, this idea stems from more general thinking that dietary increases in the availability of appropriate precursor substances may significantly increase the synthesis and release of a number of neurotransmitters, including serotonin, dopamine, and acetylcholine (106,234). These precursor studies were far-reaching in their potential functional implications because they raised the possibility that precursors might have significant psychopharmacological effects and might be useful in treating certain clinical conditions. In fact, modest therapeutic success has been claimed in certain syndromes (e.g., tardive dyskinesia, parkinsonism, etc.) using precursor manipulation of the cholinergic and dopaminergic neurotransmitter systems (50,55).

The impetus for specific interest in precursor loading of the cholinergic system can be traced to independent publications from two different research laboratories, which reported in 1975 that increases in the availability of peripheral choline could increase acetylcholine levels in brain (45,111). Within a very short span of time an intense interest in the biochemical and clinical significance of this observation developed, in conjunction with a heated debate over the reliability, interpretation, and functional significance of the *in vitro* observations. Although the development of research and thinking has been reviewed previously (23,24) and will not be the subject of this chapter, a general review of the controversy that emerged during this past decade might be useful.

From the early confusion and controversy, two primary schools of thought emerged. One contended that increases in brain choline levels cause a concomitant increase in the synthesis (and presumably release) of presynaptic acetylcholine. Their arguments were as follows: Acetylcholine is known to be synthesized in cholinergic neurons by the enzyme choline acetyltransferase (CAT) (109,124,125). Two substrates are required, acetyl coenzyme A (acetyl CoA) and choline (109,124,125). Acetyl CoA is made from the intraneuronal metabolism of glucose, pyruvate, and other precursors (117,188). Choline, on the other hand, cannot be produced by *de novo* synthesis (5,124) (except possibly in extremely small amounts) (6,95,96,130). Thus in order to achieve quantities sufficient for manufacture of required acetylcholine, choline must be carried into the brain via the circulatory system and ultimately transported into the cholinergic neurons where synthesis of acetylcholine takes place (110,237). Since the synthesizing enzyme, CAT, is well below saturation (109) and adequate quantities of acetyl CoA can be manufactured intraneuronally, the availability of circulating choline is a rate-limiting step in synthesis of acetylcholine. Accordingly, increasing the plasma levels of choline should produce an increase in the amount of acetylcholine synthesized (45,211,235). The major initial empirical finding supporting this conclusion was an increase in brain tissue levels of acetylcholine following precursor loading.

However, others noted that choline is taken up into cholinergic neurons via a sodium-dependent, high-affinity choline uptake system (HACU) that is normally saturated (96,136,207). Thus, increasing the amount of circulating choline could be expected to do little to increase the amount of choline reaching the intraneuronal manufacturing site, and would, therefore, have little effect on the amount of acetylcholine synthesized (88,92,125,153). They concluded that any changes observed in neurochemical markers with choline loading cannot be due to increased acetylcholine release. An alternative interpretation of the existing data was suggested, involving the notion that choline exerts a weak, but direct, agonist effect on muscarinic receptors in the brain (141), as was already documented for the peripheral nervous system. This possibility was quickly supported by direct evidence of a central agonist effect of choline both in neurochemical binding studies (179,208) and in electrophysiological studies of the microiontophoretic application of choline on cholinoreceptive neurons in the hippocampus (135) and cortex (134,135).

Although this controversy continued for the better part of the decade, within the last 2 to 3 years a number of papers have been published that resolve much of the controversy. These studies demonstrate that choline can indeed positively affect cholinergic function, but that this primarily occurs under conditions of high demand. For example, in the peripheral nervous system, extra choline in combination with phrenic nerve stimulation resulted in an increase of 132% in perfused acetylcholine (224). In addition, other studies using cholinergic synaptosomal preparations have shown that potassium stimulation increases the incorporation of added choline into acetylcholine (166). Further, the existence of a low-affinity choline uptake system, which becomes operative only under such conditions of increased demand, has been empirically demonstrated (224). Finally, when choline chloride was added to the incubation medium of cortical minces stimulated by potassium, release of acetylcholine was accelerated and the normal depletion of acetylcholine (due to persistent potassium stimulation) was prevented (166). Recent evidence also indicates that the effects of dietary choline have physiological relevance. For example, cholinergic transmission in the mollusk was found to be augmented with choline enrichment, as evidenced by an increase in the amplitude of the cholinergic junction potential (14). This was presumably due to an increase in transmitter release that followed increases in neurotransmitter stores. Taken together, these more recent studies suggest that (a) extra amounts of exogenous choline can indeed increase cholinergic function; (b) under certain conditions this occurs via an increase in synthesis and release of acetylcholine; (c) these effects of choline on acetylcholine are most likely to be revealed under conditions of increased neuronal activity, involving increased cholinergic demand; and (d) if extra exogenous choline is not made available under those conditions, acetylcholine stores are rapidly used up, ultimately restricting the amount available for continued synaptic release.

Despite the apparent resolution of this controversy, what remains unclear is the psychopharmacological (i.e., functional) significance of cholinergic precursor loading. Much of this interest, especially at the clinical level, has been directed toward the possibility of treating Alzheimer's patients with large doses of choline or lecithin. Almost from the inception of the cholinergic hypothesis, clinicians were eager to test the corollary that cholinomimetics might be effective in the treatment of memory problems associated with Alzheimer's disease and aging. The vast majority of these studies with cholinomimetics adopted a precursor therapy approach, because of the above assumption that extra cholinergic precursors would enhance cholinergic function, in addition to a wide margin of safety, and relatively loose government regulations associated with their use. This was in spite of the lack of any *in vivo* data indicating an improvement in tasks of memory in senescent animals.

To date, nearly three dozen independent clinical studies have been published on the effects of cholinergic precursors in geriatric memory (reviewed in ref. 23,24). Duration of treatment has ranged from a few days to several months, using a wide range of doses of choline and lecithin. The patient population has varied from mildly impaired elderly volunteers to severely demented, institutionalized patients, clinically diagnosed as having Alzheimer's disease (see ref. 23). These studies do not generally provide support for the notion that cholinergic precursor therapy represents a viable therapeutic approach to geriatric cognition. Although certain investigators claim that positive trends seem to exist in some small subpopulation of the subjects, generally the effects of the precursors are far from impressive, particularly in controlled, double-blind studies. Further, some of the authors who reported encouraging or positive trends in the earliest studies have since retracted these claims after completing more thorough, controlled investigations. Certainly, the subtle and inconsistent clinical effects with choline and lecithin are not even as impressive as the controversial results obtained with more conventional cholinomimetics (discussed below).

There are many possible explanations for the lack of clinical efficacy of cholinergic precursors. In fact, it had been noted long before the long list of negative clinical studies had accumulated, that certain assumptions inherent in this rationale, especially when applied to geriatric patients, had never been tested and may not be true (21,27).

These involve issues concerning the overall functional condition of the cholinergic system in aged brain and its ability to utilize extra exogenous choline in a functionally meaningful manner. Indeed, recent observations of decreased high-affinity choline uptake in Alzheimer's brain (200a), and of reduced acetyl CoA production (183), presynaptic neuronal degeneration (38,172,214,215,228–230,232), and numerous other disturbances in both aging and Alzheimer's disease provide empirical support for this caution.

Moreover, these studies with cholinergic precursors, and the consistent failure to reverse the memory disturbances in geriatric animals or humans, represent a good example of how significant loss of time and resources might be prevented in future clinical trials. Certainly, the state of the art in this area now seems sufficiently advanced so that scores of clinical trials need no longer be conducted only on the basis of controversial *in vitro* data, derived from tissue preparations of nonaged (i.e., young) rat and mice brains. Rather, a more rational approach would be to try

first to integrate data from relevant neurochemical studies with data obtained from appropriate *in vivo* animal models. Once such a synthesis occurs, the collective results and implications of these animal findings can be more effectively employed to help evaluate new treatment possibilities and direct novel clinical protocols.

As we continue to generate data, perceptions gained from the benefit of hindsight make this approach seem less and less viable as a therapeutic approach. However, the possible prophylactic benefits (25,27,42,147,149) of this treatment remain essentially untested in humans, and it so happens that some of the more intriguing animal work suggests that precursor prophylaxis may be beneficial. One important methodological advantage that rodents provide is that they progress through the aging process at a relatively rapid rate. One paper published several years ago attempted to exploit this characteristic when studying the ability of choline to modulate the onset of age-related behavioral deficits (27). It had previously been observed that, among other things, aged C57B1/6J mice exhibited impairment of the retention of a passive avoidance response (presumed memory loss as indicated by control tests), decreased motor activity in a novel closed-field environment (presumed decreased exploration), and failure on a rod-walking task (presumed loss of psychomotor/vestibular/kinesthetic function) (19,68). Although support existed for choline's rate-limiting role in acetylcholine synthesis, and independent evidence existed that enhancing cholinergic activity should help reduce memory loss in elderly patients, the vast majority of studies using choline failed to demonstrate these effects, as discussed above. These data seemed to be at odds with other approaches to cholinergic manipulation (e.g., anticholinesterases and muscarinic agonists), where small but reliable improvements had been observed in similar animal tests (see below). It was therefore reasoned that certain of the cholinergic dysfunctions in aged brains might militate against choline's effects on acetylcholine synthesis, creating a situation where increased choline availability may no longer be sufficient to induce a reliable change in cholinergic transmission in aged subjects. Despite this, it might still be possible to decrease the rate at which the memory impairments appear with age by increasing the availability of dietary choline earlier in the animal's life span. In other words, even though it might be difficult to *reverse* existent age-related neurochemical dysfunctions with choline or lecithin, it might be possible to *retard* the onset of these changes by proper stimulation of the cholinergic system, if treatment were initiated while the system is still operating efficiently. This approach necessarily required that the subjects be given altered amounts of choline before the onset of the age-related behavioral deficits (and the presumed cholinergic deficiencies) and that the regimen be continued for durations extending into a meaningful part of the subject's life span.

In order to address this question, retired breeder mice (9.5 months old at the start of this study) were placed on purified diets that were either deficient in free choline, had normal amounts, or were enriched in choline. In a second similar study, choline was supplemented in the animals' drinking water. In each study, the diets (or water) were given *ad lib* for a period of 4.5 months, after which time the mice were tested for effects on retention of the passive avoidance task, as well as for effects on psychomotor coordination and closed-field activity. Although little or no difference was observed in psychomotor coordination or activity, a striking effect was observed on retention of the inhibitory avoidance task (19).

The results of this study suggest that chronic manipulation of choline was able to modulate the rate at which selective, age-related behavioral impairments developed. Moreover, other studies have since replicated and extended the potentially positive, prophylactic effects of extra exogenous choline (20,65,103,144,162). Collectively, these studies in rodents indicate that the most effective results from precursor therapy might be expected to occur under conditions where the neurobehavioral losses have not yet become severely manifested. Alternatively, very long treatment regimens may be required. At the same time, however, other preliminary reports suggest that improvement with choline and lecithin may not necessarily depend on either of these two conditions. In one study, significant improvement in learning and memory was achieved in 17-month-old mice that had already begun to exhibit reliable age-related deficits (144). In another study, modest improvement in the performance of aged mice was obtained after only several days of precursor treatment, supplemented with vitamin E (103).

It is noteworthy, however, that in the only published account in which Alzheimer's patients were given precursor therapy over a reasonably long period of time, patients placed on lecithin for 3 months apparently showed no further deterioration, unlike patients not given long-term treatment (42). More recently, another study has likewise suggested that choline might provide prophylactic benefits for the cognitive symptoms of Alzheimer's disease (149). However, this conclusion is weakened by *post hoc* reasoning to account for the fact that the patients who showed the most significant effects were those who were the poorest compliers with the dosing regimen. Thus, in order to conclude that lecithin had therapeutic, prophylactic effects, the authors have to speculate that either: (a) the noncompliers in their study represented a unique subgroup that exhibits preferential positive effects, or (b) the dose of lecithin used in their study was too high and beyond the therapeutic window of efficacy, therefore fortuitously favoring the noncompliers. Regardless of the accuracy of this interpretation, the available proof for supporting or rejecting the concept of prophylactic effects of choline or lecithin on age-related memory loss is yet to be obtained. Certainly more attention to the possibility of retarding the rate at which Alzheimer's patients deteriorate via dietary precursor treatment is needed. However, progress in this area may require a shift of focus from the symptoms of the disease to the etiological variables causing it. The frustrating limitations of animal models in this area are well acknowledged and it remains to be seen whether data from animals will help clarify these issues or only add to the confusion. In addition, prophylactic choline treatment may represent an area where far greater benefits might be gained by *retarding* specific consequences of advanced, *nondiseased* aging, as compared to treating or slowing the cognitive symptoms of *Alzheimer's disease*. Relatively little effort has been directed

toward this question, and it is one that the animal data can address most easily.

Finally, it should be noted that despite the intriguing possibilities suggested by the above data, a cautionary word should be raised regarding the interpretation of the mechanisms involved. One must recognize that none of the studies cited in rodents or humans have confirmed that the behavioral effects observed with choline or lecithin are due to changes in cholinergic function. Indeed, as pointed out in the first study demonstrating positive prophylactic effects of choline on behavior (27), the neurochemical results of long-term choline manipulation may not be limited to the cholinergic system, for other important roles of choline, including phospholipid synthesis, are as well characterized. It is therefore possible that altering the availability of choline may affect more general neurotransmitter mechanisms, possibly involved with membrane phenomena, such as receptor recognition sites or secondary messengers. In fact, empirical support for possible noncholinergic mechanisms of action of choline comes from two independent sources. In the first, it has been reported that adult mice maintained on choline-enriched diets until middle age have greater numbers of cortical synaptic spines than age-matched mice maintained on a choline-deficient diet (34,161). Although these changes in membrane surface were modest (5–20%), and have not been independently confirmed, they nevertheless support the suggestion that long-term choline treatment may affect brain function independently of specific cholinergic enhancement, possibly by altering membrane phenomena via choline's role in phospholipid metabolism. Furthermore, recent studies report significant reductions in learning and memory deficits when aged rodents were treated with the phospholipid phosphatidylserine (48,79). Because phosphatidylserine does not possess cholinergic precursor activity, but, like choline, participates in phospholipid metabolic pathways, these data enhance the possibility that choline's mechanism of action in these studies may be more closely linked to its role as an important constituent in phospholipid metabolism. Certainly this possibility deserves further study and leaves the whole question of precursor manipulation of cholinergic function very much open to further empirical investigation.

ATTEMPTS TO IMPROVE AGE-RELATED MEMORY WITH CHOLINOMIMETICS

The use of cholinomimetic drugs to enhance cholinergic activity as a way of improving geriatric memory has not been as extensive as the use of cholinergic precursors, but by some definitions, it has been more successful. To date, the most popular cholinomimetic has been the anticholinesterase physostigmine. Early studies with young adults reported moderate improvement on cognitive tests within a very restricted range of single doses (63). Doses outside this narrow range produced either no change in performance or marked impairment (58,61). Similar effects have also been reported with young rhesus monkeys (3,18).

Recent studies with physostigmine in aged subjects have also demonstrated reliable facilitation of performance on memory tasks (18,41,62,78,171,206). Contrary to the effects of physostigmine in young subjects, however, the optimal acute dose seems to vary dramatically among individual aged subjects [rhesus monkeys (18), cebus monkeys (21), and humans (62)]. Although there exist many possible explanations for this phenomenon, the improvement on memory tasks achieved with an anticholinesterase is consistent with a cholinergic role in the age-related memory disorders.

More recent studies suggest that the oral form of physostigmine is active (32,216) and may not require as much attention to individual differences in most effective dose (216). However, this suggestion requires confirmation (128), and there is no *a priori* reason to believe that the therapeutic effects of oral physostigmine should be more robust or consistent than those obtained with systemic injections. Indeed, a recent pharmacokinetic study directly comparing the effects of orally, versus intravenously, administered physostigmine demonstrated that orally administered physostigmine suffers particularly poor bioavailability (101,226). This was reflected by large variations in plasma levels between (young) subjects, as well as problems in absorption and/or presystematic metabolism. These problems might be expected to be exacerbated even further in aged patients. Other investigators have suggested that another anticholinesterase, tetrahydroaminoacridine (THA), may offer certain pharmacokinetic advantages for CNS indications. While the published work to date with THA is very preliminary (59), a recent study (212a) reported that chronic treatment with THA orally can produce a marked improvement in cognitive function in Alzheimer's patients. However, these promising findings need to be extended and replicated. Finally, some progress has been made in identifying and developing agents that can selectively inhibit acetylcholinesterase activity in the CNS. One example is the sulfonyl fluorides, which apparently inhibit central acetylcholinesterase, but do not inhibit butyrylcholinesterase, a peripheral acetylcholinesterase (169). Like many newly developed drugs, the clinical utility of this class awaits future testing.

It should also be noted that some investigators have attempted to enhance cholinergic function by increasing release of acetylcholine through the use of diaminopyridines (calcium uptake enhancers) (100,184). Preliminary evidence of improved performance in aged rats (64) and Alzheimer's patients (225) suggests that more attention should be given to this possibility.

The final class of cholinergics to be considered is those drugs that directly stimulate central muscarinic receptors. Recent reports that degeneration of cholinergic forebrain nuclei may account for the loss of CAT activity in Alzheimer's patients provide additional impetus for studies with cholinergic agonists. That is, if one assumes this degeneration plays a major role in the cognitive symptoms of the disease, then the most effective means available to treat the deficit would be to compensate for the loss of cholinergic input to the cortex and hippocampus by stimulating the surviving postsynaptic receptors with direct muscarinic agonists. Certainly, drugs requiring functionally intact, presynaptic cholinergic terminals (such as cholinergic precursors and anticholinesterases) should be less capable of improving cholinergic tone or restoring the balance of the CNS than

are drugs that interact with postsynaptic cholinergic receptors. Although relatively few studies with muscarinic agonists have been performed, preliminary tests have provided empirical (albeit modest) support for using cholinergic stimulants to improve geriatric memory. When the direct muscarinic agonist arecoline was tested in aged monkeys, not only was significant improvement obtained in a delayed recall task (21), but also the dose-response effects were more consistent from monkey to monkey than those observed with physostigmine. Similar results have also been reported with Alzheimer's patients (41). Clearly, additional clinical tests are required.

By way of contrast, other tests evaluating the dopamine receptor agonist, apomorphine, and the GABA receptor agonist, muscimol, have failed to produce any significant effects in aged monkeys (22). Conflicting results with the α-adrenergic agonist clonidine have been reported in aged monkeys (7,22) and the potential utility of this class of drugs awaits further testing. Taken together, these initial tests in aged monkeys and Alzheimer's patients suggest that muscarinic agonists may provide a more effective means of treating the memory loss associated with aging and dementia than that provided by anticholinesterases, cholinergic precursors, or agonists that act on other neurotransmitter receptors. However, none of these possibilities can be excluded conclusively at this time. Clearly, work in this area is still in an emerging state of development, and the pharmacological studies that support the superiority of cholinergic agonists remain sparse and tentative, requiring additional tests and comparisons.

Whatever the positive results that have been claimed or obtained with cholinergic agents, one must recognize that they are extremely subtle, quite variable, and offer little or no significant therapeutic relief in daily living situations. Although a tenable explanation for the lack of clinically significant effects certainly includes the likelihood that multiple neurochemical factors are involved in the memory problems, other more basic pharmacologic factors may also be responsible. Foremost among these are the pharmacokinetic properties of the available cholinergics tested to date, including extremely short half-lives, lack of specificity to the CNS, poor passage through the blood-brain barrier, high incidence of adverse side effects, and extremely narrow therapeutic windows. Although any one of these shortcomings would singly or collectively be expected to dramatically limit the effectiveness of a pharmaceutical agent intended to treat a CNS disorder, these problems are particularly severe in the available cholinomimetics. For example, the half-lives of physostigmine, arecoline, and most of the other cholinomimetics that have been tested are merely several minutes long (61,174). Further, existing cholinergic agents have little specificity for the intended target organ, the brain. Moreover, many available cholinomimetics have difficulty passing the blood-brain barrier, have very steep dose-response curves, and have very narrow therapeutic windows. Incidence of adverse side effects is particularly high, in large part because of the undesirable properties of the cholinergics just described. In fact, when one considers the essential criteria for use of a drug to treat any age-related neurobehavioral disturbance, it is clear that the available cholinergic agents satisfy very few. Thus, until pharmacodynamically suitable cholinergic agents are available, it should not be surprising that clinical efforts remain so disappointing. Recent reports of measurable improvement occurring in activities of daily living when the partial cholinergic agonist bethanechol is chronically infused into the ventricles of the brains of Alzheimer's patients (108) lend additional support to this position.

Finally, perhaps the greatest area of excitement during the next decade of cholinergic psychopharmacology will be in the development of truly novel cholinergic drugs. To be sure, the cholinergic agents currently available are quite crude when considered within the context of recent advances in our understanding of cholinergic function. The development of new drugs with greater specificity or selectivity for brain regions and/or receptor subclasses, with nontraditional mechanisms of action, or with the ability to induce greater or more specific second messenger effects, will both provide valuable research tools and have potentially greater therapeutic value.

For example, recent studies suggest the existence of at least two broad classes of muscarinic agonists (90,91). Although differences in these two classes are not revealed by conventional methods of receptor-ligand binding systems (28,89,90), they can be discriminated by their ability to stimulate receptor-activated, intramembranal turnover of phosphatidate and phosphatidylinositol, which is considered to be a probable second-messenger event (1,74,90). One class (class A) stimulates inositol phospholipid turnover by two to three times control levels, whereas the other class (class B) is only partially active, stimulating turnover by only 10 to 15%. Moreover, class B agonists actually block the maximal effects of class A agonists when the two are combined. Thus, this information and associated phenomena provide a clear direction and an available measurement for developing unique muscarinic agonists with improved specificity.

Of course there exist important empirical questions to be answered regarding the physiological effects of increased agonist-induced inositol phospholipid turnover and its relationship to more practical therapeutic goals. However, recent preliminary evidence suggests that potential functional advantages may indeed exist with agonists that have increased effects on inositol phospholipid turnover. Previous work had established that relatively small structural variations in oxotremorine could produce large changes in the enhanced phospholipid turnover in brain tissue (90). From a different perspective, other work had demonstrated that aged rats exhibit a robust deficit in retention of a single-trial passive avoidance task (30,104,148,177,242), and that muscarinic agonists produce reliable (albeit modest) improvement (26).

Using aged rats in this task, we recently compared the effects of oxotremorine with two close analogs of oxotremorine (oxotremorine-2 and oxotremorine-M). Both oxotremorine-2 and oxotremorine-M are structurally similar to oxotremorine, but differ in the number of methyl groups attached to the side chain (two or three, respectively). More importantly, the three compounds differ dramatically in their ability to stimulate turnover of phosphatidate, with oxotremorine-M being most effective, oxotremorine-2 being modestly effective, and oxotremorine only weakly effective. The results of this behavioral comparison clearly revealed the superior effects of the two analogs (25), raising the possibility that muscarinic agonists that are able to induce larger biochemical signals between the receptor site and the eventual physiological response may be more efficacious in improving overall cholinergic function and possibly reducing cognitive disturbances associated with old age, Alzheimer's disease, and other clinical conditions characterized, in part, by a central cholinergic deficiency.

Of course, drugs with superior effects on phosphatidyl inositol turnover provide just one example of how newly emerging ideas on cholinergic function can be applied to help develop different and possibly superior cholinergic drugs. Not only should new drugs developed over the next decade provide us with opportunities to understand cholinergic function more fully, but one might also expect that more satisfying symptomatic treatments may become available for certain clinical disorders. The past generation of progress in research on the psychopharmacology of the cholinergic system has raised a number of interesting questions. However, more importantly, it has set the stage for the next generation of activity, which promises to produce many truly exciting answers.

ACKNOWLEDGMENTS

The authors gratefully acknowledge the help of Ms. Rhonda Sheppard, Dr. Karen Miner, Ms. Carmela Nardella, and Ms. Ruth McCormick in various phases of the preparation of this manuscript.

REFERENCES

1. Abdel-Latiff, A. A. (1983): Metabolism of phosphoinositides. In: *Handbook of Neurochemistry, Vol. 3,* edited by A. Lajtha, pp. 91–131. Plenum Press, New York.
2. Ahlenius, S., and Larsson, K. (1985): Central muscarinic receptors and male rat sexual behavior: Facilitation by oxotremorine but not arecoline or pilocarpine in methscopolamine pretreated animals. *Psychopharmacology,* 87:127–129.
3. Aigner, T. G., and Mishkin, M. (1986): The effects of physostigmine and scopolamine on recognition memory in monkeys. *Behav. Neural Biol.,* 45:81–87.
4. Alzheimer, A. (1907): Uber eine eigenartige Erkrankung der Hirnrinde. *Allg. z. Psychiatr.,* 64:146–148.
5. Ansell, G. B., and Spanner, S. (1977): The source of choline for acetylcholine synthesis. In: *Advances in Behavioral Biology, Vol. 24: Cholinergic Mechanisms and Psychopharmacology,* edited by D. J. Jenden, pp. 431–445. Plenum Press, New York.
6. Aquilonius, S. M., Ceder, G., Lying-Tunnell, U., Malmlund, H. O., and Schuberth, J. (1975): The arteriovenous differences of choline across the brain of man. *Brain Res.,* 99:420–433.
7. Arnsten, A. F. T., and Goldman-Rakic, P. S. (1985): Alpha 2-adrenergic mechanisms in prefrontal cortex associated with cognitive decline in aged nonhuman primates. *Science,* 230:1273–1276.
8. Arnsten, A. F. T., and Goldman-Rakic, P. S. (1985): Catecholamines and cognitive decline in aged nonhuman primates. *Ann. NY Acad. Sci.,* 444:218–234.
9. Askew, W. E., Kimball, A. P., and Ho, B. T. (1974): Effect of tetrahydrocannabinols on brain acetylcholine. *Brain Res.,* 69:375–378.
10. Bacq, Z. M. (1983): Chemical transmission of nerve impulses. In: *Psycho- and Neuro-Pharmacology, Vol. 1,* edited by M. J. Parnham and J. Bruinvels, pp. 49–102. Elsevier, New York.
11. Baker, T. L., and Dement, W. C. (1985): Canine narcolepsy-cataplexy syndrome: Evidence for an inherited monoaminergic-cholinergic imbalance. In: *Brain Mechanisms of Sleep,* edited by D. J. McGinty et al., pp. 199–234. Raven Press, New York.

12. Barbeau, A., Gordon, J. H., and Wurtman, R. J., eds. (1979): *Nutrition and the Brain, Vol. 5: Choline and Lecithin in Brain Disorders.* Raven Press, New York.

13. Barr, P. J., Meyers, T. C., and Clemens, L. G. (1984): Cholinergic facilitation of lordosis in progesterone desensitized female rats. *Soc. Neurosci. Abstr.,* 10:823.

14. Barry, S. R., and Gelperin, A. (1982): Exogenous choline augments transmission at an identified cholinergic synapse in terrestrial mollusk *Limax Masimus. J. Neurophysiol.,* 48:439–450.

15. Bartus, R. T. (1978): Short-term memory in the rhesus monkey: Effects of dopamine blockade via acute haloperidol administration. *Pharmacol. Biochem. Behav.,* 9:353–357.

16. Bartus, R. T. (1978): Evidence for a direct cholinergic involvement in the scopolamine-induced amnesia in monkeys: Effects of concurrent administration of physostigmine and methylphenidate with scopolamine. *Pharmacol. Biochem. Behav.,* 9:833–836.

17. Bartus, R. T. (1979): Four stimulants of the central nervous system: Effects on short term memory in young versus aged monkeys. *J. Am. Geriatr. Soc.,* 27:289–297.

18. Bartus, R. T. (1979): Physostigmine and recent memory: Effects in young and aged nonhuman primates. *Science,* 206:1087–1089.

19. Bartus, R. T. (1980): Cholinergic drug effects on memory in cognition in animals. In: *Aging in the 1980's: Psychological Issues,* edited by L. W. Poon, pp. 168–184. American Psychological Association, Washington, D.C.

20. Bartus, R. T., and Dean, R. L. (1985): Developing and utilizing animal models in the search for an effective treatment for age-related memory disturbances. In: *Normal Aging, Alzheimer's Disease and Senile Dementia,* edited by C. G. Gottfries, pp. 231–267. University of Brussels Press, Brussels.

21. Bartus, R. T., Dean, R. L., and Beer, B. (1980): Memory deficits in aged Cebus monkeys and facilitation with central cholinomimetics. *Neurobiol. Aging,* 1:145–152.

22. Bartus, R. T., Dean, R. L., and Beer, B. (1983): An evaluation of drugs for improving memory in aged monkeys: Implications for clinical trials in humans. *Psychopharmacol. Bull.,* 19:169–194.

23. Bartus, R. T., Dean, R. L., and Beer, B. (1984): Cholinergic precursor therapy for geriatric cognition: Its past, its present and a question of its future. In: *Nutrition in Gerontology,* edited by J. M. Ordy, D. Harman, and R. Alfin-Slater, pp. 191–225. Raven Press, New York.

24. Bartus, R. T., Dean, R. L., Beer, B., and Lippa, A. S. (1982): The cholinergic hypothesis of geriatric memory dysfunction. *Science,* 217:408–417.

25. Bartus, R. T., Dean, R. L., and Fisher, S. K. (1986): Cholinergic treatment for age related memory disturbances: Dead or barely coming of age? In: *Treatment Development Strategies for Alzheimer's Disease,* edited by T. Crook, R. T. Bartus, S. Ferris, and S. Gershon, pp. 421–450. Mark Powley Associates, Madison, Connecticut.

26. Bartus, R. T., Dean, R. L., III, Flicker, C., and Beer, B. (1983): Behavioral and pharmacological studies using animal models of aging: Implications for studying and treating dementia of Alzheimer's type. In: *Banbury Report 15: Biological Aspects of Alzheimer's Disease,* edited by R. Katzman, pp. 207–218. Cold Spring Harbor Laboratory, Cold Spring Harbor, NY.

27. Bartus, R. T., Dean, R. L., Goas, J. A., and Lippa, A. S. (1980): Age-related changes in passive avoidance retention: Modulation with dietary choline. *Science,* 209:301–303.

28. Bartus, R. T., Dean, R. L., Pontecorvo, M. J., and Flicker, C. (1985): The cholinergic hypothesis: A historical overview, current perspective, and future directions. *Ann. Acad. Sci.,* 444:332–358.

29. Bartus, R. T., Fleming, D., and Johnson, H. R. (1978): Aging in the rhesus monkey: Debilitating effects on short term memory. *J. Gerontology,* 33:858–871.

30. Bartus, R. T., Flicker, C., and Dean, R. L. (1983). Logical principles for the development of animal models of age-related memory impairments. In: *Assessment for Geriatric Psychopharmacology,* edited by T. Crook, S. Ferris, and R. T. Bartus, pp. 263–299. Mark Powley Associates, New Canaan, CT.

31. Bartus, R. T., and Johnson, H. R. (1976): Short term memory in the rhesus monkey: Disruption from the anticholinergic scopolamine. *Pharmacol. Biochem. Behav.,* 5:39–46.

32. Beller, S. A., Overall, J. E., and Swann, A. C. (1985): Efficacy of oral physostigmine in primary degenerative dementia: A double-blind study of response to different dose levels. *Psychopharmacology,* 87:147–151.

33. Bermudez-Rattoni, F., and Garcia, J. (1984): The role of hippocampal cholinergic activity in taste-potentiated odor aversion learning. *Soc. Neurosci. Abstr.,* 10:256.

34. Bertoni-Freddari, C., Mervis, R. F., Giuli, C., and Pieri, C. (1985): Chronic dietary choline modulates synaptic plasticity in the cerebellar glomeruli of aging mice. *Mech. Ageing Dev.,* 30:1–9.

35. Botticelli, L. J., and Wurtman, R. J. (1979): β-Endorphin administration increases hippocampal acetylcholine levels. *Life Sci.,* 24:1799–1804.

36. Botwinick, J. (1973): *Aging and Behavior.* Springer, New York.

37. Bruni, J. F., and Meites, J. (1978): Effects of cholinergic drugs on growth hormone release. *Life Sci.,* 23:1351–1358.

38. Candy, J. M., Perry, R. H., Perry, E. K., Irving, D., Blessed, G., Fairbairn, A. F., and Tomlinson, R. L. (1983): Pathological changes in the nucleus of Meynert in Alzheimer's and Parkinson's diseases. *J. Neurosci.,* 54:277–289.

39. Casanueva, F., Betti, R., Frigerio, C., Cocchi, D., Mantegazza, P., and Muller, E. E. (1980): Growth hormone-releasing effect of an enkephalin analog in the dog: Evidence for cholinergic mediation. *Endocrinology,* 106:1239–1245.

40. Chapouthier, G., Lecanuet, J. P., and Evel, A. (1982): Brain cholinergic metabolism during imprinting in chicks. *Behav. Brain Res.,* 5:95–96.

41. Christie, J. E. (1982): Physostigmine and arecoline infusions in Alzheimer's disease. In: *Alzheimer's Disease: A Report of Progress in Research,* edited by S. Corkin, K. L. Davis, J. H. Growdon, E. Usdin, and R. J. Wurtman, pp. 413–420. Raven Press, New York.

42. Christie, J. E., Blackburn, I. M., Glen, A. I. M., Zeisel, S., Shering, A., and Yates, C. M. (1979): Effects of choline and lecithin on CSF choline levels and cognitive function in patients with pre-senile dementia of the Alzheimer type. In: *Nutrition and the Brain, Vol. 5: Choline and Lecithin and Brain Disorders,* edited by A. Barbeau, J. H. Growdon, and R. J. Wurtman, pp. 377–387. Raven Press, New York.

43. Clark, W. G., and Clark, Y. L. (1980): Changes in body temperature after administration of acetylcholine, histamine, morphine, prostaglandins and related agents. *Neurosci. Behav. Rev.,* 4:175–240.

44. Clemmesen, L., Mikkelsen, P. L., Lund, H., Bolwig, T. G., and Rafaelsen, O. J. (1984): Assessment of the anticholinergic effects of antidepressants in a single-dose cross-over study of salivation and plasma levels. *Psychopharmacology,* 82:348–354.

45. Cohen, E. L., and Wurtman, R. J. (1975): Brain acetylcholine: Increases after systemic choline administration. *Life Sci.,* 16:1095–1102.

46. Cooper, D. O., Schmidt, D. E., and Barrett, R. J. (1983): Strain specific cholinergic changes in response to stress analysis of a time dependent avoidance variation. *Pharmacol. Biochem. Behav.,* 19:457–462.

47. Corkin, S., Davis, K. L., Growdon, J. H., Usdin, E., and Wurtman, R. J., eds. (1982): *Aging, Vol. 19: Alzheimer's Disease: A Report of Progress in Research.* Raven Press, New York.

48. Corwin, J., Dean, R. L., Bartus, R. T., Rotrosen, J., and Watkins, D. L. (1985): Behavioral effects of phosphatidylserine in the aged Fischer 344 rat: Amelioration of passive avoidance deficits without changes in psychomotor task performance. *Neurobiol. Aging,* 6:11–15.

49. Costa, L. G., and Murphy, S. D. (1984): Cholinergic and opiate involvement in the antinociceptive effect of DFT. *Soc. Neurosci. Abstr.,* 10:1183.

50. Cotzins, G. C., VanWoert, M. H., and Schiffer, L. M. (1967): Aromatic amino acids and modification of parkinsonism. *N. Engl. J. Med.,* 276:374–379.

51. Coyle, J. T., Price, D. L., and DeLong, M. R. (1983): Alzheimer's disease: A disorder of cortical cholinergic innervation. *Science,* 219:1184–1190.

52. Dale, H. H. (1933): Nomenclature of fibres in the autononomic system and their effects. *J. Physiol.,* 80:10–11.

53. DaRocha, M. J. A., Franci, C. T., and Antunes-Rodrigues, J. (1985): Participation of cholinergic and adrenergic synapses of

the medial septal area in the natriuretic and kaliuretic responses to intraventricular hypertonic saline. *Physiol. Behav.,* 34:23–28.

54. Davies, P. (1981): Theoretical treatment possibilities for dementia of the Alzheimer's type: The cholinergic hypothesis. In: *Strategies for the Development of an Effective Treatment for Senile Dementia,* edited by T. Crook and S. Gershon, pp. 19–32. Mark Powley Associates, New Canaan, CT.

55. Davis, K. L., and Berger, P. A. (1978): Pharmacological investigations of the cholinergic imbalance hypotheses of movement disorders and psychosis. *Biol. Psychiatry,* 13:23–49.

56. Davis, K. L., and Berger, P. A., eds. (1979): *Brain Acetylcholine and Neuropsychiatric Disease.* Plenum Press, New York.

57. Davis, K. L., Faull, K. F., Hollister, L. E., Barchas, J. D., and Berger, P. A. (1981): Alterations in cerebrospinal fluid dopamine metabolites following physostigmine infusion. *Psychopharmacology,* 72:155–160.

58. Davis, K. L., Hollister, L. E., Overall, J., Johnson, K., and Train, K. (1976): Physostigmine: Effects of cognition and affect in normal subjects. *Psychopharmacologica,* 51:23–27.

59. Davis, K. L., Mohs, R. C., Davis, B. M., Levy, M., Horvath, T. B., Rosenberg, G. S., Ross, A., Rothpearl, A., and Rosen, W. (1982): Cholinergic treatment in Alzheimer's disease: Implications for future research. In: *Aging, Vol. 19: Alzheimer's Disease: A Report of Progress in Research,* edited by S. Corkin, K. L. Davis, J. H. Growdon, E. Usdin, and R. J. Wurtman, pp. 483–494. Raven Press, New York.

60. Davis, K. L., Mohs, R. C., Davis, B. M., Levy, M., Ronsberg, G. S., Horvath, T. H., DeNigris, Y., Ross, A., Decker, P., and Rothpearl, A. (1981): Cholinomimetic agents in human memory: Clinical studies in Alzheimer's disease and scopolamine dementia. In: *Strategies for the Development of an Effective Treatment for Senile Dementia,* edited by T. Crook and R. S. Gershon, pp. 53–69. Mark Powley Associates, New Canaan, CT.

61. Davis, K. L., Mohs, R. C., Davis, B. M., Rosenberg, G. S., Horvath, T. H., and DeNigris, Y. (1981): Cholinomimetic agents in human memory: Preliminary observations in Alzheimer's disease. In: *Cholinergic Mechanisms: Phylogenetic Aspects, Central and Peripheral Synapses, and Clinical Significance,* edited by G. Pepeu and H. Ladinsky, pp. 929–936. Plenum Press, New York.

62. Davis, K. L., Mohs, R. C., and Tinklenberg, J. R. (1979): Enhancement of memory by physostigmine. *N. Engl. J. Med.,* 301:946.

63. Davis, K. L., Mohs, R. C., Tinklenberg, J. R., Pfefferbaum, A., Hollister, L. E., and Kopell, B. S. (1978): Physostigmine: Improvement of long term memory processes in normal humans. *Science,* 201:272–274.

64. Davis, H. P., Idowu, A., and Gibson, G. E. (1983): Improvement of 8-arm maze performance in aged Fischer 344 rats with 3,4-diaminopyridine. *Exp. Aging Res.,* 9:211–214.

65. Davis, H. P., and Trombetta, L. (1984): Behavioral and neuropathological effects of differential choline diets in 24 month old C57B1/6J mice. *Soc. Neurosci., Abstr.,* 10:776.

66. Dean, R. L., and Bartus, R. T. (1987): Behavioral models of the aged non-human primate. In: *Handbook of Psychopharmacology, Vol. 20: Psychopharmacology of the Aging Nervous System,* edited by L. L. Iversen, S. D. Iversen, and S. H. Snyder. Plenum Press, New York (in press).

67. Dean, R. L., Beer, B., and Bartus, R. T. (1982): Drug-induced memory impairments in non-human primates. *Neurosci. Abstr.,* 8:322.

68. Dean, R. L., Scozzafava, J., Goas, J. A., Regan, B., Beer, B., and Bartus, R. T. (1981): Age-related differences in behavior across the life span of the C57B1/6J mouse. *Exp. Aging Res.,* 7:427–451.

69. DeSouza, H., and Palermo-Neto, J. (1982): A quantitative study of cholinergic-dopaminergic interactions in the central nervous system. *Pharmacology,* 24:222–229.

70. Deutsch, J. A. (1971): The cholinergic synapse and the site of memory. *Science,* 174:788–794.

71. Deutsch, J. A., Hamburg, M. D., and Dahl, H. (1966): Anticholinesterase-induced amnesia and its temporal aspects. *Science,* 151:221–223.

72. Domino, E. F. (1981): Cannabinoids and the cholinergic system. *J. Clin. Pharmacol.,* 21:249S–255S.

73. Douglas, R. J. (1967): The hippocampus and behavior. *Psychol. Bull.,* 67:416–442.

74. Downes, C. P. (1983): Inositol phospholipids and neurotransmitter-receptor signalling mechanisms. *Trends Neurosci.,* 6:313–316.

75. Drachman, D. A. (1977): Memory and cognitive function in man: Does the cholinergic system have specific role? *Neurology,* 27:783–790.

76. Drachman, D. A. (1983): How normal aging relates to dementia: A critique and classification. In: *Aging of the Brain,* edited by D. Samuel, S. Algeri, S. Gershon, V. E. Grimm, and G. Toffano, pp. 19–31. Raven Press, New York.

77. Drachman, D. A., and Leavitt, J. (1974): Human memory and the cholinergic system: A relationship to aging? *Arch. Neurol.,* 30:113–121.

78. Drachman, D. A., and Sahakian, B. J. (1980): A memory cognitive function in the elderly: Preliminary trial of physostigmine. *Arch. Neurol.,* 37:383–385.

79. Drago, F., Canonico, P. L., and Scapagnini, U. (1981): Behavioral effects of phosphatidylserine in aged rats. *Neurobiol. Aging,* 2:209–213.

80. Dubois, B., Ruberg, M., Javoy-Agid, F., Ploska, A., and Agid, Y. (1983): A subcortico-cortical cholinergic system is affected in Parkinson's disease. *Brain Res.,* 288:213–318.

81. Dundee, J. W., and Pandit, S. K. (1972): Anterograde amnesic effects of pethidine, hyoscine and diazepam in adults. *Br. J. Pharmacol.,* 44:140–144.

82. Dunn, A. J., and Vigle, G. (1985): Grooming behavior induced by ACTH involves cerebral cholinergic neurons and muscarinic receptors. *Neuropharmacology,* 24:329–332.

83. Eccles, J. C. (1957): *The Physiology of Nerve Cells.* Johns Hopkins University Press, Baltimore.

84. Eccles, J. C., Fatt, P., and Koketsu, K. (1954): Cholinergic and inhibitory synapses in a pathway from motor-axon collaterals to motorneurons. *J. Physiol. (Lond.),* 126:524–526.

85. Enberg, G., and Svensson, T. H. (1980): Pharmacological analysis of a cholinergic receptor mediated regulation of brain norepinephrine neurons. *J. Neural Transm.,* 49:137–150.

86. Ferkany, J. W., and Enna, S. J. (1980): Interaction between GABA agonists and the cholinergic muscarinic system in rat corpus striatum. *Life Sci.,* 27:143–149.

87. Fernando, J. C. R., Hoskins, B., and Ho, I. K. (1985): Rapid induction of supersensitivity to muscarinic antagonist-induced motor excitation by continuous stimulation of cholinergic receptors. *Life Sci.,* 37:883–892.

88. Fischer, A., and Hanin, I. (1980): Choline analogs as potential tools in developing selective animal models of cholinergic hypofunction. *Life Sci.,* 27:1615–1634.

89. Fisher, S. K., and Bartus, R. T. (1985): Regional differences in the coupling of muscarinic receptors to inositol phospholipid hydrolysis in guinea pig brain. *J. Neurochem.,* 45:1085–1095.

90. Fisher, S. K., Figueiredo, J. C., and Bartus, R. T. (1984): Differential stimulation of inositol phospholipid turnover in brain by analogs of oxotremorine. *J. Neurochem.,* 43:1171–1179.

91. Fisher, S. K., Flinger, P. D., and Agranoff, B. W. (1983): Muscarinic agonist binding and phospholipid turnover in brain. *J. Biol. Chem.,* 258:7358–7363.

92. Flentge, F., and Van den Berg, C. J. (1979): Choline administration and acetylcholine in brain. *J. Neurochem.,* 24:729–734.

93. Flicker, C., Bartus, R. T., Crook, T., and Ferris, S. H. (1984): Effects of aging and dementia upon recent visuospatial memory. *Neurobiol. Aging,* 5:75–83.

94. Fox, D. A., Wright, A. A., and Costa, L. G. (1982): Visual acuity deficits following neonatal lead exposure: Cholinergic interactions. *Neurobehav. Toxicol. Teratol.,* 4:689–694.

95. Freeman, J. J., Choi, R. L., and Jenden, D. J. (1975): Plasma choline: Its turnover and exchange with brain choline. *J. Neurochem.,* 24:729–734.

96. Freeman, J. J., and Jenden, D. J. (1976): The source of choline for acetylcholine synthesis in brain. *Life Sci.,* 19:949–962.

97. Fuhrmann, G., Durkin, T., Thiriet, G., Kempf, E., and Ebel, A. (1985): Cholinergic neurotransmission in the central nervous system of the Snell Dwarf mouse. *J. Neurosci.,* 13:417–430.

98. Gauss, C. J. (1906): Gerburten im kunstlichem Dammerschlaf. *Arch. Gynakol.,* 78:579–631.

99. Ghoneim, M. M., Hinrichs, J. V., and Mewaldt, S. P. (1984): Dose-response analysis of the behavioral effects of diazepam: I. Learning and memory. *Psychopharmacology,* 82:291–295.

100. Gibson, G. E., and Peterson, C. (1983): Pharmacologic models

of age-related deficits. In: *Assessment in Geriatric Psychopharmacology,* edited by T. Crook, S. H. Ferris, and R. T. Bartus, pp. 323–343. Mark Powley Associates, New Canaan, CT.

101. Gibson, M., Moore, T., Smith, C. M., and Whelpton, R. (1985): Physostigmine concentrations after oral doses. *Lancet,* 2:695–696.

102. Gilad, G. M., Finkelstein, Y., Koffler, B., and Rabey, J. M. (1984): Dynamic changes in hippocampal cholinergic synaptic mechanisms after stress or corticosterone treatment. *Soc. Neurosci. Abstr.,* 10:95.

103. Golczewski, J. A., Kiramoto, R. N., and Ghanta, V. K. (1982): Enhancement of maze learning in old C57B1/6J mice by dietary lecithin. *Neurobiol. Aging,* 3:301–305.

104. Gold, P. E., and McGaugh, J. L. (1975): Changes in learning and memory during aging. In: *Advances in Behavioral Biology, Vol. 16: Neurobiology of Aging,* edited by J. M. Ordy and F. R. Brizee, pp. 145–148. Plenum Press, New York.

105. Gratton, A., and Wise, R. A. (1984): The substrate for medial forebrain bundle self-stimulation contains a sub-population of fast cholinergic-fibers. *Soc. Neurosci. Abstr.,* 10:309.

106. Growdon, J. H. (1979): Neurotransmitter precursors in the diet: Their use in the treatment of brain diseases. In: *Nutrition and the Brain, Vol. 3: Disorders of Eating: Nutrients in Treatment of Brain Disease,* edited by R. J. Wurtman and J. J. Wurtman, pp. 177–181. Raven Press, New York.

107. Hanin, I., Jenden, D., and Pepeu, G., eds. (1986): *Dynamics of Cholinergic Function.* Raven Press, New York.

108. Harbaugh, R. E., Roberts, D. W., Coombs, D. W., Saunders, R. L., and Reeder, T. M. (1984): Preliminary report: Intracranial cholinergic drug infusion in patients with Alzheimer's disease. *Neurosurgery,* 15:514–518.

109. Haubrich, D. R., and Chippendale, T. J. (1977): Regulation of acetylcholine synthesis in nervous tissue. *Life Sci.,* 20:1465–1478.

110. Haubrich, D. R., Gerber, N. H., and Pflueger, A. B. (1979): Choline availability and the synthesis of acetylcholine. In: *Nutrition and the Brain, Vol. 5: Choline and Lecithin in Brain Disorders,* edited by A. Barbeau, J. H. Growdon, and R. J. Wurtman, pp. 57–71. Raven Press, New York.

111. Haubrich, D. R., Wang, P. F. L., Clody, D. E., and Wedeking, P. W. (1975): Increase in rat brain acetylcholine induced by choline and deanol. *Life Sci.,* 17:975–980.

112. Hennig, C. W., and McIntyre, J. F. (1984): An explanation of cholinergic effects on tonic immobility in chickens. *Bull. Psychon. Soc.,* 22:271.

113. Herz, A. (1960): Die Gedentung der Gahung fur die Wirkung von Scopolamin und ahnlichen Substanzen auf Gedengte Reaktionen. *Z. Biol.,* 112:104–112.

114. Hollister, L. E. (1968): *Chemical Psychoses.* Charles Thomas, Springfield, IL.

115. Holmstedt, B. (1975): Pages from the history of research on cholinergic mechanisms. In: *Cholinergic Mechanisms,* edited by P. G. Waser, pp. 1–21. Raven Press, New York.

116. Horita, A., Carino, M. A., and Lai, H. (1985): ACTH fragment 1-24 induced arousal is mediated by a septohippocampal cholinergic mechanism. *Fed. Proc.,* 44:721.

117. Hrdina, P. D. (1974): Metabolism of brain acetylcholine and its modification by drugs. In: *Drug Metabolism Reviews, Vol. 3,* edited by F. J. Dicarlo, pp. 89–129. Marcel Dekker, New York.

118. Huygens, P., Baratti, C. M., Gardella, J. L., and Filinger, E. (1980): Brain catecholamine modifications: The effects on memory facilitation induced by oxotremorine in mice. *Psychopharmacology,* 69:291–294.

119. Iversen, S. D. (1973): Brain lesions and memory in animals. In: *The Physiological Basis of Memory,* edited by J. A. Deutsch, pp. 139–198. Academic Press, New York.

120. Iversen, S. D. (1976): Do hippocampal lesions produce amnesia in animals? *Int. Rev. Neurobiol.,* 19:1–49.

121. Janowsky, D. S., and Risch, S. C. (1984): Cholinomimetic and anticholinergic drugs used to investigate an acetylcholine hypothesis of affective disorders and stress. *Drug Dev. Res.,* 4:125–142.

122. Janowsky, D. S., Risch, S. C., Judd, L. L., Huey, L. Y., and Parker, D. C. (1984): Cholinergic super-sensitivity in affect disorder patients: Behavioral and neuro-endocrine observations. *Soc. Neurosci. Abstr.,* 10:851.

123. Jenden, D. J., ed. (1977): *Cholinergic Mechanisms and Psychopharmacology.* Plenum Press, New York.

124. Jenden, D. J. (1979): An overview of choline and acetylcholine metabolism in relation to the therapeutic uses of choline. In: *Nutrition and the Brain, Vol. 5: Choline and Lecithin in Brain Disorders,* edited by A. Barbeau, J. H. Growdon, and R. J. Wurtman, pp. 13–24. Raven Press, New York.

125. Jenden, D. J. (1979): The neurochemical basis of acetylcholine precursor loading as a therapeutic strategy. In: *Brain Acetylcholine and Neuropsychiatric Disease,* edited by K. L. Davis and P. A. Berger, pp. 483–513. Plenum Press, New York.

126. Jenner, P., Marsden, C. D., and Rupniak, N. M. J. (1982): Cholinergic manipulation of perioral movements induced by the chronic administration of neuroleptic drugs to rats. *Br. J. Pharmacol.,* 77:309P.

127. Johnson, K. M., and Dewey, W. L. (1978): Effects of -THC on the synaptosomal uptake of ^{3}H-Tryptophan and ^{3}H-Choline. *Pharmacology,* 17:83–87.

128. Jotkowitz, S. (1983): Lack of clinical efficacy of chronic oral physostigmine in Alzheimer's disease. *Ann. Neurol.,* 14:690–691.

129. Kaufman, L. S., Pfaff, D. W., and McEwen, B. S. (1984): Cholinergic mechanisms of lordosis in rats in the basomedial hypothalamus as revealed by intracranial application of scopolamine. *Soc. Neurosci. Abstr.,* 10:822.

130. Kewitz, H., and Pleul, D. (1976): Synthesis of choline from ethanolamine in rat brain. *Proc. Natl. Acad. Sci. USA,* 73:2181–2185.

131. Klemm, W. R. (1984): Catalepsy requires intact cholinergic function but can be caused by apomorphine. *Soc. Neurosci. Abstr.,* 10:1094.

132. Klemm, W. R. (1985): Evidence for a cholinergic role in haloperidol-induced catalepsy. *Psychopharmacology,* 85:139–142.

133. Kohl, R. L., and Homick, J. L. (1983): Motion sickness: A modulatory role for the central cholinergic nervous system. *Neurosci. Biobehav. Rev.,* 7:73–85.

134. Krnjevic, K., and Reinhardt, W. (1979): Choline excites cortical neurons. *Science,* 206:1321–1323.

135. Krnjevic, K., Reinhardt, W., and Ropert, N. (1982): Choline as an acetylcholine agonist in the mammalian neocortex and hippocampus. In: *Aging, Vol. 19: Alzheimer's Disease: A Report of Progress in Research,* edited by S. Corkin, K. L. Davis, J. H. Growdon, E. Usdin, and R. J. Wurtman, pp. 334–344. Raven Press, New York.

136. Kuhar, M. J. (1978): Characteristics and significance of sodium dependent, high affinity choline uptake. In: *Advances in Behavioral Biology, Vol. 24: Cholinergic Mechanisms and Psychopharmacology,* edited by D. J. Jenden, pp. 447–456. Plenum Press, New York.

137. Kuhar, M. J., and Yamamura, H. I. (1975): Light autoradiographic localization of cholinergic muscarinic receptors in rat brain by specific binding of a potent antagonist. *Nature,* 253:560–561.

138. Kumakura, K., Guidotti, A., Yang, T.-Y. T., Saiani, L., and Costa, E. (1980): A role for the opiate peptides that presumably coexist with acetylcholine in splanchnic nerves. In: *Neural Peptides and Neuronal Communication,* edited by E. Costa and M. Trabucchi, pp. 571–580. Raven Press, New York.

139. Kuribara, H. (1982): Strain differences to the effects of central acting drugs on Sidman avoidance response in Wistar and Fischer 344 rats. *Pharmacol. Biochem. Behav.,* 17:425–430.

140. Ladinsky, H., Consolo, S., Bellantuono, C., and Garattini, S. (1981): Interaction of benzodiazepines with known and putative neurotransmitters in the brain. In: *Handbook of Biological Psychiatry, Vol. 4,* edited by H. M. Van Pragg, M. H. Lader, O. J. Rafaelsen, and E. J. Sachar, pp. 825–858. Marcel Dekker, New York.

141. Ladinsky, H., Consolo, S., and Pugnetti, P. (1979): A possible central muscarinic receptor agonist role for choline in increasing rat striatal acetylcholine content. In: *Nutrition and the Brain, Vol. 5: Choline and Lecithin in Brain Disorders,* edited by A. Barbeau, J. H. Growdon, and R. J. Wurtman, pp. 227–232. Raven Press, New York.

142. Ladinsky, H., Consolo, S., Tirelli, A. S., and Forloni, G. L. (1980): Evidence for noradrenergic mediation of the oxotremorine-induced increase in acetylcholine content in rat hippocampus. *Brain Res.,* 187:494–498.

143. Lambrechts, W., and Parkhouse, J. (1961): Postoperative amnesia. *Br. J. Anesthesiol.,* 33:397–404.

144. Leathwood, P. D., Heck, E., and Mauron, J. (1982): Phosphati-

dylcholine and avoidance performance in 17 month old SEC/1REJ mice. *Life Sci.,* 30:1065–1071.

145. Lehmann, J., and Langer, S. Z. (1982): Muscarinic receptors on dopamine terminals in the cat caudate nucleus: Neuromodulation of [³H]dopamine release *in vitro* by endogenous acetylcholine. *Brain Res.,* 248:61–69.

146. Leventer, S. M., and Johnson, K. M. (1983): Effects of phencyclidine on the release of radioactivity from rat striatal slices labeled with tritium labeled choline. *J. Pharmacol. Exp. Ther.,* 225:332–336.

147. Levy, R., Little, A., Chuaqui, P., and Reith, M. (1983): Early results from double blind, placebo controlled trial of high dose phosphatidylcholine in Alzheimer's disease. *Lancet,* 1:987–988.

148. Lippa, A. S., Pelham, R. W., Beer, B., Critchett, D. J., Dean, R. L., and Bartus, R. T. (1980): Brain cholinergic function and memory in aged rats. *Neurobiol. Aging,* 1:10–19.

149. Little, A., Levy, R., Chuaqui-Kidd, P., and Hand, D. (1985): A double blind, placebo controlled trial of high-dose lecithin in Alzheimer's disease. *J. Neurol. Neurosurg. Psychiatry,* 48:736–742.

150. Lloyd, K. G., Garrigou, D., and Broekkamp, C. I. E. (1982): Action of mono-aminergic cholinergic and gamma-aminobutyric acid-ergic compounds in the olfactory bulbectomized rat. In: *Advances in the Biosciences, Vol. 40: New Vistas in Depression,* edited by S. Z. Langer, et al., pp. 179–186. Pergamon Press, New York.

151. Longo, V. G. (1966): Behavioral and electroencephalographic effects of atropine and related compounds. *Pharmacol. Rev.,* 18:965–996.

152. Lukyanov, A. S., Sidorov, S. S., and Frolov, O. Y. (1984): Optomotor reaction of the carp *Cyprinus-carpio cyprinidae* in phenol intoxication. *Vopr. Ikhtiol.,* 24:316–320.

153. MacIntosh, F. C. (1979): Are acetylcholine levels related to acetylcholine release? In: *Nutrition and the Brain, Vol. 5: Choline and Lecithin in Brain Disorders,* edited by A. Barbeau, J. H. Growdon, and R. J. Wurtman, pp. 201–217. Raven Press, New York.

154. Marriott, J. G., and Abelson, J. S. (1980): Age differences in short-term memory in test-sophisticated rhesus monkeys. *Age,* 3:7–9.

155. Marriott, J. G., Abelson, J. S., and Bartus, R. T. (1979): Diazepam impairment of delayed-response performance in young and old rhesus monkeys. *Neurosci. Abstr.,* 5:1053.

156. Mason, S. T., and Fibiger, H. C. (1979): Possibly behavioral function for noradrenaline-acetylcholine interaction in brain. *Nature,* 277:396–397.

157. Mayer, S. E. (1980): Neurohumoral transmission and the autonomic nervous system. In: *The Pharmacological Basis of Therapeutics,* 6th ed., edited by A. H. Gilman, L. S. Goodman, and A. Gilman, pp. 56–90. Macmillan, New York.

158. McMillan, D. E. (1977): Behavioral pharmacology of the tetrahydrocannabinols. In: *Advances in Behavioral Pharmacology, Vol. 1,* edited by T. Thompson and P. B. Dews, pp. 2–35. Academic Press, New York.

159. Medin, D. L. (1969): Form perception and pattern reproduction by monkeys. *J. Comp. Physiol. Psychol.,* 68:412–419.

160. Medin, D. L., O'Neil, P., Smeltz, E., and Davis, R. T. (1973): Age differences in retention of concurrent discrimination problems in monkeys. *J. Gerontol.,* 28:63–67.

161. Mervis, R. F., and Bartus, R. T. (1981): Modulation of pyramidal cell dendrite spine population in aging mouse neocortex: Role of dietary choline. *J. Neuropathol. Exp. Neurol.,* 40:313.

162. Mervis, R. F., Horrocks, L. A., Wallace, L. J., and Naber, E. (1984): Influence of chronic choline-containing diets on neurobehavioral parameters in the C57B1 mouse. *Soc. Neurosci. Abstr.,* 10:976.

163. Mewaldt, S. P., and Ghoneim, M. M. (1978): The effects and interactions of scopolamine, physostigmine and methamphetamine on human memory. *Pharmacol. Biochem. Behav.,* 10:205–210.

164. Meyers, B., and Domino, E. F. (1964): The effect of cholinergic blocking drugs on spontaneous alteration in rats. *Arch. Int. Pharmacodyn.,* 150:3–4.

165. Meyers, B., Roberts, D. H., Riciputi, R. H., and Domino, E. F. (1964): Some effects of muscarinic cholinergic blocking drugs on

behavior and the electrocorticogram. *Psychopharmacology,* 5:289–300.

166. Millington, E. R., and Goldberg, A. M. (1982): Precursor dependence of acetylcholine release from rat brain *in vitro. Brain Res.,* 243:263–270.

167. Moore, A. F., and Drexler, A. P. (1982): A cholinergic link in the centrally mediated actions of angiotensin II. *Drug Dev. Res.,* 2:241–250.

168. Morgan, W. W., and Pfeil, K. A. (1979): Evidence for a cholinergic influence on catecholaminergic pathways terminating in the anterior and medial basal hypothalamus. *Brain Res.,* 173:47–56.

169. Moss, D. E., Rodriguez, L. A., Selim, S., Ellett, S. O., Devine, J. V., and Steger, R. W. (1985): The sulfonyl fluorides: CNS selective cholinesterase inhibitors with potential value in Alzheimer's disease. In: *Proceedings of the Fifth Tarbox Parkinson's Disease Symposium: The Norman Rockwell Conference on Alzheimer's Disease,* edited by J. T. Hutton and A. D. Kenny, pp. 337–350. Alan R. Liss, New York.

170. Motles, E., Infante, C., and Gonzalez, M. (1983): Rotational behavior in the cat induced by electrical stimulation of the pulvinar lateralis posterior nucleus complex: Role of the cholinergic system. *Exp. Neurol.,* 82:43–54.

171. Muramoto, O., Sugishita, M., Sugota, H., and Toyokura, Y. (1979): Effects of physostigmine on constructional and memory tasks in Alzheimer's disease. *Arch. Neurol.,* 37:501–503.

172. Nakano, I., and Hirano, A. (1982): Loss of large neurons of the medial septal nucleus in an autopsy case of Alzheimer's disease. *J. Neuropathol. Exp. Neurol.,* 41:341.

173. Nicoletta, P., Pochiero, M., Losi, E., and Caputi, A. P. (1983): Interaction between renin angiotensin system and cholinergic system in brain. *Neuropharmacology,* 22:1269–1276.

174. Nutt, J. G., Tamminga, C. A., Eisler, T., and Chase, T. N. (1979): Clinical experience with a cholinergic agonist in hyperkinetic movement disorders. In: *Nutrition and the Brain, Vol. 5, Choline and Lecithin in Brain Disorders,* edited by A. Barbeau, J. H. Growdon, and R. J. Wurtman, pp. 317–324. Raven Press, New York.

175. Ohta, H., Nakamura, S., Watanabe, S., and Ueki, S. (1985): Effect of L-glutamate injected into the posterior hypothalamus on blood pressure and heart rate in unanesthetized and unrestrained rats. *Neuropharmacology,* 24:445–452.

176. Oomura, Y., and Aou, S. (1984): Catecholaminergic and cholinergic involvement in reward related responses in monkey orbitofrontal cortex. In: *Neurology and Neurobiology, Vol. 12: Modulation of Sensorimotor Activity During Alterations in Behavioral States,* edited by R. Bandler, pp. 269–290. Alan R. Liss, New York.

177. Ordy, J. M., and Schjeide, O. A. (1973): Univariate and multivariate models for evaluating long-term changes in neurobiological development, maturity, and aging. In: *Progress in Brain Research, Vol. 40: Neurobiological Aspects of Maturation and Aging,* edited by D. H. Ford, pp. 25–51. Elsevier, New York.

178. Overstreet, D. H. (1986): Selective breeding for increased cholinergic function: Development of a new animal model of depression. *Biol. Psychiatry,* 21:49–58.

179. Palacios, J. M., and Kuhar, M. J. (1979): Choline: Binding studies provide some evidence for a weak, direct agonist action in brain. *Mol. Pharmacol.,* 16:1084–1088.

180. Pandit, S. K., and Dundee, J. W. (1970): Preoperative amnesia: The incidence following the intramuscular injection of commonly used premedicants. *Anesthesia,* 25:493–499.

181. Panksepp, J., Sahley, T. L., and Normansell, L. N. (1984): Cholinergic control of social play. *Soc. Neurosci. Abstr.,* 10:1177.

182. Pepeu, G., and Ladinsky, H., eds. (1981): *Cholinergic Mechanisms: Phylogenetic Aspects, Central and Peripheral Synapses, and Clinical Significance.* Plenum Press, New York.

183. Perry, E. K., Perry, R. H., Tomlinson, B. E., Blessed, G., and Gibson, P. H. (1980): Coenzyme A-acetylating enzymes in Alzheimer's disease: Possible cholinergic "compartment" of pyruvate dehydrogenase. *Neurosci. Lett.,* 18:105–110.

184. Peterson, C., and Gibson, G. E. (1983): Amelioration of age-related neurochemical and behavioral deficits by 3,4-diaminopyridine. *Neurobiol. Aging,* 4:25–30.

185. Pilc, A., Rogoz, Z., and Skuza, G. (1982): Histidine induced

bizarre behavior in rats: Possible involvement of central cholinergic system. *Neuropharmacology*, 21:781–786.

186. Plech, A. (1981): Psychopharmacological effects of cholinomimetic agents administered into hippocampus and various hypothalamic areas in the rat. *Pol. J. Pharmacol. Pharm.*, 33:415–420.

187. Powers, J. S., Decoskey, D., and Kahrilas, P. J. (1981): Physostigmine for treatment of delirium tremens. *J. Clin. Pharmacol.*, 21:57–60.

188. Quastel, J. H. (1978): Source of the acetyl group in acetylcholine. In: *Advances in Behavioral Biology, Vol. 24: Cholinergic Mechanisms and Psychopharmacology*, edited by D. J. Jenden, pp. 411–430. Plenum Press, New York.

189. Quirion, R., Richard, J., and Dam, T. V. (1985): Evidence for the existence of serotonin type-2 receptors on cholinergic terminals in rat cortex. *Brain Res.*, 333:345–349.

190. Reisberg, B., Ferris, S. H., and Crook, T. (1982): Signs, symptoms and course of age-associated cognitive decline. In: *Aging, Vol. 19: Alzheimer's Disease: A Report of Progress in Research*, edited by S. Corkin, K. L. Davis, J. H. Growdon, E. Usdin, and R. J. Wurtman, pp. 177–182. Raven Press, New York.

191. Richardson, J. S., Miller, P. S., Lemay, J. S., Jyu, C. A., Neil, S. G., Kilduff, C. J., and Keegan, D. L. (1985): Mental dysfunction and the blockade of muscarinic receptors in the brains of the normal elderly. *Prog. Neuropsychopharmacol. Biol. Psychiatry*, 9:651–654.

192. Richmond, G., and Clemmens, L. G. (1984): Midbrain involvement in cholinergic facilitation of feminine sexual behavior. *Soc. Neurosci. Abstr.*, 10:822.

193. Riopelle, A. J., and Rogers, C. M. (1963): Behavior of chimpanzees of differing ages. *Act. Nerv. Super.*, 5:260–263.

194. Robinson, S. E., Malthe-Sorenssen, D., Wood, P. L., and Commissiong, J. (1979): Dopamine control of the septal-hippocampal cholinergic pathway. *J. Pharmacol. Exp. Ther.*, 208:476–479.

195. Rolinski, Z., and Herbut, M. (1981): Role of the cholinergic system in foot shock induced mouse aggression. *Pol. J. Pharmacol. Pharm.*, 33:177–184.

196. Romney, D. M., and Angus, W. R. (1984): A brief review of the effects of diazepam on memory. *Psychopharmacol. Bull.*, 20:313–316.

197. Russel, R. W., and Jenden, D. J. (1981): Behavioral effects of deanol or hemicholinium and their interaction. *Pharmacol. Biochem. Behav.*, 15:285–288.

198. Scatton, B., and Bartholini, G. (1980): Modulation of cholinergic transmission in the rat brain by GABA. *Brain Res. Bull.*, 5(Suppl. 2):223–229.

199. Sessler, F. M., Salhi, M. D., and Clugnet, M. C. (1983): Ontogeny of anti-cholinergic effects on water intake by new born rats. *Neurosci. Lett.*, (Suppl. 14):S340.

200. Sethy, V. H. (1979): Regulations of striatal acetylcholine concentrations by D_2-dopamine receptors. *Eur. J. Pharmacol.*, 60:397–398.

200a. Sims, N. R., Bowen, D. M., Allen, S. J., Smith, C. C. T., Neary, D., Thomas, D. J., and Davidson, A. N. (1983): Presynaptic cholinergic dysfunction in patients with dementia. *J. Neurochem.*, 40:503–509.

201. Sitaram, N., and Gillin, M. C. (1979): Acetylcholine: Possible involvement in sleep and analgesia. In: *Brain Acetylcholine and Neuropsychiatric Disease*, edited by K. L. Davis and P. A. Berger, pp. 311–343. Plenum Press, New York.

202. Sitaram, N., Weingartner, H., and Gillin, M. C. (1979): Choline chloride and arecoline: Effects on memory and sleep in man. In: *Nutrition and the Brain, Vol. 5: Choline and Lecithin in Brain Disorders*, edited by A. Barbeau, J. W. Growdon, and R. J. Wurtman, pp. 367–375. Raven Press, New York.

203. Sithichocke, N., and Marotta, S. F. (1978): Cholinergic influences on hypothalamic-pituitary-adrenocortical activity of stressed rats: An approach utilizing agonists and antagonists. *Acta Endocrinol.*, 89:726–736.

204. Sladek, C. D., and Joynt, R. J. (1979): Characterization of cholinergic control of vasopressin release by the organ-cultured rat hypothalamo-neurohypophysial system. *Endocrinology*, 104:659–663.

205. Smith, C. M., and Swash, M. (1978): Possible biochemical basis of memory disorder in Alzheimer's disease. *Ann. Neurol.*, 3:471–473.

206. Smith, C. M., and Swash, M. (1979): Physostigmine in Alzheimer's disease. *Lancet*, 1:42.

207. Speth, R. C., and Yamamura, H. I. (1979): Sodium-dependent high-affinity neuronal choline uptake. In: *Nutrition and the Brain, Vol. 5: Choline and Lecithin in Brain Disorders*, edited by A. Barbeau, J. H. Growdon, and R. J. Wurtman, pp. 129–139. Raven Press, New York.

208. Speth, R. C., and Yamamura, H. I. (1979): On the ability of choline and its analogues to interact with muscarinic cholinergic receptors in the rat brain. *Eur. J. Pharmacol.*, 58:197–201.

209. Stahl, S. M., and Berger, P. A. (1982): Cholinergic and dopaminergic mechanisms in Tourette syndrome. In: *Advances in Neurology, Vol. 35: Gilles De La Tourette Syndrome*, edited by A. J. Friedhoff and T. N. Chase, pp. 141–150. Raven Press, New York.

210. Stepien, L. S., Cordeau, J. P., and Rasmussen, T. (1960): The effect of temporal lobe and hippocampal lesions on auditory and visual recent memory in monkeys. *Brain Res.*, 83:470–489.

211. Strittmatter, H., Juckisch, R., and Hertting, G. (1982): Role of dopamine receptors in the modulation of acetylcholine release in the rabbit hippocampus. *Naunyn Schmiedebergs Arch. Pharmacol.*, 321:195–200.

212. Sulkowski, A. (1980): Marijuana "high": A model of senile dementia? *Perspect. Biol. Med.*, 23:209–214.

212a. Summers, W. K., Majovski, L. V., Marsh, G. M., Tachiki, K., and Kling, A. (1986): Oral tetrahydroaminoacridine in long-term treatment of senile dementia, Alzheimer type. *N. Engl. J. Med.*, 315:1241–1245.

213. Sunderland, T., Tariot, P., Murphy, D. L., Weingartner, H., Mueller, E. A., and Cohen, R. M. (1985): Scopolamine challenges in Alzheimer's disease. *Psychopharmacology*, 87:247–249.

214. Tagliavini, F., and Pilleri, G. (1983): Basal nucleus of Meynert: A neuropathological study in Alzheimer's disease, simple senile dementia, Pick's disease and Huntington's chorea. *J. Neurol.*, 62:243–260.

215. Tagliavini, F., and Pilleri, G. (1983): Neuronal counts in basal nucleus of Meynert in Alzheimer's disease and in simple senile dementia. *Lancet*, 1:469–470.

216. Thal, L. J., and Fuld, P. A. (1983): Memory enhancement with oral physostigmine in Alzheimer's disease. *N. Engl. J. Med.*, 308:720.

217. Van-Abeelen, J. H. F., and Boersma, H. J. L. M. (1984): A genetically controlled hippocampal transmitter system regulating exploratory behavior in mice. *J. Neurogenet.*, 1:153–158.

218. Vecsei, L., Bollok, I., and Telegdy, G. (1983): The effect of somatostatin on the active avoidance behavior and open field activity on haloperidol phenoxybenzamine and atropine pretreated rats. *Acta Physiol. Hung.*, 62:205–212.

219. Vizi, E. S. (1980): Modulation of cortical release of acetylcholine by noradrenaline released from nerves arising from the rat locus coeruleus. *Neuroscience*, 5:2139–2144.

220. Vizi, E. S., Harsing, L. G., Jr., and Zsilla, G. (1981): Evidence of the modulatory role of serotonin in acetylcholine release from striatal interneurons. *Brain Res.*, 212:89–99.

221. Warren, J. M., and Akert, G. K., eds. (1964): *The Frontal Granular Cortex and Behavior*. McGraw Hill, New York.

222. Waser, P. G. (1975): *Cholinergic Mechanisms*. Raven Press, New York.

223. Weaver, D. R., and Clemens, L. G. (1984): Analysis of the nicotinic cholinergic facilitation of lordosis. *Soc. Neurosci. Abstracts*, 10:823.

224. Wecker, L., and Goldberg, A. M. (1981): Regulation of acetylcholine releasing during increased neuronal activity. In: *Advances in Behavioral Biology, Vol. 24: Cholinergic Mechanisms*, edited by G. Pepeu and H. Ladinsky, pp. 451–461. Plenum Press, New York.

225. Wessling, H., Agoston, S., Van Dam, G. B. P., Pasma, J., DeWitt, D. J., and Havinga, H. (1984): Effects of 4-aminopyridine in elderly patients with Alzheimer's disease. *N. Engl. J. Med.*, 310:988–989.

226. Whelpton, R., and Hurst, P. (1985): Bioavailability of oral physostigmine. *N. Engl. J. Med.*, 313:1293–1295.

227. Whitehouse, J. M. (1964): Effects of atropine on discrimination learning in the rat. *J. Comp. Physiol. Psychol.*, 57:13–15.

228. Whitehouse, P. J., Price, D. L., Clark, A. W., Coyle, J. T., and DeLong, M. R. (1981): Alzheimer's disease: Evidence for selective

loss of cholinergic neurons on the nucleus basalis. *Ann. Neurol.,* 10:122–126.

229. Whitehouse, P. J., Price, D. L., Struble, R. G., Clark, A. W., Coyle, J. T., and DeLong, M. R. (1981): Alzheimer's disease and senile dementia: Loss of neurons in the basal forebrain. *Science,* 215:1237–1239.

230. Whitehouse, P. J., Struble, R. G., Clark, A. W., and Price, D. L. (1982): Alzheimer's disease: Plaques, tangles and the basal forebrain. *Ann. Neurol.,* 12:494.

231. Widman, M., Tucker, S., Brase, D. A., and Dewey, W. L. (1985): Cholinergic agents antinociception without morphine type dependence in rats. *Life Sci.,* 36:2007–2016.

232. Wilcock, G. K., Esiri, M. M., Bowen, D. M., and Smith, C. C. T. (1983): The nucleus basalis in Alzheimer's disease: Cell counts and cortical biochemistry. *Neuropathol. Appl. Neurobiol.,* 9:175–179.

233. Wood, P. L., and Stotland, L. M. (1980): Actions of enkephalin, and partial agonists analgesics on acetylcholine turnover in rat brain. *Neuropharmacology,* 19:975–982.

234. Wurtman, R. J. (1979): Precursor control of transmitter synthesis. In: *Nutrition and the Brain, Vol. 5: Choline and Lecithin in Brain Disorders,* edited by A. Barbean, J. H. Growdon, and R. J. Wurtman, pp. 1–12. Raven Press, New York.

235. Wurtman, R. J., and Fernstrom, J. D. (1976): Control of brain neurotransmitter synthesis by precursor availability and nutritional state. *Biochem. Pharmacol.,* 25:1691–1696.

236. Wurtman, R. J., Hefti, F., and Melamed, E. (1981): Precursor control of neurotransmitter synthesis. *Pharmacol. Rev.,* 32:315–335.

237. Wurtman, R. J., and Zeisel, S. H. (1982): Brain choline: Its sources and effects on the synthesis and release of acetylcholine. In: *Aging, Vol. 19: Alzheimer's Disease: A Report of Progress in Research,* edited by S. Corkin, K. L. Davis, J. H. Growdon, E. Usdin, and R. J. Wurtman, pp. 303–313. Raven Press, New York.

238. Yamamura, H. I., Kuhar, M. J., Greenberg, D., and Snyder, S. H. (1974): Muscarinic cholinergic receptor binding: Regional distribution in monkey brain. *Brain Res.,* 66:541–546.

239. Yamamura, H. I., Kuhar, M. J., and Synder, S. H. (1974): *In vivo* identification of muscarinic cholinergic receptor binding in rat brain. *Brain Res.,* 80:170–176.

240. Yamamura, H. I., and Snyder, S. H. (1974): Postsynaptic localization of muscarinic cholinergic receptor binding in rat hippocampus. *Brain Res.,* 78:320–326.

241. Zornetzer, S. F. (1985): Catecholamine system involvement in age-related memory dysfunction. *Ann. NY Acad. Sci.,* 444:242–254.

242. Zornetzer, S. F., Thompson, R., and Rogers, J. (1982): Rapid forgetting in aged rats. *Behav. Neural Biol.,* 36:49–60.

Psychopharmacology:
The Third Generation of Progress,
edited by Herbert Y. Meltzer.
Raven Press, New York © 1987.

CHAPTER 23

Chemistry and Biochemical Pharmacology of Cholinergic Neurons

Donald J. Jenden

During the past decade it has been established that changes in cholinergic function play a major role in the cognitive decline in senescence and more particularly in senile dementia of the Alzheimer type (SDAT) (15,16,37,106). This has stimulated a good deal of research on the mechanisms that might be involved, on models in which some of the pathological changes of SDAT are simulated, and on new approaches to the pharmacological enhancement of cholinergic function that might find therapeutic application in SDAT. In this review a brief summary is presented of current concepts of the regulation of acetylcholine (ACh) synthesis, storage, and release, and the sites of action of agents that alter these processes, emphasizing attempts that have been made to generate models of SDAT and pharmacological approaches that may lead to its effective treatment.

SYNTHESIS OF ACh

There are several excellent reviews of the processes involved in ACh synthesis (71,80,136,137). Choline acetyltransferase (CAT) is a soluble cytoplasmic enzyme that catalyzes the transfer of an acetyl group from acetyl coenzyme A (AcCoA) to choline (Ch). The activity of this enzyme is considerably greater than the maximal rate at which ACh synthesis probably occurs: inhibitors have little effect on ACh levels or synthesis (4,26,73,75). It seems unlikely that CAT plays a regulatory role in ACh synthesis and the concentrations of the four reactants are probably close to equilibrium, at least under resting conditions.

Neither of the precursors is freely available in the cytosol, but must be admitted from other functional compartments by processes that probably regulate the synthesis of ACh. Ch is admitted to cells by at least two distinguishable transport mechanisms: a relatively low-affinity ($K_T \sim 100$ μM) process common to all cells, including erythrocytes, and a Na^+-dependent high-affinity system located primarily, if not exclusively, on cholinergic terminals, where it is under normal circumstances closely coupled to ACh synthesis. ACh synthesis in perikarya seems to be subserved by the low-affinity Ch transport system (132). Uptake of Ch through the high-affinity transport system appears to be accelerated by conditions that stimulate release, including neuronal impulse flow (72,111,128,144). It is not clear whether this is due to an active regulation, mediated perhaps by the inhibition of Ch transport by ACh acting on the inner surface of the membrane, or the passive result of a change in the electrochemical gradient of Ch across the membrane. This could result from depletion of cytosolic Ch due to the net synthesis of ACh to replace that which was released or transported into vesicles. If CAT is present in a large excess and the reaction it catalyzes is normally close to equilibrium (105), the release of AcCoA from mitochondria could cause a shift in the cytosolic equilibrium that would favor the entry of Ch from the extracellular space through the high-affinity Ch transport system (66,137).

AcCoA is generated in mitochondria by the enzyme complex pyruvate dehydrogenase (PDH). This requires pyruvate as a substrate, which is normally provided by glycolysis. Oxygen is also required to maintain NAD^+ in the oxidized state. Little is known about the mechanisms by which AcCoA is released from brain mitochondria, but there is evidence that it can be triggered by Ca^{2+} (18,107).

Most of the ACh in nerve terminals is contained in vesicles that can be seen by electron microscopy and purified by density gradient centrifugation. They clearly play a role in storage of ACh, and are generally believed to mediate evoked release by exocytosis, although some believe that release occurs from a soluble cytoplasmic compartment by a gating mechanism in the plasma membrane (44) while vesicles play only a secondary storage role. Clearly, transport of ACh into vesicles could also play a role in the regulation of its synthesis, since the resulting depletion of cytosolic ACh would shift the equilibrium maintained by CAT, reducing the Ch concentration and increasing the inward electrochemical gradient of Ch across the membrane. Increased uptake of Ch could also result from disinhibition of the Ch transporter by a lower concentration of ACh acting on the inner side of the membrane.

PHARMACOLOGICAL INTERFERENCE WITH ACh SYNTHESIS

Compounds that interfere with ACh synthesis are of interest as probes of the regulatory mechanisms involved, and as means of producing experimental hypocholinergic states that may be of value as models of spontaneous human diseases. In the latter context they are considered further in Experimental Models of Hypocholinergic States below.

Inhibitors of Ch Transport

Hemicholinium-3 is one of several related compounds originally studied by Schueler and his colleagues (78,125,137) and found to produce a slow neuromuscular block that could be antagonized by Ch. It is now generally believed to be a potent and relatively specific inhibitor of high-affinity Ch transport (57,58), which as a consequence also inhibits ACh synthesis. The possibility that it is a competing substrate has not been ruled out, and it has been proposed that it might be stored and released as a false transmitter, either as the parent compound (79) or as the acetate ester (110). However, it is relatively ineffective as an inhibitor of the vesicular transport of ACh (2). [³H]Hemicholinium-3 has recently been used in ligand-binding studies of the high-affinity Ch transport system (138,139). A series of monoquaternary compounds has

recently been described as inhibitors of the high-affinity Ch transport system (77); one of these is reported to be more potent than hemicholinium-3. All the potent inhibitors of high-affinity Ch transport that have so far been described are quaternary ammonium compounds and must be injected intraventricularly to have an effect on the brain *in vivo*. When hemicholinium-3 is injected intraventricularly it produces profound depletion of ACh, with hyperreactivity that is characteristic of a hypocholinergic state (49,50,114). However, the behavioral effects of hemicholinium have not been completely characterized, and its effects are relatively short-lived because it is a reversible inhibitor. An analog of hemicholinium-3 has recently been described (130,131) that spontaneously forms a reactive intermediate in aqueous solution and will presumably react covalently with the carrier, resulting in sustained interference with cholinergic function. This and similar compounds are likely to be of value in producing experimental models of hypocholinergic states (see Storage and Release of ACh), and also for autoradiography and emission tomography of cholinergic terminals.

False Transmitters

Many Ch analogs have been described (96) which meet the criteria of precursors to false transmitters (74), although it was not until 1979 that it was shown by quantitative analytical techniques that a false transmitter could be synthesized and released by cholinergic terminals (34). These precursors compete with Ch for the high-affinity transport system and CAT, and their acetates compete with ACh for transport into vesicles and in release. Some of the best-documented of these are summarized in Table 1. As a result of this competition, the uptake, acetylation, storage, and release of ACh are impaired. Cholinergic transmission is impeded because the potency of the false transmitter is less (for those presently known) than that of ACh. These compounds have been used as experimental tools for studying the regulation of presynaptic mechanisms (9,35,64,152), the subcellular origin of released ACh (20,140,145,147), and as a means of selectively modifying cholinergic function *in vivo* (56,93,129).

The pharmacological results of replacing Ch with a false precursor depend not only on the facility with which the

TABLE 1. *Activities of some representative false transmitters at cholinergic receptors, relative to ACh*

Compound	Relative activity (ACh = 1)		Refs.
	Muscarinic	Nicotinic	
Acetylmonoethylcholine	0.4	0.2	12,63
Acetyldiethylcholine	0.002	0.003	12,63
Acetyltriethylcholine	0.0005	0.0002	12,63
Acetylpyrrolidinecholine	0.3	0.03	29,33,141
Acetylhomocholine	0.02	0.2	13
Acetyl-*N*-aminodeanol	0.03	0.2	99

Data have been rounded to one significant figure.

precursor is handled by presynaptic mechanisms, but also on the efficacy and affinity of the acetylated product at both nicotinic and muscarinic receptors, and the speed with which it is removed by acetylcholinesterase. If an analog is not well incorporated into presynaptic metabolism, it may still interfere with transmission if the acetylated product has a high affinity and low efficacy, since it will then antagonize the action of released ACh. For *in vivo* studies directed toward the central nervous system, it is clearly desirable that an effect on transmission at central muscarinic sites should occur without substantial interference with neuromuscular transmission. For chronic studies it is also necessary that the role of Ch in phospholipid metabolism not be compromised because of the toxic effects that are likely to ensue.

As in the case of Ch transport inhibitors, particular interest attaches to false transmitters with the potential of reacting covalently with macromolecules required for transport, acetylation, storage, and release. Early studies were directed toward choline mustard (β-chloroethyl-β-hydroxyethyl-methylamine) and the reactive aziridinium ion cyclocholine (68,102,115–120), which forms spontaneously in neutral aqueous solution. This and several related compounds are substrates and irreversible inhibitors of Ch transport and CAT. The ethyl homolog is also a potent irreversible inhibitor of choline dehydrogenase and choline kinase, and causes an increase in plasma levels of Ch that is presumably due to reduced renal and hepatic clearance (10,11). This compound, β-chloroethyl-β-hydroxyethyl-ethylamine, has been extensively studied by Hanin, Fisher, and their colleagues as a means of producing an experimental model of Alzheimer's disease (46,59,60,76,81–83,122–124,143) and was given the code name AF 64. Its pharmacological properties are very similar to those of choline mustard, but the aziridinium ion (AF 64 A) is somewhat less potent and more stable than choline mustard aziridinium ion (119). The question of selectivity for cholinergic neurons is clearly important, whether the compounds are used as biochemical probes or to generate an experimental model. AF 64 A, like cyclocholine, is not completely specific for cholinergic neurons (86,122), pre-

sumably because it is taken up through the low-affinity Ch transport system that all cells possess. It is not clear from published data whether AF 64 A is more selectively toxic to cholinergic neurons than cyclocholine.

STORAGE AND RELEASE OF ACh

There is strong evidence that the stimulation-evoked release of ACh is mediated by vesicle exocytosis and recycling (147,150,151), although it has also been proposed that evoked release occurs from a free cytoplasmic pool of ACh through gates in the plasma membrane (44,65), vesicles serving only a reserve storage function. Since vesicles in *Torpedo* electric organ contain ACh at a concentration of 0.5 to 0.6 M (101,142), it is clear that ACh must be actively transported into them. The mechanism responsible for this transport has recently been elucidated (2,103). It is driven by an outward proton gradient that is generated by a bicarbonate-activated Ca^{2+}- or Mg^{2+}-ATPase. The ACh transporter appears to be distinct from the ATPase, since it can be uncoupled by mitochondrial uncouplers and diffusible bases such as ammonia (2), can be inhibited by thiol reagents without affecting the ATPase, and functions under passive conditions without ATP (24). The pharmacological properties of the ACh transport system have been investigated (3). Table 2 summarizes the effects of some of the compounds investigated by Anderson et al. (3). Clearly, AH 5183 [2-(4-phenylpiperidino)cyclohexanol] is the most potent and specific inhibitor of vesicular ACh transport. It had been predicted some 15 years earlier to exert this action by Marshall (84) because of the pharmacological characteristics of the neuromuscular block it produced. AH 5183 has been shown to be a potent inhibitor of ACh release (25,87,88; B. Collier and S. A. Welner, *personal communication;* D. J. Jenden, *unpublished observations*), but appears to leave part of the vesicular pool of ACh unaffected (B. Collier and S. A. Weiner, *personal communication;* D. J. Jenden, *unpublished observations*). This suggests that different subpopulations of vesicles are involved in storage and release functions. Many years ago Whittaker

TABLE 2. *Activities of representative cholinergic drugs as inhibitors of vesicular ACh transport*

Compound	Primary action	ED_{50} (M) Vesicular ACh transport	ED_{50} (M) Primary action
AH 5183	—	4×10^{-8}	—
ACh	Multiple	2×10^{-4}	—
Ch	Multiple	2×10^{-2}	—
Hemicholinium-3	Choline transport inhibitor	3×10^{-4}	6×10^{-8} (112)
N-Hydroxyethyl-4-(1-naphthylvinyl)-pyridinium	CAT inhibitor	5×10^{-6}	6×10^{-7} (28)
Physostigmine	AChE inhibitor	3×10^{-4}	6×10^{-8} (5)
Oxotremorine	Muscarinic agonist	1×10^{-5}	5×10^{-7} (149)
Atropine	Muscarinic antagonist	1×10^{-5}	2×10^{-9} (149)
Nicotine	Nicotinic agonist	3×10^{-4}	8×10^{-5} (89)
Tubocurarine	Nicotinic antagonist	1×10^{-5}	1×10^{-7} (89)

Data for vesicular transport inhibition from (3).

and his colleagues proposed that a specific subfraction of vesicles from rat brain is concerned with evoked release (1,8).

The availability of potent and specific inhibitors of vesicular transport of ACh appears certain to advance our understanding of the possible role of the vesicle in regulating ACh synthesis and in mediating ACh release. These compounds may also provide specific biochemical probes for the anatomic localization of cholinergic nerve terminals by autoradiography or emission tomography.

EXPERIMENTAL MODELS OF HYPOCHOLINERGIC STATES

The discovery of a cholinergic deficit in senescence and more specifically in SDAT led naturally to attempts to produce an experimental model of SDAT in animals by interfering with cholinergic function. A model of this kind may be of value in studies of the pathogenesis of SDAT and in the initial evaluation of possible therapeutic approaches. Some limited success has been achieved. It has long been known that anticholinergics impair short-term memory, and that the elderly are particularly susceptible to this effect. Reversal of the effects of antimuscarinic agents by physostigmine (43) supported the conclusion that these effects were due to impaired cholinergic transmission, and led to clinical studies of physostigmine in SDAT (41,134), with modest success.

Hypoxia and hypoglycemia would be expected on theoretical grounds to interfere with ACh synthesis, since both oxygen and glucose are required for the production of AcCoA in brain. Loss of memory and impaired judgment are characteristic clinical features of hypoxia in pathological states or in altitude sickness. Gibson and his colleagues have described some neurochemical and behavioral sequelae of hypoxia and hypoglycemia and have shown that these are at least in part due to impaired release and turnover of ACh (52,54). The behavioral deficit can be partially corrected with physostigmine (53).

As experimental models of SDAT, both anticholinergic drug treatment and mild hypoxia are limited by their reversibility, which contrasts with the progressive and apparently irreversible course of SDAT. Moreover, the latter is known to be associated with a presynaptic lesion of cholinergic projections to the cortex, postsynaptic receptors remaining essentially unchanged (38,100). Attention has therefore been directed to lesions of the basal forebrain nuclei projecting to the cortex. Excitotoxin lesions are clearly preferable to electrolytic lesions because they spare axons of passage. Such lesions result generally in a marked reduction in cortical cholinergic markers and impairment of memory (47,70,109,121). However, the lesion is not specifically cholinergic and hence does not permit an evaluation to be made of the role of cholinergic projections in the behavioral sequelae. For this reason there is a good deal of interest in combining the anatomic specificity achievable by microinjection with the biochemical specificity of compounds directed toward cholinergic neurons. Of these the alkylating Ch analog AF 64 has been most investigated (see False Transmitters). Typically, injection

into a target area such as the dorsal hippocampus produces a sustained loss of cholinergic markers (22,83), associated with behavioral alterations characteristic of a hypocholinergic state (22,124). Within a certain dose range, the effects are relatively selective for cholinergic neurons (83,122). It remains to be established whether AF 64 is more specific or more reliable than other alkylating Ch analogs. Considerably greater specificity might be expected of alkylating analogs of hemicholinium (130,131); (see Inhibitors of Ch Transport), but it is not clear whether these compounds are cytotoxic as AF 64 is, and the effects may disappear earlier or more completely.

Chronic administration of a false transmitter is an attractive alternative to these methods for the generation of experimental models resembling SDAT. In addition to the role it serves as a precursor of ACh in cholinergic neurons, Ch is a precursor for phosphatidylcholine synthesis in all cells. At least 80% of the Ch turnover in the brain is in phospholipid metabolism (30). Based on the working hypothesis that the specific degeneration of cholinergic neurons in SDAT could be due to a competition between these two pathways, a Ch analog was sought that was less efficiently utilized in both pathways, which would exacerbate the competition and perhaps elicit its expression in young animals. A similar hypothesis has recently been advanced by Wurtman and his colleagues (148). N-Aminodeanol appears to be a suitable compound for this purpose. Methods for its analysis have been developed (98). It has been shown to be taken up by the high-affinity Ch transport system in competition with Ch and acetylated by CAT. The product is stored in synaptic vesicles and released by stimulation in the presence of Ca^{2+} (91,94,95,97,99). The acetate ester has only 4% of the potency of ACh at muscarinic receptors (99,126), but it is sufficiently active at nicotinic sites to prevent severe neuromuscular weakness in chronic feeding experiments. It is incorporated into lipids in competition with Ch, and serves (poorly) as a methyl donor (92). Chronic dietary administration of N-aminodeanol to rats in place of dietary Ch led to impaired performance on a passive avoidance task, hyperreactivity, and other signs of a cholinergic deficit (93). No direct signs of toxicity were produced. Extended studies of chronic dietary administration are now in progress.

ENHANCEMENT OF CHOLINERGIC FUNCTION

Inhibitors of acetylcholinesterase are a classic means of promoting cholinergic transmission. If the intended site of action is in the central nervous system, the agent must be nonpolar, and physostigmine is the only commonly used agent that meets this requirement. Physostigmine has been shown to improve performance on memory tasks (40) and to yield modest benefit in SDAT (17,31,133). Unfortunately its duration of action is short because of hydrolysis. There is a natural reluctance to experiment with the more potent long-acting cholinesterase inhibitors. Physostigmine itself has other actions on cholinergic systems in addition to the inhibition of acetylcholinesterase (127), and its hydrolysis product eseroline has discrete pharmacological properties of its own (27), which may complicate the interpretation of experimental and clinical data. Finally, the effects of physostigmine or other cholinesterase inhibitors are not limited to the intended sites of action in the hippocampus and neocortex. Peripheral side effects can be prevented with methylatropine or some other quaternary antimuscarinic compound, but actions at other sites in the brain are likely to result in disturbances of posture, movement, mood, sleep, and endocrine balance. Even under optimal conditions, cholinesterase inhibitors can have little or no effect if, as in advanced SDAT, most of the cholinergic terminals have already degenerated.

Some of these drawbacks can be circumvented by using a direct muscarinic agonist instead of a cholinesterase inhibitor. Arecoline has been reported to improve memory in aging monkeys (14). Agents of greater specificity will be required for clinical use. Although there is considerable interest in subtypes of muscarinic receptor referred to as M_1 and M_2 (62), the nature of the difference is unclear (23,48,55,85), and only marginal selectivity has so far been achieved among muscarinic agonists sufficiently nonpolar to enter the central nervous system.

Since early reports of Cohen and Wurtman (32) and Haubrich et al. (61), there has been a great deal of interest in the use of Ch or phosphatidylcholine (lecithin) to promote the synthesis, storage, and release of ACh. From many conflicting reports and the controversy that ensued, it appears that this precursor loading strategy may have an enabling effect on ACh synthesis at certain sites, primarily under conditions of sustained activation (67,69,135). Studies of Ch or lecithin in SDAT have been disappointing (15,16,37), but it is possible that there is a subset of patients who may respond, at least to the extent that deterioration is slowed or prevented. There is some indication that Ch levels and transport in erythrocytes may be helpful in identifying this subgroup (6,7,42,51,90).

ACh release can be enhanced by aminopyridine derivatives that increase Ca^{2+} entry by prolonging membrane depolarization associated with the action potential (21). These compounds appear to be effective in reducing a cholinergically mediated deficit in aging and other experimental models (39,54,104), but the clinical effect of 4-aminopyridine in SDAT was equivocal (146). Release is under normal circumstances closely coupled to synthesis, and Ca^{2+} entry appears to activate both (see above); however, no studies have so far appeared describing effects of aminopyridines on ACh synthesis. If they do promote synthesis, a combination of Ch and an aminopyridine deserves a trial, since these appear to be the conditions under which a precursor loading effect is observed; moreover, in the absence of additional Ch, an existing Ch deficiency could be intensified (148).

Rapid adaptation to pharmacological intervention characterizes cholinergic systems. This is most clearly seen in the tolerance that develops to organophosphates (108), which depends at least in part on down-regulation of postsynaptic receptors (19,45). There is evidence that presynaptic changes contribute to the adaptation (113), and it seems likely that the efficiency of receptor coupling mechanisms may change in response to sustained pharmacological challenge. These adaptive processes, while clearly serving a protective function, will tend to frustrate any attempt to induce a sustained enhancement of cholinergic function in SDAT. Research is clearly needed on the mechanisms involved in these adaptive responses. If they can be controlled pharmacologically, other means of functional enhancement will be more effective, and may even become unnecessary.

ACKNOWLEDGMENTS

Some of the research described in this chapter was supported by USPHS Grant MH-17691. We thank Nelly Canaan for expert editorial assistance and Dr. B. Collier for permission to cite unpublished work.

REFERENCES

1. Agoston, D. V., Kosh, J. W., Lisziewicz, J., and Whittaker, V. P. (1985): J. Neurochem., 44:229–305.
2. Anderson, D. C., King, S. C., and Parsons, S. M. (1982): Biochemistry, 21:3037–3043.
3. Anderson, D. C., King, S. C. and Parsons, S. M. (1983): Mol. Pharmacol., 24:48–54.
4. Aquilonius, S. M., Frankenberg, L., Stensio, K. E., and Winbladh, B. (1971): Acta Pharmacol. Toxicol., 30:129–140.
5. Augustinsson, K.-B., and Nachmansohn, D. (1939): J. Biol. Chem., 179:543–559.
6. Barclay, L. L., Blass, J. P., Kopp, U., and Hanin, I. (1982): N. Engl. J. Med., 307:501.
7. Barclay, L. L., Kheyfets, S., and Zemkov, A. (1985): Neurology, 35 (Suppl. 218).
8. Barker, L. A., Dowdall, M. J., and Whittaker, V. P. (1972): Biochem. J., 130:1063–1080.
9. Barker, L. A., and Mittag, T. W. (1975): J. Parmacol. Exp. Ther., 192:86–94.
10. Barlow, P., and Marchbanks, R. M. (1984): J. Neurochem., 43:1568–1573.
11. Barlow, P., and Marchbanks, R. M. (1985): Biochem. Pharmacol., 34:3117–3122.
12. Barlow, R. B., Scott, K. A., and Stephenson, R. P. (1963): Br. J. Pharmacol., 21:509–522.
13. Barrass, B. C., Brimblecombe, R. W., Rich, P., and Taylor, J. V. (1970): Br. J. Pharmacol., 39:40–48.
14. Bartus, R. T., Dean, R. L., and Beer, B. (1980): Neurobiol. Aging, 1:145–152.
15. Bartus, R. T., Dean, R. L., Beer, B., and Lippa, A. S. (1982): Science, 217:408–417.
16. Bartus, R. T., Dean, R. L., Fontecorvo, M. J., and Flicker, C. (1985): Ann. NY Acad. Sci., 444:332–358.
17. Beller, S. A., Overall, J. E., and Swann, A. C. (1985): Psychopharmacology, 87:147–151.
18. Benjamin, A. M., and Quastel, J. H. (1981): Science, 213:1495–1496.
19. Bito, L. Z., and Dawson, M. J. (1970): J. Pharmacol. Exp. Ther., 175:673–684.
20. Boksa, P., and Collier, B. (1980): Neuroscience, 5:1517–1532.
21. Bowman, W. C. (1982): Trends Pharmacol. Sci., 3:183–185.
22. Brandeis, R., Pittel, Z., Lachman, C., Heldman, E., Dachir, S., Levy, A., Hanin, I., Fisher, A., and Luz, S. (1986): In: Alzheimer's and Parkinson's Disease: Strategies for Research and Development, edited by A. Fisher, I. Hanin, and C. Lachman, pp. 469–477. Plenum Press, New York.
23. Brown, J. H., Goldstein, D., and Masters, S. B. (1985): Mol. Pharmacol., 27:525–531.
24. Carpenter, R., Koenigsberger, R. S., and Parsons, S. M. (1980): Biochemistry, 19:4373–4379.
25. Carroll, P. T. (1985): Brain Res., 358:200–209.
26. Carson, V. G., Jenden, D. J., Cho, A. K., and Green, R. (1976): Biochem. Pharmacol., 25:195–199.

27. Carson, V. G., Jenden, D. J., Booth, R. A., and Roch, M. (1977): In: *Soc. Neurosci. Abstr.,* 3:404.
28. Cavallito, C. J., Yun, H. S., Kaplan, T., Smith, J. C., and Foldes, F. F. (1970). *J. Med. Chem.,* 13:221–224.
29. Cho, A. K., Jenden, D. J., and Lamb, S. I. (1972): *J. Med. Chem.,* 15:391–394.
30. Choi, R. L., Freeman, J. J., and Jenden, D. J. (1975): *J. Neurochem.,* 24:735–741.
31. Christie, J. E., Schering, A., Ferguson, J., and Glen, A. M. (1981): *Br. J. Psychiatry,* 138:46–50.
32. Cohen, E. L., and Wurtman, R. J. (1975): *Life Sci.,* 16:1095–1102.
33. Collier, B., Barker, L. A., and Mittag, T. W. (1976): *Mol. Pharmacol.,* 12:340–344.
34. Collier, B., Boksa, P., and Lovat, S. (1979): *Prog. Brain Res.,* 49:107–121.
35. Collier, B., Lovat, S., Ilson, D., Barker, L. A., and Mittag, T. W. (1977): *J. Neurochem.,* 29:331–339.
36. Corkin, S., Growdon, J. H., Davis, K. L., Usdin, E., and Wurtman, R. J., eds. (1982): *Alzheimer's Disease: A Report of Progress in Research.* Raven Press, New York.
37. Coyle, J. T., Price, D. L., and DeLong, M. R. (1983): *Science,* 219:1184–1190.
38. Davies, P., and Verth, A. W. (1978): *Brain Res.,* 13:385–392.
39. Davis, H. P., Idown, A., and Gibson, G. E. (1983): *Exp. Aging Res.,* 9:211–214.
40. Davis, K. L., and Mohs, R. C. (1982): *Am. J. Psychiatry,* 139:1421–1424.
41. Davis, K. L., Mohs, R. C., Tinklenberg, J. R., Pfefferbaum, A., Hollister, L. E., and Kopell, B. S. (1978): *Science,* 20:272–274.
42. Domino, E. F., Minor, L., Duff, I. F., Tait, S., and Gershon, S. (1982): In: *Alzheimer's Disease: A Report of Progress in Research,* edited by S. Corkin, J. H. Growdon, K. L. Davis, E. Usdin, and R. J. Wurtman, pp. 393–398. Raven Press, New York.
43. Drachman, D. A. (1978): In: *Alzheimer's Disease: Senile Dementia and Related Disorders,* edited by R. Katzman et al., pp. 141–148. Raven Press, New York.
44. Dunant, Y., and Israel, M. (1979): *Trends Neurosci.,* 2:130–132.
45. Ehlert, F. J., Kokka, N., and Fairhurst, A. S. (1980): *Mol. Pharmacology,* 17:24–30.
46. Fisher, A., Mantione, C. R., Abraham, D. J., and Hanin, I. (1982): *J. Pharmacol. Exp. Ther.,* 222:140–145.
47. Flicker, C., Dean, R. L., Watkins, D. L., Fisher, S. K., and Bartus, R. T. (1983): *Pharmacol. Biochem. Behav.,* 18:973–982.
48. Flynn, D. D., and Potter, L. T. (1985): *Proc. Natl. Acad. Sci. USA,* 82:580–583.
49. Freeman, J. J., Choi, R. L., and Jenden, D. J. (1975): *J. Neurochem.,* 24:729–734.
50. Freeman, J. J., Macri, J. R., Choi, R. L., and Jenden, D. J. (1979): *J. Pharmacol. Exp. Ther.,* 210:91–97.
51. Friedman, E., Sherman, K. A., Ferris, S. H., Reisberg, B., Bartus, R., and Schneck, M. K. (1981): *N. Engl. J. Med.,* 304:1490–1491.
52. Gibson, G. E., and Blass, J. P. (1976): *J. Neurochem.,* 27:37–42.
53. Gibson, G. E., Pelmas, C. J., and Peterson, C. (1983): *Pharmacol. Biochem. Behav.,* 18:909–916.
54. Gibson, G. E., and Peterson, C. (1983): In: *Assessment in Geriatric Psychopharmacology,* edited by T. Crook, S. Ferris, and R. T. Bartus, pp. 323–343. Mark Powley Assoc., New Canaan, Connecticut.
55. Gil, D. W., and Wolfe, B. B. (1985): *J. Pharmacol. Exp. Ther.,* 232:608–616.
56. Glick, S. D., Crane, A. M., Barker, L. A., and Mittag, T. W. (1975): *Neuropharmacology,* 14:561–564.
57. Guyenet, P., Lefresne, P., Rossier, J., Beaujouin, J. C., and Glowinski, J. (1973): *J. Mol. Pharmacol.,* 9:630–639.
58. Haga, T., and Noda, H. (1973): *Biochim. Biophys. Acta,* 291:564–575.
59. Hanin, I., Coyle, J. T., De Groat, W. C., Fisher, A., and Mantione, C. R. (1983): In: *Banbury Report: Biological Aspects of Alzheimer's Disease,* edited by R. Katzman, pp. 243–253. Cold Spring Harbor Laboratory, Cold Spring Harbor, New York.
60. Hanin, I., Mantione, C. R., and Fisher, A. (1982): In: *Alzheimer's Disease: A Report of Progress in Research,* edited by S. Corkin, K. L. Davis, J. H. Growdon, E. Usdin, and R. J. Wurtman, pp. 267–270. Raven Press, New York.
61. Haubrich, D. R., Wang, P. F. L., Clody, D. E., and Wedeking, P. W. (1975): *Life Sci.,* 17:975–980.
62. Hirschowitz, B. I., Hammer, R., Giachetti, A., Keirns, J. J., and Levine, R. R. (1984): *Trends Pharmacol. Sci. (Supp 1.).*
63. Holton, P., and Ing, H. R. (1949): *Br. J. Pharmacol.,* 4:190–196.
64. Ilson, D., Collier, B., and Boksa, P. (1977): *J. Neurochem.,* 28:371–381.
65. Israel, M., Dunant, Y., and Manaranche, R. (1979): *Prog. Neurobiol.,* 13:237–275.
66. Jenden, D. J. (1979): In: *Nutrition and the Brain, Vol. 5,* edited by A. Barbeau, J. H. Growdon, and R. J. Wurtman, pp. 13–24. Raven Press, New York.
67. Jenden, D. J. (1979): In: *Brain Acetylcholine and Neuropsychiatric Disease,* edited by K. L. Davis and P. A. Berger, pp. 483–513. Plenum Press, New York.
68. Jenden, D. J., Parker, T., Roch, M., Macri, J., and Fainman, F. (1976): *Fed. Proc.,* 35:697.
69. Jenden, D. J., Weiler, M. H., and Gundersen, C. B. (1982): In: *Alzheimer's Disease: A Report of Progress in Research,* edited by S. Corkin, K. L. Davis, J. H. Growdon, E. Usdin, and R. J. Wurtman, pp. 315–326. Raven Press, New York.
70. Johnston, M. U., McKinney, M., and Coyle, J. T. (1981): *Exp. Brain Res.,* 43:159–172.
71. Jope, R. S. (1979): *Brain Res. Rev.,* 1:313–344.
72. Jope, R. S., Weiler, M. H., and Jenden, D. J. (1978): *J. Neurochem.,* 30:949–954.
73. Kasa, P., Szepesy, G., Gulya, K., Bansaghy, K., and Rakonizay, Z. (1982): *Neurochem. Int.,* 4:185–193.
74. Kopin, R. J. (1965): *Annu. Rev. Pharmacol.,* 8:377–394.
75. Krell, R. D., and Goldberg, A. M. (1975): *Biochem. Pharmacol.,* 24:391–396.
76. Levy, A., Kant, G. J., Meyerhoff, J. L., and Jarrard, L. E. (1984): *Brain Res.,* 305:169–172.
77. Lindberg, B., Crona, K., and Dahlbom, R. (1984): *Acta Pharm. Suec.,* 21:271–294.
78. Long, J. P., and Schueler, F. W. (1954): *J. Am. Pharm. Assoc.,* 43:79–86.
79. MacIntosh, F. C. (1961): *Fed. Proc.,* 20:562–568.
80. MacIntosh, F. C., and Collier, B. (1976): In: *Handbuch der Experimentellen Pharmakologie, Vol. 42,* edited by G. V. R. Born, O. Eichler, A. Farah, H. Herken, and A. D. Welch, pp. 99–228. Springer-Verlag, Berlin.
81. Mantione, C. R., Fisher, A., and Hanin, I. (1981): *Science,* 213:579–580.
82. Mantione, C. R., Fisher, A., and Hanin, I. (1984): *Life Sci.,* 35:33–41.
83. Mantione, C. R., Zigmond, M. J., Fisher, A., and Hanin, I. (1983): *J. Neurochem.,* 41:251–255.
84. Marshall, I. G. (1970): *Br. J. Pharmacol.,* 38:503–516.
85. Mash, D. C., Flynn, D. D., and Potter, L. T. (1985): *Science,* 228:1115–1117.
86. McGurk, S. R., and Butcher, L. L. (1985): *Fed. Proc.,* 44:897.
87. Melega, W. P., and Howard, B. D. (1984): *Proc. Natl. Acad. Sci. USA,* 81:6535–6538.
88. Michaelson, D. M., and Burstein, M. (1985): *FEBS Lett.,* 188:389–393.
89. Michaelson, D., Vandlen, R., Bode, J., Moody, T., Schmidt, J., and Raftery, M. A. (1974): *Arch. Biochem. Biophys.,* 165:796–804.
90. Miller, B. L., Jenden, D. J., Cummings, J. L., Read, S., Rice, K., and Benson, D. F. (1986): *Life Sci.,* 38:485–490.
91. Newton, M. W., Crosland, R., and Jenden, D. J. (1984): In: *IUPHAR 9th International Congress of Pharmacology,* London, 1984. Abstracts, p. 294P. Macmillan Press Ltd., London.
92. Newton, M. W., Crosland, R. D., and Jenden, D. J. (1985): *J. Pharmacol. Exp. Ther.,* 235:157–161.
93. Newton, M. W., Crosland, R. D., and Jenden, D. J. (1986): *Brain Res,* 7:316–320.
94. Newton, M. W., and Jenden, D. J. (1983): *Trans. Am. Soc. Neurochem.,* 14:90.
95. Newton, M. W., and Jenden, D. J. (1985): *J. Pharmacol. Exp. Ther.,* 235:135–146.

96. Newton, M. W., and Jenden, D. J. (1986): *Trends Pharmacol. Sci.,* 7:316–320.
97. Newton, M. W., Ringdahl, B., and Jenden, D. J. (1982): *Fed. Proc.,* 41:1323.
98. Newton, M. W., Ringdahl, B., and Jenden, D. J. (1983): *Anal. Biochem.,* 130:88–94.
99. Newton, M. W., Ringdahl, B., and Jenden, D. J. (1985): *J. Pharmacol. Exp. Ther.,* 235:147–156.
100. Nordberg, A., Larsson, C., Adolfson, R., Alafuzoff, I., and Winblad, B. (1983): *J. Neural. Transm.,* 56:13–19.
101. Ohsawa, K., Dowe, G. H. C., Morris, S. J., and Whittaker, V. P. (1979): *Brain Res.,* 161:447–457.
102. Parker, T. S., Macri, J. R., and Jenden, D. J. (1976): *Proc. West. Pharmacol. Soc.,* 19:79–86.
103. Parsons, S. M., Carpenter, R. S., Koenigsberger, R., and Rothlein, J. E. (1982): *Fed. Proc.,* 41:2765–2768.
104. Peterson, C., and Gibson, G. E. (1983): *Neurobiol. Aging,* 4:25–30.
105. Potter, L. T., Glover, V. A. S., and Saelens, J. K. (1968): *J. Biol. Chem.,* 243:3864–3870.
106. Price, D. L., Cork, L. C., Struble, R. G., Whitehouse, P. J., Kitt, C. A., and Walker, L. C. (1985): *Ann. NY Acad. Sci.,* 444:287–295.
107. Ričny, J., and Tuček, S. (1983): *Gen. Physiol. Biophys.,* 2:27–37.
108. Rider, J. A., Ellinwood, L. E., and Coon, J. M. (1952): *Proc. Soc. Exp. Biol. Med.,* 81:455–459.
109. Ridley, R. M., Baker, H. F., Drewett, B., and Johnson, J. A. (1985): *Psychopharmacology,* 86:438–443.
110. Rodriguez de Lores Arnaiz, G., Zieher, L. M., and De Robertis, E. (1970): *J. Neurochem.,* 17:221–229.
111. Roskoski, R. (1978): *J. Neurochem.,* 30:1357–1361.
112. Rothlein, J. E., and Parsons, S. M. (1979): *J. Neurochem.,* 33:1189–1194.
113. Russell, R. W., Booth, R. A., Jenden, D. J., Roch, M. R., and Rice, K. M. (1985): *J. Neurochem.,* 45:293–299.
114. Russell, R. W., and Jenden, D. J. (1981): *Pharmacol. Biochem. Behav.,* 15:285–288.
115. Rylett, R. J., and Colhoun, E. H. (1977): *J. Neurosci.,* 3:414.
116. Rylett, R. J., and Colhoun, E. H. (1978): *Can. Fed. Biol. Soc.,* 21:2.
117. Rylett, R. J., and Colhoun, E. H. (1979): *J. Neurosci.,* 32:553–558.
118. Rylett, R. J., and Colhoun, E. H. (1980): *J. Neurochem.,* 34:713–719.
119. Rylett, R. J., and Colhoun, E. H. (1982): *Abstr. Soc. Neurosci.,* 8:773.
120. Rylett, R. J., and Colhoun, E. H. (1984): *J. Neurol.,* 43:787–794.
121. Salamone, J. D., Beart, P. M., Alpert, J. E., and Iversen, S. D. (1984): *Behav. Brain Res.,* 13:63–70.
122. Sandberg, K., Hanin, I., Fisher, A., and Coyle, J. T. (1984): *Brain Res.,* 293:49–55.
123. Sandberg, K., Sandberg, P. R., and Coyle, J. T. (1984): *Brain Res.,* 299:339–343.
124. Sandberg, K., Sandberg, P. R., Hanin, I., Fisher, A., and Coyle, J. T. (1984): *Behav. Neurosci.,* 98:162–165.
125. Schueler, F. W. (1960): *Int. Rev. Neurobiol.,* 2:77–97.
126. Schueler, F. W., and Calvin, H. (1951): *Arch. Int. Pharmacodyn.,* 88:351–360.
127. Shaw, K.-P., Aracava, Y., Akaike, A., Daly, J. W., Rickett, D. L., and Albuquerque, E. X. (1985): *Mol. Pharmacol.,* 28:527–538.
128. Simon, R. J., and Kuhar, M. J. (1975): *Nature,* 225:162–163.
129. Slater, P. (1968): *Life Sci.,* 7:833–837.
130. Smart, L. A. (1981): *Neuroscience,* 81:1765–1770.
131. Smart, L. A. (1983): *J. Med. Chem.,* 26:104–107.
132. Suskiw, J. B., Beach, R. L., and Pilar, G. R. (1976): *J. Neurochem.,* 26:1123–1136.
133. Thal, L. J., and Fuld, P. A. (1983): *N. Engl. J. Med.,* 308:720.
134. Thal, L. J., Masur, D. M., Fuld, P. A., Sharpless, N. S., and Davies, P. (1983): In: *Banbury Report. Biological Aspects of Alzheimer's Disease, Vol. 15,* edited by R. Katzman, pp. 461–469. Cold Spring Harbor Laboratory, Cold Spring Harbor, New York.
135. Trommer, B. A., Schmidt, D. E., and Wecker, L. (1982): *J. Neurochem.,* 39:1704–1709.
136. Tuček, S. (1984): *Prog. Biophys. Mol. Biol.,* 44:1–46.
137. Tuček, S. (1985): *J. Neurochem.,* 44:11–24.
138. Vickroy, T. W., Roeske, W. R., Gehlert, D. R., Wamsley, J. K., and Yamamura, H. I. (1985): *Brain Res.,* 329:368–373.
139. Vickroy, T. W., Roeske, W. R., and Yamamura, H. I. (1984): *Life Sci.,* 35:2335–2343.
140. von Schwarzenfeld, I. (1979): *Neuroscience,* 4:477–493.
141. von Schwarzenfeld, I., and Whittaker, V. P. (1977): *Br. J. Pharmacol.,* 59:69–74.
142. Wagner, J. A., Carlson, S. S., and Kelley, R. B. (1978): *Biochemistry,* 17:1199–1206.
143. Walsh, T. J., Tilson, H. A., DeHaven, D. L., Mailman, R. B., and Fisher, A. (1984): *Brain Res.,* 321:91–102.
144. Weiler, M. H., Jope, R. S., and Jenden, D. J. (1978): *J. Neurochem.,* 31:789–796.
145. Welner, S. A., and Collier, B. (1984): *J. Neurochem.,* 43:1143–1151.
146. Wesseling, H., Agoston, S., Van Dam, G. B. P., Pasma, J., De Wit, D. J., and Havinga, H. (1984): *N. Engl. J. Med.,* 310:988–989.
147. Whittaker, V. P., and Lugmani, Y. A. (1980): *Gen. Pharmacol.,* 11:7–14.
148. Wurtman, R. J., Blustajn, J. K., and Maire, J.-C. (1985): *Neurochem. Int.,* 7:369–372.
149. Yamamura, H. I., and Snyder, S. H. (1974): *Proc. Natl. Acad. Sci. USA,* 71:1725–1729.
150. Zimmerman, H., and Denston, C. R. (1977): *Neuroscience,* 2:695–714.
151. Zimmerman, H., and Denston, D. R. (1977): *Neuroscience,* 2:715–730.
152. Zimmerman, H., and Dowdall, M. J. (1977): *Neuroscience,* 2:731–739.

Psychopharmacology:
The Third Generation of Progress,
edited by Herbert Y. Meltzer.
Raven Press, New York © 1987.

CHAPTER 24

Cholinergic Receptor Heterogeneity

Mark Watson, William R. Roeske, and Henry I. Yamamura

Much recent progress in our understanding of the neurobiology of cholinergic receptors is traceable to technical revolutions in the biological sciences that have occurred in the last decade. The ongoing application of modern gene technology to fundamental problems in neuropsychopharmacology, coupled with advances in the handling of membrane-bound proteins by biochemists and the development of patch-clamp techniques to measure currents through single-ion channels, suggests we may soon be studying receptor-effector mechanisms by reconstitution of entire signal transduction chains from isolated, purified components. We will focus in this chapter on our efforts to comprehend the heterogeneity observed among cholinergic receptors, with emphasis on muscarinic acetylcholine receptors (mAChR).

Although acetylcholine (ACh) has long been considered as a neurotransmitter in the CNS, the mechanistic aspects of its specific receptors and receptor subtypes associated with distinct physiological responses to ACh remain elusive. It has been well established that there are two major types of ACh receptors—nicotinic and muscarinic. Though nicotine blocks nicotinic ACh receptors (nAChR) following an initial stimulation, it is the prototypical agonist, whereas *d*-tubocurarine (curare) specifically antagonizes nAChRs. Similarly, the potent agonist muscarine stimulates, and atropine selectively blocks, mAChRs.

NICOTINIC RECEPTORS

The nAChR was the earliest neurotransmitter receptor to become known as a distinct molecular entity, the first to be isolated and purified, and also the first to be reconstituted in acceptor membrane systems in an active form.

Thus, more is known about the nAChR complex than any other receptor-transduction unit. The pentameric nAChR protein is believed to be composed of four heterologous subunits, two α and one each of β, γ, and δ (10,12,27). Although there is a great degree of structural homology in the amino acid sequences of each of these four polypeptides, Numa (43) and his colleagues demonstrated that each is encoded by a different gene. Knowledge of the secondary structure of these subunits has permitted the proposed design of a three-dimensional model (45). Changeux and his co-workers (10) have proposed a model to explain the conformational transitions of the nAChR within the context of the classical allosteric model. Lindstrom and his associates (32) employed a massive library of monoclonal antibodies to characterize functional nAChR subunits and conformational changes during synaptogenesis, as well as to localize and to purify the nAChR.

Yet the nAChR in the mammalian CNS has received comparatively little attention, in contrast to other tissues. Since the electric organ provides such a rich source of nAChR, much of our knowledge stems from these studies. Elapid neurotoxins such as α-bugarotoxin (α-BGTX) (39) and *Naja naja siamensis* α-toxin (48) were widely used to label the nAChR. However, nonspecific binding was extremely high and the physiological relevance of neurotoxin binding sites has been questioned, since α-BGTX has little, if any, nAChR antagonist activity in most mammalian systems. Although α-neurotoxins block activation of nAChR at the neuromuscular junction, they exert little effect at chick sympathetic ganglion cells, Renshaw cells, chromaffin cells, and in the PC 12 cell line. α-BGTX, the most potent nAChR antagonist in muscle, has not been convincingly demonstrated in physiological studies to be an antagonist at the mammalian CNS nAChR. Moreover, like the endogenous agonist ACh, the classical nAChR antagonists decamethonium and hexamethonium are only weak inhibitors of α-toxin binding, and the ganglionic blockers mecamylamine and hexamethonium are weak in displacing [^{3}H]nicotine from rat brain membranes, although they are potent inhibitors of ACh-induced depolarization in microiontophoretic studies of the mammalian CNS. Thus, the lack of good correlation between binding and function has impeded real growth in our understanding of the mammalian CNS nAChR.

While the search continues for more suitable specific antagonists of the nAChR, many investigators have proposed the existence of multiple nAChR binding sites in efforts to explain such discrepancies (41). An affinity reagent, 4-(N-maleimido) benzyltrimethylammonium, was used to obtain data that suggest that ACh binds two CNS nAChR sites whereas α-BGTX inhibits at only one of these sites (33). Numerous reports suggest that a second physiologically relevant site for curare exists on the ion channel responsible for gating, and two curare binding sites have been reported in the mammalian CNS (42). Goyal and Rattan (23) have suggested that nAChRs in autonomic ganglia be termed N_1 based on the presumably selective nicotinic agonist effects of dimethylphenylpiperazinium and the greater effectiveness of hexamethonium in blocking ganglionic transmission than in blocking motor endplates, and that the nAChR in skeletal muscle be termed N_2 based on the presumably selective nicotinic agonist effects of phenyltrimethylammonium and the selective blocking of the motor endplate by decamethonium. However, although Dale characterized the ganglionic effects of ACh as nicotine-like, many ACh-induced effects at autonomic ganglia are mimicked by pilocarpine and muscarine and blocked by atropine, but not hexamethonium or decamethonium. Thus, it has been widely believed and recently demonstrated by direct binding studies (54) that mAChR, as well as nAChR, is present on neurons in autonomic ganglia.

Today, as initially described by Dale at the turn of the century, the only clear and uniformly accepted distinction between cholinergic receptors is the classic delineation of mAChR and nAChR. In addition to discrete distributions and selective agonists and antagonists that characterize these receptors, numerous other features such as a typically slow onset and prolonged response generally distinguish mAChR-induced effects from the rapid onset and fleeting effects observed at the nAChR. Despite the tremendous accumulation of knowledge regarding the nAChR, a great deal of further evidence is necessary in order to firmly establish the existence of nAChR subtypes and the molecular nature of similarities and differences that may exist between them. In addition, there is comparatively little data relating the CNS nAChR with specific functions or behaviors. In contrast, there is little structural data and more specific functional data on the CNS mAChR, which is by far the predominant ACh receptor in the mammalian brain.

MUSCARINIC RECEPTORS

Background

A variety of vertebrate cells show responses, both excitatory and inhibitory, to ACh. Numerous investigative techniques, from biochemical to behavioral, have demonstrated that ACh-induced activation of mAChRs may induce diverse effects on learning, memory, attention, mood, nociception, thermoregulation, motor function, emotion, sleep, and neuroendocrine function (26). Not long ago there was widespread agreement that these responses were mediated by a homogeneous mAChR population that differed only in their regulatory properties and effector coupling mechanisms (4,15). Now, compelling evidence from pharmacological and biochemical studies strongly suggests there exist subclasses of mAChRs.

Characterization of Muscarinic Receptors

The development of radioligand binding techniques that used antagonists of high specificity and specific activity permitted the direct measurement of mAChR binding sites, providing data on the quantitation, distribution, pharmacologic specificity, and modulation of mAChR. Excellent quantitative agreement existed between values for antagonist affinity in binding studies of the CNS and the ileum as well as between pharmacologically determined values for antagonism of guinea pig ileal smooth muscle contraction (64,65). Although complexities in antagonist binding were reported under certain nonphysiological conditions (5,15), antagonists were widely believed to bind to a uniform population of sites as predicted by the Langmuir isotherm. Only agonists were believed capable of binding to a heterogeneous population of sites (5,15). Agonists also displayed a greater sensitivity to guanine nucleotide modulation. This was characterized by a decrease in the relative percentage of receptors in the high-affinity agonist state to a uniform low affinity in the presence of guanine nucleotides. Thus, affinity states of the mAChR were previously believed to reflect interconvertible conformational states of one receptor protein (5,15). The mAChR in the CNS has recently been reviewed (6,16,37,47,51,55,59,60).

Nonclassical Selective Antagonists

Although scattered reports implied the possible existence of two mAChRs, they attracted little interest. Nonclassical mAChR antagonists such as 4-diphenylacetoxy-N-methyl-piperidine (4-DAMP) had revealed complexities in functional tests (3) and the existence of mAChR subtypes had been suggested based on comparative pharmacologic studies of intestinal contraction and K$^+$ efflux (9). An M$_1$(intramural ganglia)/M$_2$(smooth muscle) subclassification was proposed to explain the discriminating effects of the novel ganglionic mAChR stimulant McN-A-343 [3-(m-chlorophenylcarbamoyloxy)-2-butynyltrimethylammonium chloride] seen in the lower esophageal sphincter of the opossum (23). However, the complex binding (24) and functional (7) profile of a new nonclassical mAChR antagonist, pirenzepine (PZ), attracted widespread interest in the molecular nature of mAChR heterogeneity.

Striking differences in the regional distribution of high-affinity [^{3}H]PZ binding in the CNS and periphery emerged when contrasted with the classical antagonist [^{3}H]-(−)quinuclidinyl benzilate ([^{3}H](−)QNB) (54–62), suggesting that [^{3}H]PZ may be used to study putative M$_1$ mAChR mechanisms. Additional physiological studies verified that basic pharmacologic differences exist between putative M_1 mAChR sites that [³H]PZ labels with high affinity (<20 nM) and lower-affinity PZ sites. We identified cortical high-affinity [³H]PZ binding (56,61) and showed putative M_1 selectivity by [³H]PZ in the functionally relevant human stellate ganglion (54), visualizing these sites by light microscopic autoradiography (67). Additional studies confirmed the selectivity of [³H]PZ and the lack of effect of guanine nucleotides on its binding in homogenates (6,31,34,35,44). Autoradiographic studies in the rat and human CNS further confirmed our initial reports (13,55). Moreover, results from in vitro [³H]PZ binding in homogenates correlate well with studies in vivo, showing a large proportion of high-affinity [³H]PZ sites in tissues sensitive to the antimuscarinic action of PZ and a low proportion of [³H]PZ sites in tissues where PZ shows little effect. The discrete localization of putative mAChR subtypes may be crucial to the elucidation of specific functions that may be selectively mediated by these subtypes, and the relationships between them. The results of our autoradiographic studies in which agonist as well as putative M_1 and M_2 mAChR subtypes in the CNS were visualized using [³H]hemicholinium-3 ([³H]HC-3), [³H](+)cismethyldioxolane ([³H](+)CD), [³H]PZ, and [³H]-(−)QNB have recently been reviewed (55). High densities of putative M_1 sites (high-affinity [³H]PZ binding sites) were seen in the cerebral cortex, corpus striatum, hippocampus, and ganglia, whereas low-affinity sites (putative M_2 sites) predominate in the cerebellum, pons-medulla, and certain other CNS areas (6,13,31,35,44,60,66).

Recently, another novel mAChR antagonist, AF-DX 116 (11-[[2-[(diethylamino)methyl]-1-piperidinyl]-acetyl]-5,11-dihydro-6H-pyrido[2,3-b][1,4]benzodiazepine-6-one) was synthesized at Dr. Karl Thomae GmbH (Biberach, F.R.G.). This compound showed selectivity for putative M_2 muscarinic receptors (Table 1). Confirming the work of Giachetti et al. (21) and Hammer et al. (25), our data demonstrate the low affinity of AF-DX 116 in the cerebral cortex and the higher affinity of this compound for the cardiac putative M_2 subtype (55,57).

Relationships Between Subpopulations

We recently compared the binding affinities of numerous agonists and antagonists in inhibiting [³H]PZ and [³H]-(−)QNB binding in the rat cerebral cortex and heart (57,62). Although K_i values in both tissues showed good agreement with affinity values obtained in functional assays (Table 1), several important distinctions became evident. K_i values for agonists were dissimilar in these tissues unless guanine nucleotides were present (62). In contrast, K_i values of antagonists were generally unaffected by guanine nucleotides and were similar for classical antimuscarinics between these tissues (57). However, PZ showed the greatest selectivity for putative M_1 sites and most other antagonists showed some M_1 selectivity. (PZ > dexetimide = scopolamine > atropine > levetimide = (−)QNB.) Only AF-DX 116 showed selectivity for putative M_2 muscarinic receptors (Table 1). Although the inverse selectivity of PZ and AF-DX 116 remains to be confirmed, it is interesting that each compound is better fitted to a two-site model in the rat cerebral cortex (55,57). PZ inhibits approximately 64% of [³H](−)QNB-labeled cortical homogenates with high affinity and AF-DX 116 inhibits approximately 31% of these sites with high affinity (57). In homogenates of cloned cells of the human neuroblastoma cell line (SH-SY5Y), both PZ and AF-DX 116 also show significant two-site fits, with 41 and 46%, respectively, showing high affinity (55). Thus, AF-DX 116 appears to be an approximately 10-fold selective M_2 antagonist.

In contrast to agonists, selectivity of antagonists appears to be independent of guanine nucleotide modulation (51,52,55,57,59–62). Thus, whereas potent classical mAChR agonists, such as carbamylcholine, show a quantitatively small (relative to cardiac) but reliable shift to lower affinity on the putative M_1 cerebral cortical mAChR labeled with [³H]PZ, the selectivity of PZ is apparently not dependent on coupling to a guanine nucleotide-binding protein or to a low-affinity agonist state (61,62). We therefore noted that mAChR heterogeneity sensed by agonists and antagonists does not appear to be the same (57,59,62). Inhibition studies of agonists versus [³H]PZ-labeled mAChR binding sites in rat cerebral cortex yielded Hill values less than unity. This suggested there are multiple agonist affinity states for the binding sites showing high affinity for [³H]PZ (56,62). This has been confirmed for numerous agonists such as carbamylcholine by two-site analysis of these data. Moreover, the highest-affinity agonist states in rat cerebral cortex and heart also show different structure-binding relationships in mAChR of these tissues (51–53,60). Thus,

TABLE 1. Comparison of apparent K_i values for selected muscarinic antagonist compounds

Antagonist	PZ cortex[a]	QNB cortex[b]	QNB heart[b] K_i (nM)	Selectivity ratio[c]	Pharmacologic affinity constant (nM)[d]
Scopolamine	0.40	0.26	2.1	5.4	0.3–1.0
Atropine	0.28	0.22	1.1	4.2	0.3–1.0
Dexetimide	0.25	0.20	1.3	5.4	0.06–2.0
Levetimide	900	840	850	0.94	>2000
(−)QNB	0.049	0.076	0.069	1.4	0.01–0.20
Pirenzepine	11	18	400	37	4.0–630
AF-DX 116	532	176	39	0.07	100–30,000

Modified from refs. 57 and 59.
[a] Assays in modified Krebs phosphate buffer at 25°C using 0.1 nM [³H]PZ for 1 hr.
[b] Assays in modified Krebs phosphate buffer at 25°C using 0.1 nM [³H](−)QNB for 2 hr.
[c] Determined by dividing K_i values vs. [³H](−)QNB in heart by those vs. [³H]PZ in cortex.
[d] Note that these divergent values are the result of assays in different tissues.

PZ, as well as other drugs, reveals differences in mAChRs when the highest-affinity agonist state is selectively labeled. Despite the apparent reciprocity of agonist and antagonist heterogeneity in many CNS areas such as the cerebral cortex and cerebellum, the lack of absolute correlation between distributions of agonist states and [³H]PZ binding in certain areas suggests that heterogeneity sensed by PZ may be distinct from heterogeneity sensed by agonists. Since many ligands appear to show some selectivity for both agonist states and putative M_1 and M_2 subtypes (55,57,62), concern for the relative selectivity for each type of heterogeneity is necessary to insure proper interpretation of these complexities (51,59).

Relationship of Putative Muscarinic Subtypes to Effector Coupling

Since mAChRs mediate the stimulation of phosphoinositide (PI) (40) breakdown and inhibition of adenylate cyclase activity, investigators have turned to these responses in attempts to identify if they are specific functional correlates of the putative mAChR subtypes. We previously speculated that the putative M_1 mAChR may be coupled to PI turnover whereas the M_2 mAChR may be coupled to inhibition of adenylate cyclase. PZ distinguishes putative mAChR subtypes in the rat cerebral cortex based on the good correlation of the high-affinity K_i value for PZ in studies of PI breakdown and its K_i value in binding studies (22,46). PZ inhibits carbamylcholine-stimulated phosphatidic acid synthesis in cholinergically enriched rat synaptosomes of the rat cerebral cortex and corpus striatum with high affinity, whereas studies of cyclic AMP production in the CNS and peripheral tissues show PZ to be of low affinity (55). There has been growing sentiment that PI hydrolysis is linked to the putative M_1 mAChR.

Numerous concerns regarding the heterogeneous cellular content of tissue homogenates can be circumvented by performing studies in cultured clonal cell lines (1,2,17,38). However, whereas both mAChR agonist-induced PI hydrolysis and direct mAChR agonist-induced inhibition of adenylate cyclase activity can be observed in NG108-15 neuroblastoma × glioma cells, and both high- (<10 nM) and low- (>100 nM) affinity PZ binding sites can be seen in homogenates of NG108-15 cells (2), only the low-affinity site is seen in the intact cell preparation (18). Thus, the question of whether there are two putative mAChR subtypes and the possible relationship between differential affinities for PZ and these responses in NG108-15 cells remains unclear.

Anterior pituitary mouse tumor cells (AtT-20/D16-16) have been widely used in the study of neuroendocrine function, and mAChRs were shown to be inversely coupled to adenylate cyclase in these cloned cells. We determined that intact AtT-20/D16-16 cells bind most mAChR antagonists in a similar manner to homogenates of NG108-15 neuroblastoma-glioma cells and rat cerebral cortex, and that they also show mAChR-mediated stimulation of PI turnover (1). Thus, these cells allow the simultaneous study of both responses. Whereas atropine was equipotent in these responses, PZ showed 40-fold greater affinity for

reversing carbamylcholine-stimulated PI turnover than for antagonizing the inhibition of cyclic AMP formation. K_i values were in good agreement with previously reported values in the rat brain for these responses and together suggest PZ can distinguish between these two responses in vivo (1,59). As may be predicted from binding data, our studies of carbamylcholine-stimulated PI turnover in human neuroblastoma SH-SY5Y cells also show PZ to be an extremely potent competitive antagonist with a K_i value of approximately 10 nM (63). In contrast, AF-DX 116 was a very weak competitive antagonist in inhibiting this response, with a K_i value of approximately 30 μM. Interestingly, mAChR agonists vary in their ability to increase the breakdown of inositol phospholipids, a property that may be related to the complexities of mAChR agonist binding to the receptor. Only carbamylcholine and ACh were found to be full agonists, whereas pilocarpine (17%), oxotremorine (16%), and McN-A-343 (8%) acted as weak agonists of low efficacy. These data suggest the SH-SY5Y cell line is well suited for studying putative M_1 mAChR effector studies.

The cardiac mAChR is inversely coupled to a macromolecular membrane complex by which it can inhibit intracellular cyclic AMP production, and enzymatically dissociated rat heart cells can provide estimates of pharmacologic parameters for drugs that interact selectively with mAChRs to inhibit (−)isoproterenol-induced cyclic AMP generation. This (−)isoproterenol response is very rapid, highly potent, of great magnitude, and fully reversible by ACh and other full mAChR agonists (e.g., cismethyldioxolane, carbamylcholine, carbamyl-β-methylcholine, oxotremorine-M). Partial agonists such as pilocarpine and the putative M_1 selective ganglionic stimulant 4-(m-chlorophenylcarbamyloxy)-2-butynyltrimethylammonium chloride [McN-A-343] also show potent inhibitory effects. Interestingly, carbamylcholine, unlike ACh, produces a shallow Hill value. In studies with ACh, atropine was 1,000-fold more potent than PZ. These results suggest that agonist affinity states of putative M_2 mAChRs may mediate the cyclic AMP response in whole cardiac cells and that PZ has low affinity versus this response in the periphery as well as in the CNS (55,59).

In this regard, our data show a good correlation ($r = 0.70$) with mAChR agonist-induced effects on adenylate cyclase activity and the low-affinity (K_L) agonist state for these agonists determined in inhibition studies of [³H](−)QNB-labeled cardiac homogenates, also noted previously (5,14). Moreover, as might be expected (5,14), the potency of GTP in reducing mAChR agonist affinity (largely by reducing the percentage of mAChR sites in the high-affinity state) ($r = 0.78$) and the K_L/K_H ratio calculated versus [³H](−)QNB-labeled cardiac homogenates ($r = 0.82$) both show good agreement with the efficacy of each agonist. Interestingly, it has been suggested that PI hydrolysis is not linked to putative M_1 mAChRs in the heart (8). However, in the rat cerebral cortex, both K_i and K_L values for mAChR agonists versus [³H]PZ-labeled sites in membranes show excellent correlation ($r > 0.9$) with their respective K_{act} (half-maximal concentration for activation) values in PI turnover studies in this tissue. The potency of GTP-induced shifts to lower affinity versus [³H](−)QNB-labeled ($r = 0.80$) and versus [³H]PZ-labeled cerebral cortical homogenates ($r = 0.88$) also demonstrates a good correlation with their efficacy in PI turnover studies. The possible involvement of another G-protein (20) in the PI cycle has already been hypothesized (11). As might be expected from the apparent presence of dual effectors in the cerebral cortex, the potency of the GTP-induced shift ($r = 0.86$) and the K_L/K_H ratio ($r = 0.61$) versus [³H](−)QNB-labeled mAChR binding sites both correlate with the efficacy of these agonists in adenylate cyclase assays as well. The K_L values for agonists versus [³H](−)QNB also are in excellent agreement ($r > 0.9$) with the K_{act} for adenylate cyclase in the cerebral cortex.

However, recent data suggest PI breakdown may also be linked to the putative M_2 mAChR (19,29). In contrast to the high affinity of PZ for inhibiting PI breakdown in rat cerebral cortex and corpus striatum, there are regional differences in K_i values for PZ in the guinea pig CNS. Although no differences were seen in PZ inhibition of [³H](−)QNB binding, PZ displayed lower affinity in the guinea pig neostriatum than in the cerebral cortex and hippocampus. Species and regional differences may be attributed to functionally distinct mAChR subtypes or to regional differences in the efficiency of mAChR coupling to PI breakdown. Nonetheless, mAChR-mediated hydrolysis of inositol phospholipids produces two critical intracellular messengers, inositol triphosphate (IP₃) and diacylglycerol. The future study of PI turnover may prove to be a suitable functional correlate for the eventual production of more selective and therapeutically useful neuropsychopharmacological drugs.

Ontogeny, Aging, and Alzheimer's Disease

Radioligand binding techniques have been used to study mAChR ontogeny in the CNS and the periphery. There is a differential ontogeny of agonist affinity states in selected brain regions of the rat (28). However, the results of our studies show a similar K_d value for the putative M_1 selective antagonist [³H]PZ during postnatal ontogeny, suggesting that the same population of high-affinity mAChR is labeled at all ages (17). The rapid rise in [³H]PZ binding between birth and 21 days corresponds to the rapid increase in cerebral cortical size and dendritic proliferation that occurs between birth and 30 days of age. As with [³H](−)QNB, approximately 10% of the total adult [³H]PZ binding is present at birth with over 90% present by day 28.

Numerous investigators have reported age-related alterations in mAChRs based on studies employing various methods (4). Decreases in mAChR density have been reported in many CNS regions in several species. The results of our aging studies in rats also show a substantial loss of mAChRs in many CNS areas. [³H](−)QNB binding is greatly reduced, particularly in areas rich in mAChR such as the cerebral cortex, hippocampus, and corpus striatum, and [³H]PZ binding is also significantly reduced in these and other areas (68). There is an apparent link between diminished learning capabilities and the natural aging process, and the possibility of a further association of this phenomenon with altered or diminished CNS muscarinic function has recently been reviewed (4). Facilitation

of memory by cholinomimetic agents, particularly in the elderly, and the pharmacologic alleviation of apparent memory dysfunction by physostigmine and cholinergic agonists are among the many lines of evidence that support cholinergic involvement in both aging and senile dementia of the Alzheimer's type (SDAT).

There are numerous reports of damage to cholinergic pathways in postmortem brain samples from patients who suffered from SDAT. Damage to the ascending projections to the hippocampus and the cerebral cortex and severe reductions in the activity of the ACh-synthesizing enzyme choline acetyltransferase (ChAT) have frequently been correlated with the severity of the symptoms of SDAT. Similarly, Parkinson's disease patients suffering from dementia show similar signs, and although cholinergic agonists are of only marginal value to most of these patients, cholinergic antagonists can produce severe disruptions of learning and memory in animals and humans. Selective losses of mAChRs have previously been reported in SDAT, yet whereas some have confirmed these findings, others have often failed to do so. Conceivably, this may be due to a selective loss of an as yet undefined mAChR subtype. A selective loss in the putative M_2 mAChR has recently been reported (44); however, these findings await further confirmation. Moreover, proportions of putative M_1 and M_2 mAChR subtypes were ascertained indirectly, rather than by [³H]PZ, and these investigators also equated agonist affinity states for carbamylcholine with putative M_1 and M_2 mAChR subtypes as defined by PZ, which may not necessarily be the case. Our preliminary data in postmortem human brain homogenates have thus far failed to uncover a consistent significant alteration in putative mAChR binding site subtypes. We are presently examining additional normal human and SDAT brain using quantitative autoradiographic methods to ascertain whether certain discrete areas within a specific tissue such as the cerebral cortex or hippocampus may show a difference in mAChR subpopulations.

Based on the results of our animal studies employing bilateral nucleus basalis magnocellularis (Meynert) lesions, we have found a reduction in the number of mAChR binding sites in the highest affinity state for agonists (58). We speculated that the highest affinity state labeled by [³H](+)CD is more closely associated with presynaptic nerve terminals (50,55,58). In contrast, PZ and (−)QNB appear to label predominantly postsynaptic neuronal elements (50,55,58). If the postsynaptic mAChR is intact in SDAT, this offers the potential for treatment with selective mAChR agonists. Novel agonists with greater M_1 selectivity than McN-A-343 and an ability to penetrate the blood-brain barrier would be of great therapeutic potential.

CONCLUDING REMARKS

Although a great deal remains to be learned about the biochemical, physiological, and behavioral implications of mAChR activation in the CNS, radioligand binding studies have proved to be very useful in providing information on the initial aspects of drug-receptor interaction. Overwhelming evidence dictates that binding sites identified by

[³H](−)QNB represent physiologically relevant mAChRs, and a similar case may increasingly be made for the binding of putative M_1-selective antagonists such as PZ and putative M_2-selective antagonists such as AF-DX 116. It is evident that nonclassical antagonists, like agonists, differentiate mAChR subpopulations on the basis of affinity, and that the mAChR recognition site may be an extremely complex protein that can couple to numerous signal amplification schemes (PI hydrolysis, adenylate cyclase) by different molecular mechanisms.

The existence of two mAChRs remains to be established. AF-DX 116 and PZ both show selectivity in the rat cerebral cortex and heart, labeling an inverse proportion of high- and low-affinity sites. In inhibition studies of [³H](−)QNB binding (57), the K_H (high-affinity dissociation constant) of AF-DX 116 in the cortex is nearly identical to the overall K_i of AF-DX 116 in cardiac homogenates, thus suggesting that putative M_2 sites in these tissues are the same. However, K_L values of PZ in cortical homogenates do not appear to be equal to K_i values for PZ in cardiac membranes. Although AF-DX 116 and PZ may discriminate mAChRs differently, one may be tempted to speculate that these data reflect the possible existence of putative M_1 and M_2 mAChRs, each possessing multiple agonist and antagonist affinity states. Yet differences in coupling could also produce these results. We should also recall that much biochemical data (e.g., gel electrophoresis) strongly suggests that there is only one recognition site, and there is an apparent lack of structural diversity among numerous tissues and species (49). The demonstration of the ability of [³H]PZ to label at least as many mAChR sites as [³H](−)QNB in the cortex under certain conditions is indicative of the complex regulatory capabilities of these putative subtypes (57). The 30- to 150-fold selectivity one may obtain for PZ suggests multiple antagonist affinity states exist, but a consistent emergence of at least two- to fivefold selectivity for PZ and AF-DX 116 may serve to remind us to exercise caution, rather than overlook the possible existence of two mAChR binding sites (57). PZ binding affinity between cortical putative M_1 and M_2 mAChRs, between intact NG108-15 and astrocytoma 1321N1 cells, and net selectivity differences between inhibition of PI and cyclic AMP in the cortex after subtracting the relative selectivity of atropine all show two- to fivefold selectivity of PZ (18,22). Thus, although one may predict that PZ binding affinities for putative M_1 and M_2 mAChRs may be differentially altered by digitonin solubilization and that the apparent selectivity of PZ may thus be altered, we should also recall that the differences consistently observed in membranes in many laboratories are in good agreement with similar differences seen in various physiological whole tissue studies and in biochemical assays of mAChR function (57).

Although the basis of the heterogeneity evidenced by PZ and AF-DX 116 is not clear, it seems unlikely that differences in apparent receptor density resulting from differential antagonist-induced isomerization (35) or from hydrophilic properties may fully account for their selective properties (30). Far more likely are differences in intrinsic structure of the primary recognition proteins or in environmental constraints imposed on putative mAChR subtypes. Either different amino acid sequences or different cell-specific posttranslational alterations, including phosphorylation, glycosylation, or acylation, may alter mAChR structure. Alternatively, and even more likely, environmental factors such as differential membrane-induced conformational constraints imposed by lipids or different effector components such as those for cyclic AMP, cyclic GMP, PI, K^+, or Ca^{2+} channels may alter affinity. These possibilities are not necessarily mutually exclusive. Structural properties of a recognition protein or other mAChR-complex associated protein may predispose an mAChR to couple to one of several potential effector molecules. Moreover, combined effects of the aforementioned would be multiplicative, and thus cells would be capable of producing selectivity of a far greater magnitude. Cellular machinery could, with only modest alteration, produce different mAChRs to allow fine modulation of cell function.

FUTURE VISTAS

Future solubilization studies will allow not only the sequencing of mAChR proteins, but also the study of mAChR recognition site interaction with other membrane components. Receptors must be removed from their natural membrane environment in an "active" form, retaining their biologic activity, in order that they can eventually be purified. A lack of abundant source and the relative instability of the mAChR have combined to slow progress in this area. Although concerns over heterogeneity of mAChRs have further complicated interpretation of this type of data, they have also prompted renewed interest in the problem. Despite some evidence to the contrary (49), since differences may be traceable to intrinsic differences in mAChR binding site proteins themselves, numerous laboratories have been actively seeking to solubilize and purify mAChR binding sites.

Many proposed differences in putative mAChR subtypes are outlined in Table 2, thus summarizing the M_1/M_2 concept. Regulatory influences of guanine nucleotides, sulfhydryl reagents, and ions differ among subtypes (51,55,57,59,61,62). It could be useful to elucidate their mechanism of interaction with each putative subtype, since they could be important endogenous regulators of mAChR function.

Clinically useful selective mAChR antagonists are presently available and will increasingly be made available. Therapeutic and untoward effects of mAChR drugs may be mediated by independent mAChR subpopulations that may be pharmacologically exploited to provide more highly selective and highly efficacious new agents. Our understanding of the molecular basis of putative M_1 and M_2 mAChR subtypes is growing rapidly, with mAChRs being solubilized, purified, and reconstituted. There is little doubt that sequencing techniques will soon yield amino acid sequences for these putative mAChR subtypes. These investigations and the cautious interpretation of radioligand binding studies of selective compounds such as PZ and AF-DX 116, done in parallel with studies of effectors under identical assay conditions and/or with biobehavioral studies, provide promising probes for the investigation of the etiologies and treatments of CNS disorders such as SDAT.

TABLE 2. *Characteristics of putative mAChR subtypes*

Characteristic	M_1	M_2
Tissue distribution		
Cerebral cortex, striatum, hippocampus, ganglia	+++	+
Heart, ileum, pons-medulla, cerebellum, pancreas	+	+++
High-affinity drug binding		
Agonists: McN-A-343, pilocarpine	+++	++
Carbamycholine, ACh	++	+++
Cis-methyldioxolane, oxotremorine, oxotremorine-M	++	++
Antagonists: (−)QNB	+++	+++
N-methylscopolamine, atropine, scopolamine, dexetimide, trihexyphenidyl	+++	++
Pirenzepine	+++	+
AF-DX 116	+	+++
Regulators of high-affinity agonist binding		
Guanine nucleotides	↓	↓↓↓
Monovalent cations (Na^+)	↓↓	↓↓
Divalent cations (low [Mg^{2+}])	0(?)	↑
Divalent cations (high [Mg^{2+}])	↓	↓↓
N-ethyl maleimide, p-chloromercuribenzoate	↑↑	↓↓↓
Effector systems		
Phosphatidylinositol turnover	+++	+(?)
Adenylate cyclase	+(?)	+++
Guanylate cyclase, CNS K^+ channel (M-channel)	++(?)	0(?)
Tissue responses		
Ileum: smooth muscle contraction	0(?)	+++
Sympathetic ganglia: excitatory transmission	+++	0(?)
Heart: contractility, rate	0(?)	+++
Gastric acid secretion	+++	0(?)
CNS-mediated passive avoidance learning	+++	0(?)
Pancreatic juice, amylase, insulin release	0(?)	+++

Modified from ref. 59.

ACKNOWLEDGMENTS

M.W. is a recipient of an Individual National Research Service postdoctoral fellowship award from the NIMH and a postdoctoral fellowship award and a Research Grant-in-Aid from the AHA, Arizona Affiliate. These studies were supported by USPHS grants MH-30626, MH-27257, HL-29565, program project grant HL-20984, an RSDA Type II (MH-00095) from NIMH to H.I.Y. and an RCDA (HL-00776) from NHLBI to W.R.R.

REFERENCES

1. Akiyama, K., Vickroy, T. W., Watson, M., Roeske, W. R., Reisine, T. D., Smith, T. L., and Yamamura, H. I. (1986): *J. Pharmacol. Exp. Ther.*, 236:653–661.
2. Akiyama, K., Watson, M., Roeske, W. R., and Yamamura, H. I. (1984): *Biochem. Biophys. Res. Commun.*, 119:289–297.
3. Barlow, R. B., Berry, K. J., Glenton, P. A. M., Nikolaou, N. M., and Soh, K. S. (1976): *Br. J. Pharmacol.*, 58:613–620.
4. Bartus, R. T., Dean, R. L., III, Bear, B., and Lippa, A. S. (1982): *Science*, 217:408–417.
5. Birdsall, N. J. M., Hulme, E. C., and Burgen, A. S. V. (1980): *Proc. R. Soc. Lond. (B) Biol. Sci.*, 207:1–12.
6. Birdsall, N. J. M., Hulme, E. C., and Stockton, J. S. (1984): *Trends Pharmacol. Sci. (Suppl.)*, 1:4–8.
7. Brown, D. A., Forward, A., and Marsh, S. (1980): *Br. J. Pharmacol.*, 71:362–364.
8. Brown, J. H., and Brown-Masters, S. (1984): *Trends Pharmacol. Sci.*, 5:417–419.
9. Burgen, A. S. V., and Spero, L. (1968): *Br. J. Pharmacol.*, 34:99–115.
10. Changeux, J.-P., et al. (1983): *Cold Spring Harbor Symp. Quant. Biol.*, 48:35–52.
11. Cockcroft, S., and Gomperts, B. D. (1985): *Nature,* 314:534–536.
12. Conti-Tronconi, B. M., and Raftery, M. A. (1982): *Annu. Rev. Biochem.*, 51:491–530.
13. Cortes, R., Probst, A., Tobler, H.-J., and Palacios, J. M. (1986): *Brain Res.*, 362:239–253.
14. Ehlert, F. J. (1985): *Mol. Pharmacol.*, 28:410–421.
15. Ehlert, F. J., Roeske, W. R., and Yamamura, H. I. (1981): *Fed. Proc.*, 40:153–159.
16. Ellis, J., and Hoss, W. (1985): *Int. Rev. Neurobiol.*, 26:151–199.
17. Evans, R. E., Watson, M., Yamamura, H. I., and Roeske, W. R. (1985): *J. Pharmacol. Exp. Ther.*, 235:612–618.
18. Evans, T., Smith, M. M., Tanner, L., and Harden, T. K. (1984): *Mol. Pharmacol.*, 26:395–404.
19. Fisher, S. K., and Bartus, R. T. (1985): *J. Neurochem.*, 45:1085–1095.
20. Florio, V. A., and Sternweis, P. C. (1985): *J. Biol. Chem.*, 260:3477–3483.
21. Giachetti, A., Micheletti, R., and Montagna, E. (1986): *Life Sci.*, 38:1663–1672.
22. Gil, D. W., and Wolfe, B. B. (1985): *J. Pharmacol. Exp. Ther.*, 232:608–616.
23. Goyal, R. K., and Rattan, S. (1978): *Gastroenterology*, 74:598–619.
24. Hammer, R., Berrie, C. P., Birdsall, N. J. M., Burgen, A. S. V., and Hulme, E. C. (1980): *Nature*, 283:90–92.
25. Hammer, R., Giraldo, E., Schiavi, G. B., Monferini, E., and Ladinsky, H. (1986): *Life Sci.*, 38:1653–1662.
26. Karczmar, A. G. (1978): In: *Cholinergic Mechanisms in Psychopharmacology (Adv. Behav. Biol., 24)*, edited by D. J. Jenden, pp. 679–708. Plenum Press, New York.

27. Karlin, A. (1980): *Cell Surface Rev.,* 6:191–260.
28. Kuhar, M. J., Birdsall, N. J. M., Burgen, A. S. V., and Hulme, E. C. (1980): *Brain Res.,* 184:373–383.
29. Lazareno, S., Kendall, D. A., and Nahorski, S. R. (1985): *Neuropharmacology,* 24:593–595.
30. Lee, J.-H., and Fakahany, E. E. (1985): *J. Pharmacol. Exp. Ther.,* 233:707–714.
31. Lin, S.-C., Olsen, K. C., Okazaki, H., and Richelson, E. (1986): *J. Neurochem.,* 46:274–279.
32. Lindstrom, J. (1985): In: *Neurotransmitter Receptor Binding,* edited by H. I. Yamamura, S. J. Enna, and M. J. Kuhar, pp. 123–152. Raven Press, New York.
33. Lukas, R. J., and Bennet, E. L. (1980): *J. Neurochem.,* 33:1151–1157.
34. Luthin, G. R., and Wolfe, B. B. (1984): *J. Pharmacol. Exp. Ther.,* 228:648–655.
35. Luthin, G. R., and Wolfe, B. B. (1984): *Mol. Pharmacol.,* 26:164–169.
36. Mash, D. C., Flynn, D. D., and Potter, L. T. (1985): *Science,* 228:1115–1117.
37. McKinney, M., and Richelson, E. (1985): *Annu. Rev. Pharmacol. Toxicol.,* 24:121–146.
38. McKinney, M., Stenstrom, S., and Richelson, E. (1985): *Mol. Pharmacol.,* 27:223–225.
39. McQuarrie, C., Salvaterra, P. M., De Blas, A., Routes, J., and Mahler, H. R. (1976): *J. Biol. Chem.,* 251:6335–6339.
40. Michell, R. H., Kirk, C. J., Jones, L. M., Downes, C. P., and Creba, J. A. (1981): *Philos. Trans. R. Soc. Lond. (B) Biol. Sci.,* 296:123–137.
41. Morley, B. J., Farley, G. R., and Javel, E. (1983): *Trends Pharmacol. Sci.,* 4(5):225–227.
42. Nordberg, A., and Larsson, C. (1980): *Acta Physiol. Scand. (Suppl.),* 479:19–23.
43. Numa, S., et al. (1983): *Cold Spring Harbor Symp. Quant. Biol.,* 48:57–70.
44. Potter, L., Flynn, D. D., Hanchett, H. E., Kalinoski, D. L., Luber-Narod, J., and Mash, D. C. (1984): *Trends Pharmacol. Sci. (Suppl.),* 1:22–31.
45. Raftery, M. A., et al. (1983): *Cold Spring Harbor Symp. Quant. Biol.,* 48:21–33.
46. Smith, T. L., and Yamamura, H. I. (1985): *Biochem. Biophys. Res. Commun.,* 130:282–285.
47. Sokolovsky, M. (1984): *Int. Rev. Neurobiol.,* 25:139–183.
48. Speth, R. C., Chen, F. M., Lindstrom, J. M., Kobayashi, R. M., and Yamamura, H. I. (1977): *Brain Res.,* 131:350–355.
49. Venter, J. C. (1983): *J. Biol. Chem.,* 258:4842–4848.
50. Vickroy, T. W., Watson, M., Leventer, S. M., Roeske, W. R., Hanin, I., and Yamamura, H. I. (1985): *J. Pharmacol. Exp. Ther.,* 235:577–582.
51. Vickroy, T. W., Watson, M., Roeske, W. R., and Yamamura, H. I. (1984): *Fed. Proc.,* 43:2785–2790.
52. Vickroy, T. W., Watson, M., Yamamura, H. I., and Roeske, W. R. (1984): In: *Neurotransmitter Receptors: Mechanisms of Action and Regulation (Adv. Exp. Med. Biol.,* 175), edited by S. Kito, T. Segawa, K. Kuriyama, H. I. Yamamura, and R. W. Olsen, pp. 99–114. Plenum Press, New York.
53. Vickroy, T. W., Yamamura, H. I., and Roeske, W. R. (1984): *J. Pharmacol. Exp. Ther.,* 229:747–755.
54. Watson, M., Roeske, W. R., Johnson, P. C., and Yamamura, H. I. (1984): *Brain Res.,* 290:179–182.
55. Watson, M., Roeske, W. R., Vickroy, T. W., Smith, T. L., Akiyami, K., Gulya, K., Duckles, S. P., Serra, M., Adem, A., Nordberg, A., Gehlert, D. R., Wamsley, J. K., and Yamamura, H. I. (1986): *Trends Pharmacol. Sci. (Suppl.),* 2:46–55.
56. Watson, M., Roeske, W. R., and Yamamura, H. I. (1982): *Life Sci.,* 31:2019–2023.
57. Watson, M., Roeske, W. R., and Yamamura, H. I. (1986): *J. Pharmacol. Exp. Ther.,* 237:419–427.
58. Watson, M., Vickroy, T. W., Fibiger, H. C., Roeske, W. R., and Yamamura, H. I. (1985): *Brain Res.,* 346:387–391.
59. Watson, M., Vickroy, T. W., Roeske, W. R., and Yamamura, H. I. (1985): *Prog. Neuropsychopharmacol. Biol. Psychiatry,* 9:569–574.
60. Watson, M., Vickroy, T. W., Roeske, W. R., and Yamamura, H. I. (1987): In: *Perspectives in Psychopharmacology,* Earl Usdin Festschrift Volume, edited by J. Barchas and W. Bunney. Alan R. Liss, New York (*in press*).
61. Watson, M., Yamamura, H. I., and Roeske, W. R. (1983): *Life Sci.,* 32:3011–3022.
62. Watson, M., Yamamura, H. I., and Roeske, W. R. (1986): *J. Pharmacol. Exp. Ther.,* 237:411–418.
63. Watson, M., Roeske, W. R., and Yamamura, H. I. (1986): *The Pharmacologist,* 28:156.
64. Yamamura, H. I., and Snyder, S. H. (1974): *Mol. Pharmacol.,* 10:861–876.
65. Yamamura, H. I., and Snyder, S. H. (1974): *Proc. Natl. Acad. Sci. USA,* 71:1725–1729.
66. Yamamura, H. I., Watson, M., and Roeske, W. R. (1983): In: *CNS Receptors: From Molecular Pharmacology to Behavior,* edited by P. Mandel and F. V. DeFeudis, pp. 331–336. Raven Press, New York.
67. Yamamura, H. I., Watson, M., Wamsley, J. K., Johnson, P. C., and Roeske, W. R. (1984): *Life Sci.,* 35:753–757.
68. Watson, M., Yamamura, H. I., and Roeske, W. R. (1987): (*in preparation*).

Psychopharmacology:
The Third Generation of Progress,
edited by Herbert Y. Meltzer.
Raven Press, New York © 1987.

CHAPTER 25

Alpha and Beta Adrenoceptors in Brain

Aaron Janowsky and Fridolin Sulser

CHARACTERIZATION AND LOCALIZATION OF ADRENOCEPTORS IN BRAIN

Using pharmacological techniques, two subtypes of alpha and beta adrenoceptors have been identified in the CNS (12,49). Throughout the brain, beta$_1$ adrenoceptors are the major subtype, except in the cerebellum, where beta$_2$ adrenoceptors are predominant (64,73,82). High concentrations of beta adrenoceptors are localized in the superficial layers of the neocortex, nucleus accumbens, olfactory tubercles, substantia nigra, nucleus interpeduncularis, subiculum, and pia mater (82). The localization of beta adrenoceptors does not strictly correlate with the distribution of presynaptic noradrenergic terminals. Thus, the striatum, which does not receive noradrenergic input from the locus coeruleus, contains nevertheless a high density of beta adrenoceptors that are functionally not distinguishable from beta adrenoceptors in brain areas that receive noradrenergic input (*unpublished results* from this laboratory). Studies aimed at the localization of striatal beta adrenoceptors in dopaminergic nerve terminals have yielded conflicting results (13,89,134). Recent electron microscopic immunocytochemical localization of beta adrenoceptors has shown that the adrenoceptor molecules appear to be clustered at postsynaptic junctions of norepinephrine (NE) neurons in brain whereas only a small proportion of the immunoreactivity appears to be associated with nonneuronal structures (113). The subpopulation of beta adrenoceptors involved in neuronal function appears to be primarily of the beta$_1$ subtype (64), suggesting that the bulk of beta$_2$ adrenoceptors are probably localized in glial cells and possibly cerebral blood

vessels. The finding that kainic acid-induced lesions of nerve cell bodies in the striatum cause only a loss of beta$_1$ adrenoceptors (74) is consistent with such a view. As in peripheral tissues, both beta$_1$ and beta$_2$ adrenoceptors are coupled via guanine nucleotide regulatory proteins (N proteins) to adenylate cyclase in a stimulatory manner. The current status of the molecular interactions between the various components of the adenylate cyclase system (receptor, N proteins, adenylate cyclase) and the pivotal role of the guanine nucleotide regulatory proteins in receptor cyclase coupling has been authoritatively reviewed (26,52,92,95).

Alpha$_1$ and alpha$_2$ adrenoceptors may share structural components (104). Alpha$_2$ adrenoceptors are localized both pre- and postsynaptically, whereas alpha$_1$ adrenoceptors appear to be exclusively located postsynaptically. Alpha$_2$ adrenoceptors localized at presynaptic nerve endings function as autoreceptors controlling the release of NE. Very recent evidence suggests there are two distinct subtypes of alpha$_2$ adrenoceptors (11). The physiological role of postsynaptic alpha$_2$ adrenoceptors in brain remains to be elucidated. Alpha$_2$ adrenoceptors are pharmacologically distinguished from postjunctional alpha$_1$ adrenoceptors by a much greater affinity for the antagonist yohimbine as compared to the alpha$_1$-selective antagonist prazosin and by a rather selective high affinity for clonidine. Alpha$_2$ adrenoceptors in peripheral tissues and in neuroblastoma $\times$ glioma hybrid cells are linked to adenylate cyclase in an inhibitory way (38). Evidence for such a coupling to adenylate cyclase via an inhibiting guanine nucleotide regulatory protein, N$_i$, in brain is sparse and mostly indirect

(7). Recent evidence from experiments utilizing solubilized alpha$_2$ adrenoceptors from brain indicates that the partially purified recognition site is associated with a guanine nucleotide-binding regulatory protein (59). Alpha$_1$ adrenoceptor activation causes phosphoinositide hydrolysis and the formation of second messengers such as diacyglycerol and inositol trisphosphate.

Over the last several years, information about the structure of alpha and beta adrenoceptors in peripheral tissues has become available (103,125–127).

Although photoaffinity labeling techniques have provided evidence that the mammalian beta adrenoceptor-binding subunit resides on a peptide of $M_r \cong 62,000$, regardless of whether it is of the beta$_1$ or beta$_2$ subtype, clearly definable differences in their peptide maps could be identified (111).

Target site analysis of the rat liver alpha$_1$ adrenoceptor has indicated that the intact membrane-bound receptor has an average molecular mass of 160,000 daltons, and target site analysis of the human platelet alpha$_2$ adrenoceptor has generated data suggesting similarity in size and structure to the alpha$_1$ adrenoceptor (127).

FUNCTIONAL ASPECTS OF ADRENOCEPTORS IN BRAIN: COUPLING TO BIOCHEMICAL EFFECTOR SYSTEMS

Beta Adrenoceptors and Their Coupling to Adenylate Cyclase

Both beta$_1$ and beta$_2$ adrenoceptors in brain are coupled to adenylate cyclase in a stimulatory way, thus generating the second messenger cyclic adenosine monophosphate (cyclic AMP). The noradrenergic cyclic AMP generating system has been thoroughly characterized in slices of the rat limbic forebrain (67,91), the rat hypothalamus (83), and in vesicular preparations of rat limbic forebrain (32). The stimulatory effects of NE and isoproterenol at saturating concentrations are nonadditive, thus excluding the possibility of separate catecholamine receptor-coupled adenylate cyclase systems. Moreover, the results suggest that isoproterenol activates a subpopulation of beta adrenoceptors, whereas NE activates two populations of receptors, one with beta characteristics and the other noradrenergic receptors that are not beta in nature (67,91). In general, alpha adrenoceptor agonists exert little or no stimulatory effect on brain adenylate cyclase (32,83,91,97,106) and may inhibit the activation of the enzyme by NE (67,100,106,128). Recent results from experiments utilizing the pineal gland indicate that alpha$_1$ adrenoceptor activation potentiates both beta adrenoceptor-mediated stimulation of serotonin-N-acetyltransferase (47) and cyclic AMP production (46). Studies by Sugden et al. (115) suggest that an activation of the calcium phospholipid-dependent protein kinase C is responsible for this synergistic interaction between alpha$_1$ and beta adrenoceptors. The activation of protein kinase C may stimulate the rapid phosphorylation of a component of the NE receptor-coupled adenylate cyclase system, resulting in a change in sensitivity to NE.

Rodbell et al. (93) have provided the first evidence that guanine nucleotides such as GTP are essential for hormone stimulation of adenylate cyclase. Guanine nucleotides reduce the affinity of agonists but not of antagonists for beta adrenoceptors. The unique property of beta adrenoceptor agonists is their ability to stabilize the high-affinity guanine nucleotide-sensitive state of the receptor, which represents an essential intermediate step for the activation of the enzyme (20). Guanine nucleotides reduce the fraction of the agonist-occupied receptors in the high-affinity state and, at maximal concentrations, convert all of the agonist-occupied receptors to the lower-affinity state (43). This explains the guanine nucleotide-induced shift of agonist competition curves which results in higher IC_{50} values for agonists. Though the GTP effect on agonist beta adrenoceptor binding can be taken as an index of the capacity for coupling between beta adrenoceptors and guanine nucleotide regulatory proteins (27), this effect is variable with different target membranes and is somewhat more difficult to demonstrate in membrane preparations from brain tissue (28,80). The N proteins that regulate adenylate cyclase activity are members of a larger family of homologous nucleotide-binding proteins and may represent branch points for transduction of information across the plasma membrane. The N proteins may regulate proteins other than the catalytic unit of adenylate cyclase (26). At the molecular level, catecholamine receptor-coupled adenylate cyclase systems function as highly efficient kinetic amplification systems, and thus small changes in receptor number or second messengers will be amplified through the cascade of cyclic AMP protein kinase-mediated phosphorylation processes (16,131).

Beta Adrenoceptors and Phospholipid Methylation

The methylation of membrane phospholipids in brain has been shown to be enhanced by catecholamines (50,135). Moreover, Zawad and Brown (135) have shown that the catecholamine-stimulated methylation of membrane phospholipids in brain is blocked by propranolol but not by phentolamine, thus indicating that the action is beta adrenoceptor mediated. Recent results from our laboratory demonstrate that S-adenosyl-L-methionine (SAMe) can modulate the phospholipid methyltransferase response to isoproterenol in brain. Thus, at low SAMe concentrations, isoproterenol inhibited methyltransferase I, whereas at high SAMe concentrations that favor phospholipid methyltransferase II, isoproterenol stimulated phospholipid methylation in a dose-dependent manner. Since the enzymatic methylation of phospholipids plays a key role in the transduction of receptor-mediated signals through membranes (29), small changes in phospholipid methylation within the discrete microenvironment of surface membrane receptors could affect their density and function.

Alpha$_1$ Adrenoceptors and Their Linkage to Phosphoinositide Hydrolysis

Activation of alpha$_1$ adrenoceptors in preparations from brain and peripheral tissues stimulates the metabolism of inositol phospholipids and the production of inositol trisphosphate and 1,2-diacylglycerol. These putative second messengers are involved in intracellular calcium mobilization and protein kinase C activation, respectively (6,78). In brain, the pathway from receptor activation to enzyme stimulation is somewhat obscure, but a number of steps have been characterized. Allison and Blisner (2) have demonstrated the inhibition of myoinositol 1-phosphatase by lithium, and the lithium-induced amplification of the agonist-stimulated accumulation of inositol phosphate (IP) has been described by Berridge et al. (5). Thus, NE and phenylephrine stimulate the production of IP in slices of cerebral cortex (9,65,99) and hippocampus (33) and the incorporation of ^{32}P into inositol phospholipids (1,30). Epinephrine and NE are full agonists, and phenylephrine and methoxamine are partial agonists in stimulating the "PI response" (41). In addition, the ability of agonists to stimulate IP accumulation (EC_{50} values) closely resembles their IC_{50} values in displacing the specific binding of [^3H]prazosin, suggesting a close correlation between alpha$_1$ adrenoceptor occupancy and agonist-induced IP accumulation.

The role of guanine nucleotide-binding proteins in the alpha$_1$ adrenoceptor-stimulated turnover of inositol phospholipids in brain has, as yet, not been described, but evidence from experiments involving a number of different tissue preparations suggests that guanine nucleotides may be involved in linking the alpha$_1$ adrenoceptor recognition site to the activation of phospholipase C.

U'Prichard and Snyder (124) have reported that agonist-sensitive alpha adrenoceptor-binding sites in calf brain membranes are altered by guanyl nucleotides, and recent reports indicate that a guanine nucleotide-binding protein, resembling that found in the beta adrenoceptor-coupled adenylate cyclase system, may be involved in signal generation by receptors linked to Ca^{2+} mobilization in mast cells (15). In addition Nakamura and Ui (75) have demonstrated the pertussis toxin (IAP)-catalyzed ADP-ribosylation of a protein that resembles the alpha subunit of the guanine nucleotide regulatory protein involved in the inhibition of adenylate cyclase (N_i) (39,72). The ADP-ribosylation is correlated with an inhibition of receptor-mediated IP accumulation. In addition, IAP has been shown to (a) inhibit alpha adrenoceptor-mediated inositol phospholipid turnover in rat adipocytes (70), (b) decrease the affinity of alpha adrenoceptor for agonists, and (c) abolish guanine nucleotide effects on alpha adrenoceptor binding sites in neuroblastoma $\times$ glioma cells (48). Results from other laboratories suggest that the effect of IAP is receptor and tissue specific (8,58).

Alpha$_2$ Adrenoceptors and Their Coupling to Adenylate Cyclase

Alpha$_2$ adrenoceptor function has been linked to inhibition of adenylate cyclase activity in a number of tissue preparations (22,53). In brain preparations, however, the effects of alpha$_2$ adrenoceptor agonists such as clonidine on adenylate cyclase activity are controversial. Kitamura et al. (45), using rat brain membrane preparations, were unable to demonstrate inhibition of "basal" adenylate cyclase activity but demonstrated a clonidine-induced in-

hibition of forskolin/GTP-stimulated activity. Treatment of the membrane preparation with pertussis toxin attenuated the clonidine-induced inhibition. ADP-ribosylation of N_i reduced the clonidine binding affinity to alpha$_2$ adrenoceptors in cortical membranes (79). Thus, the guanine nucleotide regulatory protein, N_i, may be involved in alpha$_2$ adrenoceptor-mediated inhibition of adenylate cyclase activity in brain (40). How the alpha$_2$ adrenoceptor-mediated inhibition of adenylate cyclase is linked to the physiological effects of alpha$_2$ adrenoceptor stimulation remains to be determined.

REGULATION OF DENSITY AND FUNCTION OF ADRENOCEPTORS IN BRAIN

Pharmacologic studies with drugs that alter the synaptic availability of NE and serotonin (5HT) have probably provided the most conclusive insights into the regulation of central NE receptor systems. Thus, a decrease in the synaptic availability of NE caused by either reserpine or 6-hydroxydopamine (6OHDA) causes supersensitivity of the NE-sensitive adenylate cyclase, accompanied by an increased density of beta adrenoceptors. Clinically effective antidepressants, however, elicit subsensitivity of the NE-sensitive adenylate cyclase linked to a decrease in beta adrenoceptor density (118). Generally, an increase in the responsiveness of alpha$_1$ adrenoceptor systems, often linked to an increased alpha$_1$ adrenoceptor density, parallels the antidepressant-induced down-regulation of beta adrenoceptors (55). Treatment with antidepressant drugs also causes changes in the number and function of alpha$_2$ adrenoceptors in various areas of the CNS (107). The observed sensitivity changes of the NE receptor-coupled adenylate cyclase system—supersensitivity and subsensitivity, respectively—are of the homologous type, i.e., only responses to NE and the beta adrenoceptor agonist isoproterenol are affected, whereas responses to other hormones, e.g., adenosine, are unaltered. The analysis of saturation isotherms indicates that changes in NE receptor numbers are the consequence of an increase or decrease of the B_{max} value of binding sites without changes in the K_d values. Although the basic phenomena of regulation in NE receptor number and function are firmly established in the CNS, because of the complexity of brain tissue the analysis of the molecular mechanisms of NE receptor regulation and function has been accomplished almost entirely in peripheral model systems.

Importance of NE Signal Input for the Regulation of Adrenoceptors and the Sensitivity of NE Receptor-Coupled Effector Systems in Brain

Of the various regulatory changes involving adrenoceptors in brain, changes in the regulation by antidepressant drugs have been the most extensively studied phenomena (14,24,117). The available evidence indicates that an unhindered synaptic availability of NE at the receptor is one prerequisite for down-regulation of beta adrenoceptors and the development of neurohormonal subsensitivity by, e.g., desipramine (36,37,101,102,133). However, it is not the increased synaptic availability of NE *per se,* but the interaction of the endogenous agonist NE with the receptor, that is required for the decrease in neurohormonal responsiveness to NE and the down-regulation of beta adrenoceptors. The formation of the ternary high-affinity state of the receptor—as postulated in peripheral systems (20)—seems to be a prerequisite not only for the activation of adenylate cyclase but also for the process of antidepressant-induced homologous *in vivo* desensitization. Whether the antidepressant-induced desensitization of central noradrenergic beta adrenoceptor systems involves a two-step phenomenon—uncoupling of receptors from the guanine nucleotide regulatory protein followed by loss of receptors—as has been demonstrated in nonneuronal tissue (23,31,114)—is not established. The use of conventional methods to probe coupling mechanisms following treatment with antidepressants, e.g., the determination of GTP-induced shifts of agonist competition binding curves, has not revealed changes in the interconversion of the high-affinity state of the receptor to a form that recognizes the agonist NE with lower affinity (80; *unpublished results* from this laboratory). The potential antidepressant clenbuterol, a beta adrenoceptor agonist, appears to be an exception, as chronic administration of this drug impairs the coupling of beta adrenoceptors with N_s, the guanine necleotide regulatory protein that is linked to adenylate cyclase stimulation (80). However, when Okada et al. (81) studied the time course for activation of adenylate cyclase by the nonhydrolyzable nucleotide Gpp(NH)p in membrane preparations from normal animals and from animals treated chronically with DMI, they found that the isoproterenol-induced facilitation of the release of GDP from N_s in exchange for Gpp(NH)p was suppressed in cortical membranes from animals with more than 1 day of treatment with DMI, even at a time when no significant changes were observed in the number of beta adrenoceptors. These results are compatible with the notion that DMI-like drugs may modify the coupling between the receptor and the N protein. Consequently, the *in vivo* desensitization process of the NE receptor-coupled adenylate cyclase system in brain may also involve a two-step phenomenon.

In peripheral systems, the early process of desensitization involving the uncoupling reaction is characterized by conversion of the beta adrenoceptor to a form that (a) does not effectively activate adenylate cyclase; (b) binds beta adrenoceptor agonists with low affinity and is not affected by GTP; and (c) binds beta adrenoceptor antagonists normally (114). Two major mechanisms for beta adrenoceptor desensitization have been suggested. First, results on the desensitization of turkey erythrocyte beta adrenoceptors by the agonist isoproterenol in a cell-free system have provided evidence for the role of receptor phosphorylation: (a) full coupling of the receptor-adenylate cyclase system and cyclic AMP generation are required for agonist-induced desensitization; (b) the beta adrenoceptor undergoes phosphorylation during the desensitization process (109); and (c) multiple protein kinase systems, including cyclic AMP-dependent protein kinase, protein kinase C, and Ca^{2+}/calmodulin-dependent kinase, are capable of regulating beta adrenoceptor function via phosphorylation reactions (76). It is noteworthy that phosphorylation of purified mammalian beta adrenoceptors by cyclic AMP-dependent protein kinase at two serine residues has recently been shown to lead to reduced beta adrenoceptor-N_s coupling (4), further emphasizing the pivotal role of protein kinase-mediated phosphorylation processes in the regulation of the function of neuronal systems. An alternate mechanism of agonist-induced desensitization of beta adrenoceptor systems has been studied in detail in frog erythrocytes (110). In this preparation, desensitization of the beta adrenoceptor-coupled adenylate cyclase system appears to involve the sequestration of the beta adrenoceptor away from other components of the adenylate cyclase system into internalized vesicles in which they are not degraded and from where they can recycle to the cell surface (110). At this time, we can only speculate which one of these mechanisms or combination of mechanisms is operative in the antidepressant-induced *in vivo* desensitization of beta adrenoceptor systems in brain. Updated comprehensive reviews on the molecular mechanisms of beta adrenoceptor desensitization are available (27,105).

The role of NE neuronal input in the regulation of $alpha_1$ adrenoceptor-mediated inositol phospholipid turnover has recently been described. Effects of lesions of ascending noradrenergic neurons on the characteristics of $alpha_1$ adrenoceptor recognition sites appear to depend on the methods used to destroy the catecholaminergic fibers, the brain region being studied, and the radioligand used to measure specific $alpha_1$ adrenoceptor binding sites. Thus, injecting 6OHDA into the fimbria (71) or into the dorsal bundle (17,122) causes very little change in the specific binding of [^{3}H]WB4101 in the hippocampus. Intracerebroventricular administration of the neurotoxin (120) or dorsal bundle lesions (123), however, cause an increase in the density of specific [^{3}H]WB4101 binding sites in the cortex.

Intracerebroventricular administration of 6OHDA causes an increase in NE-stimulated IP accumulation in hippocampus (34), a decrease in the EC_{50} for NE-stimulated IP accumulation in the cortex, and an increase in the maximal response to phenylephrine. These changes are not correlated with a statistically significant change in specific [^{3}H]prazosin binding, but a lesion-induced increase in a "receptor reserve" could explain the results (41). Thus, the ligand-binding assays may not accurately reflect changes in receptor-mediated events. Conversely, the lesion-induced increase in the response to agonists may reflect changes at a site in the metabolic pathway that is distal to the $alpha_1$ adrenoceptor recognition site.

Radioligand-binding studies indicate that some tricyclic antidepressants *in vitro* are antagonists at $alpha_1$ adrenoceptor [^{3}H]WB4101 binding site(s) (121,122) and will block the $alpha_1$ adrenoceptor-mediated turnover of PI in rat pineal (108). Following chronic administration of a variety of antidepressants, however, no consistent change is observed in the density of [^{3}H]WB4101 binding sites in a membrane preparation from cerebral cortex (84,119). Dietary lithium supplements, however, caused an increase in the maximal number of [^{3}H]WB4101 binding sites (94) and the density of $alpha_1$ adrenoceptors was also increased in hippocampal membranes prepared from rats that had been treated chronically with amitriptyline (88). These reports suggest that binding assays involving a single concentration of radioligand or a single brain region may not detect anti-depressant-induced changes in alpha$_1$ adrenoceptors. In addition, displacement of radiolabeled alpha$_1$ adrenoceptor antagonists by increasing concentrations of agonist may be required to detect antidepressant-induced changes in the affinity of the binding site (61). This is the case, in fact, for the beta adrenoceptor recognition site (57).

Recent reports indicate that alpha$_1$ adrenoceptor-mediated events are, in fact, "up-regulated" following chronic anti-depressant administration. Thus, iontophoretic application of NE to the facial nucleus of rats that have been treated with antidepressants is associated with an enhanced electro-physiological response (62) and behavioral correlates of alpha$_1$ adrenoceptor stimulation are also enhanced (44,63,86).

Chronic administration of antidepressants for a clinically relevant time period has been reported to have no effect on NE-stimulated inositol phospholipid turnover in slices of cerebral cortex (42), though preliminary results by Jan-owsky et al. (*unpublished observations*) suggest that there might be regional differences in the responsiveness following antidepressants.

The Corequirement of Intact Serotonergic Neurons for Normal Function of Adrenoceptors in Brain and Their Regulation by Antidepressant Treatments

Ever since Dahlström and Fuxe (19) first mapped the pathways of noradrenergic and serotonergic neurons in brain, the morphological organization of cortical mono-amine systems has suggested a biomolecular linkage of these transmitter systems in neocortical information pro-cessing (51,54). Experiments conducted in animals with specific lesions of serotonergic neurons and psychophar-macological studies with antidepressant drugs have provided new support for this aminergic link at the level of adreno-ceptors. Thus, selective lesions of 5HT neurons with the neurotoxin 5,7-dihydroxytryptamine (5,7-DHT) significantly increase the density of beta adrenoceptors in various brain areas (35,112). In frontal cortex, limbic forebrain, and hippocampus, Scatchard analysis of saturation isotherms indicates that the increase in the density of beta adrenocep-tors following 5,7-DHT lesions is due to an increase in the B_{max} value without changes in the K_d values (35,112) whereas in the striatum the marked increase in the B_{max} value of beta adrenoceptors following lesions is accompanied by a slight but significant increase in the K_d value for the antagonist dihydroalprenolol (DHA) (*unpublished results* from this laboratory). In contrast to beta adrenoceptor antagonist binding, the interaction of beta adrenoceptors with agonists is markedly altered in brain tissue from animals lesioned with 5,7-DHT. Thus, the inhibition of [^{3}H]DHA binding by isoproterenol in cortical, limbic, and striatal preparations of animals lesioned with 5,7-DHT is shifted, resulting in IC$_{50}$ values five- to sixfold greater than those obtained in receptor preparations from brains of control animals (57). Moreover, the density of beta adre-noceptors cannot be down-regulated by various antidepres-sant drugs in brain membrane preparations from animals with selective lesions of serotonergic neurons (10,21,35,77).

A reduction in the synaptic availability of 5HT by *p*-chlorophenylalanine (PCPA) has also been shown to prevent DMI from down-regulating cortical beta adrenoceptors (56,87), though negative data have also been obtained (77). In our laboratory, PCPA nullified within 2 days—despite the continuous administration of DMI—the decrease in the density of beta adrenoceptors but did not significantly alter the attenuation of the NE-sensitive adenylate cyclase (56). As in cortical tissue from animals with 5,7-DHT-induced lesions, PCPA causes a five-fold decrease in agonist affinity of beta adrenoceptors but does not alter antagonist affinity. Interestingly, 5-hydroxytryptophan coadministered with PCPA converts a DMI-resistant to a DMI-responsive beta adrenoceptor population and shifts the markedly re-duced agonist affinity of beta adrenoceptors toward control values (56). Recent analysis of binding data using a two-site model for kinetics suggests that the administration of 5,7-DHT actually has little or no effect on the antidepressant induced changes in the regulation of the high affinity [^{3}H]-DHA binding site, but the number of low affinity sites may be increased. Antidepressant induced changes in beta ad-renoceptor stimulated cyclic AMP accumulation parallel changes in the high affinity binding site (*submitted*). The changes reported in agonist properties of beta adrenoceptors following impairment of serotonergic neuronal input are reminiscent of beta adrenoceptors that have been (partially) uncoupled from the guanine nucleotide regulatory protein. The molecular basis of the regulation of the number and function of beta adrenoceptors by 5HT neurons remains to be elucidated.

Preliminary results obtained by Janowsky, Labarca, and Paul (*unpublished observations*) indicate that serotonergic deafferentation causes an up-regulation of alpha$_1$ adreno-ceptor-mediated IP accumulation. Effects of lesions of the median raphe nucleus on alpha$_1$ adrenoceptor binding characteristics have recently been described. Consolo et al. (18) have demonstrated the lesion-induced increase in a [^{3}H]WB4101-labeled alpha$_1$ adrenoceptor binding site in the hippocampus. The effects of the lesion can be reversed by chronic infusion of 5HT and the ligand binding is regulated by guanine nucleotides (132). The [^{3}H]WB4101 binding site is apparently not radiolabeled by [^{3}H]prazosin, since lesions of ascending serotonergic neurons do not alter [^{3}H]prazosin binding in either the cerebral cortex or hip-pocampus (112). Thus, both [^{3}H]WB4101 and [^{3}H]DHA may be labeling site(s) that are regulated by the availability of 5HT.

Role of Endocrine Factors in the Regulation of Adrenoceptors in Brain

Alterations in circulating steroid hormone levels can alter noradrenergic receptor sensitivity and/or density of NE receptors in brain. The sensitivity of the NE receptor-coupled adenylate cyclase system is significantly enhanced 2 weeks after adrenalectomy in rat cortex and limbic forebrain (68,69). This increase in sensitivity is restricted to the non-beta component of NE receptors, since no change was observed in either the cyclic AMP response to isoproterenol or in the B_{max} or K_d values of beta adrenoceptors. The increase in sensitivity is not seen in adrenal-demedullated animals, is reversed by corticosterone, and occurs without a change in the activity of adenylate cyclase or phosphodiesterase. The increase in sensitivity is mimicked by hypophysectomy, thus indicating that the change in noradrenergic receptor sensitivity is the consequence of a decrease in the level of circulating corticosterone (66). Inhibition of corticosterone synthesis by metopyrone mimics the effect of adrenalectomy on noradrenergic receptor sensitivity in brain, and like the effect of adrenalectomy, it is reversed by corticosterone (90). Other studies have implicated sex steroid hormones in the regulation of either sensitivity or density of beta adrenoceptors in brain (129,130). Since receptors for both glucocorticoids and sex steroids are present in brain tissue (60,96) and a strong glucocorticoid receptor immunoreactivity has been shown to be predominantly located in both NE and 5HT nerve cell bodies in the brainstem (25), it is tempting to speculate that steroid hormones may regulate the linked 5HT/NE receptor-coupled adenylate cyclase system via modulation of genomic expression of one or the other of the multiple presynaptic or postsynaptic components of central adrenoceptor systems (regulation of mRNA transcription).

A number of reports in the literature indicate that thyroid hormones are also involved in the regulation of central beta adrenoceptors (3,85). Whereas hyperthyroidism is generally associated with increased beta adrenoceptor density and/or sensitivity, hypothyroidism is associated with a decrease in beta adrenoceptor density and/or function. A desensitization of the NE receptor-coupled adenylate cyclase system linked to a down-regulation of its beta adrenoceptor population in rat cerebral cortex following prolonged treatments with triiodothyronine or thyroxine has recently been reported (98).

CONCLUSIONS AND FUTURE DIRECTIONS IN CENTRAL ADRENOCEPTOR RESEARCH

Since the identification of alpha and beta adrenoceptors and their subtypes in the CNS by radioligand binding studies, our understanding of the regulation of recognition and action function (closely linked biological responses) of these receptors has increased enormously. The importance of the endogenous agonist NE, the corequirement of 5HT for the regulation of density and agonist affinity of beta and alpha$_1$ adrenoceptors *in vivo,* and the role of endocrine modulators of central adrenergic receptor number and function have been discussed. Studies with antidepressant drugs have provided additional evidence for the biomolecular link of aminergic receptor systems in brain and a rational basis for the clinically relevant "serotonin/norepinephrine link hypothesis" of affective disorders (116).

Potentially exciting new directions of central adrenoceptor research include (a) the exploration of the interaction of second messengers generated by agonist activation of alpha$_1$, 5HT, and beta adrenoceptors for transmembrane signaling and changes in receptor sensitivity and number; (b) purification of central NE receptors, determination of their structure, and eventual cloning of the genes; (c) elucidation of the genomic expression of steroid hormones in NE and 5HT neurons, i.e., modification of the transcription of hormone-sensitive genes by modifying mRNA concentrations; (d) studies on the relationship of receptor structure, function, and regulation (or lack of regulation) to the pathophysiology of various mental and other CNS diseases.

ACKNOWLEDGMENTS

Research from our laboratories has been supported by USPHS grant MH-29228, a grant from Hoffman-La Roche, the Vanderbilt University Department of Psychiatry, and the Tennessee Department of Mental Health and Mental Retardation. We wish to thank Ms. Lynne Lindsey for the typing of the manuscript.

REFERENCES

1. Abdel-Latif, A. A., Yau, S.-J., and Smith, J. P. (1974): *J. Neurochem.,* 22:383–393.
2. Allison, J. H., and Blisner, M. E. (1976): *Biochem. Biophys. Res. Commun.,* 68:1332–1338.
3. Atterwill, C. K., Bunn, S. J., Atkinson, D. J., Smith, S. L., and Heal, D. J. (1984): *J. Neural Transm.,* 59:43–55.
4. Benovic, J. L., Pike, L. J., Cerione, R. A., Staniszewsky, C., Yoshimasa, T., Codina, J., Caron, M. J., and Lefkowitz, R. J. (1985): *J. Biol. Chem.,* 260:7094–7101.
5. Berridge, M. J., Downes, C. P., and Hanley, M. R. (1982): *Biochem. J.,* 206:587–595.
6. Berridge, M. J., and Irvine, R. F. (1984): *Nature,* 312:315–321.
7. Bousquet, P., Rouot, B., and Schwartz, J. (1983): *Trends Pharmacol. Sci.,* 4:206–208.
8. Boyer, J. L., García, A., Posadas, C., and García-Sáinz, J. A. (1984): *J. Biol. Chem.,* 259:8076–8079.
9. Brown, E., Kendall, D. A., and Nahorski, S. R. (1984): *J. Neurochem.,* 42:1379–1387.
10. Brunello, N., Barbaccia, M. L., Chuang, D. M., and Costa, E. (1982): *Neuropharmacology,* 21:1145–1149.
11. Bylund, D. B. (1985): *Pharmacol. Biochem. Behav.,* 22:835–843.
12. Bylund, D. B., and U'Prichard, D. C. (1983): *Int. Rev. Neurobiol.,* 24:343–422.
13. Chang, R. S. L., Tran, V. T., and Snyder, S. H. (1980): *Brain Res.,* 190:95–110.
14. Charney, D. S., Menkes, D. B., and Heninger, G. R. (1981): *Arch. Gen. Psychiatry,* 38:1160–1180.
15. Cockroft, S., and Gomperts, B. D. (1985): *Nature,* 314:534–536.
16. Cohen, P. (1982): *Nature,* 296:613–620.
17. Consolo, S., Ladinsky, H., Forloni, G. L., and Grombi, P. (1982): *Life Sci.,* 30:1113–1120.
18. Consolo, S., Wang, J. X., Forloni, G. L., Mocchetti, I., Racagni, G., and Ladinsky, H. (1985): *Life Sci.,* 37:449–460.
19. Dahlström, A., and Fuxe, K. (1964): *Acta Physiol. Scand.,* 62(*Suppl. 232*):5–55.
20. DeLean, A., Stadel, J. M., and Lefkowitz, R. J. (1980): *J. Biol. Chem.,* 255:7108–7117.
21. Dumbrille-Ross, A., and Tang, S. W. (1983): *Psychiatry Res.,* 9: 207–215.
22. Fain, J. N., and García-Sáinz, A. (1980): *Life Sci.,* 26:1183–1194.
23. Fishman, P. H., Mallorga, P., and Tallman, J. F. (1981): *Mol. Pharmacol.,* 20:310–318.
24. Frazer, A., and Lucki, I. (1982): In: *Typical and Atypical Antidepressants,* edited by E. Costa and G. Racagni, pp. 69–90. Raven Press, New York.
25. Fuxe, K., Härfstrand, A., Agnati, L. F., Yu, Z. Y., Cintra, A., Wikström, A. C., Okret, S., Cantoni, E., and Gustafsson, J. A. (1985): *Neurosci. Lett.,* 60:1–6.
26. Gilman, A. G. (1984): *Cell,* 36:577–579.
27. Harden, T. K. (1983): *Pharmacol. Rev.,* 35:5–32.
28. Hegstrand, L. R., Minneman, K. P., and Molinoff, P. B. (1979): *J. Pharmacol. Exp. Ther.,* 210:215–221.

29. Hirata, F., and Axelrod, J. (1980): *Science,* 209:1082–1090.
30. Hokin, L. E., and Hokin, M. R. (1958): *J. Biol. Chem.,* 233:818–826.
31. Homburger, V., Lucas, M., Cantau, B., Barabe, J., Penit, J., and Bockaert, J. (1980): *J. Biol. Chem.,* 255:10436–10444.
32. Horn, A. S., and Phillipson, O. T. (1976): *Eur. J. Pharmacol.,* 37:1–11.
33. Janowsky, A., Labarca, R., and Paul, S. M. (1984): *Life Sci.,* 35:1953–1961.
34. Janowsky, A., Labarca, R., and Paul, S. M. (1984): *Eur. J. Pharmacol.,* 102:193–194.
35. Janowsky, A., Okada, F., Manier, D., Applegate, C. D., and Sulser, F. (1982): *Science,* 218:900–901.
36. Janowsky, A. J., Steranka, L. R., Gillespie, D. D., and Sulser, F. (1982): *J. Neurochem.,* 39:290–292.
37. Johnson, R. W., Reisine, T., Spotnitz, S., Wiech, N., Ursillo, R., and Yamamura, H. I. (1980): *Eur. J. Pharmacol.,* 67:123–127.
38. Kahn, D. J., Mitrius, J. C., and U'Prichard, D. C. (1982): *Mol. Pharmacol.,* 21:17–26.
39. Katada, T., Bokoch, G. M., Northup, J. K., Ui, K., and Gilman, A. G. (1984): *J. Biol. Chem.,* 259:3568–3577.
40. Kawahara, R. S., and Bylund, D. B. (1985): *J. Pharmacol. Exp. Ther.,* 233:603–610.
41. Kendall, D. A., Brown, E., and Nahorski, S. R. (1985): *Eur. J. Pharmacol.,* 114:41–52.
42. Kendall, D. A., and Nahorski, S. R. (1985): *J. Pharmacol. Exp. Ther.,* 233:473–479.
43. Kent, R. S., DeLean, A., and Lefkowitz, R. J. (1980): *Mol. Pharmacol.,* 17:14–23.
44. Kitada, Y., Miyauchi, T., Kanazawa, Y., Nakamichi, H., and Satoh, S. (1983): *Neuropharmacol.,* 22:1055–1060.
45. Kitamura, Y., Nomura, Y., and Segawa, T. (1985): *J. Neurochem.,* 45:1504–1508.
46. Klein, D. C., Averback, D. A., and Weller, J. L. (1981): *Proc. Natl. Acad. Sci. USA,* 78:4625–4629.
47. Klein, D. C., Sugden, D., and Weller, J. L. (1983): *Proc. Natl. Acad. Sci. USA,* 80:599–603.
48. Kurose, H., Katada, T., Amano, T., and Ui, M. (1983): *J. Biol. Chem.,* 258:4870–4875.
49. Lands, A. M., Luduena, F. P., and Buzzo, H. J. (1967): *Life Sci.,* 6:2241–2249.
50. Leprohon, C. D., Blusztajn, J. K., and Wurtman, R. J. (1983): *Proc. Natl. Acad. Sci. USA,* 80:2063–2066.
51. Levitt, P., Rakic, P., and Goldman-Rakic, P. (1984): *Neurol. Neurobiol.,* 10:41–59.
52. Limbird, L. E. (1981): *Biochem. J.,* 195:1–13.
53. Limbird, L. E. (1983): *Trends Pharmacol. Sci.,* 4:135–138.
54. Lindvall, O., and Björklund, A. (1984): *Neurol. Neurobiol.,* 10:9–40.
55. Maj, L. (1984): *Proc. IUPHAR 9th Int. Congress of Pharmacology,* 3:137–143. Macmillan Press, London.
56. Manier, D. H., Gillespie, D. D., Steranka, L. R., and Sulser, F. (1984): *Experientia,* 40:1223–1226.
57. Manier, D. H., Okada, F., Janowsky, A. J., Steranka, L. R., and Sulser, F. (1983): *Eur. J. Pharmacol.,* 86:137–139.
58. Masters, S. B., Martin, M. W., Harden, T. K., and Brown, J. H. (1985): *Biochem. J.,* 227:933–937.
59. Matsui, H., Asakura, M., Tsukamoto, T., Imafuku, J., Ino, M., Saitoh, N., Miyamura, S., and Hasegawa, K. (1985): *J. Neurochem.,* 44:1625–1632.
60. McEwen, B. S. (1979): In: *Reviews of Neuroscience, Vol. 4,* edited by D. M. Schneider, pp. 1–30. Raven Press, New York.
61. Menkes, D. B., Aghajanian, G. K., and Gallager, D. W. (1983): *Eur. J. Pharmacol.,* 83:35–41.
62. Menkes, D. B., Aghajanian, G. K., and McCall, R. B. (1980): *Life Sci.,* 27:45–55.
63. Menkes, D. B., Kehne, J. H., Gallager, D. W., Aghajanian, G. K., and Davis, M. (1983): *Life Sci.,* 33:181–188.
64. Minneman, K. P., Dibner, M. D., Wolfe, B. B., and Molinoff, P. B. (1979): *Science,* 204:866–868.
65. Minneman, K. P., and Johnson, R. D. (1984): *J. Pharmacol. Exp. Ther.,* 230:317–323.
66. Mobley, P. L., Manier, D. H., and Sulser, F. (1983): *J. Pharmacol. Exp. Ther.,* 226:71–77.
67. Mobley, P. L., and Sulser, F. (1979): *Eur. J. Pharmacol.,* 60:221–227.
68. Mobley, P. L., and Sulser, F. (1980): *Nature,* 286:608–609.
69. Mobley, P. L., and Sulser, F. (1980): *Eur. J. Pharmacol.,* 65:321–323.
70. Moreno, F. J., Mills, I., García Sáinz, J. A., and Fain, J. N. (1983): *J. Biol. Chem.,* 258:10938–10943.
71. Morrow, A. L., Loy, R., and Creese, I. (1983): *Proc. Natl. Acad. Sci. USA,* 80:6718–6722.
72. Murayama, T., and Ui, M. (1983): *J. Biol. Chem.,* 258:3319–3326.
73. Nahorski, S. R. (1981): *Trends Pharmacol. Sci.,* 2:95–98.
74. Nahorski, S. R., Howlett, D. R., and Redgrave, P. (1979): *Eur. J. Pharmacol.,* 60:249–252.
75. Nakamura, T., and Ui, M. (1985): *J. Biol. Chem.,* 260:3584–3595.
76. Nambi, P., Peters, J. R., Sibley, D. R., and Lefkowitz, R. J. (1985): *J. Biol. Chem.,* 260:2165–2177.
77. Nimgonakar, V. L., Goodwin, G. M., Davies, C. L., and Green, A. R. (1985): *Neuropharmacology,* 24:279–283.
78. Nishizuka, Y. (1984): *Nature,* 308:693–698.
79. Nomura, Y., Kitamura, Y., and Segawa, T. (1985): *J. Neurochem.,* 44:364–369.
80. O'Donnell, J. M., and Frazer, A. (1985): *J. Pharmacol. Exp. Ther.,* 234:30–36.
81. Okada, F., Tokumitsu, Y., and Ui, M. (1986): *J. Neurochem.,* 47:454–459.
82. Palacios, J. M., and Kuhar, M. J. (1982): *Neurochem. Int.,* 4:473–490.
83. Palmer, G. C., Sulser, F., and Robison, G. A. (1973): *Neuropharmacology,* 12:327–338.
84. Peroutka, S. J., and Snyder, S. H. (1980): *Science,* 210:88–90.
85. Perumal, A. S., Halbreich, U., and Barkai, A. I. (1984): *Neurosci. Lett.,* 48:217–221.
86. Plaznik, A., Danysz, W., and Kostowski, W. (1984): *Eur. J. Pharmacol.,* 101:305–306.
87. Racagni, G., and Brunello, N. (1984): *Trends Pharmacol. Sci.,* 5:527–531.
88. Rehavi, M., Ramot, O., Yavetz, B., and Sokolovsky, M. (1980): *Brain Res.,* 194:443–453.
89. Reisine, T. D., Nagy, J. I., Beaumont, K., Kibiger, H. C., and Yamamura, H. I. (1979): *Brain Res.,* 177:241–252.
90. Roberts, V. J., Singhal, R. L., and Roberts, D. C. S. (1984): *Eur. J. Pharmacol.,* 103:235–240.
91. Robinson, S. E., Mobley, P. L., Smith, H. E., and Sulser, F. (1978): *Naunyn Schmiedebergs Arch. Pharmacol.,* 303:175–180.
92. Rodbell, M. (1980): *Nature,* 284:17–22.
93. Rodbell, M., Kraus, H. M., Poke, S. L., and Birnbaumer, L. (1971): *J. Biol. Chem.,* 246:1872–1876.
94. Rosenblatt, J. E., Pert, C. E., Tallman, J. F., Pert, A., and Bunney, W. E. (1979): *Brain Res.,* 160:186–191.
95. Ross, E. M., and Gilman, A. G. (1980): *Annu. Rev. Biochem.,* 49:533–564.
96. Sar, M., and Stumpf, W. E. (1981): *Nature,* 289:501–502.
97. Sawaya, M. C., Dolphin, A., Jenner, P., Marsden, C. D., and Meldrum, B. S. (1977): *Biochem. Pharmacol.,* 26:1877–1884.
98. Schmidt, B. H., and Schultz, J. E. (1985): *J. Pharmacol. Exp. Ther.,* 233:466–472.
99. Schoepp, D. D., Knepper, S. M., and Rutledge, C. O. (1984): *J. Neurochem.,* 43:1758–1761.
100. Schultz, J., and Kleefeld, G. (1979): *Pharmacology,* 18:162–167.
101. Schweitzer, J. W., Schwartz, R., and Friedhoff, A. J. (1979): *J. Neurochem.,* 33:377–379.
102. Scott, J. A., and Crews, F. T. (1983): *J. Pharmacol. Exp. Ther.,* 224:640–646.
103. Shorr, R. G. L., Heald, S. L., Jeffs, P. W., Lavin, T. N., Strohsacker, M. W., Lefkowitz, R. J., and Caron, M. C. (1982): *Proc. Natl. Acad. Sci. USA,* 79:2778–2782.
104. Shreeve, S. M., Fraser, C. M., and Venter, J. C. (1985): *Proc. Natl. Acad. Sci. USA,* 82:4842–4846.
105. Sibley, D. R., and Lefkowitz, R. J. (1985): *Nature,* 317:124–129.
106. Skolnick, P., and Daly, J. W. (1975): *Mol. Pharmacol.,* 11:545–551.
107. Smith, C. B., and Hollingsworth, P. J. (1984): In: *Proc. IUPHAR*

9th Int. Congress of Pharmacology, 3:131–136. Macmillan Press, London.

108. Smith, T. L., and Hauser, G. (1979): *Biochem. Pharmacol.,* 28: 1759–1763.

109. Stadel, J. M., Nambi, P., Shorr, R. G. L., Lawyer, D. T., Carn, M. G., and Lefkowitz, R. J. (1983): *Proc. Natl. Acad. Sci. USA,* 80:3173–3177.

110. Stadel, M. M., Strulovici, B., Nambi, P., Lavin, T. N., Briggs, M. M., Caron, M. G., and Lefkowitz, R. J. (1983): *J. Biol. Chem.,* 258:3032–3038.

111. Stiles, G. L., Strasser, R. H., Caron, M. G., and Lefkowitz, R. J. (1983): *J. Biol. Chem.,* 258:10689–10694.

112. Stockmeier, C. A., Martino, A. M., and Kellar, K. J. (1985): *Science,* 230:323–325.

113. Strader, C. D., Pickel, V. M., Loh, T. H., Stocksacker, M. W., Shorr, R. G. L., Lefkowitz, R. J., and Caron, M. J. (1983): *Proc. Natl. Acad. Sci. USA,* 80:1840–1844.

114. Su, Y. F., Harden, T. K., and Perkins, J. P. (1980): *J. Biol. Chem.,* 255:7410–7419.

115. Sugden, D., Vanecek, J., Klein, D. C., Thomas, T. P., and Anderson, W. B. (1985): *Nature,* 314:359–361.

116. Sulser, F. (1985): In: *Psychiatry,* edited by P. Pichot, P. Berner, R. Wolf, and K. Thau, pp. 411–416, Vol. 2. Plenum Publishing Corp., New York.

117. Sulser, F., Gillespie, D. D., Mishra, R., and Manier, D. H. (1984): *Ann. NY Acad. Sci.,* 430:91–101.

118. Sulser, F., and Mobley, P. L. (1981): In: *Neuroreceptors: Basic and Clinical Aspects,* pp. 55–83. John Wiley and Sons, Ltd., New York.

119. Tang, S. W., and Seeman, P. (1980): *Naunyn Schmiedebergs Arch. Pharmacol.,* 311:255–261.

120. U'Prichard, D. C., Bechtel, W. D., Rouot, B. M., and Snyder, S. H. (1979): *Mol. Pharmacol.,* 16:47–60.

121. U'Prichard, D. C., Greenberg, D. A., Sheehan, P. P., and Snyder, S. H. (1978): *Science,* 199:197–198.

122. U'Prichard, D. C., Greenberg, D. A., and Snyder, S. H. (1976): *Mol. Pharmacol.,* 13:454–473.

123. U'Prichard, D. C., Reisine, T. D., Mason, S. T., Fibiger, H. C., and Yamamura, H. I. (1980): *Brain Res.,* 187:143–154.

124. U'Prichard, D. C., and Snyder, S. H. (1978): *J. Biol. Chem.,* 253: 3444–3452.

125. Venter, J. C. (1984): In: *Monoclonal and Anti-Idiotypic Antibodies: Probes for Receptor Structure and Function,* edited by Venture, J. C., Fraser, C. M., and Lindstrom, J., pp. 117–139, Vol. 4. Alan R. Liss, New York.

126. Venter, J. C., and Fraser, C. M. (1983): *Trends Pharmacol. Sci.,* 4:256–258.

127. Venter, J. C., Horne, P., Eddy, B., Gregnski, R., and Fraser, C. M. (1984): *Mol. Pharmacol.,* 26:196–205.

128. Vetulani, J., Leith, N. J., Stawarz, R. J., and Sulser, F. (1977): *Experientia,* 33:1490–1492.

129. Wagner, D. A., and Davies, J. N. (1980): *Brain Res.,* 201:235–239.

130. Wagner, H. R., Crutcher, K. A., and Davies, J. N. (1979): *Brain Res.,* 171:147–151.

131. Walsh, D. A., and Ashby, C. S. (1973): *Recent Prog. Horm. Res.,* 29:329–359.

132. Wang, J.-X., Consolo, S., Vinci, R., Forloni, G. L., and Ladinsky, H. (1985): *Life Sci.,* 36:255–270.

133. Wolfe, B. B., Harden, T. K., Sporn, J. R., and Molinoff, P. B. (1978): *J. Pharmacol. Exp. Ther.,* 207:446–457.

134. Zahniser, N. R., Minneman, K. P., and Molinoff, P. B. (1979): *Brain Res.,* 178:589–595.

135. Zawad, J. S., and Brown, F. C. (1984): *Biochem. Pharmacol.,* 33: 3799–3805.

Psychopharmacology:
The Third Generation of Progress,
edited by Herbert Y. Meltzer.
Raven Press, New York © 1987.

CHAPTER **26**

Biochemical Properties of CNS Dopamine Receptors

Ian Creese

In 1978 I authored a review on this same topic for *Psychopharmacology: A Generation of Progress* (19). This was 6 years after the discovery that dopamine (DA) could stimulate cyclic AMP production in the brain and 3 years after the first studies of radioligand binding to DA receptors had been successfully undertaken. At the end of that review I asked the question "What, then, is the exact relationship between the DA-sensitive adenylate cyclase and the [^{3}H]DA and [^{3}H]haloperidol binding sites of the DA receptor?" Research has progressed sufficiently far now, I think, to answer this question.

By 1978 two ligands, the agonist, [^{3}H]DA, and the antagonist, [^{3}H]haloperidol, had been used in radioligand binding experiments. Both radioligands labeled sites that were enriched in the striatum, the densest and largest DA terminal area, and both had the pharmacological characteristics expected of DA receptors. For example, DA was the most potent neurotransmitter candidate that acted as a competitive inhibitor of both ligands, whereas classic DA receptor antagonists, the antipsychotic neuroleptic drugs, were more potent competitors than any other class of pharmacological agents. However, the pharmacological specificity of the binding sites for these two ligands differed in specific details. Briefly summarized, dopaminergic agonists were more potent at inhibiting [^{3}H]DA binding than they were at inhibiting [^{3}H]haloperidol binding, whereas dopaminergic antagonists were more potent at inhibiting [^{3}H]haloperidol than [^{3}H]DA binding.

Radioligand binding studies and their analysis have become a great deal more sophisticated today than then, using nonlinear least squares curve fitting computer programs such as LIGAND (65). Even before their use, however, it was noted that in the competition experiments

discussed above, there were complex binding interactions occurring. For example, when the agonist apomorphine competed for [^{3}H]DA binding, the resultant competition curve had a pseudo-Hill slope of 1, indicating that both apomorphine and the radioligand were interacting with a homogeneous set of binding sites. However, when apomorphine competed for [^{3}H]haloperidol binding, the competition curve was more shallow, indicating that the law of mass action was not being followed and that the binding of the ligands was not occurring to a homogeneous population of binding sites. The interpretation of these data was not obvious, especially when the results of studies of the DA-sensitive adenylate cyclase were also considered. For example, DA had been shown to stimulate adenylate cyclase activity, but half maximal stimulation required high, micromolar concentrations. Whereas phenothiazine neuroleptics were potent competitive antagonists of DA-stimulated adenylate cyclase activity, the butyrophenone neuroleptics such as haloperidol were much weaker than would be expected from their *in vivo* clinical and antidopaminergic activity in animals (reviewed in ref. 43). Thus, the nanomolar affinity of the binding sites for [^{3}H]DA did not correlate with DA's ability to stimulate adenylate cyclase activity. Similarly, haloperidol was 100-fold more potent at its binding site than was its ability to inhibit DA stimulation of adenylate cyclase activity. It thus appeared that potentially three pharmacologically distinct putative DA receptors were being identified, or a single DA receptor could exist in a number of pharmacologically distinguishable states. Furthermore, only affinity to compete for [^{3}H]-haloperidol binding sites was predictive of the *in vivo* activities of numerous neuroleptics as antipsychotic drugs or of their antidopaminergic activity in animals (15,76).

This observation suggested that the [³H]haloperidol binding site was "the" DA receptor that was central to most of the behavioral effects attributed to DA receptor activity.

The past eight years of research have clarified the previous data. Stated briefly, it is now clear that there are two major DA receptor subtypes: D_1 receptors, which are linked to the stimulation of adenylate cyclase, and D_2 receptors, which are linked to the inhibition of this enzyme. This nomenclature, originally suggested by Spano, has been generally accepted (46). [³H]Haloperidol and the more recently used butyrophenone [³H]spiperone (also called [³H]spiroperidol) bind specifically to the D_2 receptor. It is interesting to note that D_2 receptors escaped biochemical detection until they were first characterized in radioligand binding studies! ³H-Agonists such as [³H]dopamine, [³H]apomorphine, and N-[³H]propylnorapomorphine (NPA) bind to both D_1 and D_2 receptors. Some antagonists, such as [³H]flupentixol, also bind to both D_1 and D_2 receptors. Although the binding of antagonists follows mass action kinetics at each receptor subtype, the binding of agonists is complex because both the D_1 and D_2 receptors exist in two affinity states for agonists. This property results from the association of both receptors with guanine nucleotide binding proteins (generically referred to as N), which act as intermediaries between the receptors and the adenylate cyclase. With such complex binding characteristics it is not surprising that it has taken a number of years to clarify the biochemical and radioligand binding properties of DA receptors. This summary description is amplified in Table 1.

On top of these now understood biochemical complexities, the recent advent of *selective* D_1 receptor agonists and antagonists has again confused our understanding of the behavioral properties of DA receptors. Previously, it was demonstrated that the affinities of agonists and antagonists at D_2 receptors were predictive of many, if not all, biochemical and behavioral dopaminergic responses (73,75). This left the D_1 receptor (which is present in many brain regions at much higher concentrations than D_2 receptors) without a function, leading some to question its reality as a receptor in the first place (50). However, it is now clear that many of the functions that have been ascribed to D_2 receptors can also be stimulated or antagonized by drug interactions at D_1 receptors (reviewed in ref. 10).

I will now highlight some of the research of the past decade which has clarified our understanding of DA receptor biochemistry and function.

THE D_1 DOPAMINE RECEPTOR

The discovery that cyclic AMP was a second messenger for many hormone systems in the periphery stimulated the research that lead to the demonstration that DA could stimulate cyclic AMP production in the CNS (47). Although not a response of great magnitude (maximal stimulation generally no more than double basal activity), it is a robust phenomenon and can be demonstrated in all areas that receive a DA terminal field, as well as in dopaminergic cell body areas. A specific phosphoprotein, DARPP-32, appears to be phosphorylated in response to D_1 receptor activation (86).

Although [³H]flupentixol labels D_2 as well as D_1 receptors in striatum, it can be used to label selectively D_1 receptors by including in the assays a concentration of unlabeled spiperone, which blocks [³H]flupentixol binding to D_2 but not to D_1 receptors (40,54). The competitions of dopaminergic antagonists for D_1 receptor-specific [³H]flupentixol binding to rat striatal membranes exhibit pseudo-Hill slope factors close to 1, and curves model best to a single homogeneous binding site. The absolute potencies of 20 dopaminergic antagonists to inhibit D_1 receptor-specific [³H]flupentixol binding have been compared to their abilities to inhibit DA-stimulated adenylate cyclase activity, and the two potencies show an impressive correlation ($r = 0.95$; $p < 0.001$) (54). A novel benzazepine, SCH23390, has recently been identified as a selective D_1 receptor antagonist (42). It has subnanomolar affinity for D_1 receptors and is more than 100-fold weaker at D_2 receptors (23,41). It has been radiolabeled to high specific activity and is now the optimal D_1 receptor radioligand (8,36). Some structurally related compounds have proven to be potent and selective D_1 agonists, typified by the partial agonist SKF38393 (78). Most DA agonists stimulate adenylate cyclase activity with micromolar affinities, and ergot alkaloids have been described as partial agonists or antagonists with submicromolar to micromolar potencies. Early radioligand binding studies reported that the affinities of dopaminergic agonists to inhibit [³H]flupentixol binding were also micromolar (41). However, detailed studies of agonist binding to ³H-antagonist-labeled D_1 receptors have revealed a heterogeneity of agonist binding states. In contrast to antagonist/[³H]flupentixol curves, agonist/[³H]flupentixol curves exhibit heterogeneous characteristics with pseudo-Hill coefficients much less than 1, and which are best described by a two-site fit (52). Thus, although [³H]flupentixol labels all sites with equal affinity, agonists discriminate two affinity binding states termed R_H, which has high nanomolar affinity (K_H), and R_L, which has low micromolar affinity (K_L). A striking correlation has been observed between the percent maximal response (relative intrinsic activity) found for the agonists examined versus their ratio of K_L/K_H values. Literature estimates of the K_{act} for agonist stimulation of adenylate cyclase activity correlates with estimates of K_L determined from binding assays (52).

Guanine nucleotides such as GTP have been demonstrated to regulate agonist-receptor interactions in a variety of hormone and neurotransmitter systems, particularly those which regulate adenylate cyclase activity (72). In these systems, GTP acts to reduce agonist affinity for the receptor. GTP generally exerts no effect on antagonist binding. In the presence of 0.3 mM GTP, DA/[³H]flupentixol or [³H]SCH23390 curves are shifted to the right and steepened (36,54,77). Computer analyses of curves in the presence of GTP show that the major effect is to reduce the %R_H. GTP has no effect on [³H]antagonist affinity or B_{max}. Taken together, these data suggest that the high- and low-affinity agonist binding components found in competition experiments represent partially interconvertible states of a single D_1 receptor (54).

Interconversion of agonist binding states has now been proposed for several other monoaminergic receptors (for review see ref. 55), including the D_2 DA receptor of brain and pituitary (79). These studies have proposed a generalized

TABLE 1. *Dopamine receptor subtypes*

D$_1$ (Synonyms D-1, DA$_1$ in the periphery)

Agonist stimulation leads to increased cAMP formation followed by phosphorylation of intracellular proteins including dopamine and adenosine 3'5'monophosphate-regulated phosphoprotein (DARPP-32).

Receptor/adenylate cyclase interaction is mediated by a guanine nucleotide-binding regulatory protein, N$_s$. Receptor-binding affinity of agonists is dependent on the degree of association of R and N$_s$, which is regulated by GTP and by divalent cations.

$$R_H \underset{Ca^{2+} \text{ or } Mg^{2+}}{\overset{GTP}{\underset{\leftarrow}{\rightarrow}}} R_L$$

(high agonist affinity)　(low agonist affinity)

"D$_3$"

R$_H$ represents the D$_1$ dopamine receptor in association with N$_s$. This association is facilitated by divalent cations and perhaps agonist binding to R. The binding of GTP to N$_s$ dissociates the D$_1$ dopamine receptor from N$_s$ to give R$_L$. Antagonists have identical affinity for R$_H$ and R$_L$.

Agonist affinity for R$_L$ correlates with agonist potency in stimulating cyclic AMP production. The binding site identified directly in radioligand studies with ^{3}H-agonists (R$_H$) corresponds to the binding site previously termed "D$_3$".

Selective (partial) agonist: SKF 38393
Selective antagonist: SCH23390

Location and function of D$_1$ receptors

Central nervous system: postsynaptic to dopamine neuron terminals and dendrites in CNS (i.e., striatum, nucleus accumbens, olfactory tubercle, substantia nigra, etc.). Function: unclear.

Vertebrate retina: in the teleost localized specifically to horizontal cells. Function: unknown.

Bovine parathyroid gland. Function: increase parathyroid hormone release.

Vascular smooth muscle (canine renal and mesentery vascular bed most used model system). Function: vascular relaxation.

SKF38393 stimulates grooming and some types of stereotypic motor behavior patterns in rodents. SCH23390 can block these behaviors and induce catalepsy. SCH23390 can also block behaviors stimulated by D$_2$ agonists in normal rats. This suggests a functional interaction between D$_1$ and D$_2$ dopamine receptors on the same neurons, or, alternatively, between convergent neuronal systems activated by D$_1$ and D$_2$ dopamine receptors, respectively. D$_1$ dopamine receptors are reduced in Huntington's chorea, increased in some Parkinson's disease patients, and maybe decreased in schizophrenia where their linkage with adenylate cyclase may be modified.

Relative selectivity of some popular agonists and ergot alkaloids.

Selective D$_1$ SKF38393 ≥ SKF82526 (Fenoldopam) ≫ Apomorphine = Dopamine = ADTN > (−)N-propylnorapomorphine > Bromocryptine > Pergolide ≫ Quinpirole (LY171555) Selective D$_2$

Relative selectivity of some popular antagonists

Selective D$_1$ SCH23390 ≫ α-Flupentixol = Fluphenazine = (+)Butaclamol = Chlorpromazine > Haloperidol > Pimozide > Spiperone > Domperidone > (−)Sulpiride Selective D$_2$.

D$_2$ (Synonyms D-2, DA$_2$ in the periphery)

Agonist stimulation leads to decreased cyclic AMP formation. Receptor/adenylate cyclase interaction is mediated by a guanine nucleotide-binding regulatory protein, N$_i$. Receptor binding affinity of agonists is dependent on degree of association R with N$_i$. This is regulated by GTP and mono- and divalent cations.

$$R_H \underset{Ca^{2+} \text{ or } Mg^{2+}}{\overset{\substack{GTP \\ Na^+}}{\underset{\leftarrow}{\rightarrow}}} R_L$$

(high agonist affinity)　(low agonist affinity)

"D$_4$"

R$_H$ represents the D$_2$ dopamine receptor in association with N$_i$. This association is facilitated by divalent cations and perhaps agonist binding to R. The binding of GTP to N$_i$ or the presence of Na$^+$ dissociates the D$_2$ dopamine receptor from N$_i$ to give R$_L$. Antagonists have identical affinity for R$_H$ and R$_L$.

Agonist affinity for R$_H$ correlates best with potency at inhibiting adenylate cyclase and prolactin release in the pituitary. Agonist affinity for R$_L$ correlates best with potency in increasing striatal acetylcholine levels or decreasing striatal adenylate cyclase activity. R$_H$ was previously termed D$_4$ by Seeman and R$_L$, D$_2$. This nomenclature has fallen into disuse. However, Schwartz has termed the dopamine receptor in the pituitary D-2 but feels a distinct subclass is present in the striatum and enriched in the olfactory bulb. This site has extra high affinity for sulpiride and other benzamides and he terms it D-4. This site may correspond to previously identified ^{3}H-butyrophenone binding sites, which are not GTP sensitive.

Selective agonist: Quinpirole (LY171555)
Selective antagonist: Spiperone

Location and function of D$_2$ receptors

Pituitary gland: anterior lobe mammotrophs. Function: inhibit cyclic AMP and prolactin release. May also regulate Ca^{2+} channels and phosphoinosital turnover.

Intermediate lobe melanotrophs. Function: inhibit cyclic AMP and αMSH release.

Striatum: Cholinergic interneurons. Function: inhibit acetylcholine release.

Dopamine nerve terminals. Function: autoreceptors, inhibit dopamine release and modulate dopamine turnover.

Substantia nigra: dopamine neuron soma. Function: inhibit dopamine neuron firing.

Carotid body. Function: depress spontaneous chemosensory discharge.

Chemosensitive trigger zone. Function: emesis.

Sympathetic nerve terminals in many tissues. Function: inhibit norepinephrine release.

Activation of CNS D$_2$ dopamine receptors leads to increased motor activity and stereotyped motor behavior. In humans, psychosis with stereotyped behavior and thinking patterns can also develop. D$_2$ and mixed D$_2$/D$_1$ dopamine receptor antagonists are antipsychotic and can produce Parkinson's disease-like rigidity in humans or catalepsy in animals. CNS D$_2$ dopamine receptors are increased in schizophrenics and in patients with Parkinson's disease who are not treated with L-dopa. D$_2$ dopamine receptors are decreased in the striatum of patients with Huntington's chorea.

ternary complex model modified from the original models of Boeynaems and Dumont (9) and Jacobs and Cuatrecasas (44). Such models involve, in a simplified form, a two-step process and three components for ligand binding:

$$L + R \rightarrow LR$$

$$LR + N \rightarrow LRN$$

where N is the third membrane component, a guanine nucleotide binding protein. In this model both agonists or antagonists (L) participate in the first step, but only agonists induce a conformational change in the receptor (R) such that the second reaction takes place. Agonists have higher affinity for the "ternary complex" (LRN) than they do for the binary complex (LR). Thus the complex of agonist, receptor, and guanine nucleotide binding protein represents the R_H state seen in the membranes. The proportion of total receptor represented as R_H may be limited by equilibrium constraints or N/R stoichiometry or both factors. The binding of GTP to N promotes instability of the ternary complex and a concomitant reduction or dissipation of R_H. The formation of the ternary complex with N_s ultimately leads to stimulation (or with N_i to inhibition) of adenylate cyclase activity (24,48).

THE D_2 DOPAMINE RECEPTOR

In contrast to D_1 receptors, D_2 receptors are now functionally classified as inhibiting adenylate cyclase activity upon agonist occupation. Whereas most brain areas contain both D_1 and D_2 receptors, D_2 receptors are the sole subtype in the anterior and intermediate pituitary glands, and in neither of these tissues does DA elicit its physiological effects through the stimulation of cyclic AMP synthesis. Indeed, Kebabian and colleagues (13,63,64) have elegantly shown that in the intermediate pituitary DA inhibits the β-adrenergic agonist-stimulated synthesis of cyclic AMP, leading to a diminution of hormone release, whereas in the anterior pituitary DA inhibits basal and vasoactive intestinal peptide stimulation of adenylate cyclase (25,70). Although DA inhibition of adenylate cyclase activity in the CNS went unobserved for many years, the advent of SCH23390 has allowed the stimulation of D_1 receptors to be blocked, allowing the smaller magnitude D_2 inhibition to be uncovered (68). This inhibition is only a few percent of basal and must be amplified for easy study, either by a partial membrane purification (69) or by increasing basal activity with forskolin (7,87). D_2 receptor activation can also reduce the D_1 receptor-stimulated efflux of cyclic AMP from striatal slices in vitro (81).

The pharmacological profile of D_2 receptors is also clearly distinct from that of D_1 receptors (Table 1). Agonists consistently demonstrate higher affinities in eliciting a biochemical or physiological response at most D_2 receptors than at D_1 receptors. Apomorphine is a potent agonist with full intrinsic activity at D_2 receptors, in contrast to its partial agonist activity at D_1 receptors. Similarly, various dopaminergic ergots (e.g., bromocriptine, lisuride, lergotrile) are full, potent (effective at nanomolar concentrations) agonists at D_2 receptors compared to their weak, partial

agonist or antagonist activity at D_1 receptors. Phenothiazines and thioxanthenes are potent antagonists of D_2 receptors, although because of their equally high affinity for D_1 receptors, they are not useful for discriminating between the receptor subtypes. In contrast, butyrophenones and related drugs (e.g., domperidone, pimozide) are very potent antagonists of D_2 receptors but exhibit only weak affinity for D_1 receptors. Similarly, substituted benzamides (e.g., sulpiride, metaclopramide) have high to moderate affinity at D_2 receptors but are inactive at D_1 receptors.

In pituitary membranes, the radiolabeled butyrophenone [³H]spiperone binds exclusively to DA receptors. Analysis of saturation data indicates a homogeneous population of binding sites. Antagonist competition curves exhibit monophasic, mass-action characteristics with pseudo-Hill coefficients equal to 1. In contrast, agonist competition curves with [³H]spiperone exhibit pseudo-Hill coefficients of less than unity and the data are best explained by a two-state binding model. Interestingly, the two states are present in membranes in approximately equal proportions. In the presence of GTP, agonist curves shift to the right and their slopes steepen (pseudo-Hill coefficient = 1). Computer analysis of these data now indicates a single homogeneous population of binding sites, for which the affinity for the agonist is not significantly different from its K_L value of the control curve. We also characterized the binding of the radiolabeled agonist [³H]NPA to D_2 receptors in bovine anterior pituitary membranes. One of the more striking findings with this radioligand is that its B_{max} is approximately 50% that of [³H]spiperone, suggesting that [³H]NPA labels only the high-affinity agonist state (R_H) seen in agonist/[³H]spiperone curves. This is further supported by the finding that agonist/[³H]NPA competition curves are homogeneous, with single affinities that do not differ significantly from the K_H values obtained from the corresponding agonist/[³H]spiperone curve. Furthermore, saturating concentrations of GTP completely abolish the specific [³H]NPA binding to pituitary membranes (79). These and similar observations suggest that a modification of the ternary complex model is applicable to the pituitary D_2 receptor (14,79,88). In contrast to D_1 receptors, agonists' K_H values at D_2 receptors correlate with their potencies to inhibit adenylate cyclase activity and prolactin release (58).

Several lines of evidence suggest that the majority of high-affinity binding sites for [³H]butyrophenones in the striatum are identical to the D_2 pituitary receptor (18,75). It should be noted that [³H]spiperone has high affinity for serotonergic receptors and these must be "masked" with S-2 antagonists, such as ketanserin, for selective D_2 receptor labeling (31). The K_D for [³H]spiperone binding to DA receptors in striatum is in excellent agreement with the value obtained in bovine anterior pituitary. As in pituitary, ³H-agonist ligands can, under appropriate conditions, label these same sites with high affinity (5,29), and the affinity of agonists is partially reduced by guanine nucleotides with a specificity similar to that of pituitary (20,89,90). Pertussis toxin, which interacts with N_i, abolishes the ability of GTP to affect agonist binding (28,49). Striatal kainic acid lesion, which destroys the intrinsic striatal neurons, removes about 50% of the D_2 receptors (74). Some of the remaining D_2 receptors appear, from lesion studies, to be located on the presynaptic terminals of the cortical input to the striatum and may regulate glutamate release. These D_2 receptors are less sensitive to GTP than the D_2 receptors in the pituitary or on the intrinsic striatal neurons (21). Other studies suggest that such receptors may have higher affinity for certain benzamide antagonist ligands and demonstrate a different regional localization (80). Since these "discriminant" benzamides have a somewhat different behavioral profile from classic D_2 receptor antagonists, these binding sites may be identifying another subtype of DA receptor. There is also some recent evidence that some D_2 receptors may be coupled to calcium channels or phosphoinosital turnover and not adenylate cyclase (61).

IDENTIFICATION OF BINDING SITES LABELED WITH AGONIST RADIOLIGANDS

In addition to studies of agonist interactions with DA receptors labeled by ^{3}H-antagonists, ^{3}H-agonists have been used to directly label dopaminergic receptors/recognition sites in the brain. ^{3}H-Agonist ligands label both the high-affinity agonist binding site of the D_2 receptor and an additional site previously termed D_3 (75). Competition by the potent D_2 receptor antagonists spiperone or domperidone for radiolabeled agonist high-affinity binding sites demonstrates markedly biphasic curves. The portion of ^{3}H-agonist binding for which these antagonists exhibit subnanomolar affinity identifies high-affinity agonist binding to the D_2 receptor, whereas the portion of ^{3}H-agonist binding inhibited by submicromolar concentrations of these antagonists defines the D_3 binding site (51,75). Early studies by Nagy et al. (66) and Sokoloff et al. (80) suggested that the D_3 binding site represents presynaptic DA autoreceptors, since removal of nigrostriatal terminals by 6-hydroxydopamine (6-OHDA) decreased D_3 binding. However, such decreased D_3-specific binding is an artifact of depleting endogenous DA, and D_3 binding sites are entirely postsynaptically located in striatum. 6-OHDA-induced lesions, as well as removing DA terminals, also produce a concomitant depletion of striatal DA. Importantly, acute reserpinization, which depletes DA but without loss of DA terminals, also produces decreases in the number of D_3 binding sites similar to those produced by 6-OHDA denervation (6,51). Preincubating membranes in vitro from reserpine-treated animals with either DA (100 nM) or the supernatant from a membrane preparation of a normal striatum reverses the loss in D_3 binding. This effect is specific for DA agonists, as catechol or isoproterenol is ineffective in reversing this loss. Similarly, preincubating striatal membranes from 6-OHDA-denervated striata with DA also reverses the lesion-induced loss in D_3 ^{3}H-agonist binding. Thus, the loss in D_3 binding seen after these two treatments appears to result from the depletion of striatal DA. Furthermore, D_3 binding sites must be postsynaptic to the nigrostriatal terminals, since the addition of DA to 6-OHDA-lesioned striata, which lack DA terminals, produces normal levels of D_3 binding. Studies of binding in striata after kainic acid lesion support this hypothesis, since D_3 binding is decreased by 75% after this treatment, which removes striatal cell bodies.

Why membrane preparation in the presence of endogenous DA increases subsequent D_3 binding is not known, but must result from the stabilization of high-affinity agonist binding sites. Since D_1 receptors demonstrate a high-affinity agonist-binding state, we investigated whether D_3 binding sites could represent ^{3}H-agonist binding to the high-affinity, R_H, state of the D_1 receptor (52). To test this hypothesis, it was first necessary to characterize radiolabeled agonist binding to D_3 binding sites selectively. D_3 binding sites show clear stereoselectivity in interacting with dopaminergic antagonists such as butaclamol and thioxanthenes. However, unlike the D_2 receptor, antagonists such as spiroperidol, pimozide, and domperidone are relatively weak (K_i values 0.1–5 μM), whereas substituted benzamide neuroleptics such as sulpiride and metaclopramide are virtually inactive. This profile of antagonist rank order potencies is very similar to those seen for the D_1 receptor identified either by ^{3}H]flupentixol or ^{3}H]SCH23390 binding or by DA activation of adenylate cyclase. Indeed, impressive correlations are seen among antagonist inhibition constants for all three measures. An impressive correlation also exists between the K_H agonist affinity estimates from agonist/^{3}H]flupentixol competitions and agonist affinities for D_3-specific ^{3}H]DA binding sites. These results strongly support the hypothesis that D_3 binding sites are the high-affinity agonist binding state (R_H) of the D_1 receptor (52).

RECEPTOR REGULATION

Regardless of the means by which high-affinity D_1 receptor agonist binding sites are measured, the sites comprised only 15 to 40% of the number of sites that can be labeled by ^{3}H-antagonists. Such limits on the formation of the agonist R_H state may reflect either equilibrium constraints on the formation of the ternary complex or a functional stoichiometric limitation of N_s relative to R. The normal ratios of N_s/R in the membrane can be varied by the peripheral administration of the irreversible protein-modifying reagent, N-ethoxycarbonyl-1-ethoxy-1,2-dihydroquinoline (EEDQ) which irreversibly inactivates DA receptors (30). After in vivo EEDQ treatment, although there is a great decrease in the number of D_1 receptors and DA stimulation of adenylate cyclase activity, there is no change in the %R_H for DA/^{3}H]SCH23390 competitions, suggesting that its formation must, at least, be limited by equilibrium determinants. Importantly, no change in the stimulation of adenylate cyclase above basal activity is observed in the presence of the putative N_s effectors: GTP, guanosine 5'-(β-γ-imido)triphosphate (Gpp(NH)p), and NaF. Likewise, stimulation by forskolin, which acts directly at the catalytic subunit, is unchanged. Thus, peripherally administered EEDQ acts in a receptor-specific manner [its D_1 receptor effects can be blocked by prior administration of SCH23390 but not spiperone (35,59)], but leaves N_s and the catalytic subunit of adenylate cyclase functionally intact. Thus, peripheral EEDQ administration may be used as a tool to assess the stoichiometry of D_1 receptor/effector interactions by progressively blocking increasing numbers of receptors and monitoring adenylate cyclase activity. Interestingly, we found that approximately 40% of D_1 receptor binding sites may be lost without a significant reduction in the V_{max} of

DA-stimulated adenylate cyclase activity. Thus, these data suggest that the D_1 receptor population itself is not a stoichiometrically limiting factor in agonist stimulation of adenylate cyclase, i.e., there are "spare" receptors (35,37).

This finding has important neurophysiologic implications. Receptor occupancy is determined by transmitter (or drug) concentration. Since only approximately 60% occupancy of the normal D_1 receptor population is required for maximal effector stimulation, the transmitter concentration necessary to elicit full stimulation ($\sim 2 \times K_D$) is considerably less than that concentration necessary for 100% receptor occupancy ($100 \times K_D$). The existence of these "spare" receptors, then, enhances neurotransmission by reducing the effective concentration of DA required to diffuse across the synaptic cleft to achieve a full response.

DA receptors are dynamic macromolecules under the influence of a large variety of factors; they appear to be subject to regulatory mechanisms of up and down regulation similar to those that modulate other neurotransmitter and hormone receptors (17). The pharmacological manipulation of these regulatory mechanisms may prove to be a sensitive means of therapy in the numerous psychiatric and neurological diseases in which DA system dysfunction has been implicated. Furthermore, disruptions of the normal regulatory mechanisms may be etiologic in neurologic and psychiatric diseases and the side effects of neuroleptic drugs. Interestingly, since EEDQ irreversibly modifies both D_1 and D_2 receptors it can be utilized to determine a measure of DA receptor turnover rate by determining the rate at which new receptors appear after EEDQ treatment. We have already demonstrated that chronic DA depletion increases receptor turnover, whereas the natural aging process leads to both absolute decreases in receptor number and reductions in the turnover rates of both D_1 (67) and D_2 receptors (32,53).

BEHAVIORAL AND BIOCHEMICAL INTERACTIONS OF D_1 AND D_2 RECEPTORS

Neuroleptics administered to rodents *in vivo* induce catalepsy, suppress conditioned avoidance responses and learned responses for positive reinforcers, and antagonize the hyperactivity and stereotypy responses elicited by DA agonists. These responses are elicited by both D_2 receptor antagonists and mixed D_1/D_2 receptor antagonists and are generally predictive of antipsychotic activity. Consequently, these behavioral effects have been used by the pharmaceutical industry as screens for potential new antipsychotic drugs (45). Neuroleptics are also generally antiemetic and have been shown to induce hyperprolactinemia by blocking DA receptors in the anterior pituitary. Since this tissue lacks D_1 receptors, it is clear that hyperprolactinemia is a pure D_2-receptor-mediated response. Whereas SCH23390 is a selective D_1 receptor antagonist, it surprisingly mimics some of the behavioral effects previously associated with D_2 receptor antagonists—such as blocking agonist-induced stereotypy and hyperactivity, as well as inducing catalepsy (12,38,42,57; reviewed in ref. 10). However, SCH23390 neither antagonizes emesis nor produces hyperprolactinemia,

indicating that SCH23390 administered *in vivo* is probably not acting as an antagonist at D_2 receptors.

That SCH23390 can induce these neuroleptic behavioral effects without blockade of D_2 receptors suggests that D_1 and D_2 receptors may have similar behavioral functions and that SCH23390 may be an effective antipsychotic agent. Why might this be important—certainly more than enough neuroleptics already exist? A major side effect of the chronic neuroleptic administration used in treating schizophrenia is tardive dyskinesia, characterized by uncontrollable movements of the mouth, tongue, and extremities. The chronic treatment of animals with neuroleptics does not usually result in such obvious dyskinetic movements (85), but it does produce an enhanced sensitivity to the motoric effects of DA agonists (83). An increase in the number of D_2 receptors is concomitantly produced (18). Since chronic treatment with either D_2-receptor-selective or mixed D_1/D_2-receptor-selective antagonists produces identical behavioral supersensitivity, but D_2-receptor-selective antagonists cause a *selective* D_2 receptor up-regulation, it has been concluded that the increase in D_2 receptors is both necessary and sufficient for the production of the enhanced behavioral sensitivity to DA agonists (27,56). It has therefore been suggested that the side effect of tardive dyskinesia may result from a selective D_2 receptor up-regulation, although this has not yet been directly shown in biochemical studies of drug-treated schizophrenic brains (22). If chronic treatment with the D_1-receptor-selective antagonist SCH23390 does not increase D_2 receptor number, it may therefore lack the liability to produce tardive dyskinesia. Indeed, we found that after treating rats chronically with SCH23390 (0.5 mg/kg/day for 21 days), striatal D_1 receptors were significantly increased whereas no change was observed in the D_2 receptor population (16).

Interestingly, although the D_1 receptor B_{max} was increased over 20% by the chronic SCH23390 treatment, DA stimulation of adenylate cyclase activity was enhanced by a smaller amount (9–13%). However, this increase most probably reflected an overall increase in guanine nucleotide-stimulated enzyme activity, suggesting that "N" was, in some manner, up-regulated with the receptor. Since we have demonstrated the existence of spare D_1 receptors in control rats, it is not surprising that an approximately 20% increase in D_1 receptors after chronic SCH23390 treatment did not increase the V_{max} of stimulated adenylate cyclase activity. Receptor up-regulation probably does not act directly to increase maximal cyclic AMP production, but rather supersensitivity is manifested by reducing the effective transmitter (or drug) concentration necessary to induce the same maximal response.

Unlike chronic neuroleptic treatment, where neither an increase nor a decrease in spontaneous locomotor activity was observed (82), rats chronically treated with SCH23390 exhibited a more than twofold higher level of spontaneous locomotor activity. Again, in contrast to classic neuroleptics where tolerance develops to their cataleptogenic effects after chronic treatment (26), rats receiving chronic administration of SCH23390 for 21 days demonstrated no tolerance to its cataleptogenic action. This suggests that the neuronal network through which chronic SCH23390 elicits its effects is different from and is not regulated in the same manner as the neuronal network through which classic neuroleptics exert their effects. Other research supports this hypothesis. After treatment with either D_1- or D_2-receptor-selective agonists, unilaterally 6-OHDA-lesioned rats demonstrate contralateral circling behavior (3,4,33,34), and reserpinized or bilaterally 6-OHDA-lesioned animals demonstrate hypermotility and oral stereotypy (1,2). In these cases, although similar behaviors were induced by the D_1 and D_2 receptor agonists, behaviors induced by D_2 receptor agonists were blocked only by D_2 receptor antagonists and, similarly, D_1 receptor antagonists only blocked D_1 receptor agonist responses. These data suggest that although D_1- and D_2-receptor-mediated behaviors may be overtly similar or even identical, they are independently modulated and can be distinguished from each other through these various pharmacologic treatments.

In concert with these data, the chronically SCH23390-treated rats responded to the selective D_1 receptor agonist, SKF38393, with potentiated locomotor behavior. The rats also showed a more intense stereotypy response to SKF38393 than did the chronic saline-treated rats. Unlike mixed D_1/D_2 receptor agonists, SKF38393 induced stereotyped grooming in both groups of rats. However, grooming quickly diminished in the control rats, but the chronic SCH23390-treated rats continued to groom and/or show stereotyped sniffing and rearing in one location over the first hour in response to SKF38393.

Surprisingly, a similar potentiation in locomotor activity and stereotypy was observed in chronically SCH23390-treated rats after treatment with quinpirole (LY171555), the selective D_2 receptor agonist (84). Quinpirole initially induced intense stereotyped sniffing and rearing in one location in both groups. Between 50 and 80 min postinjection, some of the chronic SCH23390-treated rats were also showing stereotyped licking of the cage, although none of the control rats showed this response. A peak in locomotor stimulation at 140 min corresponded to the transition from stereotyped behavior in one location to locomotor activity. Surprisingly, locomotor activity was quickly attenuated in the chronically SCH23390-treated rats, and each rat "instantaneously" went from "sniff/locomotion" to "freezing" in position. This frozen posture was maintained for 5 to 10 min before the rats closed their eyes and apparently went to sleep. This response may prove to be a useful model for the "on-off" phenomenon seen during DA receptor agonist treatment of Parkinson's disease. One might speculate that this troublesome side effect may result from the up-regulation of D_1 receptors seen in this disease (71).

In *in vitro* binding studies, quinpirole has extremely low affinity for D_1 receptors, suggesting that it is unlikely that this drug might elicit these behaviors through D_1 DA receptors *in vivo*. Thus, the behavioral effects of a D_2 receptor agonist are potentiated after a selective D_1 receptor up-regulation. Certainly this is an anomalous response, given that SCH23390 has no *direct* effect on D_2 receptors *in vivo*. Paralleling the results presented herein, it has been demonstrated that although SCH23390 acts as a D_1 receptor antagonist, inducing catalepsy in rats, pretreatment with selective D_2 receptor agonists can prevent this response in a dose-dependent manner (60). Likewise, the behavioral effects of the D_1 receptor agonist SKF38393 could be partially reversed by the selective D_2 receptor antagonist metaclopramide (62). Breese and Mueller (11) have demonstrated that SCH23390 antagonism of locomotor activity induced by quinpirole seen in control rats may be prevented by 6-OHDA or reserpine treatment. That is, this D_1/D_2-DA receptor interaction is dependent on the integrity of catecholamine-containing neurons. These behavioral data, then, suggest that D_1- and D_2-receptor-activated neuronal systems are not functionally isolated. Rather, the behavioral data presented herein suggest that although the networks through which D_1 and D_2 receptors mediate behavioral effects appear to be functionally independent (i.e., separate, parallel systems), these systems are interactive in their modulation of motor function. Such observations, I am sure, will be the focus of the next decade of DA receptor research.

ACKNOWLEDGMENTS

I.C. is the recipient of an RSDA, ADAMHA MH00316. Supporting grants include the Scottish Rite Schizophrenia Research Program and the ADAMHA MH32990. I would like to thank A. Norman and E. Hess for their scientific contributions and Paula Martin for manuscript preparation.

REFERENCES

1. Arnt, J. (1985): *Eur. J. Pharmacol.*, 113:79–88.
2. Arnt, J. (1985): *Life Sci.*, 37:717–723.
3. Arnt, J., and Hyttel, J. (1984): *Eur. J. Pharmacol.*, 102:349–354.
4. Arnt, J., and Hyttel, J. (1985): *Psychopharmacology*, 85:346–352.
5. Bacopoulos, N. G. (1982): *Biochem. Pharmacol.*, 31:3085–3091.
6. Bacopoulos, N. G. (1984): *Life Sci.*, 34:307–315.
7. Battaglia, G., Norman, A. B., Hess, E. J., and Creese, I. (1985): *Neurosci. Lett.*, 59:177–182.
8. Billard, W., Ruperto, V., Crosby, G., Iorio, L. C., and Barnett, A. (1984): *Life Sci.*, 35:1885–1893.
9. Boeynaems, J. M., and Dumont, J. E. (1980): In: *Outlines of Receptor Theory*, pp. 226–242. Elsevier/North-Holland, Amsterdam.
10. Breese, G. R., and Creese, I., eds. (1986): *Neurobiology of Central D_1 Dopamine Receptors.* Plenum Press, New York.
11. Breese, G. R., and Mueller, R. A. (1985): *Eur. J. Pharmacol.*, 113:109–114.
12. Christensen, A. V., Arnt, J., Hyttel, J., Larsen, J. J., and Svendsen, O. (1984): *Life Sci.*, 34:1529–1540.
13. Cote, T. E., Grewe, C. W., and Kebabian, J. (1981): *Endocrinology*, 108:420–426.
14. Cote, T. E., Grey, E. A., and Sekura, R. D. (1984): *J. Biol. Chem.*, 259:8693–8698.
15. Creese, I., Burt, D. R., and Snyder, S. H. (1976): *Science*, 192:481–483.
16. Creese, I., and Chen, A. (1985): *Eur. J. Pharmacol.*, 109:127–128.
17. Creese, I., and Sibley, D. R. (1981): *Annu. Rev. Pharmacol. Toxicol.*, 21:357–391.
18. Creese, I., Sibley, D. R., Hamblin, M. W., and Leff, S. (1983): *Annu. Rev. Neurosci.*, 6:43–71.
19. Creese, I., and Snyder, S. H. (1978): In: *Psychopharmacology: A Generation of Progress*, edited by M. A. Lipton, A. DiMascio, and K. F. Killam, pp. 377–388. Raven Press, New York.
20. Creese, I., Usdin, T. B., and Snyder, S. H. (1979): *Mol. Pharmacol.*, 16:69–76.

21. Creese, I., Usdin, T. B., and Snyder, S. H. (1979): *Nature,* 278: 577–578.
22. Cross, A. J., Crow, T. J., Ferrier, I. N., Johnstone, E. C., McCreadie, R. M., Owen, F., Owens, D. G. C., and Poulter, M. (1983a): *J. Neural Transm. (Suppl.),* 18:265–272.
23. Cross, A. J., Marshal, R. D., Johnson, J. A., and Owen, F. (1983b): *Neuropharmacology,* 22:1327–1329.
24. De Lean, A., Stadel, J. M., and Lefkowitz, R. J. (1980): *J. Biol. Chem.,* 255:7108–7117.
25. Enjalbert, A., and Bockaert, J. (1983): *Mol. Pharmacol.,* 23:576–584.
26. Ezrin-Waters, C., and Seeman, P. (1977): *Eur. J. Pharmacol.,* 41: 321–327.
27. Fleminger, S., Rupniak, N. M. J., Hall, M. D., Jenner, P., and Marsden, C. D. (1983): *Biochem. Pharmacol.,* 32:2921–2927.
28. Fujita, N., Nakahiro, M., Fukuchi, I., Saito, K., and Yoshida, H. (1985): *Brain Res.,* 333:231–236.
29. Hamblin, M. W., and Creese, I. (1982): *Life Sci.,* 30:1587–1595.
30. Hamblin, M. W., and Creese, I. (1983): *Life Sci.,* 32:2247–2255.
31. Hamblin, M. W., Leff, S. E., and Creese, I. (1984): *Biochem. Pharmacol.,* 33:877–887.
32. Henry, J. M., and Roth, G. S. (1984): *Life Sci.,* 35:899–904.
33. Herrera-Marschitz, M., and Ungerstedt, U. (1984): *Eur. J. Pharmacol.,* 98:165–176.
34. Herrera-Marschitz, M., and Ungerstedt, U. (1985): *Eur. J. Pharmacol.,* 109:349–354.
35. Hess, E. J., Battaglia, G., Norman, A. B., and Creese, I. (1985): *Soc. Neurosci. Abstr.,* 11:313.
36. Hess, E. J., Battaglia, G., Norman, A. B., Iorio, L. C., and Creese, I. (1986): *Eur. J. Pharmacol.,* 121:31–38.
37. Hess, E. J., and Creese, I. (1986): In: *Neurobiology of Central D_1 DA Receptors,* edited by G. R. Breese and I. Creese, pp. 29–52. Plenum Press, New York.
38. Hoffman, D. C., and Beninger, R. J. (1985): *Pharmacol. Biochem. Behav.,* 22:341–342.
39. Hyttel, J. (1980): *Psychopharmacology,* 67:107–109.
40. Hyttel, J. (1984): In: *VIIIth International Symposium on Medicinal Chemistry,* edited by R. Dahlbom and J. L. G. Nilsson, pp. 426–439. Swedish Pharmaceutical Press, Stockholm.
41. Hyttel, J. (1984): *Neuropharmacology,* 23:1395–1401.
42. Iorio, L. C., Barnett, A., Leitz, F. H., Houser, V. P., and Korduba, C. A. (1983): *J. Pharmacol. Exp. Ther.,* 226:462–468.
43. Iversen, L. L. (1975): *Science,* 188:1084–1089.
44. Jacobs, S., and Cuatrecasas, P. (1976): *Biochem. Biophys. Acta,* 433:482–495.
45. Janssen, P. A. J., and Van Brever, W. F. M. (1978): In: *Handbook of Psychopharmacology,* edited by L. L. Iversen, S. D. Iversen, and S. H. Snyder, pp. 1–31. Plenum Press, New York.
46. Kebabian, J. W., and Calne, D. B. (1979): *Nature,* 277:93–96.
47. Kebabian, J. W., Petzold, G. L., and Greengard, P. (1972): *Proc. Natl. Acad. Sci. USA,* 79:2145–2149.
48. Kent, R. S., De Lean, A., and Lefkowitz, R. J. (1980): *Mol. Pharmacol.,* 17:14–23.
49. Kuno, T., Shirakawa, O., and Tanaka, C. (1983): *Biochem. Biophys. Res. Commun.,* 115:325–330.
50. Laduron, P. M. (1983): *Dopamine Receptors Am. Chem. Soc. Symp. Series 224,* edited by J. W. Kebabian and C. Kaiser, pp. 22–28. American Chemical Society Press, Washington, DC.
51. Leff, S. E., and Creese, I. (1983): *Nature,* 306:586–589.
52. Leff, S. E., and Creese, I. (1985): *Mol. Pharmacol.,* 27:184–192.
53. Leff, S. E., Gariano, R., and Creese, I. (1984): *Proc. Natl. Acad. Sci. USA,* 81:3910–3914.
54. Leff, S. E., Hamblin, M. W., and Creese, I. (1985): *Mol. Pharmacol.,* 27:171–183.
55. Limbird, L. E. (1981): *Biochem. J.,* 194:1–13.
56. Mackenzie, R. G., and Zigmond, M. J. (1985): *Eur. J. Pharmacol.,* 113:159–165.
57. Mailman, R. B., Schulz, D. W., Lewis, M. H., Staples, L., Rollema, H., and Dehaven, D. L. (1984): *Eur. J. Pharmacol.,* 101:159–160.
58. McDonald, W. M., Sibley, D. R., Kilpatrick, B. F., and Caron, M. C. (1984): *Mol. Cell. Endocrinol.,* 36:201–209.
59. Meller, E., Bohmaker, K., Goldstein, M., and Friedhoff, A. J. (1985): *J. Pharmacol. Exp. Ther.,* 233:656–662.
60. Meller, E., Kuga, S., Friedhoff, A. J., and Goldstein, M. (1985): *Life Sci.,* 36:1857–1864.
61. Memo, M., Carboni, E., Trabucchi, M., Carruba, M. O., and Spano, P. F. (1985): *Brain. Res.,* 347:253–257.
62. Molloy, A. G., and Waddington, J. L. (1985): *Eur. J. Pharmacol.,* 108:305–308.
63. Munemura, M., Cote, T. E., Tsuruta, K., et al. (1980): *Endocrinology,* 1683–1686.
64. Munemura, M., Eskay, R. L., and Kebabian, J. W. (1980): *Endocrinology,* 106:1795–1803.
65. Munson, P. J., and Rodbard, D. (1980): *Anal. Biochem.,* 107:220–239.
66. Nagy, J. I., Lee, T., Seeman, P., et al. (1978): *Nature,* 274:278–281.
67. Norman, A. B., Battaglia, G., and Creese, I. (1985): *Soc. Neurosci. Abstr.,* 11:457.
68. Onali, P., Olianas, M. C., and Gessa, G. L. (1984): *Eur. J. Pharmacol.,* 99:127–128.
69. Onali, P., Olianas, M. C., and Gessa, G. L. (1985): *Mol. Pharmacol.,* 28:138–145.
70. Onali, P., Schwartz, J. P., and Costa, E. (1981): *Proc. Natl. Acad. Sci. USA,* 78:6531–6534.
71. Raisman, R., Cash, R., Ruberg, M., Javoy-Agid, F., and Agid, Y. (1985): *Eur. J. Pharmacol.,* 113:476–468.
72. Rodbell, M. (1980): *Nature,* 284:17–22.
73. Schachter, M., Bedard, P., Debono, A. G., et al. (1980): *Nature,* 286:157–159.
74. Schwarcz, R., Creese, I., Coyle, J. T., et al. (1978): *Nature,* 271: 766–768.
75. Seeman, P. (1980): *Pharmacol. Rev.,* 32:229–313.
76. Seeman, P., Lee, T., Chau-Wong, M., and Wong, K. (1976): *Nature,* 261:717–719.
77. Seeman, P., Ulpian, C., Grigoriadis, D., Pri-Bar, I., and Buchman, O. (1985): *Biochem. Pharmacol.,* 34:151–154.
78. Setler, P. E., Sarau, H. M., Zirkle, C. L., and Saunders, H. L. (1978): *Eur. J. Pharmacol.,* 50:419.
79. Sibley, D. R., DeLean, A., and Creese, I. (1982): *J. Biol. Chem.,* 257:6351–6361.
80. Sokoloff, P., Redouane, K., Brann, M., Martres, M.-P., and Schwartz, J.-C. (1980): *Naunyn Schmiedebergs Arch. Pharmacol.,* 329:236–243.
81. Stoof, J. C., and Kebabian, J. W. (1981): *Nature,* 294:366–368.
82. Tarsy, D., and Baldessarini, R. J. (1974): *Neuropharmacology,* 13: 927–940.
83. Tarsy, D., and Baldessarini, R. J. (1984): *Annu. Rev. Med.,* 35: 605–623.
84. Tsuruta, K., Frey, E. A., Grewe, C. W., Cote, T. E., Eskay, R. L., and Kebabian, J. W. (1981): *Nature,* 292:463–465.
85. Waddington, J. L., Cross, A. J., Gamble, S. J., and Bourne, R. C. (1983): *Science,* 220:530–532.
86. Walaas, S. I., and Greengard, P. (1984): *J. Neurosci.,* 4:84–98.
87. Weiss, S., Sebben, M., Garcia-Sainz, J. A., and Bockaert, J. (1985): *Mol. Pharmacol.,* 27:595–599.
88. Wreggett, K. A., and DeLean, A. (1984): *Mol. Pharmacol.,* 26: 214–227.
89. Wreggett, K. A., and Seeman, P. (1984): *Mol. Pharmacol.,* 25:10–17.
90. Zahniser, N. R., and Molinoff, P. B. (1978): *Nature,* 275:453–455.

Psychopharmacology:
The Third Generation of Progress,
edited by Herbert Y. Meltzer.
Raven Press, New York © 1987.

CHAPTER 27

γ-Aminobutyric Acid (GABA) Receptors and Their Association with Benzodiazepine Recognition Sites

S. J. Enna and Hanns Möhler

A number of amino acids are considered neurotransmitter candidates (34). Those receiving the most intense scrutiny have been glutamic and aspartic acids, compounds that induce excitatory responses in the mammalian central nervous system, as well as γ-aminobutyric acid (GABA) and glycine, which are classified as inhibitory neurotransmitters. The majority of information relating to amino acid neurotransmitters has derived from studies with GABA, since more is known about its synthesis, metabolism, and pharmacological characteristics. Thus, investigators have at their disposal agents that inhibit GABA degradation and reuptake, as well as direct-acting GABA receptor agonists and antagonists (35,43). These tools have made it possible to characterize more fully the properties of GABAergic synapses as compared to other amino acid substances.

Interest in GABA has also been stimulated by suggestions that this transmitter system may be affected in a variety of central nervous system disorders, such as Huntington's disease, epilepsy, and Parkinson's disease (59,81,88). Moreover, manipulation of GABAergic transmission may have a beneficial effect in the treatment of anxiety and depression, and it has been hypothesized that GABAergic drugs may be useful in the management of schizophrenia (89).

Because GABA is present in relatively high concentrations in all areas of the mammalian brain and spinal cord (45), this transmitter system is considered a prime target for new psychotherapeutic agents. However, the extensive distribution of GABA has hindered the development of GABAergic drugs, since they tend to have a generalized effect on central nervous system function. Accordingly, to develop more selective agents it is necessary to identify differences among the various GABAergic synapses in brain, such as

pharmacologically and functionally distinct GABA receptors. This approach has met with some success in that two distinct GABA receptors have now been proposed (10,36). These sites, designated GABA$_A$ and GABA$_B$, differ with regard to their substrate specificity, ionic characteristics, and biochemical properties. One of the more important distinctions is that the GABA$_A$ receptor is associated with the neuronal membrane recognition site for benzodiazepines, a discovery that has provided new insights into the mechanism of action of this drug class (108). Although less is known about GABA$_B$ receptors, data suggest they serve to modulate receptor function for other neurotransmitters (65). The aim of the present report is to summarize current concepts relating to the pharmacological and functional properties of GABA receptor sites and their relationship to benzodiazepines. Particular emphasis is placed on evaluating these data from the perspective of psychopharmacology. Readers desiring a more detailed discussion of individual topics are urged to consult any of a number of monographs and reviews (26,37,39,41,47,107).

GABA$_A$ RECEPTORS

The initial data suggesting a neurotransmitter role for GABA in mammalian systems were derived from electrophysiological studies (30). These findings indicated that GABA causes a hyperpolarizing response in virtually all neuronal cells when applied at sufficient concentrations. Because of this apparent lack of selectivity, early investigators were reluctant to assign a neurotransmitter role for GABA. This attitude changed with the discovery of agents (bicuculline and picrotoxin) capable of inhibiting selectively the hyperpolarizing response to GABA (28). Since both of these compounds are rather potent convulsants, this finding confirmed the suggestion that GABA serves as an inhibitory transmitter substance.

Electrophysiological studies also revealed that the hyperpolarizing response to GABA is due to a change in chloride conductance (29,102). Since for most neurons the extracellular concentration of chloride exceeds that in the cytoplasm, GABA$_A$ receptor activation appears to facilitate the entry of this anion, increasing the firing threshold of the cell.

During the past decade ligand binding assays have made it possible to obtain more detailed knowledge of the biochemical and pharmacological properties of GABA$_A$ receptors (40). These investigations have indicated that GABA$_A$ receptor binding sites are located in virtually all regions of the central nervous system, from the retina to the spinal cord. Ligand binding data have also revealed that the brain contains a number of kinetically distinct GABA$_A$ receptors (44,46). Although it was initially believed that the site possessing the highest affinity for GABA normally mediates the response to this transmitter, more recent studies have suggested that a lower affinity receptor may be most closely associated with the effector system (3,17,66,103). These initial electrophysiological and biochemical studies demonstrated that the GABA$_A$ receptor consists of at least two basic components: the GABA$_A$ receptor recognition site and an associated ion channel (Fig. 1).

A number of substances have been found to selectively influence the GABA$_A$ receptor components (Fig. 1). Direct-acting agonists for the GABA$_A$ recognition site include muscimol, THIP (4,5,6,7-tetrahydroisoxazolo[5,4-c]pyridine-3-ol), and isoguvacine (69). Competitive antagonists for this site are bicuculline, securinine, and SR-95103 (2-[carboxy-3'-propyl]-3-amino-4-methyl-6-phenylpyridazinium) (6,20,44). In general, GABA$_A$ receptor agonists are central nervous system depressants, muscle relaxants, and

possess some antinociceptive properties, whereas the receptor antagonists are convulsants (38).

Drugs have also been found that directly modify the functioning of the chloride ion channel (Fig. 1). Included in this group are picrotoxin, TBPS (*tert*-butylbicyclophosphorothionate), and TBOB (4-*tert*-butyl-1-[4-cyanophenyl]-bicycloorthocarboxylate) (19,98,104). Selective binding sites for these chloride channel agents have been described using radiolabeled derivatives. All three appear to bind to the same site, and under the proper conditions, all can influence the binding of GABA$_A$ receptor agonists, indicating an allosteric relationship between the chloride channel and recognition site components (86,96). Inasmuch as these substances are convulsants, they are considered chloride channel antagonists.

A variety of centrally active drugs influence ligand attachment to the chloride channel binding site, including sedative-hypnotics, anticonvulsants, and some nonbenzodiazepine anxiolytics (62,105). Although none of these agents competitively interact with the picrotoxin site, their binding component seems to be more intimately associated with the chloride channel than with the GABA$_A$ receptor recognition site. Such findings indicate that GABA$_A$ receptor function can be pharmacologically manipulated in a variety of ways.

THE BENZODIAZEPINE RECOGNITION SITE

A major advance in understanding the mechanism of action of anxiolytics was the discovery of benzodiazepine binding sites in the mammalian central nervous system (77,97). Evidence that these sites mediate the responses to this drug class was provided by the finding that the relative affinities of benzodiazepines for this site paralleled their relative potencies in behavioral tests predictive of anxiolytic and anticonvulsant activity (13,78). A direct association

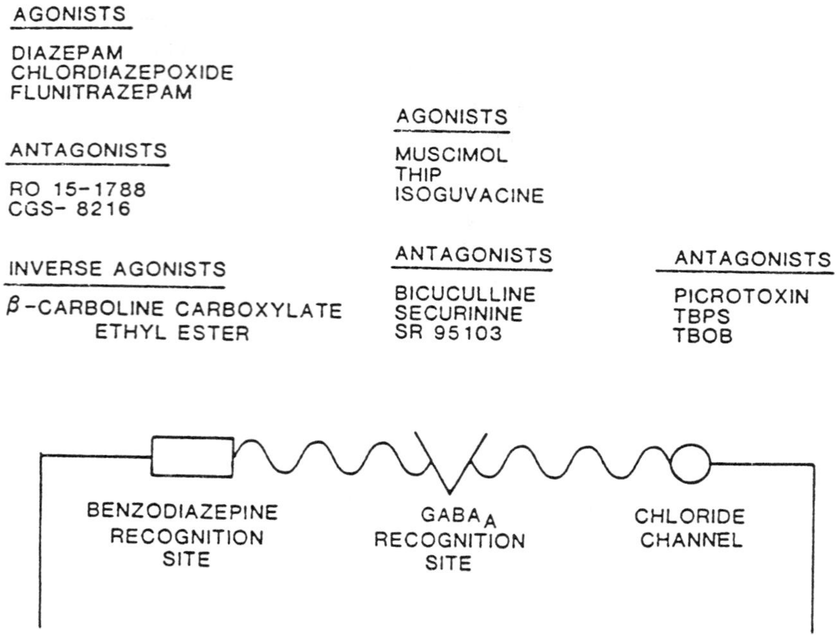

AGONISTS

DIAZEPAM
CHLORDIAZEPOXIDE
FLUNITRAZEPAM

ANTAGONISTS

RO 15-1788
CGS- 8216

INVERSE AGONISTS

β -CARBOLINE CARBOXYLATE
ETHYL ESTER

AGONISTS

MUSCIMOL
THIP
ISOGUVACINE

ANTAGONISTS

BICUCULLINE
SECURININE
SR 95103

ANTAGONISTS

PICROTOXIN
TBPS
TBOB

FIG. 1. Schematic representation of the components associated with GABA$_A$ receptors. Agents interacting at each site are listed above the individual components.

BENZODIAZEPINE RECOGNITION SITE   GABA$_A$ RECOGNITION SITE   CHLORIDE CHANNEL between the benzodiazepine binding component and GA-BA$_A$ receptors was suggested from biochemical experiments showing that activation of the GABA$_A$ recognition site enhances the affinity of benzodiazepine receptors in brain (25,66,101). Autoradiographic studies have confirmed this affiliation by demonstrating that benzodiazepine binding sites are generally found in close proximity to GABAergic synapses (79,80). These data confirm earlier electrophysiological results indicating that the benzodiazepines enhance GABAergic transmission (21–23,51,54,56,73,99). Of particular importance was the discovery that most, if not all, benzodiazepine binding sites are associated with GABA$_A$ receptors (79,93). However, additional GABA$_A$ receptor sites appear to exist that are devoid of a benzodiazepine component (106); it is unknown whether these sites are located synaptically. The effects of benzodiazepines contrast with the barbiturates, which enhance GABAergic transmission by acting at chloride channels as well as depressing excitatory transmission, thereby exerting a more generalized effect on nervous system function (54,83,105).

Electrophysiological studies have revealed that the benzodiazepines increase the probability of opening of chloride channels in response to GABA (99), an action which may account for the pharmacological and therapeutic actions of these drugs (2,55). The dose-response curve for the GABA-induced change in chloride conductance is shifted to the left in the presence of benzodiazepines, with no change in the maximal response (23). This indicates that benzodiazepines enhance GABA$_A$ receptor function only at synapses where the GABA concentration is insufficient to open all available chloride channels, but do not promote receptor function beyond that which can be obtained with GABA itself. This may explain why the benzodiazepines have a more favorable therapeutic index as compared to other central nervous system depressants which, at high doses, may depress neuronal function beyond the normal range.

When considering a general mechanism of action of benzodiazepines it is important to recall that unless the receptor is activated by GABA the benzodiazepines are ineffective (23,54,56). This suggests that benzodiazepines enhance GABA$_A$ receptor function only at GABAergic synapses while having no influence on extrasynaptic GABA$_A$ sites. This may explain the more selective actions of the benzodiazepines as compared to drugs acting directly at the GABA recognition site, since the latter may stimulate or inhibit GABA$_A$ sites regardless of their neuroanatomical location.

Three types of benzodiazepine receptor ligands have been identified (Fig. 1). Agents such as diazepam, chlorodiazepoxide, and flunitrazepam are classified as benzodiazepine receptor agonists, since they enhance GABA$_A$ receptor function. Also included in this group are nonbenzodiazepine tranquilizers (53) such as certain triazolopyridazines, e.g., CL 218872 (71); cyclopyrrolones, e.g., zopiclone (7); phenylquinolinones, e.g., PK 8165 (70); pyrazoloquinolinones, e.g., CGS 9896 (111); and some β-carbolines, e.g., ZK 93423 (72). Other substances, such as β-carboline carboxylate ethyl ester, produce effects opposite to those found with the benzodiazepine receptor agonists and are therefore referred to as inverse agonists (14,15). Binding studies indicate that agonists and inverse agonists attach to the same or overlapping sites on the benzodiazepine binding component (75). This was also demonstrated by the discovery of a third class of ligand, benzodiazepine receptor antagonists (5,50,52,60,75). These are represented by RO 15-1788, an imidazobenzodiazepinone (60). RO 15-1788 is largely devoid of pharmacological effects but competitively interacts at the benzodiazepine binding site to block the actions of either the receptor agonists or inverse agonists. Thus these three types of ligands affect GABA-dependent gating of the chloride channel with positive, negative, or zero intrinsic efficacy. Compounds have recently been synthesized that possess both agonist and antagonist properties. Such partial agonists may be even safer and more selective as anxiolytic drugs.

Phylogenetic studies reveal that benzodiazepine binding sites are present in vertebrate but not invertebrate species, suggesting a late evolutionary appearance (85). This indicates an important physiological role for the receptor and points to the possibility of an endogenous ligand for this site. Clearly, the identification of such a compound would provide important information with regard to the biological mechanisms regulating anxiety, seizure threshold, and sleep. Although numerous investigators have attempted to isolate such a substance, no compound is as yet universally accepted as the endogenous benzodiazepine receptor ligand. Interest is presently focused on a peptide, diazepam binding inhibitor (DBI), which has been extracted from brain and has properties similar to those of inverse agonists (1,24,49). DBI has an affinity constant of 1 μM for the benzodiazepine binding site. Since DBI is present in only some GABA neurons, it may serve as a ligand for only a select group of benzodiazepine receptors. Moreover, DBI is found in nonGABAergic neurons, suggesting that it may also serve some function unrelated to the benzodiazepine site (1).

Although the identification of a specific binding site for benzodiazepines strongly suggests the presence of an endogenous ligand, it does not prove its existence. Attempts to demonstrate the physiological effects of an endogenous ligand by inhibiting its receptor interaction with the benzodiazepine antagonist RO 15-1788 have been inconclusive thus far.

Studies have uncovered a variety of benzodiazepine agonists that differ in their pharmacological profiles (53). Some possible explanations for these differences include the presence of benzodiazepine receptor subclasses, only some of which mediate anxiolytic actions whereas others are important for sedative and muscle relaxant effects (61,68,74). However, there is no direct evidence supporting the existence of molecularly distinct benzodiazepine receptors, making it conceivable that the heterogeneity suggested from binding studies reflects different conformations of a single benzodiazepine site (57,80). On the other hand, differences in pharmacological profiles may be due to variations in intrinsic efficacy and in the extent of receptor reserve among neurons. For example, it is possible that neurons associated with anxiety or epileptic activity have a higher receptor reserve than those controlling alertness or muscle tone. Full agonists would produce a maximal affect when all receptors are activated on cells having no receptor reserve, whereas partial agonists would display only limited activity. In contrast, partial agonists may yield a maximal response in those cells possessing a significant amount of receptor reserve.

Although many questions remain about the molecular structure of the GABA receptor complex, there is sufficient information to propose a working model (Fig. 2). Receptor purification experiments indicate that the GABA$_A$/benzodiazepine moiety is a glycoprotein containing two subunits, with the α-subunit having a molecular weight of 50 kD and the β-subunit 55 kD. A tetrameric α/β arrangement is suggested by comparing the molecular weights of the subunits with the native receptor (76,80,94,95). The α/β structure accommodates not only the binding sites for GABA and benzodiazepines, but also the TBPS binding site (95), which is associated with the chloride channel (98) (Fig. 1). Electrophysiological studies suggest the presence of two GABA recognition sites for each GABA$_A$-receptor-associated chloride channel (90).

Little is known about the precise location of the various ligand binding sites on the GABA$_A$ receptor domain. Photoaffinity labeling suggests that the binding sites for the benzodiazepines and GABA are present on the α-subunit, although they may also be located on the β-subunit in a state that is not generally labeled (76,94). The exact location of the binding sites for barbiturates and picrotoxin is unknown. It is conceivable that these may be present on subunit interfaces.

Although the present model is consistent with the majority of experimental data, recent findings indicate that its design will have to be modified. For instance, it appears that an additional protein is present in certain purified receptor preparations (92). Furthermore, the target size of the radiation-inactivated TBPS binding site appears to be exceptionally large as compared to the size of the GABA/benzodiazepine complex (84). This might be explained by the presence of an additional subunit of 62 to 80 kD (γ-subunit) in the receptor complex (80). More precise information on the structure, synthesis, and assembly of the receptor will be forthcoming with the isolation of GABA$_A$ receptor genes. This development will also provide DNA probes to identify those cells which express GABA$_A$ receptors.

The intimate association between the benzodiazepine binding site and GABA$_A$ receptors suggests that disorders such as epilepsy, anxiety, and insomnia might result from a deficit in GABA$_A$ receptor function, or in the activity of selected GABAergic neurons. Indeed, it has been suggested that GABAergic transmission is altered in the vicinity of epileptic foci, suggesting that inhibitory influences may be insufficient to prevent the generalized spread of paroxysmal discharges (16). It is also possible that a defect in the GABAergic control of certain excitatory stimuli might contribute to anxiety, a hypothesis based on the finding that inverse agonists induce anxiety in human subjects (31). As for insomnia, it has been found that sleep latency is prolonged by the benzodiazepine inverse agonists and is diminished by benzodiazepine agonists, suggesting an involvement of GABAergic systems in the etiology of some sleep disorders. More definitive information with regard to these issues may soon be obtained with positron emission tomography using benzodiazepine ligands as the emitting isotopes (33,91).

GABA$_B$ RECEPTORS

β-p-Chlorophenyl GABA (baclofen) was designed as a centrally active GABA receptor agonist (8). However, the electrophysiological response to baclofen is resistant to blockade by bicuculline and picrotoxin, suggesting that its effects are mediated by an action other than direct activation of GABA$_A$ receptors (18). Recently it has been found that baclofen induces some responses that are mimicked by GABA, indicating that it may be a selective agonist for a receptor subgroup (GABA$_B$ receptors) that are resistant to the classical GABA$_A$ receptor antagonists (11,12,65).

Ligand binding assays suggest that the GABA$_B$ binding site is associated with divalent cations, in particular calcium (41). Functional assays indicate that the GABA$_B$ site may

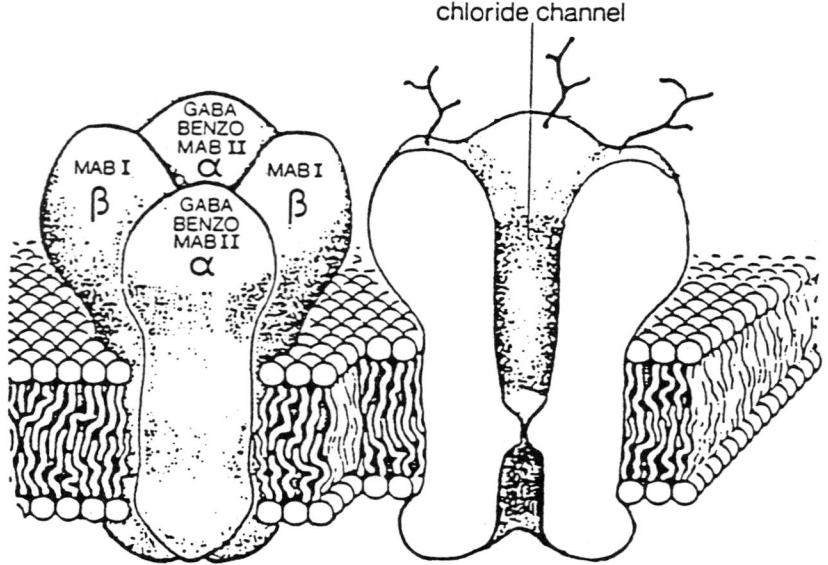

chloride channel

FIG. 2. Structural model of the GABA$_A$/benzodiazepine receptor/chloride channel complex. The α and β symbols indicate subunits differentiated on the basis of their molecular weights (50 and 55 kD, respectively). MAB I and MAB II are distinct epitopes recognized by subunit-specific monoclonal antibodies. Photolabeling studies indicate that the GABA$_A$ and benzodiazepine (Benzo) binding sites are located on the MAB II subunits, although the precise location of each binding domain remains unknown.

be important for regulating neurotransmitter release and may be associated with second messenger production in brain (9,38,42,44). Like the GABA$_A$ binding site, GABA$_B$ receptors are widely distributed throughout the central nervous system (63). Unlike GABA$_A$ receptors, the GABA$_B$ site is not associated with chloride ion channels or benzodiazepines (9). A major hindrance to the characterization of GABA$_B$ receptors is the absence of potent and selective antagonists for this site. Indeed, the existence of GABA$_B$ receptors will remain a matter of dispute until selective antagonists are found.

One action attributed to GABA$_B$ receptors is a regulatory role with respect to second messenger responses in brain (Fig. 3) (58,64,65,109). Although neither baclofen nor GABA have any direct effect on cyclic AMP production themselves, both agents amplify the production of this second messenger when brain tissue is exposed to a neurotransmitter that directly stimulates the accumulation of this cyclic nucleotide. For example, a saturating concentration of isoproterenol causes an eightfold increase in cyclic AMP production in rat brain cerebral cortical slices. In the presence of baclofen or GABA, isoproterenol-stimulated cyclic AMP accumulation is over 20-fold higher than basal levels, indicating that GABA$_B$ receptor activation amplifies the second messenger response to the β-adrenergic agonist. Similar results were obtained when cyclic AMP production was activated by norepinephrine, vasoactive intestinal peptide, or adenosine (65). Importantly, selective GABA$_A$ receptor agonists such as isoguvacine and THIP are inactive in this regard, and the response to baclofen is insensitive to blockade by bicuculline or picrotoxin (64,65). These findings suggest that the second messenger response to baclofen is mediated by a GABA receptor distinct from GABA$_A$ sites. Thus GABA, through an action at GABA$_B$ receptors, may serve to modulate the receptor responses to a variety of neurotransmitters in brain.

Experiments conducted to define the biochemical properties of GABA$_B$ receptors indicate that the amplification phenomenon is totally dependent on the presence of extracellular calcium ion (32,64). Moreover, it appears that stimulation of GABA$_B$ receptors may result in the activation of phospholipase A$_2$, a calcium-dependent enzyme that catalyzes the conversion of phospholipids to arachidonic acid (Fig. 3). Although arachidonic acid is rapidly converted to prostaglandins and a variety of hydroperoxy derivatives, these metabolites do not seem to contribute to the augmentation response (32). This suggests that arachidonate, or some other fatty acid, may mediate the GABA$_B$ receptor-induced augmentation of cyclic AMP production. In this regard it is interesting that arachidonic acid is capable of activating C kinase (82), an enzyme known to phosphorylate a variety of intracellular proteins. In platelets C kinase phosphorylates a GTP-binding protein (G$_I$) known to inhibit adenylate cyclase activity (67). Therefore it is conceivable that by stimulating the formation of arachidonic acid, GABA$_B$ receptor activation reduces the influence of G$_I$ on adenylate cyclase, thereby enhancing the responsiveness of the neurotransmitter receptor-coupled cyclic AMP generating system. This model must be considered highly speculative, however, until more direct evidence is provided that phospholipase A$_2$ is activated by GABA$_B$ agonists and that G$_I$ is phosphorylated following exposure to baclofen.

The finding that GABA may act as a neuromodulator has significant implications with regard to psychotherapeutics. For example, the monoamine theory of depression suggests that this disorder is secondary to an alteration in brain noradrenergic and serotonergic transmission (48). Since the transmitters for both systems are associated with cyclic AMP production in brain, it is conceivable that some forms of depression may be due to a GABA$_B$ receptor dysfunction that diminishes the responsiveness of the norepinephrine and serotonin receptors. In this case a GABA$_B$

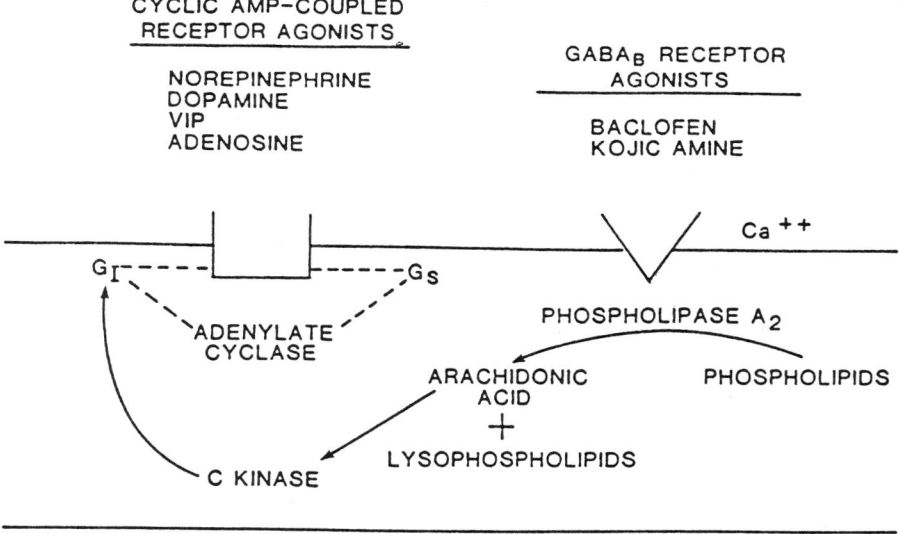

FIG. 3. Schematic representation of the components proposed for the GABA$_B$ receptor system. In this model the GABA$_B$ receptor is in the vicinity of recognition sites for cyclic AMP-coupled transmitter systems. G$_I$ and G$_S$ represent inhibitory and stimulatory guanine nucleotide binding proteins, respectively. Agonists for the two receptor recognition sites are listed above each component.

agonist may be beneficial in the treatment of affective illness either alone or in combination with standard medications. A recent study has indicated that coadministration of baclofen with imipramine facilitates the appearance of a neurochemical response thought to be related to the therapeutic efficacy of antidepressants (42).

Schizophrenia appears to be associated with excessive dopaminergic tone in critical areas of the brain (87). Inasmuch as one type of dopamine receptor (D_1) is associated with adenylate cyclase, it is conceivable that some symptoms of schizophrenia may be due to enhanced $GABA_B$ receptor activity. That is, an overactive $GABA_B$ receptor system may amplify dopaminergic responses even though dopamine turnover may be unaltered. This makes it conceivable that $GABA_B$ receptor antagonists might have antipsychotic potential. While highly speculative, such theories are consistent with the present information and serve to illustrate why continued research on GABA receptors may lead to the development of novel therapeutic agents.

CONCLUSIONS

Early studies on the chemical nature of synaptic transmission concentrated on presynaptic events, since there were few biochemical methods for studying postsynaptic mechanisms. Because of this emphasis a great deal was learned about the actions of drugs that influence the concentration or turnover of neurotransmitter substances. For example, psychopharmacological agents were found to modify the storage (reserpine), release (amphetamine), metabolism (pargyline), or reuptake (imipramine) of monoamines. It has become possible in recent years to examine directly the interaction of drugs with synaptic receptor sites (110). This has led to the discovery that some psychoactive drugs act by directly stimulating (lysergic acid diethylamide) or inhibiting (haloperidol) transmitter receptors (4,27). Moreover, it has been found that direct stimulation or inhibition of receptor recognition sites are not the only ways to modify receptor function (62,65,100). Thus it appears that transmitter receptors are macromolecular complexes containing a family of interacting sites, each of which may be manipulated for therapeutic gain.

This concept developed in part as a consequence of research on GABA receptors. One of the initial breakthroughs came with the discovery that certain GABA receptor antagonists, such as picrotoxin, selectively alter receptor function by acting on a component other than the recognition site. Of special interest to psychopharmacologists was the discovery that benzodiazepines facilitate GABAergic transmission by attaching to a receptor component physically distinct from the GABA binding site. This demonstrated that by acting on receptor components separate from the recognition site drugs can exert subtle effects on neurotransmitter systems.

Work during the past decade has revealed that the benzodiazepine component of the $GABA_A$ receptor has characteristics that distinguish it from classical neurotransmitter receptor recognition sites. Thus, not only have substances been found that activate (diazepam and chlorodiazepoxide) and inhibit (RO 15–1788) this site, but there are also agents evoking a response totally opposite from diazepam (inverse agonists).

The concept that neurotransmitter receptors may be subtly manipulated by drugs was reinforced by the discovery that GABA, through an action at $GABA_B$ receptors, may act as a neuromodulator rather than a neurotransmitter. In this case the GABA binding site appears to be affiliated with neurotransmitter receptors that are directly coupled to the cyclic AMP generating system. Thus, receptor responses are a function not only of the amount of transmitter released but also of receptor responsiveness, which appears to be under the control of modulating substances.

Such findings have implications with regard to defining the biological abnormalities associated with mental illness. Because it has been difficult to identify neurochemical lesions associated with most psychiatric diseases, it appears that neurotransmitter synthesis, storage, and release may not be dramatically altered in these conditions. The discovery that receptor activity may be continuously regulated by neuromodulators and receptor site-associated components makes it conceivable that some forms of mental illness are secondary to an alteration in these regulatory systems. Thus, studies on GABA neurotransmission have not only yielded insights with regard to the characteristics of this receptor, they have also provided new perspectives with regard to receptor mechanisms, the etiology of psychiatric illness, and the development of novel therapeutic agents.

ACKNOWLEDGMENTS

Preparation of this manuscript was made possible in part by support from the National Science Foundation (BNS-82-15427), the United States Air Force, and Bristol-Myers Inc. S.J.E. is the recipient of a U.S.P.H.S. Research Scientist Development Award (MH-00501).

REFERENCES

1. Alho, H., Costa, E., Ferrero, P., Fujimoto, M., Cosenza-Murphy, D., and Guidotti, A. (1985): *Science,* 229:179–182.
2. Barker, J. L., Gratz, E., Owen, D. G., and Study, R. E. (1984): In: *Actions and Interactions of GABA and Benzodiazepines,* edited by N. G. Bowery, pp. 203–216. Raven Press, New York.
3. Barker, J. L., and Mathers, D. L. (1981): *Science,* 212:358–360.
4. Bennett, J. P., and Snyder, S. H. (1976): *Mol. Pharmacol.,* 12: 373–389.
5. Bernard, P., Bergen, K., Sobiski, R., and Robson, R. D. (1981): *Pharmacologist,* 23:150.
6. Beutler, J. A., Karbon, E. W., Brubaker, A. N., Malik, J., Curtis, D. R., and Enna, S. J. (1985): *Brain Res.,* 330:135–140.
7. Blanchard, J. C., Boireau, A., Garret, C., and Joulou, L. (1979): *Life Sci.,* 24:2417–2420.
8. Bowery, N. G. (1982): *Trends Pharmacol. Sci.,* 3:400–403.
9. Bowery, N. G. (1983): In: *The GABA Receptors,* edited by S. J. Enna, pp. 177–213. Humana Press, Clifton, NJ.
10. Bowery, N. G., Doble, A., Hill, D. R., Hudson, A. L., Shaw, J., and Turnbull, M. J. (1982): In: *Presynaptic Receptors: Mechanism and Function,* edited by J. Belleroche, pp. 174–194. Ellis Horwood, Chichester.
11. Bowery, N. G., Doble, A., Hill, D. R., Hudson, A. L., and Turnbull, M. J. (1980): *Br. J. Pharmacol.,* 70:77P.
12. Bowery, N. G., Hill, D. R., and Hudson, A. L. (1983): *Br. J. Pharmacol.,* 78:191–206.
13. Braestrup, C. (1982): *Lancet,* 2:1030–1034.

14. Braestrup, C., Schmiechen, R., Neff, G., Nielsen, M., and Petersen, E. N. (1982): *Science,* 216:1241–1243.
15. Braestrup, C., Schmiechen, R., Nielsen, M., and Petersen, E. N. (1982): In: *Pharmacology of Benzodiazepines,* edited by E. Usdin, P. Skolnick, J. F. Tallman, D. Greenblatt, and S. M. Paul, pp. 71–86. Macmillan Press, London.
16. Browne, T. R. (1982): In: *Pharmacology of Benzodiazepines,* edited by E. Usdin, P. Skolnick, J. F. Tallman, D. Greenblatt, and S. M. Paul, pp. 329–337. Macmillan Press, London.
17. Browner, M., Ferkany, J. W., and Enna, S. J. (1981): *J. Neurosci.,* 1:514–518.
18. Calne, D. B. (1976): In: *Clinical Neuropharmacology,* edited by H. L. Klawans, pp. 137–145. Raven Press, New York.
19. Casida, J. E., Palmer, C. J., and Cole, L. M. (1985): *Mol. Pharmacol.,* 28:246–253.
20. Chambon, J.-P., Feltz, P., Heulme, M., Restle, S., Schlichter, R., Biziere, K., and Wermuth, C. (1985): *Proc. Natl. Acad. Sci. USA,* 82:1832–1836.
21. Chan, C. Y., and Farb, D. H. (1985): *J. Neurosci.,* 5:2365–2373.
22. Choi, D. W., Farb, D. H., and Fischbach, G. D. (1977): *Nature,* 269:342–344.
23. Choi, D. W., Farb, D. H., and Fischbach, G. D. (1981): *J. Neurophysiol.,* 45:621–631.
24. Costa, E., Corda, M. G., and Guidotti, A. (1983): *Neuropharmacology,* 22:1481–1492.
25. Costa, E., Corda, M. G., Wise, B., Konkel, D., and Guidotti, A. (1982): In: *Pharmacology of Benzodiazepines,* edited by E. Usdin, P. Skolnick, J. F. Tallman, D. Greenblatt, and S. M. Paul, pp. 111–120. Macmillan Press, London.
26. Costa, E., DiChiara, G., and Gessa, G. L., eds. (1981): *GABA and Benzodazepine Receptors.* Raven Press, New York.
27. Creese, I., Burt, D., and Snyder, S. H. (1976): *Science,* 192:481–483.
28. Curtis, D. R., Duggan, A., Felix, D., and Johnston, G. A. R. (1971): *Brain Res.,* 32:69–96.
29. Curtis, D. R., Hosli, L., Johnston, G. A. R., and Johnston, I. H. (1968): *Exp. Brain Res.,* 5:235–258.
30. Curtis, D. R., and Watkins, J. C. (1965): *Pharmacol. Rev.,* 17:347–391.
31. Dorrow, R., Horowski, R., Paschelke, G., Amin, M., and Braestrup, C. (1983): *Lancet,* 2:98–99.
32. Duman, R. S., Karbon, E. W., Harrington, C., and Enna, S. J. (1986): *J. Neurochem.,* 47:800–810.
33. Ehrin, E., Johnston, P., Stone-Elander, S., Nilsson, J. L., Person, A., Tarde, L., Sedvall, G., Litton, J. E., Eiksson, L., and Widen, L. (1984): *Acta Pharm. Suec.,* 21:183–188.
34. Enna, S. J. (1979): *Annu. Rev. Med. Chem.,* 14:41–50.
35. Enna, S. J. (1981): In: *Neuropharmacology of Central Disorders,* edited by G. C. Palmer, pp. 507–537. Academic Press, New York.
36. Enna, S. J. (1983): In: *The GABA Receptors,* edited by S. J. Enna, pp. 1–23. Humana Press, Clifton, NJ.
37. Enna, S. J., ed. (1983): *The GABA Receptors.* Humana Press, Clifton, NJ.
38. Enna, S. J. (1985): In: *Psychiatry Update, Vol. IV,* edited by J. T. Coyle, pp. 67–82. American Psychiatric Association Press, New York.
39. Enna, S. J. (1986): In: *GABA and Benzodiazepine Receptors,* edited by R. F. Squires. CRC Press, Boca Raton, FL (*in press*).
40. Enna, S. J., and Gallagher, J. P. (1983): *Int. Rev. Neurobiol.,* 24:181–212.
41. Enna, S. J., and Karbon, E. W. (1986): In: *Benzodiazepine/GABA Receptors and Chloride Channels: Structural and Functional Properties,* edited by R. W. Olsen and J. C. Venter, pp. 41–56. Alan R. Liss, New York.
42. Enna, S. J., Karbon, E. W., and Duman, R. S. (1985): In: *GABA and Mood Disorders,* edited by P. O. Morselli and K. G. Lloyd, pp. 23–31. Raven Press, New York.
43. Enna, S. J., and Maggi, A. (1979): *Life Sci.,* 24:1727–1738.
44. Enna, S. J., and Snyder, S. H. (1977): *Mol. Pharmacol.,* 13:442–453.
45. Fahn, S. (1976): In: *GABA in Nervous System Function,* edited by E. Roberts, T. Chase, and D. Tower, pp. 169–188. Raven Press, New York.
46. Falch, E., and Krogsgaard-Larsen, P. (1982): *J. Neurochem.,* 38:1123–1129.
47. Fonnum, F., ed. (1978): *Amino Acids as Chemical Transmitters.* Plenum Press, New York.
48. Fuller, R. W. (1981): In: *Antidepressants: Neurochemical, Behavioral and Clinical Perspectives,* edited by S. J. Enna, J. B. Malick, and E. Richelson, pp. 1–12. Raven Press, New York.
49. Guidotti, A., Forchetti, C. M., Corda, M. G., Konkel, D., Bennett, C. D., and Costa, E. (1983): *Proc. Natl. Acad. Sci. USA,* 80:3531–3535.
50. Haefely, W. (1984): In: *Actions and Interactions of GABA and Benzodiazepines,* edited by N. G. Bowery, pp. 263–285. Raven Press, New York.
51. Haefely, W. (1985): In: *Psychopharmacology 2, Part I: Preclinical Psychopharmacology,* edited by D. G. Graham-Smith, pp. 92–162. Elsevier, Amsterdam.
52. Haefely, W. (1985): *Pharmacopsychiatry,* 18:163–166.
53. Haefely, W., Kyburz, E., Gerecke, M., and Möhler, H. (1985): *Adv. Drug Res.,* 14:165–322.
54. Haefely, W., and Polc, P. (1983): In: *Anxiolytics,* edited by J. B. Malick, S. J. Enna, and H. I. Yamamura, pp. 113–145. Raven Press, New York.
55. Haefely, W., and Polc, P. (1986): In: *Benzodiazepine/GABA Receptors and Chloride Channels: Structural and Functional Properties,* edited by R. W. Olsen and J. C. Venter, pp. 97–133. Alan R. Liss, New York.
56. Haefely, W., Polc, P., Schaffner, R., Keller, H. H., Pieri, L., and Möhler, H. (1978): In: *GABA-Neurotransmitters,* edited by P. Krogsgaard-Larsen, P. J. Scheel-Kruger, and H. Kofod, pp. 357–375. Munksgaard, Copenhagen.
57. Haring, P., Stahli, C., Schoch, P., Takacs, B., Staehelin, T., and Möhler, H. (1985): *Proc. Natl. Acad. Sci. USA,* 82:4837–4841.
58. Hill, D. R., and Dolphin, A. C. (1984): *Neuropharmacology,* 23:829–830.
59. Hornykiewicz, O., Lloyd, K. G., and Davidson, L. (1976): In: *GABA in Nervous System Function,* edited by E. Roberts, T. Chase, and D. Tower, pp. 479–485. Raven Press, New York.
60. Hunkeler, W., Möhler, H., Pieri, L., Polc, P., Bonetti, E. P., Cumin, R., Schaffner, R., and Haefely, W. (1981): *Nature,* 290:514–516.
61. Johnson, R. W., Tallman, J. F., Squires, R., and Yamamura, H. I. (1983): In: *Anxiolytics: Neurochemical, Behavioral and Clinical Perspectives,* edited by J. B. Malick, S. J. Enna, and H. I. Yamamura, pp. 93–112. Raven Press, New York.
62. Johnston, G. A. R. (1983): In: *The GABA Receptors,* edited by S. J. Enna, pp. 107–128. Humana Press, Clifton, NJ.
63. Karbon, E. W., Duman, R. S., and Enna, S. J. (1983): *Brain Res.,* 274:393–396.
64. Karbon, E. W., Duman, R. S., and Enna, S. J. (1984): *Brain Res.,* 306:327–332.
65. Karbon, E. W., and Enna, S. J. (1985): *Mol. Pharmacol.,* 27:53–59.
66. Karobath, M., and Sperck, G. (1979): *Proc. Natl. Acad. Sci. USA,* 76:1004–1006.
67. Katada, T., Gilman, A. G., Watanabe, Y., Bauer, S., and Jacobs, K. H. (1985): *Eur. J. Biochem.,* 151:431–437.
68. Klepner, C. A., Lippa, A. S., Benson, D. I., Sano, M. C., and Beer, B. (1979): *Pharmacol. Biochem. Behav.,* 11:457–462.
69. Krogsgaard-Larsen, P. (1981): *J. Med. Chem.,* 24:1377–1383.
70. LeFur, G., Mizoule, J., Burgevin, M. C., Ferris, O., Heulme, M., Gauthier, A., Gueremy, C., and Uzan, A. (1981): *Life Sci.,* 28:1439–1448.
71. Lippa, A. S., Coupet, E. N., Greenblatt, C. A., Klepner, C. A., and Beer, B. (1979): *Pharmacol. Biochem. Behav.,* 11:99–106.
72. Loscher, W., Schneider, H., and Kehr, W. (1985): *Eur. J. Pharmacol.,* 114:261–266.
73. MacDonald, R., and Barker, J. L. (1978): *Nature,* 271:563–564.
74. Martin, I. L., Brown, C. L., and Doble, A. (1984): In: *Actions and Interactions of GABA and Benzodiazepines,* edited by N. G. Bowery, pp. 167–178. Raven Press, New York.
75. Möhler, H. (1984): In: *Actions and Interactions of GABA and Benzodiazepines,* edited by N. G. Bowery, pp. 155–166. Raven Press, New York.

76. Möhler, H., Battersby, M. K., and Richards, J. G. (1980): *Proc. Natl. Acad. Sci. USA,* 77:1666–1670.
77. Möhler, H., and Okada, T. (1977): *Science,* 198:849–851.
78. Möhler, H., and Richards, J. G. (1983): In: *Anxiolytics: Neurochemical, Behavioral and Clinical Perspectives,* edited by J. A. Malick, S. J. Enna, and H. I. Yamamura, pp. 15–40. Raven Press, New York.
79. Möhler, H., Richards, J. G., and Wu, J.-Y. (1981): *Proc. Natl. Acad. Sci. USA,* 78:1935–1938.
80. Möhler, H., Schoch, P., Richards, J. G., Haring, P., Takacs, B., and Stahli, C. (1986): In: *Benzodiazepine/GABA Receptors and Chloride Channels,* edited by R. W. Olsen and J. C. Venter, pp. 285–298. Alan R. Liss, New York.
81. Morselli, P. L., and Lloyd, K. G. (1983): In: *The GABA Receptors,* edited by S. J. Enna, pp. 306–336. Humana Press, Clifton, NJ.
82. Murakami, K., Chan, S. Y., and Rauttenburg, A. (1985): *Proc. Soc. Neurosci.,* 11:927.
83. Nicoll, R. (1978): In: *Psychopharmacology: A Generation of Progress,* edited by M. A. Lipton, A. DiMascio, and K. F. Killam, pp. 1337–1348. Raven Press, New York.
84. Nielsen, M., and Braestrup, C. (1983): *Eur. J. Pharmacol.,* 91:321–322.
85. Nielsen, M., Braestrup, C., and Squires, R. F. (1978): *Brain Res.,* 141:342–346.
86. Olsen, R. W., and Snowman, A. M. (1982): *J. Neurosci.,* 2:1812–1823.
87. Pearlson, G., and Coyle, J. T. (1983): In: *Neuroleptics: Neurochemical, Behavioral and Clinical Perspectives,* edited by J. T. Coyle and S. J. Enna, pp. 297–324. Raven Press, New York.
88. Reisine, T. D., Fields, J. Z., Yamamura, H. I., Bird, E., Spokes, E., Schreiner, P., and Enna, S. J. (1977): *Life Sci.,* 21:335–344.
89. Roberts, E. (1972): *Neurosci. Res. Prog.,* 10:468–482.
90. Sakmann, B., Hamill, O. P., and Bormann, J. (1983): *J. Neural Transm. (Suppl.),* 18:83–95.
91. Samson, Y., Hantraye, P., Baron, J. C., Soussaline, F., Comar, D., and Maziere, M. (1985): *Eur. J. Pharmacol.,* 110:247–251.
92. Schoch, P., Haring, P., Takacs, B., Stahli, C., and Möhler, H. (1984): *J. Recept. Res.,* 4:189–200.
93. Schoch, P., Richards, J. G., Haring, P., Takacs, B., Stahli, C.,

Staehelin, T., Haefely, W., and Möhler, H. (1985): *Nature,* 314:168–170.
94. Sieghart, W., and Karobath, M. (1980): *Nature,* 286:285–287.
95. Sigel, E., and Barnard, E. A. (1984): *J. Biol. Chem.,* 259:7219–7223.
96. Skerritt, J. H., Willow, M., and Johnston, G. A. R. (1982): *Neurosci. Lett.,* 29:63–66.
97. Squires, R. F., and Braestrup, C. (1977): *Nature,* 266:732–734.
98. Squires, R. F., Casida, J. E., Richardson, M., and Saedrup, E. (1983): *Mol. Pharmacol.,* 23:326–336.
99. Study, R. E., and Barker, J. L. (1981): *Proc. Natl. Acad. Sci. USA,* 78:7180–7184.
100. Tallman, J. F., and Gallagher, D. W. (1979): *Pharmacol. Biochem. Behav.,* 10:809–813.
101. Tallman, J. F., Thomas, J. W., and Gallagher, D. W. (1978): *Nature,* 274:384–385.
102. ten Bruggencate, G., and Engberg, I. (1968): *Brain Res.,* 11:446–450.
103. Thampy, K. G., and Barnes, E. M. (1984): *J. Biol. Chem.,* 259:1753–1757.
104. Ticku, M. K., Ban, M., and Olsen, R. W. (1978): *Mol. Pharmacol.,* 14:391–402.
105. Trifiletti, R. R., Snowman, A., and Snyder, S. H. (1984): *Mol. Pharmacol.,* 26:470–476.
106. Unnerstall, J. R., Kuhar, M. J., Niehoff, D. L., and Palacios, J. M. (1981): *J. Pharmacol. Exp. Ther.,* 218:797–804.
107. Usdin, E., Skolnick, P., Tallman, J. F., Greenblatt, D., and Paul, S. M., eds. (1982): *Pharmacology of Benzodiazepines.* Macmillan Press, London.
108. Willow, M., and Johnston, G. A. R. (1983): *Int. Rev. Neurobiol.,* 24:15–48.
109. Wojcik, W. J., and Neff, N. H. (1984): *Mol. Pharmacol.,* 25:24–28.
110. Yamamura, H. I., Enna, S. J., and Kuhar, M. J., eds. (1985): *Neurotransmitter Receptor Binding,* 2nd ed. Raven Press, New York.
111. Yokoyama, N., Ritter, B., and Neubest, A. D. (1982): *J. Med. Chem.,* 25:337–339.

Psychopharmacology:
The Third Generation of Progress,
edited by Herbert Y. Meltzer.
Raven Press, New York © 1987.

CHAPTER 28

Histamine Receptors

Jack Peter Green

To the extent that any substance can be affirmed to be a neuroregulator in brain (47,118,123,168), one can now make this assertion about histamine (126). The delay in recognizing a role of histamine in brain may appear surprising since it was unequivocally shown to be present in brain synaptosomes over 20 years ago (19,89), and before then, evidence suggested that histamine may function in brain (55). This evidence has steadily mounted (49,51,56,57,59,79,81,126,139–144). One reason for delay in acceptance of a neuroregulatory role for histamine was the absence of a method to reveal histaminergic cell bodies and nerve endings *in situ,* a need that was met by the development of immunocytochemical methods (see ref. 126). The second impediment was also a methodological one—the lack of methods to measure the metabolites of histamine, a necessity for accurate measurements of histamine turnover; several methods were recently developed and applied for this purpose (see refs. 61, 126, 136). Probably underlying the relatively sparse activity in developing methods to probe a histaminergic system, as compared with the intense activity in studying other biogenic amines, is the genesis of research on histamine. From its discovery, the dominant concern has been to learn its role in peripheral diseases, an interest provoked by its powerful effects in producing bronchoconstriction and hypotension. In 1966 Dale (30) stated, "It cannot, indeed, be doubted that it has been with this mainly pathological aspect of its significance, that an overwhelming majority of the experiments dealing with the functions of histamine have hitherto been concerned." In contrast, early in the histories of other biogenic amines—acetylcholine, norepinephrine, serotonin, and dopamine—they were postulated to function in the nervous system.

It is ironic in the face of this history that it was histamine that stimulated the development of the psychotropic drugs and hence of modern biological psychiatry. For the phenothiazines were developed as antihistamines (i.e., histamine H_1-antagonists) and observed to produce in patients an unusual effect on mood (91,153). From the phenothiazines evolved—again because of alert clinical observation—the antidepressant drugs (96). It is now known that many of these and other types of psychotropic drugs react with both histamine H_1 and histamine H_2 receptors (57,81,126,132,133), but which of the pharmacological effects of these drugs rest on these interactions is not known.

A comprehensive review of histamine and the nervous system has appeared (81). The functions that histamine may regulate in the brain have been reviewed (57,59,79, 81,103,142–144,163). Its putative roles in specific neural processes have also been reviewed. These include thermal regulation (29,101), cerebral circulation (41,63,64), cardiovascular regulation (125,134), drinking and feeding behavior (94,99,100), emesis (13), self-stimulating, conditioning, motor activity (81,142,144), analgesia (135), sleep and wakefulness (81,107,134), and neuroendocrine regulation (39,134,161). Functions have also been inferred from the effects of histamine antagonists; since the antagonists, notably the H_1 antagonists, block other receptors and presynaptic sites not related to histamine (57,81,126), the effects of antagonists can only offer suggestions of the functions of histamine. Electrophysiological studies of histamine have been reviewed (65,126,165). Several recent reviews have appeared on histamine receptors in brain (51,57,81,126), and the effector mechanisms associated with the receptors have been reviewed (126).

THE HISTAMINE H_1 RECEPTOR

Mammalian brain has the highest density of H_1 binding sites of any organ studied as measured with labeled pyrilamine, i.e., mepyramine (24). Binding with either pyrilamine or the antidepressant drug doxepin suggested a low-affinity site as well as a high-affinity site (25,66,71, 87,157,160), but the latter site may be attributable to artifacts that can occur in binding assays (1,22,156,164). The K_D values of H_1 antagonists in binding appeared to differ slightly among species (25,71,87), and in different organs within the same species (24,25). The affinities of H_1 antagonists for the H_1 receptor linked to contraction of the guinea pig ileum and for the H_1 binding sites in guinea pig small intestine correlated with their affinities for guinea pig brain membranes (69,72). Species differed in the density of the H_1 binding sites in brain regions (25,71,157,160): e.g., in rat the cerebellum was lowest, the hypothalamus highest; in guinea pig, the cerebellum was highest, the basal ganglia lowest. In monkey, the frontal cortex was highest, the pons lowest, and the cerebellum had about half the density of sites as the frontal cortex (15). In humans, the frontal, parietal, cingulate, and temporal cortices were highest, the cerebellum among the lowest (25,87). In mice *in vivo* the distribution of labeled pyrilamine in brain was similar to the B_{max} of different brain regions as measured *in vitro*, and the potencies (ED_{50}) of H_1 antagonists in competing for labeled pyrilamine were similar to their affinities for the H_1 receptor (129,130). In similar experiments *in vivo*, the H_1 antagonists decreased the amount of labeled pyrilamine in the particulate fraction of brain; the potencies of some H_1 antagonists in this effect were similar to their affinities for the H_1 receptor (36). Treatment of the mature guinea pig with pyrilamine did not alter the B_{max} or K_D of H_1 binding sites in membranes from different brain regions or in intestinal smooth muscle (70), but treating rat pups with diphenydramine or pyrilamine increased the B_{max} of H_1 binding sites in whole brain and hypothalamus (152).

The regional distribution of the H_1 binding sites in rat brain (25) was not related to the distribution of histamine, or the histamine metabolite *tele*-methylhistamine, or the enzymes that form and methylate histamine (81), or the histamine metabolite *tele*-methylimidazoleacetic acid (92). Such discordance between the distribution of a transmitter and its binding site is not uncommon (40,95,147); e.g., serotonin (5-HT) binding sites were observed by radioautography in regions where 5-HT was not shown (104). The ontogeny of the H_1 binding site in rat brain (151,159) also differs from the ontogeny of histamine content and histidine decarboxylase activity (81).

Radioautography of guinea pig brain slices (120,122) showed high density of the H_1 binding site in the molecular layer of the cerebellum. In hippocampus, the dentate gyrus was notably rich in H_1 binding sites; CA4 had greater densities than CA1, CA2, or CA3 (122). On the other hand, rat showed high densities in CA3 of the hippocampus and in the subiculum (120). The hypothalamus showed high density in the supraoptic and suprachiasmatic nuclei, ventromedial nucleus, and the nucleus premammilaris ventralis; some of these sites may be related to functions of histamine, e.g., sites at which intraventricularly injected histamine may act to alter food and water intake, body temperature, and hormone secretion, as summarized by Palacios et al. (120). High densities in structures associated with the auditory system (120) may relate to the impairment of auditory vigilance occurring with H_1 blockers in humans (124). Radioautography of the monkey spinal cord showed

H_1 binding sites in layers I and II of the dorsal horn, in the motor neurons of the ventral horn, and in dorsal root ganglion cells (113,114). Some ganglion cells had both H_1 binding sites and opiate binding sites (113,114). The cat spinal cord appeared not to have H_1 binding sites in the motor neurons in the ventral horn, but showed high density of H_1 binding sites immediately lateral to the central canal, which, as emphasized (145), may be associated with the transmission of sensory stimuli. Histamine is known to activate afferent pathways (81). Membranes of guinea pig spinal cord (69) and cultured cells of rat spinal cord (77) also have H_1 binding sites.

It is highly likely that both neurons and glia have H_1 binding sites. In guinea pig, injections of kainate into the cerebellum produced a decrease in H_1 binding sites in the molecular layer, observations suggesting that the receptors there are associated with neurons (121). Dorsal root section halved the density of H_1 binding sites in layers I and II, as observed by radioautography (114). Cultured neurons of rat spinal cord showed, by radioautography, H_1 binding sites (77). Other experiments (26) imply that nonneuronal cells in the rat also have H_1 binding sites: H_1 binding by striatal homogenates was unaltered after injection of 6-hydroxydopamine into the substantia nigra, by hemisection of the brainstem, or by ablation of the cerebral cortex; binding by hippocampal homogenates was not affected after medial forebrain lesions or transection of the fimbria and fornix; kainate injection into the hippocampus produced a transient fall in H_1 binding, which returned to normal 15 days after the lesion. The inference (26) that some of the H_1 binding sites are on glial cells has received support. Cultured astrocytes from rat showed H_1 binding sites (77) that, electrophysiological studies suggest, are responsive H_1 receptors (78). Human astrocytoma cells showed high-affinity binding sites for pyrilamine, and the binding was appropriately reduced by two H_1 antagonists (111). The H_1 binding site is an H_1 receptor, as histamine stimulated the turnover of phosphoinoside and Ca^{2+} efflux in these cells, effects that were inhibited by an H_1 antagonist (111).

The H_1 binding sites are sensitive to phospholipases A and C and to proteolytic enzymes (24). Binding of H_1 agonists has sensitivities similar to those shown by agonists to some other binding sites (23). Na^+ and GTP decrease affinity of histamine for the binding sites, as measured with labeled pyrilamine, and their effects are additive. Affinities of H_1 agonists are enhanced by manganese and magnesium but not by calcium; none of these chemicals influenced the affinities of antagonists (23). Treatment of guinea pig cerebellar membranes with N-ethylmaleimide (52,170) had no effect on the binding of H_1 antagonists but increased the affinities of full agonists, less so of partial agonists. Other sulfhydryl active reagents—iodoacetic acid, iodoacetamide, p-chloromercuriphenylsulfonic acid and mersalyl—were ineffective (170). Membranes from beef aorta showed decreased H_1 binding after treatment with N-ethylmaleimide, which also reduced the contractile response of the rabbit aorta to histamine (20). The difference in the effect of N-ethylmaleimide on brain and aortic membranes could be attributable to the differences in concentrations that were used. In studies of the brain membranes, the concentration was 2 or 5 mM (170); on aortic membranes, the maximal effect of N-ethylmaleimide was seen at 10 μM, and the effect decreased with higher concentrations (20). Treatment with dithiothreitol increased the binding of labeled pyrilamine to aortic membranes and increased the affinity of histamine for the membranes (20). As was shown for the H_1 receptor in several tissues (38), dithiothreitol also increased the sensitivity of the rabbit aorta (20) and the guinea pig ileum (38) to the contractile effect of histamine. The potentiating effect of dithiothreitol on the ileum was reversed by a sulfhydryl-oxidizing reagent (38). The EC_{50} values of other histamine agonists on the ileum were reduced by dithiothreitol, which had much less effect on the contractions produced by acetylcholine and 5-HT (38). Dithiothreitol did not prevent desensitization of the ileum to histamine (38).

Desensitization of the ileum by histamine agonists is due to an effect on the H_1 receptor, for after desensitization, pyrilamine produced less of a shift in the dose-response curve (14). In murine cerebral cortical slices, where stimulation of the H_1 receptor increases glycogenolysis, desensitization of this effect to histamine was reflected in the shift of the EC_{50} of histamine with no change in its E_{max}, and a decrease in the B_{max} of the binding of pyrilamine with no change in its K_D (131). On a neuroblastoma cell, where stimulation of the H_1 receptor increases cyclic GMP formation and phosphoinositide turnover, the desensitization was not reflected in the EC_{50} value of histamine but in the E_{max} (155). On these cells, histamine desensitization was prevented by pyrilamine (155). The histamine-stimulated increase in cyclic AMP formation in guinea pig cerebral cortical slices showed desensitization, which was ascribed to increased phosphodiesterase activity (137).

A digitonin extract of guinea pig brain retained sensitivities to Na^+, divalent cations (53), and N-ethylmaleimide (170), but not to GTP (53). As estimated by gel filtration, the digitonin-solubilized H_1 binding material from guinea pig and rat brain had molecular weights of approximately 430,000 daltons, which may be exaggerated by bound digitonin (158). Target size analysis of the H_1 binding site in bovine and human cerebral cortex showed both to be 160,000 daltons (97).

As recently reviewed (81,126), stimulation of the H_1 receptor in various neural tissues is associated with increased formation of cyclic AMP, cyclic GMP, increased phosphoinositide turnover, and ion shifts. In brain slices of different mammalian species, histamine increases cyclic AMP formation (31,86). Stimulation of the H_1 receptor in conventionally prepared homogenates did not increase cyclic AMP formation (27,62,68,102), but in a cell-free preparation containing large vesicular sacs (27,128) or synaptoneurosomes (75), stimulation of the H_1 receptor increased cyclic AMP formation. In guinea pig brain slices, by the use of antagonists in concentrations over a range sufficient to do a Schild plot on the H_1 antagonist, which showed competitive antagonism (119), it was demonstrated that the H_1 receptor is associated with increased cyclic AMP formation. The increased cyclic AMP formation on stimulation of H_1 receptor depends on stimulation of the H_2 receptor (119) and/or on the presence of adenosine (2,32,34); treatment of brain slices with adenosine deaminase abolished the cyclic AMP response to H_1 stimulation (72,138).

Histamine-stimulated cyclic GMP formation in mouse neuroblastoma cells is linked to the H_1 receptor, as clearly revealed by the effects of antagonists (155). Histamine increases the cyclic GMP content too of cerebral cortical slices of rabbit (98) and guinea pig (138) and of rat pineal body (117) and bovine superior cervical ganglion (149). Since this effect of histamine requires Ca^{2+} (138,149), it is relevant to note that histamine increases Ca^{2+} influx in membranes of smooth muscle containing the H_1 receptor (162). Increased glycogenolysis after H_1 receptor stimulation in mouse cortical slices (130) and in chick brain (42) could also be mediated by increased cytosolic Ca^{2+} (130), which, in turn, could rest on H_1 stimulation of the turnover of the phosphoinositides.

Increased turnover of phosphoinositides in brain and in many other tissues and cells is associated with stimulation of many receptors, including the H_1 receptor (10,12,73,105,115). Hydrolysis of the phosphoinositides produces both inositol phosphates and a 1,2-diacylglycerol, mainly 1-stearoyl-2-arachidonyl-sn-glycerol. In many cells, inositol-1,4,5-triphosphate has been shown to elevate cytosolic Ca^{2+} (12,105). Recently, other inositol polyphosphates have been characterized in tissue (106), which may also release Ca^{2+} from its intracellular stores (18) by binding to an intracellular receptor (148). At least one of these compounds, inositol-1,3,4,5-tetrakisphosphate, which is formed on muscarinic stimulation, may be precursor of inositol-1,4,5-triphosphate (8). Ca^{2+} and diacylgylcerol are required for maximal activation of protein kinase C (10,12,73,115).

The first indication that histamine influenced phosphoinositide turnover was in measurements of phosphate incorporation into phospholipids in rat brain *in vivo* after intracisternal injections of histamine, an effect that was blocked by H_1 antagonists (44,150,151). In slices of cerebral cortex of rat (11) and guinea pig (74), histamine stimulated the turnover of phosphoinositides. In slices of cerebral cortex of both guinea pig (33) and rat (17), the effects of agonists and antagonists showed that the H_1 receptor is linked to phosphoinositide turnover, and the response to histamine in different regions of the guinea pig brain reflected the density of H_1 binding sites (21,33). Histamine increased both phosphoinositide turnover and Ca^{2+} efflux in a human astrocytoma cell, an effect mediated by the H_1 receptor (111). In rat cerebral cortical slice, this response to histamine, in contrast to agonists for other receptors, was dependent on extracellular Ca^{2+} (90). On hippocampal slices, the effect of histamine (and of carbachol and of K^+) on phosphoinositide turnover is reduced by excitatory amino acids, e.g., N-methylaspartate, which did not influence the analogous action of norepinephrine (9). These differences in the effects of agonists for different receptors may be additional evidence of different pools of phosphoinositides for different receptors (10). The effects of Li^+ may also suggest different pools of phosphoinositides. In rat cerebral cortical slices, Li^+ did not increase the accumulation of total inositol phosphates produced by histamine stimulation, whereas Li^+ greatly increased the accumulation produced by stimulating the muscarinic, α_1-adrenergic, and 5-hydroxytryptamine receptors (17). The effect of Li^+ also varied with species. Li^+ enhanced histamine-stimulated accumulation of inositol-1-phosphate in guinea pig cerebral cortical slices (33) but not in rat cerebral cortical slices (17). In guinea pig, hippocampal slices were also responsive to Li$^+$ but cerebellar slices were not (33).

The efflorescent state (106) of the work on receptor-linked phosphoinositide turnover makes any statement about the system short-lived and inadequate. It has become clear, however, that phosphoinositide turnover yields more than one second messenger and that products of the phosphoinositides influence other second messengers. On neuroblastoma cells (146), stimulation of the H$_1$ receptor increases phosphoinositide turnover, thereby releasing arachidonate, and the histamine stimulation also increases cyclic GMP formation. Both effects were blocked not only by H$_1$ antagonists but by quinacrine, which inhibits phospholipase A$_2$, one of the enzymes that releases arachidonate. The increased cyclic GMP formation was also blocked by inhibitors of the lipoxygenase pathway of arachidonate metabolism, suggesting that a product(s) of arachidonate (e.g., hydroxyeicosatetraenoic acids, leukotrienes) influences the cyclic GMP response (146). In some cells, it is known that protein kinase C, which is activated on turnover of phosphoinositides, activates guanylate cyclase (see ref. 82). An increase in cyclic AMP and cyclic GMP formation may influence turnover of phosphoinositides (12,115,154). In guinea pig cortical slices, activation of protein kinase C increases the chloroadenosine-stimulated accumulation of cyclic AMP by either histamine or norepinephrine (76). Some of the interactions may be shown to rest on guanine nucleotide-binding proteins, which have been shown to regulate turnover of phosphoinositides (12,16,67) and mobilization of Ca^{2+} (12,54,105). In turn, products of phosphoinositide turnover can influence the state of the guanine nucleotide-binding proteins (83). Arachidonate produced by phosphoinositide turnover influences many enzymes, including adenylate cyclase and guanylate cyclase (see ref. 171), and causes the release and extrusion of Ca^{2+} from some cells (93,169). Not only does phosphoinositide turnover affect ion fluxes, but ion fluxes might also alter the biochemical effector mechanism. In rat hippocampal slices, the effect of some amino acids in inhibiting the stimulation of phosphoinositide turnover required Na$^+$, and the EC$_{50}$ values of the amino acids in inhibiting the receptor-mediated effect were identical to the EC$_{50}$ values for stimulation of receptor-stimulated Na$^+$ flux, an agreement that may suggest (9) that the effect of the amino acids may be secondary to altered intracellular Ca^{2+} produced by the Na$^+$ flux.

THE HISTAMINE H$_2$ RECEPTOR

H$_2$ binding sites have only recently been described in brain and some other tissues with the use of labeled tiotidine (43,48,85,133). In early work with labeled cimetidine, the binding did not reflect the H$_2$ receptor (see ref. 48). [^{3}H]Tiotidine labeled the H$_2$ receptor in some regions of the guinea pig brain (48) with K_D not different from that on the functioning receptor, and other H$_2$ antagonists inhibited the binding with K_D values consonant with those for the functioning receptor. The highest density was seen in the striatum (116). Failure to show specific binding of [^{3}H]tiotidine to the H$_2$ receptor in other tissues, e.g., rat

cerebral cortex, rat uterus, guinea pig atrium, guinea pig gastric mucosa (48), and guinea pig hippocampus (102), may be due to the high nonspecific binding of tiotidine, for other evidence shows that all these tissues have the H$_2$ receptor.

The H$_2$ receptor is linked to adenylate cyclase in many tissues, including brain (84). In guinea pig brain homogenates the H$_2$ receptor is directly linked to stimulation of adenylate cyclase activity as shown by the relative EC$_{50}$ values of agonists and the K_D values of a series of H$_2$ antagonists (62,68,102). In guinea pig brain, activity was highest in homogenates of the hippocampus and neocortex; other regions of the guinea pig brain (and whole rat brain) showed either little or nondetectable responses (60,68,80), even where electrophysiological studies show evidence of the presence of the H$_2$ receptor (see refs. 65, 126). Homogenates of monkey brain showed H$_2$-linked adenylate cyclase, and in this species too the neocortex and hippocampal formation, notably the subiculum, showed greatest activity (112). In neonatal chicks, which lack a blood-brain barrier to histamine, peripheral injections of histamine increased cyclic AMP levels in brain, an effect that was blocked by an H$_2$ antagonist but not an H$_1$ antagonist (108,109). Chick brain slices, especially slices from the cerebral hemispheres, responded to histamine with increased cyclic AMP formation, and the response was blocked by H$_2$ antagonists (110). The synaptic membranes of guinea pig cerebral cortex were especially rich in the H$_2$ receptor (88), a finding that suggested that the receptor is associated with neurons. Kainate lesions in guinea pig hippocampus almost abolished histamine-stimulated cyclic AMP formation in hippocampal slices (50). The H$_2$-linked cyclase may also be present in glial cells, for histamine stimulated cyclic AMP formation in astrocytoma cells (28).

At least in the myenteric plexus of the guinea pig ileum, stimulation of the H$_2$ receptor resulted in contractions that were due to acetylcholine, 5-HT, a peptide(s), and a cyclooxygenase product(s) of arachidonate metabolism (7). These findings could indicate another site of convergence of H$_2$ and H$_1$ receptors (see above) and a means of interaction of neuroregulators.

The H$_2$ receptor in some peripheral cells has been shown to be desensitized. Desensitization of human leukemic cells with dimaprit, which had a half-time of about 2.5 hr and was blocked by cimetidine, was not accompanied by a loss of tiotidine binding sites, suggesting that the receptor was not internalized but rather uncoupled from the cyclase (85). Desensitization of a human gastric cancer cell had a half-life of 20 min and was observed in the isolated membranes as well (127).

New work (167) supports a molecular mechanism for H$_2$ receptor activation that derived from quantum chemical calculations (166). The proton relay mechanisms, based on the tautomerism of the imidazole ring (166), had been shown to apply to other H$_2$ agonists including dimaprit (59).

THE HISTAMINE H$_3$ RECEPTOR

A third histamine receptor that controls histamine release from presynaptic sites has been described (3). Slices of rat brain were incubated with labeled histidine, and the effects of histamine agonists and antagonists in inhibiting the potassium-evoked release of labeled histamine were determined. Histamine inhibited release, and the inhibition was blocked by impromidine (an H_2 agonist) and burimamide (an H_2 antagonist) in a competitive manner, as shown by Schild plots, both yielding pA_2 values of 7.5 (3). The potencies of other compounds in this system differed from potencies on the H_1 and H_2 receptors, including the EC_{50} value of histamine itself, which was 40 nM, lower than its EC_{50} values for the H_1 and H_2 receptors (3–6). Release of histamine increased with increasing external Ca^{2+}, as did the inhibitory effect of histamine, which was also diminished with increasing depolarizing stimuli (5). Slices of the cerebral cortex, striatum, hippocampus, and hypothalamus, all of which are known to have histaminergic terminals, were similarly responsive, and kainate lesions of the striatum did not influence the response (5). Synaptosomes from cerebral cortex responded to histamine with the same EC_{50} as did slices and to impromidine with the same K_D as did slices (5). It is important to emphasize that these findings were on endogenous histamine, i.e., histamine that the slices formed from histidine. On cerebral cortical slices that had been incubated with exogenous, i.e., preformed, histamine, the effect of histamine on the depolarization-induced release was not seen (5). There is evidence too in peripheral tissues that exogenous histamine does not mix with the pool of endogenous histamine (35,45,46,58).

ACKNOWLEDGMENT

The author's original work cited here was supported by a grant (MH 31805) from the National Institute of Mental Health.

REFERENCES

1. Aceves, J., Mariscal, S., Morrison, K. E., and Young, J. M. (1985): *Br. J. Pharmacol.,* 84:417–424.
2. Al-Gadi, M., and Hill, S. J. (1985): *Br. J. Pharmacol.,* 85:877–888.
3. Arrang, J.-M., Garbarg, M., and Schwartz, J.-C. (1983): *Nature,* 302:832–837.
4. Arrang, J.-M., Garbarg, M., and Schwartz, J.-C. (1985): *Adv. Biosci.,* 51:143–153.
5. Arrang, J.-M., Garbarg, M., and Schwartz, J.-C. (1985): *Neuroscience,* 15:553–562.
6. Arrang, J.-M., Schwartz, J.-C., and Schunack, W. (1985): *Eur. J. Pharmacol.,* 117:109–114.
7. Barker, L. A., and Ebersole, J. (1982): *J. Pharmacol. Exp. Ther.,* 221:69–75.
8. Batty, I. R., Nahorski, S. R., and Irvine, R. F. (1985): *Biochem. J.,* 232:211–215.
9. Baudry, M., Evans, J., and Lynch, G. (1986): *Nature,* 319:329–331.
10. Berridge, M. J. (1984): *Biochem. J.,* 220:345–360.
11. Berridge, M. J., Downes, C. P., and Hanley, M. R. (1982): *Biochem. J.,* 206:587–595.
12. Berridge, M. J., and Irvine, R. F. (1984): *Nature,* 312:315–321.
13. Bhargava, K. P., Palit, G., and Dixit, K. S. (1982): *Adv. Biosci.,* 33:115–126.
14. Bielkiewicz, B., and Cook, D. A. (1984): *Gen. Pharmacol.,* 15:51–54.
15. Bielkiewicz, B., and Cook, D. A. (1985): *Can. J. Physiol. Pharmacol.,* 63:756–759.
16. Blackmore, P. F., Bocckino, S. B., Waynick, L. E., and Exton, J. H. (1985): *J. Biol. Chem.,* 260:14477–14483.
17. Brown, E., Kendall, D. A., and Nahorski, S. R. (1984): *J. Neurochem.,* 42:1379–1387.
18. Burgess, G. M., Irvine, R. F., Berridge, J. J., Mckinney, J. S., and Putney, J. W., Jr. (1984): *Biochem. J.,* 224:741–746.
19. Carlini, E. A., and Green, J. P. (1963): *Br. J. Pharmacol.,* 20:264–277.
20. Čarman-Kržan, M. (1984): *Agents Actions,* 14:561–565.
21. Carswell, H., Daum, P. R., and Young, J. M. (1985): *Adv. Biosci.,* 51:27–38.
22. Carswell, H., and Nahorski, S. R. (1982): *Eur. J. Pharmacol.,* 81:301–307.
23. Chang, R. S. L., and Snyder, S. H. (1980): *J. Neurochem.,* 34:916–922.
24. Chang, R. S. L., Tran, V. T., and Snyder, S. H. (1979): *J. Neurochem.,* 32:1653–1663.
25. Chang, R. S. L., Tran, V. T., and Snyder, S. H. (1979): *J. Pharmacol. Exp. Ther.,* 209:437–442.
26. Chang, R. S. L., Tran, V. T., and Snyder, S. H. (1980): *Brain Res.,* 190:95–110.
27. Chasin, M., Mamrak, F., and Samaneigo, S. G. (1974): *J. Neurochem.,* 22:1031–1038.
28. Clark, R. B., and Perkins, J. P. (1971): *Proc. Natl. Acad. Sci. USA,* 68:2757–2760.
29. Clark, W. G., and Lipton, J. M. (1985): *Neurosci. Biobehav. Rev.,* 9:479–552.
30. Dale, H. H. (1966): *Handb. Exp. Pharmacol.,* 18; Part 1:xxvi–xxxv.
31. Daly, J. (1977): *Cyclic Nucleotides in the Nervous System,* pp. 97–99. Plenum Press, New York.
32. Daly, J., McNeal, E., Partington, C., Neuwirth, M., and Creveling, C. R. (1980): *J. Neurochem.,* 35:326–327.
33. Daum, P. R., Downes, C. P., and Young, J. M. (1984): *J. Neurochem.,* 43:25–32.
34. Daum, P. R., Hill, S. J., and Young, J. M. (1982): *Br. J. Pharmacol.,* 77:347–357.
35. Day, M., and Green, J. P. (1962): *Biochem. Pharmacol.,* 11:1043–1048.
36. Diffley, D., Tran, V. T., and Snyder, S. H. (1980): *Eur. J. Pharmacol.,* 64:177–181.
37. Dismukes, R. K., Rogers, M., and Daly, J. W. (1976): *J. Neurochem.,* 26:785–790.
38. Donaldson, J., and Hill, S. J. (1986): *Br. J. Pharmacol.,* 87:191–199.
39. Donoso, A. O., and Alvarez, E. O. (1984): *Trends Pharmacol. Sci.,* 5:98–100.
40. Dryer, S. E. (1985): *Trends Neurosci.,* 8:522.
41. Edvinsson, L., and MacKenzie, E. T. (1977): *Pharmacol. Rev.,* 28:275–348.
42. Edwards, C., Nahorski, S. R., and Rogers, K. J. (1974): *J. Neurochem.,* 22:565–572.
43. Foreman, J. C., Norris, D. B., Rising, T. J., and Weber, S. E. (1985): *Br. J. Pharmacol.,* 86:475–482.
44. Friedel, R. O., and Schanberg, S. M. (1975): *J. Neurochem.,* 24:819–820.
45. Furano, A. V., and Green, J. P. (1963): *Nature,* 109:380–381.
46. Furano, A. V., and Green, J. P. (1964): *Biochem. Biophys. Acta,* 86:596–603.
47. Gaddum, J. H. (1963): *Nature,* 197:741–743.
48. Gajtkowski, G. A., Norris, D. B., Rising, T. J., and Wood, T. P. (1983): *Nature,* 304:65–67.
49. Garbarg, M., Barbin, G., Llorens, C., Palacios, J. M., Pollard, H., and Schwartz, J.-C. (1980): In: *Neurotransmitters, Receptors and Drug Action,* edited by W. B. Essman, pp. 179–202. Spectrum, New York.
50. Garbarg, M., Barbin, G., Palacios, J. M., and Schwartz, J.-C. (1978): *Brain Res.,* 150:638–641.
51. Garbarg, M., and Schwartz, J.-C. (1985): *N. Engl. Rev. Allergy Proc.,* 6:195–200.
52. Garbarg, M., Yeramian, E., Korner, M., and Schwartz, J.-C. (1985): *Adv. Biosci.,* 51:19–25.
53. Gavish, M., Chang, R. S. L., and Snyder, S. H. (1979): *Life Sci.,* 25:783–790.
54. Gomperts, B. D. (1983): *Nature,* 306:64–66.

55. Green, J. P. (1964): *Fed. Proc.*, 23:1095–1102.
56. Green, J. P. (1970): In: *Handb. Neurochem.*, 4:221–250.
57. Green, J. P. (1983): In: *Handb. Psychopharmacol.*, 17:385–420.
58. Green, J. P., and Furano, A. V. (1962): *Biochem. Pharmacol.*, 11:1049–1053.
59. Green, J. P., Johnson, C. L., and Weinstein, H. (1978): In: *Psychopharmacology: A Generation of Progress*, edited by M. A. Lipton, A. DiMascio, and K. F. Killam, pp. 319–332. Raven Press, New York.
60. Green, J. P., Johnson, C. L., and Weinstein, H. (1979): In: *Histamine Receptors*, edited by T. O. Yellin, pp. 185–210. Spectrum, New York.
61. Green, J. P., and Khandelwal, J. K. (1985): *Adv. Biosci.*, 51:185–195.
62. Green, J. P., Johnson, C. L., Weinstein, H., and Maayani, S. (1977): *Proc. Natl. Acad. Sci. USA*, 74:5697–5701.
63. Gross, P. M. (1982): *J. Cereb. Blood Flow Metab.*, 2:3–23.
64. Gross, P. M. (1985): *Adv. Biosci.*, 51:341–349.
65. Haas, H. L. (1985): *Adv. Biosci.*, 51:215–224.
66. Hadfield, A. J., Robinson, N. R., and Hill, S. J. (1983): *Biochem. Pharmacol.*, 32:2449–2451.
67. Haslam, R. J., and Davidson, M. M. L. (1984): *J. Recept. Res.*, 4:605–629.
68. Hegstrand, L. R., Kanof, P. D., and Greengard, P. (1976): *Nature*, 260:163–165.
69. Hill, S. J., Emson, P. C., and Young, J. M. (1978): *J. Neurochem.*, 31:997–1004.
70. Hill, S. J., Hiley, C. R., and Young, J. M. (1981): *Eur. J. Pharmacol.*, 71:421–428.
71. Hill, S. J., and Young, J. M. (1980): *Br. J. Pharmacol.*, 68:687–696.
72. Hill, S. J., and Young, J. M. (1981): *Mol. Pharmacol.*, 19:379–387.
73. Hokin, L. E. (1985): *Annu. Rev. Biochem.*, 54:205–235.
74. Hollingsworth, E. B., and Daly, J. W. (1985): *Biochim. Biophys. Acta*, 847:207–216.
75. Hollingsworth, E. B., McNeal, E. T., Burton, J. L., Williams, R. J., Daly, J. W., and Creveling, C. R. (1985): *J. Neurosci.*, 5:2240–2253.
76. Hollingsworth, E. B., Sears, E. B., and Daly, J. W. (1985): *FEBS Lett.*, 184:339–342.
77. Hösli, E., and Hösli, L. (1984): *Neuroscience*, 13:863–870.
78. Hösli, L., Hösli, E., Schneider, U., and Wiget, W. (1984): *Neurosci. Lett.*, 48:287–291.
79. Hough, L. B., and Green, J. P. (1980): *Psychopharmacol. Bull.*, 16:42–44.
80. Hough, L. B., and Green, J. P. (1981): *Brain Res.*, 219:363–370.
81. Hough, L. B., and Green, J. P. (1984): *Handb. Neurochem.*, 6:145–211.
82. Houslay, M. D. (1985): *Trends Biochem. Sci.*, 10:465–466.
83. Ishac, E. J. N., and Kunos, G. (1986): *Proc. Natl. Acad. Sci. USA*, 83:53–57.
84. Johnson, C. L. (1982): In: *Pharmacology of Histamine Receptors*, edited by C. R. Ganellin and M. E. Parsons, pp. 146–216. John Wright and Sons, Bristol.
85. Johnson, C. L., and Sawutz, D. G. (1985): *Adv. Biosci.*, 51:79–88.
86. Kakiuchi, S., and Rall, T. W. (1968): *Mol. Pharmacol.*, 4:367–378.
87. Kanba, S., and Richelson, E. (1984): *Brain Res.*, 304:1–7.
88. Kanof, P. D., Hegstrand, L. R., and Greengard, P. (1977): *Arch. Biochem. Biophys.*, 182:321–334.
89. Kataoka, K., and DeRobertis, E. (1967): *J. Pharmacol. Exp. Ther.*, 156:114–125.
90. Kendall, D. A., and Nahorski, S. R. (1984): *J. Neurochem.*, 42:1388–1394.
91. Kety, S. S. (1978): *Psychopharmacology: A Generation of Progress*, edited by M. A. Lipton, A. DiMascio, and K. F. Killam, pp. 7–11. Raven Press, New York.
92. Khandelwal, J. K., Hough, L. B., and Green, J. P. (1984): *J. Neurochem.*, 42:519–522.
93. Kolesnick, R. N., and Gershengorn, M. C. (1985): *J. Biol. Chem.*, 260:707–713.
94. Kraly, F. S. (1984): *Psychol. Rev.*, 91:478–490.
95. Kuhar, M. J. (1985): *Trends Neurosci.*, 8:190–191.
96. Kuhn, R. (1970): *Discoveries in Biological Psychiatry*, edited by F. J. Ayd, Jr., and B. Blackwell, pp. 205–217. E. B. Lippincott, Philadelphia.
97. Kuno, T., Kubo, N., and Tanaka, C. (1985): *Biochem. Biophys. Res. Commun.*, 129:639–644.
98. Kuo, J.-F., Lee, T.-P., Reyes, P. L., Walton, K. G., Donnelly, T. E., and Greengard, P. (1972): *J. Biol. Chem.*, 247:16–22.
99. Leibowitz, S. F. (1979): In: *Histamine Receptors*, edited by T. O. Yellin, pp. 219–253. Spectrum, New York.
100. Leibowitz, S. F. (1980): In: *Handbook of the Hypothalamus*, edited by P. J. Morgane and J. Panksepp, 3A:299–437. Marcel Dekker, New York.
101. Lomax, P., and Green, M. D. (1981): *Fed. Proc.*, 40:2741–2745.
102. Maayani, S., Hough, L. B., Weinstein, H., and Green, J. P. (1982): *Adv. Biochem. Psychopharmacol.*, 31:133–147.
103. Mazurkiewicz-Kwilecki, I. M. (1984): *Can. J. Physiol. Pharmacol.*, 62:709–714.
104. Meibach, R. C., Maayani, S., and Green, J. P. (1980): *Eur. J. Pharmacol.*, 67:371–382.
105. Michell, R. (1983): *Trends Biochem. Sci.*, 8:263–265.
106. Michell, R. (1986): *Nature*, 319:176–177.
107. Monnier, M., Sauer, R., and Hatt, A. M. (1970): *Int. Rev. Neurobiol.*, 12:265–305.
108. Nahorski, S. R., Rogers, K. J., and Smith, B. M. (1974): *Life Sci.*, 15:1887–1894.
109. Nahorski, S. R., Rogers, K. J., and Smith, B. M. (1977): *Brain Res.*, 126:387–390.
110. Nahorski, S. R., and Smith, B. M. (1976): *Eur. J. Pharmacol.*, 40:273–278.
111. Nakahata, N., Martin, M. W., Hughes, A. R., Hepler, J. R., and Harden, T. K. (1986): *Mol. Pharmacol.*, 29:188–195.
112. Newton, M. V., Hough, L. B., and Azmitia, E. C. (1982): *Brain Res.*, 239:639–643.
113. Ninkovic, M., and Hunt, S. P. (1985): *Neurosci. Lett.*, 53:133–137.
114. Ninkovic, M., Hunt, S. P., and Gleave, J. R. W. (1982): *Brain Res.*, 241:197–206.
115. Nishizuka, Y., Takai, Y., Kishimoto, A., Kikkawa, U., and Kaibuchi, K. (1984): *Recent Prog. Horm. Res.*, 40:301–345.
116. Norris, D. B., Gajtkowski, G. A., and Rising, T. J. (1984): *Agents Actions*, 14:543–545.
117. O'Dea, R. F., and Zatz, M. (1976): *Proc. Natl. Acad. Sci. USA*, 73:3398–3402.
118. Orrego, F. (1979): *Neuroscience*, 4:1037–1057.
119. Palacios, J. M., Garbarg, M., Barbin, G., and Schwartz, J.-C. (1978): *Mol. Pharmacol.*, 14:971–982.
120. Palacios, J. M., Wamsley, J. K., and Kuhar, M. J. (1981): *Neuroscience*, 6:15–37.
121. Palacios, J. M., Wamsley, J. K., and Kuhar, M. J. (1981): *Brain Res.*, 214:155–162.
122. Palacios, J. M., Young, W. S., and Kuhar, M. J. (1979): *Eur. J. Pharmacol.*, 58:295–304.
123. Paton, W. D. M. (1958): *Annu. Rev. Physiol.*, 20:431–470.
124. Peck, A. W., Fowle, A. S. E., and Bye, C. (1975): *Eur. J. Clin. Pharmacol.*, 8:455–463.
125. Philippu, A. (1985): *Adv. Biosci.*, 51:335–339.
126. Prell, G. D., and Green, J. P. (1986): *Annu. Rev. Neurosci.*, 9:209–254.
127. Prost, A., Emami, S., and Gespach, C. (1984): *FEBS Lett.*, 177:227–230.
128. Psychoyos, S. (1978): *Life Sci.*, 23:2155–2162.
129. Quach, T. T., Duchemin, A. M., Rose, C., and Schwartz, J.-C. (1979): *Eur. J. Pharmacol.*, 60:391–392.
130. Quach, T. T., Duchemin, A. M., Rose, C., and Schwartz, J.-C. (1980): *Neurosci. Lett.*, 17:49–54.
131. Quach, T. T., Duchemin, A. M., Rose, C., and Schwartz, J.-C. (1981): *Mol. Pharmacol.*, 20:331–338.
132. Richelson, E. (1985): *Adv. Biosci.*, 51:237–247.
133. Rising, T. J., and Norris, D. B. (1985): *Adv. Biosci.*, 51:61–67.
134. Roberts, F., and Calcutt, C. R. (1983): *Neuroscience*, 9:721–739.
135. Rumore, M. M., and Schlichting, D. A. (1985): *Life Sci.*, 36:403–416.
136. Saeki, K., Oishi, R., and Nishibori, M. (1985): *Adv. Biosci.*, 51:173–184.
137. Schultz, J., and Daly, J. W. (1973): *J. Biol. Chem.*, 248:860–866.

138. Schwabe, U., Ohga, Y., and Daly, J. W. (1978): *Naunyn Schmiedebergs Arch. Pharmacol.,* 302:141–151.
139. Schwartz, J.-C. (1975): *Life Sci.,* 17:503–518.
140. Schwartz, J.-C. (1979): *Life Sci.,* 25:895–912.
141. Schwartz, J.-C., Barbin, G., Garbarg, M., Pollard, H., and Rose, C. (1976): *Adv. Biochem. Psychopharmacol.,* 15:111–126.
142. Schwartz, J.-C., Barbin, G., Baudry, M., Garbarg, M., and Martres, M. P. (1979): In: *Current Developments in Psychopharmacology, Vol. 5,* edited by W. B. Essman and L. Valzelli, pp. 173–261. Spectrum, New York.
143. Schwartz, J.-C., Barbin, G., Duchemin, A. M., Garbarg, M., Llorens, C., Pollard, H., Quach, T. T., and Rose, C. (1982): In: *Pharmacology of Histamine Receptors,* edited by C. R. Ganellin and M. E. Parsons, pp. 351–391. John Wright and Sons, Bristol.
144. Schwartz, J.-C., Barbin, G., Duchemin, A.-M., Garbarg, M., and Pollard, H. (1981): In: *Neuropharmacology of Central Nervous System and Behavioral Disorders,* edited by G. C. Palmer, pp. 539–570. Academic Press, New York.
145. Seybold, V. S. (1985): *Brain Res.,* 342:291–296.
146. Snider, R. M., McKinney, M., Forray, C., and Richelson, E. (1984): *Proc. Natl. Acad. Sci. USA,* 81:3905–3909.
147. Snyder, S. H., and Bennet, J. P., Jr. (1976): *Annu. Rev. Physiol.,* 38:153–178.
148. Spät, A., Bradford, P. G., McKinney, J. S., Rubin, R. P., and Putney, J. W., Jr. (1986): *Nature,* 319:514–516.
149. Study, R. E., and Greengard, P. (1978): *J. Pharmacol. Exp. Ther.,* 207:767–778.
150. Subramanian, N., Whitmore, W. L., Seidler, F. J., and Slotkin, T. A. (1980): *Life Sci.,* 27:1315–1319.
151. Subramanian, N., Whitmore, W. L., Seidler, F. J., and Slotkin, T. A. (1981): *J. Neurochem.,* 36:1137–1141.
152. Subramanian, N., Whitmore, W. L., and Slotkin, T. A. (1981): *J. Neurosci.,* 1:674–678.
153. Swazey, J. P. (1974): *Chlorpromazine in Psychiatry: A Study of Therapeutic Innovation.* MIT Press, Cambridge.
154. Takai, Y., Kikkawa, U., Kaibuchi, K., and Nishizuka, Y. (1984): In: *Advances in Cyclic Nucleotide and Protein Phosphorylation Research, Vol. 18,* edited by P. Greengard and G. A. Robinson, pp. 119–158. Raven Press, New York.
155. Taylor, J. E., and Richelson, E. (1979): *Mol. Pharmacol.,* 15:462–471.
156. Taylor, J. E., and Richelson, E. (1980): *Eur. J. Pharmacol.,* 67:41–46.
157. Taylor, J. E., and Richelson, E. (1982): *Eur. J. Pharmacol.,* 78:279–285.
158. Toll, L., and Snyder, S. H. (1982): *J. Biol. Chem.,* 257:13593–13601.
159. Tran, V. T., Freeman, A. D., Chang, R. S. L., and Snyder, S. H. (1980): *J. Neurochem.,* 34:1609–1613.
160. Tran, V. T., Lebovitz, R., Toll, L., and Snyder, S. H. (1981): *Eur. J. Pharmacol.,* 70:501–509.
161. Tuomisto, J., and Mannisto, P. (1985): *Pharmacol. Rev.,* 37:249–332.
162. Uchida, M. (1980): *Eur. J. Pharmacol.,* 64:357–360.
163. Wada, H., Watanabe, T., Yamatodani, A., Maeyama, K., Itoi, N., Cacabelos, R., Seo, M., Kiyono, S., Nagai, K., and Nakagawa, H. (1985): *Adv. Biosci.,* 51:225–235.
164. Wallace, R. M., and Young, J. M. (1983): *Mol. Pharmacol.,* 23:60–66.
165. Weinreich, D. (1985): *Adv. Biosci.,* 51:205–214.
166. Weinstein, H., Chou, C. L., Johnson, C. L., Kang, S., and Green, J. P. (1976): *Mol. Pharmacol.,* 12:738–745.
167. Weinstein, H., Mazurek, A. P., Osman, R., and Topiol, S. (1986): *Mol. Pharmacol.,* 29:28–33.
168. Werman, R. (1966): *Comp. Biochem. Physiol.,* 18:745–746.
169. Wolf, B. A., Turk, J., Sherman, W. R., and McDaniel, M. L. (1986): *J. Biol. Chem.,* 261:3501–3511.
170. Yeramian, E., Garbarg, M., and Schwartz, J.-C. (1985): *Mol. Pharmacol.,* 28:155–162.
171. Zeitler, P., and Handwerger, S. (1985): *Mol. Pharmacol.,* 28:549–554.

Psychopharmacology:
The Third Generation of Progress,
edited by Herbert Y. Meltzer.
Raven Press, New York © 1987.

CHAPTER 29

Opioid Receptors

Gavril W. Pasternak

Opiates have long been used for the relief of pain. Unlike anesthetics, opiates relieve the subjective "hurt" without altering objective sensations. Attempts to develop effective analgesics lacking the side effects of the naturally occurring opiates have led to the synthesis of literally thousands of derivatives and the establishment of extensive structure-activity relationships. Based on these studies, pharmacologists predicted that the opiates acted through specific receptors within the nervous system. Indeed, tentative "maps" of the active binding site of the "opiate receptor" were suggested long before these sites were biochemically demonstrated (5,76). It was obvious, even then, that the receptors had endogenous substrates and that the opiates were probably mimicking these endogenous substances. The enkephalins, the first endogenous opioid peptides, were initially identified in 1975 (31,64,91). Since then a number of peptides with opioid activities have been identified, such as β-endorphin, dynorphin, and α-neoendorphin (for a review, see 18).

Opiate receptor multiplicity is an old concept, having first been suggested by Martin (47) on the basis of the interactions between morphine and the mixed agonist-antagonist nalorphine (29,39). This original concept, termed Receptor Dualism, was then expanded on the basis of detailed studies of a series of opiates in the chronic spinal dog (48). Based on the different pharmacological profiles of several opiates, Martin suggested three distinct classes of receptors, which he named μ (morphine), κ (ketocyclazocine), and σ (SKF10,047 or *N*-allylnormetazocine). Thus, classical pharmacological approaches provided the first evidence for the concept of opiate receptor multiplicity long before their demonstration biochemically.

OPIATE BINDING STUDIES

Opiate binding sites were first reported in 1973 (74,85,90). Although the different laboratories utilized different ligands, their results were remarkably similar. Binding was highly stereospecific and the ligand possessed affinities in the nanomolar range. Unlabeled opiates inhibited binding with rank orders of potency very similar to those observed *in vivo* (Table 1). The only notable exception was codeine, which was far less effective in binding studies than *in vivo*. However, codeine's actions *in vivo* result from its *O*-demethylation to form morphine, which does not take place under binding conditions. Thus, even this "exception" still argued for the relevancy of binding. Perhaps the most persuasive argument for the importance of these binding sites was their high selectivity for only opiate compounds. In detailed testing of literally dozens of centrally active nonopiate compounds, none inhibited radiolabeled opiate binding at concentrations over 100-fold greater than those needed for opiates.

Investigators have long used the guinea pig ileum assay to study opiate actions (71). In this bioassay, opiates inhibit the electrically induced contraction of the longitudinal muscle through the inhibition of acetylcholine release. Thus, correlating opiate binding in the plexus of ileum with the bioassay was an important issue in confirming the relevance of these binding sites. In a detailed series of experiments, Creese and Snyder (16) compared the actions of a number of opiates in both the binding and bioassays. In brief, they reported that the relative affinity of the various compounds in binding studies correlated extremely well with their potency in the bioassays.

TABLE 1. Competition of [^3H]naloxone binding by a series of opiates

Drug	IC$_{50}$ value (nM)
(−)Etorphine	0.3
(−)Levallorphan	1
(−)Levorphanol	2
(−)Nalorphine	3
(−)Morphine	7
(−)Cyclazocine	10
(−)Naloxone	10
(−)Methadone	30
(+)Methadone	300
(+)3-Hydroxy-N-allylmorphinan	7,000
(+)Dextrorphan	8,000
(−)Codeine	20,000

Note that dextrorphan is the optical isomer of levorphanol and (+)3-hydroxy-N-allylmorphinan is the inactive (+)isomer of (−)levallorphan (74).

Discrimination of Agonist and Antagonist Binding: The Sodium Effect

The opiate system with its large number of agonists and antagonists offered a major advantage in the study of agonist and antagonist actions at the receptor level. Soon after the initial studies, we reported dramatic differences in the actions of sodium ions on the binding characteristics of a number of radiolabeled opiate agonists and antagonists (73). While examining the binding of [^3H]naloxone, I noted that sodium salts markedly increased binding and suggested to Adele Snowman, a technician in the laboratory, that she should try it with [^3H]dihydromorphine, which had just become available, in the hope that its binding would also be increased. When she found dramatic decreases in [^3H]dihydromorphine binding, several heated arguments ensued. The controversy was settled by testing both ^3H-ligands together. We then examined a number of other pairs of agonists and antagonists and concluded that this was a general action of sodium ions on agonists and antagonists (Table 2). Saturation studies verified an increase in the number of sites as opposed to changes in affinity.

TABLE 2. Effect of sodium ions on [^3H]opiate binding

Radioligand	Change in binding produced by sodium
Agonists	
Dihydromorphine	−70%
Oxymorphone	−44%
Levorphanol	−38%
Antagonists	
Nalorphine	+45%
Naloxone	+145%
Levallorphan	+29%

Binding was determined in the presence and absence of sodium chloride (100 mM) (73).

Others have reported similar results (86). Thus, the opiate system was the first to demonstrate the ability of sodium ions to discriminate between agonist and antagonist binding.

Guanine nucleotides, particularly GTP, also produce similar actions on the binding of opiate agonists and antagonists (6,11,13,14). Again, agonist binding was far more sensitive. In addition, the inhibition of agonist binding was far greater in the presence of both GTP and sodium than with either alone.

Other ions and treatments also influence agonist and antagonist binding differentially (Table 3). Divalent cations, such as manganese and magnesium, facilitate agonist binding, particularly in the presence of sodium ions (66). Indeed, manganese appears to lower the sensitivity of radiolabeled agonist binding to sodium ions. In full concentration studies manganese shifted the inhibition of opiate binding by sodium to the right. Reagents, particularly those reacting with sulfhydryl groups, and enzymes such as trypsin and chymotrypsin, also affect agonist and antagonist binding differently (67,69,94). In general, these treatments enhance the sensitivity of agonist binding to sodium ions, lowering agonist binding more effectively than antagonist binding.

Although these early studies employed ligands with primarily μ selectivity, similar findings have been reported with the other classes of opiate receptors (51,52,84). However, more detailed investigations of reagents and divalent cations on these additional receptor classes are still needed.

TABLE 3. Discrimination between agonist and antagonist binding

Treatment	Agonist binding	Antagonist binding	Refs.
Ions			
Monovalent			73,86
Sodium	Decrease	Increase	
Potassium	Sl. decrease	Sl. decrease	
Lithium	Decrease	Increase	
Divalent			66
Magnesium	Increase	Little change	
Manganese	Increase	Little change	
Calcium	Little change	Little change	
Enzymes			67
Trypsin	Decrease	Little change	
Chymotrypsin	Decrease	Little change	
Phospholipase A	Decrease	Little change	
Reagents			69,94
N-Ethylmaleimide	Decrease	Little change	
Iodoacetamide	Decrease	Little change	
Mercuriacetate	Decrease	Little change	
Mersalyl acid	Decrease	Little change	
Nucleotides			6,11,13,14
GTP	Decrease	Little change	

This table reviews the actions of a number of treatments on the binding of opiate agonists and antagonists. Note that differential effects are observed at low concentrations of the treatments. The enzymes and reagents, for example, will markedly depress antagonist binding at sufficiently high concentrations.

The pattern of these actions is consistent with those observed in other receptor systems coupled through N proteins to effectors such as cyclase. Indeed, much work now suggests that the δ receptors in cell lines do modulate cyclase activity through the N_i protein.

Multiplicity of Opioid Binding Sites

After the discovery of the enkephalins, peptapeptides with morphine-like actions (31,64,91), Kosterlitz and co-workers soon reported that the relative potency of morphine and the enkephalins differed in the guinea pig ileum and mouse vas deferens bioassays (45). Using radiolabeled enkephalins and opiates, investigators soon identified separate binding sites for morphine and the enkephalins, which were named μ and δ, respectively (Table 4; 8,45). These sites differed in many respects. Foremost, they bound opiates and opioid peptides with very different specificities. Compounds potent at μ sites competed radiolabeled δ ligands quite poorly whereas those active at δ sites had a correspondingly low affinity for μ receptors. In addition, these morphine-preferring μ sites and the enkephalin-selective δ ones also were located in different regions of the brain (7).

Cross-protection studies also argued strongly for distinct classes of binding sites (79,87). Both phenoxybenzamine and the reagent N-ethylmaleimide inhibit radiolabeled opiate binding irreversibly. Occupation of the binding site with an opiate, however, can protect it from inactivation. In these studies, membranes were preincubated with opiates or opioid peptides with either μ or δ selectivity and the membranes treated with phenoxybenzamine or the reagent. In brief, both laboratories found no cross protection between the two classes of compounds. That is, each class of ligand protected only the binding of other radioligands of its own class but not the other. These findings also constituted strong evidence for discrete μ and δ binding sites.

Multiple μ Receptors

Even before the discovery of the enkephalins, binding data had suggested the presence of more than one class of site. Using the radiolabeled antagonist naloxone and the

TABLE 4. *Discrimination between μ and δ binding in the rat CNS*

Compound	IC$_{50}$ value (nM)		IC$_{50}$ ratio (δ/μ)
	δ	μ	
Morphine	35	0.5	70
Naloxone	15	0.8	19
[Met^5]enkephalin	4	10	0.4
[Leu^5]enkephalin	3.2	25	0.14
[D-Ala^2,D-Leu^5]enkephalin	1.5	6	0.25

IC$_{50}$ values were determined against δ binding (^{125}I[D-Ala^2,D-Leu^5]enkephalin) and μ binding ([^{3}H]naloxone). (Adapted from ref. 8.)

TABLE 5. *Approximate K$_D$ values for μ$_1$, μ$_2$, and δ binding*

Ligand (nM)	Approximate K$_D$ value		
	μ$_1$	μ$_2$	δ
Morphine	0.4	9	70
Dihydromorphine	0.2	3	n.d.
[D-Ala^2,D-Leu^5]enkephalin	0.5	50	6

n.d., Not determined.

agonist dihydromorphine, we identified a novel, very high-affinity binding component (68). Our laboratory has studied this binding component extensively over the past few years. At first, we thought that this component simply represented a conformational change, but this is not the case. Data from our laboratory as well as others now suggests that this high-affinity binding component, which we have termed the μ$_1$ site, represents a distinct receptor that binds opiates such as morphine and the enkephalins with similar, very high affinities (46,92,96,100). We proposed that morphine and the enkephalins label three sites: the common, high-affinity μ$_1$ site; the morphine-selective μ$_2$ site; and the enkephalin-preferring δ site (Table 5; Fig. 1; ref. 96).

Conceptually, our hypothesis of μ$_1$ sites differs from other neurotransmitter receptor systems. Most receptor systems are divergent with a single transmitter labeling a number of receptor subtypes. However, the μ$_1$ site might be considered as an example of convergence. It represents a common binding site for a number of different opiates and opioid peptides, which binds them far more potently than their respective selective sites.

Evidence supporting this concept of a common high-affinity binding site for opiates and opioid peptides comes from a variety of experimental approaches. These include standard biochemical and competition studies (27,46,55,92),

BINDING OF MORPHINE AND ENKEPHALIN IN THE BRAIN

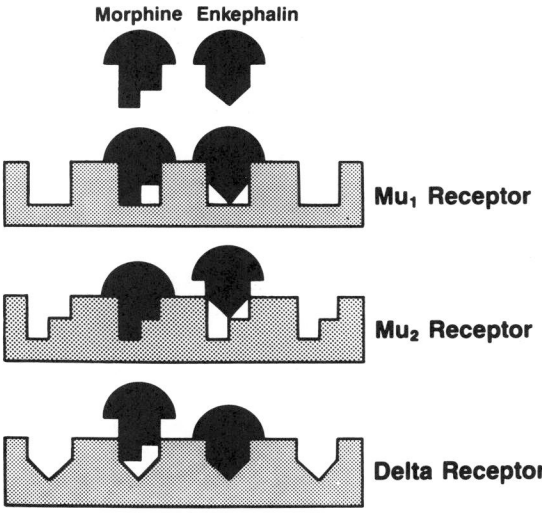

FIG. 1. Schematic representation of μ$_1$, μ$_2$, and δ binding sites.

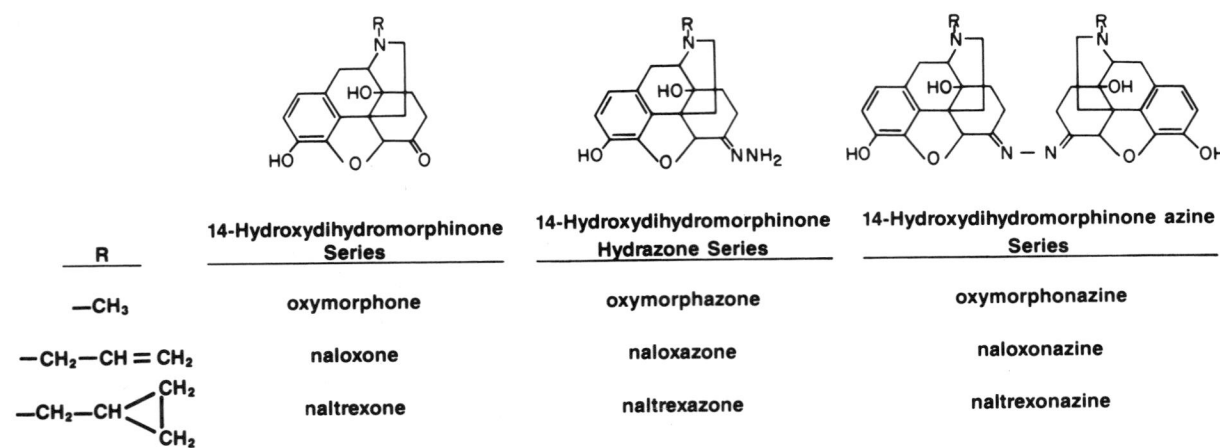

R	14-Hydroxydihydromorphinone Series	14-Hydroxydihydromorphinone Hydrazone Series	14-Hydroxydihydromorphinone azine Series
—CH₃	oxymorphone	oxymorphazone	oxymorphonazine
—CH₂—CH=CH₂	naloxone	naloxazone	naloxonazine
—CH₂—CH(CH₂)(CH₂)	naltrexone	naltrexazone	naltrexonazine

FIG. 2. Structures of a series of opiate hydrazones and azines.

as well as comparisons of the developmental appearance (70,106), phylogenetic (55), and regional distributions (24,53,54,107) of the μ_1 site with the classical morphine-selective (μ_2) and δ sites.

The 10-fold greater affinity of this high-affinity binding component coupled with its low binding capacity quickly distinguished it from the sites originally reported in 1973. However, they also resulted in a number of technical difficulties in studying its binding. Typically, μ_1 binding is overwhelmed by binding to the other subtypes, which are present in far greater numbers. Even though the percentage of μ_1 sites occupied is greater than either μ_2 or δ sites at a fixed concentration of radioligand, μ_1 binding usually represents less than 30% of total specific binding, since binding is the product of the percentage occupancy and the total number of sites (B_{max}). Indeed, under some experimental conditions, μ_1 binding cannot be easily detected at all. Using sophisticated computer analysis programs with complex statistical analysis, Rodbard and Munson have examined the question of a common, high-affinity binding site in detail (46). In brief, their results support the existence of μ_1 sites. Similarly, Toll and Loew also confirm the presence of these sites using computer analysis (92). The

more recent development of a highly selective μ_1 binding assay in which over 75% of total specific binding corresponds to μ_1 sites (15) may overcome these technical problems.

Our understanding of this binding component has been greatly facilitated by the development of several μ_1-selective affinity labels, naloxazone and naloxonazine (Fig. 2; refs. 26,65). Both compounds irreversibly inhibited the high-affinity binding component of a large series of radiolabeled opioid peptides, opiates, and antagonists (27,56,58–63,96,105), implying that they labeled a common site. This hypothesis was supported by competition studies as well. Morphine inhibited the binding of radiolabeled enkephalin in a biphasic manner (Fig. 3; refs. 8,27,56,96). A portion of binding was lowered by morphine at concentrations under 1 nM, whereas the remainder was far less sensitive. Treating the tissue with either naloxazone or naloxonazine, which eliminated the higher-affinity binding component of radiolabeled enkephalin binding, also abolished the morphine-sensitive binding, suggesting that the high-affinity binding component of radiolabeled enkephalin was highly sensitive to morphine inhibition. In additional saturation experiments, morphine at 1 nM also inhibited the higher-affinity component of radiolabeled enkephalin binding far

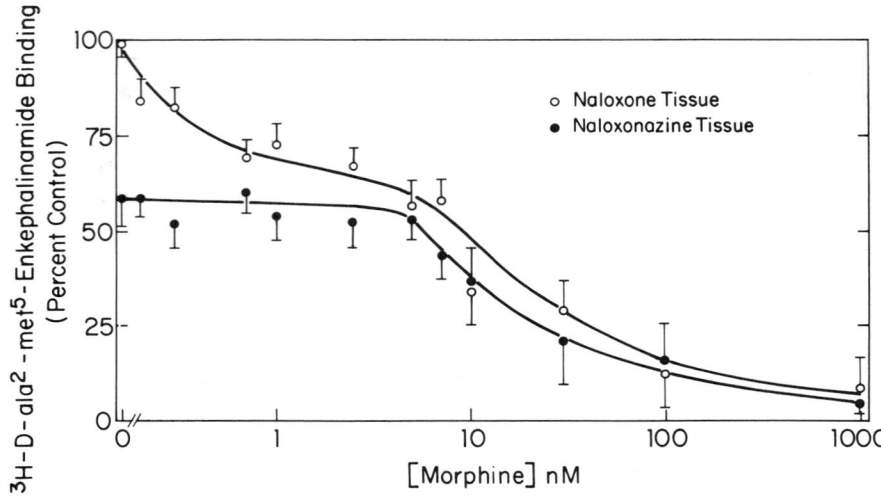

FIG. 3. Inhibition of radiolabeled enkephalin binding by morphine. Tissue was treated with either naloxone (○) or naloxonazine (●; 50 nM each) and then washed extensively to remove reversibly bound ligand. The tissue treated with naloxone provided control binding since naloxone is totally reversible. [³H][D-Ala²,Met⁵]enkephalinamide binding was then determined in the presence of various concentrations of morphine. (From ref. 26.)

more effectively than the lower-affinity component. Together, these binding studies implied that the higher-affinity binding component of radiolabeled enkephalin binding, with its greater sensitivity toward morphine, corresponded to a common, high-affinity binding for opiates and enkephalins.

A major question surrounding the μ_1 site has been its relationship to the classical μ and δ sites. The evidence reviewed above was most consistent with a common high-affinity site for both morphine and the enkephalins, yet other experiments clearly demonstrated selective sites for morphine and the enkephalins (7,8,45). Could the lower-affinity components observed in the saturation experiments represent the selective binding sites? (Note that these "low-affinity" sites still bound opiates and opioid peptides quite well with K_D values under 10 nM.) This question was addressed directly by examining the ability of opiates and enkephalins to inhibit binding in tissue whose high-affinity sites had been blocked by naloxazone treatment. After elimination of the high-affinity sites, the remaining sites selectively bound either morphine or the enkephalins (96). Together, these results led us to propose three morphine and enkephalin binding sites in the central nervous system. Other experimental approaches were also consistent with this hypothesis, including developmental, phylogenetic, and regional studies (24,55,70,106,107).

κ Receptors

Martin's original studies examining a series of opiates in the chronic spinal dog characterized the actions of ketocyclazocine, a benzomorphan. Based on these results, Martin suggested a distinct receptor for this class of compound, which he termed κ. More recently, Goldstein and co-workers reported a novel opioid peptide, which they named dynorphin (22). Subsequent results suggest that dynorphin is the natural ligand for the κ site (12). Neuropharmacological evidence supports the existence of κ sites, including discriminative effects and sensitivity toward naloxone reversal (32,57,83,97,99,101).

Binding approaches designed to demonstrate κ sites were difficult, but successful. Due to the instability of natural peptides, most investigators have successfully employed a number of synthetic opiates, such as ethylketocyclazocine and bremazocine (9,10,33,34,37,49,58,75,78,95). However, some of these investigations were difficult to interpret, since these radioligands also labeled a number of different receptor subtypes in addition to κ sites, and the density of κ sites varied dramatically among species, with relatively low levels in rat brain and high levels in guinea pig brain. The demonstration of predominantly κ sites in the guinea pig cerebellum (78) promises to provide an important experimental advance in the characterization of this receptor subtype.

σ Receptors

The pharmacological profile of *N*-allylnormetazocine (SKF10,047) also led Martin to propose selective receptors for this compound, termed σ. These sites have been implicated in psychotomimetic actions (20,28,36,48,82). Much controversy surrounds this category. First, the dextro isomers are often more active than the levo isomers, the opposite of classical opiate stereospecificity. In addition, much evidence suggests that σ opiates might actually be labeling a phencyclidine (PCP) receptor (89,93,108,109).

ε Receptors

Selective sites for β-endorphin have also been proposed on the basis of both bioassays (80,81) and binding approaches (23,30,35,40). Autoradiographic studies of [³H]β-endorphin binding also suggest the presence of distinct ϵ sites (23). However, the cross binding of radiolabeled β-endorphin to both μ and δ sites greatly complicated the interpretation of both the binding and the autoradiographic results.

REGIONAL DISTRIBUTION OF OPIATE BINDING SITES

The first detailed study examined the binding of [³H]dihydromorphine in various regions of monkey and human brain (38). This report firmly established the correlation of opiate binding sites with gray matter and demonstrated a strong association of opiate binding sites with the limbic system. Areas with particularly high levels of binding included the amygdala, hypothalamus, thalamus, caudate, and periaqueductal gray. Autoradiographic studies of opiate binding in rat brain confirmed this distribution (1–4,17,72). The binding in the striatum was particularly interesting. Instead of a diffuse labeling, a number of "patches" or clusters of high levels of binding sites were noted.

Following the development of radiolabeled enkephalin derivatives suitable for binding, Goodman and co-workers compared the distribution of δ and μ receptors in rat brain (25), confirming previous studies using homogenate binding (7). Although these studies were not quantitative, the differences in patterns were quite convincing (Table 6). For example, in the cortex, μ sites were localized to laminae I and IV whereas δ sites were found in laminae II, III, and V. In addition, μ ligands labeled the streaks and clusters in the striatum whereas δ compounds yielded a diffuse labeling, increasing in density from medial to lateral areas.

The distribution of multiple μ receptors has also been examined using both grain counting (53,54) and novel computerized digital subtraction techniques (24). These studies confirmed the previous distribution of δ sites and total μ sites. However, they also revealed the distribution of μ_1 sites within the brain. The μ_1 sites had a high distribution within the medial thalamus, periaqueductal grey, the clusters of the striatum, superior colliculus, and median raphe. The relationship of μ_1 sites to areas known to be important in mediating opiate analgesia was particularly striking. Most impressive, however, were the observations in the CXBK strain of mouse, which is relatively insensitive to morphine analgesia, that the density of μ_1 sites was far lower in brain regions associated with mor-

TABLE 6. *Regional distribution of μ and δ binding sites*

Predominantly μ	Predominantly δ	μ and δ
Cortex: laminae I & IV	Cortex: laminae II & V	Cortex: lamina VI
Streaks and clusters in corpus striatum	Diffuse labeling in corpus striatum	N. tractus solitarius
Thalamus	Amygdala	Vagus fibers
Hypothalamus	N. accumbens	N. ambiguus
Hippocampus pyramidal cell layer	Olfactory tubercle	Sub. gelatinosa
Periaqueductal gray	Pontine nuclei	
Interpeduncular nucleus		
Inferior colliculus		
Median raphe		

From ref. 25.

phine's analgesic response, including the periaqueductal gray, whereas other subtypes were not changed (53).

CORRELATION OF BINDING SITES WITH PHARMACOLOGICAL ACTIONS

Analgesia

Based on his studies in the chronic spinal dog, Martin proposed that μ sites mediated this important opiate effect (48). Studies with both naloxazone and naloxonazine support the association of analgesia with μ sites and further suggest that μ_1 sites are responsible for these actions (27,41–44,58–63,105,106). Blockade of μ_1 sites *in vivo* shifts the dose-response curve for morphine analgesia over 12-fold to the right in mice (42,62,63) and fourfold in rats (43). The analgesic activities of a number of other opiates and opioid peptides were also significantly attenuated, consistent with binding studies demonstrating their affinity for μ_1 sites. Thus, these studies suggest a role for μ_1 sites in supraspinal opioid analgesia.

The receptor mechanisms of opioid analgesia at the spinal cord level appear to be quite different from supraspinal ones. Yaksh and co-workers have examined the potency of a variety of opiates and opioid peptides given either intracerebroventricularly or intrathecally (102–104). In brief, he finds that the opioid peptides are far more effective than opiates intrathecally, suggesting a role of δ receptors in analgesia at the spinal cord level (19). Additional experiments support this general conclusion. δ-Active compounds are also relatively more potent than morphine after isolating spinal mechanisms through transection of the cord (42). Other investigators have proposed an important role for κ receptors in analgesia (32,97–99,101), but the interpretation of these results is complicated by the extensive cross binding of these drugs with other receptor subtypes.

Respiratory Depression

Respiratory depression is one of the most troublesome opioid side effects. Although it does not present clinically significant problems often, they can be fatal when they do

occur. The identification of multiple classes of opioid receptors raised the possibility that analgesia and respiratory depression might be mediated through different receptor mechanisms (43,44,50). Recent studies now suggest that respiratory depression is mediated through μ_2 sites, as opposed to supraspinal analgesia, which involves μ_1 sites (43,44). Whereas naloxonazine blockade of μ_1 sites shifts the analgesic dose-response curves for morphine, the dose-response curves for the elevation of pCO_2, depression of pO_2, and pH were unaffected (Fig. 4).

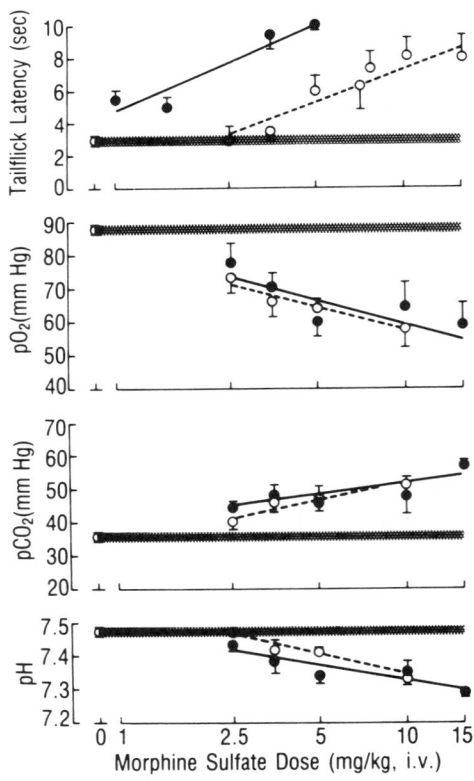

FIG. 4. Effects of naloxonazine on morphine analgesia and respiratory function. Rats were treated with naloxonazine (10 mg/kg, i.v.) and then tested 24 hr later either for analgesia in the tailflick assay or for respiratory function using chronically implanted arterial lines. (From ref. 43.)

TABLE 7. *Tentative classification of opioid actions*

μ_1-Mediated	Not μ_1-mediated
Supraspinal analgesia	Spinal analgesia (δ and/or κ)
Prolactin release	Growth hormone release (μ_2 or δ)
Acetylcholine turnover	Dopamine turnover (μ_2 and δ)
Catalepsy	Sedation (κ)
Hypothermia	Respiratory depression (μ_2)
Feeding (free and deprivation-induced)	Inhibition of guinea pig ileum contractions (μ_2 and κ)
	Bradycardia (μ_2)
	Reversal of endotoxic shock (δ)
	Feeding (deoxyglucose-induced)
	Most signs of physical dependence

Other Opioid Actions

A variety of other opioid actions have been investigated (Table 7). The peripheral bioassays, for example, have clearly implicated morphine-selective (μ_2) receptors in the peripherally mediated inhibition of intestinal transit (21). Hormone release studies have also demonstrated that morphine-induced prolactin and growth hormone release are produced through different receptor subtypes (88). Other studies examining the effects of opiates and opioid peptides on transmitter release have also established a role for μ_1 sites in the release of acetylcholine but not dopamine (97,98).

CONCLUSION

The study of opiate receptors and their endogenous peptides and the opiates has become increasingly more complex each year, tempting us to observe that the only things simple in science are scientists. Despite major advances into the mechanisms of opiate action, many more questions remain. Some are quite basic, such as the identity of the endogenous ligand for the morphine-selective μ_2 receptor. Other areas involve the effector systems mediating opiate actions at the cellular level. The binding characteristics of these compounds strongly suggest a role of N proteins, but only δ sites have been associated with cyclase. Attempts to associate the other opiate binding sites, particularly μ receptors, with phosphotidylinositol metabolism have not been successful. Finally, the concept of convergent receptor systems binding multiple classes of neurotransmitters is intriguing and needs additional study.

REFERENCES

1. Atweh, S. F., and Kuhar, M. J. (1977): *Brain Res.*, 124:53–67.
2. Atweh, S. F., and Kuhar, M. J. (1977): *Brain Res.*, 129:1–12.
3. Atweh, S. F., and Kuhar, M. J. (1977): *Brain Res.*, 134:393–405.
4. Atweh, S. F., and Kuhar, M. J. (1983): *Br. Med. Bull.*, 39:47–52.
5. Becket, A. H., and Casey, A. F. (1965): *Prog. Med. Chem.*, 4:171–218.
6. Blume, A. (1978): *Life Sci.*, 22:1843–1852.
7. Chang, K.-J., Cooper, B. R., Hazum, E., and Cuatrecasas, P. (1978): *Mol. Pharmacol.*, 16:91–104.
8. Chang, K.-J., and Cuatrecasas, P. (1979): *J. Biol. Chem.*, 254:2610–2618.
9. Chang, K.-J., Hazum, E., and Cuatrecasas, P. (1980): *Proc. Natl. Acad. Sci. USA*, 77:4469–4473.
10. Chang, K.-J., Hazum, E., and Cuatrecasas, P. (1981): *Proc. Natl. Acad. Sci. USA*, 78:4141–4145.
11. Chang, K.-J., Hazum, E., Killian, A., and Cuatrecasas, P. (1981): *Mol. Pharmacol.*, 20:1–7.
12. Chavkin, C., James, I. F., and Goldstein, A. (1982): *Science*, 215:413.
13. Childers, S. R., and Snyder, S. H. (1978): *Life Sci.*, 23:759–762.
14. Childers, S. R., and Snyder, S. H. (1980): *J. Neurochem.*, 34:583–593.
15. Clark, and Pasternak, G. W. (1986): *Soc. Neurosci.*, 12:371.
16. Creese, I., and Snyder, S. H. (1975): *J. Pharmacol. Exp. Ther.*, 194:205–219.
17. Duka, I., Schubert, P., Wuster, M., Stiber, R., and Herz, A. (1981): *Neurosci. Lett.*, 21:119–124.
18. Frederickson, R. C. A. (1984): *Endogenous Opioids and Related Derivatives in Analgesics: Neurochemical, Behavioral and Clinical Perspectives*, edited by M. J. Kuhar and G. W. Pasternak, pp. 9–68. Raven Press, New York.
19. Frederickson, R. C. A., Smithwick, E. L., Shuman, R., and Bemis, K. G. (1981): *Science*, 211:603–605.
20. Gilbert, P. E., and Martin, W. R. (1976): *J. Pharmacol. Exp. Ther.*, 198:66–82.
21. Gintzler, A. R., and Pasternak, G. W. (1983): *Neurosci. Lett.*, 39:51–56.
22. Goldstein, A., Tachibana, S., Lowney, L. I., Hunkapiller, M., and Hood, L. (1979): *Proc. Natl. Acad. Sci. USA*, 76:6666–6670.
23. Goodman, R. R., Houghten, R. A., and Pasternak, G. W. (1983): *Life Sci.*, 288:334–337.
24. Goodman, R. R., and Pasternak, G. W. (1985): *Proc. Natl. Acad. Sci. USA*, 82:6667–6671.
25. Goodman, R. R., Snyder, S. H., Kuhar, M. J., and Young, W. S. (1980): *Proc. Natl. Acad. Sci. USA*, 77:6239–6243.
26. Hahn, E. F., Carroll-Buatti, M., and Pasternak, G. W. (1982): *J. Neurosci.*, 2:572–576.
27. Hazum, E., Chang, K.-J., Cuatrecasas, P., and Pasternak, G. W. (1981): *Life Sci.*, 28:2973–2979.
28. Holtzman, S. G. (1982): *Psychopharmacology*, 77:295–300.
29. Houde, R. W., and Wallenstein, S. L. (1956): *Fed. Proc.*, 15:440–441.
30. Houghten, R. A., Chang, W. C., and Li, C. H. (1980): *J. Pept. Prot. Res.*, 16:311–320.
31. Hughes, J., Smith, T. W., Kosterlitz, H. W., Fothergill, L. A., Morgan, B. A., and Morris, H. R. (1975): *Nature*, 258:577–579.
32. Hutchinson, M., Kosterlitz, H. W., Leslie, F. M., Waterfield, A. A., and Terenius, L. (1975): *Br. J. Pharmacol.*, 55:541–546.
33. Itzhak, Y., Hiller, J. M., and Simon, E. J. (1984): *Proc. Natl. Acad. Sci. USA*, 81:4217–4222.
34. James, I. F., and Goldstein, A. (1984): *Mol. Pharmacol.*, 25:337–342.
35. Johnson, N., Houghten, R., and Pasternak, G. W. (1982): *Life Sci.*, 31:1381–1384.
36. Khazam, N., Young, G. A., El-Fakany, E. E., Hony, O., and Calligan, D. (1984): *Neuropharmacology*, 23:983–987.
37. Kosterlitz, H. W., Paterson, S. J., and Robson, L. E. (1981): *Br. J. Pharmacol.*, 73:939–949.
38. Kuhar, M. J., Pert, C. B., and Snyder, S. H. (1973): *Nature*, 245:447–451.
39. Lasagna, L., and Beecher, H. K. (1954): *J. Pharmacol. Exp. Ther.*, 112:356–363.
40. Law, P. Y., Loh, H. H., and Li, C. H. (1979): *Proc. Natl. Acad. Sci. USA*, 76:5455–5459.
41. Ling, G. S. F., Macleod, J. M., Lee, S., Lockhart, S., and Pasternak, G. W. (1984): *Science*, 226:462–464.
42. Ling, G. S. F., and Pasternak, G. W. (1983): *Brain Res.*, 271:152–156.
43. Ling, G. S. F., Spiegel, K., Lockhart, S. H., and Pasternak, G. W. (1985): *J. Pharmacol. Exp. Ther.*, 232:149–155.
44. Ling, G. S. F., Spiegel, K., Nishimura, S., and Pasternak, G. W. (1983): *Eur. J. Pharmacol.*, 86:487–488.
45. Lord, J. H., Waterfield, A. A., Hughes, J., and Kosterlitz, H. W. (1977): *Nature*, 267:495–499.

46. Lutz, R. A., Cruciani, R. A., Costa, T., Munson, P. J., and Rodbard, D. (1984): *Biochem. Biophys. Res. Commun.*, 122: 265–269.
47. Martin, W. R. (1967): *Pharmacol. Rev.*, 19:463–521.
48. Martin, W. R., Eades, C. G., Thompson, J. A., Huppler, R. E., and Gilbert, P. E. (1976): *J. Pharmacol. Exp. Ther.*, 197:517–532.
49. Maurer, R., Cortes, R., Probst, A., and Palacios, J. M. (1983): *Life Sci.*, 33(*Suppl.*):231–234.
50. McGillard, K. L., and Takemori, A. E. (1978): *J. Pharmacol. Exp. Ther.*, 207:884–891.
51. Meunier, J.-C., and Moidsand, D. (1977): *FEBS Lett.*, 77:209–213.
52. Morin, O., Caron, M. G., DeLean, A., and Labrie, F. (1976): *Biochem. Biophys. Res. Commun.*, 73:940–946.
53. Moskowitz, A. S., and Goodman, R. R. (1985): *Brain Res.* 360: 108–116.
54. Moskowitz, A. S., and Goodman, R. R. (1987): *Brain Res.* (*in press*).
55. Nishimura, S., and Pasternak, G. W. (1982): *Brain Res.*, 248: 192–195.
56. Nishimura, S. L., Recht, L. D., and Pasternak, G. W. (1984): *Mol. Pharmacol.*, 25:29–37.
57. Oka, T., Negishi, K., Uda, M., Matsumiya, T., Inazu, T., and Ucki, M. (1981): *Eur. J. Pharmacol.*, 73:235–236.
58. Pasternak, G. W. (1980): *Proc. Natl. Acad. Sci. USA*, 77:3691–3694.
59. Pasternak, G. W. (1981): *Neurology*, 31:1311–1315.
60. Pasternak, G. W. (1982): *Life Sci.*, 31:1303–1306.
61. Pasternak, G. W., Carrol-Buatti, M., and Spiegel, K. (1981): *J. Pharmacol. Exp. Ther.*, 219:192–198.
62. Pasternak, G. W., Childers, S. R., and Snyder, S. H. (1980): *J. Pharmacol. Exp. Ther.*, 214:455–462.
63. Pasternak, G. W., Childers, S. R., and Snyder, S. H. (1980): *Science*, 208:514–516.
64. Pasternak, G. W., Goodman, R., and Snyder, S. H. (1975): *Life Sci.*, 16:1765–1769.
65. Pasternak, G. W., and Hahn, E. F. (1980): *J. Med. Chem.*, 23: 674–676.
66. Pasternak, G. W., Snowman, A., and Snyder, S. H. (1975): *Mol. Pharmacol.*, 11:735–744.
67. Pasternak, G. W., and Snyder, S. H. (1974): *Mol. Pharmacol.*, 10:183–193.
68. Pasternak, G. W., and Snyder, S. H. (1975): *Nature*, 253:563–565.
69. Pasternak, G. W., Wilson, H. A., and Snyder, S. H. (1975): *Mol. Pharmacol.*, 11:340–351.
70. Pasternak, G. W., Zhang, A.-Z., and Tecott, L. (1980): *Life Sci.*, 27:1185–1190.
71. Paton, W. D. M. (1957): *Br. J. Pharmacol.*, 12:119–127.
72. Pert, C. B., Kuhar, M. J., and Snyder, S. H. (1976): *Proc. Natl. Acad. Sci. USA*, 73:3729–3733.
73. Pert, C. B., Pasternak, G. W., and Snyder, S. H. (1973): *Science*, 182:1359–1361.
74. Pert, C. B., and Snyder, S. H. (1973): *Science*, 179:1011–1014.
75. Pfeiffer, A., and Hertz, A. (1981): *Biochem. Biophys. Res. Commun.*, 101:38–44.
76. Portoghese, P. S. (1970): *Annu. Rev. Pharmacol.*, 10:51–76.
77. Quirion, R., Zajac, J. M., Morgat, J. L., and Roques, B. P. (1983): *Life Sci.*, 33(*Suppl.*):227–230.
78. Robson, L. E., Foote, R. W., Maurer, R., and Kosterlitz, H. W. (1984): *Neuroscience*, 12:621–627.

79. Robson, L. E., and Kosterlitz, H. W. (1979): *Proc. R. Soc. Lond.*, 205:425–432.
80. Schulz, R., Faase, E., Wuster, M., and Herz, A. (1979): *Life Sci.*, 24:843–850.
81. Schulz, R., Wuster, M., and Herz, A. (1981): *J. Pharmacol. Exp. Ther.*, 216:604–606.
82. Shannon, H. E. (1983): *J. Pharmacol. Exp. Ther.*, 225:144–152.
83. Sherman, G. T., and Herz, A. (1981): *Neuropharmacology*, 20: 1209–1213.
84. Simantov, R., Childers, S. R., and Snyder, S. H. (1978): *Eur. J. Pharmacol.*, 47:319–331.
85. Simon, E. J., Hiller, J. M., and Edelman, I. (1973): *Proc. Natl. Acad. Sci. USA*, 70:1947–1949.
86. Simon, E. J., Hiller, J. M., Groth, J., and Edelman, I. (1975): *J. Pharmacol. Exp. Ther.*, 192:531–537.
87. Smith, J. R., and Simon, E. J. (1980): *Proc. Natl. Acad. Sci. USA*, 77:281–284.
88. Spiegel, K., Kourides, I., and Pasternak, G. W. (1982): *Science*, 217:745–747.
89. Tam, S. W. (1983): *Proc. Natl. Acad. Sci. USA*, 80:6703–6707.
90. Terenius, L. (1973): *Acta Pharmacol. Toxicol.*, 33:377–384.
91. Terenius, L., and Whalstrom, A. (1975): *Acta Physiol. Scand.*, 94:74–81.
92. Toll, L., Keys, C., Polgar, W., and Loew, G. (1984): *Neuropeptides*, 5:205–208.
93. Vincent, J. P., Kartalovski, B., Genest, P., Kamenka, J. M., and Lazdunski, M. (1979): *Proc. Natl. Acad. Sci. USA*, 76:4678–4682.
94. Wilson, H. A., Pasternak, G. W., and Snyder, S. H. (1975): *Nature*, 253:448–450.
95. Wolozin, B. L., Nishimura, S., and Pasternak, G. W. (1982): *J. Neurosci.*, 2:708–713.
96. Wolozin, B. L., and Pasternak, G. W. (1981): *Proc. Natl. Acad. Sci. USA*, 78:6181–6185.
97. Wood, P. L., Hudgin, R. L., and Rackham, A. (1984): In: *Quo Vadis? Kappa Receptors and Their Ligands*, pp. 206–214. Clin Midy Press, Montpellier, France.
98. Wood, P. L., and Pasternak, G. W. (1983): *Neurosci. Lett.*, 37: 291–293.
99. Wood, P. L., Rackham, A., and Richard, J. (1981): *Life Sci.*, 28: 2119–2125.
100. Wood, P. L., Richard, J. W., and Thakur, M. (1982): *Life Sci.*, 31:2313–2317.
101. Woods, J. H., Smith, C. B., Medzihradsky, F., and Swain, H. H. (1979): In: *Mechanisms of Pain and Analgesic Drugs*, edited by R. F. Beers, Jr., and E. G. Bassett, pp. 429–445. Raven Press, New York.
102. Yaksh, T. L. (1978): *Brain Res.*, 153:205–210.
103. Yaksh, T. L., Huang, S. P., Rudy, T. A., and Frederickson, R. C. A. (1977): *Neuroscience*, 2:593–596.
104. Yaksh, T. L., and Rudy, T. A. (1977): *J. Pharmacol. Exp. Ther.*, 202:411–428.
105. Zhang, A.-Z., and Pasternak, G. W. (1981): *Life Sci.*, 29:843–857.
106. Zhang, A.-Z., and Pasternak, G. W. (1981): *Eur. J. Pharmacol.*, 73:29–40.
107. Zhang, A.-Z., and Pasternak, G. W. (1982): *Eur. J. Pharmacol.*, 67:323–324.
108. Zukin, R. S., and Zukin, S. R. (1981): *Life Sci.*, 29:2681–2690.
109. Zukin, S. R., and Zukin, R. S. (1979): *Proc. Natl. Acad. Sci. USA*, 76:5372–5376.

Psychopharmacology:
The Third Generation of Progress,
edited by Herbert Y. Meltzer.
Raven Press, New York © 1987.

CHAPTER **30**

Purinergic Receptors and Central Nervous System Function

Michael Williams

Neuromodulators can be conceptually differentiated from neurotransmitters inasmuch as their effects are generally considered to be more global and temporally more prolonged. In contrast, the effects of the latter agents are more transient, mediating the immediate transfer of information from one nerve cell to another in response to relatively ephemeral temporal stimuli.

Neuropeptides are considered to be the major class of neuromodulatory agents (243), and, using recombinant DNA techniques (68), many such entities have been identified which are in the process of being examined for specific physiological function(s) (188).

The factors governing the availability of neuromodulators and their precise effects also differ from the relatively simple processes of stimulus-secretion coupling and release associated with classical neurotransmitters (10). In nearly all instances, neuromodulators are considered to be cotransmitters, being released together with a more classical transmitter, e.g., cholecystokinin with dopamine (160). The neuromodulator can then modify the action of the transmitter and thereby increase the subtlety of the intercellular communication process. It is not known whether such corelease is a facet of all aspects of transmitter availability.

In the context of neuromodulatory agents, purine nucleotides and nucleosides may be considered to be the "oldest," both in terms of the history of modern pharmacological research and from a hierarchical standpoint. It is some 60 years since adenosine, in the form of its nucleotide, adenosine triphosphate (ATP), was shown to modulate cardiovascular function, causing bradycardia, coronary vasodilation and having negative inotropic actions (73). In the CNS, Feldberg and Sherwood (82) showed that ATP was a potent sedative when administered centrally. The nucleotide has also been implicated as a neurotransmitter candidate in primary afferent fibers (126,221). In separate studies over the course of two decades, Burnstock with the assistance of many co-workers (35,36) provided convincing evidence that ATP was the mediator of "nonadrenergic, noncholinergic neurotransmission" in peripheral tissues.

It is somewhat paradoxical, therefore, given this historical perspective, that the concept of purinergic neurotransmission, involving both the nucleoside, adenosine, and ATP, has taken so long to be accepted. The reasons for this have been the very ubiquity of the purine, its free levels in brain tissue being approximately 1 to 2 μM (302), and its intimate involvement in all aspects of cell function (5). Other reasons have been that the factors mediating its availability as a neuromodulator and thus controlling its specificity have not been adequately defined (253,278), and also that discrete neuronal pathways have not yet been identified. Studies related to the localization of adenosine deaminase, the enzyme that catabolizes adenosine, have pointed to a high degree of specificity in its distribution (96,178,180). In addition, antibodies to adenosine have been reported (24) to label specific areas in sections of brain tissue. However, the major evidence for regional selectivity in the actions of the purine has been related almost exclusively to the regional receptor density (100,144,145,215,241,242).

In further considering the relationship between purines and peptides as neuromodulatory agents, it is noteworthy that both are intimately involved in cellular function at a basic level and both subserve a functional role distinct from that for other, more "classical," neurotransmitters. The key position of the purines in the DNA-RNA cycle (2,51) further reinforces the hypothesis that adenosine and ATP may represent "primary" neuromodulatory agents, subserving a more global homeostatic role (276) than the peptides, which may represent a second level of sophistication in relation to neuromodulator action.

PURINES AS PHYSIOLOGICAL NEUROMODULATORS

Purines function as chemoattractants in the slime mold *Dictyastelium discoidium* (167) and in the marine shrimp *Palaemonetes pugio* (41). Taste receptors in the pufferfish (135), turbot (159), and cow (257) are also sensitive to purine nucleosides and nucleotides.

In the mammalian CNS, the impetus for examining the role of adenosine as a neuromodulator arose from studies showing that the purine was a potent stimulator of brain adenylate cyclase activity. However, of more crucial interest was the finding that the methylxanthines, caffeine and theophylline, which were used as cyclic nucleotide phosphodiesterase inhibitors, blocked the actions of adenosine on cyclic AMP formation rather than potentiating them. This led to the hypothesis that the methylxanthines were adenosine antagonists and that the central stimulant properties of caffeine might be attributable to the blockade of the sedating effects of endogenous adenosine (223).

PURINE RECEPTORS

On the basis of studies related to "nonadrenergic, noncholinergic" neurotransmission in peripheral tissues, Burnstock (36) proposed the P-1/P-2 nomenclature for purinergic receptors or "purinoceptors." Responses sensitive to adenosine were attributed to interactions with P-1 receptors (Table 1). Those sensitive to ATP were suggested to be mediated via P-2 receptors. P-1 responses could be blocked by methylxanthines and involved changes in tissue cyclic AMP levels. P-2 receptor-mediated effects were related to products of the eicosanoid pathways. To date, no consistently reliable P-2 antagonist has been described (37), although ANAPP$_3$ [3-O-(3[N-(4-azido-2-nitrophenyl)amino]propionyl) adenosine 5-triphosphate; refs. 81, 122] has proven a useful tool. Both subclasses of purinoceptor have been further subdivided. Based on extensive studies on adenylate cyclase systems in adipocytes, hepatocytes, and Leydig cell lines, Londos and Wolff (154) proposed the existence of two P-1 receptor subclasses, termed R$_i$ and R$_a$. The R designation referred to the fact that an intact ribose moeity (Fig. 1) was required for activity at the receptor, whereas the "i" and "a" subscripts described the effects of receptor activation on cyclic AMP formation: "i" was inhibitory and "a" activatory or stimulatory, and these responses were dependent on the concentration of agonist used and its structure. Thus the stable analog 2-chloroadenosine (2-CADO; Fig. 1) was more active at the R$_i$ site whereas the 5'N-ethylcarboxamido analog, NECA (Fig. 1) was more active at the R$_a$ site. Both types of receptor are on the external surface of the cell membrane, and activation of both can be blocked by methylxanthines such as theophylline, 8-phenyltheophylline (8PT), and 1,3-dipropyl-8(2-amino-4-chloro)phenylxanthine (PACPX; Fig. 1; Table 1).

A third type of adenosine recognition site modulating the activity of adenylate cyclase, termed the P site (114,155), has also been described. At this site, which is located on the catalytic subunit of adenylate cyclase, an intact purine ring is required for activity, and activation by adenosine or

TABLE 1. *Adenosine and purine receptor subtypes*

Receptor	Agonist pharmacology	Antagonist	Coupling system
A-1 (R$_i$)	CPA > CHA = R-PIA > 2-CADO > NECA > S-PIA	PACPX > 8-PT ≫ theophylline	Inhibition of adenylate cyclase ? Effects on Ca^{2+} flux
A-2 (R$_a$)	NECA > MECA > R-PIA = 2-CADO > CHA > CPA > S-PIA	Xanthines	Stimulation of adenylate cyclase
P	2'5'DDA ≫ adenosine	5'methylthioadenosine	Inhibition of adenylate cyclase
P-2$_x$	α-β-Methylene ATP = β-γ-methylene ATP > ATP = 2-methylthio ATP	ANAPP$_3$	Mediates excitation
P-2$_y$	2-Methylthio ATP ≫ ATP > α-β-methylene ATP = β-γ-methylene ATP	Weak antagonism by ANAPP$_3$	Mediates relaxation

Data from refs. 31, 38, 58, 281, 282.

Adenosine agonists

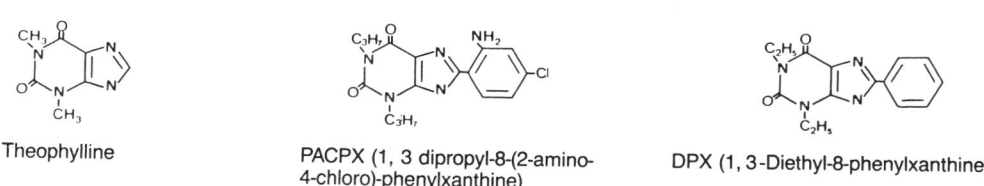

FIG. 1. Structures of adenosine agonists and antagonists.

ribose-modified analogs such as 2',5'-dideoxyadenosine (DDA; Fig. 1) results in inhibition of the enzyme. This designation should not be confused with the P-1/P-2 nomenclature. The P site is not susceptible to blockade by xanthines. Van Calker et al. (263,264), using neuroblastoma cell lines, also described two classes of adenosine receptor identical to the R_i and R_a receptors, which they termed A-1 and A-2 (Table 1). In line with the nomenclature used for central neurotransmitter receptors (288), the A-1/A-2

designation has been more widely used than the R_i/R_a system. Furthermore, based on findings that not all effects of adenosine involved cyclic AMP as a second messenger (75), the recommendation has been made (111,255) that the R_i/R_a nomenclature be replaced with the A-1/A-2 one. The criteria for this latter delineation, which involve the degree of stereoselectivity exhibited by the R and S diastereomers of N^6-phenylisopropyladenosine (PIA; Fig. 1), are shown in Table 2.

TABLE 2. New criteria for A-1 and A-2 receptor delineation

Adenosine receptor subtype	Pharmacology	Stereoselectivity
A-1	CPA > CHA > R-PIA ≫ NECA > S-PIA	R-PIA 10× >S-PIA
A-2	NECA > MECA > 2-CADO > CHA = CPA = R-PIA > A-PIA	R-PIA <10× S-PIA

These new criteria, the result of a discussion held at an INPHAR Satellite Symposium in 1984, carry no implication of the involvement of adenylate cyclase in adenosine-mediated responses.

Data from refs. 111, 255, 281.

To date no potent, selective A-2 agonists have been reported, although both NECA and 2-CADO can interact with both receptor subclasses (31,32,53,55,56,172,282,300). For the A-1 receptor, however, there are several potent, selective agonists including N^6-cyclohexyladenosine (CHA; Fig. 1; ref. 29) and N^6-cyclopentyladenosine (CPA; Fig. 1; refs. 32, 172, 282).

In contrast to the well-defined effects of adenosine in the CNS, the actions of ATP have been confounded by the high levels of ectonucleotidases in this tissue (158). Although ATP effects have been reported (82,104), these have been ascribed to the calcium-chelating properties of the polyphosphate side chain (197) or to degradation of the nucleotide to adenosine (199). However, in the dorsal horn of the spinal cord and also in the brain, ATP has distinct effects that cannot be ascribed to either calcium chelation or adenosine formation (128). It is probable, therefore, that P-2 receptors are present in both central and peripheral nervous tissue (221). The P-2 receptor has also been subdivided into P-2_x and P-2_y subclasses based on the effects of the stable ATP analogs, 2-methylthioATP and the β-γ methylene isostere of ATP (38; Table 1). The P-2_x receptor is sensitive to β-γ methylene ATP and has excitatory effects, whereas the P-2_y receptor elicits relaxation and is preferentially sensitive to 2-methylthioATP. Following from observations that the mitochondrial cofactor NAD (nicotinamide adenosine dinucleotide), a purine nucleotide, had inhibitory effects in guinea pig hippocampus (219), a relatively high-affinity binding site for NAD has been identified in rat brain (240).

ADENOSINE EFFECTS IN THE CNS

Effects on Second Messenger Systems

Adenosine is a potent modulator of CNS adenylate cyclase activity (53,55,72,223), inhibiting or stimulating the enzyme, depending on the type of receptor activated (Table 1). The purine can also potentiate the effects of other neurotransmitters, such as histamine or serotonin, on cyclic AMP production via A-2 receptor activation, eliciting large increases in the levels of the cyclic nucleotide (72). Conversely A-1 receptor activation can block the effects of cyclase-stimulating transmitters. Adenosine can block the cyclic AMP-dependent effects of norepinephrine on cardiac contractility (65). The physiological significance of such changes is, however, controversial (150,233). In the CNS, due to the low basal cyclase activity, it is not always possible to demonstrate A-1-mediated effects. It is therefore, necessary to stimulate the enzyme with the diterpene forskolin before challenging with adenosine to observe the inhibitory effects of the purine (88). Adenosine interactions with adenylate cyclase involve the N protein subunits, N_i and N_s (249), N_i being coupled to the A-1 receptor (301) and N_s to the A-2 receptor. The inhibitory effects of A-1 adenosine and γ-aminobutyric acid B (GABA$_B$) receptor activation on cerebellar Purkinje cell cyclic AMP content (293,294) have been ascribed to the sharing of a common catalytic subunit (292). The purine has no apparent direct effect on phosphatidyl inositol turnover (26) but does

appear to potentiate the effects of histamine on this second messenger system (123).

Effects on Neurotransmitter Release

Adenosine modulates the release of several neurotransmitters both *in vitro* and *in vivo*. The purine affects the release of norepinephrine, GABA, (86,112,113,124,127,253), glutamate (66), dopamine (112,170), serotonin, acetylcholine, and histamine (106a,112,225), presumably via presynaptic mechanisms. Biphasic effects of adenosine analogs on acetylcholine (247) and norepinephrine and dopamine (79) release have been reported. In cultured cerebellar neurons, Dolphin and Prestwich (67) have shown that the inhibitory effects of R-PIA on glutamate release can be converted to stimulation by treatment with pertussis toxin, which binds irreversibly to the N_i subunit to unveil the effects of the A-2-linked N_s protein.

The obligatory involvement of cyclic AMP in the effects of adenosine on transmitter release is, however, not certain (66,136,217,227,250). The physiological significance of these adenosine effects also remains unclear, especially within the framework of autoreceptor function (39). It is generally held, however, that the effects of the xanthines as central stimulants reflect an action in preventing purine inhibition of transmitter release. Mechanistically, these effects are not yet resolved, although there is evidence to suggest that alterations in potassium-evoked calcium fluxes may be involved (107,232). The purine has also been reported to interact with voltage-sensitive calcium channels (174,198). However, R-PIA cannot antagonize the positive inotropic effects of the calcium "agonist" Bay K 8644 in guinea pig papillary muscle (21).

Electrophysiological Actions of Adenosine

Adenosine and ATP depress cell firing when applied iontophoretically (76,197,228,236). This effect is antagonized by theophylline and is mediated via A-1 receptors (144,145,216). The involvement of cyclic AMP in these events is, however, not obligatory (75). Both pre- and postsynaptic effects are involved; at the presynaptic level, the purine can elicit its effects by modulating transmitter release (112,253), whereas postsynaptically, it has direct actions on cellular excitability. The ionic mechanisms for these effects appear to involve both changes in calcium influx (74,119,143,206,237) and increases in potassium conductance (107,232,259). In frog oocytes, adenosine can induce a potassium conductance change that is cyclic AMP-dependent and can be antagonized by protein kinase C activation (60).

Behavioral Effects of Adenosine

Direct administration of adenosine into the brain causes sedation (82,161). The purine alters sleep patterns (209), increasing deep sleep without significantly decreasing rapid eye movement (REM) sleep. Adenosine can also depress locomotor activity (132,245), an effect that is biphasic and may involve two distinct classes of receptor.

Adenosine is a potent anticonvulsant (77), attenuating rather than preventing postictal spiking (71). The purine can also affect food intake (148), respiration (117,273), and aggressive behavior (262) via central receptor mechanisms. Adenosine antagonists, especially caffeine, have effects opposed to those of adenosine. Caffeine is a well-known central stimulant (64), whereas a related xanthine, HWA 825 (120), has been reported to be a cognitive activator. These effects of the xanthines on behavior and on transmitter release have provided evidence for the existence of a purinergic inhibitory tone (112), and this concept has been further developed in regard to the homeostatic role of the purine in mammalian CNS function (276,278). Xanthines are potent hypothermic agents (77), and in several inbred mice strains, especially the CGA and SWR strains, these effects of the xanthines can be dissociated from their locomotor activity (40), suggesting an inherited difference in the xanthine-sensitive substrates that modulate such behaviors (231a).

Adenosine has been implicated in the actions of several classes of psychotropic agents (see below). Some components of the behavioral effects of adenosine may involve cyclic AMP as a mediator, since forskolin can depress spontaneous motor activity in mice (14).

In addition to behavioral modulation via direct effects on CNS receptor-linked systems, adenosine can also affect CNS function via its well-known actions on cardiovascular parameters (18,19). Although the doses of the purine that produce behavioral effects can be delineated from those which lower blood pressure (12,132), a good correlation has been reported for the effects of adenosine analogs on neuronal cell firing and blood pressure (200). In addition, when administered centrally, adenosine is a potent, hypotensive agent (15,226).

ADENOSINE AVAILABILITY IN THE CNS

Release

The mechanisms involved in determining the extracellular availability of adenosine have yet to be unambiguously defined (253,276,280). Stimulus-dependent, both electrical and chemical, release of purines from nervous tissue has been extensively studied (86,90,130,131,138,201,202). Calcium-dependent (139) and -independent (90) release has been described. Temporal differences have been reported to exist between purine release and that of other putative neurotransmitters (253), and recent evidence (131) suggests that stimulus-evoked adenosine release, although partially calcium dependent, is indirect, perhaps related to "neuronal nonexocytotic release" involving a carrier-mediated process.

One issue that has confounded release studies has been the form of the nucleotide that is released. Cyclic AMP, 5′-AMP, and ATP have all been considered as potential sources for extracellular adenosine (158,184,202,204). The colocalization of A-1 receptors with the enzyme 5′nucleotidase (100) has led to the suggestion that 5′-AMP is the primary source of the purine, although S-adenosyl-

homocysteine may also be a viable source (162) and may account for the large amounts of the purine that are produced in broken cell preparations (29,205,274,276). In addition, the use of tritiated purine precursors as an indication of release is another factor that can limit the usefulness of release studies (53). To define further the physiological significance of the purine, it is very important to resolve the question of purine availability in the near future.

Inactivation

The actions of extracellular adenosine can be terminated either by uptake or by deamination of the purine to inosine and hypoxanthine. High-affinity uptake processes have been reported (17,138,139,235). In rat brain tissue, both rapid and slow uptake processes occur (17), the former comprising a single site with a K_m of 0.9 μM and the latter, two sites with K_m values of 1 and 5 μM. Physiologically effective agents, such as the vasodilator dipyridamole (173), produce their effects by preventing adenosine uptake, and adenosine uptake inhibitors have also been reported to potentiate the sedative effects of the purine (50). Suggestions have also been made that the effects seen with high concentrations of several classes of psychotropic agents may be due to their actions on adenosine uptake (193,200).

Adenosine is deaminated by the enzyme adenosine deaminase (ADA), which is primarily located in the cytoplasm (207). Inhibitors of this enzyme such as deoxycoformycin have behavioral effects when administered parenterally (169,209), providing further evidence for a physiological role of the purine. Using immunocytochemical techniques, a discrete plexus of ADA-containing neurons has been described in the basal hypothalamus (180). This group of neurons innervates the striatum, amygdala, and cortex and this has been taken as additional evidence for a regionally specific role for adenosine in mammalian brain.

LABELING OF PURINE RECOGNITION SITES IN BRAIN TISSUE

The A-1 Receptor

Because of the necessity to use the catabolic enzyme ADA to remove the endogenous adenosine that obscures the nanomolar high-affinity recognition sites present in broken cell preparations (29,205), the use of [³H]adenosine as a radioligand has not been generally accepted (183,247,274), although it has been used to define recognition sites in the 108CC15 neuroblastoma × glioma cell line (239) and in rat brain membranes (239,258). More typically, the use of ADA requires stable analogs of the purine (CHA, R-PIA, CPA, 2-CADO). Of these, CHA (29,192), R-PIA (152,229), and CPA (282) are routinely used, 2-CADO (283) having been found to be unreliable as a radioligand (115). This agonist has, however, been used to label low-affinity micromolar adenosine recognition sites in rat brain (43). These are somewhat unusual in their pharmacology, adenosine being equiactive with cyclic AMP and AMP in displacing the ligand whereas the R and S enantiomers of PIA were inactive. The xanthine adenosine antagonist DPX (1,3-diethyl-8-phenylxanthine; Fig. 1) has also been used as a ligand for the A-1 receptor (11,29,165). There are no apparent regional differences in the pharmacology of A-1 receptors in rat brain (241).

The ontogeny of the A-1 receptor in mammalian brain (4,95) has been studied using autoradiographic techniques, and it has been localized to excitatory axon terminals (99). Distinct species differences in A-1 receptors have also been described (175), xanthines showing marked differences in their activity depending on the tissue studied (83,230). Since this species selectivity is not as pronounced for agonists, speculation has arisen as to the possible existence of an endogenous methylxanthine-like entity (282).

The A-1 receptor has been solubilized (94,181,251) and estimated to have a molecular weight of 280,000 daltons. Photoaffinity labeling (44,252) has identified a protein of MW 36,000 to 38,000 daltons as the ligand-binding subunit of the A-1 receptor. Using irradiation activation, this same site has been estimated to have an MW of 65,000 daltons (214).

The A-2 Receptor

As previously indicated, A-2-selective agonists are not available at this time. The A-1/A-2 agonist [^{3}H]NECA has, however, been used in striatal tissue, which is enriched in this receptor subtype (78,205), to label A-2 receptors following the selective destruction of A-1 receptors with N-ethylmaleimide (89,105,300) or their blockade by low concentrations (50 nM) of the A-1-selective ligand CPA (31,32,172). The pharmacology of NECA binding in the presence of CPA is consistent with the labeling of an A-2 receptor (Table 2). The use of the CPA/NECA labeling conditions in conjunction with quantitative autoradiography allows for a striking visualization of A-2 receptors to the striatum (242), an observation consistent with the distribution of the receptor as determined by adenylate cyclase characterization (57,78,205). Although NECA has also been found to label A-2 receptors present in the PC12 pheochromocytoma cell line (281), which is devoid of A-1 recognition sites (208), its use to label A-2 receptors in nonneuronal tissues has not been satisfactory (261). In the absence of other agents, however, NECA represents a useful tool by which to discover more selective entities.

The P Site

The selective agonist DDA (Fig. 1; 54,155) binds with relatively high affinity (K_d = 90 nM) to rat cortical and striatal membranes (187). Although binding of this ligand was insensitive to A-site effectors such as R-PIA, its displacement by 5'-methylthioadenosine was inconsistent with the labeling of a P site (54).

The Uptake Site

Adenosine uptake sites can be labeled with [^{3}H]6-(4-nitrobenzyl)thioinosine (NBI; refs. 96, 109, 110, 129, 163, 267, 268). Binding of this ligand, which has been reported to be a selective adenosine uptake inhibitor, is of exceptionally high affinity (K_d = 50 pM) in mammalian brain tissue and somewhat unexpectedly does not require the removal of endogenous adenosine to be characterized. A correlation has been reported between the regional distribution of ADA-immunoreactive neurons and NBI binding sites (179), leading to the suggestion that both indices relate to the bioavailability of adenosine.

The P-2 Receptor

Limited studies have been performed to label P-2 sites in mammalian brain tissue. The stable ATP analog AppNHp binds irreversibly with nanomolar affinity to rat brain membranes (284). ATP has been used as a ligand in rabbit bladder, binding with a K_d value of 20 nM to a recognition site that is distinct from that involving divalent-ion-regulated ATPase activity (147). ANAPP$_3$ has also been used as a radioligand for the P-2 receptor (80). The compound covalently labels two recognition sites in guinea pig vas deferens smooth muscle, which may either represent two P$_2$-type receptors or, alternatively, a P-2 receptor and some type of ectophosphohydrolase. The incubation conditions that confirmed the covalent nature of the effects of the ANAPP$_3$ photolysis product (122) did not permit the determination of any kinetic parameters for the binding site(s).

PHYSIOLOGICAL ASPECTS OF ADENOSINE RECEPTOR FUNCTION

Chronic administration of the xanthines caffeine and theophylline can increase the density of A-1 receptors in rat brain (22,85,176). Caffeine-induced up-regulation of adenosine A-1 receptors has been associated with caffeine tolerance (45). Associated changes in both benzodiazepine (22,295) and β-adrenoceptors (98) may also occur. Preliminary reports (49,269) have described minor changes in adenosine receptors in aged rats. Chronic treatment with NECA, but not R-PIA, can decrease central A-2 receptors (203), A-1 receptors being unaffected by either agonist. In gerbils, transient ischemia can cause a down-regulation of A-1 receptors in the hippocampal CA1 region (146,190), although it may be noted that this brain region is selectively destroyed following hypoxia (149). REM sleep deprivation can increase A-1 receptor density in rat brain (298).

THERAPEUTIC ASPECTS OF ADENOSINE FUNCTION IN THE CNS

Many studies have appeared in the last 5 years implicating central adenosine-mediated systems in the actions of psychotropic agents. Given the ubiquity of the purine and its effects on transmitter release it is hardly surprising that data have been obtained to relate adenosine to the mechanism of action of nearly all classes of centrally active agent. By extrapolation, possible defects in central adenosine systems have been suggested to exist in several pathophysiological disease states.

Anxiety

Given the well-known anxiogenic actions of caffeine (42,212,244,246) and the sedative effects of adenosine (82) the potential involvement of the purine in the actions of the classical benzodiazepine (BZ) anxiolytics, compounds with sedative and muscle relaxant properties, could be hypothesized. Following the discovery of a specific BZ recognition site in mammalian brain (248), considerable effort was expended, and is still continuing, in an attempt to identify an endogenous factor akin to the enkephalins at the opiate receptor. One such factor isolated from cow brain was the adenosine breakdown product, inosine (164). Inosine was a weak displacer (IC_{50} 10^{-3} M) of specific [³H]diazepam binding and in limited studies was found to block pentylenetetrazole-induced convulsions in a manner similar to that seen with diazepam. Methylxanthines, including the phosphodiesterase inhibitor isobutylmethylxanthine (IBMX) as well as 2-CADO, were also found to inhibit diazepam binding (8). However, the discovery of the β-carbolines (25), which were six orders of magnitude more active at the central BZ receptor, tended to raise some questions as to the physiological significance of the inosine interaction (108,275,287). Furthermore, there was no correlation between the effects of a series of BZ and non-BZ anxiolytics on BZ and A-1 receptor binding (286). However, it may be noted that xanthines can antagonize BZ effects in humans (7,84) in addition to antagonizing BZ effects on cell firing (199) and behavior (168,186,189). Purines are effective muscle relaxants (9,260), and it is likely that the sedative, but not the anxiolytic, actions of the BZs may be purine mediated (30). The adenosine uptake inhibitor dipyridamole can displace diazepam binding (63) and behaves as a BZ agonist *in vitro* (62). Also, the BZ inverse agonist CGS 8216 (52) can bind to the A-1 receptor (282,285), whereas the BZ antagonist Ro 15-1788 can antagonize caffeine-induced seizures in mice (266). Since BZs can inhibit adenosine uptake (296), it has been postulated that the sedative and muscle relaxant effects are due to the inhibition of uptake. The prototypic anxiolytic meprobamate may also elicit its effects via potentiation of the effects of endogenous adenosine (195). Interactions between diazepam and adenosine have been reported in peripheral tissues (134).

Epilepsy

Given the tentative relationship between adenosine and the BZs, the latter of which are used as anticonvulsants, and the fact that caffeine and theophylline have convulsant activity (212,303), the purine has also been examined in regard to a potential involvement in this disorder. Adenosine inhibits audiogenic (161), kainate, strychnine, picrotoxin, and mercaptoproprioninic acid (77) induced seizures and can raise seizure thresholds in rats. Adenosine levels in brain increase dramatically following seizure activity (290), and caffeine and theophylline can prolong the duration of kindled seizures (3,12,70). The adenosine uptake inhibitor papaverine can block kindled seizures (70), and it has been suggested, on the basis of this interaction, that adenosine is involved in the termination, but not the initiation, of

seizures (71). R-PIA can prolong postictal depression and decreases the frequency of spiking following amygdaloid-kindled (220) and pentylenetetrazol-induced (34) seizures. This latter treatment can acutely reduce A-1 receptors in rat cerebellum (297). These actions of adenosine, which are thought to be mediated via A-1 receptors, are antagonized by xanthines (177).

Both adenosine- and diazepam-related processes have been implicated in the mechanism of action of the anticonvulsant carbamazepine (165,165a,238), although the structure-activity relationship for the anticonvulsant actions of a series of carbamazepine analogs does not correlate with their ability to interact with adenosine A-1 receptors (165). Chronic carbamazepine treatment can cause an up-regulation of A-1 receptors (162), suggesting it has adenosine antagonist properties. However, these workers also reported that CHA had no effect on kindled seizures (271), and an equally valid explanation of these preliminary data, given the proposed involvement of the purine in epilepsy, would be that any agent capable of preventing convulsions, and thus the associated increases in endogenous levels of adenosine, would up-regulate receptors for the purine. Peripheral BZ receptors (248) have also been implicated in the anticonvulsant actions of carbamazepine (272). The antiepileptic actions of the CNS depressant, pentobarbital, may also be due to an interaction with A-1 receptors, although this relationship is somewhat tentative (153). The proconvulsant actions of the xanthines are further evidence for the role of endogenous adenosine in modulating CNS excitability and raise the possibility that purinergic agonists may be useful in the treatment of epileptic disorders (69,70,177).

Sleep

The hypnotic/sedative actions of adenosine are well documented (82,116,166), as are the central stimulant actions of the xanthines (212,246). Direct administration of adenosine into cat (82) and fowl brain (166) produces a sleep-like state with an EEG profile similar to that seen in deep sleep. An A-1-receptor-mediated inhibition of dopamine release is associated with R-PIA-induced deep sleep (210,210a). The marine purine 1-methylisoguanosine (MIG; ref. 9), which interacts with central A-1 receptors *in vitro* (286) and appears to produce its muscle relaxant effects via central mechanisms (33), is distinctly different from adenosine in terms of its effects on REM sleep (211), suggesting that its adenosine-like properties are selective for peripheral, rather than central, A-1 receptors. These findings may also indicate that the A-1 receptors involved in sleep have a different structure-activity profile from those previously described. In addition, the ethanol-sensitive "long-sleep" mouse is more sensitive to the sedative and hypothermic actions of R-PIA than the ethanol-insensitive "short-sleep" mouse (206). These effects are related to increases in both the affinity and the density of A-1 receptors in the "long-sleep" mouse (91).

Analgesia

Xanthines can reduce morphine analgesia (121) and also elicit a "quasimorphine withdrawal syndrome" (QMWS;

ref. 46), a response that, like that seen with the opiate antagonist naloxone, is associated with an α_2-adrenoceptor-mediated increase in norepinephrine turnover (92,218). The QMWS effects of the xanthine isobutylmethylxanthine, as well as xanthine effects on norepinephrine turnover, are antagonized by the α_2 agonist clonidine (93,103). Adenosine and clonidine have also been used to suppress opiate withdrawal (47,48,97). Since clonidine can block naloxone-precipated increases in locus ceruleus firing in dependent animals (103), it appears possible that the process of withdrawal involves hyperactive noradrenergic pathways. Adenosine agonists may, therefore, have potential use in opiate withdrawal (47). Xanthines can reverse the respiratory depressant actions of opiates (6) and may act as analgesic adjuvants (141).

The adenosine/analgesia relationship is complex, however. Theophylline has been reported to have antinociceptive activity (121,191), whereas adenosine has been found both to antagonize the analgesic actions of morphine (101) and to have antinociceptive activity (265,299). The analgesic actions of R-PIA are blocked by caffeine, but not naloxone (1). The possibility that the antinociceptive actions of the purine could be attributed to its CNS depressant activity appears unlikely in view of the fact that barbiturates are devoid of antinociceptive activity (182). However, given the nature of the analgesic paradigms used in animal models, muscle relaxation (9) could be an important component of such activity. Another explanation for the conflicting data could be the existence of systems that are responsive to different receptor subtypes.

Depression

Antidepressants, based on their effects on cyclic AMP accumulation (224) and their ability to potentiate the depressant effects of adenosine (256), have been suggested to produce certain of their therapeutic effects via purinergic-related mechanisms (194,222,254). Chronic electroconvulsive therapy (ECT), a procedure used in the treatment of depression, can increase A-1 receptor density in rat, an effect that has been related to the increase in seizure threshold associated with such treatment in humans (185). However, neither chronic antidepressant (287) nor lithium (185) treatment was found to alter A-1 receptor density, making the relationship between adenosine and antidepressant therapy somewhat obscure. The atypical antidepressant trazodone is, however, a weak (10^{-6}M) adenosine deaminase inhibitor (234), and minor effects of other antidepressants, including nortriptyline, clomipramine, iprindole, amoxapine, and viloxazine, on adenosine uptake have been reported (296).

Mood Regulation

Adenosine has been reported to have interactions with the psychotomimetic phencyclidine (PCP; ref. 27) and with alcohol (59,91,206), both agents being potent mood regulators. The effects of adenosine in antagonizing PCP-related drug discrimination were subsequently found (28) to be related to the effects of the purine on PCP bioavailability.

An additional interrelationship between adenosine and alcohol is based on the effects of alcohol in long-sleep and short-sleep mice. In addition, theophylline has been reported to attenuate the duration of alcohol-induced sleep and motor incoordination, whereas chronic treatment alters A-1 receptors in rat brain (59).

Miscellaneous Disease States

Purinergic mechanisms have been implicated in dopamine-induced effects on rotational behavior (87) and in the phenomenon of apomorphine-induced self-mutilation (106). This latter phenomenon has been related to the involvement of the basal ganglia in Lesch-Nyhan syndrome (151), and it is of interest that large doses of caffeine can elicit a self-destructive behavior similar to that observed with this syndrome (23). The lesion in Lesch-Nyhan syndrome is a deficit in the enzyme hypoxanthine-guanine phosphoribosyltransferase (HRGPTase). However, in the caffeine model, the activity of this enzyme is actually increased (171), from which finding it has been suggested that the HRGPTase deficit is coincidental and that the primary lesion is associated with dopaminergic hyperactivity. The marked density of A-2 receptors in the striatum (57,142,205,215,242), coupled with the tentative PCP/adenosine relationship, PCP having been shown to produce schizophrenic-like symptoms (157), suggests that purinergic mechanisms may play a role in schizophrenia. Furthermore, adenosine agonists have been reported to have an antipsychotic profile in certain animal models (118), whereas caffeine effects in the CNS have been related to selective interactions with dopaminergic systems (102). The adenosine-containing transmethylation product, S-adenosyl-L-homocysteine, which has sedative effects in rats (156), is currently being evaluated as a neuroleptic (231).

The α_2-receptor agonist clonidine can also induce self-mutilation behavior in mammals (213), an effect enhanced by theophylline and partially antagonized by adenosine (133). The use of clonidine and adenosine in the treatment of morphine withdrawal (47,97) and reports suggesting that clonidine is an adenosine antagonist (256) and *vice versa* (137), and that the purine can regulate α-adrenoceptor-mediated events (140,270), provide strong evidence for an interrelationship between the two receptors. Furthermore, the two compounds have been linked in their effects on aggressive behavior (125,262). It is of interest to note that opiate receptors (morphine), α_2-adrenoceptors (clonidine), and A-1 receptors (adenosine) all have similar inhibitory effects on adenylate cyclase activity at the molecular level (72).

PURINERGIC DRUGS?

It is apparent that adenosine has a multitude of effects on CNS function. Extrapolation of such actions to a potential role in normal tissue function has led to the implication of the purine in the effects of a wide variety of psychotropic agents, which in turn has suggested that endogenous adenosine is an important effector agent in the etiology of the disease states for which such drugs are used.

Given the plethora of effects of adenosine and the suggestion (244,276) that the purine subserves a homeostatic role, it would appear somewhat difficult to invoke tissue-specific action and thus search for novel agents with therapeutic potential. However, nearly all the compounds available are either purines or xanthines (58), and it is possible that these agents, because of their structure, are relatively nonselective and are thus ubiquitous in their actions. The relationship between adenosine-mediated changes in cardiovascular function (20) and cerebral blood flow (13,196,289–291) is, however, an additional factor to be considered within the context of specificity. Such compounds may be useful in global CNS disease states, such as aging, and in addition, based on the unique localization of high-affinity A-2 receptors to the caudate, disorders associated with this brain region may be treatable with such purinergic modulatory agents.

Research in the area of purinergic pharmacology is, to a certain degree, in its infancy. Several lines of evidence indicate that there are both species (83,175) and tissue (279,280) differences in A-1 receptors. More recently, several adenosine agonists have been shown to have mixed agonist/antagonist activities (16), and nonxanthine adenosine antagonists have been described (52,61,282a).

The increased interest in the area of adenosine research, both chemical and biological, coupled with concerns related to the clarification of endogenous adenosine availability, will help resolve the issue of purine receptor selectivity and within the next decade may result in the use of mimics or antagonists of this neuromodulatory agent in the treatment of human disease states.

REFERENCES

1. Ahlijanian, M., and Takemori, A. E. (1985): *Eur. J. Pharmacol.,* 112:171–179.
2. Alberts, B., Bray, D., Lewis, J., Raff, M., Roberts, K., and Watson, J. D. (1983): *Molecular Biology of the Cell.* Garland, New York.
3. Albertson, T. E., Bowyer, J. F., and Paule, M. G. (1982): *Life Sci.,* 31:1597–1601.
4. Aoki, C. (1985): *Dev. Brain Res.,* 22:125–133.
5. Arch, J. R. S., and Newsholme, E. A. (1978): *Essays Biochem.,* 14:88–123.
6. Arnanada, J. V., and Thurman, T. (1970): *Clin. Perinatol.,* 6:87–108.
7. Arvidsson, S. B., Ekstrom-Jodal, B., Martinell, S. A. G., and Niemand, D. (1982): *Lancet, 2:*1467.
8. Asano, T., and Spector, S. (1979): *Proc. Natl. Acad. Sci. USA,* 76:977–981.
9. Baird-Lambert, J., Marwood, J. F., Davis, L. P., and Taylor, K. M. (1980): *Life Sci.,* 26:1069–1077.
10. Baker, P. F. (1972): *Prog. Biophys. Mol. Biol.,* 24:177–224.
11. Barnes, E. M., and Thampy, K. G. (1982): *J. Neurochem.,* 39:647–652.
12. Barraco, R. A., Aggarawal, A. K., Phillis, J. W., Moore, M. A., and Wu, P. H. (1984): *Neurosci. Lett.,* 48:139–144.
13. Barraco, R. A., Coffin, V. L., Altman, H. T., and Phillis, J. W. (1983): *Brain Res.,* 272:392–395.
14. Barraco, R. A., Phillis, J. W., and Altman, H. J. (1985): *Gen. Pharmacol.,* 16:521–524.
15. Barraco, R. A., Aggarawal, A. K., Phillis, J. W., Moron, M. A., and Wu, P. H. (1986): *Neurosci. Lett.,* 48:139–144.
16. Bazil, C. W., and Minneman, K. P. (1985): *Pharmacologist,* 27:219(Abstr. 580).
17. Bender, A. S., Wu, P. H., and Phillis, J. W. (1980): *J. Neurochem.,* 35:629–640.
18. Berne, R. M. (1963): *Am. J. Physiol.,* 204:317–322.
19. Berne, R. M. (1980): *Circ. Res.,* 46:807–813.
20. Berne, R. M., Knabb, R. M., Ely, S. W., and Rubio, R. (1983): *Fed. Proc.,* 42:3136–3142.
21. Bohm, M., Burmann, H., Meyer, W., Nose, M., Schmitz, W., and Scholz, H. (1985): *Naunyn Schmiedebergs Arch. Pharmacol.,* 329:447–450.
22. Boulenger, J. P., Patel, J., Post, R. M., Parma, A. M., and Marangos, P. J. (1983): *Life Sci.,* 32:1135–1142.
23. Boyd, E. M., Dolman, M., Knight, L. M., and Sheppard, E. P. (1965): *Can. J. Physiol. Pharmacol.,* 43:995–1007.
24. Braas, K. M., Newby, A. C., and Snyder, S. H. (1985): In: *Adenosine: Receptors and Modulation of Cell Function,* edited by V. Stefanovich, K. Rudolphi, and P. Schubert, pp. 59–71. IRL Press, Oxford.
25. Braestrup, C., Nielsen, M., and Olsen, C. E. (1980): *Proc. Natl. Acad. Sci. USA,* 77:2288–2292.
26. Brown, E., Kendall, D. A., and Nahorski, S. R. (1984): *J. Neurochem.,* 42:1379–1387.
27. Browne, R. G., and Welch, W. M. (1982): *Science,* 217:1157–1158.
28. Browne, R. G., Welch, W. M., Kozlowski, M. R., and Duthu, G. (1983): In: *Phencyclidine and Related Arylcyclohexylamines: Present and Future Applications,* edited by T. M. Kamonka, E. F. Domino, and P. Geneste, pp. 639–666. NPP Books, Ann Arbor, MI.
29. Bruns, R. F., Daly, T. W., and Snyder, S. H. (1980): *Proc. Natl. Acad. Sci. USA,* 77:5547–5551.
30. Bruns, R. F., Katims, J. J., Annau, Z., Snyder, S. H., and Daly, J. W. (1983): *Neuropharmacology,* 22:1523–1529.
31. Bruns, R. F., Lu, G. H., and Pugsley, T. A. (1984): *Soc. Neurosci. Abstr.,* 10:282.4.
32. Bruns, R. F., Lu, G. H., and Pugsley, T. A. (1985): In: *Adenosine: Receptors and Modulation of Cell Function,* edited by V. Stefanovich, K. Rudolphi, and P. Schubert, pp. 51–58. IRL Press, Oxford.
33. Buckle, P. J., and Spence, I. (1981): *Naunyn Schmiedebergs Arch. Pharmacol.,* 316:64–68.
34. Burley, E. S., and Ferrendelli, J. A. (1984): *Fed. Proc.,* 43:2521–2524.
35. Burnstock, G. (1972): *Pharmacol Rev.,* 24:509–581.
36. Burnstock, G. (1978): In: *Cell Membrane Receptors for Drugs and Hormones,* edited by R. W. Straub and L. Bolis, pp. 107–118. Raven Press, New York.
37. Burnstock, G., and Buckley, N. J. (1985): In: *Methods in Pharmacology, Vol. 6: Methods in Adenosine Research,* edited by D. M. Paton, pp. 193–212. Plenum, New York.
38. Burnstock, G., and Kennedy, C. (1985): *Gen. Pharmacol.,* 16:433–440.
39. Carlsson, A. (1975): In: *Pre and Postsynaptic Receptors,* edited by E. Usdin and W. E. Bunney, Jr., pp. 49–67. Marcel Dekker, New York.
40. Carney, J. M., Logan, L., McMaster, S. B., and Scale, T. M. (1985): In: *Adenosine Receptors and Modulation of Cell Function,* edited by V. Jrefanovich, K. Rudolphit, P. Schubert, pp. 199–208. IRL Press, Oxford.
41. Carr, E. S., and Thompson, H. W. (1983): *J. Comp. Physiol.,* 153:47–53.
42. Charney, D. S., Galloway, M. P., and Heninger, G. R. (1984): *Life Sci.,* 35:135–144.
43. Chin, J. H., Mashman, W. E., and DeLorenzo, R. J. (1985): *Life Sci.,* 36:1751–1760.
44. Choca, J. I., Kwatra, M. M., Hosey, M. M., and Green, R. D. (1985): *Biochem. Biophys. Res. Commun.,* 131:115–121.
45. Chou, D. T., Khan, S., Forde, J., and Hirsh, K. R. (1985): *Life Sci.,* 36:2347–2358.
46. Collier, H. O. J., Cuthbert, N. J., and Francis, D. L. (1981): *Fed. Proc.,* 40:1513–1518.
47. Collier, H. O. J., Plant, J. T., Tucker, J. F., and Von Uexkulla, A. (1984): *Br. J. Pharmacol.,* 81:131p.
48. Collier, H. O. J., and Tucker, J. F. (1983): *Nature,* 302:618–621.
49. Corradetti, R., Kiedrowski, L., Nordstrom, O., and Pepeu, G. (1984): *Neurosci. Lett.,* 49:143–146.

50. Crawley, T. N., Patel, J., and Marangos, P. J. (1981): *Life Sci.*, 29:2623–2630.
51. Crick, F. (1971): *Nature*, 234:25–27.
52. Czernik, A., Petrack, B., Kalinsky, H. J., Psychoyos, S., Cash, W. D., Tsai, C., Rinehart, R. K., Granat, F. R., Lovell, R. A., Brundish, D. E., and Wade, R. (1982): *Life Sci.*, 30:363–372.
53. Daly, J. W. (1982): *J. Med. Chem.*, 25:197–204.
54. Daly, J. W. (1983): In: *Regulatory Function of Adenosine*, edited by R. M. Berne, T. W. Rall, and R. Rubio, pp. 97–113. Martinus Nijhoff, Boston.
55. Daly, J. W. (1985): *Adv. Cyclic Nucleotide Prot. Phosphorylation Res.*, 19:29–46.
56. Daly, J. W. (1985): In: *Purines: Pharmacology and Physiological Roles*, edited by T. W. Stone, pp. 5–15. Macmillan, London.
57. Daly, J. W., Butts-Lamb, P., and Padgett, W. (1983): *Cell Mol. Neurobiol.*, 3:69–80.
58. Daly, J. W., Padgett, W., Shamim, M. T., Butts-Lamb, P., and Waters, J. (1985): *J. Med. Chem.*, 28:487–492.
59. Dar, M. S., Mustafa, S. J., and Wooles, W. R. (1983): *Life Sci.*, 33:1363–1371.
60. Dascal, N., Lotan, I., Gillo, B., Lester, H. A., and Lass, Y. (1985): *Proc. Natl. Acad. Sci. USA*, 82:6001–6005.
61. Davies, L. P., Brown, D. J., Chen Chow, S., and Johnston, G. A. R. (1983): *Neurosci. Lett.*, 41:189–194.
62. Davies, L. P., Chow, S. C., and Johnston, G. A. R. (1984): *Eur. J. Pharmacol.*, 97:325–329.
63. Davies, L. P., Cook, A. F., Poonian, M., and Taylor, K. M. (1980): *Life Sci.*, 26:1089–1094.
64. Dews, P. B. (1984): *Caffeine.* Springer-Verlag, Berlin.
65. Dobson, T. G., Jr. (1983): *Circ. Res.*, 52:151–160.
66. Dolphin, A. C., and Archer, E. R. (1983): *Neurosci. Lett.*, 43:49–54.
67. Dolphin, A. C., and Prestwich, S. A. (1985): *Nature*, 316:148–150.
68. Douglass, J., Civelli, O., and Herbert, E. (1984): *Annu. Rev. Biochem.*, 53:665–715.
69. Dragunow, M. (1986): *Trends Pharmacol. Sci.*, 7:128–130.
70. Dragunow, M., and Goddard, G. V. (1984): *Exp. Neurol.*, 84:654–665.
71. Dragunow, M., Goddard, G. V., and Laverty, R. (1985): *Epilepsia*, 26:480–487.
72. Drummond, G. I. (1984): *Cyclic Nucleotides in the Nervous System.* Raven Press, New York.
73. Drury, A. N., and Szent-Gyorgi, A. (1929): *J. Physiol.*, 68:213–237.
74. Dunwiddie, T. V. (1984): *J. Physiol. (Lond.)*, 350:545–556.
75. Dunwiddie, T. V., and Fredholm, B. B. (1984): *Naunyn Schmiedebergs Arch. Pharmacol.*, 326:294–301.
76. Dunwiddie, T. V., and Hoffer, B. J. (1980): *Br. J. Pharmacol.*, 69:59–68.
77. Dunwiddie, T. V., and Worth, T. (1982): *J. Pharmacol. Exp. Ther.*, 220:70–76.
78. Ebersolt, C., Premont, T., Prochiantz, A., Perez, M., and Bockaert, T. (1983): *Brain Res.*, 267:123–126.
79. Ebstein, R. P., and Daly, J. W. (1982): *Cell. Mol. Neurobiol.*, 2:193–204.
80. Fedan, J. S., Hogaboom, G. K., O'Donnell, J. P., Jeng, C. J., and Guillory, R. J. (1985): *Eur. J. Pharmacol.*, 108:49–61.
81. Fedan, J. S., Hogaboom, G. K., O'Donnell, J. P., and Westfall, D. P. (1985): In: *Methods in Pharmacology, Vol. 6: Methods Used in Adenosine Research*, edited by D. M. Paton, pp. 279–292. Plenum, New York.
82. Feldberg, W., and Sherwood, S. L. (1954): *J. Physiol. (Lond.)*, 123:148–167.
83. Ferkany, J. W., Valentine, H. L., Stone, G. A., and Williams, M. (1986): *Drug Dev. Res.*, 9:85–93.
84. File, S. E., Bond, A. J., and Lister, R. G. (1982): *J. Clin. Psychopharmacol.*, 2:102–106.
85. Fredholm, B. B. (1982): *Acta Physiol. Scand.*, 115:283–286.
86. Fredholm, B. B., and Hedqvist, P. (1980): *Biochem. Pharmacol.*, 29:1635–1643.
87. Fredholm, B. B., Herrera-Marschitz, M., Jonzon, B., Lindstrom, K., and Ungerstedt, U. (1983): *Pharmacol. Biochem. Behav.*, 19:535–541.
88. Fredholm, B. B., Jonzon, B., and Lindstrom, K. (1983): *Acta Physiol. Scand.*, 117:461–463.
89. Fredholm, B. B., Lindgren, E., and Lindstrom, K. (1985): *Br. J. Pharmacol.*, 86:509–513.
90. Fredholm, B. B., and Vernet, L. (1978): *Acta Physiol. Scand.*, 104:502–504.
91. Fredholm, B. B., Zahniser, N. R., Weiner, G. R., Proctor, W. R., and Dunwiddie, T. V. (1985): *Eur. J. Pharmacol.*, 111:133–136.
92. Galloway, M. P., and Roth, R. H. (1983): *J. Neurochem.*, 40:246–251.
93. Galloway, M. P., and Roth, R. H. (1983): *J. Pharmacol. Exp. Ther.*, 227:1–8.
94. Gavish, M., Goodman, R. R., and Snyder, S. H. (1982): *Science*, 215:1633–1635.
95. Geiger, J. D., LaBella, F. S., and Nagy, J. I. (1984): *Dev. Brain Res.*, 13:97–104.
96. Geiger, J. D., LaBella, F. S., and Nagy, J. I. (1985): *J. Neurosci.*, 5:735–740.
97. Gold, M. S., Pottash, A. C., Sweeney, D. R., and Kleber, H. D. (1980): *JAMA*, 243:343–346.
98. Goldberg, M. R., Curatolo, P. W., Tung, C. S., and Robertson, D. (1982): *Neurosci. Lett.*, 31:47–52.
99. Goodman, R. R., Kuhar, M. J., Hester, L., and Snyder, S. H. (1983): *Science*, 220:967–969.
100. Goodman, R. R., and Snyder, S. H. (1982): *J. Neurosci.*, 2:1230–1241.
101. Gourley, D. R. H., and Beckner, S. K. (1973): *Proc. Soc. Exp. Biol. Med.*, 144:774–780.
102. Govoni, S., Petkov, V. V., Montefusco, O., Missale, C., Battaini, F., Spano, P. F., and Trabucchi, M. (1984): *J. Pharm. Pharmacol.*, 36:458–460.
103. Grant, S. J., and Redmond, D. E. (1982): *Eur. J. Pharmacol.*, 85:1054–1061.
104. Green, H. N., and Stoner, H. B. (1950): *Biological Actions of the Adenosine Nucleotides.* Lewis, London.
105. Green, R. D. (1984): *J. Neurosci.*, 4:2472–2476.
106. Green, R. D., Proudfit, H. K., and Yeung, S.-M. H. (1982): *Science*, 218:58–61.
106a. Govoni, S., Petkov, V. V., Montefusco, O., Missale, C., Battaini, F., Spano, P. F., and Trabucchi, M. (1984): *J. Pharm. Pharmacol.*, 36:458–460.
107. Haas, H. L., and Greene, R. W. (1984): *Pflugers Arch.*, 402:244–247.
108. Haefely, W., Kyburz, E., Gereck, M., and Mohler, H. (1985): *Adv. Drug. Res.*, 14:165–322.
109. Hammond, J. R., and Clanachan, A. S. (1983): *J. Neurochem.*, 45:527–535.
110. Hammond, J. R., Paterson, A. R. P., and Clanachan, A. S. (1981): *Life Sci.*, 29:2207–2214.
111. Hamprecht, B., and Van Calker, D. (1985): *Trends Pharmacol. Sci.*, 6:153–154.
112. Harms, H. H., Wardeh, G., and Mulder, A. H. (1978): *Eur. J. Pharmacol.*, 49:305–309.
113. Harms, H. H., Wardeh, G., and Mulder, A. H. (1979): *Neuropharmacology*, 18:577–580.
114. Haslam, R. J., Davidson, M. L., and Desjardins, J. W. (1978): *Biochem. J.*, 176:83–95.
115. Haubrich, D. R., Williams, M., Yarbrough, C. C., and Wood, P. L. (1981): *Can. J. Physiol. Pharmacol.*, 59:897–900.
116. Haulica, I., Aradei, L., Bransteau, D., and Topoliceanu, F. (1973): *J. Neurochem.*, 21:1019–1020.
117. Hedner, T., Hedner, J., Wessberg, P., and Jonason, J. (1982): *Neurosci. Lett.*, 33:147–151.
118. Heffner, T. G., Downs, D. A., Bristol, J. A., Bruns, R. F., Harrigan, S. E., Moos, W. H., Sledge, K. L., and Wiley, J. N. (1985): *Pharmacologist*, 21:293.
119. Henon, B. K., and McAfee, D. A. (1983): *J. Physiol. (Lond.)*, 336:607–620.
120. Hindmarch, I., and Subhan, Z. (1985): *Drug Dev. Res.*, 5:379–386.
121. Ho, I. K., Lo, H. H., and Way, E. L. (1973): *J. Pharmacol. Exp. Ther.*, 185:336–346.
122. Hogaboom, G. K., O'Donell, J. P., and Fedan, J. S. (1980): *Science*, 208:1273–1276.
123. Hollingsworth, E. B., De La Cruz, R. A., and Daly, J. W. (1986): *Eur. J. Pharmacol.*, 122:45–50.

124. Hollins, C., and Stone, T. W. (1980): *Br. J. Pharmacol.,* 69:107–112.
125. Holloway, W. R., Jr., and Thor, D. H. (1985): *Pharmacol. Biochem. Behav.,* 22:421–426.
126. Holton, F. A., and Holton, P. (1954): *J. Physiol. (Lond.),* 126:124–140.
127. Jackisch, R., Strittmatter, H., Lasakov, L., and Hertting, G. (1984): *Naunyn Schmiedebergs Arch. Pharmacol.,* 327:319–325.
128. Jahr, C. E., and Jessell, T. M. (1983): *Nature,* 304:730–733.
129. Jarvis, S. M., and Young, J. D. (1980): *Biochem. J.,* 190:377–383.
130. Jhamandas, K., and Dumbrille, A. (1980): *Can. J. Physiol. Pharmacol.,* 58:1262–1278.
131. Jonzon, B., and Fredholm, B. B. (1985): *J. Neurochem.,* 44:217–224.
132. Katims, J. J., Annau, Z., and Snyder, S. H. (1983): *J. Pharmacol. Exp. Ther.,* 22:167–173.
133. Katsuragi, T., Ushijima, I., and Furukawa, T. (1984): *Pharmacol. Biochem. Behav.,* 20:943–946.
134. Kenakin, T. P. (1982): *J. Pharmacol. Exp. Ther.,* 222:752–758.
135. Kiyohara, S., Hidaka, I., and Tamura, T. (1975): *Bull. Jpn. Soc. Sci. Fish.,* 41:383–391.
136. Kobayashi, K., Kuroda, Y., and Yoshioka, M. (1981): *J. Neurochem.,* 36:86–91.
137. Kulkarni, S. K., and Mehta, A. K. (1984): *Life Sci.,* 34:2273–2277.
138. Kuroda, Y., and McIlwain, H. (1973): *J. Neurochem.,* 21:889–900.
139. Kuroda, Y., and McIlwain, H. (1974): *J. Neurochem.,* 22:691–699.
140. Lai, R. T., Watanabe, Y., Kamino, Y., and Yoshida, H. (1984): *Life Sci.,* 34:409–418.
141. Laska, E. M., Sunshine, A., Mueller, F., Elvers, W. B., Siegel, C., and Rubin, A. (1984): *JAMA,* 251:1711–1718.
142. Lee, C. M. (1985): *Neurosci. Lett.,* 59:41–45.
143. Lee, K. S. (1985): In: *Adenosine: Receptors and Modulation of Cell Function,* edited by V. Stefanovich, K. Rudolphi, and P. Schubert, pp. 169–177. IRL Press, Oxford.
144. Lee, K. S., Reddington, M., Schubert, P., and Kreutzberg, G. (1983): *Neurosci. Lett.,* 37:81–85.
145. Lee, K. S., Schubert, P., Reddington, M., and Kreutzberg, G. W. (1983): *Brain Res.,* 260:156–159.
146. Lee, K. S., and Tetzlaff, W. (1985): *Soc. Neurosci. Abstr.,* 11:260(Abstr. 75.19).
147. Levin, R. M., Jacoby, R., and Wein, A. J. (1983): *Mol. Pharmacol.,* 23:1–7.
148. Levine, A. S., and Morley, J. E. (1982): *Science,* 217:77–79.
149. Levine, S., and Payan, H. (1966): *Exp. Neurol.,* 16:255–262.
150. Linden, J., Hollen, C. E., and Patel, A. (1985): *Circ. Res.,* 56:728–735.
151. Lloyd, K. G., Hornykiewicz, O., Davidson, L., Shannak, K., Farley, I., Goldstein, M., Shibuya, M., Kelley, W. N., and Fox, I. (1981): *N. Engl. J. Med.,* 305:1106–1111.
152. Lohse, M. J., Lenschow, V., and Schwabe, U. (1984): *Naunyn Schmiedebergs Arch. Pharmacol.,* 326:1–9.
153. Lohse, M. J., Lenschow, V., and Schwabe, U. (1984): *Naunyn Schmiedebergs Arch. Pharmacol.,* 326:69–74.
154. Londos, C., and Wolff, J. (1977): *Proc. Natl. Acad. Sci. USA,* 74:5482–5486.
155. Londos, C., Wolff, J., and Cooper, D. M. F. (1983): In: *Regulatory Function of Adenosine,* edited by R. M. Berne, T. W. Rall, and R. Rubio, pp. 17–32. Martinus Nijhoff, Boston.
156. Louis-Coindet, J., Sarda, N., Pacheco, H., and Jouvet, M. (1984): *Brain Res.,* 294:239–245.
157. Luisada, P. V. (1978): In: *Phencyclidine (PCP) Abuse: An Appraisal,* edited by R. C. Petersen and R. C. Stillman, NIDA Res. Monograph 21, pp. 241–253. US Government Printing Office, Washington, DC.
158. MacDonald, W. F., and White, T. D. (1984): *Prog. Neuropsychopharmacol. Biol. Psychiatry,* 8:487–494.
159. Mackie, A. M., and Adron, S. W. (1978): *Comp. Biochem. Physiol.,* 60A:79–83.
160. Magistretti, P. J., and Schorderet, M. (1984): *Nature,* 308:280–282.
161. Maitre, M., Ciesielski, L., Lehmann, A., Kempt, E., and Mandel, P. (1974): *Biochem. Pharmacol.,* 23:2807–2816.
162. Marangos, P. J., and Boulenger, J. P. (1985): *Neurosci. Biobehav. Rev.,* 9:421–430.
163. Marangos, P. J., Patel, J., Clark-Rosenberg, R., and Martino, A. M. (1982): *J. Neurochem.,* 39:184–191.
164. Marangos, P. J., Paul, S. M., Parma, A. M., Goodwin, F. K., Syapin, P. K., and Skolnick, P. (1979): *Life Sci.,* 24:851–858.
165. Marangos, P. J., Post, R. M., Patel, J., Zander, A., Parma, A., and Weiss, S. (1983): *Eur. J. Pharmacol.,* 93:175–182.
165a. Marangos, P. J., Weiss, S. R. B., Montgomery, P., Patel, J., Narang, P. K., Cappabianca, A. M. and Post, R. M. (1985): *Epilepsia,* 26:493–498.
166. Marley, E., and Nistico, G. (1972): *Br. J. Pharmacol.,* 46:619–636.
167. Mato, J. M., Jastorff, B., Morr, M., and Konijn, T. M. (1978): *Biochim. Biophys. Acta,* 544:309–314.
168. Mattila, M. J., Pavla, E., and Savolainen, K. (1982): *Med. Biol.,* 60:121–123.
169. Mendelson, W. B., Kuruvilla, A., Watlington, T., Goehl, K., Paul, S. M., and Skolnick, P. (1983): *Psychopharmacology,* 76:126–129.
170. Michaelis, M. L., Michaelis, E. K., and Myers, S. L. (1979): *Life Sci.,* 24:2083–2092.
171. Minana, M. D., Portoles, M., Jorda, A., and Grisolia, S. (1984): *J. Neurochem.,* 43:1556–1560.
172. Moos, W. H., Szotek, D. S., and Bruns, R. F. (1985): *J. Med. Chem.,* 28:1383–1384.
173. Moritaki, H. (1983): In: *Physiology and Pharmacology of Adenosine Derivatives,* edited by J. W. Daly, Y. Kuroda, J. W. Phillis, H. Shimizu, and M. Ui, pp. 197–207, Raven Press, New York.
174. Murphy, K. M. M., and Snyder, S. H. (1982): In: *Calcium Entry Blockers, Adenosine and Neurohumors: Recent Advances,* edited by G. F. Merill and H. R. Weiss, pp. 295–306. Urban and Schwarzenberg, Baltimore.
175. Murphy, K. M. M., and Snyder, S. H. (1982): *Mol. Pharmacol.,* 22:250–257.
176. Murray, T. F. (1982): *Eur. J. Pharmacol.,* 82:113–114.
177. Murray, T. F., Sylvester, D., Schutz, C. S., and Szot, P. (1985): *Neuropharmacology,* 24:761–766.
178. Nagy, J. I., and Daddona, P. E. (1985): *Neuroscience,* 15:799–813.
179. Nagy, J. I., Geiger, J. D., and Daddona, P. E. (1985): *Neurosci. Lett.,* 55:47–53.
180. Nagy, J. I., Labella, L. A., Buss, M., and Dadonna, P. E. (1984): *Science,* 224:166–168.
181. Nakata, H., and Fujisawa, H. (1983): *FEBS Lett.,* 158:93–97.
182. Neal, M. J. (1965): *Br. J. Pharmacol. Chemother.,* 24:170–176.
183. Newman, M. E. (1983): *Neurochem. Int.,* 5:21–35.
184. Newman, M. E., and McIlwain, H. (1977): *Biochem. J.,* 164:131–137.
185. Newman, M., Zohar, J., Kalian, M., and Belmaker, R. H. (1984): *Brain Res.,* 291:188–192.
186. Niemand, D., Martinell, S., Arvidsson, S., Svedmyr, N., and Ekstrom-Jodal, B. (1984): *Lancet,* 1:463–464.
187. Nimit, Y., Law, S., and Daly, J. W. (1982): *Biochem. Pharmacol.,* 31:3279–3287.
188. O'Donohue, T. L., Millington, W. R., Handelmann, G. E., Contreras, P. C., and Chronwall, B. M. (1985): *Trends Pharmacol. Sci.,* 6:305–308.
189. Okuma, T., Matsuoka, H., Matsue, Y., and Toyomura, K. (1982): *Psychopharmacology,* 76:201–208.
190. Ondera, H., and Kogure, K. (1985): *Brain Res.,* 345:406–408.
191. Paazlow, G., and Paazlow, C. (1973): *Acta Pharmacol. Toxicol.,* 32:22–32.
192. Patel, J., Marangos, P. J., Stivers, J., and Goodwin, F. K. (1982): *Brain Res.,* 237:203–214.
193. Phillis, J. W. (1984): *Prog. Neurobiol. Biol. Psychiatry,* 8:494–502.
194. Phillis, J. W. (1984): *Br. J. Pharmacol.,* 83:567–575.
195. Phillis, J. W., and DeLong, R. E. (1984): *Eur. J. Pharmacol.,* 101:295–297.
196. Phillis, J. W., DeLong, R. E., and Towner, J. K. (1985): *J. Cereb. Blood Flow Metab.,* 5:295–299.
197. Phillis, J. W., Edstrom, T. P., Kostopoulos, G. K., and Kirkpatrick, J. R. (1979): *Can. J. Physiol. Pharmacol.,* 57:1289–1312.

198. Phillis, J. W., Swanson, T. H., and Barraco, R. A. (1984): *Neurochem. Int.,* 6:693–699.
199. Phillis, J. W., and Wu, P. H. (1981): *Prog. Neurobiol.,* 16:187–239.
200. Phillis, J. W., and Wu, P. H. (1983): In: *Regulatory Function of Adenosine,* edited by R. M. Berne, T. W. Rall, and R. Rubio, pp. 419–437. Martinus Nijhoff, Boston.
201. Phillis, J. W., Ziang, Z. G., Chelack, B. J., and Wu, P. H. (1980): *Pharmacol. Biochem. Behav.,* 13:421–427.
202. Pons, F., Bruns, R. F., and Daly, T. W. (1980): *J. Neurochem.,* 34:1319–1323.
203. Porter, N. M., Clark, F. M., Green, R. D., and Radulovacki, M. (1985): *Soc. Neurosci. Abstr.,* 11:171.18.
204. Potter, P., and White, T. D. (1980): *Neuroscience,* 5:1351–1356.
205. Premont, T., Perez, M., and Bockaert, T. (1977): *Mol. Pharmacol.,* 13:662–670.
206. Proctor, W. R., and Dunwiddie, T. V. (1984): *Science,* 224:519–521.
207. Pull, I., and McIlwain, H. (1974): *Biochem. J.,* 144:37–41.
208. Rabe, C. S., and McGee, R., Jr. (1983): *J. Neurochem.,* 41:1623–1634.
209. Radulovacki, M., Miletich, R. S., and Green, R. D. (1982): *Brain Res.,* 246:178–180.
210. Radulovacki, M., Virus, R. M., Druricec-Nedelson, M., and Green, R. D. (1983): *Brain Res.,* 271:392–395.
210a.Radulovacki, M., Virus, R. M., Djuricec-Nedelson, M. and Green, R. D. (1984): *J. Pharmacol. Exp. Ther.,* 228:268–274.
211. Radulovacki, M., Virus, R. M., Rapoza, D., and Crane, R. C. (1985): *Neuropharmacology,* 24:547–549.
212. Rall, T. W. (1985): In: *The Pharmacological Basis of Therapeutics,* 7th ed., edited by A. G. Gilman, L. S. Goodman, T. W. Rall, and F. Murad, pp. 589–603. Macmillan, New York.
213. Razzak, A. M., Fujiwara, M., and Ueki, S. (1977): *Jpn. J. Pharmacol.,* 27:145–152.
214. Reddington, M. (1985): In: *Adenosine: Receptors and Modulation of Cell Function,* edited by V. Stefanovich, K. Rudolphi, and P. Schubert, pp. 181–189. IRL Press, Oxford.
215. Reddington, M., Erfurth, A., and Lee, K. S. (1985): *J. Neurochem.,* S41C.
216. Reddington, M., Lee, K. S., and Schubert, P. (1982): *Neurosci. Lett.,* 28:275–279.
217. Reddington, M., and Schubert, P. (1979): *Neurosci. Lett.,* 14:37–42.
218. Reinhard, J. F., Jr., Galloway, M. P., and Roth, R. H. (1983): *J. Pharmacol. Exp. Ther.,* 226:764–769.
219. Richards, C. D., Snell, C. R., and Snell, S. H. (1983): *Br. J. Pharmacol.,* 79:553–558.
220. Rosen, J. B., and Berman, R. F. (1985): *Exp. Neurol.,* 90:549–557.
221. Salter, M. W., and Henry, J. L. (1985): *Neuroscience,* 15:815–825.
222. Sattin, A. (1981): In: *Chemisms in the Brain,* edited by R. Rodnight, H. S. Bachelard, and W. S. Stahl, pp. 265–275. Churchill Livingstone, Edinburgh.
223. Sattin, A., and Rall, T. W. (1970): *Mol. Pharmacol.,* 6:13–23.
224. Sattin, A., Stone, T. W., and Taylor, D. A. (1978): *Life Sci.,* 23:2621–2626.
225. Sawynok, T., and Jhmandas, K. H. (1976): *J. Pharmacol. Exp. Ther.,* 197:379–390.
226. Schoener, E. P., Cambell, W. R., Barraco, R. A., and Marcantonio, D. R. (1985): *Soc. Neurosci. Abstr.,* 11:61.5.
227. Schoffelmeer, A. N. M., Wardeh, G., and Mulder, A. H. (1985): *Naunyn Schmiedebergs Arch. Pharmacol.,* 330:74–76.
228. Schubert, P., and Mitzdorf, V. (1979): *Brain Res.,* 172:186–190.
229. Schwabe, U., and Trost, T. (1981): *Naunyn Schmiedebergs Arch. Pharmacol.,* 313:179–187.
230. Schwabe, U., Ukena, D., and Lohse, M. T. (1985): *Naunyn Schmiedebergs Arch. Pharmacol.,* 320:212–221.
231. *Scrip* (1985): September 18, 1985, p. 22.
231a.Seale, T. W., Roderick, T. H., Johnson, P., Logan, L., Rennert, O. M., and Carney, J. M. (1987): *Pharmacol. Biochem. Behav.* (*in press*).
232. Segal, M. (1982): *Eur. J. Pharmacol.,* 79:193–199.
233. Seitelberger, R., Schutz, W., Schlappack, O., and Raberger, G. (1984): *Naunyn Schmiedebergs Arch. Pharmacol.,* 325:234–239.

234. Sheid, B. (1985): *Res. Commun. Chem. Pathol. Pharmacol.,* 47:149–152.
235. Shimizu, H., Tanaka, S., and Kodama, T. (1972): *J. Neurochem.,* 19:687–698.
236. Siggins, G., and Schubert, P. (1981): *Neurosci. Lett.,* 23:55–60.
237. Silinsky, E. M. (1985): In: *Purines: Pharmacology and Physiological Roles,* edited by T. W. Stone, pp. 67–74. Macmillan, London.
238. Skeritt, J. H., Davies, L. P., and Johnston, G. A. R. (1982): *Eur. J. Pharmacol.,* 82:195–197.
239. Snell, C. R., and Snell, P. H. (1983): *Br. J. Pharmacol.,* 83:791–798.
240. Snell, P. H., Snell, C. R., and Richards, C. D. (1985): *Eur. J. Pharmacol.,* 116:121–127.
241. Snowhill, E. W., and Williams, M. (1985): *J. Neurochem.,* 44:S88A.
242. Snowhill, E. W., and Williams, M. (1985): *Soc. Neurosci. Abstr.,* 11:171.2.
243. Snyder, S. H. (1985): *Sci. Am.,* 253:132–141.
244. Snyder, S. H. (1985): *Annu. Rev. Neurosci.,* 8:103–124.
245. Snyder, S. H., Katims, J. J., Annau, Z., Bruns, R. F., and Daly, J. W. (1981): *Proc. Natl. Acad. Sci. USA,* 78:3260–3264.
246. Snyder, S. H., and Sklar, P. (1984): *J. Psychiatr. Res.,* 18:91–106.
247. Spignoli, G., Pedata, F., and Pepeu, C. (1984): *Eur. J. Pharmacol.,* 97:341–342.
248. Squires, R. F. (1984): *Handb. Neurochem.,* 6:261–306.
249. Stadel, T. M., DeLean, A., and Lefkowitz, R. J. (1982): *Adv. Enzymol.,* 53:1–43.
250. Standert, F. G., and Dretchen, K. C. (1979): *Fed. Proc.,* 38:2183–2192.
251. Stiles, G. L. (1985): *J. Biol. Chem.,* 260:6728–6732.
252. Stiles, G. L., Daly, D. T., and Olsson, R. A. (1985): *J. Biol. Chem.,* 260:10806–10811.
253. Stone, T. W. (1981): *Neuroscience,* 6:523–555.
254. Stone, T. W. (1983): In: *Regulatory Function of Adenosine,* edited by R. M. Berne, T. W. Rall, and R. Rubio, pp. 467–477. Martinus Nijhoff, Boston.
255. Stone, T. W. (1985): In: *Purines: Pharmacology and Physiological Roles,* edited by T. W. Stone, pp. 1–4. Macmillan, London.
256. Stone, T. W., and Taylor, D. A. (1979): *Neurosci. Lett.,* 11:93–97.
257. Torii, K., and Cagan, R. H. (1980): *Biochim. Biophys. Acta,* 627:313–323.
258. Traversa, U., Puppini, P., deAngelis, L., and Vertua, R. (1984): *Pharmacol. Res. Commun.,* 16:589–603.
259. Trussell, L. O., and Jackson, M. B. (1985): *Proc. Natl. Acad. Sci. USA,* 82:4857–4861.
260. Turski, L., Schwarz, M., Turski, W. A., Ikonomidou, C., and Sontag, K. H. (1984): *Eur. J. Pharmacol.,* 103:99–105.
261. Ukena, D., Bohme, E., and Schwabe, U. (1984): *Naunyn Schmiedebergs Arch. Pharmacol.,* 327:36–42.
262. Ushijima, I., Katsuragi, T., and Furukawa, T. (1984): *Psychopharmacology,* 83:335–339.
263. Van Calker, D., Muller, M., and Hamprecht, B. (1978): *Nature,* 276:839–841.
264. Van Calker, D., Muller, M., and Hamprecht, B. (1979): *J. Neurochem.,* 33:999–1005.
265. Vapaatalo, H., Onken, D., Neuvonen, P. J., and Westermann, E. (1975): *Arzneim. Forsch.,* 25:407–410.
266. Velluci, S. V., and Webster, R. A. (1984): *Eur. J. Pharmacol.,* 97:289–293.
267. Verma, A., Houston, M., and Marangos, P. J. (1985): *J. Neurochem.,* 45:596–603.
268. Verma, A., and Marangos, P. J. (1985): *Life Sci.,* 36:283–291.
269. Virus, R. M., Baglajewski, T., and Radulovacki, M. (1984): *Neurobiol. Aging,* 5:61–62.
270. Watanabe, Y., Lai, R. T., and Yoshido, H. (1983): *Eur. J. Pharmacol.,* 86:265–269.
271. Weiss, S. R. B., Post, R. M., Marangos, P. J., and Patel, J. (1985): *Neuropharmacology,* 24:635–638.
272. Weiss, S. R. B., Post, R. M., Patel, J., and Marangos, P. J. (1985): *Life Sci.,* 36:2413–2419.
273. Wessberg, P., Hedner, J., Hedner, T., Persson, B., and Jonason, T. (1985): *Eur. J. Pharmacol.,* 106:59–61.
274. Williams, M. (1981): In: *Chemisms in the Brain,* edited by R.

Rodnight, H. S. Bachelard, and W. S. Stahl, pp. 78–88. Churchill Livingstone, Edinburgh.

275. Williams, M. (1983): *J. Med. Chem.*, 26:619–628.

276. Williams, M. (1984): *Trends Neurosci.*, 7:164–168.

277. Williams, M. (1984): *Handb. Neurochem.*, 6:1–26.

278. Williams, M. (1986): In: *Receptor Binding in Drug Research*, edited by R. A. O'Brien, pp. 235–259. Marcel Dekker, New York.

279. Williams, M. (1987): In: *Receptor Pharmacology and Function*, edited by M. Williams, R. A. Glennon, and M. W. M. Timmermans. Marcel Dekker, New York (*in press*).

280. Williams, M. (1985): In: *Adenosine: Receptors and Modulation of Cell Function*, edited by V. Stefanovich, K. Rudolphi, and P. Schubert, pp. 73–85. IRL Press, Oxford.

281. Williams, M., Abreu, M., Jarvis, M. J., and Noronha-Blob, L. (1987): *J. Neurochem.*, 48:498–502.

282. Williams, M., Braunwalder, A., and Erickson, T. E. (1986): *Naunyn Schmiedebergs Arch. Pharmacol.*, 332:179–183.

282a. Williams, M., Francis, J. E., Ghai, G. R., Braumalder, A. F., Psychoyos, S., Stone, G. A., and Cash, W. D. (1987): *J. Pharmacol. Exp. Ther.*, Vol. 241 (*in press*).

283. Williams, M., and Risley, E. A. (1980): *Proc. Natl. Acad. Sci. USA*, 77:6892–6896.

284. Williams, M., and Risley, E. A. (1980): *Fed Proc.*, 39:1009.

285. Williams, M., and Risley, E. A. (1982): *Arch. Int. Pharmacodyn. Ther.*, 260:50–53.

286. Williams, M., Risley, E. A., and Huff, J. L. (1981): *Can. J. Physiol. Pharmacol.*, 59:897–900.

287. Williams, M., Risley, E. A., and Robinson, J. L. (1983): *Neurosci. Lett.*, 35:47–51.

288. Williams, M., and U'Prichard, D. C. (1984): *Annu. Rep. Med. Chem.*, 19:283–292.

289. Winn, H. R., Morii, J., and Berne, R. M. (1985): *Ann. Biomed. Eng.*, 13:321–323.

290. Winn, H. R., Rubio, R., and Berne, R. M. (1979): *Circ. Res.*, 45:486–492.

291. Winn, H. R., Rubio, R., and Berne, R. M. (1981): *J. Cereb. Blood Flow Metab.*, 1:239–244.

292. Wojcik, W. J., Cavalla, D., and Neff, N. H. (1985): *J. Pharmacol. Exp. Ther.*, 232:62–66.

293. Wojcik, W. J., and Neff, N. H. (1983): *J. Neurochem.*, 41:759–763.

294. Wojcik, W. J., and Neff, N. H. (1984): *Mol. Pharmacol.*, 25:24–28.

295. Wu, P. H., and Coffin, V. L. (1984): *Brain Res.*, 294:186–189.

296. Wu, P. H., and Phillis, J. W. (1984): *Neurochem. Int.*, 6:613–632.

297. Wybenga, M. P., Murphy, M. G., and Robertson, H. A. (1981): *Eur. J. Pharmacol.*, 75:79–80.

298. Yanik, G., Porter, N. M., and Radulovacki, M. (1985): *Soc. Neurosci. Abstr.*, 11:171.17.

299. Yarbrough, C. C., and McGuffin-Clineschmidt, B. V. (1981): *Eur. J. Pharmacol.*, 76:137–144.

300. Yeung, S.-M. H., and Green, R. D. (1984): *Naunyn Schmiedebergs Arch. Pharmacol.*, 325:218–225.

301. Yeung, S.-M. H., Frame, L. T., Venter, J. C., and Cooper, D. M. F. (1985): In: *Purines, Pharmacology and Physiological Roles*, edited by T. W. Stone, pp. 203–214. VCH Publications, Florida.

302. Zetterstrom, T., Vernet, L., Ungerstedt, U., Tossman, U., Jonzon, B., and Fredholm, B. B. (1982): *Neurosci. Lett.*, 29:111–115.

303. Zwillich, C. W. (1975): *Ann. Int. Med.*, 82:784–787.

Psychopharmacology:
The Third Generation of Progress,
edited by Herbert Y. Meltzer.
Raven Press, New York © 1987.

CHAPTER 31

Serotonin Receptors

Stephen J. Peroutka

Physiologists have been aware of an endogenous vasoconstrictor substance since the middle of the nineteenth century. The factor was present in the serum of clotted blood and was often referred to as "vasotonin." Rapport et al. (119) and a group of Italian scientists (33) independently succeeded in identifying the compound as "serotonin" or 5-hydroxytryptamine (5-HT). The initial discovery of 5-HT in the central nervous system was made by Twarog and Page (142). Histochemical studies identified the raphe nuclei as the main 5-HT-containing cell bodies in the brain. The characterization of specific synthesis, release, and storage mechanisms for 5-HT confirmed that the biogenic amine is a central neurotransmitter.

The role of 5-HT in the central nervous system has been extensively studied using a variety of techniques. In particular, receptor site analysis has been a productive approach to the understanding of the actions of 5-HT and related agents since the differentiation of M and D receptors by Gaddum and Picarelli in 1957 (45). However, it has become clear that multiple 5-HT receptors exist in the central nervous system. For example, at least four 5-HT binding site subtypes have been differentiated by ^{3}H-ligand techniques in brain homogenates (36,44,61,73, 105,106,113,116). Anatomic studies have confirmed that a variety of serotonergic recognition sites, with distinct regional localizations, exist in the central nervous system (10,62,99,100,104,148). Neurophysiologically, the variability of effects of 5-HT and related agents has also led to a hypothesis of multiple 5-HT receptors in the central nervous system (89,123).

This chapter will focus on the use of radioligand binding techniques to characterize 5-HT receptor subtypes in brain membranes. The data derived from these studies will then be compared with the effects of 5-HT and related agents as measured in a variety of physiologic systems. Thus, an attempt will be made to define functional correlates of 5-HT binding sites in order that these membrane recognition sites can be considered "5-HT receptors." Vascular (107,143) and other peripheral 5-HT receptors (42,120) will not be discussed in this chapter.

RADIOLIGAND BINDING STUDIES OF 5-HT RECEPTORS

Preliminary Binding Studies

The first successful radioligand analysis of 5-HT receptors was reported by Bennett and Aghajanian (5). The binding of d-[^{3}H]lysergic acid diethylamide (d-LSD) was saturable, reversible, stereoselective, and displayed high affinity ($K_D = 7.5$ nM) for its membrane recognition site. The binding sites also displayed appropriate regional variations, since brain regions with the highest density of receptors were areas known to receive a dense projection of 5-HT neuronal terminals. These findings were soon extended and confirmed by other laboratories (6,79).

The second radioligand used to label 5-HT receptors was [^{3}H]5-HT (7,41,93). Like [^{3}H]LSD binding, the [^{3}H]5-HT binding was saturable, stereoselective, and displayed appropriate regional variations. However, important discrepancies were noted between the binding of [^{3}H]LSD and [^{3}H]5-HT. At the time, Bennett and Snyder (7) suggested that [^{3}H]5-HT and [^{3}H]LSD did not label the same membrane recognition site but rather two different "states" of the same receptor.

Radioligand analysis of 5-HT receptors was considerably advanced by the finding that [³H]spiperone could also be used to label presumed 5-HT recognition sites (75). Previously, [³H]spiperone had been considered a pure dopaminergic ligand. However, in the rat frontal cortex, where dopamine receptors are sparse, [³H]spiperone was found to label a receptor that appeared to be "serotonergic" in the sense that 5-HT antagonists were the most potent displacers of the ligand. However, 5-HT and related tryptamines were extremely weak displacers of [³H]spiperone. The ability of [³H]spiperone to label 5-HT receptors was quickly confirmed by other laboratories (19,118).

Differentiation of 5-HT₁ and 5-HT₂ Receptors

Thus, marked differences were noted between the binding characteristics of [³H]5-HT, [³H]LSD, and [³H]spiperone (113). If each ligand labeled the same membrane recognition site, then unlabeled drugs should be equipotent in displacing [³H]5-HT, [³H]LSD, and [³H]spiperone. This pattern is observed with d-LSD displacement of the three ligands. A K_i value of approximately 10 nM is observed with d-LSD competition studies against each of these three ligands. In marked contrast, 5-HT is approximately three orders of magnitude more potent in displacing [³H]5-HT (3.8 nM) than [³H]spiperone (2,700 nM). Its apparent K_i for [³H]LSD binding is 110 nM, a value that is intermediate between its affinity for [³H]5-HT- and [³H]spiperone-labeled sites. Furthermore, the Hill slope for 5-HT displacement of [³H]LSD but not of [³H]5-HT or [³H]spiperone binding is significantly less than unity (113). The converse pattern is observed with spiperone displacement of the three radioligands. For example, spiperone is extremely potent against [³H]spiperone binding (0.51 nM) yet has 1,400-fold less affinity for total [³H]5-HT-labeled sites (730 nM). In addition, its apparent K_i for [³H]LSD binding is 18 nM, but the displacement curve is biphasic with a "plateau" occurring between 10 and 30 nM spiperone.

Given the results outlined above and the fact that no correlation exists between drug potencies for ³H-5-HT- and ³H-spiperone-labeled "serotonergic" receptors, Peroutka and Snyder (113) concluded that at least two distinct 5-HT membrane recognition sites exist in the central nervous system. The sites labeled by [³H]5-HT were designated "5-HT₁ receptors" and those labeled by [³H]spiperone were designated "5-HT₂ receptors." Since [³H]LSD had equal affinity for both sites, it was proposed that this ligand could be used to label both 5-HT₁ and 5-HT₂ receptors.

5-HT₁ Receptor Subtypes

However, 5-HT₁ binding sites labeled by [³H]5-HT were soon shown to be heterogeneous. Nonsigmoidal displacement of [³H]5-HT by spiperone led to the suggestion that sites with high affinity ($K_i = 2–13$ nM) for spiperone should be designated 5-HT₁A sites whereas sites with relatively low affinity for spiperone ($K_i = 35$ μM) should be designated 5-HT₁B sites (105). These two subtypes have different regional localizations and have been identified in many species (130). Autoradiographic studies have also confirmed the ability of spiperone to differentiate at least two types of sites labeled by [³H]5-HT (23). More recently, a third subtype of 5-HT₁ binding sites has been identified in the choroid plexus and cortex of various species (102,103,109,146). In the past few years, the availability of selective and novel agents has greatly facilitated the analysis of 5-HT₁ binding site subtypes. A summary of the currently accepted 5-HT receptor classification system is presented in Table 1. A summary of drug potencies at each of the four known 5-HT binding site subtypes is provided in Table 2. These data are discussed in greater detail in the following section.

TABLE 1. *Characteristics of 5-HT₁A, 5-HT₁B, 5-HT₁C, and 5-HT₂ receptors*

	5-HT₁A	5-HT₁B	5-HT₁C	5-HT₂
Radiolabeled by	[³H]5-HT [³H]8-OH-DPAT [³H]TVX Q 7821 [³H]WB 4101 [³H]Buspirone [³H]PAPP	[³H]5-HT ¹²⁵I-CYP	[³H]5-HT [³H]Mesulergine ¹²⁵I-LSD	[³H]Spiperone [³H]Mesulergine ¹²⁵I-LSD [³H]Ketanserin [³H]Mianserin ¹²⁵I-Methyl-LSD
High-density regions	Raphe nuclei Hippocampus	Dorsal subiculum Globus pallidus Substantia nigra	Choroid plexus	Layer IV cortex
Potent pharmacologic agents	5-HT 8-OH-DPAT 5-MeDMT TVX Q 7821 Buspirone RU 24969	5-HT RU 24969 TFMPP	5-HT Mesulergine Mianserin Methysergide	Ketanserin Spiperone Mesulergine Mianserin Methysergide Ritanserin Cyproheptadine

TFMPP, 1-(M-trifluoromethylphenyl)piperazine
CYP, cyanopindolol

TABLE 2. *Drug affinities for 5-HT$_{1A}$, 5-HT$_{1B}$, 5-HT$_{1C}$, and 5-HT$_2$ receptors*

Drug	K_i (nM)			
	5-HT$_{1A}$	5-HT$_{1B}$	5-HT$_{1C}$	5-HT$_2$
Tryptamines				
5-Hydroxytryptamine	2.2	7.6	11	2,700
5-Methoxytryptamine	2.5	15	25	2,700
Bufotenine	5.0	52	110	840
Novel agonists				
8-OH-DPAT	1.0	24,000	7,200	15,000
Isapirone	2.9	52,000	9,000	10,000
Buspirone	15	68,000	110,000	2,100
RU 24969	2.5	0.38	150	1,000
Ergots				
d-LSD	3.9	170	100	13
Metergoline	13	52	100	2.1
Methysergide	25	520	62	2.6
Antagonists				
Spiperone	130	47,000	4,800	0.51
Mianserin	800	10,000	110	4.8
Cyproheptadine	110	840	2,600	2.0

K_i values were determined from IC$_{50}$ values as calculated from log-probit analysis. Data given are from refs. 109, 111, 113 and unpublished observations.

Characteristics of 5-HT$_{1A}$, 5-HT$_{1B}$, 5-HT$_{1C}$, and 5-HT$_2$ Binding Sites

A number of radioligands have been shown to label the 5-HT$_{1A}$ binding site. Based on spiperone-displaceable [^{3}H]5-HT binding, 5-HT$_{1A}$ sites were found to predominate in the hippocampus, septum, and cerebral cortex (23). The 5-HT$_{1A}$ site can be more directly labeled with [^{3}H]8-hydroxy2-(di-*n*-propylamino)tetralin (8-OH-DPAT) (50,54,61,108), [^{3}H]TVX Q 7821 (24), [^{3}H]buspirone (90), and [^{3}H]1-(2-(4-aminophenyl)ethyl)-4-(3-trifluoromethylphenyl)-piperazine (PAPP) (3). In addition, [^{3}H]WB 4101, previously considered a selective α_1-adrenergic radioligand, has been demonstrated to label the 5-HT$_{1A}$ site (96). Regardless of the ^{3}H-ligand used to label the site, it displays high and selective affinity for 8-OH-DPAT, 5-methoxydimethyltryptamine (5-MeDMT), TVX Q 7821, and buspirone. The 5-HT$_{1A}$ site is densely present in the CA1 region and dentate gyrus of the hippocampus and in the raphe nuclei (23,47,83,100). In addition, the fact that 5,7-dihydroxytryptamine-induced lesions of the raphe system cause a loss of [^{3}H]8-OH-DPAT binding in the striatum but not hippocampus has led Hamon and colleagues to hypothesize that [^{3}H]8-OH-DPAT also labels a presynaptic 5-HT autoreceptor (50,54).

The putative 5-HT$_{1B}$ site has been more difficult to characterize. Sills et al. (134) defined 5-HT$_{1B}$ binding as specific [^{3}H]5-HT binding in the presence of 1 mM GTP and 2,000 nM spiperone. They concluded that RU 24969 and TFMPP were selective 5-HT$_{1B}$ agents. In fact, their data show that both RU 24969 and TFMPP are essentially equipotent versus [^{3}H]5-HT binding regardless of whether 2,000 nM spiperone is added to the binding assay. Moreover, they concluded that methysergide was 30-fold "selective" for 5-HT$_1$ subtypes but

were not able to determine whether the "high" affinity component represented 5-HT$_{1A}$ or putative 5-HT$_{1B}$ sites. More recently, the 5-HT$_{1B}$ site has been labeled in rat brain with ^{125}I-cyanopindolol (60,61,101). The ^{125}I-cyanopindolol site has high affinity for 5-HT and RU 24969 and relatively low affinity for *d*-LSD and 8-OH-DPAT. The highest densities of 5-HT$_{1B}$ sites in rat brain are found in the caudate nucleus, superior colliculus, lateral geniculate body, subiculum, and substantia nigra (100). Recent data from our laboratory have shown that this site is also labeled by [^{3}H]5-HT in rat frontal cortex (109). Moreover, the 5-HT$_{1B}$ site appears to be species specific in that it is present in rat and mouse brain but not in guinea pig, cow, chicken, turtle, frog, or human brain membranes (57).

The 5-HT$_{1C}$ site was first characterized in membranes from pig choroid plexus and cortex (102,103). The site was labeled by both [^{3}H]5-HT and [^{3}H]mesulergine. Independently, Yagaloff and Hartig (146) labeled the site with ^{125}I-LSD in the rat choroid plexus. The site has high affinity for 5-HT, methysergide, and mianserin and relatively low affinity for RU 24969. These pharmacological characteristics are also shared with the putative 5-HT$_{1C}$ site identified in rat cortex (61,109). Another 5-HT$_1$ subtype site having low affinity for RU 24969 has been identified in the bovine striatum (108). The relationship between putative 5-HT$_{1C}$ sites in rat, bovine, and pig brain is currently being investigated in this laboratory.

In contrast, [^{3}H]spiperone, [^{3}H]LSD, [^{3}H]mianserin, [^{3}H]ketanserin, [^{3}H]mesulergine, ^{125}I-LSD, and N_1-methyl-2-^{125}I-LSD can be used to label the 5-HT$_2$ binding site (13,29,55,56,59,65,72,75,76,116). Serotonergic antagonists have high affinity for this site whereas 5-HT and related tryptamines are markedly less potent. The number of 5-HT$_2$, but not 5-HT$_1$, binding sites can be decreased by chronic treatment with antidepressant drugs (114,115). The highest level of 5-HT$_2$ binding in human brain is in the cerebral cortex and caudate, with all other brain regions having substantially fewer binding sites (63,131). The 5-HT$_2$ site has been extensively studied using [^{3}H]spiperone and [^{3}H]ketanserin. Using cinanserin-displaceable [^{3}H]spiperone to define binding to 5-HT$_2$ sites, the highest density of specific binding was observed in lamina IV of the neocortex (98). Similarly, a moderate amount of 5-HT$_2$ binding in rat brain was found in lamina IV of the cortex whereas a high density of specific binding was identified in the striatum (104,135).

PHYSIOLOGIC MODELS OF CENTRAL 5-HT RECEPTORS

Although radioligand techniques provide a rapid and sensitive measure of drug potencies at specific membrane recognition sites, they cannot differentiate the agonist versus antagonist properties of drugs, relative efficacy of agents, or drug interactions with other receptor sites involved in a specific physiologic response. This type of pharmacologic information can only be derived from physiologic experiments. In the following section, a number of physiologic models will be analyzed for possible relationships to 5-HT$_{1A}$, 5-HT$_{1B}$, 5-HT$_{1C}$, and 5-HT$_2$ binding sites. As shown in Table 3, a number of investigators have proposed that a relationship does indeed exist between various physiologic systems and radioligand binding sites. As will be described below, the suggested relationships have been based on the similarities between drug potencies in various physiological systems and their affinities for radioligand binding sites.

Serotonin-Sensitive Adenylate Cyclase

A 5-HT-sensitive adenylate cyclase in mammalian brain was first detected in newborn rats (144,145). Subsequent studies confirmed that half-maximal stimulation of the enzyme occurred at micromolar concentrations of 5-HT (30,31). Classical 5-HT antagonists also interacted with the enzyme at micromolar concentrations. An extensive analysis of the anatomic, developmental, and pharmacologic properties of this preparation has shown clearly that activation of this particular adenylate cyclase is not related to 5-HT$_1$ or 5-HT$_2$ binding sites (77,92,93).

However, a markedly different type of 5-HT-sensitive adenylate cyclase has been detected by Fillion and co-workers (37–40). Using a radioimmunoassay technique that detects femtomole quantities of cyclic AMP, they have described a cyclase that is stimulated by nanomolar concentrations of 5-HT. The effect of 5-HT is antagonized by classical 5-HT antagonists, but only at micromolar concentrations or higher. The cyclase system is primarily located in purified synaptic membranes, in contrast to a low-affinity 5-HT cyclase system which is present in glial cell membranes and glial cell cultures. The effects of lesion studies also support an association between the 5-HT$_1$ binding site and the high-affinity 5-HT cyclase system (37,39). A similar type of 5-HT-sensitive adenylate cyclase has been analyzed in rat hippocampal membranes (4) and in the NCB-20 hybrid clonal cell line (9). In a recent study using guinea pig hippocampal membranes, a 5-HT-sensitive adenylate cyclase could also be stimulated by nanomolar concentrations of two 5-HT$_{1A}$-selective agents, 5-carboxamido-tryptamine and 8-OH-DPAT (133). These preliminary results suggest that the 5-HT$_{1A}$ receptor may mediate activation of this cyclase.

Radioligand binding data also support an association between 5-HT$_1$ receptors and a 5-HT-sensitive adenylate cyclase. Regulation of neurotransmitter binding by guanine nucleotides often reflects an association of the agonist binding site with an adenylate cyclase (78,81,122). Thus, GTP and GDP, but not GMP, inhibit the binding of [^{3}H]5-HT to brain homogenates (82,110). In addition, guanine nucleotides significantly reduce agonist potencies for [^{3}H]5-HT binding sites, whereas antagonist potencies are not affected by nucleotides. Similar but more potent effects of guanine nucleotides have recently been observed at 5-HT$_{1A}$ sites labeled by [^{3}H]8-OH-DPAT (128). Furthermore, guanine nucleotides have a profound synergistic effect on 5-HT-sensitive cyclase systems (4,38,82,92). In summary, an association between the 5-HT$_1$ binding site and the high-affinity adenylate cyclase system is supported both by the pattern of pharmacological interactions at the cyclase in certain systems and by the effects of guanine nucleotides on [^{3}H]5-HT binding.

However, it must be emphasized that this relationship is extremely dependent on the cyclase system being studied.

TABLE 3. *Proposed functional correlates of 5-HT binding site subtypes*

5-HT$_{1A}$
Adenylate cyclase stimulation
CA1 and raphe cell inhibition
Canine basilar artery contractions
Forepaw treading, tremor, head-weaving
Facilitation of ejaculation and/or seminal emissions
Hypothermia
Hypotensive effects
5-HT$_{1B}$
"Autoreceptor"
5-HT$_{1C}$
Phosphoinositide turnover
5-HT$_2$
5-Hydroxytryptophan- or mescaline-induced head twitches
Tryptamine-induced seizures
Contraction of vascular smooth muscle
Classical "D" receptors
Rat forepaw edema
Discriminative cue properties
Contraction of bronchial smooth muscle
Platelet shape changes and aggregation
Phosphoinositol turnover
Smooth muscle prostacyclin synthesis
Hyperthermia
Neurophysiologic excitation of neuronal firing

For example, the 5-HT-sensitive cyclase located both on glial membranes (39) and in monkey cortex (1) has an EC_{50} value in the micromolar range. The effect of 5-HT can be blocked by nanomolar concentrations of 5-HT antagonists and certain neuroleptics. In addition, under certain assay conditions, guanine nucleotides have been shown to affect the binding of [^{3}H]spiperone and [^{3}H]ketanserin to 5-HT$_2$ receptors (69,132,137). As a result, indirect evidence also supports a possible linkage of the 5-HT$_2$ receptor, in certain systems, with an adenylate cyclase.

Phosphoinositide Turnover

Besides adenylate cyclase, phosphoinositide turnover is believed to be a common "second messenger" in the transduction of neurotransmitter signals to the cell interior (8,95). 5-HT has been shown to increase phosphoinositide turnover in the mammalian central nervous system (11,15,16,70). The hydrolysis of phosphoinositides may modulate a number of intracellular processes, including calcium flux, increased arachidonate metabolism, and increased cyclic GMP and protein kinase C production. Analysis of 5-HT-induced inositol phospholipid hydrolysis in rat cerebral cortex (16,70) suggests that this event may occur as a result of 5-HT$_2$ receptor activation. For example, the response to 5-HT is blocked by nanomolar concentrations of ketanserin and phosphoinositide turnover is not affected by 8-OH-DPAT. The rat thoracic aorta (91,124), cultured bovine aortic smooth muscle cells (17), and platelets (20) are three additional systems in which 5-HT appears to modulate phosphoinositide turnover via a receptor that is similar to the 5-HT$_2$ binding site. In addition, preliminary studies have shown that the 5-HT$_{1C}$ site may also mediate 5-HT-induced phosphoinositide turnover in rat choroid plexus (125).

However, a correlation with 5-HT$_2$ sites cannot be established in many regions of rat brain. For example, ketanserin only partially inhibits the response to 5-HT in the hippocampus and limbic forebrain (16). Moreover, ketanserin is much less potent in this region than in the cerebral cortex. As a result, the pattern of drug interactions with phosphoinositide turnover varies from region to region (70). Taken together, these observations suggest that besides the 5-HT$_2$ site, another 5-HT receptor may mediate phosphoinositide turnover. This putative 5-HT receptor does not appear to have been identified by radioligand techniques.

5-HT "Autoreceptors"

Neurotransmitters are stored in synaptic vesicles located in the nerve terminal. Depolarization of the neuron by potassium or electrical stimulation causes release of the prestored neurotransmitter. The release can be inhibited by 5-HT and related agonists, presumably through a "presynaptic autoreceptor." Initial studies analyzed [^{3}H]5-HT release from rat hypothalamic synaptosomes or cortical slices (12,35,49). In both systems, nanomolar concentrations

of 5-HT inhibited [^{3}H]5-HT release. Slightly higher concentrations of methiothepin and metergoline were able to block the action of 5-HT. However, micromolar concentrations of cyproheptadine, methysergide, and mianserin had no effect on the action of exogenous 5-HT. Metergoline and methiothepin were also the most potent inhibitors of [^{3}H]5-HT release following potassium-evoked depolarization of rat raphe nuclei and hypothalamic slices (18,32).

Direct comparisons have been made between the pharmacologic interactions at "autoreceptors" and 5-HT$_1$ binding sites. Using rat hypothalamic synaptosomes, the inhibitory effect of nanomolar concentrations of 5-HT was blocked by methiothepin (IC_{50} = 3.8 nM) and quipazine (IC_{50} = 670 nM). Seven other 5-HT antagonists, including spiperone, cyproheptadine, and cinanserin, had no effect on the system at micromolar concentrations (84). In a separate study of eight agonists, a significant correlation was found between potassium-evoked release of [^{3}H]5-HT from hypothalamic synaptosomes and agonist affinities for the 5-HT$_1$ binding site (85).

Engel and co-workers have compared the potencies of 14 indole derivatives at "autoreceptors" with their affinity for 5-HT$_1$ binding sites (27). A significant correlation between the 5-HT$_1$ binding site and the 5-HT "autoreceptor" was found using either electrical stimulation to induce release of [^{3}H]5-HT from rat cortical slices or overflow of [^{3}H]norepinephrine from strips of canine saphenous vein. Furthermore, agonist interactions in each of these two systems were significantly correlated (r = 0.83). More recently, Engel and colleagues (26) have expanded their analysis in view of recent data on 5-HT$_1$ binding site subtypes. No significant correlations were observed between drug potencies at the 5-HT "autoreceptor" and their affinities for 5-HT$_{1C}$ or 5-HT$_2$ binding sites. Significant correlations were obtained with drug affinities for both 5-HT$_{1A}$ and 5-HT$_{1B}$ sites. However, selective 5-HT$_{1A}$ drugs such as 8-OH-DPAT and TVX Q 7821 had no effect on the autoreceptor and therefore were not used in the calculation of the correlation coefficient. As a result, extensive pharmacologic analyses of 5-HT "autoreceptors" support the hypothesis that the receptor which mediates release of 5-HT and certain other neurotransmitters from presumed nerve terminals is mediated by the 5-HT$_{1B}$ site.

Neurophysiologic Effects of 5-HT

The neurophysiologic effects of iontophoretically applied 5-HT and related agents have also led to the concept that multiple 5-HT receptors exist in the central nervous system (53,121,123). 5-HT produces either inhibition or excitation of cell firing when microiontophoretically applied to single neurons. When 5-HT inhibits cell firing rates, the action is invariably mimicked by both LSD and methysergide. By contrast, the classical antagonists have no effect on cell inhibition produced by 5-HT. Only a single antagonist, metergoline, has been shown to antagonize the inhibitory effect of 5-HT (126). The comparatively higher potency of LSD versus 5-HT in inhibiting raphe neurons versus nonraphe cells has been cited as evidence that at least two types of inhibitory receptor are present in neurons. However, the ratio of potencies in the two neuronal groups is only 2.74 (123).

5-HT-induced excitation, on the other hand, is invariably blocked by 5-HT antagonists such as cyproheptadine and cinanserin. In addition, both methysergide and LSD are also antagonists of 5-HT-induced cellular excitation. Neither drug has any known 5-HT mimetic action in terms of neuronal excitation. Furthermore, 5-HT-induced excitation is much less common than 5-HT-induced inhibition. Although direct comparisons with radioligand binding data have not been made, the pharmacologic characteristics of 5-HT-induced cellular inhibition and excitation may correspond with 5-HT$_1$ and 5-HT$_2$ binding sites, respectively (111).

The hippocampus may be an ideal region in which to study 5-HT receptor function at the cellular level. The structure has a high density of 5-HT$_{1A}$ sites, particularly in the dentate gyrus and CA1 region (83,100) and is particularly amenable to neurophysiological analysis. Bath application of 5-HT$_{1A}$-selective agents such as 8-OH-DPAT, TVX Q 7821, and buspirone decreases the amplitude of the field potential recorded in the pyramidal cell layer of CA1 after stimulation of Schaffer collaterals in the stratum radiatum (112). The 5-HT$_2$-selective antagonist ketanserin has no independent effect and does not affect the action of the 5-HT$_{1A}$-selective drugs. Intracellular studies have shown that 5-HT markedly hyperpolarizes CA1 pyramidal cells (15–20 mV). By contrast, buspirone causes only a modest (1–2 mV) hyperpolarization of CA1 pyramidal neurons (2). These preliminary studies suggest that analysis of the hippocampal actions of selective 5-HT receptor subtype agents may yield important information on the physiological effects of these drugs.

Behavioral Studies

A complex behavioral hyperactivity results after central 5-HT stimulation with drugs such as 5-hydroxytryptophan (5-HTP) (51,64). The syndrome includes resting tremor, forepaw treading, flattened body posture, head-weaving, hindlimb abduction, Straub tail, and head-twitching. Attempts have been made to correlate each of the behavioral components with 5-HT$_1$ and/or 5-HT$_2$ binding sites. Drug antagonism of the "head-shake" or "head-twitch component" of the syndrome has clearly been related to a blockade of the 5-HT$_2$ receptors (14,73,77,111,147). Likewise, tryptamine-induced seizure activity could be prevented by antagonists in a manner consistent with antagonism of the 5-HT$_2$ receptor (75).

However, analysis of other behavioral components of the syndrome has shown that only metergoline and methysergide block the entire set of behaviors (80). In contrast, relatively high concentrations of ketanserin and pipamperone are needed to block 5-HTP-induced forepaw treading, head-weaving, tremor, hindlimb abduction, extended posture, or Straub tail. These findings suggested that the more subtle components of the 5-HT behavioral "syndrome," as

opposed to the "head-twitch," may be related to activation of 5-HT$_1$ receptors.

The recent development and characterization of 5-HT$_{1A}$-selective agents may clarify the role of 5-HT receptor subtypes in the mediation of specific behaviors. The results of behavioral studies with 8-OH-DPAT and 5-MeODMT indicate that forepaw treading and flattened body posture may be regarded as behavioral correlates of 5-HT$_{1A}$ receptor activation (88,138–141). The effects of 8-OH-DPAT, 5-MeODMT, buspirone, and TVX Q 7821 on the 5-HT behavioral syndrome were recently examined (136). 8-OH-DPAT, 5-MeODMT, and buspirone induce hindlimb abduction, flattened body posture, and Straub tail. TVX Q 7821 induces only a slight flattening of body posture. By contrast, 8-OH-DPAT and 5-MeODMT, but not buspirone or TVX Q 7821, also induce forepaw treading, head-weaving, and tremor. However, both buspirone and TVX Q 7821 antagonize the induction of these three behaviors by 8-OH-DPAT or 5-MeODMT. These data show that 8-OH-DPAT and 5-MeODMT are "full agonists" in relation to six components of the 5-HT behavioral syndrome. Buspirone and TVX Q 7821, on the other hand, act as "antagonists" in relation to forepaw treading, head-weaving, and tremor. Therefore, these data suggest that specific components of the 5-HT behavioral syndrome are mediated by 5-HT$_{1A}$ receptors.

Other behavioral effects have been attributed to specific 5-HT receptor subtypes. Two independent behavioral studies of the discriminative cue properties of 5-HT agonists have concluded that this behavioral response may be mediated by 5-HT$_2$ receptors (43,48). In male rats, 5-HT$_{1A}$-selective agonists appear to facilitate seminal emissions and/or ejaculations (71).

Other Systems

Methysergide and bromo-LSD, but not spiperone or ketanserin, inhibit the antinociceptive effects of intrathecal 5-HT. This finding was attributed to mediation of the spinal effects of 5-HT by 5-HT$_1$ receptors (129). Tachycardia induced by 5-HT in the spinal cat has also been attributed to 5-HT$_1$ receptors (127). In studies utilizing tryptamine derivatives, the hypotensive potencies in pentobarbitone-anesthetized rats correlate with their affinity for 5-HT$_1$ sites (67,68). Furthermore, similar studies with 8-OH-DPAT and RU 24969 suggest that the 5-HT$_{1A}$ site may mediate these hypotensive effects (25). The hypothermic effects of 8-OH-DPAT and RU 24969 also have been attributed to 5-HT$_{1A}$ receptor activation (52,88,141).

Antagonism of 5-HT-induced forepaw edema in the rat by 22 antagonists correlated with drug affinity for 5-HT$_2$ sites labeled by [³H]spiperone (97). Similarly, drug antagonism of tracheal smooth muscle contraction and *in vivo* bronchoconstriction is consistent with mediation by 5-HT$_2$ sites (74), as is contraction of the guinea pig ileum (28). The dose-dependent pressor response that occurs after administration of 5-HT to pithed normotensive rats can also be blocked in a manner consistent with 5-HT$_2$ receptor activation (66). 5-HT induction of platelet shape changes and aggregation may also be mediated by 5-HT$_2$ receptors (21,22,46,117). 5-HT$_2$ receptors have also been implicated in the regulation of aldosterone production (86).

FUTURE STRATEGIES FOR FURTHER DIFFERENTIATION OF 5-HT RECEPTOR SUBTYPES

In the present report, evidence is provided from a variety of biochemical, anatomic, and physiologic studies that multiple 5-HT receptors exist in the central nervous system. At the present time, the differentiation of 5-HT receptors into 5-HT$_{1A}$, 5-HT$_{1B}$, 5-HT$_{1C}$, and 5-HT$_2$ subtypes appears to be the most relevant classification system. Indeed, a number of physiologic functional correlates of these "5-HT binding sites" have been proposed (Table 3). For many of the suggested correlates, significant correlations have been documented between drug potencies in various physiologic systems and affinities for specific binding site subtypes.

Recently, the development of selective 5-HT$_1$ agonists such as 8-OH-DPAT (58,87) and RU 24969 (34) has greatly facilitated research into the analysis of 5-HT$_1$ binding site subtypes. Further advancement in the understanding of the physiologic effects of 5-HT should have important implications. To the basic scientist, characterization of specific 5-HT receptors would greatly clarify the role of 5-HT in the central nervous system. Clinically, 5-HT has been implicated in a number of human disorders such as anxiety, depression, migraine, vasospasm, and epilepsy. Analysis of 5-HT receptor subtypes and their functional role in the central nervous system should greatly elucidate the pathophysiological basis of many of these human diseases.

REFERENCES

1. Ahn, H. S., and Makman, M. H. (1978): *Life Sci.*, 23:507–512.
2. Andrade, R., and Nicoll, R. A. (1985): *Soc. Neurosci. Abstr.*, 11:597.
3. Asarch, K. B., Ransom, R. W., and Shih, J. C. (1985): *Soc. Neurosci. Abstr.*, 11:1257.
4. Barbaccia, M. L., Brunello, N., Chuang, D. M., and Costa, E. (1983): *J. Neurochem.*, 40:1671–1679.
5. Bennett, J. L., and Aghajanian, G. K. (1974): *Life Sci.*, 15:1935–1944.
6. Bennett, J. P., Jr., and Snyder, S. H. (1975): *Brain Res.*, 94:523–544.
7. Bennett, J. P., Jr., and Snyder, S. H. (1976): *Mol. Pharmacol.*, 12:373–389.
8. Berridge, M. J. (1984): *Biochem. J.*, 220:345–360.
9. Berry-Kravis, E., and Dawson, G. (1983): *J. Neurochem.*, 40:977–985.
10. Biegon, A., Rainbow, T. C., and McEwen, B. S. (1982): *Brain Res.*, 242:197–204.
11. Brown, E., Kendall, D. A., and Nahorski, S. R. (1984): *J. Neurochem.*, 42:1379–1387.
12. Cerrito, F., and Raiteri, M. (1979): *Eur. J. Pharmacol.*, 57:427–430.
13. Closse, A. (1983): *Life Sci.*, 32:2485–2495.
14. Colpaert, F. C., and Janssen, P. A. J. (1983): *Neuropharmacology*, 22:993–1000.
15. Conn, P. J., and Sanders-Bush, E. (1984): *Neuropharmacology*, 8:993–996.
16. Conn, P. J., and Sanders-Bush, E. (1985): *J. Pharmacol. Exp. Ther.*, 234:195–203.
17. Coughlin, S. R., Moskowitz, M. A., Antoniades, H. N., and Levine, L. (1981): *Proc. Natl. Acad. Sci. USA*, 78:7134–7138.
18. Cox, B., and Ennis, C. (1982): *J. Pharm. Pharmacol.*, 34:438–441.
19. Creese, I., and Snyder, S. H. (1978): *Eur. J. Pharmacol.*, 49:201–202.
20. De Chaffoy de Courcelles, D., Leysen, J. E., De Clerck, F., Van Belle, H., and Janssen, P. A. (1985): *J. Biol. Chem.*, 260:7603–7608.
21. De Clerck, F. F., and Herman, A. G. (1983): *Fed. Proc.*, 42:228–232.
22. De Clerck, F., Xhonneux, B., Leysen, J., and Janssen, P. A. (1984): *Thrombosis Res.*, 33:305–321.
23. Deshmukh, P. P., Yamamura, H. I., Woods, L., and Nelson, D. L. (1983): *Brain Res.*, 288:338–343.
24. Dompert, W. U., Glaser, T., and Traber, J. (1985): ^{3}H-TVX Q 7821: *Naunyn Schmiedebergs Arch. Pharmacol.*, 328:467–470.
25. Doods, H. N., Kalkman, H. O., De Jonge, A., Thoolen, M., Wilffert, B., Timmermans, P., and Van Zwieten, P. A. (1985): *Eur. J. Pharmacol.*, 112:363–370.
26. Engel, G., Gothert, M., Hoyer, D., Schlicker, E., and Hillenbrand, K. (1986): *Naunyn Schmiedebergs Arch. Pharmacol.*, 357:1–7.
27. Engel, G., Gothert, M., Muller-Schweinitzer, E., Schlicker, E., Sistonen, L., and Stadler, P. A. (1983): *Naunyn Schmiedebergs Arch. Pharmacol.*, 324:116–124.
28. Engel, G., Hoyer, G., Kalkman, H. O., and Wick, M. B. (1984): *J. Recept. Res.*, 4:113–126.
29. Engel, G., Muller-Schweinitzer, E., and Palacios, J. M. (1984): *Naunyn Schmiedebergs Arch. Pharmacol.*, 325:328–336.
30. Enjalbert, A., Bourgoin, S., Hamon, M., Adrien, J., and Bockaert, J. (1978): *Mol. Pharmacol.*, 14:2–10.
31. Enjalbert, A., Hamon, M., Bourgoin, S., and Bockaert, J. (1978): *Mol. Pharmacol.*, 14:11–23.
32. Ennis, C., and Cox, B. (1982): *Neuropharmacology*, 21:41–44.
33. Erpsamer, V., and Asero, B. (1952): *Nature*, 168:800–801.
34. Euvrard, C., and Boissier, J. R. (1980): *Eur. J. Pharmacol.*, 63:65–72.
35. Farnebo, L. O., and Hamberger, B. (1974): *J. Pharmac. Pharmacol.*, 26:642–644.
36. Fillion, G. (1983): *Handb. Psychopharmacol.*, 17:139–166.
37. Fillion, G., Beaudoin, D., Fillion, M., Rousselle, J. C., Robaut, C., and Netter, Y. (1983): *J. Neural Transm. (Suppl.)*, 18:307–317.
38. Fillion, G., Beaudoin, D., Rousselle, J. C., Deniau, J. M., Fillion, M. P., Dray, F., and Jacob, J. (1979): *J. Neurochem.*, 33:567–570.
39. Fillion, G., Beaudoin, D., Rousselle, J. C., and Jacob, J. (1980): *Brain Res.*, 198:361–374.
40. Fillion, G., Rousselle, J. C., Beaudoin, D., Pradelles, P., Goiny, M., Dray, F., and Jacob, J. (1979): *Life Sci.*, 24:1813–1822.
41. Fillion, G. M. B., Rousselle, J., Fillion, M., Beaudoin, D. M., Goiny, M. R., Deniau, J., and Jacob, J. J. (1978): *Mol. Pharmacol.*, 14:50–59.
42. Fozard, J. R. (1984): *Neuropharmacology*, 23:1473–1486.
43. Friedman, R. L., Barrett, R. J., and Sanders-Bush, E. (1983): *Soc. Neurosci. Abstr.*, 9:335.
44. Fuller, R. W. (1984): *Monogr. Neural Sci.*, 10:158–181.
45. Gaddum, J. H., and Picarelli, Z. P. (1957): *Br. J. Pharmacol. Chemother.*, 12:323–328.
46. Geaney, D. P., Schachter, M., Elliot, J. M., and Grahame-Smith, D. G. (1984): *Eur. J. Pharmacol.*, 97:87–93.
47. Glaser, T., Rath, M., Traber, J., Zilles, K., and Schleicher, A. (1986): *Brain Res.*, 358:129–136.
48. Glennon, R. A., Young, R., and Rosecrans, J. A. (1983): *Eur. J. Pharmacol.*, 91:189–196.
49. Gothert, M. (1980): *Naunyn Schmiedebergs Arch. Pharmacol.*, 314:223–230.
50. Gozlan, H., El Mestikawy, S., Pichat, L., Glowinski, J., and Hamon, M. (1983): *Nature*, 305:140–142.
51. Green, A. R. (1984): *Neuropharmacology*, 23:1521–1528.

52. Gudelsky, G. A., Koenig, J. I., and Meltzer, H. Y. (1985): *Abstr. Am. Soc. Neuropsychopharmacol.,* 24:64.
53. Haigler, H. J, and Aghajanian, G. K. (1977): *Fed. Proc.,* 36:2159–2164.
54. Hall, M. D., El Mestikawy, S., Emerit, M. B., Pichat, L., Hamon, M., and Gozlan, H. (1985): *J. Neurochem.,* 44:1685–1696.
55. Hartig, P. R., Kadan, M. J., Evans, J. J., and Krohn, A. M. (1983): *Eur. J. Pharmacol.,* 89:321–322.
56. Hartig, P. R., Scheffel, U., Frost, J. J., and Wagner, H. N. (1985): *Life Sci.,* 37:657–664.
57. Heuring, R. E., Schlegel, J. R., and Peroutka, S. J. (1986): *Eur. J. Pharmacol.,* 122:279–282.
58. Hjorth, S., Carlsson, A., Lindberg, P., Sanchez, D., Wikstrom, H., Arvidsson, L. E., Hacksell, U., and Nilsson, J. L. G. (1982): *J. Neural Transm.,* 55:169–188.
59. Hoffman, B. J., Karpa, M. D., Lever, J. R., and Hartig, P. R. (1985): *Eur. J. Pharmacol.,* 110:147–148.
60. Hoyer, D., Engel, G., and Kalkman, H. O. (1985): *Eur. J. Pharmacol.,* 118:1–12.
61. Hoyer, D., Engel, G., and Kalkman, H. O. (1985): *Eur. J. Pharmacol.,* 118:13–23.
62. Hoyer, D., Pazos, A., Probst, A., and Palacios, J. M. (1986): *Brain Res.,* 376:85–96.
63. Hoyer, D., Pazos, A., Probst, A., and Palacios, J. M. (1986): *Brain Res.,* 376:97–107.
64. Jacobs, B. L. (1976): *Life Sci.,* 19:777–786.
65. Kadan, M. J., Krohn, A. M., Evans, M. J., Waltz, R. L., and Hartig, P. R. (1984): *J. Neurochem.,* 43:601–606.
66. Kalkman, H. O., Batink, H. D., Thoolen, M. J. M. C., Timmermans, P. B. M. W. M., and Van Swieten, P. A. (1983): *Biochem. Pharmacol.,* 32:2111–2113.
67. Kalkman, H. O., Boddeke, H. W. G. M., Doods, H. N., Timmermans, P. B. M. W. M., and Van Zwieten, P. A. (1983): *Eur. J. Pharmacol.,* 91:155–156.
68. Kalkman, H. O., Engel, G., and Hoyer, G. (1984): *J. Hypertension,* 2:143–145.
69. Kendall, D. A., and Nahorski, S. R. (1983): *J. Pharmacol. Exp. Ther.,* 227:429–434.
70. Kendall, D. A., and Nahorski, S. R. (1985): *J. Pharmacol. Exp. Ther.,* 233:473–479.
71. Kwong, L. L., Smith, E. R., Davidson, J. M., and Peroutka, S. J. (1986): *Behav. Neurosci.,* 100:664–668.
72. Leysen, J. E. (1981): *J. Physiol. (Paris),* 77:351–362.
73. Leysen, J. (1983): *Med. Biol.,* 61:139–143.
74. Leysen, J. E., de Courcelles, D. C., De Clerck, F., Niemegeers, J. E., and Van Nueten, J. M. (1984): *Neuropharmacology,* 23:1493–1501.
75. Leysen, J. E., Niemegeers, C. J. E., Tollenaere, J. P., and Laduron, P. M. (1978): *Nature,* 272:163–166.
76. Leysen, J. E., Niemegeers, C. J. E., Van Nueten, J. M., and Laduron, P. M. (1982): *Mol. Pharmacol.,* 21:301–314.
77. Leysen, J. E., and Tollenaere, J. P. (1982): *Annu. Rev. Med. Chem.,* 17:1–10.
78. Limbird, L. E. (1981): *Biochem. J.,* 195:1–13.
79. Lovell, R. A., and Freedman, D. X. (1976): *Mol. Pharmacol.,* 12:620–630.
80. Lucki, I., Nobler, M. S., and Frazer, A. (1984): *J. Pharmacol. Exp. Ther.,* 228:133–139.
81. Maguire, M. E., Ross, E. M., and Gilman, A. G. (1977): *Adv. Cyclic Nucleotide Res.,* 8:1–83.
82. Mallat, M., and Hamon, M. (1982): *J. Neurochem.,* 38:151–161.
83. Marcinkiewicz, M., Verge, D., Gozlan, H., Pichat, L., and Hamon, M. (1984): *Brain Res.,* 291:159–163.
84. Martin, L. L., and Sanders-Bush, E. (1982): *Neuropharmacology,* 21:445–450.
85. Martin, L. L., and Sanders-Bush, E. (1982): *Naunyn Schmiedebergs Arch. Pharmacol.,* 321:165–170.
86. Matsuoka, H., Ishii, M., Goto, A., and Sugimoto, T. (1985): *Am. J. Physiol.,* 249:E234–E238.
87. Middlemiss, D. N., and Fozard, J. R. (1983): *Eur. J. Pharmacol.,* 90:151–153.
88. Middlemiss, D. N., Neill, J., and Tricklebank, M. D. (1985): *Br. J. Pharmacol.,* 85:251P.
89. Montigny, C. D. de, Blier, P., and Chaput, Y. (1984): *Neuropharmacology,* 23:1511–1520.
90. Moon, S. L., and Taylor, D. P. (1985): *Soc. Neurosci. Abstr.,* 11:114.
91. Nakaki, T., Roth, B. L., Chuang, D. M., and Costa, E. (1985): *J. Pharmacol. Exp. Ther.,* 234:442–448.
92. Nelson, D. L., Herbet, A., Adrien, J., Bockaert, J., and Hamon, M. (1980): *Biochem. Pharmacol.,* 29:2455–2463.
93. Nelson, D. L., Herbet, A., Bourgoin, S., Glowinski, J., and Hamon, M. (1978): *Mol. Pharmacol.,* 14:983–995.
94. Nelson, D. L., Herbet, A., Enjalbert, A., Bockaert, J., and Hamon, M. (1980): *Biochem. Pharmacol.,* 29:2445–2453.
95. Nishizuka, Y. (1984): *Science,* 225:1365–1369.
96. Norman, A. B., Battaglia, G., Morrow, A. L., and Creese, I. (1985): *Eur. J. Pharmacol.,* 106:461–462.
97. Ortmann, R., Bischoff, S., Radeke, E., Buech, O., and Delini-Stula, A. (1982): *Naunyn Schmiedebergs Arch. Pharmacol.,* 321:265–270.
98. Palacios, J. M., Niehoff, D. L., and Kuhar, M. J. (1981): *Brain Res.,* 213:277–289.
99. Palacios, J. M., Probst, A., and Cortes, R. (1983): *Brain Res.,* 274:150–155.
100. Pazos, A., Cortes, R., and Palacios, J. M. (1985): *Brain Res.,* 346:205–230.
101. Pazos, A., Engel, G., and Palacios, J. M. (1985): *Brain Res.,* 343:403–408.
102. Pazos, A., Hoyer, D., and Palacios, J. M. (1984): *Eur. J. Pharmacol.,* 106:531–538.
103. Pazos, A., Hoyer, D., and Palacios, J. M. (1984): *Eur. J. Pharmacol.,* 106:539–546.
104. Pazos, A., and Palacios, J. M. (1985): *Brain Res.,* 346:231–249.
105. Pedigo, N. W., Yamamura, H. I., and Nelson, D. L. (1981): *J. Neurochem.,* 36:220–226.
106. Peroutka, S. J. (1984): *Neuropharmacology,* 23:1487–1492.
107. Peroutka, S. J. (1984): *Biochem. Pharmacol.,* 33:2349–2353.
108. Peroutka, S. J. (1985): *Brain Res.,* 344:167–171.
109. Peroutka, S. J. (1986): *J. Neurochem.,* 47:529–540.
110. Peroutka, S. J., Lebovitz, R. M., and Snyder, S. H. (1979): *Mol. Pharmacol.,* 16:700–708.
111. Peroutka, S. J., Lebovitz, R. M., and Snyder, S. H. (1981): *Science,* 212:827–829.
112. Peroutka, S. J., Mauk, M. D., and Kocsis, J. D. (1987): *Neuropharmacol. (in press).*
113. Peroutka, S. J., and Snyder, S. H. (1979): *Mol. Pharmacol.,* 16:687–699.
114. Peroutka, S. J., and Snyder, S. H. (1980): *Science,* 210:88–90.
115. Peroutka, S. J., and Snyder, S. H. (1980): *J. Pharmacol. Exp. Ther.,* 215:582–587.
116. Peroutka, S. J., and Snyder, S. H. (1983): *Fed. Proc.,* 42:213–217.
117. Pletscher, A., and Affolter, H. (1983): *J. Neural Transm.,* 57:233–242.
118. Quik, M., Iversen, L. L., Lardner, A., and Mackay, A. V. P. (1978): *Nature,* 274:513–514.
119. Rapport, M. M., Green, A. A., and Page, I. H. (1948): *J. Biol. Chem.,* 176:1243–1251.
120. Richardson, B. P., Engel, G., Donatsch, P., and Stadler, P. A. (1985): *Nature,* 336:126–131.
121. Roberts, M. H. T., and Straughan, D. W. (1967): *J. Physiol. (Lond.),* 193:269–294.
122. Rodbell, M. (1980): *Nature,* 284:17–21.
123. Rogawski, M. A., and Aghajanian, G. K. (1981): *J. Neurosci.,* 1:1148–1154.
124. Roth, B. L., Nakaki, T., Chuang, D. M., and Costa, E. (1984): *Neuropharmacology,* 23:1223–1225.
125. Sanders-Bush, E., and Conn, P. J. (1985): *Abstr. Am. Col. Neuropsychopharmacol.,* 24:62.
126. Sastry, B. S. R., and Phillis, J. W. (1977): *Can. J. Physiol. Pharmacol.,* 55:130–133.
127. Saxena, P. R., Mylecharane, E. J., and Heiligers, J. (1985): *Naunyn Schmiedebergs Arch. Pharmacol.,* 330:121–129.
128. Schlegel, J. R., and Peroutka, S. J. (1986): *Biochem. Pharmacol.,* 35:1943–1949.

129. Schmauss, C., Hammond, D. L., Ochi, J. W., and Yaksh, T. L. (1983): *Eur. J. Pharmacol.*, 90:349–357.
130. Schnellmann, R. G., Waters, S. J., and Nelson, D. L. (1984): *J. Neurochem.*, 42:65–70.
131. Schotte, A., Maloteaux, J. M., and Laduron, P. M. (1983): *Brain Res.*, 276:231–235.
132. Shannon, M., Battaglia, G., Glennon, R. A., and Titeler, M. (1984): *Eur. J. Pharmacol.*, 102:23–29.
133. Shenker, A., Maayani, S., Weinstein, H., and Green, J. P. (1985): *Eur. J. Pharmacol.*, 109:427–429.
134. Sills, M. A., Wolfe, B. B., and Frazer, A. (1984): *J. Pharmacol. Exp. Ther.*, 231:480–487.
135. Slater, P., and Patel, S. (1983): *Eur. J. Pharmacol.*, 92:297–298.
136. Smith, L. M., and Peroutka, S. J. (1986): *Pharmacol. Biochem. Behav.*, 24:1513–1519.
137. Titeler, M., Battaglia, G., and Shannon, M. (1984): *Soc. Neurosci. Abstr.*, 9:334.
138. Tricklebank, M. D. (1985): *Trends Pharmacol. Sci.*, 6:403–407.
139. Tricklebank, M. D., Forler, C., and Fozard, J. R. (1984): *Eur. J. Pharmacol.*, 106:271–282.
140. Tricklebank, M. D., Forler, C., Middlemiss, D. N., and Fozard, J. R. (1985): *Eur. J. Pharmacol.*, 117:15–24.
141. Tricklebank, M. D., Middlemiss, D. N., and Neill, J. (1986): *Neuropharmacology*, 25:877–886.
142. Twarog, B. M., and Page, I. H. (1953): *Am. J. Psychiatry*, 175:157–161.
143. Van Nueten, J. M., Janssens, W. J., and Vanhoutte, P. M. (1985): *Pharmacol. Res. Commun.*, 17:585–608.
144. Von Hungen, K., Roberts, S., and Hill, D. F. (1974): *J. Neurochem.*, 22:811–819.
145. Von Hungen, K., Roberts, S., and Hill, D. F. (1975): *Brain Res.*, 84:257–267.
146. Yagaloff, K. A., and Hartig, P. R. (1985): *J. Neurosci.*, 5:3178–3183.
147. Yap, C. Y., and Taylor, D. A. (1983): *Neuropharmacology*, 22:801–804.
148. Young, W. S., III, and Kuhar, M. J. (1980): *Eur. J. Pharmacol.*, 62:237–239.

Psychopharmacology:
The Third Generation of Progress,
edited by Herbert Y. Meltzer.
Raven Press, New York © 1987.

CHAPTER 32

Receptor Mapping in Psychopharmacology

Michael J. Kuhar and Nick E. Goeders

Receptor mapping is the quantitative description of the distribution of specific receptors for drugs and neurotransmitters in brain and in other tissues using primarily histochemical or imaging techniques. The basic methodologies and the justification for using this approach have been discussed previously (9–14). The purpose of this chapter is to briefly describe receptor mapping, to mention some recent advances in the field, and to point out potential applications in psychopharmacology. Receptor mapping is an important discipline in psychopharmacology, since most psychopharmacological agents act either directly or indirectly through receptors.

Receptor mapping developed in parallel to the development of biochemical techniques for receptor binding. Since radiolabeled ligands were used in biochemical studies of receptor binding, autoradiography has been the main approach used in receptor mapping (see Fig. 1). Since most ligands bind reversibly, techniques for the prevention or the minimization of diffusion are used (30,32). Like most histochemical techniques, receptor mapping is effective at the light microscopic level and has the very significant advantages of high sensitivity and anatomical resolution. The technique has been well described (13).

RECENT ADVANCES

Important recent advances in receptor mapping include the development of quantitative methods for analyzing autoradiograms and the application of positron emission tomography (PET). Another notable development is the immunohistochemical localization of receptors. However, there are only a few studies of this type, partly because of the difficulty in obtaining antibodies to receptors, which must be at least partially purified for antibody production.

Quantitative Autoradiography

Autoradiography is a very precise technique which can be quantified. Grain counting, densitometry, and photometry are well established ways of quantification (29). Since counting grains, for example, is extremely laborious, the application of computerized image analysis to this problem has been well received (1,7,16,24). For example, one image analysis system that has been recently developed is relatively cheap, fast, user friendly, and versatile (24). It is a TV camera-based system with a modified IBM personnel computer. The system can color code images to enhance contrast, modify images, subtract one image from another, average densities in any region, include and process autoradiographic standards to get precise quantitative data, and tabulate, store, and calculate data. The system can count autoradiographic grains at high magnification or it can analyze optical densities on a less magnified image. Equipment such as this has had a significant impact on the field. Tasks can be accomplished in only a small fraction of the time that was required just a couple of years ago. There are some special difficulties when using tritiated ligands, although methods for dealing with these problems have been described (for review see 15).

PET Scanning of Receptors

Although light microscopic autoradiographic receptor mapping techniques have been very useful, they are, obviously, invasive procedures. The generation of a receptor map with human tissue requires the surgical removal, or removal at autopsy, of the tissues of interest. However, with the use of PET, receptors can be visualized in the living human brain.

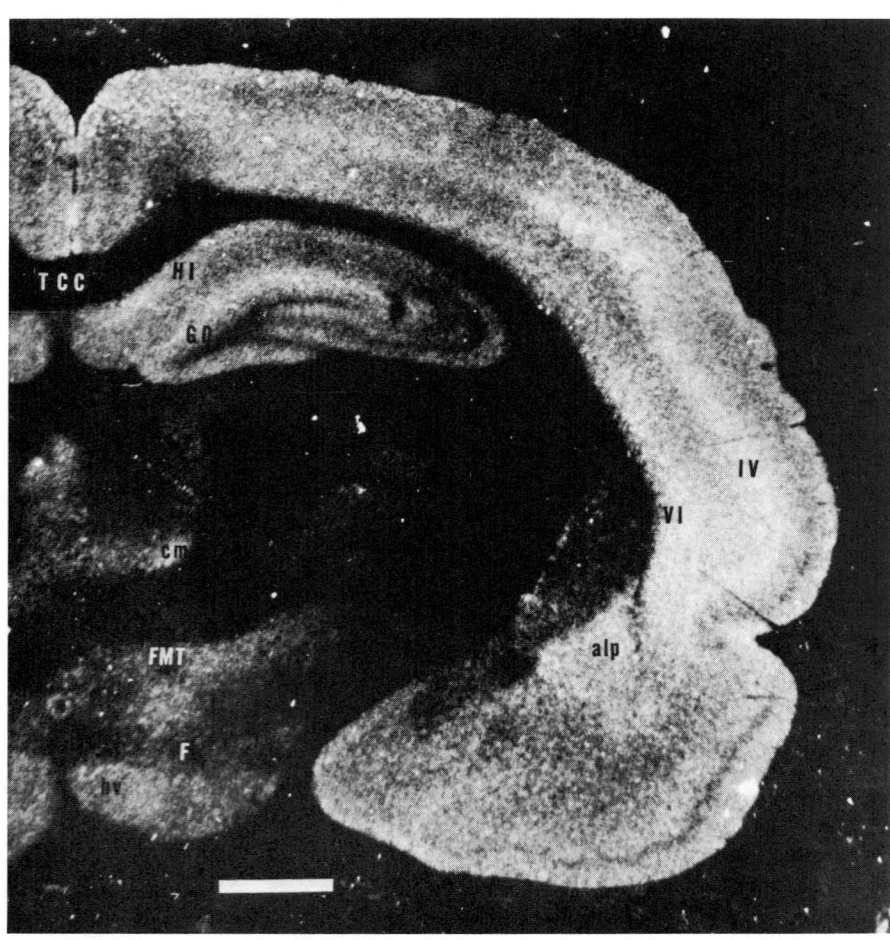

FIG. 1. Example of neurotransmitter receptor autoradiogram represented as a darkfield photomicrograph of benzodiazepine receptors in the rat brain labeled with [^{3}H]flunitrazepam. High densities of receptors are located in laminae IV and VI of the cortex, the nucleus amygdaloideus lateralis, pars posterior (alp), and parts of the hippocampal formation (GD and HI). Bar = 1,000 μm. (From ref. 38.)

PET is a procedure whereby the distribution of positron-emitting isotopes can be calculated after the detection of radiation caused by positron emissions (27). Thus, the distribution and density of receptors in the living human brain can be determined following the *in vivo* labeling of specific receptors with drugs containing positron-emitting isotopes (Fig. 2). Several receptors have been identified in humans by this approach (4,5,34,36).

We have known for several years from autopsy studies that receptors in human brain are changed or altered in neuropsychiatric disease (20). PET scanning makes it feasible to assess the degree of receptor change in these diseases in clinical populations more completely. For example, more than one measurement can be made, and measurements can be made before, during, and after treatment, and at different stages of the disease process. The ability to obtain these kinds of data may have a profound impact on our understanding of receptors in neuropsychiatric disease.

A potential drawback in PET studies is that PET scanning is limited to resolution in the millimeter range. If greater resolution is needed, then it is possible to apply light microscopic autoradiographic receptor mapping techniques to the problem, since the autoradiographic approach has resolution in the micron range. Thus, the highly versatile clinical PET studies can be complemented by high-resolu-

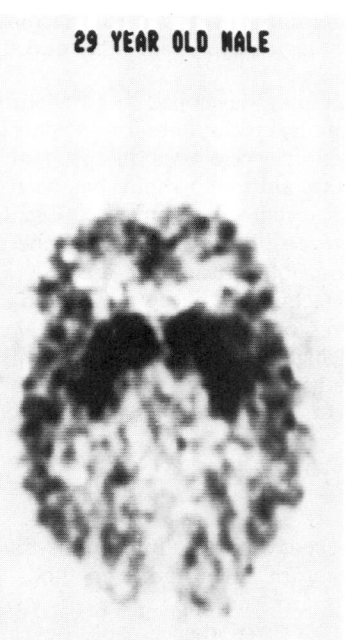

FIG. 2. Example of a PET scan of D$_2$ dopamine and S$_2$ serotonin receptors in the human brain labeled with [^{11}C]3-*N*-methylspiperone. (From ref. 36.)

tion autoradiographic studies provided suitable tissues are available.

RECEPTOR MAPPING IN PSYCHOPHARMACOLOGY

Receptor mapping has several important uses. From a pharmacological point of view, receptor mapping identifies the potential sites of drug action. In other words, this procedure helps identify the specific neuronal circuits or brain regions that are affected by certain drugs. Since drugs can have multiple physiological effects, it is not surprising that drug receptors are found in many areas of the brain. Receptor mapping studies have therefore helped to explain the multiple effects of drugs from a neuroanatomical point of view (for reviews see 9, 14).

Since receptors are highly concentrated to neurons rather than to other cell types in the brain, changes in receptors are thought to reflect changes in neuronal function. Thus, receptor mapping has been used as a neuropathological tool (3,22,33,35). Autoradiographic techniques can be used with tissue obtained at autopsy, or PET scanning can be used in living clinical populations. Since receptors are changed in neuropsychiatric disorders, it is possible that at least some of these disorders result from receptor changes. Thus, the ability to measure receptors in these situations may develop important new information on the etiology of some diseases.

The receptors for many psychotropic drugs have been studied (Table 1). Thus, basic information on the distribution and possibly the effects of many psychotropic drugs has been developed (for reviews see 9, 14). However, much of this information is from animals, and a great deal of work remains to be done both in humans and in a more detailed fashion. While receptor mapping is very powerful, the existing methods have several limitations (13,14). For example, although autoradiographic techniques permit

studies with the light microscope, they still have limits on resolution. It is not possible to easily identify the specific cell types that contain receptors by existing autoradiographic techniques. Also, it is not feasible to distinguish between functional and nonfunctional receptors or between surface receptors and interior receptors. Finally, receptor mapping techniques that are currently available are dependent mainly on receptor binding. Therefore, a given receptor can only be visualized when one has a high-affinity ligand for that receptor. It may not be possible to identify receptors for which only low-affinity ligands are available. Since light microscopic studies are limited in resolution, it is obvious that ultrastructural techniques are also needed. Because of existing ligands, autoradiographic studies are the most feasible at this point in time. However, electron microscopic autoradiography has substantial limitations in resolution and other more specific techniques are required. Perhaps immunohistochemical techniques at the electron microscopic level will provide the needed information. In any case, there is a great need for relatively easy and accurate electron microscopic techniques for localizing receptors.

PET scanning studies of receptors are relatively recent so there has not yet been enough time to accumulate significant quantities of data on various disease states. However, it has been found that receptors for neuroleptic drugs decline with increasing age in normal volunteers (36). The significance of this effect is unknown but could be quite important since the magnitude of the decline is relatively large. Also, there are indications of changes in receptors in certain disease states (3,22,35). But even aside from the issue of detecting changes in diseases, the notion that we can develop information on the distribution of drug receptors in humans is quite important, because, as mentioned above, regional studies are a key to understanding how drugs exert their effects.

SUMMARY

In the past decade, receptor mapping techniques have been developed and are now as common and popular as many other histochemical procedures. The most recent advances in the field have facilitated rapid and accurate quantitation. Another recent advance has been the very elegant application of PET scanning to receptor mapping in living human subjects. Receptor mapping is important in psychopharmacology for many reasons, primarily since receptor maps help to develop an understanding of how drugs exert their effects. Also, since the identification of receptor changes will increase our understanding of neuropsychiatric disorders, the ability to measure these receptors with a high degree of anatomical resolution in clinical populations indicates that we will be able to develop significant new knowledge in this area of study.

TABLE 1. *Examples of psychotropic drug receptors visualized autoradiographically*

Drug	Refs.
Nicotinic cholinergic	2
	18
Neuroleptic	25
	1
	23
	6
	8
LSD	19
	26
	31
Benzodiazepine	37,38
	39
	17
	28

See text for discussion.

REFERENCES

1. Altar, C. A., Walter, R. J., Neve, K. A., and Marshall, J. F. (1984): *J. Neurosci. Methods,* 10:173–188.
2. Clarke, P. B. S., Schwartz, R. D., Paul, S. M., Pert, C. B., and Pert, A. (1984): *Soc. Neurosci. Abstr.,* 10:733.

3. De Souza, E. B., Whitehouse, P. J., Kuhar, M. J., Price, D. L., and Vale, W. W. (1986): *Nature,* 319:593–595.
4. Eckelman, W. C., Reba, R. C., Rzeszotarski, W. J., Gibson, R. E., Hill, T., et al. (1984): *Science,* 223:291–293.
5. Frost, J. J., Wagner, H. N., Dannals, R. F., Ravert, H. T., Links, J. M., et al. (1985): *J. Comput. Assist. Tomogr.,* 9:231–236.
6. Gehlert, D. R., and Wamsley, J. K. (1984): *Eur. J. Pharmacol.,* 98:311–312.
7. Goochee, C., Rasband, W., and Sokoloff, L. (1980): *Ann. Neurol.,* 7:359–370.
8. Jastrow, T. W., Richfield, E., and Gnegy, M. E. (1984): *Neurosci. Lett.,* 51:47–53.
9. Kuhar, M. J. (1981): *Trends Neurosci.,* 4:6064.
10. Kuhar, M. J. (1982): In: *Receptor-Binding Radiotracers, Vol. 1,* edited by W. C. Eckelman, pp. 37–50. CRC Press, Boca Raton, FL.
11. Kuhar, M. J. (1982): In: *Handbook of Psychopharmacology, Vol. 15,* edited by S. D. Iversen, L. L. Iversen, and S. H. Snyder, pp. 299–320. Plenum Press, New York.
12. Kuhar, M. J. (1983): In: *Handbook of Chemical Neuroanatomy, Vol. 1: Methods in Chemical Neuroanatomy,* edited by A. Bjorklund and T. Hokfelt, pp. 398–415. Elsevier, Amsterdam.
13. Kuhar, M. J. (1985): In: *Neurotransmitter Receptor Binding,* 2nd ed., edited by H. I. Yamamura, S. J. Enna, and M. J. Kuhar, pp. 153–176. Raven Press, New York.
14. Kuhar, M. J., De Souza, E. B., and Unnerstall, J. R. (1986): *Annu. Rev. Neurosci.,* 9:27–59.
15. Kuhar, M. J., and Unnerstall, J. R. (1985): *Trends Neurosci.,* 8: 49–53.
16. Kuhar, M. J., Whitehouse, P. J., Unnerstall, J. R., and Loats, H. (1984): *Soc. Neurosci. Abstr.,* 10:558.
17. Lo, M. M. S., Niehoff, D. L., Kuhar, M. J., and Snyder, S. H. (1983): *Neurosci. Lett.,* 39:37–44.
18. London, E. D., Waller, S. B., and Wamsley, J. K. (1985): *Neurosci. Lett.,* 53:179–184.
19. Meibach, R. C., Maayani, S., and Green, J. P. (1980): *Eur. J. Pharmacol.,* 67:371–382.
20. Olsen, R. W., Reisine, T., and Yamamura, H. I. (1980): *Life Sci.,* 27:801–808.
21. Orzi, F., Kenney, C., Jehlo, J., and Sokoloff, L. (1983): *J. Cereb. Blood Flow Metab.,* 3:577–578.
22. Palacios, J. M. (1982): *Brain Res.,* 243:173–175.
23. Palacios, J. M. (1984): In: *Catecholamines: Neuropharmacology and Central Nervous System—Theoretical Aspects,* edited by E. Usdin, pp. 73–84. Alan R. Liss, New York.
24. Palacios, J. M., Niehoff, D. L., and Kuhar, M. J. (1981): *Neurosci. Lett.,* 25:101–105.
25. Palacios, J. M., Niehoff, D. L., and Kuhar, M. J. (1981): *Brain Res.,* 213:277–289.
26. Palacios, J. M., Probst, S., and Cortes, R. (1983): *Brain Res.,* 274: 150–155.
27. Raichle, M. E. (1979): *Brain Res. Rev.,* 1:47–68.
28. Richards, J. G., and Mohler, H. (1984): *Neuropharmacology,* 23: 233–242.
29. Rogers, A. W. (1979): *Techniques of Autoradiography.* Elsevier Scientific Publishing Co., Amsterdam.
30. Roth, L. J., and Stumpf, W. E. (1969): In: *Autoradiography of Diffusible Substances.* Academic Press, New York.
31. Seybold, V. S., and Elde, R. P. (1984): *J. Neurosci.,* 4:2533–2542.
32. Stumpf, W. E., and Roth, L. G. (1966): *J. Histochem. Cytochem.,* 14:274–287.
33. Uhl, G. R., and Kuhar, M. J. (1984): *Nature,* 309:350–352.
34. Wagner, H. N., Burns, H. D., Dannals, R. F., Wong, D. F., Langstrom, B., et al. (1983): *Science,* 221:1264–1266.
35. Whitehouse, P. J., Wamsley, J. K., Zarbin, M. A., Price, D. L., Tourtellote, W. W., et al. (1983): *Ann. Neurol.,* 14:8–16.
36. Wong, D. F., Wagner, H. N., Dannals, R. F., Links, J. M., Frost, J. J., et al. (1984): Effects of age on dopamine and serotonin receptors measured by positron tomography in the living human brain. *Science,* 226:1393–1396.
37. Young, W. S., III, and Kuhar, M. J. (1979): *Nature,* 280:393–395.
38. Young, W. S., III, and Kuhar, M. J. (1980): *J. Pharmacol. Exp. Ther.,* 212:337–346.
39. Young, W. S., III, Niehoff, D. L., Kuhar, M. J., Beer, B., and Lippa, A. S. (1981): *J. Pharmacol. Exp. Ther.,* 216:425–430.

Psychopharmacology:
The Third Generation of Progress,
edited by Herbert Y. Meltzer.
Raven Press, New York © 1987.

CHAPTER 33

Inositide-Linked Second Messengers in the Central Nervous System

R. Michael Snider, Stephen K. Fisher, and Bernard W. Agranoff

Although the information processing role of the nervous system has been thoroughly studied from the behavioral and electrophysiological standpoint, the underlying biochemistry that subserves these functions is only now becoming understood. The observed high metabolic rate and alterations in regional metabolism confirm and extend our knowledge regarding the coupling of brain metabolism and function. Although much of brain energetics can be accounted for by ion fluxes related to conduction of the nerve impulse, it becomes increasingly evident that utilization of energy also reflects synaptic events related to neurotransmitter production and the intervening steps that ultimately lead to effector action, including the generation of second messengers. The importance of the latter agents in the nervous system became apparent with the elucidation of cyclic adenosine 3',5'-monophosphate (cyclic AMP)-mediated actions. High levels of adenylate cyclase and phosphodiesterase found in the brain indicated rapid cyclic AMP turnover. More recently, it has been demonstrated that a wide variety of neurotransmitters produce their effects via the receptor-mediated phosphodiesteratic breakdown of phosphatidylinositol bisphosphate (PIP$_2$) into two products, each of which has second messenger properties, as is detailed in this chapter.

Although the significance of inositol lipid (phosphoinositide)-related neurotransmitter effects is rapidly evolving, a number of conclusions can already be drawn. First, as was foreseen 10 years ago (43), receptor-ligand interactions that stimulate phosphoinositide lipid turnover share the property that the concentration of intracellular calcium ion $[Ca^{2+}]_i$ is elevated as an obligatory step in receptor-effector coupling.

Secondly, there is virtually no overlap between the cyclic AMP-mediated neurotransmitter actions and those mediated by phosphoinositide phosphodiesterase. These two second messenger classes may nevertheless share some commonality, for example in the use of G-type proteins to couple the receptor and second messenger enzymes.

Third, the presently known neurotransmitters appear to act by one of three possible consequences of receptor activation: direct ionic mechanisms (e.g., nicotinic cholinergic and GABAergic agents), cyclic AMP-mediated reactions, or phosphoinositide-phosphodiesterase linked actions. Cyclic GMP formation occurs via receptor activation in the nervous system apparently as a consequence of phosphoinositide phosphodiesterase activation, although alternate routes of cyclic GMP generation remain possible. In any event, it appears unlikely that yet another major second messenger system will be found, inasmuch as presently known neurotransmitter actions appear to be mediated by one or another of these three mechanisms.

INOSITIDE-RELATED RECEPTOR ACTIVATION

Inositide Cycle

The concept that phospholipids play a dynamic role in receptor-mediated cell responses was first proposed by the

Hokins on the basis of labeling studies in both pancreas and brain (32). Results of these experiments indicated that radioactive orthophosphate ($^{32}P_i$) was rapidly incorporated into two quantitatively minor phospholipids, phosphatidate (PA) and phosphatidylinositol (PI), whereas little or no label was associated with the quantitatively major phospholipids such as phosphatidylcholine or phosphatidylethanolamine. Furthermore, addition of acetylcholine (ACh) selectively enhanced [^{32}P]PA and [^{32}P]PI labeling, whereas atropine blocked the stimulation, suggesting a biological role for the effect. The increase in ^{32}P labeling of PA and PI observed in the presence of ACh is not accompanied by a corresponding increase in the incorporation of either [^3H]glycerol or [^3H]glucose. This result indicates that the

^{32}P-labeling effect is not attributable to a net increase in lipid synthesis, but rather is due to the stimulated turnover and reutilization of preexisting lipid. It is now known that ^{32}P label enters a cycle at the level of diacylglycerol (DAG) kinase, with the subsequent formation of PA. PI is formed from PA by way of a liponucleotide intermediate, cytidine diphosphodiacylglycerol (CDP-DAG). The latter is also labeled, but is ordinarily not detected due to its low steady-state concentration. PI, once formed, may then be either phosphodiesteratically cleaved to DAG and inositol monophosphate (IP), thus completing a PA-PI cycle, or, alternatively, may undergo phosphorylation at the 4' of the inositol ring to yield phosphatidylinositol 4-phosphate (PIP). At this point, PIP can be cleaved phosphodiesteratically,

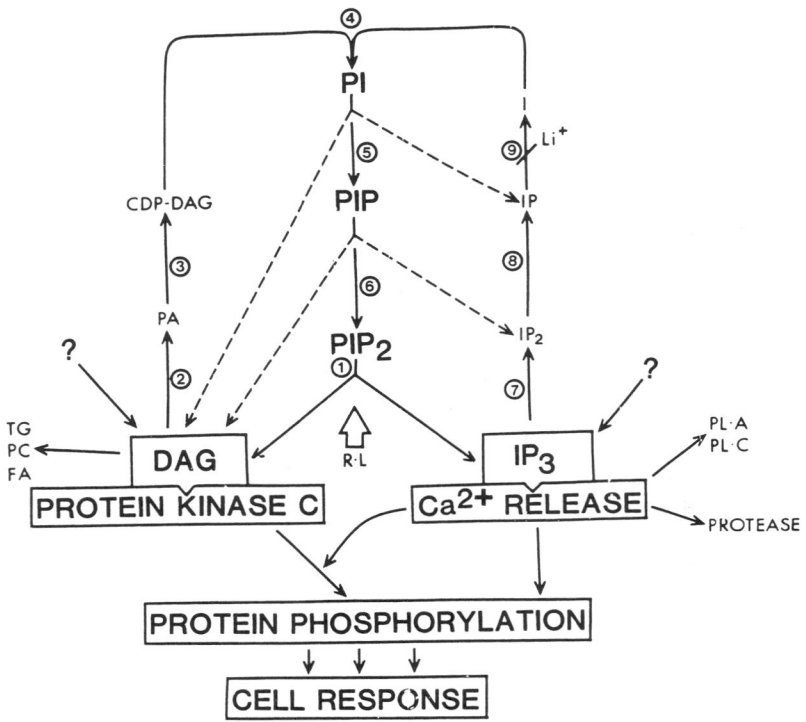

FIG. 1. Representation of the phosphoinositide labeling turnover cycle and second messenger production. Receptor-ligand (R · L) interaction results in activation of a phosphodiesterase that cleaves PIP$_2$ (step 1). Diacylglycerol release is part of the cycle depicted on the left. It is then phosphorylated by diglyceride kinase (step 2) to PA, which then reacts with CTP to form CDP-DAG (step 3). This liponucleotide then reacts with inositol under the action of PI synthase to form PI (step 4). PI is further phosphorylated by PI kinase (step 5) to PIP, and thence by PIP kinase (step 6) to PIP$_2$, completing the phosphoinositide turnover cycle. DAG activates protein kinase C (PK-C), in a calcium- and phospholipid-dependent reaction. The conversion of DAG to PA may be considered as part of the "off" reaction which removes DAG from its second messenger system. Other possible fates of DAG include loss of fatty acids (FA) by the action of a lipase, conversion to phospholipids such as PC by reaction with CDP-choline, or acylation by acyl CoA to form triglyceride (TG). While small amounts of TG are present in brain, there appears to be a rapidly turning over pool. As described in the text, the possibility must be considered that DAG can also arise from sources (?) other than phosphoinositide turnover. Breakdown of PIP$_2$

leads also to the formation of 1,4,5-IP$_3$, constituting an additional second messenger system. IP$_3$ reacts with a receptor in the endoplasmic reticulum to release Ca^{2+}. Thus, the IP$_3$ and DAG second messenger systems interreact, since PK-C is activated by Ca^{2+}. Ca^{2+} may also catalyze phosphorylation reactions independent of PK-C, as indicated by the *vertical arrow*. Other possible actions of Ca^{2+} that can participate in the cell response include the activation of phospholipase A$_2$, of other phospholipase C-type reactions than the phosphoinositide phosphodiesterase, and activation of proteases. The possibility that IP$_3$ is released by an as yet unspecified mechanism (?) must also be considered. This might be the case, for example, in skeletal muscle, in which it has been shown that IP$_3$ simulates Ca^{2+} release, even though there is no known phosphoinositide-linked receptor activation. IP$_3$ is inactivated by a 5'-phosphohydrolase (step 7) to IP$_2$, then to IP, which is subsequently converted to inositol by an inositol monophosphate phosphatase (step 9), completing the inositol phosphate cycle depicted on the right. Reaction 9 is blocked by Li$^+$. The phosphoinositide phosphodiesterase appears to act on both PI and PIP as well as on PIP$_2$ (*dotted arrows*).

or alternatively, again be phosphorylated, at the 5' position, to yield phosphatidylinositol 4,5-bisphosphate (PIP$_2$). PIP and PIP$_2$ are collectively termed the polyphosphoinositides. The products of their cleavage (in addition to DAG) are inositol bis- and trisphosphates (IP$_2$ and IP$_3$), respectively.

The increased labeling of PA and PI stems from increased availability of DAG. Although the source of DAG that emanates from receptor-ligand interaction was long considered to be PI (33), current evidence strongly suggests that the initial event is PIP$_2$ breakdown, which occurs via a phospholipase C type cleavage to yield DAG and IP$_3$ (1,9). The latter then undergoes rapid dephosphorylation to IP$_2$, then to IP, and finally to free inositol, which is then available for the resynthesis of PI (Fig. 1). In many instances, detection of the release of water-soluble inositol phosphates is complicated by the action of intracellular phosphatases. The cycle in which PIP$_2$ is broken down and resynthesized is metabolically expensive in that for each mole of PIP$_2$ recycled, 3 mol of ATP and 1 mol of CTP are consumed. The operation of this futile cycle, like that of cyclic AMP turnover, supports the notion that a significant fraction of the high rate of metabolism characteristic of brain may be for the support of amplification and regulation of chemical signals.

Neural Preparations That Support Enhanced Phosphoinositide Turnover

Enhanced phosphoinositide turnover is seen in whole brain (*in vivo*), brain slices, subcellular fractions (nerve ending preparations), and also in cultured cells of neural origin such as human astrocytoma N1321 cells, murine neuroblastoma N1E-115, and rat pituitary (GH$_3$) cells (15). Dissociated cells from "CNS-related" tissues, such as pineal and anterior pituitary, also support enhanced phosphoino-

sitide turnover. In the peripheral nervous system, stimulated turnover has been observed in adrenal medulla and sympathetic ganglia (Table 1).

Measurement of Enhanced Phosphoinositide Turnover

Three methods of assessing receptor-mediated increases in phosphoinositide turnover following ligand addition have been used: (a) an increased incorporation of added ^{32}P$_i$ into PA and PI, (b) an increased breakdown of ^{32}P- or ^{3}H-prelabeled PIP and/or PIP$_2$, and (c) an increased release of [^{3}H]inositol phosphates from prelabeled lipids (Table 1). Method a is the traditional technique and has yielded much useful information. Provided that care is taken to assess concurrently the possible incorporation of other lipid precursors to exclude the possibility of *de novo* lipid labeling, the method provides a convenient measure of phosphoinositide turnover. However, it is the secondary, restorative phase of the PA-PI cycle that is being measured by ^{32}P$_i$ incorporation, several steps away from the phosphodiesteratic site of receptor-ligand interaction. The use of a prelabeling paradigm (method b) has facilitated identification of polyphosphoinositide breakdown as the primary site of receptor-ligand interaction. However, the effects are often modest and are difficult to quantitate due to competing processes of lipid breakdown and resynthesis. Furthermore, the results do not differentiate between an inhibition of lipid synthesis and an enhanced lipid breakdown. The currently favored method for measurement of phosphoinositide turnover (method c above) is the enhanced release of inositol phosphates from tissue lipids prelabeled with [^{3}H]inositol, following stimulated phosphodiesteratic cleavage. Inositol phosphates are normally rapidly hydrolyzed by phosphatases, rendering their detection difficult or impossible unless Li$^+$ is present, in which case IP accumulates.

TABLE 1. *Neuroeffector-linked inositide turnover*

Preparation	^{32}P Increased PA/PI	^{32}P Decreased PIP/PIP$_2$	^{3}H Increased IP
Whole brain (*in vivo*)	+		
Brain slices or minces	+		+
Subcellular fractions			
Nerve ending preparations	+	+	
Synaptic plasma membranes		+	
Dissociated cells or slices			
Adrenal medulla	+	+	+
Pineal	+		+
Pituitary	+		
Superior cervical ganglion	+		+
Cell lines			
Neuroblastoma	+		+
Astrocytoma			+
GH$_3$ pituitary cells		+	+
PC-12 cells	+		+

For details, see ref. 15 and references therein.

Li$^+$ specifically blocks inositol 1-phosphatase (ref. 28; see Second Messenger Products: IP$_3$ below). The stimulated release of IP$_3$ is difficult to directly demonstrate in the CNS, presumably due to high phosphatase activity in this tissue. However, the results from the CNS have been interpreted to suggest that as in other tissues, carbon flow through PIP$_2$ occurs prior to phosphodiesteratic cleavage, and that the IP that accumulates in brain is derived from IP$_3$.

Pharmacological Characteristics of Receptor-Stimulated PPI Turnover

Although fifteen pharmacologically distinct nervous system receptors have been shown to be coupled to phosphoinositide turnover (Table 2), most detailed information has been obtained for the muscarinic cholinergic, α_1-adrenergic, and 5-HT$_2$ receptors. Muscarinic cholinergic receptors (mAChRs) are particularly enriched in the CNS, and with the notable exception of the cerebellum, mAChR-mediated phosphoinositide turnover can be demonstrated in all regions. The response is potently inhibited by antagonists such as atropine or scopolamine, with K_i values similar to the dissociation constants of the mAChR-antagonist complex (15). In contrast, nicotinic antagonists are largely without effect. In addition, the relatively "pure" muscarinic agonist muscarine is able to elicit a phosphoinositide response, whereas nicotine and 1,1-dimethyl-4-phenylpiperazinium iodide (two nicotinic agonists) are inactive (15). The relatively high concentrations of muscarinic agonists required to elicit the phosphoinositide response were initially considered to argue against a role for inositol lipid turnover in cell function. However, with the advent of radiolabeled antagonists such as [^{3}H]quinuclidinyl benzilate and [^{3}H]N-methylscopolamine, it became evident that these high agonist concentrations are precisely those required to occupy all of the available mAChR sites. Thus, little or no receptor reserve appears to exist for mAChR-mediated phosphoinositide turnover (20,44). Within the category of muscarinic agonists, there are considerable differences in efficacy. A number of agonists, including ACh, carbamoylcholine, muscarine, methacholine, and oxotremorine-M (group "A"), are considerably more effective than others, e.g., oxotremorine, pilocarpine, arecoline, and bethanechol (group "B") (18,20). Group B agonists can block the stimulatory effects of group A agonists, indicating that they are partial agonists. This differential ability of muscarinic agonists to enhance phosphoinositide turnover is related to the propensity for the agonist to bind or not to bind to multiple affinity forms of the mAChR. Regional differences in the coupling characteristics of mAChRs have also been observed in both guinea pig and rat brain (16,40). For example, in the guinea pig neostriatum, full agonists such as oxotremorine-M and carbamoylcholine are 6- to 29-fold more potent than in the cerebral cortex. In addition, partial agonists such as oxotremorine or bethanechol are markedly more effective in the neostriatum. The seemingly convenient classification of the phosphoinositide response as a function of either M$_1$ or M$_2$ subtypes (i.e., pirenzepine-sensitive or -insensitive, respectively) does not appear to be warranted in the CNS, since characteristics of both M$_1$ and M$_2$ responses are evident in various brain regions. Moreover, the differential effects of pirenzepine on the phosphoinositide responses are not readily predicted from the binding affinities of pirenzepine in these tissues (16). These results serve to emphasize the importance of measurement of a functional response of muscarinic receptor activation, such as phosphoinositide turnover, in addition to radioligand binding studies, when characterizing a given receptor population.

The adrenergic phosphoinositide response in the CNS is a function of the α_1-receptor subtype. This conclusion is based on the ability of phenylephrine, an α_1-agonist, to elicit an increase in phosphoinositide turnover, and the

TABLE 2. *Neuroreceptors linked to inositide turnover*

Receptor	*In vivo*	Brain slices	Nerve ending preparations	Transformed cells[a]	Dissociated cells or slices[b]
Muscarinic cholinergic	+	+	+	+	+
α_1-Adrenergic	+	+	+	+	+
H$_1$-histaminergic	+	+		+	
5-HT$_2$-serotonergic		+			
ACTH$_{1-24}$			+		
β-Endorphin			+		
Substance P		+			+
Substance K		+			
V$_1$-vasopressin		+			+
TRH				+	
CCK		+			
Neurotensin		+		+	+
Bradykinin				+	
Nerve growth factor					+
Glutamate		+			

[a] Neuroblastoma, GH$_3$ pituitary cells, astrocytoma, or PC-12 cells.
[b] Superior cervical ganglion, adrenal medulla, or pineal cells.
For details, see ref. 15 and references therein. For details of glutamate receptor involvement, see refs. 49, 60.

selective inhibitory effect of prazosin, an α_1-antagonist (58). In contrast, clonidine, an α_2-agonist, is largely without effect, and the α_2-antagonist yohimbine fails to block norepinephrine-stimulated phosphoinositide turnover. As is the case for the mAChR, there are few spare receptors, if any, for the α_1-mediated response (37). The addition of serotonin (5-HT) to slices of cerebral cortex elicits increased phosphoinositide turnover characteristic of the 5-HT$_2$ receptor, in that the 5-HT$_1$ agonist 8-hydroxy-2(di-N-propylamino)tetralin is without effect, and the potent 5-HT$_2$ antagonist ketanserin blocks the response (13,38). The identity of the phosphoinositide-coupled 5-HT receptor in other brain areas such as hippocampus and limbic forebrain is less certain, since ketanserin has little effect. Moreover, there is no correlation between regional differences in 5-HT$_2$ binding sites as determined by [^{3}H]ketanserin binding and the magnitude of 5-HT-induced phosphoinositide turnover (13). The histaminergic response in the CNS appears to be mediated through H$_1$ receptors, since inclusion of the H$_1$ antagonist pyrilamine blocks the response, whereas the H$_2$ antagonist cimetidine does not (64). Furthermore, the H$_1$ agonist 2-(2-pyridyl)ethylamine mimics the effect of histamine, whereas addition of the H$_2$ agonist 4-methyl histamine is ineffective.

Only recently has the ability of neuropeptides to enhance phosphoinositide turnover been established. The magnitude of these effects in the CNS is relatively modest. Nevertheless, involvement of substance P, substance K, neurotensin, vasopressin, and cholecystokinin (CCK) receptors in the CNS and bradykinin in neuroblastoma $\times$ glioma hybrid cells has been documented (15,70). Recently (and unexpectedly) glutamate receptors were found to be coupled to phosphoinositide turnover in fetal brain (49,60). Both quisqualate and N-methyl-D-aspartate receptor subtypes appear to be primarily involved.

Signal Transduction at Inositide-Linked Receptors; Role of Guanine Nucleotide Binding Proteins

The mechanism whereby the agonist-receptor interaction results in an activation of phosphoinositide phosphodiesterase (phosphoinositide-specific phospholipase C) has long remained unresolved. Recent findings, principally from nonneural preparations, raise the possibility that signal transduction at phosphoinositide-linked receptors, like that at adenylate cyclase-linked receptors, is mediated by guanine nucleotide binding proteins (G-proteins). This is based on the following observations: (a) Addition of GTP or its nonhydrolyzable analog guanylylimido diphosphate regulates agonist binding to vasopressin V$_1$ (11), α_1-adrenergic (27), thyrotropin-releasing hormone (TRH) (30), and f-Met-Leu-Phe receptors (62). (b) Addition of GTPγS to permeabilized mast cells results in histamine release—a response normally associated with receptors coupled to phosphoinositide hydrolysis (24). (c) GTP addition to a cell-free preparation from the fly salivary gland potentiates serotonin-induced release of IP$_3$ (41). (d) Direct activation of PIP$_2$ phosphodiesterase by added guanine nucleotides has been demonstrated in neutrophil membranes (12) and recently in rat cortex membranes (25). These results collec-

tively support a role for G-proteins in the coupling of receptors to phosphoinositide hydrolysis. The identity of the relevant G-protein(s) is as yet unknown, but in the neutrophil (45,51), mast cell (47), and HL-60 cell (10), the N$_i$ protein has been implicated on the basis of experiments with pertussis toxin. The latter ADP-ribosylates N$_i$ and uncouples the receptor from phosphoinositide hydrolysis. However, this result was not confirmed in studies of the mAChR response in embryonic chick heart and astrocytoma cell (42). In brain, both N$_s$ and N$_i$ proteins are present as well as an additional substrate for the pertussis toxin, the N$_o$ protein. Since this latter protein constitutes 1 to 2% of total brain protein, its possible role in signal transduction at phosphoinositide-linked receptors merits further attention (63).

Cellular and Subcellular Localization of Enhanced Phosphoinositide Turnover

Neuronal Versus Glial

Glia may exceed neurons in number in the adult mammalian brain by severalfold and thus constitute a possible major site for enhanced phosphoinositide turnover. Early experiments designed to determine the relative contribution made by the two cell types indicated that stimulated inositol lipid turnover could be detected in both neuronal- and glial-enriched fractions in response to the addition of muscarinic cholinergic, α_1-adrenergic, and 5-HT$_2$-serotonergic stimuli (2,68). This result is somewhat surprising in view of the predominantly neuronal localization of these receptors, as inferred from radioligand binding techniques, and the fact that the muscarinic phosphoinositide response is attenuated in preparations from ibotenate-lesioned hippocampus (19). Furthermore, Crews and colleagues (26) have recently noted that muscarinic cholinergic and α_1-adrenergic responses are considerably greater for neuronal cells than for glial cells in primary culture. However, Pearce et al. (54) have recently observed that significant stimulation of phosphoinositide turnover is observed in astrocyte-enriched fractions obtained from newborn rat cortex in response to the addition of several neurotransmitters. We conclude that although the phosphoinositide response appears to be predominantly neuronal, contributions from glia are also possible. It is perhaps relevant that both astrocytic and neuronal tumor cell lines exhibit large phosphoinositide responses.

Subcellular Locus

Two experimental approaches have been taken to determine the subcellular localization of the phosphoinositide response. In the first approach (a), neural preparations are labeled in the presence of ^{32}P$_i$ or [^{3}H]inositol, exposed to an appropriate stimulus, and subcellular fractions prepared and analyzed for changes in lipid labeling. A second approach (b) involves localization of the effect in isolated subcellular fractions that mediate stimulated labeling of PA and PI. Studies involving approach (a) have failed to clearly indicate the primary site of stimulated phosphoinositide turnover, since an initial loss of labeled lipid (presumably from the plasma membrane) is followed by a rapid reequilibration of lipid throughout the cell. From the second approach (b), localization of the muscarinic phosphoinositide response to a nerve ending fraction has been reported by two groups (57,69). Current evidence suggests that the active component in the nerve ending preparation is derived from postsynaptic dendritic processes rather than presynaptic nerve endings (17,19).

Pre- Versus Postsynaptic

Although both presynaptic and postsynaptic receptors could conceivably be coupled to phosphoinositide turnover, the available evidence from three experimental preparations—the superior cervical ganglion, pineal gland, and hippocampus—all points to a postsynaptic location for the receptors involved. Thus (a) surgical lesion of the afferent presynaptic cholinergic input to the hippocampus or superior cervical ganglion does not result in a loss of cholinergic-mediated phosphoinositide turnover (17,31); (b) chemical lesion of the adrenergic inputs to either the hippocampus or a CNS-related tissue, the pineal, fails to reduce the α_1-mediated responses in these two tissues (6,35); (c) the phosphoinositide response can be observed in pineal cell cultures that are essentially free of presynaptic nerve endings (61), as well as in cultured astrocytoma and neuroblastoma cell lines; and (d) lesion of postsynaptic structures in the hippocampus with the excitatory neurotoxin ibotenate results in a loss of muscarinic stimulated PA and PI labeling in the absence of any reduction in choline acetyltransferase activity, a presynaptic cholinergic marker (17,19). The predominantly postsynaptic localization of the phosphoinositide response is at odds with a claimed presynaptic distribution of protein kinase C (PK-C) (22), but accords well with the reported localization of Ca^{2+}/calmodulin-dependent protein kinase II (53).

SECOND MESSENGER PRODUCTS

IP_3

Although the relationship between stimulated phosphoinositide turnover and Ca^{2+} mobilization has long been recognized (43), the mechanism has only recently been clarified, in large part due to the work of Berridge and collaborators that implicated the PIP_2 hydrolysis product inositol 1,4,5-trisphosphate (IP_3) (9). IP_3 interacts with its putative receptor on the endoplasmic reticulum, stimulating release of bound stores of Ca^{2+}. Moreover, when exogenous IP_3 is added to permeabilized cells or is microinjected into intact cells, a transient change in $[Ca^{2+}]_i$ is detected which mimics that produced by hormone or neurotransmitter stimulation. Such changes have been determined with Ca^{2+}-selective electrodes, the fluorescent probe quin-2, and by $^{45}Ca^{2+}$ efflux (9). The IP_3-Ca^{2+} signal is rapidly terminated by the action of a specific 5'-phosphomonoesterase, which converts IP_3 to the inactive inositol 1,4-bisphosphate (IP_2). Further phosphatase actions convert the resulting inositol

phosphates to free inositol, which can be reused for PI synthesis (Fig. 1).

At present, a number of variations on this theme are being investigated experimentally. The possibility that a 1,2 (cyclic) $4,5$-IP_3 is the initial product of phosphodiesterase cleavage is under investigation (67). Since $1,4,5$-IP_3 is active in mobilizing Ca^{2+}, the question arises of whether the cyclic derivative is more active than $1,4,5$-IP_3 or, alternatively, whether it is inactive. In addition, there is evidence for the presence of the isomer $1,3,4$-IP_3 (34), which is presumed to be inactive in Ca^{2+} mobilization. The origin and significance of $1,3,4$-IP_3 is the subject of considerable speculation. Recent indications that it is derived from the tetrakisphosphate $1,3,4,5$-IP_4 (4) raise a further question: Is the IP_4 cleaved from an as yet unidentified PIP_3, or from some other source?

Diacylglycerol

The other product of PIP_2 hydrolysis, DAG, serves to activate PK-C, thus providing a possible link between phosphoinositide turnover and protein phosphorylation. PK-C is highly enriched in the CNS, and much of the enzyme is associated with synaptic plasma membranes (50). In contrast, in most other tissues, the enzyme is localized predominantly in the soluble fraction, in an inactive form. PK-C activity depends on Ca^{2+}, DAG, and the presence of a phospholipid, preferably phosphatidylserine, for full activity. The DAG produced following PIP_2 breakdown increases the affinity of PK-C for Ca^{2+}, such that concentrations of the cation as low as 10^{-7} M fully activate the enzyme. PK-C is a prime target for the stimulatory action of phorbol esters such as 12-O-tetradecanoyl phorbol-13-acetate (TPA), a known tumor-promoting agent. TPA possesses a DAG-like structure and, like DAG, lowers the affinity of PK-C for Ca^{2+}. Phorbol esters, like DAG, do not appear to directly activate the enzyme by binding to PK-C, but participate in a quaternary complex along with Ca^{2+} and phosphatidylserine.

The possibility that DAG production during PIP_2 hydrolysis can serve in an inhibitory feedback mechanism comes from recent experiments in which the phorbol esters have been shown to inhibit the agonist-induced release of inositol phosphates in brain slices (39), human astrocytoma cells (52), and in PC-12 pheochromocytoma cells (66). By means of the inhibitory effect on stimulated phosphoinositide turnover, the phorbol esters also block Ca^{2+} mobilization. Although the mechanism of inhibition remains uncertain, one possible explanation is that TPA (through PK-C) induces phosphorylation of a protein involved in signal transduction (G-protein), and hence functionally "uncouples" the receptor from PIP_2 phosphodiesterase. It should be stressed that although PK-C itself is relatively abundant, little is known of the nature of its protein substrates. Gispen and colleagues have proposed that the membrane protein B_{50} may be one such substrate. In the presence of PK-C, phosphorylation of B_{50} results in an inhibition of PIP kinase (23,65). Addition of corticotropin (1–24) tetracosapeptide (ACTH) inhibits B_{50} phosphorylation, thereby reducing the inhibition of PIP kinase, and resulting in a net increase in PIP_2 synthesis. Thus DAG, acting through PK-C, may regulate the concentration of PIP_2 in neural membranes through at least two distinct mechanisms: inhibition of receptor-mediated phosphodiesteratic breakdown of PIP_2, and modulation of PIP kinase activity. Of special interest in the CNS is the recent realization that proteins termed B_{50}, GAP 43 (5,29,59) (a growth-associated axonally transported protein), PP 46 (36) (a growth cone component), and F1 (48) (a protein phosphorylated in long-term potentiation in hippocampal slices) may be identical. The findings point directly to the importance of PK-C, and less directly to phosphoinositide turnover, in complex cellular events unique to neuroplasticity.

Since the DAG moiety shared by PI, PIP, and PIP_2 is enriched in stearate in the sn-1 position and in arachidonate in the sn-2 position, it is tempting to speculate that the arachidonate in the DAG released in phosphoinositide breakdown serves as a source of eicosanoids. It is by no means certain that this is the case, however. In order for the phosphoinositide labeling cycle to be truly regenerative, significant loss of DAG should not occur. Sources of DAG other than phosphoinositide cleavage would yield DAG molecules not of the stearoyl arachidonoyl type. Such DAGs can serve as substrate for the regenerative pathway DAG → PA → CDP·DAG → PI. At some point, however, deacylation-reacylation steps would be necessary to restore the stearoyl arachidonoyl species.

In view of the selective enrichment of the stearoyl-arachidonoyl species in the inositol lipids, the lack of specificity of various DAGs in activating PK-C is puzzling. Although one of the fatty acids must be unsaturated for full activity, it can be in either the sn-1- or sn-2 position, and fatty acids other than arachidonate are fully effective (46). The possibility remains that protein kinase C can operate independently of phosphoinositide turnover. Were this so, the lack of fatty acid specificity in the DAG stimulation would be explained as well as reported localization of protein kinase C. Possible alternate intracellular sources of DAG are the breakdown of PA by PA phosphatase, and phospholipids such as PC. The latter can serve as a source of DAG in a number of ways: by the action of a PC-specific phospholipase C, as a product of the transfer of phosphorylcholine to ceramide in sphingomyelin biosynthesis, or by reversal of the CDP-choline:DG transferase reaction.

RELEVANCE TO DRUG ACTION

Lithium

Lithium has long been used in the treatment of manic depressive disorders, despite little knowledge of its underlying mechanism of action (21). The presence of Li^+ in the CNS at therapeutically relevant concentrations (1–10 mM) selectively inhibits inositol 1-phosphatase and results in the accumulation of IP and a decrease in free myo-inositol. This could lead to decreased PI synthesis and could thereby constitute the molecular basis of its therapeutic action (3). Since the blood-brain barrier is relatively impermeable to inositol, it is not unreasonable that the phosphoinositide response in brain indeed may be limited by intracellular inositol availability. Li^+ may thus be expected to perturb the activity of those receptors that are coupled to Ca^{2+} mobilization through phosphoinositide turnover. It is further possible that Li^+ would exert little effect in quiescent cells undergoing normal rates of receptor activation, but would attenuate the response in hyperactive cells. In this way, Li^+ may function as a regulatory cellular "calcistat" affecting primarily active or hyperactive cells (8).

Psychotherapeutic Drug Interactions

Psychotherapeutic drugs, especially tricyclic antidepressants and neuroleptics, are known to act as competitive antagonists at several phosphoinositide-linked neurotransmitter receptor sites in the brain, including the mAChR, histamine H_1, α_1-adrenergic, and 5-HT_2 receptors (55,56).

Measurements of stimulated phosphoinositide metabolism thus may serve as a marker for determining the activation of these receptor systems in brain (14). Although research on the involvement of phosphoinositide turnover in receptor-effector coupling has constituted a major advance in understanding brain mechanisms, important questions remain to be answered. These include whether there is an up- or down-regulation of relevant receptors subsequent to drug treatment in vivo, and the nature of the relationship between altered receptor number and the generation of messengers. The relative involvement of pre- and postsynaptic receptors in mediating altered responsiveness following drug treatment remains to be determined. A further question concerns the relative contribution of neurons and glia to the therapeutic response.

Interventive Strategies

From the standpoint of drug development, one must look to receptor activation, because extracellular sites are more accessible to drugs than intracellular sites, and also because the intracellular second messenger systems are shared by multiple receptor types, and are therefore likely to be much less specific targets. Nevertheless, identification and development of agents that block one or another of the numbered steps in Fig. 1 would be particularly useful in dissecting out regulatory aspects of this complex, dual second messenger system. At present, there is not a good in vivo blocker of the inositide phosphodiesterase (step 1). Elsewhere in the lipid regenerative cycle, the liponucleotide synthesis step (step 3) would appear to be very amenable for disruption because of its rate-limiting nature. At the level of PI synthase (step 4), inositol analogs might prove effective. PI kinase (step 5) and PIP kinase (step 6) appear to be regulated steps, both in regard to negative feedback (protein kinase C) and positive feedback (oncogene products) (7).

Pharmacological manipulation of inositide turnover via the inositol phosphates may be the basis of useful agents, as has already been proposed for the basis of the therapeutic action of Li^+. Blockade of IP_3 breakdown would prolong its Ca^{2+} mobilizing action. Agents that compete with IP_3 at its binding site are expected to antagonize Ca^{2+} release. IP_3 analogs that penetrate cells have not been described, and the high negative charge of the molecule poses a serious challenge. Whether any such agents would have usefulness as therapeutic agents is questionable; that they would be useful as experimental agents for the further elucidation of this novel second messenger system is very likely.

REFERENCES

1. Abdel-Latif, A. A. (1983): In: *Handbook of Neurochemistry, Vol. 3*, edited by A. Lajtha, pp. 91–131. Plenum, New York.
2. Abdel-Latif, A. A., Yau, S.-J., and Smith, J. P. (1974): *J. Neurochem.*, 22:383–393.
3. Allison, J. H., Blisner, M. E., Holland, W. H., Hipps, P. P., and Sherman, W. R. (1976): *Biochem. Biophys. Res. Commun.*, 76:664–670.
4. Batty, I. R., Nahorski, S. R., and Irvine, R. F. (1985): *Biochem. J.*, 232:211–215.
5. Benowitz, L. I., and Lewis, E. R. (1983): *J. Neurosci.*, 3:2153–2163.
6. Berg, G. R., and Klein, D. C. (1972): *J. Neurochem.*, 19:2519–2532.
7. Berridge, M. J. (1984): *Biotechnology*, 2:541–546.
8. Berridge, M. J., Downes, C. P., and Hanley, M. R. (1982): *Biochem. J.*, 206:587–595.
9. Berridge, M. J., and Irvine, R. F. (1984): *Nature*, 312:315–321.
10. Brandt, S. J., Dougherty, R. W., Lapetina, E. G., and Niedel, J. E. (1985): *Proc. Natl. Acad. Sci. USA*, 82:3277–3280.
11. Cantau, B., Keppens, S., de Wulf, H. D., and Jard, S. (1980): *J. Recept. Res.*, 1:137–168.
12. Cockcroft, S., and Gomperts, B. D. (1985): *Nature*, 314:534–536.
13. Conn, P. J., and Sanders-Bush, E. (1985): *J. Pharmacol. Exp. Ther.*, 234:195–203.
14. Downes, C. P. (1983): *Trends Neurosci.*, 6:313–316.
15. Fisher, S. K., and Agranoff, B. W. (1985): In: *Phospholipids in Nervous Tissues*, edited by J. Eichberg, pp. 241–295. John Wiley, New York.
16. Fisher, S. K., and Bartus, R. T. (1985): *J. Neurochem.*, 45:1085–1095.
17. Fisher, S. K., Boast, C. A., and Agranoff, B. W. (1980): *Brain Res.*, 189:284–288.
18. Fisher, S. K., Figueiredo, J. C., and Bartus, R. T. (1984): *J. Neurochem.*, 43:1171–1179.
19. Fisher, S. K., Frey, K. A., and Agranoff, B. W. (1981): *J. Neurosci.*, 1:1407–1413.
20. Fisher, S. K., Klinger, P. D., and Agranoff, B. W. (1983): *J. Biol. Chem.*, 258:7358–7363.
21. Gerbino, L., Oleshansky, M., and Gershon, S. (1978): In: *Psychopharmacology: A Generation of Progress*, edited by M. A. Lipton, A. DiMascio, and K. F. Killam, pp. 1261–1275. Raven Press, New York.
22. Girard, P. R., Mazzei, G. J., Wood, J. G., and Kuo, J. F. (1985): *Proc. Natl. Acad. Sci. USA*, 82:3030–3034.
23. Gispen, W. H., Leunissen, J. L. M., Oestreicher, A. B., Verkleij, A. J., and Zwiers, H. (1985): *Brain Res.*, 328:381–385.
24. Gomperts, B. D. (1983): *Nature*, 306:64–66.
25. Gonzales, R. A., and Crews, F. T. (1985): *Abstracts from Second International Symposium on Subtypes of Muscarinic Receptors*, Abstract No. 19.
26. Gonzales, R. A., Feldstein, J. B., Crews, F. T., and Raizada, M. K. (1985): *Brain Res.*, 345:350–355.
27. Goodhardt, M., Ferry, N., Geynet, P., and Hanoune, J. (1982): *J. Biol. Chem.*, 257:11577–11583.
28. Hallcher, L. M., and Sherman, W. R. (1980): *J. Biol. Chem.*, 255:10896–10901.
29. Heacock, A. M., and Agranoff, B. W. (1982): *Neurochem. Res.*, 7:771–788.
30. Hinkle, P. M., and Kinsella, P. A. (1984): *J. Biol. Chem.*, 259:3445–3449.
31. Hokin, L. E. (1966): *J. Neurochem.*, 13:179–184.
32. Hokin, L. E., and Hokin, M. R. (1955): *Biochim. Biophys. Acta*, 18:102–110.
33. Hokin, M. R., and Hokin, L. E. (1964): In: *Metabolism and Physiological Significance of Lipids*, edited by R. M. C. Dawson and D. N. Rhodes, pp. 423–434. John Wiley and Sons, New York.
34. Irvine, R. F., Letcher, A. J., Lander, D. J., and Downes, C. P. (1984): *Biochem. J.*, 223:237–243.
35. Janowsky, A., Labarca, R., and Paul, S. M. (1984): *Eur. J. Pharmacol.*, 102:193–194.
36. Katz, F., Ellis, L., and Pfenninger, K. H. (1985): *J. Neurosci.*, 5:1402–1414.
37. Kendall, D. A., Brown, E., and Nahorski, S. R. (1985): *Eur. J. Pharmacol.*, 114:41–52.
38. Kendall, D. A., and Nahorski, S. R. (1985): *J. Pharmacol. Exp. Ther.*, 233:473–479.
39. Labarca, R., Janowsky, A., Patel, J., and Paul, S. M. (1984): *Biochem. Biophys. Res. Commun.*, 123:703–709.
40. Lazareno, S., Kendall, D. A., and Nahorski, S. R. (1985): *Neuropharmacology*, 24:593–595.
41. Litosch, I., Wallis, C., and Fain, J. N. (1985): *J. Biol. Chem.*, 260:5464–5471.
42. Masters, S. B., Martin, M. W., Harden, T. K., and Brown, J. H. (1985): *Biochem. J.*, 227:933–937.
43. Michell, R. H. (1975): *Biochim. Biophys. Acta*, 415:81–147.
44. Michell, R. H., Jafferji, S. S., and Jones, L. M. (1976): *FEBS Lett.*, 69:1–5.
45. Molski, T. P. P., Naccache, P. H., Marsh, M. L., Kermode, J., Becker, E. L., and Sha'afi, R. L. (1984): *Biophys. Res. Commun.*, 124:644–650.
46. Mori, T., Takai, Y., Yu, B., Takahashi, J., Nishizuka, Y., and Fujikara, T. (1982): *J. Biochem.*, 91:427–431.
47. Nakamura, T., and Ui, M. (1985): *J. Biol. Chem.*, 260:3584–3593.
48. Nelson, R. B., and Routtenberg, A. (1985): *Exp. Neurol.*, 89:213–224.
49. Nicoletti, F., Meek, J. L., Chuang, D. M., Iodarola, M., Roth, B. L., and Costa, E. (1985): *Fed. Proc.*, 44(Abstr. 480).
50. Nishizuka, Y. (1984): *Science*, 225:1365–1370.
51. Okajima, F., and Ui, M. (1984): *J. Biol. Chem.*, 259:13863–13871.
52. Orellana, S. A., Solski, P. A., and Brown, J. H. (1985): *J. Biol. Chem.*, 260:5236–5239.
53. Ouimet, C. C., McGuinness, T. L., and Greengard, P. (1984): *Proc. Natl. Acad. Sci. USA*, 81:5604–5608.
54. Pearce, B., Cambray-Deakin, M., Morrow, C., Grimble, J., and Murphy, S. (1985): *J. Neurochem.*, 45:1534–1540.
55. Richelson, E., and Nelson, A. (1984): *Eur. J. Pharmacol.*, 103:197–204.
56. Richelson, E., and Nelson, A. (1984): *J. Pharmacol. Exp. Ther.*, 230:94–102.
57. Schacht, J., and Agranoff, B. W. (1972): *J. Biol. Chem.*, 247:771–777.
58. Schoepp, D. D., Knepper, S. M., and Rutledge, C. O. (1984): *J. Neurochem.*, 43:1758–1761.
59. Skene, J. H. P., and Willard, M. (1981): *J. Cell Biol.*, 89:86–95.
60. Sladeczek, F., Pin, J.-P., Recasens, M., Bockaert, J., and Weiss, S. (1985): *Nature*, 317:717–719.
61. Smith, T. L., Eichberg, J., and Hauser, G. (1979): *Life Sci.*, 24:2179–2184.
62. Snyderman, R. (1984): *Fed. Proc.*, 43:2743–2748.
63. Sternweis, P. C., and Robishaw, J. D. (1984): *J. Biol. Chem.*, 259:13806–13813.
64. Subramanian, N., Whitmore, W. L., Seidler, F. J., and Slotkin, T. A. (1980): *Life Sci.*, 27:1315–1319.
65. Van Dongen, C., Zwiers, H., Oestreicher, A. B., and Gispen, W. H. (1985): In: *Phospholipids in the Nervous System, Vol. 2: Physiological Roles*, edited by L. A. Horrocks, J. N. Kanfer, and G. Porcellati, pp. 49–59. Raven Press, New York.
66. Vicentini, L. M., Ambrosini, A., DiVirgilo, F., Pozzan, T., and Meldosi, J. (1985): *J. Cell Biol.*, 100:1330–1333.
67. Wilson, D. B., Connolly, T. M., Bross, T. E., Majerus, P. W., Sherman, W. R., Tyler, A. N., Rubin, L. J., and Brown, J. E. (1985): *J. Biol. Chem.*, 260:13496–13501.
68. Woelk, H., Kanig, K., and Peiler-Ichikawa, K. (1974): *J. Neurochem.*, 23:1057–1063.
69. Yagihara, Y., and Hawthorne, J. N. (1972): *J. Neurochem.*, 19:355–367.
70. Yano, K., Higashida, H., Inoue, R., and Nozawa, Y. (1984): *J. Biol. Chem.*, 259:10201–10207.

Psychopharmacology:
The Third Generation of Progress,
edited by Herbert Y. Meltzer.
Raven Press, New York © 1987.

CHAPTER **34**

Patch-Clamp Studies of Ion Channels

Barry S. Pallotta

Ion channels are specialized macromolecules that provide a pathway for ion flow across the plasma membrane. Channels are immensely talented since they must recognize specific stimuli (agonist molecules or changes in membrane potential) and then open an internal "gate" to allow passage of particular ions. Recognition of the correct agonist is thought to involve binding to a closely coupled receptor site, whereas "gating" involves a sequence of conformational changes of the channel protein initiated by the agonist binding and/or changes in the membrane electric field. These functions appear to be performed by single macromolecules, since the properties of voltage-activated Na^+ channels or acetylcholine (ACh)-activated channels accompany the reinsertion of these glycoproteins into lipid bilayers (49,70). The advent of the patch-clamp technique for recording the ion flow through individual channels in small patches of membrane (52) has brought a better understanding of many of the properties of ion channels (33), and an appreciation for the diversity of physiologic functions which they perform.

One consequence of the widespread use of the patch clamp is an increase in the number of known ion channels and their responsibilities in maintaining normal cell function. In addition to their traditional role in excitable membranes, which required a response to an agonist or changes in membrane potential, ion channels now appear in secretory cells (see review 58), Schwann and glial cells (see review 27), T-lymphocytes (see review 6), erythrocytes (see review 63), and macrophages (24). Some of the ion channels found in these diverse cell types are "classical" because they appear identical to channels well described in excitable tissues, whereas in several preparations channels have been found whose function is not yet obvious. In addition to surface membranes, ion channels are also found in internalized membranes such as T-tubules (41) and sarcoplasmic reticulum (67) of skeletal muscle.

Neurotransmitters have been shown to affect the activity of surface membrane ion channels. In some cases the agonist regulates channel activity by binding to a receptor site closely associated with the ion channel itself. In other cases the agonist affects channel activity indirectly via an intracellular second messenger or metabolite that modulates channel activity. In this brief review, a few of the channel properties that appear fundamental to channel function will be described, with emphasis on those channels which are affected by neurotransmitters. Voltage-activated channels share many characteristics with the ligand-gated channels (33), except that they are capable of sensing changes in the membrane electric field instead of (or in some cases, in addition to) an agonist molecule.

SINGLE-CHANNEL RECORDING

The modern patch-clamp amplifier is an extremely sensitive amplifier that converts the relatively small ion currents (10^{-11} amp or less) that flow through the individual ion channel into measurable voltages. The channel current is directed into the patch-clamp amplifier by an extracellular glass microelectrode, cleverly tapered and firepolished to sit on and then adhere to the cell membrane. It is within the approximately 0.5-μm aperture of this electrode that one or more ion channels are often trapped. Details of patch clamping methods are found in (15,59,68).

The recent prosperity of the patch clamp arises from the tendency for the cell membrane to adhere or seal so tightly to the mouth of the electrode that "leakage" resistances on the order of 10^9 or 10^{10} ohm are not uncommon (thus the term "gigaseal" is often prefixed to "patch clamp") (31). This incredible electrical resistance greatly improves the ability of the patch clamp to resolve ever smaller channel currents, and as described below, the mechanical stability of the glass-membrane seal allows the experimenter considerable control over the ion channel being studied.

Upon sealing an electrode to the cell membrane, one can record from the ion channels trapped by the electrode in this "on-cell" configuration, or tear the 5- to 20-μm^2 membrane patch (60) from the cell so that either its inside surface ("inside-out patch") or outside surface ("outside-out patch") is in contact with the bath (31). The inside-out patch is especially useful for studying channels that are regulated by intracellular agonists, whereas the outside-out configuration is used for channels sensitive to extracellular agonists. In both excised patch configurations, the experimenter has complete control over the ionic environment on both sides of the excised patch. The presence of only one (or a few) active channel macromolecules in a patch, combined with the patch clamp amplifier's control of the voltage gradient across the patch, results in one of the best-controlled and simplest biological systems.

In some respects, the tremendous resolving power of the patch clamp is also one of its disadvantages. Physiologically important responses (e.g., action potentials), which require the interaction between two or more types of ion channels, are difficult to reconstruct from recordings obtained from only a single macromolecule or type of channel (17). A practical limitation to the technique is that the cell membranes must be freed of connective tissue by enzyme treatments unless the cells have been maintained or grown in culture. When the desired ion channels reside in relatively inaccessible membranes such as sarcoplasmic reticulum, those membranes might be inserted into lipid bilayers (see reviews 39,47). This reconstitution offers the advantage that the composition of the lipid bilayer is known.

PROPERTIES OF ION CHANNELS

Patch-clamp recordings from single ion channels can only distinguish between two groups of channel confor-

mations. "Open states" are conformations that conduct ions through the channel, whereas "closed states" are conformations that are nonconducting. The importance of these distinctions arises from the widely held view that the function of ion channels is to allow, under certain conditions, the movement of specific ions through the plasma membrane. Thus, the amount of time spent in the conducting state(s) and the identities of the ions allowed to cross the membrane are of recognized importance. As a result, many of the measurements described in the literature pertain to two properties of the channel: gating and selective permeability. Several of the common characteristics of single-channel recordings are illustrated in Figure 1, which was recorded from a membrane patch that contained only one Ca^{2+}-activated K$^+$ channel (a common channel activated by intracellular free Ca^{2+} and which preferentially conducts K$^+$ over Na$^+$).

Gating Kinetics of Ion Channels

Gating refers to the opening and closing of the channel as it makes transitions between its different conformational (or at least, kinetically distinguishable) states. As shown in Figure 1, the transitions between open and closed states often occur on a submillisecond time scale. One quantitative measure of gating is the average duration of the individual channel openings, or of the individual closings. These two measurements will yield the percent open time (or dividing by 100, the open probability), which is a measure of how active the channel is under the specified conditions. It is also apparent from the figure that the individual openings are often grouped together into "bursts." Within each burst are brief, downward "flickers," which are usually assumed to arise from complete closures of the channel that were too brief for the patch clamp to follow completely (12). The flickers thus divide the burst into a number of individual openings. The bursts also contain longer duration shut times ("gaps within bursts"), and bursts are separated from each other by much longer shut times called "gaps between bursts." Quantitative descriptions of burst kinetics often rely on an assumed kinetic scheme (10) in which the bursts arise from multiple openings and closings initiated by a single agonist occupancy; i.e., the agonist remains bound during the burst (10,12,44). It is significant to note also that most (if not all) the known agonist-activated channels demonstrate burst kinetics.

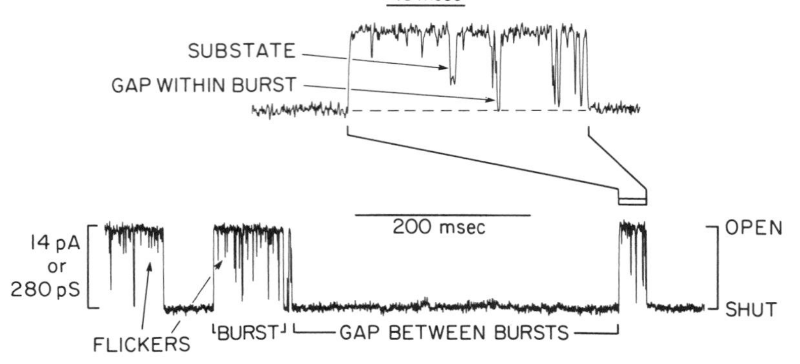

FIG. 1. Single-channel currents and patch-clamp jargon. **Bottom** trace shows a continuous single-channel current recorded from a Ca^{2+}-activated K$^+$ channel attached to a 1321N1 astrocytoma cell that had been K$^+$-depolarized. **Upper** trace shows the rightmost burst on an expanded time scale to illustrate the fine structure of a burst. Both traces were obtained by digitizing (100 μsec/sample) the original current record which had been stored on FM tape. +50 mV. (S. A. Oglesby and B. S. Pallotta, unpublished).

Determining Molecular Mechanism

One remarkable aspect of single-channel recording is that the conformational transitions between the open and closed states of a single macromolecule can be resolved. Open states have been further partitioned by amplitude and duration. Some open states share a common amplitude (or conductance), but may widely differ from each other in duration. Another set of open states is distinguished by their reduced amplitudes (see Conductance Substates: Partially Open or Partially Shut). Since the amount of time the channel dwells in the open state is determined by the rate of closing, and the closed times are determined by the rate of opening, the durations of the open and closed intervals provide important information about the rates of transition between the open and closed states (9,10). As is apparent in Figure 1, however, the durations of successive openings, closing, and even burst durations are different each time they occur, so that statistical methods must be used to extract the underlying rate constants (10). Frequency histograms of the open or closed times can also be used to determine the number of open and closed states (2,10,12), although information about the interconversions between the states must be derived by methods that correlate the appearance of particular open times with closed times (36,38,57).

Ion Permeability

The amplitude of the individual channel currents is a measure of the channel's permeability. Although the durations of the openings are all different in Figure 1, the channel opens to almost the same current level each time. In the figure, this current (14 pA, where 1 pA = 10^{-12} ampere) is equal to approximately 10^8 charges/sec flowing through the channel. If one prefers to picture ion channels as enzymes that catalyze ion permeation through the membrane (42,62), then these currents suggest that channels possess most impressive turnover numbers compared to "carriers" (33).

The rate with which a channel can transport ions (i.e., the current) is proportional to the concentration of charge-carrying ions in the bulk aqueous medium, the voltage gradient across the channel, and the permeability of the channel. Conductance (or its reciprocal, resistance) is a proportionality constant that relates the amount of current that flows through a channel to the applied voltage. As one would expect for a simple resistor, over much of the commonly applied voltage range the current increases linearly with the applied voltage. The slope of a straight line fitted to this current-voltage relation is the channel's conductance, but unlike the simple resistor, channel conductance also varies with the concentration of the permeant ion(s). The Ca^{2+}-activated K^+ channel shown in the figure has a "large" conductance (280 pS, where 1 picosiemen = 10^{-12} ohm^{-1}), whereas a dopamine-agonist-activated Cl^- channel is considered "small" at approximately 12 pS (51). The current-voltage relation is apparently more complex for channels activated by glycine (28) or γ-aminobutyric acid (GABA) (30), since considerable curvature (or "rectification") was observed.

Ion Selectivity

The ability of a channel to allow movement of specific ions results from interactions between the channel and the ions in the bulk aqueous environment. This "ion selectivity" is important since the identity of the permeant ion(s) in large part determines the channel's physiologic function. No channel is absolutely specific for only one ion, although some channels are quite specific for certain ones. One of the Ca^{2+}-activated K^+ channels, for example, allows passage of K^+ and Rb^+ while Na^+ is hardly permeant at all (3,74). In contrast, the nicotinic ACh-activated channel of skeletal muscle is known to pass more than 50 different cations (22). The ability to distinguish between different ions demonstrates that channels do not act as simple gated holes in the membrane but must interact with potentially permeant ions. Additional evidence for significant ion-channel interactions is that single-channel conductances increase and then saturate as the concentration of permeant ions is increased (3,16,34).

Conductance Substates: Partially Open or Partially Shut?

One surprising aspect of channel behavior is the appearance of conductance substates (32). A substate is a conformation of the channel that is neither fully conducting (open) nor fully closed. The upper trace of Figure 1 shows a clear interval where the fully open channel shuts only partway and dwells in this "substate" for several milliseconds. Since the substates occur only during bursts of openings, the substates are not artifacts arising from the activity of another channel in the patch. In addition to Ca^{2+}-activated K^+ channels in astrocytoma cells (Fig. 1) and skeletal muscle (2), substates have been observed in nicotinic ACh-activated channels (32), GABA-activated channels from bovine chromaffin cells (4) and mouse spinal neurons (30), glycine-activated channels in spinal neurons (30), and a serotonin-sensitive K^+ channel in *Aplysia* neurons (65).

The physiologic significance of the conductance substates is not clear, considering their relatively small conductance and the amount of time the channel spends in such a state. This latter consideration is especially troublesome since it is difficult to determine what fraction of the flickers during a burst arise from short-lived occupancies in a conductance substate as opposed to brief complete closures. Auerbach and Sachs (1) estimated that at least 15% of all flickers of the nicotinic ACh-activated channel from chick skeletal muscle were to a conductance substate that had only 10% of the full-open conductance.

THE SINGLE-CHANNEL VIEW OF AGONISTS AND ANTAGONISTS

Inferences about drug-receptor interactions have often been drawn from experiments involving large numbers of receptors or channels and where the measured response was perhaps far removed from the agonist-binding step. Patch-clamp resolution of individual ion channels has shortened the conceptual distance between binding and response, since we can directly observe many of the conformational transitions that underlie the classic pharmacological actions of agonists and antagonists. Thus, our perspective of drug-receptor interactions has shifted from that of the population to that of the individual receptor or channel itself (7,9).

Effects of Agonist Concentration

Single-channel conductances are not affected by agonist concentration except in instances of fast channel block by the agonist (see below). Instead, increasing the concentration of an agonist causes a channel to spend a larger fraction of its time in the open state until the channel is open almost 100% of the time or it desensitizes (see below). This increase in open time reflects changes in the frequency of bursting, the burst durations, and/or the lifetimes of the individual openings during each burst. Hill slopes of the concentration dependence of the percent open time suggest that several channel types require that two or more agonist molecules bind on or near the channel for opening. This group includes channels activated by glutamate (26), GABA (4), and a Ca^{2+}-activated K^+ channel (2). However, the Ca^{2+}-activated K^+ channel might open occasionally after binding only one Ca^{2+} (2), whereas the nicotinic ACh-activated channel can open in the absence of agonist (35) or after binding either one or two ACh molecules (12,20,36,66).

Effects of Different Agonists on Gating

It is often assumed that at least one agonist molecule remains bound to the receptor-channel complex while it is opening and closing during a burst, and evidence supporting this view comes from the effects of different agonists on channel gating. For the gating to vary with the agonist, the channel molecule would have to remember which agonist had activated it; otherwise, the channel would open and close with the same rates irrespective of the agonist type. The simplest mechanism that would retain information about the agonist molecule would be one in which the agonist remained bound throughout the gating process (33).

Changes in gating with agonist have been observed with glutamate-activated channels in locust muscle, where openings evoked by quisqualate were approximately twice the duration of openings in the presence of glutamate (18,25). The number of openings in each burst also appeared to vary with the agonist (19), and at a given concentration the rates at which these channels were opened also varied with the agonist (25). Similar results were found for a nicotinic ACh-activated channel: both the burst durations and individual open times within the bursts were a function of the cholinergic agonist (43,66).

Single-Channel Conductance Does Not Differ with Agonist

In contrast to the different gating kinetics observed with different agonists, the single-channel conductances of the nicotinic ACh-activated channel in muscle (8,43) or the glutamate-activated channel of locust muscle (18,25) did not vary with agonist type. However, high concentrations of agonists such as ACh or carbachol caused the single-channel conductance to appear reduced (11) because of an extremely fast type of channel block that could not be fully resolved by the patch-clamp amplifier. Thus, it appears that only the gating kinetics of these channels varies with the agonist.

Partial Agonists

The classical concept of agonist efficacy addresses the mechanism(s) whereby some agonists are more effective than others at evoking a response. A partial agonist, for example, cannot evoke as large a response as a full agonist despite very high concentrations. The single-channel correlate of partial agonism has been observed with the classical competitive antagonist d-tubocurarine (dTC), which can both open nicotinic channels (50,71) and then block them (71). Thus dTC qualifies as a partial agonist on two counts. First, dTC competitively antagonizes the agonist ACh, while alone it demonstrates weak agonist properties by evoking brief channel openings. Second, the openings induced by dTC are also subject to block by the drug, thus insuring that a full response could not be reached. At sufficiently high concentrations, even full agonists such as ACh, carbachol, and suberyldicholine will block the nicotinic channel and therefore perform as partial agonists (11,66).

Channel Blockers

Of the several pharmacologic mechanisms that describe how a drug might interact with a receptor and decrease its responsiveness to agonist, blockade of the open channel is the most dramatic at the single-channel level. Here, we envision that the blocking drug enters the open channel mouth and physically plugs the opening. Depending on how long the blocker sits in the channel, the currents recorded in the presence of such a blocker take on a very characteristic appearance.

If the blocker dwells within the channel for a relatively long time compared to the normal channel shut times, then the openings will appear grouped or clustered together by silent periods of up to several seconds duration. This type of block of a Ca^{2+}-activated K^+ channel reconstituted into lipid bilayers has been observed in the presence of Ba^{2+} (73) and charybdotoxin (48).

Blockers that dissociate within a few milliseconds of binding will cause the channel openings to now appear as bursts of very brief openings separated from each other by flickers as the drug blocks and unblocks. This behavior has been observed with the nicotinic ACh-activated channel in the presence of the charged lidocaine-derivative QX-222 (53) or uncharged benzocaine (56), and with Mg^{2+} block of glutamate-induced channel openings in mouse central neurons (55).

A third type of blocker effect appears if the blocker binds and dissociates very rapidly compared to channel opening and closing rates. In this case, the openings appear to have normal durations, but are noisier (more flickers) and of apparently reduced conductance. The conductance appears reduced because the individual blocked periods are too brief for the patch-clamp amplifier to follow, and as a result the patch clamp reports a reduced current amplitude. Block of a Ca^{2+}-activated K^+ channel by Na^+ is apparently this fast type (45,74), as is the apparent reduction of nicotinic channel conductance observed at high concentrations of full agonists (11,66).

Desensitization

The onset of desensitization is characterized by a time-dependent decline in a macroscopic response despite the sustained presence of an agonist. At the single-channel level, desensitization onset is signaled by the appearance of relatively long (perhaps tens of seconds) silent periods following application of an agonist (61). These silent periods end abruptly as the channel apparently recovers from closed desensitized state(s) and continues to open and close at a rate determined by the agonist concentration until the next silent period occurs. As a result of the long silent periods, the percent open time of the individual channels is reduced, which in turn decreases the responsiveness of the cell. In addition to the nicotinic ACh-activated channel (61), desensitization has been observed for Ca^{2+}-activated K^+ channels (57), and channels activated by glutamate (26), GABA (30), and glycine (30).

SENSITIVITY OF ION CHANNELS TO SECOND MESSENGERS AND METABOLITES

The ion permeabilities of the plasma membranes of a number of different preparations are sensitive to intracellular cyclic AMP or Ca^{2+} (see review 37). The ion channels that contribute to these conductances are now being identified, as these channels might provide a link between membrane excitability and metabolic events. Sensitivity to second messengers also allows a particular channel to respond to both intra- and extracellular stimuli, thus enabling some ion channels to play more than one role in cellular homeostasis.

Channels Regulated by Intracellular ATP

A K^+-selective channel whose activity is inhibited by millimolar concentrations of ATP has been described in cardiac muscle from guinea pig and rabbit (54), rat pancreatic B cells (13), and surface membrane of frog skeletal muscle (69). ATP-mediated inhibition does not appear to require ATP metabolism since the nonmetabolizable analog adenylylimidodiphosphate (AMP-PNP) was equally effective (13,69). In contrast to this inhibitory effect of ATP, Ca^{2+}-selective channels from rabbit sarcoplasmic reticulum incorporated into lipid bilayers are activated by millimolar ATP on the cytoplasmic side of the channel (67). Whereas this Ca^{2+} channel appears to play a major role in the efflux of Ca^{2+} from sarcoplasmic reticulum during excitation-contraction coupling, the ATP-regulated K^+ channels might

help maintain the resting potential during metabolically stressful periods that deplete intracellular ATP.

Channels Regulated by Cyclic AMP

When serotonin is applied to *Aplysia* sensory neurons, K^+-selective channels in the plasma membrane become inactive for as long as serotonin is present. Similar behavior is evoked by intracellular injection of cyclic AMP (65), and most of these effects are also observed when excised inside-out patches of membrane are exposed to purified catalytic subunit of cyclic AMP-dependent protein kinase (64). These results suggest that channel regulation by extracellular serotonin involves intracellular cyclic AMP, and probably phosphorylation of an intracellular site on or near the channel by a protein kinase.

Relatively long-lasting (minutes) increases in the activity of low-conductance (40–60 pS) Ca^{2+}-activated K^+ channels from *Helix* have been produced by catalytic subunit of cyclic AMP-dependent protein kinase applied to either membrane patches or channels incorporated into lipid bilayers (23). A larger conductance Ca^{2+}-activated K^+ channel (107 pS) is also apparently modulated by cyclic AMP in chick kidney cell culture since channel activity was increased by extracellular application of forskolin (29).

Regulation of a voltage-activated Ca^{2+}-selective channel by phosphorylation is also implied by the effects of cyclic AMP on channel activity in cultured heart cells. Addition of 8-bromocyclic AMP to the solution bathing the cells approximately doubled the Ca^{2+} channel activity during the depolarizing voltage steps required to activate this channel (5). Similar results were obtained when intracellular cyclic AMP was increased with the beta-adrenergic agonist isoproterenol. Voltage-activated Ca^{2+} channels might be another example of a channel regulated by phosphorylation of a site on or near the channel protein.

Channels Regulated by Intracellular Ca^{2+}

Considering the common roles that intracellular Ca^{2+} plays as a second or even third messenger, it is significant that a number of ion channels have been identified that are activated by micromolar concentrations of Ca^{2+} at the intracellular surface (see reviews 40,63). As the number of extracellular receptors that are linked to the regulation of intracellular Ca^{2+} increases it seems likely that the number of roles played by the Ca^{2+}-activated channels will also increase.

A variety of preparations contain a large-conductance (250–320 pS) K^+-selective channel that is sensitive to both membrane voltage and micromolar Ca^{2+} (see reviews 39,40). In the pancreatic B cell this channel is also modulated by intracellular H^+ (14). On-cell patch recordings from lacrimal glands have demonstrated activation of these channels by extracellular application of carbachol (72). The response was independent of extracellular Ca^{2+} and abolished by the presence of atropine or by dialyzing the cell interior with ethyleneglycol bis(aminoethylether)tetraacetate (EGTA), suggesting that activation of muscarinic receptors mobilized Ca^{2+} from a cytoplasmic Ca^{2+} store. Thyrotropin-releasing hormone (TRH) applied to rat growth hormone pituitary tumor cells also stimulated activity of a large-conductance Ca^{2+}-activated K^+ channel which, in excised patches, did not respond to directly applied TRH (21). Similarly, a Ca^{2+}-activated cation channel of moderate conductance (35 pS) is activated in pancreatic acinar cells by extracellular application of cholecystokinin or ACh (46). Both these results suggest that channel activation was a consequence of agonist-mediated increases in intracellular Ca^{2+}.

SUMMARY

Many types of ion channels normally inhabit the plasma membrane, where they gate the flow of selected ions across the membrane in response to specific stimuli. Ultimately, these ionic currents perform functions as diverse as the cell types in which channels have been found. Patch-clamp studies have revealed much detailed information about the properties of ion channels, while the ability to resolve conformational changes in the presence of ligands has contributed to a better understanding of drug-receptor interactions. Since ion channels are sensitive to membrane potential, extracellular agonists, and/or intracellular metabolites, they might provide a molecular basis for cellular integration of intra- and extracellular signaling pathways.

ACKNOWLEDGMENT

The author's unpublished work was supported by NIH grant GM32211.

REFERENCES

1. Auerbach, A., and Sachs, F. (1983): *Biophys. J.,* 42:1–10.
2. Barrett, J. N., Magleby, K. L., and Pallotta, B. S. (1982): *J. Physiol. (Lond.),* 331:211–230.
3. Blatz, A. L., and Magleby, K. L. (1984): *J. Gen. Physiol.,* 84:1–23.
4. Bormann, J., and Clapham, D. E. (1985): *Proc. Natl. Acad. Sci. USA,* 82:2168–2172.
5. Cachelin, A. B., de Peyer, J. E., Kokubun, S., and Reuter, H. (1983): *Nature,* 304:462–464.
6. Chandy, K. G., Decoursey, T. E., Cahalan, M. D., and Gupta, S. (1985): *J. Clin. Immunol.,* 5:1–6.
7. Colquhoun, D. (1981): *Trends Pharm. Sci.,* 2:212–217.
8. Colquhoun, D., Gardner, P., and Ogden, D. C. (1983): *J. Physiol. (Lond.),* 345:139P.
9. Colquhoun, D., and Hawkes, A. G. (1977): *Proc. R. Soc. Lond. B.,* 199:231–262.
10. Colquhoun, D., and Hawkes, A. G. (1981): *Proc. R. Soc. Lond. B.,* 211:205–235.
11. Colquhoun, D., and Ogden, D. C. (1984): *J. Physiol. (Lond.),* 353:90P.
12. Colquhoun, D., and Sakmann, B. (1981): *Nature,* 294:464–466.
13. Cook, D. L., and Hales, C. N. (1984): *Nature,* 311:271–273.
14. Cook, D. L., Ikeuchi, M., and Fujimoto, W. Y. (1984): *Nature,* 311:269–271.
15. Corey, D. P. (1983): *Neurosci. Comment.,* 1:99–110.
16. Coronado, R., Rosenberg, R. L., and Miller, C. (1980): *J. Gen. Physiol.,* 76:425–446.
17. Cranefield, P. F. (1983): *Am. J. Physiol.,* 245:H901–H910.
18. Cull-Candy, S. G., Miledi, R., and Parker, I. (1981): *J. Physiol. (Lond.),* 321:195–210.
19. Cull-Candy, S. G., and Parker, I. (1983): In: *Single-Channel Recording,* edited by B. Sakmann and E. Neher, pp. 389–400. Plenum Press, New York.
20. Dionne, V. E., and Leibowitz, M. D. (1982): *Biophys. J.,* 39:253–261.
21. Dubinsky, J. M., and Oxford, G. S. (1985): *Proc. Natl. Acad. Sci. USA,* 82:4282–4286.
22. Dwyer, T. M., Adams, D. J., and Hille, B. (1980): *J. Gen. Physiol.,* 75:469–492.
23. Ewald, D., Williams, A., and Levitan, I. B. (1985): *Nature,* 315:503–506.
24. Gallin, E. K. (1984): *Biophys. J.,* 46:821–825.
25. Gration, K. A. F., Lambert, J. J., Ramsey, R. L., Rand, R. P., and Usherwood, P. N. R. (1981): *Brain Res.,* 230:400–405.
26. Gration, K. A. F., Lambert, J. J., Ramsey, R. L., and Usherwood, P. N. R. (1981): *Nature,* 291:423–425.
27. Gray, P. T. A., and Ritchie, J. M. (1985): *Trends Neurosci.,* 8:411–415.
28. Gray, R., and Johnston, D. (1985): *J. Neurophysiol.,* 54:134–142.
29. Guggino, S. E., Suarez-Isla, B. A., Guggino, W. B., and Sacktor, B. (1985): *Am. J. Physiol.,* 249:F448–F455.
30. Hamill, O. P., Bormann, J., and Sakmann, B. (1983): *Nature,* 305:805–808.
31. Hamill, O. P., Marty, A., Neher, E., and Sigworth, F. J. (1981): *Pflugers Arch.,* 391:85–100.
32. Hamill, O. P., and Sakmann, B. (1981): *Nature,* 294:462–464.
33. Hille, B. (1984): *Ionic Channels of Excitable Membranes.* Sinauer Associates, Sunderland, MA.
34. Horn, R., and Patlak, J. (1980): *Proc. Natl. Acad. Sci. USA,* 77:6930–6934.
35. Jackson, M. B. (1984): *Proc. Natl. Acad. Sci. USA,* 81:3901–3904.
36. Jackson, M. B., Wong, B. S., Morris, C. E., Lecar, H., and Christian, C. N. (1983): *Biophys. J.,* 42:109–114.
37. Kostyuk, P. G. (1984): *Neuroscience,* 13:983–989.
38. Labarca, P., Rice, J. A., Fredkin, D. R., and Montal, M. (1985): *Biophys. J.,* 47:469–478.
39. Latorre, R., Alvarez, O., Cecchi, X., and Vergara, C. (1985): *Annu. Rev. Biophys. Chem.,* 14:79–111.
40. Latorre, R., Coronado, R., and Vergara, C. (1984): *Annu. Rev. Physiol.,* 46:485–495.
41. Latorre, R., Vergara, C., and Hidalgo, C. (1982): *Proc. Natl. Acad. Sci. USA,* 79:805–809.
42. Läuger, P. (1983): In: *Single-Channel Recording,* edited by B. Sakmann and E. Neher, pp. 177–189. Plenum Press, New York.
43. Leibowitz, M. D., and Dionne, V. E. (1984): *Biophys. J.,* 45:153–163.
44. Magleby, K. L., and Pallotta, B. S. (1983): *J. Physiol. (Lond.),* 344:605–623.
45. Marty, A. (1983): *Pflugers Arch.,* 396:179–181.
46. Maruyama, Y., and Petersen, O. H. (1982): *Nature,* 300:61–63.
47. Miller, C. (1983): In: *Current Methods in Cellular Neurobiology, Vol. III,* edited by J. L. Barker and J. F. McKelvy, pp. 1–37. John Wiley & Sons, New York.
48. Miller, C., Moczydlowski, E., Latorre, R., and Phillips, M. (1985): *Nature,* 313:316–318.
49. Montal, M., Labarca, P., Fredkin, D. R., and Suarez-Isla, B. A. (1984): *Biophys. J.,* 45:165–174.
50. Morris, C. E., Wong, B. S., Jackson, M. B., and Lecar, H. (1983): *J. Neurosci.,* 3:2525–2531.
51. Murphy, R. B., and Vodyanoy, V. (1984): *Biophys. J.,* 45:22–23.
52. Neher, E., and Sakmann, B. (1976): *Nature,* 260:799–802.
53. Neher, E., and Steinbach, J. H. (1978): *J. Physiol. (Lond.),* 277:153–176.
54. Noma, A. (1983): *Nature,* 305:147–148.
55. Nowak, L., Bregestovski, P., Ascher, P., Herbet, A., and Prochiantz, A. (1984): *Nature,* 307:492–495.
56. Ogden, D. C., Siegelbaum, S. A., and Colquhoun, D. (1981): *Nature,* 289:596–598.
57. Pallotta, B. S. (1985): *J. Physiol. (Lond.),* 363:501–516.
58. Petersen, O. H., and Maruyama, Y. (1984): *Nature,* 307:693–696.
59. Sakmann, B., and Neher, E., eds. (1983): *Single-Channel Recording.* Plenum Press, New York.
60. Sakmann, B., and Neher, E. (1983): In: *Single-Channel Recording,* edited by B. Sakmann and E. Neher, pp. 37–51. Plenum Press, New York.

61. Sakmann, B., Patlak, J., and Neher, E. (1980): *Nature,* 286:71–73.
62. Scarborough, G. A. (1985): *Microbiol. Rev.,* 49:214–231.
63. Schwarz, W., and Passow, H. (1983): *Annu. Rev. Physiol.,* 45:359–374.
64. Shuster, M. J., Camardo, J. S., Siegelbaum, S. A., and Kandel, E. R. (1985): *Nature,* 313:392–395.
65. Siegelbaum, S. A., Camardo, J. S., and Kandel, E. R. (1982): *Nature,* 299:413–417.
66. Sine, S. M., and Steinbach, J. H. (1984): *Biophys. J.,* 45:175–185.
67. Smith, J. S., Coronado, R., and Meissner, G. (1985): *Nature,* 316:446–449.
68. Smith, T. G., Lecar, H., Redman, S. J., and Gage, P. W., eds. (1985): *Voltage and Patch Clamping with Microelectrodes.* American Physiological Society, Bethesda, MD.
69. Spruce, A. E., Standen, N. B., and Stanfield, P. R. (1985): *Nature,* 316:736–738.
70. Tanaka, J. C., Eccleston, J. F., and Barchi, R. L. (1983): *J. Biol. Chem.,* 258:7519–7526.
71. Trautmann, A. (1982): *Nature,* 298:272–275.
72. Trautmann, A., and Marty, A. (1984): *Proc. Natl. Acad. Sci. USA,* 81:611–615.
73. Vergara, C., and Latorre, R. (1983): *J. Gen. Physiol.,* 82:543–568.
74. Yellen, G. (1984): *J. Gen. Physiol.,* 84:157–186.

Psychopharmacology:
The Third Generation of Progress,
edited by Herbert Y. Meltzer.
Raven Press, New York © 1987.

CHAPTER 35

Excitotoxins

Joseph T. Coyle

In recent years, there has been a progressive increase in clinical and fundamental research into several disorders that lie at the interface between neurology and psychiatry, such as Alzheimer's disease (13), Huntington's disease (67), and temporal lobe epilepsy (49). All these disorders are characterized by damage to and degeneration of certain sets of neurons in brain and are often associated with psychiatric symptoms of clinical significance. In essence, these disorders might be considered experiments of nature that allow for heuristically useful correlations between selective neuronal loss and behavioral symptoms in humans. Furthermore, the rapid expansion in the identification of neurotransmitter systems in brain has led to the exploitation of postmortem synaptic neurochemical and immunocytochemical analyses to characterize the neurotransmitter systems affected in these disorders.

To understand better the role of neuronal systems affected by these neurodegenerative disorders, animal studies can prove quite helpful. However, the selective pattern of neuronal degeneration characteristic of these disorders is poorly reproduced in experimental animals with traditional lesion methods such as thermal coagulation or surgical extirpation. These techniques cause damage not only to the neurons of interest but also to axons of passage or of termination and nonneuronal elements that are located in the area. However, over the last decade, the excitotoxin lesion method has largely supplanted these nonspecific destructive lesions and has allowed for the development of a number of animal models of these neuropsychiatric disorders that have aided greatly in our understanding of their pathophysiology (15). This chapter will review the historical background, mechanisms of action, methodologic considerations, and practical application of the excitotoxin lesion technique.

HISTORICAL BACKGROUND

The excitotoxin lesion technique derived from observations originally made 30 years ago by Lucas and Newhouse (42) on the cytotoxic effects of systemically administered glutamic acid on the retina of neonatal mice. These investigators were examining the possible therapeutic effects of treatment with glutamic acid in preventing a hereditary degeneration of the neural retina. Contrary to their expectations, they found that administration of glutamic acid to the control neonatal mice caused an acute degeneration of the neurons in the inner layers of the retina. Subsequent studies revealed that not only retinal interneurons, but also neurons with cell bodies located in the arcuate nucleus of the hypothalamus and in the circumventricular organs, which lie outside the blood-brain barrier, were vulnerable to the neurotoxic effects of monosodium glutamate (MSG) systemically administered to the neonatal rodent (56).

Olney (57,58) carried out ultrastructural studies of the evolution of the MSG lesion in the mouse retina and arcuate nucleus and demonstrated that massive swelling of neuronal dendrites and perikarya represented the initial neuropathologic alterations. Notably, axons passing through arcuate or even terminating on affected neurons remained impervious to MSG. Glutamate and structurally related acidic amino acids had been shown to have potent neuroexcitatory effects (17,33) and to cause influx of sodium and water and efflux of potassium in cerebral cortical slices incubated *in vitro* (30). In a structural activity relation study in the arcuate nucleus of the neonatal rat, Olney et al. (60) demonstrated an excellent correlation between neuroexcitatory potency and neurotoxic effects of a large series of analogs of glutamate administered systemically. He concluded that the neurotoxic effects of these agents result from their depolarizing action, which caused influx of sodium and water into the dendrites bearing "glutamate" receptors. Since axons and terminal elements presumably do not possess these excitatory receptors, Olney reasoned that they were insensitive. Accordingly, he coined the term "excitotoxins" for these substances that appeared to kill neurons on the basis of their excitatory effects.

Neurophysiologists have identified a number of conformationally restricted or synthetic analogs structurally related to glutamate whose neuroexcitatory effects are much more potent than glutamate itself (Fig. 1). These substances include kainic acid, isolated from the seaweed *Digenea simplex* (72), ibotenic acid, isolated from the mushroom *Amanita muscaria* (34), quisqualic acid, isolated from the quisqualis nut of Laos (73), and the synthetic derivative, *N*-methyl-D-aspartic acid (NMDA). While it was initially thought that these analogs were merely potent agonists at the "glutamate receptor," recent studies have indicated that pharmacologically, neuroanatomically, and physiologically distinct receptors mediate their responses (24,85). These excitatory receptors have been separated into at least three subtypes designated on the basis of the most potent agonist, i.e., the kainate receptor, the quisqualate receptor, and the NMDA receptor.

Systemic treatment with excitotoxins to create brain lesions, with the exception of kainate, suffers from the obvious limitation that the lesions occur primarily in those few areas of the brain with a deficient blood-brain barrier; furthermore, neuronal vulnerability is relatively restricted to the early postnatal period. To produce precisely localized, perikaryal specific lesions, Coyle and Schwarcz (14) first described the neurotoxic consequences of direct infusion of the potent glutamate analog, kainic acid, in the rat striatum (Fig. 2). Neurochemical and histologic studies established that the injection of kainic acid caused a

selective degeneration of neurons with cell bodies intrinsic to the striatum but spared extrinsic axons passing through or terminating in the region (12). In subsequent studies, it was shown that several other potent excitatory analogs of glutamate also exhibited selective neuronal toxicity after direct intracranial injection (69,93). However, in keeping with current understanding of several excitatory amino acid receptor subtypes, it became apparent that the analogs, ibotenic acid, quisqualic acid, and NMDA, caused different patterns of neurotoxicity than kainic acid (89). Currently, the two most commonly used excitotoxins for *in situ* lesions in brain are kainic acid and ibotenic acid (15).

GLUTAMIC ACID

Perinatal systemic administration of MSG to rodents continues to be a widely exploited technique for lesioning neurons intrinsic to the arcuate nucleus of the hypothalamus (53). Although there is considerable variation among the treatment protocols utilized in different laboratories, there is little dispute that systemic administration of MSG causes a striking loss of neuronal perikarya within the arcuate nucleus of the hypothalamus of infant rodents. The lowest effective doses are in the range of 0.5 g/kg administered orally and 0.35 g/kg administered subcutaneously in 10-day-old mice. Maximal lesions are observed after doses of 2 to 5 g/kg repeated every 2 days for the first 10 days after birth; this paradigm causes an 80 to 90% destruction of all arcuate neuronal perikarya. Aside from the circumventricular organs and the cingulate cortex (64), extrahypothalamic brain regions appear to be largely unaffected by repeated administration of high doses of MSG.

Since the arcuate nucleus constitutes an essential center for modulating neuroendocrine function (87), it is not

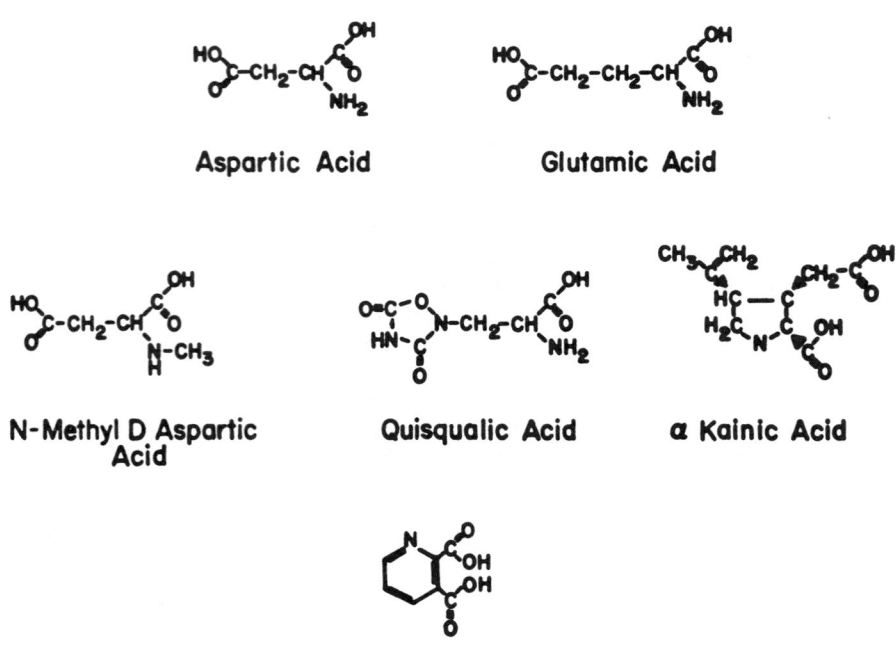

Aspartic Acid

Glutamic Acid

N-Methyl D Aspartic Acid

Quisqualic Acid

α Kainic Acid

Quinolinic Acid

FIG. 1. Structures of the major endogenous and exogenous excitotoxins.

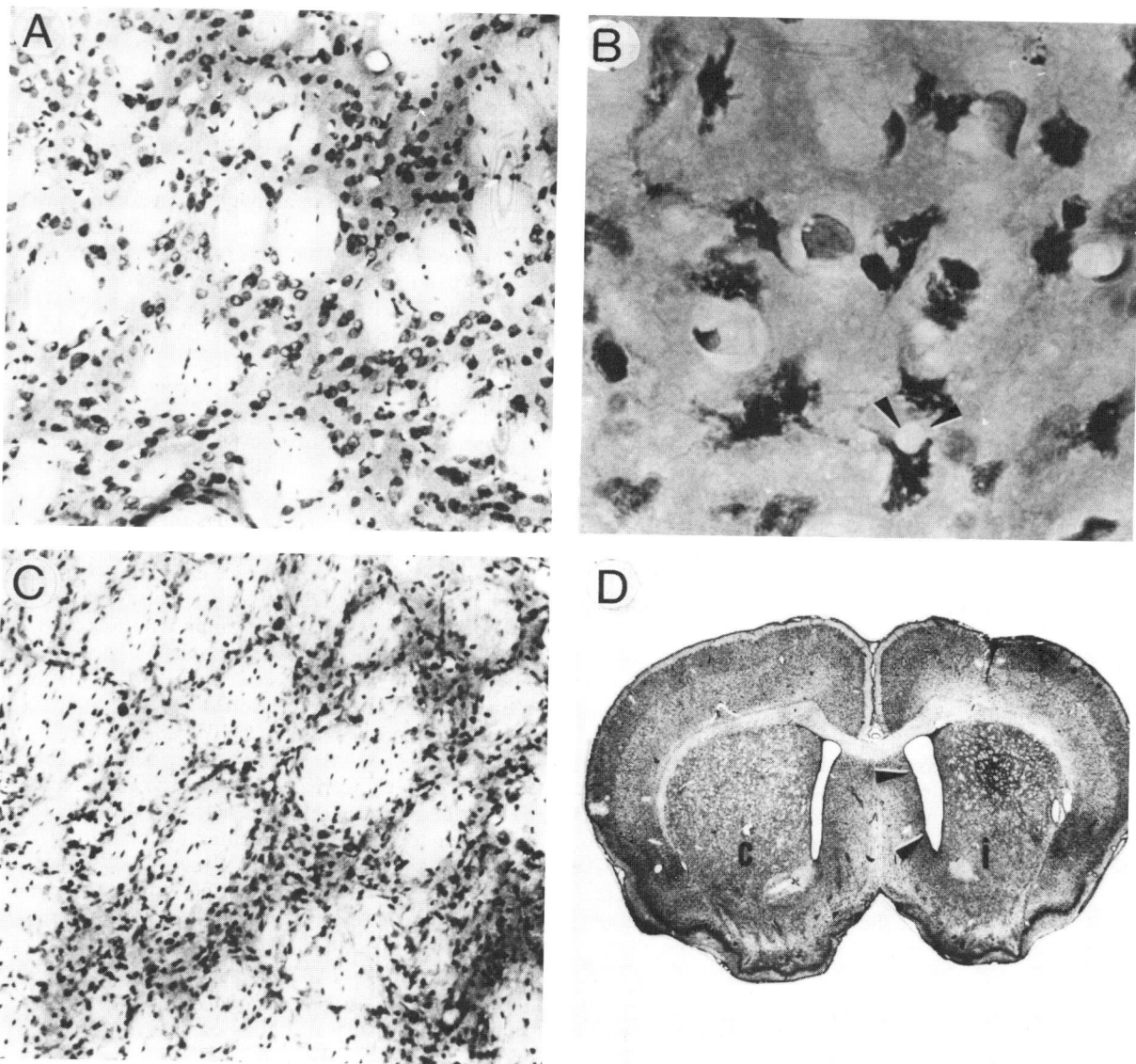

FIG. 2. Evolution of excitotoxin lesion after intrastriatal injection of kainic acid. **A:** Nissl-stained section through the normal rat striatum. Note the numerous small Golgi II neurons interspersed between the myelinated internal capsule fibers. **B:** Higher-power view of a Nissl-stained section 24 hr after intrastriatal injection of 2.3 nmol of kainic acid. Note the severe karyorrhexis of the neuronal nuclei and the floccular, edematous appearance of the neuropil. **C:** Nissl-stained section through the rat striatum (same magnification as in A) 10 days after 2.3 nmol kainate injection. Note the complete absence of neuronal perikarya and the striking astrocytic response that spares the internal capsule fibers. **D:** Low-power photomicrograph of the forebrain showing the kainate-injected (i) and control (c) striatum.

unexpected that destruction of the arcuate neurons would produce severe deficits in the function of various neuroendocrine systems. Adult animals treated with MSG during infancy are obese, stunted in linear growth, and sterile. Consistent with this, they exhibit reduced content of growth hormone and luteinizing hormone in the anterior pituitary (52,65), elevation of serum prolactin in males (54), increased plasma corticosterone levels (59), and hypothyroidism (19).

MSG lesions of the arcuate nucleus have been exploited to identify neuronal pathways that originate within the nucleus. With the use of MSG lesions, it was demonstrated that substantial portions of brain α-melanocyte-stimulating hormone (21), adrenocorticotropic hormone, β-lipotrophin, and β-endorphin (8,38) neuronal systems have their primary source in neuronal perikarya located within the arcuate nucleus. In contrast, the lesioned animals do not exhibit concomitant decrease of these peptide hormones in the pituitary, thus differentiating at least two different cellular populations. Furthermore, neurochemical analysis of MSG-induced lesions of the arcuate have demonstrated arcuate reductions in the levels of dopamine and in the specific activity of choline acetyltransferase, a marker for cholinergic neurons (53). Accordingly, MSG lesions have successfully been employed as a strategy to unravel hypothalamic microcircuitry and the involvement of specific neurotransmitter systems in neuroendocrine function.

The regulation of neurotransmitter and neurohormonal release in the arcuate nucleus has been addressed by acute, systemic treatment with subtoxic doses of glutamate or related excitatory amino acid analogs in adult rats (82). In accordance with the excitotoxin hypothesis, challenge doses of the acidic amino acids should excite those neurons which degenerate after treatment with large amounts of the excitotoxins because they bear the appropriate receptors. With the provocative paradigm, doses of the excitatory amino acid analogs, which are less than 25% of those causing cytotoxicity, are administered acutely and the alterations in serum levels of hormones are measured immediately afterwards. Elevations in serum luteinizing hormone, testosterone, and prolactin and decreases in serum growth hormone have been observed. Furthermore, Olney (59) has examined the effects of combined acute treatment with MSG and inhibitory amino acid neurotransmitters such as γ-aminobutyric acid (GABA) and taurine in examining controls of the hypothalamic-pituitary-gonadal axis.

KAINIC ACID

Kainic acid is a dicarboxyl-containing pyrrolydine that was isolated because of its ascaricidal properties from the seaweed, *Digenea simplex,* which grows off the coast of Japan. Neurophysiologic studies indicate that it is 30- to 100-fold more potent than glutamic acid as a neuronal excitant (5). Structural activity studies of the stereoisomers and analogs of α-kainic acid have revealed a remarkable degree of specificity for its effects (Table 1). The isopropylene

side chain, in particular, plays a critical role in its activity, since reduction of the double bond in dihydrokainic acid or reversal of its spatial orientation in α-allo-kainic acid markedly attenuates the neuroexcitatory effects. In contrast, domoic acid, which has a more extended side chain, is more potent than kainic acid. Blockade of the ring nitrogen by alkylation or esterification of the carboxyl groups also markedly attenuates the activity of the compound. α-Keto-kainate, which has a ketone group substituted for the methylene group, retains approximately 10% of the activity of the parent compound. Ligand binding studies with [3H]kainic acid have revealed receptor recognition sites on neuronal membranes in mammalian CNS with structural activity characteristics that correspond closely with those identified by the neurophysiologic studies (39). These sites, which can be divided into high-affinity and low-affinity components, exhibit an uneven regional and laminar distribution within the brain (83), and have a broad phylogenetic distribution (40). Since the excitatory effects of kainic acid are not antagonized by drugs that block the excitation produced by quisqualic acid or NMDA (84), it appears that kainic acid acts at a receptor distinctly different from those responsive to these other agonists.

The neurotoxic effects of kainic acid appear to be mediated by the same receptors responsible for its neuroexcitatory effects in mammalian neurons (74). Thus, structure-activity studies of the neurotoxic action indicate a close correlation between a neurophysiologic potency and the neurotoxic effects of analogs when injected into the rat striatum (69,90). Kainate lesions result in a marked reduction in the receptor sites labeled by [3H]kainate, consistent with their localization on vulnerable neurons (7,39). Furthermore, the development of neuronal vulnerability to locally injected kainic acid in the striatum coincides with the ontogenetic increase in the receptor binding sites of [3H]kainic acid (9). Recent autoradiographic studies suggest

TABLE 1. *Neurotoxic and electrophysiologic potency of kainate analogs in the striatum versus [3H]kainate receptor affinity*

Compound	K_I at KA receptor (nM)	Physiologic potency [X]/[Glu]	Toxic potency [X]/[KA]
Domoic acid	13[a]	36–109	1
α-Kainic acid	21	18–54	1
α-Keto kainic acid	430	≅10	40
α-Kainic acid diethylester	1,040	<1	≫50
Dihydrokainic acid	7,400[a]	0.06–0.8	≫50
α-Allo kainic acid	>10,000	0.5–2	50
L-Glutamic acid	722[a]	1	≫100
Quisqualic acid	610	22–90	>50 (est.)
Ibotenic acid	9,400	2–7	40
N-Methyl-D-aspartic acid	>10,000	4–12	120

Specific binding of [3H]kainic acid was performed in the rat cerebellum with displacement curves consisting of 10 or more concentrations of drug. Neurotoxicity was based on the reductions in the presynaptic markers for cholinergic and GABAergic neurons following stereotaxic injection into the rat corpus striatum (69,90). Physiologic potency is derived from the values for mammalian neurons of Biscoe et al. (5).

[a] Hill coefficient significantly less than 1.

that the density of kainate receptors correlates with neuronal sensitivity to its neurotoxic effects (25,83).

Kainic acid is disproportionately more potent as a neurotoxin than other glutamate analogs, which act at different receptors such as quisqualic acid and NMDA (90). This violation of the relationship between excitatory potency and neurotoxic effects across receptor agonists points to the unique feature of the neurotoxicity related to receptor activation. A striking aspect of the neurotoxic effects of kainic acid noted early on in its use was the marked variation in neuronal vulnerability (12,94). Certain neurons in close proximity to the injection site were spared, whereas other neurons, in some cases quite distant from the primary lesion, degenerated. Extreme examples are the CA3-4 pyramidal cells in the hippocampal formation, which degenerate in the rat after striatal injection of kainic acid (12), and the mesencephalic nucleus of nerve V, which is impervious to direct injection (10). This uneven neuronal vulnerability stands in contrast to a more uniform neurotoxic effect of analogs that interact with NMDA or quisqualate receptors (90).

Several studies have shown that prior ablation of major excitatory afferents eliminates or markedly attenuates the neurotoxic effects of kainic acid in several brain regions including the striatum (6,45), hippocampus (36), and optic tectum (81). For example, in the rat, decortication, which causes degeneration of the excitatory striatal afferents from cortex, protects against the neurotoxic effects of intrastriatally injected kainate. Notably, this lesion does not result in a marked reduction of density of [³H]kainate receptor sites in striatum (7), nor does it affect striatal neuronal sensitivity to the excitatory effects of iontophoretically applied kainic acid (46). Thus, there appears to be a dissociation between neuronal excitation and vulnerability to kainic acid, which indicates that excitation *per se* cannot entirely account for the neuronal degeneration induced by kainic acid.

An important feature of kainic acid is its striking convulsant properties. Systemic (61), intraventricular (51), or intracerebral (71) injection of kainic acid precipitates a prolonged episode of seizures with prominent limbic characteristics. The marked sensitivity of the rat to kainic acid-induced limbic seizures is associated with an unusual proclivity of the agent to cause degeneration of neurons within the hippocampus, amygdaloid nuclei, and pyriform cortex (3). Prior treatment with anticonvulsants such as diazepam and barbiturates that interfere with seizure spread markedly attenuates the neurotoxic action of kainic acid within the limbic system (92,93). These observations have led to the suggestion that the neurotoxic effects of kainic acid within the limbic system are a direct consequence of the persistent seizures. Nadler and colleagues have developed an impressive array of evidence supporting this hypothesis based on studies of the effects of selective lesions that transect component circuits in the limbic system, and lesions that prevent the propagation of seizures within the limbic system that interfere with the distant damage, especially that involving the particularly vulnerable CA3–4 pyramidal cells (50).

When considered *in toto,* these studies indicate that the mechanisms of neurotoxicity of kainic acid are complex

and probably indirect. Receptors responsive to kainic acid are an important determinant for neuronal vulnerability. The activity of excitatory afferents, many of which are thought to be glutamatergic, appears to modulate neuronal sensitivity in many areas. Kainic acid is metabolically rather inert and therefore capable of diffusing widely throughout the brain (94). Kainate's enhancement of excitatory neurotransmission at presynaptic (22) and postsynaptic (72) sites leads to seizures and increases neuronal vulnerability in distant areas to which it may diffuse; consequently, it is difficult to separate completely the "convulsant" effects of kainic acid from its direct action on vulnerable neurons. Neuronal degeneration precipitated by kainate is associated with an increase in glucose utilization (88), a depletion of high-energy phosphates (66), and accumulation of calcium (4). Whether these acute metabolic alterations are the proximate cause or a consequence of the neurodegenerative process remains unclear at present.

IBOTENIC ACID

Ibotenic acid, an isoxazole extracted from the mushroom *Amanita muscaria* (27), was the first of the heterocyclic amino acids whose neuroexcitatory properties were described (34). Although ibotenic acid contains only one carboxyl group, the hydroxyl group renders it sufficiently acidic to act as a potent excitant like other dicarboxylic amino acids. Nonenzymatic or enzymatic decarboxylation of ibotenic acid yields muscimol, a potent GABA agonist; this byproduct may account in part for reports of the inhibitory effects of ibotenate (55). In neurophysiologic studies, ibotenate has been characterized as an agonist at the NMDA receptor (47). Thus, the excitatory effects of ibotenate are blocked by the NMDA antagonists, α-amino-phosphono-valeric acid (APV) and α-amino-phosphono-heptanoic acid (APH) (80).

Although 20-fold less potent than kainate, the neurotoxic effects of ibotenate appear to be more direct, since they do not seem to be sensitive to prior deafferentation of the injected brain region. Thus, in the hippocampal formation, transection of the perforant pathway (37) or the fornix-fimbria (36), either of which protects the hippocampal granule cells from kainate, has no influence on ibotenic-induced degeneration of granule cells in the area dentata. Furthermore, ibotenate generally produces much more uniform lesions, affecting virtually all neurons within its circumference. Unlike kainate, ibotenate causes extensive lesions when injected into the striatum or hippocampal formation of the neonatal rat (78). Finally, in contrast to kainate, ibotenate exhibits a much lower propensity for causing seizures in doses within its neurotoxic range (1). The reason for this remains unclear because NMDA, which appears to act at the same receptor, produces striking seizures at doses associated with neurotoxic effects.

CLINICAL IMPLICATIONS OF EXCITOTOXINS

The investigation of the neurotoxic effects of striatal injection of kainic acid was prompted by the interest in the development of an animal model for Huntington's disease (HD). HD is a neurodegenerative disorder transmitted as an autosomal dominant which is characterized by psychiatric symptoms, a choreoathetotic movement disorder, and progressive dementia, which typically have their onset in midlife (67). The caudate and putamen bear the brunt of the neuropathology in HD with a progressive degeneration predominantly affecting the Golgi type II striatal neurons. Numerous neurochemical and histologic parallels have been demonstrated between the striatal kainate lesion in the experimental animal and HD (11). These include similar qualitative and quantitative reductions in pre- and postsynaptic markers for striatal cholinergic, GABAergic, and peptidergic neurons with the exception of somatostatin (2). Although the kainate-lesioned rat does not develop a choreiform movement disorder, rats with bilateral striatal kainate lesions exhibit abnormalities in locomotion (32), impairments in learning and memory (20), disruption of diurnal activity (43), weight loss (68), and altered sensitivity to dopaminergic drugs (44) that share features with the symptoms of HD. Notably, transplantation of fetal striatum into the kainate-lesioned adult striatum reverses certain behavioral impairments (18).

The striking parallels have raised the question whether excitotoxin mechanisms may play a fundamental role in the pathophysiology of HD. Postmortem studies have revealed significant losses of [³H]kainate and [³H]glutamate receptors in caudate and putamen, indicating that neurons enriched in these receptors are affected by the neuronal degeneration in HD (28,41). The antispastic agent baclofen, which acts at GABA$_B$ receptors, inhibits the evoked release of glutamate from glutamatergic terminals. In a prospective study, Shoulson (75) is determining whether prophylactic administration of baclofen retards the progression of the symptoms of HD by preventing excitotoxin-induced neuronal degeneration in the caudate-putamen.

The fact that compounds having excitotoxic effects act through receptors normally present in brain has raised the question whether excitotoxin mechanisms might be involved in the pathophysiology of a number of neurodegenerative disorders. Although glutamic acid and aspartic acid have been hypothesized to be the endogenous neurotransmitters that act upon these receptors, the neurotoxic effects of intracerebral injection of these two amino acids are extremely weak in the adult brain. This lack of potency presumably reflects the high activity of uptake and metabolic processes for the acidic amino acids located both on neuronal elements and on glia. Thus, Kohler and Schwarcz (35) have demonstrated that prior lesion of the glutamatergic afferents from the enterorhinal cortex to hippocampus results in the development of sensitivity of dentate granule cells to infused glutamate.

In this regard, cerebellar injection of kainic acid produces a selective pattern of neuronal degeneration that resembles the neuropathology of hereditary spinocerebellar degeneration (31). Plaitakis et al. (62) have found in one form of hereditary olivopontocerebellar (OPC) degeneration that the activity of the enzyme glutamine synthetase, which is involved in glutamate metabolism, is reduced in leukocytes of affected individuals. Serum glutamate levels are elevated and increase further upon an oral load with glutamate. The authors speculate that persistent and excessive stimulation of glutamate receptors might be responsible for the neuronal degeneration in OPC. Notably, elevations in serum glutamate have recently been described in another adult onset neurodegenerative disorder, amyotrophic lateral sclerosis (63).

Quinolinic acid, a metabolite of tryptophan in the synthesis pathway for nicotinic acid, has been shown to exert neuronal excitatory effect through activation of NMDA-type receptors (79). Schwarcz and his colleagues have demonstrated that intrastriatal injection of quinolinic acid produces perikaryal specific degeneration of striatal neurons that reproduces the histologic and neurochemical pathology of HD similar to kainate (70). Notably, like kainate, the neurotoxic effects of quinolinate require the integrity of excitatory afferents in the striatum and exhibit delayed maturational appearance. Unlike kainate, but consistent with the purported action of quinolinate at NMDA receptors, coadministration of the NMDA receptor antagonist APH acid, antagonizes the neurotoxic effects of quinolinate. Quinolinate is found in brain, where it has an uneven regional distribution, as does its catabolic enzyme (48). However, quinolinic acid phosphoribosyltranferase appears to be localized primarily in glia. As the levels of quinolinate and the activity of its degradative enzyme, quinolinic acid phosphoribosyl transferase, do not appear to be remarkably altered in HD, the etiologic role of quinolinate in the neurodegenerative process of HD remains unclear (26).

The aspects of excitotoxin mechanisms with the most direct clinical relevance concern the recent evidence of their role in selective neuronal degeneration associated with persistent seizures, hypoxemia, and hypoglycemia. As noted above, systemic or intracerebral injection of kainic acid produces a prolonged episode of seizures associated with selective degeneration of certain classes of limbic neurons, especially those in the CA3–4 pyramidal cells (51). Other types of persistent seizures produced by electrical stimulation (77) or pharmacologic treatment (29) by drugs not directly activating glutamate receptors also produce limbic neuronal degeneration. Notably, glutamate receptor antagonists exhibit powerful anticonvulsant properties in experimental models of epilepsy (16). Hypoxemia produces a delayed neuronal degeneration that evolves over several hours and is initially associated with dendritic and somal swelling similar to that seen with excitotoxin lesions. Local injection of APH in the hypoxemic area markedly reduces the extent of neuronal damage, suggesting that release of endogenous excitatory amino acid neurotransmitters activating NMDA receptors is critically involved in this phenomenon (76). Similarly, severe hypoglycemia is associated with extensive neuronal degeneration in brain. Weiloch (85) has demonstrated that prior removal of glutamatergic afferents or local injection of APH into the striatum markedly reduces the extent of neuronal damage associated with insulin-induced hypoglycemia (86). Taken together, the results of these studies suggest that endogenous substances, whose release is precipitated by persistent seizures, anoxia, and hypoglycemia, activate glutamate receptors and thereby precipitate an excitotoxin form of neuronal degeneration. These findings have important neuropsychopharmacologic implications, since they point to new therapeutic strategies

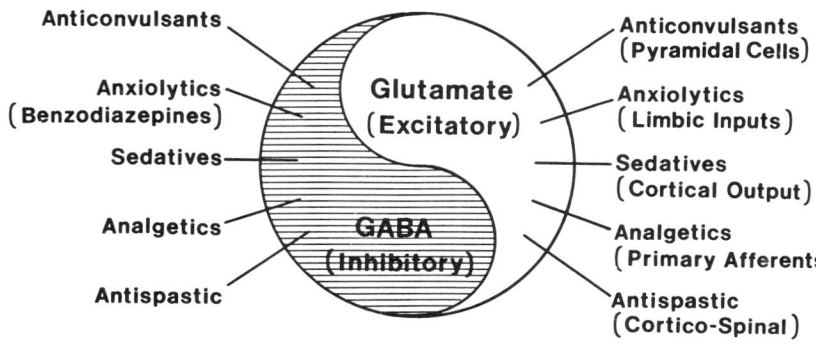

FIG. 3. Potential pharmacology of drugs inhibiting excitatory amino acid neurotransmission.

that could restrict neuronal damage resulting from status epilepticus, stroke-anoxia, and hypoglycemia.

CONCLUSIONS

The receptors responsible for the excitotoxic effects of NMDA, quisqualate, and kainate also serve as the primary mediators of excitatory neurotransmission in the brain. Whereas glutamate and aspartate are considered the endogenous neurotransmitters that act at these receptors, acidic peptides such as *N*-acetyl-aspartyl glutamate may also serve as endogenous agonists (23,91). These excitatory neuronal systems appear to be counterbalanced by the predominant inhibitory neurotransmitter, GABA. Ironically, the minor structural modification catalyzed by glutamate decarboxylase converts the major excitatory amino acid, glutamate, to the major inhibitory neurotransmitter, GABA. This Ying-Yang relationship between glutamate and GABA (Fig. 3) suggests that pharmacologic manipulations that inhibit glutamatergic neurotransmission may have effects analogous to those drugs that potentiate GABAergic neurotransmission. Thus, antagonists at the excitatory receptor subtypes may have therapeutic effects not only in preventing excitotoxin-mediated neurodegeneration but also as antiepileptics, analgetics, sedatives, and anxiolytics. Brain glutamatergic systems represent a relatively unexplored area of neuropsychopharmacology that promises to offer major therapeutic benefits in the next generation of psychopharmacologic drugs.

ACKNOWLEDGMENT

J.T.C. is the recipient of NIMH RSDA Type II MH-00125. The careful secretarial assistance of Alice Trawinski is gratefully acknowledged.

REFERENCES

1. Aldino, C., French, E. D., and Schwarcz, R. (1983): *Exp. Brain Res.,* 51:36–44.
2. Beal, M. F., Marshall, P. E., Bird, G. D., Landes, M. D., and Martin, J. B. (1985): *Brain Res.,* 361:135–145.
3. Ben-Ari, Y., Tremblay, E., and Ottersen, O. P. (1980): *Neuroscience,* 5:515–528.
4. Berdichevsky, E., Riveros, N., Sanchez-Armass, S., and Orrego, F. (1983): *Neurosci. Lett.,* 36:75–80.
5. Biscoe, T. J., Evans, R. H., Headley, P. M., Martin, M. R., and Watkins, J. C. (1976): *Br. J. Pharmacol.,* 58:373–382.
6. Biziere, K., and Coyle, J. T. (1978): *Neurosci. Lett.,* 8:303–310.
7. Biziere, K., and Coyle, J. T. (1979): *J. Neurosci. Res.,* 4:383–398.
8. Bodnar, R. J., Abrams, G. M., Zimmermann, E. A., Krieger, D. T., Nicholson, G., and Kizer, J. S. (1980): *Neuroendocrinology,* 30:280–284.
9. Campochiaro, P., and Coyle, J. T. (1978): *Proc. Natl. Acad. Sci. USA,* 75:2025–2029.
10. Colonnier, M., Geriade, M., and Landry, P. (1979): *Brain Res.,* 172:522–556.
11. Coyle, J. T., Ferkany, J. W., and Zaczek, R. (1983): *Neurobehav. Toxicol. Teratol.,* 5:617–624.
12. Coyle, J. T., Molliver, M. E., and Kuhar, M. J. (1978): *J. Comp. Neurol.,* 180:301–324.
13. Coyle, J. T., Price, D. L., and DeLong, M. R. (1983): *Science,* 219:1184–1190.
14. Coyle, J. T., and Schwarcz, R. (1976): *Nature,* 263:244–246.
15. Coyle, J. T., and Schwarcz, R. (1983): In: *Handbook of Chemical Neuroanatomy, Vol. 1: Methods in Chemical Neuroanatomy,* edited by A. Bjorklund and T. Hokfelt, pp. 508–527. Elsevier, New York.
16. Croucher, M. J., Collins, J. F., and Meldrum, B. S. (1982): *Science,* 216:899–901.
17. Curtis, D. R., and Watkins, J. C. (1963): *J. Physiol. (Lond.),* 166:1–14.
18. Deckel, A. W., Robinson, R. G., Coyle, J. T., and Sanberg, P. R. (1983): *Eur. J. Pharmacol.,* 93:287–288.
19. Dhindsa, K. S., Omran, R. G., and Bhup, R. (1981): *Acta. Anat.,* 109:97–102.
20. Divac, I., Markowitsch, H. J., and Pritzel, M. (1978): *Brain Res.,* 151:523–532.
21. Eskay, R. L., Brownstein, M. J., and Long, R. T. (1979): *Science,* 205:827–829.
22. Ferkany, J. W., Zaczek, R., and Coyle, J. T. (1982): *Nature,* 298:757–759.
23. ffrench-Mullen, J. M. H., Koller, K., Zaczek, R., Coyle, J. T., Hori, N., and Carpenter, D. O. (1985): *Proc. Natl. Acad. Sci. USA,* 82:3897–3900.
24. Foster, A. C., and Fagg, G. E. (1984): *Brain Res. Rev.,* 7:103–164.
25. Foster, A. C., Mena, E. E., Monaghan, D. T., and Cotman, C. W. (1981): *Nature,* 289:73–75.
26. Foster, A., Whetsell, W. O., Bird, E. D., and Schwarcz, R. (1985): *Brain Res.,* 336:207–214.
27. Good, R., Muller, G. F. R., and Eugster, C. H. (1965): *Helv. Chim. Acta,* 48:927–930.
28. Greenamyre, J. T., Penney, J. B., Young, A. B., D'Amato, C., Hicks, S. P., and Shoulson, I. (1985): *Science,* 227:1496–1499.
29. Griffiths, T., Evans, M. C., and Meldrum, B. S. (1984): *Neuroscience,* 12:557–567.
30. Harvey, J. A., and McIlwain, H. (1968): *Biochem. J.,* 108:269–274.
31. Herndon, R. M., and Coyle, J. T. (1977): *Science,* 198:71–72.
32. Hruska, R. E., and Silbergeld, E. K. (1979): *Life Sci.,* 25:181–194.

33. Johnston, G. A. R., Curtis, D. R., Davies, J., and McCulloch, R. N. (1974): *Nature,* 248:804–805.
34. Johnston, G. A. R., Curtis, D. R., DeGroat, W. C., and Duggan, A. W. (1968): *Biochem. Pharmacol.,* 17:2488–2489.
35. Kohler, C., and Schwarcz, R. (1981): *Brain Res.,* 211:485–491.
36. Kohler, C., Schwarcz, R., and Fuxe, K. (1979): *Brain Res.,* 175:366–371.
37. Kohler, C., Schwarcz, R., and Fuxe, K. (1979): *Neurosci. Lett.,* 15:223–228.
38. Krieger, D. T., Liotta, A. C., Nicholson, G., and Kizer, J. S. (1979): *Nature,* 278:562–563.
39. London, E. D., and Coyle, J. T. (1979): *Mol. Pharmacol.,* 15:492–505.
40. London, E. D., Klemm, N., and Coyle, J. T. (1980): *Brain Res.,* 192:463–476.
41. London, E. D., Yamamura, H. I., Bird, E. D., and Coyle, J. T. (1980): *Biol. Psychiatry,* 16:155–162.
42. Lucas, D. R., and Newhouse, J. P. (1957): *AMA Arch. Ophthalmol.,* 58:193–204.
43. Mason, S. T., and Fibiger, H. C. (1979): *Neuropharmacology,* 18:403–408.
44. Mason, S. T., Sanberg, P. R., and Fibiger, H. C. (1978): *Science,* 200:352–355.
45. McGeer, E. G., McGeer, P. L., and Singh, K. (1978): *Brain Res.,* 139:381–383.
46. McLennan, H. (1980): *Neurosci. Lett.,* 18:313–316.
47. McLennan, H., and Lodge, D. (1979): *Brain Res.,* 169:83–90.
48. Moroni, F., Lombardi, G., Carla, V., and Moniti, G. (1984): *Brain Res.,* 295:352–356.
49. Nadler, J. V. (1981): *Life Sci.,* 29:2031–2042.
50. Nadler, J. V., and Cuthbertson, G. J. (1980): *Brain Res.,* 195:47–56.
51. Nadler, J. V., Perry, B. W., and Cotman, C. W. (1978): *Nature,* 271:676–677.
52. Nagasawa, H., Yanai, R., and Kikuyama, S. (1974): *Acta Endocrinol.,* 75:249–259.
53. Nemeroff, C. B. (1981): In: *Nutrition and Behavior,* edited by S. A. Miller, pp. 177–211. Franklin Institute Press, Philadelphia.
54. Nemeroff, C. B., Grant, L. D., Bissette, G., Ervin, G. N., Harrell, L. E., and Prange, A. J., Jr. (1977): *Psychoneuroendocrinology,* 2:179–196.
55. Nielson, E. O., Schousboe, A., Hansen, S. H., and Krogsgaard-Larsen, P. (1985): *J. Neurochem.,* 45:725–731.
56. Olney, J. W. (1969): *Science,* 164:719–721.
57. Olney, J. W. (1969): *J. Neuropathol. Exp. Neurol.,* 28:455–474.
58. Olney, J. W. (1971): *J. Neuropathol. Exp. Neurol.,* 30:75–90.
59. Olney, J. W. (1979): In: *Glutamic Acid: Advances in Biochemistry and Physiology,* edited by L. J. Filer, Jr., S. Garattini, M. R. Kare, W. A. Reynolds, and R. J. Wurtman, pp. 287–319. Raven Press, New York.
60. Olney, J. W., Ho, O. L., and Rhee, V. (1971): *Exp. Brain Res.,* 14:61–76.
61. Olney, J. W., Rhee, V., and Ho, O. L. (1974): *Brain Res.,* 77:507–512.
62. Plaitakis, A., Berl, S., and Yahr, M. (1982): *Science,* 216:193–196.
63. Plaitakis, A., and Caroscio, J. T. (1985): *Ann. Neurol.,* 18:161.
64. Rascher, K. (1981): *Cell Tissue Res.,* 220:239–250.
65. Redding, T. W., Schally, A. V., Arimura, A., and Wakabayashi, I. (1971): *Neuroendocrinology,* 8:245–255.
66. Retz, K. C., and Coyle, J. T. (1982): *J. Neurochem.,* 38:196–203.
67. Sanberg, P. R., and Coyle, J. T. (1984): *CRC Crit. Rev. Clin. Neurobiol.,* 1:1–44.
68. Sanberg, P. R., and Fibiger, H. C. (1979): *Exp. Neurol.,* 66:444–466.
69. Schwarcz, R., Scholz, D., and Coyle, J. T. (1978): *Neuropharmacology,* 17:145–151.
70. Schwarcz, R., Whetsell, W. O., and Mangano, R. M. (1983): *Science,* 219:316–318.
71. Schwarcz, R., Zaczek, R., and Coyle, J. T. (1978): *Eur. J. Pharmacol.,* 50:209–220.
72. Shinozaki, H., and Konishi, S. (1970): *Brain Res.,* 24:368–371.
73. Shinozaki, H., and Shibuya, I. (1974): *Neuropharmacology,* 13:665–672.
74. Shinozaki, H., and Shibuya, I. (1974): *Neuropharmacology,* 13:1057–1065.
75. Shoulson, I. (1983): In: *Excitotoxins,* edited by K. Fuxe, P. Roberts, and R. Schwarcz, pp. 343–353. Macmillan, London.
76. Simon, R. P., Swan, J. H., Griffiths, T., and Meldrum, B. (1984): *Science,* 226:850–852.
77. Sloviter, R. S. (1983): *Brain Res. Bull.,* 10:675–697.
78. Steiner, H. X., McBean, G. J., Kohler, C., Roberts, P. J., and Schwarcz, R. (1984): *Brain Res.,* 307:117–124.
79. Stone, T. W., and Perkins, M. N. (1981): *Eur. J. Pharmacol.,* 72:411–412.
80. Stone, T. W., Perkins, M. N., Collins, J. F., and Curry, K. (1981): *Neuroscience,* 6:2249–2252.
81. Street, P., Stella, M., and Cuenod, M. (1980): *Brain Res.,* 187:47–57.
82. Terry, L. C., Epelbaum, J., Brazeau, P., and Marin, J. B. (1977): *Fed. Proc.,* 36:500.
83. Unnerstall, J. R., and Wamsley, J. K. (1983): *Eur. J. Pharmacol.,* 86:361–371.
84. Watkins, J. C., and Evans, R. H. (1981): *Annu. Rev. Pharmacol. Toxicol.,* 21:165–204.
85. Weiloch, T. (1985): *Science,* 228:681–683.
86. Weiloch, T., Engelsen, B., Westerberg, E., and Auer, R. (1985): *Neurosci. Lett.,* 56:25–32.
87. Weindl, A. (1973): In: *Frontiers in Neuroendocrinology,* edited by L. Martini and W. F. Ganong, pp. 1–32. Oxford University Press, London.
88. Wooten, G. F., and Collins, R. (1980): *Brain Res.,* 201:173–184.
89. Zaczek, R., Collins, J. F., and Coyle, J. T. (1981): *Neurosci. Lett.,* 24:181–186.
90. Zaczek, R., and Coyle, J. T. (1982): *Neuropharmacology,* 21:15–26.
91. Zaczek, R., Koller, K., Cotter, R., Heller, D., and Coyle, J. T. (1983): *Proc. Natl. Acad. Sci. USA,* 80:1116–1119.
92. Zaczek, R., Nelson, M., and Coyle, J. T. (1978): *Eur. J. Pharmacol.,* 52:323–327.
93. Zaczek, R., Nelson, M., and Coyle, J. T. (1981): *Neuropharmacology,* 20:183–199.
94. Zaczek, R., Simonton, S., and Coyle, J. T. (1980): *J. Neuropathol. Exp. Neurol.,* 39:245–264.

Psychopharmacology:
The Third Generation of Progress,
edited by Herbert Y. Meltzer.
Raven Press, New York © 1987.

CHAPTER **36**

Ethylcholine Aziridinium (AF64A; ECMA) and Other Potential Cholinergic Neuron-Specific Neurotoxins

Israel Hanin, Abraham Fisher, Heide Hörtnagl, Steven M. Leventer, Pamela E. Potter, and Thomas J. Walsh

GENERAL OVERVIEW

As information has been generated over the years demonstrating the importance of specific neurotransmitters in the etiology of various neuropsychiatric diseases, there has been a concurrent surge of interest in developing and/or identifying neurotoxins, which could be used to ablate, selectively, particular neurotransmitter systems *in vivo.*

Such agents would be extremely valuable on two levels. On the one hand they could be used to mimic specific neurotransmitter deficits shown to occur in certain disease states [e.g., dopamine in Parkinson's disease; acetylcholine (ACh) in Alzheimer's disease], and thus attempt to reproduce the biochemical abnormality. In this case, the neurotoxin-treated animal might serve as an animal model of a disease state, provided that the animal also exhibits the behavioral correlates of the disease being mimicked. Such a model could be used in the search for new therapeutic approaches that could ultimately be applied in the clinic.

Second, neuron-specific neurotoxic agents could serve as chemical probes for the study of basic mechanisms pertaining to the synthesis and metabolism of the affected neurotransmitter system, *in vivo.* Moreover, they could give valuable insight into changes occurring in the intact animal, subsequent to destruction of an endogenous neurotransmitter system. This information would be extremely important for understanding regulatory factors occurring *in vivo,* and could provide information relevant for appropriate therapeutic strategies.

Available Neurotoxins for Various Neurotransmitter Systems

A number of neurotoxins that are selective for particular neurotransmitter systems are presently available. These compounds all bear a striking structural resemblance to the neurotransmitter substances that they affect. Thus, 6-hydroxydopamine (6HDA) is structurally analogous to norepinephrine (NE) and dopamine (DA); 5,7-dihydroxytryptamine (5,7-DHT) structurally resembles 5-hydroxytryptamine (5-HT), etc. It would appear that this structural resemblance is necessary for the selectivity of action of these compounds for specific neurotransmitters; conceivably the nerve terminal selectively attracts/accumulates the neurotoxin because of this structural similarity. Once the substance is sequestered at the nerve terminal, it induces its neurotoxicity at this site.

Available Cholinergic Neurotoxins

There has long been a need for a specific cholinergic neurotoxin, for several reasons. On the one hand, a neurotoxin that would induce a selective cholinergic hypofunction might conceivably be utilized to develop an animal model of Alzheimer's disease, a devastating illness in which a cholinergic hypofunction has been implicated (6,8,16, 18,19,24,27,38,60,65,73,77,78). On the other hand, access to a selective cholinergic neurotoxin would provide a useful tool with which one could selectively perturb the cholinergic system *in vivo,* and study the consequences of such perturbation at the level of the neuron, the organ system, and the entire animal.

Under normal circumstances the rate of neuronal metabolism and turnover of ACh is extremely rapid—much faster than any of the other known neurotransmitters. As a result, the cholinergic system generally is highly resistant to insult. For this reason, studies of events at the cholinergic nerve terminal have been difficult, particularly when conducted in the intact mammalian system. Available pharmacological agents that have been able to perturb the cholinergic system *in vivo,* whether as agonists (e.g., cholinesterase inhibitors, pilocarpine, arecoline, oxotremorine, etc.) or antagonists (e.g., atropinic agents, hemicholinium-3, etc.), have a limited period of action (hours or fractions thereof). Such agents have been useful as tools in evaluating acute responses and changes at the cholinergic nerve terminal. However, when one wants to study the consequence of long-term cholinergic perturbation *in vivo,* these agents are of less use. A long-acting neurotoxin would be extremely valuable for this purpose. Furthermore, it could simulate the condition believed to exist in the case of Alzheimer's disease, i.e., a long-term, persistent cholinergic hypofunction in the central nervous system.

Several agents have been referred to as "cholinergic neurotoxins" in the past. Primarily these are high-molecular-weight compounds (8,000–150,000), usually polypeptide in structure, which are extracted from different nonmammalian species, including bacteria (*Botulinum* toxin, tetanus toxin), snakes (α-bungarotoxin, notexin, α-cobratoxin, etc.), arachnids (black widow spider venom, scorpion venom), and others (32).

Generally, the molecular mechanism of action of these substances is not well understood, although it has been suggested that they affect both storage and release of ACh as well as other neurotransmitters. Moreover, some of these neurotoxins also are known to act at receptor (nicotinic) sites. Although they exert anticholinergic action, they are not selective for the cholinergic system; other neurotransmitter systems are also affected. In addition, their effect is generally not permanent.

These toxins, therefore, do not qualify as selective cholinotoxins, which could be used to induce an irreversible perturbation of the central cholinergic system *in vivo.* Ethylcholine mustard aziridinium (see chemical structures below), on the other hand, does appear to fulfill many of the essential requirements for such a cholinotoxic substance.

The next section of this chapter will deal with our current information (as of February 1986) regarding the mode of action of this compound *in vivo.*

ETHYLCHOLINE MUSTARD AZIRIDINIUM (AF64A; ECMA)

Rationale for Structure of the Compound

The catecholamine- and indoleamine-specific neurotoxins are structurally similar to the neurotransmitters that they

FIG. 1. Structures of AF64A and choline.

affect. Taking a cue from this phenomenon, we sought to induce selective cholinotoxicity *in vivo* using a cytotoxic structural analog of choline. It occurred to us that an aziridinium analog of choline might be appropriate for this purpose, due to the known cytotoxic properties of the aziridinium moiety. Theoretically, the cholinergic nerve terminal would not distinguish between this substance and endogenous choline, and would accumulate the cytotoxic agent *in vivo.* Once in the nerve terminal, the substance would exert its cytotoxic action, and thus destroy the cholinergic terminal from within.

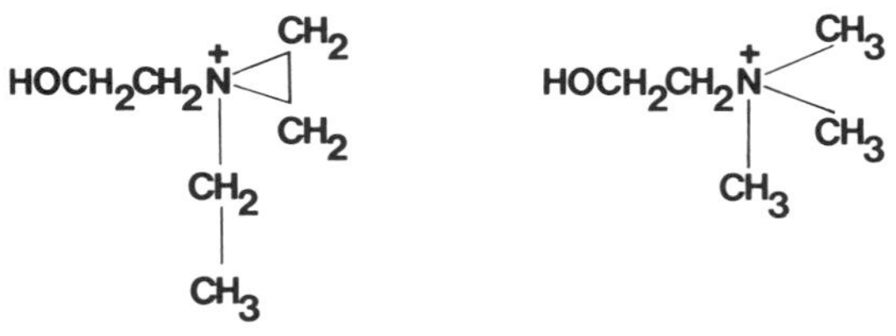

When we set out to conduct these studies in 1980, we were encouraged by earlier reports from the laboratories of Dr. Colhoun and his coinvestigators (15,67) demonstrating, *in vitro,* that several aziridinium analogs of choline are potent inhibitors of the high-affinity uptake of choline (HAChT), the step in the synthetic cycle believed to be rate limiting for the synthesis of ACh (25,34,40,41). Utilizing Dreiding models it appeared to us that the ethylcholine aziridinium compound would be closer in three-dimensional structure to choline than the methyl analog (21), and hence would conceivably be more accessible to choline binding and uptake sites at the cholinergic nerve terminal. We consequently set out to synthesize and test this compound, designated as AF64A, in experimental animals *in vivo.*

Overview of Findings to Date

The data have been classified according to specific experimental disciplines that have been used to study AF64A action, namely, neurotransmitter-related, neurochemical, electrophysiological, neuroanatomic, and behavioral studies. This is followed by some general statements critically evaluating our current overall understanding of the mode of action of AF64A, and suggesting further avenues of investigation.

Neurotransmitter-Related Effects

The consequence of AF64A treatment *in vivo* has been evaluated on a number of neurotransmitter systems, although the bulk of this work has focused on cholinergic mechanisms. The following will be an overview of the effects of AF64A on specific central nervous system neurotransmitters. Neurotransmitter and precursor as well as metabolite levels, uptake and release of precursors and products, activity of enzymes for synthesis and degradation of the neurotransmitters, and turnover of the neurotransmitter substances will be described.

Acetylcholine and choline. AF64A treatment *in vivo* attenuates cholinergic function. This conclusion is based on data obtained employing a number of diverse neurochemical approaches, following intracerebral (into specific brain areas, e.g., hippocampus, striatum, substantia nigra, nucleus basalis of Meynert, etc.) or intraventricular (icv) administration of AF64A. Specifically, AF64A treatment in rats results in a significant reduction in (a) ACh levels (7,23,33,43,48,54,64,83), (b) choline acetyltransferase (ChAT) activity (1,4,7,13,23,43,50,62,69,81), (c) acetylcholinesterase (AChE) activity (2,43), (d) HAChT (23,48,50), and (e) ACh release from hippocampal slices (43,44,64). These effects are dose dependent, take some time (2–3 days) to develop, reach a plateau (about 7 days after initial treatment with a single dose of the substance; 43), and are long lasting (some of these effects persist up to a year; the longest time period studied to date in rats; 44).

These observations conclusively indicate a reduction in function of cholinergic nerve terminals. They do not tell us, however, whether the reduction is due to diminution of function, or actual destruction of nerve terminals. For an answer to this question one must employ neuroanatomic techniques of investigation (see below).

Levels of choline, the precursor of ACh, are not altered following administration of doses of AF64A necessary to induce the cholinergic hypofunction described above (23,83). Also, AF64A does not appear to have any significant effect on muscarinic receptor binding, either *in vivo* (23,80) or *in vitro* (28). An *in vivo* study in rats injected icv with AF64A (3 nmol per side; 7 or 21 days) indicated that such treatment had no effect on high-affinity binding of either quinuclidinyl benzilate, cis-methyl-dioxolane, or pirenzepine, all selective probes of muscarinic binding sites, in several brain regions of the AF64A-treated rats. In the same tissues, however, radiolabeled hemicholinium binding was significantly reduced, implying that HAChT is indeed selectively inhibited in the AF64A-treated animal (83). *In vitro,* on the other hand, some selectivity of action for AF64A was shown vis-a-vis M_1 (pirenzepine sensitive) as opposed to M_2 (quinuclidinyl benzilate sensitive) binding sites in cerebral cortex (28). However, extremely high doses of the substance had to be employed in order to achieve such inhibition, as compared with oxotremorine.

Since the cholinergic system interacts with other neurotransmitter systems *in vivo,* these other systems might also be perturbed, secondary to the cholinergic hypofunction induced by AF64A. Our most recent findings suggest that this is the case (31,64). These findings will be described in the narrative which follows on other neurotransmitter systems. Alternatively, AF64A might have a direct toxic action on these other neurotransmitter systems in a nonspecific manner. Indeed, some investigators have suggested that AF64A has a nonselective effect on noncholinergic neurotransmitter systems *in vivo* (3,33,45,75,81). Cholinoselective doses of AF64A to be used for administration into particular brain regions have yet to be determined in a careful, dose-dependent manner. This issue is discussed further in Practical Considerations of AF64A Lesions.

Dopamine. When AF64A was administered icv, in doses up to 5 nmol per ventricle, we observed a transient effect on dopaminergic mechanisms in the striatum. Levels of both DA and its biometabolites, dihydroxyphenylacetic acid (DOPAC) and homovanillic acid (HVA), were reduced at 4 days following AF64A administration. The levels returned to normal by 7 days post-AF64A (31). We believe that this effect is secondary to that of AF64A on the cholinergic system.

When AF64A was administered directly into selected brain areas, it became apparent that there is a variable sensitivity to AF64A in different brain areas. Thus, intrastriatal administration of up to 8 nmol AF64A, while significantly lowering ChAT activity, had only a transient effect on tyrosine hydroxylase (TH) activity, and on DA levels or uptake in this brain region (70). On the other hand, doses of only 0.02 and 0.2 nmol AF64A, administered in the nucleus basalis of Meynert in rats, resulted in a significant reduction in ChAT activity in the ipsilateral cortex, with no effect on DA (and 5-HT) levels in this same brain region (1). Fourteen days following administration of 3 nmol AF64A directly into the substantia nigra, however, striatal DA levels were found to be reduced by 50% (45). It should be noted in the latter case, however, that extensive damage was also found to be present at the site of injection of AF64A, suggesting that the effects observed were probably nonspecific, due to administration of too high a dose of the neurotoxic compound.

Norepinephrine. The effect of AF64A administration on central adrenergic mechanisms is similar to that shown for DA; namely, it is minimal, at doses that exert significant effects on the cholinergic system. As was the case with DA, icv doses of up to 2 nmol AF64A, bilaterally, caused transient reductions of NE (at 4 days) in hippocampus and cortex. By 7 days, NE levels had returned to normal. The reductions in hippocampal and cortical NE levels were longer lasting following bilateral icv treatments with either 3 or 5 nmol AF64A. However, they too were transient and eventually returned to normal within 2 to 4 weeks (31). In fact, up to 15 nmol AF64A has been administered icv to rats, bilaterally, with no apparent effect on NE levels 3 months later, although significant depletions in cholinergic markers in the same brain regions of these experimental animals still remained (83).

GABA. The effect of AF64A treatment on γ-aminobutyric acid (GABA) mechanisms has also been explored by several investigators. In the study described above for DA, in which up to 8 nmol AF64A was administered directly into the striatum, there was only a minimal and transient effect of the compound on striatal activity of glutamate decarboxylase (GAD), the enzyme necessary for GABA synthesis. Moreover, GABA levels and uptake were not affected in striatal synaptosomes (70). On the other hand, when AF64A was administered directly into the interpeduncular nucleus (at doses of 1–30 nmol), there was a reduction of GAD activity and of synaptosomal GABA uptake in the interpeduncular nucleus, within 24 hr, even at the 1 nmol dose level (81). This effect returned to normal by 2 days post-AF64A administration while ChAT levels still remained significantly attenuated. Whether or not this transient effect of AF64A on GAD activity and synaptosomal GABA uptake is secondary to the concurrently observed reduction in ChAT activity in the same tissue, and whether in the long term the effect on ChAT is reversible, still has to be determined.

Serotonin. Following bilateral icv injections of AF64A to rats, at doses ≥2 nmol per ventricle, we observed a reduction in levels of 5-HT and an elevation of its biometabolite 5HIAA, in hippocampus, hypothalamus, and cortex. The effect was maximal around 7 days after treatment, and then began to recover toward normal. Turnover of 5-HT, as reflected in the ratio of 5-hydroxyindoleacetic acid (5HIAA)/5-HT levels, was increased when compared to controls, suggesting that the activity of serotonergic neurons was increased secondary to removal of inhibitory cholinergic input. The effect was dose dependent (to date we have tested doses between 1 and 10 nmol per side). The parameters measured approached, but did not actually reach normal levels by 28 days postinjection in animals treated with ≥2 nmol AF64A (31). In another study, however (after 120 days), 5-HT and 5HIAA levels were normal, even after pretreatment with a much higher icv dose of the compound (15 nmol AF64A, bilaterally), indicating a recovery of serotonergic function, whereas hippocampal as well as cortical levels of ACh were still significantly lower than normal in the same brain regions (83).

Administration of AF64A into the dorsal hippocampus (2 nmol, 5 days; ref. 50) or into the nucleus basalis of Meynert (0.02 and 0.2 nmol, 7 and 14 days; ref. 1) had no effect on 5-HT uptake in the hippocampus or on 5-HT levels in the ipsilateral cortex, respectively.

It would appear from these findings that the serotonergic system is more susceptible to the effects of AF64A administration than are the other neurotransmitter systems mentioned. However, while the perotonergic system eventually recovers from the initial effect of AF64A administration, the cholinergic mechanism remains attenuated.

Other neurotransmitters. To our knowledge, only the above neurotransmitter systems have been investigated in AF64A-related studies. It would be most interesting to evaluate the effect of AF64A administration on other putative neurotransmitter substances that may interact with the cholinergic system *in vivo,* for example, somatostatin, polypeptides, excitatory amino acids, and various enkephalinergic systems. Hopefully these will be the subject of future investigations.

Neurochemical Effects

A number of studies have dealt with the neurochemical consequences of AF64A treatment *in vitro.* The effect of AF64A has been studied on the high-affinity system for choline transport into the nerve terminal and on various enzymes relevant to neuronal function *in vivo,* including ChAT, the enzyme responsible for the synthesis of ACh.

High-affinity transport of choline. Using rat forebrain synaptosomes *in vitro,* Rylett and Colhoun have shown that a number of mustard analogs of choline, including the ethylcholine mustard (=AF64A) will inhibit, selectively, the high-affinity transport system for choline (67). This effect was shown to be due to alkylation of the uptake system. The inhibition, in their hands, was irreversible for some of the analogs tested, but not for AF64A.

Curti and Marchbanks have studied the same question, using guinea pig cortical synaptosomes (17). According to their findings, both choline influx and choline efflux are inhibited by AF64A. This effect is competitively inhibited by pretreatment with choline or hemicholinium-3, probably due to interaction of these compounds at the same site as that affected by AF64A. Finally, kinetic studies indicated that the rate of inhibition of the high-affinity transport system for choline is dose dependent. It is a first-order reaction with the choline carrier at low concentrations (5–500 μM) of AF64A, but apparently is due to translocation of the choline carrier to an outward-facing conformation at higher concentrations of AF64A (>2 mM), hence inhibiting inward choline transport into the synaptosomes.

Choline acetyltransferase. ChAT is quite resistant to AF64A treatment. Millimolar doses of the toxin are necessary to inhibit ChAT activity *in vitro* (5,23). The reported reduction of ChAT activity *in vivo* (1,4,7,13,23, 43,50,62,69,81) thus is probably secondary to a possible neuron-destructive effect of AF64A, via some other mechanism. AF64A is, however, acetylated by ChAT (apparent $K_m = 5.1$ mM; ref. 49) to a cholinesterase-degradable product. It is possible, then, that AF64A may be converted to a neurotoxic false transmitter in the cholinergic nerve terminal.

Other enzymes. AF64A is a potent inhibitor of several choline-related enzymes, when these are studied in partially purified form. The list includes choline dehydrogenase (5), choline kinase, and AChE (72). Under identical conditions AF64A treatment (100 μM, 30 min at 37°C) had minimal effect on enzymes that are not choline related, e.g., lactate dehydrogenase, chymotrypsinogen, carboxypeptidase A, and alcohol dehydrogenase (72).

Key phospholipids, including phosphatidylcholine, phosphatidylethanolamine, and phosphatidylserine were also decreased in cell culture (neuroblastoma × glioma hybrid cell line NG-108-15), following exposure of the cells to 50 μM AF64A for 24 hr (71,72). Pretreatment with choline reduced this effect of AF64A on phospholipid concentration.

Electrophysiological Effects

Electrophysiological studies at the intact animal level, as well as at the level of the isolated muscle, are beginning to reveal some interesting findings regarding possible mechanisms and sites of AF64A action *in vivo.*

In the anesthetized cat superior cervical ganglion-nictitating membrane preparation, the site of action of AF64A was localized to the presynaptic cholinergic portion of the ganglion, following intracarotid administration of the toxin (47). Moreover, this treatment led to a progressive depression of electrically stimulated impulse transmission at the neuromuscular junction of the tongue, which was more pronounced at higher frequencies, implying progressive depletion of the ACh available for release. Adrenergic transmission was unaffected in the same preparation.

A presynaptic site of action for AF64A at the cholinergic nerve terminal has also been supported by the findings of McArdle and coinvestigators, utilizing the soleus nerve-muscle preparation from mice treated with AF64A (52). In this study AF64A treatment caused a marked reduction in frequency of miniature endplate potentials and in amplitude of endplate potentials, but not in the amplitude of the miniature endplate potentials. The results imply a reduction in the number of quanta released in response to a nerve action potential. This effect was reversed following treatment with the potassium channel blocker 3,4-diaminopyridine, suggesting to the authors that the effect of AF64A is presynaptic, via disruption of the ionic process underlying transmitter release.

AF64A treatment (20 nmol, icv) also affected generalized electrophysiological sleep patterns in rats. Three months posttreatment the toxin induced in young animals a sleep profile similar to that seen in aged rats (>30 months). Treated animals had longer rapid eye movement (REM) latencies, shorter sleep times, and a higher proportion of slow-wave sleep (42). The significance of these observations is yet to be established.

Neuroanatomic Effects

Several reports on neuroanatomic studies with AF64A have recently appeared, with variable results. AF64A treatment, in some cases, has been shown to exert a selective action on cholinergic neurons, with minimal concurrent "nonspecific" tissue destruction (7,26,36,54,58,69). In other reports AF64A has been shown to actually induce lesions in the brain, at the site of administration (3,33,45,75,76). Because of this discrepancy, some discordance exists in the literature with regard to the selectivity of action of AF64A at cholinergic nerve terminals.

A review of the literature illustrates this assertion. For example, it has been reported that the icv dose of AF64A that will induce an apparently selective cholinergic deficiency, without concurrent gross nonspecific tissue damage at or around the site of drug administration is ≤3 nmol bilaterally (36), or ≤5 nmol unilaterally (26). On the other hand, 1.5 nmol AF64A, administered icv, was demonstrated, in one investigator's hands (33), to produce nonspecific tissue destruction. Similarly, 8 nmol of AF64A, administered directly into the striatum (69), 2 ng into the substantia nigra (54), 1 nmol into the dorsal hippocampus (7), and 0.1 nmol into the nucleus basalis of Meynert (53) have been reported to produce a cholinergic deficiency, and only small and insignificant lesions at or around the site of AF64A injection. On the other hand, other investigators have found tissue degenerative effects of AF64A administration following its administration at a dose of 1 nmol in the striatum (76), 3 nmol in the substantia nigra (45), 1 nmol in the medial septum (75), and 0.073 nmol in the substantia innominata/medial globus pallidus (3).

This discordance may be partially attributed to questions of purity of the starting material (acetoxy-ethylcholine mustard) used to prepare the AF64A solution and in the method of preparing the aziridinium analog from the mustard (see extensive discussion of these points by Fisher and Hanin, ref. 22). However, even when the purest compound is prepared and used, one must be extremely cautious about the dose of substance employed. AF64A is a cytotoxic agent by virtue of its aziridinium moiety. As such, it would be expected to inflict damage to membranes and tissues, when administered at too high a dose, or in too concentrated a solution at a particular locus of action. Moreover, one must be aware of the possibility that toxicity due to AF64A may be different at different loci in the brain. Hence, as illustrated above, an "effective" concentration at one site may not be appropriate at another locus in the central nervous system.

More extensive studies, utilizing concurrent neurochemical, neuroanatomic, and behavioral studies in the same animals, should yield valuable insight into the question and extent of cholinotoxicity induced by AF64A.

Behavioral Effects

The integrity of the cholinergic system has been shown to be essential for memory. Pharmacological manipulations that alter central cholinergic activity have also been shown to affect the capacity to remember and to learn. Thus, atropine has been shown to induce memory deficits in normal subjects (20). On the other hand, the cholinesterase inhibitor physostigmine has been shown, in some cases, to improve memory function in patients with Alzheimer's disease (57,78, but see 12,35,84). Based on this information, plus the fact that Alzheimer's disease has been associated strongly with a central cholinergic deficit (6,8,16,18, 19,24,27,60,65,73,77), we and others have studied the effect of AF64A treatment in rats on subsequent memory and learning capacity.

A variety of behavioral tests have been employed in animals treated with AF64A. In general, a deficit in cognitive function has been observed. However, whether or not this effect is due to a selective cholinotoxicity induced by AF64A is still being debated in the literature. Here again, for the same reasons mentioned above with regard to the large range of doses used, the results must be interpreted with caution, taking doses and site of AF64A administration into account. The following summarizes behavioral consequences of AF64A administration in different sites in the brain.

Icv administration. Various doses of AF64A have been employed in these studies, using both rats and mice. The results obtained will be summarized separately below, according to the species used.

Rats. Walsh and coinvestigators (83), in their earlier studies, administered 7.5 and 15 nmol AF64A, bilaterally, to their experimental animals. Subsequently, however, they have employed a lower (3 nmol per side) dose, with essentially similar results (82). Jarrard et al. (33) have employed 1.5 or 3 nmol, bilaterally. Brandeis and coinvestigators (9) have administered either 3 or 5 nmol AF64A, bilaterally, and Casamenti and coinvestigators (13) have used 32 nmol AF64A, unilaterally administered.

In all four laboratories, rats were shown to exhibit decrements in performance in the step-through passive avoidance task. Jarrard, Walsh, and Brandeis and their respective coinvestigators also conducted studies using the eight-arm radial maze paradigm.

According to Jarrard et al., complex place and cue tasks indicated that injected animals were impaired in reference memory only on the place task, but working memory was impaired on both tasks. However, Jarrard's group claims that their results are comparable to those seen following fimbria-fornix lesions. Since some degeneration of the fimbria-fornix area was evident in their AF64A-treated rats, they claim that the results are due to nonspecific destructive effects of AF64A. It should be noted, however, that neurochemical studies in these same animals showed a selective cholinotoxicity, with no effect on NE or DA levels in the hippocampus and striatum, respectively.

Walsh's studies indicated that AF64A treatment resulted in impaired performance in a delayed match-to-nonsample task that required the explicit use of working memory. Neurochemical analyses indicated a selective decrease in ACh levels, with no concurrent effect on concentrations of catecholamines, indolamines, their metabolites, or choline, in various brain regions. In these same rats, histological analysis revealed that AF64A did not damage the hippocampus, fimbria-fornix, septum, or caudate nucleus.

Brandeis and her coinvestigators also found a significant impairment in radial arm maze performance in AF64A-treated rats. Interestingly, pretreatment with the cholinesterase inhibitor physostigmine (0.1 mg/kg intraperitoneally, 15 min prior to testing) did not improve performance of rats in this test, although it improved significantly their response in the passive avoidance paradigm, at an intraperitoneal dose of 0.06 mg/kg. Careful optimization of the dose will be attempted in order to explore this further.

Brandeis et al. have also tested their rats in the Morris water maze test. Again, the AF64A-treated animals showed longer escape latencies than the controls, indicating an impairment in memory of the AF64A-treated rats. Physostigmine pretreatment caused a tendency toward improvement, although this effect was not statistically significant. These results were not due to any inhibitory effect on the animal's mobility, since motility measures in these animals showed no differences in open field behavior between AF64A-treated and control rats.

Mice. Caulfield and coinvestigators (14) have administered 0.5 nmol ECMA, whereas Pope et al. (62) have used 30 nmol in their mice. In both studies the toxin was injected unilaterally, icv.

Pope and coinvestigators noted a significant retention deficit in one-trial passive avoidance retention, 21 days following treatment with the toxin. Caulfield et al., on the other hand, did not observe any clear effects of drug treatment on passive avoidance learning, 7 days posttraining, at subtoxic (≤1.5 nmol) doses of the compound.

Intrastriatal administration. Sandberg and her coinvestigators have explored the consequences of AF64A administration directly into the striatum of rats (8 nmol, bilaterally administered; ref. 70). At least 5 weeks after surgery, these investigators found a significant impairment in acquisition of retention of a passive avoidance response, and an increase in spontaneous nocturnal, but not daytime, locomotor activity, when compared with controls. There was no significant difference in sensitivity to electric shock in the treated compared to the control animals. These findings were observed in the presence of concurrent significant

reductions in striatal ChAT activity, without any change in striatal GAD activity. The lesion produced by AF64A treatment was small, and was restricted to the striatum. The data thus were interpreted as demonstrating a role of the striatal cholinergic system in complex behavioral processes and in locomotor behavior.

Stwertka and Olson (76) have demonstrated that unilateral AF64A injection (1 or 2 nmol/ml, 5 days post AF64A) will induce robust ipsilateral rotation in response to amphetamine and apomorphine treatment in rats. This effect was not seen in vehicle-treated control animals. Histological (Nissl stain) analysis revealed, however, regions of necrosis in the striatum and along the cannula tract, prompting the investigators to suggest that caution should be employed in interpreting these behavioral effects vis-a-vis cholinergic neurotoxicity.

Intrahippocampal administration. Bailey and coinvestigators (4) have administered 5 nmol AF64A, bilaterally, into the dorsal hippocampus of rats. Such treatment resulted, within 1 and 2 weeks posttreatment, in an impairment of multitrial passive avoidance learning and two-way active avoidance in a shuttle box paradigm. This was combined with a significant hyperactivity. No concurrent neurochemical analyses were conducted in these studies.

Walsh and Hanin (82) have also examined the behavioral as well as the neurochemical consequences of bilateral intrahippocampal AF64A administration (0.25, 1.0, and 4.0 nmol per side) in rats. Acquisition of the eight-arm radial maze task was significantly impaired in the 1.0- and 4.0-nmol-treated groups. In these same animals, there was a significant, dose-related decrease in ChAT activity, but no change in levels of NE, DA, 5-HT, and their respective metabolites, in the same tissue extracts.

Recently, Blaker and Goodwin (7) have explored the effect of unilateral administration of 1 nmol AF64A into the dorsal hippocampus. This treatment led to a significant attenuation of ChAT activity and ACh levels at the injection site. Rats treated with AF64A exhibited a significant behavioral deficit in the continuous reinforcement, food-reinforced lever press schedule, as well as in the eight-arm radial maze paradigm. The authors concluded that even relatively minor, localized cholinergic deficits confined to the hippocampus can produce significant learning and memory impairments in the rat.

Medial septum and nucleus basalis of Meynert administration. Administration of AF64A (1 nmol) in the nucleus basalis of Meynert (bilaterally) and in the medial septum (one midline injection) of rats resulted, after 10 to 14 days, in a variety of behavioral effects. The nucleus basalis-lesioned animals did not become habituated to a novel environment as well as controls and showed impaired passive and active avoidance behavior, as well as worsened navigational performance in a water maze task. There was, however, no evidence of motor impairment in these animals. Administration of AF64A into the medial septum, on the other hand, had no effect on habituation to a novel environment, or on passive and active avoidance behavior. Behavior in the water maze test was, however, impaired, and treated animals exhibited a reversal learning deficit similar to that seen following lesions of the hippocampus (75).

The behavioral data reported indicate profound performance reductions in tasks requiring memory, learning, and habituation. Whether these effects were due to a selective cholinotoxic effect of AF64A or to nonspecific lesions of the toxin must be established, in view of the fact that the dose of AF64A used in some of these studies was considerably above the "appropriate" range referred to earlier in this chapter.

General Comments

The above summarizes the evidence to date regarding the effects of AF64A administration on a variety of parameters *in vivo*. Clearly, much information is still needed regarding the mode of action of this compound. It is especially important to determine the conditions of AF64A treatment (dose, time, site, and mode of administration) to achieve cholinospecificity at the neurochemical, biochemical, and neuroanatomic levels. This would provide a firmer basis for the accurate interpretation of studies utilizing AF64A. In the meantime, the data that have been obtained are encouraging and merit further investigation.

OTHER AZIRIDINIUM ANALOGS OF CHOLINE

AF64A is one of several aziridinium analogs of choline that have been synthesized and studied to date. Since many of these analogs have not yet been studied in detail, their effectiveness as specific cholinotoxins is not yet established. Nevertheless, the data gained using these compounds have yielded valuable information concerning their possible mode of action.

Close Structural Analogs of AF64A

Rylett, Colhoun, and Clement (15,66,67) have comprehensively investigated a variety of aziridinium analogs of choline. In general, these investigators found that these compounds were toxic when given intravenously to anesthetized mice and rats; this effect was presumably mediated via presynaptic inhibition of the phrenic nerve and contraction of the diaphragm. This inhibition appeared to occur as a result of irreversible inhibition of the high-affinity choline transport system in rat forebrain synaptosomes, leading to a subsequent carrier-mediated inhibition of ChAT activity and inhibition of ACh synthesis. The effects were dose dependent and differed for each analog tested. Structure-activity considerations indicated that the hydroxyl moiety is important for inhibition of the HAChT and that the aziridinium moiety renders compounds possessing such a structure irreversible in their binding capacity with the HAChT system.

Mistry and his coinvestigators have synthesized and conducted some preliminary experiments with the *n*-propyl, isopropyl, cyclopropyl, *n*-butyl, and isobutyl analogs of AF64A. The compounds were tested *in vitro* for their abilities to inhibit the HAChT system and to interact with the muscarinic receptor (as measured by displacement of

quinuclidinyl benzilate). For the choline uptake studies it was found that increasing the chain length reduced the IC_{50} value, whereas branching or cyclization of the propyl analogs produced compounds with activity similar to that of AF64A. Muscarinic receptor binding activity was not significantly different from that seen with AF64A, except in the case of the cyclopropane derivative. This compound was 40 times more effective than AF64A in displacing quinuclidinyl benzilate from mouse whole brain synaptosomes *in vitro* (56). Studies evaluating the relative biological effect of these various compounds *in vivo* are in progress.

Hemicholinium Analog

Hemicholinium is a very potent, albeit reversible, inhibitor of HAChT *in vivo*. Since the aziridinium moiety of AF64A is presumably the active principle in the toxicity of AF64A, it was of interest to evaluate the extent to which the bisaziridinium analog of hemicholinium would be cholinotoxic to animals *in vivo*.

Smart first reported on this compound, which he had synthesized and tested on HAChT in rat brain synaptosomes (74). He observed a significant and irreversible inhibition of choline uptake, which was interpreted as being due to alkylation of sites involved in the high-affinity reversible binding of hemicholinium, which also are the sites for HAChT.

We have also synthesized this compound and have evaluated its effects *in vivo*. Although the compound was indeed a potent inhibitor of HAChT *in vitro* ($IC_{50} = 1.34 \times 10^{-8}$ M), its effects on the cholinergic system *in vivo* were less striking. Its LD_{50} was high (80 nmol, administered icv). Unlike in studies with AF64A, after such a dose there was no effect of the treatment, up to 10 days following the injection, on hippocampal, cortical, or striatal ChAT activity. Furthermore, although HAChT was reduced to 44% of control within 2 hr of injection, it had recovered to 83% of control values within 2 days, and remained at that level for the duration of the experiment (10 days). Finally, choline levels were doubled and ACh levels somewhat reduced within 2 hr following injection, but both returned to normal levels within 2 days in all three brain regions studied. All these results are different from those observed with AF64A under similar circumstances. This points to a transient mode of action of the hemicholinium aziridinium compound on cholinergic mechanisms *in vivo* (63). The reasons for this difference in action vis-a-vis the mode of action of AF64A have yet to be established.

PRACTICAL CONSIDERATIONS OF AF64A LESIONS

By virtue of its molecular structure, AF64A is a cytotoxic substance. The aziridinium moiety imparts to it strong irreversible alkylating properties which, at high enough concentrations, could destroy tissue in a nonspecific manner. Cavitary lesions and gliosis are quite common as a result of administration of not just AF64A, but other commonly used neurotoxins. Examples are available in the literature that illustrate this destructive effect following administration of 6HDA (10,11,30,37,51,61,68,79), 5,6- or 5,7-DHT (46), and kainic acid (29,39,55,59). Only through careful selection of dose are major nonspecific lesions and unwanted side effects avoided when using these various neurotoxins.

One should anticipate certain morphologic changes secondary to neuronal destruction induced by a selective neurotoxin. It is not unusual that gliosis, tissue shrinkage, and even ventricular enlargement (if the substance is administered in the ventricle) will be evident, leading to some structural deformation induced by the toxin. It is more important that the extent of the lesion is minimal, and neurochemically selective.

For this reason, we have emphasized throughout this chapter the importance, when using AF64A, of establishing the appropriate concentration and mode of administration in order to obtain selective neurotoxicity at a given site. Both neurochemical and histologic analyses should be conducted simultaneously. Results from such investigations might begin to explain the differences reported in the literature regarding the nature and selectivity of action of AF64A *in vivo*.

SUMMARY AND CONCLUSIONS

Progress in our understanding of cholinergic mechanisms *in vivo* has traditionally lagged behind the other neurotransmitter systems. It is therefore not surprising that, although we have selective neurotoxins for the other major neurotransmitters, the cholinergic system still is in the developmental phase in this regard.

Selective cholinergic neurotoxicity *in vivo* is difficult to achieve, because of the rapid regenerative powers of the cholinergic system and the unique synthetic chemistry of this molecule, in that its precursor is also the product of its destruction. Moreover, the development of an effective and potent selective cholinotoxin is difficult because our knowledge about endogenous cholinergic mechanisms is less developed than that of the other neurotransmitter systems.

Of the various substances studied to date as selective cholinotoxins, AF64A shows considerable promise. As would be expected, there are still key experiments that must be conducted to ascertain that this substance does indeed induce selective cholinotoxicity *in vivo*. Once a selective *in vivo*-acting cholinotoxin is developed, we will have available to us an invaluable pharmacological tool with a wide range of possible applications.

ACKNOWLEDGMENTS

Some of the work described in this review was supported by NIMH grants MH26320 and MH34893, by the UCB Pharmaceutical Secteur S.A., and by the Max Kade Foundation.

REFERENCES

1. Arbogast, R. E., and Kozlowski, M. R. (1984): *Soc. Neurosci. Abstr.,* 10:1185.
2. Arst, D. S., Berger, T. W., Fisher, A., and Hanin, I. (1983): *Fed. Proc.,* 42:657.
3. Asante, J. W., Cross, A. J., Deakin, J. F. W., Johnson, J. A., and Slater, H. R. (1983): *Br. J. Pharmacol.,* 573P.
4. Bailey, E. L., Overstreet, D. H., and Crocker, A. D. (1985): *Proc. Austr. Neurosci. Soc. Mtg.,* 1985.
5. Barlow, P., and Marchbanks, R. M. (1984): *J. Neurochem.,* 43: 1568–1573.
6. Bartus, R. T., Dean, R. L., Beer, B., and Lippa, A. S. (1982): *Science,* 217:408–417.
7. Blaker, W. D., and Goodwin, S. D. (1986): *Fed. Proc.,* 45:920.
8. Bowen, D. M., Francis, P. T., and Palmer, A. M. (1986): In: *Alzheimer's and Parkinson's Diseases: Strategies for Research and Development,* edited by A. Fisher, I. Hanin, and C. Lachman, pp. 53–61. Plenum Press, New York.
9. Brandeis, R., Pittel, Z., Lachman, C., Heldman, E., Luz, S., Dachir, S., Levy, A., Hanin, I., and Fisher, A. (1986): In: *Alzheimer's and Parkinson's Diseases: Strategies for Research and Development,* edited by A. Fisher, I. Hanin, and C. Lachman, pp. 469–477. Plenum Press, New York.
10. Butcher, L. L., Eastgate, S. M., and Hodge, G. K. (1984): *Naunyn Schmiedebergs Arch. Pharmacol.,* 285:31–40.
11. Butcher, L. L., Hodge, G. K., and Schaeffer, J. C. (1975): In: *Chemical Tools in Catecholamine Research,* edited by G. Jonsson, T. Malmfors, and C. Sachs, pp. 83–90. American Elsevier, New York.
12. Caltagirone, C., Gainotti, G., and Massulo, C. (1982): *Int. J. Neurosci.,* 16:247–249.
13. Casamenti, F., Bracco, L., Pedata, F., and Pepeu, G. (1986): In: *Dynamics of Cholinergic Function,* edited by I. Hanin, pp. 1137–1143. Plenum Press, New York.
14. Caulfield, M. P., May, P. J., Pedder, E. K., and Prince, A. K. (1983): *Proc. Br. Pharmacol. Soc.*
15. Clement, J. G., and Colhoun, E. H. (1975): *Can. J. Physiol. Pharmacol.,* 53:264–272.
16. Coyle, J. T., Price, D. L., and DeLong, M. R. (1983): *Science,* 219:1184–1190.
17. Curti, D., and Marchbanks, R. M. (1984): *J. Membr. Biol.,* 82: 259–268.
18. Davies, P. (1979): *Brain Res.,* 171:318–327.
19. Davis, K. L., and Yamamura, H. I. (1978): *Life Sci.,* 23:1729–1734.
20. Drachman, D. A. (1977): *Neurology,* 27:783–790.
21. Fisher, A., and Hanin, I. (1980): *Life Sci.,* 27:1615–1634.
22. Fisher, A., and Hanin, I. (1986): *Annu. Rev. Pharmacol. Toxicol.,* 26:161–181.
23. Fisher, A., Mantione, C. R., Abraham, D. J., and Hanin, I. (1982): *J. Pharmacol. Exp. Ther.,* 222:140–145.
24. Francis, P. T., Palmer, A. M., Sims, N. R., Bowen, D. M., Davison, A. N., Esiri, M. M., Neary, D., Snowden, J. S., and Wilcock, G. K. (1985): *N. Engl. J. Med.,* 313:7–11.
25. Freeman, J. J., and Jenden, D. J. (1976): *Life Sci.,* 19:949–962.
26. Gaal, G., Potter, P. E., Harsing, L. G., Jr., Kakucska, I., Fisher, A., Hanin, I., and Vizi, E. S. (1984): In: *Regulation of Transmitter Function: Basic and Clinical Aspects,* edited by E. S. Vizi and K. Magyar, pp. 295–300. Akademiai Kiado, Budapest.
27. Growdon, J. H., and Wurtman, R. J. (1983): In: *Banbury Report: Biological Aspects of Alzheimer's Disease,* edited by R. Katzman, pp. 451–459. Cold Spring Harbor Laboratory, Cold Spring Harbor, New York.
28. Gulya, K., Fisher, A., Hanin, I., and Yamamura, H. I. (1986): *Fed. Proc.,* 45:921.
29. Herndon, R. M., Coyle, J. T., and Addics, E. (1980): *Neuroscience,* 5:1013–1026.
30. Hokfelt, T., and Ungerstedt, U. (1973): *Brain Res.,* 60:269–297.
31. Hörtnagl, H., Potter, P. E., and Hanin, I. (1986): *Fed. Proc.,* 45: 923.
32. Hucho, F., and Ovchinnikov, Y. A., eds. (1983): *Toxins As Tools in Neurochemistry.* Walter de Gruyter, Berlin, New York.
33. Jarrard, L. E., Kant, G. J., Meyerhoff, J. L., and Levy, A. (1984): *Pharmacol. Biochem. Behav.,* 21:273–280.
34. Jope, R. S. (1979): *Brain Res. Rev.,* 1:313–344.
35. Jotkowitz, S. (1983): *Ann. Neurol.,* 14:690–691.

36. Kasa, P., Farkas, P., Szerdahelyi, P., Rakonczay, Z., Fisher, A., and Hanin, I. (1984): In: *Regulation of Transmitter Function: Basic and Clinical Aspects,* edited by E. S. Vizi and K. Magyar, pp. 289–293. Akademiai Kiado, Budapest.

37. Kelly, P. H., Joyce, E. M., Minneman, K. P., and Phillipson, O. T. (1977): *Brain Res.,* 122:382–387.

38. Kitt, C. A., Price, D. L., Struble, R. G., Cork, L. C., Wainer, B. H., Becker, M. W., and Mobley, W. C. (1984): *Science,* 226:1443–1445.

39. Krammer, E. B., Lischka, M. F., Karobath, M., and Schonbeck, G. (1979): *Brain Res.,* 177:577–582.

40. Kuhar, M. J. (1973): *Life Sci.,* 13:1623–1634.

41. Kuhar, M. J., and Murrin, L. C. (1978): *J. Neurochem.,* 30:15–21.

42. Lehr, E., Kuhn, F. J., and Hinzen, D. H. (1984): *Soc. Neurosci. Abstr.,* 10:775.

43. Leventer, S., McKeag, D., Clancy, M., Wulfert, E., and Hanin, I. (1985): *Neuropharmacology,* 24:453–459.

44. Leventer, S. M., Wulfert, E., and Hanin, I. (1987): *Neuropharmacology (in press).*

45. Levy, A., Kant, G. J., Meyerhoff, J. L., and Jarrard, L. E. (1984): *Brain Res.,* 305:169–172.

46. Lorens, S. A., Gulberg, H. C., Hole, K., Kohler, C., and Srebro, B. (1976): *Brain Res.,* 100:97–113.

47. Mantione, C. R., DeGroat, W. C., Fisher, A., and Hanin, I. (1983): *J. Pharmacol. Exp. Ther.,* 225:616–622.

48. Mantione, C. R., Fisher, A., and Hanin, I. (1981): *Science,* 213:579–580.

49. Mantione, C. R., Fisher, A., and Hanin, I. (1984): *Life Sci.,* 35:33–41.

50. Mantione, C. R., Zigmond, M. J., Fisher, A., and Hanin, I. (1983): *J. Neurochem.,* 41:251–255.

51. Marshall, J. F., and Gotthelf, T. (1979): *Exp. Neurol.,* 65:398–411.

52. McArdle, J. J., Argentieri, J. M., Gargano, D., Hanin, I., and Fisher, A. (1985): *Pharmacologist,* 27:210.

53. McGurk, S. R., and Butcher, L. L. (1985): *Fed. Proc.,* 44:897.

54. McRae-Deguerce, A., Dulluc, J., and Geffard, M. (1985): *Soc. Neurosci. Abstr.,* 11:744.

55. Meibach, R. C., Brown, L., and Brooks, F. H. (1978): *Brain Res.,* 148:219–223.

56. Mistry, J. S., Abraham, D. J., and Hanin, I. (1986): *J. Med. Chem.,* 29:376–380.

57. Mohs, R. C., Davis, B. M., Johns, C. A., Mathe, A. A., Greenwald, B. S., Howath, T. B., and Davis, K. L. (1985): *Am. J. Psychiatry,* 142:28–33.

58. Morgan, I. G., and Millar, T. J. (1986): *Trends in Pharmacol. Sci.,* 7:265–266.

59. Nagy, J. I., Vincent, S. R., Lehmann, J., Fibiger, H. C., and McGeer, E. G. (1978): *Brain Res.,* 149:431–441.

60. Perry, E. K., Tomlinson, B. E., Blessed, G., Bergman, K., Gibson, P. H., et al. (1978): *Br. Med. J.,* 2:1457–1459.

61. Poirier, L. J., Langelier, P., Roberge, A., Bouncher, R., and Kitsikis, A. (1972): *J. Neurol. Sci.,* 16:401–416.

62. Pope, C. N., Englert, L. F., and Ho, B. T. (1985): *Pharmacol. Biochem. Behav.,* 22:297–299.

63. Potter, P. E., Happe, H. K., Leventer, S., Fisher, A., and Hanin, I. (1986): *Trans. Am. Soc. Neurochem.,* 17:233.

64. Potter, P. E., Harsing, L. G., Jr., Kakucska, I., Gaal, G., Vizi, E. S., Fisher, A., and Hanin, I. (1985): *Fed. Proc.,* 44:897.

65. Richter, J. A., Perry, E. K., and Tomlinson, B. E. (1980): *Life Sci.,* 26:1683–1689.

66. Rylett, B. J., and Colhoun, E. H. (1979): *J. Neurochem.,* 32:553–558.

67. Rylett, B. J., and Colhoun, E. H. (1980): *J. Neurochem.,* 34:713–719.

68. Sachs, C., and Jonsson, C. (1975): *Biochem. Pharmacol.,* 24:1–8.

69. Sandberg, K., Hanin, I., Fisher, A., and Coyle, J. T. (1984): *Brain Res.,* 293:49–55.

70. Sandberg, K., Sanberg, P. R., Hanin, I., Fisher, A., and Coyle, J. T. (1984): *Behav. Neurosci.,* 98:162–165.

71. Sandberg, K., Schnaar, R. L., Hanin, I., and Coyle, J. T. (1982): *Soc. Neurosci. Abstr.,* 8:516.

72. Sandberg, K., Schnaar, R. L., McKinney, M., Hanin, I., Fisher, A., and Coyle, J. T. (1985): *J. Neurochem.,* 44:439–445.

73. Sims, N. R., Bowen, D. M., Allen, S. J., Smith, C. C. T., Neary, D., Thomas, D. J., and Davison, A. N. (1983): *J. Neurochem.,* 40:503–509.

74. Smart, L. (1981): *Neuroscience,* 6:1765–1770.

75. Spencer, D. G., Jr., Horvath, E., Luiten, P., Schuurman, T., and Traber, J. (1985): In: *Senile Dementia of the Alzheimer Type,* edited by J. Traber and W. H. Gispen, pp. 325–342. Springer-Verlag, Berlin, Heidelberg.

76. Stwertka, S. A., and Olson, G. L. (1986): *Life Sci.,* 38:1105–1110.

77. Terry, R. D., and Davies, P. (1983): In: *Aging of the Brain,* edited by D. Samuel, E. Giacobini, G. Filogamo, G. Giacobini, and A. Vernadakis, pp. 47–59. Raven Press, New York.

78. Thal, L. J., Fuld, P. A., Masur, D. M., and Sharpless, N. S. (1983): *Ann. Neurol.,* 13:491–496.

79. Ungerstedt, U. (1971): In: *6-Hydroxydopamine and Catecholamine Neurons,* edited by T. Malmfors and H. Thoenen, pp. 101–128. North-Holland, Amsterdam.

80. Vickroy, T. W., Watson, M., Leventer, S. M., Roeske, W. R., Hanin, I., and Yamamura, H. I. (1985): *J. Pharmacol. Exp. Ther.,* 231:577–582.

81. Villani, L., Contestabile, A., Poli, A., Migani, P., and Fonnum, F. (1984): *Neurosci. Lett. (Suppl.),* 18:S228.

82. Walsh, T. J., and Hanin, I. (1986): In: *Alzheimer's and Parkinson's Diseases: Strategies for Research and Development,* edited by A. Fisher, I. Hanin, and C. Lachman, pp. 461–467. Plenum Press, New York.

83. Walsh, T. J., Tilson, H. A., DeHaven, D. L., Mailman, R. B., Fisher, A., and Hanin, I. (1984): *Brain Res.,* 321:91–102.

84. Wettstein, A. (1983): *Ann. Neurol.,* 13:210–212.

Psychopharmacology:
The Third Generation of Progress,
edited by Herbert Y. Meltzer.
Raven Press, New York © 1987.

CHAPTER 37

Neurotoxins Affecting Biogenic Aminergic Neurons

Irwin J. Kopin

Alterations in neuronal function that follow administration of drugs usually result from chemical interactions of the agent or its metabolites with molecular constituents involved in the initiation or propagation of nerve impulses or in the processes involved in the formation, storage, release, receptor activation, or termination of action of chemical neurotransmitters (or modulators). These effects are generally transient since they are dependent on the presence of the active molecules or may be reversed when irreversibly inactivated enzymes or other components of the neurotransmission system are resynthesized.

Studies of the electron microscopic localization of drugs that accumulate at sympathetic nerve terminals led to the discovery that such drugs may be toxic and cause selective destruction of the terminals. Extension of the studies to analogs of these compounds led to the discovery of related compounds that exert similar toxic effects with specificity varying according to their accessibility to or affinity for the various biogenic amine uptake sites. Thus, 6-hydroxydopamine and its analogs, guanethidine and the bretylium-analogs, DSP-4 and xylamine, and the dihydroxytryptamines were all discovered in relation to known drugs. The interactions of these toxins with neurotransmitters and their effects have been studied solely in experimental animals.

An exception to this, MPTP (1-methyl-4-phenyl-1,2,3,6-tetrahydropyridine), was first encountered as a contaminant of an illicit narcotic which, after self-administration by some drug addicts, produced a parkinsonian syndrome in humans. The mechanisms of tissue specificity and cellular toxicity of this latest addition to the biogenic amine neurotoxins are related to those of the earlier known toxins.

It is the purpose of this chapter to review the present state of knowledge of neurotoxins that are specific for neurons characterized by their release of biogenic amine neurotransmitters and to indicate the importance of the discovery of these agents for further research in the neurosciences.

GENERAL CONSIDERATIONS

Before discussing individual neurotoxins, it is useful to consider mechanisms that are involved in cellular toxicity and to identify factors that contribute to the specificity of the toxin for particular types of cells.

Mechanisms of Cellular Toxicity

The introduction of a foreign chemical substance into the cellular environment may result in one or more chemical reactions that alter the physiological processes in the cell. The initial reaction may be harmless or may severely injure the cell and cause it to die. The mechanisms responsible for cell death are frequently obscure, but physiochemical changes that disrupt membranes, inhibit enzymes (particularly those concerned with energy-producing reactions), deplete cofactors, or block regulatory mechanisms have been cited as the bases for chemically induced toxicity (see, e.g., ref. 6).

Free radical (a molecule with an odd number of electrons) formation and propagation have been implicated as a mode of action for many toxins, as well as for ionizing radiation

(21,63). The metabolic conversion of a compound to a free radical frequently involves its reaction with a reduced cofactor, e.g., nicotinamide adenine dinucleotide phosphate (NADP·H)-cytochrome C (P_{450}) reductase or other flavin reductases. Free radicals can cycle by interacting with cellular constituents which are easily oxidized [sulfides, catechols, Fe(III), etc.] and which in turn can partially reduce oxygen to its free radical, superoxide (O_2^-).

Each cell has a variety of mechanisms for preventing the accumulation of excess free radicals that could potentially disrupt its function by attacking vulnerable targets. Some of the major free radical cellular defenses and targets are listed in Table 1. The combined actions of superoxide dismutase (SOD) and catalase result in conversion of superoxide back into oxygen as a result of the following reactions:

$$O_2^- + 2H^+ \xrightarrow{SOD} H_2O_2$$

$$H_2O_2 \xrightarrow{Catalase} H_2O + \tfrac{1}{2}O_2$$

Spontaneous or enzymatically catalyzed reactions of hydrogen peroxide with other reducing agents, e.g., glutathionine, ascorbic acid, etc., also serve to reduce the levels of potentially damaging oxidative species. These reactions prevent accumulation of H_2O_2 which could give rise to toxicity.

The reaction of H_2O_2 with Fe(II) can result in formation, from $O_2\cdot$, of a potent oxidant, the hydroxide radical (OH·):

$$Fe(III) + O_2^- \rightarrow Fe(II) + O_2$$

$$Fe(II) + H_2O_2 \rightarrow Fe(III) + OH^- + OH\cdot$$

A variety of molecules can be attacked by OH·. Those which result in harmless products are considered to be scavengers, whereas those resulting in cell injury are regarded as targets (Table 1). The vulnerability of particular cells to injury is also dependent, however, on a variety of factors that are peculiar to that cell population.

Factors Influencing Selective Vulnerability

The production of irreversible injury to a given population of cells may be dependent on the properties of the cells as well as attributes of the organism of which they are part. Species, environmental factors such as nutritional status, presence of infections, season of the year, oxygenation, etc., may influence the fate of an administered drug or the

TABLE 1. *Cellular free radical defenses and targets*

Cellular defenses	Target molecules
Superoxide dismutase	Polyunsaturated lipids
Catalase	Nucleotide bases (DNA, RNA)
Glutathione peroxidase	Proteins
	Aromatic amino acids
Glutathione	Methionine
Ascorbate	Cysteine-cystine
α-Tocopherol	Histidine
β-Carotene	
Uric acid	Carbohydrates (glycoproteins)

capacity of the organism to chemically alter the compound. The toxic dose level of the substance and its accessibility to the vulnerable cells may depend on blood flow, intercellular barriers (e.g., blood-brain barrier), or specific transport mechanisms, all of which differ with age or region. The cellular enzymes or small molecules that regulate the ability of cells to inactivate (or activate) drugs or free radical intermediates, the cellular constituents that serve as defenses against toxicity or as target molecules, and the relative rates of toxic damage and capacity of the cell to repair the damage or replace essential molecules are important factors, but frequently have not been clearly defined. Such factors will vary in importance, but must be considered in assessing contributors to specific vulnerability of cells to any toxin.

Neurons that contain biogenic amines as neurotransmitters have been found to be specific targets for several toxins. The toxic mechanisms and the role of several factors in determining target specificity have been suggested and will be discussed in relation to each of these compounds.

SPECIFIC NEUROTOXINS THAT AFFECT BIOGENIC AMINERGIC NEURONS

There are several compounds which have been found to selectively damage some biogenic amine-containing neurons. The selective vulnerability of these neurons appears related to their ability to concentrate amines by a specific uptake process, but the mode of toxicity of the different compounds is not identical. Each compound and its analogs will be discussed separately.

6-Hydroxydopamine

Thoenen and Tranzer (61) have reviewed the early developments in the discovery of the toxic effects of 6-hydroxydopamine. It had first been suggested that this compound might be formed *in vivo* by the autoxidation or metabolism of dopamine, but this speculation has never been substantiated. It was soon demonstrated, however, that 6-hydroxydopamine administration produced a long-lasting depletion of tissue stores of norepinephrine. During the course of studies designed to examine by electron microscopy the localization in sympathetic neurons of various phenylethylamine derivatives, it was discovered that 12 to 72 hr after administration of 6-hydroxydopamine, the adrenergic nerve terminals of all peripheral tissues examined were in various stages of degeneration. The high selectivity for adrenergic neurons was most clearly evident in tissues such as the iris where adrenergic, but not cholinergic, nerve terminals were affected. Blockade of toxicity by drugs (e.g., desipramine) that block amine uptake into noradrenergic neurons prevents the toxicity, suggesting accumulation of the toxin in adrenergic terminals may be responsible for its specificity. Neither reserpine (which blocks storage in amine granules) nor monoamine oxidase inhibitors prevent the toxic effects—the latter even has a potentiating effect. Since 6-hydroxydopamine does not readily penetrate the blood-brain barrier, the brain is unaffected by the systemically administered neurotoxin.

When 6-hydroxydopamine is administered in sufficiently high doses to adult rats, the sympathetic nerve terminals degenerate, but the cell bodies in the sympathetic ganglia remain intact. The completeness of the involvement of peripheral sympathetic nerve terminals varies among tissues and species, as does the time required for regeneration of the sympathetic nerve terminals. In neonatal rats and mice, in contrast to adults, the whole adrenergic neuron, including the cell body, undergoes degeneration.

When administered intracerebroventricularly, 6-hydroxydopamine affects both dopaminergic and noradrenergic nerve terminals. There are regional differences in the effectiveness of the neurotoxin. These differences appear to be related to the relative vulnerability of the nerve terminals as well as to differences in accessibility of the amine to the region. Cell bodies are more resistant to the neurotoxin, but may be destroyed when it is administered locally, directly into the region, e.g., substantia nigra. Aminergic neuronal cell death leads to virtually complete degeneration of the nerve terminals, but retrograde degeneration of cell bodies after destruction of the terminals might be slight. In brain, unlike the peripheral sympathetic nerves, there is little regeneration of destroyed axons for as long as 2 years after toxin administration. Selectivity of dopaminergic or noradrenergic nerve terminal destruction by 6-hydroxydopamine has been obtained by use of drugs that block uptake of the neurotoxin into the terminals that are to be preserved. For example, pretreatment with desipramine prevents toxic destruction of noradrenergic neurons, but does not interfere with the destruction of dopaminergic terminals.

In examining the antioxidation products of 6-hydroxydopamine, Blank et al. (5) also studied the 6-amino analog, which is also readily oxidized. Both 6-hydroxy- and 6-amino-dopamine can be oxidized and undergo ring closure to form 5,6-dihydroxyindole. Since 6-amino-dopamine was found to be about as toxic as 6-hydroxydopamine (39), it was suggested that 5,6-dihydroxyindole might play a role in the toxicity. A variety of other amino analogs (3-, 4-, or 6-amino-) of 6-hydroxydopamine were found to be about equipotent in causing adrenergic nerve terminal degeneration (62), suggesting that the redox potential and affinity for the amine pump are determinants of toxicity. The relative impotence of 6-hydroxynorepinephrine as a neurotoxin is consistent with its low affinity for the amine uptake system (57).

Several possible mechanisms have been proposed to explain the neurotoxicity of 6-hydroxydopamine. The specificity for catecholaminergic neurons is almost certainly related to its selective uptake, and there is general agreement that autoxidation is important. The differences among the various proposed mechanisms relate to the role of the products of the autoxidation and the cellular targets that are responsible for the ultimate degenerative process. Thoenen and Tranzer (61) first suggested that the quinone product might bind covalently to nucleophilic groups of macromolecules and, by denaturing these, severely damage biologically important processes. The reactive products of partial reduction of oxygen (H_2O_2, $O_2\cdot$, and $OH\cdot$) are formed during the autoxidation of 6-hydroxydopamine and its amine analogs (14,29,60), and these have also been implicated in the mechanism of toxicity by the reactions with targets described above.

The amino acid precursor of 6-hydroxydopamine, 6-hydroxydopa, when administered intravenously, is able to penetrate the blood-brain barrier and its decarboxylation to 6-hydroxydopamine is probably responsible for its toxicity. Noradrenergic neurons appear to be more selectively destroyed by 6-hydroxydopa (30), but the reason for this selectivity is not clear.

Dihydroxytryptamines

The discovery of 6-hydroxydopamine-selective neurotoxicity based on its accumulation in catecholaminergic neurons led to the initiation of studies of comparable hydroxylated tryptamines that might accumulate and be selectively toxic in serotonergic neurons. It was soon found that 5,6- and 5,7-dihydroxytryptamine were indeed accumulated in serotonin-containing neurons and caused axonal degeneration (see review by Bjorkland et al., ref. 4). These amines, particularly the 5,7-derivative, are also taken up into catecholaminergic neurons and have some toxic effects that limit their specificity. The 5,6 analog is more widely useful, but neither of the dihydroxytryptamines reliably causes cell death, although secondary neuronal degeneration is occasionally seen. The axon terminals of brain serotonergic neurons degenerate, but reinnervation occurs after varying lengths of time. The effects on spinal cord serotonin are more lasting. When high doses of 5,6- (or 5,7-) hydroxytryptamine are administered, its toxicity is evident in many cellular components and specificity is lost.

Guanethidine

Many strongly basic compounds inhibit the responses to peripheral sympathetic nerve stimulation without blocking the effects of administered norpinephrine. Guanethidine (which possesses a strongly basic guanidine moiety) and bretylium (a quaternary amine) are generally considered typical of such drugs, which block release of norepinephrine from sympathetic nerve endings. Both are selectively accumulated in noradrenergic neurons by the specific amine uptake process. Guanethidine (but not bretylium) can also displace norepinephrine at its storage site and be released by sympathetic nerve stimulation as a "false transmitter." Both drugs are believed to have a local anesthetic effect at the sympathetic nerve terminals resulting in their blockade of norepinephrine release.

In 1971 it was discovered that chronic treatment with high doses of guanethidine destroys adrenergic nerves in adult (9) and newborn (20) rats. Subsequent histological studies *in vivo* and *in vitro* have suggested that there are several stages of the effects of guanethidine (25). The first changes observed *in vitro* occur in the mitochondria and ribosomes of the cell body, but no damage to axonal mitochondria is seen. Guanethidine had been shown to block oxidative phosphorylation in isolated rat liver mitochondria (49); extragranular localization of the drug in the cell body, in contrast to its granular localization in the axon, appears to be responsible for the selective cell body mitochondrial damage with sparing of axonal mitochondria (40). The second phase is characterized by retraction of the axons with organelle and myeloid whirls accumulating in the cell body and proximal regions of its processes. This is attributed to retrograde emptying into the cell body of axonal contents during axonal retraction. The third phase is degeneration of the cell bodies, presumably as a consequence of interference with mitochondrial function (25).

Chronic treatment with guanethidine has been used to produce permanent sympathectomy in rats and has been claimed to be superior to immunosympathectomy or 6-hydroxydopamine treatment, with sparing of central adrenergic neurons (38). The age of the animals appears to be important since the avoidance of brain involvement requires adequate development of the blood-brain barrier, and susceptibility of the peripheral neurons to the toxic effects appears to be greater in young than in old animals.

DSP-4

In 1976 Ross (56) reported that a tertiary alkylating analog of bretylium, N-(2-chloroethyl)-N-ethyl-2-brom benzylamine (DSP-4), produces long-term depletion of norepinephrine in the brain and heart. Jaim-Etchaverry and Zieher (32) showed that the peripheral sympathetic neurons were affected relatively transiently, whereas the neurotoxic effects in brain persisted. The cell bodies of the locus ceruleus are not destroyed by the toxin, although the projection areas are selectively damaged (17). The toxin appears to alkylate norepinephrine uptake sites (46). The debrominated analog of DSP-4, xylamine, also appears to have long-term effects on norepinephrine uptake sites and to deplete brain norepinephrine (18) but does not appear to cause axonal degeneration. These compounds appear to have their major effects by inhibiting release of norepinephrine and depleting the stores of the amine. They have little effect on dopaminergic neurons and only minor effects on serotonergic neurons. They have, however, been reported to bind to opiate receptors (64), so that complete specificity for noradrenergic mechanisms cannot always be assumed.

MPTP

As indicated earlier, biogenic amine neurotoxins were first encountered in experimental animals during studies of compounds known to be or suspected of being accumulated selectively in these neurons because of the amine uptake mechanism. Toxicity with these substances has not been reported in humans. MPTP, however, was first encountered as a neurotoxin in humans.

In 1979 it was reported that a severe parkinsonian syndrome with biochemical and histological evidence of localized destruction of the substantia nigra had resulted from the self-administration by a young drug addict of a mixture of compounds obtained during the attempted synthesis of a meperidine analog (16). Among the three candidate compounds was MPTP (1-methyl-4-phenyl-1,2,3,6-tetrahydropyridine), and this compound again surfaced in relation to similar cases in California (1,44) and in several young chemists who had been exposed to large quantities of MPTP (8,43). Shortly after the discovery of MPTP toxicity in humans, an animal model of Parkinson's disease was successfully obtained in monkeys (7). These observations have sparked, during the last several years, a flurry of investigations to determine the range of species that are susceptible to the toxin, the extent of neuronal involvement in the various species, the metabolic fate and disposition of MPTP and its metabolites, the mechanisms involved in its specificity and toxicity, and the possible implications of these in relation to the etiology and/or pathogenesis of Parkinson's disease. In the following summary only highlights will be mentioned, since more detailed reviews are available (41,51).

Acute Behavioral and Biochemical Effects of MPTP

In almost all species in which the effects of MPTP have been studied, the drug produces acute transient behavioral changes. The effects were first observed in rats soon after MPTP was first encountered (16). Within seconds after intravenous administration of 10 to 20 mg/kg MPTP, there appear patterns of behavior reminiscent of the "serotonin syndrome" (31), characterized by hunched posture, splayed hind limbs, erect (Straub) tail, profuse salivation, piloerection, proptosis, and retropulsion with clonic movements of the forelegs (12,13). This syndrome can be prevented or reversed by administration of a serotonin antagonist, methysergide; marked hyperactivity replaces the "serotonin syndrome."

Similar acute behavioral effects are seen in monkeys, dogs, mice, and other species. Humans who have taken MPTP report a burning sensation at the injection site, a metallic or medicinal taste, blurred or dimmed vision, and occasionally hallucinations (1,42). The acute effects are soon dissipated, but if the dose is sufficiently large or if several doses are administered, in some species a parkinsonian movement disorder develops (see below).

During the acute phase, alterations in biogenic amines and their metabolites in rat and mouse brain appear to reflect diminished serotonin and dopamine metabolism. Levels of serotonin increase and the deaminated metabolites of both dopamine and serotonin decrease. This could be due to diminished amine release by a direct action of MPTP or indirectly as a result of receptor stimulation, or might reflect inhibition of monoamine oxidase. Norepinephrine release, however, appears to be enhanced both in brain and at peripheral sympathetic nerve endings. Brain 3-methoxy-4-hydroxy-phenylglycol (MHPG) levels increase while norepinephrine levels decline (19). Plasma norepinephrine levels are elevated (13) and its stores are decreased in heart, blood vessels, and adrenal medulla (22).

In rhesus monkeys, the ventricular cerebrospinal fluid (CSF) levels of homovanillic acid (HVA), 5-hydroxy indoleacetic acid (5HIAA), and MHPG decline during the first day after MPTP administration and remain low for several weeks. The acute, transient syndromes due to MPTP are clearly different from the chronic toxic effects, which appear to occur only in some species and seem to be far more specific in targeting specific neurons for destruction.

Species Specificity for Chronic MPTP Toxicity

Although the acute effects of MPTP are similar among a wide variety of species, there are striking differences in the vulnerability to the chronic toxic effects. In primates, including rhesus (7), squirrel monkeys (45), marmoset (35), etc., there develops over a period ranging from 3 days to 3 weeks, increasingly severe bradykinesia, stooped posture, rigidity, episodes of "freezing," and some tremor. The degree of motor impairment that finally develops may vary from minimal symptoms to severe parkinsonism. This variability in severity of the persistent motor effects may be related to the observation that over 80% of the dopaminergic neurons must be destroyed to elicit significant behavioral deficits. The dog, which has neuromelanin, also is susceptible to MPTP toxicity (36).

The biochemical effects observed are consistent with destruction of the nigrostriatal dopamine neurons. Whereas CSF levels of 5HIAA and MHPG return almost to normal, levels of HVA remain low (7).

Attempts to produce a parkinsonian model in rats (12), guinea pigs (12), and cats (58) have not met with success. High doses of MPTP may produce transient motor effects, but biochemical and histological evidence for damage sufficiently extensive to result in a persistent parkinsonian syndrome has not been obtained.

Mice, however, do appear to be affected (24,27), and in some strains relatively low doses of MPTP (20 mg/kg) have produced marked decreases in brain dopamine, which persist for long periods, but there appear to be strain differences in sensitivity to MPTP (26). In this species, however, the lesions are not confined to the nigrostriatum. Dopamine levels in the nucleus accumbens (52) and norepinephrine levels in the striatum and frontal cortex are depressed (24). There is, however, a gradual return, over months, of brain catecholamine levels in mice (23). Frogs, salamanders (2), and leeches (47) have also been reported to be sensitive to the effects of MPTP, causing dopamine depletion and motor behavioral retardation.

Mechanisms of MPTP Neurotoxicity

Factors that contribute to MPTP toxicity include its metabolism to a toxic quaternary pyridinium derivative, MPP^+, the accumulation of MPP^+ by the amine uptake system in dopaminergic (and noradrenergic) neurons, formation of free radical intermediates possibly with the involvement of neuromelanin as a donor or an index of vulnerability, and properties of the involved neurons that diminish their capacity to prevent or repair the toxic injury. These factors vary considerably among species and may account for the selectivity of MPTP toxicity for only certain neurons in some species.

Metabolism of MPTP. MPTP is rapidly oxidized (Fig. 1) in many tissues to form the pyridinium derivative, MPP^+ (50), which persists in monkey brain (for up to 20 days) but is rapidly removed from rodent brain (37). Monoamine oxidase-B (MAO-B), which is present mostly in astrocytes and serotonergic neurons, is the enzyme mainly responsible for their oxidation (11), and inhibition of MAO-B prevents MPTP toxicity (28,50).

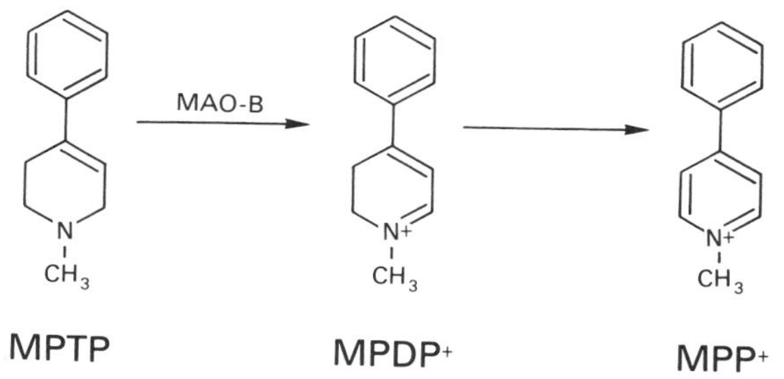

FIG. 1. Metabolism of MPTP.

Concentration of MPP^+ in catecholaminergic neurons. MPP^+ has a high affinity for both dopamine and norepinephrine uptake sites (33,34). Both MPTP (48) and MPP^+ (16a) bind to neuromelanin and this may provide a reservoir for monitoring relatively high levels of MPP^+ for prolonged periods in neurons containing the pigment.

Free radical cycling of MPP^+. MPP^+, like the related defoliant, paraquat, can accept an electron and form a free radical which can be reduced by oxygen to generate superoxide ($O_2 \cdot$). Using spin-trapping techniques, MPP^+ has been shown to stimulate superoxide and hydroxyl ion formation, but not as efficiently as paraquat (59). Superoxide, dismutase, catalase, and ethanol inhibited the formation of toxic radicals. Corsini et al. (15) showed that inhibition of superoxide dismutase potentiates the toxic effects of MPP^+ in mice, and Poirier and Barbeau (55) found that MPP^+ could inhibit NADH-cytochrome C reductase. Furthermore, the recent reports that antioxidants such as glutathionine, ascorbic acid, α-tocopherol, etc. may diminish MPTP toxicity in mice (54) are consistent with the hypothesis of free radical involvement. Neuromelanin, which is a redox polymer containing free radicals, has also been implicated as a participant in MPP^+ free radical cycling (41).

MPTP toxic mechanism. The hypothesized sequence of events involved in MPTP toxicity is shown diagrammatically in Fig. 2. MPTP is converted to MPP^+ in astrocytes (or serotoninergic neurons) containing MAO-B. The product leaves these neurons by an unknown mechanism (perhaps via an ion channel) and is concentrated by the catecholamine uptake mechanism into specific neurons. Neurons containing dopamine neuromelanin appear to be most vulnerable, perhaps because the pigment, which exists as a redox polymer, can potentiate free radical formation. The free radicals generate superoxide and other reactive molecules that react with proteins involved in the essential processes, e.g., mitochondrial functions, resulting in cell death. Nicklas et al. (53) showed that MPP^+ inhibits NADH-linked oxidation by brain mitochondria, so that free radical mechanisms may not be solely responsible for the toxic actions of MPP^+.

MPTP Toxicity and Parkinson's Disease

The highly specific neurotoxicity of MPTP in humans and primates, which results in a well-defined chemical lesioning of the nigrostriatal dopaminergic neurons and produces a clinical syndrome strikingly similar to spontaneous Parkinson's disease, has enhanced our understanding of the function of the basal ganglia in movement disorders

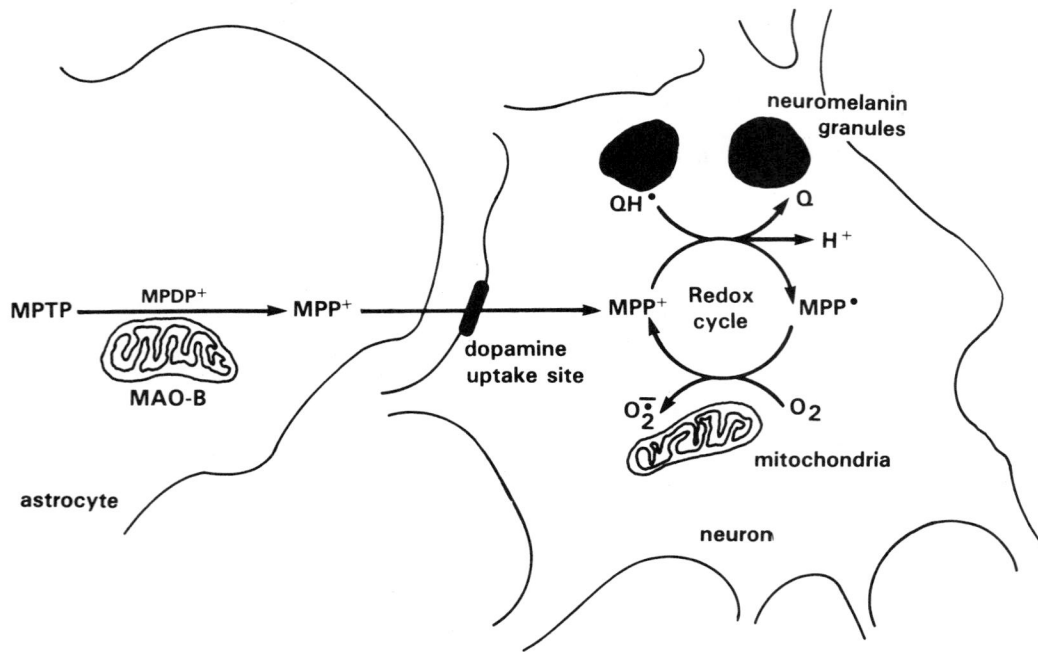

FIG. 2. Mechanisms of MPTP toxicity.

and stimulated new approaches to investigating the pathogenesis and therapy of Parkinson's disease.

First, it is now clear that most symptoms in Parkinson's disease can be attributed to the involvement of the nigrostriatal pathway in the degenerative process. Although the locus ceruleus and other brain regions may be involved in the degenerative process of Parkinson's disease, in MPTP toxicity these regions appear to be spared. In fact, in patients with MPTP toxicity, the CSF levels of MHPG, the major metabolite of norepinephrine, are elevated, whereas in Parkinson's disease MHPG levels in CSF tend to be lower than normal (8). In both Parkinson's disease and MPTP toxicity, levels of HVA in CSF are much lower than normal.

Relatively extensive involvement of the dopaminergic neurons is required before symptoms of the movement disorder become clinically detectable. Using positron emission tomography (PET) to localize the accumulation of ^{18}F-dopamine after administration of ^{18}F-dopa, Calne et al. (10) demonstrated in clinically normal subjects who had been exposed to a single dose of MPTP a decrease in caudate nucleus dopaminergic function. If the decrease in dopamine content of the brain that occurs during aging continues or is accelerated in these subjects, it might be expected that they will develop a parkinsonian syndrome at a relatively young age.

Since Parkinson's disease is not a genetic disorder, the occurrence of toxins in food, chemical wastes, and agricultural aids has been suggested as a possible etiological factor in the development of spontaneous Parkinson's disease. Several groups of investigators are searching for environmental substances that might promote effects similar to MPTP. Since smokers are believed to have a lower incidence of Parkinson's disease, it is possible that tobacco smoke

contains a substance that protects the neurons against such an environmental toxin.

The specific vulnerability of the nigrostriatal neurons to MPTP toxicity might be related to the vulnerability of these neurons to other agents that promote degeneration. Drugs such as deprenyl, which block the neurotoxicity of MPTP, could be beneficial in retarding the progress of the spontaneous degenerative disorder. Birkmayer et al. (3) have claimed that deprenyl administration prolongs the efficacy of L-dopa responsivity in patients with Parkinson's disease.

The animal models of Parkinson's disease also are valuable for development of new therapeutic agents. MPTP-treated animals respond to L-dopa and dopamine agonists and would be useful in evaluating new drugs. Furthermore, the MPTP animal models provide important experimental tools with which to investigate neuronal plasticity and regeneration as well as neuronal implants. There have already been two claims that implantation of fetal brain tissue into brains of MPTP parkinsonian monkeys produced improvement in the clinical syndrome produced by the toxin.

Thus, the tragedy of accidental induction of a severe movement disorder after inadvertent administration of MPTP in young drug addicts and chemists has led to the discovery of an important new research tool and stimulated new approaches to the therapy of Parkinson's disease.

SUMMARY

The amine uptake processes responsible for terminating the actions of biogenic amine neurotransmitters are relatively nonspecific and are also responsible for accumulation of a variety of related substances in biogenic amine-containing neurons. In high concentration some of these substances interfere with essential physiological processes by disrupting membranes, inhibiting enzymes, depleting vital cofactors, etc. The molecular events frequently involve formation of free radicals, directly by quinone formation (6-hydroxydopamine) or after metabolism to a reactive compound (MPP^+ from MPTP). These free-radical-generating substances result in excess production of oxidative species (superoxide, hydrogen peroxide, and hydroxyl radicals) which directly or indirectly damage mitochondria or other essential cell components at a rate that exceeds the capacity of the cell to repair the injury, resulting in cell death.

While these neurotoxins have provided useful pharmacological tools to study the role of the biogenic amine-containing neurons in normal physiology, the striking parkinsonian syndrome produced in primates after MPTP administration and attended by the selective destruction of the nigrostriatal dopaminergic neurons has had an important impact on Parkinson's disease research. First, this model provides a useful means for assessing new therapeutic agents and for developing surgical implantation techniques to determine how to replace successfully degenerated dopaminergic neurons. Second, attention has been redirected at determining the basis for the specific vulnerability of neurons to environmental factors in the pathogenesis of degenerative processes in the hope that by appropriate treatment these processes might be arrested or restored.

Future research on neurotoxins and the mechanism of their actions, as well as the animal models of disease states, promises to provide the basis for exciting new advances in therapy of neuropsychiatric disorders.

REFERENCES

1. Ballard, P. A., Tetrud, J. W., and Langston, J. W. (1985): *Neurology,* 35:949.
2. Barbeau, A., Dallaire, L., Buu, N. T., Veilleux, F., Boyer, H. de, Lanney, L. E., Irwin, I., Langston, E. B., and Langston, J. W. (1985): *Life Sci.,* 36:1125–1134.
3. Birkmayer, W., Knoll, J., Reiderer, P., and Youdim, M. B. H. (1983): *Mod. Probl. Pharmacopsychiatry,* 19:170–176.
4. Bjorklund, A., Baumgarten, H.-G., and Nobin, A. (1984): *Adv. Biochem. Psychopharmacol.,* 10:17.
5. Blank, C. L., Kissinger, P. T., and Adams, R. N. (1972): *Eur. J. Pharmacol.,* 19:391–394.
6. Bridges, J. W., Benford, D. J., and Hubbard, S. A. (1983): *Ann. NY Acad. Sci.,* 407:42–63.
7. Burns, R. S., Chiueh, C. C., Markey, S. P., Ebert, M. H., Jacobowitz, D. M., and Kopin, I. J. (1983): *Proc. Natl. Acad. Sci. USA,* 80:4546–4550.
8. Burns, R. S., LeWitt, P. S., Ebert, M. H., Pakkenberg, H., and Kopin, I. J. (1985): *N. Engl. J. Med.,* 312:1418–1421.
9. Burnstock, G., Evans, B., Gannon, B. J., Heath, J. W., and James, V. (1971): *Br. J. Pharmacol.,* 43:295.
10. Calne, D. B., Langston, J. W., Martin, W. R. W., Stoessl, A. J., Rugh, T. J., Adam, M. J., Pate, B. D., and Schulzer, M. (1985): *Nature,* 317:246.
11. Chiba, K., Trevor, A., and Castagnoli, N., Jr. (1984): *Biochem. Biophys. Res. Commun.,* 120:574–578.
12. Chiueh, C. C., Markey, S. P., Burns, R. S., Johannessen, J. N., Jacobowitz, D. M., and Kopin, I. J. (1984): *Psychopharmacol. Bull.,* 20:548–553.
13. Chiueh, C. C., Markey, S. P., Burns, R. S., Johannessen, J. N.,

14. Cohen, G., and Heikkila, R. E. (1984): *J. Biol. Chem.,* 8:2447–2452.
15. Corsini, G. U., Pintus, S., Chiueh, C. C., Weiss, J. F., and Kopin, I. J. (1985): *Eur. J. Pharmacol.,* 119:127–128.
16. Davis, G. C., Williams, A. C., Markey, S. P., Ebert, M. H., Caine, E. D., Beichert, C. M., and Kopin, I. J. (1979): *Psychiatry Res.,* 1:249–254.
16a. D'Amato, R. J., Lipman, Z. P., and Snyder, S. H. (1986): *Science,* 231:987.
17. Delini-Stula, A., Mogilnicka, E., Hunn, C., and Dooley, D. J. (1984): *Pharmacol. Biochem.,* 20:613–618.
18. Dudley, M. W., Butcher, L. L., Kammerer, R. C., and Cho, A. K. (1981): *J. Pharmacol. Exp. Ther.,* 217:834–840.
19. Enz, A., Hefti, F., and Frick, W. (1984): *Eur. J. Pharmacol.,* 101:37–44.
20. Eranko, O., and Eranko, L. (1971): *Histochem. J.,* 3:451.
21. Freeman, B. A., and Crapo, J. D. (1982): *Lab. Invest.,* 47:412–426.
22. Fuller, R. W., Hahn, R. A., Shoddy, H. D., and Wikel, J. H. (1984): *Biochem. Pharmacol.,* 33:2957–2960.
23. Hallman, H., Lange, J., Olson, L., Stromberg, I., and Jonsson, G. (1985): *J. Neurochem.,* 44:117–127.
24. Hallman, H., Olson, L., and Jonsson, G. (1984): *Eur. J. Pharmacol.,* 97:133–136.
25. Heath, J. W., Hill, C. E., and Burnstock, G. (1984): *J. Neurocytol.,* 3:263–276.
26. Heikkila, R. E. (1985): *Eur. J. Pharmacol.,* 117:131–133.
27. Heikkila, R. E., Hess, A., and Duvoisin, R. C. (1984): *Science,* 224:1451–1453.
28. Heikkila, R. E., Manzino, L., Cabbat, F. S., and Duvoisin, R. C. (1984): *Nature,* 311:467–469.
29. Heikkila, R. E., Mytilineou, C., Cote, L. J., and Cohen, G. (1983): *J. Neurochem.,* 21:111–116.
30. Jacobowitz, D., and Kostrzewa, R. (1971): *Life Sci.,* 10:1329–1342.
31. Jacobs, B. L. (1976): *Life Sci.,* 19:777–782.
32. Jaim-Etcheverry, G., and Zieher, L. M. (1980): *Brain Res.,* 188:513–523.
33. Javitch, J. A., D'Amato, R. J., Strittmatter, S. M., and Snyder, S. H. (1985): *Proc. Natl. Acad. Sci. USA,* 82:2173–2177.
34. Javitch, J. A., and Snyder, S. H. (1984): *Eur. J. Pharmacol.,* 106:455–456.
35. Jenner, P., Rapniak, N. M., Rose, S., Kelly, E., Kilpatrick, G., Lees, A., and Marsden, C. D. (1984): *Neurosci. Lett.,* 50:85–90.
36. Johannessen, J. N., Chiueh, C. C., Bacon, J. P., Garrick, N. A., Murphy, D. L., Burns, R. S., Weise, V. K., Kopin, I. J., and Markey, S. P. (1985): *Soc. Neurosci. Abstr.,* 11:631.
37. Johannessen, J. N., Chiueh, C. C., Burns, R. S., and Markey, S. P. (1985): *Life Sci.,* 36:219–224.
38. Johnson, E. M., Jr., O'Brien, F., and Werbitt, R. (1976): *Eur. J. Pharmacol.,* 37:45–54.
39. Jonsson, G., and Sachs, C. (1973): *J. Neurochem.,* 21:117–224.
40. Juul, P. (1973): *Acta Pharmacol. (Kbh.),* 33:79–80.
41. Kopin, I. J., Markey, S. P., Burns, R. S., Johannessen, J. N., and Chiueh, C. C. (1985): In: *Recent Developments in Parkinson's Disease,* edited by S. Fahn, pp. 165–173. Raven Press, New York.
42. Langston, J. W. (1985): *Life Sci.,* 36:201–206.
43. Langston, J. W., and Ballard, P. (1983): *N. Engl. J. Med.,* 309:310.
44. Langston, J. W., Ballard, P., Tetrud, J. W., and Irwin, I. (1983): *Science,* 219:949–980.
45. Langston, J. W., Forno, L. S., Robert, C. S., and Irwin, I. (1984): *Brain Res.,* 292:390–394.
46. Lee, C. M., Javitch, J. A., and Snyder, S. H. (1982): *J. Neurosci.,* 2:1515–1525.
47. Lent, C. M. (1987): *Brain Res. (in press).*
48. Lyden, A., Bondesson, U., Larsson, B. S., Lindquist, N. G., and Olsson, L. I. (1985): *Acta Pharmacol. Toxicol. (Copenh.),* 57:130–135.
49. Malmquist, J., and Oates, J. A. (1968): *Biochem. Pharmacol.,* 17:1845–1854.

Pert, A., and Kopin, I. J. (1984): *Eur. J. Pharmacol.,* 100:189–194.

50. Markey, S. P., Johannessen, J. N., Chiueh, C. C., Burns, R. S., and Herkenham, M. A. (1984): *Nature,* 311:464–467.
51. Markey, S. P., and Schmuff, N. R. (1987): *Med. Res. Rev. (in press).*
52. Melamed, E., Rosenthal, J., Globus, M., Cohen, O., Frucht, Y., and Uzzan, A. (1985): *Eur. J. Pharmacol.,* 114:97–100.
53. Nicklas, W. J., Vyas, I., and Heikkla, R. E. (1985): *Life Sci.,* 36: 2503–2508.
54. Perry, T. L., Yong, V. W., Clavier, R. M., Jones, K., Wright, J. M., Foulks, J. G., and Wall, R. A. (1985): *Neurosci. Lett.,* 60: 109–114.
55. Poirier, J., and Barbeau, A. (1985): *Neurosci. Lett.,* 62:7–11.
56. Ross, S. B. (1976): *Br. J. Pharmacol.,* 58:521–527.
57. Sachs, C. (1972): *Eur. J. Pharmacol.,* 20:149–155.
58. Schneider, J. S., Yuwiler, A., and Markham, C. H. (1985): *Soc. Neurosci. Abstr.,* 11:1160.
59. Sinha, B. K., Singh, Y., and Krishna, G. (1986): *Biochem. Biophys. Res. Commun.,* 135:583–588.
60. Sullivan, S. G., and Stern, A. (1981): *Biochem. Pharmacol.,* 30: 2279–2285.
61. Thoenen, H., and Tranzer, J. P. (1973): *Annu. Rev. Pharmacol.,* 13:169–180.
62. Tranzer, J. P., and Thoenen, H. (1973): *Experientia,* 29:314–315.
63. Trush, M. A., Mimnaugh, E. G., and Gram, T. E. (1982): *Biochem. Pharmacol.,* 31:3335–3346.
64. Wilkinson, M., Jacobson, W., and Wilkinson, D. A. (1985): *Brain Res. Bull.,* 14:493–495.

Psychopharmacology:
The Third Generation of Progress,
edited by Herbert Y. Meltzer.
Raven Press, New York © 1987.

CHAPTER **38**

Neurotoxicity of Methamphetamine and Related Drugs

Lewis S. Seiden and George A. Ricaurte

Methamphetamine (MA) (N-methyl-β-phenylisopropylamine), synthesized by Ogata (87), is one of the most potent indirectly acting sympathomimetic amines known. MA effects on the autonomic nervous system include cardiovascular stimulation, bronchodilatation, mydriasis, and other effects mediated by α- and β-adrenergic receptors (70). In the central nervous system, actions of MA typically lead to psychomotor activation, anorexia, hypodypsia, respiratory stimulation, hyperthermia, and, in humans, lessened fatigue and a euphoric sense of well-being (45). Due to their euphoric and antifatigue effects, MA and related psychomotor stimulant drugs are readily self-administered by humans as well as by a variety of experimental animals (109). Self-administration of MA by humans and other primates has led to the definition of MA as a positively reinforcing drug. The powerful reinforcing property of MA is seen when rhesus monkeys given unlimited access to intravenous MA self-administer a lethal dose (57).

Although the high abuse liability of MA and its congeners has long been recognized, it is only in the last decade that a concerted effort has been made to determine whether any long-lasting neurotoxic effects result from long-term or high-dose MA administration. This effort to assess the neurotoxic properties of MA and related compounds was largely prompted by epidemics of MA abuse that occurred between 1950 and 1970 in Japan (12), Great Britain (62), Sweden (55,58), and the United States (3,44,66), as well as by the observation that prolonged use of relatively high doses of MA and related drugs induced a psychotic state that closely resembled paranoid schizophrenia (8,20,21,24,25,60,120).

This chapter will review data collected over the last 10 years indicating that MA and some of its congeners exert toxic effects on brain dopamine (DA) and serotonin (5-hydroxytryptamine; 5-HT) neurons in experimental animals. First, the selectivity, determinants, and molecular mechanisms underlying the neurotoxic effects will be detailed. Second, the absence of gross behavioral alterations thus far found in MA-treated animals will be considered, and reasons why overt behavioral abnormalities do not uniformly occur will be outlined. Finally, the implications of MA-induced neurotoxicity in the study of neurodegenerative disease will be discussed.

BACKGROUND

Even before studies aimed specifically at assessing the neurotoxic properties of amphetamines were undertaken, there were two sets of published reports indicating that amphetamines might be toxic to brain DA and 5-HT neurons. The first set showed that parachloroamphetamine (PCA) and other halogenated amphetamine derivatives produced a marked and persistent reduction in brain 5-HT metabolites and levels, as well as a decrease in the number of 5-HT uptake sites (37–39,90,104,105). Although the basis for these long-lasting 5-HT neurochemical deficits was not clear initially (40,50,73,88,107), it was later concluded that PCA caused 5-HT nerve terminal destruction (33,46,106,108). Although the possibility that amphetamine itself might be toxic seems to have been considered, the observation that an equal dose of amphetamine did not produce comparable 5-HT deficits to PCA led many investigators to conclude that neurotoxicity was a unique property of PCA and not necessarily a property of amphetamine or all of its congeners (34).

The second set of early studies hinting at a neurotoxic action of amphetamines showed that MA suppressed striatal tyrosine hydroxylase (TH) activity. Results from these studies indicated that MA caused decreased neostriatal TH activity for as long as 1 week beyond the period of drug administration (28,63,64). This effect was antagonized by DA receptor blockers (14) as well as by γ-aminobutyric acid (GABA) transaminase inhibitors (52) and it was postulated that the decrease in TH activity was due to stimulation of DA receptors in the striatum causing inhibition of TH activity through a striatonigral feedback pathway (41,42,52). We will now review data that show persistent decrease in TH activity is due to DA terminal destruction by MA.

DOPAMINERGIC NEUROTOXICITY

Documentation

Effects of MA and Related Drugs on Nerve Terminals

In 1975, Seiden, Fischman, and Schuster (113) reported that rhesus monkeys repeatedly administered high doses of MA had a depletion of caudate DA that lasted for at least 6 months beyond the period of drug administration. Although this long-lasting DA depletion strongly suggested that MA might be toxic to DA terminals in the striatum, the prolonged depletion was not sufficient to demonstrate neurotoxicity. A long-lasting DA depletion could be caused by (a) a residual metabolite of the drug (as had been demonstrated with reserpine), (b) a metabolic alteration of DA neurons that did not involve cellular morphological destruction, or (c) a frank neurodegenerative effect of MA.

An important finding regarding which of these processes was at work was provided by Ellison and co-workers (26). These investigators showed that continuous amphetamine exposure caused not only a persistent decrease in neostriatal TH activity, but also induced appearance of brightly fluorescent swollen axons in the neostriatum. Since similar axonal swellings were known to occur after administration of 6HDA, a documented DA neurotoxin (1), these authors (26) proposed that amphetamine might damage DA nerve fibers. This suggestion was supported by the subsequent finding that amphetamine and MA reduced the number but not the affinity of DA uptake sites (86,125,132). DA nerve terminal destruction by MA was then demonstrated with the silver degeneration method of Fink and Heimer (94,101). Other studies followed which showed that amphetamine also destroyed DA terminals (72,93).

Effects on Cell Bodies

The evidence at present to suggest that MA and amphetamine destroy dopaminergic cell bodies in the substantia nigra is not convergent. Fink-Heimer sections through the substantia nigra indicate that in the same rats that showed dense terminal degeneration in the neostriatum, there was no sign of cell body degeneration (94). There was also no evidence of cell loss in paraffin sections through the substantia nigra of comparably treated rats killed 2 weeks after drug treatment (94). Nwanze and Jonsson (86) have also reported that DA cell bodies in the substantia nigra of mice continuously administered amphetamine are not affected. It should be noted, however, that in the studies cited above rats had only approximately a 50% DA depletion. Another set of data shows a larger DA depletion might be associated with cell loss. One recent preliminary report suggests this may be the case (126). Unfortunately, in primates, where a larger DA depletion can be consistently produced, the substantia nigra has not yet been examined.

Differences Between Terminal Fields

Not all DA terminal fields seem to be equally affected by MA. DA terminals in the striatum are the most severely affected, whereas the DA terminals in the hypothalamus appear spared (26,84,99). DA terminals in the nucleus accumbens, olfactory area, and frontal cortex are only minimally affected (84,99). The basis for these regional differences is at present unclear. Known differences in DA uptake systems in these areas (22,82,121) may be responsible, although the mechanism underlying this and its relationship to MA-induced toxicity remain speculative (114).

Selectivity to DA and 5-HT Systems

MA induces neurotoxicity at doses several times its behaviorally effective dose. Therefore, the issue of selectivity to specific CNS neurons is critical. The neurotoxic action of MA appears to be selective rather than part of a general nonspecific toxic reaction in the CNS. There are several lines of evidence to support this. First, other neuronal systems in the striatum are not altered by large doses of MA. Doses of MA that cause a profound reduction in striatal TH activity and DA levels do not alter the activity of either choline acetyltransferase or glutamate decarboxylase, indicating that cholinergic and GABAergic neurons are not destroyed by MA (54). Second, NE levels in various regions of the rat brain are not altered by MA (132,133). Third, DA neurotoxicity can be prevented with DA uptake blockers (35,53,101,124). If DA terminal destruction produced by MA were due to a nonspecific insult such as ischemia (71) or inhibition of protein synthesis (17,103), it seems highly unlikely that neurotoxic specificity of the type described above would be observed.

Two observations of considerable interest were made while investigating the selectivity of MA's DA neurotoxic action. First, 5-HT neurons were also affected by MA administration. Second, a group of somatosensory cortical neurons also appeared to be damaged by MA. Both of these toxic effects of MA are described in detail below.

Determinants

Dose and Duration of Exposure

The DA neurotoxic effect of MA has been shown to be related to dose (101,132) and duration of exposure (89). High doses of MA and amphetamine are generally required to induce DA neurotoxicity in primates and rodents. The need for high doses appears to be related to two factors: (a) the relatively short half-life of these two amphetamines (119) and (b) the apparent need for the drug to persist at its site of action for several hours. The importance of dose and duration was elucidated by Ellison et al. (26), who demonstrated DA neurotoxicity with a much lower dose of amphetamine by administering it continuously in subcutaneously implanted silicone pellets. This finding, which was soon confirmed by other investigators using osmotic minipumps (86,125), led Fuller and Hemrick-Luecke (35) to show that a single dose of amphetamine was sufficient to produce DA neurotoxicity if it was coadministered with iprindole, a drug that inhibits amphetamine metabolism and thereby increases its duration of action (32). These findings were extended to MA (89,101), and it became apparent that DA neurotoxicity was dependent not only on dose but also on persistence of drug at its site of action for several hours.

Route of Administration

Route of administration influences duration of drug action by determining *rate* of drug entry into the bloodstream (43). Accordingly, MA administered intraperitoneally is less effective than MA administered subcutaneously (unpublished observation). MA given intravenously is effective in monkeys but it must be administered very frequently (every 3 hr) and in high doses (113,131). MA infused directly in brain for several hours produces DA neurotoxicity (114).

Stereospecificity

Comparison of the toxic properties of S(+) amphetamine (*d*-amphetamine) and R(−) amphetamine (*l*-amphetamine) has revealed that *d*-amphetamine is approximately seven times more potent than *l*-amphetamine in iprindole-treated rats (123). This marked difference is not due to differences in concentrations or half-lives of the isomers in brain tissue (123).

Age

Sensitivity to the neurotoxic effects of MA is influenced by the age of the animal. Neonatal (7-day-old) rats develop smaller long-lasting DA depletions than young mature (60-day-old) rats given an equivalent amount of MA (75). This is in contrast to DA neurotoxicity induced by 6HDA, which is more pronounced in neonatal rats (77,81). Of note is that sensitivity to the DA neurotoxic effect of MA does not appear to continue to increase with age. Older mice (8–12 months of age) do not develop larger DA depletions than young mature mice (6–8 weeks of age) given an equivalent amount of MA (96). Older mice and rats (L. S. Seiden, unpublished observation) are, however, more sensitive to the lethal effect of MA.

Species

Long-lasting DA neurochemical deficits following either MA or amphetamine administration have now been demonstrated in several species, including rats (36,52,53,132), mice (86,125), guinea pigs (133), cats (69), and rhesus monkeys (113,131). There is at present no direct evidence that DA neurotoxicity occurs in humans as a consequence of use or abuse of amphetamines. Nonetheless, the striking species generalization found thus far suggests that humans taking high frequent doses of MA may be at risk (see below).

Although detailed studies comparing sensitivity of different species to neurotoxic effects of amphetamines have not been performed, available evidence suggests that mice are less sensitive than rats (101,125), and that cats may be quite sensitive (69). In general, primates appear to be the most sensitive of the animals tested (131). These results must be interpreted with caution, however, as routes and schedules of administration have not always been constant. In comparing species sensitivities, it will be important to consider not only absolute doses required to produce neurotoxicity but also the ratio of toxic dose to behaviorally active dose.

Environmental Conditions

MA effects on DA neurons are influenced by the environment. Ambient temperature, for example, markedly increases long-term DA depletions induced by MA (97). By contrast, aggregation augments the 5-HT neurotoxic effect of MA but has little or no effect on DA neurotoxicity (97).

Mechanisms

Of particular interest is the recent observation that a single large dose of MA induces formation of 6HDA in the striatum of the rat brain (114). MA's toxic effects on DA neurons depend on the integrity of the cytoplasmic pool. Two predisposing factors have been suggested to be responsible for DA neurotoxicity: (a) massive DA release and (b) monoamine oxidase inhibition by large doses of MA (114). Given these two conditions, Seiden and Vosmer (114) hypothesized that endogenous DA (previously released by MA) was nonenzymatically converted in the synaptic cleft to 6HDA, which then is accumulated by the DA terminals and causes the terminal to degenerate (78). A substance found in the caudate nucleus of MA-treated rats has a retention time identical to that of 6HDA. That such a nonenzymatic conversion can in fact take place has been previously demonstrated *in vitro* (115,117). Given the significance of the finding of *in vivo* formation of 6HDA, it will be important to insure that the substance found in the caudate nucleus of MA-treated rats is in fact 6HDA. Such efforts are in progress using gas chromatographic and mass spectrometric methods to confirm the identity of this substance as 6HDA. Endogenous formation of 6HDA from DA is an important general finding because it suggests that neurotoxins can be formed from substances present in the brain. This raises the possibility that neurotoxins may be found under other conditions (such as stress) and that the endogenous neurotoxins may be responsible for the loss of terminals that occurs with aging (116).

Pharmacological observations are consistent with the notion that 6HDA formed from endogenous DA mediates DA terminal destruction by MA. First, α-methyl-para-tyrosine blocks the DA neurotoxic effect of MA (53,129). Second, reserpine (which increases many of the pharmacological effects of MA) augments the DA neurotoxicity of MA (93,129). Third, pargyline a monoamine oxidase (MAO) inhibitor that also augments the pharmacological effects of MA also increases DA neurotoxicity after MA (also see 11). Fourth, DA uptake blockers such as amfonelic acid prevent DA terminal destruction by MA (95) and amphetamine (35,124), perhaps by blocking uptake of extraneuronally formed 6HDA into DA terminals. Fifth, DA receptor blockers (haloperidol, chlorpromazine) also block MA engendered neurotoxicity (13), perhaps by blocking the DA uptake pump (especially at the relatively high concentrations that have been employed). Sixth, ascorbic acid has been shown to attenuate the DA neurotoxic effect of MA (128). It is possible that ascorbate does so by interfering with the nonenzymatic conversion of endogenous DA into 6HDA. These observations strongly suggest that DA is essential for the expression of the MA neurotoxicity to DA terminals (112,114).

Not all of the pharmacologic influences that have been reported to date are readily explained by the scheme proposed above. Aminooxyacetic acid, for example, is a GABA transaminase inhibitor that also protects against MA-induced DA neurochemical alterations, yet it has no known effect on DA synthesis, uptake, or release. Also, the finding that methylphenidate, another psychomotor stimulant drug that releases and blocks the reuptake of DA (27,51), does not induce DA neurotoxicity (see below) is not consistent with the above scheme. However, this may be related to the fact that methylphenidate is approximately 10 times less potent than amphetamine at releasing DA and releases DA from the vesicular pool rather than the cytoplasmic pool (83).

Other Psychomotor Stimulants

Cathinone is the principal psychoactive alkaloid in khat leaves, which are chewed throughout eastern Africa and the Arab peninsula. Structurally cathinone resembles amphetamine and has similar neurochemical and behavioral effects (61). Studies indicate cathinone can also be toxic to DA neurons (130). As noted above, methylphenidate lacks DA neurotoxic activity (131,134).

Duration of DA Deficits

In primates, the depletion of caudate DA induced by methamphetamine appears to be permanent. Rhesus monkeys killed as long as 6 months after the last MA injection show no sign of DA recovery (113). Indeed, monkeys sacrificed almost 4 years after MA treatment still show a large depletion of caudate DA (L. S. Seiden, unpublished observation).

In rodents, the data are a bit more complicated. No recovery of DA was observed over an 8-week period in either rats treated with MA (132) or mice treated with amphetamine (86). In fact, in rats a depletion of caudate DA has been found in rats as long as 6 months after MA administration (10). By contrast, some authors have found partial recovery of TH activity over a 110-day period (84) and of DA uptake over an 8-week period (86). Thus there appears to be recovery of some but not all DA terminal markers. However, it should be noted that in Nwanze and Jonsson's study, the number of DA uptake sites was not quantified by means of kinetic analysis, raising the possibility that the partial recovery was due to an increase in affinity rather than number of uptake sites. Morgan and Gibb's (84) determination of TH activity is open to the same criticism. This caveat aside, it seems that in rodents there is no recovery of DA concentration, but there is partial recovery of TH activity and DA uptake after treatment with amphetamines. Nwanze and Jonsson (86) have speculated that this may be related to regenerative sprouting and that regenerating nerve fibers have a lower concentration of DA. This interesting hypothesis awaits validation.

SEROTONERGIC NEUROTOXICITY

Documentation

Nerve Terminals

As noted above, the toxic effect of MA on 5-HT nerve terminals was discovered while investigating the selectivity of MA's effect on DA neurons. MA-treated rats were found to have not only a large long-lasting depletion of DA, but also an even larger and equally long-lasting depletion of 5-HT in certain brain regions (99). This depletion was associated with loss of 5-HT uptake sites (99), a decrease in the concentration of brain 5-hydroxyindoleacetic acid (5-HIAA) (99), and a reduction in tryptophan hydroxylase activity (5,52,53). These findings suggested that MA was also toxic to 5-HT nerve terminals. Moreover, the fact that the neurochemical deficits in the 5-HT system were larger than those observed in the DA system indicated that 5-HT neurons were more sensitive than DA neurons to the toxic effect of MA (52,53,99). It should be noted that direct morphologic evidence of 5-HT terminal destruction by MA has yet to be presented. However, given recent data on methylenedioxyamphetamine (MDA) (92) demonstrating concomitant depletions of 5-HT in association with degenerating terminals in the striatum of rats, it seems likely that the same is true of MA. Acute effects of chronic MA administration on 5-HT systems have also been described (89).

Cell Bodies

There is no evidence at present that MA destroys serotonergic cell bodies in the brainstem raphe nuclei. However, Harvey and colleagues (49,50) and others (9,80,85) have previously reported that some of the halogenated amphetamine derivatives selectively destroy 5-HT cell bodies in the ventrolateral mesencephalic tegmentum (B-9 cells according to Dahlstrom and Fuxe, ref. 21). Since these reports have been disputed (73), it will be of interest to determine whether 5-HT cell body degeneration occurs after MA and other MA congeners with 5-HT neurotoxic activity.

Regional Differences

5-HT terminals in various brain regions appear sensitive to the toxic effect of MA. 5-HT nerve terminals in the hippocampus, cerebral cortex, amygdala, and striatum are all severely affected by MA (84,99). The least affected terminals are those in the hypothalamus (99). A small 5-HT depletion occurs in the brainstem (99). It is unclear whether this is due to axonal, dendritic or cell body damage.

Determinants

5-HT terminal destruction by MA is dose related (99) and dependent on the persistence of MA at its site of action for several hours (89). Neonatal rats are less vulnerable than young mature rats to the 5-HT neurotoxic effect of MA (75). This contrasts with reports that neonatal rats are more sensitive than young mature rats to the toxic effect of dihydroxytryptamines (11,76). 5-HT neurotoxicity following MA administration has now been observed in rats (52,53,99) rhesus monkeys (91), and mice (G. A. Ricaurte, unpublished observation).

Mechanisms

Preliminary data indicate that 5,6-dihydroxytryptamine (5,6-DHT) derived from 5-HT may be involved in the 5-HT neurotoxic action of MA. Using high-performance liquid chromatography (HPLC) methods, a substance has been identified in the brain of rats given a single large dose of MA that has the exact same retention time as 5,6-DHT (4), a known 5-HT neurotoxin (6,7). This finding raises the possibility that 5-HT released by MA is converted to 5,6-DHT and that this compound is taken back up into 5-HT terminals, which are subsequently destroyed. Consistent with this proposal is the finding that 5-HT uptake blockers protect against the 5-HT neurotoxic effect of MA (52,53,111). The mechanisms underlying MA-induced endogenous formation of 5,6-DHT are not known. A puzzling observation is that, PCPA, a 5-HT synthesis inhibitor (64), does not block the 5-HT neurotoxic effect of MA (4,110), since this suggests that the 5,6-DHT formed in the presence of MA originates from something other than 5-HT. Another puzzling finding is that 5-HT neurotoxicity induced by MA is blocked by AMT (52,53). As AMT has no effect on 5-HT metabolism, this suggests that either TH or catecholamines are somehow involved in the 5-HT neurotoxic action of MA.

Other Amphetamines

The 5-HT neurotoxic effect of amphetamine is not as potent as that of MA (101,125; K. J. Axt, unpublished data). In our laboratory, this was first noted during experiments in which amphetamine and MA were being given continuously by means of osmotic minipumps. Under these conditions, both MA and amphetamine produced a persistent DA depletion, but neither affected 5-HT levels on a long-term basis (101). At first the failure of MA to reduce 5-HT levels seemed puzzling, since 5-HT neurons were thought to be more sensitive than DA neurons to the toxic effect of MA (52,53,84,99). Then it became apparent that MA's failure to produce 5-HT toxicity when given continuously was probably related to the fact that slow continuous infusion allowed for peripheral conversion of MA to amphetamine, which was not as potent a toxin to 5-HT fibers. This was later confirmed using large repeated doses of amphetamine. Even very high doses of amphetamine (50 mg/kg given three times at 8-hr intervals) produced only a minimal long-lasting effect on 5-HT terminal markers.

Whereas amphetamine shows little 5-HT neurotoxic activity, other amphetamine analogs have now been identified which are more potent 5-HT neurotoxins than MA. The potency of the toxic effect is measured by considering the behaviorally affected dose (B) relative to the toxic dose (T). Thus, T/B could be considered as the toxic index. With MA, T/B is 50 to 100; but with other compounds to be discussed below, T/B is 2 to 4.

MDA is one of a number of ring-substituted amphetamines with hallucinogenic activity (79) that has been widely abused (56,102,118). Neurochemical and morphological evidence has been presented indicating that MDA is toxic to central 5-HT neurons (92). MDMA is another hallucinogenic amphetamine analog that appears to possess 5-HT neurotoxic activity (136). One striking feature about both MDA and MDMA is that they produce very large 5-HT deficits at much lower doses than MA (92,127). Another is that neither MDA or MDMA produces DA neurotoxicity at low doses. Thus, substitution on the phenyl ring alters the spectrum of toxic action of the amphetamine molecule and greatly enhances its 5-HT neurotoxic activity. Another ring-substituted amphetamine that appears to possess potent 5-HT neurotoxic activity is fenfluramine (18,47,48). Fenfluramine is currently used in the treatment of autistic children and efforts need to be directed at determining whether or not similar toxicity occurs in humans. The toxic potential of other ring-substituted amphetamines used or abused by humans also needs to be evaluated.

SOMATOSENSORY NEUROTOXICITY

Silver degeneration studies using the Fink-Heimer method (29) have revealed that MA causes degeneration of cell bodies located in a highly restricted region of the cerebral cortex (laminae III and IV of somatosensory cortical area 2, as defined by Krieg, ref. 67). In silver preparations, the neurons affected by MA have intensely argyrophilic perikarya and dendritic arbors that appear beaded; when silver sections are counterstained with cresyl violet, it can be seen that these neurons are often surrounded by glial cells, suggesting phagocytosis (94,95). The features described above suggest these neurons are undergoing degeneration. Similar toxic effects on somatosensory cortical neurons are produced by PCA and 5,6-DHT, but not 6HDA (D. Commins, unpublished observation). Recently MDA and MDMA have also been found to produce toxicity to cortical neurons (L. S. Seiden, unpublished observation). The possibility that these may be amine-producing uptake-dependent (APUD) cells is being evaluated. Somatosensory neurotoxicity induced by MA is blocked by AMT (18,19), an inhibitor of tyrosine hydroxylase (122).

CONSEQUENCES

Rats and Monkeys

Although during and immediately after the period of MA administration animals (both rats and rhesus monkeys) are clearly under the influence of the psychomotor stimulant action of the drug, several weeks later they appear entirely normal (30,31,74,100). To the best of our knowledge, no permanent overt behavioral disturbance has yet been adequately documented in animals previously intoxicated with MA. This probably relates to the fact that damage of DA and 5-HT terminal projections by MA is subtotal, rarely involving more than 70% of either projection system. Preservation of apparently normal function in the face of partial denervation may also result from related compensatory processes. Remaining nerve fibers may increase turnover of their transmitter or regrow portions that have been damaged or sprout collateral terminals from undamaged fibers (100).

Although no overt changes have been recorded, MA-treated animals display an altered sensitivity to various pharmacological agents believed to act through central DA systems. For example, rhesus monkeys trained to respond for food on a differential reinforcement for low rate (DRL) schedule show increased sensitivity to the disruptive effect of haloperidol, as well as a decreased sensitivity to the effects of apomorphine and MA (30). Similar observations have been made in rats using locomotor activity as a behavioral endpoint (74). Recently, Ando (2) has reported sensitivity changes to dopaminergic agents in rhesus monkeys tested for fine motor control, and Woolverton has found that rhesus monkeys previously intoxicated with MA tend to later self-administer higher doses of MA (133). Thus, although MA-treated animals may display no gross behavioral disturbance, they clearly show an altered sensitivity to various drugs that exert their effects through central DA systems. It seems likely that this altered sensitivity to dopaminergic agents is related to the subtotal destruction of DA neurons. Whether there are similar changes in sensitivity to serotonergic agents as a result of 5-HT nerve terminal destruction is not known. It would appear that

pharmacological challenge will prove to be a useful way of detecting partial, clinically inapparent, damage of neurons in the CNS.

Humans

Whether abuse of MA and related drugs produces neurotoxic changes in humans is not yet known. One factor to bear in mind is that doses of amphetamines required to produce neurotoxicity in animals have generally been high, ranging from 10 to 100 mg/kg depending on the particular amphetamine, its route and schedule of administration, as well as the particular species in question. The fact that primates are generally more sensitive than rodents (see above) obviously raises concerns, as does the fact that, as tolerance develops, individuals self-administer increasingly higher doses of amphetamines (59). Nonetheless, at present there is no clear indication that dopaminergic, serotonergic, or somatosensory cortical neurons are destroyed by amphetamines in humans. If neuronal damage does occur, it must be of insufficient size to produce clinically apparent signs, as there is little in the medical literature to suggest damage to DA, 5-HT, or somatosensory systems.

If MA is toxic to DA neurons in humans, its toxic effect is probably limited to DA terminals, as no reports have appeared of MA-induced Parkinsonian syndrome similar to that produced by 1-methyl-4-phenyl-1,2,3,6-tetrahydropyridine (MPTP), a recently described toxin that causes degeneration of DA cells in the substantia nigra (68) (I. J. Kopin, *this volume*). Partial destruction of dopaminergic neurons may not be without consequence, however, as it may predispose individuals to developing Parkinson's disease at an earlier age (15,16). Studies are needed to determine whether the neurotoxic effects of MA and related drugs found in animals generalize to humans, and, if they do, to ascertain the long-term consequences of this toxicity.

SUMMARY AND CONCLUSIONS

Studies over the last 10 years have generated rather compelling evidence that MA and some of its analogs destroy central dopaminergic and serotonergic nerve terminals, as well as a subset of as yet chemically unidentified somatosensory cortical neurons in a variety of experimental animals. Of the three neuronal elements damaged by MA, serotonergic neurons appear to be the most sensitive, particularly to ring-substituted amphetamines such as MDA and MDMA. Although these amphetamine analogs have not yet been shown to exert similar neurotoxic effects in humans, it seems that caution is warranted in their use. From a theoretical standpoint, perhaps the most significant aspect of the studies reviewed above is the clue they provide regarding the basis of neurodegenerative diseases involving central DA and 5-HT neurons. Specifically, the observation that MA can induce conversion of endogenous DA and 5-HT into 6HDA and 5,6-DHT, respectively, suggests that in normal animals there may be alternate metabolic pathways which, if activated, lead to formation of toxic DA and 5-HT metabolites. Endogenously formed toxins may thus be at the basis of neurodegenerative disorders such as Parkinson's disease. Are there conditions other than MA administration that promote formation of endogenous neurotoxins? Can other neurotransmitters be metabolized into toxic compounds? Can aberrant metabolic pathways be blocked? These are difficult questions, which hopefully studies over the coming decade will answer.

REFERENCES

1. Anden, N., Dahlstrom, A., Fuxe, K., and Larsson, K. (1965): *Am. J. Anat.*, 116:329–334.
2. Ando, K., Johanson, C. E., Seiden, L. S., and Schuster, C. R. (1985): *Pharmacol. Biochem. Behav.*, 22:737–743.
3. Angrist, B. M., and Gershon, S. (1969): *Semin. Psychiatry*, 1: 195–203.
4. Axt, K. J., Commins, D. L., and Seiden, L. S. (1985): *Soc. Neurosci. Abstr.*, 11:1193.
5. Bakhit, C., Morgan, M. A., Peat, M. A., and Gibb, J. W. (1981): *Neuropharmacology*, 20:1135–1140.
6. Baumgarten, H. G., Bjorklund, A., Lachenmeyer, L., Nobin, A., and Stenevi, U. (1971): *Acta Physiol. Scand.(Suppl.)*, 373:7–15.
7. Baumgarten, H. G., Evetts, K., Holman, R., Iversen, L., Vogt, M., and Wilson, G. (1972): *J. Neurochem.*, 19:1587–1597.
8. Bell, D. S. (1965): *Br. J. Psychiatry*, 111:701–708.
9. Bertilsson, L., Koslow, S., and Costa, E. (1975): *Brain Res.*, 91: 348–350.
10. Bittner, S. E., Wagner, G. C., Aigner, T. G., and Seiden, L. S. (1981): *Pharmacol. Biochem. Behav.*, 14:481–486.
11. Breese, G. R., and Traylor, T. D. (1971): *Br. J. Pharmacol.*, 42: 88–89.
12. Brill, H., and Hirose, T. (1969): *Semin. Psychiatry.*, 1:179–194.
13. Buening, M. K., and Gibb, J. W. (1974): *Eur. J. Pharmacol.*, 26: 30–34.
14. Calne, D. B., and Langston, J. W. (1983): *Lancet*, 2:1457–1459.
15. Calne, D. B., Langston, J. W., Martin, W., Stoessel, A., Ruth, T., Adam, M., and Schulzer, M. (1985): *Nature*, 317:246–248.
16. Carenzi, A., and Casacci, F. (1977): In: *Adv. Biochem. Psychopharmacol., Vol. 16*, edited by E. Costa and G. Gessa, pp. 583–587. Raven Press, New York.
17. Clineshmidt, B., Totaro, J., McGuffin, J., and Pflueger, A. (1976): *Eur. J. Pharmacol.*, 35:211–214.
18. Commins, D., and Seiden, L. S. (1986): *Brain Res.*, 365:15–20.
19. Commins, D., Seiden, L. S., and Schuster, C. R. (1984): *Soc. Neurosci. Abstr.*, 10:1199.
20. Connell, P. H. (1958): *Amphetamine Psychosis*. Chapman and Hall, Ltd., London.
21. Dahlstrom, A., and Fuxe, K. (1964): *Acta Physiol. Scand.*, 62(Suppl. 232):1–55.
22. Demarest, K. T., and Moore, K. E. (1979): *Brain Res.*, 171:545–551.
23. Eison, M. S., Ellison, G., and Eison, A. S. (1981): *J. Pharmacol. Exp. Ther.*, 218:237–241.
24. Ellinwood, E. H. (1967): *J. Nerv. Ment. Dis.*, 144:273.
25. Ellinwood, E. H. (1968): *Int. J. Neuropsychiatry*, 4:45–67.
26. Ellison, G. M., Eison, H., Huberman, H., and Daniel, F. (1978): *Science*, 201:276–278.
27. Ferris, R. M., Tang, F., and Maxwell, R. (1972): *J. Pharmacol. Exp. Ther.*, 181:407–416.
28. Fibiger, H. C., and McGeer, P. L. (1971): *Eur. J. Pharmacol.*, 16:176–180.
29. Fink, R. P., and Heimer, L. (1967): *Brain Res.*, 4:369–374.
30. Finnegan, K. T., Ricaurte, G. A., Seiden, L. S., and Schuster, C. R. (1982): *Psychopharmacology*, 77:43–52.
31. Fischman, M. W., and Schuster, C. R. (1977): *J. Pharmacol. Exp. Ther.*, 201:593–605.
32. Freeman, J. J., and Sulser, F. (1972): *J. Pharmacol. Exp. Ther.*, 183:307–315.
33. Fuller, R. W. (1978): *Ann. NY Acad. Sci.*, 305:147–159.
34. Fuller, R. W. (1978): *Ann. NY Acad. Sci.*, 305:178–201.
35. Fuller, R. W., and Hemrick-Luecke, S. (1980): *Science*, 209:305–307.
36. Fuller, R. W., and Hemrick-Luecke, S. (1982): *Neuropharmacology*, 21:433–438.
37. Fuller, R. W., Hines, C. W., and Mills, J. (1965): *Biochem. Pharmacol.*, 14:483–488.
38. Fuller, R. W., Perry, K. W., and Molloy, B. B. (1975): *Eur. J. Pharmacol.*, 33:119–124.
39. Fuller, R. W., and Snoddy, H. D. (1974): *Neuropharmacology*, 13:85–90.
40. Gal, E. M., Christiansen, P. A., and Yunger, L. M. (1975): *Neuropharmacology*, 14:31–39.
41. Gibb, J. W., and Hotchkiss, A. J. (1978): In: *Catecholamines: Basic and Clinical Frontiers*, edited by E. Usdin, I. Kopin, and J. Barchas, pp. 1125–1127. Pergamon Press, New York.
42. Gibb, J. W., and Kogan, F. J. (1979): *Naunyn Schmiedebergs Arch. Pharmacol.*, 310:185–187.
43. Goldstein, A., Aronow, L., and Kalman, S. (1974): *Principles of Drug Action*. John Wiley and Sons, New York.
44. Griffith, J. (1966): *Am. J. Psychiatry*, 123:560.
45. Gunne, L. M. (1977): In: *Drug Addiction II*, edited by W. R. Martin, pp. 248–275. Springer Verlag, New York.
46. Harvey, J. A. (1978): *Ann. NY Acad. Sci.*, 305:289–304.
47. Harvey, J. A., and McMaster, S. E. (1975): *Commun. Psychopharmacol.*, 1:217–228.
48. Harvey, J. A., and McMaster, S. E. (1977): *Commun. Psychopharmacol.*, 1:3–17.
49. Harvey, J. A., McMaster, S. E., and Fuller, R. W. (1977): *J. Pharmacol. Exp. Ther.*, 202:581–589.
50. Harvey, J. A., McMaster, S. E., and Yunger, L. (1975): *Science*, 187:841–843.
51. Heikkila, R. E., Orlanski, H., and Cohen, G. (1975): *Biochem. Pharmacol.*, 24:847–852.
52. Hotchkiss, A. J., and Gibb, J. W. (1980): *Eur. J. Pharmacol.*, 66: 204–205.
53. Hotchkiss, A. J., and Gibb, J. W. (1980): *J. Pharmacol. Exp. Ther.*, 214:257–262.
54. Hotchkiss, A. J., Morgan, M. E., and Gibb, J. W. (1979): *Life Sci.*, 25:1377–1378.
55. Inghe, G. (1969): In: *Abuse of Central Stimulants*, edited by F. Sjoqvist and M. Tottie, pp. 187–219. Almqvist and Wiksell, Stockholm.
56. Jackson, B., and Reeds, A. (1970): *JAMA*, 211:830–832.
57. Johanson, C. E., Balster, R. L., and Bonese, K. (1976): *Pharmacol. Biochem. Behav.*, 4:45–51.
58. Jonsson, L., and Gunne, L. (1970): In: *Amphetamines and Related Compounds*, edited by E. Costa and S. Garattini, pp. 929–936. Raven Press, New York.
59. Kalant, H., LeBlanc, A., and Gibbins, R. J. (1971): *Pharmacol. Rev.*, 23:135–181.
60. Kalant, O. (1966): *The Amphetamines: Toxicity and Addiction*. Charles C. Thomas, Springfield, IL.
61. Kalix, P., and Braenden, O. (1985): *Pharmacol. Rev.*, 37:149–164.
62. Kiloh, L. A., and Brandon, S. (1962): *Br. Med. J.*, 2:40.
63. Koda, L. Y., and Gibb, J. W. (1973): *J. Pharmacol. Exp. Ther.*, 185:42–48.
64. Koe, B. K., and Weissman, A. (1966): *J. Pharmacol. Exp. Ther.*, 154:499–516.
65. Kogan, J. F., Nichols, W. K., and Gibb, J. W. (1976): *Eur. J. Pharmacol.*, 36:363–371.
66. Kramer, J. C., Fischman, V. S., and Littlefield, D. C. (1967): *JAMA*, 201:305–309.
67. Krieg, W. S. (1964): *J. Comp. Neurol.*, 84:221–333.
68. Langston, J. W. (1985): *Trends Neurosci.*, 8:79–83.
69. Levine, M. S., Hull, C. D., Garcia-Rill, E., Erinoff, L., Buchwald, A., and Heller, A. (1980): *Brain Res.*, 194:263–268.
70. Lewander, T. (1977): In: *Drug Addiction II*, edited by W. R. Martin, pp. 33–181. Springer Verlag, New York.
71. Lindvall, O., Ingvar, M., and Stenevi, U. (1981): *Brain Res.*, 211: 211–216.
72. Lorez, H. (1981): *Life Sci.*, 28:911–916.
73. Lorez, H., Saner, A., and Richards, J. G. (1978): *Brain Res.*, 146:188–194.
74. Lucot, J., Wagner, G. C., Schuster, C. R., and Seiden, L. S. (1980): *Pharmacol. Biochem. Behav.*, 13:409–414.

75. Lucot, J., Wagner, G. C., Schuster, C. R., and Seiden, L. S. (1982): *Brain Res.*, 247:181–183.

76. Lytle, L. D., Jacoby, J. H., Nelson, M. F., and Baumgarten, H. G. (1974): *Life Sci.*, 15:1203–1217.

77. Lytle, L. D., Shoemaker, W. J., Cottman, K., and Wurtman, R. J. (1972): *J. Pharmacol. Exp. Ther.*, 183:56–64.

78. Malforms, T., and Thoenen, H., eds. (1971): *6-Hydroxydopamine and Catecholamine Neurons.* North Holland, Amsterdam.

79. Marquardt, G., DiStefano, V., and Ling, L. (1978): In: *Psychopharmacology of Hallucinogens*, edited by R. Stillman and R. Willette, pp. 84–98. Pergamon Press, New York.

80. Massari, V., and Gottesfeld, J. (1977): *Fed. Proc.*, 36:105.

81. Miller, F., Heffner, T., Kotake, C., and Seiden, L. S. (1981): *Brain Res.*, 229:123–132.

82. Missale, C., Castelletti, L., Govoni, S., Spano, P., Trabucchi, M., and Hanbauer, I. (1985): *J. Neurochem.*, 45:51–56.

83. Moore, K. E., Chieuh, C., and Zeldes, G. (1977): In: *Cocaine and Other Stimulants*, edited by E. H. Ellinwood and M. M. Kilbey, pp. 143–160. Plenum Press, New York.

84. Morgan, M. E., and Gibb, J. W. (1980): *Neuropharmacology*, 19:989–995.

85. Neckers, L., Bertilsson, L., Koslow, H., and Meek, J. (1975): *J. Pharmacol. Exp. Ther.*, 196:333–338.

86. Nwanze, E., and Jonsson, G. (1981): *Neurosci. Lett.*, 26:163–168.

87. Ogata, A. (1919): *J. Pharm. Soc. Jpn.*, 451:751–764.

88. Parli, C. J., and Schmidt, B. (1975): *Res. Commun. Chem. Pathol. Pharmacol.*, 10:601–604.

89. Peat, M. A., Warren, P. F., and Gibb, J. W. (1983): *J. Pharmacol. Exp. Ther.*, 225:126–131.

90. Pletscher, A. G., Bartholini, H., Bruderer, W., and Gey, K. (1964): *J. Pharmacol. Exp. Ther.*, 145:344–350.

91. Preston, K., Wagner, G., Seiden, L. S., and Schuster, C. (1985): *Brain Res.*, 338:243–248.

92. Ricaurte, G. A., Bryan, G., Strauss, L., Seiden, L. S., and Schuster, C. R. (1985): *Science*, 229:986–988.

93. Ricaurte, G. A., Fuller, R. W., Perry, K. W., Seiden, L. S., and Schuster, C. R. (1983): *Neuropharmacology*, 22:1165–1169.

94. Ricaurte, G. A., Guillery, R. W., Seiden, L. S., Schuster, C. R., and Moore, R. Y. (1982): *Brain Res.*, 235:93–103.

95. Ricaurte, G. A., Guillery, R. W., Seiden, L. S., and Schuster, C. R. (1984): *Brain Res.*, 291:378–382.

96. Ricaurte, G. A., Irwin, I., Forno, L. S., DeLanney, L. E., Langston, E., and Langston, J. W. (1987): *Brain Research*, 403:43–51.

97. Ricaurte, G. A., Malpas, P., Seiden, L. S., and Schuster, C. R. (1987): (*in preparation*).

98. Ricaurte, G. A., Malpas, P., Seiden, L. S., and Schuster, C. R. (1983): *Soc. Neurosci. Abstr.*, 9:424.

99. Ricaurte, G. A., Schuster, C. R., and Seiden, L. S. (1980): *Brain Res.*, 193:153–160.

100. Ricaurte, G. A., Seiden, L. S., and Schuster, C. R. (1983): *Neuropharmacology*, 22:1383–1388.

101. Ricaurte, G. A., Seiden, L. S., and Schuster, C. R. (1984): *Brain Res.*, 303:359–364.

102. Richards, R. N. (1972): *Can. Med. Assoc. J.*, 105:256–259.

103. Roel, L., Moskowitz, M., Rubin, D., Markovitz, D., Lyttle, L., Munro, H., and Wurtman, R. J. (1978): *J. Neurochem.*, 31:341–345.

104. Sanders-Bush, E., Bushing, J. A., and Sulser, F. (1972): *Eur. J. Pharmacol.*, 20:385–388.

105. Sanders-Bush, E., Bushing, J. A., and Sulser, F. (1975): *J. Pharmacol. Exp. Ther.*, 192:33–41.

106. Sanders-Bush, E., and Massari, V. J. (1977): *Fed. Proc.*, 36:2149–2153.

107. Sanders-Bush, E., Gallagher, D., and Sulser, F. (1974): In: *Adv. Biochem. Psychopharmacol., Vol. 10*, edited by E. Costa, G. Gessa, and M. Sandler, pp. 185–194. Raven Press, New York.

108. Sanders-Bush, E., and Steranka, L. R. (1978): *Ann. NY Acad. Sci.*, 305:208–221.

109. Schuster, C. R. (1981): In: *Handbook of Experimental Pharmacology, Vol. 55*, edited by F. Hoffmeister and G. Stille, pp. 587–605. Springer-Verlag, Berlin, Heidelberg.

110. Schmidt, C. J., and Gibb, J. W. (1983): *Fed. Proc.*, 42:879.

111. Schmidt, C. J., and Gibb, J. W. (1985): *Neurochem. Res.*, 10:637–648.

112. Schmidt, C. J., Ritter, J. K., Sonsalla, K. P., Hanson, G. R., and Gibb, J. W. (1985): *J. Pharmacol. Exp. Ther.*, 233:539–543.

113. Seiden, L. S., Fischman, M. W., and Schuster, C. R. (1975/76): *Drug Alcohol Depend.*, 1:215–219.

114. Seiden, L. S., and Vosmer, G. (1984): *Pharmacol. Biochem. Behav.*, 21:29–31.

115. Senoh, S., Creveling, C., Undenfriend, S., and Witkop, B. (1959): *J. Am. Chem. Soc.*, 81:6236–6243.

116. Senoh, S., and Witkop, B. (1959): *J. Am. Chem. Soc.*, 81:6222–6235.

117. Senoh, S., Witkop, B., Creveling, C., and Undenfriend, S. (1959): *J. Am. Chem. Soc.*, 81:1768–1771.

118. Simpson, D. L., and Rumack, B. H. (1981): *Arch. Int. Med.*, 141:1507–1510.

119. Smith, R. L., and Dring, L. G. (1970): In: *Amphetamines and Related Compounds*, edited by E. Costa and S. Garattini, pp. 121–139. Raven Press, New York.

120. Snyder, S. H. (1972): *Arch. Gen. Psychiatry*, 27:169–179.

121. Snyder, S. H., and Coyle, J. T. (1969): *J. Pharmacol. Exp. Ther.*, 165:78–86.

122. Spector, S., Sjoerdsma, A., and Undenfriend, S. (1965): *J. Pharmacol. Exp. Ther.*, 147:86–95.

123. Steranka, L. R. (1981): *Eur. J. Pharmacol.*, 76:443–446.

124. Steranka, L. R. (1982): *Brain Res.*, 234:123–136.

125. Steranka, L. R., and Sanders-Bush, E. (1980): *Eur. J. Pharmacol.*, 65:439–443.

126. Trulson, M. E., Cannon, M. S., Faegg, T. S., and Raese, J. D. (1985): *Soc. Neurosci. Abstr.*, 11:1203.

127. Virus, R., Commins, D. L., Vosmer, G., Woolverton, W., Schuster, C., and Seiden, L. S. (1986): *Fed. Proc.*, 45:1066.

128. Wagner, G. C., Carrelli, R. M., and Jarvis, M. F. (1985): *Res. Commun. Chem. Pathol. Pharmacol.*, 47:221–228.

129. Wagner, G. C., Lucot, J. B., Schuster, C. R., and Seiden, L. S. (1983): *Brain Res.*, 270:285–288.

130. Wagner, G. C., Preston, K., Ricaurte, G. A., Schuster, C. R., and Seiden, L. S. (1982): *Drug Alcohol Depend.*, 9:279–284.

131. Wagner, G. C., Ricaurte, G. A., Johanson, C. E., Schuster, C. R., and Seiden, L. S. (1980): *Neurology*, 30:547–550.

132. Wagner, G. C., Ricaurte, G. A., Seiden, L. S., Schuster, C. R., Miller, R. J., and Westley, J. (1980): *Brain Res.*, 181:151–160.

133. Wagner, G. C., Ricaurte, G. A., Schuster, C. R., and Seiden, L. S. (1979): *Drug Alcohol Depend.*, 4:435–438.

134. Wagner, G. C., Schuster, C. R., and Seiden, L. S. (1981): *Pharmacol. Biochem. Behav.*, 14:117–119.

135. Woolverton, W. L., Cervo, L., and Johanson, C. E. (1984): *Pharmacol. Biochem. Behav.*, 21:737–741.

136. Woolverton, W. L., Virus, R. B., Kamien, J. B., Nencini, P., Johanson, C. E., Seiden, L. S., and Schuster, C. R. (1985): *American College of Neuropharmacologists Annual Meeting, 1985* (Abstr.).

Psychopharmacology:
The Third Generation of Progress,
edited by Herbert Y. Meltzer.
Raven Press, New York © 1987.

CHAPTER **39**

Neuropeptides in Brain and Pituitary: Overview

Huda Akil and Stanley J. Watson

STAGES IN THE MATURATION OF NEUROPEPTIDES AND THEIR REGULATION

During the past decade, one of the most exciting growth areas in neurobiology has been the realization that peptides, previously construed to be classical hormones, play an important role as neurotransmitters and neuromodulators. The fact that the central nervous system is enriched with these substances, expressing almost every peptide found in peripheral tissues, has dramatically altered the face of neurosciences at many levels. Most notably, it has changed our conception of synaptic transmission, particularly with regard to the old notion that one neuron communicates with its neighbors via a single transmitter. The multiplicity of chemical messages between neurons is particularly well exemplified by the multiplicity of messages coded within a single peptide, the multiplicity of peptides coded within a single gene, and the multiplicity of genes expressed within a single neuron. The study of neuropeptides has also altered the way neuroscientists study the brain at a practical level. Peptide research has greatly encouraged the use of certain approaches and tools in the hands of neuroscientists, in particular, the rapid incorporation of the techniques of molecular biology to discover and sequence novel peptides, or to study the gene expression and regulation of the peptides at the transcriptional and translational levels.

The recent advances in molecular neurobiology are due to the fact that in order to understand the formation or biogenesis of any peptide, one needs to go back to the level of the gene and the specific messenger RNA (see Fig. 1). Peptides, like proteins, are encoded in the genome by specific DNA sequences (Fig. 1a), which are then transcribed to RNA only in those cells which express that particular gene. The RNA directly copied from the DNA (so-called heteronuclear RNA) (Fig. 1b) is not mature and has to be further processed by the cell to form messenger RNA (mRNA) (Fig. 1c,d). The latter is then translated into protein by the ribosomal machinery, forming the precursor (Fig. 1e–g). The factors that control which gene is expressed, the rate at which it is transcribed and processed, and the rate at which the resulting mRNA is translated are intricate and complexly regulated by a number of cellular and physiological events. Thus, a great deal of regulatory biology can take place before the protein precursor comes into being. The precursor, in turn, may code for a number of peptides, some with known biological activity and others with unknown functions. However, the full precursor itself is rarely biologically active. It needs to be further altered by specific protein-modifying enzymes (Fig. 1h,i), to produce the final peptide products of the cells. These posttranslational modifications are critical in determining the nature of the biological activity, and the metabolic stability of the products (Fig. 1j). These processing steps in the maturation of the precursor can vary between tissues that express the same gene, and even within brain, between cell groups expressing the same precursor.

Once the precursor is translated and packaged into granules or vesicles, it is transported toward the terminals to be secreted. Posttranslational processing may take place either in the cell body, on the way to the terminals, or in the terminals themselves, depending on the rate of the enzymatic reactions necessary for the maturation of the end-products. In either case, the material is eventually ready for secretion from the mature granule. However, there are a number of regulatory controls at that level. The notion of releasable pools is reasonably well established for endocrine tissues. Although the concept of releasable pools has been demonstrated for classical neurotransmitters in brain, it has not been well studied for neuropeptides in the brain and represents an area of future growth. Numerous

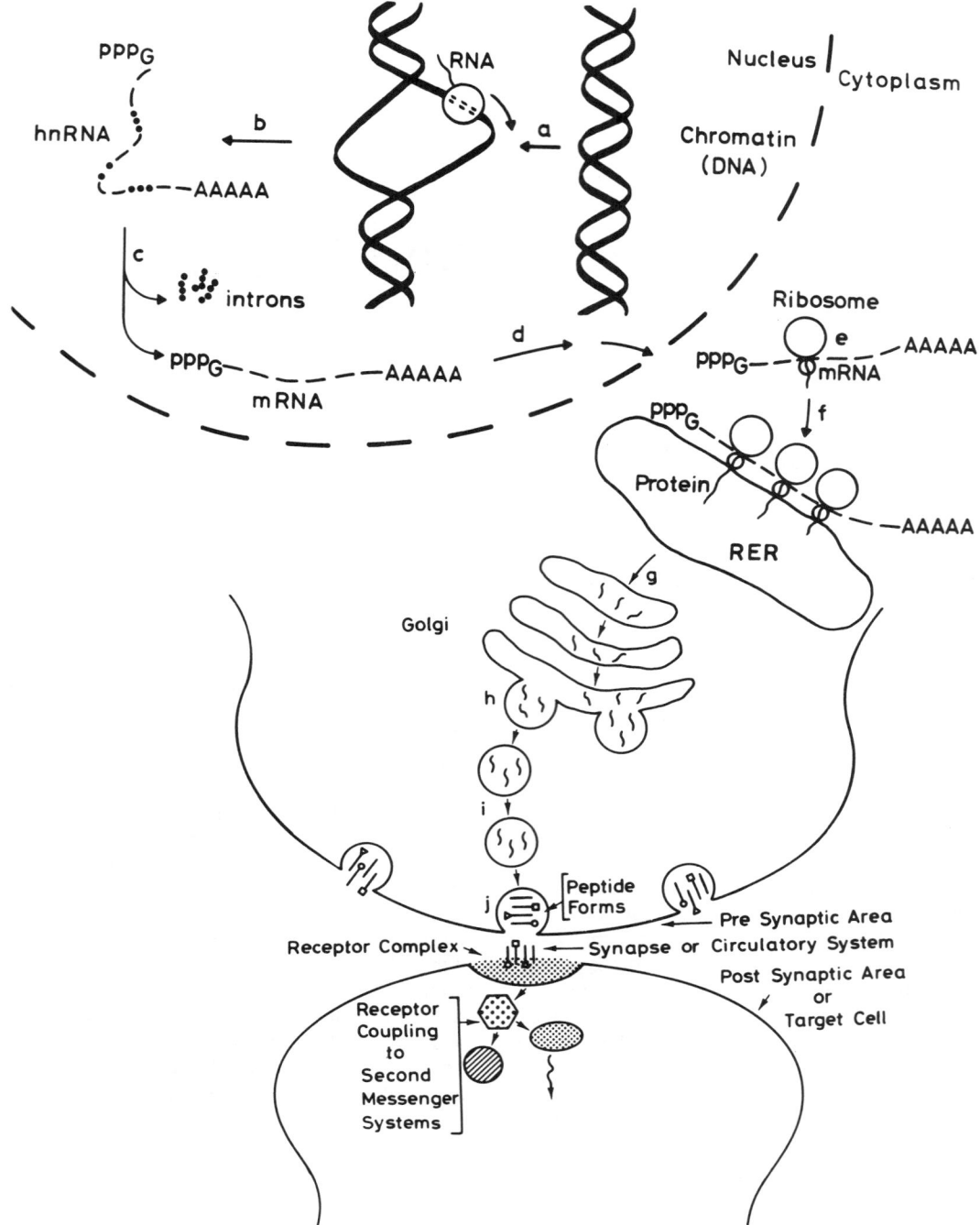

FIG. 1. Steps in the production of neuropeptides and their postsynaptic effects. **a:** Genomic transcription. **b:** Production of immature mRNA, known as "heterologous nuclear RNA" (hnRNA). **c:** Removal of intronic regions, 5' capping and 3' polyadenylation. **d:** Mature mRNA. **e:** Translation of mRNA into prepropeptide. **f:** Cleavage of signal peptide. **g:** Core glycosylation of propeptide (precursor). **h,i,j:** Cleavage of propeptide precursor into peptide; posttranslational modification of peptides into final active form. The postsynaptic area is composed of several receptor types, their interaction and coupling to second messenger systems, prior to altering the receptive cell activity.

factors can regulate the amount and rate of secretion, including the magnitude, duration, and pattern of the stimulus triggering the secretory episode, the amount of peptide stored in the cells or in a particular releasable pool, the speed with which the depleted stores can be replenished, and various feedback mechanisms that may amplify or terminate the secretory episode.

When liberated from their cells of origin, neuropeptides may act on nearby targets in the case of brain, or on distant targets in the case of endocrine signaling. It should be noted here, that the secretory granules will often store multiple products from a given precursor which, upon secretion, may have different targets (Fig. 1j). Furthermore, a peptide family can be copackaged with a classical neurotransmitter, allowing complex patterns of synaptic interactions. Even after a peptide has been released, it can be further broken down into fragments that may be devoid of biological activity at one target, but maintain biological activity on another target. This type of selectivity is evidently brought about by specific receptor mechanisms, which may recognize different portions of the peptide. Furthermore, multiple receptors to different products secreted from a given granule may interact (Fig. 1, "receptor complex"), allowing for coordinate actions of the end-products. To date, numerous types of interactions have been described, including examples of additivity, synergism, physiological antagonism, or modulatory effects wherein one product can set a threshold for the response of the target, or terminate its own secretion and that of its cosecreted companions through autoreceptor mechanisms.

Given this complexity, it is critical to bear in mind the overall physiological effect of a given peptide system, whether one is studying neuronal or hormonal actions. Thus, the complexity at the cellular level requires the coupling of peptide studies with careful physiological and behavioral approaches, in order to evaluate which of the many possible functional options are indeed put into play by the body. The combination of an understanding of all the potential regulatory points, and the normal functioning of the system, is then the framework within which one can study dysregulation or malfunction of the system in pathological conditions.

ORGANIZATION OF THE NEUROPEPTIDE SECTION OF THIS VOLUME

This section of the volume is organized along the lines outlined above, describing the stages of functional maturation of the neuropeptide message. Thus, these chapters start with the question of expression—which cells express a particular product, and along which pathways. This is followed by a chapter dealing directly with the molecular biology of gene expression and regulation. The third chapter focuses on the cotranslational and posttranslational events that yield the final peptide end-products. The fourth chapter is then concerned with the complex interactions that multiple products have on postsynaptic receptors. The fifth chapter deals with the whole organism, describing behavioral events resulting from peptide activation. And the final chapter is concerned with the search for novel peptide transmitters.

The issue of which neurons express which peptide(s) is being covered by Dr. T. Hokfelt, who has pioneered the use of immunohistochemistry in the central nervous system. His summary amply demonstrates the need to study neuropeptides within an anatomical context, since peptides can be identified biochemically in a particular brain region, but may arise from either local neurons or from distant perikarya. The issue of coexistence of multiple peptides, or of peptides and classical neurotransmitters, is particularly well addressed by this approach. Indeed, immunohisto-

chemistry was the major tool that yielded the first glimpse of coexistence of neuromodulators and has provided the neurobiologist with model systems within which to study the multiple types of interactions made possible by cotransmission.

At a more cellular level, the chapter of Dr. E. Herbert and his colleagues addresses the first stages of peptide expression—transcription of a gene to a specific messenger RNA, and the subsequent translation of that message into the proper protein precursor. The molecular biological approach to the study of neuropeptides leads to two major types of achievement: (a) identification of novel peptide genes, or characterization of full precursor sequences of known peptides, and (b) studying the regulatory biology of peptides at the level of gene expression. Although Dr. Herbert's group has contributed handsomely in both areas, the current chapter will emphasize the regulatory biology. Using opioid peptides as their model, this group of workers has been addressing several key questions in gene expression and regulation: What are the factors that regulate whether a gene is expressed in a certain tissue and the rate at which it is transcribed? What physiological mechanisms interact at the level of the gene to control such expression? Which components of the gene are key to this regulatory biology? What is the molecular basis of posttranslational modification by specific processing enzymes? These and other issues are addressed by the use of newer, more sophisticated molecular genetics tools, which allow the study of not only the genes themselves, but the expression of their final products.

The next stage of maturation, after a gene is transcribed, is the maturation of the peptide precursor. Some of these maturational processes occur concomitantly with translation, whereas others follow translation by varying periods of time. Thus, these processes are termed cotranslational and posttranslational, respectively. The work of Drs. Eipper, Mains, and their colleagues exemplifies the importance of these processes in producing the final, biologically active peptide products. Having set the pace in this area of research, they expertly describe the richness, complexity, and flexibility of the cotranslational and posttranslational processing. In particular, the idea that two different tissues can express the same precursor and yet yield an entirely different set of end-products is pivotal to studying neuropeptides. Plasticity of the cell biology, at this level, may be expressed not only with regional differences, but also with differences over time. Thus, it is conceivable that the regulation of posttranslational events may yield a unique mix of end-products in a particular region depending on the recent history of the animal. This would permit the chemical message to be altered in time as well as in space, providing the brain with yet unexplored types of flexibility in coding.

The secreted peptides exert their actions through unique recognition sites, the receptors. As mentioned above, receptor occupancy can lead to a number of possible biochemical and functional consequences, including a primary effect such as excitation or inhibition of the target cell, or to modulatory effects that modify the actions of another transmitter. This latter mode of action is newly discovered and relatively unexplored. The research of Drs. Costa, Guidotti, and their co-workers exemplifies the excitement of modern neurobiology, which continuously challenges older and simplistic ideas of communication in the brain. Their chapter describes a novel and unique example of such an interaction between peptides and γ-aminobutyric acid (GABA), a classical small-molecule inhibitory transmitter most abundant in the central nervous system. This important body of work demonstrates the current richness intrinsic to the study of peptide neurobiology, wherein the effort to understand neuromodulation has led to the discovery, purification, and subsequent sequencing of a unique and exciting peptide family—benzodiazepine binding inhibitors.

Dr. van Ree's contribution examines brain-behavior interactions of peptides, leading us to consider their net effects. Dr. van Ree and the Utrecht group led the way for the exploration of peptide actions on brain functions. At a time when the targets of hormones such as corticotropin (ACTH) and vasopressin were thought to be primarily peripheral, the Utrecht group under the leadership of D. de Wied, along with the New Orleans group of A. Kastin and A. Schally, were demonstrating that peptides act on the brain to modulate such phenomena as attention, learning, memory, and motivation. Dr. van Ree's chapter uses examples from opioid and neurohypophyseal peptides to demonstrate the richness of coding of the peptides at a behavioral level. The idea of multiple codes, of subtle interactions of modulatory effects, was first put forth based on such behavioral observations and predated the biochemical findings, which have since given it ample support.

Finally, the contribution from Dr. J. Barchas and his colleagues opens a window into the future. Although the past decade has witnessed an explosion in peptide biology, much remains to be learned about the existence of yet to be described substances with important biological functions. Furthermore, precursors with known structures may be processed in unsuspected ways, giving rise to products with unique biological activities. Dr. Barchas' group has contributed handsomely to the discovery of novel processing products of opioid precursors and the investigation of their unique functions. This group has now embarked on the exciting journey of discovering novel peptide families using sophisticated strategies, including the use of molecular biological tools, immunological tools, and peptide chemical tools. The strategies and logistics for using this powerful combination of approaches are detailed in the last chapter of this section.

FUNCTIONAL IMPLICATIONS: ENDOGENOUS DEPRESSION AS AN EXAMPLE

A better understanding of peptide anatomy, cell biology, regulation, and function carries important implications for both neurobiology and biological psychiatry. The study of peptide dysregulation in endogenous depression constitutes an example of the interface between the two disciplines of peptide and psychiatric research. The original body of work by several groups—Bunney and co-workers, Sachar and co-workers, and Carroll and co-workers—centered around the measurement of the stress steroids, the corticosteroids generated from the adrenal gland, and indicated that the hypothalamo-pituitary-adrenal (HPA) axis was functioning abnormally in patients suffering from a major depressive disorder of the endogenous type. However, since steroid secretion is controlled by the peptide ACTH, and since ACTH secretion is in turn regulated by secretagogues which are themselves peptides, such as CRF (corticotropin-releasing factor) and vasopressin, the investigator in this field is suddenly thrust in the midst of understanding peptidology in order to attempt to elucidate the cause(s) of dysregulation in the HPA axis of endogenously depressed subjects. Although we do not plan to summarize here the current thinking on the HPA axis and endogenous depression, we shall use this as a working example of how we can approach such a problem given the recent advances in peptide biology.

An underlying assumption in the depression literature is that the HPA dysregulation represents the consequence of a higher-order disruption in the limbic system. However, until recently, we have measured the last step in the axis, i.e., steroidogenesis, and assumed that it directly mirrors the preceding cascade of events, including secretion from the pituitary, stimulation of that secretion by the specific factors such as CRF and vasopressin, and the limbic control of the secretagogues, the presumed site of disruption. More recent work on this problem has attempted to move up the axis, at least to the level of the pituitary, and examine the control of ACTH and its cosynthesized peptide, β-endorphin. In doing so, the investigator faces the need for understanding peptide regulation at the level of the corticotrophs. How does the level of the peptides reflect what is really going on in the gland? If indeed the system is chronically overly stimulated, is it likely to store more material in a chronic way? Is it likely to secrete more peptide when activated? Conversely, since, in the endogenously depressed subject, the corticotrophs are often bathed in higher than normal levels of steroids, do the negative feedback mechanisms place an upper limit on secretion? Since the pituitary of a depressed patient may be subjected to two opposing influences—increased stimulation by secretagogues and increased negative feedback by steroids—which of these two opposing factors will control its moment-to-moment activity? When and how does the system recover, if it ever does? All of these questions touch upon issues of peptide regulation, from the gene to the end-product. They are likely to draw directly on our basic understanding of how the ACTH/β-endorphin precursor is controlled by factors such as secretory rates, circadian rhythms, negative feedback, and interactions with other factors, such as sex steroids. Although we can only measure secretion of the relevant peptides into the bloodstream, we can now do so in conjunction with measurement of the steroids, or following negative challenge with dexamethasone or positive challenges with CRF. Such studies are currently ongoing, but a thoughtful interpretation of the results will always profit from a more complete understanding of the regulatory biology of ACTH/β-endorphin in the anterior lobe. Thus, animal studies examining short-term and longer-term control of this system, at the level of secretion, processing, translation, and transcription, are of direct relevance to the human experiments.

A more direct examination of the hypothesis that the HPA dysregulation originates in the limbic system would require that we move closer to that system by at least studying the hypothalamus. In order to directly test the hypothesis of an increased drive of the HPA in endogenous depression, one would need to measure the amount of CRF or vasopressin liberated into the portal system—not a practical approach in the human. However, thanks to the recent advances in CRF research we can address the question indirectly. Is there evidence of up- or down-regulation of the CRF receptors as evidenced by challenge studies? Are there any effects of CRF or vasopressin peptide antagonists? Are there any changes in the level of CRF or vasopressin mRNA in the brains of depressed subjects as measured in postmortem studies? Some of these questions are currently being addressed, while others are awaiting some technical advances but should be easily addressed in the foreseeable future.

Such an approach, coupling the depression research to a better understanding of peptide biology, may or may not result in tangible clinical advances for helping endogenously depressed subjects. However, it is likely to be most fruitful for both the peptidologist and the biologically oriented psychiatrist. The peptidologist has occasion to study and possibly understand a naturally occurring example of peptide dysregulation, where the problem is subtle (unlike a tumor) and is possibly reversible. The biological psychiatrist can achieve a greater understanding of the mechanisms underlying the observed disruption, and may have to revise the assumptions as to the nature and primary site of the dysregulation. In either case, we can hopefully achieve a more accurate and exciting perception of brain function.

We hope that as the reader moves through each chapter in this section, the concepts outlined above are helpful in linking the basic biology with the problems seen in mental and neurological illnesses. As we move into the 1986–1995 decade, many of the basic biological ideas and tools presented here will be increasingly actively applied to brain diseases.

DEDICATION

We dedicate this section on Neuropeptides to the memory of Dr. Edward Herbert, a superb scientist and a dear friend.

Psychopharmacology:
The Third Generation of Progress,
edited by Herbert Y. Meltzer.
Raven Press, New York © 1987.

CHAPTER **40**

Study of the Regulation of Expression of Neuropeptide Genes by Gene Transfer Methods

Edward Herbert, Audrey Seasholtz, Michael Comb, Gary Thomas, and Barbara Thorne

In the past 20 years a variety of neuropeptides have been discovered that mediate specific behavioral responses in animals. These peptides are the messenger molecules that convert neural signals into physiological responses. They function as hormones in the circulatory system and/or neurotransmitters or neuromodulators in the nervous system. After release from the neuron or endocrine gland, these peptides combine with receptors on postsynaptic neurons or on target cells to initiate an intracellular cascade of events leading to an electrical or chemical response. All of these processes must be defined at a molecular level in order to achieve a more complete understanding of behavior. In the past decade, new methods in molecular biology have provided us with the tools necessary to begin to define these processes.

The impact of molecular biology on neuroscience is perhaps most apparent in the study of the opioid peptides. Since the discovery of Met- and Leu-enkephalin by Hughes et al. (27) in 1975, more than 16 peptides have been isolated that exhibit opioid activity. Recombinant DNA technology has revealed that all the opioid peptides identified thus far are derived from three different genes, and therefore, three different precursor proteins: proopiomelanocortin (POMC) (43,58), proenkephalin (10,19,45), and prodynorphin (31) (see Fig. 1). Each polyprotein precursor undergoes specific proteolytic cleavages and posttranslational modifications to produce multiple bioactive peptides. For example, POMC gives rise to β-endorphin, adrenocorticotropin (ACTH), and melanocyte-stimulating hormone (MSH).

Proenkephalin (proenkephalin A) is processed to Met- and Leu-enkephalin as well as a variety of larger enkephalin-containing peptides. Processing of prodynorphin (proenkephalin B) yields α- and β-neoendorphin and dynorphin A- and dynorphin B-related peptides.

These opioid polyprotein precursors can be cleaved to form different sets of biologically active peptides in the different tissues where they are expressed. For example, POMC is processed to $ACTH_{1-39}$, β-lipotropin, and an N-terminal fragment in the rat anterior pituitary, whereas the intermediate lobe contains predominantly α-MSH, corticotropin-like intermediate lobe peptide (CLIP), β-endorphin, and acetylated derivatives of β-endorphin (39,52). Similarly, proenkephalin is cleaved to form different peptides in different tissues. In the bovine adrenal medulla the major products of proenkephalin processing appear to be the higher-molecular-weight peptides (>1,000 daltons) (32). The free pentapeptides, Met- and Leu-enkephalin, comprise less than 5% of the total enkephalin-containing peptide pool in the adrenal gland (57). In contrast, the major products of proenkephalin processing in some areas of the brain (i.e., caudate nucleus) are free enkephalins and syn-enkephalin, the amino-terminal fragment of proenkephalin (36,37).

Regulation of synthesis and release of the opioid peptides is also tissue specific. In the rat anterior pituitary POMC-derived peptides are subject to positive regulation by corticotropin-releasing factor (CRF) and negative feedback by glucocorticoids (50,51). In contrast, release of these

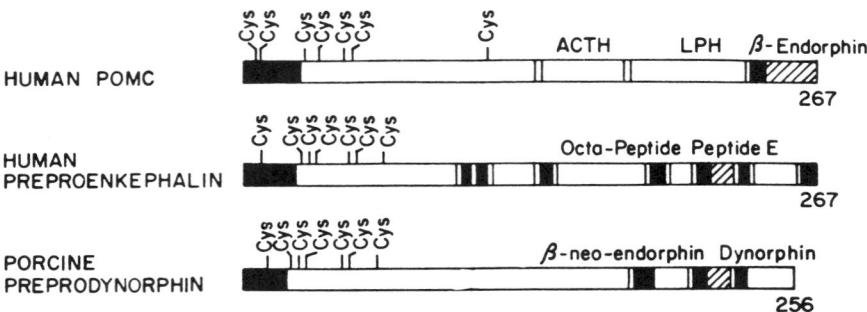

FIG. 1. Schematic representation of the three opioid polyprotein precursors. The black box at the amino terminus represents the signal sequence. The black boxes in the precursors indicate enkephalin sequences, and pairs of basic amino acid residues are indicated by a bar. (From ref. 24.)

peptides in the rat neurointermediate lobe is not affected by glucocorticoids, but is negatively controlled by dopaminergic compounds (53).

The release and synthesis of proenkephalin are also differentially regulated in a variety of tissues. Chronic administration of haloperidol causes a twofold increase in Met-enkephalin immunoreactivity in rat striatum and globus pallidus, but not in hypothalamus, septum, or medulla oblongata, where it is also expressed (55). In rat adrenal medulla, neural input regulates the release of enkephalin-containing peptides (35). In cultures of bovine adrenal medulla chromaffin cells, the levels of enkephalin peptides and proenkephalin mRNA are dramatically increased by treatment with cyclic AMP analogs (49) or activators of adenylate cyclase (14). At present we know very little about the mechanisms involved in the action of these agents. Do these compounds cause an activation or repression of transcription of the opioid genes? What are the molecular mechanisms involved in the tissue-specific regulation of gene expression?

The advances in molecular biology in the past 5 years have provided us with the tools to examine these questions. The development of improved molecular cloning techniques has allowed the preparation of very large complementary DNA (cDNA) libraries, which can be used to isolate cDNA clones for very low-abundance mRNAs. After the appropriate cDNA has been identified, it can be used to isolate the corresponding gene. Using these methods the cDNA and genes for a variety of neuroendocrine peptide precursors have been isolated and sequenced. The availability of these cloned genes and the development of new methods that permit their efficient transfer into eukaryotic cells have revolutionized the field of gene regulation, allowing us to begin to dissect the molecular mechanisms involved in the regulation of gene expression.

MOLECULAR CLONING

Recombinant DNA technology has been used to determine the complete amino acid and nucleic acid structure of a variety of neuropeptide precursor molecules (12). The general cDNA cloning procedure is described below. Poly A mRNA (either total or partially enriched mRNA fraction) is enzymatically transcribed by reverse transcriptase into cDNA. Oligo(dT), which hybridizes to the poly A region of the RNA, is used to prime the reaction. The single-stranded (ss) cDNA molecules are then incubated with

DNA polymerase to convert them to a double-stranded (ds) form (using a hairpin loop at the 3' end of the first DNA strand as primer). After digestion of the ds cDNA with the single-strand-specific nuclease S1 to remove the hairpin loop, the ds cDNA molecules can be inserted into a plasmid or bacteriophage λ vector by a variety of different cloning methods. These chimeric molecules are then introduced into bacterial cells with the resultant production of a "library" of cDNA clones. Several different approaches that can be used to screen the library to identify the clone of interest are described below. Once the clone is identified, the nucleic acid and amino acid sequences of the precursor molecules can be determined by DNA sequencing of the cDNA insert. This general procedure can be modified in many ways, and a complete discussion of these modifications is beyond the scope of this chapter.

The isolation of cDNA clones for a number of neuropeptide mRNA species has been difficult due to the low concentration of the corresponding mRNA in the total mRNA population (<0.01% of the total poly A mRNA population in complex tissues). The frequency with which cDNA clones of a specific mRNA will be found in a cDNA library is generally proportional to the abundance of that species in the mRNA population. Therefore, to isolate cDNA clones of very rare mRNAs, one must construct very large cDNA libraries representative of complex poly A mRNA populations. In these cases, bacteriophage λ vectors are often preferred over plasmid vectors due to the high efficiency and reproducibility of *in vitro* packaging of λ DNA as a method for introducing DNA sequences into *Escherichia coli*. The two λ vectors most commonly used are λgt10 and λgt11. Libraries cloned into λgt10 are useful for screening with nucleic acid probes. The second λ vector, λgt11, is an expression vector capable of producing a protein specified by the cDNA insert. Hence, these libraries can be screened by a variety of methods including antibody or ligand probes.

Once the cDNA library has been constructed, one must isolate the cDNA clone of interest. A variety of screening methods have been developed and the method of choice is usually dependent on the concentration of the precursor mRNA in the total poly A mRNA population. Synthetic oligonucleotides complementary to specific regions of the polyprotein mRNA have been used as hybridization probes for detecting rare cDNA clones. When hybridization is carried out under the proper conditions, the radiolabeled oligonucleotide probe will bind selectively to its complementary nucleotide sequences and the location of the hybridizing cDNA clone can be detected by autoradiography. This approach can be used to detect virtually any cDNA clone of interest, provided that peptide sequence information is available.

Specifically primed cDNA libraries have also been used to detect cDNA clones corresponding to low-abundance mRNA. In this approach, an oligonucleotide probe corresponding to a sequence in the 3′ region of a specific mRNA is used to prime the synthesis of cDNA from a total mRNA population. The resulting cDNA library is greatly enriched for the cDNA clone of interest. A second oligonucleotide probe that recognizes a specific 5′ region of the polyprotein mRNA is used as a hybridization probe to detect the correct specifically primed cDNA clone. This cDNA clone can then serve as a highly specific probe in the screening of oligo (dT)-primed cDNA libraries. One can also use this approach to obtain the sequence of the 5′ end of very long mRNAs. These methods have been used to isolate cDNA clones for a variety of neuropeptides including two of the opioid peptide precursors, proenkephalin (45) and prodynorphin (31). The isolated cDNA clones were used not only to determine the sequence of the protein precursor, but also to isolate the opioid peptide precursor genes.

Genomic libraries consist of large genomic DNA fragments (10–20 kb in length) which have been inserted into specially constructed λ phage vectors (34). These chimeric molecules are packaged into viable λ phage particles and used to infect bacteria. The resultant genomic library is screened by plaque hybridization using the cDNA clone or an oligonucleotide as a hybridization probe (2). This method has been used to isolate the genes for the opioid peptide precursors POMC (4,7,13,44,59,61), proenkephalin (9,46, 54), and prodynorphin (6,25). The structures of the three genes show striking similarities (see Fig. 2). All three genes have large 3′ exons that contain the nucleotides coding for all of the biologically active peptides and the majority of the N-terminal portion of the precursors. Several kilobases upstream (5′) a smaller exon contains sequences coding for the remainder of the amino-terminal portion of the precursor molecule and a few bases of 5′ untranslated sequences.

The remaining sequences coding for 5′ untranslated regions of the mRNA are farther upstream on one (POMC) or two (proenkephalin and prodynorphin) exons.

GENE TRANSFER METHODS

The availability of cDNA clones for a variety of neuropeptides allows one to examine the effects of various regulators on neuropeptide mRNA levels and transcription rates. Using the cloned neuropeptide genes, one can examine the molecular mechanisms involved in the regulation of expression at a variety of levels using gene transfer methods. Transcriptional regulation appears to be controlled by a variety of cis-acting and trans-acting regulatory elements. The DNA sequences involved in cis-acting transcriptional regulation are quite diverse in function and structure, and act in the general stimulation of transcription (promoters and enhancers), tissue-specific gene expression, or the induction (or repression) of transcription by the action of specific agents. The trans-acting regulatory elements are often specific protein factors that interact with the cis-acting DNA sequences. Methylation patterns may also play a role in controlling the transcriptional activity of a gene. Gene transfer techniques can also be used to examine the sequences in the gene or cDNA that provide signals for posttranslational modification, processing, and secretion. By constructing specifically mutated genes and analyzing their expression in a variety of expression systems, it is now possible to determine the role of specific DNA sequences in different aspects of gene expression.

Gene transfer experiments can be divided into two major categories: (a) stable transfections and (b) transient assay systems. To study stably transfected cell lines, one isolates a clone of eukaryotic cells that has integrated the foreign gene into its chromosomal DNA. The major advantage of this system is the ability to isolate stably transfected cell lines that can be grown indefinitely in culture and used to study a variety of regulatory phenomena. The gene of interest can be introduced into the eukaryotic cells by

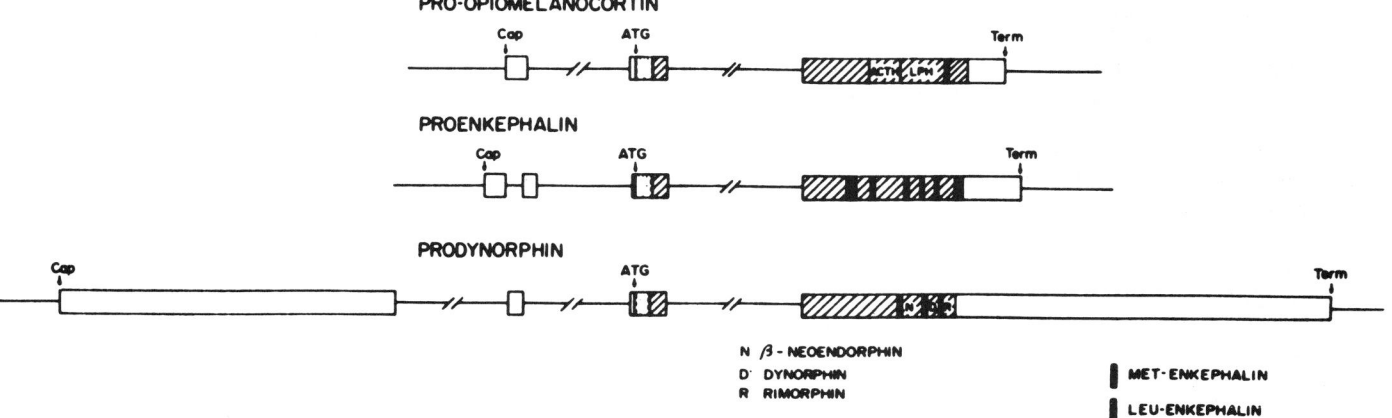

FIG. 2. Structural comparison of the human POMC, proenkephalin, and prodynorphin genes. Lines represent introns and boxes represent exons. Cap shows the start of transcription and term indicates the mRNA 3′ end. ATG indicates the initiator methionine. (From ref. 24.)

several different methods: (a) chemical methods such as the calcium phosphate precipitation method or the diethylaminoethyl (DEAE)-dextran method; (b) physical methods such as microinjection or electroporation; (c) viral-mediated DNA transfer; and (d) fusion of DNA-containing membranous vesicles such as liposomes, envelopes of Sendai virus particles, or protoplasts to cells (1).

The calcium phosphate precipitation method (16) is the most widely used procedure, but is somewhat limited at the present time in the range of target cells that give high transfer efficiency. Microinjection or fusion techniques can be used to introduce the gene of interest into almost any mammalian cell. The microinjection of fertilized mouse embryos has facilitated regulation studies in transgenic animals. Both RNA and DNA viruses have also been used very successfully as gene transfer vectors. However, all of the long-term assay systems (regardless of the method used for gene transfer) suffer one limitation: an inability to control the region of the genome into which the introduced gene is integrated. Thus, different clones carrying the same gene may show significant variability in RNA and protein production depending on differences in location of the foreign gene in the host.

The second gene transfer approach involves the use of transient expression systems. In these systems, the foreign gene or cDNA is introduced into eukaryotic cells and its expression is assayed within a few hours to days. The advantages of these assays are simplicity and rapidity. Furthermore, because the transferred molecules remain episomal, the problems associated with random chromosomal integration can be avoided. The major disadvantages are the relatively low levels of expression and the inability to conduct experiments over more than a few days. A variety of transient systems are presently available. In the first system the control region of the gene of interest is fused to the coding sequence of a gene that is readily assayed by enzymatic means, such as E. coli chloramphenicol acetyltransferase or herpes thymidine kinase. With this type of system one can assay the transcriptional activity of the foreign gene by a simple and rapid enzymatic assay. A second transient assay utilizes the Xenopus oocyte. Xenopus oocytes will efficiently transcribe and translate an injected gene and can therefore be used to study transcriptional regulation and posttranslational processing. A third transient assay system involves the use of vaccinia virus as a gene transfer vector. Vaccinia is a cytoplasmic virus with a broad host range and is therefore well suited for examining the role of specific DNA sequences in controlling the processing and secretion of a protein in different cell lines and possibly normal cells as well.

We are currently using these gene transfer techniques to study the regulation and expression of the human proenkephalin gene and mouse POMC gene. A mouse anterior pituitary tumor cell line (AtT-20) has been transfected with the human proenkephalin gene and the characteristics of several of the isolated clones will be discussed. The expression of proenkephalin in three transient systems will also be discussed: (a) proenkephalin fusion genes, (b) Xenopus oocytes, and (c) vaccinia virus. By studying the expression and regulation of the wild-type human proenkephalin gene and a variety of site-specific mutants in both the stably transfected cell lines and a variety of transient expression

systems, we hope to gain a better understanding of the DNA sequences involved in the expression and control of this gene and of the protein sequences required for correct processing and secretion of bioactive peptides.

Stably Transfected Cell Lines

The human proenkephalin gene has been introduced and expressed in AtT-20 cells in order to study the transcriptional regulation of this gene and to elucidate the mechanisms underlying processing of proenkephalin (8). The AtT-20 cell line was selected as the host system for these studies for several reasons: (a) these cells do not express proenkephalin; (b) they possess well-developed secretory vesicles and store and release large amounts of ACTH and β-lipotropin (β-LPH); and (c) they respond to physiological regulators and process POMC in a manner similar to that of anterior pituitary cells in vivo. Therefore, these cells provide a well-characterized secretory pathway in which to examine the processing and chemical modifications of neuropeptide precursors.

A recombinant plasmid containing the human proenkephalin gene ligated to pBR322 was introduced into AtT-20 cells by cotransformation with pRSVneo, a plasmid containing the neo gene, which confers resistance to the aminoglycoside drug G418 and therefore acts as a dominant selectable marker (see Fig. 3). Stable transformants containing one or more copies of the human proenkephalin gene integrated into the mouse chromosomal DNA expressed a 1.45-kb mRNA identical in size to authentic human proenkephalin mRNA. Primer extension experiments demonstrated that the human proenkephalin transcripts initiated at the same site as human pheochromocytoma proenkephalin transcripts. Thus, the control signals present in the human proenkephalin gene such as the promoter, RNA splice sites, and poly A addition sites are directing the expression of normal mature proenkephalin mRNA in the AtT-20 cells.

Analysis of protein extracts from AtT-20 transformants using a radioimmunoassay specific for Met-enkephalin demonstrated that these cells synthesize proenkephalin protein and cleave it to form free Met-enkephalin. This result suggests that the processing enzymes present in AtT-20 cells can also recognize and efficiently process the cleavage sites flanking the Met-enkephalin sequences in the proenkephalin precursor. The secretion of Met-enkephalin from these cells was also examined. Treatment of cells with CRF resulted in a twofold stimulation of secretion of both ACTH and Met-enkephalin immunoreactivity. Therefore, these stably transformed cell lines will be very useful for studying the molecular mechanisms involved in processing and secretion of the proenkephalin protein in addition to the transcriptional regulation of the gene.

Transient Expression Systems

Fusion Genes

In these studies the putative regulatory region of a gene is linked to an enzymatic reporter function which is readily assayed in eukaryotic cells. The amount of enzyme activity

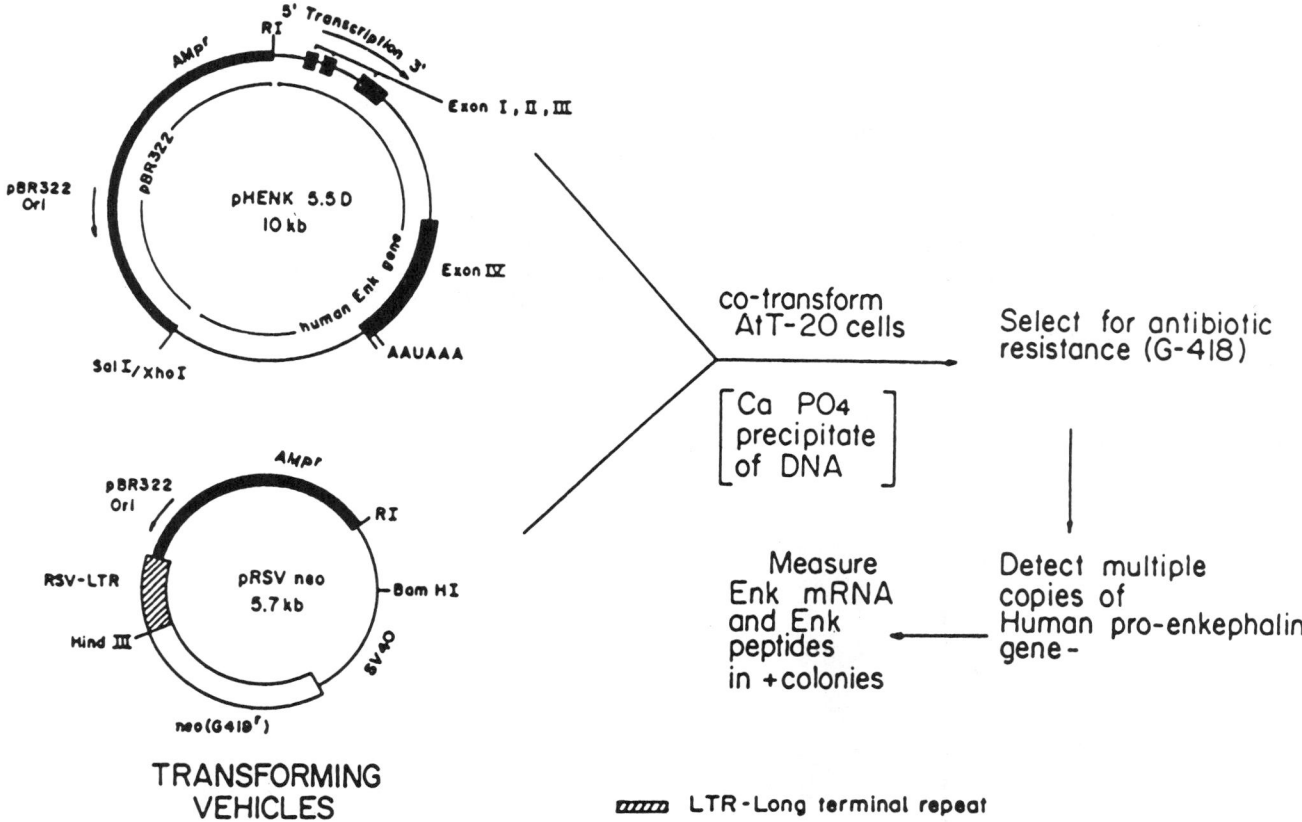

FIG. 3. Strategy for the introduction of the human proenkephalin gene into the mouse anterior pituitary tumor cell line AtT-20. (From ref. 8.)

reflects the amount of protein produced under the control of the linked regulatory region and thus provides a direct indication of the level of gene expression. The *E. coli* chloramphenicol acetyltransferase (CAT) reporter function developed by Gorman et al. (15) was selected for our studies because (a) CAT activity is easily and sensitively assayed; and (b) there is no interfering endogenous activity since CAT activity is not present in mammalian or avian cells. By fusing the 5′ end of the human proenkephalin gene to the coding region of the CAT gene, we can analyze the efficiency of the proenkephalin gene promoter, map transcriptional control elements, and test for elements of the gene required for cell-specific expression following transfection into mammalian cells.

The fusion gene (pENKAT-12) contains the first 403 base pairs (bp) of the human proenkephalin gene (200 bp of 5′ flanking regions and 203 bp of human proenkephalin DNA including exon I, intron A, and exon II) fused to the CAT gene. The 3′ untranslated sequences, poly A addition sites, and 3′ flanking sequences of the human proenkephalin gene were also placed 3′ to the CAT gene (see Fig. 4). In this fusion gene plasmid, CAT expression is driven by the linked human proenkephalin promoter and utilizes both 5′ and 3′ human proenkephalin control signals. The plasmid DNA was transfected into eukaryotic cells by the calcium phosphate precipitation method (16). The cells were harvested and lysed with Triton X-100 (0.5%) at 24 to 48 hr posttransfection and the cell extracts were then assayed for

CAT activity. The transient expression of pENKAT-12 was examined in a variety of cell lines: rat adrenal PC-12 cells, mouse pituitary AtT-20 cells, human HeLa cells, mouse L cells, and monkey kidney CV-1 cells. Relatively high levels of CAT expression were demonstrated in all the tested cell

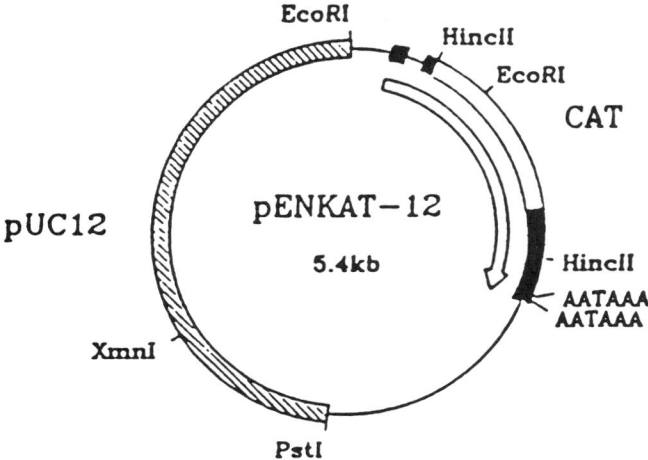

FIG. 4. Structure of the human proenkephalin/CAT fusion gene construct. The shaded region represents puc12 sequences. The solid line and black boxes represent human proenkephalin 5′ and 3′ sequences and the open box represents the CAT gene coding sequence.

lines, with values ranging between 20 and 80% of the level of expression directed by RSVcat, a plasmid containing the strong Rous sarcoma virus promoter in front of the CAT gene. Thus, the 5′ 403 bp of the human proenkephalin gene contains an efficient promoter region capable of directing high levels of CAT expression. However, this plasmid shows little tissue- or species-specific expression, suggesting that the transfected gene may not contain the DNA sequences responsible for normal tissue-specific expression. This finding is not totally unexpected since the sequences responsible for cell-specific expression of several other genes have been located several hundred bp upstream of the normal mRNA start site.

The ENKAT-12 plasmid was also examined in these transient assays to identify potential regulators of the human proenkephalin gene. Several groups have reported

that proenkephalin mRNA levels are regulated by cyclic AMP analogs (49) or activators of adenylate cyclase (14). Cyclic AMP is thought to act as a second messenger system in transcriptional regulation of eukaryotic genes. Activation of adenylate cyclase by a variety of different mechanisms causes increased levels of intracellular cyclic AMP. Increased cyclic AMP concentrations cause increased cyclic AMP-dependent protein kinase activity, and changes in protein phosphorylation may be responsible for modulation of gene transcription. Thus, activators of adenylate cyclase, analogs of cyclic AMP (8BrcAMP), or phosphodiesterase inhibitors (IBMX) which prevent breakdown of intracellular cyclic AMP may all affect gene transcription by a similar second messenger system.

When cyclic AMP regulators were added to the media 18 hr after pENKAT-12 transfections, an increase in CAT

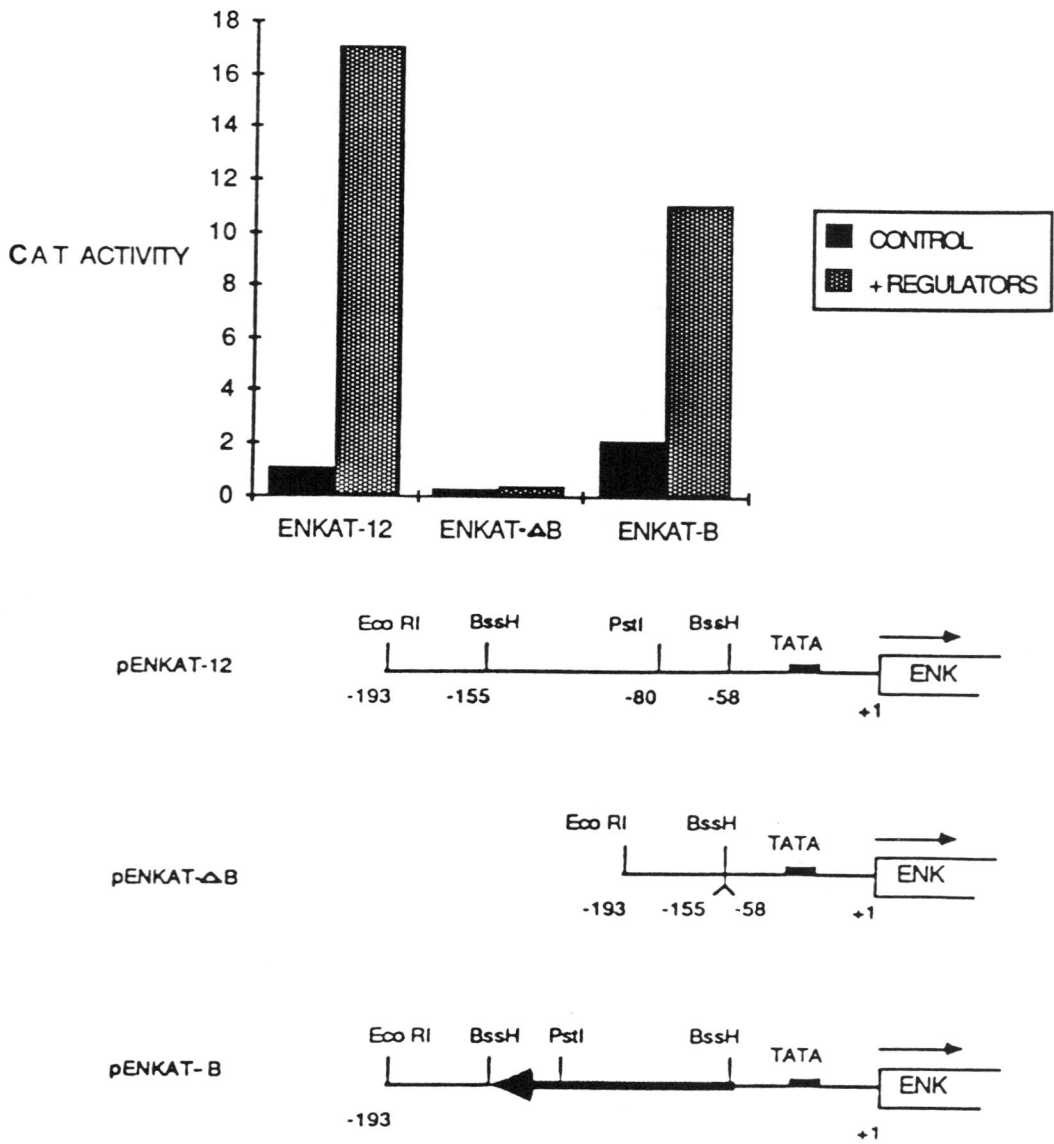

FIG. 5. Construction and analysis of deletion and reinsertion mutants in the promoter region of pENKAT-12. The **top** graph shows the relative CAT activities for each construct in the absence and presence of regulators (1.0 mM 8BrcAMP, 0.5 mM IBMX). The activity of pENKAT-12 in the absence of regulators was arbitrarily assigned the value of 1.0.

activity was observed (M. Comb, unpublished results). 8BrcAMP (1.0 mM) alone caused a fivefold increase in CAT activity, whereas 8BrcAMP and IBMX (0.5 mM) together caused an 18-fold increase in CAT expression. These data suggest a clear role for cyclic AMP as a second messenger involved in mediating proenkephalin gene expression. Cholera toxin and forskolin, other stimulators of adenylate cyclase, also produced increases in ENKAT-12-directed CAT expression.

To localize the DNA sequences in the proenkephalin gene that were responsible for the cyclic AMP transcriptional regulation, several plasmids were constructed that contained deletions or insertions in the 5' flanking region of the human proenkephalin gene. Plasmid ENKAT ΔB lacks the DNA sequence from −58 to −155 bp upstream of the human enkephalin cap site. Transfections with this plasmid gave a severalfold reduction in basal CAT activity and no induction with cyclic AMP analogs (see Fig. 5). Reinsertion of the −58 to −155 sequence into the plasmid but in the opposite orientation (ENKAT-B) restored both the basal and the regulated expression. Thus, the −58 to −155 bp region of the 5' flanking sequence of the gene contains sequences required for both basal and regulated expression, and these sequences can work in an orientation-independent fashion.

It was also exciting to find that this region of the proenkephalin gene was capable of conferring cyclic AMP regulation on a different promoter. The DNA sequence from −58 to −155 bp upstream of the human proenkephalin cap site was fused to a POMC-CAT fusion gene containing only 84 bp upstream from the POMC cap site. The POMC-CAT fusion gene expresses low basal CAT activity and shows very slight (twofold) increases in CAT activity in response to cyclic AMP. However, fusion of the −58 to −155 bp sequence from the human proenkephalin gene 5' to the 84 bp of upstream sequences in the POMC-CAT

construct showed increases of basal expression and conferred a large (>20-fold) induction by cyclic AMP. This finding suggests that this region of the human proenkephalin 5' flanking sequence is sufficient to confer cyclic AMP inducibility on an intact heterologous promoter.

In order to map the exact location of the DNA sequences responsible for cyclic AMP regulation, a series of 5' deletion mutants has been constructed using Bal 31 exonuclease (A. Seasholtz, unpublished results). Figure 6 diagrams the mutants that have been selected for further study because they span the 5' flanking region of the gene in increments of 10 to 15 bp. These deletions have all been subcloned into the ENKAT-12 plasmid and used for transfections. The region responsible for cyclic AMP regulation has been mapped to the sequences between −107 and −71 bp from the mRNA cap site. This sequence can now be examined more fully with site-specific mutagenesis and used to search for trans-acting proteins which may be involved in these regulatory processes.

Oocytes

We are also using the *Xenopus* oocyte system to examine transcriptional regulation. The oocyte will express, regulate, process, and secrete the product of an injected gene in a manner determined by its recognition of the control signals in the DNA sequence of the gene. This system has been used to locate transcriptional control signals in the 5' flanking sequences of the herpes thymidine kinase gene (40) and the Moloney murine sarcoma virus long terminal repeat (17), and a transcriptional control element in the sea urchin H2A histone gene (18). Two important features of the oocyte system are (a) the transcription of the injected gene can be assayed within a few hours of injection because of highly efficient expression of the gene, and (b) the

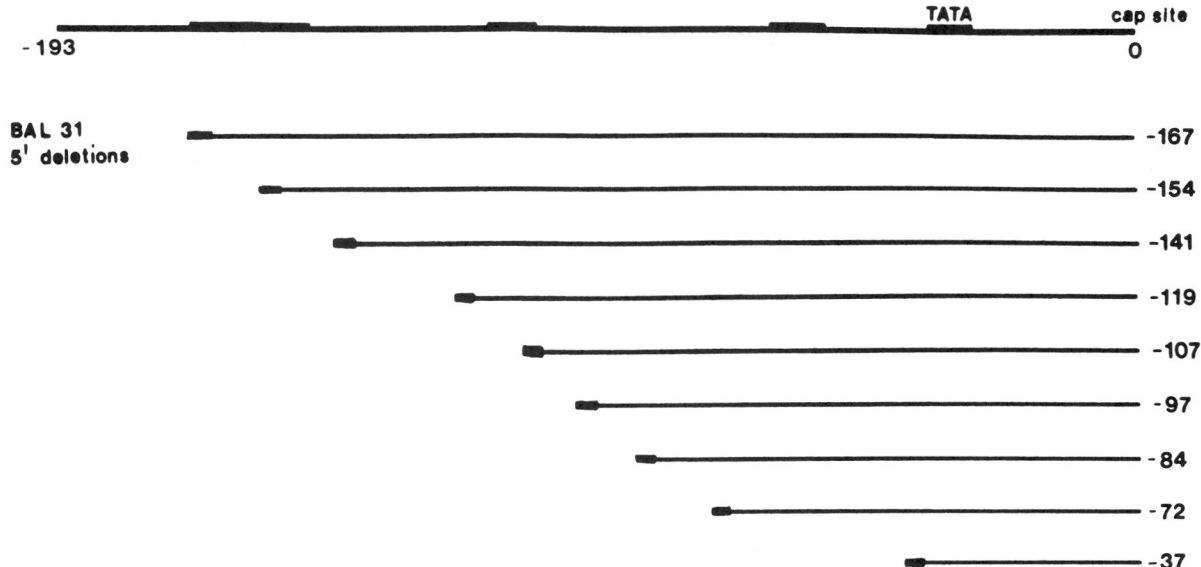

FIG. 6. Schematic representation of the 5' deletion mutants of the human proenkephalin gene. These mutants were constructed using Bal 31 exonuclease; the extent of the deletions was determined by dideoxyribonucleotide sequencing. The small boxes at the 5' ends represent the Eco RI linkers. The cap site of the mRNA molecule was assigned the +1 position.

injected DNA is neither replicated nor integrated into the host DNA. Since oocytes are highly active in RNA synthesis, they provide a convenient and efficient system for studying the transcriptional activity of wild-type and mutated genomic sequences. By quantitation of the transcripts produced from the wild-type and altered genes, the exact DNA sequences involved in some of the transcriptional regulatory processes can be determined. It is important to note that intronic DNA sequences can also be tested for control elements in the oocyte system, whereas some of these regions cannot be easily examined using the CAT-fusion gene system.

The transcription of the wild-type human proenkephalin gene (pHEnk 5.5) in *Xenopus* oocytes has been examined in our laboratory. The techniques used for injection of the DNA and isolation of RNA have been reviewed (20,21). Very briefly, 5 to 10 ng of DNA (pHEnk 5.5) was injected into the nucleus of mature oocytes (stage V or VI) using a microinjection pipette, a micromanipulator, and a manually controlled syringe. After 24 to 48 hr, the oocyte RNA was isolated and used for primer extension and Northern analyses. Primer extension experiments have unambiguously shown that all of the human proenkephalin transcripts in the injected oocytes were initiated at the same site as wild-type proenkephalin transcripts from human pheochromocytoma. Northern analysis has demonstrated that the majority of the proenkephalin transcripts produced in oocytes injected with pHEnk 5.5 are approximately 1.45 kb, the same size as human pheochromocytoma proenkephalin RNA, whereas no proenkephalin transcripts can be detected in uninjected oocytes. Thus, the injected oocytes are efficiently and accurately transcribing the human proenkephalin gene.

Further studies on the regulation of the human proenkephalin gene will be conducted in the oocytes using 5′ deletion mutants of the human proenkephalin gene. These mutants will be used to localize positive transcriptional control elements and to look for regulatory elements. *Xenopus* oocytes have been shown to exhibit responses to cyclic AMP (11) and will therefore provide a complementary system to the CAT/fusion genes for examining the transcriptional regulation of the wild-type and mutated proenkephalin genes. Thus, by using these two transient expression systems, we hope to gain a better understanding of the role of certain conserved sequences in the 5′ flanking DNA for transcriptional control of the human proenkephalin gene.

Vaccinia Virus

Vaccinia virus has recently been introduced as a eukaryotic cloning and expression vector (26,38,47). When compared to other expression vector systems, vaccinia has some decided advantages. For instance, plasmid expression vectors can only be used with certain cell types amenable to transfection techniques, and even then, only a small portion of the cells will take up and express the gene of interest (42). In contrast, vaccinia has a very broad host range and since it is a virus one can synchronously infect (and hence express an inserted gene) in virtually 100% of a cell population. Retroviruses, papovaviruses, and adenoviruses

have also been used as viral vector systems. Although these viruses are useful as vectors for many kinds of experiments, they have the disadvantage that they all replicate in the nucleus of the infected cells using the host cells' enzymatic machinery. This necessitates that foreign genes be placed in the proper context with respect to promoters, enhancers, splice junctions, polyadenylation sites, and transport signals. Using the vaccinia system, many of these considerations are circumvented as viral mRNA biogenesis occurs in the cytoplasm of infected cells and is carried out by viral enzymes directed by apparently unique regulatory signals (60). Therefore, if the cDNA for a gene of interest is inserted downstream from a vaccinia promoter, it will be rapidly transcribed (within a few minutes) and expressed at high levels in the host cell cytoplasm. This system has proven very useful then for examining the expression of neuropeptide precursors, such as proenkephalin and POMC, in a variety of different cell lines to address questions regarding the posttranslational maturation of these proteins and the characterization of enzymes that normally catalyze the processing events.

To achieve this goal, a recombinant vaccinia virus was constructed that contains and expresses the human proenkephalin (hPE) cDNA (Fig. 7). A second recombinant virus that expresses the mouse POMC cDNA was also constructed and designated VV:mPOMC. Four different cell lines were infected with either VV:hPE or VV:mPOMC. Two of the cell lines, AtT-20 and GH_4C_1 (rat pituitary), contain a full complement of secretory organelles. The other two cell lines, BSC-40 (African green monkey kidney cells) and Ltk⁻ (mouse fibroblast), do not contain stored granules typical of secretory cells. Twenty-four hours after infection, cell extracts and culture media were collected and the amount of Met-enkephalin or ACTH was quantitated by radioimmunoassay. The results are shown in Table 1. Infection of all cell types with either VV:hPE or VV:mPOMC resulted in the production of significant levels of Met-enkephalin and ACTH immunoreactivity (IR) in the respective fractions from both the cells and culture medium within 24 hr following infection.

In order to determine how effectively hPE was processed into smaller enkephalin-containing peptides (ECPs), acetic acid extracts of cells and culture medium from each cell type were next resolved on a TSK-125 high-performance liquid chromatography (HPLC) sizing column. Following peptide separation, each fraction was assayed for Met-enkephalin IR after sequential digestion with trypsin and carboxypeptidase B. Analysis of BSC-40 cells revealed two prominent peaks of Met-enkephalin IR following infection with VV:hPE. The IR material in peak 1 eluted with an apparent molecular weight of 28 kD. The IR material in the slower-migrating peak 2 eluted with an apparent molecular weight of 16 kD. Identical results were obtained for Ltk⁻ cells (data not shown). In order to determine whether one or both of these forms were secreted, a small aliquot of the culture medium was also analyzed. Only one prominent peak of Met-enkephalin IR was detected. This IR material coeluted exactly with that in peak 1.

GH_4C_1 rat pituitary cells, which possess a stored secretory granule population (56), exhibited an identical processing profile to that observed in BSC-40 cells. Interestingly,

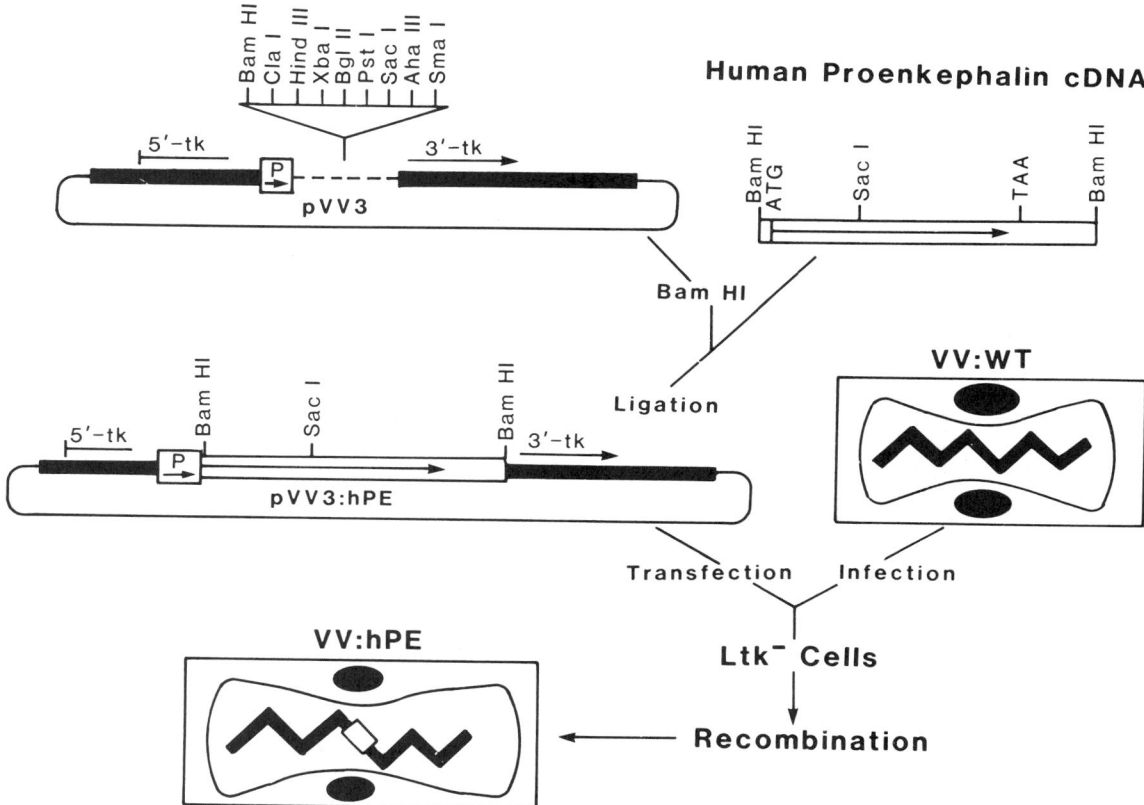

FIG. 7. Construction of VV:hPE. Synthetic BamH1 linkers were added to the ends of the 918-bp Hinc II fragment containing the entire coding region of hPE and ligated into the BamH1 cloning site of the VV recombination plasmid pVV3. The plasmid pVV3 contains the VV thymidine kinase gene interrupted by the constitutive VV 7.5K promoter adjacent to a multiple cloning site. Insertion of a foreign DNA into any of the multiple cloning sites places it under the control of the 7.5K promoter. One such plasmid, which contained the hPE insert in the correct orientation for expression with respect to the 7.5K promoter, was designated pVV3:hPE. Purified pVV3:hPE was next transfected into Ltk⁻ cells infected with 0.05 pfu/cell wild-type VV. Homologous recombination between the pVV3:hPE and VV:wild-type thymidine kinase genes resulted in the insertion of the hPE DNA into the VV genome. Recombinant VV:hPE was purified by plaque hybridization techniques.

GH₄C₁ cells, which secrete growth hormone and prolactin, efficiently process human preproparathyroid hormone (pre-proPTH) to PTH by cleavage of the prohormone at a tribasic amino acid sequence (Lys-Lys-Arg) flanking the *N*-terminus of PTH (22). Perhaps the inability of GH₄C₁ cells to cleave the dibasic amino acid sequences in hPE may be attributed to a high degree of endopeptidase specificity for the basic amino acid cleavage sequences in the precursor protein.

In contrast to the above cell types, AtT-20 cells infected with VV:hPE exhibit five major peaks of Met-enkephalin IR. Peaks 1 and 2 coeluted exactly with peaks 1 and 2 of Met-enkephalin IR from each of the other cell lines infected with VV:hPE. The presence of peaks 1 and 2 in each cell type studied shows that the modification responsible for their separation on the sizing column is common to many cell types, and therefore would occur at a point in the secretory pathway prior to packaging of the precursor into secretory granules. Peaks 3 and 4 eluted with an apparent molecular weight of 4,500 and 2,500 daltons. The slowest migrating peak, 5, coeluted with purified Met-enkephalin. Analysis of the media from VV:hPE-infected AtT-20 cells revealed two major peaks of secreted Met-enkephalin IR.

The faster-migrating peak coeluted with peak 1 of the cell sample and the slower-migrating peak coeluted with peak 5 and purified Met-enkephalin.

The size distribution of Met-enkephalin IR observed following infection of AtT-20 cells with VV:hPE is in excellent agreement with the size distribution of Met-enkephalin IR in AtT-20 cells stably transfected with the human proenkephalin gene (8). This argues that the presence of vaccinia virus infection does not alter the cellular protein maturation pathway. Purification and identification of each of the processing intermediates will be necessary in order to determine the proteolytic maturation pathway of human proenkephalin. Future experiments employing pulse-chase techniques with radiolabeled amino acids will allow for the characterization of the temporal order of production of each of the processing intermediates.

The coelution of the cellular and secreted 28-kD protein suggested that it was bona fide human proenkephalin. The secreted form was therefore purified to homogeneity by chromatofocusing followed by two rounds of reverse phase HPLC. The *N*-terminal sequence was determined for the first 20 amino acid residues (E. Weber, IABR, Oregon Health Sciences University) and found to be E-?-S-Q-D-?-

TABLE 1. *Production of Met-enkephalin and ACTH-IR by different cell types*

	pmol Met-enkephalin IR/10^6 cells			
	BSC-40 0.5 pfu/cell	AtT-20 5 pfu/cell	GH4Cl 5 pfu/cell	Ltk⁻ 5 pfu/cell
MI	—	—	—	—
VV:WT	—	0.1	—	—
VV:hPE				
Cell	19.4	10.1	43.6	7
Medium	180	36	79	43
	pmol ACTH-IR/10^6 cells			
MI	—		—	—
VV:WT	—		—	—
VV:mPOMC				
Cell	2.6		3.7	1.2
Medium	22		9.2	4.4

Parallel cultures of BSC-40, AtT-20, GH4Cl, and L cells grown in 28-cm^2 plates were either mock infected (MI), or infected with the indicated titer of wild-type vaccinia virus, VV:hPE or VV:mPOMC for 24 hr. Following infection, the cells were resuspended in 1 M acetic acid pH 1.9, headed to 100°C for 15 min and sonicated. Culture media were immediately placed at −70°C. For a Met-enkephalin IR determination, proportionate amounts (based on cell number) of each cell lysate were lyophilized and resuspended in 400 μl 50 mM Tris pH 8.0, 2 mM $CaCl_2$ containing 20 μg/ml trypsin TPCK (Cooper Biomedical). Culture media were digested with an equal volume of the trypsin solution. Following trypsin digestion, samples were treated with 2 μg/ml carboxypeptidase B (Sigma) and heated to 100°C for 15 min. Samples were next assayed for Met-enkephalin IR using a Met-enkephalin-specific antiserum (RB4, S. Sabol). Optimal virus titer and time of infection for each cell line were previously determined (data not shown). For ACTH-IR determination, lysates were assayed as previously described (23) using antiserum Henrietta. Note that proenkephalin contains six sequences of Met-enkephalin and POMC contains one sequence of ACTH.

A-T-?-S-Y-R-L-V-R-P-A-?-I-N. (Question marks denote undetected >PhNCS-AAs in those cycles.) Assuming these are cysteine residues, which are undetectable by this analysis, the sequence conforms exactly to amino acid residues 25–44 of human preproenkephalin determined by cDNA sequence analysis. This demonstrates that the infected cells are able to accurately cleave the signal peptide terminating at Ala$_{24}$. The levels of secreted proenkephalin from BSC-40 cells (1 μg/10^6 cells after 24 hr of infection) demonstrate that recombinant vaccinia virus can be readily used as an expression vector for the production of hPE as a substrate for *in vitro* processing experiments and perhaps structural determinations.

Another potential use of the vaccinia virus expression system would be to remove a specific gene product from the cell, such as a putative processing enzyme or an endogenous prohormone. Recent experiments have shown that introduction of an antisense mRNA (ss RNA complementary to a specific mRNA) into a cell can dramatically reduce the ability of that mRNA to direct protein synthesis (28,33,48). Close to maximal inhibition can be obtained with RNA complementary only to the 5′ untranslated region (29,41).

In order to determine if RNA transcribed from a recombinant vaccinia virus containing antisense POMC mRNA sequences could reduce or prevent the synthesis of the POMC protein, the following recombinant virus was constructed. Ninety-two bp of the 5′ untranslated region of mouse POMC cDNA were cloned into the plasmid pVV3 (see Fig. 7) in the antisense orientation with respect to the VV promoter. Homologous recombination was used as before to insert this into the VV genome. This construct, VV:5′ mCOMP, was then used to infect AtT-20 cells, which produce very high levels of endogenous POMC.

Preliminary results show a 40% reduction in ACTH immunoreactivity 24 hr after infection with VV:5′ mCOMP as compared with mock-infected cells, or cells infected with wild-type vaccinia virus. Conditions for optimizing the inhibition of endogenous POMC production are currently being examined. If >90% reduction can be obtained, a single recombinant VV could then be constructed that directs the synthesis of two separate RNAs. One RNA would contain the 5′ antisense sequences complementary to the 5′ untranslated region of the native POMC mRNA. The second VV-encoded RNA would contain a POMC mRNA lacking the native 5′ untranslated sequence but containing point mutations at and around sites of post-translational processing. Such a system, which would block the synthesis of the native POMC protein while generating mutant POMC proteins, would be invaluable for studying the structural requirements of hormone precursors for accurate cleavage *in vivo*.

Given the extremely high levels of POMC mRNA in AtT-20 cells (5), it may not be feasible to produce sufficient antisense message to adequately lower POMC levels, but the technique could still easily prove capable of sufficiently reducing (or eliminating) production of a somewhat less abundant protein, such as an enzyme responsible for post-translational processing.

FUTURE DIRECTIONS

Gene transfer methods have provided us with the tools for elucidating the molecular mechanisms involved in regulation of gene expression. New techniques are continually being examined in hopes of overcoming some of the limitations of the present procedures. Some inherent limitations to gene regulation studies with stably transformed cell lines are (a) low efficiency of transfer, (b) multiple gene copy insertion, and (c) random integration site of the foreign DNA in chromosomal DNA.

Recent gene transfer studies with RNA viruses (retroviruses) have demonstrated that these viral vectors have several distinct advantages over other systems: (a) Up to 100% of the cells can be infected and will express the viral and exogenous genes, and (b) the viral DNA and foreign DNA will be integrated as a single copy at a single, but random, site (1). Therefore, by inserting a foreign gene into a retroviral vector and packaging of that RNA into an infectious retrovirus particle, one can infect appropriate host cells at almost 100% efficiency. However, the integrated exogenous gene is now contained in the middle of a viral sequence that may also affect the regulation of the foreign gene.

Transgenic animals offer another approach for these studies. The injection of a foreign gene into a fertilized egg is an efficient method of gene transfer. Transgenic animals also provide an opportunity to examine the cell- and tissue-specific expression of the foreign gene in an organism. However, transgenic animals often contain more than one copy of the foreign gene and the site of chromosomal integration cannot be controlled.

Another viral system is currently being studied that offers several advantages over conventional gene transfer techniques. Bovine papilloma viral vectors can stably transform cultured rat and mouse cells while being maintained exclusively as unintegrated extrachromosomal plasmids. Thus, this viral system offers unique advantages of both stably transfected cell lines and transient expression systems. The bovine papilloma viral-transformed cell lines are stable and can be used for repeated experiments, whereas the bovine papilloma viral vector containing the exogenous gene is maintained in a homogeneous environment since it does not integrate into the chromosomal DNA (3). Different hybrid plasmids containing bovine papilloma virus sequences and pBR322 sequences are currently being constructed that can transform cells at high efficiency and serve as shuttle vectors between eukaryotic cells and bacterial cells (3).

Clearly the optimal system for gene transfer experiments would allow efficient transfer of the gene of interest into the cell type of choice and would also direct the DNA to a predetermined chromosomal location. Integration of a cloned gene to its natural site on the chromosome is possible in yeast, which undergo homologous recombination at a relatively high frequency. Previous work has suggested that homologous site-specific integration occurs at low levels in higher eukaryotes. However, recent studies show a relatively high frequency of homologous recombination in mammalian cells between endogenous and introduced SV40 genomes, possibly via a double-stranded gap repair mechanism (30). Hopefully, further studies on recombination in higher eukaryotes will yield efficient methods for site-specific integration of exogenous genes into chromosomal DNA in gene transfer experiments.

CONCLUSIONS

The availability of cloned genes and the development of gene transfer methods have given us the opportunity to examine the molecular mechanisms involved in the regulation of expression at almost every level: transcription, translation, processing, and secretion. By using a variety of gene transfer approaches to study regulation, we will be able to examine each level of regulation in detail. By then integrating the information we have learned from each system, we hope to be able to gain a more complete understanding of the complex mechanisms involved in the regulation of neuroendocrine peptides.

ACKNOWLEDGMENTS

We are grateful to Leslie Williams for expert preparation of the manuscript. A.F.S. was supported by postdoctoral fellowship F32DA05261 from NIDA. G.T. is the recipient of a Damon Runyon-Walter Winchell postdoctoral fellowship DRG 797. The research performed in E. Herbert's laboratory was supported by research grants AM37231 and AM37274 from the National Institutes of Health and research grant DA04154 from the National Institute on Drug Abuse.

REFERENCES

1. Anderson, W. F. (1984): *Science,* 226:401–409.
2. Benton, W. D., and Davis, R. W. (1977): *Science,* 196:180–182.
3. Campo, M. S. (1985): In: *DNA Cloning, Vol. II,* edited by D. M. Glover, pp. 213–238. IRL Press, Washington, D.C.
4. Chang, A. C. Y., Cochet, M., and Cohen, S. (1980): *Proc. Natl. Acad. Sci. USA,* 77:4890–4894.
5. Civelli, O., Birnberg, N., and Herbert, E. (1982): *J. Biol. Chem.,* 257:6783–6787.
6. Civelli, O., Douglass, J., Goldstein, A., and Herbert, E. (1985): *Proc. Natl. Acad. Sci. USA,* 82:4291–4295.
7. Cochet, M., Chang, A. C. Y., and Cohen, S. N. (1982): *Nature,* 297:335–339.
8. Comb, M., Liston, D., Martin, M., Rosen, H., and Herbert, E. (1985): *EMBO J.,* 4:3115–3122.

9. Comb, M., Rosen, H., Seeburg, P., Adelman, J., and Herbert, E. (1983): *DNA,* 2:213–229.
10. Comb, M., Seeburg, P. H., Adelman, J., Eiden, L., and Herbert, E. (1982): *Nature,* 295:663–666.
11. Dascal, N., Lotan, I., Gillo, B., Lester, H., and Lass, Y. (1985): *Proc. Natl. Acad. Sci. USA,* 82:6001–6005.
12. Douglass, J., Civelli, O., and Herbert, E. (1984): *Annu. Rev. Biochem.,* 53:665–715.
13. Drouin, J., and Goodman, H. M. (1980): *Nature,* 288:610–613.
14. Eiden, L. E., Giraud, P., Affolter, H.-U., Herbert, E., and Hotchkiss, A. J. (1984): *Proc. Natl. Acad. Sci. USA,* 81:3949–3953.
15. Gorman, C. M., Moffat, L. F., and Howard, B. M. (1982): *Mol. Cell. Biol.,* 2:1044–1051.
16. Graham, F. L., and Van Der Eb, A. J. (1973): *Virology,* 52:456–467.
17. Graves, B. J., Eisenman, R. N., and McKnight, S. L. (1985): *Mol. Cell. Biol.,* 5:1948–1958.
18. Grosschedl, R., and Birnstiel, M. L. (1980): *Proc. Natl. Acad. Sci. USA,* 77:1432–1436.
19. Gubler, U., Seeburg, P., Hoffman, B. J., Gage, L. P., and Udenfriend, S. (1982): *Nature,* 295:206–208.
20. Gurdon, J. B., and Melton, D. A. (1981): *Annu. Rev. Genet.,* 15: 189–218.
21. Gurdon, J. B., and Wickens, M. P. (1983): *Methods Enzymol.,* 101:370–386.
22. Hellerman, J. G., Cone, R. C., Potts, J. T., Rich, A., Mulligan, R. C., and Kornberg, H. M. (1984): *Proc. Natl. Acad. Sci. USA,* 81:5340–5344.
23. Herbert, E., Allen, R. G., and Paquette, T. C. (1978): *Endocrinology,* 102:218–226.
24. Herbert, E., Civelli, O., Douglass, J., Martens, G., and Rosen, H. (1985): In: *Biochemical Action of Hormones, Vol. XII,* pp. 1–36. Academic Press, New York.
25. Horikawa, S., Takai, T., Toyosato, M., Takahashi, H., Noda, M., Kakidani, H., Kubo, T., Hirose, T., Inayama, S., Hayashida, H., Miyata, T., and Numa, S. (1983): *Nature,* 306:611–614.
26. Hruby, D., Thomas, G., Herbert, E., and Franke, C. (1986): *Methods Enzymol.,* 124:295–309.
27. Hughes, J., Smith, T. W., Kosterlitz, H. W., Fothergill, L. A., Morgan, B. A., and Morris, H. R. (1975): *Nature,* 258:577–579.
28. Izant, J. G., and Weintraub, H. (1984): *Cell,* 36:1007–1015.
29. Izant, J. G., and Weintraub, H. (1985): *Science,* 229:345–352.
30. Jasin, M., deVillier, J., Weber, F., and Schaffner, W. (1985): *Cell,* 43:695–703.
31. Kakidani, H., Furutani, Y., Takahashi, H., Noda, M., Morimoto, Y., Hirose, T., Asai, M., Inayama, S., Nakanishi, S., and Numa, S. (1982): *Nature,* 298:245–249.
32. Kilpatrick, D. L., Taniguchi, T., Jones, B. N., Stern, A. S., Shively, J. E., Hullihan, J., Kimura, S., Stein, S., and Udenfriend, S. (1981): *Proc. Natl. Acad. Sci. USA,* 78:3265–3268.
33. Kim, F. K., and Wold, B. S. (1985): *Cell,* 42:129–138.
34. Lawn, R. M., Fritsch, E. F., Parker, R. C., Lake, G. B., and Maniatis, T. (1978): *Cell,* 15:1157–1163.
35. Lewis, R. V., Stern, A. S., Kilpatrick, D. L., Gerber, L. D., Rossier, J., Stein, S., and Udenfriend, S. (1981): *J. Neurosci.,* 1:80–82.
36. Liston, D. R., Bohlen, P., and Rossier, J. (1984): *J. Neurochem.,* 43:335–341.
37. Liston, D. R., Vanderhaeghen, J. J., and Rossier, J. (1983): *Nature,* 302:62–65.
38. Mackett, M., Smith, G. L., and Moss, B. (1982): *Proc. Natl. Acad. Sci. USA,* 79:7415–7419.
39. Mains, R. E., and Eipper, B. A. (1979): *J. Biol. Chem.,* 254:7885–7894.
40. McKnight, S. L., and Kingsbury, R. (1982): *Science,* 217:316–324.
41. Melton, D. A. (1985): *Proc. Natl. Acad. Sci. USA,* 82:144–148.
42. Mulligan, R. C., and Berg, P. (1980): *Science,* 209:1422–1427.
43. Nakanishi, S., Inove, A., Kita, T., Nakamura, M., Chang, A. C. Y., Cohen, S. N., and Numa, S. (1979): *Nature,* 278:423–427.
44. Nakanishi, S., Teranishi, Y., Noda, M., Notake, M., Watanabe, Y., and Numa, S. (1980): *Nature,* 287:752–753.
45. Noda, M., Furutani, Y., Takahashi, H., Toyosato, M., Hirose, T., Inayama, S., Nakanishi, S., and Numa, S. (1982): *Nature,* 295: 202–206.
46. Noda, M., Teranishi, Y., Takahashi, H., Toyosato, M., Notake, M., Nakanishi, S., and Numa, S. (1982): *Nature,* 297:431–434.
47. Panicali, D., and Paoletti, E. (1982): *Proc. Natl. Acad. Sci. USA,* 79:4927–4931.
48. Pestka, S., Daugherty, B. L., Jung, V., Hotta, K., and Pestka, R. K. (1984): *Proc. Natl. Acad. Sci. USA,* 81:7525–7528.
49. Quach, T. T., Tang, F., Kageyama, H., Guido, A., Meek, J. L., Costa, E., and Schwartz, J. P. (1984): *Mol. Pharmacol.,* 26:255–260.
50. Rivier, C., Brownstein, M., Soiess, J., Rivier, J., and Vale, W. (1982): *Endocrinology,* 110:272–278.
51. Rivier, C., and Vale, W. (1983): *Endocrinology,* 113:1422–1426.
52. Roberts, J. L., Budarf, M. L., Baxter, J. D., and Herbert, E. (1979): *Biochemistry,* 18:4907–4915.
53. Rosa, P. A., Policastro, P., and Herbert, E. (1980): *J. Exp. Biol.,* 89:215–237.
54. Rosen, H., Douglass, J., and Herbert, E. (1984): *J. Biol. Chem.,* 259:14309–14313.
55. Tang, F., Costa, E., and Schwartz, J. P. (1983): *Proc. Natl. Acad. Sci. USA,* 80:3841–3844.
56. Tixier-Vidal, A. (1975): In: *The Anterior Pituitary,* edited by A. Tixier-Vidal and M. G. Farquahar, pp. 181–230. Academic Press, New York.
57. Udenfriend, S., and Kilpatrick, D. (1983): *Arch. Biochem. Biophys.,* 221:309–323.
58. Uhler, M., and Herbert, E. (1983): *J. Biol. Chem.,* 258:257–261.
59. Uhler, M., Herbert, E., D'Eustachio, P., and Rubble, F. D. (1983): *J. Biol. Chem.,* 258:9444–9453.
60. Weir, J. P., and Moss, B. (1983): *J. Virol.,* 46:530.
61. Whitfeld, P. L., Seeburg, P. H., and Shine, J. (1982): *DNA,* 1:133–143.

Psychopharmacology:
The Third Generation of Progress,
edited by Herbert Y. Meltzer.
Raven Press, New York © 1987.

CHAPTER 41

Cotranslational and Posttranslational Processing in the Production of Bioactive Peptides

Betty A. Eipper, Victor May, Edward I. Cullen, Sheryl M. Sato, Adavi S. N. Murthy, and Richard E. Mains

The number of small peptides thought to play roles in the nervous and endocrine systems has increased tremendously over the past few years. Each of these small peptides is initially synthesized as part of a larger, biologically inactive precursor. Understanding the processes involved in converting precursors into products is essential to understanding how these peptides function in physiological and pathological states. In this brief review, we hope to provide the reader with an appreciation of some of the elegant posttranslational processing mechanisms that play a key role in the functioning of peptides in the nervous and endocrine systems. Given the restricted length of this review, only a few key citations will be given for each research group whose work we discuss.

For the purposes of organization, the multiple steps included in cotranslational and posttranslational processing have been divided into three temporal categories: (a) early steps occurring largely before major endoproteolytic cleavage events, such as removal of the signal peptide, protein folding, disulfide bond formation, glycosylation, hydroxylation of lysine, phosphorylation, and sulfation; (b) major endoproteolytic cleavages; and (c) later modifications such as exoproteolytic trimming, α-N-acetylation, α-amidation, and formation of pyroglutamic acid. When possible we have drawn on studies of purified processing enzymes and have tried to take into account the fact that these modifi-

cations occur at specific subcellular locations from the cisternae of the rough endoplasmic reticulum (RER) through the various subcompartments of the Golgi and into secretory granules.

PRECURSORS

The ground rules for thinking about the biosynthesis of bioactive peptides are set by the structures of the precursors and the sequences of the product peptides (Fig. 1). Although analysis of the large number of precursor structures now known allows one to formulate some general rules for prohormone processing, formation of products occurs in a tissue-specific and developmentally regulated fashion and one must identify the major products in the tissue of interest. In general, products derived from every region of a precursor are found in close to equimolar amounts; neither neurons nor endocrine cells seem to degrade major regions of a precursor. Precursors are generally synthesized with an amino-terminal signal or leader sequence that is rapidly cleaved off. Major endoproteolytic cleavage sites are often marked by pairs of basic amino acids, although not all pairs are cleaved and certain cleavages occur at single basic residues and other sites. The biologically active peptides can be situated anywhere within the precursor and

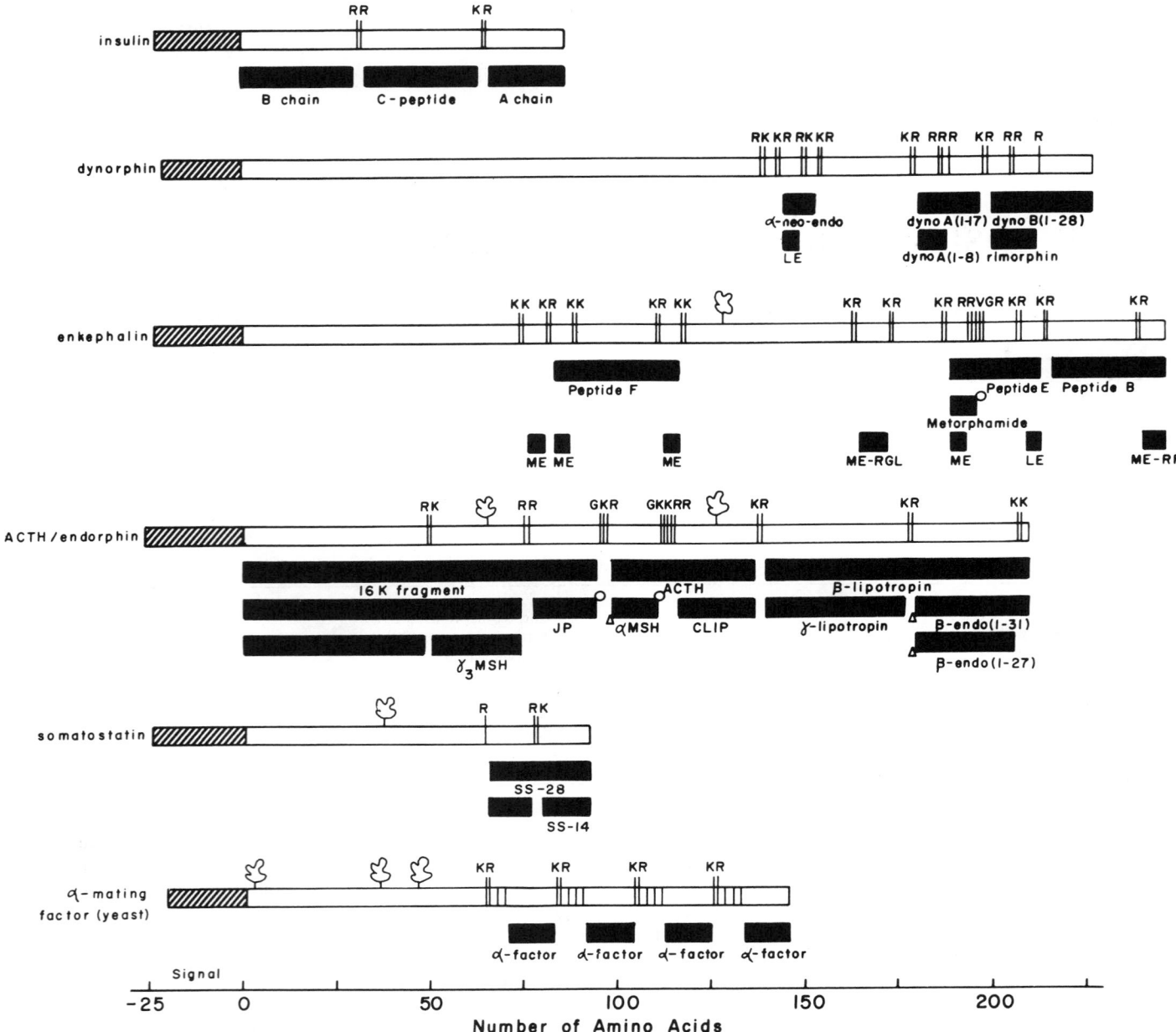

FIG. 1. Biologically active peptides: structures of selected precursors and some of their products. Data are from the following references: rat insulins (30,164), rat dynorphin (28,78), rat enkephalin (146), rat ACTH/endorphin (37,110), rat somatostatin (171), and yeast α-mating factor (91). Where the first residue of the proprotein has not been determined by peptide analysis, the signal cleavage site has been assumed to follow the usual rules (110). The standard single-letter code for amino acids was used: R, arginine; K, lysine; G, glycine; L, leucine; F, phenylalanine. Symbols are also included for sites of α-N-acetylation (△), α-amidation (○), and N-linked glycosylation (♧). Abbreviations: dyno, dynorphin; LE, leucine-enkephalin; ME, methionine-enkephalin; JP, joining peptide; αMSH, α-melanotropin; CLIP, corticotropin-like intermediate lobe peptide; β-endo, β-endorphin; SS, somatostatin. Metorphamide is also known as adrenorphin. Dyno B(1–28) in rat corresponds to dyno B(1–29) (leumorphin) in beef. As noted in the text, α-N-acetylation does occur with dyno and LE in some tissues.

a single precursor may contain peptides with different bioactivities or multiple copies of similar bioactive peptides.

In Fig. 1, there are many examples of tissue-specific processing of precursors to smaller peptides. For example, in the case of the corticotropin (ACTH)/endorphin precursor, the cleavage within ACTH(1–39) to form α-melano-tropin [α-N-acetyl-ACTH(1–13)NH₂] and corticotropin-like intermediate lobe peptide (CLIP) occurs in the intermediate pituitary and in the arcuate nucleus of the hypothalamus, but not to any great extent in the anterior pituitary of the adult rat. Similarly, NH₂-terminal acetylation of ACTH(1–13)NH₂ and β-endorphin occurs in the intermediate pituitary but not to any great extent in the anterior pituitary or arcuate nucleus (43). Cleavage of proenkephalin to various enkephalin-sized peptides goes nearly to completion in the brain, yet the adrenal medulla contains primarily the larger peptides diagrammed (47). It is important to consider the tissue specificity of processing when searching for the enzymes responsible for the processing.

CELLULAR EVENTS IN PEPTIDE PROCESSING

As outlined in Fig. 2, peptide hormone precursors are synthesized on membrane-bound ribosomes and the nascent polypeptide chains are inserted into the lumen of the RER. For most secreted, soluble proteins this vectorial synthesis requires the intervention of the signal peptide, a signal recognition particle (SRP), and an SRP receptor (or docking protein) (58,178). Recombinant DNA approaches to studying secretion have shown that presence of a signal peptide is the major determinant of secretion into the lumen of the RER, but other aspects of protein structure can also be important (23,56). In general the amino-terminal 20 to 40 amino acids constitute the signal peptide and are cleaved off. However, for several proteins there is good evidence for the existence of a noncleaved internal signal peptide necessary for transport into the lumen of the RER; both the Phe-Met-Arg-Phe-NH$_2$ precursor in *Aplysia* and the α-factor precursor in yeast appear to lack a cleavable NH$_2$-terminal signal peptide (21,155). The initial attachment of Asn-linked oligosaccharide chains occurs during or within

a few minutes after vectorial synthesis of the nascent chain into the lumen of the RER (144).

The precursors are next transported to the cis side of the Golgi apparatus (Fig. 2). Significant maturation of the molecules occurs during transport to the trans side of the Golgi, where packaging into secretory granules occurs (45,56,132,151). Estimates of the time required for newly synthesized proteins to reach secretory granules vary from 25 to 150 min for different proteins (15,45,132,151). For most precursors, biosynthetic processing begins in the Golgi and continues in secretory granules. Whether the initial endoproteolytic cleavages begin in the Golgi or are confined to secretory granules is a point of current debate. Although it would be simpler for a cell to transport intact precursors into granules and only then begin to cleave them (55,86), the bulk of current experimental data from biochemical and electron microscopic studies argues for the occurrence of endoproteolytic cleavages in the Golgi (59,69,101, 124,129,130,164). The subcellular location of the various processing steps may not be the same in all cell types (45). There is mounting evidence that initial cleavage events may occur while precursors are membrane associated (101,124,125,129). Experiments with pancreatic β cells grown in noncleavable analogs of Lys and Arg demonstrate that proteolytic processing is not essential to the subcellular sorting process (130). At least two pharmacologically distinguishable events occur during secretion from granules: movement of the granules to the membrane and release by exocytosis (25).

One key unanswered question concerns how cells sort secretory peptides into secretory granules and not into

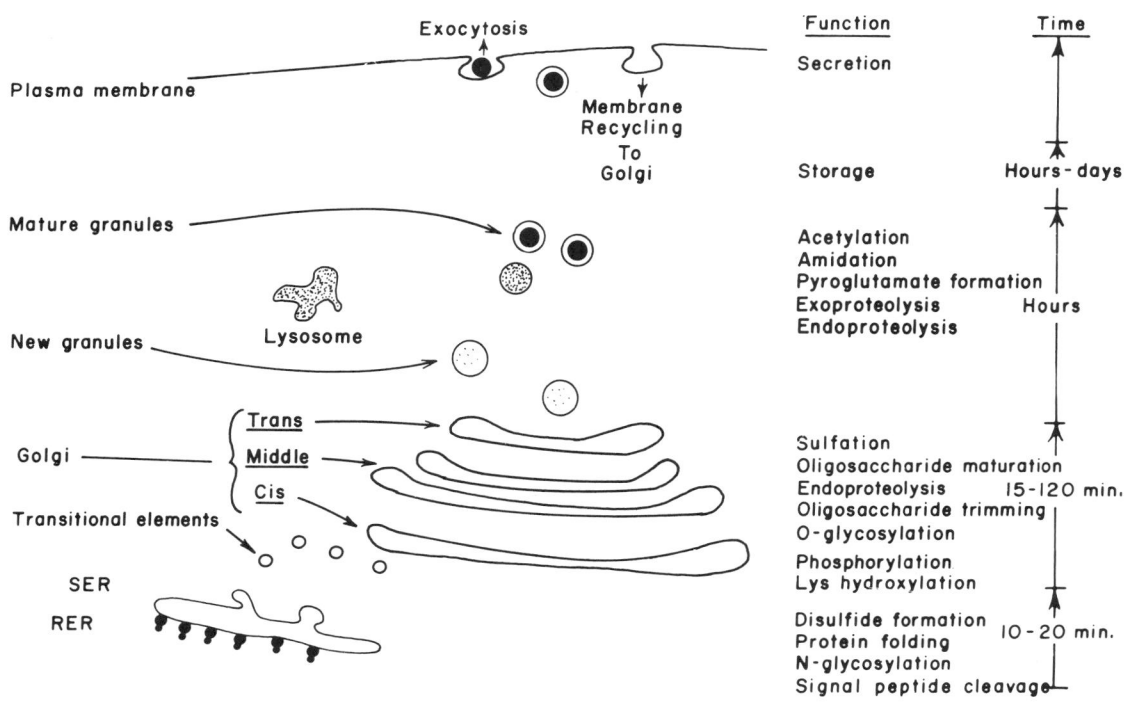

FIG. 2. Intracellular events in peptide processing. The events in the cell, from synthesis of the protein precursor on membrane-bound ribosomes through to secretion, are depicted schematically. (Adapted from refs. 45, 55, 56, 86, 101, 129, 132, 151, 164.)

TABLE 1. *Guidelines for identification of processing enzymes*

1. Precise knowledge of biosynthetic pathway from precursor to products in tissue under study
2. Purification *to homogeneity* of candidate enzyme; measurement of kinetic parameters
3. Demonstration that the purified enzyme can carry out the correct reaction on the correct substrate under the correct conditions
4. Evidence that the candidate enzyme occurs in the correct subcellular location
5. Demonstration that specific inhibition or deletion of the candidate enzyme blocks the processing step in the intact cell

lysosomes or an unregulated secretory pathway (45,56,86). Another key unanswered question concerns whether cells not normally producing peptides for storage and secretion (e.g., fibroblasts) can process precursors correctly, store product peptides, and release them in response to a stimulus. Current reports have not reached a consensus (72,82,86,181).

It is generally agreed that the later steps in posttranslational processing occur within secretory granules. The interior of these granules contains high concentrations of product peptides (1–100 mM) (55), other proteins, metals, and cofactors and presents an environment difficult to mimic in test tube studies. There is wide agreement that many mature secretory granules have an internal pH of 5.5 to 6.0 and maintain a positive membrane potential with respect to the cytoplasm (55,76,101,103), but secretory granules from the parotid gland have an internal pH of 6.8 (7). The transmembrane pH gradient of secretory granules is not crucial to the secretory process (76). Secretory granules contain millimolar levels of ascorbate and possibly other reducing agents, and possess membrane enzymes capable of transmembrane electron transfer (95,123,150,163,172). It is clear that new granules are different in electron density and sedimentation properties from older, mature granules (69,101,126). New and more mature granules also appear to be functionally different since proteolytic processing of proinsulin and amidation of peptides change with the age of the secretory granules studied (61,164). Clearly more work will be necessary to clarify the conditions under which processing enzymes must function.

The cell biological studies of peptide processing help to provide us with a set of guidelines for further studies of prohormone biosynthetic processing enzymes (Table 1).

EARLY EVENTS

During transit through the RER and Golgi, precursor proteins are subjected to various modifications including N- and O-linked glycosylation, phosphorylation, and sulfation. None of these modifications is unique to bioactive peptides. Although particular amino acid sequences are required for modifications of this type to occur, not all potential modification sites are utilized, and their utilization may vary among species, tissues, and developmental stages.

Some of these posttranslational modifications affect biological activity, while the function of others is unclear. We will not discuss protein folding and disulfide bond formation, which seem to be determined by the primary structure of the precursor (85,164). Formation of hydroxylysine residues is believed to fall in this group of modifications (6,124).

Glycosylation

In this section we will provide a brief overview of the synthesis of glycoproteins and discuss some recent results concerning the importance of glycosylation in glycoprotein sorting, secretion, and function (excellent reviews include 38,45,88,152). Oligosaccharide chains on proteins are either N-linked or O-linked; N-linked oligosaccharides are joined to glycoproteins at Asn residues that are part of the consensus sequence Asn-X-Ser/Thr whereas O-linked oligosaccharides are joined at Ser or Thr residues, often in regions of high proline content.

The N-linked glycoproteins become glycosylated cotranslationally or immediately posttranslationally when a fairly large oligosaccharide ($Glc_3Man_9GlcNAc_2$) is transferred *en bloc* from a lipid-linked precursor (dolichol phosphate) to the nascent peptide backbone just as it enters the lumen of the RER (88,144). Synthesis of the lipid-linked precursor involves stepwise addition of sugar residues to the phosphate end of the dolichol phosphate. In the first group of reactions, monosaccharides are transferred to the dolichol phosphate from nucleotide sugars such as UDP-GlcNAc that are located in the cytoplasm. At about the time that the precursor attains the structure $Man_5(GlcNAc)_2$-P-P-dolichol, the orientation of the precursor changes so that the oligosaccharide moiety is transferred into the lumen of the RER (161). On the inside of the lumen, additional sugars are added to the growing precursor from monosaccharide esters of dolichol phosphate until the lipid-linked precursor attains its final structure: $Glc_3Man_9(GlcNAc)_2$-P-P-dolichol. All N-linked oligosaccharides begin with this structure. After the oligosaccharide is transferred to the Asn-residue of the nascent glycoprotein, all three glucose residues and usually one mannose are removed while the glycoprotein is still in the RER. For secretory proteins with oligosaccharide chains of the complex type, further processing occurs in the Golgi complex and involves sequential removal of outer mannose residues and ordered addition of N-acetylglucosamine, galactose, and sialic acid or sulfate. Specific glycosyl transferases are now used as markers for the cis, middle, and trans subcompartments of the Golgi complex (Fig. 2) (38,45).

O-Linked oligosaccharides are formed directly on protein acceptors in the Golgi complex by the sequential addition of monosaccharides from sugar nucleotides such as UDP-GalNAc, UDP-Gal, and CMP-sialic acid to Ser and Thr residues (152). Uncombined α subunits of pituitary glycoprotein hormones and the β subunit of hCG are all O-glycosylated (134,152).

The factors determining whether a given site is glycosylated and what type of oligosaccharide chain is attached are not completely clear. Statistical analyses of known glycosylation sites indicate that complex oligosaccharides occur most frequently within the first 110 amino acids of a glycoprotein whereas high-mannose oligosaccharides predominate after the first 200 residues; protein folding may limit processing at later sites (88,136). In addition, secretory rate may affect the length of time a precursor is exposed to the relevant processing activities.

Overall protein structure also affects glycosylation. When immunoglobulin light chains containing amino acid analogs such as β-hydroxyleucine and 4-thiaisoleucine were synthesized in tumor cells, oligosaccharide chains were attached to the peptide backbone and the glycoprotein was secreted into the medium, but the high-mannose oligosaccharides were no longer processed into complex chains (66). Variants of vesicular stomatitis virus (VSV) and murine leukemia virus that possess slightly altered protein backbones were synthesized with different oligosaccharide chains when grown in the same cell (81,147).

Oligosaccharide moieties clearly play a role in sorting glycoproteins into the correct subcellular compartment. Recombinant DNA techniques and *in vitro* mutagenesis have permitted studies on the effects of single amino acid changes on the processing of a single secretory protein (56,68). A hybrid gene was constructed in which sequences coding for growth hormone were spliced to sequences for the VSV membrane glycoprotein (68). When transfected into appropriate host cells, this gene produced a nonglycosylated membrane-bound version of growth hormone. The hybrid growth hormone was sequestered into the lumen of the RER and was transported to the Golgi complex but not to the cell surface. When a consensus sequence for glycosylation was produced by *in vitro* mutagenesis, the resulting glycoprotein was transported to the cell surface.

The N-linked glycosylation of the α and β subunits of thyroid-stimulating hormone (TSH) is thought to be necessary in order to prevent intracellular aggregation and degradation of the TSH subunits and to allow the subunits to attain the correct conformation for dimer formation (184). The α and β subunits containing high-mannose oligosaccharide chains begin to combine in the RER; the processed oligosaccharide chains on the α and β subunits are believed to be different and maturation of the chains occurs at different rates (145). O-Linked oligosaccharides may also influence the extent of dimer formation (134). Enzymatic removal of O-linked oligosaccharides from α subunits permits recombination with free β subunits of luteinizing hormone (LH), an event not seen with O-glycosylated α subunits.

The effect of glycosylation on the biological activity of final product peptides seems to vary in different cases. Terminal sialic acid and galactose residues play an important role in determining hepatic clearance and plasma half-lives of glycoproteins (8). Evidence from several laboratories has shown conclusively that the oligosaccharide moieties of glycoprotein hormones such as human chorionic gonadotropin (hCG), TSH, and LH play key roles in the ability of these hormones to elicit responses from target tissues (12,87,153). For example, sequential removal of the sialic acid, galactose, N-acetylglucosamine, and mannose residues from hCG results in a progressive decrease in the ability of the molecules to stimulate steroidogenesis (119). In addition, hCG has been chemically deglycosylated under conditions that do not change the peptide backbone. Deglycosylated

hCG binds to physiological receptors more tightly than native hCG (87,153). However, deglycosylated hCG retains less than 8% of its ability to activate adenylate cyclase and has less than 0.5% of its ability to stimulate steroid production and therefore acts as an effective antagonist to native hCG. At least in this case, the oligosaccharide moiety is involved in coupling the hormone-receptor complex to adenylate cyclase. In rat and mouse, ACTH(1–39) is glycosylated on an Asn residue in the C-terminal region; the ability of ACTH to stimulate steroidogenesis in isolated adrenal cortical cells is virtually unaffected by this modification (110). The biosynthetic processing of pro-ACTH/endorphin to ACTH(1–39) is also unaltered by blockade of glycosylation with tunicamycin (73).

Phosphorylation

Phosphorylation and dephosphorylation of Ser, Thr, and Tyr residues by specific protein kinases and phosphatases is a widely utilized regulatory mechanism. Only a few bioactive peptides are known to occur in phosphorylated forms, and there is no indication that the phosphorylation is reversible. In mouse, rat, and human pituitary as well as in the rat hypothalamus, ACTH and CLIP contain a phosphoserine residue (14,39,43,108). The extent of phosphorylation at this site is both species and tissue specific and varies from 30 to 90%. The biological activity of ACTH is unaffected by phosphorylation (14). The phosphorylation site in pro-ACTH/endorphin is of the type recognized by Golgi enzymes known as casein kinases (Ser/Thr-X-acidic), and a type I casein kinase-like activity has been detected in rat pituitary (14). Phosphorylation of this type would be expected to occur shortly after N-linked glycosylation. In bovine and human parathyroid explants, 10 to 20% of the parathyroid hormone is phosphorylated on a Ser residue in the N-terminal region of the molecule, but which of the potential Ser residues is phosphorylated is not yet known (140). Many other hormones have potential sites for this kind of phosphorylation.

Naturally occurring forms of ovine growth hormone containing phosphotyrosine have been identified (97). The *in vitro* phosphorylation of Tyr residues in gastrin, angiotensin, and growth hormone by the epidermal growth factor receptor kinase has been demonstrated, but there is no evidence to suggest that this type of phosphorylation occurs *in vivo* (9,10,185).

Sulfation

Tyrosine sulfate was first discovered in the protein backbone of fibrinopeptide B and until recently it was thought that this modification was peculiar to fibrinogens, fibrins, and a few small peptides such as gastrin and CCK (16,75). It has recently been shown that the sulfation of protein tyrosyl residues is widespread but appears to be restricted to secretory proteins (75). A recent study of proteins secreted from hepatoma cells has shown that although all sulfated proteins may be secreted, not all secreted proteins are sulfated (100). Of 15 identified proteins examined after secretion from [^{35}S]O$_4$-labeled hepatoma cells, only seven contained radioactive sulfate and only three contained Tyr sulfate. The other four sulfated proteins were glycoproteins and were likely sulfated on their oligosaccharide chains. No clear function has yet been assigned to the sulfation of Tyr in these large secretory proteins.

Peptides containing Tyr sulfate include cholecystokinin (CCK), gastrin, and leucine-enkephalin (141,174). Essentially all of the CCK produced in the gut and in the CNS is sulfated; nonsulfated CCK is unable to stimulate pancreatic enzyme secretion or gallbladder emptying. Only about half of the antral gastrin is sulfated; unsulfated gastrin can stimulate gastric acid secretion as well as sulfated gastrin. Between 10 and 20% of the leucine-enkephalin in the corpus striatum is sulfated, and in this case sulfation destroys the known biological activity of the peptide (174).

Interesting developmental changes in the degree of sulfation of gastrin occur. In the neonatal rat pancreas, which is the primary source of gastrin in the newborn animal, gastrin is transiently expressed in a fully sulfated form, which has CCK-like activity (22). A postnatal decline in pancreatic gastrin is accompanied by an increase in intestinal CCK. A similar situation may exist in the newborn human (4). Thus, sulfation of gastrin may be used to impart a CCK-like function to gastrin in the newborn. The degree of sulfation of gastrin is increased in patients with Zollinger-Ellison syndrome and decreased in patients with hypergastrinemia, gastric ulcer, or pernicious anemia; the extent of proteolytic processing to lower-molecular-weight forms of gastrin changes in parallel with degree of sulfation (5).

The N-acetylglucosamine, N-acetylgalactosamine, and mannose residues of the N-linked oligosaccharide moieties of glycoproteins and glycopeptides can also be sulfated (88). Oligosaccharide sulfation can occur to variable extents; only 3% of hen egg albumin is sulfated, whereas all of the heparan sulfate proteoglycan is sulfated (186,187). Both of the oligosaccharide chains of rat intermediate pituitary pro-ACTH/endorphin (18,79), as well as the oligosaccharide chains of the α and β subunits of ovine and bovine LH, can be sulfated (13,133). The functional significance of sulfated oligosaccharide chains is not clear.

Histochemical evidence indicates that sulfation occurs in the trans cisternae of the Golgi apparatus (46). Although sulfotransferases responsible for sulfating secretory proteins have not yet been purified, initial steps have been taken to characterize enzymatic activities capable of sulfating both Tyr residues and oligosaccharide chains. Phosphoadenosine 5'-phosphosulfate (PAPS) is the universal sulfate donor believed to be a cosubstrate for sulfotransferases involved in posttranslational processing of proteins and oligosaccharides (99). PAPS is synthesized in the cytoplasm, but is translocated into Golgi-containing preparations from rat liver and chick embryo chondrocytes (70,157). A sulfotransferase activity from adrenal medulla which is specific for luminal, Tyr-containing macromolecules has been studied using [^{35}S]PAPS, detergent-treated Golgi membranes, and a synthetic sulfate acceptor (poly Glu$_{62}$Ala$_{30}$Tyr$_8$) (94). The sulfotransferase activity studied has a high affinity (K_m = 300 nM) for this acidic sulfate acceptor, in keeping with the finding that the amino acid sequences surrounding naturally occurring Tyr sulfates contain acidic amino acid

residues (94). A sulfotransferase activity specific for luminal oligosaccharides has been studied in microsomal vesicles from chick embryo chondrocytes using [^{35}S]PAPS and p-nitrophenyl-β-D-galactosaminide or chondroitin oligosaccharides (70).

ENDOPROTEOLYTIC CLEAVAGES

Despite much work, there is as yet no consensus on the properties of endoproteolytic processing enzymes. In fact, many major questions remain to be answered. Is there one generic "prohormone convertase" or are there many? Are there endoproteases uniquely associated with prohormone processing? Do inhibitors or activators of proteases play an important role in controlling processing? Are there labile signals used transiently to mark the cleavage sites on a precursor? Where in the cell do the various cleavage events occur?

One fact that has made the study of biosynthetic processing proteases difficult is that there doesn't need to be much of a biosynthetic cleavage enzyme to achieve the biosynthetic rates observed (47,164). If the converting enzyme in pancreatic β cells were as active as pancreatic trypsin, in vivo rates of proinsulin conversion could be obtained with one molecule of protease per 10,000 to 100,000 molecules of proinsulin (164), or roughly one enzyme molecule per granule. All evidence points to the Golgi and secretory granules as the sites of processing, but lysosomes contain so much proteolytic activity that even a minor lysosomal contamination could mask the real posttranslational processing activity (51,131,135,164). The enzymes involved in extracellular generation of bioactive peptides (e.g., angiotensin-converting enzyme) and in peptide inactivation (e.g., aminopeptidases) play essential roles in the proper functioning of peptidergic systems, but are outside the scope of this review (101,104,131).

In many cases, pairs of basic amino acids are important cleavage sites. In a mutant proalbumin (proalbumin Lille), the normal -Arg-Arg- cleavage site is replaced by -His-Arg-; this site is not cleaved in vivo, but both the mutant and normal site are easily cleaved in vitro by incubation with trypsin (1). Two paired basic amino acid processing sites in bovine pro-ACTH/endorphin have been replaced by single basic amino acids in the murine precursors, and proteolytic cleavage no longer proceeds to any extent at these single basic sites. In theory, the initial endoproteolytic cleavage could occur between or at either side of the pair of basic amino acids; the actual sites are not generally known and need not be the same for all precursors. Except for proinsulin, very little is known of the biosynthetic intermediates that occur; it is only clear that both basic amino acids are generally gone from the final products. The question is an important one, since the site of the initial endoproteolytic cleavage dictates what other enzymes are needed to generate final products.

Pairs of basic amino acids would be expected to occur on the surface of globular proteins, and structural analyses suggest that unprocessed paired basic sequences occur in a rigid conformation whereas processed sites occur in regions that do not have ordered secondary structures (57). Precursors are not generally available in large quantity, making the necessary structural studies difficult, but by using a semisynthetic prooxytocin/neurophysin molecule, it was demonstrated that oxytocin interacted with neurophysin in the precursor and that correct disulfide bond formation was favored in the intact prohormone (85). Utilization of intact, nondenatured precursors for the identification of the initial endoproteolytic cleavage enzymes is probably essential (32).

Work from many different laboratories has led to the identification of many different endoprotease activities potentially important in proteolytic processing of prohormones. No consensus has yet been reached on the properties of these enzymes, and none fulfill all of the criteria in Table 1. Hence, we will simply summarize data from a few systems so that the variety of approaches and answers can

be appreciated (Table 2; for more detailed reviews see 35,51,55,101,104,131,135,164). Endoproteases are generally subdivided based on their structures and mechanisms of action; major types include serine proteases [inhibited by diisopropylfluorophosphate (DFP)], sulfhydryl proteases [inhibited by thiol blocking reagents such as iodoacetic acid and p-chloromercuribenzoate (PCMB)], metalloproteases [inhibited by chelators such as ethylenediaminetetraacetate (EDTA) and o-phenanthroline], and acid proteases (acidic pH optimum, inhibited by pepstatin A). It has been predicted that the simple proteases essential for digestive functions have evolved into specialized prohormone-processing proteases with a high degree of substrate specificity (122). Proteolytic enzymes pose a potential hazard to cells, since, if uncontrolled, they could destroy many proteins. Two principal regulatory mechanisms have evolved to solve

TABLE 2. *Properties of selected candidate processing endoproteases*

Source (ref.)	Type	pH optimum	Assay	Inhibitors
Islet secretory granules				
Rat (35,164)	Thiol	5.5–6.5	Proinsulin to insulin	PCMB (not DFP)
Anglerfish (124,125)	Thiol	4.5–5.5	Proinsulin, proglucagon, prosomatostatin to insulin, glucagon, somatostatin	Leupeptin, antipain, PCMB (not DFP, EDTA, SBTI, TLCK)
Adrenal chromaffin granules				
Bovine (98)	Serine	8	Endogenous substrate to Met-enk (RIA); peptides E and F to smaller products (within and to COOH-terminal of paired basics)	DFP, SBTI, LBTI (not leupeptin, PCMS, TLCK, o-phenanthroline)
Bovine (116)	Serine	7.5–9.5	Leu-enkephalin-KRFA-NH₂ to Leu-enkephalin-K (between basics; Lys-Arg specific)	DFP (not leupeptin, iodoacetic acid, TLCK, EDTA)
Bovine (118)	Thiol	5.5	Proenkephalin to Met-enkephalin (RIA) (cleaves at both sides of consecutive basics)	Iodoacetic acid, PCMB, leupeptin, TPCK, TLCK (not PMSF, DFP, SBTI, EDTA)
Pituitary				
Rat int granules (27)	Thiol	5	Pro-ACTH/endorphin to multiple products (to COOH-terminal side of some Arg)	Pepstatin A, leupeptin, PCMB (not DFP, TLCK)
Bovine int granules (102)	Acid (possibly)	4–4.5	Pro-ACTH/endorphin to multiple products (within and to COOH-side of Lys-Arg in pro-ACTH/endorphin)	Pepstatin A, leupeptin (partial) (not PCMB, DFP, PMSF, TLCK, EDTA)
Rat int (137,138)	Serine	8	Kininogen conversion to bradykinin (RIA) and D-Pro-Phe-Arg-p-nitroanilide to p-nitroaniline	DFP, PMSF, aprotinin (not SBTI)
Yeast (52,84)	Thiol	7–7.5	BOC-Gln-Arg-Arg-MCA to amino-methyl coumarin (cleaves to COOH-terminal of pair)	Iodoacetic acid, EDTA, or EGTA (restored by Ca²⁺), leupeptin, antipain (not PMSF, TLCK, TPCK, pepstatin)
(117)	Serine	7.5	Leu-enkephalin-RRFA-NH₂ conversion to Leu-enkephalin-R (between basics; also does Lys-Arg, and Arg-Lys)	DFP, PMSF (not iodoacetic acid, PCMB, leupeptin, TLCK, EDTA)

Abbreviations: BOC, butoxycarbonyl; EGTA, ethylene glycol-bis(β-aminoethyl ether) tetraacetic acid; KRFA, Lys-Arg-Phe-Ala; LBTI, lima bean trypsin inhibitor; MCA, methyl coumaric acid; PCMS, parachloromercurisulfonate; PMSF, phenylmethylsulfonyl fluoride; RRFA, Arg-Arg-Phe-Ala; SBTI, soybean trypsin inhibitor; TLCK, tosyl lysine chloromethyl ketone; TPCK, tosyl phenylalanine chloromethyl ketone; PCMB, parachloromercuribenzoate; DFP, diisopropylfluorophosphate; EDTA, ethylene diamine tetraacetic acid; RIA, radioimmunoassay; -K, -Lys.

this problem: inactive protease precursors (zymogens) are activated at the appropriate time and place by limited proteolysis; proteases are inactivated by forming complexes with protein inhibitors or by changes in pH (122). It is not yet clear what role these mechanisms play in prohormone processing.

The production of insulin from proinsulin by pancreatic β cells has served as a model for other prohormone systems (Fig. 1). Cathepsin B-like thiol proteases have been implicated in the endoproteolytic cleavage of proinsulin (35,154,164) (Table 2). Cathepsin B and its precursor forms are found in insulin secretory granules as well as in lysosomes and the cathepsin B precursors are secreted into the medium along with insulin in response to glucose stimulation (154). Although cathepsin B itself does not exhibit the desired specificity, the precursor forms of the enzyme appear to be more specific for paired basic amino acid sequences. Studies on anglerfish islet secretory granules also demonstrate the importance of soluble and membrane-associated thiol proteases with acidic pH optima in the conversion of proglucagon, prosomatostatin, and proinsulin to product peptides (124,125). In anglerfish islets, newly synthesized proinsulin, proglucagon, and prosomatostatin are largely membrane associated (125).

In anglerfish, but apparently not in mammals (171), there are two prosomatostatin genes containing slightly different somatostatin-14 (SS-14) sequences at their COOH-termini (Fig. 1); both precursors contain an -Arg-Lys- sequence preceding the SS-14-like peptide and a single Arg preceding the SS-28-like peptide. However, pro-SS-I is processed to SS-14 whereas pro-SS-II gives rise to SS-28; interestingly, this SS-28 contains a 5-hydroxylysine residue (6,124,162). Enzymatic activity capable of cleaving at Arg-Lys to convert pro-SS-I to SS-14 is found only in anglerfish pancreatic secretory granules and is membrane associated; it is not found in microsomes (124). By contrast, enzymatic activity capable of cleaving after Arg to convert pro-SS-II to SS-28 is found in both microsomes and secretory granules (where it is soluble) (124). All of the anglerfish processing activities show optimal activity at pH 5 and are inhibited by thiol reagents. Processing of prosomatostatin to SS-28 and SS-14 occurs in a tissue-specific fashion in mammals. Neurosecretory vesicles from rat brain hypothalamus and cerebral cortex contain a loosely membrane-associated thiol protease with neutral pH optimum that cleaves at the Arg-Lys site in SS-28 to produce both the amino-terminal 12-amino-acid peptide and SS-14; prosomatostatin is not cleaved by this activity (64,65).

Adrenal chromaffin granules provide a rich source of processing enzymes presumably involved in converting proenkephalin into the smaller product peptides found in the gland (Fig. 1), and both thiol and serine proteases have been identified in chromaffin granule extracts (Table 2). A soluble 20,000-dalton serine protease with neutral pH optimum that cleaves peptides E and F (Fig. 1) preferentially over shorter substrates was partially purified from chromaffin granules; with some substrates this enzymatic activity shows a preference for cleavage between pairs of basic amino acids, whereas with other substrates it cleaves to the COOH-terminal side of the pairs of basic amino acids (98) (Table 2). A similar soluble serine protease with a neutral pH optimum exhibited substrate specificity suggesting that it

may be involved in proenkephalin processing (116). This enzyme activity shows a preference for cleavage within a -Lys-Arg- sequence in various enkephalin-containing peptide substrates but does not cleave at the -Arg-Arg-, -Arg-Lys-, or single Arg sites in endogenous opioid peptides such as metorphamide and α-neoendorphin (Fig. 1) (116). The same group of investigators previously identified a soluble 220,000-dalton thiol protease with an acidic pH optimum that converted proenkephalin into methionine enkephalin, presumably by the concerted removal of pairs of basic amino acids (118) (Table 2).

Secretory granules from bovine and rat neural, intermediate, and anterior pituitary have been used to study the initial endoproteolytic cleavage of biosynthetically labeled mouse and toad pro-ACTH/endorphin (26,27,101,102). Bovine intermediate pituitary was found to contain a 70,000-dalton glycoprotein that cleaves mouse pro-ACTH/endorphin either within -Lys-Arg- sequences or to the COOH-terminal of -Lys-Arg- sequences (Table 2) (102). This enzyme activity has an acidic pH optimum and appears most closely related to the acid protease group. It also cleaves proinsulin at paired basic sites, but does not cleave smaller peptides such as ACTH(1–39), which has a -Lys-Lys-Arg-Arg- site. Similar enzymatic activity occurs in a membrane-bound form. Rat intermediate pituitary secretory granules were found to contain a somewhat similar activity that cleaved to the COOH-terminal side of paired basic residues in toad pro-ACTH/endorphin. Soluble and membrane-associated endoproteolytic activity differed slightly in substrate specificity (27).

Cleavage at single basic amino acids clearly occurs in the processing of precursors such as propressophysin, prosomatostatin, pro-CCK, pro-Phe-Met-Arg-Phe-NH$_2$, and prodynorphin (31,44,101,124,142,155) (Fig. 1). Both soluble and membrane-bound enzymatic activities capable of cleaving the Thr-Arg bond in Dyno B(1–29) (leumorphin) (Fig. 1) have been identified in crude rat brain membranes (31). Proteolytic cleavage is brought about by a neutral thiol protease, although localization of this activity to secretory granules has not been demonstrated (31). In separate studies, the naturally occurring COOH-terminal fragment of Dyno B(1–29) was purified and shown to lack an NH$_2$-terminal Arg residue (44); participation of an aminopeptidase would be required to generate this product after the endoproteolytic cleavage described.

Kininogenases are serine proteases that produce kinins from kininogens by cleaving at specific Lys and Arg residues and include enzymes with a high degree of specificity, such as the kallikreins, and less specific proteases, such as trypsin. The biosynthesis of several peptide growth factors (nerve growth factor and epidermal growth factor) involves the action of kallikrein-like enzymes, and the role of similar enzymes in the posttranslational processing of smaller bioactive peptides, especially at single basic amino acid sites, has received considerable attention (17,36,93,138). Kallikrein-like proteases cleave at one or a few positions in their natural substrates and show a preference for positively charged amino acids, with a strong bias for Arg over Lys. In the mouse genome there are 25 to 30 genes coding for kallikrein-like sequences (113). High levels of granule-associated, particulate, glandular kallikrein-like activity have been found in rat intermediate pituitary; antibodies to rat urinary kallikrein inhibited the activity (138) (Table 2). In the intermediate pituitary of the rat, over 90% of the kallikrein-like activity occurs in a latent form that can be activated by trypsin, and levels of latent kallikrein-like activity were increased following treatment of rats with dopamine receptor blockers, a treatment expected to stimulate hormone production in that tissue (137). Kallikrein-like activity is present in a corticotropic tumor cell line, and a unique kallikrein-like gene is expressed at high levels in these cells and in the mouse neurointermediate pituitary (36). Little is known about the ability of any kallikrein-like enzymes to cleave prohormones. Purified glandular kallikrein cleaves BAM-22P, a methionine-enkephalin containing peptide similar to peptide E (Fig. 1), primarily at the Arg-Arg bond following the methionine-enkephalin sequence (139). Another serine-type proteolytic activity, plasminogen activator, is secreted from pancreatic β cells in parallel with insulin (177) and occurs in a subset of anterior pituitary somatotropes (90).

Yeast produce bioactive peptides from larger precursor molecules and thus provide a simple system in which to identify processing enzymes. Two quite distinct candidate endoproteolytic processing enzymes have been identified in yeast (Table 2). Genetic manipulations were used to identify, purify, and sequence a Ca^{2+}-dependent, calpain-like thiol protease whose function is required for endoproteolytic cleavage of pro-α-factor (52,84). This 105,000-dalton membrane-bound protease exhibits a neutral pH optimum and cleaves small synthetic peptides to the COOH-terminal side of pairs of basic amino acids, with a preference for cleavage after Arg residues. In addition, a soluble 43,000-dalton serine protease with a neutral pH optimum that cleaves between consecutive basic amino acids has also been purified from yeast cell lysates (117) (Table 2). This yeast enzyme cleaves several synthetic enkephalin-containing peptides between paired basic amino acids with no detectable cleavage at single basic amino acids in the same substrates; this yeast enzyme resembles an enzymatic activity identified by the same investigators in chromaffin granules (116). The two yeast enzymes are clearly different, and use of a simple system such as yeast should make it possible to understand the functional roles of both enzymes in prohormone processing.

Much work remains to be done on the characterization and purification of endoproteolytic processing enzymes. Early proteolytic cleavage events appear to be membrane associated. Recent work indicates that cleavage between the members of a pair of basic amino acids almost certainly occurs in some cases and cleavage at single basic amino acids does not appear to be uncommon. Further progress in this important but difficult area will require more knowledge of the cellular details of biosynthetic pathways, precise characterization of preparations of subcellular organelles, careful application of selective pharmacological agents, and clever use of the emerging approaches of molecular genetics.

LATE EVENTS

The late events in peptide processing occur almost exclusively in secretory granules. These events can often be tissue specific and have distinct effects on biological activity. The late events in processing can also be rather slow, some requiring days to reach their final stage. One late event we will only mention is the formation of pyroglutamic acid residues at the N-terminus of peptides; N-terminal Gln residues, when exposed after an endoproteolytic cleavage, are thought to form pyroglutamic acid by a nonenzymatic process (143,158).

Carboxypeptidases

Most of the prohormone-processing pathways known require the removal of basic amino acids from the COOH-terminus of biosynthetic intermediates. The participation of a carboxypeptidase B-like processing enzyme (CPB) was initially demonstrated with proinsulin biosynthetically labeled with [^{3}H]arginine. In both isolated and lysed granule preparations, proinsulin was processed to insulin and C-peptide, with the release of free [^{3}H]arginine, and islets were shown to contain a soluble metalloenzyme somewhat similar to pancreatic CPB (164).

Purification and Characterization of Carboxypeptidase H

Recently, a CPB-like activity thought to be involved in the processing of proenkephalin was identified in adrenal chromaffin granules (49,77). Lysosomes contain a large amount of CPB-like activity, but cobalt was shown preferentially to stimulate a CPB-like activity found primarily in chromaffin granules. Early studies demonstrated that the chromaffin granule-associated CPB-like activity was stimulated more than 10-fold by 1 mM $CoCl_2$, had a pH optimum of 5.5 to 6.0, and was inhibited by EDTA, o-phenanthroline, and cadmium ions. It differed from lysosomal and pancreatic CPB and plasma carboxypeptidase N in molecular weight, pH optimum, and inhibitor profile, suggesting that the chromaffin granule-associated CPB-like activity was a unique carboxypeptidase. This enzyme has subsequently been designated carboxypeptidase H (CPH) (also carboxypeptidase E and enkephalin convertase) (104).

High levels of CPH activity were found in the adrenal medulla, brain, and pituitary in both soluble and membrane-bound forms. Soluble CPH has been purified to apparent homogeneity from all three tissues (50). The purification scheme utilized affinity chromatography on columns of concanavalin A and p-aminobenzyl-L-arginine and gel filtration. The complete purification of soluble CPH from extracts of pituitary required a 2,800-fold enrichment, while complete purification from brain and adrenal medulla both required over a 100,000-fold enrichment. Soluble CPH purified from all three tissues appears to be identical and has the same specific activity, same apparent molecular weight [50,000 on sodium dodecyl sulfate (SDS)-polyacrylamide gel electrophoresis], and same kinetic properties. Consistent with the early characterizations, purified CPH is stimulated approximately 10-fold by cobalt and two- to three-fold by nickel, and is inhibited by copper, cadmium, EDTA, o-phenanthroline, p-chloromercuriphenyl sulfonic acid, and mercuric chloride. Iodoacetamide, N-ethylmaleimide, and phenylmethylsulphonyl fluoride have no effect on CPH. With these properties, CPH appears to be a thiol-metalloprotease. The membrane-bound form of CPH has also been purified and possesses similar kinetic characteristics (169). The molecular weight of the membrane-bound form is slightly larger (52,000–53,000), suggesting that it may contain modifications or additional sequences that anchor it to membranes.

Purified CPH shows a three- to five-fold preference for Arg over Lys as the *C*-terminal amino acid. Its activity is highest with Ala as the penultimate amino acid, and the rate constant (kcat/K_m) is 15- to 80-fold higher with Ala than with Gly, Leu, or Ile (50). With synthetically prepared enkephalins containing a *C*-terminal Arg, purified CPH removes the basic amino acid without further degrading the enkephalin produced (49).

Benzylsuccinic acid, an inhibitor of carboxypeptidase A and CPB, has no effect on CPH. However, several dicarboxylic acid analogs of Arg and Lys, originally prepared as active site inhibitors of carboxypeptidases, exhibit more potent effects on CPH than on other known carboxypeptidases (48). The high specificity of these inhibitors, most notably GEMSA (guanidinoethylmercaptosuccinic acid; K_i = 8 nM), has permitted an accurate determination of CPH levels and distribution in different tissues.

Distribution of Carboxypeptidase H

Localization of CPH by measurement of cobalt-stimulable CPB-like enzyme activity and by quantitation of [^{3}H]GEMSA binding in homogenates has given similar results. High levels of CPH activity have been found in the adrenal medulla, the anterior and neurointermediate lobes of the pituitary, the brain, AtT-20 mouse corticotropic tumor cells, and a rat insulinoma (34,50,104,109). Unlike cobalt-insensitive carboxypeptidase activity, which is homogeneously distributed in the brain, CPH activity displays a heterogeneous regional distribution; a 10-fold regional variation has been demonstrated with the highest activities in the hypothalamus, thalamus, corpus striatum, hippocampus, and midbrain. Cortical regions contain intermediate levels of activity, and low levels of CPH activity are found in the cerebellum and brainstem (49).

In membrane and soluble fractions of tissue homogenates, [^{3}H]GEMSA binding is specific and saturable, with a K_d of approximately 6 nM (167), and the tissue distribution of [^{3}H]GEMSA binding nearly parallels that of CPH activity. The high affinity of GEMSA for CPH makes [^{3}H]GEMSA particularly well suited for localizing CPH in discrete brain regions using *in vitro* autoradiographic techniques. Autoradiograms of [^{3}H]GEMSA binding to rat brain sections show direct correlations with CPH levels in different nuclei of the CNS (104). Since the technique relies on unfixed cryosections, soluble CPH is not retained and the results reflect only the distribution of membrane-bound CPH (104). Even with this limitation, CPH is observed to be heterogeneously localized to distinct brain regions with high densities in the median eminence, various nuclei of the hypothalamus, hippocampus, lateral septum, the interpeduncular nucleus, and the nucleus of the solitary tract (105). Comparison of the distribution of CPH with the localization of neuroendocrine peptides suggests that CPH is not associated with any one particular neurotransmitter system but is most likely involved in several peptidergic pathways.

Regulation of Carboxypeptidase H

Although the subcellular distribution, substrate specificity, kinetics, and tissue distribution of CPH all strongly implicate CPH in the processing of neuropeptide precursors, direct demonstration of CPH involvement in forming the final peptide products remains to be tested (criterion 5, Table 1). The observation that cells secrete CPH concomitantly with hormone in response to secretagogues is consistent with the location of the enzyme in granules and its physiological relevance. In corticotropic tumor cells, CPH is secreted in parallel with hormone in response to isoproterenol, barium, or CRF (Fig. 3); the CRF-stimulated release of hormone and CPH is acutely inhibited by glucocorticoids (109).

Purification of CPH has made it possible to investigate regulation of this activity. On long-term treatment of corticotropic tumor cells with dexamethasone, cellular levels of hormone decrease while CPH levels remain unchanged (109). In other studies using [^{3}H]GEMSA autoradiography, treatment of rats with a dopaminergic antagonist to increase intermediate pituitary levels of ACTH/endorphin peptides did not affect pituitary CPH (104). Neither adrenalectomy nor dexamethasone treatment, which increase and decrease anterior pituitary ACTH/endorphin synthesis, respectively, alters [^{3}H]GEMSA binding in the pituitary. CPH in the rat adrenal medulla is not altered on treatment with reserpine, hypophysectomy, or splanchnic nerve denervation (166). These studies imply that levels of CPH are not closely regulated and, consistent with the failure to see peptide processing intermediates bearing COOH-terminal basic

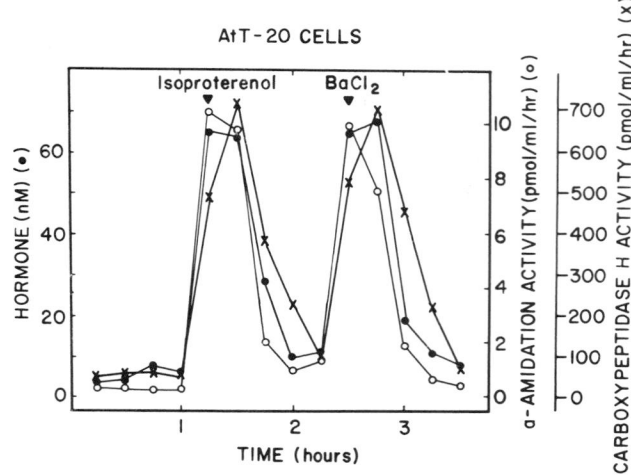

FIG. 3. Stimulation of AtT-20 secretion with isoproterenol and barium chloride. A column containing AtT-20 cells attached to Cytodex beads was perfused with medium that contained isoproterenol (1 μM) or BaCl₂ (0.2 mM) for the indicated 15-min period and samples were assayed for 16 K fragment immunoactivity (●), PAM activity (○), and carboxypeptidase H activity (×). (From ref. 109.)

amino acids, the rate-limiting step in the biosynthesis of neuropeptides is not likely to be a carboxypeptidase.

Aminopeptidases

Aminopeptidases are exopeptidases that remove amino acid residues from the amino terminus of peptides. Several candidate endoproteases are thought to cleave between pairs of basic amino acids (see above), and formation of final products would require removal of an N-terminal Lys or Arg residue. Although a role for aminopeptidases in the biosynthesis of peptides is not established, their role in the degradation of peptides such as Met-enkephalin is well documented (67). A rat brain aminopeptidase thought to be involved in enkephalin degradation has a neutral pH optimum, is activated by cobalt, zinc, and calcium, and is inhibited by EDTA and bestatin (74,80). A membrane-associated aminopeptidase activity that releases Arg and Met-enkephalin from Arg-Tyr-Gly-Gly-Phe-Met was recently detected in bovine neural and intermediate pituitary secretory granules (54). It had a pH optimum of 6.0 and was stimulated by addition of cobalt or zinc, inhibited by the addition of EDTA, and unaffected by endoprotease inhibitors such as leupeptin, pepstatin A, phenylmethylsulfonyl fluoride, and p-chloromercuribenzensulfonate. An anglerfish islet activity with similar properties, but which is not stimulated by cobalt and exhibits a pH optimum of 6.7, has recently been reported (106). Several peptides lacking amino-terminal basic residues were not substrates for these enzyme activities, and both appear to be distinct from previously characterized aminopeptidases.

Dipeptidylaminopeptidases remove dipeptides from the NH_2-terminus of their substrates and are essential for the synthesis of yeast α-mating factor (83) and melittin, a 26-amino-acid lytic peptide that is a major component of honeybee venom (89). In yeast, an exoprotease that cleaves on the carboxyl side of repeating -X-Ala- sequences removes the spacer regions of pro-α-mating factor, resulting in the production of bioactive α-mating factor (Fig. 1). Mutants that lack this activity produce biologically inactive α-mating factors with the spacer sequences attached. The yeast enzyme, called dipeptidylaminopeptidase A, is a membrane-bound, heat-stable, serine protease that is inhibited by diisopropylfluorophosphate (83). Honeybee venom glands contain a similar exoprotease that cleaves on the carboxyl side of -X-Y- sequences, where X is Ala, Glu, or Asp and Y is Pro or Ala. This enzyme cleaves sequentially the first 11 amino acid pairs of promelittin, resulting in the synthesis of bioactive melittin. The honeybee venom gland enzyme is similar in its properties to dipeptidylpeptidase IV, an enzyme that has been characterized in the brush border membranes of the hog kidney. The honeybee dipeptidylpeptidase is a soluble serine protease, which is inhibited by DFP and has an acidic pH optimum (89). No mammalian dipeptidyl aminopeptidases specifically involved in prohormone processing have yet been identified.

Acetylation

Acetylation, like most of the posttranslational processing steps discussed, is not unique to secretory proteins or bioactive peptides. Acetylation and deacetylation of certain Lys-ε-NH_2 groups in histones H2A, H2B, H3, and H4, have been implicated in gene regulation (149). Many proteins (for example, actin, cytochrome C, lactate dehydrogenase) are acetylated at their N-termini as they are synthesized, and in a few cases acetylation may affect protein turnover; in general, the functional significance of this modification is unclear (173).

Only a few bioactive peptides occur in acetylated forms, but acetylation is a powerful determinant of biological activity. Peptides derived from pro-ACTH/endorphin are subject to acetylation at two sites: the N-terminal Ser of α-melanotropin (αMSH) can be α-N-acetylated and O-acetylated and the N-terminal Tyr of β-endorphin can be α-N-acetylated (110). Similar to the proteolytic processing of the ACTH/endorphin precursor molecule, acetylation occurs in a tissue-specific fashion (Fig. 1). In the anterior pituitary and hypothalamus, neither site is extensively acetylated; in contrast, in the intermediate pituitary, both sites are highly acetylated and the major product peptides are α-N-acetyl-ACTH(1–13)NH_2 or αMSH and α-N,O-diacetyl-αMSH plus α-N-acetyl-β-endorphin-related peptides (24,43,59,188). The acetylation state of α- and γ-endorphin parallels that of β-endorphin; in the anterior pituitary, hypothalamus, and thalamus they are mostly nonacetylated whereas in the intermediate pituitary, hippocampus, and septum they are largely α-N-acetylated (182,183).

Acetylation can either increase or decrease biological activity, depending on the peptide and the bioassay. Acetylation of β-endorphin decreases the ability of the peptide to bind to μ and δ opiate receptors more than 1,000-fold (3). The analgesic potency of α-N-acetyl-β-endorphin is dramatically reduced, so that at concentrations 100 to 200 times the threshold dose for β-endorphin, N-acetylated-β-endorphin has no effect in tail-flick latency tests (29). In contrast, mono- and diacetylated αMSH are approximately five-fold more potent than desacetyl-αMSH in both in vivo and in vitro lipolytic action and 40-fold more potent in affecting melanocyte darkening (148). αMSH has also been found to be more effective than ACTH(1–13)NH_2 in improving performance in visual discrimination tests and in inducing excessive grooming behavior (127). These results have been largely attributed to a five- to 10-fold increase in the rate of degradation of desacetyl-αMSH in comparison to αMSH. However, the bioactivity of the different forms of αMSH is not determined simply by resistance to proteolysis, since desacetyl-αMSH is more potent than αMSH in blocking opiate receptor binding and opiate-induced analgesia (128).

Acetylation is known to occur in only a few other peptide systems. Approximately 20% of the dynorphin(1–8) in the neurointermediate pituitary is acetylated on its N-terminal Tyr; the high-molecular-weight forms of dynorphin and dynorphin(1–17) are not acetylated (160). Approximately a quarter of the leucine-enkephalin in the neurointermediate pituitary is acetylated, whereas Leu-enkephalin peptides in the hypothalamus, striatum, midbrain, and pons-medulla are not acetylated (159). Some 5% of the growth hormone in the anterior pituitary is acetylated, but the functional significance remains unclear (96). Tissue-specific acetylation of peptides may prove to be one of the mechanisms adopted by cells to modify the effect of some of the various peptides generated during the processing of multipotential precursors.

Acetyltransferases

As indicated above, acetylation is not limited to bioactive peptides, and acetyltransferase activities capable of transferring the acetyl group from acetyl-CoA to protein acceptors have been described in a variety of tissues including liver, oviduct, lens, kidney, lung, heart, anterior and neurointermediate pituitary, and brain (33). An acetyltransferase involved in the acetylation of αMSH or β-endorphin would be expected to occur in secretory granules (Fig. 2), since much of the proteolytic cleavage of pro-ACTH/endorphin has been shown to take place in secretory granules. Biosynthetic labeling experiments have shown that acetylation of β-endorphin begins approximately 1.5 hr after translation and that more than 80% of the acetylation process takes place in secretory granules (59). Consistent with these results, immunocytochemical studies employing an antiserum specific for the acetylated N-terminus of αMSH have demonstrated staining in the maturing secretory granules of intermediate pituitary cells and not in newly formed granules or Golgi stacks (165).

In the rat neurointermediate pituitary only approximately a fifth of the acetyltransferase activity is associated with secretory granules; rat anterior pituitary does not contain significant amounts of granule-associated acetyltransferase activity (60). The granule-associated acetyltransferase activity in bovine intermediate pituitary is soluble and exhibits a pH optimum of 7 (60). Substrates for the enzyme include peptides related to both αMSH and β-endorphin but not CLIP or lysine-rich histones. The K_m of the granule-associated acetyltransferase for various peptide substrates varies from 10 to 300 μM. The acetylation of ACTH(1–8) is competitively inhibited by β-endorphin, suggesting that the same enzyme acetylates both αMSH and β-endorphin-related peptides (60).

Acetyl-CoA is synthesized in the cytosol and it is not yet clear how it gains entry into granules to serve as a substrate for the acetyltransferase. The K_m of the granule-associated acetyltransferase for acetyl-CoA is 8 μM (60); the concentration of acetyl-CoA in secretory granules is not known. Acetyl-CoA is actively transported into rat liver Golgi vesicles in a time-, temperature-, protein-, and concentration-dependent manner (176). In theory, secretory granules could take up acetyl-CoA or utilize acetyl-CoA previously packaged into the granules. In liver lysosomes a membrane-bound acetyltransferase binds cytosolic acetyl-CoA and shuttles the acetyl group into the lumen where substrate acetylation takes place (11).

Regulation of Neuropeptide Acetylation

Acetylation of pro-ACTH/endorphin-related peptides clearly affects the biological activity of the product peptides and could function as a regulatory mechanism. However, little is yet known about factors affecting acetylation; there is no indication that acetylation of β-endorphin or αMSH is reversible (59). When rats are chronically stressed, intermediate pituitary synthesis and release of endorphin are increased; cellular and secreted levels of α-N-acetyl-β-endorphin(1–31) are selectively increased (2), consistent with

previous observations that α-N-acetylation of β-endorphin proceeds more rapidly than COOH-terminal shortening (59,107). Long-term cultures of rat intermediate pituitary cells show a slight decline in extent of β-endorphin acetylation, which may be restored to *in vivo* levels on treatment with dopaminergic compounds (71).

Amidation

About half of all known bioactive peptides are α-amidated at their COOH-terminus. Amidation is generally essential for the biological activity of the peptide. Synthetic CRF terminating with -Ala instead of -Ala-NH$_2$ is at least 1,000-fold less potent (175). COOH-terminal amidation is one of the few processing steps that appears to be uniquely associated with the production of bioactive peptides. A chemical assay for peptides containing an α-amide led to the purification and characterization of several novel bioactive peptides, including neuropeptide Y (NPY), peptides YY (PYY) and HI (PHI) (170). The signal for α-amidation appears to be an -X-Gly sequence at the COOH-terminus of the peptide. In promelittin, -Gln-Gly occurs at the COOH-terminus and no proteolytic cleavage is required to reveal the amidation site (92). The action of a carboxypeptidase B-like enzyme would be required to convert the COOH-terminal -Ala-Gly-Lys-OH of ovine pro-CRF into the -Ala-NH$_2$ of CRF (53). In many other prohormones, endoproteolytic cleavage at a single basic amino acid or at a pair of basic amino acids followed by a carboxypeptidase B-like cleavage is required. Small amounts of presumed biosynthetic intermediates of the type -X-Gly have been identified in gastric antrum (168).

Purification and Characterization of Amidation Activity

Use of a synthetic substrate, D-Tyr-Val-Gly, permitted identification of a soluble enzymatic activity in porcine pituitary secretory granules that was capable of producing D-Tyr-Val-NH$_2$ (19). The enzyme showed a preference for neutral amino acids such as Val, Phe, or Gly at -X- and a strict requirement for Gly (or D-Ala) at the COOH-terminus. Peptides terminating in α-amides of uncharged amino acids are much more common than peptides terminating in α-amides of charged amino acids (19,110). The amide nitrogen was shown to arise from the α-NH$_2$ group of Gly and glyoxylate was shown to be produced from Gly (19). Subsequent studies demonstrated the presence of a similar soluble, secretory-granule-associated α-amidation activity in rat anterior, intermediate, and neural pituitary and bovine intermediate pituitary (40,62). In contrast to the situation with endoproteolytic activity, carboxypeptidase B-like activity, or acetyltransferase activity, very little amidation activity is associated with subcellular organelles other than secretory granules (40). Amidation activity was stimulated by the addition of ascorbate (vitamin C) and copper, and inhibited by the addition of divalent metal chelators or removal of molecular oxygen (40). The enzyme was tentatively identified as a peptidyl-glycine α-amidating monooxygenase (PAM) catalyzing the following reaction (42):

D-Tyr-Val-Gly + O$_2$ + ascorbate →

D-Tyr-Val-NH$_2$ + glyoxalate + dehydroascorbate + H$_2$O

Similar activity has been identified in thyroid, brain, submandibular gland, serum, and cerebrospinal fluid (20,42,179,180). PAM activity bears marked similarities to dopamine β-hydroxylase, the enzyme that converts dopamine into norepinephrine.

Extracts of bovine neurointermediate pituitary secretory granules and frozen bovine neurointermediate pituitary contain multiple forms of PAM activity differing in apparent molecular weight (54,000 and 38,000) and in charge (121). The lower-molecular-weight form of PAM activity, PAM-B, was purified 21,000-fold using metal chelate affinity chromatography, substrate affinity chromatography, and gel filtration (121). The activity of purified PAM-B was still inhibited by chelators such as diethyldithiocarbamate and could be restored by addition of copper, but no other divalent metals. The activity of the purified enzyme was still dependent on the presence of molecular oxygen and was stimulated by the addition of ascorbate; the amount of ascorbate consumed was approximately equimolar to the amount of amidated peptide produced. The requirement for ascorbate was not strict, and dopamine, DOPA, and synthetic biopterin analogs could partially replace ascorbate. The purified enzyme continued to exhibit broad substrate specificity and was capable of producing peptides terminating with amidated Pro, Trp, Val, or Glu (120).

It is interesting to compare the properties of PAM and carboxypeptidase H, two posttranslational processing enzymes presumably functioning in the same subcellular organelle. Both have K_m values for their peptide substrates in the 5 to 500 μM range. In tissues containing both activities (e.g., rat anterior pituitary and AtT-20 cells), the amount of carboxypeptidase H activity far exceeds the amount of PAM activity. Both enzymes occur in a soluble form, but the pH optima for the two enzymes differ, with PAM-B showing optimal activity at pH 8.5 and carboxypeptidase H showing optimal activity at pH 5.6. Both enzymes require the presence of a particular divalent metal, as do many of the candidate endoproteases.

Regulation of α-Amidation

Consistent with the soluble nature of both enzymes, corticotropic tumor cells secrete carboxypeptidase H and PAM activity in parallel with pro-ACTH/endorphin-derived peptides in response to secretagogues such as CRF (109) (Fig. 3); inhibition of hormone secretion by addition of cobalt or short-term treatment with dexamethasone brought about a parallel decline in secretion of hormone and both processing enzymes. PAM activity in serum appears to represent secretion from a number of different tissues (111,179).

In corticotropic tumor cells treated with glucocorticoids for 8 days, cellular levels of hormone fell to one-third of control levels, as expected (109). Levels of PAM activity in

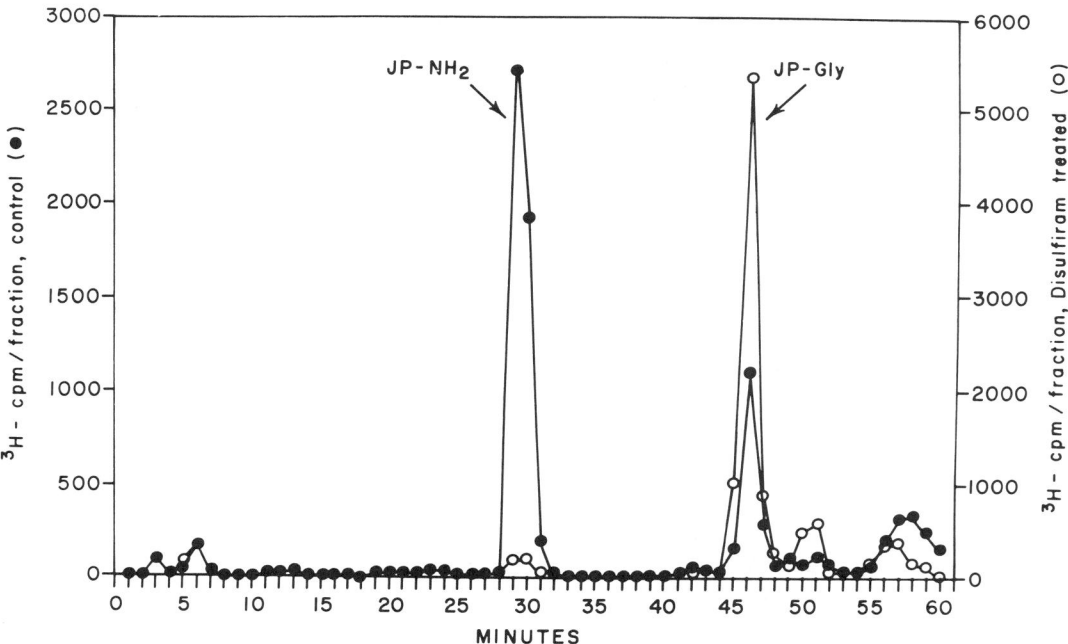

FIG. 4. Disulfiram (Antabuse) treatment of rats: effects on peptide α-amidation. Subcutaneous injections of vehicle (0.9% NaCl/0.5% Tween-80) or disulfiram (4 mg/kg emulsified in vehicle; similar to the therapeutic dose in humans of 250 mg/day) were given to adult male rats (200 g) at 38 and 14 hr before sacrifice. Each intact neurointermediate pituitary was incubated in 50 μl complete serum-free tissue culture medium containing 100 μM ascorbate and 100 μM [^{3}H]proline (32 Ci/mmol) for 6 hr, followed by 2 hr in 200 μl complete nonradioactive medium containing 400 μM proline. Individual neurointermediate pituitaries were extracted, joining peptide-sized material was prepared by high-performance liquid chromatography (HPLC) gel filtration, and one-quarter of the material was analyzed by reversed-phase HPLC (41).

cell extracts showed a parallel decline, while levels of carboxypeptidase H, total cell protein, and various cytosolic, mitochondrial, and lysosomal marker enzymes were unaltered. Levels of PAM activity are regulated differently in different tissues. For example, treatment of rats with dopaminergic agonists or antagonists brought about parallel changes in intermediate pituitary content of αMSH and PAM activity (111). Plasma PAM activity is elevated in patients with medullary carcinoma of the thyroid (179), and cerebrospinal fluid levels of PAM activity are diminished in patients with Alzheimer's disease (114).

In several cases, cells in culture have been shown to lose their ability to produce amidated products (63,156). The effect of ascorbate on purified PAM suggested that inclusion of ascorbate in the culture medium might restore the ability of cultured cells to produce amidated products. Addition of serum levels of ascorbate to the culture medium used for rat intermediate pituitary cells did restore amidation of both αMSH and joining peptide (Fig. 1) to near control levels (61,115). Corticotropic tumor cells grown in the absence of ascorbate contain no ascorbate and yet produce significant amounts of amidated joining peptide, suggesting that in intact cells, as in the test tube, other factors can substitute for ascorbate (41).

The dependence of purified PAM on copper suggested that manipulation of available copper might lead to alterations in the ability of cells and tissues to produce amidated peptides. In AtT-20 cells treated with the relatively selective copper chelator, diethyldithiocarbamate, a Gly-extended form of joining peptide is synthesized and secreted instead of amidated joining peptide (112). In rats treated chronically with Antabuse (a dimer of diethyldithiocarbamate used clinically to treat alcoholism), the intermediate pituitary contained primarily Gly-extended forms of αMSH and joining peptide (Fig. 4), and the anterior pituitary contained Gly-extended joining peptide (112). In this case we can see how knowledge about the properties of a processing enzyme has already offered insights into understanding the effects of a widely used pharmacological agent.

FUTURE DIRECTIONS

The criteria for identification of processing enzymes are difficult to satisfy, but progress has been made. As more candidate enzymes are purified and more cellular pathways of processing are established, the tools needed to address the remaining questions will become available. Use of highly specific antisera, improved methods of peptide separation and characterization, advanced enzyme purification techniques, active-site-directed reagents, and genetic engineering will play essential roles. With this knowledge, we will be able to manipulate these processing steps and get on to the task of understanding the functions of the peptides and how their production, secretion, and actions are regulated.

ACKNOWLEDGMENTS

This work was supported by grants DA-00097, DA-00098, AM-32948, AM-32949, AM-07269, AM-07360, DA-00266, and the McKnight Foundation.

REFERENCES

1. Abdo, Y., Rousseaux, J., and Dautrevaux, M. (1981): *FEBS Lett.*, 131:286–288.
2. Akil, H., Shiomi, H., and Matthews, J. (1985): *Science*, 227:424–426.
3. Akil, H., Young, E., and Watson, S. J. (1981): *Peptides*, 2:289–292.
4. Andersen, B. N., Abramovich, D., Brand, S. J., Petersen, B., and Rehfeld, J. F. (1985): *Regul. Pept.*, 10:329–338.
5. Andersen, B. N., Petersen, B., and Borch, K. (1985): *Digestion*, 31:17–24.
6. Andrews, P. C., Hawkes, D., Shively, J. E., and Dixon, J. E. (1984): *J. Biol. Chem.*, 259:15021–15024.
7. Arvan, P., Rudnick, G., and Castle, J. D. (1984): *J. Biol. Chem.*, 259:13567–13572.
8. Ashwell, G., and Harford, J. (1982): *Annu. Rev. Biochem.*, 51:531–554.
9. Baldwin, G. S., Burgess, A. W., and Kemp, B. E. (1982): *Biochem. Biophys. Res. Commun.*, 109:656–663.
10. Baldwin, G. S., Grego, B., Hearn, M. T. W., Knesel, J. A., Morgan, F. J., and Simpson, R. J. (1983): *Proc. Natl. Acad. Sci. USA*, 80:5276–5280.
11. Bame, K. J., and Rome, L. H. (1985): *J. Biol. Chem.*, 260:11293–11299.
12. Beck-Peccoz, P., Amr, S., Menezes-Ferreira, M. M., Faglia, G., and Weintraub, B. D. (1985): *N. Engl. J. Med.*, 312:1085–1090.
13. Bedi, G. S., French, W. C., and Bahl, O. P. (1982): *J. Biol. Chem.*, 257:4345–4355.
14. Bennett, H. P., Brubaker, P. L., Seger, M. A., and Solomon, S. (1983): *J. Biol. Chem.*, 258:8108–8112.
15. Berman, P. W. (1985): In: *Current Communications in Molecular Biology*, edited by M. J. Gething, pp. 85–89. Cold Spring Harbor Laboratory, Cold Spring Harbor, NY.
16. Bettelheim, F. R. (1954): *J. Am. Chem. Soc.*, 76:2838–2839.
17. Bothwell, M. A., Wilson, W. H., and Shooter, E. M. (1979): *J. Biol. Chem.*, 254:7287–7294.
18. Bourbonnais, Y., and Crine, P. (1985): *J. Biol. Chem.*, 260:5832–5837.
19. Bradbury, A. F., Finnie, M. D. A., and Smyth, D. G. (1982): *Nature*, 298:686–688.
20. Bradbury, A. F., and Smyth, D. G. (1983): In: *Peptides*, edited by V. J. Hruby and D. H. Rich, pp. 249–252. Pierce Chemical Company, Rockford, IL.
21. Brake, A. J., Brenner, C., Najarian, R., Labourn, P., and Merryweather, J. (1985): In: *Current Communications in Molecular Biology*, edited by M. J. Gething, pp. 103–108. Cold Spring Harbor Laboratory, Cold Spring Harbor, NY.
22. Brand, S. J., Andersen, B. N., and Rehfeld, J. F. (1984): *Nature*, 309:456–458.
23. Brand, S. J., Bornstein, W. A., Potts, J. T., Jr., and Kronenberg, H. M. (1985): *Endocrinology*, 116:95a.
24. Browne, C. A., Bennett, H. P. J., and Solomon, S. (1982): *Anal. Biochem.*, 124:201–208.
25. Burgoyne, R. D., Geisow, M. J., and Barron, J. (1982): *Proc. R. Soc. Lond.*, 216:111–115.
26. Chang, T. L., Gainer, H., Russell, J. T., and Loh, Y. P. (1982): *Endocrinology*, 111:1607–1614.
27. Chang, T. L., and Loh, Y. P. (1984): *Endocrinology*, 114:2092–2099.
28. Civelli, O., Douglass, J., Goldstein, A., and Herbert, E. (1985): *Proc. Natl. Acad. Sci. USA*, 82:4291–4295.
29. Deakin, J. F. W., Dostrovsky, J. O., and Smyth, D. G. (1980): *Biochem. J.*, 189:501–506.
30. DeHaen, C., Swanson, E., and Teller, D. C. (1976): *J. Mol. Biol.*, 106:639–661.
31. Devi, L., and Goldstein, A. (1985): *Biochem. Biophys. Res. Commun.*, 130:1168–1176.
32. Dignam, S. S., and Setlow, P. (1980): *J. Biol. Chem.*, 255:8408–8412.
33. Dixon, J. E., and Woodford, T. A. (1984): *Methods Enzymol.*, 106:170–179.
34. Docherty, K., and Hutton, J. C. (1983): *FEBS Lett.*, 162:137–141.
35. Docherty, K., and Steiner, D. F. (1982): *Annu. Rev. Physiol.*, 44:625–638.

36. Douglass, J., Ranney, K., Uhler, M., Little, G., and Herbert, E. (1984): In: *Molecular Biology of Development,* edited by E. H. Davidson, and R. A. Firtel, pp. 573–588. Alan R. Liss, New York.

37. Drouin, J., and Goodman, H. M. (1980): *Nature,* 288:610–613.

38. Dunphy, W. G., and Rothman, J. E. (1985): *Cell,* 42:13–21.

39. Eipper, B. A., and Mains, R. E. (1982): *J. Biol. Chem.,* 254:4907–4915.

40. Eipper, B. A., Mains, R. E., and Glembotski, C. C. (1983): *Proc. Natl. Acad. Sci. USA,* 80:5144–5148.

41. Eipper, B. A., Park, L. P., Keutmann, H. T., and Mains, R. E. (1986): *J. Biol. Chem.,* 261:8686–8694.

42. Emeson, R. B. (1984): *J. Neurosci.,* 4:2604–2613.

43. Emeson, R. B., and Eipper, B. A. (1986): *J. Neurosci.,* 6:837–849.

44. Evans, C. J., Barchas, J. D., Esch, F. S., Bohlen, P., and Weber, E. (1985): *J. Neurosci.,* 5:1803–1807.

45. Farquhar, M. G. (1985): *Annu. Rev. Cell. Biol.,* 1:447–488.

46. Farquhar, M. G., and Palade, G. E. (1981): *J. Cell Biol.,* 91:77s–103s.

47. Fleminger, G., Ezra, E., Kilpatrick, D. L., and Udenfriend, S. (1983): *Proc. Natl. Acad. Sci. USA,* 80:6418–6421.

48. Fricker, L. D., Plummer, T. H., Jr., and Snyder, S. H. (1983): *Biochem. Biophys. Res. Commun.,* 111:994–1000.

49. Fricker, L. D., and Snyder, S. H. (1982): *Proc. Natl. Acad. Sci. USA,* 79:3886–3890.

50. Fricker, L. D., and Snyder, S. H. (1983): *J. Biol. Chem.,* 258:10950–10955.

51. Friedman, T. C., Orlowski, M., and Wilk, S. (1984): *Endocrinology,* 114:1407–1412.

52. Fuller, R. S., Brake, A. J., Julius, D. J., and Thorner, J. (1985): In: *Current Communications in Molecular Biology,* edited by M. J. Gething, pp. 97–102. Cold Spring Harbor Laboratory, Cold Spring Harbor, NY.

53. Furutani, Y., Morimoto, Y., Shibahara, S., Noda, M., Takahishi, H., Hirose, T., Asai, M., Inayama, S., Hayashida, H., Miyata, T., and Numa, S. (1983): *Nature,* 301:537–540.

54. Gainer, H., Russell, J. T., and Loh, Y. P. (1984): *FEBS Lett.,* 175:135–139.

55. Gainer, H., Russell, J. T., and Loh, Y. P. (1985): *Neuroendocrinology,* 40:171–184.

56. Garoff, H. (1985): *Annu. Rev. Cell. Biol.,* 1:403–405.

57. Geisow, M. J., and Smyth, D. G. (1980): In: *The Enzymology of Post-translational Modification of Proteins, Vol. 1,* edited by R. B. Freedman and H. C. Hawkins, pp. 259–287. Academic Press, London.

58. Gilmore, R., and Blobel, G. (1985): In: *Current Communications in Molecular Biology,* edited by M. J. Gething, pp. 29–32. Cold Spring Harbor Laboratory, Cold Spring Harbor, NY.

59. Glembotski, C. C. (1982): *J. Biol. Chem.,* 257:10493–10500.

60. Glembotski, C. C. (1982): *J. Biol. Chem.,* 257:10501–10509.

61. Glembotski, C. C. (1984): *J. Biol. Chem.,* 259:13041–13048.

62. Glembotski, C. C. (1985): *Arch. Biochem. Biophys.,* 241:673–683.

63. Glembotski, C. C., Eipper, B. A., and Mains, R. E. (1983): *J. Biol. Chem.,* 258:7299–7304.

64. Gluschankof, P., Morel, A., Gomez, S., Nicolas, P., Fahy, C., and Cohen, P. (1984): *Proc. Natl. Acad. Sci. USA,* 81:6662–6666.

65. Gomez, S., Gluschankof, P., Morel, A., and Cohen, P. (1985): *J. Biol. Chem.,* 260:10541–10545.

66. Green, M. (1982): *J. Biol. Chem.,* 257:9039–9042.

67. Green, C., Giros, B., and Schwartz, J. C. (1985): *Neuropeptides,* 5:485–488.

68. Guan, J.-L., Machamer, C. E., and Rose, J. K. (1985): *Cell,* 42:489–496.

69. Gumbiner, B., and Kelly, R. B. (1981): *Proc. Natl. Acad. Sci. USA,* 78:318–322.

70. Habuchi, O., and Conrad, H. E. (1985): *J. Biol. Chem.,* 260:13102–13108.

71. Ham, J., and Smyth, D. G. (1984): *FEBS Lett.,* 175:407–411.

72. Hellerman, J. G., Cone, R. G., Potts, J. T., Rich, A., Mulligan, R. C., and Kronenberg, H. M. (1984): *Proc. Natl. Acad. Sci. USA,* 81:5340–5344.

73. Herbert, E., Phillips, M., and Budarf, M. (1981): *Methods Cell Biol.,* 23:101–118.

74. Hersh, B. L. (1985): *J. Neurochem.,* 44:1427–1435.

75. Hille, A., Rosa, P., and Huttner, W. B. (1984): *FEBS Lett.,* 177:129–134.

76. Holz, R. W., Senter, R. A., and Sharp, R. R. (1983): *J. Biol. Chem.,* 258:7506–7513.

77. Hook, V. Y. H., and Eiden, L. E. (1984): *FEBS Lett.,* 172:212–218.

78. Horikawa, S., Takai, T., Toyosato, M., Takahashi, H., Noda, M., Kakidani, H., Kubo, T., Hirose, T., Inayama, S., Hayashida, H., Miyata, T., and Numa, S. (1983): *Nature,* 306:611–614.

79. Hoshina, H., Hortin, G., and Boime, I. (1982): *Science,* 217:63–64.

80. Hui, K. S., Wang, Y. J., and Lajtha, A. (1983): *Biochemistry,* 22:1062–1067.

81. Hunt, L. A., Davidson, S. K., and Golemboski, D. B. (1983): *Arch. Biochem. Biophys.,* 226:347–356.

82. Igarashi, T., Okazaki, T., Gaz, R. D., Potts, J. T., Jr., and Kronenberg, H. M. (1985): *Endocrinology,* 116:162a.

83. Julius, D., Blair, L., Brake, A., Sprague, G., and Thorner, J. (1983): *Cell,* 32:839–852.

84. Julius, D., Brake, A., Blair, L., Kunisawa, R., and Thorner, J. (1984): *Cell,* 37:1075–1089.

85. Kanmera, T., and Chaiken, I. M. (1985): *J. Biol. Chem.,* 260:8474–8482.

86. Kelly, R. B. (1985): *Science,* 230:25–32.

87. Keutmann, H. T., McIlroy, P. J., Bergert, E. R., and Ryan, R. J. (1983): *Biochemistry,* 22:3067–3072.

88. Kornfeld, R., and Kornfeld, S. (1985): *Annu. Rev. Biochem.,* 54:631–644.

89. Kreil, G., Haiml, L., and Suchanek, G. (1980): *Eur. J. Biochem.,* 111:49–58.

90. Kristensen, P., Nielsen, L. S., Grondahl-Hansen, J., Andresen, P. B., Larsson, L.-I., and Dano, K. (1985): *J. Cell Biol.,* 101:305–311.

91. Kurjan, J., and Herskowitz, I. (1982): *Cell,* 30:933–943.

92. Lane, C. D., Champion, J., Haiml, L., and Kreil, G. (1981): *Eur. J. Biochem.,* 113:273–281.

93. Lazure, C., Seidah, N. G., Thibault, G., Boucher, R., Genest, J., and Chretien, M. (1981): *Nature,* 292:383–384.

94. Lee, R. W. H., and Huttner, W. B. (1985): *Proc. Natl. Acad. Sci. USA,* 82:6143–6147.

95. Levine, M., Morita, K., and Pollard, H. (1985): *J. Biol. Chem.,* 260:12942–12947.

96. Lewis, U. J., Singh, R. N. P., Tutwiler, G. F., Sigel, M. B., VanderLaan, E. F., and VanderLaan, W. P. (1980): *Recent Prog. Horm. Res.,* 36:477–504.

97. Liberti, J. P., Antoni, B. A., and Chlebowski, J. F. (1985): *Biochem. Biophys. Res. Commun.,* 128:713–720.

98. Lindberg, I., Yang, H.-Y. T., and Costa, E. (1984): *J. Neurochem.,* 42:1411–1419.

99. Lipmann, F. (1958): *Science,* 128:575–580.

100. Liu, M. C., Yu, S., Sy, J., Redman, C. M., and Lipmann, F. (1985): *Proc. Natl. Acad. Sci. USA,* 82:7160–7164.

101. Loh, Y. P., Brownstein, M. J., and Gainer, H. (1984): *Annu. Rev. Neurosci.,* 7:189–222.

102. Loh, Y. P., Parish, D. C., and Tuteja, R. (1985): *J. Biol. Chem.,* 260:7194–7205.

103. Loh, Y. P., Tam, W. W. H., and Russell, J. T. (1984): *J. Biol. Chem.,* 259:8238–8245.

104. Lynch, D. R., and Snyder, S. H. (1986): *Annu. Rev. Biochem.,* 55:773–799.

105. Lynch, D. R., Strittmatter, S. M., and Snyder, S. H. (1984): *Proc. Natl. Acad. Sci. USA,* 81:6543–6547.

106. Mackin, R. B., Mackin, J. A., and Noe, B. D. (1985): *Endocrinology,* 116:69a.

107. Mains, R. E., and Eipper, B. A. (1981): *J. Biol. Chem.,* 256:5683–5688.

108. Mains, R. E., and Eipper, B. A. (1983): *Endocrinology,* 112:1986–1995.

109. Mains, R. E., and Eipper, B. A. (1984): *Endocrinology,* 115:1683–1690.

110. Mains, R. E., Eipper, B. A., Glembotski, C. C., and Dores, R. M. (1983): *Trends Neurosci.,* 6:229–285.

111. Mains, R. E., Myers, A. C., and Eipper, B. A. (1985): *Endocrinology,* 116:2505–2515.

112. Mains, R. E., Park, L. P., and Eipper, B. A. (1986): *J. Biol. Chem.,* 261:11938–11941.
113. Mason, A. J., Evans, B. A., Cox, D. R., Shine, J., and Richards, R. I. (1983): *Nature,* 303:300–307.
114. May, C., Kay, A., Wand, G., Eipper, B. A., Ney, R., Rapoport, S., and Cutler, N. (1985): *Am. Acad. Neurol. 37th Meeting,* V35(*Suppl.* 1):216 (Abstr. 1).
115. May, V., and Eipper, B. A. (1985): *J. Biol. Chem.,* 260:16224–16231.
116. Mizuno, K., Kojima, M., and Matsuo, H. (1985): *Biochem. Biophys. Res. Commun.,* 128:884–891.
117. Mizuno, K., and Matsuo, H. (1984): *Nature,* 309:558–560.
118. Mizuno, K., Miyata, A., Kangawa, K., and Matsuo, H. (1982): *Biochem. Biophys. Res. Commun.,* 108:1235–1242.
119. Moyle, W. R., Bahl, O. P., and Marz, L. (1975): *J. Biol. Chem.,*; 250:9163–9169.
120. Murthy, A. S. N., Keutmann, H. T., and Eipper, B. A. (1987): *Molecular Endocrinology* (in press).
121. Murthy, A. S. N., Mains, R. E., and Eipper, B. A. (1986): *J. Biol. Chem.,* 261:1815–1822.
122. Neurath, H. (1985): *Fed. Proc.,* 44:2907–2913.
123. Njus, D. (1983): *J. Auton. Nerv. Syst.,* 7:35–40.
124. Noe, B. D., Debo, G., and Spiess, J. (1984): *J. Cell. Biol.,* 99:578–587.
125. Noe, B. D., and Moran, M. N. (1984): *J. Cell. Biol.,* 99:418–424.
126. Nordmann, J. J., and Norris, S. J. (1984): *Proc. Natl. Acad. Sci. USA,* 81:180–184.
127. O'Donohue, T. L., Handelmann, G. E., Chaconas, T., Miller, R. L., and Jacobowitz, D. M. (1981): *Peptides,* 2:333–344.
128. O'Donohue, T. L., Handelmann, G. E., Miller, R. L., and Jawbowitz, D. M. (1982): *Science,* 215:1125–1127.
129. Orci, L., Halban, P., Amherdt, M., Ravazzola, M., Vassalli, J. D., and Perrelet, A. (1985): *J. Cell. Biol.,* 99:2187–2192.
130. Orci, L., Ravazzola, M., and Perrelet, A. (1984): *Proc. Natl. Acad. Sci. USA,* 81:6743–6746.
131. Orlowski, M. (1983): *Mol. Cell Biochem.,* 52:49–74.
132. Palade, G. (1975): *Science,* 189:347–358.
133. Parsons, T. F., and Pierce, J. G. (1980): *Proc. Natl. Acad. Sci. USA,* 77:7089–7093.
134. Parsons, T. F., and Pierce, J. G. (1984): *J. Biol. Chem.,* 259:2662–2666.
135. Pelaprat, D., Seidah, N. G., Sikstrom, R. A., Lambelin, P., Hamelin, J., Lazure, C., Cromlish, J. A., and Chretien, M. (1984): *Endocrinology,* 115:581–590.
136. Pollack, L., and Atkinson, P. H. (1983): *J. Cell. Biol.,* 97:293–300.
137. Powers, C. A. (1985): *Biochem. Biophys. Res. Commun.,* 127:668–672.
138. Powers, C. A., and Nasjletti, A. (1983): *Endocrinology,* 112:1194–1200.
139. Prado, E. S., Prado de Carvalho, L., Araujo-Viel, M. S., Ling, N., and Rossier, J. (1983): *Biochem. Biophys. Res. Commun.,* 112:366–373.
140. Rabbini, S. A., Kermer, R., Bennett, H. P., and Goltzman, D. (1984): *J. Biol. Chem.,* 259:2949–2955.
141. Rehfeld, J. F. (1981): *Am. J. Physiol.,* 240:E255–E266.
142. Rehfeld, J. F., Hansen, H. F., Larsson, L.-I., Stengaard-Pedersen, K., and Thorn, N. A. (1984): *Proc. Natl. Acad. Sci. USA,* 81:1902–1905.
143. Richter, K., Kawashima, E., Egger, R., and Kreil, G. (1984): *EMBO J.,* 3:617.
144. Robbins, P. W. (1985): In: *Current Communications in Molecular Biology,* edited by M. J. Gething, pp. 109–114. Cold Spring Harbor Laboratory, Cold Spring Harbor, NY.
145. Ronin, C., Stannard, B. S., Rosenblum, I. L., Magner, J. A., and Weintraub, B. D. (1984): *Biochemistry,* 23:4503–4510.
146. Rosen, H., Douglass, J., and Herbert, E. (1984): *J. Biol. Chem.,* 259:14309–14313.
147. Rossner, M. R., Grinna, L. S., and Robbins, P. W. (1980): *Proc. Natl. Acad. Sci. USA,* 77:67–71.
148. Rudman, D., Hollins, B. M., Kutner, M. H., Moffitt, S. D., and Lynn, M. J. (1983): *Am. J. Physiol.* 244:E47–E54.
149. Ruiz-Carrillo, A., Wangh, L. J., and Allfrey, V. G. (1975): *Science,* 190:117–128.
150. Russell, J. T. (1984): *J. Biol. Chem.,* 259:9496–9507.
151. Sabatini, D. D., Kreibich, G., Morimoto, T., and Adesnik, M. (1982): *J. Cell. Biol.,* 92:1–22.
152. Sadler, J. E. (1984): In: *Biology of Carbohydrates, Vol. 2,* edited by V. Ginsburg and P. W. Robbins, pp. 199–288. John Wiley and Sons, New York.
153. Sairam, M. R., and Manjunath, P. (1983): *J. Biol. Chem.,* 258:445–449.
154. San Segundo, B., Chan, S. J., and Steiner, D. F. (1985): *Proc. Natl. Acad. Sci. USA,* 82:2320–2324.
155. Schaefer, M., Picciotto, M. R., Kreiner, T., Kaldany, R. R., Taussig, R., and Scheller, R. H. (1985): *Cell,* 41:457–467.
156. Schwartz, T. W., and Tager, H. S. (1981): *Nature,* 294:589–591.
157. Schwarz, J. K., Capasso, J. M., and Hirschberg, C. B. (1984): *J. Biol. Chem.,* 259:3554–3559.
158. Seeburg, P. H., and Adelman, J. P. (1984): *Nature,* 311:666–668.
159. Seizinger, B. R., Hollt, V., and Herz, A. (1981): *Biochem. Biophys. Res. Commun.,* 101:289–297.
160. Seizinger, B. R., Hollt, V., and Herz, A. (1982): *J. Neurochem.,* 39:143–148.
161. Snider, M. D., and Rogers, O. C. (1984): *Cell,* 36:753–761.
162. Spiess, J., and Noe, B. D. (1985): *Proc. Natl. Acad. Sci. USA,* 82:277–281.
163. Srivastava, M., Duong Le, T., and Fleming, P. J. (1984): *J. Biol. Chem.,* 259:8072–8075.
164. Steiner, D. F., Docherty, K., and Carroll, R. (1984): *J. Cell. Biochem.,* 24:121–130.
165. Stoeckel, M. E., Schimchowitsch, S., Garaud, J. C., Schmitt, G., Vaudry, H., and Porte, A. (1983): *Cell Tissue Res.,* 230:511–515.
166. Strittmatter, S. M., Lynch, D. R., de Souza, E., and Snyder, S. H. (1985): *Endocrinology,* 117:1667–1674.
167. Strittmatter, S. M., Lynch, D. R., and Snyder S. H. (1984): *J. Biol. Chem.,* 259:11812–11817.
168. Sugano, K., Aponte, G. W., and Yamada, T. (1985): *J. Biol. Chem.,* 260:11724–11729.
169. Supattapone, S., Fricker, L. D., and Snyder, S. H. (1984): *J. Neurochem.,* 42:1017–1023.
170. Tatemoto, K., Carlquist, M., and Mutt, V. (1982): *Nature,* 296:659–660.
171. Tavianini, M. A., Hayes, T. E., Magazin, M. D., Minth, C. D., and Dixon, J. E. (1984): *J. Biol. Chem.,* 259:11798–11803.
172. Thorn, N. A., Christensen, B. L., Jeppensen, C., and Nielsen, F. S. (1985): *Acta Physiol. Scand.,* 124:87–92.
173. Tsunasawa, S., and Sakiyama, F. (1984): *Methods Enzymol.,* 106:165–170.
174. Unsworth, C. D., Hughes, J., and Morley, J. S. (1982): *Nature,* 295:519–522.
175. Vale, W., Spiess, J., Rivier, C., and Rivier, J. (1981): *Science,* 213:1394–1397.
176. Varki, A., and Diaz, S. (1985): *J. Biol. Chem.,* 260:6600–6608.
177. Virji, M. A. G., Vassalli, J.-D., Estensen, R. D, and Reich, E. (1980): *Proc. Natl. Acad. Sci. USA,* 77:875–879.
178. Walter, P., Siegel, V., Lauffer, L., Garcia, P. D., Ullrich, A., and Harkins, R. (1985): In: *Current Communications in Molecular Biology,* edited by M. J. Gething, pp. 21–23. Cold Spring Harbor Laboratory, Cold Spring Harbor, NY.
179. Wand, G. S., Ney, R. L., Baylin, S., Eipper, B. A., and Mains, R. E., (1985): *Metabolism,* 34:1044–1051.
180. Wand, G. S., Ney, R. L., Mains, R. E., and Eipper, B. A. (1985): *Neuroendocrinology,* 41:482–489.
181. Warren, T. G., and Shields, D. (1984): *Cell,* 39:547–555.
182. Weigant, V. M., Verhoef, J., Burbach, J. P. H., and van Amerongen, A. (1983): *Life Sci.,* 33 (*Suppl.* 1):125–128.
183. Weigant, V. M., Verhoef, J., Burbach, J. P. H., van Amerongen, A., Gaffori, O., Sitsen, J. M. N., and de Wied, D. (1985): *Life Sci.,* 36:2277.
184. Weintraub, B. D., Stannard, B. S., and Meyers, L. (1983): *Endocrinology,* 112:1331–1345.
185. Wong, T. W., and Goldberg, A. R. (1983): *J. Biol. Chem.,* 258:1022–1025.
186. Yamashita, K., Ueda, I., and Kobata, A. (1983): *J. Biol. Chem.,* 258:14144–14147.
187. Yanagishita, M., and Hascall, V. C. (1983): *J. Biol. Chem.,* 258:12857–12864.
188. Zakarian, S., and Smyth, D. G. (1982): *Nature,* 296:250–252.

Psychopharmacology:
The Third Generation of Progress,
edited by Herbert Y. Meltzer.
Raven Press, New York © 1987.

CHAPTER **42**

Distribution of Neuropeptides With Special Reference to Their Coexistence With Classical Transmitters

T. Hökfelt, O. Johansson, V. Holets, B. Meister, and T. Melander

The volume *Psychopharmacology: A Generation of Progress,* edited by Lipton et al. (104), summarized the progress in the psychopharmacology field presented at the ACNP meeting in 1977, and this included eleven papers on neuropeptides (17,54,60,93,126,131,148,149,161,176,177), which represented a fairly small proportion of the 149 articles published in that volume. Since then an increasing interest has been focused on neuropeptides. Thanks to the rapid development in biochemical technology, numerous new peptides and peptide families have been discovered, and the introduction of recombinant DNA technology has further expanded this capacity, especially with regard to defining peptide precursor molecules.

The neuropeptide research was strongly influenced by the structural characterization of several hypothalamic releasing and inhibiting hormones by Guillemin, Schally, Vale, and their collaborators, and the demonstration that thyrotropin-releasing hormone (TRH) (19,127), luteinizing hormone-releasing hormone (LHRH) (3,151), and growth hormone release-inhibiting hormone [GHR-IF; somatostatin (SOM)] (15) were all small peptides. Moreover, these peptides were not restricted to the basal hypothalamus and the median eminence, i.e., areas where they could serve as hormones transported to the anterior pituitary according to the classical concept of Green and Harris (see 56), but

could also be seen in widespread areas in the central and peripheral nervous system (see 17,60). This suggested that these peptides may have roles in addition to that of hormones controlling anterior pituitary hormone secretion. The field was also greatly stimulated by the discovery of the enkephalins by Hughes, Kosterlitz, and collaborators (82), two pentapeptides representing endogenous ligands for the opiate receptors which had been discovered some years earlier (144,156,173). It is impressive that subsequently, in less than 10 years, a fairly complete view has been obtained of the biochemistry and immunohistochemistry not only of enkephalins but also of two further opioid peptide families, the derivatives of proopiomelanocortin and the dynorphin peptides and of their precursor molecules and genes (see 91).

In 1977, when the articles for the *Psychopharmacology* volume were written, a fairly good overview had been obtained of the distribution of several peptides in the nervous system. In addition to LHRH, TRH, and SOM, there was also information on peptides such as substance P (SP), enkephalins, angiotensin II, vasoactive intestinal polypeptide (VIP), cholecystokinin (CCK), oxytocin, and vasopressin (see 17,60). It had, for example, been recognized that some of these peptides, such as SOM, VIP, and CCK, had particularly numerous cell bodies in cortical areas,

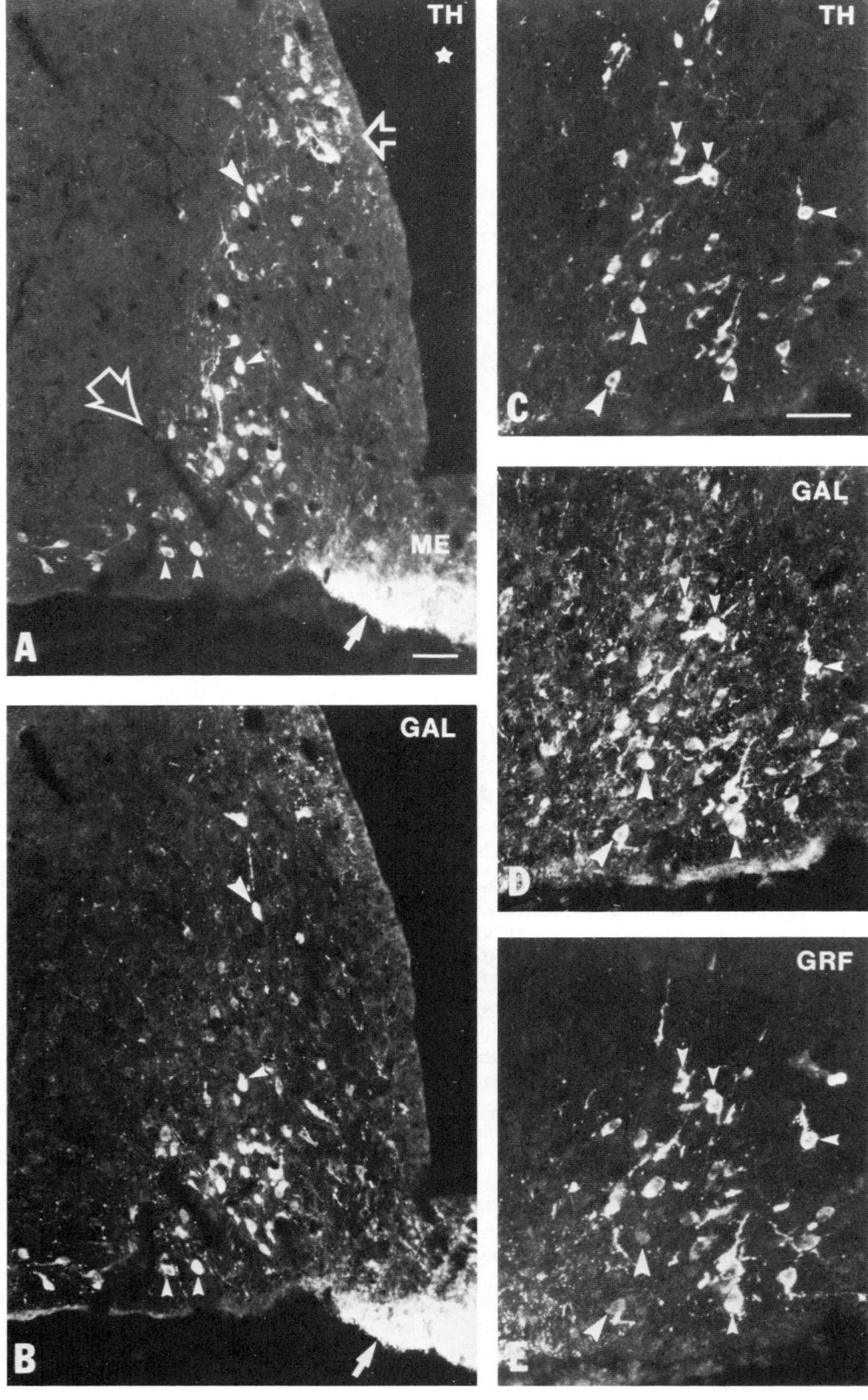

whereas other peptides, such as SP, had a fairly poor representation in these regions. Moreover, it had been observed that some brain areas were particularly rich in peptides, for example, several nuclei in the hypothalamus, the central amygdaloid nucleus, the septal area, the dorsal vagal complex, and the dorsal horn of the spinal cord. In fact, many of the peptide fibers seen in the dorsal horn originated in cell bodies in spinal ganglia, i.e., they belonged to primary sensory neurons. A variety of peptides were also found in the peripheral autonomic nervous system and in the gastrointestinal tract.

It seems reasonable to state that the general idea at that time was that peptide-containing neurons represented novel systems separate from the ones studied in detail up till then, for example, the dopamine (DA), norepinephrine or noradrenaline (NA), 5-hydroxytryptamine (5-HT), and amino acid systems, in spite of the fact that many peptides showed considerable overlap in their distribution with some of these compounds. A major obstacle in the initial immunohistochemical studies was the difficulty of demonstrating peptides in cell bodies. Not until experimental procedures were developed, above all the use of the mitosis inhibitor colchicine (see 9,34,35,59,61,68), was this problem solved, allowing reproducible demonstration of peptide-containing cell bodies in many brain areas. The larger size of cell bodies, as compared to nerve endings, made it easier to compare distribution patterns and possible identity of different chemically defined neuron populations. A major result of such comparative studies was the finding that, in fact, different peptides could be observed to be present in neurons also containing a classical transmitter, such as norepinephrine. The first example of such a coexistence between a classical transmitter and a peptide was observed in the peripheral nervous system, where some noradrenergic neurons in sympathetic ganglia contained a somatostatin-like peptide (62). Subsequently, many coexistence combinations have been observed in neuronal systems both in the periphery and in brain and spinal cord. This raises many issues with regard to mechanisms and physiology of chemical transmission. One conclusion can, however, be drawn already at this stage: if coexistence is a general phenomenon, then involvement of neuropeptides has to be analyzed against the background of the well-documented framework of knowledge of chemical transmission via classical transmitters.

The field of neuropeptides has grown explosively, and it is here not possible to give a reasonable account of peptide-containing neurons. This article will therefore focus on

selected findings, primarily on the phenomenon of coexistence of multiple messengers, especially the fact that the neuropeptides are found in the same neurons as classical transmitters (see 28,32,67,72,73,136,146). First, we would like to give an overview of the distribution of a few, selected central peptide systems and discuss them in relation to various coexistence situations with classical transmitters. We would also like to underline the complexity and multiplicity of neuronal peptides and coexistence situations by discussing a single brain nucleus, the hypothalamic arcuate nucleus. Subsequently we will summarize some general views of coexistence. We will, however, begin with some methodological aspects.

ASPECTS OF METHODOLOGY

Histochemical Mapping Techniques

The tracing of neurons on the basis of their transmitter or transmitter-related compound, for example, a synthesizing enzyme, or of neuropeptides, was initially carried out with several types of techniques. Thus presumptive cholinergic neurons were analyzed with acetylcholinesterase histochemistry (94,95,102,154,155) and catecholamines and 5-HT were mapped with formaldehyde-induced fluorescence (Falck-Hillarp) (23,36,37,45). Autoradiography has also been used extensively (see 38). Subsequently, immunohistochemical techniques have been employed, both the original indirect immunofluorescence method of Coons and collaborators (see 30) and important modifications using peroxidase as marker molecule (6,129,164). With these approaches, mapping of numerous peptides has been carried out, describing the detailed distribution of cell bodies, nerve endings, and to some extent their axonal projections. Since peptide levels are low in axons, it is difficult to follow these structures within the brain tissue. Therefore novel techniques, whereby retrograde tracing (100) is combined with immunohistochemistry, can be used to define peptide-containing projections (see 77,157).

Demonstration of Multiple Antigens in Cells

Immunohistochemistry also offers many advantages for analyzing multiple antigens in single neurons (Fig. 1). In fact, most of the information on coexistence has been obtained with this technique. At least three different approaches can be used.

FIG. 1. A–E. Immunofluorescence micrographs of the arcuate nucleus-median eminence complex after incubation with antisera to tyrosine hydroxylase (TH) (**A, C**), galanin (GAL) (**B, D**), and growth hormone-releasing factor (GRF) (**E**). **A** and **B** represent the same section, which has been processed for the double-labeling technique with mouse monoclonal antibodies to TH and rabbit polyclonal antibodies to GAL followed by FITC- and rhodamine-labeled secondary antibodies. **C** and **D** show a higher magnification of the arcuate nucleus of a section incubated in the same way as described in **A** and **B**. **E** shows the same section as **C** and **D** after elution of the TH and GAL antibodies and restaining with GRF antiserum. **A, B:** Many cell bodies in the ventral group (*large open arrow*) contain both TH- and GAL-like immunoreactivity. In the dorsal group (*small open arrow*) most cell bodies are only TH positive, but the *large arrowhead* points to a double-labeled cell. The *large arrow* points to nerve terminals in the external layer of the median eminence. **C–E:** Many cell bodies (*small arrowheads*) contain both TH-, GAL-, and GRF-like immunoreactivities. Some cells (*large arrowheads*) seem to lack GRF-LI. Bars indicate 50 μm. **A** and **B** as well as **C–E** have the same magnification.

With the *adjacent section method* serial sections are cut and incubated with different primary antisera. This method is useful for analysis of cell bodies, and the results are dependent on section thickness—the thinner the sections, the more reliably can a single cell body be identified throughout several sections. With this approach no interference between different antisera can occur, and thus cross reactivity problems will not be encountered. The disadvantages are mainly difficulties in unequivocally establishing identity between cell profiles in the adjacent sections, and the fact that coexistence in small structures such as nerve endings cannot be analyzed.

Second, with the *elution-restaining method* (Fig. 1), as first described by Nakane (128), the staining pattern of one antibody is photographed, and then elution is carried out with acid solutions, for example acid potassium permanganate ($KMnO_4$) (174). The sections are then processed for a second antiserum, and the new staining pattern photographed and compared with the first one. When used with proper controls to establish complete removal of primary antibodies, the method allows secure identification of double-labeled cells. However, the elution procedure may damage antigens in the sections so that restaining cannot be carried out and negative results should therefore be interpreted with caution.

With antisera raised in different species, a third approach can be used, the *direct double-staining method* (Fig. 1). The section is incubated with a mixture of two antisera raised, for example, in guinea pig and rabbit. As secondary antibody one can then use, for example, red fluorescent tetramethylrhodamine isothiocyanate (TRITC, rhodamine) conjugated donkey antirabbit antibodies and green fluorescent fluorescein isothiocyanate (FITC) conjugated swine anti-guinea pig antibodies. This approach offers many advantages, since coexistence can be analyzed directly in the microscope by switching between proper filter combinations, and since it often is possible to demonstrate coexistence also in fibers.

If more than two antigens are to be analyzed, one may use, as stated above, the adjacent section method with thin sections. A further possibility is to combine, for example, the direct double-staining technique with the elution-restaining method (Fig. 1).

Specificity-Sensitivity

Immunohistochemistry represents a powerful histochemical method but has problems with regard to specificity and sensitivity. Questions concerning *specificity* arise with all immunological approaches, but are especially prominent for immunohistochemical methods, where often high concentrations of antibody are used. However, even at higher dilutions the antibodies may react with peptides or proteins containing a similar amino acid sequence. Also *sensitivity* represents a serious problem in immunohistochemistry, and quality of antiserum and choice of fixation method are important. Negative results should therefore be interpreted with caution and future experiments will probably demonstrate occurrence of peptides and transmitters in more systems than so far assumed.

CENTRAL NEUROPEPTIDE DISTRIBUTION AND COEXISTENCE

Distributional maps of several peptides have been published giving detailed information on distribution of cell bodies and fibers in the central nervous system, mainly of the rat, but also other species have been analyzed. Less detailed information is available with regard to the exact projections of these peptide neurons, but such information is now accumulating rapidly. It is beyond the scope of this article to provide information on all these peptide systems, but such information can be found, for example, in books edited by Krieger et al. (98) and Björklund and Hökfelt (11). Here we would like to sketch the distribution of three peptides, SP, SOM, and galanin (GAL) and briefly indicate the distribution of neurons containing these peptides on a schematic, sagittal section (Figs. 2–4). On these maps we will also indicate the so far described coexistence situations with classical transmitters for these peptides. Subsequently we would like to contrast this with a diagram of the distribution of central catecholamine neurons and on this diagram indicate coexistence situations with peptides (Fig. 5).

A more complete description of coexistence situations observed is given in Table 1. So far only a small proportion of all central neurons have been shown to contain both classical transmitters and a peptide(s). This may reflect the actual situation, but, on the other hand, it seems highly likely that further exploration, using novel markers for classical transmitters and for new peptides, will reveal that coexistence is even more common than shown so far. It is important to note that in many systems multiple peptides have been observed together with a classical transmitter, but that there are also many neurons containing multiple peptides without apparent presence of a classical transmitter. Whether this indicates that some neurons do not contain a classical transmitter, or whether it has not been possible to demonstrate the appropriate transmitter remains to be shown. It should also be noted that other types of compounds than the classical transmitters and peptides may serve as transmitters and may be involved in coexistence situations. For example, increasing support for purines as transmitters has been presented (20,21), and ATP may coexist with both a peptide (neuropeptide Y, NPY) and classical transmitter (norepinephrine) in sympathetic neurons in the vas deferens (see 21,166).

Substance P and Coexisting Classical Transmitters

SP was originally isolated by von Euler and Gaddum (181) from both intestinal tissues and brain. It was structurally characterized by Chang et al. (24), and initial studies were focused on its role in primary sensory neurons (68,168,169). Immunohistochemical studies revealed widespread distribution in the central nervous system (33,69,105). More recently it has been recognized that the mammalian brain also contains other types of tachykinins, one of which is formed from the same precursor molecule (90,92,124,130,171). A careful comparative analysis of possible differences in distribution between these various tachy-

TABLE 1. *Immunohistochemical evidence for coexistence of classical transmitters and peptides in the central nervous system (selected cases)*

Classical transmitter	Peptide[a]	Brain region (species)	Refs.
Dopamine	CCK	Ventral mesencephalon (rat, cat, mouse, monkey, human?)	76, 78, 79
	Neurotensin	Ventral mesencephalon (rat)	63
		Hypothalamic arcuate nucleus (rat)	63, 84
Norepinephrine	Enkephalin	Locus ceruleus (cat)	29, 101
	NPY	Medulla oblongata (man, rat)	43, 71, 74
		Locus ceruleus (rat)	43
	Vasopressin	Locus ceruleus (rat)	22
Epinephrine	Neurotensin	Medulla oblongata (rat)	63
	NPY	Medulla oblongata (rat)	43
	Substance P	Medulla oblongata (rat)	106
	Neurotensin	Solitary tract nucleus (rat)	63
5-HT	Substance P	Medulla oblongata (rat, cat)	25, 26, 70, 89, 107
		Spinal cord (rat)	142
	TRH	Medulla oblongata (rat)	89
	Substance P + TRH	Medulla oblongata (rat)	89
	CCK	Medulla oblongata (rat)	118
	Enkephalin	Medulla oblongata, pons (cat)	53, 83
		Area postrema (rat)	5
ACh	Enkephalin	Superior olive (guinea pig)	2
		Spinal cord (rat)	97
	Substance P	Pons (rat)	179
	VIP	Cortex (rat)	41
	Galanin	Basal forebrain (rat)	123
	CGRP	Medullary motor nuclei (rat)	170
GABA	Motilin(?)	Cerebellum (rat)	27
	Somatostatin	Thalamus (cat)	133
		Cortex, hippocampus (rat, cat, monkey)	57, 87, 152, 160
	CCK	Cortex (cat, monkey)	57, 160
	NPY	Cortex (cat, monkey)	57
	Galanin	Hypothalamus (rat)	121
	Enkephalin	Retina (chicken)	182
		Ventral pallidum (rat)	184
	Opioid peptide	Basal ganglia (rat)	134
Glycine	Neurotensin	Retina (turtle)	183

[a] This column contains the peptide against which the antiserum used for immunohistochemistry was raised. The exact structure of the peptide coexisting with the classical transmitter has mostly not been defined.

kinins in the central nervous system has so far not been carried out with immunohistochemical techniques.

In the rat brain, SP neurons have a wide distribution with cell bodies in many nuclei. The map shown in Fig. 2 is based on the paper by Ljungdahl et al. (105), but in that paper only a few cells were seen in the caudate nucleus and none in the arcuate nucleus. More recently, Kohno et al. (96) and Tsuruo et al. (175) have, however, demonstrated numerous cell bodies in these two nuclei, respectively, and their results are included here. The cortical representation of SP is comparatively poor. Major SP immunoreactive cell groups are found in the septal area, nucleus accumbens, bed nucleus of the stria terminalis, and caudate nucleus.

The latter neurons give rise to a descending pathway terminating with very dense fiber networks in the zona reticulata of the substantia nigra. SP-positive cell bodies are also seen in many hypothalamic nuclei, especially in the most ventral aspects of the ventromedial nucleus but also in the perifornical region and in the dorsomedial nucleus. The amygdaloid nucleus, especially the central and medial nuclei, contain many SP-positive cell bodies. A large collection of small SP-immunoreactive neurons is seen in the medial habenular nucleus, and these cells give rise to axons that via the fasciculus retroflexus project to the interpeduncular nucleus. The periaqueductal central gray, including the Edinger-Westphal nucleus, is rich in

Substance P

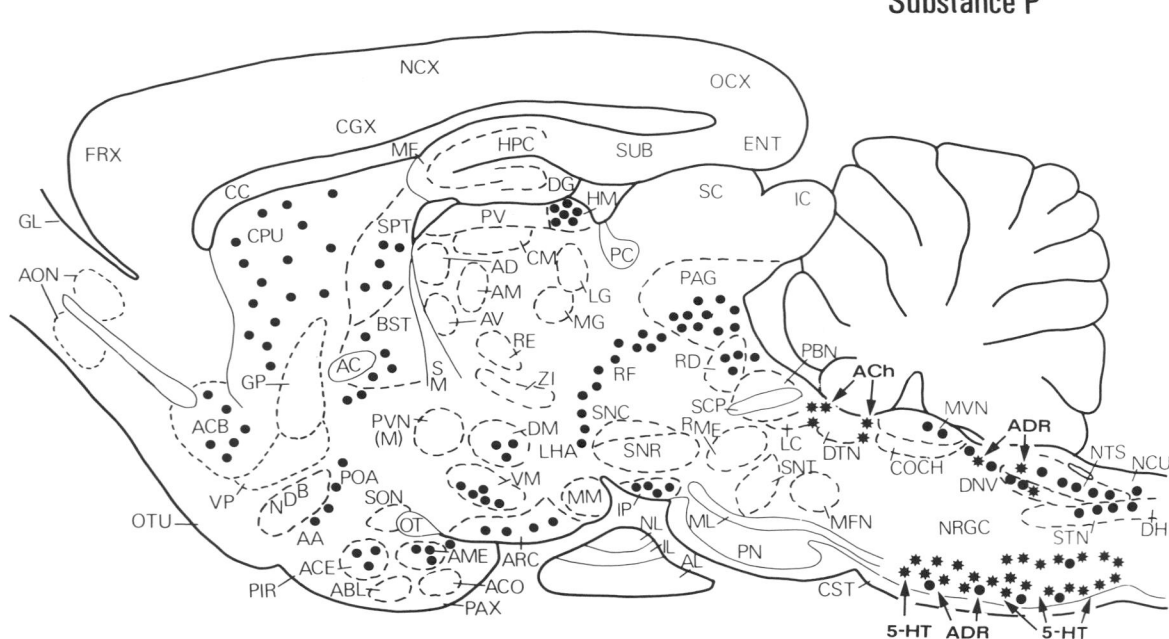

FIG. 2. Schematic illustration of distribution of major substance P-positive cell groups (*dots*) in a sagittal section of the rat brain. This map represents multiple parasagittal levels through the rat brain and was reconstructed using the rat brain atlas of Paxinos and Watson (140), and has been redrawn after Khachaturian et al. (91). Cell groups shown also to contain a classical transmitter are indicated by a *star*. The type of coexisting classical transmitter is indicated by abbreviations and arrows. Abbreviations for this Figure as well as Figs. 3–5 are as follows: AA, anterior amygdala; ABL, basolateral nucleus of amygdala; AC, anterior commissure; ACB, nucleus accumbens; ACE, central nucleus of amygdala; ACO, cortical nucleus of amygdala; AD, anterodorsal nucleus of thalamus; AL, anterior lobe of pituitary; AM, anteromedial nucleus of thalamus; AMB, nucleus ambiguus; AME, medial nucleus of amygdala; AON, anterior olfactory nucleus; ARC, arcuate nucleus; AV, anteroventral nucleus of thalamus; BST, bed nucleus of stria terminalis; CC, corpus callosum; CGX, cingulate cortex; CM, central-medial nucleus of thalamus; COCH, cochlear nucleus complex; CPU, caudate-putamen; CST, corticospinal tract; DH, dorsal horn of spinal cord; DG, dentate gyrus; DM, dorsomedial nucleus of hypothalamus; DNV, dorsal motor nucleus of vagus; DTN, dorsal tegmental nucleus; ENT, entorhinal cortex; FN, fastigial nucleus of cerebellum; FRX, frontal cortex; GL, glomerular layer of olfactory bulb; GP, globus pallidus; HM, medial habenular nucleus; HPC, hippocampus; IC, inferior colliculus; IL, intermediate lobe of pituitary; IP, interpeduncular nuclear complex; LC, nucleus locus ceruleus; LG, lateral geniculate nucleus; LHA, lateral hypothalamic area; LRN, lateral reticular nucleus; MF, mossy fibers of hippocampus; MFN, motor facial nucleus; MG, medial geniculate nucleus; ML, medial lemniscus; MM, medial mammillary nucleus; MNT, mesencephalic nucleus of trigeminal tract; MVN, medial vestibular nucleus; NCU, nucleus cuneatus; NCX, neocortex; NDB, nucleus of diagonal band; NL, neural lobe of pituitary; NRGC, nucleus reticularis gigantocellularis; NRPG, nucleus reticularis paragigantocellularis; NTS, nucleus tractus solitarii; OCX, occipital cortex; OT, optic tract; OTU, olfactory tubercle; PAG, periaqueductal gray; PAX, periamygdaloid cortex; PBN, parabrachial nucleus; PC, posterior commissure; PIR, piriform cortex; PN, pons; POA, preoptic area; PP, perforant path; PV, periventricular nucleus of thalamus; PVN(M), paraventricular nucleus (pars magnocellularis); PVN(P), paraventricular nucleus (pars parvocellularis); RD, nucleus raphe dorsalis; RE, nucleus reuniens of thalamus; RF, reticular formation; RM, nucleus raphe magnus; RME, nucleus raphe medianus; SC, superior colliculus; SCP, superior cerebellar peduncle; SM, stria medullaris thalami; SNC, substantia nigra (pars compacta); SNR, substantia nigra (pars reticulata); SNT, sensory nucleus of trigeminal tract (main); SON, supraoptic nucleus; SPT, septal nuclei; STN, spinal nucleus of trigeminal tract; SUB, subiculum; VM, ventromedial nucleus of hypothalamus; VP, ventral pallidum; ZI, zona incerta.

SP-positive cell bodies, as are the medullary raphe nuclei and adjacent areas that project to the spinal cord and numerous medullary nuclei. Cell bodies are also found in areas such as the dorsal vagal complex, the spinal trigeminal nucleus, and the dorsal horn of the spinal cord. The wide distribution of SP-positive terminal networks will not be discussed here, but we will only make one point. It is important to note that in a particular nucleus the SP-immunoreactivity may have several different origins. Thus, for example, in the dorsal horn of the spinal cord, overlapping fiber networks may come from three different types of neurons: (a) primary afferents of dorsal root ganglion cells, (b) local spinal neurons, and (c) descending bulbospinal neurons (see 105). This fact will, of course, make the analysis of the physiological significance of SP in this area difficult.

The major coexistence combination involving SP is found in the medulla oblongata (Fig. 2), where a considerable proportion of the 5-HT raphe neurons contain SP-like immunoreactivity (LI) (26,70,89,142). It is, however, clear that different subgroups of the medullary 5-HT neurons contain varying proportions of this peptide, alternatively varying levels. For example, in the nucleus raphe pallidus a large proportion of all 5-HT neurons exhibit SP-LI, whereas this proportion is fairly low in the superficial neurons underlying the pyramidal tract (medullary arcuate nuclei) (89). Many of these 5-HT neurons also contain a TRH-like peptide (72,89). However, the most rostral proportion of the medullary-pontine 5-HT raphe complex seems to lack both SP- and TRH-LI. Another peptide that may coexist in these neurons is a proctolin-like peptide (81) as well as CCK-LI (118). In the medulla oblongata SP cells in the ventrolateral medulla oblongata also contain the epinephrine-synthesizing enzyme PNMT (64,106). To a certain extent these cells also contain NPY-LI (43,64). In the pons, SP neurons in the lateral dorsal tegmental nucleus as well as in the central tegmental field contain the acetylcholine (ACh)-synthesizing enzyme choline acetyltransferase, suggesting coexistence of SP and ACh (179). It is obvious that the vast majority of SP-positive cell bodies in the rat central nervous system so far seem to lack a coexisting peptide (Fig. 2).

Somatostatin and Coexisting Classical Transmitters

Growth hormone release-inhibiting activity was first observed in the hypothalamus by Krulich et al. (99), and some years later Brazeau et al. (15) identified this activity as a tetradecapeptide and termed it SOM. More recently it has been realized that additional forms of SOM exist, especially an amino-terminal-extended form (SOM-28) (see 98). Numerous immunohistochemical studies have dealt with the distribution of SOM-positive neurons in the nervous system (Fig. 3), and a general agreement on its wide distribution exists (see, e.g. 10,46,88,178).

Briefly, high numbers of SOM-positive cell bodies were found in most cortical areas including the neocortex, pyriform cortex, hippocampus, and amygdaloid cortex; subcortical structures such as caudate nucleus and nucleus accumbens; hypothalamic nuclei, especially the anterior periventricular hypothalamic region, ventromedial hypothalamic nucleus, arcuate nucleus, and zona incerta. More caudally, SOM-immunoreactive cells were seen in the periaqueductal central gray, bed nucleus of the stria terminalis, entopeduncular nucleus/internal capsule, medial geniculate body, in relation to the lateral lemniscus, pontine reticular nuclei, nucleus cochlearis dorsalis, and within the solitary tract nucleus as well as in the dorsal horn of the spinal cord.

SOM has so far been shown to coexist with few classical transmitters. Such coexistence situations mainly involve γ-aminobutyric acid (GABA) and are located in cortex and hippocampus (Fig. 3) as well as in the thalamus of the cat (57,87,133,152,160).

Galanin and Coexisting Classical Transmitters

Recently a novel peptide, GAL, has been isolated from porcine small intestine (172). Immunohistochemical studies have revealed a wide distribution in the central nervous system (Fig. 4) (120,123,150,158).

GAL-positive cell bodies were seen in many areas; for example, the telencephalon, bed nucleus of the stria terminalis, nucleus of the diagonal band and the septum, as well as the central amygdaloid nucleus contained high numbers of positive cell bodies. In the hypothalamus

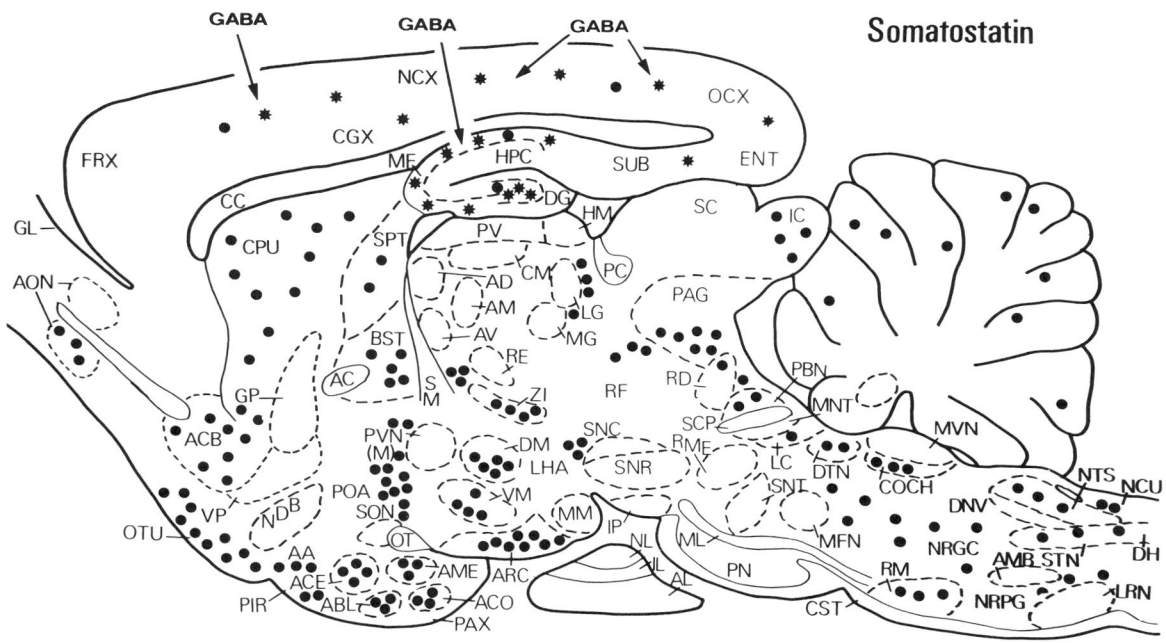

FIG. 3. Schematic illustration of distribution of major groups of somatostatin-positive neurons in a sagittal section of the rat brain. For further details see figure legend to Figure 2 on page 406.

Galanin

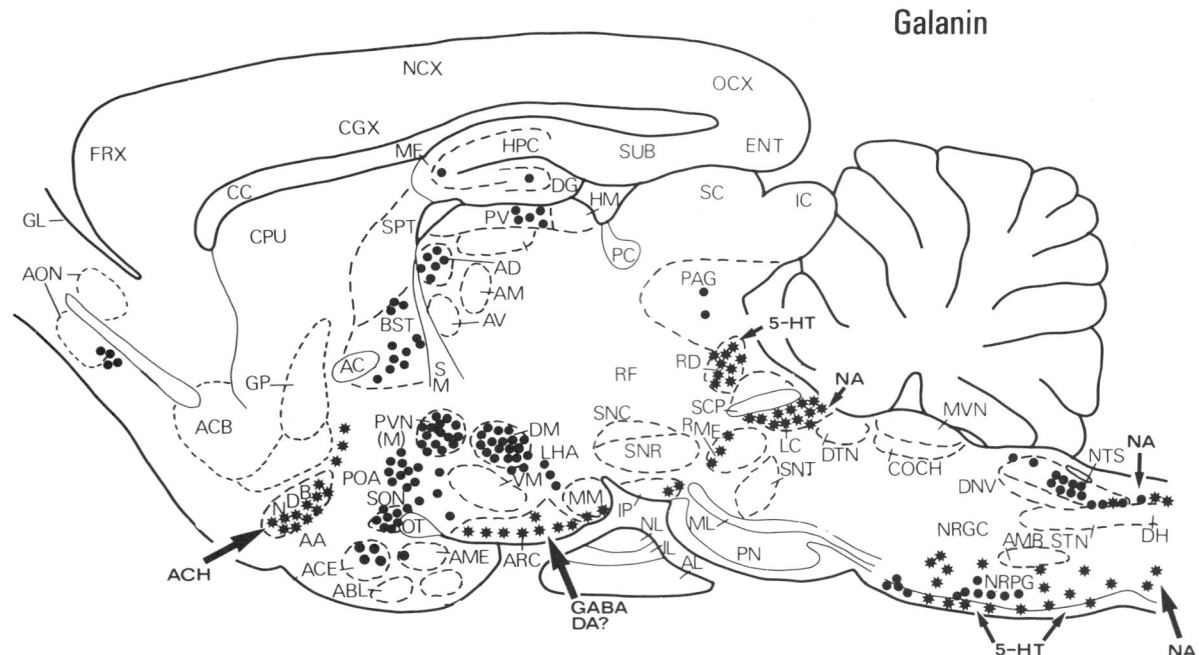

FIG. 4. Schematic illustration of distribution of major galanin-positive cell groups in a sagittal section of the rat brain. For further details see figure legend to Figure 2 on page 406.

particularly high numbers were seen, especially in the preoptic nuclei, arcuate nucleus, periventricular nucleus, dorsomedial nucleus, medial forebrain bundle area, and the various magnocellular nuclei. More caudally, the locus ceruleus and solitary tract nucleus contained numerous GAL-positive cell bodies, as did the caudal spinal trigeminal nucleus and the dorsal horn of the spinal cord.

GAL has been found to be involved in numerous coexistence situations (Figs. 1 and 4) (121–122). In the basal forebrain many GAL neurons in the diagonal band-septum complex contain choline acetyltransferase. GAL-positive neurons in the arcuate nucleus are GAD and tyrosine hydroxylase positive, and in the tuberal and caudal magnocellular nuclei GAD and GAL coexist. Furthermore, a large proportion of the noradrenergic cell bodies in the A6 and A4 cell groups contained GAL-LI. GAL-positive cell bodies in the mesencephalic/pontine and medullary raphe nuclei contained to a large extent 5-HT.

Catecholamine Neurons and Coexisting Peptides

A general feature encountered in the histochemical analysis of coexistence systems has been that a certain type of combination is limited to subpopulations of systems. Above we have shown that only a small proportion of the three peptide systems so far have been shown to contain a particular classical transmitter. Similarly, if we view classical transmitter systems, only a part of such a system, for example the catecholamine neurons, contains a certain peptide (Fig. 5). For example, coexistence of DA and CCK-LI has been observed in the mesencephalic but not in the hypothalamic dopamine neurons (76,78,79). Instead, several hypothalamic (and a few mesencephalic) DA neurons are neurotensin immunoreactive (63). Some epinephrine neurons may contain a CCK-like peptide (78). Furthermore, the proportion of neurons containing both DA and CCK varies considerably among the different mesencephalic subnuclei. Similar findings have been made in the analysis of peptides in other central catecholamine cell groups (43) (for definition of nomenclature, see 36,66,75). Thus, most NA neurons of the A1 group as well as most epinephrine neurons of the C1, C2, and C3 groups contain "neuropeptide tyrosine" (NPY)-LI, and it is present in about 25% of the neurons in locus ceruleus (43,80). So far no NPY-LI has been observed in DA neurons. It appears therefore as if central neurons containing a classical transmitter can be subdivided into subclasses on the basis of presence or absence of a certain peptide.

The most striking example in this respect may, however, be the prevertebral ganglia in the guinea pig, where three distinct subpopulations of neurons have been found, containing somatostatin-, NPY-, and VIP-LI, respectively, and they are located in different territories of the ganglion (103,113). They seem to have different targets for their projections and different functions (31,48). Although less distinctly, differential projections of subpopulations of transmitter-identified neurons containing a certain peptide may also occur in the central nervous system. For example, NA locus ceruleus neurons containing NPY seem to project preferentially to hypothalamic areas, whereas the neurons projecting to cortex and spinal cord lack this peptide more often (80). Thus, the type of combination of messenger molecules may be related to function and/or projection site.

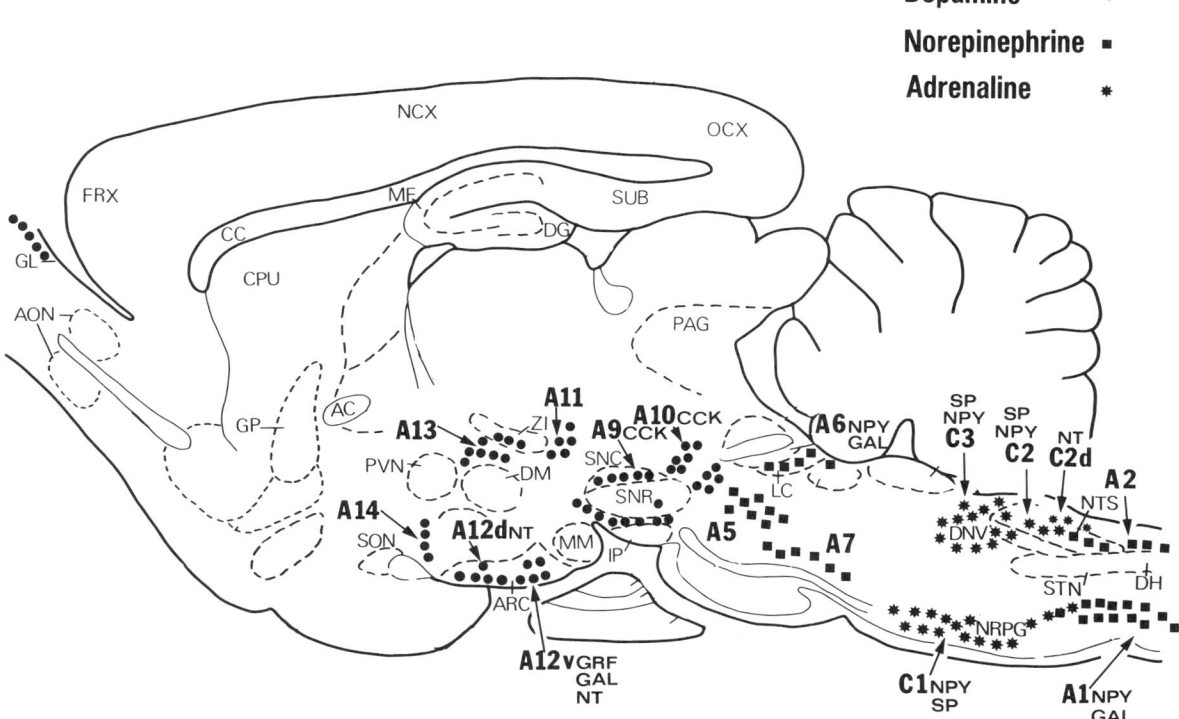

FIG. 5. Schematic illustration of distribution of dopamine, norepinephrine, and adrenaline cell groups in a sagittal section of the rat brain. The nomenclature of the different cell groups (A1, A2 . . . , C1 . . .) according to refs. 36, 66, and 75. Coexisting peptides are indicated by abbreviation adjacent to code for cell group. Note that no peptide has so far been described in several groups.

Hypothalamus—A Region Rich in Peptides and Coexistence Situations

As indicated above, peptides have a wide distribution within the central nervous system, but show particularly high concentrations in certain areas. As an example of richness in peptides and coexistence situations, we would like to mention the hypothalamus. The immunohistochemical analysis has revealed that the magnocellular neurons of the supraoptic and paraventricular nuclei are particularly rich in peptides. These neurons were first shown to contain oxytocin and vasopressin, the first chemically characterized peptides (39,40), and were analyzed in detail by the Scharrers and Bargmann (see 8), who termed them neurosecretory cells. Subsequently these neurons were shown to contain a multiplicity of further peptides, including enkephalin-like peptides and dynorphin (see 18). The parvocellular paraventricular neurons are also rich in peptides, and they include corticotropin-releasing factor (CRF), enkephalin-like peptide, neurotensin, CCK, and peptide histidine isoleucine (PHI) (see 167). Interestingly, these neurons have so far not been shown to contain a classical transmitter. Whether this type of neurosecretory cell, releasing its content directly into blood vessels, in fact lacks classical transmitter or whether the proper marker has not been found, remains to be shown. A third hypothalamic nucleus rich in peptides is the arcuate nucleus, which has been shown to contain neurotensin, growth hormone releasing factor (GRF), GAL, dynorphin, NPY, ACTH/β-endorphin, Met-enkephalin, Met-enkephalin-Arg-Gly-Leu (enkephalin octapeptide), and SOM, and in many cases these peptides coexist with the classical transmitters DA and/or GABA (Fig. 1) (see 44). In a similar way one could go through many other areas in the central nervous system and find extremely complex and rich representation of peptide in neuronal populations, often together in various combinations with classical transmitters. Needless to say, it will be an extremely complex task to reveal the physiological significance, if any, of these histochemical and biochemical findings.

COEXISTENCE—GENERAL CONSIDERATIONS

The finding that peptides coexist with classical transmitters and perhaps other types of messenger molecules raises a number of questions, particularly concerning the physiological role of this arrangement. *If* peptides can act as transmitters, the implications are that neurons release more than one messenger compound at their nerve endings. In this case, how do these compounds interact in causing a physiological response? And what is the purpose of releasing more than one compound? On the other hand, it can be argued that since these neurons apparently already have a transmitter such as NA, which could "take care" of the transmission process, it would be relevant to look for functions of peptides other than such immediately related to the synaptic transmission. In fact, SP, one of the peptides for which a transmitter role has been advocated (137,143,159), has been shown to exert effects on mitotic division in vascular smooth muscular cells *in vitro* (132). Evidence for other types of involvements of peptides has also been obtained.

The idea of ascribing an auxiliary role in chemical transmission to peptides or functions other than transmitters is attractive from many points of view, not least from aspects of the basic properties of peptide metabolism. It is well accepted that classical transmitters are produced by an extremely efficient biochemical machinery. Although this machinery differs between various types of transmitters, they all have one ability in common; the transmitter can be produced locally in the nerve endings, i.e., close to the site of their release. This provides an efficient and rapid way to replace transmitter "lost" during synaptic release. Moreover, it is also well accepted that several of the classical transmitters such as the catecholamines, 5-HT, and the amino acids all can be taken up by efficient reuptake mechanisms at their cell membrane (see 85). In this way replacement of released transmitter can occur not only via new synthesis, but also by reuptake. In marked contrast, peptides are generally accepted to be produced from larger precursor molecules, which are enzymatically split into the active fragments, principally as first described for insulin by Steiner et al. (162).

The implication of this type of biosynthesis is that each peptide molecule released at the nerve endings has to be replaced by transport from the cell body, which represents the sole source for protein synthesis (see 49). (It may be mentioned, however, that it cannot be excluded that in some cases, especially for smaller peptides, enzymatic local synthesis may occur, nor has it been completely ruled out that reuptake of peptides can occur.) In view of the considerable length of the axon, replacement by axonal transport would take considerable time, in spite of the fact that peptides are known to be transported by fast axonal flow (16,50,52). The peripheral branch of a primary sensory neuron in humans may be almost 100 centimeters long, and with a transport velocity of 5 mm/hr, it would take many days to provide replacement in this system. Since peptide levels are not particularly high, in fact peptide concentrations are often several orders of magnitude lower than for the catecholamines (see 14), this long transport time does not seem to be compensated for by excessive stores. In conclusion, a neuron relying only on a peptide as transmitter would have to represent, in terms of function and dynamics, a different neuron from the ones using amino acid or monoamines as transmitters. Instead, a more attractive view seems to us to be that peptides often have auxiliary messenger functions or are not immediately involved in the chemical transmission process. In agreement with this view, evidence that has accumulated so far indicates that peptides and classical transmitters cooperate in causing a physiological response, whereby the peptides may enhance or counteract the action of the classical transmitter (see 112).

COEXISTENCE—SOME GENERAL FEATURES

Species Variability

In many cases the same coexistence situations can be found in several species (for refs. see 65). For example, the 5-HT/SP/TRH systems in the medulla oblongata projecting to the spinal cord have been seen in the rat, cat, monkey, and human. DA/CCK coexistence has been seen in rat, mouse, cat, and monkey but not in guinea pig. These findings suggest that coexistence combinations often are maintained in various mammalian species, but that distinct differences also can be encountered.

Mechanisms for Release of Coexisting Messengers

Studies on the cat salivary gland have given evidence for differential release of peptide and classical transmitter (see 108,110,112). To try to understand the underlying mechanisms, we have studied their subcellular storage sites. It is well known that most nerves contain at least two types of vesicles, small synaptic vesicles with a diameter of 500 Å and larger vesicles, often containing an electron-dense core and having a diameter of about 1,000 Å. In peripheral and central noradrenergic neurons both types of vesicles may store NA (58). In contrast, most electron microscopic immunocytochemical studies have indicated that peptides are exclusively stored in the large-type vesicles (see 145).

To further substantiate this view, we have employed fractionation and centrifugation techniques and compared the subcellular distribution of coexisting compounds in the submandibular salivary gland of the cat, where ACh and VIP coexist in parasympathetic nerves, and in rat vas deferens, where NA and NPY are present together in the sympathetic nerves. The results indicate that in both tissues the peptide (VIP and NPY, respectively) can be observed in the high-density fraction, whereas the classical transmitters appear both in heavy and light fractions. This suggests that peptides in these tissues are exclusively stored in the large vesicles, whereas ACh and NA are present both in small and large vesicles (47,109), and provides a morphological basis for differential release, which according to our hypothesis is frequency coded (see 112). Thus, at low frequencies small vesicles are selectively activated, resulting in release of only the classical transmitter; at high nerve pulse activity the large vesicles will release their content of classical transmitter and peptide.

Coexistence and Plasticity

Coexistence situations seem to represent fairly stable phenomena in the sense that they can be demonstrated in a reproducible manner with immunohistochemical techniques in a particular species and also, as discussed above, often in several species. An interesting question is, however, to what extent phenotypy of coexistence can be influenced. It has been shown in several laboratories that during development, peripheral neurons may change their expression of transmitters both *in vitro* and *in vivo* (13,139,147). This may occur also in adult animals *in vivo* under certain experimental conditions, as shown in studies on the rat iris (12). This tissue contains sympathetic noradrenergic nerves, a proportion of which contain NPY-LI, as well as cholinergic nerves (without a known peptide) and sensory neurons containing, for example, SP. Removal of the superior cervical ganglia causes a rapid and virtually complete disappearance of noradrenergic nerves as demonstrated with formaldehyde-induced fluorescence, and this disappearance is irreversible (117). However, analysis of long-term sympathectomized irides with immunohistochemistry revealed TH-positive networks and NPY-immunoreactive fibers were also encountered (12). These fibers were largely absent after parasympathectomy, indicating that cholinergic nerves under these experimental conditions can acquire sympathetic markers (12). Furthermore, these findings in general terms suggest possibilities of plasticity in the expression of phenotypy also in adult animals, and that they involve not only markers for the classical transmitter but also that a coexisting peptide can be parallelly expressed.

FUNCTIONAL ASPECTS OF COEXISTENCE

The best evidence for a functional significance of coexistence of several messengers comes from studies on the cat salivary gland and rat vas deferens (see 108,110,112), as well as from studies on autonomic ganglia in the bullfrog (86). There are some clues that similar mechanisms to those seen in the periphery may also operate in the central nervous system.

Postsynaptic Interactions

The cat salivary gland receives a parasympathetic innervation containing ACh and VIP (114) and two populations of sympathetic fibers containing NA and NA plus NPY, respectively (116). Experiments by Lundberg, Änggård, and collaborators (see 110) on this tissue have shown that peptide and classical transmitter interact in a cooperative way and enhance each others effects on blood flow and secretion. Thus, ACh induces both secretion and increase in blood flow, whereas VIP has no apparent effect on secretion but can by itself increase blood flow. VIP can, however, potentiate ACh-induced secretion, which possibly is related to findings that VIP can markedly change the binding characteristics for cholinergic agonists to membrane fragments from the salivary gland (111). ACh and VIP infused together produce additive effects on blood flow.

It seems likely that the well-known atropine-resistant vasodilation in the salivary gland is induced by VIP. Both NA and NPY cause vasoconstriction (115), whereby NA causes a rapid, short-lasting effect and NPY a slow, long-lasting decrease in blood flow. Thus, with regard to circulatory effects the coexisting peptides in both the parasympathetic and sympathetic nerves cooperate with their respective classical transmitters. We have suggested that the classical transmitters are released already at low impulse activity, causing rapid effects with a short duration on blood flow and secretion. In contrast, the effects induced by the peptides have a slow onset and long duration and

seem to be induced at high stimulation frequencies (see 108) or alternatively when nerves are stimulated with trains of impulses (42).

Also in the central nervous system multiple messengers may interact postsynaptically in a cooperative way. Here TRH and 5-HT coexist in medullary neurons (Table 1) known to project to the spinal cord, giving rise to nerve endings in the ventral horns (89). Barbeau and Bedard (7) have demonstrated that intravenously administered TRH can markedly activate the stretch reflex in chronically spinalized rats, and the same effects could be observed with the 5-HT precursor, 5-hydroxytryptophan, as shown earlier by Andén et al. (4). The effects of TRH could be blocked by a 5-HT antagonist. Thus, 5-HT and TRH may act on the same or on two closely related (coupled?) receptor sites, possibly on motoneurons. Cooperativity between TRH and 5-HT at the spinal cord level has also been observed in studies of sexual behavior (55).

Presynaptic Interactions

A presynaptic interaction between coexisting messengers has been demonstrated both in the periphery and in the central nervous system. Thus, in the rat vas deferens, which contains NA and NPY in sympathetic nerves, NPY in a dose-dependent manner inhibits the electrically induced contraction of vas deferens, probably due to inhibition of release of NA (1,116,135,165). In the cat central nervous system DA and CCK-LI coexist in nerve endings in the caudate-putamen, arising from neurons in the substantia nigra of the ventral mesencephalon (78). The effects of CCK peptides were analyzed on basal and electrically evoked tritium outflow from striatal slices preloaded with tritiated DA. Sulfated, but not unsulfated CCK-7 and CCK-8, in very low concentrations, inhibited tritium outflow (119). It may be speculated that the inhibitory effect exerted by the two peptides in the two different systems discussed above may serve to prevent excessive release of the colocalized catecholamines.

Mitchell and Fleetwood-Walker (125) analyzed the effect of TRH and SP on potassium-induced 5-HT release from slices of the spinal cord. After addition of cold 5-HT in a concentration known to inhibit 5-HT release, SP, but not TRH, counteracted this inhibition. This indicates that SP acts on the presynaptic inhibitory 5-HT receptor, resulting in an enhanced 5-HT release and strengthening 5-HT transmission in the spinal cord. It is therefore possible that two peptides, SP and TRH, are released together with 5-HT and cooperate with the amine to enhance transmission, but in two different ways, SP by a presynaptic action and TRH, as discussed above, by a postsynaptic action.

CONCLUDING REMARKS

In this article we convey the idea that neurons in the periphery and in the central nervous system produce, store, and perhaps release more than one type of messenger molecule. This adds to our previous view of chemical transmission that multiple messenger molecules may interact at pre- and postsynaptic sites in the transmission process to cause a full physiological response. In addition to transmitter substances such as ACh, GABA, and catecholamines, neuropeptides may also be involved in such coexistence situations. In fact, the main role of peptides in the nervous system may be as auxiliary messengers.

It is interesting to compare neuronal transmitter storage sites with the storage compartments for hormones in endocrine cells (Fig. 6), which early were shown to contain both peptide hormones and biogenic amines (see 138,141) and which in the adrenal gland more recently have been shown to contain, for example, opioid peptides and catecholamines in the same storage vesicles (see 153,163,180). As indicated in Fig. 6, the morphological appearance of these storage sites in endocrine cells seems to be fairly homogeneous, representing essentially "large-type" vesicles, although with a larger diameter as compared to the large vesicles seen in neurons. In contrast, the neuronal storage sites are of at least two types, small synaptic vesicles (diameter 500 Å) and large dense-core vesicles (diameter 1,000 Å). As discussed above these vesicles may differentially store peptides and amines, whereby the small vesicles only contain the classical transmitter and the large ones both classical transmitter and peptide. This may provide a means

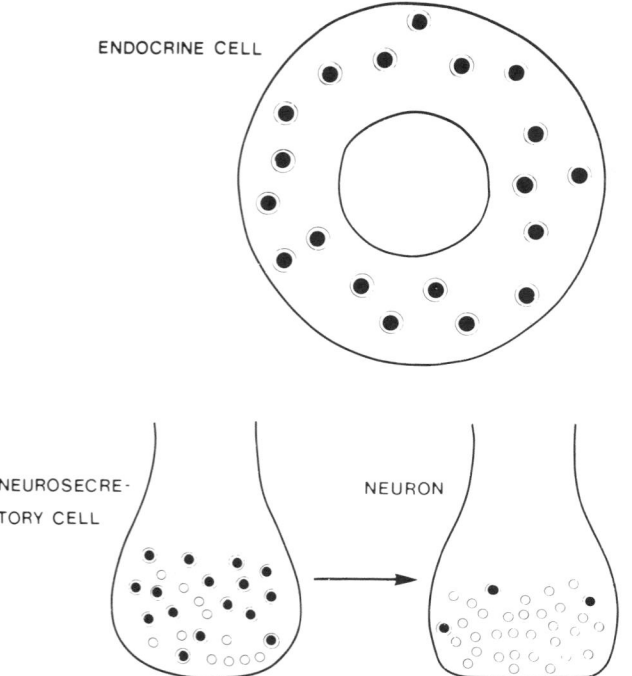

FIG. 6. Schematic illustration of storage vesicles in an endocrine cell and in nerve endings of a neurosecretory cell and of a neuron. The endocrine cell contains only one population of large vesicles, probably storing both peptides and a biogenic amine. In nerve endings there are at least two populations of vesicles, large-sized vesicles with a dense core storing classical transmitter and peptide, and small vesicles containing only classical transmitter. The proportion of large vesicles appears larger in neurosecretory nerve endings than in endings of normal neurons. For further details see text.

for differential release of the two types of messenger molecules. On this basis it could be postulated that endocrine cells are not able to differentially release their amines and peptide hormones, unless, of course, there are intragranular mechanisms that allow selective release of one of the costored compounds. It is tempting to speculate that, in a phylogenetic perspective, the appearance of small vesicles in neurons is related to the demand by the nervous system for faster communication as compared to the endocrine system. This new type of vesicle, the small synaptic vesicles, therefore perhaps developed with the task of storing and releasing exclusively classical transmitters for fast transmission. Interestingly, the neurosecretory cells first described by Bargmann and Scharrer (8), representing an intermediate between endocrine cells and neurons, often contain a higher proportion of large dense-core vesicles than neurons, releasing their messengers at more or less well-defined synapses (Fig. 6).

Although the coexistence phenomenon has been documented extensively with immunohistochemical techniques, our understanding of its functional significance and of the mechanism of interaction between the putative messengers is still rudimentary. Studies in the peripheral nervous system suggest that classical transmitters and peptides are, indeed, coreleased and may interact in a cooperative way on the effector cells. Other types of interactions have also been observed; for example, a coexisting peptide may inhibit the release of the classical transmitter. Therefore, interaction between different messengers released from the same nerve endings may be of several types and may, in a general sense, provide mechanisms for differential responses and for increasing the amount of information transferred at synapses.

It is important to note that the peptides, as discussed above, do not necessarily have to be involved in the process of transmitting nerve impulses between neurons or to effector cells at synapses, but may also have other roles, for example, exerting trophic effects or inducing other types of long-term events in neurons and effector cells. Indeed, it may be argued that the fact that peptides are present in neurons, which already contain a transmitter substance, may provide a basis for "allowing" peptides to exert other types of functions.

Multimessenger transmission may represent a principle for increasing capacity for information transfer in the nervous system. Since this capacity already appears enormous when considering just the number of neurons and their nerve endings in the mammalian nervous system, one may wonder why the nervous system should require additional mechanisms. However, our neuronal machinery has a "hard-to-imagine" capacity and, in spite of the apparent redundancy of neurons and nerve endings, transmission via multiple messengers may be necessary to achieve the outstanding performance of our brain.

Finally, a word of caution should be expressed here. There is, indeed, a discrepancy between the extensive immunohistochemical information and the meager physiological evidence for a functional role(s) of coexisting messengers. The importance of peptides is today in many cases difficult to evaluate, and it is likely that some are more important than others. For example, peptides are probably the main messengers for information transfer from the brain to the pituitary gland, as hypothalamic releasing and inhibiting hormones. In other neurons they may act as auxiliary messengers. It could also be considered that peptides may have played more important roles in lower species, but may have been replaced as important functional messengers by small molecule transmitters. In fact, it cannot be excluded that peptides in several cases are carried along more or less as "silent passengers." Thus, although considerable advances have been made in the neuropeptide field since 1978 when the first volume on *Psychopharmacology: A Generation of Progress* was published, much work lies ahead. Hopefully histochemical techniques will continue to represent valuable tools in these efforts, for example, by analyzing the cellular localization of neuropeptide mRNA with *in situ* hybridization (see 51).

ACKNOWLEDGMENTS

This research was supported by grants from the Swedish Medical Research Council (04X-2887, 14X-7162, 12P-6965), Knut and Alice Wallenbergs Stiftelse, Petrus and Augusta Hedlunds Stiftelse, and Magnus Bergvalls Stiftelse. We thank Ms. W. Hiort, Ms. S. Nilsson, and Ms. A. Peters for excellent technical assistance. Some results in this review article are in part taken from ongoing collaborative research with colleagues as indicated by the papers referred to (see reference list). We thank in particular Professor A. Claudio Cuello, Department of Pharmacology and Therapeutics, McGill University, Montreal, Canada, for tyrosine hydroxylase monoclonal antibodies. Dr. Åke Rökaeus, Department of Pharmacology, Karolinska Institutet, Stockholm, Sweden, for GAL antiserum, and Dr. Wylie Vale, The Salk Institute, California, for GRF antiserum. These antisera were used in Fig. 1. We also thank Dr. S. Watson, Department of Psychiatry, The University of Michigan, Michigan for allowing us to reproduce templates for Figs. 2–5.

REFERENCES

1. Allen, J. M., Tatemoto, K., Polak, J. M., Hughes, J., and Bloom, S. R. (1982): *Neuropeptides,* 3:71–77.
2. Altschuler, R. A., Parakkal, M. H., and Fex, J. (1983): *Neuroscience,* 9:621–630.
3. Amoss, M., Burgus, R., Blackwell, R., Vale, W., Fellows, R., and Guillemin, R. (1971): *Biochem. Biophys. Res. Commun.,* 44:205–210.
4. Andén, N.-E., Jukes, M., and Lundberg, A. (1964): *Nature,* 202:1222–1223.
5. Armstrong, D. M., Miller, R. J., Beaudet, A., and Pickel, V. M. (1984): *Brain Res.,* 310:269–278.
6. Avrameas, S. (1969): *Immunochemistry,* 6:43–47.
7. Barbeau, H., and Bédard, P. (1981): *Neuropharmacology,* 20:477–481.
8. Bargmann, W., and Scharrer, B. (1951): *Am. Sci.,* 39:255–259.
9. Barry, J., Dubois, M. P., and Poulain, P. (1973): *Z. Zellforsch. Mikrosk. Anat.,* 146:351–366.
10. Bennett-Clarke, C., Romagnano, M. A., and Joseph, S. A. (1980): *Brain Res.,* 188:473–486.
11. Björklund, A., and Hökfelt, T., eds. (1985): *Handbook of Chemical Neuroanatomy, Vol. 4.* Elsevier, Amsterdam.
12. Björklund, H., Hökfelt, T., Goldstein, M., Terenius, L., and Olson, L. (1985): *J. Neurosci.,* 5:1633–1643.
13. Black, I. B., Adler, J. E., Dreyfus, C. F., Jonakait, G. M., Katz, D. M., LaGamma, E. F., and Markey, K. M. (1984): *Science,* 225:1266–1270.
14. Bloom, F. E. (1979): In: *Central Regulation of the Endocrine System,* edited by K. Fuxe, T. Hökfelt, and R. Luft, pp. 173–187. Plenum Press, New York.
15. Brazeau, P., Vale, W., Burgus, R., Ling, N., Butcher, M., Rivier, R., and Guillemin, R. (1973): *Science,* 179:77–79.
16. Brimijoin, S., Lundberg, J. M., Brodin, E., Hökfelt, T., and Nilsson, G. (1980): *Brain Res.,* 191:443–478.
17. Brownstein, M. J. (1978): In: *Psychopharmacology: A Generation of Progress,* edited by M. A. Lipton, A. DiMascio, and K. F. Killam, pp. 397–403. Raven Press, New York.
18. Brownstein, M. J., and Mezey, E. (1986): In: *Coexistence of Neuronal Messengers: A New Principle in Chemical Transmission (Progr. Brain Res.),* edited by T. Hökfelt, K. Fuxe, and B. Pernow, Vol. 68, pp. 161–168. Elsevier, Amsterdam.
19. Burgus, R., Dunn, T. F., Desiderio, D., Ward, D. N., Vale, W., and Guillemin, R. (1970): *Nature,* 226:321–325.
20. Burnstock, G. (1976): *Neuroscience,* 1:239–248.
21. Burnstock, G. (1985): *TINS,* 8:5–6.
22. Caffé, A. R., and van Leeuwen, F. W. (1983): *Cell Tissue Res.,* 233:23–33.
23. Carlsson, A., Falck, B., and Hillarp, N.-Å. (1962): *Acta Physiol. Scand.,* 56(*Suppl. 56*):1–28.
24. Chang, M. M., Leeman, S. E., and Niall, H. D. (1971): *Nature New Biol.,* 232:86–87.
25. Chan-Palay, V. (1979): *Anat. Embryol.,* 156:241–254.
26. Chan-Palay, V., Jonsson, G., and Palay, S. L. (1978): *Proc. Natl. Acad. Sci. USA,* 75:1582–1586.
27. Chan-Palay, V., Nilaver, G., Palay, S. L., Beinfeld, M. C., Zimmerman, E. A., Wu, J.-Y., and O'Donohue, T. L. (1981): *Proc. Natl. Acad. Sci. USA,* 78:7787–7791.
28. Chan-Palay, V., and Palay, S. L., eds. (1984): *Coexistence of Neuroactive Substances in Neurons.* John Wiley & Sons, New York.
29. Charnay, Y., Léger, L., Dray, F., Bérod, A., Jouvet, M., Pujol, J. F., and Dubois, P. M. (1982): *Neurosci. Lett.,* 30:147–151.
30. Coons, A. H. (1958): In: *General Cytochemical Methods,* edited by J. F. Danielli, pp. 399–422. Academic Press, New York.
31. Costa, M., and Furness, J. B. (1984): *Neuroscience,* 13:911–919.
32. Cuello, A. C., ed. (1982): *Co-Transmission.* Macmillan, London and Basingstoke.
33. Cuello, A. C., and Kanazawa, I. (1978): *J. Comp. Neurol.,* 178:129–150.
34. Dahlström, A. (1968): *Eur. J. Pharmacol.,* 5:111–113.
35. Dahlström, A. (1971): *Acta Neuropathol.* (*Suppl. 5*):226–237.
36. Dahlström, A., and Fuxe, K. (1964): *Acta Physiol. Scand.,* 62(*Suppl. 232*):1–55.
37. Dahlström, A., and Fuxe, K. (1965): *Acta Physiol. Scand.,* 64(*Suppl. 247*):5–36.
38. Descarries, L., and Beaudet, A. (1983): In: *Handbook of Chemical Neuroanatomy, Vol. 1: Methods in Chemical Neuroanatomy,* edited by A. Björklund and T. Hökfelt, pp. 286–364. Elsevier, Amsterdam.
39. Du Vigneaud, V., Lawler, H. C., and Popenoe, E. A. (1953): *J. Am. Chem. Soc.,* 75:4880–4881.
40. Du Vigneaud, V., Ressler, C., Swan, J. M., Roberts, C. W., Katsoyannis, P. G., and Gordon, S. (1953): *J. Am. Chem. Soc.,* 75:4879–4880.
41. Eckenstein, F., and Baughman, R. W. (1984): *Nature,* 309:153–155.
42. Edwards, A. V., Järhult, J., Andersson, P. O., and Bloom, S. R. (1982): In: *Systemic Role of Regulatory Peptides,* edited by S. R. Bloom, J. M. Polak, and E. Lindenlaub, pp. 145–148. Schattauer, Stuttgart.
43. Everitt, B. J., Hökfelt, T., Terenius, L., Tatemoto, K., Mutt, V., and Goldstein, M. (1984): *Neuroscience,* 11:443–462.
44. Everitt, B. J., Meister, B., Hökfelt, T., Melander, T., Terenius, L., Rökaeus, Å., Theodorsson-Norheim, E., Dockray, G., Edwardson, J., Cuello, A. C., Elde, R. P., Goldstein, M., Hemmings, H., Ouimet, C., Walaas, I., Greengard, P., Vale, W., Weber, E., and Wu, J.-Y. (1986): *Brain Res. Rev.,* 11:97–155.
45. Falck, B., Hillarp, N. Å., Thieme, G., and Torp, A. (1962): *J. Histochem. Cytochem.,* 10:348–354.

46. Finley, J. C. W., Maderdrut, J. L., Roger, L. J., and Petrusz, P. (1981): *Neuroscience,* 6:2173–2192.
47. Fried, G., Terenius, L., Hökfelt, T., and Goldstein, M. (1985): *J. Neurosci.,* 5:450–458.
48. Furness, J. B., Costa, M., Emson, P. C., Håkanson, R., Moghimzadeh, E., Sundler, F., Taylor, J. L., and Chance, R. E. (1983): *Cell Tissue Res.,* 234:71–92.
49. Gainer, H., Loh, Y. P., and Sarne, Y. (1977): In: *Peptides in Neurobiology,* edited by H. Gainer, pp. 183–219. Plenum Press, New York.
50. Gamse, R., Lembeck, F., and Cuello, A. C. (1979): *Naunyn Schmiedebergs Arch. Exp. Pathol. Pharmakol.,* 306:37–44.
51. Gee, C. E., Chen, C.-L. C., Roberts, J. L., Thompson, R., and Watson, S. J. (1983): *Nature,* 306:374–377.
52. Gilbert, R. F. T., Emson, P. C., Fahrenkrug, J., Lee, C. M., Penman, E., and Wass, J. (1979): *J. Neurochem.,* 27:37–44.
53. Glazer, E. J., Steinbusch, H., Verhofstad, A., and Basbaum, A. I. (1981): *J. Physiol. (Paris),* 77:241–245.
54. Goldstein, A. (1978): In: *Psychopharmacology: A Generation of Progress,* edited by M. A. Lipton, A. DiMascio, and K. F. Killam, pp. 1557–1563. Raven Press, New York.
55. Hansen, S., Svensson, L., Hökfelt, T., and Everitt, B. J. (1983): *Neurosci. Lett.,* 42:299–304.
56. Harris, G. (1955): *Neural Control of the Pituitary Gland.* Edward Arnold, London.
57. Hendry, S. H. C., Jones, E. G., DeFelipe, J., Schmechel, D., Brandon, C., and Emson, P. C. (1984): *Proc. Natl. Acad. Sci. USA,* 81:6526–6530.
58. Hökfelt, T. (1968): *Z. Zellforsch.,* 91:1–74.
59. Hökfelt, T., and Dahlström, A. (1971): *Z. Zellforsch.,* 119:460–482.
60. Hökfelt, T., Elde, R., Johansson, O., Ljungdahl, Å., Schultzberg, M., Fuxe, K., Goldstein, M., Nilsson, G., Pernow, B., Terenius, L., Ganten, D., Jeffcoate, S. L., Rehfeld, J., and Said, S. (1978): In: *Psychopharmacology: A Generation of Progress,* edited by M. A. Lipton, A. DiMascio, and K. F. Killam, pp. 39–66. Raven Press, New York.
61. Hökfelt, T., Elde, R., Johansson, O., Terenius, L., and Stein, L. (1977): *Neurosci. Lett.,* 5:25–31.
62. Hökfelt, T., Elfvin, L.-G., Elde, R., Schultzberg, M., Goldstein, M., and Luft, R. (1977): *Proc. Natl. Acad. Sci. USA,* 74:3587–3591.
63. Hökfelt, T., Everitt, B. J., Theodorsson-Norheim, E., and Goldstein, M. (1984): *J. Comp. Neurol.,* 222:543–559.
64. Hökfelt, T., Foster, G. A., Johansson, O., Schultzberg, M., Holets, V., Ju, G., Skagerberg, G., Palkovits, M., Skirboll, L., Stolk, J., U'Prichard, D., and Goldstein, M. (1987): In: *International Symposium on Brain Epinephrine,* edited by J. M. Stolk, D. U'Prichard, and K. Fuxe. Oxford University Press, New York *(in press).*
65. Hökfelt, T., Holets, V. R., Staines, W., Meister, B., Melander, T., Schalling, M., Schultzberg, M., Freedman, J., Björklund, H., Olson, L., Lindh, B., Elfvin, L.-G., Lundberg, J. M., Lindgren, J. Å., Samuelsson, B., Terenius, L., Post, C., Everitt, B., and Goldstein, M. (1986): In: *Coexistence of Neuronal Messengers: A New Principle in Chemical Transmission (Progr. Brain Res.),* edited by T. Hökfelt, K. Fuxe, and B. Pernow, Vol. 68, pp. 33–70. Elsevier, Amsterdam.
66. Hökfelt, T., Johansson, O., and Goldstein, M. (1984): In: *Handbook of Chemical Neuroanatomy, Vol. 2: Classical Transmitters in the CNS, Part I,* edited by A. Björklund and T. Hökfelt, pp. 157–276. Elsevier, Amsterdam.
67. Hökfelt, T., Johansson, O., Ljungdahl, Å., Lundberg, J. M., and Schultzberg, M. (1980): *Nature,* 284:515–521.
68. Hökfelt, T., Kellerth, J.-O., Nilsson, G., and Pernow, B. (1975): *Brain Res.,* 100:235–252.
69. Hökfelt, T., Kellerth, J.-O., Nilsson, G., and Pernow, B. (1975): *Science,* 190:889–890.
70. Hökfelt, T., Ljungdahl, Å., Steinbusch, H., Verhofstad, A., Nilsson, G., Brodin, E., Pernow, B., and Goldstein, M. (1978): *Neuroscience,* 3:517–538.
71. Hökfelt, T., Lundberg, J. M., Lagercrantz, H., Tatemoto, K., Mutt, V., Lundberg, J. M., Terenius, L., Everitt, B. J., Fuxe, K., Agnati, L. F., and Goldstein, M. (1983): *Neurosci. Lett.,* 36:217–222.
72. Hökfelt, T., Lundberg, J. M., Schultzberg, M., Johansson, O., Ljungdahl, Å., and Rehfeld, J. (1980): In: *Neural Peptides and Neuronal Communication,* edited by E. Costa and M. Trabucchi, pp. 1–23. Raven Press, New York.
73. Hökfelt, T., Lundberg, J. M., Skirboll, L., Johansson, O., Schultzberg, M., and Vincent, S. R. (1982): In: *Co-Transmission,* edited by A. C. Cuello, pp. 77–126. Macmillan, London and Basingstoke.
74. Hökfelt, T., Lundberg, J. M., Tatemoto, K., Mutt, V., Terenius, L., Polak, J., Bloom, S., Sasek, C., Elde, R., and Goldstein, M. (1983): *Acta Physiol. Scand.,* 117:315–318.
75. Hökfelt, T., Mårtensson, R., Björklund, A., Kleinau, S., and Goldstein, M. (1984): In: *Handbook of Chemical Neuroanatomy, Vol. 2: Classical Transmitters in the CNS, Part I,* edited by A. Björklund and T. Hökfelt, pp. 277–379. Elsevier, Amsterdam.
76. Hökfelt, T., Rehfeld, J. F., Skirboll, L., Ivemark, B., Goldstein, M., and Markey, K. (1980): *Nature,* 285:476–478.
77. Hökfelt, T., Skagerberg, G., Skirboll, L., and Björklund, A. (1983): In: *Handbook of Chemical Neuroanatomy, Vol. 1: Methods in Chemical Neuroanatomy,* edited by A. Björklund and T. Hökfelt, pp. 228–285. Elsevier, Amsterdam.
78. Hökfelt, T., Skirboll, L., Everitt, B. J., Meister, B., Brownstein, M., Jacobs, T., Faden, A., Kuga, S., Goldstein, M., Markstein, R., Dockray, G., and Rehfeld, J. (1985): In: *Neuronal Cholecystokinin,* edited by J. J. Vanderhaeghen and J. Crawley, Vol. 448, pp. 255–274. *Ann. NY Acad. Sci.,* New York.
79. Hökfelt, T., Skirboll, L., Rehfeld, J. F., Goldstein, M., Markey, K., and Dann, O. (1980): *Neuroscience,* 5:2093–2124.
80. Holets, V., Hökfelt, T., Terenius, L., Rökaeus, Å., and Goldstein, M. (1987): *Neuroscience (submitted).*
81. Holets, V. R., Hökfelt, T., Ude, J., Eckert, M., and Hansen, S. (1984): *Soc. Neurosci. Abstr.,* 10:692.
82. Hughes, J., Smith, T. W., Kosterlitz, H. W., Fothergill, L. A., Morgan, B. A., and Morris, H. R. (1975): *Nature,* 258:577–579.
83. Hunt, S. P., and Lovick, T. A. (1982): *Neurosci. Lett.,* 30:139–145.
84. Ibata, Y., Fukui, K., Okamura, H., Kawakami, T., Tanaka, M., Obata, H. L., Isuto, T., Terubayashi, H., Yanaihara, C., and Yanaihara, N. (1983): *Brain Res.,* 269:177–179.
85. Iversen, L. L. (1967): *The Uptake and Storage of Noradrenaline in Sympathetic Nerves.* Cambridge University Press, Cambridge.
86. Jan, Y. N., and Jan, L. Y. (1983): *TINS,* 6:320–325.
87. Jirikowski, G., Reisert, I., Pilgrim, C., and Oertel, W. H. (1984): *Neurosci. Lett.,* 46:35–39.
88. Johansson, O., Hökfelt, T., and Elde, R. (1984): *Neuroscience,* 13:265–339.
89. Johansson, O., Hökfelt, T., Pernow, B., Jeffcoate, S. L., White, N., Steinbusch, H. W. M., Verhofstad, A. A. J., Emson, P. C., and Spindel, E. (1981): *Neuroscience,* 6:1857–1881.
90. Kangawa, K., Minamino, N., Fukuda, A., and Matsuo, H. (1983): *Biochem. Biophys. Res. Commun.,* 114:533–540.
91. Khachaturian, H., Lewis, M. E., Schäfer, M. K.-H., and Watson, S. J. (1985): *TINS,* 8:111–119.
92. Kimura, S., Okada, M., Sugita, Y., Kanazawa, I., and Munekata, E. (1983): *Proc. Jpn. Acad.,* 59B:101–104.
93. Kizer, J. S., and Youngblood, W. W. (1978): In: *Psychopharmacology: A Generation of Progress,* edited by M. A. Lipton, A. DiMascio, and K. F. Killam, pp. 465–486. Raven Press, New York.
94. Koelle, G. B. (1954): *J. Comp. Neurol.,* 100:211–235.
95. Koelle, G. B., and Friedenwald, J. S. (1949): *Proc. Soc. Exp. Biol. Med.,* 70:617–622.
96. Kohno, J., Shiosaka, S., Shinoda, K., Inagaki, S., and Tohyama, M. (1984): *Brain Res.,* 308:309–317.
97. Kondo, H., Kuramoto, H., Wainer, B. H., and Yanaihara, N. (1985): *Brain Res.,* 335:309–314.
98. Krieger, D. T., Brownstein, M. J., and Martin, J. B., eds. (1983): *Brain Peptides.* John Wiley, New York.
99. Krulich, L., Dhariwal, A. P. S., and McCann, S. M. (1968): *Endocrinology,* 83:783–790.
100. LaVail, J. H., and LaVail, M. M. (1972): *Science,* 176:1416–1417.
101. Léger, L., Charnay, Y., Chayvialle, J. A., Bérod, A., Dray, F., Pujol, J. F., Jouvet, M., and Dubois, P. M. (1983): *Neuroscience,* 8:525–546.
102. Lewis, P. R., and Shute, C. C. D. (1967): *Brain,* 90:521–540.

103. Lindh, B., Hökfelt, T., Elfvin, L.-G., Terenius, L., Fahrenkrug, J., Elde, R., and Goldstein, M. (1986): *J. Neurosci.,* 6:2371–2383.
104. Lipton, M. A., DiMascio, A., and Killam, K. F., eds. (1978): *Psychopharmacology: A Generation of Progress.* Raven Press, New York.
105. Ljungdahl, Å., Hökfelt, T., and Nilsson, G. (1978): *Neuroscience,* 3:861–943.
106. Lorenz, R. G., Saper, C. B., Wong, D. L., Ciaranello, R. D., and Loewy, A. D. (1985): *Neurosci. Lett.,* 55:255–260.
107. Lovick, T. A., and Hunt, S. P. (1983): *Neurosci. Lett.,* 36:223–228.
108. Lundberg, J. M. (1981): *Acta Physiol. Scand.,* 112(*Suppl.* 496): 1–57.
109. Lundberg, J. M., Fried, G., Fahrenkrug, J., Holmstedt, B., Hökfelt, T., Lagercrantz, H., Lundgren, G., and Änggård, A. (1981): *Neuroscience,* 6:1001–1010.
110. Lundberg, J. M., Hedlund, B., Änggård, A., Fahrenkrug, J., Hökfelt, T., Tatemoto, K., and Bartfai, T. (1982): In: *Systemic Role of Regulatory Peptides,* edited by S. R. Bloom, J. M. Polak, and E. Lindenlaub, pp. 93–119. Schattauer, Stuttgart and New York.
111. Lundberg, J. M., Hedlund, B., and Bartfai, T. (1982): *Nature,* 295:147–149.
112. Lundberg, J. M., and Hökfelt, T. (1983): *TINS,* 6:325–333.
113. Lundberg, J. M., Hökfelt, T., Änggård, A., Terenius, L., Elde, R., Markey, K., and Goldstein, M. (1982): *Proc. Natl. Acad. Sci. USA,* 79:1303–1307.
114. Lundberg, J. M., Hökfelt, T., Schultzberg, M., Uvnäs-Wallensten, K., Köhler, C., and Said, S. (1979): *Neuroscience,* 4:1539–1559.
115. Lundberg, J. M., and Tatemoto, K. (1982): *Acta Physiol. Scand.,* 116:393–402.
116. Lundberg, J. M., Terenius, L., Hökfelt, T., Martling, C. R., Tatemoto, K., Mutt, V., Polak, J., Bloom, S., and Goldstein, M. (1982): *Acta Physiol. Scand.,* 116:477–480.
117. Malmfors, T. (1965): *Acta Physiol. Scand.,* 64(*Suppl.* 248):1–93.
118. Mantyh, P. W., and Hunt, S. P. (1984): *Brain Res.,* 291:49–54.
119. Markstein, R., and Hökfelt, T. (1984): *J. Neurosci.,* 4:570–575.
120. Melander, T., Hökfelt, T., and Rökaeus, Å. (1986): *J. Comp. Neurol.,* 248:475–517.
121. Melander, T., Hökfelt, T., Rökaeus, Å., Cuello, A. C., Oertel, W., Verhofstad, A., and Goldstein, M. (1986): *J. Neurosci.,* 6: 3640–3654.
122. Melander, T., Hökfelt, T., Rökaeus, Å., Tatemoto, K., and Mutt, V. (1984): *Soc. Neurosci. Abstr.,* 10:694.
123. Melander, T., Staines, W. A., Hökfelt, T., Rökaeus, Å., Eckenstein, F., Salvaterra, P. M., and Wainer, B. H. (1985): *Brain Res.,* 360: 130–138.
124. Minamino, N., Kangawa, K., Fukuda, A., and Matsuo, H. (1984): *Neuropeptides,* 4:157–166.
125. Mitchell, R., and Fleetwood-Walker, S. (1981): *Eur. J. Pharmacol.,* 76:119–120.
126. Moss, R. L. (1978): In: *Psychopharmacology: A Generation of Progress,* edited by M. A. Lipton, A. DiMascio, and K. F. Killam, pp. 431–440. Raven Press, New York.
127. Nair, R. M. G., Barrett, J. F., Bowers, C. Y., and Schally, A. V. (1970): *Biochemistry,* 9:1103–1106.
128. Nakane, P. K. (1968): *J. Histochem. Cytochem.,* 16:557–560.
129. Nakane, P. N., and Pierce, G. B. (1967): *J. Cell Biol.,* 33:307–311.
130. Nawa, H., Hirose, T., Takashima, H., Inayama, S., and Nakanishi, S. (1983): *Nature,* 306:32–36.
131. Nicoll, R. A. (1978): In: *Psychopharmacology: A Generation of Progress,* edited by M. A. Lipton, A. DiMascio, and K. F. Killam, pp. 103–118. Raven Press, New York.
132. Nilsson, J., von Euler, A. M., and Dalsgaard, C.-J. (1985): *Nature,* 315:61–63.
133. Oertel, W. H., Graybiel, A. M., Mugnaini, E., Elde, R. P., Schmechel, D. E., and Kopin, E. J. (1983): *J. Neurosci.,* 3:1322–1332.
134. Oertel, W. H., and Mugnaini, E. (1984): *Neurosci. Lett.,* 47:233–238.
135. Ohhashi, T., and Jacobowitz, D. M. (1983): *Peptides,* 4:381–386.
136. Osborne, N. N. (1983): In: *Dale's Principle and Communication Between Neurones,* edited by N. N. Osborne, pp. 83–94. Pergamon Press, Oxford and New York.
137. Otsuka, M., and Takahashi, T. (1977): *Annu. Rev. Pharmacol. Toxicol.,* 17:425–439.
138. Owman, C., Håkanson, R., and Sundler, F. (1973): *Fed. Proc.,* 32:1785–1791.
139. Patterson, P. H. (1978): *Annu. Rev. Neurosci.,* 1:1–17.
140. Paxinos, G., and Watson, C. (1982): *The Rat Brain in Stereotaxic Coordinates.* Academic Press, New York.
141. Pearse, A. G. E. (1969): *J. Histochem. Cytochem.,* 17:303–313.
142. Pelletier, G., Steinbusch, H. W., and Verhofstad, A. (1981): *Nature,* 293:71–72.
143. Pernow, B. (1983): *Pharmacol. Rev.,* 35:85–141.
144. Pert, C. B., and Snyder, S. H. (1973): *Science,* 179:1011–1014.
145. Pickel, V. (1985): In: *Handbook of Chemical Neuroanatomy, Vol. 4,* edited by A. Björklund and T. Hökfelt, pp. 72–92. Elsevier, Amsterdam.
146. Potter, D. D., Furshpan, E. J., and Landis, S. C. (1981): *Neurosci. Commun.,* 1:1–9.
147. Potter, D. D., Landis, S. C., and Furshpan, E. J. (1980): *Ciba Found. Symp.,* 83:123–138.
148. Prange, A. J., Jr., Nemeroff, C. B., and Lipton, M. A. (1978): In: *Psychopharmacology: A Generation of Progress,* edited by M. A. Lipton, A. DiMascio, and K. F. Killam, pp. 441–458. Raven Press, New York.
149. Renaud, L. P. (1978): In: *Psychopharmacology: A Generation of Progress,* edited by M. A. Lipton, A. DiMascio, and K. F. Killam, pp. 423–430. Raven Press, New York.
150. Rökaeus, Å., Melander, T., Hökfelt, T., Lundberg, J. M., Tatemoto, K., Carlquist, M., and Mutt, V. (1984): *Neurosci. Lett.,* 47:161–166.
151. Schally, A. V., Arimura, A., Baba, Y., Nair, R. M. G., Matsuo, J., Redding, T. W., Debeljuk, L., and White, W. F. (1971): *Biochem. Biophys. Res. Commun.,* 43:393–399.
152. Schmechel, D. E., Vickrey, B. G., Fitzpatrick, D., and Elde, R. P. (1984): *Neurosci. Lett.,* 47:227–232.
153. Schultzberg, M., Lundberg, J. M., Hökfelt, T., Terenius, L., Brandt, J., Elde, R., and Goldstein, M. (1978): *Neuroscience,* 3: 1169–1186.
154. Shute, C. C. D., and Lewis, P. R. (1965): *Nature,* 205:242–246.
155. Shute, C. C. D., and Lewis, P. R. (1967): *Brain,* 90:497–520.
156. Simon, E. J., Hiller, J. M., and Edelman, I. (1973): *Proc. Natl. Acad. Sci. USA,* 70:1947–1949.
157. Skirboll, L., Hökfelt, T., Norell, G., Philipson, O., Kuypers, J. G. J. M., Bentivoglio, M., Catsman-Berrevoets, C. E., Visser, T. J., Steinbusch, H., Verhofstad, A., Cuello, A. C., Goldstein, M., and Brownstein, M. (1984): *Brain Res. Rev.,* 8:99–127.
158. Skofitsch, G., and Jacobowitz, D. M. (1985): *Peptides,* 6:509–546.
159. Snyder, S. (1980): *Science,* 209:976–983.
160. Somogyi, P., Hodgson, A. J., Smith, A. D., Nunzi, M. G., Gorio, A., and Wu, J.-Y. (1984): *Neuroscience,* 14:2590–2603.
161. Stein, L. (1978): In: *Psychopharmacology: A Generation of Progress,* edited by M. A. Lipton, A. DiMascio, and K. F. Killam, pp. 569–581. Raven Press, New York.
162. Steiner, D. F., Cunningham, D., Spigelman, L., and Aten, B. (1967): *Science,* 157:697–700.
163. Stern, A. S., Lewis, R. V., Kimura, S., Rossier, J., Stein, S., and Udenfriend, S. (1980): *Arch. Biochem. Biophys.,* 205:606–613.
164. Sternberger, L. A., Hardy, P. H., Jr., Cuculis, J. J., and Meyer, H. G. (1970): *J. Histochem. Cytochem.,* 18:315–324.
165. Stjärne, L., and Lundberg, J. M. (1984): *Acta Physiol. Scand.,* 120:477–479.
166. Stjärne, L., and Lundberg, J. M. (1986): In: *Coexistence of Neuronal Messengers: A New Principle in Chemical Transmission (Progr. Brain Res.),* edited by T. Hökfelt, K. Fuxe, and B. Pernow, Vol. 68, pp. 263–278. Elsevier, Amsterdam.
167. Swanson, L. W., Sawchenko, P. E., and Lind, R. W. (1986): In: *Coexistence of Neuronal Messengers: A New Principle in Chemical Transmission (Progr. Brain Res.),* edited by T. Hökfelt, K. Fuxe, and B. Pernow, Vol. 68, pp. 169–190. Elsevier, Amsterdam.
168. Takahashi, T., Konishi, S., Powell, D., Leeman, S. E., and Otsuka, M. (1974): *Brain Res.,* 73:59–69.
169. Takahashi, T., and Otsuka, M. (1975): *Brain Res.,* 87:1–11.
170. Takami, K., Kawai, Y., Shiosaka, S., Lee, Y., Girgis, S., Hillyard, C. J., MacIntyre, I., Emson, P. C., and Tohyama, M. (1985): *Brain Res.,* 328:386–389.

171. Tatemoto, K., Lundberg, J. M., Jörnvall, M., and Mutt, V. (1986): *Nature, Biochem. Biophys. Res.,* 128:947–953.

172. Tatemoto, K., Rökaeus, A., Jörnvall, H., McDonald, R. J., and Mutt, V. (1983): *FEBS Lett.,* 164:124–128.

173. Terenius, L. (1973): *Acta Pharmacol. Toxicol.,* 32:317–320.

174. Tramu, G., Pillez, A., and Leonardelli, J. (1978): *J. Histochem. Cytochem.,* 26:322–324.

175. Tsuruo, Y., Kawano, H., Nishiyama, T., Hisano, S., and Daikoku, S. (1983): *Brain Res.,* 289:1–9.

176. Udenfriend, S., and Stein, S. (1978): In: *Psychopharmacology: A Generation of Progress,* edited by M. A. Lipton, A. DiMascio, and K. F. Killam, pp. 459–463. Raven Press, New York.

177. Vale, W., Rivier, C., Rivier, J., and Brown, M. (1978): In: *Psychopharmacology: A Generation of Progress,* edited by M. A.

Lipton, A. DiMascio, and K. F. Killam, pp. 403–421. Raven Press, New York.

178. Vincent, S. R., McIntosh, C. H. S., Buchan, A. M. J., and Brown, J. C. (1985): *J. Comp. Neurol.,* 238:169–186.

179. Vincent, S. R., Satoh, K., Armstrong, D. M., and Fibiger, H. C. (1983): *Nature,* 306:688–691.

180. Viveros, O. H., Diliberto, E. J., Hazum, E., and Chang, K.-J. (1979): *Mol. Pharmacol.,* 16:1101–1108.

181. Von Euler, U. S., and Gaddum, J. H. (1931): *J. Physiol. (Lond.),* 72:74–87.

182. Watt, C. B., Su, Y. T., and Lam, D. M.-K. (1984): *Nature,* 311:761–763.

183. Weiler, R., and Ball, A. K. (1984): *Nature,* 311:759–761.

184. Zahm, D. S., Zaborszky, L., Alones, V. E., and Heimer, L. (1985): *Brain Res.,* 325:317–321.

Psychopharmacology:
The Third Generation of Progress,
edited by Herbert Y. Meltzer.
Raven Press, New York © 1987.

CHAPTER 43

Multiple Behavioral Effects of Neuropeptides: Past and Future Developments

Jan M. Van Ree and David De Wied

During the past decade there has been growing interest in peptide research. A variety of techniques have been used, including behavioral analyses. Although the basic concept that peptides can modulate nerve functions had already been advanced, the discovery in the mid-1970s that brain and pituitary tissues contain peptides with a morphine-like action (the so-called endorphins) made research in the peptide field increasingly attractive. The idea of peptide modulation of brain functions was first suggested by the observation that removal of the pituitary or parts of this endocrine organ reduced the ability of rats to acquire or to maintain a conditioned avoidance response, and that the behavioral deficits could be corrected by the hormonal peptides produced by the extirpated gland (1,10). Pituitary peptides, e.g., adrenocorticotropic hormone (ACTH) and vasopressin, also influence behavior in intact animals (10,39). Studies of the behavioral effects following endocrine manipulations, e.g., removal of the adrenals, and of the consequences of giving synthetic peptide hormone fragments led to the postulate that not only were these behavioral effects the result of a direct action of peptide and other hormones on the CNS, but that the effects were independent of the classical endocrine effects of these hormones. Whereas classical endocrine effects ("intrinsic activity") are only exerted by the whole or at least a major part of the hormone molecule, small segments of the molecule, which are devoid of the endocrine activities of the parent hormone, can mimic the behavioral effect of the hormone (10,17). The brain was thus shown to be a target organ for pituitary hormones, hormone fractions, and peptides related to them. Peptide molecules affecting the nervous system or present in neural tissue have been designated as neuropeptides (16). We now know that pituitary hormones and a large number

of other peptide molecules are formed throughout the brain. All these are found in peptidergic pathways that link a variety of brain systems.

Neuropeptides are derived from precursor molecules, which may be either pituitary hormones with classical endocrine effects or biologically inactive molecules. Enzymatic processing of the precursor molecules results in the generation of biologically active peptides that may influence brain function. These peptide hormones in turn are susceptible to enzymatic activity, yielding other peptide hormone fragments. This cascade of neuropeptides modulates brain functions. The changing bioavailability of the various neuropeptides, probably controlled by enzymatic processing, allows the peptidergic systems to play a unique role in the regulation of brain homeostatic mechanisms. The way in which information is encoded in peptide molecules can be compared with human language. The different amino acids present in a peptide can be regarded as the letters of the alphabet. Placing letters in a random order yields units without meaning for communication, but a specific sequence of letters creates useful, recognizable words. Removal of one or more letters from a word with a certain meaning can produce words with comparable or totally different meanings (e.g., brightness → bright → right). One word can have two or more meanings, depending on the context in which it is used, and in this resembles the inherent multiple effects of certain peptides. On the other hand, there may exist various words, all expressing the same meaning, which may be comparable to the redundancy present in peptide molecules.

The search for novel neuropeptides, the central action of neuropeptides, and the role of neuropeptides in altering or modulating human behavior are reviewed here. The examples will be derived mainly from the proopiomelanocortin system and the neurohypophyseal hormones. Proopiomelanocortin is present, e.g., in the anterior and intermediate parts of the pituitary, and in peptidergic pathways with cell bodies in the nucleus arcuatus and with terminals in structures of the midbrain limbic system and the lower brainstem (30). Proteolytic enzymatic processing of proopiomelanocortin results in the formation of ACTH and the fat-mobilizing hormone β-lipotropin (β-LPH). ACTH from the intermediate lobe of the pituitary can be processed to α-melanocyte-stimulating hormone (α-MSH) and ACTH from brain, further to a number of other fragments (74). The N-terminal portion of proopiomelanocortin contains an amino acid sequence that resembles α-MSH and has been designated as γ_2-MSH (41). The non-opiate-like β-LPH is the precursor molecule of β-endorphin, a neuropeptide with opiate-like action. β-Endorphin, in turn is the precursor molecule for the opioid peptides α- and γ-endorphin and for a number of nonopioid peptides (6). The neural lobe of the pituitary is the store for the hormones vasopressin and oxytocin, and these can be released to the bloodstream in response to specific stimuli. Both hormones are formed predominantly in cell bodies of hypothalamic nuclei and are transported within axons to the neurosecretory terminals in the posterior pituitary. Vasopressin and oxytocin are, however, also present in distinct neuronal pathways with terminals spread throughout the brain, e.g., in areas of the limbic system, hypothalamus, brainstem, and spinal cord (8). Brain enzymes are especially efficient at converting these hormones to a number of smaller neuropeptides (4,7).

SEARCH FOR NOVEL BEHAVIORAL ACTIONS OF NEUROPEPTIDES

To investigate the significance of neuropeptides for brain function and for initiating behavioral responses, human aspects included, three different research approaches, i.e., physiological, pharmacological, or pathological, can be followed. The physiological approach determines peptide effects on physiological processes that result in behavioral changes. Alterations in the environment trigger sensory perception mechanisms, thus generating information that is transported to the central nervous system, among other targets. This information and other inputs into the brain are integrated at different levels and may ultimately activate or inhibit brain output systems, including motor systems, thus eliciting behavioral changes.

Three aspects of the physiological process can be distinguished, i.e., the relations between environment and behavior, between environment and brain processes, and between brain processes and behavior. The original work of Pavlov (48) and Skinner (51) emphasized the importance of environmental stimuli for the behavior of individuals. Classical conditioning, in which a certain stimulus is conditioned to elicit a characterized behavioral response, and operant conditioning, dealing with a behavioral response (operant) that is maintained or increased when it elicits or is followed by a stimulus (this stimulus is referred to as the reinforcer), are methods now in frequent use in behavioral pharmacol-

ogy and peptide research. When another, neutral stimulus is repeatedly associated with the primary stimulus implicated in the behavioral response, this neutral stimulus can also function as the effective stimulus for the behavioral response. It is therefore designated as the conditioned stimulus or conditioned reinforcer. These behavioral techniques were used in the initial studies on neuropeptides. Acquisition and extinction of conditioned avoidance responses were shown to be improved by treatment with peptides related to ACTH and vasopressin (10,13,58). Operant behavior, including brain stimulation reward and drug self-administration, is affected by these peptides (13,58,61).

Studies using classical and operant conditioning as test procedures remain to be incorporated in peptide research, since environmental stimuli, conditioned or not conditioned, determine most, if not all, behaviors of normal individuals. Neuropeptides may be released or generated by environmental stimuli and may relay information from the environment to the output systems, or may modulate brain processes involved in the transport of this information. There is evidence that certain environmental stimuli can mobilize brain neuropeptides. Thus, the social interaction of rats tested in dyadic encounters is accompanied by the release of brain endorphins (46). Also passive avoidance conditioning leads to the release of vasopressin in the brain (34). However, the data available at present are limited and are difficult to interpret because of questionable specificity of stimulus and neuropeptide. It is difficult to imagine that one stimulus releases one neuropeptide, which transports the information to one output system. It is more likely that a set of stimuli evokes activity in a number of brain peptidergic neurons, resulting in the generation and release of a variety of neuropeptides that modulate the enhancement or depression of the ongoing activity of pathways implicated in the behavioral output system. If the processes underlying the transmission of information from the environment to behavior are to be understood, more attention should be directed to the identification of changes in the brain, including those in the neuropeptide system, in response to precisely characterized environmental stimuli and situations.

Studies involving neuropeptides should include measurements not only of peptide content but also of the turnover of the neuropeptides, of the activity of enzymes involved in the generation of neuropeptides, and of the level and turnover of the precursor molecules and the processes leading to the production of these molecules, e.g., activity of mRNA. The validity of such an approach is demonstrated by the finding that altering the "milieu interieur" affects precursor production; e.g., salt loading increases the mRNA level in the nucleus supraopticus and nucleus paraventricularis of the hypothalamus (5).

The relation between brain processes and behavior has been studied in greater detail than that between environment and brain processes. The microinjection technique was found particularly useful to study both the significance of a brain structure or a process for a given behavioral response and the involvement of neuropeptides in forming the response. For example, applying neuropeptides into the cerebrospinal fluid (CSF) system or directly into a brain region can elicit a behavioral response. ACTH-neuropeptides induce excessive grooming, stretching, yawning, and penile erection when injected into the CSF (2,23). Intracerebroventricular application of γ-type endorphins, as with neuroleptics, induces a grasping response (14). Peptides may also modulate a response evoked by environmental stimuli: β-endorphin injected into the CSF or the periaqueductal gray results in antinociception (54,63); injection into the nucleus accumbens of γ-type endorphins attenuates passive avoidance behavior (32). Also, the activation of certain brain systems by drugs applied to specific sites can be modulated by neuropeptides. An example of this is the antagonism of the apomorphine-induced hypoactivity by γ-type endorphins injected directly into the nucleus accumbens (59). Studies such as these can reveal the site of action of neuropeptides in the brain for eliciting a certain behavioral effect, or allow the different behavioral effects of a given neuropeptide to be separated and the mode of action of neuropeptides to be understood. Immunocytochemistry is a tool for localizing brain peptidergic pathways and binding sites for peptides. The tool is especially useful when modern imaging techniques are used and may well contribute to the search for the site(s) of peptide action.

The pharmacological approach compares the effects of peptides and of psychoactive drugs. A variety of psychoactive drugs have been used for many centuries to influence the brain function of healthy individuals and patients. These drugs include naturally occurring substances and the many psychoactive drugs that have been synthetized during the last decades. In the course of developing these drugs and of elucidating their mode of action, both their interactions with behavioral responses and their molecular site of action, i.e., their binding sites and receptors, have been studied in detail. The test systems used to study the behavioral effects of psychoactive drugs can also be used to search for novel actions of neuropeptides. The best illustration of this method is the comparison of the effect of endogenous opioids with that of morphine-related drugs. However, the presence of these endogenous peptides was first shown *in vitro,* in binding assays and tissue preparations. The endorphins, especially β-endorphin, mimic most effects of morphine: a single injection of β-endorphin induces antinociception, excessive grooming, temperature changes, immobilization, and muscular rigidity, among other effects (3,24,63). The typical effects of morphine-like drugs after repeated administration, i.e., development of tolerance, physical dependence, and self-administration (addiction), have also been observed with β-endorphin (63,69,75). The resemblance of certain behavioral effects of γ-type endorphins and neuroleptics, α-type endorphins and psychostimulant drugs, and β-endorphin- (10–16) and antidepressants (14,15,57,62) also illustrates the results of these comparative experiments. Such studies can be useful for classifying peptides with certain categories of drugs. However, almost none of the peptides thus studied induce a spectrum of behavioral effects similar to that of the psychoactive drugs. The peptides usually mimic only part of the behavioral action of the drugs. The comparison of behavioral effects may nevertheless be fruitful, in particular in the search for possible therapeutic applications of neuropeptides.

The third type of studies, using the "pathological approach," concentrates on pathophysiology and pathology. Behavior can be disturbed by, e.g., alteration in the normal input to the brain (environmental stimuli), by alterations in the brain substrates involved in a particular behavior, and by changes in the output systems. Manipulation of the environment of animals can lead to dramatic changes in their behaviors. As a result, the animals may show a variety of relatively new behavioral patterns, some of which may resemble abnormal behavior of humans. Rats can be conditioned to jump onto a pole in order to avoid an unpleasant stimulus. During extinction, when nonresponding is not followed by the unpleasant stimulus, the response is no longer relevant. Prolonged training results in resistance to extinction, and the resistance can be overcome by treatment with certain neuropeptides, e.g., γ-type endorphins (14). More innate behaviors are also susceptible to environmental changes imposed on rats before and during testing in behavioral procedures. Thus, short-term (7 days) social isolation increases the social interactions of rats tested in dyadic encounters, whereas social behavior is decreased when rats adapted to a low light environment are tested under intense illumination. Both these disturbances in social behavior can be restored by giving the rats the ACTH-(4–9) analog ORG 2766 (42). Environmentally induced behavioral alterations deserve further study, as stimuli may eventually be found that can activate certain characterized pathways or systems in the brain. These specific stimuli could then be used in humans to investigate the existence, or the extent, of damage to certain brain systems. Psychometric tests designed to collect information about the different stages of information processing currently apply methods of this type (52).

Manipulation of brain systems can result in behavioral deficits. Electrically or chemically induced lesions have frequently been employed to achieve this. Application of the neurotoxic drugs 6-hydroxydopamine (6-OHDA) or more recently 1 methyl-4-phenyl-1,2,3,6,tetrahydropyridine (MPTP) (37) into the substantia nigra, the region of the cell body of the nigrostriatal pathway, leads to behavioral changes resembling those observed in parkinsonism patients. The lesioning methods have been used in peptide research, e.g., injection of monosodium glutamate in newborn rats, which destroys the cell bodies of the proopiomelanocortin system in the nucleus arcuatus of the hypothalamus (33). The brain neuropeptide systems can be altered more specifically by injecting antibodies to a certain neuropeptide into well-defined brain regions. Thus, when antibodies to vasopressin are injected into the hippocampus, among other areas, passive avoidance behavior is attenuated (31,73). Chronic treatment with γ-endorphin antibodies into the nucleus accumbens leads to behavioral changes similar to those observed in schizophrenic patients (70,72). Although experiments such as these are useful to link a neuropeptide present in a certain brain region with a behavioral response, more experiments and different tools, e.g., monoclonal antibodies, are needed before definite conclusions can be drawn.

There is almost no information about the changes in output systems concerned with neuropeptides and their effects on behavior. Prevention of a certain behavioral response, and the consequences of this for brain processes and the effectiveness of neuropeptides would be possible directions of investigation. Some understanding of the mechanisms implicated in behavioral plasticity, e.g., behavioral switching could then be gained. The information would be relevant for the design of animal models of certain psychiatric syndromes (38). Experiments using animals with genetic defects instead of normal animals with induced behavioral disturbances could be very useful for finding the significance of various peptides for brain functions. Such genetically defective animals could also be used as models for a psychopathological syndrome. A genetic mutation resulting in a defect in a neuropeptide system may thus contribute to the study of the physiological and pathological aspects of neuropeptide actions. As an example, the homozygous Brattleboro rat with diabetes insipidus, in which the deletion of a single base from the DNA structure leads to the lack of vasopressin synthesis (50), suffers from endocrine and behavioral disturbances. Certain aspects of memory processes are disrupted in these rats, and these deficits can be restored by giving vasopressin and related peptides (11,12,58,73). This supports the ideas that vasopressin and peptides related to it are physiologically implicated in memory processes and that decreased bioavailability of vasopressin may result in memory disturbances. However, it should be kept in mind when interpreting these experiments that one hormone or neuropeptide system is involved in a variety of physiological processes. In addition, variation may be present in the expression of the altered gene material, which may affect the seriousness of the behavioral deficit. Malfunction of a neuropeptide system can be due to a defect in the neuropeptide gene structure, but it can also be the result of alterations in the molecular mechanism expressing the genes. These alterations could be due to genetic variation or, eventually, be somehow experimentally induced.

SEARCH FOR NOVEL NEUROPEPTIDES

There are several methods used for characterizing novel neuropeptides in the brain. Both the peptides and the precursor molecules can be isolated from brain and pituitary tissue and subsequently chemically characterized. More recently it has become possible to characterize the DNA and the mRNA sequences that determine the peptide structure. Some knowledge of the actions of enzymes present in the brain may allow the occurrence of putative neuropeptides to be predicted. The discovery of γ-MSH in proopiomelanocortin (41) and the finding of a peptide present in the precursor molecule of luteinizing hormone-releasing hormone (LHRH), which inhibits the release of prolactin (44), are direct consequences of applying existing information about these enzymes. A cascade of processes is involved in the expression of genetic information into biologically active neuropeptides, i.e., transcription of a gene into precursor RNA, splicing of precursor RNA resulting in production of mRNA, translation of mRNA in peptide precursors, and enzymatic processing of these precursors and of the peptides generated. These various processes are beginning to be better understood and it can be expected that in the next decade studies on DNA sequencing and the processes involved in gene expression will make many peptide sequences available for physiological

and pharmacological research. These experiments contrast strongly with earlier ones in which a characterized effect on behavior (e.g., conditioned avoidance response) or on an isolated tissue preparation *in vitro* (e.g., mouse vas deferens) was used to guide the isolation of a peptide (desglycinamide vasopressin and enkephalins, respectively) (27,35). Research of this latter type, involving both behavioral effects and work on binding sites for peptides and drugs, particularly applying the modern imaging techniques, still has a role to play in the search for novel neuropeptides. The approaches mentioned to search for novel behavioral actions should allow physiology and pharmacology to meet the challenge of linking in a useful way behavior and the many peptides present in the body.

Experiments on structure-activity relationships are one of the tools used to discover novel neuropeptides. The concept of neuropeptides is in fact partly based on results of such experiments, e.g., the finding that ACTH and α- and β-MSH have similar effects on conditioned avoidance behavior (10); the discovery of the different behavioral effects of α-, β-, and γ-endorphin, which are at least partly comparable to effects induced by psychostimulants, opiates, and neuroleptics, respectively (14,57).

The *in vitro* generation of peptides from precursor molecules may also help to uncover novel neuropeptides. Thus, incubation of brain synaptosomal membranes with β-endorphin results in the formation of γ-endorphin, subsequently, of α-endorphin and a number of nonopioid, behaviorally active fragments of α- and γ-endorphin (6). Similarly, incubation of vasopressin or oxytocin leads to the accumulation of fragments that have more potent and selective actions on certain brain functions than have the parent hormones (4,7,9,21). Incubation of ACTH yields fragments, not all of whose effects on behavior have been found (74).

If the DNA sequencing approach or the *in vitro* generation of peptides from precursors is to be used to predict the occurrence of peptides in the body, it becomes increasingly important to know the mode of action of the enzymes involved. Research on enzymatic activity as aimed at the generation of peptides may thus contribute to the discovery of novel peptides.

SEARCH FOR THE MODE OF BEHAVIORAL ACTION OF NEUROPEPTIDES

Several of the behavioral effects of peptides can be described as modulation of ongoing activity rather than as induction of activity. These effects are only present when brain pathways are activated or inhibited by certain stimuli. This could mean that in such cases peptides do not function as neurotransmitters in the reflex-like pathway from environmental stimuli to behavioral responses. A given stimulus may, however, also lead to activation of certain neuropeptide systems with, as a result, enhancement or lessening of the evoked activity in the pathway concerned, e.g., through an increase or a decrease in transmitter release. For example, the training and testing of animals for conditioned avoidance behavior is accompanied by the release of hormones (e.g., ACTH, vasopressin). These hormones and their fragments may modulate the acquisition or maintenance of the behavioral response. The modulatory action of neuropeptides may be exerted at all levels of neurons: in the cell body, by interaction with the expression of genetic information and the synthesis of enzymes and transmitter precursors; in nerve axons, by interaction with electrical activity and the transport systems; in the nerve terminal, by interaction with the synthesis and metabolism of neurotransmitters, the release and reuptake processes, and the fluidity of membranes; postsynaptically by interference with the postsynaptic receptors and the processes in the membrane involved in the translation of the activation of the neurotransmitter receptors.

Although peptidergic pathways are present in the brain, suggesting the existence of presynaptic and postsynaptic elements of these pathways, including postsynaptic receptor systems, it is not clear whether all effects of peptides can be explained by a neurotransmitter-like action. It is well possible that peptides also have a hormone-like action, implying that after their release peptides are transported via body fluids to their site of action, at a distance from the site of their release. A hormone-like action could be the underlying mechanism of the trophic action of certain neuropeptides, possibly contributing to their influence on plasticity of neurons and of behavior. More information about the significance of neuropeptides for plasticity will probably become available in the near future.

The differential effects of a neuropeptide on neurons are also illustrated by electrophysiological data showing that vasopressin, applied iontophoretically to neurons in the lateral septum, can excite some of these neurons, indicating a neurotransmitter-like effect. In addition vasopressin induces a marked, long-lasting increase in the response to excitatory amino acids, this in turn suggesting a neuromodulatory influence (28).

The localization of a neuropeptide may determine to a certain extent which processes in neurons will be influenced by this peptide. Proopiomelanocortin and neurohypophyseal hormones are present together with these peptides in peptidergic systems with cell bodies located in the hypothalamus and with terminals widespread throughout the brain. Other peptides, however, are colocalized with a neurotransmitter and are coreleased with the transmitter (e.g., CCK-8-related peptides in dopaminergic terminals) (26). It is reasonable to assume that these latter peptides primarily modulate the action of the neurotransmitters on post- and presynaptic membranes. The peptides just mentioned, e.g., ACTH, β-endorphin, and vasopressin, may have a multifaceted action on nerve functions. These peptides may modulate not only the activity of classical neurotransmitters but also that of neuropeptides that are more locally available, thus influencing neurotransmitter activity directly and indirectly.

Different neuropeptides may be involved in the activity of one particular neurotransmitter system. For example, CCK-8 and related peptides affect some dopaminergic systems in the nucleus accumbens in the same way as do the nonopioid γ-type endorphins: the hypoactivity induced by low doses of apomorphine is antagonized by these peptides when they are injected into the nucleus accumbens (64). This, however, does not mean that the mode of action of these different peptides is the same, but it suggests that

more than one peptide is involved in the control of the dopaminergic system activated by low doses of apomorphine.

A variety of neuropeptides may control one specific neurotransmitter system; each neuropeptide may have multiple actions on that system, and some of the various actions may be shared by different peptides. These rather complicated control systems are relevant to considerations of peptides and human psychopathology, because the functional lack of one peptide could easily be compensated by other peptides, resulting in normal functioning of the system. This situation illustrates not only the complexity of the brain but also the efficiency of the maintenance of brain homeostasis.

Brain homeostasis can also be achieved through other ways of functioning characteristic of peptide systems, i.e., repetition of a certain peptide sequence, redundancy of the information present in peptide molecules, and involvement of peptides in balance systems. Examples of the repetition of a certain peptide sequence are the sequences Met/Leu-enkephalin and ACTH-(4–10). Such a repetition may be present in one molecule [proopiomelanocortin for ACTH-(4–10), Met-enkephalin in proenkephalin] or across molecules (Met-enkephalin in proopiomelanocortin and proenkephalin). The reason for this repetition is unknown, but it somehow contributes to preserve information for survival during evolution, genetic drift, or damage to the individual. Thus, when a certain sequence is repeated in peptide molecules, the information encoded in the sequence may be very important for the function of the molecules.

The redundancy of information present in peptide molecules means that a certain effect can be elicited by different peptides. The principle that there are synonyms for a specific idea is a useful analogy from language. These peptides may or may not be closely related and it is usually unlikely that a single receptor system mediates the induced effects. Although two or more peptides may share some actions on one system, these peptides may have quite different effects on other systems. For example, β-endorphin has opiate-like effects and γ_2-MSH has opposite effects, thus resembling an opiate antagonist, whereas ACTH-(1–24) and ACTH-(4–10) share some actions with γ_2-MSH and others with β-endorphin (56). That one item of information is present in different peptide molecules may be relevant for the resistance of the brain to stimuli that could potentially disturb brain homeostasis. The duplication may also be of value for coping with a changing environment.

The principles of isomorphism and functional antagonism, as illustrated by the action of β-endorphin, γ_2-MSH, and ACTH-(1–24), are also important for the balance systems in the brain and contribute to homeostasis of brain function. Functional antagonism and opposing effects are quite common in the peptide field. This applies to peptides from one precursor molecule as well as from different molecules. For example, γ_2-MSH can antagonize certain opiate-like effects of β-endorphin (56), a peptide that, like γ_2-MSH, is present in proopiomelanocortin (41); some fragments of γ-endorphin, i.e., α-type and γ-type endorphins, induce opposite effects in a number of behavioral test procedures (57); vasopressin and oxytocin affect some aversively motivated and rewarded behaviors in opposite ways (11,58,61). More or less closely related peptides may thus elicit opposite effects, which suggests that they are implicated in certain balance systems involved in brain homeostasis.

A particular peptide can elicit different behavioral effects. These effects may, however, be closely related, because the brain processes affected by the peptide function as a continuum. It is well known that opium and morphine induce antinociception and euphoria. This latter feeling may be critical for the dependence-creating properties of the two substances. Attempts to separate the antinociceptive and dependence-inducing actions by synthesizing morphine-related drugs have so far been hardly successful. In fact, animal studies have shown that there is a positive correlation between the potency of opiate agonists to maintain self-administration, an experimental model of addiction (55), and their potency to exert morphine-like actions, e.g., antinociception, and suppress morphine withdrawal (68,76). Thus, the antinociceptive and dependence-inducing actions of opiate agonists may both be linked in some way and mediated by similar kinds of receptor systems. The same may hold for endorphins, for β-endorphin in particular. β-Endorphin induces antinociception and is self-administered by animals (63,69). Physiologically, β-endorphin may be implicated in pain, both physical and mental, and in euphoria, i.e., a feeling of well-being (18,25,47,53,67). The inherent reinforcing properties of β-endorphin, as demonstrated by its self-administration, may lead to the development of dependence on behaviors associated with its release. This property may be the underlying mechanism of certain addictive habits. Pain and suffering may be linked somehow to euphoria and addiction and endorphins, especially β-endorphin, may play a role in this postulated continuum.

The effects of neuropeptides may last only as long as the peptides are available, but may sometimes be longer lasting, extending beyond the time when the peptides are present in the body. The latter possibility may be the result of the interaction of peptides with certain brain processes aimed at long-term effects, e.g., learning and memory processes. The long-term effect of vasopressin and oxytocin, for example, may be due to their facilitating and attenuating effects, respectively, on certain memory processes (11). Peptides may also induce changes in the brain that are of variable duration. These changes may be induced by a single treatment or may appear after repeated treatment. The effects following repeated treatment with the peptides are of interest for two reasons. First, the neuropeptides are physiologically permanently available, a situation that may be mimicked by chronic treatment only. Second, the current treatment of psychiatric diseases with psychoactive drugs (neuroleptics and antidepressants) and the "experimental" treatment with neuropeptides, e.g., γ-type endorphins and vasopressin-related peptides in schizophrenia and memory disturbances, respectively, show that the beneficial effects are mainly observed after repeated treatment. The mechanism underlying the effects of repeated treatment may be super- and subsensitivity, as has also been proposed for, e.g., the antidepressant effects of antidepressants. Peptides can indeed act in this way, as testified by the finding that γ-type endorphins antagonize apomorphine-induced hypomotility after a single treatment, but enhance the apo-

morphine effect after repeated administration (59,66). This latter effect resembles the supersensitivity that can be induced by repeated treatment with neuroleptics. Processes such as super- and subsensitivity should thus be taken into account in discussions of the mode of neuropeptide action.

MEANING FOR HUMAN BEHAVIOR

Although human subjects and experimental animals differ markedly as to living environment and behavior, the basic principles implicated in behavioral regulation may differ less. This could permit certain effects of behaviorally active peptides in animals to be reproduced in humans. Here, as in the search for novel behavioral actions of neuropeptides, three approaches can be followed, i.e., a physiological, a pharmacological, and a pathological approach.

The physiological approach includes finding the significance of a peptide for a certain brain function in both animals and humans, and finding whether this peptide is of benefit when the specific function is disturbed. Behavioral experiments in animals showed that neuropeptides related to vasopressin facilitate memory processes (11). These peptides may have a similar effect in humans, as indicated by clinical studies with volunteers (29,65). A beneficial effect of vasopressin neuropeptides has been reported in some, but not all, patients with memory disturbances, especially when the memory deficits were mild (29,65). The effect in animals of peptides related to ACTH, including the ACTH-(4–9) analog ORG 2766, has been interpreted as being exerted on, e.g., motivation, attention, and concentration (13). Such effects have also been reported in humans (49). In addition, ORG 2766 showed effects on mood and social behavior of elderly people. This finding prompted a number of studies on the influence of this peptide on social behavior in experimental animals (19,42,43).

The pharmacological approach involves, first, a comparison of the effects of peptides with the effects of known psychoactive drugs in experimental animals. There follows a search for these peptide effects in humans. There are several illustrations of this type of approach. Endorphins mimic the antinociceptive action of opiates in animals. These peptides exert a similar effect in a certain category of patients with pain (45). In animals, γ-type endorphins and CCK-8-related peptides induce effects that are in part comparable to effects of neuroleptics. The same peptides have a beneficial effect on the psychotic symptoms of some schizophrenic patients (40,70,71).

Thus, the physiological and the pharmacological approach both suggest that at least some peptides may have comparable actions in animals and humans. However, there is only limited information available about peptide effects in humans, and moreover the reported effects are still equivocal. The latter problem may be related to the lack of homogeneity of the disorders in the patient populations treated, to the lack of sensitivity of measures applied to evaluate the peptide effects, or to variations in the treatment variables. We need more sophisticated tools both to delineate groups of patients with a similar pathology and to monitor any beneficial effects of treatment. The target patient populations for the different neuropeptides are not yet well defined. Human studies dealing with peptides should be stimulated in order to try and understand the significance of peptides for human behavior.

The third approach deals with pathophysiology and pathology. It includes the induction of the same pathology in animals as is present in patients. Information about the pathological process in patients with abnormal behavior is, however, almost unavailable. The search for information about these processes includes postmortem studies (e.g., brain levels of neuropeptides), sophisticated psychological testing, and biochemical studies (e.g., brain imaging using nuclear magnetic resonance or positron emission tomography (PET)-scan techniques, which will eventually include the measurement of neuropeptides). This search could eventually lead to some insight into the pathology of abnormal behavior. This insight would be a basis for designing animal models of certain categories of patients. When these models become available, the influence of the various neuropeptides can be analyzed and predictions made for a possible beneficial effect in patients. The existing animal model of drug addiction, the self-administration of drugs (55), is an example of the usefulness of the process. Vasopressin-related peptides decreased the heroin intake of rats during acquisition of heroin self-administering behavior (60). These peptides had some beneficial effects in heroin addicts during methadone detoxification therapy (20).

Certain peptide effects in healthy humans and in patients have been reported, but the observed effects are subtle rather than dramatic. This may be related to the bioavailability of the peptides at the site of action, or to the test procedures used to evaluate the effects and also to the lack of information about the real target population of patients. Subtlety may also be inherent in the mode of peptide action on behavior. The modulatory action of peptides, the control of a certain brain system by a variety of neuropeptides, the repetition of peptide sequences, the redundancy of information present in peptides, and the involvement of peptides in balance systems all may contribute to quench the behavioral effects of a certain peptide.

It must nevertheless be kept in mind that effects of peptides on certain human behaviors have been reported. There is thus a good reason to continue these investigations. Many neuropeptides are present in the human brain and their levels have been shown to decrease in certain psychopathological syndromes. Improving or altering the bioavailability of peptides in the brain after their administration could result in a more pronounced effect of peptides. Some factors enhancing the peptide effects could be the route of administration, which certainly affects bioavailability in the brain; procedures to attenuate the rate of metabolism or facilitate transport through the blood-brain barrier; synthesis of structurally related peptides with increased bioavailability due to resistance to metabolic degradation and increased penetration into the brain (e.g., the ACTH-(4–9) analog ORG 2766). Most human studies to date have concentrated on the neurotransmitter-like action of neuropeptides rather than on their hormonal actions, although the latter may contribute to the trophic influences. These trophic effects may be of significance for neuronal and behavioral plasticity. They may also underlie the reported beneficial effects of ACTH-related peptides on peripheral nerve regeneration in animals after crushing and on recovery from brain damage and in similar conditions seen in aging rats (22,36). Thus, animal and human studies on neuropeptides may fairly soon move in the direction of effects on neuronal plasticity, e.g., in the case of brain damage, and on behavioral plasticity, e.g., the decrease of mental functions as observed in elderly people.

REFERENCES

1. Applezweig, M. H., and Baudry, F. D. (1955): *Psychol. Rep.*, 1: 417–420.
2. Bertolini, A., Gessa, G. L., and Ferrari, W. (1975): In: *Sexual Behavior: Pharmacology and Biochemistry*, edited by M. Sandler and G. L. Gessa, pp. 247–257. Raven Press, New York.
3. Bloom, F., Segal, D., Ling, N., and Guillemin, R. (1976): *Science*, 194:630–632.
4. Burbach, J. P. H., Bohus, B., Kovács, G. L., Van Nispen, J. W., Greven, H. M., and De Wied, D. (1983): *Eur. J. Pharmacol.*, 94: 125–131.
5. Burbach, J. P. H., De Hoop, M. J., Schmale, H., Richter, D., De Kloet, E. R., Ten Haaf, J. A., and De Wied, D. (1984): *Neuroendocrinology*, 39:582–584.
6. Burbach, J. P. H., De Kloet, E. R., Schotman, P., and De Wied, D. (1981): *J. Biol. Chem.*, 256:12463–12469.
7. Burbach, J. P. H., Kovács, G. L., De Wied, D., Van Nispen, J. W., and Greven, H. M. (1983): *Science*, 221:1310–1312.
8. Buijs, R. M., De Vries, G. J., Van Leeuwen, F. W., and Swaab, D. F. (1983): *Progr. Brain Res.*, 60:101–122.
9. De Jong, W., Gaffori, O., Van Ree, J. M., and De Wied, D. (1985): In: *Vasopressin*, edited by R. W. Schrier, pp. 189–194. Raven Press, New York.
10. De Wied, D. (1969): In: *Frontiers in Neuroendocrinology*, edited by W. F. Ganong and L. Martini, pp. 97–140. Oxford University Press, New York.
11. De Wied, D. (1984): In: *Neurobiology of Learning and Memory*, edited by G. Lynch, J. L. McGaugh, and N. M. Weinberger, pp. 289–312. Guildford Press, New York.
12. De Wied, D., Bohus, B., and Van Wimersma Greidanus, Tj. B. (1975): *Brain Res.*, 85:1152–1156.
13. De Wied, D., and Jolles, J. (1982): *Physiol. Rev.*, 62:976–1059.
14. De Wied, D., Kovács, G. L., Bohus, B., Van Ree, J. M., and Greven, H. M. (1978): *Eur. J. Pharmacol.*, 49:427–436.
15. De Wied, D., Van Ree, J. M., and Greven, H. M. (1980): *Life Sci.*, 26:1575–1579.
16. De Wied, D., Van Wimersma Greidanus, Tj. B., and Bohus, B. (1974): In: *International Congress Series* no. 359, pp. 653–658. Excerpta Medica, Amsterdam.
17. De Wied, D., Witter, A., and Greven, H. M. (1975): *Biochem. Pharmacol.*, 24:1463–1468.
18. Dum, J., Gramsch, C., and Herz, A. (1983): *Pharmacol. Biochem. Behav.*, 18:443–447.
19. File, S. E. (1981): *Peptides*, 2:255–260.
20. Fraenkel, H. M., Van Beek-Verbeek, G., Fabriek, A. J., and Van Ree, J. M. (1983): *Alcohol Alcoholism*, 18:331–335.
21. Gaffori, O., Burbach, J. P. H., Kovács, G. L., Van Ree, J. M., and De Wied, D. (1987): *J. Pharmacol. Exp. Ther.* (in press).
22. Gispen, W. H., and De Wied, D. (1985): In: *Normal Aging, Alzheimer's Disease and Senile Dementia*, edited by C. G. Gottfries, pp. 37–44. Editions de l'Université de Bruxelles, Brussels.
23. Gispen, W. H., and Isaacson, R. L. (1981): *Pharmac. Ther.*, 12: 209–246.
24. Gispen, W. H., Wiegant, V. M., Bradbury, A. F., Hulme, E. C., Smyth, D. G., Snell, C. R., and De Wied, D. (1976): *Nature*, 264: 794–795.
25. Henry, J. L. (1982): *Neurosci. Biobehav. Rev.*, 6:229–245.
26. Hökfelt, T., Johansson, O., Ljungdahl, A., Lundberg, J. M., and Schultzberg, M. (1980): *Nature*, 284:515–521.
27. Hughes, J., Smith, T. W., Kosterlitz, H. W., Fothergill, L. A., Morgan, B. A., and Morris, H. R. (1975): *Nature*, 258:577–579.

28. Joëls, M., and Urban, I. J. A. (1984): *Brain Res.,* 311:201–209.
29. Jolles, J. (1983): *Prog. Brain Res.,* 60:169–182.
30. Khachaturian, H., Lewis, M. E., Schäfer, M. K.-H., and Watson, S. J. (1985): *TINS,* March:8:111–119.
31. Kovács, G. L., Buijs, R. M., Bohus, B., and Van Wimersma Greidanus, Tj. B. (1982): *Physiol. Behav.,* 28:45–48.
32. Kovács, G. L., Telegdy, G., and De Wied, D. (1982): *Neuropharmacology,* 21:451–454.
33. Krieger, D. T., Kiotta, A. S., Nicholson, G., and Kizer, J. (1979): *Nature,* 278:562–563.
34. Laczi, F., Gaffori, O., De Kloet, E. R., and De Wied, D. (1983): *Brain Res.,* 280:309–315.
35. Lande, S., Witter, A., and De Wied, D. (1971): *J. Biol. Chem.,* 246:2058–2062.
36. Landfield, P. W., Baskin, R. K., and Pitler, T. A. (1981): *Science,* 214:581–584.
37. Langston, J. W. (1985): *Trends Neurosci.,* 8:79.
38. Matthysse, S. (1986): *Prog. Brain Res.,* 65:259–270.
39. Mirsky, I. A., Miller, R., and Stein, M. (1953): *Psychosom. Med.,* 15:574–588.
40. Nair, N. P. V., Lal, S., and Bloom, D. M. (1986): *Prog. Brain Res.,* 65:237–258.
41. Nakanishi, S., Inoue, A., Kita, T., Nakamura, M., Chang, A. C. Y., Cohen, S. N., and Numa, S. (1979): *Nature,* 278:423–427.
42. Niesink, R. J. M., and Van Ree, J. M. (1983): *Science,* 221:960–962.
43. Niesink, R. J. M., and Van Ree, J. M. (1984): *Life Sci.,* 34:961–970.
44. Nikolics, K., Mason, A. J., Szónyi, E., Ramachandran, J., and Seeburg, P. H. (1985): *Nature,* 316:511–517.
45. Oyama, T., Jin, T., Yamaya, R., Ling, N., and Guillemin, R. (1980): *Lancet,* 1:122–124.
46. Panksepp, J., and Bishop, P. (1981): *Brain Res. Bull.,* 7:405–410.
47. Panksepp, J., Herman, B. H., Vilberg, T., Bishop, P., and De-Eskinazi, F. G. (1980): *Neurosci. Biobehav.,* 4:473–487.
48. Pavlov, I. P. (1927): *Conditioned Reflexes,* edited by G. Anrep. Oxford University Press, London.
49. Pigache, R. M., and Rigter, H. (1981): In: *Frontiers of Hormone Research, Vol. 8,* edited by Tj. B. Van Wimersma Greidanus and L. H. Rees, pp. 193–207. Karger, Basel.
50. Schmale, H., and Richter, D. (1984): *Nature,* 308:705–709.
51. Skinner, B. F. (1938): *The Behavior of Organisms.* Appleton-Century-Crofts, New York.
52. Sternberg, S. (1975): *Q. J. Exp. Psychol.,* 27:1–32.
53. Terenius, L. (1978): In: *Characteristics and Function of Opioids,* edited by J. M. Van Ree and L. Terenius, pp. 143–158. Elsevier-North Holland Biomedical Press, Amsterdam.
54. Tseng, L.-F., Wei, E. T., Loh, H. H., and Li, C. H. (1980): *J. Pharmacol. Exp. Ther.,* 214:328–332.
55. Van Ree, J. M. (1979): *Neuropharmacology,* 18:963–969.
56. Van Ree, J. M., Bohus, B., Csontos, K. M., Gispen, W. H., Greven, H. M., Nijkamp, F. P., Opmeer, F. A., De Rotte, A. A., Van Wimersma Greidanus, Tj. B., Witter, A., and De Wied, D. (1981): *Life Sci.,* 28:2875–2888.
57. Van Ree, J. M., Bohus, B., and De Wied, D. (1980): In: *Endogenous and Exogenous Opiate Agonists and Antagonists,* edited by E. Leong Way, pp. 459–462. Pergamon Press, New York.
58. Van Ree, J. M., Bohus, B., Versteeg, D. H. G., and De Wied, D. (1978): *Biochem. Pharmacol.,* 27:1793–1800.
59. Van Ree, J. M., Caffé, A. M., and Wolterink, G. (1982): *Neuropharmacology,* 21:1111–1117.
60. Van Ree, J. M., and De Wied, D. (1977): *Eur. J. Pharmacol.,* 43:199–202.
61. Van Ree, J. M., and De Wied, D. (1983): In: *The Neurobiology of Opiate Reward Processes,* edited by J. E. Smith and J. D. Lane, pp. 109–145. Elsevier Biomedical Press, Amsterdam.
62. Van Ree, J. M., and De Wied, D. (1985): In: *Endocoids,* edited by H. Lal, F. Labella, and J. Lane, pp. 277–284. Alan R. Liss, New York.
63. Van Ree, J. M., De Wied, D., Bradbury, A. F., Hulme, E. C., Smyth, D. G., and Snell, C. R. (1976): *Nature,* 264:792–794.
64. Van Ree, J. M., Gaffori, O., and De Wied, D. (1983): *Eur. J. Pharmacol.,* 93:63–78.
65. Van Ree, J. M., Hijman, R., Jolles, J., and De Wied, D. (1985): *Prog. Neuropsychopharmacol. Biol. Psychiatry,* 9:551–559.
66. Van Ree, J. M., Innemee, H., Louwerens, J. W., Kahn, R. S., and De Wied, D. (1982): *Neuropharmacology,* 21:1095–1101.
67. Van Ree, J. M., and Niesink, R. J. M. (1983): *Life Sci.,* 33:611–614.
68. Van Ree, J. M., Slangen, J. L., and De Wied, D. (1978): *J. Pharmacol. Exp. Ther.,* 204:547–557.
69. Van Ree, J. M., Smyth, D. G., and Colpaert, F. (1979): *Life Sci.,* 24:495–502.
70. Van Ree, J. M., Verhoeven, W. M. A., Claas, F. H. J., and De Wied, D. (1986): *Prog. Brain Res.,* 65:221–235.
71. Van Ree, J. M., Verhoeven, W. M. A., and De Wied, D. (1985): In: *Antipsychotics, Vol. 3,* edited by G. D. Burrows, T. Norman, and B. Davies, pp. 27–46. Elsevier Science Publishers, Amsterdam.
72. Van Ree, J. M., Wolterink, G., Fekete, M., and De Wied, D. (1982): *Neuropharmacology,* 21:1119–1127.
73. Van Wimersma Greidanus, Tj. B., Van Ree, J. M., and De Wied, D. (1983): *Pharmacol. Ther.,* 20:437–458.
74. Wang, X.-C., Burbach, J. P. H., Verhoef, J., and De Wied, D. (1983): *J. Biol. Chem.,* 258:7942–7947.
75. Wei, E., and Loh, H. (1976): *Science,* 193:1262–1263.
76. Young, A. M., Swain, H. H., and Woods, J. H. (1981): *Psychopharmacology,* 74:329–335.

Psychopharmacology:
The Third Generation of Progress,
edited by Herbert Y. Meltzer.
Raven Press, New York © 1987.

CHAPTER **44**

Neuropeptides as Cotransmitters: Modulatory Effects at GABAergic Synapses

E. Costa and A. Guidotti

COEXISTENCE OF NEUROMODULATORS IN THE SAME AXON

The studies of Guillemin and Schally and those of their collaborators led to the isolation and chemical characterization of three hypothalamic peptide hormones, thyrotropin-releasing hormone (TRH), luteinizing hormone-releasing hormone (LHRH), and growth hormone release-inhibiting factor (somatostatin) (2,8,9,41). With the development of appropriate immunochemical and immunohistochemical technology, it was possible to document the presence of these peptides in neurons of hypothalamic and other brain nuclei (2,8,9,36). Similar work was carried out with a number of peptides such as substance P, enkephalins, endorphins, vasoactive intestinal peptide (VIP), and avian pancreatic polypeptide (APP) (for a review see ref. 30). Though the physiological role of these peptides is still not fully clarified, several lines of direct and indirect experimentation indicate that in certain neurons they act either as transmitters or as cotransmitters (15).

The term cotransmitter implies that in some synapses, transaction of information involves a number of chemical signals rather than only one signal as stated by Dale's law. The validity of this tenet, which was inaccurately ascribed to Sir Henry Dale, is presently questioned by the discovery of the coexistence of two or more putative neurotransmitters

in the same axon. Because coexistence could be shown to be associated to corelease in a few instances, the possibility that Dale's law should be abrogated is entertained by several neuroscientists.

Neurochemically, one can characterize four types of neurotransmitter coexistence (35).

Type 1 neurons contain multiple putative neurotransmitters derived from the same prohormone. At least four different neuromodulators are encoded in proenkephalin and the four neuromodulators are expressed in the same neuron (Leu⁵ and Met⁵-enkephalin, Met⁵-enkephalin-Arg⁶-Phe⁷ and Leu⁵-enkephalin octapeptide). Another example is the endorphinergic neuronal system, where the prohormone proopiomelanocortin encodes for β-endorphin, γ-melanocyte-stimulating hormone (γ-MSH), and corticotropin (ACTH).

Type 2 neurons contain two or more putative neurotransmitter peptides derived from different genes, each expressing a different precursor specific for each of the coexisting neuropeptides. Typical examples are neurons in medulla with substance P and TRH, and neurons in central gray with substance P and cholecystokinin.

Type 3 neurons contain multiple putative neurotransmitters which are both neuropeptides and nonpeptides. Typical examples are neurons of spinal cord with serotonin and substance P, or with serotonin and TRH.

Type 4 neurons contain multiple nonpeptide putative neurotransmitters. Typical examples are arcuate nucleus neurons with γ-aminobutyric acid (GABA) and dopamine, and midbrain neurons with GABA and serotonin.

The above classification requires an operational definition of the terms transmitter and cotransmitter. A transmitter is a neuromodulator that (a) is synthesized and stored in a neuron, alone or in association with other neuromodulators; (b) is released extraneuronally on stimulation; (c) mimics the responses elicited by stimulation of the neuron that stores the transmitter by activating the same signal transduction mechanism through the same specific recognition site. Conversely, cotransmitter is a neuromodulator that (a) is synthesized and stored in neurons where it coexists with other cotransmitters and with one or more transmitters; (b) is released extraneuronally on stimulation; (c) does not mimic responses elicited by stimulation of the neurons where it is stored; but (d) modulates the responses and the signal transduction elicited by nerve stimulation or applications of the coexisting transmitter. Usually, in given synapses, pertinent transmitter(s) and cotransmitter(s) act on contiguous specific recognition sites. Whereas the transmitter recognition site is directly coupled with and activates a signal transduction mechanism, the cotransmitter recognition site functions as an allosteric modulatory site for the transmitter recognition site or for the device coupling the transmitter recognition site with the transducer mechanism. In relation to GABAergic receptor modulation, the question then arises, can all the classic nonpeptide neurotransmitters (amines and amino acids) be included in the type 3 or 4 neurons of the above-mentioned classification? Until quite recently there was no evidence for the coexistence of GABA with a neuromodulatory peptide. Now that such evidence is available (10,13,28,36), we can identify new subclasses of GABAergic neurons, each with specific neurochemical, functional, and pharmacological profiles. This possibility is enhanced by the existence of GABA$_A$ and GABA$_B$ receptors, each with specific pharmacological profiles, cotransmitter systems, and signal transduction mechanisms (7).

TRANSMITTER AND COTRANSMITTER RECEPTORS AS SUPRAMOLECULAR ENTITIES

At one time transmitter receptors were conceived as simple monomolecular entities embedded in the phospholipid bilayers of neuronal membranes, endowed with specific recognition sites for the transmitter, and operative in triggering specific response in the postsynaptic cell (3,46). At that time, a major focus in receptor studies was the structural complementarity of the chemical configuration of the recognition site and of the transmitter. On the basis of studies of chemical structure complementarity, specific transmitter receptor agonists and antagonists were discovered that soon became important pharmacological tools to further our understanding of receptor function. It is not surprising that a major goal of neuropharmacology was that of developing drugs blocking or stimulating specific receptors. In a way, classical neuropharmacology was conceived as a chemotherapy of receptor dysfunction; drugs were developed that specifically inhibit or stimulate a receptor function. With the discovery by Sutherland and his associates (39) that adenylate cyclase operates in signal transduction at adrenergic and other transmitter receptors and the subsequent report by Rodbell (40) that GTP modulates transmitter-mediated cyclase activation, specific GTP-dependent receptor coupling proteins were discovered. Thus, receptors slowly became supramolecular structures including at least three intrinsic structural characteristics: a recognition site for the transmitter, a coupling system, and a signal transducer system.

We do not attempt to classify possible families of receptors on the basis of their functional characteristics because our knowledge is still too sketchy. However, for the sake of communication we would like to indicate two major classes of transmitter receptors: those with ionophoric, and those with enzymatic signal transduction mechanisms. Ionophore-linked receptors are formed by polymeric proteins that form the lining of transmitter-regulated ion channels that allow the passage of specific ions through the cell membrane. A transmitter recognition site is located in one of the monomeric polypeptide chains forming the ionophore. The tertiary structure of the chain(s) can change when a specific ligand binds to this recognition site. These tertiary structure changes lead to the formation of specific membrane pores that allow specific transmembrane ion fluxes according to the ion concentration gradient. Since the intracellular ion steady-state changes generated by these fluxes trigger specific changes in the protoplasmic enzymes adjacent to the cell membranes, phosphorylation or other covalent modifications of specific membrane proteins may ultimately be responsible for the changes in cell function. Some channels require depolarization to respond to the transmitter (voltage-dependent ion channels).

The receptors with enzyme-linked signal transduction function are also supramolecular entities with an allosteric site for the regulation of transmitter-elicited activation of the specific enzymes. At the level of present understanding, three major enzymes that are coupled to transmitter recognition sites in signal transduction can be delineated as models: adenylate cyclase, guanylate cyclase, and a specific phosphodiesterase. The latter, by acting on phosphatidylinositol diphosphate (PIP$_2$), generates inositol triphosphate (IP$_3$) and diacylglycerol (DG) (3,4). Though our understanding might still be far from complete, the number of transducing systems seems to be small in comparison to the sophistication of the communication being handled at various brain synapses. The multiplicity of messages operative in the modulation of transmitter receptor function not only adds refinement in the regulation of communication but extends specificity of control beyond the limits imposed by the apparently small variety of transducer systems available. From a pharmacological standpoint, this modulation offers a rare opportunity to let nature be a determining element of the research strategy. Thus, future drug developments may not have to achieve a blockade of receptor function by occupying transmitter recognition sites with molecules of high intrinsic activity; rather, new drug targets may be the mechanisms of allosteric modulation of receptor function. The number of untoward side effects generated by the chemotherapy of transmitter recognition sites exemplified by the antipsychotics that block dopamine receptors may be reduced when drugs will act at the cotransmitter recognition sites, modulating, rather than permanently injuring, transmitter function. In molecular terms, the enzymatic processes that are activated in signal transduction depend on a series of interactions among the various protein constituents of the supramolecular structure. The endpoint of each interaction is to generate conformational changes in the protein next in line. As a result of these changes, the enzymatic activity of specific membrane enzymes is enhanced. These enzymes, by using membrane components (PIP_2) or typical intermediate metabolism products (ATP or GTP) as a substrate, generate second messengers such as cyclic AMP, cyclic GMP, IP_3, and DG operative in the signal propagation to various subcellular compartments. The second messengers, IP_3 and DG, result from a cannibalism of phospholipid plasma membrane constituents (34). Thus phospholipids, once thought to be inert cell constituents, are gradually becoming substrates that yield formation of second messengers. Hence, a plasma membrane constituent becomes the starting material for the synthesis of important cellular modulators. In this novel scenario phospholipids and glycolipids, in addition to being the structural components that separate the protoplasm of two cells, have become operative in receptor modulation or vectors of intracellular signal diffusion. The interaction between signal recognition and transducer protein is mediated by a family of proteins that are not active unless they bind guanosine triphosphate (GTP), and are therefore termed G proteins (40). This family of proteins may not be the only class of receptor coupling devices. For instance, in GABA receptors, GABA modulin, a basic neuronal membrane protein (24,49), may be the coupling device. In the receptors for dicarboxylic excitatory amino acids a Mg^{2+}-binding protein might be operative in receptor modulation. There are three fundamental steps in enzyme-linked receptor function: signal recognition, amplification, and transduction; cotransmitters modulate phase 1, 2, or 3, but can initiate only phase 2. In contrast, the transmitter initiates the chain of events, but cannot modulate the intensity of the final response, for it depends in part on G protein amplification and cotransmitter modulation. Two or more types of G protein appear to be involved; one of them is stimulatory (G_S) and the other is inhibitory (G_I) (40). The activity of the complex of any G protein and GTP is ended by the hydrolysis of the GTP to GDP. In the pathways where cyclases or phosphodiesterase are operative, the final message is one of protein phosphorylation by specific protein kinase activated by either cyclic AMP or cyclic GMP, DG, and Ca^{2+}. The latter is currently considered as a second messenger being released from the endoplasmic reticulum and other intracellular particles by IP_3 (45).

Cl^- IONOPHORE IN SIGNAL TRANSDUCTION AT $GABA_A$ SYNAPSES

GABA receptors mediate neuronal inhibition and can be subdivided into two major receptor classes termed $GABA_A$ and $GABA_B$ (7). $GABA_A$ recognition sites are coupled to Cl^- ionophores, which are activated by GABA, muscimol isoguvacine, and THIP (4,5,6,7-tetrahydroisoxazolo [5,4-c] pyridin-3-Ol), but not by baclofen. $GABA_A$ receptor activation is facilitated by benzodiazepines and inhibited by bicuculline. Using a series of benzodiazepine derivatives, the anxiolytic and spasmolytic activity is related to their affinity for specific synaptic recognition sites and to their capacity to allosterically increase the B_{max} of GABA binding to $GABA_A$ recognition sites and their ability to increase the probability for Cl^- channel openings (16,26). GABA recognition sites are also inhibitory, but are linked to K^+ or Ca^{2+} channels, are activated by GABA and baclofen but not by muscimol and THIP, and their activity is neither facilitated by benzodiazepines nor inhibited by bicuculline (7). There is a reciprocal relationship between GABA and benzodiazepine when one studies the binding of one compound in the presence of the other. GABA lowers the K_D of benzodiazepine binding and benzodiazepines enhance B_{max} of GABA binding (22). $GABA_A$ receptors also have another modulatory binding site located in the GABA receptor-ion channel complex, which accepts as preferred ligand [^3H]dihydropicrotoxinin, and [^{35}S]t-butyl bicyclophorothionate (TBPS) and some barbiturates (21,37,48). The coupling of these Cl^- channel modulatory sites to the GABA-receptor complex is supported by studies of the Cl^--dependent modulation and of the picrotoxin modulation of GABA and benzodiazepine binding to their recognition sites (17,48). The pharmacological specificity of these test tube interactions has been supported by electrophysiological studies of the GABA modifications of facilitated Cl^- currents in whole cell patch-clamping studies by benzodiazepines and barbiturates (47). GABA activates opening bursts of Cl^- ionophores, which are not caused by either barbiturates or benzodiazepines, but which facilitate GABA action. Facilitation of GABA-mediated Cl^- ionophore activation by benzodiazepines and barbiturates can be differentiated because barbiturates decrease the slope of extinction of GABA-activated Cl^- currents in patch-clamp studies in whole cells. In contrast, benzodiazepines enhance the intensity and decrease the extinction slope of Cl^- currents elicited by GABA. One interpretation of these findings is that benzodiazepines prolong the bursts by increasing the probability of channel openings by GABA whereas barbiturates increase the opening time of the Cl^- channels.

Schoch et al. (42) have developed monoclonal antibodies directed against the $GABA_A$-receptor complex. A clear colocalization of high-affinity GABA and benzodiazepine binding sites on the same protein complex was shown by immunoprecipitation of [^3H]muscimol and [^3H]flunitrazepam binding sites. Binding of benzodiazepines to the precipitated receptor could be stimulated by micromolar concentrations of GABA, which indirectly suggests that a low-affinity GABA binding site is located in the receptor purified by immunoprecipitation. This brings up the question of whether high- or low-affinity recognition sites have physiological importance. The question, in our view, is still unresolved, because binding studies *in vitro* express an equilibrium that never occurs in neurotransmission; hence it may be difficult to compare the results of binding and physiological experiments on neurotransmission. In addition, immunoprecipitation experiments also demonstrated the presence of TBPS binding sites on the same structural complex (5). The use of specific monoclonal antibodies recognizing either 50- or 55-K subunits showed that complete immunoprecipitation of a purified receptor preparation can be obtained irrespective of the antibody used (27). This suggests that the receptor contains a mixing of the 50- and 55-K subunits. Moreover, the use of these antibodies demonstrated that both subunits are present in the GABA receptor of cerebellum as well as in any other brain structure tested. Hence, GABA$_A$ receptor is homogeneous in the different regions of rat brain. The distinction of subpopulation of GABA$_A$ receptors on the basis of the presence of 50- or 55-K subunits cannot be made. This distinction cannot be made histologically using [³H]muscimol, [³H]Ro15-1788, the monoclonal antibodies, or [³⁵S]TBPS. Finally, using electron microscopy and monoclonal antibodies, it could be further stressed that GABA$_A$ receptors are located on synaptic membranes (27,42).

ENDOCOIDS FOR THE BENZODIAZEPINE/β-CARBOLINE BINDING SITES

The search for putative endocoids that act as ligands for the benzodiazepine/β-carboline (BZ/BC) binding sites has not been an easy task due to the lack of specific and reliable detection methods. Traditionally, endocoids of the opiate peptide family have been studied by investigating whether tissue or biological fluid extracts could displace a radioactive ligand of opioid receptors from its specific binding site. Although this has been the initial method adopted to search for a putative endogenous ligand for the benzodiazepine binding site (4,25,32,44), the complexity of the interactions among GABA/BZ/BC recognition sites located in the ionophore complex has made it increasingly clear that [³H]benzodiazepine binding to crude synaptic membranes lacks the specificity required to monitor the purification of a putative endocoid for these binding sites. Besides the several methodological pitfalls inherent to binding studies in general, one particular complication in the case of [³H]BZ and [³H]BC displacement studies is the already mentioned allosteric interaction between the different binding sites in the GABA/BZ, BC/Cl⁻ ionophore receptor complex (16,22).

In searching for endocoids displacing specific ligands from the BZ/BC binding sites, a number of important characteristics of the intrinsic ligand must be evaluated, including its intrinsic activity, potency, and profile. These characteristics may resemble that of benzodiazepines, thereby relieving anxiety, inhibiting convulsions, and amplifying GABA signal transduction, or may mimic the 3-carboxylic acid esters of β-carbolines, causing anxiety, facilitating convulsions, and restricting GABA signal transduction. Should the endocoid be a polypeptide, the binding to crude synaptic membrane preparations may be hampered by the presence of peptidases. In fact, early studies (23) have shown that brain extracts contained a peptide, which was termed DBI (diazepam binding inhibitor) because it displaces [³H]BZ and [³H]BC. To circumvent the technical problems inherent in the peptide nature of the putative endocoid, we had to modify the assay procedure to make it more appropriate for a peptide.

Binding Technology to Monitor the Purification of the Endocoid

Ligand binding to primary cultures of CNS cells has been used as the method to monitor the endocoid peptide during purification. The granule cells were prepared from 8-day-old rats as described by Gallo et al. (21). This culture consists of an almost pure population of morphologically defined and functionally viable granule cells with few (2–3%) GABAergic neurons and scattered (4%) glial cells. The intact monolayer of granule cells in culture revealed the presence of a classic GABA/BZ/BC/Cl⁻ ionophore complex. The cell culture binding sites for [³H]flunitrazepam ([³H]F) and β-[³H]carboline-3-carboxylate methylester ([³H]BCCM) are saturable (B_{max} = 500 and 450 fmol/mg prot, respectively) and possess a high-affinity binding site (apparent K_d = 10 and 3 nM, respectively). GABA (from 10^{-6} to 10^{-4} M) increases [³H]F and decreases [³H]BCCM binding in a dose related manner. We elected to use granule cell in primary cultures to monitor the purification of the endocoid for the following reasons: (a) the peptidase activity of intact granule cell culture media is lower than in the media of crude synaptic membrane preparations; (b) the granule cell culture binds BC with high affinity and specificity whereas BZ displaces BC with low affinity and a Hill slope smaller than the unit; (c) granule cell cultures are practically free of DBI immunoreactive peptides, and immunohistochemically, only few (less than 1%) unidentified cells (perhaps oligodendrocytes) can be stained reliably with rat DBI antibody. Moreover, by using primary culture of brain neurons one can conduct the same cell binding studies and electrophysiological recording and evaluate the intrinsic activity of the putative ligands. To this end we have monitored GABA-mediated Cl⁻ currents on primary cultures of patch-clamped cerebellar granule cells (50) or spinal cord neurons (6). Benzodiazepines and β-carboline derivatives, which bind with high affinity to the domain for the allosteric regulation of GABA receptors, increased or decreased the probability for GABA to activate Cl⁻ ionophore opening bursts (6,50).

Behavioral Technology to Elucidate Biological Profile of the Endocoid

The rat conflict paradigm has predictive value for anxiolytic activity of drugs acting at the GABA/BZ, BC/Cl⁻ ionophore receptor complex. In this model a positive or appetitive stimulus is coupled with a negative or aversive stimulus. Depending on the respective intensity of the positive and negative stimuli, the animal behavior will show varying degrees of responsiveness. A conflict test that is simple and reliable and does not involve animal training is the Vogel's test (51). In this test, water-deprived rats are placed in a chamber with a water source. In the absence of punishment, rats usually lick at the water spout almost without interruption for the 3-min test period, totaling approximately 25 licking periods of 3 sec each. During the conflict session, following each 3 sec of continuous licking, an electric shock of 0.2 sec duration is delivered through the drinking tube. If a high-intensity current (1 mA) is used, the animal behavior is almost completely suppressed. These experimental conditions are normally used to study anxiolytic drugs that exert an anticonflict effect. In contrast, by using an aversive stimulus of low intensity (current of 0.3 mA), the Vogel paradigm became suitable to evaluate drugs for their ability to suppress punished behavior. These experimental conditions are used to study anxiogenic drugs that exert a "proconflict effect" (11). According to their effects on the conflict test, the ligands for benzodiazepine receptors can be classified into three categories: (a) ligands that possess anticonflict action (anxiolytic benzodiazepines); (b) ligands that possess proconflict action (anxiogenic β-carbolines); (c) ligands that possess neither proconflict nor anticonflict actions but antagonize the actions of proconflict and anticonflict drugs; these ligands are classified as antagonists.

A facilitation of GABAergic transmission participates in the anticonflict action of benzodiazepines (12). In contrast, the behavioral proconflict action of β-carboline derivatives is mediated by a decrease in the GABA receptor function (13). Thus, the Vogel test in rat can be a useful tool to identify the biological profile of putative endocoids for the BZ/BC recognition sites and to determine their intrinsic activity.

IDENTIFICATION OF A DIAZEPAM BINDING INHIBITOR PEPTIDE: AN ENDOCOID FOR THE BZ/BC RECOGNITION SITE ENDOWED WITH β-CARBOLINE-LIKE ACTION

The existence of an endocoid that modulates the BZ-GABA receptor complex was suggested by the early observation (25) that brain extracts contained a peptide that produced an increase of the K_d binding of diazepam without influencing its B_{max}. Recently, we (23) have been successful in isolating a neuropeptide from brain that has affinity for the β-carboline recognition sites present on cerebellar granule cells in primary culture (20), decreases in an Ro15-1788-reversible fashion the GABA-induced increase in Cl⁻ conductance in primary culture of mouse spinal cord (6), and induces proconflict responses (blocked by pretreatment with Ro15-1788) when injected intracerebroventricularly in rats subjected to conflict-punishment test (23).

Biochemistry of DBI

DBI is a 105-amino-acid peptide originally extracted from rat (23) and more recently extracted from human brain (18). DBI was extracted by homogenizing the brain in 10 volumes of hot (90°C) 1 N acetic acid and was purified to homogeneity by using gel filtration, ammonium sulfate fractionation, and reverse-phase high-performance liquid chromatography (HPLC) using different columns

and solvent systems. The purity of DBI was established by the presence of a single band of protein in acid urea or sodium dodecyl sulfate (SDS) polyacrylamide gel electrophoresis, or by the presence of a single UV (210 nm) absorbing peak by three different column systems on HPLC. The sequence of DBI could not be determined by the Edmond degradation method due to the blockage of the amino terminus. We circumvented this obstacle by fragmenting the peptide with CNBr or trypsin digestion. By combining the sequence of DBI fragments generated with these two procedures we obtained partial information on the sequence of 78 out of 105 amino acid residues of DBI. The sequence of the carboxyl terminal fragment was determined and partial sequence of the middle fragments was obtained. Computer analysis revealed that the sequences obtained by DBI digestion are not present in any other known peptide, indicating that DBI belong to a novel family of endogenous peptides.

The information obtained with CNBr and trypsin digestion allowed for the synthesis of complementary DNA probes, which by a nick translation process were converted into a radioactive probe and used to hybridize specific complementary mRNA inserted in clones of specific vectors. This mRNA was then converted into the cDNA and read to obtain the amino acid sequence of DBI. The partial sequence of rat brain DBI known up-to-date is: 27 K-L-R-G-K-R-L-K-T-Q-P-T-D-E-E-M-L-F-I-Y-S-H-F-K-Q-A-T-V-G-D-V-N-T-D-R-P-G-L-L-D-L-K-G-K-A-R-W-D-S-W-N-K-L-K-G-T-S-K-E-N-A-M-K-T-Y-V-E-K-V-E-E-L-K-K-K-Y-G-I COOH 105.

Pharmacology of DBI

Using binding to cerebellar granular cells, it was confirmed (20) that DBI displaces [³H]BZ from their binding on the cell surface with a K_1 in the micromolar concentration range (Table 1). However, it was also observed that DBI potency in displacing [³H]BC was higher than that for the displacement of [³H]BZ. In a group of binding experiments we tested whether the potency of DBI in displacing the binding of the imidazobenzodiazepine ([³H]Ro15-1788) shifts in the presence of GABA. As reported by Mohler et al. (33), [³H]Ro15-1788 binding was unchanged by GABA in the incubation medium, whereas the displacement of [³H]Ro15-1788 by anxiolytic benzodiazepines, but not the anxiogenic β-carbolines, was potentiated by GABA. In this binding test DBI functions as a β-carboline in that it displaces [³H]Ro15-1788 in a GABA-independent manner (14).

The most direct approach to test whether DBI has a pharmacological profile similar to that of the classical benzodiazepines or to that of the classical β-carbolines was to test the modulation by DBI of the GABA-mediated Cl⁻ channel opening studied electrophysiologically.

When DBI was tested in mouse spinal cord neurons grown in primary culture and patch-clamped for the recording of the whole-cell Cl⁻ current generated by GABA, this peptide, which is devoid, *per se,* of an action on the Cl⁻ ionophores that are modulated by GABA, reduced the intensity of the GABA-generated Cl⁻ currents (6,31) (see

TABLE 1. *Pharmacological properties of DBI and synthetic peptide fragments of DBI*

Name	AA sequence	MW	ED$_{30}$ for proconflict activity (nmol/i.c.v.)	Inhibition of [^{3}H]BCCM binding K_i (μM)	Tonic-convulsion (nmol/i.c.v.)
DBI	104 residues	11,000	10	5.2	—
ODN	QATVGDNTDRPGLLDLK	1,882	2.9	1.5	>200
OP	RPGLLDLK	881	11	6	125
HEP	PGLLDLK	745	48	10	250
HEX	GLLDLK	665	65	12	300
NP	PGLLDLKGK	939	—	21	400
EDP	PGLLDLKGKAK	1,138	—	16	400
ODN-NH$_2$	QATVGDNPD RPGLLDLK-NH	1,881	>100	>50	—
	WDSWNKLK	1076	—	>50	—
	FIYSHFK	940	>100	>50	—
	TYVE	595	>100	>50	—

DBI, diazepam binding inhibitor; ODN, octadecaneuropeptide; OP, octapeptide; HEP, heptapeptide; HEX, hexapeptide; NP, nonapeptide; and EDP, endadecaneuropeptide.
Data from ref. 20.

Fig. 1). This inhibition is similar to that observed by methyl 6,7-dimethoxy-4-ethyl-beta-carboline-3-carboxylate (DMCM) or other β-carboline 3-carboxyl esters and appeared to be mediated via an occupancy of the BZ/BC recognition site. This is because it is blocked by pretreatment with Ro15-1788 (6).

Because DBI appears to interact with the GABA/BZ/BC/Cl$^-$ ionophore complex in a fashion similar to the anxiogenic β-carbolines, we attempted to clarify whether DBI affects the behavior of rats operating in a Vogel conflict-punishment test in a fashion similar to that of anxiolytic benzodiazepines or anxiogenic β-carbolines. Rats receiving i.c.v. increasing doses of DBI (from 5 to 100 nmol) have a lower threshold for the stimulus that suppresses behavior, thereby evincing a clear proconflict effect (Table 1), which is blocked by Ro15-1788 (23). In addition, DBI failed to elicit any anticonflict action and actually blocked the anticonflict action of diazepam (14,23). Similarly to the proconflict action of the β-carbolines (12), the action of DBI is potentiated by a decrease of the GABAergic tone induced by pretreatment of the animals with subconvulsive doses of isoniazid, which reduce the GABA brain stores by 45% or more.

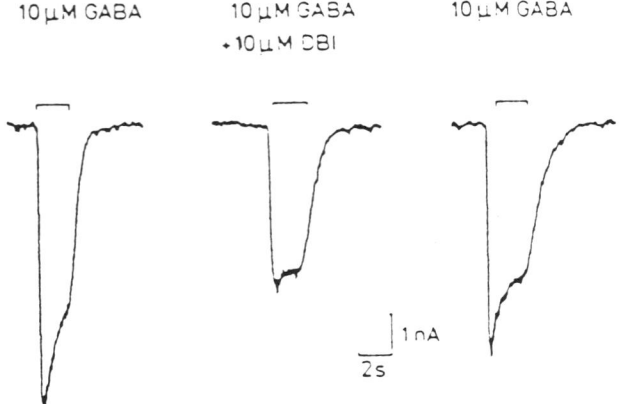

FIG. 1. Effect of DBI on GABA-induced whole cell currents in primary culture of mouse spinal cord neurons. (From ref. 6.)

PHYSIOLOGICAL RELEVANCE OF DBI

The finding that an endogenous peptide causes a proconflict action as a result of its binding to the allosteric modulatory site of GABA receptor is not sufficient to claim that this allosteric site has physiological significance. The question of whether DBI fulfills some of the criteria to be considered a physiologically relevant modulatory agent or cotransmitter operative in GABAergic transmission therefore remained unresolved. The criteria to be satisfied before claiming that DBI encodes for a GABA cotransmitter important in the modulation of rat behavior in conflict situations are (a) DBI should be present in synaptic terminals; (b) DBI should coexist with GABA or be stored in non-GABAergic axon terminals innervating GABA receptors; (c) DBI should be released extraneuronally on stimulation of the nervous tissue; (d) a specific mRNA should be present in the nervous tissue for the synthesis of DBI. In fact, its formation could be artefactual.

Brain Distribution, Histochemical, and Subcellular Studies

Antibodies were raised against rat DBI to study its distribution and cell location in rat brain. DBI-like immunoreactive material was present in high content in the arcuate nucleus of the hypothalamus (350 pmol/mg prot) and was almost undetectable in the anterior pituitary (approx. 10 pmol/mg prot) of rats. The DBI content of several brain areas is reported in Table 2.

When rat brain homogenates were fractionated by differential centrifugation, the pattern of distribution in mitochondrial, microsomal, and synaptosomal fractions was quite uneven. Relatively high percentages of DBI-like immunoreactivity were found in the mitochondrial and synaptosomal fractions, whereas less than 30% was found in the microsomal fraction.

Histochemical Studies

Immunohistochemical studies using DBI antiserum 1/40,000 coupled with peroxidase reaction revealed intense

TABLE 2. *Regional distribution of DBI-like immunoreactivity in rat brain*

Region	Immunoreactivity (pmol/mg prot)
Hypothalamus	
Arcuate nucleus	350 ± 24
Ventral medial nucleus	190 ± 14
Supraoptic nucleus	170 ± 14
Dorsal medial nucleus	150 ± 20
Posterior nucleus	120 ± 16
Cerebellum	230 ± 13
Hippocampus	
(CA$_2$-CA$_3$)	95 ± 12
Ammon's horn	109 ± 6.3
Cortex	
Frontal	45 ± 3.6
Parietal	57 ± 8.1
Occipital	44 ± 9.0
Caudate-putamen	54 ± 7.2
Globus pallidus	71 ± 10
Nucleus accumbens	60 ± 8.1
Olfactory tubercle	89 ± 6.3
Substantia nigra	93 ± 10
Dorsal raphe nucleus	142 ± 25
Periaqueductal gray	181 ± 15

DBI antiserum was obtained from rabbits injected with purified rat DBI. The antiserum was directed toward the NH$_2$ terminal portion of DBI and shows no cross reactivity with other endogenous basic proteins and neuropeptides. The sensitivity of the antiserum (1/10,000 dilution) was adjusted to detect 50 fmol DBI.

Data from ref. 1.

immunoreactivity in axons and cell bodies of many brain regions. As expected by radioimmunoassay, a dense network of immunoreactivity was detected in many hypothalamic nuclei, in particular in the arcuate nucleus. The corpus amygdaloideus, the hippocampus, and the cerebellum pre-

sented a marked immunoreactivity (1). This image was mostly given by fibers; cell bodies were not very abundant.

A few cell bodies were visualized in the normal brain but immunoreactive cell bodies were easily visualized after rats were injected i.c.v. with colchicine.

In the hippocampus, DBI immunoreactivity was located in a palisade of cells beneath the granule cell layer in an area where GABA-containing basket neurons predominate (Fig. 2B). The pyramidal cells are also immunoreactive with DBI antibodies in rats pretreated with colchicine (Fig. 2A), and this immunoreactivity disappears as a result of cell body lesions elicited by kainic acid. In the cortex, after colchicine treatment, immunoreactivity was virtually absent in the white matter and in the exterior cortical layer, but was very dense in cells of cortical layers 5 and 6 (Fig. 2B).

To ascertain whether DBI was associated with GABA in any hippocampal cell type, we have used primary cultures from fetal animals (13). We could detect that DBI and glutamic acid decarboxylase (GAD) (a marker for GABAergic neurons) coexist in some small-size neurons (Fig. 3). However, not all GABAergic neurons contain DBI immunoreactivity, and conversely, not all neurons that have DBI also contain GAD (Fig. 3).

Because some of the hippocampal cells that contain DBI immunoreactivity are pyramidal neurons which are presumably not GABAergic, it can be inferred that DBI is not exclusively located in GABAergic neurons.

In the cerebellum DBI immunoreactivity was dense in fibers of the molecular layer. The Purkinje cells failed to show DBI immunoreactivity, but their cell bodies were densely innervated by DBI-positive axons and were surrounded by small immunoreactive cells (basket or Bergam cells or both) (1).

In the granule cell layer of the cerebellum, neurons containing DBI (presumably Golgi cells) were sparse. Overall, the DBI immunoreactivity in this brain area is reminiscent of that reported for GABA. Taken together, these findings suggest that in many brain neurons DBI coexists with GABA. However, the relatively low density of DBI-

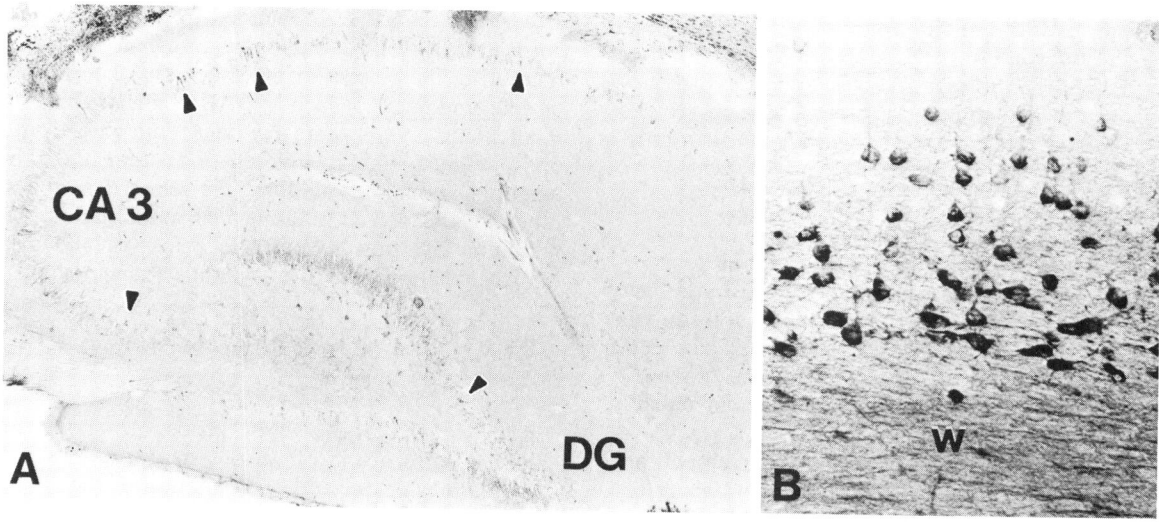

FIG. 2. DBI immunostaining in hippocampus (A) and cortex (B) of colchicine-treated rats (colchicine, 70 μg i.c.v.). **A:** DBI-positive cells (*arrowheads*) in all CA areas and in the dentate gyrus (DG). **B:** DBI positive cells in VI layer of cortex (W, white matter). (From ref. 13, modified.)

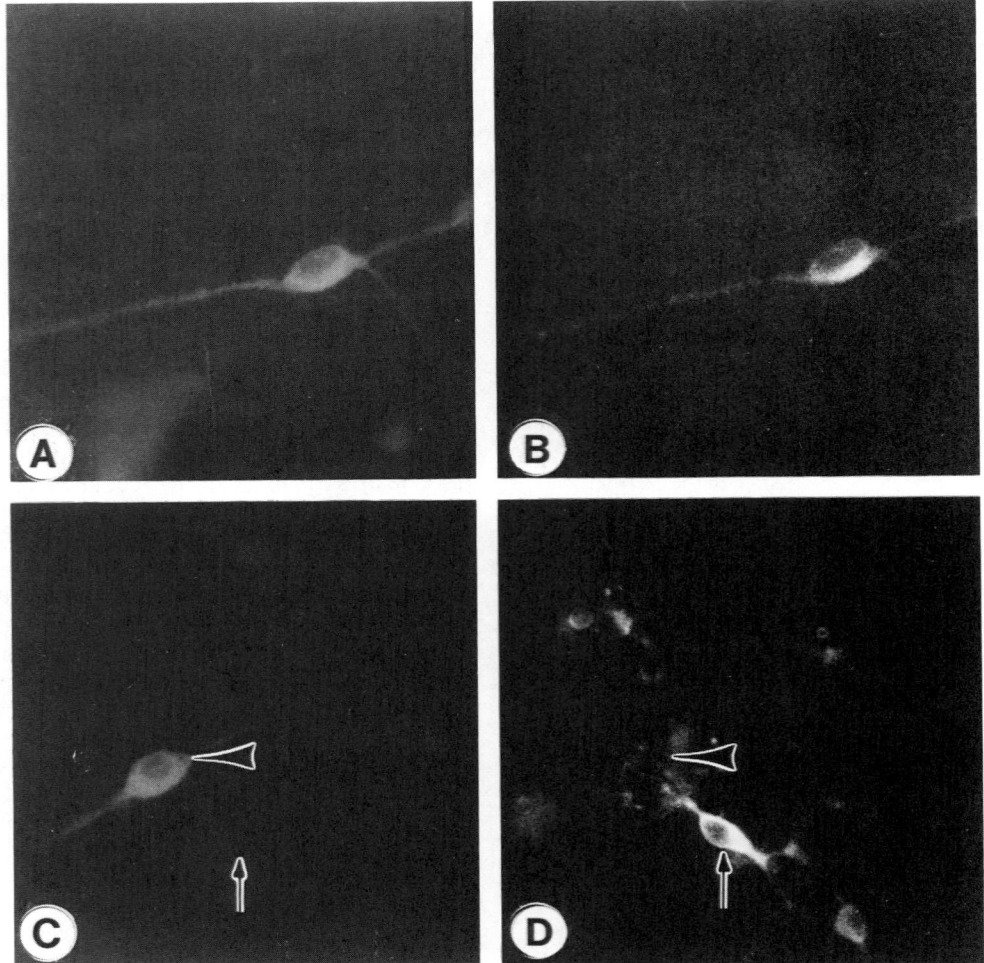

FIG. 3. Fluorescence micrographs from primary cultures of hippocampal cells. **A:** DBI immunostaining. **B:** The same cell double-stained with GAD antiserum showing the labeling in the same cell. **C:** DBI positive cell (*broad arrow*) that is not labeled with GAD antiserum. **D:** GAD immunoreactive cell (*long arrow*), not labeled with DBI antiserum in C. (From ref. 13.)

containing neurons in brain structures rich in GABAergic neurons, such as striatum, Purkinje cell layers of the cerebellum, and substantia nigra, suggests that GABAergic neurons can be divided into two classes: those in which DBI coexists with GABA and those devoid of DBI immunoreactivity.

Release of DBI from Various Preparations

One of the criteria that must be fulfilled to propose that DBI might represent a physiologically relevant cotransmitter is to show that it can be released extraneuronally on cell depolarization. A demonstration of this can be obtained with rat brain slices perfused *in vitro* and depolarized by K^+ or veratridine.

The basal release rate of DBI from hippocampal or hypothalamic slices can be increased by three to four times by depolarizing concentrations of K^+ or by 5×10^{-7} M veratridine, and this DBI release can be prevented by lowering Ca^{2+} content or by the addition of tetrodotoxin.

A DBI release was also obtained from primary cultures of cortical cells. These data are similar to those obtained measuring the release of other putative neurotransmitters or neuromodulators (such as GABA, enkephalins, substance P, etc.) and corroborate the idea emerging from several lines of independent investigations that DBI, or some posttranslational metabolites, are released in the synaptic junction and act as putative neuromodulators. More experiments are now required to prove beyond any doubt the participation of DBI in synaptic transmission.

mRNA Hybridization Techniques to Study DBI Dynamic Equilibrium

The availability of cDNA probes generated from the cloning of precursors of various neuropeptides has led to many studies on the *in vivo* regulation of the transcription rate for specific neuropeptide genes. Hybridization analyses, including *in situ* histochemical studies, have attempted to estimate the dynamic equilibrium of neuropeptides (43).

From these estimations, inferences can be made as to their participation in neuronal function. In fact, the dynamic state of transmitter neuropeptides might also reflect changes in the activity of the neurons that store these neuromodulators. Moreover, detection by *in situ* hybridization of a mRNA for a specific peptide precursor is the most reliable histochemical demonstration that the peptide precursor is expressed in that neuron. Using the partial amino acid sequence information of DBI to prepare artificial radioactive probes for specific amino acid sequences and a rat hypothalamic mRNA library, Seeburg and Gray (Genetech, San Francisco, CA), Brosius (Columbia University, New York), and Mocchetti (Fidia-Georgetown Institute for the Neurosciences, Washington, D.C.) obtained several clones of cDNA complementary to rat mRNA for DBI. In addition to helping consolidate information for the amino acid sequence of DBI, these clones have revealed diversity in the gene family of DBI. This diversity may suggest that DBI may be expressed in a variety of structurally related neuropeptides associated with differential evolution of the DBI gene family and differential mRNA splicing.

While this research is unfolding, cDNA clones of DBI are used as tools to examine the brain DBI location and document DBI participation in brain function. DBI mRNA content of rat brain areas was measured after Northern blot hybridization with a 250-bp cDNA probe. The results obtained so far demonstrate a good correlation between DBI-like immunoreactivity and DBI mRNA content, with the following rank order: hypothalamus > cerebellum > brainstem > hippocampus > striatum > cerebral cortex. *In situ* hybridization studies conducted by Roberts (Columbia University, New York) and Alho (Fidia-Georgetown Institute for the Neurosciences, Washington, D.C.) showed that in the molecular layer of cerebellum, high density of DBI immunoreactivity is paralleled by high density of mRNA, which hybridizes with DBI-cDNA probe as well.

These data suggest that areas of the brain rich in DBI content also have the machinery to synthesize the peptide or one of its immediate precursors, offering the possibility to initiate studies on the changes in the regulation of DBI biosynthesis elicited by repeated drug administration or by exposure of the animal to conflict situations.

IS DBI A PRECURSOR FOR SMALLER NEUROPEPTIDES MODULATING GABA TRANSMISSION?

DBI contains 105 amino acid residues and is larger than any other peptide considered to act as a putative transmitter or modulator of nerve impulses. Since all the neuroregulatory peptides result from posttranslational modification of high-molecular-weight precursors, it made sense to entertain the possibility that DBI might be a precursor of one or more small-molecular-weight modulatory peptides. In the DBI sequence many DBI fragments are flanked by one or two basic amino acids; hence it can be hypothesized that DBI might function as a neuromodulator/precursor.

To decide whether the biological activity of DBI resides in the entire peptide or if DBI may function as a precursor for smaller peptides that contain the biologically active domain of the molecule, we began to examine the binding activity and the proconflict action of various DBI fragments (19,20). Trypsin digestion of DBI generates an octadecaneuropeptide (ODN), QATVGDVNTDRPGLLDLK, which loses the capacity to interact with the DBI antibodies but maintains the ability to inhibit BC binding and is more active than DBI itself in lowering the punishment threshold for the suppression of drinking in thirsty rats operating in a conflict situation. The proconflict action of ODN is antagonized by the imidazobenzodiazepine Ro15-1788; thus it can be suggested to be mediated by occupancy of BC binding sites.

The pharmacological properties associated with the ODN sequence were confirmed by comparing the activity of ODN generated from tryptic digestion of DBI with that of ODN obtained by synthesis.

The biological activity of ODN requires the presence of the free COOH in the terminal lysine, for its α-amidation abolishes ODN biological activity (Table 1).

Preliminary results suggest that ODN may occur naturally in brain, as a result of "*in vivo*" posttranslational modification of DBI. Using a rabbit antiserum raised against the synthetic ODN to perform immunoaffinity chromatography combined with reverse-phase HPLC, we have detected at least three major molecular forms of ODN-like immunoreactivity in rat brain. One of these forms, with an HPLC profile similar to that of authentic ODN, yielded a single 18-amino-acid sequence identical to that of ODN (20). However, we cannot exclude the possibility that the endogenous ODN-like material contains some extra amino acid residues at the COOH or NH_2 terminal site. In spite of these uncertainties in the amino acid composition of the natural ODN-like peptide, it is interesting that ODN antibodies immunochemically stain the same brain areas and the same cells that are stained by DBI antibodies. This suggests that processing of DBI to a smaller peptide with epitopes similar to that of ODN can occur intraneuronally *in vivo*.

In order to determine the minimal amino acid sequence of ODN necessary to express its biological activity, we have initiated pharmacological studies on the structure-activity relationship of some synthetic fragments of ODN. As shown in Table 1, the biological activity of some carboxyl terminal fragments, including the last 8, 7, and 6 amino acids, decreases with the number of amino acid residues. However, when the ODN carboxyl terminal lysine is amidated (ODN-NH_2) or the carboxyl terminus of ODN fragments is extended, the proconflict activity and the ability to displace BC decrease dramatically, or are abolished (Table 1). The characteristics of the ODN sequence are presently under investigation.

Fragments of ODN, including the last six to eight amino acid residues closest to the carboxyl terminus, induce convulsions when injected in rats i.c.v.; ODN fails to elicit convulsions (Table 1). Thus, it remains to be determined whether DBI is a precursor for various polypeptide domains having diversified pharmacological profiles. Therefore it cannot be excluded that, among others, certain peptide fragments of DBI may mimic the pharmacological action of the anxiolytic benzodiazepines.

TABLE 3. *Partial amino acid sequence of human and rat DBI*

Human	QATVGDINTERPGMLDFTGKAKWDAWNELKTKPSDEEMLFIYGHYK-COOH
Rat	QATVGDVNTDRPGLLDLKGKAKWDSWNKLKTQPTDEEMLFIYSHYK-COOH

Data from ref. 18. Differences in amino acid composition between human and rat DBI are underlined.

HOMOLOGIES AND DIFFERENCES BETWEEN RAT AND HUMAN DBI

The clinical notion that benzodiazepines ameliorate anxiety states, a frequent symptom of affective illness, has suggested that alterations in the modulation of GABA receptors might be operative in affective disorders.

The demonstration that specific and high-affinity recognition sites for benzodiazepines coupled to GABA recognition sites exist in human brain (38) has suggested that this tissue may possess its own endocoids, which modulate the allosteric regulatory sites located in GABA$_A$ receptors. In order to establish whether a peptide similar to rat DBI is present in human cortex or cerebellum, both tissues were extracted and purified as reported for rat brain DBI.

The DBI-like material purified from human brain applied to a Bondapack C_{18} reverse-phase column emerges as a single UV-absorbing peak with a retention time identical to that of authentic rat DBI. When this material is applied to a 15% SDS-PAGE, it produces a single band staining with Coomassie blue with migration characteristics identical to those of rat brain DBI. Furthermore, DBI-like material purified to homogeneity from human brain has an amino acid composition similar to that of rat DBI. It does not contain cysteine, it has two methionine residues, and it is rich in lysine residues. When human DBI was tested for its ability to displace [^{3}H]BCCM, it was found to inhibit this binding with a potency similar to that of rat DBI.

Trypsin digestion of human DBI followed by HPLC analysis yields eight major peptide fragments. Of these fragments four are identical to four fragments obtained by trypsin digestion of rat DBI. However, the other four fragments have different retention times in the two species. We compared the amino acid sequence of three tryptic fragments of human and rat brain DBI. The sequences of the peaks produced by the tryptic digest of human DBI are similar but not identical to the amino acid sequences of rat DBI (see Table 2). This similarity extends to the ODN sequence (Table 3).

Since ODN is not found in any other mammalian polypeptide with the exception of rat DBI (23), it can be suggested that the homology between rat and human DBI extends to its biological activity. When purified human DBI was injected intracerebroventricularly into rats, it produced behavioral inhibition in the Vogel conflict-punishment test identical to that elicited by rat DBI.

DBI IN HUMAN BRAIN AND CEREBROSPINAL FLUID

In order to study DBI content in the CSF and brain of human subjects, we immunized rabbits with human DBI and compared these antisera with those directed against rat DBI. We found that human DBI has an affinity 100-fold lower than rat DBI for antisera raised against rat DBI. In contrast, antisera directed against human DBI have low affinity for rat DBI but high affinity for the homologous antigen.

Using an antiserum against human DBI, as little as 50 μl of CSF or 50 μg of brain-tissue is sufficient for the determination of DBI-like immunoreactivity.

The DBI was measured in a few postmortem or bioptic samples obtained from different human brain areas. These samples were frozen immediately after removal and then extracted with hot (90°C) 1 N acetic acid. The ranking order of DBI content in human brain areas resembles that of rat brain. High content was found in cerebellar cortex followed by amygdala, hippocampus, and striatum.

To shed some light on the possible role of DBI in the expression of peculiar behavioral patterns ranging from anxiety to response to stress and aggression, it became of particular interest to investigate the possible modification of DBI content in the CSF of patients suffering from various psychiatric diseases including endogenous depression, schizophrenia, and dementia of Alzheimer type.

The DBI content in the CSF of a group of 73 subjects ranging from 30 to 60 years of age was between 0.5 and 3 pmol/ml. It was higher in males than in females under the age of 50 and it was also higher in 23 patients (5 male and 17 female) with severe endogenous depression and marked anxiety. These data suggest that the higher DBI content found in CSF of depressed patients might be a trait of endogenous depression. It is impossible to rationalize this finding because the number of patients studied is not high enough. Moreover, we do not know how to interpret the increase of spinal fluid content of DBI in functional terms. A high content could indicate a decreased utilization or an increased synthesis; additional information on DBI mRNA content or biologically active peptide content is required.

CONCLUSION

GABAergic synapses appear to contain specific benzodiazepine recognition sites that allosterically modulate the receptor for the primary transmitter. DBI, a brain peptide with 105 amino acid residues, was isolated, purified, sequenced, measured, and cloned. This peptide fulfills many of the requirements expected to be present in an endogenous modulator of GABA receptors. However, the data available are not sufficient to conclude that this peptide or one fragment produced from DBI is the endogenous modulator of GABA$_A$ receptors. Modulation of these receptors appears to have a role in the regulation of behavioral responses during conflict situations. It appears that this system may be altered in affective disorders. The characteristics and physiological significance of these alterations require further investigation.

REFERENCES

1. Alho, H., Costa, E., Ferrero, P., Fujimoto, M., Cosenza-Murphy, D., and Guidotti, A. (1985): *Science,* 229:179–182.
2. Amoss, M., Burgus, R., Blackwell, R., Vale, W., Fellows, R., and Guillemin, R. (1971): *Biochem. Biophys. Res. Commun.,* 44:205–210.
3. Ariens, E. J. (1954): *Arch. Int. Pharmacodyn.,* 99:32–49.
4. Asano, T., and Spector, S. (1978): *Proc. Natl. Acad. Sci. USA,* 76:977–981.
5. Barnard, E. A., Stephenson, F. A., Sigel, E., Mamalaki, G., and Bilbe, G. (1984): *Neuropharmacology,* 23:813–814.
6. Bormann, J., Ferrero, P., Guidotti, A., and Costa, E. (1985): *Regul. Pept., (Suppl.* 4):33–38.
7. Bowery, N. G., Price, G. W., Hudson, A. L., Hill, D. R., Wilkin, G. P., and Turnbull, M. J. (1984): *Neuropharmacology,* 23:219–231.
8. Brazeau, P., Vale, W., Burgus, R., Ling, N., Butcher, M., Rivier, J., and Guillemin, R. (1973): *Science,* 179:77–79.
9. Burgus, R., Dunn, T. F., Desiderio, D., Ward, D. N., Vale, W., and Guillemin, R. (1980): *Nature,* 226:321–325.
10. Chan-Palay, V., Nilaver, G., Palay, S. L., Beinfeld, M. C., Zimmerman, E. A., Wu, J. Y., and O'Donohue, T. L. (1981): *Proc. Natl. Acad. Sci. USA,* 78:7787–7791.
11. Corda, M. G., Blaker, W. D., Mendelson, W. B., Guidotti, A., and Costa, E. (1983): *Proc. Natl. Acad. Sci. USA,* 80:2072–2076.
12. Corda, M. G., Costa, E., and Guidotti, A. (1983): In: *Benzodiazepine Recognition Ligands: Biochemistry and Pharmacology,* edited by G. Biggio and E. Costa, pp. 121–127. Raven Press, New York.
13. Costa, E., Alho, H., Santi, M. R., Ferrero, P., and Guidotti, A. (1985): In: *Progress in Brain Research,* Vol. 68, pp. 343–356. Elsevier Science Publisher B.D.
14. Costa, E., Corda, M. G., and Guidotti, A. (1983): *Neuropharmacology,* 22:1481–1492.
15. Costa, E., Forchetti, C. M., Guidotti, A., and Wise, C. M. (1983): In: *Dale's Principle and Communications Between Neurons,* edited by N. N. Osborne, pp. 161–177. Pergamon Press, Oxford and New York.
16. Costa, E., and Guidotti, A. (1979): *Annu. Rev. Pharmacol. Toxicol.,* 19:531–545.
17. Costa, T., Rodbard, D., and Pert, C. (1979): *Nature,* 227:315–317.
18. Ferrero, P., Conti-Tronconi, B. M., and Guidotti, A. (1986): In: *GABAergic Transmission and Anxiety (Advances in Biochemical Pharmacology, Vol. 41),* edited by G. Biggio and E. Costa, pp. 177–185. Raven Press, New York.
19. Ferrero, P., Guidotti, A., Conti-Tronconi, B. M., and Costa, A. (1984): *Neuropharmacology,* 23:1359–1362.
20. Ferrero, P., Santi, M. R., Conti-Tronconi, B., Costa, E., and Guidotti, A. (1986): *Proc. Natl. Acad. Sci. USA,* 81:827–831.
21. Gallo, V., Wise, B. D., Vaccarino, F., and Guidotti, A. (1985): *J. Neurosci.,* 5:2432–2436.
22. Guidotti, A., Corda, M. G., Wise, B. C., Vaccarino, F., and Costa, E. (1983): *Neuropharmacology,* 22:1471–1479.
23. Guidotti, A., Konkel, D., Bennett, C. D., and Costa, E. (1983): *Proc. Natl. Acad. Sci. USA,* 80:3531–3535.
24. Guidotti, A., Konkel, D. R., Ebstein, B., Corda, M. G., Wise, B. C., Krutzsch, J. L., Meek, J., and Costa, E. (1982): *Proc. Natl. Acad. Sci. USA,* 79:6084–6088.
25. Guidotti, A., Toffano, G., and Costa, E. (1978): *Nature,* 257:553–555.
26. Haefely, W., Pieri, L., Polc, P., and Schaffner, R. (1981): In: *Handbook of Experimental Pharmacology, Vol. 55: Psychotropic Agents,* edited by F. Hoffmeister and G. Stille, pp. 13–262. Springer-Verlag, Berlin.
27. Haring, P., Stahli, C., Schoch, B., Takacs, B., Staehelin, T., and Mohler, H. (1985): *Proc. Natl. Acad. Sci. USA,* 82:4827–4841.
28. Henry, S. H. C., Jones, E. G., Defelipe, J., Schmechel, D., Brandon, C., and Emson, P. C. (1984): *Proc. Natl. Acad. Sci. USA,* 81:6526–6530.
29. Hokfelt, H., Elde, R., Fuxe, K., Johansson, O., Ljungdahl, A., Goldstein, M., Luft, R., Efendic, S., Nilsson, G., Terenius, L., Ganten, D., Jeffcoate, S. L., Rehfeld, J., Said, S., Perez de la Mora, M., Possani, L., Tapia, R., Teran, L., and Palacois, R. (1978): In: *The Hypothalamus,* edited by S. Reichlin, R. J. Baldasserini, and J. B. Martin, pp. 69–135. Raven Press, New York.
30. Lundberg, J. M., and Hokfelt, H. (1983): *Trends Neuroscience,* 6:325–333.
31. McDonald, R. L., Weddle, M. G., and Gross, R. A. (1986): In: *GABAergic Transmission and Anxiety (Advances in Biochemical Pharmacology, Vol. 41),* edited by G. Biggio and E. Costa, pp. 67–78. Raven Press, New York.
32. Mohler, H., Polc, P., Cumin, R., Pieri, L., and Ketter R. (1979): *Nature,* 278:563–565.
33. Mohler, H., and Richards, J. G. (1981): *Nature,* 294:763–765.
34. Nishizuka, Y. (1984): *Science,* 225:1365–1370.
35. O'Donohue, T. L., Millington, W. R., Handelmann, W. R., Contreras, P. C., and Chronwall, B. M. (1985): *Trends Pharmacol. Sci.,* 6:305–308.
36. Oertel, W. H., Graybiel, A. M., Mugnaini, E. L., Schmeckel, D. E., and Kopin, I. J. (1983): *J. Neurosci.,* 3:1322–1332.
37. Olsen, R. W. (1982): *Annu. Rev. Pharmacol. Toxicol.,* 22:245–277.
38. Reisine, T. D., Wastek, G. J., Speth, R. G., Bird, E. D., and Yamamura, H. I. (1979): *Brain Res.,* 165:183–187.
39. Robison, G. A., Butcher, R. W., and Sutherland, E. W. (1968): *Am. Rev. Biochem.,* 37:149–174.
40. Rodbell, M. (1980): *Nature,* 284:17–22.
41. Schally, A. V., Arimura, A., Baba, Y., Nair, R. M. G., Matsuo, J., Redding, T. W., Debeljuk, L., and White, W. F. (1971): *Biochem. Biophys. Res. Commun.,* 43:393–399.
42. Schoch, P., Richards, J. G., Haring, P., Takals, B., Sthali, C., Staehelin, T., Haefely, W., and Mohler, H. (1985): *Nature,* 314:168–171.
43. Schwartz, J. P., and Costa, E. (1986): *Annu. Rev. Neurosci.,* 9:277–304.
44. Skolnick, P., Marangos, P., and Goodwin, F. K. (1978): *Life Sci.,* 23:1473–1480.
45. Spat, A., Bradford, P. G., McKinney, J. S. M., Rubin, R. P., and Putney, J. W. (1986): *Nature,* 319:514–516.
46. Stephenson, R. P. (1956): *Br. J. Pharmacol.,* 11:379–393.
47. Study, R. E., and Barker, J. L. (1981): *Proc. Natl. Acad. Sci. USA,* 78:7180–7184.
48. Ticku, M. K. (1983): *Life Sci.,* 33:2363–2375.
49. Vaccarino, F., Conti-Tronconi, B. M., Pannula, P., Guidotti, A., and Costa, E. (1985): *J. Neurochem.,* 44:278–289.
50. Vicini, S., Wroblewski, J. T., and Costa, E. (1986): *Neuropharmacology,* 25:207–211.
51. Vogel, J. R., Beer, B., and Clody, D. E. (1971): *Psychopharmacologia,* 21:1–7.

Psychopharmacology:
The Third Generation of Progress,
edited by Herbert Y. Meltzer.
Raven Press, New York © 1987.

CHAPTER 45

The Search for Neuropeptides

Jack D. Barchas, Kazuhiko Tatemoto, Kym F. Faull, Christopher J. Evans, Karen L. Valentino, and James H. Eberwine

The search for neuropeptides has several dimensions. Some of these deal with chemical and biological issues: what specific compounds are we searching for, what methods should be used, how sensitive are the assay and other analytical procedures, how do we determine the true physiological roles of the new substances, how are they related to behavior, and finally, can they be used to develop an improved psychopharmacology? In this chapter we consider questions from each of these realms. We start by considering the fundamental issue of the strategy adopted in the search for new compounds. We then consider some of the methods that are used and the ways in which they might be expanded. This includes a discussion of chemical assays specific for structural features of peptides, analytical tools such as mass spectrometry, immunological techniques, methods used in biochemical neuroanatomy including *in situ* hybridization, and the tools of molecular neurobiology. The chapter has as its central underlying theme the importance of identifying bioactive neuropeptides, determining their physiological interrelationships, and developing a clearer sense of the biochemical and anatomical mosaic of these substances. From such information may develop a dramatically different set of approaches to psychopharmacology.

ISSUES OF STRATEGY

The Study of Neuropeptides in the Perspective of Psychopharmacology

Contemporary neuropsychopharmacology is profoundly influenced by our knowledge of neuroregulators—substances that may act as neurotransmitters or neuromodulators (8,22). Most of the effective agents that have been found to date, either through serendipity or through design, act via the aminergic systems. Substances that act on the dopamine system, as either receptor agonists or antagonists, provide a good example of such a phenomenon. The therapeutic importance of these agents has been proven for movement disorders on the one hand and psychoses on the other. Yet even with these widely studied agents, it is clear that both our understanding of the true mechanism of action and our treatments of the conditions are still inadequate.

Having started from single neuroregulator hypotheses of severe mental disorders, there is now a growing movement toward hypotheses that consider multiple neuroregulators. Again, the dopamine system provides an example of this phenomenon. The use of dopamine antagonists provides a form of treatment of some psychoses, but is inadequate in others. Dopamine may be involved in the action of the antipsychotics without being the primary biochemical lesion in psychoses. In some ways, the situation may be analogous to the problem of our understanding of Parkinson's disease prior to the discovery of dopamine, when treatment was based on agents that antagonized the effects of acetylcholine. We now know that in this case the disease involves, at least in part, an imbalance between the two systems, with the primary lesion being in the dopaminergic system. The psychoses may be another case in which multiple neuroregulators are involved. For example, one could hypothesize that there may be two or more neuroregulators involved and that the role of dopamine might be analogous to the role of acetylcholine in Parkinson's disease—a relative

437

excess or an increased receptor sensitivity due to a relative underfunctioning of some other, known or unknown, system.

Conceptions dealing with multiple neuroregulators and their patterns of release make the study of known, but relatively unstudied, neuroregulators, as well as the search for unknown neuroregulators, of considerable importance. There are many examples of relatively understudied neuroregulators. They include the trace amines, β-phenylethylamine and para-tyramine for example, brain epinephrine, prostaglandins, and derivatives of known substances, such as the tryptolines, which are chemical condensation products of indoleamines.

Among the neuroregulators for which there is untapped potential for future developments in psychopharmacology, there may be none that are of greater importance than the neuropeptides (51). There is, as yet, only a fragmentary understanding of the physiological and biochemical roles of the bioactive neuropeptides, although it is clear that they probably play an important role in the control of behavioral and physiological functioning either as neurotransmitters or as neuromodulators. Their patterns of processing and regulation are still at the earliest stages of investigation. It is already clear that there are many different peptides in the brain and it is likely that there are more to be identified. These neuropeptides are of interest not only at a basic science level, but they also have potential importance in the development of new therapeutic agents. Neuropeptides, either in chemically modified forms or as reverse-engineered materials, may form a future base for new psychopharmacologic entities, just as compounds that impact on biogenic amine mechanisms currently form the foundation of psychopharmacology. It is not mere speculation to assert that neuropeptide research will have a fundamental impact on future developments in psychopharmacology, and a consideration of the strategies available in this relatively new but actively growing field is both timely and relevant.

Available Approaches for the Search for Novel Bioactive Neuropeptides

Among the traditional approaches that are still used in the search for neuroactive peptides is the so-called hypothetical-deductive approach. This has been successful because it has permitted the detection of substances whose action was predicted through knowledge of effects on a neuroendocrine or other physiological process. In this way a particular releasing factor or inhibiting factor, for example, can be clearly postulated and then sought (89).

Other traditional approaches have utilized specific pharmacological effects. Such bioactivities are not necessarily related to the brain and often involve receptors in peripheral tissues. A search for the substance in brain can then follow. In this case there are fewer constraints on the true physiological role of the target molecule, and the underlying postulate can be quite broad, e.g., that there might be a neuropeptide that affects blood pressure, or that acts on a model system such as the melanocyte (35).

With all approaches, the key to the method of search for a new compound is the assay endpoint. Indeed, every method of search involves a fundamental hypothesis of the existence of a specific substance. The traditional approaches have been oriented toward a biological activity. However, based on new technologies, several nontraditional approaches have now emerged that are contributing in a major way to the development of the field. These approaches rely on pharmacological activity, a chemical reaction, antibody recognition, or reading of a gene code. The emphasis in our laboratory is on these nontraditional approaches and we present some details of each to give an idea of the potential they represent.

CHEMICAL, ANALYTICAL, AND IMMUNOLOGICAL TECHNIQUES USED IN THE CHARACTERIZATION OF NOVEL NEUROPEPTIDES

Chemical Detection Approach

This approach to the search for unknown neuroregulators or neuromodulators takes advantage of a particular chemical structure, and in this way is radically different from the traditional approaches, which are frequently specific for compounds that elicit a biological activity. The approach of using a particular chemical structure as the assay endpoint permits a broad search for compounds that do not necessarily produce a response in the traditional assays. For example, many neuropeptides are characterized by a specific chemical alteration such as acetylation, phosphorylation, or amidation. The amidated structure is particularly interesting: in mammalian tissues it is known to occur only in neuroactive or hormonally active peptides. Furthermore, about half of the known neuropeptides and hormonal peptides contain this unique chemical feature. It is therefore reasonable to assume that many hitherto unrecognized neuropeptides and hormonal peptides also will contain this chemical feature. In this section we describe some of the findings that have arisen subsequent to the development of a specific chemical detection method for the C-terminal amidated structure. Based on the success of this approach, it is predicted that additional methods for detecting other posttranslational covalent modifications to peptide structure may prove valuable in the search for neuropeptides.

The Rationale for the Search for Amidated Peptides

A large proportion of mammalian hormonal and neural peptides contain a C-terminal amidated chemical group (Table 1). Studies have shown that the mechanism of C-terminal amidation involves enzymatic conversion of a glycine residue to the amide group during posttranslational processing (11). The C-terminal amide seems to be important for biological function, since the loss of this structure frequently results in the loss or modification of bioactivity (67,84).

Methodology of the Chemical Assay

In the chemical method that is used for the detection of amidated peptides (75,80), the C-terminal portion of the peptide is cleaved off enzymatically and converted to the

TABLE 1. *C-Terminal amide structures of the known peptide hormones and neuropeptides (mammalian)*

α-Melanotropin	-Lys-Pro-Val-NH$_2$
Calcitonin	-Gly-Ala-Pro-NH$_2$
Calcitonin gene-related peptide	-Lys-Ala-Phe-NH$_2$
Cholecystokinin	-Met-Asp-Phe-NH$_2$
Corticotropin-releasing factor	-Asp-Ile-Ala-NH$_2$
Galanin	-Gly-Leu-Ala-NH$_2$
Gastrin	-Met-Asp-Phe-NH$_2$
Gastrin-releasing peptide	-His-Leu-Met-NH$_2$
Gonadoliberin	-Arg-Pro-Gly-NH$_2$
Growth hormone-releasing factor	-Ala-Arg-Leu-NH$_2$
Metorphamide	-Arg-Arg-Val-NH$_2$
Neurokinin A	-Gly-Leu-Met-NH$_2$
Neurokinin B	-Gly-Leu-Met-NH$_2$
Neuromedin B	-His-Phe-Met-NH$_2$
Neuropeptide Y	-Gln-Arg-Tyr-NH$_2$
Oxytocin	-Pro-Leu-Gly-NH$_2$
Pancreatic polypeptide	-Pro-Arg-Tyr-NH$_2$
Peptide HI	-Ser-Leu-Ile-NH$_2$
Peptide YY	-Gln-Arg-Tyr-NH$_2$
Secretin	-Gly-Leu-Val-NH$_2$
Substance P	-Gly-Leu-Met-NH$_2$
Thyrotropin-releasing hormone	-Glu-His-Pro-NH$_2$
Vasoactive intestinal peptide	-Ile-Leu-Asn-NH$_2$
Vasopressin	-Pro-Arg-Gly-NH$_2$

fluorescent dansyl derivative, which is then extracted and identified, as illustrated in Fig. 1.

The systematic search for new peptides with the C-terminal amide structure using the chemical detection technique has resulted in the isolation of several important neuropeptides. Using this chemical approach, the peptides were isolated without any prior knowledge of their biological activity. Yet, without exception, each of the newly isolated peptide amides was subsequently found to be biologically active with important neural and/or hormonal properties (75,78). Thus, with this approach, the isolation of unknown peptides of mammalian origin with the C-terminal amide structure has led to finding several new neuroactive or hormonally active peptides. Preliminary results have shown that there are many other unknown peptide amides remaining to be isolated from the brain. Clearly, many more important neuropeptides remain to be discovered, and this and other chemical techniques may be examples of ways in which they will be recognized and then characterized.

Examples of Neuropeptides Found by the Chemical Assay Method

A number of examples can be given of peptides discovered using the chemical assay method. For several of those peptides there is already evidence that they may be important in neurobiology and thereby ultimately in neuropsychopharmacology.

A C-terminal tyrosine-amide-containing peptide was detected in brain extracts and subsequently isolated and characterized (77). This peptide, called neuropeptide Y (NPY), is now known to be widely distributed in both the central and peripheral nervous systems. NPY is present in brain in a concentration higher than any other known neuropeptide (2). The coexistence of NPY and catecholamines in neurons of the central (24,36) and peripheral (49) nervous system has been demonstrated using immunohistochemical techniques, suggesting physiological interactions between the amines and NPY.

More recently, a variety of possible physiological functions of central NPY have been documented. Central administration of NPY has resulted in a three- to tenfold increase in food intake (15,45,72,73), suggesting that NPY is a potent stimulator of eating and thus may play a functional role in the control of feeding behavior. Intraventricular administration of NPY suppresses copulatory behavior in rats (42). NPY injection into the third ventricle of ovariectomized rats leads to a dramatic reduction in plasma luteinizing hormone (LH) (17,53). NPY also stimulates the secretion of LH, growth hormone (GH), and follicle-stimulating hormone from perfused pituitary cells (53). Finally, injection of NPY into the suprachiasmatic region of the hypothalamus induces a shift in the circadian rhythm of rats and hamsters (1,99), suggesting a role as a chemical messenger regulating the light/dark cycle entrainment of circadian rhythms.

Peptide HI (PHI) is a C-terminal isoleucine amide-containing peptide, originally isolated from gut (76) and subsequently from brain (79), which has potent prolactin-releasing activity (40,94) and potentiates the action of corticotropin-releasing hormone (CRH) (83). Interestingly, PHI inhibits the binding of vasoactive intestinal peptide (VIP) to its receptors and stimulates cyclic AMP production *in vitro* (9,82). Since the biological spectrum of PHI is very similar to that of VIP, it is possible that both PHI and VIP

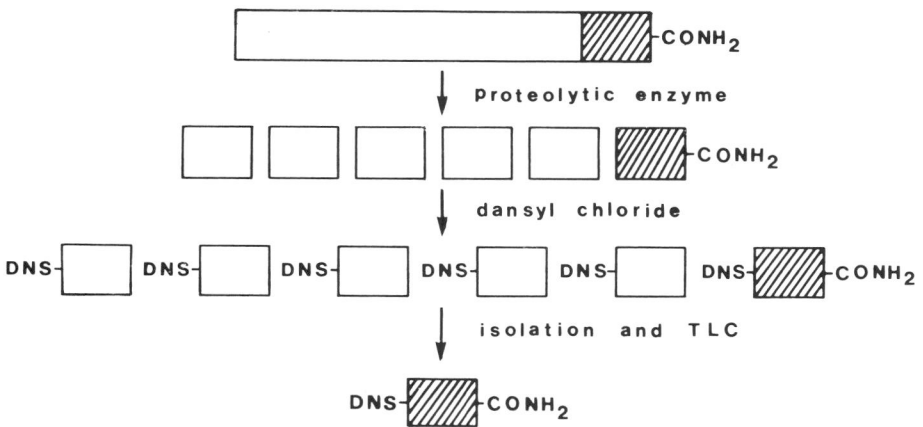

FIG. 1. The principle of the chemical detection of peptides based on the C-terminal amide group.

exhibit their biological activities through common receptors (78).

Another peptide found by the chemical assay method, galanin, a *C*-terminal alanine-amide-containing peptide, has few structural similarities with other known peptides and may belong to a hitherto unknown peptide family. Immunohistochemical studies indicate that galanin occurs not only in the intestine, from which it was originally isolated, but also in the brain (mainly in the hypothalamo-pituitary region, ref. 63). The effects of galanin in a variety of physiological systems are currently under active investigation.

The finding of brain cholecystokinin-58 (CCK-58), a *C*-terminal phenylalanine amide-containing peptide, demonstrates some of the advantages of the chemical assay approach. The brain contains high concentrations of this peptide, which is an extended form of CCK-8, the only other form of CCK that was thought to be expressed in brain (20). The new form of CCK was found to be composed of 58 amino acids (81), and recent results suggest that there may be differential posttranslational modification of the CCK precursor between the brain and intestine, and also between different regions of the central nervous system, which give rise to the different forms of CCK. In contrast to other forms of CCK, CCK-58 selectively increases dopamine turnover in certain CCK-positive dopamine nerve terminals (29), suggesting that CCK-58 may have different neural actions from other forms of CCK.

Mass Spectrometric Approaches

In the context of promising areas for future analytical developments relevant to the search for neuropeptides, it is appropriate to draw particular attention to mass spectrometric (MS) techniques. Relatively recent developments, particularly the development of fast atom bombardment mass spectrometry (FAB/MS) by Barber and his colleagues (4,6,7), have dramatically revolutionized the use of mass spectrometry for polar and thermally labile compounds of higher molecular weight, including peptides.

Fast atom bombardment mass spectrometry involves the dissolution of the sample in a liquid matrix and its introduction directly into the ion source of the mass spectrometer. It is bombarded with a beam of high-energy atoms or ions such as those from argon or xenon. This bombardment leads to the expulsion of ionized molecules from the matrix. Molecules of a molecular weight even higher than that of insulin (5) can be studied in an appropriate instrument. Relatively routine analyses of substances with a molecular weight up to 8,000 are now possible (61)—an event previously considered impossible for a mass spectrometer. The method is particularly useful for compounds with a molecular weight over 500 daltons where the chemical background is diminished. Demonstrating the important role of technology and of the instrument maker's art, the technique has resulted in the development of a new generation of mass spectrometers with extended mass ranges (32).

In the search for new neuropeptides and their subsequent characterization, FAB/MS has important attributes. The technique is particularly valuable for determining precise molecular weights. Whereas other methods are necessary for absolute structural determination, FAB/MS provides a degree of certitude and can speed the course of work. However, FAB/MS is unlikely to completely replace the traditional methods of peptide characterization such as sequencing and amino acid analysis, but the speed and relatively relaxed requirements for purity make it an invaluable complement to these techniques.

Another important virtue of FAB/MS is its sensitivity. The literature contains examples where amounts as small as 10 pmol have been analyzed by the technique (66). Further, the remaining sample can often be salvaged. One particularly valuable capability of the method may be in facilitating the purification process. The FAB/MS method can be used with impure extracts and thus one would monitor the target substance through various purification steps. One can also use FAB/MS to conveniently characterize products and derivatives produced by microchemical and enzymic reactions without prior separation of the products.

Another important aspect of the use of FAB/MS is for the characterization of peptides blocked at one of the terminal groups (66). Such covalently modified molecules are inaccessible to traditional sequencing techniques. Other uses may involve the identification of unusual and repetitive amino acids. These can also be vexing and difficult to study with conventional sequencing methods. Another valuable use involves identification of covalent modifications that might not be detected by conventional sequencing techniques (18). FAB/MS also provides the potential for obtaining some sequence information (56). This is an area that will require more development, including compilation of suitable computer programs to realize its ultimate potential. However, one can anticipate that the combination of traditional sequencing methods and those of FAB/MS might prove complementary in assuring the structure of a novel, previously unrecognized substance, particularly one with covalent modifications. Finally, another potential involves quantitative measurements of targeted peptides (19).

Yet another set of methods related to those just described involves another new method, tandem mass spectrometry (MS/MS). In this method, ions are separated from a mixture by the first mass spectrometer, and then selected primary ions are decomposed by collision with a gas. The resulting daughter ions are analyzed by the second mass spectrometer. This technique can be used with any of the ionization methods employed in mass spectrometry, including fast atom bombardment.

The MS/MS technique can enhance the amount of structural information that can be obtained regarding a particular compound. In the case of peptides, the method may prove to be particularly useful in providing sequence information, because recent results have shown the pattern of daughter ions provides immediate sequence information that is only ambiguous in the case of residues that have the same nominal masses, such as leucine and isoleucine.

It is clear that mass spectrometry has enormous promise that is only being partially realized today in the case of neuropeptide chemistry. The pioneering efforts that led to the fast atom bombardment technique are hampered in widespread utilization because of the expense of the apparatus and the relatively few centers where research dealing with its limits can be undertaken. The problems of instrument scarcity and the few available persons experienced in their use are highlighted by the MS/MS technique. In that instance, each of the applications is currently still in the earliest stages of development, since so few of the instruments exist or are being used for projects related to neurobiology and psychopharmacology of neuroregulators. It is clear that mass spectrometry centers constitute a valuable resource not only for the application of the method for the solution of current problems, but also for development of new approaches as tools in the study of new compounds.

Antibodies as Probes for New Peptides

Neurobiology has made good use of the specificity of antibodies as tools to study peptide neuroregulators. Immunocytochemistry is an invaluable technique to analyze the cellular localization of certain peptides in tissue. Radioimmunoassay and other immunoassays have been extensively employed to identify peptides in tissue extracts, enabling further characterization and quantification. Here we will describe the use of antisera to identify new endogenous peptides.

Antibodies can be generated to many classes of molecules if appropriately presented to the immune system. Among the compounds to which antisera have been generated are various hormones, peptides, proteins, and glycosolated proteins. For many of the smaller molecules, antisera can only be generated when the haptens are covalently coupled to macromolecules. For example, in raising antipeptide sera, the peptide is generally coupled chemically to a protein (usually keyhole limpet protein or thyroglobulin) and injected together in an emulsion with a stimulant of the immune system (Freund's adjuvant).

Depending on the application, two main forms of antibodies are employed for biochemical studies: polyclonal antibodies, which consist of the total sum of all the responses to the antigen, and monoclonal antibodies, which contain one homogeneous antibody population. In the search for new peptides, polyclonal antisera are perhaps the more valuable. However, because the antigenic determinants are a clearly defined amino acid sequence, their use as probes in the search for novel neuropeptides inevitably carries with it the restriction that this approach is most likely to identify molecules belonging to the same general family as the hapten employed in the antibody production.

Novel Peptides from cDNA Clones of Neuroactive Peptide Precursors

One approach to using antisera to discover new peptides has been the consequence of the progress in molecular biology. Sequencing of cDNA clones corresponding to the messenger RNA of many neuroactive precursors allows the prediction of the primary protein sequence. Many neuroactive precursors contain multiple neuroactive peptides, sometimes with considerably different activities. For example, proopiomelanocortin (POMC) from the pituitary contains adrenocorticotropic hormone, β-endorphin, and three melanocyte-stimulating-hormone (MSH)-"like" sequences (57). The entire protein sequence of POMC deduced from the cDNA sequence enables the prediction of processing products that could be generated from the precursor. Processing of neuroactive precursors in general follows some well-defined ground rules. Paired basic residues (especially lysyl-arginine residues) are favored cleavage sites. Processing also commonly occurs at single arginine residues. In both instances the basic residues are eliminated, since they are not found on either fragment except where the cleavage is adjacent to a proline residue. Cleavages rarely occur at amino acids other than basic residues. If a cleavage occurs leaving a C-terminal glycine, this amino acid is invariably decarboxylated to form the amidated peptide. Amidated peptides often, although not always, represent the biologically active forms (see ref. 50 for a review of neuropeptide processing).

The consequence of such rules is that the structure of peptide-processing products can be predicted from the precursor sequence. Synthetic peptides can be made to these predicted sequences, antisera raised to the peptides, and the endogenous forms of the immunoreactivity characterized in tissue. In the opiate field, this approach has been widely employed, since the precursors have gene-duplicated bioactive fragments; for example, in proenkephalin there are no less than eight copies of the enkephalin sequence, all preceded by pairs of basic residues (60).

Amidorphin was discovered using this antibody approach (70). The sequence of amidorphin in the precursor molecule (Fig. 2) illustrates many of the salient features of predicting a processing product from a precursor sequence. The sequence is flanked on both ends by lysyl-arginine residues, and although there is a paired basic residue after the N-terminal enkephalin sequence, this is known to be less susceptible to cleavage by the processing enzymes. The cleavage at the C-terminus results in a C-terminal glycine which is converted to the amide. The peptide corresponding to residues 104 to 149 of proenkephalin was synthesized by solid phase peptide synthesis. Polyclonal antisera were

```
100                104
XX-Phe-Met-LYS-ARG-Tyr-Gly-Gly-Phe-Met-LYS-LYS-Met-Asp-Glu-Leu-Tyr-Pro-Leu-Glu-
                                                           149                  155
                   Val-Glu-Glu-Glu-Ala-Asn-Gly-Gly-Glu-Val-Leu-Gly-LYS-ARG-Tyr-Gly-Gly-XX
```

FIG. 2. Amino acid sequence of proenkephalin residues 100–155. Amidorphin was postulated to exist as the sequence comprising residues 104–149 which would result from cleavages occurring at the two lysyl-arginine sequences 102–103 and 152– 154 with decarboxylation of the C-terminal glycine to form a C-terminal leucine amide. The peptide underlined in the figure was used for antisera generation.

raised in rabbits to the thyroglobulin-conjugated peptide. Using a radioimmunoassay (RIA) developed from this antiserum, the peptide could be isolated from tissue extracts, subsequently purified, and sequenced.

Using such antibody-related methods, a number of peptides in addition to amidorphin have been identified from opioid precursors: namely, synenkephalin (46) from proenkephalin, prodynorphin C-fragment from prodynorphin (23), and γ-MSH from proopiomelanocortin (57). Although some of these fragments have no known biological functions, they can be extremely useful markers of expression or release of the precursor. Synenkephalin is an example of a peptide that has been used extensively for such studies.

Identification of Posttranslational Products of Known Neuroactive Peptides

Antibodies can also be utilized to search for products of bioactive neuropeptides. Many neuroactive peptides are stored in several forms, the ratio of which may change considerably in different tissues. This can have dramatic influence on the biological activity. For example, β-endorphin in the intermediate lobe of the pituitary is predominantly found as the α-N-acetyl derivative, whereas in the anterior lobe and brain, the nonacetlyated forms predominate (71,91). The consequence of α-N-acetylation of either enkephalins or endorphins is to completely obliterate their opioid properties. Shortening of peptides can also alter biological activity. The conversion of β-endorphin 1–31 to β-endorphin 1–27 can have a marked effect on the analgesic potency of this peptide (30).

Antibodies are powerful tools for the study of posttranslational processing, especially when combined with modern chromatographic techniques, such as high-performance liquid chromatography (HPLC). A very good example of the discovery of a novel peptide using antisera to a known biological peptide was gastrin-releasing peptide 18–27 in brain (54,65). Gastrin-releasing peptide (GRP) was originally isolated from the gut as GRP 1–27. Antisera raised both to a synthetic C-terminal fragment (GRP 18–27) and to an N-terminal fragment (GRP 1–17) were used in RIAs to detect immunoreactive material in brain. However, when this immunoreactive material was investigated chromatographically, it was found to be predominantly of smaller molecular weight than GRP 1–27. Subsequently, HPLC studies showed the immunoreactive material corresponded to GRP 18–27 and the N-terminal fragments generated from GRP 1–27 by cleavage at a single arginine residue. Similar studies have led to the identification of CCK 1–8, dynorphin A 1–8, substance P 5–11, and α-N-acetyl β-endorphin 1–26. Antisera can also be useful in the detection of precursors or large-molecular-weight proteins possessing sequences of neuroactive peptides; recognition of CCK 58 (25) and dynorphin 32 (26) in tissues are two examples where this approach has been successful.

Antisera Directed to Biologically Active Portions of the Molecule

Many neuropeptide receptors accept molecules of different structure but with some common primary core features. It is often found that receptors or receptor families have multiple endogenous ligands. For example, there are about 20 different known endogenous opioid peptides, all with Tyr-Gly-Gly-Phe at the N-terminus and various C-terminal extensions. Antisera directed to the N-terminal structures would provide a method of screening for any opioid peptides found in tissue and possibly of isolating novel opioid peptides. It is nature's quirk that this N-terminal opioid core sequence is not antigenic. However, there is a trick whereby the N-terminus can be chemically derivitized by acetylation, a simple modification that directs the antigenic response to this portion of the molecule. The antibodies raised to these acetylated endorphins do not recognize the nonacetylated endorphins (91). However, the opiate-active core can be identified by prior α-N-acetylation with acetic anhydride followed by assay using the antisera specific for the α-N-acetyl, Tyr-Gly-Gly-Phe-X sequence. In this way it is possible to have a very sensitive and specific assay for peptides with the opioid core at the N-terminus. This procedure can be used for immunohistochemical localization of peptides as well as RIA. An example of the successful use of this approach was the identification and subsequent characterization of endorphins in shark pituitary (48). It would be anticipated that this and similar approaches could be extremely useful in the identification of other families of neuroactive peptides.

Identification of Neuropeptides Across Species

Many neuroactive peptides have been isolated from lower species such as amphibians and mollusks, since these creatures often have considerably higher and more localized peptide concentrations than mammals. Bombesin, isolated from the frog skin, and cardioexcitatory peptide (FMRF-NH$_2$), isolated from the mollusk, are examples of such peptides. Antibodies raised to both of these nonmammalian peptides showed beautiful immunostaining patterns in rat brain. The assumption made from these staining patterns was that these peptides or very similar peptides are present in rat brain. However, the problem (or in some cases, the joy) of antisera is that they are not totally specific for the sequence injected. Immunocytochemical studies can be very misleading since they are noncompetitive and generally use very high concentrations of polyclonal antisera. An antiserum raised to a given peptide may have low affinity for some other endogenous peptide, and consequently give very intense immunostaining. For this reason, RIA results that require competition of a labeled peptide for endogenous antigen are generally more reliable, especially when coupled to chromatography. There have been a number of studies of the bombesin-like and FMRF-NH$_2$-like immunoreactivity in mammalian brain. The bombesin immunoreactivity has been found to be GRP 18–27 (65). Antibodies raised to FMRF-NH$_2$ give a very extensive staining pattern in rat brain (92). However, the staining pattern is almost identical to NPY. Since NPY has a very similar C-terminus to FMRF-NH$_2$, the staining pattern can be explained by a cross reactivity with the antiserum. However, a peptide that may contribute to a portion of the FMRF-NH$_2$ immunostaining in rat brain has been recently isolated and characterized (96).

These studies illustrate how antibodies can lead to the discovery of new peptides, although caution should be exercised when using them as the sole criterion for peptide identification.

Application of Biochemical Neuroanatomy to the Search for Novel Peptides

Few research fields have been more radically transformed from an anticipated base than neuroanatomy. The changes from earlier conceptions are perhaps best paralleled by physics at its apparently stable preatomic phase, only to be radically altered by later discoveries. Similarly, conceptions of neuroanatomy, based on traditional architectonic and pathway-tracing techniques, have been dramatically changed by the discovery of new transmitters and their pathways, both from area to area and within local circuits. The methodologies of biochemical neuroanatomy have come to be important in the search for neuropeptides, and several new methods are emerging that may give us further insight into the organization of the brain.

By taking advantage of the specificity of the antibody-antigen interaction and by using antisera directed to different regions of the targeted neuropeptide in combination with carefully designed controls to rule out nonspecific staining, the field of immunohistochemistry has developed into a sophisticated art that has permitted the accurate neuroanatomical localization and mapping of many neuropeptide systems in the CNS. These techniques have been important for mapping the pathways of single substances, and have been cleverly extended to show colocalization of neuropeptides and classical neurotransmitters in specific neurons (37,39). In fact this latter application has in large part been important for initiating the question of how neurotransmitters and neuropeptides interact in the CNS. Immunohistochemical techniques combined with more traditional anatomical pathway-tracing methods (retrograde transport) have provided a powerful means of determining the projections of these peptide-containing neurons.

A particularly important technique that has only recently been applied to the central nervous system is that of *in situ* hybridization (90). The method permits precise anatomical localization of a specified nucleic acid sequence. A nucleic acid probe is developed that targets a specific nucleic acid product by complementary base-pairing, and the probe can then be hybridized to the nucleic acid in a tissue section. Originally, the focus was on the detection of DNA targets, but prime use has now centered about the detection of RNA, particularly messenger RNA (mRNA). Although a particular mRNA can be present in extremely low concentrations, the method is able to detect just a few molecules per cell. In this sense, it is more powerful than other molecular biology techniques because it confers a degree of anatomical localization.

The use of *in situ* hybridization for the localization of mRNA is potentially important for studies of all neuropeptides. Although there may be many different mRNA molecules in brain, the ability to locate with subcellular precision a specific mRNA molecule involved in the translation of a specific neuropeptide and to study the colocalization of this mRNA species with mRNAs of other neuropeptides, is an exciting development. This possibility has only arisen because of the specificity of complementary base-pairing between a nucleic acid probe and complementary mRNA and because of the relative ease and rapidity with which nucleic acid probes can now be developed.

The significance of the technique is enhanced by its remarkable sensitivity. A more commonly used procedure, that of Northern blotting, involves the extraction of RNA from tissue, and after a series of steps, transferring the RNA to nitrocellulose paper and detecting it with a labeled nucleic acid probe. This procedure is very sensitive, and an important step in determining in which tissues a given mRNA may be distributed throughout the organism. It cannot, however, give the kind of cellular resolution that *in situ* hybridization can provide, which is particularly important in studies of the nervous system.

A key utilization of the *in situ* method may be in facilitating studies of the functional significance and dynamic regulatory processes involving neuropeptides. By permitting studies in subpopulations of cells, it enhances the possibility that researchers can study core neurobiological questions, including those of differentiation, development, and aging, at the level of gene expression. For psychopharmacology, the technique may provide a particularly valuable means of determining the pattern of changes in association with various psychopharmacological agents.

However, *in situ* hybridization is not likely to completely replace the more traditional immunohistochemical approaches, but rather the two approaches are likely to be used in parallel. Because the techniques complement each other, they can be used for self-verification of data. Immunohistochemistry provides information regarding the presence of a particular product. *In situ* hybridization techniques provide information as to whether the gene is being expressed in the cells where the product is found. If both the peptide and its mRNA are found in the same cell, there is strong evidence that the cell is the place where the peptide is synthesized. In cases where posttranslational modification of peptides occurs, *in situ* hybridization can be used to detect the message for the precursor, but immunocytochemical studies will be necessary to determine which peptide is present in that particular cell.

Use of Molecular Biology in the Characterization of Novel Neuropeptides

There are three main areas in the study of peptide hormones and neurotransmitters in which the application of molecular biology techniques has supplemented and expanded on information generated by use of traditional protein techniques. These areas are (a) the study of peptide precursor structure and processing, (b) identification of novel peptides, and (c) insight into how expression of these peptides is regulated. For the purpose of this chapter we will examine these three areas individually.

The Study of Peptide Precursor Structure and Processing

Having isolated a novel peptide hormone, the first step generally in trying to determine the nature of its protein precursor is to make antibodies directed against the peptide in hopes of using these antibodies to isolate the precursor. A major problem that often ensues from using this approach is that antisera made to purified peptides are generally directed to the carboxyl terminus of the peptide so if the peptide is posttranslationally modified the antisera may not recognize the peptide in precursor form. This problem can sometimes be solved by chemically synthesizing peptides corresponding to the midregion of the peptide and then using antisera directed at the midregion peptide to isolate the precursor. This isolation scheme presumes that the precursor is in sufficiently high abundance to be isolated, purified, and sequenced. This unfortunately is often not the case.

An alternative approach to determining the nature of the peptide precursor is to isolate the cDNA or gene clone coding for the peptide precursor. Having the clone enables one to sequence the coding region and translate it into the corresponding amino acids so that the primary structure of the precursor protein is known. There are many methods in use for the cloning of peptide hormone cDNAs, ranging from "plus-minus" differential screening (87) to the screening of cDNA expression libraries in bacteria with antibodies specific for the peptide hormone of interest (44,98).

The most common method of isolating clones corresponding to a particular peptide hormone has been to make oligonucleotide sequences corresponding to a portion of the peptide amino acid sequence and to use this as a hybridization probe to screen either a cDNA or genomic DNA library. A decision that must be made in utilizing this approach is what region (N-terminal or C-terminal amino acids) of the peptide is to be utilized to make the oligonucleotide. This decision is complicated by the degeneracy of codon usage such that an amino acid can be encoded by as few as one codon (methionine and tryptophan) or as many as six codons (leucine, serine, and arginine). This often makes it impossible to predict the exact oligonucleotide sequence that corresponds to the peptide's amino acid sequence. This problem has been addressed by making either "mixed" oligonucleotides or a "long" oligonucleotide.

For a mixed oligonucleotide, every possible oligonucleotide sequence corresponding to the amino acid sequence is synthesized, pooled, and used as a screening probe (97). These generally range in size from 8 to 25 nucleotides. Alternatively, a "long" oligonucleotide can range in length from 30 to 100 nucleotides and, because of its length, affords a hybrid between the probe and its corresponding cDNA. The sequence of long oligonucleotide is chosen by utilizing the most frequently used codon choice (in the species from which the clone is being isolated) in place of the degeneracy in the hope that any mismatches that occur will be compensated for by long stretches of homology between the probe and target clone (68,85).

Several cDNA clones corresponding to peptide hormones have been isolated using a variety of these techniques, included among which are gastrin (97), thyrotropin-releasing hormone (TRH) (44), enkephalin (16,34), dynorphin (14,41), CRH (28), gonadotropin-releasing hormone (GnRH) (68), NPY (55), somatostatin (27,31), vasopressin, neurophysin (43), POMC (57), LH (13), GH (69), human chorionic gonadotropin (10), insulin (86), substance P (58), growth hormone-releasing hormone (33,52), atrial natriuretic factor (95,100), and angiotensin (12).

The information to be gleaned from having the cDNA sequence of several peptide precursor proteins has made it possible to discern specific sequences that are signals for posttranslational modifying enzymes. For instance, it is presumed since many bioactive peptides are flanked by dibasic amino acids that there are trypsin-like and carboxypeptidase B-like enzymes that are responsible for cleaving the peptide from the precursor (21). Although not all dibasic amino acids are cleaved, such a high percentage of them are that it is possible to predict the presence of previously unknown peptide hormones solely on the presence of flanking dibasic amino acids, which will be discussed in the next section.

Additional consensus sequences that have been discovered upon examination of precursor peptide sequences are N-linked glycosylation sites [asparagine-X-threonine/serine (21)] and amidation signals [X-glycine-basic amino acid (11)]. Two other areas in which having cDNA sequence information available has had an impact are precursor processing and generation of antibodies. Precursor processing studies have been facilitated because one can radioactively label specific amino acids in the protein precursor and then, using immunoprecipitation and/or RIA, examine the time-course of precursor proteolysis. It is also possible to synthesize polypeptides from different regions of the precursor protein, which can then be used to generate region-specific antibodies. These antibodies can facilitate both processing studies and cell biology experiments to examine protein trafficking.

Identification of Novel Peptides

There are many examples of presumptive novel peptide hormone identification based on examination of protein precursor sequence. A recent example that may be of physiological significance is the discovery that prolactin inhibiting factor (PIF) is synthesized as part of the same mRNA and precursor protein as GnRH (68). The initial suggestion that PIF may be a naturally occurring peptide was made after the observation, made possible by cDNA sequencing, that there were two potential peptide-coding regions contained within the GnRH protein. These were identified by virtue of there being dibasic amino acids flanking both of the peptide regions. The unknown peptide was synthesized and used in bioassays to determine its presumptive function and to raise antibodies. These studies combined to show that PIF has the most potent prolactin-inhibiting action of any previously discovered peptide (59).

Different criteria were used to identify calcitonin gene-related peptide (CGRP), a novel neuropeptide, as a product of the calcitonin gene (64). Using the cDNA clone for calcitonin as a hybridization probe, multiple bands were seen on Northern gel analysis showing that there was more than a single RNA species hybridizing to the calcitonin cDNA. On examination of the gene structure, it was suggested that the HnRNA for calcitonin is differentially spliced in a tissue-specific manner to yield different size mature mRNAs, one coding for calcitonin and the other for CGRP. These mRNAs, although substantially unique, do contain some coding regions in common, thus permitting cross hybridization. Unlike the PIF-GNRH example, CGRP is produced by the same gene that makes calcitonin, yet the two peptides are not made concomitantly. Using antibodies made to CGRP, mapping studies have localized CGRP to brain neural pathways associated with sensing stimuli.

Insight into Peptide Regulation

An insight that often comes from the discovery of an unknown peptide hormone within the cDNA precursor of a known peptide hormone is a knowledge of how the new peptide is regulated. This is possible because peptides derived from the same protein precursor in the same cell type have been found to be coregulated.

This can be illustrated by the POMC hormone system, for which much hormonal regulation data is available. In the anterior pituitary corticotroph the major products of POMC processing are β-lipotropin (β-LPH), endorphin, and corticotropin (ACTH), which are costored and secreted (93). The secretion of both of these hormones is decreased in response to glucocorticoids (62) and increased in response to CRH (88). In the intermediate lobe melanotroph, where α-MSH and β-endorphin are the major products of protein processing, one again finds the peptides are costored and coreleased, yet both hormones are nonresponsive to glucocorticoid modulation. The differential response of the POMC system to glucocorticoids is dictated by the cell type in which the various peptide products are produced, yet the peptides generated from the POMC precursor in each cell type are regulated in an analogous fashion.

This form of coregulation has been shown to occur for many peptide hormones, such as α-neo-endorphin and dynorphin from the proenkephalin B prohormone (47), leucine enkephalin and methionine enkephalin from the proenkephalin A prohormone (74), and, most recently, N-terminal peptide and somatostatin from the somatostatin prohormone (3). For the recently cloned GnRH prohormone this general rule would predict that in any cell which produces both GnRH and PIF, PIF will be regulated by the same agents that are known to modulate GnRH. With the ability to make such predictions, one can perform appropriate and interesting endocrine regulation experiments without the trial and error that is necessary when no knowledge of how a peptide hormone is regulated is available.

CONCLUSION

The search for bioactive neuropeptides and investigations of their biological functions will be a critical factor in the continued development of psychopharmacology. From this type of information whole new classes of pharmacological agents acting as either neuropeptide agonists or antagonists may be expected to emerge.

A variety of techniques will be utilized in the search for neuropeptides, and, in our view, each has validity. These will include the more traditional approaches for substances with specific and predicted actions, on the one hand, and less traditional open searches using immunological techniques and chemical assays, on the other. Each of these methods has already yielded important information. It is clear that molecular biology has begun to make a significant contribution in the study of peptide hormones. The combination of these methods is particularly powerful; thus, the discovery of a new peptide by one of many different methods can then lead to the cloning of the gene for the precursor protein and the potential discovery of a new family of neuroregulators or hormones.

Once the critical step of discovery of bioactive agents has been accomplished, and biological activity demonstrated, the next step is the extension of that knowledge into therapeutics. For psychopharmacological agents a host of additional developments will then become necessary. At a theoretical level there will be fundamental questions as to the nature of the physiological and behavioral effects: What are the implications of comodulation for therapeutics? For example: Can we develop a rational psychopharmacological agent on the basis of a substance that may be a modulator rather than a primary transmitter? Can we develop agents that will act as agonists or antagonists to a given neuropeptide system? Can these agonists and antagonists be delivered to the appropriate receptor sites? Ultimately, can we reverse-engineer a molecule that may not even be a neuropeptide but that can pass the blood-brain barrier and act on an appropriate neuropeptide receptor—an equivalent of morphine? These and other questions, including the possibility of administration of multiple substances that may act on these interacting systems, will pose exciting challenges to the neuropsychopharmacologists of the future.

Yet before we get to therapeutics, we must first define the endogenous entities and their receptors. The ultimate power of the techniques used for the isolation and characterization of neuropeptides will come when we have a table of elements of bioactive neuropeptides that can be used in physiological and pharmacological investigation of the function and interrelationship of neuropeptides in various areas of the brain. At that point, peptide chemistry, molecular neurobiology, and biochemical neuroanatomy will be used in conjunction with electrophysiological and pharmacological methods to provide critical information directly relevant to behavior and to psychopharmacology. It is from such information that an important facet of the neuropsychopharmacology of the future will be constructed.

ACKNOWLEDGMENTS

The work of the authors at Stanford has been supported in part by NIMH 23861, NIDA 01207, the ONR, and the MacArthur Foundation.

REFERENCES

1. Albers, H. E., and Ferris, C. F. (1984): *Neurosci. Lett.,* 50:163–168.
2. Allen, Y. S., Adrian, T. E., Allen, J. M., Tatemoto, K., Crow, T. J., Bloom, S. R., and Polak, J. M. (1983): *Science,* 221:877–879.

3. Aron, D. C., and Roos, B. A. (1986): *Endocrinology,* 118:218–222.
4. Barber, M., Bordoli, R. S., Elliott, G. J., Sedgwick, R. D., and Tyler, A. N. (1982): *Anal. Chem.,* 54:645A–657A.
5. Barber, M., Bordoli, R. S., Elliott, G. J., Tyler, A. N., Bill, J. C., and Green, B. N. (1984): *Biomed. Mass Spectrom.,* 11:182–187.
6. Barber, M., Bordoli, R. S., Sedgwick, R. D., and Tyler, A. N. (1981): *Nature,* 293:270–275.
7. Barber, M., Bordoli, R. S., Sedgwick, R. D., and Tyler, A. N. (1981): *J. Chem. Soc. Chem. Commun.,* 95:325–327.
8. Barchas, J. D., Akil, H., Elliott, G. R., Holman, R. B., and Watson, S. J. (1978): *Science,* 200:964–973.
9. Bataille, D., Gespach, C., Laburthe, M., Amiranoff, B., Tatemoto, K., Vauclin, N., Mutt, V., and Rosselin, G. (1980): *FEBS Lett.,* 114:240–242.
10. Boorstein, W. R., Vanvakopoulis, N. C., and Fiddes, J. C. (1982): *Nature,* 300:419–422.
11. Bradbury, A. F., Finnie, M. D. A., and Smyth, D. G. (1982): *Nature,* 298:686–688.
12. Campbell, D. J., Bouhn, K. J., Menard, J., and Corvol, P. (1984): *Nature,* 308:206–208.
13. Chin, W. W., Godine, J. E., Klein, D. R., Chang, A. S., Tan, L. K., and Habener, J. F. (1983): *Proc. Natl. Acad. Sci. USA,* 80:4649–4653.
14. Civelli, O., Douglass, J., Goldstein, A., and Herbert, E. (1985): *Proc. Natl. Acad. Sci. USA,* 82:4291–4295.
15. Clark, J. T., Kalra, P. S., Crowley, W. R., and Kalra, S. P. (1984): *Endocrinology,* 115:427–429.
16. Comb, M., Seeburg, P. H., Adelman, J., Eiden, L., and Herbert, E. (1982): *Nature,* 295:663–666.
17. Crowley, W. R., Tessel, R. E., O'Donohue, T. L., Adler, B. A., and Kalra, S. P. (1985): *Endocrinology,* 117:1151–1155.
18. Dell, A., Etienne, T., Panico, M., Morris, H. P., Vinson, G. P., Whitehouse, B. J., Barber, M. N., Bordoli, R. S., Sedgwick, R. D., and Tyler, A. N. (1982): *Neuropeptides,* 2:233–240.
19. Desiderio, D. M. (1984): *Analysis of Neuropeptides by Liquid Chromatography and Mass Spectrometry.* Elsevier, Amsterdam.
20. Dockray, G. J., Gregory, R. A., Hutchson, J. B., Harris, J. J., and Runswick, M. J. (1978): *Nature,* 274:711–713.
21. Eipper, B. A., and Mains, R. E. (1980): *Endocr. Rev.,* 1:1–27.
22. Elliott, G. R., and Barchas, J. D. (1986): In: *American Handbook of Psychiatry, Vol. VIII,* edited by P. A. Berger and H. K. H. Brodie, pp. 34–63. Basic Books, New York.
23. Evans, C. J., Barchas, J. D., Esch, F. S., Bohlen, P., and Weber, E. (1985): *J. Neurosci.,* 5:1803–1807.
24. Everitt, B. J., Hokfelt, T., Terenius, L., Tatemoto, K., Mutt, V., and Goldstein, M. (1984): *Neuroscience,* 11:443–462.
25. Eysselein, V. E., Reeve, J. R., Jr., Shively, J. E., Miller, C., and Walsh, J. H. (1984): *Proc. Natl. Acad. Sci. USA,* 81:6565–6568.
26. Fischli, W., Goldstein, A., Hunkapiller, M. W., Hood, L. E. (1982): *Life Sci.,* 31:1769–1772.
27. Funckes, C. L., Minth, C. D., Deschenes, R., Magazin, M., Tavianini, M. A., Sheets, M., Collier, K., Weith, H. L., Aron, D. C., Roos, B. A., and Dixon, J. E. (1983): *J. Biol. Chem.,* 258:8781.
28. Furutani, Y., Morimoto, Y., Shibahara, S., Noda, M., Takahashi, H., Hirose, T., Asai, M., Inayama, S., Hayashida, H., Miyata, T., and Numa, S. (1983): *Nature,* 301:537–540.
29. Fuxe, K., Agnati, L. F., Vanderhaeghen, J. J., Tatemoto, K., Andersson, K., Eneroth, P., Harfstrand, A., von Euler, G., Toni, R., Goldstein, M., and Mutt, V. (1985): In: *Neuronal Cholecystokinin,* edited by J. J. Vanderhaeghen and J. N. Crawley. *Ann. NY Acad. Sci.,* 448:231–254.
30. Geisow, M. J., Deakin, J. F. W., Dostrovsky, J. O., and Smyth, D. G. (1977): *Nature,* 269(5624):167–168.
31. Goodman, R. H., Aron, D. C., and Roos, B. A. (1983): *J. Biol. Chem.,* 258:5570.
32. Green, B. N., and Bordoli, R. S. (1986): In: *Mass Spectrometry in Biomedical Research,* edited by Simon Gaskell. John Wiley and Sons (*in press*).
33. Gubler, U., Monahan, J. J., Lomedico, P. T., Bhatt, R. S., Collier, K. J., Hoffman, B. J., Bohlen, P., Esch, F., Ling, N., Zeytin, F., Brazeau, P., Poonian, M. S., and Gage, L. P. (1983): *Proc. Natl. Acad. Sci. USA,* 80:4311–4314.

34. Gubler, U., Seeburg, P., Hoffman, B. J., Gage, L. P., and Udenfriend, S. (1982): *Nature,* 295:206–208.
35. Harris, J. I., and Lerner, A. B. (1957): *Nature,* 179:1346–1347.
36. Hokfelt, T., Fahrenkrug, J., Tatemoto, K., Mutt, V., Werner, S., Terenius, L., and Chang, K. J. (1983): *Proc. Natl. Acad. Sci. USA,* 80:895–898.
37. Hokfelt, T., Vincent, S., Dalsgaard, C.-J., Skirboll, L., Johansson, O., Schultzberg, M., Lundberg, J. M., Rosell, S., Pernow, B., and Jancso, G. (1982): *Ciba Found. Symp.,* 91:84–106.
38. Jensen, R. T., Tatemoto, K., Mutt, V., Lemp, G. F., and Gardner, J. D. (1981): *Am. J. Physiol.,* 4:G498–G502.
39. Johansson, O., Hokfelt, T., Pernow, B., Jeffcoate, S. L., White, N., Steinbusch, H. W. M., Verhofstad, A. A. J., Emson, P. C., and Spindel, E. (1981): *Neuroscience,* 6:1857–1881.
40. Kaji, H., Chihara, K., Abe, H., Minamitani, N., Kodama, H., Kita, T., Fujita, T., and Tatemoto, K. (1984): *Life Sci.,* 35:641–648.
41. Kakidani, H., Furutani, Y., Takahaski, H., Noda, M., Morimoto, Y., Hirose, T., Asai, M., Inayama, S., Nakanishi, S., and Numa S. (1982): *Nature,* 298:245–249.
42. Kalra, S. P., Allen, L. G., Clark, J. T., Crowley, W. R., and Kalra, P. S. (1986): In: *Neural and Endocrine Peptides and Receptors,* edited by T. W. Moody, pp. 353–363. Plenum Press, New York.
43. Land, H., Schutz, G., Schmale, H., and Richter, D. (1982): *Nature,* 295:299–303.
44. Lechan, R. M., Wu, P., Jackson, I. M. D., Wolf, H., Cooperman, S., Mandel, G., and Goodman, R. H. (1986): *Science,* 231:159–161.
45. Levine, A. S., and Morley, J. E. (1984): *Peptides,* 5:1025–1029.
46. Liston, D. R., Vanderhaeghen, J.-J., and Rossier, J. (1983): *Nature,* 302:62–65.
47. Lorenz, R. G., Evans, C. J., and Barchas, J. D. (1985): *Life Sci.,* 37:1523–1528.
48. Lorenz, R. G., Tyler, A. N., Faull, K. F., Makk, G., Barchas, J. D., and Evans, C. J. (1986): *Peptides,* 7:119–126.
49. Lundberg, J. M., Hokfelt, T., Tatemoto, K., and Terenius, L. (1984): In: *Catecholamines,* edited by E. Usdin, pp. 179–189. Alan R. Liss, New York.
50. Mains, R. E., Eipper, B. A., Glembotski, C. C., and Dores, R. M. (1983): *Trends Neurosci.,* 6:229–235.
51. Martin, J., and Barchas, J. D., eds. (1986): *Neuropeptides in Neurologic and Psychiatric Disease, Vol. 64.* Raven Press, New York.
52. Mayo, K. E., Vale, W., Rivier, J., Rosenfeld, M. G., and Evans, R. M. (1983): *Nature,* 306:86–88.
53. McDonald, J. K., Lumpkin, M. D., Samson, W. K., and McCann, S. M. (1985): *Proc. Natl. Acad. Sci. USA,* 82:561–564.
54. Minamino, N., Kangawa, K., and Matsuo, H. (1983): *Biochem. Biophys. Res. Commun.,* 114:541–548.
55. Minth, C. D., Bloom, S. R., Polak, J. M., and Dixon, J. E. (1984): *Proc. Natl. Acad. Sci. USA,* 81:4577–4581.
56. Morris, H. R., Panico, M., Barber, M., Bordoli, R. S., Sedgwick, R. D., and Tyler, A. (1981): *Biochem. Biophys. Res. Commun.,* 101:623–631.
57. Nakanishi, S., Inoue, A., Kita, T., Nakamura, M., Chang, A. C. Y., Cohen, S. N., and Numa, S. (1979): *Nature,* 278:423–427.
58. Nawa, H., Hirose, T., Takashima, H., Inayama, S., and Nakanishi, S. (1983): *Nature,* 306:32–36.
59. Nikolics, K., Mason, A. J., Szonyi, E., Ramachandran, J., and Seeburg, P. H. (1985): *Nature,* 316:611–617.
60. Noda, M., Furatani, Y., Takahashi, H., et al. (1982): *Nature,* 295:202–206.
61. Richter, W. J., Raschdorf, F., and Maerk, W. (1985): In: *Mass Spectrometry in the Health and Life Sciences,* edited by A. L. Burlingame and N. Castagnoli, Jr., pp. 193–208. Elsevier, Amsterdam.
62. Roberts, J. L., Chen, C.-L. C., Eberwine, J. H., Evinger, M. J. Q., Gee, C., Herbert, E., and Schachter, B. S. (1982): In: *Recent Progress in Hormone Research,* edited by R. O. Gresp, pp. 227–256, Academic Press, New York.
63. Rokaeus, A., Melander, T., Hokfelt, T., Lundberg, J. M., Tatemoto, K., Carlquist, M., and Mutt, V. (1984): *Neurosci. Lett.,* 47:161–166.

64. Rosenfeld, M. G., Amara, S. G., Roos, B. A., Ong, E. S., and Evans, R. M. (1981): *Nature,* 290:63–65.
65. Roth, K. A., Evans, C. J., Lorenz, R. G., Weber, E., Barchas, J. D., and Chang, J.-K. (1983): *Biochem. Biophys. Res. Commun.,* 112:528–536.
66. Roth, K. A., Makk, G., Beck, O., Faull, K. F., Tatemoto, K., Evans, C. J., and Barchas, J. D. (1985): *Regul. Pept.,* 12:185–199.
67. Rudinger, J. (1969): In: *Progress in Endocrinology,* edited by C. Gual and F. J. G. Ebling, pp. 419–424. Excerpta Medica Foundation, Amsterdam.
68. Seeburg, P. H., and Adelman, J. P. (1984): *Nature,* 311:666–668.
69. Seeburg, P. H., Shine, J., Martial, J. A., Baxter, J. D., and Goodman, H. M. (1977): *Nature,* 270:486.
70. Seizinger, B. R., Liebisch, D. C., Gramsch, C., Herz, A., Weber, E., Evans, C. J., Esch, F. S., and Bohlen, P. (1985): *Nature,* 313:57.
71. Smyth, D. G., Massey, D. E., Zakarian, S., and Finnie, M. D. A. (1979): *Nature,* 279:252–254.
72. Stanley, B. G., and Leibowitz, S. F. (1984): *Life Sci.,* 35:2635–2642.
73. Stanley, B. G., and Leibowitz, S. F. (1985): *Proc. Natl. Acad. Sci. USA,* 82:3940–3943.
74. Tang, F., Costa, E., and Schwartz, J. P. (1983): *Proc. Natl. Acad. Sci. USA,* 80:3841–3844.
75. Tatemoto, K. (1982): In: *Systematic Role of Regulatory Peptides* (*Symposia Medica Hoechst,* 18), pp. 507–535. F. K. Schattauer Verlag, Stuggart-New York.
76. Tatemoto, K., and Mutt, V. (1981): *Proc. Natl. Acad. Sci. USA,* 78:6603–6607.
77. Tatemoto, K. (1982): *Proc. Natl. Acad. Sci. USA,* 79:5485–5489.
78. Tatemoto, K. (1983): *Biomed. Res.,* 4(Suppl.):1–6.
79. Tatemoto, K., Carlquist, M., McDonald, T. J., and Mutt, V. (1983): *FEBS Lett.,* 153:248–252.
80. Tatemoto, K., and Mutt, V. (1978): *Proc. Natl. Acad. Sci. USA,* 75:4115–4119.
81. Tatemoto, K., Jornvall, H., Siimesmaa, S., Hallden, G., and Mutt, V. (1984): *FEBS Lett.,* 174(2):289–293.
82. Taton, G., Chatelain, P., Delhaye, M., Camus, P. C., De Neef, P., Waelbroeck, M., Tatemoto, K., Robberecht, P., and Christophe, J. (1983): *Peptides,* 3:897–900.
83. Tilders, F. J. H., Tatemoto, K., and Berkenbosch, F. (1984): *Endocrinology,* 115:1633–1635.
84. Tracy, H. J., and Gregory, R. A. (1964): *Nature,* 204:935–938.
85. Ullrich, A., Ber, J. R., Chen, E. Y., Herrera, R., Petruzzelli, L. M., Dull, T. J., Gray, A., Coussens, L., Liao, Y. C., and Tsubokawa, M. (1985): *Nature,* 313:756–761.
86. Ullrich, A., Shine, J., Chirgwin, J., Pictet, R., Tischer, E., Rutter, W. J., and Goodman, H. M. (1977): *Science,* 196:1313–1318.
87. Unterman, R. D., Lynch, K. R., Nakhasi, H. L., Dolan, K. P., Hamilton, J. W., Cohn, D. V., and Feigelson, P. (1981): *Proc. Natl. Acad. Sci. USA,* 78:3478–3482.
88. Vale, W., Rivier, C., Yang, L., Minick, S., and Guillemin, R. (1978): *Endocrinology,* 106:1910.
89. Vale, W., Spiess, J., Rivier, C., and Rivier, J. (1981): *Science,* 213:1394–1397.
90. Valentino, K. L., Eberwine, J. H., and Barchas, J. D. (1987): *In Situ Hybridization: Applications to Neurobiology.* Oxford University Press, New York (*in press*).
91. Weber, E., Evans, C. J., and Barchas, J. D. (1981): *Biochem. Biophys. Res. Commun.,* 103:982–989.
92. Weber, E., Evans, C. J., Samuelsson, S. J., and Barchas, J. D. (1981): *Science,* 214:1248–1252.
93. Weber, E., Martin, R., and Voight, K. H. (1979): *Life Sci.,* 25:1111–1118.
94. Werner, S., Hulting, A.-L., Hokfelt, T., Eneroth, P., Tatemoto, K., Mutt, V., and Wunsch, E. (1983): *Neuroendocrinology,* 37:476–478.
95. Yamanaka, M., Greenberg, B., Johnson, L., Seilhamer, J., Brewer, M., Friedemann, T., Miller, J., Atlas, S., Laragh, J., Lewicki, J., and Fiddes, J. (1984): *Nature,* 309:719–722.
96. Yang, H.-Y. T., Fratt, W., Majane, E. A., and Costa, E. (1985): *Proc. Natl. Acad. Sci. USA,* 82:7757–7761.
97. Yoo, O. J., Powell, C. T., and Agarwal, K. L. (1982): *Proc. Natl. Acad. Sci. USA,* 79:1049–1053.
98. Young, R. A., and Davis, R. W. (1983): *Proc. Natl. Acad. Sci. USA,* 80:1194–1198.
99. Zini, I., Pich, E. M., Fuxe, K., Lenzi, P. L., Agnati, L. F., Mutt, V., Tatemoto, K., and Moscara, M. (1984): *Acta Physiol. Scand.,* 122:71–77.
100. Zivin, R. A., Condra, J. H., Dixon, R. A. F., Seidah, N. G., Chretien, M., Nemer, M., Chamberland, M., and Drouin, J. (1984): *Proc. Natl. Acad. Sci. USA,* 81:6325–6329.

Psychopharmacology:
The Third Generation of Progress,
edited by Herbert Y. Meltzer.
Raven Press, New York © 1987.

CHAPTER 46

Properties and Substrates of Mammalian Memory Systems

Michel Baudry and Gary Lynch

The search for neurobiological processes that subserve memory should probably begin with the question of what we mean by memory. Although it is commonly discussed as though it were a monolithic phenomenon, there is increasing evidence suggesting that memory is a composite of subsystems and that these may have different properties and substrates. Psychologists have long been aware that the principles governing learning can differ strikingly depending on the type of material to be memorized. For example, the relative efficiency of massed versus spaced training trials varies according to the problem given to the subject. More recently, cognitive psychologists have developed the argument that humans use two quite different memory systems in everyday life. Several such dichotomizations have been proposed (e.g., episodic versus semantic, data versus procedural), but in common they invoke a distinction between the learning system used for rules ("how to drive a car") and that for individual bits of information (e.g., faces, names). Studies with brain-damaged patients have added a small, though dramatic, body of evidence in favor of this separation of memory into multiple systems (89). Patients with temporal lobe, and in particular hippocampal, damage are reported to experience a great deal of difficulty in storing new memories about events and objects in their environments but nonetheless are able to learn and retain the procedures needed to solve complex puzzles, although they do not consciously remember having learned those rules (22). Animal studies also point to the existence of multiple memory systems. O'Keefe and Nadel (72), drawing on an extensive literature, argue that rats use one type of memory to negotiate mazes when forced to rely on intra-

maze cues and quite a different system when allowed to use extramaze (spatial) stimuli. Hippocampal lesions appear to leave the first system relatively intact but eliminate the second. An elegant series of behavioral and neurobehavioral experiments by Mishkin and colleagues has led to the conclusion that monkey brain contains separable memory systems, one of which is concerned with "habits" and the other with data (63).

These distinctions all concern a very stable type of memory, but the possible existence of memory types with very different durations should also be noted. Thus, arguments for qualitatively different short- and long-term systems have been made by psychologists at various times during this century (15,60). Recently, the idea of a "working memory" that deals with sequences of recent events and decays steadily over hours or days has received considerable attention; this form of memory, it is argued, is qualitatively distinct from a "reference" memory that persists for indefinite periods. Rats are known to remember moves they have made in a maze for several hours but not longer, although the memory of the organization of the maze lasts much longer (73).

In summary, and at the risk of greatly oversimplifying matters, it appears that the brain uses one type of memory system to form rules or procedures and possibly employs these to store specific information or data; there is reason to suspect that the latter, and possibly the former, possess short- and long-term variants. Future studies may reveal that these differences are more apparent than real and that comparable cellular and psychological processes are involved in all types of memory; alternatively, it may prove to be the case that the list of memory systems is longer than that sketched here. But the procedural/data and short/long-term distinctions at the least provide a framework within which to describe experiments on the cellular bases of learning and memory.

The present chapter is chiefly concerned with the cellular triggers and substrates of the stable forms of "data" memory. In the first sections we attempt to define some properties of this memory that can be used to constrain ideas about the cellular mechanisms responsible for it. This is followed by a discussion of synaptic plasticity and of a specific hypothesis about its relationship to behavioral memory. The final section of the review takes up the very difficult question of how to test biochemical hypotheses concerned with memory.

SOME INFERENCES ABOUT THE CIRCUITRIES AND SUBSTRATES RESPONSIBLE FOR MEMORY

Memory has a number of properties, many of them available to introspection, that can be used to define the neurobiological processes that produce it. Moreover, certain of these characteristics can be used in efforts to identify neuronal systems with designs appropriate for memory operations, something that is needed for tests of neurobiological mechanisms.

A salient characteristic of the memory system is its associativity: as noted by a number of theorists, virtually anything in memory can be associated with anything else. This requirement places strong constraints on ideas about the design of the neuronal networks that carry out memory operations, a point that is elaborated below. Memory also has very peculiar (at least to a biologist) temporal properties: it is formed by events lasting seconds or fractions of seconds and yet can persist for years. The capacity of the system is also remarkable. Attempts to estimate how many "bits" of information can be stored by humans in the space of a few days have led to values on the order of 10^{11} or more (see 28 for a discussion). Note also that the retrieval of information does not noticeably slow with the acquisition of ever greater quantities of information. This seems to indicate that memories are not stored as lists of steadily increasing length and that memory operations are likely to occur in very short sequences in a number of different sites.

A number of theorists have noted that the extreme associativity and parallel operation of memory require a system that is highly interconnected but with a low degree of order (28,40,45), leading most to conclude that it involves matrices of axons and dendrites linked in an essentially random fashion. Experimental studies have demonstrated that sizable numbers of synapses must be active in a near-simultaneous manner for a neuron to be brought to its spiking threshold; therefore, we can imagine that the memory system involves combinatorial rules in quasi-random systems. If this line of argument is correct, then it is likely that synaptic modification is used to encode memory: if larger anatomical units were to change, then inputs that were totally unrelated to a learned combination would

experience a changed relationship to a target cell. The idea that synapses are the sites of the modification underlying storage is also convenient, since it helps to explain the vast capacity of the memory system (i.e., there are orders of magnitude more synapses than neurons). For years, the Hebb synapse (39) has been the cellular model of such associative mechanisms, but it clearly fails to take into account neuroanatomical constraints determined by the nature of converging pathways. It seems more logical to assume the existence of mechanisms by which activation of two separate inputs converging on the same target neurons (even at fairly long distance on the dendritic tree) results in concerted changes at these synaptic contacts. These types of mechanisms in turn require cellular processes capable of integrating various chemical or physiological signals possibly generated at fairly long distances. Recent data using hippocampal CA_1 pyramidal cells do indeed suggest the existence of such mechanisms (47). Moreover, the existence of complex interactions of different chemical signals at the level of second messenger systems might provide the necessary integrating device to accomplish those concerted changes.

The temporal parameters of memory point to a number of features that must be exhibited by the neurobiological process that encodes it. Rapid acquisition implies that the triggering event must itself be very brief. This then presumably acts directly or indirectly on some additional process that produces a lasting modification of the synapse. Conversely, the extreme persistence of memory forces us to search for a change that itself is remarkably constant. Simple posttranslational modifications of proteins seem unlikely simply because these are often reversible, and in any event proteins are not thought to have half-lives anywhere near as long as memory (note, however, that protein modifications could serve as the substrates of short-term memories). This argument has led a number of investigators to hypothesize that memory is stored by structural modifications of the synapse (24,30,36,83). This in turn raises the additional problem that local modifications need to be made stable and long-lasting in spite of continuous turnover of the individual proteins contributing to synaptic structure. Such a stability would certainly be more difficult to achieve if these proteins exhibit a high turnover rate. It might thus be highly desirable to modify those elements of the synaptic contacts that exhibit a relatively slow turnover rate, which could be accomplished by decreasing the activity of degradative systems present in the dendrites. In this regard, it is interesting to note that we recently found the existence of a negative correlation between the activity of calcium-dependent proteases (which are a major source of proteolytic activity in mammalian brains at neutral pH) and brain size, suggesting that as neurons get larger and the number of synaptic contacts they support increases, there is a concomitant decrease in proteolytic activity and thus a slower turnover rate of the proteins constituting synaptic contacts (12,56).

Summarizing these arguments, we assume that associative memory involves changes in the ultrastructure of synapses in a low-order combinatorial matrix and that the physiological patterns that produce these effects do so through a rapidly appearing, transient process.

POTENTIAL CELLULAR MECHANISMS UNDERLYING MEMORY

Long-Term Potentiation

The discovery of hippocampal long-term potentiation (LTP) provided direct experimental evidence for the existence of physiological plasticity matching several of the criteria described immediately above. Long-term potentiation is an increase in the amplitude of excitatory postsynaptic potentials (elicited by single pulse stimulation of axons) and is produced by very brief (<1 sec) bursts of high-frequency stimulation of axons (95). The effect has been reported to last for weeks and thus fulfills the all-important conditions of brief triggering event and extreme persistence. Moreover, LTP is highly selective in that only those synapses on a cell that have experienced the high-frequency bursts are potentiated by it. The potentiation effect has another property that makes it an attractive candidate for a memory mechanism: it requires the interaction (or "cooperativity") of a number of simultaneously active synapses (61). Thus, associativity is intrinsic to LTP.

Recent studies indicate that the LTP phenomenon is somewhat more complex than originally thought. Racine and co-workers (79) have convincingly demonstrated that two types of potentiation follow a series of extended (200-msec) bursts of high-frequency (400 sec^{-1}) stimulation, one ("LTP 1") with a half-life of 1 to 4 hr and the second ("LTP 2") with a half-life of 3 to 7 days. Moreover, they present evidence that these may have different cellular substrates. Barnes (6) has reported data that suggest that potentiation can last for days or weeks depending on the number of stimulation bursts. It is tempting to imagine that these different effects are reflections of the processes responsible for certain forms of short- and long-term memory; at a minimum, they show that physiological analogs of these behavioral phenomena are to be found in hippocampus and probably elsewhere.

The occurrence of multiple forms of potentiation does raise problems in comparing the results of experiments using different preparations or paradigms, since one is not certain that what is labeled as LTP is in all cases the same phenomenon. As with memory itself, it may be necessary to begin developing categories of potentiation with appropriate defining characteristics rather than to proceed with the assumption that any form of synaptic facilitation lasting for more than a few minutes is "LTP."

Triggering Processes

Identification of Ca^{2+} as the Critical Second Messenger

As discussed, the identification of the cellular mechanisms underlying memory is complicated by the probable existence of different forms of memory characterized by different time courses and cellular and anatomical localizations. In addition, synapses contain a bewildering array of biochemical mechanisms with the potential for altering synaptic transmission for varying periods of time. Fortunately, two discoveries made during the last 5 years have provided strong evidence concerning the identity of the initial events responsible for the activity-dependent modification of synaptic efficacy, at least as manifested in hippocampal long-term potentiation. First, Lynch et al. (55) showed that intracellular injection of the calcium chelator EGTA in CA$_1$ pyramidal cells did not result in major alterations of synaptic responses induced by stimulation of the Schaffer-commissural pathway (except for the suppression of the Ca^{2+}-dependent hyperpolarization that normally follows the EPSP) but totally prevented the formation of LTP. This result strongly suggests that the triggering event for potentiation is an influx of calcium into the postsynaptic elements. Second, it is generally agreed that glutamate is the excitatory transmitter used by the pathways exhibiting the LTP phenomenon, and several groups have reported that selective blockers of a subtype of glutamate receptors (the so-called NMDA receptor, which is preferentially activated by the glutamate analog N-methyl-D-aspartate) blocked the induction of LTP in the CA$_1$ field of hippocampus without disturbing synaptic transmission (23,38,66,97). There is a strong possibility that these two sets of findings are related. The NMDA receptor exhibits a peculiar voltage dependence such that the ionic channel associated with it is blocked by magnesium at normal resting membrane potential but not when the membrane is depolarized to about −30 mV (59,71). Thus, the existence of this voltage- and transmitter-dependent receptor provides an amplification mechanism by which brief trains of high-frequency stimulation can result in very large depolarization restricted to the activated synapses. Moreover, recent experiments seem to indicate that the ionic channel associated with the NMDA receptor prefers Ca^{2+} to other cations, thus providing a molecular mechanism for augmenting the influx of Ca^{2+} into postsynaptic elements during high-frequency stimulation. However, this mechanism may not be absolutely necessary for producing a large influx of calcium in postsynaptic elements, and different types of synapses could well use different mechanisms (e.g., high concentrations of voltage-dependent calcium channels) to achieve a similar result. Nevertheless, it is interesting that the NMDA receptors are widely distributed in telencephalic structures and virtually absent in nontelencephalic structures (64), a finding with clear implications concerning the operation of different excitatory synapses.

In any event, these two sets of findings strongly suggest that Ca^{2+} is the critical second messenger involved in triggering LTP and that the initial sets of events leading to LTP occur postsynaptically.

Effects of Calcium

Although Ca^{2+} is implicated in the regulation of a large number of cellular processes, we are concerned here with the possible contributions of some of these to changes in synaptic efficacy (see Fig. 1). The amplitude and duration of the changes in intracellular calcium concentrations determine not only the amplitude and duration of the changes elicited by Ca^{2+}-dependent processes but also their natures, since different processes have different thresholds for calcium (80). A useful distinction at this point consists in separating

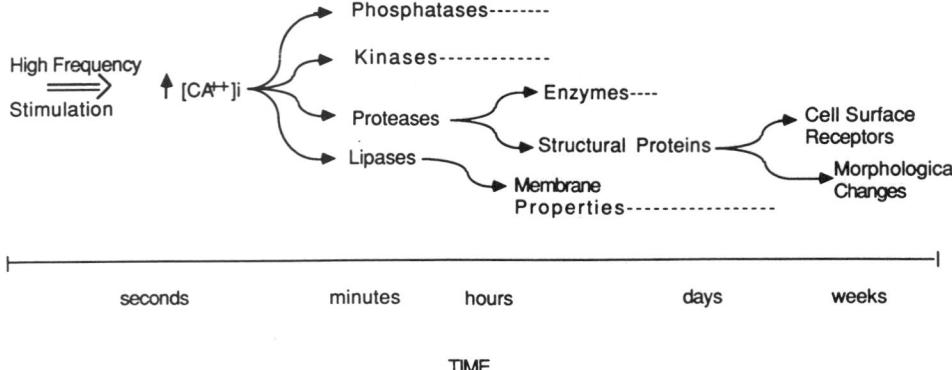

FIG. 1. Schematic representation of some of the effects of calcium. Following high-frequency stimulation, calcium concentration in postsynaptic elements is postulated to increase and to activate various calcium-dependent processes (see text). Also indicated on this scheme (*bottom line*) are approximate time courses (visualized with *dotted lines*) for the various processes.

those calcium-dependent processes that have reversible effects from those that are likely to have irreversible effects. In the former category, covalent modifications of proteins offer means for modifying various aspects of synaptic functions for the duration of this modification. In this category, phosphorylation reactions have been widely discussed as ideal candidates, although direct evidence concerning the nature of their functional roles is still somewhat sparse (69). It is clear that the synaptic complex possesses a full set of the different forms of protein kinases [cyclic AMP dependent, Ca^{2+}–calmodulin dependent, especially the type II, and Ca^{2+}-dependent/phospholipid-dependent kinase (kinase C)]. These kinases have been shown to phosphorylate a wide range of synaptic proteins including synapsin I, microtubule-associated proteins, phosphatase inhibitors, and possibly ionic channels and transmitter receptors. Experiments using invertebrate preparations indicate that activation of kinases leads to changes in a variety of membrane ionic currents including the Ca^{2+}, K^+, and Ca^{2+}-dependent K^+ currents (2,44). In hippocampal pyramidal neurons, kinase C activation by phorbol esters blocks the slow afterhyperpolarization (which is presumably mediated by the alteration of a Ca^{2+}-dependent K^+ channel) (5) and a voltage-dependent Cl^- channel (57). Translocation of kinase C from the soluble fraction to membranes has also been recently reported as a result of high-frequency stimulation of the perforant path (1).

Thus, a transient rise in calcium concentration in postsynaptic elements is likely to result in a complex set of alterations of phosphoproteins resulting in a variety of functional modifications of synaptic functions. Because of the relatively fast turnover of phosphate groups on protein substrates, these alterations are transitory and by themselves can account for modifications lasting from seconds to minutes, possibly hours. Some longer-lasting changes in phosphorylation could be provided by mechanisms such as the translocation discussed above, for which molecular turnover might be required for the elimination of the change in activity. In addition, because most of the kinases are capable of autophosphorylation, and in some cases autophosphorylation represents a positive feedback, it has

been proposed that alterations in kinase activity through phosphorylation could provide a self-sustaining and thus long-lasting change in enzyme activity (24,51). Nonetheless, the rate of protein turnover is likely to preclude phosphorylation itself from being the substrate of memories lasting for weeks. Other effects of phosphorylation could, however, be quite persistent. Several cytoskeletal proteins are substrates for kinases, raising the possibility that covalent modifications might produce structural changes in the synaptic complex. Thus, for example, changes in the state of phosphorylation of microtubule-associated protein II might regulate microtubule polymerization or their susceptibility to proteolytic degradation (see below).

A second category of calcium-dependent processes results in irreversible alterations of lipids or proteins and is therefore more likely to be responsible for longer-lasting modifications of synaptic function following transient changes in intracellular calcium concentrations. Calcium-dependent lipases potentially could perturb the lipid domain of the membrane sufficiently to modify protein–lipid interactions, possibly resulting in long-lasting alterations in cell surface receptor distributions or functions. Calcium-dependent proteases are also attractive candidates for a mechanism to translate brief changes in calcium concentrations into long-lasting and possibly permanent changes in synaptic structure and function (53). Two forms of this category of enzymes have been identified in a variety of tissues including brain; they differ by their sensitivity to calcium, with a low-threshold form (calpain I or μCANP) being activated by micromolar calcium concentrations and a high-threshold form (calpain II or mCANP) activated by low-millimolar calcium concentrations (68). Recently, we found that the low-threshold form is preferentially associated with synaptosomes (84) and synaptic membranes, whereas the high-threshold form is mostly soluble. The localization of calpain I in dendritic spines and postsynaptic densities has been confirmed by immunohistochemical techniques at the electron microscopic level (77). Moreover, we also detected the existence in brain membranes of a phenomenon reported in erythrocytes, namely, a calcium-dependent translocation of the enzyme from the soluble compartment to membranes

(62,78). Substrates of this protease include protein kinase C and most of the proteins constituting the cell cytoskeleton (e.g., neurofilament proteins, microtuble-associated proteins, tubulin, actin, and brain spectrin) (10,58,81,85,98). Interestingly, partial proteolytic degradation of kinase C by calpain results in the formation of an active kinase (kinase M) that does not require calcium and phospholipids for activity (42), which could provide another means for producing long-lasting alterations in protein phosphorylation as a result of a transient rise in calcium concentrations.

Brain spectrin, like its counterpart in erythrocytes, is a filamentous protein constituted of two polypeptide chains, α and β, organized as a tetramer $(\alpha\beta)_2$, which forms a network underlying the plasma membrane, attached to the membranes via interactions with ankyrin-like proteins (see 35 for a review). Brain spectrin also binds calmodulin and actin and possibly forms a ternary complex with actin and the brain analog of protein 4.1 of erythrocyte membranes (13,16,17). Interestingly, it was recently shown that synapsin and protein 4.1 are immunologically related (3), a fact that raises the additional possibility that phosphorylation of synapsin might regulate the interaction of brain spectrin with the membrane. Brain spectrin is rapidly degraded by calpain I with the formation of a relatively stable degradation product with a MW of about 150,000 (85), which is also present in isolated postsynaptic densities (19), suggesting that calcium-dependent proteolysis of brain spectrin occurs *in situ* in postsynaptic membranes. Brain spectrin is also a phosphoprotein, but so far the functional role of such a covalent modification is not known; it is conceivable that it also modifies spectrin's susceptibility to proteolysis and/ or its association with other cytoskeletal elements. Similar considerations are also applicable to neurofilament proteins and microtubule-associated proteins.

Although we are only beginning to understand the complex interactions among these different cytoskeletal elements, it remains that a transient activation of calpain in postsynaptic elements can be expected to result in major modifications in the cell cytoskeleton and in the distribution of cell surface receptors as well as in the ultrastructural organization (see below). It is important to note here that the synergistic interactions among various biochemical processes (for instance, phosphorylation and proteolysis) might well be required to provide the optimal amplitude

of the changes and that there might exist a continuum of changes depending on the amplitude and duration of the calcium signals.

Regulation of Calcium Levels

Since calcium is a critical second messenger involved in triggering the activity-dependent changes in synaptic efficacy, factors involved in its regulation can play an indirect role in modulating the amplitude and duration of the changes triggered by physiological events. Three main systems are involved in cellular calcium regulation: calcium pumps located in plasma membranes, the endoplasmic reticulum, and mitochondria (Fig. 2). The relative contribution of each of these systems is still a matter of controversy and probably varies depending on the cellular localization as well as the amplitude of the calcium signals (80). Several factors acting on one or another of these systems have been identified, any of which could be mobilized as a result of the primary stimulating event or the "state" of the system at the time of the primary event. As mentioned, the primary event triggers an influx of calcium via an activation of transmitter-gated or voltage-dependent (or both) calcium channels, and the characteristics of these channels might well be modulated by a variety of effectors including membrane potential, phosphorylating enzymes, and the neurotransmitter and cotransmitters released during the primary event.

Calcium is extruded from the cell by an ATP-dependent calcium pump located in the plasma membrane. The activity of this pump is regulated by the amount of phosphatidylinositol-4,5-biphosphate (PI-P_2) (76). Since a large number of transmitters or hormones stimulate phosphatidylinositol (PI) turnover (14), it follows that the amount of PI-P_2 present in the plasma membranes and therefore the activity of the calcium pump at any time will reflect the integration of a large number of chemical signals impinging on the same target neuron. We recently reported that excitatory amino acids, unlike the majority of hormones or neurotransmitters, do not stimulate PI turnover but rather inhibit the stimulation elicited by various aminergic agonists such as acetylcholine and histamine while having no effect on the stimulation elicited by adrenergic agonists

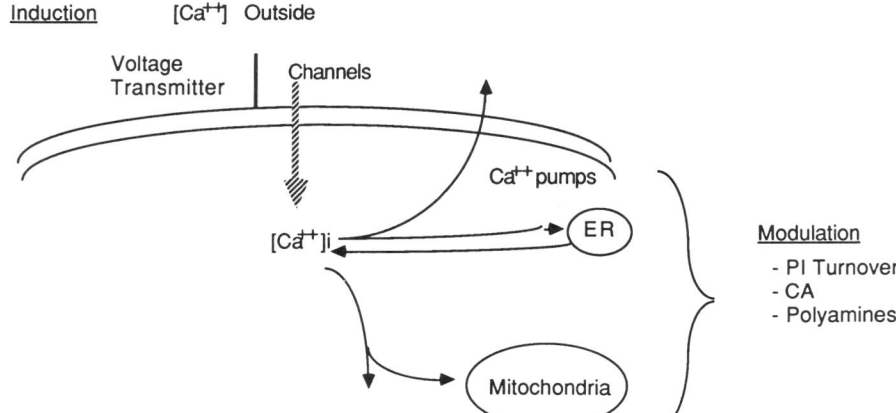

Induction   [Ca⁺⁺] Outside

Voltage Transmitter   Channels

Ca⁺⁺pumps

[Ca⁺⁺]i   ER

Modulation
- PI Turnover
- CA
- Polyamines

Mitochondria

FIG. 2. Schematic representation of various mechanisms regulating calcium concentration in postsynaptic elements. Induction refers to the triggering events that initiate an influx of calcium in the postsynaptic elements, whereas modulation refers to the various factors that can modify the duration and amplitude of the changes in intracellular calcium concentration.

(11). Stimulation of PI turnover results in the generation of two breakdown products, inositol triphosphate (IP$_3$) and diacylglycerol, which respectively induce the release of calcium from endoplasmic reticulum and stimulate protein kinase C (14). Again, the amount of IP$_3$ generated at a given time will reflect the integration of different chemical signals and will determine the extent of intracellular calcium released from the endoplasmic reticulum.

Although the current status of understanding of the role of mitochondria in calcium regulation suggests that these organelles might not play a critical role in the regulation of intracellular calcium concentrations under resting conditions, their influence probably is critical in determining the rate at which intracellular calcium returns to normal following a large increase in intracellular calcium. This is because the maximal velocity of the mitochondrial calcium uptake system is 100-fold higher than those of the calcium pumps located in plasma membranes or in endoplasmic reticulum. Moreover, several factors have been shown to modulate the rate of calcium cycling by the mitochondria, and these factors might therefore also influence the extent and duration of the rise in intracellular calcium following a calcium influx. In several systems it has been shown that adrenergic agonists can induce a release of calcium from mitochondria, although the mechanism underlying this effect is not yet totally clear (34). More recently it was found that polyamines markedly stimulate the rate of calcium uptake in mitochondria from brain (42a), as had been reported for mitochondria in hepatocytes (70). Half-maximal stimulation was observed at a spermine concentration of 0.1 mM, and, given that endogenous levels of spermine correspond to a concentration of about 0.3 mM, it is not unlikely that these compounds serve as endogenous modulators of mitochondrial calcium transport. Moreover, the amount/activity of ornithine decarboxylase, the rate-limiting enzyme in polyamine synthesis, has been shown to be dramatically altered by a wide range of treatments or factors, such as hormones, growth factors, and intense electrical stimulation, with a corresponding increase in endogenous levels of polyamines (50,65,74,75). In summary, there are a set of known mechanisms that can regulate the rate at which increased calcium levels return to normal following a transient disturbance.

Modulation Versus Induction Mechanisms

The picture that emerges from these studies, complex as it may be, strongly suggests that the triggering mechanisms for synaptic changes involve a sequence of biochemical processes and that various regulatory mechanisms can be superimposed at each level. This description of the triggering mechanisms accounts for several features of synaptic plasticity. First, it provides an explanation for the considerable variability in results obtained by various groups using different paradigms to elicit physiological plasticity. One can readily imagine that variations in the pattern of stimulations (duration, frequency) have differential effects on one or the other biochemical events constituting the essential sequence leading to functional modifications. Second, it clearly accounts for the existence of different time courses

of synaptic plasticity that result from the simultaneous activation of biochemical processes with different time courses. This has obvious implications for the distinction between short-term and long-term memory. Moreover, this interpretation provides a useful framework to determine whether there is a continuum between memories of different duration as opposed to existence of parallel mechanisms. Third, the concept of modulation also incorporates the notion that the state of the system at the time of the triggering stimulus, or even during the transitory period that follows this stimulus, plays a critical role in determining the extent and duration of the ultimate changes in synaptic transmission. Factors such as arousal state, hormonal conditions, dietary state, etc., which have often been implicated in the modulations of memory processes (60), can all be reflected as alterations in one or several parameters that participate in the chain of events. In addition, manipulation of the system after the triggering stimulus has taken place could affect critical parts of intermediate duration and modify the extent of the final modification. Finally, this scheme makes it clear that interpretation of pharmacological manipulations should be done carefully in view of the difficulty of dissociating modulating reactions and induction reactions.

Substrates of Lasting Changes

The previous section identified dynamic processes that might be set in motion by the triggering stimulus, but it left unanswered the question of the nature of the permanent (or quasipermanent) traces responsible for the very long-lasting (weeks or months) changes in synaptic efficacy. As noted, the time course of memory probably exceeds by far the half-life of most proteins and therefore cannot be accounted for by simple covalent modification of proteins. Long-term potentiation studies, again, have demonstrated the existence of forms of plasticity that have durations suitable for a memory substrate. In the following sections we briefly review the evidence regarding these stable modifications and consider their possible relationships with the activation of calcium-dependent proteases (Fig. 3).

Changes in Glutamate Binding Sites

As mentioned earlier, glutamate appears to be the major excitatory neurotransmitter in mammalian CNS and, as is the case for most neurotransmitters, several types of receptors have been identified using a variety of biochemical and physiological techniques (7,9,32). One subtype is the NMDA receptor, but, although it is synaptically localized at excitatory synapses (27), it does not appear to be the receptor activated by low-frequency stimulation of afferent pathways, at least in hippocampus. It has been generally assumed that this latter receptor is preferentially activated by another glutamate analog, quisqualate. Binding studies using different ligands have also identified several types of binding sites, and although there is not yet a perfect agreement between the classifications of glutamate receptors derived from binding studies and electrophysiological studies, there is nonetheless a large body of data indicating that

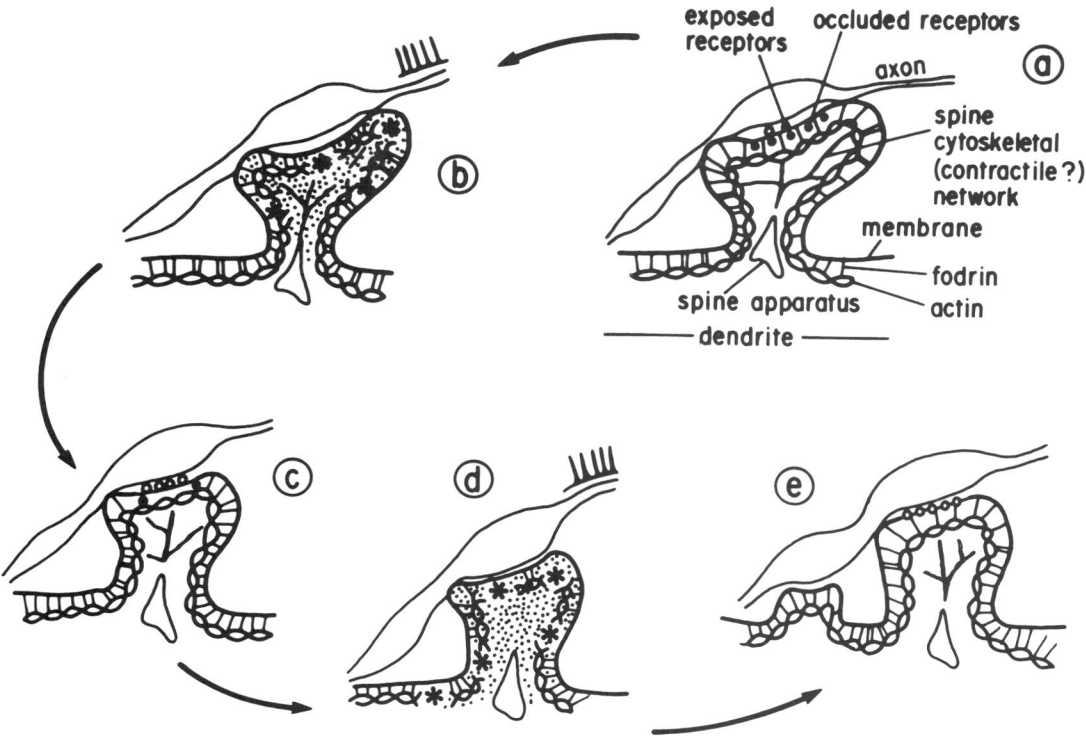

FIG. 3. A possible mechanism for the activity-dependent changes in dendritic spine morphology. In **a** are represented different elements of the cytoskeleton as well as synaptic glutamate receptors. In **b**, a brief burst of high-frequency stimulation results in the opening of calcium channels (see text) and in a rise in the intracellular calcium concentration followed by the activation of calpain and the partial proteolysis of various cytoskeletal proteins. This induces **c**, the loosening of the structure of the spine and an increase in the number of glutamate receptors. In **d**, subsequent bursts of high-frequency stimulation produce a larger depolarization and a larger influx of calcium. Under these conditions, calcium ions might be able to reach larger domains of the postsynaptic elements, possibly resulting in the formation of additional contacts **e**.

[3]H-glutamate labels a category of binding sites that could correspond to the quisqualate synaptic glutamate receptor.

Studies have been conducted to determine if changes in the number of binding sites occur with the induction of LTP. This involved preparing "minislices" containing a subfield of hippocampus and *in vitro* stimulation of approximately 30 contiguous sites; these procedures were used in an effort to potentiate the largest possible fraction of synapses contained in the tissue. Following the physiological phase of the experiments, the minislices were homogenized, and crude synaptosomal membrane fractions were prepared and assayed for glutamate binding. The induction of LTP produced about a 30% increase in the binding of ^{3}H-glutamate, whereas high-frequency stimulation that did not cause LTP was without effect on binding (54). Other laboratories have also reported an increase in glutamate binding in hippocampus following intense, high-frequency stimulation (82). These experiments thus provided a biochemical correlate of LTP and one that might well be responsible for the increased postsynaptic responses that define the effect.

It was then possible to ask if calcium and any of the processes it initiates produce similar effects on subcellular fractions enriched in synapses. This proved to be the case: calcium in low-micromolar concentrations caused an irreversible increase in binding that appeared to be caused by an increase in the number, as opposed to the affinity, of the binding sites (8). This effect of calcium was totally blocked by inhibitors of calcium-dependent proteases and was also blocked by antibodies against brain spectrin (10,86). This suggests that the calcium-induced increase in the number of glutamate receptor binding sites results from the activation of calpain and the resulting degradation of brain spectrin. Blocking either calpain activity or brain spectrin degradation prevents the increase in glutamate receptor binding. In addition, exogenous calpain augments the calcium-induced increase in glutamate receptor binding as well as the calcium-induced degradation of brain spectrin (9a). This situation is reminiscent of the role of spectrin in a variety of cells where it is generally agreed that spectrin is involved in the regulation of the distribution of cell surface receptors. In particular, spectrin has been shown to participate in the capping of cell surface receptors (49,22a). Moreover, it was recently proposed that calpain-induced degradation of spectrin-like proteins is responsible for the uncovering of fibrinogen receptors in blood platelets stimulated by thrombin or ADP (4).

In the case of glutamate receptors, two possible interpretations have been proposed. In the first, brain spectrin would serve to regulate the movement of receptor molecules in the lipid bilayer, and calpain-mediated degradation of the spectrin network would result in the uncovering of glutamate receptors previously in a configuration not accessible to the ligand (9). In this case, the modification in the number of glutamate receptors could become permanent if it is further assumed that the spectrin degradation is also accompanied by a permanent modification of the membrane structure that allows for an increase in the number of insertion sites for new molecules of receptors. A second interpretation is a generalization to the glutamate receptors of the properties exhibited by the cholinergic receptors (21). In this case, it is assumed that glutamate receptors can exist in two configurations with markedly different affinities for glutamate and that the transition between these two configurations is regulated via interaction with the underlying spectrin network. Calpain-induced degradation of spectrin would shift the equilibrium between these two configurations and increase the number of receptors in the active configuration (7). Here also, the change in the number of glutamate receptors requires some permanent modification of the organization of the spectrin network to become permanent. Although much remains to be done to establish firmly the nature of the modifications in glutamate receptors elicited by calpain activation, these results indicate that this enzyme has profound effects on the properties of membrane proteins.

Structural Changes in Dendritic Spines

Changes in the shape of dendritic spines have also been found in hippocampal pyramidal neurons following the induction of LTP (20,29,48,96). These consist in a reduction in the variability of the length of postsynaptic densities and spine head area, effects that are best interpreted as a shift of the dendritic spine head from an ellipsoidal to a spherical shape. As discussed previously, the fact that most cytoskeletal proteins are substrates of calpain provides a possible mechanism by which increase in calcium concentration and the resulting activation of calpain induce a transient perturbation of the spine cytoskeleton (87). Depending on the extent and duration of calpain activation as well as the various phosphorylation reactions that are postulated to accompany calcium influx and to modify the state of phosphorylation of cytoskeletal proteins, a certain fraction of these cytoskeletal proteins could be degraded, resulting in a transient loosening of the cytoskeletal structure. As a consequence, the spine head would tend to adopt the most thermodynamically stable configuration. Since most of the cytoskeletal elements are self-assembling, the remaining elements would reorganize themselves once the levels of calcium return to a level below the threshold for calpain activation. Since the altered configuration is the most stable, this reorganization, once in place, could be maintained in spite of turnover of the individual molecules that constitute the spine.

Again, this interpretation is in agreement with the role of calpain and cytoskeletal elements in peripheral tissues. For instance, it has been shown that erythrocytes and blood platelets can reversibly and sometimes irreversibly modify their shapes. In the case of erythrocytes, activation of calpain and the resulting degradation of spectrin and band 3 have been shown to correlate well with the accompanying transition from discocyte to echinocyte (87). This transition was shown to be related to the transient detachment of the spectrin network from its sites of attachment in the plasma membrane (43). Similarly, activated platelets modify their shape from smooth diskoid to convoluted spherical. This reaction involving complex phosphorylation reactions can occur reversibly through calcium-dependent microtubule depolymerization but appears to be irreversible once calpain is activated and spectrin-like proteins are degraded (33). Although it is conceivable that the dendritic spine shape change can occur and be maintained despite protein turnover, recent findings have suggested the possibility that local protein synthesis might be involved in the long-term stabilization of the new structural organization. Polyribosomes have long been reported to be present in dendritic elements, often located at the base of the spines. Various groups have reported that high-frequency stimulation of presynaptic afferents results in an increase in the state of aggregation of polyribosomes and have suggested that such stimulation results in the translation of specific messenger RNA coding for some subset of synaptic proteins (94,96). Again whether this mechanism participates in modulation or in direct induction remains to be determined.

Changes in the Number of Synaptic Contacts

The induction of LTP is also accompanied by an increase in the number of certain types of synapses. This effect was first detected for spineless or shaft contacts (i.e., synapses on the branches of the dendrites without spines) and has been replicated twice with the additional observation that short, stubby ("sessile") spines also increase in number (20,96). It is possible that some part of this effect reflects some type of altering of spines beyond the point of shape change and that some of the added contacts are on inhibitory interneurons; resolution of these and related points will require three-dimensional reconstruction of serial sections.

The increase in contacts appears rapidly (before 15 min, the earliest time tested) and persists apparently unchanged through the longest measurement period (8 hr); this effect, though not large, is relatively robust, since it has been found both in slices and in anesthetized animals. Given the speed with which the synapses form, it is highly probable that this reflects the existence of local interactions of the type seen in growth cones in tissue culture. It is not implausible that the biochemical processes proposed above as the agents responsible for shape change could, if carried to an extreme degree, result in process extension and contact formation. Again, there are other examples of such rapid modification of cell structure. Platelets proceed through a shape change phase to filopodia extension and finally aggregation; as noted above, there is evidence that increased intracellular calcium concentration and activation of calcium-dependent kinase and protease play crucial roles in this sequence.

TESTING OF SPECIFIC HYPOTHESES

Anatomical Issues

One of the greatest challenges facing behavioral neurobiology is finding ways in which to test hypotheses concerning the cellular mechanisms of memory. Presumably, we should like to (a) carry out physiological, anatomical, and chemical tests on synapses to determine if the changes predicted by the hypotheses actually occur during learning (correlation) and (b) determine if treatments that affect critical variables in the various hypotheses have selective effects on the encoding of information (manipulation). There are two quite formidable anatomical obstacles to correlational experiments. First, it would be necessary to identify synaptic populations that contain the elements affected by a learning episode, and efforts in this direction have had a long and frustrating history. Thus, although there is good reason to suspect that neocortex is the site of associative memory storage, the extreme complexity of this brain region makes it an unlikely area in which to locate the pertinent synapses. Second, there is the extreme likelihood that the number of synapses affected by a learning episode is but a very small percentage of the field within which they are contained. It can be expected, therefore, that any chemical or structural effects associated with learning will be greatly diluted by neighboring unchanged contacts.

The manipulative (typically pharmacological) approach does not necessarily confront these problems and has been widely used in studies of mammalian memory; nonetheless, it does have its own set of difficulties. Chief among these is selectivity. Memory, as we have noted elsewhere (53), can be viewed as a higher-order process of the brain; that is, memory presumably involves either an exaggeration of normal CNS functions or an addition of a normally quiescent mechanism to those functions. It follows then that any manipulation that at all disturbs the coordinated operation of brain circuitry could potentially interfere with memory. This difficulty is especially severe for hypotheses that invoke cellular events that are probably vital to the moment-to-moment operation of neurons (e.g., protein phosphorylation). Behavioral controls for unwanted "primary" effects are not easily designed, in part because we are not so familiar with the activities of laboratory animals that subtle deviations from the norm can be detected.

An alternative approach to the problem of control would be to observe the physiology of the circuits, or better still the synapses, involved in memory and then test if a given manipulation selectively interferes with the modification of those synapses. Thus, rather than dealing with the immense complexity of behavior and the admitted difficulty of detecting subtle disturbances, any number of which could influence memory, we might hope to restrict our field of observation to the site at which the pertinent changes actually occur. The reason this approach is not widely attempted relates to the points raised above; namely, how does one find the cortical synapses involved in memory and then measure physiological events associated with them?

Olfactory System as a Model

Not all telencephalic cortex is as complicated as the neocortex. Some of the regions that together constitute the hippocampal formation have a straightforward and well-described anatomy consisting of a dense layer of cell bodies and one or two adjacent cell-free dendritic zones containing discrete layers of terminals from known afferents. Moreover, the physiology of many of the major synaptic connections in hippocampus has been intensively studied over the past decade, and much is known about the firing characteristics of different types of cells during various behaviors. However, it has proven difficult to identify the types of signals the hippocampus samples and, related to this, the role that it plays in behavior. Thus, although there is reason to assume that hippocampus and related cortical structures are involved in "data"-type memory in humans, controversies continue about their functions in laboratory animals. Clearly, as first documented by a number of investigators starting with O'Keefe and Nadel (72), the hippocampus is crucial for spatial behavior, but whether this is because it stores "maps" of the environment (72) or "working" memories of sites just visited (73) or performs some other functions remains controversial. It is also the case that the hippocampus is connected to the sensory (with the exception noted below) and motor systems of the brain by a tortuous and poorly understood series of connections. Because of this, it is difficult to construct hypotheses about its functions from anatomical data, and therefore ideas about its roles in behavior must be drawn largely from correlative (recording) and manipulative (lesions) studies of behavior. It is difficult to incorporate such ideas and behavioral tests of them in a larger neurobiological context.

Olfactory cortex (pyriform/lateral entorhinal cortex) is more complex than most of the subdivisions of hippocampus but is much more accessible for functional analyses. It is composed of three layers of cells, the outermost of which has a simple and well-defined anatomy (Fig. 4). Moreover, the dominant input to the cortex terminates in this layer and arises solely from the mitral cells of the olfactory bulb. Since these latter neurons are themselves directly innervated by the receptor cells for odors, it follows that pyriform-entorhinal cortex is only two synapses removed from the physical stimulus for the olfaction. Clearly then, the pyriform cortex must first and foremost serve a primary role in representing and processing information about odorants.

The neuroanatomy of the pyriform cortex provides some compelling ideas about what that role might be and, moreover, bears some surprising resemblances to that expected for an associative memory system. The axons of the lateral olfactory tract (LOT) ramify throughout the pyriform with little if any topography between bulbar and cortical areas; the layer II target cells in the pyriform in turn generate a recursive feedback system that lacks any obvious topographic rules (37,52). Since we can assume that a collection of synapses must be cojointly activated to bring a pyriform neuron to its firing threshold, it appears that the afferent axons and dendrites of this cortical area form a quasirandom combinatorial network; this system presumably sacrifices information about which part of the bulb was stimulated by a given odor but allows for the association of inputs from disparate parts of the bulb. As discussed above, associativity is a key element of the memory system. Note also that the evidence from neuroanatomy points to the conclusion that odors are likely to be "represented" in the pyriform cortex as combinations of cells responding to a given odor; the number of potential combinations in the pyriform cortex, assuming that a sizable percentage of the

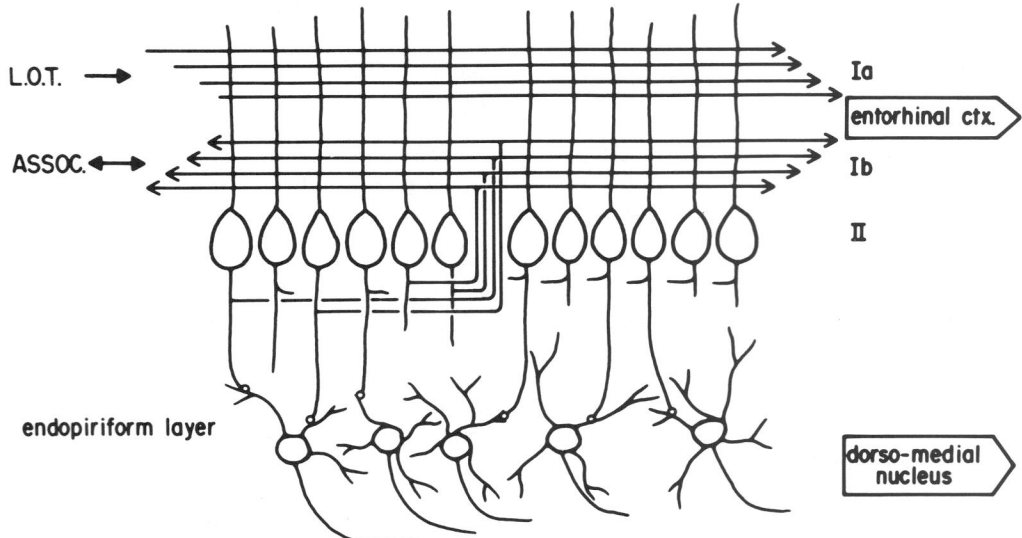

FIG. 4. Schematic representation of the organization of the pyriform cortex. The lateral olfactory tract (LOT) generates an extensive terminal field in layer Ia and forms synaptic contacts on neurons whose cell bodies are located in layer II; the axons of these neurons send collaterals in layer Ib, forming a dense associational system, as well as in the deep layer of the pyriform cortex (the endopyriform nucleus).

total population participates in any given odor, is thus immense.

Assuming that they possess the requisite plasticity, even the early stages of the olfactory projections through telencephalon can be seen to possess fundamental features needed for association and storage capacity. However, associativity in the sense used here refers to elements of a stimulus rather than the linking together of central representations of peripheral events, which is the sense that associativity is typically used in memory research. It is indeed interesting that olfactory cortex, or more precisely its lateral entorhinal cortical wing, projects massively into hippocampus, a region that also receives auditory, visual, and probably motoric information. It is not implausible then that associations between odor and nonolfactory representations occur in the hippocampus, although it is certainly the case that hippocampus has functions beyond and in addition to this. In all, the anatomy of the olfactory paths from bulb through pyriform and into hippocampus constitutes a series of simple cortical stages that seem capable of representing and associating environmental cues that are of great importance, at least to most nonprimate mammals. Given the relative simplicity and repetition that characterize the system, it may be possible to locate populations of synapses containing elements that have been influenced by learning and then to conduct neurobiological studies of the learning process.

The first step in this would be to determine if olfactory memory actually possesses the characteristics proposed above and then to test if other features, including the data and procedural aspects of memory, are also present. A number of experiments pertinent to this have been conducted. Slotnick and co-workers reported that the performance of rats on successive reversal tasks involving odors steadily improved over days until reversals were achieved in only a few trials and suggested that rats acquire "learning sets" for odors in much the same way as primates do for visual cues (88). This indicates that rapid acquisition of olfactory learning does occur and that multiple types of memory (i.e., learning the task versus learning the reversal for a given day) are also present (Table 1).

Experimental Results

Behavioral Approach

Experiments in our laboratories using mazes as well as simple operants have been directed specifically at the issues of rapid acquisition, capacity, duration, and types of memory involved in olfaction (U. Staubli *unpublished data*). The design is relatively simple: rats are trained over days on two odor discriminations with a new pair of novel cues used each day. The animals learn the first discrimination very slowly (up to hours depending on the odors) but improve over days until after 4 to 6 days they are able to master a new discrimination in fewer than five trials; i.e., virtually one-trial learning. It seems that, as in Slotnick's

TABLE 1. *Properties of olfactory memory in the rat*

Human-like neurology
Combinatorial
Involves two processes subserved by different anatomical systems
Rapid acquisition
Long duration
Large capacity
Blocked by calpain inhibitor

experiments, the rats learn something about the problem over days and then make use of this information to deal with each novel discrimination. We suggest that the first type of learning is "procedural" whereas the second requires a "data" memory system. Although learning is rapid in these paradigms, it nonetheless has great stability, since the rats remember previously learned odors even after delays of several weeks. Moreover, the capacity of the system must be very large, since the rats are able to learn new discriminations each day for a month and then to exhibit excellent recall of any of the elements in the group (U. Staubli and G. Lynch, *unpublished data*).

Many of the odors used in these experiments were composites of three chemicals, suggesting that some stage of the olfactory circuitry carries out associations of disparate cues. That this can occur beyond the bulbar level is suggested by recent and elegant work by Mouly et al. (67), who demonstrated that rats respond to stimulation of multiple points in the bulb as though a single odor were present. Moreover, researchers in our laboratories have demonstrated that rats are capable of distinguishing between two composite odors with considerable overlap but do not recognize the not-in-common elements when these are given alone (that is, an odor composed of chemicals ABC is distinguished from one with BCD, but A versus D is treated as though it were a new problem). These last experiments point to the conclusion that complex odors are treated as unitary cues by the olfactory system, an operation that would be predicted for a quasirandom combinatorial system.

In addition to these purely behavioral considerations, the "neurology" of olfactory memory matches that expected for a cortical memory system. It will be recalled that hippocampal damage in humans produces a "rapid forgetting" syndrome in which data items are retained for only a very brief period, although preinjury memories and procedural memory were less affected. Lesions of the connections from olfactory cortex to hippocampus reproduce much of this effect in rats that have prelesion training on olfactory discriminations (93). Thus, the animals are able to learn new discrimination problems if the trials are given with short intervals (1–3 min) between them but are severely impaired if 10-min intertrial delays are used (normal rats have no difficulty with this). Moreover, if rats are trained to criterion with short intervals but then are retested 10 min later, they give no evidence of the prior learning experience. Since the rats rapidly learn new discriminations, it can be concluded that the memories formed on problems acquired before surgery must be at least reasonably intact.

Pharmacological Approach

Attempts to use the olfactory system to test the cellular hypotheses about memory storage began with pharmacological manipulations of calpain. As a first step, the calpain inhibitor leupeptin was slowly infused over days into the lateral ventricles of rats from subdermal osmotic minipumps, and feeding, drinking, body temperature, and two forms of spontaneous activity were measured. The highest concentrations of drug (estimated ventricular concentration of 50–

100 μM) produced disturbances in the activity patterns of some of the animals, but lower dosages (10–50 μM) did not affect the control measures. However, even the lowest drug concentration caused an impairment in acquisition of a novel odor discrimination by rats with extensive predrug training in successive discriminations (91). This deficit appeared to be quite selective: rats performed normally in the task with the exception that learning was slow or absent. Moreover, they were able to locate food using familiar odor cues. The effect of leupeptin on memory was not restricted to olfaction; the animals were also impaired on a spatial memory test involving an eight-arm radial maze (90). In those experiments, the rats were also given extensive predrug experience and, under the influence of leupeptin, still ran into alley arms, retrieved food, and gave other evidence of normal behavior. The effect on memory acquisition was not obtained when a drug that blocks several proteases but not calpain was administered.

We then asked if leupeptin affected other types of memory. The drug was administered as above, and the rats were tested for inhibitory and active avoidance conditioning. In these tasks the rat must either refrain from moving (inhibitory avoidance) or move quickly (active avoidance) in order to avoid a mild foot shock. In contrast to olfactory and spatial maze learning, avoidance conditioning does not require training over days and instead occurs with a single trial in the case of the inhibitory problem or five to 10 trials for active avoidance. Memory was tested on the following day. Leupeptin, even at the highest concentrations, had little if any influence on acquisition and retention of shock avoidance (90).

These studies do support the idea that calpain is involved in memory storage but also indicate that this is not universal and in particular that some other cellular process is responsible for shock-avoidance learning. There is a sizable literature showing that avoidance conditioning is blocked by protein synthesis inhibitors (26,31); whether this is caused by protein synthesis inhibition or by some other effect of the drugs is controversial, but the basic finding that the drugs suppress the retention of learned avoidance responses has been reported several times. However, we have found that protein synthesis inhibitors do not interfere with the acquisition or retention of specific olfactory memories (92). Together, these results produce a double dissociation of memory, with leupeptin causing deficits in one form but not the other and protein synthesis inhibitors producing the opposite pattern.

Electrophysiological Approach

The next stage in the analysis of the substrates of olfactory memory is to exploit the relative simplicity of the underlying anatomy in an attempt to find synaptic fields that contain elements affected by learning. With this information it may be possible to ask if leupeptin or other drugs directed at various elements of the cellular hypothesis act selectively on synaptic modification and leave untouched normal synaptic functioning. There are, however, major difficulties: (a) odors are difficult to use as cues that could be expected to produce synchronous synaptic field potentials, and (b) given the vast storage capacity of the olfactory memory system, it is extremely unlikely that the learning of a single discrimination will influence more than a small percentage of synapses in a terminal field. In an effort to obviate these problems, experiments have been initiated using electrical stimulation of the lateral olfactory tract in place of odors in a successive olfactory discrimination problem. In this way it is possible to sample the strength of those synapses in pyriform cortex that clearly must have been involved in representing the learned cues. The rats were first trained on a series of odor discriminations before attempts were made to substitute electrical stimulation; the rats did not respond well behaviorally to single pulses to LOT but did behave as though an odor were present when short bursts of pulses were applied with the bursts occurring at 5/sec. Moreover, they quickly learned to discriminate between "positive" and "negative" electrodes. The size of the monosynaptic extracellular responses in pyriform cortex to single pulses was measured before and after a learning episode; in a great majority of cases these responses were potentiated after learning, an effect that did not dissipate over 24 hr. The responses to control electrodes (i.e., electrodes that were not used as "cues") did not change during or after the learning episodes (80a).

One of the most surprising results from this series of experiments was that the patterned stimulation used as an odor did not produce potentiation when used outside the learning task. Apparently the learning situation in some way exerts an influence on the pyriform cortex such that patterns of electrical activity are able to impress an extremely stable potentiation of synapses. These experiments may be providing clues about the interaction of the "procedural" and "data" memory systems in that prior learning acquired over several days seems to be needed to produce plasticity in response to a particular datum (in this case an "electric odor"). It should also be noted that the stimulation pattern that proved effective as an "odor" closely resembles endogenous activity patterns found throughout the hippocampus and related structures and has been found to be optimal for inducing LTP in hippocampus (41). From the above results, it appears that this pattern serves not only as an information-coding device but also as a signal for synapses to increase their relative strengths. Finally, we should not overlook the fact that the electrical odor experiments provide us with our first experimental evidence that a group of cortical synapses in a defined larger population actually changes their synaptic strength selectively during learning.

Returning now to our major theme, the electric odor paradigm should allow a second, more molecular description of the relationship between a particular pharmacological manipulation and the process that encodes memory. That is, the paradigm permits us to study drug effects on control behaviors (e.g., activity) and learning and at the same time to analyze its effects on control and "plastic" aspects of synaptic transmission.

Can the preparation also be used to study if biochemical effects predicted by various hypotheses occur? The "electrical" odor paradigm pinpoints the locus of a group of synapses that change with learning, but it does not inform us of the percentage of the total population that is affected, although we can assume that this is not large. It may be possible, however, to use several electrodes in the LOT to train the rats on a series of discriminations and then remove the pyriform cortex, dissect the pertinent dendritic field, and conduct biochemical assays. Note that this could be done only for the more persistent biochemical (anatomical) consequences of learning; very transient effects would not be detected by this approach. In any event, the electrical odor paradigm, by solving the problem of localizing "memory" synapses, brings into sharp focus the problems associated with using correlational measures to test ideas about the chemistry of memory; this is a clear advance and should prompt efforts to find solutions to the now-defined experimental difficulties.

CONCLUSIONS

Considerable progress has been accomplished in our undertanding of the properties and mechanisms of learning during the past 5 to 10 years. At the phenomenological level, various paradigms have been developed allowing a more precise definition of the characteristics of different memory systems as well as their localizations in different brain structures. In particular, the previously existing gap between experimental psychologists studying the neuropsychology of learning and memory in humans and those concerned with other mammalian species seems to be closing; if so, then we may hope for the formulation of general rules for learning and memory that are applicable to humans and yet testable in animals. At the cellular level, a variety of biochemical mechanisms exhibiting the requisite properties of molecular and temporal integration of several chemical signals have been identified. Moreover, these mechanisms can account for the existence of several time courses for changes in efficacy of synaptic transmission ranging from seconds to days and weeks. A precise mapping of the distribution of the different molecular elements constituting these mechanisms in different types of neurons and neuronal pathways should allow the formulation of specific hypotheses concerning their participation in the different types of memory. Testing of specific hypotheses, although still remaining a major problem, may become more rigorous with the identification in the mammalian nervous system of the neural networks, and possibly the synapses, responsible for the storage of specific information. Finally, an understanding of the structures and adaptive properties of neural networks (especially cortical networks) is slowly emerging. Should it be totally accomplished in the next decade, it would result in a fundamental scientific revolution.

ACKNOWLEDGMENTS

This research was supported by grants BNS 81-12-156 from the National Science Foundation to M. Baudry and AFOSR 85-NL-105 to G. Lynch. The authors wish to thank Jackie Porter for her skillful assistance in preparing the manuscript.

REFERENCES

1. Akers, R. F., Lovinger, D. M., Colley, P. A., Linden, D. J., and Routtenberg, A. (1986): *Science,* 231:587–589.
2. Alkon, D. (1984): *Science,* 226:1037–1045.
3. Baines, A. J., and Bennett, V., (1985): *Nature,* 315:410–413.
4. Baldassare, J. J., Bakshian, S., Knipp, M. A., and Fisher, G. J. (1985): *J. Biol. Chem.,* 260:10531–10535.
5. Baraban, J. M., Snyder, S. H., and Alger, B. E. (1985): *Proc. Natl. Acad. Sci.,* 82:2538–2542.
6. Barnes, C. A. (1979): *J. Comp. Physiol. Psychol.,* 93:74–104.
7. Baudry, M. (1986): In: *Excitatory Amino Acids,* edited by P. J. Roberts, J. Storm-Mathisen, and H. Bradford. Macmillan, London *(in press).*
8. Baudry, M., and Lynch, G. (1979): *Nature,* 282:748–750.
9. Baudry, M., and Lynch, G. (1984): In: *Neurobiology of Learning and Memory,* edited by G. Lynch, J. McGaugh, and N. Weinberger, pp. 431–447. The Guilford Press, New York, London.
9a. Baudry, M., and Lynch, G. (1986): *(unpublished observations).*
10. Baudry, M., Bundman, M., Smith, E., and Lynch, G. (1981): *Science,* 212:937–938.
11. Baudry, M., Evans, J., and Lynch, G. (1986): *Nature,* 319:329–331.
12. Baudry, M., Simonson, L., Dubrin, R., and Lynch, G. (1986): *J. Neurobiol.,* 17:15–28.
13. Bennett, J., and Davis, J. (1981): *Proc. Natl. Acad. Sci U.S.A.,* 78:7550–7554.
14. Berridge, M. J., and Irvine, R. F. (1984): *Nature,* 312:315–321.
15. Bloch, V., and Laroche, S. (1984): In: *Neurobiology of Learning and Memory,* edited by G. Lynch, J. McGaugh, and N. Weinberger, pp. 249–260. The Guilford Press, New York.
16. Branton, D., Cohen, C. M., and Tyler, J. (1981): *Cell,* 24:24–32.
17. Burridge, K., Kelly, T., and Mangeat, P. (1982): *J. Cell. Biol.,* 95:478–486.
18. Canellakis, E. S., Viceps-Madore, D., Kyriakidis, D. A., and Heller, J. S. (1979): *Curr. Top. Cell. Regul.,* 15:155–202.
19. Carlin, R. K., Bartelt, D. C., and Siekevitz P. (1983): *J. Cell Biol.,* 96:443–448.
20. Chang, F. L. F., and Greenough, W. T. (1984): *Brain Res.,* 309:35–46.
21. Changeux, J. P., Devillers-Thiery, A., and Chemouilli, P. (1984): *Science,* 225:1335–1345.
22. Cohen, N., and Squire, L. R. (1980): *Science,* 210:207–209.
22a. Colaco, C. A. L. S., and Lazarides, E. (1983): *Proc. Natl. Acad. Sci. U.S.A.,* 80:1626–1630.
23. Collingridge, G. L., Kehl, S. J., and McLennan, H. (1983): *J. Physiol. (Lond.)* 334:33–46.
24. Coss, R. G., and Perkel, D. H. (1985): *Behav. Neural Biol.,* 44:151–185.
25. Crabtree, B. (1985): *FEBS Lett.,* 187:193–195.
26. Dunn, A. J. (1976): *Molecular and Functional Neurobiology,* edited by W. H. Gispen, pp. 347–387. Elsevier, Amsterdam.
27. Fagg, G. E., and Matus, A. (1984): *Proc. Natl. Acad. Sci. U.S.A.,* 81:6876–6880.
28. Feldman, J. A. (1981): In: *Parallel Models an Associative Memory,* edited by G. E. Hinton and J. A. Anderson, pp. 49–82. Lawrence Erlbaum, Hillsdale, NJ.
29. Fifkova, E., and Van Harreveld, A. (1975): *J. Neurocytol.,* 6:211–380.
30. Fifkova, E., and Delay, R. (1982): *J. Cell Biol.,* 95:345–350.
31. Flood, J. F., Jarvik, M. E., Bennett, E. L., Orme, A. E., and Rosenszweig, M. R. (1977): *Behav. Biol.,* 20:168–183.
32. Foster, A. C., and Fagg, G. E. (1984): *Brain Res. Rev.,* 7:103–164.
33. Fox, J. E. B., Goll, D. E., Reynolds, C. C., and Phillips, D. R. (1985): *J. Biol. Chem.,* 260:1060–1066.
34. Goldstone, T. P., Duddridge, R. J., and Crompton M. (1983): *Biochem. J.,* 210:463–472.
35. Goodman, S. R., and Zagon, I. S. (1985): *Brain Res. Bull.,* 13:813–832.
36. Greenough, W. (1984): *Trends Neurosci.,* 7:229–233.
37. Haberly, L. B. (1985): *Chem. Senses,* 10:219–238.
38. Harris, E. W., Ganong, A. H., and Cotman, C. W. (1984): *Brain Res.,* 323:132–137.
39. Hebb, D. O. (1949): *The Organization of Behavior.* John Wiley & Sons, New York.
40. Hinton, G. E., and Anderson, J. A. (1981): *Parallel Models of Associative Memory.* Lawrence Erlbaum, Hillsdale, NJ.
41. Hopfield, J. J. (1982): *Proc. Natl. Acad. Sci. U.S.A.,* 79:2554–2558.
42. Inoue, M., Kishimoto, A., Takai, Y., and Nishizuka, Y. (1977): *J. Biol. Chem.,* 252:7610–7616.
42a. Jensen, J., Lynch, G., and Baudry, M. (1987): *J. Neurochem. (in press).*
43. Jinbu, Y., Sato, S., Nakao, M., Tsukita, S., and Ishikawa, H. (1984): *Biochim. Biophys. Acta.* 773:237–245.
44. Kandel, E. R., and Schwartz, J. H. (1982): *Science,* 218:433–443.
45. Kohonen, T. (1984): *Self-Organization and Associative Memory.* Springer-Verlag, Berlin.
46. Larson, J., Wong, D., and Lynch, G. (1986): Patterned stimulation at the theta frequency is optimal for the induction of hippocampal long-term potentiation. *Brain Res.,* 368:347–350.
47. Larson, J., and Lynch, G. S. (1986): *Science,* 232:985–988.
48. Lee, K., Schottler, F., Oliver, M., and Lynch, G. (1980): *J. Neurophysiol.,* 44:247–258.
49. Levine, J., and Willard, M. (1983): *Proc. Natl. Acad. Sci. U.S.A.,* 80:191–195.
50. Lewis, M. E., Laksmanan, J., Nagaiah, K., McDonnell, P. C., and Guroff, G. (1978): *Proc. Natl. Acad. Sci. U.S.A.,* 75:1021–1023.
51. Lisman, J. E. (1985): *Proc. Natl. Acad. Sci. U.S.A.,* 82:3055–3057.
52. Lynch, G. (1986): *Synapses, Circuits and the Beginnings of Memory.* MIT Press, Cambridge *(in press).*
53. Lynch, G., and Baudry, M. (1984): *Science,* 224:1057–1063.
54. Lynch, G., Halpain, S., and Baudry, M. (1982): *Brain Res.,* 244:101–111.
55. Lynch, G., Larson, J., Kelso, S., Barrionuevo, G., and Schottler, F. (1983): *Nature,* 305:719–721.
56. Lynch, G., Larson, J., and Baudry, M. (1986): *Treatment Development Strategies for Alzheimer's Disease.* Mark Powley Associates, Inc., pp. 119–149.
57. Madison, D. V., Malenka, R. C., and Nicoll, R. A. (1986): A voltage-dependent chloride current in hippocampal pyramidal cells is blocked by phorbol esters. *Biophys. J. (in press).*
58. Malik, M. N., Meyers, L. A., Iqbal, K., Sheikh, A. M., Scotto, I., and Wisniewski, H. M. (1981): *Life Sci.,* 29:795–802.
59. Mayer, M. L., Westbrook, G. L., and Guthrie, P. B. (1984): *Nature,* 309:261–263.
60. McGaugh, J. L. (1966): *Science,* 153:1351–1358.
61. McNaughton, B. L., Douglas, R. M., and Goddard, G. V. (1978): *Brain Res.,* 157:277–293.
62. Melloni, E., Pontremoli, S., Michetti, M., Sacco, O., Sparatore, B., Salamino, F., and Horecker, B. L. (1985): *Proc. Natl. Acad. Sci. U.S.A.,* 82:6435–6439.
63. Mishkin, M., Malamut, B., and Bachevalier, J. (1984): *Neurobiology of Learning and Memory,* edited by G. Lynch, J. L. McGaugh, and N. Weinberger, pp. 65–78. Guilford Press, New York.
64. Monaghan, D., Holets, V. R., Toy, D. W., and Cotman, C. W. (1983): *Nature,* 306:176–178.
65. Morris, G. M., Seidler, F. J., and Slotkin, T. A. (1983): *Life Sci.,* 32:1565–1571.
66. Morris, R. G. M., Anderson, E., Lynch, G., and Baudry, M. (1986): *Nature,* 319:774–776.
67. Mouly, A. M., Vigouroux, M., and Holley, A. (1985): *Behav. Brain Res.,* 17:45–58.
68. Murachi, T., Tanaka, K., Hatanaka, M., and Murakami, T. (1981): *Adv. Enzyme Regul.* 19:407–424.
69. Nestler, E. J., Walaas, S. I., and Greengard, P. (1984): *Science,* 225:1357–1364.
70. Nicchitta, C. V., and Williamson, C. V. (1984): *J. Biol. Chem.,* 259:12978–12983.
71. Nowak, L., Bregestovski, P., Ascher, P., Herbet, A., and Prochiantz, A. (1984): *Nature,* 307:462–465.
72. O'Keefe, J., and Nadel, L. (1978): *The Hippocampus as a Cognitive Map.* Oxford University Press, London.
73. Olton, D. S., Becker, J. T., and Handelmann, G. E. (1979): *Behav. Brain Sci.* 2:313–365.
74. Pajunen, A. E. I., Hietala, O. A., Virransalo, E. L., and Piha, R. S. (1978): *J. Neurochem.,* 30:281–283.

75. Pegg, A. E., and McCann, P. P. (1982): *Am. J. Physiol.*, 243: C212–C221.
76. Penniston, J. T. (1982): *Ann. N.Y. Acad. Sci.*, 402:296–303.
77. Perlmutter, L., Siman, R., Gall, C., Baudry, M., and Lynch, G. (1987): *(submitted)*.
78. Pontremoli, S., Salamino, F., Sparatore, B., Michetti, M., Sacco, D., and Melloni, E. (1985): *Biochim. Biophys. Acta*, 831:335–339.
79. Racine, R. J., Milgram, N. W., and Hafner, S. (1983): *Brain Res.*, 260:217–231.
80. Rasmussen, H., and Barrett, P. O. (1984): *Physiol. Rev.*, 64:938–984.
80a. Roman, F., Staubli, U., and Lynch, G. (1987): *Brain Res. (in press)*.
81. Sandoval, I. V., and Weber, K. (1978): *Eur. J. Biochem.*, 92:463–470.
82. Savage, D. P., Werling, L. L., Nadler, J. V., and McNamara, J. O. (1982): *Eur. J. Pharmacol.*, 85:255–256.
83. Siekevitz, P. (1985): *Proc. Natl. Acad. Sci. U.S.A.*, 82:3494–3498.
84. Siman, R., Baudry, M., and Lynch, G. (1983): *J. Neurochem.*, 41: 950–956.
85. Siman, R., Baudry, M., and Lynch, G. (1984): *Proc. Natl. Acad. Sci. U.S.A.*, 81:3276–3280.
86. Siman, R., Baudry, M., and Lynch, G. (1985): *Nature*, 315:225–227.
87. Siman, R., Baudry, M., and Lynch, G. (1987): In: *Dynamic Aspects of Neocortical Functions*, edited by G. Edelman, W. M. Cowan, and W. Gall, John Wiley & Sons, New York *(in press)*.
88. Slotnick, B. M., and Katz, H. M. (1974): *Science*, 185:796–798.
89. Squire, L. R. (1982): *Annu. Rev. Neurosci.*, 5:241–251.
90. Staubli, U., Baudry, M., and Lynch, G. (1984): *Behav. Neural Biol.*, 40:58–69.
91. Staubli, U., Baudry, M., and Lynch, G. (1985): *Brain Res.*, 337: 333–336.
92. Staubli, U., Faraday, R., and Lynch, G. (1985): *Behav. Neural Biol.*, 43:287–297.
93. Staubli, U., Ivy, G., and Lynch, G. (1985): *Proc. Natl. Acad. Sci. U.S.A.*, 81:5885–5887.
94. Steward, O., and Fass, B. (1983): *Prog. Brain Res.*, 58:131–136.
95. Teyler, T. J., and Discenna, P. (1984): *Brain Res. Rev.*, 7:15–28.
96. Wenzel, J., and Matthies, H. (1985): In: *Memory Systems of the Brain*, edited by N. Weinberger, J. McGaugh, and G. Lynch, pp. 150–170. The Guilford Press, New York.
97. Wigstrom, H., and Gustasfsson, B. (1984): *Neurosci. Lett.* 44:327–332.
98. Zimmerman, U. J. P., and Schlaepfer, W. W. (1984): *Prog. Neurobiol.*, 23:63–78.

Psychopharmacology:
The Third Generation of Progress,
edited by Herbert Y. Meltzer.
Raven Press, New York © 1987.

CHAPTER **47**

Experience, Neurotransmitter Plasticity, and Behavior

I. B. Black, J. E. Adler, C. F. Dreyfus, W. J. Friedman, E. F. LaGamma, and A. H. Roach

One critical question in the brain sciences concerns the plastic mechanisms that allow the nervous system to function physiologically and perform some of its more spectacular feats such as learning and memory. In fact, do neurons and their networks change with experience? Can we identify, if only provisionally, underlying molecular mechanisms? Indeed, what would such molecular mechanisms look like? Alternatively, what are the probabilities that cognitive function simply cannot be understood at the molecular level and that higher-order processes alone hold the key to comprehending brain function? Could it not be usefully argued that inquiries relating molecules to mind are at best premature and perhaps misleading? One might submit that even a few tentative steps relating molecular to cognitive function would represent a meaningful contribution.

In fact, information emerging from numerous laboratories over the past several years suggest that an understanding of plasticity at the molecular level may provide insights into mind and brain function. The extraordinary (a) specificity, (b) selectivity, and (c) precision that are characteristic of mental function derive, in part, from these properties at the molecular level. Specifically, a subset of neuroactive molecules exhibit characteristics that are central to mind function.

Neurotransmitters, the agents of neural communication, occupy a pivotal role in such considerations. These intercellular signals govern physiologic function of the nervous system and, simultaneously, exhibit a number of characteristics critical for cognitive function. A number of transmitter molecules are capable of transducing extraneuronal information into altered function and thereby encode, store, and transmit environmental information. Consequently, these molecules serve simultaneously as intercellular phys-iological regulators and symbols representing extraneuronal stimuli [4]. In this manner transmitter molecules interrelate a variety of levels of neural function from environment to genome, molecule, synapse, neuron, and system and on to behavior and cognitive function.

Extensive experimental evidence now indicates that transmitter functions, governed by specific regulatory molecules, are constantly undergoing marked plastic responses with altered neuronal experience. Further, these changes account for a number of behavioral patterns associated with learning and memory, discussed in this chapter. Additionally, the transmitter changes are relatively longterm with respect to inciting stimuli and tend to be progressively enhanced with repetition and duration of stimulus, thereby exhibiting mnemonic characteristics. A number of specific stimuli evoking these changes have already been identified. In summary, neurons and their transmitters are not simply invariant components of an extensive hard-wired cognitive network. Rather, transmitter mechanisms are in constant flux, reflecting internal and external influences impinging on the neuron.

The recent realizations that neurons use multiple, colocalized transmitters that may be independently regulated [5] have added an entirely new combinatorial dimension to our understanding of neural plasticity. Consequently, in addition to the complexity of 10^{11} neurons, each with approximately 10^4 interconnections, each neuron may be capable of expressing an ever-changing, complex transmitter repertoire. Concepts of reverberating circuits, growth of new cell assemblies, neosynaptogenesis, and neurogenesis with ongoing neuronal turnover [17,19,20,38,39] must now be complemented by concepts of plasticity within the individual neuron and at the single synapse. Transmitters and their molecular regulators constitute some of the basic units of neural plasticity and brain function.

What intracellular mechanisms transduce environmental information into altered transmitter metabolism and expression and, consequently, into altered neural function? Evidence summarized in this chapter indicates that extracellular stimuli may alter the levels of messenger RNA (mRNA) coding for transmitter molecules, perhaps by altering gene readout itself, thereby altering transmitter function. Additional fine tuning occurs through posttranslational processing and biochemical regulation of the final product. In summary, environmental events appear to alter transcription of specific genes, leading to altered transmitter states of certain neuronal subpopulations.

In turn, the remarkable specificity, selectivity, and precision that characterize neuronal, synaptic, and systems function derive in large part from the combinatorial character of individual neurons and their assemblies. Ongoing studies indicate that at least 50 different amine, acetylcholine, amino acid, purine, and peptide transmitters are present in the nervous system, and the list continues to expand. Moreover, individual neurons use multiple transmitters that are differentially regulated by extracellular signals. Consequently, the single neuron expresses multiple combinatorial states in response to environmental signals. In this chapter we focus on several model systems to illustrate how specific experiences differentially regulate different colocalized transmitter systems. The resultant distinct transmitter states serve to encode different environmental stimuli.

CATECHOLAMINERGIC PLASTICITY IN SYMPATHETIC NEURONS: A MODEL SYSTEM

It is now well recognized that peripheral sympathetic neurons express a number of transmitters in addition to the classical norepinephrine. For example, extensive evidence indicates that this population also elaborates acetylcholine (16,24,34,35), substance P (5), somatostatin (22), and VIP (vasoactive intestinal peptide; 28) under appropriate conditions *in vivo* and *in vitro*. This is of particular interest

in the present context, since sympathetic responses to specific environmental stimuli have been well characterized physiologically, and since the system is easily accessible for biochemical and molecular genetic analysis after experimental manipulation. Consequently, it is convenient to move from environmental stimulus to plastic transmitter response to altered physiologic function using this relatively well-defined system.

It has long been known that environmental stress increases sympathetic impulse activity, resulting in physiologic components of the classical "fight or flight" behavioral repertoire. The molecular plasticity associated with this environmental-behavioral complex is being analyzed in detail, defining relationships among the environmental, physiologic, molecular, and behavioral levels of neural function. For example, extensive studies indicate that environmental stress, eliciting increased impulse activity in sympathetics, transsynaptically induces tyrosine hydroxylase (TH), the rate-limiting enzyme in catecholamine biosynthesis (32,33). Increased impulse activity releases presynaptic acetylcholine, which interacts with postsynaptic nicotinic receptors (Fig. 1). Available evidence suggests that transmembrane Na^+ influx attendant to depolarization is necessary for TH induction (8).

We utilized a cDNA probe (29) complementary to TH mRNA to define mechanisms underlying TH induction in sympathetic neurons (6). The sympathetic system was reflexly activated by administering reserpine to rats, and the sympathetic superior cervical ganglion (SCG) was examined (32,33). As expected, reserpine treatment increased TH activity approximately threefold after 3 days of treatment ($p < 0.001$). The TH mRNA was examined in parallel sets of ganglia by dot blot analysis using the pTH.4 cDNA probe. In fact, control ganglia exhibited detectable levels of TH mRNA, whereas reserpine treatment evoked a threefold rise (6). Consequently, transsynaptic induction of TH is accompanied by elevated TH message.

To determine whether transsynaptic stimulation itself elicited the rises in TH and TH mRNA, rats were subjected to unilateral ganglion denervation (decentralization) surgically, and the contralateral ganglion served as a control. One week postoperatively, animals were divided into two groups, one treated with reserpine and the other with

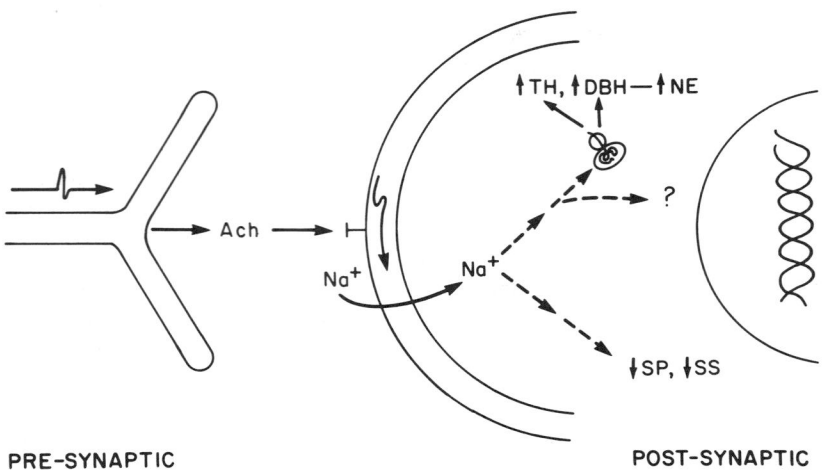

FIG. 1. Schematic representation of the transsynaptic regulation of neurotransmitter traits in sympathetic neurons. Presynaptic impulses release acetylcholine (Ach), which interacts with postsynaptic nicotinic receptors, eliciting transmembrane sodium ion (Na^+) influx. These molecular events biochemically induce TH and dopamine-β-hydroxylase (DBH), resulting in elevated synthesis of norepinephrine (NE) in the postsynaptic neuron. Simultaneously, SP and somatostatin (SS) are decreased. (Reprinted from Black, ref. 4.)

PRE-SYNAPTIC   POST-SYNAPTIC

vehicle, as above. This regimen resulted in four groups of ganglia: (a) intact, vehicle; (b) intact, reserpine; (c) denervated, vehicle; (d) denervated, reserpine. Each group of ganglia was used to determine TH activity, and parallel groups were used for RNA dot hybridization and Northern blot analysis.

As anticipated, reserpine increased TH in control ganglia, and decentralization completely blocked this rise. Moreover, by dot hybridization, reserpine treatment caused a 2.4-fold increase in TH mRNA in intact ganglia but an insignificant 26% change in denervated ganglia (6).

The results of RNA dot hybridization were confirmed and extended by Northern blot analysis (Fig. 2). The cDNA probe for TH hybridized to a single band of approximately 1,900 nucleotides, which was the same size in all ganglia and corresponded to the migration of TH mRNA previously observed from rat pheochromocytoma cells and adrenal (29). Moreover, reserpine treatment elicited a clear increase in TH mRNA, which was prevented by ganglion decentralization. Densitometric analysis of the Northern blot revealed no difference between the intact control group and the decentralized control and, once again, revealed a significant increase in TH mRNA in the intact group only (6).

These results indicate that induction of TH in the SCG elicited by reserpine is accompanied by an increase in TH mRNA. The observations are consistent with recent work indicating that reserpine increases TH mRNA in adrenal medulla and brain (30). Our findings extend previous results by indicating that elevation of TH mRNA is prevented by denervation, which is known to prevent TH induction. Consequently, transsynaptic stimulation may sequentially increase message and TH activity. Thus, transsynaptic increases in impulse activity may induce TH by increasing cellular levels of specific TH message. We do not yet know whether the increase in TH mRNA arises from an increased rate of transcription itself and/or decreased TH mRNA degradation (stabilization).

It is now quite clear, however, that the transsynaptic induction of the rate-limiting enzyme in catecholamine synthesis, a form of quantitative plasticity, is associated with elevated TH mRNA levels. Consequently, sympathetic plasticity elicited by transsynaptic stimulation appears to be regulated at the level of mRNA and potentially at the level of gene readout.

More generally, it is now clear that increased impulse activity, and thus extracellular information, may be represented in the neuron by elevated transmitter regulatory molecules, increased specific mRNA, and, potentially, elevated gene readout. These mechanisms may thereby convert environmental language to neural language.

Having initially defined some of the molecular mecha-

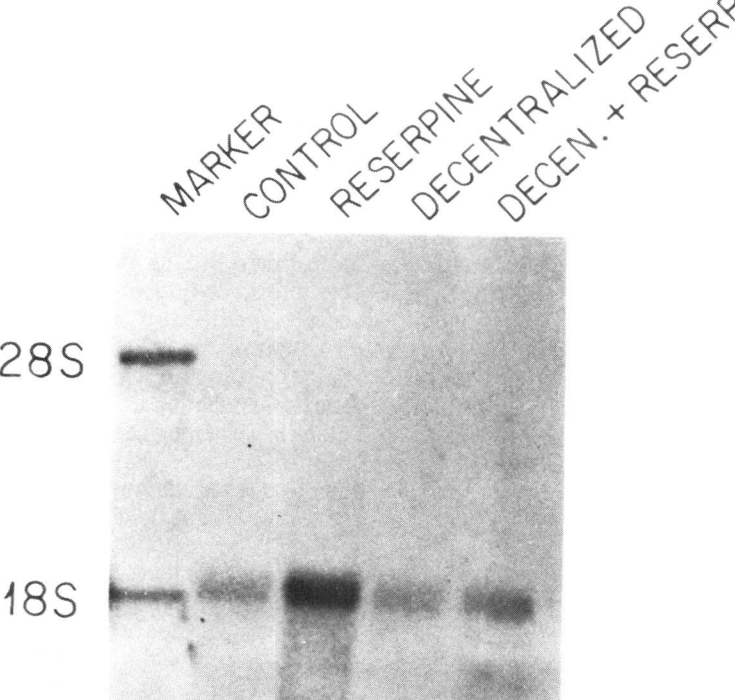

FIG. 2. Northern blot analysis of TH mRNA in ganglia. An aliquot of 5 µg of total RNA was denatured and separated by electrophoresis in 1.1% agarose gels containing formaldehyde. The RNA was transferred to nitrocellulose, probed with pTH.4, and exposed to X-ray film for 2 days. "Marker" lane consists of 18 S and 28 S rRNAs; "control" was vehicle treated, intact; "reserpine" signifies reserpine treatment, intact; "decentralized" was vehicle treated; "decen. + reserpine" was denervated and reserpine treated. (Reprinted from Black et al., ref. 6.)

nisms underlying this transduction, we may characterize the relationship between environmental information and neuronal representation in greater detail. Specifically, can we delineate the kinetics of TH induction? May such knowledge indicate some of the rules by which environmental events are converted to intraneuronal information? Can we thereby gain further insight into the role that plasticity plays in behavioral function?

In fact, the kinetics of TH induction have been defined in detail and exhibit a number of mnemonic characteristics. Environmental stress and sympathetic activation evoke a two- to three-fold increase in sympathetic TH activity within 2 days, and activity remains elevated for at least 3 days after cessation of increased impulse activity. Further, direct electrical nerve stimulation for 30 to 90 min elevates enzyme molecule number for at least 3 days (10,41,42). Thus, a brief stimulus elicits a long-term neuronal molecular change, providing the temporal amplification required of a neural memory system.

Tyrosine hydroxylase induction exhibits another notable characteristic associated with mnemonic phenomena: repetitive stimuli elicit a far greater increase in TH activity than a single stimulus. In one set of experiments, rats were treated with the pharmacologic agent reserpine, which mimics environmental stress by increasing sympathetic impulse flow (32). A single injection elicited a 2.5-fold increase in TH in 3 days. In contrast, repeated daily treatment caused a fivefold rise after 5 days. These results were paralleled by direct electrical stimulation of the preganglionic trunk. Stimulation at 10 Hz for only 10 min increased enzyme activity by 25% 3 days later, whereas stimulation for 60 min increased activity by 73% (41). Thus, repetition and increased stimulus duration are associated with an increase in the magnitude of TH induction, as would be predicted for a molecular memory function.

In summary, brief environmental experiences, stress, or nerve stimulation lasting minutes alters a functionally critical transmitter regulatory molecule for days. Repetition and enhanced stimulus duration increase and prolong this effect. Consequently, short-term environmental stimuli cause relatively long-term alterations of neuronal molecular function. A number of the pivotal mechanisms that transduce experience into altered neural function have been identified, and the resultant molecular changes have been characterized kinetically, conforming to specific behaviors and functions.

Environmental stress leads to (a) increased presynaptic sympathetic impulse activity, (b) acetylcholine release, (c) postsynaptic nicotinic receptor stimulation, (d) sympathetic depolarization, (e) transmembrane Na^+ influx, (f) elevated TH mRNA, (g) increased TH molecule number and activity, and (h) enhanced norepinephrine synthesis. In turn, this environmental–molecular cascade is associated with the physiologic "fight or flight" behavioral repertoire.

The physiological effects of sympathoadrenal activation are well characterized and include mydriasis, lid lag, piloerection, tachycardia, increased cardiac output, redistribution of blood flow away from viscera and to striated muscle, generally increased blood pressure, and increased respiratory minute volume (36).

What other long-term plastic changes are elicited by increased impulse activity in sympathetic neurons? How is the combinatorial potential of this neuronal population manifested?

SUBSTANCE P IN SYMPATHETIC NEURONS

To characterize further the spectrum of transmitter plasticity in sympathetic neurons, we examined the regulation of substance P (SP) in some detail.

In initial studies we found that the adult rat superior cervical sympathetic ganglion (SCG) contained low but detectable levels of SP and that ganglion denervation (decentralization) elicited significant elevation of the peptide (23). Moreover, pharmacologic blockade of ganglionic transmission reproduced the effects of denervation, suggesting that transsynaptic impulses, through the interaction of acetylcholine with postsynaptic nicotinic receptors and depolarization, normally decreased SP (23). Conversely, as expected, agents that reflexly increased sympathetic impulse flow significantly depressed ganglion SP below normal, basal levels.

To elucidate underlying molecular mechanisms, we explanted ganglia to culture, allowing experimentation without the confounding, uncontrolled variables encountered *in vivo*. Explantation (and consequent denervation) resulted in a striking, 20-fold rise in SP by 24 hr and a 50-fold rise after 48 hr (21). The marked elevation in SP provided a unique opportunity to localize SP in the SCG. In fact, immunocytochemical examination indicated that the vast majority of the principal sympathetic neurons expressed SP (7,21). These neurons simultaneously expressed the noradrenergic and SP phenotypes (7).

Having localized SP to the sympathetic neurons, we were in a position to examine mechanisms underlying the rise in culture. Inhibition of protein synthesis completely blocked the elevation of SP on explantation, whereas inhibition of RNA synthesis partially inhibited the increase. Consequently, it appears that both protein and RNA synthesis were necessary for the elevation of SP (21,22).

The above studies were performed with neonatal ganglia, since immature ganglia are more conveniently cultured than mature ganglia. However, we were particularly interested in determining whether mature and developing neurons exhibit similar plastic regulatory mechanisms. We succeeded in culturing mature ganglia and investigated regulation of SP (1). To determine whether depolarization inhibited the increase of SP, we cultured ganglia in the presence of veratridine, which increases sodium ion influx by binding to sodium channels (40). The alkaloid completely blocked the increase in SP (Fig. 3), reproducing the effects of impulse activity *in vivo*. Further, addition of tetrodotoxin, which antagonizes the effect of veratridine on sodium channels (9,15), blocked the effects of veratridine on SP. Similar results were obtained with neonatal ganglia (21). These observations suggest that depolarization, through the mediation of sodium ion influx, suppresses SP in sympathetic neurons. Previous studies had indicated that this effect did not simply reflect release of the peptide (22) but rather inhibition of net synthesis (synthesis less catabolism).

In summary, our *in vivo* and culture studies, viewed in conjunction, indicate that (a) presynaptic impulse activity,

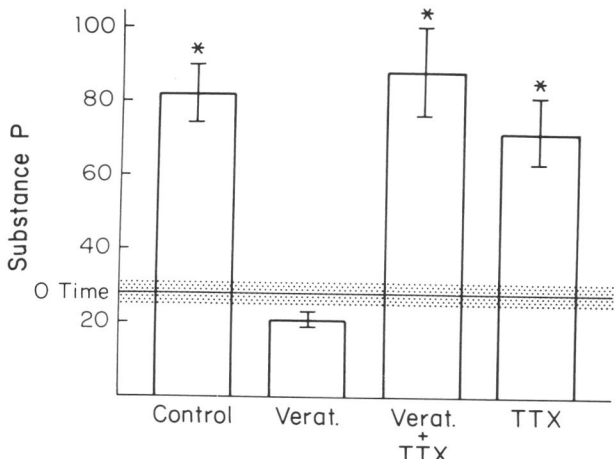

FIG. 3. Effect of membrane depolarization on adult ganglia. Superior cervical ganglia from 6-month-old rats were cultured in serum-supplemented medium in the presence of veratridine (5×10^{-5} M), tetrodotoxin (10^{-7} M), or both. After 48 hr, the ganglia were examined for substance P content, which is expressed as mean picograms per ganglion ± standard error (SE) for eight ganglia. *Line* and *stippled bar* represent mean substance P content ± SE for freshly dissected ganglia. Verat., veratridine; TTX, tetrodotoxin. *Differs from zero time and veratridine at $p < 0.01$ (one-way analysis of variance; Newman-Keuls test). (Reprinted from Black et al., ref. 5.)

(b) release of acetylcholine, (c) interaction with nicotinic receptors, (d) depolarization, and (e) sodium ion influx suppress net synthesis of SP in neonatal and mature sympathetic neurons. Note, however, that this same sequence of events induces catecholaminergic TH in the very same neurons (Fig. 1). Consequently, impulse activity is apparently represented in different ways by different transmitter systems in the same neurons. This combinatorial capability exhibits the specificity, selectivity, and precision required for complex representational function. The same or similar extraneuronal events are stored in multiple molecular species through different processes.

We have begun to analyze molecular genetic mechanisms underlying SP plasticity, using cloned cDNA copies of mRNAs for the preprotachykinins (PPT mRNA), the precursors of SP (37). We used the culture system described above to analyze specific message levels. In culture, PPT mRNA increased significantly by RNA blot analysis after only 6 hr, well before the rise in SP is detectable at 12 hr. The increase in PPT mRNA was maximal at 24 hr, preceding the major rise in SP (at 4 days). Camptothecin and actinomycin D, inhibitors of RNA synthesis that had previously been shown to prevent the increase in SP, also prevent the elevation of PPT mRNA. Further, veratridine depolarization also prevented the rise in PPT mRNA, reproducing effects on SP itself. Finally, tetrodotoxin, which prevents veratridine effects on Na$^+$ channels, simultaneously prevented the effects of veratridine on SP and PPT mRNA (7).

The sequential increases in PPT mRNA and SP and the effects of RNA synthesis inhibitors suggest that increased

SP is attributable to altered expression of the PPT gene. Moreover, the foregoing experiments suggest that depolarization alters the pattern of PPT gene expression. We are presently attempting to determine whether increased SP is, in fact, caused by enhanced gene readout and/or increased stabilization of message.

It is apparent that depolarizing stimuli exert differential effects on noradrenergic and peptidergic transmitter systems localized to SCG sympathetic neurons. Moreover, these plastic effects are manifested at the level of mRNA, perhaps by altering gene readout. In turn, these complex transduction mechanisms endow the neuron with remarkable plasticity, resulting in the representation of environmental stimuli by multiple transmitter states. Consequently, even the relatively primitive sympathetic neuron exhibits a complex, combinatorial transmitter representational network capable of receiving, encoding, storing, and transmitting information. Additional studies indicate that other peripheral neuroendocrine cells also contain colocalized neurohumoral signals that are independently regulated by extracellular stimuli. For example, adrenal medullary cells contain opioid peptide and catecholaminergic systems that are differentially regulated by impulse activity (25). In medullary cells, as in sympathetic neurons, critical transduction mechanisms occur at the level of mRNA (26,27). It is apparent, consequently, that plastic transmitter mechanisms are widespread in the periphery. It was of particular interest to determine whether similar plastic phenomena occur in brain neurons and whether we can begin to understand the molecular bases of higher functions.

TRANSMITTER PLASTICITY IN THE BRAIN

To initiate studies of brain neurons, it is necessary to choose a model system that fulfills a number of criteria. First, the system must contain well-characterized transmitters that are amenable to sensitive and accurate measurement. Second, the system should, ideally, thrive in tissue culture, allowing analysis of molecular mechanisms under rigorously controlled conditions. Finally, the role of the system in brain function should be at least partially characterized, ultimately permitting correlation of molecular mechanisms with brain function. The noradrenergic neurons of the pontine nucleus locus coeruleus met these criteria.

The locus coeruleus is composed of bilateral nuclei, each consisting of approximately 1,400 neurons, lying laterally in the pons, below the floor of the fourth ventricle. The neurons project throughout the neuraxis, innervating the cerebral cortex rostrally, cerebellar Purkinje cells and cortex superiorly, and spinal neurons inferiorly (31).

The classic work of Bloom and colleagues has suggested that the locus, which is activated by multimodal somatosensory stimuli, globally biases central neurons, setting levels of vigilance or alertness and orienting the CNS to either environmental or internal demands (2). According to this view, the locus subserves an arousal–attentional function.

Tyrosine hydroxylase plays a role in locus function analogous to that already described in the periphery. Moreover, the rate-limiting enzyme is influenced by environmental stimuli. For example, the same pharmacologic agents that induce TH in sympathetic neurons also induce the enzyme in the locus *in vivo* (Fig. 4). However, from experiments in the whole animal, it is difficult to ascertain whether depolarization per se is the factor that regulates TH. To approach this issue, we grew coeruleal neurons in culture (13). The mouse locus was explanted on embryonic day 12, grown in basal medium for 1 week, and then subjected to veratridine depolarization for 7 days (11,12,14). Veratridine exposure significantly increased TH activity above that in cultures of the contralateral control locus, and this effect was blocked by tetrodotoxin (Fig. 5). Further, depolarizing concentrations of K^+ reproduced the effect of veratridine, suggesting that depolarization itself increased TH activity. Immunoblot analysis indicated that the increase in TH catalytic activity was entirely attributable to an increase in enzyme protein (12). Finally, morphometric analysis indicated that veratridine did not significantly alter TH-positive cell number, suggesting that depolarization

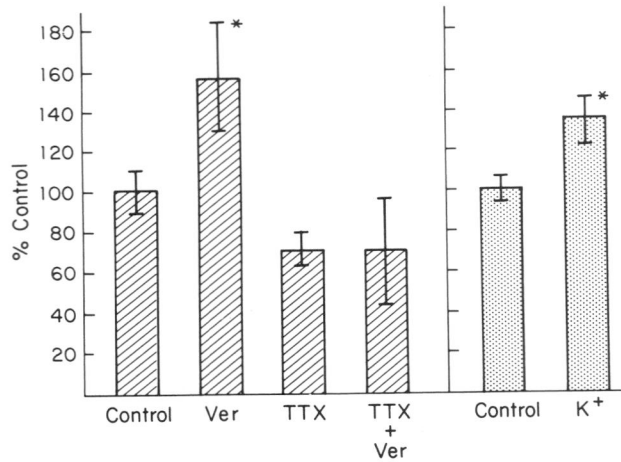

FIG. 5. Effects of depolarizing agents on TH activity in the brain nucleus locus coeruleus. E-12 cultures were grown for 1 week and then exposed to the indicated agents for 7 days. In the **left panel,** cultures were exposed to veratridine (Ver, 1.5 μM) or tetrodotoxin (TTX, 0.1 μM) or both. In the **right panel,** cultures were exposed to K^+ (20 mM). Cultures were rinsed well in cold Hanks balanced salt solution and dissected free of the collagen-coated coverslips for TH assay. Each sample in each group consisted of two cultures. At least seven such samples were included in each group in the **left panel** and 24 in the **right panel.** Results are expressed as percentages of the appropriate vehicle-exposed control. Control values were 8.9 ± 0.99 pmole of dopa per locus pair per hour (mean ± SE) for the **left panel** and 15.8 ± 1.12 for the **right.** *Differs from control, TTX, and TTX + Ver groups at $p < 0.01$ (one-way analysis of variance, Newman–Keuls test). (Reprinted from Black et al., ref. 5.)

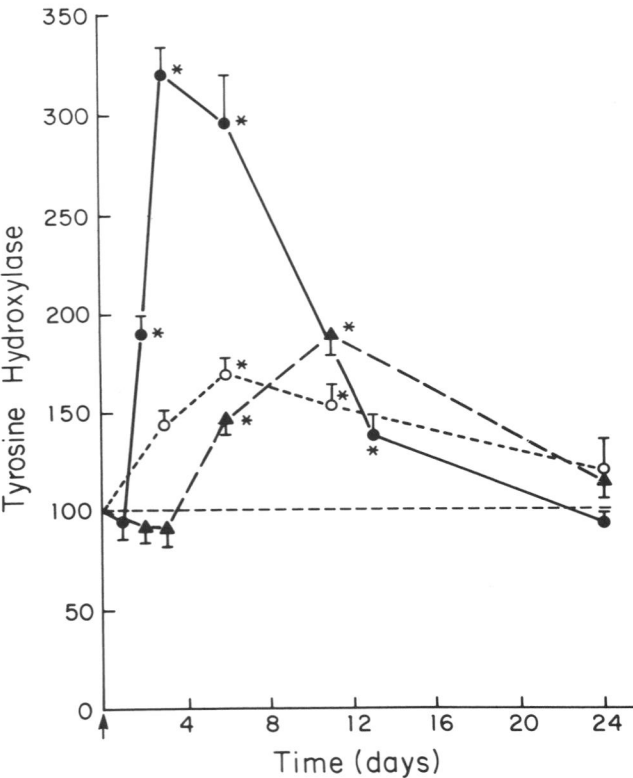

FIG. 4. Time course of the increases in tyrosine hydroxylase activity in locus coeruleus, cerebellum, and frontal cortex after reserpine treatment. Rats were treated with reserpine, 10 mg/kg s.c. at time zero (*arrow*), or with saline. At varying times after injection, groups of six control and six reserpine-treated animals were killed, and enzyme activity was assayed in the indicated areas. Results are expressed as percentage of respective controls ± SEM (*vertical bars*). Thus, "100" represents enzyme activity in controls, which was 692.5 ± 52.56 pmol/pair·hr for locus coeruleus, 80 ± 6.7 fmole/μg protein·hr for frontal cortex, and 25 ± 1.2 fmole/μg protein·hr for cerebellum. *Differs from respective control at $p < 0.001$. (Reprinted from Black, ref. 3.)

increased TH per neuron rather than increasing the number of neurons. In aggregate, these observations suggest that depolarization causes induction of TH in brain locus neurons, as in the periphery. It is apparent that brain neurons exhibit plasticity in response to external stimuli, paralleling properties of peripheral neurons. More specifically, it is logical to conclude that increased presynaptic impulse activity with consequent locus depolarization induces TH, resulting in elevated norepinephrine biosynthesis, target stimulation, and resultant orientation of multiple CNS targets to environmental exigencies.

In this manner, TH, as only one example, serves to interrelate several distinct levels of brain function and behavior. Viewed somewhat differently, TH simultaneously serves physiologic as well as representational roles in brain as in the periphery. What are the temporal characteristics of TH elevation in the brain? Might such information provide additional insights and even lead to predictions regarding locus and behavioral function? In fact, after a brief inciting stimulus, Th induction in locus perikarya and subsequent axonal transport over centimeter distances lead to prolonged elevation of enzyme in locus terminals in the frontal cortex (Fig. 4). The frontal terminals are thus capable of synthesizing and releasing increased norepinephrine for days to weeks after the precipitating environmental stimulus. In principle, then, TH provides temporal amplification in brain as in the periphery. This rather straight-forward observation concerning the kinetics of enzyme induction and transport at the molecular level may have profound behavioral consequences. Prolonged elevation of TH in locus frontal terminals suggests that the frontal cortex target may be, potentially, biased towards environmental exigencies for a period of weeks after enzyme induction in cell bodies of the pons. Consequently, a single constellation of environmental events, by inducing locus TH, may result in enhanced arousal and attention for weeks. This prediction is testable in a number of behavioral and physiological paradigms.

More generally, it is apparent that knowledge of the kinetics of action and reaction of transmitter molecules may lead to new insights and testable predictions regarding behavioral function. Moreover, this knowledge may lead to a more complete understanding of systems and behavioral function and help to integrate multiple levels of function in the brain. By understanding the mechanisms by which environmental and internal states alter transmitter-related molecules such as TH, we will gain a clearer understanding of the process of transduction from environmental to neural language. Further, the molecular basis for specificity, selectivity, and precision in mental processing may become clearer. Finally, it may be possible to determine how molecules in multiple-transmitter systems encode, store, and transmit behavioral information.

ACKNOWLEDGMENTS

This work was supported by NIH grants NS 10259, HD 12108, NS 29788, and HL 00756 and aided by a grant from the American Parkinson Disease Association. I.B.B. is the recipient of a McKnight Research Project Award. C.F.D. is the recipient of a Teacher-Scientist Award from the Andrew Mellon Foundation. A.R. is the recipient of a postdoctoral fellowship from the Medical Research Council of Canada.

REFERENCES

1. Adler, J. E., and Black, I. B. (1984): *Science,* 225:1499–1500.
2. Aston-Jones, G., and Bloom, F. E. (1981): *J. Neurosci.,* 1:876–886.
3. Black, I. B. (1975): *Brain Res.,* 95:170–176.
4. Black, I. B. (1984): *Brain, Behav. Evol.,* 24:35–46.
5. Black, I. B., Adler, J. E., Dreyfus, C. F., Jonakait, G. M., Katz, D. M., LaGamma, E. F., and Markey, K. M. (1984): *Science,* 225:1266–1270.
6. Black, I. B., Chikaraishi, D., and Lewis, E. J. (1985): *Brain Res.,* 339:151–153.
7. Bohn, M. C., Kessler, J. A., Adler, J. E., Markey, K. A., Goldstein, M., and Black, I. B. (1984): *Brain Res.,* 298:378–381.
8. Bonisch, H., Otten, U., and Thoenen, H. (1980): *Naunyn-Schmiedebergs Arch. Pharmacol.,* 313:199–203.
9. Catterall, W. A., and Nirenberg, M. (1973): *Proc. Natl. Acad. Sci. U.S.A.,* 70:3759–3763.
10. Chalazonitis, A., and Zigmond, R. E. (1980): *J. Physiol. (Lond.),* 300:525–538.
11. Dreyfus, C. F., Friedman, W. J., Markey, K. A., and Black, I. B. (1986): *Brain. Res.,* 379:216–222.
12. Dreyfus, C. F., Gillies, M. A., Goldstein, M., and Black, I. B. (1985): *Soc. Neurosci. Abstr.,* 11:947.
13. Dreyfus, C. F., Markey, K. A., Goldstein, M., and Black, I. B. (1983): *Dev. Biol.,* 97:48–58.
14. Dreyfus, C. F., Markey, K. A., and Black, I. B. (1984): *Soc. Neurosci. Abstr.,* 10:13.
15. Evans, M. H. (1973): *Int. Rev. Neurobiol.,* 15:83–166.
16. Furshpan, E. J., MacLeish, P. R., O'Lague, P. H., and Potter, D. D. (1976): *Proc. Natl. Acad. Sci. U.S.A.,* 73:4225–4229.
17. Hebb, D. O. (1949): In: *The Organization of Behavior.* John Wiley & Sons, New York, London.
18. Hökfelt, T., Johansson, O., Ljungdahl, A., Lundberg, J. M., and Schultzberg, M. (1980): *Nature,* 284:515–521.
19. Horn, G., Rose, S. P. R., and Bateson, P. P. G. (1973): *Science,* 181:506–514.
20. Kandel, E. R., and Schwartz, J. H. (1982): *Science,* 218:433–443.
21. Kessler, J. A., Adler, J. E., Bohn, M. C., and Black, I. B. (1981): *Science,* 214:335–336.
22. Kessler, J. A., Adler, J. E., Bell, W. O., and Black, I. B. (1983): *Neuroscience,* 9:309–318.
23. Kessler, J. A., and Black, I. B. (1982): *Brain Res.,* 234:182–187.
24. Ko, C.-P., Burton, H., Johnson, M., and Bunge, R. P. (1976): *Brain Res.,* 117:461–485.
25. LaGamma, E. F., Adler, J. E., and Black, I. B. (1984): *Science,* 224:1102–1104.
26. LaGamma, E. F., White, J. D., Adler, J. E., Krause, J. E., McKelvy, J. F., and Black, I. B. (1985): *Soc. Neurosci. Abstr.,* 11:1142.
27. LaGamma, E. F., White, J. D., Adler, J. E., Krause, J. E., McKelvy, J. F., and Black, I. B. (1986): *Proc. Natl. Acad. Sci. U.S.A.,* 82:8252–8255.
28. Landis, S. C. (1983): *Fed. Proc.,* 42:1633–1638.
29. Lewis, E. J., Tank, A. W., Weiner, N., and Chikaraishi, D. M. (1983): *J. Biol. Chem.,* 258:14632–14637.
30. Mallet, J., Faucon Biquet, N., Buda, M., Lamouroux, A., and Samolyk, D. (1983): *Cold Spring Harbor Symp. Quant. Biol.,* 48:305–308.
31. Moore, R. Y., and Bloom, F. E. (1979): *Annu. Rev. Neurosci.,* 2:113–168.
32. Mueller, R. A., Thoenen, H., and Axelrod, J. (1969): *J. Pharmacol. Exp. Ther.,* 169:74–79.
33. Mueller, R. A., Thoenen, H., and Axelrod, J. (1969): *Mol. Pharmacol.,* 5:463–469.
34. Patterson, P. H., and Chun, L. L. Y. (1974): *Proc. Natl. Acad. Sci. U.S.A.,* 71:3607–3610.
35. Patterson, P. H., and Chun, L. L. Y. (1977): *Dev. Biol.,* 56:263–280.
36. Pick, J. (1970): In: *The Autonomic Nervous System—Morphological, Comparative, Clinical and Surgical Aspects,* p. 483. J. B. Lippincott, Philadelphia.
37. Roach, A. H., Adler, J. E., Krause, J., and Black, I. B. (1985): *Soc. Neurosci. Abstr.,* 11:669.
38. Thompson, R. F., Berger, T. W., and Madden, J. IV (1983): *Annu. Rev. Neurosci.,* 6:447–492.
39. Tsukahara, N. (1981): *Annu. Rev. Neurosci.,* 4:351–380.
40. Ulbricht, W. (1964): *Ergeb. Physiol.,* 61:18–70.
41. Zigmond, R. E., and Chalazonitis, A. (1979): *Brain Res.,* 164:137–152.
42. Zigmond, R. E., Chalazonitis, A., and Joh, T. (1980): *Neurosci. Lett.,* 20:61–65.

Psychopharmacology:
The Third Generation of Progress,
edited by Herbert Y. Meltzer.
Raven Press, New York © 1987.

CHAPTER **48**

Brain Tissue Transplantation in Animal Models of Extrapyramidal Motor Dysfunction

William J. Freed and Richard Jed Wyatt

It has been known for many years that brain tissue from embryonic animals, as well as other tissues including endocrine organs, tumors, and peripheral tissues, survive transplantation into the brain. In many experiments, tissues have been found to survive transplantation into the brain more readily than when transplanted into peripheral sites (4). Nevertheless, methods of producing functional alterations in the host brain by transplantation of brain tissue were not found until quite recently. Development of functional brain tissue transplantation as an area of investigation corresponds to the relatively recent description of specific anatomical–biochemical systems in the brain with defined functional properties, such as the nigrostriatal dopamine system, to which brain tissue transplantation could be applied.

The corpus striatum, consisting of the caudate nucleus and the putamen, has an important role in the control of motor function. In Parkinson's disease, where the dopamine-containing cells of the substantia nigra (SN) pars compacta die, the loss of the dopamine-containing projections of these cells to the striatum results in profound motor deficits (5,63,70). These deficits consist primarily of difficulty in initiating and controlling movement, and tremor. Animal models of this disorder can be produced by destroying the dopamine-containing cells of the SN either with stereotactic injection of the neurotoxin 6-hydroxydopamine in small animals (101–103) or by systemic administration of the neurotoxic drug *N*-methyl-4-phenyl-1,2,3,6-tetrahydropyridine (MPTP) in primates (15,70). Huntington's chorea is a second disorder associated with impaired functioning of the corpus striatum. The neuropathological and behavioral manifestations of this disease are, however, quite different from those of Parkinson's disease. In Huntington's disease, cells intrinsic to the striatum die rather than lose their innervation, and the primary manifestation of this disorder is the appearance of choreiform movements. In this chapter, research on the application of brain tissue transplantation to animal models of these two disorders, and potentially to human subjects, is reviewed.

INTRAOCULAR GRAFTING STUDIES AND MATURATION OF TRANSPLANTED SN

Much of the technology for studies of intracerebral transplantation of monoamine-containing brain nuclei was developed in a series of experiments by Olson, Seiger, and Hoffer in which various tissues were transplanted to the anterior chamber of the eye (61,78,79,92,93). The immunological properties of the anterior eye chamber are similar to those of the brain (4,85,86), and the growth of tissue transplanted to the anterior eye chamber can be monitored by external observation. Innervation of the host iris by the graft can also be studied.

In their initial experiments, Olson and his colleagues transplanted various tissues, such as sympathetic ganglia, fetal locus coeruleus, and fetal cerebellar cortex, to the anterior eye chamber. In these studies, techniques for the dissection and transplantation of embryonic brain mono-amine-containing neurons were developed (78,93), and growth properties and interactions of these tissues with the host iris were investigated (61,79,92,93). For example, intraocular locus coeruleus grafts were found to reinnervate about one-third of the host iris. When a second iris was then transplanted to the eye chamber, the locus coeruleus graft completely innervated the second iris (79,92). Complete innervation of the host iris could be induced by sensory, but not by sympathetic, denervation of the iris (79,92). Thus, sensory denervation of the iris has a trophic effect on the growth of locus coeruleus neurites.

In more recent experiments, Olson and colleagues have employed the transplantation of more than one embryonic brain region to the anterior eye chamber to investigate developmental and trophic interactions between brain regions. For example, grafts of locus coeruleus, tectum, and brainstem nuclei were found to stimulate the growth of cerebral cortex grafts (13). Olson and his colleagues (80) reported that embryonic SN grafts in the eye chamber can innervate grafts of caudate–putamen or cerebral cortex also placed into the anterior eye chamber. When target brain regions—such as caudate–putamen—were transplanted into eye chambers that contained SN grafts that had already been allowed to mature, dopamine-containing neurite growth was reinitiated, and the target grafts were reinnervated (80). Thus, even mature SN neurons were found to be capable of generating a vigorous growth response in the presence of a denervated target tissue.

Thus, the state of maturity of transplanted SN neurons is not of primary importance in the ability of these cells to generate dopaminergic neurites. This has also been observed in another situation, when embryonic SN were transplanted to the colliculus, far from the striatum, and allowed to mature. When sciatic nerve "bridges"—which are very conducive to neurite growth—were later implanted, bridging the gap between the denervated striatum and the nonmatured grafts, vigorous outgrowth of dopaminergic neurites from the matured grafts was initiated (52). Thus, transplanted SN neurons are capable of generating new neurites even after they have matured.

FUNCTIONAL EFFECTS OF EMBRYONIC BRAIN GRAFTS IN THE NIGROSTRIATAL DOPAMINE SYSTEM

The first experiments in which brain tissue grafts were employed to produce functional alterations in the host animal involved the rotational behavior model of nigrostriatal dopaminergic function developed by Ungerstedt (101–103). In this experimental model, rats first receive unilateral lesions of the SN by stereotactic administration of 6-hydroxydopamine. The dopaminergic projection to the caudate–putamen ipsilateral to the SN lesion degenerates, leading to the development of supersensitivity to dopamine agonists in the caudate–putamen ipsilateral to the lesion. When these lesioned animals are given the dopamine receptor agonist apomorphine, the supersensitive dopamine receptors in the caudate–putamen ipsilateral to the lesion

are stimulated to a greater degree than the dopamine receptors on the normal side. This causes rotational behavior away from the lesioned side. When animals are given amphetamine, which stimulates dopamine release from presynaptic terminals, only the normal caudate–putamen is stimulated because the presynaptic terminals on the lesioned side have degenerated. This results in rotational behavior toward the side of the lesion. Amphetamine-induced rotational behavior thus provides a means of behaviorally assaying the relative excess of releasable dopamine in the normal striatum as compared with the denervated side. Apomorphine-induced rotational behavior provides an assay of the striatal (i.e., the host) response to the denervation.

It was appreciated, in the first experiments, that it would be necessary to transplant the embryonic SN immediately adjacent to the striatum in order to obtain a reinnervation, because newly generated neurites would be unlikely to traverse long distances. Two transplantation techniques were initially employed to accomplish this. In the first, embryonic SN was transplanted to the lateral ventricle, which is immediately adjacent to the striatum. Embryonic SN transplanted to the lateral ventricle show excellent survival and produce a partial dopaminergic reinnervation of the dorsal–medial caudate–putamen adjacent to the grafts. Both amphetamine- and apomorphine-induced rotational behavior are decreased by SN grafts in the lateral ventricle (33,43,47,83).

The second technique that has been used to transplant embryonic SN to the striatum involves the use of previously prepared "transplantation cavities." A small area of the cerebral cortex and corpus callosum overlying the striatum is removed by aspiration. After a period of time, embryonic SN is transplanted into the cavity (6,95). Implanted brain tissues show excellent survival under these conditions, which has been attributed in part to the formation of a vascular bed in the cavity and in part to the secretion of trophic substances by injured brain tissue adjacent to the transplantation cavity (76). The SN grafts implanted into such cavities also partially reinnervate the striatum and reduce rotational behavior induced by apomorphine and amphetamine (6,9,23,26,27).

In both of these transplantation paradigms, ventricular and cavity-implanted grafts, the reductions in amphetamine-induced rotation are usually found to be greater than the reductions in apomorphine-induced rotation. The reductions in apomorphine-induced rotational behavior are a reflection of the long-term influence of the graft on the host, specifically on the host striatal dopamine receptors. The fact that apomorphine-induced rotation is only decreased but not eliminated suggests that the influence of the grafts on the host brain is only partial. Amphetamine-induced rotational behavior, on the other hand, may be entirely eliminated or even reversed in direction (24,43). This may reflect the presence of an excess of dopamine in the grafts and their processes, the release of which can be stimulated by amphetamine. Histochemical and biochemical studies confirm that grafted SN contain excess amounts of dopamine in comparison with the normal SN (41,47). On the other hand, it has also been suggested that transplanted dopaminergic neurons are abnormally hypersensitive to dopamine (58), perhaps because some of the mechanisms that normally control these neurons are lost.

On the other hand, several studies suggest that many of the properties of transplanted SN neurons are similar to those of normal SN neurons. Grafted SN neurons show spontaneous activity similar to that of normal SN neurons and are normally inhibited by dopamine agonists and excited by dopamine antagonists (108). Spiroperidol autoradiography studies, which directly measure dopamine receptors, have shown that dopaminergic supersensitivity in the striatum is markedly reduced by substantia nigra grafts, but only in those parts of the striatum that are reinnervated (43,45). Recent studies by Hoffer and his colleagues (62) using *in vivo* electrochemistry have shown that concentrations of dopamine in the striatum are increased in correspondence with the areas of reinnervation, consistent with earlier studies using measurements of dopamine in punch samples (47) and studies demonstrating increased striatal dopamine turnover in animals that had received SN grafts (88).

DISSOCIATED CELLS

The ability of dopamine-containing processes from an embryonic SN graft implanted in a single site adjacent to the striatum to penetrate into the striatum is limited. One approach that has been used to obtain a more complete reinnervation is the implantation of grafts into several sites within the striatum. Although some investigators have obtained good survival of intraparenchymal brain grafts (17,19,21), embryonic SN implanted directly into brain tissue does not survive well (95). When, however, the embryonic brain tissue is dissociated into individual cells and injected directly into the host brain tissue (11), reasonably good graft survival occurs, and reinnervation of the striatum is comparable to that obtained by other techniques (8,89). Embryonic SN implanted by this method has been found to produce large decreases and in some cases reversals in the direction of amphetamine-induced rotational behavior (24). In the studies of Dunnett and his colleagues (24,25), grafts implanted into more than one site within the striatum were found to be more effective than a single graft, verifying the hypothesis that the dissociated cell transplantation technique would be an effective method of increasing the behavioral efficacy of embryonic SN grafts.

The dissociated-cell transplantation technique has recently been employed by two groups (3,87) in primates that have received MPTP-induced nigrostriatal damage. Although only preliminary results have thus far been reported, both studies suggest that this transplantation technique may be quite effective in reducing motor deficits in these animals.

OTHER BEHAVIORAL MODELS

Spontaneous motor asymmetry, without drug injections, has been described in animals with unilateral SN lesions (27). Animals with unilateral SN lesions have a strong tendency to make contralateral arm choices in a T-maze and tend to turn spontaneously toward the side of the lesion when given some activating stimulus, such as a mild tail pinch. Dunnett and his colleagues have reported that this spontaneous locomotor asymmetry is also reduced by SN grafts, either as dissociated cells or as grafts in cortical lesion sites (24,27).

Another technique that has been extensively employed to measure the functional status of the nigrostriatal system is the measurement of sensorimotor neglect (72,73). Normal rats respond to tactile, visual, and olfactory stimuli by orienting and sometimes biting or grasping directed toward the stimulus. Rats with unilateral lesions of the SN tend to ignore sensory stimuli contralateral to the lesion; this has been called sensorimotor neglect. Dunnett and his colleagues have reported that SN grafts situated in cortical cavities close to dorsomedial parts of the striatum do not decrease the sensorimotor neglect of animals with SN lesions (27). When SN grafts were situated so that ventral–lateral parts of the striatum were reinnervated, sensorimotor neglect was decreased, with little or no effect on spontaneous and drug-induced motor asymmetry (24,29). When grafts are placed in both dorsomedial and ventral–lateral striatum, using the dissociated-cell technique, both forms of behavioral deficit can be alleviated (29).

When the SN is lesioned bilaterally rather than unilaterally, animals develop profound aphagia and adipsia in addition to akinesia and other behavioral deficits such as rigidity and impaired grooming (102; also cf. 99). Initial studies reported that SN grafts had no effect or only slight effects on the aphagia and adipsia after bilateral SN lesions, even though in some experiments the akinesia observed in the bilaterally lesioned animals was decreased (28). Even when SN grafts were placed into multiple locations in the striatum of animals with bilateral SN lesions, alleviating the akinesia and sensorimotor impairments, animals remained completely adipsic and lost weight rapidly, although modest increases in amounts of food eaten were observed (25). On the other hand, when the usual experimental paradigm is reversed, so that animals receive SN grafts as neonates and *subsequently* receive bilateral SN lesions, the aphagia and adipsia, as well as the akinesia, are markedly reduced (41,91). Thus, in general, it is more difficult to influence the aphagia and adipsia than other manifestations of SN lesions.

There have also been reports of other behavioral effects of SN grafts. For example, Fray and his colleagues (49) reported that rats will press a lever to initiate electrical stimulation of SN grafts; i.e., they will "self-stimulate" SN brain grafts. Electrodes were implanted either into the SN grafts or into cortical tissue grafts in the cortical cavities. Rats with electrodes in SN grafts responded at higher rates than controls. Rates of responding were as high as one per 6 sec, which has been interpreted as suggesting that the SN grafts are not acting merely through nonspecific release of catecholamines into the cerebrospinal fluid (also see ref. 41).

Another behavioral study of SN grafts (51) involved tests of motor coordination in aged rats that had received grafts of dissociated SN cells into the striatum or grafts of dissociated septal cells into the hippocampus. The SN grafts significantly improved the motor coordination of the aged rats, as evidenced by an increased ability to walk across a narrow bridge to reach a safe platform. Animals with septal grafts were unaffected, and there were no changes of general behavioral activity or ability to hang from a wire, a general measure of weight and strength of the animals.

Lesions of the mesolimbic dopaminergic neurons, which innervate the nucleus accumbens, produce, rather than motor impairments, inactivity, a lack of exploratory behavior, decreases in amphetamine-induced hyperactivity, and an increased responsivity to apomorphine. Nadaud and his colleagues (75) have studied the effects of dissociated embryonic SN grafted to the nucleus accumbens of animals with lesions of the mesolimbic dopaminergic neurons. These grafts increased exploratory behavior, spontaneous activity, and responses to amphetamine. The hyperactive responses to apomorphine were only slightly affected. Herman et al. (58,59) have also reported that normal animals with grafts of dopaminergic neurons in the striatum and nucleus accumbens are hyperreactive to amphetamine. Grafted animals were found to respond to lower doses of amphetamine than controls and also showed prolonged responses to amphetamine.

ADRENAL MEDULLA GRAFTS

One of the primary goals of brain tissue transplantation experiments is the development of a procedure that could be applicable to human patients with Parkinson's disease. One of the potential obstacles to human application would be the source of donor tissue if embryonic tissue were required, and alternate sources of tissue are therefore needed. Olson (77) had found that adrenal chromaffin cells grafted to the anterior eye chamber developed neurite-like processes that partially reinnervated the host iris. Adrenal chromaffin cells also contain dopamine (94,109) and develop neurite-like processes when exposed to nerve growth factor in tissue culture (100,104,105).

When adrenal medulla was transplanted to the lateral ventricle, the chromaffin cells developed some coarse neurite-like processes, although these processes did not reinnervate the host brain (42,44). These grafts did, however, contain large amounts of catecholamines, which appeared to diffuse into the host brain in fluorescence histochemical studies (33,42). Apomorphine-induced rotational behavior was decreased by these intraventricular adrenal medulla grafts (44). Measurements of catecholamines showed that intraventricular adrenal medulla grafts contained high concentrations of dopamine (42). Concentrations of dopamine in grafted adrenal medulla were increased relative to the concentrations of epinephrine and norepinephrine (33,42). Thus, adrenal medulla grafts appear to function not by reinnervating the host brain but simply by producing dopamine, which enters into the host brain by diffusion.

Unfortunately, adrenal medulla does not survive particularly well when implanted directly into the tissue of the striatum (37–39,97). Without additional manipulations, the average number of surviving chromaffin cells reported by Freed et al. (39) was 200, and in the Stromberg et al. (97) study, an average of 127 cells per animal survived. These numbers represent only very small fractions of the numbers of cells initially implanted. In the case of adrenal medulla

grafts, there does not appear to be an advantage in the use of dissociated cells. Numbers of dissociated chromaffin cells surviving transplantation into the striatum are moderate, and the surviving chromaffin cells appear to produce only small amounts of catecholamines (82).

There may be several methods through which the numbers of adrenal chromaffin cells surviving intrastriatal implantation can be increased (105). Stromberg et al. (97) have reported that nerve growth factor (NGF) infusions substantially increase the numbers of chromaffin cells that survive intrastriatal implantation as well as increasing the behavioral efficacy of these grafts. In these experiments, nerve growth factor was chronically infused into the striatum using osmotic minipumps and dialysis fibers.

One final factor that appears to influence the efficacy of adrenal medulla grafts is the age of the donor. When the donors of adrenal medulla tissue are young adult animals, the grafts are generally found to be behaviorally effective. Adrenal medulla grafts obtained from aging rat donors (1 or 2 years of age) are ineffective when implanted into the lateral ventricle (33). When implanted directly into the striatum, grafts obtained from 2-year-old donors were behaviorally effective although slightly less effective than tissue obtained from young donors (37,39). This suggests that there may be a decrease in the ability of chromaffin tissue from aging donors to shift catecholamine production in favor of dopamine after transplantation, although this hypothesis has not been directly tested. The age of the donors of adrenal medulla tissue may, however, become an issue for transplantation studies in human patients.

Adrenal medulla has been successfully transplanted into the striatum of primates, although the numbers of surviving cells are also small (74). In initial studies, adrenal medulla was autologously transplanted into the striatum by needle injection. In the most successful animals, numbers of surviving cells were similar to the numbers of chromaffin cells surviving implantation into the rat striatum. In the first three animals implanted, fewer than 20 surviving cells were found. In the best animals, between 100 and 600 surviving chromaffin cells were found. More recently, we have investigated the survival of chromaffin cells implanted into cortical cavities of primates. Numbers of surviving cells were considerably greater, in excess of 1,000 per implant site (110).

Intraparenchymal implantation of adrenal medulla has also been attempted in human patients with Parkinson's disease (1,2). In the first two patients, chromaffin tissue was implanted into a single site in the striatum. The tissue was embedded into a steel spring, and the spring was ejected into the brain by forcing it through a window in the side of a large (2.5 mm diameter) needle with a wedge-shaped stylette. The purpose of the spring was to allow the graft to be found subsequently in case it had to be destroyed because of adverse side effects. Transient improvements were observed in both of these initial patients, but these improvements disappeared within a few days. Measurements of catecholamines in the cerebrospinal fluid also showed very transient elevations, suggesting that the grafted cells may have survived for only a few days. Stromberg et al. (96) and Herrera-Marchitz et al. (60) had, in fact, previously reported that most adrenal chromaffin cells transplanted to the striatum die within a few hours after transplantation and that during this time the grafted cells produce pronounced behavioral effects consistent with the release of catecholamines from the dying cells. The short-term survival of the grafts in the human patients was not because of immunlogical rejection of the grafts, as these grafts were autologous, obtained by removal of one adrenal medulla from the recipient patients. Two additional patients have subsequently received adrenal medulla grafts with some minor modifications of the procedure, including omission of the steel spring. Improvements in these patients were again transitory, although they lasted for about 2 months rather than only for a few days (87a). Perhaps, with additional improvements in the transplantation procedure, lasting clinical improvement can be produced by adrenal medulla transplantation. It should be noted, however, that no study has yet demonstrated behavioral efficacy of adrenal medulla grafts in a model of Parkinson's disease in primates or other higher animals. At the present time, intraventricular transplantation allows the most consistent long-term survival of adrenal medulla grafts, although the prospects for behavioral efficacy of intraventricular grafts in larger species are still in doubt.

PHEOCHROMOCYTOMA CELLS

The PC12 pheochromocytoma cell line was developed from a rat adrenal medullary tumor (55). PC12 cells contain only norepinephrine and dopamine and contain neither epinephrine nor its synthetic enzyme, as do adrenal chromaffin cells (54,55). PC12 cells have therefore been considered a possible alternative to adrenal medulla for transplantation into the brain.

Jaeger (67) reported that PC12 cells implanted into the brain of immature rat hosts (4–12 days of age) survive and continue to proliferate for up to 2 months. Hefti and coworkers (57), on the other hand, investigated the transplantation of PC12 cells into the brains of mature Wistar rats and found that the cells survived for only 1 to 2 weeks and degenerated thereafter. During the 2 weeks that the cells survived, a reduction in apomorphine-induced rotational behavior was produced. It is unclear in this experiment whether the cells were rejected or simply degenerated; however, since the PC12 cell line is derived from a different rat strain than the Wistar hosts (106), graft rejection is certainly a possibility. Another study (46), also using mature hosts, reported that transplanted PC12 cells were rejected in some recipients after about 2 to 3 weeks, similar to the time course of rejection reported by Hefti et al. (57). Rejection appeared to occur only in those animals in which the cells continued to proliferate. In other recipients, the grafted PC12 cells did not proliferate after transplantation, and in these animals complete rejection of the grafts did not occur. Although there was a gradual decrease in the number of surviving cells, small numbers of cells did survive for as long as 4 months.

Thus, small numbers of PC12 cells can survive for

extended periods after transplantation into the brain. It is possible that some manipulation could be developed that would permit extended survival of larger numbers of cells after transplantation. For example, alternative cell lines might be employed, or the cells might be provided with a source of extracellular matrix to stabilize the cells. Nerve growth factor is also known to inhibit division and promote differentiation of PC12 cells (55), so that treatment of PC12 cells with NGF after transplantation might also be effective in promoting long-term survival of the grafted cells.

MECHANISMS OF ACTION

How is a brain graft, which may innervate only 10 to 25% of the host striatum, able to produce a functional improvement in the behavior of animals with SN lesions? Do the neurites from SN grafts develop synaptic contacts with host neurons, or do they function only through nonspecific release of dopamine? These issues have been the object of recent investigations by several groups, who have examined the anatomy and physiology of SN grafts.

Apomorphine-induced rotational behavior does not develop until there is approximately a 90% complete denervation of the striatum. One might reason that if the reinnervation of the striatum produced by a SN graft brings the total amount of dopaminergic innervation of the striatum above this 10% "threshold," the rotational behavior may disappear. The SN grafts do not, however, produce an overall 10% reinnervation of the striatum but instead produce a more or less complete reinnervation within a very restricted anatomical area. This may be an entirely different situation.

Substantia nigra grafts contain dopaminergic cells similar to those of the normal SN, with some properties resembling those of immature SN cells (47,68). These cells produce neurites that enter into the host striatum, and the degree of production of these neurites is associated with the degree of reductions in rotational behavior (6). It is also apparent, however, that diffuse release of dopamine from grafts, as in the case of adrenal medulla grafts, is capable of decreasing rotational behavior (41,44).

Do SN grafts, then, also release dopamine from their neurites in a diffuse manner, or do these neurites form synaptic contacts within the host brain? By use of tyrosine hydroxylase immunocytochemistry to distinguish graft-derived neurites from neurites endogenous to the host, it has recently been possible to identify synaptic contacts between graft-derived neurites and host neurites in the striatum (48,71). Tyrosine-hydroxylase-labeled axons derived from the grafted SN have been observed to form synaptic contacts with unlabeled host dendrites, similar to the synapses formed by normal SN dopaminergic neurites. Mahalik et al. (71) also reported that graft-derived tyrosine-hydroxylase-labeled dendrites form synaptic contacts with host axons, although these were only seen within a relatively restricted area, no more than about 0.5 mm from the grafts. A very interesting observation reported by Freund and co-workers (48) was that tyrosine-hydroxylase-labeled axons formed dense basket-like hyperinnervations of striatal giant cells, which appear to be cholinergic interneurons. Similar dopaminergic innervations of these interneurons are not observed in normal rats. Freund and his colleagues (48) suggested that these abnormal hyperinnervations may serve as a type of "amplification" mechanism, which could allow a graft innervating only a small part of the host striatum to produce a substantial behavioral effect.

Stromberg and her colleagues (98) have investigated the electrophysiological influence of SN grafts on the host striatum by comparing properties of striatal neurons within 1.0 mm of the graft to "distal" neurons more than 2.0 mm from the graft. The firing rates of these distal neurons were elevated (average 13.4 spikes/sec), presumably because of the loss of the inhibitory dopaminergic innervation. Neurons close to the grafts fired at a reduced and more normal average rate of 4.9 spikes/sec. Phencyclidine, an indirect dopamine agonist that requires the presence of dopamine terminals for activity, was much more effective in inhibiting the activity of neurons close to the graft as compared with the "distal" neurons.

This study, most importantly, supports the idea that the reinnervation of the striatum, although anatomically restricted, is quantitatively substantial because most neurons in the reinnervated area within 1.0 mm from the graft were affected. The direct sphere of influence of the grafts did not appear, however, to extend beyond this 2.0-mm range through secondary connections or other influences, at least by electrophysiological criteria.

LIMITS OF DOPAMINERGIC NEURITE GROWTH

A single SN graft, whether implanted into the lateral ventricle, cortical cavities, or directly into the striatum as dissociated cells, reinnervates only part of the striatum (6,12,43,47). The depth of penetration of catecholaminergic neurites from a SN graft in the lateral ventricle into the striatum may reach nearly 1 mm in 3 weeks, but even after nearly 2 years, depths of penetration rarely exceed 1.5 mm (33,34,38). The depth of neurite penetration is not altered by chronic treatment with haloperidol or estrogen (38) or ganglioside G_{M1} (34). Brain injury does, however, increase the growth of neurites from SN grafts. Animals received cortical aspiration lesions and after 10 days received SN grafts in the lateral ventricle. Depth of neurite penetration was increased in the animals that had received the cortical lesions, but only in the most dorsal one-fourth of the caudate–putamen immediately underneath the cortical lesion (38; *unpublished data*). The 10-day interval between cortical lesioning and SN grafts was chosen to coincide with the optimal time for secretion of neuronotrophic substances from brain lesion sites (76). Thus, brain injury may have a trophic effect of the growth of SN dopaminergic neurites. It is also possible that in cavity transplantation experiments, the brain injury induced in the process of making the cortical cavities has a stimulatory effect on the growth of graft-derived neurites.

IMMUNOLOGY

It is generally recognized that tissues transplanted into the brain have an increased likelihood of surviving rejection compared with similar tissues transplanted to peripheral sites. This increased tendency for grafts of foreign tissues to survive in the brain and certain other sites is known as "immunological privilege" (4). The brain does not, however, afford total protection from rejection under all circumstances; depending on the degree of genetic disparity between donor and host and the nature of the transplanted tissue, grafts to the brain can sometimes be rejected (4,86).

Animals of most common laboratory strains used in brain grafting studies are not inbred and are not genetically identical. Inbred strains, in which all members of the strain are identical to each other, are developed by repeated brother–sister mating over many generations. From a transplantation standpoint, such inbred strains are analogous to identical twins in humans, and virtually any tissue will survive transplantation from one individual of the strain to another. Commonly used inbred laboratory rat strains are, for example, Fisher 344, ACI, and Brown–Norway. Individuals of these inbred strains are called syngeneic or isogeneic with respect to other individuals of the same strain and allogeneic with respect to individuals of other genetically different strains. Grafts between isogeneic individuals are called isografts, and grafts between allogeneic individuals are termed allografts.

Most common randomly bred laboratory rat strains, such as the Sprague–Dawley and Long–Evans, are not genetically homogeneous, and individuals of these strains may have more than one major histocompatibility group. Tissues transplanted from one individual to another of these strains will usually behave in the same way as allografts. Tissues transplanted from one individual to another of the same species, as in the case of randomly bred strains, are termed homografts. Homografts differ from allografts only in that, for homografts, there is a possibility that donor and host will be genetically matched by chance. Other terms employed to describe grafts are heterograft for grafts between different species and autograft when a single individual serves as host and as donor.

Most initial experiments on brain grafts employed randomly bred strains of rats, and in many of these experiments excellent graft survival was reported. For example, embryonic SN grafts survive in nearly 100% of recipient animals whether implanted into the lateral ventricle, cortical cavities, or into brain tissue as dissociated cells (6,33,36,47). These grafts survive for extended periods; for example, in one experiment, surviving intraventricular grafts were found in all animals examined 15 to 20 months after transplantation, at which time nearly 50% of the graft recipients used in the experiment had died of age-related diseases such as tumors (43). There were no histological signs of graft rejection or deterioration, even in grafts examined after long survival times. Thus, intraventricular brain grafts are essentially permanently integrated into the host brain, even in randomly bred strains of rats.

As has been mentioned, there is some uncertainty about the degree of genetic disparity between donor and host when randomly bred strains are employed as a model to investigate graft survivability. The degree of protection from rejection can be much better defined when inbred strain animals are employed. We have found that interstrain allografts of embryonic SN or adrenal medulla were, to some degree, protected from rejection, using inbred F344 hosts and Brown–Norway donors. Embryonic brain grafts and adrenal medulla grafts survived for extended periods, as long as 7 months, without rejection. Whether these grafts were studied for sufficiently long periods to insure that rejection would never occur is unclear. Rejection of the grafts within 2 weeks could be provoked, however, by peripheral sensitization induced through skin grafting. The presence of a brain graft did not alter the duration of survival of a skin allograft, and antibodies directed at Brown–Norway histocompatibility antigen were not found in the serum of animals that had received Brown–Norway brain grafts (33). This study suggests that brain grafts can be rejected but normally survive because they fail to sensitize the host immune system.

Brain tissue has been reported to contain very little of the histocompatibility antigens that are primarily responsible for graft rejection, although blood vessels in the brain do appear to contain some of these antigens (56,90,107). Although brain grafts can be rejected after peripheral sensitization with other tissues, the degree to which the immunological privilege of the brain depends on the lack of antigenicity of brain tissue has not been established. Two studies have reported survival of adrenal medulla heterografts (69,84).

There is also evidence that partial survival of heterologous SN grafts can occur. Bjorklund and his colleagues (10) have investigated the transplantation of mouse SN into rat cortical cavities. Dopamine-containing neurons were found adjacent to the cortical cavities in 10 of 18 rats examined. The bulk of the graft, i.e., the solid piece of tissue in the cavity, was not found in any of the animals. It appears, then, that the major part of the graft did not survive, but transplanted neurons appear to have survived in the brain adjacent to the graft. In a subsequent experiment by Brundin and his colleagues (14), dissociated SN cells from mouse donors were transplanted into the striatum of rats, and some of the recipients were treated with the immuno-suppressant drug cyclosporin. Cyclosporin treatment greatly increased the number of surviving cells; more than 300 surviving cells were found in each of the cyclosporin-treated rats, whereas the largest number of surviving cells found in any vehicle-treated rat was less than 200. Since small numbers of cells were found in three of the seven vehicle-treated rats, it appears that some of the grafted cells survived in these rats even though many cells had been rejected when there was no immunosuppression. Perhaps brain tissues grafted deep within brain sites are not easily reached by the effector cells of the immune system, even in rats that have been sensitized as evidenced by rejection of parts of the grafted tissues. If so, this would be an unusual situation in the literature on the properties and mechanisms of immunological privilege (4). Most of the literature suggests that immunological privilege is related to abnormal presentation of antigens to the immune system

(4,85,86). These recent studies (10,14), however, suggest that the possibility of inaccessibility of brain grafts to immune effector mechanisms should be considered further.

HUNTINGTON'S CHOREA MODELS

Parkinson's disease is characterized by a loss of the dopaminergic innervation of the striatum. In Huntington's disease, another debilitating motor disorder, neurons within the striatum die rather than lose their inputs. An animal model of Huntington's disease can be produced in animals by stereotactic injection of the neurotoxins kainic acid or ibotenic acid directly into the striatum (16). These neurotoxins result in a loss of striatal neurons accompanied by behavioral abnormalities such as hyperactivity (16). Deckel and his colleagues (18,22) and Isacson and his colleagues (64–66) have investigated the transplantation of embryonic striatal tissue into the striatum of animals with these striatal lesions. Deckel and co-workers (19,21,22), using solid tissue fragments, and Isacson and co-workers (64), using dissociated cells, found that the grafted tissues showed excellent survival after transplantation into the striatum and formed large, well-delineated masses. These grafts contain neurons resembling normal striatal neurons, although connectivity between grafts and host brain has not been described (22). These grafts reduced the locomotor hyperactivity that is present in these lesioned animals (18,20,66). Locomotor hyperactivity induced by stimulants was not affected (18). Isacson and his colleagues have also reported that striatal grafts partially normalize the altered cerebral glucose metabolism that is seen in various brain regions after the ibotenic acid lesions (66).

These studies differ from most studies of brain tissue transplantation in that the tissues were transplanted to the same location as the lesion. In these studies, it is suspected that the transplants might have restored local circuits that were interrupted by the lesion rather than replacing a longer pathway. Alternatively, the transplants might simply release a chemical substance that interacts with the host brain, or they could even be exerting some mechanical or trophic influence on the surrounding tissues. Even though the reasons for the behavioral effects of these grafts are unknown, this is a very interesting area for future exploration.

CONCLUSIONS

Since the initial observations that functional improvements could be induced in animals with SN lesions by brain grafts (9,27,47,83), a number of reports have verified this initial observation (3,24–26,31–33,43,51,58,59,75, 81,87,97) and contributed to an explanation of the mechanisms by which these grafts exert their functional effects (43,48,62,68,71,98). Several experiments have reported additional behavioral effects of SN grafts, including effects on other behavioral abnormalities induced by SN lesions and lesions of the mesolimbic dopamine system, behavioral effects in aging animals, and effects in normal animals without lesions (23,24,29,49,51,58,59,75). Thus, it has been essentially established that brain grafts can be employed to produce a functionally significant replacement to the dopaminergic innervation of the striatum.

There have been a number of reports that brain grafts can be functionally effective in several other systems, in particular the septohippocampal cholinergic system and several neuroendocrine systems (7,30,40,50,53). Nevertheless, brain tissue transplantation is probably only applicable to a very restricted set of neuronal systems, which have properties resembling the nigrostriatal dopamine system. These properties include innervation of a relatively restricted brain region and simple circuitry that is not dependent on reciprocal innervation or other complex interactions (35,40). Whether the ultimate scope of applicability of brain tissue grafting has yet been reached is doubtful. On the other hand, there are probably very few brain systems that are as conducive to brain grafting as the nigrostriatal system and the septohippocampal cholinergic system that have not yet been studied.

Part of the attraction of the nigrostriatal system as an area for application of brain grafting is its relevance to Parkinson's disease. Parkinson's disease is a severe and common disorder, and an effective treatment procedure derived from brain grafting experiments could find wide applicability. The disorder is relatively well understood, and most of the symptomology can be ascribed to degeneration of this single relatively restricted system, consisting of the SN dopaminergic neurons and the dopaminergic innervation of the striatum (5,15,63). Development of an understanding of the mechanisms of action of SN and adrenal medulla grafts, finding more effective transplantation techniques and improving current techniques, development of other alternative procedures, elucidating the immunology of brain grafts, and development of procedures for use in primates are the challenges for this field over the next decade and are the areas of study that are most likely to lead to an effective human therapy.

REFERENCES

1. Backlund, E.-O., Granberg, P.-O., Hamberger, B., Sedvall, G., Seiger, A., and Olson, L. (1985): *Neural Grafting in the Mammalin CNS,* edited by A. Bjorklund and U. Stenevi, pp. 551–556. Elsevier, Amsterdam.
2. Backlund, E.-O., Granberg, P.-O., Hamberger, B., Knutsson, E., Martenson, A., Sedvall, G., Seiger, A., and Olson, L. (1985): *J. Neurosurg.,* 62:169–173.
3. Bakay, R. A. E., Barrow, D. L., Schiff, A., and Fiandaca, M. (1985): *Soc. Neurosci. Abstr.,* 11:1160.
4. Barker, C. F., and Billingham, R. E. (1977): *Adv. Immunol.,* 25:1–54.
5. Bernheimer, H., Birkmayer, W., Hornykiewicz, O., Jellinger, K., and Seitelberg, K. (1973): *J. Neurol. Sci.,* 20:415–455.
6. Bjorklund, A., Dunnett, S. B., Stenevi, U., Lewis, M. E., and Iversen, S. D. (1980): *Brain Res.,* 199:307–333.
7. Bjorklund, A., Gage, F. H., Schmidt, R. H., Stenevi, U., and Dunnett, S. B. (1983): *Acta Physiol. Scand. [Suppl.],* 522:59–66.
8. Bjorklund, A., Schmidt, R. H., and Stenevi, U. (1980): *Cell Tissue Res.,* 212:39–45.
9. Bjorklund, A., and Stenevi, U. (1979): *Brain Res.,* 177:555–560.
10. Bjorklund, A., Stenevi, U., Dunnett, S. B., and Gage, F. H. (1982): *Nature,* 298:652–654.
11. Bjorklund, A., Stenevi, U., Schmidt, R. H., Dunnett, S. B., and Gage, F. H. (1983): *Acta Physiol. Scand. [Suppl.],* 522:1–7.
12. Bjorklund, A., Stenevi, U., Schmidt, R. H., Dunnett, S. B., and Gage, F. H. (1983): *Acta Physiol. Scand. [Suppl.],* 522:9–18.
13. Bjorklund, H., Seiger, A., Hoffer, B., and Olson, L. (1982): *Dev. Brain Res.,* 6:131–140.
14. Brundin, P., Nilsson, O. G., Gage, F. H., and Bjorklund, A. (1985): *Exp. Brain Res.,* 60:204–208.
15. Burns, R. S., Markey, S. P., Phillips, J. M., and Chiueh, C. C. (1984): *Can. J. Neurol. Sci.,* 11(Suppl. 1):166–184.
16. Coyle, J. T., and Schwarcz, R. (1983): In: *Handbook of Chemical Neuroanatomy, Vol. 1,* edited by A. Bjorklund and T. Hokfelt, pp. 508–527. Elsevier, Amsterdam.
17. Das, G. D. (1985): In: *Neural Grafting in the Mammalian CNS,* edited by A. Bjorklund and U. Stenevi, pp. 11–123. Elsevier, Amsterdam.
18. Deckel, A. W., Moran, T. H., and Robinson, R. O. (1985): *Soc. Neurosci. Abstr.,* 11:616.
19. Deckel, A. W., Moran, T. H., Coyle, J. T., Sandberg, P. R., and Robinson, R. G. (1987): *Brain Res. (in press).*
20. Deckel, A. W., Robinson, R. G., Coyle, J. T., and Sandberg, P. R. (1983): *Eur. J. Pharmacol.,* 93:287–288.
21. Deckel, A. W., and Robinson, R. G. (1986): *Exp. Neurol.,* 91:212–218.
22. DiFiglia, M., Schiff, L., and Deckel, W. A. (1985): *Soc. Neurosci. Abstr.,* 11:365.
23. Dunnett, S. B., Bjorklund, A., Gage, F. H., and Stenevi, U. (1985): In: *Neural Grafting in the Mammalian CNS,* edited by A. Bjorklund and U. Stenevi, pp. 451–469. Elsevier, Amsterdam.
24. Dunnett, S. B., Bjorklund, A., Schmidt, R. H., Stenevi, U., and Iversen, S. D. (1983): *Acta Physiol. Scand. [Suppl.],* 522:29–37.
25. Dunnett, S. G., Bjorklund, A., Schmidt, R. H., Stenevi, U., and Iversen, S. D. (1983): *Acta Physiol. Scand. [Suppl.],* 522:39–47.
26. Dunnett, S. B., Bjorklund, A., and Stenevi, U. (1983): *Trends Neurosci.,* 6:266–270.
27. Dunnett, S. B., Bjorklund, A., Stenevi, U., and Iversen, S. D. (1981): *Brain Res.,* 215:147–161.
28. Dunnett, S. B., Bjorklund, A., Stenevi, U., and Iversen, S. D. (1981): *Brain Res.,* 229:209–217.
29. Dunnett, S. B., Bjorklund, A., Stenevi, U., and Iversen, S. D. (1981): *Brain Res.,* 229:457–470.
30. Dunnett, S. B., Low, W. C., Iversen, S. D., Stenevi, U., and Bjorklund, A. (1982): *Brain Res.,* 251:335–348.
31. Dymecki, J., Poltorak, M., Pucilowski, O., Markiewicz, D., and Kostowski, W. (1985): *Neuropathol. Pol.,* 23:181–189.
32. Dymecki, J., Pucilowski, O., Dyr, W., Markiewicz, D., Poltorak, M., Kostowski, W., Hauptmann, M., and Lipinska, B. (1985): *Neuropathol. Pol.,* 23:287–295.
33. Freed, W. J. (1983): *Biol. Psychiatry,* 18:1205–1267.
34. Freed, W. J. (1985): *Brain Res. Bull.,* 14:91–95.
35. Freed, W. J. (1985): *Neurobiol. Aging,* 6:153–156.
36. Freed, W. J. (1985): In: *Neural Grafting in the Mammalian CNS,* edited by A. Bjorklund and U. Stenevi, pp. 31–40. Elsevier, Amsterdam.
37. Freed, W. J., and Cannon-Spoor, H. E. (1984): *Soc. Neurosci. Abstr.,* 10:666.
38. Freed, W. J., Cannon-Spoor, H. E., and Krauthamer, E. (1985): In: *Neural Grafting in the Mammalian CNS,* edited by A. Bjorklund and U. Stenevi, pp. 491–504. Elsevier, Amsterdam.
39. Freed, W. J., Cannon-Spoor, H. E., and Krauthamer, E. (1986): *J. Neurosurg.,* 65:664–670.
40. Freed, W. J., de Medinaceli, L., and Wyatt, R. J. (1985): *Science,* 227:1544–1552.
41. Freed, W. J., Hoffer, B. J., Olson, L., and Wyatt, R. J. (1984): In: *Neural Transplants,* edited by J. R. Sladek, Jr., and D. M. Gash, pp. 373–406. Plenum Press, New York.
42. Freed, W. J., Karoum, F., Spoor, L., Olson, L., Morihisa, J., and Wyatt, R. J. (1983): *Brain Res.,* 269:184–189.
43. Freed, W. J., Ko, G. N., Niehoff, D. L., Kuhar, M. J., Hoffer, B. J., Olson, L., Cannon-Spoor, H. E., Morihisa, J. M., and Wyatt, R. J. (1983): *Science,* 222:937–939.
44. Freed, W. J., Morihisa, J. M., Spoor, E., Hoffer, B. J., Olson, L., Seiger, A., and Wyatt, R. J. (1981): *Nature,* 292:351–352.

45. Freed, W. J., Olson, L., Ko, G. N., Morihisa, J. M., Niehoff, D., Stromberg, I., Kuhar, M., Hoffer, B. J., and Wyatt, R. J. (1985): In: *Neural Grafting in the Mammalian CNS*, edited by A. Bjorklund and U. Stenevi, pp. 471–489. Elsevier, Amsterdam.

46. Freed, W. J., Patel-Vaidya, U., and Geller, H. M. (1986): *Exp. Brain Res.*, 63:557–566.

47. Freed, W. J., Perlow, M. J., Karoum, F., Seiger, A., Olson, L., Hoffer, B. J., and Wyatt, R. J. (1980): *Ann. Neurol.*, 8:510–519.

48. Freund, T. F., Bolam, J. P., Bjorklund, A., Stenevi, U., Dunnett, S. B., Powell, J. F., and Smith, A. D. (1985): *J. Neurosci.*, 5: 603–616.

49. Fray, P., Dunnett, S. B., Iversen, S. D., Bjorklund, A., and Stenevi, U. (1983): *Science*, 219:416–419.

50. Gage, F. H., Bjorklund, A., Stenevi, U., and Dunnett, S. B. (1985): In: *Neural Grafting in the Mammalian CNS*, edited by A. Bjorklund and U. Stenevi, pp. 585–594. Elsevier, Amsterdam.

51. Gage, F. H., Dunnett, S. B., Stenevi, U., and Bjorklund, A. (1983): *Science*, 221:966–969.

52. Gage, F. H., Stenevi, U., Carlstedt, T., Foster, G., Bjorklund, A., and Aguayo, A. J. (1985): *Exp. Brain Res.*, 60:584–589.

53. Gash, D. M., Collier, T. J., and Sladek, J. R., Jr. (1985): *Neurobiol. Aging*, 6:131–150.

54. Greene, L. A., and Rein, G. (1977): *Brain Res.*, 129:247–263.

55. Greene, L. A., and Tischler, A. S. (1976): *Proc. Natl. Acad. Sci. U.S.A.*, 73:2424–2428.

56. Hart, D. N. J., and Fabre, J. W. (1981): *J. Exp. Med.*, 154:347–361.

57. Hefti, F., Hartikka, J., and Schlumpf, M. (1985): *Brain Res.*, 348:283–288.

58. Herman, J.-P., Choulli, K., and Le Moal, M. (1985): *Exp. Brain Res.*, 60:521–526.

59. Herman, J. P., Nadaud, D., Choulli, K., Taghzouti, K., Simon, H., and Le Moal, M. (1985): In: *Neural Grafting in the Mammalian CNS*, edited by A. Bjorklund and U. Stenevi, pp. 519–527. Elsevier, Amsterdam.

60. Herrera-Marschitz, M., Stromberg, I., Olsson, D., Ungerstedt, U., and Olson, L. (1984): *Brain Res.*, 297:53–61.

61. Hoffer, B., Seiger, A., Ljungberg, T., and Olson, L. (1974): *Brain Res.*, 79:165–184.

62. Hoffer, B., Rose, G., Gerhardt, G., Stromberg, I., and Olson, L. (1985): In: *Neural Grafting in the Mammalian CNS*, edited by A. Bjorklund and U. Stenevi, pp. 437–447. Elsevier, Amsterdam.

63. Hornykiewicz, O. (1966): *Pharmacol. Rev.*, 18:925–964.

64. Isacson, O., Brundin, P., Dawbarn, D., Kelly, P. A. T., Gage, F. H., Emson, P. C., and Bjorklund, A. (1985): In: *Neural Grafting in the Mammalian CNS*, edited by A. Bjorklund and U. Stenevi, pp. 539–549. Elsevier, Amsterdam.

65. Isacson, O., Brundin, P., Gage, F. H., and Bjorklund, A. (1985): In: *Advances in Behavioral Biology, Vol. 28, Brain Plasticity, Learning, and Memory*, edited by B. E. Will, P. Schmitt, and J. C. Dalrymple-Alford, pp. 519–535. Plenum Press, New York.

66. Isacson, O., Brundin, P., Kelley, P. A. T., Gage, F. H., and Bjorklund, A. (1984): *Nature*, 311:458–460.

67. Jaeger, C. B. (1985): *Exp. Brain Res.*, 59:615–624.

68. Jaeger, C. B. (1985): *J. Comp. Neurol.*, 231:121–135.

69. Kamo, H., Kim, S. U., McGeer, P. L., and Shin, D. H. (1985): *Neurosci. Lett.*, 57:43–48.

70. Langston, J. W., Forno, L. S., Rebert, C. S., and Irwin, I. (1984): *Brain Res.*, 292:390–394.

71. Mahalik, T. J., Finger, T. E., Stromberg, I., and Olson, L. (1985): *J. Comp. Neurol.*, 240:60–70.

72. Marshall, J. F., and Gotthelf, T. (1979): *Exp. Neurol.*, 65:398–411.

73. Marshall, J. F., and Teitelbaum, P. (1974): *J. Comp. Physiol. Psychol.*, 86:375–395.

74. Morihisa, J. M., Nakamura, R. K., Freed, W. J., Mishkin, M., and Wyatt, R. J. (1984): *Exp. Neurol.*, 84:643–653.

75. Nadaud, D., Herman, J. P., Simon, H., and Le Moal, M. (1984): *Brain Res.*, 304:137–141.

76. Nieto-Sampedro, M., Manthorpe, M., Barbin, G., Varon, S., and Cotman, C. W. (1983): *J. Neurosci.*, 3:2219–2229.

77. Olson, L. (1970): *Histochemie*, 22:1–7.

78. Olson, L., and Seiger, A. (1972): *Z. Zellforsch.*, 135:175–194.

79. Olson, L., Seiger, A., and Alund, M. (1978): *Med. Biol.*, 56:23–27.

80. Olson, L., Seiger, A., Hoffer, B., and Taylor, D. (1979): *Exp. Brain Res.*, 35:47–67.

81. Olson, L., Stromberg, I., Herrera-Marschitz, M., Ungerstedt, U., and Olson, L. (1985): In: *Neural Grafting in the Mammalian CNS*, edited by A. Bjorklund and U. Stenevi, pp. 505–518. Elsevier, Amsterdam.

82. Patel-Vaidya, U., Wells, M. R., and Freed, W. J. (1985): *Cell Tissue Res.*, 240:281–285.

83. Perlow, M. J., Freed, W. J., Hoffer, B. J., Seiger, A., Olson, L., and Wyatt, R. J. (1979): *Science*, 204:643–647.

84. Perlow, M. J., Kumakura, K., and Guidotti, A. (1980): *Proc. Natl. Acad. Sci. U.S.A.*, 77:5278–5281.

85. Raju, S., and Grogan, J. B. (1971): *Transplant. Proc.*, 3:605–608.

86. Raju, S., and Grogan, J. B. (1977): *Transplant Proc.*, 9:1187–1191.

87. Redmond, D. E., Roth, R. H., Elsworth, J. D., Sladek, J. R., Collier, T. J., Deutch, A. Y., and Haber, S. (1986): *Lancet*, pp. 1125–1127.

87a. *Science News* (1985): *Sci. News*, 128:276.

88. Schmidt, R. H., Bjorklund, A., and Stenevi, U., Dunnett, S. B., and Gage, F. H. (1983): *Acta Physiol. Scand. [Suppl.]*, 522:19–28.

89. Schmidt, R. H., Bjorklund, A., and Stenevi, U. (1981): *Brain Res.*, 218:347–356.

90. Schnitzer, J., and Schachner, M. (1981): *J. Neuroimmunol.*, 1: 429–456.

91. Schwarz, S., and Freed, W. J. (1986): *Exp. Brain Res.*, 65:449–454.

92. Seiger, A., and Olson, L. (1977): *Exp. Brain Res.*, 29:15–44.

93. Seiger, A., and Olson, L. (1977): *Cell Tissue Res.*, 179:285–316.

94. Snyder, S. R., Sahar, D., Prasad, A. L. N., and Fahn, S. (1977): *Life Sci.*, 20:1077–1086.

95. Stenevi, U., Bjorklund, A., and Svendgaard, N.-A. (1976): *Brain Res.*, 114:1–20.

96. Stromberg, I., Herrera-Marschitz, M., Hultgren, L., Ungerstedt, U., and Olson, L. (1984): *Brain Res.*, 297:41–51.

97. Stromberg, I., Herrera-Marschitz, M., Ungerstedt, U., Ebendal, T., and Olson, L. (1985): *Exp. Brain Res.*, 60:335–349.

98. Stromberg, I., Johnson, S., Hoffer, B., and Olson, L. (1985): *Neuroscience*, 14:981–990.

99. Teitelbaum, P., and Epstein, A. N. (1962): *Psychol. Rev.*, 69:74–90.

100. Tischler, A. S., Perlman, R. L., Nunnemacher, G., Morse, G. M., DeLellis, R. A., Wolfe, H. J., and Sheard, B. E. (1982): *Cell Tissue Res.*, 225:525–542.

101. Ungerstedt, U. (1971): *Acta Physiol. Scand. [Suppl.]*, 367:69–93.

102. Ungerstedt, U. (1971): *Acta Physiol. Scand. [Suppl.]*, 367:95–122.

103. Ungerstedt, U. (1976): *Pharmacol. Ther. B*, 2:37–40.

104. Unsicker, K., Krisch, B., Otten, U., and Thoenen, H. (1978): *Proc. Natl. Acad. Sci. U.S.A.*, 75:3498–3502.

105. Unsicker, K., Skaper, S. D., and Varon, S. (1985): *Dev. Brain Res.*, 17:117–129.

106. Warren, S., and Chute, R. N. (1972): *Cancer*, 29:327–331.

107. Whelan, J. P., and Lampson, L. A. (1985): *Soc. Neurosci. Abstr.*, 11:1105.

108. Wuerthele, S. M., Freed, W. J., Olson, L., Morihisa, J., Spoor, L., Wyatt, R. J., and Hoffer, B. J. (1981): *Exp. Brain Res.*, 44: 1–10.

109. Wurtman, R. J., and Axelrod, J. (1966): *J. Biol. Chem.*, 241: 2301.

110. Wyatt, R. J., de Medinaceli, L., and Freed, W. J. (1986): In: *The 1986 Sandoz Lectures in Gerontology: Dimensions in Aging*, edited by M. Bengener, M. Ermini, and H. B. Stähelin, pp. 143–160. Academic Press, London.

Psychopharmacology:
The Third Generation of Progress,
edited by Herbert Y. Meltzer.
Raven Press, New York © 1987.

CHAPTER **49**

Genetics of Affective Illness[1]

Elliot S. Gershon, Wade Berrettini, John Nurnberger, Jr.,
and Lynn R. Goldin

Once evidence is developed that a disorder is inherited (by which we mean a disorder with genetic components to vulnerability), this knowledge can become the basis of clinical research into the etiology and definition of the disorder. Such evidence invites study of families to test the validity of specific hypotheses on the mode of transmission and on the location of any major gene(s), as well as tests of pathophysiological hypotheses.

Furthermore, epidemiological clinical genetic studies can be used to identify the spectrum of clinical diagnoses that are cotransmitted, and can define the diagnostic criteria that most powerfully distinguish the inherited entity from nonfamilial and noncotransmitted forms of psychopathology. The inherited spectrum of diagnoses in the affective disorders appears to include schizoaffective, bipolar, and unipolar disorders, and may also include cyclothymic disorder, anorexia, and suicide. Unipolar disorder may be clinically heterogeneous, including a separate form which is cotransmitted with alcoholism, as discussed below. This has obvious importance for biologic studies, to predict which relatives should have a pathophysiologic vulnerability or chromosomal linkage marker and which should not.

It is worth emphasizing that epidemiologic studies of diagnosis, including pedigree studies, do *not* illuminate by themselves some of the more important genetic issues: Is there biologic heterogeneity, what is the pathophysiologic inherited process in an illness, where on the gene map is the disease locus (or loci), and what are the gene defects?

The types of epidemiologic genetic diagnostic evidence that have been reported are twin studies, adoption studies, and family studies.

TWIN STUDIES OF BIPOLAR AND UNIPOLAR AFFECTIVE DISORDERS

As noted elsewhere (43), the difference between monozygotic (MZ) and dizygotic (DZ) concordance in numerous twin studies of affective illness over a 50-year period is a strong argument for heritability. Bertelsen et al. (9,10) reported on a study using the Danish Twin Register. This register comprises all same-sex twins born between 1870 and 1920. One hundred ten twin pairs in which one or both had manic-depressive illness (by Kraepelinian criteria, which include unipolar cases) were ascertained. The concordance for MZ twins was 0.67 and for DZ twins was 0.20. Concordance (pairwise) was higher for bipolar MZ probands (0.79) than for unipolar MZ probands (0.54), whereas DZ rates were similar (0.24 and 0.19, respectively). Concordance relates to severity of illness in this way: Bipolar I probands, 80% concordance in MZ twins; bipolar II, 78% concordance; unipolar with three or more episodes of depression, 59% concordance; unipolar with fewer than three episodes, 33% concordance. The unipolar data may reflect a population with fewer episodes that may not have passed through the age of risk yet.

Further analysis of concordant pairs for polarity reveals 11 unipolar/unipolar, 14 bipolar/bipolar, and 7 unipolar/bipolar, suggesting some genetic specificity for polarity, but also that unipolar and bipolar can be associated with the

---

[1] This chapter includes updated revision of materials originally published in ref. 95.

same genetic makeup. These data most clearly demonstrate the inherent ambiguity in biological comparisons of bipolar versus unipolar patients. At least a substantial proportion of unipolar patients have the same genetic and biologic vulnerability of bipolar patients. Family study data and mathematical models of observed distribution of diagnoses in families support the same conclusion. What causes some patients to display mania or hypomania at some point in the course of their mood disorders, whereas others never do, is a crucial unanswered question.

ADOPTION STUDIES

Adoption data are of unique importance in demonstrating that prenatal and perinatal events are sufficient to predispose a person to an illness.

Mendlewicz and Rainer (89) reported on 29 bipolar adoptees. They found 31% affective disorder (including spectrum disorder) in the biologic parents of these probands, higher than biologic or adoptive parents of normal adoptees (2 and 9%, respectively).

Schulsinger et al. (118) and Kety (73) reported on an adoption study of suicide. Biologic relatives of 71 adoptees with affective disorder had significantly more suicides (15/381 or 3.9%) than adoptive relatives of those probands (1/168 or 0.6%) or biological or adoptive relatives of control adoptees (1/353 or 0.3%, and 1/166 or 0.6%, respectively).

"Nonpsychiatric" suicide, defined as suicide with no preceding psychiatric hospitalization, also appears to be genetically transmitted in this Danish adoption study. It is not clear from their published data whether this entity is independent of affective disorders.

Von Knorring et al. (141) reported an adoption study from Sweden which included 56 probands with a wide range of affective disorder, mostly "unipolar" and "nonpsychotic depression," and matched adopted and nonadopted controls. Probands and relatives were diagnosed through records of the Swedish health insurance system, with additional records requested as indicated from psychiatric hospitals and clinics throughout Sweden. The investigators found no concordance of psychopathology between biologic parents and adoptees, with the possible exception of more affective disorder in biological mothers of female adoptees with affective disorder.

The Swedish study is not necessarily a failure to replicate the Danish adoption study. Suicide, the key outcome variable in the Danish study, could be entirely missed in the Swedish study. Untreated psychiatric disorders and disorders treated privately or under nonpsychiatric guise could be missed, since subjects were not examined. Nonetheless, this study does cast some doubt on the genetic transmissibility of nonbipolar major depression. It is possible that some of the included cases in the von Knorring study represent a nongenetic form of depression. In a Danish adoption study of depression (including bipolars) based on hospital and suicide records, the biological relatives of affective patients had more affective disorders than similar control relatives only if neurotic depression and affective reactions are excluded (74). The literature on adoption in affective disorders must be considered spotty, and further reports are awaited.

FAMILY STUDIES

Major Affective Disorders

By family studies we mean case-controlled studies of illness in relatives of patients or normal controls. The key questions that can be answered by morbid risk estimates from family studies are whether bipolar illness is transmitted independently of unipolar illness (and other forms of affective disorder), whether specific genetic models fit the familial segregation of illness, and what is the familial concentration of bipolar and other affective disorders in the population. Independence is assessed by studying the cross prevalence, which is defined as the prevalence of one illness in relatives of patients with a second illness. If two illnesses are independent, the cross prevalences are the same as the population prevalences. If they are not, either or both of the cross prevalences may be higher.

It is well known that widely discrepant estimates have been reported for morbid risk of different forms of affective disorder in relatives of patients, as reviewed elsewhere (95). The discrepancies appear to be largely due to differences in diagnostic procedures and criteria, and to population differences. But could the inconsistencies reflect a basically unreliable methodology? Using recently developed family study procedures and criteria, good reliability of diagnosis is routinely attained in collaborative studies, and very similar prevalences in relatives can be found, as evidenced by the similarity of findings in the collaborative study of Gershon et al. (50) and Weissman et al. (144).

The prevalences from that study, and a related study on anorexia, are shown in Fig. 1.

The diagnostic criteria for major depression are far from resolved; two recurrent issues are number of episodes and degree of impairment required for the diagnosis. A comparison of familial vs nonfamilial depression can be rationally made: We examined depressed relatives [by *Diagnostic and Statistical Manual of Mental Disorders,* 3rd ed. (DSM-III) criteria for major depressive disorder] of identified patients with schizoaffective, bipolar, and unipolar illness, and compared them with depressed relatives of normal controls (49). Two characteristics were associated with the familial depressions: First, the presence of observable and significant impairment or incapacitation in performance of

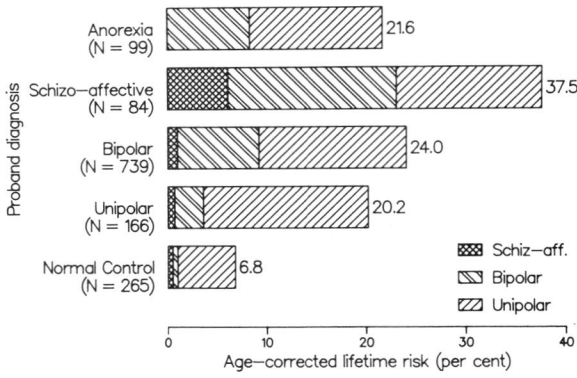

FIG. 1. Morbid risk of different forms of affective disorder in relatives of patients. (Data from refs. 46 and 50.)

the person's major life role, and second, the presence of multiple episodes of depression. These criteria, particularly the first, may prove useful in distinguishing the inherited form of major depressive disorder on clinical grounds.

Within studies with good reliability and using quite similar procedures, it has been possible to demonstrate cultural factors leading to differences in diagnostic rates in family studies (50), of which the recently observed cohort effect is the most striking.

The cohort effect observed in mood disorders, whereby persons born in decades starting approximately 1940 have higher lifetime prevalence of depression than persons born earlier, has been observed in epidemiological studies and in families of affective patients (64,76,129). Surprisingly, this is true for mania as well as for depression (1,103,116). We have reanalyzed our family study data (50) to give a graphic portrayal of this effect in relatives of bipolar patients, where the post-1940 cohorts have higher rates of both bipolar and unipolar disorder than the earlier cohorts (45). This finding cannot be due to gene frequency changes over such a short period, or to selective effects on reproductive fitness. Whatever the cause, it interacts with the familial vulnerability, since the rate remains elevated in relatives of patients.

Despite the variability in absolute observed rates, there are consistencies in within-study comparisons done by numerous investigators. First, the rate of affective illness is consistently several times higher in relatives of affectively ill patients than in relatives of controls. This is evidence for a strong familial contribution to diagnostic variance within the population. Second, in nearly all studies there is a great deal of unipolar illness in relatives of bipolar patients, although the reverse is generally not found. This implies at least partial genetic overlap between bipolar and unipolar illness, as do the twin data.

Are there genetic differences between clinically defined subdivisions of bipolar disorder? Dunner et al. (27) defined patients who have had hypomania but not mania as bipolar II (BP II). It is generally agreed that this category appropri-ately includes only patients who have also had major depression. Even with this stipulation, BP II is most difficult to diagnose reliably. It appears that BP II patients tend to have more BP II and unipolar relatives and fewer BP I relatives than do BP I patients (Table 1). This suggests that BP II is genetically somewhere between BP I and unipolar.

Related Disorders in Relatives of Affective Patients

A clinical genetic spectrum of affective disorders can be constructed by comparing prevalence of illness in relatives of patients versus relatives of controls. Based on such data, in addition to unipolar illness, schizoaffective disorder and cyclothymic personality may be considered part of the spectrum of bipolar illness, as reviewed elsewhere (95). In addition, anorexia and bulimia are associated with familial affective disorder (46).

Unipolar illness has been reported to be heterogeneous, especially with regard to association of alcoholism with a subgroup of cases (146).

Childhood depression is not clearly increased in children (up to age 17) of affective patients in controlled studies, but the number of children studied is modest (7,47). However, if children or adolescents hospitalized for severe depression are studied, there is increased affective disorder and alcoholism among their adult relatives (130).

Taken together, these studies can be interpreted to suggest that the most severely depressed children and adolescents, referred for treatment to psychiatric facilities, appear to be familially related to adults with affective disorders, but that such cases are not found with great statistical frequency among the children of adult affective disorder patients. The age of onset of the adult form of major depression, as suggested by Puig-Antich, may well extend into the pre-pubertal period. The childhood form of major depression as detected on survey interviews, which is clinically less severe than the adult form, may not be increased in offspring of patients with affective disorders.

TABLE 1. Comparison of affective disorders in relatives of bipolar I and bipolar II patients

Probands	Schizoaffective (SA)	Bipolar BP I	Bipolar BP II	Unipolar (UP)	N
BP I					
Angst et al. (2)	0.9	1.8[a]		6.6	225
Gershon et al. (50)	1.1	4.5	4.1	14.0	441
Fieve et al. (35)		3.6	1.5	6.4[b]	760
Coryell et al. (17)		2.9	2.5	22.7	278
BP II					
Angst et al. (2)	2.6	3.4[a]		14.8	176
Gershon et al. (50)	0.6	2.6	4.5	17.3	157
Fieve et al. (35)		0.7	4.2	11.1[b]	549
Coryell et al. (17)		0.9	9.8	21.4	111

[a] BP I or BP II not specified.
[b] Includes "UP other."

MODE OF GENETIC TRANSMISSION

Specific genetic hypotheses can be tested on clinical diagnostic data in patients and relatives, or by combining diagnostic data with chromosomal linkage markers or pathophysiologic vulnerability markers in the members of a pedigree.

Pedigree and Segregation Analyses of Clinical Diagnosis

Single Autosomal Locus Models

Elston and Stewart (32) developed a general model for single locus inheritance that allows estimation of the maximum likelihood that a particular (set of) pedigree(s) would be found under each of the different types of transmission subsumed in the model. The likelihoods of each transmission mode can be compared with each other and with the most general case, which is a powerful way of ruling out possible transmission modes or specific parameter values. This model is applicable to multigenerational families, variable age of onset, and different conditions of pedigree ascertainment (30,31,33). This likelihood approach can also be used to test both major locus and polygenic components of inheritance (77,93).

Goldin et al. (56,60) have tested the power of the combined model to detect single locus transmission in simulated pedigrees, with and without a linked marker. Under certain parameter values, when there is incomplete penetrance and/or phenocopies, the power of these models to detect single gene transmission is reduced. Linkage under these conditions was only detectable at very small recombination frequencies; if the recombination fraction was 15%, linkage was not detectable. Thus, failure to detect single locus inheritance by use of segregation analyses should not be considered to rule out this mode of inheritance.

For traits with simple Mendelian inheritance, Botstein et al. (11) suggest that 150 properly spaced linkage markers can scan the entire genome. With respect to complex traits such as affective disorders, whose inheritance is clearly not simple Mendelian, perhaps several hundred more closely spaced markers would be needed to scan for a single gene disease locus. This is only now becoming possible, with the new availability of DNA variants as linkage markers (restriction fragment length polymorphisms: RFLPs).

Prior to the development of this complete linkage map, mathematical analysis of segregation of illness in pedigrees has been the technique used to test for single gene locus inheritance of illness. Segregation analyses of affective disorders in family data have been generally inconsistent with single major locus transmission even when using models that allow for incomplete penetrance, variable age of onset, and ascertainment of families through affected individuals. This has been found in multiple data sets (13,14,18,136). We performed similar analyses on a large sample of families of patients treated at the National Institute of Mental Health (59). Transmission was not consistent with single locus models even if families were

analyzed according to the proband diagnostic subtype (schizoaffective, SA; bipolar, BP; or unipolar, UP) or by subtypes according to some extreme value of a biological trait in the proband ("low" platelet monoamine oxidase, MAO; "low" CSF 5-hydroxyindoleacetic acid, 5HIAA; and positive antidepressant response to lithium).

Transmission of psychiatric disorders can also be modeled as a multifactorial illness. Such an illness would be the end result of a large number of liability factors, both genetic and environmental, that act additively to produce susceptibility. At a certain threshold level of susceptibility, a person becomes ill. The genetic liability factors can be modeled either as a single major locus or as a large number of genes (polygenic inheritance). These models can be tested based on the prevalences of the disease in relatives compared to the population prevalence. Reich et al. (108) extended this model to include multiple thresholds so that one could hypothesize that two or more disorders with increasing severity shared the same liability factors. That is, the model can test whether the transmission of different diagnostic entities fits a single dimension of underlying vulnerability. A polygenic model with separate thresholds for UP, BP, and SA illness was consistent with our family data (40,50) and other data (127). Here, SA disorder can be placed on the same continuum as BP and UP disorders as an extreme form of affective disorders. That is, relatives of probands with SA disorder in our study had the highest risk for affective illness. However, other family studies do not find the highest risk in relatives of SA patients (2,5). This may be due to different criteria for SA disorder or to sampling variations. It appears that the multiple threshold model is powerful for determining whether or not a group of diagnoses share genetic liability factors, but it does not determine whether the genetic liability is polygenic or single major locus. In addition, these analyses have all combined prevalence rates for different generations. In one study, when prevalences for different generations were separated, both major locus and polygenic threshold models were rejected (103). This was due to the higher prevalences of illness in younger generations (cohort effect, see above) found in these data. T. Reich (106) has demonstrated that if this generational difference is accounted for by environmental factors, then the familial concentration of affective illness still fits polygenic inheritance.

It can be concluded that within the limits of current model detection, homogeneous single locus transmission is not consistent with the segregation of affective disorders in families. Polygenic models do seem to be consistent with the data. This does not exclude the existence of single loci for affective disorder, since simulation studies (56,60) have shown that certain types of single major locus inheritance are not detectable by segregation analysis, although the major locus for the trait *can* be detected if there is a closely linked genetic marker locus. Thus, analysis of linkage of a presumed susceptibility locus to genetic marker locus is a powerful method for detecting a disease susceptibility locus, as well as for ruling out its existence. Until the application of a complete panel of linkage markers to the major psychiatric disorders has been performed, the possibility of an undetected single major locus in these disorders is not ruled out.

Linkage Markers

Unquestionably, the major impetus to linkage studies in psychiatric illness has come from the mapping of the Huntington's disease locus by Gusella et al. (63), which was made possible by the vast increase in linkage markers resulting from recombinant DNA technology (11). In addition, a large number of new markers have been identified by high-resolution two-dimensional electrophoresis of proteins (61,62,98). These methods have greatly increased the proportion of the genome currently accessible to linkage studies. The power of the pedigree linkage method lies in its scanning of the chromosomal fragment, adjacent to the polymorphism, which is genetically transmitted along with the polymorphic locus. This allows definitive conclusions to be drawn about the presence or absence of a disease locus within a chromosomal region encompassing several million base pairs.

The weakness of linkage methods in psychiatric illness is that the inheritance of these illnesses is clearly complex, and does not fit simple or even fairly complex models of segregation applied to pedigrees, as discussed above. Complex inheritance and genetic heterogeneity of an illness weaken the power of linkage analyses, making it necessary to study more markers and more families to detect a single gene producing illness vulnerability, and in some instances making it impractical to detect single loci (see ref. 92). But this does not make the search necessarily hopeless; the example of diabetes mellitus, long thought of as a multifactorial disease without detectable single gene components, is instructive. Because of the finding of linkage and association to single genes [the human leukocyte antigen (HLA) and insulin structural gene] this illness is now known to have major forms with single locus determinants of vulnerability (117).

X-Chromosome Markers

Based on their earlier family studies, which were compatible with X-chromosome transmission of BP illness, Winokur and his colleagues (107,148) presented evidence using genetic linkage markers to support this hypothesis. A larger series of informative families was later reported by Mendlewicz and his co-workers (84–86). Combining their and Winokur's data, they concluded that in families of BP patients, affective illness is closely linked to protan and deutan color blindness, and that linkage to the Xg blood group is also present. Since families were excluded from analysis if there was apparent father-son transmission, these authors qualified their conclusion as being applicable to a subgroup of patients with BP illness.

These reported data are problematic, and the presence of linkage may be seriously questioned, as we have reviewed elsewhere (76). The chief problem is that the reported close linkage of BP illness to both Xg and the protan-deutan region of the X chromosome is not compatible with the known large chromosomal map distance between the Xg locus and the protan-deutan region.

We have not been able to replicate either of these linkages in our data. For both Xg and protan-deutan color blindness, close linkage to affective illness could be ruled out (53,79). The pedigrees were not heterogeneous with each other; there were no instances of single pedigrees strongly suggesting linkage to either marker. In studying large pedigrees among the Amish, with affective disorder and color blindness present, Kidd et al. (75) did not report linkage between the two conditions.

Mendlewicz et al. (87), on the other hand, reported eight new families in Belgium suggesting linkage to color blindness in at least one of the families.

The studies from our group and the original study from Mendlewicz and co-workers (84–86) were done at comparable research settings 200 miles apart in the northeastern United States in clinics with predominantly white patients, so it is improbable that population differences account for the discrepancy. The two color blindness linkage series are the most opposite. Each of the two studies is statistically significant by the lod score test, but they support opposite conclusions. Both are statistically homogeneous. Baron et al. (6), Mendlewicz (83), and Risch and Baron (110) have proposed that heterogeneity accounts for these differences, but we find this difficult to accept. Methodologic errors in diagnostic or ascertainment procedures could have produced the unique homogeneity of the 1972 to 1974 pedigree series of Mendlewicz et al., and that would explain why the strikingly positive results are not replicated either in our series or in the later series of Mendlewicz et al. (87).

This is not to say that linked pedigrees do not exist. Our own pedigree series on red-green color blindness and bipolar illness is small enough (six pedigrees) so that a proportion of all pedigrees in reality might be linked and still none might show up in our series. Strongly positive, multigenerational, individual pedigrees for the red-green color blindness region have been reported by Winokur et al. (147), Mendlewicz et al. (87), and Baron (4). Del Zompo et al. (20) reported two pedigrees with possible linkage of affective illness to the color blindness region, and Kidd et al. (75) found no linkage present in an Amish pedigree. However, these reports were not part of large pedigree-series studies, which can provide assurance of independent, systematic, and unbiased ascertainment and diagnostic procedures.

Mendlewicz et al. (88) reported a family with linkage between manic depressive illness and glucose-6-phosphate dehydrogenase (G6PD) deficiency, a marker on the X chromosome, very close to the red-green color blindness loci. DNA probes for this region of the X chromosome now exist (102). It may serve to make virtually all pedigrees informative for linkage, and lead to a resolution of the controversy.

Linkage Markers: Autosomal

HLA associations with BP affective illness have been reported, but statistical significance has been lacking, the reports are not compatible with each other, and later reports did not support the presence of any association, as reviewed elsewhere (57). Within pedigrees, genetic heterogeneity of illness can be expected to be minimal or absent. Linkage of HLA to affective illness in bipolar families could be definitively ruled out in the data of Targum et al. (135).

Smeraldi et al. (128) applied the identical by descent method to HLA types in sib pairs where both had affective illness, and noted increased concordance suggesting a possible linkage.

Turner and King (137) analyzed five pedigrees for linkage to HLA, and proposed that BP illness is a heterogeneous condition with 10 to 30% not HLA linked and most of the rest linked to HLA on chromosome 6. Their assignment of phenotypes is confusing to us, and may have been based on other than diagnostic factors, as we read the description of the "inclusion in the taxon" procedure.

Weitkamp et al. (145) concluded that a major susceptibility gene for depression is located in the HLA region based on the increased sharing of common HLA types in ill pairs of siblings in 20 families, when their sample was subdivided by sibship size and number affected. Goldin et al. (55) have argued that this criterion for dividing a sample is not theoretically sound. Their new data on 18 families combined with 9 families previously published by Targum from the same study, did not support the hypothesis of a relationship of the HLA locus to depression. In two separate studies, Suarez and Croughan (131) and Suarez and Reich (132) also did not replicate this linkage. Although heterogeneity could again be claimed as an explanation of non-replication, it appears more parsimonious to consider this linkage not generally present.

Goldin et al. (59) and Goldin and Gershon (57) did linkage studies of 21 autosomal markers to affective illness, and found no suggestive linkages.

These studies cover perhaps 22% of the genome, and all the positive linkage reports are controversial.

Restriction Fragment Length Polymorphisms

The introduction of polymorphisms defined by Southern blot location of digestion fragments of DNA for a specific gene has revolutionized clinical genetics, starting with the initial demonstration of an RFLP associated with sickle cell hemoglobin by Kan and Dozy (72). The number of new RFLPs has increased exponentially; at the present time, it is estimated that about 50% of the genome is mappable. With the availability of great increases in the number of available markers, largely through the DNA methodology of RFLPs, geneticists expect the entire human genome to be mappable. The multiplicity of markers will also contribute to resolution of the scientific controversies since several closely linked loci can be used to verify a disease marker location, and the problem of finding families informative for a particular polymorphism will be less pressing.

There are two types of RFLP that can be used in linkage studies. The first type is a random single-copy DNA sequence, whose gene product, if any, need not be of interest. Since the number of RFLP markers needed to cover the entire human genome is as small as 150, the use of any single marker in a linkage study with disease can be a tangible contribution to scientific knowledge; this approach was strikingly successful in Huntington's disease (63). The second type of RFLP is one related to a prior hypothesis on pathophysiology. Here, the structural genes for the

neuropeptides and for the ligand-binding proteins of receptors offer current investigative opportunities in neuropsychiatric illness. Of course, the second type of gene also serves as a random marker for the region around it for several million base pairs, so the justification for trying a particular gene in a linkage study need not be compelling *a priori*. But we would emphasize that there are pathophysiologic hypotheses that cannot be otherwise investigated, such as a hypothesis that there is a difference in the structural gene for a neuroreceptor associated with an illness.

As of this writing, these recombinant DNA approaches are just starting to appear in the literature. Gerhard et al. (39), studying an Amish pedigree with BP and UP relatives, reported a possible linkage of affective disorder to the insulin-Ras 1 oncogene region of chromosome 11. Feder et al. (34) reported no association of proopiocortin (POMC) polymorphisms with affective illness or schizophrenia. Detera-Wadleigh et al. (21) reported that somatostatin gene RFLPs are not associated with or closely linked to affective disorder.

POTENTIAL ETIOLOGIC MARKERS

An important difference between a linkage marker and a risk factor (vulnerability marker) is that linkage is necessarily an event that occurs in relation to a single genetic locus, whereas a risk factor may be polygenically determined or be the result of complex interactions between several loci.

The current status of selected putative heritable risk factors is displayed in Table 2.

Enzymes of Catecholamine Metabolism

The specific enzymes of catecholamine metabolism that can be assayed in peripheral blood, and which appear to be identical to brain enzymes in humans, are plasma dopamine beta-hydroxylase (DBH), erythrocyte catechol-*O*-methyltransferase (COMT), and platelet monoamine oxidase (MAO). All three have heritable activity in humans and have been studied extensively in affective disorders, as reviewed elsewhere (44,58). For plasma DBH activity, our data suggest dominant inheritance with a polygenic background (54). The mathematical demonstration of a single locus was confirmed by linkage to the ABO locus (58). There do not appear to be patient-control differences for this activity, and the inheritance of affective illness is independent of the major locus controlling activity (44,58). Erythrocyte COMT activity appears also to have single-gene inheritance, with dominant transmission, on a polygenic background (54,58). Earlier reports of patient-control differences have not been confirmed, and the segregation of COMT activity and affective illness in families appears to be independent (44).

Platelet MAO activity has been subject to the most intense investigation in clinical psychiatry, without being definitively related to the inheritance of any psychiatric disorder. A single-locus, two-allele determinant of platelet

TABLE 2. *Current status of proposed genetic vulnerability markers for affective illness*

Finding	Criteria				
	Patients differ from controls	State independent	Heritable	Segregates with illness	Refs.
Enzymes of monoamine metabolism					
Plasma DBH	No	Yes	Yes—single locus	No	
Erythrocyte COMT	No	Yes	Yes—single locus	No	Gershon et al. (44)
Platelet MAO	Yes (most studies)	Yes	Yes—single locus	No	Rice et al. (109)
Monoamine and amino acid metabolites					
CSF 5HIAA	Yes (most studies)	Conflicting data	No	Unknown	Van Praag & de Haan (138) Sedvall et al. (119)
Membrane transport					
Lithium erythrocyte plasma ratio	Yes (some studies)	Possible	Yes	No (most data)	Dorus et al. (22,25) Nurnberger et al. (97) Shaughnessy et al. (120)
Platelet [³H]IMI	Yes	No	Possibly	No data	Berrettini et al. (8) Mellerup et al. (81) Langer (78) Suranyi-Cadotte et al. (133) Friedl & Propping (36)
CNS protein polymorphism					
Duarte Pc 1 brain protein	Yes	Presumably	Yes—single locus	No data	Comings (16)
Neurotransmitter receptor and pharmacologic response studies					
Muscarinic cholinergic					
Early induction of REM sleep by arecoline muscarinic agonist	Yes	Yes	Possibly	Possibly	Sitaram et al. (126) Nurnberger et al. (96) Jones et al. (70) Sitaram et al. (125)
Adrenergic					
Platelet α₂ adrenoceptor	Possibly (conflicting data)	No	Yes	No data	Siever et al. (121) Kafka et al. (71) Propping and Friedl (104) Healy et al. (65) Garcia-Sevilla et al. (37,38) Wood and Coppen (149)
Lymphoblast β-Receptor	Possibly (conflicting data)	Yes	Yes	Almost no data	Daiguji et al. (19) Wright et al. (150) Berrettini et al. (8a)

MAO activity was observed in segregation analysis of a large set of family data (109). It has been claimed that there are multiple alleles, rather than two, based on the distribution of activity in a Swedish sample, but family data have not been available to corroborate this (15).

Platelet MAO has been reported decreased in BP patients by some, but not all, investigators (see review in ref. 51; also 28, 41, 134). Pandey et al. (99) report that low MAO sorts with illness in BP and alcoholic relations of BP probands. Von Knorring et al. (142) reported increased BP disorders in relatives of high platelet MAO activity depressed patients, but increased neurotic depression and alcoholism in relatives of patients with low platelet MAO. Gershon et al. (44,52) reported that low MAO does not sort with affective illness in relatives of low-MAO probands. The differences between these studies remain to be explained.

Central nervous system metabolites of serotonin and dopamine are measurable in CSF, without interference from the peripheral sources of these metabolites. 5-Hydroxyindoleacetic acid, the principal metabolite of serotonin in CSF, was bimodally distributed in two series of depressed patients (3,139). A substantial proportion of depressed patients studied have reduced 5HIAA in CSF, although not all studies show significant patient-control differences, as reviewed elsewhere (41). Sedvall et al. (119) have demonstrated a significant correlation in CSF 5HIAA between twins, but there was no MZ-DZ difference, which suggests nongenetic control. Van Praag and de Haan (138) compared family history of patients with persistent reduced 5HIAA to patients with normal 5HIAA, and found higher depressive admissions in relatives of the reduced 5HIAA group. But the family study data are presented without diagnostic definitions or estimates of the number of relatives at risk, and no families have yet been studied for concordance or discordance of CSF metabolites in ill relatives.

Monoamine-Related Binding Sites on Peripheral Cells

The [³H]imipramine ([³H]IMI) binding site in platelets apparently is similar to, or associated with, a serotonin transport protein. This system resembles the serotonin uptake system in brain (100,101,105). Initial reports of reduced binding in depression raised interest in density of sites or their affinity to ligand as possible trait markers in affective illness (12). Variation in B_{max} for [³H]IMI binding is highly correlated in MZ twins, suggesting that this is a heritable characteristic (36). We and others have observed that binding is not decreased in euthymic medication-free BP patients (8,78,81,133). The weight of evidence, then, does not support [³H]IMI binding B_{max} as a genetic vulnerability marker.

β-Receptor density on lymphoblasts is reduced in bipolar patients and relatives in the work of Wright (150), but only a few ill relatives have been studied. These also had decreased density, whereas most well relatives did not. A recent study has not confirmed a patient-control difference (8a).

Recent data on changed density and affinity of α_2 receptors on platelets in depression have stimulated genetic hypotheses (37), but no genetic evidence has been reported.

Although muscarinic receptors on fibroblasts were reported to exist, and to be more dense in bipolar illness (94), these results have not been replicable (48,80,140).

Cation Transport Parameters

Alterations in cell membranes have been proposed as a source of vulnerability to affective disorder (66,82).

Dorus and co-workers (23-26) have demonstrated genetic control of the intracellular:extracellular Li ratio. In a complex analysis, a major gene for elevated Li ratio, associated with bipolar illness, was reported by these authors (22). However, the analysis depended on assumptions about the ratio in ill persons whose blood was not studied, based on

correlations observed in relatives who were studied. This was not borne out in their subsequent work (120).

Egeland et al. (29) found no relation between Li-Na countertransport and BP or UP affective illness in an Amish pedigree. Waters et al. (143) also found no abnormality in Na-Li countertransport flow in ill individuals in bipolar illness pedigrees. Nor did we find differences between patients and controls, often controlling for amount of time off lithium (96).

Cholinergic Functional Measurements

The cholinergic hypothesis in affective disorders originated in the observation of a consistency in the psychological effects of cholinomimetic and anticholinergic agents (67). With advances in the anatomical and functional knowledge of acetylcholine (ACh) in brain, clinical investigative interest focused on two central muscarinic cholinergic functions: the initiation of rapid eye movement (REM) sleep periods, and the release of the anterior pituitary hormone corticotropin (ACTH) and β-endorphin (which share the same precursor molecule). Both functions are thought to be anatomically localized to the cholinergic neuronal groupings of the medulla, which project to the hypothalamus and thalamus (90,91).

Cholinomimetic agents cause secretion of ACTH and β-endorphin; conversely, the muscarinic antagonist atropine, injected into hypothalamus, inhibits ACTH release, as reviewed elsewhere (68). Janowsky and Risch demonstrated increased sensitivity to cholinomimetic-induced β-endorphin and ACTH release in depressed patients, as compared with normal controls (69,111-115). However, this cholinergic neuroendocrine response has not been demonstrated to be state independent or under genetic control.

REM sleep induction offers another investigative opportunity. Sitaram and Gillin demonstrated that REM sleep initiation is physiologically under muscarinic cholinergic control, and responds as predicted to pharmacologic stimulation, blockade, or alterations in receptor sensitivity (122-124). Patients with affective disorders, whether depressed or euthymic, were more sensitive than normal to cholinergic REM induction (70,126).

Sitaram and Gillin speculated that this increased sensitivity might reside at the receptor level, since the cholinergic agonist used was a direct agonist, arecoline. Furthermore, they speculated that this was a genetic vulnerability characteristic in affective disorders, since it was state independent. Nurnberger et al. (97) demonstrated that REM induction values are highly correlated in normal MZ twins, suggesting that they are under genetic control.

Duarte Protein

Comings (16) reported experiments using a two-dimensional protein electrophoretic technique by which he identified a mutant protein, Pc 1 Duarte (Pc for perchloric acid extract) with an increased frequency in brain specimens taken at autopsy from individuals with affective disorder and/or alcoholism. Controls ($N = 152$) showed a frequency of 31.6% carrying the abnormal protein, whereas the frequency for depressed and alcoholic individuals ($N = 42$)

was 61.9%. In the bipolar patients ($N = 11$), the frequency of the Duarte protein was 72.7%.

CONCLUSION

The heritability of the major psychiatric disorders is evident from clinical studies, but the mode of transmission and identification of a transmitted defect have not been demonstrated. With new developments in molecular genetics, and new techniques for clinical investigation of the CNS, progress towards these goals may be expected.

REFERENCES

1. Angst, J. (1985): *Psychopathology,* 18:140–154.
2. Angst, J., Frey, R., Lohmeyer, B., and Zerbin-Rudin, E. (1980): *Hum. Genet.,* 55:237–254.
3. Asberg, M., Thoren, P., Traskman, L., Bertilsson, L., and Ringberger, V. (1976): *Science,* 191:478–480.
4. Baron, M. (1977): *Arch. Gen Psychiatry,* 34:721–725.
5. Baron, M., Gruen, R., Asnis, L., and Kane, J. (1982): *Acta Psychiatr. Scand.,* 65:253–262.
6. Baron, M., Rainer, J. D., and Risch, N. (1981): *J. Affective Disord.,* 3:141–157.
7. Beardslee, W. R., Bemporad, J., Keller, M. B., and Klerman, G. L. (1983): *Am. J. Psychiatry,* 140:825–832.
8. Berrettini, W. H., Nurnberger, J. I., Jr., Post, R. M., and Gershon, E. S. (1982): *Psychiatry Res.,* 7:215–219.
8a. Berrettini, W. H., Cappellari, C. B., Nornberger, J. I., Jr., and Gershon, E. S. (1987): *Neuropsychobiology (in press).*
9. Bertelsen, A. (1979): In: *Origin, Prevention and Treatment of Affective Disorders,* edited by M. Schou and E. Stromgren, pp. 227–239. Academic Press, London.
10. Bertelsen, A., Harvald, B., and Hauge, M. (1977): *Br. J. Psychiatry,* 130:330–351.
11. Botstein, D., White, R. L., Skolnick, M., and Davis, R. W. (1980): *Am. J. Hum. Genet.,* 32:314–331.
12. Briley, M. S., Langer, S. Z., Raisman, R., Sechter, D., and Zarifian, E. (1980): *Science,* 209:303–305.
13. Bucher, K. D., and Elston, R. C. (1981): *J. Psychiatr. Res.,* 16:53–63.
14. Bucher, K. D., Elston, R. C., Green, R., Whybrow, P., Helzer, J., Reich, T., Clayton, P., and Winokur, G. (1981): *J. Psychiatr. Res.,* 16:65–78.
15. Cloninger, C. R., von Knorring, L., and Oreland, L. (1985): *Psychiatry Res.,* 15:133–143.
16. Comings, D. E. (1979): *Nature,* 277:28–32.
17. Coryell, W., Endicott, J., Reich, T., Andreasen, N., and Keller, M. (1984): *Br. J. Psychiatry,* 145:49–54.
18. Crowe, R. R., Namboodiri, K. K., Ashby, H. B., and Elston, R. C. (1981): *Neuropsychobiology,* 7:20–25.
19. Daiguji, M., Meltzer, H. Y., Tong, C., U'Pritchard, D. C., Young, M., and Kravitz, H. (1981): *Life Sci.,* 29:2059–2064.
20. Del Zompo, M., Bocchetta, A., Goldin, L. R., and Corsini, G. U. (1984): *Acta Psychiatr. Scand.,* 70:282–287.
21. Detera-Wadleigh, S., Berrettini, W. H., DeLisi, L. E., Nurnberger, J. I., Goldin, L. R., and Gershon, E. S. (1985): In: *Proceedings of the IVth World Congress of Biological Psychiatry,* edited by C. Shagass, pp. 67–69. Elsevier, New York.
22. Dorus, E., Cox, N. J., Gibbon, R. D., Shaughnessy, R., Pandey, G. N., and Colinger, C. R. (1983): *Arch. Gen. Psychiatry,* 40:545–552.
23. Dorus, E., Pandey, G. N., and Davis, J. M. (1975): *Arch. Gen. Psychiatry,* 32:1097–1102.
24. Dorus, E., Pandey, G. N., Frazer, A., and Mendels, J. (1974): *Arch. Gen. Psychiatry,* 31:463–465.
25. Dorus, E., Pandey, G. N., Shaughnessey, R., and Davis, J. M. (1979): *Biol. Psychiatry,* 14:989–994.
26. Dorus, E., Pandey, G. N., Shaughnessey, R., and Davis, J. M. (1980): *Arch. Gen. Psychiatry,* 37:80–81.
27. Dunner, D. L., Dwyer, T., and Fieve, R. R. (1976): *Compr. Psychiatry,* 17:447–451.
28. Edwards, D. J., Spiker, D. G., Kupfer, D. J., Foster, F. G., Neil, J. F., and Abrams, L. (1978): *Arch. Gen. Psychiatry,* 35:1443–1446.
29. Egeland, J. A., Kidd, J. R., Frazer, A., Kidd, K. K., and Neuhauser, B. S. (1984): *Am. J. Psychiatry,* 141:1049–1054.
30. Elston, R. C. (1973): *Hum. Hered.,* 23:105–112.
31. Elston, R. C., and Sobel, E. (1979): *Am. J. Hum. Genet.,* 31:62–69.
32. Elston, R. C., and Stewart, J. (1971): *Hum. Hered.,* 21:523–542.
33. Elston, R. C., and Yelverton, K. C. (1975): *Am. J. Hum. Genet.,* 27:31–45.
34. Feder, J., Gurling, H. M. D., Darby, J., and Cavalli-Sforza, L. L. (1985): *Am. J. Hum. Genet.,* 37:286–294.
35. Fieve, R. R., Go, R., Dunner, D. L., and Elston, R. (1984): *J. Psychiatr. Res.,* 4:425–446.
36. Friedl, W., and Propping, P. (1984): *Psychiatry Res.,* 11:279–285.
37. Garcia-Sevilla, J., Gulmon, J., Garcia-Vallejo, P., and Fuster, M. J. (1986): *Arch. Gen. Psychiatry,* 43:51–57.
38. Garcia-Sevilla, J. A., Zis, A. P., Hollingsworth, M. A., Greden, J. F., and Smith, C. B. (1981): *Arch. Gen. Psychiatry,* 38:1327–1333.
39. Gerhard, D. S., Egeland, J. A., Pauls, D. L., Kidd, J. R., Kramer, P. L., Housman, D., and Kidd, K. K. (1984): *Am. J. Hum. Genet.,* 36(4):3S.
40. Gershon, E. S., Baron, M., and Leckman, J. F. (1975): *J. Psychiatr. Res.,* 12:301–317.
41. Gershon, E. S., Belmaker, R. H., Ebstein, R., and Jones, W. Z. (1977): *Arch. Gen. Psychiatry,* 34:731–734.
42. Gershon, E. S., and Bunney, W. E., Jr. (1976): *J. Psychiatr. Res.,* 13:99–117.
43. Gershon, E. S., Bunney, W. E., Jr., Leckman, J. F., van Eerdewegh, M., and Debauche, B. A. (1976): *Behav. Genet.,* 6:227–261.
44. Gershon, E. S., Goldin, L. R., Lake, C. R., Murphy, D. L., and Guroff, J. J. (1980): In: *Enzymes and Neurotransmitters in Mental Disease,* edited by E. Usdin, P. Sourkes, and M. B. H. Youdim, pp. 281–299. John Wiley & Sons Ltd., London.
45. Gershon, E. S., Hamovit, J. R., Guroff, J. J., and Nurnberger, J. N. (1987): *Arch. Gen. Psychiatry (in press).*
46. Gershon, E. S., Hamovit, J. R., Schreiber, J. L., Dibble, E. D., Kaye, W., Nurnberger, J. I., Jr., Andersen, A., and Ebert, M. (1983): In: *Childhood Psychopathology and Development,* edited by S. B. Guze, F. J. Earls, and J. E. Barrett, pp. 279–286. Raven Press, New York.
47. Gershon, E. S., McKnew, D., Cytryn, L., Hamovit, J., Schreiber, J., Hibbs, E., and Pellegrini, D. (1985): *J. Affective Disord.,* 8:283–291.
48. Gershon, E. S., Nadi, N. S., Nurnberger, J. I., Jr., and Berrettini, W. H. (1985): *N. Engl. J. Med.,* 312:862.
49. Gershon, E. S., Weissman, M. M., Guroff, J. J., Prusoff, B. A., and Leckman, J. F. (1986): *J. Affect. Dis.,* 11:125–131.
50. Gershon, E. S., Hamovit, J., Guroff, J. J., et al. (1982): *Arch. Gen. Psychiatry,* 39:1157–1167.
51. Gershon, E. S., Targum, S. D., Kessler, L. R., Mazure, C. M., and Bunney, W. E., Jr. (1977): In: *Progress in Medical Genetics, Vol. 2,* edited by A. G. Steinberg, A. G. Bearn, A. G. Motulsky, and B. Childs, pp. 101–164. W. B. Saunders Co., Philadelphia.
52. Gershon, E. S., Targum, S. D., Leckman, J. F., Guroff, J. J., and Murphy, D. L. (1979): *Psychopharmacol. Bull.,* 15:27–30.
53. Gershon, E. S., Targum, S. D., Matthysse, S., and Bunney, W. E., Jr. (1979): *Arch. Gen. Psychiatry,* 36:1423–1434.
54. Goldin, L. R. (1985): *Genet. Epidemiol.,* 2:317–325.
55. Goldin, L. R., Clerget-Darpoux, F., and Gershon, E. S. (1982): *Psychiatry Res.,* 7:29–45.
56. Goldin, L. R., Cox, N. J., Pauls, D. L., Gershon, E. S., and Kidd, K. K. (1984): *Genet. Epidemiol.,* 1:285–296.
57. Goldin, L. R., and Gershon, E. S. (1983): *Psychiatr. Dev.,* 4:387–418.
58. Goldin, L. R., Gershon, E. S., Lake, C. R., Murphy, D. L., McGinniss, M., and Sparkes, R. S. (1982): *Am. J. Hum. Genet.,* 34:250–263.
59. Goldin, L. R., Gershon, E. S., Targum, S. D., Sparkes, R. S., and McGinniss, M. (1983): *Am. J. Hum. Genet.,* 35:274–287.

60. Goldin, L. R., Kidd, K. R., Matthysse, S., and Gershon, E. S. (1981): In: *Genetic Research Strategies in Psychobiology and Psychiatry*, edited by E. S. Gershon, S. Matthysse, R. D. Ciaranella, and X. O. Breakefield, pp. 305–317. Boxwood Press, Pacific Grove, CA.

61. Goldman, D., Goldin, L. R., Rathnagiri, P., O'Brien, S. J., Egeland, J. A., and Merril, C. R. (1985): *Am. J. Hum. Genet.*, 37:898–911.

62. Goldman, D., and Merril, C. (1983): *Am. J. Hum. Genet.*, 35:827–837.

63. Gusella, J. F., Wexler, N. S., Conneally, P. M., Naylor, S. L., Anderson, M. A., Tanzi, R. E., Watkins, P. C., Ottina, K., Wallace, M. R., Sakaguchi, A. Y., Young, A. B., Shoulson, I., Bonilla, E., and Martin, J. B. (1983): *Nature*, 306:234–238.

64. Hagnell, O., Lanke, J., Rorsman, B., et al. (1982): *Psychol. Med.*, 12:279–289.

65. Healy, D., Carner, P. A., and Leonard, B. E. (1982): *J. Psychiatr. Res.*, 17:251–260.

66. Hokin-Neaverson, M., Spiegel, D. A., and Lewis, W. C. (1974): *Life Sci.*, 15:1739–1748.

67. Janowsky, D. S., El-Yousef, M. K., and Davis, J. M. (1972): *Lancet*, 2:632.

68. Janowsky, D. S., and Risch, S. C. (1984): *Drug Dev. Res.*, 4:125–142.

69. Janowsky, D. S., Risch, S. C., Parker, D. C., Huey, L. Y., and Judd, L. L. (1982): In: Proceedings of the 13th Collegium Internationale Neuro-Psychopharmacologicum Congress, Jerusalem, Israel, June (Abstr.).

70. Jones, D., Kelwala, S., Bell, J., Dube, S., Jackson, E., and Sitaram, N. (1985): *Psychiatry Res.*, 14:99–110.

71. Kafka, M. S., van Kammen, D. P., Kleinman, J. E., Nurnberger, J. I., Jr., Siever, L. J., Uhde, T. W., and Polinsky, R. J. (1980): *Commun. Psychopharmacol.*, 4:477–486.

72. Kan, Y. W., and Dozy, A. M. (1978): *Proc. Natl. Acad. Sci. USA*, 75:5631–5635.

73. Kety, S. S. (1979): *Sci. Am.*, 241:202–218.

74. Kety, S. S. (1985): Presented at the IVth World Congress of Biological Psychiatry, Philadelphia, September 12.

75. Kidd, K. K., Egeland, J. L., Molthan, L., Pauls, D. L., Kruger, S. D., and Messner, K. H. (1984): *Am. J. Psychiatry*, 141:1042–1048.

76. Klerman, G. L., Lavori, P. W., Rice, J., Reich, T., Endicott, J., Andreasen, N. C., Keller, M. B., and Hirschfield, R. M. A. (1985): *Arch. Gen. Psychiatry*, 42:689–695.

77. Lalouel, J. M., and Morton, N. E. (1981): *Hum. Hered.*, 31:312–321.

78. Langer, S. Z., Galzin, A. M., Lee, C. R., and Schoemaker, H. (1986): In: *Antidepressants and Receptor Function*, edited by R. Porter, G. Bock, and S. Clark, pp. 3–29. John Wiley and Sons, London.

79. Leckman, J. F., Gershon, E. S., McGinniss, M. H., Targum, S. D., and Dibble, E. D. (1979): *Arch. Gen. Psychiatry*, 36:1435–1441.

80. Lenox, R. H., Hitzemann, R. J., Richelson, E., Kelsoe, J. R., Gillin, J. C., Janowsky, D. S., Brown, J. H., Risch, S. C., and Lumkin, B. (1985): *N. Engl. J. Med.*, 312:861–862.

81. Mellerup, E. T., Plenge, P., and Rosenberg, R. (1982): *Psychiatry Res.*, 7:221–227.

82. Mendels, J., and Frazer, A. (1973): *J. Psychiatr. Res.*, 10:9–18.

83. Mendlewicz, J. (1981): *Arch. Gen Psychiatry*, 38:719.

84. Mendlewicz, J., and Fleiss, J. L. (1974): *Biol. Psychiatry*, 9:261–294.

85. Mendlewicz, J., Fleiss, J. L., and Fieve, R. R. (1972): *JAMA*, 222:1624–1627.

86. Mendlewicz, J., Fleiss, J. L., and Fieve, R. R. (1975): In: *Genetics and Psychopathology*, edited by R. R. Fieve, D. Rosenthal, and H. Brill, pp. 219–232. Johns Hopkins University Press, Baltimore.

87. Mendlewicz, J., Linkowski, P., Guroff, J. J., and van Praag, H. M. (1979): *Arch. Gen. Psychiatry*, 36:1442–1449.

88. Mendlewicz, J., Linkowski, P., and Wilmette, J. (1980): *Br. J. Psychiatry*, 137:337–342.

89. Mendlewicz, J., and Rainer, J. D. (1977): *Nature*, 268:327–329.

90. Mesulam, M. M., Mufson, E. J., Levey, A. I., and Wainer, B. H. (1983): *J. Comp. Neurol.*, 214:170–197.

91. Mesulam, M. M., Mufson, E. J., Wainer, B. H., and Levey, A. I. (1983): *Neuroscience*, 10:1185–1201.

92. Morton, N. E., Crow, J. F., and Muller, H. J. (1956): *Proc. Natl. Acad. Sci. USA*, 42:855–863.

93. Morton, N. E., and Maclean, C. J. (1974): *Am. J. Hum. Genet.*, 26:489–503.

94. Nadi, N. S., Nurnberger, J. I., and Gershon, E. S. (1984): *N. Engl. J. Med.*, 311:225–230.

95. Nurnberger, J. I., Jr., and Gershon, E. S. (1984): In: *Neurobiology of Mood Disorders*, edited by R. Post and J. Ballenger, pp. 76–101. Williams and Wilkins, Baltimore.

96. Nurnberger, J. I., Jr., Pandey, G., Gershon, E. S., and Davis, J. M. (1983): *Psychiatry Res.*, 9:201–206.

97. Nurnberger, J. I., Jr., Sitaram, N., Gershon, E. S., and Gillin, J. C. (1983): *Biol. Psychiatry*, 18:116–117.

98. O'Farrell, P. H. (1975): *J. Biol. Chem.*, 250:4007–4021.

99. Pandey, G. N., Dorus, E., Schumacher, R., Gaviria, M., Val, E., and Davis, J. M. (1979): Presented at the 34th Annual Convention and Scientific Meeting, Society of Biological Psychiatry, Chicago, Palmer House, May 10–13.

100. Paul, S. M., Rehavi, M., Rice, K. C., Ittah, Y., and Skolnick, P. (1981): *Life Sci.*, 28:2753–2760.

101. Paul, S. M., Rehavi, M., Skolnick, P., and Goodwin, F. K. (1981): In: *Biological Markers in Psychiatry and Neurology*, edited by I. Hanin and E. Usdin, pp. 193–204. Pergamon Press, London.

102. Persico, M. G., Toniolo, D., Nobile, C., D'Urso, M., and Luzzatto, L. (1981): *Nature*, 294:778–780.

103. Price, R. A., Kidd, K. K., Pauls, D. L., Gershon, E. S., Prusoff, P. A., Weissman, M. M., and Goldin, L. R. (1985): *J. Psychiatr. Res.*, 19:533–546.

104. Propping, P., and Friedl, W. (1983): *Hum. Genet.*, 64:105–109.

105. Rehavi, M., Ittah, Y., Rice, K. C., Skolnick, P., Goodwin, F. K., and Paul, S. M. (1981): *Biochem. Biophys. Res. Commun.*, 99:954–959.

106. Reich, T. (1984): Remarks at meeting of Consortium on Childhood Depression, Boston, September 13.

107. Reich, T., Clayton, P. J., and Winokur, G. (1969): *Am. J. Psychiatry*, 125:1358–1369.

108. Reich, T., James, J. W., and Morris, C. A. (1972): *Ann. Hum. Genet.*, 36:163–184.

109. Rice, J., McGuffin, P., Goldin, L. R., Shaskan, E. G., and Gershon, E. S. (1984): *Am. J. Hum. Genet.*, 36:36–43.

110. Risch, N., and Baron, M. (1982): *Ann. Hum. Genet.*, 46:153–166.

111. Risch, S. C., and Janowsky, D. S. (1983): In: *Neurobiology of the Mood Disorders*, edited by B. M. Post and J. C. Ballenger, pp. 652–663. Williams and Wilkins, Baltimore.

112. Risch, S. C., Janowsky, D. S., Judd, L. L., and Huey, L. Y. (1982): *Psychopharmacol. Bull.*, 18:211–216.

113. Risch, S. C., Janowsky, D. S., Siever, L. J., Judd, L. L., Huey, L. Y., Beckman, K. A., Cohen, R. M., and Murphy, D. C. (1982): *Psychopharmacol. Bull.*, 18:21–25.

114. Risch, S. C., Kalin, N. H., and Janowsky, D. S. (1981): *J. Clin. Psychopharmacol.*, 1:186–192.

115. Risch, S. C., Kalin, N. H., Janowsky, D. S., Cohen, R. M., Pickar, D., and Murphy, D. L. (1983): *Science*, 222:75.

116. Robins, L. N., Helzer, J. E., Weissman, M. M., Orvaschel, H., Gruenberg, E., Burke, J. D., and Regier, D. A. (1984): *Arch. Gen. Psychiatry*, 41:949–958.

117. Rotter, J. I. (1981): *Am. J. Hum. Genet.*, 33:835–851.

118. Schulsinger, F., Kety, S. S., Rosenthal, D., and Wender, P. H. (1979): In: *Origin, Prevention, and Treatment of Affective Disorders*, edited by M. Schou and Stromgren, pp. 277–287. Academic Press, London.

119. Oxenstierna, G., Edman, G., Iselius, L., Oreland, L., Ross, S. B., and Sedvall, G. (1986): *J. Psychiatr. Res.*, 20:19–29.

120. Shaughnessy, R., Greene, S. C., Pandey, G. N., and Dorus, E. (1985): *Biol. Psychiatry*, 20:451–460.

121. Siever, L. J., Kafka, M. S., Targum, S., and Lake, C. R. (1984): *Psychiatry Res.*, 11:287–302.

122. Sitaram, N., and Gillin, J. C. (1980): *Biol. Psychiatry*, 15:925–955.

123. Sitaram, N., Gillin, J. C., Mendelson, W. B., and Wyatt, R. J. (1977): *Brain Res.,* 122:562–567.

124. Sitaram, N., Gillin, J. C., and Moore, A. M. (1978): *Arch. Gen. Psychiatry,* 35:1239–1242.

125. Sitaram, N., Jones, D., Dube, S., Bell, J., and Rivard, P. (1985): Presented at IVth World Congress of Biological Psychiatry, Philadelphia, September 13.

126. Sitaram, N., Nurnberger, J. I., Jr., Gershon, E. S., and Gillin, J. C. (1980): *Science,* 208:200–202.

127. Smeraldi, E., Negri, R., Heimbuch, R. C., and Kidd, K. K. (1981): *J. Affective Disord.,* 3:173–182.

128. Smeraldi, E., Negri, F., Melica, A. M., and Scorza-Smeraldi, R. (1978): *Tissue Antigens,* 12:270–274.

129. Solomon, M. I., and Hellon, C. P. (1980): *Arch. Gen. Psychiatry,* 37:511–513.

130. Strober, M. (1984): In: *An Update on Childhood Depression,* edited by E. Weller, American Psychiatric Press, Washington, DC.

131. Suarez, B. K., and Croughan, J. (1982): *Psychiatry Res.,* 7:19–27.

132. Suarez, B. K., and Reich, T. (1984): *Arch. Gen Psychiatry,* 41:22–27.

133. Suranyi-Cadotte, B. E., Wood, P. L., Vasavan Nair, N. P., and Schwartz, G. (1982): *Eur. J. Pharmacol.,* 85:357–358.

134. Takahaski, S. (1977): *Folia Psychiatr. Neurol. Jpn.,* 31:37–48.

135. Targum, S. D., Gershon, E. S., Van Eerdewegh, M., and Rogentine, N. (1979): *Biol. Psychiatry,* 14:615–636.

136. Tsuang, M. T., Faraone, S. V., and Fleming, J. A. (1985): *Br. J. Psychiatry,* 146:268–271.

137. Turner, W. J., and King, S. (1981): *Biol. Psychiatry,* 16:417–439.

138. Van Praag, H. M., and de Haan, S. (1979): *Psychiatry Res.,* 1:219–224.

139. Van Praag, H., and Korff, J. (1971): *Psychopharmacologia,* 19:148.

140. Van Riper, D. A., Absher, M. P., and Lenox, R. H. (1985): *J. Clin. Invest.,* 76:882–886.

141. von Knorring, A.-L., Cloninger, C. R., Bohman, M., and Sigvardsson, A. (1983): *Arch. Gen Psychiatry,* 40:943–950.

142. von Knorring, L., Perris, C., Oreland, L., Eisemann, M., Holmgren, S., and Perris, J. (1985): *Psychiatry Res.,* 15:271–279.

143. Waters, B., Thankar, J., and Lapierre, Y. (1983): *Neuropsychobiology,* 9:94–98.

144. Weissman, M. M., Gershon, E. S., Kidd, K. K., Prusoff, B. A., Leckman, J. F., Dibble, E., Hamovit, J., Thompson, W. D., Pauls, D. L., and Guroff, J. J. (1984): *Arch. Gen. Psychiatry,* 41:13–21.

145. Weitkamp, L. R., Stancer, H. C., Persad, E., Flood, C., and Guttormsen, S. (1981): *N. Engl. J. Med.,* 305:1301–1306.

146. Winokur, G. (1972): *Compr. Psychiatry,* 13:3–8.

147. Winokur, G., Clayton, P., and Reich, T. (1969): *Manic Depressive Illness.* CV Mosley Co., St. Louis.

148. Winokur, G., and Tanna, V. L. (1969): *Dis. Nerv. Syst.,* 30:87–94.

149. Wood, K., and Coppen, A. (1983): *J. Affective Disord.,* 5:253–258.

150. Wright, A. F., Loudon, J. B., Hampson, M. E., Crichton, D. N., and Steel, C. M. (1984): *Clin. Neuropharmacol. (Suppl. 1),* 7:194–195.

Psychopharmacology:
The Third Generation of Progress,
edited by Herbert Y. Meltzer.
Raven Press, New York © 1987.

CHAPTER **50**

Role of Noradrenergic Mechanisms in the Etiology of the Affective Disorders

Larry J. Siever

The original catecholamine hypothesis of the affective disorders (16,138) postulated that depression is characterized by a deficiency of functional norepinephrine, whereas mania is characterized by an excess of functional norepinephrine. More recent tempering and refinement of this hypothesis has placed more emphasis on possible disturbances in the regulation of the noradrenergic system's function as a phasic affective/arousal system (45). A dysregulated noradrenergic system may contribute importantly to the vegetative and anxiety-related symptoms of the affective disorders (9,142). The focus for investigation of this system has correspondingly begun to shift from measurements of basal concentrations of norepinephrine and its metabolites in body fluids to the assessment of changes in these indices over time and in response to environmental and pharmacologic manipulations.

These newer strategies permit the evaluation of the dynamic responsiveness of the noradrenergic system. Psychopharmacologic challenge studies with agents that enhance noradrenergic activity presynaptically can evaluate the net functional activity of the system, whereas biochemical/hormonal responses to challenge with specific agonists can provide an index of adrenergic receptor responsiveness. Receptor number and physiologic responsiveness may also be measured by *in vitro* studies of peripheral tissues using specific agonists or antagonists as ligands or physiologic probes. Thus, whereas earlier studies focused solely on presynaptic events of the noradrenergic system, e.g., avail-

ability of norepinephrine in the synaptic cleft, using indices of noradrenergic release/metabolism, more recent studies have also emphasized postsynaptic aspects of this system, e.g., responsiveness of adrenergic receptors on postsynaptic neurons (148).

There has been an increasing recognition of the interaction of the noradrenergic systems with other neurotransmitter systems such as the serotonergic, dopaminergic, and cholinergic systems. The noradrenergic system cannot, therefore, be considered in isolation from other neurotransmitter systems, and any role it plays in the pathophysiology of depression is almost certainly a part of a constellation of neurotransmitter abnormalities.

In this chapter, the function of the noradrenergic system in humans will be briefly discussed followed by a review of both more classical and newer challenge and receptor studies of the noradrenergic system in depression. These will be discussed with a view toward understanding what role a dynamic dysfunction of the noradrenergic system might play in the pathophysiology of depression.

FUNCTION OF THE NORADRENERGIC SYSTEM IN HUMANS

The noradrenergic system seems to serve a global modulatory function in enhancing arousal and orientation to novel and/or potentially threatening stimuli (7,45,120). The locus ceruleus, the major site of noradrenergic neuronal cell bodies, thus fires in a phasic manner, signaling shifts in global states in response to specific environmental stimuli. It serves an executive function mediating parallel changes in peripheral sympathetic activity (34,40,63) as well as modulating cortical information processing by enhancement of the signal-to-noise ratio of other neuronal systems. Basal firing of postsynaptic neurons may be depressed by norepinephrine while other specifically excitatory or inhibitory signals to these postsynaptic neurons are augmented (7,45,167). In this way, the signal responses to significant or unanticipated incoming stimuli are highlighted, facilitating the appropriate processing and organization of responses to the stimuli. The locus ceruleus is relatively quiescent during vegetative functions such as feeding, grooming, and sleep when orientation to external stimuli is reduced, and increases markedly when novel stimuli are presented (7). Thus, it appears that the locus ceruleus integrates information from incoming sensory stimuli and from internal physiologic processes to appropriately modulate sympathetic arousal and vigilance to the environment (63), a process consistent with the affective registration of internal and external events.

Thus the noradrenergic system appears to function as a phasic affective arousal system that might plausibly play a role in the prominent disturbances of vegetative function associated with the affective and anxiety disorders. Patients with affective disorders may exhibit a dysphoric hyperarousal that appears dissociated from active, goal-directed behavior, as well as anergic and vegetative symptoms. It is conceivable that inappropriate increases in a poorly modulated noradrenergic system might contribute to the anxiety and dysphoria associated with the affective disorders. Conversely, decreases in noradrenergic activity, possibly secondary to depletion of a dysregulated noradrenergic system, could easily be seen as mediating anergic and vegetative symptoms (142). Although these relationships are far from established, our current understanding of the function of the noradrenergic system derived from these preclinical studies provides a useful heuristic context for the clinical studies of noradrenergic function in affective disorders described below.

STUDIES OF NOREPINEPHRINE AND ITS METABOLITES IN BIOLOGIC FLUIDS

There has been an increasing attention to the methodology and interpretation of metabolic studies in the past decade based on preclinical data that have increased our understanding of the interconversion of norepinephrine metabolites and the estimation of central and peripheral contributions to these measures (69,94,118).

Urinary Noradrenergic Metabolites

The earliest studies designed to test the catecholamine hypotheses of the affective disorders measured norepinephrine and its metabolites in 24-hr urine collections. However, a number of methodologic issues in metabolic studies highlighted in the last decade have significantly influenced the interpretation of such studies. First, the proportion of the most frequently measured noradrenergic metabolite, 3-methoxy-4-hydroxyphenylglycol (MHPG), that derives from the brain may be considerably lower than originally estimated, as MHPG from the brain may be further metabolized in the periphery to vanillylmandelic acid (VMA) (69). However, several studies suggest that peripheral and central noradrenergic activity may change in concert under a variety of circumstances (34,40,63). Thus, an index of total body noradrenergic activity may be a physiologically appropriate measure to assess possible dysfunction of this system in depression, but may be limited in value under pathological circumstances where central and peripheral activity are dissociated as, for example, in orthostatic hypotension or pheochromocytoma (69). Second, the assumption implicit in the early metabolite studies that concentrations of noradrenergic metabolites parallel the activity of noradrenergic neurons by reflecting the release of norepinephrine may not always be warranted. The concentration of norepinephrine and/or its metabolites also depends on the total volume of distribution and the clearance of these substances by rates of reuptake into noradrenergic neurons, metabolism, and excretion (118). These constituents of norepinephrine clearance may vary widely between individuals and thus conceivably could be a substantial source of variation between subject populations (118). Therefore, studies utilizing small amounts of labeled norepinephrine infused into the bloodstream allow calculation of clearance and can thus be helpful in quantifying this possible source of variance (45). Thirdly, clinical and demographic variables such as gender, age, diet, tobacco use, caffeine intake, medication status, time of day, state of activity, and position may influence concentrations of norepinephrine and its metabolites in bodily fluids and thus must be carefully controlled in clinical studies (117).

Most studies over the past decade, including those attempting to control for these potentially artifactual variables, have tended to support earlier studies suggesting decreased 24-hr urinary excretion of MHPG in depressed patients, particularly bipolar depressed patients, compared to controls, although discrepant results have been reported (121). Longitudinal studies of bipolar patients studied in both the manic and the depressed state have continued to suggest an increased MHPG excretion in the manic compared to the depressed state (115,118). Studies of unipolar patients have yielded more variable results, with most studies explicitly comparing unipolar and bipolar patients indicating increased urinary MHPG excretion in the unipolar patients compared to bipolar patients (118,139). Low values of urinary MHPG in acutely depressed patients have been reported to approach normal values following clinical recovery in the same patient (113). Thus, urinary MHPG concentrations appear to be partially state dependent in affective disorder patients, with relatively low concentrations particularly identified in acutely depressed bipolar patients.

Recently, however, a multicenter collaborative study (70) reported no difference in urinary MHPG excretion in depressed patients (including both unipolars and bipolars) compared to controls, but did find increased urinary excretion of the norepinephrine metabolites, VMA and normetaphrine. These results might suggest increases in peripheral and perhaps central noradrenergic activity in some forms of depression. It is difficult to compare the collaborative study with early studies reported in the literature as assay techniques, and patient populations may have changed considerably. Patients studied more recently in academic settings may more likely be refractory to classical antidepressant treatments than in prior decades when these medications were less widely utilized. Some evidence suggests that patients who are relatively refractory to antidepressant treatment may have higher urinary excretion of MHPG (137). Thus, recent studies may be more likely to suggest high concentrations of noradrenergic metabolites in depression than earlier studies, which often focused primarily on treatment-responsive bipolar depressed patients.

These results cumulatively suggest that average presynaptic noradrenergic activity may be decreased in some forms of bipolar depression and increased in mania and some forms of unipolar depression, whereas changes in MHPG excretion in individual patients may be associated clinical state changes. However, limitations of measurements of urinary metabolite excretion for delineating the dynamics of the noradrenergic system have stimulated the development of additional approaches to assess noradrenergic activity in the affective disorders.

Plasma Norepinephrine Concentrations

In the last decade, an attempt has been made to characterize conveniently obtained plasma indices of noradrenergic activity in depressed patients and controls. Concentrations of plasma norepinephrine reflect the activity of the sympathetic nervous system under a variety of conditions, including standing, immersion of the hands into cold water, and mental arithmetic (77). Sympathetic activity depends on a variety of other neurotransmitter systems, including the serotonergic system and cholinergic system, so that alterations in plasma norepinephrine need not necessarily reflect a primary disturbance in central noradrenergic neurons. However, evidence that peripheral sympathetic and central noradrenergic activity may be regulated in parallel fashion (34,40,63) has rekindled interest in plasma norepinephrine as a measure of noradrenergic function in humans.

The increased understanding of central regulation of sympathetic outflow has prompted further investigation of earlier findings that plasma catecholamine was elevated in depressed patients compared to normals (169). Several studies in the last decade using radioenzymatic and radioactive tracer assay techniques have replicated the finding of elevated plasma norepinephrine concentrations in patients with major depressive disorder (42,76,87,125). This elevation seems partially due to increased norepinephrine release (42). Depressed patients with melancholia (by history or concurrently) have higher lying and supine plasma norepinephrine concentrations than other depressed or dysthmic patients, and bipolar melancholics have lower values than unipolar melancholics (125). Unipolar dexamethasone nonsuppressors have significantly higher lying plasma norepinephrine concentrations than dexamethasone suppressors (125). In another study, bipolar depressive patients had lower supine norepinephrine levels than either unipolar

depressed patients or normal controls (129). The variance in plasma norepinephrine has also been reported to be greater in depressed patients than in normal controls, in the absence of differences between the means (151). Although these studies are partially discrepant, they suggest that sympathetic nervous system activity may be abnormal in many depressed patients in heterogeneous fashion, with a significant subgroup, particularly unipolar melancholic patients with dexamethasone nonsuppression, showing hyperactivity.

Plasma MHPG Concentrations

Plasma MHPG is derived from the release of norepinephrine from peripheral and central noradrenergic neurons. A number of studies suggest that plasma MHPG concentrations parallel concentrations in brain and CSF in animals and humans (82). This measure has the advantage of allowing more frequent sampling intervals than urinary measures, permitting continuous monitoring of plasma concentrations, and is more convenient and comfortable for the patient to obtain than CSF measures. It may be measured as the free or unconjugated form or as the total of conjugated and unconjugated forms. It is relatively stable for a particular individual (87), has a circadian rhythm (38), and appears to have a genetic component (65,82). Measurements of plasma MHPG may be particularly useful for longitudinal, psychopharmacologic challenge, and circadian studies requiring multiple, frequent samples. However, when central and peripheral noradrenergic activities are dissociated, plasma MHPG concentrations may be difficult to interpret (69). Under other circumstances, its relative stability and partially central origin make it an appealing and convenient measure to assess noradrenergic activity in humans.

Concentrations of plasma-free MHPG from morning blood samples have not been found to be significantly different between depressed patients and controls (25,66, 148,161), although the plasma MHPG concentrations may tend to be higher in depressed patients than controls (66,148). The variance of free plasma MHPG in a group of depressed patients was reported to be greater than that of controls, suggesting the possibility of subgroups of patients with both high and low values (148). Plasma MHPG is higher in affective disorder patients in the manic phase of their illness than in these same patients in the depressed state or than in normal controls (54,65). Total plasma MHPG sampled over 24 hr has a higher average value in the morning in depressed patients compared to controls, as well as circadian rhythm disturbances described later in this chapter (38,55). The results of studies of plasma MHPG parallel those of other studies of noradrenergic metabolites in depression, suggesting increased variance in the depressed group, with high values often observed in manic and some unipolar patients, whereas low values are more frequent in bipolar patients.

CSF Norepinephrine Concentrations

CSF norepinephrine has attracted recent interest as a possibly more valid measure of central noradrenergic activity than plasma or urinary measures. Patients with high plasma norepinephrine concentrations from a pheochromocytoma do not show corresponding increases in CSF concentrations, suggesting that CSF norepinephrine receives little contribution from plasma norepinephrine (172). In patients with cerebral vasospasm, concentrations of CSF norepinephrine may be high, raising the possibility that a substantial proportion of CSF norepinephrine may partially derive from arterial release rather than brain release (172). Furthermore, gradient studies suggest a contribution to CSF norepinephrine from spinal cord noradrenergic neurons. However, the relative proportions of the various sources of CSF norepinephrine have not been established. Although how closely CSF norepinephrine reflects brain noradrenergic activity remains unclear, CSF norepinephrine derives from CNS noradrenergic neurons, and thus lends itself as a tool to understand central noradrenergic activity in depression.

Depressed patients have been reported to have significantly increased CSF norepinephrine in comparison to normal controls but not to neurologic controls (115). CSF norepinephrine concentrations after probenecid correlate highly with baseline (nonprobenecid) CSF norepinephrine concentrations and are also elevated in manic compared to depressed patients. CSF norepinephrine concentrations do not seem related to activity but have been associated with anxiety, atypical presentation, and increased frequency and duration of hospitalization in depressed patients (115). On the other hand, another study found no difference between CSF norepinephrine concentrations in depressed patients and controls, in contrast to the finding that CSF epinephrine was decreased in depressed patients in the same study (30). Lower concentrations of CSF norepinephrine have also been observed in depressed patients, particularly bipolar patients, compared to controls (128). In summary, evidence does not consistently suggest significant differences in CSF norepinephrine between depressed patients and controls, but does suggest a high degree of variability or heterogeneity of values of CSF norepinephrine among depressed patients. Increased CSF norepinephrine may be associated with mania and atypical depression, whereas decreased CSF norepinephrine may be associated with some forms of bipolar depression.

CSF MHPG Concentrations

As MHPG is the major metabolite of brain norepinephrine, CSF MHPG has been evaluated in depressed patients and controls as a possible reflection of brain noradrenergic activity. CSF MHPG also receives a contribution from spinal cord, although the lumbar contribution may derive from terminals extending from brain neuronal cell bodies (115). CSF MHPG will also vary as a function of concentrations of plasma MHPG (69). However, simultaneous determinations of CSF and plasma MHPG may permit correction for the peripheral contribution to CSF MHPG (69).

Although most studies have found no difference in CSF MHPG concentrations between depressed patients and controls, CSF MHPG has been reported to be lower in some populations of depressed patients than controls (115).

CSF MHPG has also been demonstrated to be higher in manics than in comparable controls, but not consistently (68,115). Thus, the variability of values of CSF MHPG in affective disorder patients is similar to that found for other measures of noradrenergic metabolite in biologic fluids, but does suggest increases associated with agitation and mania and decreases in some forms of depression.

Relationship Between Noradrenergic Metabolites and Indices of Hypothalamic-Pituitary-Adrenal Activity

Concurrent measurements of indices of noradrenergic activity and indices of hypothalamic-pituitary-adrenal (HPA) activity have been utilized to better understand the relationship between HPA hyperactivity and the function of the noradrenergic system in depression. Animal evidence suggests that the noradrenergic system plays both an inhibitory and an excitatory role in the regulation of adrenal activity both through the HPA axis and through direct sympathetic innervation of the adrenal glands (8,109). Inhibitory influences of the noradrenergic system on stress-induced increases in HPA activity mediated by x-adrenergic receptors have been documented, as have excitatory influences at both the hypothalamus and the pituitary (8). The latter are mediated by β_2-adrenergic and α_1-adrenergic receptors at the pituitary (8). Corticotropin-releasing factor may in turn influence noradrenergic neuronal firing and receptor responsiveness (162). The relationship between the noradrenergic system and the HPA axis seems to depend both on the basal activity of the HPA axis and the relative responsiveness of different adrenergic receptor subtypes, both of which may vary in different clinical conditions.

Several studies suggest differences in the relationship of noradrenergic activity and cortisol secretion in normal subjects compared to depressed patients. In one study, a negative correlation between urinary free cortisol (UFC) and MHPG excretion was observed in normal subjects, whereas a positive correlation between these two variables was observed in depressed subjects (124). Other studies of depressed patients have found positive correlations between concentrations of baseline or postdexamethasone plasma MHPG and postdexamethasone serum cortisol concentrations (64,126) or between plasma norepinephrine concentrations and serum cortisol concentrations (125). An association between low urinary MHPG excretion and high pre- and postdexamethasone cortisol concentrations, however, has also been reported (37). These studies, in general, suggest an association of increased noradrenergic activity, at least in the sympathetic nervous system, and cortisol hypersecretion in depression that might be mediated via the HPA axis or sympathetic innervation. These studies, in conjunction with the results of studies of cortisol responses to adrenergic challenges, which suggest a defective central adrenergic inhibition of HPA activity, implicate a predominance of excitatory noradrenergic influences over inhibitory influences on adrenal cortisol secretion in depressed patients.

Studies of Postmortem Brain

Concentrations of norepinephrine and its metabolites as well as synthetic and metabolic enzymes affecting noradrenergic activity and radioligand binding to specific nor-adrenergic receptor subtypes can be measured in postmortem brains. These parameters have been usually measured in brains of suicides rather than in specifically diagnosed depressed patients. In general, no differences in brain norepinephrine or MHPG concentrations have been found between suicide (14,35,37,92,114) or depressed patients and controls (35), although recently decreases in brain norepinephrine concentrations associated with increases in β-adrenergic receptor binding have been reported (92). At this point, data from postmortem studies in specifically depressed patients are sparse, but such studies represent an avenue of investigation requiring further exploration.

Conclusions Regarding Noradrenergic Metabolite Studies

Current available evidence does not suggest uniform increases or decreases in norepinephrine or its metabolites in biologic fluids of depressed patients and controls. However, results of studies to date are consistent with some forms of bipolar depression being associated with decreased noradrenergic release/metabolism, and some forms of unipolar depression, as well as mania, being associated with increased noradrenergic release/metabolism (139,148). In the case of unipolar depression, increased noradrenergic output may be associated with reduced postsynaptic and possibly presynaptic adrenergic receptor responsiveness (see next section) (148). The heterogeneity of depressive disorders with respect to noradrenergic activity may thus account for the increased variance of these metabolites sometimes observed in depressed patients. The state-dependence of noradrenergic metabolite concentrations (113,116) raises the possibility that the increased variance in noradrenergic metabolite concentrations in depression may also reflect a less tightly buffered or dysregulated noradrenergic system (142).

STUDIES REFLECTING ADRENERGIC RECEPTOR RESPONSIVENESS

β-Adrenergic Receptors in Peripheral Tissues

In an attempt to characterize the sensitivity of adrenergic receptors, receptor number has been evaluated directly in peripheral tissues. β-Adrenergic receptor number can be evaluated directly in peripheral tissues such as the lymphocyte, leukocyte, or fibroblast by the measurement of binding of specific radiolabeled antagonists to the β-adrenergic receptor. A reduced number of β-adrenergic receptors in human lymphocytes has been found in depressed patients compared to controls (43). However, studies are discrepant with reports of increase (59) and no difference (32,91,173) in β-adrenergic receptor binding in the lymphocytes of depressed patients compared to controls and decreases with antidepressant treatment (59). Although studies have been somewhat inconsistent, there is thus increasing evidence for reduced β-adrenergic sensitivity in peripheral tissues of depressed patients. The extent to which this represents

down-regulation secondary to increased concentrations of circulating norepinephrine has yet to be clarified. These results contrast with the preliminary reports of increases in β-adrenergic receptor binding in postmortem studies of suicide patients (92,170).

Measures of in vitro responsiveness of β-adrenergic receptors in peripheral tissues to exogenous norepinephrine or isoproterenol, a β-adrenergic agonist, have the advantage of assessing the receptor's functional responsiveness. These compounds generate an increase in cyclic-adenosine-3,5-monophosphate (cyclic AMP) due to coupling of the β-adrenergic receptor (as well as to other as yet undefined adrenergic receptors in the case of norepinephrine) to adenylate cyclase via a GTP-coupled stimulatory protein to adenylate cyclase. Thus, the magnitude of the cyclic AMP response to agonist provides an index of the responsiveness of the receptor. There is evidence for decreased in vitro responses to isoproterenol concentrations of 10^{-4} M and 10^{-5} M (43) in the lymphocytes of depressed patients compared to controls. Decreased cyclic AMP responses to 10^{-5} M isoproterenol in depressed patients compared to controls, attributable to a subgroup of the depressed patients with psychomotor agitation, have been observed despite a lack of difference in receptor number or affinity between groups. Receptor number was correlated with isoproterenol-induced cyclic AMP stimulation in this study (91). No difference in the adenylate cyclase response to isoproterenol, however, was observed between alprazolam responders and non-responders (101). Studies of the functional responsiveness of β-adrenergic receptors parallel, but are more consistent than, ligand binding studies in suggesting reduced responsiveness of this receptor on the lymphocyte.

Decreased cyclic AMP responses to 10^{-4} M isoproterenol were also reported in the leukocyte (111). Decreased maximal binding of transformed lymphocytes has been found in manic-depressive patients and their ill relatives in three of five families of these patients, raising the possibility of a genetic component to the reduced binding (168). Tissue cultures of skin fibroblasts derived from skin biopsies in euthymic bipolar patients and their relatives as well as normal controls have been assayed for cyclic AMP responses to isoproterenol stimulation (11). No significant differences were observed between any of these groups. Therefore, the generalizability of the finding of reduced β-adrenergic sensitivity in the lymphocyte to other tissues, the extent to which the binding alterations reflect changes in ambient conditions, as well as the state-dependence and genetics of β-adrenergic sensitivity all remain to be clarified. The applicability of these studies to the CNS β-adrenergic receptors as yet remains unclear, especially in light of the increased β-adrenergic receptor number reported to be associated with suicide (92,170).

α-Adrenergic Receptors in Peripheral Tissues

α_2-Adrenergic receptors located on platelet membranes mediate responses to circulating epinephrine and norepinephrine. The platelet, therefore, affords a convenient peripheral tissue for the evaluation of α_2-adrenergic receptor sensitivity. The α_2-adrenergic receptor on the platelet is pharmacologically similar to α_2-adrenergic receptors found in the brain, so that the measurement of α_2-adrenergic receptors on the platelet might conceivably have implications for the assessment of central α_2-adrenergic receptor function.

The number of α_2-adrenergic receptors as measured by radiolabeled agonists such as clonidine, which preferentially label high-affinity sites (18), has been reported to be increased in depressed patients compared to controls (39,47). However, the binding to platelets of yohimbine or rauwolscine, α_2-adrenergic antagonists that label a larger pool of α_2-adrenergic receptors but may not label all of the high-affinity sites (18), has consistently not been different between depressed patients and controls (20,36,84,114,157). Dihydroergocryptine (DHE) is an α_2-adrenergic antagonist, which labels more sites than yohimbine, including high-affinity α_2-adrenergic and other uncharacterized sites. Tritiated DHE also binds to more sites in the platelets of depressed patients than controls in some (59,146), but not all, studies (166). An inverse correlation between plasma norepinephrine concentrations and platelet α_2-adrenergic receptor binding has been reported (130), but not consistently (146).

Because ligand binding studies cannot assess the functional activity of adrenergic receptors, physiologic responsiveness of these receptors has been measured. The physiologic responsiveness of the platelet α_2-adrenergic receptor as measured by inhibition of prostaglandin E_1 (PGE_1)-stimulated cyclic AMP production was initially not found to be different between depressed patients and controls (103,163), whereas more recent studies using submaximal doses of norepinephrine demonstrated a significant lower stimulatory response to PGE_1 or PGD_2 and inhibitory response to norepinephrine or epinephrine in depressed patients compared to controls (100,101,146). Other studies have found normal cyclic AMP responses to PGE_1 stimulation or norepinephrine inhibition (84) or increased platelet aggregation in response to epinephrine (46). The inhibitory response to norepinephrine did not correlate with either receptor number or concentrations of circulating norepinephrine in the depressed patients in one study (146), whereas in another study both stimulatory and inhibitory responses to agonist were inversely correlated with urinary catecholamine concentrations (102). Receptor number may thus not consistently parallel receptor responsiveness in pathologic situations and might conceivably be increased as a compensatory response to post-receptor coupling defects. Decreases in α_2-adrenergic receptor responsiveness might thus reflect such a post-receptor abnormality or, alternatively, a desensitized high-affinity site, secondary to increased circulating catecholamines (102,146). As α_2-adrenergic receptors may be regulated differently in the brain and platelet (58), it is not clear how these results may be extrapolated to central α_2-adrenergic receptors.

Psychopharmacologic Challenge Strategies to Assess Adrenergic Receptor Responsiveness

Responses to acute administration of pharmacologic agents known to increase noradrenergic activity at postsynaptic receptor sites have been utilized to assess the functional activity of the noradrenergic system in depression. Challenges with specific receptor agonists also permit an indirect evaluation of central adrenergic receptor responsiveness in depression. In the last 10 years, such studies have employed increasingly selective challenge agents for such assessments.

Growth Hormone Responses

Growth hormone (GH) increases in response to a variety of challenges that enhance noradrenergic activity, including dextroamphetamine (79), methyl-amphetamine (12,121), L-dopa (95), insulin-induced hypoglycemia (133), desipramine (76,77), and clonidine (78). The GH response to all of these agents may be antagonized by α-adrenergic antagonists, more specifically in most cases by α_2-adrenergic antagonists (141,145), suggesting that the α_2-adrenergic receptor may be the common mediator of the GH responses to these challenges. Studies utilizing less selective noradrenergic agents such as the amphetamine derivatives have suggested a reduced GH response to their administration in acute and/or depressed patients compared to normal or psychiatric controls in some studies (4,80), but not others (26,28,57,107,108). Similarly, the GH response to L-dopa in depressed patients initially appeared to be reduced (131,133), but this finding was not consistently replicated (53,88). The GH response to insulin-induced hypoglycemia, which also depends on the degree of hypoglycemia as well as on α-adrenergic receptor and perhaps serotonergic receptor responsiveness (13), was reported to be diminished in earlier studies (53,132) but not in the large-scale and more recent NIMH collaborative study (69). However, these studies are difficult to interpret due to the substantial proportion of depressed patients with an inadequate hypoglycemic response to insulin (71,106). Bipolar patients may evidence an enhanced GH response to both L-dopa (51) and insulin-induced hypoglycemia (132) in the depressed phase and reduced responses in the manic phase (22,48). Several studies have suggested that the GH response to insulin remains blunted in depressed patients following antidepressant treatment (21,53) and in medication-free remitted unipolar patients (67). These studies with relatively less selective challenges cumulatively raise the possibility that α-adrenergic receptors are less responsive in depressed patients, particularly unipolar patients, than in controls, but variability in the GH response to these less selective agents is relatively great. They hint at the possibility of an increased α-adrenergic receptor responsiveness in bipolar depressed patients and the persistence of decreased α-adrenergic receptor responsiveness in remitted unipolar depressed patients.

Desipramine selectively blocks the reuptake of norepinephrine and stimulates GH by an α_2-adrenergic facilitatory effect (75). The GH response to desipramine has been reported to be reduced in depressed patients compared to controls in most studies, although its specificity for endogenous depression remains controversial (6,19,72,74,98). These results are consistent with decreased α_2-adrenergic receptor responsiveness and/or enhanced α-adrenergic receptor responsiveness.

The GH response to the most selective α-adrenergic challenge, clonidine, a specific α_2-adrenergic agonist, has been consistently demonstrated to be reduced in depressed patients, particularly endogenously depressed patients, compared to matched normal controls, reactive depressive patients, and schizophrenic patients (3,24,29,85,96,155). Among depressed patients, the GH response to clonidine does not correlate with such possible artifacts as age, sex, weight loss, or number of days since medication discontinuation, but does correlate with endogenicity (27). The blunted GH response is unaltered by long-term antidepressant treatment with desipramine (23,50) or clorgyline (150) and has been reported to be blunted in preliminary studies of unmedicated remitted depressed patients (48,61,140). These results are consistent with the possibility that reduced α_2-adrenergic receptor responsiveness represents a state-independent or trait characteristic of many depressed patients.

Cortisol Responses

Depressed patients demonstrate abnormal cortisol responses to noradrenergic challenges compared to normal or other psychiatric controls. Attenuated increases in cortisol in response to intravenous methylamphetamine have been observed in acute compared to remitted depressed patients (28) and endogenous compared to reactive depressives (26). Actual decreases in plasma cortisol concentrations in response to dextroamphetamine were reported in depressed patients in comparison to increases reported in controls in some studies (134,135), but this finding was not replicated in another study of acute depressed patients (44) or of remitted bipolar patients (107). Relatively decreased cortisol responses to amphetamine have also been observed in depressed outpatients (159). The distribution of cortisol responses to amphetamine in depressed patients may in fact be bimodal (56). As the effects of norepinephrine on the HPA axis are complex and may include α_1-adrenergic and β-adrenergic excitatory influences as well as α_2-adrenergic inhibitory effects (74,121), these studies are difficult to interpret, but are partially consistent with a reduced response to amphetamine in depressed patients.

Plasma cortisol does not change in response to clonidine, the α_2-adrenergic agonist, in normal subjects (78,153), but does significantly decrease in depressed patients with hypercortisolemia (153), consistent with the possibility that α_2-adrenergically mediated inhibitory effects may only be important when baseline cortisol concentrations are elevated. Baseline cortisol concentrations are inversely correlated with plasma MHPG responses to clonidine, raising the possibility that the hypercortisolemia of depression may in part be related to decreased α_2-adrenergic receptor responsiveness and that the exogenously administered clonidine may override this subsensitivity, reducing elevated basal cortisol concentrations (153). Parallel results have been reported in which the cortisol increase in response to yohimbine was greater in depressed patients than controls, also consistent with the possibility of decreased α_2-adrenergic receptor responsiveness in depression (119). As α_2-adrenergic agonists have inhibitory effects on stimulated cortisol secretion, these results suggest reduced central noradrenergic inhibitory constraints on cortisol secretion. Decreased central

inhibition may contribute to unopposed excitatory noradrenergic influences on cortisol release, accounting for the correlations between peripheral noradrenergic indices and cortisol concentrations described previously (64,125).

Noradrenergic Metabolite and Other Responses

Plasma MHPG and norepinephrine responses have been measured in response to the α_2-adrenergic agonist, clonidine. The plasma MHPG response to clonidine has been reported to be decreased in response to intravenous (152), although not to oral (24), clonidine, raising the possibility that α_2-adrenergic receptors inhibitory to noradrenergic firing/release are reduced in responsiveness in depression. Decreased plasma norepinephrine responses to clonidine have also been reported in depressed patients compared to controls (96). Heart rate (152), but not blood pressure (24,29,152), decrements in response to clonidine have been reported to be reduced in depressed patients compared to controls.

Behavioral Responses

Euphoria and activation frequently are associated with amphetamine administration in normal subjects and depressed patients (145). Remitted bipolar patients with low basal plasma MHPG concentrations have increased excitation responses to amphetamine as compared to those patients with high basal plasma MHPG responses, an association opposite in direction to the expected positive correlation observed in normal subjects (107). These results raise the possibility that abnormalities in adrenergic receptor responsiveness (e.g., decreased responsiveness in patients with high plasma MHPG concentrations) may alter the expected normal relationship between basal plasma MHPG and the behavioral response to amphetamine.

Clonidine reduces anxiety, particularly in anxious bipolar patients (148), whereas sedation responses to clonidine may be decreased (62) or unchanged (29) in depressed patients compared with controls.

General Conclusions Regarding Challenge Studies

The studies described, although discrepant in many specifics, present a substantial body of evidence that α_2-adrenergic receptor responsiveness is reduced in at least a subpopulation of depressed patients. Results have been relatively more consistent for the more easily interpretable paradigms using selective agonists such as clonidine than for challenges with effects on multiple neurotransmitter systems such as amphetamine and its derivatives, or insulin-induced hypoglycemia. The relatively more consistent blunting of GH responses to clonidine than to amphetamine in the same patients (143) suggests that responses to a more selective agent might be expected to yield clearer differences between depressed patients and controls.

The GH response to adrenergic challenges has been most consistently decreased of all response parameters in studies of depressed patients. Although GH release is modulated by multiple neurotransmitter receptors, postsynaptic α_2-adrenergic receptors apparently mediate the major excitatory influence of norepinephrine on GH release and are the only specific receptor system activated by all these diverse challenges. Thus, these results are consistent with the hypothesis that α_2-adrenergic receptors are less responsive in depressed patients than in controls. However, the role of variables distal to aminergic receptors in the hypothalamus, such as availability for release of growth hormone-releasing factor (GRF), somatostatin, or GH itself, must be considered. Relative depletion of GH at the level of the pituitary cannot easily account for these findings in the face of the normal GH responses to other challenges stimulating GH release that are not mediated by α_2-adrenergic receptors, such as apomorphine or GRF, in depressed patients (2,33,88,110). Reductions in CSF somatostatin in depressed patients (127), argue against excessive somatostatin inhibitory influences contributing to blunted GH responses.

Reduced α_2-adrenergic receptor responsiveness might result from an intrinsic defect in the α_2-adrenergic binding site, alterations in its coupling to second messenger effectors such as adenylate cyclase, or impairment in its regulation (142,146). The first possibility is rendered unlikely by the inconsistent results of platelet binding studies discussed previously, although these studies are possibly consistent with a coupling defect distal to the α_2-adrenergic receptor (101,146). Persistent down-regulation of the α_2-adrenergic receptor secondary to episodically increased noradrenergic release interacting with a more generalized alteration in the plasticity of receptor availability might be more consistent with reports implicating altered receptor responsiveness in other neuronal systems, such as the serotonergic (60,97,147) and cholinergic (123,156) systems.

Several of these studies also hint that a subgroup of bipolar depressed patients may evidence increased GH responses to clonidine. It is intriguing to speculate that increased adrenergic receptor responsiveness associated with decreased noradrenergic availability might contribute to the susceptibility of such patients to switch to mania (17,154). Such a model is also consistent with the observed decreases in indices of noradrenergic release/metabolism in bipolar depressed patients. An increased GH response to clonidine in preclinical studies is associated with pharmacologic manipulations decreasing presynaptic norepinephrine activity and inducing supersensitivity of α_2-adrenergic receptors (41). Thus, an augmented GH response may reflect an increased capacity for up-regulation of adrenergic receptors in the face of decreased norepinephrine availability that might distinguish bipolar from unipolar patients. This possibility invites further investigation.

The studies of cortisol responses to adrenergic challenges, although more difficult to interpret, tend to support a contribution of reduced α_2-adrenergic receptor responsiveness to the hypercortisolemia of depression, whether via a dampened inhibitory role for norepinephrine at postsynaptic α-adrenergic sites or a disinhibited presynaptic release of norepinephrine on other excitatory adrenergic postsynaptic receptors. Alterations in other neurotransmitter systems stimulating the HPA axis as well as abnormalities distal to the hypothalamus, e.g., in pituitary responsiveness to CRF

or adrenal responsiveness to ACTH, may play a role in the abnormal cortisol responses to adrenergic challenges.

Studies of biochemical and physiologic responses to these agents, such as the plasma MHPG response to clonidine, deserve further exploration. Some studies suggest that α_2-adrenergic receptors inhibitory to noradrenergic firing/release that may be located presynaptically may also be reduced in their responsiveness in depressed patients. Decreased responsiveness of inhibitory presynaptic receptors may have implications for the control of norepinephrine release under stimulated conditions, contributing to disinhibition of noradrenergic output and the observed variability in basal, time-dependent, and stimulus-dependent noradrenergic activity (142). Increased plasma MHPG concentrations are modestly correlated with blunted GH responses to clonidine (155), supporting such an association between reduced receptor responsiveness and increased noradrenergic output, particularly in unipolar patients (148). Such an association might reflect receptor down-regulation secondary to increased noradrenergic release, also suggested by some of the platelet α_2-adrenergic receptor studies (101,102,130), as well as reduced α_2-adrenergically mediated inhibitory constraints on noradrenergic release (142).

These studies have not yet yielded results suggesting that any of these agents will be useful as a diagnostic test, although this possibility cannot be ruled out. However, the blunted GH response to clonidine has also been reported in preliminary studies of obsessive-compulsive patients (144) and panic disorder/agoraphobic patients (149), suggesting that this finding may extend beyond the boundaries of classically defined affective disorder. Nevertheless, blunted GH responses to clonidine are not associated with schizophrenia (78,96), reactive depression (27,29,96), or stressful medical illness (81). These studies suggest that the blunted GH response to clonidine is not a nonspecific response to stress, and may reflect a noradrenergic abnormality common to both the anxiety and affective disorders, overlapping disorders with common phenomenologic, familial, biologic, and treatment-response features (83,104,149).

It remains to be determined whether the altered responses to adrenergic challenges observed in the acute state of depression may also be found in remitted depressed patients. Preliminary studies indicate that this may be the case (140,148). These studies are compatible with the possibility that the blunted GH responses to clonidine may be a correlate of a susceptibility to depressive illness that may, under circumstances of stress, contribute to the overt dysregulation of noradrenergic release/metabolism apparent in acute depression (142).

Studies of Melatonin

The monitoring of nighttime melatonin by urinary collection of melatonin metabolites or by serial sampling of plasma melatonin concentrations permits an indirect monitor of postsynaptic noradrenergic activity. Melatonin release is stimulated by noradrenergic neurons in the sympathetic superior cervical ganglion via postsynaptic β-adrenergic receptors in the pineal gland. Thus, measures reflecting total melatonin secretion throughout the night provide an index of net noradrenergic activity mediated by β-adrenergic receptors in the pineal system. Melatonin secretion as reflected in the excretion of 6-hydroxymelatonin is reduced in depressed patients comparably to controls (10,14,31, 86,99,136), suggesting reduced net noradrenergic activity in this system in depression.

DYNAMIC NONPHARMACOLOGIC STRATEGIES

Studies of Circadian and Ultradian Rhythms

The noradrenergic system has been demonstrated to show a circadian rhythm in primates and humans (171). Studies of the rhythm of urinary noradrenergic metabolite excretion in depression have reported relatively low concentrations of the noradrenergic metabolite, VMA, without the expected circadian rhythm observed in controls (122). A significant phase advance in the circadian rhythm of urinary MHPG excretion in depressed patients compared to controls has also been observed (165), but did not reach significance in another study (49). In the latter study, a desynchronized pattern characterized the depressed patients. In a case report, an erratic pattern of urinary MHPG excretion that was desynchronized from temperature and VMA excretion in an acutely depressed bipolar patient normalized when that patient achieved remission (112).

A more recent study measuring serial samples of plasma total MHPG suggested a phase shift in the acrophase of the rhythm in depressed patients that appeared to be a function of more prominent 12-hr than 24-hr periodicity in these patients (38,55). Erratic, unexplained peaks were also observed in both this study and another preliminary study (140), consistent with the possibility of higher frequency, "noisy" periodicities. Thus, in depressed patients, there appears to be a relative loss of normal circadian periodicities with a phase advance and/or higher frequency periodicities, suggesting an alteration in the time-dependent regulation of the noradrenergic system (142).

Responses to Naturalistic Stressors

Another dynamic approach to the assessment of the noradrenergic system in depression is the evaluation of the response of this system to environmental stimuli. Thus, in normal humans stimuli such as change in position to standing, immersion of the hand in cold water, or low-level shocks will increase concentrations of plasma or urinary norepinephrine and/or its metabolites (15,77,164). Exaggerated norepinephrine response to orthostatic challenge in depressed patients suggests inefficiency of the noradrenergic system (128). Environmental changes that do not produce changes in noradrenergic measures in normal subjects, such as withdrawal from a low-monoamine diet (105) or physical exercise (52,105), will alter urinary MHPG excretion in depressed patients. Conversely, relatively discrete and specific environmental stimuli that do produce adrenergic responses in normal subjects, such as low-intensity shock, mental arithmetic, venipuncture, or cold pressor challenge, do not produce as robust responses

in depressed patients (1,15,89). These studies suggest that the noradrenergic system may be less efficient, i.e., less selectively responsive to discrete environmental stimuli (142).

CONCLUSIONS

Over the last 10 years, studies of the function of the noradrenergic system in depression have shifted from studies of concentrations of noradrenergic metabolites in biologic fluids to more dynamic assessment strategies, such as the use of pharmacologic challenges, serial sampling techniques, and specific environmental stressors in order to evaluate the response characteristics of this system in affective disorder patients and controls. These strategies also permit the evaluation of responsiveness of adrenergic receptors, which may importantly influence presynaptic release as well as the efficiency of responses to norepinephrine at postsynaptic receptors.

Studies of noradrenergic metabolite concentrations continue to suggest that the release/metabolism of norepinephrine may be reduced in many bipolar depressed patients, whereas they are increased in at least a subgroup of unipolar depressed patients as well as in manic patients. However, studies are not entirely consistent in this regard. The data available may be more compatible with defective regulation of the noradrenergic system, as suggested by studies of the time-dependent and stimulus-dependent regulation of this system. Thus, average levels of noradrenergic activity may differ between unipolar and bipolar depressed patients, but both groups may be characterized by impaired responsiveness of this system, resulting in a less efficient, poorly modulated system.

The results of adrenergic challenge studies implicate a reduction in central α_2-adrenergic receptor responsiveness. Reduced α_2-adrenergic receptor responsiveness may contribute to a dysregulation of norepinephrine release/metabolism. Studies of peripheral tissues suggest that intrinsic alterations in α_2-adrenergic receptor binding may be less likely than the possibility that the observed abnormalities reflect defects distal to the receptor site or a maladaptive plasticity of these receptors in the CNS. Studies of the β-adrenergic receptor are less numerous, but some neuroendocrine as well as postmortem data might be consistent with increased β-adrenergic receptor responsiveness, whereas peripheral studies suggest reductions in β-adrenergic receptor responsiveness. The α_2-adrenergic and β-adrenergic receptor systems may be reciprocally regulated (90), consistent with reports suggesting increased central β-adrenergic and reduced α_2-adrenergic receptor sensitivity in depression. It may be useful then to explore the mutual regulation of these two receptor systems in depressed patients.

The interaction of neurotransmitter or neuromodulator systems must be considered in the evaluation of any single neurotransmitter system's role in the affective disorder. For example, an intact serotonergic system is required for x-adrenergic receptor desensitization following antidepressant treatment (160), and conversely, noradrenergic influences are necessary for antidepressant-induced changes in the serotonergic system (68). The activity of the locus ceruleus is modulated not only by adrenergic but also by opiate, prostaglandin, and cholinergic receptor sites (158). Thus, disturbances in one neuromodulator system may impact on the regulation of other systems in interactive or reciprocal fashion, so that "primary" and "secondary" disturbances may be difficult to determine at this point in our knowledge of the pathophysiology of depression.

It may be more useful to consider what possible pathologic role the noradrenergic system plays in depression, e.g., relationship to disturbances in vegetative function, arousal, and anxiety, rather than considering that alterations in the noradrenergic system must be etiologic to all the psychobiologic disturbances observed in depression. Similarities and differences between the specific character of apparently impaired noradrenergic function in anxiety and affective disorders require clarification. To address these questions, multiple strategies addressing noradrenergic function and that of other related systems in the same population are required. Longitudinal studies of the same patients across the acute unmedicated phase, antidepressant treatment phase, and unmedicated remitted phase may help to differentiate state-dependent changes implicated in the overt pathology of depression and state-independent abnormalities that might reflect the susceptibility to the biologic dysregulation associated with acute depression (142). Studies of the noradrenergic system in the last decade have moved in these directions but, at this point, have raised more questions than can currently be answered and thus suggest avenues for further exploration over the next decade.

REFERENCES

1. Ackenheil, M., Albus, M., Mullen, F., et al. (1979): In: *Catecholamines: Basic and Clinical Frontiers, Vol. II,* edited by E. Usdin, I. J. Kopin, and J. Barchas, pp. 1937–1939. Pergamon Press, New York.
2. Amsterdam, J. D., Winokur, A., Luck, I., Snyder, P., Harris, R. I., Caroff, S., and Rickels, K. (1982): *Psychoneuroendocrinology,* 7:177–184.
3. Ansseau, M., Schaeyvert, M., Dumont, A., Legross, J. J., and Frank, G. (1984): *Psychiatry Res.,* 12:261–272.
4. Arato, M., Rihmer, Z., Banki, C. M., and Grof, P. (1983): *Prog. Neuropsychopharmacol. Biol. Psychiatry,* 7:715–718.
5. Ashcroft, G. W., Dow, R. C., Yates, C. M., and Pullar, I. A. (1976): In: *CNS and Behavioral Pharmacology, Vol. 3,* edited by S. Tuomisto and M. K. Paasonen, pp. 277–284. University of Helsinki, Finland.
6. Asnis, G. M., Halbreich, U., Rabinovich, H., Puig-Antich, S., and Ryan, N. D. (1985): Abstracts of the IVth World Congress of Biological Psychiatry, Philadelphia, 212.5, p. 137.
7. Aston-Jones, G., and Bloom, F. E. (1981): *J. Neurosci.,* 1:887–900.
8. Axelrod, J., and Reisine, T. D. (1984): *Science,* 224:452–459.
9. Ballenger, J., Post, R., Jimerson, D., Lake, C. R., and Zuckerman, M. (1984): In: *Neurobiology of Mood Disorders,* edited by R. M. Post and J. C. Ballenger, pp. 481–501. Williams and Wilkins, Baltimore.
10. Beck-Friis, J., Von Rosen, D., Kjellman, B. F., Ljunggren, J., and Welterberg, L. (1984): *Psychoendocrinology,* 9:261–274.
11. Berrettini, W. H., Bardakjian, J., Barnett, A. L., Nurnberger, J. I., and Gershon, S. (1986): In: *Antidepressants and Receptor Function. CIBA Foundation Symposium 123,* pp. 30–35. John Wiley and Sons, New York.
12. Besser, G. M., Butler, P. W. P., Landon, J., and Rees, L. (1969): *Br. Med. J.,* 4:528–530.
13. Bivens, C. H., Lebovitz, H. E., and Feldman, J. M. (1973): *N. Engl. J. Med.,* 289:236–239.
14. Brown, R. P., Kocsis, J. H., Caroff, S., Amsterdam, J., Winokur, A., Stokes, P. E., and Frazer, A. (1985): *Am. J. Psychiatry,* 142:811–816.
15. Buchsbaum, M. S., Muscettola, G., and Goodwin, F. K. (1981): *Neuropsychobiology,* 7:212–224.
16. Bunney, W. E., Jr., and Davis, J. M. (1965): *Arch. Gen. Psychiatry,* 13:483–494.
17. Bunney, W. E., Jr., Post, R. M., Anderson, A. C., and Kopanda, R. T. (1977): *Commun. Psychopharmacol.,* 1:393–405.
18. Bylund, B. B., and U'Prichard, D. C. (1983): *Int. Rev. Neurobiol.,* 24:343–431.
19. Calil, H. M., Lesicur, P., Gold, P. W., Brown, C. M., Zavadil, A. P., and Potter, W. Z. (1984): *Psychiatry Res.,* 13:231–242.
20. Campbell, I. C., McKernan, R., Checkely, S. A., Glass, I. B., Thompson, C., and Shur, E. (1985): *Psychiatry Res.,* 14:17–31.
21. Carroll, B. J. (1972): In: *Depressive Illness: Some Research Studies,* edited by B. Davis, B. J. Carroll, and R. M. Mowbray, pp. 23–202. Charles C Thomas, Springfield, IL.
22. Casper, R. C., Davis, J. M., Pandey, G. N., Garver, D. L., and Dekirmenjian, H. (1977): *Psychoneuroendocrinology,* 2:105–113.
23. Charney, D. S., Heninger, G. R., and Sternberg, D. E. (1982): *Psychiatry Res.,* 17:135–138.
24. Charney, D. S., Heninger, G. R., Sternberg, E. E., Halsted, K., McGiddings, S., and Landis, H. (1982): *Arch. Gen. Psychiatry,* 39:290–294.
25. Charney, D. S., Heninger, G. A., Sternberg, D. E., and Roth, R. H. (1981): *Psychiatry Res.,* 5:2117–2129.
26. Checkley, S. A. (1979): *Psychol. Med.,* 9:107–116.
27. Checkley, S. A., and Corn, T. H. (1985): Abstracts of the IVth World Congress of Biological Psychiatry, Philadelphia, 212.11.
28. Checkley, S. A., and Crammer, J. L. (1977): *Br. J. Psychiatry,* 131:582–586.
29. Checkley, S. A., Slade, A. P., and Shur, E. (1981): *Br. J. Psychiatry,* 138:51–55.
30. Christensen, N. S., Vestergaard, P., Sorenson, J., and Rafaelson, O. J. (1980): *Acta Psychiatr. Scand.,* 61:178–182.
31. Claustrat, B., Chazot, G., Brun, J., Jordon, D., and Sassolas, G. (1984): *Biol. Psychiatry,* 19:1215–1228.
32. Cooper, S. J., Kelly, J. G., and King, D. J. (1985): *Br. J. Psychiatry,* 147:23–29.
33. Corn, T. H., Hale, A. S., Thompson, C., Bridges, P. K., and Checkley, S. A. (1984): *Br. J. Psychiatry,* 144:636–639.
34. Crawley, J. M., Hattox, S. E., Maas, J. N., and Roth, R. H. (1978): *Brain Res.,* 141:380–384.
35. Crow, T., Cross, A. J., Cooper, S. J., Deakin, J. F. W., Ferrier, I. N., Johns, J. A., Joseph, J. A., Joseph, M. H., Owen, F., Poulter, M., Lofthouse, R., Corsellis, J. A. N., Chambers, D. R., Blessed, G., Perry, E. K., Perry, R. H., and Tomlinson, B. E. (1984): *Neuropharmacology,* 128:1561–1569.
36. Daiguji, M., Meltzer, H. Y., Tong, C., U'Prichard, D. C., Young, M., and Kravitz, H. (1981): *Life Sci.,* 29:2059–2064.
37. Davis, K. L., Hollister, L. E., Mathé, A., Davis, B. M., Rothpearl, A. B., Faull, K. F., Hsieh, J. Y.-K., Barchase, J. D., and Berger, P. A. (1981): *Am. J. Psychiatry,* 138:1555–1562.
38. DeMet, G. M., Halaris, A. E., Gwirtsman, H. E., Reno, R. M., and Becker, P. I. (1982): *Psychopharmacol. Bull.,* 18:221–223.
39. Doyle, M. C., George, A. J., Ravindran, A. V., and Philpoh, R. (1985): *Am. J. Psychiatry,* 12:1489–1490.
40. Elam, M., Yao, T., Svensson, T. H., and Thorn, P. (1984): *Brain Res.,* 290:281–287.
41. Eriksson, E., Eden, S., and Modigh, K. (1982): *Psychopharmacology,* 77:327–331.
42. Esser, M., Turbott, J., Shwartz, R., Leonard, P., Bobik, A., Skews, H., and Jackman, G. (1982): *Arch. Gen. Psychiatry,* 39:296–300.
43. Extein, J., Tallma, J., Smith, C. C., and Goodwin, F. K. (1979): *Psychiatry Res.,* 1:191–197.
44. Feinberg, M., Greden, J. F., and Carroll, B. J. (1981): *Psychoneuroendocrinology,* 6:355–357.
45. Foote, S. L., Bloom, F. E., and Aston-Jones, G. (1983): *Physiol. Rev.,* 63:844–914.
46. Garcia-Sevilla, J. A., Guimon, P., Garcia-Vellejo, P., and Fuster, M. J. (1986): *Arch. Gen. Psychiatry,* 43:51–57.
47. Garcia-Sevilla, J. A., Zis, A. D., Hollingsworth, P. J., Greden, J. F., and Smith, C. B. (1981): *Arch. Gen. Psychiatry,* 38:1327–1333.
48. Garver, D. L., Pandey, G. N., Dekirmenjian, H., and Deleon-Jones, F. (1975): *Am. J. Psychiatry,* 132:1149–1154.

49. Giedke, H., Gaertner, H. J., and Mahal, A. (1982): *Acta Psychiatr. Scand.,* 66:243–253.
50. Glass, I. B., Checkley, S. A., Shur, E., and Dawling, S. (1982): *Br. J. Psychiatry,* 141:372–376.
51. Gold, P. W., Goodwin, F. K., Wehr, T., Rebar, R., and Sack, R. (1976): *Lancet,* 2:1308–1309.
52. Goode, D. J., Dekirmenjian, H., Meltzer, H. Y., and Maas, T. W. (1973): *Arch. Gen. Psychiatry,* 29:391–396.
53. Gruen, P. H., Sachar, E. J., Altman, N., and Sassin, J. (1975): *Arch. Gen. Psychiatry,* 32:31–33.
54. Halaris, A. E. (1978): *Am. J. Psychiatry,* 135:493–494.
55. Halaris, A., and DeMet, E. (1985): Abstracts of the IVth World Congress of Biological Psychiatry, Philadelphia, 134.5.
56. Halbreich, V., Sachar, E. J., Asnis, G. M., Nathan, R. S., and Halperin, F. S. (1981): *Psychoneuroendocrinology,* 6:223–229.
57. Halbreich, V., Sachar, E. J., Asnis, G. M., Quitkin, F., Nathan, R. M., Halpern, F. S., and Klein, D. F. (1982): *Arch. Gen. Psychiatry,* 39:189–192.
58. Hamilton, C. A., Jones, C. R., Mishra, N., Barr, S., and Reid, J. L. (1985): *Brain Res.,* 347:350–353.
59. Healy, D., Carney, P. A., and Leonard, B. E. (1982/83): *J. Psychiatr. Res.,* 17:251–260.
60. Heninger, G. R., Charney, D. S., and Sternberg, D. E. (1984): *Arch. Gen. Psychiatry,* 41:398–402.
61. Hoehe, M., Valido, G., and Matussek, N. (1986): Proceedings of the IVth World Congress of Biological Psychiatry (*in press*).
62. Horton, R. (1986): In: *Antidepressants and Receptor Function. CIBA Foundation Symposium 123,* pp. 84–95. John Wiley and Sons, New York.
63. Jacobs, B. L. (1987): In: *Psychopharmacology: The Third Generation of Progress,* edited by H. Y. Meltzer and I. Davis. Raven Press, New York (*in press*).
64. Jimerson, D. C., Insel, T. R., Reus, V. I., and Kopin, I. J. (1983): *Arch. Gen. Psychiatry,* 40:173–176.
65. Jimerson, D. C., Nurnberger, J. I., Post, R. M., Gershon, E. S., and Kopin, I. J. (1981): *Arch. Gen. Psychiatry,* 38:1287–1290.
66. Jimerson, D. C., Sun, C. L., Yamaguchi, L., and Kopin, I. J. (1979): In: *Catecholamines: Basic and Clinical Frontiers,* pp. 912–929. Pergamon Press, New York.
67. Kathol, R. G., Sherman, B. M., Winokur, G., Lewis, G., and Schlesser, M. (1983): *Psychiatry Res.,* 9:99–106.
68. Kellar, K. J., and Cascio, C. S. (1983): Abstracts of Annual Meeting of the Society of Neurosciences, 209.1.
69. Kopin, I. J., Gordon, E. K., Jimerson, D. C., and Polinsky, D. J. (1983): *Science,* 219:73–75.
70. Koslow, S. H., Maas, J. W., Bowden, C. L., Davis, J. M., Hanin, I., and Javaid, J. (1983): *Arch. Gen. Psychiatry,* 40:999–1010.
71. Koslow, S. H., Stokes, P. E., Mondels, J., Ramsey, A., and Casper, R. (1982): *Psychol. Med.,* 12:45–55.
72. Laakman, G., and Benkert, O. (1978): *Neuroendokrinol. Psychopharmak. Forsch.,* 28:1277–1280.
73. Laakman, G., Benkert, O., Neulinger, E., Werger, K. V., and Erhardt, F. (1978): *Arzneimittelforsch.,* 28:1292–1294.
74. Laakman, G., Wittman, M., Schoen, H. W., Zykan, K., Weiss, A., Meissner, R., Mueller, O. A., and Stalla, G. K. (1987): *Psychoneuroendocrinology* (*in press*).
75. Laakman, G., Zykan, K., Schoen, H. W., Weiss, A., Wittman, M., Meissner, R., and Blaschke, D. (1987): *Psychoneuroendocrinology* (*in press*).
76. Lake, C. R., Pickar, D., Ziegler, M., et al. (1982): *Am. J. Psychiatry,* 139:1315–1318.
77. Lake, C. R., Zeigler, M. G., and Kopin, I. J. (1976): *Life Sci.,* 18:1315–1326.
78. Lal, S., Tolis, G., Martin, J. B., Brown, G. M., and Guyda, H. (1975): *J. Clin. Endocrinol. Metab.,* 41:827–832.
79. Langer, G., Heinze, G., Rein, B., and Matussek, N. (1976): *Arch. Gen. Psychiatry,* 33:1471–1475.
80. Langer, G., and Matussek, N. (1977): *Psychoneuroendocrinology,* 11:191–196.
81. Lechin, F., Vander Dijs, B., Jakobowicz, D., Camero, R. E., Villa, S., Lechin, E., and Gomez, F. (1985): *Neuroendocrinology,* 40:253–261.
82. Leckman, J. F., and Maas, J. W. (1984): In: *Neurobiology of Mood Disorders: Plasma MHPG,* edited by R. M. Post and J. C. Ballenger, pp. 529–538. Williams and Wilkins, Baltimore.
83. Leckman, J. F., Weissman, M. M., Merikangas, K. R., Pauls, D. L., and Prusoff, B. A. (1983): *Arch. Gen. Psychiatry,* 40:1055–1060.
84. Lenox, R. H., Ellis, J. E., Van Riper, D. A., Ehrlich, Y. H., Peyser, J. M., Shipley, J. E., and Weaver, L. A. (1983): In: *Frontiers in Neuropsychiatric Research,* edited by E. Usdin, M. Goldstein, and A. Friedhopp, p. 331. Macmillan, London.
85. Lenox, R. H., Shipley, J. E., Peyser, J. M., Weaver, L. A., Armstrong, C. B., and Ashikaga, T. (1983): New Research Abstracts of the American Psychiatric Association, NR 32.
86. Lewy, A. J., Wehr, T. A., Gold, P. W., and Goodwin, F. K. (1979): In: *Catecholamines: Basic and Clinical Frontiers, Vol. 2,* edited by E. Usdin, I. J. Kopin, and J. Barchas, pp. 1173–1175. Pergamon Press, New York.
87. Louis, W. J., Doyle, A. E., and Anavekar, S. N. (1975): *Clin. Sci. Mol. Med.,* 48:2395–2425.
88. Maany, I., Mendels, J., Frazer, A., and Brunswick, D. (1979): *Neuropsychobiology,* 5:282–289.
89. Maas, J. W., Dekirmenjian, H., and Fawcett, S. (1971): *Nature,* 230:330–331.
90. Maggi, A., U'Prichard, D. C., and Ennas, S. J. (1986A): *Science,* 207:645–647.
91. Mann, J. J., Brown, R. P., Halper, J. P., Sweeney, J. A., Kacsis, J. H., Stokes, P., and Bilzekian, J. P. (1985): *N. Engl. J. Med.,* 313:715–720.
92. Mann, J. J., McBride, A., and Stanley, M. (1987): *Ann. NY Acad. Sci.* (*in press*).
93. Manome, T., Wantanabe, A., Kaneko, M., Numala, Y., Hoshino, Y., Kano, T., and Kumashiro, H. (1985): Abstracts of Panels and Posters presented at the Annual Meeting of the American College of Neuropsychopharmacology.
94. March, G., Sjoquist, B., and Anggard, E. (1981): *J. Neurochem.,* 36:1181–1185.
95. Massala, A., Delitalia, G., Alagna, S., and Devilla, L. (1977): *Clin. Endocrinol.,* 7:253–256.
96. Matussek, N., Ackenheil, M., Hippius, H., Muller, F., Schroder, H., Schuttes, H., and Wasilewski, B. (1980): *Psychiatry Res.,* 2:25–36.
97. Meltzer, H. Y., Umberkoman-Witta, B., Robertson, A., Tricou, B. J., Lowy, M., and Perline, R. (1984): *Arch. Gen. Psychiatry,* 41:366–374.
98. Mendlewicz, J., and Gilles, C. (1985): Abstracts of the IVth World Congress of Biological Psychiatry, Philadelphia, 212.2.
99. Mendlewicz, J., Linkowski, P., Branchey, L., Weinberg, U., Weitzman, E. D., and Branchey, M. (1979): *Lancet,* 2:1362.
100. Mitrius, J. C., Micuni, M., Arora, R. C., Meltzer, H. Y., and U'Prichard, D. C. (1983): *Neurosci. Abstr.,* 9:990.
101. Mooney, J. J., Schatzberg, A. F., Cole, J. O., Kizuka, P. P., and Schildkraut, J. J. (1985): *J. Psychiatr. Res.,* 19:65–75.
102. Mooney, J. J., Schildkraut, J. J., Schatzberg, A. F., Gershon, B., Pappalardo, K., and Cole, J. O. (1986): American Psychiatric Association, New Research Programs and Abstracts, Washington, DC, NR, 165.
103. Murphy, D. L., Donelly, C., and Moskowitz, J. (1974): *Am. J. Psychiatry,* 131:1389–1391.
104. Murphy, D. L., Siever, L. J., and Insel, T. R. (1985): *Prog. Neuropharmacol. Biol. Psychiatry,* 9:3–13.
105. Muscettalo, G., Wehr, T., and Goodwin, F. K. (1977): *Am. J. Psychiatry,* 134:914–916.
106. Nathan, R. S., Sachar, E. J., Asnis, G. M., Halbreich, U., and Halpern, F. S. (1981): *Psychiatry Res.,* 4:291–300.
107. Nurnberger, J. I., Gershon, E. S., Sitaram, N., Gillin, C., Brown, G., Elbert, M., Gold, P., Jimerson, D. C., and Hessler, L. (1981): *Psychopharmacol. Bull.,* 17:80–82.
108. Nurnberger, J. I., Simmons-Alling, S., Kessler, L., Jimerson, D. C., Schreiber, J., Hollander, E., Tamminga, C. A., Nadi, N. S., Goldstein, D. S., and Gershon, E. S. (1984): *Psychopharmacology,* 84:200–204.
109. Ottenweiler, J. E., and Meer, A. H. (1982): *Endocrinology,* 111:1334–1338.
110. Palazidou, E., Corn, T. H., Bean, J., and Checkley, S. A. (1985): Abstracts of the IVth World Congress of Biological Psychiatry, Philadelphia, 233.4.
111. Pandey, G. N., Dykson, M. W., Garver, D. L., and Davis, J. M. (1979): *Am. J. Psychiatry,* 136:675–678.

112. Pflug, B., Engelman, W., and Gaertner, H. S. (1982): *J. Neural Transm.* 53:213–215.
113. Pickar, D., Sweeney, D. R., Maas, J. W., and Heninger, R. (1978): *Arch. Gen. Psychiatry,* 35:1378–1383.
114. Pimoule, C., Briley, M. S., Gay, C., Loo, H. Sechter, D., Zaifian, E., Raisman, R., and Langer, S. Z. (1983): *Psychopharmacology,* 79:308.
115. Post, R. M., Jimerson, D. C., Ballenger, J. C., Lake, C. R., Uhde, T. W., and Goodwin, F. K. (1984): In: *Neurobiology of Mood Disorders,* edited by R. M. Post and J. C. Ballenger, pp. 539–553. Williams and Wilkins, Baltimore.
116. Post, R. M., Stoddard, F. J., Gillin, J. C., Buschbaum, M. S., Runkle, D. C., Black, K. E., and Bunney, W. E. (1977): *Arch. Gen. Psychiatry,* 34:470–477.
117. Potter, W. Z., Muscettola, G., and Goodwin, F. K. (1983): In: *MHPG Basic Mechanisms and Psychopathology,* edited by J. W. Maas, pp. 145–165. Academic Press, New York.
118. Potter, W. Z., Ross, R. J., and Zavadil, H. P. (1985): In: *Catecholamines in Psychiatric Disorders,* edited by C. R. Lake and M. G. Ziegler, pp. 213–233. Butterworth, Boston.
119. Price, L. H., and Heninger, G. R. (1985): American Psychiatric Association, 138th Annual Meeting, New Research Program and Abstracts, NR 85.
120. Redmond, D. E., and Huang, Y. H. (1979): New evidence for a locus ceruleus—norepinephrine connection with anxiety. *Life Sci.,* 25:2149–2162.
121. Rees, L., Butler, P. W. P., Gosling, C., and Besser, G. M. (1970): *Nature,* 228:565–566.
122. Reiderer, P., Birkmayer, W., Newmayer, E., Ambrozi, L., and Linauer, W. (1974): *J. Neural Transm.,* 35:23–45.
123. Risch, S. C., Siever, L. J., Gillin, J. C., Janowsky, D. J., Sitaram, N., Weker, J., Cohen, R. M., and Murphy, D. L. (1983): *Psychopharmacol. Bull.,* 19:696–698.
124. Rosenbaum, A. H., Maruta, T., Schatzberg, A. F., Oraulak, P. J., Jiang, N. S., Cole, J. D., and Schildkraut, J. J. (1983): *Am. J. Psychiatry,* 140:314–318.
125. Roy, A., Pickar, P., Linnoila, M., and Potter, W. Z. (1985): *Arch. Gen. Psychiatry,* 42:1181–1185.
126. Rubin, A. L., Price, L. H., Charney, D. S., and Heninger, G. R. (1985): *Psychiatry Res.,* 15:5–15.
127. Rubinow, D. R. (1986): *Biol. Psychiatry,* 21:341–365.
128. Rudorfer, M. V., Lesieur, P., Ross, R. J., Linnoila, M., and Potter, W. Z. (1983): New Research Abstracts, American Psychiatric Association, Annual Meeting, NR 46.
129. Rudorfer, M. V., Ross, R. J., Linnoila, M., Sherer, M., and Potter, W. Z. (1985): *Arch. Gen. Psychiatry,* 42:1186–1192.
130. Sacchetti, E., Conte, G., Pennati, A., Vita, A., Alciati, A., and Cazzullo, C. L. (1985): *J. Psychiatr. Res.,* 19:579–586.
131. Sachar, E. J., Altman, N., Gruen, P. H., Glassman, A., Halpern, F. S., and Sassin, J. (1975): *Arch. Gen. Psychiatry,* 32:502–503.
132. Sachar, E. J., Finkelstein, J., and Hellman, L. (1971): *Arch. Gen. Psychiatry,* 25:263–269.
133. Sachar, E. J., Frantz, A. B., Altman, N., and Sassin, J. (1973): *Am. J. Psychiatry,* 130:1362–1367.
134. Sachar, E. J., Halbreich, U., Asnis, G. M., Nathan, R. S., and Halpern, F. S. (1981): *Arch. Gen. Psychiatry,* 38:1113–1123.
135. Sachar, E. J., Halbreich, U., Asnis, M., Nathan, R. S., Halpern, F. S., and Ostrow, L. (1981): *Arch. Gen. Psychiatry,* 38:1113–1117.
136. Sack, R. L., and Lewy, A. J. (1986): *Biol. Psychiatry,* 21:406–410.
137. Schatzberg, A. F., Rosenbaum, A. H., Orsulak, P. J., Rhote, W. A., Marita, T., Kruger, E. R., Cole, J. O., and Schildkraut, J. J. (1981): *Psychopharmacology,* 75:34–38.
138. Schildkraut, J. J. (1965): *Am. J. Psychiatry,* 122:509–522.
139. Schildkraut, J. J., Orsulak, P. J., Schatzberg, A. F., Gudeman, J. E., Cole, J. O., Rohde, W. A., and LaBrie, R. A. (1978): *Arch. Gen. Psychiatry,* 35:1427–1433.
140. Siever, L. J., Coccaro, E. F., Adan, F., Mohs, R. C., and Davis, K. L. (1986): In: *New Perspectives in Depression Research,* edited by H. Hippius, N. Matussek, and G. R. Klerman, pp. 189–195. Springer-Verlag, Berlin.
141. Siever, L. J., Coccaro, E. F., and Davis, K. L. (1987): In: *Hormones and Depression,* edited by U. Halbreich and R. Rose. Raven Press, New York (*in press*).
142. Siever, L. J., and Davis, K. L. (1985): *Am. J. Psychiatry,* 142:1017–1031.
143. Siever, L. J., Insel, T. R., Hamilton, J. A., Aloi, J., and Murphy, D. L. (1985): *Psychiatry Res.,* 16:79–82.
144. Siever, L. J., Insel, T. R., Jimerson, D. C., Lake, C. R. Aloi, J., and Murphy, D. L. (1983): *Br. J. Psychiatry,* 142:184–187.
145. Siever, L. J., Insel, T. R., and Uhde, T. W. (1981): *J. Clin. Psychopharmacol.,* 1:190–206.
146. Siever, L. J., Kafka, M. S., Targum, S., and Lake, C. R. (1984): *J. Psychiatr. Res.,* 11:287–302.
147. Siever, L. J., Murphy, E. L., Slater, S., de la Vega, E., and Lipper, S. (1984): *Life Sci.,* 34:1029–1039.
148. Siever, L. J., and Uhde, T. W. (1984): *Biol. Psychiatry,* 19:131–156.
149. Siever, L. J., Uhde, T. W., Insel, T. R., Kay, W. H., Jimerson, D. C., Lake, C. R., Kafka, M. S., Targum, S., and Murphy, D. L. (1985): *Neuropsychopharmacol. Biol. Psychiatry,* 9:15–24.
150. Siever, L. J., Uhde, T. W., Insel, T. R., Roy, B. I., and Murphy, D. L. (1980): *Psychiatry Res.,* 7:139–144.
151. Siever, L. J., Uhde, T. W., Jimerson, D. C., Lake, C. R., Kopin, I. J., and Murphy, D. L. (1986): *Psychiatry Res.,* 19:59–73.
152. Siever, L. J., Uhde, T. W., Jimerson, D. C., Lake, C. R., Silberman, E. R., Post, R. M., and Murphy, D. L. (1984): *Am. J. Psychiatry,* 141:733–741.
153. Siever, L. J., Uhde, T. W., Jimerson, D. C., Post, R. M., Lake, C. R., and Murphy, D. L. (1984): *Arch. Gen. Psychiatry,* 41:63–68.
154. Siever, L. J., Uhde, T. W., and Murphy, D. L. (1984): In: *Neurobiology of Mood Disorders,* edited by R. M. Post and J. C. Ballenger, pp. 502–518. Williams and Wilkins, Baltimore.
155. Siever, L. J., Uhde, T. W., Silberman, E. Jimerson, D. C., Aloi, J. A., Post, R. M., and Murphy, D. L. (1982): *Psychiatry Res.,* 6:171–183.
156. Sitaram, N., Nurnberger, J. L., Jr., Gershon, E. S., and Gillin, J. C. (1980): *Science,* 208:200–202.
157. Stahl, S. M., Lemoine, P. M., Ciaranello, R. D., and Berger, P. A. (1983): *Psychiatry Res.,* 10:157–164.
158. Starke, K. (1981): *Annu. Rev. Pharmacol. Toxicol.,* 21:7–30.
159. Stewart, J. W., Quitkin, F., McGrath, P. J., Liebowitz, M. R., Harrison, W., Rabkin, J. G., Novacenko, H., Push-Antich, T., and Asnis, G. M. (1984): *Psychiatry Res.,* 12:195–206.
160. Sulser, F., Gillespie, D. D., and Manier, D. H. (1984): *Clin. Neuropharmacol.,* 7(Suppl. 1):304–305.
161. Sweeney, D. R., Leckman, J. F., Maas, J. W., Hattox, S., and Heninger, G. R. (1980): *Arch. Gen. Psychiatry,* 37:1100–1103.
162. Valentine, R. J., Foote, S. L., and Koslow, S. H. (1985): Abstracts of Panels and Posters presented at the Annual Meeting of the American College of Neuropsychopharmacology, Nashville.
163. Wang, Y.-C., Pandey, G. N., Mendels, J., and Frazer, A. (1974): *Psychopharmacologia,* 36:291.
164. Ward, M. M., Mefford, I. N., Parker, S. D., Chesney, M. A., Barr-Taylor, C., Keegan, D. L., and Barchas, J. D. (1983): *Psychosom. Med.,* 45:471–486.
165. Wehr, T. A., Muscettola, G., and Goodwin, F. K. (1980): *Arch. Gen. Psychiatry,* 37:257–263.
166. Wood, K., and Coppen, A. (1982): In: *Advances in Biochemical Psychopharmacology, Vol. 32,* edited by E. Costa and C. Racagni, pp. 13–19.
167. Woodward, P. J., Moises, H. C., Waterhouse, B. D., Hoffer, B. J., and Freeman, R. (1979): *Fed. Proc.,* 38:2109–2116.
168. Wright, A. F., Crichton, D. N., Loudon, J. B., Marsden, J. E. N., and Steel, C. M. (1984): *Ann. Hum. Genet.,* 48:201–214.
169. Wyatt, R. J., Portnoy, B., Kupfer, D. J., Snyder, F., and Engelman, K. (1971): *Arch. Gen. Psychiatry,* 24:65–70.
170. Zanko, M. T., and Biegon, A. (1983): Abstracts of Annual Meeting, Society for Neuroscience, Boston, p. 719.
171. Ziegler, M. G., Lake, C. R., Wood, J. H., et al. (1977): *Nature,* 266:656–658.
172. Ziegler, M. G., Milano, A. J., and Hull, E. (1985): In: *The Catecholamines in Psychiatric and Neurologic Disorders,* edited by C. R. Lake and M. G. Ziegler, pp. 37–53. Butterworth Publishers, Boston.
173. Zohar, J., Bannet, J., Drummere, D., Fisch, R., Epstein, R. P., and Belmaker, R. H. (1983): *Biol. Psychiatry,* 18:553–560.

Psychopharmacology:
The Third Generation of Progress,
edited by Herbert Y. Meltzer.
Raven Press, New York © 1987.

CHAPTER 51

Role of Dopamine Mechanisms in the Affective Disorders

David C. Jimerson

Although the original catecholamine hypothesis of affective illness focused largely on norepinephrine (24,142), accumulating neurochemical and pharmacologic evidence suggests that functional dopamine activity is reduced in some subgroups of depressed patients, and increased in manic patients. Recent studies have particularly focused on the possible role of altered dopamine receptor activity in these syndromes. This chapter is organized into separate discussions of recent investigations pertaining to dopamine function in depression and mania. When possible from the data available, findings are presented separately for unipolar and bipolar depression, delusional and nondelusional depression, and retarded and agitated depression. Limited space precludes discussion of the numerous interactions of brain dopamine systems with other neurotransmitters and neuromodulators that have been implicated in affective illness (especially norepinephrine, serotonin, acetylcholine, γ-aminobutyric acid (GABA), and endogenous opiates).

DEPRESSION

Clinical Effects of Dopamine Agonists and Antagonists

The neurotransmitter hypotheses of depression derived largely from indirect pharmacologic evidence of behavioral and mood effects of neurotransmitter active drugs in laboratory animals and humans. Initial studies with the catecholamine precursor L-dopa documented a modest antidepressant effect in patients with psychomotor retardation (28,169). Low pretreatment levels of the major dopamine metabolite homovanillic acid (HVA) in cerebrospinal fluid (CSF) were predictive of favorable clinical response (169). A differential mood response to L-dopa was also reported according to diagnostic subtype, such that hypomanic symptoms were much more prominent in bipolar than in unipolar depressed patients (113). Administration of methylamphetamine or methylphenidate resulted in transient mood-elevating effects in one-half to two-thirds of depressed patients (75,84,134,148), whereas the remaining patients felt worse. This range of mood responses to psychomotor stimulant drugs does not differentiate depressed patients from healthy controls (74,116). Preinfusion levels of CSF HVA were not predictive of behavioral responses (80), but patients with bipolar depression had a consistently euphoric response to amphetamine, whereas some patients with unipolar illness manifested distinct postamphetamine dysphoria (148).

Development of relatively selective postsynaptic dopamine receptor agonists suitable for clinical trials presented a new opportunity for assessing the potential antidepressant effects of increased central dopamine function. In a double-blind trial with piribedil, Post et al. (125) reported measurable antidepressant effects in 12 of 16 patients, with substantial improvement in four of these subjects. Low pretreatment levels of CSF HVA were predictive of greater clinical improvement during drug treatment. Similar antidepressant effects of piribedil were reported by Angrist et al. (6) in one of two depressed patients, and by Shopsin and Gershon (146) in an open trial in seven patients, although dysphoric effects became prominent over time in the latter trial. Antidepressant effects have also been observed with the dopamine agonist bromocriptine (19,35,115,149,164,174).

Antidepressant responses to bromocriptine were not correlated with CSF levels of HVA (115). Silverstone (149) reported that five patients with bipolar depression showed a clearer antidepressant response to bromocriptine (with two of the five developing manic symptoms) than did five patients with unipolar depression. It is of note that several newer antidepressant drugs proven effective in large clinical trials, including nomifensine and bupropion, have prominent effects on dopamine systems (138).

To the extent that dopamine precursors and dopamine agonists have an antidepressant effect (possibly most marked in patients with bipolar depression), it is pertinent to inquire whether dopamine antagonists result in symptoms of depression. There are numerous reports of depressive states in patients receiving neuroleptics, and evidence for rebound improvement in mood and even hypomania following neuroleptic withdrawal, as reviewed by Randrup et al. (131). Beneficial effects of neuroleptics sometimes seen in depression are usually associated with low dose treatment (131,182), in comparison to the higher doses effective in mania and schizophrenia, and have generally been studied in anxiety-depressive states rather than in major, endogenous depressions (135). Atypical neuroleptics such as sulpiride reported to be effective in depression have a distinctive neurochemical profile, with activating effects associated with preferential blockade of presynaptic dopamine receptors (77). The clinically accepted combination of neuroleptics with antidepressants in delusional/psychotic depression (61) may involve differential effects on dopamine pathways modulating mood and cognitive function.

Cerebrospinal Fluid Studies

Measurement of HVA in CSF has provided one of the most direct means for assessing brain dopamine function in clinical studies (78,123). Consistent with the hypothesis of decreased dopamine turnover in depression, five of six studies with a medication-free period of at least 10 days showed evidence for reduced CSF HVA in patients in comparison to controls (16,17,23,65,86,119). Similar results were reported in another recent study with some patients drug-free for long periods (10). Recent results from NIMH studies utilizing gas chromatography-mass spectrometry and high pressure liquid chromatography show a trend for lower HVA values in patients with major depression in comparison to healthy controls (R. M. Post, *personal communication,* November 1986). The substantial variability in other studies may be related not only to the limited duration of medication withdrawal, but also to other methodological limitations including nonavailability of age- and sex-matched healthy control groups (3,11,15,22,58,83,118,151,156,162,166,168,170,173). Sedvall et al. (143) reported family study data indicating that low CSF HVA might be a state-independent variable related to depression. Bipolar patients studied during a euthymic phase did not, however, have altered CSF HVA in comparison to controls (18).

There is little evidence for a difference in CSF HVA levels between unipolar and bipolar depressed patients (78), although the number of bipolar patients studied is too small to consider this a definitive conclusion. Initial reports suggesting that low HVA values were most common in retarded depressed patients (15,168) were not replicated in later studies (15,65,173). In the NIMH collaborative study, low HVA levels were most marked in older male patients (86). In a recent study Roy et al. (136) showed that CSF levels of HVA were significantly lower in 15 medication-free patients with a major depressive episode with melancholia than in a combined group of 13 patients with a nonmelancholic depressive episode or dysthymic disorder, although a normal control group was not available for comparison.

Increased dopamine turnover, as reflected in increased HVA levels in the CSF and periphery, has been noted in patients with delusional/psychotic depression. Sweeney et al. (160) reported that a small subgroup of delusional unipolar patients had significantly higher levels of CSF HVA [and a lower 3-methoxy-4-hydroxyphenylglycol (MHPG)/HVA ratio] than nondelusional depressed patients. Agren and Terenius (4) reported that 22 medication-free patients with major depression and a history of psychosis/hallucinations had significantly higher HVA than 111 patients without a history of psychosis. Similar results were observed by Aberg-Wistedt and colleagues (2) in eight delusional depressed patients who, in comparison to 42 nondelusional depressed patients, had significantly elevated CSF HVA and HVA/5-hydroxyindoleacetic acid (5HIAA) ratio (as well as elevated levels of 5HIAA). Elevated plasma HVA levels have been noted in female depressed patients with delusions (44). Psychotic symptoms developing in patients treated with antidepressants have been associated with increases in urinary or plasma HVA (63,97).

Neuroendocrine Studies of Dopamine Function

The tuberoinfundibular pathway originates in cell bodies in arcuate and periventricular nuclei of the hypothalamus and releases dopamine into the hypothalamic-hypophyseal portal system, resulting in tonic inhibition of prolactin release (49,68,94). Dopamine agonists stimulate growth hormone release through effects at both the hypothalamus and the anterior pituitary gland (89,90,98,106). Other neuroregulators influence prolactin and growth hormone secretion, with norepinephrine in particular playing a major role in the latter case (30,46). Decreased presynaptic dopamine release in depression could result in decreased neuroendocrine responses to dopamine precursors and increased responses to postsynaptic receptor agonists (reflecting compensatory receptor up-regulation). Conversely, a primary decrease in postsynaptic dopamine receptor function could result in blunted neuroendocrine responses to both dopamine precursors and receptor agonist drugs. Caution is required in making inferences about mesolimbic and mesocortical dopamine function from responses in the tuberoinfundibular pathway, since these separate dopamine systems are likely to be regulated differently (7,53,88).

Clinical studies of prolactin regulation in depressed patients have provided little consistent evidence for altered dopamine activity. Although prolactin levels have been reported to be low during depression (14,79), there are also reports of increased (73,102,111,140) or normal (9,34,51,55,71,108,122) prolactin levels in depression. Prolactin responses in depressed patients have been reported as not different from controls following L-dopa (109), bromocriptine (39), amphetamine (116), and apomorphine (79). Although there are relatively few data comparing unipolar and bipolar depression, there are reports of low baseline prolactin levels (111) and increased prolactin suppression (62) in bipolar patients. Meltzer et al. (108) reported a correlation between depression ratings and apomorphine-induced prolactin suppression in a mixed psychiatric population, although this relationship did not reach significance among the depressed patients.

Growth hormone responses to apomorphine were not significantly different for depressed patients and controls (29,57,79,99,108). Growth hormone responses to amphetamine (which may largely reflect noradrenergic influence; refs. 47, 104) were reported normal in three of four studies in depression (30,31,93,116). Two of three studies reported normal growth hormone responses to L-dopa in depression (62,109,139).

Hypothermic responses to apomorphine are mediated through central dopamine systems (129) and may provide a nonpituitary correlate of neuroendocrine responses. Cutler et al. (40) observed normal hypothermic response to apomorphine in depression.

Taken as a whole, the neuroendocrine data reviewed in this section do not provide support for altered dopamine-mediated responses in the tuberoinfundibular system in depression. It is pertinent to mention the observation of state-dependent dyskinesias in medication-free patients with affective illness. Increased severity of extrapyramidal symptoms in depression in comparison to mania suggests the possibility of up-regulated dopamine receptors in the nigrostriatal system in the depressive phase (41). This finding may be related to the observation that depressed patients may have an increased vulnerability to neuroleptic-induced tardive dyskinesia (43). These observations illustrate the caveat that changes in another dopamine system (here the nigrostriatal) are not necessarily reflected in dopamine-mediated neuroendocrine responses.

Antidepressants as Dopamine-Active Drugs

Preclinical studies have demonstrated that chronic treatment with antidepressant drugs results in a number of neurochemical and behavioral changes involving brain dopamine function (158,179–181). Antidepressant drugs inhibit the neuronal reuptake of dopamine, but this effect is less potent and more variable than effects on the other neurotransmitters (52,70,130,133,176). Serra et al. (144) reported that chronic treatment with antidepressant drugs decreased the sensitivity of dopamine autoreceptors, based on behavioral and biochemical data. Chiodo and Antelman (8,32,33) found that treatment of rats with tricyclic antidepressants, monoamine oxidase inhibitors, and electroconvulsive therapy (ECT) all inhibited the electrophysiologic response of single dopamine neurons to low doses of apomorphine, consistent with autoreceptor subsensitivity. Subsequent investigators failed to find decreases in autore-

ceptor activity utilizing similar neurochemical, electrophysiological, and behavioral approaches (45,72,101,154,177). Studies of chronic antidepressant treatments have reported varying effects on receptor binding (85,96,105,120,163). Moreover, antidepressant treatment did not alter dopamine turnover in rat brain (157). Studies of CSF HVA levels in depressed patients treated with a range of antidepressant drugs have shown variable or absent changes in levels of the metabolite with drug treatment (12,20,21,42,110, 119,126,128,147,165). Pretreatment CSF HVA values are not predictive of clinical response to classical antidepressant treatments (100), although low CSF HVA levels predicted response to zimelidine (1) and nomifensine (171).

Recent studies (with some qualifications; refs. 67, 105) have suggested that chronic antidepressant treatment results in increased sensitivity of postsynaptic dopamine receptor function in mesolimbic/mesocortical pathways, as reflected in increased locomotor, neurochemical, and behavioral responses (50,103,117,152–154). The tendency for antidepressant drugs to induce hypomanic or manic episodes in bipolar patients may be a result of drug-induced postsynaptic receptor supersensitivity (26).

Nonpharmacologic antidepressant treatments may also involve increased functional activity in brain dopamine pathways. Thus, ECT has been reported to increase responsiveness to dopamine agonists (48,66,67,112,154,178). Rapid eye movement (REM) sleep deprivation increased dopamine function in laboratory rats (145,167), although total sleep deprivation decreased the growth hormone response to apomorphine in healthy human volunteers (92). In depressed patients, Gerner and associates (60) reported that relatively low baseline levels of CSF HVA were predictive of greater antidepressant response to sleep deprivation.

MANIA

Clinical Effects of Dopamine Agonists and Antagonists

Initial support for a role of increased dopamine function in the etiology of mania derived from pharmacological observations with dopamine agonists and antagonists. Thus, the activating and mood-elevating effects of amphetamine and related psychomotor stimulants in humans, as well as excited psychotic states resulting from chronic amphetamine administration (5), had behavioral similarities to mania, and these effects could be blocked by dopamine antagonists (69,82,116,175). Administration to depressed patients of dopamine precursors and agonists, including L-dopa, amphetamine, piribedil, and bromocriptine, could result in hypomania or mania, most clearly in patients with bipolar depression (59,81,113). [In contrast, however, a double-blind study of bromocriptine at moderate doses showed no clinical effects in manic patients (81).] Behavioral excitation and hypomania following amphetamine withdrawal has been proposed as a model for mania resulting from drug-induced supersensitivity of dopamine receptors (25).

Considerable data link the clinical efficacy of neuroleptic drugs in mania to dopamine receptor blockade (130). Selective inhibition of norepinephrine synthesis by inhibition of dopamine β-hydroxylase was without effect in mania

(141). Although classical neuroleptic drugs affect a number of neurotransmitter systems, the importance of effects on dopamine was substantiated by reports that the relatively selective dopamine receptor antagonists pimozide (38,127) and cis-clopenthixol (114) were efficacious in controlled studies in mania. In the study by Cookson et al. (36), clinical response to pimozide was paralleled by a progressive increase in prolactin, with later evidence indicating that neuroleptic treatment resulted in altered pharmacologic responsiveness of the tuberoinfundibular dopamine system to acute neuroleptic challenge, possibly reflecting similar neuroleptic-induced changes in forebrain dopamine pathways. Consistent with preclinical reports that low doses of dopamine receptor agonists preferentially activate inhibitory presysnaptic receptors, low doses of piribedil had antimanic effects in two patients (124).

Cerebrospinal Fluid Studies

Studies by Banki (15), Vestergard et al. (173), and Swann et al. (159) showed elevated HVA levels in manic patients in comparison to controls. A similar trend toward elevated CSF HVA levels in mania was observed by Gerner et al. (58), and in recent data from the NIMH group (R. M. Post, *personal communication,* November, 1986). Possible methodologic issues (as reviewed elsewhere; refs. 78, 123) may have contributed to variability in earlier reports (13,150). Alterations in other metabolite levels have also been noted in these studies (e.g., elevated 5HIAA in female manic patients studied by Swann et al., ref. 159), consistent with the proposal that several related neurotransmitters may be altered in mania.

Neuroendocrine Studies

Neuroendocrine studies have not shown altered tuberoinfundibular dopamine function in mania, although the number of patients studied is small. Thus, baseline levels of prolactin (37,108) and apomorphine-induced suppression of prolactin (108) were normal in mania. Resting growth hormone levels were not elevated in manic patients (37,76). Growth hormone responses to apomorphine were normal (108) or blunted (56) in manic patients. Meltzer et al. (108) reported a trend toward a negative correlation of the growth hormone response with ratings of severity of delusions.

Lithium Effects on Brain Dopamine Systems

In line with a "second generation" hypothesis focusing on the possible role of supersensitive catecholamine receptors in the switch from depression into mania (25,27), there has been substantial recent research on the effects of lithium on dopamine receptor mechanisms. Studies of the effects of chronic lithium treatment on brain dopamine receptor binding in normal animals yielded variable results (reviewed in ref. 25). In volunteers lithium pretreatment had no effect on growth hormone responses to apomorphine or prolactin responses to haloperidol (91).

Recent preclinical data suggest that lithium may block neuroleptic- or denervation-induced supersensitivity of brain dopamine receptors. Biochemical (121,172), electrophysiological (54), and behavioral (87,155,161) studies in rodents have demonstrated this stabilizing effect of lithium treatment, although the results have not been replicated in all studies (95,107,132). In another model, the behavioral effects of agonist-induced sensitization were not blocked by lithium pretreatment (137). In psychiatric patients treated with lithium, the apomorphine-induced suppression of plasma prolactin was blunted whereas growth hormone responses were unaltered (64). Given the weight of the preclinical evidence indicating that behavioral measures of dopamine receptor supersensitivity are reduced by lithium pretreatment (27,161), further studies are needed to test this concept in humans.

OVERVIEW OF DOPAMINE IN DEPRESSION AND MANIA

The hypothesis of decreased dopamine function in depression is supported by evidence for low CSF levels of HVA and therapeutic responses to dopamine agonists. Additional aspects of dopamine dysregulation have been demonstrated in bipolar and delusional subgroups of depressed patients. Evidence for increased dopamine function in mania includes the efficacy of selective dopamine antagonists, and the precipitation of mania in bipolar patients by dopamine agonists. Recent preclinical studies suggest that mechanisms of action of antidepressant drugs and lithium involve prominent effects on regulation of forebrain postsynaptic dopamine receptors.

ACKNOWLEDGMENT

The author wishes to thank Dr. Robert Post for his continued scientific support of this work.

REFERENCES

1. Aberg-Wistedt, A., Ross, S. B., Jostell, K.-G., and Sjoquist, B. (1982): *Acta Psychiatr. Scand.,* 66:66–82.
2. Aberg-Wistedt, A., Wistedt, B., and Bertilsson, L. (1985): *Arch. Gen. Psychiatry,* 42:925–926.
3. Agren, H. (1980): *Psychiatry Res.,* 3:211–223.
4. Agren, H., and Terenius, L. (1985): *J. Affective Disord.,* 9:25–34.
5. Angrist, B., Schweitzer, J., Friedhoff, A., Gershon, S., Hekimian, L., and Floyd, A. (1969): *Int. Pharmacopsychiatry,* 2:125–139.
6. Angrist, B., Thompson, H., Shopsin, B., and Gershon, S. (1975): *Psychopharmacologia,* 44:273–280.
7. Annunziato, L. (1979): *Neuroendocrinology,* 29:66–76.
8. Antelman, S. M., and Chiodo, L. A. (1981): *Biol. Psychiatry,* 16:717–727.
9. Arana, G., Boyd, A. E., III, Reichlin, S., and Lipsitt, D. (1976): *Psychosom. Med.,* 39:193–197.
10. Asberg, M., Bertilsson, L., Martensson, B., Scalia-Tomba, G.-P., Thoren, P., and Traskman-Bendz, L. (1984): *Acta Psychiatr. Scand.,* 69:201–219.
11. Ashcroft, G. W., Blackburn, I. M., Eccleston, D., Glen, A. I. M., Hartley, W., Kinloch, N. E., Lonergan, M., Murray, L. G., and Pullar, I. A. (1973): *Psychol. Med.,* 3:319–325.

12. Ashcroft, G. W., Eccleston, D., Murray, G., Glen, A. I. M., Crawford, T.-B., Pullar, I. A., Shields, P. J., Walter, D. S., Blackburn, I. M., Connechan, J., and Longeran, M. (1972): *Lancet,* 2:573–577.

13. Ashcroft, G. W., and Glen, A. I. M. (1974): *Adv. Biochem. Pharmacol.,* 11:335–339.

14. Asnis, G. M., Nathan, R. S., Halbreich, U., Halpern, F. S., and Sachar, E. J. (1980): *Am. J. Psychiatry,* 137:1117–1118.

15. Banki, C. M. (1977): *J. Neurochem.,* 28:255–257.

16. Banki, C. M., Molnar, G., and Fekete, I. (1981): *Arch. Psychiatr. Nervenkr.,* 229:345–353.

17. Berger, P. A., Faull, K. F., Kilkowski, J., Anderson, P. J., Kraemer, H., Davis, K. L., and Barchas, J. D. (1980): *Am. J. Psychiatry,* 137:174–180.

18. Berrettini, W. H., Nurnberger, J. I., Jr., Scheinin, M., Seppala, T., Linnoila, M., Narrow, W., Simmons-Alling, S., and Gershon, E. S. (1985): *Biol. Psychiatry,* 20:257–269.

19. Bouras, N., and Bridges, P. K. (1982): *Curr. Med. Res. Opin.,* 8: 150–153.

20. Bowden, C. L., Koslow, S. H., Hanin, I., Maas, J. W., Davis, J. M., and Robins, E. (1985): *Clin. Pharmacol. Ther.,* 37:316–324.

21. Bowers, M. B. (1972): *Psychopharmacology,* 23:26–33.

22. Bowers, M. B. (1974): *J. Nerv. Ment. Dis.,* 158:325–330.

23. Brodie, H. K. H., Sack, R., and Siever, L. (1973): In: *Serotonin and Behavior,* edited by J. Barchas and E. Usdin, pp. 549–627. Academic Press, New York.

24. Bunney, W. E., Jr., and Davis, J. M. (1965): *Arch. Gen. Psychiatry,* 13:483–494.

25. Bunney, W. E., Jr., and Garland, B. L. (1982): *Pharmacopsychiatry,* 15:111–115.

26. Bunney, W. E., Jr., Goodwin, F. K., Murphy, D. L., House, K., and Gordon, E. K. (1972): *Arch. Gen. Psychiatry,* 27:304–308.

27. Bunney, W. E., Jr., Post, R. M., Andersen, A. E., and Kopanda, R. T. (1977): *Commun. Psychopharmacol.,* 1:393–405.

28. Butcher, L. L., and Engel, J. (1969): *Brain Res.,* 15:233–241.

29. Casper, R. C., Davis, J. M., Pandey, G. N., Garver, D. L., and Dekirmenjian, H. (1977): *Psychoneuroendocrinology,* 2:105–113.

30. Checkley, S. A. (1979): *Psychol. Med.,* 9:107–116.

31. Checkley, S. A., and Crammer, J. L. (1977): *Br. J. Psychiatry,* 131:582–586.

32. Chiodo, L. A., and Antelman, S. M. (1980): *Eur. J. Pharmacol.,* 66:255–256.

33. Chiodo, L. A., and Antelman, S. M. (1980): *Science,* 210:799–801.

34. Cole, E. N., Groom, G. V., Link, J., O'Flanagan, P. M., and Seldrup, J. (1976): *Postgrad. Med. J.,* 52(*Suppl.* 3):93–100.

35. Colonna, L., Petit, M., and Lepine, J. P. (1979): *J. Affective Disord.,* 1:173–177.

36. Cookson, J. C., Moult, P. J. A., Wiles, D., and Besser, G. M. (1983): *Psychol. Med.,* 13:279–285.

37. Cookson, J. C., Silverstone, T., and Rees, L. (1982): *Br. J. Psychiatry,* 140:274–279.

38. Cookson, J., Silverstone, T., and Wells, B. (1981): *Acta Psychiatr. Scand.,* 64:381–397.

39. Coppen, A., and Ghose, K. (1978): *Psychopharmacology,* 59: 171–177.

40. Cutler, N. R., Post, R. M., and Bunney, W. E., Jr. (1979): *Commun. Psychopharmacol.,* 3:375–382.

41. Cutler, N. R., Post, R. M., Rey, A. C., and Bunney, W. E., Jr. (1981): *N. Engl. J. Med.,* 304:1088–1089.

42. Dahl, L.-E., Lundin, L., Le Fevre Honore, P., and Dencker, S. J. (1982): *Acta Psychiatr. Scand.,* 66:9–17.

43. Davis, K. L., Berger, P. A., and Hollister, L. E. (1976): *Psychopharmacol. Commun.,* 2:125–130.

44. Devanand, D. P., Bowers, M. B., Jr., Hoffman, F. J., Jr., and Nelson, J. C. (1984): *Psychiatry Res.,* 15:1–4.

45. Diggory, G. L., and Buckett, W. R. (1984): *Eur. J. Pharmacol.,* 105:257–263.

46. Durand, D., Martin, J. B., and Brazeau, P. (1977): *Endocrinology,* 100:722–728.

47. Estler, C. J. (1975): *Adv. Pharmacol. Chemother.,* 13:305–357.

48. Evans, J. P. M., Grahame-Smith, D. G., Green, A. R., and Tordoff, A. F. C. (1976): *Br. J. Pharmacol.,* 56:193–199.

49. Ferland, L., Labrie, F., Cusan, L., Dupont, A., Lepine, J., Beaulieu, M., Denizeau, F., and Lemay, A. (1980): In: *Endocrine Functions of the Brain,* edited by M. Motta, pp. 271–296. Raven Press, New York.

50. Fibiger, H. C., and Phillips, A. C. (1981): *Science,* 214:683–685.

51. Francis, A. F., Williams, P., Williams, R., Link, J., Cole, E. N., and Hughes, D. (1976): *Postgrad. Med. J.,* 52(*Suppl.* 3):87–91.

52. Friedman, E., Fung, F., and Gershon, S. (1977): *Eur. J. Pharmacol.,* 42:47–51.

53. Friend, W. C., Brown, G. M., Jawahir, G., Lee, T., and Seeman, P. (1978): *Am. J. Psychiatry,* 135:839–841.

54. Gallagher, D. W., Pert, A., and Bunney, W. E. (1978): *Nature,* 273:309–312.

55. Garfinkel, P. E., Brown, G. M., Warsh, J. J., and Stancer, H. C. (1979): *Psychoneuroendocrinology,* 4:13–20.

56. Garver, D. L., Pandey, G. M., Dekirmenjian, H., and DeLeon-Jones, F. (1975): *Am. J. Psychiatry,* 132:1149–1154.

57. Garver, D. L., Pandey, G. N., Hengeveld, C., and Davis, J. M. (1977): *Psychopharmacol. Bull.,* 13:61–63.

58. Gerner, R. H., Fairbanks, L., Anderson, G. M., Young, J. G., Scheinin, M., Linnoila, M., Hare, T., Shaywitz, B. A., and Cohen, D. J. (1984): *Am. J. Psychiatry,* 141:1533–1540.

59. Gerner, R. H., Post, R. M., and Bunney, W. E., Jr. (1976): *Am. J. Psychiatry,* 133:1177–1180.

60. Gerner, R. H., Post, R. M., Gillin, J. C., and Bunney, W. E., Jr. (1979): *J. Psychiatr. Res.,* 15:21–40.

61. Glassman, A. H., and Roose, S. P. (1981): *Arch. Gen. Psychiatry,* 38:424–427.

62. Gold, P. W., Goodwin, F. K., and Wehr, T. (1976): *Lancet,* 2: 1308–1309.

63. Golden, R. N., James, S. P., Sherer, M. A., Rudorfer, M. V., Sack, D. A., and Potter, W. Z. (1985): *Am. J. Psychiatry,* 142: 1459–1462.

64. Goodnick, P. J., and Meltzer, H. Y. (1983): *J. Clin. Psychopharmacol.,* 3:239–243.

65. Goodwin, F. K., Post, R. M., Dunner, D. L., and Gordon, E. K. (1973): *Am. J. Psychiatry,* 130:73–79.

66. Green, A. R., Heal, D. J., and Grahame-Smith, D. G. (1977): *Psychopharmacology,* 52:195–200.

67. Green, A. R., Heal, D. J., Johnson, P., Laurence, B. E., and Nimgaonkar, V. L. (1983): *Br. J. Pharmacol.,* 80:377–385.

68. Gudelsky, G. A. (1981): *Psychoneuroendocrinology,* 6:3–16.

69. Gunne, L., and Anggard, E. (1973): *J. Pharmacokinet. Biopharm.,* 1:481–495.

70. Halaris, A. E., and Freedman, D. X. (1975): In: *Biology of the Major Psychoses,* edited by D. X. Freedman, pp. 247–258. Raven Press, New York.

71. Halbreich, U., Grunhaus, L., and BenDavid, M. (1979): *Arch. Gen. Psychiatry,* 36:1183–1186.

72. Holcomb, H. H., Bannon, M. J., and Roth, R. H. (1982): *Eur. J. Pharmacol.,* 82:173–178.

73. Horrobin, P. F., Mtabji, J. P., and Karmali, R. A. (1976): *Postgrad. Med. J.,* 52(*Suppl.* 3):79–85.

74. Hurst, P. M., Radlow, R., Weidner, M. F., and Ross, S. (1973): *Psychol. Rep.,* 33:683–694.

75. Janowsky, D. S., El-Yousef, M. K., Davis, J. M., and Sekerke, H. J. (1973): *Arch. Gen. Psychiatry,* 28:185–191.

76. Janowsky, D. S., Judd, L., Huey, L., Roitman, N., and Parker, D. (1979): *Psychopharmacology,* 65:95–97.

77. Jenner, P., and Marsden, C. D. (1982): *Adv. Biochem. Psychopharmacol.,* 32:85–103.

78. Jimerson, D. C., and Berrettini, W. (1985): In: *Pathochemical Markers in Major Psychoses,* edited by H. Beckmann and P. Riederer, pp. 129–143. Springer-Verlag, Berlin.

79. Jimerson, D. C., Cutler, N. R., Post, R. M., Rey, A., Gold, P. W., Brown, G. M., and Bunney, W. E., Jr. (1984): *Psychiatry Res.,* 13:1–12.

80. Jimerson, D. C., and Post, R. M. (1984): In: *The Neurobiology of the Mood Disorders,* edited by R. M. Post and J. C. Ballenger, pp. 619–628. Williams and Wilkins, Baltimore.

81. Johnson, J. M. (1981): *Am. J. Psychiatry,* 138:980–982.

82. Jonsson, L.-E., Anggard, E., and Gunne, L.-M. (1971): *Clin. Pharmacol. Ther.,* 12:889–896.

83. Kasa, K., Otsuki, S., Yamamoto, M., Sato, M., Kuroda, H., and Ogawa, N. (1982): *Biol. Psychiatry,* 17:877–883.
84. Kiloh, L. G., Neilson, M., and Andrews, G. (1974): *Br. J. Psychiatry,* 125:496–499.
85. Klimek, V., Nielsen, M., and Maj, J. (1985): *Eur. J. Pharmacol.,* 109:131–132.
86. Koslow, S. H., Maas, J. W., Bowden, C. L., Davis, J. M., Hanin, I., and Javaid, J. (1983): *Arch. Gen. Psychiatry,* 40:999–1010.
87. Kozlowski, M. R., Neve, K. A., Grishman, J. E., and Marshall, J. F. (1983): *Brain Res.,* 267:301–311.
88. Lal, H., Brown, W., Drawbaugh, R., Hynes, M., and Brown, G. (1977): *Life Sci.,* 20:101–106.
89. Lal, S., De la Vega, C. E., and Sourkes, T. L. (1973): *J. Clin. Endocrinol. Metab.,* 37:719–724.
90. Lal, S., Guyda, H., and Bikadoroff, S. (1977): *Science,* 44:766–770.
91. Lal, S., Nair, N. P. V., and Guyda, H. (1978): *Acta Psychiatr. Scand.,* 57:91–96.
92. Lal, S., Thavndayil, J., Nair, N. P. V., Etienne, P., Rastogi, R., Schwartz, G., Pulman, J., and Guyda, H. (1981): *J. Neural Transm.,* 50:39–45.
93. Langer, G., Heinze, G., Reim, B., and Matussek, N. (1976): *Arch. Gen. Psychiatry,* 33:1471–1475.
94. Leblanc, H., Lachelin, G. C. L., Abu-Fadil, S., and Yen, S. S. C. (1976): *Psychol. Rep.,* 43:668–674.
95. LeDouarin, C., Oblin, A., Fage, D., and Scatton, B. (1983): *Eur. J. Pharmacol.,* 93:55–62.
96. Lee, T., and Tang, S. W. (1982): *Psychiatry Res.,* 7:111–119.
97. Linnoila, M., Karoum, F., and Potter, W. Z. (1983): *Arch. Gen. Psychiatry,* 40:1015–1017.
98. Maany, I., Frazer, A., and Mendels, J. (1975): *Biomed. Mass Spectrom.,* 40:162–163.
99. Maany, I., Mendels, J., Frazer, A., and Brunswick, D. (1979): *Neuropsychobiology,* 5:282–289.
100. Maas, J. W., Koslow, S. H., Katz, M. M., Bowden, C. L., Gibbons, R. L., Stokes, P. E., Robins, E., and Davis, J. M. (1984): *Am. J. Psychiatry,* 141:1159–1171.
101. MacNeil, D. A., and Gower, M. (1982): *Nature,* 298:302.
102. Maeda, K., Kato, Y., Ohgo, S., Chihara, K., Yoshimoto, Y., Yamaguchi, N., Kuromaru, S., and Imura, H. (1975): *J. Clin. Endocrinol. Metab.,* 40:501–505.
103. Maj, J., Rogoz, G., Skuza, G., and Sowinska, H. (1984): *J. Neural Transm.,* 60:273–282.
104. Marantz, R., Sachar, E. J., Weitzman, E., and Sassin, J. (1976): *Endocrinology,* 99:459–465.
105. Martin-Iverson, M. T., Leclere, J.-F., and Fibiger, H. C. (1983): *Eur. J. Pharmacol.,* 94:193–201.
106. McCann, S. M., and Ojeda, S. R. (1976): In: *Reviews of Neuroscience,* edited by S. Ehrenpreis and I. J. Kopin, pp. 91–110. Raven Press, New York.
107. McIntyre, I. M., Kuhn, C., Demitrou, S., Fucek, F. R., and Stanley, M. (1983): *Psychopharmacology,* 81:150–154.
108. Meltzer, H. Y., Kolakowska, T., Fang, V. S., Fogg, L., Robertson, A., Lewine, R., Strahilevitz, M., and Busch, D. (1984): *Arch. Gen. Psychiatry,* 41:512–519.
109. Mendlewicz, J., Linkowski, P., and Brauman, H. (1977): *Lancet,* 1:653.
110. Mendlewicz, J., Pinder, R. M., Stulemeijer, S. M., and Van Dorth, R. (1982): *J. Affective Disord.,* 4:219–226.
111. Mendlewicz, J., van Cauter, E., and Linkowski, P. (1980): *Life Sci.,* 27:2015–2024.
112. Modigh, K. (1975): *J. Neural Transm.,* 36:19–32.
113. Murphy, D. L., Brodie, H. K. H., Goodwin, F. K., and Bunney, W. E., Jr. (1971): *Nature,* 229:135–136.
114. Nolen, W. A. (1983): *J. Affective Disord.,* 5:91–96.
115. Nordin, C., Siwers, B., and Bertilsson, L. (1981): *Acta Psychiatr. Scand.,* 64:25–33.
116. Nurnberger, J. L., Jr., Gershon, E. S., Simmons, S., Ebert, M., Kessler, L. R., Dibble, E. D., Jimerson, S. S., Brown, G. M., Gold, P., Jimerson, D. C., Guroff, J. J., and Storch, F. I. (1982): *Psychoneuroendocrinology,* 7:163–176.
117. O'Donnell, J. M., and Seiden, L. S. (1984): *J. Pharmacol. Exp. Ther.,* 229:629–635.
118. Oreland, L., Wiberg, A., Asberg, M., Traskman, L., Sjostrand, L., Thoren, P., Bertilsson, L., and Tybring, G. (1981): *Psychiatry Res.,* 4:21–29.
119. Papeschi, R., and McClure, D. J. (1971): *Arch. Gen. Psychiatry,* 25:354–358.
120. Peroutka, S., and Snyder, S. H. (1980): *Science,* 210:88–90.
121. Pert, A., Rosenblatt, J. E., Sivit, C., Pert, C. B., and Bunney, W. E., Jr. (1978): *Science,* 201:171–173.
122. Polleri, A., Murialdo, G., Masturzo, P., Martucci, N., Palese, N., Agnoli, A., and Gasparetto, B. (1979): In: *Neuroendocrine Correlates in Neurology and Psychiatry,* edited by E. E. Muller and A. Agnoli, pp. 225–261. Elsevier/North Holland Biomedical Press, Amsterdam.
123. Post, R. M., Ballenger, J. C., and Goodwin, F. K. (1980): In: *Neurobiology of Cerebrospinal Fluid,* edited by J. H. Wood, pp. 685–717. Plenum Press, New York.
124. Post, R. M., Gerner, R. H., Carman, J. S., and Bunney, W. E., Jr. (1976): *Lancet,* 1:203–204.
125. Post, R. M., Gerner, R. H., Carman, J. S., Gillin, J. C., Jimerson, D. C., Goodwin, F. K., and Bunney, W. E., Jr. (1978): *Arch. Gen. Psychiatry,* 35:609–615.
126. Post, R. M., and Goodwin, F. K. (1974): *Arch. Gen. Psychiatry,* 25:234–239.
127. Post, R. M., Jimerson, D. C., Bunney, W. E., Jr., and Goodwin, F. K. (1980): *Psychopharmacology,* 67:297–305.
128. Potter, W. R., Scheinin, M., Golden, R. N., Rudorfer, M. V., Cowdry, R. W., Calil, H. M., Ross, R. J., and Linnoila, M. (1985): *Arch. Gen. Psychiatry,* 42:1171–1177.
129. Quock, R. M., Carino, M. A., and Horita, A. (1975): *Life Sci.,* 16:525–532.
130. Randrup, A., and Braestrup, C. (1977): *Psychopharmacology,* 53:309–314.
131. Randrup, A., Munkvad, I., Fog, R., Gerlach, J., Molander, L., Kjellberg, B., and Scheel-Kruger, J. (1975): *Curr. Dev. Psychopharmacol.,* 2:205–248.
132. Reches, A., Jackson-Lewis, V., and Fahn, S. (1984): *Psychopharmacology,* 82:330–334.
133. Richelson, E., and Pfenning, M. (1984): *Eur. J. Pharmacol.,* 104:277–286.
134. Roberts, J. M. (1959): *J. Ment. Sci.,* 105:703–713.
135. Robertson, M. M., and Trimble, M. R. (1982): *J. Affective Disord.,* 4:173–193.
136. Roy, A., Pickar, D., Linnoila, M., Doran, A. R., Ninan, P., and Paul, S. M. (1985): *Psychiatry Res.,* 15:281–292.
137. Rubin, E. H., and Wooten, G. F. (1984): *Psychopharmacology,* 84:217–220.
138. Rudorfer, M. V., Golden, R. N., and Potter, W. Z. (1984): *Psychiatr. Clin. North Am.,* 7:519–534.
139. Sachar, E. J., Altman, N., Gruen, P. H., Glassman, A., Halpern, F. S., and Sassin, J. (1975): *Arch. Gen. Psychiatry,* 32:502–503.
140. Sachar, E. J., Frantz, A. G., Altman, N., and Sassin, J. (1973): *Am. J. Psychiatry,* 130:1362–1367.
141. Sack, R. L., and Goodwin, F. K. (1974): *Arch. Gen. Psychiatry,* 31:649–654.
142. Schildkraut, J. J. (1965): *Am. J. Psychiatry,* 122:509–522.
143. Sedvall, G., Fyro, B., Gullberg, B., Nyback, H., Wiesel, F.-A., and Wode-Helgodt, B. (1980): *Br. J. Psychiatry,* 136:366–374.
144. Serra, G., Argiolas, A., Klimek, V., Fadda, F., and Gessa, G. L. (1979): *Life Sci.,* 25:415–424.
145. Serra, G., Melis, M. R., Argiolas, A., Fadda, F., and Gessa, G. L. (1981): *Eur. J. Pharmacol.,* 72:131–135.
146. Shopsin, B., and Gershon, S. (1978): *Neuropsychobiology,* 4:1–14.
147. Sievers, B., Ringberger, V., Tuck, J. R., and Sjoqvist, F. (1977): *Clin. Pharmacol. Ther.,* 21:194.
148. Silberman, E. K., Reus, V. I., Jimerson, D. C., Lynott, A. M., and Post, R. M. (1981): *Am. J. Psychiatry,* 138:1302–1307.
149. Silverstone, T. (1984): *Lancet,* 1:903–904.
150. Sjostrom, R. (1973): *J. Clin. Pharmacol.,* 6:75–80.
151. Sjostrom, R. (1973): *Acta Univ. Upsaliensis,* 154:5–35.
152. Smialowski, A., and Maj, J. (1985): *Psychopharmacology,* 86:468–471.

153. Spyraki, C., and Fibiger, H. C. (1981): *Eur. J. Pharmacol.,* 74: 195–206.
154. Spyraki, C., Papadopoulou, Z., Kourkoubas, A., and Varonos, D. (1985): *Naunyn Schmiedebergs Arch. Pharmacol.,* 329:128–134.
155. Staunton, D. A., Magistretti, P. J., Showmaker, W. J., and Bloom, F. E. (1982): *Brain Res.,* 232:391–400.
156. Subrahmanyam, S. (1975): *Brain Res.,* 87:355–362.
157. Sugrue, M. F. (1980): *Life Sci.,* 26:423–429.
158. Sugrue, M. F. (1983): *Pharmacol. Ther.,* 21:1–33.
159. Swann, A. C., Secunda, S., Davis, J. M., Robins, E., Hanin, I., Koslow, S. H., and Maas, J. W. (1983): *Am. J. Psychiatry,* 140: 396–400.
160. Sweeney, D., Nelson, C., Bowers, M., Maas, J., and Heninger, G. (1978): *Lancet,* 2:100–101.
161. Swerdlow, N. R., Lee, D., Koob, G. F., and Vaccarino, F. J. (1985): *J. Pharmacol. Exp. Ther.,* 235:324–329.
162. Takahashi, S., Yamane, H., Kondo, H., Tani, N., and Kato, N. (1974): *Folia Psychiatr. Neurol. Jpn.,* 28:347–354.
163. Tang, S. W., Seeman, P., and Kwan, S. (1981): *Psychiatry Res.,* 4:129–138.
164. Theohar, C., Fischer-Cornelssen, K., Brosch, H., Fischer, E. K., and Petrovic, D. (1982): *Arzneimittelforsch.,* 32:783–789.
165. Traskman, L., Asberg, M., Bertilsson, L., Cronholm, B., Mellstrom, B., Neckers, L. M., Sjoqvist, F., Thoren, P., and Tybring, G. (1979): *Clin. Pharmacol. Ther.,* 26:600–610.
166. Traskman, L., Asberg, M., Bertilsson, L., and Sjostrand, L. (1981): *Arch. Gen. Psychiatry,* 38:631–636.
167. Tufik, S. (1981): *J. Pharm. Pharmacol.,* 33:732–733.
168. Van Praag, H. M., and Korf, J. (1971): *Psychopharmacologia,* 19:199–203.
169. Van Praag, H. M. S., and Korf, J. (1975): *Pharmakopsychiatrie,* 8:322–326.
170. Van Praag, H. M., Korf, J., and Schut, D. (1973): *Arch. Gen. Psychiatry,* 28:827–831.
171. van Sheyen, J. D., Van Praag, H. M., and Korf, J. (1977): *Br. J. Clin. Pharmacol.,* 4:179S–184S.
172. Vermier, T., Goodale, D. B., and Long, J. P. (1980): *J. Pharm. Pharmacol.,* 32:665–666.
173. Vestergaard, P., Sorensen, T., Hoppe, E., Raphaelsen, O. J., Yates, C. M., and Nicolaou, N. (1978): *Acta Psychiatr. Scand.,* 58:88–96.
174. Waehrens, J., and Gerlach, J. (1981): *J. Affective Disord.,* 3:193–202.
175. Wald, D., Ebstein, R. P., and Belmaker, R. H. (1978): *Psychopharmacology,* 57:83–87.
176. Waldmeier, P. C. (1982): *J. Pharm. Pharmacol.,* 34:391–394.
177. Welch, J., Kim, H., Fallon, S., and Liebman, J. (1982): *Nature,* 298:301–302.
178. Wielosz, M. (1981): *Neuropharmacology,* 20:941–945.
179. Willner, P. (1983): *Brain Res. Rev.,* 6:211–224.
180. Willner, P. (1983): *Brain Res. Rev.,* 6:225–236.
181. Willner, P. (1983): *Brain Res. Rev.,* 6:237–246.
182. Young, J. P. R., Hughes, W. C., and Lader, M. (1976): *Br. Med. J.,* 1:1116–1118.

Psychopharmacology:
The Third Generation of Progress,
edited by Herbert Y. Meltzer.
Raven Press, New York © 1987.

CHAPTER **52**

The Serotonin Hypothesis of Depression

Herbert Y. Meltzer and Martin T. Lowy

Serotonin (5-HT) has occupied a central place in current theories of the etiology of depression and, to a lesser extent, mania, for nearly two decades. It has been proposed that decreased serotonergic activity may increase vulnerability to affective disorders or may, in fact, produce depression (145). An alternative view that excessive serotonergic activity may cause depression has also been put forward (10,153). Early research concentrated on the possibility of decreased output of 5-HT as the cause of depression or mania, or as a factor increasing vulnerability to these disorders (43,105). In the last decade, increased understanding of the 5-HT reuptake process and identification of multiple subtypes of pre- and postsynaptic 5-HT receptors have suggested these mechanisms as primary etiological factors and critical to an understanding of the action of antidepressant drugs and electroconvulsive treatment (ECT), particularly their relatively slow rate of bringing about clinical response. The importance of considering interactions of 5-HT with other neurotransmitters that may also contribute to the pathophysiology of depression and mania, especially norepinephrine (NE), dopamine (DA), acetylcholine, and γ-aminobutyric acid (GABA) has also received particular attention.

This chapter will discuss the highlights of recent research on these issues with a view toward clarifying the role of the serotonergic system in the pathophysiology of affective disorders.

EFFECT OF SEROTONIN ON SOMATIC FUNCTIONS RELEVANT TO DEPRESSION

According to Vogt (208), 5-HT plays a key role in homeostasis, helping the organism to modulate excessive stimuli of a wide variety, make appropriate responses, and thus ward off feelings of fear, helplessness, and ensuing depression. Serotonin is usually thought to have an inhibitory influence on behavior (208) or a general modulatory effect (5). The widespread distribution of serotonergic terminals in the brain is the basis for the ability of 5-HT to influence nearly every brain function investigated. The effect of 5-HT is usually inhibitory, either directly or by stimulation of GABAergic or other inhibitory neurons (208). Serotonin has been implicated in the control of numerous specific behaviors (19). For 5-HT to have importance for the etiology of depression or mania, it must have a significant role, direct or indirect, in the regulation of those somatic processes that are disturbed in the mood disorders: e.g., mood, sleep, sexual activity, appetite, circadian rhythms, neuroendocrine function, body temperature, anxiety, motor activity, cognitive function, etc. The role of 5-HT in some of the behaviors affected during depression will now be reviewed.

Mood

A recent controlled trial in normal volunteers of the effect on mood of ingestion of amino acid mixtures that were (a) tryptophan-free, (b) balanced, or (c) tryptophan-loaded showed that the tryptophan-free mixture produced a mild depression of mood at 5 hr, when plasma tryptophan levels were at their nadir (221). Two studies have reported that L-tryptophan loading produced mood elevations in normals (37,182), and three reported negative results (47,73,111). The direct-acting 5-HT agonist m-chlorophenylpiperazine (m-CPP) produced a significant increase in activation-euphoria ratings in 14 normal volunteers (141). In general, these results suggest serotonergic activity may be relevant to mood.

Appetite

Decreased appetite is a frequent symptom of major depression. However, some depressed patients, particularly those with seasonal affective disorder, show increased appetite, particularly for carbohydrates (170). Increased serotonergic activity is generally associated with decreased food intake (27). This conclusion is based on the ability of 5-HT precursors, agonists, uptake inhibitors, and releasers to decrease food intake. Conversely, decreasing 5-HT activity, through 5-HT antagonists or some but not all lesions of 5-HT neurons, may lead to increased food intake and weight gain. Part of the discrepancy between the role of 5-HT in appetite regulation and the hyposerotonin hypothesis of depression may be due to the incomplete knowledge of the complex ways in which 5-HT modulates food intake. For example, the 5-HT_{1A} agonist 8-hydroxy-2-(di-n-propylamine)tetralin (8-OH-DPAT) has been shown to increase food intake (61), possibly by stimulating 5-HT autoreceptors that diminish 5-HT release. Increased stimulation of 5-HT_{1A} autoreceptors could cause appetite loss in depression by ultimately decreasing serotonergic neurotransmission (20). However, conclusions about the role of 5-HT in regulation of physiological functions based on administration of exogenous agents may not be valid (133,219).

Sleep Studies

Sleep disturbances are one of the most common symptoms of depression. The effect of 5-HT on sleep function has been reviewed in detail (163). Increased 5-HT activity is believed to promote total sleep time. Inhibition of 5-HT synthesis with parachlorophenylalanine (PCPA) produces insomnia (174), whereas tryptophan improves sleep in some, but not all, studies (77). Thus, decreased availability of 5-HT could very well contribute to insomnia. Pharmacological studies provide more evidence for an effect of 5-HT on sleep architecture in relation to depression. Decreased

latency to rapid eye movement (REM) is the sleep abnormality most characteristic of major depression (104). That this could be related to decreased 5-HT is suggested by the findings that increasing the availability of 5-HT by fenfluramine (66) or zimelidine (168), a selective 5-HT uptake blocker, lengthens REM latency.

Sexual Function

Loss of sexual interest is another classical somatic symptom sometimes associated with depression. Serotonin, in general, has an inhibitory effect on release of gonadal hormones and sexual behavior (122). This is based on observations that drugs which enhance 5-HT activity suppress sexual function, whereas depletion of brain 5-HT by PCPA or 5,7-dihydroxytryptamine facilitates sexual behavior. The decrease in libido during depression may also be a secondary phenomenon, e.g., due to loss of interest, motor retardation, etc.

Pain

Increased pain sensitivity is a common complaint among depressed patients; approximately 50% of depressed patients report pain as a symptom (209). A large amount of experimental evidence suggests that 5-HT is involved in antinociception (169). For example, increases in serotonergic activity produce analgesia in both laboratory animals and patients with chronic pain, which may be related to an interaction with an endogenous opiate system (169). Thus, it would appear that the putative decrease in brain serotonergic activity in depressed patients could contribute to the increased self-reports of pain in depression.

Circadian Rhythms

Several lines of evidence suggest that disturbances in circadian rhythms occur in some patients with affective disorders (214). The suprachiasmatic nucleus, a critical brain structure involved in circadian rhythms, is richly innervated with 5-HT neurons. Central 5-HT content (165) and 5-HT receptors (33) have a well-established circadian rhythm that may mediate the circadian rhythm of various hormones, particularly the hypothalamic-pituitary-adrenal (HPA) axis (98). Serotonergic abnormalities could be related to the flattened circadian cortisol rhythm present in depressed patients (173).

Body Temperature

Temperature elevations and probable shifts in the time of nocturnal minimal temperature have been reported in patients with affective disorder (14). There is strong evidence that 5-HT affects body temperature in rats (74). Stimulating 5-HT_1 receptors may lower temperature whereas stimulating 5-HT_2 receptors enhances body temperature (74). Thus, the observed changes in temperature in depressed patients may be due to diminished activity of 5-HT_1 receptors or increased 5-HT_2 activity.

Comment

In addition to the functions already described, 5-HT has an important role in regulating neuroendocrine function, which may be disturbed in depression, especially the HPA axis (128), motor activity (136), anxiety (84), memory (7), and aggression (199). It is also of interest to note that stress is associated with increased presynaptic (92) and postsynaptic (93) serotonergic activity. Failure of serotonergic neurotransmission to respond to stress adequately could be a factor in depression. Recent findings that a new class of anxiolytic drugs, e.g., buspirone, are potent 5-HT$_{1A}$ agonists (158) and that buspirone may have some antidepressant action (176) provide additional support for the 5-HT hypothesis of depression. The increasing evidence that anxiety and depressive disorders lie on a continuum (8) and that 5-HT, along with NE, may be important to both should have a powerful shaping influence on future research. In all these areas, decreased serotonergic activity is most consistent with the symptoms of depression.

Thus decreased serotonergic activity is consistent with many of the changes in mood and somatic function observed in depressed patients, e.g., depressed mood, insomnia, decreased REM latency, disturbed circadian rhythms, abnormal neuroendocrine function, anxiety, inability to cope with stress, decreased motor activity, etc. However, decreased serotonergic activity may or may not be consistent with the observed changes in appetite, sexual behavior, and temperature regulation usually present in depression. It is possible that in depression, persistent stress leads to a failure of the adaptive mechanisms dependent on serotonergic activity. A mixture of increased as well as decreased pre- or postsynaptic serotonergic activity may be present in depression. The independent regulation of various 5-HT-dependent behaviors, based on anatomical specificity, receptor differences, and local control mechanisms, has been discussed by Ogren and Johansson (154). Other neurotransmitters, e.g., NE or acetylcholine, which are affected by 5-HT, or which directly affect some of the behaviors discussed in this section, no doubt also contribute to the symptomatology of depression.

ANIMAL MODELS OF DEPRESSION

Animal models of depression have been extensively used to test hypotheses of the neurobiology of depression, the mechanisms of action of antidepressants, and to screen for new antidepressants. Intracranial self-stimulation (ICSS) (e.g., behavioral despair), chronic stress, learned helplessness, primate separation, and olfactory bulb lesions appear to be the most promising models (86,216). These are discussed in detail in Chapter 70, *this volume*. Various types of evidence indicate that dysfunction of the serotonergic system occurs in many of these models. The evidence for a central role of a 5-HT deficit or 5-HT–catecholamine interaction in these models is perhaps clearest for olfactory bulbectomy (36). Self-stimulation in the median raphe is dependent on intact serotonergic neurotransmission (132). It is also noteworthy that learned helplessness decreases [^{3}H]imipramine binding (IB) in rat cortex but not septum or hippocampus

(180). It should be noted that some animal models of depression are more consistent with increased rather than decreased serotonergic activity (31,80). The available evidence from animal models of depression appears to be most consistent with the hyposerotonergic hypothesis.

CEREBROSPINAL FLUID 5-HYDROXYINDOLEACETIC ACID

Information about the turnover of 5-HT in brain is of critical importance for understanding serotonergic activity in depression and the effect of treatment thereon. The levels of 5-hydroxyindoleacetic acid (5-HIAA), the major metabolite of 5-HT, in cerebrospinal fluid (CSF) have been used as the indicator of central serotonergic activity. Lumbar CSF 5-HIAA concentrations have been reported to be correlated with brain 5-HIAA in humans (189). However, it is estimated that half the concentration of lumbar 5-HIAA comes from spinal cord (17,220). Tryptophan loading increases 5-HIAA in lumbar as well as cisternal (220) and ventricular (100) CSF. There are pronounced gradients in CSF 5-HIAA related to differences in height that must be considered in interpreting CSF 5-HIAA concentrations (17,25). Some studies suggest sex effects must also be considered (101). However, these findings are controversial, and stress effects related to environmental factors may have important influence on CSF 5-HIAA levels (75). No evidence for any effect of prior drug treatment on CSF 5-HIAA was found by Asberg et al. (13). Probenecid treatment to block the egress of 5-HIAA from the CSF has been suggested as a means of obtaining an estimate of the rate of transport of 5-HIAA within the CSF (64), but the usefulness of this method has been challenged (47).

Despite increased awareness of the factors affecting CSF 5-HIAA levels, there is still significant disagreement about whether its levels are lower in depression *per se*. Two of the more comprehensive recent studies (6,13) have reported significantly lower CSF 5-HIAA levels in a combined group of hospitalized, drug-free unipolar and bipolar depressed patients compared to normal controls. However, no differences in CSF 5-HIAA between unmedicated depressed patients and controls were noted in many other studies (18,172,207), including those with probenecid pretreatment (21,99). Finally, increased CSF 5-HIAA in depressed and manic female patients, but no differences between male depressives and controls, has also been reported (101). Increased CSF 5-HIAA levels were also reported in eight delusional depressed patients compared to 42 nonpsychotic depressed patients (4). CSF 5-HIAA remained fairly stable in seven depressed patients from one episode to another and in 16 normal volunteers studied over a 1- to 3-month period (197). However, in 11 of the 18 depressed patients studied, CSF 5-HIAA increased after recovery, but these were the patients whose initial 5-HIAA levels were low. It was proposed that this may be a subgroup with a less stable 5-HT system (197). The evidence for the stability of CSF 5-HIAA levels between illness and recovery in depression is mixed (197). Normal CSF levels of 5-HIAA were reported in 25 lithium-treated euthymic bipolar patients (24).

The reasons for these discrepancies do not appear to be

assay differences. The control or comparison group 5-HIAA levels in most studies are quite similar. The care with which standard conditions for obtaining lumbar CSF were observed appears similar. Methods of diagnosis and severity of illness appear comparable. It has been suggested that low CSF 5-HIAA is related to some aspect of depression such as suicide (see Chapter 65, *this volume*) and that the discrepancies between studies may be due to the proportion of such patients in any given study. A positive correlation between ventricular enlargement and ventricular 5-HIAA levels in depressed patients undergoing stereotactic subcaudate tractotomy has been reported (187). Other factors such as polarity, psychosis, endogenous features, retardation/agitation, stress, sleep disturbances, amino acid imbalances, etc., may also contribute to differences. It seems unlikely that determination of CSF 5-HIAA will serve as a biological marker for depression, although it appears to have some merit as a measure of central serotonergic activity. Positron emission tomography may provide a more accurate, regional estimate of central serotonergic activity.

A number of studies have examined the relationship between CSF 5-HIAA and depressive symptomatology other than suicide (6,16,18,51,106,172). Some studies have reported positive correlations between CSF 5-HIAA and depressive symptoms (6,106,172), others no effect or the opposite (6,51).

Both low and high CSF 5-HIAA levels have been reported to predict clinical response to antidepressant drugs (90). Van Praag et al. (205) reported that low 5-HIAA predicted response to 5-HTP. Maas et al. (120) found that low CSF 5-HIAA predicted a good clinical response to imipramine but not amitriptyline, and Aberg-Wistedt et al. (3) reported that it predicted response to zimelidine, a 5-HT uptake blocker. Imipramine and amitriptyline decreased CSF 5-HIAA levels, but the magnitude of the difference did not relate to clinical response (28). There is mixed evidence for the effect of ECT on CSF 5-HIAA levels (82).

It is difficult to draw any firm conclusions on 5-HT turnover in depression from the extensive research with CSF 5-HIAA, except that no finding is robust enough to achieve widespread replication, despite increasing sophistication about the variables that affect it. The stability of CSF 5-HIAA levels in controls and depressed patients suggests it is not spontaneous fluctuations in these levels that account for the discrepancies in various studies. It seems likely that not yet identified factors affect CSF 5-HIAA levels. Further research to identify the factors may be necessary before valid findings will be obtained. It is also likely that multiple neurotransmitter metabolites and neuromodulators will have to be accounted for to reliably ascertain the significance of any one neurotransmitter system.

PLASMA TRYPTOPHAN

There has been extensive recent investigation of the possibility that the availability of tryptophan in brain may contribute to the deficiency of 5-HT in depression. Since tryptophan hydroxylase (TH) is the rate-limiting step in the synthesis of 5-HT from the essential amino acid tryptophan, and TH is not normally saturated by its substrate, changes in brain tryptophan levels could influence the rate of 5-HT synthesis. Studies in recent years have focused on the importance of total vs free (unbound) plasma tryptophan and the ratio of tryptophan to large neutral amino acids that compete with tryptophan for transport via a carrier across the blood-brain barrier (155).

There have been about 25 studies of the concentration of free tryptophan in depression. Half of the studies report significantly lower levels of plasma free tryptophan in depressed patients (137). Total plasma tryptophan levels are not decreased in depression (138,139). There is no difference in the diurnal rhythm in plasma tryptophan levels between depressed patients and normal controls (49). Carbamazepine, which has both antidepressant and antimanic effects, increases both total and free tryptophan (160). Neither free nor total plasma tryptophan levels predict clinical response to L-tryptophan with or without tricyclic antidepressants (41,196).

Administration of one of the amino acids, e.g., leucine, isoleucine, valine, tyrosine, and phenylalanine, that compete with tryptophan for brain transport can decrease brain tryptophan and 5-HT under some conditions (65). However, there is other evidence that changes in levels of these amino acids within the physiological range do not significantly affect brain tryptophan levels (70,175). DeMeyer et al. (52) found an inverse correlation between Hamilton Depression Rating Scale (HDRS) scores and the ratio of plasma tryptophan to five neutral amino acids in 18 unmedicated unipolar depressed patients studied over a 4-day period. This study, while carefully controlled, is remarkable because of the marked improvement of the depressed patients over a very brief period with no somatic treatment. Moller et al. (139) found that a low tryptophan/neutral amino acid ratio predicted a better response to L-tryptophan. However, there was considerable overlap in the plasma tryptophan/amino acid ratio between the full patient sample and normal controls. These results are consistent with a previous study from the same authors (138) in which four depressed responders to L-tryptophan had the lowest plasma tryptophan/amino acid ratio. Joseph et al. (87) found that the tryptophan/amino acid ratio did differentiate depressives from normal controls. Although the ratio was unrelated to response to the overnight dexamethasone suppression test, it did help predict, along with 1600 hr post dexamethasone cortisol levels, the HDRS scores. Citalopram was found to increase the plasma tryptophan/neutral amino acid ratio during a clinical trial, suggesting increased 5-HT synthesis might be a result (22).

Abnormalities of tryptophan metabolism must be considered as a possible cause of a 5-HT deficiency in depression. Two studies of plasma tryptophan following oral tryptophan administration over the subsequent 6 hr found no differences between depressed patients and normal controls (81,140). However, Smith and Stromgren (183) found significantly lower serum tryptophan levels following an oral tryptophan load in a 6-hr study in 13 depressed patients, endogenous type, compared to 13 volunteers. Some patients were receiving psychotropic drugs. This difference persisted after a clinically effective course of ECT. We have observed significant differences in the pharmacokinetics of plasma tryptophan following intravenous tryptophan, 100 mg/kg, in depressed patients (103). We noted a larger volume of distribution and a longer half-life in the depressed patients. This suggested less tryptophan was available to the depressed patients and a slower rate of utilization by some or all of its metabolic pathways, including tryptophan hydroxylase.

In summary, abnormalities of tryptophan availability and its conversion to 5-HTP appear to be a promising area for further exploration of why serotonergic activity may be decreased in some depressions.

SEROTONIN UPTAKE AND IMIPRAMINE BINDING IN PLATELETS

The blood platelet has many features in common with 5-HT neurons (186). Many studies have reported decreased platelet 5-HT uptake in unmedicated depressed patients (44,124,193,198). This is mainly due to a decrease in the number of uptake sites (V_{max}). Manic patients also have decreased V_{max} (124). The number of uptake sites remains decreased after recovery in unipolar depressed patients (44,177) but has been reported to be normal in recovered manic patients off lithium (72). Chronic administration of lithium increases V_{max} (45). V_{max} is most decreased in bipolar depressed patients (124). No significant relationship between V_{max} and severity of depression has been reported. There is too much overlap between V_{max} of depressed patients and normal controls and other types of psychiatric patients for it to be of value as a diagnostic tool by itself, but it may be of use in combination with other markers, such as the Dexamethasone Suppression Test (DST) (126) or IB. Serotonin uptake in platelet did not predict response to zimelidine or desipramine (2).

There is no evidence that decreased V_{max} without any change in affinity for 5-HT (K_m) is an artifact of drug treatment. It appears to be robust evidence of a 5-HT abnormality in affective disorders, but its significance is unclear. The decrease in the number of uptake sites would, if it occurred in the CNS, be associated with less 5-HT uptake and more 5-HT at the synapse. This would ordinarily be expected to have an antidepressant effect unless it led to a selective stimulation of 5-HT autoreceptors, which would decrease 5-HT synthesis and release. Otherwise, decreased V_{max} might be construed as an adaptive response to restore serotonergic function toward normal.

Platelet imipramine binding (IB) has been reported to be decreased in depressed patients in many studies (29,125,157,194,210). The decrease in IB is due to a decrease in the number of IB sites, B_{max}. The IB site modulates 5-HT uptake. A decrease in B_{max} should lead to increased 5-HT uptake and, if present in brain, might contribute to decreased 5-HT. No significant correlation between decrease in V_{max} of 5-HT uptake and B_{max} of IB has been found in any study. Unlike the decreased number of 5-HT uptake sites, the B_{max} of IB has been found to normalize in recovered depressed (194) and bipolar patients (23).

IB sites in brain are located mainly on 5-HT nerve terminals (178). These appear to be particularly rich in the substantia nigra and the ventral tegmental area (67). This suggests the possibility that IB sites may have an important influence on brain dopaminergic function via their effect on 5-HT uptake. B_{max} of IB has been reported to be decreased in the frontal cortex of suicides (190) and the hippocampus and occipital cortex of depressed patients (159). These findings were not replicated in another study (156). Chronic administration of antidepressant drugs decreases the number of rat brain IB sites (95). This raises the possibility that decreased IB in brains of suicides may be an artifact of drug treatment. The finding that drug treatment produces down-regulation of brain IB sites and that untreated depressives show the same type of change suggests the decrease in B_{max} in depressed patients may, like the decrease in V_{max}, also be an adaptive response. ECT has no effect on IB in rat cortex but does increase the number of IB sites in platelet membranes (1).

Decreased platelet 5-HT uptake and IB provide new biochemical evidence for a serotonergic abnormality in major affective disorders. The postmortem studies of B_{max} are too preliminary to allow confidence about their validity. Further studies are indicated to determine whether brain 5-HT uptake in depression is, in fact, abnormal and whether it is increased or decreased. Regional differences are, of course, possible.

NEUROENDOCRINE STUDIES

Since the secretion of hormones can be influenced by 5-HT, various agents that affect serotonergic activity have been administered to patients with affective disorders in an effort to assess central serotonergic systems and the effect of somatic treatments on these systems. These agents include amino acid precursors of 5-HT, fenfluramine, and direct-acting 5-HT agonists such as m-CPP or MK-212.

The cortisol response to oral D,L-5-hydroxytryptophan (D,L-5-HTP), 200 mg, has been reported to be enhanced in unmedicated depressed and manic patients (129). This increase is associated with increased plasma corticotropin (ACTH) levels, suggesting a hypothalamic or pituitary response to the 5-HTP. No differences in plasma 5-HTP or 5-HIAA levels were found. The cortisol response to 5-HTP was inversely correlated with CSF 5-HIAA levels in the depressed patients (102). These findings suggest the enhanced 5-HTP-induced increase in cortisol in affective disorders could be due to stimulation of supersensitive 5-HT receptors. Both 5-HT$_{1A}$ and 5-HT$_2$ receptors stimulate cortisol secretion in humans (127); it is not clear whether only one of these or other types might be involved. 5-HT$_2$ receptors appear to be involved in mediating the prolactin (PRL) and cortisol, but not the growth hormone (GH) response, to insulin hypoglycemia (161). Increased numbers of 5-HT$_2$ receptors have been reported in the brains of suicide completers (188). However, the latter findings were not replicated by Owen et al. (156). These authors also found normal 5-HT$_1$ receptor density and brains of suicide completers. The 5-HTP-induced increase in cortisol was enhanced by treatment with lithium carbonate, whereas treatment with tricyclic antidepressants normalized the response (128).

Heninger et al. (79) have administered L-tryptophan, 100 mg/kg i.v., to unmedicated depressed patients and normal controls and found a diminished PRL response. Following treatment with desipramine or amitriptyline, the PRL response was normalized (38). A diminished PRL and GH response to tryptophan was also found by Koyama and Meltzer (103), but after covarying out differences in plasma tryptophan levels, which were lower in the depressed patients, only the GH response was diminished in the depressed patients. Diminished GH response could be due to a diminished conversion of tryptophan to 5-HTP and hence 5-HT, to subsensitive 5-HT receptors, or to some nonserotonergic mechanism by which such large doses of L-tryptophan stimulate PRL secretion. The 5-HT antagonist cyproheptadine did not consistently block the PRL or GH response to L-tryptophan (47); it did block the GH but not the PRL response to the 5-HT agonist N,N-dimethyltryptamine (H. Y. Meltzer et al., *unpublished data*). Further studies with more specific and potent 5-HT$_2$ antagonists are needed to clarify the issue of the mechanism of the L-tryptophan-induced increase in endocrine secretion. It is curious that no cortisol response was observed, since direct-acting 5-HT agonists, e.g., quipazine, have a greater effect on cortisol than PRL or GH secretion (129). It is also possible that PRL and cortisol are controlled by separate serotonergic systems that differ in their overall pattern of function, both pre- and postsynaptically. There is evidence that the 5-HT-dependent increases in prolactin and corticosterone in the rat are mediated by different neural mechanisms (200).

The PRL response to fenfluramine has been reported to be decreased in depressed patients (181). No difference between manic-depressives in remission and normal controls in the fall in cortisol levels during fenfluramine administration has been reported (143). Prolonged lithium treatment enhances the cortisol (143) and PRL (142) responses to fenfluramine. These discrepancies between the results of fenfluramine and precursors are possibly due to differences in the mechanism of action of fenfluramine and differences in regulation of PRL and the HPA axis. The ACTH and cortisol responses to fenfluramine in humans are blocked by cyproheptadine (110). The corticosterone response to fenfluramine is not serotonergically mediated, whereas the PRL response is at least partially so (200).

Studies with direct-acting 5-HT agonists such as MK-212 and *m*-CPP indicate potent effects on cortisol and ACTH in normal volunteers (118,141). There are as yet insufficient data comparing the cortisol responses in depressed or manic patients and normal controls with either of these agents.

There is also evidence linking the failure to suppress cortisol after dexamethasone to an abnormality in the serotonergic system (32,116,123,150). The HPA axis may, in turn, have marked effects on serotonergic neurotransmission, especially 5-HT receptor sensitivity and 5-HT uptake (12,34).

The results of neuroendocrine studies appear to be promising, but there are many pitfalls in such studies. It is necessary to use a variety of probes together with determination of plasma levels of the probes to adequately assess pre- and postsynaptic serotonergic mechanisms. Possible interactions with other neurotransmitters that influence hormone secretion and clearance must be considered. The available evidence suggests that there are 5-HT abnormalities in the hypothalamus in patients with affective disorders, most likely a decrease in 5-HT-dependent mechanisms.

EFFECT OF SEROTONIN PRECURSORS IN DEPRESSION

Tryptophan

There has been relatively minimal additional investigation of the antidepressant effects of L-tryptophan alone or in combination with other antidepressants since this topic was reviewed in this series (145). It is generally agreed that tryptophan alone is not as effective as standard antidepressant drugs in most clinical trials (35). In the studies reviewed by Cole et al. (42), 48 of 136 tryptophan-treated patients (35%) improved, a rate no better than that due to placebo treatment. Although tryptophan alone was as effective as antidepressant alone in several double-blind studies (41,119), the absence of a placebo group makes interpretation difficult. However, one recent study compared 115 depressed patients from five general practice settings in a 12-week double-blind study comparing L-tryptophan, amitriptyline, the combination, and placebo. All three active treatments were superior to placebo (196). This study suggests tryptophan is effective in the treatment of mild depression, possibly due to its mood-elevating or sleep-inducing effects.

L-Tryptophan potentiated the action of a tricyclic antidepressant or monoamine oxidase inhibitor (MAOI) in eight of 13 trials (15). However, this improvement was mainly in patients treated with MAOIs rather than tricyclic antidepressants. The latter group of studies suffered from small sample size, short duration, and questionable methods of sample selection and data analysis. Reversible neurologic toxicity may occur with the combination of tryptophan and an MAOI (195). L-Tryptophan did not enhance the rapidity of response to ECT (96). It should be noted that all patients responded to ECT in this study. L-Tryptophan has been found to have an inhibitory effect on seizure duration (166), which may counteract any ECT potentiating effect it has. Since ECT enhances the sensitivity of 5-HT$_2$ receptors, it is disappointing that tryptophan was not more effective in potentiating ECT. It could be that L-tryptophan is not the rate-limiting factor in 5-HT synthesis during ECT. In summary, tryptophan, as a treatment for major depression, appears to be effective mainly in conjunction with MAOIs. The failure of tricyclics and ECT to be potentiated by tryptophan suggests that caution is in order before attributing the ability of tryptophan to potentiate MAOIs to a serotonergic mechanism. It is possible that the effect of tryptophan on catecholamines may be more relevant to this action.

5-Hydroxytryptophan

There have been relatively few controlled studies of L-5-HTP, alone or in combination with an MAOI, a peripheral decarboxylase inhibitor, or a reuptake blocker, in major depression. Earlier studies, most of which were positive, have been reviewed by van Praag (202,203). Important post-1978 studies will be discussed here. Administration of 5-HTP with a peripheral decarboxylase inhibitor was as effective as 5-HTP plus the MAOI deprenyl in treating a mixed group of unipolar and bipolar depressions, but only the latter treatment was superior to placebo, producing improvement within 1 week for most improvers (131). Van Hiele (201) administered L-5-HTP plus carbidopa on an open basis to 99 previously refractory outpatient depressives. Previous treatments were continued. Of these 99, 43 responded by complete recovery and eight by partial recovery. Twenty-five of 44 endogenous depressions responded. Fifteen of the 24 responders showed hypomanic symptoms that responded to dosage reduction or, in two cases, lithium. In a controlled double-blind study of a subtherapeutic dose of chlorimipramine and L-5-HTP or placebo (146), a clear benefit of L-5-HTP was found in both endogenous and reactive depressions of both sexes ($N = 24$). L-5-HTP was particularly effective in relieving anxiety symptoms, which is of interest in regard to another study reporting a significant antianxiety effect of L-5-HTP in anxiety disorders (88) and evidence reviewed earlier for the role of 5-HT in anxiety. In several open and double-blind studies of L-5-HTP vs imipramine, Angst et al. (9) could find no difference in the two treatments in severely depressed hospitalized patients not selected for being treatment refractory. Kaneko et al. (89), in an uncontrolled study, also reported a rapid antidepressant effect of L-5-HTP alone in 10 of 18 hospitalized depressed patients. In a double-blind study of three groups of eight endogenous depressed patients given L-tryptophan, tryptophan plus L-5-HTP, or nomifensine for 3 weeks, the combination of tryptophan plus 5-HTP was superior to both other treatments (164). However, in a controlled crossover study of L-5-HTP alone vs tranylcypromine in refractory depressed patients, no evidence of an antidepressant effect of L-5-HTP could be found (149). In all, the evidence is fairly consistent for an antidepressant action of 5-HTP in combination with other antidepressants that might reasonably be expected to potentiate the effects of 5-HT. A controlled trial of antidepressant effects of the combination of lithium plus 5-HTP would be of interest. There is no evidence that unipolar or bipolar depressives differ in their response to 5-HTP.

Of considerable additional interest is the prophylactic use of 5-HTP in unipolar and bipolar disorder. In the only published study, van Praag and de Haan (204) compared the incidence of relapse in a crossover design of 1-year periods of placebo vs 5-HTP plus carbidopa, in two groups of 10 depressed patients. 5-HTP significantly reduced the number of relapses. Response was related to low CSF 5-HIAA levels. 5-HTP treatment was less effective than lithium in bipolar but not unipolar patients. If confirmed, these findings indicate that serotonergic activity is relevant to the vulnerability to become affectively ill.

The 5-HT precursors, tryptophan and 5-HTP, both appear to have an adjunctive role in the treatment of depression. Their efficacy might be due to secondary effects on other neurotransmitters, e.g., DA and NE, but the most parsimonious explanation of their efficacy is their ability to facilitate 5-HT synthesis and release. Documented enhancement of brain serotonergic activity, possibly through positron emission tomography, by the precursors, or blockade of their potentiating effect by selective 5-HT antagonists, would help to confirm the importance of 5-HT in depression.

Fenfluramine

A single dose of fenfluramine has been reported to produce a transient improvement in depression in some patients with major depression (213). No studies of fenfluramine as a treatment of depression have been carried out, possibly because of the potential toxic effects of this agent.

CLINICAL STUDIES OF "SPECIFIC" SEROTONIN UPTAKE BLOCKERS

Research on the mechanism of action of antidepressants was once dominated by the hypothesis that blockade of biogenic amine uptake was of critical importance. It is now known that in vitro studies may give erroneous impressions of specificity because active metabolites may show a different uptake blocking profile and because of as yet poorly understood effects on amine uptake processes through facets other than competitive or noncompetitive inhibition of the 5-HT transporter (121).

The classical tertiary tricyclic antidepressant drugs such as imipramine and amitriptyline are approximately equally active in vivo as inhibitors of 5-HT and NE uptake as indicated by effects of plasma from patients treated with these agents on the uptake of both biogenic amines by rat brain synaptosomes in vitro. The secondary amines derived from these drugs by metabolism, desipramine, and nortriptyline are relatively more potent as NE uptake inhibitors but still block 5-HT uptake into blood platelets (3). The view that uptake inhibition is crucially relevant to antidepressant drug action has faded because a number of effective antidepressants have minimal effects on 5-HT, NE, or DA uptake and are not MAOIs [e.g., iprindole and mianserin (222)] and because the time course of uptake blockade is much faster than the onset of antidepressant action.

Much effort has been expended to develop drugs that have a relatively high selectivity for inhibition of 5-HT uptake compared to NE uptake in vivo. This requires that the metabolites of these agents also be selective. Such agents were thought to be of value to test the hypothesis that 5-HT rather than NE might be the most relevant to the etiology of depression, i.e., that 5-HT might be involved in specific types of depressions or related to specific depressive syndromes. However, this approach assumed that these agents affected biogenic amine neurotransmitters only through their effect on uptake mechanisms. This is now known to be incorrect. Chronic administration of some 5-HT uptake blockers, e.g., zimelidine, will down-regulate β-adrenergic receptor binding sites (171) or produce a significant reduction in the sensitivity of the NE-coupled adenylate cyclase in rat forebrain (135). On the other hand, fluoxetine and citalopram, even more specific 5-HT uptake blockers than zimelidine, do not down-regulate β-adrenergic receptor binding sites (83,134). Despite the difference in effect on β-adrenergic receptors, all three drugs are clinically effective (2,83,112,211). Zimelidine has been shown to significantly reduce urinary 3-methoxy-4-hydroxyphenylglycol (MHPG) excretion, as did desipramine (113), leading to the suggestion of a mechanism common to both. Citalopram, another specific 5-HT blocker, was found to increase levels of homovanillic acid (HVA) (major metabolite of DA) in CSF and decrease levels of MHPG (major metabolite of NE) in CSF (22).

The issue of the effectiveness of specific 5-HT uptake blockers vis-a-vis uptake blockers that are more specific for NE uptake has been explored extensively. No significant difference in overall efficacy was found in two studies comparing zimelidine and desipramine (2,112). Of special interest is the finding of Aberg-Wistedt et al. (3) that low CSF 5-HIAA and HVA predicted better response to zimelidine. On the other hand, CSF MHPG levels were significantly higher in patients who responded to desipramine. Aberg-Wistedt et al. concluded that low 5-HT might be related to better response to 5-HT uptake blockers. However, Dahl et al. (48) found no relation between clinical response to femoxetine, another specific uptake blocker, and CSF 5-HIAA levels. Lingjaerde et al. (112) noted that nonresponders to zimelidine usually responded rapidly to desipramine and vice versa. In the absence of a random assignment to remain on the initial drug, it is difficult to conclude much from this potentially important strategy. Lingjaerde et al. (112) found a positive correlation between improvement and platelet 5-HT uptake in zimelidine-treated patients and not in the desipramine-treated patients, but Aberg-Wistedt et al. (3) found the opposite.

Nystrom et al. (152) found that the uptake of 5-HT by rat synaptosomes was less when incubated in plasma from female responders to zimelidine compared to zimelidine and maprotiline nonresponders, but no different when incubated in plasma from maprotiline responders. Knudsen et al. (97) found no difference in efficacy between nomifensine and zimelidine. Nystrom and Hallstrom (151) found no difference in the rate of response of mood, anxiety, retardation, or endogenous symptoms between maprotiline, an NE uptake blocker, and zimelidine, and concluded there was no relation of NE or 5-HT to any specific aspect of depression. They did find that responders to maprotiline had fewer prior episodes and fewer years since the first episode, whereas the zimelidine-treated patients who had more previous episodes and longer duration since the first episode responded better.

Walinder et al. (211) reported that the antidepressant effect of zimelidine was not potentiated by L-tryptophan, whereas many previous studies have shown that L-tryptophan potentiates the antidepressant effects of tricyclic antidepressants, e.g., chlorimipramine (212). They noted no difference in CSF 5-HIAA or HVA levels between responders and nonresponders. They did note a rapid response to zimelidine in some patients. Zimelidine has been withdrawn from clinical use because it produced Guillain-Barré syndrome in some users, but other specific 5-HT uptake blockers, e.g., fluoxetine, fluvoxamine, citalopram, and sertraline, are at various stages of clinical development throughout the world. In general, double-blind clinical studies of these drugs, e.g., citalopram (60), fluoxetine (40), fluvoxamine (59), femoxetine (48,167), and indalpine (147), show no significant difference between these drugs and comparison drugs that have a less specific effect on 5-HT uptake, e.g., desipramine or amitriptyline, or no effect, e.g., mianserin.

Overall, the results of clinical studies with specific 5-HT uptake blockers have not helped to clarify the role of 5-HT in depression. Their unquestionable efficacy does not necessarily mean that 5-HT is involved in depression or their antidepressant action. They have helped to rule out β-receptor down-regulation, which most do not produce as a necessary component of antidepressant action. The absence of any evidence that 5-HT uptake blockers that are not 5-HT antagonists exacerbate depression would seem to argue against the thesis of Ogren et al. (153) that a 5-HT excess is involved in depression. This depends on the view that the 5-HT uptake blockers will enhance 5-HT neurotransmission by prolonging the effect of 5-HT, but it must also be noted that these agents can diminish 5-HT neuronal firing, synthesis, and release via the feedback effect of released 5-HT on autoreceptors and perhaps postsynaptic receptors (55). Various preclinical studies have shown specific 5-HT blockers will enhance the functional effects of exogenous 5-HTP, but this does not necessarily apply to endogenous 5-HT, whose release in depression may, in fact, be seriously impaired. Future studies of the effect of 5-HT uptake blockers on specific symptoms will be of interest but may not clarify the role of 5-HT in depression unless accompanied by evidence showing 5-HT uptake blockade *per se* is more important to their efficacy than now appears to be the case.

LITHIUM CARBONATE POTENTIATION OF ANTIDEPRESSANT TREATMENT

DeMontigny et al. (58) reported that eight nonpsychotic unipolar major depression patients who were nonresponders following at least 3 weeks of treatment with a tricyclic antidepressant showed a significant improvement within 48 hr of beginning lithium carbonate treatment. Similar results have been reported with psychotic depressives and unipolar as well as bipolar depression (117,162). Lithium may also potentiate the antidepressant effects of MAOIs (148). Two controlled studies of the ability of lithium to enhance the action of antidepressants have been carried out (57,78). Using various research designs, supplemental lithium carbonate treatment was more effective than placebo in antidepressant-treated patients. Lithium had no such synergistic effect in placebo-treated patients. Clinical response to antidepressants plus lithium often occurs within 7 to 14 days rather than within 48 hr as first reported. These results have been supported by a number of case reports. Although no entirely negative studies have been reported, this may be merely selective publication, and some degree of reservation about the robustness of this phenomenon is still warranted. However, the impact of the combination is evident in that mania or hypomania has been noted shortly after lithium addition (117). This is analogous to the triggering of a manic episode by antidepressant treatment. The enhancement of antidepressant drug action by lithium could be due to lithium-induced enhancement of serotonergic neurotransmission (26). Evidence that lithium can enhance pre- and postsynaptic serotonergic activity has been reviewed elsewhere (126), but it is also possible that the enhancement by lithium could be related to potentiation or inhibition of other neurotransmitters, e.g., DA or NE, or a simple additive effect (78). Lithium has also been reported to decrease the plasma concentration of neutral amino acids that compete with tryptophan for entry into the brain, which might further stimulate 5-HT synthesis as discussed previously (108).

MANIC REACTIONS FOLLOWING ENHANCED SEROTONERGIC ACTIVITY: THE ROLE OF 5-HT IN MANIA

There are numerous reports of hypomania or mania or mania following L-tryptophan or 5-HTP. Wirz-Justice (218) noted seven of 12 studies in nonpsychiatric subjects in which either precursor produced disinhibition, mild to moderate euphoria, or, in one case, hypomania. Mania following L-tryptophan has also been reported in other studies (68,71,144), in six of 25 elderly unipolar depressed patients treated with chlorimipramine (206) and following treatment with antidepressants plus lithium (117). Case reports of mania during treatment with specific 5-HT blockers, e.g., fluoxetine (179), chlorimipramine, and citalopram (215), have been reported. As previously mentioned, hypomanic reactions occurred in 15 of 24 depressed patients given L-5-HTP plus carbidopa, in addition to various antidepressants that had previously been ineffective (201). However, L-tryptophan may also have antimanic effects, although this is controversial (40). This apparent paradox suggests that an interaction of 5-HT with other factors may determine whether 5-HT will depress or elevate mood. There are no reports of 5-HT-stimulating drugs worsening mania in subjects who are hypomanic or manic. These results indicate that a serotonergic stimulus can trigger a manic reaction, but they do not allow one to conclude that 5-HT itself is the immediate cause of mania. The switch from depression to mania is not specific for serotonergic drugs. The serotonergic stimulus may, while moving a person out of depression, provide a stimulus to some other system that is more directly related to manic symptoms. Future studies of the use of 5-HT antagonists to prevent or treat the switch process would be of interest.

EFFECT OF CHRONIC ANTIDEPRESSANTS ON SEROTONERGIC NEUROTRANSMISSION

Determination of the effects of antidepressant treatment on central serotonergic mechanisms must consider the variety of pre- and postsynaptic receptor mechanisms that affect neurotransmission, e.g., firing of 5-HT neurons, 5-HT synthesis, release, reuptake, MAO activity, autoreceptor induced-inhibition of 5-HT release, postsynaptic receptor sensitivity, direct stimulation of postsynaptic receptors (e.g.,

by a metabolite) or 5-HT receptor antagonism (e.g., amitriptyline). The multiplicity of effects can either synergize or counteract each other and these relationships can change over time as receptor-mediated tolerance develops, drug metabolism changes, and compensatory mechanisms develop. Moreover, the effects on different serotonergic systems may vary from one brain region to the other and across species. Therefore, extrapolation from preclinical studies is hazardous and mainly should be viewed as revealing possibilities that may be relevant to clinical findings. Clinical studies are most useful, especially if there is a relationship between clinical response and any putative change in serotonergic mechanisms.

There has been extensive investigation of the effects of antidepressant treatment on serotonergic mechanisms. This has been reviewed by deMontigny (56) and Willner (217) in great detail and will only be briefly summarized here. Acutely many antidepressants block 5-HT uptake or metabolism. Although this tends to increase 5-HT at the synapse, it also reduces the rate of 5-HT neuron firing and 5-HT synthesis, probably due to feedback on 5-HT autoreceptors. Some antidepressants also block 5-HT$_2$ receptors, e.g., mianserin, amitriptyline, trazodone. The net effect on 5-HT activity is, however, a potentiation. None of these acute effects appear to be relevant to clinical response.

Chronic administration of desipramine, imipramine, and related antidepressants decreases 5-HT levels and 5-HT turnover. The effects of 5-HT on most behaviors due to postsynaptic receptor stimulation are enhanced by antidepressant drug treatment despite down-regulation or no change in 5-HT$_2$ or 5-HT$_1$ ligand binding. However, chronic treatment with the 5-HT uptake blocker citalopram may decrease some responses to 5-HT agonists (11). Inositol phosphate as a second messenger for 5-HT$_2$ receptors has been intensively investigated recently. Chronic treatment with imipramine or iprindole produced a greater loss of 5-HT-induced inositol phospholipid hydrolysis than specific [^{3}H]ketanserin binding (91). Antidepressant treatments also affect NE, DA, GABA, acetylcholine and various neuropeptides (39). These effects may be as important as, or more relevant than, effects on 5-HT mechanisms. It can be concluded that consideration of the effect of antidepressants is compatible with the importance of 5-HT in depression but does not identify it as of singular importance for their action and does not illuminate the role of 5-HT in the etiology of depression.

ELECTROCONVULSIVE TREATMENT

There is little question that ECT is the most effective form of treatment for psychotic depression or severe nonpsychotic depression. ECT increased 5-HT content in several brain regions after a single shock or multiple shocks (63). There is conflicting evidence as to whether ECT decreases or increases 5-HT turnover as revealed by changes in CSF 5-HIAA levels (217). However, there is good evidence that chronic ECT produces functional increases in 5-HT neurotransmission subsequent to the administration of 5-HT precursors or direct agonists (63). This enhancement requires intact 5-HT and NE neurotransmission, and is blocked by

PCPA, 5-HT antagonists, or lesions of noradrenergic neurons. Chronic ECT increases the number of 5-HT$_2$ receptors in rat frontal cortex, an effect blocked by lesions of 5-HT neurons (191). Six ECT treatments increased the responsiveness of hippocampal neurons to 5-HT (54). Blood platelet but not cortical [^{3}H]IB sites are increased after ECT (1).

There is surprisingly little study of the effect of ECT on serotonergic mechanisms in humans. There are mixed reports of decreased CSF 5-HIAA after ECT (113). ECT decreased urinary 5-HIAA output (114). The significance of decreased urinary 5-HIAA is unknown.

Although this evidence strongly suggests ECT affects serotonergic systems, it also affects many other neurotransmitters, e.g., down-regulation of β-adrenergic receptors (109).

INTERACTION OF SEROTONIN WITH NORADRENERGIC, DOPAMINERGIC, AND GABA NEURONS

It is highly likely that neurotransmitters other than 5-HT also play an important role in the etiology of depression. Other chapters in this section consider the role of NE, DA, and acetylcholine in the etiology of affective disorders and the mechanism of action of mood-altering drugs (Chapters 50,51,53, this volume). There is also extensive evidence for the role of GABA in the action of antidepressant drugs (115). These neurotransmitters may have an independent role, act entirely or partially through 5-HT neurons, or be strongly affected by 5-HT neurons. All these mechanisms may, in fact, be significant for different behaviors, be relevant at different phases of the evolution of an episode of illness and its resolution, and differ among individuals. Species differences in the interactions of neurotransmitters may make it very hazardous to extrapolate from animal to human studies.

It is beyond the scope of this review to detail the many interactions between 5-HT neurons and other biogenic amine neurotransmitters. Only a few highlights and general principles can be cited.

Perhaps the most important interactions are between 5-HT and NE. Both systems clearly can influence the activity of each other through well-defined pathways between the midbrain raphe and locus ceruleus. Chronic antidepressant treatment or ECT effects on noradrenergic mechanisms require an intact NE system. Both α- and β-adrenergic drugs can affect 5-HT release, turnover, and receptors. It is possible, for example, that the ability of β-adrenergic blockers to produce depression may be related to their antagonism to 5-HT receptors. Lesions of 5-HT neurons up-regulate β-adrenergic receptors (192) and prevent the down-regulation of β-adrenergic receptors in the cortex of rats treated with desipramine (85).

There is considerable evidence that 5-HT inhibits various dopaminergic neuronal tracts. We have reviewed this evidence elsewhere (130). Fuxe et al. (69) have identified IB sites on the cell bodies of DA neurons, suggesting that 5-HT uptake or the endogenous ligand of the IB site may be important for the control of these DA neurons. There is

evidence that repeated administration of tryptophan, 5-HTP, MAOIs, and some tricyclic antidepressants inhibits the firing of 5-HT neurons (53). Eccleston (62) has proposed that some antidepressants act by removing the inhibitory effect of 5-HT on catecholaminergic neurons. Serotonin inhibits acetylcholine release from rat striatum by a presynaptic receptor-mediated mechanism (67). The possibility that increased cholinergic activity may produce depression is discussed by Janowsky (Chapter 53, this volume). It is possible this might be due, in part, to decreased serotonergic activity. Drugs acting as GABA receptors modulate the 5-HT-induced head twitch in mice (76) and the release of 5-HT (185). The importance of these interactions is discussed further in the conclusion of this chapter.

SEROTONIN AND ORGANIC BRAIN DISEASES

Some clues as to the possible role of 5-HT in mood regulation may be obtained from a consideration of the psychopathology of organic brain diseases with abnormalities of various kinds of 5-HT metabolism. Familial abnormalities of tryptophan metabolism, associated with high levels of plasma tryptophan, and markedly increased urinary 5-HIAA levels among other abnormalities of indole metabolism, are associated with depression and affective lability (184). Depressive symptoms are common in Alzheimer's disease, Parkinson's disease, Huntington's chorea, and multiple sclerosis. There is evidence of serotonergic hypofunction in all four disorders (e.g., 50,94). Several cases of stupor associated with low plasma tryptophan levels and presumably decreased brain 5-HT have been reported in carcinoid syndrome and L-dopa-treated Parkinson's disease (107). The depressive syndrome that occurs in some cancer patients has been hypothesized to relate to an autoimmune reaction that affects serotonergic neurotransmission but no direct evidence to support this interesting idea has yet been developed (30).

CONCLUSIONS

The hypothesis that 5-HT plays a major role in depression (and mania) cannot be rejected after this last decade of intensive research. Direct investigation of the serotonergic system in depressed patients has provided some biochemical (platelet 5-HT uptake and IB) and neuroendocrine (5-HTP-cortisol, tryptophan-GH) evidence that there is an abnormality of 5-HT in depression. Other serotonergic measures, such as amino acid ratios, CSF 5-HIAA, and measures of brain 5-HT, 5-HIAA, IB sites, and 5-HT$_2$ receptors, have also provided some support for the 5-HT hypothesis of depression. However, negative data of this type are less telling because of our still limited appreciation of the factors affecting these measures and problems in studying a full range of informative subjects with valid techniques. The same caution, of course, needs to be maintained with the positive findings noted above, especially the neuroendocrine evidence, but the weight of the positive studies seems, at the present time, to provide a fairly strong case for the hypothesis that serotonergic neurotransmission is disturbed in affective disorders. Psychopharmacologic studies have provided considerable support for the hyposerotonemia hypothesis, especially the more recent evidence that precursors such as tryptophan and 5-HTP have some supplementary antidepressant action. There is intriguing evidence that the lithium-enhancement of antidepressant drugs is due to the promotion of serotonergic activity, although it cannot be ruled out that there are other factors which account for this effect.

Some progress is apparent in determining what the primary defect or defects in serotonergic mechanisms in depression may be. The leading candidates for biochemical mechanisms of decreased serotonergic activity appear to be decreased availability of tryptophan compared to other pathways, excessive competition from other amino acids for entry of tryptophan into the brain, decreased conversion of tryptophan to 5-HT because of insufficient tryptophan hydroxylase activity, decreased firing of 5-HT neurons due to autoreceptor supersensitivity or adrenergic influences, increased reuptake of 5-HT, and decreased postsynaptic 5-HT receptor responsivity. There is no compelling reason why only one of these mechanisms may be responsible for too little serotonin activity. It is possible that each may be important for different patients; various combinations may be relevant in others. It is tempting to speculate that a combination of factors, none of which alone may be abnormal, could produce a net decrease in serotonergic activity. These possibilities need to be explored in further clinical studies.

We have previously discussed the evidence for interactions between 5-HT, NE, DA, GABA, and acetylcholine. Serotonin-opioid and other peptide interactions are also well-known and may be relevant. Further clinical research must consider these interactions through research designs that emphasize concomitant longitudinal assessment of various transmitter systems. Both peripheral and central mechanisms are potential targets for such investigations.

It is to be hoped that with another decade of research, we will attain definitive information as to which subtypes of affective disorders have a 5-HT abnormality, which disturbed functions are related to 5-HT, and to what extent 5-HT abnormalities are primary or secondary. Future studies must concentrate on longitudinal investigation of patients ranging from mildly to severely depressed, prior to and during treatment, as well as following remission and withdrawal of drugs. Such studies will permit identification of state-dependent and state-independent abnormalities that could be responsible for vulnerability. Defects in the regulation of many processes that comprise serotonergic neurotransmission, in relation to other neurotransmitter systems, may emerge as the most important factor in the etiology of depression.

ACKNOWLEDGMENTS

Supported in part by USPHS MH 41684, MH 41683, MH 41594, Research Scientist Award, MH 47808, and a grant from the Cleveland Foundation. The assistance of Diane Mack and Craig Stockmeier, Ph.D., in preparation of this manuscript is greatly appreciated.

REFERENCES

1. Abel, M. S., Clody, D. E., Wennogle, L. P., and Meyerson, L. R. (1985): *Biochem. Pharmacol.*, 34:679–683.
2. Aberg-Wistedt, A. (1982): *Acta Psychiatr. Scand.*, 66:50–65.
3. Aberg-Wistedt, A., Ross, S. B., Jostell, K.-G., and Sojquist, B. (1982): *Acta Psychiatr. Scand.*, 66:66–82.
4. Aberg-Wistedt, A., Wistedt, B., and Bertilsson, L. (1985): *Arch. Gen. Psychiatry*, 42:925–926.
5. Aghajanian, G. K. (1981): In: *Serotonin Neurotransmission and Behavior*, edited by B. L. Jacobs and A. Gelperin, pp. 156–185. MIT Press, Cambridge.
6. Agren, H. (1980): *Psychiatry Res.*, 3:211–224.
7. Altman, H. J., Nordy, D. A., and Ogren, S. O. (1984): *Psychopharmacology*, 84:496–502.
8. Angst, J., and Dobler-Mikola, A. (1985): *Eur. Arch. Psychiatr. Neurol. Sci.*, 235:179–186.
9. Angst, J., Woggon, B., and Schoepf, J. (1977): *Arch. Psychiatr. Nervenkr.*, 224:175–186.
10. Aprison, M. H., Takahashi, R., and Tachiki, K. (1977): In: *Neuropharmacology and Behavior*, edited by B. Haber and M. Aprison, pp. 23–53. Pergamon Press, New York.
11. Arnt, J., Fredricson Overo, K., Hyttel, J., and Olsen, R. (1984): *Psychopharmacology*, 84:457–465.
12. Arora, R. C., and Meltzer, H. Y. (1986): *Eur. J. Psychiatry*, 123:415–419.
13. Asberg, M., Bertilsson, L., Martensson, B., Scalla-Tomba, G.-P., Thoren, P., and Traskman-Bendz, L. (1984): *Acta Psychiatr. Scand.*, 69:201–219.
14. Avery, D. H., Wildschiodtz, G., and Rafaelsen, O. J. (1982): *J. Affective Disord.*, 4:61–71.
15. Baldessarini, R. J. (1984): *Psychopharmacol. Bull.*, 20:224–239.
16. Banki, C. M., and Molnar, G. (1981): *Biol. Psychiatry*, 16:753–762.
17. Banki, C. M., and Molnar, G. (1981): *Psychiatry Res.*, 5:23–32.
18. Banki, C. M., Vojnik, M., and Molnar, G. (1981): *J. Affective Disord.*, 3:81–89.
19. Barchas, J., and Usdin, E. (1973): In: *Serotonin and Behavior*. Academic Press, New York.
20. Bendotti, C., and Samanin, R. (1986): *Eur. J. Pharmacol.*, 121:147–150.
21. Berger, P. A., Faull, K. F., Kilkowski, J., Anderson, P. J., Kraemer, H., Davis, K. L., and Barchas, J. D. (1980): *Am. J. Psychiatry*, 137:174–180.
22. Berkenstedt, L., Edman, G., Flyckt, L., Hagenfeldt, L., Sedvall, G., and Wiesel, F. A. (1985): *Psychopharmacology*, 87:253–259.
23. Berrettini, W. H., Nurnberger, J. I., Jr., Post, R. M., and Gershon, E. S. (1982): *Psychiatry Res.*, 7:215–219.
24. Berrettini, W. H., Nurnberger, J. I., Scheinin, M., Seppala, T., Linnoila, M., Narrow, W., Simmons-Alling, S., and Gershon, E. S. (1985): *Biol. Psychiatry*, 20:257–269.
25. Bertilsson, L., Asberg, M., Lantto, O., Scalia-Tomba, G., Traskman-Bende, L., and Tybring, G. (1982): *Psychiatry Res.*, 6:77–83.
26. Blier, P., and de Montigny, C. (1985): *Eur. J. Pharmacol.*, 113:69–77.
27. Blundell, J. E. (1984): *Neuropharmacology*, 23:1537–1551.
28. Bowden, C. L., Koslow, S. H., Hanin, I., Maas, J. W., Davis, J. M., and Robins, E. (1985): *Clin. Pharmacol. Ther.*, 37:316–324.
29. Briley, M. S., Langer, S. Z., Raisman, R., Sechter, D., and Zarifran, E. (1980): *Science*, 209:303–305.
30. Brown, J. H., and Paraskevas, F. (1982): *Br. J. Psychiatry*, 141:227–232.
31. Brown, L., Rosellini, R. A., Samuels, O. B., and Riley, E. P. (1982): *Pharmacol. Biochem. Behav.*, 17:877–883.
32. Brown, W. A., Arato, M., and Shrivastava, R. (1986): *Am. J. Psychiatry*, 143:88–90.
33. Bruinink, A., Lichtensteiger, W., and Schlumpf, M. (1983): *Life Sci.*, 33:31–38.

34. Buckett, W. R., and Luscombe, G. P. (1984): *Br. J. Pharmacol.,* 81:132.
35. Byerley, W. F., and Risch, S. C. (1985): *J. Clin. Psychopharmacol.,* 5:196–206.
36. Cairncross, K. D., Cox, B., Forster, C., and Wren, A. F. (1979): *Psychoneuroendocrinology,* 4:253–272.
37. Charney, D. S., Heninger, G. R., and Reinhard, J. F. (1982): *Psychopharmacology,* 77:217–222.
38. Charney, D. S., Heninger, G. R., and Steinberg, D. E. (1984): *Arch. Gen. Psychiatry,* 41:398–404.
39. Charney, D. S., Mendes, D. B., and Heninger, G. R. (1981): *Arch. Gen. Psychiatry,* 38:1160–1180.
40. Chouinard, G., Young, S. N., and Annable, L. (1985): *Biol. Psychiatry,* 20:546–557.
41. Chouinard, G., Young, S. N., Annable, L., and Sourkes, T. L. (1979): *Acta Psychiatr. Scand.,* 59:395–414.
42. Cole, J. O., Hartmann, E., and Brigham, P. (1980): *McLean Hosp. J.,* 5:37–71.
43. Coppen, A., Prange, A. J., Hill, C., Whybrow, P. C., and Noguera, R. (1972): *Arch. Gen. Psychiatry,* 26:474–478.
44. Coppen, A., Swade, C., and Wood, K. (1978): *Clin. Chim. Acta,* 87:165–168.
45. Coppen, A., Swade, C., and Wood, K. (1980): *Br. J. Psychiatry,* 136:235–238.
46. Cowdry, R. W., Ebert, M. H., van Kammen, D. P., Post, R. M., and Goodwin, F. K. (1983): *Biol. Psychiatry,* 18:1287–1299.
47. Cowen, P. J., Gadhvi, H., Gosden, B., and Kolakowska, T. (1985): *Psychopharmacology,* 86:164–169.
48. Dahl, L.-E., Lunden, L., LeFevre Honore, P., and Dencker, S. J. (1982): *Acta Psychiatr. Scand.,* 66:9–17.
49. Dam, H., Mellerup, E. T., and Rafaelsen, O. J. (1984): *Acta Psychiatr. Scand.,* 69:190–196.
50. Davidson, D., Pullar, A. I., Mawdsley, C., Kinloch, N., and Yates, C. M. (1977): *J. Neurol. Neurosurg. Psychiatry,* 40:741–745.
51. Davis, K. L., Hollister, L. E., Mathe, A. A., Davis, B. M., Rothpearl, A. B., Faull, K. F., Hsiech, J. Y., Barchas, J. D., and Berger, P. A. (1981): *Am. J. Psychiatry,* 138:1555–1562.
52. De Meyer, M. K., Shea, P. A., Hendrie, H. C., and Yoshimura, N. N. (1981): *Arch. Gen. Psychiatry,* 38:642–646.
53. deMontigny, C. (1981): *J. Physiol. (Paris),* 77:455–461.
54. deMontigny, C. (1984): *J. Pharmacol. Exp. Ther.,* 228:230–234.
55. deMontigny, C., Blier, P., Caille, G., and Kouassi, E. (1981): *Acta Psychiatr. Scand.,* 63:79–90.
56. deMontigny, C., Blier, P., and Chaput, Y. (1984): *Neuropharmacology,* 23:1511–1520.
57. deMontigny, C., Cournoyer, G., Morissette, R., Langlois, R., and Caille, G. (1983): *Arch. Gen. Psychiatry,* 40:1327–1334.
58. deMontigny, C., Greenberg, F., Mayer, A., and Deschennes, J.-P. (1981): *Br. J. Psychiatry,* 138:252–256.
59. deWilde, J., and Doogan, D. P. (1982): *J. Affective Disord.,* 4:249–259.
60. deWilde, J., Mertens, C., Fredricson Overo, K., and Hopfner Petersen, H. E. (1985): *Acta Psychiatr. Scand.,* 72:89–96.
61. Dourish, C. T., Hutson, P. H., and Curzon, G. (1985): *Psychopharmacology,* 86:197–204.
62. Eccleston, D. (1981): *Br. J. Psychiatry,* 138:257–258.
63. Essman, W. B. (1986): *Ann. NY Acad. Sci.,* 462:99–104.
64. Faull, K. F., Kraemer, H. C., Barchas, J. D., and Berger, P. A. (1981): *Biol. Psychiatry,* 16:879–899.
65. Fernstrom, J. D., and Wurtman, R. J. (1972): *Science,* 414–416.
66. Fornal, C., and Radulovacki, M. (1983): *J. Pharmacol. Exp. Ther.,* 225:667–674.
67. Fuxe, K., Calza, L., Benfenati, F., Zini, I., and Agnati, L. F. (1983): *Proc. Natl. Acad. Sci. USA,* 80:3836–3840.
68. Gaylord, J. J., Parker, A. L., Phillips, E. M., and Roswell, A. R. (1973): *Br. J. Psychiatry,* 122:597–598.
69. Gillet, G., Ammor, S., and Fillion, G. (1985): *J. Neurochem.,* 45:1687–1691.
70. Gillman, P. K., Bartlett, J. R., Bridges, P. K., Hunt, A., Patel, A. J., Kantamaneni, B. D., and Curzon, G. (1981): *J. Neurochem.,* 37:410–417.
71. Goff, D. C. (1985): *Am. J. Psychiatry,* 142:1487–1488.
72. Goodnick, P. J., and Meltzer, H. Y. (1984): *Biol. Psychiatry,* 19:891–898.
73. Greenwood, M. H., Lader, M. H., Kantamenemi, B. D., and Curzon, G. (1975): *Br. J. Clin. Pharmacol.,* 2:165–172.
74. Gudelsky, G. A., Koenig, J. I., and Meltzer, H. Y. (1986): *Neuropharmacology,* 25:1307–1313.
75. Guthrie, S. K., Berrettini, W., Rubinow, D. R., Nurnberger, J. I., Bartko, J. J., and Linnoila, M. (1986): *Acta Psychiatr. Scand.,* 73:315–321.
76. Handley, S. L., and Singh, L. (1985): *Br. J. Pharmacol.,* 86:297–303.
77. Hartmann, E. (1983): *J. Psychiatr. Res.,* 17:107–113.
78. Heninger, G. R., Charney, D. S., and Sternberg, D. E. (1983): *Arch. Gen. Psychiatry,* 40:1335–1342.
79. Heninger, G. R., Charney, D. S., and Steinberg, D. E. (1984): *Arch. Gen. Psychiatry,* 41:398–402.
80. Hingtgen, J. N., Fuller, R. W., Mason, N. R., and Aprison, M. H. (1985): *Biol. Psychiatry,* 20:592–597.
81. Hoes, M. J. A. J. M., Loeffen, T., and Vree, T. B. (1981): *Psychopharmacology,* 75:350–353.
82. Hoffmann, G., Linkowski, P., Kerkhofs, M., Desmedt, D., and Mendlewicz, J. (1985): *Psychiatry Res.,* 16:199–206.
83. Hyttel, J., Fredricson Overo, K. F., and Arnt, J. (1984): *Psychopharmacology,* 83:20–27.
84. Iversen, S. D. (1984): *Neuropharmacology,* 23:1553–1560.
85. Janowski, A., Okada, F., Manier, D. H., Applegate, C. D., and Sulser, F. (1982): *Science,* 218:900–901.
86. Jesberger, J. A., and Richardson, J. S. (1985): *Biol. Psychiatry,* 20:764–784.
87. Joseph, M., Brewerton, T., Reus, V., and Stebbins, G. (1984): *Psychiatry Res.,* 11:185–192.
88. Kahn, S., and Westenberg, H. G. M. (1985): *J. Affective Disord.,* 8:197–200.
89. Kaneko, M., Kumashiro, H., Takahashi, Y., and Hoshino, Y. (1979): *Neuropsychobiology,* 5:232–241.
90. Kelwala, S., Jones, D., and Sitoram, N. (1983): *Prog. Neuropsychopharmacol. Biol. Psychiatry,* 7:229–240.
91. Kendall, D., and Nahorski, S. R. (1985): *J. Pharmacol. Exp. Ther.,* 233:473–479.
92. Kennett, G. A., and Joseph, M. (1981): *Neuropharmacology,* 20:39–43.
93. Kennett, G. A., Kickinson, S. L., and Curzon, G. (1985): *Brain Res.,* 330:253–263.
94. Kienzl, E., Riederer, P., Jellinger, K., and Wessemann, W. (1981): *J. Neural Transm.,* 51:113–122.
95. Kinnier, W. J., Chuang, D. M., Gyunn, G., and Costa, E. (1981): *Neuropharmacology,* 20:411–419.
96. Kirkegaard, C., Moller, S. E., and Bjorum, N. (1978): *Acta Psychiatr. Scand.,* 58:457–462.
97. Knudsen, P., Bjorndal, N., Johnson, T., and Pfeiffer-Petersen, K. (1984): *Neuropsychobiology,* 11:236–242.
98. Kordon, C., Hery, M., Szafarczyk, A., Ixart, G., and Assenmachet, I. (1981): *J. Physiol. (Paris),* 77:489–496.
99. Korf, J., van den Burg, W., and van den Hoofdakker, R. H. (1983): *Psychiatr. Clin.,* 16:1–16.
100. Koskiniemi, M., Laakso, J., Kieurne, T., Laipo, M., and Harkoven, M. (1985): *Acta Neurol. Scand.,* 71:127–132.
101. Koslow, S. H., Maas, J. W., Bowden, C. L., Dairs, J. M., Hanin, I., and Javaid, J. (1983): *Arch. Gen. Psychiatry,* 40:999–1014.
102. Koyama, T., Lowy, M. T., and Meltzer, H. Y. (1987): *Am. J. Psychiatry* (in press).
103. Koyama, T., and Meltzer, H. Y. (1986): In: *New Results in Depression Research,* edited by H. Hippius, pp. 169–188. Springer-Verlag, Berlin.
104. Kupfer, D. J. (1978): In: *Animal Models in Psychiatry and Neurology,* edited by I. Hanin and E. Usdin, pp. 181–188. Pergamon Press, New York.
105. Lapin, I. P., and Oxenkrug, G. F. (1969): *Lancet,* 1:132–136.
106. Leckman, J. F., Charney, D. S., Nelson, C. R., Heninger, G. R., and Bowers, M. B., Jr. (1981): In: *Recent Advances in Neuropsychopharmacology,* edited by B. Angrist, G. D. Burrows, M. Lader, O. Lingjaerde, G. Sedvall, and D. Wheatley, pp. 289–297. Pergamon Press, Oxford.

107. Lehmann, J. (1982): *Acta Psychiatr. Scand. (Suppl.),* 300:1–57.
108. Leighton, W. P., Rosenblatt, S., and Chanley, J. P. (1983): *Psychiatry Res.,* 8:33–40.
109. Lerer, B. (1984): *Biol. Psychiatry,* 19:361–383.
110. Lewis, D. A., and Sherman, B. M. (1984): *J. Clin. Endocrinol. Metab.,* 58:455–462.
111. Lieberman, H. R., Corkin, S., Spring, B. J., Growdon, J. H., and Wurtman, R. J. (1983): *J. Psychiatr. Res.,* 17:135–145.
112. Lingjaerde, O., Bratfos, O., Bratlid, T., and Haugi, J. O. (1983): *Acta Psychiatr. Scand.,* 68:22–30.
113. Linnoila, M., Karoum, F., Dalil, H. M., Kopin, I. J., and Potter, W. Z. (1982): *Arch. Gen. Psychiatry,* 39:1025–1028.
114. Linnoila, M., Litoritz, G., Scheinin, M., Chang, M.-D., and Cutler, N. R. (1984): *Biol. Psychiatry,* 19:79–84.
115. Lloyd, K. G., and Pilc, A. (1985): *J. Pharmacol. Exp. Ther.,* 235:191–199.
116. Lopez-Ibor, J. J., Saiz-Ruiz, J., and Perez de los Cobos, J. C. (1985): *Neuropsychobiology,* 14:67–74.
117. Louie, A. K., and Meltzer, H. Y. (1984): *J. Clin. Psychopharmacol.,* 4:316–321.
118. Lowy, M. T., Robertson, A. G., Koenig, J. I., and Meltzer, H. Y. (1987): *(submitted for publication).*
119. Lundberg, D., Ahlfors, H. G., Dencker, S. J., Fruensgaard, K., Hausten, S., Jensen, K., Ose, E., and Pihkansam, T. A. (1979): *Acta Psychiatr. Scand.,* 60:287–294.
120. Maas, J. W., Kocsis, J. H., Bowden, C. L., Davis, J. M., Redmond, D. E., Hanin, I., and Robins, E. (1982): *Psychol. Med.,* 12:37–43.
121. Manias, B., and Taylor, D. A. (1983): *Eur. J. Pharmacol.,* 95:305–309.
122. McEwen, B. S., and Parsons, B. (1982): *Annu. Rev. Pharmacol. Toxicol.,* 22:555–598.
123. McIntyre, I. M., Oxenkrug, G. F., Stanley, M., and Gershon, S. (1984): *Brain Res.,* 309:156–158.
124. Meltzer, H. Y., Arora, R. C., Baber, R., and Tricou, B. J. (1981): *Arch. Gen. Psychiatry,* 38:1325–1326.
125. Meltzer, H. Y., Arora, R. C., Robertson, A. G., and Lowy, M. T. (1984): *Clin. Neuropharmacol.,* 7:320–321.
126. Meltzer, H. Y., Arora, R. C., Tricou, B. J., and Fang, V. S. (1983): *Psychiatry Res.,* 8:41–48.
127. Meltzer, H. Y., and Gudelsky, G. A. (1987): In: *Buspirone: Mechanisms and Clinical Aspects,* edited by G. Tunnicliff, A. Eison, and D. Taylor *(in press).*
128. Meltzer, H. Y., Lowy, M. T., Robertson, A., Goodnick, P., and Perline, R. (1984): *Arch. Gen. Psychiatry,* 41:391–402.
129. Meltzer, H. Y., Umberkoman-Wiita, B., Robertson, A., Tricou, B. J., Lowy, M. T., and Perline, R. (1984): *Arch. Gen. Psychiatry,* 41:366–374.
130. Meltzer, H. Y., Young, M., Metz, J., Fang, V. S., Schyve, P. M., and Arora, R. C. (1979): *J. Neural Transm.,* 45:165–175.
131. Mendlewicz, J., and Youdin, M. B. H. (1980): *J. Affective Disord.,* 2:137–146.
132. Miliaressis, E. (1977): *Pharmacol. Biochem. Behav.,* 7:177–180.
133. Millhorn, D. E., Eldridge, F. L., Waldrop, T. G., and Klingler, L. E. (1983): *Brain Res.,* 264:349–354.
134. Mishra, R., Janowsky, A., and Sulser, F. (1979): *Eur. J. Pharmacol.,* 60:379–382.
135. Mishra, R., Janowsky, A., and Sulser, F. (1980): *Neuropharmacology,* 19:983–987.
136. Modigh, K. (1972): *Psychopharmacologia,* 23:48–54.
137. Moller, S. E., Kirk, L., Brandrup, E., Hollnagel, M., Kaldan, B., and Odum, K. (1983): *Adv. Biol. Psychiatry,* 10:30–46.
138. Moller, S. E., Kirk, L., and Fremming, K. H. (1976): *Psychopharmacology,* 49:205–213.
139. Moller, S. E., Kirk, L., and Honore, P. (1980): *J. Affective Disord.,* 2:47–59.
140. Moller, S. E., Kirk, L., and Honore, P. (1982): *Psychopharmacology,* 76:79–83.
141. Mueller, E. A., Murphy, D. L., and Sunderland, T. (1985): *J. Clin. Endocrinol. Metab.,* 61:1179–1184.
142. Muhlbauer, H. D. (1984): *Pharmacopsychiatry,* 17:191–193.
143. Muhlbauer, H. D., and Muller-Oerlinghausen, B. (1985): *J. Neural Transm.,* 61:81–94.
144. Murphy, D. L., Baker, M., Goodwin, F. K., Miller, H., Kotin, J., and Bunney, W. E., Jr. (1974): *Psychopharmacology,* 34:11–20.
145. Murphy, D. L., Campbell, I., and Costa, J. L. (1978): In: *Psychopharmacology: A Generation of Progress,* edited by M. A. Lipton, A. DiMascio, and K. F. Killam, pp. 1234–1248. Raven Press, New York.
146. Nardini, M., De Stefano, R., Iannuccelli, M., Borghesi, R., and Battistini, N. (1983): *Int. J. Clin. Pharm. Res.,* 111:239–250.
147. Naylor, G. J., and Martin, B. (1985): *Br. J. Psychiatry,* 147:306–309.
148. Nelson, J. C., and Byck, R. (1982): *Br. J. Psychiatry,* 141:85–86.
149. Nolen, W. A., Van de Putte, J. J., Dijken, W. A., and Kamp, J. S. (1985): *Br. J. Psychiatry,* 147:16–22.
150. Nuller, J. L., and Ostroumova, M. N. (1980): *Acta Psychiatr. Scand.,* 61:169–177.
151. Nystrom, C., and Hallstrom, T. (1985): *Acta Psychiatr. Scand.,* 72:6–15.
152. Nystrom, C., Ross, S. B., Hallstrom, T., and Kelder, D. (1986): *Acta Psychiatr. Scand.,* 73:133–138.
153. Ogren, S. O., Fuxe, K., Agnati, L. F., Gustafsson, J. A., and Holm, A. C. (1979): *J. Neural Transm.,* 45:85–103.
154. Ogren, S.-O., and Johansson, C. (1985): *Psychopharmacology,* 86:12–26.
155. Oldendorf, W. H. (1971): *Am. J. Physiol.,* 221:1629–1639.
156. Owen, F., Chambers, D. R., Cooper, S. J., Crow, T. J., Johnson, J. A., Hofthouse, R., and Poulter, M. (1986): *Brain Res.,* 362:185–188.
157. Paul, S. M., Rehavi, M., Skolnick, P., Ballenger, J. C., and Goodwin, F. K. (1981): *Arch. Gen. Psychiatry,* 38:1315–1317.
158. Peroutka, S. J. (1985): *Biol. Psychiatry,* 20:971–979.
159. Perry, E. K., Marshall, E. F., Blessed, G., Tomlinson, B. E., and Perry, R. H. (1983): *Br. J. Psychiatry,* 142:188–192.
160. Pratt, J. A., Jenner, P., Johnson, A. L., Shorvon, S. D., and Reynolds, E. H. (1984): *J. Neurol. Neurosurg. Psychiatry,* 47:1131–1133.
161. Prescott, R. W. G., Kendall-Taylor, P., Weightman, D. R., Watson, M. J., and Ratcliffe, W. A. (1984): *Clin. Endocrinol.,* 20:137–142.
162. Price, L. H., Conwell, Y., and Nelon, J. C. (1983): *Am. J. Psychiatry,* 140:318–322.
163. Puizillout, J. J., Gaudin-Chazal, G., Sayadi, A., and Vigier, D. (1981): *J. Physiol. (Paris),* 77:415–424.
164. Quadbeck, H., Lehmann, E., and Tegeler, J. (1984): *Neuropsychobiology,* 11:111–115.
165. Quay, W. B., and Meyer, D. C. (1978): In: *Serotonin in Health and Disease, Vol. 2,* edited by W. B. Essman, pp. 159–204. Medical and Science Books, New York.
166. Raotma, H. (1978): *Acta Psychiatr. Scand.,* 57:253–258.
167. Reebye, P. N., Yiptong, C., Samsoon, J., Schulsinger, F., and Favricus, J. (1982): *Pharmacopsychiatry,* 15:164–169.
168. Reyes, R. B., Hill, S. Y., and Kupfer, D. J. (1983): *Psychopharmacology,* 80:214–216.
169. Roberts, M. H. T. (1984): *Neuropharmacology,* 23:1529–1536.
170. Rosenthal, N. E., Sack, D. A., Gillin, J. C., Lewy, A. J., Goodwin, F. K., Davenport, Y., Mueller, P. S., Newsome, D. A., and Wehr, T. A. (1984): *Arch. Gen. Psychiatry,* 41:72–80.
171. Ross, S. B., Hall, H., Renyi, A. L., and Westerlund, D. (1981): *Psychopharmacology,* 72:219–225.
172. Roy, A., Pickar, D., Linnoila, M., Doran, A. R., Ninan, P., and Paul, S. M. (1985): *Psychiatry Res.,* 15:281–292.
173. Sachar, E. J., Hellman, J., Roffwarg, H. P., Halpern, F. S., Fukushima, D. K., and Gallagher, T. F. (1973): *Arch. Gen. Psychiatry,* 28:19–24.
174. Sallanon, M., Janin, M., Buda, C., and Jouvet, M. (1983): *Brain Res.,* 268:95–104.
175. Sarna, G. S., Tricklebank, M. D., Kantemaneni, B. D., Hunt, A., Patel, A. J., and Curzon, G. (1982): *J. Neurochem.,* 39:1283–1290.
176. Schweizer, E. E., Amsterdam, J., Rickels, K., Kaplan, M., and Droba, M. (1986): *Psychopharmacol. Bull.,* 22:183–191.

177. Scott, M., Reading, H. W., and Loudon, J. B. (1979): *Psychopharmacology,* 60:131–135.
178. Sette, M., Raisman, R., Briley, M., and Langer, S. Z. (1981): *J. Neurochem.,* 37:40–42.
179. Settle, E. C., Jr., and Settle, G. P. (1984): *Am. J. Psychiatry,* 141: 280–281.
180. Sherman, A. D., and Petty, F. (1984): *J. Affective Disord.,* 6:25–32.
181. Siever, L. J., Murphy, D. L., Slater, S., de la Vega, E., and Lipper, S. (1984): *Life Sci.,* 34:1029–1039.
182. Smith, B., and Prockop, D. J. (1962): *N. Engl. J. Med.,* 267: 1338–1341.
183. Smith, D. F., and Stromgren, L. S. (1981): *Pharmacopsychiatry,* 14:135–138.
184. Snedden, W., Mellor, C. S., and Martin, J. R. (1983): *Clin. Chim. Acta,* 131:247–256.
185. Soubrie, P., Montastruc, J.-L., Bourgoin, S., Reisine, T., Artaud, F., and Glowinski, J. (1981): *Eur. J. Pharmacol.,* 69:483–488.
186. Stahl, S. M. (1977): *Arch. Gen. Psychiatry,* 34:509–516.
187. Standish-Barry, H. M. A. S., Bouras, N., Hale, A. S., Bridges, P. K., and Bartlett, J. R. (1986): *Br. J. Psychiatry,* 148:386–392.
188. Stanley, M., and Mann, J. J. (1983): *Lancet,* 1:214–216.
189. Stanley, M., Traskman-Bendz, L., and Dorovin-Zis, K. (1985): *Life Sci.,* 37:1279–1286.
190. Stanley, M., Virgilio, J., and Gershon, S. (1982): *Science,* 216: 1337–1339.
191. Stockmeier, C. A., and Kellar, K. J. (1986): *Life Sci.,* 38:117–127.
192. Stockmeier, C. A., Martino, A. M., and Kellar, K. J. (1985): *Science,* 230:323–325.
193. Suranyi-Cadotte, B. E., Quiron, R., Nair, N. P. V., Lafaille, F., and Schwartz, G. (1985): *Life Sci.,* 36:795–799.
194. Suranyi-Cadotte, B. E., Wood, P. L., Vasavan Nair, N. P., and Schwartz, G. (1982): *Eur. J. Pharmacol.,* 85:357–358.
195. Thomas, J. M., and Rubin, E. H. (1984): *Am. J. Psychiatry,* 141: 281–283.
196. Thompson, J., Rankin, H., Ashcroft, G. W., Yates, C. M., McQueen, J. K., and Cummings, S. W. (1982): *Psychol. Med.,* 12:741–751.
197. Traskman-Bendz, L., Asberg, M., Bertilsson, L., and Thoren, P. (1984): *Acta Psychiatr. Scand.,* 69:333–342.
198. Tuomisto, J., and Tukianen, E. (1976): *Nature,* 262:596–598.
199. Valzelli, L. (1981): *Int. Pharmacopsychiatry,* 16:39–48.
200. Van der Kar, L. D., Karteszi, M., Bethea, C. L., and Ganong, W. F. (1985): *Neuroendocrinology,* 41:380–384.
201. van Hiele, L. J. (1980): *Neuropsychobiology,* 6:230–240.
202. van Praag, H. M. (1981): *Biol. Psychiatry,* 16:291–310.
203. van Praag, H. M. (1984): *Psychopharmacol. Bull.,* 20:599–602.
204. van Praag, H. M., and de Haan, S. (1981): *Acta Psychiatr. Scand. (Suppl. 290),* 63:191–201.
205. van Praag, H. M., Korf, J., Dols, L. C. W., and Schut, T. (1972): *Psychopharmacologia,* 25:14–21.
206. van Scheyen, J. D., and van Kamman, D. P. (1979): *Arch. Gen. Psychiatry,* 36:560–565.
207. Vestergaard, P., Sorensen, T., Hoppe, E., Rafaelsen, O. J., Yates, C. M., and Nicolaaou, N. (1978): *Acta Psychiatr. Scand.,* 58:88–96.
208. Vogt, M. (1982): In: *Biology of Serotonergic Neurotransmission,* edited by N. N. Osborne, pp. 229–316. John Wiley & Sons, Chichester.
209. von Knorring, L., Perris, C., Oreland, L., Eisemann, M., Eriksson, U., and Perris, H. (1984): *J. Neural Transm.,* 60:1–9.
210. Wagner, A., Aberg-Wistedt, A., Asberg, M., Ekquist, B., Martensson, B., and Montero, D. (1985): *Psychiatry Res.,* 16:131–139.
211. Walinder, J., Carlsson, A., and Persson, R. (1981): *Acta Psychiatr. Scand.,* 63:179–190.
212. Walinder, J., Carlsson, A., Persson, R., and Wallin, L. (1980): *Acta Psychiatr. Scand.,* 280:243–249.
213. Ward, N. G., Ang, J., and Pavinich, G. (1985): *Biol. Psychiatry,* 20:1090–1097.
214. Wehr, T. A., and Goodwin, F. K. (1981): In: *American Handbook of Psychiatry, Vol. 7,* 2nd ed., edited by S. Arieti and H. K. H. Brodie, pp. 46–74. Basic Books, New York.
215. White, K., Keck, P. E., Jr., and Lipinski, J. (1986): *Compr. Psychiatry,* 27:211–214.
216. Willner, P. (1984): *Psychopharmacology,* 83:1–16.
217. Willner, P. (1985): *Psychopharmacology,* 85:387–404.
218. Wirz-Justice, A. (1977): *Jpn. J. Clin. Med.,* 34:49–53.
219. Wolf, W. A., and Kuhn, D. M. (1984): *Brain Res.,* 295:356–359.
220. Young, S. N., and Gauthier, S. (1981): *J. Neurol. Neurosurg. Psychiatry,* 44:323–327.
221. Young, S. N., Smith, S. E., Pihl, R. O., and Ervin, F. R. (1985): *Psychopharmacology,* 87:173–177.
222. Zis, A. P., and Goodwin, F. K. (1979): *Arch. Gen. Psychiatry,* 36:1097–1107.

Psychopharmacology:
The Third Generation of Progress,
edited by Herbert Y. Meltzer.
Raven Press, New York © 1987.

CHAPTER **53**

Role of Acetylcholine Mechanisms in the Affective Disorders

David S. Janowsky and S. Craig Risch

Considerable information suggests a role for acetylcholine in the pathogenesis of the affective disorders. As proposed by Janowsky et al. (25), depression may be a manifestation of cholinergic predominance, whereas mania, conversely, may be due to a relative adrenergic predominance. In the years since 1972, when this hypothesis was first proposed, information further supporting a role for adrenergic-cholinergic interactions in the regulation of mood and affective disorders has accumulated, and some data have surfaced that are inconsistent (31).

BEHAVIORAL EFFECTS OF CHOLINOMIMETIC DRUGS

Animal Studies and Models

Many behavioral models of depression have been developed in animals, including the hypoactivity model, the learned helplessness model, the chronic stress model, and the behavioral despair or forced swim model (22,37). It is possible that alterations in cholinergic systems may contribute to the behavioral states induced by such models.

Centrally active cholinomimetic drugs, administered to a variety of animal species, consistently produce behavioral inhibitory effects including lethargy and hypoactivity, as well as causing a decrease in self-stimulation (25,26)—all

variables that have been considered to be animal models of depression. These phenomena are reversible with centrally active sympathetic agents, thus supporting a role for a balance between adrenergic and cholinergic factors in the regulation of motoric behaviors (25,26).

Recently, interest has focused on the increased cholinergic sensitivity that can be induced by selective breeding for anticholinesterase sensitivity (16,52) as a potential model of the cholinergic supersensitivity proposed to exist in human affective disorder patients.

Two lines of rats have been bred that appear to be cholinergically supersensitive. The Roman High Avoiding (RHA) and Roman Low Avoiding (RLA) strains of rats were selectively bred to differ in their ability to learn an active avoidance response (22); and the Flinders Sensitive Line (FSL) and Flinders Resistant Line (FRL) strains of rats were bred to differ in sensitivity to the cholinomimetic anticholinesterase diiosopropylfluorophosphate (DFP) (51,53).

A number of studies have reported differences in sensitivity to cholinergic agonists in these two lines. The RHA strain has been reported to be more sensitive to the behavioral effects of oxotremorine and physostigmine (36). Also, FSL rats, developed by Overstreet and Russell in Australia, exhibit increased sensitivity to the cholinomimetics physostigmine and DFP, and to muscarinic agonists. Also, they have decreased body weight, decreased locomotor activity, and increased numbers of hippocampal and striatal muscarinic acetylcholine receptors. Furthermore, the FSL rat is less active and more sensitive to the induction of behavioral immobility following a forced swim test, a behavior considered analogous to depression by many researchers (49,52). In addition, Overstreet et al. (50) have now found that when normal rats develop up-regulated muscarinic receptors due to withdrawal of chronic scopolamine treatment, they also show a greater degree of behavioral immobility in a forced swim test, compared to control animals, and have greater cholinomimetic (arecoline)-induced elevations in serum cortisol. Conversely, anticholinergic drugs reduce behavioral immobility in the forced swim test and have been reported to reduce the effects of inescapable shock, the procedure commonly used to produce learned helplessness (22).

Effects on Manic Symptoms of Cholinomimetics

If aberrant mood is due to an imbalance between adrenergic and cholinergic factors, it is logical to expect that increases in central cholinergic activity might decrease manic symptoms. Several studies have shown that centrally active cholinergic agonists and cholinesterase inhibitors possess antimanic properties. In a study by Rowntree et al. (57) the centrally active cholinesterase inhibitor DFP was given to manic-depressive patients and normals. The normal subjects and remitted manic-depressives developed irritability, lassitude, depression, apathy, and slowness and/or poverty of thoughts. Two patients who were hypomanic at the time of the study improved with DFP and continued euthymic after its administration, and one hypomanic patient became less manic and was minimally depressed after each of two courses of DFP, but relapsed on DFP withdrawal.

More recently Janowsky et al. (27) found that the centrally active cholinesterase inhibitor physostigmine caused a dramatic but brief reduction in hypomanic and manic symptoms in bipolar patients. Neither placebo nor neostigmine, a noncentrally active cholinesterase inhibitor, produced such changes. After physostigmine administration, the manics became significantly less talkative, active, euphoric, happy, grandiose, and friendly and showed a decrease in flight of ideas on the Beigel Murphy Mania Rating Scale. The effects of physostigmine lasted from 20 to 90 min (27). Modestin et al. (39,40) subsequently also reported a lessening of manic symptoms following infusion of physostigmine, but not neostigmine; and Davis et al. (8) reported that physostigmine caused dramatic antimanic effects, particularly in patients with low levels of hostility and/or irritability. Carroll et al. (4) and Shopsin et al. (58) also reported a decrease in euphoria and mobility in manics after physostigmine infusion. More recently, Berger et al. reported pilot data suggesting that RS86, a relatively specific muscarinic (M_1) agonist, may have significant antimanic effects (2).

Although most data to date are supportive of cholinomimetic agents exerting an antimanic effect, some authors have reported effects only on the affective and motoric components of mania, and no effects on the grandiose thinking and expansiveness that accompanies mania (4,58). Skeptics of the possibility that cholinomimetics exert antimanic effects point out that manic patients, treated with centrally acting cholinomimetic drugs, still continue to show grandiosity and to have manic delusions.

Mania-Rebounding Effects of Cholinomimetics

In addition to antagonism of motoric behaviors, there is evidence that when the cholinergic system is activated, there may be a later compensatory antagonistic activation of the adrenergic system. Fibiger et al. (19) demonstrated that the increase in cholinergic activity caused by the administration of physostigmine leads to an eventual increase in locomotion in rats, as presumed adrenergic mechanisms begin to exert effects. This activating effect becomes apparent as the cholinergic predominance induced by physostigmine decreases, and is exaggerated if a centrally acting anticholinergic agent is given at the beginning of the hyperactivity phase.

As with the work of Fibiger et al., there is some evidence that a behavioral rebound following physostigmine infusion also can occur in humans. A case of rebounding into mania was noted by Rowntree et al. (57), and Shopsin et al. (58) demonstrated rebounding into hypermania in two of three manic patients given physostigmine. In these patients a marked postphysostigmine exacerbation or intensification of the manic state was observed. However, "rebounding" in humans has not generally been observed following physostigmine infusion.

Depression-Inducing Effects of Cholinomimetics

Probably the most convincing evidence that acetylcholine is involved in the etiology of the affective disorders comes from the observation that these agents can rapidly induce a depressed mood. In addition to observations of depression-induction caused by DFP (57) and insecticides (21), Janowsky et al. (27) found induction and/or intensification of depressive symptoms in a subset of the actively ill bipolar manic patients given physostigmine described above, as well as worsening of depression in groups of unipolar depressed and schizoaffective-depressed patients (24). Similarly, Davis et al. (8) and Modestin et al. (39,40) showed an increase in depression in manic patients given physostigmine. In addition, Risch et al. (56) and Nurnberger et al. (44–46) found that depressed patients given the direct cholinergic agonist arecoline also developed depression and other forms of negative affect, including hostility and anxiety. Physostigmine also caused a depressed mood in a majority of euthymic bipolar patients maintained on lithium (47).

In addition, Risch et al. (54) found statistically significant increases in self- and observer-rated negative affect on the Brief Psychiatric Rating Scale (BPRS), Profile of Mood States (POMS), and Activation-Inhibition Rating Scales in normals receiving intravenous physostigmine or arecoline. Likewise, Mohs et al. (41) reported severe depression occurring in Alzheimer's patients receiving the cholinergic agonist oxotremorine. Also, El-Yousef et al. (18) reported that normals, having smoked marijuana, became profoundly depressed after receiving physostigmine, an effect that was atropine-reversible. Similarly, Davis et al. (11) noted severe depression in a volunteer receiving physostigmine who had surreptitiously smoked marijuana before receiving physostigmine.

Evidence supportive of a role for acetylcholine in the phenomenology of affective disorders also comes from descriptions of the anergic-inhibitory behavioral effects of centrally acting cholinesterase inhibitors, which induce a psychomotor retardation which is very similar to that occurring in endogenous depression. Thus, Rowntree et al. (57) and Modestin et al. (39,40), studying normals, depressives, and manics, and Gershon and Shaw (21), observing normals, all reported that cholinesterase inhibitors exerted anergic and behavioral-inhibitory effects, as did Janowsky et al. (24) in their physostigmine-treated subjects.

Depressed moods have also been observed in subjects receiving presumptive acetylcholine precursors, including deanol, choline, and lecithin. Davis et al. (10) and Tamminga et al. (63) found that depressive symptoms occurred in some schizophrenic patients who were treated with choline, a phenomenon that was atropine-reversible. In a subgroup of cases, it was noted that depressed mood was a side effect of choline or lecithin treatments employed to try to reverse the memory deficits of Alzheimer's disease (1). Also, Casey (6) observed that a depressed mood and, in some cases, a paradoxical hypomania occurred in some deanol-treated tardive dyskinesia and other movement-disordered patients. Thus, precursors of acetycholine may induce a depressed mood—a finding that is consistent with the adrenergic-cholinergic imbalance hypothesis.

Conversely, Cohen et al. (7) reported that lecithin can cause mild but measurable antimanic effects in manic patients. Similarly, Cohen et al. (unpublished data) have found oral physostigmine, given over a period of days, to exert antimanic effects.

Anticholinergic Withdrawal Phenomena

In addition to the mood-depressing and inhibitory effects of cholinomimetics, antidepressant and antiparkinsonian agent-treated patients may develop some aspects of depression, including a depressed mood, anxiety, withdrawal, agitation, and insomnia soon after discontinuing these medications. These symptoms are preventable and/or reversible with anticholinergic treatment, and may represent the unmasking of muscarinic receptor hypersensitivity. This issue has been elaborated upon in detail by Dilsaver et al. (12–14), who proposed the concept of "cholinergic overdrive," consisting of anxiety, nausea, agitation, and sometimes depression. Cholinergic overdrive occurred after discontinuation of anticholinergic tricyclics and antiparkinsonian drugs and after anticholinergic drug withdrawal combined with marijuana intoxication (14). Dilsaver attributes cholinergic overdrive to the unmasking of up-regulated cholinergic receptors occurring secondary to withdrawal of antimuscarinic blockade, and proposes that such "overdrive" may also activate noradrenergic receptors, leading to induction of arousal and manic symptoms in some cases (13).

DIFFERENTIAL EFFECTS OF CHOLINOMIMETICS IN AFFECT DISORDER PATIENTS

Behavioral Supersensitivity

Patients with affective disorders may be relatively more sensitive to the negative affect and inhibitory effects of cholinomimetics. Janowsky et al. (24) noted that those patients with depression, mania, or schizoaffective disorders, as compared to those schizophrenics without a significant mood component to their illness, become significantly more sad and depressed after receiving physostigmine. Oppenheimer et al. (47) likewise observed that a significant percentage of euthymic bipolar patients receiving lithium became depressed after receiving physostigmine, whereas normal controls who received physostigmine alone did not become depressed. Furthermore, Janowsky et al. (30) found that rater-evaluated behavioral inhibition and self-rated anxiety, depression, hostility, confusion, and elation subscales showed significantly greater increases in affect disorder patients than in other psychiatric patient groups or normals after physostigmine infusion. However, nonaffective disorder subjects and normals receiving physostigmine also do develop depression and other negative affect to some extent, and differences between affective disorder patients and controls are not profound. Also, differential behavioral sensitivity was not seen in a group of euthymic affective disorder patients given arecoline (46).

The possibility that physostigmine may behaviorally differentiate patients with affective disorder diagnoses has received further support from the work of Edelstein et al. (17). These investigators used physostigmine to differentiate schizophrenic patients who were responsive to lithium carbonate therapy from those who were not. They found that patients who responded to physostigmine with a clearing of psychotic symptoms were significantly more likely to respond to a trial of lithium, presumably because they represented an affective disorder variant. Finally, Casey (6) noted that those patients with a strong history of affective disorder selectively showed increased affective symptoms while receiving the presumed acetylcholine precursor deanol.

Cholinomimetic Effects on Sleep Parameters

Although not as specific as previously believed, major depression is generally associated with a series of characteristic sleep changes, including decreased rapid eye movement (REM) latency and increased REM density. In parallel with these characteristics of depression, cholinergic agonists generally cause a shortening of REM latency and an increase in REM density (60,61). In addition, Sitaram et al. (60,61) have shown that induction of muscarinic up-regulation by the withdrawal of chronic scopolamine leads to shortening of REM latency and an increase in REM density.

Furthermore, Sitaram et al. (60,61) have found that REM latency shortened significantly more following arecoline infusion in patients with an affective disorder episode or a family history of affective disorder than in normals

(60), a finding not replicated by Gillin et al. (*unpublished data*) in a recent study.

This presumed hypersensitivity appears to be genetically linked, as noted in monozygotic twin studies in which arecoline is administered to paired twins (46), and as observed in the recent work of Sitaram et al., in which affectively ill members of the families of affectively ill patients showed exaggerated shortening of REM latency after arecoline infusion (60).

Berger et al. (2) also found that supershortening of REM latency in endogenous depressives occurred following administration of the long-acting oral muscarinic agonist, RS86. Possibly related to all of the above findings, Berger et al. (3) also found that physostigmine induced arousal and awakening from sleep more frequently in affective disorder patients than in normals.

NEUROHORMONAL EFFECTS OF CHOLINOMIMETIC DRUGS: CHANGES IN HPA FUNCTION

Another characteristic of depression is the activation of the hypothalamic-pituitary-adrenal (HPA) axis. A variety of studies have shown that increased cortisol, corticotropin (ACTH), and β-endorphin secretion occurs in depressed patients. As with behavioral and sleep parameters, there is evidence from a variety of studies that cholinomimetic drugs may elevate serum ACTH, cortisol, and β-endorphin secretion (55). Several recent clinical studies (9,15,29,55,56) have documented the effects of cholinomimetics on neuroendocrine activity in humans. Physostigmine and arecoline infusions significantly increase serum ACTH, cortisol, and β-endorphin levels in normals and in psychiatric patients. Also, physostigmine reverses the dexamethasone-induced suppression of cortisol in normals, which occurs naturally in some depressives (5,15). Furthermore, affective disorder patients seem to show significantly greater increases in β-endorphin and ACTH levels after physostigmine infusion (55).

Thus, it appears that physostigmine-induced increases in HPA activity occur, and that these parallel other phenomena noted in endogenous depression, such as increased cortisol secretion, cortisol resistance to suppression by dexamethasone, and elevated ACTH and β-endorphin levels.

Although considerable converging animal and human evidence suggests that depression-relevant stress hormones are activated by cholinomimetics, some caution is indicated in interpreting these findings. First, cholinomimetic drugs could cause their behavioral and neuroendocrine effects by inducing nausea, or by causing a syndrome akin to motion sickness (9).

However, several observations have been made that are inconsistent with such an etiology for physostigmine's mode of action. In a small subgroup of psychiatric patients, physostigmine infusion caused increased negative affect, anergia, and increased pulse and blood pressure without causing any nausea or emesis whatsoever, although light-headedness and dizziness did occur (D. S. Janowsky et al., *unpublished observations*). Also, arecoline given to normals and affective disorder patients caused affective changes, as well as increases in ACTH, cortisol, and β-endorphin, whereas nausea only rarely occurred (54–56). In addition, Fulton et al. (20) have shown that low doses of arecoline can increase serum cortisol and ACTH levels, while causing no other side effects.

ADRENOMEDULLARY AND CARDIOVASCULAR EFFECTS OF CHOLINOMIMETIC DRUGS

A recent series of investigations have shown that groups of patients with major depressive disorders often have increased urinary epinephrine excretion and, to a lesser extent, increased norepinephrine excretion. As with many parameters, physostigmine infusion causes similar effects in humans and in animals. Administration of physostigmine to normals and affect disorder patients causes profound increases in serum epinephrine levels, and slight increases in serum norepinephrine levels (35). Furthermore, Janowsky et al. (35) have demonstrated a blunting of the epinephrine response to physostigmine in affective disorder patients.

Several studies have suggested that depressed patients may have increased pulse rates and blood pressure levels. Similarly, physostigmine and arecoline have been shown to increase pulse rate and blood pressure levels in subjects treated with peripherally acting anticholinergic drugs. These changes can be profound and appear, as with cholinomimetic-induced increases in epinephrine release, to be due to muscarinic activation of centrally mediated sympathetic outflow (28,32).

MONOAMINE-ACETYLCHOLINE INTERACTIONS

A pharmacologic-behavioral model for naturally occurring adrenergic-cholinergic regulation of mood may be found in the interactions and reciprocal effects of psychostimulants (which increase catecholaminergic activity) and cholinomimetics (which increase cholinergic activity).

Methylphenidate-induced psychostimulation in humans is rapidly antagonized by physostigmine but not by neostigmine. Conversely, physostigmine's inhibitory-depressant effects can be reversed by methylphenidate (23,26). Possibly related to the ability of physostigmine to antagonize methylphenidate-induced psychomotor stimulation is the observation that physostigmine caused a rapid, dramatic drop in the norepinephrine metabolite serum 3-methoxy-4-hydroxyphenylglycol (MHPG) in a manic patient, presumably reflecting a drop in CNS noradrenergic activity. This phenomenon was associated with induction of a tearful depressed state and an improvement in manic symptoms (48).

Furthermore, a reciprocal relationship apparently may exist between a subject's response to a psychostimulant and his separate response to a cholinomimetic agent. A negative correlation was noted between amphetamine-induced behavioral excitation and the ability of arecoline, given on another occasion, to decrease REM latency (46). Similarly, Siever et al. (59) showed that in a mixed group of affective disorder and normal subjects, those with the most dramatic physostigmine- and arecoline-induced anergy and negative affect showed a blunted growth hormone response to the noradrenergic agonist clonidine (presumably a reflection of decreased noradrenergic responsiveness).

CENTRAL MUSCARINIC REGULATION OF CHOLINOMIMETIC EFFECTS

Several studies have attempted to better understand the mechanisms by which the behavioral, cardiovascular, and neuroendocrine effects of cholinomimetic drugs occur. In early studies, Janowsky et al. (27) and Modestin et al. (39,40) noted that the noncentrally acting cholinesterase inhibitor, neostigmine, like placebo, did not exert any behavioral effects, thus suggesting a central effect for physostigmine's manifestations. More recently, Janowsky et al. (32) noted that the increase in blood pressure, pulse rate, serum epinephrine, ACTH, cortisol, and prolactin, as well as the anergia and negative affect caused by physostigmine, occurs via a central mechanism, since no such changes occur with neostigmine. Furthermore, Janowsky et al. (32) have now noted that the behavioral, cardiovascular, and neuroendocrine effects of physostigmine can be blocked by the centrally acting anticholinergic drug scopolamine, but not by the noncentrally acting anticholinergic methscopolamine. This suggests a central muscarinic mechanism for physostigmine's action.

MOOD EFFECTS OF ANTIADRENERGIC AGENTS

Observations exist that many sympatholytic-antihypertensive medications, including alphamethyldopa, propranolol, clonidine, and reserpine, which can cause depression, also have significant cholinomimetic properties (25). In humans the CNS side effects of reserpine and other antiadrenergic-cholinomimetic antihypertensives are similar to those of centrally active cholinergic agents, and include mood depression, vivid nightmares, lethargy, and sleepiness. With respect to antipsychotic drugs, Van Putten and May (64) have shown that these agents, which block central dopamine and increase acetylcholine turnover, can cause some of the components of depression in selected patients, effects that can be reversed with centrally active anticholinergic drugs.

MUSCARINIC RECEPTORS IN AFFECTIVE DISORDER PATIENTS

Several recent studies have suggested a difference among affective disorder and normal subjects with respect to muscarinic receptor binding. Nadi et al. (42) reported that fibroblasts grown in culture from affective disorder patients and their mood-disordered relatives have more muscarinic binding sites than controls. Similarly, Meyerson et al. (38)

noted that samples from the frontal cortex of individuals who committed suicide had more muscarinic receptor binding activity than matched brains from people dying from accidents or murder. Unfortunately, however, as noted in the *New England Journal of Medicine* (43), Kelsoe, Richelson, Lennox, and their respective co-workers have not been able to replicate the fibroblast receptor findings described above; and others (34,62) have not been able to find increased muscarinic binding in the brains of suicides. Generally, the evidence suggests that muscarinic binding in fibroblasts and brain is not altered in affective disorder patients, at least in the studies reported to date.

MOOD EFFECTS OF CENTRALLY ACTIVE ANTICHOLINERGIC AGENTS

As reviewed elsewhere, there is evidence evolving that centrally active anticholinergic drugs may have mood-elevating properties, although this evidence is generally anecdotal and uncontrolled (28,31). As noted by Jellinec in 1981 and Smith in 1980, antiparkinsonian drugs used to treat drug-induced parkinsonian symptoms have been reported to cause feelings of euphoria associated with a sense of well-being, increased sociability, and a reversal of depressed mood. Furthermore, one report by Coid and Strong in 1982 suggested that the anticholinergic agent procyclidine caused a switch into mania in a bipolar patient.

In addition, several reports suggest that high doses of atropine and other anticholinergics such as ditran may alleviate depression, and one report suggests that the tricyclic-antidepressant-induced central anticholinergic syndrome may alleviate depression. Also, Jimerson et al. in 1982 reported that trihexylphendyl may have antidepressant properties; and Kasper et al. (33) observed antidepressant effects with the anticholinergic drug biperidin, especially in patients with endogenous depression who had a nonsuppressing dexamethasone suppression test. In spite of the above-reviewed positive evidence, it must be stressed that many effective antidepressant medications, such as mianserin and trazodone, lack antimuscarinic properties yet can alleviate depression. To answer this incongruity, Janowsky et al. (31) have reviewed evidence suggesting that increased noradrenergic activity occurring secondary to tricyclics may inhibit cholinergic neurotransmission via a presynaptic mechanism.

DISCUSSION

As reviewed above, considerable evidence suggests that the cholinergic nervous system, alone or interacting in concert with other neurotransmitters, may have an important role in the regulation of affect. Nevertheless, as with all currently proposed biologic hypotheses of the etiology of affective disorders, there exist alternative explanations, as well as some data that are inconsistent with the hypothesis in question.

It is possible that pharmacologically induced changes in acetylcholine may be the cause of perturbations in other systems than the cholinergic nervous system. Pharmacologically induced acetylcholine alterations could cause a "model depression" by perturbing other potential governing neurotransmitters in affect disorder patients (for example, GABA, serotonin, dopamine, or norepinephrine) (31), but at the same time, endogenous acetylcholine may not actually cause depression. Furthermore, obviously, the fundamental problem in depression could be a relatively low level of norepinephrine or serotonin activity, relative to normal acetylcholine activity, a situation that could explain all the above observations under the scope of a balance hypothesis.

However, even if cholinomimetics can only cause a "model depression," with such components as low mood, psychomotor depression, elevated ACTH, cortisol, β-endorphin, epinephrine levels, and pulse rates, understanding how this presumed pharmacologic phenomenon occurs may ultimately offer a window into understanding the pathophysiology of affective disorders, and may have useful treatment implications. Thus, at the least, understanding the "downstream" implications of the mood-depressant and other "depression-like" effects of cholinomimetics may give clues to the actual neurobiology of affective disorders. Alternatively, it is not beyond possibility that acetylcholine actually is involved in the etiology of the expression of affective disorders, alone or acting through other relevant neurotransmitters.

Finally, at a more general level, as reviewed by Janowsky and Risch in 1984 (28), all the above reviewed information is consistent with a role for acetylcholine in the overall regulation of the effects of stress, of which depression may be but one possible outcome. Supportive of this concept is evidence from animal studies that central acetylcholine turnover increases with stress, and that this effect is exaggerated in a strain of stress-sensitive rats (28). Furthermore, blood pressure and pulse rate increases, increases in neurohormones including epinephrine, ACTH, cortisol, β-endorphin, prolactin, growth hormone, and vasopressin, and increases in anxiety, depression, fatigue, hostility, and analgesia frequently occur following exposure to naturally occurring nonpharmacologic aversive stressors, as well as following cholinomimetic administration. Such parallels thus suggest that acetylcholine may be a major modulator of the more general behavioral, neuroendocrine, and cardiovascular manifestations of stress.

REFERENCES

1. Bajada, S. (1982): In: *Alzheimer's Disease: A Report of Progress,* edited by S. Corkin, K. Davis, and J. Growden, pp. 427–432. Raven Press, New York.
2. Berger, M., Hochli, D., Zulley, J., Lauer, C., and von Zerssen, D. (1985): *Lancet,* 1:1385–1386.
3. Berger, M., Lund, R., Bronisch, T., and von Zerssen, D. (1983): *Psychiatry Res.,* 10:113–123.
4. Carroll, B. J., Frazer, A., Schless, A., and Mendels, J. (1973): *Lancet,* 1:427–428.
5. Carroll, B. J., Greden, J. F., Haskett, R., Feinberg, M., Albala, A., Martin, F., Rubin, R., Heath, B., Sharp, P., McLeod, W., and McLeod, M. (1980): *Acta Psychiat. Scand. (Suppl),* 280:183–199.
6. Casey, D. E. (1979): *Psychopharmacology,* 62:187–191.
7. Cohen, B. M., Lipinsky, J. F., and Altesmar, R. F. (1982): *Am. J. Psychiatry,* 138:1162–1164.
8. Davis, K. L., Berger, P. A., and Hollister, L. E. (1978): *Arch. Gen. Psychiatry,* 35:119–122.
9. Davis, K. L., and Davis, B. M. (1979): In: *Brain Acetylcholine and Neuropsychiatric Disease,* edited by K. L. Davis and P. A. Berger, pp. 445–458. Plenum Press, New York.
10. Davis, K. L., Hollister, L. E., and Berger, P. A. (1979): *Am. J. Psychiatry,* 136:1581–1584.
11. Davis, K. L., Hollister, L. E., and Overall, J. (1976): *Psychopharmacology,* 51:23–27.
12. Dilsaver, S. C., and Greden, J. R. (1984): *Biol. Psychiatry,* 19:237–256.
13. Dilsaver, S. C., and Greden, J. R. (1984): *Brain Res. Rev.,* 7:29–48.
14. Dilsaver, S. C., and Greden, J. R. (1984): *J. Clin. Psychopharmacol.,* 3:157–164.
15. Doerr, P., and Berger, M. (1983): *Biol. Psychiatry,* 18:261–268.
16. Driscoll, P., and Battig, K. (1982): In: *Genetics of the Brain,* edited by I. Lieblich, pp. 96–123. Elsevier, Amsterdam.
17. Edelstein, P., Schultz, J. R., Hirschowitz, J., Kanter, D. R., and Garver, D. L. (1981): *Am. J. Psychiatry,* 138:1078–1081.
18. El-Yousef, M., Janowsky, D. S., Davis, J. M., and Rosenblatt, J. E. (1973): *Br. J. Addict.,* 68:321–325.
19. Fibiger, H. D., Lynch, G. S., and Cooper, H. P. (1971): *Psychopharmacology,* 20:366–382.
20. Fulton, C. L., Rush, A. J., Charles, G. A., Orsulak, P. J., Fairchild, C. J., and Crowley, G. T. (1985): Abstracts of the American College of Neuropsychopharmacology Annual Meeting, Hawaii, p. 47, No. 11.
21. Gershon, S., and Shaw, F. H. (1961): *Lancet,* 1:1371–1374.
22. Goldman, M. E., and Erickson, C. K. (1983): *Neuropharmacology,* 22:1215–1222.
23. Janowsky, D. S., El-Yousef, M. K., and Davis, J. M. (1973): *Am. J. Psychiatry,* 130:1370–1376.
24. Janowsky, D. S., El-Yousef, M. K., and Davis, J. M. (1974): *Psychosom. Med.,* 36:248–257.
25. Janowsky, D. S., El-Yousef, M. K., Davis, J. M., and Sekerke, H. J. (1972): *Lancet,* 2:6732–6735.
26. Janowsky, D. S., El-Yousef, M. K., Davis, J. M., and Sekerke, H. J. (1972): *Psychopharmacologia,* 27:295–303.
27. Janowsky, D. S., El-Yousef, M. K., Davis, J. M., and Sekerke, H. J. (1973): *Arch. Gen. Psychiatry,* 28:542–547.
28. Janowsky, D. S., and Risch, S. C. (1984): *Drug Dev. Res.,* 4:125–142.
29. Janowsky, D. S., Risch, S. C., Huey, L. Y., Judd, L. L., and Rausch, J. (1983): *Peptides,* 4:775–784.
30. Janowsky, D. S., Risch, S. C., Judd, L. L., Huey, L. Y., and Parker, D. C. (1981): *Psychopharmacol. Bull.,* 17:129–132.
31. Janowsky, D. S., Risch, S. C., Judd, L. L., Huey, L. Y., and Parker, D. C. (1985): In: *Central Cholinergic Mechanism and Adaptive Dysfunction,* edited by M. M. Singh, D. M. Warburton, and H. Lal, pp. 309–353. Plenum, New York.
32. Janowsky, D. S., Risch, S. C., Kennedy, B., Ziegler, M., and Huey, L. Y. (1986): *Psychopharmacology,* 89:150–154.
33. Kasper, S., Moises, H. W., and Beckman, H. (1981): *Pharmacopsychiatry,* 14:195–198.
34. Kaufman, C. A., Gillin, J. C., Hill, B., O'Laughlin, T., Phillips, I., Gleinman, J. E., and Wyatt, R. J. (1984): *Psychiatry Res.,* 12:47–56.
35. Janowsky, D. S., Risch, S. C., Ziegler, M. G., Gillin, J. C., Huey, H. L., and Rausch, J. (1986): *Am. J. Psych.,* 143:919–921.
36. Martin, J. R., Overstreet, D. H., Driscoll, P., and Battig, K. (1981): *Psychopharmacology,* 72:135–142.
37. McKinney, W. T. (1984): *Psychiatr. Dev.,* 2:77–96.
38. Meyerson, L. R., Wennogle, L. P., Abel, M. S., Coupet, J., Lippa, A., Rauh, C., and Beer, B. (1982): *Pharmacol. Biochem. Behav.,* 17:159–163.
39. Modestin, J. J., Hunger, J., and Schwartz, R. B. (1973): *Arch. Psychiatrie Nervenkr.,* 218:67–77.
40. Modestin, J. J., Schwartz, R. B., and Hunger, J. (1973): *Pharmacopsychiatria,* 9:300–304.
41. Mohs, R., Hollander, E., Haroutunian, V., Davidson, M., Horvath, T., and Davis, K. L. (1985): Abstracts of the IVth World Congress of Biological Psychiatry, Philadelphia, 518:3.

42. Nadi, N. S., Nurnberger, J. L., and Gershon, E. S. (1984): *N. Engl. J. Med.,* 311:225–230.
43. *N. Engl. J. Med.* (1985): 312:861–862.
44. Nurnberger, J., Gershon, E. S., Sitaram, N., Gillin, J. C., Brown, G., Ebert, M., Gold, P., Jimerson, D., and Kessler, L. (1982): *Psychopharmacol. Bull.,* 17:80–82.
45. Nurnberger, J., Jimerson, D. C., Simmons, S., Tamminga, C., Nadi, N. S., and Gershon, E. S. (1982): Presented at Society of Biological Psychiatry 13th Annual Convention, Toronto.
46. Nurnberger, J., Jimerson, D. C., Simmons-Alling, S., Tamminga, C., Nadi, N. S., Lawrence, D., Sitaram, N. S., Gillin, J. C., and Gershon, E. S. (1983): *Psychiatry Res.,* 9:191–200.
47. Oppenheimer, G., Ebstein, R., and Belmaker, R. (1979): *J. Psychiatr. Res.,* 14:133–138.
48. Ostrow, D. (1985): *J. Clin. Psychol.,* 46(10, Sec. 2):25–30.
49. Overstreet, D. H. (1986): *Biol. Psychiatry,* 21:49–58.
50. Overstreet, D. H., Janowsky, D. S., Gillin, J. C., Shiromani, P., and Sutin, E. (1986): *Biol. Psychiatry,* 21:657–664.
51. Overstreet, D. H., and Russell, R. W. (1982): *Psychopharmacology,* 78:150–154.
52. Overstreet, D. H., and Russell, R. W. (1984): *Behav. Neurol. Biol.,* 40:227–238.
53. Overstreet, D. H., and Russell, R. W. (1986): *Behav. Neurol. Biol.,* 40:227–238.
54. Risch, S. C., Cohen, P. M., Janowsky, D. S., Kalin, N. H., Insel, T. R., and Murphy, D. L. (1981): *J. Psychiatr. Res.,* 4:89–94.
55. Risch, S. C., Janowsky, D. S., Kalin, N. H., Cohen, R. M., Aloi, J. A., and Murphy, D. L. (1982): In: *Biological Markers in Psychiatry and Neurology,* edited by I. Hanin and E. Usdin, pp. 269–278. Pergamon Press, Oxford.
56. Risch, S. C., Siever, L. J., and Gillin, J. C. (1983): *Psychopharmacol. Bull.,* 19:696–698.
57. Rowntree, D. W., Neven, S., and Wilson, A. (1950): *J. Neurol. Neurosurg. Psychiatry,* 13:47–62.
58. Shopsin, B., Janowsky, D. S., and Davis, J. M. (1975): *Neuropsychobiology,* 1:180–187.
59. Siever, L. J., Risch, S. C., and Murphy, D. L. (1981): *Psychiatry Res.,* 5:108–109.
60. Sitaram, N., Jones, D., Dube, S., Bell, J., and Rivard, P. (1985): Abstracts of the IVth World Congress of Biological Sciences, Philadelphia, 518.6.
61. Sitaram, N., Nurnberger, J., and Gershon, E. S. (1982): *Am. J. Psychiatry,* 139:571–576.
62. Stanley, M. (1983): New Research Abstracts of the Annual Meeting of the American Psychiatry Association, Washington, DC.
63. Tamminga, C., Smith, R. C., Change, S., Haraszti, J. S., and Davis, J. M. (1976): *Lancet,* 2:905.
64. Van Putten, T. V., and May, P. A. (1978): *Arch. Gen. Psychiatry,* 35:1101–1107.

Psychopharmacology:
The Third Generation of Progress,
edited by Herbert Y. Meltzer.
Raven Press, New York © 1987.

CHAPTER 54

Mechanism of Action of Antidepressant Treatments: Implications for the Etiology and Treatment of Depressive Disorders

George R. Heninger and Dennis S. Charney

Recent research on the mechanism of action of antidepressant treatments has led to major revisions of the earlier concepts of the pathogenesis of depression and the mechanism of action of antidepressant treatments (ADT) (20). The hypothesis that depression was a result of a monoamine deficiency has not been verified by studies of monoamine and monoamine metabolite levels in plasma, urine, and CSF of depressed patients (60). The monoamine deficiency hypothesis was in part based on the premise that the therapeutic action of ADT was a consequence of an increased availability of synaptic norepinephrine (NE) or serotonin (5-HT) secondary to high-affinity reuptake inhibition and/or decreased catabolism (60). However, this hypothesis does not account for the large temporal discrepancy between the rapid drug-induced biochemical effects on amine uptake and catabolism, which occur within hours, and the antidepressant response, which occurs after at least 7 to 14 days of treatment (90,91). There is an extremely wide range in the inhibitor constants (K_i) of effective ADTs on monoamine uptake, and some effective ADTs such as iprindole and mianserin do not inhibit amine uptake or exhibit monoamine oxidase inhibitor (MAOI) activity to a significant extent (104). In addition, reuptake inhibitors such as amphetamine or cocaine are not effective antidepressant treatments (91,97).

Studies of monoamine turnover in laboratory animals following long-term ADT demonstrate no consistent changes across a wide spectrum of compounds or electroconvulsive therapy (ECT) (118). The decrease in turnover observed following acute administration of compounds that inhibit reuptake of NE or 5-HT appears to be secondary to inhibitory feedback mechanisms involving presynaptic autoreceptors (117). With many compounds, long-term administration results in "adaptive changes" that result in no net change in turnover or even "paradoxical" increases in metabolite levels. For example, although acute desipramine (DMI) reduces the NE metabolite 3 methoxy-4-hydroxy-phenylglycol (MHPG) in most brain areas, following chronic DMI administration, MHPG is increased 5 hr following the last dose in hippocampus and thalamus (83). In clinical studies consistent drug effects on NE metabolism are not observed (20). Thus, clear decreases in plasma MHPG levels are seen with drugs that are known to inhibit NE reuptake, but not with drugs that have no NE uptake blocking properties (19,98). There is some evidence that the total urinary excretion of NE metabolites is decreased with drugs that inhibit NE uptake, such as DMI, and this is also seen with ECT (64). Zimelidine also has this effect, but it is not clear if this is due to NE or 5-HT blocking properties (blood levels of norzimelidine, NE uptake-blocking metabolite of zimelidine, are higher than the parent compound). There is more consistency in the pattern of change of 5-HT metabolites. When CSF of depressed patients is obtained before and after treatment, 5-hydroxyindoleacetic acid (5-HIAA) is observed to decrease following all of the ADTs that are known to inhibit monoamine uptake as well as the MAOI drugs. These changes have also been seen with the more specific 5-HT reuptake-blocking drugs (20,127). The ADT-induced 5-HIAA changes do not relate to clinical response. Thus, there do not appear to be consistent changes in NE or 5-HT turnover that can easily account for the therapeutic mechanism of action of all or even most of the currently used antidepressant treatments.

LONGER-TERM ADAPTIVE CHANGES IN MONOAMINE RECEPTOR SYSTEMS

The lack of correspondence between ADT-induced changes in monoamine metabolism and antidepressant effects has focused current research on the problem of ADT-induced adaptive modifications in monoamine and other neurotransmitter receptor systems. Recent advances in basic neuroscience research have led to a vastly improved understanding of the possible neurobiologic mechanisms that could be implicated in long-term effects of ADT. There has been an improved understanding of the regulation of monoamine neurotransmission resulting from the integration of data obtained from studies of radioligand receptor binding, pharmacological characterization of adenylate cyclase and other second messenger production, single-unit electrophysiologic recordings, and pharmacologic evaluation in neurotransmitter-behavioral paradigms, all of which, together, provide a more integrated concept of possible ADT effects on receptor regulation and function. Changes in receptor sensitivity of monoamine or other neurotransmitter systems have been observed following all ADTs, and the time course of these receptor changes more closely approximates the delay in clinical antidepressant effects seen in patients.

ANTIDEPRESSANT TREATMENT AND RECEPTOR SENSITIVITY IN LABORATORY ANIMALS

Norepinephrine-Stimulated Cyclic AMP Accumulation

Adenosine-3,5-monophosphate (cyclic AMP) is a nucleotide that acts within the cell as a second messenger to mediate the physiologic actions of several central neurotransmitters at the postsynaptic level (94). Alterations in neurotransmitter stimulation of cyclic AMP production have been demonstrated to reflect changes in the receptor mechanisms involved in the transduction of effects. *In vitro* NE is particularly active in stimulating the accumulation of cyclic AMP, and this has been shown to be in part a β-receptor-mediated effect (94). A number of investigations have evaluated the effects of ADT on the functional sensitivity of the cyclic AMP generating system to NE agonists in brain slices (20,82,129). In Table 1 it can be seen that

TABLE 1. Summary of effects of long-term administration of antidepressant treatments on measures of monoamine receptor sensitivity[a]

[a] Symbols used: ↑, increase; ↓, decrease; 0, no change; —, not tested; averaged over different brain areas and different drugs. Not all drugs were tested in all brain areas; mixed results are indicated when different drugs of the same class produced different effects, and when the same drug produced different effects in different brain areas.

[b] Includes trazodone, iprindole, and buproprion.

across all of the drug categories of proven antidepressant efficacy listed, except for the specific 5-HT uptake blockers, there is a decrease in the NE-stimulated accumulation of cyclic AMP following long-term treatment. The effect appears to be dependent on the time of drug exposure and is not just related to drug accumulation in brain. This finding is consistent with the hypothesis that ADTs that increase synaptic NE levels secondary to reuptake blockade or decreased catabolism cause compensatory decreases in β-receptor sensitivity and decreased cyclic AMP response to NE. However, the fact that iprindole, an effective ADT that does not block NE uptake or alter brain NE levels, also produces subsensitivity to NE in this model indicates that other factors are also involved (129). The observation that tricyclic drugs, atypical ADTs, MAOIs, and ECT all reduce NE-stimulated cyclic AMP accumulation in brain has stimulated considerable research into assessing neurotransmitter receptor binding properties as well as the mechanisms involved in the transduction of receptor binding into cyclic AMP production.

Neurotransmitter-Receptor Binding

The utilization of radioligand binding to study receptor affinity and number over the past 10 years has led to a large number of studies investigating the effects of acute and longer-term administration of ADTs on these measures in a number of brain areas. In 1976 it was initially found that chronic ADT reduced the density of β-adrenoceptors in homogenates of whole rat brain (123). This finding has been replicated many times with many different ADTs across numerous brain areas (20,129). In Table 1 it can be seen that, except for most 5-HT uptake inhibitors (i.e., citalopram, fluoxetine, paroxetine, and alaproclate), all forms of ADT studied (including sleep deprivation (1)) produce a decrease in β-receptor number. The importance of this finding is strengthened by the fact that a decrease in binding is observed following long-term but not short-term or acute treatment. Treatment with a variety of other psychotropic agents, including most antipsychotics, anxiolytics, and amine uptake inhibitors, is ineffective in reducing β-receptor binding (20). An exception is the finding that amphetamine has been reported to reduce β-receptor density, and the effective antidepressant drug mianserin fails to reduce binding (20,82). It is of interest to note that mianserin does have the ability to desensitize the NE-stimulated cyclic AMP in brain slices. Mianserin may reduce the cyclic AMP response to NE via a non-β mechanism, since β-receptors mediate possibly less than half the cyclic AMP response to NE (84).

There has been much more variability in the findings reported for α-adrenergic binding following ADT. Thus, most studies have found no change in α_1-receptor density following ADT (20), although recently, utilizing prazosin as a ligand, some investigators have shown some drugs and ECT to produce an increase (120,121). There are reports of super-high-affinity sites that increase in density after chronic DMI, amitriptyline (AMI), or iprindole treatment (79). Whether other ADTs will affect the super-high-affinity site has not yet been extensively studied.

α_2-Adrenergic receptor binding studies have primarily used clonidine as the ligand, and receptor numbers have been reported to increase, decrease, or be unchanged following most ADTs. In general, the largest changes in α_2 binding have been found following DMI and other NE uptake blocking drugs, as well as MAOI compounds (28,29). In comparison to the robust consistency in the β-receptor system, it appears that long-term ADT with a variety of drugs does not produce consistent changes in α_2 binding.

In recent years there has been considerable research directed toward identifying and characterizing different types of 5-HT receptors. Initial studies labeled 5-HT_1 receptors with lysergic acid diethylamide (LSD) and 5-HT_2 receptors with spiroperidol. More recently, more selective 5-HT_1 ligands have been utilized to differentiate 5-HT_{1a} and 5-HT_{1b} receptors (80,95,96). In general, the 5-HT_1 binding has not consistently varied across a large number of ADTs studied, including ECT. In contrast, 5-HT_2 binding has been consistently demonstrated to be decreased by long-term ADT (20,32,37). It is of considerable interest that ECT has been the one treatment reported to clearly increase binding at this site (44,58). The increase in 5-HT_2 binding with ECT contrasts to the robust regularity of decreased 5-HT_2 binding with all the other ADTs. Presently, this discrepancy remains unexplained.

The recently identified imipramine binding site related to the 5-HT uptake system has been studied in animals receiving ADT. In general, there is a decrease in the number of these sites following long-term treatments with most drugs and ECT (39,50). The functional consequences of changes in the number of these binding sites relative to the efficiency of 5-HT uptake remain to be elucidated.

The effects of ADT on other neurotransmitter receptors, including acetylcholine and dopamine, have also been studied. In general, there has been little consistent change in the number of these receptors following long-term ADTs. This lends credence to the specificity of the effects observed with the β-, α_1-, and 5-HT_2 receptor binding studies.

It is important to note that receptor number, as measured by binding studies, and functional changes are not always correlated. Thus, in the rat spinal cord, denervation results in an excellent correlation of increased receptor number to increased physiologic responsivity (5). However, in the same system, chronic ADT results in increased physiologic responsivity without concomitant changes in receptor number (79). Thus, ADTs may be affecting coupling factors that are important in transducing the events associated with receptor binding into physiologic responsiveness of the cells. An example of this is the alteration by mianserin of isoproterenol-stimulated cyclic AMP accumulation but not of β-receptor binding (82). It is also of considerable importance that there is a strong interaction of the NE and 5-HT systems. The β-receptor down-regulation is clearly dependent on an intact 5-HT system (115), and evidence has been presented that lesions of the NE system also prevent the ADT-induced increase in 5-HT_2 sensitivity (43). One difficulty is the inability to identify a clear physiologic or behavioral role for the β-receptor system in brain. Similarly, the function of the 5-HT_2 receptor system is not clearly delineated; thus it has been difficult to fully evaluate the physiologic and behavioral effects of ADT on these systems.

Neurophysiologic Sensitivity to Neurotransmitters

Neurophysiologic studies from single neurons have been conducted following long-term ADT. Iontophoretic administration of neurotransmitters, as well as systemic administration of transmitter agonists and antagonists, has been utilized to characterize the effects of long-term ADT on single-unit physiologic sensitivity. In Table 1 it can be seen that in the noradrenergic system the α_1-receptors appear to demonstrate the most consistent change following ADT (2,20). In contrast, presynaptic α_2-receptors studied on the locus ceruleus do not demonstrate as consistent a change across a spectrum of ADT (20). Because of the difficulties in conducting these studies, a large number of brain areas have not been studied with all forms of ADT. In the brain areas where the physiologic responses are thought to be mediated by β-receptors, NE responsiveness has been found to be diminished by most treatments (2,88,89). However, in the hippocampus, where NE responses are apparently also mediated by β-receptors, no significant changes in sensitivity in NE were detected after treatment with a variety of tricyclic drugs (2,89).

The effects of long-term ADT on the 5-HT system appear somewhat more consistent in that many excitatory responses, consistent with stimulation of the 5-HT receptors, are potentiated by most ADTs, including ECT (33), except for 5-HT uptake blockers and the MAOI corgyline (2,13,20). The increased sensitivity to 5-HT occurs with drugs that are not antagonists of the 5-HT system. 5-HT uptake blockers do produce the expected decreased postsynaptic sensitivity, but there is some evidence that overall transmission is increased due to a concurrent and possibly greater decrease in sensitivity of the inhibitory presynaptic 5-HT$_1$ autoreceptors (12–14,34). Thus, both 5-HT uptake blockers and MAOIs have been shown to decrease sensitivity of presynaptic 5-HT autoreceptors, which results in an ADT-induced increase in 5-HT transmission when electrical stimulation is applied to the ascending 5-HT tracks (14). This would result in an overall increase in efficiency of 5-HT transmission following these two types of ADT. The increased postsynaptic responses to 5-HT following chronic tricyclic antidepressants and ECT would also increase 5-HT transmission (11,14,33).

Dopamine (DA) presynaptic subsensitivity has been reported to occur following long-term ADT, including ECT (25,116,125,126). This subsensitivity has been reported to occur after just 2 days of treatment (24). However, this has not been found by other investigators (69). The receptor binding studies show no clear consistent effects of ADTs on DA binding; however, if ADTs induced decreased DA presynaptic sensitivity, this could augment the postsynaptic DA sensitivity seen on behavioral tests so that following ADT there would be an overall increase in DA transmission.

Behavioral Effects of Long-Term ADT Treatment

The effects of long-term ADT described above are certainly very important in understanding possible mechanisms. However, it is clear that ADTs have multiple effects at the cellular and subcellular levels, and many of these effects may not be robust enough to be evident at the behavioral level. The study of the effects of long-term ADT on overall integrated functioning may provide the best data as to the net effects of ADTs on the function of monoamine-mediated systems. This approach has been pursued by the development of behavioral models that are thought to reflect the sensitivity of NE, 5-HT, and DA systems. The use of relatively high doses of clonidine and/or apomorphine to produce increases in activity and aggression before and during chronic ADT treatment has allowed some evaluation of the NE (presumably α_1) and DA (presumably postsynaptic DA) systems during this treatment. In Table 1 it can be seen that most antidepressant treatments except 5-HT uptake inhibitors potentiate this presumably α_1-type-mediated behavior (70,72). Also, the response to apomorphine is potentiated by most tricyclic antidepressant treatments (4,71,73,128). In contrast, the salbutamol-induced inhibition of exploratory behavior or isoproterenol-induced drinking (β-receptor effect) is reduced by most antidepressant treatments (40,74,100,102). Several behavioral models of 5-HT receptor activation in the rat have been identified (27,41,68). Long-term ADT, including ECT, reduced the hypothermic response to a 5-HT$_1$ agonist (27,41), although ECT was found to increase the hypothermic response in another study (122). Long-term ADT has more mixed effects on the preserved 5-HT$_2$ responses, with one study reporting an increase (36); another study, however, reports that many drugs produced a decrease but ECT produced an increase (38,42,67,93). Thus, one of the more consistent effects of most behavioral ADT studies is the augmentation of NE α_1 and postsynaptic DA effects with a concomitant decrease in NE β- and 5-HT$_1$-receptor-mediated behaviors. One of the problems in these studies involves the fact that the behaviors often were studied 24 or more hours following the last antidepressant treatment when blood levels were very low. This raises the question of how relevant these studies might be to clinical studies where patients are continually exposed to relatively high drug levels.

Effects of ADT on Other Neurotransmitter Systems

A recent finding of considerable interest is that long-term administration of a large number of ADTs, including MAOI and ECT, produces an up-regulation of γ-aminobutyric acid$_B$ (GABA$_B$) binding in rat frontal cortex (65). Thus the antidepressant activity of GABA mimetics could result from direct stimulation of GABA receptors, whereas ADTs could work via a combination of up-regulation and endogenous stimulation of GABA receptors (8,65). Since there are data suggesting that GABA$_B$ agonists may modulate neurotransmitter function by altering a component of the cyclic AMP system beyond the transmitter recognition site, this may be an area where ADT effects on monoamine and GABA neurotransmission interact (56).

The antihistaminic effects of many ADTs have been recognized for some time, but this is thought to relate primarily to side effects, such as sedation, since this effect is shared by many antihistamines and antipsychotics that are not antidepressants (30). Long-term ADT produces inconsistent changes in H$_1$ histamine receptor binding, which suggests that alteration of histamine receptor function is not a major therapeutic effect of ADTs (9,92,107,131).

The relative potency of tricyclic antidepressants on the modulation of the sensitivity of opiate receptors does not correlate with ADT clinical efficiency (3,51,108), although modest increases in naloxone binding have been observed following many ADTs (3). Repeated ECT alters biosynthesis of enkephalin (49,130), down-regulates opioid receptors (85), and demonstrates cross sensitivity to morphine tolerance (66), which indicates that alterations in the opioid system are more relevant for ECT. Research on the effects of long-term ADT on other aspects of opioid neurotransmission is in its early stages, and this may be an important area for future research.

Neuronal sensitivity to substance P is increased after long-term treatment with several ADTs, but it is decreased after repeated ECT (53–55). Repeated ECT increases thyrotropin-releasing hormone (TRH) levels in rat brain, and a wide range of other ADTs also increase TRH and its *ex vivo* release in the CNS (10,61,63). Thus ADT effects on neuropeptides indicate that this is an important area for future research.

Summary of Laboratory Animal Studies

The ADT-induced decrease in β-receptor densities and NE-stimulated cyclic AMP response is the most consistent finding across all the ADTs studied, and this correlates well with ADT-induced blunting of physiologic and behavioral responses to β-agonists. Even though increased NE α_1 binding has not been reported by all investigators, the ADT-induced increase in physiologic and behavioral responses to α_1 stimulation indicates that increased sensitivity of α_1-receptor systems is also an important effect of ADT. The inconsistent ADT-induced changes in 5-HT$_2$ binding and behavioral responses to 5-HT agonists do not correlate with the increased physiologic responses to 5-HT agonists identified in electrophysiologic investigations. Also, the lack of ADT-induced changes in DA receptors does not relate to the ADT-induced decrease in presynaptic and increase in postsynaptic responses to DA agonists. The physiologic and therapeutic significance of GABA$_B$ receptor up-regulation and histamine receptor down-regulation remains to be established.

PATIENT STUDIES OF ADT EFFECTS ON RECEPTOR SENSITIVITY

Although many long-term effects of ADT treatment have been demonstrated in laboratory animals, the clinical relevance of these findings remains to be definitively demonstrated. Almost all of the studies have been conducted in healthy laboratory animals, and ADTs produce rather small changes in mood and behavior of healthy human subjects. This contrasts with the large ADT-induced changes in mood and behavior of depressed patients. There are large pharmacokinetic differences between species, and many rat studies have been done 24 hr after the last ADT dose when blood levels have dropped to near zero, whereas patients

have demonstrated clear dose-response curves for blood levels for many of the drugs studied. In addition, since the animal studies have demonstrated many different effects of ADTs, it is not clear which of these are important and meaningful in the clinical situation for explanation of the antidepressant effects in patients. Human studies are limited for ethical reasons to the use of interventions that are not harmful. Thus, all of the procedures and many of the compounds utilized in the animal studies described above are not possible in depressed patients. Postmortem receptor binding studies in humans may provide some information as to the possible abnormalities in the monoamine receptor systems of patients, but studies of ADT using this method are very difficult because of problems of drug dosage, treatment duration, agonal effects, and postmortem changes. Studies of ADT effects on monoamine receptors on blood elements are possible, but such studies have all the problems associated with peripheral effects (e.g., changes in plasma epinephrine, NE, cortisol, etc.) and the obvious problem that only brain has the relevant biologic mechanisms for the complex regulation and interaction of receptors. Since peripheral catecholamine administration does not alter cerebral β-receptor density, it is unlikely that ADT-induced changes in regulation of receptors in blood elements would be a reliable model of the changes occurring in brain (81).

An alternative strategy has been to administer a clinically safe neurotransmitter agonist or antagonist before and during long-term ADT and to assess the effect of this neurotransmitter challenge on measured variables. Table 2 lists the studies where this method has been applied. Obviously, there are many possible pitfalls in this method. If the sensitivity of the synapses distal to the one initially stimulated is altered, then the interpretation of the test is confounded. Many of the pathways (e.g., light to inhibit melatonin secretion) are long and complex and only partially understood. Thus, even though a neurotransmitter agonist or antagonist may demonstrate a patient control difference or an effect of ADT, it is not assured that this does reflect abnormalities or drug effects on the neurotransmitter receptor system studied. However, even with these difficulties, the human studies that have been conducted generally support the findings described in the animal experiments mentioned above.

Noradrenergic Receptors

The α_2-adrenergic receptor agonist clonidine has been administered to depressed patients, and the responses of plasma MHPG, blood pressure, heart rate, sedation, growth hormone, and cortisol have been assessed. The clonidine-induced drop in plasma MHPG was found to be slightly increased in depressed patients in one study using i.v. clonidine (113), but not different from controls in the study using oral clonidine (15). Clonidine-induced decreases in blood pressure and increases in sedation have been found to be normal in all of the studies of depressed patients (15,23). The growth hormone response to clonidine is decreased and the cortisol response to clonidine is increased in depressed patients. These two hormonal responses are thought to result from postsynaptic actions of clonidine

TABLE 2. *Clinical evaluation of receptor sensitivity in depressed patients[a]*

Receptor type/ receptor stimulus	Location	Effect of stimulus on variable	Receptor sensitivity (patient vs controls)	Effect of ADT treatment	Change in sensitivity
NE-α_2					
Clonidine	Pre	↓ Plasma MHPG	Normal or decreased	DMI	↓
				AMI	↓
				MIA	0
				TRZ	0
	Pre/post	↓ Blood pressure	Normal	DMI	↓
				AMI	↓
				MIA	0
				TRZ	0
				MAOI	↓
	Pre/post	↑ Sedation	Normal	AMI	↓
				MIA	0
				TRZ	0
	Post	↑ Growth hormone	Decreased	DMI	0
				AMI	0
				MIA	0
				TRZ	0
				MAOI	0
	Post	↓ Cortisol	Increased	—	—
Yohimbine	Pre	↑ Plasma MHPG	Normal	—	—
	Pre/post	↑ BP	Increased	—	—
	Post	↑ Cortisol	Decreased	—	—
NE-α_1					
Phenylephrine	Post	↑ Dilation iris	Normal	MAOI	↑
Amphetamine	Post	↑ Corticosteroids	Decreased	TCA	0
				ECT	0
NE-β					
Light	Post	↓ Nighttime melatonin	Decreased	DMI	↑
5-HT					
Tryptophan	Pre/post	↑ Prolactin	Decreased	DMI	↑
				AMI	↑
				MAOI	↑
5-HTP	Pre/post	↑ Cortisol	Increased	TCA	↓
				MAOI	↑
Fenfluramine	Pre/post	↑ Prolactin	Decreased	—	—

[a] Symbols: ↑, increase; ↓, decrease; 0, no change; —, not tested. DMI, Desipramine; AMI, amitriptyline; MIA, mianserin; TRZ, trazodone; TCA, tricyclic drugs; MAOI, monoamine oxidase inhibitors; ECT, electroconvulsive treatment.

(35,99,114). Long-term treatment with a variety of ADTs listed in Table 2 indicates that those drugs which are thought to augment synaptic NE (inhibit NE reuptake and MAOI) generally produce a decrease in the clonidine-induced response of MHPG, blood pressure, and sedation (16,19,112). Mianserin and trazodone, which do not have clear effects on NE uptake, do not change the response to clonidine of these variables (18,98). The blunted growth hormone response found in depressed patients has not been normalized by a variety of ADTs and would appear to be a more stable trait measure (35). The relatively normal function of the presynaptic α_2-receptor as measured by clonidine was also observed in the yohimbine test, where the increase in plasma MHPG is normal in depressed patients (46). Since there is evidence that the postsynaptic α_2-receptor is inhibitory to cortisol release, the increased cortisol following yohimbine would be interpreted as a decreased sensitivity of this receptor (99).

The α_1-receptor has been studied in the iris, and the phenylephrine-induced dilation of the iris, which is mediated by an α_1-receptor, has been shown to be increased following MAOIs (109). It has been difficult to identify other more central measures of α_1 function. There is some evidence that α_1-receptors are stimulatory to corticosteroid release, and the corticosteroid response to amphetamine has been found to be decreased in depressed patients, but this is not affected by tricyclic drug administration or ECT (22,105).

Given the strength of the animal data, it would be extremely important to study β-receptor function in depressed patients (6). One of the few β-receptor-related measures available for the study in humans has involved the use of light to inhibit melatonin secretion. Since β-receptors are the last in a number of synapses regulating light effects on melatonin secretion, receptor changes earlier in the neuronal chain leading to the β-receptor on the pineal could affect the results. The light-induced decrease in nighttime melatonin is increased in bipolar patients (62). DMI increases nighttime melatonin levels (105,119, but not found by all investigators: 31,79). This would suggest that β-receptor function is decreased in depression and is increased by DMI treatment. This contrasts with studies in rats where long-term DMI treatment decreases β-receptor function and melatonin levels (48). There appear to be important differences in the effects of long-term DMI treatment on healthy rats and depressed humans.

Serotonergic Receptors

In the serotonergic system, the 5-HT precursors tryptophan and 5-hydroxytryptophan (5-HTP) have been utilized to stimulate serotonergic receptors. The prolactin response to i.v. tryptophan in depressed patients has been observed to be decreased, and this has been reversed toward normal with DMI, AMI, and MAOI treatment (17,47). In contrast, the cortisol response to 5-HTP has been found to be increased in depressed patients, and this is decreased with tricyclic antidepressant treatment, although it is increased with MAOI treatment (75–77). It is of some importance that tryptophan does not alter cortisol secretion and 5-HTP does not alter prolactin secretion. The reasons for this are currently unexplained, since it is clear from a number of animal and human studies that serotonergic agonists release both cortisol and prolactin. The prolactin response to fenfluramine has been shown to be blunted in depressed patients, but this has not been studied with ADT treatment (111). The blunted prolactin response to tryptophan and fenfluramine and the increased cortisol response to 5-HTP could result from presynaptic abnormalities in uptake of the 5-HT precursor, or it could involve the release of 5-HT (this is the process by which fenfluramine increases 5-HT). The prolactin and cortisol responses are presumed to result from stimulation of postsynaptic 5-HT receptors. It has not yet been possible to stimulate the 5-HT presynaptic autoreceptors in a manner analogous to that done with clonidine and yohimbine for the α_2 NE receptors.

As a test of the DA system in depressed patients, bromocriptine has been used to inhibit prolactin secretion. A course of ECT treatment was found to increase the inhibitory effect of bromocriptine on prolactin release in one study but not in another (7,26). Tests of other DA receptor systems have not yet been developed.

Summary of Patient Studies

There is little evidence of abnormality in the presynaptic α_2-adrenergic receptor in depressed patients, and an ADT-induced subsensitivity of this receptor is observed only with ADTs that block NE uptake. Postsynaptic α_2 function appears to be impaired in depressed patients and has not been found to revert toward normal with a number of ADTs. The α_1- and the β-receptor have been insufficiently studied for any conclusion to be made regarding their abnormality in depression. The ADT-induced changes in hormonal responses to 5-HT precursors are variable, and

since these responses involve both presynaptic and postsynaptic processes, at present more specific tests of 5-HT function in humans are needed.

COMMENT

A Common Mechanism of Action of ADTs

The central question on antidepressant mechanisms is whether changes in receptor sensitivity reflect a common mechanism by which all ADTs produce therapeutic effects. In a general sense, the current evidence reviewed above supports this hypothesis, since all ADTs have been shown to produce some form of delayed changes in receptor sensitivity in laboratory animals. What is not clear, however, is whether all ADTs act uniformly on one type of receptor or on one neurotransmitter system. An additional question involves whether different types of depressive illness respond differently to separate aspects of ADT (e.g., are different ADTs better for certain types of depression?).

In the animal studies, the most consistent finding is the reduced cyclic AMP response to NE and the decreased β-receptor binding. There is also physiologic and some behavioral evidence suggesting that this is behaviorally relevant. However, the role of β-receptors in regulating human behavior is not clear, and it is known that many β-receptors exist on neuroglial cells. The confirmation of the importance of β-receptor down-regulation may need to wait until more effective methods for assessing β-receptor function in patients are developed.

One of the more consistent findings across both the animal and patient studies is the role of postsynaptic α-receptors. The impaired growth hormone response to clonidine is a very reliable and clearly defined abnormality in depression. If postsynaptic α-receptors are implicated in inhibition of cortisol secretion, this could also be strong evidence in support of postsynaptic α_2-receptor system abnormalities in patients. In the animal studies, most ADTs increase the physiologic and behavioral sensitivity of postsynaptic α_1-receptors. It has not been possible to test this in the central nervous system of patients.

In the clinical data there is evidence for both increased and decreased 5-HT function in depression. With the methods available it has not been possible to separate out the pre- and postsynaptic factors that might explain these discrepancies. The physiologic and some of the behavioral studies indicate that ADTs increase serotonergic function. The role of the 5-HT$_2$ receptors is not fully understood, and the functional implication of the decrease in 5-HT$_2$ receptor binding seen with almost all ADTs remains to be clarified. The use of new more specific 5-HT agonists in clinical studies may help clarify these problems.

The role of dopamine in depression has been recently reviewed (124,126). There is not as strong and consistent evidence of the primary involvement of the dopaminergic system in the pathogenesis of depression and the mechanism of action of ADT. However, similar to the postsynaptic α_1 system, there are some data from animal studies that ADTs do potentiate overall dopaminergic function.

Multiple Mechanisms of Actions of ADTs

An overview of all the data from animal and patient studies does not yet point to a single effect of ADTs on receptor sensitivity that is necessary and sufficient for antidepressant efficacy. At present it would appear that different receptor mechanisms are involved. The different effects on separate receptor mechanisms could have a similar end result, i.e., a net improvement in overall transmission. For example, in the 5-HT system, the slowly developing subsensitivity of the presynaptic 5-HT$_1$ autoreceptors following 5-HT uptake blocking drugs and MAOIs results in increased overall efficiency of 5-HT function following electrical stimulation. The other ADTs that do not work through this mechanism appear to sensitize postsynaptic 5-HT receptors, and through this mechanism they also could increase 5-HT transmission. Similarly, it is possible that some compounds (those blocking NE uptake) produce decreased sensitivity of the α_2-receptor (or block it directly, e.g., mianserin) and thereby augment NE function; this would secondarily reduce β-receptor sensitivity. Other treatments could directly alter postsynaptic α_1 sensitivity.

There remain, however, considerable problems in interpretation of the receptor changes. For example, in the β-receptor system the ADT down-regulation of β sensitivity would suggest that depression is accompanied by an abnormally increased β-receptor sensitivity which is normalized by ADT; however, an opposing concept would suggest that β-receptor function is subsensitive in depressed patients and that it is further down-regulated as a consequence of increased synaptic NE, which is necessary to augment the originally impaired overall function. The opposite effects of long-term ADT on α- and β-receptors do not necessarily have to be seen as incompatible. Many reciprocal regulations of these receptors have been observed, and thus the effects induced by long-term ADT may serve to correct a disorder of regulation in which the balance between α- and β-receptor sensitivity is more important than just the absolute effects of either system (45). Complex interactions between NE and 5-HT systems during long-term ADT have also been put forth to explain ADT effects (45,103,110).

Even though at the neurochemical level it would appear that ADTs act via multiple mechanisms, it is important to recognize that at the clinical level the lack of specificity of clinical effects suggests that the different treatments share some aspect of a final common mechanism. The nature of that mechanism remains to be elucidated.

Treatment Implications

Although it has been proposed that subtypes of depression exist that respond potentially to different ADTs (e.g., amitriptyline vs imipramine), in general there have been few studies demonstrating clear differences between patients in their response to treatment. Alternatively, the data may be better interpreted as demonstrating a factor of responsiveness-unresponsiveness to any form of ADT, as opposed to patients responding to one type of treatment vs another.

In addition to possibly more fully understanding the

pathogenic sequences involved in depression, a better knowledge of ADT effect on receptor sensitivity could lead to the improved efficacy of current treatments. Previously studied possibilities include the following:

1. The use of combined α_2-adrenergic antagonists and NE uptake blocking drugs to rapidly reduce β-receptors (6,32,57). A trial of DMI and yohimbine has been conducted, and the combination was not found to be any better than DMI alone (21).

2. The use of thyroid hormone to increase α-adrenergic function. There have been a number of reports that thyroid hormone accelerates and potentiates the effect of a variety of ADTs, and receptor sensitization may indeed be the mechanism involved (see review, *this volume*).

3. If most ADTs increase postsynaptic 5-HT sensitivity, then ADTs in combination with augmentation of presynaptic 5-HT function would lead to a faster ADT response. When lithium, which has been shown to augment presynaptic 5-HT function, is added to ADT, there is an augmentation of the ADT response. This has been hypothesized but not demonstrated to be dependent on long-term ADT treatment. There are, however, studies indicating that lithium may potentiate ADTs as early as during the first week of treatment (see review, *this volume*).

Implications for the Future: Development of New Treatments

Even though at the present time it is not possible to clearly document abnormalities in the regulations of monoamine receptor systems as the cause of depressive illness, the findings reviewed in the other chapters of this volume and the data on ADT reviewed above suggest that dysregulation of receptor systems may play a critical role in the pathogenesis of depression. The mechanisms involved in the receptor-mediated transduction of the neurotransmitter signal are increasingly better understood. The possible effects of ADTs acting more directly on receptor–N-protein coupling are being investigated (86,87), as well as second messenger effects (52,59,101). Of considerable interest is the possible use of drugs that inhibit phosphodiesterase, thus directly elevating cyclic AMP levels by a mechanism not directly involving receptors (101). The rapid progress of neuroscience will certainly provide many new possibilities. With the use of these increasingly available new methods an improved understanding of the mechanism of action of ADT is expected.

SUMMARY

There is preclinical evidence that all ADTs produce changes in monoamine receptor sensitivity, and the time course of these changes is similar to the time course of therapeutic actions of ADT. Long-term ADT has been found to reduce β-adrenergic sensitivity and the cyclic AMP response to NE. ADTs have also been found to enhance responses to α-adrenergic, serotonergic, and, to some extent, dopaminergic stimulation. Initial clinical data indicate that postsynaptic NE α_1- and α_2-receptor systems may be subsensitive in depressed patients, but that presynaptic NE α_2-receptor systems are relatively normal. These abnormalities do not clearly improve with ADTs. There is some evidence that the serotonergic system is abnormal in depressed patients, and that this is normalized with ADTs. Thus, the data provide support for the hypothesis that alterations in the sensitivity of receptor systems are involved in the pathogenesis of depression, and that effective ADTs act to alter this abnormality. The data also suggest, however, that ADTs may act at the neurochemical level through different mechanisms. How these separate neurochemical effects interact to bring about an antidepressant response remains to be elucidated.

REFERENCES

1. Abel, M. S., Villegas, F., Abreu, J., Gimino, F., Steiner, S., Beer, B., and Meyerson, L. R. (1983): *Brain Res. Bull.*, 11:729–734.
2. Aghajanian, G. K. (1981): In: *Neuroreceptors: Basic and Clinical Aspects*, edited by E. Usdin, W. E. Bunney, and J. M. Davis, pp. 27–35. John Wiley & Sons, Chichester.
3. Antkiewicz-Michaluk, L., Rokosz-Pelc, A., and Vetulani, J. (1984): *Eur. J. Pharmacol.*, 102:179–181.
4. Arnt, J., Overo, K. F., Hyttel, J., and Olsen, R. (1984): *Psychopharmacology*, 84:457–465.
5. Astrachan, D. I., Davis, M., and Gallager, D. W. (1983): *Brain Res.*, 260:81–90.
6. Avorn, J., Everitt, D. E., and Weiss, S. (1986): *JAMA*, 255:357–360.
7. Balldin, J., Granerus, A. K., Lindstedt, G., Modigh, K., and Walnder, J. (1982): *Psychopharmacology*, 876:371–376.
8. Bartholini, G., Lloyd, K. G., and Morselli, P. L. (1985): In: *GABA and Mood Disorders: Animal and Clinical Studies*. Raven Press, New York.
9. Beckmann, H., and Schmaub, M. (1983): *Arch. Psychiatr. Nervenkr.*, 233:59–70.
10. Bennett, G. W., Green, A. R., Lighton, C., and Marsden, C. A. (1986): *Br. J. Pharmacol.*, 99:129–139.
11. Blier, P., and deMontigny, C. (1980): *Naunyn Schmiedebergs Arch. Pharmacol.*, 314:123–128.
12. Blier, P., and deMontigny, C. (1983): *J. Neurosci.*, 3:1270–1278.
13. Blier, P., and deMontigny, C. (1985): *Neuroscience*, 16:949–955.
14. Blier, P., deMontigny, C., and Tardif, D. (1984): *Psychopharmacology*, 84:242–249.
15. Charney, D. S., Heninger, G. R., and Sternberg, D. E. (1982): *Arch. Gen. Psychiatry*, 39:290–294.
16. Charney, D. S., Heninger, G. R., and Sternberg, D. E. (1983): *Br. J. Psychiatry*, 142:265–270.
17. Charney, D. S., Heninger, G. R., and Sternberg, D. E. (1984): *Arch. Gen. Psychiatry*, 41:359–365.
18. Charney, D. S., Heninger, G. R., and Sternberg, D. E. (1984): *Br. J. Psychiatry*, 144:407–416.
19. Charney, D. S., Heninger, G. R., Sternberg, D. E., Redmond, D. E., Leckman, M. D., Maas, J. W., and Roth, R. H. (1981): *Arch. Gen. Psychiatry*, 38:1334–1340.
20. Charney, D. S., Menkes, D. B., and Heninger, G. R. (1981): *Arch. Gen. Psychiatry*, 38:1160–1180.
21. Charney, D. S., Price, L. H., and Heninger, G. R. (1986): *Arch. Gen. Psychiatry*, 43:1155–1161.
22. Checkley, S. A. (1978): *Psychol. Med.*, 8:1–9.
23. Checkley, S. A., and Shure, E. (1981): *Br. J. Psychiatry*, 138:51–55.
24. Chiodo, L. A., and Antelman, S. M. (1980): *Nature*, 287:451–454.
25. Chiodo, L. A., and Antelman, S. M. (1980): *Science*, 210:799–801.
26. Christie, J. E., Whalley, L. J., Brown, N. S., and Dick, H. (1982): *Br. J. Psychiatry*, 40:268–273.
27. Cohen, R. M., Aulakh, C. S., and Murphy, D. L. (1983): *Eur. J. Pharmacol.*, 94:175–179.
28. Cohen, R. M., Campbell, I. C., Dauphin, M., Tallman, J. F., and Murphy, D. L. (1982): *Neuropharmacology*, 21:293–298.
29. Cohen, R. M., Ebstein, R. P., Daly, J. W., and Murphy, D. L. (1982): *J. Neurosci.*, 2:1588–1595.
30. Coupet, J., and Szuchs-Myers, V. A. (1981): *Eur. J. Pharmacol.*, 74:149–155.
31. Cowen, P. J., Green, A. R., Grahame-Smith, D. G., and Braddock, L. E. (1985): *Br. J. Clin. Pharmacol.*, 19:799–805.
32. Crews, F. T., Scott, J. A., and Shorstein, N. H. (1983): *Neuropharmacology*, 22:1203–1209.
33. deMontigny, C. (1984): *J. Pharmacol. Exp. Ther.*, 228:230–234.
34. deMontigny, C., Blier, P., and Chaput, Y. (1984): *Neuropharmacology*, 23:1511–1520.
35. Eriksson, E. (1985): In: *Experimental Psychoneuroendocrinology: Brain Alpha 2 Adrenoceptor Function and Growth Hormone Release*. Med. Press, Goteborg, Sweden.
36. Friedman, E., Cooper, T. B., and Dallob, A. (1983): *Eur. J. Pharmacol.*, 89:69–76.
37. Fuxe, K., Ogren, S. O., Agnati, L. F., Benfenati, F., Fredholm, B., Andersson, K., Zini, I., and Eneroth, P. (1983): *Neuropharmacology*, 22:389–400.
38. Fuxe, K., Ogren, S. O., Agnati, L. F., Eneroth, P., Holm, A. C., and Andersson, K. (1981): *Neurosci. Lett.*, 21:57–62.
39. Gentsch, C., Lichtsteiner, M., and Feer, H. (1984): *J. Neural Transm.*, 59:257–264.
40. Goldstein, J. M., Knoblock-Litwin, L. C., and Malick, J. B. (1985): *Arch. Pharmacol.*, 329:355–358.
41. Goodwin, G. M., DeSouza, R. J., and Green, A. R. (1985): *Nature*, 317:531–533.
42. Goodwin, G. M., Green, A. R., and Johnson, P. (1984): *Br. J. Pharmacol.*, 83:235–242.
43. Gravel, P., and deMontigny, C. (1983): *Abstr. Soc. Neurosci.*, 429.
44. Green, A. R., Heal, D. J., Johnson, P., Laurence, B. E., and Nimgaonkar, V. L. (1983): *Br. J. Pharmacol.*, 80:377–385.
45. Harrison-Read, P. E. (1981): *Trends Neurosci.*, 4:32–34.
46. Heninger, G. R., Charney, D. S., and Price, L. H. (1987): (submitted for publication).
47. Heninger, G. R., Charney, D. S., and Sternberg, D. E. (1984): *Arch. Gen. Psychiatry*, 41:398–402.
48. Heydorn, W. E., Brunswick, D. J., and Frazer, A. (1982): *J. Pharmacol. Exp. Ther.*, 222:534–543.
49. Hong, J. S., Yoshikawa, K., Kanamatsu, T., McGinty, J. F., Mitchell, C. L., and Sabol, S. L. (1985): *Neuropeptides*, 5:557–560.
50. Hrdina, P. D. (1983): *Psychiatry Res.*, 11:271–278.
51. Isenberg, K. E., and Cicero, T. J. (1984): *Eur. J. Pharmacol.*, 103:57–63.
52. Johnson, R. D., and Minneman, K. P. (1985): *Brain Res.*, 341:7–15.
53. Jones, R. S. G., Mondadori, C., and Olpe, H. R. (1985): *Neuropharmacology*, 24:627–633.
54. Jones, R. S. G., and Olpe, H. R. (1983): *Eur. J. Pharmacol.*, 87:171–172.
55. Jones, R. S. G., and Olpe, H. R. (1984): *Br. J. Pharmacol.*, 81:659–664.
56. Karbon, E. W., and Enna, S. J. (1984): *Mol. Pharmacol.*, 27:53–59.
57. Keith, R. A., Howe, B. B., and Salama, A. I. (1985): *J. Pharmacol. Exp. Ther.*, 236:356–363.
58. Kellar, K. J., and Bergstrom, D. A. (1983): *Neuropharmacology*, 22:401–406.
59. Kendall, D. A., and Nahorski, S. R. (1984): *J. Pharmacol. Exp. Ther.*, 233:473–479.
60. Koslow, J. H., Maas, J. W., Bowden, C. L., et al. (1983): *Arch. Gen. Psychiatry*, 40:999–1010.
61. Kubek, M. J., and Sattin, A. (1984): *Life Sci.*, 34:1149–1152.
62. Lewy, A. J., Wehr, T. A., Goodwin, F. K., Newsome, D. A., and Rosenthal, N. E. (1981): *Lancet*, 1:383–384.
63. Lighton, C., Bennet, G. W., and Marsden, C. A. (1985): *Neuropharmacology*, 24:401–406.

64. Linnoila, M., Guthrie, S., Lane, E. A., Karoum, F., Rudorfer, M., and Potter, W. Z. (1986): *Psychiatry Res.,* 17:229–239.
65. Lloyd, K. G., Thuret, F., and Pilc, A. (1985): *J. Pharmacol. Exp. Ther.,* 235:191–199.
66. Lucas Belenky, G., and Holaday, J. W. (1981): *Life Sci.,* 29:553–563.
67. Lucki, I., and Frazer, A. (1982): *Psychopharmacology,* 77:205–211.
68. Lucki, I., Nobler, M. S., and Frazer, A. (1983): *J. Pharmacol. Exp. Ther.,* 228:133–139.
69. MacNiell, D. A., and Gower, M. (1982): *Nature,* 298:302.
70. Maj, J., Mogilnicka, E., Klimek, V., and Kordecka-Magiera, A. (1981): *J. Neural Transm.,* 52:189–197.
71. Maj, J., Rogoz, Z., Skuza, G., and Sowinska, H. (1982): *J. Neural Transm.,* 55:19–25.
72. Maj, J., Rogoz, Z., Skuza, G., and Sowinska, H. (1984): *Pol. J. Pharm. Pharmacol.,* 36:127–130.
73. Martin-Iverson, M. T., Leclere, J. F., and Fibiger, H. C. (1983): *Eur. J. Pharmacol.,* 94:193–201.
74. Mason, S. T., and Angel, A. (1983): *Psychopharmacology,* 81:73–77.
75. Meltzer, H. L. (1984): *Arch. Gen. Psychiatry,* 41:366–378.
76. Meltzer, H. L. (1984): *Arch. Gen. Psychiatry,* 41:379–390.
77. Meltzer, H. L. (1984): *Arch. Gen. Psychiatry,* 41:391–398.
78. Mendlewicz, J. (1983): *Lancet,* 2:283.
79. Menkes, D. B., Aghajanian, G. K., and Gallager, D. W. (1983): *Eur. J. Pharmacol.,* 87:35–41.
80. Middlemiss, D. N., and Fozard, J. R. (1983): *Eur. J. Pharmacol.,* 90:151–153.
81. Minneman, K. P., Wolfe, B. B., and Molinoff, P. B. (1982): *Brain Res.,* 252:309–314.
82. Mishra, R., Janowsky, A., and Sulser, F. (1980): *Neuropharmacology,* 19:983–987.
83. Miyauchi, T., Kitada, Y., and Satoh, S. (1982): *Neuropsychopharmacol. Biol. Psychiatry,* 6:137–142.
84. Mobley, P. L., and Sulser, F. (1979): *Eur. J. Pharmacol.,* 60:221–227.
85. Nakata, Y., Chang, K. J., Mitchell, C. L., and Hong, J. S. (1985): *Brain Res.,* 346:160–163.
86. Newman, M. E., Solomon, H., and Lerer, B. (1986): *J. Neurochem.,* 46:1667–1669.
87. O'Donnell, J. M., and Frazer, A. (1985): *J. Pharmacol. Exp. Ther.,* 234:30–36.
88. Olpe, H. R., Schellenberg, A., and Jones, R. S. G. (1984): *J. Neural Transm.,* 60:265–271.
89. Olpe, H. R., Schellenberg, A., and Steinmann, M. W. (1981): *Eur. J. Pharmacol.,* 72:381–385.
90. Oswald, I., Brezinova, V., and Dunleavy, D. L. F. (1972): *Br. J. Psychiatry,* 120:673–677.
91. Overall, J. E., Hollister, L. E., Pokorny, A. D., et al. (1962): *Clin. Pharmacol. Ther.,* 3:16–22.
92. Pandey, G. N., Krueger, A., Sudershan, P., and Davis, J. M. (1982): *Life Sci.,* 30:921–927.
93. Pawlowski, L., and Melzacka, M. (1986): *Psychopharmacology,* 88:279–284.
94. Perkins, J. P. (1983): In: *Current Topics in Membranes and Transport,* edited by D. M. F. Cooper, pp. 85–108. Academic Press, New York.
95. Peroutka, S. J. (1985): *Brain Res.,* 344:167–171.
96. Peroutka, S. J., and Snyder, S. H. (1981): *Science,* 212:287–289.
97. Post, R. M., Kopin, J., and Goodwin, F. K. (1974): *Am. J. Psychiatry,* 131:511–517.
98. Price, L. H., Charney, D. S., and Heninger, G. R. (1986): *Psychopharmacology,* 89:38–44.
99. Price, L. H., Charney, D. S., Rubin, A. L., and Heninger, G. R. (1986): *Arch. Gen. Psychiatry,* 43:849–858.
100. Przegalinski, E., Baran, L., and Siwanowicz, J. (1983): *Psychopharmacology,* 80:355–359.
101. Przegalinski, E., Baran, L., Siwanowicz, J., Nowak, G., Antkiewicz-Michaluk, L., and Vetulani, J. (1985): *J. Neural Transm.,* 64:211–226.
102. Przegalinski, E., Siwanowicz, J., Begajska, K., and Baran, L. (1984): *J. Pharm. Pharmacol.,* 36:626–628.
103. Racagni, G., and Brunello, N. (1984): *Trends Pharmacol. Sci.,* 5:128–134.
104. Richelson, E., and Pfenning, M. (1984): *Eur. J. Pharmacol.,* 104:277–286.
105. Sachar, E. J., Asnis, G., and Nathan, S. (1980): *Arch. Gen. Psychiatry,* 37:755–757.
106. Sack, R. L., and Lewy, A. J. (1986): *Biol. Psychiatry,* 21:406–410.
107. Savard, P., Merand, Y., and Dupont, A. (1982): *Prog. Neuropsychopharmacol. Biol. Psychiatry,* 6:449–454.
108. Scuvee-Moreau, J. J., and Svensson, T. H. (1982): *J. Neural Transm.,* 54:51–63.
109. Shur, E., and Checkley, S. (1982): *Br. J. Psychiatry,* 140:181–184.
110. Siever, L. J., and Davis, K. L. (1985): *Am. J. Psychiatry,* 142:1017–1031.
111. Siever, L. J., Kafka, M. S., Targum, S., and Lake, C. R. (1984): *Psychiatry Res.,* 11:287–302.
112. Siever, L. J., Uhde, T. W., Insel, T. R., Roy, B. F., and Murphy, D. L. (1982): *Psychiatry Res.,* 7:139–144.
113. Siever, L. J., Uhde, T. W., and Jimerson, D. C. (1984): *Am. J. Psychiatry,* 141:733–741.
114. Siever, L. J., Uhde, T. W., and Jimerson, D. C. (1984): *Arch. Gen. Psychiatry,* 41:63–68.
115. Stockmeier, C. A., Martino, A. M., and Kellar, K. J. (1985): *Science,* 230:323–325.
116. Stolz, J. F., and Marsden, C. A. (1982): *Eur. J. Pharmacol.,* 79:17–22.
117. Sugrue, M. F. (1983): *J. Neural Transm.,* 57:281–295.
118. Sugrue, M. F. (1983): *Pharmacol. Ther.,* 13:219–247.
119. Thompson, C., Checkley, S. A., Corn, T., Franey, C., and Arendt, J. (1983): *Lancet,* 1:735.
120. Vetulani, J., Antkiewicz-Michaluk, L., and Rokosz-Pelc, A. (1984): *Brain Res.,* 310:360–362.
121. Vetulani, J., Antkiewicz-Michaluk, L., Rokosz-Pelc, A., and Pilc, A. (1983): *Brain Res.,* 275:392–395.
122. Vetulani, J., Lebrecht, U., and Pilc, A. (1981): *Eur. J. Pharmacol.,* 76:81–85.
123. Vetulani, J., Stawarz, R. J., Dingell, J. V., et al. (1976): *Naunyn Schmiedebergs Arch. Pharmacol.,* 293:109–114.
124. Willner, P. (1983): *Brain Res. Rev.,* 6:211–224.
125. Willner, P. (1983): *Brain Res. Rev.,* 6:225–236.
126. Willner, P. (1983): *Brain Res. Rev.,* 6:237–246.
127. Willner, P. (1985): *Psychopharmacology,* 85:387–404.
128. Willner, P., Towell, A., and Montgomery, T. (1984): *Eur. J. Pharmacol.,* 98:397–406.
129. Wolfe, B. B., Harden, T. K., Sporn, J. R., et al. (1978): *J. Pharmacol. Exp. Ther.,* 207:446–457.
130. Yoshikawa, K., Hong, J.-S., and Sabol, S. L. (1985): *Proc. Natl. Acad. Sci. USA,* 82:589–593.
131. Zawilska, J., and Nowak, J. Z. (1986): *Agents Actions,* 18:222–225.

Psychopharmacology:
The Third Generation of Progress,
edited by Herbert Y. Meltzer.
Raven Press, New York © 1987.

CHAPTER 55

Monoamine Oxidase Inhibitors as Antidepressants: Implications for the Mechanism of Action of Antidepressants and the Psychobiology of the Affective Disorders and Some Related Disorders

Dennis L. Murphy, Charanjit S. Aulakh, Nancy A. Garrick, and Trey Sunderland

The monoamine oxidase (MAO) inhibitors were the first true antidepressants discovered. The mood-elevating properties of iproniazid observed in tuberculosis patients led to successful trials of this MAO inhibitor in depressed patients which were reported in the late 1950s. The preexisting knowledge that MAO was an important enzyme in the metabolism of brain catecholamines and serotonin, coupled with later information that acute, high-dose administration of MAO inhibitors with different chemical structures uniformly led to rapid elevations in brain monoamine concentrations, spawned the hypothesis that enhancement of brain monoaminergic function was a key element in the mechanism of action of antidepressant treatments.

While increasing evidence from studies of additional MAO inhibitors, tricyclics, and other antidepressants has continued to bolster the proposition that antidepressants most likely act through brain monoaminergic system changes, a derivative hypothesis, that patients with affective disorders have derangements in monoaminergic function, has remained far more controversial. Originally formulated primarily on the basis of interpretations from what was

known about the behavioral effects of drugs that altered brain catecholamines or indoleamines, conclusive, direct evidence of a simple monoamine deficit state underlying depression (or a state of monoamine excess in mania) has never been found. Nonetheless, as revealed in other chapters in this volume, variants of this hypothesis linking brain monoamine dysfunction to the development of affective disorders continue to thrive, and hypotheses regarding other major and minor (or "trace") neurotransmitters, including acetylcholine, γ-aminobutyric acid (GABA), phenylethylamine, octopamine, and others have evolved.

There is a major weakness in logic in attempting to reason from what a drug does in any one neurotransmitter system to proposing an abnormality in that system as important to an illness which responds to treatment with that drug. There are examples throughout clinical pharmaceutics of drugs that act through mechanisms that are unconnected or very distant from the primary disease state. On the other hand, there are clear examples where drug mechanisms have provided valuable clues to etiology or at least to common, intermediate pathways in disease processes.

However, in neuropsychopharmacology, one has only to look at the complex and checkered history of our 30 to 40 years of study of antidepressant, neuroleptic, and antianxiety drug-derived hypotheses to become profoundly cautious in this approach.

The point here is that there seems only a distant likelihood of establishing a linkage between a disorder and a brain biochemical change by studying therapeutic drug actions. However, given the vicissitudes and many limitations in naturalistic human psychobiological investigations, clues from what therapeutic drugs do or do not do may be of help in narrowing the search or opening new horizons for more definitive studies, and it is the proposition of this chapter that clinical and basic studies of MAO-inhibiting antidepressants have provided some interesting clues worth pursuing in trying to understand (a) the psychobiology of the affective disorders, (b) how drugs that are useful in treating the affective disorders work, and, perhaps, (c) the relationship of the affective disorders to other psychiatric diagnostic entities.

MAO INHIBITORS: THERAPEUTIC EFFICACY

A necessary prerequisite to the assessment of the potential usefulness of the psychobiological consequences of MAO inhibitor administration in deriving some hypotheses regarding their mechanisms of action and their implications for depressive disorders is the question of how therapeutically effective the MAO inhibitors are, and what patient subgroups respond to them.

A survey of recent, major, double-blind, random-assignment studies of MAO inhibitors available for prescription in the United States accomplished during the 1980s reveals that phenelzine, tranylcypromine, and isocarboxazid continue to be found more effective than placebo and, in general, equally as effective as the standard tricyclic antidepressants (Table 1), confirming the earlier conclusions of a 1979 review (62). Moreover, these MAO inhibitors were demonstrated to be as effective as the tricyclics in all recent controlled studies of typical populations of depressed patients meeting current diagnostic criteria (Table 1) as in those patients with so-called atypical depression (Table 1). This is a major finding, which would appear to contradict quite widely held clinical lore that "atypical" patients are preferentially responsive to MAO inhibitors, whereas typical depressed patients respond best to tricyclics and related heterocyclic agents.

A core problem here may be that different patient characteristics were chosen to define the atypical subgroups both in the early studies and in some of the more recent studies (Table 2). High anxiety, hysteroid features, and reversed vegetative signs (e.g., oversleeping, overeating, feeling better in the morning) or some more discrete similar symptoms such as panic have sometimes been found to occur more frequently in responders to phenelzine than in nonresponders to this or other MAO inhibitors (24,53,64). Nonetheless, many attempts to validate the existence of a

TABLE 1. *Recent double-blind, random-assignment trials with MAO inhibitors[a]*

Study	Patient N and criteria	Results
Depressed patients meeting standard diagnostic criteria		
Davidson et al., 1981 (10)	N = 43 Feighner (PD, SD)	Phenelzine = imipramine (81 mg/day) (144 mg/day)
Davidson and Turnbull, 1983 (12)	N = 29 RDC (MDD, MD, SD)	Isocarboxazid (73%) > placebo (21%) (50 mg/day)
Giller et al., 1982 (19)	N = 43 DSM-III (MDE) Ham-D ≥ 20	Isocarboxazid (60%) ≫ placebo (18%) (inc 7/7 melancholia)
White et al., 1984 (80)	N = 122 RDC (MDD)	Tranylcypromine (68%) = nortriptyline (62%) (44 mg/day) (109 mg/day) Both TCP and NT ≫ placebo (42%)
"Atypical" depressed patients		
Paykel et al., 1982 (55)	N = 131 Non-severe depression and mixed anxiety depression	Phenelzine = amitriptyline (1.0 mg/kg/day) (2.5 mg/kg/day) Both P and AMI ≫ placebo
Zisook et al., 1985 (82)	N = 69 Atypical but RDC (M/mDD), nonmelancholic HAM-D > 20	Isocarboxazid > placebo (43%) (44 mg/day)
Liebowitz et al., 1984 (29)	N = 60 Atypical HAM-D > 10	Phenelzine (69%) ≥ imipramine (43%) (74 mg/day) P ≥ IMI ≥ placebo
Kayser et al., 1985 (24)	N = 47 14 HD, 33 non-HD; all RDC (M/mDD), HAM-D = 25	Non-HD: P (79%) = AMI (79%) HD: Phenelzine (100%) > amitriptyline (60%) (60 mg/day) (150 mg/day)

[a] HAM-D, Hamilton depression rating scale score; RDC, research diagnostic criteria for major (MDD), minor (mDD), or secondary (SD) depression; Feighner criteria for primary (PD) or secondary (SD) depressive disorder (13); DSM-III, criteria for major depressive episode (MDE) (71); HD, hysteroid dysphoria; percentages in parentheses under Results indicate the proportion of patients rated as improved.

subgroup of depressed patients with atypical characteristics have not been successful, and consistent response differences between atypical and typical depressed patient groups to MAO inhibitors versus tricyclics have not been found (11,54) (Table 1).

This information from studies in the 1980s has served to diminish the relevance of atypical symptoms in considerations of the efficacy of MAO inhibitors. In fact, several of these recent studies have drawn specific attention to evidence that patients meeting criteria for severe depression, including very high Hamilton depression scale scores and melancholic symptoms, and treatment-resistant, rapid-cycling bipolar patients respond well to MAO inhibitors (19,31,48,60). Additionally, the MAO inhibitors, like the tricyclics, have been found to be quite broad-spectrum therapeutic agents, with efficacy not only in depression but also in patients with primary anxiety, bulimia, the chronic pain syndrome, attention deficit disorder, panic disorder, and possibly obsessive-compulsive disorder (44,49). In some of these disorders, responses to MAO inhibitors or tricyclics have been found to be independent of the presence or absence of coexistent or "secondary" depressive symptoms. This has raised interesting questions regarding what onto-genic associations might exist among these disorders with quite different primary symptomologic presentations (44,49). Alternatively, these findings have led to speculations regarding the multiple effects of these drugs on different neurotransmitter systems, and the possibility that, for example, a serotonergic system change may be more responsible for therapeutic changes in one disorder, whereas noradrenergic consequences may be important in another (49). Whatever the answer, the evidence from clinical studies that MAO inhibitors, tricyclics, and related agents have generally similar efficacy across similar patient populations has reinforced the search for common mechanisms of action for their antidepressant and other therapeutic effects.

The quest toward defining key components in how antidepressants work has been aided, in the case of the MAO inhibitors, by progress made in the last decade that

TABLE 2. *Atypical depression: Some descriptive criteria used to evaluate responses to MAO-inhibiting antidepressants*

Characteristics of iproniazid responders: Absence of morning worsening, early awakening, and self-reproach; presence of evening worsening, hysterical symptoms, tremor, and history of worsening with ECT; also, long illness, phobic and generalized anxiety, fatigue (78).

Criteria for phenelzine response prediction in atypical depression: Psychic and somatic anxiety, initial insomnia (as compared to criteria for phenelzine response prediction in typical depression: suicidal ideation, weight loss, depressed mood, agitation, retardation, guilt, hallucinations, nihilistic delusions) (64).

Criteria for atypical depression in phenelzine trials: Increased eating, increased sleep, sensitivity to rejection (lifelong), reactivity of mood, and loss of energy ("leaden paralysis") (62).

TABLE 3. *Antidepressant effects of selective MAO inhibitors: Double-blind, randomized trials*

Selective MAO-A inhibitors		Ref.
Clorgyline	> Amitriptyline	23
	= Imipramine	79
	> Pargyline	31
Moclobemide	> Placebo	4
	= Clomipramine	26
	= Amitriptyline	50
Selective MAO-B inhibitors		
Deprenyl	= Placebo	38
	> Placebo	39

has delineated two major MAO isoenzymes, MAO-A and MAO-B. These enzymes act preferentially on different substrates for MAO (i.e., MAO-A more actively deaminates serotonin and norepinephrine, and MAO-B preferentially deaminates phenylethylamine and dopamine in humans). Highly selective agents which more readily inhibit one form of the enzyme (e.g., clorgyline or moclobemide for MAO-A, and deprenyl or pargyline in low doses for MAO-B) have provided some refinement in considering which neurotransmitter systems may be involved in their clinical effects, since there is now quite substantial evidence that MAO-A inhibitors are more effective antidepressants than MAO-B inhibitors, as had originally been postulated following the first direct comparison of an MAO-A inhibitor versus an MAO-B inhibitor (31,46,48). As indicated in Table 3, which lists all of the double-blind, random-assignment studies conducted with selective inhibitors, MAO-A inhibiting agents have been found to be more consistently effective antidepressants (six of six studies) than selective or partially selective MAO-B inhibitors [one of three studies, when one report which directly contrasted pargyline with clorgyline (31) is included]. Two additional studies of deprenyl did not use a fully controlled design with a comparison group and with random-assignment, double-blind procedures. Both described beneficial effects, one with a very rapid onset of antidepressant and stimulant effects in the first week of treatment (35). Half the patients in this study were bipolar. In the other study, antidepressant effects in a group of "atypical" depressed patients were not observed at low doses of deprenyl (10 mg/day) but did occur at higher doses (20–30 mg/day) (61).

BIOCHEMICAL CONSEQUENCES OF MAO INHIBITOR ADMINISTRATION THAT ARE POSSIBLY RELEVANT TO THEIR CLINICAL EFFECTS

There is substantial evidence that the behaviorally relevant effects of MAO inhibitors depend on their primary action [i.e., inactivation of the MAO isoenzymes together with the secondary, adaptational consequences of this inactivation (45–48,58)]. A sequence of neurochemical and physiological changes occurs immediately following MAO inhibitor treatment, many of which are sustained. These include elevation of the concentration of many monoamines in brain and other tissues, including serotonin, norepinephrine, and dopamine, as well as even greater relative changes in the so-called trace amines, which include phenylethylamine, tryptamine, and tyramine. Apparent adaptational events to the increased intraneuronal and intrasynaptic amine concentrations then follow, involving reductions in the firing rates of neurons in the locus ceruleus and the raphe nuclei, feedback-induced reductions in amine synthesis, and, somewhat later, alterations in the number and the responsivity of many neurotransmitter receptors or binding sites (3,45–47).

This sequence of changes in amines, amine turnover, and neuronal electrophysiologic activity and receptors has been well delineated in animal studies, particularly in the rat, and is summarized elsewhere (45). In addition, multiple adaptive changes in amine binding sites and receptors that follow MAO inhibitor administration in rodents have been described in the present decade. A summary of the major findings in this important area is presented in Table 4.

Unfortunately, there are major gaps in knowledge that limit the conclusions that can be drawn from separate measurements of changes in neurotransmitter binding sites or receptors and changes in amine concentration or turnover. Even within one neurotransmitter system, there is evidence that agonists for receptor subtypes will, under some circumstances, act in an opposing fashion (e.g., α- vs β-adrenoceptors, and 5-HT_1 vs 5-HT_2 receptors). There is some evidence that MAO-inhibitor-induced down-regulation

in adrenoceptors may be temporally different for β- vs α-receptors (8). There are only a few studies in which binding site numbers, second messenger (e.g., cyclic AMP) concentrations, and physiological changes believed to result from the same neurotransmitter have been measured contemporaneously (3,7,8). However, even in these investigations, knowledge is lacking about regional amine concentrations and the input from other neurotransmitter systems that are known to be affected by the MAO inhibitors and that are known to be capable of influencing the course of receptor changes (e.g., the apparent influence of serotonergic input on antidepressant drug-induced adrenoceptor down-regulation).

For these reasons, it is necessary to pay particular attention to evidence of changes in the net output of functions mediated by specific neurotransmitter systems to evaluate the meaningfulness of more isolated components (e.g., binding site B_{max} changes) in neurotransmitter system responses to chronic MAO inhibitor administration. Some examples of experiments in which relatively selective agonists for serotonergic or noradrenergic receptors have been administered to rodents chronically treated with selective MAO-A or MAO-B inhibitors (and, in a few cases, where these results have been compared to those obtained with nonselective MAO inhibition) are presented in Table 5. As indicated, there are some quite striking examples where responses to serotonin and a selective serotonergic agonist are decreased by chronic treatment with the MAO-A inhib-

TABLE 4. *Studies of changes in brain neuronal receptor binding sites accompanying chronic treatment for 5–21 days with MAO inhibitors*

Receptor	Drug	Change	Ref.
Adrenergic binding sites			
β	Nialamide, 7–21 days	Reduced	15, 77
	Tranylcypromine, 16 days	Reduced	15
	Phenelzine, 21 days	Reduced	8
	Pargyline, 11–21 days	Reduced	41, 56, 62, 77, 81, 83
	Pargyline, 21 days	No change	8
	Deprenyl, 10–21 days	Reduced	42, 83
	Deprenyl, 14 days	No change	40
	Clorgyline, 21 days	Reduced	8
α_1	Pargyline, 21 days	No change	56
	Clorgyline, 10–21 days	Reduced	8
α_2	Clorgyline, 10–21 days	Reduced	8
	Pargyline, 14 days	Reduced	72
Serotonergic binding sites			
5-HT_1	Nialamide, 5–16 days	Reduced	15, 25, 68
	Pargyline, 21 days	Reduced	56
	Clorgyline, 5 days	Reduced	25, 26
5-HT_2	Tranylcypromine, 21 days	Reduced	27
	Pargyline, 21 days	Reduced	56
	Deprenyl, 21 days	No change	83
Other binding sites			
Dopaminergic	Pargyline, 21 days	No change	56
Muscarinic	Pargyline, 21 days	No change	56
Imipramine	Pargyline, 21 days	No change	83
	Deprenyl, 21 days	Increased	83
$GABA_B$	Pargyline, 18 days	Increased	32
Desmethylimipramine	Pargyline, 18 days	Increased	73
	Iproniazid, 18 days	Increased	73

TABLE 5. *Some examples of changes in physiologic functions following selective MAO-A or MAO-B inhibitors given chronically to rodents*[a]

Physiologic function	MAO inhibitors		Ref.
	Clorgyline	Deprenyl or pargyline (low dose)	
Serotonin-related changes			
5HT-induced reduction in cortical neuron firing rates	Decreased	NC	51
m-CPP (5-HT$_{1B}$ agonist)-induced changes			
Food intake reduction	Decreased	—	6
Sedation	Decreased	—	
Limb abduction and head movements	Decreased	—	
8-OH-DPAT (5-HT$_{1A}$ agonist)-induced hypothermia	NC (but decreased by clorgyline plus deprenyl)	NC	21
Norepinephrine-related changes			
Hypothalamic self-stimulation	Increased	NC	1, 20
Clonidine attenuation of hypothalamic self-stimulation	Decreased	NC	1
Clonidine-induced hypotension	Decreased	Minor reduction	22
Pressor responses to sympathetic stimulation or tyramine	Increased	NC	7, 14
Locomotor activity in mice following			
L-dopa	Increased	NC	18
Amphetamine	Increased	NC	
Phenylethylamine	NC	Increased	
Vas deferens responses to clonidine or tyramine	Increased	NC	14

[a] NC, No change; —, no data.

itor clorgyline, but not with the MAO-B inhibitor deprenyl. These results match quite well the evidence for reduced numbers of serotonin binding sites (both 5-HT$_1$ and 5-HT$_2$ subtypes) observed after clorgyline or nonselective MAO inhibitors but not after chronic treatment with *l*-deprenyl, as reviewed in Table 4. Similarly, there are some examples of experiments in which noradrenergically mediated responses (hypothalamic self-stimulation, sympathetic stimulation) or responses elicited by selective noradrenergic agonists such as clonidine are altered by chronic treatment with clorgyline but not deprenyl (Table 5). Conversely, locomotor responses to phenylethylamine, a preferential substrate for MAO-B, were enhanced by deprenyl, but not by chronic clorgyline administration (Table 5). These investigations of physiological and behavioral endpoints have proved very useful in validating some of the concepts derived from more discrete biochemical studies in animals, and have provided some of the impetus for the selective agonist challenge strategy used to evaluate the functional status of central neurotransmitter systems in humans receiving MAO inhibitors, as described below.

EVIDENCE FROM STUDIES IN HUMANS REGARDING NEUROTRANSMITTER SYSTEM CHANGES DURING TREATMENT WITH MAO INHIBITORS AND THEIR RELATIONSHIP TO CLINICAL RESPONSE AND POSSIBLE PSYCHOBIOLOGICAL DYSFUNCTION IN DEPRESSION

Only limited psychobiological information is available from studies of patients receiving MAO inhibitors. However,

if one accepts the evidence briefly reviewed above and elsewhere (36,44–48,62) that (a) MAO inhibitors are effective antidepressants; (b) MAO-A inhibitors are apparently more effective antidepressants than MAO-B inhibitors when used in isoenzyme-selective dosage regimens; and (c) there may be some parallels [despite species differences in brain MAO (16)] between the sequential biochemical and physiological responses to MAO inhibitors observed in animals and in the less detailed data from humans, some propositions regarding specific neurotransmitter system involvement in MAO-inhibitor-induced behavioral responses can be considered.

The Noradrenergic System

Although mean cerebrospinal fluid (CSF) norepinephrine was not significantly altered by treatment with clorgyline or the partially selective MAO-B inhibitor pargyline, a positive correlation between CSF norepinephrine and improvement in depression was observed in a small study (33). Quite large reductions in CSF, plasma, and urinary concentrations of 3-methoxy-4-hydroxyphenylglycol (MHPG), a major metabolite of norepinephrine, uniformly occur with MAO inhibitor treatment, although these changes in individual patients do not correlate with antidepressant responses to either phenelzine or clorgyline (2,65).

The substantially greater reductions in MHPG after clorgyline (80–85%) than after deprenyl (9–40%) parallel the greater antidepressant efficacy of clorgyline than deprenyl, as do the relatively greater reductions in "total" norepinephrine metabolite excretion (the sum of MHPG, vanylmandelic acid, and normetanephrine) following low-

or high-dose clorgyline (70–75%) vs low-dose deprenyl (24%) (30,74; D. L. Murphy et al., *unpublished data*). Reductions in plasma norepinephrine concentrations and in blood pressure are significantly correlated with antidepressant and antianxiety responses in patients treated with clorgyline (65), adding further indirect but highly suggestive evidence to the prominent noradrenergic system changes observed in animals to suggest that this neurotransmitter system may be importantly involved in the mechanisms underlying therapeutic efficacy (30,31,45–48,59).

It is noteworthy that the dominant change in the noradrenergic system, at least in the periphery, is a dampening of all indices of sympathetic outflow and noradrenergic function, which may have some direct relevance to the prominent antianxiety effects of these agents (31,47,63). One direct assessment in patients of the adrenergic receptor changes previously observed in animals did find a reduction in the hypotensive response to the selective α_2-adrenoceptor agonist clonidine during chronic but not acute clorgyline treatment (69), suggesting a direct parallelism in noradrenergic functional changes. Specific assessment of β- or α-adrenoceptor function in patients has not yet been accomplished, which is unfortunate because there is more suggestive evidence from animals relating down-regulation of these receptors to both MAO inhibitor and tricyclic antidepressant efficacy.

Despite the predominant dampening of noradrenergic function observed in patients, several controlled studies of the pressor and catecholamine release responses to tyramine indicate that there is increased stored norepinephrine available for release during MAO inhibitor treatment, and that this change is also greater for clorgyline than for deprenyl or low-dose pargyline (57,59,74). This change thus is also in parallel with the relative clinical efficacy of these selective MAO inhibitors. It also helps confirm that a basic effect of MAO inhibition in animals, an increased store of monoamines (in this case, norepinephrine), is present and is sustained in humans, and that this norepinephrine change is more prominent with MAO-A inhibitors.

The Serotonergic System

CSF and urinary concentrations of the major serotonin metabolite, 5-hydroxyindoleacetic acid (5-HIAA), are reduced during MAO inhibitor treatment, and these changes are greater following clorgyline than with deprenyl or pargyline (34,75). Changes in 5-HIAA were not correlated with clinical improvement during clorgyline treatment (47). Unfortunately, CSF serotonin concentrations have not yet been studied.

Increased morning plasma prolactin concentrations were found during clorgyline and high-dose pargyline treatment; these changes are consistent with increased hypothalamic serotonin output (70). L-Tryptophan-induced prolactin elevations were also increased during tranylcypromine treatment (5). Increased plasma and CSF melatonin release during clorgyline but not deprenyl treatment has been observed in rats, monkeys, and humans (44,52) and has been interpreted as being likely to represent an increased availability of serotonin for conversion to melatonin in the

pineal gland. It may also represent a discrete enhancement of α- or β-adrenoceptor activity, since pineal function has been thought to be predominantly regulated via adrenergic mechanisms, at least in rats. A catecholamine-stimulating effect produced by MAO-A inhibition would be an exception to the bulk of the data reviewed above, suggesting decreased sympathetic outflow during clorgyline administration.

Other evidence somewhat akin to that from tyramine studies in the catecholamine system suggests that a capacity for exaggerated responses in some serotonergically mediated functions is present during MAO inhibitor administration (9,28,40). Neuromuscular responses with some resemblance to the "serotonin syndrome" of behaviors in rodents have been reported when clomipramine was given too soon after discontinuation of clorgyline (9). Similar responses were elicited when L-tryptophan was administered during tranylcypromine treatment (5).

The Dopaminergic System

Reductions in concentrations of the major metabolite of dopamine, homovanillic acid (HVA), in CSF produced by clorgyline treatment are smaller than those in MHPG or 5-HIAA (34). Changes in this metabolite did not correlate with clinical response. CSF dopamine concentrations have not yet been measured after selective MAO inhibitor treatment, but would be of interest.

Deprenyl treatment led to approximately equivalent reductions in HVA (75) as those produced by clorgyline. *In vitro* data suggest that dopamine deamination is chiefly accomplished by MAO-B in human and nonhuman primate brain (16), and a greater HVA reduction might have been expected after deprenyl. However, in a model study in monkeys, deprenyl's effects on CSF HVA did not exceed those of clorgyline (17; N. A. Garrick et al., *unpublished data*) in keeping with the clinical study data. As deprenyl was not clinically effective as an antidepressant in the low doses that completely inhibited platelet MAO-B activity, and as pargyline was less clinically effective than clorgyline when given in doses that produced greater reductions in HVA than did clorgyline (34) (and also completely inhibited platelet MAO activity), an important role of dopamine in the action of MAO-inhibiting antidepressants seems unlikely.

Other Monoamines

A deficit in phenylethylamine (66), an alteration in octopamine or other trace amines that might function as false transmitters (43,67), and a lack of tyramine-mediated norepinephrine release (39) have been suggested as possible contributions to depression or to be consequences of MAO inhibitor treatment. Urinary phenylethylamine and phenylethanolamine concentrations were found to be markedly increased by pargyline and deprenyl but were essentially unchanged by clorgyline (48). Again, like the dopamine metabolism results, these changes seem counter to the differential clinical efficacy data, suggesting that an important role for the phenylethylamines in antidepressant action, and probably in depression, is unlikely to exist.

Octopamine in platelets and *p*-tyramine in urine are modestly increased to an approximately equivalent extent by clorgyline, pargyline and, in the case of tyramine, by deprenyl (48). The expected elevations in octopamine after MAO inhibitor administration could contribute to the reductions in catecholamine output reviewed above. The equivalent changes in *p*-tyramine after both the MAO-A and MAO-B selective inhibitors do not parallel the greater efficacy of the MAO-A inhibitors as antidepressants, arguing against direct changes in tyramine availability as an integral component of antidepressant actions. Relative changes in the urinary excretion of *p*-tyramine are much smaller than the increased sensitivity to tyramine observed with MAO-A inhibitors (48,57). This is in keeping with the proposal that tyramine supersensitivity is more a function of the increased availability of norepinephrine in sympathetic nerve endings than an alteration in tyramine degradation following MAO inhibition (47,48,57,74).

CONCLUSIONS

In summary, it would seem that recent evidence from carefully controlled, comparative clinical studies in the 1980s indicates that MAO inhibitors are effective both in typical, tricyclic-responsive depressed patients and in so-called atypical depressed patients. Therefore, "atypically" is less of an issue in considering drug choice for particular depressed patients. The overlapping spectrum of efficacy suggests that considerations of antidepressant drug mechanisms of action should comparatively examine MAO inhibitors and the tricyclics for the possibility of some commonalities in final effects. However, as discussed elsewhere, the effectiveness of antidepressants in patients without primary affective disorder (49) and the possibility of different properties of some of these agents—including possible different clinical efficacy spectra for different MAO inhibitors, such as phenelzine vs clorgyline (44–48)—also argue for looking for differences as well as commonalities.

The studies with substrate-selective MAO inhibitors have refocused attention on the likelihood of a primary involvement of the noradrenergic and serotonergic neurotransmitter systems and their interactions in the mediation of the antidepressant and antianxiety effects of the MAO inhibitors. The comparative investigations of MAO-A vs MAO-B inhibitors have emphasized the far tighter linkage of MAO-A inhibitors than MAO-B inhibitors with therapeutic effects in patients with affective disorders and related psychiatric disorders.

Although the newer selective MAO inhibitors have provided valuable new ways to explore clinical and biochemical hypotheses, the currently available MAO inhibitors have a number of liabilities and side effects, and there is definitely room for improvement. It may well be that some of the reversible MAO-A inhibitors undergoing early clinical study such as moclobemide or brofaremine may prove to be effective and easier to use (since dosage titration will be easier) and also may lessen the liability of tyramine-related hypertension reactions. Likewise, prodrugs such as MDL 72-394, which, when given with a peripheral decarboxylase inhibitor, will produce selective MAO-A inhibition in the brain but not the periphery (37), should also increase the safety factor.

The MAO-B-selective inhibitors, although apparently not as effective as MAO-A inhibitors, are nonetheless agents with some interesting properties. They have beneficial effects in Parkinson's disease and may yet have a place in treating depression when used in higher, non-MAO-B-selective doses. Deprenyl has also been reported to lengthen the lifespan of parkinsonian patients receiving it as an adjunct to L-dopa, and, in animals, it blocks the neuronal damage produced by the parkinsonian toxin MPTP. Preliminary data suggest deprenyl may have some modest beneficial effects in Alzheimer's dementia (76). As with the MAO-A inhibitors, there are also new reversible MAO-B inhibitors and prodrug MAO-B agents under development, providing similar opportunities to gain new knowledge and, hopefully, therapeutic advantages in the future.

REFERENCES

1. Aulakh, C. S., Cohen, R. M., Pradhan, S. N., and Murphy, D. L. (1983): *Brain Res.,* 270:383–386.
2. Beckman, H., and Murphy, D. L. (1977): *Neuropsychobiology,* 3:49–55.
3. Campbell, I. C., Gallager, D. W., Hamburg, M. A., Tallman, J. F., and Murphy, D. L. (1985): *Eur. J. Pharmacol.,* 3:355–364.
4. Casacchia, M., Carolei, A., Barba, C., and Rossi, A. (1985): In: *Monoamine Oxidase and Disease: Prospects for Therapy with Reversible Inhibitors,* edited by K. F. Tipton, P. Dosterf, M. Strulin-Benedett, C. T. Dollery, C. J. Fowler, and E. Zarifian, pp. 607–608. Academic Press, London.
5. Charney, D. S., and Heninger, G. R. (1985): *Life Sci.,* 113:678–683.
6. Cohen, R. M., Aulakh, C. S., and Murphy, D. L. (1983): *Eur. J. Pharmacol.,* 94:175–179.
7. Cohen, R. M., Campbell, I. C., Yamaguchi, I., Pickar, D., Kopin, I. J., and Murphy, D. L. (1982): *Eur. J. Pharmacol.,* 80:155–160.
8. Cohen, R. M., Ebstein, R. P., Daly, J. W., and Murphy, D. L. (1982): *J. Neurosci.,* 2:1588–1595.
9. Cohen, R. M., Pickar, D., and Murphy, D. L. (1980): *Am. J. Psychiatry,* 37:105–106.
10. Davidson, J., McLeod, M. N., Turnbull, C. D., and Miller, R. D. (1981): *J. Clin. Psychiatry,* 42:183–189.
11. Davidson, J., and Pelton, S. (1985): *Psychiatry Res.,* 17:87–95.
12. Davidson, J., and Turnbull, C. (1983): *J. Affective Disord.,* 5:183–189.
13. Feighner, J. P., Robins, E., Guize, S., Woodruff, R. A., Winokur, G., and Munoz, R. (1972): *Arch. Gen. Psychiatry,* 16:57–63.
14. Finberg, J. P. M., and Youdim, M. B. H. (1985): *Br. J. Pharmacol.,* 85:541–546.
15. Frazer, A., and Lucki, I. (1982): *Adv. Biochem. Psychopharmacol.,* 31:69–90.
16. Garrick, N. A., and Murphy, D. L. (1980): *Psychopharmacology,* 72:27–33.
17. Garrick, N. A., Scheinin, M., Chang, W.-H., Linnoila, M., and Murphy, D. L. (1984): *Biochem. Pharmacol.,* 33:1423–1427.
18. Gianutsos, G., Carlson, G. M., and Godfrey, J. G. (1983): *Pharmacol. Biochem. Behav.,* 19:263–268.
19. Giller, E., Bialos, D., Riddle, M., Sholomskas, H., and Harkness, L. (1982): *Psychiatry Res.,* 6:41–48.
20. Greenshaw, A. J., Juorio, A. V., and Boulton, A. A. (1985): *Brain Res. Bull.,* 15:183–189.
21. Gudelsky, G. A., Koening, J. I., Jackman, H., and Meltzer, H. Y. (1986): *Psychopharmacology,* 90:403–407.
22. Gutkind, J. S., and Enero, M. A. (1984): *Naunyn Schmiedebergs Arch. Pharmacol.,* 327:189–192.
23. Herd, J. A. (1969): *Clin. Trials,* 6:219–225.
24. Kayser, A., Robinson, D. S., Nies, A., and Howard, D. (1985): *Am. J. Psychiatry,* 142:486–488.

25. Kellar, K. T., Cascio, C. S., and Butler, T. A. (1981): *Eur. J. Pharmacol.*, 69:515–518.
26. Larsen, J. K., Mikkelsen, P. L., and Holm, P. (1985): In: *Monoamine Oxidase and Disease: Prospects for Therapy with Reversible Inhibitors*, edited by K. F. Tipton, P. Dosterf, M. Strulin-Benedett, C. T. Dollery, C. J. Fowler, and E. Zarifian, p. 609. Academic Press, London.
27. Lee, C. M., Javitch, J. A., and Snyder, S. H. (1983): *Science*, 220:626–629.
28. Lieberman, J. A., Kane, J. M., and Reife, R. (1985): *J. Clin. Psychopharmacol.*, 5:221–228.
29. Liebowitz, M., Quitkin, F., Stewart, J., McGrath, P. J., Harrison, W., Rabkin, J., Tricano, E., Markowitz, J. S. D., and Klein, D. F. (1984): *Arch. Gen. Psychiatry*, 41:469–677.
30. Linnoila, M., Karoum, F., and Potter, W. Z. (1982): *Arch. Gen. Psychiatry*, 39:513–516.
31. Lipper, S., Murphy, D. L., Slater, S., and Buchsbaum, M. S. (1979): *Psychopharmacology*, 62:123–128.
32. Lloyd, K. G., Thuret, F., and Pilc, A. (1985): *J. Pharmacol. Exp. Ther.*, 235:191–199.
33. Major, L. F., Lake, C. R., Lipper, S., Lerner, P., and Murphy, D. L. (1979): *Prog. Neuropsychopharmacol.*, 3:535–542.
34. Major, L. F., Murphy, D. L., Lipper, S., and Gordon, E. (1979): *J. Neurochem.*, 32:229–231.
35. Mann, J., and Gershon, S. (1980): *Life Sci.*, 26:872–882.
36. McDaniel, K. D. (1986): *Clin. Neuropharmacol.*, 9:207–234.
37. McDonald, I. A., Lacoste, J. M., Bey, P., Palfreyman, M. G., and Zreika, M. (1985): *J. Med. Chem.*, 28:186–193.
38. Mendelewicz, J., and Youdim, M. B. H. (1983): *Br. J. Psychiatry*, 142:508–511.
39. Mendis, N., Pare, C. M. B., Sandler, M., Glover, V., and Stern, M. (1981): *Psychopharmacology*, 73:87–90.
40. Meyerson, L. R., Ong, H. H., Martin, L. L., et al. (1980): *Pharmacol. Biochem. Behav.*, 19:943–948.
41. Minneman, K. P., Wolfe, B. B., and Molinoff, P. B. (1982): *Brain Res.*, 252:309–314.
42. Mishra, R., Gillespie, D. D., Youdim, M. B. H., and Sulser, F. (1984): *Psychopharmacology*, 81:220–223.
43. Murphy, D. L. (1972): *Am. J. Psychiatry*, 129:141–148.
44. Murphy, D. L., Aulakh, C. S., and Garrick, N. A. (1986): In: *Depression, Antidepressants and Receptor Sensitivity*, pp. 106–125. Pitman Publishing Co., London.
45. Murphy, D. L., Garrick, N. A., Aulakh, C. S., and Cohen, R. M. (1984): *J. Clin. Psychiatry*, 45:37–43.
46. Murphy, D. L., Lipper, S., Campbell, I. C., Major, L. F., Slater, S. L., and Buchsbaum, M. S. (1979): In: *Monoamine Oxidase: Structure, Function and Altered Functions*, pp. 457–475. Academic Press, New York.
47. Murphy, D. L., Lipper, S., Pickar, D., Jimerson, D., Cohen, R. M., Garrick, N. A., Alterman, I. S., and Campbell, I. C. (1981): In: *Monoamine Oxidase Inhibitors: The State of the Art*, pp. 189–205. John Wiley and Sons, New York.
48. Murphy, D. L., Pickar, D., Jimerson, D., Cohen, R. M., Garrick, N. A., Karoum, F., and Wyatt, R. J. (1981): In: *Clinical Pharmacology in Psychiatry*, pp. 307–316. Macmillan Press, London.
49. Murphy, D. L., Siever, L. J., Insel, T. R., and Cohen, R. M. (1985): *Prog. Neuropsychopharmacol. Biol. Psychiatry*, 9:3–13.
50. Norman, T. R., Ames, D., Burrows, G. D., and Daview, B. (1985): *J. Affective Disord.*, 8:19–35.
51. Olpe, H. R., and Schellenberg, A. (1980): *Eur. J. Pharmacol.*, 63:7–13.
52. Oxenkrug, C. F., McCauley, N., McIntyre, I. M., and Filipowicz, C. (1985): *J. Neural Transm.*, 61:265–269.
53. Paykel, E. S. (1979): *Br. J. Psychiatry*, 134:572–581.
54. Paykel, E. S., Parker, R. R., Rowan, P. R., Rao, B. M., and Taylor, C. N. (1983): *Psychol. Med.*, 13:131–139.
55. Paykel, E. S., Rowan, P. R., Parker, R. R., and Bhat, A. V. (1982): *Arch. Gen. Psychiatry*, 39:1041–1049.
56. Peroutka, S., and Snyder, S. H. (1980): *Science*, 210:89–90.
57. Pickar, D., Cohen, R. M., Jimerson, D. C., Lake, C. R., and Murphy, D. L. (1981): *Psychopharmacology*, 74:8–12.
58. Pletcher, A., Gay, F. K., and Burkand, W. B. (1966): *Handbook Exp. Pharmacol.*, 19:593–735.
59. Potter, W. Z., Karoum, F., and Linnoila, M. (1983): *Prog. Neuropharmacol. Biol. Psychiatry*, 8:153–161.
60. Potter, W. Z., Murphy, D. L., Wehr, T. A., Linnoila, M., and Goodwin, F. K. (1982): *Arch. Gen. Psychiatry*, 39:505–510.
61. Quitkin, F. M., Liebowitz, M. R., and Stewart, J. W. (1984): *Arch. Gen. Psychiatry*, 41:777–781.
62. Quitkin, F., Rifkin, A., and Klein, D. F. (1979): *Arch. Gen. Psychiatry*, 36:749–760.
63. Robinson, D. S., Johnson, C. A., Nies, A., Corcella, J., Cooper, T. B., Albright, D., and Howard, D. (1983): *J. Clin. Psychopharmacol.*, 3:282–287.
64. Robinson, D. S., Nies, A., Ravaris, L., and Lamborn, K. R. (1973): *Arch. Gen. Psychiatry*, 29:407–413.
65. Roy, B. F., Murphy, D. L., Lipper, S., Siever, L., Alterman, I. S., Jimerson, D., Lake, C. R., and Cohen, R. M. (1987): *J. Clin. Psychopharmacol. (in press)*.
66. Sabelli, H. C., and Mosnaim, G. (1974): *Am. J. Psychiatry*, 131:695–699.
67. Sandler, M., Ruthven, C. R., Goodwin, B. L., and Reynolds, G. P. (1979): *Nature*, 278:357–358.
68. Savage, D. D., Mendels, J., and Frazer, A. (1980): *Neuropharmacology*, 19:1063–1070.
69. Siever, L. J., Uhde, T. W., and Murphy, D. L. (1981): *Psychiatry Res.*, 6:293–302.
70. Slater, S., Lipper, S., Shilling, D. J., and Murphy, D. L. (1977): *Lancet*, 2:275–276.
71. Spitzer, R., Endicott, J., and Robins, E. (1978): *Arch. Gen. Psychiatry*, 35:773–782.
72. Sugrue, M. F. (1982): *Naunyn Schmiedebergs Arch. Pharmacol.*, 320:90–96.
73. Sulser, F., Vetulani, J., and Mobley, P. (1978): *Biochem. Pharmacol.*, 27:257–261.
74. Sunderland, T., Mueller, E. A., Cohen, R. M., Jimerson, D. C., Pickar, D., and Murphy, D. L. (1985): *Psychopharmacology*, 867:432–437.
75. Sunderland, T., Tariot, P., Cohen, R. M., Newhouse, P. A., Mellow, A. M., Mueller, E. A., and Murphy, D. L. (1987): *Psychopharmacology, (in press)*.
76. Tario, P., et al. (1987): *Arch. Gen. Psychiat. (in press)*.
77. Vetulani, J., Stawarz, R. J., and Sulser, F. (1976): *J. Neurochem.*, 27:661–666.
78. West, E. D., and Dally, P. J. (1959): *Br. Med. J.*, 1:1491–1494.
79. Wheatley, D. (1970): *Br. J. Psychiatry*, 117:547–550.
80. White, K., Razani, J., Cadow, B., Gelfand, R., Parlmer, R., Simpson, G., and Sloane, R. B. (1984): *Psychopharmacology*, 82:258–262.
81. Wolfe, B. B., Harden, T. K., Sport, J. R., et al. (1978): *J. Pharmacol. Exp. Ther.*, 207:446–457.
82. Zisook, S., Braff, D. L., and Click, M. A. (1985): *J. Clin. Psychopharmacol.*, 5:131–137.
83. Zsilla, G., Barbaccia, M. L., Gandolfi, O., Knoll, J., and Costa, E. (1983): *Eur. J. Pharmacol.*, 89:111–117.

Psychopharmacology:
The Third Generation of Progress,
edited by Herbert Y. Meltzer.
Raven Press, New York © 1987.

CHAPTER **56**

Mechanisms of Action of Lithium in Affective Illness: Basic and Clinical Implications

William E. Bunney, Jr., and Blynn L. Garland-Bunney

ABSTRACT

The introduction of lithium (Li) as a treatment for manic-depressive illness more than 35 years ago (28) has stimulated much research into its clinical efficacy and possible modes of action. A recent study estimated that there are more than 12,000 publications on the subject of Li in medicine and approximately 1,000 more reports are added each year (143). This review will explore the basic and clinical effects of Li on several systems, including (a) electrolytes and ion channels; (b) neurotransmitters, including serotonin (5-hydroxytryptamine; 5-HT), dopamine (DA), norepinephrine (NE), acetylcholine (ACh), and γ-aminobutyric acid (GABA); and finally (c) second messenger systems such as cyclic AMP and phosphatidylinositol (PI). The relevance of Li-associated changes observed in these systems will be discussed. Accumulated data thus far suggest a convergence of consistent evidence that Li may enhance serotonergic activity and decrease cholinergic activity, block the development of the behavioral manifestations of dopaminergic supersensitivity, and inhibit both second messenger systems, cyclic AMP and PI. It is proposed that enhancement of serotonergic activity may, in part, be responsible for the acute and prophylactic efficacy of Li treatment in depression and a decrease in cholinergic activity, DA interactions and inhibition of two second messenger systems may relate to the antimanic actions.

CLINICAL EFFICACY: A BRIEF REVIEW

Li is now well established as the treatment of choice in the prophylaxis of manic-depressive illness and is also used in the acute treatment of mania. Schou (152) estimated that 0.1 to 0.2% of the worldwide depressed population with proper access to medical care are currently administered Li.

Overall, there is general agreement that Li prophylaxis is more effective than placebo in the prevention of manic and depressive episodes (8,10,40,136), although some studies report a greater prophylactic effect against manic recurrences (46,137,138). In the treatment of acute mania, more than 100 published reports involving 3,000 patients in 20 countries indicate that Li is effective in 60% of patients (135). This effect appears to be independent of age, sex, and duration of illness in patients who did not improve with antidepressant treatment alone (77,162).

More recently, Li in combination with antidepressants has been shown to be effective (7,48,50,51,87,106,139,133).

PHYSICAL CHEMISTRY AND TRANSPORT

Li is a monovalent cation and is the smallest of the alkali metals. Thus, it has the highest electrical field density of this group and, accordingly, the largest energy of hydration (energy required to strip off water molecules). This last property is an important variable that affects the rate of passage of ions and that might account for the rapidity of the passage of Li through the sodium channels (185a).

The physicochemical similarities of the Li ion to four other cations found in mammalian cells (Na^+, K^+, Ca^{2+}, and Mg^{2+}) may provide clues to its mechanism of action, as these ions appear to compete with one another in cellular systems where these cations are recognized. Li has been shown to affect systems that normally interact with functional ammonium groups of the biogenic amines and related compounds (88a).

Interaction of Li with Other Electrolytes and Ion Channels

Animal Studies

Li is thought to be transported through ion-carrying channels of cell membranes. A study of the interaction of Li^+, sodium, and potassium with ion channels suggests that the larger the interactional energy between cation and ligand, the easier is the ion passage through the channel. Li was shown to have the largest energy of interaction, followed by sodium and potassium. In addition, it was found that Li is capable of penetrating the sodium channels just about as well as sodium, but that both Li and sodium fail to pass through the potassium channel. Factors such as interactional energy and the diameters of the ions (Li is close in size to sodium) explain the passage of Li through the sodium channels but do not fully explain why Li fails to penetrate the potassium channel (119).

Other possible cellular sites where interactions between Li and other cations might occur are on receptor sites which are maximally sensitive to changes in the concentration of other cations. For example, Li could compete for calcium binding sites and affect calcium-dependent release of a neurotransmitter or alter calcium-dependent cyclic AMP production (186).

Possible effects of Li on cellular functions include (a) the alteration of cellular proteins; (b) Li's influence on cellular carriers (64); and (c) more recently, the selective effect of Li on astrocytes, which are thought to have influences on impulse traffic in neurons. For example, therapeutic doses of Li were found to increase extracellular potassium by the Na^+/K^+-ATPase on astrocytes but not on neurons (88,184).

LiCl was shown to produce a slowing of reequilibration of intracellular calcium concentrations after depolarization-induced calcium loads in snail neurons, suggesting that this effect could have two consequences. In a highly active neuron, a decrease in calcium reequilibration may lead to increased intracellular calcium levels and thereby produce hyperpolarization which would slow down the discharge frequency. In a less active neuron, the single calcium-transient would become more prominent for calcium-binding structures. It is hypothesized that this mechanism could explain changes in neuronal activity under chronic Li treatment (3).

In view of the above evidence, it appears that a possible mechanism of action of Li may be its capability of substituting or successfully competing with other ions. Li alone or in combination with neurotransmitters may stabilize some aspects of the membrane receptors.

Clinical Studies

Recent clinical studies used to probe electrolyte abnormalities in affective illness include studies of the effects of Li on transport mechanisms, on the sodium pump, and on calcium ions.

Li ion transport has been the subject of genetic studies in families of bipolar patients. Dorus et al. (53) suggest the presence of a polymorphism at an autosomal gene locus, where one allele is associated with elevated red blood cell Li ion ratios and vulnerability to affective disorders. Inter-individual variability in the Li ion ratio (the ratio of the red blood cell to the plasma Li ion concentration) may be determined by variability in a Li-sodium ion counterflow mechanism. Members of 120 normal families and first-degree relatives of 31 bipolar patients were included in this study. Results suggested that the allele at the major locus resulting in elevated Li ion ratios was associated with an increased likelihood of psychiatric hospitalization among relatives of bipolar patients. The implication of this finding is that there may be a genetic defect in the Li-sodium counterflow mechanism which operates through a Li-sodium ion exchange system that maintains the uneven distribution of the Li ion across red blood cell membranes by extruding it from the cells.

Li transport mechanisms were studied in erythrocytes in bipolar patients on prophylactic Li and in healthy control subjects (150). The mechanisms studied included Li-sodium countertransport, Li-potassium co-transport, and passive Li efflux. Results indicated that the maximal velocity of Li-sodium countertransport measured at saturating intracellular concentrations was lower in bipolars than in controls. No differences were found between the groups on other measures. The values for Li transport were not related to age, duration of treatment, hypertension, or obesity. However, lower values were found in patients with Li-induced thyroid enlargement. These results provide additional evidence for a possible variation in transport mechanisms in bipolar patients (150).

A research strategy to investigate Li's effect on the sodium pump was used in manic patients. Li therapy has been associated with increases in erythrocyte Na^+/K^+-ATPase in manic-depressive patients, a response that has not been reported to occur in normal subjects (121,123). Additional evidence suggests that the rise in Na^+/K^+-ATPase may be correlated with prophylactic response (79,122). Using digoxin, an antagonist of Na^+/K^+-ATPase activity, Chambers et al. (35) showed in a double-blind, placebo-controlled study that patients treated with Li/placebo had significantly greater improvement in their symptoms than those patients treated with Li/digoxin, suggesting that the effect of inhibiting the membrane cation carrier is to reduce the response to Li. An earlier study revealed that digoxin treatment, alone, was not correlated with mood changes in mania (124). In an effort to find the mechanism of action, Cooper et al. (39) assessed sodium pump activity using ^{86}Rb uptake in erythrocytes. Six healthy volunteers were treated with Li for 2 weeks. Digoxin (0.75 mg i.v.) was administered before and after Li treatment, and results indicated no significant changes in serum electrolyte interactions, possibly suggesting that Li may act through an alternate mechanism.

A recent study investigated fibroblasts as an alternative model to study Li transport. No differences in Li transport between manic-depressive patients and controls were reported (22).

Evidence from CSF calcium studies in bipolar patients show highest calcium values in bipolar depression or catatonic stupor, lowest calcium values in mania or catatonic excitement, and intermediate values in euthymia (34). Li and other drug therapies (CBZ (134)) and verapamil (62) and ECT (33) have been shown to modify intraneuronal calcium.

BASIC AND CLINICAL EFFECTS OF Li ON NEUROTRANSMITTERS

The relevance of animal investigations for the study of the effect of Li on neurotransmitters requires special consideration in terms of acute versus chronic treatment, dosages necessary to reach equivalent therapeutic levels in humans, and the sensitivity measurements of biochemical and behavioral changes related to Li administration.

Serotonin

Animal Studies

There is increasing evidence that Li alters the 5-HT system and that this interaction may play a role in Li's mode of action in the acute and prophylactic treatment of manic-depressive illness. In 1979, Yuwiler et al. (188) studied the effects of Li on 5-HT metabolism and reported that the effects are dose-dependent and appear to change with duration of treatment. Short-term treatment of 3 to 5 days was shown to increase brain 5-HT turnover (128,132,171), increase brain tryptophan levels (128), and increase the concentration of brain 5-hydroxyindoleacetic acid (5-HIAA) (128). Following continuous treatment, blood tryptophan levels return to normal (153), but brain tryptophan (145,153) and 5-HIAA (38,164) remain elevated and conversion of labeled tryptophan to 5-HT and 5-HIAA (140) is accelerated. Some proposed mechanisms of action include an increased "high-affinity" 5-HT uptake of tryptophan into synaptosomes (31,109,188), with increases in the synthesis and turnover of 5-HT (31,109,132) and increases in 5-HIAA levels may result from an impairment in the storage mechanisms within 5-HT terminals (38). Although there is increasing evidence that Li may have serotonergic agonist effects, some studies reported Li-induced decreases in 5-HT brain concentrations (2,6,164).

In a series of studies, Blier and DeMontigny (19) used electrophysiological recordings to measure the effect of Li on the 5-HT system. Short-term Li did not affect the responsiveness of the postsynaptic neurons to 5-HT nor the electrical activity of the 5-HT neurons but was reported to enhance the efficacy of the ascending (presynaptic) 5-HT system.

In other animal studies, the effect of Li on the 5-HT system was investigated following the administration of a monoamine oxidase inhibitor (MAOI), pheniprazine. Increases in 5-HT and decreases in 5-HIAA were similar in both Li and control groups, compatible with similar rates of 5-HT synthesis and degradation (20). Another group of investigators administered the tryptophan hydroxylase inhibitor α-propyldopacetamide (H22/54) and reported decreases in 5-HT in chronically (44) but not acutely (43) Li-treated animals as compared to controls. Collard (37) stimulated the raphe nucleus in rats and showed that forebrain 5-HIAA increased following 10 days of Li treatment as well as in control animals, but that chlorimipramine was unable to block the 5-HIAA increase in the Li group. Treiser et al. (176) reported that chronic Li increased basal and potassium chloride release of endogenous 5-HT from the hippocampus but not the cortex. They hypothesize that Li may be able to stabilize 5-HT transmission with the interaction of two opposing processes: an increase in 5-HT levels and a decrease in the number of 5-HT receptors. This is in partial agreement with a recent review which concluded that chronic Li (within the therapeutic range) induces 5-HT agonist effects (118).

In a set of behavioral studies, Smith (166) showed that short-term administration of Li was associated with a decrease in locomotor activity in rats. When Li was combined with pargyline, an MAOI, a 5-HT-dependent behavioral syndrome resulted. Smith (166) concluded that the enhancement of 5-HT processes plays a role in the effects of Li.

Clinical Studies

Meltzer et al. (113,114,115) reported an increase in serum cortisol levels following the administration of 5-hydroxytryptophan (5-HTP) and used this finding as a probe to study the effects of Li on 5-HTP-induced cortisol response. Seven manic patients were administered 5-HTP before and after approximately 3 to 4 weeks of Li treatment. There was a significant decrease in 5-HTP-induced cortisol response in the unmedicated group as compared to the Li-treated group. The authors conclude that the enhancement of the 5-HTP response during Li treatment could be due to an effect of Li on pre- and postsynaptic mechanisms that augment 5-HT activity. In addition, nearly significant correlations between drug-free 5-HTP-induced cortisol changes and clinical ratings (GAS; SADS-C) suggest that manic patients with the largest initial changes in cortisol levels were the least psychiatrically ill or manic at the time of the on-treatment study. Also, patients who responded best to Li treatment had the smallest treatment-associated change (increase) in cortisol levels. Meltzer et al. (113) feel that these results, along with other known 5-HT/Li interactions, may indicate that manic patients have supersensitive 5-HT receptors prior to Li treatment and that these receptors become even more responsive to 5-HT after Li treatment, i.e., increasing 5-HT activity has an antimanic effect. In a previous study, this same group (114) showed that platelet 5-HT uptake in patients with bipolar depression was inhibited after 2 to 3 weeks of treatment with Li, thus strengthening the argument that if similar mechanisms occurred in the hypothalamus, the observed enhancement of 5-HTP-induced increases in serum cortisol following Li treatment could possibly be explained. Studies in depressed patients (113,115) showed that antidepressants other than Li decreased the 5-HTP-cortisol response—an effect opposite to that of Li, but which Meltzer (113) speculates may be a sign that Li is acting at a variety of pre- and postsynaptic mechanisms.

Narasimhachari and Ettigi (120) reported that platelet 5-HT, serum 5-HT, and serum tryptophan levels were all increased following the administration of Li in depressed patients as compared to normal controls. Other studies in patients have shown that chronic Li doses increase platelet 5-HT (41,114), although acute treatment may have the opposite effect (114).

The addition of Li to antidepressant medication in depressed patients who are nonresponsive to antidepressant medication alone has inspired new research. Two double-blind, placebo-controlled studies measured the rate of response in tricyclic-resistant patients who had Li added to their treatment regimen. One study (48) reported a significant clinical improvement within 48 hr, whereas the second study showed a small but significant improvement during the first 2 days and a greater rate of improvement from days 7 to 12 (85). In an open study, DeMontigny et al. (49) studied seven patients with major unipolar depression. All patients were shown to be nonresponders to iprindole, a tricyclic drug that does not affect 5-HT or NE reuptake processes. Iprindole was administered for a 3-week period. When Li was added to the regimen there was a marked and rapid alleviation of symptoms in all seven patients, which took place within 48 hr. In view of these results and preclinical data (19), the authors (49) suggest that an enhanced release of 5-HT on sensitized target neurons might underlie the rapid antidepressant response.

In summary, it appears from both many consistent animal and clinical studies that Li may enhance 5-HT activity. There is also increasing evidence that pretreatment with antidepressants might be associated with 5-HT supersensitivity responses, which when Li is added might result in a more rapid antidepressant response in otherwise treatment-resistant patients. We feel that these findings are more relevant to Li's actions in depression than in mania. However, other neurotransmitter systems need to be carefully evaluated.

Norepinephrine

Animal Studies

The effects of Li on NE levels appear to be severalfold. Li administration is first associated with an increase in labeled NE uptake in rat brain synaptosomes (30,36,101). After 7 days of Li treatment, NE levels return to baseline; at 21 days of treatment [^{3}H]NE levels uptake levels are again increased and return to baseline levels by day 42. Observations through day 70 revealed no further changes (30). Cameron and Smith (30) compared high and low doses of Li administration and found that high doses (2.5–15 mEq/kg) resulted in earlier increases in [^{3}H]NE uptake (16 hr) than did low doses (1.25 mEq/kg). Surprisingly, however, high-dose animals returned to baseline levels within 1 week, whereas those treated with low doses resumed normal levels by day 14.

Regional effects of Li on NE in rat brain have also been reported. Ahluwahlia and Singhal (1) described significant decreases in pons-medulla, hippocampus, and midbrain as compared to controls. There was no reported alteration in the NE metabolite MOPEG during or after Li withdrawal (1).

One would predict that the administration of α-methyl-paratyrosine (AMPT), an inhibitor of catecholamine synthesis, might alter Li responses. However, results revealed no changes in the rate of degradation or in NE levels in Li-treated rats as compared to controls (20).

Clinical Studies

The effect of Li on NE metabolism in patients with primary major depression was studied in one unipolar and four bipolar females (104). Li was shown to significantly reduce 24-hr urinary NE and turnover of normetanephrine, 3-methoxy-4-hydroxyphenylglycol (MHPG), and vanillyl mandelic acid (VMA). This is in agreement with an earlier study by Schildkraut (151), who reported decreases in NE measures in one bipolar patient; however, Beckmann et al. (12) reported increases in urinary MHPG in Li treatment-responsive patients.

Psychostimulant drugs, such as methylphenidate and amphetamine produce euphoria in man (180). Two double-blind, placebo-controlled studies have demonstrated an attenuation of the euphoric response to these drugs by Li pretreatment (90,181).

GABA

Chronic Li was administered to rats, and brain levels of GABA and related GABA enzymes were compared to those of control rats on a Li-free diet. Results indicated increases of GABA levels in limbic striatum, thalamus-hypothalamus, hippocampus, midbrain, pons, and cerebellum (172).

Dopamine

Animal Studies

Studies on the chronic administration of Li in animals suggest that Li may differentially affect DA pathways. Corrodi et al. (44) reported increased DA turnover in tuberoinfundibular neurons, whereas Ahlwahlia and Singhal

(1) showed decreased DA levels in pons-medulla and midbrain regions; two studies reported increases (63,107) decreases (69) or no change (142) in DA metabolites in striatum.

A chronic study of Li treatment in rats examined DA control of prolactin release in the terminal regions of tuberoinfundibular and tuberohypophyseal neurons and anterior pituitary gland. DOPAC levels were also monitored in this region. Results indicated that there were significant increases in DOPAC and a significant decrease in plasma and anterior lobe prolactin levels, suggesting that Li may be associated with increased release of DA from the hypothalamus (98).

Another research strategy involved the effect of chronic Li administration on haloperidol-induced increases in DA metabolism. Results indicated no effect of Li in the striatum (112,142), nucleus accumbens (142), or frontal cortex (142).

The DA synthesis blocker, AMPT, was shown to produce behavioral dopaminergic supersensitivity (78) in rats. Several studies have shown AMPT-induced decreases in DA levels (78,144). Li was shown to enhance the DA decrease (18) or have no effect (20,141A) on AMPT-induced DA changes.

Clinical Studies

The effect of Li treatment on DA turnover was investigated by Linnoila et al. (105) in a retrospective longitudinal study of one unipolar and seven bipolar women. Results indicated that Li decreased the amount of DA and its metabolites (DOPAC, HVA) in all of the patients. The authors hypothesize that this reduction might play a role in blocking, delaying, or reducing the intensity of the switch process from depression to mania.

Acetylcholine

Animal Studies

There is some suggestion that acute Li decreases brain ACh (100), but it appears that this effect may be temporary. In a series of studies Jope (93) investigated the acute and chronic effects of LiCl injections (10 mmol/kg i.p.). Short-term effects were correlated with a reduction in ACh synthesis in rat brain cortex followed by an increase in ACh utilization 24 hr later. After 10 days of treatment with the same dose of Li, there was a continued increased rate of ACh synthesis. Also, the high-affinity transport of $[^2H]4$-choline and its conversion to $[^2H]4$-ACh was significantly activated in synaptosomes in the striatum as compared to other brain areas. Jope (93) suggests that the stimulating effect of LiCl on the cholinergic system may play a significant role in the therapeutic effects of neuropsychiatric disorders.

Clinical Studies

Treatment with Li was associated with significant increases in red blood cell (RBC) choline levels. A recent review (82) showed that this effect is independent of psychiatric diagnosis and does not correlate with Li levels; its relationship to treatment response and its clinical significance are unclear. Plasma choline concentrations, in contrast, change only slightly with Li treatment. Gutterman et al. (82) studied RBC choline levels in 26 Li-treated affectively ill patients as compared to normal controls and found increased RBC choline levels in the patients. This finding is in agreement with that of Jope et al. (94) and Shea et al. (157).

Dopamine Receptors

Animal Studies

DA supersensitivity has been associated with increases in response to DA agonists. It has been proposed that the apparent proliferation of receptors following chronic blockade of DA transmission may be causally related to supersensitivity (27,45).

There is now substantial evidence to suggest that Li may be effective in blocking the development of the behavioral manifestations of DA supersensitive receptors. The first groups to report the attenuating effects of Li on DA-related behavioral sensitivity was that of Klawans et al. (96,97), who treated rats with haloperidol and noted a prolonged decrease in threshold for apomorphine (APO)-induced stereotypical behavior. The supersensitive responses were effectively blocked in those animals concurrently treated with Li (97). Similar findings were reported by Pert et al. (129), who demonstrated that long-term haloperidol treatment in rats produced a significant increase in sensitivity to the locomotor and stereotypic effects of APO and could be effectively blocked by pretreatment with Li.

Electrophysiological data utilizing single-unit recording demonstrated evidence of supersensitive presynaptic receptors in the zona compacta of the substantia nigra following chronic haloperidol. Supersensitive responses were measured by decreasing firing rates after iontophoretically applied DA or systemically administered APO. These presynaptic effects were blocked by chronic Li (72).

A study designed to test pre- and postsynaptic DA behavioral supersensitivity in rats was completed by Verimer et al. (182). Following chronic haloperidol treatment, both low (0.004 mg/kg) and high (0.016 mg/kg) doses of APO were administered. Results indicated that low doses (presynaptic) produced sedation, whereas high doses (postsynaptic) induced increases in locomotor activity. Concurrent administration of Li/haloperidol blocked both responses, possibly suggesting that Li may be capable of preventing the development of both pre- and postsynaptic receptor changes.

Thus far, it appears that Li is effective in blocking the development of neuroleptic-induced DA behavioral supersensitivity. However, there is some evidence that Li may be only partially effective or perhaps incapable of blocking the development of DA supersensitivity induced by other methods. Mailman et al. (108) also administered 6-hydroxydopamine (6-OHDA) to rats and demonstrated increases in locomotor activity in response to APO. Although they reported that this effect could not be blocked by chronic Li treatment, several subsequent studies revealed that Li may have a transient effect on the development of

TABLE 1. *Effect of lithium on the development of behavioral manifestations of dopaminergic supersensitivity*

Study	Animal	Intervention	Challenge	Effect of Li on behavior
Mailman et al., (108)	Rat	Haloperidol	Apomorphine	↓ Locomotor activity
Pert et al., (129)	Rat	Haloperidol	Apomorphine	↓ Locomotor activity ↓ Stereotypy
Klawans et al., (96,97)	Rat, guinea pig	Haloperidol	Apomorphine	↓ Stereotypy
Verimer et al., (182)	Rat	Haloperidol	Apomorphine	↓ Locomotor Activity
Gallager et al., (72)	Rat	Haloperidol	Apomorphine	↓ Cell firing rates
Allikmets et al., (4)	Rat	Haloperidol	Apomorphine	↓ Stereotypy aggression
Meller & Friedman (112)	Rat	Haloperidol	Apomorphine	↓ Stereotypy
Rosenblatt et al., (146)	Rat	Haloperidol	Apomorphine	↓ Locomotor activity
Staunton et al., (167,168)	Rat	Haloperidol	Apomorphine	↓ Weak suppression of stereotypy NS locomotor
Bloom et al., (21)	Rat	Haloperidol	Apomorphine	↓ Weak suppression of stereotypy NS locomotor
Pittman et al., (131)	Rat	Haloperidol	Apomorphine	↓ Weak suppression of stereotypy
Calil & Rodrigues (29)	Rat	Haloperidol	Apomorphine	↑ Stereotypy NS aggression

NS, not significant.

lesion-induced supersensitivity. Gruenthal et al. (81) noted no differences in contralateral rotations in the Li-treated groups as compared to controls following 1 week of Li treatment. However, there was a suppression in the apomorphine-induced contralateral rotations 3 and 12 hours after the lst Li injection as compared to control rats. Gardner et al. (74) reported only partial suppression (65%) of 6-OHDA-induced rotational behavior in Li-treated rats after APO, and this effect disappeared by 4 weeks. In a crossover study, Kozlowski et al. (99) showed that 6-OHDA injections were associated with a large decrease in contralateral orientation to somatosensory stimuli in both Li-treated and control rats at 3 days. However, at 4 weeks, animals in the control group showed significantly greater contralateral orientation than the Li group but had a 40% increase in orientation that was evident 5 days after termination of Li, which plateaued at 3 to 4 weeks. These results suggest that Li's effect on 6-OHDA-induced changes may be incomplete and reversible.

As reviewed above, studies of the effects of Li on the behavioral responses following the administration of 6-OHDA have suggested that Li is capable of attenuating supersensitivity (74,99) or has no effect (81,160,168). Swerdlow (170) reported that Li is capable of altering behavioral responses to stimulation of both supersensitive nigrostriatal and supersensitive mesolimbic DA receptors. They note that alterations were dependent on the anatomical location of the DA receptors that were stimulated.

Nucleus accumbens-6-OHDA-treated animals on Li showed lower levels of locomotor activity than controls. Li was also shown to produce "less constrained" stereotypy responses in the substantia nigra-6-OHDA-treated animals

than in controls. These results suggest that chronic dietary Li modifies postsynaptic mechanisms to suppress elements of the behavioral manifestations of supersensitive mesolimbic and nigrostriatal DA activity in the absence of a presynaptic terminal. Swerdlow et al. (170) speculate that mania may involve the activation of some postsynaptic element of the forebrain DA systems and that the therapeutic actions of Li may result from a decrease in this pathological overactivity.

Other measures of DA receptor activity have been studied. Prolactin (PRL) secretion was used as a measure of DA receptor supersensitivity in the tuberoinfundibular system and was measured after treatment with haloperidol. Tanimoto et al. (173) showed that rats had longer-lasting inhibition of PRL secretion produced by APO as compared to controls. The DA supersensitivity was observed on the fifth day after the last haloperidol injection and disappeared by the 33rd day. Treatment with Li/haloperidol for a period of 2 weeks resulted in the inhibition of PRL-lowering action at day 5 after withdrawal, possibly indicating that the supersensitivity of DA receptors in the pituitary may be decreased by Li.

Reches et al. (142) studied the effect of prophylactic Li on haloperidol-induced presynaptic DA receptor supersensitivity in the striatum and nucleus accumbens. The response was estimated by its effect on the accumulation of DOPAC following the administration of γ-butyrolactone (GBL) in the presence of a dopa decarboxylase inhibitor. Chronic Li did not attenuate this neuroleptic-induced presynaptic DA receptor supersensitivity.

The effect of Li on DA receptor binding has been studied in rat brain using [³H]spiroperidol and measuring changes in receptor number and affinity. Haloperidol treatment is associated with an increase in the number of DA receptors. Several studies have demonstrated that if Li is administered prior to the development of supersensitivity it is capable of blocking the rise in the number of DA receptors (129,146); however, other investigators were unable to replicate these results (21,131,168). In addition, Li was ineffective in preventing 6-OHDA-induced increases in DA receptors (21,99,168).

Although it appears that Li in some manner affects the development of supersensitivity, it may be critical to review the effect of Li treatment alone on DA receptors. One study demonstrated that Li decreased DA receptor binding in the rat striatum (146), but other studies were unable to support these findings (12,130,160,174), although Tanimoto et al. (174) did report significant decreases in DA binding in the rat limbic forebrain following acute and chronic Li treatment. However, it has been shown that chronic Li may selectively reduce the affinity of DA agonists but not antagonists for DA receptor sites in the neostriatum in rats. Furthermore, Bloom et al. (21) noted that simultaneous treatment with haloperidol and denervation with 6-OHDA produced additive increases in DA receptor sites.

DA agonist supersensitivity was shown to be induced by amphetamine. Three days of Li pretreatment enhanced stereotypy when relatively low test doses of amphetamine were used. However, in the presence of higher doses of amphetamine, Li's effects were diminished or absent (149).

Enhancement of behavioral responses by Li administration was also reported by Friedman et al. (68), who administered reserpine to rats and reported supersensitivity of stereotypic responses to APO. Pretreatment with Li increased the stereotypy response, suggesting that drugs may have different mechanisms of action associated with the induction of supersensitivity.

Other effects of Li on supersensitivity have also been reported. Chronic haloperidol was shown to enhance amphetamine-induced locomotor activity, and this effect was reported to be attenuated by Li. Treatment with Li alone, without haloperidol, did not block the amphetamine-induced locomotor activity (131).

Another method used to induce DA supersensitivity is that of rapid eye movement (REM) sleep deprivation (32,145,179). Rodrigues et al. (145) REM-deprived rats and then measured stereotypy and aggressive behavioral responses to APO challenges. Pretreatment with Li was shown to block the increased stereotypy and to partially prevent aggressive-induced behaviors.

A proposed mechanism of action of Li is that it blocks behavioral DA supersensitivity by preventing haloperidol-induced increases in DA receptors. A number of studies on the effects of Li on the DA receptor have been completed (9,21,112,129,131,146,168), but there is no general agreement as to the relationship between haloperidol-induced increases in DA receptors and the role of Li.

Lesioning studies of the dopaminergic pathways in rat brain may provide other possible clues as the effects of Li on DA supersensitivity. Three (74,81,170) out of four studies reported that Li was capable of suppressing lesion-induced (6-OHDA) DA behavioral supersensitivity. The postsynaptic DA receptor was suggested as a possible site

of Li action in that Li decreased locomotor activity in the absence of presynaptic DA terminals (170). However, DA receptor binding studies were unable to provide additional clues for the specific mode of Li action (see Bloom et al., (21) for review).

Other models used to test Li's effect on DA behavioral supersensitivity have provided interesting data. Drugs other than haloperidol, such as reserpine (68,111), amphetamine (149), and fluphenazine (149), have suggested varied effects of Li on DA supersensitivity. REM-sleep deprivation-induced DA supersensitivity (145) and intracranial self-stimulation studies (155,156) have provided additional data that Li is able to suppress DA behavioral supersensitivity responses.

In conclusion, there is convincing data to suggest that Li is effective in preventing the development of neuroleptic-induced dopaminergic behavioral manifestations of supersensitivity (Table 1). However, the mechanism of action of Li has not yet been identified.

The time of Li administration may be critical in the modification of DA supersensitivity. A number of studies noted a lack of effect if Li was administered after supersensitivity was induced (21,81,97,167). Other experimental variables which may be important in the interpretation of data include length of drug administration, time off treatment, and dose of the challenge drugs. For example, behavioral effects of Li/drug combinations appeared to be extremely sensitive to variations in APO doses.

Norepinephrine Receptors

Animal Studies

The effect of chronic Li on α- and β-adrenergic receptors has been the focus of many studies, as it is thought these receptors may play an important role in affective disorders. There are varied reports of the effect of drug-induced changes in adrenergic receptor sensitivity, although it appears that Li may differentially affect the development of subsensitivity and supersensitivity. In two studies, Li was reported to be ineffective in blocking the development of β subsensitivity. Rosenblatt et al. (147) found that Li failed to prevent the development of imipramine-induced subsensitivity of β-receptors. Pert et al. (130) demonstrated that Li blocked the development of both α and β supersensitivity after depletion of NE by 6-OHDA. Trieser and Kellar (177) indicated that although Li did not block α supersensitivity, it did block the development of reserpine-induced β supersensitivity in rat cortex. However, these results were not in agreement with those of Mailman et al. (108), who failed to show that Li blocked the development of 6-OHDA-induced β supersensitivity. A study completed in mice showed that chronic Li treatment blocked the behavioral phenomena induced by isolation. However, the number and affinity of β-receptors in the mouse brain (excluding cerebellum) were unchanged by either isolation or Li (67).

Using the cerebellum as a model system in the rat, Schultz et al. (154) conducted a series of studies of the effects of chronic Li on Purkinje cells. They concluded that there is NE involvement in the mechanism of action of Li and that there may be long-term adaptive mechanisms, since acute Li has opposite effects to that of chronic Li treatment on firing rates. However, binding studies were unable to show any effect on β-receptor sites in cerebellum (107,154).

Studies involving Li treatment alone showed varied results. Rosenblatt et al. (147) reported that Li treatment increased α binding and decreased β-receptor binding in whole brain homogenates. This is in partial agreement with the investigations of Trieser and Kellar (177), who reported Li-induced decreases in β-receptors in rat cortex, although they could not detect changes in α-receptors. They suggested that the differences may be related to the brain area studied. However, in a later investigation, Maggi and Enna (107) reported no significant changes in β-receptor binding ([^{3}H]DHA) in rat cerebral cortex, cerebellum, or hypothalamus. Another group of investigators has reported decreased [^{3}H]DHA (β-receptor) binding in rat frontal cortex following chronic Li treatment (187). Electrophysiological studies revealed a moderately enhanced responsivity to iontophoretically applied NE in rat cerebellum following chronic Li treatment (154).

Clinical Studies

In humans the binding of [^{3}H]clonidine in platelets was measured in depressed patients treated with Li. Results showed a decrease in the high-affinity binding site of the α_2-receptor and an increase in epinephrine-induced platelet aggregation responses, suggesting that Li induces a down-regulation of the platelet α_2-receptors in depressed patients (73). In another clinical study, Belmaker (13) reported that Li was unable to block the development of subsensitive β-receptors induced by salbutamol (β_2-agonist) in 11 depressed patients.

In summary, it appears that Li is unable to block induced down-regulation of β-receptors but has varied effects on the development of α and β supersensitivity.

Serotonin Receptors

Animal Studies

The ability of chronic Li administration to modify tricyclic antidepressant-induced supersensitivity development in cells receiving 5-HT input was investigated using microiontophoretic techniques. In these experiments chronic chlorimipramine or imipramine administration resulted in a significant increase in the sensitivity of the hippocampal pyramidal cells to iontophoretically applied 5-HT. This supersensitivity was not blocked by concurrent administration of Li (71). Friedman et al. (68) reported that Li was unable to block reserpine-induced 5-HT supersensitivity but enhanced the reserpine-elicited sensitization. Chronic Li treatment alone was shown to be correlated with a decrease in the number of 5-HT receptor sites in hippocampus (107,174,176,178) and striatum (107,178) and no change in cortex (107,174,178) or hypothalamus (107). However,

in vitro treatment did not affect 5-HT receptors (107,177). Tanimoto et al. (174) also showed that chronic Li treatment markedly decreased the affinity of 5-HT receptors in the hippocampus but not in the cerebral cortex.

An unexpected finding of the effect of Li on the 5-HT-2 receptor was demonstrated using [^{3}H]ketanserin in rat frontal cortex. Battaglia et al. (11) showed that LiCl was approximately fivefold more potent than NaCl or KCl in lowering the apparent affinity of serotonin for the 5-HT-2 receptor. Yamawaki et al. (187) reported that chronic Li treatment decreased the density of 5-HT-2 but not 5-HT-1 receptors in rat frontal cortex, and decreased 5-HT-1 receptors in hippocampus. This group did not report any findings on changes in receptor affinities.

In concluding, the data suggest varied responses to Li administration that may be due to changes in receptor binding, affinity, or regional specificity, and more recently, studies have indicated the differential response of 5-HT-1 and 5-HT-2 receptors to Li interventions.

Cholinergic-Muscarinic Receptor Binding

Several studies have measured the effect of Li on the regulation of muscarinic receptors in rat brain. Results indicate that Li may increase [^{3}H]QNB (quinuclidinyl benzilate) binding to muscarinic-cholinergic receptors in rat brain (95,102,103) or have no effect (107). In human caudate nucleus, Tollefson and Senogle (175) reported that Li reduced the affinity of [^{3}H]QNB for the receptor in patients who had no history of psychiatric disease or drug abuse.

Using cholinergic drugs, the effect of Li on up- and down-regulation of muscarinic-cholinergic receptors was assessed. Levy et al. (103) showed that Li pretreatment completely abolished the increase in [^{3}H]QNB binding induced by atropine but was unable to block the decrease in binding induced by DFP (diisopropyl fluorophosphate, a cholinesterase inhibitor), suggesting that Li pretreatment may be successful in blocking supersensitivity but is ineffective in blocking subsensitivity. However, Lerer et al. (102), using scopolamine, reported increased binding in cortex, striatum, and hippocampus. Concurrent treatment with Li and scopolamine was unable to block the development of scopolamine-induced supersensitivity.

In behavioral studies, chronic Li was reported to enhance the cholinergic-mediated responses, pilocarpine-induced hypothermia, and catalepsy, whereas the combined Li/scopolamine treatment was associated with a greater response than that induced by scopolamine alone. Lerer et al. (102) conclude that a likely explanation for Li's effects is a presynaptic action of Li with increased ACh turnover and release and a postsynaptic effect of scopolamine on the receptor.

In a comprehensive review of Li's effects on muscarinic receptor binding parameters, Dilsaver (52) hypothesizes that Li's antimanic, antidepressant, and anticycling efficacy may depend on its cholinotropic properties, which may play an important role in cholinergic-monoaminergic interactions and mechanisms.

GABA Receptors

After 3 weeks of Li treatment there was a significant decrease in low-affinity [^{3}H]GABA sites in the corpus striatum (68%) and hypothalamus (36%). Acute treatment (2 days) did not affect GABA receptor binding in the brain regions studied. Also, Li had no effect on *in vitro* [^{3}H]GABA binding, indicating that the decreases were not due to the presence of Li in the brain tissue (107).

EFFECTS OF Li ON SECOND MESSENGER SYSTEMS

Cyclic AMP

Animal Studies

There is increasing evidence to suggest that Li may exert some of its therapeutic actions by inhibiting adenylate cyclase within the central nervous system (15,54,57, 59,65). At clinically relevant levels, Li has been shown to inhibit NE-induced cyclic AMP (14,58,65,127,141). When rats were tested after 21 and 42 days following Li withdrawal, there was no evidence of NE-stimulated cyclic AMP supersensitivity in cortex or hypothalamus (58), as might have been expected following chronic inhibition of the Li system. Belmaker et al. (15) notes that adenylate cyclase differs from tissue to tissue, and therefore a "therapeutic target" adenylate cyclase might be more sensitive to Li inhibition at a specific dose. This group suggests that a prime candidate for the target adenylate cyclase is NE-sensitive adenylate cyclase, which appears to be inhibited at lower doses than DA-sensitive adenylate cyclase (75,141). In addition, Belmaker et al. (15) suggest that some of the toxic side effects related to Li administration may, in fact, be correlated with inhibition of other adenylate cyclase systems and vasopressin (ADH)-sensitive cyclase.

Reches et al. (141), using guinea pig brain, studied the effects of therapeutic Li levels on NE- and DA-induced accumulations of cyclic AMP. These investigators showed that it may be possible to simultaneously stimulate DA-sensitive accumulations in the caudate nucleus while inhibiting NE-induced cyclic AMP in the cortex. However, Walker et al. (183) earlier reported no effect of Li on DA-sensitive adenylate cyclase.

Hermoni et al. (87), who showed that low-dose Li pretreatment blocked reserpine-induced increases in NE stimulated cyclic AMP in rat cortex. These results suggest that low-dose prophylactic treatment, although incapable of directly inhibiting NE-sensitive adenylate cyclase, is capable of blocking a possible index of reserpine-induced supersensitivity.

More recently, Okada (126) measured the effects of chronic Li on the β-adrenergic-adenylate cyclase system of rat cerebral cortex. The authors conclude that following 2 weeks of Li treatment, the function of the guanine nucleotide regulatory component of adenylate cyclase may be suppressed. Another study (76) provided further evidence that Li may possibly interfere with adenylate cyclase both on the GTP protein and on the catalytic subunit.

Also, behavioral research in mice suggest that adenosine-stimulated cyclase may be a possible site of Li action (84).

Clinical Studies

Li has been shown to act on nonneuronal adenylate cyclases, such as those processes that affect polypeptide hormones. In a number of systems it has been shown that Li interacts with cyclic AMP-mediated processes that are regulated by polypeptide hormones. This is apparently true in the kidney, thyroid (165), and central nervous system. Nephrogenic and central diabetes insipidus occur in patients treated with Li carbonate. Nephrogenic diabetes insipidus is the most common condition. Li may act by lowering hormone induced increases in cyclic AMP levels produced by the release of ADH. However, Forrest (66) has found that Li-induced polyuria in rats is completely unresponsive to ADH and only partially responsive to cyclic AMP, which suggests a dysfunction both before and after the metabolic steps involved in cyclic AMP production. Thus, in part, Li may act only in part in this system by inhibiting ADH-induced increases in cyclic AMP levels.

Some individuals treated chronically with Li also develop a nontoxic goiter and hypothyroidism. Again, Li may act by inhibition of adenyl cyclase in the thyroid. Thyroid-stimulating hormone activates adenylate cyclase to produce cyclic AMP, which then mediates the release of thyroxin. Other studies, however, suggest that Li may also act at a step beyond adenylate cyclase, perhaps directly on the calcium-dependent endocytotic release process for thyroxin, as Li has been observed to decrease the accumulation of colloid droplets from which thyroglobulin is released.

In humans the stimulation of platelet adenylate cyclase and cyclic AMP production by prostaglandin E-1 has been shown to be markedly inhibited by NE (56). Li antagonizes both the NE and the prostaglandin E-1 responses, with higher concentrations of Li required in acute *in vitro* experiments than in chronic treatment studies (25,26). Li treatment is also associated with decreasing plasma cyclic GMP elevations in normal subjects challenged with epinephrine (16) and has been shown to attenuate the increase in plasma cyclic AMP response to epinephrine (13). Chronic Li does not prevent the subsensitivity of β-adrenergic adenylate cyclase induced by salbutamol treatment (190), although it blocks the plasma cyclic AMP response to this selective β-agonist (14). Using human platelets and lymphocytes, Ebstein (60) showed that human membrane adenylate cyclase is extremely sensitive to very low concentrations of Li (0.5 mM) and inhibits epinephrine-induced rises in plasma cyclic AMP (56).

In the human brain, one study reported that cortex has a more sensitive NE adenylate cyclase system than that in the rat (159). In another study, Belmaker et al. (15) surgically removed human brain tumors, isolated the healthy tissue, and then assayed for NE-sensitive adenylate cyclase activity in seven patients. Results indicated that therapeutic levels of Li were capable of inhibiting NE-adenylate cyclase in frontal cortical and temporal gray matter. Newman et al. (125) also showed that Li inhibited adenylate cyclase in the human brain.

Phosphoinositide System

The PI system is thought to act as a second messenger, and there is increasing evidence that one mode of action of Li is to alter PI-linked receptors, thereby modulating neuronal and hormonal responses. Briefly, the PI cycle can be described as follows: Receptor stimulation triggers the cleavage of phosphatidylinositol-bis-phosphate, giving rise to diacylglycerol and inositol triphosphate. In turn, inositol triphosphate mobilizes intracellular calcium, while diacylglycerol activates protein kinase C by enhancing its affinity for calcium, which stimulates protein kinase C activity. Phosphatase enzymes sequentially remove phosphate from inositol triphosphate, giving rise to free inositol, which is then reconverted to phosphatidylinositol-bis-phosphate.

Li is thought to slow down the PI cycle by inhibiting phosphatase activity and, in turn, building up various inositol phosphates. As a result of phosphatase inhibition in rat cerebral cortex, there is a decrease in myo-inositol and an increase in myo-inositol-1 phosphatase levels, which Sherman et al. (158) describe as the "lithium effect." *In vitro* research has shown that the Li effect takes place at Li concentrations low enough to be therapeutically relevant (83) and that it can be attenuated by muscarinic-cholinergic antagonists and mimicked to a degree by cholinomimetics (5).

Several studies have shown that Li is capable of enhancing the responses of PI-linked receptors. In the smooth muscle system, Menkes et al. (117) demonstrated that the combination of atropine/Li resulted in a longer-lasting relaxation response as compared to Li treatment alone. In two other studies in rat cerebral cortex, the addition of Li to centrally acting cholinomimetics and other agonists *in vivo* resulted in greater phosphate level increases as compared to Li treatment alone (89,158). These data suggest, according to Menkes et al., that Li at therapeutic concentrations alters the physiological responses of neurotransmitters that stimulate the PI cycle, thus dampening the neurotransmitter response. They speculate that neurotransmitters affected would involve all those known to act via the PI cycle, including NE, 5-HT, ACh, and histamine. A recent investigation demonstrated that Li stimulated the release of corticotropin (ACTH) via the PI system (189). It has been suggested that Li may differentially affect PI metabolism of PI-linked receptors, thus providing a possible model for regional neuronal effects (17,158).

EFFECTS OF Li ON PROTEIN SYNTHESIS

Chronic Li administration has been shown to affect protein synthesis as measured by polysomal translation *in vitro*. Rats were treated for 6 weeks with intragastric intubation of either 150 mg/kg/day or 225 mg/kg/day of Li. At the lower dose (serum level, 1.0–1.5 mEq/liter), protein synthesis was stimulated in the brain, whereas at the higher dose (serum level, 1.5–2.0 mEq/liter), protein synthesis was shown to be inhibited (148).

EFFECTS OF Li ON THE OPIATE SYSTEM

Locomotor responses to morphine in chronic Li-treated rats were shown to be enhanced, possibly suggesting that Li could be acting to produce an increased sensitivity to morphine at opioid peptide receptors. Additional data suggest that these sites may be located in the midbrain DA systems (61). Previous animal studies have shown consistent, dose-dependent increases in brain enkephalin following chronic Li treatment (21,80).

DISCUSSION AND SUMMARY

At the present time, we are unable to integrate the mode of action of Li into one theory that would explain its antimanic and antidepressant effect. Eventually, knowledge concerning Li's interaction with various cations and ionophore complexes may provide a unified theory of the mode of action of Li in depression and mania. However, it does seem useful to develop, from the large number of studies of the effect of Li on neurotransmitter and receptor systems, two separate theories of Li's mode of action as related to depression and mania. From the many studies, a few very consistent bodies of data emerge and are summarized below.

Possible Mode of Action of Li in Depression

The many reports concerning the effects of Li converge to suggest that Li has a serotonergic enhancing action. There is a good deal of data to suggest that such an action would have an antidepressant effect. The following evidence supports this hypothesis. Most of the effective antidepressants, including tricyclics, MAOIs, and electroconvulsive therapy (ECT) are associated with the down-regulation of β-receptors. It has been shown in both animal (23,24,55,91) and human (161,163) studies that an intact serotonin system is necessary in order to down-regulate β-receptors.

In animals, if one depletes 5-HT stores, tricyclics are incapable of down-regulating β-receptors (69,70,110,169), whereas in humans an antidepressant response to either MAOIs or tricyclic antidepressants can be reversed by blocking the synthesis of serotonin at the rate-limiting step with PCPA (161,163). Furthermore, in some patients, Li added to tricyclics can produce an immediate therapeutic response (48,49). Finally, the serotonin precursor, tryptophan, plus MAOI, seems to have a synergistic effect in producing a more rapid therapeutic response (42,116,181).

In summary, a number of animal and clinical studies document serotonergic enhancing activity of Li, which would be compatible with an antidepressant action. Furthermore, in a number of animal studies, Li alone was associated with a down-regulation of β-receptors (147,178). Tricyclics and MAOIs affect β-receptors; thus the interaction of Li and the possible testing of selective β_1 and β_2 agonists in humans should prove useful in the future.

Possible Mode of Action of Lithium in Mania

(a) A large body of data documents that Li blocks behavioral manifestations in the development of supersensitive DA receptors. (b) There is also a consistent literature that Li has a muscarinic-cholinergic enhancing action. These data are compatible with the observations of Janowsky (92) and Davis (47) that physostigmine could produce acute remission in manic symptomatology. (c) A large number of studies document the consistent effect of Li in inhibiting second messenger cyclic AMP-mediated processes. (d) There are intriguing observations that Li produces an inhibition of the phosphoinositol phosphatase, leading to a buildup in phosphates that could result in dampening of the effects of the neurotransmitters.

ACKNOWLEDGMENT

We would like to acknowledge the excellent library research assistance of Sarju Bhaskerrao Patel.

REFERENCES

1. Ahluwalia, P., and Singhal, R. L. (1980): *Br. J. Pharmacol.,* 71: 601–607.
2. Ahluwalia, P., and Singhal, R. L. (1981): *Neuropharmacology,* 20:483–487.
3. Aldenhoff, J. B. (1985): *Abstr. IVth World Congr. Biol. Psychiatry,* p. 440.
4. Allikmets, L. H., Stanley, M., and Gershon, S. (1979): *Life Sci.,* 25:165–170.
5. Allison, J. H. (1978): In: *Cyclitols and Phosphoinositides,* edited by W. W. Wells and F. Eisenberg, Jr., pp. 507–509. Academic Press, New York.
6. Arora, R. C., Fessler, R. G., and Meltzer, H. Y. (1983): *Prog. Neuropsychopharmacol. Biol. Psychiatry,* 7:39–45.
7. Ayd, F. J. (1984): *Psychiatr. Ann.,* 14:549–550.
8. Brastrup, P. C., Poulsen, J. C., Schou, M., Thomsen, K., and Amidsen, A. (1970): *Lancet,* 2:326–330.
9. Banay-Schwartz, M., Wajda, I. J., Manigault, I., DeGuzman, T., and Lajtha, A. (1982): *Neurochem. Res.,* 7:179–189.
10. Baron, M., Gershon, E. S., Rudy, V., Jonas, W. Z., and Buchsbaum, M. (1975): *Arch. Gen. Psychiatry,* 32:659–668.
11. Battaglia, G., Shannon, M., and Titeler, M. (1983): *Life Sci.,* 32: 2597–2601.
12. Beckmann, H., St-Laurent, J., and Goodwin, F. K. (1975): *Psychopharmacologia,* 42:277–282.
13. Belmaker, R. H. (1981): *Biol. Psychiatry,* 16:333–350.
14. Belmaker, R. H. (1985): *Abstr. IVth World Congr. Biol. Psychiatry,* p. 449.
15. Belmaker, R. H., Hamburger-Bar, R., Newman, M., and Bannet, J. (1984): In: *Current Trends in Lithium and Rubidium Therapy,* edited by G. U. Corsini, pp. 59–75. MTP Press, Lancaster.
16. Belmaker, R. H., Kon, M., Ebstein, R. P., and Dasberg, H. (1980): *Biol. Psychiatry,* 15:3–8.
17. Berridge, M. J., Downes, C. P., and Hanley, M. R. (1982): *Biochem. J.,* 212:849–858.
18. Beuthin, F. C., Miya, T. S., Blake, D. E., and Bousquet, W. F. (1972): *J. Pharmacol. Exp. Ther.,* 131:446–456.
19. Blier, P., and DeMontigny, C. (1983): *Neurosci. Soc. Abstr.,* p. 428.
20. Bliss, E. L., and Ailion, J. (1970): *Brain Res.,* 24:305–310.
21. Bloom, F. E., Baetge, G., Deyo, S., Ettenberg, A., Koda, L., Magistretti, P. J., Shoemaker, W. J., and Staunton, D. A. (1983): *Neuropharmacology,* 22:359–365.
22. Breslow, R. E., DeMuth, G. W., and Weiss, C. (1985): *Biol. Psychiatry,* 20:58–65.
23. Brunello, N., Barbaccia, M. L., Chuang, D. M., and Costa, E. (1982): *Neuropharmacology,* 21:1145–1149.
24. Brunello, N., Moccheti, I., Volterra, A., Cuomo, V., and Racagni, G. (1985): *Psychopharmacol. Bull.,* 21:379–384.
25. Bunney, W. E., Jr., and Murphy, D. L. (1976): *Neurosci. Res. Prog. Bull.,* 14:111–207.
26. Bunney, W. E., Jr., Pert, A., Rosenblatt, J., Pert, C. B., and Gallager, D. (1979): *Arch. Gen. Psychiatry,* 36:898–901.
27. Burt, D. R., Creese, I., and Snyder, S. H. (1977): *Science,* 196: 326–328.
28. Cade, J. F. J. (1949): *Med. J. Aust.,* 36:349–352.
29. Calil, H. M., and Rodrigues, F. C. (1984): In: *Current Trends in Lithium and Rubidium Therapy,* edited by G. U. Corsini, pp. 72–92. MTP Press, Lancaster.
30. Cameron, O. G., and Smith, C. B. (1980): *Psychopharmacology,* 67:81–85.
31. Cappeliez, P., White, N., and Duhamel, J. R. (1982): *Neuropsychobiology,* 8:129–134.
32. Carlini, E. A. (1983): *Rev. Pure Appl. Pharmacol. Sci.,* 4:1–25.
33. Carman, J. S., Post, R. M., Goodwin, F. K., and Bunney, W. E., Jr. (1977): *Biol. Psychiatry,* 12:5–7.
34. Carman, J. S., and Wyatt-Knowles, E. S. (1985): *Abstr. IVth World Congr. Biol. Psychiatry,* p. 442.
35. Chambers, C. A., Smith, A. H., and Naylor, G. J. (1982): *Psychol. Med.,* 12:57.
36. Colburn, R. N., Goodwin, F. K., Bunney, W. E., Jr., and Davis, J. M. (1967): *Nature,* 215:1395–1397.
37. Collard, K. J. (1978): *Br. J. Pharmacol.,* 62:137–142.
38. Collard, K. J., and Roberts, M. H. T. (1977): *Neuropharmacology,* 16:671–673.
39. Cooper, S. J., Kelly, J. G., Johnston, G. D., King, D. J., Copeland, S., and McDevitt, D. G. (1985): *Abstr. IVth World Congr. Biol. Psychiatry,* p. 107.
40. Coppen, A., Peet, M., and Bailey, J. (1963): *Psychiatr. Neurol. Neurochir.,* 76:500–510.
41. Coppen, A., Rao Rana, V. A., and Bishop, M. (1980): *J. Affective Disord.,* 2:311–315.
42. Coppen, A., and Wood, K. (1982): *Adv. Biochem. Psychopharmacol.,* 34:249–258.
43. Corrodi, H., Fuxe, K., Hokfelt, T., and Schou, M. (1967): *Psychopharmacologia,* 11:345–353.
44. Corrodi, H., Fuxe, K., and Schou, M. (1969): *Life Sci.,* 8:643–651.
45. Creese, I., Burt, D. R., and Snyder, S. H. (1977): *Science,* 197: 596–598.
46. Cundall, R. L., Brooks, P. N., and Murray, L. G. (1972): *Psychol. Med.,* 2:308–311.
47. Davis, K. L., Berger, P. A., Hollister, L. E., and DeFraites, E. (1978): *Arch. Gen. Psychiatry,* 35:119–122.
48. DeMontigny, C., Cournoyer, G., Morissette, R., and Caille, G. (1983): *Arch. Gen. Psychiatry,* 40:1327–1334.
49. DeMontigny, C., Elie, R., and Caille, G. (1985): *Am. J. Psychiatry,* 142:220–223.
50. DeMontigny, C., Greenberg, F., and Mayer, H. (1981): *Br. J. Psychiatry,* 138:252–256.
51. DeMontigny, C., Tan, A.-T., and Caille, G. (1981): Presented at Society for Neuroscience, 11th Annual Meeting, Los Angeles, p. 646.
52. Dilsaver, S. C. (1984): *Biol. Psychiatry,* 19:1551–1565.
53. Dorus, E., Cox, N. J., Gibbons, R. D., Shaughnessy, R., Pandey, G. N., and Cloninger, R. (1983): *Arch. Gen. Psychiatry,* 40:545–552.
54. Dousa, T., and Hechter, O. (1970): *Life Sci.,* 9:765–770.
55. Dumbrille-Ross, A., and Tang, S. W. (1983): *Psychiatry Res.,* 9: 207–215.
56. Ebstein, R. (1976): *Nature,* 259:411–413.
57. Ebstein, R. P., and Belmaker, R. H. (1979): In: *Lithium: Controversies and Unresolved Issues,* edited by T. B. Cooper, S. Gershon, N. S. Kline, and M. Schou, pp. 703–729. Excerpta Medica, Amsterdam.

58. Ebstein, R. P., Hermoni, M., and Belmaker, R. H. (1980): *J. Pharmacol. Exp. Ther.*, 213:161–167.
59. Ebstein, R. P., Reches, A., and Belmaker, R. H. (1978): *J. Pharm. Pharmacol.*, 30:122–123.
60. Ebstein, R. P., Zeevi, S., Moscovich, D. G., Newman, M. E., and Lerer, B. (1985): *Abstr. IVth World Congr. Biol. Psychiatry*, p. 65.
61. Ehlers, C. L., and Koob, G. F. (1985): *Prog. Neuropsychopharmacol. Biol. Psychiatry*, 9:133–142.
62. Emrich, H. M., and Dose, M. (1985): *Abstr. IVth World Congr. Biol. Psychiatry*, p. 442.
63. Eroglu, L., Hizel, A., and Koyuncuoglu, H. (1981): *Psychopharmacology*, 73:84–86.
64. Eroglu, L., Keyer-Uysal, M., and Baykara, S. (1984): *Arzneimforsch. Drug Res.*, 34:762–763.
65. Forn, J., and Valdecasas, F. (1971): *Biochem. Pharmacol.*, 20:2773–2779.
66. Forrest, J. N. (1974): *J. Clin. Invest.*, 53:1115–1123.
67. Frances, H., Maurin, Y., LeCrubier, Y., and Puech, A. (1981): *Eur. J. Pharmacol.*, 72:337–341.
68. Friedman, E., Dallob, A., and Levine, G. (1979): *Life Sci.*, 25:1263–1266.
69. Friedman, E., and Gershon, S. (1973): *Nature*, 243:520–521.
70. Friedman, E., Shopsin, B., and Goldstein, M. (1974): *J. Pharm. Pharmacol.*, 26:995–997.
71. Gallager, D. W., and Bunney, W. E., Jr. (1979): *Naunyn Schmiedebergs Arch. Pharmacol.*, 307:129–134.
72. Gallager, D. W., Pert, A., and Bunney, W. E., Jr. (1978): *Nature*, 273:309–312.
73. Garcia-Sevilla, J. A., Guimon, J., Garcia-Vallejo, P., and Fuster, M. J. (1986): *Arch. Gen. Psychiatry*, 43:51–57.
74. Gardner, E. L., Hirschhorn, I., Seeger, T. F., Weiss, M., and Makman, M. H. (1980): *Soc. Neurosci. Abstr.*, 6:546.
75. Geisler, A., and Klysner, R. (1978): *Life Sci.*, 23:635–636.
76. Geisler, A., and Mork, A. (1985): *Abstr. IVth World Congr. Biol. Psychiatry*, p. 180.
77. Gerbino, L., Oleshansky, M., and Gershon, S. (1978): In: *Psychopharmacology: A Generation of Progress*, edited by M. A. Lipton, A. DeMascio, and K. F. Killam, pp. 1261–1275. Raven Press, New York.
78. Geyer, M. A., and Segal, D. S. (1973): *Psychopharmacologia*, 29:131–140.
79. Glen, A. I. M. (1978): In: *Lithium in Medical Practice*, edited by F. N. Johnson and S. Johnson, pp. 183–192. MTP Press, Lancaster.
80. Gillin, J. C., Hong, J. S., Yang, H.-Y. T., and Costa, E. (1978): *Proc. Natl. Acad. Sci. USA*, 75:2991–2993.
81. Gruenthal, M. (1980): *Soc. Neurosci. Abstr.*, 6:546.
82. Gutterman, D. E., Correa, E. I., DePaulo, J. R., Jr., and Coyle, J. T. (1985): *Am. J. Psychiatry*, 142:493–495.
83. Hallcher, L. M., and Sherman, W. R. (1980): *J. Biol. Chem.*, 255:10896–10901.
84. Hamburger-Bar, R., Robert, M., Newman, M., and Belmaker, R. H. (1986): *Pharmacol. Biochem. Behav.*, 24:9–13.
85. Heninger, G. R., Charney, D. S., and Sternberg, D. E. (1983): *Arch. Gen. Psychiatry*, 40:1335–1344.
86. Heninger, G. R., Charney, D. S., and Sternberg, D. E. (1984): *Arch. Gen. Psychiatry*, 41:398–402.
87. Hermoni, M., Lerer, B., Ebstein, R. P., and Belmaker, R. H. (1980): *J. Pharm. Pharmacol.*, 32:510–515.
88. Hertz, L., and Richardson, S. (1984): *TIPS* (July), 272–276.
88a. Hille B, (1974): *Neurosci Res. Prog. Bull.*, 14:161–164.
89. Honchar, M. P., Olney, J. W., and Sherman, W. R. (1983): *Science*, 220:323–325.
90. Huey, L. Y., Janowsky, D. S., Judd, L. L., Abrams, A., Parker, D., and Clopton, P. (1981): *Psychopharmacology*, 73:161–164.
91. Janowsky, A., Okada, R., and Manier, D. H. (1982): *Science*, 218:900–901.
92. Janowsky, D. S., El-Yousef, M. K., and Davis, J. M. (1973): *Arch. Gen. Psychiatry*, 28:542–547.
93. Jope, R. S. (1979): *J. Neurochem.*, 33:487–495.
94. Jope, R. S., Jenden, D. J., and Erlich, B. E. (1980): *Proc. Natl. Acad. Sci. USA*, 77:6144–6146.
95. Kafka, M., Wirz-Justice, A., Naber, D., Marangos, P., O'Donohue, T., and Wehr, T. (1982): *Neuropsychobiology*, 8:41–50.
96. Klawans, H. L., and Rubovits, R. (1972): *J. Neural Transm.*, 33:235–246.
97. Klawans, H. L., Weiner, W. J., and Nausieda, P. A. (1976): *Prog. Neuropsychopharmacol.*, 1:53–60.
98. Koyama, T., Koenig, J. I., Meltzer, H. Y., and Gudelsky, G. A. (1985): *Soc. Neurosci. Abstr.*, 11:658.
99. Kozlowski, M. R., Neve, K. A., Grisman, J. E., and Marshall, J. F. (1983): *Brain Res.*, 267:301–311.
100. Krell, R. D., and Goldberg, A. M. (1973): *Biochem. Pharmacol.*, 22:3289–3291.
101. Kuriyama, K., and Speken, R. (1970): *Life Sci.*, 9:1213–1220.
102. Lerer, B. (1985): *Biol. Psychiatry*, 20:20–40.
103. Levy, A., Zohar, J., and Belmaker, R. H. (1982): *Neuropharmacology*, 21:1199–1201.
104. Linnoila, M., Karoum, F., and Potter, W. Z. (1983): *Arch. Gen. Psychiatry*, 40:1015–1017.
105. Linnoila, M., Karoum, F., Rosenthal, N., and Potter, W. Z. (1983): *Arch. Gen. Psychiatry*, 40:677–680.
106. Lipinski, J. F., and Pope, H. G. (1982): *Am. J. Psychiatry*, 139:948.
107. Maggi, A., and Enna, S. J. (1980): *J. Neurochem.*, 34:888–892.
108. Mailman, R. B., Kilts, C. D., Mueller, R. A., Harden, T. K., and Breese, G. R. (1980): *Fed. Proc.*, 39:1007.
109. Mandell, A. J., and Knapp, S. (1976): *Neuropsychopharmakol.*, 9:116–126.
110. Manier, D. H., Gillespie, D. D., and Sulser, F. (1984): *Experientia*, 40:1223–1226.
111. McIntyre, I. M., Kuhn, C., Demitriou S., Fucek, F. R., and Stanley, M. (1983): *Psychopharmacology*, 81:150–154.
112. Meller, E., and Friedman, E. (1981): *Eur. J. Pharmacol.*, 76:25–29.
113. Meltzer, H. Y. (1984): *Ann. NY Acad. Sci.*, 430:115–137.
114. Meltzer, H. Y., Arora, R. C., and Goodnick, P. (1983): *J. Affective Disord.*, 5:215–221.
115. Meltzer, H. Y., Lowy, M., Robertson, A., Goodnick, P., and Perline, R. (1984): *Arch. Gen. Psychiatry*, 41:391–397.
116. Mendlewicz, J., and Youdim, M. B. H. (1980): *J. Affective Disord.*, 2:137–146.
117. Menkes, H. A., Baraban, J. M., Freed, A. N., and Snyder, S. H. (1986): *Proc. Natl. Acad. Sci. USA*, 5727–5730.
118. Muller-Oerlinghausen, B. (1985): *Pharmacopsychiatry*, 18:214–.
119. Nagata, C., and Aida, M. (1984): *J. Theor. Biol.*, 110:569–585.
120. Narasimhachari, N., and Ettigi, P. (1985): *Abstr. IVth World Congr. Biol. Psychiatry*, p. 180.
121. Naylor, G. J., Dick, D. A. T., Dick, E. G., and Moody, J. P. (1974): *Psychopharmacologia*, 37:81–86.
122. Naylor, G. J., Dick, D. A. T., Dick, E. G., Worrall, E. P., Peet, M., Dick, P., and Boardman, L. J. (1976): *Psychol. Med.*, 6:659–663.
123. Naylor, G. J., Smith, A., Boardman, L. J., Dick, D. A. T., Dick, E. G., and Dick, P. (1977): *Psychol. Med.*, 7:229–233.
124. Naylor, G. J., Worrall, E. P., Dick, P., Peet, M., Watson, Y., and Stewart, M. (1975): *Lancet*, 2:639–640.
125. Newman, M., Klein, H., Bismaker, B., Feinsod, M., and Belmaker, R. H. (1983): *Brain Res.*, 278:380–381.
126. Okada, F. (1985): *Abstr. Am. Coll. Neuropharmacol.*, p. 165.
127. Palmer, G. C., Robinson, G. A., Manian, A. A., and Sulser, F. (1972): *Psychopharmacology*, 23:201–211.
128. Perez-Cruet, J., Murphy, D. L., and Bunney, W. E., Jr. (1971): *Clin. Res.*, 19:735.
129. Pert, A., Rosenblatt, J. E., Sivit, C., Pert, C. B., and Bunney, W. E., Jr. (1978): *Science*, 201:171–173.
130. Pert, C. B., Pert, A., Rosenblatt, J. E., Tallman, J. F., and Bunney, W. E., Jr. (1979): In: *Catecholamines: Basic and Clinical Frontiers*, edited by E. Usdin, I. J. Kopin, and J. D. Barchas, pp. 583–585. Pergamon Press, New York.
131. Pittman, K. J., Jakubovic, A., and Fibiger, H. C. (1984): *Psychopharmacology*, 82:371–377.
132. Poitou, P., Geurinot, F., and Bohoun, C. (1974): *Psychopharmacologia*, 38:75–80.
133. Post, R. M., and Uhde, T. W. (1984): *Arch. Gen. Psychiatry*, 41:210.
134. Post, R. M., Uhde, T. W., Rubinow, D. R., Joffe, R. T., and

Gold, P. W. (1985): *Abstr. IVth World Congr. Biol. Psychiatry,* p. 449.

135. Prien, R. F. (1978): In: *Lithium: Controversies and Unresolved Issues,* edited by T. B. Cooper, S. Gershon, N. S. Kline, and M. Schou, pp. 3–29. Excerpta Medica, Amsterdam.
136. Prien, R. F. (1983): In: *Treatment of Depression: Old Controversies and New Approaches,* edited by P. J. Clayton and J. E. Barrett, pp. 105–114. Raven Press, New York.
137. Prien, R. F., Caffey, E. M., Jr., and Klett, C. J. (1971): *Dis. Nerv. Syst.,* 32:521–531.
138. Prien, R. F., Caffey, E. M., Jr., and Klett, C. J. (1973): *Arch. Gen. Psychiatry,* 28:337–341.
139. Puszet, P. J. (1982): *Pharmabulletin,* p. 65.
140. Rastogi, R. B., and Singhal, R. L. (1977): *J. Pharmacol. Exp. Ther.,* 201:92–102.
141. Reches, A., Ebstein, R. P., and Belmaker, R. H. (1978): *Psychopharmacology,* 58:213–216.
141a. Reches, A., Hassan, M., Jackson, V., and Fahn, S. (1983): *Life Sci.,* 33:157–160.
142. Reches, A., Jackson-Lewis, V., and Fahn, S. (1984): *Psychopharmacology,* 82:330–334.
143. Redmann, B., and Jefferson, J. W. (1985): *Wis. Med. J.,* 84:23–26.
144. Redmond, D. E., Maas, J. W., Kling, A., and Dekirmenjian, H. (1971): *Psychosom. Med.,* 33:97–113.
145. Rodrigues, F. C., Zwicker, A. P., and Calil, H. M. (1985): *J. Pharm. Pharmacol.,* 37:210–211.
146. Rosenblatt, J. E., Pert, A., Layton, B., and Bunney, W. E., Jr. (1980): *Eur. J. Pharmacol.,* 67:321–322.
147. Rosenblatt, J. E., Pert, C. B., Tallman, J. F., Pert, A., and Bunney, W. E., Jr. (1979): *Brain Res.,* 160:186–191.
148. Rosnowska, M., and Tewari, S. (1983): *Research Monograph,* 10:319–322.
149. Rubin, E. H., and Wooten, G. F. (1984): *Psychopharmacology,* 84:217–220.
150. Rybakowski, J., and Strzyzewski, W. (1985): *Abstr. IVth World Congr. Biol. Psychiatry,* p, 182.
151. Schildkraut, J. J. (1974): *J. Nerv. Ment. Dis.,* 158:348–360.
152. Schou, M. (1982): *Pharmacopsychiatria,* 15:128–130.
153. Schubert, J. (1973): *Psychopharmacologia,* 32:301–311.
154. Schultz, J. E., Siggins, G. R., Schocker, F. W., Turck, M., and Bloom, F. E. (1981): *J. Pharmacol. Exp. Ther.,* 216:28–38.
155. Seeger, T. F., and Gardner, E. L. (1979): *Soc. Neurosci. Abstr.,* 2259:662.
156. Seeger, T. F., Gardner, E. L., and Bridger, W. H. (1981): *Brain Res.,* 215:405–409.
157. Shea, P. A., Small, J. G., and Hendrie, H. C. (1981): *Biol. Psychiatry,* 16:825–830.
158. Sherman, W. R., Munsell, L. Y., Gish, B. G., and Honchar, M. P. (1985): *J. Neurochem.,* 44:798–807.
159. Shimizu, H., Tanaka, S., Suzuki, T., and Matsukado, Y. (1971): *J. Neurochem.,* 18:1157–1161.
160. Shoemaker, W. J., Staunton, D. A., Magistretti, P. J., McCoy, F. B., and Bloom, F. E. (1980): *Soc. Neurosci. Abstr.,* 20:1.
161. Shopsin, B., Friedman, E., and Gershon, S. (1976): *Arch. Gen. Psychiatry,* 33:811–819.

162. Shopsin, B., and Gershon, S. (1971): In: *Brain Chemistry and Mental Disorders,* edited by B. T. Ho and W. M. McIsaac, p. 319. Plenum Press, New York.
163. Shopsin, B., Gershon, S., Goldstein, M., Friedman, E., and Wilk, S. (1975): *Psychopharmacol. Commun.,* 1:239–247.
164. Shukla, G. S. (1985): *Prog. Neuropsychopharmacol. Biol. Psychiatry,* pp. 153–156.
165. Singer, I., and Rotenberg, D. (1973): *N. Engl. J. Med.,* 289:254–260.
166. Smith, D. F. (1985): *Abstr. IVth World Congr. Biol. Psychiatry,* p. 181.
167. Staunton, D. A., Magistretti, P. J., Shoemaker, W. J., and Bloom, F. E. (1982): *Brain Res.,* 160:186–191.
168. Staunton, D. A., Magistretti, P. J., Shoemaker, W. J., Deyo, S., and Bloom, F. E. (1982): *Brain Res.,* 232:401–412.
169. Sulser, F. (1984): *Neuropharmacology,* 23:255–261.
170. Swerdlow, N. R., Lee, D., Koob, G. F., and Vaccarino, F. J. (1985): *J. Pharmacol. Exp. Ther.,* 235:324–329.
171. Tagliamonte, A., Tagliamonte, P., Perez-Cruet, J., Stern, S., and Gessa, G. L. (1971): *J. Pharmacol. Exp. Ther.,* 177:475–480.
172. Tamura, T., Kaiya, H., Yamashita, M. et al. (1985): *Abstr. IVth World Congr. Biol. Psychiatry,* p. 199.
173. Tanimoto, K., Maeda, K., and Chihara, K. (1982): *Brain Res.,* 245:163–166.
174. Tanimoto, K., Maeda, K., and Terada, T. (1983): *Brain Res.,* 265:148–151.
175. Tollefson, G. D., and Senogles, S. (1983): *Biol. Psychiatry,* 18:467–479.
176. Treiser, S. L., Cascio, C. S., O'Donohue, T. L., Thoa, N. B., Jacobowitz, D. M., and Keller, K. J. (1981): *Science,* 213:1529–1531.
177. Treiser, S., and Kellar, K. J. (1979): *Eur. J. Pharmacol.,* 58:85–86.
178. Treiser, S., and Kellar, K. J. (1980): *Eur. J. Pharmacol.,* 64:183–185.
179. Tufik, S. (1981): *J. Pharm. Pharmacol.,* 33:732–733.
180. van Kammen, D. P., and Murphy, D. L. (1975): *Psychopharmacology,* 44:215–224.
181. van Praag, H. M. (1982): *Adv. Biochem. Psychopharmacol.,* 34:259–286.
182. Verimer, T., Goodale, D. B., and Long, J. P. (1980): *J. Pharm. Pharmacol.,* 32:665–666.
183. Walker, J. B. (1974): *Biol. Psychiatry,* 8:245–251.
184. Walz, W., Hertz, E., and Hertz, L. (1983): *Prog. Neuropsychopharmacol. Biol. Psychiatry,* 7:697–702.
185. Williams, R. J. P. (1976): *Neurosci. Res. Prog. Bull.,* 14:145–151.
185a. Winkler, R. (1974): *Neurosci. Res. Prog. Bull.,* 14:139–142.
186. Wood, K. (1985): *J. Affective Disord.,* 8:215–223.
187. Yamawaki, S., Hotta, I., and Sarai, K. (1985): *Abstr. IVth World Congr. Biol. Psychiatry,* p. 267.
188. Yuwiler, A., Bennett, B. L., Brammer, G. L., and Geller, E. (1979): *Biochem. Pharmacol.,* 28:2709–2712.
189. Zatz, M., and Reisine, T. (1985): *Soc. Neurosci. Abstr.,* 11:657.
190. Zohar, J., Lerer, B., Ebstein, R. P., and Belmaker, R. H. (1982): *Biol. Psychiatry,* 17:343–350.

Psychopharmacology:
The Third Generation of Progress,
edited by Herbert Y. Meltzer.
Raven Press, New York © 1987.

CHAPTER 57

Mechanisms of Action of Carbamazepine and Related Anticonvulsants in Affective Illness

Robert M. Post

The use of carbamazepine and related anticonvulsants has evolved in the past decade so that these treatments now represent alternative or adjunctive modalities for the lithium-resistant, bipolar manic-depressive patient. As described elsewhere in detail (63,74–76,79), there is now substantial evidence that carbamazepine has acute antimanic and longer-term prophylactic effects in the treatment of bipolar affective disorder. In both open and double-blind studies, some 60% of patients appear to show a substantial clinical response. Moreover, four double-blind studies indicate that carbamazepine shows a similar magnitude and time course of acute antimanic efficacy to that achieved with classical neuroleptics with a comparable or lesser incidence of side effects. Preliminary evidence suggests that carbamazepine may also have acute antidepressant properties (75), although the frequency and magnitude of response compared to classical antidepressant modalities requires further investigation.

Although the other anticonvulsants have been less well studied, five reports have indicated an antimanic and/or prophylactic effect of sodium valproate, particularly when used in combination with lithium carbonate. A double-blind study of Chouinard (8) suggests that the anticonvulsant clonazepam may also have acute antimanic effects. The anticonvulsant alprazolam appears to have clinically useful effects only in depression, as it, like tricyclics and monoamine oxidase inhibitors (MAOIs), has been reported to induce or exacerbate mania. The putative γ-aminobutyric acid (GABA) agonist progabide, which is marketed in Europe as an anticonvulsant, has been reported to have acute antidepressant and possible antimanic properties. Although early literature suggested that phenytoin might have useful effects in the treatment of manic-depressive patients (32,35), controlled studies have not yet been performed, and Freyhan (19) reported a series of patients who were doubtful responders to phenytoin, although he observed one patient who responded positively on four occasions and showed relapses on four other occasions following drug discontinuation. Acetazolamide, a carbonic anhydrase inhibitor anticonvulsant, has been reported to have positive effects on some atypical affectively ill patients who respond to lithium or carbamazepine (24).

Finally, we must add electroconvulsive therapy (ECT) to the list of putative anticonvulsant agents. We and others have found that electroconvulsive seizures (ECS) in experimental animals exert potent anticonvulsant effects against amygdala-kindled and other types of seizures (66,67). These experimental data support the literature earlier in this century suggesting that ECT may have clinically useful anticonvulsant properties in the treatment of some epileptic patients. Thus, a series of anticonvulsant agents in addition to carbamazepine may emerge as useful treatments of affective illness, and a consideration of their common and different mechanisms of action may give important clues to their actions in affective illness and its underlying neurochemical aberrations.

In attempting to ascertain which mechanism of action of carbamazepine may be important to its effects in manic-depressive illness, several clinical and biological perspectives offer possible theoretical leverage. These include (a) the time course of onset of clinical efficacy of carbamazepine; (b) comparison of carbamazepine with lithium, the classical agent for the acute and prophylactic treatment of manic and depressive illness; (c) comparison and contrast of carbamazepine with other anticonvulsants which do or do not share therapeutic effects in manic-depressive illness; and (d) the use of carbamazepine in pharmacological and electrophysiological animal models.

(a) The onset of the acute antimanic effects of carbamazepine occurs quite early in the course of treatment, often within the first several days or within the first week. Thus, the time course of this action is more akin to, but slower than that seen in the treatment of epilepsy or trigeminal neuralgia. In contrast, the acute antidepressant properties of carbamazepine appear to evolve more slowly after a lag of 1 to 2 weeks, as is often seen with other antidepressant modalities. Thus, acute biochemical and physiological effects of carbamazepine seen in animals could account for its antimanic efficacy but are less likely to be associated with its antidepressant effects.

(b) Preliminary evidence suggests that either a different subgroup of patients or those in a different stage of the longitudinal course of their manic-depressive illness may respond to carbamazepine in contrast to lithium carbonate. Although relatively poorer response to lithium has been associated with more severe and dysphoric mania and a rapidly cycling course of illness, it is just these same variables that appear to be associated with better response to carbamazepine (63,84). Therefore, these clinical distinctions suggest that one might be searching for differential biochemical and physiological effects of carbamazepine compared to lithium, even though the two agents share a generally similar clinical profile of efficacy in the acute and prophylactic treatment of manic-depressive illness.

(c) In a similar fashion, considerably more data are required in order to elucidate whether a series of anticonvulsants share a similar spectrum of clinical efficacy or whether different agents are effective in different patients or subtypes of affective illness. The preliminary data in individual case studies suggest that patients may be differentially responsive to anticonvulsant agents and not generally responsive to all drugs in a given class. For example, Post et al. (64) found that an intensively studied bipolar patient responded to carbamazepine during a series of double-blind clinical trials but showed no evidence of response to two other anticonvulsants, i.e., valproic acid and phenytoin. In contrast, we have observed other patients who appear to show inadequate prophylactic response to carbamazepine and who respond well to valproic acid. These data suggest that instead of looking for common mechanisms of action that might be associated with their anticonvulsant properties, potentially different effects of agents in this series may be importantly involved in their efficacy in the treatment of manic-depressive patients. We might also ask whether anticonvulsants with a different clinical profile in epilepsy are more particularly effective in the treatment of manic-depressive illness. Preliminary evidence indicates that agents which are effective in treating

temporal lobe epilepsy (complex partial seizures) are also effective in manic-depressive illness, although we are not aware of clinical trials of petit mal agents such as ethosuximide in affective illness. Similarly, we are not aware of systematic clinical trials of intravenous barbiturates for acute mania.

(d) Finally, we might use findings regarding the differential efficacy of anticonvulsants in different stages of amygdala kindling to ask whether carbamazepine and other psychotropic agents might not also be differentially effective in manic-depressive illness according to the stage of its evolution.

In assessing what biochemical mechanisms may be important in the therapeutic effects of carbamazepine, it is important to note that, as in epilepsy, effective blood levels appear to be between 4 and 12 μg/ml. This corresponds to approximately 17 to 51 μmol/liter. Side effects (particularly those such as dizziness, ataxia, dysarthria, diplopia, and sedation) occur at highly individualized doses and blood levels but are generally more prominent at levels beyond 12 to 14 μg/ml. Thus, one would want to observe biochemical effects in animals within this clinically effective range. This is normally accomplished by doses of 10 to 20 mg/kg i.p. in the rat, a dose tolerated with relatively little sedation or ataxia in most instances. However, many biochemical effects in animals are observed only at doses of 25 to 50 mg/kg and thus raise the question of their relevance for clinical efficacy as opposed to side effects. Parenthetically, the half-life of carbamazepine in the rat is on the order of $\frac{1}{2}$ hr, whereas that in humans is approximately 35 hr acutely (7). With chronic treatment, hepatic enzymes are induced, the metabolism of carbamazepine proceeds more rapidly, and the half-life in humans decreases to 10 to 20 hr. Similar enzyme induction occurs in the rat and, thus, it becomes quite difficult to administer this drug chronically to rats, particularly given its insolubility. It is also of relevance that carbamazepine-10,11-epoxide is a major metabolite of carbamazepine in humans but only represents approximately 25% of the parent compound. In contrast, this ratio is reversed in the rat, and levels of epoxide are four times higher than carbamazepine itself following chronic administration (45). Thus, the biochemical effects of the epoxide would be particularly prominent in a species such as the rat and might confound biochemical interpretations.

Nonetheless, it is likely that the epoxide may share some of the properties of the parent compound, since this agent is itself a potent anticonvulsant and has recently been shown to be effective in the treatment of trigeminal neuralgia (102). Its efficacy in the treatment of manic-depressive patients remains to be demonstrated. However, a series of clinical trials of a related carbamazepine derivative, which is also an anticonvulsant, the keto derivative of carbamazepine, oxcarbazepine, has been reported by Emrich and associates (15) and others to be effective in treatment of manic-depressive patients, thus suggesting the possibility that a series of active carbamazepine congeners may each be active in epilepsy, trigeminal neuralgia, and manic-depressive illness. Comparison and contrast of the biochemical effects of a series of carbamazepine analogs that are not effective in epilepsy may also be of considerable use in attempting to elucidate the important mechanisms of action for affective illness.

This latter point raises a further complexity and caveat in the assessment of the biochemical effects of carbamazepine. Adequate animal models of manic-depressive illness are either not yet available or the existing ones are cumbersome and unreliable. In contrast, study of the anticonvulsant effects of carbamazepine offers precise qualitative and quantitative measures to assess, such as seizure stage, duration, and afterdischarge duration. Thus, the mechanisms of *anticonvulsant* action of carbamazepine are more readily discernible, but it remains to be demonstrated whether these same mechanisms will also be important to carbamazepine's efficacy in manic-depressive illness.

BIOCHEMICAL EFFECTS OF CARBAMAZEPINE

Noradrenergic Effects

Carbamazepine exerts complex effects on noradrenergic mechanisms. Its blockade of norepinephrine reuptake is weaker than that of imipramine (84), and Quattrone et al. (85) have found that 10 mg/kg of carbamazepine was not sufficient to block norepinephrine reuptake *in vivo* in rats, as evidenced by its inability to protect against the effects of 6-hydroxydopamine (6-OHDA). Carbamazepine also blocks stimulated-induced release of norepinephrine in a synaptosomal and in a rabbit ear artery preparation (84). DeLorenzo et al. (11) also reported that carbamazepine inhibits norepinephrine secretion induced by calcium-calmodulin. Carbamazepine increases the firing of the locus ceruleus at clinically relevant doses (3–30 mg/kg i.p.) (55). Only high levels of carbamazepine (50–100 mg/kg) increased 3-methoxy-4-hydroxyphenylglycol (MHPG) sulfate in rat brain (43,50). At the same time, 100 mg/kg dose decreased several measures of norepinephrine turnover (43). Palmer et al. (56) and Lewin and Bleck (38) also reported that carbamazepine inhibited noradrenergic-stimulated cyclic AMP production. Yet, carbamazepine does not downregulate β-adrenergic receptor density, as do a variety of other antidepressant compounds (45; Joffe, Sulzer, and Post, *unpublished data,* 1985).

Noradrenergic mechanisms appear important to the anticonvulsant effects of carbamazepine. Depletion of norepinephrine induced by 6-OHDA impairs the anticonvulsant effects of this drug (86,87). Although Crunelli et al. (10) found that clonidine would reverse the anticonvulsant effects of carbamazepine on maximum induced ECS, we have observed that the α_2-antagonist, yohimbine, partially blocks the anticonvulsant effects of carbamazepine on amygdala-kindled seizures (S. R. B. Weiss and R. M. Post, *unpublished data,* 1986). Thus, although α_2-noradrenergic mechanisms may be implicated in the anticonvulsant effects of carbamazepine, the type of effect appears to differ across these two seizure models. It also remains to be demonstrated whether carbamazepine's effects on noradrenergic mechanisms are important to its effects on manic-depressive

illness. It is of interest that carbamazepine, in contrast to a variety of other tricyclic antidepressants, does not decrease cerebrospinal fluid (CSF) MHPG (70). In four manic patients studied after probenecid, carbamazepine decreased these elevated levels of CSF norepinephrine (63), perhaps consistent with its effects in decreasing stimulated-induced release in animals (11,84).

Serotonin

Serotonergic lesions or depletions do not appear to affect carbamazepine's anticonvulsant effects (9,86). Moreover, although carbamazepine increases plasma total and free tryptophan in humans (81), it does not increase brain tryptophan levels in rat or brain levels of 5-hydroxyindoleacetic acid (5-HIAA) except at toxic doses (100 mg/kg) (14,49,82). In humans, we found no effect of carbamazepine on CSF levels of 5-HIAA (62). Thus, the selective increase in plasma tryptophan by carbamazepine in contrast to other anticonvulsants, including phenytoin and phenobarbital (81), leaves open the possibility that this effect could account for some aspect of carbamazepine's psychotropic properties, such as those involving impulsivity and aggression (60).

Dopaminergic and Cholinergic Effects

Although carbamazepine has a time course and magnitude of antimanic effects that parallel those of classical neuroleptics which block dopamine receptors (62,79), a variety of evidence indicates that carbamazepine does not act via this mechanism of receptor blockade. There is no evidence that carbamazepine inhibits binding of [³H]spiroperidol (44) or blocks stimulant-induced hyperactivity in animals (8) or euphoria in humans (37). Rather than increasing dopamine turnover and increasing levels of homovanillic acid (HVA) in rat brain, carbamazepine appears to decrease dopamine turnover (106), consistent with our findings of decreased probenecid-induced accumulations of HVA in affectively ill patients treated with carbamazepine (69). We also found that baseline levels of HVA during a medication-free interval were inversely correlated with the degree of antidepressant response to carbamazepine (69), a finding reported in association with a variety of antidepressant modalities including sleep deprivation, levodopa, nomifensine, and some tricyclic antidepressants.

The lack of blockade of dopamine receptors is associated with a similar lack of acute parkinsonian side effects on longer-term tardive dyskinesia (69,88) often associated with neuroleptic treatment. Moreover, the lack of dopamine receptor blockade by carbamazepine offers an additional theoretical rationale for the use of carbamazepine in combination with neuroleptics, since the two agents would apparently be acting by dissimilar biochemical mechanisms.

In clinically relevant doses, carbamazepine does not block reuptake of dopamine *in vivo* since it is insufficient to protect dopaminergic neurons from the effects of 6-OHDA in a fashion similar to that of nomifensine (85).

Barros et al. (2a) reported that, compared to 92% for tyramine, carbamazepine released 62% of accumulated [^{3}H]-dopamine in striatal slices *in vitro* and suggested that carbamazepine may act presynaptically on striatal neurons through enhancement of dopamine release. These data are consistent with those of Kowalik et al. (34a) indicating that carbamazepine increased dopamine, but not norepinephrine or epinephrine, concentrations in cerebroventricular perfusates, and a report of increased dopamine, but not norepinephrine or serotonin, in brain slices (34b). Moreover, acute carbamazepine potentiated apomorphine-induced stereotypy, but chronically inhibited it (2b); carbamazepine also blocked the development of dopamine supersensitivity to apomorphine after chronic haloperidol treatment or rapid eye movement (REM) sleep deprivation (2b).

Carbamazepine increases levels of acetylcholine selectively in rat striatum, while the precursor choline was decreased (8a). Carbamazepine also decreases calcium-calmodulin release of acetylcholine from synaptic vesicles (11). Carbamazepine is 3,000- and 100,000-fold weaker than amitriptyline on muscarinic receptors (human caudate) and on H$_1$ histamine receptors (murine neuroblastoma), respectively (Elliot Richelson, *personal communication,* 1985).

GABA Mechanisms

There is no consistent effect of carbamazepine on levels of GABA in rat brain or human CSF (78). Bernasconi et al. (4) reported that carbamazepine (as well as valproic acid, propranolol, and lithium) decreased GABA turnover. Although the effects were more prominent in hippocampus than in cortex, they appeared only at high doses of carbamazepine; the ED$_{50}$ for hippocampal effects was 75 mg/kg, p.o. This effect on turnover does not appear to be related to a direct GABA effect, as carbamazepine does not bind at GABA receptors (44), alter chloride flux (2), release GABA (98), or alter GABA responses electrophysiologically (42).

Terrence et al. (100) postulated that GABA$_B$ mechanisms may be important to the effects of carbamazepine in trigeminal neuralgia. Not only is baclofen an effective treatment for trigeminal neuralgia, but it produces electrophysiological effects similar to carbamazepine in a trigeminal nucleus model in the cat. The inactive *l*-isomer of baclofen blocks the physiological effect of carbamazepine in this animal model, further implicating GABA$_B$ mechanisms.

However, we have not observed similar effects in our studies of the effects of carbamazepine on amygdala-kindled seizures. In contrast to the trigeminal nucleus model, we did not find that *l*-baclofen (10 mg/kg) was an effective anticonvulsant or that *d*-baclofen (10 mg/kg) was able to block the anticonvulsant effects of carbamazepine (S. R. B. Weiss and R. M. Post, *unpublished data,* 1986). Thus, it is unlikely that GABA$_B$ mechanisms are involved in carbamazepine's anticonvulsant effects, but they could be important to its effects in trigeminal neuralgia (100) or even affective illness, particularly in light of the recent data of Lloyd (39) indicating that a variety of antidepressant modalities all significantly increase GABA$_B$ receptor binding in frontal cortex of rats. Acute carbamezapine does not directly affect GABA$_B$ binding, however (N. G. Bowery, *personal communication,* 1984).

Central and "Peripheral-Type" Benzodiazepine Receptor Mechanisms

Biochemically, carbamazepine is more potent in displacing "peripheral-type" (P-type) benzodiazepine binding in brain utilizing the ligand [^{3}H]Ro5-4864 than in inhibiting the classical or central-type benzodiazepine binding, as assessed by [^{3}H]diazepam or [^{3}H]β-carboline (44). Consistent with these biochemical data are the recent physiological findings of Weiss et al. (111,113) assessing anticonvulsant mechanisms on amygdala-kindled seizures in the rat. Weiss and colleagues observed that anticonvulsant effects of carbamazepine and its -10,11-epoxide were inhibited by Ro5-4864, whereas the anticonvulsant effects of diazepam were unaltered by Ro5-4864. Conversely, the anticonvulsant effects of diazepam were blocked by the antagonists of central benzodiazepine receptor sites, Ro-15-1788 and B-CCM, both of which were without effect on the anticonvulsant effects of carbamazepine. Although high doses of Ro5-4864 are not selective for the P-type site and also displace binding from [^{3}H]picrotoxinin sites, PK-11195 (a compound with opposite effects from Ro5-4864) is highly selective for the P-type site. We found that PK-11195 reversed the effects of Ro5-4864 on the ability of carbamazepine to act as an anticonvulsant (111,113).

These data suggest that, in contrast to diazepam, the P-type benzodiazepine sites are important to carbamazepine's anticonvulsant effects. Since the P-type site has recently been linked to "anxiogenic" properties in animal models (47), it remains a possibility that interactions of carbamazepine with this binding site may be important not only to the anticonvulsant effects of this compound, but also to some aspects of its psychotropic properties. Since clonazepam acts exclusively at central-type benzodiazepine receptors, it is likely that its mechanism of anticonvulsant and antimanic efficacy differs from that of carbamazepine.

In contrast to central-type benzodiazepine binding, which is associated with a GABA receptor and the chloride ionophore, initial evidence suggests that the P-type benzodiazepine receptor is more closely linked to a calcium channel mechanism. These findings implicating P-type benzodiazepine mechanisms in carbamazepine's anticonvulsant efficacy become all the more intriguing in relationship to recent clinical data suggesting possible antimanic effects of calcium channel antagonists such as verapamil (12,13).

Adenosine Mechanisms

Carbamazepine, in contrast to a variety of other anticonvulsants, significantly inhibits binding of adenosine agonists and antagonists to their receptors (44,96,97,99,108). Although this effect occurs at clinically relevant concentrations (25 μmol), there is little direct evidence that it is related to the anticonvulsant properties of carbamazepine. There was no relationship between the ability of carbamazepine analogs to displace adenosine binding in rat brain membranes and oral ED_{50} values of these compounds on maximum ECS in mice (44). Moreover, anticonvulsant effects of carbamazepine were not reversed by high doses of adenosine receptor antagonists such as caffeine and theophylline in our studies of amygdala kindling (112).

Although on the basis of contrasting effects of carbamazepine and caffeine on anxiety and seizures, one would postulate that carbamazepine might have adenosine agonist properties exclusively, there is substantial evidence to the contrary. Chronic administration of carbamazepine to rats, like that of caffeine, causes up-regulation of adenosine receptors (45). Carbamazepine is more potent in displacing antagonist than agonist binding, and its effects are not affected by GTP (44,97,108). Carbamazepine also inhibits adenosine-mediated cyclic AMP accumulation (38,97,108). Phillis (58) also reported that carbamazepine weakly inhibited the agonist effects of adenosine on single-unit firing. Marangos et al. (*unpublished data,* 1986) also found that carbamazepine showed an adenosine antagonist profile on binding affected by temperature (facilitation at low temperature) and GppNHp.

Nonetheless, there are some data suggesting agonist properties of carbamazepine, in that theophylline blocks the inhibition by carbamazepine of guinea pig ileum contractions and blocks the anticonvulsant effects of carbamazepine on tonic extension induced by pentylenetetrazol seizures (97). Moreover, carbamazepine does not potentiate caffeine-induced running behavior in rats (S. R. B. Weiss, L. A. Post, and R. M. Post, *unpublished data,* 1985). Thus, carbamazepine appears to have complex effects (possibly mixed agonist-antagonist properties) on adenosine receptor mechanisms, which may be further elucidated by defining its effects on A_1 versus A_2 systems (20). The adenosine-like effects of carbamazepine could account for a variety of effects of carbamazepine on other neurotransmitter systems. These might include the blockade of norepinephrine reuptake and release and blockade of glutamate efflux, each of which has been reported to occur with adenosine analogs. The adenosine antagonist-like effects could be related to the ability of carbamazepine (like caffeine, ref. 103) to induce escape from dexamethasone suppression (92).

Glutamate

Skerritt et al. (97) and Olpe et al. (54) reported that carbamazepine does not potently displace [^{3}H]glutamate binding. S. Nadi, Ph.D. (*personal communication,* 1985), has found an effect of carbamazepine on binding in freshly prepared rat brain membranes by [^{3}H]4-aminophosphonobutyric acid, another putative marker for glutamate receptors. Carbamazepine does reduce L-[^{3}H]glutamate efflux induced by potassium and veratridine from hippocampal slices with a threshold concentration of 10 μmol (54). Vogler and Zieglgansberger (104) found that carbamazepine inhibited both spontaneous and L-glutamate-evoked firing in extracellular recordings from single cortical neurons in halothane-anesthetized rats. These studies suggest that carbamazepine may have indirect, but important, effects on inhibition of glutamate release. Such an effect on an excitatory neurotransmitter could be relevant to carbamazepine's clinical profile, either in epilepsy or affective illness.

Calcium Concentrations and Calcium Channel Fluxes

We have found that carbamazepine significantly decreases serum calcium (27) but not CSF calcium (76); the effects of carbamazepine on intracellular calcium fluxes remain to be further elucidated. However, a variety of data suggest that the carbamazepine may alter calcium fluxes indirectly through systems that have themselves been closely associated with calcium. As noted above, carbamazepine has important effects on adenosine, P-type benzodiazepine receptors, and $GABA_B$ mechanisms, all of which have been closely associated with calcium channels or fluxes (76). Winkel and Lux (116) reported that clinically relevant concentrations of carbamazepine reduced calcium currents to 30% of normal in voltage-clamped helix neurons. Alterations in calcium mechanisms remain an important candidate for carbamazepine's psychotropic effects, particularly in light of recent data suggesting that calcium channel blockers such as verapamil may exert positive effects in affective illness (12,13).

Sodium Channel Effects of Carbamazepine

Schauf (95) reported that relatively high concentrations of carbamazepine reduced sodium and potassium conductances in voltage-clamped *Myxicola* giant neurons. More recently, Willow and Catterall (114) found that clinically relevant concentrations of both phenytoin and carbamazepine inhibited binding of [^{3}H]batrachotoxin-A20-α-benzoate, a ligand that binds to type 2 sodium channels, which regulate sodium channel activation. Two groups have subsequently documented the physiological relevance of this binding. Willow et al. (115) and McDonald et al. (42), working with mouse neuroblastoma cells and mouse neurons in primary dissociated cell culture, respectively, found that carbamazepine inhibited sodium currents (half maximal inhibition at 30 μmol) and that this effect became more substantial under conditions of depolarization and rapid neuronal firing.

These findings may be of considerable import in light of the observations that depolarization and fast firing are conditions found in epileptic foci. Willow et al. (115) make the argument that the increasing effects of carbamazepine and phenytoin on stabilization of sodium fluxes under these conditions could provide a mechanism for the anticonvulsant efficacy of these agents without their inhibiting normal neuronal processes. In light of these data and various hypotheses about alterations in intracellular sodium in affective disorders, this effect of carbamazepine also remains a candidate for its psychotropic properties.

Naylor et al. (52) reported that carbamazepine reversed the inhibition of sodium-potassium-ATPase produced by vanadate in erythrocytes of patients with affective illness.

Cyclic Nucleotides

Carbamazepine decreases concentration of cyclic AMP in brain (16,17,41,53) or in CSF (51). Palmer et al. (56) reported that carbamazepine was the only anticonvulsant tested that decreased steady state levels of cyclic AMP in cerebral cortex in the cerebellum, although all anticonvulsants tested decreased pentylenetetrazol-induced increases of cyclic AMP studied *in vivo*. In tissue slices from mouse cortex, carbamazepine decreased cyclic AMP accumulations induced by norepinephrine, adenosine, potassium, veratridine, and ouabain (56). In a broken-cell preparation of mouse and rat cerebral cortex, Palmer (56) found that carbamazepine also inhibited dopamine-induced and norepinephrine-induced accumulations of cyclic AMP. These findings were consistent with the earlier observations of Lewin and Bleck (38) that carbamazepine potently inhibited norepinephrine-induced cyclic AMP accumulation in rat cortical slices. Ferendelli and Kinscherf (18) and Palmer et al. (57) reported that carbamazepine decreased accumulations of cyclic GMP induced by veratridine and ouabain, respectively.

We found no effect of carbamazepine on baseline levels of cyclic AMP and cyclic GMP, although probenecid-induced accumulations of cyclic GMP were significantly reduced during carbamazepine treatment, with a similar trend for accumulations of cyclic AMP (62). Since lithium has potent effects on this second messenger system (117) and alterations in cyclic nucleotides have been postulated in both affective illness and epilepsy, this system remains an important candidate for carbamazepine's spectrum of clinical activity.

Opiate Mechanisms

In light of carbamazepine's effects in trigeminal neuralgia and its ability to enhance opiate-induced running activity in mice (34), we were interested in possible interactions of carbamazepine with opiate mechanisms. Utilizing an opiate-binding receptor assay, we observed no effect of carbamazepine on this measure of total opioid substances in CSF of 17 patients (65). We also found carbamazepine did not affect baseline or morphine-induced tail-flick or paw-lick (hotplate) latencies in the rat, either with acute or chronic treatment with carbamazepine for 10 days (79, A. Pert and S. R. B. Weiss, *unpublished data,* 1985). Thus, the mechanism of the carbamazepine-induced facilitation of opiate-induced running activity in mice, and any potential effect of carbamazepine on discrete opiate subsystems in brain, remain to be further elucidated.

Vasopressin

In contrast to lithium, which antagonizes the effects of vasopressin by inhibiting adenylate cyclase, carbamazepine appears to enhance the effects of vasopressin, perhaps acting as a direct vasopressin agonist (6). Gold et al. (21) reported that carbamazepine and lithium have opposite effects on the plasma vasopressin response to hypertonic saline. Lithium increases the plasma vasopressin response whereas carbamazepine diminishes it, possibly because of its vasopressin agonist-like effects. These differential effects of carbamazepine and lithium have direct implications for side effects and potential psychotropic effects. Carbamazepine remains an alternative agent which will not produce diabetes insipidus, although it will not reverse lithium-induced diabetes insipidus. However, carbamazepine has been associated with the induction of hyponatremia (27), particularly at high blood levels in older patients (31,36), and several instances of water intoxication have been reported (1).

It remains to be demonstrated whether the essentially opposite effects of lithium and carbamazepine on vasopressin function may relate to a differential profile of effects on cognitive functioning. Preliminary data suggest that carbamazepine, at least compared to other anticonvulsants, has a profile of less cognitive impairment both clinically in patients with seizure disorders (101) and in an animal model of reversal of ECS-induced amnesia in mice (48).

Substance P

Although this peptide has been reported to be altered in the CSF of affectively ill patients compared with controls (89), Kaiya et al. (30) and Berrettini et al. (5) have not confirmed these findings. Nonetheless, Jones et al. (29) have reported that chronic carbamazepine administration increases the sensitivity of neurons in the cingulate cortex of the rat to substance P. This effect is paralleled by chronic administration of a variety of other antidepressant modalities including desipramine, chlorimipramine, trimipramine, zimeldine, oxaprotiline, and tranylcypromine. However, chronic but not acute ECT decreases substance P sensitivity and the inactive (−) isomer of oxaprotiline has the same increased effect as the (+) isomer, indicating that there is not yet a close relationship between substance P changes and psychotropic effects. Mitsushio et al. (46) have also reported that chronic administration of carbamazepine increases levels of substance P-like immunoreactivity in rat brain.

Effects on Somatostatin

Rubinow et al. (91,93) found that carbamazepine significantly decreased somatostatin in the CSF of affectively ill patients. Decreases in brain somatostatin by carbamazepine have been reported in amygdala-kindled animals (22), although we were unable to show an effect on brain somatostatin in naive rats given carbamazepine in their diet for 12 days (109). Effects of carbamazepine could interact with an underlying perturbation of somatostatin mechanisms in either affective disorders or epilepsy. Rubinow et al. (91) reported that depressed patients showed decreases in CSF somatostatin with normalization upon recovery or the switch into mania. As summarized elsewhere (68), five other studies have reported related findings of decreases in CSF somatostatin in depression compared with other psychiatric patients or controls. Kato et al. (33) reported that a series of five amygdala-kindled seizures increased brain somatostatin for up to 2 months following last seizure. Moreover, inhibition of somatostatin function with cysteamine or injection of somatostain antibodies was associated with anticonvulsant effects in amygdala-kindled, lidocaine-kindled (23), and CRF-induced seizures (Weiss et al., 1985, *unpublished data*).

The relationship of carbamazepine's decreases in somatostatin in CSF of affectively ill patients, or in brains of kindled animals but not in normal animals, remains to be elucidated. Another anticonvulsant, valproic acid, did not share this effect of carbamazepine on brain somatostatin, even though it had a potent antikindling effect (22). It is also of interest that lithium does not produce decreases in CSF somatostatin parallel to that of carbamazepine (5,93), yet neuroleptics have been reported to decrease somatostatin in CSF (D. R. Rubinow et al., *personal communication*) and in rat brain (3). Since decreases in somatostatin have been consistently reported in brain and CSF of Alzheimer's patients, and depleting somatostatin in hippocampus has induced learning and memory defects (107), we would wonder whether carbamazepine might alter cognitive, affective, or seizure processes in part through effects on this neuropeptide system. Finally, since somatostatin is a major inhibitory neuromodulator of the hypothalamic-pituitary-adrenal axis, it is possible that carbamazepine's ability to decrease CSF somatostatin is related to the hypercortisolism observed during carbamazepine treatment, as described below.

Hypothalamic-Pituitary-Adrenal (HPA) Axis

Carbamazepine increases urinary excretion of free cortisol in normal volunteers (40) and in patients with affective illness (94). Moreover, it induces escape from dexamethasone suppression (83,92). Although it appears to decrease levels of dexamethasone (93), the finding of increases in urinary free cortisol excretion suggests that this pharmacokinetic effect of carbamazepine is not sufficient to explain the hypercortisolism. Although carbamazepine may be associated with an increased secretion of corticotropin (ACTH) in response to corticotropin-releasing factor (CRF) (P. W. Gold, M. A. Kling, et al. *unpublished data,* 1985), the mechanism of carbamazepine's influence on the HPA axis in general and cortisol metabolism in particular remains to be further delineated. Carbamazepine induces minimal basal elevations in prolactin without changes in growth hormone or gonadal steroids (26,63). Carbamazepine increases arginine-induced prolactin secretion without affecting those induced by TRH. These findings are opposite to those observed with lithium, where arginine-induced prolactin secretion is normal but that following thyrotropin-releasing hormone (TRH) is increased (26).

Hypothalamic-Pituitary-Thyroid (HPT) Axis

Like lithium carbonate, carbamazepine decreases circulating levels of 3,5,3'-triiodothyronine (T_3) and thyroxine (T_4). However, in contrast to lithium, which often induces substantial elevations in thyroid-stimulating hormone (TSH) and associated hypothyroidism that requires supplemental treatment with thyroid hormone, carbamazepine induces minimal changes in basal TSH levels and does not induce clinical hypothyroidism (90) (only two cases had been reported in the world literature up to 1984).

Whereas lithium enhances the TSH response to TRH, carbamazepine blunts this response (25,26,28). Joffe et al. (28) recently postulated that the ability of a series of agents to decrease thyroid function (lithium, carbamazepine, ECT) could paradoxically be related to their psychotropic properties in affectively ill patients.

SUMMARY AND CONCLUSIONS

Carbamazepine and lithium share a common clinical profile of acute and prophylactic effects in manic and depressive illness (63,72–74). However, these drugs may have a different clinical profile of effects in that carbamazepine appears to have better antimanic effects in those patients in whom lithium is less effective, i.e., those with more severe mania, more disphoric mania, and more rapid cycling illness (77,79). Carbamazepine also has clinically important effects in pain syndromes such as trigeminal neuralgia and in the treatment of a variety of seizure disorders (80), particularly those thought to be related to temporal lobe and limbic system dysfunction. Lithium and carbamazepine also have quite divergent side effects on many systems, including white count, the induction of diabetes insipidus (20), hypothyroidism (90), hyponatremia (28), or hypocalcemia (28). Although carbamazepine and lithium share their ability to decrease GABA turnover (at least in high doses) and inhibit adenylate cyclase stimulated by a variety of ligands, they show differing biochemical, neuroendocrine, and neuropeptide effects in almost every system that we have examined. Thus, just as lithium is a relatively "dirty" drug with a panoply of biochemical effects, none of which has been definitively linked to its therapeutic efficacy in manic-depressive illness, carbamazepine also affects a multiplicity of biological systems with no one system clearly being linked to its psychotropic profile.

However, several neurotransmitter-neuropeptide candidates appear closely associated with the anticonvulsant properties of carbamazepine. It is likely that noradrenergic mechanisms are involved in its anticonvulsant effects, possibly those involving α_2-noradrenergic mechanisms. P-type benzodiazepine mechanisms appear to be excellent candidates for carbamazepine's anticonvulsant effects in light of convergent biochemical and electrophysiological data. Convergent data also implicate stabilization of sodium channel fluxes in the anticonvulsant effects of carbamazepine. Among the peptides, somatostatin is the most likely candidate to be involved in carbamazepine's anticonvulsant actions, although the evidence for this is indirect and preliminary.

Since these mechanisms are the most likely candidates for carbamazepine's anticonvulsant effects, there is some likelihood that they might also be involved in its psychotropic properties. There is no converging evidence in this regard, except in the few patients studied, where carbamazepine decreased CSF levels of norepinephrine in manic patients, possibly consistent with its ability to decrease norepinephrine release in a variety of preparations and to decrease norepinephrine turnover. Since we have previously observed CSF norepinephrine to be elevated in manic patients, compared to other psychiatric populations and normal volunteer controls (61,68), there does appear to be some evidence of a preliminary pharmacological convergence with a putative biochemical alteration observed in the manic syndrome that carbamazepine has been used to treat.

Carbamazepine's lack of dopamine receptor blockade rules out this mechanism for its antimanic effects, but its dopaminergic profile is also associated with its lack of induction of tardive dyskinesia. Carbamazepine's ability to increase plasma tryptophan could be related to its effects on impulse disorders and aggression, if not to its profile of effects on affective illness. While speculative, this remains an easily testable proposition in light of the accessibility of plasma tryptophan measures in a variety of patient populations. GABA_B properties of carbamazepine would appear more closely associated with its antinociceptive effects in paroxysmal pain syndromes than with its anticonvulsant effects. The potent effects of carbamazepine on adenosine receptors are particularly intriguing, since they are unique to this agent among the anticonvulsants and could account for some of the diverse biochemical and clinical effects of carbamazepine. It is possible that carbamazepine's ability to act like caffeine in some respects (displacing binding of adenosine analogs and up-regulating adenosine receptors with chronic administration) could account for carbamazepine's ability to induce escape from dexamethasone suppression, as has been reported for caffeine (103).

Several biochemical effects of carbamazepine do not appear to be shared by other anticonvulsant agents. These include the ability to increase firing of the locus ceruleus, increase plasma tryptophan, displace adenosine receptor binding, act at P-type benzodiazepine receptors, and exert vasopressin-like effects. To the extent that psychotropic effects of carbamazepine eventually are shown to differ from those of other anticonvulsant agents, all of these systems would remain important candidates for this aspect of carbamazepine's clinical profile.

We have reviewed the electrophysiological effects of carbamazepine elsewhere (63,71,79,80). Suffice it to say that there is little direct evidence that the ability of carbamazepine to stabilize dysfunction in limbic system structures (an initial rationale for the use of carbamazepine in affectively ill patients) is, in fact, related to its clinical effects in manic and depressive illness. Nonetheless, we have used the ability of carbamazepine to inhibit a variety of seizure types, particularly amygdala-kindled seizures, to elucidate possible mechanisms of action of this drug. Moreover, we have recently discovered that carbamazepine not only appears to be differentially effective in different types of kindling paradigms, but is differentially effective as a function of the stage of kindling. For example, although carbamazepine is effective in inhibiting the development of amygdala kindling in cat and monkey (105), it is ineffective in blocking the development of amygdala kindling in the rat (80,110). At the same time, it is a highly effective anticonvulsant on completed amygdala-kindled seizures in the rat. Conversely, carbamazepine is highly effective in inhibiting the development of cocaine and lidocaine-kindled seizures in the rat but is not effective in suppressing these seizures once they are fully developed (S. R. B. Weiss and R. M. Post, *unpublished data*, 1986). Pinel (60) has previously demonstrated differential effectiveness of phenytoin and diazepam as a function of stage of kindling as well. He found that diazepam was effective on the development and completed kindled seizure phase, but was without effect on spontaneous seizures that occur late in kindling and as a result of the induction of multiple seizures. Conversely, phenytoin is a weak anticonvulsant for the early stages of kindling, whereas it is effective in blocking the late-occurring seizures of the spontaneous variety (60).

These data would appear to suggest an important principle that may be relevant not only for the treatment of epilepsy, but also for affective illness; that is, that the efficacy of pharmacological interventions such as carbamazepine may differ as a function of stage of evolution of the illness. There is preliminary evidence that this might be the case for affective illness where lithium appears useful in the early and intermediate stages of the illness, but is less effective in the late stages associated with rapid or continuous cycling. In these instances, carbamazepine and related anticonvulsants offer effective adjunctive or alternative treatment. It remains to be demonstrated whether carbamazepine would be equally effective early in the course of affective illness (67a).

Further clinical data are required in order to choose among the possibilities that lithium and carbamazepine responders (a) considerably overlap, (b) constitute substantially different subgroups, or (c) may vary as a function of course of illness. The answer to these questions will not only have considerable clinical import, but should help in the elucidation of which mechanisms of these agents are critically involved in their therapeutic actions in manic-depressive illness. Finally, it is hoped that by comparing and contrasting the biological effects of carbamazepine not only with lithium but with other "unimodal" treatments of mania and depression such as neuroleptics or tricyclic antidepressants, progress can be made in elucidating important biological disturbances underlying affective illness.

REFERENCES

1. Ashton, M. G., Ball, S. G., Thomas, T. H., and Lee, M. R. (1979): *Br. Med. J.*, 1:1134–1135.
2. Barker, J. L., Owen, D. G., and Segal, M. (1984): *Neurosci. Lett.* 47:313–318.
2a. Barros, H. M., Braz, S., and Leite, J. R. (1986): *Epilepsia*, 27:534–537.
2b. Barros, H. M., and Leite, J. R. (1986): *Eur. J. Pharmacol.*, 123:345–349.
3. Beal, M., and Martin, J. (1984): *Neurosci. Lett.*, 47:125–130.
4. Bernasconi, R. (1982): In: *Basic Mechanisms in the Action of Lithium* (Proceedings of a Symposium held at Schloss Ringberg, Bavaria, October 4–6, 1981), pp. 183–192. Excerpta Medica, Amsterdam.
5. Berrettini, W. H., Golden, L. R., Nurnberger, J. I., Jr., and Gershon, E. S. (1985): *J. Psychiatr. Res.*, 18:329–350.
6. Berrettini, W. H., Post, R. M., Worthington, E. K., and Casper, J. B. (1982): *Life Sci.*, 30:425–432.
7. Bertilsson, L. (1978): *Clin. Pharmacokinet.*, 3:128–143.
8. Chouinard, G., Young, S. N., and Annable, L. (1983): *Biol. Psychiatry*, 18:451–466.
8a. Consolo, S., Bianchi, S., and Ladinsky, H. (1976): *Neuropharmacology*, 15:653–657.
9. Crunelli, V., Bernasconi, S., and Samanin, R. (1979): *Psychopharmacology*, 66:79–85.
10. Crunelli, V., Cervo, L., and Samanin, R. (1981): In: *Neurotransmitters, Seizures, and Epilepsy*, edited by P. L. Morselli, K. G. Lloyd, W. Loscher, B. Meldrum, and E. H. Reynolds, pp. 195–202. Raven Press, New York.
11. DeLorenzo, R. J. (1983): In: *Status Epilepticus*, edited by A. V. Delgado-Escueta, C. G. Wasterlain, D. M. Treimean, and R. J. Porter, pp. 325–338. Raven Press, New York.

12. Dose, M., and Emrich, H. M. (1985): Abstract, IVth World Congress of Biological Psychiatry, Sept. 8–13, 1985, Philadelphia, p. 442, No. 612.8.

13. Dubovsky, S. L., and Franks, R. D. (1983): *Biol. Psychiatry,* 18: 781–797.

14. Elhwuegi, A. (1978): *Br. J. Pharmacol.,* 64:407P.

15. Emrich, H. M., Dose, M., and von Zerssen, D. (1985): *J. Affective Disord.,* 8:243–250.

16. Ferrendelli, J. A., Gross, R. A., Kinscherf, D. A., and Rubin, E. H. (1979): In: *Neuropharmacology of Cyclic Nucleotides,* edited by G. Palmer, pp. 211–227. Urban & Schwarzenberg, Baltimore.

17. Ferrendelli, J. A., and Kinscherf, D. A. (1977): *Epilepsia,* 18: 525–531.

18. Ferrendelli, J. A., and Kinscherf, D. A. (1979): *Ann. Neurol.,* 5: 533–538.

19. Freyhan, F. A. (1945): *Arch. Neurol. Psychiatry,* 53:370–374.

20. Gold, P. W., Ballenger, J. C., Robertson, G. L., Weingartner, H., Rubinow, D. R., Hoban, M. C., Goodwin, F. K., and Post, R. M. (1984): In: *Neurobiology of Mood Disorders,* edited by R. M. Post and J. C. Ballenger, pp. 323–339. Williams & Wilkins, Baltimore.

21. Gold, P. W., Robertson, G. L., Ballenger, J. C., Kaye, W., Chen, J., Rubinow, D. R., Goodwin, F. K., and Post, R. M. (1983): *J. Clin. Endocrinol. Metab.,* 57:952–957.

22. Higuchi, T., Kato, N., Noguchi, T., Friesen, H. G., and Wada, J. A. (1986): In: *Kindling III,* edited by J. A. Wada, pp. 375–392. Raven Press, New York.

23. Higuchi, T., Sikand, G. S., Kato, M., Wada, J. A., and Friesen, H. G. (1983): *Brain Res.,* 288:359–362.

24. Inoue, H., Hazama, H., Hamazoe, K., Ichikawa, M., Omura, F., Fukuma, E., Inoue, K., and Umezawa, Y. (1984): *Folia Psychiatr. Neurol. Jpn.,* 38:425–436.

25. Joffe, R. T., Gold, P. W., Uhde, T. W., and Post, R. M. (1984): *Psychiatry Res.,* 12:161–166.

26. Joffe, R. T., Post, R. M., Ballenger, J. C., Rebar, R., and Gold, P. W. (1986): *Epilepsia,* 27:156–160.

27. Joffe, R. T., Post, R. M., and Uhde, T. W. (1986): *Psychol. Med.,* 16:331–335.

28. Joffe, R. T., Roy-Byrne, P. P., Uhde, T. W., and Post, R. M. (1984): *Biol. Psychiatry,* 19:1685–1691.

29. Jones, R. S., Mondadori, C., and Olpe, H. R. (1985): *Neuropharmacology,* 24:627–633.

30. Kaiya, H., Tamura, Y., Adachi, S., Moriuchi, I., Namba, M., Tanaka, M., Yoshida, H., Yanaihara, N., and Yanaihara, C. (1981): *Psychiatr. Res.,* 5:11–21.

31. Kalff, R., Houtkooper, M., Meyer, J., Geodhart, D., Augusteijn, R., and Meinardi, H. (1984): *Epilepsia,* 25:390–397.

32. Kalinowsky, L., and Putnam, T. (1943): *Arch. Neurol. Psychiatry,* 49:414–423.

33. Kato, N., Higuchi, T., Friesen, H. G., and Wada, J. A. (1983): *Life Sci.,* 32:2415–2422.

34. Katz, R. J., and Schmaltz, K. (1979): *Psychopharmacology,* 65: 65–68.

34a. Kawalik, S., Levitt, M., Barkai, A. (1984): *Psychopharmacology,* 83:169–171.

34b. Keneko, S., Kurahashi, K., Mori, A., Hill, R. G., and Taberner, P. V. (1981): *Exerpta Medica,* 548:318–319.

35. Kubanek, J. L., and Rowell, R. C. (1946): *Dis. Nerv. Syst.,* 7: 47–50.

36. Lahr, M. B. (1985): *Clin. Pharmacol. Ther.,* 37:693–696.

37. Lerer, B., Moore, N., Meyendorff, E., Cho, S. R., and Gershon, S. (1985): Abstract IVth World Congress of Biological Psychiatry, Sept. 8–13, 1985, Philadelphia, p. 120, No. 204.4.

38. Lewin, E., and Bleck, V. (1977): *Epilepsia,* 18:237–242.

39. Lloyd, K. G., Thuret, E. W., and Pilc, A. (1986): In: *GABA and Mood Disorders: Experimental and Clinical Research, L.E.R.S. Monograph Series,* edited by G. Bartholini, K. G. Lloyd, and P. L. Morselli, pp. 33–42. Raven Press, New York.

40. London, D. R. (1980): In: *Advances in Epileptology, XI Epilepsy International Symposium,* edited by R. Carger, F. Angeleri, and J. K. Penry, pp. 399–405. Raven Press, New York.

41. Lust, W. D., Kupferberg, J. H., Yonekawa, W. D., Penry, J. K., Passonneau, J. V., and Wheaton, A. B. (1978): *Mol. Pharmacol.,* 14:347–356.

42. MacDonald, R. L., McLean, M. J., and Skerritt, J. H. (1985): *Fed. Proc.,* 44:2634–2639.

43. Maitre, L., Baltzer, V., Mondadori, C., Olpe, H. R., Baumann, P. A., and Waldmeier, P. C. (1984): In: *Anticonvulsants in Affective Disorders,* edited by H. M. Emrich, T. Okuma, and A. Muller, pp. 3–13. Excerpta Medica, Amsterdam.

44. Marangos, P. J., Post, R. M., Patel, J., Zander, K., Parma, A., and Weiss, S. (1983): *Eur. J. Pharmacol.,* 93:175–182.

45. Marangos, P. J., Weiss, S. R. B., Montgomery, P., Patel, J., Narang, P. K., Cappabianca, A. M., and Post, R. M. (1985): *Epilepsia,* 26:493–498.

46. Mitsushio, H., Takashima, M., and Toru, M. (1984): Proc. 14th C.I.N.P. Congress, Abstract F-4.

47. Mizoule, J., Gauthier, A., Uzan, A., Renault, C., Dubroeucq, M. C., Gueremy, C., and Le Fur, G. (1985): *Life Sci.,* 36:1059–1068.

48. Mondadori, C., and Classen, W. (1984): *Acta Neurol. Scand.,* 99: 125–129.

49. Morselli, P. L., Baruzzi, A., Gerna, M., Bossi, L., and Porta, M. (1977): *Br. J. Clin. Pharmacol.,* 4:535–540.

50. Morselli, P. L., Calderini, G., Consolazione, A., Riva, E., and Altamura, C. (1977): In: *Advances in Epileptology,* edited by H. Meinardi and A. J. Rowan, pp. 176–182. Swets & Zeitlinger BV, Amsterdam.

51. Myllyla, V. V. (1976): *Eur. Neurol.,* 14:97–107.

52. Naylor, G. (1985): *J. Affective Disord.,* 8:91–93.

53. Nistico, G. (1977): *Int. J. Clin. Pharmacol. Biopharm.,* 15:19–22.

54. Olpe, H.-R., Baudry, M., and Jones, R. S. G. (1985): *Eur. J. Pharmacol.,* 110:71–80.

55. Olpe, H., and Jones, R. (1983): *Eur. J. Pharmacol.,* 91:107–110.

56. Palmer, G. C., Jones, D. J., Medine, M. A., and Stavinoha, W. B. (1979): *Epilepsia,* 20:95–104.

57. Palmer, G. C., Palmer, S. J., and Legendre, J. L. (1981): *Exp. Neurol.,* 71:601–614.

58. Phillis, J. W. (1984): *Epilepsia,* 25:765–772.

59. Pinel, J. P. J. (1981): *Exp. Neurol.,* 72:559–569.

60. Post, R. M. (1986): In: *The Limbic System: Functional Organization and Clinical Disorders,* edited by B. K. Doane and K. E. Livingston, pp. 229–249. Raven Press, New York.

61. Post, R. M., Ballenger, J. C., Reus, V. I., Lake, C. R., Lerner, P., and Bunney, W. E., Jr. (1978): *APA New Research Abstracts,* No. 7.

62. Post, R. M., Ballenger, J. C., Uhde, T. W., and Bunney, W. E., Jr. (1984): In: *Neurobiology of Mood Disorders,* edited by R. M. Post and J. C. Ballenger, pp. 777–816. Williams & Wilkins, Baltimore.

63. Post, R. M., Ballenger, J. C., Uhde, T. W., Smith, C., Rubinow, D. R., and Bunney, W. E., Jr. (1982): *Biol. Psychiatry,* 17:1037–1045.

64. Post, R. M., Berrettini, W., Uhde, T. W., and Kellner, C. (1984): *J. Clin. Psychopharmacol.,* 4:178–185.

65. Post, R. M., Pickar, D., Naber, D., Ballenger, J. C., Uhde, T. W., and Bunney, W. E., Jr. (1981): *Psychiatry Res.,* 5:59–66.

66. Post, R. M., Putnam, F. W., Contel, N. R., and Goldman, B. (1984): *Epilepsia,* 25:234–239.

67. Post, R. M., Putnam, F., Uhde, T. W., and Weiss, S. R. B. (1986): In: *Electroconvulsive Therapy: Clinical and Basic Research Issues. Annals of the N.Y. Academy of Sciences,* edited by S. Malitz and H. A. Sacheim, pp. 376–388. New York Academy of Sciences, New York.

67a. Post, R. M., Rubinow, D. R., and Ballenger, J. C. (1986): *Br. J. Psychiatry,* 149:191–201.

68. Post, R. M., Rubinow, D. R., and Gold, P. W. (1987): In: *Neuropeptides in Psychiatric and Neurological Disease,* edited by C. B. Nemeroff. Johns Hopkins University Press, Baltimore (in press).

69. Post, R. M., Rubinow, D. R., Uhde, T. W., Ballenger, J. C., Lake, C. R., Linnoila, M., and Reus, V. (1985): *Psychopharmacology,* 87:59–63.

70. Post, R. M., Rubinow, D. R., Uhde, T. W., Ballenger, J. C., and Linnoila, M. (1985): *Arch. Gen. Psychiatry,* 43:392–396.

71. Post, R. M., and Uhde, T. W. (1983): *Epilepsia,* 24:S97–S108.

72. Post, R. M., and Uhde, T. W. (1985): *Psychiatr. J. Univ. Ottawa,* 10:205–219.

73. Post, R. M., and Uhde, T. W. (1986): In: *Aspects of Epilepsy and Psychiatry,* edited by M. R. Trimble and T. G. Bolwig, pp. 177–212. John Wiley & Sons, New York.

74. Post, R. M., Uhde, T. W., Joffe, R. T., Roy-Byrne, P. P., and Kellner, C. (1985): In: *The Psychopharmacology of Epilepsy,* edited by M. R. Trimble, pp. 141–171. John Wiley & Sons, Chichester, England.

75. Post, R. M., Uhde, T. W., Roy-Byrne, P. P., and Joffe, R. T. (1986): *Am. J. Psychiatry,* 143:29–34.

76. Post, R. M., Uhde, T. W., Rubinow, D. R., Gold, P. W., and Joffe, R. T. (1985): Abstract IVth World Congress of Biological Psychiatry, Sept. 8–13, 1985, Philadelphia, p. 364, No. 506.5.

77. Post, R. M., Uhde, T. W., Roy-Byrne, P. P., and Joffe, R. T. (1987): *Psychiatric Res. (in press).*

78. Post, R. M., Uhde, T. W., Rubinow, D. R., Joffe, R. T., Roy-Byrne, P. P., and Weiss, S. R. B. (1986): In: *GABA and Mood Disorders, L.E.R.S.,* Vol. 4, edited by G. Bartholini et al., pp. 201–214. Raven Press, New York.

79. Post, R. M., Uhde, T. W., Rubinow, D. R., and Weiss, S. R. B. (1987): In: *Mania: New Research and Treatment,* edited by A. Swan. APA Press, Washington, DC (*in press*).

80. Post, R. M., Weiss, S. R. B., and Pert, A. (1984): *Prog. Neuropsychopharmacol. Biol. Psychiatry,* 8:425–434.

81. Pratt, J. A., Jenner, P., Johnson, A. L., Shorvon, S. D., and Reynolds, E. H. (1984): *J. Neurol. Neurosurg. Psychiatry,* 47:1131–1133.

82. Pratt, J. A., Jenner, P., and Marsden, C. D. (1985): *Neuropharmacology,* 24:59–68.

83. Privitera, M. R., Greden, J. F., Gardner, R. W., Ritchie, J. C., and Carroll, B. J. (1982): *Biol. Psychiatry,* 17:611–620.

84. Purdy, R. E., Julien, R. M., Fairhurst, A. S., and Terry, M. D. (1977): *Epilepsia,* 18:251–257.

85. Quattrone, A., Annunziato, L., Aguglia, K., and Preziosi, P. (1981): *Arch. Int. Pharmacodyn. Ther.,* 252:180–185.

86. Quattrone, A., Crunelli, V., and Samanin, R. (1978): *Neuropharmacology,* 17:643–647.

87. Quattrone, A., and Samanin, R. (1977): *Eur. J. Pharmacol.,* 41:333–336.

88. Reynolds, E. H. (1975): In: *Complex Partial Seizures and Their Treatment. Advances in Neurology, Vol. 11,* edited by J. K. Penry and D. D. Daly, pp. 345–353. Raven Press, New York.

89. Rimon, R., Le Greves, P., Nyberg, F., Heikkila, L., Salmela, L., and Terenius, L. (1984): *Biol. Psychiatry,* 19:509–516.

90. Roy-Byrne, P. P., Joffe, R. T., Uhde, T. W., and Post, R. M. (1984): *Arch. Gen. Psychiatry,* 41:1150–1153.

91. Rubinow, D. R., Gold, P. W., Post, R. M., Ballenger, J. C., and Cowdry, R. (1984): In: *Neurobiology of Mood Disorders,* edited by R. M. Post and J. C. Ballenger, pp. 369–387. Williams & Wilkins, Baltimore.

92. Rubinow, D. R., Post, R. M., Gold, P. W., Ballenger, J. C., and Reichlin, S. (1985): *Psychopharmacology,* 85:210–213.

93. Rubinow, D. R., Post, R. M., Gold, P. W., and Uhde, T. W. (1984): *Psychopharmacol. Bull.,* 20:590–594.

94. Rubinow, D. R., Post, R. M., Gold, P. W., and Uhde, T. W. (1986): *Psychopharmacology,* 88:115–118.

95. Schauf, C. L., Davis, F. A., and Marder, J. (1974): *J. Pharmacol. Exp. Ther.,* 189:538–543.

96. Skerritt, J. H., Davies, L. P., and Johnston, G. A. R. (1982): *Eur. J. Pharmacol.,* 82:195–197.

97. Skerritt, J. H., Davies, L. P., and Johnston, G. A. R. (1983): *Epilepsia,* 24:634–642.

98. Skerritt, J. H., and Johnston, G. A. R. (1983): *Clin. Exp. Pharmacol. Physiol.,* 10:527–533.

99. Skerritt, J., Johnston, G., and Chow, S. (1983): *Epilepsia,* 24:643–650.

100. Terrence, C. F., Sax, M., Fromm, G. H., Chang, C.-H., and Yoo, C. S. (1983): *Pharmacology,* 27:85–94.

101. Thompson, P., Huppert, F., and Trimble, M. (1980): *Acta Neurol. Scand.,* 62:75–81.

102. Tomson, T., and Bertilsson, L. (1984): *Arch. Neurol.,* 41:598–601.

103. Uhde, T. W., Bierer, L. M., and Post, R. M. (1985): *Arch. Gen. Psychiatry,* 42:737–738.

104. Vogler, J., and Zieglgansberger, W. (1985): Abstracts, IVth World Congress of Biological Psychiatry, Philadelphia, Sept. 8–13, 1985, p. 441, No. 612.5.

105. Wada, J. A. (1977): *Arch. Neurol.,* 34:389–395.

106. Waldmeier, P. C., Baumann, P. A., Fehr, B., De Herdt, P., and Maitre, L. (1984): *J. Pharmacol. Exp. Ther.,* 231:166–172.

107. Walsh, T. J., Emerich, D. F., Winocur, A., Banki, C., Bissette, G., and Nemeroff, C. B. (1985): Abstracts, Society for Neuroscience, 15th Annual Meeting, Dallas, Oct. 20–25, 1985, p. 621, No. 182.7.

108. Weir, R. L., Padgett, W., Daly, J. W., and Anderson, S. H. (1984): *Epilepsia,* 25:492–498.

109. Weiss, S. R. B., Nguyen, T., Rubinow, D. R., Helke, C. J., Narang, P. K., Post, R. M., and Jacobowitz, D. M. (1987): *J. Neural. Trans. M. (in press).*

110. Weiss, S. R. B., and Post, R. M. (1987): *Clin. Neuropharmacol. (in press).*

111. Weiss, S. R. B., Post, P. M., Marangos, P. J., and Patel, J. (1986): In: *Kindling III,* edited by J. Wada, pp. 375–392. Raven Press, New York.

112. Weiss, S. R. B., Post, R. M., Marangos, P. J., and Patel, J. (1985): *Neuropharmacology,* 24:635–638.

113. Weiss, S. R. B., Post, R. M., Patel, J., and Marangos, P. S. (1985): *Life Sci.* 36:2413–2419.

114. Willow, M., and Catterall, W. A. (1982): *Mol. Pharmacol.,* 22:627–635.

115. Willow, M., Kuenzel, E. A., and Catterall, W. A. (1984): *Mol. Pharmacol.,* 25:228–234.

116. Winkel, R., and Lux, H. D. (1985): Abstracts, IVth World Congress of Biol. Psychiatry. Philadelphia, Sept. 8–13, 1985, p. 441, #612.6.

117. Zohar, J., Ebstein, R. P., and Belmaker, R. H. (1982): In: *Basic Mechanisms in the Action of Lithium,* edited by H. M. Emrich, J. B. Aldenhoff, and H. D. Lux, pp. 154–166. Excerpta Medica, Amsterdam.

Psychopharmacology:
The Third Generation of Progress,
edited by Herbert Y. Meltzer.
Raven Press, New York © 1987.

CHAPTER **58**

Neurochemical and Other Neurobiological Consequences of ECT: Implications for the Pathogenesis and Treatment of Affective Disorders

Bernard Lerer

The past decade has witnessed an impressive resurgence of scientific interest in electroconvulsive therapy (ECT). A series of impeccably controlled clinical trials has definitively established the antidepressant efficacy of the treatment and has defined the induced seizure as its major therapeutic element (e.g., 14,46). ECT techniques have been considerably refined, with issues such as electrode placement, stimulus waveform, and dosage subjected to rigorous scrutiny (e.g., 86,135). The characteristics, severity, and persistence of ECT-induced memory impairment have been carefully defined (e.g., 123), and technical as well as pharmacological methods of prevention and treatment have been explored (e.g., 76,135). Studies on the mechanism of action of ECT are, however, the most relevant to the biology of affective disorders and are therefore the primary focus of this chapter.

CLINICAL CONSIDERATIONS CRITICAL TO ECT MECHANISMS

A review of the basic mechanisms of ECT must take into account clinical attributes of the treatment that are critical to an effective integration of relevant research findings. The most important considerations are the following:

1. The central therapeutic role of the induced seizure. This is strongly supported by Ottoson's (102) pioneering studies showing a reduction in therapeutic efficacy by chemical attenuation of the induced seizure and by the superior antidepressant efficacy of "real" ECT as compared to that of simulated treatment (e.g., 14,46). The fact that seizures induced by nonelectrical means (e.g., fluorythyl) are therapeutically effective (36) further strengthens the original contention of Cerletti and Bini (17) that "the electricity itself is of little importance . . . the important and fundamental factor is the epileptic-like seizure no matter how it is obtained."

2. The clinical spectrum of ECT. This is substantially different from that of the chemical antidepressants. In addition to its antidepressant action, ECT is also effective in the acute treatment of mania (121), in some cases of schizophrenia (36), and in the prevention of affective recurrences (57). In this respect ECT more closely resembles lithium than it does the tricyclic antidepressants (72). A further important difference is the specific therapeutic efficacy of ECT in psychotic depression, a syndrome that does not respond to tricyclic antidepressants without neu-

roleptic supplementation (106). Parallels between the basic mechanisms of ECT and those of chemical antidepressants should therefore not be too rigorously demanded.

3. Clinical factors related to the technique of ECT administration. Some important correlates should be considered. For example, unilateral ECT is effective in a significant number of depressed patients (135). In the treatment of mania, however, bilateral treatment may be specifically indicated (121). The optimum frequency of ECT administration and the number of treatments required in order to achieve remission are further considerations. Clinical experience and research findings suggest that alterations in brain function induced by ECT evolve over a period of time and are not accelerated by increasing the frequency of treatment administration (70). Animal models that parallel the clinical context are therefore of considerable importance.

MAJOR THEORIES OF ECT ACTION

Psychological Theories

Historically, these theories have focused either on psychodynamic explanations or on a putative link between the amnestic effects of ECT and its therapeutic action (91). Psychodynamic theories tended to be strongly linked to punitive or regression-inducing aspects, lost considerable ground with the introduction of anesthetic and muscle relaxant-modified ECT (15), and were further weakened by the demonstration of superior efficacy for "real" versus simulated treatments (e.g., 14,46). With regard to amnestic effects, no correlation between the degree of ECT-induced memory impairment and therapeutic efficacy has been demonstrated. Furthermore, technical advances such as unilateral electrode placement and the use of pulsed stimuli have considerably reduced amnestic but not therapeutic effects (135).

Neurophysiological Theories

The physiological sequelae of grand mal seizures are numerous, as might be expected of so major a neurometabolic event. It is therefore not surprising that a significant body of data has accumulated regarding ECT effects on neurophysiological parameters such as the permeability of the blood-brain barrier, regional cerebral blood flow, and brain electrical activity (see 75). These studies have, however, not yet yielded comprehensive theoretical formulations. A recent research direction provides an intriguing new approach (114). Threshold for seizure induction is known to increase during a series of ECT administrations. It has been suggested that this anticonvulsant property of ECT may be correlated with its antidepressant efficacy and that suppression of neurometabolic activity may underlie both effects (114). Alterations in regional cerebral blood flow during ECT support this hypothesis (109), and recent advances in brain imaging techniques should yield further information. The precise relationship between seizure threshold increases and therapeutic response remains, however, to be definitively established.

Neuroendocrine Theories

Affective illness, particularly depression, is associated with significant vegetative symptoms, most of which are hypothalamically mediated and reversed by ECT (36). It has therefore been suggested that ECT may act via a direct effect on the hypothalamus, possibly by the release of specific hypothalamic peptides (37). ECT induces a significant increase in prolactin levels immediately following the seizure (137). Corticotropin (3) and neurophysin (137) levels are also acutely increased by ECT, whereas other pituitary hormones such as growth hormone (GH) and thyroid-stimulating hormone (TSH) are not affected (137). These effects are acutely related to the seizure, and longer-term alterations in basal hormone levels have not been demonstrated. Studies on the interrelationship between clinical response to ECT and the dexamethasone suppression test are another important line of investigation. Although reversal of this state marker is usually observed, correlations with clinical response and implications for subsequent relapse remain controversial (26). Thus, although ECT is clearly associated with hypothalamic-pituitary activation, it is still unclear whether this is a primary therapeutic mechanism or merely a correlate of clinical response.

Neurochemical Theories

The major emphasis of most recent research on ECT mechanisms has been on the effects of the treatment on the regulation and function of brain neurotransmitters and their pre- and postsynaptic receptor sites (see 19,38,68,75). These findings have been primarily derived from studies in rodents. In this review, preclinical observations will be integrated with available evidence from neuroendocrine challenge studies and other clinically applicable strategies (71). Interactions between the different neurotransmitters and neuromodulators affected by ECT will be emphasized and implications for mechanism of action will be considered.

Effects of ECS and ECT on the major monoamines in rodents and humans are summarized in Tables 1 and 2.

NEUROTRANSMITTER SYSTEMS AFFECTED BY ECT

Serotonin

Presynaptic Effects

Although a single electroconvulsive shock (ECS) tends to increase serotonin levels in rat brain (32), most studies suggest no significant effect of chronic administration (38,68). Potassium-evoked serotonin release from rat cortical synaptosomes is also unchanged by repeated ECS (92). One study of serotonin uptake reported decreased maximal velocity (V_{max}) after both single and chronic ECS (92), whereas another (60) found no significant change in this parameter. [^{3}H]Imipramine binding, a putative marker for the serotonin uptake site, is also inconsistently affected (60,65).

In patients treated with ECT, cerebrospinal fluid (CSF) levels of 5-hydroxyindoleacetic acid (5-HIAA) are variably

TABLE 1. *Effects of chronic ECS on the major monoamine neurotransmitters: rodent studies[a]*

	Norepinephrine	Serotonin	Dopamine	Refs.[b]
Presynaptic effects				
Turnover	↑	0 ↑	0	34, 68, 93
Uptake	↓↑[c]	↓ 0[d]	—	60, 92
Release	0 ↑	0	—	31, 92
Receptor effects				
Presynaptic				
Behavioral	↓ (α_2)	—	↓	48, 107, 117
Electrophysiological	—	—	↓	21
Binding	↓ (α_2)[e]	—	—	107
Postsynaptic				
Behavioral	↑ (α_2)	↑ (5-HT$_2$)	↑	38, 93, 133
Electrophysiological	0 (β)	↑	—	17, 20
Binding	0 ↑ (α_1)[f]	0 (5-HT$_1$)	0 (D$_2$)	13, 131
	↓ (β)	↑ (5-HT$_2$)		59, 103, 132
2nd Messengers				
Cyclic AMP	↓↑[g]	—	0 ↑[h]	38, 48, 134
Polyphosphoinositide (PPI)	—	—	—	

[a] ↑, Increased; ↓, decreased; ↑↓, increases and decreases reported; 0, no change; —, no studies or not applicable.

[b] Representative references given; for full citations see text.

[c] V_{max} and K_m both reduced. Different interpretations of net effect on uptake possible.

[d] [^{3}H]Imipramine binding reported as decreased (65) or unchanged (60).

[e] [^{3}H]Clonidine binding labels both pre- and postsynaptic α_2-receptors.

[f] [^{3}H]WB1011 and [^{3}H]DHE binding unchanged (13), α_1-specific [^{3}H]prazosin binding increased (131).

[g] Decreased in whole-cell preparations (99,134), increased in membrane preparations (89,99).

[h] No change in DA-sensitive cyclic AMP accumulation (38); enhanced behavioral response to dibutyryl cyclic AMP in nucleus accumbens (48).

TABLE 2. *Effect of chronic ECT on the major monoamine neurotransmitters: human studies[a]*

	Norepinephrine	Serotonin	Dopamine	Refs.[b]
Plasma	NE ↓	—	HVA 0	24, 80
	MHPG 0			80
Urine	NE ↓	5-HIAA ↓	HVA 0	78, 79, 81
	Normetanephrine ↓			79
CSF[c]	MHPG 0 ↓	5-HIAA ↓↑ 0	HVA 0 ↑	50, 68
Receptors	Platelet α_2 ↓ 0	Platelet imipramine ↓ 0	—	24, 64, 122
	Lymphocyte β_2 0			24
Neuroendocrine	GH/clonidine 0	PRL/TRH ↑	PRL/APO 0 ↑	120
				23, 25
				27
			GH/APO 0 ↑[d]	8, 23
			PRL/metham 0	120
Other	Sedation/clonidine 0	—	Activation/Metham 0	120

[a] PRL, Prolactin; APO, apomorphine; Metham, methamphetamine. Other abbreviations explained in text. Symbols as in Table 1.

[b] Representative references given; for full citations see text.

[c] Includes studies with and without probenecid loading.

[d] Degree of reduction in GH levels by apomorphine.

altered (see 50,68), whereas a reduction in urinary 5-HIAA output has been reported (81). Effects on platelet [³H]imipramine binding sites are similarly inconsistent (64). Overall, ECT does not appear to alter presynaptic serotonin availability to an extent consistent with its postsynaptic effects in this system.

Receptor Effects

Enhancement of behavioral and functional responsiveness to a variety of serotonergic agents has been consistently reported after repeated ECS, including alternate day treatments (see 38,68). These effects require intact serotonergic transmission and are blocked by serotonin synthesis inhibition or receptor blockade prior to each ECS (41). Chemically induced convulsions result in a similar increase in serotonin-mediated behavior, which is not present after chronic subconvulsive shocks (43,101).

Electrophysiological studies of serotonin receptor responsiveness have also shown increased sensitivity after chronic ECS (30). This finding, demonstrated by iontophoretic application of serotonin agonists to hippocampal pyramidal neurons, is common to ECS and a series of antidepressant agents. The ECS effect was demonstrable after three times weekly ECS for 2 weeks and was not present in rats administered subconvulsive shocks.

An important influence of cortical noradrenergic innervation on the ECS-induced enhancement of serotonin-mediated behavior has been demonstrated. Green and Deakin (42) showed that lesioning of ascending noradrenergic pathways abolished the ECS-induced enhancement of serotonergic responses. This enhancement was also abolished by pretreatment with the norepinephrine (NE) synthesis inhibitor α-methylparatyrosine (AMPT) (41).

It is noteworthy that chronic administration of GABA agonists such as progabide and baclofen enhances serotonergically mediated behavior in a similar fashion to ECS (44,90). Baclofen is a relatively pure γ-aminobutyric acid-B (GABA$_B$) agonist, indicating the specific involvement of this GABA receptor subtype. Although progabide has putative antidepressant properties, enhanced serotonin-mediated responses have also been demonstrable after agents such as diazepam, which lack antidepressant effects, but not after carbamazepine, which does have mood-stabilizing properties (44,90).

Radioligand binding ([³H]serotonin) to receptors of the 5-hydroxytryptamine-1 (5-HT$_1$) subtype is not altered by repeated ECS (e.g., 6,13). However, up-regulation of cortical 5-HT$_2$ receptors (labeled by [³H]spiperone) is a consistent finding (59,132). There is strong evidence that the behavioral serotonergic responses that are enhanced by ECS are mediated via serotonin receptors of the 5-HT$_2$ subtype (103,132). As in the case of the behavioral responses, the ECS-induced increase in 5-HT$_2$ receptor number is dependent on intact serotonergic and noradrenergic innervation and is blocked by concurrent inhibition of NE and serotonin synthesis and by lesioning of ascending serotonergic pathways (39,60). 5-HT$_2$ receptor number is also increased by GABAergic agents, which, as described above, enhance behavioral serotonergic responses mediated via the 5-HT$_2$ receptor subtype (90).

Neuroendocrine Studies

There are few human studies directly referable to ECT effects on brain serotonin function. Coppen et al. (25) demonstrated that the prolactin response to thyrotropin-releasing hormone (TRH), which is thought to be serotonergically mediated, was enhanced following a series of ECT. Enhanced prolactin responses to intravenous L-tryptophan challenge have been demonstrated following chronic tricyclic antidepressant (TCA) administration (18), but results following ECT are not yet available.

Discussion

With regard to functional serotonergic responsiveness, ECS effects parallel those reported for a series of antidepressant agents, including compounds such as desmethylimipramine that do not block serotonin uptake. For antidepressants, however, this finding is dependent on withdrawal of the antidepressant agent and a time lapse of 18 to 24 hr before testing. Recent reports suggest that when animals are tested while still on antidepressant treatment, serotonergically mediated behaviors are attenuated rather than enhanced (39). This latter finding is consistent with the observation that cortical [³H]spiperone-labeled 5-HT$_2$ receptor number is reduced following antidepressant treatment (39). It therefore appears that ECT and antidepressant effects on serotonergic neurotransmission may be diametrically opposite. Electrophysiological studies do indicate enhanced serotonergic responsiveness following both ECS and antidepressants (30). However, in the case of antidepressants these studies were conducted following treatment withdrawal, and it remains to be demonstrated whether the finding exists in animals studied while receiving antidepressants.

The indoleamine hypothesis of affective disorder postulates a reduction in the central availability of serotonin (95). Central serotonergic responsiveness is enhanced by ECT, which implies a reversal of this pathological state. The potentially attractive conclusion that increased serotonergic function is an effect common to both ECT and antidepressant administration is, however, not supported by available data. Differences in the clinical spectrum of the two treatments may be of importance in explaining this discrepancy if it is not resolved on the preclinical level.

Norepinephrine

Presynaptic Effects

Most reported studies indicate that repeated ECS administration increases the synthesis and utilization of NE in rodent brain (e.g., 61,93). The activity of tyrosine hydroxylase, the rate-limiting enzyme in catecholamine biosynthesis, is also enhanced (96). Studies with synaptosomal preparations suggest that both the affinity constant (K_m) and V_{max} of NE uptake are increased by alternate-day ECS for 10 days (92). This finding may be interpreted as indicating reduced uptake (because of the decreased affinity) or the opposite (in view of the V_{max} change). However, studies with an *in vivo* model of NE uptake support a reduction following repeated ECS (93). Potassium-evoked release of NE from synaptosomal preparations has been reported as increased (31) or unchanged (92) following repeated ECS. The discrepant findings may be due to differing calcium concentrations used in the medium, increased release being demonstrable in the presence of low levels of the ion (31).

Early studies in humans reported an immediate increment in plasma NE and epinephrine concentrations after ECT (36). These findings were probably due to sympathetic nervous system activation in response to the seizure. Linnoila et al. (80) recently showed no significant increment in plasma free 3-methoxy-4-hydroxyphenylglycol (MHPG) immediately following the seizure. A further study that examined urinary NE, normetanephrine, and vanillyl mandelic acid (VMA) output following 12 ECTs showed a significant reduction in the first two parameters and a trend toward reduced whole-body NE turnover (79). A reduction in plasma NE levels during a course of ECT has been reported by Cooper et al. (24), who found that high baseline levels fell in parallel with clinical recovery. One study reported a reduction in CSF MHPG levels after a series of ECT, but others found this parameter unchanged (68). Interpretation of these findings in terms of the effects of ECS on central NE turnover is complex. They do, however, support the role of plasma NE levels as a state marker for depression and an index of treatment response.

The net effect of repeated ECS on NE would, however, appear to be one of increased synaptic availability of the neurotransmitter, an effect consistent with the receptor effects discussed below.

Receptor Effects

β-Adrenoceptors. One of the most consistently replicable effects of repeated ECS in rodents is a reduction in β-adrenoceptor number in the cortex following chronic treatment (e.g., 13,103). This finding has been reported after spaced ECS (three times weekly for 4 weeks) (66) and is persistent for up to 7 days following the last treatment (58). Reduced responsiveness to NE of the β-adrenoceptor-linked cyclic AMP generating system has been demonstrated in parallel (134). β-Adrenoceptor down-regulation is common to ECS and a variety of antidepressant agents of different classes (134).

An important influence of serotonergic innervation on β-adrenoceptor down-regulation by antidepressant treatment has recently been demonstrated. Lesioning of ascending serotonergic pathways has been shown by a number of groups to prevent the β-adrenoceptor down-regulating effect of both TCAs (16,55) and ECS (39). Stockmeier et al. (125) have shown recently that specific lesioning of the raphe nuclei or of serotonin axons induces highly significant increases in cortical β-adrenoceptor number and NE-sensitive cyclic AMP responses, an effect not observed by the other groups. These findings suggest that serotonin axons may directly regulate β-adrenoceptor number and function. Prevention by serotonergic lesioning of antidepressant-induced β-adrenoceptor down-regulation could be explained on the basis of this mechanism.

It is interesting to note that GABA agonists such as progabide, which have the same effects as ECS on serotonergic responses and serotonin receptor number (39,44), do not affect β-adrenoceptors in a parallel fashion. Progabide does not reduce β-adrenoceptor number after chronic administration, although it and other GABAergic agents enhance serotonin-mediated behavior and increase $5-HT_2$ receptor number (44). Progabide does, however, attenuate clonidine-induced sedation (44), an effect in common with ECS and indicative of subsensitivity of presynaptic $α_2$-adrenoceptors (see below). The down-regulating effect of ECS on β-adrenoceptors would therefore appear to be a finding highly specific to agents with antidepressant activity.

$α_1$-Adrenoceptors. Earlier studies that used WB 4101 as the radioligand suggested that α-adrenoceptors are unchanged by repeated ECS (13). This ligand is, however, not specific for $α_1$ sites. Using the specific $α_1$ ligand [³H]prazosin, Vetulani et al. (131) found an ECS-induced increase in $α_1$-receptor number in the cortex and hippocampus. Similar effects were reported for a variety of chemical antidepressant agents (130). The same group has also reported increased post-decapitation convulsions which may be a functional correlate of the increase in $α_1$ receptor number (132), following repeated ECS and antidepressants.

$α_2$-Adrenoceptors. Adrenoceptors of the $α_2$ subtype are located both pre- and postsynaptically. Those located presynaptically inhibit NE release and putatively underlie the sedation and hypothermia induced by low-dose clonidine administration (63). Repeated ECS attenuates both the sedative and hypothermic effects of clonidine (47,107). This $α_2$-receptor subsensitivity is also induced by spaced ECS and by a number of chemical antidepressant agents (130). Release studies from our laboratory are consistent with these behavioral parameters. Repeated but not single ECS was found to attenuate inhibition of NE release by clonidine in cortical synaptosomal preparations (31). Reduction by clonidine of MHPG SO_4 levels is also attenuated by ECS (47).

[³H]Clonidine binding, which does not select between pre- and postsynaptically located $α_2$-receptors, is affected in a complex fashion by repeated ECS. Pilc and Vetulani (107) have reported a loss of high-affinity [³H]clonidine binding sites without change in the low-affinity sites. Smith et al. (122), studying [³H]clonidine and [³H]yohimbine binding to $α_2$-adrenoceptors on human blood platelets, found a significant reduction in B_{max} for both ligands following chronic ECT administration. This finding was not, however, confirmed by Cooper et al. (24), who also found no effect of ECT on lymphocyte $β_2$-adrenoceptors. $α_2$-Adrenoceptor studies are, however, generally suggestive of subsensitivity of these receptors and an effect of ECT to enhance the availability of NE for interaction with postsynaptic recognition sites.

Effects Distal to the Receptor

The receptor-adenylate cyclase complex is now known to be composed of three components—the receptor (R), a guanyl nucleotide-binding subunit (N) mediating transfer of the signal to the catalytic unit (C), and the catalytic unit itself. Menkes et al. (89) reported that both ECS and a series of antidepressant agents enhanced the responsiveness of the N protein to stimulation by the nonhydrolyzable GTP analog, GPP NHp, and by sodium fluoride. A recent study from our laboratory examined the effect of single and repeated ECS on adenylate cyclase activity in both membrane and whole-cell (slice) preparations from rat cortex (99). In the membrane preparation, chronic ECS significantly increased adenylate cyclase activity in response to GppNHp (activating the N protein) and to forskolin and manganese (which activate the C unit). These findings confirmed the report of Menkes et al. (89) with regard to chronic ECS effects distal to the receptor. In the slice preparation, we observed, as has been previously reported (134), reduced cyclic AMP production in response to NE, but we also found reduced responsiveness to activation of the C unit with forskolin. This latter finding (which was opposite to that observed with forskolin in the membrane preparation) emphasizes the difference in effects observed in the two preparations. The findings in slice preparations would support an ECS-induced reduction in signal amplification distal to the receptor (a finding congruent with the observed reduction in β-adrenoceptor number following chronic ECS). The findings in the membrane preparation, now reported by two groups (89,99), would suggest an opposite effect. The difference in effects may be a function of the preparations used, the slice preparation possibly being more physiologically relevant. Resolution of this issue may depend on the development of tools other than forskolin that can be used in intact cell preparations to stimulate those portions of receptor-cyclase complex distal to the receptor.

Neuroendocrine Studies

Blunted GH responses to the α_2-adrenergic agonist clonidine have been demonstrated in depressed patients by a number of groups (see 71). No alteration in this response was observed in patients studied by Slade and Checkley (120) 24 hr after a series of ECT administrations. A posttreatment difference in the sedative effect of clonidine was also not observed. Checkley et al. (20) have suggested that anesthetic effects may delay the manifestation of a blunted response to clonidine. McWilliam et al. (88) did observe blunting of the GH response to clonidine in baboons tested 24 hr after the last of a series of photically induced seizures unaccompanied by anesthesia. The same investigators also found enhancement of the GH response in baboons tested 2 weeks after a series of ECS administered under anesthesia (20). Further studies are required to elucidate this question.

Discussion

ECT effects on brain NE function are highly relevant to the classical theories linking this neurotransmitter and affective illness (116). The effects of ECT on brain NE systems are suggestive, overall, of enhanced presynaptic availability. However, recognition sites for NE are affected in a complex fashion, with β- and possibly α_2-adrenoceptors down-regulated and α_1-receptor number and sensitivity apparently increased. Vetulani and Antkiewicz-Michaluk (130) have suggested an integrated hypothesis encompassing these effects. In brief, the α_2- and α_1-adrenoceptor changes are viewed as representing a shift of effect between the inhibitory function of the α_2 sites and the postsynaptic excitatory effects of the α_1 sites. β-Adrenoceptor down-regulation is explained as compensatory or homeostatic in nature. These suggestions are consistent with much but not all of the available data. Further elucidation of the effect of ECT on signal amplification processes distal to the receptor is needed.

Dopamine

Presynaptic Effects

Brain content of dopamine (DA) and the synthesis rate of this neurotransmitter are unchanged following a series of ECS administered to rats daily for 7 to 10 days (34,93). This contrasts with reports that DA synthesis is accelerated by a single ECS (33). Studies in patients receiving ECT have revealed no immediate alterations in plasma homovanillic acid (HVA) following seizure induction (80) and no longer-term changes in CSF HVA levels (68), urinary HVA excretion, or whole-body dopamine turnover after chronic treatment (78).

Receptor Effects

Postsynaptic receptors. A variety of DA-mediated behavioral responses, including hyperactivity, stereotypy, and circling in rats with unilateral nigrostriatal lesions, are enhanced by daily ECT over 7 to 10 days (38,94). Reports disagree, however, as to whether ECS at a less frequent, more clinically equivalent schedule induces behavioral DA supersensitivity (42,69). Enhancement of DA-mediated behavioral responses by repeated ECS is dependent on intact noradrenergic but not serotonergic innervation. Lesioning of ascending NE pathways, as well as pretreatment with the catecholamine synthesis inhibitor AMPT, has been shown to attenuate the DA behavioral supersensitivity induced by repeated ECS (41,42). No attenuation was observed after serotonin depletion by means of parachlorophenylalanine (PCPA) pretreatment (41).

The behavioral findings referable to DA receptors have not been paralleled by biochemically measurable receptor changes. DA-sensitive adenylate cyclase activity (38) and [³H]spiperone binding to striatal DA receptors (6,13,69) are unchanged following chronic ECS. ECS-induced enhancement of DA-mediated behaviors may, however, be correlated with biochemical changes distal to the receptor. Heal and Green (48) showed that ECS enhanced behavioral responses to injections of dibutyryl cyclic AMP into the nucleus accumbens. Dibutyryl cyclic AMP acts "beyond" the postsynaptic DA receptor and increases DA function even in the presence of a DA antagonist (49).

Presynaptic receptors. Studies of ECS effects on presynaptic DA receptors suggest that these sites are rendered subsensitive by chronic treatment. After daily ECS for 10 days, Serra et al. (117) found a reduced hypoactive response to low-dose apomorphine. This effect is thought to be mediated via presynaptic DA receptors. Chiodo and Antelman (21) used single-unit electrophysiological techniques to study the effect of ECS on DA autoreceptor sensitivity in the substantia nigra. Six daily ECS significantly reduced the ability of low-dose apomorphine to inhibit the spontaneous discharge of nigral DA neurons. Single ECS had no immediate effect but was found to induce significant autoreceptor subsensitivity after a treatment-free interval of 7 days. Antelman and colleagues have also reported similar findings after acute administration of a tricyclic antidepressant (22) and a monoamine oxidase inhibitor (4). These findings are of interest because of their implication that the antidepressant effects of ECT may be dependent on the first treatment rather than the full series, a suggestion recently raised on the clinical level by Rich and Black (111). It should, however, be noted that at least two groups have been unable to demonstrate DA autoreceptor subsensitivity following antidepressant treatment (85,136). Further studies are required to resolve this issue.

Neuroendocrine Studies

Neuroendocrine probes are an obvious tool for investigating ECT effects on DA receptors in humans and have been used by a number of investigators. In general, DA agonists induce increases in plasma GH and decreases in plasma prolactin (113). Slade and Checkley (120) found no enhancement of the GH response to methamphetamine following ECT in depressed patients. There was also no enhancement of the euphoric and stimulant effects of methamphetamine (120). Balldin et al. (8) found that apomorphine-induced suppression of prolactin secretion was significantly enhanced by ECT, a finding not replicated by Christie et al. (23). Neither Balldin et al. (8) nor Christie et al. (23) could show enhancement of GH responses to apomorphine following a course of ECT, although Costain et al. (27) reported such an effect. All the above studies measured GH responses to apomorphine 24 hr after the last of a series of ECT. The suggestion that anesthetic effects may delay the manifestation of changed neuroendocrine responses following ECT (20) could shed some light on these inconsistent findings.

Discussion

Although some theoretical formulations have suggested a role for DA in the pathogenesis of affective disorders (108), this neurotransmitter has, in general, been less emphasized than the other monoamines. Moreover, the induction of DA supersensitivity might logically be expected to exacerbate conditions such as psychotic depression or mania, which are ameliorated by DA blockade with neuroleptic drugs. However, ECS effects on signal amplification distal to the DA receptor remain to be evaluated.

An important clinical correlate of DA receptor supersensitivity following repeated ECS should be stressed. There are now a number of reports suggesting that ECT may significantly improve the symptoms of Parkinson's disease even in patients nonresponsive to L-dopa (e.g. 53,94,139). This may be a clinical correlate of the DA receptor supersensitivity observed following ECS in rodents. In this regard, it would be important to establish whether the antiparkinsonian and mood-elevating effects of ECT are indeed dissociated, as suggested in one report (139) but not supported in another (53).

Acetylcholine

Brain cholinergic function has been closely linked to the pathogenesis of affective disorders (56,119) as well as being strongly implicated in normal and disturbed memory function (9). Since ECT has significant effects on both mood and memory, posttreatment alterations in central cholinergic function are of potential importance.

Presynaptic Effects

There is little evidence for cumulative changes in presynaptic cholinergic mechanisms following repeated ECS. Neither high-affinity choline uptake nor choline acetyltransferase (ChAT) activity are significantly altered in rat brain following chronic treatment (6). There is, however, evidence indicative of acute release of acetylcholine during the induced seizure. Single ECS is associated with a significant intra- or immediately postictal reduction in acetylcholine levels (e.g., 83). ChAT (83) and acetylcholinesterase (1) activities are acutely increased following ECS. Acute release of acetylcholine during seizures is also suggested by human data showing increased CSF acetylcholine levels following pentylenetetrazol-induced or epileptic convulsions and evidence for cholinergically related electroencephalogram (EEG) slowing following ECT (35).

Receptor Effects

Dashieff et al. (28) found a highly significant reduction in [^{3}H]quinuclidinyl benzilate ([^{3}H]QNB) binding to hippocampal muscarinic cholinergic receptors after four ECS daily over 4 days. Lerer et al. (67,73,74) have observed that repeated but not single ECS induces a small but significant reduction in cortical muscarinic receptor number. Lerer et al. (73) also demonstrated that concurrent ECS administration reversed the significant increase in cortical [^{3}H]QNB binding caused by chronic atropine administration. A possible functional correlate of ECS-induced reductions in muscarinic receptor binding had been demonstrated by Green et al. (40) and was confirmed by Stanley and Lerer (124). ECS was shown by both groups to induce subsensitive cataleptic responses to the muscarinic agonist pilocarpine, although a clear time-course relationship with muscarinic cholinergic receptor down-regulation could not be demonstrated (124).

Discussion

Central cholinergic overactivity may be an important factor in the pathogenesis of major depression (56,119). Induction of muscarinic cholinergic receptor subsensitivity represents a possible mechanism for the reversal by ECT of depressed mood (67). A possible relationship to ECT-induced memory impairment has also been studied (67,74). This suggestion is supported by the finding that memory function in rats is impaired by chronic administration of physostigmine, which also down-regulates muscarinic receptors (84).

ECS-induced down-regulation of cortical muscarinic cholinergic receptors is, however, small in magnitude and has not been demonstrable in some studies (29,58). Further preclinical investigation using agonist rather than antagonist binding is indicated. Neuroendocrine and other applicable challenges have not yet been utilized to determine whether alterations in muscarinic receptor sensitivity are demonstrable in humans following ECT. ECS effects on signal amplification distal to the muscarinic receptor also remain to be investigated.

Endogenous Opioids

Repeated ECS administered to rats significantly increases metenkephalin levels in the caudate nucleus, hypothalamus, and limbic areas (45,54), and dynorphin levels in the hippocampus (110). ECT in humans has been shown to induce an acute rise in plasma β-endorphin levels (2). There is considerable evidence derived from behavioral, EEG, and autonomic paradigms that ECS increases endogenous opioid activity in rodents (see 12,52). A single ECS significantly enhances cataleptic and antinociceptive responses in rats and these effects are blocked by pretreatment with the opioid antagonist naloxone. Postical EEG slow-wave activity following ECS closely resembles that induced by intracerebroventricular injection of opioid peptides and is reversed by naloxone administration (127). ECS-induced increases in heart rate and arterial pressure and reduction in respiratory rate are blocked by doses of naloxone that do not affect these parameters preictally (10).

Although repeated ECS might be expected to induce tolerance to these opioid-mediated effects, the reverse, i.e., sensitization, has been observed. Repeated ECS results in a progressive enhancement of postictal catalepsy and antinociceptive responses (11,127). These enhanced responses are not blocked by naloxone administration, contrary to the effects observed following a single ECS (127). A similar pattern of naloxone effect has been observed with regard to the ECS-induced EEG changes (127). Repeated ECS administration also results in cross sensitivity to the cataleptic and antinociceptive effects of morphine challenge (11). The converse has also been demonstrated, i.e., cross sensitization of morphine-tolerant rats to the opioid-like effects of ECS (11). These findings, consistently reported by Holaday and colleagues (12,52), have not been completely replicated by some investigators (129).

Holaday et al. (52) have concluded that the enhanced opioid-like effects induced by repeated ECS are most logically attributable to alterations in postsynaptic receptor sites for these peptides. Both repeated ECS and chronic morphine administration were found by Holaday et al. (51,52) to significantly increase the number of [³H]D-Ala²-D-Leu⁵ enkephalin ([³H]DADLE), [³H]diprenorphine, and [³H]morphine binding sites in membranes from whole rat brain. These findings suggest an overall increase in binding sites without respect to opioid receptor subtype. However, Antkiewicz-Michaluk et al. (5) reported that following chronic ECS, only [³H]DADLE binding (labeling predominantly δ-opioid receptors) was increased, and this finding was limited to the cortex, whereas [³H]naloxone binding (labeling both μ- and δ-receptors) was decreased in the striatum to a small (15%) but significant extent. More recently, Nakata et al. (97) found reductions in both δ- and μ-opioid receptors in the hypothalamus, hippocampus, and caudate nucleus but not in frontal cortex or brainstem. Methodological issues such as ligand concentration and presence or absence of cations may explain these discrepant results. The receptor changes putatively underlying ECS-induced enhancement of opioid-mediated behavioral responses remain, therefore, to be conclusively defined.

Anticonvulsant Effects

Opioid peptides have been shown in a number of studies to have anticonvulsant effects and may mediate the increase in seizure threshold induced postictally by ECS and other convulsant agents (126). In a recent study, Tortella and Long (128) demonstrated that CSF transferred from ECS-treated rats to the lateral ventricles of naive rats raised the threshold for fluorythyl-induced seizures in the recipient animals. This effect was blocked by naloxone pretreatment of the recipient animals. An endogenous opioid substance released during the seizure may exert this anticonvulsant action.

Seizure threshold in ECT-treated patients and rats subjected to ECS is modified by a number of factors, including GABA and adenosine (see below). The interactive relationship of these various factors remains to be clarified. If, as has been suggested (114), alterations in seizure threshold are important in the antidepressant action of ECT, these considerations may have considerable implications for the mechanism of action of the treatment.

Discussion

The effects of repeated ECS on endogenous opioid systems are strongly indicative of enhanced responsiveness following chronic treatment, although the biochemical mediation of these effects has yet to be established. Other than the increase in plasma β-endorphin levels observed immediately following ECT in humans (e.g., 2), this issue has not yet been directly addressed in clinical studies. The preclinical findings would imply that exogenous opioid agents should be effective in the treatment of affective disorders. This question remains to be addressed clinically in a controlled fashion. Endogenous opioids may, however, be indirectly implicated in the mechanism of action of ECT via their effects on other neurotransmitter systems (e.g., inhibition of DA release) or via their anticonvulsant effects. These possibilities remain to be definitively studied.

GABA

Brain GABA function is intimately linked to the induction and generalization of seizures (138). The epileptogenic potential of GABA antagonists has been consistently demonstrated, and GABA agonists block both spontaneous and induced seizures (138). Repeated ECS has been reported to increase GABA levels in the caudate nucleus and nucleus accumbens and to decrease GABA synthesis rate in these regions (40). This combination of effects is interpreted as suggesting decreased release of the neurotransmitter. The findings referred to were demonstrated in rats examined 24 hr after the last of 10 daily treatments and were not induced by single ECS or subconvulsive shocks (45).

Increases in both [^{3}H]diazepam and [^{3}H]GABA binding to cortical sites have been reported in the early postictal period (104,112). This may account for the increase in seizure threshold regularly observed following spontaneous and induced seizures. Persistent GABA receptor changes have not been demonstrated using nonspecific GABA ligands such as [^{3}H]muscimol or in [^{3}H]diazepam binding (7,29) [with the exception of one study (87) that found increases in hippocampal [^{3}H]diazepam binding 24 hr after 17 daily ECS administrations]. Recently, however, Lloyd et al. (82) reported a persistent increase in GABA$_B$ sites following chronic ECT and antidepressant administration, suggesting a specific role for this GABA receptor subtype.

The possible modulating influence of GABA function on monoamine-mediated responses affected by ECS should again be noted. In parallel with ECS, GABA agonists increase both serotonin-mediated responses and 5-HT$_2$ receptor number (15). GABA mechanisms may, in addition to their pivotal role in seizure induction, be more strongly implicated in antidepressant mechanisms than had been previously thought.

Other Neurotransmitters and Neuromodulators

Adenosine

Newman et al. (100) reported that chronic but not single ECS increased [^{3}H]cyclohexyladenosine binding in rat cerebral cortex. The anticonvulsant action of adenosine may be mediated via the A$_1$ adenosine receptor subtype, which is labeled by this ligand. Newman et al. (100) therefore suggested that an increase in adenosine receptor number may underlie the well-recognized increase in seizure threshold that occurs during a course of ECT. An early clinical trial with caffeine sodium benzoate administered preictally suggested that administration of an adenosine antagonist may indeed lower seizure threshold and increase seizure length (118). ECS effects on A$_2$ adenosine receptors (measured in cortical slices by cyclic AMP accumulation in response to 2-chloro-adenosine) are inconsistent, both increased (115) and decreased (100) responses having been reported.

Thyrotropin-Releasing Hormone

This endogenous peptide has been reported to have antidepressant properties (98). It has also been shown to interact with both serotonergic and dopaminergic systems (77). Two groups have studied the effect of ECS on brain TRH levels, results differing with the area studied. Kubek et al. (62) found significant increases in the hippocampus, pyriform cortex, and amygdala after repeated ECS but not after single ECS or subconvulsive shocks. Lighton et al. (77) found significant reductions in TRH content of the nucleus accumbens and lumbar spinal cord after repeated but not single ECS and decreased TRH release from nucleus accumbens slices. These differing findings require further investigation.

CONCLUSIONS

The fact that a series of electrically induced seizures may so effectively alleviate the most severely disturbed mood states is one of the most intriguing phenomena in biological psychiatry. Of the major theories seeking to explain this remarkable clinical effect, neurochemical mechanisms have been the most intensively investigated. ECT induces significant alterations in most of the major neurotransmitters and neuromodulators or their recognition sites. However, the challenge of defining which of these effects are related to mechanism of action and which are irrelevant epiphenomena has yet to be adequately met.

Parallels between ECS and antidepressant effects on brain NE function have been consistently demonstrated; yet findings in the serotonergic system presently suggest a diametrically opposite action. DA effects may explain the antiparkinsonian action of ECT but are more difficult to correlate with mood-stabilizing or antipsychotic actions. Cholinergic effects may be related to the amnestic adverse effects of the treatment but could theoretically be linked to antidepressant action as well. Endogenous opioid effects appear to have major functional consequences but are less easily interpreted in terms of mechanism of action. Effects on GABA and adenosine systems may be more closely related to the mechanism of seizure induction than to therapeutic mechanisms but remain to be conclusively evaluated in this regard.

Studies on the interaction between the various neurotransmitters have highlighted critical interrelationships with regard to ECS-induced changes. Further studies are likely to add support to the view that a single neurotransmitter is unlikely to be exclusively implicated in the pathogenesis and treatment of affective disorders. Similarly, the wide clinical spectrum of ECT makes it illogical to seek a single neurochemical action that underlies its manifold clinical effects.

The animal models used in preclinical ECS studies have been considerably refined, and comparisons of chronic ECS effects with those of single treatments, subconvulsive shocks, and, to a lesser extent, other convulsant agents, are regularly encompassed. Clinically relevant, spaced schedules of ECS administration are, however, infrequently used and could be important in defining preclinical effects that are pertinent to mechanism of action. Comparisons of unilateral ECS administration with those of bilateral treatment have also not received sufficient attention. Similarly, relative effects of different waveforms and stimulus intensity remain to be explored. These considerations could be of critical importance in relating preclinical ECS effects to the therapeutic action of ECT.

Studies in humans have thus far yielded only minimal support for most of the hypotheses tested and in some cases ostensibly contradictory results. Human studies are a critical avenue for future research; present indirect methodology may ultimately be replaced by brain imaging techniques that accurately reflect neurotransmitter and receptor function in humans. It should then be easier to determine which of the neurochemical effects of ECT are most closely linked to clinical response or adverse effects.

The interface between ECT and the biology of affective illness has been an actively productive research area. Interest is likely to be intensified as novel preclinical and clinical techniques are applied. Results obtained could further advance our understanding of the biological mechanism of ECT and the pathogenesis of disorders that are alleviated by this unique treatment.

REFERENCES

1. Adams, H. E., Hoblit, P. R., and Sulker, P. D. (1969): *Physiol. Behav.,* 4:113–116.
2. Alexopoulos, G. S., Inturrisi, C. E., Lipman, R., Frances, R., Haycox, J., Dougherty, J. H., and Rossier, J. (1983): *Arch. Gen. Psychiatry,* 40:181–183.
3. Allen, M. J. P., Denney, D., Kendall, J. W., and Blachly, P. H. (1974): *Am. J. Psychiatry,* 131:1225–1228.
4. Antelman, S. M., Chiodo, L. A., and DeGiovanni, L. A. (1982): In: *Typical and Atypical Antidepressants: Molecular Mechanisms,* edited by E. Costa and G. Racagni, pp. 121–132. Raven Press, New York.
5. Antkiewicz-Michaluk, L., Rokosz-Pelc, A., and Vetulani, J. (1984): *Naunyn Schmiedebergs Arch. Pharmacol.,* 328:87–89.
6. Atterwill, C. K. (1980): *J. Neurochem.,* 35:729–734.
7. Atterwill, C. K. (1984): In: *ECT: Basic Mechanisms,* edited by B. Lerer, R. D. Weiner, and R. H. Belmaker, pp. 79–88. John Libbey, London.
8. Balldin, J., Granerus, A. K., Lindstedt, G., Modigh, K., and Walinder, J. (1982): *Psychopharmacology,* 76:371–376.
9. Bartus, R. T., Dean, R. L., Beer, B., and Lippa, A. S. (1982): *Science,* 217:407–417.
10. Belenky, G. L., and Holaday, J. W. (1979): *Brain Res.,* 177:414–417.
11. Belenky, G. L., and Holaday, J. W. (1981): *Life Sci.,* 29:553–563.
12. Belenky, G. L., Tortella, F. C., Hitzemann, R. J., and Holaday, J. W. (1984): In: *ECT: Basic Mechanisms,* edited by B. Lerer, R. D. Weiner, and R. H. Belmaker, pp. 89–97. John Libbey, London.
13. Bergstrom, D. A., and Kellar, K. J. (1979): *Nature,* 278:464–466.
14. Brandon, S., Cowley, P., McDonald, C., Neville, P., Palmer, R., and Wellstood-Eason, S. (1984): *Br. Med. J.,* 228:22–25.
15. Brown, J. P. (1984): In: *ECT: Basic Mechanisms,* edited by B. Lerer, R. D. Weiner, and R. H. Belmaker, pp. 164–177. John Libbey, London.
16. Brunello, N., Barbaccia, M. L., Chuang, D.-M., and Costa, E. (1982): *Neuropharmacology,* 21:1145–1149.
17. Cerletti, V., and Bini, L. (1938): *Boll. Acad. Med. Roma,* 64:136–138.
18. Charney, D. S., Heninger, G. R., and Sternberg, D. E. (1984): *Arch. Gen. Psychiatry,* 41:359–365.
19. Charney, D. S., Menkes, D. B., and Heninger, G. R. (1981): *Arch. Gen. Psychiatry,* 38:1160–1180.
20. Checkley, S. A., Meldrum, B. S., and McWilliam, J. R. (1984): In: *ECT: Basic Mechanisms,* edited by B. Lerer, R. D. Weiner, and R. H. Belmaker, pp. 101–106. John Libbey, London.
21. Chiodo, L. A., and Antelman, S. M. (1980): *Science,* 210:799–801.
22. Chiodo, L. A., and Antelman, S. M. (1980): *Nature,* 287:451–454.
23. Christie, J. E., Whalley, L. J., Brown, N. S., and Dick, H. (1982): *Br. J. Psychiatry,* 133:416.
24. Cooper, S. J., Kelly, J. G., and King, D. J. (1985): *Br. J. Psychiatry,* 147:23–29.
25. Coppen, A., Rao, V. A., Bishop, M., Abou-Saleh, M. T., and Wood, K. (1980): *J. Affective Disord.,* 2:311–315.
26. Coryell, N., and Zimmerman, M. (1983): *Biol. Psychiatry,* 18:21–27.
27. Costain, D. W., Cowen, P. J., Gelder, M. G., and Grahame-Smith, D. G. (1982): *Lancet,* 2:400–404.
28. Dashieff, R. M., Savage, D. D., and McNamara, J. O. (1982): *Brain Res.,* 235:327–334.
29. Deakin, J. F. W., Owen, F., Cross, A. J., and Dashwood, M. J. (1981): *Psychopharmacology,* 73:345–349.
30. DeMontigny, C. (1984): *J. Pharmacol. Exp. Ther.,* 228:230–234.
31. Ebstein, R. P., Lerer, B., Shlaufman, M., and Belmaker, R. H. (1983): *Cell. Mol. Neurobiol.,* 3:191–201.
32. Engel, J., Hanson, L. C. F., and Roos, B. E. (1971): *Psychopharmacologia,* 20:197–200.
33. Engel, J., Hanson, L. C. F., Roos, B. E., and Strombergsson, L. E. (1968): *Psychopharmacologia,* 13:140–144.
34. Evans, J. P. M., Grahame-Smith, D. G., Green, A. R., and Tordoff, A. F. C. (1976): *Br. J. Pharmacol.,* 56:193–199.
35. Fink, M. (1966): *J. Nerv. Ment. Dis.,* 142:475–484.
36. Fink, M. (1979): *Convulsive Therapy: Theory and Practice.* Raven Press, New York.
37. Fink, M., and Ottosson, J. O. (1980): *Psychiatry Res.,* 2:49–61.
38. Grahame-Smith, D. G., Green, A. R., and Costain, D. W. (1978): *Lancet,* 1:245–256.
39. Green, A. R. (1985): *Acta Pharmacol. Toxicol. (Suppl.),* 56:128–137.
40. Green, A. R., Bloomfield, M. R., Atterwill, C. K., and Costain, D. W. (1979): *Neuropharmacology,* 18:447–451.
41. Green, A. R., Costain, D. W., and Deakin, J. W. F. (1980): *Neuropharmacology,* 19:907–914.
42. Green, A. R., and Deakin, J. F. W. (1980): *Nature,* 285:232–233.
43. Green, A. R., Heal, D. J., and Grahame-Smith, D. G. (1977): *Psychopharmacology,* 52:195–200.
44. Green, A. R., Johnson, P., Mountford, J. A., and Nimgaonkar, V. L. (1985): *Br. J. Pharmacol.,* 84:337–346.
45. Green, A. R., Peralta, E., Hong, J. S., Mao, C. C., Atterwill, C. K., and Costa, E. (1978): *J. Neurochem.,* 31:607.
46. Gregory, S., Shawcross, C. R., and Gill, D. (1985): *Brit. J. Psychiatry,* 146:520–524.
47. Heal, D. J., Akagi, H., Bowdler, J. M., and Green, A. R. (1981): *Eur. J. Pharmacol.,* 75:231–237.
48. Heal, D. J., and Green, A. R. (1978): *Neuropharmacology,* 17:1085–1087.
49. Heal, D. J., Phillips, A. G., and Green, A. R. (1978): *Neuropharmacology,* 17:265–267.
50. Hoffman, G., Linkowski, P., Kerkhofs, M., Desmedt, D., and Mendlewicz, J. (1985): *Psychiatry Res.,* 16:199–206.
51. Holaday, J. W., Hitzemann, R. J., Curell, J., Tortella, F. C., and Belenky, G. L. (1982): *Life Sci.,* 31:2209–2212.
52. Holaday, J. W., Tortella, F. C., Long, J. B., Belenky, G. L., and Hitzemann, R. J. (1986): In: *Ann. NY Acad. Sci.: Electroconvulsive Therapy: Clinical and Basic Research Issues,* edited by H. Sackeim and S. Malitz, pp. 124–139. New York Academy of Sciences, New York.
53. Holcomb, H. H., Sternberg, D. E., and Heninger, G. R. (1983): *Biol. Psychiatry,* 18:865–873.
54. Hong, J. S., Gillin, J. C., Yang, H.-Y. T., and Costa, E. (1979): *Brain Res.,* 177:273.

55. Janowsky, A., Okada, F., Manier, A. H., Applegate, C. D., and Sulser, F. (1982): *Science,* 218:900–901.
56. Janowsky, D. S., El-Yousef, M. K., Davis, J. M., and Sekerke, H. J. (1972): *Lancet,* 2:6732–6735.
57. Karliner, W., and Werheim, H. K. (1965): *Am. J. Psychiatry,* 121:113–115.
58. Kellar, K. J., Cascio, C. S., Bergstrom, D. A., Butler, J. A., and Iadarola, P. (1981): *J. Neurochem.,* 37:830–836.
59. Kellar, K. J., Cascio, C. S., Butler, J. A., and Kurtzke, R. N. (1981): *Eur. J. Pharmacol.,* 69:515–518.
60. Kellar, K. J., Stockmeier, C. A., and Gomez, J. M. (1985): *Acta Pharmacol. Toxicol. (Suppl.),* 56:138–145.
61. Kety, S. S., Javoy, F., Thierry, A.-M., Julou, L., and Glowinski, J. (1977): *Proc. Natl. Acad. Sci. USA,* 58:1249–1254.
62. Kubek, M. J., Meyerhoff, J. L., Hill, T. G., Norton, J. A., and Sattin, A. (1985): *Life Sci.,* 36:315–320.
63. Langer, S. Z. (1974): *Biochem. Pharmacol.,* 23:1793–1800.
64. Langer, S. Z., and Raisman, R. (1983): *Neuropharmacology,* 22:407–413.
65. Langer, S. Z., Zarifian, E., Briley, M., Raisman, R., and Sechter, D. (1981): *Life Sci.,* 29:211–220.
66. Lerer, B. (1984): *Biol. Psychiatry,* 19:361–383.
67. Lerer, B. (1985): *Biol. Psychiatry,* 20:20–40.
68. Lerer, B., and Belmaker, R. H. (1982): *Biol. Psychiatry,* 17:497–511.
69. Lerer, B., Jabotinsky-Rubin, K., Bannet, J., Ebstein, R. P., and Belmaker, R. H. (1982): *Eur. J. Pharmacol.,* 80:131–134.
70. Lerer, B., and Shapira, B. (1986): *Convulsive Therapy,* 2:141–144.
71. Lerer, B., and Sitaram, N. (1983): *Prog. Neuropsychopharmacol. Biol. Psychiatry,* 7:309–333.
72. Lerer, B., Stanley, M., and Belmaker, R. H. (1984): In: *ECT: Basic Mechanisms,* edited by B. Lerer, R. D. Weiner, and R. H. Belmaker, pp. 67–78. John Libbey, London.
73. Lerer, B., Stanley, M., Demetriou, S., and Gershon, S. (1983): *J. Neurochem.,* 41:1680–1683.
74. Lerer, B., Stanley, M., McIntyre, I., and Altman, H. (1984): *Life Sci.,* 35:2659–2664.
75. Lerer, B., Weiner, R. D., and Belmaker, R. H., eds. (1984): *ECT: Basic Mechanisms.* John Libbey, London.
76. Lerer, B., Zabow, T., Egnal, N., and Belmaker, R. H. (1983): *Biol. Psychiatry,* 18:821–824.
77. Lighton, C., Marsden, C. A., Bennett, G. W., Minchin, M., and Green, A. R. (1984): *Neuropharmacology,* 23:963–966.
78. Linnoila, M., Karoum, F., and Potter, W. Z. (1983): *Arch. Gen. Psychiatry,* 40:1015–1017.
79. Linnoila, M., Karoum, F., Rosenthal, N., and Potter, W. Z. (1983): *Arch. Gen. Psychiatry,* 40:677–680.
80. Linnoila, M., Litovitz, G., Scheinin, M., Chang, M.-D., and Cutler, N. A. (1984): *Biol. Psychiatry,* 19:79–84.
81. Linnoila, M., Miller, T. L., Bartko, J., and Potter, W. Z. (1984): *Arch. Gen. Psychiatry,* 41:688–692.
82. Lloyd, K. G., Thuret, F., and Pilc, A. (1985): ECT, antidepressants and the GABA-B receptor. *Abstracts of the IV World Congress of Biological Psychiatry,* Philadelphia.
83. Longoni, R., Mulas, A., Novak, B. O., Pepeu, I. M., and Pepeu, G. (1976): *Neuropharmacology,* 15:283–286.
84. Loullis, C. C., Dean, R. L., Lippa, A. S., Meyerson, L. P., Beer, B., and Bartus, R. T. (1983): *Pharmacol. Biochem. Behav.,* 18:601–604.
85. MacNeil, D. A., and Gower, M. (1982): *Nature,* 298:302.
86. Malitz, S., Sackeim, H. A., and Decina, P. (1981): *Psychiatr. J. Univ. Ottawa,* 7:126–134.
87. McNamara, J. O., Peper, A. M., and Patrone, V. (1980): *Proc. Natl. Acad. Sci. USA,* 77:3029–3032.
88. McWilliam, J. R., Meldrum, B. S., and Checkley, S. A. (1981): *Psychoneuroendocrinology,* 6:77–79.
89. Menkes, D. B., Rasenick, M. M., Wheeler, M. A., and Bitensky, M. W. (1983): *Science,* 219:65.
90. Metz, A., Goodwin, G. M., and Green, A. R. (1985): *Neuropharmacology,* 24:357–360.
91. Miller, D. H. (1967): *Br. J. Psychiatry,* 113:301–311.
92. Minchin, M. C. W., Williams, J., Bowdler, J. M., and Green, A. R. (1983): *J. Neurochem.,* 40:765–768.
93. Modigh, K. (1976): *Psychopharmacology,* 49:179–185.
94. Modigh, K., Balldin, J., Eriksson, E., Granerus, A.-K., and Walinder, J. (1984): In: *ECT: Basic Mechanisms,* edited by B. Lerer, R. D. Weiner, and R. H. Belmaker, pp. 18–27. John Libbey, London.
95. Murphy, D. L., Campbell, I., and Costa, J. L. (1978): In: *Psychopharmacology: A Generation of Progress,* edited by M. A. Lipton, A. DiMascio, and A. F. Killam, pp. 1235–1247. Raven Press, New York.
96. Musacchio, J. M., Julou, L., Kety, S. S., and Glowinski, J. (1969): *Proc. Natl. Acad. Sci. USA,* 63:1117–1119.
97. Nakata, Y., Chang, K. J., Mitchell, C. L., and Hong, J. S. (1985): *Brain Res.,* 346:160–163.
98. Nemeroff, C. B., Loosen, P. T., Bissette, G., Manberg, P. J., Wilson, I. C., Lipton, M. A., and Prange, A. J., Jr. (1979): *Psychoneuroendocrinology,* 3:279–310.
99. Newman, M. E., Salomon, H., and Lerer, B. (1986): *J. Neurochem,* 46:1667–1669.
100. Newman, M., Zohar, J., Kalian, M., and Belmaker, R. H. (1984): *Brain Res.,* 291:188–192.
101. Nutt, D. J., Green, A. R., and Grahame-Smith, D. G. (1980): *Neuropharmacology,* 19:897–900.
102. Ottoson, J. O. (1960): *Acta Psychiatr. Neurol. Scand. (Suppl. 145),* 35:1–141.
103. Pandey, G. N., Heinze, W. J., Brown, B. D., and Davis, J. M. (1979): *Nature,* 280:234–235.
104. Paul, S. M., and Skolnick, P. (1978): *Science,* 202:892–893.
105. Peroutka, S. J., Lebovitz, R. M., and Snyder, S. H. (1981): *Science,* 212:827–829.
106. Perry, P. J., Morgan, D. E., Smith, R. E., and Tsuang, M. T. (1982): *J. Affective Disord.,* 4:195–200.
107. Pilc, A., and Vetulani, J. (1982): *Eur. J. Pharmacol.,* 80:109–113.
108. Post, R. M., Jimerson, D. C., Bunney, W. E., Jr., and Goodwin, F. K. (1980): *Psychopharmacology,* 67:297–305.
109. Prohovnik, I., Sackeim, H. A., Decina, P., and Malitz, S. (1986): In: *Ann. NY Acad. Sci.: Electroconvulsive Therapy: Clinical and Basic Research Issues,* edited by S. Malitz and H. A. Sackeim, pp. 249–262. New York Academy of Sciences, New York.
110. Przewlocki, R., Lason, W., Stach, R., Kacz, D., Stala, L., and Przewlocki, B. (1981): In: *Advances in Endogenous and Exogenous Opioids,* edited by H. Takagi, pp. 238–240. Kodansja, Tokyo.
111. Rich, C. L., and Black, N. A. (1985): *Psychiatry Res.,* 16:147–154.
112. Ross, S. M., and Craig, C. R. (1982): *Life Sci.,* 31:2499–2505.
113. Sachar, E. J., Gruen, P. H., Altman, N., Halpern, F. S., and Frantz, A. G. (1976): In: *Hormones, Behavior and Psychopharmacology,* edited by E. J. Sachar, pp. 161–176. Raven Press, New York.
114. Sackeim, H. A., Decina, P., Prohovnik, I., Malitz, S., and Resor, S. R. (1983): *Biol. Psychiatry,* 18:1301–1310.
115. Sattin, A. (1981): In: *Chemisms of the Brain,* edited by R. Rodnight, H. S. Bachelard, and W. L. Stahl, pp. 265–275. Churchill Livingstone, Edinburgh.
116. Schildkraut, J. J. (1965): *Am. J. Psychiatry,* 122:509–522.
117. Serra, G., Argiolas, A., Fadda, F., Melis, M. R., and Gessa, G. L. (1981): *Psychopharmacology,* 73:194–196.
118. Shapira, B., Zohar, J., Newman, M., Drexler, H., and Belmaker, R. H. (1985): *Convulsive Therapy,* 1:58–60.
119. Sitaram, N., and Gillin, J. C. (1980): *Biol. Psychiatry,* 15:925–955.
120. Slade, A. P., and Checkley, S. A. (1980): *Br. J. Psychiatry,* 137:217–221.
121. Small, J. G., Small, I. F., Milstein, V., Kellams, J. J., and Klapper, M. H. (1985): *Biol. Psychiatry,* 20:125–134.
122. Smith, C. B., Hollingsworth, P. J., Garcia-Sevilla, J. A., and Athanasios, P. Z. (1983): *Prog. Neuropsychopharmacol. Biol. Psychiatry,* 7:241–247.
123. Squire, L. R. (1977): *Am. J. Psychiatry,* 134:997–1001.

124. Stanley, M., and Lerer, B. (1985): *Convulsive Therapy,* 1:158–166.
125. Stockmeier, C. A., Martino, A. M., and Kellar, K. J. (1985): *Science,* 230:323–325.
126. Tortella, F. C., Cowan, A., and Adler, M. W. (1984): *Neuropharmacology,* 23:749–754.
127. Tortella, F. C., Cowan, A., Belenky, G. L., and Holaday, J. W. (1981): *Eur. J. Pharmacol.,* 76:121–128.
128. Tortella, F. C., and Long, J. B. (1985): *Science,* 228:1106–1107.
129. Urca, G., Nof, A., Weissman, B. A., and Sarne, Y. (1983): *Brain Res.,* 260:271–277.
130. Vetulani, J., and Antkiewicz-Michaluk, L. (1985): *Acta Pharmacol. Toxicol. (Suppl.),* 56:55–65.
131. Vetulani, J., Antkiewicz-Michaluk, L., Rokosz-Pelc, A., and Pilc, A. (1983): *Brain Res.,* 275:392–395.
132. Vetulani, J., Lebrecht, U., and Pilc, A. (1981): *Eur. J. Pharmacol.,* 76:81–85.
133. Vetulani, J., and Pilc, A. (1982): *Eur. J. Pharmacol.,* 85:269–275.
134. Vetulani, J., and Sulser, F. (1975): *Nature,* 257:495–496.
135. Weiner, R. D., Rogers, H. J., Welch, C. A., Davidson, J. R. J., Miller, R. D., Weir, D., and Cahill, J. F. (1984): In: *ECT: Basic Mechanisms,* edited by B. Lerer, R. D. Weiner, and R. H. Belmaker, pp. 139–147. John Libbey, London.
136. Welch, J., Kim, H., Fallon, S., and Liebman, J. (1982): *Nature,* 298:301–302.
137. Whalley, L. J., Dick, H., Watts, A. G., Christie, J. E., Rosie, R., Levy, G., Sheward, W. J., and Fink, G. (1982): *Lancet,* 2:1064–1068.
138. Wood, J. D. (1975): *Prog. Neurobiol.,* 5:77–95.
139. Young, R. C., Alexopoulos, G. S., and Shamoian, C. A. (1985): *Biol. Psychiatry,* 20:566–569.

Psychopharmacology:
The Third Generation of Progress,
edited by Herbert Y. Meltzer.
Raven Press, New York © 1987.

CHAPTER 59

Hypothalamic-Pituitary-Adrenal Axis in Affective Disorders

Peter E. Stokes and Carolyn R. Sikes

During the last half-century, investigators have focused on the biological regulation of behavior by two interacting systems: the nervous system and the endocrine system. As we shall see, it is indeed difficult to elaborate on one system without discussing the collaboration of the other. The hypothalamic-pituitary adrenocortical (HYPAC) system is a neuroendocrine axis that exemplifies this intimate interrelationship between the nervous system and the endocrine system.

For years, the pituitary was thought to function relatively independently of the central nervous system. We now know, however, that the hypothalamus acts to functionally integrate the activities of the brain and pituitary gland. Current concepts about the control of the pituitary gland have been derived from a number of divergent experimental approaches, such as electrical stimulation and lesioning (62,69), pituitary stalk transection (60,145), pituitary transplantation (70,134,180), and *in vitro* preparations (65,162). More recently, certain releasing factors, such as corticotropin-releasing hormone (CRH), have been identified with regard to chemical structure (196), and in some cases, even synthesized.

Taken together, these studies have demonstrated that neural regulation of the pituitary is achieved by peptide secretion from hypothalamic neurosecretory cells. These cells can be considered transducers (203) that translate neuronal signals from higher centers in the brain into secretory activity. It is important to remember that no sharply anatomically defined brain region has been shown alone to regulate a specific anterior pituitary hormone. Rather, each of the hypothalamic neurosecretory cells seems to be responsive to a variety of *pathways* utilizing a particular neurotransmitter [serotonin, dopamine, norepinephrine, γ-aminobutyric acid (GABA), etc.]. Furthermore, since tropic hormones are released under a variety of conditions (e.g., basal release, circadian release, stress-induced release, etc.), it seems likely that different neurotransmitters are implicated under each of these circumstances. Thus, each of the neurosecretory cells may have binding sites for several chemical transmitters, arriving via various anatomical pathways, and excited or inhibited by different stimuli.

Although structurally and functionally similar in many ways to the classic neuron, the axons of the hypophyseal

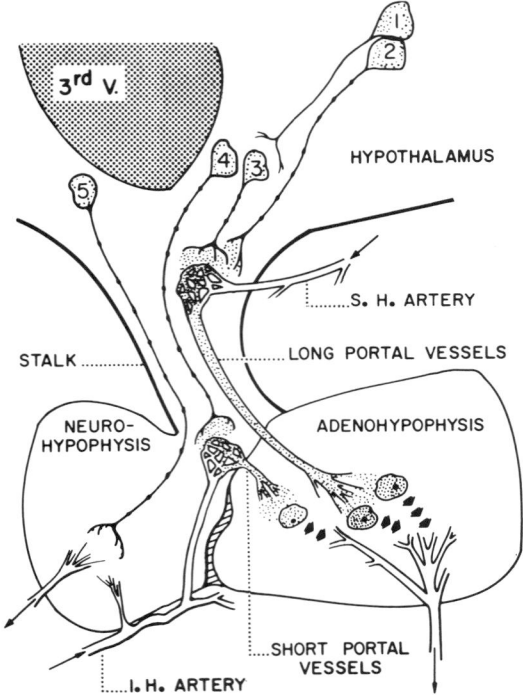

FIG. 1. Neural control of pituitary gland. This figure summarizes the types of neural inputs into pituitary regulation. Neuron 5 represents the peptidergic neurons of the supraoptico-hypophysial and paraventriculo-hypophysial tracts, with hormone-producing cell bodies in the hypothalamus and nerve terminals in the neural lobe. Neurons 3 and 4 are the peptidergic neurons of the tubero-hypophysial tract, which secrete the hypophysiotropic hormones into the substance of the median eminence in anatomical relationship to the primary plexus. Neuron 3 ends in the median eminence. Neuron 4 ends low in the stalk. Neuron 1 represents a monoaminergic neuron ending in relation to the cell body of the peptidergic neuron. Neuron 2 represents a monoaminergic neuron ending on terminals of the peptidergic neuron to give axoaxonic transmission as proposed by Schneider and McCann (171a). Neurons 1 and 2 are the functional links between the remainder of the brain and the peptidergic neuron. (From ref. 52.)

neurosecretory cells of the HYPAC system terminate on the capillaries of the microportal circulatory system, located in the pituitary stalk. Hypothalamic peptides, specifically CRH in the case of the HYPAC axis, are thus released into the portal system of the pituitary stalk. From here CRH travels to a relatively distal site in the pituitary to act on pituitary corticotropes, causing synthesis and release of adrenocorticotropic hormone (ACTH), for example.

It is now generally accepted that the central nervous system regulates HYPAC activity in at least three specific ways. First a "set point" is maintained by long- and short-loop feedback systems. Second, "higher" neural centers regulate the circadian periodicity of HYPAC activity. Last, a number of physical and psychological stresses, ultimately mediated via the limbic system and reticular formation, can stimulate HYPAC activation. These mechanisms of CNS control will be discussed in more detail in subsequent sections.

HISTORICAL DEVELOPMENTS LINKING HYPAC HYPERACTIVITY TO PSYCHOPATHOLOGY

Since the turn of the century, numerous reports have documented the psychopathology associated with Cushing's syndrome or disease (see 200 for review). The psychiatric disturbances in Cushing's disease can occur early in its course, and include a broad spectrum of depressive symptoms ranging from mild dysphoria and overreactions to stress, to profoundly depressed mood with anhedonia, mood-congruent delusions, neurovegetative signs, and suicidality (158,200). Other mental disturbances have also been noted, such as elation, euphoria, hyperactivity, and even full-blown mania (71). These symptoms are apparently unrelated to the gross catabolic changes of late stage disease.

Reports of psychiatric disturbances observed in medical patients on prolonged corticosteroid therapy provide additional support for the link between affective illness and HYPAC dysfunction (57,116). The initial psychological response included elation, grandiosity, mild delirium, excessive energy, and in some cases, hypomania. Usually, however, it was not long before these patients lost their mild euphoria, and in some instances, depression developed even though steroid treatment continued with large pharmacologic doses of cortisone (200). Similar findings have been reported for ACTH when administered in pharmacological doses that produced pronounced and protracted hypercortisolemia (57,116). Steroid or ACTH administration also produces behavioral changes in animals (201).

Although the earlier studies seem to provide suggestive evidence for a link between endocrine and behavioral perturbations, observations were generally not well quantified. Moreover, the heuristic value of these findings was limited by the state of clinical, physiological, and technological knowledge available at the time. These data did, however, suggest the potential value of exploring the nature and extent of HYPAC dysfunction during periods of emotional arousal and/or affective disturbance. Research in this area closely followed the biochemical revolution in endocrinology in the 1940s and 1950s. With the advent of wet chemical (spectrophotometric) techniques for the measurement of urinary excretory products of adrenocortical hormone secretion, it became possible to quantitate urinary, and then plasma, glucocorticoids. It soon became apparent that not only "organic" disease of the endocrine system (such as Cushing's syndrome), but also "psychological" stimuli (such as stressful life events) caused detectable, though modest and transient, increases in circulating plasma corticosteroids in most people (146).

Shortly thereafter, in the late 1950s and 1960s, it was observed that depressed patients showed even more remarkable and protracted elevations in plasma corticosteroids (9,11,20,40,55). However, the extent of HYPAC hyperfunction in depressed patients and its significance as a biological marker were generally not appreciated.

By the late 1960s and early 1970s, however, further reports (21,185) confirmed and extended these findings in larger numbers of psychiatric patients. At this time, many investigators still considered these HYPAC abnormalities to be only the result of HYPAC activation sometimes observed with the nonspecific stress of psychosis (157) or novelty effects of hospitalization (119). It later became obvious, however, that nonspecific stress could not account for the remarkable HYPAC abnormalities observed (18,185,188). Furthermore, depression was found to coexist with other state-dependent HYPAC abnormalities, in particular, resistance to dexamethasone suppression (26,184,185). Since this time, a vast amount of data deriving from many laboratories has clearly documented a number of striking abnormalities of the HYPAC system in affective illness.

In parallel with these developments, there were major advances in our understanding of endocrine physiology, neuroanatomy, and clinical endocrinology that provided further information about the structural/functional relationships within the HYPAC system, and thus about the function of the HYPAC system in psychopathological states. The following review touches on some of these advances in neuroendocrine anatomy and physiology.

BIOCHEMISTRY AND PHARMACOLOGY OF THE HYPAC AXIS

Glucocorticoid Synthesis

Adrenocortical steroidogenesis is accomplished by enyzmatic stepwise modification of cholesterol taken up from the blood, or synthesized from acetate within the adrenocortical cells. The fetal cortex is ACTH responsive and fetal pituitary absence is associated with atrophy of the cortex. ACTH stimulates increased cholesterol uptake and synthesis in the cortex as well as increased synthesis of pregnenolone from cholesterol, the rate-limiting step in ACTH-induced adrenocortical hormone production. The adrenal cortex synthesizes cortisol as the major glucocorticoid in humans, and as a closely related byproduct, much smaller amounts of corticosterone. Cortisol is by several criteria the more potent of the two glucocorticoids. Mineralocorticoids (aldosterone) are synthesized in the outer (glomerulosa) layer of cortical cells. Androgens, mainly dehydroepiandrosterone (DHEA), a small amount of which is converted to a classical potent androgen (testosterone), and minute amounts of estrogen are also produced in the adrenal cortex, almost as byproducts of glucocorticoid synthesis. Only cortisol and perhaps aldosterone are necessary for maintenance of life.

Without question, the major and essential stimulus for normal adrenocortical cell growth and secretion of steroids is ACTH. This hormone precipitates cell steroidogenesis and growth by binding to specific cell receptors near or on the cell membrane. By producing a variety of synthetic modifications of the ACTH molecule, it has become apparent that the first 24 amino acids at the N-terminal portion of the native 39-amino-acid peptide are the only essential portions of the molecule for maximal adrenocortical steroidogenesis. The shortest N-terminal fragment with some residual steroidogenic activity contains only 10 amino acids. It has been shown that minor alterations such as selected amino acid substitution or removal of the NH_2 group will remarkably impair or eliminate steroidogenic potency. Various fragments of the ACTH molecule have been found to exist in human plasma. These fragments may be assayable by radioimmunoassay, but may also be biologically inactive. Some of the current and past difficulties found in trying to correlate changes in plasma cortisol concentration with coincident changes in ACTH may be accounted for by this finding.

Plasma Binding and Metabolism of Glucocorticoids

Normally, the enzymatic transformation of cholesterol to cortisol occurs very rapidly. Therefore, only the final products are secreted in significant amounts from the adrenal cortex into the blood. Once secreted into the blood, cortisol is largely bound in a reversible (noncovalent), but tight, association, with an α_1-globulin termed "transcortin" or "corticosteroid-binding globulin" (CBG). The CBG-bound cortisol accounts for approximately 75% or slightly more of the total. Another 15% is loosely bound to albumin, and approximately 10% (or somewhat less) is present in plasma as free cortisol. It is this latter material which is immediately biologically active because it can diffuse easily across the capillary beds of the body and bathe all tissue cells, in all organs. If total plasma cortisol levels rise above approximately 20 to 25 μg%, the normal level of CBG is totally saturated (177). Further cortisol increments result in sharp elevations of the biologically active plasma free cortisol, as well as increases in cortisol loosely bound to albumin. The reversibility of cortisol binding to CBG also allows a continued, though decreasing, amount of free plasma cortisol to be made readily available during periods of secretory inactivity, or when total plasma cortisol falls to abnormally low levels, such as in adrenocortical insufficiency. CBG concentration is normally very constant and shows no diurnal variation, although the concentration may vary from individual to individual (39). No effect of gender or age has been found, though in an initial study (100) it was suggested that unipolar depressed patients had slightly lower cortisol-binding capacity, but this has not been subsequently confirmed. Disease states (nephrotic syndrome) can produce low CBG concentrations by a massive urinary loss of plasma protein, resulting in low total plasma cortisol, though free cortisol remains within the normal range, and continues its negative feedback role. Special physiological conditions, such as pregnancy or treatment with estrogens, induce an estrogen-dependent increased CBG production by the liver. This can result in a two- to threefold increase in total plasma cortisol with relatively little, though some, increase in the concentration of free plasma cortisol.

The free fraction or unbound fraction of plasma cortisol is that portion readily available for metabolic degradation, as well as for activation of specific effects on selected target tissues and cells. The major tissue accounting for cortisol degradation in humans is the liver, with much smaller amounts being enzymatically inactivated by muscle, intestines, connective tissue, fibroblasts, and lymphocytes. Although numerous (and minor) metabolic pathways exist for the inactivation of adrenocortical steroids, the major one involves serial, enzymatically determined steps. The most important initial reaction involves reduction of the "A" ring of the basic cyclopentophenanthrene steroid nucleus, resulting in the biologically inactive dihydrocortisol. Dihydrocortisol is rapidly converted to tetrahydrocortisol and further conjugated to form the glucuronide, or in smaller amounts, sulfate salt. All these compounds are hormonally inactive. The conversion to the polar glucuronide from the nonpolar native cortisol makes the compound more readily filterable through the glomerular membrane into the urine, its major route of excretion in humans. Small amounts of cortisol are converted to cortisone and similar enzymatic degradation of cortisone then occurs. The three other major compounds secreted by the adrenal cortex (aldosterone, corticosterone, and "androgens," especially DHEA) are mainly deactivated in the same manner as described for cortisol. However, much of DHEA is conjugated to sulfate rather than glucuronide, and is the principal precursor of so-called urinary or plasma 17-ketosteroids. Less than 0.5% of the total daily adrenocortical secretion of approximately 20 mg of cortisol appears in the urine as active nonmetabolized free cortisol. When there is excess adrenal secretion of cortisol such that the total capacity of CBG is exceeded, then increasing and elevated amounts of free cortisol in plasma do cross the glomerular membrane and are present in the urine.

Effects of Drugs on the HYPAC System

There are many chemical agents that are capable of producing notable perturbations or inhibition of HYPAC activity. Common substances of interest medically are alcohol, morphine, anesthetics, etc. These are outside the purview of this chapter and are discussed elsewhere (189). More important for the investigator studying HYPAC function in humans are the effects of a number of prescription or over-the-counter drugs that may have been ingested prior to the period of testing. For example, barbiturates are well-documented inducers of liver microsomal enzymes that are capable of increasing the metabolic degradation of dexamethasone. It has been shown that dexamethasone suppression test suppressors can be converted to nonsuppressors within 3 days of pentobarbital administration (but *not* benzodiazepines) in doses sufficient to produce mild daytime sedation and anxiolysis (186). Diphenylhydantoin (DPH) also interferes with the normal metabolism of cortisol via several mechanisms (92).

The prior administration of antidepressants or neuroleptics has apparently little direct effect on basal or stimulated HYPAC function, in spite of the effects of these drugs on CNS monoamines, including norepinephrine and serotonin, both of which seem to be important in the control of CRH release. Chronic administration of antidepressants in depressed patients with HYPAC hyperactivity usually results in a gradual return to normal HYPAC activity, either preceding or coincident with the return to euthymia (77). Sudden or abrupt withdrawal of tricyclic antidepressants (TCAs) may be associated with rebound changes in central monoamines and possibly altered HYPAC function (59).

CONTROL OF HYPOTHALAMIC AND PITUITARY ACTIVITY

The Nature of CRH and Hypothalamic Influences

CRH activity has been found in both hypothalamic and extrahypothalamic sites with bioassay (204). Extrahypothalamic CRH seems to differ from median eminence CRH in its potency and duration of action, and may be implicated in HYPAC activation during periods of prolonged stress (175). Hypothalamic CRH has been reported to increase within 2 to 4 min following acute stress (166), and CRH, in general, has been implicated in modification of various behaviors (12). The effects of CRH on the pituitary release of ACTH can be blocked by a number of substances, including substance P (89), somatostatin (197), and prostaglandins (199), as well as glucocorticoid administration.

Vasopressin has been known for many years to possess CRH-like activity (170). Vasopressin apparently acts by increasing ACTH release, as shown with posterior pituitary extracts and recently by enhanced ACTH release after combined CRH and vasopressin compared to CRH alone (56). Furthermore, adrenal insufficiency in humans is associated with increased vasopressin secretion, and this rapidly reverts to normal with replacement doses of glucocorticoids (1).

ACTH Release

ACTH is synthesized primarily in the anterior pituitary, though it may also be elaborated in the hypothalamus, amygdala, placenta, and certain tumors. The pituitary gland does not store large amounts of ACTH, though considerable amounts of the precursor molecule, proopiomelanocortin (POMC), are present. ACTH production is the result of specific stepwise cleavage of the precursor POMC (66), which also results in molecular equivalent amounts of β-endorphin. The major stimulus to production of pituitary POMC and ACTH is CRH.

ACTH secretion involves the interaction of a number of control factors including feedback mechanisms, circadian rhythms, and stress. Within minutes after activation of CRH release, the entire HYPAC axis responds, producing increases in peripheral plasma cortisol (86). Vasopressin enhances the release of ACTH and is probably important in initiating steroidogenesis, especially in response to strong stimuli. The pituitary is capable of producing and secreting very large amounts of ACTH chronically, without exhaustion. This phenomenon can be observed in states of chronic adrenocortical insufficiency and in the metyrapone test, which gives an estimate of the pituitary response to chemically induced, reversible adrenocortical insufficiency.

Extrahypothalamic Control of ACTH Release

As previously mentioned, the hypothalamus is related structurally and functionally to nuclei in the forebrain, midbrain, and limbic system. If all neural pathways to the medial basal hypothalamus are surgically severed in the rat, producing a hypothalamic island, plasma corticosterone levels remain steady and elevated, but diurnal rhythm is lost (67). Thus, extrahypothalamic mechanisms do not appear to be necessary for basal HYPAC activity. Recent studies, however, have demonstrated their role in regulation of ACTH release in response to physiological demands. In general, those areas found to contain glucocorticoid feedback receptors are those which have been implicated in HYPAC regulation via stimulation or lesion studies in animals.

The ascending reticular activating system (ARAS), a region involved in maintaining arousal, appears to exert both inhibitory and facilitory influences on the HYPAC system, which are probably mediated via different neural pathways (192). For example, stimulation of the ARAS was shown to result in increased ACTH release when HYPAC activity was low, and decreased release during HYPAC activation. Ganong (49) reported that bilateral destruction of the amygdaloid nuclei in the dog reduced the ACTH response to immobilization stress, but not to gut traction. Furthermore, stimulation of the anteromedial amygdala results in HYPAC activation, whereas similar stimulation to the basolateral amygdala has the opposite effect (178), thus illustrating the importance of functional localization within each of these classically recognized extrahypothalamic anatomical regions, and showing differential distribution of receptors within anatomically defined nuclei [consistent with work by McEwen and others (122–124)]. Finally, HYPAC activation in response to *prolonged* amygdaloid stimulation is not maintained, although the system is functionally able to respond further (163).

Hippocampal lesioning results in chronically elevated basal levels of plasma corticosterone (154), suggesting a tonic inhibitory influence on HYPAC activity. However, similar to the ARAS, the influence of the hippocampus appears to depend on the prior functional activity of the HYPAC system. For example, the stress-induced release of ACTH is blocked by hippocampal stimulation (42), but resting pituitary adrenocortical activity is facilitated (98). Transection of the fornix, which contains hippocampal/hypothalamic projections, has been shown to transiently abolish the circadian periodicity of corticosterone in the rat (128).

The role of brain centers in HYPAC regulation remains to be elucidated further, and such studies may prove particularly useful in the search for neurobiological underpinnings of affective disorder.

Neurotransmitter Regulation of CRH/ACTH Release

Most of the putative neurotransmitters have been identified in the median eminence of the hypothalamus. To date, however, the specific effects of a given neurotransmitter on CRH/ACTH release remain controversial. It has already been noted that ACTH secretion occurs under a variety of conditions, and that many neurotransmitter pathways involved in CRH release impinge on the specialized neurosecretory cells within the hypothalamus. Therefore, although many studies point to the importance and involvement of a *particular* neurotransmitter, the picture emerging is a complex one.

In general, cholinergic pathways have been found to be associated with ACTH release *in vivo* and *in vitro*. Evidence that norepinephrine (NE) plays an inhibitory role in CRH/ACTH release comes from neuropharmacological manipulations of catecholaminergic pathways. However, there is also evidence to suggest a role of NE in facilitation of ACTH release. Although serotonin (5-hydroxytryptamine; 5-HT) pathways have been implicated in the control of HYPAC secretion, the issue of whether 5-HT is excitatory or inhibitory to ACTH release has not been satisfactorily resolved. A number of other substances, such as GABA, histamine, and various peptides have been examined as possible regulators of CRH/ACTH release. At present, there are no substantive data to support or refute their role in HYPAC regulation. A more detailed discussion of neuroregulation of CRH is given by Gold and Rubinow in Chapter 61 (*this volume*). For a comprehensive review of currently available evidence and controversies in the area of neurotransmitter regulation of CRH/ACTH release, see Jones et al. (152).

NEUROPHYSIOLOGY OF HYPAC FUNCTION

Feedback

The hypothalamus from the optic chiasm to the mamillary bodies contributes to activation of CRH-mediated ACTH release from the pituitary (13). Thus graded lesions within this hypothalamic area produce graded defects in the pituitary adrenal response. Further pituitary ACTH release results from electrical stimulation over a similar wide area of the ventral hypothalamus (37). These findings underscore the widespread hypothalamic input into the control of these vital secretions, in contrast to the relatively localized hypothalamic centers for gonadotropin-releasing factors.

There is now clear and recurrent evidence that the concentration of CRH in the median eminence region is increased after adrenalectomy and decreased with exogenous glucocorticoid treatment, as initially demonstrated over 20 years ago. Evidence for a short loop feedback effect of ACTH on the hypothalamic median eminence secretion of CRH has also been available for many years. Adrenalectomized animals show increased median eminence CRH concentration, and hypophysectomy increases this further. Treatment of these adrenalectomized/hypophysectomized animals with ACTH decreases the median eminence CRH concentration to levels observed with adrenalectomy alone (130). Furthermore, adrenalectomized rats treated with ACTH have histological changes consistent with short loop feedback effects of ACTH on median eminence CRH secretion, such as alterations in median eminence cell nuclei (79) and increases in median eminence neurosecretory material.

Prior to the 1970s, conclusions about the secretion of CRH were generally derived from measurements of cortisol and bioassay of ACTH. ACTH has only recently been measurable by direct radioimmunoassay rather than bioassay, and plasma samples often reveal more immunoassayable than bioassayable ACTH. This would suggest that biologically inactive ACTH fragments, or precursors, in plasma are included in the immunoassayable ACTH.

The HYPAC axis, like all the neuroendocrine axes, has feedback loops that help to maintain an intrinsic homeostatic system. Feedback processes in the HYPAC axis are generally inhibitory, i.e., the target gland regulates its own secretion (cortisol) by depressing the release of the corresponding tropic (ACTH) and releasing (CRH) hormones. All available evidence suggests that positive feedback does not appear to play a pivotal role, since surgical isolation of the medial basal hypothalamus results in tonic secretion of corticosterone (67). Rather, *disinhibition* of negative feedback mechanisms occurs when circulating cortisol concentrations decrease, and this process is responsive to both rate of change and absolute level. Thus, the corticotropes (pituitary cells secreting ACTH) are programmed to halt ACTH secretion above a certain "set point," and resume secretion when corticosteroid concentrations fall below a certain level. The HYPAC system is essentially a closed loop system. However, this reciprocal system would tend to damp out if were not for added positive inputs from other brain centers that activate the system. For example, a prime drive source is the brain oscillator that induces the circadian rhythm of the HYPAC axis and is linked to temperature and sleep-wake cycle. Additionally, a variety of physical and psychological stimuli (e.g., stress, endocrine disease) acting through neural pathways that finally impinge on hypothalamic CRH secretory cells may enhance or restrict CRH release or modulate feedback processes via alterations in "set point."

Perhaps the earliest work showing negative feedback from the adrenal cortex to the pituitary was performed by Ingle in the 1930s (80). Adrenocortical extracts injected into rats resulted in adrenocortical atrophy, but combinations of anterior pituitary and adrenocortical extracts did not produce adrenal atrophy. Sayers and Sayers (168) showed that corticosteroids can produce an immediate (now called "fast"), as well as a delayed, inhibition of ACTH release. These same experiments also demonstrated that HYPAC response to a stressful stimulus was proportional to the intensity of that stimulus and was inhibited when corticosteroids were administered before the stimulus. The physiological relevance of this feedback effect in humans was perhaps first clearly demonstrated by James and co-workers (83). This group reported that infusion of cortisol at a rate equal to the endogenous production rate in humans (20–25 mg/day) produced no increase in the total urinary excretion of 17-OHCS, which were largely derived metabolically from cortisol. This finding suggests negative feedback mechanisms with the ability to compensate for exogenous administered corticosteroid by equivalent decrements in endogenous production. Further evidence for a negative feedback mechanism comes from the observation that plasma ACTH levels are promptly and persistently elevated after adrenalectomy in rats and humans, and are reduced to normal with replacement therapy. In adrenalectomized animals or in humans, ACTH release after stress is greatly exaggerated above that observed in intact animals or humans.

It is now clear that ACTH secretion is regulated by two distinct forms of feedback. The first is a fast, rate-sensitive feedback occurring within minutes of an increase or rise in plasma corticosteroids (cortisol in humans). The second feedback is termed "delayed" or "proportional" feedback, which occurs some time after corticosteroid administration, when plasma levels may still be high or are declining or have reached lower levels. The fast feedback component is transient, lasting less than 10 min in some animal species, and is initiated by a sudden increase in glucocorticoid concentration impinging on the rate-sensitive mechanisms in the pituitary and/or CNS. It is followed by a silent period during which feedback is relatively inactive, and stressful stimuli may produce some release of ACTH. The silent period ends with the beginning of the delayed or proportional feedback control. This response is progressive in its inhibitory effects on the functioning of the HYPAC system and persists at least as long as corticosteroid levels are elevated.

In humans, the rate of increase of plasma corticosteroid necessary to initiate fast feedback is much greater than normal in individuals with Cushing's disease, but somewhat reduced in those with autonomous adrenocortical tumors. "Paradoxical" (positive) fast or rate-sensitive feedback has also been shown to occur, for reasons that are not clear, in some patients with pituitary-dependent Cushing's disease during the first 15 min of cortisol infusion. Removal of the pituitary adenoma does not correct this abnormality, but 1 week of administration of the serotonin antagonist cyproheptadine does (110). This effect of cyproheptadine on the early feedback abnormality may be caused by a direct inhibition of ACTH release from the pituitary microadenoma. Cyproheptadine has been shown to inhibit ACTH secretion from pituitary tumors *in vitro* as well as in ectopic ACTH syndrome (111). However, a direct inhibitory effect of cyproheptadine on central serotonergic pathways cannot be ruled out, even though animal data indicate that serotonin pathways mediate late corticosteroid feedback inhibition of ACTH secretion rather than early rate-sensitive feedback.

Many steroids have little or no effect on fast feedback inhibition, but glucocorticoids such as cortisol and corticosterone are both active in humans (90). Negative feedback effects of various steroids may occur at different sites. Moreover, the effects of various glucocorticoids may not be identical because of different regional cellular and nuclear uptakes in brain and pituitary. Fast and delayed feedback sites are probably different in type and location, both regionally and intracellularly (e.g., cell membrane and cytosol as genome).

Further data supporting the presence of a rate-sensitive fast feedback mechanism in humans are obtained from infusion of saline and cortisol alternately over many hours (36). ACTH secretion was inhibited during intervals when plasma cortisol levels were rising, but resumed when cortisol levels plateaued, whether high or low in the physiological range. There was no correlation between inhibition of ACTH secretion and *absolute* level of circulating cortisol or total dose of cortisol administered. In humans, initiation of fast feedback is also relatively slower in onset, perhaps up to 30 min, whereas it is much shorter in the rat (a period of seconds or minutes) (36,86). These studies also provide evidence for a difference between rat and human in terms of the onset of the delayed or proportional feedback inhibition. In the rat it occurs within approximately 2 hr, but in humans the time to onset may be considerably longer.

It should be noted that the data for feedback function in humans are based on studies done under basal conditions. At the present there is little direct evidence showing fast feedback (inhibition) to be present in a physiologically revelant manner in humans during conditions of stress. Some of the difficulties in ascertaining the effects of steroids on HYPAC function are related to procedural differences. It is more and more evident that considerations of dosage, frequency of administration, and time of subsequent testing of the HYPAC axis are important in defining fast versus delayed feedback effects. The response of the system to corticosteroid may also be considerably different with regard to acute stressful stimuli versus chronic ones, such as depression.

There are some stresses to which the HYPAC response is not suppressible by any dose of short-term administration of steroids. Examples of these steroid-resistant stressors are gut traction at laparotomy or severe hemorrhage that occurs at a rate above a certain minimum (33). It has long been known that protracted administration of steroids rapidly produces atrophy of the adrenal cortex and diminution of pituitary ACTH and hypothalamic CRH. Studies by Liddle et al. (115) showed the hierarchical recovery of the HYPAC system in individuals who had been exposed to chronically high autonomous steroid output from adrenal tumors. It was many months before ACTH secretion returned, and some months thereafter before adrenal cortisol secretion was manifest. Consequently, it should not be surprising,

from this and prior animal studies, that repeated and protracted high-dose steroid administration inhibits the HYPAC response to any subsequent stress. In fact, partial inhibition of the HYPAC response to stress after a short-term, but repeated, administration of steroid has been shown (176). Specifically, large doses of dexamethasone, applied over 1 day, reduced steroid-resistant stresses to suppressible ones. These kinds of changes may be reflective of early involution or atrophy of the HYPAC system. Some data are now available to support this conclusion. It has been shown (50) that dexamethasone pretreatment does not alter the concentration of mRNA translation for ACTH precursors in mouse pituitary tumor cells in culture until after the dexamethasone treatment continues for approximately 6 to 12 hr. After that time, there is evidence for decreased mRNA activity. Thereafter ACTH production will progressively fail and ACTH reserves might become rapidly exhausted in vivo. In fact, adrenal atrophy in rats has been observed after 24 hr of continued treatment with dexamethasone (34). Moreover, hypothalamic implants of dexamethasone cause hypothalamic CRH and pituitary ACTH concentrations to fall rapidly (28).

The sites of feedback activity by corticosteroids are multiple and still have not been fully mapped out in humans. Glucocorticoids do have an immediate feedback effect on ACTH release from dispersed pituitary cells in vitro (179), suggesting the existence of fast feedback mechanisms at this level. However data collected from in vivo studies suggest that the fast feedback effects of steroids are probably mediated at sites above the pituitary. Moreover, the work of McEwen and co-workers (125) and Sapolsky and co-workers (165) suggests that at least in the rat, steroid receptors in the hippocampus are very important in the suppression of HYPAC activity. Binding of corticosteroids to pituitary, hypothalamus, septum, and hippocampus has been identified, but there is no compelling evidence to suggest that these areas play a role in negative feedback (123).

Recent data (164) have shown that the number of receptors and cells in the hippocampus decreases in aged rats, while circulating plasma corticosterone levels simultaneously increase. This resonates with current data from human studies that reveal a positive correlation between advancing age and plasma cortisol levels, as well as increased incidence of dexamethasone suppression test (DST) nonsuppression (4,53,187). Sapolsky (164) has suggested that administration of exogenous steroid has in fact caused hippocampal cell loss in non-aged rats. The implication here is that the cells that are sensing the circulating corticosteroid and influencing negative feedback are in some way adversely affected by steroid per se. Perhaps a high concentration of steroids within the receptor-laden cells in some way produces enhanced catabolic and finally lethal effects on those cells, similar to the effects observed on tissues in general, when subjected to persistent high glucocorticoid levels.

The initial mechanism by which corticoids exert a feedback effect appears to involve release of CRH (and perhaps ACTH). Onset of fast feedback can occur very rapidly in some species (within minutes of glucocorticoid administration), suggesting an effect on release of hormone, perhaps

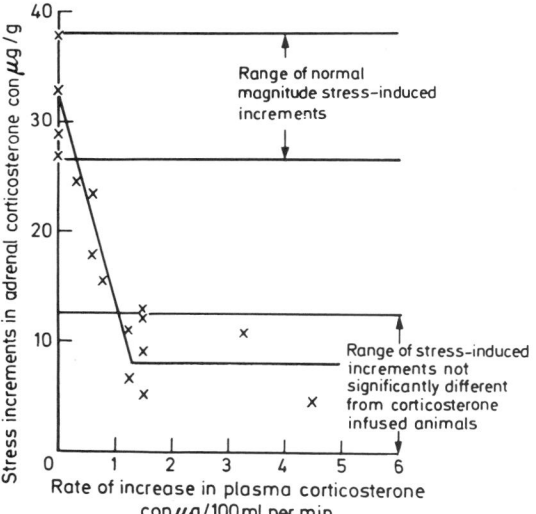

FIG. 2. Relationship between magnitude of the stress response and the rate of increase of plasma corticosterone. (From ref. 88.)

occurring at the cell membrane. It has been shown that during initial stages of corticosteroid inhibition of CRH release, there is an increase in the tissue content of CRH, as though synthesis were continuing (86). Delayed corticosteroid feedback is clearly associated with a reduction in CRH synthesis as well as release (87). This inhibition of release can be observed within 1 to 2 hr, but reduction in synthesis of CRH, a clear genome effect (observed decrease in mRNA), requires at least 6 hr and is not maximal until 48 hr (151).

The neural pathways that mediate steroid feedback inhibition are not yet clear. It does appear that noradrenergic neural input is necessary for fast feedback, since destruction of noradrenergic neurons by pretreatment with 6-hydroxydopamine prevents the (expected) fast feedback effect of corticosterone on histamine-induced CRH synthesis (95). The current concept is that the steroid-nonsuppressible HYPAC responses are transmitted via steroid-resistant neural pathways. There may in addition be an effect of glucocorticoids at the cell bodies in the hypothalamus or on the final neurons having an input into the CRH peptidergic neurosecretory neurons.

Delayed feedback also appears to involve corticosteroid action at the level of the hypothalamus and pituitary, probably both simultaneously. After prolonged or repeated treatment with large doses of glucocorticoids, the HYPAC response to both steroid-sensitive and initially steroid-resistant stimuli is inhibited. This treatment results in suppression of hypothalamic CRH and pituitary ACTH production and content (33). The combined affect of glucocorticoids on hypothalamic *and* pituitary activity is shown by earlier work demonstrating greater inhibition of ACTH secretion when glucocorticoids are placed in the hypothalamus rather than the pituitary (28,179).

The role of monoamine neurotransmitter systems on release of CRH may be species-specific (e.g., dog vs rat vs human) and is not completely understood in humans (51,95). NE and possibly epinephrine appear inhibitory to CRH release in the rat and dog (51). ACTH release can be inhibited by nanogram amounts of NE injected into the third but not into the fourth ventricle. Intracarotid clonidine, a centrally active α-adrenergic agonist, inhibits ACTH secretion when given in systemically ineffective doses. α-Adrenergic blockers injected into the third ventricle can prevent this. Stimulation of ascending noradrenergic (and adrenergic) pathways in the brainstem is associated with inhibition of ACTH release (152). Most evidence suggests that NE acts postsynaptically to inhibit CRH/ACTH release. This central α-adrenergic inhibition of CRH/ACTH release is less clear in other species, but apparently is present in the rat and the human. The potential importance of species differences is demonstrated in studies of *un*anesthetized dogs. Here L-dopa, which would be expected to produce mainly noradrenergic postsynaptic activation, caused stimulation of adrenal glucocorticoids. This was prevented by prior administration of pimozide, a centrally acting DA receptor blocker, suggesting that central dopaminergic mechanisms are important to the control of ACTH release in the dog (51). No clear evidence for this dopaminergic effect exists in humans. The role of *serotonin* in CRH/

ACTH release is disputed. Serotonin has been thought to be important in control of the circadian rhythm of ACTH release (169), and others have proposed a serotonergic inhibition of CRH release in view of the decrease in plasma cortisol and ACTH after administration of the serotonin blocker cyproheptadine in patients with Cushing's syndrome (110).

Brain Glucocorticoid Receptors

In 1968 McEwen (124) reported greater uptake and retention of tritiated corticosteroid in the hippocampus of adrenalectomized rats than in other brain areas, such as the hypothalamus, cortex, pituitary gland, or septum, or than in the plasma, and subsequently these findings were extended in subhuman primates. The uptake and retention of corticosterone were particularly evident in Ammon's horn and the granule neurons of the dentate gyrus of the hippocampus. The specific retention of corticosteroid in the hippocampus was subsequently explained by the discovery of the presence of soluble and cell nuclear macromolecules with a high affinity for corticosterone (63).

It is notable that at high levels of corticosterone, brain nuclear retention of the steroid may occur in glial cells. It is clear from the time course of *in vivo* labeling studies with tritiated corticosterone that cytosol receptor binding precedes cell nuclear receptor binding as the macromolecular cytosol-bound corticosterone is transferred gradually to nuclear binding sites. Dexamethasone does not have the affinity for the CBG-like cytosol receptor, and though high concentrations can get into the cell, the dexamethasone is not retained selectively by the hippocampus. Dexamethasone is found in large amounts in the pituitary (38) and can label the pituitary even in the presence of corticosterone, unless very high levels of the latter steroid are present. Interestingly, tritiated dexamethasone radioactivity has been found to be highest near the cerebral ventricles, indicating that this steroid may in part enter the brain by diffusion from the ventricle. Glial cells are probably glucocorticoid targets, and thus it appears that the initial diffuse uptake of dexamethasone throughout the brain is probably a reflection of glial cell uptake, whereas the subsequent regional variations in uptake of corticosterone retention are dependent on presence of selective uptake and nuclear retention in particular brain areas, e.g., hippocampus. It should be noted, however, that even brain areas that do not retain corticosterone on autoradiography show glucocorticoid receptors on biochemical assay (136). Interestingly, the effects of corticosterone on GABA uptake in the hippocampus are such as to inhibit transmission within the hippocampus, decreasing GABA uptake. These electrical effects of the steroid could be a byproduct of their action on the genome (44).

Corticosterone appears to inhibit hippocampal function. The specificity of hippocampal steroid uptake is evident in those behavioral studies that reveal corticosterone to be effective in changing behavior in animals while dexamethasone is not (127). Hippocampal uptake of corticosterone is associated with a rapid decrease in electrical activity and inhibition of high-affinity GABA uptake in the hippocampus. Thus, McEwen has suggested that the influence of hippocampal uptake of corticosterone may be opposite to the normal action of the dorsal bundle, which increases selective attention. The hippocampus also has an effect on HYPAC function, as demonstrated by the fact that lesions of the hippocampus, much like fornix transection, reduce the negative feedback effects of steroids on HYPAC activity. Overall, one might at this point conclude that steroid uptake in the hippocampus tends to act like hippocampal ablation, in that hippocampal function is suppressed.

It has been recently shown (171) that peripheral lymphocytes from patients with adrenocortical insufficiency have fewer binding sites and increased binding affinity for glucocorticoids. Replacement with usual doses of cortisone produced a decrease in binding affinity toward normal but no change in receptor number, at least over the time interval studied. Since glucocorticoid receptors are present in many cells, there may be similar changes in the human brain, specifically the hippocampus.

The behavioral or nonendocrine effects of various HYPAC system secretions, as well as their specific endocrine functions within the axis, are further demonstrated by recent data showing that CRH-specific receptors exist in the rat forebrain. There are also nonendocrine behavioral effects of CRH given by intracerebroventricular (ICV) administration that underscore the role of this peptide in behavior (113).

Circadian Rhythm of the HYPAC Axis

The circadian rhythm of the HYPAC axis occurs in a variety of animal species, including humans and other primates. The limbic (hippocampal-fornix) system is intimately related to this rhythm. Transection of the fornix will at least temporarily disrupt the circadian rhythm (128), as will administration of parachlorophenylalanine (pCPA) (169). This latter finding demonstrates that serotonergic pathways influence the circadian periodicity of the HYPAC axis. In fact, there is also a circadian pattern in the CNS content of serotonin, which suggests the existence of an endogenous CNS pacemaker controlling HYPAC cyclicity (169). Interestingly, in the rat brain this serotonin circadian rhythm matures at the same time as the appearance of a diurnal HYPAC rhythm.

Circadian rhythmicity and the HYPAC stress response appear to be dissociable systems, since the control of the circadian rhythm appears developmentally later in the rat pup than the HYPAC stress response (112). Furthermore, in animals with anterior hypothalamic lesions sufficient to remove the circadian rhythm, the stress response can still be elicited (34).

Although the circadian rhythm of the HYPAC axis is endogenous, its phase can be entrained by several zeitgebers. This rhythm is altered to a persistent low level following protracted continuous light exposure, and is phase-shifted by food and water restriction (97). Additionally, sleep/wake patterns are known to influence its rhythmicity, although the 24-hr periodicity is generally resistant to short-term

changes in the sleep/wake cycle. Hypothalamic circadian CRH levels continue in the absence of ACTH (191,202) and corticosteroid feedback (106), though the CRH concentration may be altered.

The currently recognized HYPAC circadian rhythm, consisting of a sequence of irregular bursts of release of ACTH and cortisol, was first described in 1970 from studies in humans (73). Subsequent studies indicated that the pattern of pulsatile release of cortisol roughly relates to immediately prior ACTH pulses, although there is not always a one-to-one relationship. It should be noted that in normal healthy individuals, a steady-state level of cortisol is not present for any long period during the day. Furthermore, there is considerable variability in secretory output, duration, and latency of secretory episodes, not only between individuals, but also in a given individual on different days. In general, however, the pattern of cortisol release shows increasing secretory episodes early in the morning hours, with decreasing secretion in the late afternoon and evening in healthy subjects. The increased frequency and duration of the cortisol bursts during the early morning hours (just prior to awakening) and until about 10:00 a.m. results in a gradual accumulation of plasma cortisol due to its prolonged plasma half-life (approximately 60 min). The HYPAC system uses this frequency modulation at the hypothalamic CRH level to produce frequency and amplitude modulation of severalfold at the pituitary and adrenal level (95).

Early studies in humans showed that there was also a nyctohemeral rhythm to adrenal responsiveness to exogenous ACTH, with greater early morning steroid secretion (135,140). Later work with submaximal ACTH administration confirmed this day-night adrenal cortical sensitivity difference in rats, revealing both adrenal gland cyclic AMP and plasma corticosteroid response to be approximately 2.5 times greater just before onset of darkness in these nocturnal animals. However, persistent maximal adrenal stimulation with exogenous ACTH produces the same response morning and night. In rats this adrenal gland rhythm persists for 1 or 2 days without ACTH (postdexamethasone) showing dissociation of adrenal gland ACTH rhythms in vivo similar to that reported in organ culture (195) and hypophysectomized fishes (195). There is also some evidence for at least "partially autonomous" CRH-independent ACTH secretion via the pituitary gland (95).

The circadian rhythm and responsiveness of the HYPAC axis appear to be influenced by extrapituitary non-ACTH mechanisms, though the phase of this rhythm is controlled by a CNS oscillator probably located in the suprachiasmatic nucleus. The presence of extrapituitary mechanisms has been suggested by the preservation of plasma corticosteroid rhythms in hypophysectomized killifish (182) and in hypophysectomized rats implanted with beeswax pellets containing slowly and constantly released ACTH and thyroxine (182), as well as by persistent daily rhythms in adrenal cyclic AMP and cyclic GMP in hypophysectomized rats (64). These rhythms can be abolished by autotransplantation of the adrenal (202) and more convincingly by transection of the spinal cord at T_5 or T_7, but not by low spinal cord transection at L_1 (137). These findings support prior work showing a neural connection between the hypothalamus and the adrenal gland that mediates compensatory adrenal hypertrophy (43). Some data suggest similar mechanisms in humans, and factors other than ACTH secretion appear to be important in the rhythms and responsiveness of the adrenal cortex (47). In ACTH-deficient patients, the prolonged infusion of small "subthreshold" amounts of ACTH was associated with "marked oscillations" of plasma cortisol concentration, even though the "occasional" measured plasma ACTH values were "less than 15 ng/ml." Thus far the data suggesting a *clear* dissociation between ACTH and cortisol secretion in man are less than compelling, though of great interest. Such neural connections are also suggested by the observation that the number of adrenal glands (none, one, or two) remaining in an animal is inversely related to the level of ACTH observed after a stimulus activation of that HYPAC system or the amount of administered glucocorticoid needed to inhibit the ACTH release.

PATHOLOGY OF THE HYPAC AXIS IN AFFECTIVE ILLNESS

Circadian Rhythm Disturbances

Before 1970, attempts to examine rhythmic disturbances of corticosteroid secretion in affective illness were limited by infrequent blood sampling, and thus actually reflected altered *diurnal variation* in HYPAC activity (e.g., 11,17,30,121). Moreover, these early investigations were conducted before the complexity of the normal 24-hr cortisol secretory pattern had been revealed (73). Sampling of plasma cortisol levels at 20-min intervals revealed that compared to normals, depressed patients had more secretory episodes, secreted more cortisol per episode, spent more time in active secretion, and actively secreted cortisol during nighttime periods when adrenal activity in normals is quiescent (160). These abnormalities reverted to a more normal pattern following successful treatment. Subsequent studies suggested a phase advance in the daily nadir of cortisol secretion (84,141), but others reported conflicting results (206). Despite HYPAC hypersecretion in depressed patients, the morning peak and evening trough in cortisol concentrations are generally preserved. Only in a few severely depressed individuals does the circadian profile become flattened. However, the normal diurnal variation in cortisol secretion appears blunted, due to relatively heightened evening activity.

Recently, disturbances in the temporal pattern of cortisol and corticotropin secretion have been related to abnormalities in feedback inhibition, as detected by the DST (96,141). In one study, DST nonsuppressors were found to have not only higher mean UFC circadian levels than controls while depressed, but also elevated *circannual* levels of cortisol excretion when clinically recovered (96). These results, however, were based on a small sample.

It has been suggested that elevated plasma cortisol and resistance to DST suppression in depressed patients are secondary to excessive ACTH secretion by the pituitary; however, limited basal sampling of ACTH (6) and postdexamethasone (0800, 1600, 2300) sampling of ACTH (45,148)

suggest conflicting findings. Recently, some studies employing multiple circadian sampling have revealed that postdexamethasone ACTH in depressed patients is elevated relative to controls, regardless of DST status (141). Furthermore, the amplitude and duration of ACTH secretory pulses were greater in the depressed group, and the cortisol rhythm was phase-advanced. Similar findings were reported by Linkowski et al. (117); however, normal and depressed subjects did not differ in mean 24-hr ACTH concentration. Taken together, these observations suggest that HYPAC hypersecretion in some depressed patients is related to changes in pulse amplitude, rather than pulse frequency.

Few studies have systemically examined HYPAC circadian rhythm disturbances during the manic phase, though other related rhythms, such as 3-methoxy-4-hydroxyphenylglycol (MHPG) (198), have been examined. Although some basal studies report no significant change in cortisol production or urinary excretion of 17-OHCS (159), others note loss of diurnal variation in plasma cortisol (142). In one study, 24-hr monitoring of cortisol and aldosterone levels in manic patients did, however, reveal elevated levels of aldosterone, but no apparent change in integrated concentration of cortisol (2).

At present it is not clear whether these circadian disturbances represent (a) dysfunction of the main circadian pacemaker ("master clock"); (b) desynchronization of only some physiological functions such that they are no longer entrained to environmental cues and are discordant with other rhythms; or (c) an epiphenomenon derived from depressive symptomatology (e.g., disrupted sleep, appetite, and activity levels).

Basal vs Dynamic Tests

In assessing the status of a hormonal system, it is often useful to obtain both *basal* (resting) measures and *dynamic* measures (stimulation/suppression tests) of the system's function. The latter methods enable us to assess the functional capacity of the system, its reserve capacity, and its ability to respond to stress, as well as the integrity of negative feedback mechanisms. In a system that incorporates several functionally interdependent organs like the HYPAC axis (brain-pituitary-adrenal cortex), the need for both types of measures is increased.

Basal Tests

Severe endogenous depression is frequently accompanied by altered HYPAC activity. These abnormalities have been reflected by changes in basal levels of cortisol, ACTH, and CRH, measured in blood (plasma), urine, saliva, and cerebrospinal fluid. In consequence alterations in circadian or nyctohemeral rhythms can ensue (*vide supra*).

PLASMA CORTISOL AND PLASMA ACTH

Plasma Cortisol

In many, but not all, patients with endogenous depression, basal plasma cortisol levels have been found to be elevated over control values. Since Board and his colleagues (8) reported increased mean plasma 17-OHCS levels in depressed patients, a number of researchers have reported significant effects of diagnostic category on *basal* cortisol measures, including morning plasma cortisol, urine free cortisol, and CSF cortisol (24,25,187), and others have replicated and extended these findings. Moreover, a correlation between severity of depression and elevation of plasma cortisol has been shown, with a decrease in plasma levels as depressive symptoms subside.

As previously mentioned, these HYPAC disturbances do not appear to be the result of undifferentiated emotional arousal. Plasma abnormalities have been extensively reviewed (21,27,156) and thus will not be detailed here.

Elevated plasma cortisol provides increased tissue exposure to biologically active cortisol. After plasma CBG becomes saturated, unbound cortisol levels increase exponentially. Measurement of plasma free cortisol levels in depression has generally not proven fruitful because of methodologic and interpretational difficulties. Preliminary evidence, however, suggests that plasma free cortisol may be elevated in some depressed patients (27), but not to the same extent as that seen in Cushing's disease. At present, integrated levels of free cortisol present in the urine and CSF seem to provide better estimates of tissue exposure to unbound cortisol.

The nature of cortisol production in the manic state has been less extensively investigated. Manic bipolar patients have been found to have elevated (142,187), normal (159), and low (55) levels of plasma cortisol. These inconsistencies may in part arise from differences in clinical state, activity level, sleep/wake disturbances, and limited plasma sampling.

Although elevated basal plasma cortisol appears to provide a useful biological marker, the complex nature of HYPAC physiology prevents us from drawing any simplified conclusions about its etiology. The disturbance could clearly occur at any of several levels of the HYPAC axis or the CNS. Not to be downplayed either are the *effects* of cortisol hypersecretion on the HYPAC axis itself, on other physiological systems, and on brain and behavioral variables.

Plasma ACTH

Over the years it has been speculated that changes in cortisol release parallel similar changes in ACTH release by the pituitary. However, recent studies suggest that changing plasma cortisol levels are *not always* directly linked to concomitant pituitary ACTH secretion (74). Moreover, paradoxical feedback responses to cortisol have been reported for ACTH (48). Initial uncontrolled studies (6) found normal basal plasma ACTH levels in endogenous depression, though many values were in the upper part of the normal range. Subsequent systematic studies reported no difference in ACTH levels between cortisol suppressors and nonsuppressors postdexamethasone (45,132,205), but in some cases a correlation between plasma ACTH and plasma cortisol was noted (101). However, contradictory evidence also exists, and recent findings indicate that ACTH is indeed elevated in cortisol nonsuppressors (76,94,148). Discrepancies may be due to differences in

frequency of blood sampling, since ACTH is secreted episodically and has a very short half-life. Recent studies (see Circadian Rhythm of the HYPAC Axis), employing more frequent sampling over a 24-hr period, may help clarify this issue (117,141). Also questionable is the validity of the ACTH radioimmunoassays, since not all immunoassayable ACTH is biologically active (172).

Urine Glucocorticoids

While measurement of adrenal corticoids in plasma provides a fairly accurate minute-by-minute description of HYPAC functioning, urinary assessments provide an integrated measure of HYPAC activity over time. Many, but not all early studies conducted before 1970, reported elevated urinary excretion of cortisol metabolites (17-hydroxycorticosteroids or 17-OHCS, and 17-ketogenic steroids or 17-KGS) in patients suffering from depression (19,108,119). In manic bipolar patients, however, 17-OHCS and 17-KGS were usually normal (20,155).

There has long been evidence to suggest that urinary 17-OHCS and 17-KGS do not always correlate well with plasma indices (31,153). In fact, the urinary 17-OHCS excretion reflects less than 50% of total cortisol secretion (82), and both 17-OHCS and 17-KGS determinations are affected by a number of factors (82,143). Moreover, in stress situations, 17-OHCS excretion has been found to underestimate the actual degree of HYPAC activation (99). Measurements of urinary free cortisol (UFC), have in many studies, replaced 17-OHCS or 17-KGS as a more sensitive measure of HYPAC activity. UFC, which reflects the physiologically active free portion of plasma cortisol, has been shown to be elevated in many endogenously depressed patients compared to normals and other psychiatric populations (24,187). UFC levels in hypomanic and manic bipolar patients have also been studied, but findings are less consistent. While some investigators suggest that only severely psychotic manics show elevated UFC levels, others have observed state-related *lowered* 24 hour mean UFC values in a number of patients during the manic phase (183). In general, the amount of free urinary cortisol has been found to correlate well with other indices of HYPAC function. While normals secrete very small amounts of UFC, this increases exponentially with increasing rates of cortisol secretion, and thus its measurement can provide useful information in cases of HYPAC hyperactivity.

Saliva

Recently, measurement of saliva cortisol concentration has been suggested as a noninvasive alternative to blood measurements in normal and depressed individuals (150). There are, however, some caveats to be taken into consideration (109). First, saliva cortisol levels are only 4 to 6% of the *total* found in plasma, because only the unbound portion enters the saliva. Thus, colorimetric and fluorimetric assays are generally not sensitive enough, and commercial kits formulated for direct RIA must be modified. In addition, some of the cortisol transported from blood to saliva is rapidly converted to cortisone by 11β-hydroxysteroid de-hydrogenase present in the salivary glands, so that saliva cortisol levels are between 60 and 100% of plasma *free* cortisol (14). Furthermore, there is a time lag between plasma levels of cortisol and corresponding saliva levels, which may vary from individual to individual (68), though a high correlation with serum cortisol level was reported in a small group of subjects. Poland and Rubin (144) found higher saliva cortisol levels in dexamethasone escapers, but a large variation in the pre- and postdexamethasone saliva/serum cortisol ratio. These results suggest that at present, saliva cortisol levels are not an unequivocal substitute for blood determinations of cortisol.

Cerebrospinal Fluid Measures

CRH, ACTH, and cortisol have all been found in measurable quantities in human cerebrospinal fluid (CSF), but cortisol has been the most extensively studied. Early investigations of CSF cortisol concentrations reported either *lower* CSF cortisol in the depressed patients (122) or no difference between depressed patients and controls with neurologic disorders (85). Subsequent studies, employing more improved methodology, found significantly higher CSF cortisol levels in depressives than in normal controls and other psychiatric groups (25,54,187,194). Moreover, many of these investigators also concurrently validated their findings with peripheral cortisol measurements in plasma and urine. These results have a number of implications. First, CSF cortisol may provide a relatively *stable* integrated measure of HYPAC activity, as opposed to plasma levels, which are subject to minor and rapid perturbations. Second, anatomical and physiological studies have provided indirect evidence to suggest that cortisol in CSF may play an active role in CNS function. For example, the CSF may function as a reservoir by which free cortisol feeds back on regions implicated in HYPAC regulation. Additionally, several circumventricular areas appear to contain corticosteroid-responsive tissue which may be sensitive to CSF cortisol concentrations. Furthermore, electron microscopic studies suggest that CSF cortisol may have direct access to the hypophyseal portal system via active transport (103). Finally, high CSF levels of cortisol may act to alter neurotransmitter levels within the brain (173).

Centrally derived ACTH has also been detected in CSF by radioimmunoassay (91). However, CSF concentrations of ACTH have not yet been extensively and completely systematically assessed in affective disorder patients, though preliminary studies are currently being presented at international conferences.

Recently, the presence of immunoreactive CRH (I-CRH) has been demonstrated in human CSF (193). In order to elucidate further the role of extrapituitary mechanisms in HYPAC function, Nemeroff and co-workers (133) measured the concentration of I-CRH in the CSF of depressed patients, normal volunteers, and patients with schizophrenia or dementia. The depressed patients showed significantly elevated levels of I-CRH compared to normals and other patient groups; however, no relationship was observed between CSF I-CRH concentrations and peripheral plasma cortisol measures either pre- or postdexamethasone.

Although these studies are suggestive, evidence is still too preliminary to draw conclusions regarding an association between HYPAC products in the CSF and psychiatric symptoms. Further studies must be conducted to assess the functional significance of these hormones in the CSF of normals and psychiatric patients.

Brain Tissue

Based on CSF findings, one might expect brain tissue levels of glucocorticoids to show elevations as well. However, two studies of suicide brains reported a 40% *reduction* of both cortisol and corticosterone compared to controls who died suddenly (15,16). Interpretation of suicide brain studies is often difficult, because of prior drug ingestion and unknowns regarding functional state of the HYPAC system prior to death. Such findings may also have limited clinical significance until more is known about the postmortem decay of HYPAC hormones, especially ACTH and CRH, in brain tissue. This is a current area of much investigation.

STIMULATION TESTS

In the past, a variety of stimuli have been used by endocrinologists and psychobiologists to produce stimulation of the HYPAC axis. As the understanding of the physiology of this axis has increased, so has the availability of more specific stimuli to the axis, as well as more precise and specific assays for measuring the resulting response. Moreover, we are now able to stimulate rather precisely at several functional and anatomical levels of the HYPAC axis in order to observe the response of the axis to these maneuvers.

Most recently, for example, the availability of purified CRH (either ovine or human) has allowed precise and specific stimulation at the level of the pituitary, using the ACTH and cortisol responses as measures of the effectiveness of this stimulus.

CRH Stimulation Test

Ovine CRH (oCRH) produces specific and prompt ACTH release *in vivo* in rats and humans without producing serious side effects (32). Ovine CRH has a prolonged half-life and produces prolonged stimulation of the HYPAC axis compared to the rapidly degraded human CRH, though studies to date have not established whether the continued presence of biologically active oCRH in the blood is essential for sustained ACTH release, or results from initial activation of adenylcyclase in the pituitary corticotropes with continued ACTH release unrelated to ongoing plasma levels of oCRH.

Prior administration of glucocorticoids inhibits the sensitivity of pituitary corticotropes to CRH. Consequently stimulation tests for purposes of assessing the HYPAC axis should optimally be done during periods of quiescence of the axis, such as in the late afternoon or evening. Single injections of exogenous CRH alter the normal HYPAC circadian rhythm and produce fluctuations in HYPAC activity for a number of hours thereafter.

Human CRH has been shown to produce only a transient HYPAC response, less consistently related to diagnostic category (75,77). Depressed patients were found (58) to have an attenuated ACTH response to administered oCRH as compared to normals, whereas patients with Cushing's disease had exaggerated release of ACTH in response to oCRH. This finding in Cushing's disease patients occurred in the face of basal hypercortisolemia, supporting the concept that glucocorticoid negative feedback is inadequately operative in patients with Cushing's disease. It should be noted, however, that almost all the patients studied thus far have had confirmed microadenomata of the pituitary gland. Consequently, although inadequate negative feedback appears to be present in these patients, hyperfunction of the adenoma by itself may be considered a source of overdrive for the HYPAC system, as well as a site of increased sensitivity to the actions of CRH. Although the difference in response to administered oCRH is generally present between depressed patients and those with Cushing's disease, it should be noted that there was a good degree of overlap in ACTH response: About one-quarter of the depressed patients had peak ACTH responses in the cushingoid range, and approximately one-quarter of the patients with Cushing's disease had ACTH responses that were within the range of patients with primary depressive disorder.

See Chapter 61, *this volume,* for further details on the CRH stimulation test.

Vasopressin Stimulation Tests

In the past vasopressin has been considered possibly to be the primary ACTH releaser (120). Recent evidence, beginning with the isolation and characterization of CRH, has shown clearly that this latter peptide is the primary releaser of ACTH. However, there is a close interrelationship between vasopressin and CRH. This is, in part, characterized by their normally close anatomical localization in subdivisions of the paraventricular nucleus of the hypothalamus (102,167), and recent reports suggesting that after adrenalectomy and loss of glucocorticoid feedback, there is co-localization of CRF in cells that normally stain for vasopressin alone and are apparently those that deliver vasopressin to the hypothalamus. Vasopressin has been shown to potentiate the effects of CRH on ACTH release (35,118).

Vasopressin concentration in the pituitary hypophyseal portal system can get extremely high during severe stress, and may reach levels a thousand times greater than that found in peripheral blood (where it is a few picograms per milliliter). During adrenal insufficiency, peripheral vasopressin concentrations increase, as does ACTH (72). This increase in peripheral vasopressin may be the result of activity of the parvocellular neurons, although some of this may be derived from a second vasopressin system, which is located in the supraoptic nucleus. This latter vasopressin system has axons that project directly to the posterior (neuro) hypophysis and is apparently not inhibited by glucocorticoid feedback, as are the parvocellular vasopressin and CRH-containing neurons. In states of reduced glucocorticoid feedback, vasopressin concentration in the parvocellular neurons increases in parallel to CRH (167).

Administration of a moderately large dose of vasopressin has generally been associated with a prompt increment in plasma ACTH and cortisol in control subjects. Administration to a small group of depressed patients, however, yielded mixed results, with only half the patients showing an ACTH and cortisol release (105). It may be that vasopressin is important in the release of ACTH only under severe stress conditions. Recent evidence suggests that the CNS pathways sensitive to glucocorticoid feedback are those that control CRH release without any modulation from vasopressin. Although these neuronal systems may be blocked by feedback from elevated glucocorticoid levels, the so-called "steroid-resistant" neuronal pathways discussed previously remain operative, and it has been proposed that these systems include vasopressin release (perhaps along with CRH). Thus in the condition of elevated glucocorticoid negative feedback, stimuli sufficient to produce the release of vasopressin from the parvocellular nuclei may play an important role in the secretion of pituitary ACTH. For example, recently it was found that in a state of dexamethasone suppression (i.e., glucocorticoid excess), neither lysine vasopressin nor CRH produced significant HYPAC activation in normals (5). However, when these two secretagogues were administered together in dexamethasone-suppressed normals, there was a prompt and marked increase in plasma ACTH and cortisol levels. These investigators suggested that both vasopressin and CRH are thus necessary for escape of the HYPAC system in the postdexamethasone suppressed state of depressed patients. Prior work (118) had demonstrated this potentiation by vasopressin of CRH action on ACTH release under baseline conditions without dexamethasone.

Obviously, further studies of this interesting vasopressin effect on HYPAC function are needed. Now that lysine vasopressin is available, it is possible to conduct such studies without the attendant risk of induced hypertension, angina, or other untoward cardiovascular effects that often accompanied the use of arginine vasopressin in stimulation studies.

ACTH Stimulation Test

The ACTH stimulation test was developed in the 1950s to assess adrenocortical responsiveness to exogenous animal-derived natural ACTH. Some years later, the availability of the synthetic 1–24-amino-acid peptide subunit of natural ACTH provided advantages over the natural hormone. These advantages included chemical purity and assay by weight, much diminished incidence of immune reactions, and ease of intramuscular or intravenous administration due to the synthetic peptide's high water solubility. The adrenal response to the natural and the shorter-chain synthetic 1–24 ACTH was identical. Thus, the latter has become the standard for testing via intramuscular injections, intravenous infusions, or intravenous bolus administration, using plasma hydrocortisone response to the ACTH as a measure of adrenocortical function.

It is now clear that an intact HYPAC system will show an initial adrenocortical response to exogenous ACTH similar to the release induced by endogenous ACTH in response to appropriate environmental stimuli. The subsequent second or third response can vary remarkably, however, because in the endogenous situation a variety of feedback inhibitions occur at the hypothalamic and pituitary level (and, to a lesser degree, at the adrenocortical level). The subsequent adrenocortical responses can therefore be variable, and also depend on the force and time of repetition (or lack) of sufficient stimulus, as discussed previously. Exogenous ACTH, on the other hand, while producing negative feedback on pituitary endogenous ACTH release, will *continue* to drive the steroidogenesis and secretion from adrenocortical cells. Given sufficient duration and magnitude, exogenous ACTH administration can induce adrenocortical hypertrophy and, ultimately, hyperplasia. Conversely, the absence of ACTH will rapidly allow a gradual decay or atrophy of the intracellular machinery necessary for steroidogenesis, and with sufficient time (probably only days in humans) actual cellular involution and glandular atrophy can occur. It is because of this atrophy that adrenocortical insufficiency is well diagnosed by the ACTH stimulation test, which reveals a characteristically subnormal response in terms of slope of plasma cortisol increment, peak level, and total area under the curve over time. On the other hand, if the adrenal cortex has been driven by "excessive" ACTH, due to slight but continuous increments of ACTH over time, or large periodic boluses (or both), then additional exogenous ACTH will drive steroidogenesis to levels above that observed in the normal HYPAC axis. For example, one could postulate that patients with affective disease and basal increments in steroid production (best reflected by increased 24-hr UFC) will most reliably show hyperresponsiveness to exogenous ACTH. It is also clear, from a consideration of the physiological hierarchy of the HYPAC axis, that one may see increased cortisol production from exogenous stimulation at levels above the adrenal cortex, including both pituitary and hypothalamic (CRH) levels.

Recently, some interesting studies performed by Amsterdam et al. (3), using cosyntropin (ACTH α 1–24), revealed significantly higher cortisol response to infused ACTH and prior postdexamethasone plasma cortisol values. These authors suggest that hypersecretion of cortisol during depression might result, at least in part, from adrenocortical hyperresponsiveness. Prior ACTH stimulation tests in depression have used different methods so that comparisons with the current studies are difficult to make. However, prior data are generally consistent with Amsterdam's current conclusions. Endo (41) studied adrenocortical response to an i.v. bolus of ACTH in the postdexamethasone state and found a greater cortisol response during depression, as compared to after recovery. Similarly, Bridges (10) administered ACTH intramuscularly after dexamethasone, and found that DST nonsuppressors had a higher 30-min post-ACTH cortisol level than did DST suppressors. However, others (174) reported no differences in the response to intramuscular ACTH in depressed patients before and after recovery. In considering these data it should be borne in mind that intramuscular ACTH responses may be more variable than intravenous administration. Furthermore, different ACTH doses were used, and sampling at 30-min postintramuscular administration may be an inadequate time interval. Carpenter and Bunney (21) found no difference between depressed patients and healthy controls in

terms of cortisol response to prolonged 4-hr infusion of pharmacological amounts of ACTH. Amsterdam (3) suggested that the use of a 4-hr ACTH infusion may have produced down-regulation of the adrenocortical ACTH receptors and, hence, masked the potentially greater response of the depressed patients. This seems unlikely, since the increased cortisol response in the depressed patients was probably due to prior endogenous priming of the adrenal cortex by endogenous ACTH. In other words, down-regulation should have already occurred. An alternative explanation might rest on the fact that the pharmacological doses used by Carpenter and Bunney (21) and the prolonged 4-hr infusion may have been sufficient to allow the normals to reach maximal secretory response comparable to those particular depressed patients. Furthermore, the relatively lower metabolic clearance rate of cortisol reported by Carpenter et al. (21) in the normals (as compared to the depressed patients) may have allowed relatively greater accumulation of plasma cortisol in these ACTH-stimulated individuals (as compared to plasma cortisol in the depressed patients, who had higher metabolic clearance rates). Further studies are needed to investigate the apparent heightened responsiveness of the adrenal cortex to ACTH in patients who are depressed, and we would hypothesize that clear evidence for adrenocortical hyperfunction and hypertrophy will be found.

Insulin Hypoglycemia

Another standard procedure that produces pituitary release of ACTH in a relatively quantitative manner is insulin-induced hypoglycemia or the insulin tolerance test (ITT). This is a sensitive and standard test of the functional status of the HYPAC system. Rapidly induced hypoglycemia following bolus i.v. injection of 0.1 unit of insulin produces a strong stress response via the CNS, stimulating CRH and thus ACTH secretion. The mechanism involved in insulin hypoglycemia is complex, but in part related to glucose-sensitive cells, probably located in multiple areas of the CNS, including the hypothalamus and sympathetic nervous system. For example, glucose infusions into the hypothalamus can blunt or minimize neuroendocrine responses to systemic hypoglycemia in animals. Furthermore, HYPAC axis activation and adrenocortical secretion in response to hypoglycemia require an intact pituitary. It has been suggested that, at least in the rat, peripheral circulating catecholamines released in response to the hypoglycemia contribute to HYPAC response during the hypoglycemia, as well as during other severe stressors (126). Moreover, these investigators speculate that circulating catecholamines act directly on the pituitary and do not require an intact, functional hypothalamus. However, this may not be so in normal humans (29,189) or in depressed patients (189), where infusions of catecholamines within the physiological range have not been associated with HYPAC activation. Controversy about this issue continues (147).

The cortisol response to hypoglycemia in normals is reported to be fairly reproducible within the same individual unless there is a significant change in glucose nadir between tests. However, extensive test-retest comparisons have not yet been done. The HYPAC axis response occurs late in the induced hypoglycemic phase (60–90 min following insulin injection) just prior to the rise in plasma glucose from its nadir. In normals, there is a clear dose-response of blood sugar and of the HYPAC axis to doses of insulin up to 0.1 unit/kg body weight, and perhaps up to as much as 0.15 unit/kg body weight (61).

A number of studies have evaluated HYPAC response to insulin hypoglycemia in depressed patients. A diminished cortisol response to hypoglycemia has been observed in psychotic depressives compared to normals and neurotic depressives (where the response was actually exaggerated), despite similar minimum glucose levels (138). Other studies (23) of depressed patients before treatment with electroconvulsive therapy (ECT) have also found impaired HYPAC response to hypoglycemia. However, the minimum blood glucose levels were lower on recovery from depression than during illness, whereas the mean plasma cortisol response was less during illness than after treatment. The impaired HYPAC responses to insulin hypoglycemia were also associated with an abnormal DST in the same patients. Two other studies (41,161) reported a normal cortisol response to hypoglycemia with no difference between depressed and recovered states, although both studies noted more profound hypoglycemia during the recovered phase. This resistance to insulin-induced hypoglycemia in depressed patients was reported extensively by Mueller et al. (131) and subsequently commented on by Koslow et al. (104) during measurements of growth hormone response to insulin-induced hypoglycemia, where these authors also noted that hormone release was inversely related to the postinsulin glucose nadir.

These findings suggest that some depressed patients may have an impaired HYPAC response to insulin hypoglycemia, although this finding is by no means consistent or clearly established. The inverse relationship between insulin-induced glucose nadir and concomitant HYPAC response is still a confounding factor not adequately controlled. For example, if there is truly such an inverse relationship, then the data showing no difference between hormone response in the depressed vs recovered condition should be reinterpreted. That is to say there actually is a difference in hormone release in these two states (relatively greater in the depressed), since hypoglycemia was more profound in the recovered patients (41,161). Moreover, the impairment may be associated with other known HYPAC abnormalities, such as cortisol hypersecretion and resistance to the feedback inhibition by dexamethasone.

Pyrogen Test

Injection of bacterial pyrogens also stimulates pituitary ACTH release, but this test is used less frequently than insulin hypoglycemia, since the sites and mechanisms of pyrogen action are not well understood, and there is considerable distress associated with the test.

RU-486 Glucocorticoid-Receptor Blocker Stimulation Tests

Recently a synthetic steroid hormone antagonist acting at the receptor level has become available (manufactured by Roussel-Uclaf, Paris, France). Studies in nonhuman primates (72) revealed that RU-486 is a potent releaser of ACTH and arginine vasopressin and cortisol after a single dose. It has recently been demonstrated that RU-486 will antagonize the negative pituitary feedback of nocturnal endogenous cortisol rise and produce a persistent and protracted (hours-long) increase in ACTH and cortisol secretion (7). Thus the HYPAC system reacts as though the increased circulating cortisol were in fact not present. This response is due to the blockade of glucocorticoid receptors (necessary to detect the negative feedback of the increased plasma cortisol) by RU-486. In a similar manner, the suppressive effect of exogenously administered dexamethasone could be inhibited by appropriate doses of RU-486 given concomitantly. In normal men, RU-486 given alone led to a dose-dependent increase in plasma ACTH, β-endorphin, and cortisol (50). The data available suggest that RU-486 is a competitive antiglucocorticosteroid in humans (as well as an antiprogesterone) and that it probably acts at the glucocorticosteroid receptor. Increasing doses of dexamethasone can overcome the effects of RU-486; thus any state of clinical hypocortisolism induced by administration of RU-486 could be reversed by corticosteroid administration. Further studies of this interesting compound are obviously indicated, and are in progress.

Metyrapone Test

The metyrapone test was introduced as a measure of pituitary adrenal reserve by Liddle et al. (114). Since then, the test has been performed in many different ways. The test uses the 11-β-hydroxylase inhibitor to prevent the hydroxylation of 11-deoxycortisol (compound S) to cortisol within the adrenal cortex. Inhibition of synthesis of cortisol decreases negative feedback effects on CRH/ACTH release, and the increased ACTH further stimulates adrenocortical steroidogenesis within the glucocorticoid synthetic chain up to the point of formation and secretion of 11-deoxycortisol from the adrenal cortex. The 11-deoxycortisol can be measured in peripheral blood by newer techniques, or indirectly as described in the initial methodology by the increase in total urinary 17-OHCS that can be observed. Metabolites of 11-deoxycortisol become major contributors to the spectrophotometrically determined chromatogens that make up urinary 17-OHCS after 11-β-hydroxylase blockade of the adrenal cortex.

In 1970 it was shown that in 30 normals and 11 patients with adrenal insufficiency the single-dose metyrapone test was equivalent to the standard metyrapone test (93). This finding eliminated the need for the difficult and protracted four-dose, 24-hr administration of metyrapone and the collection of pre- and postdose 24-hr urine samples. Subsequently, Spiger (181) applied the methodology for measuring plasma 11-deoxycortisol to the simplified test procedure. In the current simplified test, a single standard dose of metyrapone (between 2 and 3 g), based on body weight, is given in the late evening (2300–2400 hr) and a single blood sample obtained the next morning at 0800 hr. Using this simple test, adrenocortical hyporesponse to the administration of metyrapone is demonstrated by low plasma levels of 11-deoxycortisol (the morning after metyrapone) similar to the early reports of low urinary 17-OHCS following 24-hr administration of metyrapone.

Early studies with the metyrapone test performed on depressed patients did not reveal clearly abnormal responses of the HYPAC axis (21,81) when urinary 17-OHCS was measured, though a relatively decreased response was reported in depressed males with initially high basal 17-OHCS levels. These results and the frequent difficulties with gastrointestinal upset (nausea secondary to the metyrapone) plus difficulty with 24-hr urine collections caused the test to fall into relative disuse in psychoendocrine studies. More recently one group (46) has reported on the single-dose metyrapone test comparing plasma 11-deoxycortisol (HYPAC) response in depressed patients vs schizophrenics. They found an essentially normal distribution of plasma 11-deoxycortisol in both diagnostic groups postmetyrapone. Depressed patients with DST nonsuppression had higher postmetyrapone 11-deoxycortisol levels than suppressors, though this barely reached statistical significance. However, it is important to note that Holsboer (78) has reported variable HYPAC responses to metyrapone as regards cortisol, 11-deoxycortisol, and ACTH. In another report, the same group noted that in a small group of schizophrenic patients the 11-deoxycortisol levels were state related and returned to normal as the patients improved (139). Finally, the same investigators (129) reported on 10 depressed males and 10 age-matched healthy controls. One of the depressed subjects had an inadequate plasma 11-deoxycortisol response following the single overnight metyrapone test. These investigators suggested that *hypo*activity of the HYPAC axis might be an occasional finding in depressed patients. Although these are intriguing findings, it is important to note that the response of the HYPAC system to the blockade of cortisol synthesis with metyrapone is variable, and some 4% or more of normals have "an inadequate rise of plasma 11-deoxycortisol after metyrapone" (181). Furthermore, with the extensive evaluation of HYPAC activity performed over the last 20 or 30 years in psychiatric patients, there have not come to light incidences of HYPAC *hypo*function other than in those patients with coincident primary endocrine disease (e.g., nonfunctional pituitary tumors, Addison's disease). Most stimulation tests and perhaps those like the metyrapone test in particular, suffer from the large variability both between and within patients in response to the same stimulus applied at different times. Perhaps the variable response in the metyrapone test is secondary to variation in rate or completeness of absorption of the metyrapone given orally, as well as individual differences in sensitivity to adrenocortical 11-β-hydroxylase inhibition. Future metyrapone studies should consider measurements of plasma metyrapone levels and assess plasma ACTH or β-endorphin levels as well as 11-deoxycortisol levels before and after stimulus. At the very least, and as indicated by prior reports (129), it is essential that considerably larger numbers of patients be studied with carefully matched controls, and that attention be given to test-retest reliability.

Paradoxical ACTH Response to Glucocorticoids

It has been demonstrated that the abnormal HYPAC function in patients with Cushing's disease is associated in most cases studied with a paradoxical and transient *increased* release of ACTH during the initial minutes of an infusion of hydrocortisone (cortisol) or dexamethasone (83,107,149). This paradoxical response to increased exogenously applied glucocorticoid negative feedback is more pronounced in Cushing's patients after bilateral adrenalectomy, in which basal ACTH levels are even more clearly elevated in spite of usual and clinically adequate replacement doses of hydrocortisone or cortisone (48). This finding suggests that the small paradoxical response observed preadrenalectomy in these patients is the result of inhibition of that response by the then circulating high levels of plasma cortisol. These interesting and provocative findings stimulated interest in examining the HYPAC response to infusion of glucocorticoids in patients with primary depression. An initial report (149) found that one of four depressed patients infused with glucocorticoids showed a similar transient paradoxical release of ACTH. Carr et al. (22) subsequently reported that two of 10 depressed patients showed a mild transient paradoxical increase in plasma ACTH during glucocorticoid infusion. However, other reports confirming these findings have not yet appeared. Recent *data* from our laboratory (*unpublished*) have only found examples of possible paradoxical HYPAC response in two of 14 cases thus far studied by infusion of hydrocortisone or dexamethasone. At this point no final conclusion can be reached as regards the possibility of paradoxical HYPAC response in patients with primary depression. It would appear, however, that if present in depressives the incidence must be far lower than that observed recently in patients with Cushing's disease. No data are available on the presence or absence of pituitary microadenoma either pre- or postadrenalectomy in the earlier studies of the Cushing's patients with paradoxical response (48). The paradoxical response may be explained by the phenomenon of periodic hormonogenesis, not specifically related to the administration of the glucocorticoid. All reports have shown a late clear suppressive effect of the infused glucocorticoid on ACTH secretion, after the initial episode of paradoxical response. However, there may be a slower rate of (delayed feedback) inhibition of ACTH secretion in these individuals who show paradoxical increase initially. Fehm (79) speculated that the normal negative rapid feedback mechanism in Cushing's disease is converted into a positive one, by an unexplained phenomenon, whereas the delayed feedback mechanism remains intact.

CONCLUDING REMARKS

From this overview it can be seen that measures of the HYPAC axis have the continuing potential for contributing to our understanding of the pathogenesis of psychopathology in affective illness. Further, they hold promise as possible biological markers of specific classes of affective illness. Although our understanding of the physiology/pharmacology of the HYPAC system is far from complete, the studies performed by psychobiologists have contributed to the increase in our knowledge of the function and significance of the neuroendocrine system in healthy and affectively disturbed individuals.

ACKNOWLEDGMENTS

Research from this laboratory was supported in part by National Institute of Mental Health Research Grant 1-R01-MH38677-01 and by a grant from the Hexter Foundation. The authors wish to acknowledge the competent assistance of Maxine Y. Greene.

REFERENCES

1. Ahmed, A. B. J., George, B. C., Gonzalez-Auvert, C., and Dingman, J. F. (1967): *J. Clin. Invest.,* 46:111–123.
2. Akesode, A., Hendler, N., and Kowarski, A. A. (1976): *Psychoneuroendocrinology,* 1:419–426.
3. Amsterdam, J. D., Winokur, A., Abelman, E., Lucki, I., and Rickels, K. (1983): *Am. J. Psychiatry,* 140:907–909.
4. Asnis, G. N., Sachar, E. J., Halbreich, U., Nathan, J. S., Novacenho, H., and Ostrow, L. C. (1981): *Psychosom. Med.,* 43:235–246.
5. Bardeleben, U. von (1986): *Life Sci.,* 37:1613–1618.
6. Berson, S., and Yalow, R. (1968): *J. Clin. Invest.,* 47:2725–2751.
7. Bertagna, X., Bertagna, C., Luton, J.-P., Husson, J.-M., and Girard, F. (1984): *J. Clin. Endocrinol. Metab.,* 59:25–28.
8. Board, F., Persky, H., and Hamburg, D. A. (1956): *Psychosom. Med.,* 18:324–333.
9. Board, F., Wadeson, R., and Persky, H. (1957): *Arch. Neurol. Psychiatry,* 78:612–620.
10. Bridges, P. K. (1973): *Psychiatr. Neurol. Neurochir.,* 76:335–344.
11. Bridges, P. K., and Jones, M. T. (1966): *Br. J. Psychiatry,* 112:1257–1261.
12. Britton, D. R., Koob, G. F., Rivier, J., and Bak, W. (1982): *Life Sci.,* 31:363–367.
13. Brodish, A. (1963): *Endocrinology,* 73:727–735.
14. Brooks, F. S., and Brooks, R. V. (1984): In: *Immunoassays of Steroids in Saliva,* edited by G. F. Read, pp. 322–326. Alpha Omega Publishing, Cardiff.
15. Brooksbank, B. W. L., Brammall, M. A., Cunningham, A. E., Shaw, D. M., and Camps, F. E. (1972): *Psychol. Med.,* 2:56–65.
16. Brooksbank, B. W. L., Brammall, M. A., and Shaw, D. M. (1973): *Steroids Lipids Res.,* 4:162–183.
17. Brooksbank, B. W. L., and Coppen, A. (1967): *Br. J. Psychiatry,* 113:395–404.
18. Brown, W. A., and Shuey, I. (1980): *Arch. Gen. Psychiatry,* 37:747–751.
19. Bunney, W. E., Jr., Mason, J. W., and Hamburg, D. A. (1965): *Psychosom. Med.,* 27:299–308.
20. Bunney, W. E., Jr., Mason, J. W., Roatch, J. E., and Hamburg, D. A. (1965): *Am. J. Psychiatry,* 122:72–80.
21. Carpenter, W. T., and Bunney, W. E., Jr. (1971): *Am. J. Psychiatry,* 128:31–40.
22. Carr, D. B., Wool, C., Lydiard, R. B., Fisher, J., Belenberg, A., and Klerman, G. (1984): *Am. J. Psychiatry,* 141:590–592.
23. Carroll, B. J. (1969): *Br. Med. J.,* 3:27–28.
24. Carroll, B. J., Curtis, G. C., Davies, B. M., Mendels, J., and Sugerman, A. A. (1976): *Psychol. Med.,* 6:43–50.
25. Carroll, B. J., Curtis, G. C., and Mendels, J. (1976): *Psychol. Med.,* 6:235–244.
26. Carroll, B. J., Martin, F. I. R., and Davies, B. M. (1968): *Br. Med. J.,* 3:285–287.
27. Carroll, B. J., and Mendels, J. (1976): In: *Hormones, Behavior, and Psychology,* edited by E. J. Sachar, pp. 193–224. Raven Press, New York.
28. Chowers, I., Conforti, N., and Feldman, S. (1967): *Neuroendocrinology,* 2:193–199.
29. Clutter, W. E., Bier, D. M., Shah, S. D., and Cryer, P. E. (1980): *J. Clin. Invest.,* 66:94–101.
30. Conroy, R. T., Hughes, B. D., and Mills, J. N. (1968): *Br. Med. J.,* 3:405–407.
31. Cope, C. L., and Black, E. G. (1959): *Br. Med. J.,* 2:1117–1122.
32. Copinschi, G., Beyloos, M., Bosson, D., Desir, D., Golstein, J., Robyn, C., Linkowski, P., Mendlewicz, J., and Franckson, J. R. M. (1983): *J. Clin. Endocrinol. Metab.,* 57:1287–1291.
33. Dallman, M. F. (1979): In: *Interaction Within the Brain-Pituitary-Adrenocortical System,* edited by M. T. Jones, B. Gillham, M. F. Dallman, and S. Chattopadhyay, pp. 149–162. Academic Press, London.
34. Dallman, M. F., Engeland, W. C., Rose, J. C., Wilkinson, C. W., Shinsako, J., and Siedenburg, F. (1978): *Am. J. Physiol.,* 235:R210–R218.
35. Dallman, M. F., Makara, G. B., Robert, J. L., Levin, N., and Blum, M. (1983): *Endocrinology,* 117:2190–2197.
36. Daly, J. R., Reader, S. C. J., Alaghband-Ladeh, J., and Halsmann, P. (1979): In: *Interaction Within the Brain-Pituitary-Adrenocortical System,* edited by M. T. Jones, B. Gillham, M. F. Dallman, and S. Chattopadhyay, pp. 181–188. Academic Press, London.
37. D'Angelo, S. A., Snyder, J., and Grodin, J. M. (1964): *Endocrinology,* 75:417–427.
38. DeKloet, E. R., Wallach, G., and McEwen, B. S. (1975): *Endocrinology,* 96:568–609.
39. Doe, R. P., Fernandez, R., and Seal, U. S. (1964): *J. Clin. Endocrinol.,* 24:1029–1039.
40. Doig, R. J., Mummery, R. V., and Wills, M. R. (1966): *Br. J. Psychiatry,* 112:1263–1267.
41. Endo, M., Endo, J., Nishikubo, M., Yamaguchi, T., and Hatotani, N. (1974): In: *Psychoneuroendocrinology,* edited by N. Hatotani, pp. 22–31. Karger, Basel.
42. Endroczi, E., Lissak, K., Bohus, B., and Kovacs, S. (1959): *Acta Physiol. Hung.,* 16:17–22.
43. Engeland, W. C., and Dallman, M. F. (1975): *Neuroendocrinology,* 19:352–362.
44. Etgen, A. M., Martin, M., Gilbert, R., and Lynch, G. (1980): *J. Neurochem.,* 35:598–602.
45. Fang, V. S., Tricou, B. J., Robertson, A., and Meltzer, H. (1981): *Life Sci.,* 29:931–938.
46. Fava, G. A., Carson, S. W., Perini, G. I., Morphy, M. A., Molnar, G., and Jusko, W. J. (1984): *J. Affective Disord.,* 6:241–247.
47. Fehm, H. L., Klein, E., Holl, R., and Voigt, K. H. (1984): *J. Clin. Endocrinol. Metab.,* 58:410–414.
48. Fehm, H. L., Voigt, K. L., Lang, R. E., Beinert, K. E., Kummer, G. W., and Pfeiffer, E. F. (1977): *N. Engl. J. Med.,* 297:904–907.
49. Fullerton, D. T., Wenzel, F. J., Lohrenz, F. N., and Fahs, H. (1968): *Arch. Gen. Psychiatry,* 19:674–681.
50. Gaillaird, R. C., Riondel, A., Muller, A. F., Herrmann, W., and Baulieu, E. E. (1984): *Proc. Natl. Acad. Sci. USA,* 81:3879–3882.
51. Ganong, W. F. (1980): *Fed. Proc.,* 39:2923–2929.
52. Gay, V. L. (1972): *Fertil. Steril.,* 23:50–63.
53. Georgotas, A., Stokes, P. E., Krakowski, M., Fanelli, C., and Cooper, T. (1984): *Biol. Psychiatry,* 19:685–693.
54. Gerner, R. H., and Wilkins, J. N. (1983): *Am. J. Psychiatry,* 140:92–94.
55. Gibbons, J. L., and McHugh, P. R. (1962): *J. Psychiatr. Res.,* 1:162–171.
56. Gillies, G., Linton, E. A., and Lowry, P. J. (1982): *Nature,* 299:355–357.
57. Glaser, G. H. (1953): *Psychosom. Med.,* 15:280–291.
58. Gold, P. W., Loriaux, L., Roy, A., Kling, M. A., Calabrese, J. R., Kellner, C. H., Nieman, L. K., Post, R. M., Pickar, D., Gallucci, W., Avgerinos, P., Paul, S., Olfield, E. H., Cutter, G. B., Jr., and Chrousos, G. P. (1986): *N. Engl. J. Med.,* 314:1329–1335.
59. Greden, J. F., Gardner, R., King, D., Grunhaus, L., Carroll, B. J., and Kronfol, Z. (1983): *Arch. Gen. Psychiatry,* 40:493–500.
60. Green, J. D., and Harris, G. W. (1947): *J. Endocrinol.,* 5:136–146.
61. Greenwood, F. C., Landon, J., and Stamp, T. C. B. (1966): *J. Clin. Invest.,* 45:429–436.
62. Groot, J. de, and Harris, G. W. (1950): *J. Physiol. (Lond.),* 111:335–346.
63. Grosser, B. I., Stevens, W., and Reed, D. J. (1973): *Brain Res.,* 57:387–395.
64. Guillemant, J., Guillemant, S., and Reinberg, A. (1980): *Experientia,* 36:367–368.
65. Guillemin, R., and Rosenberg, B. (1955): *Endocrinology,* 57:599–607.
66. Guillemin, R., Vango, J., Rossier, J., Minick, S., Ling, N., Rivier, C., Vale, W., and Bloom, F. (1977): *Science,* 197:1367–1369.
67. Halasz, B., Slusher, M. A., and Gorski, R. A. (1967): *Neuroendocrinology,* 2:43–55.

68. Hanada, K., Yamada, N., Shimoda, K., Takahashi, K., and Takahashi, S. (1985): *Psychoneuroendocrinology,* 10:193–201.
69. Harris, G. W. (1948): *J. Physiol. (Lond.),* 107:418–429.
70. Harris, G. W., and Jacobsohn, D. (1952): *Proc. R. Soc. (Biol.),* 139:263–276.
71. Haskett, R. F. (1985): *Am. J. Psychiatry,* 142:911–916.
72. Healy, D. L., Chrousos, G. P., Schulte, H. M., Williams, R. F., Gold, P. W., Baulieu, E. E., and Hodgen, G. D. (1983): *J. Clin. Endocrinol. Metab.,* 57:863–865.
73. Hellman, L., Fujinori, N., Curti, J., Weitzman, E. D., Kream, J., Roffwang, H., Ellman, S., Fukushima, D. K., and Gallagher, T. F. (1970): *J. Clin. Endocrinol.,* 30:411–422.
74. Holaday, J. W., Martinez, H. M., and Natelson, B. H. (1977): *Science,* 198:56.
75. Holsboer, F., Bardeleben, U. von, Gerken, A., Staller, G. K., and Muller, O. A. (1984): *N. Engl. J. Med.,* 311:1127.
76. Holsboer, F., Doerr, H. G., Gerken, A., Muller, D., and Sippell, W. G. (1984): *Psychiatr. Res.,* 11:15–23.
77. Holsboer, F., Gerken, A., Stalla, G. K., and Muller, D. A. (1985): *Biol. Psychiatry,* 20:276–286.
78. Holsboer, F., Muller, O. A., Winter, K., Doerr, H. G., and Sippell, W. G. (1983): *Psychopharmacology,* 80:85–87.
79. Ifft, J. D. (1966): *Neuroendocrinology,* 1:350–357.
80. Ingle, D. J., and Kendall, E. C. (1937): *Science,* 86:245–252.
81. Jakobson, T., Sternback, A., Strandstrom, L., and Rimon, R. (1966): *J. Psychosom. Res.,* 9:363–367.
82. James, V. H. T., and Landon, J., eds. (1968): *Mem. Soc. Endocrinol.,* 17.
83. James, V. H. T., Landon, J., and Fraser, R. (1968): *Mem. Soc. Endocrinol.,* 17:141–158.
84. Jarrett, D. B., Coble, P. A., and Kupfer, D. J. (1983): *Arch. Gen. Psychiatry,* 40:506–511.
85. Jimerson, D. C., Post, R. M., von Kommen, D. P., Skyler, J. S., Brown, G. L., and Bunney, W. E., Jr. (1980): *Am. J. Psychiatry,* 137:979–980.
86. Jones, M. T. (1979): In: *The Adrenal Gland,* edited by V. H. T. James, pp. 93–130. Raven Press, New York.
87. Jones, M. T., Gillham, B., DiRenzo, G., Beckford, V., and Holmes, M. C. (1981): *Front. Horm. Res.,* 8:12–43.
88. Jones, M. T., Gillham, B., Greenstein, B. D., Beckford, U., and Holmes, M. C. (1982): In: *Adrenal Actions on the Brain,* edited by D. Ganten and D. Pfaff, pp. 45–68. Springer-Verlag, New York.
89. Jones, M. T., Gillham, B., Homes, M. C., and Buckingham, J. C. (1978): *J. Endocrinol.,* 76:183–184.
90. Jones, M. T., and Tiptaft, E. M. (1977): *Br. J. Pharmacol.,* 59: 35–41.
91. Jordan, R. M., Kendall, J. W., Seaich, J. L., Allen, J. P., Paulsen, C. A., Kerber, C. W., and Vanderlaon, W. P. (1976): *Ann. Intern. Med.,* 85:49–55.
92. Jubiz, W., Meikle, A. W., Levinson, R. A., Mizutani, S., West, C. D., and Tyler, F. H. (1970): *N. Engl. J. Med.,* 283:11–14.
93. Jubiz, W., Meikle, A. W., West, C. D., and Tyler, F. H. (1970): *Arch. Intern. Med.,* 125:472–474.
94. Kalin, N. H., Weiler, S. J., and Shelton, S. E. (1982): *Psychiatr. Res.,* 7:87–92.
95. Kaneko, M., Hiroshige, T., Shinsako, J., and Dallman, M. F. (1980): *Am. J. Physiol.,* 239:R309–R316.
96. Kathol, R. G. (1985): *J. Affective Disord.,* 8:137–145.
97. Kato, H., Saito, M., and Suda, M. (1980): *Endocrinology,* 106: 918–921.
98. Kawakami, M., Seto, K., Kimura, F., and Yanase, D. (1971): In: *Influence of Hormones on the Central Nervous System,* edited by D. H. Ford, pp. 107–120. Karger, Basel.
99. Kehlet, H., and Binder, C. (1973): *J. Clin. Endocrinol. Metab.,* 36:330–333.
100. King, D. J. (1973): *Psychol. Med.,* 3:53–65.
101. Kirkegaard, C., and Carroll, B. J. (1980): *Psychiatry Res.,* 3:253–264.
102. Kiss, J. Z., Mezey, E., and Skirboll, E. (1984): *Proc. Natl. Acad. Sci. USA,* 81:1854–1858.
103. Knigge, K. M., and Scott, D. E. (1970): *Am. J. Anat.,* 129:223–244.
104. Koslow, S. H., Stokes, P. E., Mendels, J., Ramsey, A., and Casper, R. (1982): *Psychol. Med.,* 12:45–55.

105. Krahn, D. D., Meller, W. H., Shafer, R. B., and Morley, J. E. (1985): *Biol. Psychiatry,* 20:918–921.
106. Krieger, D. T., and Gewirtz, G. P. (1974): *J. Clin. Endocrinol. Metab.,* 39:46–52.
107. Krieger, D. T., Howanitz, P. J., and Frantz, A. G. (1976): *J. Clin. Endocrinol. Metab.,* 42:260–272.
108. Kurland, H. D. (1964): *Arch. Gen. Psychiatry,* 10:554–560.
109. Landon, J., Smith, D. S., Perry, L. A., and Al-Ansari, A. A. K. (1984): In: *Immunoassays of Steroids in Saliva,* edited by G. F. Read, pp. 300–307. Alpha Omega Publishing, Cardiff.
110. Lankford, H. V., Tucker, S. G., and Blackard, W. G. (1981): *N. Engl. J. Med.,* 305:1244–1248.
111. Leveston, S. A., McKeel, D. W., Buckley, P. J., Deschryver, K., Greider, M. H., Jaffe, B. M., and Daughaday, W. H. (1981): *J. Clin. Endocrinol. Metab.,* 53:682–689.
112. Levin, R., and Levine, S. (1975): *Am. J. Physiol.,* 229:E1397–E1399.
113. Levine, A. S., Rogers, B., Kneip, J., Grace, M., and Morley, J. E. (1983): *Neuropharmacology,* 22:337–339.
114. Liddle, G. W., Estep, H. E., Kendall, J. W., Williams, C. W., and Torres, A. W. (1959): *J. Clin. Endocrinol. Metab.,* 19:875–894.
115. Liddle, G. W., Island, D., and Meadoir, C. K. (1962): *Recent Prog. Horm. Res.,* 18:125–166.
116. Lidz, T., Carter, J. D., Lewis, B. I., and Surratt, C. (1952): *Psychosom. Med.,* 14:363–377.
117. Linkowski, P., Mendlewicz, J., Leclercq, R., Brasseur, M., Hubain, P., Golstein, J., Copinschi, G., and van Cauter, E. (1985): *J. Clin. Endocrinol. Metab.,* 61:429–438.
118. Liu, J. H., Muse, K., Contreras, P., Gibbs, D., Vale, W., Rivier, J., and Yen, S. S. (1983): *J. Clin. Endocrinol. Metab.,* 57:1087–1089.
119. Mason, J. W., Sachar, E. J., Fishman, J. R., Hamburg, D. A., and Handlon, J. H. (1965): *Arch. Gen. Psychiatry,* 13:1–8.
120. McCann, S. H., and Flaberland, P. (1957): *Proc. Soc. Exp. Biol. Med.,* 102:319–325.
121. McClure, D. J. (1966): *J. Psychosom. Res.,* 10:189–195.
122. McClure, D. J., and Cleghorn, R. A. (1970): In: *Science and Psychoanalysis,* edited by J. H. Masserman, pp. 12–19. Grune & Stratton, New York.
123. McEwen, B. S. (1977): *Ann. NY Acad. Sci.,* 297:568–579.
124. McEwen, B. S., Weiss, J. M., and Schwartz, L. (1968): *Nature,* 220:911–912.
125. McEwen, B. S., Weiss, J. M., and Schwartz, L. S. (1969): *Brain Res.,* 16:227–241.
126. Mezey, E., Reisine, T. D., Brownstein, M. J., Palkovits, M., and Axelrod, J. (1984): *Science,* 226:1085–1087.
127. Micco, D. J., Jr., and McEwen, B. S. (1980): *J. Comp. Physiol. Psychol.,* 94:624–633.
128. Moberg, G. P., Scapagnini, V., deGroot, J., and Ganong, W. F. (1971): *Neuroendocrinology,* 7:11–15.
129. Morphy, M. A., Fava, G. A., Perini, G. I., and Molnar, G. (1985): *Prog. Neuropsychopharmacol. Biol. Psychiatry,* 9:187–191.
130. Motta, M., Mangili, M., and Martini, L. (1965): *Endocrinology,* 77:392–395.
131. Mueller, P. S., Heninger, G. R., and McDonald, R. K. (1969): *Arch. Gen. Psychiatry,* 21:587–593.
132. Nasr, S. J., Pandey, G., Altman, E. G., Gibbons, R., Gaviria, F. M., and Davis, J. M. (1983): *Biol. Psychiatry,* 18:571–574.
133. Nemeroff, C. B., Widerlov, E., Bissette, G., Walleus, H., Karlsson, I., Ekland, K., Kitts, C. D., Loosen, P. T., and Vale, W. (1984): *Science,* 226:1342–1344.
134. Nitkovitch-Winer, M. B., and Everett, J. W. (1959): *Endocrinology,* 65:357–368.
135. Nugent, C. A., Eik-Nes, K., Kent, H. S., Samuels, L. T., and Tyler, F. H. (1960): *J. Clin. Endocrinol. Metab.,* 20:1259–1268.
136. Olpe, H.-R., and McEwen, B. S. (1976): *Brain Res.,* 105:121–128.
137. Ottenweller, J. F., and Meier, A. H. (1982): *Endocrinology,* 111: 1334–1338.
138. Perez-Reyes, M. (1972): In: *Recent Advances in the Psychobiology of the Depressive Illnesses,* edited by T. Williams, M. Katz, and J. Shield, Jr., pp. 131–135. Government Printing Office, Washington, DC.

139. Perini, G. I., Fava, G. A., Morphy, M. A., Carson, S. W., Molnar, G., and Jusko, W. J. (1984): *J. Affective Disord.*, 7:265–272.

140. Perkoff, G. T., Eik-Nes, K., Nugent, C. A., Fred, H. L., Nimer, R. A., Rush, L., Samuels, L. T., and Tyler, F. H. (1959): *J. Clin. Endocrinol. Metab.*, 19:432–443.

141. Pfohl, B., Sherman, B., Schlecte, J., and Stone, R. (1985): *Arch. Gen. Psychiatry*, 42:897–903.

142. Platman, S. R., and Fieve, R. R. (1968): *Arch. Gen. Psychiatry*, 18:591–594.

143. Poe, R. O., Rose, R. M., and Mason, J. W. (1970): *Psychosom. Med.*, 32:369–378.

144. Poland, R. E., and Rubin, R. T. (1982): *Life Sci.*, 30:177–181.

145. Popa, G. T., and Fielding, U. (1933): *J. Anat.*, 67:227–232.

146. Price, D. B., Thaler, M., and Mason, W. (1957): *Arch. Neurol. Psychiatry*, 77:646–656.

147. Reisine, T. D., Mezey, E., Palkovits, M., Brownstein, M. J., and Axelrod, J. (1986): *Science*, 231:502.

148. Reus, V. I., Joseph, M. S., and Dallman, M. F. (1982): *N. Engl. J. Med.*, 306:238–239.

149. Reus, V. I., Joseph, M., and Dallman, M. F. (1983): *Peptides*, 4: 785–788.

150. Riad-Fahmy, D., Read, G. F., Walker, R. F., and Griffiths, K. (1982): *Endocr. Rev.*, 3:367–395.

151. Roberts, J. L., Budarf, M. L., Baxter, J. D., and Herbert, E. (1979): *Biochemistry*, 18:4907–4915.

152. Rose, J. C., Goldsmith, P. C., Holland, F. J., Kaplan, S. L., and Ganong, W. F. (1976): *Neuroendocrinology*, 22:352–362.

153. Rosner, J. M., Cos, J. J., Biglieri, E. G., Hane, S., and Forsham, P. H. (1963): *J. Clin. Endocrinol. Metab.*, 23:820–827.

154. Rubin, R. T., Mandell, A. J., and Crandall, P. H. (1966): *Science*, 153:767–768.

155. Rubin, R. T., Young, W. M., and Clark, B. R. (1968): *Psychosom. Med.*, 30:162–171.

156. Rubinow, D. R., Post, R. M., Gold, P. W., Ballenger, J. C., and Wolff, E. A. (1984): In: *Neurobiology of Mood Disorders*, edited by R. M. Post and J. C. Ballenger, pp. 271–289. Williams & Wilkins, Baltimore.

157. Sachar, E. J. (1967): *Arch. Gen. Psychiatry*, 17:554–567.

158. Sachar, E. J. (1975): In: *American Handbook of Psychiatry*, edited by M. Reiser, pp. 299–313. Basic Books, New York.

159. Sachar, E. J., Hellman, L., Fukushima, D. K., and Gallagher, T. F. (1972): *Arch. Gen. Psychiatry*, 26:137–139.

160. Sachar, E. J., Hellman, L., Roffwarg, H. P., Halpern, F. S., Fukushima, D. K., and Gallagher, T. F. (1973): *Arch. Gen. Psychiatry*, 28:19–24.

161. Sachar, E. J., Finkelstein, J., and Hellman, L. (1971): *Arch. Gen. Psychiatry*, 25:263–269.

162. Saffran, M., Schally, A. V., and Benfey, B. G. (1955): *Endocrinology*, 57:439–444.

163. Saleman, M., Peck, L., and Egdahl, R. H. (1970): *Neuroendocrinology*, 6:361–367.

164. Sapolsky, R. M., Krey, L. C., and McEwen, B. S. (1983): *Brain Res.*, 289:235–240.

165. Sapolsky, R. M., Krey, L. C., and McEwen, B. S. (1984): *Endocrinology*, 114:287–292.

166. Sato, T. F., Sato, M., Shinsako, J., and Dallman, M. F. (1975): *Endocrinology*, 97:265–274.

167. Sawchenko, P. E., Swanson, L. W., and Vale, W. W. (1984): *Proc. Natl. Acad. Sci. USA*, 81:1883–1887.

168. Sayers, G. T., and Sayers, M. A. (1948): *Endocrinology*, 40:265–273.

169. Scapignini, U., Moberg, G. P., Van Lon, G. R., de Groot, J., and Ganong, W. F. (1971): *Neuroendocrinology*, 7:90–96.

170. Scharrer, E., and Scharrer, B. (1954): *Recent Prog. Horm. Res.*, 10:183–240.

171. Schlecte, J. A., and Sherman, B. M. (1982): *J. Clin. Endocrinol. Metab.*, 54:145–149.

171a.Schneider, H. P. G., and McCann, S. M. (1970): *Endocrinology*, 86:1127–1133.

172. Schoneshofer, M., Fenner, A., and Molmar, I. (1981): *Clin. Chem.*, 27:1875–1877.

173. Schubert, D., La Corbine, M., and Klier, G. G. (1980): *Brain Res.*, 190:67–69.

174. Sclare, A. B., and Grant, J. K. (1972): *Scott. Med. J.*, 17:7–8.

175. Simpson, C. W., Hamlet, M., and Brodish, A. (1980): *Neuroendocrinology*, 31:210–214.

176. Sirett, N. E., and Gibbs, F. P. (1969): *Endocrinology*, 85:355–359.

177. Slaunwhite, W. R., Lockie, G. N., Back, N., and Sandberg, A. A. (1962): *Science*, 135:1062–1063.

178. Slusher, M. A., and Hyde, J. E. (1961): *Endocrinology*, 69:1080–1084.

179. Smelik, P. G. (1977): *Ann. NY Acad. Sci.*, 297:580–588.

180. Smith, P. E. (1963): *Endocrinology*, 73:793–806.

181. Spiger, M., Jubiz, W., Meikle, A. W., West, C. D., and Tyler, F. H. (1975): *Arch. Intern. Med.*, 135:698–700.

182. Srivastava, A. K., and Meier, A. H. (1972): *Science*, 177:185–186.

183. Stoddard, F. J., Post, R. M., and Bunney, W. E., Jr. (1977): *Br. J. Psychiatry*, 130:72–78.

184. Stokes, P. E. (1970): Abstracts of the 52nd Meeting of the Endocrine Society, St. Louis.

185. Stokes, P. E. (1972): In: *Psychobiology of Depressive Illness*, edited by T. Williams and M. Katz, pp. 199–220. U.S. Government Printing Office, Washington, DC.

186. Stokes, P. E., and Stoll, P. M. (1974): Abstracts of the Annual Meeting of the Society for Neuroscience, St. Louis.

187. Stokes, P. E., Stoll, P. M., Koslow, S. H., Maas, P. W., Davis, J. M., Swann, A. C., and Robins, E. (1984): *Arch. Gen. Psychiatry*, 41:257–267.

188. Stokes, P. E., Stoll, P. M., Mattson, M. R., and Sollod, R. N. (1976): In: *Hormones, Behavior, and Psychopathology*, edited by E. Sachar, pp. 225–229. Raven Press, New York.

189. Stokes, P. E., Stoll, P. M., Skerry, J. E., and Silbersweig, D. (1986): Abstracts of the Annual Meeting of the Society of Biological Psychiatry, Washington, DC.

190. Suzuki, T. (1983): *Physiology of Adrenocortical Secretion*. Karger, Basel.

191. Takebe, K., Sakakura, M., and Mashimo, K. (1972): *Endocrinology*, 90:1515–1520.

192. Taylor, A. N. (1969): *Brain Res.*, 13:234–246.

193. Tomori, N., Suda, T., Tozawa, F., Demura, H., Shizumi, K., and Mouri, T. (1983): *J. Clin. Endocrinol. Metab.*, 57:1305–1307.

194. Traskman, L., Tybring, G., Asberg, M., Bertilsson, L., Lantto, O., and Schalling, D. (1980): *Arch. Gen. Psychiatry*, 37:761–767.

195. Ungar, F., and Halberg, F. (1962): *Science*, 137:1058–1060.

196. Vale, W., Spiess, J., Rivier, C., and Rivier, J. (1981): *Science*, 213:1394–1397.

197. Voigt, K. H., Fehm, H. L., Lang, R. E., and Walter, R. (1976): *Life Sci.*, 21:739–746.

198. Wehr, T. A., Muscettola, G., and Goodwin, F. K. (1980): *Arch. Gen. Psychiatry*, 37:257–263.

199. Weidenfeld, J., Siegal, R. A., Conforti, N., and Chowers, I. (1980): *Neuroendocrinology*, 31:81–84.

200. Whybrow, P. W., and Hurwitz, T. (1976): In: *Hormones, Behavior, and Psychopathology*, edited by E. J. Sachar, pp. 125–143. Raven Press, New York.

201. Wied, D. de (1969): In: *Frontiers in Neuroendocrinology*, edited by W. F. Ganong and L. S. Martini, pp. 97–140. Oxford University Press, London.

202. Wilkinson, C. W., Shinsako, J., and Dallman, M. F. (1981): *Endocrinology*, 109:162–169.

203. Wurtman, R. J. (1970): In: *The Neurosciences*, edited by F. O. Schmitt, pp. 530–538. The Rockefeller University Press, New York.

204. Yasuda, N., and Greer, M. A. (1976): *Clin. Res.*, 24:103.

205. Yerevanian, B. I., and Woolf, P. D. (1983): *Psychiatr. Res.*, 9: 45–51.

206. Zerssen, D. von, Barthelmes, H., Dirlich, G., Doerr, P., Emrich, H. M., von Lindern, L., Lund, R., and Pirke, K. M. (1985): *Psychiatr. Res.*, 16:51–63.

Psychopharmacology:
The Third Generation of Progress,
edited by Herbert Y. Meltzer.
Raven Press, New York © 1987.

CHAPTER 60

Clinical Use of the Dexamethasone Suppression Test in Psychiatry

George W. Arana and Ross J. Baldessarini

The dexamethasone suppression test (DST) is the most extensively evaluated biological test in psychiatry. The relative simplicity and low cost of the DST and improved assays of corticosteroids, combined with a reawakening of a more descriptive psychiatric nosology in the last decade (3), have produced a virtual explosion of publications on the DST in the 1980s following a seminal report by Carroll and his colleagues (20).

The test is usually performed by giving a small dose (1–2 mg) of the long-acting synthetic steroid, dexamethasone, at bedtime and obtaining serum samples at one or more times on the following day (typically midafternoon and late evening); a test is considered "positive" (nonsuppression) if the concentration of cortisol exceeds an experimentally defined criterion, typically between 4 and 6 μg/dl (40–60 ng/ml; 110–165 nM). Although there has been a great deal of interest in the application of the DST in clinical psychiatry, especially in the evaluation of major affective disorders, its clinical use requires considerable care (19). Moreover, several aspects of its biological basis and interpretation remain to be further clarified.

FACTORS INFLUENCING DST OUTCOME

Physiological and Pharmacological Factors

The proposal that the DST might reflect altered function of the limbic system or hypothalamus in severe depression or melancholia with a high degree of specificity remains controversial. Complex interactions among adrenal steroids, corticotropin (ACTH), corticotropin releasing factor (CRF), and various neurotransmitters that regulate CRF release may be involved in DST outcome (45,57). One indication of the complexity of the DST phenomenon is that available data are in conflict as to the correspondence of ACTH concentrations and either pre- or postdexamethasone cortisol levels in affective illnesses (4,35,47,50). Also, the relationships of altered ultradian and circadian rhythms of activity and sleep to similar changes in neuroendocrine function in psychiatric disorders need further study.

The pharmacology of dexamethasone and its actions on the hypothalamic-pituitary-adrenal (HPA) axis, although incompletely understood, also may have an impact on DST outcome. For example, several recent reports suggest that levels of the exogenous steroid can vary by up to 10-fold between individuals and may be 35 to 55% lower in some DST(+) patients so as to covary with the test outcome (4). If individual or illness-related differences in absorption or metabolism of the exogenous suppressing agent can influence the outcome of the DST, it may be useful to assay plasma dexamethasone and cortisol concentrations simultaneously (38). Even less is known about the status of metabolism of endogenous corticosteroids in psychiatric illnesses, although such alterations can occur in certain medical illnesses (33) and as a result of some medical treatments (20,22). Whether such pharmacokinetic factors exert an important influence on the outcome of the DST in psychiatric populations is not clear.

In general, there are many pharmacological, medical, and other clinical variables that may alter the outcome or interpretation of the DST in psychiatric populations. Many of these are summarized in Table 1.

Effects of Technique on DST Outcome

The rate of nonsuppression of cortisol following dexamethasone administration in depressed patients (test sensitivity) is dependent on the dose of dexamethasone em-

TABLE 1. *Factors that may influence the DST[a]*

Technical factors
    Compliance with oral dose of dexamethasone
    Characteristics of assay for cortisol (specificity, linearity)

Physiological factors
    Functional status of limbic, hypothalamic, and pituitary, in
        adrenal systems and response to exogenous steroids
    Pharmacokinetics of dexamethasone
    Metabolism of ACTH and cortisol in psychiatric disorders
    Altered circadian and ultradian biorhythms

Clinical factors
    Nonspecific stress effects (e.g., hospitalization, medical
        illness, ECT within 24 hr)
    Effects of treatment with and withdrawal from
        psychotropic drugs or other agents (alcohol, sedatives,
        anticonvulsants, antidepressants, steroids)
    Acute major medical illnesses (fever, cancer, recent
        seizures, etc.)
    Endocrine disorders
    Changes in diet or weight
    Altered sleep and activity
    Age < 18 and >60 years

[a] Discussions of these factors are available elsewhere (4,5,14,15,17–20,22,48,62). Most of these conditions lead to "false positive" DST outcomes; some are not firmly established.

ployed. Test sensitivity in over 5,000 patients apparently suffering from major depression and given 1 mg of dexamethasone averaged 44%, and for over 300 apparently clinically similar patients given 2 mg, the rate averaged 31% (5). Occasionally, and perhaps more often in outpatients, artifactual nonsuppression can occur because the patient failed to take the dexamethasone. Several proposals for confirming compliance include use of parenteral dexamethasone (41), adding a readily detected marker such as a urine-coloring dye or a small dose of a lithium salt, or assay of a morning sample of serum to confirm early depression of cortisol output, but the best simple method of maximizing compliance is careful clinical monitoring of dexamethasone administration.

Some information on DST results vs the time of blood sampling for the assay of cortisol in psychiatric populations is available. Studies of normal subjects and various medically ill patients suggest that 1 mg of dexamethasone strongly suppresses cortisol in more than 90% of such subjects for at least 24 hr (58). Studies based on comparisons of depressed and normal subjects suggest that specificity (suppression in normal or other comparison subjects) is not lost appreciably at sampling times up to 24 hr following a bedtime dose of 1 mg of dexamethasone (20,57). Although full suppression may occur during the first 12 hr, afternoon and evening samples are most likely to show escape from normal suppression by dexamethasone (20,47,57). Sampling later than 24 hr would increase the risk of artifactual nonsuppression. Sampling more than twice (between 12 and 24 hr) for assay of cortisol seems to add little to test sensitivity (20,57).

As the criterion of plasma cortisol level for nonsuppression is lowered, sensitivity rises, but specificity falls correspond-

ingly (1). The trade-off between sensitivity and specificity is an empirical matter to be determined in each set of circumstances. A test criterion for plasma cortisol ≥ 5.0 μg/dl (50 ng/ml or 138 nM) applied between 8 and 24 hr after 1 to 2 mg of dexamethasone given at 11 p.m. has usually provided relatively high specificity (presumably false-positive results average <10% in normal subjects), while providing moderate sensitivity (approximately 40–50%) in patients with major or melancholic depression (20,57). If the criterion is raised to 6 or 7 μg/dl (165 or 193 nM), specificity (in normals) can be increased further only slightly, but there is a 20 to 30% loss of test sensitivity in depressed patients (15,57).

The method of assay of cortisol may have an effect on rates of nonsuppression in the DST, and results of various assays require careful standardization to assure accuracy, especially at levels of cortisol of 4 to 10 μg/dl (5,20,40,51,59). In studies involving nearly 2,200 depressed patients, the rates of nonsuppression of cortisol averaged between 45 and 50% with either a competitive protein binding assay or a radioimmunoassay (RIA) (5).

CLINICAL STUDIES OF DST IN PSYCHIATRY

General Approach

We recently reviewed literature on the use of the DST in psychiatric patients with particular emphasis on the large body of information published recently on its role in diagnosis, prediction of treatment outcome, and clinical course (5). The clinical reports reviewed were screened for diagnostic methods, medications being taken, time and dose of dexamethasone administered, time that blood samples were drawn for cortisol assay, and method of assay employed.

Studies included followed RDC, *Diagnostic and Statistical Manual of Mental Disorders,* 3rd edition (DSM-III), or apparently equivalent objective criteria. Most of the accepted reports (>150) used a plasma cortisol criterion of ≥5 μg/ dl (rarely 4 or 6 μg/dl) to define nonsuppression and a dose of dexamethasone of 1 mg (rarely 2 mg). Most reports assayed cortisol in 4 p.m. and 11 p.m. venous blood samples obtained the day after dexamethasone administration, but several included an 8 a.m. sample or used only a single sampling time. When several publications were available from the same investigators and may have included some of the same subjects, we attempted to rely on the latest publication or that reporting the largest number of patients, although it was not always clear which patients were reported more than once in this large and complex literature.

Sensitivity of the DST in Major Affective Disorders

Overall, the sensitivity of the DST in reports on over 5,000 patients averaged 44% nonsuppression among cases with major depressive illnesses (5). The sensitivity of the DST averaged 46% in over 1,000 patients with a DSM-III diagnosis of major depressive disorder and 41% in a similar number of patients with an RDC diagnosis of major depressive illness, indicating that results obtained with these two common diagnostic methods can be pooled.

DST sensitivity averaged significantly higher in elderly patients (aged >60 years) with depressive illnesses (64.5%) (2,5,20,24,25,37,57) than in all adult patients (44%) or young patients (aged <18 years; 34%). It is not yet proved that this tendency for older depressed patients to have somewhat higher rates of nonsuppression in the DST represents an important pathophysiological or nosological feature of patients in that age group. Adequate evaluation of the risk of relatively high postdexamethasone levels of cortisol in normal elderly persons and children remains to be carried out, although some preliminary reports suggest that such an increase may occur in older patients (51), especially following 0.5 mg of dexamethasone (44). If some loss of specificity proves to be a problem in the elderly, it might be increased by increasing the dose of dexamethasone or the criterion level of cortisol (51); conversely, it may be possible to increase sensitivity in young depressed patients by lowering the dose or criterion. Clearly, application of DST to demented or delirious elderly patients results in high, spurious rates of nonsuppression (5,12,31,37,48).

Severity of affective illness may also influence the outcome of the DST. Available data involving assessment of the severity of affective illness by clinical rating scales suggest a moderate relationship between higher depression scores and nonsuppression of cortisol (5,15,24,25,32). Some findings also suggest that higher rates of cortisol nonsuppression are found among depressed patients with endogenous or melancholic features (14,23). There is a particularly striking increase in the rank order of DST sensitivity reported in grief reaction (10%), dysthymia (23%), major depression (44%), melancholia (50%), and psychotic affective disorders (psychotic depression plus mixed bipolar disorder, 69%) (see 5). Although such subcategories may be influenced by severity (61), the results may also reflect qualitative pathophysiologic variables.

Attempts to improve the subtyping of major depressive illnesses have included at least 12 reports (see 5), involving nearly 900 depressed patients, on the congruence of cortisol nonsuppression with family history criteria. DST(+) cases were somewhat more common among depressed patients with a family history of depression in first-degree relatives (47%) than in sporadic cases (38%) or those with a family history of alcoholism (27%) (5,53). The distinction between bipolar depression (38%) or mania (48%) and major depression overall (44%) has suggested only small differences in rates of cortisol nonsuppression (5), but requires further study.

Specificity of the DST for Major Depression

A particularly controversial aspect of the DST in psychiatry is its specificity (true-negative rate, or adequate suppression among those lacking the index diagnosis, calculated as 100% minus the false-positive rate) when patients with major depression or apparently related conditions are compared with normal controls or other diagnostic groups. One reason for such controversy is suspicion that available clinical methods of subtyping affective disorders are likely

to yield biologically heterogeneous groups. Factors such as signs and symptoms, age of onset, course of illness, family history, treatment response, and possibly personality characteristics may need to be combined with biological descriptors to yield biomedically coherent groups, even if they cut across currently proposed clinical phenotypes, such as the bipolar-nonbipolar distinction and the melancholic vs dysthymic or endogenous vs nonendogenous subtypes. Nevertheless, the application of such biological tests as the DST to clinical nosology requires caution if the biological index is not stable as a state marker and is influenced by severity or acuteness of illness per se or by nonspecific aspects of illness due to stress; or if the biological index does not correspond strongly with external validating criteria, such as family history, treatment response, or course of illness.

Specificity of the DST (5) is consistently high (92.8 ± 2.5% [±SEM] in 32 studies) with respect to normal controls, due to the low rate of false-positive nonsuppression of cortisol (7.2%) in over 1,100 normal subjects, and so readily distinguishes patients with major depression from normal persons. Similarly high specificity can be obtained when normal subjects are pooled with nonpsychiatrically ill medical or neurological patients (91% in nearly 1,300 patients). For clinical application in supporting psychiatric differential diagnosis, the specific distinction between depression and normality has limited importance.

The specificity of the DST has been reported to be ≥87% in several other psychiatric groups, including normal persons during bereavement (91%) and patients with anxiety, panic, or phobic disorders (88%), or schizophrenia (87%). Specificity is somewhat lower in dysthymic disorder or nonendogenous depression (77%), although the distinction of this group from major depression may be unreliable. When control subjects and patients with psychiatric disorders other than major depression were pooled (over 2,000 cases), the apparent specificity of the DST was 86.5% (Table 2).

Acute psychosis or mania (5,6) and dementia (12,31,48) are apparently especially hard to differentiate from major depression by use of the DST and were found to yield values of specificity of 52 to 65%. That is, as presently performed, the DST may not be effective in resolving clinical difficulties sometimes encountered in differentiating these diagnoses from major depression or melancholia. An alternative view is that some of these severe disorders and even some cases of dysthymia may have pathophysiological features in common with melancholia. Nevertheless, the possible scientific or clinical utility of modifying of the clinical concept of major affective disorders requires further experimental evaluation.

Other comparisons may have greater clinical utility, however. For example, nonsuppression in the DST seems to have impressive power to distinguish psychotic-affective patients from other clinically relevant groups (5,6,52). Psychotic affective disorders would include illnesses diagnosed as major depression or mania, with features of psychosis, and so include patients with "dysphoric" mania or mixed manic-depressive states, severe mania with psychotic features, as well as cases of severe (especially agitated) depression with psychotic features. Representative data on such patients suggest a DST(+) rate of 69% (Table 2).

TABLE 2. *Rates of nonsuppression in the DST in representative clinical groups[a]*

Group	Subjects (N)	Nonsuppression rate (%)
Controls		
Normal	1,130	7
Normal + nonpsychiatric patients	1,269	8[b]
Major depression patients		
Young (<18 years)	205	34
Elderly (>60 years)	183	64
Familial	265	47
Sporadic	379	38
All adult major depression	4,411	43
Bipolar	110	38
Melancholic or endogenous	583	50
Psychotic[c]	150	67
Mixed bipolar (manic-depressive)[c]	41	78
Psychiatric comparison patients		
Anxiety disorders (inc. panic and phobias)	74	8[b]
Schizophrenia	260	13[b]
Minor depression (dysthymic disorder or nonendogenous)	238	23[b]
Acute or atypical psychoses[d]	69	34[b]
Dementia	174	41
Mania[e]	137	41[b]

[a] Specific references are provided elsewhere (5), but the primary data have been reanalyzed for this table.

[b] As a representative estimate of overall specificity of the DST in comparisons vs normal subjects or patients with psychiatric disorders other than major depression, the categories indicated ([b]) yield an overall specificity of 86.5%.

[c] Pooled psychotic affective cases (N = 191) yield a rate of nonsuppression of 69.4%.

[d] Includes schizophreniform, schizoaffective, and atypical psychosis.

[e] Excludes a study with no DST(−) RDC manics among 60 patients tested at 8 a.m.

A striking separation of psychotic-affective patients from (chronic) schizophrenics was found (positive predictive power, PPP-50[1] = 84%) (5). Psychotic affective patients were not quite as clearly distinguished by the DST from patients with dysthymia (PPP-50 = 75%), but the distinction from normal controls was clear (PPP-50 = 90%). Psychotic affective patients were also not as clearly distinguished by

[1] PPP-50 is the calculated predictive power of a positive DST, assuming a prevalence of the index illness among those tested of 50% (PPP-50). This measurement (11) is closely related to the specificity of a test and represents the chance that a positive test result will be associated with the index condition (rate of index diagnosis or true-positive test results among all positive test results). This measure is useful in comparing index and comparison diagnoses at the same prevalence.

the DST from a combination of those with an "atypical" psychosis or schizoaffective disorder (combined, as they have very few distinguishing features in DSM-III; PPP-50 = 67%), and these categories may overlap with the psychotic affective disorders.

These observations indicate that the DST is relatively effective in distinguishing psychotic-affective patients from chronic schizophrenics (or normals) but less effective in separating the former from patients with other acute psychotic disorders, mania, or even dysthymia. The failure of nonsuppression of cortisol to distinguish psychotic-affective cases clearly from others with acute psychoses, mania, or even dysthymia, may suggest a shared pathophysiology or similar stress responses among these clinical disorders.

Additional possible diagnostic uses of the DST include the confirmation of clinical diagnoses of probable major depression, potentially amenable to antidepressant treatment, either occurring alone (primary depression) or associated with another illness (secondary depression). Although such an approach to differentiating depression from dementia in the elderly has been disappointing, encouraging preliminary findings have been reported in chronic pain patients (34). As another example, several studies have found DST nonsuppression in 64% of stroke (including aphasic) patients with signs of major depression vs 20% of similar, usually elderly, patients without evidence of depression (5,26,36,49). These various comparisons of rates of nonsuppression of cortisol secretion in the DST are summarized in Table 2.

Treatment Response and DST Status

In addition to its possible clinical utility in supporting certain differential diagnoses, the DST might aid the clinician by predicting short-term treatment response. We found 19 recent reports in which over 500 depressed patients were tested with the DST and treated with an antidepressant or electroconvulsive therapy (ECT). Eight of these, selected on the basis of the adequacy of the reported criteria of diagnosis, treatment, and response, yielded a total of 319 patients (5). Of those who were initially DST(+), 76% responded to treatment, whereas only 64% of those initially DST(−) responded comparably well (Table 3). A similar difference occurred among the seven reports of this group that involved only an antidepressant [10.5% difference, favoring the DST(+) cases]. The difference in treatment response rates between DST(+) and DST(−) cases of major depression varied considerably between studies (16,43); moreover, the overall effect was small (ca 11%) and not statistically significant (Table 3). Another recent review of many of the same studies came to the same conclusion and suggested that the DST does not add to current clinical methods for recommending treatment (28). Other preliminary observations, however, suggest that there may be an excess of responses to a placebo among DST(−) depressed patients (46,56). These observations suggest that differences between DST(+) and (−) depressed patients in responsiveness to thymoleptic or placebo treatment may exist and are interesting from a research perspective, but require further study to assess their possible clinical utility in

TABLE 3. *DST to predict treatment response and outcome in depression*

Criterion	N	Proportion meeting criterion DST(+)	DST(−)	Ratio
Favorable initial antidepressant response[a]	308	120/159 (75.5%)	103/160 (64.4%)	1.17
Poor outcome at follow-up[b]	136	34/44 (77.3%)	19/101 (18.8%)	4.11

[a] Successfully treated cases (antidepressants, lithium salts, ECT) among those initially DST(+) or (−) in eight studies meeting stringent selection criteria reviewed in detail elsewhere, including one study with some cases treated with ECT (5). The overall difference was small (11.1%) and not significant by chi-squared for pooled data (χ^2 for main effect = 1.61, $p = 0.20$) as recommended by Mantel and Haenszel.

[b] Indicate cases with poor outcome (including suicide) among initially DST(+), treatment-responsive cases in which DST remained or again became positive. The data are based on 13 reports (see 4) involving a mean ($\pm$SD) of 10.5 ± 8.4 subjects per study. The difference is 4.1-fold. Analysis of the 10 studies appropriate for the Mantel-Haenszel χ^2 method indicates a statistically significant difference ($\chi^2 = 28.2, p = 1.18 \times 10^{-8}$).

predicting treatment response in primary major depression or in major depression associated with other medical or psychiatric diagnoses.

Even if DST(+) patients with major depression, as a group, are somewhat more likely to respond to adequate medical treatment, it does not follow that treatment should be any less vigorous in DST(−) cases. Excessive reliance on DST nonsuppression to guide treatment selection may lead to unfavorable outcomes. For example, severe cases of depression with psychotic features, while having high rates of cortisol nonsuppression (Table 2), may respond preferentially to the addition of a neuroleptic agent (55) or ECT (42) to antidepressant treatment. Moreover, some cases of bipolar disorder (with a high rate of cortisol nonsuppression) may be worsened by use of an antidepressant alone without other mood-stabilizing or antipsychotic treatment; examples include induction or worsening of mania in mixed bipolar and bipolar depressive disorders, which are not always easily differentiated from major depression (9,29).

Other proposed uses of the DST are to monitor the progress of treatment. Hypothetically, conversion of the DST response from positive to negative might correspond with or predict a favorable clinical response. However, in some cases the DST reportedly normalizes rapidly before appreciable change in depression ratings occurs (13), perhaps especially after ECT (21). Reanalysis of one recent report (30) indicates that, over the first month of antidepressant treatment, postdexamethasone cortisol levels fell by 67 and 71% (nonsignificant difference) in treatment-responsive and nonresponsive cases, respectively, whereas depression ratings of the same groups fell by 80 and 32% (highly significant). Although normalization may help to predict eventual clinical

response (30), this proposal seems unwarranted without more compelling evidence that treatment of nonresponsive patients fails to normalize the DST. If the DST normalizes while patients are still depressed, one might question the generality of its validity as a "state marker" of major depression.

An additional potential role of the DST is to help in predicting or following outcome in major depression. At least 13 reports provide data on DST results and clinical outcome of 144 depressed patients (5). Poor outcome was defined variously in these reports but included early relapse or suicidal behavior within several months of initial DST assessment and treatment. Overall, of DST(+) depressed patients who subsequently converted to and maintained normal cortisol suppression, only 19% had a poor clinical outcome, but 77% of those who continued to be, or again became, DST(+) had a poor or fatal outcome (Table 3). Although there may be a greater likelihood of relapse or suicide in depressive illness if the DST remains or soon again becomes positive, these provocative findings are based on small numbers of cases per study, are largely anecdotal or incidental, and are not definitive. At least one prospective, controlled study has been undertaken in depressed patients followed for 6 to 12 months; preliminary results suggest only moderate differences in the rate of poor outcome between treated depressed patients who were persistently DST(+) and those who became DST(−) (E. D. Peselow, *personal communication*, June 1985).

CONCLUSIONS

The DST has had unprecedentedly intensive investigation among biological tests proposed for clinical use in psychiatry. Its study has involved hundreds of reports and thousands of patients since the 1970s. Although many important technical aspects of conducting the test appear to be well accepted and validated, additional technical information is needed, including clarification of whether suspected individual and illness-related variation in the bioavailability or pharmacokinetics of dexamethasone may influence DST outcome. Even if there is no systematic difference in the absorption or elimination of dexamethasone between normal and psychiatric populations, marked interindividual differences in plasma dexamethasone suggest that the sensitivity and specificity of the DST might be improved by factoring dexamethasone levels into test interpretations. There also may be advantages in the development of a modified test involving other exogenous and index steroids, such as monitoring corticosterone levels after administering cortisol (7,39,60).

The application of the DST in psychiatry continues to be of considerable scientific, pathophysiologic, and nosologic interest (5,8,10,17–20,23). The limited sensitivity of the DST in major depression (even with melancholic features) to about half of the patients reported is striking and consistent but poorly explained. It does not seem to be due entirely to sampling bias, because of transient ultradian peaks in cortisol secretion that occur even following dexamethasone in many depressed patients (54).

The DST may be sufficiently specific as to have some

diagnostic value in psychiatry. Rates of nonsuppression are relatively low in anxiety disorders or dysthmic disorder, and low in schizophrenia compared to psychotic affective conditions (Table 2). The test may help to support clinical differentiation of these disorders. The additional suggestion that nonsuppression responses may emerge during follow-up of some depressed patients somewhat earlier than clinically apparent changes in mood or behavior requires investigation.

A fundamental concern about the DST is whether it is an expression of altered regulation of the HPA axis at the level of limbic-hypothalamic interactions. Relations among the various components of the HPA axis are complex, and the hypothesis concerning contributions of brain pathophysiology to DST outcome in psychiatric patients requires further validation. The additional old question whether responses in this basic alarm system (27), as in the central and peripheral sympathetic systems (8), may be relatively nonspecific concomitants of the distress of acute, severe emotional disorder remains open.

Gains from the intensive study of the DST in recent years include a growing understanding of the physiology and pharmacology of the HPA axis and a greater appreciation of appropriate methods and standards by which to evaluate medical "tests" in psychiatry, including application of the principles of conditional probability and decision theory (17–19,26). In conclusion, neither uncritical enthusiasm nor excessive skepticism about the DST is warranted. Evidence to date should encourage investigators to pursue refinement of the DST or other tests of HPA functioning to increase their predictive power and clinical utility. Experience with this testing method in psychiatry strongly encourages the search for additional relatively simple biological measures to help validate the diagnosis and objective categorization of psychiatric patients and to aid in predicting treatment responses and longer-term prognosis.

ACKNOWLEDGMENTS

This work was supported, in part, by a Research Administration grant of the USVA and by USPHS (NIMH) awards and grants MH-47370, MH-31154, and MH-36224. The manuscript was prepared by Mrs. B. Bradley.

REFERENCES

1. Aggernaes, H., Kirkegaard, C., Krog-Meyer, I., Kijne, B., Larsen, J. K., Lund-Laursen, A., Lykke-Olesen, L., Mikkelsen, P. L., Rasmussen, S., and Bjorum, N. (1983): Acta Psychiatr. Scand., 67:258–264.
2. Alexopoulos, G. S., Young, R. C., Kocsis, J. H., Brockner, N., Butler, T. A., and Stokes, P. E. (1984): Biol. Psychiatry, 19:1567–1571.
3. American Psychiatric Association (1980): Diagnostic and Statistical Manual, Third Edition (DSM-III). American Psychiatric Association, Washington, DC.
4. Arana, G. W., and Baldessarini, R. J. (1987): In: Hormones and Depression, edited by U. Halbreich and R. Rose. Raven Press, New York (in press).
5. Arana, G. W., Baldessarini, R. J., and Ornsteen, M. (1985): Arch. Gen. Psychiatry, 42:1193–1204.
6. Arana, G. W., Barreira, P. J., Lipinski, J. F., Schachter, H., Cohen, B. M., and Ornsteen, M. (1985): Proc. Am. Psychiatr. Assoc. Annu. Meeting, Dallas, May, p. 60 (NR 96).
7. Arana, G. W., Wilens, T. E., and Baldessarini, R. J. (1985): Psychoneuroendocrinology, 10:49–60.
8. Baldessarini, R. J. (1983): Biomedical Aspects of Depression and Its Treatment. American Psychiatric Press, Washington, DC.
9. Baldessarini, R. J. (1985): In: Chemotherapy in Psychiatry: Principles and Practice, pp. 130–234. Harvard University Press, Cambridge.
10. Baldessarini, R. J., and Arana, G. W. (1985): J. Clin. Psychiatry, 46:25–29.
11. Baldessarini, R. J., Finklestein, S. P., and Arana, G. W. (1983): Arch. Gen. Psychiatry, 40:569–573.
12. Balldin, J., Gottfries, G. G., Karlsson, I., Lindstedt, G., Langstrom, G., and Walinder, J. (1983): Br. J. Psychiatry, 143:277–281.
13. Berger, M., and Klein, H. E. (1984): Eur. Arch. Psychiatr. Neurol. Sci., 234:137–146.
14. Berger, M., Pirke, K.-M., Doerr, P., Krieg, J. C., and von Zerssen, D. (1983): Arch. Gen. Psychiatry, 40:585–586.
15. Berger, M., Pirke, K. M., Doerr, P., Krieg, J. C., and von Zerssen, D. (1984): Br. J. Psychiatry, 145:372–382.
16. Brown, W. A., and Shuey, I. (1980): Arch. Gen. Psychiatry, 37:747–751.
17. Carroll, B. J. (1982): Br. J. Psychiatry, 140:292–304.
18. Carroll, B. J. (1985): J. Clin. Psychiatry, 46:13–24.
19. Carroll, B. J. (1986): J. Clin. Psychiatry, 47(Suppl. 1):10–12.
20. Carroll, B. J., Feinberg, M., Greden, J. F., Tarika, J., Albala, A. A., Haskett, R. F., James, N. M., Kronfol, Z., Lohr, N., Steiner, M., deVigne, J. P., and Young, E. (1981): Arch. Gen. Psychiatry, 38:15–22.
21. Coryell, W., and Zimmerman, M. (1983): Biol. Psychiatry, 18:21–27.
22. Crapo, L. (1979): Metabolism, 28:955–977.
23. Davidson, J. R., Lipper, S., Zung, W. W., Strickland, R., Krishnan, K. R., and Mahorney, S. (1984): Am. J. Psychiatry, 141:1220–1223.
24. Davis, K. L., Davis, B. M., Mathé, A. A., Mohs, R. C., Rothpearl, A. B., Levy, M. I., Gorman, L. K., and Berger, P. (1984): Am. J. Psychiatry, 141:872–874.
25. Feinberg, M., and Carroll, B. J. (1984): Arch. Gen. Psychiatry, 41:1080–1085.
26. Finklestein, S. P., Benowitz, L. I., Baldessarini, R. J., Arana, G. W., Levine, D., Woo, E., Bear, D., Moya, K., and Stoll, A. L. (1982): Ann. Neurol., 12:463–468.
27. Friedman, S. B., Mason, J. W., and Hamburg, D. A. (1963): Psychosom. Med., 25:364–376.
28. Gitlin, M. J., and Gerner, R. H. (1986): J. Clin. Psychiatry, 47:16–21.
29. Goodwin, F. K. (1983): McLean Hosp. J., 8:1–16.
30. Greden, J. F., Gardner, R., King, D., Grunhaus, L., Carroll, B. J., and Kronfol, Z. (1983): Arch. Gen. Psychiatry, 40:393–500.
31. Jenike, M., and Albert, M. S. (1984): J. Am. Geriatr. Soc., 32:441–444.
32. Kasper, S., and Beckmann, H. (1983): Acta Psychiatr. Scand., 68:31–37.
33. Krieger, D. T. (1979): In: Endocrinology, Vol. 2, edited by L. J. Degroot, G. F. Cahill, L. Martini, D. H. Nelson, W. D. Odell, J. T. Potts, E. Steinberger, and A. I. Wiregrad, pp. 1139–1156. Grune & Stratton, New York.
34. Krishnan, K. R., France, R. D., Pelton, S., McCann, U. D., Manepalli, A. N., and Davidson, J. R. (1985): Biol. Psychiatry, 20:957–964.
35. Linkowski, P., Mendlewicz, J., Leclercq, R., Brasseur, M., Hubain, P., Golstein, J., Copinschi, G., and Van Cauter, E. (1985): J. Clin. Endocrinol. Metab., 61:429–438.
36. Lipsey, J. R., Robinson, R. G., Pearlson, G. D., Rao, K., and Price, T. R. (1985): Am. J. Psychiatry, 142:318–323.
37. McKeith, I. G. (1984): Br. J. Psychiatry, 145:389–393.
38. Meikle, A. W. (1982): Clin. Endocrinol., 16:401–408.
39. Meikle, A. W., Stanchfield, J. B., West, C. D., and Tyler, F. H. (1974): Arch. Intern. Med., 134:1068–1071.
40. Meltzer, H. Y., and Fang, V. S. (1983): Arch. Gen. Psychiatry, 40:501–505.
41. Mendlewicz, J., Charles, G., and Franckson, J. M. (1982): Br. J. Psychiatry, 141:464–470.

42. Minter, R. E., and Mandel, M. R. (1979): *J. Nerv. Ment. Dis.*, 162:726–733.
43. Nelson, W. H., Orr, W. W., Stevenson, J. M., and Shane, S. R. (1982): *Arch. Gen. Psychiatry*, 39:1033–1036.
44. Oxenkrug, G. F., Pomara, N., McIntyre, I. M., Branconnier, R. J., Stanley, M., and Gershon, S. (1983): *Psychiatry Res.*, 10: 125–130.
45. Pepper, G. M., and Krieger, D. T. (1984): In: *Neurobiology of Mood Disorders*, edited by R. M. Post and J. C. Ballenger, pp. 245–270. Williams & Wilkins, Baltimore.
46. Peselow, E. D., Stanley, M., and Fieve, R. R. (1985): *Proc. Annu. Meeting Am. College Neuropsychopharmacology*, Maui, HI, December, p. 124.
47. Pfohl, B., Sherman, B., Schlechte, J., and Stone, R. (1985): *Arch. Gen. Psychiatry*, 42:897–903.
48. Raskind, M., Peskind, E., Rivard, M., Veith, R., and Barnes, R. (1982): *Am. J. Psychiatry*, 139:1468–1471.
49. Redding, M., Orto, L., Willensky, P., Fortuna, I., Day, N., Steiner, S. F., Gehr, L., and McDowell, F. (1985): *Arch. Neurol.*, 42:209–212.
50. Reus, V. I., Joseph, M., and Dallman, M. (1983): *Peptides*, 4:785–788.
51. Rosenbaum, A. H., Schatzberg, A. F., MacLaughlin, R. A., Snyder, K., Jiang, N.-S., Ilstrup, D., Rothschild, A. J., and Kliman, B. (1984): *Am. J. Psychiatry*, 141:1550–1555.
52. Rothschild, A. J. (1985): *McLean Hosp. J.*, 10:68–83.
53. Schlesser, M. A., Winokur, G., and Sherman, B. M. (1980): *Arch. Gen. Psychiatry*, 37:737–743.
54. Sherman, B., Pfohl, B., and Winokur, G. (1984): *Arch. Gen. Psychiatry*, 41:271–275.
55. Spiker, D. G., Weiss, J. C., Dealy, R. S., Griffin, S. J., Hanin, I., Neil, J. F., Perel, J. M., Rossi, A. J., and Soloff, P. H. (1985): *Am. J. Psychiatry*, 142:430–436.
56. Srivastava, R. V., Schwimmer, R., Brown, W. A., and Arito, M. (1985): *Proc. Am. Psychiatr. Assoc. Annu. Meeting*, Dallas, May, p. 59 (NR 94).
57. Stokes, P. E., Stoll, P. M., Koslow, S. M., Maas, J. W., Davis, J. M., Swann, A. C., and Robins, E. (1984): *Arch. Gen. Psychiatry*, 41:257–267.
58. Tourigny-Rivard, M.-F., Raskind, M., and Rivard, D. (1981): *Biol. Psychiatry*, 16:1177–1184.
59. Wilens, T. E., Arana, G. W., Baldessarini, R. J., and Cremens, C. (1983): *Psychiatry Res.*, 8:199–206.
60. Wilens, T. E., Ritchie, J. C., and Carroll, B. J. (1984): *Psychoneuroendocrinology*, 9:45–56.
61. Zimmerman, M., Coryell, W., and Pfohl, B. (1986): *Am. J. Psychiatry*, 143:98–100.
62. Zimmerman, M., Pfohl, B. M., and Coryell, W. H. (1984): *Biol. Psychiatry*, 19:923–928.

Psychopharmacology:
The Third Generation of Progress,
edited by Herbert Y. Meltzer.
Raven Press, New York © 1987.

CHAPTER 61

Neuropeptide Function in Affective Illness: Corticotropin-Releasing Hormone and Somatostatin as Model Systems

Philip W. Gold and David R. Rubinow

HISTORICAL OVERVIEW

The past decade has revealed that the brain is the most prolific of all endocrine organs, producing scores of neuropeptide hormones within and beyond the boundaries of the endocrine hypothalamus. It is extraordinary that this concept of the brain as a gland was first advanced in 400 B.C. by Hippocrates (152), but that so little had been learned about the endocrine functions of the brain over the next 2,350 years. For instance, 500 years passed after Hippocrates' pronouncement before one of the principal target tissues of the neurohormones was inadvertently identified by Galen, which he mistook for a mucous (pituita) secretion of the brain (80,123). Sixteen hundred more years passed until the hypothalamic-pituitary system of portal vessels was described by Lieutaud (71), and another 200 until its functional significance was alluded to by Harris in 1948 (56). By 1955 Saffron and Schally obtained the first convincing evidence of the existence of an endocrine function for the brain, when they showed that hypothalamic fragments possessed remarkable corticotropin releasing properties when incubated with pituicytes *in vitro* (118). It is on this foundation, spanning many years, that the most recent decade in neurohormone research was initiated in 1976 by the awarding of the Nobel Prize in medicine and physiology to Guillemin and Schally for determining the structure of two representative hypothalamic anterior pituitary releasing hormones, thyrotropin-releasing hormone (TRH) and luteinizing hormone-releasing hormone (LHRH).

The past decade of neuropeptide research has fulfilled much of the promise heralded by the recognition of Guillemin and Schally by the Nobel Committee. Indeed, most of the major concepts regarding neuropeptide physiology and function that many now take for granted have emerged out of the investigations of the past decade. For instance, once the sequence of several hypothalamic hormones was known, it became possible to demonstrate that many were synthesized and distributed in multiple brain regions lying outside of the hypothalamus. Such a widespread distribution of the neurohormones in brain provided the primary supporting evidence for the principle that the brain, in contrast to most other organs, was the principal target of its own secretions. Moreover, this principle, along with the discovery that brain hormones exerted relatively long-lasting effects at minute concentrations, helped to explain subsequent observations that neuropeptides could act to organize the activity of multiple nerve cell aggregates located disparately throughout the central nervous system to promote the execution of complex behavioral and physiological processes. For instance, extensive aggregates of corticotropin-releasing hormone (CRH) cell bodies and terminal fields were found not only in the hypothalamus, but also in the amygdala, the cortex, and in close association with the central autonomic system and the locus ceruleus (12,82). This distribution of CRH within and beyond the boundaries of the hypothalamus provided an anatomic context for the observation that CRH can simultaneously activate and coordinate not only neuroendocrine but also metabolic (15), circulatory (16), and behavioral responses (14,138,142) that are adaptive in stressful situations. Hence, in the rat, intracerebroventricular (ICV) administration of CRH leads not only to activation of the HPA axis (50), but also to activation of the sympathetic nervous system and to several behavioral changes characteristic of the stress response, including decreased feeding (14) and sexual behavior (133), assumption of a freeze posture in a foreign environment (140), and increased exploration in familiar surroundings (140).

The work of the past decade has been distinguished not only by studies that began to elucidate the distribution and biological actions of neuropeptides, but also by studies exploring the regulation of their synthesis and release. For instance, of particular interest to psychiatry were the observations starting in the mid-1970s that the biogenic amines thought to play an important role in the pathophysiology of affective disorder also influenced the functional activity of all of the known hypothalamic hormones. Conversely, hypothalamic hormones were shown to significantly influence transsynaptic neurotransmitter functional activity. These concepts were dramatized by the demonstration that neuropeptides and biogenic amine neurotransmitters such as cholecystokinin and dopamine were often colocalized in the same neuron. Not unexpectedly, neurohormones were also shown to be intimately connected to one another's activity, and examples of the colocalization of two or more neurohormones in the same cell body also became commonplace. For example, following adrenalectomy, CRH and vasopressin are found to be colocalized in cell bodies of the paraventricular nucleus. Parenthetically, this colocalization of CRH and vasopressin during glucocorticoid deficiency probably has functional significance, since CRH and vasopressin have been shown to exert a synergistic rather than an additive effect on pituitary ACTH secretion (47).

The unraveling of the details associated with neuropeptide synthesis and metabolism has revealed many additional layers that can be interwoven into the complex and often subtle interplay between neuropeptides, physiology, and behavior. For instance, the genes that code for the amino acid sequence of neuropeptides almost always code for families of large precursor peptides, which are cleaved to form one or more biologically active moieties. For example, the sequences of ACTH and β-endorphin are contained within the sequence of a large precursor peptide, proopiomelanocortin (68). Following stimulation by CRH, these two peptides are released in equivalent amounts by the pituitary into the systemic circulation (55). Guillemin suggested that during stress ACTH might be elaborated for metabolic adaptation and β-endorphin for behavioral adaptation (55). Cleavage at specific sites of a large precursor represents only one form of posttranslational processing. Other posttranslational events include methylation, amidation, or alteration of the sequence of a posttranslational fragment to produce a product with enhanced, diminished, or antithetical biologic activity compared with the original posttranslational product. For example, removal of the N-terminal glutamine from TRH results in a compound that, compared to TRH, has opposite effects on prolactin release, as well as more powerful activating properties in terms of reversing ethanol-induced narcosis. As a corollary, it also became apparent that small differences in the structure of two different peptides can produce profound differences in activity. This was first convincingly established when a series of studies showed that vasopressin and oxytocin, which differ by only two amino acids, display opposite effects on learning and memory, reaction time, and nerve conductance. Parenthetically, such structural differences not only can determine the specificity of receptor interactions, but also can influence the susceptibility of a peptide to degradation to an inactive form, hence affecting the potency and duration of action of the parent peptide or posttranslational product.

In light of these complex effects and interrelationships, it is not surprising that clinical and preclinical investigators have begun to explore the potential role of neuropeptides in the symptom complex of major psychiatric syndromes such as primary affective disorder. The remainder of this chapter will focus on a series of clinical studies examining the potential relevance of two hormones to the syndrome of affective illness, namely, CRH and somatostatin. Each of these hormones illustrates many of the general principles that we have come to associate with neuropeptide function. For instance, each was initially identified in the hypothalamus and principally recognized for its role in modulating anterior pituitary activity. Subsequently, however, each has been found to be widely distributed outside the hypothalamus and to regulate a variety of physiologic and behavioral activities that may be of relevance to major neuropsychiatric disorders. Moreover, both show an intimate association with biogenic amine neurotransmitters and other peptides of potential interest to psychiatry, such as vasopressin and the endogenous opiates. Finally, each of these peptides derives from a larger prohormone and can undergo extensive posttranslational modifications with implications for a multiplicity of biological actions.

CORTICOTROPIN-RELEASING HORMONE

CRH is a 41-amino-acid peptide first isolated from ovine hypothalami by Vale et al. in 1981. It possesses greater *in vivo* and *in vitro* corticotropin (ACTH) releasing potency than any previously identified synthetic or endogenous peptide (146). Shortly thereafter, Schally et al. described the sequence of porcine CRF (120) and Rivier et al. that of rat CRH (rCRH) (109). Finally, Furitani et al. sequenced the genes of both ovine CRH (oCRH) and human CRH (hCRH) and deduced the amino acid sequence of the corresponding peptides (43). Surprisingly, rCRH and hCRH appeared to be chemically identical. Moreover, oCRH and h/rCRH are also structurally similar, both containing 41 amino acids and showing 83% homology.

The sequencing and subsequent synthesis of CRH was of great potential importance to biological psychiatrists, representing the best opportunity available to investigate the central component of the hypothalamic-pituitary-adrenal axis, which is hyperactive not only in depression (19,117) but also in anorexia nervosa (45), alcoholism (141), and obsessive-compulsive neurosis (66). An additional clinically relevant aspect of this hypercortisolism is that in depression and alcoholism it can be so severe that these illnesses can be difficult to distinguish from early or mild Cushing's disease; hence, each of these psychiatric entities has been referred to colloquially by some endocrinologists as pseudo-Cushing's states. Additional reasons for psychiatric interest in CRH were the observations, as noted earlier, that CRH is the principal signal for the elaboration of both ACTH and β-endorphin from their common precursor (77), and that it can coordinate a series of physiological and behavioral responses adaptive during stressful situations (14–16,50,133,140). Recent studies also show that CRH given via the intraventricular route to the rat stimulates the locus ceruleus (147), produces markedly aggressive behavior, and induces limbic seizures that facilitate the development of electrically kindled seizures from the amygdala (150).

Given CRH's significant role in hypothalamic-pituitary-adrenal (HPA) regulation and its intriguing effects on CNS function, this peptide has been studied extensively in volunteers and in patients with major psychiatric and neuroendocrine disorders, despite the fact that its sequence has been known for less than 4 years. In volunteers, many questions have been addressed, such as the physiological relevance of CRH to pituitary-adrenal function in humans, as well as the differential biological effects and pharmacokinetics of oCRH and hCRH under varying conditions. Some of the questions asked of clinical populations include the following: (a) Can CRH help determine whether hypercortisolism in depression reflects an alteration in the setpoint for feedback inhibition of cortisol on ACTH secretion at a pituitary locus, versus the possibility of an alteration in the secretion of endogenous CRH? (b) Can CRH help in the differential diagnosis of the various hypercortisolemic psychiatric syndromes? (c) Can CRH help determine whether depression and Cushing's disease share common pathophysiological mechanisms or aid in their differential diagnosis? (d) Is CRH of potential relevance to the symptom complex of major psychiatric illnesses such as depression?

RELEVANCE OF CRH TO HUMAN PITUITARY-ADRENAL FUNCTION

To explore CRH's physiological relevance in normal volunteers, Avgerinos et al. compared naturalistically occurring ACTH pulses to those induced by human CRH administration. It was noted that spontaneous endogenous ACTH and cortisol secretory episodes (isolated during normal circadian studies) were identical to those induced by hCRH administration in a dose of 1 μg/kg (Avgerinos et al., *unpublished observations*). To further explore a role for hCRH in normal pituitary-adrenal function, our group also administered hCRH to patients with hypothalamic CRH deficiency to see if this peptide could restore normal pituitary-adrenal function. It was noted that eight 1-μg/kg pulses of hCRH given over 24 hr in a temporal sequence designed to mimic naturally occurring ACTH pulses restored the normal pulse frequency and amplitude of ACTH and

cortisol secretion and produced urinary free cortisol excretion rates in the normal range (6). This study also showed that the ACTH response to hCRH was enhanced in the early morning, suggesting that the pituitary corticotroph cell shows a circadian rhythm in its response to CRH. In addition to these studies, which have ascertained the relevance of CRH to basal and circadian ACTH and cortisol secretion, Avgerinos et al. also attempted to assess the relationship of CRH to pituitary-adrenal function during stress. This study, which showed that frequent pulses of hCRH given at 30- to 90-min intervals during the night produced ACTH secretory episodes that were much smaller in amplitude than those following insulin-induced hypoglycemia, suggested that stress-induced ACTH secretion requires factors other than CRH (Avgerinos et al., *unpublished observations*). Putative factors that may underlie these extra-CRH influences on stress-induced ACTH secretion include the catecholamines and arginine vasopressin, both of which are known to increase during hypoglycemia and other forms of stress.

DEVELOPMENT OF A CLINICALLY APPLICABLE CRH STIMULATION PARADIGM

To ascertain the clinical applications of CRH, several studies in volunteers have been conducted to assess the following questions: (a) Which peptide, oCRH or hCRH, might be best suited for acute challenges of the pituitary adrenal axis? (b) What dose should be administered in these studies and for how long should hormonal samples be obtained? (c) What time of day would be best suited for performance of this test? To answer these questions, pharmacokinetic and dose-response studies have been conducted with both oCRH and hCRH. Some of these studies were performed at different times of day to correspond to periods when the adrenal axis is normally quiescent or more active.

In both primates and humans, Schulte noted the lowest maximal stimulatory dose for cortisol secretion after oCRH administration was 1 μg/kg (128). In similar dose-response studies with hCRH in nonhuman primates and humans, Schuermeyer et al. also noted dose-dependent increases in plasma ACTH and cortisol concentrations (124,125). Moreover, the ACTH and cortisol responses to hCRH were of much shorter duration than those following oCRH. Accordingly, comparisons of the integrated secretory responses of both ACTH and cortisol following hCRH administration indicate that oCRH is at least five times more potent than hCRH (124,125). These long-lasting effects of oCRH on ACTH secretion can be accounted for by differences in their rate of clearance from human plasma. Hence, a comparison of the metabolic clearance rate of these two peptides in human volunteers reveals that hCRH is cleared from plasma 10 times more rapidly than oCRH. On the basis of their studies showing the relatively slower clearance and more prolonged biological effects of oCRH, Gold et al. elected to use this peptide to characterize the functional integrity of the pituitary corticotroph cell in clinical populations (48–52). It was reasoned that the extra information provided by a pulse of oCRH might provide the kind of additional information that could be helpful in exploring the pathophysiology of HPA function in different patient subgroups. Parenthetically, the short half-life of hCRH renders it far more suitable than oCRH for studying ACTH pulsatile secretion. In applying the oCRH stimulation paradigm in the morning and the evening, it was noted that the responses to this peptide were significantly greater in the evening than in the morning (78). This is presumably due to the relatively quiescent state of the axis in the evening, when the responses to exogenous CRH would not be inhibited as much by glucocorticoid negative feedback. Moreover, the evening represents a time in which responses to exogenous CRH are less likely to be interfered with by naturally occurring ACTH pulsatile episodes.

CLINICAL STUDIES WITH OVINE CRH IN PATIENTS WITH MAJOR PSYCHIATRIC DISORDERS

The first major finding utilizing CRH in psychiatry was made by Gold et al., who noted that a group of 12 drug-free depressed patients showed a significantly attenuated ACTH response to oCRH (50). This finding, replicated now in a large series of depressed patients (52) (see Fig. 1), was further replicated several months later in a preliminary study by Holsboer et al., who administered hCRH rather than oCRH (63). Because hCRH is a much weaker stimulus to ACTH secretion than oCRH, it may be less suitable for clinical studies. Indeed, Gold et al. have been unable to replicate the finding of blunted ACTH responses to hCRH in a group of 15 depressed patients, despite the fact that these same patients showed a marked attenuation in their ACTH responses to oCRH (*unpublished observation*). In light of this fact, these authors recommend the use of oCRH rather than hCRF for diagnostic testing in psychiatry.

The finding of an attenuated ACTH response to oCRF in depressed patients suggested that the pituitary corticotroph cell in these subjects was appropriately restrained by the negative feedback effects of elevated cortisol levels. This hypothesis is supported by the finding of a significant negative correlation between basal cortisol levels and the ACTH response to CRH in depression (52). These findings, suggestive of appropriate pituitary corticotroph cell function in depression, led Gold et al. to postulate that the hypercortisolism of this disorder reflects a defect at or above the hypothalamus, which resulted in the hypersecretion of CRH (48–50,52). Indirect evidence for this assertion has come from their study in which oCRH was administered as a continuous infusion to normal volunteers for 24 hr (126). This effort to replicate a situation of excessive availability of CRH at the pituitary corticotroph cell in normals produced 24-hr ACTH and cortisol secretory patterns which mimic those seen in depressed patients, in which the normal circadian pattern was preserved. Moreover, the 24-hr infusion of CRH elevated the 24-hr urinary free cortisol excretion rate in normals to levels typically seen in depression (i.e., 100–250 μg/day). In further support of a hypothesis of increased CRH secretion in depression are the data of Nemeroff et al., showing increased levels of CRH in the CSF of depressed patients (89). Moreover, Roy

et al. have noted in depressed patients that although the level of hCRH measured in the CSF was not elevated, it was positively correlated with the post-dexamethasone cortisol levels (113).

An inspection of the ACTH and cortisol responses to CRH in depression (see Fig. 1) reveals other salient features of HPA dysfunction in depressed patients (48–50,52). For instance, depressed patients showed a robust total and free cortisol response to the very small amount of ACTH released during CRH stimulation (48–50,52). In fact, the free cortisol response during CRH administration was even greater in depressed patients than it was in controls (52). It was surmised from these data that the adrenal cortex in depression had grown hyperresponsive to ACTH, a phenomenon that is known to occur during chronic stress in experimental animals (130) or after the experimental administration of repeated doses of ACTH

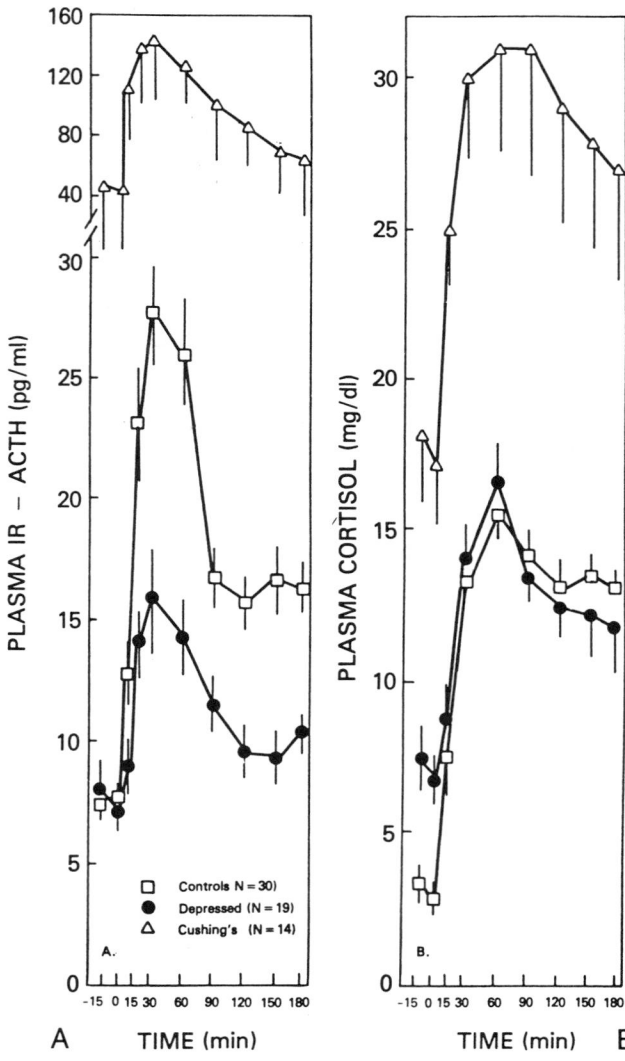

FIG. 1. Comparison of plasma ACTH (**A**) and cortisol (**B**) responses to CRH in controls and patients with Cushing's disease and depression. All data expressed as mean ± 1 SEM.

to volunteers. This concept of adrenocortical hyperresponsiveness to ACTH in depression is supported by the data of Amsterdam et al., who showed that depressed patients manifested an exaggerated cortisol response to exogenously administered ACTH (2).

Although Gold et al. noted that at the time of CRH testing depressed patients were hypercortisolemic, it is noteworthy that their basal early evening ACTH levels remained in the normal range. It was theorized that this "normal" plasma ACTH in depression most likely reflects a normal corticotroph cell caught in the balance between forces (i.e., negative feedback exerted by a hyperactive adrenal cortex from below and a predominating excess of CRH drive from above). Hence, the corticotroph cell, though restrained by normal negative feedback to secrete at a rate that produces ACTH levels in the normal range, is nevertheless sufficiently driven by CRH to promote excessive cortisol secretion by hyperplastic adrenals. Parenthetically, according to the above model, depressed patients presumably would have shown elevated levels of plasma ACTH in the beginning of their illness before a functional adrenal hypertrophy could have supervened. A schematic diagram of this proposed model of HPA regulation in depression is shown in the first three panels of Fig. 2.

The idea that depressed patients may secrete ACTH pulses of normal amplitude but at a more frequent rate than controls is supported by the preliminary data of Kling and Gold (unpublished), who examined the 24-hr profile of ACTH secretion in affective illness. These data reveal that depressed patients showed an increased number of normal-amplitude ACTH pulses in association with an equal number of cortisol secretory episodes whose amplitude was somewhat higher than normal. It should be noted, however, that some depressed patients showed an increased amplitude of ACTH pulses confined to the early morning surge.

Gold et al. have also administered CRH to other psychiatric patients whose illness is characterized by hypercortisolism. For instance, it was noted that drug-free, chronically underweight patients with anorexia nervosa also showed blunted ACTH responses to CRH negatively correlated with the degree of basal hypercortisolism (12). The finding of a pattern of HPA dysfunction in anorexia nervosa similar to that found in depression is compatible with data that suggest that anorexia nervosa and depression may lie

on a pathophysiologic continuum. For instance, data show that many patients with anorexia nervosa are depressed and show strong family histories for depression (45). To support the suggestion of a pathophysiological similarity between the two illnesses, it was noted, concordant with data indicating excessive endogenous CRH secretion in depression, that patients with anorexia nervosa show frank elevation in the level of CRH in the CSF (Kaye and Gold, unpublished observations). Of significance is the fact that these data indicate a strong positive correlation between the degree of depression in anorexia nervosa and the magnitude of elevation of the CSF CRH (Kaye and Gold, unpublished observation). Parenthetically, patients with panic-anxiety disorders also showed basal hypercortisolism and attenuated ACTH responses to CRH, whereas drug-free psychotic schizophrenic patients showed normal basal cortisol and ACTH and their responses to CRH (115), as well as normal levels of CRH in the CSF (70).

In addition to clarifying some aspects of the pathophysiology of hypercortisolism in psychiatric disorders characterized by hypercortisolism, CRH has also been shown to have clinical utility as an aid in the differential diagnosis between depression and early or mild Cushing's disease. Hence, Gold et al. showed that in a direct comparison with depressed patients, patients with Cushing's disease had a markedly higher response to exogenous oCRH (52). In fact, only four of 25 patients with Cushing's disease showed net ACTH responses to oCRH that were below the highest response seen in 32 depressed patients. The finding of exaggerated ACTH responses to oCRH in Cushing's disease (21,52,76,86,94) suggests that in contrast to depression, the pituitary corticotroph cell is much less responsive to glucocorticoid feedback. On the other hand, several lines of evidence suggest that in contrast to depression, in which a hyperactive CRH neuron is postulated, the hypothalamic CRH neuron in Cushing's disease is suppressed by high cortisol levels (52), including recent data that CSF CRH is much lower in Cushing's disease than in depressed patients or controls (Kling and Gold, unpublished observations). A schematic diagram of the proposed differential pathophysiology of hypercortisolism in depression and Cushing's disease is shown in the four panels of Fig. 2.

Whether CRH plays a role in any human disease apart from the rare cases of Addison's disease secondary to trauma- or tumor-induced CRH deficiency remains to be established. However, we have previously noted that its

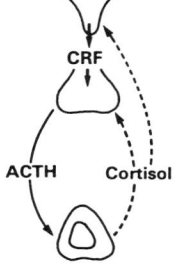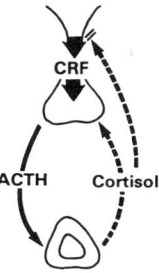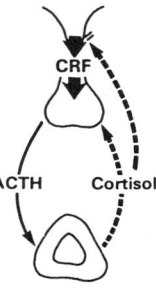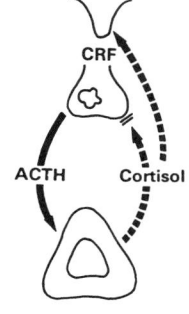

NORMAL   **EARLY DEPRESSION**   **LATE DEPRESSION**   **CUSHING'S DISEASE**

FIG. 2. Schematic representation of a hypothetical model depicting the functional status of the HPA axis in depression and Cushing's disease.

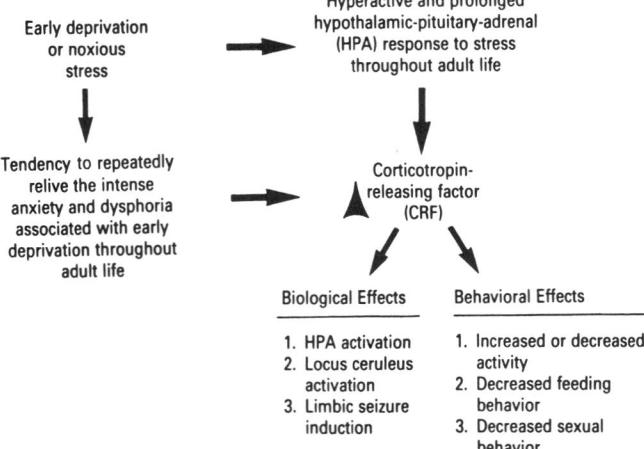

FIG. 3. Schematic representation of a hypothetical model of depression. This model suggests that the putative effect of early deprivation in increasing the vulnerability to depression may be translated biologically via regulatory peptides such as CRH.

possible involvement in depression is intriguing in light of the following four sets of findings taken from the disciplines of developmental psychology, clinical psychiatry, and neurophysiology: (a) Laboratory animals subjected to maternal deprivation during the neonatal period show significant hyperactivity of the HPA axis during stress throughout adult life (reviewed in 50). Hence, such animals presumably show a permanent change in the responsivity of their CRF neurons. (b) Clinical experience suggests that a history of early deprivation produces a diathesis to depression and a tendency to relive the intense anxiety and dysphoria associated with this early deprivation throughout adult life whenever a significant frustration or important loss occurs. Thus, such individuals also seem prone to a hyperresponsivity of their CRH neurons intermittently throughout life (32). (c) CRH given ICV to experimental animals not only stimulates the HPA axis (50) but also activates the locus ceruleus (147), produces decreased eating (14) and sexual behavior (133), and causes significant changes in activity (3). (d) CRH has been reported to induce limbic seizures that cross sensitize with electrically kindled seizures (150). These findings, taken together, suggest that a CRH model of depression could help integrate dynamic formulations that take into account early losses and subsequent internal and external stress as factors that can predispose to or precipitate major depression, and the observations that depressed subjects often show hypercortisolism, significant anxiety, anorexia, diminished libido, hypo- or hyperactivity, and respond at times to limbic anticonvulsants. A schematic representation of this model is shown in Fig. 3. That changes in CRH may be related to depressive symptomatology is also supported by empirical observations that depression is perhaps the only major symptom presented in a substantial number of patients with each of the various psychiatric disorders characterized during their course by sustained or episodic hypercortisolism.

SOMATOSTATIN

Somatostatin is a tetradecapeptide that has influenced neuropeptide research over the last decade and has additionally assumed an increasingly important role in investigations of neuropsychiatric disorders. Much information about the distribution and regulation of neuropeptides was derived from early studies with somatostatin. Dual peptidergic regulation of anterior pituitary function was demonstrated as somatostatin was identified as a hypothalamic hormone that inhibited rather than stimulated the release of growth hormone from the pituitary (13). Somatostatin, like substance P, was established as one of the first of a now long list of "brain-gut" hormones that are extensively distributed throughout the central nervous and gastrointestinal systems (17,75). Somatostatin was found to colocalize in neurons with classical neurotransmitters (30,62,122), a phenomenon that is currently recognized to be the rule rather than the exception for peptide hormones. Finally, somatostatin demonstrated the manifold regulatory activities of a peptide hormone; i.e., somatostatin acts as a neurohormone (a blood-borne neurosecretory product) at the pituitary, as a neurotransmitter or neuromodulator in the central nervous system, and as a hormone, paracrine secretion (local regulator), or autocrine secretion (self-regulator) in the periphery (37,100).

A variety of evidence suggests a role for somatostatin in the modulation of central nervous system activity as well as in the pathophysiology of certain neuropsychiatric disorders. Thus, somatostatin is located in a widespread and discrete fashion throughout the central nervous system, that displays neurophysiologic effects, interacts with other brain peptides and neurotransmitters, produces a variety of behavioral effects following local and ICV administration, and manifests disease-related alterations in the CSF and brain in a number of CNS disorders.

Neuronal cell bodies containing somatostatin-like immunoactivity have been identified in a variety of brain regions including the preoptic and periventricular nuclei, nucleus accumbens, amygdala, hippocampus, neocortex, locus ceruleus, striatum, and septal nuclei (17,32,42,74). Several somatostatin pathways in the brain have been described on the basis of lesion studies; most somatostatin-containing neurons in the median eminence originate in the periventricular hypothalamus, whereas the amygdala is the source of somatostatin fibers in the striatum and ventromedial hypothalamus (5,26,38,40,96,119).

As is the case with most other neuropeptides, the somatostatin tetradecapeptide is a cleavage product of a larger propeptide. Thus, preprosomatostatin (116 amino acids), prosomatostatin (92 amino acids), somatostatin-28 (a 28-amino-acid N-terminal extension of somatostatin-14), and somatostatin-12 (1–12) have all been identified, with all but somatostatin-12 (1–12) N-terminal extensions of somatostatin-14 and thus cross-reactive with antibodies directed toward the midregion or C-terminal of the tetradecapeptide (8,18,53). These tetradecapeptide-related peptides have biological activities and potencies as well as regions of distribution that are distinguishable from somatostatin-14 (81,83,84). Finally, specific, saturable, high-affinity binding sites for somatostatin have been detected in brain tissue (69,105,137), with particularly high concentrations in the cerebral cortex, hippocampus, septum, amygdala, and locus ceruleus (70,144). Recent studies suggest that several forms of the somatostatin-14 receptor exist in addition to distinct receptors for the somatostatin-related peptides (104,138,144).

Given the extensive distribution of somatostatin and somatostatin receptors throughout the brain, the manifold CNS regulatory properties of somatostatin are not surprising. Neurophysiologic studies employing both in vitro and microiontophoretic techniques have revealed both excitatory and inhibitory actions of somatostatin on central neurons in several brain regions (33,91,103). These ostensibly contradictory findings may reflect unusual dose- and time-related characteristics of the response to somatostatin. Consistent with this hypothesis is the description by Delfs and Dichter (29) of a biphasic dose-related response of neurons to somatostatin application, with low doses increasing and high doses inhibiting or not affecting action potential generation. In addition to the selective CNS distribution and neurophysiologic actions of somatostatin, evidence in support of the role of somatostatin as a neuromodulator if not a neurotransmitter includes its localization in synaptic granules and neuronal terminal regions (39), calcium-dependent release from neuron terminals (65), degradation by enzymes found in brain extracts (78), and binding to specific brain receptors (137). Further, somatostatin secretion is intimately related to the regulation of classical neurotransmitters and other neuropeptides.

Somatostatin increases the turnover of aminergic (norepinephrine, dopamine, serotonin) and cholinergic neurotransmitters (44,79), with inhibition of acetylcholine release (24), stimulation of serotonin release (141), and both stimulation and inhibition of norepinephrine release (54,145) reported. In turn, somatostatin release is decreased by γ-aminobutyric acid (GABA) (111) and is stimulated by dopamine (87) and (muscarinic) acetylcholine (111). Discrepancies in reported effects of neurotransmitters on somatostatin appear to reflect differences in brain regions and methods utilized. The regulatory potential of somatostatin is suggested by its colocalization in neurons with an ever-increasing list of neuroactive substances or their markers, including dopamine β-hydroxylase (62), acetylcholinesterase (30), glutamic acid decarboxylase (122), and neuropeptide Y (20).

A variety of hormones have been observed to stimulate (neurotensin, substance P, glucagon, somatomedin A, growth hormone, secretin, T_3) or inhibit (vasoactive intestinal peptide, VIP) the release of somatostatin from the hypothalamus (99). The secretion of an impressive array of hormones appears to be inhibited by somatostatin in a site-dependent fashion, with somatostatin most clearly involved in the physiological regulation of basal and stimulated growth hormone and TSH secretion. Reisine and colleagues have recently identified several mechanisms by which somatostatin interferes with stimulated ACTH secretion following application of CRF, isoproterenol, and VIP to pituitary cell culture (59,102). These mechanisms include inhibition of adenylate cyclase through guanine inhibitory protein activation (102), reduction of cytosolic free calcium

and interference with calcium mobilization (121), enhancement of the permeability of cells to potassium (which also may reduce accumulation of intracellular calcium) (95), and inhibition of protein phosphorylation (J. Patel, personal communication; 34).

A variety of behavioral alterations have been observed following somatostatin administration. Thus, ICV somatostatin produces sleep disturbances (decreased total and rapid eye movement sleep) (58,106), dose-related biphasic alterations in locomotor activity (stimulation with low doses and inhibition with high doses) (108), eating disturbances (increased or dose-related biphasic intake) (3,72,107), and analgesia (58), perhaps consistent with the putative or partial agonist activity of somatostatin at the opiate receptor (98,142).

Studies of somatostatin in neurologic disorders have described increases in CSF somatostatin accompanying inflammatory or destructive CNS lesions with reduced levels reported in senile dementia (93), Parkinson's disease (36), and multiple sclerosis during relapse (136). Dramatic reductions in somatostatin in the CSF, cerebral cortex, and subcortical structures have been observed in Alzheimer's disease (28,88,131,151), and the somatostatin neurons have been described as the major locus of development of neurofibrillary tangles and plaques in this disorder (85,110). Additionally, the reductions in somatostatin have been found to be correlated with decreased choline acetyltransferase and with the severity of the dementia in Alzheimer's (27,134), all of which suggests a prominent role for somatostatin in the pathophysiology of Alzheimer's. Studies of CSF somatostatin in Huntington's dementia are contradictory (7,25), although postmortem studies have reported marked increases in somatostatin-like immunoreactivity in the caudate and nucleus accumbens of Huntington's patients (4,89).

Studies of CSF somatostatin in several psychiatric populations have been performed. Gerner and Yamada (46) and Rubinow et al. (115) reported significant reductions in CSF somatostatin in depressed patients compared with normal controls. Lower levels in patients with anorexia and higher levels in patients during mania were also observed by Gerner and Yamada, although these findings were not replicated by others (115; Kaye et al., unpublished manuscript).

Depression-related reductions in CSF somatostatin have also been observed in several subsequent studies. Black et al. (11) reported lower ventricular CSF somatostatin levels in depressed patients studied prior to cingulotomy compared with hydrocephalic patients, with values in the depressed patients also significantly lower than those seen in the lumbar CSF of normal controls. Bissette et al. (10) observed significantly lower CSF somatostatin values in depressed patients as well as patients with dementia and schizophrenia compared with normal volunteers. A group of depressed patients studied during their worst week of depression was reported by Agren and Lundqvist (1) to show significantly lower somatostatin levels than a group of depressed patients studied more than 2 months following their most depressed week. Sunderland et al. (unpublished manuscript) have described reduced CSF somatostatin levels in depressed patients and patients with Alzheimer's disease compared with age-matched controls; values in the Alzheimer's patients were also significantly lower than those observed in patients with depression. Finally, a group of schizophrenic patients studied by Doran et al. (35) had CSF somatostatin values that were comparable to normal values obtained in the same laboratory during a different assay run.

Postmortem studies of somatostatin in patients with depression have not been performed, whereas reports of reductions in several brain areas in patients with schizophrenia have not been consistent (41,89). These studies may be complicated by the recent description of rapid reductions in brain somatostatin within the first 6 hr following death (135).

As can be seen in Fig. 4, significant differences in CSF somatostatin concentration were observed (35,114,115) among groups of patients with affective illness, schizophrenics, and normal controls (ANOVA, $F = 3.90$, $df = 5$, $p < 0.005$); depressed patients demonstrated significantly lower levels of CSF somatostatin (42.3 ± 3.2 pg/ml) than schizophrenics (65.2 ± 4.0 pg/ml) ($t = 4.38$, $p < 0.001$), patients with affective illness during the improved state (61.3 ± 5.4 pg/ml) ($t = 3.08$, $p < 0.01$), or normal volunteers (62.1 ± 5.4 pg/ml) ($t = 3.10$, $p < 0.01$). No other significant differences were observed. Somatostatin levels were not predicted by age, gender, or severity of depression.

Although the evidence in support of depression-related reductions of CSF somatostatin is increasingly convincing, the meaning of this finding is at present unclear and requires further knowledge of the source and regulation of CSF somatostatin. A variety of indirect evidence reviewed elsewhere (114) suggests that CSF somatostatin reflects brain secretion, with cerebral somatostatin entering the CSF through nerve terminals located adjacent to the third ventricle (67) or in the periventricular organs (149) and by cellular diffusion via the Virchow-Robbins spaces of the brain. Nonetheless, somatostatin is secreted by a variety of

different cells within the neuroaxis, preventing determination of the cell type or brain area responsible for the depression-related reductions in CSF somatostatin.

Given the number of neuropsychiatric disorders characterized by reduced CSF somatostatin levels, it seems likely that these CSF alterations reflect central neurotransmitter or neuropeptide abnormalities. Of particular interest with respect to this hypothesis are studies by A. Doran et al. (*unpublished manuscript*) and D. R. Rubinow et al. (116) showing reductions in CSF somatostatin occurring during treatment with the neuroleptic fluphenazine or with carbamazepine, respectively. The fluphenazine-related reductions appear consistent with the dopamine-blocking effects of fluphenazine and with the ability of other dopamine-blocking agents to reduce somatostatin-like immunoreactivity in a variety of brain regions (6). No mechanism for carbamazepine-induced reductions of CSF somatostatin has been identified, although alterations of central neurotransmitter or neuropeptide activity by this medication are most likely. Carbamazepine has been reported to blunt electrical stimulation-induced elevations in brain somatostatin in rats (60), although an absence of effect on basal somatostatin in various brain regions has also been observed (S. R. Weiss et al., *unpublished data*). Nonetheless, reports of long-term increases in somatostatin in brain regions following kindling (66) and inhibition of kindled seizures following administration of somatostatin-depleting agents (61) suggest that the anticonvulsant effects of carbamazepine may relate to its ability to reduce CSF somatostatin.

A possible way in which reduced CSF somatostatin levels may reflect or contribute to other physiological abnormalities in depression has been described by Doran et al. (35). These authors observed a significant inverse relationship between CSF somatostatin levels and maximum postdexamethasone plasma cortisol; further, this relationship between low CSF somatostatin and escape from dexamethasone suppression was observed in both depressed and schizophrenic patient groups. Somatostatin has been observed to

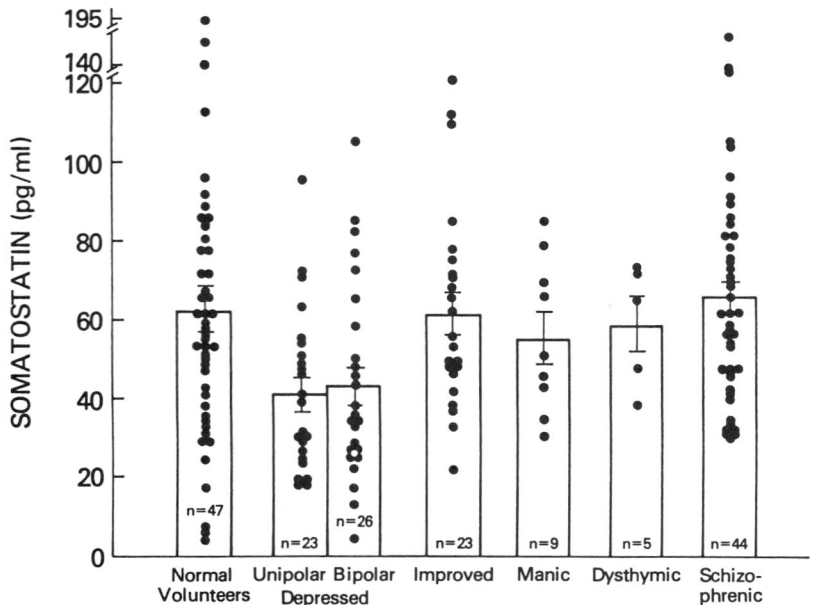

FIG. 4. CSF somatostatin in normal volunteers and in medication-free patients with affective illness and schizophrenia.

reduce stimulated ACTH secretion from the pituitary following administration of a variety of secretagogues (59) and has further been shown to reduce stress-induced CRH secretion (16). Thus, the findings of Doran et al. may represent reduced hypothalamic somatostatin-induced ACTH disinhibition or may reflect a more central neurotransmitter or neuropeptide abnormality that results in both reduced CSF somatostatin secretion and disinhibited ACTH secretion. The observed relationship between CSF somatostatin and response to dexamethasone clearly requires replication; preliminary results of a study by C. B. Nemeroff et al. (*personal communication, 1985*) show a similar relationship in normal volunteers but not in depressed patients, whereas Agren and Lundqvist (1) found no relationship employing a variant of the dexamethasone suppression test. Nonetheless, further investigation of the role of somatostatin in the physiologic and behavioral dysregulations of depression may prove profitable.

Future studies of somatostatin in neuropsychiatric disorders will capitalize on the availability of neuroscience and molecular genetics techniques that have developed over the last decade. Chromatographic characterization of CSF and brain somatostatin will permit further delineation of the specific somatostatin-related peptide fragments that may be selectively dysregulated in different neuropsychiatric disorders. Passive immunization studies may clarify the physiologic consequences of reduced CSF somatostatin. Similarly, development of somatostatin antagonists and long-acting agonists that will gain access to the brain will allow precise determination of the role of somatostatin in central nervous system activity. Sequencing of the human somatostatin gene (132) and mRNA permits an unparalleled view of the processes resulting in alterations in hormonal concentration and has already demonstrated that, at least during development, gene expression may be transiently turned on or off (82). Transfection of the rat preprosomatostatin gene into mice resulted in somatostatin synthesis by organs that do not normally produce somatostatin (73) and offers a potential means for identifying the consequences of the presence of altered forms or concentrations of somatostatin. Through these and other means of altering the activity of somatostatin and somatostatin-related peptides, a clear understanding of the significance of somatostatin dysregulation in depression and other neuropsychiatric disorders will emerge. Similar techniques applied to the study of CRH and other neurohormones promise significant advancement in our understanding of the physiology of central peptide systems and their relevance to the pathophysiology of neuropsychiatric disorders.

REFERENCES

1. Agren, H., and Lundqvist, G. (1984): *Psychoneuroendocrinology,* 9:233–248.
2. Amsterdam, J. D., Winokur, A., Abelman, E., Lucki, I., and Rickels, K. (1983): *Am. J. Psychiatry,* 140:907–909.
3. Aponte, G., Leung, P., Gross, D., and Yamanda, T. (1984): *Life Sci.,* 35:741–746.
4. Beal, M. F., Bird, E. D., Langlais, P. J., and Martin, J. B. (1984): *Neurology,* 34:663–666.
5. Beal, M. F., Domesick, V. B., and Martin, J. B. (1985): *Brain Res.,* 330:309–316.
6. Beal, M. F., and Martin, J. B. (1984): *Neurosci. Lett.,* 47:125–130.
7. Beal, M. F., and Martin, J. B. (1987): *Neurology (in press).*
8. Benoit, R., Bohlen, P., Esch, F., and Ling, N. (1984): *Brain Res.,* 311:23–29.
9. Benoit, R., Ling, N., Alford, B., and Guillemin, R. (1982): *Biochem. Biophys. Res. Commun.,* 107:944–950.
10. Bissette, G., Walleus, H., Widerlov, E., Karlsson, I., Eklundt, K., Loosen, P. T., and Nemeroff, C. B. (1984): *Abstracts of the 14th Annual Meeting of the Society for Neuroscience,* Vol. 10 (Part 2), p. 1093, Abstract No. 319.11.
11. Black, P. M., Ballantine, H. T., Carr, D. B., Beal, M. F., and Martin, J. B. (1984): *39th Annual Convention of the Society of Biological Psychiatry,* p. 177, Abstract No. 135.
12. Bloom, F. E., Battenberg, E. L. F., Rivier, J., and Vale, W. (1982): *Regul. Pept.,* 4:43–48.
13. Brazeau, P., Vale, W., Burgus, R., Ling, N., Butcher, M., Rivier, J., and Guillemin, R. (1973): *Science,* 197:77–79.
14. Britton, D. R., Koob, G. F., Rivier, J., and Vale, W. (1982): *Life Sci.,* 31:363–367.
15. Brown, M. R., Fisher, L. A., Spiess, J., Rivier, C., Rivier, J., and Vale, W. (1982): *Endocrinology,* 111:928–931.
16. Brown, M. R., Rivier, C., and Vale, W. (1984): *Endocrinology,* 114:1546–1549.
17. Brownstein, M., Arimura, A., Stao, H., Schally, A. V., and Kizer, J. S. (1975): *Endocrinology,* 96:1456–1461.
18. Cannon, W. B. (1929): *Physiol. Rev.,* 9:399–431.
19. Carroll, B. J., Curtis, G. C., and Mendels, J. (1976): *Arch. Gen. Psychiatry,* 33:1039–1044.
20. Chronwall, B. M., Chase, T. N., and O'Donohue, T. L. (1984): *Neurosci. Lett.,* 50:213–217.
21. Chrousos, G. P., Schulte, H. M., Oldfield, E. H., Gold, P. W., Cutler, G. B., Jr., and Loriaux, D. L. (1984): *N. Engl. J. Med.,* 310:622–627.
22. Chrousos, G. P., Schulte, H. M., Oldfield, E. H., Gold, P. W., Cutler, G. B., Jr., and Loriaux, D. L. (1984): *J. Clin. Endocrinol. Metab.,* 58:1064–1067.
23. Chrousos, G. P., Schulte, H. M., Oldfield, E. H., Niemann, L., Gold, P. W., and Loriaux, D. L. (1984): *N. Engl. J. Med.,* 311: 472–473.
24. Cohen, N., Rosing, E., Wiley, K., and Slater, P. (1978): *Life Sci.,* 23:1659–1664.
25. Cramer, H., Kohler, J., Oepen, G., Schomburg, G., and Schrotev, E. (1981): *J. Neurol.,* 225:183.
26. Crowley, W. R., and Terry, L. C. (1980): *Brain Res.,* 200:283–291.
27. Davies, P. (1981): Read before the International Study Group on the Pharmacology of Memory Disorders Associated with Aging, Zurich, April 1.
28. Davies, P., and Terry, R. D. (1981): *Neurobiology,* 2:9–14.
29. Delfs, J. F., and Dichter, M. A. (1983): *J. Neurosci.,* 3:1176–1188.
30. Delfs, J. F., Zhu, C.-H., and Dichter, M. A. (1984): *Science,* 223: 61–63.
31. DeSouza, E. B., Perrin, M. H., Insel, T. R., Rivier, J., Vale, W. W., and Kuhar, M. J. (1984): *Science,* 224:1449–1451.
32. Dierickx, K., and Vandesande, F. (1979): *Cell Tissue Res.,* 201: 349–359.
33. Dodd, J., and Kelly, J. S. (1978): *Nature,* 273:674–675.
34. Dokas, L. A., Klis, M., Liauw, A., and Coy, D. H. (1983): *Abstracts, Society for Neuroscience,* Vol. 9, Abstract No. 171.4.
35. Doran, A., Rubinow, D. R., Roy, A., and Pickar, D. (1987): *Arch. Gen. Psychiatry,* (in press).
36. Dupont, E., Christensen, S. E., Hansen, A. P., Olivarius, B. deF., and Orskov, H. (1982): *Neurology,* 32:312–314.
37. Efendic, S., and Luft, R. (1980): *Ann. Clin. Res.,* 12:87–94.
38. Elde, R. P., Hokfelt, T., Johannsson, O., Efendic, S., and Luft, R. (1976): *Neuroscience,* 2:759.
39. Epelbaum, J., Brazeau, P., Tsang, D., Brawer, J., and Martin, J. B. (1977): *Brain Res.,* 126:309–323.
40. Epelbaum, J., Willoughby, J. O., Brazeau, P., and Martin, J. B. (1977): *Endocrinology,* 101:1495–1502.
41. Ferrier, I. N., Cross, A. J., Johnson, J. A., Roberts, G. W., Crow,

T. J., Corsellis, J. A., Lee, Y. C., O'Shaughnessy, D., Adrian, T. E., McGregor, G. P., Baracese-Hamilton, A. J., and Bloom, S. R. (1983): *J. Neurol. Sci.,* 62:159–170.

42. Finley, J. C. W., Maderdrut, J. L., Roger, L. J., and Petrusz, P. (1981): *Neuroscience,* 6:2173–2192.

43. Furutani, Y., Morimoto, Y., Shibahara, S., and Numa, S. (1983): *Nature,* 301:537–540.

44. Garcia-Sevilla, J., Magnusson, T., and Carlsson, A. (1978): *Brain Res.,* 155:159–164.

45. Gerner, R. H., and Gwirtsman, H. E. (1981): *Am. J. Psychiatry,* 138:650–653.

46. Gerner, R. H., and Yamada, T. (1982): *Brain Res.,* 238:298–302.

47. Gillies, G. E., Linton, E. A., and Lowry, P. J. (1982): *Nature,* 299:355–357.

48. Gold, P. W. (1985): *Ann. Intern. Med.,* 102:346–350.

49. Gold, P. W., and Chrousos, G. P. (1985): *Psychoneuroendocrinology,* 10:401–419.

50. Gold, P. W., Chrousos, G. P., Kellner, C. H., Post, R. M., Schulte, H. M., and Loriaux, D. L. (1984): *Am. J. Psychiatry,* 141:619–627.

51. Gold, P. W., Gwirtsman, H., Avgerinos, P. C., Kaye, W., Jimerson, D. C., Ebert, M., Loriaux, D. L., and Chrousos, G. P. (1987): *N. Engl. J. Med.,* 314:1335–1342.

52. Gold, P. W., Loriaux, D. L., Roy, A., Kellner, C. H., Post, R. M., Pickar, D., Avgerinos, P. C., Paul, S. M., Schulte, H. M., Oldfield, E. H., Cutler, G. B., Jr., and Chrousos, G. P. (1987): *N. Engl. J. Med.,* 314:1329–1335.

53. Goodman, R. H., Aron, D. C., and Roosa, B. A. (1983): *J. Biol. Chem.,* 258:5570–5573.

54. Gothert, N. (1980): *Nature,* 288:86–88.

55. Guillemin, R., Vargo, T., Rossier, J., Minick, S., Ling, N., Rivier, C., Vale, W., and Bloom, F. (1977): *Science,* 197:1367–1369.

56. Harris, G. W. (1948): *Physiol. Neur.,* 28:134–179.

57. Havlicek, V., Rezek, M., and Friesen, H. (1976): *Pharmacol. Biochem. Behav.,* 5:73–77.

58. Havlicek, V., Rezek, M., Leybin, L., and Friesen, H. (1977): *Fed. Proc.,* 36:363.

59. Heisler, S., Reisine, T., Hook, V., and Axelrod, J. (1982): *Proc. Natl. Acad. Sci. USA,* 79:6502–6507.

60. Higuchi, T. (1987): In: *IIIrd International Kindling Symposium,* edited by J. A. Wada. Raven Press, New York (*in press*).

61. Higuchi, T., Sikand, G. S., Kato, N., Wada, J. A., and Friesen, H. G. (1983): *Brain Res.,* 288:359–362.

62. Hokfelt, T., Elfvin, L. G., Elde, R., Schultzberg, M., Goldstein, M., and Luft, R. (1977): *Proc. Natl. Acad. Sci. USA,* 74:3587–3591.

63. Holsboer, F., Gerken, A., Stalla, G. K., and Muller, O. A. (1984): *N. Engl. J. Med.,* 311:1127.

64. Insel, T. R., Kalin, N. H., Guttmacher, L. B., Cohen, R. M., and Murphy, D. L. (1982): *Psychiatry Res.,* 6:153–160.

65. Iversen, L. L., Iversen, S. D., Bloom, F., Douglas, C., Brown, M., and Vale, W. (1978): *Nature,* 273:161–163.

66. Kato, N., Higuchi, T., Friesen, H. G., and Wada, J. A. (1983): *Life Sci.,* 32:2415–2422.

67. Knigge, K. M., Bennett-Clarke, C., Burchanowski, B., Joseph, S. A., Romagnano, M. A., and Sternberger, L. A. (1980): In: *Endocrine Functions of the Brain,* edited by M. Motta, pp. 195–206. Raven Press, New York.

68. Lamberts, S. W., Verleun, T., Oosterom, R., DeJong, F., and Hackens, W. H. L. (1984): *J. Clin. Endocrinol. Metab.,* 58:298–303.

69. Leitner, J. W., Rifkin, R. M., Maman, A., and Sussman, K. E. (1979): *Biochem. Biophys. Res. Commun.,* 87:919–927.

70. Leroux, P., and Pelletier, G. (1984): *Peptides,* 5:503–506.

71. Lieutaud, J. (1742): *Essais Anatomique Contenant L'Histoire Exact de Toutes les Parties Qui Composert le Corps de L'Homme, Avec la Maniere de Dissequer.* Huart, Paris.

72. Lotter, E. C., and Woods, S. C. (1977): *Diabetes,* 26(*Suppl.* 1):358.

73. Low, M. J., Hammer, R. E., Goodman, R. H., Habener, J. F., Palmiter, R., and Brinster, R. (1987): *Cell (in press).*

74. Luft, R., Efendic, S., and Hokfelt, T. (1978): *Diabetologia,* 14:1–13.

75. Luft, R., Efendic, S., Hokfelt, T., Johansson, O., and Arimura, A. (1974): *Med. Biol.,* 52:423–430.

76. Lytras, N., Grossman, A., Perry, L., Tomlins, S., Wass, J. A. H., Coy, D. H., Schally, A. V., Rees, L. H., and Besser, G. M. (1983): *Clin. Endocrinol.,* 20:71–84.

77. Maines, R. E., Eipper, B. A., and Lind, N. (1977): *Proc. Natl. Acad. Sci. USA,* 74:3014–3018.

78. Marks, N., and Stern, F. (1975): *FEBS Lett.,* 55:220–224.

79. Matthe-Sorenssen, D., Wood, P. L., Cheney, D. L., and Costa, E. (1978): *J. Neurochem.,* 31:685–691.

80. Medvei, V. C. (1982): *A History of Endocrinology.* MTP Press, Boston.

81. Meyer, C. A., Murphy, W. A., Redding, T. W., Coy, D. H., and Schally, A. V. (1980): *Proc. Natl. Acad. Sci. USA,* 77:6171–6174.

82. Montminy, M. R., Childers, H., Lechian, R. M., Forte, S., Wolfe, H., and Goodman, R. H. (1985): *Abstracts of the 67th Annual Meeting of the Endocrine Society,* Baltimore, p. 57.

83. Morrison, J. H., Benoit, R., Magistretti, P. J., and Bloom, F. E. (1983): *Brain Res.,* 262:344–351.

84. Morrison, J. H., Benoit, R., Magistretti, P. J., Ling, N., and Bloom, F. E. (1982): *Neurosci. Lett.,* 34:137–142.

85. Morrison, J. H., Rogers, J., Scherr, S., Benoit, R., and Bloom, F. E. (1985): *Nature,* 314:90–92.

86. Nakahara, M., Shibasaki, T., Shizume, K., Kiyosawa, Y., Odagiri, E., Suda, T., Yamaguchi, H., Tsushima, T., Denura, H., Maeda, T., Wakagayashi, I., and Ling, N. (1983): *J. Clin. Endocrinol. Metab.,* 57:963–968.

87. Negro-Vilar, A., Ojeda, S. R., Arimura, A., and Mccann, S. (1978): *Life Sci.,* 23:1493–1498.

88. Nemeroff, C. B., Bissette, G., Busby, W. H., Youngblood, W. W., Rossor, M., Roth, M., and Kizer, J. S. (1983): *Neurosci. Abstr.,* 9:1052.

89. Nemeroff, C. B., Youngblood, W. W., Manber, P. J., Prange, A. J., and Kizer, J. S. (1983): *Science,* 221:972–975.

90. Nemeroff, C. B., Widerlov, E., Bissette, G., Walleus, H., Karlsson, I., Eklund, K., Kilts, C., and Loosen, P. (1984): *Science,* 226:1342–1344.

91. Olpe, H. R., Balcar, V. J., Bittiger, H., Ring, K., and Sieber, P. (1980): *Eur. J. Pharmacol.,* 63:127–133.

92. Olschowka, J. A., O'Donohue, T. L., Mueller, G. P., and Jacobowitz, D. M. (1982): *Peptides,* 3:995–1015.

93. Oran, J. J., Edwardson, J., and Millard, P. H. (1981): *Gerontology,* 27:216–223.

94. Orth, D. N., DeBold, C. R., DeCherney, G. S., Jackson, R. V., Alexander, A. N., Rivier, J., Rivier, C., Spiess, J., and Vale, W. (1982): *J. Clin. Endocrinol. Metab.,* 55:1017–1019.

95. Pace, C. S., and Tarvin, J. T. (1981): *Diabetes,* 30:836–842.

96. Palkovits, M., Tapia-Arancibia, L., Kordon, C., and Epelbaum, J. (1982): *Brain Res.,* 250:223–228.

97. Pieters, G. F. F. M., Hermus, A. R. M. M., Smals, A. G. H., Bartelink, A. K. M., Benraad, T. H. J., and Kluppenborg, P. W. C. (1983): *J. Clin. Endocrinol. Metab.,* 57:513–515.

98. Pugsley, T. A., and Lipmann, W. (1978): *Res. Commun. Chem. Pathol. Pharmacol.,* 21:153–156.

99. Reichlin, S. (1981): In: *Neurosecretion and Brain Peptides,* edited by J. B. Martin, S. Reichlin, and K. L. Bick, pp. 573–597. Raven Press, New York.

100. Reichlin, S. (1983): *N. Engl. J. Med.,* 309:1495–1501.

101. Reichlin, S. (1983): *N. Engl. J. Med.,* 309:1556–1563.

102. Reisine, T. (1984): *Clin. Neuropharmacol.,* 7(*Suppl.* 1):56–57.

103. Renaud, L. P., Martin, J. B., and Brazeau, P. (1975): *Nature,* 255:233–235.

104. Reubi, J. C. (1984): *Neurosci. Lett.,* 49:259–263.

105. Reubi, J. C., Perrin, M., Rivier, J., and Vale, W. (1981): *Life Sci.,* 28:2191–2198.

106. Rezek, M., Havlicek, V., Hughes, K. R., and Friesen, H. (1976): *Pharmacol. Biochem. Behav.,* 5:73–77.

107. Rezek, M., Havlicek, V., Hughes, K. R., and Friesen, H. (1976): *Neuropharmacology,* 15:499–504.

108. Rezek, M., Havlicek, V., Hughes, K. R., and Friesen, H. (1977): *Neuropharmacology,* 16:157–162.

109. Rivier, C., and Vale, W. (1983): *Nature,* 305:325–327.

110. Robbins, R. J., Sutton, R. E., and Reichlin, S. (1982): *Brain Res.,* 243:377–386.

111. Roberts, G. W., Crow, T. J., and Polak, J. M. (1985): *Nature,* 314:92–94.
112. Roy, A., Pickar, D., Chrousos, G. P., Paul, S. M., and Gold, P. W. (1987): *Am. J. Psychiatry (in press).*
113. Roy, A., Pickar, D., Doran, A., Paul, S. M., Chrousos, G. P., and Gold, P. W. (1987): *Am. J. Psychiatry (in press).*
114. Rubinow, D. R. (1987): *Biol. Psychiatry (in press).*
115. Rubinow, D. R., Gold, P. W., Post, R. M., Ballenger, J. C., Cowdry, R. W., Bollinger, J., and Reichlin, S. (1983): *Arch. Gen. Psychiatry,* 40:409–412.
116. Rubinow, D. R., Post, R. M., Gold, P. W., Ballenger, J. C., and Reichlin, S. (1985): *Psychopharmacology,* 85:210–213.
117. Sachar, E. J., Hellman, L., Fukashima, D. K., and Gallagher, T. F. (1970): *Arch. Gen. Psychiatry,* 23:289–298.
118. Saffran, M., Schally, A. V., and Bentey, B. G. (1955): *Endocrinology,* 57:439–444.
119. Sakanaka, M., Shiosaka, S., Takatsuki, K., Inagati, S., Takagi, H., Senba, E., Kawai, Y., Matsuzaki, T., and Tohyama, M. (1981): *Brain Res.,* 221:231–242.
120. Schally, A. V., Chang, R. C., Arimura, A., Redding, T. W., Fishback, J. B., and Vigh, S. (1981): *Proc. Natl. Acad. Sci. USA,* 78:5197–5201.
121. Schlegel, W., Wuarin, F., Wollheim, C. B., and Zahnd, G. R. (1984): *Cell Calcium,* 5:223–236.
122. Schmechel, D. E., Vickrey, B. G., Fitzpatrick, D., and Elde, R. P. (1984): *Neurosci. Lett.,* 47:227–232.
123. Schneider, C. V. (1660): *Liber Primus de Catarrhis.* T. Merii and E. Schumacheri, Wittembergae.
124. Schuermeyer, T. H., Avgerinos, P. C., Gold, P. W., Tomai, T. P., Gallucci, W. T., Cutler, G. B., Jr., Loriaux, D. L., and Chrousos, G. P. (1984): *J. Clin. Endocrinol. Metab.,* 59:1103–1108.
125. Schuermeyer, T. H., Gold, P. W., Gallucci, W. T., Tomai, T. P., Cutler, G. B., Jr., Loriaux, D. L., and Chrousos, G. P. (1985): *Endocrinology,* 117:300–306.
126. Schulte, H. M., Chrousos, G. P., Gold, P. W., Booth, J. D., Oldfield, E. H., Cutler, G. B., Jr., and Loriaux, D. L. (1985): *J. Clin. Invest.,* 75:1781–1785.
127. Schulte, H. M., Chrousos, G. P., Gold, P. W., Oldfield, E. H., Hoban, M. C., Culter, G. B., Jr., and Loriaux, D. L. (1983): *Acta Endocrinol. (Suppl.),* 253:32.
128. Schulte, H. M., Chrousos, G. P., Oldfield, E. H., Gold, P. W., Cutler, G. B., Jr., and Loriaux, D. L. (1984): *J. Clin. Endocrinol. Metab.,* 56:192–197.
129. Schulte, H. M., Chrousos, G. P., Oldfield, E. H., Gold, P. W., Cutler, G. B., Jr., and Loriaux, D. L. (1987): *Horm. Res. (in press).*
130. Selye, H. (1936): *Nature,* 138:32.
131. Serby, M., Richardson, S. B., Twente, S., Siekierski, J., and Rotrosen, J. (1983): *Abstracts of the Annual Meeting of the American College of Neuropsychopharmacology,* San Juan, p. 84.
132. Shen, L. P., and Rutter, W. J. (1984): *Science,* 224:168–171.
133. Shibahara, S., Morimoto, Y., Furutani, Y., and Neuma, S. (1983): *EMBO J.,* 2:775–779.
134. Soininen, H. S., Jolkkonen, J. T., Reinikainen, K. R., Halonen, T. O., and Riekkinen, P. J. (1984): *J. Neurol. Sci.,* 63:167–172.
135. Sorensen, K. V. (1984): *Biomed. Pharmacother.,* 38:458–461.
136. Sorensen, K. V., Christensen, S. E., Dupont, E., Hansen, A. P., Pedersen, E., and Orskov, H. (1980): *Acta Neurol. Scand.,* 61:186–191.
137. Srikant, C. B., and Patel, Y. C. (1981): *Proc. Natl. Acad. Sci. USA,* 78:3930–3934.
138. Srikant, C. B., and Patel, Y. C. (1981): *Nature,* 294:259–260.
139. Stokes, P. E. (1973): *Ann. NY Acad. Sci.,* 215:77–83.
140. Sutton, R. E., Koob, G. F., LeMoal, M., Rivier, J., and Vale, W. (1982): *Nature,* 297:331–333.
141. Tanaka, S., and Tsujimoto, A. (1981): *Brain Res.,* 208:219–222.
142. Terenius, L. (1976): *Eur. J. Pharmacol.,* 38:211–213.
143. Tran, V. T., Beal, M. F., and Martin, J. B. (1985): *Science,* 288:492–495.
144. Tran, V. T., Uhl, G. R., Perry, D. C., Manning, D. C., Vale, W. W., Perrin, M. H., Rivier, J. E., Martin, J. B., and Snyder, S. H. (1984): *Eur. J. Pharmacol.,* 101:307–309.
145. Tsujimoto, A., and Shokichi, T. (1980): *Life Sci.,* 28:903–910.
146. Vale, W., Spiess, J., Rivier, C., and Rivier, J. (1981): *Science,* 213:1394–1397.
147. Valentino, R., Foote, S. L., and Aston-Jones, G. (1983): *Brain Res.,* 220:363–367.
148. Von Luschka, H. (1860): *Der Hirnanhan u. die Steissdruese des Menschen.* G. Reimer, Berlin.
149. Weindl, A., and Sofroniew, M. V. (1982): In: *Advances in Biochemical Psychopharmacology,* edited by J. B. Martin, S. Reichlin, and K. L. Bick, pp. 303–320. Raven Press, New York.
150. Weiss, S. R., Post, R. M., Gold, P. W., Chrousos, G. P., and Pert, A. (1987): *Brain Res.,* 372:345–351.
151. Wood, P. L., Etienne, P., Lal, S., Gauthier, S., Cajal, S., and Nair, N. P. V. (1982): *Life Sci.,* 31:2073–2079.
152. Zuingerus, T. (1669): *Commentarii Hippocratis.* Episcopiorum Opear, Basileae.

Psychopharmacology:
The Third Generation of Progress,
edited by Herbert Y. Meltzer.
Raven Press, New York © 1987.

CHAPTER 62

The Hypothalamic-Pituitary-Thyroid Axis in Affective Disorders

Arthur J. Prange, Jr., James C. Garbutt, and Peter T. Loosen

The concept is venerable that thyroid hormones play a role in mental disorders. In 1850 Sir John Simon emphasized this point of view when he wrote, "In the case of the thyroid gland, there are strong reasons for believing that (functional changes) may reciprocate with similar differences in the nourishment of the brain" (68). More than a century later aspects of the reciprocal relationship between the thyroid gland and the brain are being elucidated at an accelerating rate. Progress in this area of psychoendocrinology, as in all other areas of psychoendocrinology, depended on progress in neurophysiology. A milestone was reached some 16 years ago when Guillemin (24) and Schally (65), working independently, announced the chemical structure of thyrotropin-releasing hormone (TRH). This discovery proved that the anterior pituitary gland is influenced by the brain; it led to the identification of other so-called hypothalamic hypophysiotropic hormones; it demonstrated a site where, and a mechanism by which, the two great communicating systems of the organism, the nervous system and the endocrine system, themselves communicate.

ENDOCRINE DYNAMICS

It is necessary here to furnish a guide for the material to follow by outlining the main features of the hypothalamic-pituitary-thyroid (HPT) axis. TRH (pGlu-His-Pro-NH$_2$) is released from nerve terminals in the median eminence of the hypothalamus into the portal venous system and is transported therein to the anterior pituitary gland, where it binds to membrane receptors, inducing release of thyroid-stimulating hormone (TSH, thyrotropin) (23). TSH, after release into the general circulation, reaches the thyroid gland, causing the synthesis and release of the thyroid hormones, L-tetraiodothyronine (T_4, thyroxine) and L-triiodothyronine (T_3). T_4 is the main secretion. Thyroid hormones exert metabolic effects: increased oxygen consumption, heat production, and synthesis of new protein. In addition to these effects and to their negative feedback actions on the pituitary gland, thyroid hormones penetrate brain and exert a medley of actions (10).

The regulation of thyroid state is not the province only of the hypothalamus and the pituitary. The thyroid gland itself plays a role: When iodine is scarce, the gland secretes relatively more T_3 than T_4. Thus, while using three iodine atoms instead of four, and saving 25% on a raw material, the gland produces a molecule, T_3, that is several times more potent (62). Peripheral tissues also regulate thyroid state, by enzymatically converting T_4 to T_3. In fact, the major source of T_3 is not the thyroid gland directly, but the transformation of its chief product T_4 (26). In an extreme view, T_4 can be regarded merely as a prohormone for T_3; however, T_4 itself does have intrinsic metabolic effects (26). T_4 can be converted not only to T_3, but also to "reverse" T_3. T_3 is L-3,3',5-triiodothyronine; it is potent. Reverse T_3 (rT_3) is L-3,3',5'-triiodothyronine; it is thought to be metabolically inert (5).

The simple tripeptide, TRH, has complicated endocrine actions. (Its complicated *non*endocrine, i.e., behavioral, actions will be mentioned below.) TRH releases not only TSH but also prolactin (PRL) and, in certain pathological states, growth hormone (GH) as well, each of which is also influenced by one or more other factors. Even the release of TSH is not a simple function of stimulation by TRH; it is potently influenced by negative feedback from thyroid hormones. In addition, two other hormones clearly inhibit TRH-induced release of TSH: somatostatin, which also inhibits GH release, and cortisol. Gonadal steroids, neurotensin, dopamine, cholecystokinin, vasoactive intestinal polypeptide, and other neuromodulators also influence the TSH response (50).

It is now commonplace to measure TSH and total T_3 and total T_4 directly, and in the case of T_4 to derive a value that is proportional to the fraction of the hormone that is free. One can regard the anterior pituitary as algebraically summing the relevant information that reaches it and secreting TSH as an appropriate response, often amplifying signals of imbalance. Thus, in mild hypothyroidism, T_3 and T_4 may be only slightly reduced but TSH elevations may be substantial. In the converse situation, basal TSH levels are somewhat less revealing, as there is less room, as it were, for TSH to fall than to rise.

Useful as it may be, the measurement of TSH and of thyroid hormones may leave certain questions unanswered. What is the locus of any fault that may exist? What is the significance of minor changes? The ability to evoke TSH secretion by TRH administration has contributed to the solution of these problems. To perform a TRH stimulation test, one simply measures TSH at baseline and 30 min after TRH injection, measurement at additional times yielding only little more information. In humans the peak TSH response is proportional to TRH doses from 0.006 to 0.4 mg intravenously (26). In primary (thyroidal) hypothyroidism, TSH baseline values are high; TSH response to TRH is exaggerated. In secondary (pituitary) hypothyroidism, baseline TSH is low; TSH response is deficient. In tertiary (hypothalamic) hypothyroidism, the existence of which is controversial, TSH baseline values would be low; TSH response would be normal or exaggerated.

DESCRIPTIVE ASPECTS OF THYROID-BRAIN RECIPROCITY

Mental Changes in Patients with Thyroid Disorders

Hyperthyroid Patients

Many studies have described the frequency and quality of psychological changes in patients with thyroid disease (77,79). In hyperthyroidism a typical depression syndrome is generally not observed. Clearly dysphoric, these patients complain of anxiety, fatigue, and irritability (77,79). Severe mental disorder is uncommon, though delirium may occur.

Hypothyroid Patients

In myxedema, psychological disturbance is common. In addition to organic symptoms, which may be the psycho-logical counterpart of a lowered metabolic rate, there may occur delusions and auditory hallucinations, usually persecutory (34). In milder states of hypothyroidism, depression and impairment of cognitive function are the common mental sequelae (77,79).

Subclinical Hypothyroidism

On prima facie grounds it would seem likely that hypothyroidism, rather than being an all-or-none condition, must be a graded disorder. This concept, old as it is, was revived in part by the demonstration by our group that a small dose of a thyroid hormone would enhance the therapeutic effects of tricyclic antidepressants (TCAs) in many patients, all of whom were euthyroid by usual criteria (see below). But can a truly euthyroid patient profit from a thyroid hormone? Some patients' ankle reflex time accelerated and remained accelerated during the 4 weeks of T_3 administration, suggesting that "replacement," however subtle, had taken place; in other patients (also responsive in an antidepressant fashion), ankle reflex time was unchanged. The question of subclinical hypothyroidism was moot because only crude measures of thyroid hormones (protein-bound iodine and the like) were available. With the introduction of accurate assays for all hormones of the HPT axis, the determination of the true thyroid state of depressed patients (and other mental patients) became possible.

Evered et al. (13) and Wenzel et al. (75) proposed definitions of stages of primary (thyroidal) hypothyroidism: from subclinical hypothyroidism (grade 3) to overt (grade 1) (Table 1).

Using this scheme, Gold and his colleagues (19) reported that 19 of 250 patients with depression or anergia could be classified as having grade 2 or grade 3 hypothyroidism, whereas by traditional standards these patients would have been considered euthyroid. Cowdry et al. (7) have reported very high rates of grades 2 and 1 hypothyroidism in rapidly cycling bipolar patients, many of whom were taking lithium.

The fact that hypothyroidism is frequently secondary to an autoimmune process offers an additional dimension to the search for subtle changes within the HPT axis. Hypothyroid patients, more often than normal people, have elevated antithyroid antibodies (antithyroglobulin, antimicrosomal, or both). Like the presence of hypothyroidism and of depression, the presence of elevated antithyroid antibodies is more common in women and increases with age. In their studies of psychiatric patients, Gold et al. (20) reported that 60% of patients with grades 2 or 3 hypothyroidism had detectable titers of antimicrosomal antibodies.

TABLE 1. *Stages of primary hypothyroidism*

	Grades		
	3	2	1
TSH response to TRH	↑	↑	↑
Basal TSH level	Normal	↑	↑
T_4 and T_3 levels	Normal	Normal	↓

Recently, Nemeroff et al. (54) showed that 20% of depressed patients admitted consecutively to a mental hospital had antithyroid antibodies of one or the other kind.

The clinical significance of antithyroid antibodies in the absence of overt thyroid disease in psychiatric patients (or other people) is presently unclear. In psychiatric patients, the reported rates may not differ greatly from those seen in a normal population (22). Factors that have been associated with the progression of symptomless autoimmune thyroiditis to hypothyroidism include high antibody titers, persistence of antibodies over time, and the presence of elevated TSH. Lithium may induce antithyroid antibodies; clearly it increases preexisting titers (4,9). Furthermore, patients with antithyroid antibodies may be more likely than others to develop overt hypothyroidism when given lithium (51).

How best to define the stages of subclinical hypothyroidism and how to integrate them with the body of data pertaining to blunted (not exaggerated) TSH responses (see below) will require longitudinal study. Success in such efforts could provide answers to important questions. Do patients usually progress from one stage to another? At what stage are mental symptoms likely and symptoms of what kind? In whom should lithium be used with special caution? Is a thyroid hormone indicated for patients at some stages and can it be sufficient treatment for mental symptoms? Is it possible to predict who will benefit most from use of a thyroid hormone as an adjunct to a TCA?

HPT Changes in Patients with Mental Disorders

Basal Values of Thyroid Hormones

There exists a consensus that thyroid dysfunction is somewhat higher in a psychiatric population, regardless of specific diagnosis, than in a general population. However, McLarty et al. (47) found an incidence of only 0.5% hypothyroidism and 0.7% hyperthyroidism in 1,200 psychiatric inpatients. A much more common finding has been the occurrence of transient hyperthyroxinemia. This has been reported to occur in anywhere from 4 to 38% of acute psychiatric admissions and may be accompanied by other HPT axis changes such as a reduced TSH response to TRH (69). As the term itself implies, transient hyperthyroxinemia tends to subside within a few weeks. Morley (50) has reported that amphetamine abuse can cause hyperthyroxinemia.

Assessment of the 24-hr secretion of TSH has revealed a reduced output in some patients with major depression that is associated with a lower TSH response to TRH in some instances (32). Furthermore, it has been reported that the normal nightly rise in TSH is reduced in major depression, especially in the acute state of illness (32,73).

TSH Response to TRH

Although depressed patients only infrequently show frank thyroid disease, on testing they often reveal a clear abnormality in the HPT axis. Their peak TSH response to the intravenous injection of TRH is subnormal or, to use the word that has become customary, "blunted." This finding by itself would suggest the presence of hyperthyroidism; in hyperthyroidism, elevated levels of thyroid hormones exert increased negative feedback on the anterior pituitary and thus blunt the pituitary TSH response to a stimulus such as TRH. However, the vast majority of psychiatric patients in whom a blunted TSH response has been demonstrated are *not* hyperthyroid; they are euthyroid by all usual criteria of history, physical examination, and chemical testing; they do not, as a group, show the transient hyperthyroxinemia seen in some newly admitted patients (see above). The phenomenon of the blunted TSH response to TRH in mental patients has been recently reviewed in detail (43,45), and only its salient features require mention here.

Because the criteria for blunting and the dose of TRH have varied between studies, so inevitably has the reported incidence of blunting. However, it is conservative to state, based on the study of hundreds of patients in scores of studies, that about 25% of depressed patients, after receiving a dose of TRH that for normal subjects is supramaximal, will show a TSH maximum rise over baseline of <5 $\mu IU/$ml serum. Among depressed patients, blunting does not seem to be a function of sex, age, or polarity, though each of these parameters could be studied further with profit.

There is slight evidence to suggest that a blunted TSH response may be related to chronicity of the depression process (45). If this proves to be the case, it would bear implications for the mechanism of the blunted response. Blunting might well be a reflection of down-regulation of TRH receptors on pituitary thyrotrophs from chronic overstimulation (perhaps tending toward recovery from the depression process) by hypothalamic TRH. Nevertheless, the mechanism of the blunted TSH response must presently be regarded as unknown (43,45). In this connection, it is well to recall that the TSH response to TRH is physiologically regulated by a host of factors, within and without the HPT axis, at the hypothalamic, pituitary, and peripheral levels. There need not be a single pathway to the common endpoint of a blunted TSH response. However this may be, a word must be directed to what the mechanism is not. Cortisol is often elevated in depression, and elevated cortisol is among the factors that can blunt the TSH response. However, direct evidence shows that only uncommonly is elevated cortisol the cause of a blunted response in depressed patients (14).

Among psychiatric patients, the blunted TSH response is not limited to depressed patients. It occurs with increased frequency in alcoholic men in a state of acute alcohol withdrawal (women have not been extensively tested), and at a rate similar to that in depressed patients in alcoholic men who have been abstinent for extended periods (46). Borderline patients often show blunting (16), and this is another in a series of biological findings that places them closer to affective disordered patients than to schizophrenic patients, who rarely show blunting. Manic patients sometimes show the phenomenon. In patients with anorexia nervosa the peak TSH response may be delayed, but it is usually normal in magnitude. In reviewing our data to date we found that about 4% of normals show TSH blunting (44). It is interesting that the lifetime prevalence rate for major affective disorder in the general population is about 4 to 6% (63).

From the foregoing it is obvious that the specificity and sensitivity of the TRH test are such as to render it of little *psycho*diagnostic value. The state-trait status of the blunted TSH response is also obscure. We have found blunting in 26% of ill depressed patients and in 16% of remitted depressed patients (44). Unfortunately, these figures are based on samplings of populations rather than on longitudinal study of the same patients. Nevertheless, it is clear from our work and the work of others (43–45) that in depression, as in alcoholism, blunting may or may not persist into recovery. Because the incidence in people fated to become depressed is unknown, one cannot be sure that it is *ever* a trait marker. It *might* be a trait marker in, say, 16% of depressed patients, with another 10% or so acquiring the phenomenon as a state marker (by whatever mechanism); alternatively, in the extreme case, blunting might *never* be a trait marker before the first attack. It might simply persist in some patients *after* an attack and thus become an *acquired* trait marker, an endocrine scar as it were.

The above remarks notwithstanding, the blunted TSH response is not without present and potential value. Kirkegaard et al. were the first to suggest that blunting might have prognostic utility (29). They tested unselected depressed patients before and after a course of ECT, which, in the event, always induced clinical remission. Whether blunted or not, some patients showed an enhanced TSH response to TRH after recovery from depression and some did not. To a statistically significant degree it was the former group, as compared to the latter, who avoided depressive relapse within 6 months. Kvist and Kirkegaard (35) reported similar data using sleep deprivation as the therapeutic modality. Langer et al. (38) showed, with TCAs as the therapeutic modality, that patients who gain in TSH responsiveness tend to be those who have shown the greatest antidepressant response.

The TSH response has other uses. When positive (i.e., blunted), the test may help differentiate mania from schizophrenia, as Extein et al. (15) have suggested. It may help clarify the diagnostic problem that sometimes attends borderline patients. Moreover, the explication of the means by which blunting can occur is sure to clarify the role that thyroid state may play in the pathogenesis of depression and in the recovery process. In a general way, the identification of a clear HPT fault in a large minority of depressed, alcoholic, and borderline patients demands further investigation of HPT dynamics. It also begins to provide a rational basis for the therapeutic use in psychiatry of HPT axis hormones, which heretofore have been employed only empirically.

Euthyroid Sick Syndrome

The euthyroid sick syndrome (ESS) is a disorder of thyroid economy that is characterized by an elevation in rT_3, a reduction in T_3, and minimal changes in T_4 and TSH. This pattern can occur in a wide range of medical illnesses, in starvation and after certain pharmacological interventions (e.g., glucocorticoids and amiodarone) (72). One study has revealed that a component of the ESS,

elevated rT_3, is present in some depressed patients (42). Contrariwise, it has been reported that rT_3 is not elevated in depression but instead varies over the course of illness, diminishing with recovery (31,33). It has generally been observed that psychiatric patients do not exhibit significant reductions in T_3 even when rT_3 is elevated. A factor requiring study is the role that weight loss may play in the development of ESS in affective disorders.

Although the reasons for the development of the ESS are not certain, it is generally thought that the increase in rT_3 (calorigenically inactive) and the decrease in T_3 (calorigenically potent) are an attempt on the part of the organism to minimize catabolism during the stress of illness. The occurrence of the ESS in depression suggests that the process can have a central as well as a peripheral origin.

THERAPEUTIC ASPECTS OF THYROID-BRAIN RECIPROCITY

TRH

TRH is widely distributed within and, to a lesser extent, outside the nervous system. It is phylogenetically older than the thyroid gland, which, of course, is limited to vertebrates. The view is widely held that TRH has served many important functions and has only recently acquired the task of adjusting TSH secretion by the pituitary. Its old functions might be expected to be biologically harmonious with its new ones (53); Metcalf and Dettmar (48) have referred to TRH as an endogenous ergotropic substance. That in animals TRH exerts behavioral effects that are not mediated by hormonal effects is incontrovertible. These myriad effects have often been reviewed, most recently by Kalivas and Prange (28).

The question of behavioral effects of TRH in humans is controversial. Prange et al. first reported that, in a series of women with unipolar depression, the intravenous injection of TRH caused an antidepressant response that was prompt, partial, and brief. One day after injection, patients were approximately 50% improved; they relapsed to baseline severity in approximately 1 week. Quickly following this report, many studies of TRH in depression were performed. Usually addressing the question of whether TRH is an antidepressant competitive with standard agents and utilizing a variety of designs, populations, dosage schedules, routes of administration, outcome measures, and the like, the studies are difficult to summarize, but *in toto* they can be regarded as equivocal at best (56).

Prange et al. (57) reported that TRH had immediate beneficial effects in some schizophrenic patients. We also reported that, more often than placebo injection, TRH injection produced a sense of relaxation and well-being in normals (81), a result confirmed by Betts et al. (3). Thus a trial of TRH in anxious patients may be indicated. There is, indeed, no reason to believe that the behavioral effects of TRH are disease specific. TRH has been used experimentally in Japan and Italy to treat coma from head injury, a procedure that takes its origin in part from an early demonstration that the tripeptide will awaken rodents from barbiturate-induced sleep without altering barbiturate blood levels (55).

TSH

In light of the plethora of behavioral effects attributed to most anterior pituitary peptides (59), most notably adrenocorticotropic hormone, it has been striking to note that virtually nothing has been published about behavioral effects of TSH. This pituitary peptide, like certain others, may be synthesized in hypothalamus as well as pituitary or at least reach the former site from the latter (49). Recently TSH has been reported to exert an effect on temperature regulation in rodents independent of its endocrine effects (39).

In early work our group gave depressed women TSH (10 IU i.m.) or saline injection the day before all patients began a standard imipramine (IMI) regimen. The patients who received TSH improved much faster than their controls (56). An adequate explanation, of course, is the thyroid stimulation (see below) caused by TSH. However, the possibility cannot be discounted that the pituitary hormone exerted a direct behavioral effect as well.

T_3 to Accelerate TCA Action

Piqued by a clinical observation, encouraged by preliminary findings in animals, and later supported by additional laboratory work (56,60), our group proposed that T_3, used as an adjunct, might ameliorate one of the chief drawbacks of TCA treatment, viz., slow onset of therapeutic action. In a series of controlled trials we found that T_3, 25 μg per day orally, did in fact greatly accelerate the therapeutic response in women, all of whom were euthyroid. Later trials in the United Kingdom by Coppen et al. (6) and by Wheatley (76), performed in inpatients and outpatients, respectively, confirmed the finding. Generalizing from the array of trials that have been performed, one can conclude that T_3 greatly accelerates the onset of therapeutic action of IMI or amitryptyline (and probably of other TCAs, though this has not been systematically demonstrated) in euthyroid women whether they show the unipolar or bipolar form of the disorder, whether they are agitated or motorically retarded, and whether they are pre- or postmenopausal (though only a small number of the latter have been studied) (56,60). In all studies, drug side effects were not increased. Indeed, they were decreased, but this observation is probably an artifact of the enhanced efficacy of T_3-TCA treatment. In clinical trials many items, e.g., headache, that are noted as side effects are also noted as depression symptoms.

Does T_3 alone exert an antidepressant effect? With the leadership of the late Ian Wilson (80), our group performed a study to test this question, but the results were inconclusive. Doses of T_3 alone that began to exert a therapeutic effect also began to exert a toxic effect. If T_3 alone is an antidepressant (in euthyroid patients), its therapeutic index must be slight. However, one can now speculate whether the use of a β-blocker such as atenolol, which penetrates brain only poorly, would allow T_3 to exert useful central effects while blocking peripheral side effects.

A word is needed about the mechanism of action of T_3. Early animal work suggested, and a study by Garbutt et al. (17) proved, that T_3 does not alter serum levels of IMI or of its metabolic derivative, desipramine. In 1972, guided entirely by inferential evidence, we suggested that transmitter receptor sensitivity might be important in affective disorders and that thyroid hormones might enhance central noradrenergic receptors (61), a theme later elaborated by Whybrow and Prange (78). Direct evidence to support it continues to accrue (58,71).

T_3 to Convert TCA Failures to Successes

A second drawback of TCA treatment is its occasional failure. Even when usual causes of failure have been eliminated and even after a trial of 5 weeks or so, TCAs fail to produce substantial improvement in, say, 20% of depressed patients. In a double-blind study involving 12 TCA-failed patients, drawn from two inpatient units of the National Institute of Mental Health, Goodwin et al. (21) showed that T_3, 25 μg, added to the TCA regimen then in use, promptly converted nine patients to successes. Men and women, bipolar and unipolar patients, profited equally. All earlier studies, most of them less systematic, had yielded almost identical results. Two careful studies by Banki (1,2) addressed an important clinical point: Will the addition of T_3 to a TCA regimen in failed patients accomplish something not obtainable by simply increasing the TCA dose? Banki randomly assigned a large series of failed patients to one of two treatments: the addition of T_3 or an increase in TCA. The former maneuver was much more effective than the latter.

Since the use of T_3 to convert TCA failures was announced, de Montigny et al. (8) and Heninger et al. (25) have shown that a similar effect can be obtained by the addition of lithium. Because both T_3 and lithium will convert most failures, there must be a substantial number of patients for whom either treatment will be successful. A nice question then arises: How can a "prothyroid" treatment (T_3) and an "antithyroid" treatment (lithium) achieve the same result? Of course, both agents produce a variety of nonmetabolic effects: The net effect of T_3 is "proadrenergic"; the net effect of lithium is "proserotonergic." With offsetting metabolic effects and with complementary neurotransmitter effects, T_3 and lithium together might comprise a splendid antidepressant treatment.

T_4

As stated earlier, many tissues, including brain, convert T_4 to T_3. Thus, in the absence of some rare defect in conversion, T_4 ought to produce about the same effects as T_3. In our initial studies we chose T_3 in preference to T_4 for two reasons: It acts faster, and it disappears faster (half-life approximately 12 hr versus half-life approximately 7 days). Thus, if toxicity were encountered one could stop T_3 and regain safety quite promptly. In later studies we persisted in using T_3 mainly to provide comparability between studies. Nonetheless, we have been informed by several clinicians that they use T_4 as we have used T_3, with excellent results. Indeed, when the hormone is given once daily, the T_4 effect may be smoother because of its longer half-life. On a weight basis, two to four times as much T_4 as T_3 is needed; daily doses employed thus are 50 to 100 μg.

The above observations are relevant to the recent work of Joffe, Post, and colleagues (27). They have suggested that an antidepressant effect can be produced by reducing the thyroid state of brain. They suggest that the antidepressant effects of lithium and carbamazine are, at least in part, due to their antithyroid effects. The antidepressant effects of adjunctive T_3 do not contradict this hypothesis, in their view, because T_3 administration leads to a reduction in T_4 levels, causing less T_4 to be available to brain (for conversion *in situ* to T_3). To confirm or refute this formulation, we think it is critical to establish in controlled studies whether small doses of T_4, like small doses of T_3, will in fact amplify the antidepressant effects of TCA.

T_4, in hypermetabolic amounts, has recently been reported to exert mood-stabilizing effects in rapid-cycling bipolar patients (70).

THYROID-DRUG INTERACTIONS

Lithium

Among psychotropic drugs, lithium clearly has the most profound effects on thyroid function. Early in the history of its use, it was found that lithium caused some patients to develop overt hypothyroidism. Because lithium is used in patients at high risk for depression and because hypothyroidism may mimic depression, predispose to it, or aggravate it, this observation is important to clinicians. Many, if not all, subjects given lithium will show mild, transient reductions in T_4 and T_3 and corresponding elevations in TSH. In most instances thyroid function will not be reduced because the HPT axis will homeostatically maintain, via TSH stimulation of the thyroid gland, normal levels of thyroid hormones. However, from 4 to 10% of lithium-treated patients will develop overt hypothyroidism, whereas as many as 30% will show an elevated TSH (12,67). Not surprisingly, the incidence of overt hypothyroidism after lithium treatment is more common in women and in patients with preexisting antithyroid antibodies or an exaggerated TSH response to TRH (40,51). Thyroxine replacement permits continued use of lithium and, in fact, may even reduce lithium exacerbation of underlying thyroiditis (4).

Carbamazepine

Carbamazepine, a tricyclic anticonvulsant increasingly used in bipolar disorder, has been reported to have consistent but relatively mild antithyroid effects. Significant reductions in T_4 and T_3 have been noted, as have mild elevations in TSH (64). Apparently the development of overt hypothy-

roidism after carbamazepine is extremely rare, and the effect of carbamazepine on antithyroid antibodies is, to our knowledge, unknown.

TCAs

TCAs, structurally similar to carbamazepine, have not been found to alter levels of T_4 or T_3 (41). The effects of TCAs on the TSH response to TRH are less certain, though it is clear that TCAs do not induce clinically significant changes in basal TSH. Kirkegaard et al. (30) reported that acute intravenous infusion of IMI did not alter the TSH response to TRH. Studies in which TCAs were given for longer times have revealed that the TSH response may be increased or unchanged (36). One study has reported that nomifensine, a nontricyclic antidepressant drug with pro-dopaminergic properties, can *reduce* the TSH response in normals (18). As Krog-Meyer, Kirkegaard, and colleagues have noted (36), given the observations that the TSH response to TRH may increase with recovery from depression, it becomes important to sort out TCA effects on the HPT axis versus TCA effects on the depressive illness.

Neuroleptics

Neuroleptics, because of their dopamine receptor-blocking actions, would be predicted to increase TSH secretion. In fact, in normal subjects the acute administration of the dopamine blockers metoclopramide or domperidone does increase the TSH response to TRH (74). Clinical studies with neuroleptics have been less consistent. Nader et al. (52) found no changes in basal TSH or in TRH test results in schizophrenic patients chronically treated with neuroleptics. At least one group has noted that some neuroleptics may *reduce* TSH response, presumably because of their α-adrenoreceptor blocking properties (37).

Benzodiazepines

In general, benzodiazepines have not been noted to alter the HPT axis, though they have not been extensively studied in this regard. Drugs of this class given acutely have been shown not to change the TSH response to TRH (30). However, it has been reported recently that benzodiazepines bind to the TRH receptor (66), and this binding has been shown to inhibit certain biochemical effects of TRH, e.g., the *in vitro* hydrolysis of phosphatidylinositol 4,5-bisphosphate (11). Two considerations—the order of potency of a series of benzodiazepines and the high concentrations required—imply that the TRH receptors addressed by benzodiazepines are different from the high-affinity receptors that account for the drugs' antianxiety effects.

β-Blockers

Propranolol, which has been used experimentally in anxiety disorders and in schizophrenia, influences both thyroid hormone effects and T_4 metabolism. It blocks β-adrenoreceptor stimulation and it inhibits the conversion of T_4 to T_3 (72).

SUMMARY AND CONCLUSIONS

Early in life the thyroid gland is necessary for maturation. Throughout life it contributes to the regulation of a variety of functions, including brain functions, while the brain contributes to the regulation of thyroid hormone secretion. For this purpose, the brain hormone principally involved is TRH. Its endocrine actions and its behavioral actions appear harmonious. Within the HPT axis, TRH probably influences the set-point of the anterior pituitary gland, i.e., the range beyond which the pituitary and the thyroid gland, in concert, defend against too much or too little thyroid activity, in relation to total psychobiological needs.

New approaches to the study of brain-thyroid relationships have produced a variety of findings and the description of several syndromes. The details of none of these are clear, and the relationships between findings, at any time in populations or across time in individuals, are also obscure. What does emerge from these data are certain important themes. HPT disorders, especially hypothyroidism, may contribute to several mental disorders, prominently, but probably not exclusively, depression. When such disorders occur, from whatever concatenation of causes, whether or not thyroid dysfunction has been among them, the HPT axis may be invoked as a remedial force. Beyond these generalizations a trenchant clinical point can be made: The psychopharmacologist often, if only inadvertently, becomes a psychoendocrinologist. As a common instance, neuroleptics elevate PRL levels. However, lithium and carbamazepine, nearly as reliably, lower thyroid hormone levels. The situation is symmetrical: Thyroid hormones affect the brain transmitter systems to which psychotropic drugs are addressed. In this sense, drugs that address either the brain or the thyroid gland reinforce the venerable concept of their reciprocal relationship.

REFERENCES

1. Banki, C. M. (1975): *Orv. Hetil.,* 116:2543–2547.
2. Banki, C. M. (1977): *Eur. J. Clin. Pharmacol.,* 11:311–315.
3. Betts, T. A., Smith, J., Pidd, S., Macintosh, J., Harvey, P., and Funicane, J. (1976): *Br. J. Clin. Pharmacol.,* 3:469–473.
4. Calabrese, J. R., Gulledge, A. D., Hahn, K., Skwerer, R., Kotz, M., Schumacher, O. P., Gupta, M. K., Krupp, N., and Gold, P. W. (1985): *Am. J. Psychiatry,* 142:1318–1321.
5. Chopra, I. J., Sack, J., and Fisher, D. A. (1975): In: *Perinatal Thyroid Physiology and Disease,* edited by D. A. Fisher and G. N. Burrow, pp. 33–48. Raven Press, New York.
6. Coppen, A., Whybrow, P. C., Noguera, R., Maggs, R., and Prange, A. J., Jr. (1972): *Arch. Gen. Psychiatry,* 26:234–241.
7. Cowdry, R. W., Wehr, T. A., Zis, A. P., and Goodwin, F. K. (1983): *Arch. Gen. Psychiatry,* 40:414–420.
8. de Montigny, C., Cournoyer, G., Morissette, R., Langlois, R., and Caille, G. (1983): *Arch. Gen. Psychiatry,* 40:1327–1334.
9. Deniker, P., Eyguem, A., Bernheim, R., Loo, H., and Delarue, P. (1978): *Neuropsychobiology,* 4:270–275.
10. Dratman, M. B., and Crutchfield, F. L. (1981): In: *The "Low T3 Syndrome,"* edited by R. D. Hesch, pp. 115–126. Academic Press, New York.
11. Drummond, A. H. (1985): *Biochem. Biophys. Res. Commun.,* 127:63–70.
12. Emerson, C. H., Dison, W. L., and Utiger, R. D. (1973): *J. Clin. Endocrinol. Metab.,* 36:338–346.
13. Evered, D. C., Ormston, B. J., Smith, P. A., Hall, R., and Bird, T. (1973): *Br. Med. J.,* 1:657–662.
14. Extein, I., Pottash, A. L. C., and Gold, M. S. (1981): *Psychiatry Res.,* 4:49–53.
15. Extein, I., Pottash, A. L. C., and Gold, M. S. (1982): *Arch. Gen. Psychiatry,* 39:77–81.
16. Garbutt, J. C., Loosen, P. T., Tipermas, A., and Prange, A. J., Jr. (1983): *Psychiatry Res.,* 9:107–113.
17. Garbutt, J., Malekpour, B., Brunswick, D., Jonnalgadda, M. R., Joliff, I., Podolak, R., Wilson, I. C., and Prange, A. J., Jr. (1979): *Am. J. Psychiatry,* 136:980–982.
18. Giusti, M., Mazzocchi, G., Mignone, D., Tarditi, W., and Giordano, G. (1983): *J. Endocrinol. Invest.,* 6:125–129.
19. Gold, M. S., Pottash, A. L. C., and Extein, I. (1981): *JAMA,* 245:1919–1925.
20. Gold, M. S., Pottash, A. L. C., and Extein, I. (1982): *Psychiatry Res.,* 6:261–269.
21. Goodwin, F. K., Prange, A. J., Jr., Post, R. M., Muscattola, G., and Lipton, M. A. (1981): *Am. J. Psychiatry,* 139:334–338.
22. Gordin, A., Maatela, J., Miettinen, A., Helenius, T., and Lambert, B.-A. (1979): *Acta Endocrinol.,* 90:33–42.
23. Grant, G., Vale, W., and Guillemin, R. (1972): *Biochem. Biophys. Res. Commun.,* 46:28–34.
24. Guillemin, R. (1978): *Science,* 202:390–402.
25. Heninger, G. R., Charney, D. S., and Sternberg, D. E. (1983): *Arch. Gen. Psychiatry,* 40:1335–1342.
26. Ingbar, S. H., and Woeber, K. A. (1974): In: *Textbook of Endocrinology,* edited by R. H. Williams, pp. 117–247. W. B. Saunders, Philadelphia.
27. Joffe, R. T., Roy-Byrne, P. P., Udhe, T., and Post, R. M. (1984): *Biol. Psychiatry,* 19:1685–1691.
28. Kalivas, P. W., and Prange, A. J., Jr. (1987): In: *Peptide Hormones: Effects and Mechanisms of Action,* edited by A. Negro-Vilar and P. M. Conn. CRC Press, Boca Raton, FL (*in press*).
29. Kirkegaard, C. (1981): *Psychoneuroendocrinology,* 6:189–212.
30. Kirkegaard, C., Bjorum, N., Cohn, D., Faber, J., Lauridsen, U. B., and Nerup, J. (1977): *Psychoneuroendocrinology,* 2:131–136.
31. Kirkegaard, C., and Faber, J. (1981): *Acta Endocrinol.,* 96:199–207.
32. Kjellman, B. F. (1983): Thesis, Karolinska Institute Department of Psychiatry and Medicine, St. Goran's Hospital, Stockholm, and Department of Psychiatry, University of Linkoping, Stockholm, Sweden.
33. Kjellman, B. F., Ljunggren, J.-G., Beck-Friis, J., and Wetterberg, L. (1983): *Psychiatry Res.,* 10:1–9.
34. Klaiber, E. L., Broverman, D. M., Vogel, W., and Kobayashi, Y. (1976): In: *Psychotropic Action of Hormones,* edited by T. M. Itil, G. Laudahn, and W. M. Herrman, pp. 135–154. Spectrum Publishing Company, New York.
35. Kvist, J., and Kirkegaard, C. (1980): *Acta Psychiatr. Scand.,* 62:494–502.
36. Krog-Meyer, I., Kirkegaard, C., Kijne, B., Lumholta, B., Smith, E., Cykke-Olesen, L., and Bjorum, N. (1985): *Psychiatry. Res.,* 15:145–151.
37. Lamberg, B.-A., Linnoila, M., Fogelholm, R., Olkinuora, M., Kotilainen, P., and Saarinen, P. (1977): *Neuroendocrinology,* 24:90–97.
38. Langer, G., Resch, F., Aschauer, M. S., Koinig, G., Schonbeck, G., and Dittrich, R. (1984): *Neuropsychobiology,* 11:213–218.
39. Lin, M. T., Chu, P. C., and Leu, S. Y. (1983): *Neuroendocrinology,* 37:206–211.
40. Lindstedt, G., Nilsson, L.-A., Walinder, J., Skott, A., and Ohman, R. (1977): *Br. J. Psychiatry,* 130:452–458.
41. Linnoila, M., Gold, P., Potter, W. E., and Wehr, T. A. (1981): *Psychiatry Res.,* 4:357–360.
42. Linnoila, M., Lamberg, B.-A., Potter, W. Z., Gold, P. W., and Goodwin, F. K. (1982): *Psychiatry Res.,* 6:271–276.
43. Loosen, P. T. (1985): *Psychoneuroendocrinology,* 10:237–260.
44. Loosen, P. T., Garbutt, J. C., and Prange, A. J., Jr. (1987): *Pharmacopsychiatry* (*in press*).

45. Loosen, P. T., and Prange, A. J., Jr. (1982): *Am. J. Psychiatry,* 139:405–416.
46. Loosen, P. T., Wilson, I. C., Dew, B. W., and Tipermas, A. (1983): *Am. J. Psychiatry,* 130:1145–1149.
47. McLarty, D. G., Ratcliffe, W. A., Ratcliffe, J. G., Shiminins, J. G., and Goldberg, A. (1978): *Br. J. Psychiatry,* 133:211–218.
48. Metcalf, G., and Dettmar, P. (1981): *Lancet,* 1:586.
49. Moldow, R. L., and Yalow, R. S. (1978): *Life Sci.,* 22:1859–1864.
50. Morley, J. E. (1981): *Endocr. Rev.,* 2:396–436.
51. Myers, D. H., Carter, R. A., Burns, B. H., Armond, A., Hussain, S. B., and Chengapa, U. K. (1985): *Psychol. Med.,* 15:55–61.
52. Naber, D., Ackenheil, M., and Laakmann, G. (1980): *Adv. Biochem. Psychopharmacol.,* 24:419–423.
53. Nemeroff, C. B., and Prange, A. J., Jr. (1978): *Arch. Gen. Psychiatry,* 35:999–1010.
54. Nemeroff, C. B., Simon, J. S., Haggerty, J. J., and Evans, D. L. (1985): *Am. J. Psychiatry,* 142:840–843.
55. Prange, A. J., Jr., Breese, G. R., Cott, J. M., Martin, B. R., Cooper, B. R., Wilson, I. C., and Plotnikoff, N. P. (1974): *Life Sci.,* 14:447–455.
56. Prange, A. J., Jr., Loosen, P. T., Wilson, I. C., and Lipton, M. A. (1984): In: *Neurobiology of Mood Disorders,* edited by R. M. Post and J. C. Ballenger, pp. 311–322. Williams & Wilkins, Baltimore.
57. Prange, A. J., Jr., Loosen, P. T., Wilson, I. C., Meltzer, H. Y., and Fang, V. S. (1979): *Arch. Gen. Psychiatry,* 36:1086–1093.
58. Prange, A. J., Jr., and Mason, G. A. (1985): *IVth World Congr. Biol. Psychiatry,* Abstract II 414.2.
59. Prange, A. J., Jr., Nemeroff, C. B., Lipton, M. A., Breese, G. R., and Wilson, I. C. (1978): In: *Handbook of Psychopharmacology,* edited by L. L. Iversen, S. D. Iversen, and S. H. Snyder, pp. 1–107. Plenum Press, New York.
60. Prange, A. J., Jr., Wilson, I. C., Breese, G. R., and Lipton, M. A. (1976): In: *Hormones, Behavior and Psychopathology,* edited by E. J. Sachar, pp. 15–19. Raven Press, New York.
61. Prange, A. J., Jr., Wilson, I. C., Knox, A. E., McClane, T. K., Breese, G. R., Martin, B. R., Alltop, L. B., and Lipton, M. A. (1972): *J. Psychiatr. Res.,* 9:187–205.
62. Robbins, J., Rall, J. E., and Groden, P. (1974): In: *Duncan's Disease of Metabolism: III, Endocrinology,* edited by P. K. Bondy and L. E. Rosenberg, pp. 1009–1104. W. B. Saunders, Philadelphia.
63. Robins, L. N., Helger, J. E., Weissman, M. M., Orvaschel, H., Gruenberg, E., Burke, J. D., and Regier, D. A. (1984): *Arch. Gen. Psychiatry,* 41:949–958.
64. Roy-Byrne, P. P., Joffe, R. T., Uhde, T. W., and Post, R. M. (1984): *Arch. Gen. Psychiatry,* 41:1150–1153.
65. Schally, A. V. (1978): *Science,* 202:18–28.
66. Sharif, N., and Burt, D. (1984): *J. Neurochem.,* 43:742–746.
67. Shopsin, B., and Gershon, S. (1973): In: *Lithium: Its Role in Psychiatric Research and Treatment,* edited by S. Gershon and B. Shopsin, pp. 107–146. Plenum Press, New York.
68. Simon, Sir John (1845): *The Physiological Essay on the Thymus Gland.* H. Renshaw, London.
69. Spratt, D., Pont, A., Miller, M., McDongall, I., Bayer, M., and McLaughlin, W. (1982): *Am. J. Med.,* 73:41–47.
70. Stancer, H. C., and Persad, E. (1982): *Arch. Gen. Psychiatry,* 39:311–312.
71. Sulser, F. (1984): In: *Frontiers in Biochemical and Pharmacological Research in Depression,* edited by E. Usdin, pp. 249–261. Raven Press, New York.
72. Wartofsky, L., and Burman, K. D. (1982): *Endocr. Rev.,* 3:164–217.
73. Weeke, A., and Weeke, J. (1978): *Acta Psychiatr. Scand.,* 57:281–289.
74. Wenzel, K. W., and Doring, J. (1982): *Acta Endocrinol.,* 101:550–554.
75. Wenzel, K. W., Meinhold, H., Raffenberg, M., Adlkofer, F., and Schleusener, H. (1974): *Eur. J. Clin. Invest.,* 4:141–148.
76. Wheatley, D. (1972): *Arch. Gen. Psychiatry,* 26:229–233.
77. Whybrow, P. C., and Prange, A. J., Jr. (1981): *Arch. Gen. Psychiatry,* edited by E. J. Sacher, pp. 125–142. Raven Press, New York.
78. Whybrow, P. C., and Prange, A. J., Jr. (1981): *Arch. Gen. Psychiatry,* 38:106–113.
79. Whybrow, P. C., Prange, A. J., Jr., and Treadway, C. R. (1969): *Arch. Gen. Psychiatry,* 20:48–63.
80. Wilson, I. C., Prange, A. J., Jr., and Lara, P. P. (1974): In: *The Thyroid Axis, Drugs, and Behavior,* edited by A. J. Prange, Jr., pp. 49–62. Raven Press, New York.
81. Wilson, I. C., Prange, A. J., Jr., Lara, P. P., Alltop, L. B., Stikeleather, R. A., and Lipton, M. A. (1973): *Arch. Gen. Psychiatry,* 29:15–21.

Psychopharmacology:
The Third Generation of Progress,
edited by Herbert Y. Meltzer.
Raven Press, New York © 1987.

CHAPTER 63

Opioid Peptides in Affective Disorders

Philip A. Berger and Charles B. Nemeroff

One of the most exciting advances in the recent history of neurochemistry is the discovery of opioid receptors and the endogenous opioid peptides or endorphins. Neither of these discoveries was serendipitous. Classical pharmacology with its preparation of opiate agonists and antagonists in active and inactive stereoisomer forms was an enormous stimulus to opiate research (32,34). The extreme potency as well as the stereospecificity of certain opioid compounds such as etorphin led some investigators to suggest, as early as the 1950s, that these opiate drugs might act through specific opioid receptors (11,13). When the classical opiate pharmacological armamentarium was combined with the availability of techniques for producing drugs tagged with radioisotopes, it was possible to propose a paradigm for the search for these opiate receptors. This paradigm may have first been proposed by Avram Goldstein (33).

In 1973 three groups of investigators led by Terenius in Sweden, Simon in New York, and Pert and Snyder in Baltimore reported highly specific opiate receptors in mammalian brain (63,75,78). Following this discovery, numerous investigators suggested that brain opiate receptors must be the target of a naturally occurring endogenous opioid substance (11,13).

A second observation also led to the search for endogenous opioid compounds. In 1972 Akil et al. (3) reported that analgesia could be produced by electrical stimulation of certain areas in the brains of rats and, eventually, cats, monkeys, and humans. This analgesia is comparable in efficacy to opiate analgesia for both acute and chronic pain (55) and is commonly referred to as stimulation-produced analgesia (SPA). In studying SPA, Akil and colleagues were able to show that the analgesia produced provided excellent pain relief, while not interfering with normal function over a broad set of measures. Perhaps most interesting, the analgesia could be partially reversed by the potent opioid antagonist naloxone (3,4). The ability of naloxone to par-

tially reverse SPA led to the conclusion that the electrical stimulation released an endogenous material that seemed to be acting on the opiate receptor to produce pain control. This observation suggested that SPA was mediated in part by a natural substance with actions like those of morphine. This substance would have to be an endogenous opioid compound (11,13).

The first endogenous opioids discovered were two small peptides of five amino acids named methionine-enkephalin (met-ENK) and leucine-enkephalin (leu-ENK) by their discoverers, Hughes and Kosterlitz (39). Since then, numerous opioid peptides have been discovered and characterized in mammalian brain. There has also been an explosion of research on the possible role of these numerous endorphins or endogenous opioids.

Soon after the discovery of met- and leu-ENK, it was possible to demonstrate several important characteristics of their action that suggested they functioned as putative neurotransmitters. Not only were they stored intravesicularly and had well-demonstrated interaction with specific binding sites, but they also exhibited rapid release and degradation. The demonstration of enkephalin release was first carried out in humans, rather than animals, since enkephalin-like material was detected in human cerebrospinal fluid (CSF) (5,6,82). The animal work on SPA had already been extended to the clinical situation, and SPA was used to relieve chronic intractable pain in humans (68). During neurosurgery, when these patients were electrically stimulated, enkephalin-like material increased in the CSF from the third ventricle (5). Enkephalin degradation was demonstrated in several studies that suggested the presence of a specific membrane-bound enzyme, now known as enkephalinase, which degrades enkephalin and has a high affinity for the compound (53,76).

In their first reports on the enkephalins, Hughes and Kosterlitz pointed out that the structure of met-ENK appeared within the larger pituitary peptide, β-lipotropin (47). Several groups of investigators simultaneously recognized that β-lipotropin contained at least three compounds, including β-, γ-, and α-endorphin, which are active endorphins in their own right (16,20,36,48). β-Endorphin was soon shown to be located in the corticotrophic cells of the anterior lobe of the pituitary gland and in all cells of the intermediate lobe of the pituitary gland (15). Since adrenocorticotropic hormone (ACTH) is also present in these two cell types, there was an obvious association between β-endorphin, β-lipotropin, and ACTH in the pituitary. Soon several investigators were able to demonstrate that β-lipotropin and ACTH immunoreactivity occurred within precisely the same granules in pituitary cells using electron microscope techniques. This suggested a common biosynthetic origin for ACTH, β-endorphin, and β-lipotropin. Shortly after, Mains and co-workers (52) and Roberts and Herbert (71) used a mouse pituitary tumor line to demonstrate that all three substances, ACTH, β-endorphin, and β-lipotropin, were made from the same precursor molecule, the 31,000-dalton precursor now known as proopiomelanocortin (POMC).

Opioid peptides, distinct from both the enkephalins and β-endorphin, were discovered by Goldstein and colleagues at Stanford (34) and Matsuo and colleagues in Japan (56). Goldstein et al. called the peptide they discovered dynorphin and found that it included the full structure of leu-ENK as its first five amino acids. Matsuo and colleagues described two endorphins, now known as α- and β-neoendorphin, which share with dynorphin a common N-terminal leu-ENK sequence. Preliminary immunohistochemical studies have located dynorphin and α-neoendorphin almost exclusively in the posterior pituitary, unlike β-endorphin and POMC, which occur in the intermediate lobe and anterior lobe of the pituitary. Dynorphin and α-neoendorphin are also distributed in the brain separately from enkephalin. This suggested that these two endorphins, dynorphin and α-neoendorphin, are part of a separate endorphin system from both enkephalin and β-endorphin.

Using cDNA technology, Numa's group in Japan (44) were then able to discover and elucidate the structure of a precursor protein for dynorphin and the neoendorphins. This prohormone contains not only dynorphin and the neoendorphins, but also a separate dynorphin-like endorphin that is now called dynorphin-B. The discovery of a common precursor for dynorphin and the neoendorphin was anticipated by Weber and associates (83), who demonstrated that dynorphins and the neoendorphins are located in the same cells of the hypothalamus.

A third endorphin family has also been identified by the work of several investigators. This family is the enkephalin family, whose precursor is proenkephalin. The structure of proenkephalin was also defined and sequenced using cDNA technology by Numa's group at the University of Kyoto (44). This enkephalin family contains more than met-ENK and leu-ENK. cDNA sequencing demonstrates that the adrenal precursor contains four copies of met-ENK and one copy each of leu-ENK, methionine-enkephalin-Arg[6]-Phe[6] (heptapeptide), and methionine-enkephalin-Arg[6]-Gly[7]-Leu[8] (octapeptide) (72).

To summarize, in studying the possible role of endorphins in affective disorders or other type of psychopathology, we are faced with at least three major endogenous opioid systems in the brain that are intimately associated with pain, affect, and endocrine changes. Each of these endorphin systems is enormously complex in its own right. As described above, there are three completely different opioid families whose precursors have now been defined as three distinct precursors, each with a molecular weight of approximately 28,000 to 30,000 daltons. Each of these precursors has been characterized and sequenced; however, many years of research will be required to determine the activity and possible physiological and pathophysiological roles of these opioid peptide families.

The task is even more complex because of the existence of multiple opioid receptors. The first evidence for the existence of multiple opioid receptors was reported by Martin and co-workers (31,54), who performed classical pharmacological studies in dogs. Based on Martin's results, three types of opioid receptors were postulated, which Martin named for the prototype drugs used in the studies: μ from morphine, κ from ketocyclazocine, and σ from SKF 10047 (13,74).

Subsequent to Martin's work, Kosterlitz and colleagues provided the first evidence of an additional opiate receptor that prefers enkephalins (50). Since this receptor appeared to be the predominant receptor type present in the mouse vas deferens, which is an important *in vitro* bioassay system for opioids, it was named the δ receptor (for deferens). The other *in vitro* bioassay system, the guinea pig ileum, was found to have mainly Martin's μ receptor (74). Recent studies suggest that morphine and β-endorphin show high affinity for both μ and δ receptors. Dynorphin seems to bind to κ receptors, whereas the enkephalins show the highest affinity for δ receptors. Although this is a simplification, it gives some idea of the complications in trying to determine the role of opioid receptors and endogenous opioids in both normal and abnormal physiology (13,74).

Thus, whereas endorphins are putative brain neurotransmitters or neuromodulators, they are also pituitary and adrenal hormones and are known to exist in the peripheral nervous system and the gastrointestinal tract (38). The peripheral targets for the endorphins remain to be determined and their primary brain functions need to be defined. Whereas the complexity of endorphins speaks to their importance in physiology and behavior, it creates severe logistical problems for clinical research. For example, it is extremely difficult to influence one endorphin system or one set of opioid receptors using pharmacological tools without affecting the other systems and receptors. Thus, enkephalin analogs are likely to be recognized at brain sites and perhaps also at peripheral sites, both of which normally interact only with β-endorphin. Opioid antagonists will block endogenous opioid effects indiscriminately, although possibly with differential efficacy. Thus, research on the possible role of endorphins in affective disorders and other types of psychopathology must proceed and be interpreted with extreme caution.

Before considering the role of endorphins in psychiatric disorders, one should carefully compare the neurobiology of neuropeptides with that of the more well-studied mono-amines. One major difference between these two classes of neuroregulators is their mode of biosynthesis. Neuropeptides are synthesized by protein synthesis in ribosomes in the perikaryon (usually as a large prohormone) and, after packaging, are transported down the axon to the nerve terminal, where they are subsequently released in active form. In contrast, monoamines are synthesized largely in the nerve terminal region by a series of well-characterized enzymatic steps from an amino acid precursor. The mode of inactivation of these two classes of neuroregulators is also quite different: Peptides are inactivated by enzymes (peptidases) (35,51), whereas monoamines are removed from the synaptic cleft largely by transmitter reuptake into the presynaptic terminal. The physiological consequences of monoamine release are brief, whereas the action of neuropeptides such as the endorphins can be quite sustained.

In this chapter, three strategies for evaluating the possible role of opioid peptides in affective disorders are considered. First, studies in postmortem brain tissue and CSF have been conducted to determine whether the integrity or activity of endorphin-containing systems and their receptors is altered in affective disorders. Second, studies in which endorphins, endorphin analogs, and nonpeptide opioid agonists have been administered to humans to evaluate their potential therapeutic use in affective disorders are reviewed. Finally, the effects of opioid and endorphin receptor antagonists on the behavior and mood of patients with affective disorders are reviewed in detail.

There are, of course, problems with each of these approaches. In both types of studies, several potentially confounding variables must be carefully evaluated; these include patient age and sex, and drug effects. Such considerations increase the likelihood that alterations in endorphin concentration (or receptor number) are related to patient diagnosis and not to these artifacts. In postmortem tissue studies, stability of the opioid peptide to be measured must be taken into consideration, as well as agonal state, postmortem delay, and cause of death. In CSF and postmortem studies, the time of day and date the sample is obtained may be important because of possible circadian and circannual rhythms in the concentrations of certain neurotransmitters and their metabolites, including endorphins (81). In general, neuropeptides are remarkably stable in postmortem brain tissue and CSF. However, the complexity of endorphin neurobiology is demonstrated by the presence of multiple forms of certain endorphins that have been found in brain and CSF as described above.

The studies in which endorphins, endorphin analogs, and nonpeptide opioid agonists have been administered to patients as potential therapeutic agents have been quite problematical. It is unclear at this time whether endorphins penetrate the blood-brain barrier in appreciable quantities after systemic injection, and therefore, any subsequent effects observed may not be due to direct endorphin action on the CNS. Studies of endorphins as putative pharmacotherapeutic agents must be judged with the same rigor as any other pharmacological trial. Ideally, investigations should be prospective, randomized, placebo-controlled, double-blind studies with large numbers per group con-ducted by clinically experienced investigators. The endorphin antagonist studies are also not without problems. The duration of action of these antagonists is relatively brief, and at higher doses, these antagonists may have agonist actions and produce effects on nonopioid systems (73).

Wherever possible in this chapter, the review of a reported finding includes a report of the specificity of the antiserum used to measure an endorphin. This detailed description of methodology is justified, since differences in methodology may well explain discrepant reports in the literature. Second, inclusion of methodological considerations increases their visibility, and this should have a positive effect on the quality of studies in biological psychiatry.

MEASURING ENDORPHIN CONCENTRATIONS IN AFFECTIVE DISORDERS

The earliest measurement of endorphins in affective disorders was accomplished by Terenius and colleagues from Sweden (80). In this pilot report, the CSF concentration of opioid activity in 13 manic-depressive patients was measured by radioreceptor assay with [³H]dihydromorphine as the trace ligand during manic, euthymic, and depressed stages of their illness. No diagnostic criteria were described, and lithium treatment was continued during the study. No statistical comparison was sought, since no normal controls were included. The CSF was filtered and chromatographed on Sephadex G-10; two fractions with opiate receptor activity were isolated, fractions I and II. Met-ENK coeluted with fraction II; fraction I activity tended to be highest during the manic phase; and no correlations between fraction II concentrations and mental state were evident.

In another early study by the same group (79), case histories of five depressed women treated subcutaneously with 4.8 mg naloxone three times per day were presented. No diagnostic criteria were provided; a variety of tricyclic and anxiolytic drug treatments were continued during the trial; and no normal controls or statistical analyses were included. CSF was obtained at least twice, and up to four times, per patient over a 12-month period, and CSF opioid activity was measured by a radioreceptor assay using [³H]dihydromorphine as the radioactive ligand, as described above. No effect of naloxone on fraction II opioid concentrations was observed, but fraction I concentrations seemed to decrease with continued naloxone treatment.

These early uncontrolled studies are very difficult to interpret because of the absence of controls and the inability to characterize what opioid peptide(s) comprise fraction I. In a later study by Terenius and colleagues (49), 19 normal controls were compared to four manic-depressive patients. No data were included on the age or sex of these manic-depressive patients, the diagnostic criteria used to classify them, or their current medication status. Radioreceptor assay of the CSF fractions after Sephadex G-10 filtration revealed slightly higher levels of fraction I opioid activity in the manic phase when compared to the euthymic or depressed phases of the illness.

Recently, the Swedish group led by Terenius (1) attempted to assess the possibility of seasonal variation in fraction I opioid concentrations of unipolar and bipolar depressed patients. The patient population consisted of 62 unipolar patients and 32 bipolar patients who satisfied Research Diagnostic Criteria (RDC) (14) and who were medication-free, except for benzodiazepines, for at least 10 days prior to lumbar puncture. The fraction I concentrations of opioid activity were adjusted for sex, age, height, and weight values by analysis of covariance and plotted according to time of year. No control subjects were used for comparison, and no patient was assessed more than once, rendering interpretation of the findings difficult.

Naber et al. (57,58) and Pickar et al. (65) from the National Institute of Mental Health (NIMH) have compared the concentrations of endogenous opioid activity and immunoreactive β-endorphin concentrations in CSF of 41 normal volunteers and 35 unipolar and 13 bipolar patients (RDC criteria) (14). Patients were drug-free for at least 14 days before CSF collection. The NIMH group used ^{3}H-[D-Ala^2] enkephalin-(L-Leu-amide) (8) as the competing ligand in the radioreceptor assay for opioid activity and an antiserum to β-endorphin that exhibited significant cross reactivity with β-lipotropin. Two-way analysis of variance failed to reveal significant differences between the controls and either depressed group or any effect due to sex in either opioid activity or β-endorphin immunoreactivity. The same NIMH group has determined whether carbamazepine alters CSF opioid activity in a study of 13 depressed, three manic, and one euthymic patient (RDC criteria) (14). Patients were drug-free for 10 days before the first sample of CSF was obtained, and they were then treated with 200 to 400 mg/day carbamazepine for an average of 33 days before a second CSF sample was obtained. No significant carbamazepine-induced difference in CSF opioid activity was detected.

Gerner et al. (29,30) compared CSF β-endorphin concentrations in nine normal controls and in 19 unipolar and eight bipolar depressed patients (RDC criteria) (14) who were free of antidepressant medication for at least 7 days. The antisera used to measure β-endorphin cross reacted equally with β-lipotropin (β-LPH). Column chromatography of pooled CSF fractions showed β-LPH in a molar ratio of 1.3:1 with β-endorphin. The use of analysis of variance failed to reveal statistically significant differences in the mean CSF concentrations of β-endorphin immunoreactivity between either group of depressed patients and controls.

Brambilla et al. (18) measured β-LPH and β-endorphin immunoreactivity in the plasma of 35 psychiatric controls and nine unipolar primary affective disorder (RDC criteria) and seven secondary affective disorder patients who were drug-free for 10 days. The plasma concentration of both β-LPH and β-endorphin immunoreactivity was significantly increased ($p < 0.001$, Student's t-test) in the secondary affective disorder patients, whereas only β-LPH plasma immunoreactivity was significantly increased ($p < 0.001$) in the primary affective disorder patients.

Alexopoulas et al. (7) and Inturrisi et al. (40) reported the effect of the first and second electroconvulsive therapy (ECT) treatment of plasma β-endorphin concentrations in 11 depressed patients (RDC criteria) (14) and 16 neurological controls. Patients were drug-free for at least 10 days before ECT, and blood was drawn immediately before and

15 min after each ECT treatment. Plasma was extracted with talc, acetone, and HCl, and the antiserum to β-endorphin had approximately 25% cross reactivity to β-LPH. The concentration of plasma β-endorphin-like immunoreactivity increased approximately threefold ($p < 0.05$, two-tailed t-test) after each ECT treatment and returned to initial values within 48 hr.

Janowsky et al. (42) reported a recurrence of depressive symptomatology in patients with a history of depression following the infusion of the cholinesterase inhibitor physostigmine. Several investigators have reported that intravenous physostigmine infusion has antimanic properties and can reverse mania even to the point of inducing depression for a period of 1 to 3 hr (22,41). In an investigation with normal volunteers performed by Risch et al. (70), the physostigmine-induced mood changes, particularly the depressive components, were reported to be significantly correlated with elevations in plasma β-endorphin concentrations. The plasma β-endorphin assay was performed with radioimmunoassay (RIA) kits employing rabbit antiserum to synthetic human β-endorphin, which were supplied by New England Nuclear Corporation. The antibody for β-endorphin has 50% cross reactivity with β-lipotropin, but less than 0.1% cross reactivity with α-endorphin and α-melanocyte-stimulating hormone (α-MSH) and less than 0.004% cross reactivity with leu-ENK and met-ENK. Within-assay variability for β-endorphin is approximately 5%, and between-assay variability is approximately 9%. Sensitivity varies from 25 to 50 pg/ml. The physostigmine-induced mood changes that correlated with β-endorphin concentrations included an increase in depression, hostility, and confusion and a decrease in arousal and mania. However, the mood and behavioral changes were not correlated with peak increases in cortisol. This study suggests that a cholinergically mediated β-endorphin pathway may exist and that this pathway is hyperactive in depression.

In another investigation by Risch and colleagues (69) using the same β-endorphin RIA described above, the morning plasma concentrations of β-endorphin immunoreactivity were reported to be significantly higher in a group of depressed patients meeting RDC criteria than in age- and sex-matched normal controls and psychiatric patients without affective disorders. Using the same assay, this investigator also reported that the physostigmine-stimulated release of β-endorphin was significantly greater in depressed patients diagnosed by RDC (69).

Dexamethasone has been used to suppress the secretion of ACTH and, hence, of cortisol in investigations of depressed patients. Since ACTH and β-endorphin can arise from the same prohormone (POMC), dexamethasone might also suppress the release of β-endorphin-like immunoreactivity into plasma. A subgroup of depressed patients have an abnormality of the hypothalamic-pituitary-adrenal axis that results in a decreased ability of dexamethasone to suppress pituitary ACTH secretion and, hence, adrenal cortisol secretion. This is the basis of the dexamethasone suppression test (DST). Akil (2) has reported that a subgroup of depressed patients failed to decrease plasma β-endorphin-like immunoreactivity in response to dexamethasone.

In Akil's preliminary report, depressed patients were

divided into four groups: The first group consisted of patients in whom dexamethasone decreased both cortisol and β-endorphin-like immunoreactivity, as it does in normal controls; the second group had a suppression of cortisol but not a suppression of β-endorphin-like immunoreactivity in plasma; the third group had a failure to suppress cortisol but did suppress β-endorphin-like immunoreactivity following dexamethasone administration; and finally, a fourth group failed to suppress either cortisol or β-endorphin-like immunoreactivity in response to the dexamethasone (2). If these results can be replicated, these four groups of depressed patients should be carefully evaluated for differences in clinical phenomenology, biochemical correlates, or pharmacological responses.

TREATMENT OF AFFECTIVE DISORDERS WITH ENDORPHINS AND ENDORPHIN ANALOGS

Studies of β-Endorphin Administration in Affective Disorders

The New York Study

The first investigation of β-endorphin in affective disorders was performed by Kline and Lehmann using a single-blind design (46). Choh Hao Li of the University of California San Francisco School of Medicine provided the β-endorphin for this study. These investigators gave 1.8 and 9 mg of β-endorphin to a patient with unipolar depression and two doses of 9 mg to a patient with bipolar depression. Both patients were reported to experience improvement in their depression. The unipolar patient was markedly activated and had increased spontaneity. The bipolar patient also had increased spontaneity and diminished guilt and suicidal urges. However, in both patients, the effects were transient and disappeared by the end of the first few hours following the injection. It is difficult to evaluate this single-blind study with only two patients.

The Switzerland Study

Another early single-blind investigation of β-endorphin in patients with affective disorders was performed by Angst et al. (9) and also used β-endorphin synthesized by Choh Hao Li (48). In this investigation, six hospitalized depressed female patients were chosen for symptoms that had been stable for at least 8 days. Each patient received 10 mg of β-endorphin in a single dose, slowly injected intravenously over 5 min. Four of the patients had bipolar depression, whereas two of the patients had unipolar depression. In all cases, antidepressant medication was stopped at least 3 days prior to the β-endorphin infusion. Changes in subjective state were measured using visual analog scales and the Zung rating scale (9).

In three of the six patients, a switch into hypomania or mania was observed during or after the trial. In one bipolar patient, this change seemed to be induced by sleep deprivation, which was provoked by the withdrawal of the sleeping medication (sedative hypnotic) she had used before the trial. This patient exhibited dysphoric hypomania for a few days and then relapsed. In the second case, a unipolar depressed patient, a clear hypomanic state developed in the afternoon and evening after the β-endorphin injection and was followed by a relapse into depression the next day. The patient was reported to be overactive, talkative, and euphoric. The third patient, who had bipolar depression, switched into a manic episode the day after the trial. This manic episode was severe and required haloperidol treatment for a few weeks. Angst et al. (9) concluded that the switch into hypomania or mania observed in three of six cases of depression was "of some interest, but should not be over-interpreted." Angst and colleagues believe that other factors, such as poor sleep the night before the experiment, withdrawal of previous medication, and distress induced by the study, may also have induced the change in psychiatric status (9). Thus, it is difficult to evaluate this single-blind study with a small number of patients.

The Los Angeles Study

Gerner et al. at UCLA gave β-endorphin to ten depressed patients in a double-blind, placebo-controlled crossover study (28). The β-endorphin, supplied by Choh Hao Li, was infused at a constant rate over a 30- to 35-min time period. This slow infusion was used because of the UCLA group's observation that rapid infusions might produce side effects that would interfere with the maintenance of the double-blind nature of the study. Subjects in this investigation were rated by self-rating scales that consisted of 100 mm visual analog scales using the dimensions of depression, anxiety, hopelessness, and feeling good or bad. Day-to-day changes were measured using the Brief Psychiatric Rating Scale (BPRS) (28).

The condition of depressed patients was described as significantly improved 2 to 4 hr after the β-endorphin infusion when compared to placebo. The investigators describe a typical effect of β-endorphin as including "bright facial expression, decreased psychomotor retardation, increased social integration and less depressed speech content." These positive effects decreased during the day following the infusion. Thus, no patient showed long-term improvement following β-endorphin administration, and no patient had evidence of a hypomanic response of the type described by Angst et al. (9,28).

The NIMH Washington Study

Pickar et al. at the NIMH gave 4 to 15 mg β-endorphin to four depressed patients in a double-blind, placebo-controlled study (65). The β-endorphin in this investigation was supplied by Choh Hao Li. The mean dose of β-endorphin for depressed subjects was 0.15 mg/kg given in a solution with concentrations of either 2 or 4 mg/ml. The compound was infused by an intravenous line by bolus injection at a rate of 1 ml per minute. Individual physician raters recorded pertinent clinical observations and completed the BPRS at baseline and at regular intervals for 4 hr following the infusion. The BPRS was also given each morning for 5 consecutive days after the placebo and β-endorphin administrations.

One of the depressed patients was given 10 mg of β-endorphin, 5 mg of methadone, and placebo. This patient showed prolactin stimulation and decreased cortisol in response to both β-endorphin and methadone, but not in response to placebo. However, the effects of β-endorphin on both prolactin and cortisol were less prolonged than the response to methadone. Comparison of the BPRS change scores for placebo and β-endorphin indicated that β-endorphin did not cause significant behavioral or mood changes in the four depressed subjects. Thus, the NIMH group (65) was unable to find the transient improvement in their four depressed patients that was reported by the UCLA group in 10 depressed patients (9,65), nor did they find the hypomanic response reported by Angst et al. (9,28).

The Japan Intrathecal Study

One of the major problems in β-endorphin investigations has been the extent to which β-endorphin crosses the blood-brain barrier to reach opioid receptors in the brain. One way around this problem may be to administer β-endorphin into CSF rather than intravenously. Profound analgesic effects of β-endorphin were observed by Oyama et al. after the intrathecal administration of the peptide by lumbar puncture in 14 patients with intractable pain due to disseminated cancer (60). The β-endorphin used in this study was synthesized by Nicholas Ling and Roger Guillemin of the Salk Institute. Drowsiness and transient mild confusion were observed in some patients, and no electroencephalographic (EEG) abnormalities were observed. Interestingly, these patients had previously required very large and frequent doses of morphine and obtained only partial pain relief. The authors referred to a study by Wang et al., where intrathecally injected morphine produced analgesia in eight patients with intractable pain (77). The duration of the analgesia produced by morphine was shorter than Oyama's reported observed analgesia with β-endorphin. The Oyama studies indicate that the receptor mechanisms for endogenous and exogenous opiates are not necessarily identical (59,60). Thus, intrathecal administration of β-endorphin may be necessary to obtain efficient analgesic effects.

In continued investigation by Oyama, prolonged analgesia was also observed in all of 14 obstetrical patients who received 1 mg of intrathecally administered β-endorphin at the time of delivery (61). Labor pains in all patients disappeared within 3.5 min after β-endorphin was injected, and the time of the uterine contractions remained unchanged. The women reported the analgesic effects for as long as 12 to 32 hr after completion of labor. During the period of pain relief, there was no evidence of muscle rigidity or catatonia, and all the women were alert except for three who reported feeling drowsy. The studies by Oyama did not describe the psychological effects of intrathecal β-endorphin in great detail (60,61). However, in the study with pain patients, three of the 14 patients did

report experiencing euphoria, and all 14 patients experienced somnolence in addition to pain relief (60).

The NIMH Washington Intrathecal Case Report

Several other investigators have also administered intrathecal β-endorphin and observed both its psychological effects and its effects on pain relief (23). In general, intrathecal β-endorphin produces analgesia and side effects that closely resemble those of morphine. However, intrathecal β-endorphin may produce prolonged analgesia and psychological side effects in addition to those produced with morphine (23,27,66). Pickar et al. (66) gave a patient with disseminated malignancy 3 mg of synthetic β-endorphin intrathecally. This patient had a rapid decrease in pain, but later developed a striking behavioral syndrome characterized by confusion, elation, hypomanic/manic behavior, and psychosis, which lasted for 2 days.

Summary of the Studies on β-Endorphin in Affective Disorders

Thus, although the effects of β-endorphin in depressed patients have not been consistently produced, there does seem to be preliminary evidence that the antidepressant effects of a single dose of β-endorphin occur transiently, if at all. It is important to remember that an antidepressant of established efficacy such as imipramine would not demonstrate efficacy using the single-dose design. For this reason, future studies of β-endorphin in affective disorders should use repeated administration of β-endorphin in the same patient or should use the intrathecal route.

As described above, intrathecal β-endorphin injection appears to have prolonged pharmacological activity. When given intrathecally, the compound can produce prolonged analgesia and, sometimes, behavioral effects. Since some patients developed euphoria or elation, which suggests that the intrathecal administration route may be an important strategy for studying the behavioral effects and therapeutic usefulness of β-endorphin in affective disorders. However, the serious behavioral disturbance reported by Pickar et al. (66) in their patient given 3 mg of β-endorphin intrathecally suggests that such investigations should use lower doses and should be performed cautiously, with an awareness of the possibility that the β-endorphin might produce a transient manic psychosis.

A Study of an Endorphin Analog in Affective Disorders

The effects of the stable met-ENK analog FK-33-824 in depressed patients (International Classification of Diseases, ICD) (14) have been evaluated in an open study (45) using the Hamilton Rating Scale for Depression. Nine depressed patients received 0.5 mg of the peptide on day 1 and 1.0 mg on day 2. No beneficial effects of FK-33-824 were reported (45). This study is difficult to interpret because of the small number of subjects and the open design.

Studies with Nonpeptide Opioid Compounds in Affective Disorders

Since the time of Hippocrates, opium has been considered one of the most powerful and efficacious psychoactive drugs (24). Because of the potent antianxiety, sedative, and tranquilizing effects of opium, Emil Kraepelin recommended the "opium cure" in 1901 for patients with agitated depression. The treatment consisted of slowly increasing and later decreasing doses of opium. Reports of this opium treatment state that addiction never became a problem in these patients. In addition, although no standardized evaluations were performed and the studies were not controlled, the opium treatment was described as effective (24). However, because of the effective heterocyclic antidepressant and monoamine oxidase inhibitor treatments of depression, the opium treatment has never been reevaluated using modern psychopharmacological methods.

In an uncontrolled investigation, Extein et al. (25) reported only slight antidepressant activity of 5.0 mg of morphine in 10 patients with major depressive disorder and no effect of 5.0 mg of methadone in comparison to placebo in six depressed patients in a double-blind investigation.

A mixed agonist/antagonist opiate, cyclazocine, has also been reported in uncontrolled studies to be useful for the treatment of depression. Fink and co-workers treated 10 severely depressed patients with 1.0 to 3.0 mg/day of cyclazocine and reported 50% reduction in depressed mood and apathy (26). Unfortunately, the putative antidepressant activity of cyclazocine has not been evaluated in a double-blind investigation.

In another preliminary investigation, Emrich et al. (24) gave buprenorphine, a nonpeptide partial opiate receptor agonist with potent analgesic properties, to 10 patients with endogenous depression. This clinical trial of buprenorphine was a double-blind, placebo-controlled study with an A-B-A design. The authors report a significant reduction in depressive symptoms as measured by a 40% reduction in mean Hamilton Depression Rating Scale scores within 3 days of buprenorphine treatment (0.4 mg/day; given as two 0.2 mg sublingual tablets per day) (24).

TREATMENT OF AFFECTIVE DISORDERS WITH ENDORPHIN ANTAGONISTS

As described above, several investigators have hypothesized that depression is a state of opioid deficiency, and they have therefore tested β-endorphin, the enkephalin analog FK-33-824, and opiate agonists as potential therapeutic agents in depression. Others, in contrast, have used the opiate antagonists, particularly naloxone, as potential drugs to treat depression or mania, with the idea that one of these affective disorders might be associated with hyperactivity of the endorphin systems. These studies have been the subject of recent comprehensive reviews (12,17,62).

The consensus of several studies appears clear; naloxone either has no effect or exacerbates the symptoms of patients with major depression (21,79). In a recent study, Cohen et

al. (19) investigated the effects of 2 mg/kg naloxone i.v. in six depressed inpatients and eight controls in a double-blind paradigm. The opioid antagonist produced a significant worsening in the signs and symptoms of depression in the patient group, without any noticeable effect in normal controls.

In contrast to the lack of effect or the exacerbation reported after naloxone treatment in depressed patients are the salutary effects reported after naloxone administration in patients with mania. Davis et al. (21) observed a clear antimanic effect of 0.4 to 30 mg naloxone i.v. in one of four patients. The following year, Judd and colleagues (43) treated eight manic patients with 20 mg naloxone i.v., and four exhibited a clear reduction in symptoms. Janowsky et al. (10) observed similar effects. A World Health Organization (WHO) Collaborative Study (64,67), performed in six participating countries, was unable to confirm these findings. In this WHO study (67), 0.3 mg naloxone administered s.c. was found to have no beneficial effect in 26 manic patients. One obvious difference between the different trials of naloxone in mania is the dose of the drug tested. High doses of naloxone seem necessary for the antimanic effects, if any, of naloxone.

Captopril is not a peptide receptor antagonist, but is an inhibitor of angiotensin-converting enzyme and enkephalinase, one of the enzymes that is probably involved in the metabolic degradation of enkephalins. Zubenko and Nixon (84) recently reported that three depressed patients exhibited substantial mood elevation after oral captopril treatment. The small number of subjects and the lack of placebo control make this investigation difficult to interpret; nevertheless the finding is important enough to suggest a controlled double-blind trial of captopril in depression.

CONCLUSION

The number of known neurotransmitters and neuromodulators has increased enormously in the last few years. However, few of these newly discovered brain chemicals have so rapidly affected research in biological psychiatry as have the endorphins. This may be because exogenous opiates clearly alter mood and affect and because some exogenous opiates, particularly the mixed agonist antagonists, produce hallucinations and bizarre thought content (37,54). Exogenous opiates have also been used in the past as treatments for psychiatric disorders, including affective disorders, with variable success. Furthermore, addiction to morphine or heroin is a psychiatric and social problem with both physiological and psychological roots and manifestations. Finally, opiate analgesics on one hand, and street and illegal opiate use on the other, are closely associated with the concepts of pleasure and pain, concepts that lie at the core of many psychological theories of normal and abnormal behavior including the affective disorders, depression, and mania.

In spite of the large amount of research generated, a firm link between the endorphins and the pathophysiology of affective disorders has not been made. There are, however, some intriguing preliminary findings that will require further investigation. The report from the Swedish group led by Terenius (49,79) of altered opioid fractions in affective disorders will require further investigation. An important step in this investigation will obviously be the determination of which endogenous opiates comprise fraction I and fraction II. This will allow more specific testing of the Swedish group's preliminary findings using specific RIAs for the endorphins contained in these uncharacterized fractions.

The reports of Risch and colleagues (69,70) suggesting a greater sensitivity in depressed patients to the physostigmine-induced release of β-endorphin are also an important finding that may connect acetylcholine and endorphin hypotheses of the pathophysiology of at least a subgroup of patients with affective disorders. This finding is made more intriguing by the correlation reported between the physostigmine-induced depressive syndromes in normal controls and elevations in plasma β-endorphin concentrations induced by physostigmine.

The preliminary report from Akil and colleagues (2) suggests that a β-endorphin counterpart of the DST may prove to be a useful technique for subdividing patients with biological depression into different subtypes. Akil's work tentatively divides depressed patients into four groups. If these results can be replicated and extended, these four groups may prove to have different clinical phenomenology and biochemical correlates, or, even more important, different pharmacological responses.

The studies with β-endorphin in affective disorders are disappointing. Intravenous β-endorphin is clearly not an effective treatment for depression. One of the main problems with this investigation has been a failure to characterize the amount of β-endorphin that crosses the blood-brain barrier to interact with brain opioid receptors. The intrathecal studies by Oyama and colleagues (59–61) are intriguing and do suggest that β-endorphin can have an effect, not only on analgesia, but also on mood. The single case report from Pickar and colleagues at the NIMH is even more interesting (66). Although anecdotal, the fact that a syndrome with many of the features of manic psychosis developed in a patient who received 3 mg β-endorphin intrathecally should be further evaluated. This striking case report suggests that endogenous opiates may indeed be involved in the pathophysiology of manic psychosis. Nevertheless, it is hard to picture that the intrathecal administration of any compound will ever be a standard treatment for affective disorders.

Neither the endorphin analogs nor the nonpeptide opioid compounds seem to have clinically useful antidepressant activity. However, before giving up entirely on the notion of the use of exogenous nonpeptide opiates in depression, a careful prospective double-blind clinical trial should probably be carried out with methadone or another opium derivative.

Further trials with the mixed agonist-antagonist buprenorphine are needed in order to confirm and extend the finding of Emrich and colleagues (24). Their preliminary double-blind, placebo-controlled study suggests that buprenorphine is an effective antidepressant, at least for some patients. It is disappointing that there are no reports of attempted replication of this potentially important finding.

Naloxone appears either to have no effect or to exacerbate the symptoms of patients with major depression. Understanding the mechanism of naloxone exacerbation of depression may help connect the endorphins to the pathophysiology of this disorder. The effects of naloxone in mania are intriguing but have been difficult to replicate. If naloxone has any antimanic effects, it would appear that high doses are required and that only some patients respond (10,43,67). Further studies with naloxone in manic patients are needed.

The use of captopril as a possible inhibitor of enkephalinase, one of the enzymes involved in the metabolism of enkephalins, is an interesting strategy for the treatment of depression. However, the positive report of Zubenko and Nixon (84) is based on only three subjects in an uncontrolled study. Before one can draw any conclusions about the use of an enzyme inhibitor in affective disorders, a controlled, double-blind trial of captopril in depression is needed.

There are several methodological considerations that are applicable to future investigations with the endorphins. All studies on concentrations of endorphins in biological fluids must include a carefully defined group of control subjects matched to the study group on important confounding variables such as age, sex, activity, diet, and drug status. One of the causes of discrepant reports in the literature may be the use of poorly characterized and described RIAs. Future reports should include data on recovery of exogenously added peptides in every assay system, particularly those that use an extraction method. In addition, when describing an RIA, the sensitivity and specificity should be carefully described. This should include information on the amino acid sequence of the molecule that is recognized by the antiserum and information on how much cross reactivity is exhibited by other peptides containing homologous sequences. It is also important to know that a variety of other peptides, including those with dissimilar structures, do not cross react with the antiserum. Finally, it is necessary in evaluating a particular RIA to know the concentration at which one observes 50% displacement of trace ligand (IC_{50}), the minimal detectable concentration (sensitivity, picograms per tube), and the inter- and intraassay coefficients of variation.

When working with uncharacterized tissue sources of immunoreactivity, attempts should be made to identify the nature of the immunoreactivity. Several chromatographic methods are available for this problem and the exact method chosen usually depends on the quantity of the starting material.

In pharmacological trials with endorphins or endorphin and opioid antagonists, the standards of accurate and sensitive pharmacological investigations must be applied. Investigations should be prospective, placebo-controlled, double-blind studies using patients diagnosed by a standard nosological classification method and rated with quantitative instruments for cross-sectional symptom assessment.

These suggestions for improved methodology are not intended to detract from the studies performed to date. Anecdotal case reports and preliminary uncontrolled trials with new compounds are important and often represent pioneering work. The development and use of new assays described in this chapter are at the forefront of efforts to understand the biological basis of psychopathology in affective disorders. Thus, these suggestions are intended to provide guidelines for future study designs in an attempt to reduce the contradictions and discrepancies that are obvious in cross-study comparisons, such as those made in this review. Such a retrospective examination of studies from a variety of investigators using different techniques and patient populations should eventually reveal important, diagnostically dependent group differences in endorphin concentrations or psychopharmacological responses to endorphins that will help characterize the probable role of endorphins in the pathophysiology of affective disorders.

Since the discovery of the endorphins, an enormous number of innovative investigations have taken place. This exponentially increasing body of data should be viewed as preliminary findings and in the next decade should yield data that are relevent to our understanding of the biological basis of psychiatric disorders such as depression and mania. Certainly, advances in biological psychiatry and psychopharmacology in the endorphin field are dependent on advances in neuropeptide molecular biology and physiology. Advances in both basic science and clinical studies of the endorphins should have an enormous impact on our understanding of the physiological and pathophysiological role of these interesting compounds.

ACKNOWLEDGMENTS

Dr. Berger is supported by a grant from the NIMH, MH-30854, to the Norris Mental Health Clinical Research Center at Stanford University and a grant from the Research Service of the Veterans Administration to the Schizophrenia Biologic Research Center at the Palo Alto Veterans Administration Medical Center. Dr. Berger currently holds the Kenneth T. Norris, Jr., Professorship in Psychiatry and Behavioral Sciences. Dr. Nemeroff is supported by NIMH MH-39415 and MH-40524 and grants from the Schizophrenia Research Foundation and the Gorrell Family Psychiatric Research Fund. Dr. Nemeroff is the recipient of a Nanaline H. Duke Fellowship from Duke University. We are grateful to Christie Price and Pamela Elliott for manuscript preparation.

REFERENCES

1. Agren, H., and Terenius, L. (1983): *Psychiatry Res.,* 10:303–311.
2. Akil, H. (1983): Abstracts presented at the Annual Meeting of the American College of Neuropsychopharmacology, p. 57.
3. Akil, H., Mayer, D. J., and Liebeskind, J. C. (1972): *C. R. Seances Acad. Sci. (D),* 274:3603.
4. Akil, H., Mayer, D. J., and Liebeskind, J. C. (1976): *Science,* 191:961–962.
5. Akil, H., Richardson, D. E., Hughes, J., and Barchas, J. D. (1978): *Science,* 201:463–465.
6. Akil, H., Watson, S. J., Sullivan, S., and Barchas, J. D. (1978): *Life Sci.,* 23:121–126.
7. Alexopoulos, G. S., Inturrisi, C. E., Lipman, R., Frances, R., Haycox, J., Dougherty, J. N., and Rossier, J. (1983): *Arch. Gen. Psychiatry,* 40:181–183.
8. Anderson, L. T., David, R., Bonnet, K., and Dancis, J. (1979): *Life Sci.,* 24:905–910.
9. Angst, J., Autenrieth, V., Brem, F., Koukkou, M., Meyer, H., Stassen, H. H., and Storck, U. (1979): In: *Endorphins in Mental Health Research,* edited by E. Usdin, W. E. Bunney, Jr., and N. S. Kline, pp. 518–528. Macmillan Press, London.
10. Beckwith, B. E., Petros, T., Kanaan-Beckwith, S., Cook, D. L., Hoag, R. J., and Ryan, C. (1982): *Peptides,* 3:627–630.
11. Berger, P. A. (1975): In: *An Introduction to Treatment in Psychiatry: Crisis Clinic Consultation,* edited by C. P. Rosenbaum and J. Beebe, pp. 161–171. McGraw-Hill, New York.
12. Berger, P. A. (1983): In: *Mind and Medicine: Emotions in Health and Illness,* edited by L. Temoshok, C. Van Dike, and L. S. Vegans, pp. 153–166. Grune and Stratton, New York.
13. Berger, P. A., Watson, S. J., Akil, H., and Barchas, J. D. (1986): In: *Neuropeptides: Implications for Neurologic and Psychiatric Diseases,* edited by J. Martin and J. Barchas. Raven Press, New York (*in press*).
14. Berner, P., Gabriel, G., Katschnig, H., Kieffer, W., Lenz, G., and Simhandl, C. (1983): *Diagnostic Criteria for Schizophrenia and Affective Disorders.* World Psychiatric Association, American Psychiatric Press, Washington, D.C.
15. Bloom, F. E., Battenberg, E., Rossier, J., Ling, N., Leppaluoto, J., Vargo, T. M., and Guillemin, R. (1977): *Life Sci.,* 20:43–48.
16. Bradbury, A. F., Feldberg, W. F., Smyth, D. G., and Snell, C. (1976): In: *Opiates and Endogenous Opioid Peptides,* edited by H. W. Kosterlitz. Elsevier/North Holland Press, Amsterdam.
17. Brambilla, F., Genazzani, A. R., and Facchinetti, F. (1984): In: *Psychoneuroendocrine Dysfunction,* edited by N. S. Shah and A. G. Donald, pp. 309–329. Plenum Press, New York.
18. Brambilla, F., Genazzani, A. R., Facchinetti, F., Parrini, D., Petraglia, F., Sacchetti, E., Scarone, S., Guastella, A., and D'Antona, N. (1981): *Psychoneuroendocrinology,* 6:321–330.
19. Cohen, M. R., Cohen, R. M., Pickar, D., Sunderland, T., Mueller, E. A., III, and Murphy, D. L. (1984): *Biol. Psychiatry,* 19:825–832.
20. Cox, B. M., Goldstein, A., and Li, C. H. (1976): *Proc. Natl. Acad. Sci. USA,* 73:1821–1823.
21. Davis, G. C., Bunney, W. E., Jr., De Fraites, E. G., Kleinman, J. E., van Kammen, D. P., Post, R. M., and Wyatt, R. J. (1977): *Science,* 197:74–77.
22. Davis, K., Berger, P. A., Hollister, L. E., and De Fraites, E. G. (1978): *Arch. Gen. Psychiatry,* 35:119–222.
23. De Conno, F., Li, C. H., Muller, E. E., Panerai, A. E., Ripamonti, C., and Ventafridda, V. (1984). Abstract presented at the IVth World Congress on Pain of the International Association for the Study of Pain, Seattle.
24. Emrich, H. M., Vogt, P., and Herz, A. (1981): In: *Biological Psychiatry,* edited by C. Perns, G. Strüwe, and B. Jansson, pp. 380–385. Elsevier/North-Holland, Amsterdam.
25. Extein, I., Pickar, D., Gold, M. S., Gold, P. W., Pottash, A. L. C., Sweeney, D. R., Ross, R. J., Rebard, R., Martin, D., and Goodwin, F. K. (1981): *Psychopharmacol. Bull.,* 17:29–33.
26. Fink, M., v. Simeon, J., Itil, T. M., and Freedman, A. M. (1970): *Clin. Pharmacol. Ther.,* 11:41–48.
27. Foley, K., Kourides, I. A., and Inturrisi, C. E. (1979): *Proc. Natl. Acad. Sci. USA,* 76:5377–5381.
28. Gerner, R. H., Catlin, D. H., Gorelick, D. A., Hui, K. K., and Li, C. H. (1980): *Arch. Gen. Psychiatry,* 37:642–647.
29. Gerner, R. H., Gorelick, D. A., Catlin, D. H., and Sharp, B. (1981): In: *Biological Psychiatry,* edited by C. Perris, G. Strüwe, and B. Jansson, pp. 386–389. Elsevier, Amsterdam.
30. Gerner, R. H., and Sharp, B. (1982): *Brain Res.,* 237:244–247.
31. Gilbert, P. E., and Martin, W. R. (1976): *J. Pharmacol. Exp. Ther.,* 198:66–82.
32. Goldstein, A. (1978): In: *Psychopharmacology: A Generation of Progress,* edited by M. A. Lipton, A. Dimascio, and K. F. Killam, pp. 1557–1563. Raven Press, New York.
33. Goldstein, A., Lowney, L. I., and Pal, B. K. (1971): *Proc. Natl. Acad. Sci. USA,* 68:1742–1747.
34. Goldstein, A., Tachibana, S., Lowney, L. I., Hunkapiller, M., and Hood, L. (1979): *Proc. Natl. Acad. Sci. USA,* 76:6666–6670.
35. Griffiths, E. C., McDermott, J. R., and Smith, A. I. (1977): *Proc. Natl. Acad. Sci. USA,* 74:1291–1294.
36. Guillemin, R., Ling, N., and Burgus, R. (1976): *C. R. Seances Acad. Sci. (D),* 282:783–785.
37. Gunne, L. M., Lindström, L., and Terenius, L. (1977): *J. Neural. Transm.,* 40:13–19.

38. Hokfelt, T. (1987): In: *Advances in Biochemical Pharmacology: Regulation and Function of Neuropeptides,* edited by E. Costa and E. M. Trabucchi. Raven Press, New York (*in press*).

39. Hughes, J., Smith, T. W., Kosterlitz, H. W., Fothergill, L. A., Morgan, B. A., and Morris, H. R. (1975): *Nature,* 258:577–579.

40. Inturrisi, C. E., Alexopoulas, G., Lipman, R., Foley, K., and Rossier, J. (1982): *Ann. NY Acad. Sci.,* 413:413–423.

41. Janowsky, D. S., El-Yousef, K., Davis, J. M., and Sekerke, H. I. (1973): *Arch. Gen. Psychiatry,* 28:542–547.

42. Janowsky, D. S., Khaled, M. K., and Davis, J. M. (1974): *Psychosom. Med.,* 36:248–257.

43. Judd, L. L., Janowsky, D. S., Segal, D. S., and Huey, L. Y. (1978): In: *Characteristics and Function of Opioids,* edited by J. M. van Ree and L. Terenius, pp. 173–174, Elsevier/North Holland, Amsterdam.

44. Kakidani, H., Furutani, Y., Takahashi, H., Noda, M., Morimoto, Y., Hirose, T., Asai, M., Inayama, S., Nakanishi, S., and Numa, S. (1982): *Nature,* 298:245–249.

45. Klein, H., Jungkunz, G., Nedopil, N., Ruther, E., and Spiegel, R. (1981): In: *Biological Psychiatry,* edited by C. Perris, G. Strüwe, and B. Jansson, pp. 390–393. Elsevier, Amsterdam.

46. Kline, N. S., and Lehmann, H. E. (1979): In: *Endorphins in Mental Health Research,* edited by E. Usdin, W. E. Bunney, Jr., and N. S. Kline, pp. 500–517. Macmillan, London.

47. Li, C. H., Barnafi, L., Chretien, M., and Chung, D. (1965–66): *Excerpta Medica,* 3:111–112.

48. Li, C. H., and Chung, D. (1976): *Proc. Natl. Acad. Sci. USA,* 73:1145–1148.

49. Lindström, L. H., Widerlöv, E., Gunne, L. M., Wahlström, A., and Terenius, L. (1978): *Acta Psychiatr. Scand.,* 57:153–169.

50. Lord, J. A. H. (1977): *Nature,* 267:495–499.

51. MacKay, A. (1981): *Trends Neurosci.,* 4:9–11.

52. Mains, R. E., Eipper, B. A., and Ling, N. (1977): *Proc. Natl. Acad. Sci. USA,* 74:3014–3018.

53. Malfroy, B., Swerts, J. P., Guyon, A., Roques, B. P., and Schwartz, J. C. (1978): *Nature,* 276:523–526.

54. Martin, W. R., Eades, G. G., Thompson, J. A., Huppler, R. E., and Gilbert, P. E. (1976): *J. Pharmacol. Exp. Ther.,* 197:518–532.

55. Mayer, D. J., Wolfle, T. L., Akil, H., Carder, B., and Liebeskind, J. C. (1971): *Science,* 174:1351–1354.

56. Minamino, M., Kangawa, K., Chino, N., Sakakibara, S., and Matsuo, H. (1981): *Biochem. Biophys. Res. Commun.,* 99:864–870.

57. Naber, D., Pickar, D., Post, R. M., van Kammen, D. P., Ballenger, J., Rubinow, D., Waters, R. N., and Bunney, W. E., Jr. (1981): In: *Biological Psychiatry,* edited by C. Perris, G. Struwe, and B. Jansson, pp. 372–375. Elsevier, Amsterdam.

58. Naber, D., Pickar, D., Post, R. M., van Kammen, D. P., Waters, R. N., Ballenger, J. C., Goodwin, F. K., and Bunney, W. E., Jr. (1981): *Am. J. Psychiatry,* 138:1457–1462.

59. Oyama, T., Fukushi, S., and Jin, T. (1982): *Can. Anaesthes. Soc. J.,* 29:24.

60. Oyama, T., Jin, T., and Yamaya, R. (1980): *Lancet,* 1:122–124.

61. Oyama, T., Matsuki, A., Taneichi, T., Ling, N., and Guillemin, R. (1980): *Am. J. Obstet. Gynecol.,* 137:613–616.

62. Pert, A., Pert, C. B., Davis, G. C., and Bunney, W. E., Jr. (1981): In: *Handbook of Biological Psychiatry, Vol. IV: Brain Mechanisms and Abnormal Behavior-Chemistry,* edited by H. M. van Praag, M. H. Lader, O. J. Rafaelsen, and E. J. Sacher, pp. 547–582. Marcel Dekker, New York.

63. Pert, C. B., and Snyder, S. H. (1973): *Science,* 179:1011–1014.

64. Pickar, D., and Bunney, W. E. (1981): In: *Biological Psychiatry,* edited by C. Perris, G. Strüwe, and B. Jansson, pp. 394–397. Elsevier, Amsterdam.

65. Pickar, D., Davis, G. D., Schulz, S. C., and Bunney, W. E., Jr. (1981): *Am. J. Psychiatry,* 138:160–166.

66. Pickar, D., Dubois, M., and Cohen, M. R. (1984): *Am. J. Psychiatry,* 141:103–104.

67. Pickar, D., Naber, D., Post, R. M., van Kammen, D. P., Kaye, W., Rubinow, D. R., Ballenger, J. C., and Bunney, W. E., Jr. (1982): *Ann. NY Acad. Sci.,* 398:399–412.

68. Richardson, D. E., and Akil, H. (1977): *J. Neurosurg.,* 47:184–194.

69. Risch, S. C. (1982): *Biol. Psychiatry,* 17:1071–1079.

70. Risch, S. C., Cohen, R. M., Janowsky, D. S., Kalin, N. H., and Murphy, D. L. (1980): *Science,* 209:1545–1546.

71. Roberts, J. L., and Herbert, E. (1977): *Proc. Natl. Acad. Sci. USA,* 74:5300–5304.

72. Rossier, J. (1982): *Nature,* 298:221–222.

73. Savoldi, F. (1984): In: *Central and Peripheral Endorphins: Basic and Clinical Aspects,* edited by E. E. Muller and A. R. Gerazzani, pp. 333–338. Raven Press, New York.

74. Simon, E. J. (1984): *Roche Receptor,* 1:1–6.

75. Simon, E. J., Hiller, J. M., and Edelman, I. (1973): *Proc. Natl. Acad. Sci. USA,* 70:1947–1949.

76. Sullivan, S., Akil, H., and Barchas, J. D. (1978): *Commun. Psychopharmacol.,* 2:525–531.

77. Tamminga, C. A., Tighe, P. J., Chase, T. N., De Fraites, E. G., and Schaffer, M. H. (1981): *Arch. Gen. Psychiatry,* 38:167–168.

78. Terenius, L. (1973): *Acta Pharmacol. Toxicol.,* 33:377–384.

79. Terenius, L., Wahlström, A., and Agren, A. (1977): *Psychopharmacology,* 54:31–33.

80. Terenius, L., Wahlström, A., Lindström, L. H., and Widerlöv, E. (1976): *Neurosci. Lett.,* 3:157–162.

81. Von Graffenried, B., del Pozo, E., Roubicek, J., Krebs, E., Poldinger, W., Burmeister, P., and Kerp, L. (1978): *Nature,* 272:729–730.

82. Wahlstrom, A., Johansson, L., and Terenius, L. (1976): In: *Opiates and Endogenous Opioid Peptides,* edited by H. W. Kosterlitz, pp. 49–56. Elsevier/North Holland Press, Amsterdam.

83. Weber, E., Roth, K. A., and Barchas, J. D. (1982): *Proc. Natl. Acad. Sci. USA,* 79:3062–3066.

84. Zubenko, G. S., and Nixon, R. A. (1984): *Am. J. Psychiatry,* 141:110–111.

Psychopharmacology:
The Third Generation of Progress,
edited by Herbert Y. Meltzer.
Raven Press, New York © 1987.

CHAPTER 64

Sleep and Affective Disorders

Charles F. Reynolds, III, J. Christian Gillin, and David J. Kupfer

The application of electroencephalographic (EEG) sleep measures in clinical psychiatry, as well as the role of such measures in the psychobiology of depression, has received intensive investigation during the past decade. As we have previously reviewed this literature (34,43), available evidence suggests that EEG sleep studies have utility both in the diagnostic confirmation and in the differential diagnosis of depression. Thus, studies using EEG sleep variables have demonstrated acceptable sensitivity (range 61.0–90%) and specificity (range 72–100%) for different EEG sleep measures, in diverse settings, and across various comparison groups (56). Similarly, the studies have suggested that the diagnostic confidence of an abnormal EEG sleep study is relatively high (range 83–100%) in the confirmation and differential diagnosis of depression.

EEG sleep measures may be useful also for distinguishing diagnostic subtypes of depression. A number of investigators have compared EEG sleep in patients classified as endogenously or nonendogenously depressed (for example, 16,47) and have reported that REM latency is significantly lower in endogenous depressives than in nonendogenously depressed patients. In this same context, delusional depression represents a special subtype of endogenous depression, with a significantly poorer response to tricyclic antidepressants and often with greater psychomotor disturbance. It is now clear that delusional depressives are more likely to have extremely short, sleep-onset REM latencies and to generate less REM sleep than nondelusional depressives, even after allowing for the effects of age, severity, and psychomotor disturbance (57).

Another application of EEG sleep studies with both theoretical and clinical interest is for the differential diagnosis of severe character disorder and primary depressive disorders. Thus, there is a growing body of research suggesting that a portion of this heterogeneous group may have a concurrent affective disorder responsive to antidepressant chemotherapy (2,44).

Although EEG sleep measures have already shown considerable promise in the differential diagnosis of depression from nonaffective disorders and in the delineation of depressive subtypes, nonetheless, it is apparent that different sets of EEG sleep criteria are necessary to differentiate endogenous from nonendogenous depression, anxiety disorder, dementia, schizophrenia, etc. Thus, improving diagnostic accuracy based on sleep measures remains a priority for psychiatric sleep research.

In addition to their utility for distinguishing depression from nonaffective disorders and for distinguishing between subtypes of major depression, EEG sleep measures may also be useful in monitoring the neurophysiological effects of tricyclic antidepressants in the prediction of treatment response. All-night sleep recordings during drug treatment have shown that a number of tricyclic antidepressants produce rapid suppression of REM sleep, and that patients who eventually have a satisfactory clinical response show a greater REM sleep suppression during the first 2 nights of drug administration than do nonresponders (for review, see 29).

A final application of sleep measures lies in the assessment of treatment course beyond the immediate response to the acute episode. There is considerable interest in ascertaining the residual sleep abnormalities in depressed patients during remission. The hypothesis is that those individuals who are at high risk for relapse or for the onset of a new episode will demonstrate sleep abnormalities no different from the acute episode or abnormalities found somewhere between the acute episode and the normal state.

Progress in this area of psychobiological research has not been limited to a broadening of the empirical data base, however. Indeed, considerable progress on the conceptual front has also taken place with respect to the development of testable hypotheses in the pathophysiology of depression (for review, see 18). This progress has been evidenced by the publication of several different models conceptualizing the pathophysiology of depression as evidenced by EEG sleep changes. Such models, which have also attempted to account for the growing body of neurochemical, biological rhythms, and developmental data, are already determining current directions of research in this area and are likely to bear upon future efforts. In general, it may be said that sleep research in the psychobiology of depression is moving away from its previously descriptive emphasis on baseline or unchallenged sleep, towards using naturalistic and pharmacologic probes, in order to test specific hypotheses. In addition, sleep measures are being increasingly integrated with other types of psychobiological measures obtained concurrently on the same patient, such as measures of psychomotor activity, neuroendocrine secretory activity, and 24-hr core body-temperature rhythms.

Within this broad context, we will first review progress in methodology that has made possible advances in psychiatric sleep research during the past decade, followed by a brief review of the current consensus regarding sleep abnormalites and affective disorders. These considerations will include a review of differential diagnosis based on sleep neurophysiological data. After an overview of these descriptive data, we will review arguments bearing on the issue of whether sleep abnormalities are epiphenomenal to depression or in fact reflect the basic etiopathogenesis of depression. This question will lead to further neurobiological considerations of the sleep disturbances in depression, including current hypotheses about cholinergic-aminergic imbalance in depression (36), phase advance (60), and process "S" deficiency (8). We will then conclude with a brief consideration of future directions for research in this area.

METHODOLOGIC ADVANCES

Progress in sleep research in the affective disorders has been facilitated by increasing sensitivity to methodological issues and to sources of unwanted variance (29). Studies that have been performed in the 1970s and early to mid-1980s have been assisted by increased diagnostic precision, such as the implementation of research diagnostic criteria and the development of better operationalized diagnostic criteria in most categories, particularly in the affective disorders. These developments have made it somewhat easier to select patients for research studies. To date, studies of sleep in affective disorders have generally focused on more severely ill samples with endogenous or melancholic depressions.

Second, the importance of ruling out concurrent medical or neurological syndromes before psychobiological investigation has been recognized. Thus, depressed patients in research studies undergo meticulous medical and neurologic evaluation before being judged protocol-eligible. The importance of this point is illustrated by studies of medical depressive syndromes (27), which have been shown to have diminished rapid eye movement (REM) sleep and rapid eye movement density, compared with primary major depressive illness.

Third, although little controversy now exists concerning whether patients should be studied on any type of psychotropic medication, it is not clear how long the drug-free

period should be. Nonetheless, an accepted compromise position has been the use of a 2-week drug-free period. REM latency and other EEG sleep measures show little change over time in inpatients receiving placebo pharmacotherapy (11), suggesting that these measures appear to have high test-retest reliability over 2- to 6-week intervals. In this same context, recent proposals to use cognitive behavioral therapy (CBT) in the treatment of depressives seem particularly promising with respect to the research goal of understanding what types of EEG sleep abnormality might persist in clinically recovering patients *not* exposed to antidepressant drugs. The advantage conferred by this approach is that it permits one to examine the stability or lability of sleep measures before, during, and after depression, solely as a function of clinical state change, without the potentially confounding effects of a somatic intervention.

Fourth, recent studies have dealt with the issue of entrainment and novelty in a more sophisticated manner than earlier studies. Many recent studies have actually been conducted in the hospital room where patients have resided for several weeks before the investigation. This procedure has led to a considerable amount of entrainment; therefore, issues raised in the early 1970s on adaptation and the stress of the first period of studies are not as prominent. Nevertheless, even though adaptation has been made easier, because current approaches often include simultaneous measurement of several variables, such as the conduct of sleep, neuroendocrine, and biochemical studies, investigators have had to remain sensitive to possible effects of intensive experimental manipulation and, indeed, to interactions among tests.

Finally, increasing reliance on the computer for characterizing phasic phenomena, such as the temporal distribution of REM or EEG delta waves, has led to finer-grained descriptions of pathophysiologic events during depression, and, hence, to more sophisticated hypotheses concerning regulation and dysregulation of sleep in depression.

EEG SLEEP ABNORMALITIES AND AFFECTIVE DISORDERS

Approximately 90% of patients with major depressive illness experience some form of EEG-verified sleep disturbance (29). The most predictable sleep abnormalities of endogenous depression include (a) sleep continuity disturbances (i.e., prolonged sleep latency, nocturnal awakenings, and early morning awakening); (b) diminished slow wave sleep (stages 3 and 4), with a shift of EEG delta activity from the first to the second non-REM (NREM) sleep period; (c) an abbreviated first NREM sleep period leading to more rapid appearance of the first REM sleep period; and (d) altered intranight temporal distribution of REM sleep, with increased REM sleep time and REM activity earlier in the night.

Whereas sleep continuity disturbances and diminished slow wave sleep are relatively nonspecific correlates of psychiatric disorder *per se,* the abbreviation of the first NREM period, the redistribution of EEG delta activity from the first NREM period to the second NREM period, and the increased density of rapid eye movements in the first REM period are relatively more specific to endogenous depression, compared with Alzheimer's dementia, schizophrenia, or generalized anxiety disorder (41,42,44,45).

It is now also clear that there are important interactions between age and disease in determining the sleep characteristics of major depressive disorders (23,31). Specifically, the sleep changes that characterize depression also occur, though to a lesser extent, during the course of normal aging itself. It is particularly the age-dependent increase in wakefulness after sleep onset and a decrease in slow wave sleep that characterize both normal aging and depressive illnesses. At the same time, however, it is not yet firmly established from published data whether REM sleep latency itself shortens during the course of normal aging, and if so, how robust a trend this may be. On the other hand, the tendency for REM sleep periods to become progressively longer during the night is also significantly less in healthy middle-aged and older persons than in young adults. That is to say, the capacity to sustain REM sleep inhibition during the first half of the night appears to be diminished by advancing age and, to a much greater extent, by the presence of a depressive illness. It is precisely the shortening of REM sleep latency and the altered intranight temporal distribution of REM sleep (with greater amounts of earlier REM sleep) that most specifically characterize the sleep of patients with major depressive disorders.

During the past 5 years, additional data on the sleep of childhood, young-adult, middle-aged, and elderly depressives have been published, and these data lend further support to the concept of an interaction between aging and disease in determining the sleep abnormalities of depression. In a large study of prepubertal children with major depressive illness, Puig-Antich (39a) has reported few differences between the sleep of depressed children and healthy controls matched for age, sex, and pubertal status. On the other hand, when the depressed children were studied during clinical remission, their REM latency showed a shortening compared to the controls (39). More recently, Lahmeyer (35) has suggested that the sleep of adolescents with major depression is characterized by a constellation of findings similar to that of adult major depressives, particularly shortening of REM latency or first NREM sleep period. In a recent comparison of automated REM and slow-wave sleep analysis in young-adult and middle-aged depressed subjects, average REM counts were significantly higher in the middle-age depressives, an effect due primarily to the first REM period (30). For average delta counts, the opposite was true, with young-adult depressives having significantly greater average delta counts in all NREM periods, but primarily during the first and second NREM periods. At the other end of the life cycle, it has been demonstrated that very short REM latencies, prolonged first REM periods, and extreme sleep maintenance difficulty reliably characterize the sleep of elderly nonbipolar and nondelusional, but predominantly endogenous elderly depressives (41). One of the more interesting findings to emerge from these studies has been the high frequency of sleep-onset REM periods (SOREMPs) in elderly endogenous depressives, where approximately 43% of REM latency values are less than 10 min. This finding stands in contrast to rates of 1.4% in healthy controls and 17% in nondepressed Alzheimer demented patients. Like middle-aged depressives, elderly depressives show a redistribution of EEG delta activity from first to second NREM period, in contrast to healthy controls and Alzheimer patients, where peak delta counts per minute occur in the first NREM sleep period (40).

As previously noted, REM latency and other EEG sleep measures show little change over time in inpatients not receiving pharmacotherapy, in the absence of clinical change (11). Moreover, the findings of Hauri (24), Schulz (49), and Cartwright (9), taken together, suggest that chronic sleep abnormalities including reduced REM latency may well persist beyond the clinically symptomatic period. Thus, although further prospective data are necessary for the complete resolution of this issue, it appears that REM latency is reduced and stable in depression, in remission, and during the acute episode. If this finding is confirmed in larger samples of drug-free remitted depressives, the question then arises to whether abnormal REM latency can be viewed as an indicator of continued vulnerability to depression, a consequence of depression that remits more slowly than the clinical episode itself, and/or a potential predictor of depression in people who are unaffected but at risk.

In this context, longitudinal evaluation of change in clinical and biologic data may shed some light on neurobiological mechanisms of response to treatment. Most effective somatic treatments are known, for example, to produce alterations in REM sleep, and, with respect to treatment with tricyclic antidepressants, suppression of REM indices appears to be significantly correlated with both clinical response and plasma drug levels (33,50,51). Vogel (59) has proposed that REM suppression is the key mechanism underlying treatment response (i.e., antidepressants work because they are REM suppressants), a suggestion based not only on the polysomnographic effects of efficacious antidepressant drugs, but also on the antidepressive effectiveness of REM sleep deprivation in endogenously ill patients.

Data published during the last 5 years have shown that EEG sleep measures are useful in monitoring the neurophysiological effects of tricyclic antidepressants and in the prediction of treatment response. All-night sleep recordings during drug treatment have shown that amitriptyline, desimipramine, and zimelidine all produce rapid suppression of REM sleep, as evidenced by REM latency prolongation, REM activity reduction, and REM percent decrease (50,51). Concurrently, there appears to be a redistribution of REM density into the second REM period. Tonic aspects of REM sleep, such as REM sleep latency and REM percent, tend to remain suppressed for weeks or longer during maintenance treatment. In contrast, tolerance to REM activity suppression appears to develop over several weeks of treatment, as evidenced by a return of phasic REM activity.

Concurrent with suppression of REM sleep time and activity, as well as redistribution of REM activity from first to second REM period, both amitriptyline and zimelidine appear to strengthen delta activity and density in the first NREM period, thereby normalizing the distribution of EEG delta activity during the night (32). Thus, antidepressant drug effects appear to be most evident during the first NREM-REM cycle of the night. Moreover, patients who respond to amitriptyline tend to show a greater REM sleep suppression than do nonresponders, as well as a greater prolongation of the first NREM period, during the first 2 nights of drug administration (33). In other words, final clinical response is significantly correlated with the extent of acute REM percent reduction and prolongation of REM latency during the first 2 nights of amitriptyline treatment.

The importance of monitoring the acute effects of antidepressants on EEG sleep has to do not only with the ability to predict treatment response. Increasingly, sleep research in this area is characterized by the use of antidepressants with more specific neuropharmacologic activity, such as desimipramine (which is a relatively specific noradrenergic reuptake blocker) and zimelidine or fluvoxamine (which are relatively specific serotonin reuptake blockers). The use of more specific pharmacologic probes, which are at the same time potent antidepressants, will permit one to test hypotheses concerning monoamine abnormalities in the pathogenesis of depression and in the sleep-wake dysregulation of depression.

As noted above, specific sleep changes appear to characterize subtypes of depression. Thus, for example, Rush et al. (47) were able to distinguish endogenous versus nonendogenous depressed outpatients with a diagnostic confidence of 83%, by using a REM latency cutoff score of 60 min or less for the endogenous depressives. Similarly, Akiskal and Tashjian (2) were able to classify correctly by diagnosis outpatients with primary depression versus either outpatients with secondary depression, nondepressed psychiatric, or healthy controls, with a diagnostic confidence of 90%. These investigators used a REM latency cutoff score of 70 min or less on 2 consecutive nights. Reynolds and colleagues (1942) were able to show successful separation of outpatients with primary depression from outpatients with generalized anxiety disorder with a 90% diagnostic confidence, by using REM latency and REM percentage in a discriminant function analysis.

Delusional depression represents a special subtype of endogenous depression, with a significantly poorer response rate to tricyclic antidepressants and often greater psychomotor disturbance. In a recent study of sleep in delusional depressives, comparison of pretreatment EEG sleep measures in delusional and nondelusional depressives indicated that the delusionals had significantly decreased generation of REM sleep and REM activity (about 20% less than nondelusionals), but higher frequency of sleep onset REM periods (52 vs 31% of patients), than did nondelusional depressives, even after controlling for the effects of age, severity, and agitation (57).

Regarding the distinction of unipolar versus bipolar affective disorders, sleep efficiency tends to be reduced in unipolar depression compared to bipolar depression (13); however, phase of illness needs to be considered when discussing hypersomnia in bipolar depression. For example, patients in a mixed state of bipolar disorder often have significant hyposomnia and sleep continuity disturbance. Conversely, sleep studies of anergic unipolar depressives are often similar to those of bipolar patients, with both showing evidence of hypersomnia (such as elevated sleep efficiency). Short REM latency has been reported in all series studying bipolar depressives to date. The difference in sleep efficiency between unipolar and bipolar depressives may parallel differences between these groups in psychomotor activity levels because bipolar depressives tend to show lower levels of daytime and nocturnal activity than do unipolar depressives.

Another application of sleep studies with both theoretical and clinical interest is for the differential diagnosis of severe character disorder and primary depressive symptomatology. One of the earliest publications in this area was that of Akiskal and colleagues (1), who compared pretreatment EEG sleep in five characterologic depressives who subsequently responded to tricyclic antidepressants, with the sleep of eight nondepressed controls, and seven characterologic depressives who did not respond to tricyclics. The investigators found that REM latency was reduced to a mean of 58 min in the drug-responder group, indistinguishable from that of unipolar depressive controls. The sleep of patients with borderline personality disorder also tends to be similar in many regards to the sleep of age-matched nonborderline primary depressives (44). The similarity of sleep measures suggests that, in some patients, there may be a relation between borderline personality and the affective spectrum of disorders.

A basic question inspired by the large body of empirical data on sleep changes in depression is whether these abnormalities are primary or secondary changes. That is, do sleep changes represent epiphenomena, or do they reflect the basic biological changes associated with, and perhaps responsible for, the presence of affective disorder? Similarly, as we shall review below, available data suggest that the sleep abnormalities of depression may result from perturbations in several neurotransmitter systems.

ARE THE SLEEP ABNORMALITIES OF DEPRESSION EPIPHENOMENA?

What is the significance of these sleep changes in depression at a more basic level? Is it possible that they are merely epiphenomena or nonspecific changes and without major importance for etiology or pathophysiology? There appear to be three major approaches to this issue. The first has to do with diagnostic sensitivity and specificity, which is addressed elsewhere in this chapter. If these changes were pathognomonic of depression, the relationship would be more straightforward than it now appears. As yet, however, the sleep disturbances of depression do not appear to be completely specific in all studies.

The second approach asks whether manipulations of sleep can induce depression in normal subjects. The answer appears to be no. No one has convincingly demonstrated that partial or complete sleep deprivation, selective sleep stage deprivation (i.e., REM sleep or delta sleep), or alterations in the timing of sleep induce true depression in normal volunteers. To be sure, individuals experiencing loss of sleep or jet lag may feel dysphoric or even miserable but they do not usually display the signs and symptoms of major depressive disorder. Although early experiments in the 1960s initially claimed that REM deprivation might have psychopathological consequences, these conclusions are no longer accepted. Furthermore, it is possible to induce many of the sleep abnormalities of depression (i.e., short REM latency, increased REM density, etc.) in normal subjects without producing mood disturbances. Such sleep changes have been associated with pharmacological treatments (i.e., cholinomimetic agonists, withdrawal from repeated anticholinergic administration), recovery sleep following selective REM deprivation, sleep during free-running experiments (i.e., short REM latency typically occurs), and phase shifts of sleep time (i.e., morning naps typically have short REM latency). From these observations, one can conclude that sleep disturbances do not cause depression. Furthermore, the physiological mechanisms causing short REM latency or other characteristic sleep disturbances may reflect a common final pathway that can be reached by a number of different routes.

The third approach is to ask whether manipulations of sleep can induce normality in depressed patients. In this case, the answer appears to be yes. Several different sleep manipulations have been reported to have antidepressant effects (17) (Table 1).

Selective REM deprivation by the awakening method was reported by Vogel et al. (59) to be clinically effective in endogenous depressives. He compared REM deprivation with controlled awakenings from NREM sleep. Following approximately 2 to 3 weeks of REM deprivation, endogenously depressed patients showed significant clinical improvement. Seventeen of 34 patients were discharged from the hospital as a result of this treatment. NREM awakenings had no significant effect. Furthermore, patients with reactive depression showed no clinical change with either REM deprivation or NREM awakenings. Unfortunately, no one has attempted to replicate this heroic study.

Total sleep deprivation is the best-documented of the "sleep therapies" of depression (see review in 17). Approximately 40 to 60% of depressed patients show an antidepressant response, usually beginning approximately 4 to 6 a.m. Although there is considerable overlap in the clinical characteristics of responders and nonresponders, responders more often tend to be endogenous, to have diurnal mood variation (worse in morning), to have more depressive-like sleep patterns before sleep deprivation, to be dexamethasone nonsuppressors, and to have elevated nocturnal core body temperature. The clinical specificity of total sleep deprivation treatment may not be narrow, however, since it has been reported to help schizophrenic patients suffering from a postpsychotic depression. The mechanism of this antidepressant effect remains unknown. Unfortunately from a clinical point of view, the effects of sleep deprivation are frequently transient, i.e., once the recovered patient returns to sleep, he or she usually wakes up depressed again. Some data suggest, for example, that brief naps can immediately reverse the antidepressant effects of total sleep deprivation (28,46). From a research point of view, however, it is fascinating that depression can be "turned on and off" with sleep manipulations.

Partial sleep deprivation has also been reported to have antidepressive effects. Limited evidence suggests that partial sleep deprivation in the last half of the night is superior to partial sleep deprivation in the first half of the night.

A fifth approach has been to advance bedtime, usually by about 6 hr. After maintaining patients on this new schedule for several days, clinical improvement has been reported in some (48,61) but not all studies (15).

Finally, a combination of partial sleep deprivation and advance of the bedtime has been reported to have antidepressant effects in both hospitalized patients with major depressive disorder (D. Sack, *personal communication*, 1985) and in women with premenstrual depression (B. L. Parry, *personal communication*, 1985).

Are the clinical benefits of the various manipulations of sleep nonspecific? So many sleep manipulations apparently have antidepressant effects, it might be argued that any change in sleep could be helpful, perhaps as a response to the stress of "treatment." It should be emphasized, however, that this was not true in the study of Vogel et al. They claimed specificity for both the type of sleep manipulation (REM deprivation vs NREM awakenings) and for diagnostic group (endogenous vs reactive depressive). In addition, partial sleep deprivation appears to be better in the latter half of the night than the first.

The fact that some sleep manipulations, but not all, have dramatic clinical benefits in some depressed patients suggests that sleep changes are not mere epiphenomena of depression. Sleep appears to be intimately involved in the pathophysiology of affective disorders.

TABLE 1. *"Sleep therapies" of depression*

Treatment	Duration of Rx	Length of benefits	Comments
REM deprivation	2–3 weeks	Months	Best for endogenous patients. Not useful for reactive patients. NREM awakenings not beneficial.
Total sleep deprivation	Benefits may begin by 4–6 a.m.	Typically until next sleep	Seems best in severe endogenous patients, with diurnal mood swings. Reported to help postpsychotic depression in schizophrenia
Partial sleep deprivation	Several hours	Typically until next sleep	Partial sleep deprivation in last half of night may be better. Few published reports
Phase advance of bedtime	Several days	Weeks	Few published reports. One study claimed no benefits
Phase advance of bed plus partial sleep deprivation	Several days	Weeks	Reported to work in hospitalized depressives and premenstrual depression

THEORETICAL MODELS OF SLEEP DISTURBANCE IN DEPRESSION

Various theoretical interpretations or models have been proposed to explain the sleep disturbances, mood changes, neuroendocrine abnormalities, and other signs and symptoms of depression. Three of the major current hypotheses are reviewed here (see also 18).

First, some of the sleep and other changes may reflect neurotransmitter abnormalities implicated in depression, particularly an increased ratio of cholinergic to aminergic neurotransmission (20,36). These suggestions are consistent with the cholinergic-aminergic imbalance hypothesis, originally proposed by Janowsky et al. (25). Most of the original evidence was based on pharmacological interpretations of how drugs induced or improved depression. For example, physostigmine, an anticholinesterase, and arecoline, a muscarinic agonist, both induced depressive-like mood changes in normal volunteers and in depressed patients (for further discussion, see Chapter 53, *this volume*). More recently, as far as the sleep aspects of depression are concerned, it has been demonstrated in both animals and humans that REM latency can be shortened by cholinomimetic drugs and prolonged by anticholinergic agents (52). In animals, REM sleep or its components can be triggered by intracerebral administration of carbachol, oxotremorine, neostigmine, and other cholinergic agonists in selected areas of the brainstem. In humans REM latency has been shortened by oral administration of RS-86, a muscarinic agonist, before bed (55), and by intravenous administration of physostigmine or arecoline during the first NREM period. Scopolamine blocks the REM-inducing effects of arecoline. Furthermore, a model of muscarinic supersensitivity in normal volunteers, induced by three daily administrations of scopolamine for 3 mornings, mimicked many of the major sleep disturbances of depression: short REM latency, increased REM density, reduced total sleep time and sleep efficiency (20). Depressed mood was not produced.

Although less well established, other pharmacological data suggest that REM sleep is under inhibitory control of the aminergic systems. REM sleep has been induced or increased by administration of thymoxamine, an α-receptor antagonist (37), reserpine (12), and α-methyl-*para*-tyrosine, an inhibitor of tyrosine hydroxylase (53).

Some evidence from sleep studies indicates that depressed patients show a supersensitive REM induction compared with normal controls or patients with anxiety disorders, following administration of arecoline (14,26,54) or RS-86 (6). Berger et al. (5) also reported that depressed patients are more likely to awaken to an infusion of physostigmine than normal controls. Further evidence is needed to confirm these findings.

The second model is the phase-advance hypothesis, originally implied by F. Snyder in a discussion of Weitzman et al. (63) and later elaborated by Weitzman et al. (64), Papousek (38), and Wehr et al. (62). This idea is based on chronobiological considerations, namely, that there is a phase advance of the circadian "clock" governing the daily rhythms of REM sleep, core body temperature, and cortisol. Some theoreticians have proposed that these three biological rhythms are controlled by a "strong oscillator" or brain

clock. Thus, the depressed patient who goes to bed at midnight is like the normal patient who goes to bed at 6 a.m. It is known that such changes in bedtime will shorten REM latency and produce other sleep changes characteristic of depression.

Attempts to test the phase advance hypothesis have had mixed results. It is not clear that short REM latency actually indicates a phase advance of the strong oscillator. Furthermore, the circadian temperature rhythm is not clearly advanced, although depressed patients may be relatively "hot" at night compared with controls (4,58).

The third model of current interest is based on the two-process hypothesis of sleep regulation proposed by Borbely (7). This hypothesis postulates that sleep is regulated by a homeostatic process (process S), which increases with duration of wakefulness, and a circadian process (process C), which alters circadian sleep propensity. According to the S-deficiency hypothesis of depression, process S is deficient or accumulates too slowly during wakefulness in depression (8). This accounts for the loss of stage 3 and 4 sleep and of power density in the delta frequency band in depression. Furthermore, it is postulated that NREM sleep processes exert an inhibitory effect on REM sleep, thus accounting for short REM latency in depression. The beneficial effects of total and partial sleep deprivation are accounted for by increased time to strengthen process S.

All three of these models account for some of the known data but not all of it. Both the cholinergic-aminergic imbalance and the phase advance hypothesis can account empirically for the short REM latency of depression, whereas the S-deficiency hypothesis has not experimentally demonstrated this yet. Neither the phase advance hypothesis nor the S-deficiency hypothesis easily explains depressed mood, whereas the cholinergic-amergic imbalance hypothesis has empirical data that are consistent with depressed-like mood, although not entirely convincing. The cholinergic-aminergic imbalance hypothesis also offers an interpretation of hypercortisolemia in depression, whereas the other two models have not yet produced firm empirical evidence for this. Furthermore, studies on body temperature rhythms, cortisol secretion, and circadian REM latency have not yet convincingly demonstrated a phase advance of the strong oscillator. As far as the beneficial effects of sleep deprivation are concerned, the two-process model was formulated with this issue in mind. To explain these observations, the phase advance hypothesis postulates a "depressogenic" period during the 24-hr cycle, which is phase advanced into the sleep period during depression when sleep induces depression. The cholinergic-aminergic imbalance hypothesis does not readily explain the sleep therapies.

On the other hand, the phase advance hypothesis is potentially the most testable of the three hypotheses at this time. Although the current evidence of circadian rhythm disturbances in depression is weak, all the clinical data on patients have been accumulated under entrained conditions. Even under the best of experimental conditions, it is difficult to determine phase. With the possibility of studying depressed patients under free-running conditions, it will be easier to estimate phase, amplitude, and cycle length of circadian processes in various psychopathological states.

The other two models—the cholinergic-aminergic imbalance hypothesis and the two-process Model—may be more difficult to assess fully. It is not easy to measure directly the physiological processes postulated to be relevant. Central cholinergic transmission is even more difficult to quantify in humans than aminergic transmission. Process S is more of a concept at this time than an identified substance or physiological process and is currently inferred from EEG analysis. Nevertheless, the integration of theory and clinical observation has been an advance that will benefit both clinical studies and basic science.

LIMITATIONS AND FUTURE DIRECTIONS

The psychobiological research summarized in this chapter illustrates an evolution from a purely descriptive focus to the formulation of testable hypotheses relating abnormalities in several domains to models of pathophysiology in depression. The testing of such hypotheses has necessarily involved the use of a variety of experimental manipulations, both pharmacologic and naturalistic, to understand possible underlying mechanisms. As we have reviewed, examples of such experimental manipulation have included the use of more or less specific pharmacologic probes, sleep deprivation, REM deprivation, and circadian rhythm engineering. For example, as previously mentioned, studies by Sitaram et al. (54) have tested the cholinergic supersensitivity hypothesis of affective disorders by infusing the cholinergic muscarinic agent, arecoline, during the second NREM sleep period. The differential REM induction responsivity of some depressive patients to arecoline can be viewed within the context of a hypothesized imbalance between cholinergic and monoaminergic activity, as recently reviewed by McCarley (36).

Another example of such hypothesis-driven research has attempted to link the sleep neurophysiological abnormalities of depression to disturbances of biological rhythms. Indeed, a number of features of depressive illness have suggested that abnormalities in the control of endogenous circadian rhythms are involved in the phenotypic expression of depression, such as the circadian mood change in depression, the early occurrence of wake onset in depression, seasonal variation in depressive symptoms, a short REM sleep latency and long first REM period, and other evidence suggesting a phase advance of temperature, cortisol secretion, activity, and neurotransmitter metabolites. Thus, total sleep deprivation, partial sleep deprivation (particularly in the latter half of the night), selective REM sleep deprivation, and phase advance shifts of the daily sleep wake cycle have all been reported to result in a transient remission of depressive symptoms in about half the patients studied. This improvement, usually noted on the first day following treatment, lasts for a period of days to months, depending upon the nature of the manipulation. In this chapter we have reviewed several theories that have been put forth to explain these clinical observations, including the hypothesis that REM sleep deprivation transiently reverses an imbalance between cholinergic and adrenergic neurotransmitter symptoms (23), as well as hypotheses derived from Borbely's two-process model of sleep regulation (7).

Further sleep research in depression will probably continue to move beyond a largely descriptive (and passive) emphasis to the testing of specific hypotheses and predictions derived from models of the pathophysiology of depression. These models are and will be variously neurochemical, chronobiological, genetic, and developmental in nature. The use of pharmacologic and naturalistic probes will help to further characterize the physiology of depressed patients during illness and remission, and under conditions of "disequilibrium," such as following sleep deprivation, REM deprivation, or the administration of specific serotonergic antidepressant drugs.

At the same time, however, if one is to understand further whether the sleep abnormalities of depression are part of a larger 24-hr circadian rhythm disturbance, investigations will have to include 24-hr measures of sleep-wake activity, psychomotor activity, and probably core body-temperature rhythm. A complementary point of view would suggest at the same time that more intensive investigative efforts be focused on the first 100 min of sleep at night, since it is the first NREM-REM cycle that seems to show the greatest deviation in depressive patients from normal controls. Thus, efforts to further characterize this part of the 24-hr cycle, with respect to age, gender, and responses to physiologic, hormonal, pharmacologic, and naturalistic probes, are strongly warranted and appear to be very promising.

ACKNOWLEDGMENTS

This work was supported by NIMH Grants 30915, 24652 (Dr. Kupfer), 00295, and 37869 (Dr. Reynolds); and by a grant from the John D. and Catherine T. MacArthur Foundation Research Network on the Psychobiology of Depression.

REFERENCES

1. Akiskal, H. S., Rosenthal, T. L., Haykal, R. F., Lemmi, H., Rosenthal, R. H., and Scott-Strauss, A. (1980): *Arch. Gen. Psychiatry,* 37:777–783.
2. Akiskal, H. S., and Tashjian, R. (1983): *Hosp. Community Psychiatry,* 34:822–830.
3. Akiskal, H. S., Yerevanian, B. I., David, G. C., King, D., and Lemmi, H. (1984): *Am. J. Psychiatry,* 142:192–197.
4. Avery, D. H., Widschiodtz, G., and Rafaelson, D. J. (1982): *J. Affective Disord.,* 4:61–71.
5. Berger, M., Lund, R., Bronisch, T., and van Zerssen, D. (1983): *Psychiatry Res.,* 10:113–123.
6. Berger, M., Hoch, D., Zulley, J., Lauer, C., and von Zerssen, D. (1985): *Lancet,* 1:1385–1386.
7. Borbely, A. A. (1982): *Hum. Neurobiol.,* 1:195–204.
8. Borbely, A. A., and Wirz-Justice, A. (1982): *Hum. Neurobiol.,* 1: 205–210.
9. Cartwright, R. D. (1983): *Arch. Gen. Psychiatry,* 40:197–201.
10. Chambers, W., Tabrizima, M. A., and Weitzman, E. D. (1982): *Arch. Gen. Psychiatry,* 39:932–939.
11. Coble, P. A., Kupfer, D. J., Spiker, D. G., Neil, J. F., and McPartland, R. J. (1979): *J. Affective Disord.,* 1:131–138.
12. Coulter, J. D., Lester, B. K., and Williams, H. L. (1971): *Psychopharmacologia,* 19:134–147.
13. Detre, T. P., Himmelhoch, J., and Swartzburg, M. (1972): *Am. J. Psychiatry,* 128:1303–1305.

14. Dube, S., Kumar, N., Ettedgui, E., Pohl, R., Jones, D., and Sitaram, N. (1985): *Biol. Psychiatry,* 20:408–418.
15. Elsenga, S., and van den Hoffdakker, R. H. (1983): *Sleep,* 12:326.
16. Feinberg, M., Gillin, J. C., Carroll, B. J., Greden, J. F., and Zis, A. P. (1982): *Biol. Psychiatry,* 17:305–316.
17. Gillin, J. C. (1983): *Biol. Psychiatry,* 7:351–364.
18. Gillin, J. C., and Borbely, A. A. (1985): In: *Trends Neurosci.,* 8: 537–542.
19. Gillin, J. C., Duncan, W. C., Murphy, D. L., Post, R. M., Wehr, T. A., Goodwin, F. K., Wyatt, R. J., and Bunney, W. E. (1981): *Psychiatry Res.,* 4:73–78.
20. Gillin, J. C., Duncan, W. C., Pettigrew, K. D., Frankel, B. L., and Snyder, F. (1979): *Arch. Gen. Psychiatry,* 36:85–90.
21. Gillin, J. C., and Sitaram, N. (1984): *Psychol. Med.,* 14:501–506.
22. Gillin, J. C., Sitaram, N., and Duncan, W. C. (1979): *Psychiatry Res.,* 1:17–22.
23. Gillin, J. C., Sitaram, N., and Mendelson, W. B. (1982): *Hum. Neurobiol.,* 1:211–219.
24. Hauri, P., Chernik, D., Hawkins, D., and Mendels, T. (1974): *Arch. Gen. Psychiatry,* 31:386–391.
25. Janowsky, D. J., El-Yousef, M. K., Davis, J. M., et al. (1972): *Lancet,* 2:632–635.
26. Jones, D., Kelwala, S., Bell, J., Dube, S., Jackson, E., and Sitaram, N. (1985): *Psychiatry Res.,* 14:99–110.
27. King, D., Akiskal, H. S., and Lemmi, H. (1981): *Psychiatry Res.,* 5:267–276.
28. Knowles, J., Southmayd, S. E., Delava, N., Maclean, A. W., Cairns, J., and Letemendia, F. J. (1979): *Br. J. Psychiatry,* 135: 403–410.
29. Kupfer, D. J., and Reynolds, C. F. (1983): In: *The Origins of Depression: Current Concepts and Approaches,* edited by J. Angst, pp. 235–252. Springer-Verlag, Berlin.
30. Kupfer, D. J., Reynolds, C. F., Ulrich, R. F., and Grochocinski, V. J. (1986): *Biol. Psychiatry,* 21:189–200.
31. Kupfer, D. J., Reynolds, C. F., Ulrich, R. F., Shaw, D. H., and Coble, P. A. (1982): In: *Neurobiology of Aging: Experimental and Clinical Research,* edited by R. T. Bartus, pp. 351–360. ANKHO International, Fayetteville, NY.
32. Kupfer, D. J., Shipley, J. A., Perel, J. M., Pollack, B., Coble, P. A., and Spiker, D. G. (1987): In: *Clinical Pharmacology in Psychiatry: Selectivity in Psychotropic Drug Action—Promises or Problems?,* edited by S. G. Dahl, L. F. Gram, S. M. Paul, and W. Z. Potter, pp. 167–173. Springer Verlag, New York.
33. Kupfer, D. J., Spiker, D. G., Rossi, A., Coble, P. A., Ulrich, R. F., and Shaw, D. H. (1983): In: *Treatment of Depression: Old Controversies and New Approaches,* edited by P. Clayton and J. Barrett, pp. 31–52. Raven Press, New York.
34. Kupfer, D. J., and Thase, M. E. (1983): *Psychiatr. Clin. North Am.,* 6:3–25.
35. Lahmeyer, H. W., Poznanski, E. O., and Bellur, S. N. (1983): *Am. J. Psychiatry,* 140:1150–1153.
36. McCarley, R. W. (1982): *Am. J. Psychiatry,* 139:565–570.
37. Oswald, I., Thacore, V. R., Adam, K., Brezinova, V., and Burack, R. (1975): *J. Clin. Pharmacol.,* 2:107–110.
38. Papousek, M. (1975): *Neurol. Psychiatry,* 43:381–440.
39. Puig-Antich, J., Goetz, R., Hanlon, C., Tabrizi, M. A., Davies, M., and Weitzman, E. (1983): *Arch. Gen. Psychiatry,* 40:187–192.
39a.Puig-Antich, I., Goetz, R., Hanlon, C., Davies, M., Thompson, J.,

Chambers, W., Tabrizina, M. A., and Weitzman, E. (1982): *Arch. Gen. Psychiatry,* 39:932–939.
40. Reynolds, C. F., Kupfer, D. J., Taska, L. S., Hoch, C. C., Sewitch, D. E., and Grochocinski, V. J. (1985): *Sleep,* 8:155–159.
41. Reynolds, C. F., Kupfer, D. J., Taska, L. S., Hoch, C. C., Spiker, D. G., Sewitch, D. E., Zimmer, B., Marin, R. S., Nelson, J. P., Martin, D., and Morycz, R. (1985): *Biol. Psychiatry,* 20:431–442.
42. Reynolds, C. F., Shaw, D. H., Newton, T., Coble, P. A., and Kupfer, D. J. (1983): *Psychiatry Res.,* 8:81–89.
43. Reynolds, C. F., and Shipley, J. E. (1985): In: *Psychiatry Update,* 4:341–351.
44. Reynolds, C. F., Soloff, P. H., Kupfer, D. J., Taska, L. S., Restifo, K., Coble, P. A., and McNamara, M. E. (1985): *Psychiatry Res.,* 14:1–15.
45. Reynolds, C. F., Spiker, D. G., Hanin, I., and Kupfer, D. J. (1983): *Biol. Psychiatry,* 2:139–155.
46. Roy-Byrne, P., Uhde, T. W., and Post, R. M. (1984): In: *Neurobiology of Mood Disorders,* edited by R. M. Post, and J. C. Ballenger, pp. 817–835. Williams and Wilkins, Baltimore.
47. Rush, A. J., Giles, D. E., Roffwarg, H. P., and Parker, C. R. (1982): *Biol. Psychiatry,* 17:327–341.
48. Sack, D., Nurnberger, J., Rosenthal, N. E., Ashburn, E., and Wehr, T. A. (1985): *Am. J. Psychiatry,* 142:606–608.
49. Schulz, H., Lund, R., Cording, C., and Dirlich, G. (1979): *Biol. Psychiatry,* 14:595–600.
50. Shipley, J. E., Kupfer, D. J., Griffin, S. J., Dealy, R. S., Coble, P. A., McEachran, A. B., Grochocinski, V. J., and Ulrich, R. F. (1985): *Psychopharmacology,* 85:14–25.
51. Shipley, J. E., Kupfer, D. J., Sewitch, D. E., Coble, P. A., McEachran, A. B., and Grochocinski, V. J. (1984): *Clin. Pharmacol. Ther.,* 2:251–259.
52. Shiromani, P. J., and Gillin, J. C. (1987): In: *Neurobiology of Acetylcholine (in press).*
53. Sitaram, N., Gillin, J. C., and Bunney, W. E. (1984): In: *Neurobiology of Mood Disorders,* edited by R. M. Post and J. C. Ballenger, pp. 629–651. Williams and Wilkins, Baltimore.
54. Sitaram, N., Nurberger, J. I., Gershon, E. S., and Gillin, J. C. (1982): *Am. J. Psychiatry,* 139:571–576.
55. Spiegel, R. (1984): *Psychiatry Res.,* 11:1–13.
56. Thase, M. E., and Kupfer, D. J. (1987): In: *Advances in Human Psychopharmacology, Vol. 10,* edited by G. D. Burrows and J. S. Werry. JAI Press, Greenwich, CT *(in press).*
57. Thase, M. E., Kupfer, D. J., and Ulrich, R. F. (1987): *Arch. Gen. Psychiatry,* 43:886–893.
58. Van den Hoofdakker, R., and Beersma, D. G. M. (1985): *Psychiatry Res.,* 16:155–163.
59. Vogel, G. W., Voegel, F., McAbee, R. S., and Thurmond, A. J. (1980): *Arch. Gen. Psychiatry,* 37:247–253.
60. Wehr, T. A., and Goodwin, F. K. (1981): In: *American Handbook of Psychiatry: Vol. 7,* edited by S. Arieti and H. K. H. Brodie, pp. 46–74. Basic Books, New York.
61. Wehr, T. A., and Wirz-Justice, A. (1982): *Psychopsychiatry,* 15: 31–39.
62. Wehr, T. A., Wirz-Justice, A., Goodwin, F. K., Duncan, W., and Gillin, J. C. (1979): *Science,* 206:210–213.
63. Weitzman, E. D., Goldmacher, D., Kripke, D. F., MacGregor, P., Kream, J., and Hellman, L. (1970): *Trans. Am. Neurol. Assoc.,* 22:483–489.
64. Weitzman, E. D., Kripke, D., Goldmacher, D., et al. (1970): *Arch. Neurol.,* 22:483–489.

Psychopharmacology:
The Third Generation of Progress,
edited by Herbert Y. Meltzer.
Raven Press, New York © 1987.

CHAPTER **65**

Psychobiology of Suicide, Impulsivity, and Related Phenomena

Marie Åsberg, Daisy Schalling, Lil Träskman-Bendz, and Anna Wägner

Most research on suicide has been focused on the role of psychological and social problems as causes of self-destructive behavior. Biological factors were considered of little importance until the recent emergence of two clusters of biological variables that tend to correlate with suicidal behavior. These are associated with serotonergic neurotransmission and with certain neuroendocrine functions, particularly the release of cortisol and thyrotropin.

Interest in a possible biological involvement in some cases of suicide has been paralleled by an increased interest in similar correlates of other types of disinhibitory behavior, such as impulsive violence. In this chapter we review the evidence linking different types of disinhibition, including certain suicides and suicide attempts, to serotonin-related and neuroendocrine variables.

BIOLOGICAL MEASURES IN SUICIDAL BEHAVIOR

The biochemical investigation techniques used in the field almost entirely derived from studies of depressive illness. They include studies of brain tissue obtained at autopsy, and measurements in cerebrospinal fluid (CSF), blood platelets and plasma, and urine. Monoamines and their precursors, catabolizing enzymes, and degradation products have all been measured; and hormonal processes

thought to be controlled by monoamine neurons, and the reaction of the various systems to challenge, have been studied. The methodological difficulties in these measurements are well known and have been discussed in detail, both in this volume and elsewhere (see, e.g., ref. 13).

Studies of Brain Tissue from Suicide Victims

Monoamines and Their Metabolites

Studies of monoamines and monoamine metabolites in brains from suicide victims began to be published in the mid-1960s. It was then often assumed that those who commit suicide are depressed, and the primary goal was to collect information about depression. To some extent this approach is valid. About half of those who commit suicide are retrospectively diagnosed as having suffered from a depressive *syndrome*, whereas the majority of suicide victims have had depressive *symptoms* prior to death (22,26).

In Table 1 are summarized some controlled studies of monoamines and their metabolites in brains from suicide victims. In most of these studies, suicide victims have lower concentrations of serotonin in certain parts of the brain. Previous treatment and variations in the interval between death and autopsy may, however, have accounted for some of the differences (27). Circadian variation in serotonin

TABLE 1. *Some controlled studies of neurotransmitter-related markers in brains from suicide victims*

Author	Subjects	Tissue	Result (suicidal patients vs nonsuicidal, or controls)	
Shaw et al. (149)	22 suicides 17 controls	Hindbrain	↓ 5-HT	
Bourne et al. (28)	23 suicides 28 controls	Hindbrain	0 5-HT ↓ 5-HIAA 0 NE	
Pare et al. (120)	26 suicides 15 controls	Brainstem, caudate, hypothalamus	↓ 5-HT 0 NE 0 DA	
Lloyd et al. (93)	7 suicides 5 controls	Six raphe nuclei	↓ 5-HT 0 5-HIAA	In nuclei raphe dorsalis and centralis inf.
Grote et al. (71)	14 suicides 19 controls	Hypothalamus	0 MAO	
Gottfries et al. (68)	15 suicides 20 controls	Several brain areas	↓ MAO	
Cochran et al. (48)	19 suicides 12 controls	Several brain areas	0 5-HT	
Beskow et al. (27)	23 suicides 62 controls	Several brain areas	0 5-HT 0 NE 0 DA 0 5-HIAA 0 HVA	(Adjusted for differences in postmortem delay suicides, see text)
Meyerson et al. (103)	8 suicides 10 controls	Cortex	↑ Muscarinic receptors ↑ Imipramine receptors	
	7 suicides 9 controls	Cortex	0 β-Receptors	
Stanley et al. (154)	9 suicides 9 controls	Frontal cortex	↓ Imipramine receptors	
Kaufmann et al. (76)	8 suicides 8 controls	Cortex, hypothalamus	0 Muscarinic receptors	
Korpi et al. (80)	29 controls 30 schizophrenics (50% dead from suicide), 14 nonschizophrenic suicides	Several brain areas	↓ 5-HT 0 5-HIAA 0 TRY	Hypothalamus in nonschizophrenic subjects
Owen et al. (118)	7 suicides 18 controls	Frontal cortex	0 5-HT$_1$ receptors 0 5-HT$_2$ receptors[a] 0 5-HIAA	
Perry et al. (123)	13 suicides 10 controls	Hippocampus	↓ Imipramine receptors	
	11 suicides 16 controls	Occipital cortex	↓ Imipramine receptors	
Stanley et al. (153)	11 suicides 11 controls	Frontal cortex	↑ 5-HT$_2$ receptors[b]	
Mann and Stanley (96)	13 suicides 13 controls	Frontal cortex	0 MAO	
Paul et al. (121)	8 suicides 9 controls	Hypothalamus	↓ Imipramine receptors 0 Desipramine receptors	
Stanley (152)	22 suicides 22 controls	Frontal cortex	0 Muscarinic receptors	
Kleinman et al. (79)	19 suicides 18 controls	Caudate nucleus	0 Substance P 0 Neurotensin 0 Metenkephalin	

[a] [^{3}H]Ketanserine as ligand.
[b] [^{3}H]Spiroperidol as ligand.
Abbreviations: 5-HT, 5-Hydroxytryptamine (serotonin); NE, norepinephrine; DA, dopamine; 5-HIAA, 5-hydroxyindoleacetic acid; HVA, homovanillic acid; TRY, tryptophan; MAO, monoamine oxidase.

concentrations in the brain, particularly in the hypothalamus (41), may also lead to erroneous conclusions about group differences, if clock time of death is different in suicides and controls. However, in the study by Korpi et al. (80), where clock time of death was taken into consideration, lower hypothalamus serotonin concentrations were found in suicide victims.

The concentrations of monoamines (serotonin, dopamine, norepinephrine, and epinephrine) after death by suicide were measured in suboccipital CSF by Kauert et al. (75), who somewhat unexpectedly found *increased* serotonin concentrations in the suicide victims. It cannot be excluded, however, that this finding may reflect differences in the time of death in suicides and controls. In monkeys, CSF serotonin concentrations are almost doubled during the night, the daytime mean concentration being only 5% of the peak nocturnal concentration (64).

Monoamine Oxidase

Although the relationship between the activity of mono-amine oxidase (MAO) in brain and the function of the serotonergic system is likely to be complex (114), a positive correlation between MAO-B and serotonin turnover has been reported in human brain (2).

MAO activity in brain regions from suicide victims was found to be similar to that of controls in two studies (71,96). Gottfries et al. (68), however, found a lower MAO activity in alcoholic suicide victims than in controls, which is in line with the repeated finding of low platelet MAO activity in alcoholic subjects (see review in ref. 114).

Receptor Binding

The development of methods for studying the specific binding of drugs to brain tissue has reawakened interest in autopsy studies of suicide victims. So far, the most intensively studied ligand has been [3H]imipramine, whose binding sites are probably closely connected with the 5-HT (5-hydroxytryptamine; serotonin) uptake site. The distribution of [3H]imipramine binding sites in the brain closely parallels the distribution of serotonin neurons (70,148), whereas [3H]desipramine labels the neuronal norepinephrine uptake sites (83,84,86).

Stanley et al. (154), Perry et al. (123), and Paul et al. (121) all found lower imipramine binding in suicide victims. Paul et al. (121) also measured the density of [3H]desipramine binding sites, which did not differ from control values. In contrast, Meyerson and co-workers (103) report *increased* [3H]imipramine binding in suicide victims as compared with controls.

In addition to [3H]imipramine binding, Stanley and Mann (153) also measured postsynaptic 5-HT$_2$ binding sites with [3H]spiroperidol in their suicide cases. In agreement with a hypothesis of reduced serotonin release in suicidal patients, they found an increased number of binding sites. The correlation between [3H]imipramine binding and [3H]spiroperidol binding was negative, although nonsignificant—possibly due to the small number of subjects. Owen

et al. (118), however, found no increase in 5-HT$_2$ binding using [3H]ketanserin as a ligand.

Muscarinic binding of [3H]quinuclidinyl benzilate (QNB) was normal in the suicide victims studied by Stanley (152) and in those studied by Kaufmann et al. (76), whereas increased QNB binding in suicide victims was reported from the Meyerson et al. (103) study cited above. Results from the binding studies are summarized in Table 1.

Studies of Suicide Attempters

Serotonin-Related Measures

CSF 5-Hydroxyindoleacetic acid. In a study aimed at finding clinical correlates in a biochemical subgroup of depressed patients characterized by low CSF concentrations of 5-hydroxyindoleacetic acid (5-HIAA), Åsberg et al. (15) unexpectedly found an increased incidence of suicide attempts. Although the average CSF 5-HIAA concentration is lower in depressed patients than in healthy controls, there is evidence that this is due to the existence of a subgroup of patients with low CSF 5-HIAA (14,66,168).

In the study by Åsberg et al. (15), 40% of the patients with low CSF 5-HIAA concentration had attempted suicide during their present illness, as compared with 15% in patients with normal 5-HIAA. Moreover, the attempts were of a more determined nature with a preference for active, violent methods in the low 5-HIAA patients, whereas those in the high 5-HIAA group were confined to drug overdoses. Two deaths from suicide occurred during the study period, both in low 5-HIAA patients (14).

The relationship between CSF 5-HIAA and suicidal behavior has been confirmed by Ågren (3), who studied depressed patients and measured suicidal behavior by means of the suicide behavior scales in the Schedule for Affective Disorder and Schizophrenia (SADS). These scales do not differentiate suicidal ideation and suicidal acts. In the Åsberg et al. (14) study, there was no association between low CSF 5-HIAA and suicidal ideation, only with suicidal acts. Ågren's choice of method may thus have weakened the correlation, which nonetheless was statistically significant.

These early studies did not take into account the relationship between CSF 5-HIAA and such interference factors as sex and body height. Men tend to have lower CSF 5-HIAA concentrations than women, and they are also more prone to use violent methods if they attempt suicide. The sex factor could, however, be ruled out in a subsequent confirmatory study by Träskman et al. (159).

More recently, the relationship between 5-HIAA and suicide has been confirmed in Dutch depressed patients studied by van Praag (162), who found a very highly significant increase in suicidal behavior in patients with low probenecid-induced accumulation of 5-HIAA. In a British study of depressed patients, Montgomery and Montgomery (105) also found lower 5-HIAA concentrations in suicidal than in nonsuicidal subjects. Among depressed patients in India, Palaniappan and co-workers (119) found a significant correlation between CSF 5-HIAA concentrations and suicidal tendencies (estimated by scores on the item Suicide in the Hamilton Rating Scale). Banki and co-workers (20) found a relationship between low CSF 5-HIAA and suicide attempts in Hungarian female patients. In Banki's study, the association was confined to those who had used active methods. Lopez-Ibor et al. (95) have reported a relationship between suicide attempts and low CSF 5-HIAA in Spanish patients, irrespective of the method used in the attempt.

There is also one well-designed, nonconfirmatory study by Roy-Byrne and co-workers (135), who mainly studied treatment-resistant American patients, referred to a research center specializing in the study of depressive disorders. No significant relationship was found between CSF 5-HIAA and lifetime suicidal behavior, possibly owing to the high proportion of bipolar (manic-depressive) patients in the group. Suicidal unipolar patients tended to have lower CSF 5-HIAA than nonsuicidal unipolars. The biological correlates of suicidal behavior may thus differ in bipolar and unipolar disorder. A similar conclusion was reached by Ågren (5).

Another difference between the study of Roy-Byrne et al. (135) and those of Åsberg et al. (15) and Träskman et al. (159) is that the former considered suicidal behavior over the patients' entire life span. In the Åsberg et al. (15) study, the significant association with CSF 5-HIAA was restricted to suicidal behavior during the index illness episode. The discrepancy suggests that CSF-HIAA values may not be stable over time in suicidal individuals, a possibility that will be discussed in further detail below.

As mentioned previously, only about 50 to 60% of those who commit suicide are retrospectively diagnosed as having suffered from a depressive syndrome. Several groups have studied the relationship between suicide attempts and CSF 5-HIAA in other diagnostic categories. Träskman et al. (159) found low CSF 5-HIAA in comparison with healthy subjects in *nondepressed* suicide attempters (mainly patients with personality disorders and minor affective disorders). Brown et al. (31) studied two groups of men with *personality disorders* and found more lifetime suicidal behavior in those with low CSF 5-HIAA.

Van Praag (166) and Ninan and co-workers (108) found a similar association in *schizophrenia*. Both studies are well designed with carefully selected, matched controls. Patients with a depressive disorder superimposed on their schizophrenia were deliberately excluded from van Praag's study. Roy et al. (134), whose subjects and controls were not matched, found no difference in CSF 5-HIAA concentrations between chronic schizophrenic subjects who had attempted suicide at some time during their life, and those who had not. Lower CSF 5-HIAA concentrations were, however, reported in suicidal patients with schizophrenia than in nonmatched controls by Banki et al. (20), who also found similar relationships in *alcoholism* and *adjustment disorder*. The bulk of the evidence would thus seem to support the notion that a low concentration of 5-HIAA in CSF is associated with suicidal behavior, even beyond the realm of the affective disorders.

The CSF studies of 5-HIAA in suicide attempters are summarized in Table 2.

Monoamine Oxidase activity in platelets. Although there is little direct evidence of a correlation between platelet MAO (which is exclusively of the B-type) and brain MAO, there is a rapidly growing literature on reproducible behavioral correlates of platelet MAO activity (see, e.g., the review in ref. 114). Oreland and Shaskan (112) have suggested that platelet MAO activity in humans may reflect some innate characteristic of the serotonin system, such as its extent or capacity, rather than its activity at any given time. A weak, but significant, positive correlation between CSF 5-HIAA and platelet MAO activity was reported by Oreland et al. (115) in healthy volunteers, but not in depressed patients. On the other hand, Zuckerman et al. (185) reported a significant negative correlation between the two variables in healthy volunteers.

There is some evidence that platelet MAO activity is related to suicidal behavior. Buchsbaum and co-workers (33) found an increased frequency of psychosocial problems, including suicide attempts, in college students with very low activity of platelet MAO. Among the relatives of these students, the incidence of suicide attempts was significantly higher than among relatives of high MAO probands.

In psychiatric patients, Buchsbaum and co-workers (34) found a relationship between platelet MAO and suicide, but only in those patients who were also augmenters in averaged evoked response tests. Gottfries and co-workers (69) reported that depressed patients who had made violent suicide attempts had significantly lower platelet MAO activity than other depressives, including those who had taken drug overdoses. Oreland et al. (115) found similar platelet MAO activity in patients who had made a suicide attempt and patients who had not, but the number of patients who had used violent methods was too small to be analyzed separately.

[³H]Imipramine binding. So far, in only one study of [³H]imipramine binding have suicide attempters and non-attempters been examined separately. Wägner et al. (176), who found significantly lower platelet [³H]imipramine binding in depressed patients than in controls, report that among suicide attempters, the binding was higher in those who had used violent methods, though the difference was only marginally significant.

Postsynaptic effects. In a very interesting study of serotonin function beyond the postsynaptic receptor, Meltzer and co-workers (101) measured the response in blood cortisol concentration to administration of the serotonin precursor, 5-hydroxytryptophan. Normally, this procedure results in a slight increase in serum cortisol. The cortisol release is exaggerated in depressive illness. When the depressed patients were subdivided into those who had attempted suicide, those who had suicidal thoughts, and those who were nonsuicidal, the cortisol reaction was clearly enhanced in the attempters (100). This finding is in line with the hypothesis of a reduced release of serotonin in suicide attempters, which would tend to cause hypersensitivity of serotonin receptors.

Melatonin and magnesium. Recently, two studies have appeared in which two other biological variables, melatonin in plasma and magnesium in CSF, have been related to suicidal behavior. Since both are in certain respects related to serotonin, they will be discussed here.

Beck-Friis and co-workers (23) reported that nocturnal serum melatonin concentrations, known to be decreased

TABLE 2. *Studies of CSF 5-HIAA in relation to suicidal behavior*

Author	Subjects	Measure of suicidality	Result
Åsberg et al. (13)	68 hospitalized depressed patients	Attempted or completed suicide within index illness episode	Low 5-HIAA in the 15 attempters, particularly those using violent methods
Brown et al. (32)	22 men with personality disorder	Lifetime history of suicide attempt	Lower 5-HIAA and higher MHPG in the 11 suicide attempters
Ågren (3)	33 depressed patients	SADS suicidality scale scores	Negative correlation with 5-HIAA and MHPG
Träskman et al. (159)	30 suicide attempters (8 depressed, 22 other psychiatric disorders excluding schizophrenia and alcoholism), 45 healthy controls	Recent attempted or completed suicide	5-HIAA lower in attempters than in controls, HVA lower in depressed attempters only
Leckman et al. (85)	132 psychiatric patients	Nurses' ratings of suicidal tendencies	Negative correlation with 5-HIAA
Brown et al. (31)	12 patients with borderline personality disorder	Lifetime history of suicide attempt	Lower 5-HIAA in the 5 attempters
van Praag (165)	203 depressed patients	Recent suicide attempt	Lower CSF 5-HIAA after probenecid in the 54 suicide attempters
Palanappian et al. (119)	40 hospitalized depressed patients	Suicide item in the Hamilton Rating Scale	Negative correlation with CSF 5-HIAA and HVA
Ågren (5)	110 depressed patients	SADS suicidality scales	Negative correlation with CSF 5-HIAA and MHPG
Roy-Byrne et al. (135)	32 bipolar, 13 unipolar patients in different phases of illness	Lifetime history of suicide attempt	No association with 5-HIAA
van Praag (166)	10 nondepressed schizophrenics who attempted suicide in response to imperative hallucinations, 10 nonsuicidal schizophrenics, 10 controls	Recent suicide attempt	Lower CSF 5-HIAA after probenecid in suicide attempters
Banki et al. (20)	141 female inpatients (36 depressed, 46 schizophrenic, 35 alcoholic, 24 with adjustment disorder; 45 previously reported)	Recent suicide attempt	Negative correlation with 5-HIAA in all diagnostic groups, particularly with violent attempts; inconsistent relationships to HVA
Ninan et al. (108)	8 suicidal, 8 nonsuicidal schizophrenic patients, matched for age and sex	Lifetime history of suicide attempt	Lower 5-HIAA in suicidal patients
Lopez-Ibor et al. (95)	21 depressed patients	Suicide attempt, suicidal ideation rated on the Hamilton Scale and the AMDP system	More attempts and higher suicidality scores in patients with low 5-HIAA
Roy et al. (133)	27 depressed patients	Lifetime history of suicide attempt	Lower 5-HIAA and HVA in the 19 attempters, significant for HVA only

in depression (47,179), were closer to normal in suicidal than in nonsuicidal depressed patients. Melatonin production is dependent on vicinal lighting conditions and thought to be regulated by β-adrenergic neurotransmission. Serotonin is a precursor of melatonin, although little is known of any correlation between the concentrations of the two compounds in humans.

Banki and co-workers (21) found a relationship between low CSF concentrations of magnesium and suicide attempts.

There was a strong positive correlation between CSF magnesium and CSF 5-HIAA. Interestingly, melatonin concentrations in CSF are strongly correlated to CSF magnesium concentrations (24).

Dopamine-Related Measures

The average concentration of the dopamine metabolite, homovanillic acid (HVA), in CSF is reduced in depression

(11,125), and more consistently so than CSF 5-HIAA, to which it is strongly correlated. Whether the correlation between the two metabolites is due to their sharing the same transport mechanism, or to a functional connection between the parent amines, is not known.

Low concentrations of HVA in suicidal depressed patients have been reported by Träskman et al. (159), Montgomery and Montgomery (105), Ågren (5), and Roy et al. (133). In the Roy et al. study of 27 depressed patients, low HVA, but not low 5-HIAA concentrations in CSF, were associated with suicidal behavior at any time during the patients' life. Both 5-HIAA and HVA concentrations were associated with ultimate suicide, but the HVA association was the stronger. Banki et al. (20), on the other hand, found a less clear-cut relationship between suicide and HVA than with 5-HIAA. In particular, their depressed patients who had taken drug overdoses had significantly *higher* HVA than had nonsuicidal patients, whereas HVA was very low in violent attempters.

A similar percentage reduction is seen in both 5-HIAA and HVA concentrations in melancholia, as compared with healthy people (once confounding variables such as age, sex, and body height are controlled for; ref. 11), although the difference in HVA between patients and controls is numerically larger than the difference in 5-HIAA, and presumably easier to pick up in small-scale studies. This is probably the reason why, over a range of studies, HVA concentrations have more consistently been found to be low in depression than 5-HIAA concentrations.

Reduced HVA concentrations in the CSF may, however, be related to some aspect of the depressive (melancholic) illness rather than to suicide in general. Thus, in the Träskman et al. (159) study, only in the suicide attempters who were also depressed were HVA concentrations lower than normal, whereas those of 5-HIAA were reduced both in depressed and nondepressed attempters. Only depressive suicide attempters were included in the Montgomery and Montgomery (105), the Ågren (5), and the Roy et al. (133) studies. The failure of Ninan et al. (107) to find any difference in CSF HVA between their suicidal and nonsuicidal schizophrenic subjects is in line with a relationship between low HVA and depressive illness.

Norepinephrine and MHPG

In contrast to the evidence relating suicide to serotonin, the relationships with norepinephrine are less clear. In depressed patients, Ågren (4) reported a negative correlation between suicidal tendencies and the CSF concentration of the norepinephrine metabolite 3-methoxy-4-hydroxy-phenylglycol (MHPG). Brown and co-workers (32) found a positive correlation in subjects with personality disorders, which was not reproduced in their study (31) of borderline patients.

Ostroff and associates have measured the ratio between norepinephrine and epinephrine (the NE/E ratio) in *urine* in two studies (116,117) of mixed diagnostic groups, and found a relationship between low ratio and suicidal behavior. Within a group of suicide attempters, Prasad (127) found

that the NE/E ratio was significantly lower in those who used violent methods in the attempt.

Endocrinological Variables

The most extensively documented neuroendocrine disturbances in depressive illness are a blunted thyrotropin (TSH) response to the injection of thyrotropin-releasing hormone (TRH), and an activation of the hypothalamic-pituitary-adrenal axis. The latter is evidenced by high cortisol concentrations in blood, urine, and CSF, disturbance of their circadian and circannual rhythm, and an inability to suppress cortisol release after administration of dexamethasone. Reviews of the two areas of research have been published by Loosen and Prange (94) and Carroll (42).

The hypothalamic-pituitary-adrenal axis. In 1965 Bunney and Fawcett (35) reported that in patients who attempted or completed suicide, excretion of cortisol metabolites was unusually high prior to the event. In 1969 Bunney and co-workers (36) duplicated their findings and suggested that the measurement of cortisol might be useful in identifying people at risk for suicide. Although there has been some doubt as to the usefulness of the test for measuring suicide potential (87), very similar findings were made by Ostroff and colleagues in 1982 (116). They used urinary 24-hr excretion of cortisol rather than cortisol metabolites, and their results were confirmed by Prasad (127) in patients who used violent methods in suicide attempts compared to those who used other means. A very good separation between the two subgroups of attempters was obtained when both urinary free cortisol and the NE/E ratio were considered.

In a prospective study, Krieger (81) demonstrated a relationship between high cortisol concentrations in blood and ultimate suicide. Träskman and co-workers (160) found high CSF concentrations of cortisol in suicidal patients, but only in those who were depressed as well. Banki and co-workers (20) found no relationship between CSF cortisol and suicidal tendencies in any of the diagnostic categories studied, which agrees with the normal concentrations of cortisol in brains from suicide victims found by Brooksbank and co-workers (30).

With the introduction of the dexamethasone suppression test (DST), interest has been reawakened in the relationship between suicide and cortisol. There is fairly good agreement among investigators that the DST is abnormal in approximately 60% of patients with the melancholic subtype of major depressive disorder. There is less agreement as to whether the abnormality is specific for melancholia. Although this has been strongly claimed, for example by Carroll (42), there is much evidence to the contrary (see, e.g., ref. 25).

Carroll and co-workers (43) found abnormal DSTs more often in suicidal than in nonsuicidal patients, but the relationship was confined to patients with melancholia. Whereas Ågren (5) found no relationship between an abnormal DST and suicidal behavior measured by the SADS scales, Coryell and Schlesser (51) and Targum and co-workers (158) did find a relationship in depressed patients. Robbins and Alessi (130) found a similar relationship in adolescents, most of whom were also depressed. Banki and co-workers (20) not only found a relationship between abnormal DST and suicidal tendencies, but in their case even in schizophrenics, alcoholics, and patients with adjustment disorder.

The thyroid axis. Blunted TSH responses to injection of TRH are seen in 25 to 50% of patients with depressive disorders, and in occasional alcoholic patients (even when they have been abstinent for years). There is no correlation between cortisol suppression by dexamethasone and increase in TSH in response to TRH (9,126).

The blunted TSH response to TRH seen in depression has been associated both with an increased incidence of suicide and of suicide attempts, as reported by Linkowski and co-workers (90,91) and Kjellman et al. (78). In contrast, Banki et al. (20) reported a *higher* TSH response to TRH in suicidal than in nonsuicidal psychiatric patients. Although the reason for the discrepancy is not known, it is interesting to note that Ågren (4) found that baseline plasma TSH correlated in different directions with different suicide scales from the SADS.

Other hormones. Other endocrine abnormalities (e.g., disturbance of growth hormone release) have been described in depression, but as they have not yet been specifically associated with suicide they will not be discussed here. There is, however, some preliminary evidence of a reduction, prior to suicide, in testosterone concentrations in serum (which are lower in depressed men than in age-matched controls, according, *inter alia,* to Yesavage et al., ref. 184). A dramatic decrease in plasma testosterone in three psychiatric patients who shortly afterwards committed suicide by violent methods was found by Mason et al. (97).

Prediction of Suicide from Biological Measures

Those who commit suicide and those who merely attempt it are well known to differ in many important respects, even if there is an overlap between the two populations (155). In several studies, subsequent mortality from suicide among suicide attempters has amounted to about 2% within a year after the attempt (56). Although this is a considerable increase in suicide frequency over that of the general population, suicide is a rare event even in this group.

Estimating suicide risk and taking appropriate precautions is one of the most difficult tasks of the practising psychiatrist, and many attempts have been made to create rating scales and inventories for the purpose. Most of these have not been very successful (38,124), which may be due, at least partly, to the low base rate of suicide and other statistical problems (49).

Among a well-known risk group for suicide, namely patients who have made a suicide attempt, those with low CSF 5-HIAA were 10 times more likely to die from suicide than the remainder (159). Roy et al. (133) reported a relationship to exist between low concentrations of HVA in the CSF and subsequent suicide in depressed patients, regardless of whether previous attempts had been made.

These findings suggest that inclusion of biological variables in the clinical assessment of suicide risk might increase its precision.

Stability of Markers over Time

Related to the question of the usefulness of biological markers as predictors of suicide is their stability over a long time. Unfortunately, CSF studies of recovered depressives are necessarily rare. Such patients are often maintained on drugs for extended periods, and those who are not, even if available for lumbar puncture studies, may well be nonrepresentative of the depressed population.

A further complication in follow-up studies is that most serotonin-related variables also seem to vary seasonally. Seasonal rhythms have been shown for the serotonin concentration in the human hypothalamus (41), for the platelet serotonin uptake (10,181), and for the platelet [^{3}H]imipramine binding (54,180). There is some evidence that a seasonal rhythm, very similar to that observed for serotonin in the hypothalamus, may also exist for CSF 5-HIAA (12).

The evidence from four published follow-up studies suggests that 5-HIAA concentrations in CSF remain fairly stable over limited periods in normal subjects and in depressed patients readmitted for relapse of depression (50,125,161,164). Recovered depressives, whose 5-HIAA concentrations are normal during illness, also remain stable over prolonged periods, whereas in depressives with low 5-HIAA during illness the concentration sometimes increases with recovery, though it remains in the low range in most cases.

A possible interpretation of available data is that there is a subgroup of depressed patients, characterized by concentrations of CSF 5-HIAA that are not only low but also less stable over time. If this type of unstable serotonin system is associated with an increased vulnerability to illness, and with a further decrease in release during illness, the emergence of bimodal distributions in diseased populations is easily explained.

In line with the "instability" hypothesis are findings from two patients on whom repeated lumbar punctures were made, and who subsequently committed suicide (M. Åsberg and co-workers, *in preparation*). In both cases, there was a substantial *reduction* in CSF 5-HIAA from one puncture to the next.

Although low, and possibly unstable, CSF 5-HIAA concentrations appear to be a persistent phenomenon in an individual, there is universal agreement that the activation of the hypothalamic-pituitary-adrenal (HPA) axis is related to the state of being depressed.

Low CSF 5-HIAA: A Vulnerability Marker?

Van Praag and co-workers have suggested that low CSF 5-HIAA may be an indicator of vulnerability to depression. Supporting their view, they have found an increased incidence of depressive illness in *relatives* of patients with low

CSF 5-HIAA, as compared with those of patients with normal 5-HIAA concentrations (167). This finding is reminiscent of the observation by Sedvall and co-workers (146) that CSF 5-HIAA concentrations were lower in healthy subjects with a family history of depressive illness than in healthy subjects without such antecedents. Preliminary data from twin studies by Sedvall and co-workers (147) further support familial implication in CSF concentrations of the monoamine metabolites.

Correlations Between Markers

So far, there is little knowledge of the interrelations between the potential markers of serotonin function, in healthy and in disease states. There is an obvious advantage in clarifying these relationships, both with a view to understanding their physiological significance and for practical diagnostic purposes.

Interestingly, there are no clear-cut relationships between imipramine binding and serotonin uptake in depressed patients (129). These two possible serotonin markers may thus reflect different aspects of serotonin function. The relationships reported between CSF 5-HIAA and platelet MAO activity have not been consistent (115,185).

Monoaminergic neurons are known to be involved in the chain of events that leads to the release of many hormones, including cortisol. The details of this have not yet been worked out, but the data from the Meltzer et al. (101) study of 5-hydroxytryptophan-induced release of cortisol strongly suggest a functional connection between the serotonin system and the HPA axis.

The available data in humans do not, however, show any negative correlations between markers of the systems, such as might be expected if they reflect an identical risk factor for suicide. Thus CSF concentrations of cortisol and of 5-HIAA have been shown to correlate positively, though weakly (160), or not at all (21; Aminoff et al., *in preparation*). Both Carroll et al. (44) and Banki and Arató (17) found a positive correlation between postdexamethasone cortisol and 5-HIAA. Interpretation of the results from Carroll et al. is, however, complicated by the fact that spinal fluid was drawn after the administration of dexamethasone, which raises CSF 5-HIAA concentrations (19).

Among other potential markers of serotonin, the ratio of *l*-tryptophan to other neutral amino acids was positively correlated to postdexamethasone cortisol (74), whereas V_{max} of serotonin uptake into platelets (which is reduced in depression) tended to be negatively correlated to an abnormal DST (99).

Gold and co-workers (67) report an inverse correlation between CSF 5-HIAA concentrations and the magnitude of the TSH reaction to TRH. The negative correlation between CSF 5-HIAA and the TRH/TSH test also appears in a study by Banki and co-workers (20), where it is compatible with their finding of more normal TRH/TSH responses in suicidal than in nonsuicidal patients.

SUICIDE AND GENETICS

The possibility of a genetic basis for suicide is raised by repeated findings of associations between suicidal behavior and biological variables, some of which are assumed to be of trait, rather than state, character. The relevant twin and family studies have been reviewed by Rainer (128), who concludes that, on the whole, the empirical evidence does not favor a genetic hypothesis. Among those who attempt or commit suicide, a family history of suicide is found more often than expected (132), but this can be explained as a consequence of psychological identification, and of shared genetic vulnerability to depressive illness.

There is, however, one important exception to this generally negative series of studies. Schulsinger et al. (145) reported a significant increase in suicide mortality in biological relatives of adopted suicide victims, as compared with suicide in their adopted relatives. This increase was found when the proband was classified as schizophrenic, depressive, or psychopathic, and also in relatives of probands who, according to available records, had not been in psychiatric treatment.

AGGRESSION AND SUICIDE

In their discussion of the association between suicide attempts and low concentration of 5-HIAA in CSF, Åsberg et al. (15) suggested that aggression might be an intervening variable. This speculation was based on the association known to exist between aggression in animals and serotonin turnover (summarized in ref. 163), and the links between anger and suicide proposed by classic psychoanalytical theory (1,61). "Aggression" is a somewhat nebulous concept. The word has many meanings, and some aspects of aggression are hardly amenable to empirical study. Aggression in the sense of verbal threats or violent acts, aimed at causing injury to others or to oneself, has, however, been studied in suicidal individuals. Thus, Weissman et al. (177) found that excessive hostility was characteristic of suicidal depressed patients, and Brown et al. (31) found more overt aggressive behavior in subjects who had made suicide attempts.

One of the strongest predictors of suicide is murder. In Great Britain, a 30% suicide rate is reported after a murder. The risk of suicide is greatest in those cases where the victim is a spouse (178). (In the United States, the suicide rate after murder is lower, around 4% according to Wolfgang, 182.)

BIOLOGICAL CORRELATES OF VIOLENCE

The proneness to anger arousal varies from one individual to another, and is likely to be subject to genetic influence factors (40). Normally, aggressive behavior in humans is under strong restraint, partly as a result of socializing factors. Animal experiments suggest that decrease of serotonin turnover leads to a shift from inhibition to disinhibition or commission, particularly in situations where there is competition between activating and restraining influences (151).

Serotonin-Related Measures and Aggressive and Violent Behavior

Several studies have tested the hypothesis that aggression dyscontrol is the link between serotonin turnover and suicidal behavior. Brown and associates (32) found a life pattern of aggressive behavior in subjects with personality disorder and low CSF 5-HIAA.

Further support for a relationship between serotonin and violence came from three studies of murderers. Linnoila and co-workers (92) found lower CSF 5-HIAA in violent offenders whose crimes were unpremeditated. Lidberg et al. (89) found lower CSF 5-HIAA in those homicide offenders who had killed a spouse or a lover than in those who had killed someone of less emotional significance (usually a drinking buddy). Lidberg and co-workers (88) also found very low CSF 5-HIAA concentrations in three cases in which a suicide attempter had killed or attempted to kill his or her child.

A relationship between serotonin and aggressive behavior in alcoholics was also found by Branchey et al. (29), who studied the ratio of tryptophan to other neutral amino acids in serum. They found significantly lower ratios, compatible with a deficiency of brain serotonin, in those subjects who had been arrested for assaultive behavior than in other alcoholics or in nonalcoholic controls.

Hormones

Testosterone

As mentioned previously, preliminary evidence exists of an association between male suicide and a rapid drop from previously very high concentrations of plasma testosterone (97). There is some evidence of an association between high plasma concentrations of testosterone and violent crime in men with chromosomal deviations, but also in chromosomally normal male controls (143). In a study of juvenile delinquents, high testosterone concentrations were associated with more violent crimes, and also with verbal aggression, a liking for sports, high sensation seeking, and low conformity (98,137). Similar patterns were found in normal adolescents (111).

The connection between suicide and a drop in testosterone is particularly interesting in light of animal data associating increase in testosterone with "winning" and decrease in testosterone with "defeat" (73,77,131). Similar findings have been made in wrestlers (55).

Hypoglycemia

In a series of studies on people imprisoned for crimes of violence, Virkkunen (169,170,173,174) studied the occurrence of hyperinsulinism and exaggerated hypoglycemia after an oral glucose load. An increased reactive hypoglycemia was found in subjects with antisocial personality disorder with habitual violence, and in subjects with intermittent explosive disorder [as defined by the Diagnostic and Statistical Manual of Psychiatric Disorders, 3rd edition (DSM-III)], but not in violent offenders with paranoid or passive-aggressive personality disorder. Insulin concentrations peaked faster and declined faster in subjects with intermittent explosive disorder than in those with antisocial personality disorder (173). The antisocial subjects had lower than normal urinary excretion of free cortisol, which

was not the case in the intermittent explosive disorder cases (172).

Virkkunen (171) also studied arsonists, and found 47% of the subjects to have very low blood glucose concentrations after an oral glucose load. These subjects were habitually violent when drunk, and their acts of arson had almost always occurred while they were in a confused state following a period of poor eating and alcohol abuse (likely to induce an even more profound hypoglycemia). They were significantly more likely than normoglycemic arsonists to have made suicide attempts in connection with the fire-setting (171).

There is evidence of a reciprocal interaction between insulin and the serotonin system. Insulin increases serotonin turnover in the hypothalamus of the rat, possibly by means of an increase in the uptake of tryptophan (183), and causes a drop of free plasma tryptophan in depressed patients, but not in healthy subjects (102). Whether the insulin release produced in the glucose tolerance test is sufficient to affect central serotonin turnover in humans is not known, however.

SUICIDE AND THE BIOLOGY OF PERSONALITY

Personality (or temperament), as used in recent studies of the psychobiology of suicide and of personality correlates of biological markers, refers to some basic, assumedly innate qualities of the information-processing and arousal systems of an individual.

Dimensions of temperament can be measured by inventory scales. Dimensions related to suicide, MAO, and monoamine metabolite measures are *sensation seeking* or *monotony avoidance, impulsivity, susceptibility to fear* (anxiety), and *susceptibility to anger and irritation* (aggression). Another important personality variable in relation to suicide (Nordström et al., *in preparation;* D. Schalling et al., *in preparation*) is *psychoticism* (P) from the Eysenck EPQ inventory (57,58), which reflects schizoid, nonconforming, nonempathetic, hostile personality traits. Particularly high scores in impulsivity scales and psychoticism have been found among individuals who have made violent suicide attempts (140).

Platelet MAO Activity

A significant negative correlation was found by Schooler et al. (144) between platelet MAO activity and the Zuckerman Sensation Seeking Scales (SSS). Similar findings have been obtained by Murphy et al. (106), Perris et al. (122), von Knorring et al. (175), and Schalling and Åsberg (138). Fowler et al. (60) found higher SSS scores and lower platelet MAO activity in mountain climbers than in controls. Some other studies, e.g., by Coursey et al. (52) and Zuckerman et al. (185) have not, however, confirmed the association between MAO and sensation seeking.

In a series of studies by Schalling and co-workers (reviewed by Oreland et al., 114), low platelet MAO activity subjects have consistently scored high in two impulsiveness scales. Impulsive behavior has been observed after frontal cerebral lesions, and neuropsychological methods sensitive to frontal lesions may thus be used in order to further elucidate mediating mechanisms between platelet MAO and impulsivity.

Increased frequency of perceived perspective fluctuations in an ambiguous figure such as the Necker cube has been found after bilateral frontal lesions, and also in psychopathic subjects. In two recent studies, a low platelet MAO activity was associated with increased perspective fluctuations (D. Schalling et al., *in preparation*).

CSF Monoamine Metabolites

In comparison with the relatively large number of consistent results obtained with platelet MAO, the studies of CSF monoamine metabolites as correlates of personality dimensions are few. Brown et al. (31) gave personality inventories to their subjects in an extended study, and found an inverse relationship between CSF 5-HIAA and the Psychopathic deviate (Pd) scale from the MMPI (Minnesota Multiphasic Personality Inventory). They did not, however, find any significant relationship to self-reported aggressive feelings, as measured by the Buss Durkee Inventory (39).

Rydin and co-workers (136) compared hostility, rated on the basis of Rorschach protocols, in otherwise matched pairs of psychiatric patients with low *vis-à-vis* high CSF 5-HIAA. Low CSF 5-HIAA patients scored significantly higher not only in hostility, but also in several anxiety measures, which is in agreement with Banki's (16) findings, based on anxiety ratings.

Questionnaire studies support a relationship between low CSF 5-HIAA and impulsivity, sensation seeking, and low socialization in psychiatric patients (139). Banki and Arató (18) reported an inverse correlation between CSF 5-HIAA and the Validity scale in the Marke-Nyman Temperament Scales, suggesting high "vitality" in low 5-HIAA subjects.

Studies of healthy volunteers show a relatively consistent pattern of correlations between CSF 5-HIAA and personality dimensions. Psychasthenia and inhibition of aggression in the Karolinska Scales of Personality (KSP) and the Psychasthenia Scale from the MMPI correlated positively with the serotonin metabolite (185; D. Schalling et al., *in preparation*). Schalling et al. also found a negative correlation between CSF 5-HIAA and Psychoticism, which is in line with findings in patients by Schalling et al. (139) and with the correlation with MMPI Pd reported by Brown et al. (31).

Correlations with HVA, when reported, were generally in the same directions as with 5-HIAA, but weaker.

Results from personality studies with self-selected volunteers are difficult to generalize to the general population. A recent study of healthy men may be less vulnerable to this type of bias, however, as the subjects were recruited from a representative sample of normal young men. The relationship between high CSF 5-HIAA and Inhibition of aggression was confirmed in this group, and consistent associations were found between low CSF 5-HIAA and measures reflecting high anger expression, low fear, and high social dominance (D. Schalling et al., *in preparation*).

SUICIDE AND NEUROPSYCHOLOGY

The series of correlations described between suicide, platelet MAO activity, certain personality features and some neuropsychologic tests and brain dysfunction suggests that it might be worthwhile examining the evidence of "organicity" in suicidal patients, as well as their neuropsychological functioning.

Epilepsy

Epilepsy is known to be associated with a pronouncedly increased risk of suicidal behavior (72). Struve and co-workers (156,157) have found and duplicated an association between EEG dysrhythmia (in nonepileptic patients) and suicide attempts. Interestingly, Virkkunen (170) reports that violent offenders with EEG dysrhythmia had significantly higher mean insulin secretion after an oral glucose load.

Laterality

Left-handedness is associated with low platelet MAO activity (52,114). The finding is interesting in view of the theory of Geschwind and Behan (65) which associates left-handedness (and dyslexia and childhood hyperactivity, which are also associated with low MAO) with slow development of the left cerebral hemisphere, due to increased fetal levels of testosterone.

Left-handers are overrepresented among juvenile delinquents (6,59,82). Gabrielli and Mednick found that left-handedness predicted delinquency (62) and violence (63) in a prospective birth cohort study. Andrew (7), however, found that left-handed delinquents of either sex had committed significantly fewer violent crimes than right-handers. Since left-handers have been reported to be significantly overrepresented among (alcoholic) suicide attempters (46), it might be worth examining aggression control and suicidal behavior in relation to handedness.

Habituation

Even more subtle deviations in neuropsychological functions may be associated with suicidal behavior. Edman et al. (53) studied skin conductance habituation to auditory stimulation in suicidal patients. Suicide attempters who had used violent methods in their attempts habituated significantly more rapidly to the stimulation than did those with suicide ideation only, or those who had used nonviolent methods in the attempt. All patients who subsequently died from suicide were located in the lower mode of the number-of-responses-prior-to-habituation distribution, which was clearly bimodal.

These results may appear counterintuitive, since anxiety states are associated with a slow, rather than a rapid, skin conductance habituation, and suicide in general is associated with anxiety. However, the anxiety experienced by "violent" suicide attempters may be of a different type. Thus, violent suicide attempters were shown by Schalling et al. (140) to have close to normal questionnaire scores on "Psychic Anxiety" (a dimension of anxiety reflecting worry and anticipatory anxiousness), whereas their scores were very high on "Somatic Anxiety" (reflecting autonomic arousal and probably related to Panic Disorder). Prasad's (127) finding that violent suicide attempters differ from other attempters in catecholamine excretion may be relevant in this context.

Interestingly, habituation was not correlated with CSF 5-HIAA. Its relation to platelet MAO and other potential biochemical suicide markers is not yet known, although Mirkin and Coppen (104) reported that depressed patients who did not respond to tone stimuli had a reduced uptake of serotonin into blood platelets.

Habituation is an interesting phenomenon in relation to suicide, since it can be conceptualized as learning *not* to respond to irrelevant stimuli. On the cognitive level, habituation reflects a less extensive processing of stimuli, as they become familiar (110). In other words, rapid habituation may indicate a superficial analysis of stimuli.

Other learning processes are known to be under serotonergic control—for instance, passive avoidance learning which is impaired after lesions of serotonin neurons (109). Interestingly, deficient passive avoidance learning in humans has shown consistent relations with psychopathy (150,162).

TOWARD A PSYCHOBIOLOGICAL MODEL FOR SUICIDE

Apparently, both a low CSF 5-HIAA and an activation of the HPA axis are associated with an increased risk for suicide. The absence of reports of negative correlations between the two markers suggests that they may be independent and associated with suicide through different mechanisms.

Although the nature of these mechanisms is far from clear, available data do allow some speculation. The HPA activation, for instance, has long been regarded as an indicator of emotional stress and failing defenses (37). In animals, hypercortisolism accompanies defeat and submission (73).

Recently, strong support for the stress hypothesis was provided in a study by Ceulemans et al. (45), who found almost 50% abnormal DSTs immediately prior to surgery for herniated disks in otherwise healthy, nondepressed individuals. The nonsuppressors had higher scores in inventories for state anxiety, whereas their trait anxiety scores were similar to those of the suppressors, suggesting that anticipatory anxiety prior to surgery was indeed the reason for the HPA activation.

If the HPA activation reflects the emotional suffering and subjective helplessness associated with depressive illness, the relationship with suicide makes intuitive sense. The abnormal DST may function as an alert signal that the emotional pain is approaching unbearable levels.

With a low CSF 5-HIAA, the situation is slightly different. Low 5-HIAA concentrations also occur in mentally healthy people who have never been depressed or contemplated suicide. This has led to the hypothesis that 5-HIAA is a marker of vulnerability.

In most individuals with low CSF 5-HIAA, vulnerability will never be manifested in a suicide attempt. A suicide attempt is unlikely to occur unless the individual finds himself in a situation which he conceives of as desperate, or when he is without hope for the future. Adverse events may have created this situation, or the individual's perception of the situation may be colored by depressive illness. Previous experience of adverse events (e.g., during childhood) is liable to render the interpretation of current adversity more ominous. Whether or not this state of affairs leads to a suicide attempt is to some extent determined by the quality of the person's social support network, which may attenuate the effect of adverse events, or render the sufferings of depressive illness more tolerable.

A low-output serotonin system (or perhaps even more likely, a low-stability one) might render an individual more vulnerable to self-destructive or impulsive action in time of crisis. This characteristic of the serotonin system might have a genetic basis, or it might be acquired. There are suggestions that "learned helplessness" situations in rats may lead to functional changes in the monoamine systems (8), that prolonged social isolation in mice consistently reduces serotonin turnover (163), and that different genetic strains of animals differ in their susceptibility to these influences.

If serotonin transmission is permanently low or unstable, it is conceivable that this may be manifested in other ways than in suicidal tendencies. The often quite unpremeditated, impulsive, and violent character of many of the suicide attempts in low 5-HIAA patients suggests that they might have difficulties with impulse control, particularly perhaps in the control of aggressive impulses.

Information about neuropsychological and personality correlates of the serotonin-related suicide markers is scant but relatively consistent. Low platelet MAO activity and CSF 5-HIAA are associated with impulsiveness and psychopathy-related variables. Low CSF 5-HIAA is also associated with vitality and absence of psychaesthenic features. The pattern may differ between psychiatric patients and healthy controls, in whom an association between low CSF 5-HIAA and anger arousability, assertiveness, and social dominance is more prominent.

IMPLICATIONS FOR SUICIDE PREVENTION

The association with a heightened risk of suicide suggests that markers of serotonin and HPA activation may be valuable in a clinical context. Low concentrations of CSF 5-HIAA in suicide attempters, for instance, were connected with a 20% mortality from suicide within a year, which suggests that the combination may be one of the strongest suicide predictors hitherto identified.

A dexamethasone test is easy to perform and is unaffected by current antidepressant treatment. In contrast, spinal taps for 5-HIAA measurements require hospitalization and highly standardized procedures, and the patient must not be taking any antidepressant or neuroleptic drugs. There is an obvious need for new, more easily accessible markers of the state of the serotonin system. Nevertheless, in those centers that have access to the relevant analytical procedures, routine spinal taps may be a real help in clinical management.

A better understanding of the biological and psychological links between serotonin turnover and suicidal behavior might also open up new approaches to the prevention of suicide. Serotonin transmission can be controlled, with drugs or amino acid precursors, and possibly by dietary changes, and it would seem important to test such treatment regimens in patients with a high suicide potential. It is also plausible that an increased understanding of the psychological processes that are controlled by serotonin neurons could be used to develop more specific psychotherapeutic techniques than has hitherto been possible.

ACKNOWLEDGMENTS

Financial support was given by the Swedish Medical Research Council (5454, 4545, 7336), the Söderström-König Foundation, the Torsten and Ragnar Söderberg Foundation, the Fredrik and Ingrid Thuring Foundation, the Bank of Sweden Tercentenary Foundation, and the Karolinska Institute. Marie Skjöldebrand helped in the preparation of the manuscript.

REFERENCES

1. Abraham, K. (1927): *Versuch einer Entwicklungsgeschichte der Libido auf Grund der Psychoanalyse seelischer Störungen. Neue Arbeiten zur ärztlichen Psychoanalyse, Vol 2*, edited by S. Freud. Internationaler Psychoanalytischer Verlag, Leipzig.
2. Adolfsson, R., Gottfries, C.-G., Oreland, L., Roos, B.-E., Wiberg, Å., and Winblad, B. (1978): *Prog. Neuropsychopharmacol.*, 2:225–230.
3. Ågren, H. (1980): *Psychiatry Res.*, 3:225–236.
4. Ågren, H. (1981): *Biological Markers in Major Depressive Disorders. A Clinical and Multivariate Study*. Academic dissertation, Acta universitatis upsaliensis. Abstracts of Uppsala Dissertations from the Faculty of Medicine 405, Uppsala.
5. Ågren, H. (1983): *Psychiatr. Dev.*, 1:87–104.
6. Andrew, J. M. (1978): *J. Clin. Child Psychol.*, 7:149–150.
7. Andrew, J. M. (1980): *J. Youth Adolescence*, 9:1–9.
8. Anisman, H., Pizzino, A., and Sklar, L. S. (1980): *Brain Res.*, 191:583–588.
9. Arató, M., Rihmer, Z., Banki, C. M., and Grof, P. (1983): *Prog. Neuropsychopharmacol. Biol. Psychiatry*, 7:715–718.
10. Arora, R. C., Kregel, L., and Meltzer, H. Y. (1984): *Biol. Psychiatry*, 19:1579–1584.
11. Åsberg, M., Bertilsson, L., Mårtensson, B., Scalia-Tomba, G.-P., Thorén, P., and Träskman-Bendz, L. (1984): *Acta Psychiatr. Scand.*, 69:201–219.
12. Åsberg, M., Bertilsson, L., Rydin, E., Schalling, D., Thorén, P., and Träskman-Bendz, L. (1981): In: *Recent Advances in Neuropsycho-Pharmacology*, edited by B. Angrist, G. Burrows, M. Lader, O. Lingjaerde, G. Sedvall, and D. Wheatley D., pp. 257–271. Pergamon Press, Oxford and New York.
13. Åsberg, M., Nordström, P., and Träskman-Bendz, L. (1986): In: *Suicide*, edited by A. Roy. pp. 47–71. Williams and Wilkins, Baltimore.
14. Åsberg, M., Thorén, P., Träskman, L., Bertilsson, L., and Ringberger, V. (1976): *Science*, 191:478–480.
15. Åsberg, M., Träskman, L., and Thorén, P. (1976): *Arch. Gen. Psychiatry*, 33:1193–1197.
16. Banki, C. M. (1977): *J. Neural Transm.*, 41:135–143.
17. Banki, C. M., and Arató, M. (1983): *J. Affective Disord.*, 5:223–232.
18. Banki, C. M., and Arató, M. (1983): *Acta Psychiatr. Scand.*, 67:272–280.
19. Banki, C. M., Arató, M., Papp, Z., and Kurcz, M. (1983): *Pharmacopsychiatria*, 16:77–81.
20. Banki, C. M., Arató, M., Papp, Z., and Kurcz, M. (1984): *J. Affective Disord.*, 6:341–350.
21. Banki, C. M., Vojnik, M., Papp, Z., Balla, K. Z., and Arató, M. (1985): *Biol. Psychiatry*, 20:163–171.
22. Barraclough, B., Bunch, J., Nelson, B., and Sainsbury, P. (1974): *Br. J. Psychiatry*, 125:355–373.
23. Beck-Friis, J., Kjellman, B. F., Aperia, B., Undén, F., von Rosen, D., Ljunggren, J.-G., and Wetterberg, L. (1985): *Acta Psychiatr. Scand.*, 71:319–330.
24. Beckmann, H., Wetterberg, L., and Gattaz, W. F. (1984): *Psychiatry Res.*, 11:107–110.
25. Berger, M., Pirke, K.-M., Doerr, P., Krieg, J.-C., and von Zerssen, D. (1984): *Br. J. Psychiatry*, 145:372–382.
26. Beskow, J. (1979): *Acta Psychiatr. Scand. (Suppl.)* 277.
27. Beskow, J., Gottfries, C. G., Roos, B. E., and Winblad, B. (1976): *Acta Psychiatr. Scand.*, 53:7–20.
28. Bourne, H. R., Bunney, W. E., Jr., Colburn, R. W., Davis, J. M., Davis, J. N., Shaw, D. M., and Coppen, A. J. (1968): *Lancet*, 2:805–808.
29. Branchey, L., Branchey, M., Shaw, S., and Lieber, C. S. (1984): *Psychiatry Res.*, 12:219–226.
30. Brooksbank, B. W. L., Brammall, M. A., Cunningham, A. E., Shaw, D. M., and Camps, F. E. (1972): *Psychological Medicine* 2:56–65.
31. Brown, G. L., Ebert, M. H., Goyer, P. F., Jimerson, D. C., Klein, W. J., Bunney, W. E., and Goodwin, F. K. (1982): *Am. J. Psychiatry*, 139:741–746.
32. Brown, G. L., Goodwin, F. K., Ballenger, J. C., Goyer, P. F., and Major, L. F. (1979): *Psychiatry Res.*, 1:131–139.
33. Buchsbaum, M. S., Coursey, R. D., and Murphy, D. L. (1976): *Science*, 194:339–341.
34. Buchsbaum, M. S., Haier, R. J., and Murphy, D. L. (1977): *Acta Psychiatr. Scand.*, 56:69–79.
35. Bunney, W. E., Jr., and Fawcett, J. A. (1965): *Arch. Gen. Psychiatry*, 13:232–239.
36. Bunney, W. E., Jr., Fawcett, J. A., Davis, J. M., and Gifford, S. (1969): *Arch. Gen. Psychiatry*, 21:138–150.
37. Bunney, W. E., Jr., Mason, J. W., Roatch, J. F., and Hamburg, D. A. (1965): *Am. J. Psychiatry*, 122:72–80.
38. Bürk, F., Kurz, A., and Möller, H.-J. (1985): *Eur. Arch. Psychiatry Neurol. Sci.*, 235:153–157.
39. Buss, A. H., and Durkee, A. (1957): *J. Consult. Psychol.*, 21:343–348.
40. Buss, A. H., and Plomin, R. (1984): *Temperament: Early Developing Personality Traits*. Lawrence Erlbaum Associates, Hillsdale, NJ.
41. Carlsson, A., Svennerholm, L., and Winblad, B. (1980): In: *Biogenic Amines and Affective Disorders*, edited by T. H. Svensson and A. Carlsson, pp. 75–83. Acta Psychiatr. Scand., 61(Suppl. 280).
42. Carroll, B. J. (1982): *Br. J. Psychiatry*, 140:292–304.
43. Carroll, B. J., Greden, J. F., and Feinberg, M. (1981): In: *Recent Advances in Neuropsycho-Pharmacology*, edited by B. Angrist, G. Burrows, M. Lader, O. Lingjaerde, G. Sedvall, and D. Wheatley. Pergamon Press, New York.
44. Carroll, B. J., Greden, J. F., Haskett, R., Feinberg, M., Albala, A. A., Martin, F. I. R., Rubin, R. T., Heath, B., Sharp, P. T., McLeod, W. L., and McLeod, M. F. (1980): In: *Biogenic Amines and Affective Disorders*, edited by T. H. Svensson and A. Carlsson, pp. 183–198. Acta Psychiatr. Scand., 61(Suppl. 280).
45. Ceulemans, D. L. S., Westenberg, H. G. M., and van Praag, H. M. (1985): *Psychiatry Res.*, 14:189–195.
46. Chyatte, C., and Smith, V. (1981): *Milit. Med.*, 146:277–278.
47. Claustrat, B., Chazot, G., Brun, J., Jordan, D., and Sassolas, G. (1984): *Biol. Psychiatry*, 19:1215–1228.
48. Cochran, E., Robins, E., and Grote, S. (1976): *Biol. Psychiatry*, 11:283–294.
49. Cohen, J. (1987): *Proc. NY Acad. Sci. (in press)*.

50. Coppen, A., Prange, A. J., Jr., Whybrow, P. C., and Noguera, R. (1972): *Arch. Gen. Psychiatry*, 26:474–478.
51. Coryell, W., and Schlesser, M. A. (1981): *Am. J. Psychiatry*, 138: 1120–1121.
52. Coursey, R. D., Buchsbaum, M. S., and Murphy, D. L. (1979): *Br. J. Psychiatry*, 134:372–381.
53. Edman, G., Åsberg, M., Levander, S., and Schalling, D. (1986): *Arch. Gen. Psychiatry*, 43:586–592.
54. Egrise, D., Desmedt, D., Shoutens, A., and Mendlewicz, J. (1983): *Neuropsychobiology*, 10:101–102.
55. Elias, M. (1982): *Aggressive Behav.*, 7:215–224.
56. Ettlinger, R. (1975): *Acta Psychiatr. Scand. (Suppl. 260)*.
57. Eysenck, H. J., and Eysenck, S. B. G. (1975): *Manual of the Eysenck Personality Questionnaire.* Hodder and Stoughton, London.
58. Eysenck, H. J., and Eysenck, S. B. G. (1976): *Psychoticism as a Dimension of Personality.* Hodder and Stoughton, London.
59. Fitzhugh, K. B. (1973): *Percept. Motor Skills*, 36:494.
60. Fowler, C. J., von Knorring, L., and Oreland, L. (1980): *Psychiatry Res.*, 3:273–279.
61. Freud, S. (1917): *Trauer und Melancholie.* In: *Sigmund Freud: Gesammelte Werke*, 6th ed., *Vol. X*, 1973, edited by A. Freud, E. Bibring, W. Hoffer, E. Kris, and O. Isakower, pp. 428–446. Fischer, Frankfurt am Main.
62. Gabrielli, W. F., and Mednick, S. A. (1980): *J. Abnorm. Psychol.*, 89:654–661.
63. Gabrielli, W. F., and Mednick, S. A. (1983): *Am. Behav. Sci.*, 27:59–74.
64. Garrick, N. A., Tamarkin, L., Taylor, P. L., Markey, S. P., and Murphy, D. L. (1983): *Science*, 221:474–476.
65. Geschwind, N., and Behan, P. (1982): *Proc. Natl. Acad. Sci. USA*, 79:5097–5100.
66. Gibbons, R. D., and Davis, J. M. (1986): *Acta Psychiatr. Scand.*, 74:8–12.
67. Gold, P. W., Goodwin, F. K., Wehr, T., and Rebar, R. (1977): *Am. J. Psychiatry*, 134:1028–1031.
68. Gottfries, C.-G., Oreland, L., Wiberg, Å., and Winblad, B. (1975): *J. Neurochem.*, 25:667–673.
69. Gottfries, C.-G., von Knorring, L., and Oreland, L. (1980): *Prog. Neuropsychopharmacol.*, 4:185–192.
70. Gross, G., Göthert, M., Ender, H.-P., and Schümann, H.-J. (1981): *Naunyn Schmiedebergs Arch. Pharmacol.*, 317:310–314.
71. Grote, S. S., Moses, S. G., Robins, E., Hudgens, R. W., and Croninger, A. B. (1974): *J. Neurochem.*, 23:791–802.
72. Hawton, K., Fagg, J., and Marsack, P. (1980): *J. Neurol. Neurosurg. Psychiatry*, 43:168–170.
73. Henry, J. P., and Stephens, P. M. (1978): *Stress, Health and the Social Environment.* Springer, New York.
74. Joseph, M. S., Brewerton, T. D., Reus, V. I., and Stebbins, G. T. (1984): *Psychiatry Res.*, 11:185–192.
75. Kauert, G., Gilg, T., Eisenmenger, W., and Spann, W. (1984): Presented at the 14th Congress of the Collegium Internationale Neuro-Psychopharmacologicum, Florence, Italy.
76. Kaufmann, C. A., Gillin, J. C., Hill, B., O'Laughlin, T., Phillips, I., Kleinman, J. E., and Wyatt, R. J. (1984): *Psychiatry Res.*, 12: 47–55.
77. Keverne, E. B., Meller, R. E., and Eberhart, J. A. (1982): *Scand. J. Psychol. (Suppl.)*, 1:37–47.
78. Kjellman, B. F., Ljunggren, J.-G., Beck-Friis, J., and Wetterberg, L. (1985): *Psychiatry Res.*, 14:353–363.
79. Kleinman, J. E., Hong, J., Iadarola, M., Govoni, S., and Gillin, C. J. (1985): *Prog. Neuropsychopharmacol. Biol. Psychiatry*, 9: 91–95.
80. Korpi, E. R., Kleinman, J. E., Goodman, S. I., Phillips, I., DeLisi, L. E., Linnoila, M., and Wyatt, R. J. (1983): Presented at the meeting of the International Society for Neurochemistry, Vancouver, Canada, July 14, 1983.
81. Krieger, G. (1974): *Dis. Nerv. Syst.*, 35:237–240.
82. Krynicki, V. E. (1978): *J. Nerv. Ment. Dis.*, 166:59–67.
83. Langer, S. Z., and Raisman, R. (1983): *Neuropharmacology*, 22: 407–413.
84. Langer, S. Z., Raisman, R., and Briley, M. (1981): *Eur. J. Pharmacol.*, 72:423–424.
85. Leckman, J. F., Charney, D. S., Nelson, C. R., Heninger, G. R.,

and Bowers, M. B., Jr. (1981): *Recent Adv. Neuropsychopharmacol.*, 31:289–297.
86. Lee, C. M., and Snyder, S. H. (1981): *Proc. Natl. Acad. Sci. USA*, 78:5250–5254.
87. Levy, B., and Hansen, E. (1969): *Arch. Gen. Psychiatry*, 20:415–418.
88. Lidberg, L., Åsberg, M., and Sundqvist-Stensman, U. B. (1984): *Lancet*, 2:928.
89. Lidberg, L., Tuck, J. R., Åsberg, M., Scalia-Tomba, G.-P., and Bertilsson, L. (1985): *Acta Psychiatr. Scand.*, 71:230–236.
90. Linkowski, P., van Wettere, J. P., Kerkhofs, M., Brauman, H., and Mendlewicz, J. (1983): *Br. J. Psychiatry*, 143:401–405.
91. Linkowski, P., van Wettere, J. P., Kerkhofs, M., Gregoire, F., Brauman, H., and Mendlewicz, J. (1984): *Neuropsychobiology*, 12:19–22.
92. Linnoila, M., Virkkunen, M., Scheinin, M., Nuutila, A., Rimon, R., and Goodwin, F. K. (1983): *Life Sci.*, 33:2609–2614.
93. Lloyd, K. G., Farley, I. J., Deck, J. H. N., and Hornykiewicz, O. (1974): In: *Serotonin: New Vistas. Adv. Biochem. Psychopharmacol.*, 11, edited by E. Costa, G. L. Gessa, and M. Sandler, pp. 387–397. Raven Press, New York.
94. Loosen, P. T., and Prange, A. J. (1982): *Am. J. Psychiatry*, 139: 405–416.
95. Lopez-Ibor, J. J., Jr., Saiz-Ruiz, J., and Pérez de los Cobos, J. C. (1985): *Neuropsychobiology*, 14:67–74.
96. Mann, J. J., and Stanley, M. (1984): *Acta Psychiatr. Scand.*, 69: 135–139.
97. Mason, J. W., Giller, E. L., and Ostroff, R. B. (1984): *Curr. Clin. Pract. Ser.*, 26:215–228.
98. Mattsson, Å., Schalling, D., Olweus, D., Löw, H., and Svensson, J. (1980): *J. Am. Acad. Child Psychiatry*, 19:476–490.
99. Meltzer, H. Y., Arora, R. C., Tricou, B. J., and Fang, V. S. (1983): *Psychiatry Res.*, 8:41–47.
100. Meltzer, H. Y., Perline, R., Tricou, B. J., Lowy, M., and Robertson, A. (1984): *Arch. Gen. Psychiatry*, 41:379–387.
101. Meltzer, H. Y., Umberkoman-Wiita, B., Robertson, A., Tricou, B. J., Lowy, M., and Perline, R. (1984): *Arch. Gen. Psychiatry*, 41:366–374.
102. Menna-Perper, M., Swartzburg, W., Mueller, P. S., Rochford, J., and Manowitz, P. (1983): *Biol. Psychiatry*, 18:771–780.
103. Meyerson, L. R., Wennogle, L. P., Abel, M. S., Coupet, J., Lippa, A. S., Rauh, C. E., and Beer, B. (1982): *Pharmacol. Biochem. Behav.*, 17:159–163.
104. Mirkin, A. M., and Coppen, A. (1980): *Br. J. Psychiatry*, 137: 93–97.
105. Montgomery, S. A., and Montgomery, D. (1982): *J. Affective Disord.*, 4:291–298.
106. Murphy, D. L., Belmaker, R. H., Buchsbaum, M., Martin, N. F., Ciaranello, R., and Wyatt, K. J. (1977): *Psychol. Med.*, 7: 149–157.
107. Ninan, P. T., van Kammen, D. P., and Linnoila, M. (1985): *Am. J. Psychiatry*, 142:148.
108. Ninan, P. T., van Kammen, D. P., Scheinin, M., Linnoila, M., Bunney, W. E., Jr., and Goodwin, F. K. (1984): *Am. J. Psychiatry*, 141:566–569.
109. Ögren, S. O. (1985): *Acta Physiol. Scand.*, 125(Suppl. 544).
110. Öhman, A. (1979): In: *The Orienting Response in Humans*, edited by H. D. Kimmel, E. H. van Holst, and J. F. Orlebeke, pp. 443–471. Lawrence Erlbaum Associates, Hillsdale, NJ.
111. Olweus, D., Mattsson, Å., Schalling, D., and Löw, H. (1980): *Psychosom. Med.*, 42:253–269.
112. Oreland, L., and Shaskan, E. G. (1983): *Trends Pharmacol. Sci.*, 4:339–341.
113. Oreland, L., and von Knorring, L. (1984): *Clin. Neuropharmacol.*, 7(Suppl. 1):762–763.
114. Oreland, L., von Knorring, L., and Schalling, D. (1984): In: *Proceedings of the IUPHAR 9th International Congress of Pharmacology, London 1984, Vol. 2*, edited by W. Paton, J. Mitchell, and P. Turner, pp. 193–202. Macmillan Press, London.
115. Oreland, L., Wiberg, Å., Åsberg, M., Träskman, L., Sjöstrand, L., Thorén, P., Bertilsson, L., and Tybring, G. (1981): *Psychiatry Res.*, 4:21–29.
116. Ostroff, R. B., Giller, E., Bonese, K., Ebersole, E., Harkness, L., and Mason, J. (1982): *Am. J. Psychiatry*, 139:1323–1325.

117. Ostroff, R. B., Giller, E., Harkness, L., and Mason, J. (1985): *Am. J. Psychiatry,* 142:224–227.
118. Owen, F., Cross, A. J., Crow, T. J., Deakin, J. F. W., Ferrier, I. N., Lofthouse, R., and Poulter, M. (1983): *Lancet,* 2:1256.
119. Palaniappan, V., Ramachandran, V., and Somasundaram, O. (1983): *Indian J. Psychiatry,* 25:286–292.
120. Pare, C. M. B., Yeung, D. P. H., Price, K., and Stacey, R. S. (1969): *Lancet,* 2:133–135.
121. Paul, S. M., Rehavi, M., Skolnick, P., and Goodwin, F. K. (1984): In: *Neurobiology of Mood Disorders, Vol. 1,* edited by R. M. Post and J. C. Ballenger, pp. 846–853. Williams and Wilkins, Baltimore.
122. Perris, C., Jacobsson, L., von Knorring, L., Oreland, L., Perris, H., and Ross, S. B. (1980): *Acta Psychiatr. Scand.,* 61:477–484.
123. Perry, E. K., Marshall, E. F., Blessed, G., Tomlinson, B. E., and Perry, R. H. (1983): *Br. J. Psychiatry,* 142:188–192.
124. Pokorny, A. D. (1983): *Arch. Gen. Psychiatry,* 40:249–257.
125. Post, R. M., Ballenger, J. C., and Goodwin, F. K. (1980): In: *Neurobiology of Cerebrospinal Fluid I,* edited by J. H. Wood, pp. 685–717. Plenum Press, New York.
126. Prange, A. J., Jr., and Loosen, P. T. (1984): In: *Frontiers in Biochemical and Pharmacological Research in Depression. Adv. Biochem. Psychopharmacol.,* 39, edited by E. Usdin, M. Åsberg, L. Bertilsson, and F. Sjöqvist, pp. 127–145. Raven Press, New York.
127. Prasad, A. J. (1985): *Neuropsychobiology,* 13:157–159.
128. Rainer, J. D. (1984): *Am. J. Psychother.,* 38:329–340.
129. Raisman, R., Briley, M. S., Bouchami, F., Sechter, D., Zarifian, E., and Langer, S. Z. (1982): *Psychopharmacology,* 77:332–335.
130. Robbins, D. R., and Alessi, N. E. (1985): *Biol. Psychiatry,* 20:107–110.
131. Rose, R. M., Holaday, J. W., and Bernstein, I. S. (1971): *Nature,* 231:366–368.
132. Roy, A. (1983): *Arch. Gen. Psychiatry,* 40:971–974.
133. Roy, A., Ågren, H., Pickar, D., Linnoila, M., Doran, A. R., Cutler, N. R., and Paul, S. M. (1986): *Am. J. Psychiatry,* 143:1539–1545.
134. Roy, A., Ninan, P., Mazonson, A., Pickar, D., van Kammen, D., Linnoila, M., and Paul, S. M. (1985): *Psychol. Med.,* 15:335–340.
135. Roy-Byrne, P., Post, R. M., Rubinow, D. R., Linnoila, M., Savard, R., and Davis, D. (1983): *Psychiatry Res.,* 10:263–274.
136. Rydin, E., Schalling, D., and Åsberg, M. (1982): *Psychiatry Res.,* 7:229–243.
137. Schalling, D. (1987): In: *Biosocial Bases of Antisocial Behavior,* edited by S. Mednick and T. Moffit. Cambridge University Press, Cambridge (*in press*).
138. Schalling, D., and Åsberg, M. (1985): In: *The Biological Bases of Personality and Behavior, Vol. 1,* edited by J. Strelau, F. H. Farley, and A. Gale, pp. 181–194. Hemisphere Publishing Corp., Washington, DC.
139. Schalling, D., Åsberg, M., Edman, G., and Levander, S. (1984): *Clin. Neuropharmacol.,* 7(Suppl. 1):746–747.
140. Schalling, D., Åsberg, M., Edman, G., and Rydin, E. (1985): Presented at the 2nd Meeting of the International Society for the Study of Individual Differences, Barcelona, 1985.
141. Schalling, D., Cronholm, B., and Åsberg, M. (1975): In: *Emotions, Their Parameters and Measurement,* edited by L. Levi, pp. 603–617. Raven Press, New York.
142. Schalling, D., Edman, G., and Åsberg, M. (1983): In: *Biological Bases of Sensation Seeking, Impulsivity and Anxiety,* edited by M. Zuckerman, pp. 123–145. Laurence Erlbaum Associates, Hillsdale, NJ.
143. Schiavi, R. C., Theilgaard, A., Owen, D. R., and White, D. (1984): *Arch. Gen. Psychiatry,* 41:93–99.
144. Schooler, C., Zahn, T. P., Murphy, D. L., and Buchsbaum, M. S. (1978): *J. Nerv. Ment. Dis.,* 166:177–186.
145. Schulsinger, F., Kety, S. S., Rosenthal, D., and Wender, P. H. (1979): In: *Origin, Prevention and Treatment of Affective Disorders,* edited by M. Schou and E. Strömgren, pp. 277–287. Academic Press, London.
146. Sedvall, G., Fyrö, B., Gullberg, B., Nybäck, H., Wiesel, F.-A., and Wode-Helgodt, B. (1980): *Br. J. Psychiatry,* 136:366–374.
147. Sedvall, G., Iselius, L., Nybäck, H., Oreland, L., Oxentierna, G., Ross, S. B., and Wiesel, F. A. (1984): In: *Frontiers in Biochemical and Pharmacological Research in Depression. Adv. Biochem. Psychopharmacol.,* 39, edited by E. Usdin, M. Åsberg, L. Bertilsson, and F. Sjöqvist, pp. 79–85. Raven Press, New York.
148. Sette, M., Raisman, R., Briley, M., and Langer, S. Z. (1981): *J. Neurochem.,* 37:40–42.
149. Shaw, D. N., Camps, F. E., and Eccleston, E. G. (1967): *Br. J. Psychiatry,* 113:1407–1411.
150. Siddle, D. A. T., and Trasler, G. B. (1981): In: *Foundation of Psychosomatics,* edited by I. M. J. Christie and P. G. Mellet, pp. 283–303. Wiley, Chichester.
151. Soubrié, P. (1986): *Behav. Brain Sci.,* 9:319–334.
152. Stanley, M. (1984): *Am. J. Psychiatry,* 141:1432–1436.
153. Stanley, M., and Mann, J. J. (1983): *Lancet,* 2:214–216.
154. Stanley, M., Virgilio, J., and Gershon, S. (1982): *Science,* 216:1337–1339.
155. Stengel, E., and Cook, N. C. (1958): *Attempted Suicide.* Chapman & Hall, London.
156. Struve, F. A., Klein, D. P., Saraf, K. R., and Oaks, G. (1972): *Arch. Gen. Psychiatry,* 27:363–365.
157. Struve, F. A., Saraf, K. R., Arho, R. S., Klein, D. F., and Beche, D. R. (1977): In: *Psychopathology and Brain Dysfunction,* edited by C. Shagass, S. Gershon, and A. J. Friedhoff, pp. 199–221. Raven Press, New York.
158. Targum, S. D., Rosen, L., and Capodanno, A. E. (1983): *Am. J. Psychiatry,* 140:877–879.
159. Träskman, L., Åsberg, M., Bertilsson, L., and Sjöstrand, L. (1981): *Arch. Gen. Psychiatry,* 38:631–636.
160. Träskman, L., Tybring, G., Åsberg, M., Bertilsson, L., Lantto, O., and Schalling, D. (1980): *Arch. Gen. Psychiatry,* 37:761–767.
161. Träskman-Bendz, L., Åsberg, M., Bertilsson, L., and Thorén, P. (1984): *Acta Psychiatr. Scand.,* 69:333–342.
162. Trasler, G. (1978): In: *Psychopathic Behavior: Approaches to Research,* edited by R. D. Hare and D. Schalling, pp. 273–298. Wiley, Chichester.
163. Valzelli, L. (1981): *Psychobiology of Aggression and Violence.* Raven Press, New York.
164. van Praag, H. M. (1977): *Biol. Psychiatry,* 12:101–131.
165. van Praag, H. M. (1982): *J. Affective Disord.,* 4:275–290.
166. van Praag, H. M. (1983): *Lancet,* 2:977–978.
167. van Praag, H. M., and de Haan, S. (1979): *Psychiatry Res.,* 1:219–224.
168. van Praag, H. M., and Korf, J. (1971): *Psychopharmacologia,* 19:148–152.
169. Virkkunen, M. (1982): *Neuropsychobiology,* 8:35–40.
170. Virkkunen, M. (1983): *Br. J. Psychiatry,* 142:598–604.
171. Virkkunen, M. (1984): *Acta Psychiatr. Scand.,* 69:445–452.
172. Virkkunen, M. (1985): *Acta Psychiatr. Scand.,* 72:40–44.
173. Virkkunen, M. (1987): *Aggressive Behav.* (*in press*).
174. Virkkunen, M., and Huttunen, M. O. (1982): *Neuropsychobiology,* 8:30–34.
175. von Knorring, L., Oreland, L., and Winblad, B. (1984): *Psychiatry Res.,* 12:11–26.
176. Wägner, A., Åberg-Wistedt, A., Åsberg, M., Ekqvist, B., Mårtensson, B., and Montero, D. (1985): *Psychiatry Res.,* 16:131–139.
177. Weissman, M., Fox, K., and Klerman, G. L. (1973): *Am. J. Psychiatry,* 130:450–455.
178. West, D. J. (1965): *Murder Followed by Suicide.* Heinemann, London.
179. Wetterberg, L., Beck-Friis, L., Aperia, B., and Pettersson, U. (1979): *Lancet,* 1:1361.
180. Whitaker, P. M., Warsh, J. J., Stancer, H. C., Persad, E., and Vint, C. K. (1984): *Psychiatry Res.,* 11:127–131.
181. Wirz-Justice, A., and Richter, R. (1979): *Psychiatry Res.,* 1:53–60.
182. Wolfgang, M. E. (1958): *Patterns in Criminal Homicide.* Oxford University Press, London.
183. Yehuda, R., and Meyer, J. S. (1984): *Neuroendocrinology,* 38:25–32.
184. Yesavage, J. A., Davidson, J., Widrow, L., and Berger, P. A. (1985): *Biol. Psychiatry,* 20:222–225.
185. Zuckerman, M., Ballenger, J. C., Jimerson, D. C., Murphy, D. L., and Post, R. M. (1983): In: *Biological Bases of Sensation Seeking, Impulsivity and Anxiety,* edited by M. Zuckerman, pp. 229–248. Laurence Erlbaum Associates, Hillsdale, NJ.

Psychopharmacology:
The Third Generation of Progress,
edited by Herbert Y. Meltzer.
Raven Press, New York © 1987.

CHAPTER 66

Biological Rhythms in Psychiatry

David A. Sack, Norman E. Rosenthal, Barbara L. Parry, and Thomas A. Wehr

The observation that affective disorders recur with striking regularity (every other day, every 2 weeks, once per year (55,108,136) stimulated research into the cyclical aspects of these conditions. Rhythmic fluctuations in affective disorders could arise from an endogenous biological cycle in the systems that regulate mood or through a coupling of these systems with environmental cycles or other biological rhythms.

Endogenous biological rhythms are by definition self-sustaining and can be discriminated from passive responses to environmental changes by several characteristics. First, these variations persist when environmental conditions are held constant and the influence of all external time cues has been eliminated (*temporal isolation*). Second, the length of a biological cycle (*free-running period*), as determined in temporal isolation, must be different from the corresponding environmental cycle. For example, the human sleep-wake cycle has a period of approximately 25 hr (148), slightly longer than a solar day. If the periods of biological rhythms do not differ from the corresponding environmental cycles, one cannot be certain that subtle environmental cues are not continuing to influence the organism so as to produce a periodic pattern. Finally, since the period of a biological rhythm differs from its corresponding environmental cycle, there must be a mechanism for synchronizing the endogenous rhythm to the environment cycle, a process called *entrainment*. Light-dark transitions, duration of daylight, environmental temperature changes, and social cues are examples of recurring environmental signals or *zeitgebers* that entrain biological rhythms (103,148).

Certain forms of manic-depressive illness exhibit the formal properties of endogenous rhythms (45). When normal subjects are allowed to free-run in temporal isolation, persistent circadian variations are observed in the sleep-wake cycle, body temperature, cortisol, and a number of other variables (145,148), indicating that these rhythms are intrinsic and self-sustaining. In our laboratory we have performed similar experiments with manic-depressive patients (140). One patient, whose mood cycle was extremely rapid (approximately 6 days) during an observation period on the ward, continued to cycle between mania and depression with approximately the same frequency while in temporal isolation (see Fig. 1).

There is also evidence that manic-depressive cycles can be entrained by environmental factors. Jenner et al. (61) placed a manic-depressive who exhibited a 48-hr cycle on an artificially short day (22 hr) as part of a temporal isolation experiment. The subject, who was blind to the experimental conditions, exhibited a shortening of his mood cycle from 48 to 44 hr, the equivalent of 2 experimental (short) "days," suggesting that the mood cycle could be entrained to artificial days of varying length. Kraines (66), and Rosenthal et al. (108) have described manic-depressive patients who suffered annual recurrences of depression. In the Kraines case, the patient initially experienced summer depressions which after several years rotated to the wintertime. In Rosenthal et al. the patient's depressions recurred in the winter for many years before rotating around the year over several years. Eventually this patient returned to his previous winter pattern of depression (see

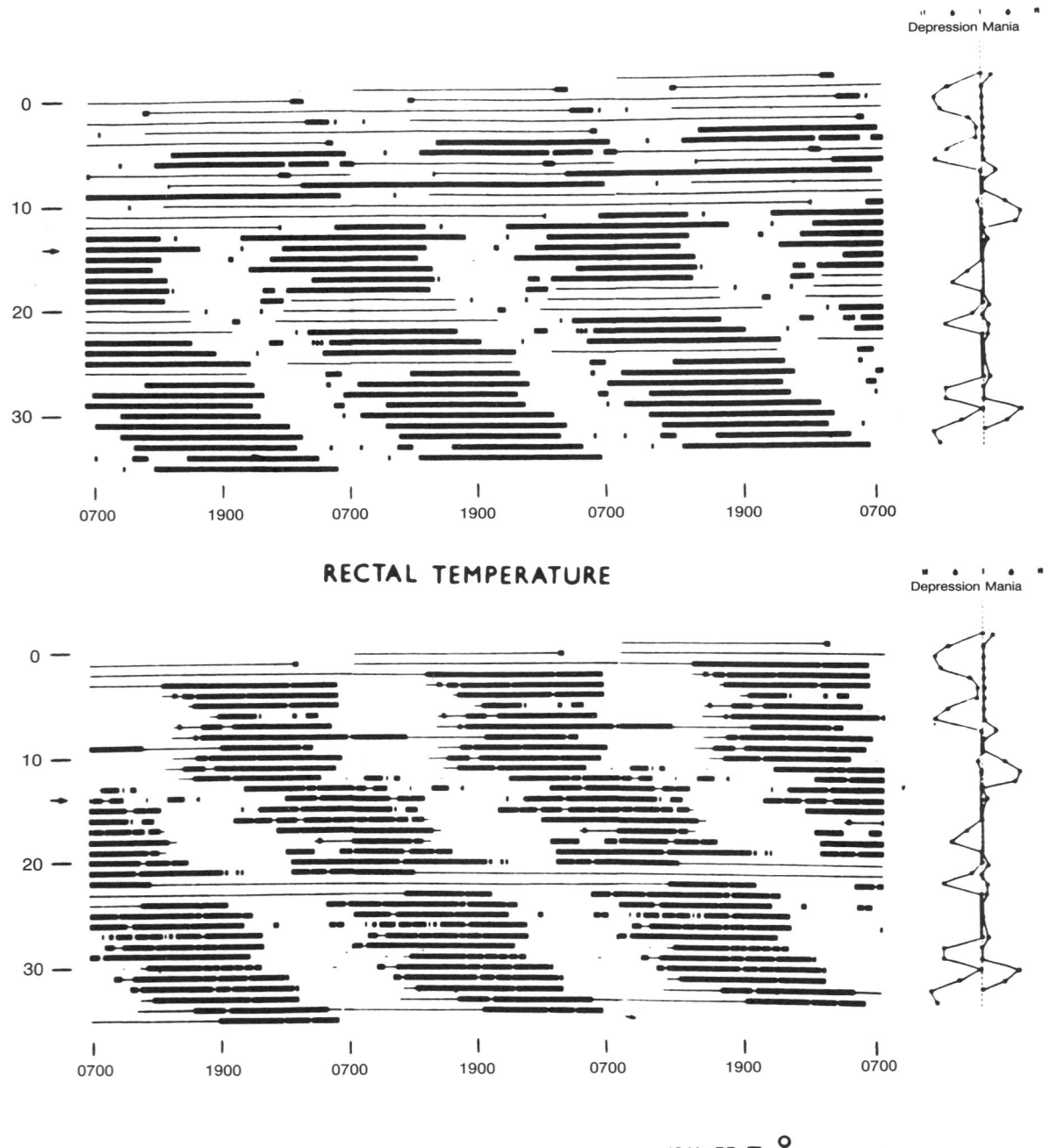

AWAKE

NURSES' RATINGS

Depression Mania

RECTAL TEMPERATURE

Depression Mania

48 Yr. BP Ⅱ ♀

Begin Isolation Day 14

FIG. 1. Sleep-wake cycle and temperature data from a rapid-cycling manic-depressive patient entrained and free-running in temporal isolation. Arrow to left indicates beginning of temporal isolation. Daily mood ratings during the experiment are shown along the right margin. Patient's mood continues to fluctuate between mania and depression while activity and temperature remain synchronized during the isolation experiment. Dark lines indicate temperature less than 37°C. (From ref. 140.)

Fig. 2). These cases suggest that the annual rhythm in mood was endogenous and was being entrained by environmental (seasonal) factors.

Clinical and epidemiological data suggest that affective syndromes may also be synchronized to other endogenous rhythms or to the environment. The tendency for depressed patients to awake late in the night and for their mood to be worse in the morning suggests an interaction between disturbed mood and circadian processes (93,99,127,139). In premenstrual syndrome there is, by definition, a close

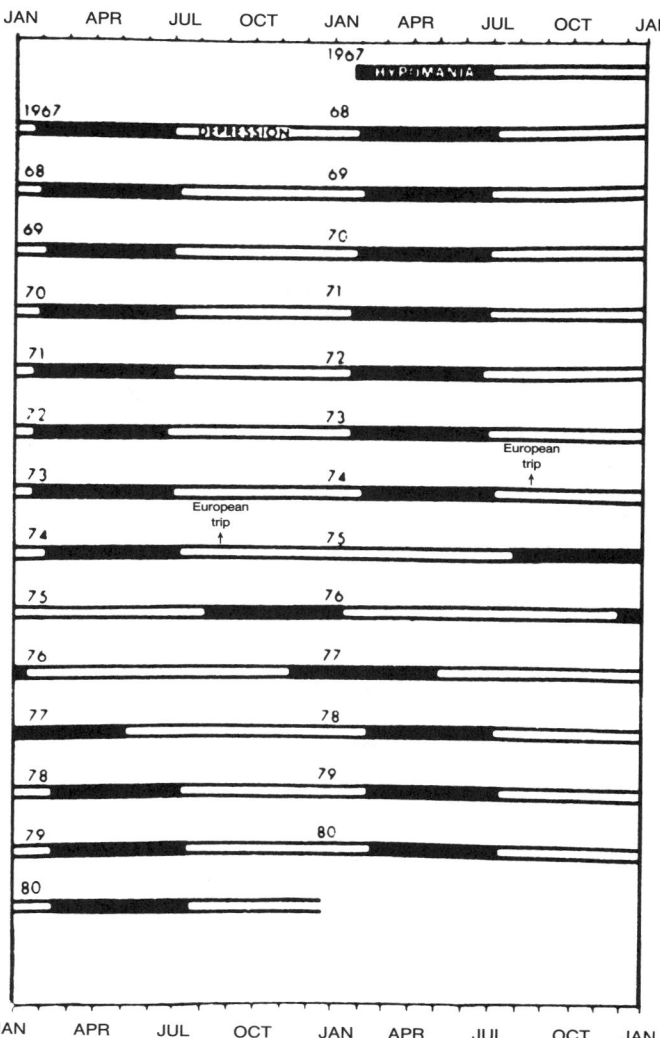

FIG. 2. After 8 years in which the patient's depressions occurred between the summer and winter solstice, the depressive episodes gradually rotated for several years before they again became associated with winter. (From ref. 111.)

relationship between a physiological cycle and alterations in mood (54). The observation that suicides occur most often in the spring (3) indicates that seasonal rhythms may also influence the course of affective disorders. In this chapter we examine the evidence that circadian, circannual, and circamenstrual processes may be involved in the pathophysiology of affective disorders.

CIRCADIAN RHYTHMS IN AFFECTIVE DISORDERS

The human circadian system has been described as consisting of two coupled biological oscillators, a strong oscillator, which controls body temperature, cortisol secretion, and rapid eye movement (REM) sleep propensity, and a weaker oscillator, which controls waking and sleeping

(144,148). This model was derived from observations of subjects living in temporal isolation, where it was noted that the rhythms in body temperature and in sleeping and waking, which are ordinarily closely associated, can become disassociated and oscillate separately, i.e., with different intrinsic periods. This process, called *internal desynchronization,* has been interpreted as evidence that these systems are regulated by separate biological clocks. More recently, Borbely (12) has proposed a two-process model of the human circadian system in which there is only one circadian oscillator. This oscillator, which regulates the threshhold for sleeping and waking, interacts with a physiological drive toward sleep, called process "S," which increases during wakefulness and is dissipated by sleep. Although a complete discussion of these models is beyond the scope of this chapter, it is worth noting that in both models the process regulating sleeping and waking is to a certain extent separable from the regulation of other circadian processes.

Several hypotheses have been advanced that attempt to explain manic-depressive cycles in terms of disturbances of the normal circadian system. Halberg (48) and others (4,69) hypothesized that manic-depressive illness could arise from internal desynchronization between the two circadian subsystems due to the fact that one oscillator is no longer being entrained to 24-hr *zeitgebers.* Wehr et al. (137) have commented on the similarity between the behavioral patterns of manic patients and the behavior of normal subjects in temporal isolation who go through long periods of wakefulness without fatigue during periods of internal desynchronization (see Fig. 3). According to the desynchronization hypothesis, switches into and out of depression would occur as the two circadian oscillators go in and out of phase with one another. Atkinson et al. (4) and Kripke et al. (69) have presented evidence suggesting that the temperature rhythm of rapid-cycling manic-depressives was not entrained to a 24-hr period but free-ran with a cycle length shorter than 24 hr. In contrast, we observed in temporal isolation no evidence of internal desynchronization in a rapid-cycling patient who continued to cycle between mania and depression (Fig. 1).

In order to explain certain characteristic sleep changes of depressed patients, i.e., short REM sleep latency, increased REM density early in the night, and reversal of the normal REM progression during the night (44), Papousek (96), Vogel (129,130), and Wehr and Goodwin (135) have hypothesized that the oscillator regulating the rhythm in REM sleep propensity may be shifted to an abnormally early time relative to sleeping and waking in depression. Since the same oscillator that regulates REM sleep also regulates the circadian rhythm in a number of other physiologic variables, Wehr and Goodwin (135) reviewed previously published circadian studies for evidence of a phase advance in depressed patients. They found that depressed patients showed advances in plasma and urinary hormones, neurotransmitter metabolites, body temperature, motor activity, and heart rate, with the magnitude of these advances ranging from 30 min to several hours.

Wehr et al. hypothesized that if a phase advance of one circadian oscillator relative to the other was etiologic in the symptomatic expression of depressive disorders, then experimental manipulations that restored a normal phase

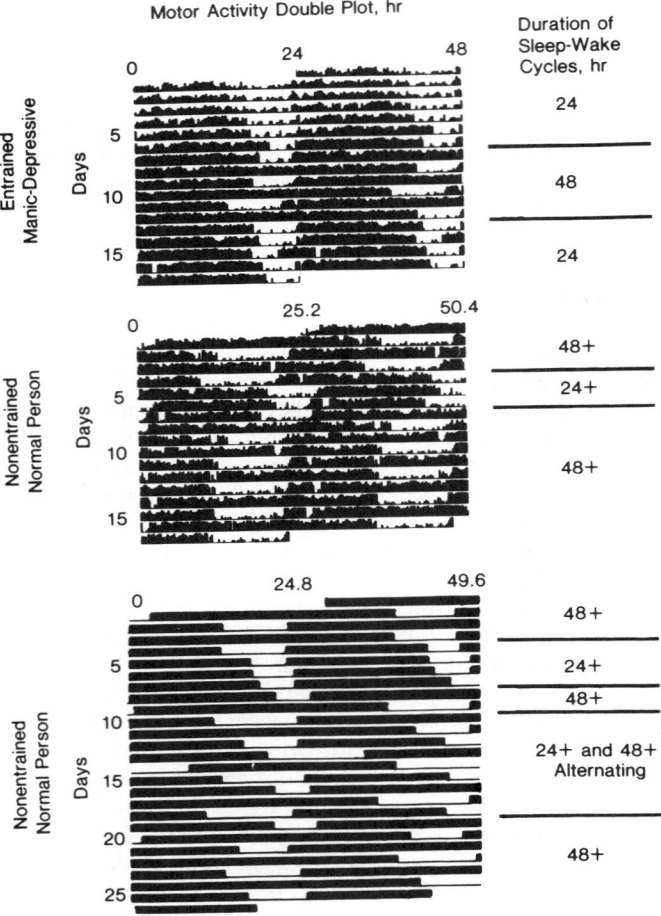

Motor Activity Double Plot, hr

Duration of Sleep-Wake Cycles, hr

FIG. 3. Double plot of motor activity of an entrained manic-depressive and a free-running (nonentrained) normal during internal desynchronization with a sleep-wake cycle of approximately 48 hr. (From ref. 137.)

relationship between the sleep-wake cycle and other circadian rhythms should have antidepressant effects (142). In order to test this hypothesis, they placed depressed patients on an experimental sleep schedule from 5 p.m. to 1 a.m. (phase-advance therapy). Consistent with their hypothesis, all four subjects improved on this regime and the antidepressant effects of this treatment have been confirmed by Sack et al. (115) and Souetre et al. (121).

Although these studies would tend to support the phase-advance hypothesis of depression, many of the studies reviewed by Wehr and Goodwin (136) suffered from serious methodological flaws. Recently more rigorous studies have appeared and it seems appropriate to review the current literature as it applies to the phase-advance hypothesis. Since the sleep abnormalities of depressed patients are extensively reviewed elsewhere in this text, we will limit our discussion to the regulation of specific hormones and body temperature.

Circadian Disturbances in the Hypothalamic-Pituitary-Adrenal Axis

Disturbances of hypothalamic-pituitary-adrenal (HPA) axis function as evidenced by increased cortisol secretion (17,20,40,113) and escape of cortisol secretion from

suppression by dexamethasone have been extensively documented in depressed patients (21). Cortisol is secreted in episodes that exhibit a circadian rhythm with peak secretion occurring in the morning shortly before waking and the nadir occurring at night, shortly after sleep onset (145). The circadian rhythm of cortisol or its metabolites has been studied in the plasma and urine of depressed patients (see Table 1). Results of eight of 14 studies performed over a 25-year period, often using different methodologies, indicated some feature of the cortisol circadian rhythm to be advanced, and nearly all reported an increase in mean secretion.

The phase of the cortisol circadian rhythm has been described in terms of its peak (acrophase), its trough (nadir), and the time at which the major nocturnal peak begins (cortisol latency), and there is evidence from circadian studies in normals that these different features of the waveform may be controlled by different physiological processes (29,30). Recent circadian studies in normals have revealed that the phase of the cortisol rhythm advances with increasing age (50,80,119). Of the studies in Table 1, only four used controls matched for age: In two other studies the authors specifically analyzed their data for the effects of age on cortisol secretion. In all of the other studies the controls were younger or their age was not stated.

If one examines only those studies in which the authors controlled the effects of age, the results are less consistent. Doig (32), sampling plasma cortisol every 3 hr, observed that the peak in cortisol secretion was shifted 3 hr earlier in seven of 10 of his depressed patients compared with surgical patients. Linkowski et al. (80) studied plasma cortisol and corticotropin (ACTH) sampled every 20 min in 18 drug-free depressed patients and seven controls of similar age and found that the cortisol nadir, but not the acrophase, was significantly advanced in the unipolar patients. Bipolar patients showed only a trend toward a significant phase advance in the cortisol nadir but showed a significant *delay* in peak cortisol secretion.

Pfohl et al. (101) reported a 2.5-hr phase advance in the cortisol nadir in a sample of predominantly unipolar depressed patients receiving psychotropic medications. Although the patients were younger than the controls, the phase advance in the patients persisted when they controlled for age. In contrast, Halbreich et al. (51) noted a 0.5-hr phase advance in the cortisol rhythm in drug-free patients but found no difference when the effects of age were controlled. One difference between these two studies is that Pfohl et al. included a higher proportion of unipolar patients (21/25 vs 20/32).

Jarret et al. (60) studied plasma cortisol secretion in 14 drug-free depressed patients and 14 controls sampled every 20 min during the night. Since the authors were primarily interested in the timing of cortisol secretion relative to sleep onset, data were presented in terms of *cortisol latency,* defined as the time after sleep onset that cortisol secretion exceeds the minimal nocturnal cortisol concentration by 2 standard deviations (a measure that is similar in phase to the cortisol peak). Although the cortisol latencies of the depressed group were shorter than those of the controls relative to sleep onset (188 min in the patients, 239 min in the controls), the timing of the cortisol rise in terms of clock hour was essentially the same in both groups (3:31

TABLE 1. Circadian corticosteroid studies[a]

First author	Ref.	Subjects No.	Subjects Age	Control No.	Control Age	Mean	Nadir	Peak	Comments
Sakai	116	12	42.5	9	30.3	—	—	D	3 normals, 6 psychiatric controls
Doig	32	10	50.9	9	49.3	Inc.	A	NC	Surgical controls
Conroy	26	6	—	10	—	Inc.	A	NC	Phase change normalizes with recovery
Sachar	113	6	55.2	8	—	Inc.	NC	C	Controls were younger; cortisol increased early in the night
Doerr	31	1	66	None		Inc.	A	NC	Depressed vs euthymic; phase advance in plasma but not in urine
Yamaguchi	154	20	36.6	10	27.4	Inc.	A	NC	Nocturnal values obtained during sleep deprivation
Branchey	13	3	50.3	None		Inc.	—	—	
Claustrat	25	11	44.5	8	27.3	Inc.	NC	D	Patients UP
Jarett	60	14	29	14	29	Inc.	—	NC	Decreased cortisol latency but time of secretion unchanged
Pfohl	101	25 21 4	42.4 UP BP	21	33.7	Inc.	A	NC	2.5-hr advance persists when age effects controlled: patients receiving TCA, lithium, and trazadone
Halbreich	51	32	42.4	72	31.2	Inc.	A	NC	Drug-free × 10 days. No phase advance when age controlled. Controls phase-advance with age
Linkowski	80	18 10 8	47.2 UP BP	7	47	Inc.	A (UP)	D (BP)	Drug free × 15 days
von Zerssen	132	10	31–69	10	26–67	Inc.	NC	NC	Urinary free cortisol

[a] Abbreviations: A, phase advance; BP, bipolar; D, phase delay; Inc., NC, no change; TCA, tricyclic antidepressants; UP, unipolar; —, not stated.

a.m. in the patients, 3:40 a.m. in the controls). Thus, the shorter *cortisol latencies* observed in the depressed patients probably resulted from their longer sleep latencies rather than from a phase advance of the cortisol rhythm defined in this way. Finally, von Zerrsen (132) examined the rhythm in urinary free cortisol in 10 patients and 10 age-matched controls and found no phase shift in either the peak or the nadir, although subjects were awakened once during the night in order to collect urine specimens and these awakenings may have altered the apparent rhythm in cortisol.

In summary, of the six studies in which the age effects on cortisol secretion were controlled for, three found a phase advance in the cortisol rhythm and three did not. Diagnostic factors may account for some of this difference, since it appears that unipolar patients are more likely than bipolar patients to show a phase advance in their cortisol rhythm (80,101). Differences could also be related to whether the peak or the nadir of the cortisol rhythm was used as a phase marker. Studies of the phase of the cortisol rhythm after transmeridian jet flights (146) and in temporal isolation (29) suggest that the cortisol nadir may be a better marker of circadian phase than the cortisol peak. When one considers the 12 studies in which the timing of the peak in cortisol secretion was examined, three report delays, eight report no change, and only one reports a phase advance.

When the nadir is examined, five of eight report a phase advance and none report a delay (Table 1).

Thus far, too few drug-free patients and age-matched controls have been studied to definitely characterize the cortisol rhythm in major depression. It seems likely that additional studies will confirm the finding of a phase advance in the cortisol nadir in endogenously depressed patients. Separate analyses of unipolar and bipolar patients are needed to further clarify the relationship between the circadian disturbance of cortisol and diagnostic subgroups. Furthermore, the different phase markers of the cortisol rhythm (peak, trough, latency) should be considered separately, since they reflect different aspects of cortisol rhythm and may be affected differently in various diagnostic subgroups.

Temperature

Body temperature exhibits a circadian rhythm with peak values occurring in the evening and lowest values occuring late in the night, usually between 3 and 6 a.m. In phase shift studies (145) and temporal isolation studies (145) the rhythm in body temperature is closely associated with the cortisol and REM sleep propensity circadian rhythms, all three of which are thought to be governed by a single circadian oscillator. Therefore, a phase disturbance in REM sleep propensity or cortisol secretion should be seen in the temperature rhythm as well. A number of authors have measured the circadian rhythm of body temperature in depressed patients either by studying a small number of subjects longitudinally or by comparing groups of depressed patients with normal controls. In the latter category some authors restudied their depressed patients following clinical recovery, and therefore these studies also provide longitudinal information (see Table 2).

Studies of depressed patients in which temperature was recorded daily over long periods of time have generally relied on oral temperature measurements (4,69,99,137). Since no measurements were obtained during sleep, these data provide information only about the temperature maxima and not the minima. Pflug found that mean body temperature was increased in affective patients and was higher during both mania and depression compared to the euthymic state. Of four subjects studied longitudinally by Pflug (99,100), three showed phase advances in their temperature maxima while depressed compared with euthymic periods (see Fig. 4). Although temperature maxima tended

TABLE 2. *Temperature*[a]

First author	Year	Patients No.	Patients Mean/age	Control No.	Control Age	Mean	Oral/ rectal	Nadir	Peak	Comments
Longitudinal studies										
Atkinson	4	3	38	—	—	—	O	—	A	
Pflug	100	1	31	—	—	Inc.	O	—	A	Included in ref. 69
Kripke	69	7	—	—	—	—	O	—	A	
Nikitopoulou	93	6	49.8	—	—	—	Axilla	*	*	Minimum occurs at more than one time during the night in depression
Wehr	139	1	49	—	—	—	O	—	A	
Pflug	100	4	46	—	—	Inc.	O	—	A	
Beersma	10	4	—			NC	R	A	NC	Mean phase of 4 recovered patients earlier when depressed
Cross-sectional studies										
Cahn	18	6	56.2	6	64.8	—	R	NC	A	3/6 advanced compared to controls
Tupin	126	11	—	5	—		O	—	NC	
Mellerup	84	55	50.5 (BP)	58	49	Inc.	O	—	A	Advanced in BP on lithium but not off lithium
Gerner	42	25	45	20	36	No diff.	O	NC	NC	Measurement obtained during sleep deprivation
Kripke	68	12	BP manic				O	—	NC	No normal controls
		12	BP depressed							
		5	UP endogenous							
		7	UP reactive							
		4	ETOH detox							
Wehr	139	10	40.0 depressed	14	21	NC	O	—	A	Significant only in manics
		8	40.0 manic				O	—	A	
Avery	5	9	50	12	52	Inc.	R	NC	NC	4/7 advanced in depression compared with recovery
Wehr	136	16	—	7	—	—	R	A	NC	Patients with bimodal temperature minima
Lee	71	10	49.1	6	41		O	—	NC	
Lund	83	7	46.1	5	42.8	—	R	NC	NC	Early minima in both patients and controls. 2/7 advanced in depression compared with recovery
von Zerssen	132	10	31–69	10	26–67	Inc.		NC	NC	

[a] Abbreviations: ETOH, ethanol; O, oral temperature; R, rectal temperature; other abbreviations as in Table 1.

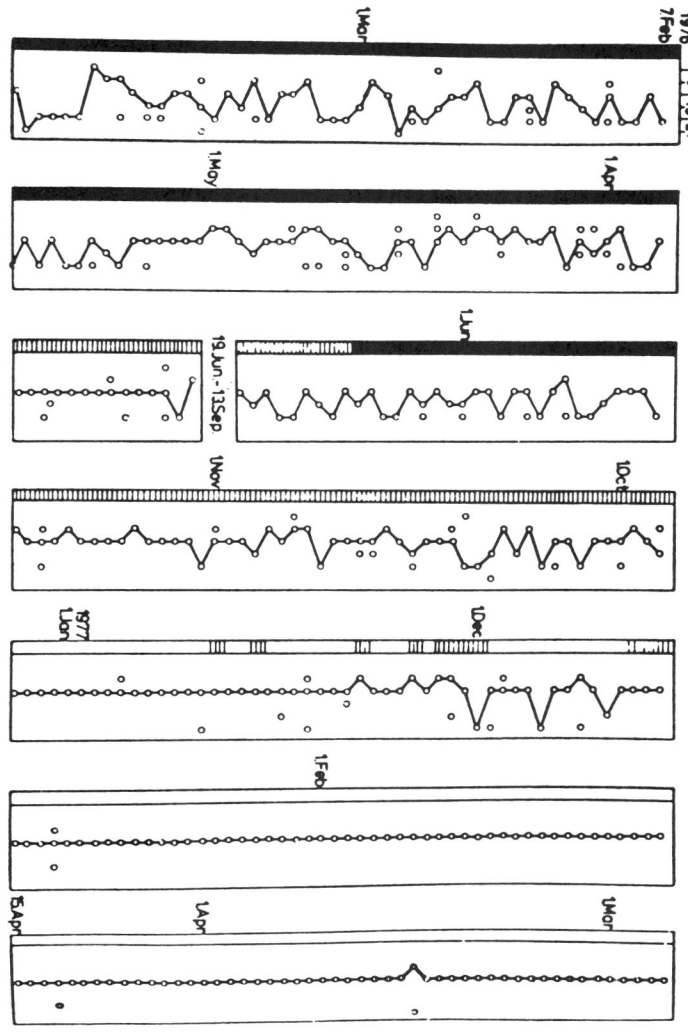

FIG. 4. Longitudinal study of the timing of the daily temperature maximum of a depressed patient plotted vertically against mood. Black bar, Depression; hatched, dysthymia; open, euthymic mood. The time of the temperature maximum is more variable and occurs earlier in depression. (From ref. 99.)

to occur earlier in depression, Pflug noted considerable day-to-day variability, with phase advances occurring during depression only about half the time. Kripke (69) and Wehr (136) both found that the timing of the temperature peak advanced during mania and was at its earliest point just prior to switches into depression. Lund et al. (83) and Avery et al. (5) studied their patients when depressed and also in the recovered state. Avery et al. found that in four of seven recovered patients the time of the temperature minimum was delayed, whereas Lund et al. found phase delays in only two of seven recovered patients.

In contrast to the longitudinal studies of body temperature, most cross-sectional studies have failed to find phase differences between patients and controls (see Table 2). Tupin et al. (126) found no difference in the phase of the temperature rhythm between controls and patients but found that the temperature rhythm was phase advanced in patients treated with lithium carbonate. Mellerup et al. (84) compared bipolar depressed patients with age-matched unipolar patients and normal controls. Both groups of depressed patients had higher mean temperatures than controls. Bipolar patients who continued to receive lithium on their usual schedule exhibited a 4-hr phase advance in

their temperature maxima compared with controls, whereas bipolars in whom lithium was delayed by 12 hr did not show a phase advance. Kripke et al. (68) compared three groups of depressed patients with a group of manic patients and a group of detoxified alcoholics and found there were no phase differences between the groups and none was phase advanced. Wehr et al. (139) compared the oral temperature rhythms of depressed and manic patients to a group of normal controls and found manics to be phase advanced compared to normals, but depressed patients showed only a trend toward phase advance. In a second study using rectal temperature measurements, Wehr et al. (136) compared 16 patients with seven young normal controls and found the distribution of temperature minima to be bimodal in the depressed patients with an early temperature minimum occurring approximately half the time, a finding consistent with the longitudinal observations of Pflug et al. (99,100). On the other hand, both Avery et al. and Lund et al. found no phase shift in their depressed patients compared with age-matched controls.

There are several possible explanations for the discrepancy between cross-sectional and longitudinal studies. Conclusions drawn from longitudinal studies have relied on the temperature maximum to determine phase, whereas cross-sectional studies that used rectal temperature measurements have usually reported on the temperature minimum. Another methodological issue is that phase advances in the temperature rhythm may be inconsistent from day to day (83,136) or may vary depending on the phase of the manic-depressive cycle, as in Kripke et al. (69) and Wehr (136). In either of these cases the results of a single night study would be less sensitive than a longitudinal study in detecting phase shifts. Finally, most patients were studied while taking psychotropic medications, and in two studies phase advances were specifically associated with lithium therapy. Lithium, monoamine oxidase inhibitors, and tricyclic antidepressants have all been shown to affect the timing of circadian rhythms in animals (38,123,141,152) and may have similar effects in humans.

Other Hormone Studies

A number of authors have investigated the circadian rhythm of the pineal hormone melatonin in depression. Melatonin plays an important role in the regulation of seasonal and circadian rhythms in animals (79), and phase disturbances in depression might be reflected in the melatonin rhythm. Melatonin has also been of interest as a system in which to test for alterations in noradrenergic activity in depression, since its nocturnal rise is mediated by β-adrenergic receptors on the pineal gland (76).

Lewy et al. (76) compared the circadian rhythm of plasma melatonin in depressed and manic bipolar patients and found that melatonin secretion occurred earlier in the depressed subjects. A number of other investigators have compared the melatonin rhythm of patients and controls, and although most studies report lower melatonin levels in depression, none have reported a phase advance in melatonin circadian rhythm (9,13,15,25,62,63,78,85,147; D. A. Sack et al., *unpublished data*). Wetterberg and Beck-Friis have noted that low melatonin levels occur most often in patients with cortisol hypersecretion, and they have hypothesized that these two abnormalities are related to one another.

Recently Touitou et al. (124) and Nair et al. (92) have reported that melatonin levels decline significantly with age and that the phase of the melatonin rhythm delays with age (92). Some (15,25), but not all (9), studies of plasma melatonin used controls that were substantially younger than patients. This would tend to bias the results toward a finding of lower levels in the patients while obscuring a possible phase advance in the melatonin rhythm. In a recent experiment we compared plasma melatonin, sampled every half-hour, in eight drug-free depressed patients and eight age-matched controls during a baseline 24-hr period and during a second 24-hr period in which subjects were sleep deprived. We found no differences in the phase, mean, or peak levels of melatonin secretion between depressed patients and controls (D. A. Sack et al., *unpublished data*).

The pituitary hormone thyrotropin (TSH) exhibits a circadian rhythm which is highest at night (28,134) but which is partially suppressed by sleep (97). Although a blunted TSH response on thyrotropin-releasing hormone

(TRH) challenge tests has been extensively described in approximately 30% of depressed patients, no difference has been observed in the basal levels of TSH between depressed patients and normal controls (81). Weeke and Weeke (133), hypothesizing that the blunted TSH responses might be associated with an abnormality of the TSH circadian rhythm, measured plasma TSH in the morning and evening in depressed patients and controls. They found that the depressed patients failed to show the normal nocturnal rise of TSH. This has since been confirmed in circadian studies of plasma TSH levels by several groups (14,46,64). Lower TSH levels were not associated with a phase advance of the TSH rhythm, although depressed patients showed more variable timing of their TSH rhythms (46,114). Low TSH levels in depression may result from elevated temperature in these patients (95).

Summary

It is difficult to draw firm conclusions about the nature of circadian rhythm disturbances in depression because the results of studies vary greatly. The present data suggest that the rhythms of temperature and cortisol are phase advanced in some depressed patients, but there is little evidence that the rhythms of other hormones are advanced. Instead it appears that the amplitude of circadian rhythms in cortisol, temperature, melatonin, and TSH are reduced and that the phase of these rhythms may be more variable in depression. The importance of phase advance in the etiology of depression is supported by the clinical efficacy of phase-advance therapy, although no studies have specifically tested for a relationship between phase advances in the cortisol-temperature-REM sleep oscillator and the clinical response to phase-advance therapy. The increased variability in hormone secretion seen in depression could also arise from an alteration in the neurotransmitters that regulate their secretion rather than from a shift in the underlying biological clock. Siever and Davis (120) have recently hypothesized that increased variability in a number of physiologic systems could arise from dysregulation of a single neurotransmitter system.

There are certain similarities between the abnormalities found in depression and the changes that occur as part of the normal aging process. The phase of the cortisol rhythm advances with age, body temperature may be higher, and the nocturnal secretion of melatonin and TSH also decreases with age. Others have commented on the similarity between the sleep of older normals and depressed patients. Gillin et al. (43) have noted that age-related changes in sleep are more marked in older depressives than in older controls, suggesting that age-related changes in the circadian system may compound the abnormalities that occur with depression.

A number of factors contribute to the lack of reproducibility in circadian studies, including small sample size, diagnostic heterogeneity, medication status, failure to age-match controls to patients, assay differences, and differences in statistical methods. Another problem in describing the phase of circadian rhythms in depressed patients is that the phase of circadian rhythms in depressed patients may be unstable rather than consistently advanced, as appears to be the case with temperature. Similarly, REM sleep parameters also vary considerably from night to night in depressives but only slightly in controls (131). To date, the circadian rhythms of plasma hormones have not been studied longitudinally for more than 1 day in depressed patients in the same clinical state and the same medication status, so it is not possible to know whether the circadian phases of these rhythms are more stable than those of temperature and REM sleep.

An additional methodological problem in clinical circadian studies is the problem of "masking" in the measurement of rhythms. The timing of a biological oscillator cannot be measured directly in humans, and the apparent changes in the phase or amplitude in the rhythm of hormones or body temperature may be caused by external and internal factors that change their levels without necessarily affecting the timing of the biological clock. These factors are responsible for what has been called masking, and they include sleep schedules, environmental temperature, physical activity, dietary habits, and lighting conditions (86,87,104,148).

Masking can be particularly problematic in depression studies, since symptoms such as weight loss, disturbed sleep, and hypoactivity might be expected to produce systematic differences in masking effects. For example, depressed patients are less active than controls during the day but are more active at night when their sleep is disturbed. Since temperature is raised by physical activity and lowered by sleep, one might suspect that the apparent differences in temperature between patients and controls could be secondary to motor retardation or disrupted sleep rather than a change in the biological clock that regulates temperature.

Minors and Waterhouse (86,87) have advocated the use of constant routines as a method for controlling for the effects of masking in circadian rhythm studies. Subjects are kept at bedrest, given equal hourly feedings, and kept continuously awake throughout the study; under these conditions it has been possible to describe what has been hypothesized to be the intrinsic component of circadian rhythms in cortisol, urinary electrolytes, and mental performance. Similar studies performed in depressives and controls could resolve some of the inconsistencies in the circadian literature and might discriminate between patient-normal differences caused by masking and those which arise from a shift in the circadian oscillator.

SEASONAL FACTORS IN AFFECTIVE DISORDERS

A relationship between the seasons and mood has been recognized since antiquity and has been the focus of systematic investigation since the nineteenth century (111). Studies of seasonality in psychiatry have examined birth patterns, hospital admissions, incidence of specific disorders, and suicide rates. In this section we review the evidence for seasonal influences in the course of affective disorders and explore possible mechanisms for this influence in a subgroup of depressed patients whose symptoms recur regularly in the winter.

The most consistent evidence that seasonal factors influence the course of affective disorders comes from studies of suicide rates. Durkheim (34) was the first to focus attention on seasonal variations in suicides, and since his seminal work a number of investigators (3) have observed a seasonal pattern in suicides with a peak occurrence in the spring. Most data are derived from northern hemisphere countries (western Europe and Japan), but Krapf (67), who studied suicide rates in Buenos Aires, Argentina, found that the suicide rate peaked in November, in late spring. These data may indicate that biological factors rather than cultural factors account for the seasonality in suicides, since Argentina has a European cultural and religious heritage. Aschoff (3) reviewed suicide data going back to the mid-nineteenth century and found that the late spring peak suicide incidence has remained remarkably consistent, but the amplitude of the annual variation in suicide has been declining since the turn of the century. Aschoff concluded that environmental factors either produce or entrain this rhythm, and he attributed the decline in amplitude to a decrease in the influence of seasonal changes in the environment, possibly because of industrialization.

Although depressions probably account for the majority of suicides (6), other psychiatric disorders contribute substantially. There is increasing evidence that suicidal behavior may be associated with certain neurochemical changes (125), which are not specifically related to affective disorders but which may occur in other violent or impulsive conditions (14). For these reasons conclusions drawn from suicide data may offer only limited insight into the seasonal variation in depression, *per se*.

Rosenthal et al. (111) reviewed the literature regarding the seasonal incidence of affective disorders. Although methodologies used in these studies and the clinical descriptions of the populations varied, a number of studies showed peaks in the hospitalization for depression in the spring and fall, whereas hospitalizations for mania were more frequent during the summer months. Diagnostic differences may account for the bimodal pattern in the seasonal occurrence of depression, since studies of bipolar patients show a bimodal distribution (1,35,39,91,107), and studies of unipolar patients (1,39) show a unimodal pattern that peaks in the spring. Eastwood and Stiasny found that "endogenous" depressives were admitted most often in the spring, but "neurotic" depressives were hospitalized most often in the fall, providing evidence that the clinical severity of depression may be an additional factor in the seasonal incidence of depression.

One problem in these data is that hospitalizations may reflect only the most severe cases and thus may be a better measure of the incidence of mania or endogenous depression than of less severe affective disorders. Another problem with these studies is the variable interval between the onset of the disorder and the time at which hospitalization occurs, which has been estimated to be approximately 1 month for mania (150) but may be several months for depression (72).

In addition to the epidemiological studies of seasonality in depression, occasional reports have appeared in the literature that describe depressed patients whose symptoms recur at a particular time of year (66,102,110). Kraepelin

(65) observed that depressions in this group frequently begin in the fall and remit by spring, and follow a less severe course than other forms of manic-depressive illness. The predictable nature of the clinical course in these patients, as well as preliminary data showing that environmental manipulations might be effective in their treatment, makes these patients valuable for studies of the seasonal aspects of affective disorders.

Seasonal Affective Disorder

Although descriptions of seasonally depressed patients have appeared sporadically in the literature, most clinicians were unfamiliar with this clinical phenomenon at the time we began our studies. For this reason we recruited patients by a variety of means, including through newspaper articles that described some of the features of previous cases. To be included in our studies patients had to meet the following criteria: (a) a history of major affective disorder, depressed, according to Research Diagnostic Criteria; (b) regularly occurring fall-winter depressions that remitted in the spring or summer for at least 2 consecutive years; and (c) absence of any other major psychiatric disorder. The clinical and demographic characteristics of patients with seasonal affective disorder (SAD) are summarized in Tables 3 and 4 (110).

Women exceeded men in our studies by a ratio of 4 to 1. Although a history of mania or hypomania was not a selection or recruitment criterion, 93% of our sample had a lifetime diagnosis of bipolar disorder (76% bipolar II; 17% bipolar I). A significant proportion of these patients (31%) had never been treated for depression, and only 10%

TABLE 3. Clinical and demographic features and family history of patients with SAD[a]

Feature	Finding
Sex	F, 86%; M, 14%
Mean ± SD age, years	36.5 ± 11.2
Mean ± SD age at onset, years	26.9 ± 13.2
Mean ± SD No. of seasonal cycles	9.5 ± 7.4
Depression milder near equator	83%
RDC diagnosis	Bipolar II, 76%
	Bipolar I, 17%
	Unipolar, 7%
Previous treatment (%)	
Antidepressants	24
Lithium carbonate	17
Thyroid	21
Hospitalization	10
ECT	0
No treatment	31
Family history[b]	
Affective disorder	69
Alcohol abuse	7
SAD	17

[a] Percentage of patients is given throughout, except as noted. Abbreviations: SAD, seasonal affective disorder; RDC, Research Diagnostic Criteria; ECT, electroconvulsive therapy.
[b] First-degree relative.

TABLE 4. Depressive symptoms of patients with SAD

Symptom	Percent of patients
Affect	
Sadness	100
Anxiety	72
Irritability	90
Physical activity decreased	100
Appetite	
Increased	66
Decreased	28
Mixed	3
No change	3
Carbohydrate craving	79
Weight	
Increased	76
Decreased	17
Mixed	3
No change	3
Sleep	
Earlier onset	79
Later waking	76
Increased sleep time	97
Change in quality (interrupted, not refreshing)	90
Daytime drowsiness	72
Decreased libido	69
Difficulties around menses	71
Work difficulties	97
Interpersonal difficulties	100

had ever been hospitalized for psychiatric treatment, which is consistent with Kraepelin's observation of a generally milder course in seasonal patients. A family history of depression was often present (69%) in first-degree relatives.

Patients with SAD report diminished activity, lethargy, decreased libido, and disturbed sleep during the winter months but also have prominent atypical vegetative features such as overeating, weight gain, hypersomnia, and a "reverse" diurnal variation in mood that worsens in the late afternoon. Unlike other patients with atypical depressions (78), SAD patients do not usually exhibit marked reactivity to psychological stimuli. Patients with SAD have normal dexamethasome suppression test (DST) responses and normal responses to TRH challenge tests (81). Electroencephalogram (EEG) sleep studies have confirmed self-reports of hypersomnia; SAD patients sleep more in the winter than in the summer. They also have higher REM density than controls in both seasons. However, we have not found that SAD patients exhibit other sleep changes associated with severe depression, such as a long sleep latency, short REM sleep latency, or early morning awakening. Thus, SAD patients differ from melancholic patients in their biological as well as clinical profiles, but resemble patients with atypical depressions.

Animal Models of SAD and the Antidepressant Effects of Light

The regular seasonal changes in SAD may be analogous to seasonal behaviors in other mammals and birds, the most widespread and conspicuous being the seasonal rhythms in reproduction. These rhythms confer an adaptive advantage on the species by insuring that offspring are born at a time when food is readily available (47). Because of the time lag involved in behaviors such as reproduction (conception must occur before the occurrence of the environmental conditions favorable to birth), many organisms have developed strategies for anticipating the environmental changes. Of the available stimuli that provide information about the seasons, the photoperiod (the illuminated part of the 24-hr day) is the most reliable and widely used in nature (47). In animals, seasonal rhythms in reproduction can be experimentally induced or suppressed by exposure to artificially short or long days (36,41,57).

Photoperiodism has been extensively studied in animals, and it appears that the effects of day length on reproduction are mediated by changes in the pattern of secretion of melatonin by the pineal gland. Light impinging on the retina sends nerve impulses along the retinohypothalamic tract to the suprachiasmatic nucleus of the hypothalamus (88). These signals are then transmitted to the pineal gland via the superior cervical ganglion, where they modify the nocturnal rise in melatonin (76). In some species longer photoperiods result in shorter durations of melatonin secretion, and it is the duration of melatonin secretion that appears to be critical in conveying information about the photoperiod to the relevant target organs. In sheep (79) and hamsters (23) it is possible to simulate the effects of photoperiod on reproduction with infusions of melatonin of appropriate duration.

The importance of photoperiodism in animals led us to consider whether artifically extending the photoperiod might have antidepressant effects in patients with SAD. Lewy et al. (77) previously demonstrated that the nocturnal secretion of melatonin is suppressed by high-intensity lighting but not by ordinary room lighting. It therefore seemed plausible that the artificial light to which patients are ordinarily exposed in their environments may be of insufficient intensity to prevent or to treat their depression but that bright light might be effective (73). This concept that the threshold for the effects of light on biological rhythms is considerably higher than the threshold for vision has been further supported by the observation of Wever (149) that the circadian rhythms of humans free running in temporal isolation can be entrained to circadian days of varying length by high-intensity lighting but not ordinary levels of artificial illumination.

After successfully treating a single patient with SAD with bright (2,500 lux) artificial light (74), we treated four groups of patients with phototherapy. In all four studies the active treatment was 2,500 lux of full-spectrum light (Vitalite) emitted from a rectangular fixture, used for approximately 5 to 6 hr per day (58,109,110). Subjects were asked to sit 3 feet away from the fixture and to glance at the lights each minute for a few seconds. A "placebo" (dim) light treatment administered in the same way was used as the control for these studies.

We found significant antidepressant effects following bright light but not dim light phototherapy in all of the above studies. More recently, others (56,75,151) have confirmed the antidepressant effects of bright light in SAD.

The clinical response to light has been remarkably similar in all of the studies. Clinical improvement occurs within the first 4 days, with full clinical remission occurring by the end of 1 week of therapy (see Fig. 5) (109). While the light treatment is continued, the antidepressant response is maintained, but relapse frequently occurs within several days following discontinuation of the light treatment. In our initial studies patients received light in the morning and in the evening. The morning treatment session usually began between 5:30 and 6:30 a.m., which was earlier than the patients' habitual wake-up time. The early timing of the morning treatment session raised the possibility that sleep deprivation (which has antidepressant effects) could have been responsible for the clinical improvement. In order to eliminate sleep deprivation as a variable, we subsequently treated a group of SAD patients with evening light alone (58), with patients maintaining their usual sleep schedules. We again found that the bright light had significant antidepressant effects but that dim light did not. This result suggests that an equivalent amount of light administered in the evening is approximately as effective as light given twice a day and that sleep deprivation is not necessary for the antidepressant effect of phototherapy. Although light treatment has been helpful in most SAD patients, some patients have not responded to phototherapy. At this time we are unable to predict which patients are most likely to benefit from this therapy.

Lewy (75) has proposed a circadian rhythm hypothesis for the syndrome of SAD. He has interpreted the hypersomnia and the reverse diurnal variation in mood seen in seasonal depressives as possible evidence of a *phase delay* in their circadian oscillator relative to the sleep-wake cycle, a pattern that is opposite to the one suggested for endogenously depressed patients (135). Based on data from primate studies that show that light administered in the morning advances certain circadian rhythms and that light administered in the evening delays them, Lewy proposed that morning phototherapy would be effective in treating SAD because it would advance the circadian rhythms to a normal phase position, but that evening light would be

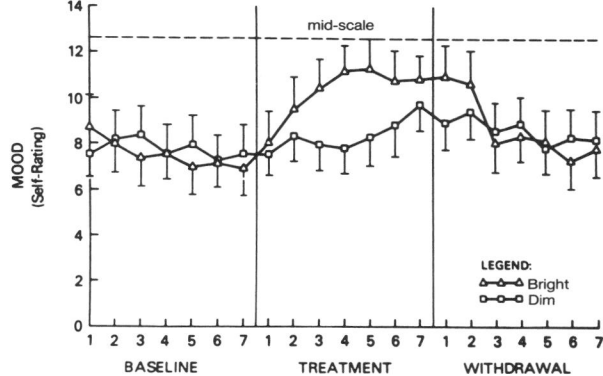

FIG. 5. Antidepressant effects of bright and dim artificial light in 15 patients with SAD as measured by mean visual analog scale (VAS). Improvement is evident following several days of bright light treatment and relapse occurs when the lights are withdrawn.

ineffective or make the symptoms worse because it would further delay the circadian rhythms. In a recent study Lewy et al. (75) treated a group of 14 SAD patients with 2 hr of light administered either in the morning or in the evening. Consistent with their prediction, patients showed significantly greater improvement when treated with morning phototherapy. This finding appears to be at odds with the finding of James et al. (58) that 5 hr of light in the evening was an effective treatment for SAD. One difference between these studies was the longer duration of light exposure in the study of James et al. (5 vs 2 hr). Thus the difference in efficacy that Lewy et al. found between morning and evening phototherapy may be relative rather than absolute.

Attempts to control for the placebo effects of a dramatic treatment such as phototherapy have not been entirely satisfactory. In our work, the response to bright light has been found to be consistently effective, whereas dim light has not. Recently, however, Wirz-Justice et al. (151) have found bright and dim light to be equally effective in the treatment of a group of SAD patients in Switzerland. Nevertheless, the consistent time course of the clinical response, and the relapse on withdrawal of phototherapy seen in our studies, would seem to make a placebo response unlikely as the sole explanation for the effects of phototherapy. As additional centers critically evaluate phototherapy, confirmatory findings would make a placebo response much less probable.

The Role of Melatonin in SAD

In view of the critical role that melatonin plays in some of the seasonal rhythms in mammals, the effective treatment of SAD by artificially extending the photoperiod immediately raises the possibility that melatonin may be responsible for the winter depressive symptoms in these patients. Effective phototherapy relies on light of sufficient intensity to suppress melatonin, whereas in most studies lower levels of light are ineffective. This finding increases the plausibility of the hypothesis that the antidepressant response to phototherapy is mediated through a reduction in the duration or timing of melatonin.

We have attempted to critically evaluate the role of melatonin in the response to phototherapy in SAD through a series of experiments. If phototherapy exerts its therapeutic effects through the suppression of melatonin, then light administered during the daytime hours, a time when melatonin is not actively secreted, should not be effective in treating depression. We recently compared the efficacy of 6 hr of phototherapy administered in the morning and evening to an equivalent amount of light administered in the middle of the day (138) and found their antidepressant effects to be approximately equal. This result indicates that suppression of melatonin is not critical for the antidepressant effects of phototherapy.

We have also explored whether exogenously administered melatonin might antagonize the antidepressant effects of phototherapy. SAD patients who had successfully been treated with phototherapy were given melatonin or placebo capsules during the phototherapy sessions. If phototherapy were acting by reducing the duration of melatonin secretion, then patients receiving melatonin but not placebo capsules would be expected to relapse into depression. Although certain symptoms, such as hypersomnia, decreased energy, hyperphagia, and carbohydrate craving, recurred while the patients were receiving melatonin but not placebo, but the mood improvement induced by phototherapy, as measured by the Hamilton rating scale, was not reversed by melatonin. This finding fails to support a central role of melatonin in SAD but might be interpreted as evidence that melatonin may have some role in the pathogenesis of specific symptoms. In a separate experiment, we further explored the role of melatonin by treating SAD with atenolol, a β-receptor antagonist that blocks the nocturnal rise of melatonin (27). Overall atenolol did not significantly reduce the severity of depression in 19 SAD patients, but a few patients who showed no change on the placebo treatment improved dramatically on atenolol.

At this time it does not appear that melatonin is central in the pathophysiology of SAD, or that phototherapy acts via photoperiodic mechanisms. Other hormones and neurotransmitters that exhibit seasonal changes may prove to be important in this syndrome. In animals prolactin and gonadotropins appear to be important in seasonal changes (33) and may play a role in SAD. The levels of the two neurotransmitters, serotonin and dopamine, exhibit seasonal variations in postmortem human brains (19), and the serotonin metabolite 5-hydroxyindoleacetic acid (5-HIAA) has a seasonal variation in human cerebrospinal fluid (82). Both of these neurotransmitters have been implicated in the etiology of mania and depression, and the seasonal changes in their levels could contribute to the seasonal pattern of SAD (122). More knowledge of the biochemical and psychophysiological correlates of phototherapy may lead to a better understanding of its mechanism of action.

PREMENSTRUAL SYNDROME: DESCRIPTION AND CHRONOBIOLOGIC ASPECTS

Premenstrual affective syndrome (PMS) is a form of rapid-cycling mood disorder that occurs in association with the menstrual cycle. The diagnosis of PMS is based not only on the nature and severity of symptoms, but also on the presence of a consistent pattern of remission and relapse of symptoms linked to specific phases of the menstrual cycle. It is desirable to base the diagnosis on prospective daily ratings over several cycles, since only 50% of retrospective reports of PMS are confirmed by daily ratings (37). Symptoms generally include irritability, changes in mood (depression, anxiety), cognitive alterations (difficulty concentrating, negative self-perception), disturbances in sleep, appetite, and energy, and other somatic disturbances (weight gain, breast swelling, and tenderness). Halbreich et al. (53) have suggested that premenstrual depressive features could be differentiated into three main subtypes characterized by (a) atypical depressive features (hypersomnia and increased appetite), (b) hostility, and (c) anxiety. These subtypes have not yet been validated.

The relation of PMS to other psychiatric syndromes is unclear. Many psychiatric illnesses (affective disorder, schizophrenia, eating disorders, anxiety disorders, and obsessive-compulsive disorders) and medical illnesses (migraine, seizures, allergies) can be exacerbated premenstrually. A link between PMS and major depressive disorder (MDD) is suggested by Halbreich and Endicott's (52) finding that 84% of women with premenstrual depressive syndrome also had a prior history of major depressive disorder and 57% of women with a lifetime diagnosis of MDD met criteria for premenstrual depressive syndrome. Comparable figures for normal subjects were 9 and 14%, respectively.

A relationship between PMS and SAD is suggested by the fact that approximately 50% of women with SAD also have PMS (110). Furthermore, we recently identified a patient with a seasonal form of PMS who suffered from severe premenstrual depressions in the fall and winter that remitted spontaneously in the spring and summer. Phototherapy in the winter alleviated her symptoms. Furthermore, the therapeutic effect of light could be blocked by simultaneous administration of melatonin. Propranolol and atenolol, which suppress melatonin secretion, had a therapeutic effect similar to that of light. Patients whose cyclic symptoms of PMS occur only in the fall and winter are analogous to patients described by Gjessing (45) whose cycles of periodic catatonia or rapid-cycling manic-depressive illness occurred only in the fall and winter.

Affective illness occurs in association with other alterations in reproductive function, such as those induced by oral contraceptives, abortion, the postpartum period, and menopause. It may be that the clinical phenomenology and biologic substrates of affective changes occurring in association with PMS are related to those associated with other aspects of reproductive function.

It is unclear whether the cyclicity of affective symptoms in PMS arises from a potentially independent mood cycle's having become synchronized or entrained by the menstrual cycle or is a direct expression of hormonal changes that are part of the menstrual cycle. The latter interpretation is supported by Muse et al. (90), who report alleviation of PMS symptoms by "medical ovariectomy" (elimination of the pulsatile release of gonadotropins required for cyclic ovarian function by chronic administration of gonadotropin-releasing hormone). On the other hand, there are reports of PMS occuring in anovulatory cycles, and oral contraceptives do not consistently eliminate PMS symptoms. There are also anecdotal reports of cyclic disturbances of mood occurring after cessation of ovarian function (oophorectomy and menopause). In these cases the cyclic programming of the hypothalamus, rather than the ovary, may be responsible for the persistent cyclicity of affective changes.

Theories of Pathophysiology

There are several theories about the pathogenesis of PMS, none of which has been substantiated (54).

Gonadal Steroids

Various studies have examined the possible role of gonadal hormones in the pathogenesis of PMS. Although no firm conclusions can be drawn because of methodological problems, these studies generally suggest a progesterone deficiency relative to estrogen in the luteal phase in those women reporting premenstrual symptoms. Exogenous estrogen has been reported to induce symptoms of PMS. The major problem with this theory as a single hypothesis for PMS is that progesterone is also deficient relative to estrogens in the follicular phase of the cycle when there is a relative absence of symptoms. Although androgens also vary with the menstrual cycle, they have not been studied in patients with PMS.

Prolactin

Some studies show an increase in prolactin in the luteal phase in PMS patients (54). One investigator found that women with PMS (of variable symptomatology) had higher prolactin levels throughout the cycle as compared to non-symptomatic women, and the levels were increased premenstrually. Bromocriptine, a dopamine agonist that lowers prolactin, has been shown to alleviate premenstrual symptoms in some studies (22).

On the other hand, not all studies show a consistent luteal elevation in prolactin in PMS (22). One modified hypothesis is that the level of prolactin in relation to estrogen and progesterone affects the type of psychological symptoms reported premenstrually, but this remains to be demonstrated.

Mineralocorticoids

Because of symptoms related to fluid retention, a mineralocorticoid hypothesis of premenstrual changes has been proposed. Progesterone causes a loss of sodium in the urine during the lueteal phase that may trigger the subsequent release of renin, angiotensin, and aldosterone. A luteal rise in renin, angiotensin, and aldosterone has been correlated with negative moods, with weight gain, and with the ratio of K/Na excreted in the urine. These findings led Janowsky et al. (59) to suggest that premenstrual mood and behavior changes might be due to central nervous system effects of angiotensin, possibly mediated by cholinergic mechanisms. Although diuretics do not generally diminish dysphoric mood, O'Brien (94) reported that the diuretic spironolactone, an aldosterone antagonist, relieved the symptoms of PMS. In contrast to these findings, women with Conn's syndrome, where aldosterone levels are also high, do not report psychological disturbance.

Prostaglandins

Prostaglandin inhibitors are effective in treating dysmenorrhea, the cramping pain associated with the onset of menses (153); whether or not these agents might also prove effective for PMS is an open question. Since prostaglandins generally increase in the luteal phase and decline during menses, this possibility has some physiologic basis but requires substantiation.

Endogenous Opiates

Since several premenstrual symptoms mimic those of narcotic withdrawal, some investigators have wondered whether a decline in endogenous opiates occurs premenstrually in association with symptomatology (105). Plasma and cerebrospinal fluid (CSF) studies of β-endorphin levels have failed to substantiate this hypothesis. In fact, when symptomatology did increase in association with β-endorphin changes premenstrually, the correlation was in a direction opposite to that predicted.

Biogenic Amines

Gonadal steroids affect brain serotonin, dopamine, norepinephrine, and acetylcholine receptors and turnover. Since these neurotransmitters are thought to play a role in regulating mood and behavior in affective disorders, researchers have also explored their possible role in premenstrual affective symptomatology. Various monoamines appear to be involved in regulating the menstrual cycle, with a prominent effect of norepinephrine (NE) on the luteinizing hormone (LH) surge. Furthermore, the following substances reflecting biogenic amine metabolism vary across the menstrual cycle: urinary and CSF 3-methoxy-4-hydroxyphenylglycol (MHPG), the central metabolite of norepinephrine, serotonin and its major metabolite 5-HIAA, and monoamine oxidase.

The specific nature of the reciprocal interactions between gonadal hormones and monoamines represents a new frontier for research on menstrual-related mood and behavior changes.

Other

A variety of other substances, such as glucocorticoids and melatonin (112), fluctuate across the menstrual cycle and may be found to play a role in the pathogenesis of PMS.

Methodologic Problems in the Study of PMS: A Chronobiologic Perspective

Studies that use single time points to determine measurements of physiological variables are inadequate to describe a biological process that varies continuously over the course of a month. To identify correlates of the menstrual cycle, spans between measurements should be no more than 7 days. A second problem is that menstrual cycle lengths vary between cycles and between individuals. In PMS research, different or inadequate methods for ascertaining menstrual cycle phase or accounting for variation in total cycle length may be responsible for inconsistency of findings. The same cycle day may reflect different menstrual cycle phases in women with different cycle lengths. Thus, reliance on external time markers rather than internal ones can increase variability due to menstrual phase differences between individuals. To standardize menstrual phase definitions, it is desirable to relate menstrual

day to menstrual stage using cytological, hormonal, or body temperature measurements. To further reduce variability due to phase differences arising from biological rhythms, month of the year should be reported, since there may be circannual changes in menstrual rhythms (106).

Variation due to circadian rhythms is often quite large and may be greater than that associated with the menstrual cycle or PMS. For example, prolactin, which has been a focus of investigation and theory in PMS, exhibits plasma levels that are many times higher during sleep at night than during wakefulness in the daytime. Studies that examine only morning (basal) prolactin values may miss important fluctuations occurring across the menstrual cycle. Twenty-four-hour profiles of variables of interest at weekly intervals throughout the menstrual cycle would provide a more sensitive measure of change in these systems and could provide new insights into interactions between the menstrual and circadian systems in PMS.

Treatment

Many treatments have been proposed for PMS but none has proven consistently effective. These treatments include diet (restriction of carbohydrates or salt), vitamins (pyridoxine), diuretics, prostaglandin inhibitors, progesterone, bromocriptine, lithium, and other conventional thymoleptic therapies (54). One methodological problem is the high placebo response rate (approximately 60%) in PMS.

Although PMS patients do not exhibit sleep disturbances similar to those occuring in major depressive disorder, we wondered whether sleep deprivation, a treatment with acute antidepressant effects, might also be effective in PMS. In a preliminary study we found that PMS patients respond to total and partial sleep deprivation (98), a finding that strengthens the link between PMS and other affective syndromes. An antidepressant response to sleep deprivation is also consistent with the hypothesis that increased prolactin secretion is involved in the pathogenesis of PMS, since sleep deprivation profoundly lowers prolactin levels. Since PMS episodes are relatively short, total or partial sleep deprivation may prove to be a viable clinical treatment for this disorder.

CONCLUSIONS

Biological rhythms appear to play a role in the clinical course and pathophysiology of affective disorders. Circadian, seasonal, and circamenstrual changes are a part of normal human physiology, and the cyclical recurrences seen in manic-depressives may reflect an interaction between the illness and other biological rhythms. The regulation of the circadian rhythms in a number of hormones and in sleep appears to be disturbed in patients with endogenous depression, and analogous disturbances in circannual and circamenstrual rhythms may be found for SAD and PMS. A chronobiological approach to these disorders has led to new therapeutic modalities such as phase-advance therapy of depression and phototherapy of SAD, but the mechanism of action of these treatments remains unknown. Further work is needed to clarify how changes associated with biological rhythms may interact with neurotransmitter and neuropeptide systems to produce symptoms in these disorders. When the pharmacology of biological rhythms is better understood, it may be possible to develop novel drug therapies that imitate the effects of phase shifts or phototherapy.

REFERENCES

1. Angst, J., Grof, P., Hippies, H., Poldinger, W., and Weis, P. (1968): In: *Symposium Bel-Air III*, Masson, Geneva.
2. Arora, R. C., Kregel, L., and Meltzer, H. Y. (1980): *Biol. Psychiatry*, 6:795–804.
3. Aschoff, J. (1981): In: *Handbook of Behavioral Neurobiology, Vol. 4*, edited by J. Aschoff, pp. 475–487. Plenum Press, New York.
4. Atkinson, M., Kripke, D. F., and Wolf, S. R. (1975): *Chronobiologia*, 2:325–335.
5. Avery, D. H., Wildschiltz, G., and Rafaelson, O. J. (1982): *J. Affective Disord.*, 4:61–71.
6. Barraclough, B. M., Bunch, J., Nebon, B., and Sawsbury, P. (1974): *Br. J. Psychiatry*, 125:355–373.
7. Beck-Friis, J., Hanssen, T., Kjellman, B. F., Ljunggren, J.-G., Unden, F., and Wetterberg, L. (1983): In: *Melatonin in Depressive Disorders: A Methodological and Clinical Study of the Pineal-Hypothalamic-Pituitary-Adrenal Cortex System*, pp. 87–89. Modik-Tryck AB, Stockholm.
8. Beck-Friis, J., Ljunggren, J.-G., Thoren, M., von Rosen, D., Kjellman, B., and Wetterberg, L. (1985): *Psychoneuroendocrinology*, 71:319–330.
9. Beck-Friis, J., von Rosen, D., Kjellman, B. F., Ljunggren, J.-G., and Wetterberg, L. (1984): *Psychoneuroendocrinology*, 9:261–277.
10. Beersma, D. G. M., vanden Hoofdakker, R. H., and van Berkestijn, H. W. B. M. (1983): *Adv. Biol. Psychiatry*, 11:114–127.
11. Bittman, E. L., Dempsey, R. J., and Karsch, R. J. (1983): *Endocrinology*, 113:2276–2283.
12. Borbely, A. A. (1982): *Hum. Neurobiol.*, 1:195–204.
13. Branchey, L., Weinberg, U., Branchey, M., Linkowski, P., and Mendlewicz, J. (1982): *Neuropsychobiology*, 8:225–232.
14. Brown, G. L., Goodwin, F. K., Ballenger, J. C., Goyer, P. F., and Major, L. F. (1979): *Psychiatry Res.*, 1:131.
15. Brown, R., Kocsis, J. H., Caroff, S., Amsterdam, J., Winokur, A., Stokes, P. E., and Frazer, A. (1985): *Am. J. Psychiatry*, 142:811–816.
16. Bunner, D. L., Morris, E., and Smallridge, R. C. (1984): *Metabolism*, 33:337–341.
17. Bunney, W. E., Jr., Hartmann, E. L., and Mason, J. W. (1965): *Arch. Gen. Psychiatry*, 12:619–625.
18. Cahn, H. A., Folk, E., and Huston, P. E. (1968): *Aerospace Med.*, 39:608–610.
19. Carlsson, A., Svennerholm, L., and Windblad, B. (1980): *Acta Psychiatr. Scand.*, 61:75–85.
20. Carroll, B. J., Curtis, G. C., Davies, B. M., Mendels, J., and Sugerman, A. A. (1976): *Psychol. Med.*, 6:43–50.
21. Carroll, B. J., Curtis, G. C., and Mendels, J. (1976): *Arch. Gen. Psychiatry*, 33:1051–1058.
22. Carroll, B. J., and Steiner, M. (1978): *Psychoneuroendocrinology*, 3:171–180.
23. Carter, D. S., and Goldman, B. S. (1983): *Endocrinology*, 113:1261–1265.
24. Christensen, P., Gram, L. F., Kragh-Sorensen, P., Christensen, L., Kristensen, C. B., Pedersen, O. L., and Thomsen, H. Y. (1985): *J. Affective Disord.*, 8:271–278.
25. Claustrat, B., Chazot, G., Brun, J., Jordan, D., and Sassolas, G. (1984): *Biol. Psychiatry*, 19:1215–1228.
26. Conroy, R. T. W. L., Hughes, B. D., and Mills, J. N. (1968): *Br. Med. J.*, 3:405–407.
27. Cowen, P. J., Fraser, S., Sammous, and Green, A. R. (1983): *Br. J. Clin. Pharmacol.*, 15:579–581.
28. Cuestro, N., and Scaglione, R. (1980): *Acta Endocrinol.*, 95:465–471.
29. Czeisler, C. A. (1978): Ph.D. Thesis, Stanford University.
30. Czeisler, C. A., Zimmerman, J. C., Ronda, J. M., Moore-Ede, M. C., and Weitzman, E. D. (1980): *Sleep*, 2:329–346.
31. Doerr, P., von Zerssen, D., Fischler, M., and Schulz, H. (1979): *J. Affective Disord.*, 1:93–104.
32. Doig, R. J., Mummery, R. V., Willis, M. R., and Elkes, A. (1966): *Br. J. Psychiatry*, 112:1263–1267.
33. Duncan, M. J., and Goldman, B. D. (1985): *Am. J. Physiol.*, 248:R664–R667.
34. Durkheim, E. (1897): *Le Suicide*. Translated (1952) as *Suicide: A Study in Sociology*, by J. A. Spaulding and C. Simpson. Routledge and Kegan Paul, London.
35. Eastwood, M. R., and Stiasny, S. (1978): *Arch. Gen. Psychiatry*, 35:769–771.
36. Elliott, J. A. (1976): *Fed. Proc.*, 35:2339–2346.
37. Endicott, J., and Halbreich, U. (1982): *Psychopharmacol. Bull.*, 18:109–112.
38. Engelmann, W., Bollig, I., and Hartmann, R. (1973): *Arzeinimittelforsch.*, 26:17.
39. Frangos, E., Athanassenas, G., Tsitourides, S., Psilolignos, P., Robos, A., Katsanou, N., and Bulgaris, C. (1980): *J. Affective Disord.*, 2:239–247.
40. Fullerton, D. T., Wenzel, F. J., Lohrenz, F. N., and Fohs, H. (1968): *Arch. Gen. Psychiatry*, 19:674–681.
41. Gaston, S., and Menaker, M. (1968): *Science*, 160:1125–1127.
42. Gerner (1979): *J. Psychiat. Res.*, 15:21–40.
43. Gillin, J. C., Duncan, W. C., Murphy, D. L., Post, R. M., Wehr, T. A., Goodwin, F. K., Wyatt, R. J., and Bunney, W. E., Jr. (1981): *Psychiatry Res.*, 4:73–78.
44. Gillin, J. C., Sitaram, N., Wehr, T. A., Duncan, W., Post, R., Murphy, D. L., Mendelson, W. B., Wyatt, R. J., and Bunney, W. E., Jr. (1984): In: *Neurobiology of Mood Disorders*, edited by R. M. Post and J. C. Ballenger, pp. 157–189. Williams and Wilkins, Baltimore.
45. Gjessing, R. R. (1976): In: *Contribution to the Somatology of Periodic Catatonia*, edited by L. R. Gjessing and F. A. Jenner, pp. 40–67. Pergamon Press, Oxford.
46. Golstein, J., Van Cauter, E., Linkowski, P., Vanhaelst, L., and Mendlewicz, J. (1980): *Life Sci.*, 27:1695–1703.
47. Gwinner, E. (1981): In: *Handbook of Behavioral Neurobiology, Vol. 4*, edited by J. Aschoff, pp. 391–408. Plenum Press, New York.
48. Halberg, F. (1968): In: *Symposium Bel-Air III*, pp. 73–126. Masson, Geneva.
49. Halbreich, U., Grunhaus, I., and Ben-David, B. (1979): *Arch. Gen. Psychiatry*, 36:1183–1186.
50. Halbreich, U., Asnis, G. M., Shindledecker, R., Zumoff, B., and Nathan, R. S. (1985): *Arch. Gen. Psychiatry*, 42:904–908.
51. Halbreich, U., Asnis, G. M., Shindledecker, R., Zumoff, B., and Nathan, R. S. (1985): *Arch. Gen. Psychiatry*, 42:909–914.
52. Halbreich, U., and Endicott, J. (1985): *Acta Psychiatr. Scand.*, 77:331–338.
53. Halbreich, U., Endicott, J., and Nee, J. (1983): *Arch. Gen. Psychiatry*, 77:535–542.
54. Hamilton, J. A., Parry, B. L., Alagna, S., Blumenthal, A., and Herz, E. (1984): *Psychiatr. Ann.*, 14:426–435.
55. Hanna, S. M., Jenner, F. A., Pearson, I. B., Sampson, G. A., and Thompson, E. A. (1972): *Br. J. Psychiatry*, 121:271–280.
56. Hellekson, C. J., Fairbanks, A. K., and Rosenthal, N. E. (1985): In: *IVth World Congress of Biological Psychiatry Abstracts*, p. 328, Philadelphia.
57. Hoffman, K. (1981): In: *Handbook of Behavioral Neurobiology, Vol. 4*, edited by J. Aschoff, pp. 449–473. Plenum Press, New York.
58. James, S. P., Wehr, T. A., Sack, D. A., Parry, B. L., and Rosenthal, N. E. (1985): *Br. J. Psychiatry*, 147:424–428.
59. Janowsky, D. S., Berens, S. C., and Davis, J. M. (1973): *Psychosom. Med.*, 35:143–153.
60. Jarett, D. B., Coble, P. A., and Kupfer, D. J. (1983): *Arch. Gen. Psychiatry*, 40:506–511.
61. Jenner, F. A., Gjessing, L. R., Cox, J. R., Davies-Jones, A.,

Hullin, R. P., and Hanna, S. M. (1967): *Br. J. Psychiatry,* 113: 895–910.

62. Kijne, B., Aggernaes, H., Fog-Moffler, F., Andersen, J. N., Kirkegaard, C., and Bjorum, N. (1982): *Psychiatry Res.,* 6:277–282.

63. Kirkegaard, C., Faber, J., Hummer, L., and Rogowski, P. (1979): *Psychoneuroendocrinology,* 4:227–235.

64. Kjellman, B. F., Beck-Friis, J., Ljunggren, J.-G., and Wetterberg, L. (1984): *Acta Psychiatr. Scand.,* 69:491–502.

65. Kraeplin, E. (1921): *Manic Depressive Insanity and Paranoia.* Translated by R. M. Barclay, edited by G. M. Robertson. E. and S. Livingstone, Edinburgh.

66. Kraines, S. (1957): *Mental Depressions and Their Treatment.* Macmillan, New York.

67. Krapf, E. E. (1937): *Revista Neurol. (Buenos Aires),* 2:107–112.

68. Kripke, D. F., Mullaney, D. J., Atkinson, M. L., Huey, L. Y., and Hubbard, B. (1979): *Chronobiologia,* 6:365–375.

69. Kripke, D. F., Mullaney, D. J., Atkinson, M., and Wolf, S. (1978): *Biol. Psychiatry,* 13:335–350.

70. Kripke, D. F., Risch, S. C., and Janowsky, D. S. (1983): *Psychiatry Res.,* 10:105–112.

71. Lee, M. A., and Taylor, M. A. (1983): *Biol. Psychiatry,* 18:1127–1132.

72. Leutold, G. H. (1940): *Arch. Psychiatr. Nervenkr.,* 111:55–61.

73. Lewy, A. J. (1984): In: *Neurobiology of Mood Disorders,* edited by R. M. Post and J. C. Ballenger, pp. 207–214. Williams and Wilkins, Baltimore.

74. Lewy, A. J., Kern, H. A., Rosenthal, N. E., and Wehr, T. A. (1982): *Am. J. Psychiatr.,* 139:1496–1498.

75. Lewy, A. J., Sack, R. L., and Singer, C. (1985): Presented at the 138th annual meeting of the American Psychiatric Association (New Research), Dallas.

76. Lewy, A. J., Wehr, T. A., Gold, P. W., and Goodwin, F. K. (1979): In: *Catecholamines: Basic Clinical Frontiers, Vol. 2,* edited by E. Usdin, I. J. Kopin, and J. Barches, pp. 1173–1175. Pergamon Press, Oxford.

77. Lewy, A. J., Wehr, T. A., Goodwin, F. K., Newsome, D. A., and Marky, S. P. (1980): *Science,* 210:1267–1269.

78. Liebowitz, M. R., Quitkin, F. M., Stewart, J. W., McGrath, P. J., Harrison, W., Rabkin, J., Tricamo, E., Markowitz, J. S., and Klein, D. F. (1984): *Arch. Gen. Psychiatry,* 41:669–677.

79. Lincoln, G. A., and Short, R. V. (1980): In: *Recent Progress in Hormone Research,* edited by R. O. Greep, pp. 1–52. Academic Press, New York.

80. Linkowski, P., Mendlewicz, J., Leclercq, R., Basseur, M., Hubain, P., Golstein, J., Copinschi, G., and Van Cauter, E. (1985): *J. Clin. Endocrinol. Metab.,* 61:429–438.

81. Loosen, P. T., and Prange, A. J. (1982): *Am. J. Psychiatry,* 139:405–415.

82. Losonsky, M. F., Mohs, R. C., and Davis, K. L. (1984): *Psychiatry Res.,* 12:79–87.

83. Lund, R., Kammerloher, A., and Dirlich, G. (1983): In: *Circadian Rhythms in Psychiatry,* edited by T. A. Wehr and F. K. Goodwin, pp. 75–88. Boxwood Press, Pacific Grove, CA.

84. Mellerup, E. T., Widding, A., Wildschiodtz, G., and Rafaelson, O. J. (1978): *Acta Pharmacol. Toxicol.,* 42:157–161.

85. Mendlewicz, J., Branchey, L., Weinberg, U., Branchey, M., Linkowski, R., and Weitzman, E. D. (1980): *Commun. Psychopharmacol.,* 4:49–55.

86. Minors, D. S., and Waterhouse, J. M. (1984): *Experientia,* 40:410–422.

87. Minors, D. S., and Waterhouse, J. M. (1984): *Chronobiol. Int.,* 1:205–216.

88. Moore, R. Y. (1978): In: *Frontiers in Neuroendocrinology, Vol. 5,* edited by F. W. Ganong and L. Martini, pp. 185–206. Raven Press, New York.

89. Mosko, S. S., Holowach, J. B., and Sassin, J. F. (1983): *Sleep,* 6:137–146.

90. Muse, K. N., Cetel, N. S., Futterman, L. A., and Yen, S. C. (1984): *N. Engl. J. Med.,* 311:1345–1349.

91. Myers, D. H., and Davies, P. (1978): *Psychol. Med.,* 8:433–440.

92. Nair, N. P. V. (1985): Presented at the 138th annual meeting of the American Psychiatric Association (New Research), Dallas.

93. Nikitopoulou, G., and Crammer, J. L. (1976): *Br. Med. J.,* 1:1311–1314.

94. O'Brien, P. M. S., Craven, D., Selby, C., and Symonds, E. M. (1979): *Br. J. Obstet. Gynaecol.,* 86:142–147.

95. O'Malley, B. P., Richardson, A., Cook, N., Parker, D. C., Pekary, A. E., and Hershman, J. M. (1976): *J. Clin. Endocrinol. Metab.,* 43:318–329.

96. Papousek, M. (1975): *Fortschr. Neurol. Psychiatr.,* 43:381–440.

97. Parker, D. C., Pekary, A. E., and Hershman, J. M. (1976): *J. Clin. Endocrinol. Metab.,* 43:318–329.

98. Parry, B. L., and Wehr, T. A. (1985): Presented at the annual meeting of the American College of Neuropharmacology.

99. Pflug, B., Engelmann, W., and Gaertner, H.-J. (1982): *J. Neural Transm.,* 53:213–215.

100. Pflug, B., Erikson, R., and Johnsson, A. (1976): *Acta Psychiatr. Scand.,* 54:254–266.

101. Pfohl, B., Sherman, B., Schlechte, J., and Stone, R. (1985): *Arch. Gen. Psychiatry,* 42:897–903.

102. Pilcz, A. (1901): *Die periodischen Geistesstorungen.* Verlag Fischer, Jena.

103. Pittendrigh, C. S. (1981): In: *Handbook of Behavioral Neurobiology, Vol. 4,* edited by J. Aschoff, pp. 95–124. Plenum Press, New York.

104. Prinz, P. N., Christie, C., Smallwood, R., Vitaliano, P., Bokan, J., Vitiello, M. V., and Martin, D. (1984): *J. Gerontol.,* 1:30–35.

105. Reid, R. L., and Yen, S. S. C. (1981): *Am. J. Obstet. Gynecol.,* 139:85–104.

106. Reinberg, A., and Smolensky, H. (1974): In: *Biorhythms and Human Reproduction,* edited by M. Ferin, F. Halberg, R. M. Richart, and R. L. Van DeWiele, pp. 241–258. John Wiley & Sons, New York.

107. Rihmer, Z. (1980): *Psychiatry Res.,* 3:247–251.

108. Rosenthal, N. E., Lewy, A. J., Wehr, T. A., Kern, H. E., and Goodwin, F. K. (1983): *Psychiatry Res.,* 8:25–31.

109. Rosenthal, N. E., Sack, D. A., Carpenter, C. J., Parry, B. L., Mendelson, W. B., and Wehr, T. A. (1985): *Am. J. Psychiatry,* 142:163–170.

110. Rosenthal, N. E., Sack, D. A., Gillin, J. C., Lewy, A. J., Goodwin, F. K., Davenport, Y., Mueller, P. S., Newsome, D. A., and Wehr, T. A. (1984): *Arch. Gen. Psychiatry,* 41:72–80.

111. Rosenthal, N. E., Sack, D. A., and Wehr, T. A. (1983): In: *Circadian Rhythms and Affective Disorders,* edited by T. A. Wehr and F. K. Goodwin, pp. 185–201. Boxwood Press, Pacific Grove, CA.

112. Roy, S. K., Ghosh, B. P., and Bhattacharjee, S. K. (1971): *J. Indian Med. Assoc.,* 57:201–204.

113. Sachar, E. J., Hellman, C., Roffwarg, H. P., Halpern, F. S., Fukushima, D. K., and Gallagher, T. F. (1973): *Arch. Gen. Psychiatry,* 28:19–24.

114. Sack, D. A., and James, S. P. (1985): Presented at the 138th annual meeting of the American Psychiatric Association (New Research), Dallas.

115. Sack, D. A., Nurnberger, J., Rosenthal, N. E., Ashburn, E., and Wehr, T. A. (1985): *Am. J. Psychiatry,* 142:606–608.

116. Sakai, C., and Coppen, A. (1980): *J. Affective Disord.,* 2:249–255.

117. Sherman, B. M., and Pfohl, B. (1985): *J. Affective Disord.,* 9:55–61.

118. Sherman, B., Pfohl, B., and Winokur, G. (1984): *Arch. Gen. Psychiatry,* 41:271–275.

119. Sherman, B., Whysham, C., and Pfohl, B. (1985): *J. Clin. Endocrinol. Metab.,* 61:439–443.

120. Siever, L., and Davis, K. (1985): *Am. J. Psychiatry,* 142:1017–1031.

121. Souetre, E., Salvati, E., Pringuey, D., and Darcourt, G. (1985): In: *IVth World Congress of Biological Psychiatry Abstracts,* p. 402, Philadelphia.

122. Swade, C., and Coppen, A. (1980): *J. Affective Disord.,* 2:249–255.

123. Tamarkin, L., Craig, C. J., Garrick, N. A., and Wehr, T. A. (1983): *Am. J. Physiol.,* 245:R215–R221.

124. Touitou, Y., Fevre, M., Bogdan, A., Reinberg, A., DePrins, J., Beck, H., and Touitou, C. (1984): *Acta Endocrinol.,* 106:145–151.

125. Traskman-Bendz, L. (1980): Depression and Suicidal Behavior. A Biochemical and Pharmacological Study. Thesis, Stockholm.

126. Tupin, J. P. (1970): *Int. Pharmacopsychiatry,* 5:227–232.

127. vanden Hoofdakker, R. H. (1980): In: *Sleep 1980. Fifth European Congress on Sleep Research,* edited by W. P. Koella, pp. 2–9. Karger, Basel.

128. Vanhaelst, L., Van Cauter, E., Degante, J. P., and Golstein, J. (1972): *J. Clin. Metab.,* 35:479–482.

129. Vogel, G. W., McAbee, R., and Barber, K. (1977): *Arch. Gen. Psychiatry,* 33:96–97.

130. Vogel, G. W., Thurmond, S., Gibbons, P., Sloan, K., and Walker, M. (1975): *Arch. Gen. Psychiatry,* 32:765–777.

131. Vogel, G. W., Vogel, C., McAbee, R. S., and Thurmond, A. J. (1980): *Arch. Gen. Psychiatry,* 37:247–253.

132. von Zerssen, D., Barthelmes, H., Dirlich, G., Doerr, P., Emrich, H. M., von Lindern, L., Lund, R., and Pirke, K. M. (1985): *Psychiatry Res.,* 16:51–63.

133. Weeke, A., and Weeke, J. (1976): *Acta Psychiatr. Scand.,* 57: 281–289.

134. Weeke, J. (1973): *Scand. J. Clin. Lab. Invest.,* 31:337–342.

135. Wehr, T. A. and Goodwin, F. K. (1981): In: *American Handbook of Psychiatry, Vol. VII,* edited by S. Arieti and H. K. H. Brodie, pp. 46–74.

136. Wehr, T. A., and Goodwin, F. K. (1983): In: *Circadian Rhythms in Psychiatry,* edited by T. A. Wehr and F. K. Goodwin, pp. 129–184. Boxwood Press, Pacific Grove, CA.

137. Wehr, T. A., Goodwin, F. K., Wirz-Justice, A., Breitmaier, J., and Craig, C. (1982): *Arch. Gen. Psychiatry,* 39:559–565.

138. Wehr, T. A., Jacobsen, F. M., Sack, D. A., Arendt, J., Tamarkin, L., and Rosenthal, N. E. (1987): *Arch. Gen. Psychiatry (in press).*

139. Wehr, T. A., Muscettola, G., and Goodwin, F. K. (1980): *Arch. Gen. Psychiatry,* 37:257–263.

140. Wehr, T. A., Sack, D. A., Duncan, W. C., Mendelson, W. B., Rosenthal, N. E., Gillin, J. C., and Goodwin, F. K. (1985): *Psychiatry Res.,* 15:327–339.

141. Wehr, T. A., and Wirz-Justice, A. (1982): *Pharmacopsychiatry,* 15:31–39.

142. Wehr, T. A., Wirz-Justice, A., and Goodwin, F. K. (1979): *Science,* 206:710–713.

143. Weitzman, E. D. (1975): In: *Behavior and Brain Electrical Activity,* edited by N. Burch and H. L. Altshuler, pp. 93–111. Plenum Press, New York.

144. Weitzman, E. D. (1982): *Hum. Neurobiol.,* 1:173–183.

145. Weitzman, E. D., Czeisler, C. A., and Moore-Ede, M. C. (1979): In: *Biological Rhythms and Their Central Mechanisms,* edited by M. Suda, O. Hayaishi, and H. Nakagawa, p. 199–207. North-Holland Biomedical Press, Amsterdam.

146. Weitzman, E. D., Goldmacher, D., Kripke, D., McGregor, P., Kream, J., and Hellman, F. (1968): *Trans. Am. Neurol. Assoc.,* 93:153–157.

147. Wetterberg, L., Beck-Friis, J., Aperia, B., and Petterson, U. (1979): *Lancet,* 2:1361.

148. Wever, R. A. (1979): *The Circadian System of Man.* Springer-Verlag, New York.

149. Wever, R. A., Polasek, J., and Wildgruber, C. M. (1983): *Pflugers Arch.,* 396:85–87.

150. Winokur, G. (1976): *Neuropsychobiology,* 2:87–93.

151. Wirz-Justice, A., Bucheli, C., Graw, P., Fisch, H.-U., Waggon, B., and Kielholz, P. (1985): Presented at the Fourth World Congress of Biological Psychiatry, Philadelphia.

152. Wirz-Justice, A., Kafka, M. S., Naber, D., Campbell, I. C., Marangos, P. J., Tamarkin, L., and Wehr, T. A. (1982): *Brain Res.,* 241:115–122.

153. Wood, C., and Jacubowicz, D. (1980): *Br. J. Obstet. Gynaecol.,* 87:627–630.

154. Yamaguchi, N., Maeda, K., and Kuromaru, S. (1978): *Folia Psychiatr. Neurol. Jpn.,* 32:479–487.

Psychopharmacology:
The Third Generation of Progress,
edited by Herbert Y. Meltzer.
Raven Press, New York © 1987.

CHAPTER **67**

Animal Models in Psychiatry

Fritz A. Henn and William T. McKinney

WHAT ARE MODELS?

The concept of animal models for psychiatric illnesses has become controversial, so some discussion of how the term should, and should not, be used is in order. Animal models should be conceptualized as experimental preparations developed in one species for the purpose of studying phenomena occurring in another species. In the case of animal models of human diseases, one seeks to develop syndromes in animals that resemble aspects of human psychopathology. In order to allow detailed study of these conditions, the models may not resemble all aspects of human disease. There will inevitably be differences, and, indeed, the study of these differences may be as important as the similarities.

There is no such thing as a single animal model for psychiatric syndrome. However, if there were, under the most ideal of circumstances, an animal model of a specific illness would be identical to the human illness in terms of etiology, symptoms, underlying mechanisms, and treatment responsiveness. No such complete model exists for any psychiatric syndrome, nor is it likely that it will. There can only be successive approximations or simulation of specific, but limited, aspects of a given syndrome. Nevertheless, there is much to be learned from a comparative approach in psychiatry, as there is in many fields of medicine, and the value of using animal models to study aspects of specific psychiatric disorders will be discussed later in this chapter.

Rarely do psychiatric illnesses have a single etiology, but rather they usually involve multiple interacting variables. Different factors appear to account for different proportions of the variance in different individuals. Consequently, it is proving difficult to develop an integrative view of most forms of human psychopathology that is data based. Such a framework has been described for human depression (2,3,63,64) and is an integrative view based partly on animal work. Multiple variables, each having a central effect as well as interacting with others, create a complex pattern that is difficult to unravel on the basis of clinical data alone. Animal models permit evaluation of the effects of these etiological variables one at a time in a systematic and controlled way. For example, from the standpoint of phenomenology, depression involves a mixture of cognitive, emotional, affective, behavioral, and physiological manifestations. A model of this disorder is useful if one or more of these factors is present and can be studied. As mentioned above, a useful model is not necessarily the reproduction of all the signs and symptoms of the illness. This is an improper conceptualization of what models should be. Models should be designed along defined and limited grounds so as to develop an experimental system in which a specific sign or symptom can be studied, or to evaluate a specific etiological theory in a way that cannot be done in humans. Another possible use for models is to evaluate the effect of a specific treatment intervention on a particular behavior. This is different from the more frequent use of models, which is to use them for drug evaluation studies in a more global sense and to validate the model on the basis of how well clinically effective drugs act on it.

Thus one can speak of the following general kinds of animal models (42):

1. Those designed to simulate a specific sign or symptom of the human disorder (behavioral similarity)
2. Those designed to evaluate a specific etiological theory
3. Those designed to study underlying mechanisms
4. Those designed to permit preclinical drug evaluations

GENERAL KINDS OF ANIMAL MODELS

Models Designed to Simulate Specific Signs or Symptoms

In this approach to animal modeling one tries to produce, in animals, certain specific aspects of the human disorder. The primary intent is not to evaluate either a specific etiological theory or treatment responsiveness. In this context, the validity of the model is judged by how closely it approximates the human condition. The reason for developing these kinds of models is to focus on the study of a particular symptom or a cluster of symptoms. The methods used to induce the behavior may or may not be those by which such behaviors are produced in humans.

An example that could be cited is stereotypic behavior. Stereotypy is a behavior that occurs in a number of psychiatric syndromes and there are a number of ways to produce this behavior in animals. Drugs can be used as well as social isolation or overcrowding. It may even be a trait-related characteristic of certain animals. This kind of animal preparation can then be used to further dissect stereotypic behavior in a particular species. Since stereotypy is an important psychopathological behavior in humans with a variety of illnesses, such studies are potentially clinically relevant. However, one does not have to equate the stereotypic behavior being studied with any one specific syndrome. Studies of the phenomena are important in their own right. More animal modeling work of just this kind needs to be done as part of an effort to develop general principles of psychopathology.

Models Designed to Test a Specific Etiological Theory

In this type of experimentation, one begins with a specific theory of a given form of psychopathology or, alternatively, with a general theory about the importance of certain variables in a number of forms of psychopathology. Typically, such theories have developed from studies of sick humans and therefore are retrospective in nature. This is an area where suitable animal preparations can play a particularly useful role. One can evaluate prospectively the effects of paradigms designed to represent certain causative theories.

The use of animals in this way obviously involves the development of paradigms that reasonably simulate theories developed from clinical research. Such experimental paradigms are now available for a number of theories. It should be emphasized that this use of animal models does not make any *a priori* assumptions about the validity of the theory. Rather, the attempt is to operationalize the theory and develop experimental paradigms to evaluate the effects of such inducing conditions. Modeling research is ideal for isolating the behavioral consequences of specified conditions. This type of research across species can provide us with an understanding of the factors that shape behavior and may contribute to a better understanding of the origins of psychopathological behavior. Models such as these are sometimes called "theory-driven" models and are distinguished from the previous kind of models involving behavioral similarities that are more atheoretical. These kinds of models are theory driven in the sense that a theory drives the development of the paradigm and the form of behavior is then subject to an analysis that may confirm, modify, or discredit the original theory.

Models Designed to Study Underlying Mechanisms

This is a complex topic at present, including two different but complementary views. It involves a discussion of what is meant by the term "mechanisms." To some the term is synonymous with neurobiological mechanisms, and the value of animal models is directly related to how easily direct studies of such underlying mechanisms can be done. There are many examples of such approaches, mostly in invertebrates and rodents. Typically, in such studies the description of social behavior is quite limited, though the neurobiological aspects will be very precise. To the developmentalist or the behaviorist the term "mechanism" might have very different meanings. Typically in such studies the behavioral descriptions, whether they be of social behavior or apparent behavior, will be quite precise, but neurobiological indices will be limited to those which can be done while still studying social behavior.

These approaches should be viewed as complementary. What often happens at present is that some approaches to animal modeling are criticized because they do not involve direct studies of underlying central mechanisms, whereas other approaches that predominantly focus on central mechanisms are criticized because they cannot, or do not, include descriptions of social behavior. There is room for both approaches. It is to be hoped that as work continues more examples of studies in which both aspects are considered will emerge.

One cannot necessarily directly transpose techniques of mechanism studies from rodents to monkeys nor, for that matter, from monkeys to humans. The study of mechanisms must be approached from different vantage points in different species and in different kinds of protocols. Each approach has advantages and disadvantages. The appropriateness of each technique of studying mechanisms must be evaluated on a number of grounds including species, economics, ethics, the kind of behavioral data desired, etc.

Models Designed to Permit Preclinical Drug Evaluation

If one is mainly interested in developing an animal model system in which drugs can be evaluated, how one induces the syndrome and even issues of behavioral similarity become secondary. One then evaluates the animal model by how well the drug effects in the model predict clinical effectiveness. However, drugs may have the same effects in two species for quite different reasons. For example, the fact that the ability of a given drug to prevent reserpine-induced sedation is correlated with its effectiveness as a clinical antidepressant does not necessarily establish the reserpine-induced sedation as a valid animal model of depression. Validity is a relative concept and has to be considered in relationship to the reasons for the development of the model in the first place. This does not make the reserpine-induced sedation model, or any other model with high empirical validity, any less important, but it does circumscribe the kinds of conclusions that can be drawn from it.

This use of models represents one of the oldest and most widely known uses. The pharmaceutical industry has pioneered in the development of such models. In an ideal empirically based model there should be no false positives and no false negatives. That is, in all instances a drug that works in the animal model should also work clinically in humans and vice versa. This goal has never been achieved nor is it likely that it will, although there are a number of paradigms that have high empirical validity for depression, for schizophrenia, and for anxiety.

ANIMAL MODELING RESEARCH IN RELATION TO OTHER APPROACHES TO PSYCHIATRIC RESEARCH

Before proceeding to a discussion of the evaluation of animal models, it may be helpful to consider the rationale for models and their role in a spectrum of approaches to psychiatric research. In this context, some additional contributions which animal models can make will be given along with their limitations.

Historically, psychiatry has relied heavily on case histories in its theory development. Starting with a sick population, etiological theories have evolved in the process of treatment. Such theories have provided a framework for understanding psychopathology, but since the development of such theories has been based on retrospective data obtained from sick patients and/or relatives, their general validity has been suspect.

The limitations of this approach have long been recognized and other research methods have been sought. Another approach that was developed was epidemiological and involved community sampling techniques. In more recent years there has been increased clinical research activity in controlled settings. Patients with specified diagnoses are carefully studied with highly developed neurological techniques and behaviorally assessed with many rating scales. Patients are studied longitudinally through the course of their illnesses.

The special contribution of animal modeling research to this spectrum of psychiatric research activity is in the ability to control inducing conditions and study the behavioral and biological effects on both a short- and long-term basis. Furthermore, the nature of the interaction among developmental, social, and biological variables in a social species can be studied in a meaningful way. In human clinical research, multiple variables interact simultaneously, and it is typically impossible to sort out these variables in any quantifiable way. It is at this interface that animal modeling research has a unique contribution to make. In animal studies the precise inducing condition is known and other variables can be kept constant.

LIMITATIONS OF ANIMAL MODELS

There are limitations in the use of animal models that must be recognized and considered in the interpretation of data. Perhaps the main one involves the generalization of results across different species. Although it is true that certain animal species have many behavioral and physical traits in common with humans, there are differences and one cannot reason directly from the results in one species to another. Not all species, even those which are phylogenetically very close, necessarily respond in the same fashion, or even in the same intensity to identical events or stimulations. This is exemplified in the research of Kaufman and Rosenblum (31,32) with pigtail (*Macaca nemestrina*) and bonnet (*Macaca radiata*) monkeys, where the two species respond differently to maternal separation.

A very important way in which the study of animal behavior can aid in the understanding of human behavior is in the description and classification of behaviors. Ethologists have contributed to the careful description and dissection of behavior into its component parts, including the context in which the behavior occurs. Psychiatrists and comparative psychologists have begun considering this issue again. We have become very descriptive with the criteria for our diagnoses. Animal behavior research can help sensitize us in this area and help with the development of improved observational techniques. For example, there are a number of highly sophisticated behavioral scoring systems for describing animals' social behavior in the field, in seminaturalistic settings, and in the laboratory. Such parameters as duration, frequency, sequence, and reciprocity can be quantified. These techniques have only rarely been used to study psychiatric patients, even though most major forms of psychopathology involve significant alterations in behavior and in patterns of social relationships.

Often in this area one is talking about the establishment of principles of animal behavior and assessment of their applicability to humans, i.e., the overlapping territories of psychiatry and ethology (19,25,27,39–41,65). This is an area where the study of animal behavior can be a special asset. Although I would in no way dismiss or underestimate the complexity of interactions in animals, one can nevertheless isolate behaviors and sets of behaviors and study them in a more controlled manner than can be done in humans. As a result it is possible to highlight certain theoretical issues. This can be an especially dangerous procedure and has been grossly misused by certain writers who, by selecting facts to fit preconceived theories and neglecting awkward cases, have tried to take a very reductionistic view of human behavior. However, with caution and concern, this snare can be circumvented and does not negate the value of this principle properly used in assessing human behavior.

Humans and their fellow primates are alike in many aspects of social behavior and physical structure. Research into animal behavior that is tempered by an awareness and consideration not only of those traits which are similar but also of those which are unique to either may provide new information and understanding of the model. This in turn may provide a more accurate means by which human behavior can be assessed and interpreted.

EVALUATION OF ANIMAL MODELS

Several investigators have written concerning evaluation of animal models (1,21,35,43,45,59). The present section draws on many of these contributions but also discusses the question of evaluation in a different framework from those presented previously.

The evaluation of an animal model should closely relate to the purposes for which the model is being developed in the first place. To cite an extreme example, a model created to screen for antidepressant drugs may have high empirical validity in that context but be completely inappropriate for studying various etiological theories. On the other hand, a model developed to evaluate a given etiological variable in depression might be completely inappropriate or impractical for drug screening. It is not a matter of one kind of modeling approach being better or worse. It is a question of why the model is being developed in the first place and how it is to be used.

Abramson and Seligman (1) point out that it is important to know the "essential" features of the model. They cite the example of inescapable electric shock. If shock itself were the important variable, then the paradigm would be relevant only to the production of psychopathology in concentration camps or other such places. On the other hand, if the shock is just a tool to induce a given state, and the issue is uncontrollable aversive events in general, then the paradigm has far-reaching significance for human psychopathology.

We and others have previously proposed that one criterion to use in evaluating animal models involves similarity of inducing conditions. That is, a given animal paradigm is or is not valid to the extent that the conditions used to produce the animal preparation are also operative in the production of the human condition. In that there are no forms of human psychopathology for which a specific etiology is known, this limits the extent to which this criterion can be used in animal modeling studies. However, we are learning new things about risk factors for some illnesses and the continued development of paradigms in which to evaluate the risk factors will be an important contribution of animal models.

Another proposed method for evaluating animal models is the requirement that they have the same underlying mechanisms as the human syndrome being modeled. This criterion is nice in theory but impractical in practice. There is no known neurobiological change for any form of human psychopathology that one could say must be present in a given animal model for that model to be valid on this ground.

In evaluating animal models, it should be kept in mind that some may model specific aspects of certain clinical disorders, whereas others model some fundamental features that are important for many forms of psychopathology. We need models in both of these areas, and it should not always be necessary to have to anchor the research to a specific syndrome. There is increasing pressure to do this, but in the long run it is shortsighted.

An additional way in which animal models are frequently evaluated regards their responsiveness to pharmacological agents. A given animal model is said to be valid or not valid to the extent that it is influenced by pharmacological agents in a like manner as in humans. This has been addressed above. One cannot make definitive statements about the validity of a given model solely on the basis of its response to drugs. This is not surprising, given possible species differences in the metabolism and neurobiological effects of drugs. These data must be considered in relationship to all the other methods for evaluating models. This is neither a necessary nor a sufficient criterion. How then are we to evaluate models? We must evaluate them in terms of their appropriateness for studying the question we are interested in; only in that light can their utility be judged.

In reality there is room and need for a plurality of animal models for a given psychiatric illness. There is no "best" model for any syndrome. An investigator should have done as thorough an experimental analysis of the model as possible, so that the critical features can be described, and choose a model appropriate to the question being asked. The focus may be on a specific response, whether it be behavioral, electrophysiological, or neurochemical, and on how this response is affected by interventions used in the treatment of certain human syndromes. The induction techniques used to produce these responses may vary without necessarily having to be identical to induction techniques thought to play a role in human disease. Until clinical research with humans pinpoints more specific etiologies, there is room for a variety of approaches in animal studies with regard to induction techniques. Such work may as a matter of fact lead to the development of improved etiological theories of clinical syndromes.

There is room and need for animal modeling studies in a variety of species. What species are appropriate depends on the questions being investigated, and we need to continue to develop different kinds of models in many species. The use of animals also allows a direct exploration of genetic factors in a specific behavioral response. This is a valuable ability, and behavioral genetics will undoubtedly play a larger and larger role in psychiatric research.

To summarize concerning evaluation, we would say that there is no universally valid animal model for any syndrome. Instead, there are animal preparations available for studying specific aspects of a number of syndromes. There are ideal criteria but these must be applied with caution depending on the function of the particular model. The realization that a diversity of models can be used to ask diverse questions represents the evolution of the field and offers a more realistic assessment of its contributions, potential, and limitations than has sometimes been present. A review of models by broad categories of psychopathology will be presented. This illustrates which tests have utility in drug screening; what models may lead to fruitful correlations between neurobiological variables and specific behavior; and what models suggest hypothesis concerning the etiology of behavioral abnormalities.

MODELS OF ASPECTS OF PSYCHIATRIC SYNDROMES

Affective Disorder

The area of depression has been the focus of the most varied studies of animal models. This has come about for two reasons. First there are a variety of theories involving stress or separation which are amenable to animal model formation. Second, the vegetative signs of depression, especially decreased learning performance, can be easily measured in animals, as can reversal of a specified behavior by antidepressant drugs; thus objective measures are readily available. A recent review of animal models of depression discusses the validity of 18 defined models (62). Of these, four have generated a considerable body of work and will briefly be reviewed here.

Separation Models

It is likely that humans and many animal species are in their most stable condition when they have developed secure social attachment systems. Disruption of such attachment systems almost invariably leads to the development of grief reactions and in some vulnerable individuals can lead to clinical depression. Many developmental, social, and neurobiological variables are thought to influence the reaction to separation. Sorting out the influence of these different variables, and how they might interact with each other, has been extremely difficult in humans. For this and other reasons investigators have turned to animal models for a more systematic study of the effects of separation.

The earliest work on maternal separation in primates began in the 1960s. Jensen and Tolman (26) reported the effects of separating pigtail macaque (*Macaca nemestrina*) infants from their mothers at the ages of 5 and 7 months for short periods of time and then reuniting them with their own or another mother. Several other laboratories performed significant investigations of separation beginning in the 1960s and continuing to the present (23,31,32,56). The behaviors seen following separation have been generally divided into two categories and labeled "protest" ("agitations") and "despair" ("depression"). The protest stage is characterized by increased vocalization, increased activity, and frantic attempts to return to the mother. In the "despair" stage, the monkeys are socially withdrawn, hypoactive, show decreased food and water intake, and exhibit an increase in self-directed behaviors such as huddling.

As researchers extended this original work on the response to maternal separation, it became apparent that the response of the infants was influenced by a number of parameters, including the species, age, and social conditions. The reaction to maternal separation is a true biobehavioral syndrome. Not only are there the significant behavioral effects summarized above, but there are also major neurobiological changes.

Reite and associates (53,54) have done a series of studies of pigtail macaque infants undergoing maternal separation. They use totally implanted multichannel biotelemetry systems and study heart rate, body temperature, and sleep physiology of the infants before, during, and after separation from their mothers. Separation is generally accomplished by removing the biological mother from a group-living situation and leaving the infant in the group. From a behavioral standpoint, they, like others, have found that attachment bonds are as central to the development of monkeys as they are to people, and that disruption of these bonds leads to serious changes. In one study, for example, they found significant increases in the infant's heart rate and body temperature immediately after maternal separation. These changes were most pronounced very early in separation and tended to diminish as the separation continued. Beginning with the first night, both the heart rate and body temperature showed marked decreases from baseline levels and the behavioral patterns became more depressive-like. During reunion both the heart rate and body temperature returned to normal, although some infants showed the lower heart rate well into the reunion. This research group has also reported an increased incidence of cardiac arrythmias as a result of maternal separation. Significant sleep changes [including increased sleep latency, more frequent arousals, less total sleep, and disruption of rapid eye movement (REM) sleep] have also been reported to occur during maternal separation.

It has been found that brief separations from the mother, or from a surrogate, result in a marked increase in the pituitary-adrenal response (10). Initially it was reported that there was identical physiological response whether the infant was separated from a mother or a surrogate. Data from a number of studies support the hypothesis that the changes are due to the separation itself rather than to housing changes. Also, the presence of a familiar animal during the separation phase does not alter the corticoid response, suggesting that the disruption of the specific attachment bond between mother and infant is the main cause of increased corticoid levels. In a later report from the same group concerning separation distress in surrogate-reared squirrel monkeys, it was shown that separation from the surrogate resulted in behavioral response but no corticoid response, whereas separation from the real mother resulted in both a behavioral and a corticoid response. In later work, it appears to be the case that infants of the highly dominant mothers are the ones that showed the greatest adrenocortical response to separation. This important research illustrates the complexity of understanding the neurobiological and behavioral changes that might accompany separation. It is important to obtain adequate baseline behavioral profiles of both the group structure and individual behavioral assessments.

In another study, desipramine has been reported to be effective in preventing the response to maternal separation in primates (24).

Additional maternal separation studies have been done using canine puppies, guinea pigs, and chicks (49). From this, research has developed a theory that brain endorphins may play a critical role in the mediation of social bonds, and that when these bonds are disrupted by separation, a syndrome much like that following narcotic withdrawal is produced. In this work, distress vocalizations are used as an index of separation. The distress vocalizations are relieved by morphine and made worse by the narcotic antagonist, naloxone, when given as single injections. A variety of opiate-like peptides have been tested and all have been reported to be effective, like morphine, in decreasing distress vocalizations in separated animals when injected (in quite low doses) into the vicinity of the fourth ventricle.

Another type of approach to separation models that has developed in recent years is the peer separation model.

Rhesus monkeys and most other primate species develop strong and complex social bonds, and paradigms have been developed that involve experimental disruption of these bonds in peers of various ages including adults. In general, the behavioral reaction to peer separation is quite similar to the reaction to maternal separation in terms of the classic protest-despair response. Furthermore, when peer groups are formed and repetitive separations are done, the response is obtainable with each separation. A number of variables can influence the nature of this response, and these have been described in a number of publications (8,44). These include age, rearing conditions, housing conditions before, during, and after each separation, and treatment with pharmacological agents. There is significant individual variability, which can be related to a number of developmental and neurobiological variables. For example, cerebrospinal fluid norepinephrine (CSF NE) appears to be a trait-related marker predicting a more severe response to separations. Animals with lower CSF NE respond to separation with more huddling and self-directed behaviors than animals with high levels. By contrast CSF homovanillic acid (HVA) and 5-hydroxyindoleacetic acid (5-HIAA) are state-related markers that reflect the behavioral response to separation no matter how this response is obtained (36).

Pharmacological agents can effect the response to peer separation (38). Imipramine will reverse the reaction to peer separation and prevent the reaction to future separations as long as the monkeys are kept on it. They return to more typical separation behavior when it is withdrawn. Amphetamine modifies the behavioral response to separation in a very similar manner to imipramine, but the overall effects of the two drugs on group social behavior can be distinguished. α-Methylparatyrosine, which lowers norepinephrine and dopamine, makes the separation response much more severe, and at doses that have no effect on animals maintained in group housing. Parachlorphenylalanine, which blocks serotonin synthesis, has no effect. Low doses of alcohol alleviate the peer separation response, whereas high doses make it worse (37).

In relationship to depression models, the rationale for separation studies in animals is that the bulk of evidence strongly suggests social separations as risk factors, and as risk factors that cut across types of depression. The animal studies represent one way of studying these risk factors. There are, of course, many other factors involved in depression; nevertheless, separations appear to be important events in vulnerable individuals and worthy of further study.

Another rationale for separation studies is that they may be prototypes for the study of stressful events in general, and of the role of stress factors in depressions. With the recent advances in our knowledge of the neurobiology of depression, it becomes increasingly important to have some experimental paradigms in which the interactions between neurobiological factors and social risk factors can be examined. In this type of animal preparation there is opportunity to control social and developmental variables and to do prospective studies of both behavioral and neurobiological parameters. The long-term effects of early alterations can be examined in a much shorter period of time. One can obtain repeated measurements of neurobiological variables, e.g., in CSF, in a manner that cannot be done in humans and in relationship to specific units of behavior. One can also evaluate the effects of drugs on the CSF parameters being studied in humans, and determine what these changes mean in relationship to specific social behaviors. There can also be clarification of the role that specific neurotransmitter systems play in influencing specific units of social behavior, including responses to separation. Humans are fundamentally social creatures, and an understanding of the social origins of psychopathology, and how these are related to neurotransmitter systems, becomes possible in this kind of preparation.

Learned Helplessness

This is a behavioral phenomenon first described by Overmier and Seligman (48), in which animals are exposed to aversive stimuli under circumstances in which they cannot control or predict these stimuli. This treatment is found to result in a long-lasting deficit in escape performance, which has been called learned helplessness. This syndrome has three features, all thought to be caused by the lack of control of the adverse stimuli: deficits in (a) motivation, (b) associative learning, and (c) emotion. The first is illustrated by the lack of attempts to escape in subsequent learning trials; the second by the lack of learning in subsequent trials; and the third by decreased vocalization and general passivity. The use of a triadic design in which there is a no-shock control, an executive animal that can control the shock, and a yoked animal that receives the same shock as the executive without control over the stimuli supports the idea that control is a crucial variable in initiating this behavior. Recently Overmier (47) suggested that other factors such as predictability also may play a role and that the phenomenon is a complex one with multiple causal inputs. The attempt to specify causative factors such as motivation and emotion, which are only very indirectly assessed, has been the source of controversy in the learned-helplessness literature. This is not surprising, since questions of etiology in both animals and humans remain uncertain. The model, though developed from a theoretical position, may be as interesting in terms of face validity and pharmacological specificity.

Face validity refers to the ability of the model to look like the human condition being modeled. Learned helplessness presents an interesting model in this regard. The model is defined via a performance deficit so that learning appears impaired, and weight loss, decreased activity, and sleep disturbance have all been reported (61). Recent studies by Overmeier (47) suggest cortisol may be specifically elevated in helpless animals. Thus the model offers a number of behavioral and physiological responses analogous to those reported in human depressive illnesses. The use of a learning task to assess "helplessness" provides a good way to screen drugs in this model. Using rats, it appears that tricyclics, monoamine oxidase inhibitors (MAOIs), novel antidepressants, and electroconvulsive therapy (ECT) reverse helplessness whereas stimulants, sedatives, and neuroleptics do not (58). The anticholinergic scopolamine and stimulants reversed a similar phenomenon in mice (4), so more work is needed on this issue. In summary, the model offers a reasonable way of inducing behavioral changes consistent with depression that can be reversed using clinically successful somatic treatments.

This suggested that a study of the mechanism of antidepressant action and the neurobiology of the behavioral change in this model might offer clues to the neurobiology of mood disorders in humans. This use of the model has led to interesting results. Weiss et al. found that animals showing deficits in escape performance have NE depletion specifically in the locus ceruleus and have implicated the α_2-receptor system in the locus ceruleus using agonists and antagonists to manipulate this system. This was confirmed in mice by Anisman and Zacharko (5), who in addition found a role for serotonin (5-HT) and acetylcholine. Recent studies by Henn et al. (22) suggest that specific alterations in the hippocampal β-receptors occur with the development of "helpless" behavior. They showed that these changes are reversed by antidepressant drug treatments and that 5-HT appears to regulate β-receptor levels in the hippocampus. This study, along with lesion studies implicating the fornix and septal regions in the behavioral alterations, points to the septal-hippocampal pathway as an important site for 5-HT regulation of NE function. This use of the model is leading to detailed hypothesis concerning the neurobiological regulation of affect which may be testable in humans.

Behavioral Despair

In this model mice or rats are forced to swim in a confined space. After a period of vigorous swimming and attempts to escape the animals become immobile. This state has been termed behavioral despair by Porsalt (51,52), who initially described it. This model is extensively used to screen drugs, and aside from a suggested relationship to learned helplessness (62) little testing of face validity has taken place. This test is a quick and convenient screen for antidepressant activity; however, a series of false positives has been reported, including anticholinergic stimulants and sedatives (50). Modification of the test to look at chronic rather than acute drug treatment and prolongation of the period of stress have been reported to improve the specificity (33). This model has been combined with inescapable shock by Weiss et al. (61) and has proven to be an easy reproducible screening test for pharmacological activity. It does not appear to offer theoretical possibilities for understanding affect, and the neurobiology of this system appears to be mediated at least in part through the NE system.

Chronic Unpredictable Stress

This model, developed by Katz et al. (30), is similar in concept to the learned helplessness model but the stresses are varied and chronic over a 3-week period. Animals are exposed to a series of aversive events over 3 weeks, including electric shock, cold water, immobilization, reversal of light-dark cycle, tail pinch, shaker stress, and other stressors. Animals are then placed in an open field situation following exposure to loud noises and bright lights. The chronically stressed animals do not have increased open-field activity after lights and noise as opposed to control animals. Treatment during the stress period with antidepressant is able to reverse this effect. The animals chronically stressed have elevated corticosterone levels and do not respond to a pleasurable stimulus (29). This model, which is more realistic in its induction, has proven to be too cumbersome for drug screening and as yet has not been studied with a view toward finding alterations in neurobiological systems. Many animals do not survive the 21-day schedule and the behavioral alterations dissipate quickly.

Models of Anxiety

In modeling anxiety there is a need to distinguish between panic attacks and more general forms of anxiety. Generalized anxiety disorders are poorly studied in comparison to panic attacks in clinical populations; however, there are two excellent animal models of generalized anxiety. The availability of a human model of panic attacks, lactate-induced anxiety (34), has lessened the animal work in this area. However, the development of anxiolytics has heightened interest in models that predict this action in humans.

Conflict model. In this most widely used model, animals receive both a reward (often food or water) and footshock when they press a lever following a period when the reward alone was the response to lever pressing. After the onset of footshock in conjunction with reward, lever pressing is markedly attenuated (18). This situation, in which both approach and avoidance components are present, is the basis of the conflict model of anxiety. This model appears operative across species from goldfish to monkeys (57). Many modifications of this design have been used, and, in general, antianxiety drugs, sedatives, and ethanol decrease the avoidance. Other classes of compounds are ineffective. The site of action again may involve the limbic circuits; both amygdala (46) and hippocampal regions (9) have been implicated. There are suggestions that GABAergic innervations of 5-HT sites in raphe are also involved in antianxiety effects of these drugs (60). Of all animal models this model may be the most sensitive pharmacologically, with very good record of responsiveness to anxiolytic compounds.

Social interaction. In this test, developed by File and Hyde (13,14), two male rats are placed in a neutral arena and the time they spend interacting, i.e. sniffing, grooming, kicking, boxing, and wrestling, is scored. The rats can be in either high or low light, and can be familiar or unfamiliar with the area. The use of increased light or an unfamiliar area leads to less social interaction, and this can be overcome by anxiolytics (12). This test is specific for anxiolytics and appears able to distinguish sedative from anxiolytic effects. The use of stimulants increases social interaction under all conditions, unlike anxiolytics. Thus, stimulants and anxiolytics may also be distinguished by this test (20). Interestingly the ootropic piracetam is anxiolytic in this test (15).

The neurobiology of this model has been studied. Small 5,7-dihydroxytryptamine lesions specifically in the dorsal raphe had an anxiolytic effect, as did lesions into the lateral septum. These effects are quite specific, and general lesions or 5-HT uptake inhibitors have no effect in this test. This model appears to have excellent pharmacological specificity and uses naturally occurring behavior. Thus it is a particularly promising model for further neurobiological studies.

Schizophrenia

The problem with models of schizophrenia in part resides in the definition of the disorder. Most generally accepted definitions involve two clusters of symptoms. The first group includes thought disorder and manifest signs of psychosis, such as hallucinations or delusions, and the second the absence of drive, and motivation and the inability to enjoy experiences. These, together with some evidence of chronicity, are the basis for the diagnosis of schizophrenia. The second group of symptoms is difficult to test in animals under the best of conditions, and they become impossible to ascertain if attempts to create psychosis have taken place. Thus we have no models that really resemble schizophrenia, but some work has been done developing models of psychosis. In general, no theory-driven models have been useful except those developed from biochemical theories of psychosis.

Drug screening has been done using models that probe the dopamine system, such as rotation or reversal of amphetamine stereotypy. The dopamine theory of schizophrenia has dominated thinking about possible models of psychosis. This is in part due to the difficulty of defining psychotic behavior such as delusional thinking in animals. Most of the approaches to psychosis involve drug manipulations of specific amine systems. The most studied model involves amphetamine intoxication.

Amphetamine Intoxication

Chronic amphetamine usage in humans has led to the description of a psychosis very similar to paranoid schizophrenia (6,7). Utilizing this observation, an animal model of psychosis has been developed. The more elegant model uses subcutaneously implanted slow-release pellets of *d*-amphetamine. When such preparations are used in rats or monkeys, a series of behavioral stages somewhat analogous to that shown by humans engaging in chronic high-dose amphetamine usage is seen (11). The animals experience an initial phase of hyperactivity followed by the development of motor stereotypies. These stereotypic behaviors become almost constant. Following this the animals enter a quiet phase which gives way to a period of what appears to be frank psychosis. They exhibit "wet dog" shakes and grooming behavior suggestive of parasitic infestation and other forms of hallucinatory-like behavior. The problems with this model are that it is impossible to verify hallucinations or delusions, and although it is helpful in understanding the effects of chronic dopamine excitation, it is not helpful in looking for other etiologies of psychosis. Other recent drug models have looked at alterations of the enkephalin system, which prompted increased dopamine activity (28). In none of these models has great attention been paid to genetic factors screening the specificity of an animal's response. This is an area where we can expect more effort.

Dementia

The area of dementia has lagged behind in the development of comprehensive animal models. As interest in dementia and particularly Alzheimer's disease grows, more studies in this area will be found. In general, early attempts involved modeling of the neuropathological lesion which is the hallmark of Alzheimer's disease. This generally has involved toxins such as aluminum; however, recent studies using brain implants may be of interest in testing the infectious theory of transmission. Flament-Durand et al. (16) in Belgium took human cortical tissue rich in neurofibrillary tangles from a brain biopsy sample and implanted it into the tissue of occipital cortex of 7-week-old rats. The human implant caused fibrous gliosis and the rat astrocytes showed twisted filaments. In general, few studies have been done looking at behavioral factors related to dementia. Friedman et al. (17) used bilateral lesions of globus pallidus with kainic acid. They found evidence of decreased cholinergic function and decreased ability in a passive avoidance task. With more precise theories concerning the anatomical sites of the memory defect in this disorder, animal studies may provide critical tests of the validity of these theories. A problem in the work on dementia is that there are no effective treatments; thus the search for possibly effective drugs is hampered by not having a reasonable screening model. In general, tests of learning are used. For example, reversal of the memory deficit induced by bilateral ECT in animals has been used to screen drugs. This area, because of the objective behavioral and neurobiological markers of the illness, should soon develop a variety of animal models.

This brief overview has suggested the range of uses and problems found in animal models. We hope it will help focus realistic research efforts and encourage the development of new models clearly specified to help answer specific questions about aspects of psychiatric illnesses.

REFERENCES

1. Abramson, L. Y., and Seligman, M. E. P. (1977): In: *Psychopathology: Experimental Methods*, edited by J. D. Maser and M. E. P. Seligman, pp. 1–26. W. H. Freeman and Co., San Francisco.
2. Akiskal, H., and McKinney, W. (1973): *Science*, 182:20–29.
3. Akiskal, H., and McKinney, W. (1975): *Arch. Gen. Psychiatry*, 32: 285–305.
4. Amisman, H., Remington, G., and Shlar, L. S. (1979): *Psychopharmacology*, 61:107–124.
5. Amisman, H., and Zacharko, R. M. (1982): *Behav. Brain Sci.*, 5: 89–137.
6. Angrist, B., and Gershon, S. (1970): *Biol. Psychiatry*, 2:95–107.
7. Bell, D. S. (1965): *Am. J. Psychiatry*, 111:701–707.
8. Bowden, D. M., and McKinney, W. T. (1972): *Dev. Psychobiol.*, 5:353–362.
9. Campbell, J., Sherman, A., and Petty, F. (1980): *Commun. Psychopharmacol.*, 4:387–391.
10. Coe, C. L., Weiner, S. G., Rosenberg, L. T., and Levin, S. (1985): In: *Psychobiology of Attachment and Separation*, edited by M. Reite and T. Field, pp. 163–199. Academic Press, Orlando, FL.
11. Ellison, G. D., and Eison, M. S. (1983): *Psychol. Med.*, 13:751–761.
12. File, S. E. (1985): *Neuropsychobiology*, 13:55–63.
13. File, S. E., and Hyde, J. R. G. (1977): *J. Pharm. Pharmacol.*, 29: 735–738.
14. File, S. E., and Hyde, J. R. G. (1978): *Br. J. Pharmacol.*, 62:19–24.

15. File, S. E., and Hyde, J. R. G. (1979): *J. Affective Disord.*, 1:227–235.
16. Flament-Durand, J., Brion, J. P., and Couck, A. M. (1984): *Experimentia*, 40:402–403.
17. Friedman, E., Leher, B., and Kuster, J. (1983): *Pharmacol. Biochem. Behav.*, 19:309–312.
18. Geller, I., and Siefter, J. (1960): *Psychopharmacologia*, 1:482–484.
19. Grant, E. C. (1965): In: *Modern Perspectives in Child Psychiatry*, edited by J. G. Howells, pp. 20–37. Oliver and Boyd, Edinburgh.
20. Guy, A. P., and Gardner, C. R. (1985): *Neuropsychobiology*, 13:194–200.
21. Hamburg, D. S. (1968): In: *Science and Psychoanalysis, Vol. 12: Animal and Human*, edited by J. H. Masserman, pp. 39–52. Grune and Stratton, New York.
22. Henn, F. A., Johnson, A., Edwards, E., and Anderson, D. (1985): *Pharmacol. Psychopharmacol. Bull.*, 21:443–446.
23. Hinde, R. A., Spencer-Booth, Y., and Bruce, M. (1966): *Nature*, 210:1021–1023.
24. Hrdina, P., Kulmiz, P. von, and Stretch, R. (1979): *Psychopharmacology*, 64:89–93.
25. Hutt, S. J. (1970): In: *Behavior Studies in Psychiatry*, pp. 1–24. Pergamon Press, New York.
26. Jensen, G. D., and Tolman, C. W. (1962): *J. Comp. Physiol. Psychol.*, 55:131–136.
27. Jones, I. H. (1971): *Aust. NZ J. Psychiatry*, 5:258–263.
28. Kalivas, P. W. (1985): 4th World Congress of Biol. Psych., Abstract No. 111.4, p. 16.
29. Katz, R. J. (1982): *Pharmacol. Biochem. Behav.*, 16:965–968.
30. Katz, R. J., Roth, K. A., and Carroll, B. J. (1981): *Neurosci. Biobehav. Res.*, 5:247–251.
31. Kaufman, I. C., and Rosenblum, L. A. (1967): *Science*, 155:1030–1031.
32. Kaufman, I. C., and Rosenblum, L. A. (1967): *Psychosom. Med.*, 29:648–675.
33. Kitada, Y., Miyauchi, T., Satoh, A., and Satoh, S. (1981): *Eur. J. Pharmacol.*, 72:145–152.
34. Klein, D. (1974): *Arch. Gen. Psychiatry*, 31:447–454.
35. Kornetsky, C. (1977): In: *Animal Models in Psychiatry and Neurology*, edited by I. Hanin and E. Usdin, pp. 1–7. Pergamon Press, New York.
36. Kraemer, G. W., Ebert, M. H., Lake, C. R., and McKinney, W. T. (1984): *Psychiatry Res.*, 11:303–315.
37. Kraemer, G. W., Lin, D. H., Moran, E. C., and McKinney, W. T. (1981): *Psychopharmacology*, 73:307–310.
38. Kraemer, G., and McKinney, W. T. (1979): *J. Affective Disord.*, 1:33–54.
39. Kraemer, S. (1977): In: *The Future of Animals, Cells, Models, and Systems in Research, Development, Education, and Testing*, pp. 76–114. National Academy of Sciences, Washington, DC.
40. Lehrman, D. S. (1974): In: *Ethology and Psychiatry*, edited by N. F. White, pp. 187–196. University of Toronto Press, Toronto.
41. McGuire, M. T., and Fairbanks, L. A. (1977): In: *Ethological Psychiatry*, edited by M. T. McGuire and L. A. Fairbanks, pp. 1–40, 211–219. Grune and Stratton, New York.
42. McKinney, W. T. (1984): *Psychiatr. Dev.*, 2:77–96.
43. McKinney, W. T., and Bunney, W. E. (1969): *Arch. Gen. Psychiatry*, 21:240–248.
44. Mineka, S., and Suomi, S. J. (1978): *Psychol. Bull.*, 85:1376–1400.
45. Mitchell, G. D. (1970): In: *Primate Behavior*, edited by L. Rosenblum, Vol. 1, pp. 196–243. Academic Press, New York.
46. Nagy, J., Zambo, K., and Decsi, L. (1979): *Neuropharmacology*, 18:573–579.
47. Overmier, J. B. (1985): In: *Affect, Conditioning and Cognition: Essays on the Determinants of Behavior*, edited by F. R. Brush and J. B. Overmier, pp. 221–227. Lawrence Erlbaum Associates, Hillsdale, NJ.
48. Overmier, J. B., and Seligman, M. E. (1967): *J. Comp. Physiol. Psychol.*, 63:28–33.
49. Panksepp, J., Vilberg, T., Bean, N. J., Coy, D. H., and Kastin, A. J. (1978): *Brain Res. Bull.*, 3:663–667.
50. Porsolt, R. D. (1981): In: *Antidepressants: Neurochemical Behavioral and Clinical Perspectives*, edited by S. J. Enna, J. B. Malick, and E. Richelson, pp. 121–139. Raven Press, New York.
51. Porsolt, R. D., Bertin, A., and Jalfre, M. (1977): *Arch. Int. Pharmacodyn.*, 229:327–336.
52. Porsolt, R. D., Le Pinchon, M., and Jalfre, M. (1977): *Nature*, 266:730–732.
53. Reite, M., and Short, R. (1983): *Prog. Clin. Biol. Res.*, 131:219–253.
54. Reite, M., and Short, R. (1983): In: *Ethopharmacology: Primate Models of Neuropsychiatric Disorders*, edited by K. A. Miczek, pp. 219–253. Alan R. Liss, New York.
55. Reite, M., Short, R., Seiler, C., and Pauley, J. D. (1981): *J. Child Psychol. Psychiatry*, 22:141–169.
56. Seay, B., Hansen, E., and Harlow, H. (1962): *J. Child Psychol. Psychiatry*, 3:123–132.
57. Sepinewall, J., and Cook, L. (1978): In: *Handbook of Psychopharmacology*, edited by L. L. Iversen, S. D. Iversen, and S. H. Snyder, pp. 345–393. Plenum Press, New York.
58. Sherman, A. D., Sacquitine, J. L., and Petty, F. (1982): *Pharmacol. Biochem. Behav.*, 16:449–454.
59. Suomi, S. J., and Immelman, K. (1983): In: *Comparing Behavior: Studying Man Studying Animals*, edited by D. W. Rajecki, pp. 203–224. Lawrence Erlbaum Associates, Hillsdale, NJ.
60. Thiebot, M. H., Jobert, A., and Soubrie, P. (1980): *Neuropharmacology*, 19:633–640.
61. Weiss, J. M., Bailey, W. H., Goodman, P. A., Hoffmann, L. J., Ambrose, M. J., Salman, S., and Charry, J. M. (1982): In: *Behavioral Models and the Analysis of Drug Action*. Proceedings of the 27th OHOLO Conference, edited by M. Y. Spiegetstein and A. Levy, pp. 195–223. Elsevier Press, Amsterdam.
62. Willner, P. (1984): *Psychopharmacology*, 83:1–16.
63. Whybrow, P. C., Akiskal, H. S., and McKinney, W. T. (1984): In: *Mood Disorders: Toward a New Psychobiology*. Plenum Press, New York.
64. Whybrow, P. C., and Parlatore, A. A. (1973): *Psychiatry Med.*, 4:351–378.
65. Zegans, L. S. (1967): *Am. J. Psychiatry*, 124:729–739.

Psychopharmacology:
The Third Generation of Progress,
edited by Herbert Y. Meltzer.
Raven Press, New York © 1987.

CHAPTER **68**

Neurochemical and Psychopharmacologic Aspects of Aggressive Behavior

Burr Eichelman

In the United States, the incidence of interpersonal violence is at an alarming level. Homicide is more common than death by bronchitis, emphysema, and asthma combined (10.3/100,000 in 1981) (126). Battery is reported as the leading cause of injury to women (83). Child abuse reports for the United States in 1981 numbered 413,000 (69). Clinicians consequently encounter with great frequency patients with aggressive and violent behavior. Whereas modification of aggressive behavior may take many forms, including social and behavioral interventions, aggressive behavior has a biological substrate. Neurochemical and pharmacologic research has developed with both animal and human subjects. As this research has progressed, there appears to be an increasing concordance between many of the animal and human findings.

Aggression can be defined as "behavior that leads to the damage or destruction of a target entity." The biological conceptualization of human aggressive disorders fits most easily into the model of a drive state seeking expression. Biological interventions can affect the development of the drive, e.g., by decreasing "frustration" or the organism's perception of frustration. The interventions can block the discharge of the drive or render the discharge less impulsive. Freud (37) hypothesized a drive state—thanatos—which was directed toward death and destruction. The drive theory of aggressive behavior was popularized by Lorenz in *On Aggression* (67). His "hydraulic theory" postulated the existence of aggressive urges which eventually "spill over" and are released. Dollard et al. in the 1930s (27) proposed a frustration-aggression theory. This theory also posited a reservoir of aggressive energy seeking release but differed from the Freudian theory in suggesting that aggressive energy was generated by frustration that developed when an organism had a goal-directed behavior interrupted, rather than developing according to some internally set rate.

HISTORICAL APPROACHES TO THE STUDY OF AGGRESSIVE BEHAVIOR

Early studies in the psychopharmacology of aggression dealt with animal models and alterations in levels of aggressive behavior induced by acute administration of drugs. A classic summary of such work is Valzelli's review published in 1967 (122). In Valzelli's article, 81 drugs were listed in six different behavioral paradigms.

Behavioral Paradigms

A traditional animal model for the study of aggression is isolation-induced fighting in mice. It was first described by Yen et al. (132) and has been well-studied by Valzelli (123). In this model male mice are isolated for 2 to 6 weeks and then placed together for fighting. The latency, duration, and intensity of fighting are measured and compared between drug-treated and control groups.

Painful stimulation (shock-induced fighting) can induce aggressive behavior of a defensive topography in rats, mice, cats, and monkeys (121). A typical paradigm for inducing this behavior in rats is to administer a 2-mA footshock of

0.5 sec duration recycled every 3 to 10 sec. A block of 50 footshocks can provide a daily test session. The frequency of fights per test period is compared between control and experimental conditions (32).

Predatory aggression models provide another series of paradigms. In these models the latency of the animal to kill its prey, the number of killer animals, or the change from nonkiller to killer status is often the experimental variable. Several species have been studied. These include cats killing rats (127) and rats killing mice (9).

Neurophysiological preparations have been developed. These include the traditional surgical preparation in the cat that induces sham rage (91). Olfactory bulb or septal lesions that induce hyperaggressive states have been used in the rat (72). Such preparations can be used to assess the antiaggressive effect of various drugs. Electrical stimulation of limbic regions has also been employed as a technique to induce aggressive behavior (59).

More recently there have been attempts to study more ethologically appropriate aggressive encounters. This has led to the study of drug effects on aggression induced by the introduction of an intruder into an established colony (82) or by studying changes in hierarchy or aggression within an established social system (89).

Drug Screening

Pharmacologic reviews cataloging drug effects with various animal models include Valzelli's monograph (122) and a comprehensive review by Miczek and Barry (77). Such studies include work with antipsychotic, anxiolytic, antidepressant, and sedative drugs as well as studies of hormones and drugs of abuse.

Empirical drug screening in animals was paralleled in the human literature in the mid-1970s by reviews that cataloged case reports and open studies of various classes of drugs. An example of such a review was published as a series of articles in Volume 160 (1975) of the *Journal of Nervous and Mental Disease.* These articles reviewed antipsychotic medications (53), stimulants (2), anxiolytics (5), anticonvulsants (79), lithium (100), and hormonal agents (11).

A Neurochemical Approach

As research into the pharmacology of aggressive behavior progressed, there developed a new approach that focused on putative neurotransmitter systems involved in aggressive behavior and attempts to localize these systems within discrete brain regions.

CURRENT APPROACHES TO THE STUDY OF AGGRESSIVE BEHAVIOR: POTENTIAL BRIDGES BETWEEN ANIMAL AND HUMAN STUDIES

As both animal and human studies relating to the biological aspects of aggressive behavior have increased, there has developed a literature from many disparate sources. The literature now points to a multiple neurotransmitter theory regarding the modulation of aggressive behavior. It also supports the notion that different types of aggressive behavior (e.g., predatory aggression, offensive affective aggression, and defensive affective aggression) have differing neurochemical and neuroanatomical substrates. In some areas of research, particularly those relating to the noradrenergic and serotonergic systems, there is a remarkable convergence of findings for animal and human research; other neurochemical and pharmacologic systems seem less closely correlated.

Aggression and the Noradrenergic System

Norepinephrine (NE) has been implicated in the neurochemistry of aggressive behavior. Reis and his co-workers showed a close linkage between NE and feline affective aggression (91). They demonstrated that stimulation of the amygdala, which induced sham rage behavior, also induced a fall in brainstem and forebrain NE, but not dopamine (DA) (91). This decrease did not occur with stimulation that failed to induce sham rage. Similarly, high decerebrating lesions that induced rage also produced a fall in brainstem NE. The depletion of NE in the brainstem following high decerebration with rage induction was proportional to the frequency of the sham rage attacks (91). When catecholamine stores were depleted using reserpine and the new synthesis of catecholamines was blocked with α-methyl-paraatyrosine, sham rage was abolished (91). Finally, rage attacks were enhanced when the cat was treated with protriptyline, a drug that blocks the reuptake of NE (91), again supporting an aggression-enhancing role for NE.

There is also a substantial literature supporting the role of NE in rodent affective aggressive behavior. Stolk et al. (110) have shown a correlation in the rat between the number of shock-induced fighting episodes and increased turnover of NE in the medulla-pons and diencephalon an hour after bouts of fighting. Drugs that are believed to enhance noradrenergic central activity, such as tricyclic antidepressants and monoamine oxidase inhibitors, enhance rodent shock-induced fighting (30). Acutely, clonidine decreases such aggressive behavior whereas piperoxane increases fighting (101), consistent with the effects of these drugs on the firing of the noradrenergic locus ceruleus (19,113). Treatment with alkali metal cations further supports a noradrenergic involvement in affective aggression. Chronic rubidium treatment in rats is associated with increased central noradrenergic turnover (111), whereas chronic lithium treatment is believed to decrease the functional availability of NE (96). Chronic rubidium treatment leads to an increase in shock-induced fighting (33,109) whereas lithium treatment has an opposite effect (33,99).

Environmental manipulation can enhance central noradrenergic metabolism and induce concomitant changes in aggressive behavior. Pedestal stress in the rat induces in a 5-day period increased brainstem tyrosine hydroxylase (TH) activity coupled with a down-regulation of cortical β-adrenergic receptors (31). This is associated with increased irritability and increased shock-induced fighting (32).

Chronic immobilization stress in the rat can increase hypothalamic TH activity and increase shock-induced fighting (62). These changes in central brain chemistry and fighting persist after the cessation of the chronic stress, long after peripheral signs of stress such as hypertension have abated (62).

Acute β-adrenergic blockade with propranolol reduces shock-induced fighting (125). In rats chronically treated with propranolol, the reduction is not sustained; rather an increase in aggressive behavior develops in those rats which develop an increase in the number of cortical β-adrenergic receptors (51). For example, such an increase develops in rats treated with l-propranolol (52) but not d-propranolol, the levostereoisomer being the one which induces supersensitivity. This increased aggression is attributed to a transient supersensitivity that develops between the chronic injections of propranolol. A similar enhancement of fighting can be seen for the first 12 hr in rats treated chronically with propranolol and then rapidly withdrawn from the drug (51).

In the human literature, Brown et al. (16) found a positive correlation between a history of aggressive behavior in a population of military personnel and their cerebrospinal fluid (CSF) levels of 3-methoxy-4-hydroxyphenylglycol (MHPG), a NE metabolite. This study suggested that central NE turnover was increased in the more aggressive individuals. In the therapeutics literature, both lithium and propranolol have been reported effective in decreasing human aggressive behavior. Lithium, reported to decrease functional NE centrally (96), has been shown by Sheard and his collaborators (103) in a double-blind study to decrease aggressive infractions in treated prisoners who maintain serum levels between 0.60 and 0.90 mEq/liter. Tupin et al. (119) corroborated Sheard's observations. Gram and Rafaelson (43) have reported lithium's efficacy in reducing aggressive behavior in psychotic children. In a more recent double-blind study, Campbell et al. (17) have demonstrated lithium to reduce aggressive behavior in children with a diagnosis of conduct disorder—aggressive type.

Since initial clinical trials, lithium has been given to many different aggressive patient populations with positive results: (a) criminal populations (103), (b) psychotic children (43), (c) personality-disordered aggressive patients (35,98), (d) paranoid schizophrenics (75), a self-mutilator (22), and (e) unipolar depressed psychiatric patients (130). Reports of lithium's efficacy in treating children have been mixed. Dostal and Zvoltsky (28) reported an effect of decreased aggression with severely retarded adolescents. Annell (3) reported a positive effect with aggressive children of mixed psychiatric diagnosis. Whitehead and Clark (128) failed to find a difference between the effects of lithium and placebo on aggressive hyperactive children.

The β-adrenergic antagonist propranolol has been reported in an increasing number of case reports and open studies to effectively reduce human episodic aggressive behavior. Elliott initially reported a clinical observation that propranolol could attenuate intermittent aggressive behavior in patients known, or suspected, to have some organic brain injury (34). This observation has now been extended by other centers that treat patients with organic brain syndromes (46,136). Aggressive behavior in Korsakoff's psychosis (135) and in organically impaired children with rage outbursts (129) is also reported to be decreased with propranolol treatment. Propranolol may also have an aggression-attenuating effect in schizophrenics when used in combination with neuroleptic agents (104,133). Blind clinical trials and a clearer definition of appropriate patient populations are needed now to confirm the open studies.

It must be noted in discussing a hypothesis of NE enhancing aggressive behavior that not all of the animal literature is in agreement. Rats treated with the neurotoxin 6-hydroxydopa to deplete brain NE but not DA or serotonin (5-HT) show enhanced shock-induced fighting with lowered brain NE levels (116). This has been attributed to a supersensitivity effect to endogenously released NE, but other explanations are possible. A second discrepant observation was reported by Geyer and Segal (39), who noted an inhibitory effect of NE acutely infused into the cerebroventricles of rats tested for shock-induced fighting.

The use in rodents of catecholaminergic neurotoxins such as 6-hydroxydopa or 6-hydroxydopamine might provide a model to further explore the role of stimulants in decreasing aggressive behavior in children with an attention deficit with hyperactivity. For example, the increased aggressive behavior observed in rats treated with the neurotoxin 6-hydroxydopamine is transiently reversed with amphetamine (115). This parallels the reports of amphetamine reducing aggressive behavior in hyperactive children, as reviewed by Allen et al. (2).

Aggression and the Serotonergic System

The predatory aggression model has been studied using drugs as modulators of the serotonergic system. Studies that lowered brain serotonin by restricting dietary tryptophan, the precursor of serotonin (41), or by blocking the synthesis of serotonin with the use of parachlorophenylalanine (pCPA), a tryptophan hydroxylase inhibitor (25), produced an induction of mouse-killing in rats. Lesions of the serotonin-containing raphe nucleus (44) and central injections of the serotonin neurotoxin 5,7-dihydroxytryptamine (14) also lower central serotonin levels and enhance predatory aggression. Conversely, administration of the serotonin precursor 5-hydroxytryptophan blocks mousekilling (60).

Comparable effects can be observed using models of affective aggression. Inhibition of tryptophan hydroxylase with a consequential lowering of brain serotonin can increase shock-induced fighting in the rat (given brief intershock intervals) (102). Similar effects can be achieved through lesions of the raphe nucleus (54) or with the use of the serotonergic neurotoxin 5,7-dihydroxytryptamine (57). Dietary tryptophan restriction can lower brain serotonin and induce increased fighting in the rat (58). Raising brain serotonin levels through dietary supplementation of tryptophan does not alter shock-induced fighting in normal rats (58). However, if brain-damaged rats (rats made more aggressive by septal lesions or neurotoxin treatment) are treated with supplementary dietary tryptophan, the increase in fighting expected as a consequence of the brain injury is blocked (56).

Initial human studies appear to be consistent with the preponderance of animal studies that show a correlation of increased aggression with lowered serotonin levels or activity. Brown et al. (16) observed an inverse relationship between CSF levels of the serotonin metabolite 5-hydroxyindoleacetic acid (5-HIAA) and rating scores of lifelong patterns of aggressive behavior in a population of military personnel. Linnoila et al. (64) also reported a correlation between low 5-HIAA levels and impulsive aggressive behavior. Yaryura-Tobias and Neziroglu (131) reported lower serotonin levels in whole blood samples of aggressive patients compared to nonaggressive patients. Aggressive behavior directed toward self may also be associated with low serotonergic activity. Asberg and her co-workers have reported an association between low brain 5-HIAA levels and violent suicide (4). Aggressive behavior in some hyperactive children has also been linked to low blood levels of serotonin (45).

The therapeutic effect of lithium reviewed earlier in this chapter could be related to its ability to increase brain tryptophan concentrations (84) and enhance serotonergic activity. Open trials of serotonin precursors have been reported successful in decreasing human aggression. Soulairac et al. (107) reported a decrease in aggressive behavior in a patient treated with the serotonin precursor 5-hydroxytryptophan. Morand et al. (80) reported an open study using 4 or 8 g of tryptophan per day to successfully treat schizophrenic patients with high Buss Durkee scores and a high lifetime frequency of aggressive behavior.

Aggression and the GABA/Benzodiazepine Systems

Most animal studies have implicated central GABAergic systems in the inhibition of aggression in various animal models. γ-Aminobutyric acid (GABA) levels in the olfactory bulbs of mouse-killing rats were lower than in nonkillers (73). GABA injections into the olfactory bulbs of rats transiently inhibited mouse killing (73). A similar effect was obtained by treating rats with N-dipropylacetate (valproate), which effectively raises brain GABA levels (73). Cannula administration of picrotoxin (a GABA antagonist) or allylglycine (an inhibitor of glutamate decarboxylase) into the olfactory bulbs of rats induces mouse-killing behavior (73). Drugs enhancing central GABA activity also decrease isolation-induced fighting in mice (87). Isolated mice have reduced numbers of GABA binding sites (24). This same role for GABA systems (i.e., GABA agonists inhibiting aggression and antagonists enhancing it) has been reported for shock-induced fighting in mice (88).

Benzodiazepines enhance central GABAergic activity (23). The pharmacologic literature includes many reports of benzodiazepines diminishing aggressive behavior. Benzodiazepines decrease isolation-induced fighting in mice (124). They attenuate aggressive behavior induced by septal lesions, lesions of the ventromedial hypothalamic nucleus, or olfactory bulbs (72). Chlordiazepoxide induces a substantial taming effect on rhesus monkeys at relatively low doses (90). Such studies have led to observations that "there is probably no other class of drugs that has been linked more directly to the inhibition of aggressive behavior" (77).

The animal studies are not uniform. Fox et al. (36) have shown that the chronic administration of diazepam can enhance aggressive behavior. This has also been demonstrated with low-dose, acute administration of chlordiazepoxide (76).

Clinically, benzodiazepines are claimed to decrease aggressive behavior in patients of many diagnostic classes. Boyle and Tobin (12) reported symptomatic improvement in "psychotic" patients treated with chlordiazepoxide. Over half of this population had organic pathology. Kalina (55) reported a decrease in aggressive behavior in prisoners reported as having schizophrenia or schizoid personality disorders who were treated with diazepam. Monroe (79) suggested that chlordiazepoxide be used in patients with an episodic dyscontrol syndrome. Oxazepam in doses of 120 or 240 mg/day was more effective than placebo and chlordiazepoxide (100 or 200 mg/day) in decreasing reported symptoms of anxiety and hostility in outpatients with a history of hostile outbursts associated with anxiety (65). Newer benzodiazepines such as clonazepam have not been studied in the treatment of aggressive behavior.

Complicating the clinical use of benzodiazepines in the treatment of violent behavior has been the reporting of paradoxical rage reactions occurring in certain patients treated with these drugs. Tobin et al. (117) reported a 3.6% incidence of rage reactions in a patient group treated with chlordiazepoxide. Enhanced aggressive behavior in patients has also been noted with other benzodiazepines (66).

Certain benzodiazepines may induce aggressive behaviors whereas others may not. This differential ability has been suggested in a review of the animal literature (26) and is suggested in a few clinical studies. Gardos et al. (38) demonstrated an increase in Buss Durkee Inventory scores of verbal hostility in healthy volunteers treated with chlordiazepoxide but not with oxazepam. In an open clinical trial of oxazepam as compared with diazepam in a prison population, fewer episodes of enhanced aggression were noted in the oxazepam group (15). Definitive answers regarding the efficacy of benzodiazepines and whether there is a difference between drugs in this class for the treatment of aggressive behavior require additional blind clinical trials.

Aggression and Other Neurotransmitter Systems

There is a substantial literature suggesting a major role for central dopaminergic mechanisms in the development of aggressive behavior. For example, L-dopa treatment induces aggressive behavior in rodents (61). The dopaminergic agonist apomorphine induces "spontaneous fighting" in rats (97). This behavior is potentiated in rats pretreated with 6-hydroxydopamine, suggesting an enhanced effect on aggression that is related to central supersensitivity (115). Dopamine antagonists tend to suppress fighting and clinically have provided the mainstay of agents used in managing aggressive behavior in psychiatric patients (53).

Acetylcholine appears to function as a neurotransmitter that enhances aggressive behavior. The cholinomimetic carbachol induces aggressive behavior in the cat when injected into the amygdala (47). Physostigmine injected into the amygdala of rats increases shock-induced fighting (93). Such fighting is suppressed with cholinergic blockade (86). In the rat, cholinergic agonists such as carbachol were shown to induce mouse-killing behavior when placed into the lateral hypothalamus of nonkilling animals (106). Similar effects were observed measuring the latency of attack time with frogs as prey, again with hypothalamically implanted carbachol (7). Other effective brain sites in the thalamus were also discovered (8). This predatory behavior could be blocked with atropine (7,106). Data suggesting cholinergic involvement in human aggressive behavior have not yet been developed.

Drugs of abuse have also been studied in the context of animal and human aggressive behavior. There is considerable animal literature on the effects of alcohol, stimulants, and hallucinogenic drugs on animal aggressive behavior which is not discussed in this chapter but can be reviewed elsewhere (77). There is also substantial literature on the effect of hormones on aggressive behavior (112). In both areas of research, however, there appears to be little overlap in the area of human therapeutics other than the preliminary trials of "antiandrogen" agents in the treatment of aggressive behavior in sexually violent males (10,11,78).

Aggression and Seizure Disorders

Electrical disturbances in the brain have been implicated as a cause of episodic human violent behavior (74), although not linked exclusively to a single neurotransmitter system. Ever since the work of Hess (52) it has been accepted that electrical brain stimulation in animals could induce aggressive behavior in the form of a predatory (127) or affective (59) attack. Recently, animal experiments studying the phenomenon of kindling have begun to report behaviors that may model portions of the dyscontrol syndrome. Cats subjected to electrical brain stimulation in limbic regions just short of inducing seizures are observed to alter defensive and predatory behavior (1). Irritability can be induced in the rat by repeated systemic injections of lidocaine, which eventually kindles generalized seizures of limbic origin. Such kindled rats exhibit marked irritability toward handling (85). Further studies of these models and their modulation with anticonvulsant drugs may provide a clearer understanding and therapeutic approach to human aggressive behavior linked to abnormal brain electrical activity.

In open trials, phenytoin has been reported to decrease violence in episodic dyscontrol patients (6,70). Human "rage reactions" have been reported attenuated by phenytoin (120). Phenytoin has been reported to reduce hostility and aggressiveness in prisoners and juvenile delinquents (92). Stephens and Shaffer (108) reported decreased anger, irritability, and anxiety in "neurotic" outpatients treated with phenytoin. In contrast, Rosenblatt et al. (94) reported that phenytoin was ineffectual in changing aggressive or hostile attitudes in child-abusing parents.

Controlled studies have been contradictory. Maletzky and Klotter (71) reported a positive effect of phenytoin on dyscontrol patients in a double-blind study. Lefkowitz (63)

and Gottschalk et al. (42) failed to find positive effects. Connors et al. (20) failed to find phenytoin effective in treating aggressive delinquents. Mixed reports of efficacy also occur regarding the use of phenytoin in schizophrenic patients (50,105).

Monroe (79) suggested that primidone either alone or in combination with chlordiazepoxide is effective in treating the human dyscontrol syndrome. Carbamazepine, a drug with anticonvulsant and psychotropic properties, has been reported in an open study to decrease violent behavior in patients with a dyscontrol syndrome (118). Hakola and Laulamaa reported a decrease in aggressive behavior in eight violent schizophrenic females (49). Neppe (81) reported improvement in aggressive behavior in eight of 11 psychiatric inpatients also treated with neuroleptic agents. Luchins (68) noted a similar effect of carbamazepine when added to ongoing neuroleptic treatment. These studies have described the use of anticonvulsants in patient populations without clearly documented epilepsy. The literature does not address the addition of specific anticonvulsants such as carbamazepine to the treatment regimen of epileptics who are also violent when their seizures are clinically controlled with other anticonvulsants.

FUTURE RESEARCH

Basic research is needed to further the understanding of the neurochemical mechanisms of aggressive behavior, particularly the interaction of multiple neurotransmitter systems which continue to be modified by environmental influences and experience (21). A more comprehensive nosology of human aggressive behavior must be developed that might include biochemical parameters and might distinguish among impulsive, controlled, drug-induced, or delusional violence. Such a nosology should lead to more predictive pharmacologic treatment.

Drug studies require the clinical research community to standardize and accept evaluation scales for in- and outpatient treatment trials that can be shared from center to center for replication of initial findings of drug efficacy. Such rating scale development is only just beginning (134). Increased support for blind and more tightly controlled studies is needed to validate the current expansion of "innovative treatment," which fails to generate a literature of solid and reproducible findings. Since many of these drug treatments cannot be completely blind due to biological indicators such as tremor or bradycardia, partially blind studies may need to be legitimized. Small research populations may require well-monitored $N = 1$ protocols (48) rather than studies composed of large population samples. The magnitude of the clinical problem of violent behavior requires a greater clinical research investment than has previously occurred.

Pharmacologically, currently available drugs merit more extensive testing. The role of serotonin in animal and human aggressive behavior suggests additional clinical trials designed to manipulate central serotonin systems, including the use of serotonin reuptake blockers used alone or in combination with serotonin precursors or lithium. New compound development should also continue. Bradford et al. (13) have been studying a new class of compounds that they have labeled "serenics," which are reported to have relatively specific antiaggressive effects in animal models.

Pharmacologic research on violence also faces social restraints. Animal research suggests that opioids (40) and marijuana (18) can decrease aggressive behavior. Users of marijuana allege that it reduces their anger and raises the threshold for violent behavior. This has been supported in a research format (95,114). However, approval to use potentially addictive or illegal drugs under present research regulations has been impossible to obtain, regardless of the potential benefits that might accrue to the individual and society in the realm of diminished violent behavior.

CONCLUSION

This chapter has reviewed the development of pharmacologic and neurochemical research on aggressive behavior in animals and humans. This chapter has not outlined a clinical pharmacologic approach to the violent patient. For this, the reader is referred elsewhere (29).

Psychopharmacologic research on aggression has evolved from the general screening of drugs to the systematic use of drugs to delineate central neurochemical mechanisms involved in aggressive behavior. Application of basic research and preliminary findings in human studies now requires an increase in controlled studies in human populations as well as the application of newer noninvasive biological assessment of violent patients in the attempt to clarify and redefine a nosology of human aggressive behavior. This challenge requires additional allocation of research resources and a keen sensitivity to the ethical issues in such research.

ACKNOWLEDGMENTS

I thank A. Hartwig for constructive review of this chapter and M. Romig for technical assistance in the preparation of the manuscript. The writing of this manuscript was supported by the Veterans Administration.

REFERENCES

1. Adamec, R., Stark-Adamec, C., and Livingston, K. E. (1981): In: *The Biology of Aggression,* edited by P. F. Brain and D. Benton, pp. 397–404. Sijthoff and Noordhoff, The Netherlands.
2. Allen, R. P., Safer, D., and Covi, L. (1975): *J. Nerv. Ment. Dis.,* 160:138–145.
3. Annell, A. L. (1969): *Psychiatr. Scand. (Suppl).,* 207:19–33.
4. Asberg, M., Traskman, L., and Thoren, P. (1976): *Arch. Gen. Psychiatry,* 33:1193–1197.
5. Azcarate, C. L. (1975): *J. Nerv. Ment. Dis.,* 160:100–107.
6. Bach-Y-Rita, G., Lion, J. R., Clement, C. E., and Ervin, R. F. (1971): *Am. J. Psychiatry,* 127:1473–1478.
7. Bandler, R. J. (1970): *Brain Res.,* 20:409–424.
8. Bandler, R. J. (1971): *Brain Res.,* 26:81–93.
9. Bandler, R. J., and Moyer, K. E. (1970): *Commun. Behav. Biol.,* 5:177–182.
10. Barry, D. J., and Cicione, J. R. (1975): *Bull. Am. Acad. Psychiatr. Law,* 3:179–184.
11. Blumer, D., and Migeon, C. (1975): *J. Nerv. Ment. Dis.,* 160:127–137.
12. Boyle, D., and Tobin, J. M. (1961): *J. Med. Soc. NJ,* 58:427–429.
13. Bradford, L. D., Olivier, B., van Dalen, D., and Schipper, J. (1984): In: *Ethopharmacological Aggression Research,* edited by K. A. Miczek, M. R. Kruk, and B. Olivier, pp. 191–207. Alan R. Liss, New York.
14. Breese, G. R., and Cooper, B. R. (1975): *Brain Res.,* 98:517–527.
15. Brown, C. R. (1979): In: *New Frontiers in Psychotropic Drug Research,* edited by S. Fielding and R. C. Effland, pp. 241–258. Futura, New York.
16. Brown, G. L., Ballanger, J. C., Minichiello, M. D., and Goodwin, F. K. (1979): In: *Psychopharmacology of Aggression,* edited by M. Sandler, pp. 131–148. Raven Press, New York.
17. Campbell, M., Small, A. M., Green, W. H., Jennings, S. J., Perry, R., Bennett, W. G., and Anderson, L. (1984): *Arch. Gen. Psychiatry,* 41:650–656.
18. Carlini, E. A. (1978): *Mod. Probl. Pharmacopsychiatry,* 13:82–102.
19. Cedarbaum, J. M., and Aghajanian, G. K. (1976): *Brain Res.,* 112:413–419.
20. Conners, C. K., Kramer, R., Rothschild, G. H., Schwartz, L., and Stone, A. (1971): *Arch. Gen. Psychiatry,* 24:156–160.
21. Cools, A. (1981): In: *The Biology of Aggression,* edited by P. F. Brain and D. Benton, pp. 405–425. Sijthoff and Noordhoff, The Netherlands.
22. Cooper, A. F., and Fowlie, H. C. (1973): *Br. J. Psychiatry,* 122:370–371.
23. Costa, E., Guidotti, A., and Mao, C. C. (1976): In: *GABA in Nervous System Function,* edited by E. Roberts, T. N. Chase, and D. B. Tower, pp. 413–426. Raven Press, New York.
24. DeFeudis, F. V., Madtes, P., Ojeda, A., and DeFeudis, P. A. (1976): *Exp. Neurol.,* 52:285–294.
25. DiChiara, G., Gamba, R., and Spano, P. F. (1971): *Nature,* 233:272–273.
26. DiMascio, A. (1973): In: *The Benzodiazepines,* edited by S. Garattini, E. Mussini, and L. O. Randall, pp. 433–440. Raven Press, New York.
27. Dollard, J., Doob, L., Miller, N., Mowrer, O., Sears, R., and Sears, R. R. (1939): In: *Frustration and Aggression.* Yale University Press, New Haven.
28. Dostal, T., and Zvolsky, P. (1970): *Int. Pharmacopsychiatry,* 5:203–207.
29. Eichelman, B. (1986): In: *The American Handbook of Psychiatry, Vol. 8,* edited by P. A. Berger and H. K. H. Brodie, pp. 651–678. Basic Books, New York.
30. Eichelman, B., and Barchas, J. (1975): *Pharmacol. Biochem. Behav.,* 3:601–604.
31. Eichelman, B., and Hegstrand, L. (1982): Presented at the Thirteenth Collegium Internationale Neuro-Psychopharmacologicum. Jerusalem.
32. Eichelman, B., and Thoa, N. B. (1973): *Biol. Psychiatry,* 6:143–164.
33. Eichelman, B., Thoa, N. B., and Perez-Cruet, J. (1973): *Pharmacol. Biochem. Behav.,* 1:121–123.
34. Elliott, F. A. (1977): *Ann. Neurol.,* 1:489–491.
35. Forssman, M., and Walinder, J. (1969): *Acta Psychiatr. Scand. (Suppl.),* 207:34–40.
36. Fox, K. A., and Snyder, R. L. (1969): *J. Comp. Physiol. Psychol.,* 69:663–666.
37. Freud, S. (1930): In: *The Standard Edition of the Complete Psychological Works of Sigmund Freud, Vol. 21,* edited by J. Strachey, pp. 64–145. Hogarth Press, London.
38. Gardos, B., DiMascio, A., Salzman, C., and Shader, R. I. (1968): *Arch. Gen. Psychiatry,* 18:757–760.
39. Geyer, M. A., and Segal, D. S. (1974): *Behav. Biol.,* 10:99–104.
40. Gianutstos, G., and Lal, H. (1978): In: *Modern Problems of Pharmacopsychiatry, Vol. 13,* edited by L. Valzelli, pp. 114–138. Karger, Basel, New York.
41. Gibbons, J. L., Barr, G. A., Bridger, W. H., and Leibowitz, S. F. (1979): *Brain Res.,* 169:139–153.

42. Gottschalk, L., Covi, L., Uliana, R., and Bates, D. (1973): *Compr. Psychiatry,* 14:503–511.

43. Gram, L. F., and Rafaelsen, O. J. (1972): *Acta Psychiatr. Scand. (Suppl.),* 48:263–260.

44. Grant, L. D., Coscina, D. V., Grossman, S. P., and Freedman, D. X. (1973): *Pharmacol. Biochem. Behav.,* 1:77–80.

45. Greenberg, A. S., and Coleman, M. (1976): *Arch. Gen. Psychiatry,* 33:331–336.

46. Greendyke, R. M., Schuster, D. B., and Wooton, J. A. (1984): *J. Clin. Psychopharmacol.,* 4:282–285.

47. Grossman, S. P. (1963): *Science,* 142:409–411.

48. Guyatt, G., Sackett, D., Taylor, D. W., Chong, J., Roberts, R., and Pugsley, S. (1986): *N. Engl. J. Med.,* 314:889–892.

49. Hakola, H. P., and Laulamaa, V. A. (1982): *Lancet,* 1:1358.

50. Haward, L. R. C. (1969): In: *Aggressive Behaviour,* edited by S. Garattini and E. B. Sigg, pp. 317–321. Excerpta Medica Foundation, Amsterdam.

51. Hegstrand, L., and Eichelman, B. (1983): *Pharmacol. Biochem. Behav.,* 19:313–320.

52. Hess, W. R. (1957): *The Functional Organization of the Diencephalon.* Grune and Stratton, New York.

53. Itil, T., and Wadud, A. (1975): *J. Nerv. Ment. Dis.,* 160:83–99.

54. Jacobs, B. L., and Cohen, A. (1976): *J. Comp. Physiol. Psychol.,* 90:102–108.

55. Kalina, R. K. (1964): *Dis. Nerv. Syst.,* 25:101–107.

56. Kantak, K. M., Hegstrand, L., and Eichelman, B. (1981): *Pharmacol. Biochem. Behav.,* 15:343–350.

57. Kantak, K. M., Hegstrand, L., and Eichelman, B. (1981): *Psychopharmacology,* 74:157–160.

58. Kantak, K. M., Hegstrand, L., Whitman, J., and Eichelman, B. (1980): *Pharmacol. Biochem. Behav.,* 12:173–179.

59. Kruk, M. R., Meelis, W., Van der Poel, A. M., and Mos, J. (1981): In: *The Biology of Aggression,* edited by P. F. Brain and D. Benton, pp. 383–395. Sijthoff and Noordhoff, The Netherlands.

60. Kulkarni, A. S. (1968): *Life Sci.,* 7:125–128.

61. Lammers, A. J. J. C., and Van Rossum, J. M. (1968): *Eur. J. Pharmacol.,* 5:103–106.

62. Lamprecht, F., Eichelman, B., Thoa, N. B., Williams, R. B., and Kopin, I. H. (1972): *Science,* 177:1214–1215.

63. Lefkowitz, M. (1969): *Arch. Gen. Psychiatry,* 20:643–651.

64. Linnoila, M., Virkkunen, M., Scheinin, M., Nuutila, A., Rimon, R., and Goodwin, F. K. (1983): *Life Sci.,* 33:2609–2614.

65. Lion, J. R. (1979): *J. Clin. Psychiatry,* 40:70–71.

66. Lion, J. R., Azcarate, C. L., and Koepke, H. H. (1975): *Dis. Nerv. Syst.,* 36:557–558.

67. Lorenz, K. (1966): *On Aggression.* Harcourt Brace Jovanovich, New York.

68. Luchins, D. J. (1983): *Lancet,* 2:766.

69. Magnuson, E. (1983): *Time,* 5 September, pp. 20–22.

70. Maletzky, B. M. (1973): *Dis. Nerv. Syst.,* 34:178–185.

71. Maletzky, B. M., and Klotter, J. (1974): *Dis. Nerv. Syst.,* 35:175–179.

72. Malick, J. B., Sofia, R. D., and Goldberg, M. E. (1969): *Arch. Int. Pharmacodyn. Ther.,* 181:459–465.

73. Mandel, P., Mack, G., and Kempf, E. (1979): In: *Psychopharmacology of Aggressive Behavior,* edited by M. Sandler, pp. 95–110. Raven Press, New York.

74. Mark, V. H., and Ervin, F. R. (1970): *Violence and the Brain.* Harper and Row, New York.

75. Martorano, J. T. (1972): *Compr. Psychiatry,* 13:533–537.

76. Miczek, K. A. (1974): *Psychopharmacologia,* 39:275–301.

77. Miczek, K. A., and Barry, J. (1976): In: *Behavioral Pharmacology,* edited by S. D. Glick and J. Goldfarb, pp. 176–257. C. V. Mosby Company, St. Louis.

78. Money, J. (1970): *J. Sex Res.,* 6:165–172.

79. Monroe, R. (1975): *J. Nerv. Ment. Dis.,* 160:119–126.

80. Morand, C., Young, S. N., and Ervin, F. R. (1983): *Biol. Psychiatry,* 18:575–578.

81. Neppe, V. M. (1982): *Lancet,* 2:334.

82. Olivier, B., van Aken, H., Jaarsma, I., van Oorschot, R., Zethof, T., and Bradford, D. (1984): In: *Ethopharmacological Aggression,* edited by K. A. Miczek, M. R. Kruk, and B. Olivier, pp. 137–156. Alan R. Liss, New York.

83. O'Reilly, J. (1983): *Time,* 5 September, pp. 23–26.

84. Perez-Cruet, J., Tagliamonte, A., Tagliamonte, P., and Gessa, G. L. (1971): *J. Pharmacol. Exp. Ther.,* 178:325–330.

85. Post, R. M. (1981): In: *Kindling 2,* edited by J. A. Wada, pp. 149–160. Raven Press, New York.

86. Powell, D. A., Milligan, W. L., and Walters, K. (1973): *Pharmacol. Biochem. Behav.,* 1:389–394.

87. Puglisi-Allegra, S., and Mandel, P. (1980): *Psychopharmacology,* 70:287–290.

88. Puglisi-Allegra, S., Simler, S., Kempf, E., and Mandel, P. (1981): *Pharmacol. Biochem. Behav.,* 14(Suppl. 1):13–18.

89. Raleigh, M. J., McGuire, M. T., Brammer, G. L., and Yuwiler, A. (1984): *Arch. Gen. Psychiatry,* 41:405–410.

90. Randall, L. O. (1960): *Dis. Nerv. Syst. (Suppl.),* 21:7–10.

91. Reis, D. J. (1972): *Res. Publ. Assoc. Res. Nerv. Ment. Dis.,* 50:266–297.

92. Resnick, O. (1967): *Int. J. Neuropsychiatry,* 3:530–547.

93. Rodgers, R. J., and Brown, K. (1976): *Aggressive Behav.,* 2:131–152.

94. Rosenblatt, S., Schaeffer, D., and Rosenthal, J. S. (1976): *Curr. Therap. Res.,* 19:332–336.

95. Salzman, C., Vanderkolk, B. A., and Shader, R. I. (1976): *Am. J. Psychiatry,* 133:1029–1033.

96. Schildkraut, J. J., Schanberg, S. M., Breese, G. R., and Kopin, I. J. (1967): *Am. J. Psychiatry,* 124:600–608.

97. Senault, B. (1970): *Psychopharmacologia,* 18:271–287.

98. Shader, R. I., Jackson, A. H., and Dodes, L. M. (1974): *Psychopharmacologia,* 40:17–24.

99. Sheard, M. H. (1970): *Nature,* 228:284–285.

100. Sheard, M. H. (1975): *J. Nerv. Ment. Dis.,* 160:108–118.

101. Sheard, M. H. (1979): In: *Catecholamines: Basic and Clinical Frontiers,* edited by E. Usdin, pp. 1690–1692. Pergamon Press, New York.

102. Sheard, M. H., and Davis, M. (1976): *Brain Res.,* 111:433–437.

103. Sheard, M. H., Marini, J. L., Bridges, C. I., and Wagner, E. (1976): *Am. J. Psychiatry,* 133:1409–1413.

104. Sheppard, G. P. (1979): *Br. J. Psychiatry,* 134:470–476.

105. Simopoulis, A. M., Pinto, A., Uhlenhuth, E. H., McGee, J. J., and de Rosa, E. R. (1974): *Arch. Gen. Psychiatry,* 30:106–111.

106. Smith, D. E., King, M. B., and Hoebel, B. G. (1970): *Science,* 167:900–901.

107. Soulairac, A., Lambinet, H., and Aymard, N. (1976): *Ann. Med. Psychol. (Paris),* 2:459–463.

108. Stephens, J. H., and Shaffer, J. W. (1970): *Pharmacologia,* 17:169–181.

109. Stolk, J., Conner, R., and Barchas, J. (1970): *Psychopharmacologia,* 22:250–260.

110. Stolk, J. M., Conner, R. L., Levine, S., and Barchas, J. D. (1974): *J. Pharmacol. Exp. Ther.,* 190:193–209.

111. Stolk, J. M., Nowack, W. J., Barchas, J. D., and Platman, S. R. (1970): *Science,* 168:501–503.

112. Svare, B. B., ed. (1983): *Hormones and Aggressive Behavior.* Plenum Press, New York.

113. Svensson, T. H., Bunney, B. S., and Aghajanian, G. K. (1975): *Brain Res.,* 92:291–297.

114. Taylor, S. P., Vardaris, R. M., Rawtich, A. B., Gammon, C. B., Cranston, J. W., and Lubetkin, A. I. (1976): *Aggressive Behav.,* 2:153–161.

115. Thoa, N. B., Eichelman, B., and Ng, K. Y. (1972): *Brain Res.,* 43:467–475.

116. Thoa, N. B., Eichelman, B., Richardson, J. S., and Jacobwitz, D. (1972): *Science,* 178:75–77.

117. Tobin, J. M., Bird, I. F., and Boyle, D. F. (1960): *Dis. Nerv. Syst.,* 21:11–19.

118. Tunks, E. R., and Dermer, S. W. (1977): *J. Nerv. Ment. Dis.,* 164:56–63.

119. Tupin, J. P., Smith, D. B., Clanson, T. L., Kim, L. I., Nugent, A., and Groupe, A. (1973): *Compr. Psychiatry,* 14:311–317.

120. Turner, W. J. (1967): *Int. J. Neuropsychiatry,* 3:8–20.

121. Ulrich, R. E., Hutchinson, R. R., and Azrin, N. H. (1965): *Psychol. Rec.,* 14:111–126.
122. Valzelli, L. (1967): *Adv. Pharmacol.,* 5:79–108.
123. Valzelli, L. (1969): In: *Aggressive Behaviour,* edited by S. Garattini and E. B. Sigg, pp. 70–76. Excerpta Medica Foundation, Amsterdam.
124. Valzelli, L., Giaconone, E., and Garattini, S. (1967): *Eur. J. Pharmacol.,* 2:144–146.
125. Vassout, A., and Delini-Stula, A. (1977): *J. Pharmacol. (Paris),* 8:5–14.
126. *Vital Statistics Report (Final Data)* (1984): Vol. 33, Suppl., 22 June, p. 27, Table 8.
127. Wasman, M., and Flynn, J. P. (1962): *Arch. Neurol.,* 6:220–227.
128. Whitehead, P. L., and Clark, L. D. (1970): *Am. J. Psychiatry,* 127:824–825.
129. Williams, D. T., Mehl, R., Yudofsky, S., Adams, S. D., and Roseman, B. (1982): *J. Am. Acad. Child Psychiatry,* 21:129–135.
130. Worrall, E. P., Moody, J. P., and Naylor, G. J. (1975): *Br. J. Psychiatry,* 126:464–468.
131. Yaryura, J. A., and Neziroglu, F. A. (1981): In: *Aggression and Violence: A Psychobiological and Clinical Approach,* edited by L. Valzelli and L. Morgene, pp. 195–210. Centro Culturale, St. Vincent.
132. Yen, C. Y., Stranger, R. L., and Millman, N. (1959): *Arch. Int. Pharmacodyn. Ther.,* 123:179–185.
133. Yorkston, N. J., Zaki, S. A., Pitcher, D. R., Gruzelier, J. H., Hollander, D., and Sergeant, H. G. S. (1977): *Lancet,* 2:575–578.
134. Yudofsky, S. C., Silver, J. M., Jackson, W., Endicott, J., and Williams, D. (1986): *Am. J. Psychiatry,* 143:35–39.
135. Yudofsky, S., Stevens, L., Silver, J., Barsa, J., and Williams, D. (1984): *Am. J. Psychiatry,* 141:114–115.
136. Yudofsky, S., Williams, D., and Gorman, J. (1981): *Am. J. Psychiatry,* 138:218–220.

Psychopharmacology:
The Third Generation of Progress,
edited by Herbert Y. Meltzer.
Raven Press, New York © 1987.

CHAPTER **69**

The Genetics of Schizophrenia: A Current Perspective

Kenneth S. Kendler

The goal of this chapter is to provide a selective, current perspective on the genetics of schizophrenia. The discussion will focus on four questions: (a) *Is schizophrenia familial?* If schizophrenia is familial, (b) *To what extent is the familial aggregation of schizophrenia due to environmental versus genetic factors?* and (c) *What is transmitted within families that predisposes to schizophrenia?* Finally, if genetic factors play an important role in the familial transmission of schizophrenia, (d) *What is their mode of genetic transmission?*

IS SCHIZOPHRENIA FAMILIAL?

In a 1967 review article, Zerbin-Rudin (66) listed 17 major family studies of schizophrenia involving first-degree relatives. Since then, at least eight further major studies have been reported. Aside from parents where, due to fertility effects, a low risk of illness would be predicted (23,48), these studies have consistently shown a risk for schizophrenia in the relatives of schizophrenics that is substantially greater than that expected in the general population.

However, nearly all of these studies had three important methodologic limitations. First, no control groups were used. Figures for population rates of schizophrenia were derived from other samples or from the literature. Second, diagnoses were made nonblind. That is, the investigator always knew that the individual being evaluated was a relative of a schizophrenic. Third, structured personal interviews and operationalized diagnostic criteria were not used. In fact, in many of the earlier studies, it is unclear

how many individuals were personally examined versus evaluated indirectly from the reports of other relatives, doctors, hospital notes, etc. (e.g., 19).

Noting the limitations of earlier studies and reporting small uncontrolled samples themselves, two recent reports (1,44) have questioned whether schizophrenia, when carefully or "narrowly" diagnosed, is indeed a familial disorder. Since 1980, four major studies meeting most or all of these methodologic criteria have been performed, which permit an evaluation of these claims.

The study of Scharfetter and Nusperli (53) included a large sample of relatives of probands with schizophrenia, schizoaffective disorder, and affective illness. Seventy percent of the living relatives were personally examined using a structured interview. Diagnoses according to the International Classification of Diseases, 9th Edition (ICD-9) criteria were made blind to knowledge about the proband's diagnosis. No normal control group was included. In the 726 first-degree relatives of schizophrenia probands, 49 cases of schizophrenia were found. This produced a morbid risk (MR, an estimate of the proportion of relatives who would be affected if they all lived through their age of risk for schizophrenia) for schizophrenia of 8.9%. The parallel figure in the relatives of the affective disorder probands was 3.3%. Although this risk is higher than would be generally expected in the population, the MR for schizophrenia was still highly significantly ($p = 0.0003$) greater in the relatives of schizophrenics than in the relatives of affective disorder probands.

In the "St. Louis-500 study," 500 probands and 1,249 first-degree relatives were personally evaluated using a structured psychiatric interview developed at Washington

University. Diagnoses of definite and probable schizophrenia were made blindly using a modification of the Feighner criteria. Of the 500 probands, 44 were diagnosed as definitely schizophrenic. The prevalence of definite and probable schizophrenia in their interviewed relatives was 3.6 and 4.5%, respectively (15). The parallel figures in the relatives of all the nonschizophrenic psychiatric probands were 0.6 and 1.1%. No normal control probands were studied. Both definite schizophrenia ($p = 0.0008$) and probable schizophrenia ($p = 0.004$) were significantly more common in the relatives of the schizophrenic than in the relatives of nonschizophrenic psychiatrically ill probands.

Baron et al. (3) personally interviewed the relatives of 90 schizophrenic and 90 matched control probands using a structured interview. Diagnoses were made blindly according to the DSM-III, except that "chronic schizoaffective disorder" was included in schizophrenia. The MR for schizophrenia was significantly greater in the relatives of the schizophrenic (5.8%) than in the relatives of the control probands (0.6%) ($p = 0.0001$).

Two reports have appeared on schizophrenia from the Iowa 500 and non-500 studies (26,60). Probands for these studies were obtained from 510 consecutive admissions to the Iowa Psychopathic Hospital from 1934 to 1944 with a chart diagnosis of schizophrenia. Controls were obtained from routine surgical admissions to the University of Iowa Hospital. In the 1970s, the probands were systematically followed up and the relatives were interviewed using a structured interview. Records from the public hospitals in Iowa were also searched. Probands and relatives were diagnosed blindly. The first report (60) was based on 200 probands diagnosed as schizophrenic from the index charts according to the Feighner criteria and 160 controls. Diagnoses in relatives were based on the consensus of three senior psychiatrists. Including relatives with only hospital records, this study found an MR for schizophrenia of 5.3% in the relatives of schizophrenics and 0.6% in the relatives of controls ($p = 0.000002$). Including only relatives with a personal interview, the parallel figures were 3.2% and 0.6% ($p = 0.003$). The second study (26) was based on 332 schizophrenic probands diagnosed from both index chart and followup information as schizophrenic by the Diagnostic and Statistical Manual of the American Psychiatric Association, 3rd edition (DSM-III) criteria and 318 control probands. Relatives were diagnosed by DSM-III criteria as well. In this larger sample using more restrictive diagnostic criteria, including relatives with only hospital records, they found an MR for schizophrenia of 3.7% in the relatives of schizophrenics and 0.2% in the relatives of controls ($p = 7.9 \times 10^{-8}$). Including only relatives with personal interviews, the parallel figures were 1.8 and 0% ($p = 0.00004$). Because of the relatively old age of the population studied in this sample, the excess mortality in schizophrenia results in an approximately 35% underestimation of MR when only living interviewed relatives are considered (26).

Results of recent family studies that have included control groups, blind diagnosis, and structured psychiatric interviews have replicated the extensive earlier literature and suggest that schizophrenia, even when "narrowly" diagnosed, is indeed a familial disorder.

TO WHAT EXTENT IS THE FAMILIAL AGGREGATION OF SCHIZOPHRENIA DUE TO GENETIC VERSUS ENVIRONMENTAL FACTORS?

Resemblance among relatives can generally be ascribed to three possible mechanisms: cultural transmission, shared environment, and genes. Cultural transmission occurs in a variety of ways but is best demonstrated by the tendency in human families for offspring to learn or model behaviors from their parents. For example, language and religious affiliation are almost certainly passed from generation to generation by cultural transmission.

Shared environment occurs when relatives cohabit together and hence share similar environmental conditions. For example, a correlation in blood pressure among relatives might in part arise from a shared high-sodium diet.

A major goal of genetic epidemiology is to discriminate for familial disorders the degree to which familial transmission is due to one of these first two mechanisms versus genes. Although sophisticated analysis of family data can begin to make this discrimination, for schizophrenia the great bulk of our knowledge about this problem comes from twin and adoption studies.

Twin studies are based on the assumptions that (a) monozygotic (MZ) and dizygotic (DZ) twins share their environment to approximately the same degree, but (b) MZ twins are genetically identical whereas DZ twins, like normal siblings, have on average only half of their genes identical by descent. Although the second of these assumptions is beyond question, the first, or "equal environment" assumption, has been a focus of considerable controversy.

Several studies have shown that measures of the social environment (e.g., sharing the same friends, attitudes of parents and teachers, etc.) are more highly correlated among young MZ than among young same-sex DZ twins (21). These results at first appear to suggest that the equal environment assumption is false. However, reflection suggests another possible interpretation. Although the similarity in environment might make MZ twins more similar, the similarity in behavior of MZ twins might *create* for themselves more similar environments. As recently reviewed (21), these two alternative hypotheses have been subject to empirical test in at least nine different studies. Consistently, these studies suggest that the environmental similarity of MZ twins is the *result* and not the cause of their behavioral similarity. Whereas most of these studies examined such traits as intelligence and personality, one specifically examined schizophrenia and found no evidence that concordance for schizophrenia was produced in MZ twins as a result of the similarity of their treatment by the environment (21). Current evidence supports the general validity of the equal environment assumption of twin studies.

Results are available from 12 major twin studies of schizophrenia (Table 1). None of these studies meet all the methodologic criteria outlined above for family studies and an additional criterion that zygosity assignment be made blind with respect to psychiatric diagnosis. Some studies come closer than others. For example, blind diagnoses by

TABLE 1. *Probandwise concordance and the coefficient of genetic determination in the major twin studies reported to date*

Senior author	Country	Year	Probandwise MZ		Concordance same-sex DZ		Coefficient of genetic determination ±SE
			N	%	N	%	
Luxenburger (38)	Germany	1928	14/22	64	0/13	0	*
Rosanoff (49)	USA	1934	25/41	61	7/53	13	.84 ± .26
			to		to		to
			50/66	76	14/60	23	.63 ± .26
Essen-Moller (9)	Sweden	1941	7/11	64	4/27	15	.87 ± .36
Kallmann (20)	USA	1946	191/245	78	59/318	19	.90 ± .13
Slater (54)	England	1953	32/41	78	14/61	23	.65 ± .23
Inouye (18)	Japan	1961	33/55	60	2/11	18	.66 ± .35
Kringlen (35)	Norway	1967	31/69	45	14/96	15	.61 ± .20
Fischer (12)	Denmark	1973	14/23	61	12/43	28	.41 ± .29
Gottesman (14)	England	1972	15/26	58	4/34	12	.86 ± .32
Tienari (57)	Finland	1975	7/21	33	6/42	14	.53 ± .33
Leonard (21)	Germany	1982	30/44	68	7/34	21	.63 ± .24
Kendler (31)	USA	1983	60/194	31	18/277	6	.91 ± .16

* Cannot be calculated.

Concordance rates are *not* age corrected. Estimates of the coefficient of genetic determination (approximately equal to "broad heritability of liability") are based on population risks for schizophrenia either provided in the study or estimated by the reviewer. For further details regarding figures in this table see refs. 21 and 31. For studies with multiple reports, the latest or most complete report was chosen for analysis.

a variety of different clinicians on summarized case records are reported from the Maudsley twin series of Gottesman and Shields (14). In the National Academy of Sciences-National Research Council (NAS-NRC) registry, psychiatric diagnoses were collected from a wide variety of clinical settings that could not possibly have been aware of any research hypotheses (31). Furthermore, it could be shown that zygosity assignment was not biased with respect to psychiatric diagnosis.

Although all these studies agree that probandwise concordance for schizophrenia (the probability of illness in the cotwin of proband twins) is much higher in MZ than in DZ twins, the absolute rates of concordance vary widely. Two factors are probably responsible for most of this variation. First, some studies employed a broader definition of schizophrenia than others. Second, some studies obtained most of their proband twins from chronically hospitalized populations, whereas others used population-based registries where milder cases would commonly occur. Twin studies have consistently found a positive relationship between concordance and severity of illness (14,31,35).

Both the diagnostic approach to schizophrenia and the method of ascertaining probands should apply equally to MZ and DZ twins. Therefore, a better method of comparing results across studies would be a summary statistic based on concordance in both MZ and DZ twins. One of the best of these is the coefficient of genetic determination or *G* as outlined by Smith (56). *G*, which is similar to the "broad heritability of liability" of quantitative genetics, is based on a multifactorial threshold model which may or may not be true for the transmission of schizophrenia. Although these results should be regarded as only one plausible way of approximating reality, there is substantial

agreement across the major twin studies of schizophrenia that the heritability of liability of schizophrenia is between 0.6 and 0.9. Twin studies consistently suggest that genetic factors play a major role in the familial transmission of schizophrenia.

Limitations of space prohibit a thorough review of adoption studies of schizophrenia. In brief, three studies have examined the risk of schizophrenia in adopted-away offspring of schizophrenics versus controls (16,50,58). All three studies found a substantial excess of schizophrenia and related disorders in the adopted-away offspring of schizophrenics versus controls. The results from Rosenthal's study (50) were of only borderline significance. However, a conservative reanalysis using DSM-III criteria which excluded many of the parents with uncertain diagnoses broadly replicated the original results (37). The results from the Finnish sample of Tienari (58) are preliminary, since this study is still in progress, and are based only on rates of "psychosis" rather than of schizophrenia *per se*.

The second major adoption strategy used for studying schizophrenia begins with ill adoptees rather than ill parents. Such studies contain two separate "experiments." A comparison of the adoptive relatives of schizophrenic and control adoptees is a test of the role of shared environment and/or cultural transmission, whereas a comparison of the biologic relatives of the two groups of adoptees is a test for the role of genes in the familial transmission of schizophrenia.

This strategy has been used by Kety and colleagues in a series of adoption studies carried out in Denmark (32–34). The first or Copenhagen sample began with 34 adoptees located in Copenhagen who received a consensus diagnosis of chronic, borderline, or acute schizophrenia. These adoptees and their matched controls had been separated from their biologic parents at an early age and raised by individuals with whom they had no biologic relationship. The first report on this series was based on hospital abstracts of all relatives located by the population and psychiatric registries available in Denmark. Schizophrenia and related disorders were significantly concentrated only in the biologic relatives of the schizophrenic adoptees (32). The next phase of this project involved the personal interviews of all available and cooperative relatives. A diagnostic review of these interviews, translated into English and reviewed blind, also indicated a substantial concentration of schizophrenia spectrum disorders only in the biologic relatives of the schizophrenic adoptees (33).

A second sample of 41 schizophrenia spectrum adoptees were located from outside of Copenhagen and have been termed the "provincial" sample. Only the first phase of this second sample, involving the blind review of hospital abstracts, has been completed (34). Results basically replicated the parallel findings from the Copenhagen sample. Schizophrenia and the spectrum disorders were significantly more common in the biologic relatives of the schizophrenic versus control probands, whereas these disorders were equally uncommon in the two groups of adoptive relatives. As of October 1985, personal interviews have been conducted with nearly all available and cooperative relatives from the provincial sample and results from their analysis should be available soon.

The interviews from the Copenhagen sample have been subject to several reanalyses. Only one has involved a reexamination of all available interviews with relatives and adoptees (25). Using DSM-III criteria, this review replicated and extended all the major earlier findings of Kety and co-workers.

Results from Kety's adoption studies have been subjected to considerable criticism from several sources (e.g., 36). A focal point of this criticism has been the analysis of the half-siblings. Because of the reproductive habits of the biologic parents of the adoptees from Copenhagen, the adoptees had relatively few full sibs but many maternal and paternal half-sibs. In most analyses, half-sibs (who are second-degree relatives) have been combined with full sibs and parents (who are first-degree relatives). An apparently anomolous result is that rates of schizophrenia spectrum pathology are higher in Kety's report in the half-sibs than in the full sibs and parents (33). Furthermore, when analyzing first-degree relatives only, Kety et al. found that the rate of schizophrenia spectrum was higher in biologic relatives of schizophrenics than in controls (13.0 vs. 7.1%), but the difference was not significant. The following points need to be considered in weighing these criticisms: (a) Combining first- and second-degree relatives in a single analysis is proper and will maximize statistical power as long as the proportion of each group of relatives is approximately equal in the families of the two groups of adoptees. This is the case in the Copenhagen sample. (b) Because the number of full sibs is so small in the sample, first-degree relatives are mostly parents. Because of the reduced fertility of individuals with schizophrenia, parents of schizophrenics will have a lower rate of schizophrenia than sibs (23,47). Therefore, rates of illness in first-degree relatives (mostly parents) should not necessarily be markedly higher than in half-siblings where fitness effects play a much smaller role. (c) In their reanalysis using DSM-III criteria, Kendler and Gruenberg (25) found higher rates of schizophrenia spectrum in first-degree than in second-degree interviewed biologic relatives of schizophrenic adoptees, and significantly higher rates of schizophrenia spectrum in biologic relatives of schizophrenic versus control adoptees when considering *either* first-degree or second-degree relatives only. Although not devoid of limitations, the Danish adoption studies of schizophrenia by Kety et al. have been tested by personal interviews, diagnostic reevaluations, and now a full replication; the initial results have been repeatedly reconfirmed.

Studies involving only MZ and DZ twins have no power to resolve the degree to which nongenetic transmission of schizophrenia may be due to cultural transmission. Adoption studies potentially have such power, particularly with respect to cultural transmission from parent to offspring (termed *vertical* cultural transmission or VCT). Before discussing these results, it is important to clarify a source of continued confusion. With some clinical justification, it has been said that schizophrenic parents may not be the most potentially schizophrenogenic. Therefore studies that show no evidence for VCT of schizophrenia do not necessarily suggest that family environment plays no role in the etiology of schizophrenia. However, if schizophrenic parents are not schizophrenogenic, then familial factors *cannot* explain why schizophrenia runs in families. In other words, if schizophrenic parents are not schizophrenogenic, why do offspring of schizophrenic parents have such an increased risk for schizophrenia?

Several adoption strategies have been used that can clarify the role of VCT in schizophrenia. First, the risk for schizophrenia in the adopted-away offspring of normal individuals reared by schizophrenic parents can be examined. Although limited by the small sample size and the small number of parents with typical schizophrenia, Wender et al. (64) found no evidence for increased rates of illness in such adoptees. Second, VCT of schizophrenia would predict that among adopted individuals who become schizophrenic, schizophrenia should be overrepresented in their adoptive parents who would culturally "transmit" schizophrenia. In Kety's Copenhagen and provincial samples (33,34), no excess cases of schizophrenia or related spectrum conditions were seen in the adoptive parents of the schizophrenic adoptees. In separate samples, Wender et al. twice studied psychopatholgy in the adoptive parents of schizophrenics (63,65). In the first of these studies, evidence was found for an excess of severe psychopathology in the adoptive parents of schizophrenics. In the second study, which the authors felt was better controlled, no such increase was found. Third, since step-siblings of schizophrenics would be exposed to the same schizophrenogenic rearing environment as the schizophrenic but lack the biologic relationship to the parents, VCT would predict an excess of schizophrenia in step-sibs of schizophrenics. Both Rudin (51) and Kallmann (19) examined step-sibs of schizophrenics and found that rates of illness were not substantially increased in this group. Finally, if schizophrenic parents in part transmit the risk for schizophrenia to their offspring culturally, then decreasing the amount of contact between schizophrenic parents and their children should decrease their risk for illness. Higgins (17) compared two small samples of offspring of schizophrenic mothers, of which one sample had been reared with their mothers and the other had been adopted away to normal parents at an early age. Rates for schizophrenia were nonsignificantly higher in the adopted-away than in the home-reared offspring. Mirsky et al. (42) examined offspring of schizophrenic parents in Israel raised either in towns in a typical nuclear family setting or on a kibbutz where parents are not directly responsible for rearing their own children. They found rates for schizophrenia and associated spectrum disorders to be nonsignificantly *higher* in the kibbutz-reared than in the town-reared offspring.

Adoption studies provide little evidence for an important role of VCT in the etiology of schizophrenia. However, there is other empirical evidence that at least suggests that family environment may play a role in the transmission of this disorder. First, Singer et al. were able to select with striking accuracy the blinded Rorschach protocols of the adoptive parents of schizophrenics from the first study of Wender (63). However, in their second study, Wender et al. (65) were unable to replicate these results. Second, in the ongoing Finnish adoption study of schizophrenia (58), a highly significant correlation was found between the global health of the adoptive family and the psychopathologic outcome of the adoptee. However, these results cannot distinguish whether disturbed families were producing disturbed adoptees or vice versa. Third, high-risk studies are beginning to produce results suggestive of a specific role for parental behavior in subsequent risk for schizophrenia spectrum disorders. For example, communication deviance, affective style, and expressed emotion of parents of a mildly to moderately disturbed teenager significantly predicted schizophrenia spectrum outcome 15 years later (13). However, since this was a nuclear family study, it remains possible that these parental measures were an index of genetic predisposition to schizophrenia in the parents rather than a measure of schizophrenogenic behavior.

Fourth, path analytic models generally support a modest role for VCT in the etiology of schizophrenia. Path analysis, which assumes a polygenic-multifactorial model, is a method that has considerable power at discriminating genetic from cultural transmission. Two related studies applied this method to schizophrenia (40,45). Both were performed on summary data sets of western European studies including twins, spouses, and first- and second-degree relatives. The second study (40) used an updated data set, examined the relationship between definite and probable schizophrenia, and took account of the heterogeneity of recurrence figures between studies. The same path analytic model was employed in both studies and is a relatively restrictive one. Finally, recurrence risks were not corrected for fitness effects. Rather, risk in parents and uncles/aunts were simply excluded from the analysis. The results of both studies were similar. The multifactorial model fit the data well. Estimates for the heritability of liability for schizophrenia ranged from .63 to .71 and were always highly statistically significant. This result is reassuringly similar to the .68 found from all major twin studies of schizophrenia as the weighted mean estimate of heritability under a multifacto-

rial-threshold model (21). The proportion of variance in liability due to transmissible environment (cultural heritability) varied between .19 and .24 and was statistically significant in most but not all analyses.

One of the reasons VCT for schizophrenia may have been hard to detect is that only certain relatively rare genotypes are sensitive to a schizophrenogenic rearing environment. Under this model, a substantial excess risk for schizophrenia would not be expected in step-sibs of schizophrenics or individuals adopted by a schizophrenic parent. This form of gene × environment interaction, which can more usefully be conceptualized as genetic control of sensitivity to the environment, has specifically been suggested by Tienari et al. (58). Their adoption design, in which both genetic liability to schizophrenia (as indexed by diagnosis of biologic parent) and rearing environment (as indexed by assessment of adoptive family) are measured, is potentially quite powerful at detecting such effects.

In summary, twin and adoption studies suggest that most of the familial aggregation of schizophrenia is due to genes. Evidence for VCT of the liability to schizophrenia is much less clear. Both twin and more general path analytic models suggest that the heritability of liability of schizophrenia is best estimated as between 60 and 70%. By contrast, if present, nongenetic familial factors appear to account for only about 20% of the variance in liability.

WHAT IS TRANSMITTED IN FAMILIES THAT PREDISPOSES TO SCHIZOPHRENIA?

On the level of psychopathological syndromes, four major hypotheses can be articulated about the form of liability to schizophrenia that is transmitted in families: (a) a general liability to all psychiatric illness; (b) a liability to poor psychosocial functioning, oddness, suspiciousness, etc.; (c) a liability to psychosis; and (d) a specific liability only to typical schizophrenia. These hypotheses are useful because each generates specific predictions about the pattern of psychopathology that should be seen in families of schizophrenics.

The first hypothesis predicts that all major forms of psychiatric illness should occur in excess in relatives of schizophrenics. The hypothesis would be consistent with the unitary hypothesis of mental disorders, which postulates that all psychiatric illness is on a single continuum with schizophrenia at the most deviant end. In his famous 1938 family study, Kallmann (19) argued for the specificity of the familial liability to schizophrenia by showing that relatives of schizophrenics had no apparent excess of nonschizoid psychopathy, alcoholism, or criminality. In the interview phase of the Copenhagen sample of the Danish adoption study, Kety et al. (33) found no excess of organic, neurotic, or affective illness or nonschizophrenia spectrum personality disorders in the biologic relatives of schizophrenic adoptees. However, in an earlier adoption study, Heston (16) found a significant excess of cases of "neurotic personality disorder" in adopted-away offspring of schizophrenic versus control mothers.

Only with the introduction of operationalized criteria could this hypothesis be fully evaluated. The crucial comparison is between relatives of schizophrenics and a sample representative of the general population. Both of the two recent family studies containing such a control group and using DSM-III criteria (3,26) found results inconsistent with this hypothesis. In both studies, no excess risk for affective illness, anxiety disorders, or alcoholism was found in the relatives of the schizophrenics versus controls. Similar results on a smaller sample size were found in the Copenhagen sample of the Danish adoption study (25) and in pilot data from the West of Ireland (K. S. Kendler et al., unpublished data). The familial liability to schizophrenia appears to possess some specificity.

Early studies argue against the fourth hypothesis that would predict that only schizophrenia should occur in excess in relatives of schizophrenics (22). For example, in accord with the third hypothesis, Rudin (51) found that in the siblings of schizophrenics, the MR for other psychotic disorders was nearly as great as for typical schizophrenia (4.1 vs. 4.5%). In accord with the second hypothesis, Kallmann (19) found in siblings and offspring of schizophrenic probands very high rates for what he termed "borderline cases" and "schizoid psychopaths," parts of what he termed the "schizophrenic disease-complex." More recently, the Danish adoption studies (32–34,50) found evidence for a genetic relationship between chronic schizophrenia and "borderline" or "uncertain" schizophrenia.

The more recent application of operationalized criteria has replicated and extended these earlier findings. Reanalyses of the Danish adoption samples (25,37) have found that, as defined by DSM-III, schizotypal, paranoid, and possibly schizoid personality disorder have a strong genetic relationship to schizophrenia. Three further investigations based on intact families have supported these findings. Two were done in New York, one employing the family history method (30) and the other utilizing direct interviews (3). Both provided strong evidence for a familial relationship between schizophrenia and schizotypal and paranoid personality disorder. The third study comes from County Roscommon, Ireland (K. S. Kendler et al., unpublished data), where pilot data also show a significantly higher risk for schizotypal and paranoid personality disorders in interviewed first-degree relatives of schizophrenic versus control probands.

Recent studies have also suggested that psychotic disorders other than schizophrenia aggregate in relatives of schizophrenics. When schizoaffective disorder is defined to exclude the mainly affective cases where the psychotic symptoms have only occurred during major affective episodes (e.g., mood-incongruent psychotic affective illness in DSM-III terms), a number of studies beginning either with schizophrenic (24,26) or with schizoaffective probands (2,27,53) suggest that schizoaffective disorder bears a genetic/familial relationship to more classic schizophrenia.

Evidence regarding the familial relationship between schizophrenia and paranoid disorder and the remitting or atypical psychoses is less clear. Three studies beginning with paranoid disorder probands (28,29,62) have found no excess risk for schizophrenia in their relatives. However, in a study beginning with schizophrenic probands, Kendler et al. (26) found a significant excess risk for paranoid disorder in their relatives. This asymmetry of results may result

from differing levels of diagnostic accuracy in probands versus secondary cases.

Previous studies have disagreed as to whether the atypical and schizophreniform psychoses are closely related to typical schizophrenia (e.g., 4) or are not (e.g., 39). Recently gathered results using DSM-III criteria are also contradictory. Sautter and Garver (52) found that lithium-responsive schizophreniform patients have little familial risk for schizophrenia or related spectrum disorders. However, in the Iowa data set, compared to relatives of controls, atypical psychoses were highly significantly more common in relatives of schizophrenics (26), and the risk for schizophrenia but not affective illness was significantly increased in relatives of schizophreniform probands (27).

Another specific test of the third hypothesis is to examine the frequency of psychotic affective illness in relatives of schizophrenics. In the Iowa data set, although relatives of schizophrenics were not at increased risk for affective illness, if affectively ill they were more than $2\frac{1}{2}$ times as likely to become psychotic as affectively ill relatives of controls (26).

In summary, results to date strongly suggest that neither hypothesis (a) nor (d) is correct. The familial predisposition to schizophrenia is neither completely nonspecific, nor highly specific. Results are available to strongly support the second hypothesis and also to provide some evidence in favor of the third hypothesis. These findings provide an increasingly complex, but informative, picture of the nature of the transmitted liability to schizophrenia.

MODE OF GENETIC TRANSMISSION OF LIABILITY TO SCHIZOPHRENIA

Although evidence in favor of a genetic contribution to schizophrenia has been available for nearly 50 years, we are still quite ignorant about the mode of transmission of this genetic liability. Early investigators nearly all favored simple mendelian models (e.g., one or two recessive loci; refs. 19, 51). With the introduction of the multifactorial threshold model by Falconer (10), the application of this model to schizophrenia (e.g., 14) gained wide acceptance. Innovations in analytic methods have recently sparked an increasing interest in more sophisticated single gene models for schizophrenia. The major problem has been that, until recently, tools that were sufficiently powerful to discriminate these varying modes of transmission were not available. Since the genes involved in schizophrenia are not fully penetrant (i.e., MZ concordance is substantially below 100%), morbidity risk figures alone provide little power to discriminate between major gene and polygene models (55). Interest has therefore recently focused on two techniques which incorporate information about family structure whose goal is to detect a single locus that substantially affect liability to illness: complex segregation analysis and linkage analysis.

Complex segregation analysis developed from relatively simple methods to determine whether the segregation ratio observed within sibships was consistent with the mendelian expectation of $\frac{1}{4}$ for a recessive disorder when both parents are normal. This method has grown considerably in complexity, and modern techniques will include estimates of gene frequency, penetrance, transmission probabilities, polygenes, common sibling environment, and variable age of onset. Despite these advances, applications of this method to schizophrenia have been few and controversial.

Four major segregation analyses of schizophrenia have been published. In brief, two of them (8,59) found evidence for vertical transmission of schizophrenia but strongly rejected a single gene model. The other two (5,48) also found strong evidence for vertical transmission of schizophrenia and found the pattern could be explained by polygenes with a relatively high heritability (.62–.82). However, in both studies a single major gene alone (5) or a single major gene with a modest polygene "background" (48) also gave a good fit to the data. These results should be regarded as very preliminary for several reasons. First, only two of these used data sets that would meet the methodologic criteria noted above for family studies (48,59). Second, only one of the studies included a specific evaluation of the schizophrenia spectrum (48). Third, only one of the analyses was based on what is widely regarded as the best current general model for segregation analysis, the "unified mixed-model," and made any attempt to correct for the major impact of reduced fitness in schizophrenia (48). Fourth, no segregation analysis of schizophrenia to date has incorporated exciting new developments, including tests for genetic heterogeneity (e.g., 43) and the incorporation of environmental risk factors into the analysis (6). Finally, the two studies based on adequately studied samples were both relatively small in size (ref. 61, 354, and ref. 48, 276 interviewed relatives). Power analyses have suggested that if a major gene strongly influences liability to a discontinuous trait like schizophrenia, its detection by complex segregation analysis is more likely to require in the range of 1,000 relatives (46).

Given the many complexities that may underlie the genetic transmission of schizophrenia, of which the most troublesome is likely to be genetic heterogeneity, the ultimate resolving power of segregation analysis remains controversial. In the wake of the scientific revolution spawned by DNA technology, and the spectacular success at locating the gene for Huntington's disease, interest has increased markedly in the application of linkage analysis to psychiatric disorders such as schizophrenia. Linkage analysis used to be limited in humans because informative markers could be found in any given pedigree for only a small proportion of the human genome. Using recently developed techniques, it is now possible to examined variability in the human genome at the level of individual DNA base pairs. The number of informative markers discovered in this way has been increasing at a nearly exponential rate. A total linkage map of the human genome is realistic within the next decade.

If a sufficient number of large pedigrees informative for schizophrenia can be found and a single gene exists that substantially influences liability to schizophrenia in at least a subset of these pedigrees, it is theoretically only a matter of screening a sufficient number of markers to locate the gene. However, even if such a gene exists, obtaining evidence for linkage in schizophrenia should prove much more difficult than for Huntington's disease. For example, it is improbable that a major gene for schizophrenia is fully penetrant. However, incomplete penetrance can both markedly reduce the power of linkage analysis and make precise estimates of recombination distance difficult or impossible (P. McGuffin and E. Sturt, in preparation).

To date, linkage studies of schizophrenia using conventional markers have been few and relatively disappointing. Elston et al. (7) reported possible linkage between schizophrenia and the group specific protein (Gc) and the immunoglobin Gm locus. Turner (61) found possible evidence for linkage between schizophrenia and human lymphocyte antigen (HLA). However, the most carefully done linkage study of schizophrenia to date (41) could replicate neither of these findings and found no evidence for linkage between schizophrenia and any other of the 17 markers examined. Given that the sample sizes of all these studies were relatively small and that only a quite small proportion of the human genome was examined, the negative results should not be too surprising.

Another application of molecular techniques to the genetics of schizophrenia is the direct examination of small sections of DNA by endonucleases. The first such report detected no abnormalities in the region of the proopiomelancortin gene in a small sample of schizophrenic patients (11).

What are we to conclude regarding the transmission of schizophrenia? First, although it has been known at least since 1916 that schizophrenia does not follow a classic mendelian pattern, it still remains possible that a single gene defect substantially *influences* liability to schizophrenia in a major proportion of cases. However, this influence has been difficult to detect for one or more of the following reasons: (a) genetic heterogeneity; (b) major environmental determinants, which can either make an individual with a normal genotype affected (e.g., a phenocopy) or render an individual with a deviant genotype unaffected (e.g., reduced penetrances); (c) nongenetic forms of familial transmission such as VCT or viral infections, which can markedly complicate the detection and estimation of genetic parameters; (d) genotype × environment interactions, such as genetic control of sensitivity to the environment, so that the genetic liability to schizophrenia is only expressed in certain environments; (e) limitations in our ability to precisely define the boundaries of "schizophrenia" phenotype, so that a number of relatives are misclassified; (f) continued practical limitations of field studies, such as the differential mortality, migration, and cooperation of affected versus unaffected relatives; and (g) more "technical" issues regarding the schizophrenia phenotype, such as reduced fitness, which are difficult to fully capture in models.

Second, Occam's razor requires that high priority be given to the detection of a possible single major gene for schizophrenia. In addition to simplicity, the demonstration of a single gene accounting for a major proportion of the liability to schizophrenia would have profound implications for our understanding of the biology of this condition. It would indicate that a single, potentially detectable biologic abnormality must play a major role in the etiology of schizophrenia.

Third, because of developments in field study methods, analytic genetic techniques, and molecular genetics, cautious optimism is now appropriate regarding our ability to detect a major gene for schizophrenia if it is present.

Fourth, the multifactorial-polygenic is conceptually appealing, mathematically simple, and fits the currently available information about schizophrenia rather well. However, acceptance of this model should be tempered by two facts. First, the model is very flexible (55), and therefore difficult to disprove. Second, from a biological perspective, the multifactorial model is a pessimistic one. If this model is correct, understanding *the* biology of schizophrenia will be as difficult as understanding *the* biology of height, a typical "polygenic" trait with a high heritability.

CONCLUSIONS

The evidence is strong that schizophrenia is a familial disorder and that the familial aggregation of schizophrenia is due largely, but not entirely, to genetic factors. Whatever the familial predisposition that operates for schizophrenia, it not only "codes" for the classic, psychotic disorder but also increases liability to "schizophrenia-like" personality disorders and probably other nonschizophrenic, nonaffective psychoses. We remain largely ignorant about the mode of transmission of the genetic liability to schizophrenia. Although previous studies have been inconclusive, newly developed methods of complex segregation and linkage analysis provide a source for cautious optimism regarding the possibility of clarifying this central issue. In addition to elucidating the mode of genetic transmission for schizophrenia, other critical questions in the genetics of schizophrenia include (a) What kinds of characteristics, behaviors, or physiologic variables do the genes for schizophrenia "code for"? (b) How does the genetic susceptibility to schizophrenia interact with environmental risk factors? (c) What are the magnitude and form of the contribution of nongenetic factors to the familial transmission of schizophrenia?

ACKNOWLEDGMENT

Preparation of this chapter was supported in part by the Department of Mental Health and Mental Retardation, Commonwealth of Virginia.

REFERENCES

1. Abrams, R., and Taylor, M. A. (1983): *Am. J. Psychiatry,* 140: 171–175.
2. Baron, M., Gruen, R., Asnis, L., and Kane, J. (1982): *Acta Psychiatr. Scand.,* 65:253–262.
3. Baron, M., Gruen, R., Rainer, J. D., Kane, J., Asnis, L., and Lord, S. (1985): *Am. J. Psychiatry,* 142:447–455.
4. Bleuler, M. (1978): *The Schizophrenic Disorders: Long-Term Patient and Family Studies* (trans. S. M. Clemens). Yale University Press, New Haven.
5. Carter, C. L., and Chung, C. S. (1980): *Hum. Hered.,* 30:350–356.
6. Eaves, L. J. (1984): *Genet. Epidemiol.,* 1:215–228.
7. Elston, R. C., Kringlen, E., and Namboodiri, K. K. (1973): *Behav. Genet.,* 3:101–106.
8. Elston, R. C., Namboodiri, K. K., Spence, M. A., and Rainer, J. D. (1978): *Neuropsychobiology,* 4:193–206.
9. Essen-Moller, E. (1941): *Acta Psychiatr. Scand.* (Suppl.):23.
10. Falconer, D. S. (1965): *Ann. Hum. Genet.,* 29:51–76.
11. Feder, J., Gurling, H. M. D., Darby, J., and Cavalli-Sforza, L. L. (1985): *Am. J. Hum. Genet.,* 37:286–294.
12. Fischer, M. (1973): *Acta Psychiatr. Scand.* (Suppl.):238.
13. Goldstein, M. J. (1985): *Acta Psychiatr. Scand.* (*Suppl.*), 319:71: 7–18.
14. Gottesman, I. I., and Shields, J. (1972): In: *Schizophrenia and Genetics: A Twin Study Vantage Point.* Academic Press, New York.
15. Guze, S. B., Cloninger, C. R., Martin, R. L., and Clayton, P. J. (1983): *Arch. Gen. Psychiatry,* 40:1273–1276.
16. Heston, L. L. (1966): *Br. J. Psychiatry,* 112:819–825.
17. Higgins, J. (1976): *J. Psychiatr. Res.,* 13:1–9.
18. Inouye, E. (1963): In: *Proceedings, Third World Congress of Psychiatry, 1961, Vol. I.* University of Toronto Press, Montreal.
19. Kallmann, F. J. (1938): *The Genetics of Schizophrenia.* J. S. Augustin, New York.
20. Kallmann, F. J. (1946): *Am. J. Psychiatry,* 103:309–322.
21. Kendler, K. S. (1983): *Am. J. Psychiatry,* 140:1413–1425.
22. Kendler, K. S. (1985): *Schizophr. Bull.,* 11:539–554.
23. Kendler, K. S. (1986): *Behav. Genet.,* 16:417–431.
24. Kendler, K. S., and Adler, D. (1984): *Am. J. Psychiatry,* 141:509–513.
25. Kendler, K. S., and Gruenberg, A. M. (1984): *Arch. Gen. Psychiatry,* 41:555–564.
26. Kendler, K. S., Gruenberg, A. M., and Tsuang, M. T. (1985): *Arch. Gen. Psychiatry,* 42:770–779.
27. Kendler, K. S., Gruenberg, A. M., and Tsuang, M. T. (1986): *Am. J. Psychiatry,* 143:1098–1105.
28. Kendler, K. S., and Hays, P. (1981): *Arch. Gen. Psychiatry,* 38: 547–551.
29. Kendler, K. S., Masterson, C. C., and Davis, K. L. (1986): *Br. J. Psychiatry,* 147:524–531.
30. Kendler, K. S., Masterson, C., Ungaro, R., and Davis, K. (1984): *Am. J. Psychiatry,* 141:424–427.
31. Kendler, K. S., and Robinette, C. D. (1983): *Am. J. Psychiatry,* 140:1551–1563.
32. Kety, S. S., Rosenthal, D., Wender, P. H., and Schulsinger, F. (1971): *Am. J. Psychiatry,* 138:302–306.
33. Kety, S. S., Rosenthal, D., Wender, P. H., Schulsinger, F., and Jacobsen, B. (1975): In: *Genetic Research in Psychiatry,* edited by R. R. Fieve, D. Rosenthal, and H. Brill, pp. 147–165. Johns Hopkins University Press, Baltimore.
34. Kety, S. S., Rosenthal, D., Wender, P., Schulsinger, F., and Jacobsen, F. (1978): In: *The Nature of Schizophrenia,* edited by L. C. Wynn, pp. 25–37. John Wiley & Sons, New York.
35. Kringlen, E. (1967): *Heredity and Environment in the Functional Psychoses: An Epidemiological-Clinical Twin Study.* Universitetsforlaget, Oslo.
36. Lidz, T., and Blatt, S. (1983): *Am. J. Psychiatry,* 140:426–434.
37. Lowing, P. A., Mirsky, A. F., and Pereira, R. (1983): *Am. J. Psychiatry,* 140:1167–1171.
38. Luxenburger, H. (1928): *Z. Gesamte Neurol. Psychiatrie,* 116: 297–326.
39. McCabe, M. S., Fowler, R. C., Cadorte, R. J., and Winokur, G. (1971): *Psychol. Med.,* 1:326–332.
40. McGue, M., Gottesman, I. I., and Rao, D. C. (1983): *Am. J. Hum. Genet.,* 35:1161–1178.
41. McGuffin, P., Festenstein, H., and Murray, R. (1983): *Psychol. Med.,* 13:31–43.
42. Mirsky, A. F., Silberman, E. K., Latz, A., and Nagler, S. (1985): *Schizophr. Bull.,* 11:150–154.
43. Moll, P. P., Berry, T. D., Weidman, W. W., Ellefson, R., Gordon, H., and Kottke, B. A. (1984): *Am. J. Hum. Genet.,* 36:197–211.
44. Pope, H. G., Jones, J. M., Cohen, B. M., and Lipinski, J. F. (1982): *Am. J. Psychiatry,* 139:826–828.
45. Rao, D. C., Morton, N. E., Gottesman, I. I., and Lew, R. (1981): *Hum. Hered.,* 31:325–333.
46. Reich, T., Rice, J., and Cloninger, C. R. (1981): In: *Genetic Research Strategies for Psychobiology and Psychiatry,* edited by E. S. Gershon, pp. 353–367. Boxwood Press, Pacific Grove, California.
47. Risch, N. (1983): *Behav. Genet.,* 13:441–451.
48. Risch, N., and Baron, M. (1984): *Am. J. Hum. Genet.,* 36:1039–1059.

49. Rosanoff, A. J., Handy, L. M., and Plesset, I. R. (1934): *Am. J. Psychiatry,* 91:247–286.
50. Rosenthal, D., Wender, P. H., Kety, S. S., Welner, J., and Schulsinger, F. (1980): *Am. J. Psychiatry,* 128:307–311.
51. Rudin, E. (1916): *Studien uber Vererburg und Entstehung Geistiger Storungen.* Springer, Berlin.
52. Sautter, F., and Garver, D. (1985): *J. Psychiatr. Res.,* 19:1–8.
53. Scharfetter, C., and Nusperli, M. (1980): *Schizophr. Bull.,* 6:586–591.
54. Slater, E. (1953): *Psychotic and Neurotic Illnesses in Twins.* Her Majesty's Stationery Office, London.
55. Smith, C. (1971): *Clin. Genet.,* 2:303–314.
56. Smith, C. (1974): *Am. J. Hum. Genet.,* 26:454–466.
57. Tienari, P. (1975): In: *Studies of Schizophrenia,* edited by M. H. Lader, pp. 29–35. Headley Brothers, Ashford, Kent.
58. Tienari, P., Sorri, A., Lahti, I., Naarala, M., Wahlberg, K., Ronkko, T., Pohjola, J., and Moring, J. (1985): *Yale J. Biol. Med.,* 58:227–237.
59. Tsuang, M. T., Bucher, K. D., and Fleming, J. A. (1982): *Br. J. Psychiatry,* 140:595–599.
60. Tsuang, M. T., Winokur, G., and Crowe, R. R. (1980): *Br. J. Psychiatry,* 137:497–504.
61. Turner, W. J. (1979): *Biol. Psychiatry,* 14:177–206.
62. Watt, J. A. G., Hall, D. J., and Olley, P. C. (1980): *Acta Psychiatr. Scand.,* 61:413–426.
63. Wender, P. H., Rosenthal, D., and Kety, S. S. (1968): In: *The Transmission of Schizophrenia,* edited by D. Rosenthal and S. S. Kety. Pergamon Press, New York.
64. Wender, P. H., Rosenthal, D., Kety, S. S., Schulsinger, F., and Welner, J. (1974): *Arch. Gen. Psychiatry,* 30:121–128.
65. Wender, P. H., Rosenthal, D., Rainer, J. D., Greenhill, L., and Sarlin, M. B. (1977): *Arch. Gen. Psychiatry,* 34:777–784.
66. Zerbin-Rubin, E. (1967): In: *Humangenetik: Ein kurzes Handbuch in funf Banden,* edited by P. E. Becker, *Band V/2,* pp. 446–513. Thieme, Stuttgart.

Psychopharmacology:
The Third Generation of Progress,
edited by Herbert Y. Meltzer.
Raven Press, New York © 1987.

CHAPTER 70

The Dopamine Hypothesis of Schizophrenia

Miklos F. Losonczy, Michael Davidson, and Kenneth L. Davis

A search for insight into the pathological basis of schizophrenia has been the focus of many major investigations in the biology of abnormal human behavior. Although yet to yield fruit in developing improved treatment for the symptoms of this disorder, the hypothesis that at least some schizophrenic individuals suffer from a relative overactivity of some (unknown) central dopaminergic systems has formed the foundation for much of the efforts in this field. This view is largely based on evidence that antipsychotic medications, although varying in many of their actions on brain tissue, have in common the ability to counteract dopamine activity in the CNS. This chapter will review the basis for the belief that antipsychotic efficacy is related to an antidopaminergic effect, and the very separate issue that an overactivity of some dopamine systems may be involved in some schizophrenic individuals.

NEUROLEPTICS: THE FOUNDATION OF THE HYPOTHESIS

A number of convergent lines of evidence have implicated dopamine receptor blockade as the site of antipsychotic action. The clinical observation that antipsychotics frequently produced motoric side effects resembling idiopathic Parkinson's disease, in which dopamine deficits had previously been established, led to the initial speculation that these side effects resulted from an antidopaminergic action of these drugs. The subsequent demonstration that neuroleptics can accelerate the turnover of dopamine, as reflected by increased levels of its metabolite, homovanillic acid (HVA), was interpreted as a negative feedback response to postsynaptic dopamine receptor blockade (17,23,24). Furthermore, neuroleptic agents were shown to inhibit some behavioral effects of apomorphine and amphetamine that were felt to reflect increased dopamine activity, presumably by preventing postsynaptic agonist effects (138). Additional support for the notion that neuroleptic action is mediated through the attenuation of dopamine activity is available from studies showing some synergistic effects of neuroleptics and drugs that inhibit dopamine synthesis (18). The discovery that neuroleptics can inhibit the binding of radiolabeled dopamine to synaptosomal preparations at very low concentrations and show stereospecific, saturable high-affinity binding to these preparations has demonstrated that dopamine receptor blockade is indeed a common pharmacological property of this class of agents (127). Finally, the demonstration that the *in vitro* potencies to displace the binding of spiroperidol from striatal membranes of a wide range of antipsychotics closely parallel the clinical antipsychotic doses has been interpreted as the strongest evidence that the site of antipsychotic action of these drugs involves dopamine blockade (27).

The understanding of the role that this blockade of dopamine receptors plays in diminishing some psychotic symptoms, however, awaits clarification of the nature of the CNS dysfunctions associated with these symptoms. As a working hypothesis, it is not unrealistic to propose that the reason dopamine receptor blockade is involved in antipsychotic action is due to its ability to reverse the effects of a primary lesion that results in the overstimulation of postsynaptic neurons. There are obvious limitations to this simplistic view. It is well established that psychotic symptoms rarely respond to neuroleptic therapy during the short time frame necessary for drug delivery to its putative site of action, but usually take weeks for measurable improvements, whereas the direct action of neuroleptics on the postsynaptic neuron is measurable in hours. Furthermore, it is the unfortunate clinical fact that a substantial number of individuals do not respond to these drugs, and few individuals have a complete remission of all symptoms following neuroleptic treatment. It is of value to note that clinical data on antipsychotic efficacy do not suggest that the psychotic symptoms of schizophrenia are in any way more responsive to these drugs than the psychotic symptoms of other diagnoses. Perhaps because of the dominant role of psychosis in the clinical picture of schizophrenia, the hypothesis of increased dopamine activity has received the greatest attention in studies focusing on this diagnostic group, although the theoretical justification for limiting studies to this group is not clear.

The indirect evidence implicating dopaminergic overactivity based on neuroleptic pharmacology has spurred considerable efforts to provide some direct evidence. The relative inaccessibility of brain tissue to chemical and physiological probes has caused considerable methodological difficulties in study designs and interpretation of results. Two basically different proposed lesions involving dopaminergic overactivity have led to two different approaches and interpretations of data. An excessive discharge of dopaminergic neurons could be responsible, which may be detectable by a local increase in HVA. Any changes in CNS HVA levels could potentially be reflected either in the cerebrospinal fluid (CSF) or in the plasma. Alternatively, dopaminergic overactivity could result from a primary defect in the control mechanisms for maintaining postsynaptic dopamine receptor homeostasis, resulting in an abnormally high concentration of receptors. Interestingly, if associated with an intact negative feedback control on presynaptic firing rates, the hypothesis of increased postsynaptic dopamine receptors, or dopamine supersensitivity, could be associated with a decrease in HVA production. Thus, nearly any change in HVA levels could be consistent with the dopamine hypothesis of schizophrenia in one form or another. Other means of evaluating dopaminergic function could also be explored, including the pharmacological or clinical impact of agents affecting the dopamine system. Additionally, the existence of a group of schizophrenics with no appreciable antipsychotic response to neuroleptics has led to the subsidiary hypothesis that any etiologically significant alteration in dopamine activity may be limited to a subgroup of schizophrenic individuals. Interpretation of any clinical studies would be considerably facilitated if a means of identifying subgroups with and without a dopamine abnormality could be determined. The remainder of this chapter will review the work that has addressed these various complementary or competing approaches to the evaluation of the dopamine hypothesis of schizophrenia.

THE SEARCH FOR MORE DIRECT EVIDENCE

Cerebrospinal Fluid Studies

Because of its physical continuity with the CNS extracellular space, the CSF has been a logical site for examinations of central dopamine turnover. However, unless one assumes that any dopaminergic abnormality is found in the same degree throughout the brain and spinal column, the concentrations of any substance of interest in the CSF may be primarily determined by factors far removed from the putative site of any dopaminergic lesion. Since the majority of work addressing this issue has centered on lumbar CSF HVA levels, a discussion of factors confounding interpretation of these levels may be useful in understanding the limitations of this technique.

It has been reasonably well established that acute changes in the firing rates of dopamine neurons induced by electrochemical or pharmacological means are correlated with local changes in the level of the major extracellular dopamine metabolite, HVA (107). The majority of centrally produced HVA appears to originate in the nigrostriatum, especially the caudate (104,151). Because the head of the caudate abuts on the lateral ventricles, it is thought to be the prime source of HVA in the CSF (151). Although direct data on the actual site (or sites) of antipsychotic and/or psychotogenic action are not yet available, most hypotheses center on mesolimbic or mesocortical regions. Complete maps of the distribution of dopamine receptors in human brains are not yet available, but recent autoradiography of brain tissue slices using the specific D-2 ligand ^{125}I-iodosulpiride suggests a distribution more widespread than conventionally believed, including sensorimotor cortex and cerebellar locations (85). However, these areas are not believed to contribute substantially to the CSF. Furthermore, there is some evidence that a measurable proportion of HVA in the lumbar CSF may originate in the spinal cord (151). Although HVA is fairly resistant to further metabolism, its levels in the CSF are very strongly influenced by the rate of its active transport out of the CSF by a carrier process believed to be concentrated in the choroid plexus but probably present throughout the CSF space, resulting in a very substantial gradient in HVA along the spinal cord (151). Levels of HVA in the lumbar space may be 50 times less than those found in the lateral ventricles (39). This gradient is so steep that there may be significant differences in spinal fluid levels taken from the L3-L4 interspace (151) compared to the L4-L5 interspace, and significant correlations have been reported for lumbar CSF HVA levels and subjects' heights (135), suggesting that active transport of HVA out of the CSF may occur at rates proportional to the surface area available. The potential impact of substantial differences in lateral ventricular area on lumbar CSF HVA levels is presently unknown. In fact, it is conceivable that the interindividual differences in the rate of HVA clearance from the CSF may be the major source of variance between individuals. This possibility is underscored by the high correlations reported by most groups between the CSF levels of the serotonin metabolite 5-hydroxyindole-acetic acid (5-HIAA) and HVA (1,66), often interpreted as reflecting a dominant effect of the common spinal pump mechanism for clearing acid metabolites. To complicate matters further, there is good evidence that neuroleptic use can elevate HVA acutely (129), although this change returns toward normal as drug use becomes chronic (106). The time course of CSF HVA following withdrawal of neuroleptics is also poorly understood, but a period of at least 2 weeks drug free is probably necessary to avoid direct neuroleptic effects on dopamine turnover. There are other factors that require control to assure that any possible group differences are not due to extraneous influences, such as possible circadian and circannual rhythms (77) or the level of prior motor activity (107).

To combat some of these problems, a technique taking advantage of the property of probenecid to block the active transport mechanisms for organic acids has been developed (39). It was hoped that the total blockade of HVA clearance from the CSF space would minimize the interindividual differences due to effects of clearance and would magnify any small differences as the continuous production of HVA could accumulate metabolite over a period of many hours. Generally, probenecid has been given orally at a dose of 100 mg/kg divided over 12 hr to ameliorate the emetic effects of this maximal dosage. Its use has yielded HVA levels as much as 10 times greater than the levels without probenecid. However, it is apparent that total blockade is not attained with this dose, since the CSF levels of proben-ecid and HVA are highly correlated, even in individuals attaining relatively high levels of probenecid. It appears that the additional variance in CSF HVA due to probenecid administration has severely compromised its utility as a means of enhancing determinations of central dopamine turnover rates. It also makes comparisons of studies done with and without probenecid problematic. The interpreta-tion of studies using probenecid is further clouded by its direct CNS effects, including nausea and vomiting.

The attempts to find differences in CSF HVA levels between groups of schizophrenic individuals and appropriate control subjects have primarily resulted in negative findings (10,12,106). However, some subgroups of schizophrenics have been reported to differ from normals in CSF HVA concentrations. High CSF HVA has been found in schizo-phrenics with family history of schizophrenia (122) or with poor premorbid sexual adjustment (71). Low values of CSF HVA have been associated with poor prognosis (13) and the presence of first rank schneiderian symptoms (12,105). A study of a mixed group of schizophrenics and first-break, never-medicated schizophreniform individuals compared to normals did find levels of CSF HVA 30% lower in both psychotic groups (75). The significance of this finding is obscured by the differences in prior motor activity of the normal subjects and the mixed psychotic group, with the latter at bed rest overnight prior to lumbar puncture, whereas the former group traveled to the hospital the morning of the study. The specificity of the results for chronic schizophrenia is also questionable in light of the fact that the majority of individuals with a first psychotic episode will not go on to develop chronic schizophrenia, yet the group of schizophreniform individuals showed equally low CSF HVA as the chronic group. However, the findings of this study are consistent with a role for postsyn-aptic dopamine receptor supersensitivity in psychotic illness, reflected by diminished CSF HVA, but other CSF studies have not supported the view that dopamine receptor su-persensitivity is generally present in schizophrenics.

It is perhaps not surprising that CSF studies have not given any conclusive evidence about abnormalities in central dopamine turnover rates in schizophrenia. It is certainly possible that this is the result of no genuine etiologically relevant disturbances in dopamine firing rates in schizo-phrenia. However, this technique is sensitive only to fairly large changes in dopamine activity in the caudate and only under extremely well-controlled conditions. Any overactivity of a dopamine system may be limited to other areas of the brain, where the impact on CSF levels of HVA may be undetectable. The possible pathophysiological heterogeneity of schizophrenia may also mask any true differences in the relatively small sample sizes studied to date.

The invasive nature of CSF studies severely limits the number of samples from a given individual, thereby making estimates of reliability of any given measurement very difficult, and rendering impossible multiple studies under different conditions that might affect dopamine activity differentially in schizophrenic individuals and normals. This severe restriction has motivated efforts to find other more easily obtained measures of central dopaminergic activity. An obvious source of information is the plasma, and a substantial body of evidence has evolved on the factors normally affecting plasma HVA (pHVA) levels. Although varying considerably from species to species, it appears that the central contribution to pHVA levels is in the neighborhood of 40% in humans (7,83). This large central contribution makes it an attractive candidate as a reflection of central activity. There are some data suggesting that manipulations of dopaminergic systems limited to the CNS are indeed reflected in changes in peripheral HVA values (36).

Plasma HVA Studies

Administration of either dopamine receptor agonists or antagonists has been shown to produce parallel changes in brain HVA and pHVA in subhuman primates and rodents via central, and not peripheral, effects (60,61). These findings suggest that measurements of pHVA concentrations may be an accurate index of brain dopamine activity, and may prove useful for studying neuropsychiatric illnesses in which dopamine abnormalities have been implicated. However, attempts to explore the pathophysiology of psychiatric illnesses by pHVA measurements are not without consid-erable methodological problems. Confounding factors af-fecting pHVA concentrations can originate from either central or peripheral dopaminergic systems. Consumption of food rich in monoamine precursors can increase pHVA concentrations in normal subjects by as much as 100% over baseline (63), and to a lesser extent physical activity (63) and chronic stress (62) also increase pHVA concentra-tions. Furthermore, based on CSF HVA studies and inves-tigations of other neurotransmitter systems, it is conceivable that age, sex, weight, circadian, and seasonal variations might have an impact on pHVA concentrations (77,101,107,125,147). Current investigations are addressing these issues in an attempt to improve the methodology employed to control potential confounding factors (33). For example, administration of the monoamine oxidase (MAO) inhibitor debrisoquin diminishes the contribution of peripheral HVA production to the total pHVA concen-trations, thus enhancing the degree to which pHVA reflects brain dopamine activity (33,36,82).

Using present techniques, some intriguing pHVA findings have already been reported in psychiatric patients. Unmedicated, severely ill schizophrenic patients appear to have higher pHVA concentrations than less severe schizophrenics (37), and elevated PHVA may be associated with a good response to haloperidol (14). Furthermore, with the help of debrisoquin it has been shown that neuroleptic treatment produces an initial increase (33) and a subsequent gradual decrement in pHVA concentrations, and these pHVA variations correlate with symptom reduction (103). If schizophrenia is a disorder characterized by dopamine receptor up-regulation, as suggested by postmortem studies, the presence of high pHVA values in the more severely ill patients could reflect a dysfunction of the negative feedback mechanisms between postsynaptic DA receptor densities and presynaptic firing rates. Several animal experiments lend support to this dysregulation hypothesis. Destruction of the mesocortical dopaminergic projections by lesioning cells in the ventral tegmental area or frontal cortex areas directly was found to induce both the expected cortical hypodopaminergia and an increase in dopamine in the mesolimbic and nigrostriatal tract. Furthermore, the increase in dopamine production was associated with increased dopamine receptor ligand binding, implying both dopamine receptor up-regulation and concurrent increased presynaptic dopamine activity (108,109). A lesion of an analogous mesocortical dopamine tract in humans might induce similar changes in the regulation of dopaminergic activity in the mesolimbic and nigrostriatal regions, rather than the predicted negative feedback inhibition between postsynaptic receptor densities and presynaptic activity. According to this notion, the most severely ill schizophrenic patients may be those with the greatest production of dopamine in the face of postsynaptic dopamine receptor up-regulation, and this could be reflected in high pHVA concentrations.

Postmortem Studies of Dopamine Receptors

Although plasma HVA determinations hold promise for further investigations of central dopamine abnormalities in schizophrenia, the traditional pathologist's approach of exploring postmortem brain tissue has been of value as the most direct approach to assessing the dopamine hypothesis in schizophrenics. This has primarily taken two different paths: determining presynaptic dopamine activity by analyzing dopamine, HVA, and/or dihydroxyphenylacetic acid (DOPAC) concentrations in a few selected brain regions, or determining dopamine receptor binding concentrations, presumably postsynaptic, in a few regions.

There are several methodological issues of considerable importance in assessing postmortem studies of schizophrenics. First, information necessary for retrospective psychiatric and medical diagnoses is of uncertain and uneven quality, usually much less complete than that used in well-controlled clinical trials. There is often considerable difficulty with the rigorous diagnosis of schizophrenia in living subjects, and this is compounded by the inability to ask specific questions of subjects postmortem. Additionally, any abnormalities involved in schizophrenia may be state dependent, possibly detectable only in clinical relapse, or may relate to specific symptom clusters. Without careful antemortem assessment

these issues are extremely difficult to address retrospectively. Another major concern in interpreting postmortem research is the potential impact of prior neuroleptic treatment on the measures of importance. Clinical and preclinical studies suggest that there may be long-lasting changes in the firing rates and postsynaptic binding of dopamine receptors following neuroleptic treatment (123). Even a single dose of neuroleptic may affect postsynaptic responsivity for weeks (15). Receptor binding studies may be influenced by residual neuroleptic levels, if samples are inadequately washed prior to analysis. The rare individual with an unambiguous diagnosis of schizophrenia who died without prior medication exposure, whose brain would be free of any potential changes due to drugs, may not be representative of typical schizophrenics. Finally, many substances in the brain are dramatically influenced by the cause of death and the time until adequate cooling of the tissues has elapsed. Postmortem studies need to control for all of these possible confounding influences.

Postmortem studies have not provided much evidence for increased presynaptic dopaminergic activity in schizophrenia. Although quite labile in postmortem brain, dopamine concentrations in the putamen and nucleus accumbens did not differ between schizophrenic and normal control subjects, whereas an increase was found in the caudate (99). However, dopamine concentrations do not correlate well with dopamine activity, and the concentrations of the two metabolites that do reflect central activity, HVA and DOPAC, were not increased in any brain regions studied (99). These negative findings have spurred efforts to explore possible changes in postsynaptic dopamine receptor densities.

There have been several independent controlled studies demonstrating increased neuroleptic binding in brains of presumably schizophrenic individuals compared to control brains (see Table 1) (28,72,84,99,124), with a single small study finding no difference in B_{max} values (111). It should be pointed out that neuroleptic binding is not identical to dopamine receptor binding, since all neuroleptics are known to bind multiple neurotransmitter receptor types, and that the relative affinity of dopamine for the two (or three or possibly more) dopamine receptor subtypes is not parallel to that of any neuroleptic (123). Generally, tritiated spiroperidol has been used in studies ascertaining putative dopamine binding levels, but it is known that this ligand has substantial affinity for serotonin receptors (102), which are present in smaller but appreciable numbers in some regions with high dopamine receptor densities. Spiroperidol is also known to bind preferentially to dopamine receptors not linked to adenylate cyclase (D-2 receptors), which may be the subclass most closely related to antipsychotic activity (27). In a study comparing the binding of D-1 (adenylate cyclase-linked) and D-2 receptors in 15 schizophrenic brains and 15 control brains, only D-2 receptor densities were elevated (28). In a large multicenter study, the distribution of spiroperidol binding was bimodal in schizophrenic brains, but not in control brains, in all three regions examined (caudate, putamen, and accumbens). Both modes were significantly elevated relative to normals, with one mode 25% above normal and the other mode 130% above (124). The evidence is quite strong that dopamine receptor densities

TABLE 1. *Postmortem studies of spiperone binding in schizophrenia*

Study	Diagnostic group	N	N "Drug-free"	"Drug-free" criterion	B_{max}	B_{max} "Drug-free"	Regions studied
Owen et al. (99)	Schizophrenics	15	5	1 yr	100%	50%	Caudate, putamen
	Controls	15	15				
Reynolds et al. (111)	Schizophrenics	12	4	3 mo	No diff	30%	Putamen
	Controls	9	9				
Lee and Seeman (72)	Schizophrenics	37	11	"Virtually never medicated"	50%	32%	Caudate, putamen
	Controls	27	27				
Mackay et al. (84)	Schizophrenics	18	4	1 mo	60%	No change	Caudate, accumbens
	Controls	30	30				
Cross et al. (28)	Schizophrenics	36	NR	NR	60%	NR	Putamen, accumbens
	Controls	32					
Seeman et al. (124)	Schizophrenics	59	8	6 mo	Bimodal 25%, 130%	35%	Caudate, putamen, accumbens
	Controls	81	76				

NR, Not reported

are indeed elevated in brains of schizophrenic individuals relative to control brains. However, the etiological significance of this finding is under considerable dispute due to the widespread exposure to neuroleptics in the schizophrenic groups.

Although the effect of neuroleptics on dopamine receptor levels in human brains is not known at present, it is reasonable to infer from many animal studies finding substantial increases in B_{max} (but not in K_d) following several weeks to months of neuroleptic administration (93,142) that similar changes may occur in schizophrenic individuals during antipsychotic treatment. The magnitude of such changes in humans remains unknown at present, but animal studies report increases of 30 to 70% in maximal spiroperidol binding values (123). This is in the range of increases found in schizophrenic brains relative to normals. The significance of this increase in neuroleptic binding in schizophrenic brains is difficult to interpret, since it could result from treatment alone, from the disease process itself, or an interaction of these two effects. Ideally, this issue could be addressed by studying randomly selected, never-medicated schizophrenic individuals, but the number of brains that have been available from these rare individuals is still quite small. Three studies have reported increases in maximal spiroperidol binding values of brains of a subgroup of schizophrenic individuals unmedicated for variable lengths of time prior to death (72,99,124), but few of those individuals had never been exposed to neuroleptics, and the magnitude of changes reported was generally smaller than that of the overall schizophrenic groups. Animal data are sparse on the time course that is required for the reversal of drug-induced dopamine receptor proliferation following discontinuation of neuroleptic administration, although it has been suggested that 6 months is insufficient to reverse the effects on D-1 receptors of 12 months of drugs (25). Human data directly addressing this issue are not yet available. One study reported that the four brains from subjects who had been drug free for at least 1 month prior to death had dopamine receptor densities the same as the control group (84), although the statistical power of the small sample studied renders any conclusion problem-

atic. It has been argued that the magnitude of the changes in spiroperidol binding found in schizophrenic brains, the specificity of the changes for D-2 receptors, and the significant positive correlation between D-2 receptor densities postmortem and the intensity of positive psychotic symptoms antemortem indicate that the increases in dopamine receptors reported in schizophrenic brains reflect the disease process rather than a response to treatment (28). However, the role of neuroleptics in the finding of increased dopamine receptors in postmortem brains of schizophrenics is yet to be clarified.

PET Studies with Dopamine Receptor-Binding Ligands

Many of the difficulties presented by examining dopamine receptor concentrations in postmortem tissue may be addressed by the recent development of positron-emitting neuroleptic ligands for use in positron emission tomography (PET scan). These agents have demonstrated stereospecific binding, with concentrations in regions known to be rich in dopamine receptors, especially the caudate and the putamen, and show extremely low levels in regions thought to be devoid of dopamine receptors, such as the cerebellum (140). Two radioisotopes have been used in such studies: carbon-11, with a physical half-life of 20 min, and fluorine-18, with a half-life of 110 min. The former is useful for its ability to clear rapidly, allowing more than one study in a day, whereas the latter has a sufficiently long half-life for studies of the kinetics of high-affinity receptor binding. Most reported work has used N-methylspiroperidol, an analog of spiroperidol that has not been used clinically, but that has similar *in vitro* characteristics and has better penetrance into the brain than spiroperidol, and is moderately more specific for D-2 (as opposed to serotonin S-2) receptors (140). More specific D-2 ligands, such as raclopride, have recently been developed (41).

Although the development of *in vivo* dopamine receptor imaging techniques holds great promise for addressing the role that dopamine receptor supersensitivity may play in schizophrenia, important methodological issues need to be addressed in developing research paradigms to explore this topic. Although the sensitivity of PET scans has improved dramatically over the last few years and may soon near the physical limits of resolution of 2 mm, present techniques effectively limit resolution to regions greater than 7 to 10 mm in diameter. For dopamine receptor studies, this limits current work to the caudate and putamen, since mesolimbic structures are too small. Although the locus of any abnormality in dopamine receptors in the pathogenesis of schizophrenia is not established, some similarity to behavioral changes associated with damage to the limbic and frontal structures has focused interest on these regions in schizophrenia (49). The caudate and putamen are known to subserve some coordinated motor functions, but their possible role in behavior has received less attention. However, evidence from animal studies suggests that destruction of dopamine neurons in the medial prefrontal cortex is followed by increased dopamine receptor binding in both mesolimbic and striatal regions, probably mediated through a recurrent loop from the frontal cortex to these areas (109). Pathological changes in the frontal lobes in some schizophrenics could similarly be associated with striatal and mesolimbic DA receptor supersensitivity. PET studies of the caudate DA receptor densities may be directly relevant for examining this hypothesis.

Other unresolved pharmacodynamic issues also affect interpretation of PET studies. The ligand selected for use either may be not sufficiently specific to identify a distinct abnormality or may simply be specific for the wrong subtype of receptor. Although the best evidence suggests that D-2 receptors are involved in antipsychotic action, there are data consistent with a facilitatory effect of D-1 receptors on D-2-mediated behavior (5). Additionally, the time course and effects of chronic neuroleptic use on dopamine receptor binding can also distort any findings. Since concomitant neuroleptic use would radically reduce any apparent radioligand binding, studies need to be conducted without any significant residual neuroleptic in the CNS. The time necessary for this to occur in humans is currently unknown, although detectable effects on serum prolactin levels are generally absent after 1 month off neuroleptics. Furthermore, the time course for resolution of any neuroleptic-induced dopamine supersensitivity to return toward normal, if it ever does, is unknown and may be at least months (25). Ideally, never previously medicated subjects should be studied to avoid the obscuring effects of drugs. Finally, there is not yet agreement on a mathematical model to translate PET scan image intensities into relevant receptor densities, although several have been proposed. The simplest method uses the ratio of image intensities in the caudate to the cerebellum at a fixed time point following injection of the radioligand (140). At best, this may be an approximation of the ratio of total to nonspecific neuroleptic binding, although the cerebellum may not be devoid of specific binding (85).

As of this writing, there are no published reports of determinations of dopamine receptors in never previously medicated schizophrenic individuals using PET scan techniques. Normative values for the ratio of caudate to cerebellar binding have been published for a wide range of ages and for both men and women (149). An interesting increase in the variance of this ratio among premenopausal women could reflect an underlying dependence on the menstrual cycle in this group, but studies directly exploring this issue are not yet available. Preliminary data in schizophrenics, most of whom have been free of neuroleptics at least 6 months, have been suggestive of an elevation of $[^{11}C]n$-methylspiperone binding (D. F. Wong, personal communication), in contrast to a small series of schizophrenics whose caudate-to-cerebellar ratios did not significantly differ from normal (150). Until enough subjects have been studied, no definite conclusions will be possible.

PHARMACOLOGICAL TESTS OF THE DOPAMINE HYPOTHESIS

Autoreceptor Approaches to Decreasing Symptoms of Schizophrenia

The existence of presynaptic receptors or autoreceptors was suggested by the observation that electrochemically identified neurons can respond to direct application of their own neurotransmitter at sites removed from any known synaptic location (16,59,69,116). Events known to be intrinsic to dopaminergic neurons, like blockade of impulse flow by γ-hydroxybutyrate (GHB) and the subsequent increase in tyrosine hydroxylation, or the electrical stimulation-induced increase in tyrosine hydroxylation, were both reversed by dopamine agonist stimulation (114,141). The biochemical, pharmacological, and functional characterization of autoreceptors (Table 2) has led to the suggestion that dopamine agonists might decrease dopamine synthesis and release via autoreceptor stimulation. Decreasing dopamine turnover and dopamine secretion by autoreceptor stimulation has been proposed as a therapeutic approach in conjunction with postsynaptic receptor blockade in those neuropsychiatric disorders in which hyperdopaminergia is suspected (88).

There is evidence that autoreceptor stimulation can affect behavior in humans. Activities thought to be related to decreasing dopamine turnover, such as sleep induction, relaxation, and reduction of abnormal movement in tardive

TABLE 2.

Characterization of dopamine autoreceptors
Present on the soma, terminal axon, and dendrites of the nigrostriatal and mesolimbic dopaminergic tract. Absent in the mesocortical and tuberoinfundibular tract
Modulate dopamine cell firing rate, synthesis, and release
Responsiveness can be modified by chronic exposure to antagonists
Reduced doses of dopamine agonists can stimulate autoreceptors without affecting postsynaptic receptors

Characterization of neurons without apparent dopamine autoreceptors
Higher cell firing rate and transmitter turnover
Diminished biochemical and electrophysiological responsiveness to dopamine agonists and antagonists
Lack of tolerance following administration of chronic antipsychotic drugs

dyskinesia, were temporarily induced in human subjects following administration of apomorphine or other dopamine agonists with presumed presynaptic dopamine selectivity (9,20,26,68,131,133). However, clinical evidence supporting an antischizophrenic effect related to autoreceptor stimulation is far from conclusive, ranging from transient improvement in some patients to absolutely no effects (see Table 3). An overview of these studies suggests that higher apomorphine doses combined with neuroleptics may be preferable (38,132).

Several anatomical and pharmacological factors need to be considered in interpreting the conflicting studies of autoreceptor stimulation in schizophrenics. An autoreceptor agonist would potentially decrease dopamine activity in the nigrostriatal and mesolimbic dopaminergic tract, but not in the mesocortical tract where autoreceptors are apparently absent (8). Furthermore, the dual effects of most dopamine agonists and antagonists on pre- and postsynaptic receptors, with opposing consequences on dopamine activity (128), are additional impediments in using dopamine agonists to decrease dopamine activity. Agonist activation of receptors could simultaneously decrease presynaptic dopamine activity and increase postsynaptic activity. Similarly, dopamine antagonists could increase presynaptic activity while decreasing postsynpatic dopamine activity. These dual and opposing effects on dopamine firing rates could produce a net decrease, increase, or no change. Interindividual pharmacokinetic differences may be expected to complicate this picture, as a given dose may yield a wide range of local apomorphine concentrations. These considerations may also partly account for conflicting pHVA findings. Attempts to replicate in humans the apomorphine-induced reduction in pHVA, reported in rat (61) and considered evidence for its ability to decrease dopamine turnover, produced positive results in some (32), but not all, clinical investigations (119).

Combined administration of dopamine agonists selective for presynaptic receptors and dopamine antagonists selective for postsynaptic receptors could resolve the problem of competing effects. Biochemical and behavioral studies have suggested that 3-(3-hydroxyphenyl) N-n-propylpiperidine (3-PPP) may be a selective autoreceptor agonist. Furthermore, the levo isomer of this racemic mixture appears to have postsynaptic antagonist properties in addition to the presynaptic agonist effect (50). Another agent of possible interest is the selective D-1 antagonist SCH23390. SCH23390 activates the firing rate of the dopaminergic neuron similar to haloperidol or sulpiride in the nigrostria-

tum, but fails to prevent the inhibition induced by apomorphine, suggesting that this agent might be a selective postsynaptic antagonist (90).

Decreasing Dopamine Activity Via Nondopaminergic Systems

Cholecystokinin

Cholecystokinin (CCK) is a gastrointestinal hormonal peptide recently identified in the mammalian brain (91). The demonstration that CCK-like peptides and dopamine coexist within mesolimbic and mesocortical dopaminergic neurons has focused interest on the possible role of CCK in schizophrenia (51,52). Preclinical experiments in rodents examining the functional interaction between CCK and dopamine indicate that CCK reduces dopamine turnover in caudate nucleus and nucleus accumbens (43) and increases striatal dopamine release (67). In addition, CCK appears to increase dopamine receptor affinity and reduce receptor density in the striatum (43,94), suggesting a neuromodulator-neurotransmitter interaction between CCK and dopamine. Investigations of dopamine-related motor behavior in rodents have demonstrated that apomorphine-induced hypomobility can be antagonized by CCK and passive avoidance behavior can be attenuated. These CCK-induced behavioral effects suggest that CCK and CCK-like peptides might possess neuroleptic-like properties and possibly antipsychotic effects (55,67,137).

The anatomical and functional association between dopamine and CCK and the presumed neuroleptic-like properties have prompted clinical investigators to examine the effect of this neuropeptide in schizophrenic individuals. Four open trials of CCK or its decapeptide analog, ceruletidide, performed in schizophrenic patients, have reported symptomatic improvement starting as soon as a few hours following the drug injection and persisting more than 2 weeks (56,92,96,97). The reported improvement was observed in both positive and negative symptoms (92). However, four double-blind controlled studies failed to demonstrate efficacy (22,55,80,86). The ability of CCK and CCK-like peptides to cross the blood-brain barrier without serious adverse effects is questionable (22). Also CCK appears to exert different and at times opposite effects on the dopaminergic activity in discrete brain areas. A better understanding of the relationship between schizophrenic symptoms and dysfunction of specific dopaminergic tracts

TABLE 3. Clinical studies utilizing putative dopamine autoreceptor agonists in schizophrenia

Study	N	DA agonist	Effect
Corsini et al. (26)	58	Apomorphine 1 mg im	Transient improvement in 21 pts
Smith et al. (126)	4	Apomorphine 1.5–6 mg sc or po	Transient improvement in 3 pts
Tamminga et al. (132)	18	Apomorphine 3 mg sc	Transient improvement in 9 pts
Hollister et al. (53)	11	Apomorphine 20 mg po	No improvement
Levy et al. (73)	24	Apomorphine 0.75 mg sc	No improvement
Cutler et al. (32)	5	Apomorphine 0.005 mg/kg	Transient improvement in 2 pts
Ferrier et al. (42)	30	Apomorphine 0.75 mg sc	No improvement
Davidson et al. (35)	9	Apomorphine 0.375 mg sc	No improvement

may eventually indicate whether a CCK-like peptide can be useful in the treatment of schizophrenia.

Des-Tyrosine-γ-Endorphin

The B-lipotropin fragment des-tyrosine-γ-endorphin (DT E, LPH62-77) has been identified in mammalian pituitary and appears to have some neuroleptic-like activity. Two clinical trials in which DT E was administered to schizophrenic patients reported moderate clinical improvement in some subjects (40,139), whereas a third study failed to observe such improvement (133). DT E administration to schizophrenic patients does not result in elevation of serum prolactin levels (89), suggesting any antipsychotic effect is not a result of direct dopamine blocking activity. Although a therapeutic role for DT E in schizophrenia is unclear at this time, there is considerable evidence suggesting that γ-endorphins may possess a possible neuroregulatory role in dopaminergic transmission.

γ-Aminobutyric Acid

The widespread inhibitory activity of γ-aminobutyric acid (GABA) on many neuronal pathways in mammalian brain has led to the suggestion that pharmacological manipulation of the GABAergic systems might affect dopamine activity and be relevant to the treatment of schizophrenics (113). *In vitro*, GABA inhibits the firing of dopamine neurons in the substantia nigra and the ventral tegmental area, which are the origins of the mesolimbic and mesocortical dopaminergic tract (148). If this inhibitory activity occurs physiologically, or could be induced pharmacologically, an increase in GABAergic activity would be of potential therapeutic value. However, the precise relationship between the GABAergic and the dopaminergic system has not been clarified, with GABA being reported to increase or decrease dopamine firing and turnover under different conditions.

At least some of the dopamine-mediated behaviors in animal studies, such as locomotor activity and catalepsy, are inhibited by GABA or GABA agonists (11,117). This relationship provides some support for the presumption that GABAergic agents might decrease dopamine activity in those patients in whom hyperdopaminergia is related to the production of schizophrenic symptoms. Baclofen, an agent with GABA-like pharmacological properties, was given in seven clinical trials to a total of 103 schizophrenic patients without any significant therapeutic effect (45).

Structurally related to GABA, GHB has been shown to inhibit impulse flow in the nigrostriatal dopaminergic pathway, increase dopamine synthesis, and decrease dopamine release (115). Based on this preclinical evidence it was postulated that a possible GHB presynaptic effect could potentiate the postsynaptic neuroleptic effect in reducing dopaminergic activity and be useful in the treatment of some schizophrenias. One open clinical trial and two double-blind controlled studies have reported minimal or no antipsychotic effect following exogenous administration of GHB (73,121,134).

Valproic acid (VPA), a clinically used anticonvulsant, has also been tried in the treatment of schizophrenic symptoms. The rationale for using VPA in schizophrenia is based on preclinical evidence indicating that VPA might increase brain GABA concentrations (21) and consequently reduce dopamine activity (143). A positive therapeutic effect of VPA was reported in two clinical trials (76,95); however, two other recent investigations reported no improvement or symptomatic worsening in schizophrenics given VPA (65,70).

Prediction of Clinical Remission Stability by Agents Increasing Dopamine Activity

Both achieving and maintaining remission in schizophrenia are facilitated by neuroleptics (64). Unfortunately, chronic neuroleptic administration has potentially irreversible adverse effects, such as tardive dyskinesia (58), in addition to extrapyramidal side effects (112). On the other hand, frequent schizophrenic relapse causes severe anguish and deterioration of an already damaged social network. These considerations call for a careful assessment of the benefits and risks of neuroleptic maintenance, in each individual patient. A clinical tool that would be able to distinguish between patients who, on withdrawal of neuroleptic medication, will experience a rapid relapse, and those who can maintain a prolonged state of remission medication free, would greatly assist the clinician in this assessment.

Several clinical studies in which schizophrenic patients in remission were challenged with indirect dopamine agonists such as amphetamine (3) or methylphenidate (74), or with L-dopa (34), indicate that neuroleptic-free patients in whom those drugs produced transient symptom activation are more likely to experience relapse within a few weeks than patients in whom dopamimetics had little or no detrimental effect. It is conceivable that schizophrenic relapse represents an episodic failure of complex feedback mechanisms in the context of vulnerability to dopaminergic dysregulation. According to this speculation, dopamine agonist activation might elicit a transient hyperdopaminergia with consequent symptomatic worsening in those schizophrenic patients in whom the dopaminergic system cannot buffer this augmentation. Conversely, those patients who have a greater reserve in their regulatory abilities would not be affected by DA agonist activation.

SUBGROUPING SCHIZOPHRENIA, OR ISOLATING THE HYPER- OR HYPODOPAMINERGIC SUBGROUP

Potential Subgrouping Variables

The richly variable clinical picture found in individuals with schizophrenia has struck many observers as evidence for multiple etiologies, and has formed the focus for many of the attempts to identify meaningful subgroups of schizophrenia. Many medical conditions have been identified that are associated in some individuals with psychiatric presentations indistinguishable from schizophrenia. It is possible that the underlying pathology is not essentially the same in all schizophrenic individuals, but due to two or more unrelated processes with similar clinical expressions. This concern has led to efforts to identify signs and symptoms of schizophrenics that could be useful in discriminating groups that may have differences in dopaminergic activity. Traditional clinical subtypes, such as catatonic, hebephrenic, paranoid, and undifferentiated, have not shown much promise as biological discriminators. Attention recently has turned to the possibility that symptoms classed as positive or negative may be useful, as well as differences in neuroanatomical measures commonly assessed by computerized axial tomography (CAT scan). Other potentially useful measures, such as differences in neuroleptic response, cognitive impairment, clinical course, premorbid function, family history for psychiatric illness, or sensitivity to the extrapyramidal side effects of neuroleptics, and presence of soft neurological signs or tardive dyskinesia, have also been suggested.

Positive and Negative Symptoms

The classification of schizophrenic symptoms into positive and negative groups has a long history and has recently been subjected to considerable debate about definition and significance. Although no scheme has yet won universal acceptance, positive symptoms are generally thought to include hallucinations, delusions, and some aspects of thought disorder, such as derailment, neologisms, or incoherence. Negative symptoms are thought to represent loss of functioning in various areas, such as social withdrawal, blunted affect, diminished motivation, psychomotor retardation, and poverty of speech. It has been hypothesized that these two groups of symptoms represent independent disease processes (19), although it is also possible that they are associated with variable manifestations of a single underlying pathological entity (31). Primarily based on the belief that neuroleptics are more effective in treating positive symptoms, it has been proposed that the hyperdopaminergic state is associated with this constellation of symptoms. The finding that D-2 receptor densities in postmortem brains of schizophrenics correlate with the antemortem intensity of positive, but not negative, symptoms is consistent with this view (28). Alternatively, patients with more positive symptoms may well have received more neuroleptics than patients with fewer positive symptoms, and may simply reflect a greater degree of neuroleptic-induced dopamine receptor proliferation. Although there is a general belief that negative symptoms are not improved by neuroleptics, there is increasing evidence that some negative symptoms may also be responsive to antipsychotic medications (46) or may improve indirectly as the positive symptoms responsible for their appearance subside (19). The ability of antipsychotics to cause akinesia, severe sedation, and diminished motor activity may also obscure ratings of negative symptoms and possible changes in negative symptoms following neuroleptic treatment.

There is also clinical and preclinical evidence that some negative symptoms may be associated with decreased central dopamine activity (87,110,129). Parkinson's disease, which is characterized by loss of dopaminergic neurons in the nigrostriatal tract, is often associated with social withdrawal and flat affect. Large doses of neuroleptics also cause Parkinson-like motor symptoms and can mimic negative symptoms. Treatment of patients with dopamine agonists has been reported to improve negative symptoms in some schizophrenic individuals. Chronic L-dopa administration may partially reverse blunted affect, emotional withdrawal, and apathy (2), whereas D-amphetamine can transiently improve negative symptoms (4).

At present, the definition, assessment, and validity of negative symptoms is an active subject of investigation. This reflects the widespread belief that dichotomizing schizophrenic symptoms by some form of a positive/negative paradigm may ultimately be useful as an etiologically relevant discriminator. Some negative symptoms may be produced by the activation of positive symptoms, and reflect a hyperdopaminergic state, whereas other negative symptoms have been associated with diminished central dopaminergic activity. These preliminary findings lend encouragement to further investigations exploring the role of deficit symptoms in schizophrenia.

Neuroimaging Techniques

The existence of ventricular enlargement in some schizophrenic individuals has been demonstrated in multiple studies using pneumoencephalography (6,48), and similar findings have been reported in the vast majority of controlled studies by CAT scan (146), although one well-controlled study has found no such difference (57). Depending on the population studied, from 10 to 50% of schizophrenics showed increases in the ventricular brain ratio (VBR), determined by dividing the area of the lateral ventricles by the area of the brain in that slice which shows the lateral ventricles most prominently. Because of several reports associating enlarged ventricles with poor response to neuroleptic treatment (81,120,144), it has been proposed that hyperdopaminergia is more likely in those individuals without ventricular enlargement (29). Evidence that subjects with ventricular enlargement are likely to show cognitive decline (47), poor treatment response, and possibly fewer positive symptoms and more negative symptoms has led to development of a typology of schizophrenia that could prove useful in discriminating subjects with abnormalities in dopamine transmission (see Table 4) (30). Several studies, however, have not found associations of enlarged VBRs with either treatment response (79,145), or negative symptoms (79,100). The absence of clearly defined criteria for designation of type I and type II schizophrenia has inhibited further assessment of the utility of this subgrouping scheme. Perhaps the most intriguing association of VBR has been the finding by several groups that ventricular size is negatively correlated with CSF HVA levels in schizophrenics (78,98,136), but perhaps not in normals (98). If this relationship is not the result of increased clearance of HVA by the larger ventricular size, it may suggest that increased presynaptic dopaminergic activity is present only in schizophrenics without evidence of structural damage. Further examination of measures of central neurotransmitter activ-

TABLE 4. *Hypothetical subtyping of schizophrenia based on CT brain imaging*

	Type I	Type II
CT brain image	Normal	Atrophic
Symptom picture	Positive	Negative
Prognosis	Good	Poor
Treatment response	Good	Poor
Intellectual impairment	None	May be present
Premorbid sociality	Normal	Poor
Etiology	Hyperdopaminergia and/or supersensitive dopamine receptors	Structural brain damage, normal dopamine function

ities in subjects with and without ventricular enlargement may eventually clarify the usefulness of subgrouping schizophrenia by CAT scan results.

The suggestion that a combination of the positive-negative symptom classification and VBR evaluations may be useful in isolating specific abnormalities in dopamine transmission in schizophrenia has been supported by some tantalizing evidence, yet no specific guidelines are available for discerning which individuals are indeed suffering from a state of hyper- or hypodopaminergia, or perhaps even both in different regions of the brain. This may well result from the complexity of the real pathophysiology, and from our limited understanding of the normal human brain, but as further evidence builds for the existence of some discriminators of dopamine activity, better understanding of the disease and treatment of schizophrenia may eventually be possible.

Summary

The dopamine hypothesis of schizophrenia is based largely on the ability of antipsychotic medications to diminish dopaminergic activity, most likely involving D-2 receptors. Postmortem studies showing a generalized elevation of D-2 receptors in the brains of schizophrenics provide some support for the dopamine hypothesis, although the possible impact of chronic neuroleptic use on dopamine receptor proliferation requires cautious interpretation of these findings. CSF studies of central dopamine turnover have not generally found abnormal dopamine activity in schizophrenics, although both high and low levels of HVA have been reported in specific subgroups. The improving methodology of pHVA determinations shows promise for this measure as a simple marker of central dopamine activity. The recent development of positron-emitting analogs of neuroleptics has made it possible to examine central dopamine receptor levels in living human subjects, using PET scan techniques. Other pharmacological tests of the dopamine hypothesis have also been explored. The administration of autoreceptor agonists to diminish presynaptic dopamine activity may prove to be useful in conjunction with neuroleptics, whereas manipulation of the neuronal systems thought to reduce dopamine firing rates, through the use of such agents as DT E, GHB, CCK, or VPA, has produced minimal effects. The possible etiological heterogeneity of schizophrenic symptoms has been the impetus for efforts to identify biologically meaningful subtypes of schizophre-

nia. The positive-negative symptom dichotomy, neuroimaging evidence of cerebral atrophy, and chronicity of symptoms are all areas of inquiry that may ultimately yield useful measures to discriminate between schizophrenics of differing etiologies. The dopamine hypothesis, now over 30 years old, continues to generate new ideas and may improve our understanding of the pathology of schizophrenia.

REFERENCES

1. Agren, H. (1983): In: *The Origins of Depression, Current Concepts and Approaches,* edited by J. Angst, pp. 297–311. Springer-Verlag, Berlin.
2. Alpert, M., and Rush, M. (1983): *Psychopharmacol. Bull.,* 196: 118–120.
3. Angrist, B., Peselow, E., Rubinstein, M., Wolkin, A., and Rotrosen, J. (1985): *Psychopharmacology,* 85:277–283.
4. Angrist, B., Rotrosen, J., and Gershon, S. (1980): *Psychopharmacology,* 72:17–19.
5. Apud, J. A., Masotto, C., Ongini, E., and Racagni, G. (1985): *Eur. J. Pharmacol.,* 112:187–193.
6. Asano, N. (1967): In: *Pneumoencephalogram Study of Schizophrenia,* edited by H. Mitsuda, pp. 209–219. Fankashoin Ltd., Tokyo.
7. Bacopolous, N. G., Hattox, S. E., and Roth, R. H. (1979): *Eur. J. Pharmacol.,* 56:225.
8. Bannon, M. J., Reinhard, J. F., Jr., Bunney, E. B., and Roth, R. H. (1982): *Nature,* 296:444–446.
9. Bassi, S., Albizzati, M. G., Frattola, L., Passerini, D., and Trabucchi, M. (1979): *J. Neurol. Neurosurg. Psychiatry,* 42:458–460.
10. Berger, P. A., Faull, K. F., Kilkowski, J., Anderson, P. J., Kraemer, H., Davis, K. L., and Barchas, J. D. (1980): *Am. J. Psychiatry,* 137:174–180.
11. Binas, B., and Carlsson, A. (1978): *Psychopharmacology,* 59:91–94.
12. Bowers, M. B., Jr. (1973): *Psychopharmacologia,* 28:309–318.
13. Bowers, M. B., Jr. (1974): *Arch. Gen. Psychiatry,* 31:50–54.
14. Bowers, M. B., Jr., Swigar, M. E., Jatlow, P. I., and Goicoecnea, N. (1984): *J. Clin. Psychiatry,* 45:248–251.
15. Campbell, A., Baldessarini, R. J., Teicher, M. H., and Kula, N. S. (1985): *Psychopharmacology,* 87:161–166.
16. Carlsson, A. (1975): In: *Pre and Postsynaptic Receptors,* edited by E. Usdin and W. E. Bunney, pp. 49–65. Marcel Dekker, New York.
17. Carlsson, A., and Lindquist, M. (1963): *Acta Pharmacol. Toxicol.,* 20:140–144.
18. Carlsson, A., Persson, T., Roos, B.-E., and Walander, J. (1972): *J. Neural Transm.,* 33:83–90.
19. Carpenter, W. T., Heinrichs, D. W., and Alphs, L. D. (1985): *Schizophr. Bull.,* 11:440–452.
20. Carroll, B. J., Curtis, G. C., and Kokman, E. (1977): *Am. J. Psychiatry,* 134:785–789.
21. Chapman, A. G., Meldrum, B. S., and Mendes, E. (1983): *Life Sci.,* 32:2023–2031.
22. Chase, T. M., Barone, P., Bruno, G., Cohen, S. L., Juncos, J.,

Knight, M., Ruggeri, S., Steardo, L., and Tamminga, C. A. (1985): *Experimental Therapeutics Branch, National Institute of Neurological and Communication Disorders and Stroke*, Bethesda, MD., pp. 553–561.

23. Chase, T. N., Schnur, J. A., and Gordon, E. K. (1970): *Neuropharmacology*, 9:265–268.
24. Clow, A., Jenner, P., and Marsden, C. D. (1978): *Life Sci.*, 23:421–424.
25. Clow, A., Theodorous, A., Jenner, P., and Marsden, C. D. (1980): *Eur. J. Pharmacol.*, 63:135–144.
26. Corsini, G. U., DelZompo, M., Manconi, S., Cianchetti, C., Mangoni, A., and Gessa, G. L. (1977): *Adv. Biochem. Psychopharmacol.*, 16:645–648.
27. Creese, L., Burt, D. R., and Snyder, S. H. (1976): *Science*, 192:481–483.
28. Cross, A. J., Crow, T. J., Ferrier, I. N., Johnstone, E. C., McCreadie, R. M., Owen, F., Owens, D. G. C., and Poulter, M. (1983): *J. Neural Transm. (Suppl.)*, 18:265–272.
29. Crow, T. J. (1980): *Br. Med. J.*, 280:66–68.
30. Crow, T. J. (1982): *Psychopharmacol. Bull.*, 18:22–29.
31. Crow, T. J. (1985): *Schizophr. Bull.*, 1:471–486.
32. Cutler, N. R., Jeste, D. V., Karoum, F., and Wyatt, R. J. (1982): *Life Sci.*, 30:753.
33. Davidson, M., Giordani, A., Mohs, R. C., and Davis, K. L. (1986): Presented at the 41st Annual Convention of the Society of Biological Psychiatry, Washington, DC, 1986.
34. Davidson, M., Keefe, R. S. C., Mohs, R. C., Horvath, T. B., and Davis, K. L. (1986): *Am. J. Psychiatry (in press)*.
35. Davidson, M., Kendler, K. S., Davis, B. M., Horvath, T. B., Mohs, R. C., and Davis, K. L. (1985): *Psychiatry Res.* 16:95–99.
36. Davidson, M., Kendler, K. S., Mohs, R. C., Hollander, E., Ryan, T., and Davis, K. L. (1987): *J. Psychiatr. Res. (in press)*.
37. Davis, K. L., Davidson, M., Mohs, R. C., Kendler, K. S., Davis, B., Johns, C. A., DeNigris, Y., and Horvath, T. B. (1985): *Science*, 227:1601–1602.
38. Davis, K. L., Horvath, T. B., Mohs, R. C., and Davis, B. M. (1985): *Arch. Gen. Psychiatry*, 42:927–928.
39. Ebert, M. H., Kartzinel, R., Cowdry, R. W., and Goodwin, F. (1980): In: *Neurobiology of Cerebrospinal Fluid*, edited by J. H. Wood, pp. 97–112. Plenum Press, New York.
40. Emrich, H. M., Loudig, M., Lerssen, D. V., Herz, A., and Kissling, W. (1980): *Lancet*, 2:1364–1365.
41. Farde, L., Hall, H., Ehrin, E., and Sedvall, G. (1986): *Science*, 231:258–261.
42. Ferrier, I. N., Johnstone, E. C., and Crow, T. J. (1984): *Br. J. Psychiatry*, 144:341–348.
43. Fuxe, K., Agnatic, L. F., Benfenati, F., Cimmino, M., Algeri, S., Hokfelt, T., and Mutt, V. (1981): *Acta Physiol. Scand.*, 113:567–569.
44. Fyro, B., Wode-Holgodt, B., Borg, S., and Sedvall, G. (1974): *Psychopharmacology*, 35:287–294.
45. Garbutt, J. C., and van Kammen, D. P. (1983): *Schizophr. Bull.*, 9:336–353.
46. Goldberg, S. C. (1985): *Schizophr. Bull.*, 11:453–456.
47. Golden, J. C., Moses, J. A., Zelazowski, R., Graber, R., Zatz, L. M., Horvath, T. B., and Berger, P. A. (1980): *Arch. Gen. Psychiatry*, 37:619–623.
48. Hang, J. O. (1962): *Acta Psychiatr. Scand.*, 38:1–114.
49. Hecaen, H., and Albert, M. L. (1975): In: *Psychiatric Aspects of Neurobiological Disease*, edited by D. F. Benson and D. Blumer, pp. 137–149. Grune and Stratton.
50. Hjorth, S. (1983): *Acta Physiol. Scand. (Suppl.)*, 517:1–52.
51. Hokfelt, T., Rehfeld, J. F., Skirboll, L., Ivemark, B., Goldstein, M., and Marley, K. (1980): *Nature*, 285:476–480.
52. Hokfelt, T., Skirboll, L., Rehfeld, J. F., Goldstein, M., Marley, K., and Dann, O. (1980): *Science*, 2093–2124.
53. Hollister, L. E., Davis, K. L., and Berger, P. S. (1980): *Commun. Psychopharmacol.*, 4:227–281.
54. Hommer, D. W., Pickar, D., Roy, A., Ninan, P., Boronow, J., and Paul, S. M. (1984): *Arch. Gen. Psychiatry*, 41:617–619.
55. Hommer, D., and Skirboll, L. (1983): *Eur. J. Pharmacol.*, 91:151–152.
56. Itoh, H., Tanoue, S., and Yagi, G. (1982): *Keio J. Med.*, 31:71–95.

57. Jernigan, T. L., Lals, L. M., Bowden, C. L., Davis, J. M., Hanin, L., and Javaid, J. (1983): *Arch. Gen. Psychiatry*, 40:999–1010.
58. Jeste, D. V. (1982): *Understanding and Treating Tardive Dyskinesia*, pp. 81–106. Guilford Press, New York.
59. Kehr, W., Carlsson, A., Lindquist, M., Malnusson, T., and Atack, C. (1972): *Pharmacol. Pharmac.*, 24:744.
60. Kendler, K. S., Heninger, G. R., and Roth, R. H. (1981): *Eur. J. Pharmacol.*, 71:321–326.
61. Kendler, K. S., Heninger, G. R., and Roth, R. H. (1982): *Life Sci.*, 30:2063–2069.
62. Kendler, K. S., Hsieh, J. Y.-K., and Davis, K. L. (1982): *Psychopharmacol. Bull.*, 18:152–155.
63. Kendler, K. S., Mohs, R. C., and Davis, K. L. (1983): *Psychiatry Res.*, 8:215–223.
64. Klein, D., and Davis, J. (1969): *Diagnosis and Drug Treatment of Psychiatric Disorders*, pp. 52–138. Williams and Wilkins, Baltimore.
65. Ko, G. N., Korpi, E. P., Freed, W. J., Zalcman, S. J., and Bigelow, L. B. (1985): *Biol. Psychiatry*, 20:209–215.
66. Koslow, S. H., Maas, J. W., Bowden, C. L., Davis, J. M., Hanin, L., and Javaid, J. (1983): *Arch. Gen. Psychiatry*, 40:999–1010.
67. Kovacs, G. L., Szabo, G., Penke, B., and Telegdy, G. (1981): *Eur. J. Pharmacol.*, 69:313–319.
68. Lal, S., and De la Vega, C. E. (1975): *J. Neurol. Neurosurg. Psychiatry*, 38:722–726.
69. Langer, S. (1973): In: *Frontiers in Catecholamine Research*, edited by S. H. Snyder and E. Usdin, p. 543–552. Pergamon Press, New York.
70. Lautin, A., Angrist, B., Stanley, M., Gershon, S., Heckl, K., and Karobath, M. (1980): *Br. J. Psychiatry*, 137:240–244.
71. Leckman, D. F., Bowers, M., Jr., and Sturges, J. S. (1981): *Am. J. Psychiatry*, 138:472–477.
72. Lee, T., and Seeman, P. (1980): *Am. J. Psychiatry*, 137:191–197.
73. Levy, M. L., Davis, B. M., Mohs, R. C., Trigos, G. C., Mathe, A. A., and Davis, K. L. (1983): *Psychiatry Res.*, 9:1–8.
74. Lieberman, J. A., Kane, J. M., and Gadaleta, D. (1984): *Am. J. Psychiatry*, 141:633–638.
75. Lindstrom, L. H. (1985): *Psychiatry Res.*, 14:265–273.
76. Linnoila, M., Viukari, M., and Hietala, O. (1976): *Br. J. Psychiatry*, 129:114–119.
77. Losonczy, M. F., Mohs, R. C., and Davis, K. L. (1984): *Psychiatry Res.*, 12:79–87.
78. Losonczy, M. F., Song, I. S., Mohs, R. C., Mathe, A. A., Davis, B. M., Davidson, M., and Davis, K. L. (1986): *Am. J. Psychiatry*, 143:1113–1118.
79. Losonczy, M. F., Song, I. S., Mohs, R. C., Small, N. A., Johns, C. A., Davidson, M., and Davis, K. L. (1986): *Am. J. Psychiatry*, 143:976–981.
80. Lostra, F., Verbanck, P., and Mendlewicz, J. (1984): *Biol. Psychiatry*, 19:871–882.
81. Luchins, D. J., Lewine, R. R. J., and Deltzer, H. Y. (1983): *Psychopharmacol. Bull.*, 19:518–522.
82. Maas, J. W., Contreras, S. A., Bowden, C. L., and Weintraub, S. E. (1985): *Life Sci.*, 36:2163–2170.
83. Maas, J. W., Hattox, S. E., and Landis, D. H. (1979): *J. Neurochem.*, 32:839–843.
84. Mackay, A. V. P., Iversen, L. L., and Rossor, M. (1982): *Arch. Gen. Psychiatry*, 39:991–997.
85. Martes, M. P., Bouthenet, M. L., Sales, N., Sokoloff, P., and Schwartz, J. C. (1985): *Science*, 752–755.
86. Mattes, J. A., Hom, W., and Rochford, J. M. (1985): *Biol. Psychiatry*, 20:533–538.
87. McKinney, W. T., Moran, E. C., Kraemer, G. W., and Prange, A. J. (1980): *Psychopharmacology*, 72:35–39.
88. Meltzer, H. Y. (1980): *Schizophr. Bull.*, 6:456–475.
89. Meltzer, H. Y., Busch, D. A., Schyve, P. M., and Fang, V. S. (1981): *Arch. Gen. Psychiatry*, 38:1138.
90. Mereu, G., Collu, M., Ongini, E., Biggio, G., and Gessa, G. L. (1985): *Eur. J. Pharmacol.*, 111:393.
91. Morley, J. E. (1982): *Life Sci.*, 30:479–493.
92. Moroji, T., Watanabe, N., Aoki, N., and Itoh, S. (1982): *Arch. Gen. Psychiatry*, 39:485–486.
93. Muller, P., and Seeman, P. (1978): *Psychopharmacology*, 60:1–11.

94. Murphy, R. B., and Schuster, D. I. (1982): *Peptides,* 3:539–543.
95. Nagao, T., Ohshimo, T., Mitsunobu, K., Sata, M., and Otskui, S. (1979): *Biol. Psychiatry,* 14:509–523.
96. Nair, N. P. V., Bloom, D. M., and Nestoros, J. N. (1982): *Prog. Neuropsychopharmacol. Biol. Psychiatry,* 6:509–512.
97. Nair, N. P. V., Bloom, D. M., Nestoros, J. N., and Schwartz, G. (1983): *Psychopharmacol. Bull.,* 19:134–136.
98. Nyback, H., Berggren, B., Hindmarsh, T., Sedvall, G., and Wiesel, F. (1983): *Psychiatry Res.,* 9:301–308.
99. Owen, F., Cross, A. J., Crow, T. J., Longden, A., Poulter, M., and Riley, G. J. (1978): *Lancet,* 2:223–226.
100. Owens, D. G., Johnstone, E. C., Crow, T. J., Frith, C. D., Jagoe, J. R., and Kreel, L. (1985): *Psychol. Med.,* 15:27–41.
101. Perlow, M. J., Ebert, M. H., Gordon, E. K., Ziegler, M. G., Lake, R. C., and Chase, T. N. (1978): *Brain Res.,* 139:101–113.
102. Petrouka, S. J., and Snyder, S. H. (1979): *Mol. Pharmacol.,* 16:549–556.
103. Pickar, D., Laborca, R., Linnoila, M., Roy, A., Hommer, D., Everett, D., and Paul, S. M. (1984): *Science,* 225:954–957.
104. Portig, P. J., and Vogt, M. (1968): *J. Physiol. (Lond.),* 194:65–69.
105. Post, R. M., Carpenter, W. T., and Goodwin, F. K. (1975): *Am. J. Psychiatry,* 32:1063–1069.
106. Post, R. M., and Goodwin, F. K. (1975): *Science,* 109:488–489.
107. Post, R. M., Kotin, J., Goodwin, F. K., and Gordon, E. K. (1973): *Am. J. Psychiatry,* 130:67–72.
108. Pycock, C. J., Carter, C. J., and Kerwin, R. W. (1980): *Neurochemistry,* 34:91–99.
109. Pycock, C. J., Kerwin, R. W., and Carter, C. J. (1980): *Nature,* 286:74–77.
110. Redmond, D. E., Maas, J. W., Kling, A., and Dekirmenjian, H. (1971): *Psychosom. Med.,* 33:97–113.
111. Reynolds, G. P., Reynolds, L. M., Riederer, P., Jellinger, K., and Gabriel, E. (1980): *Lancet,* 2:1251.
112. Rifkin, A., Quitkin, F., and Klein, D. F. (1975): *Arch. Gen. Psychiatry,* 32:672–674.
113. Roberts, E. (1976): *GABA in Nervous System Function,* pp. 515–539. Raven Press, New York.
114. Roth, R. H. (1979): *Commun. Psychopharmacol.,* 3:429–445.
115. Roth, R. H., and Surk, Y. (1970): *Biochem. Pharmacol.,* 19:3001–3009.
116. Roth, R. H., Walters, J. R., and Aghajanian, G. K. (1973): In: *Frontiers in Catecholamine Research,* edited by S. H. Snyder and E. Costa, p. 567–577. Pergamon Press, New York.
117. Scheck-Kruger, J., Christensen, A., and Azut, A. (1978): *Life Sci.,* 22:75–84.
118. Scheinin, M. (1984): *Psychopharmacol. Bull.,* 20:660.
119. Scheinin, M., Syvalahti, E. K. G., Hietala, J., Hupponen, R., Pihlajamaki, K., Seppala, O. P., and Sako, E. (1985): *Prog. Neuropsychopharmacol. Biol. Psychiatry,* 9:441–449.
120. Schultz, S. C., Sinicrope, P., Kishore, P., and Friedel, R. O. (1983): *Psychopharmacol. Bull.,* 19:510–512.
121. Schultz, S. C., van Kammen, D. P., Buchsbaum, M. S., Roth, R. H., Alexander, P., and Bunney, W. E., Jr. (1981): *Pharmacopsychiatria,* 14:129.
122. Sedvall, G. C., and Wode-Helgodt, B. (1980): *Arch. Gen. Psychiatry,* 37:1113–1116.
123. Seeman, P. (1980): *Pharmacol. Rev.,* 32:229–313.
124. Seeman, P., Ulpian, C., Bergeron, C., Riederer, P., Jellinger, K., Gabriel, E., Reynolds, G. P., and Tourtellotte, W. W. (1984): *Science,* 225:728–731.
125. Seijert, W. E., Foxx, J. R., and Butler, J. J. (1980): *Ann. Neurol.,* 8:38–42.
126. Smith, R. C., Tamminga, C., and Davis, J. M. (1977): *J. Neural Transm.,* 40:171–176.
127. Snyder, S. H. (1976): *Am. J. Psychiatry,* 133:197–202.
128. Sokoloff, P., Martres, M. P., and Schwartz, J. C. (1980): *Nature,* 288:283–286.
129. Stawarz, R. J., Hill, H., Robinson, S. E., Setler, P., Dingell, J. V., and Sulser, F. (1975): *Psychopharmacologia,* 43:125–130.
130. Syvalahti, E. K. G., Sako, E., Scheinin, M., Pihlajamaki, K., and Hietala, J. (1986): *Br. J. Psychiatry,* 148:204–208.
131. Tamminga, C. A., DeFraites, E. G., Gotts, M. D., and Chase, T. N. (1981): *Apomorphine and Other Dopaminomimetics, Vol. 2: Clinical Pharmacology,* edited by G. U. Corsini and G. L. Gessa, pp. 49–56. Raven Press, New York.
132. Tamminga, C. A., Schaeffer, M. H., Smith, R. C., and Davis, J. M. (1978): *Science,* 200:567–568.
133. Tamminga, C. A., Tighe, P. J., Chase, T. N., DeFraites, E. G., and Schaeffer, M. H. (1981): *Arch. Gen. Psychiatry,* 38:167–168.
134. Tanaka, Z., Mukai, Z., Takayanagi, Y., Muto, A., and Aizawa, H. (1966): *Folia Psychiatr. Neurol. Jpn.,* 20:9.
135. Traskman, L., Asberg, M., Bertillson, L., and Sjostrand, L. (1981): *Arch. Gen. Psychiatry,* 38:631–636.
136. van Kammen, D. P., Mann, L. S., Steinberg, D. E., Scheinin, M., Ninan, P. T., Marder, S. R., van Kammen, W. B., Reider, R. O., and Linnoila, M. (1983): *Science,* 220:974–977.
137. Van Ree, J. M., Verhoeven, W. M. A., Brouwer, G. J., and Weid, D. (1984): *Neuropsychobiology,* 12:4–8.
138. Van Rossum, J. M. (1966): *Arch. Int. Pharmacodyn.,* 160:492–494.
139. Verhoeven, W. M. A., Van Ree, J. M., De Weid, D., and Van Praag, H. M. (1981): *Arch. Gen. Psychiatry,* 38:1182–1193.
140. Wagner, H. N., Burns, H. D., Dannals, R. F., Wong, D. F., Langstrom, B., Buelfer, R., Frost, J. J., Ravert, H. T., Links, J. M., Rosenbloom, S. B., Lukas, S. E., Kramer, A. V., and Kuhar, M. J. (1983): *Science,* 221:1264–1266.
141. Walters, J. R., and Roth, R. H. (1976): *Naunyn Schmiedebergs Arch. Pharmacol.,* 296:5–14.
142. Wan, C. W., Peck, E. J., Ho, B. T., and Schoolar, J. C. (1983): *Life Sci.,* 32:1255–1262.
143. Waszczak, B., and Walters, J. (1979): *Adv. Neurol.,* 123:727–740.
144. Weinberger, D. R., Karson, C. N., Bigelow, L. B., Kleinman, J. E., Klein, S. T., Rosenblatt, J. E., and Wyatt, R. J. (1980): *Arch. Gen. Psychiatry,* 37:11–14.
145. Weinberger, D. R., Karson, C. N., Bigelow, L. B., and Wyatt, R. J. (1982): *Abstracts of the Annual Meeting of the American College of Neuropsychopharmacology,* 57.
146. Weinberger, D. R., Wagner, R. L., and Wyatt, R. J. (1983): *Schizophr. Bull.,* 9:193–212.
147. Wode-Helgodt, B., and Sedvall, G. (1978): *Commun. Psychopharmacol.,* 2:177–183.
148. Wolf, P., Olpe, H. R., Avrith, D., and Hans, H. (1978): *Experientia,* 34:73–74.
149. Wong, D. F., Wagner, H. N., Dannals, R. F., Links, J. M., Frost, J. J., Ravert, H. T., Wilson, A. A., Rosenbaum, A. E., Gjedde, A., Douglass, K. H., Petronis, J. D., Folstein, M. F., Toung, J. K. T., Burns, H. D., and Kuhar, M. J. (1984): *Science,* 226:1393–1396.
150. Wong, D. F., Wagner, H. N., Pearlson, G. D., et al. (1985): *Psychopharmacol. Bull.,* 21:595–598.
151. Wood, J. H. (1980): In: *Neurobiology of Cerebrospinal Fluid,* edited by J. H. Wood, p. 56. Plenum Press, New York.

Psychopharmacology:
The Third Generation of Progress,
edited by Herbert Y. Meltzer.
Raven Press, New York © 1987.

CHAPTER 71

Peptides in Schizophrenia

Charles B. Nemeroff, Philip A. Berger, and Garth Bissette

Study of the physiological and pathophysiological roles and actions of an increasingly large number of peptides in the CNS, as well as in nonneural tissue, has become a major focus of research for neuroscience. More than 40 peptides with possible CNS activity have been isolated and sequenced from mammalian brain (Table 1). They range in size from dipeptides (two amino acids joined by a single peptide bond) to large molecules such as corticotropin-releasing factor (CRF), which contains 41 amino acids. Detailed and comprehensive reviews of the neuroanatomical distribution and neurochemical, neurophysiological, neuropharmacological, and behavioral effects of a variety of neuropeptides have appeared (8,17,42,52,54,68,69,84, 90,92,93,106,108,110,115,122,123,132,136). Other chapters in this volume summarize some of the extensive basic and clinical investigations on neuroactive peptides. This chapter reviews the evidence that neuropeptides are involved in the pathophysiology of schizophrenia.

With a few notable exceptions, the pattern of peptide discovery has been as follows: first, a crude extract of brain (or some other tissue) is found to possess a specific biological activity. This activity is then found to be due to the presence of a peptide, and the peptide is eventually purified and sequenced. In 1931, substance P (sub P) was discovered by Von Euler and Gaddum (83), but 40 years were to pass before its chemical identity was determined. A few peptides, such as insulin, were discovered in the 1950s; however their presence in the CNS was not recognized until about 20 years later. In the 1940s and 1950s, the pioneering work of a few investigators spawned the "new" multidisciplinary field of neuroendocrinology.

For approximately 20 years, the greatest stimulus for research in neuropeptide neurobiology was the discovery that the various endocrine axes are organized in hierarchical fashion, with the CNS at the summit. The chemical regulators of anterior pituitary hormone secretion, the release and release-inhibiting factors, are now known to be neuropeptides. The chemotransmitter-portal vessel hypothesis, expounded by Harris and his colleagues (45) and others (124), postulated the presence of neurohormones that are released from nerve endings in the median eminence region of the hypothalamus and are transported from the primary capillary plexus to the adenohypophysis by the hypothalamo-hypophysial venous portal system. Once vascularly transported to the anterior pituitary, these hypophysiotropic hormones bind to specific membrane receptors, which results in the release (or inhibition of release) of one (or more) pituitary trophic hormones. Millions of sheep and pig hypothalami were extracted to eventually yield a few precious milligrams of the first hypothalamic releasing hormones to be discovered (137). These include thyrotropin-releasing hormone (TRH, a tripeptide), gonadotropin-releasing hormone (GnRH or LHRH, a decapeptide), and somatostatin (SRIF, a tetradecapeptide).

These findings have not only resulted in major diagnostic and treatment breakthroughs in clinical endocrinology, but they have had considerable impact in psychiatry as well. It is now becoming more evident that particular psychiatric disorders are often associated with robust and reproducible neuroendocrine abnormalities; these findings are described in detail in other chapters in this volume. The major reason for this chapter's review of the possible role of neuropeptides in schizophrenia rests on several distinct, but related, discoveries that have led to one major conclusion—that neuropeptides are important neuroregulators in the CNS. The neuropeptides function in the CNS as neurotransmitters

TABLE 1. *Neuropeptides identified in mammalian brain*

Adrenocorticotropin (ACTH)	Luteinizing hormone (LH)
Angiotensin	Luteinizing hormone-releasing
Bombesin (BOM)	hormone (LHRH, GnRH)
Bradykinin	Melanocyte stimulating hormone-
Calcitonin	release inhibiting factor (MIF-I)
Carnosine	α-Melanocyte-stimulating hormone
Cholecystokinin (CCK)	(α-MSH)
Corticotropin-releasing factor (CRF)	β-Melanocyte-stimulating hormone
Delta-sleep-inducing peptide (DSIP)	(β-MSH)
Dynorphin	Met-enkephalin (Met-ENK)
α-Endorphin	Neuromedin N
β-Endorphin	Neuropeptide Y
γ-Endorphin	Neurotensin (NT)
Gastrin	Oxytocin
Gastrin-releasing peptide	Prolactin (PRL)
Glucagon	Secretin
Gonadotropin-releasing hormone	Somatostatin (SRIF, GHIH)
(GnRH, LHRH)	Substance P (sub P)
Growth hormone (GH)	Thyrotropin-releasing hormone
Growth hormone-releasing factor	(TRH)
(GRF, GHRH)	Thyroid-stimulating hormone
Insulin	(thyrotropin, TSH)
Kallikrein	Vasoactive intestinal peptide (VIP)
Kytorphin	Vasopressin
Leu-enkephalin (leu-ENK)	Vasotocin

and neuromodulators and, consequently, they also modulate behavior. Moreover, some evidence is concordant with the view that alterations of specific neuropeptide-containing neurons occur in certain neuropsychiatric diseases, including schizophrenia.

Space constraints preclude a detailed discussion of the evidence that supports a neurotransmitter role for each of the more than 40 neuropeptides (see Table 1) present in the mammalian CNS.

Neuropeptides are heterogeneously distributed in the CNS. The pattern of distribution of each peptide is relatively unique. Thus, in humans and other mammals, neurotensin (NT) is found in high concentrations in hypothalamus, amygdala, nucleus accumbens, and septum (58,81). In contrast, vasoactive intestinal peptide (VIP) and cholecystokinin (CCK) are present in high concentrations in cerebral cortex, as well as in the hippocampus (71,98). Other neuropeptides, like GnRH/LHRH or growth hormone-releasing factor (GRF) have much more restricted patterns of distribution—they are found almost exclusively in the diencephalon (55,62).

Unlike the monoamines, neuropeptides, once released into the synaptic cleft, are inactivated primarily by enzymatic degradation and not by reuptake into the presynaptic terminal. Current knowledge about the transduction of the signal that occurs after neuropeptides bind to their membrane receptor(s) is also quite limited. However, electrophysiological changes in neuronal firing rates have repeatedly been observed after microiontophoretic application of neuropeptides such as NT (11,46). Finally, behavioral changes and modifications in responses to centrally acting pharmacological agents have been observed after intracerebroventricular or direct CNS administration of neuropeptides

(47,107,108). These latter findings suggest that changes in the extracellular fluid concentration of neuropeptides can produce marked physiological and pharmacobehavioral alterations.

Prior to a consideration of the role of neuropeptides in schizophrenia, it is useful to carefully compare the neurobiology of neuropeptides with that of the more well-studied monoamines. These differences, highlighted by Hughes (52), are summarized in Table 2. One major difference between these two classes of neuroregulators is their mode of biosynthesis. Neuropeptides are synthesized by protein synthesis in the perikaryon (usually as a large prohormone) and, after packaging, are transported down the axon to the nerve terminal, where they are subsequently released in active form. In contrast, monoamines are synthesized largely in the nerve terminal region by a series of enzymatic steps from an amino acid precursor. The mode of inactivation of these two classes of neuroregulators is also quite different: peptides are inactivated by enzymes (peptidases) (43,86), whereas monoamines are removed from the synaptic cleft largely by transmitter reuptake into the presynaptic terminal. The physiological consequences of monoamine release are brief, whereas the action of neuropeptides can be quite sustained.

An exciting recent finding by Hokfelt and colleagues (48) and others (53) is the convincing demonstration of colocalization of neuropeptides and monoamines. For example, compelling evidence for colocalization of CCK and dopamine (DA) has appeared (49).

Thus, a large number of neuropeptides are now known to be present in the mammalian CNS. Their unique anatomical localization and the concatenation of behavioral, electrophysiological, and pharmacological properties attrib-

TABLE 2. *Comparison of aminergic and peptidergic systems*

Neuropeptides	Amine
Biosynthesis	
Ribosomal synthesis of protein precursor and enzymatic cleavage to active products in nerve axon. Posttranslational peptide modification occurs (amidation, acetylation, sulfation)	Local synthesis in terminals via specific catabolic enzymes subject to feedback control
Storage	
Large granular vesicles. Protein carriers	Large and small vesicles, often granulated. Specific uptake and storage mechanisms in vesicles
Tissue concentrations vary from 1 to 1000 pmol/g	Tissue concentrations vary from 1 to 100 nmol/g
Release	
Calcium-dependent	Calcium dependent exocytosis Quantal
Inactivation	
Aminopeptidases Endopeptidases Carboxypeptidases	Reuptake into nerve terminal; ester hydrolysis, methylation, and deamination

From ref. 100.

uted to them make neuropeptides prime candidates for one of the classes of endogenous substances (endocoids) that modulate normal and abnormal physiology and behavior.

In this chapter, three types of evidence for the possible role of neuropeptides in the pathophysiology of schizophrenia are considered. First, studies in postmortem brain tissues and cerebrospinal fluid (CSF) have been conducted to determine whether the integrity or activity of neuropeptide-containing systems and their receptors is altered in schizophrenia. Second, studies in which peptides have been administered to human subjects with the diagnosis of schizophrenia to evaluate their potential therapeutic use are reviewed. Finally, the effects of peptide receptor antagonists on the symptoms of schizophrenic patients are reviewed in detail.

There are, of course, problems with each of these approaches. The postmortem tissue and CSF studies have recently been reviewed by Edwardson and McDermott (29) and Rossor (128), and by Post and co-workers (121), respectively. In both types of studies, several potentially confounding variables must be carefully evaluated; these include patient age and sex, and drug effects. Such considerations increase the likelihood that alterations in peptide concentration (or receptor number) are related to schizophrenia and not to these artifacts. In postmortem tissue studies, stability of the peptide to be measured must be taken into consideration, as well as agonal state, postmortem delay, and cause of death. In CSF and postmortem studies, the time of day (and year) the sample is obtained may be important because of possible circadian and circannual rhythms in the concentrations of certain neurotransmitters (e.g., melatonin and the endorphins) and their metabolites (150). In general, neuropeptides have been found to be

remarkably stable in postmortem brain tissue and CSF. However, the complexity of neuropeptide neurobiology is demonstrated by the multiple forms of certain neuropeptides that have been found in brain and CSF (134).

The studies in which peptides have been administered to schizophrenic patients as potential treatments are also quite problematical. It is unclear at this time whether neuropeptides penetrate the blood-brain barrier in appreciable quantities after systemic injection; therefore, any subsequent effects observed may not be due to direct peptide actions on the CNS. Studies of peptides as putative pharmacotherapeutic agents must be evaluated with the same rigor as any other drug trial. Ideally, there should be randomized, placebo-controlled, double-blind studies with large numbers per group and conducted by clinically experienced investigators. The peptide antagonist studies, largely limited at this time to naloxone and naltrexone, the opiate receptor blockers, also have problems. The duration of action of the antagonists is relatively brief, and at higher doses, they may have opioid agonist effects as well as effects on nonopioid systems (129).

When reviewing a reported finding in the succeeding text, the specificity of the antiserum used to measure a peptide and the method of statistical analysis employed will be described whenever possible. This detailed description of methodology is necessary since methodological differences may well explain discrepant reports in the literature. Second, inclusion of methodological considerations increases their visibility, and this can only have a positive effect on psychiatric research. Finally, the use of inappropriate statistical tests can lead investigators to incorrect conclusions and thus, the methods for data analysis must also be carefully scrutinized.

STUDIES OF NEUROPEPTIDE CONCENTRATIONS IN SCHIZOPHRENIA

Endorphin Concentrations in Schizophrenia

Terenius et al. (135) from Sweden first reported alterations in endogenous opioid peptide (endorphin) concentrations in CSF of schizophrenic patients. Their radioreceptor assay utilized [^{3}H]dihydromorphine as the ligand and measured total opioid activity without discrimination as to which particular opioid was present. In this original report, the CSF opioid activity of four chronic schizophrenic patients (ill for at least 10 years, but drug-free for 4 weeks) was compared before, and 2 and 4 weeks after, clozapine treatment. The diagnostic criteria used were not specified in this early report. The CSF was filtered and chromatographed on Sephadex G-10; two fractions with opiate receptor activity were isolated (fractions I and II). Methionine-enkephalin (Met-ENK) coeluted with fraction II, but only the concentration of fraction I was changed after neuroleptic treatment. Two of the four schizophrenic patients had elevated CSF fraction I opioid concentrations after 4 weeks of neuroleptic treatment, but no statistical test was performed on this small sample.

In a later study by the same group of Swedish investigators, Lindstrom et al. (76) reported that when CSF opioid activity, as defined with the same radioreceptor assay, was measured in nine chronic schizophrenic patients after a drug-free period of 12 months, six of the patients had higher fraction I opioid concentrations than the mean fraction I concentration of 19 normal volunteers. In addition, when retested after treatment with antipsychotic drugs (clozapine, flupenthixol, or chlorpromazine for 12 days–2 months), the schizophrenic patients with higher CSF fraction I levels exhibited values close to the mean of the normal controls. In another study (126) using the same methods, CSF fraction I opioid activity was measured in 18 drug-free acute schizophrenic patients (11 had never received neuroleptics, seven had stopped neuroleptic treatment 4 to 8 weeks before this study) and in 24 chronic schizophrenic patients who had been neuroleptic-free for at least 2 weeks. The schizophrenic patients fulfilled Feighner's criteria (3) for definite schizophrenia, and only the chronic patients whose symptoms worsened during the 2-week drug holiday were studied (nine of 12). Two of nine chronic schizophrenic patients, four of the six relapsed patients, and six of nine acute schizophrenic patients had elevated CSF fraction I opioid concentrations when compared to mean values for normal controls from the Lindstrom et al. (76) study.

In another recent study, this Swedish group (74) found that either fraction I or II CSF opioid activity was elevated above their previously published mean normal control values (76) in 72% of 53 1-week neuroleptic-free schizophrenic patients (using Bleuler's criteria) (3). These elevations did not attain statistical significance when compared to normal controls, but within the schizophrenic group, the CSF fraction I opioid activity was significantly higher in the hebephrenic ($n = 23$) than in the undifferentiated subgroup ($n = 21$). No significant correlations were noted between CSF opioid activity of either fraction I or II and duration of disease, length of neuroleptic treatment, or psychotic symptoms.

Dupont et al. (27), using a radioreceptor assay employing [^{3}H]naloxone as the radioactive ligand, found decreased CSF concentrations of opioid activity in 19 chronic schizophrenic patients when compared to nine controls. The diagnostic criteria used were not specified, and all of the schizophrenic patients were receiving neuroleptics. The CSF opioid(s) that displaced [^{3}H]naloxone binding coeluted with Met-ENK and leucine-enkephalin (Leu-ENK) on Sephadex G-25, but the decreases observed in the schizophrenic patients were reported as not significant (8), and the method of statistical analysis is not described. After incubation of CSF for 5 hr at 37°C, the schizophrenic group had no measurable immunoreactivity in CSF, whereas the mean control CSF concentration remained at 80% of preincubation levels, implying higher peptide degradative (enzymatic) activity of opioid peptides in the schizophrenic group. This latter finding has not been confirmed by Burbach et al. (13) in a study of nine schizophrenic patients and neurological controls.

The molecular nature of the opioid material in CSF is clearly an important issue. Akil et al. (1) measured CSF Met-ENK by radioimmunoassay (RIA) and opioid activity by radioreceptor assay in 10 healthy volunteers and expressed the results as picograms of Met-ENK equivalents per milliliter in order to compare the two methods directly. Both assays used [^{3}H]Met-ENK as the radiolabeled ligand; CSF was extracted with acid-methanol; and the peptides were separated using two liquid chromatography columns. Both assays found levels of Met-ENK/opioid activity that agreed with those reported for fraction II by the Swedish group of Terenius and colleagues.

In contrast, Jeffcoate et al. (57) reported on the measurement of β-endorphin by RIA in CSF of 20 control patients undergoing diagnostic lumbar punctures or pneumoencephalograms; the CSF concentrations of β-endorphin were in the same range as the opioid activity reported by Dupont et al. (27). Because almost all antisera to β-endorphin recognize β-lipotropin (β-LPH, a precursor to β-endorphin), Jeffcoate et al. separated the two immunoreactive forms on Sephadex G-25 and used an antiserum that was directed toward β-LPH, but not β-endorphin, to assess the contribution of β-LPH to the total immunoreactivity. β-Endorphin accounted for more than 90% of the immunoreactivity in all of the samples tested. These two studies (1,57) may establish a standard for normal concentrations of Met-ENK and β-endorphin in CSF, although further study is necessary. Naber and Pickar (101) have comprehensively reviewed the problems of measuring endorphins in biological fluids, including CSF.

In a preliminary report, Domschke et al. (25) presented data on the CSF concentrations of β-endorphin in five acute and seven chronic (>10 years) schizophrenic patients compared to seven normal controls and 10 patients with herniated vertebral discs. No diagnostic criteria for schizophrenia were provided and all psychiatric patients were receiving neuroleptic drug therapy. The CSF was extracted in silicic acid and acetone, and β-endorphin was estimated by RIA. Inappropriately using Student's t-test to analyze the data, this group claimed that the acute schizophrenic patients had increased, and the chronic schizophrenic patients had decreased, CSF β-endorphin concentrations, when compared to the controls.

Burbach et al. (13) compared CSF concentrations of β-endorphin and Met-ENK in nine neurologically diseased controls and nine schizophrenic patients. No diagnostic criteria were reported for the schizophrenic patients, and all were currently treated with neuroleptics. Both peptides were measured by RIA. No significant group-related differences in CSF β-endorphin or Met-ENK concentrations were observed.

Naber et al. (102,103) and Naber and Pickar (101), using a radioreceptor assay for opioid activity and an RIA for β-endorphin, studied CSF from psychiatric patients with a variety of diagnoses, including schizophrenia ($n = 27$), schizoaffective disorder ($n = 17$), depression ($n = 35$), and mania ($n = 13$), as well as from normal controls. Schizophrenic patients were diagnosed by Research Diagnostic Criteria (RDC) (6) and were medication-free for 2 weeks prior to the study. The radioreceptor assay used a Met-ENK analog, [³H]D-Ala-L-Leu-enkephalinamide (D-ALA), and the RIA used ¹²⁵I-β-endorphin as the tracer. Opiate receptor activity was significantly reduced in the schizophrenic males only ($p < 0.005$, Student's t-test, two-tailed), but β-endorphin concentrations were much lower than those reported by others. Recently, Naber et al. (100) reported that in 23 unmedicated acute schizophrenic patients, serum β-endorphin concentrations were not correlated with baseline measures of psychotic behavior, nor were they associated with the therapeutic efficacy of neuroleptics.

Emrich et al. (31,32) and Hollt et al. (50) measured the concentration of β-endorphin-like immunoreactivity by RIA in CSF and plasma of eight controls (CSF was obtained to diagnose meningitis/encephalitis and found to be negative) compared to 15 schizophrenic patients and a variety of other neurological patients. Schizophrenic patients were diagnosed by the International Classification of Disease (ICD) nomenclature (6) and were medication-free for 4 weeks. Plasma, but not CSF, β-endorphin was extracted with a silicic acid/acetone mixture. No significant concentration differences between controls and schizophrenic patients were detected in CSF or plasma.

Van Kammen et al. (138) measured both β-endorphin concentration and opioid activity in CSF from 30 schizophrenic patients; in addition, vasopressin and angiotensin I and II concentrations were assayed. The results were compared to those obtained in 52 normal controls. Schizophrenic patients fulfilled RDC criteria (6) and were drug-free for an average of 33 days before treatment. Concentrations of β-endorphin, vasopressin, and angiotensin I and II were measured by RIA using ¹²⁵I-labeled peptides, and opioid activity was assessed by radioreceptor assay with [³H]D-ALA as the radioligand. The concentration of vasopressin was found to be reduced by approximately 40% ($p < 0.01$) in the CSF of male schizophrenic patients. No differences were found in the concentrations of the other peptides including the opioid peptides.

Recently, Wen et al. (153) measured CSF Met-ENK levels in chronic schizophrenic patients ($n = 18$; duration of illness greater than 10 years) and neurological controls ($n = 18$; eight stroke, 10 headache). The schizophrenic patients were rated before CSF withdrawal according to the Brief Psychiatric Rating Scale (BPRS); no mention was made of medication status. The RIA employed recognized Met-O-enkephalin, and therefore ¹²⁵I-Met-O-enkephalin was used as the radioactive trace. All CSF samples were passed through Sep-Pak filters and oxidized with hydrogen peroxide to form Met-O-enkephalin. Recovery was estimated at 70%, and schizophrenic patients were reported to have significantly less Met-ENK present in CSF than controls ($p < 0.02$, Student's t-test). No significant correlation was seen between BPRS score and Met-ENK concentration. This group used identical biochemical methodology in a second study (78) while investigating the purported antipsychotic effects of naloxone in schizophrenic patients. They found a significant correlation between the increase in CSF Met-ENK concentrations and the naloxone-induced decrease in psychotic symptoms in seven schizophrenic patients.

Thus, at the present time, the data provided by measuring opioid peptides in CSF and plasma are contradictory and confusing and provide no compelling evidence for a significant role of endorphins in schizophrenia.

Hemodialysis and Leucine-5-β-Endorphin

Wagemaker and Cade (151) reported in 1977 that an open and uncontrolled trial of hemodialysis in schizophrenic subjects on a weekly basis produced a substantial improvement in schizophrenic symptoms. Simultaneously, they and their collaborators, Palmour et al. (114), reported the existence of a previously unknown peptide, a leucine-5-β-endorphin. The existence of leucine in position 5 of β-endorphin had not been reported in any tissue of any species prior to this report. This group further argued that the effectiveness of the hemodialysis in schizophrenia depended on the removal of leucine-5-β-endorphin from the plasma. The group offered the hypothesis that leucine-5-β-endorphin was causing schizophrenic symptoms in their patients who improved on hemodialysis. Thus, several issues were brought together in a very complex package: the issue of the clinical efficacy of hemodialysis in schizophrenia, the issue of the existence of leucine-5-β-endorphin, and the issue of whether removal of that compound by dialysis was an effective means of treating schizophrenia. To address the first issue, several studies using hemodialysis or peritoneal dialysis were carried out in medical centers across the country. To date, these studies have failed to confirm the clinical utility or efficacy of hemodialysis as a treatment for schizophrenia (33).

There are also many presentations, discussions, and case histories in the literature that report that most schizophrenic patients are not responsive to hemodialysis. However, there are some anecdotal reports in which an occasional patient is responsive to dialysis. The type of dialysis membrane, the psychological nature of the setting, and the actual diagnosis of the patient are all major concerns in evaluating the validity of these reports. In addition to the case reports,

Port et al. (120) have carried out a retrospective study of the literature on 50 schizophrenic patients who were dialysed in Veterans Administration Medical Centers because of renal problems. They found that during the course of the dialysis, 40 patients were unchanged and eight were improved. They argued that from the multiphasic character of schizophrenia and the heterogeneity of symptoms, one would expect this degree of fluctuation among 50 patients. They also argued that the kidney is much more efficient at filtering these molecules from the plasma than is the dialysis machine and therefore raised questions about the effectiveness of dialysis as a means of removing molecules of the size of β-endorphin or leucine-5-β-endorphin from plasma.

Investigations of the chemical aspects of this question have failed to yield positive results. Lewis et al. (73) studied the hemofiltrate from dialysed schizophrenics and could detect no methionine-5- or leucine-5-β-endorphin in the hemofiltrate. It should be pointed out that their level of sensitivity for detecting methionine-endorphin (β-endorphin) concentrations in normal individuals was quite low. However, the levels for schizophrenic patients reported by Palmour et al. (114) are 1000- to 10,000-fold higher than in normal individuals and should have been detected, even using the techniques of Lewis et al. (73).

The Stanford group has also addressed the problem of the possible significance of leucine-5-β-endorphin to schizophrenia (127). If schizophrenics have extremely high levels of β-endorphin or leucine-5-β-endorphin, then high levels of peptide should be obvious in the plasma of these subjects (in contrast to normal individuals) using RIAs for both methionine-5- and leucine-5-β-endorphin. The Stanford group developed an RIA to test this hypothesis. The antiserum used in this study recognized human methionine-5-β-endorphin and human leucine-5-β-endorphin equally. The binding for radioactively labeled β-endorphin is inhibited 50% by 2 fmol (7 pg) of either peptide in an assay tube. The antiserum cross reacts 30% with β-lipotropin; this has also been demonstrated in human plasma (127). In 98 patients and 42 normals, the Stanford group found surprisingly similar concentrations of endorphin-like immunoreactivity in plasma (schizophrenics, 2.8 fmol/ml average; normals, 2.4 fmol/ml). Further, the Stanford group was unable to detect leucine-5-β-endorphin in dialysate from nine schizophrenic patients (127).

Nonendorphin Neuropeptide CSF Concentrations in Schizophrenia

There have been several reports in which nonopioid peptides have been measured in the CSF of schizophrenic patients. Nemeroff, Prange, and colleagues (154) assayed CSF NT concentrations by RIA in 21 schizophrenic patients diagnosed by RDC (6) and 12 age- and sex-matched healthy volunteers. This study was undertaken because several findings in neurochemistry, neuroanatomy, and neuropharmacology have unequivocally demonstrated NT-DA interactions in the CNS (105,107,109), and because the DA hypothesis of schizophrenia remains the most viable theory concerning the pathogenesis of this disorder.

The schizophrenic patients were drug-free for at least 2 weeks, and psychiatric symptoms were assessed with the Comprehensive Psychopathological Rating Scale (CPRS) (154). Group mean CSF concentrations of NT-like immunoreactivity were not significantly different, but the schizophrenic group was shown to consist of two subgroups; one of these had very low CSF concentrations of NT-like immunoreactivity. After neuroleptic treatment, this latter subgroup exhibited normalization of CSF NT concentrations. Only one of 16 items in the CPRS was significantly correlated with the concentration of NT in CSF from the schizophrenic group: slowness of movement ($p < 0.01$). In this regard, it is of interest that all of the catatonic patients were in the low NT subgroup.

Recently, Nemeroff and Bissette in North Carolina, in collaboration with Widerlov and Lindstrom from Sweden (unpublished observations), have confirmed the decrease of NT-like immunoreactivity in the CSF of patients, but changes in NT concentration after neuroleptic treatment were not found. No such CSF NT reductions were observed in patients with major depression, anorexia-bulimia, or premenstrual syndrome (80).

Recently, in a second collaboration between the Swedish and Duke University groups (9), CSF concentrations of SRIF were measured in 10 healthy volunteers, 29 demented patients, 23 patients with major depression, and 10 schizophrenic patients (DSM-III criteria) (6). The antiserum recognized $SRIF_{1-14}$ (cyclic or linear), $SRIF_{1-25}$, and $SRIF_{1-28}$. All three psychiatric diagnostic groups had significantly reduced CSF concentrations of SRIF when compared to controls. Thus, decreases in CSF SRIF appear not to be specific to a particular disease state but may reflect cognitive impairment.

Gerner and Yamada (41) assayed CSF concentrations of immunoreactive CCK, SRIF, and bombesin (BOM) in normal healthy volunteers ($n = 29$) and patients with anorexia nervosa ($n = 23$), mania ($n = 10$), primary depression ($n = 28$), and chronic schizophrenia ($n = 13$), all ill for more than 6 months. Diagnoses were made using RDC criteria (6), and schizophrenic patients were neuroleptic-free for 14 days prior to CSF sampling. A small, but statistically insignificant, decrease in BOM-like immunoreactivity was observed in the schizophrenic patients when compared to the controls; no diagnostic group-related differences in CSF concentrations of SRIF- or CCK-like immunoreactivity were found.

In a more recent study, Gerner (39) measured BOM, SRIF, and CCK by RIA in CSF obtained from 31 normal controls, 19 schizophrenic patients from California hospitals, and 53 schizophrenic patients from the National Institute of Mental Health (NIMH). All schizophrenic patients fulfilled RDC criteria (6) and were neuroleptic-free for at least 14 days. Only the schizophrenic patients from the NIMH exhibited significant elevations in CCK and SRIF concentrations and decreases in BOM, when compared to controls. Neither CCK, SRIF, nor BOM showed any consistent change in CSF concentration after blockade of acid transport by treatment with probenecid or after treatment with the neuroleptic drug pimozide. No significant correlation was seen between CSF concentration of CCK, SRIF, or BOM and concentrations of homovanillic acid (HVA), 5-hydroxyindoleacetic acid (5-HIAA), 3-methoxy-4-hydroxyphenylglycol (MHPG), β-endorphin, tyrosine, tryptophan, γ-aminobutyric acid (GABA), or cortisol. The SRIF findings in schizophrenia are in contrast to the findings of the Duke University group in collaboration with the Swedish group (9).

Verbanck et al. (142) measured CSF CCK concentrations in control subjects and in patients with Parkinson's disease ($n = 13$), depression ($n = 30$), and schizophrenia ($n = 15$). Schizophrenic patients were diagnosed using Feighner's criteria (6). Nine patients were drug-free for 6 weeks, and six received haloperidol prior to CSF withdrawal. The antiserum used to measure CCK also recognized gastrin and cerulein, and ^{125}I-gastrin was used as the radioligand in the CCK assay. The concentration of CCK in CSF was reported to be significantly decreased in the drug-free schizophrenic patients when compared to the normal controls.

Rimon et al. (125) recently measured the concentration of sub P in CSF from 15 controls, 12 depressed patients, and 12 schizophrenic patients. Schizophrenic patients fulfilled Feighner's criteria (6) and were drug-free for 2 weeks. Samples of CSF were filtered on Sep-Pak cartridges and sub P was measured by RIA. The schizophrenic patients were reported to have significantly increased CSF concentrations of this undecapeptide. Gel electrophoresis of the sub P immunoreactivity in CSF revealed that less than 10% of the observed immunoreactivity was due to the presence of the intact sub P molecule; fragments coeluting with sub P$_{5-11}$ and sub P$_{3-11}$ represented the bulk of the immunoreactivity.

Kaya et al. (61) measured the concentration of sub P-like immunoreactivity in plasma of schizophrenic patients, normal controls, and patients with other psychiatric diagnoses. After more than 1 year of antipsychotic drug treatment, plasma sub P-like immunoreactivity was elevated when compared to controls, but this finding was observed only in the medicated schizophrenic patients.

Lindstrom et al. from Sweden (75) measured the CSF concentrations of immunoreactive delta sleep-inducing peptide (DSIP) in healthy volunteers ($n = 20$), schizophrenic patients ($n = 22$), and depressed patients ($n = 10$). Schizophrenic patients fulfilled RDC criteria (6) and were drug-free for 2 weeks before the first CSF sample was obtained. The DSIP antiserum was directed toward the N-terminal end of the DSIP molecule and ^{125}I-DSIP was used as the radioactive ligand. Schizophrenic patients had significantly lower CSF DSIP concentrations than controls, both in the drug-free state and after 4 weeks of neuroleptic treatment.

Neuropeptide Concentrations in Postmortem Brain in Schizophrenia

In addition to neuropeptide measurement in CSF, investigators have also examined postmortem brain tissue from schizophrenic patients in the hope that the neurotransmitter(s) involved in the etiology and pathogenesis of schizophrenia might be elucidated. As yet, few reports have

appeared concerning alterations in neuropeptide concentrations in postmortem brain regions of patients who had been, in life, diagnosed as schizophrenic. Indeed, few studies describing the concentrations of these peptides in the normal human brain have been conducted.

Recently, Crow and his colleagues have measured the concentrations of five neuropeptides in brain regions from 12 controls and 14 schizophrenic patients (36,37). All schizophrenic patients fulfilled Feighner's criteria (6) and were further subclassified into type I ($n = 7$) and type II ($n = 7$) based on the presence or absence of "positive" and "negative" symptoms, as described by Crow (18). The neuropeptides (NT, sub P, CCK, SRIF, and VIP) were assayed by RIA in temporal, frontal, parietal, and cingulate cortices and several subcortical regions including the hippocampus, amygdala, globus pallidus, putamen, dorsomedial thalamus, and lateral thalamus. Significant alterations were observed for CCK (reduced in temporal cortex) and sub P (increased in hippocampus) in the total group of schizophrenic patients compared to controls. Type II schizophrenic patients had significantly decreased mean concentrations of CCK in the amygdala and significantly decreased SRIF and CCK concentrations in the hippocampus; type I schizophrenic patients had elevated levels of VIP in the amygdala. No significant correlation was seen for any regional neuropeptide concentration with age, postmortem delay, or presence of neuroleptic medication.

Nemeroff et al. (111) measured the regional postmortem brain concentrations of NT, SRIF, and TRH in controls (free of neurological or psychiatric disease, $n = 50$), patients with Huntington's chorea ($n = 24$), and schizophrenic patients ($n = 46$). Schizophrenic patients were diagnosed by RDC criteria (6) and were on various neuroleptic regimens before and, in some cases, up to the time of death. All peptides were measured by RIA, and analysis of variance was utilized to determine whether significant group-related differences in a particular regional peptide concentration were present. No significant differences in NT, SRIF, or TRH concentrations were seen between controls and schizophrenic patients in the caudate nucleus, nucleus accumbens, amygdala, or hypothalamus. A significant decrease in SRIF ($p < 0.05$) and TRH ($p < 0.004$) concentrations in Brodmann's area 12 (frontal cortex) and a significant decrease ($p < 0.05$) in TRH concentration in Brodmann's area 32 (frontal cortex) were observed in the schizophrenic patients when compared to the controls; in contrast, NT content was significantly elevated ($p < 0.006$) in Brodmann's area 32 (frontal cortex) in the schizophrenic group.

Kleinman et al. (64) measured the concentration of four neuropeptides (Met-ENK, sub P, NT, and CCK) by RIA in postmortem brain regions from normal control subjects ($n = 18$), alcoholic patients ($n = 7$), opiate users ($n = 12$), suicide victims ($n = 19$), and psychotic patients ($n = 40$). The psychotic group was subdivided by RDC criteria (6) into chronic paranoid schizophrenic patients ($n = 11$), chronic undifferentiated schizophrenic patients ($n = 6$), and patients with "other" psychotic disorders (unspecified functional psychoses and affective psychoses). No significant differences between normals and psychotic patients were found in Met-ENK concentrations in nucleus accumbens, hypothalamus, globus pallidus, or putamen. Similarly, no significant group-related differences in NT concentrations in nucleus accumbens, globus pallidus, or hypothalamus were observed. Moreover, no significant differences were seen between control and psychotic patients in CCK levels in amygdala, nucleus accumbens, caudate nucleus, frontal cortex, substantia nigra, hippocampus, or temporal cortex. Met-ENK concentrations were reported to be significantly ($p < 0.05$) decreased in the caudate nucleus of chronic paranoid schizophrenics compared to other diagnostic groups or controls; sub P levels were significantly increased in the caudate nucleus of patients with psychoses when compared to diagnoses other than schizophrenia.

Biggins et al. (7) have recently measured amygdaloid concentrations of NT and TRH by RIA in normals ($n = 7$) and patients with senile dementia of Alzheimer's type ($n = 7$), depressive illness ($n = 7$), or schizophrenia ($n = 7$). No criteria were given for the diagnosis of schizophrenia, and no mention was made of medication status. No significant difference was seen in amygdaloid concentrations of TRH or NT between the four diagnostic groups. A significant positive correlation between the concentrations of TRH and NT was noted in this brain region. Total NT and TRH immunoreactivity in the amygdala was characterized on high-performance liquid chromatography (HPLC); NT immunoreactivity coeluted with the synthetic standard as a single peak, whereas TRH immunoreactivity consisted of a major peak (50%) and several minor peaks.

STUDIES USING NEUROPEPTIDES AS EXPERIMENTAL TREATMENTS FOR SCHIZOPHRENIA

β-Endorphin in Schizophrenia

The New York Study

In an early study that stimulated considerable further research, Kline et al. (66) administered 1.5 mg β-endorphin i.v. to three schizophrenic patients and reported a rapid worsening of their cognitive difficulties (e.g., more difficulty conceptualizing). Less than 2 weeks later, a second trial was conducted with higher doses of β-endorphin. One schizophrenic patient who had not responded to the previous 1-mg dose responded to 4 mg of β-endorphin i.v. by looking more energetic, smiling frequently, and speaking rapidly. He spoke of plans for the future and a new lack of fear of others. However, after 7 mg of β-endorphin i.v., he again looked fatigued and spoke in a halting manner. Two other schizophrenic patients who received 3 mg β-endorphin i.v. showed no behavioral changes.

The Stanford Study

Another investigation using β-endorphin in schizophrenic patients was accomplished by the Stanford group (5). The study design was a double-blind, crossover investigation in 10 male, drug-free veterans with the diagnosis of chronic schizophrenia who were given a single injection of 20 mg β-endorphin i.v. or placebo on three consecutive Mondays. Choh Hao Li of the University of California, San Francisco, supplied the β-endorphin. The study design was not optimal for testing the putative antischizophrenic activity of β-endorphin, since the design was a compromise due to the limited availability of β-endorphin, its expense, and the report of Kline et al. (66,67) of dramatic improvement of schizophrenic symptoms following a single injection of β-endorphin as described above.

Two investigators rated the patients' symptoms using the BPRS and the Clinical Global Impressions Scale (CGI) (15,113). Frequent ratings were performed on the day of the infusion and daily ratings were continued until the following Monday. To confirm that the β-endorphin was pharmacologically active, prolactin concentrations were measured on samples taken after the infusion by Robert T. Rubin at UCLA. Prolactin concentrations on the saline days compared to the β-endorphin days showed a statistically significant difference ($p < 0.001$) consistent with opiate activity (130). This suggests that the β-endorphin was pharmacologically active.

One schizophrenic patient was studied by Pfefferbaum et al. (117). This patient had EEG changes monitored during each infusion of β-endorphin or placebo and during one 10-mg infusion of morphine. Following the injection of either morphine or β-endorphin, spectral analysis demonstrated changes in the alpha frequency range (8 to 12 Hz). The alpha activity increased quickly and remained high for about 50 min after the morphine sulfate injection. Following the β-endorphin infusion, there was an increase in alpha activity that was similar to but faster than that produced by morphine. However, the increase following β-endorphin injection was shorter, lasting less than 30 min. There were no changes observed in alpha EEG activity after the two saline placebo injections (117). This suggests that the β-endorphin injected intravenously had some effects that parallel those of morphine on the EEG.

The CGI scores were consistent with the impressions of both staff and patients that neither could distinguish the response to β-endorphin from the response to saline. However, when the BPRS scores were analyzed, there was a statistically significant but not clinically obvious improvement following β-endorphin injection compared to placebo injection ($p < 0.05$, one-tailed test).

The Los Angeles Study

β-Endorphin was given to eight schizophrenic patients in a double-blind, placebo-controlled crossover design by Gerner et al. at UCLA (40). In this study, β-endorphin was also supplied by Choh Hao Li. The UCLA group infused β-endorphin at a constant rate over 30 to 35 min. This slow infusion was justified by the observation that in earlier studies, rapid infusion of β-endorphin had produced such symptoms as abdominal cramps, dry mouth, and dermal flushing, burning, and paresthesias. These side effects might have jeopardized the blind nature of the experimental design. Subjects in this investigation were rated by self-rating scales that consisted of 100-mm visual analog scales using the dimensions of depression, anxiety, hopelessness, and feeling good or bad. Day-to-day changes were measured using the BPRS. All investigators and raters were blind to the order of compound administration (40).

As a group, the schizophrenic subjects in the UCLA study were not significantly different after β-endorphin administration than after placebo on overall ratings. However, as a general observation, the condition of six of the eight subjects worsened after β-endorphin, whereas only one subject worsened after placebo. According to the UCLA group, the six schizophrenic subjects whose symptoms were exacerbated became more withdrawn and non-communicative and showed increased psychotic distortion of their environment. Three of the six subjects became aggressive on the day after the β-endorphin infusion. This increase in aggression was suggested to be secondary to increased hallucinatory activity. Thus, the UCLA group concluded that β-endorphin did not improve the symptoms of schizophrenia. In fact, in the UCLA study, the direction of change in the schizophrenic subjects' conditions was toward deterioration (14).

The Washington Study

Pickar et al. at the NIMH gave 4 to 15 mg β-endorphin i.v. to six schizophrenic patients in a double-blind, placebo-controlled investigation (118). The β-endorphin in this investigation was also supplied by Choh Hao Li. The mean dose of β-endorphin for schizophrenic subjects was 0.17 mg/kg given in a solution with concentrations of either 2 mg/ml or 4 mg/ml. The compound was infused intravenously at a rate of 1 ml per minute. Individual physician raters recorded pertinent clinical observations and completed the BPRS at baseline and at regular intervals for 4 hr following the infusion. The BPRS was also given each morning for 5 consecutive days after the placebo and β-endorphin administrations (118).

Comparison of the BPRS change scores for placebo and β-endorphin indicated that β-endorphin did not cause significant behavioral changes in the six schizophrenic subjects. Three of the six schizophrenic patients had behavioral changes by observation. One patient had day-long worsening, one patient had day-long improvement, and one patient had a transient worsening in response to β-endorphin. There was no indication of late-appearing therapeutic effects in the four of six schizophrenic patients who were rated for five consecutive postinfusion days. Thus, the NIMH group was unable to demonstrate a therapeutic effect of β-endorphin in six schizophrenic subjects (118).

The Hungary Study

Petho et al. gave human β-endorphin supplied by Choh Hao Li to six acute schizophrenic patients using a double-blind, parallel-groups design (116). Six patients were given 4 mg β-endorphin i.v. over a 5 min time period, while three patients were given the same volume of physiological saline solution. Symptom changes were recorded using the Factor Construct Rating Scale (FCRS). Patients were rated at baseline and at frequent intervals through the day of the infusion. They were also rated twice per week for 1 week (116).

Each of the six schizophrenic patients given β-endorphin demonstrated some change following the β-endorphin infusion. The changes were reported as an improvement in the areas of mood and activity. However, there was no improvement in specific psychotic symptoms or in the cognitive disorders of schizophrenia. The investigators concluded that there was very little evidence that β-endorphin had any influence whatsoever in relieving psychosis in these schizophrenic patients (116).

Enkephalin Analogs in Schizophrenia

The effects of a potent and stable Met-ENK analog, FK-33-824, have been studied in schizophrenia. The studies by Nedopil, Jungkunz, and co-workers have been summarized by Klein et al. (63). In an open study of nine paranoid schizophrenic patients, treatment with FK-33-824 (0.5 mg i.v. on day 1, 1.0 mg on day 2) resulted in three patients dropping out of the study because of a dramatic worsening of symptoms. However, five of the remaining six patients were improved, as evidenced by a significant decrease in BPRS scores. In contrast, in a later double-blind 2-day study (60), the effects of FK-33-824 (3 mg i.m. per day) or diazepam (20 mg i.m. per day) in 16 schizophrenic patients were evaluated. No clinical improvement was observed in any of the patients.

DTγE and DEγE in Schizophrenia

In a series of reports, De Wied, van Ree, Verhoeven, and their associates from Utrecht in the Netherlands have postulated that schizophrenia is a disorder of endorphin metabolism—an overproduction of α-type endorphins, which purportedly have amphetamine-like properties, and/or an underproduction of the γ-type endorphins, which purportedly possess neuroleptic properties. Such theoretical considerations and the preclinical data concordant with these hypotheses have led to clinical trials of des-tyrosine-γ-endorphin (DTγE) and related peptides in schizophrenic patients. DTγE is γ-endorphin with the tyrosine removed. DTγE has no opioid activity but does demonstrate some neuroleptic-like properties. In addition, Burbach and De Wied of the Utrecht group found evidence of naturally occurring DTγE in rat pituitary, rat brain, and human CSF. They also report that incubation of β-endorphin with homogenates of rat forebrain yields DTγE, suggesting that DTγE may be an endogenously formed compound (12,26). These theoretical issues and early clinical trials have been described in a series of reviews (23,139–141).

The preclinical studies with γ-endorphin fragments by the Utrecht group have been criticized on the grounds that the tests used to detect "neuroleptic activity" are atypical [e.g., the pole-jumping test and the paw-grip test (24)] when compared to standardly used tests such as facilitation of extinction of conditioned avoidance responding or blockade of the actions of dopamine (DA) agonists. Such criticisms are only partially warranted, because use of standard neuroleptic screening tests may only reveal activity of compounds with DA receptor blocking action, and these drugs may possess unwanted side effects such as extrapyramidal symptoms, and may eventually produce tardive dyskinesia. Using atypical or novel screening tests for neuroleptics may eventually produce medications useful for schizophrenia without the usual neuroleptic side effects.

γ-Endorphin derivatives with purported antipsychotic activity have been tested for antipsychotic efficacy in schizophrenic patients by the Utrecht group. In the first study (143), six schizophrenic patients were withdrawn from neuroleptic drugs 1 week prior to the clinical trial. The patients then received daily treatments with 0.5 to 1.0 mg DTγE i.m. for 10 days. All six patients were reported to show dramatic improvement, although three patients rapidly relapsed during treatment with the peptide.

In a second study by the same group (141,143), schizophrenic patients were maintained on neuroleptics during treatment with DTγE. In this double-blind, crossover-designed study, 16 patients received DTγE (1 mg i.m. daily for 16 days) or placebo. The authors reported a significant improvement after combining neuroleptic and DTγE treatment when compared to the combined neuroleptic and placebo treatment. The patients became progressively less psychotic, and hallucinations and delusions were significantly reduced. Eight patients were reported to exhibit dramatic improvements.

Further impetus for the study of DTγE was provided by the report of Metz et al. (89), who found effects of DTγE on the H-reflex in schizophrenic patients to be similar to the effects of neuroleptic drugs on the H-reflex. The H-reflex is an electrically evoked monosynaptic spinal reflex that has been correlated with the production of extrapyramidal symptoms by neuroleptics.

In contrast to these findings, Emrich and his colleagues (35), in a double-blind trial using daily injections of 2 mg DTγE i.m., found no significant antipsychotic effects of the peptide in 13 patients maintained on neuroleptic medication. Patients were maintained on neuroleptics in an attempt to replicate the conditions used by Verhoeven et al. (143). Other largely negative studies have been published, including those of Fink et al. (38), Manchandra and Hirsch (82), Tamminga et al. (133), and Meltzer et al. (88). In these studies and in the recent study by Volavka et al. (148), the antipsychotic effects of DTγE, when evident at all, were short-lived, barely attained statistical significance, and were not clinically robust.

De Wied (23) has stated that these negative results from other centers can be attributed to the fact that schizophrenia is a heterogeneous disorder; thus, only a subgroup of patients respond to DTγE. In addition, the Utrecht group has found that duration of illness, duration of last episode, and patient age correlate negatively with response to DTγE.

Recently, the Utrecht group has studied the clinical effects of des-enkephalin-γ-endorphin (DEγE), the shortest fragment of γ-endorphin with neuroleptic-like activity in preclinical studies. Similar to DTγE, DEγE has no opioid activity. Both single- and double-blind studies have been conducted (146). In a single-blind study of four patients (one neuroleptic-free), two patients received 1 mg DEγE i.m. and two received 10 mg DEγE i.m. All four patients were reported to show a marked amelioration of psychotic symptomatology, and two of these were discharged from the hospital. In the double-blind study, 19 patients were studied and received 3 mg DEγE i.m. A significant reduction in BPRS scores was associated with the peptide treatment. Two patients showed no response, four a slight to moderate response, four a moderate to marked response, and three a very marked response.

In their latest review, van Ree and De Wied (140), adding together results from several of their studies, reported that of 43 schizophrenic patients treated with DTγE and 21 treated with DEγE (total of 64 patients), 13 showed no response (<20% improvement), 19 showed a slight response (20–50% improvement), 16 showed a moderate response (50–80% improvement), and 16 showed a marked response (>80% improvement). In a recent study, Verhoeven et al. (147) treated 18 neuroleptic-free schizophrenic patients with DTγE (1 mg i.m. per day for 10 days) in a double-blind, crossover design. Six patients showed little or no response, seven exhibited a moderate response, and five a marked response. Paranoid and hebephrenic patients benefited most from DTγE treatment. Clearly, further clinical trials are warranted in this area to determine why, with few exceptions, only the Utrecht group has observed the dramatic and marked antipsychotic effects of DTγE.

Clinical Trials of Non-Endorphin Peptides in Schizophrenia

Two other neuropeptides have been tested clinically for antipsychotic effects: CCK and TRH. Based on compelling evidence of colocalization of CCK and DA in the mesolimbic system (49), the effects of treatment with CCK or a related homologous decapeptide, ceruletide, on the symptoms of schizophrenia have been studied. Moroji et al. (94–96) treated 20 chronic schizophrenic patients maintained on antipsychotic drugs with a single injection of ceruletide (0.3 or 0.6 μg/kg i.v.) and used the BPRS to rate symptoms in this open-label study. After the low dose, five of 12 patients showed improvement in mood, and one patient reported a reduction in auditory hallucinations. After the high dose of the peptide, improved mood was noted in 16 patients, and reduction in auditory hallucinations was observed in three patients. These improvements were reported to persist for 3 weeks after injection.

The effects of CCK-33 (0.3 μg/kg i.v.) in chronic schizophrenia were studied by another group (10,104). Six chronic paranoid schizophrenic patients maintained on neuroleptic drugs were studied in the first trial. In this open, uncontrolled study, CCK-33 produced a significant reduction in the BPRS score that was maintained for 6 weeks. In a second study, a single dose of CCK-8 (0.04 μg/kg i.v.) was administered to eight chronic schizophrenic patients maintained on neuroleptic drugs. A rapid improvement in psychopathology was reported, and BPRS and Present State Examination (PSE) scores were significantly reduced. In contrast, no changes in the Nurses' Observations Scale (NOSIE) were reported. Peak improvement was observed 6 days post-CCK injection.

Stimulated by these preliminary findings, three research groups have evaluated the effects of ceruletide in schizophrenia using a double-blind, placebo-controlled protocol. The results have been quite disappointing.

Hommer et al. (51) treated eight neuroleptic-treated schizophrenic patients with ceruletide with increasing i.m. doses beginning at 0.3 μg/kg twice per day to reach a final dose of 0.6 μg/kg. The peptide produced no amelioration in schizophrenic symptoms as assessed by several rating scales, including the BPRS. Albus et al. (2) have conducted both an open study (six patients) and a double-blind study (20 patients) with ceruletide. No antipsychotic effects of the peptide were observed. Finally, Mattes et al. (85) in a double-blind study of 17 chronic, neuroleptic-treated, schizophrenic patients, administered two injections of either ceruletide (0.6 μg/kg i.m.) or placebo 1 week apart. The evaluation included ratings of 29 variables related to prognosis in schizophrenia, as well as BPRS and symptom check list-90 (SCL-90) scales. No beneficial effects of the peptide were observed. Recently, Tamminga and her colleagues (personal communication) and Itoh and his colleagues (personal communication) have conducted double-blind trials of CCK in schizophrenia. No salutary effects of the peptide were reported.

The effects of TRH have been most widely studied in affective disorders, but a few studies with schizophrenic patients have been conducted. This literature has been reviewed most recently by Loosen and Prange (79) in a comprehensive treatise. In general, the results of TRH trials in schizophrenia are disappointing, with the exception of one research group. In a single-blind study, TRH was administered orally (4 mg/day) to 62 chronic, neuroleptic-treated schizophrenic patients. A beneficial effect was reported within 2 weeks in 75% of the patients (79). The studies in which TRH was administered intravenously to schizophrenic patients have been disappointing. Moreover, several investigators have reported that TRH apparently worsens the symptoms of paranoid schizophrenic patients (22,79).

TREATMENT OF SCHIZOPHRENIA WITH PEPTIDE ANTAGONISTS

The only neuropeptide antagonists that have been evaluated as putative antipsychotic agents are the opiate/opioid receptor blockers naloxone and naltrexone. Many, but not all, of the trials that have been conducted are described below, and the interested reader can refer to the comprehensive reviews of Mueser and Dysken (97) and McNichols and Martin (87). These studies are based on the hypothesis that schizophrenia is associated with excess CNS opioid activity, and that therefore opioid receptor blockade should ameliorate the symptoms of schizophrenia.

The first attempt to reverse schizophrenic symptoms with naloxone was carried out by Terenius, Gunne, and colleagues (44), based on their finding of elevated endorphin fractions in CSF described earlier in this chapter. The initial study of Gunne et al. (44) was a single-blind study in which a low dose of naloxone (0.4 mg) was given to six schizophrenic patients. Four of the six patients reported significantly decreased auditory hallucinations following naloxone, but not following saline. The beneficial effects persisted for up to 4 hr.

The original report of Gunne et al. led to several attempted replications using a double-blind crossover design that produced basically negative results. Volavka et al. (149) used 0.4 mg naloxone i.v. in seven patients and reported that naloxone had no effects on the symptoms of their schizophrenic subjects over a time period of 24 hr. Janowsky et al. (56) used 1.2 mg naloxone administered over 1 hr in a study of a heterogeneous group of patients. This group also failed to find an effect of naloxone in their eight subjects. Kurland et al. (70) administered between 0.4 and 1.2 mg naloxone and also found no statistically significant effect on their eight patients. Dysken and Davis (28), in a single-blind study, gave 20 mg naloxone to a single subject and observed no effects over a 10-min period. Lipinski et al. (77), using a double-blind crossover design, gave 1.6 mg naloxone to schizophrenic patients and reported no changes in schizophrenic symptoms. Naber et al. (99) performed a double-blind crossover study with 10 mg per day naloxone in acute and chronic schizophrenics for 5 days. Treatment over 5 days did not change the psychotic symptoms in any of the 12 patients. Another investigation using multiple doses of naloxone performed by Verhoeven and colleagues from Utrecht also failed to demonstrate positive effects of this narcotic antagonist on schizophrenic symptoms (144). Thus, in these seven investigations there is no evidence that naloxone had an effect on schizophrenic symptoms as reported by Gunne et al. (44).

There is a series of investigations that seem to support the original finding of Gunne et al. (44) suggesting that naloxone decreases schizophrenic auditory hallucinations. Davis et al. (21), in a double-blind crossover design, using low doses (0.4 mg and in a few instances 10 mg) of naloxone, studied 14 schizophrenic patients and found a change in the "unusual thought content" item on the BPRS.

In the Stanford investigation (3,152), a large number of schizophrenic subjects (1,800) were prescreened in order to find 18 patients who met the RDC and Diagnostic and Statistical Manual of the American Psychiatric Association, Third Edition (DSM-III) criteria for schizophrenia and who had constant auditory hallucinations. They were diagnosed either as chronic undifferentiated or paranoid schizophrenic, were at the same time cooperative and stable on their medication, and had at least a twice-per-hour pattern of hallucinations. In this double-blind crossover design, 10 mg of naloxone was used and the patients were followed for up to 2 days after the infusion. Under these conditions, naloxone was found to produce a statistically significant reduction of hallucinations as rated by the BPRS in these chronic hallucinating schizophrenic patients at 1½ to 2 hr after naloxone administration. The decrease was observed in patients receiving neuroleptics, as well as in patients who were drug-free.

Emrich et al. (30,32,34) reported two studies in which they evaluated the effects of naloxone on schizophrenics and other psychotic patients. Their general impression in the first study was that naloxone was effective in reducing schizophrenic hallucinations between 2 and 7 hours after administering 1.2 to 4 mg naloxone. In the second study, using much larger doses of naloxone (24.8 mg), there was a reduction in both psychotic symptoms and hallucinations. However, 24.8 mg naloxone was no more effective than 4 mg naloxone in reducing schizophrenic hallucinations. Davis et al. (20), in another double-blind study using 15 mg of naloxone, found that there was a significant reduction in unusual thought content in their schizophrenic patients. This effect tended to be most pronounced in those patients maintained on neuroleptics who had been somewhat resistant to their effects. Lehmann et al. (72) found that three of their six patients reported improved "tension" and five of five patients demonstrated improvement in their symptoms of thought disturbance and hallucinations in both single- and double-blind paradigms using 10 mg naloxone and following the patients for up to 3 hours. In this study, the diagnostic criteria used and the medication status of the patients were not described.

In a large, multicentered investigation organized and coordinated by the World Health Organization (WHO), six groups from around the world participated in a study on the effects of naloxone on schizophrenic symptoms. The WHO collaborative study found significant reductions in schizophrenic hallucinations in 32 schizophrenic subjects who were given 0.3 mg/kg naloxone subcutaneously (a typical dose for a 60-kg man would be 18 mg) (119). The reduction in schizophrenic hallucinations in the WHO study occurred in the neuroleptic-treated patients ($n = 19$), but not in the drug-free patients ($n = 13$). Another group of investigators led by Kleinman also reported positive effects of naloxone on schizophrenic symptoms in patients currently being treated with neuroleptics, but not in patients who were drug-free (65).

In a single case report, Orr and Oppenheimer (112) reported that naloxone (0.4 mg i.v.), but not placebo, produced marked reduction in auditory hallucinations and mild euphoria on three separate occasions in a 28-year-old chronic schizophrenic patient maintained on antipsychotic drugs. Jorgensen and Cappelen also report a positive effect from naloxone in a double-blind investigation in a single subject who had a positive response to naloxone in a preliminary open-label trial. In this study, the patient was reported to repeatedly experience marked temporary reduction in schizophrenic symptoms after treatment with naloxone (0.4 mg), whereas placebo had no effect (59). Lo et al. (78) gave seven patients 0.4 mg naloxone per day for 7 days and six patients saline for the same treatment period. Of the seven patients receiving naloxone, three improved, whereas only one patient receiving saline showed any improvement. The psychotic symptoms that were most reduced after naloxone treatment were conceptual disorganization and hallucinations. Finally, Cohen et al. (16)

treated four chronic unmedicated schizophrenic patients (DSM III criteria) with a high dose of naloxone (2 mg/kg i.v.) versus vehicle in a double-blind design. Three of the four patients showed improvement after naloxone as evidenced by a decrease in BPRS scales.

Thus, the investigations using naloxone to treat schizophrenic symptoms have produced inconsistent results. However, when one examines high-dose, double-blind crossover naloxone studies, which use between 4 and 25 mg naloxone in schizophrenic patients, the majority of studies report positive, if somewhat variable, results. The variability of the results and the failure of every naloxone investigation to improve schizophrenic symptoms may therefore be due to an insufficient dose of naloxone to accomplish functional blockade of all relevant opioid receptors. The positive effects may also be due to an action of high-dose naloxone on systems other than the endogenous opioid system.

The positive naloxone studies report changes in auditory hallucinations, psychotic symptoms, unusual thought content, or tension. From a clinical point of view, these would appear to be essential symptoms of schizophrenia; however, the symptoms are somewhat disconcerting to the clinical investigator, because they are not normally thought of as involving the same underlying variable. This raises questions about the validity of the measurement instruments and the consistency of the effects of naloxone. It is of interest that the effects reported in the high-dose naloxone studies have generally occurred at time points much later than one would expect from the classical pharmacology of that opiate antagonist. This raises an important theoretical question: Is the naloxone effect due to opiate receptor blockade, or is it the result of secondary or tertiary effects resulting from that blockade?

The opiate antagonist naltrexone would appear to have several advantages over naloxone in the study of the effects of opiate antagonists in schizophrenia. It can be given in large doses, in an oral form, and has a very long period of action. There have been a few attempts to study naltrexone in schizophrenia. Mueser and Dysken (97) have reviewed these studies and summarized the current literature; of 42 schizophrenics treated with naltrexone (50–800 mg orally for 2 to 6 weeks), only seven improved. Mielke and Gallant (91), in an open-label design, gave 250 mg naltrexone to three schizophrenic patients, but observed no effect. Simpson et al. (131) administered up to 800 mg of naltrexone in a single-blind study and found no effect in four patients. The Stanford group evaluated naltrexone in a single-blind paradigm (two subjects) and a double-blind paradigm (two subjects) and found mixed results. Single-blind subjects were improved on 250 mg naltrexone as measured by the BPRS scale. Of two double-blind subjects, one improved between 250 and 400 mg, and one worsened, and one subject (one of the single-blind subjects) worsened on 800 mg (4). The effects of naltrexone appear to be poorly studied but generally negative, although there is the possibility of a therapeutic window in the 250 to 400 mg range.

The general impression from results of the study of opiate antagonists in schizophrenia is one of a rather delicate, ephemeral, and inconsistent effect. Certainly, lower doses of naloxone seem to be less effective in the majority of studies. Higher-dose naloxone studies are generally positive, with the exceptions described above. However, the nature of the positive effect tends to change between measurement scales and research groups. Naltrexone does not appear to be particularly effective, although it has not been carefully evaluated. The more beneficial results with naloxone compared to naltrexone may be due to the fact that at higher doses, naltrexone reportedly has opiate agonist, as well as antagonist, properties.

In an elegant, if indirect, series of studies, Davis et al. (19) have been able to show a defect in pain response (flattened evoked response) in their schizophrenic patients. This pattern is similar to that seen in control patients on morphine. When several schizophrenic subjects were given naltrexone, their evoked responses changed so that they were more normal in appearance. This, again, is suggestive of overactivity in endogenous opioids in some schizophrenics. A broader and more extensive set of studies is needed, however. As Buchsbaum points out, the evoked potential response to pain paradigm might be useful for selecting individuals with endorphin-related schizophrenia (19).

CONCLUSION

This chapter is an attempt to provide an overview of neuropeptides in schizophrenia. In its infancy, this research field has provided results of sufficient interest to stimulate further study. Although much remains to be elucidated, a few findings seem of particular interest. There is no doubt that much of our ignorance concerning the possible role of neuropeptides in the pathogenesis of schizophrenia resides with the lack of tools necessary to assess the functional activity of neuropeptide-containing systems in the CNS. The present situation is indeed reminiscent of our understanding of monoamine systems in the 1960s. Exquisitely sensitive RIAs are now available and can usually measure as little as 0.5 pg of a peptide. However, their specificity is often not adequately studied, and the nature of the peptide immunoreactivity has frequently not been characterized.

Of particular concern is our inability to routinely measure neuropeptide turnover or biosynthesis. However, advances in molecular biology are now being applied to neuropeptide biosynthesis and processing. Only recently have structural analogs of neuropeptides been synthesized that, when radiolabeled, result in radioligands suitable to detect high-affinity binding sites for these substances in brain membranes. Simply stated, when neuropeptide concentrations are found to be altered in postmortem brain tissue or CSF in a disease such as schizophrenia, the meaning of this finding is unclear. Thus, a 50% reduction in the concentration of a neuropeptide might be due to degeneration of neuropeptide-containing neurons or, perhaps, to greatly increased utilization of neuropeptide-containing circuits so that biosynthesis cannot keep up with release. Whether CSF or tissue concentrations of neuropeptides accurately reflect extracellular fluid concentrations at relevant synaptic receptor sites in the CNS also remains to be determined.

The present literature on measurement of neuropeptides in human CSF and brain tissue is difficult to evaluate because of the existence of several potentially confounding variables. Some of these can be controlled, but others are inherent to this type of experimentation. First, we must consider the confounding effects of the use of different diagnostic criteria for schizophrenia. This problem cannot be solved at the present time, because the validity of each currently used nosological classification such as DSM III, RDC, and ICD-9 is undetermined, and also because application of the same diagnostic criteria within different research centers often results in poor interrater reliability. The inclusion of a nonpsychiatric control group is important in all future studies.

Patient drug use is an obvious confounding variable in CSF and postmortem tissue studies; therefore, this variable must be described, and, if possible, patients should be drug-free for as long a time as is practical and ethical prior to obtaining CSF or plasma for neuropeptide measurement. In the CSF studies, some researchers use one or another extraction method, whereas others assay the CSF without extraction (neat). Generally speaking, such an extraction step is unnecessary unless there are substances present that interfere with the assay or unless enzymes are present in the biological tissue or fluid that will degrade the neuropeptide under investigation. Plasma, urine, and, of course, tissue samples must be extracted because of the variety and concentration of substances they contain. Regardless of whether or not an extraction step is performed, data on recovery of exogenously added peptide should always be included.

When describing an RIA, it is necessary to explicitly state the sensitivity and specificity of the assay. This should include which region or amino acid sequence of the molecule is recognized by the antiserum and whether structures containing homologous sequences exhibit cross reactivity. It is also helpful to know that a variety of other neuropeptides (with dissimilar structures) do not cross react with an antiserum. The most pertinent information in evaluating a particular RIA is the concentration at which one observes 50% displacement of trace ligand (IC_{50}), the minimal detectable concentration (sensitivity, picograms per tube), and the inter- and intraassay coefficients of variation. In the studies discussed in this chapter, there are very few reports that supply this minimal epidemiological, drug-related, and assay information.

When working with plasma, CSF, urine, or any uncharacterized tissue source of immunoreactivity, some attempt must be made to identify the nature of the immunoreactivity. Liquid column chromatography, gel permeation chromatography, and HPLC are some of the methods that may be employed to study this problem; the method chosen usually depends on the quantity of the starting material.

It is disturbing to report that most of the studies reviewed in this chapter either contained no statistical analysis or used an inappropriate statistical test. Reports without appropriate statistical analysis should not be accepted for publication, with the exception of clinical case reports.

The criticisms outlined in this chapter are not meant to belittle or demean the research performed to date, which, in many instances is in fact pioneering work. Instead, these guidelines are intended to provide a framework for future study design so that cross-study comparison can be made with a minimum of confounding factors. In these types of human studies, it is certainly the retrospective examination of a variety of observations among different investigators and patient populations that will eventually reveal the important, diagnostically dependent, group differences.

To draw conclusions from the present literature is difficult. Although the CSF opioid peptide studies in schizophrenia have not been fruitful, the NT, CCK, and DSIP studies in similar patients showed differences worthy of additional study. The postmortem tissue measurement studies have not revealed large differences between controls and schizophrenic subjects in neuropeptide concentrations. Nevertheless, the data base is very small, and further peptide study is certainly warranted. Peptide receptor studies will provide valuable data.

As treatments for schizophrenia, neuropeptides have certainly not yet been shown to be effective. β-Endorphin is clearly not a practical treatment for schizophrenia, and the use of DTγE in schizophrenia remains quite controversial. As noted in this chapter, the Utrecht group has consistently observed antipsychotic effects of DTγE in schizophrenic patients. In open studies, CCK seemed to possess antipsychotic effects, but this has not been confirmed in double-blind studies. One must conclude that the neuropeptide treatment strategy for schizophrenia is in its infancy, and considerable work in drug design and clinical neuropsychopharmacology must take place.

The peptide antagonist studies are of considerable interest. It seems clear that naloxone reduces hallucinations and unusual thought content in a subset of schizophrenic patients. Unfortunately, these effects are fleeting, difficult to measure, and variable from investigator to investigator.

Advances in clinical neuropeptide neuropsychopharmacology must await advances in neuropeptide physiology and pharmacology. For example, basic questions relating to the passage of administered neuropeptides from the blood to brain remain unanswered. This is, of course, a flaw of most of the peptide treatment studies reviewed in this chapter; few investigators have provided relevant clinical or animal data on whether the peptide, in the dose used, actually entered the CNS and increased the peptide's concentration at relevant extracellular fluid sites in the vicinity of peptidergic receptors. If peptides have difficulty penetrating the blood-brain barrier, then drug design strategies must be appreciably altered. The entry of β-endorphin into the CNS from the vascular compartment is low, but measurable. In contrast, opiate alkaloids such as morphine and dihydromorphine are lipophilic and are, therefore, readily able to enter the brain and act at opioid receptor sites. It may be imperative to identify nonpeptidergic, lipophilic compounds that act on peptidergic receptor sites and can readily enter the CNS.

If we regard the last 15 years of research as preliminary findings, then the next decade will almost certainly witness a veritable explosion in neuropeptide research, with an emphasis on molecular biology. The impact of this research in psychiatry, especially in the area of the pathophysiology of schizophrenia, may be extremely important. Thus, the

wisest course will be to withhold conclusions on the possible role of neuropeptides in schizophrenia until more extensive basic science information is available to clarify the various clinical controversies and yield new data.

ACKNOWLEDGMENTS

Dr. Nemeroff and Dr. Bissette are supported by NIMH MH-39415 and MH-40524, and grants from the Schizophrenia Research Foundation and the Gorrell Family Psychiatric Research Fund. Dr. Nemeroff is the recipient of a Nanaline H. Duke Fellowship from Duke University. Dr. Berger is supported by a grant from the NIMH, MH-30854 to the Norris Mental Health Clinical Research Center at Stanford University, and a grant from the Research Service of the Veterans Administration to the Schizophrenia Biologic Research Center at Palo Alto Veterans Administration Medical Center. Dr. Berger currently holds the Kenneth T. Norris, Jr., Professorship in Psychiatry and Behavioral Sciences. We are grateful to Christie Price and Pamela Elliott for manuscript preparation.

REFERENCES

1. Akil, H., Watson, S. J., Sullivan, S., and Barchas, J. D. (1978): *Life Sci.,* 23:121–126.
2. Albus, M., Ackenheil, M., Munch, U., and Naber, D. (1984): *Arch. Gen. Psychiatry,* 41:528.
3. Berger, P. A., Watson, S. J., Akil, H., and Barchas, J. D. (1981): *Am. J. Psychiatry,* 138:913–918.
4. Berger, P. A., Watson, S. J., Akil, H., and Barchas, J. D. (1986): In: *Neuropeptides in Neurologic and Psychiatric Disease,* edited by J. Martin and J. Barchas, pp. 309–333. Raven Press, New York.
5. Berger, P. A., Watson, S. J., Akil, H., Elliott, G. R., Rubin, R. T., Pfefferbaum, A., Davis, K. L., Barchas, J. D., and Li, C. H. (1980): *Arch. Gen. Psychiatry,* 37:635–640.
6. Berner, P., Gabriel, G., Katschnig, H., Kieffer, W., Lenz, G., and Simhandl, C. (1983): *Diagnostic Criteria for Schizophrenia and Affective Disorders.* World Psychiatric Association, American Psychiatric Press, Inc, Washington, D.C.
7. Biggins, J., Perry, E. K., McDermott, J. R., Smith, I. A., Perry, R. H., and Edwardson, J. A. (1983): *J. Neurol. Sci.,* 58:117–122.
8. Bissette, G., Nemeroff, C. B., and MacKay, A. (1986): *Prog. Brain Res.,* 66:161–176.
9. Bissette, G., Walleus, A., Widerlov, E., Forssman, A., Karlsson, I., Eklund, K., and Nemeroff, C. B. (1984): *Arch. Gen. Psychiat.,* 43:1148–1154.
10. Bloom, D. M., Nair, N. P. V., and Schwartz, G. (1983): *Psychopharmacol. Bull.,* 19:361–363.
11. Braitman, D. J., Auker, C. R., and Carpenter, D. O. (1980): *Brain Res.,* 194:244–248.
12. Burbach, J. P. H., and De Wied, D. (1980): In: *Enzymes and Neurotransmitters in Mental Disease,* edited by E. Usdin, T. S. Sourkes, and M. B. H. Youdim, pp. 103–114. Wiley, New York.
13. Burbach, J. P. H., Loeber, J. G., Verhoef, J., de Kloet, E. R., van Ree, J. M., and De Wied, D. (1979): *Lancet,* 2:480–481.
14. Catlin, D. H., Gorelick, D., Gerner, R. H., Gui, K. K., and Li, C. H. (1980): In: *Advances in Biochemical Pharmacology: Regulation and Function of Neuropeptides,* edited by E. Costa and E. M. Trabucchi, pp. 465–472. Raven Press, New York.
15. *The Clinical Global Impressions Scale (CGI)* (1967): Psychopharmacological Research Branch of the National Institute of Mental Health, March.
16. Cohen, M. R., Cohen, R. M., Pickar, D., Sunderland, T., Mueller,

E. A., III, and Murphy, D. L. (1985): *Biol. Psychiatry,* 20:573–575.

17. Costa, E., and Trabucchi, M. (1982): *Adv. Biochem. Psychopharmacol.,* 33:1–561.

18. Crow, T. J. (1982): In: *Disorders of Neurohumoural Transmission,* edited by T. J. Crow, pp. 287–340. Academic Press, New York.

19. Davis, G. C., Buchsbaum, M. S., Van Kammen, D. P., and Bunney, W. E., Jr. (1979): *Psychiatry Res.,* 1:61–69.

20. Davis, G. C., Bunney, W. E., De Fraites, E. G., Extein, I., Goodwin, F. K., Hamilton, W., Kleinman, J., Mendelson, W., Post, R., Reces, V., Shiling, D., Van Kammen, D., Weinberger, D., Wyatt, R. J., and Li, C. H. (1978): Presented at the Annual Meeting of the American College of Neuropsychopharmacology, Maui, Hawaii, December.

21. Davis, G. C., Bunney, W. E., De Fraites, E. G., Kleinman, J. E., Van Kammen, D. P., Post, R. M., and Wyatt, J. (1977): *Science,* 197:74–77.

22. Davis, K. L., Hollister, L. E., and Berger, P. A. (1975): *Am. J. Psychiatry,* 132:9.

23. De Wied, D. (1982): In: *Brain Peptides and Hormones,* edited by R. Collu, pp. 137–147. Raven Press, New York.

24. De Wied, D., Bohus, B., van Ree, J. M., Kovacs, G. L., and Greven, H. M. (1978): *Lancet,* 1:1046.

25. Domschke, W., Dickschas, A., and Mitznegg, P. (1979): *Lancet,* 1:1024.

26. Dorsa, D. M., van Ree, J. M., and De Wied, D. (1979): *Pharmacol. Biochem. Behav.,* 10:899–905.

27. Dupont, A., Villeneuve, A., Bouchard, J. P., Bouchard, R., Merand, Y., Rouleau, D., and Labrie, F. (1978): *Lancet,* 2:1107.

28. Dysken, M. W., and Davis, J. M. (1978): *Br. J. Psychiatry,* 133:476.

29. Edwardson, J. A., and McDermott, J. R. (1982): *Br. Med. Bull.,* 38:259–264.

30. Emrich, H. M., Cording, C., Piree, S., Kolling, D., Uzerssen, D., and Herz, A. (1977): *Pharmacopsychiatria,* 10:265–270.

31. Emrich, H. M., Hollt, V., Kissling, W., Fischler, M., Heinemann, H., van Zerssen, D., and Herz, A. (1979): In: *Modulators, Mediators and Specifiers in Brain Function,* edited by Y. H. Erlich, J. Volavka, L. G. Davis, and E. G. Brunngraber, pp. 307–317. Plenum Press, New York.

32. Emrich, H. M., Hollt, V., Kissling, W., Fischler, M., Laspe, H., Heinemann, H., von Zerssen, D., and Herz, A. (1979): *Pharmacopsychiatria,* 12:269–276.

33. Emrich, H. M., Kissling, W., Fischler, M., Zerssen, D. F., Riedhammer, H., and Edel, H. H. (1979): *Am. J. Psychiatry,* 136:1095.

34. Emrich, H. M., Moller, H. J., Laspe, H., Meisel-Kosik, I., Dwinger, H., Oechsner, R., Kissling, W., and von Zerssen, D. (1979): In: *Biological Psychiatry Today,* edited by J. Obiols, C. Ballus, E. Gonzalez Monclus, and J. Pujol, pp. 798–805. Elsevier/North Holland Press, Amsterdam.

35. Emrich, H. M., Zaudig, M., Kissling, W., Dirlich, G., von Zerssen, D., and Herz, A. (1980): *Pharmacopsychiatria,* 13:290–298.

36. Ferrier, I. N., Crow, T. J., Roberts, G. W., Johnstone, E. C., Owens, D. G. C., Lee, Y., Baracese-Hamilton, A., McGregor, G., O'Shaughnessy, D., Polak, J. M., and Bloom, S. R. (1984): In: *Psychopharmacology of the Limbic System,* edited by M. R. Trimble and E. Zaritan, pp. 244–254. Oxford University Press, London.

37. Ferrier, I. N., Roberts, G. W., Crow, T. J., Johnstone, E. C., Owens, D. G. C., Lee, Y. C., O'Shaughnessy, D., Adrian, T. E., Polak, J. M., and Bloom, S. R. (1983): *Life Sci.,* 33:475–482.

38. Fink, M., Papakostas, Y., Lee, J., and Johnson, L. (1981): In: *Biological Psychiatry,* edited by C. Perris, G. Struwe, and B. Jansson, pp. 398–401. Elsevier, Amsterdam.

39. Gerner, R. H. (1984): In: *Neurobiology of Mood Disorders,* edited by R. M. Post and J. C. Ballenger, pp. 388–392. Williams and Wilkins, Baltimore.

40. Gerner, R. H., Catlin, D. H., Gorelick, D. A., Hui, K. K., and Li, C. H. (1980): *Arch. Gen. Psychiatry,* 37:642–647.

41. Gerner, R. H., and Yamada, T. (1982): *Brain Res.,* 238:298–302.

42. Goldstein, A. (1976): *Science,* 193:1081–1086.

43. Griffiths, E. C., McDermott, J. R., and Smith, A. I. (1984): *Comp. Biochem. Physiol.,* 77C:363–366.

44. Gunne, L. M., Lindstrom, L., and Terenius, L. (1977): *J. Neural. Transm.,* 40:13–19.

45. Harris, G. W. (1972): *J. Endocrinol.,* 53:ii–xxiii.

46. Henry, J. L. (1982): *Ann. NY Acad. Sci.,* 400:216–227.

47. Hoebel, B. (1984): In: *Eating and Its Disorders,* edited by A. J. Stunkard and E. Stellar, pp. 15–38. Raven Press, New York.

48. Hokfelt, T., Everitt, B. J., Theodorsson-Norheim, E., and Goldstein, M. (1984): *J. Comp. Neurol.,* 222:543–559.

49. Hokfelt, T., Rehfeld, J. F., Skirboll, L., Ivemark, B., Goldstein, M., and Markey, K. (1980): *Nature,* 285:476–478.

50. Hollt, V., Emrich, H. M., Bergmann, M., Nedopil, N., Dieterie, D., Gurland, H. J., Nussett, L., von Zerssen, D., and Herz, A. (1982): In: *Endorphins and Opiate Antagonists in Psychiatry,* edited by N. S. Shah and A. G. Donald, pp. 231–243. Plenum Press, New York.

51. Hommer, D. W., Pickar, D., Roy, A., Ninan, P., Boronow, J., and Paul, S. M. (1984): *Arch. Gen. Psychiatry,* 41:617–619.

52. Hughes, J. (1984): In: *Alzheimer's Disease: Advances in Basic Research Therapies,* edited by R. J. Wurtman, S. H. Corkin, and J. H. Growden, pp. 259–273. Plenum, Zurich.

53. Ibata, Y., Okamura, F. H., Kawakami, T., Tanaka, M., Obata, H. L., Tsuto, O. T., Terobayashi, H., Yanaihara, C., and Yanaihara, N. (1983): *Brain Res.,* 269:177–179.

54. Iversen, L. L., Iversen, S. D., and Snyder, S. H., eds. (1983): In: *Handbook of Psychopharmacology, Neuropeptides, Vol. 16,* pp. 1–577. Plenum Press, New York.

55. Jacobowitz, D. M., Schulte, H., Chrousos, G. P., and Loriaux, D. L. (1983): *Peptides,* 4:521–524.

56. Janowsky, D. S., Segal, D. S., Bloom, F., Abrams, A., and Guillemin, R. (1977): *Am. J. Psychiatry,* 134:926–927.

57. Jeffcoate, W. J., McLoughlin, L., Hope, J., Rees, L. H., Ratter, S. J., Lowry, P. J., and Besser, G. M. (1978): *Lancet,* 2:119–121.

58. Jennes, L., Stumpf, W. E., and Kalivas, P. W. (1982): *J. Comp. Neurol.,* 210:211–224.

59. Jorgensen, J. A., and Cappelen, C., Jr. (1982): *Acta Psychiatr. Scand.,* 65:370–374.

60. Jungkunz, G., Nedopil, N., and Ruther, E. (1984): *Pharmacopsychiatria,* 17:76–78.

61. Kaiya, H., Tamura, Y., Adachi, S., Moriuchi, I., Namba, M., Tanaka, M., Yashida, H., Yanaihara, N., and Yanaihara, C. (1981): *Psychiatry Res.,* 5:11–21.

62. King, J. C., Tobet, S. A., Snavely, F. L., and Arimura, A. A. (1980): *Peptides,* 1:85–100.

63. Klein, H., Jungkunz, G., Nedopil, N., Ruther, E., and Spiegel, R. (1981): In: *Biological Psychiatry,* edited by C. Perris, G. Struwe, and B. Jansson, pp. 390–393. Elsevier, Amsterdam.

64. Kleinman, J. E., Iadarola, M., Govoni, S., Hong, J., Gillin, J. C., and Wyatt, R. J. (1983): *Psychopharmacol. Bull.,* 19:375–377.

65. Kleinman, J. E., Weinberger, D. R., Rogol, A., Shiling, D. J., Mendelson, W. B., Davis, G. C., Bunney, W. E., Jr., and Wyatt, R. J. (1982): *Psychiatry Res.,* 7:1.

66. Kline, N. S., and Lehmann, H. E. (1979): In: *Endorphins in Mental Health Research,* edited by E. Usdin, W. E. Bunney, Jr., and N. S. Kline, pp. 500–517. Macmillan, London.

67. Kline, N. S., Li, C. H., Lehmann, H. E., Lajtha, A., Laski, E., and Cooper, T. (1977): *Arch. Gen. Psychiatry,* 34:1111–1113.

68. Koch, G., and Richter, D. (1983): *Biochemical and Clinical Aspects of Neuropeptides: Synthesis, Processing, and Gene Function.* Academic Press, New York.

69. Krieger, D. T., Brownstein, M. J., and Martin, J. B. (1983): *Brain Peptides,* John Wiley and Sons, New York.

70. Kurland, A. A., McCable, O. L., Hanlon, T. E., and Sullivan, D. (1977): *Am. J. Psychiatry,* 134:1408–1410.

71. Lamers, C. B., Morley, J. E., Poitras, P., Sharp, B., Carlson, H. E., Hershman, J. E., and Walsh, J. H. (1980): *Am. J. Physiol.,* 239:E232–235.

72. Lehmann, H., Vasavan Nair, N. P., and Kline, N. S. (1979): *Am. J. Psychiatry,* 136:762–766.

73. Lewis, R. V., Gerber, L. D., Stein, S., Stephen, R. L., Grosser,

B. I., Velick, S. F., and Udenfriend, S. (1979): *Arch. Gen. Psychiatry*, 36:237–239.

74. Lindstrom, L. H., Besev, G., Gunne, L. M., Sjostrom, R., Terenius, L., Wahlstrom, A., and Wistedt, B. (1982): In: *Endorphins and Opiate Antagonists in Psychiatry*, edited by N. S. Shah and A. G. Donald, pp. 245–256. Plenum Press, New York.

75. Lindstrom, L. H., Ekman, R., Walleus, H., and Widerlov, E. (1985): *Prog. Neuropsychopharmacol. Biol. Psychiatry*, 9:51–63.

76. Lindstrom, L. H., Widerlov, E., Gunne, L. M., Wahlstrom, A., and Terenius, L. (1978): *Acta Psychiatr. Scand.*, 57:153–169.

77. Lipinski, J., Meyer, R., Kornetsky, C., and Cohen, B. M. (1979): *Lancet*, 2:1292–1293.

78. Lo, C. W., Wen, H. L., and Ho, W. K. K. (1983): *Eur. J. Pharmacol.*, 92:77–81.

79. Loosen, P. T., and Prange, A. J., Jr. (1984): In: *Peptides, Hormones and Behavior*, edited by C. B. Nemeroff and A. J. Dunn, pp. 533–577. Spectrum Publishers, New York.

80. Manberg, P. J., Nemeroff, C. B., Bissette, G., Prange, A. J., Jr., and Gerner, R. H. (1983): *Soc. Neurosci. (Abstr.)*, 9:1034.

81. Manberg, P. J., Youngblood, W. W., Nemeroff, C. B., Rossor, M. N., Iversen, L. L., Prange, A. J., Jr., and Kizer, J. S. (1982): *J. Neurochem.*, 38:1777–1780.

82. Manchandra, R., and Hirsch, S. R. (1981): *Psychol. Med.*, 11:401–403.

83. Marsan, C. A., and Traczyk, W. Z. (1980): Raven Press, New York.

84. Martin, J. B. (1984): In: *Psychoneuroendocrine Dysfunction*, edited by N. S. Shah and A. G. Donald, pp. 15–40. Plenum Press, New York.

85. Mattes, J. A., Hum, W., Rochford, J. M., and Orlosky, M. (1985): *Biol. Psychiatry*, 20:533–538.

86. McKelvy, J. F. (1983): In: *Brain Peptides*, edited by D. T. Krieger, M. J. Brownstein, and J. B. Martin, pp. 117–133. Wiley Interscience, New York.

87. McNichols, L. F., and Martin, W. R. (1984): *Drugs*, 27:81–93.

88. Meltzer, H. Y., Busch, D. A., Tricon, B. J., and Robertson, A. (1982): *Psychiatry Res.*, 6:313–326.

89. Metz, J., Busch, D. A., and Meltzer, H. Y. (1981): *Life Sci.*, 28:2003–2008.

90. Meyerson, B. J. (1979): *Med. Biol.*, 57:69–83.

91. Mielke, D. H., and Gallant, D. M. (1977): *Am. J. Psychiatry*, 134:1430–1431.

92. Millar, R. P. (1981): *Neuropeptides: Biochemical and Physiological Studies*, Churchill-Livingstone, London.

93. Miller, L. H., Sandman, C. A., and Kastin, A. J. (1977): *Neuropeptide Influences on the Brain and Behavior*. Raven Press, New York.

94. Moroji, T., Watanabe, N., Aoki, N., and Itoh, S. (1982): *Int. Pharmacopsychiatry*, 17:255–273.

95. Moroji, T., Watanabe, N., Aoki, N., and Itoh, S. (1982): *Arch. Gen. Psychiatry*, 39:485–486.

96. Moroji, T., Watanabe, N., and Itoh, S. (1982): *Proceedings of the World Psychiatric Association*, pp. 165–169.

97. Mueser, K. T., and Dysken, M. W. (1983): *Schizophr. Bull.*, 9:213–225.

98. Mutt, V. (1983): In: *Brain Peptides*, edited by D. T. Krieger, M. J. Brownstein, and J. B. Martin, pp. 871–902. Wiley-Interscience, New York.

99. Naber, D., Munch, U., Wissmann, J., Grosse, R., Ritt, R., and Welter, R. (1983): *Acta Psychiatr. Scand.*, 67:265–271.

100. Naber, D., Nedopil, N., and Eben, E. (1984): *Br. J. Psychiatry*, 144:651–653.

101. Naber, D., and Pickar, D. (1983): *Psychiatr. Clin. North Am.*, 6:443–456.

102. Naber, D., Pickar, D., Post, R. M., van Kammen, D. P., Ballenger, J., Rubinow, D., Waters, R. N., and Bunney, W. E., Jr. (1981): In: *Biological Psychiatry*, edited by C. Perris, G. Struwe, and B. Jansson, pp. 372–375. Elsevier, Amsterdam.

103. Naber, D., Pickar, D., Post, R. M., van Kammen, D. P., Waters, R. N., Ballenger, J. C., Goodwin, F. K., and Bunney, W. E., Jr. (1981): *Am. J. Psychiatry*, 138:1457–1462.

104. Nair, N. V. P., Bloom, D. M., and Nestoros, J. D. (1982): *Prog. Neuropsychopharmacol. Biol. Psychiatry*, 6:509–512.

105. Nemeroff, C. B. (1986): *Psychoneuroendocrinology*, 11:15–37.

106. Nemeroff, C. B., Bissette, G., Manberg, P. J., Luttinger, D., and Prange, A. J., Jr. (1984): In: *Peptides, Hormones and Behavior*, edited by C. B. Nemeroff and A. J. Dunn, pp. 217–272. Spectrum Publishers, New York.

107. Nemeroff, C. B., Hernandez, D. E., Orlando, R. C., and Prange, A. J., Jr. (1982): *Am. J. Physiol.*, 242:342–346.

108. Nemeroff, C. B., Kalivas, P. W., Golden, R. N., and Prange, A. J., Jr. (1984): *Pharmacol. Ther.*, 24:1–56.

109. Nemeroff, C. B., Luttinger, D., Hernandez, D. E., Mailman, R. B., Mason, G. A., Davis, S. D., Widerlov, E., Frye, G. D., Kilts, C. D., Beaumont, K., Breese, G. R., and Prange, A. J., Jr. (1983): *J. Pharmacol. Exp. Ther.*, 225:337–345.

110. Nemeroff, C. B., and Prange, A. J., Jr. (1978): *Arch. Gen. Psychiatry*, 35:999–1010.

111. Nemeroff, C. B., Youngblood, W. W., Manberg, P. J., Prange, A. J., Jr., and Kizer, J. S. (1983): *Science*, 221:972–975.

112. Orr, M., and Oppenheimer, C. (1978): *Br. Med. J.*, 1:481.

113. Overall, J. E., and Gorham, D. R. (1962): *Psychol. Rep.*, 10:799–812.

114. Palmour, R. M., Ervin, F. R., Wagemaker, H., and Cade, R. (1977): Abstract, Society for Neuroscience, Anaheim, California, November, p. 320.

115. Pert, A., Pert, C. B., Davis, G. C., and Bunney, W. E., Jr. (1981): In: *Handbook of Biological Psychiatry, Vol. IV: Brain Mechanisms and Abnormal Behavior—Chemistry*, edited by H. M. van Praag, M. H. Lader, O. J. Rafaelsen, and E. J. Sacher, pp. 547–582. Marcel Dekker, New York.

116. Petho, B., Laszlo, G., Karczag, I., Borvendeg, J., Bitter, I., Barna, I., Ilona, H., Tolna, J., and Baraczka, K. (1983): *Ann. NY Acad. Sci.*, 398:460–469.

117. Pfefferbaum, A., Berger, P. A., Elliott, G. R., Tinklenberg, J. R., Kopell, B. S., Barchas, J. D., and Li, C. H. (1979): *Psychiatry Res.*, 1:83–88.

118. Pickar, D., Davis, G. D., Schulz, S. C., and Bunney, W. E., Jr. (1981): *Am. J. Psychiatry*, 138:160–166.

119. Pickar, D., Vartanian, F., and Bunney, W. E. (1982): *Arch. Gen. Psychiatry*, 39:313–319.

120. Port, F. K., Kroll, P. D., and Swartz, R. D. (1978): *Am. J. Psychiatry*, 135:743–744.

121. Post, R. M., Gold, P. W., Rubinow, D. R., Bunney, W. E., Jr., Ballenger, J. C., and Goodwin, F. K. (1983): In: *Neurobiology of Cerebrospinal Fluid*, edited by J. H. Wood, pp. 107–141. Plenum Publishing Company, New York.

122. Prange, A. J., Jr., Loosen, P. T., and Nemeroff, C. B. (1979): In: *Frontiers in Psychotropic Drug Research*, edited by S. Fielding, pp. 117–189. Futura Publishing Company, New York.

123. Prange, A. J., Jr., Nemeroff, C. B., and Lipton, M. A. (1977): In: *Psychopharmacology: A Generation of Progress*, edited by M. A. Lipton, K. F. Killam, and A. DiMascio, pp. 441–458. Raven Press, New York.

124. Reichlin, S. (1981): In: *Textbook of Endocrinology*, edited by R. H. Williams, pp. 589–671. W. B. Saunders Company, Philadelphia.

125. Rimon, R., LeGreves, P., Nyberg, F., Heikkila, L., Salmela, L., and Terenius, L. (1984): *Biol. Psychiatry*, 19:509–516.

126. Rimon, R., Terenius, L., and Kampman, R. (1980): *Acta Psychiatr. Scand.*, 61:395–403.

127. Ross, M., Berger, P. A., and Goldstein, A. (1979): *Science*, 205:1163–1164.

128. Rossor, M. (1984): *J. Psychiatr. Res.*, 18:457–465.

129. Sawynok, J., Pinskey, C., and LaBella, F. S. (1979): *Life Sci.*, 9:213–225.

130. Siegel, S. (1956): *Nonparametric Statistics for the Behavioral Sciences*. McGraw-Hill, New York.

131. Simpson, G. M., Branchly, M. H., and Lee, J. H. (1977): *Curr. Ther. Res.*, 22:909–913.

132. Snyder, S. H. (1980): *Science*, 219:976–983.

133. Tamminga, C. A., Tighe, P. J., Chase, T. N., De Frattes, G., and Schaeffer, M. H. (1981): *Arch. Gen. Psychiatry*, 38:167.

134. Terenius, L., and Nyberg, F. (1983): In: *Biochemical and Clinical Aspects of Neuropeptides: Synthesis, Processing and Gene Function*, edited by G. Kock and D. Richter, pp. 99–112.

135. Terenius, L., Wahlstrom, A., Lindstrom, L. H., and Widerlov, E. (1976): *Neurosci. Lett.,* 3:157–162.
136. Ungar, G. (1975): *Int. Rev. Neurobiol.,* 17:37–60.
137. Vale, W., and Rivier, C. (1975): In: *Handbook of Psychopharmacology, Vol. V,* edited by L. L. Iversen, S. D. Iversen, and S. H. Snyder, pp. 195–237. Plenum Press, New York.
138. Van Kammen, D. P., Waters, R. N., Gold, P., Sternberg, D., Robertson, G., Ganten, D., Pickar, D., Naber, D., Ballenger, J. C., Kaye, W. H., Post, R. M., and Bunney, W. E., Jr. (1981): In: *Biological Psychiatry,* edited by C. Perris, G. Struwe, and B. Jansson, pp. 339–344. Elsevier, Amsterdam.
139. van Praag, H. M., and Verhoeven, W. M. A. (1981): In: *Handbook of Biological Psychiatry, Part IV: Brain Mechanisms and Abnormal Behavior—Chemistry,* edited by H. M. van Praag, M. H. Lader, O. J. Rafaelson, and E. J. Sachar, pp. 511–545. Marcel Dekker, New York.
140. van Ree, J. M., and De Wied, D. (1984): In: *Central and Peripheral Endorphins: Basic and Clinical Aspects,* edited by E. E. Muiler and R. Genazzani, pp. 325–332. Raven Press, New York.
141. van Ree, J. M., Verhoeven, W. M. A., van Praag, H. M., and De Wied, D. (1978): In: *Characteristics and Functions of Opioids,* edited by J. M. van Ree and L. Terenius, pp. 181–184. Elsevier/North Holland Press, Amsterdam.
142. Verbanck, P. M. P., Lotstra, F., Gilles, C., Linkowski, P., Mendlewicz, J., and Vanderhaeghen, J. J. (1983): *Life Sci.,* 34:67–72.
143. Verhoeven, W. M. A., van Praag, H. M., Botter, P. A., Sunier, A., van Ree, J. M., and De Wied, D. (1978): *Lancet,* 2:1046–1047.
144. Verhoeven, W. M. A., van Praag, H. M., and van Ree, J. M. (1984): *Psychiatry Res.,* 12:297–312.
145. Verhoeven, W. M. A., van Praag, H. M., van Ree, J. M., and De Wied, D. (1979): *Arch. Gen. Psychiatry,* 36:294–298.
146. Verhoeven, W. M. A., van Ree, J. M., Heezius-van Bentum, A., De Wied, D., and van Praag, H. M. (1982): *Arch. Gen. Psychiatry,* 39:648–654.
147. Verhoeven, W. M. A., van Ree, J. M., Westenberg, H. G. M., Krul, J. M., Brouwer, G. J., Thijssen, J. H. H., De Wied, D., van Praag, H. M., Ceulemans, D. L. S., and Kahn, R. S. (1984): *Psychiatry Res.,* 11:329–346.
148. Volavka, J., Hui, K.-S., Anderson, B., Nemes, Z., O'Donnell, J., and Laytha, A. (1983): *Psychiatry Res.,* 10:243–252.
149. Volavka, J., Mallya, A., Baig, S., and Perez-Cruet, J. (1977): *Science,* 196:1227–1228.
150. Von Knorring, L., Almay, B. G. L., Johansson, F., Terenius, L., and Wahlstrom, A. (1982): *Pain,* 12:265–272.
151. Wagemaker, H., and Cade, R. (1977): *Am. J. Psychiatry,* 134:684–685.
152. Watson, S. J., Berger, P. A., Akil, H., Mills, M. J., and Barchas, J. D. (1978): *Science,* 201:73–76.
153. Wen, H. L., Lo, C. W., and Ho, W. K. (1983): *Clin. Chim. Acta,* 128:367–371.
154. Widerlov, E., Lindstrom, L. H., Besev, G., Manberg, P. J., Nemeroff, C. B., Breese, G. R., Kizer, J. S., and Prange, A. J., Jr. (1982): *Am. J. Psychiatry,* 139:1122–1126.

Psychopharmacology:
The Third Generation of Progress,
edited by Herbert Y. Meltzer.
Raven Press, New York © 1987.

CHAPTER 72

Biochemical Instability in Schizophrenia I: The Norepinephrine System

Daniel P. van Kammen and Joel Gelernter

It has been clear for some time that the pathophysiology of schizophrenia cannot be sufficiently explained by dopamine (DA) overactivity alone, even though the evidence is compelling. The concept of DA overactivity as the etiology of schizophrenia appears to be too simplistic; some of the data can be interpreted as indicating DA hypoactivity (16,79). There is no single neurotransmitter system proposed to date that is likely to replace DA as a major source of schizophrenic psychopathology, but studies of several other neurotransmitter systems that interact with DA activity have produced exciting results over the last 20 years. Presently, the most enduring monoaminergic findings, besides DA in schizophrenia, are noradrenergic (for review see 36, 75) and serotonergic (65,66).

One of the major problems in schizophrenia research is the episodic nature of the illness. Most evidence supports a state-dependent DA disorder or DA dysregulation (82). There is also evidence for norepinephrine (NE)-related state-dependent changes (77,82). State dependency is less well established for the serotonin (5HT) and γ-aminobutyric acid (GABA) systems, but could be present; both interact with the DA and NE systems (van Kammen and Gelertner, *next chapter*).

In this and the next chapter we will examine selectively some of the evidence linking the nondopaminergic NE, 5-HT, and GABA systems with schizophrenia, and emphasize those findings that are most frequently replicated. Rather than speculate about the primary or secondary relationship to schizophrenia, we will present the actual findings with limited discussion of the systems themselves and the assay methodologies. Since no neurotransmitter acts in isolation, we will indicate some relationships with other systems, including DA, and with clinical symptoms whenever possible (Table 1). We will advance some concepts that may facilitate the understanding of these diverse and conflicting data, such as state dependency, clinical instability, stress sensitivity, and genetic vulnerability, which may reflect dysregulation or instability of brain chemistry.

In 1971, Stein and Wise (67) proposed that anhedonia in schizophrenia was caused by a brain dopamine-β-hydroxylase (DBH) deficiency. The subsequent NE deficiency would lead to an aberrant DA metabolite with cytotoxic properties, explaining the progressive deteriorating course. Hornykiewicz suggested that NE regulates the sensitivity of the DA system (36). Since that time several authors have suggested that schizophrenia is a disorder of both DA and NE systems (36,75). Van Kammen and Antelman (75) stressed that most of the schizophrenic behaviors thought to be DA mediated can also be mediated or modified by NE (37). Antelman and co-workers (4,5) reviewed the evidence for a NE and DA interaction in the brain and concluded that during minimal stress or activation, NE modulates DA-dependent behaviors, whereas in times of stress, NE facilitates DA-dependent behaviors. When, under conditions of high stress or disturbed NE regulation, NE is unable to sustain its modulatory influence on DA, such behaviors can become deregulated. Recently, prefrontal cortical NE and DA systems have been proposed to be involved in negative and cognitive symptoms in schizophrenia.

TABLE 1. *Evidence that norepinephrine activity is involved in schizophrenia*

Brain NE and MHPG levels are increased in some brain areas

CSF NE is episodically elevated in drug-free patients (state dependent)

CSF NE and MHPG decrease with neuroleptic treatment relative to clinical improvement

Plasma NE is elevated in chronic, drug-free, and medicated patients

Decreased PGE_1-stimulated cyclic AMP production (platelets). NE inhibition is not impaired

Impaired coupling of adenyl cyclase and its catalytic unit (α_2-receptor)

Increased and decreased binding of α_2-receptor on platelets (receptor function may be subsensitive)

CSF DBH is decreased in patients with brain atrophy, good premorbid functioning, and patients with low psychosis ratings at discharge

Clonidine and *d,l*-propranolol may have antipsychotic effects in some patients (presumably, in those with increased NE activity or subsensitive adrenergic receptors)

NOREPINEPHRINE ACTIVITY IN AUTOPSY BRAINS AND RELATED TO CT SCANS

Postmortem studies of brains of schizophrenics have provided evidence for NE involvement in schizophrenia. Farley et al. (22) provided the first evidence for elevated NE in postmortems of paranoid schizophrenic patients' limbic brains, which was followed by several other groups (13,14,19). Kleinman et al. (43,44) did not report significant differences in NE, but an increase in free 3-methoxy-4-hydroxyphenylglycol (MHPG).

Wise and Stein (85) reported decreased DBH activity (see below) in the brains of nine schizophrenic patients. Cross et al. (17) could not confirm this decrease in 12 normal subjects and 12 schizophrenic patients. Brain atrophy on computerized tomographic (CT) scans is associated with decreased CSF levels of NE and DBH (78,80). Decreased CSF DBH (and homovanillic acid, HVA) levels were found in CSF of 11 schizophrenics with brain atrophy compared to 22 schizophrenics with normal head CT scans (80). A major problem in the assessment of DBH in schizophrenia autopsy studies is the lack of information on brain atrophy and the small number of brains studied.

CSF NOREPINEPHRINE

Lake et al. (47) reported elevated CSF NE levels in 35 drug-free schizophrenics compared to 29 control subjects. All three subgroups considered (paranoid, undifferentiated, and schizoaffective) had signs suggestive of generally increased noradrenergic activity, including increased heart rate and diastolic blood pressure. Kemali et al. (42) reported increased CSF and plasma NE levels in 46 drug-free schizophrenic patients. Additional evidence for increased NE levels in CSF comes from Gomes et al. (32), who found that chronic schizophrenics had significantly higher

NE levels than acute patients and a control group. Unfortunately, the 11 chronic schizophrenic patients considered here were on antipsychotic drugs at the time, as were five of the 10 acute schizophrenic patients. It is noteworthy that the studies quoted above all relied on single CSF catecholamine measurements.

Linnoila et al. (48) found that levels of NE varied from lumbar puncture (LP) to LP essentially unpredictably (up to four LPs per patient), although some of the intraindividual changes in NE values could be related to change in psychosis ratings ($r = 0.62$, $n = 9$ women, $p < 0.05$). This suggests that CSF NE levels may be state dependent. Further support for NE state dependency comes from van Kammen et al. (82,84), who found in a preliminary study that the CSF NE was higher in patients who slept less the night before the LP ($r = -0.44$, $n = 53$, $p = 0.0008$) and from Sternberg et al. (69), who demonstrated that pimozide treatment caused a significant decrease in CSF NE, relative to improvement in psychotic symptoms ($r = 0.71$, $p < 0.02$). Decreased sleep is frequently observed as a prodromal symptom early in psychotic episodes. Restoration of sleep is one of the first signs that the patient is responding to neuroleptic treatment.

Gattaz et al. (29) reported that patients who were receiving antipsychotics had elevated CSF NE, whereas drug-free patients could not be distinguished from controls by this measure. Bagdy et al. (8) reported a slight decrease in CSF NE at 2 weeks following withdrawal from long-term neuroleptic treatment. One explanation of the decreased levels following neuroleptic withdrawal in some studies may be related to changes in clinical state, because some patients temporarily improve after withdrawal (51), or, alternatively, that some neuroleptics block α-receptors, leading to an increase in NE levels, particularly in high doses (58).

If the proposed interaction of NE and DA activity exists, then CSF values should relate to each other; indeed, CSF NE correlated with CSF DA ($r = 0.64$, $n = 34$, $p < 0.001$) and $DASO_4$ ($r = 0.35$, $n = 35$, $p < 0.05$). On the other hand, MHPG and NE levels reportedly do not correlate with each other in schizophrenia as they do in affective disorder (11).

CSF NOREPINEPHRINE METABOLITES

Shopsin et al. (64) reported that schizophrenic patients had normal CSF MHPG levels, although some schizophrenic subjects had levels outside the range of control subjects. Similarly, other groups did not find CSF MHPG in acutely ill schizophrenic patients with and without probenecid to be different from those in depressed patients or in normal control subjects either (10,23,57,63). Post et al. (57) observed that MHPG levels did not change when patients went into remission, in contrast to HVA levels, which declined. On the other hand, van Kammen et al. (76) noted that CSF MHPG levels obtained prior to an amphetamine challenge test predicted the direction in change in psychosis following the *d*-amphetamine administration. Those patients with the lowest levels of MHPG tended to improve with *d*-amphetamine ($r = 0.58$, $p < 0.005$). Kopin et al. (46) reported that plasma-free MHPG was highly correlated with CSF MHPG, and suggested that free MHPG is able to cross the blood-brain barrier with relative facility. Consequently, a significant proportion of MHPG found in the CSF is thought to be of peripheral origin. In patients with cortical atrophy, CSF MHPG was decreased compared to those with normal CT scans (40 ± 13.8 vs 34 ± 5.7 ng/ml, $p = 0.055$) and correlated significantly with degree of atrophy ($r = -0.37$, $n = 22$, $p = 0.04$) (D. P. van Kammen, unpublished data). This is a much smaller difference than for CSF HVA or 5-hydroxyindoleacetic acid (5HIAA), suggestive that plasma MHPG may have contributed to the levels. CSF MHPG decreases significantly following neuroleptic treatment (e.g., chlorpromazine) in some studies (2,3,62), similar to the pimozide-related decrease in CSF NE levels (69). However, not all CSF studies have shown such a decrease in MHPG with neuroleptic treatment (30), nor has the decrease been found with all neuroleptics (86).

CSF DOPAMINE-β-HYDROXYLASE

Sternberg et al. (69) studied CSF DBH longitudinally in 30 schizophrenic and schizoaffective-schizophrenic patients, compared with 27 normal controls. The mean CSF DBH levels were not significantly different for the two groups, nor was there any relationship of DBH to age or sex. In the patient group, DBH was not related to clinical subtype, severity of psychosis, or drug treatment (pimozide). Both patient and control groups showed a wide range of DBH values. However, premorbid and present level of social and sexual function correlated with CSF DBH; better-functioning patients had lower levels. The low-DBH group had more "reactive" type schizophrenic patients (by Phillips scale), compared to more "process" schizophrenic patients in the high DBH group (71) and were less psychotic at time of discharge (antipsychotic response, ref. 70). The report of decreased CSF DBH in schizophrenic patients with brain atrophy (see above) appears to be inconsistent with this, unless low DBH has several causes (i.e., genetic and environmental) and interacts differently with DA activity.

PLASMA NOREPINEPHRINE

Ackenheil et al. (1) reported that besides evidence of elevated baseline plasma NE levels, plasma NE response to "stress" in chronic schizophrenic patients was less than in normal subjects. Zander et al. (88) reported that during neuroleptic treatment in chronic, hospitalized schizophrenic patients, plasma NE levels were significantly elevated. After a 30-day drug-free period, NE levels decreased but were still elevated above values of normal subjects. Gjerris et al. (31) reported that hypoglycemia induced significantly smaller increases in plasma NE in acute schizophrenic patients than in control subjects, suggesting subsensitive NE receptor function.

Castellani et al. (15) noted that a group of young drug-free schizophrenic patients had supine plasma NE levels similar to control subjects but standing levels were significantly more elevated. This increase in NE was felt to be consistent with decreased peripheral α_2-receptor sensitivity.

Haloperidol did not increase NE levels as did chlorpromazine, which has significantly more α_2-receptor blocking effects. When NE levels are measured in patients treated with a variety of neuroleptics, the α_2-receptor blocking effects of some of these drugs needs to be taken into account. Kemali et al. (42) reported that plasma NE levels did not correlate with central NE levels or psychopathology, in contrast to the report of Ziegler et al. (89), who observed a significant correlation between NE levels in plasma and CSF in normal controls ($r = 0.78$, $p < 0.0001$) or in depressed patients (11).

PLASMA DBH

Plasma DBH studies have not yielded consistent results and neuroleptic treatment may have an inconsistent effect. Plasma and CSF DBH levels correlate significantly, but brain atrophy may affect this relationship in schizophrenic patients (55). Plasma DBH levels were increased (52) or decreased (27) in schizophrenic, particularly in demented (53), patients, but most groups reported no differences with controls. Of interest is the biological evaluation of the schizophrenic Genain quadruplets; plasma DBH was decreased in all four schizophrenic women (20).

CYCLIC AMP STIMULATION WITH PGE$_1$ IN PLATELETS

Rotrosen et al. (ref. 59, *this volume*), Kafka and co-workers (39–41), and Pandey et al. (56) observed that the accumulation of [^{3}H]cyclic AMP in platelets of chronic schizophrenic patients in response to prostaglandin E$_1$ (PGE$_1$) stimulation was decreased (for review see Rotrosen et al., *this volume*). Decreased NE inhibition of PGE$_1$-stimulated cyclic AMP production is also observed in depression, essential hypertension, and idiopathic orthostatic hypotension. However, decreased inhibition of PGE$_1$-stimulated cyclic AMP production by NE in depressed but not in schizophrenic patients suggests that NE inhibition is mediated through a mechanism separate from cyclic AMP production induced by PGE$_1$. Consistent with these reports, the schizophrenic Genain quadruplets showed decreased PGE$_1$-stimulated cyclic AMP production (20). Adenyl cyclase activity was decreased in schizophrenic patients also. The data suggest an alteration in the adenyl cyclase catalytic unit or a dissociation between receptor, regulator unit, and adenyl cyclase.

α_2-RECEPTOR BINDING (PLATELETS)

Kafka et al. (39) reported increased [^{3}H]dihydroergocryptine ([^{3}H]DHE) binding on platelets in schizophrenia ($n = 83$), but also in depression ($n = 23$), essential hypertension ($n = 22$), and some forms of orthostatic hypotension. Because this increased binding is also observed with [^{3}H]clonidine, but not with [^{3}H]yohimbine or [^{3}H]rauwolscine, the binding site is presumably a high-affinity α_2-site. Future studies will have to resolve whether the increased receptor sites are functionally intact or desensitized. The corresponding brain studies have not been reported yet, but are under way (G. N. Ko et al., personal communications). Rice et al. (58) did not find elevated [³H]clonidine, but did find decreased [³H]yohimbine binding in drug-free schizophrenic patients. It is of interest that Holmgren et al. (34) reported that yohimbine worsened schizophrenic symptoms.

PLASMA MHPG

Plasma MHPG levels have been determined in schizophrenic patients only recently. According to Sternberg et al. (68), acute clonidine administration suppresses plasma MHPG in normal control subjects compared to placebo, but not in schizophrenic patients. Ko et al. (45) did not find differences in plasma MHPG between schizophrenics and normals.

NORADRENERGIC DRUGS

Clonidine

In recent years several small open studies have suggested an antipsychotic effect of the α_2-agonist clonidine (21,25,38) in schizophrenia. The only double-blind placebo controlled study, by Freedman et al. (26), reported that in eight patients clonidine had an antipsychotic effect equal to haloperidol. Presently, there are no CSF studies in schizophrenic patients reported. Martin et al. (54) reported that clonidine increased CSF HVA, and decreased MHPG, but did not change 5HIAA in patients with an alcohol-related amnestic syndrome. In a double-blind study of ten drug-free schizophrenic patients we noted that memory improved significantly with 5 weeks of clonidine treatment independently of improvement in psychosis, and CSF MHPG declined significantly ($p < 0.01$) (24). We found four of 13 drug-free schizophrenic patients to improve with clonidine. Since clonidine improves memory only in impaired animals (6) or humans (49), the improvement in Memory Quotient suggests prefrontal impairment in schizophrenia (as in the idea of dementia praecox). The clonidine challenge test showed higher growth hormone response in clonidine treatment responders (81).

Prazosin

Hommer et al. (35) reported that 6 weeks of treatment with the α_1-antagonist, prazosin, had no antipsychotic effect, but it increased autonomic arousal in schizophrenic patients.

d,l-Propranolol

Since Atsmon et al. (7) reported improvement with "high doses" of the β-receptor antagonist d,l-propranolol, studies have appeared with mixed results (9,12,28,33,87). Most negative studies included only 4 weeks treatment with

1,000 mg or less of d,l-propranolol alone. Treatment led to decreases in CSF 5HIAA, which may be due to an MAO-inhibiting effect of doses studied or a β-receptor effect on tryptophan hydroxylase activity (61). We noted also an increase in CSF MHPG and a lack of change in CSF HVA. Baseline CSF monoamine metabolites did not identify responders, but lymphocyte β-receptor activity ([³H]-isoproterenol binding) was lower in the patients who improved (D. P. van Kammen, unpublished data, 1980). This decreased binding may be due to increased circulating plasma NE levels. The length of treatment and the lack of clearly positive studies have greatly decreased interest in future clinical studies of d,l-propranolol.

CONCLUSIONS

As in the proposed DA disturbance, the NE system can be either over- or underactive (36,75) in schizophrenia, in different patients or by different tests. Increased NE levels in brain, CSF, and plasma appear to be associated with paranoid schizophrenia. It is conceivable that increased NE levels are associated specifically with an acute schizophrenic syndrome, response to neuroleptics and clonidine, which is similar to type I symptomatology (the proposed hyper-dopaminergic syndrome) (18). Type I symptomatology, which is episodic and state dependent, resembles paranoid schizophrenia as defined by Tsuang and Winokur (74). Chronic, clinically stable paranoid schizophrenic patients, who have developed type II symptoms, do not show these elevated levels at all (29). This supports the proposal that the variable CSF NE elevations in drug-free patients are state dependent (82). With the chronicity of the illness, state-dependent fluctuations may decrease or disappear. We propose that a dysregulation of the NE systems leads to the prepsychotic phase, exposing the DA disturbance, when NE is activated beyond the system's capacity by environmental stimulation. Such stimulation does not have to be extreme if the NE system is not well regulated—for example, in the presence of subsensitive α_2-receptor function impairing the feedback system, increased receptor binding, or decreased DBH activity (75,76). That NE is elevated in both autopsy brains and spinal fluid suggests that we are not dealing with an impairment of NE removal from the CSF.

Low plasma and CSF DBH activity have not consistently been reported in schizophrenia, and the early findings of decreased brain DBH activity could not be replicated. Unfortunately, no replications of CSF DBH studies have been attempted so far. One of the problems of all replication studies in schizophrenia is that each of the variables that correlate significantly seldom explains more than 10 to 30% of the variance. A small shift in sample composition (e.g., with respect to age, sex, height, weight, psychosis, premorbid functioning, brain atrophy, or days drug-free) can be expected to produce different CSF results (10,83). CSF NE and DBH levels did not correlate with each other in schizophrenia (83), suggesting that in schizophrenia NE is predominantly released from a nonvesicular pool, or that DBH is not necessarily rate limiting. CSF DBH, however, seems to be very stable over time and does not change

TABLE 2. *Changes in norepinephrine metabolism in schizophrenia*

	State dependent	Trait dependent	Specific for schizophrenia
NE (brain, CSF, plasma)	Yes	No	No
MHPG (brain, CSF, plasma, urine)	Partially	Yes	No
DBH (brain, CSF, plasma)	No	Yes	No
α_2-Receptor binding (platelets)	Possibly	Likely	No
Cyclic AMP production (PGE$_1$ stimulation)	?	Yes	?

All of the above variables have been found to be different in schizophrenic patients compared to normals. These abnormal findings have been observed in other psychiatric populations as well, without a full understanding of the mechanisms by which these findings are caused in a specific patient population.

with pimozide treatment. The stability of DBH suggests that state-dependent effects are not responsible for discrepant findings in DBH, but that sample composition, such as the number of patients with brain atrophy and differences in premorbid functioning, could play a major role. Presumably, in good premorbid patients with a *hyperactive* DA system, low DBH may lead to isolated psychotic episodes. Indeed, alcoholic subjects with low CSF DBH activity were more likely to experience psychotic episodes when treated with a DBH inhibitor (disulfiram) (50). On the other hand, low DBH in the presence of *decreased* DA function could lead to increasingly prolonged episodes and negative symptoms (79). At this time, interpretation of these findings of low DBH in seemingly inconsistent groups of patients has to wait.

The PGE$_1$-stimulated cyclic AMP production in platelets is another widely replicated finding in schizophrenia (39–41,56,59; Rotrosen et al., *this volume*), but its cause is not well understood. Since hypertensive and affective disorder patients seem to have a somewhat similar deficit (39), we may be dealing with a vulnerability factor for several noradrenergic-related disorders. Interestingly, many of our patients have shown labile hypertension and increased pulse rates at one time or another in drug-free conditions. Whether a similar α_2-receptor-related deficit is present in schizophrenic brains awaits further study (45a). However, potentially, a subsensitive cAMP response to PGE$_1$ could trigger a psychotic episode.

Because several different biochemical parameters are disturbed, presumably for different endogenous reasons, it is likely that some of these effects may be caused or aggravated by a variety of factors such as a membrane disorder (72), cell loss due to a viral encephalitis (73), pre- or perinatal trauma (56), or an autoimmune disorder (60). Some of the biochemical findings may be due to environmental deprivation or overstimulation, or the patient's place in his social network. These and other disturbances may interact with, contribute to, or result from a stress sensitivity, i.e., neurochemical instability, leading to schizophrenic symptoms.

In summary, subsensitive α_2 receptor activity and state-dependent increases in NE levels seem to be present in schizophrenia, although none of the noradrenergic system-related findings seem to be specific for schizophrenia particularly during prodromal states (Table 2). The clinical

and treatment implications of these findings are not fully understood, but are an important area for further studies, particularly in combination with psychophysiological, brain blood flow, and brain imaging techniques.

ACKNOWLEDGMENT

The authors thank Mrs. Rose Dombrowski for assistance with the preparation of this manuscript.

REFERENCES

1. Ackenheil, M., Albus, M., Bondy, B., Müller-Spahn, F., Munch, U., and Naber, D. (1985): In: *Pathochemical Markers in Major Psychoses,* edited by H. Beckmann and P. Rieder, pp. 78–87. Springer-Verlag, Berlin.
2. Ackenheil, M., Beckmann, H., Greil, W., Hoffmann, G., Markianos, E., and Raese, J. (1974): In: *The Phenothiazines and Structurally Related Drugs,* edited by L. S. Forrest, C. J. Carr, and E. Usdin, pp. 647–657. Raven Press, New York.
3. Alfredsson, G., Bjerkenstedt, L., Edman, G., Harnryd, C., Oxenstierna, G., Sedvall, G., and Wiesel, F.-A. (1983): *Acta Psychiatr. Scand.,* 311(Suppl.):49–74.
4. Antelman, S. M., and Caggiula, A. R. (1977): *Science,* 195:646–653.
5. Antelman, S. M., and Chiodo, L. A. (1983): In: *Stimulants: Neurochemical Behavioral and Clinical Perspectives,* edited by L. L. Iversen, S. Iversen, and S. H. Snyder, pp. 269–299. Raven Press, New York.
6. Arnsten, A. F. T., and Goldman-Rakic, P. S. (1985): *Science,* 230:1273–1276.
7. Atsmon, A., Blum, I., Steiner, M., Latz, A., and Wijsenbeek, H. (1972): *Psychopharmacology,* 27:249–254.
8. Badgy, G., Peré, A., Frecsk, E., Révai, K., Papp, Z., Fekete, M. I. K., and Arató, M. (1985): *Psychopharmacology,* 85:62–64.
9. Belmaker, R. H., Ebstein, R. P., Dasberg, H., Levy, A., Sedvall, G., and van Praag, H. M. (1979): *Psychopharmacology,* 63:293–396.
10. Berger, P. A., Faull, K. F., Kildowski, J., Anderson, P. J., Draemer, H., Davis, K. L., and Barchas, J. D. (1980): *Am. J. Psychiatry,* 137:174–180.
11. Berrettini, W. H., Nurnberger, J. I., Scheinin, M., Seppala, T., Linnoila, M., Narrow, W., Simmons-Alling, S., and Gershon, E. S. (1985): *Biol. Psychiatry,* 20:257–269.
12. Bigelow, L. B., Zalcman, S., Kleinman, J. E., Weinberger, D., Luchins, D., Tallman, J., Karoum, F., and Wyatt, R. J. (1979): In: *Catecholamines: Basic and Clinical Frontiers, Vol. 2,* edited by E. Usdin, I. J. Kopin, and J. Barchas, pp. 1851–1853. Pergamon Press, New York.
13. Bird, E. D., Spokes, E. G., and Iversen, L. L. (1979): *Brain,* 102:347–360.

14. Carlsson, A. (1980): In: *Catecholamines: Basic and Clinical Frontiers,* edited by E. Usdin, I. J. Kopin, and J. Barchas, pp. 4–19. Pergamon Press, New York.
15. Castellani, S., Ziegler, M. G., van Kammen, D. P., Alexander, P. E., Siris, S. G., and Lake, C. R. (1982): *Arch. Gen. Psychiatry,* 39:1145–1149.
16. Chouinard, G., and Jones, B. D. (1979): *Am. J. Psychiatry,* 24: 661–667.
17. Cross, A. J., Crow, T. J., Killpack, W. S., Longden, A., Owen, F., and Riley, G. J. (1978): *Psychopharmacology,* 59:117–121.
18. Crow, T. J. (1980): *Br. Med. J.,* 280:66–68.
19. Crow, T. J., Baker, H. F., Cross, A. J., Joseph, M. H., Lofthouse, R., Longden, A., Owen, F., Riley, G. J., Glover, V., and Killpack, W. S. (1979): *Br. J. Psychiatry,* 134:249–256.
20. DeLisi, L. E., Mirsky, A. F., Buchsbaum, M. S., van Kammen, D. P., Berman, K. F., Caton, C., Kafka, M. S., Ninan, P. T., Phelps, B. H., Karoum, F., Ko, G. N., Korpi, E. R., Linnoila, M., Scheinin, M., and Wyatt, R. J. (1984): *Psychiatry Res.,* 13:59–76.
21. Elizur, A., Levy, A., Favah, M., and Blum, I. (1980): *Commun. Psychopharmacol.,* 4:507–517.
22. Farley, I. J., Price, K. S., McCullough, E., Deck, J. H., Hordynski, W., and Hornykiewicz, O. (1978): *Science,* 200:456–458.
23. Faull, K. F., King, R. J., Berger, P. A., and Barchas, J. D. (1984): In: *Catecholamines: Neuropharmacology and Central Nervous System—Therapeutic Aspects,* edited by E. Usdin, A. Carlsson, A. Dahlström, and J. Engel, pp. 143–152. Alan R. Liss, New York.
24. Fields, R., van Kammen, D. P., Peters, J., Rosen, J., and Linnoila, M. (1986): (in preparation).
25. Freedman, R., Bell, J., and Kirch, D. (1980): *Am. J. Psychiatry,* 137:629–630.
26. Freedman, R., Kirch, D., Bell, J., Adler, L. E., Pecevish, M., Pachtman, E., and Denver, P. (1982): *Acta Psychiatr. Scand.,* 65: 35–45.
27. Fujita, K., Ito, T., Marata, K., Teradaira, R., Beppu, H., Nakagami, Y., Kato, Y., Nagatsu, T., and Kato, T. (1979): In: *Catecholamines: Basic and Clinical Frontiers,* edited by E. Usdin, I. J. Kopin, and J. Barchas, pp. 1940–1942. Pergamon Press, New York.
28. Gardos, G., Cole, J. O., Volicer, L., Orzack, M. H., and Oliff, A. C. (1973): *Curr. Ther. Res.,* 15:314–323.
29. Gattaz, W. F., Riederer, P., Reynolds, G. P., Gattaz, D., and Beckmann, H. (1983): *Psychiatry Res.,* 8:243–250.
30. Gattaz, W. F., Waldmeyer, P., and Beckmann, H. (1982): *Acta Psychiatr. Scand.,* 66:350–360.
31. Gjerris, A., Jensen, E., Christensen, N. J., and Rafaelsen, O. J. (1981): In: *Biological Psychiatry,* edited by C. Perris, G. Struwe, and B. Jansson, pp. 565–568. Elsevier/North Holland, Amsterdam.
32. Gomes, U. C., Shanley, B. C., Potgieter, L., and Roux, J. T. (1980): *Br. J. Psychiatry,* 137:346–351.
33. Hansen, T., Heyden, T., Sundberg, I., Alfredsson, G., Nyback, H., and Wetterberg, L. (1980): *Arch. Gen. Psychiatry,* 37:685–690.
34. Holmgren, G., Gershon, S., and Beck, L. H. (1962): *Nature,* 193: 1313–1314.
35. Hommer, D. W., Zahn, T. P., Pickar, D., and van Kammen, D. P. (1984): *Psychiatry Res.,* 11:193–204.
36. Hornykiewicz, O. (1982): *Nature,* 299:484–486.
37. Joseph, M. H., Frith, E. D., and Waddington, J. L. (1979): *Psychopharmacology,* 63:273–280.
38. Jouvent, R., Lecrubier, Y., Puech, A. J., Simon, P., and Widlocher, D. (1980): *Am. J. Psychiatry,* 137:1275–1276.
39. Kafka, M. S., Siever, L. J., Nurnberger, J. I., Uhde, T. W., Targum, S., Cooper, D. M. J., van Kammen, D. P., and Tokola, N. S. (1985): *Psychopharmacol. Bull.,* 21:599–602.
40. Kafka, M. S., and van Kammen, D. P. (1983): *Arch. Gen. Psychiatry,* 40:264–270.
41. Kafka, M. S., van Kammen, D. P., Nurnberger, J. I., Siever, L. J., Uhde, T. W., and Polinsky, R. J. (1980): *Commun. Psychopharmacol.,* 4:477–486.
42. Kemali, D., Del Vecchio, M., and Maj, M. (1982): *Biol. Psychiatry,* 17:711–717.
43. Kleinman, J. E., Bridge, P., Karoum, F., Speciale, S., Staub, R., Zalcman, S., Gillin, J. C., and Wyatt, R. J. (1979): In: *Catecholamines: Brain and Clinical Frontiers,* edited by E. Usdin, I. J. Kopin, and J. Barchas, pp. 1845–1847. Pergamon Press, New York.
44. Kleinman, J. E., Karoum, F., Rosenblatt, J., Gillin, J. C., Hong, J., Bridge, T. P., Zalcman, S., Storch, F., DelCarmen, R., and Wyatt, R. J. (1981): In: *Biological Psychiatry,* edited by C. Perris, G. Struwe, and B. Jansson, pp. 711–714. Elsevier/North Holland, Amsterdam.
45. Ko, G. N., Korpi, E. R., Freed, W. J., Zalcman, S. J., and Bigelow, L. B. (1985): *Biol. Psychiatry,* 20:209–215.
45a. Ko, G. N., Unnerstall, J. R., Kuhar, M. J., Wyatt, R. J., and Kleinman, J. E. (1986): *Psychopharmacol. Bull.,* 22:1011–1016.
46. Kopin, I. J., Gordon, E. K., Jimerson, D. C., and Polinsky, R. J. (1983): *Science,* 219:73–75.
47. Lake, C. R., Sternberg, D. E., van Kammen, D. P., Ballenger, J. C., Ziegler, M. G., Post, R. M., Kopin, I. J., and Bunney, W. E., Jr. (1980): *Science,* 207:331–333.
48. Linnoila, M., Ninan, P. T., Scheinin, M., Waters, R. N., Chang, W. H., Bartko, J., and van Kammen, D. P. (1983): *Arch. Gen. Psychiatry,* 40:1290–1294.
49. Mair, R. G., and McEntee, W. J. (1986): *Psychopharmacology,* 88:374–380.
50. Major, L. F., Lerner, P., Ballenger, J. C., Brown, G. L., Goodwin, F. K., and Lovenberg, W. (1979): *Biol. Psychiatry,* 14:337–344.
51. Marder, S. R., van Kammen, D. P., Docherty, J. P., Rayner, J., and Bunney, W. E., Jr. (1979): *Arch. Gen. Psychiatry,* 36:1080–1085.
52. Markianos, E. S., Mystrom, I., Reichel, H., and Matussek, N. (1976): *Psychopharmacology,* 50:259–267.
53. Markianos, M., and Tripodianakis, J. (1985): *Biol. Psychiatry,* 20: 98–100.
54. Martin, P. R., Ebert, M. H., Gordon, E. K., Linnoila, M., and Kopin, I. J. (1984): *Clin. Pharmacol. Ther.,* 35:322–327.
55. Meltzer, H. Y., Arora, R. C., and Metz, J. (1984): *Schizophr. Bull.,* 10:49–70.
56. Pandey, G. N., Garver, D. L., Tamminga, C., Ericksen, S., Ali, S. I., and Davis, J. M. (1977): *Am. J. Psychiatry,* 134:518–522.
57. Post, R. M., Fink, E., Carpenter, W. T., and Goodwin, F. K. (1975): *Arch Gen. Psychiatry,* 32:1063–1069.
58. Rice, H. E., Smith, C. B., and Rosen, J. (1984): *Psychiatry Res.,* 12:69–77.
59. Rotrosen, J., Miller, A. D., Mandio, D., Traficante, L. J., and Gershon, S. (1980): *Arch. Gen. Psychiatry,* 37:1047–1054.
60. Rudin, D. O. (1979): *Schizophr. Bull.,* 5:623–626.
61. Scheinin, M., van Kammen, D. P., Ninan, P. T., and Linnoila, M. (1984): *Clin. Pharmacol. Ther.,* 36:33–39.
62. Sedvall, G., Alfredsson, G., Bjerkenstedt, L., Eneroth, P., Fryö, B., Härnryd, C., and Wode-Helgodt, B. (1976): In: *The Impact of Biology on Modern Psychiatry,* edited by E. S. Gershon, R. H. Belmaker, S. S. Kety, and M. Rosenbaum, pp. 41–54. Plenum, New York.
63. Sedvall, G., Nyback, H., Oxenstierna, G., Wiesel, F. A., and Wode-Helgodt, B. (1981): In: *Recent Advances in Neuropsychopharmacology,* edited by B. Angrist, G. D. Burrows, M. Lader, O. Lingjaerde, G. Sedvall, and D. Wheatley, pp. 299–305. Pergamon Press, Oxford.
64. Shopsin, B., Wilk, S., and Gershon, S. (1973): *Arch. Gen. Psychiatry,* 28:230–233.
65. Stahl, S. M., Thornton, J. E., Simpson, M. L., Berger, P. A., and Napoliello, M. J. (1985): *Biol. Psychiatry,* 20:888–893.
66. Stahl, S., Uhr, S., and Berger, P. (1985): *Biol. Psychiatry,* 20: 1098–1102.
67. Stein, L., and Wise, C. D. (1971): *Science,* 171:1032–1036.
68. Sternberg, D. E., Charney, D. S., Heninger, G. R., Leckman, J. F., Hafstad, K. M., and Landis, H. (1982): *Arch. Gen. Psychiatry,* 39:285–289.
69. Sternberg, D. E., van Kammen, D. P., Lake, C. R., Ballenger, J. C., Marder, S. R., and Bunney, W. E., Jr. (1981): *Am. J. Psychiatry,* 138:1045–1051.
70. Sternberg, D. E., van Kammen, D. P., Lerner, P., Ballenger, J. C., Marder, S. R., Post, R. M., and Bunney, W. E., Jr. (1983): *Arch. Gen. Psychiatry,* 40:743–747.
71. Sternberg, D. E., van Kammen, D. P., Lerner, P., and Bunney, W. E., Jr. (1982): *Science,* 216:1423–1425.
72. Stevens, J. D. (1972): *Schizophr. Bull.,* 6:60–61.
73. Torrey, E. F., Yolken, R. H., and Winfrey, C. J. (1982): *Science,* 216:892–893.

74. Tsuang, M. T., and Winokur, G. (1974): *Arch. Gen. Psychiatry,* 31:43–47.

75. van Kammen, D. P., and Antelman, S. (1984): *Life Sci.,* 34:1403–1413.

76. van Kammen, D. P., Bunney, W. E., Jr., Docherty, J. P., Marder, S. R., Ebert, M. H., Rosenblatt, J. E., and Rayner, J. N. (1982): *Am. J. Psychiatry,* 139:991–997.

77. van Kammen, D. P., Malas, K. L., Sternberg, D. E., Murphy, D. L., Lerner, P., Lake, C. R., Dalton, L. A., and Bunney, W. E., Jr. (1981): *Psychopharmacol. Bull.,* 17:207–209.

78. van Kammen, D. P., Mann, L. S., Scheinin, M., van Kammen, W. B., and Linnoila, M. (1984): *Psychopharmacol. Bull.,* 20:519–522.

79. van Kammen, D. P., Mann, L. S., Seppala, T., van Kammen, W. B., and Linnoila, M. (1986): *Arch. Gen. Psychiatry.,* 43:978–983.

80. van Kammen, D. P., Mann, L. S., Sternberg, D. E., Scheinin, M., Ninan, P. T., Marder, S. R., van Kammen, W. B., Rieder, R. O., and Linnoila, M. (1983): *Science,* 220:974–977.

81. van Kammen, D. P., Peters, J., Rosen, J., van Kammen, W. B., and Nugent, N. (1986) (*in preparation*).

82. van Kammen, D. P., Rosen, J., Peters, J., Fields, R., and van Kammen, W. B. (1985): *Psychopharmacol. Bull.,* 21:497–502.

83. van Kammen, D. P., Sternberg, E. D., Hare, T. A., Waters, R. N., and Bunney, W. E., Jr. (1982): *Arch. Gen. Psychiatry,* 39:91–97.

84. van Kammen, D. P., Sternberg, D. E., Lake, C. R., and Lerner, P. (1982): In: *Frontiers of Hormone Research, Vol. 9: Cerebrospinal Fluid and Peptide Hormones,* edited by E. Rodriguez and T. B. van Wimersma Greidanus, pp. 198–212. S. Karger, Basel.

85. Wise, C. D., and Stein, L. (1973): *Science,* 181:344–347.

86. Wode-Helgodt, B., Eneroth, P., Fyrö, B., Gullberg, B., and Sedvall, G. (1977): *Acta. Psychiatr. Scand.,* 56:280–293.

87. Yorkston, N. J., Zaki, S. A., Pitcher, D. R., Gruzelier, J. H., Hollander, D., and Sergeant, H. G. S. (1977): *Lancet,* 9:575–578.

88. Zander, K. J., Fischer, B., Zimmer, R., and Ackenheil, M. (1981): *Psychopharmacology,* 33:43–47.

89. Ziegler, M. G., Lake, C. R., Post, R. M., and Kopin, I. (1976): *J. Neurochemistry,* 28:677–679.

Psychopharmacology:
The Third Generation of Progress,
edited by Herbert Y. Meltzer.
Raven Press, New York © 1987.

CHAPTER **73**

Biochemical Instability in Schizophrenia II: The Serotonin and γ-Aminobutyric Acid Systems

Daniel P. van Kammen and Joel Gelernter

The serotonin (5-HT) and γ-aminobutyric acid (GABA) systems have not received as much attention as the dopamine and norepinephrine systems in schizophrenia. The GABA system seems to be of more interest in affective disorder patients, even though studied in schizophrenia. Unfortunately, the study populations in schizophrenia have been mainly chronic patients. Although some studies suggest that lower GABA levels may be present early in the illness, recent understanding of interrelationships of GABA and 5-HT with the DA and NE (65) systems may help us to reevaluate the many repeated, but inconsistent, findings in these two systems as state-dependent phenomena. Many of the abnormalities found in the GABA system in schizophrenia may relate more specifically to certain behaviors than to the disease process itself.

After the initial hopes that endogenous hallucinogens could explain psychotic phenomena in schizophrenia (28), the 5-HT system was studied intensely, but was ultimately a less rewarding candidate for a primary role in schizophrenia. However, studies of both systems have quietly produced many interesting findings away from the dopamine limelight, as this review will show.

SEROTONIN (5-HYDROXYTRYPTAMINE, 5-HT)

Over a quarter of a century ago, 5-HT was thought to be involved in psychotic disorders (74). Since then, numerous hypotheses have been proposed, from endogenous hallucinogens and faulty methylation (27) to modulation of DA and NE activity, and from involvement in impulse control to motor activity. In one of the earlier 5-HT-related cerebrospinal fluid (CSF) studies, Bowers (8) suggested as a reason for studying 5-HT metabolism specifically in psychosis the probable serotonergic mechanism of action of the psychotomimetic lysergic acid diethylamide (LSD). Since then, the understanding of the mechanism of action of LSD's behavioral effects has changed a bit, but studies of serotonergic systems in schizophrenia have continued to be fruitful. We will discuss brain and CSF studies, which focus on 5-hydroxyindoleacetic acid (5HIAA) (the major CNS metabolite of 5-HT), as they pertain to schizophrenia and briefly to violent suicide; whole blood and platelet 5-HT studies, which led to the proposal of serotonergic abnormalities as a familial marker or "trait" in schizophrenia; and some of the recent studies of serotonergic drugs in schizophrenia. This is of particular interest because 5-HT interacts with the dopamine (DA) system.

5-HT Brain Studies

Autopsy studies of 5HIAA in the temporal cortex, hippocampus, and putamen revealed no deficit or differences in 5HIAA (33,35). However, Farley et al. (19), who analyzed several more forebrain areas, did find increased 5HIAA in the stria terminalis region of chronic schizophrenic patients. Bennett et al. (6) reported a 40 to 50% decrease in [³H]LSD binding in the cortex of schizophrenic autopsy brains. In spite of several replications by the same group, Crow et al. (14) did not find such a decrease.

CSF 5HIAA Studies

CSF 5HIAA in schizophrenia has consistently been negatively associated with states of motor activity, agitation, and arousal (8,9,39), and this has led to interest in its potential use as a marker for subtype. King et al. (38) measured CSF and platelet 5HIAA, which were both positively correlated with mannerisms and posturing (Brief Psychiatric Rating Scale, BPRS). CSF 5HIAA did not correlate with other BPRS symptoms. These authors speculated that the increased serotonergic activity seen in this type of patient could explain motor deficits such as eye tracking abnormalities. Thus, it appears that decreased serotonergic activity is partially associated with agitation or increased arousal in schizophrenic patients, whereas increased serotonergic activity is associated with mannerisms and posturing and other positive symptom items. Bowers (9) was the first author to point out possible state-dependent influences on CSF 5HIAA.

Gattaz et al. (24) found decreased 5HIAA levels in schizophrenic patients, regardless of medication status, and in paranoid patients (21). Bowers (9,10) reported that there was lower CSF 5HIAA in the acute (8) and "better prognosis" patients. Gerner et al. (25) showed a trend for increased CSF 5HIAA in chronic schizophrenics. Finally, in two studies comparing acute schizophrenic patients with controls, Post et al. (54) and Berger et al. (7) found no statistical differences in CSF 5HIAA (after probenecid).

Increased CSF 5HIAA could be a marker associated with a family history of schizophrenia, that is, a trait marker. Subjects with a family history of schizophrenia have significantly higher (43,60) or lower (60) CSF 5HIAA levels than subjects with a family history of depression; the subjects themselves did not have any "overt behavioral deviations."

Low CSF 5HIAA is associated with increased risk for violent suicide (4). Although initially demonstrated for depressed patients, this has been independently demonstrated in two schizophrenic populations with violent attempts or completed suicides, controlled for height and sex (5,51); these authors suggested that the low CSF 5HIAA relates to a vulnerability to commit violence against self or others, independent of diagnosis. The association with increased arousal in schizophrenics and the increased suicide risk (10%) and loss of impulse control in general make CSF 5HIAA worthwhile to pursue in schizophrenia.

Another interesting factor is that of brain atrophy. In several studies, an association was found between cortical atrophy or large ventricle brain ratios and reduced levels of CSF 5HIAA in schizophrenic populations (52,55,70). These results suggest a particular difficulty in interpreting studies using chronic or "type II" patients as opposed to acute or "type I" patients without clearly describing the patients. Patients with type II would be expected to have more atrophy and thus lower levels of CSF monoamine metabolites (52,55,70,71).

Whole Blood and Platelet 5-HT Studies

Whole blood and platelet 5-HT have consistently been reported to be increased in chronic schizophrenic patients (17,21,23,34,64,68). DeLisi et al. (17) reported increased whole blood 5-HT levels in schizophrenic patients with large frontal horns of lateral ventricles on computerized tomographic (CT) scans. The increased platelet 5-HT may not be explained by changed uptake mechanisms in chronic patients (3), unless other factors such as 5-HT content, imipramine binding, and platelet monoamine oxidase (MAO) are taken into account (49). Acute schizophrenic patients may resemble depressed patients in this parameter (57).

Serotonergic Drugs

Since the observation that serotonergic drugs have psychotomimetic effects, it has been proposed that antiserotonergic drugs could have antipsychotic effects. There have been two recent small studies reporting the positive effects of fenfluramine in schizophrenia, one on chronic patients (total BPRS scores) (61) and one specifically investigating its effect on negative symptoms (63). Fenfluramine decreases CSF 5HIAA in humans, and in animals it causes a decrease in whole brain 5-HT. Marder and van Kammen (unpublished data, 1978) observed improvement in two patients' psychotic symptoms only after *withdrawal* from fenfluramine.

Discussion

Serotonergic dysregulation is probably a factor in some schizophrenic patients, whether it be of primary or secondary importance (Table 1). Increased CSF 5HIAA is associated with a family history of schizophrenia, chronic illness, and motor abnormalities such as mannerisms and posturing. Low CSF 5HIAA is associated with increased levels of arousal and increased likelihood of violence to self or others, or with a more acute and good premorbid functioning illness. On the other hand, low CSF 5HIAA is also

TABLE 1. *Evidence that 5-HT activity is involved in schizophrenia*

CSF 5HIAA is lower in acute and paranoid patients and higher in chronic patients

CSF 5HIAA is negatively correlated with agitation and arousal

CSF 5HIAA is higher or lower in normals who have schizophrenic relatives

Cortical atrophy and large ventricle/brain ratios (VBRs) on CT scans are associated with lower CSF 5HIAA

Fenfluramine may decrease negative symptoms

Antipsychotic drugs affect 5-HT receptor populations directly

Whole blood and platelet 5-HT are increased in chronic schizophrenic patients

Brain 5HIAA has been reported to be increased and decreased in schizophrenia present in patients with large lateral ventricles and cortical atrophy by CT scan.

The meaning of increased whole blood or platelet 5-HT remains obscure, particularly in those with CT scan brain atrophy. One explanation may be that increased 5-HT uptake indicates less 5-HT at the receptor sites if platelet dynamics reflect neuronal mechanisms. Some animal studies may be relevant. Recently, McGuire and Raleigh (46) provided evidence that in vervet monkeys serotonergic systems enhanced grooming, approaching, and resting behaviors and reduced locomotion, being solitary, vigilance, and avoiding behaviors. These vigilant, avoiding, and solitary behaviors may find their counterpart in psychopathology in humans: they are seen in paranoid schizophrenic patients. They (46) reported that whole blood 5-HT levels are increased in dominant compared to nondominant male vervet monkeys. When animals are isolated, however, whole blood 5-HT decreases, and it rises again after 10 to 12 weeks of isolation. The behavior of the long-term isolated animals resembles that of nondominant males more closely. In humans, elevated whole blood 5-HT has been found in males with type A behavior (44) and in schizophrenics (17,21,64). The monkey studies by McGuire and Raleigh (46) clearly show that a dissociation between behavior and biological measures can occur and that the interaction between environment and individual needs to be assessed.

AMINOBUTYRIC ACID (GABA)

Roberts (56) hypothesized that decreased GABA could be involved in schizophrenia; strategies to study GABA function in schizophrenia were outlined by van Kammen (69). It has been hypothesized that the relative DA excess proposed in schizophrenia stems from a GABA deficiency (69). If this were the case, CSF GABA levels could be altered; enzymes responsible for GABA metabolism could have abnormal activity in brain or CSF; and finally, GABA-ergic drugs should have a positive effect on schizophrenic symptoms. In this section, we review GABA-related studies in schizophrenia and advance the notion that GABA activity in schizophrenia may be linked inversely with DA activity (9,10) and that GABA$_B$ agonists (e.g., baclofen) may induce psychosis resembling schizophrenic symptoms as in response to the amphetamine challenge test. However, the most robust findings linking altered CSF GABA with psychiatric illness to date are those of low GABA in depression (25,26,29). The relationship of the GABA system and schizophrenia has been reviewed extensively (18,22,47). GABA$_A$ and GABA$_B$ receptors also have a differing distribution in the CNS (18). Development of GABAergic drugs with specificity for either receptor may help to sort out the confusing behavioral reports. For further review of the GABA system, see Chapters 19, 27, and 96, in *this volume.*

CSF GABA

Several groups have looked to the CSF as a direct reflection of GABAergic activity in brain, with varying results. McCarthy et al. (45) found increased CSF GABA by radioimmunoassay (RIA) in chronic schizophrenics compared to all other groups; however, there were only seven patients in that group (compared to nine acute schizophrenics and 75 others). In a study where there was no significant difference in CSF GABA between drug-free and medicated psychotic patients, and controls, Bowers et al. (11) reported a significant negative correlation between GABA and anxiety, agitation, and conceptual disorganization. In a comparison of 30 drug-free schizophrenic patients and 39 controls (72), there was no significant difference in CSF GABA, but this was felt to be because the control subjects were older (see below). Van Kammen et al. (72) found that recently ill schizophrenics had significantly lower GABA. GABA levels increased with duration of illness. Gerner and Hare (26) and Gerner et al. (25) also found a negative correlation with age in normal and depressed subjects, but not in schizophrenic patients. Gold et al. (29) did not find any age–GABA relationship. Gerner et al. (25) did not report altered CSF GABA in their schizophrenic group either.

Plasma GABA

Plasma GABA may also reflect central function; this is supported by animal data (22). A study considering plasma GABA levels in control subjects and various psychiatric disorders (53) found no statistical difference in mean levels in schizophrenics, but an increased scatter. The validity of this method is supported by the finding of decreased plasma GABA levels also in depressed patients in whom CSF levels are known to be low. Finally, there is a report of measuring plasma GAD (glutamic acid decarboxylase, which catalyzes the synthesis of GABA from glutamic acid) in schizophrenic and other psychiatric illnesses (36). Kaiya et al. (36) found that whereas GAD levels were not statistically different between schizophrenic and control subjects, plasma GAD levels increased when the patients were given antipsychotic drugs with anticholinergics. In contrast, GAD levels were lower in depressed patients.

GABAergic Drugs

Baclofen is a GABA$_B$ receptor agonist and is used as a muscle relaxant. Since an early positive study in 1975 (20), results with this agent have been negative. Unfortunately, drugs that enhance GABA activity in the brain have been associated with inducing either schizophreniform or toxic psychosis in schizophrenic patients (16,62). Van Kammen et al. (unpublished data, 1980) observed that a chronic paranoid patient, who for years reported only occasionally a residual auditory hallucination, decompensated severely with baclofen. This agent can apparently provoke schizophrenic symptoms.

In a small double-blind trial of its effects in schizophrenia, valproic acid did not change in BPRS ratings; this study used patients refractory to antipsychotic treatment (40). Only a few patients have been studied with muscimol

(66,67; van Kammen and co-workers, unpublished data, 1979). It is of interest that Hanada et al. (30) found increased [³H]muscimol binding in schizophrenic brains. γ-Hydroxybutyrate, which like γ-butyrolactone (GBL) turns off DA neurons, showed variable antipsychotic and worsening responses, sometimes resembling amphetamine effects (59). It induced akathisia and other extrapyramidal side effects requiring anticholinergic treatment.

The results with benzodiazepines (BDZs) have been more promising. Jimerson et al. (32) found some improvement in two of five schizophrenic patients placed on high doses of diazepam. Lerner et al. (42) compared haloperidol and diazepam in acutely psychotic schizophrenics and found them about equally effective. Nestoros et al. (50) added diazepam in high doses to antipsychotic drugs in their 10-patient sample of chronic schizophrenic patients. Seven of these experienced marked or moderate improvement, and none got worse. The improvement was seen in paranoid schizophrenic patients. Wolkowitz et al. (73) found alprazolam added to antipsychotic drugs to be beneficial for both positive and negative symptoms in the two chronic schizophrenics they studied.

The largely negative results with baclofen and valproic acid contrast somewhat with the studies with BDZs. BDZs modulate GABAergic transmission, are anxiolytics, and anxiety is often a prominent feature in prepsychotic or psychotic conditions; whether this explains the results is unclear. An additional dimension has been added to GABA research by the recent characterization of an endogenous diazepam binding inhibitor (1). No reports of this compound in humans have appeared as yet.

Discussion

There is evidence of decreased CSF GABA levels in young, recently ill, and good premorbid schizophrenic patients, whereas GABA levels are increased with duration of illness and chronic neuroleptic treatment. With aging, CSF GABA levels decrease in normals, but increase in schizophrenic patients, perhaps as the patients progress from Crow's type I to type II. Bowers et al. (12) reported that increased agitation was associated with lower GABA, but higher CSF homovanillic acid (HVA) levels. Decreased CSF GABA levels in both schizophrenic and affective disorder patients suggest that these two diagnoses share some disturbances, although the differences change with progression of the illness. Certain neurological diseases are associated with decreased CSF GABA as well, e.g., Huntington's chorea, suggesting the nonspecificity of decreased CSF GABA levels. For the most part, studies relating GABA to schizophrenia have not yielded consistent results so far. Methodological difficulties abound in CSF GABA studies. In evaluating studies of plasma, CSF, or brain GABA levels, it is important to realize that GABA levels increase as the samples stay at room temperature for longer than 1 hr (31).

State-dependent changes in GABA activity cannot be excluded. The inverse relationship of GABA activity compared to decreased dopamine (DA) activity with increasing duration of illness and the increased variance in plasma

TABLE 2. *Evidence that GABA activity is involved in schizophrenia*

CSF GABA is lower in young drug-free schizophrenic patients (females and good premorbid)
CSF GABA increases with duration of illness
CSF GABA is higher in patients with negative symptoms
Plasma GABA levels fluctuate or vary more in schizophrenics than in other groups
[³H]Muscimol binding is increased in autopsy brains
GAD activity in brain, plasma, or platelets is not different in schizophrenic patients
GABA_B agonists such as baclofen worsen schizophrenic patients
Most GABA_A agonists are ineffective in schizophrenia
BDZs may decrease psychotic and negative symptoms

GABA are intriguing. GABAergic agents have largely failed to fulfill their promise of therapeutic effects in schizophrenia, with a possible exception of the BDZs. Also, we note the worsening observed with baclofen (a GABA_B agonist), which could be a diagnostic challenge test similar to that with amphetamine (2). Whether GABA_B antagonists can have antipsychotic effects remains untested.

An important factor inhibiting our understanding of GABAergic mechanisms in schizophrenia is that although GABA serves as an inhibitory neurotransmitter on a single synapse basis in some DA systems, it is also capable of the opposite effect of potentiating DA transmission (for review see 22). We are left with an unclear picture of GABA's role in schizophrenia (72). In any event, the evidence does not support a primary GABA disorder in schizophrenia (Table 2).

CONCLUSIONS

Monoamines regulate or modify many behaviors, whereas pharmacological interventions that affect monoamine activity can change these behaviors. These relationships have led to several hypotheses, but many of the biological findings in schizophrenia seem inconsistent with them. Even though previous chronic treatment with neuroleptics can be blamed for our inability to nail down a comprehensive simple neurotransmitter hypothesis, the evidence for this effect is not very strong. Besides the multiple interactions between the different systems, peripheral and central monoaminergic mechanisms may influence each other, but are not necessarily regulated the same way. Conceivably, norepinephrine (NE), 5-HT, and GABA fulfill permissive roles, regulate the environmental impact on the organism, and may affect the sensitivity of the DA system.

Many neurotransmitter systems proposed initially to be responsible for schizophrenic symptomatology have found their place in the study of major affective illness with abnormalities in both disorders: low CSF GABA and 5HIAA levels have been found most consistently in affective disorders, whereas a NE-related hypothesis for schizophrenia was soon abandoned for a decreased NE hypothesis in depression (13,58). The reviewed data of 5-HT and GABA activity suggest that unstable (acute) schizophrenic patients may biologically resemble affective disorder patients early in the illness. Meltzer et al. (48) pointed out that some biological similarities exist (e.g., in creatinine phosphokinase (CPK) and MAO activity) between the two major "functional" psychoses.

Some of these findings are not only present in schizophrenia and affective disorders [prostaglandin E_1 (PGE_1)-induced stimulation of cyclic AMP production, elevated CSF NE, decreased urinary 3-methoxy-4-hydroxyphenyl-glycol (MHPG), decreased CSF GABA], but also in hypertension (PGE_1-induced stimulation of cyclic AMP production, increased [^{3}H]dihydroergocrypine (DHE) binding), type A personality (increased whole blood 5-HT), brain atrophy (low CSF 5HIAA, NE, MHPG, and DBH), or suicide (low CSF 5HIAA). None of these findings are specific for schizophrenia; for that matter, none of the DA system-related findings are either.

The reports of increased or decreased NE, 5-HT, and GABA activity are consistent with the numerous studies indicating that schizophrenics can be subdivided into patients who are hyper- or hypoaroused (17a,41,75). Other clinical dichotomies include acute vs chronic, good neuroleptic responders vs nonresponders, patients with good premorbid vs poor premorbid functioning, patients with positive vs negative symptoms, those early in the illness vs those later in the illness, and patients with brain atrophy vs those without.

We propose yet another dichotomy: *stable vs unstable.* We suggest that the stable and unstable conditions can be defined biochemically and sometimes by drug response (2). In general, physiological variables change with psychological fluctuations, but in stable psychological states—even when they are abnormal—physiological measures remain normal. This seems to hold true for the neurochemistry as well, and may explain why so many chronic schizophrenic or remitted acute patients in stable condition show no difference in biochemical findings (24) or in response to pharmacological challenge tests compared to normals (2). With increasing chronicity most patients become more stable—less responsive to neuroleptics but also less psychotic—and may develop more negative symptoms. Antipsychotic drugs can induce temporal stability and negative symptoms too. $GABA_A$ receptors may be involved in these negative symptoms (15). Chronically hospitalized patients can become rather stable in the natural history of the disease. We expect to find clinical instability to be associated with state-dependent markers (Table 3). In stable patients normal or low values are found, whereas in unstable patients increased or normal values with increased variance are observed. We have stressed elsewhere the need for longitudinal assessment in schizophrenia to rule out state-dependent effects, even though in normal subjects the variables under study are stable (Table 3). We propose that the discrepant biological findings in schizophrenia related to the NE, 5-HT, and GABA (or DA) systems may be explained by an episodic instability in neurochemical and clinical states (37), particularly in young, good premorbid, neuroleptic-responsive schizophrenic patients. Therefore, a diverse mix of drug-free patients should be included to identify the clinical conditions associated with each variable.

The last decade has seen a cascade of new approaches and new technologies applied in the psychobiological evaluation of schizophrenia. The excitement of the 1960s and 1970s over single neurotransmitter system hypotheses has abated. Understanding how these biochemical findings relate to course, relapse, prognosis, drug response, and side effects in schizophrenia is the issue now. None of these findings by itself appears to be specific for schizophrenia. The implied dysregulation or instability of the systems may. Schizophrenia is most likely a multi-neurotransmitter-system disease, caused by a factor or factors that could be acting on any of these systems.

TABLE 3. *Changes in 5-HT and GABA metabolism in schizophrenia*

	State dependent	Trait dependent	Specific for schizophrenia
5-HT (Whole blood)	Yes	Yes	No
5HIAA (CSF)	Possibly	Yes	No
GABA (CSF, plasma)	Possibly	—	No

All of the above variables have been found to be different in schizophrenic patients compared to normals and may reflect clinical instability. These abnormal findings have been observed in other psychiatric populations as well, without a full understanding of the mechanisms by which these findings are caused in a specific patient population.

ACKNOWLEDGMENT

The authors thank Mrs. Rose Dombrowski for assistance with the preparation of the manuscript.

REFERENCES

1. Alho, H., Costa, E., Ferrero, P., Fujimoto, M., Cosenza, O., Murphy, D., and Guidotti, A. (1985): *Science,* 229:179–182.
2. Angrist, B., and van Kammen, D. P. (1984): *Trends Neurosci.,* 7: 388–390.
3. Arora, R. C., and Meltzer, H. Y. (1982): *Psychiatry Res.,* 6:327–333.
4. Åsberg, M., Bertilsson, L., Tuch, D., Cronholm, B., and Sjöqvist, F. (1972): *Clin. Pharmacol. Ther.,* 14:277–286.
5. Banki, C. M., Arato, M., Papp, Z., and Kurca, M. (1984): In: *Catecholamines: Neuropharmacology and Central Nervous System—Therapeutic Aspects,* edited by E. Usdin, A. Carlsson, A. Dahlstrom, and J. Engel, pp. 153–159. Alan R. Liss, New York.
6. Bennett, J. P., Enna, S. J., Bylund, D. B., Gillin, J. C., Wyatt, R. J., and Snyder, S. H. (1979): *Arch. Gen. Psychiatry,* 36:927–934.
7. Berger, P. A., Faull, K. F., Kildowski, J., Anderson, P. J., Draemer, H., Davis, K. L., and Barchas, J. D. (1980): *Am. J. Psychiatry,* 137:174–180.
8. Bowers, M. B. (1975): *Psychopharmacol. Commun.,* 1:655–662.
9. Bowers, M. B. (1978): In: *Biochemistry of Mental Disorders,* edited by E. Usdin and A. Mandell, pp. 191–204. Marcel Dekker, New York.
10. Bowers, M. B. (1978): *Biol. Psychiatry,* 13:375–383.
11. Bowers, M. B., Gold, B. I., and Roth, R. H. (1980): *Psychopharmacology,* 70:279–282.
12. Bowers, M. B., Heninger, G. R., and Sternberg, D. (1980): *Commun. Psychopharmacol.,* 4:177–188.
13. Bunney, W. E., Jr., and Davis, J. M. (1965): *Arch. Gen. Psychiatry,* 13:484–494.

14. Crow, T. J., Baker, H. F., Cross, A. J., Joseph, M. H., Lofthouse, R., Longden, A., Owen, F., Riley, G. J., Glover, V., and Killpack, W. S. (1979): *Br. J. Psychiatry*, 134:249–256.
15. Csernansky, J. J., Lombrozo, L., Bulbritch, G. B., and Hollister, L. O. (1984): *J. Clin. Psychopharmacol.*, 4:349–352.
16. Davis, K. L., Hollister, L. E., and Berger, P. A. (1976): *Lancet*, 1: 1245.
17. DeLisi, L. E., Neckers, L. M., Weinberger, D. R., et al. (1981): *Arch. Gen. Psychiatry*, 38:647–650.
17a. Docherty, J. P., van Kammen, D. P., Siris, S. G., and Marder, S. R. (1978): *Arch. Gen. Psychiatry*, 35:420–426.
18. Enna, S. J. (1985): In: *Psychiatry Update: Vol. 4*, edited by R. E. Hales and A. J. Frances, pp. 67–96. APA, Washington, DC.
19. Farley, I. J., Sharnak, K. S., and Hornykiewicz, O. (1980): *Adv. Biochem. Psychopharmacol.*, 21:427–433.
20. Fredericksen, P. K. (1975): *Läkartidningen*, 72:456–458.
21. Freedman, D. X., Belendiuk, K., Belendiuk, G. W., et al. (1981): *Arch. Gen. Psychiatry*, 38:655–659.
22. Garbutt, J. C., and van Kammen, D. P. (1983): *Schizophr. Bull.*, 9:336–353.
23. Garelis, E., Gillin, J. C., Wyatt, R. J., et al. (1975): *Am. J. Psychiatry*, 132:184–186.
24. Gattaz, W. F., Waldmeyer, P., and Beckmann, H. (1982): *Acta Psychiatr. Scand.*, 66:350–360.
25. Gerner, R. H., Fairbanks, L., Anderson, G. M., Young, J. G., Scheinin, M., Linnoila, M., Hare, T. A., Shaywitz, B. A., and Cohen, D. J. (1984): *Am. J. Psychiatry*, 141:1533–1540.
26. Gerner, R. H., and Hare, T. A. (1981): *Am. J. Psychiatry*, 138: 1098–1101.
27. Gillin, J. C., Kaplan, J., Stillman, R., and Wyatt, R. J. (1976): *Am. J. Psychiatry*, 153:203–208.
28. Gillin, J. C., Stoff, D. M., and Wyatt, R. J. (1978): In: *Psychopharmacology: A Generation of Progress*, edited by M. A. Lipton, A. DiMascio, and K. F. Killam, pp. 1097–1112. Raven Press, New York.
29. Gold, B. I., Bowers, M. B., Roth, R. H., and Sweeney, D. W. (1980): *Am. J. Psychiatry*, 137:362–364.
30. Hanada, S., Nishino, N., Mita, T., Kuno, T., Kuyama, T., Isoda, K., Hosomi, T., Uchida, S., Kasai, T., and Nakai, H. (1984): *Sheshin Shinkeigaku Zasshi*, 86:225–229.
31. Hare, T. A., Wood, J. H., Ballenger, J. C., and Post, R. M. (1979): *Lancet*, 8:534–535.
32. Jimerson, D. C., van Kammen, D. P., Post, R., Docherty, J., and Bunney, W. E., Jr. (1982): *Am. J. Psychiatry*, 139:489–491.
33. Joseph, M. H., Baker, H. F., Crow, T. J., Riley, G. J., and Risby, D. (1979): *Psychopharmacology*, 62:279–285.
34. Joseph, M. H., Frith, E. D., and Waddington, J. L. (1979): *Psychopharmacology*, 63:273–280.
35. Jus, A., Laskowska, D., and Zimny, S. (1958): *Ann. Med. Psychol. (Paris)*, 166:898–913.
36. Kaiya, H., Namba, M., Yoshida, H., and Nakamura, S. (1982): *Psychiatry Res.*, 6:335–343.
37. King, R., Barchas, J. D., and Huberman, B. A. (1984): *Proc. Natl. Acad. Sci. USA*, 81:1244–1247.
38. King, R., Faull, K. F., Stahl, S. M., Mefford, I. N., Thiemann, S., Barchas, J. D., and Berger, P. A. (1985): *Psychiatry Res.*, 14:235–240.
39. Kirstein, L., Bowers, M. B., and Heninger, G. R. (1976): *Biol. Psychiatry*, 11:421–434.
40. Ko, G. N., Korpi, E. R., Freed, W. J., Zalcman, S. J., and Bigelow, L. B. (1985): *Biol. Psychiatry*, 20:209–215.
41. Kornetsky, C., and Mirsky, A. F. (1966): *Psychopharmacology*, 8: 309–312.
42. Lerner, Y., Low, E., Leviton, A., and Belmaker, R. H. (1979): *Am. J. Psychiatry*, 136:1061–1064.
43. Lindström, L. H. (1985): *Psychiatry Res.*, 14:265–273.
44. Madsen, D., and McGuire, M. T. (1984): *Psychosom. Med.*, 46: 546–548.
45. McCarthy, B. W., Gomes, U. R., Neethling, A. C., Shanley, B. C., Taljaard, J. J. F., Potgieter, L., and Roux, J. T. (1981): *J. Neurochem.*, 36:1406–1408.
46. McGuire, M. T., and Raleigh, M. R. (1985): *Psychopharmacol. Bull.*, 21:458–463.
47. Meldrum, B. (1982): *Psychol. Med.*, 12:1–5.
48. Meltzer, H. Y., Busch, D., and Fang, V. S. (1981): *Psychoneuroendocrinology*, 6:17–36.
49. Meltzer, H. Y. (1985): *Adv. Biochem. Psychopharmacol.*, 40:59–68.
50. Nestoros, J. N., et al. (1980): *Science*, 209:708–718.
51. Ninan, P. T., van Kammen, D. P., Scheinin, M., Linnoila, M., Bunney, W. E., Jr., and Goodwin, F. K. (1984): *Am. J. Psychiatry*, 141:566–569.
52. Nybäck, H., Berggren, B.-M., Nyman, H., Sedvall, G., and Wiesel, F.-A. (1984): In: *Catecholamines: Neuropharmacology and Central Nervous System—Therapeutic Aspects*, edited by E. Usdin, A. Carlsson, A. Dahlström, and J. Engel, pp. 161–165. Alan R. Liss, New York.
53. Petty, S., and Sherman, A. P. (1984): *J. Affect. Dis.*, 6:131–138.
54. Post, R. M., Fink, E., Carpenter, W. T., and Goodwin, F. K. (1975): *Arch. Gen. Psychiatry*, 32:1063–1069.
55. Potkin, S. G., Weinberger, D. R., Linnoila, M., and Wyatt, R. J. (1983): *Am. J. Psychiatry*, 140:21–25.
56. Roberts, E. (1972): *Neurosci. Res. Program Bull.*, 10:468–483.
57. Rotman, A., Munitz, H., Modai, I., Tjano, S., and Wijsenbeek, H. (1980): *Psychiatry Res.*, 3:239–246.
58. Schildkraut, J. J., Gordon, E. K., and Durrel, J. J. (1965): *Psychiatry Res.*, 3:213–228.
59. Schulz, S. C., van Kammen, D. P., Buchsbaum, M. S., Roth, R. H., Alexander, P., and Bunney, W. E., Jr. (1981): *Pharmacopsychiatria*, 14:129–134.
60. Sedvall, G., Fyrö, B., Gullberg, B., Nybäck, H., Wiesel, F.-A., and Wode-Helgodt, B. (1980): *Br. J. Psychiatry*, 136:366–374.
61. Shore, D., Korpi, E. R., Bigelow, L. B., Zec, R. F., and Wyatt, R. J. (1985): *Biol. Psychiatry*, 20:329–352.
62. Simpson, G. M., Branchey, M. H., and Shrivastava, R. K. (1976): *Lancet*, 1:966–967.
63. Stahl, S., Uhr, S., and Berger, P. (1985): *Biol. Psychiatry*, 20: 1098–1102.
64. Stahl, S. M., Woo, D. J., Mefford, I. N., Berger, P. A., and Ciaranello, R. D. (1983): *Am. J. Psychiatry*, 140:26–30.
65. Stockmeier, C. A., Martin, A. M., and Kellar, K. J. (1985): *Science*, 230:323–325.
66. Tamminga, C. A., Crayton, J. W., and Chase, T. N. (1979): *Arch. Gen. Psychiatry*, 36:595–598.
67. Tamminga, C. A., Thaker, J. R., Ferraro, T. N., and Hare, T. A. (1983): *Lancet*, 2:97–98.
68. Todrick, A., Tait, A. C., Marshall, E. F., et al. (1960): *Br. J. Psychiatry*, 106:884–890.
69. van Kammen, D. P. (1977): *Am. J. Psychiatry*, 134:138–143.
70. van Kammen, D. P., Mann, L. S., Scheinin, M., van Kammen, W. B., and Linnoila, M. (1984): *Psychopharmacol. Bull.*, 20:519–522.
71. van Kammen, D. P., Mann, L. S., Seppala, T., van Kammen, W. B., and Linnoila, M. (1986): *Arch. Gen. Psychiatry*, 43:978–983.
72. van Kammen, D. P., Sternberg, E. D., Hare, T. A., Waters, R. N., and Bunney, W. E., Jr. (1982): *Arch. Gen. Psychiatry*, 39: 91–97.
73. Wolkowitz, O. M., Pickar, D., Doran, A. R., Breier, A., Tarell, J., and Paul, S. M. (1986): *Am. J. Psychiatry*, 143:85–87.
74. Woolley, D. W., and Shaw, E. (1954): *Proc. Natl. Acad. Sci. USA*, 40:228–231.
75. Zahn, T. P., Carpenter, W. T., and McGlashan, T. H. (1981): *Arch. Gen. Psychiatry*, 38:251–258.

Psychopharmacology:
The Third Generation of Progress,
edited by Herbert Y. Meltzer.
Raven Press, New York © 1987.

CHAPTER **74**

Phospholipid and Prostaglandin Hypotheses of Schizophrenia

John Rotrosen and Adam Wolkin

This chapter will review recent work relating membrane lipids and prostaglandins. Although these areas have clearly not been in the mainstream of schizophrenia research, there have been sufficient hypothetical and experimental advances to merit review. Further, pathology related to these two areas may be quite compatible with more traditional approaches to schizophrenia, e.g., membrane lipid changes may alter dopaminergic neurotransmission. The primary goal of this chapter will be to review the potential roles of membrane lipids and prostaglandins as etiopathological agents. A secondary goal will be to examine how endogenous lipids and prostaglandins may be factors in determining drug response and side effects, as well as how exogenous lipids and prostaglandins may themselves be used as therapeutic agents.

PHOSPHOLIPIDS

Although phospholipids are the major components of all cell membranes and are the source of much of a membrane's structural integrity and biophysical properties, until recently they have not received much attention from researchers in psychiatry and neuropsychopharmacology. This was due in part to the view that the phospholipids that composed the bilamellar membrane leaflet were relatively static and served only to provide a skeleton or matrix to support and structure membrane proteins. Gradually, it was recognized that the membrane lipid microenvironment surrounding these proteins had important regulatory characteristics and affected enzyme activity *per se* as well as receptor enzyme coupling, ion transport, etc. More recently it has been shown that membrane lipids have direct second messenger functions themselves, and that these may well be as important as those attributed to cyclic AMP.

In 1972, John Stevens (50) published what was perhaps the first report describing membrane lipid pathology in schizophrenia. He studied the lipid composition of erythrocyte membranes from 101 schizophrenics and compared these to 20 normal controls. Of the four major phospholipids studied, Stevens found a marked increase in phosphatidylserine (PS) in schizophrenics and associated smaller decreases in phosphatidylcholine and phosphatidylethanolamine (PE). Stevens was foresighted in his brief discussion in which he pointed out that if these membrane abnormalities extended to the brain, they "could change the electrostatic charge at the synapse and thus have an influence on the threshold and transmission of impulses." Indeed, membrane abnormalities that can be detected in formed blood elements are now known to be associated with a number of neurologic and neuromuscular disorders, including Duchenne muscular dystrophy, myotonia, Huntington's chorea, the gangliosidoses, and Friedreich's ataxia (8).

Stevens' finding of a nearly 50% increase in membrane PS in schizophrenics is particularly interesting in light of the pharmacology of PS—a pharmacology that could not have been appreciated in 1972, but which now suggests that PS has diverse membrane regulatory properties and a broad array of effects on catecholamine neurotransmission. PS is particularly highly enriched in the brain, where it comprises between 10 and 20% of the total brain phospholipid pool. PS is localized asymmetrically more on the inner, cytosolic aspect of the membrane bilayer than it is on the outer extracellular surface. From a structural viewpoint this is important because PS is acidic and negatively charged, and therefore contributes to the transmembrane electrical dipole. Likewise from a metabolic perspective this is important because of the asymmetrical localization of phospholipid methylation enzymes (23).

Many of PS's pharmacologic properties are thought to be mediated by its conversion to lysoPS, which is a very short-lived intermediate (6). Another important metabolic pathway is decarboxylation of PS to PE and subsequent sequential methylation to form phosphatidyl-*N*-mono-methylethanolamine (PME), phosphatidyl-*N*-dimethyleth-anolamine (PDE), and finally PC; the methyl donor for these reactions is *S*-adenosyl methionine (SAM). Activation of this methylation pathway has been shown in a number of different cell types to be associated with increased membrane fluidity, increased cell surface receptor exposure, and enhanced efficiency of receptor-second messenger coupling (15,23). In addition, PC formed by this pathway is preferentially used as a source of free choline as a precursor for acetylcholine (5).

When it is administered peripherally, PS elicits a number of pharmacological effects on CNS neurotransmitter function and on behavior in rodents. Leon and Toffano (42) reported that a mixed brain phospholipid preparation enhanced the turnover of brain catecholamines, and Mantovani et al. (44) and Amaducci et al. (3) showed that the same preparation stimulated the release of acetylcholine from cerebral cortex. These effects have since been demonstrated to be due to PS.

Acute treatment with PS is followed by a short-lived decrease in hypothalamic levels of norepinephrine accompanied by a marked increase in levels of its major metabolite, 3-methoxy-4-hydroxyphenylglycol (MHPG). These effects are observed at doses ranging from 5 to 50 mg/kg and suggest that PS enhances turnover of norepinephrine (39). Increased dopamine turnover in corpus striatum and increased norepinephrine turnover in cortex also occur, but at higher doses from 50 to 100 mg/kg (51). The increases in catecholamine turnover appear to ultimately affect synaptic receptors, since they elicit increases in cyclic AMP that can be blocked with appropriate receptor antagonists (51).

Casamenti et al. (9) found that *in vivo* injections of PS elicited a dose-dependent and calcium-dependent increase in acetylcholine release that was prevented by prior administration of the dopamine receptor antagonist pimozide. PS did not enhance acetylcholine release when it was added to brain slices *in vitro*. Further, the effects of PS were specific, and not shared to any significant extent by other phospholipids. They concluded that the effects of PS were mediated (at least in part) indirectly via a dopaminergic pathway.

The behavioral effects of PS in animals are somewhat diverse; whereas these effects appear to suggest therapeutic potential in treating age-related cognitive decline, certain of PS's actions might well have relevance to schizophrenia. PS enhances acquisition of shuttle box avoidance behavior, facilitates acquisition, and retards extinction of pole-jump active avoidance. Likewise, treatment with PS improves retention of a single-learning-trial passive avoidance task (11,16,56).

Drago et al. (17) noted that intellectual impairment may be a consequence of suboptimal dendritic arborization or synaptogenesis during CNS development. Further, they point out that perinatal administration of antibodies to synaptic membrane components can reduce arborization and produce later behavioral deficits in adult rats and in acquisition of normal behaviors during postnatal develop-

ment. They found that PS-treated pups showed precocious development of maturational behaviors and later showed improved acquisition of avoidance behaviors. Drago et al. suggest that PS may have trophic effects on synaptic development similar to those attributed to gangliosides, and that these effects may underlie some of PS's effects on behavioral expression.

Stevens' findings were largely ignored for nearly a decade until they were virtually replicated by Henn (22), who studied 20 schizophrenics and 15 controls. The most striking aspect of Henn's report was that when the data were analyzed by looking at the ratio of PE (decreased in schizophrenics) to PS (increased) there was almost no overlap between schizophrenics and controls. Thus, it appeared that these findings represented both a marker and a laboratory test for schizophrenia and suggested new leads with possible etiopathological implications that were compatible with the dopamine hypothesis. Unfortunately, attempts at replication in other laboratories have yielded conflicting data; in fact, findings from these other laboratories differ not only from those of Stevens and Henn, but differ among themselves. The reasons for these differences remain to be determined.

Using both thin-layer chromatography with phosphorous determination and high-performance liquid chromatography (HPLC) separation with UV detection, Lautin et al. (41) found virtually identical phospholipid ratios between schizophrenics and controls for PS, PC, PE, and SPM. Hitzeman and Garver (24) reported a small but statistically highly significant decrease in PC in schizophrenics (similar to the Stevens and Henn finding), an increase in sphingomyelin (SPM) in schizophrenics, and no changes in PS or PE. Sengupta et al. (49) reported a nearly 70% increase in erythrocyte membrane PC in schizophrenics, accompanied by a 50% decrease in PE, and a 50% increase in PS; SPM and phosphatidylinositol (PI) were identical in schizophrenics and controls. In these studies Sengupta et al. reported that schizophrenics' erythrocytes contained nearly 70% more total lipid, 110% more phospholipid, and 40% more cholesterol than did erythrocytes of controls (on a per milligram protein basis). Similar results (for both total lipid and for individual phospholipids) were reported for platelets from the same patient groups. Tolbert et al. (52) found that schizophrenics had a highly significant increase in erythrocyte PS, a decrease in PE, a trend toward a decrease in PC, and no change in SPM. Finally, Buckman et al. (7) have found a small but significant increase in PS and a decrease in PC in platelets from paranoid schizophrenics; PI and PE did not differ between schizophrenics and controls. In erythrocytes, Buckman et al. report that paranoid schizophrenics show a significant increase in PI, a trend toward an increase in PS, a significant decrease in PC, and no difference in PE compared to controls. These data are summarized in Table 1.

In spite of the lack of consistent findings in this area, a number of these laboratories have extended the basic quantitative aspects of this work by looking at biochemical, physiologic, and treatment response correlates of these membrane lipid abnormalities. Thus, Rotrosen et al. (unpublished data) have attempted to develop a model for elevated membrane PS by chronically treating rats and

TABLE 1. *Phospholipids in schizophrenics*

Author	Year	Schiz (n)	Controls (n)	Tissue	Method	PS	PE	PC	SPM	PI
Stevens	1972	101	20	RBCs	TLC	↑ (37%)	↓ (9%)	↓ (10%)	—	n.r.
Henn	1980	20	15	RBCs	TLC	↑ (43%)	↓ (10%)	↓ (9%)	—	n.r.
Sengupta	1981	26	34	RBCs	TLC	↑ (50%)	↓ (47%)	↑ (61%)	—	—
Sengupta	1981	26	34	Platelets	TLC	↑ (22%)	↓ (48%)	↑ (31%)	—	—
Lautin	1982	27	14	RBCs	TLC	—	—	—	—	n.r.
Lautin	1982	16	16	RBCs	HPLC	—	—	—	n.r.	n.r.
Hitzeman	1982	23	15	RBCs	TLC	—	—	↓ (13%)	↑ (22%)	—
Hitzeman	1984	33	35	RBCs	TLC	—	—	↓ (10%)	—	—
Hitzeman	1985	20	12	RBCs	TLC	n.r.	n.r.	↓ (11%)	n.r.	n.r.
Tolbert	1983	17	31	RBCs	TLC	↑ (20%)	↓ (14%)	↓ (4%)	—	n.r.
Buckman	1985	13	8	Platelets	HPLC	↑ (50%)	—	↓ (10%)	n.r.	—
Buckman	1985	13	8	RBCs	HPLC	↑ (25%)	—	↓ (9%)	n.r.	↑ (40%)

Notes: ↑, schiz > controls; ↓, schiz < controls; —, schiz = controls; (xx%) = % change from control value; n.r., not reported; HPLC, high-performance liquid chromatography; TLC, thin-layer chromatography; RBCs, red blood cells.

mice with serine (both by intraperitoneal injection and by a serine-enriched diet). Despite prolonged high-dose treatment, they were unable to obtain an increase in PS in either erythrocytes or synaptosomes; the other major phospholipids were not affected.

Hitzemann, Hirschowitz, and Garver (24–26) have focused primarily on the reduction of red blood cell (RBC) membrane PC, and have begun to correlate this membrane abnormality with changes in phospholipid methylation, Na$^+$-Li$^+$ counterflow, and clinical therapeutic response to lithium. On a group basis, patients whose RBCs had reduced membrane PC also showed reduced [^{3}H]PC synthesis via the phospholipid methylation pathway when exogenous [^{3}H]SAM was used as precursor. For three patient groups, schizophrenia, schizophreniform disorder, and mania, there was a rank order correlation between membrane PC levels and [^{3}H]PC formation; however, there was no correlation on an individual basis. PC levels in RBCs from manics were not statistically significantly reduced compared to controls.

In a related study schizophrenic and schizophreniform patients were evaluated for treatment response to lithium. Based on RBC PC levels these patients were divided into upper and lower quartiles. Those in the lowest PC quartile had higher 24-hr lithium ratios (increased 43%) than did those in the highest PC quartile. Differences in phospholipid methylation were also noted between eight lithium-responsive patients and 16 nonresponders. Formation of phosphatidyl-dimethylethanolamine and of PC was reduced approximately 50% in the lithium responders compared to the lithium nonresponders. These two groups, however, did not differ from each other in endogenous RBC PC levels, nor in formation of phosphatidyl-monomethylethanolamine. Thus, although the absolute differences in RBC membrane PC appear to be small (approximately 10% change from controls, and not differing at all between patient subpopulations), they are associated with marked differences in lithium transport. Reduced phospholipid methylation, not associated with differences in membrane PC, appears to define a clinically important subgroup of schizophrenic and

schizophreniform patients that is responsive to treatment with lithium.

Tolbert, Monti, and Smythies and their collaborators (2,40,46,52) have approached the reduction of membrane PC by way of their interest in enzymes of one-carbon metabolism. Kelsoe et al. (40) reported that both the V_{max} and K_m for methionine adenosyltransferase (MAT), the enzyme responsible for synthesis of SAM, are reduced in RBCs from schizophrenics compared to those from controls. More recently Tolbert et al. (52) found that the reduction in MAT was highly correlated with the reduction of membrane PC. They suggest that reduced SAM levels are insufficient to maintain phospholipid methylation, and that as a result, membrane PC levels are low. They also suggest that the reduced MAT activity might account for schizophrenics' low plasma levels of SAM that had previously been reported by Andreoli and Maffei (4), as well as the report of Ismail et al. (33) describing decreased oxidation of methionine in leukocytes from schizophrenics.

Buckman's work in this area is an extension of his studies on the selective regulatory effects of PS on type B monoamine oxidase (MAO) from various tissues. Buckman et al. (7) found a marked decrease in MAO B activity in platelets from paranoid schizophrenics compared to those from residual/undifferentiated schizophrenics or healthy controls. Further, they reported that PS inhibited MAO B activity and that the IC$_{50}$ for PS was approximately 70% greater for paranoid schizophrenics than for either of their other two populations. It is suggested that the lower sensitivity to exogenous PS seen in platelets from paranoid schizophrenics might be a result of already present inhibition by high levels of endogenous PS.

Overall, there seems to be good reason to continue to study membrane lipids in schizophrenia. It is not at all apparent why such discrepant findings have emerged from different laboratories. Potentially fruitful areas of investigation that should be pursued in future studies include (a) continued attempts to relate changes in membrane lipids to physiological functioning (e.g., lithium transport, membrane fluidity), enzyme changes (e.g., MAT, phospholipid methylation, MAO, prostaglandin synthesis), treatment response, and other clinical features, and (b) attempts to evaluate the degree to which membrane changes in RBCs and platelets extend to the CNS and to other tissues.

PROSTAGLANDINS

The prostaglandins (PGs) are a group of 20 carbon cyclopentane carboxylic acids which are synthesized from precursor fatty acids in response to a given stimulus, exert their effects *in situ,* and are rapidly metabolized both locally and in distant organs. In the CNS, gross effects of various PGs (over a range of doses) include sedation (32) (from mild tranquilization to catatonia), euphoria (31), alteration in body temperature and food intake, and actions on spinal and postural mechanisms (10). At the neuronal level, PGs are thought to have a neuromodulatory role. PG synthesis and release is enhanced by increased neural activity in a number of neurotransmitter systems. Conversely, PG release modifies synaptic events at both the pre- and postsynaptic level (see 10, 32 for references). E-type PGs have been specifically implicated in a negative feedback loop inhibiting catecholamine release (21).

The potential neuromodulatory role of PGs is of obvious relevance to neuropsychiatric disorders with putative neurotransmitter abnormalities. In 1976, Feldberg initially proposed that schizophrenia may be due to a PG excess, citing, in part, that PGE_1 produces catalepsy in animals and that elevated PGE_1 levels are seen in endotoxin-induced cataleptic states (18). Horrobin subsequently proposed that schizophrenia may reflect a PG deficiency (27–29). This hypothesis was based on a variety of circumstantial clinical and anecdotal data consistent with decreased PG function in schizophrenics, and also on *in vitro* studies of decreased PG activity in schizophrenics' platelets (*vide infra*). Theoretical support for this hypothesis in part reflected the congruence of evidence for dopaminergic hyperactivity in schizophrenia, and evidence that decreased PG activity might facilitate dopaminergic activity via decreased inhibition of DA release.

In general, a functional PG deficiency could result from a decrease in PG precursors (essential fatty acids), abnormalities in the mobilization and conversion of fatty acids to PGs or in degradative metabolism of PGs, or defects at the PG receptor complex. To date, studies addressing these components of PG system activity in schizophrenia have included (a) *in vitro* assays of PG synthesis and actions in peripheral tissues, (b) measurement of tissue PG and precursor fatty acid levels, and (c) assessment of the antipsychotic efficacy of PGs and PG precursor fatty acids.

In Vitro Assays of PG Activity

Using platelet preparations from 20 schizophrenics, 8 normals, and 18 other psychiatric subjects, Abdullah and Hamadah (1) measured the ADP-enhanced synthesis of $[^{14}C]PGE_1$ from $[^{14}C]$dihomo-gammalinolenic acid (DHLA, 20:4ω6). Basal rates of $[^{14}C]PGE_1$ synthesis were similar in all subjects. ADP greatly stimulated PGE_1 synthesis in

platelets from controls, but had absolutely no effect on PGE_1 synthesis in schizophrenics' platelets.

This report was followed by a series of studies several years later in which the ability of PGE_1 to stimulate cyclic AMP was used as an index of PG receptor sensitivity in platelets. Rotrosen et al. studied PGE_1-stimulated $[^3H]$cyclic AMP accumulation in 21 controls and 28 schizophrenics (47). Significantly less PGE_1-stimulated $[^3H]$cyclic AMP accumulation was seen in platelets from schizophrenics than in those from controls at 0.5 and 10 μM concentrations of PGE_1. Similar data have also been reported by Kafka and van Kammen (35) and in a subsequent report by Rotrosen et al. (48). Neuroleptics added *in vitro* did not alter basal or PGE_1-stimulated $[^3H]$cyclic AMP accumulation.

Decreased cyclic AMP production upon PGE_1 stimulation could potentially be the result of a defect in one of several steps in the receptor activation–adenylate cyclase stimulation–cyclic AMP production sequence. Garver et al. attempted to delineate the basis for decreased cyclic AMP production in schizophrenics (19). Using disrupted platelet preparations from 20 schizophrenics and 11 normal controls, they measured cyclic AMP generation induced either by NaF (which directly stimulates adenylate cyclase) or PGE_1. Again, schizophrenics had less PGE_1-stimulated cyclic AMP generation than did normals (by approximately 30%). However, there were no differences in NaF-induced cyclic AMP generation. These results were interpreted as "evidence for a membrane associated abnormality of either receptor or receptor-adenylate cyclase linkage in schizophrenics" (19). Kafka and van Kammen (34) also extended their earlier finding with measurements of basal and PGE_1-stimulated cyclic AMP production. As compared with 31 male controls, 28 medication-free male schizophrenics had significantly lower basal and PGE_1-stimulated cyclic AMP production in both intact and lysed platelets. In contrast to Garver, Kafka and van Kammen also observed decreased NaF-stimulated cyclic AMP production and suggested that the decrease in cyclic AMP formation in schizophrenia may be due to reduced adenylate cyclase activity.

Kaiya et al. attempted to assess responsivity to PGE_1 by measuring its effect in blocking ADP-induced platelet aggregation (37). They found no differences in ADP-stimulated aggregation between 18 controls, 18 unmedicated schizophrenics (for 3 months), and 13 treated schizophrenics. Kaiya et al. concluded that these results supported a hyposensitive PGE_1-receptor system, and might therefore be consistent with the findings above.

Measurement of PGs and Precursor Fatty Acids

Mathe et al. measured total immunoreactive PGE in CSF from eight medication-free schizophrenics (45). As compared with nine controls, schizophrenics had markedly higher total PGE levels. Gerner and Merrill also determined CSF PGE levels using 18 schizophrenics and an equal number of controls (20). They found no differences in total PGE between the two groups. However, the authors pointed out that alterations in either PGE_1 or PGE_2 conceivably could be obscured by measuring total PGE, and that total

CSF levels might not reflect localized brain alterations in PGE synthesis. Linnoila et al. examined CSF levels of PGE_2, $PGF_{2\alpha}$, and 6-keto-$PGF_{1\alpha}$ in 11 schizophrenics and 12 patients with affective disorders (43). PGE_2 was nondetectable in schizophrenics, whereas measurable levels were found in six subjects with affective disorders. F-type PGs were also undetectable in schizophrenics.

Abnormalities in PG synthesis might potentially arise from a precursor deficiency. One- and two-series PGs are synthesized from omega-6 fatty acid precursors, with the 1-series derived from DHLA and the 2-series from conversion of arachidonic acid (AA) (30). AA and DHLA are in turn derived from shorter-chain essential fatty acid (EFA) precursors according to the sequence: cis-linoleic (cLA, 18: $2\omega6$) → γ-linolenic (GLA, 18:$3\omega6$) → DHLA → AA.

Hitzemann and Garver measured fatty acid levels in the PC fraction of red cell ghosts from controls and lithium nonresponsive schizophrenics (26). Both cLA and DHLA levels were lower, whereas AA levels were threefold greater in schizophrenics. Vaddadi et al. measured RBC fatty acid levels in 16 medicated schizophrenics and 14 controls (54). Schizophrenics had significantly lower levels of cLA and AA, as well as some longer-chain fatty acids, whereas their GLA levels were higher. In collaboration with Horrobin, Wolkin et al. (unpublished data, 1983) measured fatty acids in total RBC membrane phospholipids from 10 medicated, chronic schizophrenics and 13 controls. Mean values were not significantly different for any of the 16- to 22-carbon omega-6 fatty acids that were measured.

PG and PG Precursor Supplementation

Kaiya et al. (36) initially reported the effects of daily intravenous infusions of 40 to 100 μg of PGE_1 in an open study with six schizophrenics. At 28 days, a marked decrease in Brief Psychiatric Rating Scale (BPRS) scores was observed in three patients. In a subsequent study (38), Kaiya administered 100 to 250 μg of PGE_1 for 8 to 23 days to seven schizophrenic and schizophreniform subjects. A 50% decrease in BPRS scores was noted in one schizophreniform subject and in one undifferentiated schizophrenic. The two subjects who responded to PGE_1 had quite elevated pretreatment levels of plasma PGE immunoreactivity, which decreased upon initiation of PGE_1 administration.

A hypothetical PG deficiency in schizophrenia might conceivably be corrected by increasing precursor EFA availability. Traditionally, PGs were thought to derive from EFAs (DHLA and AA) esterified to phospholipids in cell membranes. Since this fatty acid pool is comparatively large relative to dietary intake of EFAs, it seemed improbable that PG synthesis would be significantly affected by manipulation of dietary PGs. However, Crawford has recently suggested that there might be two sources of PG precursors: a structural cell membrane pool and a mobile, dietary pool. According to Crawford "the metabolic pathway would be more directly influenced in the short term by the dietary levels of EFA and other fatty acids, whereas the membrane pool of PG precursor would be expected to be that much more stable and susceptible only to long-term dietary manipulations" (14).

Vaddadi et al. first reported improvement in two chronic, refractory schizophrenics when treated with a combination of EFA supplementation (GLA 100 mg/day and cLA 700 mg/day) and penicillin (53). Subsequently, Vaddadi et al. examined the efficacy of EFA supplementation in 21 schizophrenics (54). EFA supplementation consisted of 1 g/day of DHLA. BPRS scores tended to improve with both EFA and inactive treatments; there were no significant differences between groups.

Wolkin et al. (unpublished data, 1983) have assessed the effects of GLA supplementation in 14 chronic schizophrenics on a stable neuroleptic regimen. Subjects received either GLA, 300 mg/day, or placebo on a double-blind basis. At the end of 6 weeks, there were no group differences in either BPRS, nuclear schizophrenic symptoms, or negative symptoms.

In the course of their clinical trials, both Vaddadi and Kaiya noted amelioration of dyskinetic movements in several patients. Costall and Naylor have reported that 5 days pretreatment with DHLA (100 mg/kg i.p.) abolished dopamine-induced (intrastriatal) oral dyskinesia in guinea pigs (13). This effect was blocked by aspirin, suggesting mediation through PG synthesis. Similar results have been reported with direct administration of PGs (12). These data support an antidopaminergic influence of PGE_1 and suggest a novel treatment for tardive dyskinesia.

Based on this rationale, Wolkin et al. (55) studied the effects of GLA (600 mg/day) in a placebo-controlled, double-blind study of 16 patients with mild to moderate tardive dyskinesia. Tardive dyskinesia was rated at baseline and at 6 weeks with the AIMS exam. GLA supplementation at the dose used had no effects.

The results of the studies outlined above offer modest support for PG system abnormalities in some schizophrenics. Many of the findings are contradictory, and the nature of such a disturbance remains unclear. The most consistent evidence is suggested by in vitro platelet studies. Measurement of PGE_1-stimulated cyclic AMP accumulation possibly implicates PGE_1 receptor complex dysfunction and suggests further study in order to dissect the aberrant steps in receptor stimulation.

Although EFA supplementation may affect PG synthesis and activity, the data to date do not strongly support antipsychotic efficacy for the EFA dose regimens that were used. The few reports of improvement have been from open studies, whereas double-blind, controlled studies have all been negative. In the absence of corollary measures of PG activity, it is unclear whether these EFA supplementation studies actually enhanced PG synthesis. As noted above, there are data that EFA supplementation may increase PG synthesis; however, it is unknown at what dose this effect occurs in the CNS in humans. Thus, the results of these EFA trials do not necessarily argue against a PG deficiency hypothesis.

Intravenous infusion of PGs provides a direct method by which to observe the CNS effects of increased PG availability and to test the PG deficiency hypothesis. Initial results with PGE_1 are promising, but may reflect biases inherent in uncontrolled studies. There is quite preliminary evidence that clinical response to PGE may relate to initial

PGE levels. This suggests a biological subgroup in which EFA/PG abnormalities may be of relevance.

Perhaps more exciting, both in terms of potential efficacy and therapeutic feasibility, are the findings of Costall and Naylor. Their preclinical results strongly suggest that EFAs may have specific antidyskinetic effects. Although Wolkin et al. observed no beneficial results from GLA in the treatment of tardive dyskinesia, the EFA regimen represented a lower dose and a more distal step (relative to PG synthesis) than that used by Costall and Naylor. Future studies, of theoretical and practical interest, using PGE_1 and DHLA are clearly warranted in tardive dyskinesia.

ACKNOWLEDGMENTS

This work was supported in part by the Veterans Administration. The authors wish to thank Ms. Shirley Irons for editorial assistance.

REFERENCES

1. Abdulla, Y. H., and Hamadah, K. (1975): *Br. J. Psychiatry,* 127: 591–595.
2. Alarcon, R. D., Tolbert, L. C., Monti, J. A., Morere, D. A., Walter-Ryan, W. G., Kemp, B., and Smythies, J. R. (1985): *J. Affective Disord.,* 9:297–301.
3. Amaducci, L., Mantovani, P., and Pepeu, G. (1976): *Br. J. Pharmacol.,* 56:379.
4. Andreoli, W. M., and Maffei, T. (1979): *Biol. Psychiatry,* 13:773–776.
5. Blusztajn, J. K., and Wurtman, R. J. (1981): *Nature,* 290:417–418.
6. Bruni, A., and Toffano, G. (1982): *Pharmacol. Res. Commun.,* 14:469–484.
7. Buckman, T. D., Orologas, A., and Eiduson, S. (1985): Presented at the International Society for Neurochemistry, Mantova, Italy, May 26–29.
8. Butterfield, D. A., and Markesbury, W. R. (1980): *J. Neurol. Sci.,* 97:261–271.
9. Casamenti, F., Mantovani, P., Amaducci, L., and Pepeu, G. (1979): *J. Neurochem.,* 32:529–533.
10. Coceani, F. (1974): *Arch. Gen. Intern. Med.,* 133:119–129.
11. Corwin, J., Dean, R. L., III, Bartus, R. T., Rotrosen, J., and Watkins, D. L. (1985): *Neurobiology of Aging,* 6:11–15.
12. Costall, B., Holmes, S. W., Kelly, M. E., et al. (1985): *Br. J. Pharmacol.,* 85:943.
13. Costall, B., Kelly, E., and Naylor, R. J. (1984): *Br. J. Pharmacol.,* 83:733–740.
14. Crawford, M. A. (1985): *Br. Med. Bull.,* 39:210–213.
15. Crews, F. T. (1984): In: *Brain Receptor Methodologies, Part A,* edited by P. J. Marangos, I. C. Campbell, and R. M. Cohen, pp. 217–226. Academic Press, New York, NY.
16. Drago, F., Canonico, P. L., and Scapagnini, U. (1981): In: *Neurobiology of Aging, Vol. 2,* pp. 209–213. Ankho International, Inc., USA.
17. Drago, F., Continella, G., Alloro, M. C., LoPresti, L., and Scapagnini, U. (1983): *Personal Communication.*
18. Feldberg, W. (1976): *Psychol. Med.,* 6:359–369.
19. Garver, D. L., Johnson, C., and Kanter, D. R. (1982): *Life Sci.,* 31:1987–1992.
20. Gerner, R. H., and Merrill, J. E. (1983): *Biol. Psychiatry,* 18:565–569.
21. Hedqvist, P. (1973): In: *The Prostaglandins, Vol. 1,* edited by P. W. Ramwell, pp. 101–132. Plenum Press, New York.
22. Henn, F. A. (1980): In: *Perspectives in Schizophrenia Research,* edited by C. Baxter and T. Melnachuk, p. 209. Raven Press, New York.
23. Hirata, F., and Axelrod, J. (1980): *Science,* 209:1082–1090.
24. Hitzemann, R., and Garver, D. (1982): *Psychopharmacol. Bull.,* 18:190–193.
25. Hitzemann, R., Hirschowitz, J., and Garver, D. (1984): *J. Psychiatry Res.,* 18:319–326.
26. Hitzemann, R., Mark, C., Hirschowitz, J., and Garver, D. (1985): *Biol. Psychiatry,* 20:397–407.
27. Horrobin, D. F. (1977): *Lancet,* 1:936–937.
28. Horrobin, D. F. (1978): *Psychol. Med.,* 8:43–48.
29. Horrobin, D. F. (1979): *Lancet,* 1:529–530.
30. Horrobin, D. F. (1980): *Med. Hypotheses,* 6:687–709.
31. Horrobin, D. F. (1987): *Alcohol Clin. Exp. Res.,* 11:2–9, 1987.
32. Horton, E. W. (1972): *Monogr. Endocrinol.,* 7:117–149.
33. Ismail, L., Sargent, T., Dobson, E. L., and Pollycore, M. (1978): *Biol. Psychiatry,* 13:649–660.
34. Kafka, M. S., and van Kammen, D. P. (1983): *Arch. Gen. Psychiatry,* 40:264–270.
35. Kafka, M. S., van Kammen, D. P., and Bunney, W. E. (1979): *Am. J. Psychiatry,* 136:685–687.
36. Kaiya, H. (1985): *Biol. Psychiatry,* 19:457–463.
37. Kaiya, H., Imai, H., and Murumatsu, Y. (1983): *Psychiatric Res.,* 9:309–318.
38. Kaiya, H., Takai, A., and Morita, K. (1985): In: *Clinical and Pharmacological Studies in Psychiatric Disorders,* edited by G. D. Burrows and T. R. Norman. John Libbey, London.
39. Kaiya, H., Takeuchi, K., Namba, M., Imai, A., Nakashima, S., and Nozawa, Y. (1984): *Folia Psychiatr. Neurol. Jpn.,* 38:437–444.
40. Kelsoe, J. R., Jr., Tolbert, L. C., Crews, E. L., and Smythies, J. R. (1982): *J. Neurosci. Res.,* 8:99–103.
41. Lautin, A., Mandio Cordasco, D., Segarnick, D. J., Wod, L., Mason, M. F., and Rotrosen, J. (1982): *Life Sci.,* 31:3051–3056.
42. Leon, A., and Toffano, G. (1976): *Adv. Exp. Med. Biol.,* 72:307–313.
43. Linnoila, M., Whorton, R., Rubinow, D. R., et al. (1983): *Arch. Gen. Psychiatry,* 40:405–506.
44. Mantovani, P., Pepeu, G., and Amaducci, L. (1976): *Adv. Med. Biol.,* 72:285–292.
45. Mathe, A. A., Sedvall, G., Wiesal, F. A., et al. (1980): *Lancet,* 1: 16–18.
46. Morere, D. A., Alarcon, D., Monti, J. A., Walter-Ryan, W. G., Bancroft, A. J., Smythies, J. R., and Tolbert, L. C. (1986): *J. Clin. Psychopharmacol.,* 6:155–161.
47. Rotrosen, J., Miller, A., Mandio, D., et al. (1978): *Life Sci.,* 23: 1989–1996.
48. Rotrosen, J., Miller, A., Mandio, D., et al. (1980): *Arch. Gen. Psychiatry,* 37:1047–1054.
49. Sengupta, N., Datta, S. C., and Sengupta, D. (1981): *Biochem. Med.,* 25:267–275.
50. Stevens, J. D. (1972): *Schizophr. Bull.,* 6:60–61.
51. Toffano, G., Leon, A., Mazzari, S., Savoini, G., Teolato, S., and Orlando, P. (1978): *Life Sci.,* 23:1093–1102.
52. Tolbert, L. C., Monti, J. A., O'Shields, H., Walter-Ryan, W., Meadows, D., and Smythies, J. R. (1983): *Psychopharmacol. Bull.,* 19:594–599.
53. Vaddadi, K. S. (1979): *Prostaglandins Med.,* 2:77–80.
54. Vaddadi, K. S., Gilleard, C. J., Mindham, R. H. S., et al. (1986): *J. Psychopharmacol.,* 88:362–367.
55. Wolkin, A., Jordan, B., Peselow, E., Rubinstein, M., and Rotrosen, J. (1986): *Am. J. Psychiatry,* 143:912–914.
56. Zanotti, A., Aporti, F., Toffano, G., and Valzelli, L. (1984): *Pharmacol. Res. Commun.,* 16:485–493.

Psychopharmacology:
The Third Generation of Progress,
edited by Herbert Y. Meltzer.
Raven Press, New York © 1987.

CHAPTER 75

Viral and Immune Hypotheses for Schizophrenia

Lynn E. DeLisi

THE VIRAL HYPOTHESIS OF SCHIZOPHRENIA

Most hypotheses for the etiology of schizophrenia include an interaction between environmental and genetic determinants. Whether there exist several nonspecific environmental factors (e.g., toxins, head injury, obstetrical complications, infections), any of which can, in a genetically vulnerable individual, produce schizophrenia, or whether there is one specific factor in all cases is unknown. The importance of exposure to a specific virus, or perhaps any virus that has a predilection for the central nervous system, has been proposed. Although some viruses are known to initiate behavioral disturbances, whether they are prime etiological agents for known clinically characterized psychiatric disorders is speculative. It is known that some viruses integrate into the human genome (e.g., retroviruses), and in some instances, infection of germ cells occurs, transmitting viral DNA to later generations in a mendelian fashion (61). Thus, an alternative to an interaction of a viral etiology with genetic predisposition is that specific types of viral infections (retroviral) may even explain the genetics of schizophrenia (as stated by Crow, refs. 19, 20).

Historical Origins

Reports that psychosis may be contagious date back to the nineteenth century (24,59,128,153), although this generally had been attributed to a psychological influence, as in cases of *folie à deux,* rather than to microbial transmission.

Bruce and Peebles reported in 1903 that leukocytosis and elevated body temperature were associated with acute onset of dementia praecox (13). However, the possibility that some psychoses could be virally induced was not considered until Karl Menninger identified psychoses associated with the influenza outbreaks of 1889–1892 and 1918–1919 (100,101). One-third of these, he reported, resembled dementia praecox, although usually with a better prognosis. Other early investigators (55,98) described schizophrenic symptoms as sequelae of encephalitis lethargica.

Goodall in 1932 (44), after reviewing similar observations of several investigators (67,96,102,110,116,122,126), appears to have been the first to formulate a specific viral hypothesis. In an excerpt from an address before The Royal Medico-Psychological Association he stated:

> Epidemic encephalitis, with the psycho-somatic disorders which may accompany it, may be a virus disease . . . and similarly caused, perhaps are the schizophrenic states which resemble them, katatonia especially. The same cause may be operative in the two conditions, differences in the clinical picture being due to differences in individuals, based on heredity or inborn predisposition.

It is now recognized that a number of viral encephalitides may present with, or be followed by, symptoms resembling schizophrenia (11,34,42,63,105,114,131,150). Mononucleosis, commonly caused by the Epstein-Barr virus, has occasionally been found in association with a schizophrenic-like disorder (77,115,125). Acquired Immune Deficiency Disorder (AIDS), now attributed to a retrovirus, and increasing in prevalence, is known to have associated neurologic and psychiatric symptoms (12). Whereas these reports suggest that virus infections of the central nervous system can cause schizophrenia-like symptoms, it remains to be shown that the clinical syndrome of chronic schizophrenia may be virally induced in significant numbers of individuals.

Epidemiologic Evidence

Some researchers argue that the scarcity of descriptions of what would now be regarded as schizophrenia prior to 1800, suggests that schizophrenia is a disease that has increased in prevalence (49,139), as might occur with the appearance of a new infectious agent. However, others (reviewed by Wilson, 152) conclude that there is evidence in the literature of schizophrenia dating back to antiquity.

The finding of a seasonal distribution in the birth rates of schizophrenics, a disproportionate number being born in the late winter and early spring (50,113,139,141,148), suggests that the similar seasonality of some viral infections may have an effect on perinatal brain development. This may predispose individuals toward schizophrenic illness in adult life.

Although the prevalence of schizophrenia is widely believed to be constant in different populations, reports of prevalence rates higher than expected in northern Sweden (10), western Ireland (71), and Croatia (18), while lower than expected in Papua-New Guinea (141) and Micronesia (22) remain unexplained. If present, clusters of high density of illness may represent genetic isolates, or geographic locations where a specific virus or other environmental agent is prevalent.

If temporal and geographical variations exist, and are to be explained in terms of a viral etiology, some evidence of horizontal transmission might be expected. One study from Moscow claims an increased incidence of schizophrenia among genetically unrelated individuals residing in close proximity to an already defined case of schizophrenia (69). This study, however, does not appear consistent with data from adoption studies finding increased illness in biologic relatives, but not adoptive relatives of schizophrenic probands (72).

Despite evidence from adoption studies, other findings from family studies, which can not be explained solely from a genetic viewpoint, are compatible with close contact playing a role in the development of schizophrenia (19). For example, higher concordance rates for schizophrenia in monozygotic than dizygotic twins support the genetic hypothesis (reviewed by Gottesman and Shields, 46). However, concordance rates are also higher among dizygotic twins than siblings (39), and in same-sex than in opposite-sex pairs of dizygotic twins (123), although in both instances genes are shared to the same extent. Abe (1) found the risk of schizophrenia to the second twin of monozygotic pairs increased in the 2 years following the development of illness in the first twin, with increased risk confined to twins residing together during that time. A possible explanation (proposed by Crow, 19) for these findings is that proximity (assumed to be greater in same-sex than opposite-sex dizygotic twin pairs, and in dizygotic twins than in siblings) to an affected individual increases risk for the disease. Similarly, genetic factors are known to be relevant in other diseases with established infectious etiology (e.g., tuberculosis, (66); and poliomyelitis, (56)). Even in those

disorders that appear to have clear mendelian inheritance (e.g., Huntington's chorea) it cannot be excluded that the disease is initiated by a viral infection (51).

Evidence against the occurrence of contagion comes from data on the age of onset of illness in sibling pairs with schizophrenia. If the disorder is contagious, one would expect a close association of time of onset (only separated by an unknown incubation period) if one sibling acquires illness from the other, or even closer if both acquire it from the same source regardless of their ages of onset. However, this does not appear to be the case (21). The significant correlation of actual ages of onset among sibling pairs suggests genetic or early (intrauterine) influences. This lack of evidence for contagion does not, however, rule out a viral etiology. If acquisition of the virus occurs *in utero* or close to birth, actual ages of onset in ill sibling pairs will be correlated. The season of birth effect, which has been found in association with a negative family history for illness (76), might be specifically related to this method of acquisition.

Associations with Specific Viruses

In attempts to identify a specific virus likely to be the causal agent, different experimental approaches have been employed. Past exposure to specific viruses, or the presence of active infection, as reflected in serum and CSF antibody titers has been studied. Whereas some investigations uncovered elevated antibody titers to the herpes class viruses (2,25,45,86,140,143,144), others fail to confirm these findings (74,75,117,130). No other viral antibody associations with schizophrenia have been found, although antibodies to most known viruses infecting humans have been searched for. To explore whether human retroviruses may be present in schizophrenic patients, two studies have assayed sera and/or CSF for antibodies to proteins of HTLV-I, II, III, and reverse transcriptase (30,119). These studies, however, were negative.

Even when present, elevated viral antibody titers are not evidence of definite viral infection, *per se,* but rather indicate a selective increased activity of lymphocytes able to produce these antibodies. This increased activity may be due to many factors associated with the complex functional network for immune response, including its CNS nervous system interactions, and may have little to do directly with schizophrenia. Even if specifically demonstrating viral infection, no antibody study of patients sampled serially with time shows a rise in antibody titers associated with the onset of illness. An increased susceptibility to certain viral infections might alternatively be a consequence of the degenerative aspects of the psychotic illness, or its long-term treatment. Elevated antibody titers to a variety of viruses have been shown to be present in several neurological disorders; however, the definitive studies to identify the presence of a virus remain to be completed.

Interferon Production

Another immunological index of active infection, detectable CSF interferon levels, has been reported in some

(86,111), but not all, studies (118). The observation of Libikova et al. (87) that chlorpromazine can induce a rise in interferon production in mice infected with an encephalitis virus suggests that the reported increase in patient populations might be a consequence of neuroleptic treatment. The use of interferon as a possible therapeutic agent for schizophrenia has been considered; however, the results from one small nonblind trial of intramuscularly injected interferon (15) are unconvincing.

Neuropathological Evidence

The search for neuropathological evidence of viral infection has not been successful in the majority of studies. Evidence of inflammation is lacking, and studies reporting gliosis in postmortem schizophrenic brains (40,108,133) have not been supported by others (48,120). Nevertheless, some known CNS infections lack such changes (64). Electron microscopic studies in search of viral particles have yet to be carefully done. One recently presented preliminary study from Cuba (104) describing viral-like structures in the brains of schizophrenics needs further confirmation. To date, examination of schizophrenic brains using DNA hybridization or immunohistochemical techniques to detect viral-specific nucleic acid or antigens, respectively, has not produced evidence of any of the herpes class of viruses (4,134,138). Many other classes of viruses have yet to be studied.

The presence of viral-like particles in the CSF from schizophrenic patients was first reported in the 1950s in the USSR and Italy (95,107,127). The techniques used in these studies, however, are crude and difficult to replicate.

Transmission Experiments

Attempts to transmit the unknown infectious agent have also been reported. Malis and Dolgikh (94) (reviewed in Malis, 93) observed excessive mortality of chicken embryos inoculated with serum from schizophrenic patients, although no attempt to specifically replicate this work has been reported. Tyrrell and colleagues (145) described degenerative changes in tissue cultures inoculated with CSF from some schizophrenic patients and patients with other neurological disorders. Attempts at serial passage of this cytopathic effect, however, were unsuccessful, and further studies to characterize the cytopathic agent failed to provide evidence for the presence of a replicating virus (136,137). CSF with cytopathic effects was also injected directly into the brains of marmosets in a series of controlled experiments. Subtle behavioral change appeared in the experimental animals after a delay of 2 to 3 years, whereas animals having received control CSF did not show these changes (5). One other independent study (86), but not another (103), has found similar cytopathic effects of CSF from patients with schizophrenia. A different attempt at transmission to animals using schizophrenic brain was unsuccessful (149). However, random regions from postmortem schizophrenic brain were used, the injected tissue was not screened prior to injection for evidence of any abnormality (as had been the case with the CSF studies), and behavioral assessment,

such as that of Baker and colleagues (5) was not performed, thus hampering any negative conclusions about the ability to transmit a "schizophrenia agent" at present.

THE AUTOIMMUNE AND IMMUNE DYSFUNCTION HYPOTHESES OF SCHIZOPHRENIA

Although evidence of changes in indices of immune responsiveness may support a viral etiology to schizophrenia, the complexity of the immune system, and its CNS connections, make other speculative proposals equally plausible. Dysfunction of specific components of the immune system, may, for example, explain increased susceptibility to certain viruses. If present, these viral infections may or may not be related to the actual disease pathology. Alternatively, abnormalities in CNS neuroregulator metabolism, as discussed elsewhere in this volume, may have significant effects on immune system functioning.

Increased circulating leukocytes, particularly in the acute stages of the disorder, were reported in early studies of schizophrenic patients (13,14,16,23,47,60,112,126,129), although these observations may have represented the easy spread of infectious diseases in institutional settings, and the presence of undiagnosed primary bacterial, parasitic, or viral infection.

One study of blood-forming elements in the bone marrow is not consistent with the above studies, finding a general depression of leukocytosis and decreased maturation of young neutrophils (92). Although elevated total leukocyte counts are no longer noticed, attention has focused on the subtypes of lymphocytes and a possible disproportion of the B cells, T cells, and suppressor T cells. Since these cells function together to maintain balanced immune response, more activity of one functional subtype could have an overall effect on the total response. Increased B cells, decreased T cells, and both increased and decreased suppressor cell percentages have been reported (17,26,78,79,146,156). These, however, are only preliminary findings that may be subject to long-term effects of neuroleptic medication, and have not been consistently found in all studies (70).

Another set of studies has focused on the presence of atypical lymphocytes (similar to those described in the circulation of patients with infectious mononucleosis) in peripheral blood smears from schizophrenic patients (37,58,68) and in bone marrow aspirations (57). Whereas this morphological appearance of lymphocytes may be a consequence of neuroleptic treatment (38), Hirata-Hibi finds increased numbers of these cells in patients who have never been medicated, although there have been failures to replicate this finding (29, and E. F. Torrey et al., unpublished data).

Two early reports described the presence of deficient cellular and immune responsiveness in schizophrenic patients (106,147). Although there have been no attempts to repeat these studies, other studies show decreased in vitro functioning of B and T lymphocytes (89,146) and natural killer cells (29,81). None of these findings are specific to schizophrenia, and many have been shown to be present during psychological stress in normal individuals (43). In addition, *in vitro* functional activity of lymphocytes is reduced by neuroleptics, thus complicating the interpretation of studies of chronically medicated patients (35,91).

Several studies show small subgroups of schizophrenic patients with elevated serum IgG, IgA, or IgM levels (3,33,132,135,140,156), whereas a few studies show decreased immunoglobulin levels (8,27,28,74,75), and one fails to find any differences (121). Elevated levels of IgM and IgG occur in acute response to viral infection, whereas low baseline immunoglobulin levels may result from chronic persistent infection. The heterogeneity of the populations of patients examined, as well as the variable status of patients at the time of blood sampling, may explain some of these inconsistencies. Season of study, gender, race, age, and genetic factors all are additional factors unrelated to acute immune response that influence immunoglobulin production.

Autoimmunity

An autoimmune hypothesis of neuropsychiatric disorders (that psychosis results from an allergic reaction to brain proteins) has long been considered (73). In the late 1930s, Lehmann-Facius (84,85) demonstrated that a lipid-extracted fraction of schizophrenic serum forms a precipitate with brain extract from schizophrenics. Other workers, using different techniques, have since confirmed these results.

In a series of investigations, Heath and co-workers claimed to isolate a factor ("taraxein") from schizophrenic patients that produced catatonia and abnormal brain wave tracings when injected into normal monkeys and humans. Both the behavioral changes and the EEG abnormalities resulting from taraxein injections were similar to those described in schizophrenic patients by these authors (53,54). They suggested that taraxein is an antibody directed against brain protein, and supported this with the demonstration (using an indirect immunofluorescent technique) of the presence of anti-human antibody binding to brain from schizophrenic patients incubated with schizophrenic sera, but not sera from normal controls (52). In further studies "antibrain antibodies" were prepared and injected into animals, producing behavioral and EEG abnormalities similar to those seen with taraxein injections (54). The chemical properties of taraxein have been disputed by at least one investigator (7), who fails to find evidence for its similarity to immunoglobulins, and suggests that it may be a carrier molecule for these proteins. Whereas a few investigators have reported confirmation of some portions of Heath's work (7,36,83,97,99), others have not (9,90,151), and the original investigators, unfortunately, have failed to pursue their studies further.

A few more recent studies, using different techniques, have reported increased titers of antibodies to brain tissue in schizophrenic patients (6,31,88,109). These studies conflict, however, in percentages of patients with autoantibodies, their specificity to schizophrenia, or specificity to human brain tissue. Further pursuit of this hypothesis may be promising with molecular specificity to crucial receptor proteins. One such study already reported by Lieberman et al. (88) shows increased production of antibodies to the nicotinic cholinergic receptor in schizophrenic patients.

In another approach to the detection of an autoimmune reaction to brain tissue, Jankovic et al. (62) injected normal volunteers and psychiatric patients intradermally with antigens prepared from normal human brain tissue. The subsequent delayed hypersensitivity reaction was greater in the psychiatric patients and neurologic patients with brain atrophy than in controls, suggesting prior sensitization and cellular immune recognition of brain membrane protein in these individuals. This work has not been repeated and remains controversial.

Some patients with schizophrenia also have a delayed hypersensitivity reaction to myelin basic protein (MBP) (82) and may have CSF antibodies to MBP as well (118). However, access of brain antigens to the systemic immune system may be a nonspecific result of CNS degenerative change allowing passage of proteins through the blood-brain barrier. The presence of these antibodies may thus be unrelated to the pathogenesis of schizophrenia. Antibodies to MBP are also present in other neurodegenerative disorders, such as multiple sclerosis and subacute sclerosing panencephalitis (124).

Miscellaneous other evidence of a more generalized increase in systemic autoantibody production has been published. Kolyaskina et al. (79,80) have found antibodies to lymphocytes in schizophrenic patients (antithymic antibodies). If binding of these antibodies to the surface of lymphocytes occurs *in vivo*, these could produce widespread impairment of immune function.

In addition, increased antinuclear antibody titers, the hallmark of systemic autoimmune disorders, have been found in approximately 20% of hospitalized psychiatric patients (31,41,65,156). None of these studies, however, have found antibodies to native DNA in schizophrenic patients, as is present in patients with lupus erythematosus. Increased antinuclear antibody titers among patients with psychiatric disorders are not specific to schizophrenia, and are generally thought to be related to length of pharmacologic treatment. Since one study (32) found a small group of acute schizophrenics to have elevated antinuclear antibody titers before the onset of neuroleptic treatment, this finding may be worth further pursuit as a marker of immune dysfunction in some psychiatric patients.

CONCLUSION

In summary, immunological functioning appears to be altered in some schizophrenic patients, although its meaning is obscured by the complexity of CNS-immune system interactions, the nonspecificity of these findings to one immunological function or to one clinically characterizable group of patients, and the unknown contributions of pharmacologic treatment and infectious agents to the status of this system. It is presently unknown whether any of these abnormalities are related to the etiology of schizophrenia or morbidity due to other medical diseases. If a virus is involved in the pathogenesis of schizophrenia, it might produce clinical signs of immunologic dysfunction; on the other hand, if decreased competence of the immune system is the primary defect, increased vulnerability to infectious agents might be a secondary effect. The limitations in present assay techniques, and difficulty obtaining immune function studies on a longitudinal basis in medication-free acutely ill patients, have prevented the clear delineation of a schizophrenia-associated viral or immune disorder. Although the studies reviewed here are only weakly suggestive, these remain viable hypotheses worthy of further evaluation.

ACKNOWLEDGMENT

The author gratefully acknowledges the helpful contributions, discussions, and advice received from Dr. Timothy J. Crow, Head of the Division of Psychiatry, Clinical Research Centre, Northwick Park Hospital, Harrow, England. These led to the development and completion of the following review.

REFERENCES

1. Abe, K. (1969): *Br. J. Psychiatry,* 115:519–531.
2. Albrecht, P., Torrey, E. F., Boone, E., Hicks, J. T., and Daniel, N. (1980): *Lancet,* 2:769–772.
3. Amkraut, A., Solomon, G. F., Allansmith, M., McClellan, B., and Rappaport, M. (1973): *Arch. Gen. Psychiatry,* 28:673–677.
4. Aulakh, G. S., Kleinman, J. E., Aulakh, H. S., Albrecht, P., Torrey, E. F., and Wyatt, R. J. (1981): *Proc. Soc. Exp. Biol. Med.,* 167:172–174.
5. Baker, H. F., Ridley, R. M., Crow, T. J., Bloxham, C. A., Parry, R. P., and Tyrrell, D. A. J. (1983): *Psychol. Med.,* 13:499–511.
6. Baron, M., Stern, M., Anavi, R., and Witz, J. P. (1977): *Biol. Psychiatry,* 12:199–219.
7. Bergen, J. R., Grinspoon, L., Pyle, H. M., Martinez, J. L., and Pennell, R. B. (1980): *Biol. Psychiatry,* 15:369–379.
8. Bock, E., Week, B., and Rafaelson, O. J. (1970): *Lancet,* 2:523.
9. Boehme, D. H., Cottrell, J. C., Dohan, F. C., and Hillegass, L. M. (1974): *Biol. Psychiatry,* 8:89–94.
10. Book, J. A. (1953): *Acta Genet. Statist. Med.,* 4:1–100.
11. Brierley, J. R., Corsellis, J. A. N., Hierons, R., and Nevin, S. (1960): *Brain,* 83:357–368.
12. Britton, C. (1984): Presented at The First World Conference on Virus Diseases and Mental Health, Montreal, Canada, November, 1984.
13. Bruce, L. C., and Peebles, A. M. S. (1903): *J. Ment. Sci.,* 49:614–628.
14. Bruce, L. C., and Peebles, A. M. S. (1904): *J. Ment. Sci.,* 50:409–417.
15. Cantell, K., Pulkkinen, E., Elosuo, R., and Suominen, J. (1980): *Ann. Clin. Res.,* 12:131–132.
16. Chistovich, L. (1945): Collection from the Departments of Nervous Diseases and Psychiatry, Novosibirsk. Reported in Malis, 1961, pp. 18–19.
17. Coffee, C. E., Sullivan, J. L., and Rice, J. R. (1983): *Biol. Psychiatry,* 18:113–120.
18. Crocetti, G. M., Lemkau, P. V., Kulcar, Z., and Kesic, B. (1971): *Am. J. Epidemiol.,* 94:126–134.
19. Crow, T. J. (1983): *Lancet,* 1:173–175.
20. Crow, T. J. (1984): *Br. J. Psychiatry,* 145:243–253.
21. Crow, T. J., and Done, D. J. (1986): *Psychiatry Res.,* 18:107–117.
22. Dale, P. W. (1981): *J. Psychiatr. Res.,* 16:103–111.
23. Dameschek, W. (1930): *Arch. Neurol. Psychiatry,* 24:855.
24. De Boeck, Le Dr. (1893): *Bull. Soc. Med. Ment. Belg-Gand Leipz:* 416–437.
25. DeLisi, L. E., Goldin, L. R., Nurnberger, J. I., Alling, S. S., and Gershon, E. S. (1986): In: *Proceedings of the IVth World Congress of Biological Psychiatry,* edited by C. Shagass et al. Elsevier Publishing Co., New York.
26. DeLisi, L. E., Goodman, S., Neckers, L. M., and Wyatt, R. J. (1982): *Biol. Psychiatry,* 17:1003–1007.
27. DeLisi, L. E., King, A. K., and Targum, S. (1984): *Br. J. Psychiatry,* 145:661–664.
28. DeLisi, L. E., Neckers, L. M., Weinberger, D. R., Shilling, D., and Wyatt, R. J. (1981): *Br. J. Psychiatry,* 139:513–518.
29. DeLisi, L. E., Ortaldo, J. R., Maluish, A. E., and Wyatt, R. J. (1983): *J. Neural Transm.,* 58:96–106.
30. DeLisi, L. E., and Sarin, P. (1985): *Br. J. Psychiatry,* 146:674.
31. DeLisi, L. E., Weber, R., and Pert, C. (1985): *Biol. Psychiatry,* 20:110–115.
32. DeLisi, L. E., and Wyatt, R. J. (1982): *Psychopharmacol. Bull.,* 18:158–163.
33. Domino, E. F., Krause, R. R., Thiessen, M. M., and Batsakis, J. G. (1975): *Arch. Gen. Psychiatry,* 32:717–721.
34. Drachman, D. A., and Adams, R. D. (1962): *Arch. Neurol.,* 7:45–63.
35. Ferguson, R. M., Schmidtke, J. R., and Simmons, R. L. (1978): In: *Neurochemical and Immunological Components of Schizophrenia.* (Series: Birth Defects) *Vol. 18,* pp. 379–402, edited by D. Bergsma and A. L. Goldstein. Alan R. Liss, New York.
36. Fessel, W. J. (1962): *Arch. Gen. Psychiatry,* 6:320–323.
37. Fessel, W. J., and Hirata-Hibi, M. (1963): *Arch. Gen. Psychiatry,* 9:601–613.
38. Fieve, R. R., Blumenthal, B., and Little, B. (1966): *Arch. Gen. Psychiatry,* 15:529–534.
39. Fischer, M. (1973): *Acta Psychiatr. Scand.,* 238:1–58.
40. Fisman, M. (1975): *Br. J. Psychiatry,* 126:414–422.
41. Gallien, M., Schnetzler, J. P., and Morin, J. (1975): *Ann. Med. Psychol.,* 1:237–248.
42. Glaser, G. H., Solitare, G. B., and Manuelidis, E. A. (1968): *Res. Publ. Assoc. Res. Nerv. Ment. Dis.,* 49:178–215.
43. Glaser, R., Kiecolt-Glaser, J. K., Stout, J. C., Tarr, K. L., Speicher, C. E., and Holliday, J. E. (1986): *Psychiatry Res. (in press).*
44. Goodall, E. (1932): *J. Ment. Sci.,* 78:746–755.
45. Gotlieb-Stematsky, T., Zonis, J., Arlozoroff, A., Mozes, T., Sigal, M., and Szekely, A. (1981): *Arch. Virol.,* 67:333–339.
46. Gottesman, I. I., and Shields, J. (1982): *Schizophrenia: The Epigenetic Puzzle.* Cambridge University Press, New York, London.
47. Granskaya, N. A. (1927): *J. Nevropatol. Psikhiatr.,* 20:139–148.
48. Hankoff, L. D., and Peress, N. S. (1981): *Biol. Psychiatry,* 16:945–952.
49. Hare, E. H. (1983): *Br. J. Psychiatry,* 142:439–455.
50. Hare, E. H., and Walter, S. D. (1978): *J. Epidemiol. Community Health,* 32:47–52.
51. Harper, P. S. (1977): *J. Med. Genet.,* 14:389–398.
52. Heath, R. G., and Krupp, I. M. (1967): *Arch. Gen. Psychiatry,* 16:1–9.
53. Heath, R. G., Krupp, I. M., Byers, L. W., and Liljekvist, J. I. (1967): *Arch. Gen. Psychiatry,* 16:10–23.
54. Heath, R. G., Krupp, I. M., Byers, L. W., and Liljekvist, J. I. (1967): *Arch. Gen. Psychiatry,* 16:24–33.
55. Hendrick, I. (1928): *Am. J. Psychiatry,* 84:898–1014.
56. Herndon, C. N., and Jennings, R. G. (1951): *Am. J. Hum. Genet.,* 3:17.
57. Hirata-Hibi, M., and Fessel, W. J. (1964): *Arch. Gen. Psychiatry,* 10:414–419.
58. Hirata-Hibi, M., Higashi, S., Tachibana, T., and Watanabe, N. (1982): *Arch. Gen. Psychiatry,* 39:82–87.
59. Hofbauer, B. (1846): *Osterreichische Med. Wochenschr.,* 39:1183–1188.
60. Itten, W. (1914): *Z. Ges. Neurol. Psychol.,* 24:341–377.
61. Jaenisch, R. (1976): *Proc. Nat. Acad. Sci. USA,* 73:1260–1264.
62. Jankovik, B. D., Jakulic, S., and Horvat, J. (1979): *Periodic Biol.,* 81:219–220.
63. Jelliffe, S. E. (1927): *Am. J. Psychiatry,* 6:413–465.
64. Johnson, R. T. (1982): *Viral Infections of the Nervous System.* Raven Press, New York.
65. Johnstone, E. C., and Whaley, K. (1975): *Br. Med. J.,* 28:724–725.
66. Kallman, F. J., and Reisner, D. (1943): *J. Hered.,* 34:269–276.
67. Kamman, G. R. (1930): *JAMA,* 94:1286–1288.
68. Kamp, H. V. (1962): *J. Neuropsychiatry,* 4:1–3.
69. Kasanetz, E. F. (1979): *Riv. Psicol. Anal.,* 10:193–202.
70. Kaufman, C. A., DeLisi, L. E., Torrey, E. F., Folstein, S. E., and Smith, W. J. (1987): In: *Viruses, Immunity and Mental Diseases,*

edited by E. Kustak and P. Morozov. Plenum Publishing Co., New York (*in press*).

71. Kelleher, M. J., Copeland, J. R. M., and Smith, A. J. (1974): *Psychol. Med.,* 4:460–462.

72. Kety, S. S., Rosenthal, D., Wender, P. H., and Schulsinger, F. (1968): In: *The Transmission of Schizophrenia,* edited by D. Rosenthal and S. S. Kety, pp. 345–362. Pergamon Press, Oxford.

73. Khoroshko, V. K. (1912): *Reactii Zivotnogo Organizma na Vvedenie Nervnoi Tkani (Nevrotoxini Anaphylaksia Endotoxini).* Moscow.

74. King, D. J., Cooper, S. J., Earle, J. A. P., Martin, S. J., McFerran, N. V., Rima, B. K., and Wisdom, G. B. (1985): *Br. J. Psychiatry,* 147:137–144.

75. King, D. J., Cooper, S. J., Earle, J. A. P., Martin, S. J., McFerran, N. V., and Wisdom, G. B. (1985): *Br. J. Psychiatry,* 147:145–149.

76. Kinney, D. K., and Jacobsen, B. (1978): In: *The Nature of Schizophrenia,* edited by L. C. Wynne, R. Cromwell, and S. Mattysse, pp. 38–51. Wiley, New York.

77. Klaber, M., and Lacey, J. (1968): *Br. Med. J.,* 3:124.

78. Kolyaskina, G. I. (1983): In: *Research on the Viral Hypothesis of Mental Disorders (Adv. Biol. Psychiatry, Vol. 12),* edited by P. V. Morozov, pp. 142–149. Karger Press, New York, Basel.

79. Kolyaskina, G. I. (1984): Presented at the First World Conference on Virus Diseases and Mental Health. Montreal, Canada, November, 1984.

80. Kolyaskina, G. I., Tsutsulkovskaya, M., Domashneva, I., Kielholz, P., Bunney, W., Rafaelsen, O., Heltberg, J., Coppen, A., Hippius, H., Hoecherl, H., and Vartanian, F. (1980): *Neuropsychobiology,* 6:349–355.

81. Kronfol, Z. (1985): Presented at The NIMH Workshop for Neuropsychoimmunology. Rockville, Maryland, September 27, 1985.

82. Kuritzky, A., Livni, E., Munitz, H., Englander, T., Tyano, S., Wysenbeek, H., Joshua, H., and Kott, E. (1976): *J. Neurol. Sci.,* 30:369–373.

83. Kuznetoza, N. I., and Semenov, S. F. (1961): *Zh. Nevropatol. Psikhiatr.,* 61:869–873.

84. Lehmann-Facius, H. (1937): *Klin. Wochenschr.,* 16:1646–1648.

85. Lehmann-Facius, H. (1939): *Alg. Z. Psychiatr.,* 110:232–243.

86. Libikova, H. (1983): In: *Research on the Viral Hypothesis of Mental Disorders (Adv. Biol. Psychiatry, Vol. 12),* edited by P. Morozov, pp. 20–51. Karger Press, Basel, New York.

87. Libikova, H., Stancek, D., Wiedermann, V., Hasto, J., and Breier, S. (1977): *Arch. Immunol. Ther. Exp.,* 25:641–649.

88. Lieberman, J. A., Bradley, R. J., Rubinstein, M., and Kane, J. M. (1984): *Ann. NY Acad. Sci.,* 435:444–447.

89. Liedeman, R. R., and Prilipko, L. L. (1978): In: *Birth Defects, Vol. 14,* pp. 365–377. Alan R. Liss, New York.

90. Logan, D. G., and Deodhar, S. D. (1970): *JAMA,* 212:1703–1704.

91. Lovett, C. L., Urlich, J. T., Simms, B. G., and Goldstein, A. L. (1978): In: *Neurochemical and Immunological Components of Schizophrenia (Birth Defects, Vol. 18),* edited by D. Bergsma and A. L. Goldstein, pp. 407–422. Alan R. Liss, New York.

92. Lyubovskaya, P. I., and Rokhlenko, S. Z. (1957): *Vrachebnoe Delo,* No. 12.

93. Malis, G. Yu. (1961): *Research on the Etiology of Schizophrenia (The International Behavioral Sciences Series), Chapter 7,* pp. 151–182. Consultants Bureau, New York.

94. Malis, G. Yu., and Dolgikh, S. I. (1954): *Zh. Nevropatol. Psikhiatr.,* 54:728–731.

95. Mar, G. I., and Sviadats, A. M. (1957): *Zh. Nevropatol. Psikhiatr.,* 57:1098–1100.

96. Marchand, L. (1930): *Ann. Med. Psychol.,* 88:5–36;52–53.

97. Martens, S., Vallbo, S., and Melander, B. (1959): *Acta Psychiatr. Scand. (Suppl.),* 136:361.

98. McCowan, P. K., and Cook, L. C. (1928): *Lancet,* 1:1316.

99. Meckler, L. B., Laptera, N. N., Lozovskii, D. V., and Balezinc, T. I. (1960): *Proc. Acad. Sci. USSR,* 130:1148.

100. Menninger, K. A. (1926): *Am. J. Psychiatry,* 5:469–529.

101. Menninger, K. A. (1928): *Arch. Neurol. Psychiatry,* 20:464–481.

102. Menninger von Lerchenthal, E. (1930): *Z. Ges. Neurol. Psychol.,* 125:12–19.

103. Mered, B., Albrecht, P., Torrey, E. F., Weinberger, D. R., Potkin, S. G., and Winfrey, C. J. (1983): *Lancet,* 2:919.

104. Mesa, C. S., Odelsa, N. A., and Gomez, H. (1985): *Abstracts of the IVth World Congress of Biological Psychiatry,* Philadelphia, Pennsylvania, 1985, p. 242.

105. Misra, P. C., and Hay, G. G. (1971): *Br. Med. J.,* 1:523–533.

106. Molholm, H. B. (1942): *Psychiatric Q.,* 16:565–571.

107. Morozov, V. M. (1954): *J. Neuropathol. Psychiatry,* 1954:732–734.

108. Nieto, D., and Escobar, A. (1972): In: *The Pathology of the Nervous System, Vol. 3.,* edited by J. Minckler, pp. 2654–2670. McGraw-Hill, New York.

109. Pandey, R. S., Gupta, A. K., and Chaturvedi, V. C. (1981): *Biol. Psychiatry,* 16:1123–1136.

110. Pinto-Cezar, E. (1930): Translated in *Arch. Neurol. Psychiatry,* London, December, 1930 (as quoted by Goodall, 1932).

111. Preble, O. T., and Torrey, E. F. (1985): *Am. J. Psychiatry,* 142:1184–1186.

112. Prusenko, A. I. (1915): *Zh. Nevropatol. Psikhiatr.,* 15:118–142.

113. Pulver, A. E., Stewart, W., Carpenter, W. T., and Childs, B. (1983): *Br. J. Psychiatry,* 143:389–396.

114. Raskin, D. E., and Frank, S. W. (1974): *Arch. Gen. Psychiatry,* 31:544–546.

115. Raymond, R. W., and Williams, R. L. (1948): *N. Engl. J. Med.,* 239:542–544.

116. Rehm, *Zentralbl. Ges. Neurol. Psychol.,* March, 1932 (as quoted by Goodall, 1932).

117. Rimon, R., and Halonen, P. (1977): In: *The Impact of Biology on Modern Psychiatry,* edited by E. S. Gershon, S. S. Kety, and M. Rosenbaum, pp. 105–112. Plenum Publishing Co., New York.

118. Rimon, R. H., Halonen, P., Lebon, P., Heikkila, L., Frey, H., Karhula, P., Hintikka, J., and Salmela, L. (1983): *Adv. Biol. Psychiatry,* 12:161–167.

119. Robert-Guroff, M., Torrey, E. F., and Brown, M. (1985): *Br. J. Psychiatry,* 146:326.

120. Roberts, G. W., Colter, N., Lofthouse, R., Brown, R., and Crow, T. J. (1985): *Abstracts of the IVth World Congress of Biological Psychiatry,* September 8–13, 1985, Philadelphia, Pennsylvania, p. 6.

121. Roos, R. P., Davis, K., and Meltzer, H. Y. (1985): *Arch. Gen. Psychiatry,* 42:124–128.

122. Rosenfeld, M. (1930): *Zentralbl. Ges. Neurol. Psych.,* 57:1–27.

123. Rosenthal, D. (1962): *Psychol. Bull.,* 59:401–421.

124. Ruutiainen, J., Arnadottir, T., Molnar, G., Salmi, A., and Frey, H. (1981): *Acta Neurol. Scand.,* 64:196–206.

125. Rzewuska-Szatkowska, M. (1972): *Psychiatr. Pol.,* 6:453–456.

126. Sagel, W. (1930): *Z. Ges. Neurol. Psychiatr.,* 125:436–464.

127. Scarlato, G., and Mastrogiovanni, P. D. (1956): *Acta Neurol. (Napoli),* 11:587–595.

128. Schonfeldt, M. (1894): *Arch. Psychiatr. Nervenkr.,* 26:202–266.

129. Schultz, J. H. (1913): *Dtsch. Med. Wochnschr.,* 39:1399–1402.

130. Shrikhande, S., Hirsch, S. R., Coleman, J. C., Reveley, M. A., and Dayton, R. (1985): *Br. J. Psychiatry,* 146:503–506.

131. Sobin, A., and Ozer, M. N. (1966): *J. Mount Sinai Hosp.,* 33:73–82.

132. Solomon, G. F., Allansmith, M., McClellan, B., and Amkraut, A. (1969): *Arch. Gen. Psychiatry,* 20:272–277.

133. Stevens, J. (1982): *Arch. Gen. Psychiatry,* 39:1131–1139.

134. Stevens, J. R., Langloss, J. M., Albrecht, P., Yolken, R., and Wang, Y.-N. (1984): *Arch. Gen. Psychiatry,* 41:795–804.

135. Strahilevitz, M., Fleishman, J. B., Fischer, G. W., Harris, R., and Narasimhachari, N. (1976): *Am. J. Psychiatry,* 133:772–776.

136. Taylor, G. R., Crow, T. J., Carter, G. I., and Gamble, S. J. (1986): *J. Exp. Mol. Pathol.,* 42:271–277.

137. Taylor, G. R., Crow, T. J., Ferrier, I. N., Johnstone, E. C., Parry, R. P., and Tyrrell, D. A. J. (1982): *Lancet,* 2:1166–1167.

138. Taylor, G. R., Crow, T. J., Higgins, T., and Reynolds, G. (1985): *J. Neuropathol. Exp. Neurol.,* 44:176–184.

139. Torrey, E. F. (1980): *Schizophrenia and Civilization,* Jason Aronson, New York.

140. Torrey, E. F., Peterson, M. R., Brannon, W. L., Carpenter, W. T., Post, R. M., and van Kammen, D. P. (1978): *Br. J. Psychiatry,* 132:342–348.

141. Torrey, E. F., Torrey, B. B., and Burton-Bradley, B. G. (1974): *Am. J. Psychiatry,* 131:567–573.

142. Torrey, E. F., Torrey, B. B., and Petersen, M. R. (1977): *Arch. Gen. Psychiatry,* 34:1065–1070.

143. Torrey, E. F., Yolken, R. H., and Albrecht, A. (1983): *Adv. Biol. Psychiatry,* 12:150–160.

144. Torrey, E. F., Yolken, R. H., and Winfrey, C. J. (1982): *Science,* 216:892–894.

145. Tyrrell, D. A. J., Parry, R. P., Crow, T. J., Johnstone, E. C., and Ferrier, I. N. (1979): *Lancet,* 1:839–841.

146. Vartanian, M. E., Kolyaskina, G. I., Lozovsky, D. V., Burbaeva, G. Sh., and Ignatov, S. A. (1978): In: *Neurochemical and Immunological Components of Schizophrenia (Birth Defects, Vol. 18),* edited by D. Bergsma and A. L. Goldstein, pp. 339–364. Alan R. Liss, New York.

147. Vaughan, W. T., Sullivan, J. C., and Elmadjian, F. (1949): *Psychosom. Med.,* 11:327–333.

148. Watson, C. G., Kucala, T., Tilleskjor, C., and Jacobs, L. (1984): *Arch. Gen. Psychiatry,* 41:85–90.

149. Weinberger, D. R., Kaufman, C. A., and Stevens, J. R. (1984): Presented at the First World Conference on Virus Diseases and Mental Health, Montreal, Canada, November, 1984.

150. Weinstein, E. A., Linn, L., and Kahn, R. L. (1955): *J. Mount Sinai Hosp.,* 21:341–354.

151. Whittingham, S., Mackay, I. R., Jones, I. H., and Davies, B. (1968): *Br. Med. J.,* 1:347–348.

152. Wilson, K. J. (1967): In: *Diseases in Antiquity,* edited by D. Brothwell, and A. T. Sandison, pp. 723–733. Charles C. Thomas, Springfield, IL.

153. Wollenberg, R. (1889): *Arch. Psychiatrie,* 20:62–88.

154. Wunderlich, V., Fey, F., and Sydow, G. (1980): *Arch. Geschwulstforsch.,* 50:758–762.

155. Wunderlich, V., and Zotter, S. (1982): *Exp. Pathol.,* 21:59–61.

156. Zarrabi, M. H., Zucker, S., Miller, F., Derman, R. M., Romano, G. S., Hartnett, J. A., and Varma, A. O. (1979): *Ann. Intern. Med.,* 91:194–199.

Psychopharmacology:
The Third Generation of Progress,
edited by Herbert Y. Meltzer.
Raven Press, New York © 1987.

CHAPTER 76

Brain Morphology in Schizophrenia

Richard C. Shelton and Daniel R. Weinberger

One of the more dramatic trends in schizophrenia research in the past decade has been a renaissance of interest in brain morphology. To the extent that schizophrenia has long been viewed as the most "neurological" of psychiatric disorders, it is not surprising that investigators might search for evidence of structural neuropathology. During the first half of this century, numerous laboratories around the world were engaged in neuroanatomical studies of brain tissue from schizophrenic persons. Despite many reports of positive findings, this effort did not produce conclusive evidence of replicable brain pathology that could be considered clinically relevant (53). As a result, from 1950 until the past decade, the study of brain morphology had been all but abandoned. Discoveries in neuropharmacology led researchers in new directions that appeared to hold greater promise.

Several factors have contributed to the morphological renaissance. The development of new technologies for studying brain structure during life, such as the computed tomography or CT scan, made it possible to examine large samples of carefully diagnosed patients and matched controls. The adoption of quantitative approaches to the analysis of postmortem brain tissue made it possible to appreciate subtle differences in morphology that earlier qualitative approaches might have overlooked. Last but not least, it had become increasingly apparent that current neuropsychopharmacologically based theories and treatments of schizophrenia addressed only part of the problem. In this chapter we will review the evidence from *in vivo* and postmortem anatomical studies that has made cerebral morphology a vital component of research in schizophrenia.

COMPUTERIZED TOMOGRAPHIC STUDIES

The advent of the CT scan launched the modern era of "brain imaging" in neuroscience. It is responsible for the resurgence of interest in brain morphology in schizophrenia and for compelling evidence that schizophrenia is associated with structural pathology of the brain. The CT scan technique, introduced in the early 1970s, took *in vivo* observations of brain structure a giant step beyond early radiological techniques such as pneumoencephalography. For the first time the brain could be observed in cross section in what seemed like exquisite detail.

Lateral Ventricular Enlargement

Johnstone et al. (49) published the first of now nearly 100 reports of CT scans in schizophrenia. In this study of elderly schizophrenic and control males, the size of the lateral cerebral ventricles as a function of total brain area was significantly larger in the schizophrenic patient. Over the past 10 years, lateral ventricular enlargement has become the most exhaustively studied single phenomenon in the field of schizophrenia research, and possibly the most replicable biological finding in psychiatry. The lateral ventricles are of interest in schizophrenia for two reasons: first, changes in their morphology are a nonspecific but sensitive sign of cerebral structural pathology, and second, the structures that lie adjacent to them, such as the caudate, putamen, globus pallidus, thalamus, hypothalamus, amygdala hippocampus, fornix, and corpus callosum are areas of at least theoretical relevance. Enlargement of the lateral ventricles may imply abnormalities in some of these areas. The finding of enlarged ventricles supports and extends the prodigious but often ignored earlier reports of cerebral abnormalities in schizophrenia in the pneumoencephalography literature (122).

Figure 1 summarizes studies of lateral ventricular enlargement in schizophrenia. Though clearly the positive studies outnumber the negative, the question remains: why the discrepancies? There seem to be three broad areas that

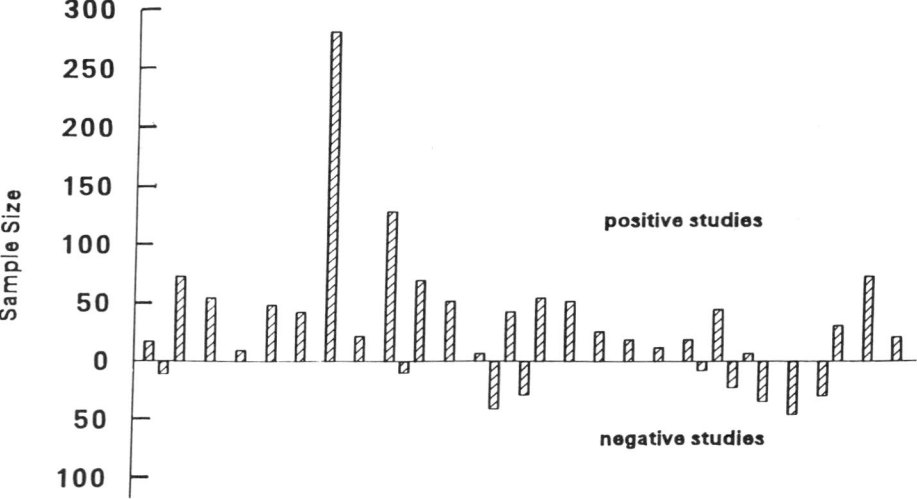

FIG. 1. Computerized tomographic studies of lateral ventricular enlargement in schizophrenia. Sample size is in numbers of schizophrenic persons per study. References, left to right (in chronological order): 49 and 50, 118, 133, 73, 129, 115, 88 and 89, 114, 95, 51, 8, 33, 3 and 4, 98, 84, 87, 46, 78 and 79, 130, 56, 137, 102, 92 and 93, 25, 63, 91, 101, 60, 107, 13, 136, 106, 66.

have influenced the outcome of the studies. The first is the method of measurement of the lateral ventricles. Most investigators have used a variation of the ventricular-brain ratio (VBR) method of Synek and Reuben (112), in which the area of the ventricles on the scan is divided by the total area of the brain. This percentage ratio is highly correlated with ventricular volume; it has been derived by using both a fixed-arm planimeter (an engineering device used for estimating the size of irregular areas) and computer-generated methods, such as summing density measurements from the scans corresponding to fluid (ventricle) and tissue (brain) (48). Simple linear methods of estimating ventricular volumes, though quite effective in detecting gross changes in conditions such as hydrocephalus, have generally been less sensitive for detecting the subtle changes in schizophrenia (105).

The second source of variability of findings is the choice of control sample. Lateral ventricular enlargement is by no means specific to schizophrenia. It is found in a number of disorders (10,105), including affective illnesses (44,51,65,81,82,94,95,100,104,110,116,117). In studies that have utilized control scans from groups with medical, neurological, or affective illnesses, differences were less commonly found than in those using normal volunteer controls (105).

Certain reports, such as those of Benes et al. (8) and Jernigan et al. (46), did not contain these problems and yet still yielded negative results. These studies illustrate the third variable affecting outcome in studies of ventricular size in schizophrenia: patient sample selection. Data from many studies suggest that the greater the representation of severely impaired patients in a sample, the more likely it is that enlarged lateral ventricles will be found. Therefore, enlargement of ventricles is more likely to be found in a sample of chronically hospitalized patients than in subjects taken from an outpatient clinic or acute treatment unit

(4,66). This qualification notwithstanding, most studies of patients not chronically hospitalized also have found larger lateral ventricles. In fact, of the three most frequently cited negative studies (8,13,46), one (13) proved to be positive when the data were reanalyzed using a more sensitive measurement technique (97), whereas another (8) was not replicated by the same research group on a new and similar patient sample that demonstrated enlarged ventricles (137).

Confounding factors that might be potential explanations for differences between schizophrenic and control samples have been investigated. The possibilities that ventricular enlargement is an artifact of sex, race, socioeconomic circumstances, and neuroleptic or electroconvulsive treatment have been excluded. In addition, age and duration of illness have also not been found to explain the findings (105). This has been interpreted to mean that the underlying pathology is relatively static (123).

Correlations have been found between relative ventricular enlargement and clinical factors such as poor premorbid adjustment (29,38,39,49,50,128), decreased response to neuroleptics (62,63,103,127), poor outcome (24,136) with persistent unemployment (92,93), a lower incidence of so-called "positive" symptoms (hallucinations, delusions, etc.) (3,63), and more "negative" symptoms (flattened affect, anergia, social isolation, etc.) (3,92,93,136). These findings support a concept of a relationship between ventricular enlargement and both severity of illness and prognosis. Further, studies by Schulz et al. (102), Weinberger et al. (130), and Nyback et al. (87), of young patients, revealed that abnormalities are present at or before onset of the illness and prior to medical therapies. In a recent 5-year follow-up study, Nasrallah et al. (76) found overall stability in VBR values in their sample, consistent with the idea that the pathology is relatively static.

Ventricular size has been found to be strongly correlated within families, especially between monozygotic twins (98).

Several investigators have found that schizophrenic probands have enlarged lateral ventricles as compared with family members, including co-twins (98,99) and other siblings (22,79,101,129). Further, Schulsinger et al. (101) and Reveley et al. (98,99) have reported a relationship between ventricular enlargement and perinatal trauma, though birth histories are hard to reliably reconstruct 30 years after the fact. The claim that large ventricles reflect "nongenetic" schizophrenia, however, has been contested (20–22).

Of particular significance to the interface of neuropsychopharmacology and brain morphology research in schizophrenia are the relationships between structural abnormalities and central neurotransmitter activity. Such associations have been investigated to a limited degree in the case of lateral ventricular enlargement. For example, DeLisi et al. (23) found a relative increase of 5-hydroxytryptophan (5-HT) in blood, and three groups (45,86,96) reported decreased cerebrospinal fluid (CSF) 5-hydroxyindole acetic acid (the primary metabolite of 5-HT) in patients with ventricular enlargement. Special importance, however, has been given to associations with central dopamine activity. Tachiki et al. (113) found that the plasma activity of monoamine oxidase-b varied proportionally with VBR in a subgroup of nonparanoid schizophrenic patients. Other investigators have looked more directly at measures of brain dopamine activity. In an investigation of the CSF dopamine metabolites homovanillic acid (HVA) and dopamine β-hydroxylase, van Kammen et al. (121) found that these constituents were reduced in patients with ventricular enlargement. Nyback et al. (86) and Jennings et al. (45) reported an inverse relationship between CSF HVA and lateral ventricular size in psychotic inpatients. Finally, in a study of blink rates (which are felt to vary directly with central dopamine activity), Kleinman et al. (54) found that blink rates were unaffected by treatment with neuroleptics in patients with significantly enlarged lateral ventricles. These latter studies, coupled with the relative unresponsiveness of patients with larger lateral ventricles to neuroleptic treatment, seem to indicate that central dopamine activity may be of somewhat lesser importance pathophysiologically in patients with ventricular enlargement as compared with those in the normal range.

Third Ventricular Enlargement

As with the lateral ventricles, the third ventricle is of interest because of adjacent structures: thalamus, hypothalamus, fornix, and habenulae. Since in pathological conditions enlargement of the third ventricle involves primarily lateral expansion, simple measurement of the maximum width has been used in most studies.

Figure 2 summarizes the third ventricle studies. As can be readily appreciated, almost all studies have found significant enlargement in schizophrenia. Furthermore, this seems to be true for the most part whether or not medical/neurological controls are used (105). Because there have been relatively few studies of the third ventricle in schizophrenia, there is limited information regarding clinicopathological correlations. Whereas length of illness usually does not correlate with lateral ventricular enlargement, there is some evidence of such correlation with third ventricle size (34,87,115), though this is not robust (13,73,106).

Increased Cortical Surface Markings

As with the lateral and third ventricles, the surface of the cerebral cortex can show changes associated with normal aging and a number of medical/neurological conditions, especially the dementias. These (presumably) atrophic processes produce thinning of the gyri and widening of the sulci, which can be demonstrated on the CT scan. Most investigators studying cortical surface markings have directly

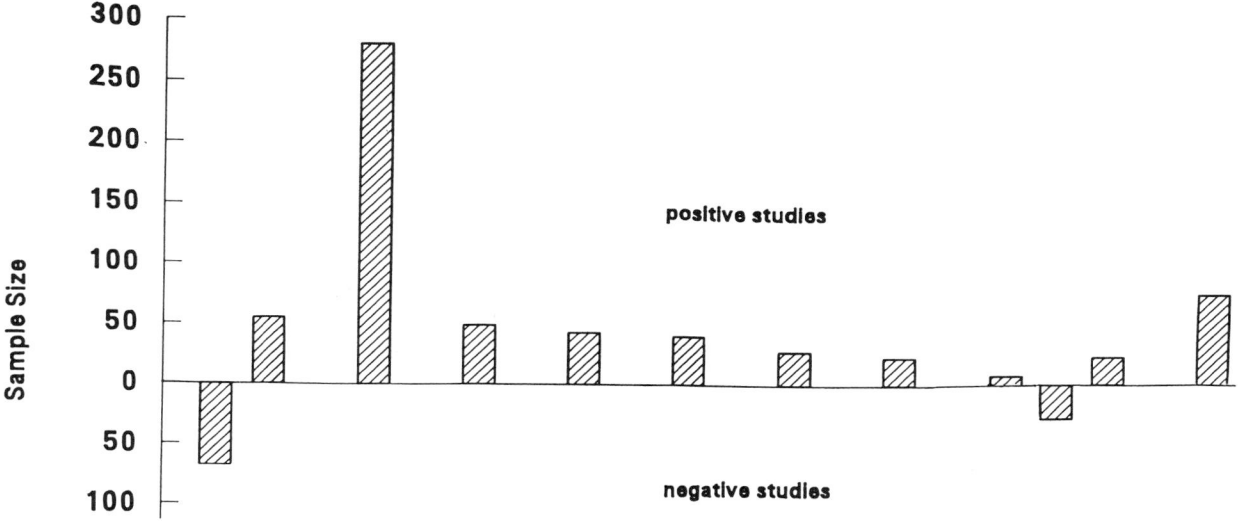

FIG. 2. Computerized tomographic studies of third ventricular enlargement in schizophrenia. Sample size is in numbers of schizophrenic persons per study. References, left to right (in chronological order): 35 and 75, 73, 114 and 115, 88 and 89, 34, 87, 27, 91, 25, 60, 13, 106.

observed the scans themselves, either rating the relative degree of increase of surface markings, or actually measuring the widths of sulci and fissures. One group (46) used a method of summing density numbers from individual points ("pixels") on each scan, corresponding to tissue (high numbers) or fluid (low values). This method yields a tissue/fluid ratio that theoretically corresponds with the degree of widening of fissures and sulci.

Figure 3 demonstrates that the majority of studies found increased cortical surface markings in schizophrenic patients as compared with controls. As with lateral ventricle studies, the sensitivity of method is somewhat reduced by utilizing medical/neurological controls (105). This is not surprising in view of the fact that many illnesses produce atrophy of the cortical surface.

Since it is unusual to find patients with increased cortical markings and no change in ventricular size, it has been difficult to examine the relationship of cortical changes alone to clinical variables. In schizophrenia, the markings do not seem to be explained by age effects (45,80,106,134) or duration of illness (80,134). At least one study found no relationship with severity of overall symptomatology, premorbid adjustment, response to medication, positive/negative symptoms, or family history (80). Two studies did, however, find a correlation between cortical surface markings and degree of cognitive impairment (80,100).

Most CT studies of the cortex have not considered the possibility that the underlying pathology may not be generalized, but rather may be localized to a particular part of the cortex. The majority of studies simply reported the changes as a whole. Takahashi et al. (114), however, reported that the most significant differences involved the sylvian fissures and frontal cortex. Tanaka et al. (115) also localized the increased cortical sulci to the frontal and temporal areas (with no findings in parietal and occipital cortex). Oxenstierna et al. (90) found excess cortical markings in the prefrontal cortex. In a recent study, Shelton et

al. (106) compared the degree of cortical surface markings in prefrontal and parietooccipital cortex and found differences between schizophrenic patients and controls only in the former. Taken as a whole, these studies do indicate the presence of cortical surface changes in schizophrenia and the possibility that the changes may be specific to the prefrontal and temporal areas. Whether these changes are primary or secondary to pathology in areas that connect with the cortex (e.g., periventricular areas, vide infra) cannot be determined from a CT scan. Furthermore, it is still unresolved whether the ventricular and cortical changes seen on CT scan are related or independent.

Other Studies

The cerebellum, located in the posterior fossa, is somewhat more poorly visualized on CT scan than the cerebrum. Because of the connections between the cerebellum (especially the vermis) and the limbic-diencephalic structures, as well as the fact that disorders of the cerebellum occasionally give rise to schizophrenia-like illnesses (41,58), several groups have investigated the issue of cerebellar pathology in schizophrenic patients (17,26,41,42,61,77,82, 84,95,130,135). Most groups found a relative excess of apparent cerebellar atrophy in the patient groups. This is also true of affective disorders. Cerebellar atrophy tends to occur in a number of illnesses, as well as with exposure to drugs and other toxins. The clinicopathological significance of cerebellar atrophy in schizophrenia, therefore, remains obscure.

Another area of investigation has been cerebral anatomical asymmetries. A substantial body of literature supports the concepts of both normal lateralization of cerebral function and localization of psychopathology in left or right hemispheres (32,40). Most normals have relatively larger right frontal and left occipital lobes. Reversal of this pattern can be seen normally, but has been seen with greater than expected frequency in disorders such as dyslexia and autism. The majority of studies (1,47,55,56,64,67–69,84,87,119,130) failed to find an excess of reversed cerebral asymmetry in schizophrenic persons. Though not a commentary on the importance of functional lateral differences, these studies do not support structural asymmetries in schizophrenia.

As X-rays pass through tissue, their energy is absorbed by internal structures resulting in a decrease of beam intensity. This reduction in energy, or "attenuation," depends on the relative densities of body structures and is a fundamental principle of X-ray imaging. Similarly, on CT scan, the individual pixel elements provide an estimate of the relative density of corresponding tissue. Investigators have looked at tissue densities on CT scans within defined areas of interest in the brains of schizophrenic persons. The early work by Golden et al. (36,37,69) assessed densities over cerebral areas without regard to fluid-filled spaces (fissures, sulci, ventricles); the reduced regional densities found in these studies probably reflected enlargement of these spaces, not differences in tissue *per se*. When smaller intracerebral regions of interest were defined, the results were mixed. Largen et al. (59) initially reported relatively increased density in the right hemisphere, but this was not

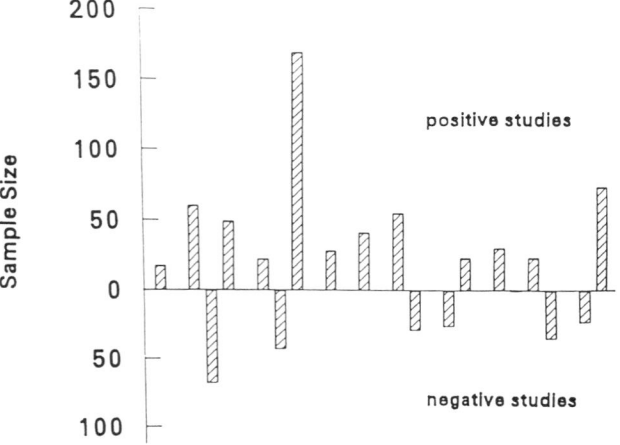

FIG. 3. Computerized tomographic studies of increased cortical surface markings ("cortical atrophy") in schizophrenia. Sample size is in numbers of schizophrenic persons per study. References, left to right (in chronological order): 50, 133, 35 and 75, 115, 95, 88 and 89, 114, 87, 84, 80 and 82, 46, 56, 27, 90, 91, 60, 13, 106.

supported by a later more conservative statistical comparison (60). Coffman et al. (18), on the other hand, reported *decreased* density in the left cerebral hemisphere, whereas a study by Kanba et al. (52) found decreases frontally and occipitally. Finally, Dewan et al. (27) indicated that there was increased tissue density in the periventricular areas in their patient sample, with no cortical differences. These discrepancies in findings, serious questions about methodology, and unclear clinopathological significance of density measures in general, make interpretations in this area highly problematic (105).

MAGNETIC RESONANCE IMAGING STUDIES

Magnetic resonance imaging (MRI) is a nonradiologic technique for examining brain morphology that grew out of methods in analytic chemistry for examining the relative concentrations of certain molecular species in solutions. The technique is based on the principle that when atoms with an odd number of nucleons (neutrons and protons) are placed in a strong magnetic field, they will tend to orient themselves along the lines of force of the magnetic field. If a brief pulse of radiofrequency energy is applied to these atoms, they will become activated and tilt out of alignment. When the pulse is discontinued, the atoms return to their original orientation in the magnetic field after emitting an element-specific radiofrequency. Depending on how the radiofrequency pulse is applied, it is possible to determine certain characteristics of the molecular environment of the atoms by calculating the time it takes them to emit their characteristic frequency ("relaxation time") (5,72,108). In order to apply these principles to a system for imaging structures in the human body, it was necessary to incorporate technological innovations in spatial signal processing and the mathematical models developed for CT.

To date, *in vivo* MRI has focused on signals retrievable from the most abundant of imageable atoms in tissue, hydrogen-1 (5,14,16). Although MRI data are in theory physiological information, hydrogen-based images are of practical value for studies of normal neuroanatomy and structural pathology. For this purpose their potential is far greater than CT because of vastly superior resolution and gray-white matter contrast, as well as the capacity to reconstruct images in all planes of anatomical cross section. The detail in images from current high-field-strength MRI machines approaches that of fresh tissue specimens.

Few MRI studies of patients with schizophrenia have appeared in the literature and most of the results have been preliminary and inconclusive. One study by Smith et al. (109) compared linear and area measurements of lateral ventricular size, cortical surface markings, lobar asymmetries, and corpus callosal thickness in 29 patients with schizophrenia and 20 normal controls and found no significant differences on any of these measures (109). Although this seems surprising in light of the CT literature, it must be viewed in the context that the same group had previously found no differences in similar quantitative measures on CT scan (59). This group did, however, report increased MRI signal intensity in both gray and white matter in their patients, a finding that is also difficult to interpret because the meaning of signal intensity in their study is unknown.

In another study, quantitative measurements were made on midsagittal images in a group of up to 38 patients and 49 normal controls (2). By dividing the corpus callosum into four segments and the groups into males and females, they were able to show that female patients had larger middle callosal segments (83). The possibility that this is a chance finding related to multiple comparisons must be considered. Another finding to emerge from this study was reduced areas of the frontal lobe, the entire cerebrum, as well as the cranium. The finding of reduced frontal lobe area may be consistent with CT studies of apparent frontal atrophy. However, the finding of smaller heads is surprising and not consistent with past literature. The interpretation of these results is difficult, in large part because of the limitations inherent in drawing conclusions about brain morphology based solely on a midsagittal image.

Mathew et al. (70) were not able to confirm either reduced brain area or increased callosal area. They did, however, report increased area of the septum pellucidum on midsagittal images, a finding that must in fact indicate ventricular enlargement, because the septum itself is not visualized in a 1-cm thick midsagittal section.

The future of MRI scanning in schizophrenia will involve morphometric study of specific nuclei and cortical areas not visualizable with CT. This technique has the potential to replicate *in vivo* the results of recent postmortem studies described below. Because of its greater resolution and safety, MRI will soon become the primary approach for imaging brain structure in psychiatric patients. Since there is no exposure to ionizing radiation, it is an ideal technique for longitudinal studies. Moreover, in the near future it will be possible to image other atoms, such as phosphorus and fluorine, that will extend MRI beyond brain structure and into physiology and pharmacology (30,43,120,138).

POSTMORTEM NEUROANATOMICAL STUDIES

Although preliminary experience with MRI has produced inconsistent findings, the results of studies with CT have been consistent and interpretable. Ventricular enlargement and dilatation of cortical sulci implicate a neuropathological process or event that caused reduced brain tissue mass. Furthermore, the weight of the CT data suggests that the pathology is static rather than progressive. As informative as this body of research findings appears to be, if the process implicated by the CT data is real, it should be observable on postmortem examination. Failure to find evidence of a pathological process consistent with the CT findings would indicate that the fixed structural pathology of the brain suggested by these findings did not exist.

Several recent controlled postmortem investigations strongly suggest that the pathology implicated by CT is real. In contrast to studies from the first half of this century, which tended to look for a qualitatively pathognomonic lesion, recent investigations have pursued more conservative goals, usually evidence that a neuropathological process has occurred at all (see Table 1). The report that most directly related to the CT data is a morphometric study by Brown et al. (15) that measured the ventricular system in

TABLE 1. *Controlled postmortem neuropathological studies in schizophrenia 1964–1985*

Study	Schizophrenic subjects/controls	Brain area	Reported abnormality
Nieto, Escobar (1972) (85)	10/3	Reticular formation, hypothalamus, periaqueductal gray, hippocampus	Gliosis
Colon (1972) (19)	3/2	Cortical areas 4, 10, 24	Decreased number of neurons (especially layers IV and V)
Miyakawa et al. (1972) (71)	5/4	Frontal cortex	Ultrastructural (EM) abnormalities, neurons, and glia
Fisman (1975) (31)	7/24	Brainstem	6/7 schizophrenics showed glial "knots" and perivascular infiltrates
Weinberger et al. (1980) (132)	12/35	Cerebellar vermis	Increased frequency of "atrophy"
Averback (1981) (6)	13/35	Nucleus ansa peduncularis (substantia innominata)	Degeneration
Dom et al. (1981) (28)	5/5	Neostriatum, nucleus accumbens	Loss of Golgi II neurons
Stevens (1982) (111)	25/48	Periventricular diencephalon, periaqueductal gray, basal forebrain	Fibrillary gliosis
Bogerts et al. (1983) (11)	6/9	Lateral substantia nigra	Decreased volume
Kovelman and Scheibel (1984) (57)	10/8	Hippocampus	Pyramidal cell disarray
Bogerts et al. (1985) (12)	13/9	Amygdala, hippocampal formation, parahippocampal gyrus, pallidum internum	Decreased volume
Benes et al. (1986) (7)	10/10	Layers VI (prefrontal), V (cingulate), III (motor)	Decreased cortical cells (neurons > glia)
Brown et al. (1986) (15)	41/29	Parahippocampal gyrus	Decreased width (also decreased brain weight and larger temporal horn of lateral ventricle)

photos of coronal sections through the mamillary bodies of 41 brains of patients with schizophrenia and 29 controls who had affective disorders and died of similar circumstances. The schizophrenia group had significantly larger ventricles, which at the temporal horns were almost twice as large. This study also found that the schizophrenia cases had slightly smaller parahippocampal gyri and lower brain weight. The morphometric studies of Bogerts et al. (11,12) are also consistent with the CT findings as well as the study of Brown et al. (15), but go one step farther in providing evidence of what brain structures are directly involved. These investigators conducted a volumetric survey of selected periventricular limbic and diencephalic nuclei in up to 13 schizophrenic and eight normal brains, all of whom died before the advent of neuroleptic medication. Several regions were significantly smaller, including the substantia nigra, the medial pallidum, amygdala, hippocampal formation and parahippocampal gyrus, and diencephalic periventricular gray. To a great extent, the findings of Bogerts et al. and of Brown et al. are mutually consistent and both are compatible with the CT data.

One carefully controlled quantitative investigation of cell numbers in the frontal cortex has found evidence of reduced neuronal populations in schizophrenia (7), especially in the prefrontal association cortex. This finding may be related to evidence from physiological cerebral imaging studies of impaired activation of prefrontal cortex (9,74,126) and is consistent with CT studies showing increased prefrontal cortical markings (106).

Other findings have been reported in studies that were less quantitative and that have yet to be replicated (6,19,28,31,57,71,85,111,132). Although the exact nature of these findings differs, their location also implicates mainly periventricular limbic and diencephalic structures, and they would also probably result in reduced tissue mass and larger cerebral ventricles. Finally, the assumption from CT that the process is static and not progressive appears to be supported by the postmortem data in that none of the postmortem findings implicate an active, degenerative disorder. Indeed, several of the findings were interpreted to be most consistent with a developmental deficit or dysplasia (7,11,12,57).

COMMENT

In less than 10 years, brain morphology has gone from being one of the least productive areas of research in schizophrenia to becoming one of its richest. As a result of new approaches to the direct examination of cerebral anatomy both during life and at postmortem, there is now virtually conclusive evidence that many patients with schizophrenia have structural pathology of the brain. Although it is impossible to definitively rule out that all the findings are epiphenomena, the evidence does not imply this conclusion.

One of the controversies that has emerged from this work is whether the structural pathology applies to only a subgroup of patients, or perhaps, identifies a distinct illness subtype (20,21). In other words, do some patients have "structural pathology schizophrenia" while others have another type (e.g., "dopamine schizophrenia")? In support of this notion are reports that ventricular enlargement on CT tends to predict a variety of poor prognostic features and also tends to show less of a correlation with aspects of the illness traditionally linked to excessive dopaminergic activity. Indeed, it has been proposed that research data in schizophrenia support the dopamine hypothesis much better if patients with large ventricles are excluded from the data sample (55). On the other hand, the distribution of ventricular sizes in almost every study has failed to suggest that the phenomenon affects only a small group of extreme outliers. Instead, it seems that ventricular size in the entire population is shifted upwards with respect to controls, similar to what one finds in studies of ventricular size in patients with Alzheimer's disease. In schizophrenia, one is just as likely to find few small ventricles as many large ones. This suggests that the pathological process exists along a continuum of severity. The correlation with prognosis and neurochemistry might also reflect this, in that the more severe the structural pathology, the poorer the outcome and the less dramatic the effect of neuropharmacological interventions.

The relationship of the structural pathology to the neurochemical aspects of schizophrenia is a matter of speculation. The structural changes could be the primary condition and the neurochemical aspects secondary, or *vice versa*. Postmortem neurochemical findings of increased dopamine receptors in basal ganglia and limbic forebrain could reflect a loss of inhibitory input to the involved dopamine terminal fields. Findings of increased concentrations of catecholamines and metabolites in periventricular nuclei could reflect a loss of nuclear mass that spares the dopamine projections (131). In the future, it may be possible to clarify these issues by conducting anatomical and neurochemical investigations on the same brain specimens.

The studies reviewed in this chapter suggest that periventricular limbic regions and prefrontal cortex are the areas of maximum pathological involvement in schizophrenia. These are the same areas implicated in most postmortem neurochemical investigations and in *in vivo* physiological studies (131). Furthermore, they are the areas that are generally thought to mediate the characteristic symptoms of schizophrenia (124). The magnitude of the pathology is not great and certainly not diagnostic either on CT scan or under the microscope. Nevertheless, its location and interaction with brain systems that normally reach physiological maturity in early adulthood (e.g., prefrontal cortex) may partially explain its devastating impact (125).

Although the CT and postmortem anatomical findings have provided information about the existence of structural pathology and some clues about its location within the brain, they do not implicate a particular etiological process. Most of the current theories about neurobiological causes of schizophrenia would be consistent with the anatomical findings. It is interesting to note, however, that the majority of the evidence favors the interpretation that an early developmental injury occurred and left a static structural deficit or that certain neuroanatomical systems failed to develop or developed in a deficient manner. Regardless of the etiology of this pathology or of its exact contribution to the pathogenesis of schizophrenia, it is difficult to escape the conclusion that the cause of this illness is related to the pathological process responsible for the morphological findings reviewed in this chapter.

ACKNOWLEDGMENTS

The authors would like to thank Mrs. Selena Cunningham for the preparation of the manuscript.

REFERENCES

1. Andreasen, N. C., Dennert, J. W., Olsen, S. A., and Damasio, A. R. (1982): *Am. J. Psychiatry*, 139:427–430.
2. Andreasen, N., Nasrallah, H., Dunn, V., Olson, S. C., Grove, W. M., Ehrhardt, J. C., Coffman, J. A., and Crossett, J. H. W. (1986): *Arch. Gen. Psychiatry*, 43:136–144.
3. Andreasen, N. C., Olsen, S. A., Dennert, J. W., and Smith, M. R. (1982): *Am. J. Psychiatry*, 139:297–302.
4. Andreasen, N. C., Smith, M. R., Jacoby, C. G., Dennert, J. W., and Olsen, S. A. (1982): *Am. J. Psychiatry*, 139:292–296.
5. Andrew, E. R. (1984): *Br. Med. Bull.*, 40:115–119.
6. Averback, P. (1981): *Arch. Neurol.*, 38:230–235.
7. Benes, F. M., Davidson, J., and Bird, E. D. (1986): *Arch. Gen. Psychiatry*, 43:31–35.
8. Benes, F., Sunderland, P., Jones, B. D., LeMay, M., Cohen, B. M., and Lipinski, J. (1982): *Br. J. Psychiatry*, 141:90–93.
9. Berman, K. F., Zec, R. F., and Weinberger, D. R. (1986): *Arch. Gen. Psychiatry*, 43:126–135.
10. Bird, J. M. (1982): *Prog. Neurobiol.*, 19:91–115.
11. Bogerts, B., Hantsch, J., and Herzer, M. (1983): *Biol. Psychiatry*, 18:952–969.
12. Bogerts, B., Meertz, E., and Schonfelt-Bausch, R. (1985): *Arch. Gen. Psychiatry*, 42:784–791.
13. Boronow, J., Pickar, D., Ninan, P. T., Roy, A., Hommer, D., Linnoila, M., and Paul, S. M. (1985): *Arch. Gen. Psychiatry*, 40:266–271.
14. Bottomley, P. A., Hart, H. R., Edelstein, W. A., Schenck, J. F., Smith, L. S., Leve, W. M., Mueller, O. M., and Redington, R. W. (1984): *Radiology*, 150:441–446.
15. Brown, R., Colter, N., Corsellis, J. A. N., Crow, T. J., Frith, C. D., Jagoe, R., Johnstone, E. C., and Marsh, L. (1986): *Arch. Gen. Psychiatry*, 43:36–42.
16. Bydder, G. M. (1984): *Br. Med. Bull.*, 40:170–174.
17. Coffman, J. A., Meffered, J., Golden, C. J., Broch, S., and Graber, B. (1981): *Lancet*, 1:666.
18. Coffman, J. A., and Nasrallah, H. A. (1984): *J. Affective Disord.*, 6:307–315.
19. Colon, E. J. (1972): *Acta Neuropathol.*, 20:1–10.
20. Crow, T. J. (1980): *Br. Med. J.*, 28:66–68.
21. Crow, T. J. (1980): *Br. J. Psychiatry*, 137:383–386.
22. DeLisi, L. E., Goldin, L. R., Hamovit, J. R., Maxwell, E., Kurtz, D., and Gershon, E. S. (1986): *Arch. Gen. Psychiatry*, 43:148–153.
23. DeLisi, L. E., Neckers, L. M., Weinberger, D. R., and Wyatt, R. J. (1981): *Arch. Gen. Psychiatry*, 38:647–650.
24. DeLisi, L. E., Schwartz, C. C., Targum, S. D., Byrnes, S. M., Cannon-Spoor, E., Weinberger, D. R., and Wyatt, R. J. (1983): *Psychiatry Res.*, 9:169–171.
25. DeMeyer, M. K., Gilmor, R., DeMeyer, W. E., Hendric, H., Edwards, M., and Franco, J. N. (1984): *J. Operational Psychiatry*, 15:2–8.

26. Dewan, M. J., Pandurangi, A. K., Lee, S. H., Ramachandran, T., Levy, B. F., Boucher, M., Yazawitz, A., and Major, L. (1983): *Psychiatry Res.*, 10:97–103.

27. Dewan, M. J., Pandurangi, A. D., Lice, S. H., Ramachandran, T., Levy, B., Boucher, M., Yazawitz, A., and Major, L. F. (1983): *Biol. Psychiatry*, 18:1133–1140.

28. Dom, R., DeSaedeleer, J., Bogerts, J., and Hopf, A. (1981): In: Proceedings of the Third World Congress of Biological Psychiatry, Stockholm. Elsevier, Amsterdam.

29. Donnelly, E. F., Weinberger, D. R., Waldman, I. N., and Wyatt, R. J. (1980): *J. Nerv. Ment. Dis.*, 168:305–308.

30. Findly, R. C., Gillies, R. J., and Shulman, R. G. (1983): *Science*, 219:1223–1225.

31. Fisman, M. (1975): *Br. J. Psychiatry*, 126:414–422.

32. Flor-Henry, P., and Gruzelier, J. H. (1983): *Laterality and Psychopathology*. Elsevier, Amsterdam.

33. Frangos, E., Anthanassenas, G., Gregoriades, A., and Kapsalakis, Z. (1982): *Enkaphalos*, 19:64–70.

34. Gattaz, W. F., Kasper, S., Kohlmeyer, K., and Beckman, H. (1981): *Fortschr. Psychiatr. Neurol.*, 49:286–291.

35. Gluck, E., Radu, E. W., and Gerhardt, P. (1980): *Neuroradiology*, 20:167–171.

36. Golden, C. J., Graber, B., Coffman, J., Berg, R., Bloch, S., and Brogan, D. (1980): *Psychiatry Res.*, 3:179–184.

37. Golden, C. J., Graber, B., Coffman, J., Berg, R. A., Newllin, D. B., and Bloch, S. (1981): *Arch. Gen. Psychiatry*, 38:1014–1017.

38. Golden, C. J., MacInnes, W. D., Ariel, R. N., Ruedrich, S. L., Chu, C.-C., Coffman, J. A., Graber, B., and Bloch, S. (1982): *J. Consult. Clin. Psychol.*, 50:87–95.

39. Golden, C. J., Moses, J. A., Zelazowski, R., Graber, B., Zatz, L. M., Horvath, T. B., and Berger, P. A. (1980): *Arch. Gen. Psychiatry*, 37:619–623.

40. Gruzelier, J. H., and Flor-Henry, P. (1979): *Hemisphere Asymmetrics of Function in Psychopathology*. Elsevier, Amsterdam.

41. Heath, R. G., Franklin, D. E., and Shraberg, D. (1979): *J. Nerv. Ment. Dis.*, 167:585–592.

42. Heath, R. G., Franklin, D. E., Walker, C. F., and Keating, J. W. (1982): *Biol. Psychiatry*, 17:569–583.

43. Hilberman, M., Subramanian, V. H., Haselgrove, J., Cone, J. B., Egan, J. W., Gyulai, L., and Chance, B. (1984): *J. Cereb. Blood Flow Metab.*, 4:334–342.

44. Jacoby, R. J., and Levy, R. (1980): *Br. J. Psychiatry*, 136:270–275.

45. Jennings, W. S., Schulz, S. C., Nasrasinhachari, N., Hamer, R. M., and Friedel, R. O. (1985): *Psychiatry Res.*, 16:87–94.

46. Jernigan, T. L., Zatz, L. M., Moses, J. A., and Berger, P. A. (1982): *Arch. Gen. Psychiatry*, 39:765–770.

47. Jernigan, T. L., Zatz, L. M., Moses, J. A., and Cardilleno, J. P. (1982): *Arch. Gen. Psychiatry*, 39:771–773.

48. Jernigan, T. L., Zatz, L. M., and Naesu, M. A. (1979): *Radiology*, 132:463–466.

49. Johnstone, E. C., Crow, T. J., Frith, C. D., Husband, J., and Kreel, L. (1976): *Lancet*, 2:924–926.

50. Johnstone, E. C., Crow, T. J., Frith, C. D., Stevens, M., Kreel, L., and Husband, J. (1978): *Acta Psychiatr. Scand.*, 57:305–324.

51. Johnstone, E. C., Owens, D. G. L., Crow, T. J., and Jagoe, R. (1981): In: *Biological Psychiatry*, edited by C. Perris, G. Struwe, and B. Jansson, pp. 237–240. Elsevier, Amsterdam.

52. Kanba, S., Shima, S., Tsukumo, D., Masuda, Y., and Asai, M. (1984): *Biol. Psychiatry*, 19:273–274.

53. Kirch, D. G., and Weinberger, D. R. (1986): In: *Handbook of Schizophrenia, Vol. 1*, edited by H. A. Nasrallah and D. R. Weinberger, Chapter 14. Elsevier, Amsterdam.

54. Kleinman, J. E., Karson, C. N., Weinberger, D. R., Freed, W. J., Berman, K. F., and Wyatt, R. J. (1984): *Am. J. Psychiatry*, 141:1430–1432.

55. Kleinman, J. E., Weinberger, D. R., Rogol, A. D., Bigelow, L. B., Klein, S. T., Gillin, J. C., and Wyatt, R. J. (1982): *Arch. Gen. Psychiatry*, 39:655–657.

56. Kling, A. S., Kurtz, N., Tachiki, K., and Orzeck, A. (1983): *J. Psychiatry Res.*, 17:375–384.

57. Kovelman, J. A., and Scheibel, A. B. (1984): *Biol. Psychiatry*, 19:1601–1621.

58. Kutty, I. N., and Prendes, J. L. (1981): *J. Nerv. Ment. Dis.*, 169:390–391.

59. Largen, J. W., Calderon, M., and Smith, R. C. (1983): *Am. J. Psychiatry*, 140:1060–1062.

60. Largen, J. W., Smith, R. C., Calderon, M., Baumgarten, R., Lu, R.-B., Schoolar, J. C., and Ravichandran, G. K. (1984): *Biol. Psychiatry*, 19:991–1013.

61. Lippman, S., Manshadi, M., Baldwin, H., Drasin, G., Rice, J., and Alrajeh, S. (1982): *Am. J. Psychiatry*, 139:667–668.

62. Luchins, D. J., Lewine, R. J., and Meltzer, H. Y. (1983): *Schizophr. Bull.*, 19:518–522.

63. Luchins, D. J., Lewine, R. R. J., and Meltzer, H. Y. (1984): *Biol. Psychiatry*, 19:29–44.

64. Luchins, D. J., and Meltzer, H. Y. (1983): *Psychiatry Res.*, 10:87–95.

65. Luchins, D. J., and Meltzer, H. Y. (1983): *Biol. Psychiatry*, 18:1197–1198.

66. Luchins, D. J., and Meltzer, H. Y. (1986): *Psychiatry Res.*, 17:7–14.

67. Luchins, D. J., Weinberger, D. R., and Wyatt, R. J. (1979): *Arch. Gen. Psychiatry*, 36:1309–1311.

68. Luchins, D. J., Weinberger, D. R., and Wyatt, R. J. (1982): *Am. J. Psychiatry*, 139:753–757.

69. Lyon, K., Wilson, J., Golden, C. J., Graber, B., Coffman, J. A., and Bloch, S. (1981): *Psychiatry Res.*, 5:33–37.

70. Mathew, R. J., and Partain, C. L. (1985): *Am. J. Psychiatry*, 142:970–971.

71. Miyakawa, T., Sumiyoshi, S., Deshimaru, M., Suzuki, T., Tomonari, H., Yasuoka, F., and Tatetsu, S. (1972): *Acta Neuropathol.*, 20:67–77.

72. Moore, W. S. (1984): *Br. Med. Bull.*, 40:120–124.

73. Moriguch, I. (1981): *Folia Psychiatr. Neurol.*, 35:55–72.

74. Morihisa, J. M., and McAnulty, G. B. (1985): *Biol. Psychiatry*, 20:3–19.

75. Mundt, C., Radu, W., and Gluck, E. (1980): *Nervenarzt*, 51:745–748.

76. Nasrallah, H. A., Andreasen, N. C., Coffman, J. A., Olson, S. C., Dunn, V. D., Ehrhardt, J. C., and Chapman, S. M. (1986): *Biol. Psychiatry*, 21:274–282.

77. Nasrallah, H. A., Jacoby, C. G., and McCalley-Whitters, M. (1981): *Lancet*, 1:1102.

78. Nasrallah, H. A., Jacoby, C. G., McCalley-Whitters, M., and Kuperman, S. (1982): *Arch. Gen. Psychiatry*, 39:774–777.

79. Nasrallah, H. A., Kuperman, S., Hamra, B. J., and McCalley-Whitters, M. (1983): *J. Clin. Psychiatry*, 44:407–409.

80. Nasrallah, H. A., Kuperman, S., Jacoby, C. G., McCalley-Whitters, M., and Hamra, B. (1983): *Psychiatry Res.*, 10:237–242.

81. Nasrallah, H. A., and McCalley-Whitters, M. (1982): *J. Affective Disord.*, 4:15–19.

82. Nasrallah, H. A., McCalley-Whitters, M., and Jacoby, G. C. (1982): *J. Clin. Psychiatry*, 43:439–441.

83. Nasrallah, H. A., Olson, S. C., McCalley-Whitters, M., Chapman, S., and Jacoby, C. G. (1986): *Arch. Gen. Psychiatry*, 43:157–159.

84. Nasrallah, H. A., Rizzo, M., Damasio, H., McCalley-Whitters, M., Kuperman, S., and Jacoby, C. G. (1982): *J. Clin. Psychiatry*, 43:307–309.

85. Nieto, D., and Escobar, A. (1972): In: *Pathology of the Nervous System, Vol. 3*, pp. 2654–2665. McGraw-Hill, New York.

86. Nyback, H., Berggren, B.-M., Hindmarsh, T., Sedvall, G., and Wiesel, F.-A. (1983): *Psychiatry Res.*, 9:301–308.

87. Nyback, H., Weisel, F.-A., Berggren, B.-M., and Hindmarsh, T. (1982): *Acta Psychiatr. Scand.*, 65:403–414.

88. Okasha, A., and Madkour, O. (1982): *Acta Psychiatr. Scand.*, 65:29–34.

89. Okasha, A., Madkour, O., and Magd, F. A. (1981): In: *Biological Psychiatry 1981*, edited by C. Perris, G. Struwe, and B. Jansson, pp. 241–245. Elsevier, Amsterdam.

90. Oxenstierna, G., Bergstrand, G., Bjerkenstedt, L., Sedvall, G., and Wik, G. (1984): *Br. J. Psychiatry*, 144:654–661.

91. Pandurangi, A. K., Dewan, M. J., Lee, S. H., Ramachandran, T., Levy, B. F., Boucher, M., Yozawitz, A., and Major, L. (1984): *Br. J. Psychiatry*, 144:172–176.

92. Pearlson, G. D., Garbacz, D. J., Breakey, W. R., Ahn, H. S., and DePaulo, J. R. (1984): *Psychiatry Res.,* 12:1–9.

93. Pearlson, G. D., Garbacz, D. J., Moberg, P. J., Ahn, H. S., and DePaulo, J. R. (1985): *J. Nerv. Ment. Dis.,* 173:42–50.

94. Pearlson, G. D., Garbacz, D. J., Tompkins, R. H., Ahn, H. S., Gutlerman, D. F., Beroff, A. E., and DePaulo, J. R. (1984): *Am. J. Psychiatry,* 141:253–256.

95. Pearlson, G. D., and Veroff, A. F. (1981): *Lancet,* 2:470.

96. Potkin, S. G., Weinberger, D. R., Linnoila, M., and Wyatt, R. J. (1983): *Am. J. Psychiatry,* 140:21–25.

97. Raz, S., Raz, N., Weinberger, D. R., Boronow, J., Pickar, D., Bigler, E. D., and Turkheimer, E. N., (1987): *Psychiatry Research* (*in press*).

98. Reveley, A. M., Reveley, M. A., Clifford, C. A., and Murray, R. M. (1982): *Lancet,* 1:540–541.

99. Reveley, A. M., Reveley, M. A., and Murray, R. M. (1984): *Br. J. Psychiatry,* 144:89–93.

100. Rieder, R. O., Donnelly, E. F., Herdt, J. R., and Waldman, I. N. (1979): *Psychiatry Res.,* 1:1–9.

101. Schulsinger, F., Parnas, J., Petersen, E. T., Schulsinger, H., Teasdale, T. W., Meduick, S. A., Moller, L., and Silverton, L. (1984): *Arch. Gen. Psychiatry,* 41:602–606.

102. Schulz, S. C., Koller, M. M., Kishore, P. R., Hamer, R. M., Gehl, J. J., and Friedel, R. O. (1983): *Am. J. Psychiatry,* 140:1592–1595.

103. Schulz, S. C., Sinicrope, P., Kishore, P., and Friedel, R. O. (1983): *Schizophr. Bull.,* 19:510–512.

104. Scott, M. Z., Golden, C. J., Ruedrich, S. L., and Bishop, R. J. (1983): *Psychiatry Res.,* 8:91–93.

105. Shelton, R. C., and Weinberger, D. R. (1986): In: *Handbook of Schizophrenia, Volume 1: The Neurology of Schizophrenia,* edited by H. A. Nasrallah and D. R. Weinberger, Chapter 9. Elsevier, Amsterdam.

106. Shelton, R. C., Weinberger, D. R., Doran, A., and Pickar, D. (1985): Presented at the Fourth World Congress of Biological Psychiatry, Philadelphia.

107. Shima, S., Kanba, S., Masuda, Y., Tsukumo, T., Kitamura, T., and Asai, M. (1985): *Acta Psychiatr. Scand.,* 71:25–29.

108. Shulman, R. G. (1983): *Sci. Am.,* 248:86–93.

109. Smith, R. C., Calderon, M., Ravichandran, G. K., Largen, J., Vroulis, G., Shvartsburd, A., Gordon, J., and Schoolar, J. C. (1984): *Psychiatry Res.,* 12:137–147.

110. Standish-Barry, H. M. A. S., Bouras, N., Bridges, P. K., and Bartlett, J. R. (1982): *Br. J. Psychiatry,* 141:614–617.

111. Stevens, J. R. (1982): *Arch. Gen. Psychiatry,* 39:1131–1139.

112. Synek, W., and Reuben, J. R. (1976): *Br. J. Radiol.,* 49:233–237.

113. Tachiki, K. H., Kurtz, W., Kling, A. S., and Hullett, F. J. (1984): *J. Psychiatr. Res.,* 18:233–243.

114. Takahashi, R., Inaba, Y., Inanaga, K., Kato, N., Kumashiro, H., Nishimura, T., Okuma, T., Otskui, S., Sakai, T., Sato, T., and Shimazono, Y. (1981): In: *Biological Psychiatry 1981,* edited by C. Perris, G. Struwe, and B. Jansson, pp. 259–268. Elsevier, Amsterdam.

115. Tanaka, Y., Hazama, H., Kawahara, R., and Kobayash, K. (1981): *Acta Psychiatr. Scand.,* 63:191–197.

116. Targum, D. S., Rosen, L. N., and Citrin, C. M. (1983): *South. Med. Assoc. J.,* 79:985–987.

117. Targum, D. S., Rosen, L. N., DeLisi, L. E., Weinberger, D. R., and Citrin, C. M. (1983): *Biol. Psychiatry,* 18:329–336.

118. Trimble, M. R., and Kingsley, D. (1978): *Lancet,* 1:278–279.

119. Tsai, L. Y., Nasrallah, H. A., and Jacoby, C. G. (1983): *Arch. Gen. Psychiatry,* 40:1286–1289.

120. Unkefer, C. J., Blazer, R. M., and London, R. E. (1983): *Science,* 222:62–65.

121. van Kammen, D. P., Mann, L. S., Sternberg, D. E., Scheinin, M., Ninan, P. T., Marler, S. R., and van Kammen, W. B. (1983): *Science,* 220:974–976.

122. Weinberger, D. R. (1982): In: *Schizophrenia as a Brain Disease,* edited by F. A. Henn and H. A. Nasrallah, pp. 148–174. Oxford University Press, New York.

123. Weinberger, D. R. (1984): *J. Psychiatr. Res.,* 18:477–490.

124. Weinberger, D. R. (1985): In: *Controversies in Schizophrenia,* edited by M. Alpert, pp. 92–109. Guilford Press, New York.

125. Weinberger, D. R. (1986): In: *Handbook of Schizophrenia, Vol. 1: The Neurology of Schizophrenia,* edited by H. A. Nasrallah and D. R. Weinberger, Chapter 19. Elsevier, Amsterdam.

126. Weinberger, D. R., Berman, K. F., and Zec, R. F. (1986): *Arch. Gen. Psychiatry,* 43:114–125.

127. Weinberger, D. R., Bigelow, L. B., Kleinman, J. E., Klein, S. T., Rosenblatt, J. E., and Wyatt, R. J. (1980): *Arch. Gen. Psychiatry,* 37:11–113.

128. Weinberger, D. R., Cannon-Spoor, E., Potkin, S. G., and Wyatt, R. J. (1980): *Am. J. Psychiatry,* 137:1410–1412.

129. Weinberger, D. R., DeLisi, L. E., Neophytides, A. N., and Wyatt, R. J. (1981): *Psychiatry Res.,* 4:65–71.

130. Weinberger, D. R., DeLisi, L. E., Perman, G. P., Targum, S., and Wyatt, R. J. (1982): *Arch. Gen. Psychiatry,* 39:778–783.

131. Weinberger, D. R., and Kleinman, J. E. (1986): In: *American Psychiatric Association Annual Review, Vol. 4,* edited by R. E. Hales and A. J. Frances, pp. 42–67. American Psychiatric Association Press, Washington, DC.

132. Weinberger, D. R., Kleinman, J. E., Luchins, D. J., Bigelow, L. B., and Wyatt, R. J. (1980): *Am. J. Psychiatry,* 137:359–361.

133. Weinberger, D. R., Torrey, E. F., Neophytides, A. N., and Wyatt, R. J. (1979): *Arch. Gen. Psychiatry,* 36:735–739.

134. Weinberger, D. R., Torrey, E. F., Neophytides, A. N., and Wyatt, R. J. (1979): *Arch. Gen. Psychiatry,* 36:935–939.

135. Weinberger, D. R., Torrey, E. F., and Wyatt, R. J. (1979): *Lancet,* 1:718–719.

136. Williams, A. O., Reveley, M. A., Kolakowska, T., Ardern, M., and Mandelbrote, B. M. (1985): *Br. J. Psychiatry,* 146:239–246.

137. Woods, B. T., and Wolf, J. (1983): *Am. J. Psychiatry,* 140:1564–1570.

138. Wyrwicz, A. M., Pszenny, M. H., Schofield, J. C., Tillman, P. C., Gordon, R. E., and Martin, P. E. (1983): *Science,* 222:428–430.

Psychopharmacology:
The Third Generation of Progress,
edited by Herbert Y. Meltzer.
Raven Press, New York © 1987.

CHAPTER **77**

Positron Emission Tomography in Schizophrenia

Monte S. Buchsbaum

Positron emission tomography (PET) studies in schizophrenia have used two main approaches: metabolic imaging with deoxyglucose or glucose, and dopamine receptor imaging with ligands for the dopamine receptor. The metabolic studies have generally shown relatively reduced metabolic rates in the frontal cortex, consistent with most studies of cerebral blood flow. Relatively low metabolic rates in the basal ganglia have also been observed in some studies. With labeled neuroleptics, brain images showing greatest uptake in the basal ganglia have been obtained, and clinical studies comparing normals and schizophrenics are still in progress. For both approaches, the problem of biological heterogeneity in schizophrenia must be fully considered so that PET can reach its potential as a tool for the understanding of the location and mechanism of drug action in brain, the selection of a particular drug for the individual patient, and ultimately an understanding of the psychopharmacology of schizophrenia.

PET imaging has the capability to survey functional activity throughout the brain and thus to bring together the disparate lines of neurochemical and behavioral approaches. It has adequate resolution to view both individual gyri of the cortex and discrete portions of the basal ganglia, so important in schizophrenia research. When PET is supplemented by the high time resolution and low cost of electrical activity mapping and the positive anatomic identification possible with magnetic resonance imaging (MRI), a comprehensive analysis of brain function in the patient is now possible.

PET, using the mathematics of X-ray CT scanning to produce slice images of any chemical that is tagged with a radioisotope, opens an almost unlimited vista of metabolic studies. Positron-emitting atoms such as ^{11}C or ^{18}F can be incorporated into sugar, amino acids, neurotransmitter precursors, or psychoactive medications. Using a combination of such radiopharmaceuticals, one could potentially reveal the anatomic area made hypermetabolic by a delusion, the distribution of synaptic receptors for a treatment medication, and the physiological effect of a drug with a repeat metabolic scan. This report reviews the initial studies of schizophrenia with PET and electrophysiological imaging and outlines some of the promise of the future.

PET SCANNER TECHNOLOGY

Positron Imaging

The PET scanner uses a ring arrangement of radiation detectors to produce slice images of the distribution of radioisotopes in the human brain (7,43,44). PET takes advantage of two properties of four positron-emitting radionuclides—^{11}C, ^{13}N, ^{15}O, and ^{18}F—their biochemical properties, and the geometry of positron decay. The first three are convenient labels of the biochemical building blocks of many cell constituents, and the fourth, ^{18}F, is a small, chemically reactive atom that can be attached to many biologically important molecules, often with little alteration in their function (53). Because of the relatively long half-life of ^{18}F, 110 min, it has been the isotope most widely used.

Positrons emitted with isotope decay interact with electrons in the brain in quite short distances (about 1 mm or less); an annihilation results and two 511,000-electron-volt photons are emitted, which travel in opposite directions at an angle of almost exactly 180 degrees. The detector crystals are located in a ring around the head. The nearly simultaneous arrival of the photons in crystals on opposite sides of the ring provides information that the positron annihilation event very likely occurred somewhere along a line joining the two crystals. This unique feature of positron decay allows great spatial precision in mathematically reconstructing the location of the density of isotopes. The single-photon tomographic system, moving a single crystal around the head, lacks the degree of precision obtained with the more complex and costly PET device.

The resolution of current commercially available PET scanners is in the range of 8 to 16 mm or about the size of the caudate nucleus. Resolution is typically reported as full-width half-maximum (FWHM). A small-diameter (>1 mm) needle filled with radioactivity and oriented axially in the scanner (as an axle of the wheel of crystals) serves to measure resolution. A PET scan shows a cross section—a circle 10 or more millimeters in diameter, intense in the center and falling off to one-half of the center value in a number of millimeters. The diameter of the circle where the count rate at the circumference is 50% of the central point is the FWHM value. In the brain, structures are not pinpoints of intensity but are globular and irregular. A structure as wide as the FWHM would have its measured value diluted by surrounding tissue about 70%. Thus, very small but sufficiently intense structures can be visualized, but their quantitative interpretation would be confounded with surrounding brain structures. The caudate and thalamus, with volumes of the order of 5 cm^3, are well measured with PET resolution of 10 mm. The internal capsule and the globus pallidus in the 2 cm^3 range are fairly well quantitated, and structures such as the substantia nigra with less than 1 cm^3 may be seen in some individuals but are poorly quantitated (33,37). Spherical structures are more reliably measured than thin or wedge-shaped ones. The cortical mantle, 4 to 6 mm thick and folded as a ribbon, appears as an irregular band; this is sufficient to see the lobes, but individual gyri have blurred margins. This dilution may be important in quantitative PET work where, for example, gray matter/white matter differences in local concentration of isotopes may be between 10 and 100%. In contrast, the X-ray transmission differences seen in CT scans between bone and air are more than 1,000-fold, allowing quite a sharp skull image to be produced. However, gray matter/white matter differences in X-ray transmission are in the range of 0.5%, accounting for the capacity of the intrinsically lower-resolution PET to reveal brain structures so dramatically in comparison to routine clinical CT.

Animal studies suffer especially from the limited resolution of PET. Whereas the caudate in humans is in the 10-mm range, in the rat it is in the 1-mm range; indeed the FWHM would include the entire brain of a rat. Large primates such as the baboon can be scanned, but the images allow only the largest structures to be visualized. PET is largely a human technique with current scanners.

Resolution is limited by, among other factors, uncertainty in how far positrons travel before encountering an electron, variation from exactly 180 degrees opposite travel, and the size of the gamma-sensitive crystal detector system. Basic positron physics limit the ultimate resolution of PET scanners to 1.5 to 2.5 mm, leaving a large improvement possible. Smaller detectors would allow more to be packed into the ring and result in more precise localization of the gamma coincidences. Shrinking the size of the assembly of crystals and their accompanying photomultiplier tubes, which detect the photon, is a soluble engineering problem.

Cyclotron Production of Positron Emitters

The small-atomic-weight isotopes used in PET have quite short half-lives (^{15}O, 2 min; ^{13}N, 10 min; ^{11}C, 20 min; and ^{18}F, 110 min). Thus, in order to have a sufficient amount of isotope for patient study, a cyclotron to produce positron emitters from stable atoms and a radiochemistry laboratory for swift synthesis of radiopharmaceuticals are essential components of each PET operation (62).

The short half-life of positron emitters keeps radiation dose to the patient relatively low. For example, typical ^{18}F doses of 5 millicuries provide whole-body doses in the 300 to 400 mR range; brain doses are less than half that of a typical CT scan. Most PET centers limit scans to no more than three for an individual. Radiation dosimetry for [^{18}F]deoxyglucose (FDG) is reviewed by Jones (32).

Imaging the Brain's Metabolic Rate

Brain work requires energy. Glucose, burned to carbon dioxide and water, serves as the source of high-energy phosphate bonds, which fuel cell repolarization and other processes (see refs. 53, 55). However, glucose itself, labeled with a positron emitter such as ^{11}C and injected into the patient's antecubital vein, would be metabolized rapidly and would begin to be breathed out as radioactive carbon dioxide before the scan could be completed. Although very rapid scanning and mathematical techniques for separating metabolic products from source and blood flow have been developed (46), most PET centers have used 2-deoxyglucose as an alternative method. The missing oxygen at the 2-position allows its metabolism by hexokinase, the first step in the glycolytic path to CO_2—but limits further steps. The cells are thus labeled in proportion to their deoxyglucose uptake, which is largely complete within the 40 min after intravenous administration and remains stable for the 40- to 120-min postinjection period necessary to complete the scan (27,52). At this point, the radioactivity is fixed in the brain, much as the latent image is fixed on a photographic film by opening and closing a camera shutter and exposing the silver in the emulsion to light. The patient can be moved to the scanner and the latent image reconstructed. Thus, the deoxyglucose scan primarily shows brain activity in the 40 min of tracer uptake, not activity during the scan. For schizophrenia research, this separation of uptake and scanning is convenient. The isotope may be injected in the comparatively controlled environment of a psychophysical test chamber with the patient participating in a task known to show deficits in schizophrenia. After completion of the task, the patient can then be moved to the scanner to acquire the image of brain metabolic rate during the task. PET scans thus show brain work associated with specific task demands to sensory, motor, and association cortex (10,48).

It is important to note that both excitatory and inhibitory cell processes require energy and both processes will be indexed by glucose uptake. Cells may also modify cell activity elsewhere with their projections. Thus, the mapping of functional deficits or neuropharmacological effects with glucose may be complex. Detailed analysis of autoradiographic changes with [¹⁴C]deoxyglucose led Sokoloff to conclude that the metabolic rate changes shown with deoxyglucose represent mainly "alterations in the metabolic activity of synaptic terminals triggered by changes in Na⁺, K⁺, ATPase activity." Areas containing large masses of axons seem far less sensitive to change (54) and may be useful as reference areas for metabolic rate comparisons.

Typical Deoxyglucose Scan Procedure

In a typical scan procedure with deoxyglucose, the patient arrives an hour before the scan. An intravenous line with a plastic cannula is inserted into a vein in each arm so that when the isotope arrives no time or isotope is lost. A psychological task may be started just before isotope injection and must continue for 30 to 40 min. A challenge drug dose would also be given at this point. The tracer deoxyglucose is then injected in one arm and a series of 1- to 2-cc blood samples withdrawn from the other arm throughout the uptake and scanning period for the measurement of glucose and deoxyglucose. This arm is usually warmed with a hot pad to increase arteriovenous shunting so that glucose and 2-deoxyglucose concentration in samples approximates that achieved with arterial sampling (42). After 30 to 40 min, 70 to 90% of the deoxyglucose has been taken up from the blood and the patient can be moved to the scanner. The patient lies on a special bed, and his head is placed into a holder to keep it still during the 3 to 15 min required to accumulate enough counts for an image. An individually fitted head holder may be made from thermosetting plastic casting material to hold the patient still during the scan and to allow the patient's head to be returned to the same position for a second scan on a later date. Now the coincidence counts are collected by the computer, from one or more rings of crystals. The patient's bed may advance the patient further into the ring to count additional slice positions.

After acquisition of the count data, the computation of the final quantitative image begins. The image is typically smoothed to remove noise. A correction is next made for the greater attenuation of radiation from central than peripheral tissue. Then, the data for deoxyglucose and glucose concentration in blood, together with their exact times, are united in a mathematical model of glucose metabolism (39,52,53) and the metabolic rate of the brain (in micromoles of glucose per 100 grams of brain tissue per minute) is calculated for each of the squares that make up the final PET picture. These numerical values are then transformed by the computer into the color images of brain activity. This transformation is linear over the range of

physiologically normal tissue; thus, raw count and metabolic rate pictures have the same appearance except that the scale is now expressed in units of rate.

METABOLIC IMAGING IN SCHIZOPHRENIA

Cortical Metabolism

Preliminary PET reports by Farkas et al. (23) in one never-medicated schizophrenic suggested a relative metabolic hypofunction of the frontal lobe. This was consistent with the pioneering studies of regional cerebral blood flow by Ingvar and Franzen (28). Using intracarotid injection of ¹³³Xe to assess regional flow, they observed that the ratio of frontal lobe to whole surface flow was reduced in patients with schizophrenia. Consistent cerebral blood flow changes in the frontal lobe have been found by Ariel et al. (2), Weinberger et al. (59), and Chabrol et al. (15), but other studies have been inconsistent or have not tested the hypothesis directly (see Weinberger, *this volume*).

In the first published controlled series with PET, eight off-medication patients with schizophrenia and six normal

PET Supraventricular Slice

Normal Controls

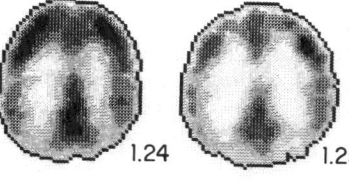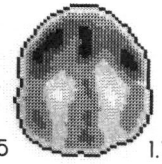

1.24   1.25   1.17 AP Ratio

Schizophrenia

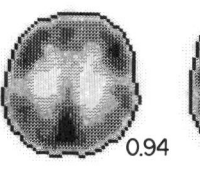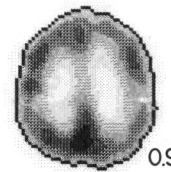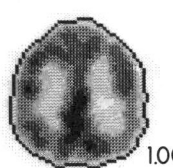

0.94   0.91   1.00

FIG. 1. PET scans with [¹⁸F]deoxyglucose in a horizontal plane parallel to and about 8 cm above the canthomeatal line. The image is scaled so that black represents the highest rate of glucose metabolism within the slice and white the lowest level. This allows comparison of relative relationships of metabolic rate across subjects. The slices show the higher rate of metabolism in the outer rim of cerebral cortex and the lower rate in the more central areas of white matter. The **upper three** brain images are from three typical normal controls and show the usual pattern of greater frontal than occipital metabolic rate. The lower three images are from three patients with schizophrenia and show higher posterior than anterior metabolic rates. The anteroposterior (AP) ratio is the frontal sector/occipital sector, as calculated in Buchsbaum et al. (8). Higher values were found in normals than in patients with schizophrenia.

TABLE 1. PET scans of different

Author	Frontal/occipital ratio			Frontal/whole slice or whole hemisphere		
	Normals	Schizophrenics	p	Normals	Schizophrenics	p
Jernigan [b] (31)	1.10	1.03	NS	1.03	0.98	NS
Buchsbaum (8)	1.08	1.02	1	1.14	1.09	1
Buchsbaum (11)	1.14	1.05	2	1.12	1.06	1
Farkas [a] (24)	1.14	1.07	3	1.11	1.05	NT
Wolkin (63)	1.09	1.04	NS	1.08	1.04	4
Kling (34)	0.79	0.74	NS	0.97	0.92	1
Wiesel [c] (61)	—	—		1.16	1.12	NT
Sheppard [d] (51)	1.1	1.0	NS	—	—	—

Analysis for right hemisphere supraventricular slice when available.
NT, Not tested; NS, not significant.
1, t-test, significant.
2, Linear trend ANOVA, significant.
3, Analysis of covariance, significant.
4, Difference for glucose metabolic rate but not tested for ratio of whole slice.
[a] Right and left combined, calculated from Tables 1–3.
[b] Automated analysis.
[c] Occipital data not given in report; frontal areas calculated from Brodmann area 9 + 10 data; CM level not given.
[d] Ratio calculated by authors to only 1 significant figure after the decimal.

controls (11) were studied. Patients rested in a darkened room with their eyes closed, to replicate the conditions of Ingvar and Franzen. The patients similarly had significantly lower frontal/whole slice glucose metabolic rate ratios (1.06) than normal controls (1.13). This was more strongly confirmed with linear trend analysis of variance, indicating the presence of a front-to-back gradient in metabolic rate in both groups, stronger in normals than in patients with schizophrenia.

A second study (Fig. 1) also found a reduced anteroposterior gradient in cerebral cortex in schizophrenia (8) as well as in patients with bipolar affective disorder. These patients received brief electrical shocks to their right forearm during tracer uptake, a task chosen because of its reported tendency to increase cerebral blood flow in the frontal lobes (29,30) and because it shows reduced pain sensitivity in schizophrenics (17). Again, group differences were most strongly statistically confirmed by linear trend analysis of variance (ANOVA); lower frontal lobe/whole slice ratios for patients with schizophrenia than for normal controls were observed but did not reach statistical significance by t-test ($p = 0.07$). Six additional studies have observed either lower or relatively lower frontal cortex metabolism in schizophrenia (see Table 1). Each study was summarized when possible from published data for the right side, frontal area at the level of the centrum semiovale, as this was the strongest finding in the initial PET study, and ratios calculated from tables in each paper. The series of studies is heterogeneous with respect to sensory conditions, analytic methods, and patient medication. Note first that the phenomenon of hyperfrontality in resting normals appears in six of eight studies; this can be seen in the frontal/occipital ratios, taking values greater than 1.0. Only the Kling study showed a ratio lower than 1.0, one of two studies in which

the subject's eyes were open. The Wiesel study did not give exactly comparable data, but a ratio of 0.99 was seen for the left side for area (6 + 8)/(39 + 40) for normal volunteers.

The lower frontal/occipital ratios in schizophrenics were seen in all seven studies, although statistically significant in only three. Frontal lobe/whole slice values were similarly lower in seven studies, significantly so in four.

Two PET studies that have not confirmed this pattern require detailed comment (51,60). Sheppard et al. (51) examined 12 normal controls and 12 patients, 6 of whom were medicated within 7 days of scanning and 2 of whom were currently medicated. Unlike the other PET studies, they scanned with ^{15}O and ^{15}O-labeled carbon dioxide; regional cerebral metabolic rate (rCMRO) and regional cerebral blood flow (rCBF) were computed. Using an image analysis technique adapted from Buchsbaum et al. (11), those investigators calculated frontal/occipital ratios, but schizophrenic/normal comparisons did not reach significance. The data are not presented in sufficient detail in this initial report to allow full comparison with the other studies, but the frontal/occipital ratio they calculated is given in Table 1. In addition to the use of different tracers, possible differences include (a) 50% of the patients were on or recently treated with neuroleptics and (b) scans were done in an open room without rigorous sensory or cognitive control. Widen et al. (60) examined six schizophrenics but only two healthy volunteers with ^{11}C-labeled glucose rather than deoxyglucose. Because they report only ratios of frontal to parietal rather than frontal to occipital lobe, and no other tabular values, their data could not be conveniently included in Table 1. In a continuation of the same series, Wiesel et al. (61) reported on 13 patients and eight volunteers. In this comparison, they found significantly reduced *brain regions in schizophrenics*

Level	Sample size schizophrenics	Test condition	Comments
Midventricular	6	Auditory vigilance task, eyes closed	Off meds
Supraventricular	16	Somatosensory stimulation, eyes resting, eyes closed	Off meds
Supraventricular	8		Off meds
Supraventricular	11	Open room	6/13 medicated
Midventricular	10	Eyes open	Off meds
"High"	6	Eyes open, lying in scanner	6/6 medicated
Brodmann 9 + 10	13	Eyes closed	Off meds
OM + 6 cm	12	Eyes closed, open room	6/12 patients not more than 7 days med free

metabolic rates in prefrontal cortex in schizophrenics (Brodmann's areas 9 and 10) but higher rates in area 6 (premotor). Anteroposterior ratios were tested for areas (6 + 8)/(39 + 40), not exactly corresponding anatomically to the frontal/occipital ratios examined in several other PET reports.

A study of the four Genain quadruplets, 50-year-old monozygotics concordant for schizophrenia but differing widely in clinical severity and lifetime history of hospitalization and neuroleptic treatment, also showed low anteroposterior ratios (12) (Fig. 2). Devous et al. (19) used single-photon tomography with ^{133}Xe and observed 43% of schizophrenics with frontal hypoperfusion compared to 11% of controls.

Relative reductions in frontal lobe protein synthesis in schizophrenia were reported by Bustany et al. (14). They used [^{11}C]L-methionine, an amino acid rapidly incorporated into neuronal and glial proteins, as a tracer and a three-compartment model to calculate the rate of local protein synthesis. Six patients with schizophrenia showed a frontal/occipital ratio of 0.80 in contrast to a ratio of 0.96 in normals (their ratio calculation, $t = 5.0$, $p < 0.001$). Patients with dementia had even lower ratios (0.64). It is of interest that whereas protein synthesis in frontal lobes of patients with schizophrenia was actually higher than in normals (although not significantly so), it is the relative ratio that reveals the significant difference and thus parallels some of the glucose metabolic rate reports of Table 1.

Consistent with these findings of relative hypofrontality, recent MRI studies by Andreasen et al. (1) reported that schizophrenics had significantly smaller frontal lobes; this was interpreted as providing "anatomic evidence for the hypofrontality hypothesis." Three other studies have examined the relationship between ventricular/brain ratio

(VBR) determined by CT scan and metabolic rate. Buchsbaum et al. (11) found a correlation of −0.42 between AP ratio and VBR, which was of marginal statistical significance ($p < 0.10$). Jernigan et al. (31) found similar and significant negative correlations (−0.56 on the right) between frontal/slice ratios and ventricular size. Lastly, Kling et al. (34) reported negative but nonsignificant regression coefficients between VBR and posterior inferior frontal and posterior superior temporal cortex.

Several methodological problems deserve note. First, glucose metabolic rate in the cortex is changed 3 to 8 μmol/100 g/min by tasks. A subject with open eyes lying in the scanner and observing the procedure would raise his parietal and occipital glucose rate, altering the anteroposterior ratio. Blindfolding or plugging the ears is a sensory manipulation possibly of quite different effect in schizophrenics and normals. Tasks that challenge particular brain areas or neurochemical systems need development.

Second, techniques for identification and definition of cortical areas need development. The glucose scale shows activity, not structure; visually drawing a line around an area of activity may exclude low-metabolic-rate cortex, altering the average. Automated and stereotaxic methods apply uniform criteria to all slices, avoid problems of subjective bias, and are transferable from investigator to investigator. The high anatomic resolution magnetic resonance scan provides an ideal method for accurate identification of structural edges on carefully matched PET scans.

Third, the finding of hypofrontality has been variably assessed by examining absolute metabolic rates in frontal cortex, frontal rates relative to whole slice, and frontal cortex relative to inferior parietal or occipital cortex.

Although absolute metabolic rates are reliable over sessions (47), they show a wide range of values in normals.

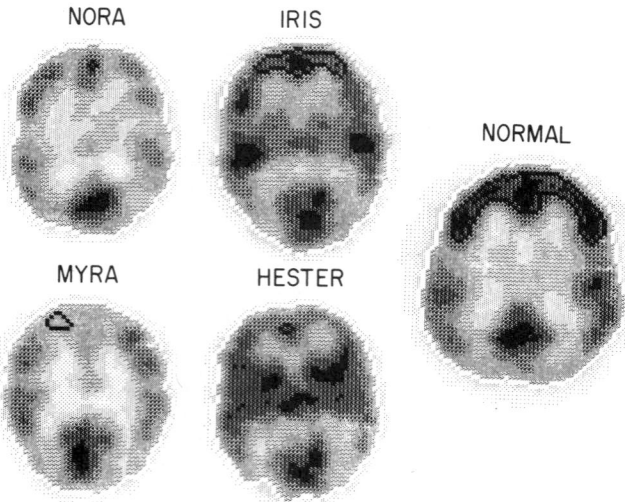

NORA   IRIS

NORMAL

MYRA   HESTER

FIG. 2. Supraventricular level PET scans in the four identical Genain quadruplets who are concordant for schizophrenia; a normal control is shown to the right for comparison. A complete area of high metabolic rate is outlined by an edge-finding algorithm in the normal; the same algorithm fails to find a similar configuration in the four other scans. The anteroposterior ratio (see Fig. 1) was also low (12).

Age, sex, and other factors that may affect whole brain metabolic rate but are irrelevant to psychopathology can be controlled for by forming ratios between brain areas. Coefficients of variation have been reported to be smaller in ratio than absolute measurements (8). Ratios may also be advantageous where two brain areas change; if schizophrenics have diminished frontal function as well as parietal or occipital increases associated with hallucinatory processes, a frontal/posterior ratio may provide an index of greater sensitivity and specificity. To date, a systematic study of reliability, sensitivity, and specificity using both measures has not been carried out.

Basal Ganglia and Neuroleptic Effects

Most studies have shown low metabolic rates in the basal ganglia of schizophrenics, which are raised by neuroleptics. Five studies (9,11,50,51,61) found significantly lower glucose metabolic rates in the basal ganglia of schizophrenics than in normal volunteers. Wolkin et al. (63) found similarly lower metabolic rates in the basal ganglia, but this difference was not statistically confirmed. The Sheppard study included some recently medicated patients, but as noted below, this might have diminished group differences rather than spuriously causing them. The only study to report higher relative metabolic rates in the basal ganglia of schizophrenics than normals is the report of Kling et al. (34) in which all patients were on neuroleptics. Relatively lower metabolic rates were also found in largely unmedicated patients with affective disorder (5,13).

Differences within portions of the basal ganglia may be important. The Sedvall study found the reduction in the lentiform nucleus but not the caudate, whereas Buchsbaum

et al. (9) found caudate to yield greater differences. Overlap in patients between the Sedvall and Wiesel samples is not specified, but the latter study has a larger sample size and also shows the lentiform decrease. One interesting consistency between Buchsbaum et al. (11), Sedvall et al. (50), Wolkin et al. (63), and Buchsbaum et al. (9) is the concordance of strongest schizophrenia/normal differences on the left side (although not statistically confirmed in all studies independently). Wolkin noted the left/right ratios significantly higher in patients with schizophrenia.

Neuroleptics tend to increase metabolic rates in the basal ganglia, consistent with a normalization of the low metabolic rates observed. In a preliminary analysis of scans in nine patients with schizophrenia on and off neuroleptic medication, we found that glucose metabolic rate in the entire brain, the temporal cortex, and the region of the basal ganglia was increased (18). Similar metabolic rate elevations have been reported by Wolkin et al. (63) and for the right but not left lentiform nucleus (60). More detailed analyses (9) revealed (Fig. 3) increases of 41% in the upper right putamen with less change in lower structures. Some associations between magnitude of change on the Brief Psychiatric Rating Scale and basal ganglia metabolic rate increase were noted both by Wolkin et al. and by Buchsbaum et al. but a larger sample is clearly needed for replication. The asymmetrical finding of larger right than left basal ganglia increases noted for putamen (9), caudate (63), and lentiform nucleus (60) deserves further study.

The increase in metabolic activity in the right upper caudate and putamen with dopamine-blocking neuroleptics suggests that dopamine as a neurotransmitter is inhibitory in these regions. Moore and Bloom (38) reported dopamine as an inhibitory neurotransmitter from data on 20 extracellularly recorded structures. The reported decrease of metabolic activity in the basal ganglia in Huntington's disease (35), also associated with a loss of dopaminergic activity, is similarly consistent.

Attention Deficit in Schizophrenia

Recent studies have indicated that certain deficits in attentional and information processing tasks are among the most consistent abnormalities found to characterize populations at heightened risk for schizophrenic disorder (3,20,40). One productive measure has been the Continuous Performance Test (CPT). This visual vigilance task involves monitoring a series of briefly presented stimuli (usually numbers or letters) that appear one at a time at a rapid serial rate and signaling by a button press each time a predesignated target stimulus is presented. Adult chronic schizophrenic patients have been shown to obtain a significantly lower percentage of correct target detections on the CPT than chronic alcoholics or normal subjects, whereas chronic alcoholics score significantly more poorly than schizophrenics and normals on the Digit-Symbol Substitution Test, a self-paced number-symbol transposition task (41). Hospitalized schizophrenic patients achieve fewer correct target detections on the CPT than hospitalized patients with either schizoaffective disorder or major affective

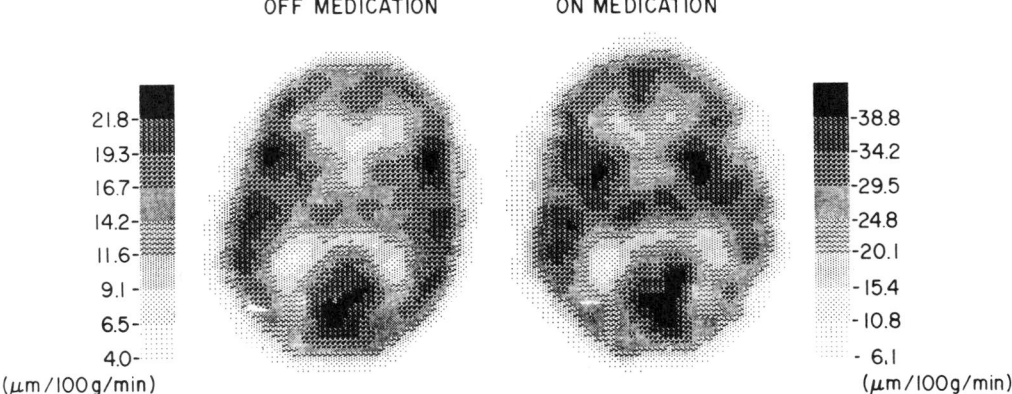

OFF MEDICATION   ON MEDICATION

21.8
19.3
16.7
14.2
11.6
9.1
6.5
4.0
(μm/100g/min)

38.8
34.2
29.5
24.8
20.1
15.4
10.8
6.1
(μm/100g/min)

FIG. 3. PET scans through the midventricular level of an 18-year-old male patient with schizophrenia 19 days drug-free **(left)** and on medication **(right)**. Note increase in region of basal ganglia, especially in the right putamen.

disorder (57). The abnormally low CPT target detection rate characterizes 40 to 50% rather than all schizophrenic inpatients (41,58). Furthermore, these poor CPT performers are more likely to have a family history of schizophrenia (58) or serious mental illness (41) than schizophrenic patients who are good CPT performers.

The CPT is especially appropriate for PET studies with FDG as it can be done for the 30 min of uptake and fills the interval with continuous vigilance activity by the subject. In a pilot investigation in normal controls, the metabolic rate of glucose was assessed in two groups of subjects. One group executed the standard CPT task for 30 min during FDG uptake. The second received no instructions except to use the flashes as a fixation point. Statistical analysis, based on exactly the same methods used previously to compare schizophrenics and normals, revealed that the CPT was associated with an increase in metabolic rate (Fig. 4) greatest in the right superior frontal gyrus—the same region (Fig. 5) in which patient/normal differences were greatest (8; see also Table 1). Data on the basal ganglia in normals and schizophrenics are not yet available, but their role may be important in sensory and attentional defects (26,36,49).

These findings of frontal and basal ganglia changes in functional activity in schizophrenia are consistent both with the dopamine theory of schizophrenia and with the psychological deficits observed in the syndrome. It should be noted at the outset that decreases in basal ganglia glucose metabolism need to be interpreted with the same caution as autopsy studies of dopamine receptor binding. Although patients in most studies were off neuroleptic medication at the time of the scan, they had still been exposed previously to neuroleptics. Nevertheless, it is of interest that the low levels of metabolism observed in these dopamine-rich areas are normalized by neuroleptics. An influence of the frontal dopamine system on the basal ganglia is suggested by the frontal cortex lesion studies of Pycock et al. (45); prefrontal lesions in the rat enhanced striatal spiperone binding. Thus, primary frontal lobe dopamine system lesions could be consistent with these findings. Recently, Benes et al. (6)

have reported lowered neuronal density in the prefrontal cortex of schizophrenics. Although the changes were not typical of neuronal degeneration, the possibility of abnormal maturation and/or perinatal insult is raised by this finding.

Both frontal cortex and the basal ganglia are involved in the modulation and maintenance of attention (see 26,49), and frontal lobe damage may produce some symptoms of behavioral disorganization not entirely unlike schizophrenia.

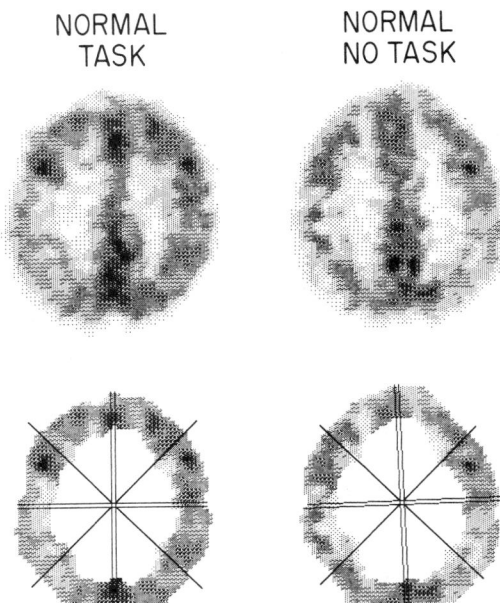

NORMAL TASK   NORMAL NO TASK

FIG. 4. PET scans at the supraventricular level as in Fig. 1, but with a higher resolution scanner, obtained at our facility at the University of California at Irvine. **Above, left:** Normal control, performing the Continuous Performance Test, a visual vigilance task. **Above, right:** Normal control, viewing the same stimuli but without performing any task. Note relatively lower glucose metabolic rate in the right frontal cortex, and compare with Fig. 1. **Below:** Images dissected by computer algorithm for statistical analysis.

NORMAL CONTROL   SCHIZOPHRENIC

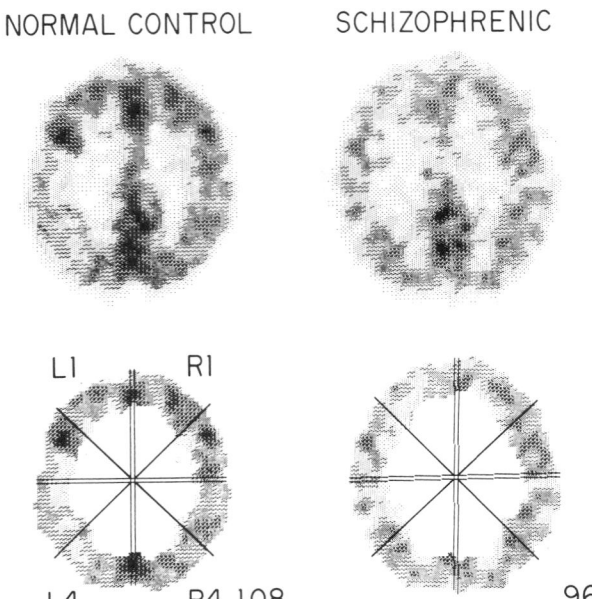

FIG. 5. Comparison of normal control and patient with schizophrenia, both performing the Continuous Performance Test. **Above:** Supraventricular level slices. **Below:** Dissection of cortical rim by computer algorithm as in Fig. 1 and computation of the anteroposterior ratio. Note reduced ratio in patient with schizophrenia.

Dopamine Receptor Binding

Comar and co-workers (16) published the first clinical PET study in psychiatry, reporting on images obtained with [^{11}C]chlorpromazine in patients with schizophrenia who had not been treated with neuroleptics for several months before the study. Since chlorpromazine has a high binding affinity for dopaminergic receptors in the brain, the PET scan values could reflect the number of receptors per unit volume, receptor affinity for the labeled compound, and the concentrations of natural receptors present. Unfortunately, other factors would also affect labeling. Neuroleptic ligands bind to receptors other than the dopamine receptor. The presence of multiple dopamine receptors with different affinities complicates the direct interpretation of the quantitative image. Metabolic products of neuroleptics that retained the ^{11}C would appear. In addition, these drugs are lipid soluble, and enter fat and myelin. Distribution in proportion to blood flow thus could be important, especially shortly after injection. The resultant image reflects all of these influences on radiolabel distribution. The images of Comar et al. are actually not unlike the FDG images produced later. A fast penetration of the labeled molecules into the brain in the first 5 to 15 min after injection was observed, with the uptake in the frontal lobe only about half of the uptake in the occipital lobe. They note the similarity of their results to the relative hypofrontality findings of Ingvar and Franzen (28) for blood flow and discuss the problems of imaging neuroleptic binding.

Wagner et al. (56) used [^{11}C]methylspiperone in PET studies. This tracer bound more selectively to the caudate than the cerebellum with a 4.4:1 ratio at 70 to 130 min. Preliminary reports of comparisons of patients with schizophrenia and normal controls have not revealed large differences (56). Large decreases in concentration of ^{76}Br-labeled bromspiperone relative to the cerebellum were found with PET in patients with progressive supranuclear palsy, an extrapyramidal disorder with loss of striatal dopamine receptors (4). This demonstrates the power of the methodology; whether diagnostic heterogeneity or biological differences obscure findings in schizophrenia remains to be determined.

Farde et al. (21,22) introduced the use of [^{11}C]raclopride, a substituted benzamide, for PET studies on dopamine D_2 receptors. The rapid association of this drug with the D_2 receptor and its low affinity for D_1 dopamine, S_2 serotonin, and α-1-adrenergic receptors make its use advantageous. They observed specific uptake of this compound in the basal ganglia of normal volunteers. A marked reduction of uptake in the basal ganglia of patients with schizophrenia who were receiving neuroleptic treatment was also found. Receptor occupancy by haloperidol was estimated to be 90% and remained high for at least 2 days after the last dose. Similar results were obtained for sulpiride. Studies comparing groups of schizophrenics and normals are not yet available.

Garnett et al. (25) used [^{18}F]L-dopa and showed caudate and frontal cortex concentration, demonstrating the versatility of PET approaches to dopamine neurochemistry in humans. Studies in patients with schizophrenia are not yet available.

FUTURE STRATEGIES

For metabolic imaging, the key scientific problem may be the selection of the task for the schizophrenic during FDG uptake. The task must exercise the brain in the area of deficit in order to reveal the differences between normals and patients. Tasks performed by patients in brain areas other than the one used by normals may prove revealing of adaptation to deficit by brain area, neurotransmitter, and cognitive strategy (see also Weinberger, *this volume*).

For receptor imaging, interpretation of the meaning of the isotope concentration numbers obtained remains an important methodological problem. Artifacts of previous and current neuroleptic exposure will need to be explored as part of these investigations.

For both approaches to schizophrenia, the problem of biological heterogeneity needs consideration. Clinical response to neuroleptics, catecholamine measures in CSF, blood, and urine, and neuroendocrine challenge tests have all indicated that considerable individual differences occur between schizophrenics. PET studies, because of their expense and technical complexity, tend to have small sample sizes and thus may be initially disappointing in schizophrenia. The data of Table 1 are typical of many biological markers. These important early studies develop the technology and prepare the research teams for the larger sample size studies to come. This later cohort of studies can address the individual who responds to neuroleptics, has low CSF homovanillic acid, dilated ventricles, attention deficits, paranoid symptoms, low platelet monoamine oxidase, or other markers of a biologically homogeneous grouping. From such studies, the use of PET scanning is the psychiatrist's and psychopharmacologist's tool to select, administer, and monitor drugs.

REFERENCES

1. Andreasen, N., Nasrallah, H. A., Dunn, V., Olson, S. C., Grove, W. M., Ehrhardt, J. C., Coffman, J. A., and Crossett, J. H. W. (1986): *Arch. Gen. Psychiatry,* 43:136–144.
2. Ariel, R. N., Golden, C. J., Berg, R. A., Quaife, M. A., Dirksen, J. W., Forsell, T., Wilson, J., and Graber, B. (1983): *Arch. Gen. Psychiatry,* 40:258–263.
3. Asarnow, R. F., Steffy, R. A., MacCrimmon, D. J., and Cleghorn, J. M. (1977): *J. Abnorm. Psychol.,* 86:267–275.
4. Baron, J. C., Maziere, B., Loc'h, C., Sgouropoulos, P., Bonnet, A. M., and Agid, Y. (1985): *Lancet,* 7:1163–1164.
5. Baxter, L. R., Phelps, M. E., Mazziotta, J. C., Schwartz, J. M., Gerner, R. H., Selin, C. E., and Sumida, R. M. (1985): *Arch. Gen. Psychiatry,* 42:441–447.
6. Benes, F. M., Davidson, J., and Bird, E. D. (1986): *Arch. Gen. Psychiatry,* 43:31–35.
7. Brownell, G. L., Budinger, T. F., Lauterbur, P. C., and McGeer, P. L. (1982): *Science,* 215:619–626.
8. Buchsbaum, M. S., DeLisi, L. E., Holcomb, H. H., Cappelletti, J., King, A. C., Johnson, J., Hazlett, E., Dowling-Zimmerman, S., Post, R. M., Morihisa, J., Carpenter, W., Cohen, R., Pickar, D., Weinberger, D. R., Margolin, R., and Kessler, R. M. (1984): *Arch. Gen. Psychiatry,* 41:1159–1166.
9. Buchsbaum, M. S., DeLisi, L. E., Holcomb, H. H., Wu, J. C., Hazlett, E., Cooper-Langston, K., and Kessler, R. M. (1987): (submitted).
10. Buchsbaum, M. S., Holcomb, H. H., Johnson, J., King, A. C., and Kessler, R. (1983): *Hum. Neurobiol.,* 2:35–38.
11. Buchsbaum, M. S., Ingvar, D. H., Kessler, R., Waters, R. N., Cappelletti, J., van Kammen, D. P., King, A. C., Johnson, J. L., Manning, R. G., Flynn, R. W., Mann, L. S., Bunney, W. E., Jr., and Sokoloff, L. (1982): *Arch. Gen. Psychiatry,* 39:251–259.
12. Buchsbaum, M. S., Mirsky, A. F., DeLisi, L. E., Morihisa, J., Karson, C. R., Mendelson, W. B., King, A. C., Johnson, J., and Kessler, R. (1984): *Psychiatry Res.,* 13:95–108.
13. Buchsbaum, M. S., Wu, J., DeLisi, L. E., Holcomb, H., Kessler, R., Johnson, J., King, A. C., Hazlett, E., Cooper-Langston, K., and Post, R. M. (1986): *J. Affective Disord.,* 10:137–152.
14. Bustany, P., Henry, J. F., Rotrou, J., Singnoret, P., Cabanis, E., Zarifian, E., Ziegler, M., Derlon, J. M., Crouzel, C., Soussaline, F., and Comar, D. (1985): In: *The Metabolism of the Human Brain Studied with Positron Emission Tomography,* edited by T. Greitz, D. H. Ingvar, and L. Widen, pp. 241–250. Raven Press, New York.
15. Chabrol, H., Guell, A., Bes, A., and Moron, P. (1986): *Am. J. Psychiatry,* 143:130.
16. Comar, D., Zarifian, E., Verhas, M., Soussaline, F., Maziere, M., Berger, G., Loo, H., Cuche, C., Kellershohn, C., and Deniker, P. (1979): *Psychiatry Res.,* 1:23–29.
17. Davis, G. C., Buchsbaum, M. S., van Kammen, D. P., and Bunney, W. E., Jr. (1979): *Psychiatry Res.,* 1:61–69.
18. DeLisi, L. E., Holcomb, H. H., Cohen, R. M., Pickar, D., Carpenter, W., Morihisa, J., King, A. C., Kessler, R., and Buchsbaum, M. S. (1985): *J. Cereb. Blood Flow Metab.,* 5:201–206.
19. Devous, M. D., Raese, J. D., Herman, J. H., Paulman, R. G., Gregory, R. R., Rush, A. J., Chehabi, H. H., and Bonte, F. J. (1985): Society of Nuclear Medicine, 32nd Annual Meeting, Houston, Texas.
20. Erlenmeyer-Kimling, L., and Cornblatt, B. (1978): *J. Psychiatr. Res.,* 14:93–98.
21. Farde, L., Ehrin, E., Eriksson, L., Greitz, T., Hall, H., Hedstrom, C. G., Litton, J. E., and Sedvall, G. (1985): *Proc. Natl. Acad. Sci.,* 82:3863–3867.
22. Farde, L., Hall, H., Ehrin, E., and Sedvall, G. (1986): *Science,* 231:258–259.
23. Farkas, T., Reivich, M., Alavi, A., Greenberg, J. H., Fowler, J. S., MacGregor, R. R., Christman, D. R., and Wolf, A. P. (1980): In: *Cerebral Metabolism and Neural Function,* edited by J. V. Passonneau, R. A. Hawkins, W. D. Lust, and F. A. Welsh, pp. 403–408. Williams and Wilkins, Baltimore.
24. Farkas, T., Wolf, A. P., Jaeger, J., Brodie, J. D., Christman, D. R., and Fowler, J. S. (1984): *Arch. Gen. Psychiatry,* 41:293–300.
25. Garnett, E. S., Firnau, G., and Nahmias, C. (1983): *Nature,* 305:137–138.
26. Goldberg, E. (1985): *Schizophr. Bull.,* 11:255–263.
27. Huang, S. C., Phelps, M. E., Hoffman, E. J., Sideris, K., Selin, C. J., and Kuhl, D. E. (1980): *Am. J. Physiol.,* 238:E69–E82.
28. Ingvar, D. H., and Franzen, G. (1974): *Acta Psychiatr. Scand.,* 50:425–462.
29. Ingvar, D. H., and Lassen, N. A. (1976): In: *Brain Metabolism and Cerebral Disorders,* edited by H. E. Himwich, pp. 181–206. Spectrum Publishers, ECAT.
30. Ingvar, D. H., Rosen, I., and Elmqvist, D. (1975): In: *Blood Flow and Metabolism in the Brain,* edited by M. Harper, B. Jennett, D. Miller, and J. Rowan, pp. 1429–1432. Churchill Livingstone, New York.
31. Jernigan, T. L., Sargent, T., III, Pfefferbaum, A., Kusubov, N., and Stahl, S. M. (1985): *Psychiatry Res.,* 16:317–329.
32. Jones, S. C., Alavi, A., Christman, D., Montanez, I., Wolf, A. P., and Reivich, M. (1982): *J. Nucl. Med.,* 23:613–617.
33. Kessler, R. M., Ellis, J. R., Jr., and Eden, M. (1984): *J. Comp. Assisted Tomogr.,* 8:514–522.
34. Kling, A. S., Metter, E. J., Riege, W. H., and Kuhl, D. E. (1986): *Am. J. Psychiatry,* 143:175–180.
35. Kuhl, D. E., Metter, E. J., Riege, W. H., and Hawkins, R. A. (1985): In: *The Metabolism of the Human Brain Studied with PET,* edited by T. Greitz, D. H. Ingvar, and L. Widen, pp. 419–432. Raven Press, New York.
36. Lidsky, T. I., Manetto, C., and Schneider, J. S. (1985): *Brain Res. Reviews,* 9:133–146.
37. Mazziotta, J. C., Phelps, M. E., Plummer, D., and Kuhl, D. E. (1981): *J. Comput. Assist. Tomogr.,* 5:734–743.
38. Moore, R. Y., and Bloom, F. E. (1978): *Annu. Rev. Neurosci.,* 1:129–169.
39. Nelson, T., Lucignani, G., Atlas, S., Crane, A. M., Dienel, G. A., and Sokoloff, L. (1985): *Science,* 229:60–62.
40. Nuechterlein, K. H. (1983): *J. Abnorm. Psychol.,* 92:4–28.
41. Orzack, M. H., and Kornetsky, C. (1966): *Arch. Gen. Psychiatry,* 14:323–326.
42. Phelps, M. E., Huang, S. C., Hoffman, E. J., Selin, C., Sokoloff, L., and Kuhl, D. E. (1979): *Ann. Neurol.,* 6:371–388.
43. Phelps, M. E., and Mazziotta, J. C. (1985): *Science,* 28:799–809.
44. Phelps, M. E., Mazziotta, J. C., Huang, S.-C., and the Division of Biophysics, Dept. of Radiological Sciences, the Lab. of Nuclear Medicine, and the Dept. of Neurology, UCLA, School of Medicine (1982): *J. Cereb. Blood Flow Metab.,* 2:113–162.
45. Pycock, C. J., Kerwin, R. W., and Carter, C. J. (1980): *Nature,* 286:74–77.
46. Raichle, M. E. (1983): *Annu. Rev. Neurosci.,* 6:249–267.
47. Reivich, M., Alavi, A., Wolf, A., Greenberg, J. H., Fowler, J., Christman, D., MacGregor, R., Jones, S. C., London, J., Shiue, C., and Yonekura, Y. (1982): *J. Cereb. Blood Flow Metab.,* 2:307–319.
48. Reivich, M., Gur, R., and Alavi, A. (1983): *Hum. Neurobiol.,* 2:25–33.
49. Schneider, J. S. (1984): *Biol. Psychiatry,* 19:1693–1710.
50. Sedvall, G., Blomquist, G., DePaulis, T., Ehrin, E., Eriksson, L., Farde, L., Greitz, T., Hedstrom, C. G., Ingvar, D. H., Litton, J.-E., Nilsson, J. L. G., Stone-Elander, S., Widen, L., Wiesel, F. A., and Wik, G. (1984): In: *Psychiatry: The State of the Art,* Vol. 2, edited by P. Pichot, P. Berner, R. Wolf, and K. Thau, pp. 305–312. Plenum Publishing Company, New York.

51. Sheppard, G., Gruzelier, J., Manchanda, R., Hirsch, S. R., Wise, R., Frackowiak, R., and Jones, T. (1983): *Lancet,* 2:1448–1452.
52. Sokoloff, L. (1977): *J. Neurochem.,* 29:13–26.
53. Sokoloff, L. (1982): In: *Advances in Neurochemistry,* edited by B. W. Agranoff and M. H. Aprison, pp. 1–82. Plenum Publishing Co., New York.
54. Sokoloff, L. (1984): In: *Metabolic Probes of CNS Activity in Experimental Animals and Man,* Vol. 1, pp. 28–71. Sinauer Associates, Sunderland, MA.
55. Sokoloff, L., Reivich, M., Kennedy, C., Des Rosiers, M. H., Patlak, C. S., Pettigrew, K. D., Sakurada, O., and Shinohara, M. (1977): *J. Neurochem.,* 28:897–916.
56. Wagner, H. N., Burns, H. D., Dannals, R. F., Wong, D. F., Langstrom, B., Duelfer, T., Frost, J., Ravert, H. T., Links, J. M., Rosenbloom, S. B., Lukas, S. E., Kramer, A. V., and Kuhar, M. J. (1983): *Science,* 221:1264–1266.
57. Walker, E. (1982): *Arch. Gen. Psychiatry,* 38:1355–1358.
58. Walker, E., and Shaye, J. (1982): *Arch. Gen. Psychiatry,* 39:1153–1156.
59. Weinberger, D. R., Berman, K. F., and Zec, R. F. (1986): *Arch. Gen. Psychiatry,* 43:114–124.
60. Widen, L., Blomqvist, G., Greitz, T., Litton, J. E., Bergstrom, M., Ehrin, E., Ericson, K., Eriksson, L., Ingvar, D. H., Johansson, L., Nilsson, J. L. G., Stone-Elander, S., Sedvall, G., Wiesel, F., and Wik, G. (1983): *Am. J. Neurol.,* 4:550–552.
61. Wiesel, F.-A., Blomquist, G., Greitz, T., Nyman, H., Schalling, D., Stome-Elander, S., Widen, L., and Wik, G. (1986): In: *Proceedings of the 4th World Congress of Biological Psychiatry,* edited by C. Shagass. Elsevier Science Publishing Co., New York.
62. Wolf, A. P. (1984): *Ann. Neurol.,* 15:519–524.
63. Wolkin, A., Jaeger, J., Brodie, J. D., Wolf, A. P., Fowler, J., Rotrosen, J., Gomez-Mont, F., and Cancro, R. (1985): *Am. J. Psychiatry,* 142:564–571.

Psychopharmacology:
The Third Generation of Progress,
edited by Herbert Y. Meltzer.
Raven Press, New York © 1987.

CHAPTER 78

Electrical Brain Activity in Psychiatric Disorders

Walton T. Roth

The last 10 years of research into psychiatric applications of human electrical brain potentials have been characterized by increasingly sophisticated computer analysis and graphic presentation of scalp-recorded electrical potentials, more attention to potentials evoked by single stimuli, and a better knowledge of the deep sources and psychological meanings of these evoked potentials. However, unlike neurology, for which brain potentials find increasing diagnostic use, psychiatry has not adopted them or any other biological measure as a part of standard diagnosis. The reasons for this are complex and controversial. I will discuss some of them later in this review, which is not intended to be exhaustive but oriented to recent trends. The review will be less than comprehensive in that it will not consider two topics in which electroencephalographic (EEG) studies have played a major role, namely, sleep disorders and normal aging.

Several organizational principles are possible for a review of EEG research in psychiatry. One could list findings by diseases, by theoretical motivations (for example, theories of arousal, epileptiform discharge, information processing, etc., as in ref. 84), by whether brain potentials are "spontaneous" or "evoked," or by EEG analysis method. I have chosen to organize this chapter in terms of EEG analysis method, since the most influential recent investigations have been associated with new or improved methodologies. However, in practice, the two main analysis methods described, spectral analysis and signal averaging, have also been associated with different theories and different amounts and types of stimulation.

SPECTRAL ANALYSIS

The earliest observers of the EEG were impressed with its rhythmic qualities, especially when the subject's eyes were closed. From the beginning this led to its description in terms of frequency spectrum. The traditional Greek-lettered bands of EEG power make sense to a human looking at a polygraph paper, and can be rated by eye, or by analog or digital Fourier analysis. Digital analysis has become cheap and easy, and the results can be displayed in impressive color topographic displays.

Basic Findings

A certain consistency can be seen in the results of EEG studies of psychiatric patients: whether absolute or relative power is considered (relative power is the fraction of total power in a given band), chronic schizophrenics compared to controls have less power in the fast alpha range (11–13 Hz), and more in the fast beta range (20–40 Hz) and theta and delta bands (0.5–8 Hz) (6,14,24,44,48,64,100). Acute schizophrenics may only show reduced alpha (24). None of these findings is specific to schizophrenia: chronic alcoholics show the same alpha, beta, theta, and delta findings (14), and demented subjects the alpha, theta, and delta findings (49,50). Demented subjects may show either decreased beta (21) or increased beta (49). In an investigation of patients with senile dementia of the Alzheimer type, theta percentage power distinguished best the degree of dementia (13).

The findings above are present in unmedicated patients and thus are not medication artifacts. However, psychoactive medications do affect the spectrum, in some cases increasing pathological deviations and in other cases reversing these deviations. Antipsychotic drugs tend to increase theta power and to decrease beta (46). Antianxiety drugs, both barbiturates and benzodiazepines, increase slow beta activity. Antidepressants, anticholinergic hallucinogens, and central cholinergic drugs all increase delta (41,46,70). In spite of some overlaps, the spectral properties of anxiolytics, antidepressants, stimulants, antipsychotics, and placebos are sufficiently distinct in normal subjects that the psychoactive properties of new compounds can be correctly predicted (47). The accuracy of assignment of new drugs to the correct category by multivariate discriminant analysis of spectral changes has been estimated to be 60%.

My references to activity in frequency bands have been to *average* power over periods of minutes. Variability over periods of seconds for total EEG power or of power divided into spectral bands has also been examined. This variability has been found to be reduced in chronic schizophrenics (33,55,56,58,94) and in acute schizophrenics while hallucinating (58). The reduction is not specific to schizophrenia, since manics show it too (94). Increased frequency variability may accompany the lower power variability (94).

Spectral analysis has been used to study episodes of psychotic behavior as transitory states rather than as manifestations of a trait. The essential design is to compare EEG spectra during periods of normal behavior to those recorded during periods of blocking, automatisms, or hallucinations. According to one group, psychotic periods are not accompanied by temporal spikes, as might be expected from the similarities between the symptoms of temporal lobe epilepsy and schizophrenia, but by a change in spectrum to a ramp-like pattern of smooth decline in power from lower to higher frequencies (99,100). However, a later single case study reports the opposite spectral change (from a ramp shape to a peaked shape) with a change from normal behavior to hallucinating (92).

Spatial Spectral Mapping and Multivariate Analysis

The results of multilead EEG recordings, which have long been standard for clinical EEG examinations, are evaluated by the trained eye of a clinician scanning a paper record from a polygraph. Automatic methods for analytic spatial and temporal mapping of EEG data have been proposed in the past, but until recently most researchers have concentrated on thorough analyses of a few leads. Now, however, there is growing interest in spatial mapping, the impetus for which comes from a combination of factors: hypotheses about specific brain regions and psychopathology, amazing advances in three-dimensional structural and metabolic imaging, and greater availability of hardware and software systems for analyzing and displaying complex data sets. A number of companies sell integrated packages that make spatial mapping possible for clinicians—packages that include EEG amplifiers, a microcomputer, storage disks, color displays, and the requisite software.

For schizophrenia, spectral analysis of multilead record-ings usually has confirmed the findings of studies with fewer leads, and, in addition, has suggested certain asymmetries—for example, that beta increases in schizophrenia are largest in the left anterior temporal area (66) or left posterior areas (65). EEG laterality findings, however, have tended to be inconsistent. For example, in one report the right-left ratio in the higher-frequency bands at temporal electrodes was less than one in schizophrenics and greater than one in depressives (26), whereas later studies found the opposite (60,106).

A general statistical problem with multilead recording is the high ratio of potentially meaningful comparisons to the number of subjects that can be practically tested. Any EEG recording contains so many data that it is tempting to compare them in many different ways; with multiple leads this temptation is overwhelming. This gives rise to post hoc possibilities of mistaking random variation for real differences. Certain multivariate procedures offer some protection against wrong inferences. A reasonably conservative classification by multivariate discriminant analysis of complexly determined features was quite accurate for distinctions such as nonpsychotic patients vs overt schizophrenics, latent schizophrenics, and manics (95).

The statistical analysis of regional differences such as right-left asymmetry has an additional pitfall: the statistical significance of asymmetries is usually calculated in such a way that it depends not only on hemispheric specialization but also on hemispheric integration (12). The more activity between regions is correlated within subjects (hemispheric integration), the more sensitive will be repeated-measure within-subject statistics (e.g., paired *t*-tests) to differences between regions. Thus, these statistics are not reliable guides to the location of right-left differences. This caveat applies to all regional measuring techniques—for example, to measurements of regional cerebral blood flow.

Spectral Artifacts

The problem of eye and muscle artifacts continues to bedevil the interpretation of EEG spectral changes. Eye movements produce slow activity in frontal EEG electrodes, and muscle tension produces beta activity over much of the scalp, particularly in posterior electrodes. Gross movement of the head artifactually enhances the slow end of the spectrum. The ordinary way to exclude these artifacts is to exclude portions of the EEG records in which voltages from the eye leads or EEG leads exceed threshold values. Unfortunately, the threshold may be less sensitive to artifact than spectral analysis, leaving an indeterminate amount of eye, muscle, and movement artifact to contaminate the EEG spectrum. Residual eye artifact, within two perfectly localized sources, may be estimated by spatial analysis of spectral voltage sources. Muscle activity, however, is diffuse, and the patterns of contraction too complex and idiosyncratic to be localized with certainty. Residual muscle artifact can be estimated best from the amount of higher-than-beta power present in spectra from scalp recordings made using electromyograph (EMG) electrodes and amplifiers with high frequency limits. Masseter and temporalis muscle artifacts can be asymmetrical and give rise to false inferences of EEG lateralization (ref. 25, p. 198).

Significance of Spectral Findings

From a practical point of view, spectral analysis tends to be insensitive and nonspecific as a diagnostic method. Neither schizophrenia nor any other mental disease can be diagnosed from the EEG spectrum of an individual patient because there is too much overlap between diagnostic groups. Part of the problem is that EEGs differ greatly from person to person, both in patients and in normals. Because of this variability, longitudinal drug studies often preselect subjects for supposedly drug-sensitive EEG features (47). Psychiatric diagnosis based on multivariate classification of patients by amplitude and frequency parameters shows some promise (95), but it is important that discriminant functions be replicated on different samples in different laboratories to avoid functions that capitalize on idiosyncratic associations. Tests that compare functions based on "all the sample but one" can be particularly misleading (29).

From a theoretical point of view, the meaning of spectral changes is ambiguous; a variety of psychological or neurophysiological interpretations are possible. We have distinguished five types of interpretations: arousal variations, cerebral insufficiency, epileptiform activity, and regional imbalances (84). None of them is fully satisfactory.

Briefly, arousal theory could explain increased delta in schizophrenics as a sign of their drowsiness during recording. Using EEG differences between eyes-closed and eyes-open recording as a basis for defining indicators of arousal, overt schizophrenics, latent schizophrenics, and manics were considered to be more aroused on several amplitude and frequency measures than controls, who in turn were more aroused than major depressives and personality disorder patients (94). This interpretation may not be justified, since eye opening and closing does more to the EEG spectrum than can plausibly be explained by changes in arousal. Furthermore, if spectral differences in psychotic patients are due to arousal, the differences will never be important for diagnosis, since arousal disturbances are secondary, variably present symptoms in psychotic diseases. Arousal interpretations are strengthened when other indices of arousal (subjective, behavioral, autonomic, hormonal) have been measured and concur with the EEG. Unfortunately, however, measurement of other arousal indices in EEG spectral studies is rare.

On the other hand, increased frontal delta in schizophrenics could be interpreted as regional "cerebral insufficiency," the same insufficiency that is manifested in metabolic imaging studies as reduced frontal glucose consumption (7), although direct comparisons of the two measures in the same subject have not yet been published. The idea that cerebral slowing was evidence of cerebral insufficiency (coined in analogy to other organ insufficiencies such as renal, pulmonary, etc.) was postulated by Engel and Romano more than 25 years ago (23). Recent findings of enlarged ventricles and sulci in schizophrenics have revived interest in diffuse organic deficits as an underlying factor in certain types of schizophrenia (reviewed in 59 and 91).

Spectral analysis is usually not sensitive to epileptic spikes, but one group has tried to associate a "ramp-like" spectrum with temporal lobe epilepsy, certain symptoms of which resemble schizophrenic symptoms (99,100). Depth electrode studies from another group have demonstrated that limbic spiking occurs concomitantly with psychotic symptoms in certain patients, although no trace of the spikes is discernible at scalp electrodes (39,40).

Spectral asymmetries are usually discussed in terms of popular theories of right and left brain specialization. Schizophrenia has been considered more a disorder of the linguistic and analytical left brain, and depression and mania disorders of the emotional right brain (25). These interpretations are suspect not only because relevant data are inconsistent, but because it is unclear what particular EEG signs mean on a neurophysiological or psychological level—whether they mean excitatory or inhibitory processes, or more or less cognitive or affective activity (57).

Future Directions for Spectral Analysis

The potential value of spectral analysis has not been exhausted by what has been done so far. First, in most studies, patients have done nothing but sit with their eyes open or closed. Largely unexplored are the effects of physical or pharmacological stimulation or of task performance on the spectra of patients. Second, many spectral and other measures of regional coupling have been developed which might be applied more widely in psychiatric populations (e.g., 30). Third, discriminant functions from one setting should be applied in other settings to various groups of patients; then the power of these measures can be rightly assessed. Fourth, more attention should be paid to the possibility that EEG spectrum does not reflect any mental disease in itself, but instead is a measure of psychological states or traits, such as anxiety, depersonalization, obsessive thinking, and anhedonia, that crosscut diseases. The state of arousal of the subject is bound to fluctuate in a recording session more than a few minutes long, and different subjects vary markedly in their fear or excitement while being recorded, factors that can be expected to have profound influence on EEG spectra. These factors may be secondary to the diagnostic question being asked, but they are of clinical value and can be ignored only at the risk of misunderstanding what individual and group differences mean.

SIGNAL AVERAGING

Rhythmic EEG activity may be transiently altered in response to stimuli (alpha blocking or alpha provocation). However, buried in the ongoing EEG are more subtle and specific electrical stimuli responses, much lower voltage than rhythmic activity. These responses are best elucidated by signal averaging, which emphasizes the time domain, rather than by spectral analysis, which emphasizes the frequency domain. Signal averaging combines EEG records from more than one presentation of the stimulus in a time-locked fashion: the first time point of the signal average is the average of the first time points of all of the separate stimulus presentations, the second time point of the average

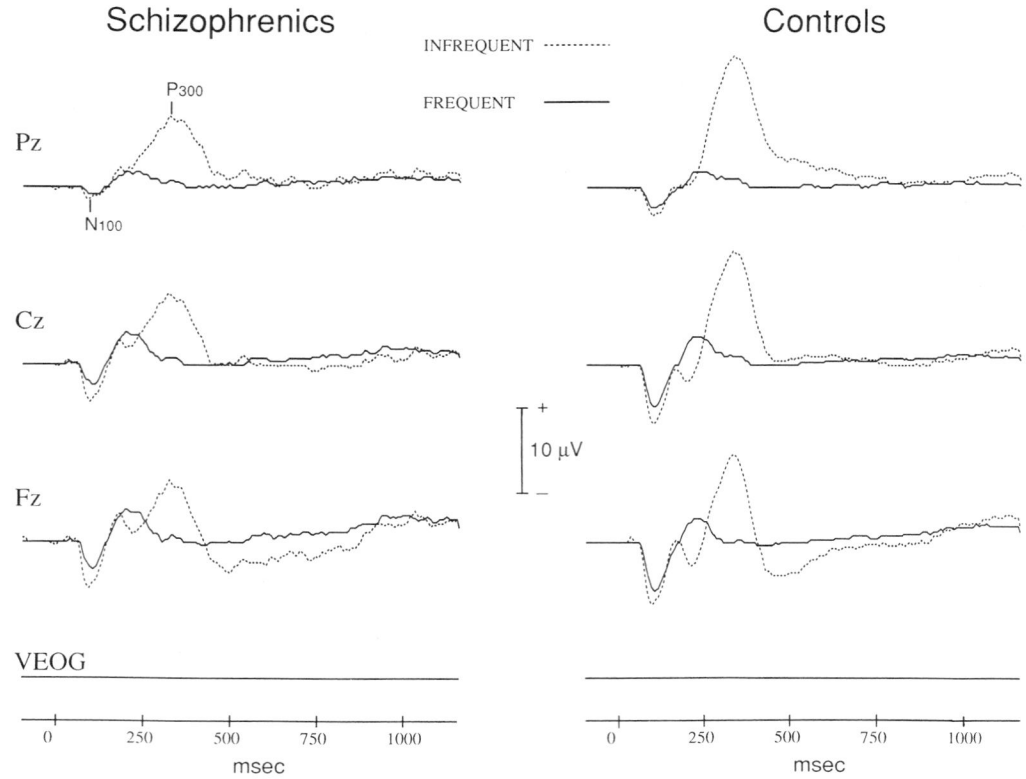

FIG. 1. Event-related potentials averaged across subjects for 24 schizophrenic patients and 28 normal controls. Averages are shown for three leads, Pz, Cz, and Fz, referenced to a thoracic electrode and for a vertical eye derivation (VEOG) of electrodes above and below the right eye. Stimuli were 80 dB (Sound Pressure Level) tone pips given at 1.5-sec intervals. The frequent stimuli were 500 Hz tone pips with a probability of occurrence of 0.80, and the infrequent stimuli were 1,000 Hz with a probability of 0.20. Two hundred and forty frequent trials and 60 infrequent trials were given to each subject. Subjects were instructed to press a button quickly to higher pitch stimuli. N100 and P300 peaks are marked on the upper left ERP average. (These data are provided by A. Pfefferbaum.)

is the average of all the second time points, etc. In signal averaging, the ongoing EEG is considered noise from which the signal must be extracted. Since this noise is not time-locked to the stimuli, its average tends towards zero as the number of samples increases. Thus, the signal-to-noise ratio improves and the various peaks and valleys of voltage become more reliable as more stimulus epochs are averaged together. The density of time points (sampling interval) for analog-to-digital conversion, and the number of stimulus events (often called "trials") depend on which evoked potential is being studied. Figure 1 illustrates ERPs to tones while subjects are performing a simple tone discrimination task. Samples were made every 5 msec, and the ERP to the infrequent target is based on 60 trials/subject. Some small, fast potentials require sampling intervals of 0.25 msec and 500 or more trials per subject.

One of the powers of signal averaging is the wide range of events that can be considered signals. Not only can any external physical stimulus or response be a signal, but internal mental operations that recur at consistent times are possible signals. Thus, "motor preparation," "expectancy," and "surprise" can be associated with the waves extracted by signal averaging. Because the signal can be any event, these waves are often termed "event-related potentials" (ERPs). Essentially, signal averaging is a method

of uncovering EEG potentials temporally correlated with any event. Another power of EEG signal averaging is the very fine temporal resolution that is possible. Other methods of studying the brain, such as metabolic imaging, do not approach its millisecond by millisecond resolution.

Computation of the signal average is just the beginning of data analysis. A method for measuring the resulting waveform must be chosen. Often this is peak-to-peak measurement or integration of voltage over regions of the signal average curve. Sometimes Principal Component Analysis or other multivariate methods are used (32). Peaks in the ERP averages or peaks in the components derived from these averages by Principal Component Analysis are commonly labeled according to their latency and polarity. Thus, N100 is a negative peak at 100 msec, and P300 is a positive peak at 300 msec. These derivative measures are then tested statistically. Like spectral measures, they can be entered into multivariate searches for diagnostic discriminators.

The usefulness of EEG signal averaging for testing sensory pathways is well established. Indeed, neurologists regularly measure evoked potentials, for example, when the diagnosis of multiple sclerosis is entertained (10). But psychiatry is less concerned with sensory pathways (except perhaps in patients with possible conversion symptoms) than with more complex cognitive or affective processes. Abnormalities in these processes may be grounded in basic neurophysiological alterations detectable in latency or amplitude properties of components of evoked potentials to simple stimuli, or they may be detectable only in components associated with the processes themselves.

Basic Findings of Signal Averaging

There is a split of opinion so deep among researchers in this area, that it is difficult to reach a consensus about what kind of experiments are worthwhile. Some researchers concentrate on components they hope are not affected by attention and motivation in order to discover basic, primary neurophysiological parameters that are deranged in the mentally ill or altered by psychotropic drugs. Others feel that such components are irrelevant to psychiatry, since they are unlikely to be affected by complex mental disturbances. A few investigators try to sidestep this controversy by ignoring both neurophysiological and psychological rationales and simply measuring a wide variety of ERPs, in the hope that multivariate statistics will make sense of the results. This agnostic, empirical approach is not completely unjustifiable, considering the scarcity of relevant neurophysiological and psychological knowledge.

I will present the findings of EEG signal averaging in psychiatry under the rubrics of "psychological" and "neurophysiological," aware of the philosophical and practical limitations of this classification. Although "psychological" investigations usually concern themselves with later components than "neurophysiological" ones, there is considerable overlap.

Psychological ERP Findings

One finding stands out as the most consistent and best established in this area: P300 amplitude is diminished in schizophrenia (e.g., 2,22,51,54,68,81,83,86,105). This finding has been reported in more than 15 studies (69), and it is not an artifact of medication (52). The P300 component has been the focus of more than 100 published studies in normal subjects, and much is known about its psychological determinants: it appears to stimuli that are surprising and task-relevant and its latency corresponds in time to the subject's ability to make those assessments (75). In almost all studies of psychiatric patients, the subjects were asked to count or to press a button to tones of a certain pitch imbedded in a series of more numerous tones with a different pitch. The interval between tones was ordinarily between 1 and 2 sec. In this task, P300 occurs almost exclusively to the target tones and only when the subject is counting or pressing the button. That is not to say that P300 elicitation always requires the subject's cooperation: it occurs automatically to loud auditory stimuli (80,82).

Since P300 amplitude is determined by both the surprising and task-relevant features of the stimulus, one can ask whether schizophrenics have become insensitive to one or both of these features. There is evidence both for and against the importance of surprise. One study reports that schizophrenic P300 amplitudes and reaction times (RTs)

vary with the microstructure of the tone sequence in the same way as control P300s and RTs, suggesting that schizophrenics make normal inferences about stimulus probability and have normal reactions to it (22). On the other hand, schizophrenics register less surprise to tones in terms of skin conductance orienting responses (4,67,88). There is also evidence for and against the importance of task relevance (87). The overall poorer counting or RT performance usually observed in schizophrenics on the P300 task may indicate that to them the targets are less task relevant, presumably because schizophrenics are less affectively involved and motivated. On the other hand, when RTs are matched between controls and schizophrenics, P300 is still smaller in the latter (2,85). But these studies did not match mean RTs, only individual ones.

P300 reduction can be alternatively explained in terms of automatic vs controlled processing. There is evidence from non-ERP experiments that schizophrenics perform poorly only when controlled processing is required (9). Returning to the P300 study mentioned in the last paragraph (22), probability inferences based on the microstructure of the sequence may be a relatively automatic feature of short-term memory, its automaticity enhanced by the simplicity of the discrimination required. Since automatic processing is intact in schizophrenia, P300 amplitude varies with the stimulus sequence. However, other aspects of the task, such as being constantly ready to use target stimuli to unleash a prepared-for, quick motor response, may require controlled processes, which are mobilized with difficulty in schizophrenia. This difficulty leads to the stimuli being effectively less task relevant and giving rise to smaller P300s independently of the position of the stimulus in the sequence. This explanation would predict that P300s automatically elicited by loud auditory stimuli would be the same size in schizophrenics and controls, a matter currently under investigation in our laboratory.

If general factors like reduced task involvement or defective controlled processing are important, one might expect smaller P300s in other psychologically impaired groups. This is indeed the case. Depressed (18), alcoholic (74), and organically impaired patients have smaller P300s (73). Among children, hyperactive (43,61) or schizophrenic children (101) have smaller P300s. This finding even extends to apparently well children of alcoholics (3), siblings of schizophrenics (89), and female undergraduates who rate themselves high on a scale of anhedonia (lacking the capacity for physical pleasure) (62). Even normal aging results in P300 reduction (71).

P300 latency in combination with P300 amplitude provides more diagnostic specificity than amplitude alone (98). In the standard paradigm described above, P300 latency is usually more prolonged by organic impairments than by so-called "functional" psychoses, whereas P300 amplitude is reduced in both disorders (for an exception, see 73). The latency prolongation in dementia is independent of etiology, appearing in Alzheimer's disease (102), Huntington's disease (37,78), and Parkinson's disease (36). Alcoholic Korsakoff syndrome may be an exception, with normal P300 latencies and amplitudes (98).

Critics have questioned whether P300 adds any information to that given by RT, since RT is also usually longer for patients in P300 paradigms whenever it is measured.

The fact is that P300 amplitude and latency are usually more sensitive to psychopathology than RT in these paradigms, probably because RT depends on multiple factors, some of which are poorly correlated with psychopathology. Experiments on normal subjects have shown that P300 latency is a measure of the time taken to evaluate the stimulus and is independent of subsequent response stages, whereas RT is dependent on both (19,75). For example, unlike P300, RT depends on whether a subject has adopted a strategy emphasizing speed or accuracy, and on motoric factors. The dissociability of RT and P300 latency is exemplified in clinical experiments comparing the effects of getting older and of methylphenidate in hyperactive children (8,35). Both aging and methylphenidate reduce RT in these children, whereas only aging shortens P300 latency. Thus, methylphenidate increases motor speed but not the speed of categorization of targets. Returning to our comparison of P300 latency in schizophrenia and dementia, one can infer that schizophrenia slows RT primarily after stimulus evaluation, whereas dementia begins to slow RT before or during that stage.

Although P300 amplitude can be said to depend on the amount of attention being paid to stimuli that elicit it, it is not as pure a measure of attention as certain earlier negative waves. P300 does not occur to frequently occurring types of stimuli in the attended channel. In a dichotic listening paradigm in which one series of tone pips is presented to one ear and another series concurrently to the other, only infrequent targets in the attended ear elicit P300s. However, both frequent and infrequent stimuli in the attended ear give rise to a frontal-central negative wave peaking at 125 msec (for a review, see ref. 42). This wave, a more general indicator of selective attention than P300, was also reduced in schizophrenics compared to controls when the intervals between stimuli were in the 500 to 1,500 msec range, but not when the intervals were 250 to 750 msec (2). Thus, schizophrenics manifested a selective attentional deficit when stimuli came more slowly.

The Contingent Negative Variation (CNV) is another ERP phenomenon that has been used to study attentional deficits in psychiatric patients. The essential CNV paradigm is a fixed foreperiod RT paradigm in which warning stimuli are followed at fixed intervals by "imperative" stimuli signaling the subject to press or not to press an RT button. Recent research has demonstrated that the CNV is made up of two relatively independent negative components: an earlier one in response to the signal properties of the warning tone and a later one that reflects motor preparation (77). These two waves are inextricably overlapped if the foreperiod is less than 2 sec, which has been the case in most clinical investigations. The general finding has been that patients have smaller CNVs and longer RTs, whether their diagnosis is schizophrenia, depression, dementia, or head trauma (20,79,97,104). In addition, patients with acute schizophrenia have a slower return of the negativity to baseline even after they have pressed the RT button, a phenomenon called Post-Imperative Negative Variation (PINV) (104). PINV might be interpreted as a slowness in demobilizing the attentional resources of motor preparation.

ERPs associated with preparation for body movement can be studied in self-paced tasks. Under those conditions,

chronic schizophrenics give a smaller negative shift (Readiness Potential or Bereitschaftpotential) immediately before the button press (11). This negative shift is equivalent to the later component of the CNV, and, as for the CNV, its reduction may indicate difficulties in mobilizing attentional resources.

Neurophysiological ERP Findings

Just as P300 has dominated psychological ERP studies, the study of augmenting-reducing or stimulus-intensity modulation has attracted the widest attention among more biologically oriented ERP investigators. Augmenting and reducing refer to a hypothetical personality dimension of over- and under-reaction to intense stimuli of any kind. An augmenter automatically turns up the gain on an internal amplifier as the intensity of stimuli increases; a reducer automatically turns down the gain. A commonly used ERP measure of this dimension is the function relating amplitudes of ERP components in the 75 to 250 msec range to light flash intensity. Certain groups of schizophrenics and affective disorder patients are reducers on this paradigm. One of the most convincing ERP augmenting-reducing experiments used as stimuli a random sequence of four intensities of shocks to the left forearm. Schizophrenics rated the higher intensity shocks as relatively less painful than did controls, and schizophrenics had corresponding smaller N120 ERPs to them (17). That endorphins have something to do with this effect was suggested by the fact that naltrexone, an opiate antagonist, tended to reverse the schizophrenic pain insensitivity and small ERPs.

The augmenting-reducing ERP literature has been criticized recently on three grounds: insufficient attention to eye-blink artifact (45), inconsistency of augmenting-reducing measures across modalities (76), and inconsistency across peaks (15). Earlier studies seemed arbitrary in selecting peaks to assess this dimension. Clearly, peaks should be selected for their fidelity in reflecting the subjective physical or affective intensity of stimuli, if the term augmenting-reducing is to be retained. That does not preclude examining other stimulus-intensity/ERP-measure functions for indications of group differences.

Another phenomenon that has attracted clinical attention is the temporal recovery of ERPs when stimuli are given in quick succession (90). Early experiments showed that somatosensory ERPs in the 20 to 30 msec range recovered full amplitude more slowly in certain groups of psychiatric patients when the interval between stimuli was less than 20 msec (93). This recovery was to some extent a state rather than trait phenomenon, since it normalized with clinical improvement in severely depressed patients. More recently, temporal recovery of ERPs to auditory stimuli has been investigated. Schizophrenics, whether on or off medication, show less recovery of P50 to clicks: the ratio of their P50 amplitude after a 0.5-sec ISI to P50 amplitude after a 10-sec inter-stimulus interval (ISI) is greater than in controls (1,28). This finding is not specific to schizophrenia but is found in clinically well first-degree relatives of schizophrenics (96) and in patients with manic depressive disease (27).

Components with latencies less than 10 msec, such as brainstem auditory ERPs, are of more clinical interest to neurologists than to psychiatrists, since these short-latency components mainly test the integrity of sensory pathways presumed to be unaltered by mental disease. Some investigators have found aberrations in brainstem potentials in autistic children (103) and in adult schizophrenics (38), whereas others have not (5,16,72). On the balance, the evidence suggests that short-latency components, at least of higher functioning patients, do not differ from those of controls.

Averaging Artifacts

As for spectral analysis, the main sources of signal averaging artifact are the eye and scalp muscles. Eye blinks or eye movements that may be triggered by stimuli give rise to potentials over the entire scalp; these potentials often have a morphology similar to, but usually of a higher voltage than brain ERP components. Instructions that might reduce these artifacts, such as looking at a fixation point or blinking only at certain times, are particularly ineffective in psychiatric patients. Avoiding eye artifacts by throwing out trials for which a suprathreshold amount of voltage is picked up from electrodes around the eye runs the risk of eliminating too many trials to maintain an adequate signal-to-noise ratio and of eliminating trials in a biased way. An alternative method is statistically removing the effect of eye artifact in individual trials (34). Time-locked contractions of scalp muscles are less of a problem than eye artifacts if stimuli are not loud or startling. Electrodermal potential or conductance artifacts are possible under certain conditions, as are electrocardiographic artifacts. The last are easily recognizable and can be minimized with proper electrode placement. Whatever the source of the artifact, it is imperative that the method of excluding it is powerful enough to remove its traces from averages, not just from single trials.

Significance of Signal-Averaging Findings

At the present time, psychologically oriented investigators have succeeded mainly in finding a consistent indicator of a general deficit, P300 amplitude. The psychological meaning of P300 reduction is not clear, but it is probably related to an inability to meet the task demands of the experiment in a sustained, efficient way. This inability may have both affective and cognitive dimensions, and is probably closely related to problems in directing and maintaining attention. On the positive side, ERPs are probably the most sensitive way known to assess this important deficit; on the negative side, ERPs do not reflect any deficits specific to any psychiatric disease. Specific indicators would be useful, since psychiatric disease entities vary in their prognosis and treatment.

Neurophysiologically oriented investigators have not produced widely replicated results, with only augmenting-reducing being studied in a significant number of laboratories. However, augmenting-reducing is at best the indicator of a personality trait rather than of any deficit produced by psychiatric disease. Furthermore, neurophysiologically oriented investigators have had difficulty in integrating their findings convincingly with any body of neurological knowledge. In contrast, the understanding of P300 in terms of the concepts of cognitive psychology has been quite successful.

However, neither cognitive psychology nor any other discipline has convincingly demonstrated specific deficits or organic lesions in schizophrenia or in any other of the nonorganic psychiatric diseases. No specific structural changes, endogenous psychotogens, or biochemical imbalances have been proven. All that has been found are nonspecific psychological (31) or structural abnormalities (63,108). Thus, EEG methods have not been more or less revealing than other research approaches.

Future Directions for Signal Averaging

Signal averaging is virtually unlimited in the kinds of stimulus situations and synchronizing events that might be used. Much remains to be explored. For example, little work has been done with olfactory pathways and their limbic system connections. Until now, the emphasis in psychological ERPs has been on "cold cognition," with little attention to motivation and emotion. There has been too sharp a dichotomy of paradigms between psychologically and nonpsychologically oriented investigators. Spontaneous shifts of attention and automatically elicited cognitive components should be investigated. Correlations should be established between ERPs and physiological and behavioral responses in non-ERP paradigms that have given abnormal results in schizophrenia, such as the skin conductance habituation paradigm and eye tracking paradigms.

More accurate accounting for the contributions of attention and motivation might enable us to get beyond effects due to the general, nonspecific deficit of mental illness. To the neurophysiologically oriented investigator, attention and motivation are artifacts, the influence of which needs to be estimated so that they do not distort the measurement of more basic neurophysiological parameters. To the psychologically oriented investigator, it would be useful if the effects of attention and motivation could be made constant across groups, or their effects parceled out statistically, so that other, perhaps more specific, psychological deficits could be detected.

Finally, coordinating ERP findings with those of other branches of neuroscience would be facilitated if the sources of ERP potentials could be localized. Magnetoencephalographic measurements give information complementary to EEG voltage measurements for source localization (53,107). Depth recording incidental to brain operations in humans or in animals is another source of important information (109).

Significance of EEG Studies of Psychiatric Disorders for Psychopharmacology

Insofar as psychopharmacology develops drugs to treat psychiatric disorders, objective methods for assessing the clinical efficacy of a treatment are important. If specific EEG signs of a psychiatric disease could be found, their reversibility by a drug could be an indication that this drug treats the disease specifically. Even nonspecific EEG signs might be used to measure the efficacy of treatment. The EEG might be better than verbal report or overt behavior in assessment because it is less influenced by observational and self-report misunderstandings and biases.

A second potential advantage of EEG measures is that they are closer to basic brain processes than verbal or gross behavioral measures and, as mentioned, their temporal resolution is better than most other biological measures. The identification of specific aberrant neurophysiological mechanisms in psychiatric illnesses might suggest new drug interventions. Of course, until now biochemistry has been the sovereign model for explaining the effectiveness of pharmacological treatments of psychiatric illnesses, but this model is not complete: biochemical processes have to be expressed neurophysiologically in order to give rise to what we call mind.

Finally, psychological mechanisms of drug action should be able to be specified more finely using a combination of EEG signal averaging and cognitive psychology paradigms. The dream of finding a specific processing stage or attentional resource that is uniquely affected by a specific drug or class of drugs is still to be realized, but there has been progress, for example, in separating the effects of drugs on motor and nonmotor stages of action sequences (8,35).

ACKNOWLEDGMENTS

Preparation of this manuscript was supported by NIMH Grant CRC30854, MH40052, and the Medical Research Service of the Veterans Administration. I thank Margaret Rosenbloom for her assistance. Dr. Pfefferbaum made helpful comments on an earlier draft.

REFERENCES

1. Adler, L. E., Pachman, E., Franks, R. D., Pecevich, M., Waldo, M. D., and Freedman, R. (1982): *Biol. Psychiatry,* 17:639–654.
2. Baribeau-Braun, J., Picton, T. W., Gosselin, J.-Y., and Quan, F. W. (1983): *Science,* 219:874–876.
3. Begleiter, H., Porjesz, B., Bihari, B., and Kissin, B. (1984): *Science,* 225:1493–1496.
4. Bernstein, A. S., Frith, C. D., Gruzelier, J. H., Patterson, T., Straube, E., Venables, P. H., and Zahn, T. P. (1982): *Biol. Psychol.,* 14:155–211.
5. Brecher, M., and Begleiter, H. (1985): *Biol. Psychiatry,* 20:199–228.
6. Buchsbaum, M. S., Coppola, R., and Cappelletti, J. (1982): In: *Positron Emission Tomography, EEG and Evoked Potential Topography: New Approaches to Local Function in Pharmaco-Electroencephalography,* edited by W. Herrmann, (*Electroencephalography in Drug Research*), pp. 193–207. Gustav Fischer, Stuttgart.
7. Buchsbaum, M. S., DeLisi, L. E., Holcomb, H. H., Cappelletti, J., King, A. C., Johnson, J., Hazlett, E., Dowling-Zimmerman, S., Post, R. M., Morihisa, J., Carpenter, W., Cohen, R., Pickar, D., Weinberger, D. R., Margolin, R., and Kessler, R. M. (1982): *Arch. Gen. Psychiatry,* 41:1159–1166.
8. Callaway, E., Halliday, R., and Naylor, H. (1983): *Arch. Gen. Psychiatry,* 40:1243–1248.
9. Callaway, E., and Naghdi, S. (1982): *Arch. Gen. Psychiatry,* 38:333–350.
10. Chiappa, K. H., and Ropper, A. H. (1982): *N. Engl. J. Med.,* 306:1140–1150, 1205–1211.
11. Chiarenza, G. A., Papakostopoulos, D., Dini, M., and Cazzullo, C. L. (1985): *Electroencephalogr. Clin. Neurophysiol.,* 61:218–228.
12. Clark, C. M., Kessler, R., and Margolin, R. (1985): *Brain Cognition,* 4:7–12.
13. Coben, L. A., Danziger, W., and Storandt, M. (1985): *Electroencephalogr. Clin. Neurophysiol.,* 61:101–113.
14. Coger, R. W., Dymond, A. M., and Serafetinides, E. A. (1979): *Arch. Gen. Psychiatry,* 36:91–94.
15. Connolly, J. F., and Gruzelier, J. H. (1982): *Psychophysiology,* 19:599–608.
16. Courchesne, E., Courchesne, R. Y., Hicks, G., and Lincoln, A. J. (1985): *Electroencephalogr. Clin. Neurophysiol.,* 61:491–502.
17. Davis, G. C., Buchsbaum, M., van Kammen, D. P., and Bunney, W. E. (1979): *Psychiatry Res.,* 1:61–69.
18. Diner, B. C., Holcomb, P. J., and Dykman, R. A. (1985): *Psychiatry Res.,* 15:175–185.
19. Donchin, E. (1981): *Psychophysiology,* 18:493–513.
20. Dongier, M., Dubrovsky, B., and Engelsmann, F. (1977): In: *Psychopathology and Brain Dysfunction,* edited by C. Shagass, S. Gershon, and A. J. Friedhoff, pp. 339–352. Raven Press, New York.
21. Duffy, F. H., Albert, M. S., and McAnulty, G. (1984): *Ann. Neurol.,* 16:439–448.
22. Duncan-Johnson, C. C., Roth, W. T., and Kopell, B. S. (1984): In: *Brain and Information: Event-Related Potentials,* edited by R. Karrer, J. Cohen, and P. Tueting. *Ann. NY Acad. Sci.,* 425:570–577.
23. Engel, G. L., and Romano, J. (1959): *J. Chronic Dis.,* 9:260–277.
24. Fenton, G. W., Fenwick, P. B. C., Dollimore, J., Dunn, T. L., and Hirsch, S. R. (1980): *Br. J. Psychiatry,* 136:445–455.
25. Flor-Henry, P. (1983): *Cerebral Basis of Psychopathology.* John Wright, Boston.
26. Flor-Henry, P., Koles, Z. J., Hovarth, B. G., and Burton, B. (1979): In: *Hemisphere Asymmetries of Function in Psychopathology,* edited by J. Gruzelier and P. Flor-Henry, pp. 189–222. Elsevier/North Holland Biomedical Press, Amsterdam.
27. Franks, R. D., Adler, L. E., Waldo, M. C., Alpert, J., and Freedman, R. (1983): *Biol. Psychiatry,* 18:989–1005.
28. Freedman, R., Adler, L. E., Waldo, M. C., Pachtman, E., and Franks, R. D. (1983): *Biol. Psychiatry,* 18:537–551.
29. Gevins, A. S. (1980): *IEEE Transactions on Pattern Analysis and Machine Intelligence,* 2:383–404.
30. Gevins, A. S., Schaffer, R. E., Doyle, J. C., Cutillo, B. A., Tannehill, R. S., and Bressler, S. L. (1983): *Science,* 220:97–99.
31. Gjerde, P. F. (1983): *Psychol. Bull.,* 95:57–72.
32. Glaser, E. M., and Ruchkin, D. S. (1976): *Principles of Neurobiological Signal Analysis.* Academic Press, New York.
33. Goldstein, L., Sugerman, A. A., Stolberg, H., Murphree, H. B., and Pfeiffer, C. C. (1965): *Electroencephalogr. Clin. Neurophysiol.,* 19:350–361.
34. Gratton, G., Coles, M. G. H., and Donchin, E. (1983): *Electroencephalogr. Clin. Neurophysiol.,* 55:468–484.
35. Halliday, R., Callaway, E., and Naylor, H. (1983): *Electroencephalogr. Clin. Neurophysiol.,* 55:258–267.
36. Hansch, E. C., Syndulko, K., Cohen, S. N., Goldberg, Z. I., Potvin, A. R., and Tourtellotte, W. W. (1982): *Ann. Neurol.,* 11:599–607.
37. Hansch, E. C., Syndulko, K., Cohen, S. N., Tourtellotte, W. W., and Potvin, A. R. (1980): *Bull. Los Angeles Neurol. Soc.,* 45:61 (Abstr.).
38. Hayashida, Y., Mitani, Y., Hosomi, H., Amemiya, M., Mifune, K., and Tomita, S. (1986): *Biol. Psychiatry,* 21:177–189.
39. Heath, R. G. (1954): *Studies in Schizophrenia.* Harvard University Press, Cambridge.
40. Heath, R. G., and Walker, C. F. (1985): *Biol. Psychiatry,* 20:669–674.
41. Herrmann, W. M. (1982): In: *Electroencephalography in Drug Research,* edited by W. M. Herrman, pp. 249–351. Gustav Fischer, Stuttgart.
42. Hillyard, S. A., and Kutas, M. (1983): *Annu. Rev. Psychol.,* 34:33–61.

43. Holcomb, P. J., Ackerman, P. T., and Dykman, R. A. (1985): *Psychophysiology,* 22:656–668.
44. Iacono, W. G. (1982): *J. Nerv. Ment. Dis.,* 170:91–101.
45. Iacono, W. G., Gabbay, F. H., and Lykken, D. T. (1982): *Biol. Psychiatry,* 17:897–911.
46. Itil, T. M. (1977): *Schizophr. Bull.,* 3:61–79.
47. Itil, T. M. (1982): In: *Electroencephalography in Drug Research,* edited by W. M. Herrmann, pp. 131–157. Gustav Fischer, Stuttgart.
48. Itil, T. M., Saletu, B., and Davis, S. (1972): *Biol. Psychiatry,* 5:1–13.
49. John, E. R. (1977): In: *Functional Neuroscience, Vol. 2: Neurometrics: Clinical Applications of Quantitative Electrophysiology,* edited by E. R. John and R. W. Thatcher, pp. 143–174. Lawrence Erlbaum Associates, Hillsdale, NJ.
50. John, E. R., Karmel, B. Z., Corning, W. C., Easton, P., Brown, D., Ahn, H., John, M., Harmony, T., Prichep, L., Toro, A., Gerson, I., Bartlett, F., Thatcher, R., Kaye, H., Valdes, P., and Schwartz, E. (1977): *Science,* 196:1393–1410.
51. Josiassen, R. C., Shagass, C., Roemer, R. A., and Straumanis, J. J. (1981): *Psychiatry Res.,* 5:147–156.
52. Josiassen, R. C., Shagass, C., Straumanis, J. J., and Roemer, R. A. (1984): *Psychiatry Res.,* 11:151–162.
53. Kaufman, L., and Williamson, S. F. (1982): *Ann. NY Acad. Sci.,* 388:197–213.
54. Levit, R. A., Sutton, S., and Zubin, J. (1973): *Psychol. Med.,* 3:487–494.
55. Lifshitz, K., and Gradijan, J. (1972): *Biol. Psychiatry,* 5:149–163.
56. Lifshitz, K., and Gradijan, J. (1974): *Psychophysiology,* 11:479–490.
57. Marin, R. S., and Tucker, G. J. (1981): *J. Nerv. Ment. Dis.,* 169:546–557.
58. Marjerrison, G., Krause, A. E., and Keogh, R. P. (1968): *Electroencephalogr. Clin. Neurophysiol.,* 24:35–41.
59. Maser, J. D., and Keith, S. J. (1983): *Schizophr. Bull.,* 9:265–283.
60. Matousek, M., Capone, C., and Okawa, M. (1981): In: *Advances in Biological Psychiatry, Vol. 6,* pp. 76–80. S. Karger, Basel.
61. Michael, R. L., Klorman, R., Salzman, L. F., Borgstedt, A. D., and Dainer, K. B. (1981): *Psychophysiology,* 18:665–667.
62. Miller, G. A. (1986): *Biol. Psychiatry,* 21:100–115.
63. Mirsky, A. F., and Duncan, C. C. (1986): *Annu. Rev. Psychol.,* 37:291–319.
64. Morihisa, J. M., and McAnulty, G. B. (1985): *Biol. Psychiatry,* 20:3–20.
65. Morihisa, J. M., Duffy, F. H., and Wyatt, R. J. (1985): *Arch. Gen. Psychiatry,* 40:719–728.
66. Morstyn, R., Duffy, F. H., and McCarley, R. W. (1983): *Electroencephalogr. Clin. Neurophysiol.,* 56:263–271.
67. Ohman, A. (1981): *Biol. Psychol.,* 2:87–145.
68. Pass, H. L., Klorman, R., Salzman, L. F., Klein, R. H., and Kaskey, G. B. (1980): *Biol. Psychiatry,* 15:9–20.
69. Pfefferbaum, A. (1986): *Cerebral Psychophysiology: Studies in Event-Related Potentials,* edited by W. C. McCallum, R. Zappoli, and F. Denoth, pp. 425–429. (*EEG Suppl.* 38). Elsevier, Amsterdam.
70. Pfefferbaum, A., Davis, K. L., Coulter, C. L., Mohs, R. C., Tinklenberg, J. R., and Kopell, B. S. (1979): *Psychopharmacology,* 62:225–233.
71. Pfefferbaum, A., Ford, J. M., Wenegrat, B. G., Roth, W. T., and Kopell, B. S. (1984): *Electroencephalogr. Clin. Neurophysiol.,* 59:85–103.
72. Pfefferbaum, A., Horvath, T. B., Roth, W. T., Tinklenberg, J. R., and Kopell, B. S. (1980): *Biol. Psychiatry,* 15:209–223.
73. Pfefferbaum, A., Wenegrat, B. G., Ford, J. M., Roth, W. T., and Kopell, B. S. (1984): *Electroencephalogr. Clin. Neurophysiol.,* 59:104–124.
74. Porjesz, B., Begleiter, H., and Garozzo, R. (1980): In: *Biological Effects of Alcohol,* edited by H. Begleiter. pp. 603–623. Plenum Press, New York.
75. Pritchard, W. S. (1981): *Psychol. Bull.,* 90:506–540.
76. Raine, A., Mitchell, D. A., and Venables, P. H. (1981): *Psychophysiology,* 18:700–708.
77. Rohrbaugh, J. W., and Gaillard, A. W. K. (1983): *Tutorials in ERP Research: Endogenous Components,* edited by A. W. K. Gaillard and W. Ritter, pp. 269–310. North Holland Publishing Company, Amsterdam.
78. Rosenberg, C., Nudleman, K., and Starr, A. (1985): *Arch. Neurol.,* 42:984–987.
79. Roth, W. T. (1977): *Schizophr. Bull.,* 3:105–120.
80. Roth, W. T., Blowers, G. H., Doyle, C. M., and Kopell, B. S. (1982): *Electroencephalogr. Clin. Neurophysiol.,* 54:132–146.
81. Roth, W. T., and Cannon, E. H. (1972): *Arch. Gen. Psychiatry,* 27:466–471.
82. Roth, W. T., Dorato, K. H., and Kopell, B. S. (1984): *Psychophysiology,* 21:466–481.
83. Roth, W. T., Horvath, T. B., Pfefferbaum, A., and Kopell, B. S. (1980): *Electroencephalogr. Clin. Neurophysiol.,* 48:127–139.
84. Roth, W. T., and Pfefferbaum, A. (1986): In: *The American Handbook of Psychiatry,* edited by P. A. Berger and H. K. H. Brodie, pp. 189–212. Basic Books, New York.
85. Roth, W. T., Pfefferbaum, A., Horvath, T. B., Berger, P. A., and Kopell, B. S. (1980): *Electroencephalogr. Clin. Neurophysiol.,* 49:497–505.
86. Roth, W. T., Pfefferbaum, A., Kelly, A. F., Berger, P. A., and Kopell, B. S. (1981): *Psychiatry Res.,* 4:199–212.
87. Roth, W. T., Tecce, J. J., Pfefferbaum, A., Rosenbloom, M., and Callaway, E. (1984): In: *Brain and Information: Event-Related Potentials,* edited by R. Karrer, J. Cohen, and P. Tueting. *Ann. NY Acad. Sci.,* 425:496–522.
88. Roth, W. T., and Tinklenberg, J. R. (1982): *Psychopharmacol. Bull.,* 18:78–83.
89. Saitoh, O., Niwa, S. I., Hiramatsu, K. I., Kameyama, T., Rymar, K., and Itoh, K. (1984): *Biol. Psychiatry,* 19:293–303.
90. Schwartz, M., and Shagass, C. (1963): *Electroencephalogr. Clin. Neurophysiol.,* 15:265–271.
91. Seidman, L. J. (1983): *Psychol. Bull.,* 94:195–238.
92. Serafetinides, E. A., Coger, R. W., and Martin, J. (1986): *Psychiatry Res.,* 17:73–75.
93. Shagass, C. (1972): *Evoked Brain Potentials in Psychiatry.* Plenum Press, New York.
94. Shagass, C., Roemer, R. A., and Straumanis, J. J. (1982): *Arch. Gen. Psychiatry,* 39:1423–1435.
95. Shagass, C., Roemer, R. A., Straumanis, J. J., and Josiassen, R. C. (1984): *Br. J. Psychiatry,* 144:581–592.
96. Siegel, C., Waldo, M., Mizner, G., Adler, L. E., and Freedman, R. (1984): *Arch. Gen. Psychiatry,* 41:607–612.
97. Spohn, H. E., and Patterson, T. (1979): *Schizophr. Bull.,* 5:581–611.
98. St. Clair, D. M., Blackwood, D. H. R., and Christie, J. E. (1985): *Br. J. Psychiatry,* 147:702–706.
99. Stevens, J. R., Bigelow, L., Denney, D., Lipkin, J., Livermore, A. H., Rauscher, F., and Wyatt, R. J. (1979): *Arch. Gen. Psychiatry,* 36:251–262.
100. Stevens, J. R., and Livermore, A. (1982): *J. Neurol. Neurosurg. Psychiatry,* 45:385–395.
101. Strandburg, R. J., Marsh, J. T., Brown, W. S., Asarnow, R. F., and Guthrie, D. (1984): *Electroencephalogr. Clin. Neurophysiol.,* 57:236–253.
102. Syndulko, K., Hansch, E. C., Cohen, S. N., Pearce, J. W., Goldberg, Z., Montan, B., Tourtellotte, W. W., and Potvin, A. R. (1982): In: *Clinical Applications of Evoked Potentials in Neurology,* edited by J. Courjon, F. Maugière, and M. Revol, pp. 279–285. Raven Press, New York.
103. Tanguay, P. E., Edwards, R. M., Buchwald, J., Schwafel, J., and Allen, V. (1982): *Arch. Gen. Psychiatry,* 39:174–180.
104. Timsit-Berthier, M. (1986): In *Cerebral Psychophysiology: Studies in Event-Related Potentials (EEG Suppl. 38),* edited by W. C. McCallum, R. Zappoli, and F. Denoth, pp. 429–438. Elsevier, Amsterdam.
105. Verleger, R., and Cohen, R. (1978): *Psychol. Med.,* 8:81–93.
106. Volavka, J., Abrams, R., Taylor, M. A., and Reker, D. (1981): In: *Advances in Biological Psychiatry, Vol. 6,* pp. 72–75. S. Karger, Basel.
107. Weinberg, H., Stroink, G., and Katila, T., eds. (1985): *Biomagnetism: Applications and Theory.* Pergamon, New York.
108. Weinberger, D. R., Torrey, E. F., Neophytides, A. N., and Wyatt, R. J. (1979): *Arch. Gen. Psychiatry,* 36:735–739.
109. Wood, C. C., McCarthy, G., Squires, N. K., Vaughan, H. G., Woods, D. L., and McCallum, W. C. (1984): *Ann. NY Acad. Sci.,* 425:681–721.

Psychopharmacology:
The Third Generation of Progress,
edited by Herbert Y. Meltzer.
Raven Press, New York © 1987.

CHAPTER 79

Prolactin and Schizophrenia

Robert T. Rubin

Considerable evidence points to the involvement of dopamine (DA), as a CNS neurotransmitter, in the pathophysiology of schizophrenia and other psychoses (12,31,43,55,59). Of importance in the link between CNS DA neurotransmission and psychotic symptomatology is the fact that most neuroleptic (antipsychotic) drugs act as postsynaptic DA receptor blockers, and this effect correlates with their therapeutic potency (48). This suggests that there may be a functional overactivity of CNS dopaminergic neurotransmission in schizophrenia and other psychoses. Whether this putative net excess of dopaminergic activity is a consequence of increased presynaptic DA release, postsynaptic DA receptor hypersensitivity, underactivity of counterbalancing neurotransmitter systems, or some combination thereof, is not known.

The direct measurement of dopaminergic activity in the human brain is not presently possible. Indirect measures, therefore, have been used in many research studies of psychoses and antipsychotic drugs; these include primarily the quantitation of DA and its metabolites in various body fluids, particularly cerebrospinal fluid. However, at best the measurement of these compounds reflects dopaminergic activity throughout the CNS, without regard to specific dopaminergic pathways. Other, more limited approaches have been to examine the functional activity of certain DA systems in psychoses such as schizophrenia, for example the nigrostriatal system (23). Because the secretion of the hormone prolactin (PRL) by the anterior pituitary gland is under the tonic inhibition of a specific CNS dopaminergic system, measurement of PRL secretion has been used as another index of DA activity in schizophrenia and its response to neuroleptic treatment. This chapter offers a selective review of this research.

DA SYSTEMS IN THE BRAIN

There are several discrete dopaminergic systems in the brain, and their function is known to a greater or lesser

extent (20,45). A brief overview of these systems will facilitate a discussion of the relationship of PRL secretion to schizophrenia.

Of perhaps greatest relevance to possible neurophysiologic mechanisms underlying schizophrenia are the mesolimbic and mesocortical DA tracts. These tracts have cell bodies lying in the ventral tegmental area of the mesencephalon, and their axons project to numerous structures including amygdala, anterior olfactory nucleus, olfactory bulb, olfactory tubercle, septal area, nucleus accumbens, and several cortical areas including cingulate and frontal cortex. Anatomically contiguous with the ventral tegmental area is the substantia nigra, containing cell bodies whose axons project densely to the neostriatrum (caudate and putamen) and also to the globus pallidus—the nigrostriatal tract. The mesolimbic and mesocortical dopaminergic systems have been proposed to act as gating or biasing circuits for the cortical control of sensory perceptual function in schizophrenia (59), much as the nigrostriatal system acts as modulating circuit for the cortical control of motor function. Together, these three tracts comprise the mesotelencephalic system (20).

The tuberoinfundibular DA (TIDA) tract is important in the regulation of PRL secretion. It is a short tract, with cell bodies in the arcuate and periventricular nuclei of the hypothalamus, and axonal projections to the neural and intermediate lobes of the pituitary and to the median eminence of the hypothalamus and the pituitary stalk. The axonal endings in the median eminence and pituitary stalk are in close proximity to the pituitary portal system, which carries blood between a bed of capillaries in these structures and the capillaries surrounding the cells of the anterior pituitary. The hypothalamic releasing and inhibiting hormones that control the secretion of the anterior pituitary hormones are produced in neurosecretory cells in the hypothalamus and transported to their target cells in the anterior pituitary by the portal system. There is considerable evidence that DA itself, produced in the TIDA neurons and transported via the portal system to the lactotrophs of the anterior pituitary, is the major PRL inhibiting factor (4,22). As the secretion of PRL is primarily under tonic inhibitory control, reduced neurotransmission in the TIDA system results in increased PRL release. This occurs consistently following the administration of neuroleptic drugs, because they block DA receptors on the lactotrophs (54).

There are some functional differences between the TIDA system and the mesotelencephalic DA system that are important when considering the relationship between PRL and schizophrenia. The TIDA system does not have neurotransmitter-mediated reciprocal neuronal feedback circuits, as does the mesotelencephalic DA system. Rather, its regulatory feedback appears to be hormonal, by PRL itself. Increased concentrations of PRL reaching the hypothalamus via the general circulation, and also likely by retrograde flow in the pituitary portal system, result in increased DA synthesis and release, with consequent inhibition of PRL secretion. DA receptors are of different types in the TIDA and mesencephalic systems (14); in the former system they are of the D_2 type, which are coupled with a decrease or have no interaction with cyclic AMP synthesis, whereas in the latter system they are of both the D_2 type and the D_1 type, which are coupled with adenylate cyclase, the enzyme that forms cyclic AMP from ATP.

Also, ovarian steroids play an important role in the regulation of PRL secretion (4,22). Estrogens have multiple actions at the level of the pituitary, including stimulating the synthesis and release of PRL and increasing the number of lactotrophs. Progesterone may have an opposing action, by increasing DA release into the portal circulation.

These functional differences between the TIDA system and the other CNS DA systems may be relevant to the differences in their response to DA receptor-blocking drugs, e.g., the more sensitive and rapid PRL response to neuroleptics compared to their antipsychotic and extrapyramidal side-effect-inducing properties. For example, in normal adult volunteers PRL secretion can be stimulated by a dose of haloperidol as low as 0.25 mg i.m. or i.v. (56), which produces no objective or subjective clinical effects and which is well below the usual i.m. clinical dose of 3.0 to 5.0 mg. A maximal PRL response can be attained by as little an amount of haloperidol as 1.5 mg i.m. or i.v. (33). Nevertheless, there is good correspondence between the relative antipsychotic potencies of several neuroleptic drugs and their PRL-releasing potencies at low doses, in both human volunteers (32) and laboratory animals (25).

Basal PRL Concentrations and PRL Responses to DA Agonists

If DA neurotransmission in the CNS indeed is increased in schizophrenia, and if this hyperactivity extends to the TIDA system, then measurement of basal circulating PRL concentrations should reveal decreases in schizophrenic patients compared to controls, analogous to the markedly reduced plasma PRL concentrations reported in patients with Huntington's chorea, in whom a predominance of DA occurs in the nigrostriatal system (24). This question has been addressed in a number of studies in which

circulating PRL levels in unmedicated patients and control subjects were compared. Most of these studies have reported negative results, i.e., no difference in mean values between the two groups and a comparable range of values in both (11,15,19,37,42,50). Whereas these studies were alike in that they did compare patients against controls, they were dissimilar in the radioimmunoassays used for PRL measurement, the number of blood samples drawn (generally single samples), and the length of time before study the patients had been off psychotropic medications (unspecified to 1 year). In one study (15) the patients remained on neuroleptic medication. The last two points are important in that (a) PRL is secreted episodically, so that there may be considerable variability in single samples, and (b) the PRL-augmenting effect of neuroleptics may be manifest from days to months after withdrawal, especially following a course of depot neuroleptics (61).

From these studies of baseline PRL in patients and controls, one might conclude that the lack of clear PRL differences indicates no alteration in CNS dopaminergic activity in schizophrenics. A few studies, however, have provided data that might indicate otherwise. These several studies have attempted to relate specific dimensions of psychopathology in schizophrenics to PRL secretion. Johnstone et al. (27) found generally normal serum PRL concentrations in 16 unmedicated, male, hospitalized, chronic schizophrenics who were tested on two occasions 2 months apart. However, within subjects there were significant negative correlations between PRL and total positive symptoms ($r = -0.54$) and between PRL and incoherence of speech ($r = -0.56$), consistent with the hypothesis that increased CNS dopaminergic activity may be responsible for the positive symptoms of schizophrenia. Similarly, Kleinman et al. (28) found normal plasma PRL concentrations in 17 unmedicated, hospitalized chronic schizophrenics, but a significant inverse relationship across subjects between PRL and total score on the Brief Psychiatric Rating Scale (BPRS) (47) ($r = -0.63$). Of interest, this negative correlation was especially strong ($r = -0.82$) for the subgroup of eight patients who had normal-sized cerebral ventricles compared to the nine patients with enlarged cerebral ventricles ($r = -0.58$); the latter correlation was not significant. Thought disturbance also was significantly negatively related to PRL in the former group ($r = -0.72$) but not in the latter group ($r = -0.37$). These data would support the notion that there is a subgroup of schizophrenics with normal ventricular size in whom CNS dopaminergic hyperactivity might be a determinant of the severity of their psychopathology. However, unexplained in this study were the clearly significant negative correlations between anxiety/depression and PRL in both groups of patients ($r = -0.78$ and -0.74, respectively).

Rinieris et al. (52) studied 35 drug-free, male, hospitalized paranoid schizophrenics during acute exacerbations of their illness and found that 17 of the 35 had delusions with a homosexual content. These 17 were similar to the other 18 patients in age, duration of illness, and overall mental state, and their serum PRL concentrations as well were not significantly different. However, the patients with homosexual delusions did have a mean serum PRL concentration significantly lower than that of 16 normal male controls, whereas the mean serum PRL of the other group of patients was not different from that of the normal controls. The differences in mean PRL were small, however, and were of marginal statistical significance, especially if the *p* values were to be corrected for the number of tests performed.

Another approach to the investigation of PRL dynamics in schizophrenic patients has been the use of challenge tests. DA receptor-blocking neuroleptics, of course, represent one such challenge and will be discussed in the next section. Of the other challenge tests, apomorphine, a DA agonist that reduces PRL secretion, has been the most commonly used. In a series of studies in which schizophrenics were compared to controls, Rotrosen et al. (53) found a suggestive blunting of PRL suppression in the patients, but varying baseline PRL values did not allow a clear difference to be discerned. This highlights the importance of having stable baseline PRL measures, since PRL secretion is increased by the stress of venipuncture and serum PRL may require more than an hour to return to baseline values (1). A further suppression of serum PRL by a DA agonist thus may be obscured by declining pretest PRL values.

Similarly, Davis et al. (15) found a blunted PRL response to apomorphine in 18 schizophrenics compared to 14 normal controls, but this difference was abolished when the PRL responses were corrected for baseline PRL (somewhat higher in the normal subjects). Davis et al. (15) also highlighted other variables, in addition to baseline hormone concentrations, that can influence PRL responses; these include age, time of day of sampling, meals, use of drugs and alcohol, overall endocrine status of the subjects, and level of current stress, e.g., whether subjects have been recently hospitalized. Clearly negative results, i.e., no difference in PRL suppression following apomorphine between schizophrenics and controls, have been reported by several other investigators (18,38,41). Meltzer et al. (41) found a positive correlation between the PRL response and measures of depression but not total BPRS, positive or negative symptoms.

The above studies are consistent in indicating that the PRL response to apomorphine is not abnormal in schizophrenic subjects. However, further studies relating this response to specific dimensions of psychopathology are indicated.

The PRL Secretory Response to Neuroleptic Drugs

As mentioned earlier, the antipsychotic potencies of most DA-blocking neuroleptic drugs correlate well with their PRL-stimulating potencies at low doses in both human subjects and laboratory animals (25,32). Considerable attention has been given to the importance of the PRL increase associated with higher, clinical doses of neuroleptic drugs (see 36, 38, 54 for reviews). Galactorrhea, the discharge of milk from the breasts of men and nonnursing women, is a side effect of neuroleptics that results from elevated circulating PRL, as will be discussed below. Proposed clinical applications of serum plasma PRL measurements, as a reflection of alterations in CNS DA activity secondary to treatment with neuroleptic drugs, include the PRL response as an index of clinical response, predicting ultimate

clinical response on the basis of an initial PRL response, and using PRL to monitor compliance with treatment (54).

PRL concentrations are increased within 30 min after a parenteral dose of neuroleptic drug (56). Following oral medication, PRL concentrations rise during the first days of treatment as the neuroleptic dose is increased (40). Because estrogen potentiates the PRL response in premenopausal women, serum hormone concentrations increase faster in women than they do in men on comparable doses of neuroleptics. Generally, at doses of most neuroleptics up to 600 mg of chlorpromazine (CPZ) equivalents per day, there is a correlation between drug dose and PRL concentration, with higher values in women (39,54). One exception might be haloperidol, for which strong correlations between PRL and doses up to 80 to 90 mg per day (roughly 3,000–4,000 CPZ equivalents per day) have been reported (8,35,49).

As mentioned above, one possible clinical application of PRL measurements in schizophrenics is as an index of therapeutic response. This is a potentially important application. Many studies have shown large interindividual differences in the blood levels of antipsychotic drugs in patients given the same drug doses, owing to different amounts absorbed and different rates of metabolism. Furthermore, serum drug concentrations themselves do not always correlate well with therapeutic response. The formation of active metabolites, such as with CPZ, and/or differences in the concentration of free (active) neuroleptic due to drug binding to serum proteins, might influence antipsychotic activity but not be reflected in serum drug concentrations, depending on the method of analysis. For example, radioimmunoassays that have been developed for haloperidol measure either the parent compound alone or the parent compound plus its reduced metabolite, depending on the antibody used (49). (Whether or not reduced haloperidol has significant antipsychotic potency at the serum concentrations in which it occurs in treated patients remains an open question.) Radioreceptor assays for neuroleptic drugs are based on *in vitro* caudate nucleus DA receptor binding and therefore theoretically should measure both a parent compound and all its "active" (i.e., DA receptor-binding) metabolites. However, receptor binding does not necessarily mean receptor blocking, and radioreceptor assays in some instances may be too nonspecific. The PRL response, as a physiologic response to the DA blocking action of neuroleptics, should reflect both active metabolites and the free (unbound) serum fraction of drug and thus might provide a type of "*in vivo* bioassay" of neuroleptic action in patients.

Toward this end, investigators have studied the relation of the time course and magnitude of the PRL responses of patients during neuroleptic treatment to the time course and magnitude of their clinical responses. Unfortunately, these studies have yielded discordant results (8,35,39,40,44,54,60). For example, Meltzer and Fang (40) found a modest but significant correlation between average serum PRL concentration and improvement in psychosis among male (*r* = +0.53) but not among female (*r* = +0.15) patients. Of importance, these investigators noted that PRL levels commonly reached a plateau within the first week of treatment, whereas psychotic behavior declined only gradually over a period of 6 to 8 weeks. These clinical observations agree with the previously noted experimental findings that the PRL response to neuroleptics is very rapid and that doses of neuroleptic drugs required for antipsychotic therapeusis are generally greater than those required for maximal stimulation of PRL. One possible refinement in methodology might be to correct PRL values for differences in serum neuroleptic values, as suggested by Swigar et al. (60), who found that the ratio of serum PRL concentration to serum neuroleptic concentration was a better predictor of clinical improvement than either measure alone. The rationale here is that correcting the PRL response for the concentration of drug provides a more accurate index of individual sensitivity to TIDA receptor blockade, and by inference to receptor blockade in other DA systems in the brain. In this regard, a correlation between the PRL response to neuroleptics and the development of extrapyramidal side effects also has been documented (51,54).

Because the doses of most neuroleptics required for antipsychotic activity exceed those doses which maximally stimulate PRL secretion, as mentioned above, individual differences in PRL secretion at clinical drug doses might be due largely to differences in maximal capacity to synthesize and secrete PRL, rather than to differences in sensitivity to DA receptor blockade. Also, PRL secretion during chronic stimulation by neuroleptics may be influenced by variables irrelevant to the antipsychotic response, such as feedback inhibition of PRL release, tolerance to the PRL elevating action of the drug, changing estrogen status of female patients, interactions among combinations of drugs given to schizophrenic patients (3,17), and the time of blood sampling for PRL measurement (21).

As previously discussed, PRL feedback inhibition appears to be mediated by a PRL-stimulated increase in DA release in the median eminence. Whether or not the usual doses of neuroleptics would be sufficiently large to block the pituitary binding of the increased amounts of DA, thereby masking PRL autoregulatory mechanisms, undoubtedly depends on the drug, its dosage, and differing physiological characteristics of the TIDA system among individuals. Tolerance of the PRL response to neuroleptics has been held by some investigators not to occur, since elevated PRL concentrations persist even after many weeks of drug treatment (18,46,54). However, other investigators have reported slowly declining PRL concentrations with chronic neuroleptic treatment, particularly in men, suggesting a slowly developing tolerance that might be masked by a treatment regimen of increasing drug dosage (6,9,10,16,34). Kolakowska et al. (29) did show such patients to be PRL-responsive to an acute neuroleptic challenge. On the other hand, following withdrawal of rats from chronic neuroleptic medication, a supersensitivity of the PRL system to inhibition by DA agonists has been demonstrated (30). Thus, the issue of tolerance to PRL stimulation during chronic neuroleptic treatment in psychotic patients remains moot. If indeed it can occur, its mechanism (e.g., change in DA receptor sensitivity vs change in PRL synthesis and/or secretion) remains to be elucidated. In some patients, PRL tolerance to neuroleptic treatment may be predictive of early relapse following drug withdrawal (9).

There are large interindividual differences in therapeutic responsiveness to neuroleptics, but as yet there are no satisfactory methods for predicting a given patient's clinical response to a specific drug. The "test dose" model, in which a patient is given an initial dose of drug and his or her short-term response is monitored, has been tried for psychotropic drugs of different classes. The PRL response to a small test dose of neuroleptic drug, were it to prove to be a reliable predictor of ultimate treatment response, would be readily applicable to clinical circumstances. However, a major problem with such a test paradigm is that there is considerable interindividual variability in PRL responses to low doses of neuroleptic drugs, even in normal subjects and with intravenous drug administration (26). Although these differences in PRL response might correlate with differences in the sensitivity of the mesolimbic and mesocortical DA systems to receptor blockade, which might be an important source of variability in therapeutic responsiveness to these drugs, a great deal of work remains to be done to calibrate the range of PRL responses in different groups of patients (e.g., men vs women) and for different subgroups of neuroleptic drugs. In essence, differences in physiologic characteristics of the TIDA system among individuals need to be clearly understood before the PRL response can be applied as a clinical test.

Finally, measurement of PRL secretion in psychotic patients has been proposed as a means of detecting noncompliance with treatment, since PRL usually returns to baseline within a few days after neuroleptics are stopped. However, this is of little practical utility, for several reasons. First, as mentioned earlier, in some patients PRL concentrations can remain elevated for 2 to 3 weeks after medication has been discontinued. Second, the PRL response occurs very rapidly, so that a single dose of medication given some hours before blood sampling will elevate PRL, even if no medication was taken for many weeks. Third, if tolerance indeed does occur, PRL concentrations may have returned to baseline despite a patient's compliance with the treatment regimen.

Clinical Effects of Neuroleptic-Induced PRL Increase

Soon after the introduction of phenothiazine neuroleptics into clinical psychiatry, the side effects of amenorrhea and galactorrhea in some women patients were noted. Galactorrhea had been reported in psychiatric patients on many different neuroleptic drugs. Apostolakis et al. (2) found galactorrhea in 50% of 200 female patients on moderate doses of various antipsychotic drugs and in 10% of male patients receiving similar treatment. Abnormally high plasma PRL activity (pigeon crop bioassay) was found in most of the cases studied. Women in the mid-childbearing age had a higher incidence of galactorrhea than younger or older women, perhaps related to estrogen enhancement of PRL secretion and PRL effects on mammary tissue.

Beumont et al. (6,7) noted neuroendocrine side effects in 15 of 16 women of childbearing age; these included amenorrhea alone, galactorrhea with irregular menses, and both galactorrhea and amenorrhea. In most of the patients, PRL was elevated. In those whose menses were normal, plasma concentrations of luteinizing hormone (LH), estradiol, and progesterone followed the normal menstrual pattern. In those who were amenorrheic, basal plasma LH concentrations were variable, midcycle LH peaks were absent, and estradiol and progesterone concentrations were in the follicular phase range. Although the neuroleptics themselves might have suppressed LH secretion by the anterior pituitary, elevated circulating PRL also is known to have an LH-suppressing effect. Beumont et al. (5) treated nine female patients who had phenothiazine-induced galactorrhea with bromocryptine, a DA agonist. Plasma PRL was decreased with treatment, but values were still above the normal range. Similarly, the galactorrhea persisted, although its severity was reduced. Amantadine, an indirect DA agonist, also has been used successfully in this regard (58).

The usual physical consequences of inappropriate lactation and possible cessation of menses in patients taking neuroleptics are obvious: breast discharge and infertility. The psychological consequences on occasion may be profound; one 15-year-old psychotic girl was reported to have developed a delusion of pregnancy following chlorpromazine-induced lactation (13). Of major concern some years ago was the possibility that neuroleptic-treated female psychiatric patients, who had increased circulating PRL for extended periods, might be at increased risk for the development of breast cancer. This concern followed upon considerable evidence that certain rodent mammary tumors are sensitive to PRL and that some human mammary tumors have PRL receptors and may be PRL-dependent. Fortunately, several epidemiologic surveys of psychiatric hospital records yielded negative results: no increased incidence of breast cancer development or mortality in patients who had been treated with neuroleptics (57). Thus, a potentially serious complication of treatment with neuroleptics has proved to be of little clinical concern.

CONCLUSIONS

While perhaps not readily apparent from this brief and necessarily selective review, a great deal of work has been done on the importance of the anterior pituitary hormone PRL for clinical psychiatry. The focus of this review has been on human studies, primarily studies of psychotic patients. Not covered has been the large number of preclinical studies in laboratory animals, which, for example, have used the PRL response as an index of DA receptor-blocking potency in the development of new, putative neuroleptic drugs.

Whether or not the measurement of PRL in psychotic patients will have any ultimate clinical utility remains to be determined. The measurement of basal PRL concentrations and PRL responses to DA agonist challenge in schizophrenics has yielded few consistent (mostly negative) results, and they add little to our understanding of the DA-overactivity hypothesis of schizophrenia. The consistent PRL increases following the administration of neuroleptic drugs are generally so sensitive and variable that they have not been a reliable and reproducible correlate of treatment response. Some patients may develop tolerance in their TIDA system to chronic neuroleptic therapy, as indicated

by declining serum PRL concentrations over time, which may be reflective of other hyperactive dopaminergic systems within the CNS and also possibly predictive of early relapse. This potential utility of PRL measurement certainly needs further study. Finally, a question for the future may be asked: Will the development of new, more highly selective mesolimbic and mesocortical DA-blocking neuroleptics (of which clozapine might be a prototype) and/or neuroleptics that work by a different pharmacologic mechanism (and thus might avoid altogether such side effects as tardive dyskinesia) render the measurement of PRL ultimately irrelevant to the study and treatment of schizophrenia?

ACKNOWLEDGMENT

The author is the recipient of National Institute of Mental Health Research Scientist Award MH47363.

REFERENCES

1. Adler, R. A., Noel, G. L., Wartofsky, L., and Frantz, A. G. (1975): *J. Clin. Endocrinol. Metab.*, 41:383–389.
2. Apostolakis, M., Kapetanakis, S., Lazos, G., and Madena-Pyrgaki, A. (1972): In: *Lactogenic Hormones*, edited by G. E. W. Wolstenholme and J. Knight, pp. 349–359. Churchill Livingstone, Edinburgh.
3. Arato, M. (1980): *Commun. Psychopharmacol.*, 4:317–322.
4. Ben-Jonathan, N. (1985): *Endocrinol. Rev.*, 6:564–589.
5. Beumont, P., Bruwer, J., Pimstone, B., Vinik, A., and Utian, W. (1975): *Br. J. Psychiatry*, 126:285–288.
6. Beumont, P. J. V., Gelder, M. G., Friesen, H. G., Harris, G. W., MacKinnon, P. C. B., Mandelbrote, B. M., and Wiles, D. H. (1974): *Br. J. Psychiatry*, 124:413–430.
7. Beumont, P. J. V., Harris, G. W., Carr, P. J., Friesen, H. G., Kolakowska, T., MacKinnon, P. C. B., Mandelbrote, B. M., and Wiles, D. (1972): *J. Psychosom. Res.*, 16:297–304.
8. Bjørndal, N., Bjerre, M., Gerlach, J., Kristjansen, P., Magelund, G., Oestrich, I. H., and Waehrens, J. (1980): *Psychopharmacology*, 67:17–23.
9. Brown, W. A., and Laughren, T. (1981): *Am. J. Psychiatry*, 138:237–239.
10. Brown, W. A., and Laughren, T. P. (1981): *Psychiatry Res.*, 5:317–322.
11. Cabranes, J. A., Fuentenebro, F., Recio, M. N., Borque, M., and Almoguera, M. I. (1982): *Int. Pharmacopsychiatry*, 17:1–7.
12. Carlsson, A. (1978): *Biol. Psychiatry*, 13:3–21.
13. Cramer, B. (1971): *Am. J. Psychiatry*, 127:136–139.
14. Creese, I., Sibley, D. R., Hamblin, M. W., and Leff, S. E. (1983): *Annu. Rev. Neurosci.*, 6:43–71.
15. Davis, B. M., Davis, K. L., Mohs, R. D., Mathe, A. A., Rothpearl, A. B., Johns, C. A., Levy, M. I., and Horvath T. B. (1985): *Arch. Gen. Psychiatry*, 42:259–264.
16. de Rivera, J. L., Lal, S., Ettigi, P., Hontela, S., Muller, H. F., and Friesen, H. G. (1976): *Clin. Endocrinol.*, 5:273–282.
17. Elizur, A., Segal, Z., Yeret, A., and Ben-David, M. (1980): *Commun. Psychopharmacol.*, 4:203–206.
18. Ettigi, P., Nair, N. P. V., Lal, S., Cervantes, P., and Guyda, H. (1976): *J. Neurol. Neurosurg. Psychiatry*, 39:870–876.
19. Ferrier, I. N., Johnstone, E. C., Crow, T. J., and Rincon-Rodriguez, I. (1983): *Arch. Gen. Psychiatry*, 40:755–761.
20. Foote, S. J. (1985): In: *Psychiatry, Vol. 3*, edited by J. O. Cavenar, Jr., Chapter 44. Lippincott, Philadelphia.
21. Goode, D. J., Meltzer, H. Y., and Fang, V. S. (1981): *Biol. Psychiatry*, 16:653–662.
22. Gudelsky, G. A. (1981): *Psychoneuroendocrinology*, 6:3–16.
23. Haase, H.-J. (1966): *Neuroleptika, Tranquilizer, und Antidepressiva in Klinik und Praxis.* Janssen, Dusseldorf.

24. Hayden, M. R., Paul, M., Vinik, A. I., and Beighton, P. (1977): *Lancet*, 2:423–426.
25. Hays, S. E., Poland, R. E., and Rubin, R. T. (1980): *J. Pharmacol. Exp. Ther.*, 214:362–367.
26. Hays, S. E., and Rubin, R. T. (1979): *Psychopharmacology*, 61:17–24.
27. Johnstone, E. C., Crow, T. J., and Mashiter, K. (1977): *Psychol. Med.*, 7:223–228.
28. Kleinman, J. E., Weinberger, D. R., Rogol, A. D., Bigelow, L. B., Klein, S. T., Gillin, J. C., and Wyatt, R. J. (1982): *Arch. Gen. Psychiatry*, 39:655–657.
29. Kolakowska, T., Braddock, L., Wiles, D., Franklin, M., and Gelder, M. (1981): *Br. J. Psychiatry*, 139:400–412.
30. Lal, H., Brown, W., Drawbaugh, R., Hynes, M., and Brown, G. (1977): *Life Sci.*, 20:101–106.
31. Langer, D. H., Brown, G. L., and Docherty, J. P. (1981): *Schizophr. Bull.*, 8:208–224.
32. Langer, G., Sachar, E. J., Gruen, P. H., and Halpern, F. S. (1970): *Nature*, 266:639–640.
33. Langer, G., Sachar, E. J., Halpern, F. S., Gruen, P. H., and Solomon, M. (1977): *J. Clin. Endocrinol. Metab.*, 45:996–1002.
34. Laughren, T. P., Brown, W. A., and Williams, B. W. (1979): *Am. J. Psychiatry*, 136:108–110.
35. Linkowski, P., Hubain, P., von Frenckell, R., and Mendlewicz, J. (1984): *Eur. Arch. Psychiatry Neurol. Sci.*, 234:231–236.
36. Meltzer, H. Y. (1980): *Psychiatr. Clin. North Am.*, 3:277–298.
37. Meltzer, H. Y., and Busch, D. (1983): *Psychiatry Res.*, 9:285–299.
38. Meltzer, H. Y., Busch, D., and Fang, V. S. (1981): *Psychoneuroendocrinology*, 6:17–36.
39. Meltzer, H. Y., Busch, D. A., and Fang, V. S. (1983): *Psychiatry Res.*, 9:271–283.
40. Meltzer, H. Y., and Fang, V. (1976): *Arch. Gen. Psychiatry*, 33:279–286.
41. Meltzer, H. Y., Kolakowska, T., Fang, V. S., Fogg, L., Robertson, A., Lewine, R., Strahilevitz, M., and Busch, D. (1984): *Arch. Gen. Psychiatry*, 41:512–519.
42. Meltzer, H. Y., Sachar, E. J., and Frantz, A. G. (1974): *Arch. Gen. Psychiatry*, 31:564–569.
43. Meltzer, H. Y., and Stahl, S. M. (1976): *Schizophr. Bull.*, 2:19–76.
44. Möller, H. J., Kissling, W., Maurach, R., Schmid, W., Doerr, P., Pirke, K., and von Zerssen, D. (1981): *Pharmakopsychiatrie*, 14:27–34.
45. Moore, R. Y., and Bloom, F. E. (1979): *Annu. Rev. Neurosci.*, 1:129–169.
46. Naber, D., Fischer, H., and Ackenheil, M. (1979): *Commun. Psychopharmacol.*, 3:59–65.
47. Overall, J. E., and Gorham, D. R. (1962): *Psychol. Rep.*, 10:799–812.
48. Peroutka, S. J., and Snyder, S. H. (1980): *Am. J. Psychiatry*, 137:1518–1522.
49. Poland, R. E., and Rubin, R. T. (1981): *Life Sci.*, 29:1837–1845.
50. Prange, A. J., Jr., Loosen, P. T., Wilson, I. C., Meltzer, H. Y., and Fang, V. S. (1979): *Arch. Gen. Psychiatry*, 36:1086–1093.
51. Rama Rao, V. A., Bishop, M., and Coppen, A. (1980): *Br. J. Psychiatry*, 137:518–521.
52. Rinieris, P., Markianos, M., Hatzimanolis, J., and Stefanis, C. (1985): *Acta Psychiatr. Scand.*, 72:309–314.
53. Rotrosen, J., Angrist, B., Gershon, S., Paquin, J., Branchey, L., Oleshansky, M., Halpern, F., and Sachar, E. J. (1979): *Br. J. Psychiatry*, 135:444–456.
54. Rubin, R. T., and Hays, S. E. (1980): *Psychoneuroendocrinology*, 5:121–137.
55. Rubin, R. T., and Marder, S. R. (1982): In: *Affective and Schizophrenic Disorders*, edited by M. R. Zales, pp. 53–100. Brunner/Mazel, New York.
56. Rubin, R. T., Poland, R. E., O'Connor, D., Gouin, P. R., and Tower, B. B. (1976): *Psychopharmacology*, 47:135–140.
57. Schyve, P., Smithline, F., and Meltzer, H. Y. (1978): *Arch. Gen. Psychiatry*, 35:1291–1301.
58. Siever, L. J. (1981): *J. Clin. Psychopharmacol.*, 1:2–7.
59. Stevens, J. R. (1973): *Arch. Gen. Psychiatry*, 29:177–189.
60. Swigar, M. E., Jatlow, P. I., Goicoechea, N., Opsahl, C., and Bowers, M. B., Jr. (1984): *Am. J. Psychiatry*, 141:1281–1283.
61. Wistedt, B., Wiles, D., and Kolakowska, T. (1981): *Lancet*, 1:1163.

Psychopharmacology:
The Third Generation of Progress,
edited by Herbert Y. Meltzer.
Raven Press, New York © 1987.

CHAPTER 80

Growth Hormone and Schizophrenia

S. Lal

Growth hormone (GH) secretion is regulated by several neurotransmitters (NTs), including dopamine (DA), norepinephrine (NE), serotonin (5-HT), acetylcholine (Ach), and γ-aminobutyric acid (GABA). A variety of drugs which affect NT function stimulate GH secretion in man (45). This has led to the use of GH responses induced by drugs or physiological stimuli to selectively evaluate specific NT systems in schizophrenia (SCZ). These studies have attempted to (a) evaluate the hypotheses that DA (69) or NE (54) function is deranged in SCZ; (b) evaluate the hypothesis that neuroleptics (NLs) alter DA receptor sensitivity (25); (c) identify subgroups of SCZ (7); (d) predict relapse (17) or therapeutic response to NLs (97) or lithium in SCZ (32); and (e) investigate the effect of psychoactive drugs and putative neuromodulators of DA neurotransmission on DA function in normal subjects (52). The assumption underlying this approach is that NT function in the hypothalamic-pituitary axis (HPA) may reflect NT function in extrahypothalamic brain areas, which may be relevant to the pathophysiology of SCZ and mode of action of antischizophrenic agents.

Interpretation of GH findings following drug stimuli requires information on (a) the selectivity of action; (b) site of action; (c) sequence of events (direct or indirect) leading to changes in circulating GH concentrations; (d) clearance of GH; (e) pharmacokinetics of administered drug; and (f) careful consideration of the physiological variables known to influence GH secretion. For many of the stimuli to be

discussed the mode of action is unclear. Prior NL treatment complicates interpretation of data. In many of the published studies consideration of key physiological variables in selecting controls or in conducting the test procedures are neglected or unspecified.

The present chapter summarizes studies on GH secretion in SCZ and provides pertinent information on the physiology of GH secretion to permit critical evaluation of published investigations.

REGULATION OF GH SECRETION

Hypothalamic-Pituitary Axis and GH Secretion

GH is synthesized, stored, and secreted by specific cells (somatotropes) located in the anterior pituitary. The major functional connection between the anterior pituitary and the hypothalamus is the pituitary portal system. There are few nerve fibers in the anterior lobe and none are involved in the control of GH secretion. GH secretion is regulated by (a) clusters of cell bodies (nuclei) within the hypothalamus which interconnect and project to the median eminence (ME) and (b) neuronal inputs to the hypothalamus from extrahypothalamic brain regions (64). The hypothalamic nuclei and ME contain a number of NT substances (DA, NE, 5-HT, GABA, Ach, epinephrine) (11). The ME receives fibers containing growth hormone-release inhibiting factor

(SRIF) (12) and growth hormone-releasing factor (GRF) (4), which act on the somatotrope after release into the pituitary portal system. NTs affect GH secretion possibly (a) by acting on SRIF and GRF secretory cells by axoaxonic interactions at the ME or axodendritic or axosomatic influences at other sites; (b) by serving as relaying stimuli of GH release from extrahypothalamic areas; or (c) by direct effect on the pituitary following release into the portal system (64). A variety of peptides, including thyrotropin releasing hormone (TRH), cholecystokinin (CCK), and opioid peptides, are found in the hypothalamus and may modulate GH secretion. The ME (and pituitary) lies outside the blood-brain barrier (114). Feedback mechanisms influence GH secretion at the level of the pituitary and/or hypothalamus.

Variables Affecting GH Secretion in Humans

A variety of factors that affect GH secretion in humans (Table 1) may influence the GH response to certain provocative stimuli. Obesity influences a broad range of stimuli (96). Of the 48 studies summarized in Table 2, only 12 specify that obese subjects were excluded and only two (57,66) give exclusion criteria for deviation from ideal body weight. Matching for weight without regard to adiposity is an insufficient control. The effect of gender varies greatly with the nature of the provocative agent (48). Activity (96) or taking a meal (93) may affect GH secretion so that tests are best done in the fasting state with the subject recumbent. To ensure basal conditions subjects are best resting for an hour in a nonstimulating environment after insertion of a cannula and before commencing baseline sampling. There is evidence for an autoregulatory mechanism (1) so that subjects with elevated GH concentrations at baseline may show a diminished response to a challenge test. The disappearance half-life of circulating GH is between 17 and 45 min (64).

TABLE 1. *Factors affecting growth hormone secretion in humans*

Spontaneous release	Elevated basal growth
Slow-wave sleep	hormone levels
Age	Smoking
Gender	Regular alcohol intake
Stage of pubertal	Amino acids
development	Arginine
Prolonged fasting	Histidine
(starvation)	Lysine
Body build	Phenylalanine
Obesity	Methionine
Altered protein intake	Hormones
Changes in plasma glucose	Glucagon
Prolonged bed rest	Antidiuretic hormone
Exercise	1-24 Adrenocorticotropin
Physical stress	hormone
Psychological stress	Sex steroids
Surgery	Glucocorticoids
Halothane anesthesia	Insulin
Electroconvulsion	Cholecystokinin
Sleep deprivation	Opioid peptides

For references see ref. 45 and text.

SPONTANEOUS AND SLEEP-ASSOCIATED GH SECRETION

In Normal Subjects

Spontaneous secretory bursts of GH secretion occur during the day and night (82). In older subjects there is a decline in the number of secretory episodes (28). The 24-hr integrated GH concentration changes with stage of puberty (highest in Tanner stage 5), declines with advancing age (115), and is decreased in the obese (68). Little is known about the NT regulation of spontaneous GH secretion.

A major secretory burst of GH occurs 30 to 60 min following sleep onset in relation to slow wave sleep (SWS). Additional minor peaks may occur in association with subsequent episodes of SWS. However, not all episodes of SWS are associated with GH release and dissociations may occur (63). Daytime naps with appearance of SWS are also associated with GH release (92). Hence, sleeping during provocation tests introduces another variable. Major influences on SWS-GH secretion are age and height/weight ratio (91). Many of the pharmacological agents that affect GH secretion have little or no effect on sleep-GH secretion, which suggests a unique regulatory mechanism for the latter (77). A negative feedback suppression of sleep GH secretion has been described (77). Some data point to an inhibitory effect of glucocorticoids (84). Evidence for an inhibitory 5-HT pathway is conflicting (45). Facilitatory muscarinic and nicotinic influences have been described. NLs have no inhibitory effect (47), which points to the absence of DA modulation.

Changes in Schizophrenia

In untreated long-term hospitalized chronic schizophrenics, Schimmelbusch et al. (101) found a decrease in basal GH concentration. However, in the majority of studies differences in basal GH levels have not been found (70). Twenty-four-hour patterns of GH secretion or 24-hr integrated GH concentrations have not been studied in SCZ. Ettigi et al. (25) noted elevated GH concentrations (≥6 ng/ml) during baseline sampling in 6 of 17 chronic schizophrenics but in none of the 21 controls. Recently, Whalley et al. (113) found elevated baseline values in 6 of 25 patients with psychosis. These observations suggest that spontaneous GH secretion may be altered in some patients with SCZ. Mendlewicz et al. (79) found an increase in 24-hr GH secretion in major affective disorder patients and questioned whether this increased GH output might account for the blunted GH responses that are obtained after some GH-provoking stimuli. In several of the studies to be discussed a blunted GH response to apomorphine (Apo) has been noted in chronic SCZ. Hence, it becomes an important area of future research to examine the 24-hr secretory pattern and total 24-hr GH output in SCZ.

A reduction in SWS has been reported in SCZ. This has led to investigations of sleep-induced GH secretion. All three studies which used EEG monitoring found an absent SWS-GH peak (Table 2). The patients reported by Vignieri

TABLE 2. *Growth hormone (GH) response in schizophrenia*

Stimulus (dose)	Diagnosis (criteria)	Gender (M:F)	Neuroleptic (NL) withdrawal	Controls	Results & comments	Ref.
Sleep	C-SCZ A-SCZ	3M 1M	10 dy	8M. Similar age range to pts	No SWS-GH peak in pts. EEG monitored	(109)
Sleep	C-SCZ	10M	On NL	5 (?M). Epileptics on NLs. Similar age range to pts	No sleep-GH peak in 2/10 SCZ & 1/5 controls. No EEG monitoring	(104)
Sleep	C-SCZ	2	On NL	None	No sleep GH peak. EEG monitored	(72)
Sleep	C-SCZ	10M	30 dy	6M. Significantly younger than pts	No SWS-GH peak in pts. EEG monitored	(35)
Apo 0.5 mg s.c.	SCZ (FDC)	10M	7–20 dy	7M. Nonpsychiatric	Bimodal distribution of GH responses in SCZ	(98) *f
Apo 0.5 mg s.c.	SCZ (FDC)	22M	1–3 wk	9M. Nonpsychiatric	Bimodal distribution of GH responses in SCZ	(99) f
Apo 0.5 mg s.c.	C & Sub-C SCZ (RDC)	25M	≥1 wk	16M. Normal + alcoholics & character disorders. Comparable mean age & body weight to pts	Bimodal distribution of GH response in SCZ	(97) f
Apo HCl 0.75 mg s.c.	SCZ (FDC)	17M	2–15 wk	21M (normal + 9 alcoholics). Comparable mean age & body weight to pts	Significant decrease in SCZ. Inverse correlation with duration of NL therapy	(25) *f
Apo HCl 0.75 mg s.c.	A + Sub-A SCZ C + Sub-C SCZ (RDC)	5M; 4F 8M; 7F	2–3 wk	4M; 4F. Nonpsychiatric. Groups not well matched for age	Acute significantly greater than chronic or controls	(94) f
Apo 0.75 mg s.c.	C-SCZ (RDC)	12 (M & F)	≥5 dy	5 (M & F)	No difference	(108) f
Apo 0.75 or 1.5 mg s.c.	A-SCZ C-SCZ	3 4	NL free	No data	No difference from controls	(73)
Apo 0.75 mg s.c.	A-SCZ (n = 5) C-SCZ + SCZ-Aff (n = 13)	7M; 11F	≥1 wk	7M; 8F. Nonpsychiatric	Ill less than 4 years significantly greater than ill more than 4 years	(71) (69) f
Apo 0.75 mg s.c.	SCZ SCZ-Aff (DSM III)	12M; 2F 3M; 5F	≥1 wk	8M; 8F. Nonpsychiatric	No difference between either SCZ or SCZ-Aff and controls	(75) f
Apo HCl 0.75 mg s.c.	C-SCZ (n = 23) A-SCZ (n = 9) SCZ-Aff (n = 18) (RDC)	M & F	≥1 wk	8M; 8F. Nonpsychiatric. Age 20–28 vs 18–55 for pts	No relation between GH response and duration of illness after correction for age	(74) f
Apo 0.75 mg s.c.	A-SCZ C-SCZ (RDC)	9M; 6F 14M; 13F	≥1 wk	8M; 8F. Nonpsychiatric	No relation between GH response and duration of illness after correction for age	(70) f
Apo 0.75 mg s.c.	C-SCZ (FDC) A-SCZ (nuclear SCZ on PSE)	15M 15M	≥1 y (n = 10); never treated (n = 5) ≥1 mo (n = 6); never treated (n = 9)	10M. Nonpsychiatric. Age 27 ± 2 vs 30.1 ± 2 in acute and 62 ± 2 in chronic pts	Significantly blunted in C-SCZ vs either A-SCZ or controls. Inversely correlated with negative symptoms	(26) f
Apo 0.75 mg s.c.	Schneider positive Schneider negative	9M; 1F 3M; 6F	≥9 mo (n = 8); never treated (n = 11)	6M; 3F. Age within 5 years of pts	Schneider positive greater than Schneider negative patients or controls	(113) f
Apo HCl 0.5 mg s.c.	C-SCZ (ICD-9)	9M; 2F	Tested on NL & at 12 & 30 dy after NL withdrawal	10M; 2F. Comparable age with pts	No difference between pts and controls	(86) *f
Apo HCl 0.003, 0.006, 0.012 mg/kg s.c.	A-SCZ Remitted SCZ (DSM III)	10M; 2F 4M; 4F	≥4 wk	9M	A-SCZ significantly greater than remitted SCZ or controls	(87) *f
Apo HCl 0.75 mg/70 kg s.c.	SCZ (n = 8) SCZ-Aff (n = 1) (RDC)	7M; 2F	Tested each 2 mo up to 14 mo after NL discontinued	7M; 2F. Nonpsychiatric. Not studied longitudinally	Exaggerated response in 5/7 blunted in 2/7 relapsing patients. Subjects not fasted	(15)
Apo HCl 0.1, 0.25, 0.75 mg/70 kg s.c.	SCZ (RDC)	10M	3–36 mo (n = 6); never treated (n = 4)	14M. Nonpsychiatric. Normal MMPI. Similar mean age to pts	Exaggerated responses to 0.1 or 0.25 mg dose in SCZ	(16)
Apo HCl 0.75 mg/70 kg s.c.	SCZ (RDC)	11M; 2F	Tested 3–17 times up to 2 y off NL	7M; 3F. Nonpsychiatric. Similar age range to pts. Longitudinally studied	8/10 relapses associated with exaggerated GH response; blunted or normal in 2/10	(17) f
Apo 0.75 mg s.c.	SCZ (n = 9) SCZ-Aff (n = 1) (RDC)	6M; 4F	≥4 wk	—	Significant negative correlation between peak GH and MAO activity (benzylamine substrate)	(61)
Apo 0.75 mg s.c.	SCZ (n = 37) SCZ-Aff (n = 3) (RDC)	24M; 16F	2 wk	—	Significant positive correlation between peak GH and MAO V_{max} (tyramine substrate)	(33) f
Apo 0.75 mg s.c.	SCZ or SCZ-Aff (RDC)	31 (M & F)	1 wk	—	GH response greater than 20 ng/ml predictive of therapeutic response to lithium	(32)

TABLE 2. (*Continued*)

Stimulus (dose)	Diagnosis (criteria)	Gender (M:F)	Neuroleptic (NL) withdrawal	Controls	Results & comments	Ref.
Apo 0.75 mg s.c.	SCZ or SCZ-Aff (Mood incongruent)	20	1 wk	Lithium responders. Mood congruent (RDC-Mania) (n = 4)	Lithium-responsive & nonresponsive SCZ greater than mood-congruent pts	(116)
Apo 0.005 or 0.01 mg/kg s.c.	SCZ or SCZ-Aff (RDC)	14M; 3F	On NL	—	No relation of GH response to therapeutic outcome	(39) f
L-Dopa 0.5 g p.o.	SCZ (FDC)	8M	7–20 dy	10M. Nonpsychiatric	No significant difference	(98) *f
L-Dopa 0.5 g p.o.	C-SCZ (RDC)	9 (M & F)	≥5 dy	11 (M & F)	Low response in 7/9 SCZ vs 2/11 controls	(108) f
L-Dopa 0.5 g + 100 mg Carbidopa p.o.	C-SCZ (RDC)	8M; 2F	≥10 dy	None	Normal GH response. After haloperidol treatment and withdrawal GH & NL response related to HLA antigen status	(7) *f
CLON 0.15 mg i.v.	C-SCZ (FDC)	13M	2–96 wk	18M. Nonpsychiatric controls	No significant difference	(54) *f
CLON 0.15 mg i.v.	SCZ (n = 10) SCZ-Aff (n = 8)	7M; 3F 3M; 5F	≥4 wk	14M; 18F. Nonpsychiatric controls	SCZ-Aff significantly lower than SCZ	(66) *f
CLON 0.15 mg i.v.	SCZ (DSM III)	26M	5 dy (n = 9) 12 dy (n = 17)	9M + 17M Nonpsychiatric controls. Matched for age with pts	Significant decrease in SCZ at 12 days vs controls	(85) *f
AmpSO₄ 0.1 mg/kg i.v.	A-SCZ C-SCZ (ICD-8)	5M; 3F	≥6 wk	11M; 10F	No significant difference	(57) *f
Methyl-PD 0.5 mg/kg i.v.	SCZ (n = 16) SCZ-Aff (n = 3) (DSM III)	11M; 8F	On NL & misc. drugs	21M; 4F. Misc. psychiatric in-patients. Not well matched with SCZ pts	Baseline GH higher in SCZ. GH response decreased in SCZ vs hospital controls	(36)
Methyl-PD 0.5 mg/kg i.v.	SCZ (n = 7) SCZ-Aff (n = 5)	9M; 3F	≥20 dy	—	Clinical outcome and GH response unrelated	(59) f
Insulin 0.1 U/kg i.v.	C-SCZ (n = 15) C-SCZ Backward (n = 7)	22M	On NL (n = 10) 7 days (n = 5) Backward pts drug free (n = 7)	8M hospitalized psychiatric controls. Drug free. Comparable mean age and weight to SCZ pts	Decreased response in backward C-SCZ vs controls	(101) *f
Insulin 0.1 U/kg i.v.	Hebephrenic (n = 15) Paranoid (n = 4) (ICD)	10M; 9F	10 dy. Retested on NLs	None. Pts aged 16–53	Variable response in hebephrenics; related to psychopathology	(8) *f
Insulin 0.1 U/kg i.v.	Hebephrenic (ICD)	15M	10 dy–1 y	10M. Hospitalized pts with sociofamilial mental retardation	No difference from controls. On repeat testing 4 SCZ no or reduced response	(6) f
Insulin 0.1 U/kg i.v.	SCZ	24 (M & F)	On NL (n = 12); Never treated (n = 12)	12M. Matched for age and gender with pts	No difference in GH response	(3)
TRH 0.2 mg i.v.	Adolescent A-SCZ (RDC)	6M	Drug free	6M. Matched for age and pubertal development. Endocrine referrals	GH response in 4/6 SCZ vs 0/6 controls	(31) f
TRH 0.2 mg i.v.	Adolescent SCZ (DSM III)	6M; 4F	On NL	6M; 4F. Age-matched with pts	GH response in 5/10 SCZ vs 0/10 controls. Positive family history of SCZ in 4/5 responders	(112) *f
TRH 0.5 mg i.v.	Adolescent SCZ (RDC)	7M	6/7 on NL	5M. Hospitalized with conduct disorder. Matched for age and puberty (Tanner stage)	GH response in 3/7 SCZ vs 0/5 controls. 3/3 responders 1/4 nonresponders positive family history for SCZ	(22) *f
TRH 0.5 mg i.v.	SCZ + SCZ-Aff (FDC)	8M; 7F	5–26 dy	8M; 7F. Age-matched with pts	No GH response in patients or controls	(95) f
TRH 0.5 mg i.v.	SCZ + SCZ-Aff (RDC)	8M; 2F	On NL	6M; 1F	GH response in 1/10 pts vs 0/7 controls	(5) f
LHRH, 0.05 mg/m² body surface i.v.	Adolescent A-SCZ (RDC)	9M	Drug free	9M. Matched for age and puberty. Endocrine referrals	GH response in 8/9 SCZ vs 0/9 controls	(30) f
Naloxone 15 mg i.v.	C-SCZ (RDC)	6M; 3F 7M; 1F	13–97 days On NL	No data	Increase in GH in both pt groups. No consistent increase in controls	(38) f
5-HTP 0.2 g p.o.	SCZ (RDC)	2M; 2F	≥2 wk	3M; 1F	No GH increase in SCZ or controls	(2) f

Abbreviations (by column): Stimulus: Doses of apomorphine (Apo) expressed either as the base or salt. CLON, clonidine; AmpSO₄, amphetamine sulfate; Methyl-PD, methylphenidate; TRH, thyrotropin-releasing hormone; LHRH, luteinizing hormone-releasing hormone; 5-HTP, 5-hydroxytryptophan. Diagnosis (criteria): SCZ, schizophrenia; C-SCZ, chronic schizophrenia; A-SCZ, acute schizophrenia; Sub-A-SCZ, subacute schizophrenia; Sub-C-SCZ, subchronic schizophrenia; SCZ-Aff, schizo-affective; RDC, Research Diagnostic Criteria; FDC, Feighner Diagnostic Criteria; ICD, International Classification of Diseases; PSE, Present State Examination. Controls: Pts, patients; MMPI, Minnesota Multi-Phasic Personality Inventory. Results & comments: SWS, slow wave sleep; MAO, monoamine oxidase. Ref.: *Subjects specified as being nonobese; f, Experiments conducted in the fasting state.

et al. (109) had a normal GH response to insulin-induced hypoglycemia (IH) which shows that the GH secretory reserve was not deficient. In the one acute schizophrenic patient, sleep peaks were observed on both nights but none was associated with SWS. None of the studies mentioned whether subjects were matched for body build with controls. It is difficult to know whether NLs restored sleep GH secretion in the patients studied by Syvalahti and Pekkarinen (104).

DOPAMINERGIC REGULATION OF GH SECRETION

The DA hypothesis of SCZ (76,102) has led to considerable interest in DA regulation of GH secretion. High concentrations of DA are found in the ME. DA cells are located in the arcuate nucleus and periventricular nuclei (and to a lesser extent in other hypothalamic areas) and send fibers to the external zone of the ME (64). DA receptors have been identified in both ME and pituitary (20). DA infusion, L-dopa, bromocriptine, and Apo stimulate GH secretion in humans, and their effect is antagonized by DA receptor antagonists (45).

APOMORPHINE–INDUCED GH SECRETION

In Normal Subjects

Many clinical studies have used Apo, a DA receptor agonist in animals (103) and humans (40), as a stimulus of GH secretion (41,48). Apo does not increase GH secretion in the conscious rat (23) or monkey (14), so that animal studies on hypothalamic-pituitary DA function must be extrapolated to humans with caution. Apo binds to DA receptors in human brain (58). In human pituitary cell culture, Apo inhibits GH secretion (62), which suggests that the stimulatory effect of Apo is not at the level of the pituitary. Clinical studies point to an effect of Apo on DA receptors within the HPA which are not linked to adenylate cyclase (89) and which lie outside the blood-brain barrier (51), or at least in part (10). The GH response to Apo is not affected by 5-HT agents. The finding that diazepam antagonizes the response is compatible with GABA modulation, but other GABAergic agents, namely, baclofen and sodium valproate, are without effect (48). Atropine (13) and pirenzepine (21) but not benztropine (46) antagonize the GH response to Apo. This may indicate that the effect of Apo on GH requires intermediation of an Ach neuron. Whether GRF plays a role in the effect of Apo is unknown. The finding that CCK peptides also antagonize the GH response to Apo (50) emphasizes the difficulty in identifying specific NT derangements in SCZ by neuroendocrine techniques.

The GH response to Apo is significantly less in women than men (24). Many normal women may show little or no GH increase (49). Birth control pills and administration of estrogens to postmenopausal women increase the response (49). Adequate studies on the effect of phase of menstrual cycle on the GH response to Apo are not available, so that matching for gender without regard to phase of menstrual

cycle is unwise. There is some evidence that circulating testosterone levels are important variables (55). The Apo-GH response declines with age (49,60). In subjects 35 to 115% above ideal body weight the response is blunted (48). At what point deviation from ideal body weight is an important variable is unclear. The response is also blunted by a glucose load (24) and is diminished after sleep deprivation (48).

The GH response to Apo is not dependent on a stress effect (46). However, nausea is a frequent side effect, especially in young adults (60), and stress is known to increase GH secretion (96). Meltzer et al. (69) reported a 70% incidence of nausea and/or vomiting in their schizophrenic population. Cleghorn et al. (15) noted an exaggerated GH response in 6 of 20 tests in which the patient was nauseated. Ferrier et al. (26) implied that nausea and vomiting were not important variables in their studies but gave no statistical data. Unfortunately, cortisol levels are rarely monitored as part of the protocol in Apo studies. The prompt occurrence of peak GH concentrations (within 30–60 min of s.c. injection), the short duration of action, the reproducibility of response in the same subjects both over short intervals (87,97) and over a period of many months (17), and relative selectivity of action are advantages over other agents.

Changes in Schizophrenia

Several investigators have reported that acute schizophrenics have a significantly greater GH response to Apo than chronic schizophrenics (26,94), remitted schizophrenics (87), or controls (16,87,94). In the studies of Meltzer and co-workers (Table 2), patients ill for less than 4 years had significantly higher GH responses than those ill more than 4 years. Neither group, however, was significantly different from controls. In chronic patients a significantly blunted response has been described by at least 2 groups (25,26), whereas others have found no difference compared with controls (86,94,108). Rotrosen et al. (98) noted both blunted and exaggerated GH responses in patients who were descriptively acutely exacerbating chronic schizophrenics. The above findings are suggestive of increased DA receptor sensitivity in acutely ill patients and blunted DA receptor function in some chronic patients. In keeping with this, patients with Schneider's First Rank Symptoms have significantly greater GH responses than psychotic patients without Schneider's First Rank Symptoms (113) or controls. Also, in longitudinal studies, Cleghorn and associates (Table 2) have shown that exaggerated GH responses (above the 99% confidence limits of controls) are often associated with relapse, as indicated by significant changes on the scale of Krawiecka and Goldberg, which measures positive symptoms in SCZ (17). Relapses were less likely to occur if the GH response was blunted or normal. Also, Meltzer et al. (74) noted a significant positive correlation between GH response and psychosis rating on the Schedule for Affective Disorders and Schizophrenia. Further, Ferrier et al. (26) found a significant negative correlation between GH increment and negative symptoms of schizophrenia. This inverse relationship was also seen in the chronic patient group alone. In contrast, Meltzer et al. (74) found a positive correlation with negative symptoms.

Whether changes in GH response are related to SCZ or to NL therapy, however, is not certain. In the study of Ettigi et al. (25) in chronically hospitalized patients, the blunted GH responses were interpreted as being a consequence of NL therapy rather than of psychosis. Friend et al. (29) reported that chronic treatment with haloperidol in the rat decreases Apo binding in the pituitary but increases Apo binding in the striatum. Unfortunately, data for the hypothalamus were not available. Autopsy data on DA receptors in the HPA of schizophrenics are not available. Rotrosen et al. (97,99), working with a transient hospital population, noted that subjects with sporadic or little NL use tended to have exaggerated GH responses to Apo whereas those on chronic high-dosage NLs had blunted responses. Unfortunately, the patients received chloral hydrate or paraldehyde for sedation, and the effect of these agents on Apo-GH secretion is unknown. Muller-Spahn et al. (86) found no relationship between GH response to Apo and duration of NL therapy or duration of illness. Meltzer et al. (74) found a significant negative correlation between duration of illness and Apo-GH response. However, this correlation disappeared when data were corrected for age. Whether there was any correlation with duration of NL therapy was unstated. Three of five chronic patients in the study of Ferrier et al. (26) who had never been treated with NLs had GH responses well below controls. The authors argued that the blunting could not be due to prior NL treatment but was related to negative symptoms, which in turn might reflect the presence of hypothalamic damage. This would be in keeping with ideas on Crow type II schizophrenia. Unfortunately, there were striking differences in age between the chronic patients on the one hand and acute patients and controls on the other (Table 2). In the study of Pandey et al. (94), age differences may also have been a confounding variable. The mean age of 7 of 15 of their chronic patients was more than double that of the acute patients; the controls were a mean of 8.4 years older than the acute patients. In the study of Whalley et al. (113) gender differences may have accounted for their findings. In the longitudinal study of Cleghorn and associates, in addition to exaggerated responses, some subjects had blunted responses associated with relapse. In the two patients who relapsed within 24 hr after Apo testing, Ettigi et al. (25) found blunted GH peaks in both subjects (3.0 and 4.0 ng/ml). Recently, Brown and Cleghorn (9) have completed studies on 13 schizophrenics for periods up to 22 months. No difference in GH responses between patients and controls was found. However, exacerbation of positive symptoms of SCZ was positively and significantly correlated with a heightened GH response in some patients. In others there was a significant inverse relationship between symptom scores and GH peak. An effect of season was also noted; the GH response in patients was lower in winter than in summer, whereas the opposite was true for the normals.

In initial studies, Rotrosen et al. (98,99) found that subjects who had an unusually high GH response to Apo subsequently failed to respond to NLs, whereas those with a low response responded to NLs. This was not confirmed (97). Meltzer et al. (69,71) found that the GH response to Apo was a weak predictor of short-term response to NL therapy. All the patients in the study of Tamminga et al. (108) were nonresponders to NL, which points to the absence of a relationship between magnitude of Apo-GH response and response to NL therapy for many patients.

Patients maintained on chronic NL treatment continue to show an antagonism to Apo (39,86). It is unclear in the study of Kolakowska et al. (39) whether the GH increase noted in a few subjects was related to Apo or to spontaneous release, as placebo was not given and peaks of some of the subjects were delayed. There was no relation between therapeutic outcome and GH response under NL treatment.

Hirschowitz et al. (32) have used the GH response to identify lithium responders. Six of 31 patients responded to lithium; all had GH responses exceeding 20 ng/ml. In contrast, only 7 out of the 25 non-lithium responders had GH peaks above 20 ng/ml. Unfortunately, selection criteria for the study excluded subjects who were nonresponders to Apo so prediction of lithium response may be of less value than hoped for. Attempts have been made to correlate GH response to Apo to a vulnerability factor for psychopathology, namely, platelet monoamine oxidase (MAO) activity. Results are conflicting. One possible reason for the discrepancy may be that 26 of the 40 patients investigated by Hitzemann et al. (33) belonged to the paranoid subtype, in contrast to only 1 of 10 of the patients examined by Malas et al. (61).

Patients with tardive dyskinesia have shown either a decreased GH response to Apo (25) or no difference (86,94,108). This consistent finding of a lack of an enhanced response suggests that there is no DA receptor supersensitivity in the HPA in tardive dyskinesia.

ANTIDOPAMINERGIC AGENTS, GH SECRETION, AND SCHIZOPHRENIA

Clinical studies with Apo provide suggestive evidence that DA function in the HPA may reflect DA function in brain regions relevant to SCZ. Chlorpromazine (42), pimozide (44), haloperidol (97), and the atypical NLs sulpiride (89) and clozapine (88) block the GH response to Apo. In contrast to other NLs, clozapine has little or no effect on prolactin (PRL) secretion and has little ability to induce parkinsonism or tardive dyskinesia. The failure to increase PRL cannot be accounted for by the intrinsic anticholinergic properties of clozapine. These observations—together with the findings that (a) Apo can increase GH in a dose that has no effect on PRL; (b) (+)-sulpiride and (−)-sulpiride increase PRL but only (−)-sulpiride antagonizes Apo-GH secretion in humans (53); (c) electroconvulsive therapy improves parkinsonism and enhances the PRL lowering effect of Apo but has no effect on Apo-GH secretion—suggest that DA receptors relevant to the antipsychotic site of NL action and the GH response to Apo, on the one hand, are pharmacologically different from DA receptors mediating extrapyramidal function and regulating PRL secretion, on the other (48,52). A dissociation in effect of drugs on Apo-GH secretion and basal PRL secretion may provide a clinical approach for screening for novel NLs which are devoid of extrapyramidal complications and which do not cause hyperprolactinemia. The location of the DA receptor mediating the GH response to Apo permits evaluation of the modulatory role of peptides and other compounds that may not cross the blood-brain barrier on central DA function in humans (50).

L-DOPA-INDUCED GH SECRETION

In Normal Subjects

L-Dopa, a precursor of DA and NE, increases the formation of both DA and NE and decreases the turnover of 5-HT. The mechanism of increase in GH secretion in humans is less well defined than with Apo. Rotrosen et al. (98) observed an inverse relation between the GH response produced by L-dopa and the GH response induced by Apo, which suggests that a mechanism other than DA may be involved. Both α-adrenergic and DA blockers as well as GABAergic agents antagonize the GH response to L-dopa (45,48). The failure of some investigators to observe an inhibitory effect of NLs can be attributed to problems in experimental design (47). The response is antagonized by pyridoxine (83) and diminished in the obese, in women, after glucose loading (48), and possibly by glucocorticoids. The GH response is much more variable in terms of the number of subjects who show an adequate GH response and in the time of onset of the peak compared with Apo (46). This, together with its lack of selectivity of action, makes L-dopa studies difficult to interpret.

Changes in Schizophrenia

The relationship of GH response, therapeutic response to NLs, and HLA antigen status found by Brambilla et al. (7) is of interest, but their findings were not statistically significant. Data obtained on psychopathological rating scales were not given. It is unclear why similar differences (or trends) between the two patient groups were not observed following initial withdrawal from NLs prior to haloperidol treatment.

AMPHETAMINE AND METHYLPHENIDATE-INDUCED GH SECRETION

In Normal Subjects

Amphetamine (19) and methylphenidate (27) increase DA and NE function. Few data are available on the pharmacology of the GH response to these agents. In the monkey, pimozide has no inhibitory effect on the GH response to amphetamine (100). Whether this implies that DA is not involved in the amphetamine-GH response in humans is unclear because of possible species differences. Langer et al. (57) observed a significant negative correlation between smoking habits and peak GH response to amphetamine. Smoking habits are seldom mentioned in clinical studies. The effect of smoking on the GH response to Apo is unknown. Patients with reactive depression have a significantly greater amphetamine-GH response than controls (57). This latter observation emphasizes the importance of careful screening of normal controls for GH studies. Inves-

tigators rarely report on methods used to select and screen normal volunteers.

Changes in Schizophrenia

There is no change in GH response to amphetamine in SCZ (57) (Table 2). Janowsky et al. (36) found a blunted GH response following methylphenidate. Unfortunately, in the latter study the patients were not well matched with suitable controls. The GH response does not show a relationship to exacerbation of schizophrenic symptoms following methylphenidate challenge (59). In patients with tardive dyskinesia the GH response to methylphenidate is decreased (59).

CLONIDINE-INDUCED GH SECRETION

In Normal Subjects

Much of the evidence supporting a role for DA in SCZ is also compatible with an alteration in NE function (54). Clonidine (CLON), an α-adrenergic agent, stimulates GH secretion in humans (56). This has led to the use of this response to evaluate α-adrenergic function in SCZ. There is good evidence in animal studies that CLON stimulates GH secretion via GRF (81) by stimulating hypothalamic (34) α_2 postsynaptic receptors (67). The mechanism involved in humans is less well established. The failure of NE to stimulate GH secretion in human pituitary monolayer cultures (107) suggests a hypothalamic site of action for CLON, which is known to bind to α_2-receptors in this region of human brain (110). The recent finding that anticholinergic agents antagonize the effect of CLON (13,21) suggests the intermediary role of a cholinergic neuron in CLON-induced GH secretion. Smoking (18) enhances the response and regular drinking of more than one liter of beer a day induces an inhibition that persists following abstinence for several weeks (65). An effect of age has been noted after oral (31) but not after i.v. administration (85). The response is decreased in postmenopausal women (66) and in women compared to men (43). The influence of phase of the menstrual cycle is unclear (65). A paradoxical decrease follows CLON administration to subjects with elevated baseline GH concentrations (111). The use of CLON as a probe of α_2-adrenergic function requires that it be a reliable stimulus of GH secretion in normals. In a review of eight studies, Lal and Guyda (43) noted that 29 of 115 normal subjects and 9 of 22 patients with a depressive neurosis had an impaired response (peak or increment <5 ng/ml).

Changes in Schizophrenia

In all three studies in SCZ (Table 2), GH responses have shown great variability. In the study of Matussek et al. (66) schizo-affective patients had significantly lower responses than schizophrenics. High GH responses tended to occur in some schizophrenics, particularly those of the paranoid type. In chronic schizophrenia no difference (54) or a diminished response has been found (85). Neither study (54,85) found a relationship between GH response and duration of illness or duration of NL treatment.

INSULIN-INDUCED GH SECRETION

In Normal Subjects

In patients with a pituitary stalk section the GH response to IH is blocked, which points to a hypothalamic site of action (45). The response is antagonized by α-blockers. Serotonergic as well as cholinergic mechanisms (78) have been implicated in the effect of IH; DA does not seem to be involved (90). In 4 of 13 studies, reviewed neuroleptics blunted the GH response to IH, whereas the remainder showed no effect (47). The response is decreased in obesity (96). Women have a greater GH response than men, but the gender difference depends on the phase of the menstrual cycle and magnitude of the hypoglycemia (80).

Changes in Schizophrenia

Beg et al. (3) found no difference in GH response to IH, and the decrease observed by Schimmelbusch et al. (101) in backward schizophrenic patients was related to a significantly lower hypoglycemic response, which in turn was related to the duration of hospitalization. Brambilla and associates (6,8) found that whereas paranoid patients had fairly stable responses to IH, the responses were much more variable in hebephrenics and seemed to depend on clinical state. The response was blunted in patients who were withdrawn from reality, apathetic, and negativistic, but hyperresponsive when the patient showed psychomotor excitement and hostility. Thus, the state of arousal appeared to influence the endocrine response. The authors suggested that onset of illness in puberty was a significant factor in the hypothalamic-pituitary dysfunction, as hebephrenics have an earlier onset of illness than paranoids. Patients were evaluated with rating scales, but no scores or statistical analysis of behavioral observations were given.

TRH AND LHRH-INDUCED GH SECRETION

In Normal Subjects

An interaction between TRH and catecholamines in GH regulation has been described in sheep pituitary *in vitro* (105). In normal subjects neither TRH nor LHRH induces GH secretion. Increases after TRH, however, have been described in endogenous depression, anorexia nervosa, and in a variety of medical conditions, including a very high percentage of cancer patients (37). Aberrant GH responses to LHRH have been less commonly observed.

Changes in Schizophrenia

TRH increases GH secretion in a number of adolescent schizophrenics but is rare in adults (Table 2). This again suggests that age of onset might be an important factor in the development of abnormalities in hypothalamic-pituitary function in SCZ. The GH response in adolescent patients was associated with a family history of SCZ. A GH increase was also noted with LHRH (30). In the study of Gil-Ad et al. (30) the reason for referral for endocrine evaluation in the control subjects was not stated. Also, criteria for matching on pubertal development were not specified. In none of the three studies in adolescents was placebo TRH (or placebo LHRH) given, so that it is unclear whether the GH peaks were spontaneous peaks or the consequence of TRH administration. It is unlikely that NLs affected the TRH-GH response, as administration of NLs for 3 months had no effect on the GH response but blunted the LHRH-GH response (30). The wide range of conditions in which an abnormal GH response to TRH is found suggests a nonspecific factor as being responsible for the alterations in HPA responsiveness in adolescent SCZ.

MISCELLANEOUS AGENTS AND GH SECRETION IN SCHIZOPHRENIA

Electroconvulsive therapy (ECT) stimulates GH secretion. α-Adrenergic mechanisms appear important in this action (45). Takahashi et al. (106) observed an increase in GH in five of six schizophrenics after ECT; the exception was an obese individual.

SUMMARY AND CONCLUSIONS

The assumption underlying GH studies in SCZ is that changes in hypothalamic-pituitary NT function may reflect NT changes in extrahypothalamic regions of brain, which may be relevant to the pathophysiology of SCZ and mode of action of antischizophrenic drugs. Interpretation of results is difficult because of the confounding effects of prior NL treatment, heterogeneity of SCZ, the complex series of events that occur in the application of a stimulus and the subsequent change in circulating GH, and the many physiological variables that influence GH secretion. Failure to control for the latter has marred several published investigations. The following trends emerge: (a) impaired SWS-GH secretion in SCZ; (b) enhanced GH response to the DA receptor agonist Apo in some acutely ill patients and a blunted or normal response in chronically ill subjects; (c) aberrant GH responses to TRH and LHRH in adolescents with SCZ; (d) absence of DA receptor supersensitivity in the HPA in tardive dyskinesia. Further studies using a longitudinal approach in carefully characterized patients and well-selected controls, also followed longitudinally, are required.

REFERENCES

1. Abrams, R. L., Grumbach, M. M., and Kaplan, S. L. (1971): *J. Clin. Invest.*, 50:940–950.
2. Ansseau, M., Doumont, A., Thiry, D., Geenen, V., and Legros, J. J. (1983): *Acta Psychiatr. Belg.*, 83:50–56.
3. Beg, A. A., Varma, V. A., and Dash, R. J. (1979): *Am. J. Psychiatr.*, 136:914–917.
4. Bloch, B., Gaillard, R. C., Brazeau, P., Lin, H. D., and Ling, N. (1984): *Regul. Pept.*, 8:21–31.

5. Braddock, L. E., and Blake, I. M. (1981): *Br. J. Psychiatr.*, 139:404–407.
6. Brambilla, F. (1980): *Acta Psychiatr. Belg.*, 80:421–435.
7. Brambilla, F., Bellodi, L., Negri, F., Smeraldi, E., and Malagoli, G. (1979): *Psychoneuroendocrinology*, 4:329–339.
8. Brambilla, F., Guerrini, A., Rovere, C., Guastalla, A., Riggi, F., and Recchia, M. (1975): *Neuropsychobiology*, 1:267–276.
9. Brown, G. M., and Cleghorn, J. M. (1985): 8th Annual Meeting, Canadian College Neuropsychopharmacol., London, Ontario, May 6–8.
10. Brown, G. M., Verhaegan, H., Van Wimersma Greidanus, T. B., and Brugmans, J. (1981): *Clin. Endocrinol.*, 15:275–282.
11. Brownstein, M. (1977): *Fed. Proc.*, 36:960–963.
12. Bugnon, C., Fellmann, D., and Bloch, B. (1977): *Cell Tissue Res.*, 183:319–328.
13. Casenueva, F. F., Villanueva, L., Cabranes, J. A., Cavezas-Cerrato, J., and Fernandez-Cruz, A. (1984): *J. Clin. Endocrinol. Metab.*, 59:526–530.
14. Chambers, J. W., and Brown, G. M. (1976): *Endocrinology*, 98:420–428.
15. Cleghorn, J. M., Brown, G. M., Brown, P. J., Kaplan, R. D., Dermer, S. W., MacCrimmon, D. J., and Mitton, J. (1983): *Br. J. Psychiatr.*, 142:482–488.
16. Cleghorn, J. M., Brown, G. M., Brown, P. J., Kaplan, R. D., and Mitton, J. (1983): *Biol. Psychiatry*, 18:875–885.
17. Cleghorn, J. M., Brown, G. M., Brown, P. J., Kaplan, R. D., and Mitton, J. (1983): *Prog. Neuropsychopharmacol. Biol. Psychiatry*, 7:545–549.
18. Coiro, V., d'Amato, L., Borciani, E., Rossi, G., Camellini, L., Maffei, M. L., Pignatti, D., and Chiodera, P. (1984): *Br. J. Clin. Pharmacol.*, 18:802–805.
19. Costa, E., Groppetti, A., and Naimzada, M. K. (1972): *Br. J. Pharmacol.*, 44:742–751.
20. Cronin, M. J., and Weiner, R. I. (1979): *Endocrinology*, 104:307–312.
21. Delitala, G., Maioli, M., Pacifico, A., Branda, S., Palermo, M., and Mannelli, M. (1983): *J. Clin. Endocrinol. Metab.*, 57:1145–1149.
22. DeMilio, L. (1984): *Br. J. Psychiatr.*, 145:649–651.
23. Durand, D., Martin, J. B., and Brazeau, P. (1977): *Endocrinology*, 100:722–728.
24. Ettigi, P., Lal, S., Martin, J. B., and Friesen, H. G. (1975): *J. Clin. Endocrinol. Metab.*, 40:1094–1098.
25. Ettigi, P., Nair, N. P. V., Lal, S., Cervantes, P., and Guyda, H. (1976): *J. Neurol. Neurosurg. Psychiatry*, 39:870–876.
26. Ferrier, I. N., Johnstone, E., and Crowe, T. J. (1984): *Br. J. Psychiatr.*, 144:349–357.
27. Ferris, R. M., Tang, F. L. M., and Maxwell, R. A. (1972): *J. Pharmacol. Exp. Ther.*, 181:407–416.
28. Finkelstein, J. W., Roffwarg, H. P., Boyar, R. M., Kream, J., and Hellman, L. (1972): *J. Clin. Endocrinol. Metab.*, 75:665–670.
29. Friend, W. C., Brown, G. M., Jawahie, G., Lee, T., and Seeman, P. (1978): *Am. J. Psychiatr.*, 135:839–841.
30. Gil-Ad, I., Dickerman, Z., Weizman, R., Weizman, A., Tyano, S., and Laron, Z. (1981): *Am. J. Psychiatr.*, 138:357–360.
31. Gil-Ad, I., Gurewitz, R., Marcovici, O., Rosenfeld, J., and Laron, Z. (1984): *Mech. Ageing Dev.*, 27:97–100.
32. Hirschowitz, J., Zemlan, F. P., and Garver, D. L. (1982): *Am. J. Psychiatr.*, 139:646–649.
33. Hitzemann, R., Hirschowitz, J., Zemlan, F., Hitzemann, B., and Garver, D. (1983): *Biol. Psychiatry*, 18:1503–1507.
34. Ishikawa, K., Suzuki, M., and Kakegawa, T. (1983): *Endocrinol. Jpn.*, 30:397–403.
35. Isidori, A., Fraioli, F., Rotolo, A., Piro, C., Conte, D., Muratorio, A., Murri, L., and Cerone, G. (1976): *Chronobiologia*, 3:39–50.
36. Janowsky, D. S., Leichner, P., Parker, D., Judd, L. L., Huey, L., and Clopton, P. (1978): *Arch. Gen. Psychiatry*, 35:1384–1389.
37. Kamijo, K., Saito, A., Kato, T., Kawasaki, K., Yachi, A., and Wada, T. (1983): *Endocrinol. Jpn.*, 30:777–782.
38. Kleinman, J. E., Weinberger, D. R., Rogol, A., Shiling, D. J., Mendelson, W. B., Davis, G. C., Bunney, W. E., and Wyatt, R. J. (1982): *Psychiatr. Res.*, 7:1–7.
39. Kolakowska, T., Gelder, M., and Fraser, S. (1981): *Br. J. Psychiatr.*, 139:408–412.
40. Lal, S. (1981): In: *Clinical Pharmacology of Apomorphine and Other Dopaminomimetics, Vol. 2*, edited by G. U. Corsini and G. L. Gessa, pp. 1–11. Raven Press, New York.
41. Lal, S., de la Vega, C. E., Sourkes, T. L., and Friesen, H. G. (1972): *Lancet*, 2:661.
42. Lal, S., de la Vega, C. E., Sourkes, T. L., and Friesen, H. G. (1973): *J. Clin. Endocrinol. Metab.*, 37:719–724.
43. Lal, S., and Guyda, H. (1987): Proc. IVth World Cong. Biol. Psychiatry, Philadelphia, Sept. 8–13 (*in press*).
44. Lal, S., Guyda, H., and Bikadoroff, S. (1977): *J. Clin. Endocrinol. Metab.*, 44:766–770.
45. Lal, S., and Martin, J. B. (1980): In: *Handbook of Biological Psychiatry, Vol. 3*, edited by H. M. Van Praag, M. H. Lader, O. J. Rafaelsen, and E. J. Sachar, pp. 101–167. Marcel Dekker, New York.
46. Lal, S., Martin, J. B., de la Vega, C. E., and Friesen, H. G. (1975): *Clin. Endocrinol.*, 4:277–285.
47. Lal, S., and Nair, N. P. V. (1980): *Dev. Endocrinol.*, 9:223–241.
48. Lal, S., and Nair, N. P. V. (1984): In: *Psychoneuroendocrine Dysfunction*, edited by N. S. Shah and A. G. Donald, pp. 485–501. Plenum Publishing Corp., New York.
49. Lal, S., Nair, N. P. V., Cervantes, P., and Guyda, H. (1980): In: *Progress in Psychoneuroendocrinology*, edited by F. Brambilla, G. Racagni, and D. deWied, pp. 295–307. Elsevier, Amsterdam.
50. Lal, S., Nair, N. P. V., Eugenio, H., Thavundayil, J., Lizondo, E., Wood, P. L., Etienne, P., and Guyda, H. (1983): *Prog. Neuropsychopharmacol. Biol. Psychiatry*, 7:537–544.
51. Lal, S., Nair, N. P. V., Iskandar, H. I., Etienne, P., Wood, P. L., Schwartz, G., and Guyda, H. (1982): *J. Neural. Transm.*, 54:75–84.
52. Lal, S., Nair, N. P. V., Iskandar, H. I., Thavundayil, J. X., Etienne, P., Wood, P. L., and Guyda, H. (1982): *Prog. Neuropsychopharmacol. Biol. Psychiatry*, 6:631–637.
53. Lal, S., Nair, N. P. V., Thavundayil, J. X., Eugenio, H., and Guyda, H. (1984): XV Int. Soc. Psychoneuroendocrinol., Vienna, July 15–19, Abstract p. 106.
54. Lal, S., Nair, N. P. V., Thavundayil, J. X., Monks, R. C., and Guyda, H. (1983): *Acta Psychiatr. Scand.*, 68:82–88.
55. Lal, S., Oravec, M., Aronoff, A., Kiely, M. E., Guyda, H., Solomon, S., and Nair, N. P. V. (1981): *J. Neural. Transm.*, 53:7–21.
56. Lal, S., Tolis, G., Martin, J. B., Brown, G. M., and Guyda, H. (1975): *J. Clin. Endocrinol. Metab.*, 41:827–832.
57. Langer, G., Heinze, G., Reim, B., and Matussek, N. (1976): *Arch. Gen. Psychiatry*, 33:1471–1475.
58. Lee, T., Seeman, P., Tourtellotte, W. W., Farley, I. J., and Hornykiewicz, O. (1978): *Nature*, 274:897–898.
59. Lieberman, J. A., Kane, J. M., Gadaletta, D., Ramos-Lorenzi, J., Bergmann, K., Wegner, J., and Novacenko, H. (1985): *Psychopharmacol. Bull.*, 21:123–129.
60. Maany, I., Frazer, A., and Mendels, J. (1975): *J. Clin. Endocrinol. Metab.*, 40:162–163.
61. Malas, K. L., van Kammen, D. P., De Fraites, E. A., Brown, G. M., and Gold, P. W. (1983): *Biol. Psychiatr.*, 18:255–259.
62. Marcowitz, S., Goodyer, C. G., Guyda, H., Gardiner, R. J., and Hardy, J. (1982): *J. Clin. Endocrinol. Metab.*, 54:6–16.
63. Martin, J. B. (1976): In: *Frontiers in Neuroendocrinology*, edited by L. Martini and W. F. Ganong, pp. 129–168. Raven Press, New York.
64. Martin, J. B. (1983): *Pediatr. Adolesc. Endocrinol.*, 12:1–26.
65. Matussek, N., Ackenheil, M., and Herz, M. (1984): *Psychoneuroendocrinology*, 9:173–177.
66. Matussek, N., Ackenheil, M., Hippius, H., Muller, M., Schroder, H. P., Schultes, H., and Wasilewski, B. (1980): *Psychiatr. Res.*, 2:25–36.
67. McWilliam, J. R., and Meldrum, B. S. (1983): *Endocrinology*, 112:234–239.
68. Meistas, M., Foster, G. V., Margolis, S., and Kowarski, A. A. (1982): *Metabolism*, 31:1224–1228.
69. Meltzer, H. Y., Busch, D., and Fang, V. S. (1981): *Psychoneuroendocrinology*, 6:17–36.
70. Meltzer, H. Y., Busch, D., and Fang, V. S. (1984): In: *Neuroendocrinology and Psychiatric Disorders*, edited by G. M. Brown, S. Reichlin, and S. Koslow, pp. 1–28. Raven Press, New York.

71. Meltzer, H. Y., Busch, D., So, R., Holcomb, H., and Fang, V. S. (1980): In: *Perspectives in Schizophrenia Research,* edited by C. Baxter and T. Melnechuk, pp. 149–176. Raven Press, New York.

72. Meltzer, H. Y., Goode, D. J., and Fang, V. S. (1978): In: *Psychopharmacology: A Generation of Progress,* edited by M. A. Lipton, A. Damascio, and K. F. Killam, pp. 509–530. Raven Press, New York.

73. Meltzer, H. Y., Goode, D. J., Fang, V. S., Schyve, P., and Young, M. (1976): *Lancet,* 2:1142.

74. Meltzer, H. Y., Koladowska, T., Fang, V. S., Fogg, L., Robertson, A., Lewine, R., Strahilevitz, M., and Busch, D. (1984): *Arch. Gen. Psychiatry,* 41:512–519.

75. Meltzer, H. Y., Perline, R., and Lewine, R. (1982): *J. Nerv. Ment. Dis.,* 170:758–765.

76. Meltzer, H. Y., and Stahl, S. M. (1976): *Schizophr. Bull.,* 2:19–76.

77. Mendelson, W. B., Jacobs, L. S., and Gillin, J. C. (1983): *J. Clin. Endocrinol. Metab.,* 56:486–488.

78. Mendelson, W. B., Lantinuga, R. A., Wyatt, R. J., Gillin, J. C., and Jacobs, L. S. (1981): *J. Clin. Endocrinol. Metab.,* 52:409–415.

79. Mendlewicz, J., Linkowski, T., Kerkhofs, N., Desmedt, D., Golstein, J., Copinschi, G., and Van Cauter, E. (1985): *J. Clin. Endocrinol. Metab.,* 60:505–512.

80. Merimee, T. J., and Fineberg, S. E. (1971): *J. Clin. Endocrinol. Metab.,* 33:896–902.

81. Miki, N., Ono, M., and Shizume, K. (1984): *Endocrinology,* 114:1950–1952.

82. Miller, J. D., Tannenbaum, G. S., Colle, E., and Guyda, H. J. (1982): *J. Clin. Endocrinol. Metab.,* 55:989–994.

83. Mims, R. B., Scott, C. L., Modebe, O., and Bethune, J. E. (1975): *J. Clin. Endocrinol. Metab.,* 40:256–259.

84. Motson, R. W., Glass, D. N., South, D. A., and Daly, J. R. (1978): *Clin. Endocrinol.,* 55:989–994.

85. Muller-Spahn, F., Ackenheil, M., Albus, M., Botschew, C., Naber, D., and Welter, D. (1986): *Psychopharmacology,* 88:190–195.

86. Muller-Spahn, F., Ackenheil, M., Albus, M., May, G., Naber, D., Welter, D., and Zander, K. (1984): *Psychopharmacology,* 84:436–440.

87. Muller-Spahn, F., Ackenheil, M., Bondy, B., May, G., and Ruther, E. (1987): Proc. IV World Cong. Biol. Psychiatry, Philadelphia, Sept. 8–13 (*in press*).

88. Nair, N. P. V., Lal, S., Cervantes, P., Yassa, R., and Guyda, H. (1979): *Neuropsychobiology,* 5:136–142.

89. Nair, N. P. V., Lal, S., Iskandar, H. I., Etienne, P., Wood, P. L., and Guyda, H. (1982): *Brain Res. Bull.,* 8:587–591.

90. Nathan, R. S., Sachar, E. J., Ostrow, L., Asnis, G. M., Halbreich, U., and Halpern, P. S. (1981): *J. Clin. Endocrinol. Metab.,* 52:807–809.

91. Othmer, E., Levine, W. R., Malarkey, W. B., Corvalan, J. C., Hayden-Otto, M. P., Fishman, P. M., and Daughaday, W. H. (1974): *Horm. Res.,* 5:156–166.

92. Othmer, E., Mendelson, W. B., Levine, W. R., Malarkey, W. B., and Daughaday, W. H. (1974): *Steroid Lipid Res.,* 5:380–386.

93. Pallotta, J. A., and Kennedy, P. J. (1968): *Metabolism,* 17:901–908.

94. Pandey, G. N., Garver, D. L., Taminga, C., Ericksen, S., Ali, S. I., and Davis, J. M. (1977): *Am. J. Psychiatr.,* 134:518–522.

95. Prange, A. J., Loosen, P. T., Wilson, I. C., Meltzer, H. Y., and Fang, V. S. (1979): *Arch. Gen. Psychiatry,* 36:1086–1093.

96. Reichlin, S. (1974): In: *Handbook of Physiology, Vol. IV, Sect. 7, Part 2,* edited by E. Knobil and W. H. Sawyer, pp. 405–447. Williams and Wilkins, Baltimore.

97. Rotrosen, J., Angrist, B., Gershon, S., Paquin, J., Branchey, L., Oleshansky, M., Halpern, F., and Sachar, E. J. (1979): *Br. J. Psychiatr.,* 135:444–456.

98. Rotrosen, J., Angrist, B. M., Gershon, S., Sachar, E. J., and Halpern, F. (1976): *Psychopharmacology,* 51:1–7.

99. Rotrosen, J., Angrist, B. M., Paquin, J., Halpern, F. S., and Sachar, E. J. (1978): *Psychopharmacol. Bull.,* 14:14–17.

100. Sachar, E. J., Gruen, P. H., Altman, N., Halpern, F. S., and Frantz, A. G. (1976): In: *Hormones, Behavior and Psychopathology,* edited by E. J. Sachar, pp. 161–175. Raven Press, New York.

101. Schimmelbusch, W. H., Mueller, P. S., and Sheps, J. (1971): *Br. J. Psychiatr.,* 118:429–436.

102. Seeman, P., Ulpian, C., Bergeron, C., Riederer, P., Jellinger, K., Gabriel, E., Reynolds, G. P., and Tourtellotte, W. W. (1984): *Science,* 225:728–773.

103. Sourkes, T. L., and Lal, S. (1975): *Adv. Neurochem.,* 1:247–299.

104. Syvalahti, E., and Pekkarinen, A. (1977): *J. Neural. Transm.,* 40:221–226.

105. Takahara, J., Arimura, A., and Schally, A. V. (1974): *Endocrinology,* 95:1490–1494.

106. Takahashi, K., Takahashi, S., Honda, Y., Shizume, K., Irie, M., Sakuma, M., and Tsushima, T. (1967): *Folia Psychiatr. Neurol. Jpn.,* 21:87–105.

107. Tallo, D., and Malarkey, W. B. (1981): *J. Clin. Endocrinol. Metab.,* 53:1278–1284.

108. Tamminga, C. A., Smith, R. C., Pandey, G., Frohman, L. A., and Davis, J. M. (1977): *Arch. Gen. Psychiatry,* 34:1199–1203.

109. Vigneri, R., Pezzino, V., Squatrito, S., Calandra, A., and Maricchiolo, M. (1974): *Neuroendocrinology,* 14:356–361.

110. Weinreich, P., and Seeman, P. (1981): *Biochem. Pharmacol.,* 30:3115–3120.

111. Weizman, A., Gil-Ad, I., Weizman, R., Hering, R., Bechar, M., Tyano, S., and Laron, Z. (1984): *Neuropsychobiology,* 12:106–111.

112. Weizman, R., Weizman, A., Gil-Ad, I., Tyano, S., and Laron, Z. (1982): *Br. J. Psychiatr.,* 141:582–585.

113. Whalley, A. J., Christie, J. E., Brown, S., and Arbuthnott, G. W. (1984): *Arch. Gen. Psychiatry,* 41:1040–1043.

114. Wislocki, G. B., and King, L. S. (1936): *Am. J. Anat.,* 58:421–472.

115. Zadick, Z., Chalew, S. A., McCarter, R. J., Meistas, M., and Kowarski, A. A. (1985): *J. Clin. Endocrinol. Metab.,* 60:513–516.

116. Zemlan, F. P., Hirschowitz, J., and Garver, D. L. (1984): *Psychiatr. Res.,* 11:317–328.

Psychopharmacology:
The Third Generation of Progress,
edited by Herbert Y. Meltzer.
Raven Press, New York © 1987.

CHAPTER 81

The Role of Drugs in the Production of Schizophreniform Psychoses and Related Disorders

Malcolm B. Bowers, Jr.

The notion that pharmacological substances can be a significant factor in the production of psychotic disorders is not a new one. J. J. Moreau, in 1845, asserted that "several natural substances" can affect the brain and lead to the production of "a well-defined mental illness, usually transitory but sometimes lengthy or even permanent" (45). It would be difficult to find a more succinct statement of our knowledge in this field even today.

Whereas a number of chemical substances can produce psychotic ideation in a grossly altered sensorium, relatively few are capable of causing such symptoms in the absence of delirium. In this regard, the classification of hallucinogenic drugs proposed by Brawley and Duffield is illustrative, and I will use some of their concepts in this review (15). Their classification is based primarily on differences in symptoms and signs following acute drug administration. For example, their class 1 includes all drugs which at relatively high doses induce toxic or metabolic disturbances, that is, organic brain syndromes accompanied by psychosis. Class 2 refers to drugs that possess potent anticholinergic properties and are capable of producing a specific delirium, the central anticholinergic syndrome. Class 3 includes substances known to produce varying degrees of a generic "psychotomimetic syndrome," usually without clouding of consciousness or delirium. This syndrome is characterized by Brawley and Duffield as including physiological evidence of increased sympathetic tone, sensory and perceptual changes, and marked alterations in mood and thinking. The substances listed in this class are lysergic acid diethylamide (LSD), the phenethylamines such as mescaline, and the indolealkyl-amines, such as psilocybin. Phencyclidine is questionably included in their class 2 (atropinic deliriants), and separate categories are proposed for cannabis compounds and the amphetamines. Therapeutic drugs that may produce psychotic disorder in a clear sensorium, including the antidepressants and L-dihydroxyphenylalanine (L-dopa), are not classified. The steroids are misplaced, in my view, in class 1.

By contrast, the criterion I will use in the present discussion requires that the drug be associated, following single or repeated use, with the occurrence of psychotic disorders whose phenomenology and clinical course may be indistinguishable from the spectrum of psychotic disorders not associated with drug use. Primary emphasis will thus be placed on those drugs which can trigger a prolonged psychotic reaction in a vulnerable individual that may persist even after the drug is no longer being used. The drugs I will include are cannabis, mescaline, LSD, amphetamine, phenylcyclidine (PCP), and certain prescribed drugs, including steroids, antidepressants, and L-dopa. [Cocaine is not included in this group, perhaps somewhat arbitrarily. It is certain that psychotic ideation may occur in individuals who are under the influence of cocaine (49,61). It is less clear that cocaine use can trigger a psychosis that persists after cessation of cocaine use.] The principal criterion proposed here is in keeping with what I believe has been a shift in thinking over the past 25 years with respect to the psychotogenic significance of these substances. In the late 1950s and early 1960s experience with some of these drugs led to proposals for drug models of mental illness and to hypotheses concerned with possible endogenous synthesis of psychotogenic compounds; more recently there has been recognition that actual use of these drugs by certain vulnerable individuals can lead to bona fide mental illness. Compounds that were thought to mimic or provide a model for psychotic disorders (psychotomimetic) are now generally recognized to be capable of producing psychotic disorders in some instances and of promoting relapse in individuals who have previously had psychotic episodes (psychotogenic).

PSYCHOTOGENIC DRUGS

Cannabis

The classic work *Hashish and Mental Illness,* written by J. J. Moreau in 1845, first became available in English translation in 1973. Moreau, whom Bo Holmstedt calls the first psychiatrist interested in psychopharmacology, possessed a rather sophisticated view regarding the role of natural substances in the production of altered mental states. In his travels throughout the Middle East, Moreau observed the variety of mental changes that could be produced by cannabis use. He postulated that cannabis produced the fundamental process of pathological arousal or excitation seen in most serious mental illness. He stated, "Excitement carries the seed of all mental pathology as the trunk of a tree, its branches, its leaves, and its flowers are contained in the grain."

The medical literature in English dealing with psychotic reactions in association with cannabis use has been increasing in the past 25 years, although "hemp insanity" has long been recognized in India (25). An early review of the clinical manifestations of cannabis intoxication by Bromberg mentioned the problem posed by the "toxic psychoses which seem usually to be the admixture of the toxic effects of the drug to a basic cyclothymic (manic-depressive) or schizophrenic reaction" (17). Bromberg, like most observers then and to the present, tended to ascribe long-lasting psychopathology secondary to cannabis as evidence for preexisting major mental illness. There was the implication that schizophrenia or manic-depressive illness was already evident and that cannabis made a rather minor causative contribution, which Bromberg explained in psychoanalytic terms in relation to "the narcissism of the individual and its changing value for the ego." However, he also mentioned the possibility that the drug produced "a true 'symptomatic' schizophrenia where the drug in its primary cerebral effects is the cause of the psychoses." Over the past 15 years there has been a significant increase in reports dealing with psychotic reactions to cannabis (7,19,36,37,51,53,55,56,60). A remarkable degree of consistency characterizes the reports themselves. Cannabis-related acute psychosis is usually described in these studies as manic-like or schizophreniform with significant agitation. Authors note that sometimes subjects appear to have relatively normal prepsychotic personalities. The presence or absence of a family history of major mental illness is not usually noted in detail. Several authors emphasize that cannabis-related psychoses respond rapidly to neuroleptic treatment. More recently

studies have appeared describing the psychotogenic effect of cannabis use in known schizophrenic patients despite adequate neuroleptic maintenance (38,57).

Mescaline

Mescaline (3-4-5 trimethoxyphenethylamine) is significant because of its importance in the history of psychotomimetic substances. This compound was isolated from peyote in 1896 and its structure determined in 1918, although some clinical studies were initiated as early as 1913. Judging from Stockings' classic paper, there can be little doubt that mescaline (200–400 mg) can produce the "psychotomimetic syndrome" in humans (54). The structural similarity between mescaline and the catecholamines, which was recognized early, probably initiated conceptual thinking regarding the possibility of endogenous psychotogens. In fact, Stockings himself hypothesized in 1940, on the basis of his observations following the administration of mescaline to himself and to other volunteers, that "the various diseases commonly known as the psychoses are all variants of the same disease process and that the causative agent is probably a toxic amine with chemical and pharmacological properties similar to those of mescaline." It is remarkable how similar Stockings' analysis of the relationship between mescaline-induced states and psychopathology was to Moreau's views concerning cannabis and mental illness.

Amphetamine

The capacity of amphetamine to produce psychotic disorders was recognized soon after it became available for clinical use and was being prescribed commonly for the treatment of shock, coma, fatigue, narcolepsy, and nonspecific states of fatigue and lassitude (62). Connell's classic monograph (24) and more recent clinical research by Griffith (34), Bell (6), Angrist and Gershon (3), and others have confirmed the psychotogenic potential of amphetamine and related compounds, and these findings have been critical for theories of the psychoses that implicate central catecholamine systems. In much of this research, rather large cumulative doses of amphetamine have been used, although clinical experience suggests that prolonged psychoses can be triggered in vulnerable individuals by low doses of amphetamine.

LSD

The synthesis and self-administration of LSD by Albert Hofmann in 1943 ushered in an era of renewed interest in drugs that produce symptoms reminiscent of the major psychoses. One factor responsible for this renewal of interest was simply the unprecedented potency of LSD in humans, a fact that made the notion of endogenous psychotoxins even more credible than before. In addition, beginning approximately in the middle of this century, the interest of the public in the recreational use of mind-altering drugs increased, as did the availability of these compounds for casual use. Initially there was a period of extensive clinical experimentation with at least two primary goals in mind. First, there was the hope that the unique disorganization of mental processes produced by LSD would contribute to the knowledge of schizophrenia and related disorders. LSD and mescaline were sometimes administered to a variety of psychiatric patient populations in rather unrestricted fashion (47). In most psychotic patients who had not been ill for long periods, these drugs intensified their psychosis. A second purpose of the early clinical research with LSD was related to its use as an adjunct to psychotherapy by means of the intense emotional experience which the drug produced. However, as early as 1955 Elkes (26) sounded a precautionary note by stating, among other concerns, that "early psychotic reactions may be aggravated by the drug." Other observers who were initially somewhat skeptical came to recognize the dangers of LSD use by certain individuals (22,23,29).

Phencyclidine (PCP)

Clinical research using PCP was first reported in the mid-1950s. As was the case with mescaline and LSD, the initial impression was that PCP caused a number of disruptive psychological symptoms but that the drug could only be seen as a "model" psychosis since it did not produce the complete clinical picture of schizophrenia (43). Nevertheless, subsequent clinical experience, following a period of increased PCP availability on the street, made it clear that PCP can produce psychotic reactions which are prolonged and which closely resemble acute psychotic episodes unrelated to drug use (27,50).

Steroids, Antidepressants, L-Dopa

The earliest reports of steroid psychosis occurred in association with the introduction of corticotropin (ACTH) and cortisol into medical practice at midcentury (21). The affective changes associated with steroid administration are often stressed but psychotic symptoms may be seen as well, as a recent review emphasizes (42). Steroid psychosis is included here because it may be characterized by schizophreniform symptoms in a clear sensorium. Further, such reactions do not necessarily abate when the steroid dose is lowered and affected patients may require treatment with neuroleptics or lithium.

Since their introduction into clinical psychiatry in the 1950s, the tricyclic antidepressants and monoamine oxidase inhibitors have been reported to have different effects in psychotic as compared to depressed patients. It is a well-recognized clinical observation that these drugs stimulate psychotic excitement in certain vulnerable individuals (48), although a recent study challenges this view (40). Stimulation of psychotic symptoms by these compounds usually occurs after approximately 1 week of drug treatment and need not be associated with disorientation.

Psychotic reactions in association with L-dopa treatment of parkinsonism were first reported about 1970 (18). Elderly subjects who may also receive anticholinergics for parkinsonism are prone to disorientation during L-dopa psychotic reactions; however, this psychosis may occur without evidence of disorientation. Other dopamine agonists used in the treatment of parkinsonism, such as bromocriptine, may also produce psychotic reactions (52).

FROM MODEL TO REALITY?

The concept of a model psychosis had been considered by Moreau with regard to cannabis and by Stockings with respect to mescaline, as noted above. However, the discovery and widespread use of LSD gave rise to renewed interest in this idea. Comparisons of drug-induced states with schizophrenic syndromes generally concluded that there were substantial differences (35,39). However, when the schizophrenic syndrome was broken down into its components, it was possible to point to similarities as well (9,11).

The concept of a model psychosis was also pursued using biochemical techniques, thanks to technical advances that were being made in the 1960s. The endogenous methylation pathways were particular objects of study since methyl groups appeared crucial for the action of several psychotomimetic drugs (20). S-Adenosylmethionine (a methyl donor) was initially considered a possible source of psychotomimetic metabolites in humans but was ruled out to a considerable degree on the basis of experimental findings (4). The possibility that dimethyltryptamine (DMT) could be an endogenous hallucinogen in humans was reviewed by Gillin et al. (31). DMT was even detectable in the urine of psychotic patients but was ultimately not thought to be etiological (46).

In the early 1970s clinicians were seeing an increasing number of patients whose drug use (usually LSD and cannabis) appeared to have triggered a psychotic state, which was prolonged and posed the same therapeutic problems as did other psychoses. The usual explanation offered was that such individuals were "latent" schizophrenics, so that the question of vulnerability to psychotic states became an important one to consider.

In general, patients with psychoses associated with hallucinogen use were younger, had somewhat better prognostic profiles, and showed more positive and fewer negative symptoms compared to psychotic patients who had not used drugs (8). On the other hand, we found that approximately half of drug-induced psychotic patients had done reasonably well at a 2- to 5-year follow-up and half had done poorly, including two suicides (10). Not all investigators have agreed on the clinical profiles of drug-induced psychotic patients, however. Breakey and co-workers (16) found that hospitalized schizophrenics who had used drugs did have better premorbid histories than those who had not but were admitted to the hospital at an earlier age. Erard et al. (27), studying first admission psychoses following PCP ingestion, reported that the PCP psychotics were younger, less anxious, and showed less religious preoccupation and depression than a comparison schizophrenic group without a history of drug use. On the whole, however, these workers were impressed with the clinical similarity between their drug and nondrug psychotics. They commented that "the most fruitful path of future theory and research in this field may be to try to understand the interface between the drug effect and the naturally occurring syndrome (e.g., schizophrenia) rather than treating the drug effect as an analogue of the syndrome." Tsuang et al. (58) studied a group of psychotic patients ill for at least 6 months who had used hallucinogens and found that they were very comparable in premorbid history and symptoms to a group of "atypical schizophrenics" who met Washington University criteria for schizophrenia but who also showed affective symptoms or muteness. Vardy and Kay (59) also reported that their LSD psychotics were quite similar to a nondrug schizophrenic comparison group with respect to phenomenology and course of illness. In general, therefore, with regard to symptoms and premorbid adjustment there is no clear consensus that major clinical differences exist between drug and nondrug psychotics.

In recent years vulnerability has come to mean more specifically genetic vulnerability, as determined through an assessment of family history. In our follow-up study we noted that the incidence of major psychiatric disorder in first-degree relatives was high (about 30%) but also approximately equal in our drug and nondrug psychotics (14). Tsuang et al. (58) noted that family history in his prolonged drug psychosis group was increased for both schizophrenia and affective disorder, just as it was in his atypical schizophrenic group. We found a reciprocal relationship in male drug psychotics between degree of drug use and family history such that psychotic males with lesser degrees of drug use had a greater incidence of major mental illness requiring hospitalization in first-degree relatives (14). One clear cohort difference between drug psychotics and nondrug psychotics that has been consistent for most studies is the preponderance of males in the drug psychosis groups. Most family assessments in reports of drug-induced psychosis have been retrospective so that more definitive conclusions must await prospective studies.

If increased hallucinogenic drug availability and use were creating new cases of schizophreniform psychoses and related disorders, an increase in the actual numbers of patients ought to be observable. With this possibility in mind, we examined data from all Connecticut state hospitals from 1967 to 1979 to see whether the incidence of psychotic disorders had changed during this period of increased hallucinogenic drug use by the general population (M. B. Bowers, unpublished data). In 1970 the diagnostic category "drug abuse" increased to 20.3% of all first admissions, compared to 2.7% in 1967. In 1970 the category "schizophrenia and paranoid disorders" represented 10.9% of all first admissions, and that figure had been a relatively constant one for several years. Beginning in 1973 (at 12.2%) this diagnostic category began to increase and rose to 24.0% of all first admissions by 1979 and has remained around 20% ever since. These data are consistent with the interpretation that in the late 1960s in Connecticut a large increase in drug abuse patients was observed as first admissions to state hospitals, followed in 3 to 5 years by a substantial increase in first admissions diagnosed as schizophrenia and paranoid disorders. Further, the state hospital data showed that this increase was age-specific; namely, it occurred in psychotic patients 15 to 34 years old and not in older psychotic patients. It seems likely that this phenomenon has played a significant role in the emergence of the so-called "young adult chronic" psychotic patients so familiar to clinicians practicing during the past 15 years. Acknowledging the limitations of this kind of data, it nevertheless suggests that hallucinogen use has created new cases of bona fide schizophreniform psychosis and related disorders in the past 15 years. Similar conclusions can be drawn from a Veterans Administration study by McLellan and co-workers (44), where patients initially diagnosed as stimulant and hallucinogen abusers required repeated inpatient admissions and received psychotic diagnoses in subsequent years (1972–1978).

Thus, it appears reasonable to propose that psychotogenic drug use may be influencing the picture of psychotic disorders seen in recent years. Assuming that genetic liability to most psychotic disorders in the schizophrenia-mania spectrum is a continuous and not a dichotomous distribution, drugs may be playing a variety of roles. In some individuals, they may simply be causing a psychosis to become manifest at an earlier age. In others they may be producing a psychotic disorder that would have remained dormant if drugs had not been used. Certainly psychotogenic drug use becomes a significant risk factor for relapse in an individual who has previously suffered a psychotic disorder. It appears that what was once a model is now in some sense a reality, and that those drugs which have been termed psychotomimetic are indeed, for some vulnerable individuals, psychotogenic.

IS THERE A UNIFYING BIOCHEMICAL THEORY?

Since the discovery of LSD, there has been an active search for a biochemical mechanism that might explain its action and that of other hallucinogens such as mescaline and psilocybin. Since the pioneering work of Freedman and Giarman (28,30) demonstrating that LSD increases serotonin levels in rat brain and by Aghajanian and co-workers (2) showing that LSD decreases the firing rate of serotonin-containing neurons in the midbrain dorsal raphé, the central serotonin system has been the main focus of preclinical studies concerning hallucinogenic drugs. A more general property has been observed more recently: namely, the ability of several hallucinogens to increase the response of certain neurons to excitatory afferent inputs (1). One theoretical problem relevant to the present review has been the linking of theories of hallucinogen mechanism of action with the neurochemical system known to be affected by antipsychotic drugs, the dopamine system. Recently subpopulations of serotonin receptors have been described that also appear to be binding sites for at least one class of antipsychotic drugs, the butyrophenones (33,41).

The central dopamine system itself has been studied less thoroughly with regard to psychotogenic drug action. Indeed, many of the drugs discussed here have been shown to augment central dopaminergic transmission in some experimental systems. Since the mesolimbic and mesocortical dopamine pathways appear to be uniquely affected by antipsychotic drugs (5), we have been interested in the effects of psychotogenic drugs on the dopamine system in these brain regions. Thus far we have shown in rats that LSD, PCP, and cannabis preferentially increase the concentration of dopamine metabolites in these regions (12,13).

Thus, the search for a final common biochemical pathway that might explain the generic effects of psychotogenic substances will continue. It is likely that multiple neuronal mechanisms can lead to a common state of pathologically excessive arousal, which may be the behavioral precursor of psychotic disorders. The so-called negative symptoms of schizophrenia could be a reflection of tonic underactivity in certain arousal pathways driven to periodic overactivity by psychotogenic drugs or other endogenous mechanisms. Such "defect states" have been described in chronic psychotogenic drug users (32). It thus seems prudent for clinicians to take psychotogenic drug use into account as a risk factor in the onset and course of schizophreniform psychoses and related disorders.

ACKNOWLEDGMENTS

This review was supported by USPHS grants MH-28216 and MH-30929, the Robert Alwin Hay Fund for Schizophrenia Research, and the Abraham Ribicoff Research Facilities of the Connecticut Mental Health Center.

REFERENCES

1. Aghajanian, G. K. (1980): *Brain Res.,* 186:492–498.
2. Aghajanian, G. K., Foote, W. E., and Sheard, M. H. (1968): *Science,* 161:706–708.
3. Angrist, B. M., and Gershon, S. (1970): *Biol. Psychiatry,* 2:95–107.
4. Baldessarini, R. J., Stramentinoli, G., and Lipinski, J. F. (1979): *Arch. Gen. Psychiatry,* 36:303–307.
5. Bannon, M. J., Reinhardt, J. F., Bunney, E. B., Jr., and Roth, R. H. (1982): *Nature,* 296:444–446.
6. Bell, D. S. (1973): *Arch. Gen. Psychiatry,* 29:35–40.
7. Bernhardson, G., and Gunne, L.-M. (1972): *Int. J. Addict.,* 7:9–16.
8. Bowers, M. B., Jr. (1972): *Arch. Gen. Psychiatry,* 27:437–440.
9. Bowers, M. B., Jr. (1973): In: *Psychopathology and Psychopharmacology,* edited by J. O. Cole, A. M. Freedman, and A. J. Friedhoff, pp. 1–14. Johns Hopkins University Press, Baltimore.
10. Bowers, M. B., Jr. (1977): *Arch. Gen. Psychiatry,* 34:832–835.
11. Bowers, M. B., Jr., and Freedman, D. X. (1966): *Arch. Gen. Psychiatry,* 15:240–248.
12. Bowers, M. B., Jr., and Hoffman, F. J., Jr. (1984): *Psychopharmacology,* 84:136–137.
13. Bowers, M. B., Jr., and Salomonsson, L. (1982): *Biochem. Pharmacol.,* 31:4093–4096.
14. Bowers, M. B., Jr., and Swigar, M. E. (1983): *Psychiatry Res.,* 9:91–97.
15. Brawley, P., and Duffield, J. C. (1972): *Pharmacol. Rev.,* 24:31–66.
16. Breakey, W. R., Goodell, H., Lorenz, P. C., and McHugh, P. R. (1974): *Psychol. Med.,* 4:255–261.
17. Bromberg, W. (1934): *Am. J. Psychiatry,* 91:303–329.
18. Celesia, G. G., and Barr, A. N. (1970): *Arch. Neurol.,* 23:193–200.
19. Chopra, G. S. (1971): *Bull. Narc.,* 23:15–22.
20. Christian, S. T., Benington, F., Morin, R. D., and Corbett, L. (1975): *Biochem. Med.,* 14:191–200.
21. Clark, L., Bauer, W., and Cobb, S. (1952): *N. Engl. J. Med.,* 246:205–216.
22. Cohen, S. (1960): *J. Nerv. Ment. Dis.,* 130:30–40.
23. Cole, J. O., and Katz, M. M. (1964): *JAMA,* 187:758–761.
24. Connell, P. H. (1958): *Amphetamine Psychosis.* Maudsley Monographs, No. 5. Oxford University Press, London.
25. Dhunjibhoy, J. E., and Bomb, B. S. (1930): *J. Ment. Sci.,* 75:254–264.
26. Elkes, C., Elkes, J., and Meyer-Gross, W. (1954): *Lancet,* 1:719.
27. Erard, R., Luisada, P. V., and Peele, R. (1980): *J. Psychedelic Drugs,* 12:235–251.
28. Freedman, D. X. (1961): *J. Pharmacol. Exp. Ther.,* 134:160–166.
29. Frosch, W. A., Robbins, E. S., and Stern, M. (1965): *N. Engl. J. Med.,* 273:1235–1239.
30. Giarman, N. J., and Freedman, D. X. (1965): *Pharmacol. Rev.,* 17:1–25.
31. Gillin, J. C., Kaplan, J., Stillman, R., and Wyatt, R. J. (1976): *Am. J. Psychiatry,* 133:203–208.
32. Glass, G. S., and Bowers, M. B., Jr. (1970): *Arch. Gen. Psychiatry,* 23:97–103.
33. Glennon, R. A., Titeler, M., and McKenney, J. D. (1984): *Life Sci.,* 35:2505–2511.
34. Griffith, J. D., Cavanaugh, J., Held, J., and Oates, J. (1972): *Arch. Gen. Psychiatry,* 26:97–100.
35. Hollister, L. E. (1962): *Ann. NY Acad. Sci.,* 96:80–92.
36. Jones, R. T. (1973): In: *Psychopathology and Psychopharmacology,* edited by J. O. Cole, A. M. Freedman, and A. J. Friedhoff, pp. 71–86. Johns Hopkins University Press, Baltimore.
37. Keup, W. (1970): *Dis. Nerv. Syst.,* 31:119–126.
38. Knudsen, P., and Vilmar, T. (1984): *Acta Psychiatr. Scand.,* 69:162–174.
39. Langs, R. J., and Barr, H. L. (1968): *J. Nerv. Ment. Dis.,* 147:163–172.
40. Lewis, J. L., and Winokur, G. (1982): *Arch. Gen. Psychiatry,* 39:303–306.
41. Leysen, J. E., Awouters, R., Kennis, L., Laduron, P. M., Vanderberk, J., and Janssen, P. A. J. (1981): *Life Sci.,* 28:1015–1022.
42. Ling, M. H. M., Perry, P. J., and Tsuang, M. T. (1981): *Arch. Gen. Psychiatry,* 38:471–477.
43. Luby, E. D., Cohen, B. C., Rosenbaum, G., Gottlieb, J. S., and Kelly, R. (1959): *Arch. Neurol. Psychiatry,* 81:363–369.
44. McLellan, A. T., Woody, G. E., and O'Brien, C. P. (1979): *N. Engl. J. Med.,* 301:1310–1314.
45. Moreau, J. J. (1973): *Hashish and Mental Illness.* Raven Press, New York.
46. Murray, R. M., Oon, M. C. H., Rodwight, R., Birley, J. L. T., and Smith, A. (1979): *Arch. Gen. Psychiatry,* 36:644–649.
47. Pennes, H. H. (1954): *J. Nerv. Ment. Dis.,* 119:95–112.
48. Pollack, M., Klein, D. F., Wilner, A., Blumberg, A., and Fink, M. (1965): In: *Recent Advances in Biological Psychiatry, Vol. III,* edited by J. Wortis, pp. 53–61. Plenum Press, New York.
49. Post, R. M. (1975): *Am. J. Psychiatry,* 132:225–231.
50. Rainey, J. M., and Crowder, M. K. (1975): *Am. J. Psychiatry,* 132:1076–1078.
51. Rottanburg, D., Ben-Arie, O., Robins, A. H., Teggin, A., and Elk, R. (1982): *Lancet,* 2:1364–1366.
52. Serby, M., Angrist, B., and Lieberman, A. (1978): *Am. J. Psychiatry,* 135:1227–1229.
53. Spencer, D. J. (1970): *Br. J. Addict.,* 65:369–372.
54. Stockings, G. T. (1940): *J. Ment. Sci.,* 86:29–47.
55. Talbott, J. A., and Teague, J. W. (1969): *JAMA,* 210:299–302.
56. Thacore, V. R., and Shukla, S. R. P. (1976): *Arch. Gen. Psychiatry,* 33:383–386.
57. Treffert, D. A. (1978): *Am. J. Psychiatry,* 135:1213–1215.
58. Tsuang, M. T., Simpson, J. C., and Kronfol, Z. (1982): *Arch. Gen. Psychiatry,* 39:141–147.
59. Vardy, M. M., and Kay, S. R. (1983): *Arch. Gen. Psychiatry,* 40:877–883.
60. Weil, A. T. (1970): *N. Engl. J. Med.,* 282:997–1000.
61. Wetli, C. V., and Fishbain, D. A. (1985): *J. Forensic Sci.,* 30:873–880.
62. Young, D., and Scoville, W. B. (1938): *Med. Clin. North Am.,* Vol. 22, May, pp. 637–646.

Psychopharmacology:
The Third Generation of Progress,
edited by Herbert Y. Meltzer.
Raven Press, New York © 1987.

CHAPTER **82**

Genetic and Neurobiological Approaches to the Pathophysiology of Autism and the Pervasive Developmental Disorders

J. Gerald Young, Leonard I. Leven, Jeffrey H. Newcorn, and Peter J. Knott

SYMPTOMS AND PROBLEMS OF CLASSIFICATION

The term "pervasive developmental disorders" accurately describes the nature of the severe childhood neuropsychiatric disorders. The designation captures the limitations of our current knowledge by indicating simply that multiple adaptive functions of the individual are affected in the developing child. For the clinical investigator attempting to unravel the neurobiological origins of these disorders, the terminology asserts the crucial role that clinical assessment and nosology play in biological research. Pervasive disorders affect a range of functional capacities in the child and typically do so unequally; individual children vary markedly along individual symptom dimensions, so that their clinical appearance differs somewhat, and their inclusion or exclusion from specific diagnostic categories is a continuous question threatening the validity of biological research on these disorders.

The occurrence of these symptoms in the developmental period assures that the symptom profile for each child will undergo a metamorphosis, inviting intermittent reexamination of the child's diagnosis. These factors lead to several perspectives on research on the most severe disorders in childhood: (a) meticulous clinical assessment is the prerequisite for authentic neurobiological research on pervasive developmental disorders; (b) arbitrary classification schemes should be simple and unpretentious when our knowledge is limited, and open to reconsideration as research provides new understanding of underlying mechanisms; and (c) biological variables should be examined in relation to symptom dimensions in addition to diagnostic categories, so that the contributions of fundamental biological systems to the regulation of observable behaviors can be recognized regardless of the diagnostic group examined at a particular time (1).

In this spirit, a review of neurobiological factors in the pervasive developmental disorders and infantile autism requires brief comments on the diagnostic features of these illnesses. This is followed by a discussion of genetic contributions to these impairments; a review of neurochemical, neuroimmunological, and electrophysiological research; and a description of the brain imaging and neuropathological studies on autism and related disorders.

Infantile autism stands as the single syndrome among the pervasive developmental disorders that has achieved a definitional status agreed on by essentially all investigators; other pervasive developmental disorders (PDD) retain the quality of residual categories, to a greater or lesser degree, because of the lack of distinctive specificity in their criteria. The diagnostic criteria for autism provide the clinical basis for neurobiological research, and these same symptoms can be examined separately in nonautistic PDD in order to establish the strength of the association between individual biological indices and specific symptoms. The essential symptoms in autism include impairments in social relatedness, cognition, sensory modulation, language, and communicative behaviors as well as a characteristic resistance to change and the presence of stereotypic involuntary movements.

Social Relatedness and Attachment Behaviors

Impaired social relatedness has been considered a fundamental symptom of autism since the first description of the syndrome by Kanner in 1943 (2). Although each of the symptoms of autism occupies the status of the primary or characteristic symptom in the syndrome at one time or another, impaired social relatedness has retained this role in the mind of the lay public and many clinicians over the decades of study of this syndrome. This reflects the fact that the other symptoms of autism also occur in large subgroups of individuals with other related disorders, including nonautistic pervasive developmental disorders, developmental language disorders, and many mental retardation syndromes. In spite of this, impaired social relatedness was not the subject of systematic investigation, as other symptoms were, until the past few years. This led to a general deemphasis of the importance of social relatedness as a subject for independent scrutiny as well as to disagreement and confusion concerning the definition, presence, and role of a deficit in social relatedness.

Social relatedness has been conceptualized as including, but not limited to, attachment behaviors. Thus, it includes those constructs related to the broad concept of attachment, such as security, dependency, sociability, and separation and reunion reactions. However, in addition, autistic children have other deficits in the social domain, including those related to nonverbal communication (social interaction, joint referencing or indicating, requesting gestures), emotional expression, social understanding, and differential social response (3–5).

Cognition

Some investigators consider a cognitive deficit to be the core symptom in autism. In this view, individuals with autism have an impairment in cognition that can be specified as an abnormality in the information-processing sequence and shown to interfere with multiple behavioral functions (including language, motoric regulation, social

behaviors, and the response to novelty). Presumably, the neural substrate for this deficit would be the target for treatment, so that identification of a core cognitive impairment would be an essential step in directing neurobiological research. Cumulative research has demonstrated the presence of cognitive dysfunction in all autistic individuals and has clarified that there are specific types of deficits characteristically present (6). One domain of current research seeks to identify specific subtypes of cognitive impairments (7).

Language and Communicative Behaviors

The relationship between developmental language disorders and autism has intrigued clinicians for many years. The two disorders share many clinical features, and it is not uncommon for the diagnoses to be confused in individual children; meticulous language assessment is essential to the evaluation of autistic patients. Some children given the diagnosis of a developmental language disorder have a longitudinal course and outcome similar to that for autistic children, particularly those whose language disorder has atypical features. This latter group fails to meet criteria for autism, but the children have autistic features such as social and play abnormalities (8,9). The strong overlap between these diagnostic categories is obvious, and the group of children residing at the boundary resists straightforward assignment of a diagnosis. This led to the proposal that the core deficit in autism might be language impairment and that the inability to organize and regulate the self through language and language-related thought might lead to subsidiary symptoms in the cognitive, social, and motor spheres (10,11).

Stereotypic Behaviors and Related Motor Phenomena

The involuntary stereotypies evident in many autistic individuals are also typical of other retarded children; similarly, other abnormal involuntary movements (such as tics) can occasionally be observed in autistic children. The lack of diagnostic specificity, the minor effects of these motor symptoms, and the responsiveness of severe stereotypies to behavior modification procedures have resulted in less investigative attention to these phenomena. Nevertheless, these repetitive movements can take the form of self-injurious behaviors and become the central target symptoms in treatment profiles for individual patients. Behavioral methods for management of self-injurious behaviors can run the gamut of frustration from ineffective procedures to aversive methods that are unacceptable to the staff and parents. Neurobiological research could make an especially crucial contribution by guiding the development of novel pharmacological treatments for self-injurious behaviors; current medications are limited in their efficacy.

Resistance to Change

The inability of the autistic child to respond to new stimuli by altering his attention to observe and explore the new phenomena in his environment has been likened to perseverative motoric behaviors. The resistance to change can be conceptually related to cognitive, attentional, and language impairments in the autistic patient and is of particular interest in relation to possible neurochemical models that might explain this inflexibility and the often accompanying catastrophic anxiety evident when novelty intrudes.

THE MATURATIONAL FRAMEWORK: NEUROGENETICS AND DEVELOPMENTAL NEUROBIOLOGY

Neurogenetic Perspectives on Pervasive Developmental Disorders

Congenital Causes of Autism: Prenatal, Perinatal, and Postnatal Factors

Etiologic heterogeneity is assumed by most investigators of the PDD because of the occurrence of the autistic syndrome in individuals with many disorders, including those with genetic, viral, and other causes. This led to the examination of many possible congenital causes for autism in an attempt to separate children with identifiable insults from those children with unknown etiology and familial aggregation of autism. However, it is important to recognize the emerging evidence that one type of genetic contribution to autism might be a vulnerability to a variety of perinatal insults, infectious and otherwise, so that the presence of the full disorder requires the interaction of both factors. Although some studies have failed to identify any prenatal or perinatal events occurring at a higher rate in autistic individuals, others have determined bleeding during pregnancy, prematurity/low birth weight, maternal age, flu-like symptoms during pregnancy, and ingestion of medications during pregnancy to be more common in the autistic group; disagreement across studies leaves this an open question requiring further research (12–15).

Two congenital factors have been observed with sufficient frequency to encourage further investigation. Several investigators have reported that minor physical anomalies are more common in autistic children, suggesting the possibility of a first-trimester insult. Other types of neuropsychiatric disorders in early childhood may share this increase in minor physical anomalies with autistic children (16). Congenital viral infections in association with autism are also well documented in the literature. Although this does not appear to be a common cause of the syndrome, the increased incidence of viral infection and exposure during pregnancy and the demonstration of the occurrence of autistic symptoms in children with congenital rubella and cytomegalovirus infections have raised questions concerning diminished immunological competence as a genetically predisposing vulnerability in families of autistic children or viral infections as risk factors requiring additional insults in the genesis of the autistic syndrome (17–20). Inadequate markers for viral penetration of the central nervous system (CNS) have hampered prior research, and further investigation is required (21).

Clinical Genetic Research on Autism and Related Disorders

"Single-gene" defects leading to an inborn error of metabolism can be associated with autistic symptoms. Cases of phenylketonuria, tuberous sclerosis, and neurofibromatosis accompanied by the autistic syndrome have been described (22). Nevertheless, the proportion of autistic cases explained on this basis is quite small using current methods, and clinical genetic research has sought to determine whether modes of inheritance can be distinguished for subgroups of autistic individuals with an unknown etiology. This research was encouraged by two factors noted by clinical investigators with substantial samples of autistic children: multiple-incidence families were identified, sometimes including twins concordant for the syndrome, and prevalence of autism among siblings of autistic probands was reported to be 2 to 3%, a rate 50 times that expected (23,24).

A study of a sample of twins sparked renewed interest in genetic contributions to autism. A concordance rate for autism of 40% in monozygous twin pairs was contrasted with a 10% concordance rate in dizygous twins (25). More recently, conceptualization of the heritable trait began to broaden, as it appeared that families of autistic children were characterized by an increased incidence of several types of psychopathology, even if no other autistic relatives were identified. Thus, the possibility of a "lesser variant" or *form fruste* of the autistic syndrome was considered, centered on the aggregation of cognitive and language impairments (23). For example, in one study 25% of the autistic probands had a parent or sibling afflicted with a language disorder or history of delayed speech (11). Another research group reported that 15.5% of the siblings of a sample of autistic children had cognitive disabilities, whereas 3% of a comparison group of Down's syndrome children were similarly diagnosed. These cognitive disabilities clustered in a few families of autistic probands and included disturbances in expressive and receptive language, specific learning disabilities, and borderline or more severe mental retardation (26). Another clinical laboratory observed an excess of subnormal intellectual functioning in siblings of autistic children and documented significantly lower verbal scores than performance scores on formal intelligence testing (27).

Findings in another sample of families of autistic children again emphasized the importance of meticulous assessment. Cognitive disabilities occurred in 19.6% of the siblings of autistic probands, and the incidence of autism in the siblings was 5.9%. These investigators found that the 10 siblings with cognitive disabilities came from 6 of 29 families; a total of 11 siblings in these six families yielded 10 siblings with a diagnosis of autism, nonspecific intellectual retardation, or a specific cognitive impairment. This aggregation occurred in the families of severely retarded autistic probands and not among siblings of higher-functioning autistic individuals. These results suggest that low-functioning, severely retarded autistic individuals may have a strong genetic vulnerability that distinguishes them from other autistic subjects (28). High-functioning autistic individuals, possibly those sometimes designated as Asperger's syndrome, might be a different subgroup of the syndrome; this requires detailed clinical evaluation to assure differentiation of subgroups (29,30) and may explain, in part, the earlier inability to identify a genetic contribution to the syndrome of autism (earlier studies were more likely to exclude severely retarded autistic children from their samples). For the severely retarded subgroup of autistic individuals, the heritable factor may be related to a general cognitive impairment.

A study of 40 pairs of autistic twins established concordance rates of 95.7% (22 of 23 pairs) for monozygotic (MZ) twins and 23.5% (four of 17) for dizygotic (DZ) twins. These rates were significantly different from the 50% concordance rate predicted by a dominant mode of inheritance with full penetrance. However, they are compatible with autosomal recessive inheritance, which predicts 100% concordance in monozygotic twins and 25% concordance in dizygotic twins. The findings fail to account for the excess of males in their twin sample (31).

A related report by these investigators described the ascertainment of 46 families with multiple incidences of autism, comprised of 41 families with two autistic probands and five with three autistic probands. Segregation analyses described a maximum likelihood estimate of the segregation ratio (0.19) that was significantly less than 0.50 (the expected value for autosomal dominant inheritance) but not significantly different from 0.25 (the anticipated value for autosomal recessive inheritance). A polygenic threshold model also tested was rejected. The findings were most consistent with a hypothesis of autosomal recessive inheritance.

Yet, these pioneering studies generated intriguing results through methods that emphasize the level of sophistication required for genetic studies of child psychiatric disorders if their results are not to be misinterpreted. The investigators emphasize that these findings apply only to the specific multiple-incidence population ascertained for this study (32). The results cannot be generalized to other multiple-incidence families or to families with only a single autistic proband. These strict limitations are derived from ascertainment procedures that spawned a unique group that may bias the data in unknown ways (members of the National Society for Autistic Children, access to this organization's newsletter, previous diagnosis, cooperation in studies at UCLA, etc.). The problems of an ascertainment bias when establishing an autosomal recessive mode of inheritance are well known: probands are included, but most unaffected heterozygotes are not. In addition to these problems of ascertainment, these were retrospective chart diagnoses from records of varying quality, not all probands had testing for fragile-X, and there was a strong preponderance of males in the sample. The possible presence of fragile-X autistic subjects or other explanations for the male preponderance were not described or adequately considered in their report.

These investigators considered an autosomal dominant mode of inheritance in autism but state that their analyses rejected it. They also excluded an X-linked recessive mechanism, although reservations about this decision are suggested above; further consideration of X-linked inheritance in autism is given below. However, a multifactorial or polygenic model, also discarded by these investigators, deserves further scrutiny. One model to be examined is a sex-dependent threshold effect. A continuously distributed liability (encompassing genetic and environmental factors) to the disorder in the population would include a threshold value for phenotypic manifestation. This threshold might be higher for females, consistent with the observed increased prevalence of autism in males. In this case, the trait would appear in a larger proportion of male relatives of female probands than in male relatives of male probands; for example, this mode of inheritance may be the basis for familial aggregation of Tourette's disorder and chronic multiple tics. Establishment of this model requires a large family study.

Another multifactorial model deserves examination. An example of this model is the first twin study in which a genetic vulnerability to cognitive and language disabilities was suggested; their findings also indicated that an environmental insult was required for full expression of the autistic syndrome. Among the MZ twins discordant for autism, the "unaffected" twin had cognitive or language impairments in five of the seven twins and no evidence of perinatal injury. However, there was evidence of perinatal injury in their autistic cotwins. This model suggests that a vulnerability to a cognitive or language impairment coupled with perinatal injury might lead to autism (24,25). Other research has indicated that mothers of autistic probands from single-incidence families had a significantly increased incidence of bleeding, flu-like symptoms, ingestion of medication, and induced labor than mothers of probands in the multiple-incidence group (15).

Chromosomal Analyses and the Fragile-X Syndrome

Evidence for chromosomal abnormalities in autism and related disorders was not compelling in early karyotype examinations. Aberrations were either absent or rare in these studies (33–36). The lack of specific diagnostic criteria for autism prior to 1980 suggests that studies of karyotypes in all childhood psychoses should be reviewed, but even this larger group of papers fails to generate consistent findings of chromosomal abnormalities. However, in a recent survey approximately half of the autistic individuals and the larger group of patients with pervasive developmental disorders had associated chromosomal abnormalities (not necessarily implying that these caused the disorder) (37).

For many years the pursuit of biological causes of infantile autism and related pervasive developmental disorders met with limited success, typically the identification of isolated patients with disorders such as congenital rubella or phenylketonuria. The demonstration of the fragile-X syndrome in some autistic individuals has encouraged optimism that application of novel technical methods will elucidate further specific biological etiologies for large subgroups of autism. X-linked mental retardation affects a population second only to Down's syndrome in size among mental retardation syndromes with a distinct etiology. Report of a constriction of the X chromosome causing instability at this site was followed by the determination that folic-acid-deficient culture media were required for expression of the fragile site (38,39). Surveys of families of patients with nonspecific X-linked mental retardation led to the identification of many individuals with this syndrome. Typical phenotypic features (other than mental deficiency) are inconsistently present, and macroorchidism is the most common. Other physical features noted have included prognathism, large ears, and narrow faces. Speech abnormalities and seizures have been observed in subgroups. A small subgroup of heterozygous women are affected and characterized by an intellectual deficit.

The fragile-X syndrome is inherited in an X-linked recessive manner, and its incidence is estimated to be 0.92 per 1,000 males (39–44). Autistic males were surveyed for this disorder because of the 4:1 male-to-female ratio and a prevalence of mental retardation in the range of 75% of the autistic population. Multiple reports have described samples of males who met rigid criteria for infantile autism and had the characteristic fragile site on the X chromosome. The prevalence of the fragile-X syndrome in the autistic population samples studied has varied but appears to constitute a significant subgroup varying from 0 to 17% of samples at different centers (37,45–48). No treatment other than preventive genetic counseling has been identified; recent trials of folic acid have produced mixed results (49).

Many types of chromosomal abnormalities have been identified in children with pervasive developmental disorders; most are rarely observed, and the clinical significance of some remains unknown (Table 1). In a recent Swedish survey, karyotypes of 66 psychotic children were examined. There were 56 mentally retarded children; 46 (40 boys and 6 girls) met strict criteria for infantile autism, and 20 were diagnosed as other psychoses (15 boys and 5 girls, a majority fulfilling criteria for childhood-onset pervasive developmental disorder). Among these children, 42% had a known organic syndrome, epilepsy, or cerebral palsy, although in only a small minority was there evidence of organicity in early childhood, when the original diagnosis had been made. A total of 47% of the psychotic children (and 48% of the autistic children) had some type of chromosomal marker or abnormality (Table 1). This is a much higher rate of abnormalities than previously reported, and the meaning is not yet clear. Several of the chromosomal abnormalities do not yet have a known base rate in the population, making it impossible to judge their significance; for others, a population frequency of less than 1% makes it obvious that these findings are quite deviant. Seventeen percent of the autistic children had the fragile-X marker (37). These investigators also noted the possibility that children with chromosomal disorders are prone to speech and language disorders (especially those with the XYY syndrome). The intriguing results of this research are difficult to interpret in isolation but encourage further investigation of chromosomal abnormalities in autism (50–59).

Biochemical Genetics and Molecular Biology

Attempts to determine a locus responsible for familial aggregation of autism are underway. An initial gene-mapping study examined 34 families (27 multiplex) through gene linkage analyses with 30 standard phenotypic gene markers. This research, assuming an autosomal recessive mode of inheritance, excluded close linkage with HLA and 19 other autosomal genetic markers. The largest positive *lod* scores (over 1.0) were obtained with haptoglobin over the entire

TABLE 1. *Chromosome abnormalities reported in the pervasive developmental disorders*

Abnormality	Reference
Autosomal aneuploidies	
46,XY + 47,XY +8 (mosaic of trisomy 8)	Burd et al. (59)
Trisomy 21	Wakabayashi (58)
	Gillberg and Wahlstrom (37)
Structural anomalies of autosomes	
fra (6) (q26)	Gillberg and Wahlstrom (37)
9h+	Gillberg and Wahlstrom (37)
fra (16) (q23)	Gillberg and Wahlstrom (37)
Sex chromosomal aneuploidies	
XXX	Wolraich et al. (36)
WY mosaicism (long Y and short Y)	Gillberg and Wahlstrom (37)
XYY	Forsius et al. (54)
	Nielsen et al. (55)
	Gillberg et al. (57)
	Gillberg and Wahlstrom (37)
Structural anomalies of sex chromosomes	
Long Y (Y = F)	Judd and Mandell (35)
	Hoshino et al. (56)
	Gillberg and Wahlstrom (37)
fra (X) (p22)	Gillberg and Wahlstrom (37)
fra (X) (q27)	Turner et al. (41)
	Brown et al. (45)
	Meryash et al. (46)
	And others

sample and with ABO in families with at least a single affected girl (60).

Screening for known genetic causes of autism is rapidly expanding, and these subgroups will be intensively investigated for biochemical abnormalities. A disorder sharing some clinical features with autism provides a model for the progress in genetic and biochemical research on autism that can be anticipated. The Lesch–Nyhan syndrome is an X-linked recessive disorder in which there is partial or complete loss of activity of an enzyme critical to purine metabolism, hypoxanthine–guanine phosphoribosyl transferase (HGPRT). The HGPRT gene is located on the long arm of the X chromosome (Xq26–27) between the loci for two marker genes and has been cloned. The symptoms of the Lesch–Nyhan syndrome include self-mutilating behavior, spasticity, and hyperuricemia as well as inconsistently present renal stones, psychomotor retardation, movement disorder, difficult swallowing, malnutrition, and pneumonia. The gene and complementary DNAs have been isolated and sequenced, and probes are now being utilized to characterize the mutations occurring in patients afflicted with the disorder. This may ultimately lead to the development of gene therapy for Lesch–Nyhan syndrome. Although our understanding of biochemical abnormalities in subgroups of autistic children lags far behind, the evolving molecular biology of the Lesch–Nyhan syndrome is an encouraging model for future advances in the understanding and treatment of autism (61,62).

Early Brain Development, Insults to the Nervous System, and Brain Plasticity

The brain more than doubles in volume during the first year of life, reaching 60% of its adult size. The 350-g brain at birth increases in weight to 1,000 g by 18 months of age; at 3 years of age the size of the brain is close to that of the adult (1,300 g) (63). This increase in size mirrors massive structural changes in the developing infant brain, and the neural events associated with the precise patterning of the neuronal network during the fetal and postnatal periods are of special interest in relation to causes of later developmental disabilities. The sequence of events leading to the eventual adult cellular structure of the brain has been mapped in considerable detail. At the early embryonic phase, the outer layer (ectoderm) of the embryo becomes a specialized tissue that develops into the spinal cord and brain. Only the rudiments of this process of neural induction are beginning to be understood. It is followed by the proliferation phase, when cells multiply in different local regions. A migration phase then transports the cells to the locations in which they will ultimately reside. The nerve cells aggregate with other similar cells in layers or nuclear masses in accord with the specific type of cell and anatomical location and attain a specific alignment and orientation amid the other cells (64).

At this time, these immature neurons initiate the process of differentiation through which they become committed to either chemical transmission or electrical, gap junction transmission; determine the neurotransmitter(s) they will release; settle on the principal ion to be used for the propagation of nerve impulses; and form the neuronal

processes that are the vehicle for their interaction with other cells (65). The neurons with their elaborated processes are then prepared to form guided, highly specific patterns of connections with multiple other nerve cells (66,67). The major phases of brain development come to an end through a regressive phase, as certain nerve cells selectively die. At a later stage in this phase, these adjustments are completed through the elimination of selected processes and synapses, while others are stabilized (68).

The timing of these maturational events in relation to simultaneous behavioral development is of fundamental interest to clinical investigators, as these timetables underlie the potential for environmental influences and the basis for brain plasticity. Some of these developmental processes have come to completion by the time of the birth of the infant: cellular proliferation and cell migration have essentially come to an end, although cellular proliferation in the cerebellum during the postnatal period may be an important exception with pathophysiological significance for developmental disorders. However, neuronal differentiation, growth of neuronal processes, formation of patterns of connectivity, and selective nerve cell death and process elimination all occur subsequent to birth (64). Myelination continues for years after the neonatal period. Little is known about their determination of the timing and form of behavioral phenomena in the first years of life, and the mapping of these relations poses an invigorating challenge to clinical developmental neurobiology (69).

Recognition of the paramount importance of these postnatal events for brain development not only suggests their vulnerability to insult but carries the hopeful prospect of a period of unusual brain plasticity that might allow compensatory processes to restore function compromised through fetal or neonatal brain injury.

NEUROCHEMICAL RESEARCH ON AUTISM

Serotonin and the Indoleamines

An abnormality in serotonergic function in infantile autism has been suggested through several investigative approaches. Hyperserotonemia in autistic and mentally retarded patients has been replicated in many clinical laboratories, and approximately one-third of autistic children have elevated blood serotonin levels (71–75). However, hyperserotonemia occurs in several medical and neuropsychiatric disorders, is not firmly associated with any behavior or symptom, and is not related to any other physiological parameter. Thus, the significance of the finding is unclear, reflecting the obscurity of its origin. Blood serotonin is carried almost entirely in platelets, and the serotonin concentration per platelet is increased; although there are morphological and functional analogies between platelets and serotonergic nerve endings, the relations between the two are speculative (76).

The first autistic subjects found to have hyperserotonemia had mixed features of autism and severe retardation, and subgroups of patients with mental retardation (with both known and unknown etiologies) have been shown to have hyperserotonemia, so it has been suggested that the finding in autistic subjects reflects diagnostic imprecision rather than a biological mechanism. However, autistic children selected on the basis of strict diagnostic criteria following intensive evaluations and followed over an extensive time period were found to have a subgroup of 40% characterized by hyperserotonemia (77). The elevation in blood serotonin is not caused by abnormalities in either platelet serotonin uptake or efflux nor by a reduction in serotonin through degradation by monoamine oxidase within the platelet (78,79). Familial clustering of blood serotonin levels may reflect genetic influences (80).

In an effort to test the hypothesis that a drug-induced reduction in blood serotonin levels in hyperserotonemic autistic children would lead to fewer symptoms and improved adaptation, two drugs were given trials. Blood serotonin levels decreased moderately following L-dopa administration, but global symptoms were unchanged (81). Fenfluramine, an anorexogenic drug known to reduce blood and brain serotonin levels, was used to treat three autistic boys. Blood serotonin levels dropped markedly in all three, accompanied by improved performance on IQ tests and decreased symptoms across a range of functional domains (82). In a subsequent study of 14 autistic patients, these investigators found that fenfluramine administration was associated with a 51% decrease in blood serotonin concentration, unchanged platelet counts, reduced symptoms in the motor, sensory, and social spheres, and a modest increase in mental age and IQ. Deterioration in clinical status occurred on return to placebo. Symptom improvement characterized patients with both normal and increased base-line blood serotonin levels. There were minimal adverse reactions to the drugs (83). Other investigators have joined in a multicenter study of fenfluramine treatment of autism. The drug consistently causes a decrease in blood serotonin levels; however, behavioral and cognitive responses are more variable, although some improvement in individual patients continues to be reported (84,85). Other neuroleptic and anticonvulsant drugs also cause a reduction in brain serotonin levels (75).

An understanding of hyperserotonemia has been complicated by the observations that (a) increased blood serotonin levels in male monkeys have a state-dependent association with active occupation of the dominant male social position (86) and (b) decreased CSF levels of 5-hydroxyindoleacetic acid (5-HIAA, the major serotonin metabolite) are related to a lower level of global function in children with autism and other severe developmental disorders (87–89). It is not clear whether this reflects etiological heterogeneity or an inadequate understanding of serotonergic function and clinical measures. In addition, serotonergic function cannot be considered in isolation but must be evaluated in relation to the activities of other neuronal systems.

Catecholamines

Dopamine: Abnormal Involuntary Movements and Cognitive Deficits

Altered dopaminergic function has been implicated as a component of behavioral impairments in autism as in other neuropsychiatric disorders in children and adults.

The strongest evidence has been that the drugs that have been most efficacious in the treatment of various symptoms in autistic individuals have been dopamine receptor blocking agents, the neuroleptics; dopamine agonists typically aggravate the symptoms (90). Increased dopaminergic function, as measured by cerebrospinal fluid levels of homovanillic acid (HVA, the major dopamine metabolite), is associated with reduced social responsiveness and attention and amplification of motoric stereotypies in autistic children (87,88,91). This is similar to the association observed between plasma HVA levels and global symptom severity in adult schizophrenic patients (92). The ratio of CSF serotonin and dopamine metabolites (5-HIAA/HVA) highlights the interactive relationship among neuronal systems and has been a useful index in both autistic children and children with Tourette's syndrome of chronic multiple tics, as a higher ratio is associated with higher functional competence in these two groups of children (87–89). On the other hand, regional depletion of dopamine in the prefrontal cortex of the rhesus monkey causes a cognitive deficit that is reversible by dopamine agonists such as L-dopa and apomorphine (93).

Norepinephrine: Dysregulation of Attention, Arousal, and Habituation

Noradrenergic indices have also been investigated in autistic subjects. Urinary free catecholamines and MHPG were significantly decreased in autistic boys compared to normal boys (94,95). These findings may be related to disturbances in attention, arousal, and cardiovascular indices in autistic patients. The breadth of functions affected by noradrenergic systems in the brain has suggested that many symptoms in autism might be influenced by the principal norepinephrine-containing neuronal system, the locus coeruleus (NE–LC system) (96). For example, there has been investigation of a possible role for NE–LC activity in attentional function, contributing to a filtering of irrelevant stimuli when attention to a specific set of stimuli is required. In rats with lesions of a portion of the NE–LC system, the dorsal bundle, extinction of certain learned responses occurs slowly, and perseveration on other tasks is observed (97,98). This combination of distractibility and perseveration matches prominent characteristics of autistic individuals and is of special interest in relation to complex features such as the resistance to change observed in autism. The NE–LC system may mediate other components of behavior such as arousal, anxiety, learning, and cardiovascular function, so it retains its position as a primary focus of investigation in autism (99).

Neuroendocrine and Neuropeptide Research in Autism

Subgroups of autistic patients show nonsuppression of cortisol levels in response to dexamethasone or blunted plasma growth hormone response to L-dopa (100,101). Further investigation of neuroendocrine mechanisms and possible hypothalamic dysregulation is a fundamental goal for neurochemical research on autism. These mechanisms may be especially important sources of dysfunction during conditions of stress (102,103).

Measurement of opioid peptide levels in the CSF of 20 autistic children and four children with other childhood psychoses gave intriguing results. The receptor assay utilized detects pools of opioid peptides in the CSF without identifying specific opioid peptides or peptide systems. This determination includes a chromatographic procedure that separates opioid activity into endorphin fractions I and II. The two childhood psychosis groups had higher mean CSF endorphin fraction II levels than the control group, and 55% of the 20 autistic patients had levels higher than the highest among the normal children. A trend toward an association between both decreased pain sensitivity and greater self-destructiveness and high fraction II levels was observed. There was no relationship between peptide levels and age, sex, or IQ (104).

Another approach to delineating the possible role of opioid peptide systems in autism has been the administration of trial doses of naltrexone, a potent, long-acting oral opiate antagonist. Low doses given to one 5-year-old nonverbal autistic boy led to a reduction in hyperactivity, impulsivity, sterotypies, and aggressiveness; in contrast to this tranquilizing effect, higher doses were stimulating, with facilitating effects on language and social behaviors (105). Another group of investigators examined the effects of naltrexone on self-injurious behaviors in a mentally retarded youth. This was based on the theory that self-injurious behavior might occur because the release of endogenous opiates following injury serves as a positive reinforcement. In this patient, naltrexone led to a 33% reduction in self-injurious behaviors, with a return to base line at the time of resuming placebo (106).

NEUROIMMUNOLOGICAL PERSPECTIVES ON AUTISM AND PERVASIVE DEVELOPMENTAL DISORDERS

A novel approach to possible causes of hyperserotonemia has suggested the presence of an antibody to brain serotonin (5-hydroxytryptamine, 5-HT) receptors in a subgroup of autistic children. Screening of children with autism for autoimmune phenomena demonstrated antibodies directed against human cortical 5-HT binding sites. A classification utilizing four discrete brain 5-HT binding site subtypes (5-HT_{1A}, 5-HT_{1B}, 5-HT_2, 5-HT_3) was applied in a study of sera and CSF from a 9-year-old girl meeting criteria for infantile autism. They characterized 5-HT binding sites in human, bovine, and rat cerebral cortex membranes and found that both pharmacological and physical characteristics of the 5-HT_1 class of receptors are conserved across these species. The 5-HT_3 binding site does not occur in rat cortical membranes.

Antibodies from the autistic girl were characterized and applied to the examination of 5-HT receptor subtypes; the antibodies were shown to block 5-HT_{1A} binding sites. Investigation of CSF from this autistic girl showed an IgG-mediated decrease in the number of 5-HT_1 binding sites. This spinal fluid inhibitory factor has a concentration four times as high as that found in serum. The antibody from the autistic girl was incubated with human, bovine, and rat cortical membranes to demonstrate that, in spite of the pharmacological and physical similarities among the 5-

HT_{1A} binding sites in these species, inhibition of 5-HT binding in the rat or bovine membranes did not occur, and there are evident differences in the antigenic domains of the 5-HT_{1A} binding protein across species. This research demonstrated the presence of autoantibodies against 5-HT binding proteins in the blood and CSF of an autistic girl; they are of the IgG class, differentiate 5-HT_{1A} from other 5-HT binding proteins, and are specific for human 5-HT_{1A} binding sites. A subgroup of autistic children may have an autoimmune disorder, and further study of 13 autistic children demonstrated seven to have circulating antibodies against human brain 5-HT receptors, whereas none were found in 13 normal children (107). A 5-HT_{1A} receptor polypeptide in rat brain has recently been identified by photoaffinity labeling, and a selective radioligand for the receptor has been synthesized, promising continued progress in this new direction for research (108,109).

Research on the cell-mediated immune response to a brain tissue antigen (human myelin basic protein) in 17 autistic children and 11 patients with similar severe disorders disclosed an abnormality in 13 of the autistic subjects and none of the comparison group. This demonstration of inhibition of macrophage migration in the autistic group was the first evidence of an autoimmune response to brain antigen in autistic children. The results appeared to be independent of drug treatment effects (110). Other researchers suggested a link between these findings and hyperserotonemia by pointing out that myelin basic protein contains a serotonin binding site in its tryptophan peptide region; this region is immunologically active and responds by activating lymphocytes. They propose theories linking myelin basic protein and serotonin in the genesis of autism (111).

Another immunological study of families of autistic children produced interesting preliminary findings. The HLA antigens of 52 sets of parents of autistic children were compared with HLA antigens of 83 sets of parents of normal children reported in the literature. Seventy-five percent of the subject groups shared at least one antigen, whereas this occurred in 22% of the control group. This significant difference raises questions concerning possible mechanisms for immune attack on the fetoplacental unit by maternal antibodies (112). In a follow-up study, 11 of 20 (55%) sets of parents of autistic children were found to share antigens, whereas 15 of 20 (75%) sets of parents of normal children shared antigens. This difference was not significant, so the findings of the first study were not supported. This led these investigators to hypothesize that autism might be an autoimmune disorder. The data gave partial support to this view, but further studies of both hypotheses are necessary (113).

RESEARCH ON NEUROANATOMICAL LOCALIZATION OF PATHOLOGY IN AUTISM

Imaging Methods Applied to Autistic Subjects

Pneumoencephalography and Computed Tomographic Brain Scanning

Pneumoencephalographic (PEG) studies suggested enlargement of the left ventricular system, particularly the left temporal horn, in developmentally disabled children. There was no relationship between severity of PEG abnormalities and either intelligence or symptom severity (114). Investigation of brain morphology by computed tomographic (CT) brain scanning in several centers indicates that a higher than usual percentage of patients with autism and related developmental disorders have abnormalities, but no distinct abnormal features occur that identify subgroups of children or correspond to symptom severity; other studies show no increase in abnormalities (115–122). Some aspects of brain structure measures on CT scan may show greater heterogeneity in autistic children (120). In summary, CT scan abnormalities vary widely in their anatomical location and features in autistic individuals (including increased ventricular size, reduced cerebral asymmetry, high-density areas, etc.), are inconsistently present, and have not been confirmed in all studies.

New Imaging Methods

Regional cerebral blood flow, measured in autistic men with the ^{133}Xe inhalation technique, showed significantly lower gray matter flow in both right and left hemispheres. A moderate correlation between gray matter flow pattern and IQ suggests that this might reflect mental retardation. Hyperfrontal flow was absent on the right side during the resting state and less prominent on the left side than in normal controls; this finding could reflect altered attentional capacities. A reduction in interhemispheric homogeneity in the sensorimotor area in the autistic men suggested an altered cognitive response to the resting state. The decline in cerebral blood flow typically observed in normals between the first and second rest states, thought to reflect habituation to the task, did not occur in the autistic subjects. This might be a further indication of both cognitive dysfunction and altered frontal lobe function and led to speculation that there was abnormal mesolimbic dopaminergic function (subcortical to frontal cortical projections) in the autistic subjects (123).

The cerebral metabolic rate for glucose was studied in autistic men and controls by positron emission tomography (PET) with ^{18}F-fluoro-2-deoxy-D-glucose (FDG) during rest without stimulation. There were no deficiencies in absolute resting cerebral metabolic rates for glucose (diffuse or focal). Diffusely elevated metabolic rates were observed in the autistic men, but there was substantial overlap with the control subjects. These autistic men had normal CT scans. The cause of the elevated glucose utilization is unknown; it has also been reported in adults with Down's syndrome. Some autistic subjects had one or more regions with extreme relative metabolic rates (124).

Magnetic resonance imaging methods have been utilized to assess only a small number of autistic individuals, and their capacity to detect pathological structures in these patients is not yet known.

Neuropathologic Studies

Very few brains from deceased autistic individuals have been evaluated by neuropathologic examination, although procedures for interinstitutional cooperation have now been established by the National Society for Autistic Children to facilitate postmortem studies. Difficult problems continue to plague this research, including diagnostic heterogeneity, varied causes of the premature death of the individuals, confounding effects of retardation, coexisting medical conditions, seizures, and medication, and varying delays prior to preparation of brain tissue for examination. A variety of abnormalities in conditions related to autism have been reported, but a lack of pathological findings has been most common (126). One laboratory reported no abnormalities following a complete neuropathologic examination of brains from four autistic and retarded individuals, one of whom had phenylketonuria (127). Another laboratory utilized meticulous cell counts in specific regions of the cerebral cortex of an autistic woman and two controls. No consistent differences in cell density (numbers of neurons and glia) were found in the primary auditory cortex, Broca speech area, and auditory association cortex (128).

Another neuropathologic approach applied a comparison microscope (allowing visualization of comparable areas side by side) to the examination of the brain of a 19-year-old retarded, autistic man and an age- and sex-matched control. Abnormalities were present in the forebrain (hippocampal complex, entorhinal cortex, septal nuclei, mamillary body), amygdala (central, medial, and cortical nuclei), neocerebellar cortex, roof nuclei of the cerebellum, and the inferior olivary nucleus. The changes observed in the forebrain-amygdala were reduced neuronal size and increased cell density, common features in an immature brain. Cerebellar abnormalities also suggested lesions occurring early in development (129).

STUDIES OF BRAIN ACTIVITY IN AUTISM: ELECTROPHYSIOLOGICAL RESEARCH

Electroencephalography

Electroencephalographic (EEG) recordings have continued as a standard component of the evaluation of autistic children. Although the EEG is utilized to exclude discrete, undetected brain pathology, it has not achieved a significant role in the specification of diagnosis or treatment except in the subgroup (approximately 25%) of autistic patients who develop seizures (130–133).

There are a higher number of EEG abnormalities in autistic patients, but the patterns of deviant records vary, and EEG–clinical correlations have failed to establish replicable subgroups. Deficient hemispheric lateralization is a possible exception, as several investigators have reported an absence of the normal left hemisphere increment in EEG voltage and activation in autistic individuals (134–136).

Event-Related Potentials

Brainstem auditory evoked responses (BAER) have been examined in autistic individuals in many clinical research laboratories in an attempt to uncover deficits in sensory modulation at the brainstem level. The brainstem transmission time (BSTT) has been reported to be prolonged in some studies but normal in others. Careful matching for age and sex should clarify these discrepant findings in future research, and prolonged BSTTs may identify a homogeneous subgroup of autistic children under those conditions (137–141). Such data may be better understood when examined in association with other indices suggesting significant brainstem pathophysiology in autism, such as impaired autonomic responsivity and abnormal vestibulo-ocular responses (142–144).

Further refinement of electrophysiological techniques for the examination of information processing in autistic individuals may illuminate poorly understood clinical phenomena. Clinical investigators have proposed that autistic children do not orient to novel information normally, whether because a response is lacking or abnormal or because a response to prior stimuli persists. The P300 component of event-related potentials is responsive to unexpected or novel stimuli, and several studies have shown that the auditory P300 is reduced in amplitude in autistic subjects (145–148). Additional research extended these findings to indicate that nonretarded autistic adolescents and young adults are able to detect novel auditory and visual information and to make simple classification decisions in relation to these stimuli. They do not misperceive the auditory and visual stimuli as insignificant or nonnovel; on the other hand, they are not hypersensitive to novel information. These results suggest that it is unlikely that differences in the ERP components of the autistic group can be attributed to poor motivation, and the abnormalities do not indicate a maturational delay.

The findings indicate that autistic individuals have a limited or selective capacity to orient to novel information, that the visual ERP abnormalities (i.e., the components affected) during performance of a sustained attention task were different from the auditory ERP abnormalities, and that classification of simple visual information may be less impaired than auditory classification processes (149). Orienting to novel information is fundamental to the development of cognitive processes, and a partial diminution of this capacity could have far-reaching effects and contribute not only to cognitive impairments but to a child's resistance to change, limited language, and oddities in social relations (150).

PERSPECTIVES: RESEARCH ON AUTISM, DEVELOPMENTAL DISORDERS, AND MENTAL RETARDATION

New perspectives promise to enrich genetic and biological studies of autism. Reconsideration of classification of the pervasive developmental disorders will improve confidence in research on these illnesses and amplify the knowledge generated by genetic and biological investigation (151,152). Extensive research in developmental neurobiology has been minimally applied to clinical studies of autism. Impaired regulation of developmental phenomena (neurotransmitter plasticity, trophic hormones, cell recognition molecules, regressive events, and myelination) may play a pathophysiological role. Abnormalities in basic behavioral dimensions

of the severe disorders of childhood will be fruitfully examined. For example, clinical research related to the neurobiology of learning and memory in childhood may clarify aspects of the loss of brain plasticity in mental retardation and the pervasive developmental disorders (153). Similarly, operational definition of the core symptom in autism, pervasive lack of responsiveness to others, will facilitate neurobiological studies of attachment behaviors. Myelination of limbic structures in the first postnatal months, the role of thalamocingulate and prefrontal structures in attachment behaviors, and identification of ensembles of neurons in the amygdala and cortex of the superior temporal sulcus of the monkey that have response selectivity for faces are examples of neurobiological phenomena that may enlighten and guide clinical research on attachment behaviors. Clinical investigation of autism, developmental disorders, and mental retardation carries the hope of alleviating great losses in human potential.

ACKNOWLEDGMENTS

We are grateful to Ms. A. Cooper for preparation of the manuscript. We are appreciative of support of research activities by the Office of Mental Retardation and Developmental Disabilities, State of New York, The Rosenstiel Foundation, and The Shulman Foundation.

REFERENCES

1. Young, J. G., Cohen, D. J., Shaywitz, S. E., et al. (1982): *Schizophrenia Bull.,* 8:205–235.
2. Kanner, L. (1943): *Nerv. Child,* 2:217–250.
3. Sigman, M., and Ungerer, J. (1984): *J. Autism Dev. Disorders,* 14(3):231–244.
4. Waters, E., and Deane, K. E. (1985): *Soc. Res. Child Dev.,* 50: 41–65.
5. Stahlecker, J. E., and Cresci Cohen, M. (1985): *Child Dev.,* 56: 502–507.
6. Rutter, M. (1983): *J. Child Psychol. Psychiatry,* 24:513–531.
7. Fein, D., Waterhouse, L., Lucci, D., and Snyder, D. (1985): *J. Autism Dev. Disorders,* 15:77–95.
8. Cohen, D. J., Caparulo, B. K., and Shaywitz, B. A. (1976): *J. Am. Acad. Child Psychiatry,* 15:606–645.
9. Paul, R., Cohen, D. J., and Caparulo, B. K. (1983): *J. Am. Acad. Child Psychiatry,* 22:525–534.
10. Rutter, M. (1968): *J. Child Psychol. Psychiatry,* 9:1–25.
11. Bartak, I., Rutter, M., and Cox, A. (1975): *Br. J. Psychiatry,* 126: 127–145.
12. Finegan, J., and Quarrington, B. (1979): *J. Child Psychol. Psychiatry,* 20:119–128.
13. Deykin, E. Y., and MacMahon, B. (1980): *Am. J. Dis. Child.,* 134:860–864.
14. Gillberg, C., and Gillberg, I. C. (1983): *J. Autism Dev. Disorders,* 13:153–166.
15. Mason-Brothers, A., Ritvo, E. R., Guze, B., Mo, A., Freeman, B. J., Funderburk, S. J., and Schroth, P. C. (1987): *J. Amer. Acad. Child Adol. Psychiatry,* 26: 39–42.
16. Campbell, M., Geller, B., Small, A. M., Petti, T. A., and Ferris, S. H. (1978): *Am. J. Psychiatry,* 135:573–575.
17. Chess, S. (1977): *J. Autism Child. Schizo.,* 7:69–81.
18. Stubbs, E. G. (1978): *J. Autism Child. Schizo.,* 8:37–43.
19. Deykin, E. Y., and MacMahon, B. (1979): *Am. J. Epidemiol.,* 109:628–638.
20. Markowitz, P. I. (1983): *J. Autism Dev. Disorders,* 13:249–253.
21. Young, J. G., Caparulo, B. K., Shaywitz, B. A., Johnson, W. T., and Cohen, D. J. (1977): *J. Am. Acad. Child Psychiatry,* 16:174–179.

22. Lowe, T. L., Tanaka, K., Seashore, M. R., Young, J. G., and Cohen, D. J. (1980): *J.A.M.A.,* 243:126–128.
23. Ritvo, E. R., Ritvo, E. C., and Brothers, A. M. (1982): *J. Autism Dev. Disorders,* 12:109–114.
24. Folstein, S. E. (1985): *Annu. Rev. Med.,* 36:415–419.
25. Folstein, S., and Rutter, M. (1977): *J. Child Psychol. Psychiatry,* 18:297–321.
26. August, G. J., Stewart, M. A., and Tsai, L. (1981): *Br. J. Psychiatry,* 138:416–422.
27. Minton, J., Campbell, M., Green, W. H., Jennings, S., and Samit, C. (1982): *J. Am. Acad. Child Psychiatry,* 21:256–261.
28. Baird, T. D., and August, G. J. (1985): *J. Autism Dev. Disorders,* 15:315–321.
29. Wing, L. (1981): *Psychol. Med.,* 11:115–129.
30. Schopler, E. (1985): *J. Autism Dev. Dis.,* 15:359–360.
31. Ritvo, E. R., Freeman, B. J., Mason-Brothers, A., Mo, A., and Ritvo, A. M. (1985): *Am. J. Psychiatry,* 142:74–77.
32. Ritvo, E. R., Spence, M. A., Freeman, B. J., Mason-Brothers, A., Mo, A., and Marazita, M. L. (1985): *Am. J. Psychiatry,* 142: 187–192.
33. Biesele, N. J., Schmid, W., and Lawlis, M. G. (1962): *Lancet,* 3: 403–405.
34. Book, J. A., Nichtern, S., and Gruenberg, E. (1963): *Acta Psychiatr. Scand.,* 39:309–323.
35. Judd, L. L., and Mandell, A. J. (1968): *Arch. Gen. Psychiatry,* 18:450–457.
36. Wolraich, M., Bzostek, B., Neu, R. L., and Gardner, L. (1970): *N. Engl. J. Med.,* 283:1231.
37. Gillberg, C., and Wahlstrom, J. (1985): *Dev. Med. Child Neurol.,* 27:293–304.
38. Lubs, H. A. (1969): *Am. J. Hum. Genet.,* 21:231–244.
39. Sutherland, G. R. (1977): *Science,* 197:265–266.
39a Jennings, M., Hall, J. G., and Hoehn, H. (1980): *Am. J. Med. Genet.,* 7:417–432.
40. Herbst, D. S. (1980): *Am. J. Med. Genet.,* 7:443–460.
41. Turner, G., Daniel, A., and Frost, M. (1980): *J. Pediatr.,* 96: 837–841.
42. Carpenter, N. J., Leichtman, L. G., and Say, B. (1982): *Am. J. Dis. Child.,* 136:392–398.
43. Blomquist, H. K., Gustavson, K.-H., Holmgren, G., Nordenson, I., and Sweins, A. (1982): *Clin. Genet.,* 21:209–214.
44. Blomquist, H. K., Gustavson, K.-H., Holmgren, G., Nordenson, I., and Palsson-Strae, U. (1983): *Clin. Genet.,* 24:393–398.
45. Brown, W. T., Jenkins, E. C., Friedman, E., Brooks, J., Wisniewki, K., Raguthu, S., and French, J. (1982): *J. Autism Dev. Disorders,* 12(3):303–309.
46. Meryash, D. L., Szymanski, L. S., and Gerald, P. S. (1982): *J. Autism Dev. Disorders,* 12:295–301.
47. Watson, M. S., Leckman, J. F., Annex, B., Breg, W. R., Boles, D., et al. (1984): *N. Engl. J. Med.,* 310:1462.
48. Pueschel, S. M., Herman, R., and Groden, G. (1985): *J. Autism Dev. Disorders,* 15:335–338.
49. Rosenblatt, D. S., Duschenes, E. A., Hellstrom, F. V., Golick, M. S., Vekemans, M. J. J., Zeesman, S. F., and Andermann, E. (1985): *Am. J. Hum. Genet.,* 37:543–552.
50. Garvey, M., and Mutton, D. E. (1973): *Arch. Dis. Child.,* 48: 937–941.
51. Leonard, M. F., Landy, G., Ruddle, F. H., and Lubs, H. (1974): *Pediatrics,* 54:208–212.
52. Bender, L., Fry, E., Pennington, B., Puck, M., Salbenblatt, J., and Robinson, A. (1983): *Pediatrics,* 71:262–267.
53. Walzer, S. (1985): *J. Child Psychol. Psychiatry,* 26:177–184.
54. Forsius, H., Kaski, U., Schroder, J., and de la Chapelle, A. (1972): *Acta Paedopsychiatr.,* 39:28–41.
55. Nielsen, K. B., Christensen, K. R., Friedrich, U., Zeuthen, E., and Østergaard, O. (1973): *J. Autism Child. Schizo.,* 3:5–26.
56. Hoshino, Y., Yashima, Y., Tachibana, R., Kaneko, M., Watanabe, M. A., and Kumashiro, H. (1979): *Fukushima J. Med. Sci.,* 26: 31–42.
57. Gillberg, C., Winnergard, I., and Wahlstrom, J. (1984): *Appl. Res. Ment. Retard.,* 5:353–360.
58. Wakabayashi, S. (1979): *J. Autism Dev. Disorders,* 9:31–36.
59. Burd, L., Kerbeshian, J., Fisher, W., and Martsolf, J. T. (1985): *J. Autism Dev. Disorders,* 15:351–352.
60. Spence, M. A., Ritvo, E. R., Marazita, M. L., Funderburk, S. J., Sparkes, R. S., and Freeman, B. J. (1985): *Behav. Genet.,* 15:1–13.
61. Wilson, J. M., Young, A. B., and Kelley, W. N. (1983): *N. Engl. J. Med.,* 309:900–909.
62. Stein, S. A., and Morrison, M. R. (1985): *Trends Neurosci.,* 8: 148–150.
63. Lemire, R. J., Loeser, J. D., Leech, R. W., and Alvord, E. C., Jr. (1975): *Normal and Abnormal Development of the Human Nervous System.* Harper & Row, New York.
64. Cowan, W. M. (1979): *Sci. Am.,* 241:112–133.
65. Black, I. B., Adler, J. E., Dreyfus, C. F., Jonakait, G. M., Katz, D. M., La Gamma, E. F., and Markey, K. M. (1984): *Science,* 225:1266–1270.
66. Levi-Montalcini, R. (1982): *Annu. Rev. Neurosci.,* 5:341–362.
67. Goodman, C. S., Bastiani, M. J., Doe, C. Q., du Lac, S., Helfand, S. L., Kuwada, J. Y., and Thomas, J. B. (1984): *Science,* 225: 1271–1279.
68. Cowan, W. M., Fawcett, J. W., O'Leary, D. D. M., and Stanfield, B. B. (1984): *Science,* 225:1258–1265.
69. Young, J. G., Cohen, D. J., Anderson, G. M., and Shaywitz, B. A. (1984): In: *The Psychobiology of Childhood: A Profile of Current Issues,* edited by L. L. Greenhill and B. Shopsin, pp. 51–84. SP Medical Scientific Books, New York.
70. Ciaranello, R. D., Vandenberg, S. R., and Anders, T. F. (1982): *J. Autism Dev. Disorders,* 12:115–145.
71. Schain, R. J., and Freedman, D. X. (1961): *J. Pediatr.,* 58:315–320.
72. Ritvo, E. R., Yuwiler, A., Geller, E., Ornitz, E. M., Saeger, K., and Plotkin, S. (1970): *Arch. Gen. Psychiatry,* 23:566–572.
73. Campbell, M., Friedman, E., De Vito, E., Greenspan, L., and Collins, P. J. (1974): *J. Autism Child. Schizo.,* 4:33–41.
74. Hanley, H. G., Stahl, S. M., and Freedman, D. X. (1977): *Arch. Gen. Psychiatry,* 34:521–531.
75. Anderson, G. M., Hoder, E. L., Volkmar, F. R., Pual, R., McPhedran, P., Minderaa, R. B., Young, J. G., Hansen, C. R., and Cohen, D. J. (1987): *Arch. Gen. Psychiatry* (in press).
76. Young, J. G., Kavanagh, M. E., Anderson, G. M., Shaywitz, B. A., and Cohen, D. J. (1982): *J. Autism Dev. Disorders,* 12(2): 147–165.
77. Young, J. G., Cohen, D. J., and Shaywitz, B. A. (1982): In: *Handbook of Psychiatry 3: Psychoses of Uncertain Aetiology,* edited by L. Wing and J. K. Wing, pp. 229–235. Cambridge University Press, Cambridge.
78. Yuwiler, A., Ritvo, E. R., Geller, E., Glousman, R., Scheiderman, G., et al. (1975): *J. Autism Child. Schizo.,* 5:83–98.
79. Cohen, D. J., Young, J. G., and Roth, J. A. (1977): *Arch. Gen. Psychiatry,* 34:534–537.
80. Kuperman, S., Beeghly, J. H. L., Burns, T. L., and Tsai, L. Y. (1985): *J. Am. Acad. Child Psychiatry,* 24(2):186–190.
81. Ritvo, E. R., Yuwiler, A., Geller, E., et al. (1971): *J. Autism Child. Schizo.,* 1:190–205.
82. Geller, E., Ritvo, E. R., Freeman, B. J., and Yuwiler, A. (1982): *N. Engl. J. Med.,* 307(3):165–168.
83. Ritvo, E. R., Freeman, B. J., Geller, E., and Yuwiler, A. (1983): *J. Am. Acad. Child. Psychiatry,* 22(6):549–558.
84. August, G. J., Raz, N., and Davis Baird, T. (1985): *J. Autism Dev. Disorders,* 15(1):97–107.
85. Klykylo, W. M., Feldis, D., O'Grady, D., Ross, D. L., and Halloran, C. (1985): *J. Autism Dev. Disorders,* 15:417–423.
86. Raleigh, M. J., McGuire, M. T., Brammer, G. L., and Yuwiler, A. (1984): *Arch. Gen. Psychiatry,* 41:405–410.
87. Cohen, D. J., Shaywitz, B. A., Johnson, W. T., and Bowers, M. B., Jr. (1974): *Arch. Gen. Psychiatry,* 31:845–853.
88. Cohen, D. J., Caparulo, B. K., Shaywitz, B. A., and Bowers, M. B. (1977): *Arch. Gen. Psychiatry,* 34:545–550.
89. Cohen, D. J., Shaywitz, B. A., Caparulo, B., Young, J. G., and Bowers, M. B., Jr. (1978): *Arch. Gen. Psychiatry,* 35:245–250.
90. Campbell, M., Anderson, L. T., Small, A. M., Perry, R., Green, W. H., and Caplan, R. (1982): *J. Autism Dev. Disorders,* 12: 167–175.
91. Gillberg, C., Svennerholm, L., and Hamilton-Hellberg, C. (1983): *J. Autism Dev. Disorders,* 13:383–396.

92. Davis, K. L., Davidson, M., Mohs, R. C., Kendler, K. S., Davis, B. M., et al. (1985): *Science,* 227:1601–1602.
93. Brozoski, T. S., Brown, R. M., Rosvold, H. E., and Goldman, P. S. (1979): *Science,* 205:929–931.
94. Young, J. G., Cohen, D. J., Brown, S. L., and Caparulo, B. K. (1978): *J. Am. Acad. Child. Psychiatry,* 17:671–678.
95. Young, J. G., Cohen, D. J., Caparulo, B. K., Brown, S. L., and Maas, J. W. (1979): *Am. J. Psychiatry,* 136:1055–1057.
96. Young, J. G., Cohen, D. J., Shaywitz, B. A., Anderson, G. M., and Maas, J. W. (1982): In: *MHPG in Psychopathology,* edited by J. Maas, pp. 193–218. Academic Press, New York.
97. Mason, S. T., and Iversen, S. D. (1978): *Brain Res.,* 1:107–137.
98. Mason, S. T., and Iversen, S. D. (1978): *Brain Res.,* 150:135–148.
99. Aston-Jones, G., Foote, S. L., and Bloom, F. E. (1984): In: *Norepinephrine,* edited by M. G. Ziegler and C. R. Lake, pp. 92–116. Williams & Wilkins, London.
100. Jensen, J. B., Realmuto, G. M., and Garfinkel, B. D. (1985): *J. Am. Child Psychiatry,* 24:263–265.
101. Deutsch, S. I., Campbell, M., Sachar, E. J., Green, W. H., and David, R. (1985): *J. Autism Dev. Disorders,* 15:205–212.
102. Ciaranello, R. D. (1980): In: *Catecholamines and Stress,* edited by E. Usdin, R. Kvetnansky, and I. J. Kopin, pp. 106–111. Elsevier Press, New York.
103. Ciaranello, R. D. (1983): In: *Stress, Coping, and Development in Children,* edited by N. Garmezy and M. Rutter, pp. 85–105. McGraw-Hill, New York.
104. Gillberg, C., Terenius, L., and Lonnerholm, G. (1985): *Arch. Gen. Psychiatry,* 42:780–783.
105. Campbell, M., Perry, R., Palij, M., Nobler, M., and Shore, H. (1985): In: *Proceedings, Annual Meeting of the American Academy of Child Psychiatry,* edited by L. Greenhill, p. 29. American Academy of Child Psychiatry, Washington, D.C.
106. Bernstein, G. A., Hughes, J. R., Mitchell, J. E., and Thompson, T. (1985): In: *Proceedings, Annual Meeting of the American Academy of Child Psychiatry,* edited by L. Greenhill, p. 33.
107. Todd, R. D., and Ciaranello, R. D. (1985): *Proc. Natl. Acad. Sci. U.S.A.,* 82:612–616.
108. Ransom, R. W., Asarch, K. B., and Shih, J. S. (1985): Identification of a 5-HTIA receptor polypeptide in rat brain by photoaffinity labeling. *Abstr. Soc. Neurosci.,* 11:1257.
109. Asarch, K. B., Ransom, R. W., and Shih, J. C. (1985): *Abst. Soc. Neurosci.,* 11:1257.
110. Weizman, A., Weizman, R., Szekely, G. A., Wijsenbeek, H., and Livni, E. (1982): *Am. J. Psychiatry,* 139:1462–1465.
111. Westall, F. C., and Root-Bernstein, R. S. (1983): *Am. J. Psychiatry,* 140:1260–1261.
112. Stubbs, E. G., Ritvo, E. R., and Mason-Brothers, A. (1985): *J. Am. Acad. Child Psychiatry,* 24(2):182–185.
113. Stubbs, E. G., Budden, S., Borzy, M., and Norman, D. (1985): In: *Proceedings, Annual Meeting of the American Academy of Child Psychiatry,* edited by L. L. Greenhill, p. 28. American Academy of Child Psychiatry, Washington, D.C.
114. Hauser, S. L., DeLong, G. R., and Rosman, N. P. (1975): *Brain,* 98:667–668.
115. Damasio, H., Maurer, R. G., Damasio, A. R., et al. (1980): *Arch. Neurol.,* 37:504–510.
116. Caparulo, B. K., Cohen, D. J., Rothman, S. D., Young, J. G., Katz, J. D., et al. (1981): *J. Am. Acad. Child Psychiatry,* 20:338–357.
117. Campbell, M., Rosenbloom, S., Perry, R., George, A. E., Kricheff, I. I., et al. (1982): *Am. J. Psychiatry,* 139:510–512.
118. Hier, D. B., LeMay, M., and Rosenberger, P. B. (1979): *J. Autism Dev. Disorders,* 9:153–159.
119. Tsai, L. Y., Jacoby, C. G., and Stewart, M. A. (1983): *Biol. Psychiatry,* 18(3):317–327.
120. Rosenbloom, S., Campbell, M., George, A. E., Kricheff, I. I., Taleporos, E., et al. (1984): *J. Am. Acad. Child Psychiatry,* 23(1):72–77.
121. Prior, M. R., Tress, B., Hoffman, W. L., et al. (1984): *Arch. Neurol.,* 41:482–484.
122. Harcherik, D. F., Cohen, D. J., Ort, S., Paul, R., Shaywitz, B. A., et al. (1985): *Am. J. Psychiatry,* 142:731–734.
123. Sherman, M., Nass, R., and Shapiro, T. (1984): *J. Autism Dev. Disorders,* 14(4):439–446.
124. Rumsey, J. M., Duara, R., Grady, C., Rapoport, J. L., Margolin, R. A., et al. (1985): *Arch. Gen. Psychiatry,* 42:448–455.
125. Gaffney, G. R., Kuperman, S., Tsai, L., and Dunn, V. (1985): In: *Proceedings, Annual Meeting of the American Academy of Child Psychiatry,* edited by L. L. Greenhill, p. 28. American Academy of Child Psychiatry, Washington, D.C.
126. Darby, J. K. (1976): Neuropathologic aspects of psychosis in children. *J. Autism Child. Schizo.,* 6:339–352.
127. Williams, R. S., Hauser, S. L., Purpura, D. P., DeLong, G. R., and Swisher, C. N. (1980): *Arch. Neurol.,* 37:749–753.
128. Coleman, P. D., Romano, J., Lapham, L., and Simon, W. (1985): *J. Autism Dev. Disorders,* 15(3):245–255.
129. Bauman, M., and Kemper, T. L. (1985): *Neurology (N.Y.),* 35:866–874.
130. Waldo, M. C., Cohen, D. J., Caparulo, B. K., Young, J. G., Prichard, J. W. et al. (1978): *J. Am. Acad. Child Psychiatry,* 17:656–670.
131. Deykin, E. Y., and MacMahon, B. (1979): *Am. J. Psychiatry,* 136:1310–1312.
132. Tanguay, P. E., and Edwards, R. M. (1982): *J. Autism Dev. Disorders,* 12:177–184.
133. Tsai, L. Y., Tsai, M. C., and August, G. J. (1985): *J. Autism Dev. Disorders,* 15(3):339–344.
134. Small, J. G. (1975): *Biol. Psychiatry,* 10:385–397.
135. Dawson, G., Warrenburg, S., and Fuller, P. (1982): *Brain Lang.,* 15:353–368.
136. Ogawa, T., Sugiyama, A., Ishiwa, S., Suzuki, M., Ishihara, T. et al. (1982): *Brain Dev.,* 4:439–449.
137. Fein, D., Skoff, B., and Mirsky, A. F. (1981): *J. Autism Dev. Disorders,* 11:303–315.
138. Tanguay, P. E., Edwards, R. M., Buchwald, J., Schwafel, J., and Allen, V. (1982): *Arch. Gen. Psychiatry,* 39:174–180.
139. Piggott, L. R., and Anderson, T. (1983): *J. Am. Acad. Child Psychiatry,* 22:6:535–540.
140. Rumsey, J. M., Grimes, A. M., Pikus, A. M., Duara, R., and Ismond, D. R. (1984): *Biol. Psychiatry,* 19(10):1403–1418.
141. Ornitz, E. M. (1985): *J. Am. Acad. Child Psychiatry,* 24:251–262.
142. Cohen, D. J., and Johnson, W. T. (1977): *Arch. Gen. Psychiatry,* 34:561–567.
143. Kootz, J. P., and Cohen, D. J. (1981): *J. Am. Acad. Child Psychiatry,* 20:692–701.
144. Ornitz, E. M., Atwell, C. T., Kaplan, A. R., and Westlake, J. R. (1985): *Arch. Gen. Psychiatry,* 42:1018–1025.
145. Small, J. G., DeMyer, M. K., and Milstein, V. (1971): *J. Autism Child. Schizo.,* 1:215–231.
146. Novick, B., Kurtzberg, A., and Vaughan, H. G., Jr. (1979): *Psychiatry Res.,* 1:101–108.
147. Novick, B., Vaughan, H. G., Jr., Kurtzberg, D., and Simson, R. (1980): *Psychiatry Res.,* 3:107–114.
148. Courchesne, E., Kilman, B. A., Galambos, R., and Lincoln, A. J. (1984): *Electroencephalogr. Clin. Neurophysiol.,* 59:238–248.
149. Courchesne, E., Lincoln, A. J., Kilman, B. A., and Galambos, R. (1985): *J. Autism Dev. Disorders,* 15:55–76.
150. Knight, R. T. (1984): *Electroencephalogr. Clin. Neurophysiol.,* 59:9–20.
151. Volkmar, F., Cohen, D. J., and Paul, R. (1986): *J. Am. Acad. Child Psychiatry,* 25:190–197.
152. Waterhouse, L., Fein, D., Nath, J., and Snyder, D. (1984): In: *DSM-III: An Interim Appraisal,* edited by G. Tischler, pp. 82–109. American Psychiatric Association, Washington.
153. Young, J. G. (1985): In: *Psychiatry, Vol. 2,* edited by R. Michels and J. O. Cavenar. J. B. Lippincott, Philadelphia.

Psychopharmacology:
The Third Generation of Progress,
edited by Herbert Y. Meltzer.
Raven Press, New York © 1987.

CHAPTER 83

Noradrenergic Hypothesis of Attention Deficit Disorder with Hyperactivity: A Critical Review

Alan J. Zametkin and Judith L. Rapoport

Several theoretical models of the pathophysiology of attention deficit disorder with hyperactivity (ADDH) have been developed over the past 20 years. Typically, these models have postulated some deficit or dysregulation of specific monoamine neurotransmitter systems. At least 10 papers have suggested different anatomical areas of CNS dysfunction. It is beyond the scope of this critique to review all the models, but a critical review of the noradrenergic hypothesis is presented as, to date, this is the strongest model based on both basic studies and clinical research.

Despite the lack of consistent differences between ADDH children and controls on noradrenergic parameters and the lack of an adequate noradrenergic animal model of ADDH, current psychopharmacological trials support a noradrenergic hypothesis in many cases, but not in all.

The noradrenergic system is often summarized as consisting of three major systems: the dorsal noradrenergic, ventral tegmental, and medulla–spinal cord systems.

DORSAL NORADRENERGIC SYSTEM

The cell bodies of this system lie in the locus coeruleus (A6, A4, A7). This blue-pigmented area in the brainstem reticular formation lies on the floor of the fourth ventricle. It is from this source that fibers ascend via the dorsal noradrenergic bundle and the medial forebrain bundle (MFB) to terminate diffusely in all areas of the cortex.

Some collateral fibers terminate on the Purkinje cells of the cerebellum. This system has an extremely wide distribution over global brain areas.

It is this system that has been suggested to play a role in arousal, affect, and attention (17).

LATERAL TEGMENTAL SYSTEM

The cell bodies of this system are found throughout the medulla and pons (A1, A2, A3, A4). The axons of this system form the diffuse ventral noradrenergic bundle, which passes to various subcortical areas, especially the hypothalamus.

MEDULLA AND SPINAL CORD

Axons originating in the locus coeruleus pass via the lateral sympathetic columns of the spinal cord to terminate at various levels of the cord. Although the role of this system is not well worked out, the axons also project throughout the cerebrum, modulating activities of many types of cells.

With an appreciation for the distribution of the noradrenergic system in the central nervous system, previous neuroanatomical hypotheses for the locus of pathology for dysfunction in ADDH children can be examined. As will become apparent, only a small number of these neuroanatomical hypotheses involve areas known to be involved in noradrenergic neurotransmission.

NEUROANATOMICAL HYPOTHESES OF ADDH

Eleven groups have speculated that specific areas of the brain may be dysfunctional in children with ADDH.

Laufer et al. (23), who provided much of the early clinical description of the syndrome of "hyperkinesis," first hypothesized that the symptoms of ADDH were caused by diencephalic dysfunction (23). The diencephalic structures that involve noradrenergic neurotransmission include median forebrain bundle and hypothalamus. Their studies using photometrazol to elicit spike-and-wave discharges on EEG represent the earliest neurophysiological attempts to localize anatomical abnormalities in this population of children. Their pioneering efforts influenced subsequent theoretical efforts and stimulated considerable research. Because the diencephalon includes thalamus, hypothalamus, subthalamus, and epithalamus, the theory of Laufer et al. included many different brain structures with an array of functions, making it difficult to test their hypotheses in any anatomically specific way.

In 1971, Satterfield and Dawson (37) proposed that the syndrome of hyperactivity was associated with lowered levels of reticular activating system excitation. The notion that these children were underaroused sparked a multitude of studies that provided inconsistent results. After review of EEG, skin conductance, and other studies of autonomic arousal, Rosenthal and Allen (1978) conclude that:

> . . . it does *not* appear that hyperkinetics exhibit lower than normal levels of an autonomic arousal, which is contradictory to the underarousal hypothesis. A second feature of the low-RAS notion is that amphetamine and methylphenidate are beneficial because they increase arousal. Indeed, the data indicate that stimulants increase tonic autonomic levels and also the magnitude of cardiac deceleration responses, but they also appear to decrease skin conductance responses. The latter effect is clearly inconsistent with the theory as proposed by Satterfield and Dawson (p. 706).

Callaway's later studies (5) with averaged evoked response further supported Rosenthal and Allen's view, reversing their own earlier hypothesis of hypoarousal in ADDH. Calloway, using event-related potentials and EEG spectra, did note differences between hyperactive and control children, but the nature of the differences in no way supported a hypothesis of either maturational lag or underarousal. Wender's hypothesis (46) focused on the limbic areas associated with positive reinforcement: the medial forebrain bundle and the hypothalamus. His theoretical work generated more interest in monoamine mechanisms and psychopharmacological trials than psychophysiological studies and neuroanatomical investigations. The medial forebrain bundle has not been studied, in most likelihood, because it lacks any selective measurable function. On the other hand, hypothalamic functioning has received indirect attention in ADDH because of the stimulants' growth suppression. Although stimulant effects on growth hormone and appetite

regulation may be "incidental effects" on structures unrelated to the pathophysiology of ADDH, the hypothalamic actions of these drugs could be a clue to an anatomically important site of drug action in these children. Any simple primary lesion of the hypothalamus is most unlikely in that most hypothalamic functions (temperature regulation, autonomic control, and appetite regulation) are not abnormal in these children.

Anatomical localization of anorexogenic drug effects with concomitant assessment of neurotransmitter functioning has been carried out in animals, delineating the hypothalamic control of food regulation. Brain monoamine projections and receptor systems of the lateral and medial hypothalamus have been well worked out (reviewed in 14, 24).

The concomitant finding of stimulant effects on growth led Aarskog, Fevang, and Klove (1) to carry out indirect tests of hypothalamic function. Growth hormone secretion is regulated by the hypothalamic growth hormone-releasing factor. Aarskog demonstrated that growth hormone (GH) was elevated from base line by chronic treatment with methylphenidate but found that the usual increase in GH after L-dopa and dextroamphetamine was diminished after chronic methylphenidate treatment. Shaywitz et al. (39) also assess GH and prolactin responses and found increases concurrent with peak methylphenidate levels. However, Greenhill et al. (13) could not document any change in nocturnal growth hormone release (thought to be the physiologically most meaningful) in children on chronic methylphenidate treatment.

In summary, Wender's hypothesized hypothalamic dysfunction has been tested only indirectly. Future testing of hypothalamic function should include studies with normal control comparison groups, a problematic approach with normal pediatric control groups.

THE NORADRENERGIC HYPOTHESIS

Kornetsky's landmark work *The Psychopharmacology of the Immature Organism* (20) first suggested a specific noradrenergic hypothesis:

> that in the overaroused organism amphetamine may act as an inhibitor of either norepinephrine synthesis or turnover or block the release of norepinephrine. . . . Since amphetamine, a sympathomimetic amine, causes a release of norepinephrine and probably an increase in rate of turnover, it might be expected that there would simply be an increase in norepinephrine causing increased hyperkinetic behavior.

Kornetsky went on to hypothesize that amphetamine may act to bind competitively to postsynaptic NE receptors, reducing noradrenergic neurotransmission. Today competitive inhibition is not described as a mechanism of action of amphetamine on noradrenergic systems, but there is certainly evidence that some drugs effective for ADDH decrease noradrenergic turnover.

Kornetsky postulated that hyperactivity was caused by an increase in noradrenergic neurotransmission. To date, only Hunt et al. (15) have speculated on specific mechanisms that might increase noradrenergic transmission, citing (a) dysregulation of pre- or postsynaptic receptor sensitivity, (b) production or synthesis defects, (c) enzyme abnormalities, (d) synthesis abnormalities, (e) synthesis inhibition as a result of autoreceptor dysfunction or long-loop feedback inhibition from hypersensitive postsynaptic receptors, (f) synthesis acceleration caused by down-regulation of post-synaptic receptors, and (g) synaptic activation from increased release.

Despite the large number of possible defects in neural communication, tools are now available to tease apart different mechanisms. For example, synthesis increase or decrease can be estimated by measuring whole-body turn-over (25). Postsynaptic receptor number can be estimated, at least for dopaminergic systems (54). Using specific pharmacologic probes such as clonidine, an α_2 presynaptic noradrenergic agonist, pre- versus postsynaptic specificity may be obtained.

As summarized above, most neuroanatomical speculation has been vague and marginally tested. Animal models of stimulant drug effects on cerebral glucose utilization have been interesting, showing large differences among stimulants. The nucleus accumbens seems to be the only common area of increased metabolism following lower doses of the stimulants amphetamine and methylphenidate (31).

Lou et al. (26) have localized areas of decreased cerebral blood flow in frontal areas in ADDH children compared to control siblings. These areas are not felt to be associated with specific neurotransmitters.

STUDIES ADDRESSING THE NORADRENERGIC HYPOTHESIS: URINE AND BLOOD STUDIES, PHARMACOLOGIC PROBES, AND BIOCHEMICAL–BEHAVIOR CORRELATIONS

Support for a noradrenergic hypothesis is mostly indirect, and studies comparing ADDH and control children on peripheral measures of urine, plasma, and blood platelets and the more central measure, CSF, have for the most part failed to find any consistent differences.

Urinary catecholamine studies have focused primarily on MHPG (3-methoxy-4-hydroxyphenylglycol, the major metabolite of NE). One laboratory reported that ADDH children excrete less MHPG than normals (41–43), with one independent replication (50). No differences were found in two other independent studies (33,45), and one study found increased MHPG excretion in ADDH (19). Thus, the data comparing MHPG in normals and ADDH children are inconsistent. In the one study showing increased excre-tion of MHPG in ADDH children, the absolute values of MHPG excretion for the ADDH group were quite com-parable to the other studies in ADDH groups, but the excretion of MHPG for the control group in that study was considerably lower than that for the other studies' control group. A possible source of artifact in urinary MHPG studies has been identified by Zametkin et al. (51–53), who found in one study that 4 weeks of treatment with stimulant medication decreased urinary MHPG ex-cretion for at least 2 weeks after medication was discontin-ued. The standard "washout" period for most of the urinary studies reported was 2 weeks only. Hence, differences found between ADDH children and normals might reflect

prior drug use, since the majority of studies reported decreased MHPG excretion in ADDH (consistent with previous drug use).

Early studies measuring endogenous MAO-B in normal and hyperactive children yielded mixed results. Shekim et al. (40) originally reported that hyperactive children have less MAO-B activity than normal controls. This finding was not replicated by Brown et al. (4). Brown et al. did find, however, that the normal decrease of MAO activity between the ages of 6 and 12 found in normal controls was not observed in his sample of 18 ADDH children. Since platelet MAO seems to decrease during childhood and adolescence (49), this is a particularly interesting finding. A relative excess of MAO in childhood would tend to decrease norepinephrine in synapses. If an excess of MAO were contributing to the symptoms of ADDH, then MAO inhibitors might be useful.

If the pathophysiology of this disorder were related to norepinephrine, there might be differences between ADDH children and normals on such peripheral measures of noradrenergic functioning as blood pressure and pulse.

One study comparing plasma NE levels in hyperactive and normal boys (28) found that medication-free ADDH children had similar plasma NE levels and blood pressures as controls while recumbent. Both groups had a similar increase in plasma NE on standing (called postural move-ment). However, the hyperactive group had significantly greater blood pressure or pressor response on standing. Although a number of interpretations are possible, Mikkel-sen speculated that

The hyperactive children released slightly less NE, but increased their blood pressure significantly more than con-trols. This could be due to increased α-adrenergic receptor sensitivity to NE. Noradrenergic nervous systems are regu-lated by presynaptic α_2 receptor feedback mechanisms, which affect both tyrosine hydroxylase activity and neuronal release of NE. Thus, increased α-receptor sensitivity might cause an imbalance with diminished NE release, exaggerated α response, and decreased β-receptor response. The hypoth-esis that α receptors might be supersensitive in hyperactive children is testable, since α_1 and α_2 receptors can be stimulated or blocked by approved drugs, and receptors are accessible in blood platelets.

Noradrenergic mechanisms involved in the pathogenesis of ADDH are also indirectly supported by the preclinical pharmacology of the stimulants. Braestrup (2) and Reigle et al. (35) demonstrated major central noradrenergic (as well as dopaminergic) effects of the stimulants.

In an extensive review of the biochemical actions of the stimulants, Kuczenski (21) noted that, among other findings, amphetamine is more potent as an uptake inhibitor of norepinephrine than of dopamine into synaptosomes and is more potent in blocking norepinephrine storage in vesicles (21, p. 44).

Further direct tests of the hypothesis might compare peripheral noradrenergic (autonomic) functioning, which could be evaluated using a number of interventions. For example, one could look for overshoot in the Valsalva maneuver or at blood pressure measurements on the tilt table, with NE level determinations made during steady state and following tilt. Other measures could include blood pressure recovery time following bolus injections of NE and pupillary diameter following epinephrine instillation in the eye. These tools for the assessment of noradrenergic function are summarized by Gotoh et al. (12).

Pharmacologic Trials Addressing the Noradrenergic Hypothesis

The noradrenergic hypothesis appears testable because of the large number of "relatively" specific noradrenergic agonists and antagonists. A number of investigators have attempted to modify noradrenergic functioning selectively by using such medications as mianserin (22), imipramine (34), desipramine (8,9), and clonidine (16). Langer's (22) study of mianserin at doses consistent with presynaptic α-adrenergic receptor blockade demonstrated no therapeutically effective changes in five subjects in spite of increased plasma NE. The trial was terminated because of postural hypotension and oversedation. Interestingly, urinary MHPG was unchanged.

Studies of tricyclic antidepressants in children with ADDH are more numerous and clinically somewhat more promising. In Rapoport's study (34) as well as the more recent work of Garfinkle et al. (9) and Donnelly et al. (8), a consistent pattern emerges; although as a class the tricyclics are not as effective as the stimulants, the moderate beneficial effect occurs within hours. Donnelly et al. (8) found that with mean daily doses of 98 mg of desipramine, classroom behavior ratings showed maximal improvement by day 3, sustained at week 2 of treatment. Of great interest is that desipramine significantly decreased urinary MHPG excretion on both day 3 and day 14. Blood concentration of the tricyclic did not correlate significantly with clinical change or with changes in MHPG excretion.

The recent work of Donnelly and Garfinkle is consistent with earlier findings. Clonidine, an α-adrenergic agonist, is currently being used in children with ADDH, also with moderate clinical improvement (16).

The antipsychotics were also studied quite extensively in children with ADDH. The majority of studies [as reviewed by Winsberg and Yepes (47)] demonstrated that such drugs as thioridizine and chlorpromazine as well as haloperidol were helpful at low doses in these children in decreasing symptoms of attention and motor restlessness. Most intriguing was the finding of Gittelman et al. (10) that thioridizine effects were additive with methylphenidate. If one hypothesizes that methylphenidate causes an acute release of dopamine and that antipsychotics are dopamine antagonists, this additive effect does not make pharmacological sense. In fact, however, this finding supports another possible mechanism of action for the antipsychotic in this disorder. It is well known that antipsychotics have significant α-adrenergic blocking characteristics. At low doses efficacious in ADDH, the basic literature (30) supports the predominant effect of the antipsychotics as being on α-adrenergic systems. Thus, the efficacy of the antipsychotics is not incompatible with, and may even support, a noradrenergic hypothesis of stimulant drug action of ADDH.

Monoamine Oxidase Inhibition

Monoamine oxidase is found in two forms, A and B, distinguished primarily by their substrate specificity (7).

Type A monoamine oxidase deaminates or deactivates norepinephrine and serotonin and normetanephrine (and dopamine in rodents) and is inhibited specifically by clorgyline. Type B MAO deaminates dopamine and phenylethylamine and is selectively inhibited by deprenyl. Tranylcypromine, like most MAOIs in clinical use, is a mixed MAO inhibitor, affecting both types of the enzyme.

As mentioned above, comparisons of platelet MAO-B in normal and hyperactive children have been inconclusive (4,40). As discussed, Brown et al. did find, however, that the normal decrease of MAO activity between the ages of 6 and 12 seen in the normal controls was not observed in his sample of 18 ADDH children.

Three MAO inhibitors have been studied in hyperactive children to date. Six children have received clorgyline, the selective MAO-A inhibitor; eight received tranylcypromine, a mixed MAO-A and -B blocker; 14 received L-deprenyl. The first two drugs had immediate and dramatic therapeutic effects for ADDH children (52,53). Unlike the antidepressant action of MAOIs in adults, effects were apparent within days of initiating treatment. Sustained attention (measured by the Continuous Performance Test) was also significantly improved. These medications were roughly comparable in effect to dextroamphetamine, which was used for comparison in the double-blind crossover study. However, clinically, the stimulant still seemed somewhat superior.

In contrast is Donnelly's ongoing study (M. Donnelly, *personal communication*) of deprenyl, a selective MAO-B inhibitor. At doses of 15 mg/day (a dose thought to inhibit selectively central MAO-B without affecting MAO-A), relatively little therapeutic effect has been observed in the first 14 patients. The relationship between the different types of MAO and their substrates is important to consider. The MAO-A inhibitor (the more potent deactivator of 5-HT and NE) works quite well; a mixed MAO-A and -B inhibitor (dopamine and norepinephrine inactivation) also was effective. Since preliminary evidence indicates that a MAO-B inhibitor (which metabolizes phenylethylamine and dopamine) is ineffective or less effective, noradrenergic metabolism seems to be the common denominator for MAO inhibitors that are effective in treating ADDH.

Studies of the MAO inhibitors are also of theoretical interest in relation to the time course of drug action in hyperactivity. It is well documented that all MAO inhibition (either A or B) is achieved within hours of drug administration. Early changes produced by clorgyline, for example, include reduced NE deamination and increased NE in the synapse. Later adaptive changes include reduced locus coeruleus firing rates and reduced α_1, α_2, and β adrenoceptors (6,29). Persistent functional changes include a decreased central sympathetic outflow with reduced plasma NE. Since the therapeutic efficacy of both clorgyline and tranylcypromine is almost immediate in hyperactivity, it is unlikely that receptor sensitivity change accounts for therapeutic action. To clarify this issue further, behavioral measurements (e.g., continuous performance testing and activity monitoring) should be made after initial single doses of MAOIs to clarify immediate versus adaptive changes in neurochemistry.

Clorgyline's efficacy is particularly interesting, as this agent, unlike tranylcypromine, lacks direct amphetamine-like sympathetic stimulation and amine transport effects across various membranes (29). The specificity of clorgyline is further supported by the work of Murphy et al. (29), showing that 5-HIAA changes were considerably smaller when compared to MHPG, for example. The "purity" of drug effects, however, is often short-lived.

It should be noted that a recent study found that clorgyline may alter dopaminergic function, at least in rodents (48). Chronic treatment elevates the endogenous DA level and might therefore be expected to down-regulate normosensitive DA receptors (27). As our clinical effects are immediate, however, the dopaminergic changes would be unrelated.

In theory, any effects of deprenyl would be hard to interpret because the drug is partially metabolized to amphetamine (18); these considerations make the preliminary unimpressive results even more striking.

Biochemical–Behavioral Correlations of MHPG

The last line of evidence supporting a role of norepinephrine is that drugs ameliorating ADDH often alter MHPG, the major metabolite of norepinephrine. The finding that dextroamphetamine reduces the urinary excretion of MHPG has been replicated by three independent groups (3,41,42,51), a rarity in clinical research.

Zametkin et al. (51) were unable to demonstrate an effect of methylphenidate on urinary MHPG in an initial study or replication (*unpublished data*). Other recent work at the NIH (8) also implicated the noradrenergic systems with significant reductions in urinary MHPG after desipramine (moderately efficacious in ADDH). On the other hand, fenfluramine, an entirely ineffective agent, also lowered MHPG excretion.

A third line of support for a noradrenergic role in the pathophysiology of ADDH is the behavioral–biochemical correlative data from a number of recent drug trials of tricyclic antidepressants and monoamine oxidase inhibitors. Although some studies using these antidepressants find significant correlations between biochemical change and behavioral improvement, certain inconsistencies are also found. Although improvement on *d*-amphetamine and DMI is correlated with MHPG, dissociation between timing and effect is noted with MAOIs (52,53).

Single Neurotransmitter Strategies

Some neurological disorders such as Parkinson's disease, a movement disorder with associated psychiatric symptomatology, have been successfully treated using a neurotransmitter precursor that is metabolized to dopamine.

Although hypotheses of selective neurotransmitter defects are attractive, it is not clear whether one can change the functioning of one transmitter without altering others. This intimate interrelationship between amine systems is clarified in basic neurophysiology, neurochemistry, neuropharmacology, and recent pharmacological work in man. For example, NE is synthesized from DA; although dopamine-β-hydroxylase, the enzyme that converts DA to NE, is not the rate-limiting step in catecholamine production, both NE and DA could feedback inhibit tyrosine hydroxylase (the rate-limiting step) (7).

Second, the noradrenergic tracts in the brain are widespread and diffuse, unlike the more specific dopaminergic systems. In the past, animal studies have focused on the ability of chronically administered antidepressants presumed to have specific actions on either NE or serotonin reuptake. In reviewing these studies as well as more recent human studies, Potter et al. (32) concludes that "specific" antidepressants such as DMI in fact alter both NE and serotonin receptor number and/or function. Thus, it may be difficult to alter one neurotransmitter system with today's "specific" agents. Even such "selective" antidepressants as desipramine (NE reuptake blocker) and zimelidine (serotonin reuptake blocker) have nonselective effects in human subjects (32). Desipramine, for example, reduced 5-HIAA, the serotonin metabolite, whereas zimelidine reduced CSF MHPG as well as 5-HIAA.

Finally, dopamine is a catecholamine with prominent effects on α- and β-adrenergic neurons, although its potency is less than that of epinephrine, norepinephrine, or isoproterenol (11). Thus, the concept of specificity may be both physiologically meaningless and untestable.

THE STIMULANTS: NORADRENERGIC EFFECTS

Dextroamphetamine, methylphenidate, and pemoline are the most effective treatments and, for the most part, benefit the same subjects. (There are rare selective responders to one or the other, but such subjects are beyond the scope of this review.) These questions remain: What systems are crucial for efficacy? Can a common mechanism of action be found in these three agents? Are there any similarities to those MAO inhibitors that are effective treatment?

The preclinical pharmacology of the three drugs shows immediate release of dopamine, although methylphenidate and dextroamphetamine release different pools of dopamine (2). A variety of studies in rat brain also implicate noradrenergic involvement, with methylphenidate and dextroamphetamine occasionally changing catecholamines in opposite directions in selected rat brain areas and in the same direction in others (35).

Dextroamphetamine is a very weak MAO inhibitor, and methylphenidate much weaker still. Preclinical studies of pemoline have focused primarily on dopaminergic effects (44) while not addressing other transmitters. The animal model of ADDH described by Shaywitz et al. (38) suggests dopaminergic involvement in the ameliorating effects of dextroamphetamine.

FUTURE DIRECTIONS

Despite the voluminous and confusing data surrounding the noradrenergic hypothesis of attention deficit disorder with hyperactivity, several key areas need clarification.

1. Differences between hyperactives and controls on the excretion of urinary MHPG should be clarified, controlling for previous drug history and activity and using children with ADDH who have never received stimulants.

2. The finding of Mikkelson et al. (28) should be replicated, demonstrating that for equivalent amount of NE release on standing, hyperactives maintain standing blood pressure more adequately than controls. If replicated, norepinephrine challenge studies could be performed on both normals and hyperactives to assess peripheral noradrenergic sensitivity.

3. Clarification of pemoline's (Cylert®) mechanism of action should be attempted, since this is the only stimulant drug (with clear-cut efficacy) that does not increase blood pressure and pulse.

4. More complex pharmacological studies using drug combinations such as β blockers and stimulants could be tried in adults with ADD-RT (residual-type) to try to dissect out the necessary and sufficient changes in the periphery to have therapeutic responses to the stimulants.

REFERENCES

1. Aarskog, D., Fevang, F. O., and Klove, H. (1977): *J. Pharmacol. Exp. Ther.,* 202:544–557.
2. Braestrup, C. (1977): *J. Pharm. Pharmacol.,* 29:463–470.
3. Brown, G. L., Ebert, M. H., Hunt, R. D., and Rapoport, J. L. (1981): *Biol. Psychiatry,* 16:779–787.
4. Brown, G. L., Murphy, D. L., Langer, D. H., Ebert, M. H., Post, R. M., et al. (1984): Paper presented at Annual Meeting of the American Academy of Child Psychiatry. Toronto, Canada.
5. Callaway, E., Holliday, R., and Naylor, H. (1983): *Arch. Gen. Psychiatry,* 11:1243–1248.
6. Campbell, I. C., Murphy, D. L., Gallager, D. W., Tallman, J. F., and Marshall, E. F. (1979): In: *Monoamine Oxidase: Structure Function and Altered Functions,* edited by S. von Korff and D. L. Murphy, pp. 517–530. Academic Press, New York.
7. Cooper, J. R., Bloom, F. E., and Roth, R. H. (1982): In: *The Biochemical Basis of Neuropharmacology,* 4th edition, pp. 109–170. Oxford University Press, New York.
8. Donnelly, M., Rapoport, J. L., Zametkin, A., and Ismond, D. (1986): *Clin. Pharmacol. Ther.,* 39:72–81.
9. Garfinkle, B. D., Wender, P. H., Sloman, L., and O'Neil, I. (1983): *J. Am. Acad. Child Psychiatry,* 22:343–348.
10. Gittelman, R., Klein, D., Katz, S., Sarf, K., and Pollack, E. (1976): *Arch. Gen. Psychiatry,* 33:1217–1231.
11. Goldberg, L. I., Volkman, P. H., and Kohli, J. D. (1978): *Annu. Rev. Pharmacol. Toxicol.,* 18:57–79.
12. Gotoh, F., Komatsumoto, S., Araki, N., and Gomi, S. (1984): *Arch. Neurol.,* 41:951–955.
13. Greenhill, L. L., Puig-Antich, J., Halpern, F., Sachar, E. J., Rubinstein, B., et al. (1980): *Pediatrics,* 66:152–153.
14. Hoebel, B. G., and Leibowitz, S. F. (1981): In: *Brain, Behavior, and Bodily Disease,* edited by H. Weiner, M. A. Hofer, and A. J. Stunkard, pp. 103–138. Raven Press, New York.
15. Hunt, R. D., Cohen, D. J., Anderson, G., and Minderra, R. (1987): In: *Attention Deficit Disorder and Hyperactivity, Vol. III,* edited by L. Bloomingdale. Spectrum, New York (in press).
16. Hunt, R. D., Minderra, R., and Cohen, D. J. (1985): *J. Am. Acad. Child Psychiatry,* 24(5):617–629.
17. Iversen, S. D. (1980): *Psychol. Med.,* 10:527–539.
18. Karoum, F., Chuange, L. W., Eislar, T., Calne, D. B., Liebowitz, M. R., et al. (1982): *Neurology (N.Y.),* 32:503–505.
19. Khan, A. U., and DeKirmenjian, H. (1981): *Am. J. Psychiatry,* 138:108–112.
20. Kornetsky, C. (1970): *Psychopharmacologia,* 17:105–136.
21. Kuczenski, R. (1983): In: *Stimulants: Neurochemical, Behavior and Clinical Perspectives,* edited by I. Crease, pp. 31–63. Raven Press, New York.
22. Langer, D. H., Rapoport, J. L., Ebert, M. H., Lake, C. R., and Nee, L. E. (1987): In: *Psychobiology of Childhood: Profiles of Current Issues,* edited by B. Shopsion and L. Greenhill. Spectrum Publications, New York (in press).
23. Laufer, M. W., Denhoff, E., and Solomons, G. (1957): *Psychosom. Med.,* 19:38–49.
24. Leibowitz, S. F. (1984): In: *Neuroendocrinology and Psychiatric Disorder,* edited by G. M. Brown, pp. 383–399. Raven Press, New York.
25. Linnoila, M., Guthrie, S., Pharm, D., Lane, E., Karoum, F., et al. (1986): *Psychiatr. Res.,* 17:229–239.
26. Lou, H. C., Henriksen, L., and Bruhn, P. (1984): *Arch. Neurol.,* 41:825–829.
27. Meller, E., Bohmaker, K., and Friedhoff, A. J. (1984): *Life Sci.,* 35:1825–1838.
28. Mikkelsen, E., Lake, C. R., Brown, G. L., Ziegler, M. G., and Ebert, M. H. (1981): *Psychiatr. Res.,* 4:157–169.
29. Murphy, D. L., Pickar, D., Cohen, R. M., Roy, B., Garrick, N. A., et al. (1982): *Clin. Pharmacol. Ther.,* 31:252–253.
30. Peroutka, S. J., Prichard, D., Greenberg, D. A., and Snyder, S. H. (1977): *Neuropharmacology,* 6:549–556.
31. Porrino, L. J., Lucignani, G., Dow-Edwards, D., and Sokoloff, L. (1984): *Brain Res.,* 307:311–320.
32. Potter, W. Z., Scheinin, M., Golden, R., Rudorfer, M., Cowdry, R. W., et al. (1985): *Arch. Gen. Psychiatry,* 42(12):1171–1177.
33. Rapoport, J. L., Mikkelsen, E. J., Ebert, M. H., Brown, G. L., Weise, V. L., et al. (1978): *J. Neurol. Ment. Dis.,* 166(10):731–737.
34. Rapoport, J. L., Quinn, P. O., Bradbard, G., Riddle, K. D., and Brooks, E. (1974): *Arch. Gen. Psychiatry,* 30:789–793.
35. Reigle, T., Isaac, W. L., and Isaac, W. (1981): *J. Pharm. Sci.,* 70:816–817.
36. Rosenthal, R. H., and Allen, T. W. (1978): *Psychol. Bull.,* 85:689–715.
37. Satterfield, J. H., and Dawson, M. E. (1971): *Psychophysiology,* 8:191–197.
38. Shaywitz, B. A., Yager, R. D., and Klopper, J. H. (1986): *Science,* 191:305–308.
39. Shaywitz, S. E., Hunt, R. D., Jatlow, P., Cohen, D. J., Young, J. G., et al. (1982): *Pediatrics,* 696:688–694.
40. Shekim, W. O., Davis, L. G., Bylund, D. B., Brunngraber, E., Fikes, L., et al. (1982): *Am. J. Psychiatry,* 139:936–938.
41. Shekim, W. O., DeKirmenjian, H., and Chapel, J. L. (1977): *Am. J. Psychiatry,* 134:1276–1279.
42. Shekim, W. O., DeKirmenjian, H., and Chapel, J. L. (1979): *Am. J. Psychiatry,* 136:667–671.
43. Shekim, W. O., Javaid, J., Dans, J. M., and Bylund, D. S. (1983): *Biol. Psychiatry,* 18:707–714.
44. Tagliamonte, S., and Tagliamonte, P. (1971): *Fed. Proc.,* 30:197–198.
45. Wender, P. (1971): *Minimal Brain Dysfunction in Children.* John Wiley & Sons, New York.
46. Wender, P. (1972): *J. Nerv. Ment. Dis.,* 155:55–71.
47. Winsberg, B. G., and Yepes, L. E. (1978): In: *Pediatric Psychopharmacology: The Use of Behavior Modifying Drugs in Children,* edited by John S. Werry, pp. 234–274. Brunner Maazel, New York.
48. Yang, H. Y. T., and Neff, N. H. (1974): *J. Pharmacol. Exp. Ther.,* 189:733–740.
49. Young, J. G., Cohen, D. J., Waldo, M. C., Feiz, R., and Roth, J. A. (1980): *Schizophrenia Bull.,* 6:324–333.
50. Yu-cun, A., and Yu-Peng, W. (1984): *Biol. Psychiatry,* 19:861–870.
51. Zametkin, A. J., Karoum, F., Linnoila, M., Rapoport, J. L., Brown, G. L., et al. (1985): *Arch. Gen. Psychiatry,* 42:251–255.
52. Zametkin, A. J., Rapoport, J. L., Murphy, D. L., Linnoila, M., and Ismond, D. (1985): *Arch. Gen. Psychiatry,* 42:963–969.
53. Zametkin, A. J., Rapoport, J. L., Murphy, D. L., Linnoila, M., Karoum, F., et al. (1985): *Arch. Gen. Psychiatry,* 42:969–973.
54. Zemlan, F. P., Hitzemann, R. J., Hirschowitz, J., and Garver, D. L. (1985): *Am. J. Psychiatry,* 142:1334–1357.

Psychopharmacology:
The Third Generation of Progress,
edited by Herbert Y. Meltzer.
Raven Press, New York © 1987.

CHAPTER 84

Affective Disorders in Children and Adolescents: Diagnostic Validity and Psychobiology

Joaquim Puig-Antich

Since this book's last edition, a substantial new body of knowledge has emerged that has made the main research question being asked a decade ago, namely, "Do affective disorders exist in children and adolescents?" obsolete. Instead, today's questions concern much more the nature of affective disorders in children and their relationship to the same phenotypic diagnoses of adult onset: major depression, dysthymia, schizoaffective disorder, cyclothymia, and bipolar illness. It should be stated at the outset that the concept of adulthood frequently carries an implicit sense of unity or uniformity, which constitutes an oversimplification. For instance, affective illnesses with onset in early adulthood are probably etiologically quite different from those of geriatric onset and even from those with onset in the mid-40s (1). Because of their importance to the current conceptualization of very early onset affective disorders, throughout this chapter, these distinctions are emphasized repeatedly. To state it in a more general way, within the phenomenological syndromic unity of the major affective disorders, there are likely to be major shifts in etiological and pathogenetic constellations not only from childhood to adulthood but also within the adult life cycle. Age of onset may be the most important variable in this regard. Therefore, a summary of the current body of knowledge on very early onset (under age 18 years) affective disorders is presented in this chapter, always in the context of what is known about affective illnesses in adults.

ADVANCES IN ASSESSMENT AND DIAGNOSIS

The steps that opened the way towards systematic research in this area were the development of reliable and valid semistructured interview techniques for the assessment of affective symptoms in youngsters (2–5) and the use of unmodified Feighner et al. (6), RDC (7), and later *DSM-III* diagnostic criteria (8–15). A comprehensive discussion of current problems and controversies in this area is beyond the scope of this chapter. Suffice it to say that the main clinical diagnostic instruments are administered in a semistructured mode and follow the symptom-by-symptom model of similar instruments for adults, on which they were based, and that most have made provision for the systematic recording of parental and of the child's information about the child's symptoms.

There is disagreement on if and how both sets of information should be integrated, with the more clinically inclined using the same interviewer separately for both informants, integrating the information symptom by symptom as it is obtained, whereas others use a different interviewer for each informant and make two types of diagnoses for each child, one according to the child's information and another according to the parent's. Obviously, which method to use should depend on the questions being asked and on the aims of each study, but this is not always apparent from the choices made. As a general rule, agreement between parent and child is usually better for objective behaviors than for inner symptoms, except when the latter are severe enough to break out into public behavior.

Reliabilities for affective symptom ratings and diagnoses vary from adequate to excellent. As expected, the more structured an instrument is administered, the higher is its reliability, and the harder to come by is the evidence of diagnostic validity for the affective disorders. It is doubtful that rigid structure can supplant the skill of a well-trained interviewer of children when it is so critical for the rater to "learn" the specific meaning attached to each key word by each particular child and when using different wordings to ask the same question is the best way to find out if a child understood the concept correctly. The study by Breslau et al. (16) comparing a structured interview against a semi-structured method ("editing") demonstrated this point. The same issue applies to self-administered questionnaires, which, even when administered to teachers (who always have a "control group" in their minds, the average child), are relatively poor in picking up affective psychopathology. When the child's self-ratings are contrasted to final diagnoses, most studies have shown too many false positives and false negatives for their efficient use for screening purposes, at least before puberty. These issues are not different than in adult patients; they just are also evident in child and adolescent affective disorders.

Contrary to earlier speculations (4–7), the evidence indicates that there are very few phenomenological changes in the syndromic pictures of depression (8–10) and mania (11,12,17) between children and adolescents (15) and between them and adults. Furthermore, the variability that does exist in affective symptoms can mostly be attributed, once the necessary adaptations in interview techniques essential to their proper assessment in this age group are taken into account, to developmental patterns in certain functions rather than to the nature of the symptoms themselves. For example, in a proportion of children (3,18) and adolescents (19) who have a major depressive disorder (MDD), evident psychotic symptoms (depressive hallucinations and delusions) have implications for a true developmental nosology. In the prepubertal years, depressive delusions are very rare; almost all psychotically depressed prepubertal children in that age group present only hallucinations. With the onset of adolescence, depressive delusions become more frequent (10), although hallucinations also occur. In contrast, among psychotically depressed adults, the pattern is that of a marked predominance of delusions. This apparent age effect suggests that the younger child's cognitive immaturity makes the development of a depressive delusional system unlikely. The fact that some other cognitive symptoms, such as hopelessness, have been found to be somewhat less prevalent in MDD children than in adolescents (15) provides some support for this hypothesis. On the other hand, the absence of a relationship between Piagetian cognitive stages and depressive symptomatology in children (20) tends to militate against it. These findings are not in and of themselves contradictory as they apply to different aspects of cognition and of depressive symptomatology. Further work in this area may

be helpful if certain psychotherapies are to be applied to depressed children.

In the last few years there have been other nosological developments in very early onset affective illness besides the description of the classical depressive and manic syndromes. One of them has been the description and validation of a chronic, relatively low-grade, protracted depressive picture, which makes up in duration what it lacks in number and severity of symptoms and has been well described among school-aged children and early adolescents as dysthymia (13,14). The prognostic importance of dysthymia in children is similar to that described for the same disorder in adults (21,22); it is the best predictor of future major depression. In addition, the potential of dysthymia to induce long-term psychosocial disability (23,24) makes its clinical recognition in youngsters very important for preventive purposes (13,14,25). The demonstration of psychosocial deficits and impairments in relationships that are associated with major depression in prepuberty (23) and their lack of full resolution in spite of pharmacologically associated affective recovery (24) echo the well-known findings concerning the social functioning of adult depressives (26–29).

Another important phenomenological aspect of affective illness in youngsters is the prevalence of bipolar clinical pictures or outcomes in this age group. Frank manic-depressive illness, including full depressive and manic episodes, has been convincingly described in adolescents for many years (11,30,31). In fact, bipolar disorder in adolescence is not rare, but it is less common and much more misdiagnosed before puberty (17), although it still should be looked at very cautiously when applied to preschoolers (3,32). Sexually provocative behavior towards adults in a prepubertal child, if prior sexual abuse can be excluded, should always make the clinician think about prepubertal hypomania. What has not been widely appreciated is that, besides full phenomenologically discrete manic episodes, mixed disorders (12), rapid cycling, hypomania, and cyclothymia (33–36) occur frequently in adolescents either spontaneously or pharmacologically triggered by antidepressants. In fact, as in young adults (37–39), it is likely that over half of the bipolar adolescents do not show typical full-fledged mania but instead display less easily diagnosable forms of the disorder. Mixed states should be considered in the differential diagnosis of any adolescent with a primary diagnosis of major depression and a secondary diagnosis of conduct disorder, because a prolonged mixed state with high irritability is highly likely to be associated with socially deviant behaviors that, if sufficiently repeated during adolescence, can be mistaken for conduct disorder. At times the initial presentation of such adolescents is as an impulsive alcohol or drug abuser; and bipolarity only becomes clear after detoxification (35).

RELATIONSHIP TO ADULT AFFECTIVE DISORDERS

At present, there is enough evidence from familial aggregation and follow-up studies, the classical validators of psychiatric diagnoses (40–42), that makes it probable that very early onset affective illness is likely to be characterized by unusually high pedigree loading for affective illness, a tendency to chronicity (dysthymia), frequent bipolar outcome in later years, a relatively high rate of depressive psychosis, and the frequent development of secondary complications (conduct disorder, alcoholism, substance abuse, and possibly, antisocial personality).

Natural History and Follow-up Studies

Kovacs' group has demonstrated the chronicity of prepubertal dysthymia and its predictive power for the development of major depression (13) and the continuity into adolescence of prepubertal depressive disorders (14). These fundamental contributions do away with the until recently commonly held belief that the depressive clinical pictures in children were transient. Even in the restricted prepubertal onset age range, Kovacs et al. (14) found a negative relationship between age at onset and frequency of future recurrences. As the characterization of affective illness in children is recent, no study has yet followed prepubertal depressive children up into adulthood, the key test of the continuity hypothesis. Preliminary results of a follow-up of adolescents with affective illness (12,43) also attest to the continuity of these disorders over time. In fact, the results of the follow-up studies of prepubertal and adolescent onset depressive disorders, cited before, are largely parallel to the results of methodologically similar studies of adult major depressives (27,28,44). It is therefore likely that continuity across ages does exist.

What is especially interesting in these follow-up studies is the high rate of bipolar outcomes. In Kovacs' study, analysis up to 6 years revealed bipolar outcome in 20% of the MDD subjects, which results in a projected rate of 37% if all subjects had been followed up for a full 6 years (17). In Strober and Carlson's data, 20% of adolescent inpatients with MDD showed a bipolar outcome in a 1- to 4-year follow-up. These findings are consistent with the relationship between affective loading of the pedigree and early age of onset, which will be reviewed shortly, and with the consistent finding of earlier age at onset for adult bipolars (II and I in this order) compared to unipolar depression (45,47). These high rates for relatively short-term bipolar outcome are substantially higher than in older adult patients (46) and are likely to continue to increase, since these youngsters have most of the period of risk for bipolar outcome left to live. The use of "unipolar" as a qualifier of major depression in children and adolescents is at least self-deceiving, as bipolar is a positive definition and unipolar is a negative one, and there is heavy transit over time in these age groups from the "unipolar" to the bipolar I or II (or unipolar II) (47). The heterogeneity of "unipolar" depression in children and adolescents is likely to be so marked as to render this category meaningless. Classifying nonbipolar depression by familial history of bipolarity may be the most reasonable approach in this age group.

Psychotic depressions are highly likely to predict bipolarity and to be associated with a family history of bipolar disorder in children (17), adolescents (12), and young adults (45,48,49). This outcome is opposite to findings on follow-up of psychotic depressions in older adults (50–53) and again emphasizes the differences between early onset and late onset affective illness.

Familial Aggregation Studies

Two main designs have been used to determine if youngsters and adults with affective disorders cluster in the same families: those that examined the first-degree relatives (offspring or siblings) under 18 years of age of adult patients with unipolar or bipolar major affective disorders ("from the top down") and those that ascertained lifetime psychiatric diagnoses of first- and second-degree relatives of child and adolescent probands with major affective illness ("from the bottom up"). The age-corrected lifetime morbidity risk for major depression in first-degree relatives of adult probands with major depression is between 0.18 and 0.30 (54–59). Within this range, morbidity risks are highest for relatives of schizoaffective and bipolar probands and lowest for relatives of unipolar late onset probands. In families of adolescent probands with major depression, the corresponding figure has been reported to be between 0.35 in relatives of inpatient probands (60) and 0.37 among adult first-degree relatives of nonbipolar, mostly outpatient adolescent major depressives (61), although it was higher among relatives of bipolar than nonbipolar probands (60). Among families of prepubertal children with major depression, the age-corrected morbidity risk for first-degree biological relatives over 16 years of age has been reported to be 0.50 (62).

These morbidity risks are not strictly comparable across age groups because of differences in control groups and methodologies, which, although similar, were not identical. Nevertheless, in all studies morbidity risks for MDD in the proband families were between two- and threefold those for controls. Data in families of adult probands cited here were obtained by the more sensitive family study method (i.e., direct interview of every available relative), whereas two out of three of the studies cited on families of child and adolescent probands were studied by the less sensitive family history method (63,64). It should be noted that the finding of higher familial aggregation among the earlier onset groups is contrary to the sensitivity of the methods used, a fact that lends credence to the hypothesis that there appears to be an inverse relationship between age of onset of the disorder and familial morbidity risks. On the other hand, more definitive conclusions should await comparison of morbidity risks for first-degree relatives between families of depressive and control child and adolescent probands obtained by the family study method. Further evidence of this inverse relationship between age of onset and family aggregation has also been found within families of depressive probands with adult onset of major depression.

Thus, onset below 20 years of age was associated with a raw rate of 24.2% of first-degree relatives affected with MDD. A rate of 17.5% was associated with onset in the third decade of life, and 11.9% in the fourth (1). In addition, there was aggregation for early onset within certain families. Little evidence of familial aggregation of affective illness was found when the proband's age of onset was over 40 years of age.

Further evidence of familial aggregation of depressive disorders is provided by studies of the child and adolescent offspring of adult MDD probands (65,66). So far, these studies indicate that the morbidity risk for major depression for offspring under age 18 years increases with parental major depression, parental assortative mating, familial loading for psychiatric disorders, parental recurrent depression, and also with parental associated diagnoses of panic disorder or agoraphobia, which increased the risk not only for major depression but also for separation anxiety in the offspring. In one study mothers are more likely to transmit these disorders than fathers (Z. Welner, *personal communication,* 1984). In another study of adult probands and relatives (56), over 50% of adult offspring of dual parental mating for major affective illness were shown to be affected. Only in one small "top down" study (67) were no differences found between offspring of adult depressives and those of controls, as both groups had unexpectedly high prevalence of psychopathology among their offspring. In a study of offspring and younger siblings of adult bipolar probands followed up for 3 years, Akiskal et al. (35) found that half the sample presented signs of bipolarity, either mania, hypomania, mixed disorder, rapid cycling, or cyclothymia. Only six of 68 remained undiagnosed throughout the study. The remainder received a diagnosis of MDD or dysthymia at some point. Eleven of these youngsters presented initially with polydrug abuse and were reclassified as either cyclothymic or dysthymic during follow-up.

Taken as a whole, the data suggest that childhood onset, adolescent onset, and young adult onset affective disorders tend to cluster in the same families and that familial aggregation for affective illness occurs mostly when these disorders begin in the first half of the life-span. Nevertheless, morbidity risks in the families of very early onset probands are raised not only for affective illness but also for other psychiatric disorders; this is especially true for alcoholism (62,68) and anxiety disorders (61,62,65). In this regard, it is interesting that in a study of adult primary major depressive probands, only age of onset of affective illness and the secondary diagnoses of alcoholism or an anxiety disorder in the proband were independently related to higher familial aggregation for major depression in relatives, whereas the presence of none of the clinical characteristics of the proband's major depressive episodes (any of the RDC depressive subtypes, recurrent depression, hospitalization, or suicidal ideation or attempts) showed evidence of any independent influence on familial aggregation for affective illness (69). Similar negative familial findings have been reported regarding the presence or absence of endogenicity in adult MDD patients (70).

The association between primary depression and secondary alcoholism in adult probands may be mediated by the associated diagnoses of panic or other anxiety disorders. Adult MDD probands with associated panic disorder also had a younger age at onset of MDD and higher proportions of associated secondary alcoholism and suicidal attempts than those without associated anxiety disorders (71). In addition, adult relatives of adult probands with major depression and panic disorder have been shown to present doubly high risks not only for major depression and panic disorder and phobia but also for alcoholism compared to relatives of MDD probands without any anxiety disorder. Furthermore, an increased risk for anxiety disorders and younger age at onset of MDD have been found in relatives of adult probands with depression and secondary alcoholism, whereas probands with depression and alcoholism had increased familial rates for both disorders, and those with only depression had no increase in familial risk for alcoholism (72).

These associations are important in this context, because anxiety disorders (13,73), conduct disorders (11,74), and drug and alcohol abuse (25,35) are frequently associated psychiatric diagnoses in affectively ill children and adolescents as well as in their families besides the increased familial risk for affective illness. The associated diagnosis of separation anxiety in prepubertal children with MDD has been found to be associated with an increase in the rate of alcoholism, but not for MDD, in the parents (73). The studies mentioned suggest that very early age of onset may be associated with more secondary diagnoses and that associated familial anxiety disorders, and perhaps bipolarity, may predispose to drug and alcohol abuse. These associations may have major long-term implications for long-term outcome. There is evidence that a secular change resulting in an increase in the prevalence of depression (65) and suicide (75,76) in young people may have taken place (77). In the presence of such a cohort effect, the interpretation of the studies reviewed in this section is more difficult.

The aggregation of child, adolescent, and young adult onset affective disorders in the same families, their high pedigree density for affective illness, together with the likely inverse relationship between density of familial aggregation for affective illness and age of onset of the proband on the one hand and rate of disorder in the offspring on the other, all strongly suggest, but do not prove, that genetic inheritance is likely to play an important role in the familial transmission of affective disease, and more so the earlier the age at onset. As the evidence for continuity among child, adolescent, and young adult onset affective disorders appears very consistent, we can only attempt to separate genetic from environmental factors in the familial transmission of affective illness by briefly reviewing the literature on adult depression. Neither adoption nor twin studies have been reported in very early onset affective illness, and well-replicated positive findings in chromosomal linkage studies have been absent. Higher concordance rates have been found for adults with major affective illness in MZ over DZ twins (54,78,79). In addition, MZ/DZ twin concordance ratios have been found to be higher for bipolar illness (4.2) than for unipolar depression (2.3) (79). This is consistent with the earlier onset of bipolar as compared to unipolar illness in adult samples (45) and with the high rate of bipolar outcome in very early onset affective illness. There is also evidence of genetic transmission from other twin studies for bipolar illness and nonbipolar major depression (age of onset not reported) (79,85), nonendogenous depression (80), and for depression and anxiety symptoms from a large study of twin volunteers (81).

The results from the only two fully reported adoption studies of affective disorders in the literature are rather consistent with the data from adult twin studies. In one study, bipolar illness in adoptees was found to be associated with affective disorders in the biological but not in the adoptive parents (82). In the other, on a sample of adult adoptees with primary and secondary (to alcoholism) unipolar depression (mean age at onset in the early 20s), associations were shown in older adoptees with psychiatric diagnoses in both adoptive and biological parents. Environmental transmission was supported, but the evidence to support genetic transmission was found to be weak (83). The secondary nature of depression in about half the sample limits the generalization of the conclusions. A third study (84) does not report age of onset, although the adoptees were in their 40s, and has a wide majority of nonbipolar affective probands. The results were inconclusive.

Therefore, the data from the adoption studies seem to be consistent in supporting the importance of genetic factors in the familial transmission of bipolar illness. The overall picture that seems to be emerging is that genetic factors are paramount in the affective disorders with onset in the first three or four decades of life, although their importance is likely to be less within that range the higher the age of onset. On the other hand, onset after the fifth decade seems not to be associated with much familial aggregation of affective illness, and it may, therefore, be related to aging or to other brain disorders. With advancing age at onset, phenocopies may become the rule.

The fact that identical twins do not have 100% concordance rates even for bipolarity suggests a causal role for nongenetic factors as well, but the studies that have investigated the role of nongenetic factors in affective disorders in youngsters have thus far found primarily negative results. Thus, there is little evidence that either marital status of the parent, size of the sibship, socioeconomic status, parental separation, divorce or marital functioning, nor familial constellation or structure plays much of a role in the causation of depressive disorders in children and adolescents. In one study (65), parental divorce was shown to have an effect, albeit minor. Nevertheless, the studies in this area have not focused primarily on cultural or environmental modes of transmission, and it is still premature to come to any conclusions regarding the interplay and mechanisms of environmental and genetic factors in the familial transmission of very early onset affective illness. A very careful study of environmental factors in conjunction with genetic studies will be key to the development of methods to identify phenocopies among early onset affective illness, which is probably one of the most important research priorities in this area. Such techniques may be critical in order to maximize sample homogeneity for future biological research.

PSYCHOBIOLOGICAL MARKERS

Since very early onset affective disorders may represent the most genetically determined form of the illness, the importance of using tools that provide a window into brain function (namely, those that are regulated by the limbic system and hindbrain, involving the same neurotransmitter systems that have been implicated in the pathophysiology of the affective disorders) should be emphasized in this group. At least some of the biological markers specific to a disorder are likely to reflect pathophysiological mechanisms. If this is found in a disorder with high familial aggregation, where genetic transmission is likely to be involved, and the abnormalities persist in recovery, then such markers may reflect genetic expression much earlier than the development of the classical phenotypic expression: clinical illness. Biological high-risk paradigms, where risk is defined on the basis of familial aggregation alone, are therefore critical for future research in this area. Other advantages of this group for psychobiological research are (a) the availability of at least three and frequently four preceding generations, (b) the relatively short life-span of the proband (which makes lifetime diagnoses more credible), (c) the lower prevalence of chronic intercurrent diseases, which become more likely with advancing age, and (d) the neuroendocrine "window into the brain" is likely to be much more "transparent" before puberty because of the low levels of sex steroid hormones.

Sleep EEG

During the Major Depressive Episode

The evidence for polysomnographic markers occurring during the episode of major depressive disorder in adults is very strong. It has been repeatedly confirmed that adult primary major depressives present decreased first REM period latency, decreased slow-wave sleep (δ) time, increased REM density, decreased sleep efficiency, and abnormal temporal distribution of REM throughout the night (86–90). The EEG sleep records of prepubertal major depressives, in spite of their multiple sleep complaints, and regardless of subtype, have not been found to differ from those of nondepressed psychiatric or normal control children (91,92). There was no decrease in slow-wave sleep, no decrease in sleep efficiency, no shortening of latency to the first REM period, no increase in REM density, and no abnormality in the temporal distribution of REM sleep during the night. Neither REM signs (or "attempts") before the first REM period nor the latency from sleep onset to the first REM attempt were different among the groups (93). Circadian abnormalities were minimal.

The virtual lack of cross-sectional sleep architecture differences in prepubertal major depressives does not necessarily prove that prepubertal and adult major depressive disorders are different conditions. This finding can alternatively be interpreted as evidence of maturational differences in sleep correlates of clinical depressive disorder at different ages. There is evidence in the data from adults that age has a fundamental influence on EEG in sleep. Several studies have found strong relationships between age and sleep measures in adult depressives (86,87,94). These age effects on sleep are so marked that norms need to be expressed by decade within the adult age range. Normative data show a progressive decrease of stage IV with age, not fully compensated by a minor increase in other NREM stages, shortening of REM latency, and a decrease in total sleep time with increasing age (87,95). We have argued (91) that the evidence at hand from studies of familial aggregation, natural history, and biological studies in children after recovery from major depression indicates that the EEG sleep findings during the episode are not likely to indicate a fundamental difference in the nature of the illness between prepuberty and adulthood. Instead, we hypothesized that the EEG sleep findings in adult depression may express the effects of an interaction between depression and age.

Preliminary findings by Lahmeyer et al. (96) showed shortened REM latency comparing 13 adolescent major depressives with 13 normal controls, but the finding is difficult to interpret because of the small sample size and because the normal controls had a mean REM latency much longer than is usual for this age group. Goetz et al. (97) have compared adolescent endogenous and nonendogenous major depressives during the episode ($N = 49$) and normal controls ($N = 40$). No differences in REM latency were found. Some sleep continuity disturbances were evident in the depressive group, including longer sleep latency and higher number of awakenings. Appleboom et al. (98) have confirmed these findings with a very similar study design. Cashman et al. (99) also found normal REM latency in adolescent depressives, but this study also found increased REM density for the first REM period in this sample compared to psychiatric controls. Puig-Antich et al. (100) found normal REM latency and first REM period density in adolescent major depressives compared to normal controls. In addition, REM latency and δ sleep were found to be highly correlated with age in the predicted direction, although there were no sex effects (97).

As we discuss later, there also is some evidence of objectively mild sleep continuity disturbances in prepubertal major depressives when their records during the episode are compared to those during the recovered state. The REM latency has also been found normal in young adults in their early 20s during MDD episodes (R. Goetz, et al., *unpublished data;* 101), but not later. In the study by Hawkins et al. (101), hypersomnia was the predominant finding. Severity of depression is unlikely to be responsible for these differences among age groups, as childhood and adolescent depressive illness is frequently quite severe judging from the high proportion of endogenous or psychotic subtypes. On the other hand, shortened REM latency has been found in older depressives with milder clinical pictures, including "atypical depressives" (102) and those with dysthymic disorders (103). The mean age of each of these two samples was in the mid-30s. The progressive decrease in REM latency and increase in REM density are age effects apparent throughout the life-span in both depressives and normals, although differences between these two groups may therefore not appear until the mid- or late 20s. The same may be true for the progressive decrease in sleep continuity measures, although here depressive/control differences appear by early adolescence.

Because normal REM latency during the MDD episode occurs in adolescence and young adulthood before the mid-20s as well as before puberty, it is unlikely that puberty effects play a significant role in EEG sleep. No significant pubertal effects on sleep EEG measures over and above age effects appear evident among normal children either (104). Instead, the mechanisms behind these child/adult differences in sleep EEG in MDD are more likely to be found in either the effects of aging or maturation or in the higher genetic loading present in very early onset affective disorders. Sleep EEG studies in adults over 30 with prepubertal or adolescent onset should clarify whether age at onset (and genetic loading) or current age is the key issue in the negative REM latency findings during the episode. Paradoxically, therefore, although the EEG sleep studies of prepubertal and adolescent major depressive episodes show different results from those of adults with the same diagnosis, the results may be quite consistent across age groups once the effects of age are taken into account. Conversely, shortened REM latency during episodes of MDD in adult depressives is probably the result of an interaction between depression and age. These age effects appear to be consistent through the life-span. The sleep EEG during the depressive episode constitutes a prime example of an age-sensitive marker.

Sleep EEG of Recovered Prepubertal Major Depressives

Twenty-eight prepubertal major depressives (endogenous and nonendogenous) were restudied when fully recovered from the depressive episode for at least 4 months and drug-free for at least 1 month (105). They were compared to their own sleep EEG measures during the episode and to the base-line sleep studies of two control groups, nondepressed psychiatric and normal. Recovered prepubertal major depressives showed significantly shorter first REM period latency and significantly greater number of REM periods. These findings were independent of the length of time between clinical recovery or drug discontinuation and restudy. Although recovered children with depression fell asleep somewhat earlier than when they were ill, no relationship was found between change in sleep onset time and change in REM latency. In addition, the sleep continuity of recovered depressives improved significantly on most relevant measures compared to the time they were clinically depressed. Therefore, shortened first REM period latency may be a marker of trait or past episode in prepubertal major depressives during the recovered state. It is open to question if shortened REM latency normalizes with the onset of a new depressive episode and if it in fact precedes the development of the first episode of depression/dysthymia in prepubertal children from families with dense aggregation for affective disorders. In a recent study, Coble et al. (P. A. Coble, *personal communication,* 1985) compared sleep EEG of normal prepubertal children with ($N = 16$) and without ($N = 16$) a positive family history for affective illness. Pedigree density for affective illness was moderate to low. Children with positive family history showed significantly higher REM densities than those without. This pilot study suggests that EEG sleep trait markers for prepubertal onset major depression may indeed exist in children.

Notwithstanding the lack of polysomnographic abnormalities, most prepubertal children in the midst of a major depressive episode experience sleep difficulties (reported by themselves and by their parents) that do not differ from those of adult depressives. On recovery, these complaints by and large disappear, along with a small but significant improvement in sleep continuity variables. These findings suggest that children are very sensitive to small sleep disruptions that in adults [except for pseudoinsomniacs (106)] would be accompanied by little or no subjective perception of sleep difficulty. The Stanford studies, which demonstrated the massive effects of sleep deprivation on daytime functioning of normal children, support this interpretation (107–111).

It is not clear whether or not the REM sleep results in recovered depressive children just summarized are at variance with adult or adolescent data. No EEG sleep data are yet available from adolescents who have recovered from an episode of major depression. Data on recovered drug-free adult depressives are contradictory. On the one hand, there are three studies that suggest normalization of REM latency in recovered adult depressives (112–114). On the other hand, a variety of pilot or ongoing formal studies that used depressives as their own controls (115–118; D. Kupfer, *personal communication, 1985*) suggest that sleep continuity measures tend to improve during recovery, whereas in many patients REM measures, especially REM period latency, tend to remain the same or improve only to a small degree. Thus, the results of longitudinal adult studies across states (depressed/nondepressed) are not wholly in agreement with comparisons with control groups in adult remitted depressive patients. Nevertheless, shortened REM latency in recovered depressive children is consistent with the increased tendency to REM advancement in recovered adult depressives after arecoline or physostigmine infusion (119–122) during the first (126) and the second NREM periods (114,124–126). This effect was blocked with pretreatment with scopolamine (127), a muscarinic receptor blocker that crosses the blood–brain barrier. Furthermore, administration of scopolamine for three consecutive mornings to nonaffective adult volunteers induces progressively shorter REM latencies and other EEG sleep changes seen in depressive illness: increased REM density and sleep latency with lower sleep efficiency and total sleep time (128,129). In view of the fact that scopolamine is a muscarinic receptor blocker and that its action lasts no longer than 6 hr (127), the progressive sleep changes are best interpreted as secondary to scopolamine-induced muscarinic supersensitivity.

These EEG sleep findings suggest that an excessive tendency to REM advancement does remain in recovered affective disorder adult patients even when abnormalities in REM latency are not demonstrable in the absence of pharmacological challenges and that cholinergic supersensitivity is likely to be a major mediator of such pathological tendency. Cholinergic supersensitivity may also mediate the shortening of REM latency found in recovered prepubertal depressives. If this hypothesis is correct, it would suggest that what is constant from age group to age group in the recovered patients is a chronic state of central muscarinic receptor supersensitivity, which in children would manifest itself spontaneously in the recovered state, probably in relationship to age differences in neuroregulatory equilibrium. An alternative, but not mutually exclusive, complementary hypothesis is that shortened REM latency is more likely to persist (in adults) or appear (in prepuberty) during the recovered state the younger the age of onset, the higher the familial aggregation, and the higher the likelihood of bipolar outcome and depressive recurrences (65).

Other mechanisms that are also likely to be involved in the regulation of REM latency in adults are the serotonergic and the noradrenergic systems. There is evidence that decreased NE activity shortens REM latency as shown by a study using the tyrosine hydroxylase blocker α-methyl-*para*-tyrosine (AMPT) which depletes NE in the CNS (126). Furthermore, drugs that cause a selective potentiation of 5-HT mechanisms, like i.v. clomipramine (D. Kupfer, *personal communication, 1985*), induce a lengthening of REM latency. Animal work concordant with these findings has been reviewed by McCarley (130), who proposed that REM regulation is dependent on the interaction of cholinergic and aminergic pathways. It is likely that developmental aspects of the function of aminergic systems may underlie the puzzling finding of normal REM latency in young people during a major depressive episode. Further research in this area is indicated.

NEUROENDOCRINE FUNCTION

Growth Hormone Secretion

Growth Hormone Response to Hypoglycemia

Prepubertal children, during an episode of endogenous major depression, have been found to hyposecrete GH in response to insulin-induced hypoglycemia (ITT) compared to nonendogenous depressive children and nondepressed psychiatric controls (131). The test could not be carried out in normal children; therefore, the possibility remains that prepubertal psychiatric patients hyposecrete GH in this test, although if this were true, endogenous depressives would still secrete significantly less than children with other psychiatric diagnoses. Preliminary replication of these results has been obtained by Meyers et al. (132). Sachar et al. (133) and Mueller et al. (134) reported diminished GH responses to ITT in adult patients suffering from depressive illness. Nevertheless, the fact that both androgens (135) and estrogens (136,137) have potentiating effects on GH responses to a variety of stimuli and the inclusion of women of different ages and menstrual status presented some difficulties in the interpretation of these results. To eliminate the variable of estrogen status, Gruen et al. (138) studied GH ITT responses in postmenopausal depressed women and postmenopausal normal controls and demonstrated GH hyposecretion in the depressive group. All normals had maximal GH values of 5 ng/ml or over, whereas in 60% of the depressives maximal GH values were under 5 ng/ml. Casper et al. (139) and Gregoire et al. (140) reported similar results: about 50% of adult depressives had absent or very low (<3.5 ng/ml) GH responses to ITT. In a more recent study, Koslow et al. (141) did not replicate these findings, but their almost 50% exclusion rate based on insufficient hypoglycemia suggests that their results could be generalized only to adult endogenous depressives with minimal insulin resistance (134,142). It is therefore likely that about one-half of unipolar endogenous patients, especially postmenopausal women, present this characteristic GH hyporesponse. There is some agreement, but meager data, that bipolar patients may secrete GH normally in this test (141,143). The pubertal potentiation of GH responsivity to most stimuli has been known (144). It is likely that only during puberty and after menopause does GH response to ITT reflect closely neuroregulatory mechanisms involved in depressive illness. In adolescence and early adulthood, these effects are probably blurred by sex hormone influence. Other examples of variability in GH responses in depression apparently dependent on the sex steroid environment are in the literature (226).

It is well known that not only phentolamine (an α-adrenergic receptor blocker) (145–147) and reserpine (148) but also serotonin receptor blockers such as methysergide (149,150) and cyproheptadine (149,151) block the GH response to ITT. Serotonergic mediation was also suggested in the study of Takahashi et al. (152) in which L-5-HTP, a relatively nonspecific serotonergic precursor on acute administration (153,154), was used as a provocative agent resulting in significant differences in GH responses between depressives and controls. In addition, neither apomorphine (a dopamine receptor agonist) (155) nor L-dopa (156) consistently produce differences in GH responses in depressives compared with controls once estrogen status is controlled. Therefore, a functional noradrenergic or serotonergic deficit in adult depressives has been hypothesized as a possible substrate for these findings. It is now likely that the ITT stimulus to glucoreceptor neurons in the hypothalamus releases GH by inhibiting hypothalamic somatostatin secretion (157–159).

Growth Hormone Secretion During Sleep

Prepubertal major depressives, regardless of endogenous features, were found to hypersecrete GH during sleep compared to normal and psychiatric controls (160). This neurohormonal abnormality may be specific to prepubertal major depressives. Most GH secreted in children during the 24-hr period is released during the first few hours of sleep in conjunction with δ sleep (161,162). This chronological association has been found in all ages at which δ sleep can be demonstrated (163). As pointed out by Mendelson (164), several instances of dissociation can be found in which pharmacological abolition of either GH secretion during sleep (164) or slow-wave sleep (165) did not affect the associated phenomenon. On the other hand, when subjects are studied in an environment free of time cues (166), and also when marked phase shifts in the sleep–wake cycle are externally imposed (167), GH secretion continues to be chronologically associated with δ sleep. This relationship between SWS and GH was not altered in depressive children compared to controls. Work carried out recently by Jarrett and D. Kupfer (*personal communication,* 1985) indicates that adult endogenous depressives hyposecrete GH during sleep, after δ sleep is controlled for. Mendlewicz et al. (168) have likewise reported that unipolar depressives do not hypersecrete GH during sleep, but they have also found a marked increase of daytime GH secretion. In our ongoing study of adolescent depression, we have so far found no significant differences in GH SWS secretion between depressives and controls, an intermediate position between the findings in prepubertal and adult depression.

Day and nighttime GH secretion increases with puberty (144). There is an age effect in GH secretion after adolescence; namely, with increasing age there is a steady decrease of both δ sleep and sleep-related GH. It is, therefore, conceivable that there may be a combination of age and pubertal effects that reverses the effect of major depression on the amount of GH secreted during sleep and on its distribution in a 24-hr period and increases daytime secretion. In prepubertal children we did not find differences in daytime secretion between controls and depressives.

Sleep GH secretion is likely to be regulated through different neurotransmitter systems than daytime GH secretion (164,169,170). Neither α_1 or β norepinephrine receptors (171) nor dopamine systems (163,172,173) seem to have any influence on sleep-related GH secretion in normal adults. Assuming that data from normal adult volunteers can be applied to prepubertal sleep–neuroendocrine regulatory mechanisms, there are three likely mechanisms of sleep GH hypersecretion in MDD children: first, a functional deficit of hypothalamic serotonin systems, because methysergide, a serotonin receptor blocker, increases sleep GH secretion (150); second, an increase in cholinergic activity, either through muscarinic receptor hypersensitivity or increase of acetylcholine release, since methoscopolamine, an antimuscarinic agent, dramatically inhibits sleep GH secretion (174); and third, through nicotinic receptor hypersensitivity, since piperidine, a nicotinic receptor agonist, increases sleep GH secretion (170).

The importance of cholinergic mechanisms as permissive or active agents in the secretion of GH cannot be overemphasized. Casanueva et al. (175) have convincingly demonstrated that muscarinic blockade by atropine blocked GH responses to clonidine, exercise, and arginine as well as GH responses to opioids (176), glucagon and arginine (177), L-dopa, apomorphine, and clonidine (178), and, to a much lesser extent, GH responses to insulin-induced hypoglycemia (174,179). Cholinergic nicotinic stimulation (170) increases GH response to ITT and to sleep. Anticholinergic agents also block GH response to hpGRF-40 (180). This suggests that anticholinergics may induce the secretion of somatostatin, which in pituitary cell cultures totally inhibits the release of GH from somatotropes when GRF is added to the culture (181), although a direct pituitary effect cannot be completely ruled out as yet.

Growth Hormone Response to Demethylimipramine

The GH response to demethylimipramine (DMI), a relatively pure presynaptic NE reuptake blocker, has been studied in prepubertal children with MDD and controls (J. Puig-Antich et al., *unpublished data*). Desmethylimipramine was given orally at either 50 or 75 mg depending on the child's weight in order to approximate 2 mg/kg. A minor secretory episode followed DMI ingestion by an average 2 hr and then remained steady for the remainder of the sampling period. No significant differences in GH response, measured by area under the curve and by a maximum increase over baseline, were found. These results are consistent with a study of GH response to 75 mg of DMI (injected i.m.) in postmenopausal women. The GH response was markedly decreased compared to younger women, and no differences were found between depressives and normals (182). On the other hand, the findings of GH hyporesponse to DMI in MDD endogenous premenopausal women and men have been replicated in several samples (183–185). This across-the-life-span pattern seems to be the exact reverse of the pattern found with ITT. As indicated above, GH response to ITT shows maximal differences between depressives and controls in prepuberty and in postmenopausal women, when sex steroids are minimal or absent, whereas they are blurred during the reproductive years. The GH response to DMI discriminates well between endogenous depressives and controls in adult males and in premenopausal women but not in prepuberty or postmenopausal women. In our ongoing adolescent study, GH response to DMI (75 mg i.m.) is significantly decreased in both endogenous and nonendogenous major depressives compared to normal controls. The low GH response to DMI before puberty and its lack of discrimination between depressives and controls further suggest that the ITT GH results in prepubertal depression may reflect dysregulation in mechanisms other than noradrenergic and/or that differences in the balance of α- and β-adrenergic receptors accompany changes in the sex steroid environment that take place during puberty and menopause.

Growth Hormone Response to Clonidine Challenge

The GH response to clonidine, an α_2-adrenergic receptor agonist, has been proposed as a potentially clinically useful and safer test than ITT for children and has been used as a standard probe of GH release in children for GH deficiency (186–189) and also as a research probe in Tourette's (190). There is high agreement in pediatric populations between GH secretion to clonidine and to ITT (191). Meyer et al. (132) have reported preliminary data on decreased GH response to a low oral dose of clonidine in children during a depressive episode. There is as yet no report in MDD adolescents during an episode of MDD. The preferred dosage is low, as used by Checkley et al. (183), in order to preserve the drug's specificity of action.

Clonidine has a very different mode of action than DMI, the GH response to which did not discriminate between prepubertal depressives and controls. The GH response to clonidine discriminates well between adult depressives and normal controls independently of the effects of age (183,192–196), although it has also been found abnormal in some anxiety disorders (197).

Growth Hormone Secretion in Recovered Prepubertal Depressives

Both sleep and ITT GH response abnormalities in prepubertal children who have suffered a major depressive episode persist in the sustained affectively recovered state, retested under drug-free conditions (198,199). Pre/post correlations for both markers are of the order of 0.8. These findings were not related to the length of time elapsed from either clinical recovery or drug discontinuation or having

recovered while on placebo only and raise again the possibility of the existence of trait markers in prepubertal major depression, subject to the same considerations and caveats described before regarding REM latency.

Data on GH secretion in recovered adolescent depressives is not available as yet. There is evidence that the GH response to ITT in recovered adult depressives may normalize (200). The GH response to DMI in adult depressives has also been reported to normalize on recovery (201). It would be important to know if age of onset of affective illness and/or degree of familial aggregation influences the findings in adult recovered depressives. There is some evidence supporting the hypothesis that MDD patients may show CNS α_2-adrenergic receptor subsensitivity as a vulnerability trait and that, therefore, low GH response to clonidine may remain abnormal in the recovered state (197). No data in recovered children or adolescents are available yet.

Interrelationships of GH and REM Latency Findings

When the findings on GH response to ITT and to sleep in our sample of prepubertal major depressive disorders (131,160,198,199) were taken together, no significant correlations were found among GH and REM latency variables in either of the control groups. On the other hand, the areas under the curve of GH–ITT and GH–sleep were significantly positively correlated in the depressives during the episode and also during the recovered state. Since low GH response to ITT is associated with depression, whereas, on the contrary, high GH response to SWS is depression related, a simple serotonin deficit alone could not explain the findings. Although the group findings appear to be a dissociation of GH responses to sleep and ITT (202), this is not true at the individual level, as both responses were positively correlated. In addition, REM latency in recovered depressive children was found to correlate positively with GH response to ITT and not with GH secretion during sleep, whereas REM latency during the episode (which was found to be normal) was not correlated with any other variable. Interestingly, episode/recovery stability of the three variables was significant in each case. In contrast, illness/recovery stability of PRL and cortisol measures was negligible.

It is likely that the predisposition to depressive illness in prepubertal children is associated with a particular constellation of neurotransmitter system dysfunction that affects a variety of hypothalamic/midbrain regulatory functions in a predictable fashion. Several investigators have proposed the notion that cholinergic/adrenergic and serotonergic balance in the CNS may mediate the affective changes in manic depressive illness (153,203,204). Thus, there is evidence for a cholinergic overdrive, probably caused by muscarinic receptor supersensitivity, as a trait or past-episode marker in major depression in adults (125,129). There is also evidence that low catecholamine activity may precipitate depressive episodes among bipolar adults (126). Serotonin deficits seem also to be associated with some depressive episodes, especially nonpsychotic suicidal depressions with familial aggregation and bipolarity (205).

Given the correlational pattern described, and given that noradrenergic changes do not affect sleep-related GH secretion (164), the evidence so far points to the serotonergic and cholinergic systems as those most likely to play a major role in the pathophysiology of these findings in prepubertal depressive disorders. In addition, changes in the catecholamine system may be related to the onset of depressive episode. These working hypotheses require further investigation and specific strategies to test them.

Biological Correlates of Suicidal Planning and Behavior in Prepubertal MDD

A functional CNS serotonin deficit may be implicated in suicidal behavior from postmortem brain studies of suicide victims (206–210) and from finding low CSF 5-HIAA in adult patients who have attempted or completed suicide across diagnostic categories including affective disorders, nonaffective schizophrenics, alcoholics, and personality disorders (211–221). Furthermore, low CSF 5-HIAA may be associated not only with suicidal behavior per se but also with a broad range of violent, impulsive behavior, including murder and arson (220,222) and patients with impulsiveness, aggression, and "monotony avoidance" (e.g., sensation seeking) independent of suicide tendencies (221). Of more interest in this context is the finding that low CSF 5-HIAA exists in normal volunteers who show positive family histories for depression (223) and that it postdates the suicidal episode (212,219,224), suggesting that this finding may be a trait marker for suicide and perhaps for aggressive behavior.

As an indirect test of the hypothesis that serotonergic mechanisms are likely to be involved in the REM sleep and GH abnormalities found in prepubertal major depressives, biological data from major depressive prepubertal children with suicidal planning or behavior were compared to those from those without. Suicidal MDD children showed significantly shorter REM latency during the catheter night than nonsuicidal MDDs, both during the episode and also after recovery. In addition, during the episode, the nonsuicidal MDD group had a significantly lower sleep efficiency as well as longer sleep latency than the suicidal MDD group. Thus, the suicidal depressive children slept significantly better than the nonsuicidal group.

Although both groups of MDD children secreted more GH during sleep than the nondepressed (normal and psychiatric) controls, the nonsuicidal MDD group secreted substantially more GH during sleep than the suicidal group. The same patterns repeated at recovery. No differences were found between suicidal and nonsuicidal MDD children during the episode on GH response to ITT, but only in the suicidal MDD group was GH response to ITT abnormally low during recovery compared to the control group. No pattern of differences in these comparisons were found with cortisol and PRL secretion.

Reexamination of the correlation patterns among GH and REM latency measures within each subgroup, suicidal and nonsuicidal MDD children, demonstrated that REM latency during the episode showed significantly divergent correlational patterns from one group to the other. In the suicidal MDD group, it was positively correlated with all measures of GH secretion, significantly so with GH response to ITT. Instead, in the nonsuicidal group, REM latency showed significant negative correlations with both GH measures. In contrast, after recovery, REM latency correlated positively with both GH measures in both groups, suicidal and nonsuicidal. These divergent patterns were not related to the significant differences in sleep latency between suicidal and nonsuicidal MDD groups and were not explained by severity of depression either. Therefore, the lack of relationship between REM latency during the episode and GH measures found in the group as a whole is related to the cancellation of two strongly divergent patterns, one within the suicidal MDD group and another within the nonsuicidal MDD group. This suggests that during the episode of depression, suicidal and nonsuicidal children are likely to differ in at least some aspects of the constellation of abnormalities of neurotransmitter systems that regulate REM latency and GH secretion. These differences are consistent with the hypothesis that a functional serotonin deficit may be present in suicidal prepubertal children. Further studies to separate the neurobiology of prepubertal affective illness from that of suicidal planning and/or behavior in this age group are in order.

Sleep-Related Melatonin Secretion

The evidence for decreased sleep-related melatonin secretion in adult depression is impressive. Several studies from different centers report a decrease of nighttime melatonin secretion in adult endogenous depressives (225, 227,231). In addition, Lewy et al. (232) have reported daytime and nighttime melatonin to be increased in mania as compared to controls, whereas sleep-related melatonin is reported decreased in bipolars during the depressed phase (230,232). More importantly, three different studies have indicated that low nighttime melatonin remains abnormal after recovery from major depression (227,229–231,233) both in bipolars and in bipolar adult patients. These findings suggest that low sleep-related melatonin may be a true trait marker for major depression in adults. Preliminary evidence from Cavallo et al. (234) indicates lower plasma melatonin levels during the night in a small sample of MDD children compared to endocrinologically normal short-stature controls. Melatonin secretion is inversely related to age, although most of the variance takes place between the first year of life and adolescence (235). Earlier claims that its decrease may be the signal to the hypothalamus to initiate the neuroendocrine events of puberty (236) have not been widely accepted after further examination. But even within the adult age span, the melatonin secretion inverse relationship with age is so strong that it has recently been proposed as an index of brain aging (237).

The adult data also indicate that suicide tendencies may be related to low melatonin secretion in major depression. Beck-Friis et al. (231) have studied the relationship between history of suicidal attempts in the current or past major depressive episodes and nighttime melatonin. They found that among suicidal depressives nighttime melatonin was indistinguishable from that of normal controls and that only among nonsuicidal depressives was nighttime melatonin significantly lower than in controls, similar to our findings on sleep-related GH secretion. The differences in nighttime melatonin in that study occurred with suicidality but not with melancholia. Brown et al. (228) hypothesize that the low melatonin findings in depression may be secondary to β-adrenergic receptor subsensitivity, in turn caused by high circulating levels of plasma NE (238–244) or by intrinsic postreceptor mechanisms (245). On the other hand, the hypothesis is consistent with normal melatonin in suicidal depressed patients, as their serotonergic deficit could induce an increase in β-adrenergic receptors as it does experimentally in rat brain (246). β-Adrenergic receptors have been found increased in the brains of suicides (245). Melatonin deserves further attention in very early onset affective illness.

Cortisol Secretion

Twenty-four-hour Plasma Cortisol

Contrary to our preliminary report on only four cases (324), we have found cortisol hypersecretion only occasionally (approximately 10% of the sample) when the circadian cortisol patterns of prepubertal children in a major depressive episode are compared to their own after recovery. In addition, no differences in 24-hr cortisol secretion were found when children with major depression were compared to psychiatric and normal control children. We found that the cortisol diurnal pattern was such in children that the lowest point was usually coincident or within 0.5 hr of sleep onset. Minor differences can occur in each serial time point among the different groups when this synchronization is not taken into account. But when the 24-hr patterns are aligned for sleep onset, there are no differences in cortisol secretion that identify the depressive groups. Therefore, the majority of these children have normal cortisol secretion during and after a major depressive episode.

Although at variance with the findings among adult endogenous depressives (247–250), these findings in children are quite consistent with the positive correlation between age and cortisol hypersecretion in adult endogenous major depressive patients (249,251) and in normal adults (252,253). Age effects are probably responsible for the substantially lower rate of spontaneous cortisol hypersecretors in prepubertal endogenous depressives compared to older adults with the same diagnosis. As in the case of sleep EEG variables, it appears that age may be at least as important as major depression in the pathophysiological mechanisms resulting in cortisol hypersecretion in older depressed patients. Preliminary data from our ongoing study suggest a low rate of cortisol hypersecretors among adolescent nonbipolar major depressives also, which provides further support for the hypothesis of interaction between depression and age in the mechanisms underlying cortisol hypersecretion in adult depressives. It should be added that the specificity of cortisol hypersecretion to major depression, as opposed to severe psychiatric disorders, is currently in question (254).

Dexamethasone Suppression Test

The published data on the dexamethasone suppression test (DST) in depressed children are contradictory. In a small outpatient controlled study of RDC endogenous prepubertal depressives the DST showed a sensitivity of 63% and a specificity versus nondepressed psychiatric disorders of 90% (255). In an uncontrolled study of 10 outpatient children with the same diagnosis, only one escaped suppression (256). Dosage was fixed (0.5 mg) in the first study and weight corrected in the second, but in fact dosage differences were minor and unlikely to explain the discrepant results. In a third study, a nonsuppression rate of 70% was found in an inpatient sample of 20 children with major depression after 1 mg of dexamethasone (257). Although the study was not controlled, samples were obtained not only at 4 p.m. but also at 8 a.m. Most 8 a.m. samples were suppressed, providing some indirect evidence that the dexamethasone pill was in fact ingested. Two other studies have addressed specificity questions. Targum et al. (258) found a 1-mg suppression rate of 89% among prepubertal inpatient conduct disorders, and Livingston et al. (259) found three of five inpatient children with separation anxiety and three of five children with major depression to escape suppression with a dose of 0.5 mg. Livingstone et al. (260) presented results from a second inpatient prepubertal sample. Escapers to 0.5 mg DST were eight of eight children with MDD and seven of ten nondepressed children with separation anxiety or overanxious disorders, whereas nine out of ten conduct disorders suppressed normally. Finally, Petty et al. (261) have studied prepubertal inpatients and reported that six of seven MDDs, five of six dysthymic disorders, three of 11 "dysphorics," and five of six nondepressed nondysphoric psychiatric disorders, including schizophrenia and conduct disorders, had positive 0.5 mg DSTs.

We did not find significant differences between children with major depression, regardless of endogenicity, and nondepressed psychiatric and normal controls using either 0.25 or 0.5 mg of dexamethasone. The protocol consisted of three consecutive 24-hr studies with sequential hourly plasma samples. The first was a base line, immediately followed the next day by another 24-hr collection after one dose of dexamethasone. Approximately 5 days later, a third study was done with the other DST dose. The order of the doses was randomized. No order effect was found. Because of children's usual earlier bedtime, dexamethasone was given at 9 p.m. In spite of good evidence of compliance including dexamethasone plasma levels, the four groups did not differ significantly in the 24-hr plasma cortisol AUCs either at base line or after either of the two dexamethasone dosages. No significant differences were found among the groups for individual blood samples at any point in time. These results indicate that 0.5-mg dexamethasone nonsuppression is unlikely to be of value in the diagnosis of prepubertal major depression. As stress has been reported to induce positive DST tests normal in adults (262,263), we studied the degree of stress reported by our patients and controls during the biological studies. Overall, the degree of stress was rather low. All studies were carried out in the same setting, outside the inpatient unit, with a great deal of individual attention.

In summary, although there are methodological problems with many of the studies, the data suggest that inpatients are substantially more likely to escape suppression than outpatients. Furthermore, there are doubts about specificity, as very high rates of escape in nondepressed inpatients have been reported. The high rate of escape among dysthymic inpatient children in the only study that has systematically looked at them suggests that severity of the disorder alone may not be a key variable. This is especially true in child psychiatry, where inpatient admission is at least as likely to be related to the degree of familial chaos as to the severity of the child's psychopathology. Overall, the data suggest that stress may be related to DST escape and that prepubertal depressives may be somewhat more vulnerable to such effect. In adolescents the pattern of DST results appears to be quite similar to that in adults: among inpatients there is a 30 to 70% escape rate (264,265; M. Strober, *personal communication*), whereas in our ongoing study we have found the rate to be very low among outpatients with major depression when tested in a relatively stress-free environment.

The early claims for the dexamethasone suppression test as a sensitive and specific test for endogenous major depression (266–268) have been considerably downsized by more recent work, reviewed by Arana et al. (269). Suffice it to say that sensitivity has been reported substantially lower for outpatient depressives [14% (270); 26% (271)], that specificity has also been found to be lower than initially thought by several groups. Any type of acute psychiatric illness necessitating inpatient admission has been found to be accompanied by DST escape (269,272,273). In some studies, rather moderate stress (262,263) and also diet-induced weight loss (274–277) have been found to induce DST escape in normals. Recent withdrawal from antidepressant medication (278) as well as variability in plasma dexamethasone levels (279,280) may also influence the results. There is good reason to believe that this variability may be partially explained by assay variation from laboratory to laboratory (281) and also by too sporadic sampling routine in the face of considerable variability in patterns of nonsuppression found when 24-hr studies have been carried out (282). Although Carroll et al. (268) found no age effects on the rate of escapers to DST 1 mg in adult endogenous depressives, the majority of the other investigators have found substantial age influences (249,251,283–287), with older patients being more likely to escape. This is consistent with the low rates of nonsuppression found in many of the studies in children and adolescents with MDD.

Three noradrenergic agents have been reported to suppress spontaneous cortisol hypersecretion in depressives and to differentiate adult MDD patients from normal controls: d-amphetamine (280,283,288,289), desmethylimipramine (290), and clonidine (291). These studies suggest that cortisol dysregulation in adult depressives is likely to reflect, at least in part, a CNS noradrenergic functional deficit. But cortisol secretion dysregulation in adult depressives is likely to be more complex than initially thought. A rather low degree of agreement has been found among different pro-

vocative challenges of HPA overactivity in adult depressives (228,249,283,292–295), suggesting that each taps different aspects of their neuroregulatory mechanisms. This suggests that the dysregulation of cortisol secretion in adult depressives is likely to be more widespread and "polytonic" (294,295) in these patients than the spontaneous plasma cortisol abnormalities and the DST alone would suggest. "Spontaneous" cortisol hypersecretion and a positive DST may be only two of the manifestations, and neither necessary, of dysregulation of CRF–ACTH–cortisol secretion during an episode of major depression.

In this regard, Meltzer et al. (153) have reported that adult patients with major depression (and also with mania) presented a significantly higher increase in plasma cortisol after oral ingestion of 200 mg of 5-hydroxytryptophan (L-5-HTP), a serotonin precursor, compared to normal controls. Contrary to the work just reviewed with catecholaminergic agents, the response to L-5-HTP was negatively correlated with base-line plasma cortisol. This correlation was significant in the controls but was weaker, although still positive, in the depressive group. Stated differently, the data suggest that this test may be more likely to reveal abnormalities of neuroregulation of CRF–ACTH–cortisol secretion in adult depressives without spontaneous evidence of cortisol hypersecretion. In combination with the data on catecholaminergic agents "correcting" cortisol hypersecretion in adult MDD, the high plasma cortisol response to L-5-HTP in some adult depressives suggests postsynaptic serotonin receptor supersensitivity, which may be secondary to a deficit in 5-HT concentration in the synapse. The data also suggest that cortisol hypersecretion may be absent in adult depressives with functional serotonin deficiency. These are likely to be nonpsychotic depressives, who have committed violent suicidal acts and have a positive family history for major affective disorder and bipolarity (205). Many of these characteristics are shared by adolescent and prepubertal depressives: loaded pedigrees, likelihood of bipolarity, and normal base-line cortisol. In this context, it is noteworthy that cortisol hypersecretion in adult bipolar depression (251) and in cyclothymia (33) may not be related to age; therefore, special attention to these diagnostic and familial factors, as well as to suicidal tendencies, stress, and other methodological issues, should be paid in future studies of the HPA axis in very early onset affective illness.

The TSH Response to TRH

The thyroid-stimulating hormone (TSH) response to thyrotropin-releasing hormone (TRH) has been found blunted in adult endogenous depressives during the episode (226,296–307). There is some evidence that this marker may be age dependent (308,309), being most useful in postmenopausal women and less useful as the age lowers. The mechanism is unknown, although increased secretion of hypothalamic somatostatin, which lowers secretion of TSH among other hormones (310), remains a possibility. Consistent with these age effects, we have found no differences in TSH response to TRH between prepubertal depressives and controls. There were no differences in magnitude of response between dosages of 2 and 7 μg/kg. Similar negative results have been reported for adolescent depressives (311).

DEVELOPMENTAL CAVEATS

It seems clear that at least three main neurotransmitter systems are involved in the dysregulation of sleep and neuroendocrine functions in adult depression. There is abundant animal and clinical evidence that during development, the balance among different neuroregulatory systems is not equivalent to that in adulthood. Thus, the maturational rates of different systems in the rat vary substantially from each other. For instance, catecholamine (CA) systems, although the earliest to begin, do not develop fully, anatomically and functionally, in the primate until the beginning of adulthood (312), whereas cholinergic (ACh) and serotonergic systems become fully developed much earlier in the postnatal period (313,314).

In humans there is clinical evidence that physiological changes in CA function in the CNS also occur with age (315,316). For example, CSF concentrations of HVA and 5-HIAA are much higher in children than in adults (315). On a more clinical level, the normally short attention span of young children and the high prevalence of attention deficit (317,318), which in many cases tends to improve over time (319,320), points to low CA function during the early years. The lack of an excitatory, elated, or euphoric response to dextroamphetamine in prepuberty (321) as well as the relative rarity of mania (322) and of elation suggest the same thing.

Although adult data on normals and patients with affective disorders are very valuable points of departure for biological research on the affective disorders of very early onset, we can not take neurobiological data in adult normal volunteers and transfer them to prepubertal children, ignoring the biological changes that take place in growth and development, puberty, and aging (323). A great deal of work in basic developmental neuroscience remains to be done. It should be evident that it will be crucial for further advances in this field to determine the normal patterns of neurotransmitter interaction in this age group and to study children at high risk for affective illness. It will also be crucial to use primate models of depressive illness in order to be able to answer the many questions that cannot be investigated in humans for ethical reasons. Thus, much closer collaboration between developmental neurobiological and behavioral studies in primates and in humans will be essential.

REFERENCES

1. Weissman, M. M., Wickramaratne, P., Merikangas, K. R., Leckman, J. F., Prusoff, B. A., et al. (1984): *Arch. Gen. Psychiatry,* 41:1136–1143.
2. Strober, M., Green, J., and Carlson, G. (1981): *Arch. Gen. Psychiatry,* 38:141–145.
3. Poznanski, E. O., Israel, M. C., and Grossmann, J. (1984): *J. Am. Acad. Child Psychiatry,* 23:105–110.
4. Kovacs, M. (1985): *Psychopharmacol. Bull.,* 21:991–994.
5. Chambers, W. J., Puig-Antich, J., Hirsch, M., Paez, P., Ambrosini, P., et al. (1985): *Arch. Gen. Psychiatry,* 42:696–702.
6. Feighner, J. P., Robins, E., Guze, S. B., et al. (1972): *Arch. Gen. Psychiatry,* 26:57–61.
7. Spitzer, R. L., Endicott, J., and Robbins, E. (1978): *Arch. Gen. Psychiatry,* 35:773–782.
8. Kupferman, S., and Stewart, M. A. (1979): *J. Affect. Disorders,* 1:213–217.
9. Puig-Antich, J., Blau, S., Marx, N., Greenhill, L. L., and Chambers, W. (1978): *J. Am. Acad. Child Psychiatry,* 17:695–707.
10. Strober, M., Green, J., and Carlson, G. (1982): *J. Affect. Disorders,* 3:281–290.
11. Carlson, G., and Strober, M. (1978): *J. Am. Acad. Child Psychiatry,* 12:138–153.
12. Strober, M., and Carlson, G. (1982): *Arch. Gen. Psychiatry,* 39: 549–558.
13. Kovacs, M., Feinberg, T. L., Crouse-Novak, M. A., Paulauskas, S., and Finkelstein, R. (1984): *Arch. Gen. Psychiatry,* 41:219–239.
14. Kovacs, M., Feinberg, T. L., Crouse-Novak, M. A., Paulauskas, S., Pollock, M., et al. (1984): *Arch. Gen. Psychiatry,* 41:643–649.
15. Ryan, N. D., Puig-Antich, J., Rabinovich, H., Robinson, D., Ambrosini, P. J., et al. (1987): (submitted).
16. Breslau, N. (1987): *J. Am. Acad. Child Psychiatry,* (in press).
17. Kovacs, M. (1985): Presented at the World Congress of Biological Psychiatry, Philadelphia, Pennsylvania.
18. Chambers, W. J., and Puig-Antich, J. (1982): *Arch. Gen. Psychiatry,* 39:921–927.
19. Strober, M., and Carlson, G. (1982): *Arch. Gen. Psychiatry,* 39: 549–558.
20. Kovacs, M., and Paulauskas, S. L. (1984): In: *Childhood Depression: New Directions for Child Development,* edited by D. Cichetti and K. Schneider-Rosen, pp. 59–79. Jossey-Bass, San Francisco.
21. Keller, M. B., Shapiro, R. W., Labori, P. W., et al. (1982): *Arch. Gen. Psychiatry,* 39:905–910.
22. Keller, M. B., Shapiro, R. W., Lavori, P. W., and Wolfe, N. (1982): *Arch. Gen. Psychiatry,* 39:911–920.
23. Puig-Antich, J., Lukens, E., Davies, M., Goetz, D., Quattrock, J., et al. (1985): *Arch. Gen. Psychiatry,* 42:500–507.
24. Puig-Antich, J., Lukens, E., Davies, M., Goetz, D., and Todak, G. (1985): *Arch. Gen. Psychiatry,* 42:511–517.
25. Kashani, J. H., Keller, M. B., Solomon, N., Reid, J. C., and Mazzola, D. (1985): *J. Affect. Disorders,* 8:153–157.
26. Weissmann, M. M., Paykel, E. S., Siegel, R., et al. (1971): *Am. J. Orthopsychiatry,* 41:391–405.
27. Paykel, E. S., Weissmann, M. M., Prussof, B., et al. (1971): *J. Nerv. Ment. Dis.,* 152:158–172.
28. Youngren, M. A., and Lewinsohn, P. M. (1980): *J. Abnorm. Psychol.,* 89:333–341.
29. Weissmann, M. M., Klerman, G. L., Paykel, E. S., et al. (1974): *Arch. Gen. Psychiatry,* 30:771–778.
30. Campbell, J. D. (1952): *J. Nerv. Ment. Dis.,* 116:424–439.
31. Carlson, G., and Strober, M. (1979): *Psychiatr. Clin. North Am.,* 2:511–525.
32. Weinberg, W. A., and Brumback, R. A. (1976): *Am. J. Dis. Child.,* 130:380–384.
33. Depue, R. A., Slater, J. F., Wolfstetter-Kausch, H., Klein, D., Goplerud, E., et al. (1981): *J. Abnorm. Psychol.,* 90:381–437.
34. Klein, D. N., Depue, R. A., and Slater, J. F. (1985): *J. Abnorm. Psychol.,* 94:115–127.
35. Akiskal, H. S., Downs, J., Jordan, P., Watson, S., Daugherty, D., et al. (1985): *Arch. Gen. Psychiatry,* 42:996–1003.
36. Klein, D. N., Depue, R. A., and Slater, J. F. (1986): *Arch. Gen. Psychiatry,* 43:441–445.
37. Akiskal, H. S., and Puzantian, V. R. (1979): *Psychiatr. Clin. North Am.,* 2:419–440.
38. Himmelhoch, J. M. (1979): *Psychiatr. Clin. North Am.,* 2:449–460.
39. Dunner, D. L. (1979): *Psychiatr. Clin. North Am.,* 2:461–468.
40. Robins, E., and Guze, S. B. (1970): *Am. J. Psychiatry,* 125:983–987.
41. Cantwell, D. P. (1975): In: *Explorations in Child Psychiatry,* edited by E. J. Anthony, pp. 57–79. Plenum Press, New York.
42. Guze, S. B. (1972): *Biol. Psychiatry,* 5:221–224.

43. Strober, M. (1983): Presented at the Annual Meeting of the American Psychiatric Association. New York, New York.
44. Keller, M. B., Lavori, P. W., Lewis, C. E., and Klerman, G. (1984): *J.A.M.A.*, 250:2199–2204.
45. Endicott, J., Nee, J., Andreasen, N., Clayton, P., Keller, M., et al. (1985): *J. Affect. Disorders*, 8:17–28.
46. Akiskal, H., Walker, P., Putantian, V. R., et al. (1983): *J. Affective Dis.*, 5:115–128.
47. Coryell, W., Endicott, J., Andreasen, N., and Keller, M. (1985): *Am. J. Psychiatry*, 142:817–821.
48. Weissman, M. M., Prusoff, B. A., and Merikangas, K. R. (1984): *Am. J. Psychiatry*, 141:892–893.
49. Endicott, J., Nee, J., Coryell, W., Keller, M., Andreasen, N., et al. (1986): *Comp. Psychiatry*, 27:1–13.
50. Coryell, W., and Tsuang, M. T. (1982): *Arch. Gen. Psychiatry*, 39:1181–1184.
51. Robinson, D. G., and Spiker, D. G. (1985): *J. Affect. Disorders*, 9:79–83.
52. Coryell, W., Lavori, P., Endicott, J., Keller, M., and Van-Eerdewegh, M. (1984): *Arch. Gen. Psychiatry*, 41:787–791.
53. Coryell, W., Endicott, J., Keller, M., and Andreasen, N. C. (1985): *J. Affect. Disorders*, 9:13–18.
54. Gershon, E. S., Bunney, W. E., Leckman, J. F., van Eerdewegh, M., and DeBauche, B. A. (1976): *Behav. Genet.*, 6:227–261.
55. Gershon, E. S., Targum, S. D., Kessler, L. R., Mazure, C. M., and Bunney, W. E. (1977): In: *Progress in Medical Genetics, Vol. II,* edited by A. G. Steinberg, A. G. Bearn, A. G. Motulsky, et al., pp. 101–164. W. B. Saunders, Philadelphia.
56. Gershon, E. S., Hanovit, J., Guroff, J. J., Dibble, E., Leckman, J., et al. (1982): *Arch. Gen. Psychiatry*, 39:1157–1167.
57. Perris, C. (1974): In: *Biological Psychiatry,* edited by J. Mendels, pp. 385–415. John Wiley & Sons, New York.
58. Weissman, N. N., Kidd, K. K., and Prusoff, B. (1982): *Arch. Gen. Psychiatry*, 39:1397–1406.
59. Weissman, M. M., Gershon, E. S., Kidd, K. K., Prusoff, J. F., Leckman, E., et al. (1984): *Arch. Gen. Psychiatry*, 41:13–21.
60. Strober, M., Burroughs, J., Salkin, B., et al. (1986): *Biol. Psychiatry*, (*in press*).
61. Puig-Antich, J., Ryan, N. D., and Larson, C. (1987): (*submitted*).
62. Puig-Antich, Goetz, D., Davies, M., et al. (1987): (*submitted*).
63. Andreasen, N. C., Endicott, J., Spitzer, R. L., and Winokur, G. (1977): *Arch. Gen. Psychiatry*, 34:1223–1229.
64. Andreasen, N. C., Rice, J., Endicott, J., Reich, T., and Coryell, W. (1986): *Arch. Gen. Psychiatry*, 43:421–429.
65. Weissman, M. M., Leckman, J. F., Merikangas, K. R., Gammon, G. D., and Prusoff, B. A. (1984): *Arch. Gen. Psychiatry*, 41:845–853.
66. Welner, Z., Welzer, A., McCray, M. D., and Leonard, M. A. (1977): *J. Nerv. Ment. Dis.*, 164:408–413.
67. Gershon, E. S., McKnew, D., Cytryn, L., et al. (1985): *J. Affect. Disorders*, 8:283–291.
68. Strober, M. (1984): In: *An Update of Childhood Depression,* edited by E. Weller, pp. 37–48. American Psychiatric Press, Washington.
69. Weissman, M. M., Merikangas, K. R., Wickramaratne, P., and Kidd, K. K. (1986): *Arch. Gen. Psychiatry*, 43:430–434.
70. Andreasen, N. C., Scheftner, W., Reich, T., Hirschfeld, R. M. A., Endicott, J., et al. (1986): *Arch. Gen. Psychiatry*, 43:246–251.
71. Leckman, J. F., Weissman, M. M., Merikangas, K. R., Pauls, D. L., and Prusoff, B. A. (1983): *Arch. Gen. Psychiatry*, 40:1055–1060.
72. Merikangas, K. R., Leckman, J. F., Prusoff, B. A., Pauls, D. L., and Weissman, M. M. (1985): *Arch. Gen. Psychiatry*, 42:367–372.
73. Puig-Antich, J., and Rabinovich, H. (1986): In: *Anxiety Disorders of Childhood,* edited by R. Gittelman, pp. 136–159. Guilford Press, New York.
74. Puig-Antich, J. (1982): *J. Am. Acad. Child Psychiatry*, 21:118–128.
75. Shaffer, D. (1985): In: *Child and Adolescent Psychiatry: Modern Approaches,* edited by M. Rutter and L. Hersov. Blackwell, pp. 698–719. London, England.
76. Brent, D., and Perper, J. (1985): Presented at the 32nd Annual Meeting of the American Academy of Child Psychiatry. San Antonio, Texas.
77. Klerman, G. L., Lavori, P. W., Rice, J., Reich, T., Endicott, J., et al. (1985): *Arch. Gen. Psychiatry*, 42:689–693.
78. Zerbin-Rudin, E. (1972): *Int. J. Ment. Health*, 1:42–62.
79. Bertelsen, A., Harvald, B., and Hauge, M. (1977): *Br. J. Psychiatry,* 130:330–357.
80. Shapiro, R. W. (1970): *Acta Jutland.*, Vol. 42.
81. Kendler, K. S., Heath, A., Martin, N. G., and Eaves, L. J. (1986): *Arch. Gen. Psychiatry*, 43:213–221.
82. Mendlewicz, J., and Ramer, J. D. (1977): *Nature,* 268:327–329.
83. Cadoret, R. J., Gorman, T. W., Heywood, E., and Troughton, E. (1985): *J. Affect. Disorders*, 9:155–164.
84. von Knorring, A. L., Cloninger, C. R., Bohman, M., and Sigvardsson, S. (1983): *Arch. Gen. Psychiatry*, 40:943–950.
85. Targensen, S. (1986): *Arch. Gen. Psychiatry*, 43:222–226.
86. Coble, P., Kupfer, D. J., Spiker, D. G., Neil, J. F., and Shaw, D. H. (1980): *Sleep Res.*, 9:165.
87. Gillin, J. C., Duncan, W., Pettigrew, K. D., Frankel, B., and Snyder, F. (1979): *Arch. Gen. Psychiatry*, 36:85–90.
88. Kupfer, D. (1976): *Biol. Psychiatry*, 11:159–174.
89. Kupfer, D., and Foster, F. G. (1979): In: *Sleep Disorders: Diagnosis and Treatment,* edited by R. L. Williams and I. Karacan, John Wiley & Sons, New York.
90. Vogel, G. W., Vogel, F., McAbee, R. S., and Thurmond, A. J. (1980): *Arch. Gen. Psychiatry*, 37:247–253.
91. Puig-Antich, J., Goetz, R., Hanlon, C., Tabrizi, M. A., Davies, M., et al. (1982): *Arch. Gen. Psychiatry*, 39:932–939.
92. Young, W., Knowles, J. B., MacLean, A. W., Boag, L., and McConville, B. J. (1982): *Biol. Psychiatry*, 17:1163–1168.
93. Goetz, R. R., Hanlon, H. S., Puig-Antich, J., and Weitzman, E. D. (1985): *Sleep*, 8:1–10.
94. Ulrich, R., Shaw, D. H., and Kupfer, D. J. (1980): *Sleep*, 3:31–40.
95. Williams, R. L., Karacan, I., and Hursch, C. J. (1974): *Electroencephalography (EEG) of Human Sleep: Clinical Applications.* John Wiley & Sons, New York.
96. Lahmeyer, H. W., Poznanski, E. O., and Bellur, S. N. (1983): *Am. J. Psychiatry*, 140:1150–1153.
97. Goetz, R., Puig-Antich, J., Ryan, N., Rabinovich, H., Ambrosini, J., et al. (1987): *Arch. Gen. Psychiatry*, 44:61–68.
98. Appleboom, Karkoff, Mendlewicz. (1986): Presented at the Annual Meeting of Belgian Association for the Study of Sleep. Brussels, Belgium.
99. Cashman, M., Coble, P., McCann, B. S., Taska, L., Reynolds, C. F., et al. (1986): *Sleep Res.*, 15:91.
100. Puig-Antich, J., Ryan, N., Larson, C., Nelson, B., Gulasky, J., et al. (1986): Presented at the Annual Meeting of the Association of Professional Sleep Societies. June 15–20, Columbus, Ohio.
101. Hawkins, D. R., Taub, J. M., and Van de Castle, R. L. (1985): *Am. J. Psychiatry*, 142:905–910.
102. Quitkin, F., Rabkin, J. G., Stewart, J., McGrath, P., Harrison, W., et al. (1985): *J. Affect. Disorders*, 8:61–67.
103. Akiskal, H. S., Lemmi, H., Dickson, H., King, H., Yerevanian, D., et al. (1984): *J. Affect. Disorders*, 6:287–295.
104. Coble, P. A., Taska, L. S., Kupfer, D. J., Spiker, D. G., Neil, J. F., et al. (1980): *Sleep Res.*, 9:165.
105. Puig-Antich, J., Goetz, R., Hanlon, C., Tabrizi, M. A., Davies, M., et al. (1983): *Arch. Gen. Psychiatry*, 40:187–192.
106. Borkovec, T. D. (1979): *Behav. Res. Ther.*, 2:27–55.
107. Anders, T., Carskadan, M., Dement, W., and Harvey, K. (1978): *Child Psychiatry Hum. Dev.*, 9:56–63.
108. Anders, T. S., Carskadan, M., and Dement, W. C. (1980): *Pediatr. Clin. North Am.*, 27:29–43.
109. Carskadan, M., Harvey, K., Duke, P., Anders, T., Citt, I., et al. (1980): *Sleep*, 2:453–460.
110. Carskadan, M. A., Harvey, K., and Dement, W. C. (1981): *Percept. Motor Skills*, 53:103–112.
111. Carskadan, M. A., Harvey, K., and Dement, W. C. (1981): *Sleep*, 4:299–312.
112. Hauri, P., Chernik, D., Hawkins, D., and Mendels, J. (1974): *Arch. Gen. Psychiatry*, 31:386–391.
113. Schulz, H., and Trojan, B. (1979): *Sleep Res.*, 8:49.
114. Sitaram, M., Nurnberger, J. I., Gershon, E. S., and Gillin, J. C. (1982): *Am. J. Psychiatry*, 139:571–576.
115. Avery, D., Wildshiodz, G., and Rafaelsen, O. (1982): *Biol. Psychiatry*, 17:463–470.

116. Kupfer, D., and Foster, F. G. (1973): *J. Nerv. Ment. Dis.*, 156: 341–348.
117. Mendels, J., and Chernik, D. A. (1973): *Sleep Res.*, 1:142.
118. Mendels, J., and Chernik, D. A. (1975): In: *The Nature and Treatment of Depression*, edited by F. F. Flach and S. C. Draghi, pp. 309–334. John Wiley & Sons, New York.
119. Gillin, J. C., Sitaram, N., Mendelson, W. B., et al. (1978): *Psychopharmacology*, 58:111–113.
120. Sitaram, B., Wyatt, R. J., Dawson, S., and Gillin, J. C. (1976): *Science*, 191:1281–1283.
121. Sitaram, N., Mendelson, W. B., Wyatt, R. J., and Gillin, J. C. (1977): *Brain Res.*, 122:562–567.
122. Sitaram, N., Moore, A. M., and Gillin, J. C. (1978): *Sleep*, 1:83–90.
123. Sitaram, N., Moore, A. M., and Gillin, J. C. (1978): *Arch. Gen. Psychiatry*, 35:1239–1243.
124. Dube, S., Kumar, N., Ettedgui, E., Pohl, R., Jones, D., et al. (1985): *Biol. Psychiatry*, 20:408–418.
125. Sitaram, M., Nurnberger, J. I., Gershon, E. S., and Gillin, J. C. (1980): *Science*, 208:200–201.
126. Sitaram, N., Gillin, J. C., and Bunney, W. E. (1984): In: *Neurobiology of Mood Disorders*, edited by R. M. Post and J. C. Ballenger, pp. 629–651. Williams & Wilkins, Baltimore.
127. Sagales, T., Erill, S., and Domino, E. F. (1975): *Clin. Pharmacol. Ther.*, 18:717–732.
128. Gillin, J. C., Sitarem, N., and Duncan, W. C. (1979): *Psychiatr. Res.*, 1:17–22.
129. Sitaram, N., Moore, A. M., and Gillin, J. C. (1979): *Psychiatr. Res.*, 1:9–16.
130. McCarley, W. (1982): *Am. J. Psychiatry*, 139:565–570.
131. Puig-Antich, J., Novacenko, H., Davies, M., Chambers, W. J., Tabrizi, M. A., et al. (1984): *Arch. Gen. Psychiatry*, 41:455–460.
132. Meyer, W. J., Richards, G. E., Cavallo, A., Holt, K. G., Hejabi, S., et al. (1986): *Pediatr. Res.*, 20:217A.
133. Sachar, E. J., Finkelstein, J., and Hellman, L. (1971): *Arch. Gen. Psychiatry*, 25:263–269.
134. Mueller, P. S., Heninger, G. R., and MacDonald, R. K. (1972): In: *Recent Advances in Psychobiology of Depressive Illnesses*, edited by T. A. Williams, M. M. Katz, and J. A. Shield, pp. 235–245. US Dept. of Health, Education, and Welfare, Washington.
135. Smals, A. E. M., Pieters, G. F. F. M., Smals, A. G. H., Benraad, T. J., Van Laarhoven, J., et al. (1986): *J. Clin. Endocrinol. Metab.*, 62:336–341.
136. Frantz, A. G., and Rabkin, M. T. (1965): *J. Clin. Endocrinol. Metab.*, 25:1470–1480.
137. Merimee, T. J., and Fineberg, S. E. (1971): *J. Clin. Endocrinol. Metab.*, 33:896–902.
138. Gruen, P. H., Sachar, E. J., Altman, N., and Sassin, J. (1975): *Arch. Gen. Psychiatry*, 32:31–33.
139. Casper, R. C., David, J. M., Pandey, G. N., Garver, D. L., and Dekirmenjian, H. (1977): *Psychoneuroendocrinology*, 2:105–113.
140. Gregoire, F., Branman, G., DeBuck, R., and Corvilain, J. (1977): *Psychoneuroendocrinology*, 2:303–312.
141. Koslow, S. H., Stokes, P. E., Mendels, J., Ramsey, A., and Casper, R. (1982): *Psychol. Med.*, 12:45–55.
142. Lewis, D. A., Kathol, R. G., Sherman, B. M., Winokur, G., and Schlesser, M. (1983): *Arch. Gen. Psychiatry*, 40:167–172.
143. Sachar, E. J., Frantz, A. G., Altman, N., and Sassin, J. (1978): *Am. J. Psychiatry*, 130:1362–1367.
144. Minuto, F., Barreca, A., Ferrini, S., Mazzochi, G., Del Monte, P., et al. (1982): *Acta Endocrinol. (Kbh.)*, 99:161–165.
145. Blackard, W. G., and Heidingsfelder, S. A. (1968): *J. Clin. Invest.*, 47:1407–1414.
146. Imura, H., Kato, Y., Ikeda, M., Morimoto, M., and Yawata, M. (1971): *J. Clin. Invest.*, 50:1069–1079.
147. Vinik, A. I., and Joubert, S. M. (1970): *Life Sci.*, 9:441–446.
148. Cavagnini, F., and Perachi, M. (1971): *J. Endocrinol.*, 51:651–656.
149. Bivens, C. H., Lebovitz, H. E., and Feldman, J. M. (1973): *N. Engl. J. Med.*, 289:236–239.
150. Mendelson, W. B., Jacobs, L. S., Reichman, J. D., Othmer, E., Cryer, P. E., et al. (1975): *J. Clin. Invest.*, 56:690–697.
151. Smythe, G. A., and Lazarus, L. (1974): *J. Clin. Invest.*, 54:116–121.
152. Takahashi, S., Kondo, H., Yoshimur, M., and Ochi, Y. (1974): In: *Psychoneuroendocrinology Workshop, Conference International Society of Psychoneuroendocrinology*, pp. 32–38.
153. Meltzer, H. Y., Unberkoman-Wilta, B., Robertson, A., Tricou, B., Lowy, M., et al. (1984): *Arch. Gen. Psychiatry*, 41:366–378.
154. van Praag, H. M. (1984): In: *Frontiers in Biochemical and Pharmacological Research in Depression*, edited by E. Usdin, et al., pp. 301–314. Raven Press, New York.
155. Frazier, A. (1975): In: *The Psychobiology of Depression*, edited by J. Mendels, pp. 7–26. Spectrum Books, New York.
156. Sachar, E. J. (1975): In: *Topics in Psychoendocrinology*, edited by E. J. Sachar, pp. 135–156. Grune & Stratton, New York.
157. Shibasaki, T., Hotta, M., Masuda, A., Imaki, T., Obara, N., et al. (1984): *J. Clin. Endocrinol. Metab.*, 60:1265–1267.
158. Seki, K., Kato, K., and Shima, K. (1986): *J. Clin. Endocrinol. Metab.*, 62:783–784.
159. Vance, M. L., Kaiser, D. L., Rivier, J., Vale, W., and Thorner, M. O. (1986): *J. Clin. Endocrinol. Metab.*, 62:591–594.
160. Puig-Antich, J., Goetz, R., Davies, M., Fein, M., Hanlon, C., et al. (1984): *Arch. Gen. Psychiatry*, 41:463–466.
161. Finkelstein, J. W., Roffwarg, H. P., Boyar, R. M., Kream, J., and Hellman, L. (1972): *J. Clin. Endocrinol. Metab.*, 35:665–670.
162. Mace, J. W., Gotlin, R. W., and Beck, P. (1972): *J. Clin. Endocrinol. Metab.*, 34:339–341.
163. Takahashi, Y., Kipais, D. M., and Daughaday, W. H. (1968): *J. Clin. Invest.*, 47:2079–2090.
164. Mendelson, W. B. (1982): *Int. Rev. Neurobiol.*, 23:367–389.
165. Rubin, R. T., Govin, P. R., Arenander, A., and Poland, R. (1973): *Res. Commun. Chem. Pathol. Pharmacol.*, 6:331–334.
166. Weitzman, E. D., Czeisler, C. A., and Moore-Ede, M. C. (1981): In: *Biological Rhythms, Sleep and Shiftwork*, edited by L. C. Johnson, W. P. Colquhoun, D. I. Tepas, et al., pp. 75–92. Spectrum Books, New York.
167. Parker, D. C., Rossman, L. G., Pakary, A. E., Hershman, J. M., Kripke, D. F., et al. (1981): In: *Biological Rhythms, Sleep, and Shiftwork*, edited by L. C. Johnson, W. P. Coloquhoun, D. I. Tepas, et al., pp. 111–132. Spectrum Books, New York.
168. Mendlewicz, J., Linkowski, P., Kerkhofs, M., Esmedt, D., Golstein, J., et al. (1985): *J. Clin. Endocrinol. Metab.*, 60:513–516.
169. Mendelson, W. B., Jacobs, L. S., Gillin, J. C., and Wyatt, R. J. (1979): *Psychoneuroendocrinology*, 4:341–350.
170. Mendelson, W. B., Latigna, R. A., Wyatt, R. V., Gillin, V. C., and Jacobs, L. S. (1981): *J. Clin. Endocrinol. Metab.*, 52:409–414.
171. Lucke, G., and Glick, S. M. (1971): *J. Clin. Endocrinol. Metab.*, 32:729–736.
172. Chihara, K., Kato, Y., Maeda, Y., Ohgo, S., and Imura, H. (1976): *Acta Endocrinol. (Kbh.)*, 81:19–27.
173. Cime, E. D., Mendelson, W. B., and Loriaux, D. L. (1979): *J. Nerv. Ment. Dis.*, 167:504–507.
174. Mendelson, W. B., Sitaram, N., Wyatt, R. J., Gillin, J. C., and Jacobs, L. S. (1978): *J. Clin. Invest.*, 61:1683–1690.
175. Casanueva, F. F., Villanueva, L., Cabranes, J. A., et al. (1984): *J. Clin. Endocrinol. Metab.*, 59:526–534.
176. Delitala, G., Grossman, A., and Besser, G. M. (1983): *J. Clin. Endocrinol. Metab.*, 55:1231.
177. Delitala, G., Frulio, T., Pacifico, A., and Maioli, M. (1982): *J. Clin. Endocrinol. Metab.*, 55:1231.
178. Delitala, G., Maioli, M., Macifico, A., Brianda, S., Palermo, M., et al. (1983): *J. Clin. Endocrinol. Metab.*, 57:1145.
179. Blackard, W. G., and Waddell, C. C. (1969): *Proc. Soc. Exp. Biol. Med.*, 131:192.
180. Massara, F., Ghigo, E., Goffi, S., Molinatti, G. M., Muller, E. E., et al. (1984): *J. Clin. Endocrinol. Metab.*, 59:1025–1026.
181. Lamberts, S. W. J., Verleun, T., and Oosterom, R. (1984): *J. Clin. Endocrinol. Metab.*, 58:250–254.
182. Matussek, N., and Laakmann, G. (1981): *Acta Psychiatr. Scand. [Suppl.]*, 63:122–126.
183. Checkley, S. A., Slade, A. P., and Shur, E. (1981): *Br. J. Psychiatry*, 138:51–55.
184. Laakman, G. (1979): In: *Neuroendocrine Correlates in Neurology and Psychiatry*, edited by E. E. Miller and A. Agnoli, pp. 263–272. North Holland, New York.
185. Laakman, G., Schoen, H. W., Blaschke, D., and Wittmann, M. (1985): *Psychoneuroendocrinology*, 10:83–93.

186. Lal, S., Tolis, G., Martin, J. B., Brown, G. M., and Guyda, H. (1975): *J. Clin. Endocrinol. Metab.*, 41:827–832.
187. Gil-Ad, I., Topper, E., and Laron, Z. (1979): *Lancet*, 2:278–279.
188. Salti, R., Galluzzi, F., Becherucci, P., Seminara, S., Calzolari, C., et al. (1981): *Helv. Paediatr. Acta*, 36:527–531.
189. Lanes, R., and Hurtado, E. (1982): *J. Pediatr.*, 100:710–714.
190. Leckman, J. F., Cohen, D. J., Gertner, J. M., Ort, S., and Harcherik, D. F. (1984): *J. Am. Acad. Child Psychiatry*, 23:174–181.
191. Health Services Human Growth Hormone Committee (1981): *Arch. Dis. Child.*, 56:952–954.
192. Charney, D. S., Heninger, G. R., Sternberg, D. E., Hastad, K., Giddings, S., et al. (1982): *Arch. Gen. Psychiatry*, 39:290–294.
193. Checkley, S., and Arendt, J. (1984): In: *Neuroendocrinology and Psychiatric Disorders*, edited by G. M. Brown, S. H. Koslow, and S. Reichlin, pp. 165–190. Raven Press, New York.
194. Siever, L. J., Pickar, D., Lake, C. R., Cohen, R. M., Uhde, T. W., et al. (1983): *J. Clin. Psychopharmacol.*, 3:39–41.
195. Matussek, N., Ackenheil, M., Hippius, H., Muller, F., Schroder, H., et al. (1980): *Psychiatr. Res.*, 2:25–36.
196. Uhde, T. W., Siever, L. J., and Post, R. M. (1984): In: *Neurobiology of Mood Disorders*, edited by R. M. Post and J. C. Ballenger, pp. 554–571. Williams & Wilkins, Baltimore.
197. Siever, L. J., and Davis, K. L. (1985): *Am. J. Psychiatry*, 142:1017–1031.
198. Puig-Antich, J., Davies, M., Novacenko, H., Tabrizi, M. A., Ambrosini, P., et al. (1984): *Arch. Gen. Psychiatry*, 41:471–475.
199. Puig-Antich, J., Goetz, R., Davies, M., Tabrizi, M. A., Novacenko, H., et al. (1984): *Arch. Gen. Psychiatry*, 41:479–483.
200. Kathol, R. G., Winokur, G., Sherman, B. M., Lewis, D., and Schlesser, M. (1984): *Psychoneuroendocrinology*, 9:57–68.
201. Calil, H. M., Lesieur, P., Gold, P. W., Brown, G. M., Zavadil, A. P. 3d, et al. (1984): *Psychiatr. Res.*, 3:231–242.
202. Hindmarsh, P. C., Smith, P. J., Taylor, B. J., Pringle, P. J., and Brook, C. G. D. (1985): *Lancet*, 2:1033–1035.
203. Janowsky, D. C., El-Yousef, M. K., and David, J. M. (1972): *Lancet*, 2:632–635.
204. Traskman, L., Asberg, M., Bertelsson, L., and Slostrand, L. (1981): *Arch. Gen. Psychiatry*, 38:631–636.
205. Meltzer, H. Y., Perline, R., Tricou, B. J., Lowy, M., and Robertson, A. (1984): *Arch. Gen. Psychiatry*, 41:379–390.
206. Bourne, H. R., Bunney, W. E., Jr., Colburn, R. W., et al. (1968): *Lancet*, 2:805–808.
207. Shaw, D. M., Camps, F. E., and Eccleston, E. G. (1967): *Br. J. Psychiatry*, 113:1407.
208. Mann, J. J., McBride, A., and Stanley, M. (1987): *Ann. N.Y. Acad. Sci.*, 114–121.
209. Stanley, M., and Mann, J. (1983): *Lancet*, 1:214–216.
210. Stanley, M., and Mann, J. J. (1987): *Ann. N.Y. Acad. Sci.*, 294–300.
211. Agren, H. (1980): *Psychiatr. Res.*, 3:225–236.
212. Asberg, M., Traskman, L., and Thoren, P. (1976): *Arch. Gen. Psychiatry*, 33:1193–1197.
213. Banki, C., Molnar, G., and Feliete, I. (1981): *Arch. Psychiatr. Nervenkr.*, 229:345–353.
214. Banki, C., Arato, M., Papp, Z., and Kurcz, M. (1984): *J. Affect. Disorders*, 6:341–450.
215. Oreland, L., Wiberg, A., Asberg, M., Traskman, L., Sjostrand, L., et al. (1981): *Psychiatr. Res.*, 1:21–29.
216. Traskman, L., Tybry, G., Asbert, M., Bertilsson, L., Lantto, O., et al. (1980): *Arch. Gen. Psychiatry*, 37:761–767.
217. van Praag, H. M. (1982): *J. Affect. Disorders*, 4:275–290.
218. Brown, G., Goodwin, F., Ballenger, J., Goyer, P., and Major, L. (1979): *Psychiatr. Res.*, 1:131–139.
219. Brown, G., Ebert, M., Goyer, P., Jimerson, D., Klein, W., et al. (1982): *Am. J. Psychiatry*, 139:741–746.
220. Linnoila, M., Roy, A., and Guthne, S. (1987): *Ann. N.Y. Acad. Sci.*, 202–220.
221. Traskman-Bendz, L., Asberg, M., and Schalling, D. (1987): *Ann. N.Y. Acad. Sci.*, 168–174.
222. Lidberg, L., Tuck, J. R., Asberg, M., Scalia-Tomba, G. B., and Bertilsson, L. (1985): *Acta Psychiatr. Scand.*, 71:230–236.
223. Sedvall, G., Fyro, B., Gullberg, B., Nybadi, H., Weisal, F. A., et al. (1980): *Br. J. Psychiatry*, 136:366–374.
224. van Praag, H. M. (1977): *Biol. Psychiatry*, 12:101–131.
225. Wirz-Justice, A., and Arendt, J. (1979): In: *Biological Psychiatry Today*, edited by J. Obiols, C. Ballus, M. E. Gonzalez, and J. Pujol, pp. 294–302. Elsevier/North Holland, Amsterdam.
226. Mendlewicz, J., Linowski, P., and Brauman, H. (1979): *Lancet*, 2:1079–1080.
227. Wetterberg, L. (1983): *Psychoneuroendocrinology*, 8:75–80.
228. Brown, G. L., and Ebert, M. H. (1985): In: *The Catecholamines in Psychiatric and Neurologic Disorders*, edited by C. R. Lake and M. G. Ziegler, pp. 185–210. Butterworth, Boston.
229. Beck-Friis, J., von Rosen, D., Kjellman, B. F., Ljunggren, J. G., and Setterberg, L. (1984): *Psychoneuroendocrinology*, 10:261–277.
230. Beck-Friis, J., Kjellman, B. F., Aperia, B., Unden, F., von Rosen, D., et al. (1985): *Acta Psychiatr. Scand.*, 71:319–330.
231. Beck-Friis, J., Ljunggren, J. G., Thoren, M., von Rosen, D., Kjellman, B. J., et al. (1985): *Psychoneuroendocrinology*, 10:173–186.
232. Lewy, A. J., Wehr, R. A., Gold, P. W., et al. (1979): In: *Catecholamines: Basic and Clinical Frontiers, Vol. 2*, edited by E. Usdin, I. J. Kopin, and J. Barchas, Pergamon Press, New York.
233. Branchey, L., Weinberg, U., Branchey, M., et al. (1982): *Neuropsychobiology*, 8:225–232.
234. Cavallo, A., Richards, G. E., Holt, K. G., Hejabi, S., Rose, R. M., et al. (1987): *J. Amer. Acad. Child Psychiat. (in press)*.
235. Waldhauser, F., Frisch, H., Waldhauser, M., Weiszenbacher, G., Ulrike, Z., et al. (1984): *Lancet*, 1:362–365.
236. Ramarkin, L., Baird, C. J., and Almeida, O. F. X. (1985): *Science*, 227:714–720.
237. Nair, N. P. V., Hariharasubramanian, Pilapil, C., Isaac, I., and Thavundayil, J. X. (1986): *Biol. Psychiatry*, 21:141–150.
238. Wyatt, R. J., Portnoy, B., Kupfer, D. J., Snyder, F., and Engelman, K. (1971): *Arch. Gen. Psychiatry*, 24:65–70.
239. Schatzberg, A. F., Orsulak, P. J., Rosenbaum, A. H., et al. (1982): *Am. J. Psychiatry*, 139:471–475.
240. Lake, C. R., Pickar, D., Ziegler, M. G., Lipper, S., Slater, S., et al. (1982): *Am. J. Psychiatry*, 139:1315–1318.
241. Esler, M., Turbot, J., Schwarz, R., Leonard, P., Bobik, A., et al. (1982): *Arch. Gen. Psychiatry*, 140:1623–1625.
242. Veith, R. C., Raskind, M. A., Barnes, R. F., Gumbrecht, G., Ritchie, J. L., et al. (1983): *Clin. Pharmacol. Ther.*, 33:763–769.
243. Rudorfer, M. V., Ross, R. J., Linnoila, M., Sherer, M. A., and Potter, W. Z. (1985): *Arch. Gen. Psychiatry*, 42:1186–1192.
244. Roy, A., Pickar, D., Linnoila, M., and Potter, W. Z. (1985): *Arch. Gen. Psychiatry*, 42:1181–1185.
245. Mann, J. J., Brown, R. P., Halper, J. P., Sweeney, J. A., Kocsis, J. H., et al. (1985): *N. Engl. J. Med.*, 313:715–720.
246. Stockmeier, C. A., Martino, A. M., and Kellar, K. J. (1985): *Science*, 18:323–325.
247. Gibbons, M. L. (1964): *Arch. Gen. Psychiatry*, 10:572–575.
248. Sachar, E. J., Hellman, L., Roffwarg, H. P., Halpern, F. S., Fukushima, D. K., et al. (1973): *Arch. Gen. Psychiatry*, 28:19–24.
249. Stokes, P. E., Stoll, P. M., Koslow, S. H., Maas, J. W., Davis, J. M., et al. (1984): *Arch. Gen. Psychiatry*, 41:257–270.
250. Linkowski, P., Mendlewicz, J., Leclercq, R., Brasseur, M., Hubain, P., et al. (1985): *J. Clin. Endocrinol. Metab.*, 61:429–438.
251. Asnis, G. M., Sachar, E. J., Halbreich, U., Nathan, R. S., Novacenko, H., et al. (1981): *Psychosom. Med.*, 43:235–242.
252. Pfohl, B., Sherman, B., Schlechte, J., and Stone, R. (1985): *Arch. Gen. Psychiatry*, 42:897–903.
253. Pfohl, B., Sherman, B., Schlechte, J., and Winokur, G. (1985): *Biol. Psychiatry*, 20:1055–1072.
254. Christie, J. E., Whalley, L. J., Dick, H., Blackwood, D. H. R., Blackfurn, M., et al. (1986): *Br. J. Psychiatry*, 148:58–65.
255. Poznanski, E. O., Carroll, B. J., Banegas, M. C., Sook, S. C., and Grossman, J. A. (1982): *Am. J. Psychiatry*, 139:321–324.
256. Geller, B., Rogol, A. D., Knitter, E. F. (1983): *Amer. J. Psychiat.*, 140:620–622.
257. Weller, E. B., Weller, B. A., Fristad, M. A., and Preskorn, S. H. (1984): *Am. J. Psychiatry*, 141:290–291.
258. Targum, S., Chastek, C., and Sullivan, A. (1981): *Psychiatr. Res.*, 5:107–108.

259. Livingston, R., Reis, C. J., and Ringdahl, I. C. (1984): *Am. J. Psychiatry,* 141:106–107.
260. Livingston, R. L., and Martin-Cannici, C. E. (1985): Presented at the American Psychiatric Association Annual Meeting. Dallas, Texas, May 18–24.
261. Petty, L. K., Asarnow, J. R., Carlson, G. A., and Lesser, L. (1985): *Am. J. Psychiatry,* 142:631–633.
262. Baumgartner, A., Graf, K. J., and Kurten, I. (1985): *Biol. Psychiatry,* 20:675–679.
263. Ceulemans, D. L. S., Westenberg, H. G. M., and van Praag, H. M. (1985): *Psychiatr. Res.,* 14:189–196.
264. Robbins, D. R., Alessi, N. E., Yanchyschyn, G. W., and Colfer, M. (1982): *Am. J. Psychiatry,* 139:942–943.
265. Extein, I., Gold, M. S., Pottash, A. L. C., and Sternbach, H. (1982): In: *Abstracts of the Collegium Internationale Neuro-Psychopharmacologicum, 13th Congress, Jerusalem, Israel, 1982,* p. 204.
266. Carroll, B. J., Curtis, G. C., and Mendels, J. (1976): *Arch. Gen. Psychiatry,* 33:1039–1044.
267. Carroll, B. J., Curtis, G. C., and Mendels, J. (1976): *Arch. Gen. Psychiatry,* 33:1051–1058.
268. Carroll, B. J., Feinberg, M., Greden, J. F., Carroll, B., Feinberg, M., et al. (1981): *Arch. Gen. Psychiatry,* 38:15–23.
269. Arana, G. W., Baldessarini, R. J., and Ornsteen, M. (1985): *Arch. Gen. Psychiatry,* 42:1193–1204.
270. Rabkin, J., Quitkin, F., Stewart, J., McGrath, P., and Puig-Antich, J. (1983): *Am. J. Psychiatry,* 140:926–928.
271. Amsterdam, J. D., Winokur, A., Caroff, S. N., and Conn, J. (1982): *Am. J. Psychiatry,* 139:287–291.
272. Arana, G. W., Wilens, T. E., and Baldesarini, R. J. (1985): *Psychoneuroendocrinology,* 10:49–60.
273. Johnson, M. V., and Singer, H. S. (1982): *Pediatrics,* 70:57–68.
274. Edelstein, C. K., Roy-Byrne, P., Fawzy, F., and Dornfield, L. (1983): *Am. J. Psychiatry,* 140:338–341.
275. Berger, M., Doerr, P., Lund, R., Bronish, T., and von Zerssen, D. (1982): *Biol. Psychiatry,* 17:1217–1242.
276. Berger, M., Krieg, C., and Pirke, K. M. (1982): *Neuroendocrinol. Lett.,* 4:177.
277. Berger, M., Pirke, K., Doerr, P., et al. (1983): *Arch. Gen. Psychiatry,* 40:585–586.
278. Dilsaver, S. C., and Greden, J. F. (1985): *Psychiatr. Res.,* 14:111–122.
279. Arana, G. W., Workman, R. J., and Baldesarini, R. J. (1984): *Am. J. Psychiatry,* 141:1619–1620.
280. Morris, H., Carr, V., Gilliland, J., and Hooper, M. (1986): *Br. J. Psychiatry,* 148:66–69.
281. Meltzer, H. Y., and Fang, V. S. (1983): *Arch. Gen. Psychiatry,* 40:501–505.
282. Sherman, B., Pfohl, B., and Winokur, G. (1984): *Arch. Gen. Psychiatry,* 41:271–278.
283. Sachar, E. J., Puig-Antich, J., Ryan, N., Asnis, G. M., Rabinovich, H., et al. (1985): *Acta Psychiatr. Scand.,* 71:1–8.
284. Lewis, D. A., Coryell Pfohl, B., Schlechte, J., and Coryell, W. (1984): *Psychiatr. Res.,* 13:213–221.
285. Halbreich, U., Asnis, G. M., Zumoff, B., Nathan, R. S., and Shindledecker, R. (1984): *Psychiatr. Res.,* 13:221–229.
286. Oxenkrug, G., Pomara, N., McIntyre, I., Branconnier, R., Stanley, M., et al. (1983): *Psychiatr. Res.,* 10:125–130.
287. Brown, W. A., and Qualls, C. B. (1981): *Psychiatr. Res.,* 4:115–128.
288. Sachar, E. J., Halbreich, U., Sanis, G. H., et al. (1981): *Arch. Gen. Psychiatry,* 38:1113–1117.
289. Stewart, J. W., Quitkin, F., McGrath, P. J., Liebowitz, M. R., Harrison, W., et al. (1984): *Psychiatr. Res.,* 12:195–206.
290. Asnis, G. M., Rabinovich, H., Ryan, N., Sachar, E. J., Nelson, B., et al. (1985): *Psychiatr. Res.,* 14:225–232.
291. Siever, L. J., Uhde, T. W., Jimerson, D. C., Post, R. M., Lake, C. R., et al. (1984): *Arch. Gen. Psychiatry,* 41:63–71.
292. Sachar, E. J., Asnis, G. M., Nathan, R. S., Halbreich, U., Tabrizi, M. A., et al. (1980): *Arch. Gen. Psychiatry,* 37:755–757.
293. Rubinow, D. R., Post, R. M., Gold, P. W., Ballenger, J. C., and Wolff, E. (1984): In: *Neurobiology of Mood Disorders,* edited by R. M. Post and J. C. Ballenger. Williams & Wilkins, Baltimore.
294. Halbreich, U., Asnis, G. M., Shindledecken, R., Zumoff, B., and Nathan, R. S. (1985): *Arch. Gen. Psychiatry,* 42:909–914.
295. Halbreich, U., Asnis, G. M., Shindledecker, R., Zumoff, B., and Nathan, R. S. (1985): *Arch. Gen. Psychiatry,* 42:904–908.
296. Amsterdam, J. D., Winokur, A., Mendels, J., et al. (1979): *Lancet,* 2:904–905.
297. Asnis, G. M., Nathan, R. S., Halbreich, U., et al. (1980): *Lancet,* 1:424–425.
298. Bjorum, N., and Kirkegaard, C. (1979): *Lancet,* 2:694.
299. Kirkegaard, C., Bjorum, N., Cohn, D., Faber, J., Lauridsen, U., et al. (1977): *Psychoneuroendocrinology,* 2:131–136.
300. Kirkegaard, C., Bjorum, N., Cohn, D., et al. (1978): *Arch. Gen. Psychiatry,* 35:1017–1021.
301. Extein, I., Pottash, A. L. C., and Gold, M. S. (1980): *N. Engl. J. Med.,* 302:923–924.
302. Extein, I., Pottash, A. L. C., and Gold, M. S. (1981): *Psychiatr. Res.,* 5:311–316.
303. Gold, M. S., Pottash, A. L. C., Ryan, N., Sweeney, D., Davies, R., and Martin, D. (1980): *Psychoneuroendocrinology,* 5:147–155.
304. Gold, M. S., Pottash, A. L., Exteen, I., Martin, D. M., Howard, E., et al. (1981): *Psychoneuroendocrinology,* 66:159–169.
305. Hollister, L. E., Kenneth, L. D., and Berger, P. A. (1976): *Arch. Gen. Psychiatry,* 33:1393–1396.
306. Loosen, P. T., and Prange, A. L., Jr. (1980): *N. Engl. J. Med.,* 303:224–225.
307. Loosen, P. T., Prange, A. J., Jr., Wilson, I. C., Lara, P. P., and Pettus, C. (1977): *Psychoneuroendocrinology,* 2:137–148.
308. McGrath, P. J., Quitkin, F. M., Stewart, J. W., Asnis, G., Novacenko, H., et al. (1984): *Psychiatr. Res.,* 12:185–193.
309. Baumgartner, A., Hahnenkamp, L., and Meinhold, H. (1986): *Psychiatr. Res.,* 17:285–294.
310. Adrian, T. E., Barnes, A. J., Long, R. G., O'Shaughnessy, D. J., Brown, M. R., et al. (1981): *J. Clin. Endocrinol. Metab.,* 53:675–681.
311. Greenberg, R., Rosenberg, G., Weisberg, L., Semlitz, L., DeMilio, L., et al. (1985): Presented at the New Research Section, 32nd Annual Meeting of the American Academy of Child Psychiatry. San Antonio, Texas.
312. Goldman-Rakic, P. S., and Brown, R. M. (1982): *Brain Res.,* 256:339–349.
313. Lidor, H. G., and Molliver, M. E. (1982): *Brain Res. Bull.,* 8:389–430.
314. Shelton, D. L., Nadler, J. V., and Cotman, C. W. (1979): *Brain Res.,* 164:263–275.
315. Siefert, W. E., Foxx, J. L., and Butler, I. J. (1980): *Ann. Neurol.,* 8:38–42.
316. Young, J. G., Kyprie, R. M., Ross, N. T., and Cohen, D. J. (1980): *J. Autism Dev. Disord.,* 10:1–13.
317. Stewart, M., Pitts, F., Craig, A., and Dieruf, A. (1966): *Am. J. Orthopsychiatry,* 36:861–867.
318. Wender, P. (1971): *Minimal Brain Dysfunction in Children.* Wiley-Interscience, New York.
319. Minde, G., Weiss, G., and Mendelson, M. (1972): *J. Am. Acad. Child Psychiatry,* 11:595–610.
320. Weiss, G., Minde, K., Werry, J., et al. (1971): *Arch. Gen. Psychiatry,* 24:409–414.
321. Rapoport, J. L., Buchsbaum, M. S., Weingartner, H., Zahn, T., Ludlow, C., et al. (1980): *Arch. Gen. Psychiatry,* 47:933–943.
322. Puig-Antich, J. (1980): *Psychiatr. Clin. North Am.,* 3(3):403–424.
323. Johnson, G. F., Hunt, G., and Gerken, A. (1984): *Psychiatr. Res.,* 13:305–314.
324. Puig-Antich, J., Marx, N., Greenhill, L., and Chambers, W. J. (1979): *Psychoneuroendocrinology,* 4:191–197.

Psychopharmacology:
The Third Generation of Progress,
edited by Herbert Y. Meltzer.
Raven Press, New York © 1987.

CHAPTER **85**

Molecular Biological Approaches to Mental Retardation

Dona L. Wong and Roland D. Ciaranello

Three percent of the population of the United States, or approximately 6.6 million individuals, suffer from mental retardation. Symptoms range from mild to severe. In cases of mild retardation, the individuals can develop social, communicative, and academic skills sufficient for self-support, but assistance may be required in situations of social and economic stress. For the profoundly retarded, the prognosis is less encouraging. These individuals require life-long institutionalization, although some may achieve very limited self-care. Motor and speech development are minimal at best.

Mental retardation should be viewed as a multidimensional disorder including biochemical, psychological, psychosocial, and educational components. In the final analysis, the psychosocial component is the major determinant of the afflicted individual's ability to function within accepted societal norms.

The American Association on Mental Deficiency broadly defines mental retardation as subaverage intellectual functioning (1). Intellectual deficiency arises during development and leads to impaired adaptive behavior. Legally, subaverage intellect has been defined as an IQ of less than 70. Based on this definition, the *DSM-III* defines four subcategories of mental retardation (2): mild, IQ 50 to 70; moderate, IQ 35 to 49; severe, IQ 20 to 34; and profound, IQ < 20.

Epidemiologic studies suggest that 80% of the mentally retarded fall into the category of mildly retarded. These individuals can be educated and are generally identified at school, where they fail to meet academic standards for performance and norms on intelligence tests. Once their formal education is completed, however, they blend into the general population, since they can acquire the necessary intellectual, social, and vocational skills for adaptive functioning. Most in this group come from the lower socioeconomic strata.

The next category, the moderately retarded, comprises 12% of the entire retarded population. These individuals are also considered trainable in that communication skills can be learned, but social consciousness is limited. The moderately retarded benefit from vocational training and, as adults, can support themselves in semiskilled or unskilled work under close supervision.

The remaining 8% of the retarded population consists of severely retarded (7%) and profoundly retarded (1%). Custodial care in a structured environment with constant supervision and aid is essential to their existence.

Over 200 factors independently or in combination have been implicated in the etiology of mental retardation. These include prenatal, perinatal, postnatal, and sociocultural factors and are summarized in Table 1. The biomedical approach seeks to identify how these factors produce specific anatomical lesions leading to altered brain tissue and consequent retardation. Changes in basic brain constituents, developmental failures in myelogenesis, neuronal migration, and impaired neural transmission may all be critical com-

TABLE 1. *Etiologic factors associated with mental retardation*

Factors	Examples
Prenatal	Inborn errors of metabolism Chromosomal aberrations Maternal illness during pregnancy Complications of pregnancy
Perinatal	Prematurity Retarded intrauterine growth Birth injury Kernicterus
Postnatal	Infection Lead poisoning Traumas Convulsive disorders Infantile spasms Febrile convulsions Cerebral palsy Heller's disease Malnutrition
Sociocultural	Familial mental retardation Medical problems Emotional and social Environmental deprivation

ponents in brain maldevelopment. The biochemical approach focuses attention on the severe and profound categories of mental retardation, since the severity implicit in brain maldevelopment leads to early diagnosis of the condition. When developmental changes can be ascribed to heritable prenatal factors such as inborn errors of metabolism and chromosomal aberrations, prenatal diagnosis, diagnostic and prognostic work, genetic counseling, and gene therapy may be viable options as a consequence of technological advances in biochemistry, genetics, and molecular biology.

To date, numerous inherited metabolic disorders and chromosomal abnormalities have been associated with mental retardation. These are summarized in Table 2. In the sections that follow, we survey four specific disorders associated with mental retardation and molecular biological approaches applied to studying these disorders. They include phenylketonuria, an inborn error of phenylalanine metabolism; Lesch–Nyhan disease, an X-linked recessive disorder related to altered purine metabolism; fragile X-linked mental retardation, a form of retardation associated with a fragile site on the X chromosome; and Down's syndrome, a chromosomal disorder primarily associated with trisomy 21. First, let us review the necessary molecular biology for understanding medical genetic approaches to these disorders.

TABLE 2. *Inherited metabolic disorders and chromosomal abnormalities associated with mental retardation*

Type	Category	Disorder
Chromosomal aberration	Autosomal disorder	Down's syndrome *Cri du chat* Trisomy 13 Trisomy 18 Trisomy 22
	Sex chromosome anomalies	Klinefelter's syndrome Turner's syndrome
Inborn metabolic disorders	Amino acid metabolism	Phenylketonuria Menke's maple syrup disease Hartnup disease Citrullinuria Hyperammonemia Argininosuccinic aciduria Idiopathic hyperglycinemia Histidinemia Homocystinuria Lowe's oculorenal dystrophy Cystathionuria Hyperolinemia Tyrosinosis Hyperlysinemia
	Fat metabolism	Cerebromacular degeneration Tay–Sachs, gangliosidosis G_{M2} Generalized gangliosidosis (G_{M1}, type 1) Juvenile gangliosidosis (G_{M1}, type 2) Niemann–Pick disease Gaucher's disease Metachromic leukodystrophy Bigler and Hsia syndrome
	Carbohydrate metabolism	Galactosemia Von Gierke's disease

MOLECULAR BIOLOGICAL APPROACHES

We do not attempt to review all the requisite biochemistry and molecular biology but simply present a sufficient overview so that the material relevant to each of the specific disorders can readily be understood by those less familiar with medical genetic approaches to studying disease. The reader is referred to other chapters in this book and other references (3,4) for a detailed explanation of the science.

All of the genetic information that ultimately defines the phenotype of an organism is encoded in its deoxyribonucleic acid (DNA). Molecular diversity in unrelated organisms results from sequence variation of the four deoxyribonucleotide building blocks, deoxyadenylic acid, deoxycytidylic acid, deoxyguanylic acid, and thymidilic acid, organized along linear polynucleotide chains. Transmission of genetic information is generally stable between parents and progeny, and thus, DNA must be accurately replicated. Accurate generation of daughter chains is provided by the replication process itself. Parent duplex chains of DNA unwind to serve as templates for the polymerization of two complementary daughter strands.

Phenotypic expression of genetically inherited DNA occurs through the processes of transcription and translation. The information encoded in specific DNA sequences is transcribed to generate a polymer of ribonucleic acids (adenylic acid, cytidylic acid, guanylic acid, and uridylic acid) or RNA. Again, DNA serves as a replicating template, but the transcript generated is a messenger RNA (mRNA). The mRNA is then translated into a specific polypeptide based on its nucleotide sequence. Each amino acid in the polypeptide is represented by three successive nucleotides, which form a codon. The amino acid sequence determines both the three-dimensional folding of the protein and its interaction with other macromolecules.

Each polypeptide is represented by a single gene. Therefore, an organism reflects a composite of all proteins encoded in its DNA and the signals regulating the synthesis of these proteins. Thus, proper timing of DNA replication, transcription, and translation as well as correct products for each of these steps are critical to the processes of differentiation, development, and adaptation. Interruption in the requisite control mechanisms or altered products can lead to either diseased states or death.

Recombinant DNA techniques now permit us to examine closely the control of gene expression and its relationship to disease. "Foreign" DNA, either genomic or complementary DNA (cDNA), can be inserted into vector chromosomes by annealing and ligating the "sticky" ends of restriction-endonuclease-treated vector and "foreign" DNA. The vector can be either a plasmid, bacteriophage, or cosmid, and the "foreign" DNA is often inserted adjacent to a promoter site to increase its expression. The vector containing inserted DNA is replicated in bacterial hosts. Thus, specific DNA can be cloned, identified, isolated, and amplified.

These recombinant cDNA clones can then be used as probes because of two critical properties of nucleic acids. First, complementary strands of DNA or DNA and RNA will hybridize by forming hydrogen bonds between their base pairs (A–T/A–U, C–G). Hybridization depends on the amount of complementarity between the strands and stringency conditions (e.g., temperature, salt concentration).

Second, DNA can be fragmented by enzymes called restriction endonucleases. Each restriction enzyme recognizes a specific sequence of bases and will cleave only at sites where the sequence exists. Gene and cDNA clones thus permit us to determine gene structure, map encoded genes, assign genes to specific chromosomes, and investigate genetic polymorphisms with or without accompanying phenotypic alterations using techniques such as Southern analysis (5) or *in situ* hybridization (6). In the case of Southern analysis, DNA fragments are separated on agarose gels, the separated polynucleotides are hybridized with radioactively labeled cDNA probes, and the banding pattern is visualized by autoradiography. In the case of *in situ* hybridization, radioactive cDNA probes can be hybridized to cell or tissue samples prepared by standard cytological methods followed by autoradiographic development to detect cross-reacting chromosomal material.

For example, the arrangement of genes at a complex locus can be determined by restriction mapping. Various restriction endonucleases are used to generate overlapping segments of DNA carrying the genes in question. The genes are aligned by ascertaining the cleavage sites for various restriction endonucleases within each fragment by hybridization to cDNA probes according to Southern analysis.

Chromosomal location of specific genes can also be assigned by hybridization of cDNA to gene fragments. By use of cDNA specific for the desired gene product, chromosome-enriched DNA libraries can be screened for the DNA fragment associated with the gene product. Somatic cell hybrids containing DNA from specific chromosomes similarly allow the assignment of gene loci to the appropriate chromosome.

Finally, genetic polymorphisms exist for many genes. In some cases, the polymorphism is recognized by accompanying phenotypic changes. In other cases, there are no obvious phenotypic changes. The mutations resulting in the polymorphism may be caused by point mutations, deletions, duplications, or translocations. In each case, the altered DNA changes in its susceptibility to restriction endonuclease cleavage. A simple point mutation, for example, can block cleavage. Thus, restriction fragment length polymorphisms (RFLP) can be used to study genetic linkage and chromosome assignment by comparing autoradiograms of normal and mutant DNA subjected to Southern analysis.

In the next sections, we discuss specific applications of the molecular biological approaches described here in furthering our understanding of the genetic etiology of diseases associated with mental retardation.

PHENYLKETONURIA

Fifty years ago, Fölling described phenylketonuria (PKU), the first of many inherited diseases in which mental retardation was linked to a biochemical disorder (7). The classic feature of PKU is elevated serum phenylalanine caused by a deficiency in liver phenylalanine hydroxylase, the enzyme converting the amino acid phenylalanine to tyrosine (Fig. 1). *In utero,* the fetal brain develops normally despite the absence of this hepatic enzyme. However, the central nervous system continues to develop for the first 5 or 6 years. During this time, the DNA, protein, and lipid

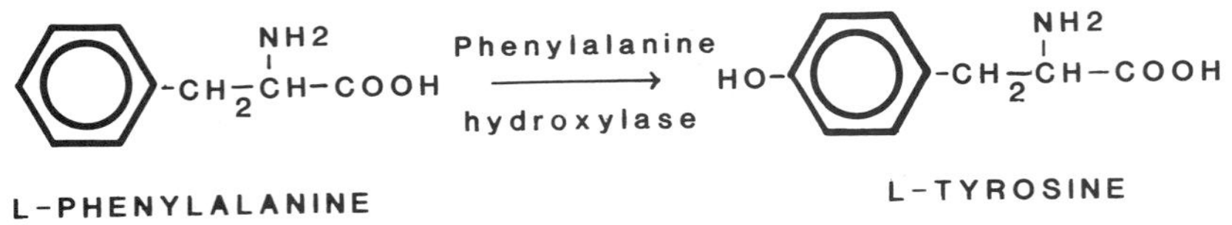

FIG. 1. Conversion of L-phenylalanine to L-tyrosine by the hepatic enzyme phenylalanine hydroxylase. This enzyme is deficient in PKU, and phenylalanine accumulates.

contents of the brain change, synaptogenesis and myelination occur, etc. Elevation of phenylalanine or its metabolites (e.g., phenylpyruvic acid, phenyllactate, phenylacetate) may cause biochemical changes that alter these processes and result in CNS maldevelopment in the neonate accompanied by subsequent retardation. Once these processes are completed, however, intellect and emotional behavior should be minimally affected by elevated phenylalanine or phenylalanine metabolites.

Prenatal or neonatal identification of this inborn error of metabolism is critical, since infants are often asymptomatic in the first year. In the absence of proper dietary control of phenylalanine, severe mental retardation is the inevitable outcome. If serum phenylalanine levels are maintained between 5.5 and 10 mg/dl, most of the adverse effects can be circumvented. However, reduction of phenylalanine to less than 5.5 mg/dl must be avoided, since this also precipitates severe retardation (8).

When dietary phenylalanine is not restricted, other symptoms develop after the first year, including eczema, convulsions, abnormal EEG, diluted pigment, decreased growth, poor coordination, hyperactivity, agitated and aggressive behavior, tremor, perceptual difficulties, and, of course, severe retardation. Early diagnosis (≤6 months) and dietary regulation allow normal cerebral development.

A mechanism that reconciles all the diverse findings associated with this disorder proposes that phenylalanine competes with other amino acids for intercellular transport. This creates a relative imbalance of the essential amino acids required for protein synthesis (9). In the case of neuronal cells, inhibition of protein synthesis and the associated effects on synaptogenesis will be devastating to the developing brain. For example, alterations in myelin synthesis in phenylketonuric patients are responsible for the observed changes in myelin constituents and CNS myelination.

In classic PKU, phenylalanine hydroxylase enzymatic activity is completely lacking. The enzyme does not appear to be synthesized, since antibody to rat liver phenylalanine hydroxylase, which cross reacts with the human enzyme, does not cross react with any liver protein in PKU patients (10). The human enzyme has been shown to consist of two nonidentical subunits of relative molecular weight 50,000 (11). Controversy exists as to whether phenylalanine hydroxylase exists as a homo- or heterodimer (12–14). However, it has been proposed that a homodimer undergoes posttranslational processing to yield nonidentical subunits (15). Recent gene-cloning studies (16) further support the existence of a single gene for the protein, with carbohydrate substitution, phosphorylation, or limited proteolysis generating differences in subunit structure.

The cloning of the gene and complementary DNA for phenylalanine hydroxylase has additionally provided essential diagnostic tools for prenatal and neonatal diagnosis of classic PKU, a disorder transmitted as an autosomal recessive. Present diagnostic procedures and dietary control have permitted most PKU patients to live normal lives. However, recombinant DNA techniques may be critical to a new variant of PKU: maternal PKU. Infants born to PKU mothers whose phenylalanine levels were not controlled during pregnancy show severe retardation and other symptoms associated with PKU. Most of these infants are heterozygotes and thus not PKU positive. However, elevated phenylalanine in the maternal blood appears to precipitate fetal brain damage, congenital heart disease, low birth weight, microcephaly, and a high incidence of hyperphenylalaninemia (9,17). With these thoughts in mind, let us now examine how modern medical genetic techniques can be applied to PKU.

Human Phenylalanine Hydroxylase Gene

Phenylalanine hydroxylase cDNA was first isolated for the rat liver enzyme using a polysomal preparation enriched in phenylalanine hydroxylase mRNA (13). Complementary DNA was synthesized from the mRNA and inserted into the PstI site of the plasmid pBr322. Positive clones were identified by differential hybridization in which cDNA was selected by its ability to hybridize with enriched messenger. Hybrid-selected translation was performed to verify the identification of the clones. Polypeptide products generated by cell-free translation of mRNA hybridizing to the cDNA clones were immunoprecipitated with phenylalanine hydroxylase antibody. The immunoprecipitated polypeptide products were analyzed by sodium dodecylsulfate polyacrylamide gel electrophoresis, and a single species was observed with a relative molecular weight of 50,000, corresponding to the estimated molecular weight of the purified monomeric rat liver enzyme. An amino acid sequence deduced from an open reading frame of the cDNA matched 17 residues in a partial amino acid sequence of the purified enzyme (18).

The rat liver cDNA clone for phenylalanine hydroxylase was then used to develop a cDNA clone for the human enzyme (19). Previous studies had established the cross reactivity of the rat liver antibody with the human enzyme. Similarly, rat phenylalanine hydroxylase cDNA was shown to cross react with human liver phenylalanine hydroxylase mRNA. Therefore, the rat cDNA was used to screen a human liver cDNA library of 40,000 transformants. Four specific clones with inserts of 0.3 to 1.4 kb were selected, and the two largest probes were used for hybridization studies with DNA isolated from normal individuals and two PKU cell lines. In these studies, all of the restriction endonucleases tested (>10) generated identical hybridization patterns, suggesting that classical PKU did not result from a deletion or rearrangement in the region specified by these two probes.

Therefore, a full-length probe for the human phenylalanine hydroxylase gene was isolated (20). A human liver λgt11 cDNA library was constructed and screened with the rat liver cDNA probe. From this library, a 2.5-kb insert was identified that approximated the length of phenylalanine hydroxylase mRNA.

Nucleotide sequence analysis of this 2,428-bp cDNA generated an amino acid sequence for human phenylalanine hydroxylase similar to that determined for the rat protein (20). Furthermore, the nucleotide sequence coded for a 51.7-kd polypeptide, close to the estimated molecular weight of the protein.

Restriction Fragment Length Polymorphism Analysis in Classical PKU

Both the partial and full-length probes have been used in RFLP analysis in classical phenylketonuria. As indicated above, no polymorphisms in the coding region of the partial cDNA probe were observed in PKU cell lines. However, when leukocyte genomic DNA from random individuals was analyzed with three restriction endonucleases, SphI, MspI, and HindIII, polymorphic patterns were observed at the phenylalanine hydroxylase locus (19). Seven allelic variants were identified, suggesting the existence of twelve haplotypes and permitting analysis of classical PKU patients and families by restriction fragment length polymorphisms.

Similarly, the full-length cDNA probe was used to screen families with one or two affected and unaffected children (21). Classical PKU was verified in affected children by testing for phenylalanine tolerance. Lymphocytes were collected from all family members, and isolated DNA was analyzed for restriction fragment length polymorphisms using SphI and HindIII and the human full-length clone described above.

In all cases, the restriction fragment pattern could be linked to the mutant allele; segregation of the mutant allele and the disease state was concordant in families with two affected siblings, and segregation was discordant between affected and unaffected siblings. Therefore, haplotype analysis may prove a very powerful diagnostic tool.

The full-length phenylalanine hydroxylase cDNA has provided additional information about PKU-associated RFLPs that may be valuable in the diagnosis of the diseased state (22). Eight restriction enzymes generated polymorphic patterns for the chromosomal gene. When these RFLP haplotypes were used to study the phenylalanine hydroxylase gene in PKU and normal families, two RFLP haplotypes were more common in 75% of the control genes, whereas two different RFLP haplotypes predominated in 75% of the PKU genes.

The Use of RFLPs for Prenatal Diagnosis

Cosmid genomic libraries were constructed from normal and PKU lymphocytic DNA (21). Southern analysis of the genomic clones using the full-length cDNA probe showed that rearrangements and deletions did not exist in the PKU gene. However, several restriction length polymorphisms were identified that distinguish normal phenylalanine hy-

droxylase genes from mutant genes. These RFLPs were used in prenatal diagnosis of two at-risk families.

DNA purified from parent and proband lymphocytes was analyzed by Southern blots to determine the restriction fragment with which the PKU allele segregated for each of the families. At 16 weeks, amniocentesis was performed, amniotic cells propagated, and the DNA isolated and analyzed for RFLPs. In the first family, the fetus was determined to be homozygous for PKU. It had the same genotype as the PKU proband and had inherited the restriction fragment segregating with the PKU allele from mother and father. In the second family, the fetus was heterozygous, hence a non-PKU child. In this case, however, the parents were of the same genotype, and the mutant phenylalanine hydroxylase genes segregated with alternative restriction fragments. Thus, a prenatal diagnosis would not have been possible if the fetus were affected or free of the PKU trait.

Chromosome Mapping of the PKU Locus

In order to map the phenylalanine hydroxylase gene, genomic DNA from mouse/human cell hybrids containing an assortment of human chromosomes were analyzed by molecular hybridization using the full-length cDNA clone for human phenylalanine hydroxylase (23). The chromosome content of each of hybrid was first determined by karyotype and isozyme analysis. Then Southern analysis was performed on DNA from these cell lines. Twelve of the hybrids showed concordant segregation of the phenylalanine hydroxylase locus and chromosome 12. More recent studies have further localized the gene to 12q2.2 to 12q24.1 (22).

Gene Expression of the PKU Locus

Gene transfer studies (16) have shown that the genetic information for phenylalanine hydroxylase is encoded in a single gene. The full-length human cDNA clone was subcloned into a eukaryotic expression vector containing the human metallothionein gene promoter (MT-II). When NIH3T3 cells, which do not express the enzyme, were transfected with this recombinant, the cells expressed phenylalanine-hydroxylase-specific mRNA by Northern analysis, immunoreactive protein by Western analysis, and enzymatic activity as measured in cell extracts, all characteristic of the normal gene. These results suggest that the human probe might be a valuable tool in future gene therapy studies.

LESCH–NYHAN SYNDROME

Lesch–Nyhan syndrome (24) was first described in 1964 as a familial disorder of uric acid metabolism and central nervous system function. The syndrome is inherited as an X-linked recessive disorder in which hypoxanthine phosphoribosyltransferase (HPRT) is virtually absent (<1%). Characteristics of the syndrome include excess uric acid production, mental retardation, and neurologic defects such as self-mutilation, muscle spasticity, and choreoathetosis.

Approximately one in 100,000 births results in this devastating disorder for which there is no cure. In most cases, life extends only into the second decade with death from either infection or renal failure.

Most Lesch–Nyhan patients are normal at birth. However, 3 to 4 months marks the beginning of developmental retardation. By the end of the first year, many of the CNS aberrations become apparent: extrapyramidal signs, fine athetoid movements of the hands and feet, dystonia and chorea, and pyramidal tract symptoms. Beyond the age of 2, compulsive self-mutilation begins. This is characterized by involuntary biting of the fingers, lips, and buccal mucosa and can only be prevented by restraining the limbs or, in severe cases, extracting the teeth. Unusually aggressive behavior is also observed, but the degree of self-mutilation and aggressive behavior varies greatly depending on the patients as well as the daily environment.

Mental retardation is very characteristic of the syndrome: IQ testing shows that most patients fall in the range of 39 to 65, although it is suspected that communication difficulties resulting from dysarthria and choreoathetosis may be partially responsible for the low IQ scores (25).

The excessive production of uric acid in Lesch–Nyhan patients results in orange uric acid crystals in the urine, a telltale sign on the diaper of an infant. However, in most cases, this clue remains unrecognized or unmentioned to the physician. If the patient progresses to uric acid nephrolithiasis, uropathy with azotemia may develop, a common cause of death in untreated cases.

The central nervous system of Lesch–Nyhan patients shows no marked changes, although decreased brain size, some demyelination, and vascular lesions have been observed in autopsied brains. Hence, the mechanism responsible for central nervous system dysfunction remains unclear. There does appear to be dysfunction of neurotransmitter systems in the basal ganglia, including dopaminergic neurons and cholinergic interneurons (26). In addition, although HPRT is present in most tissues, higher concentrations exist in the brain (27). Approximately 0.05% of brain protein is represented by this enzyme. Basal ganglia concentrations of HPRT are especially high, suggesting that salvage pathways are critical for purine production in brain tissue.

Hypoxanthine phosphoribosyltransferase is responsible for purine synthesis by the salvage mechanism (Fig. 2). The monomeric molecular weight of the enzyme ranges from 24 to 26,000, and the native enzyme is thought to exist as a tetramer (28). Under *in vitro* conditions, both dimeric and tetrameric forms have been observed, and the tetramer is thought to be a dimer of dimers.

Deficiencies in brain HPRT seem to enhance *de novo* purine synthesis, leading to purine excess (29). 5-Phosphoribosyl-1-pyrophosphate (PRPP), normally utilized by HPRT in the conversion of hypoxanthine to inosinic acid through the purine salvage pathway, activates PRPP amidotransferase instead. This accelerates *de novo* purine synthesis and leads to uric acid accumulation. Interestingly, CSF concentrations of uric acid are normal, suggesting that CNS alterations do not arise from excesses of this metabolite. However, allopurinol treatment is still recommended to minimize peripheral side effects.

Normal HPRT displays much heterogeneity, as many electrophoretic variants exist (30). Since the electrophoretic variants do not change in immunogenicity, alterations in primary structure seem unlikely. Rather, heterogeneity appears to arise from posttranslational modification, one example being deamidation of an asparagine residue at position 106. Family studies show that some structural variation does occur, since changes in thermostability, electrophoretic mobility, product and by-product inhibition, substrate specificity, and Michaelis constants have been observed. The latter supports the presence of heterogeneity at the HPRT locus. Let us now examine the molecular biological evidence for this genetic diversity.

Cloning of the Human HPRT Gene and Its cDNA

Hypoxanthine phosphoribosyltransferase is constitutively expressed at very low levels. However, two cell lines, the mouse neuroblastoma cell line NBR4 and the Chinese hamster cell line RJK159, overproduce HPRT and its corresponding mRNA, providing abundant mRNA for construction of a cDNA library (31). With mRNA as a template, complementary DNA was synthesized with reverse transcriptase. The resulting duplex was inserted into the PstI site of pBR322 by dG–dC tailing, and the transformants were grown in *E. coli*. Recombinants for HPRT were selected by differential hybridization and reconfirmed by positive selection hybridization as described above for the PKU gene. A recombinant cDNA of apparent full length was obtained with the mouse mRNA (32), whereas recombinant clones representing only 61% of the total message were obtained with the Chinese hamster mRNA. Therefore, the full-length mouse cDNA was used to isolate human recombinant DNA clones coding for HPRT by screening a human fetal liver cDNA library (33).

The human HPRT gene has also been isolated by an alternative method (34,35): HPRT-deficient mouse cells were transfected with total human DNA, and transformed cells were selected in HAT medium. Cytoplasmic extracts of cells were checked for expression of HPRT enzymatic

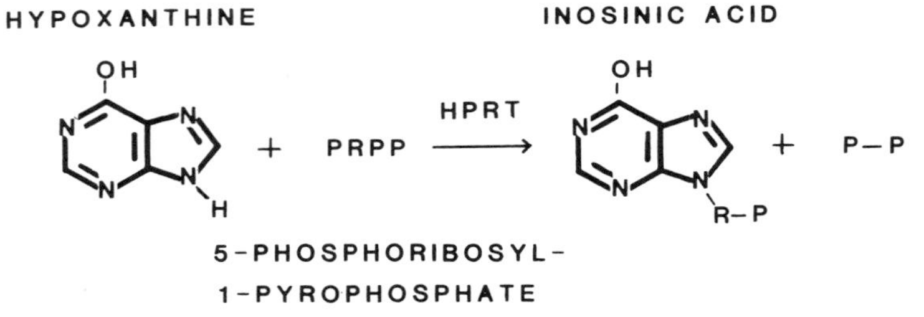

HYPOXANTHINE   INOSINIC ACID

5-PHOSPHORIBOSYL-
1-PYROPHOSPHATE

FIG. 2. Purine synthesis by the salvage mechanism catalyzed by HPRT. PRPP, 5-phosphoribosyl-1-pyrophosphate.

activity. DNA from HPRT-positive transformants was used for secondary transfection. DNA from these secondary transfectants was next hybridized to total human cDNA probes to select common bands. The common bands were cloned in pBr322, and recombinants selected by homology with human DNA and then subcloned. Subclones were identified by cross reactivity with human X chromosome DNA and hybridization with mRNA from secondary transfectants as well as human mRNA. Identification was confirmed by using the subclone to screen a cDNA library. Further verification was provided by transfection into HPRT-deficient mouse cells. Transformed cells expressed human HPRT (36).

Nucleotide sequence analysis of the human recombinant DNA generated an amino acid sequence identical to that generated for the protein with the minor exception of one less amino acid (217 instead of 218) (35). After translation, the amino-terminal methionine is cleaved, and the exposed alanine residue is acetylated. The primary sequence of HPRT shows considerable species conservation. Only seven amino acids differ between mouse and hamster and mouse and human sequences. In most cases, these amino acid changes represent a single base change.

The HPRT Gene

Recombinant cDNA clones of HPRT have been used to characterize the HPRT gene, HPRT-specific mRNA, and the steps involved in the processing of this mRNA (35,37). Whereas the structural gene consists of 34 kb, the mRNA is only 1.6 kb in length and represents only 5% of the genomic DNA. The difference in size between gene and messenger arises from eight intervening, noncoding sequences (introns) ranging in length from 100 to 10,800 bp. The coding sequences are represented by nine exons, which range in length from 77 to 593 bp.

The primary mRNA transcript is thought to be a precursor mRNA consisting of both coding and noncoding regions of the gene (35). Mature mRNA is produced by excision of the noncoding sequences to generate the 1.6-kb messenger. At the 5' end of the messenger is a noncoding region of greater than 100 bp followed by the AUG initiation codon for protein translation. The translated region, consisting of 654 bp, ensues, flanked by a termination codon and a 3' noncoding region of 589 bp. This latter noncoding region is followed by a polyadenylation signal and the polyadenylated tail.

Mapping of the HPRT Gene

Pedigree studies of families of Lesch–Nyhan patients (38,39) had originally suggested that the HPRT locus was located on the X chromosome. By use of human/rodent hybrids, this has been confirmed by showing that HPRT activity segregates with the X chromosome (40). The gene has now been specifically localized to the distal section of the X chromosome between the gene loci for PRPP synthetase and glucose-6-phosphate dehydrogenase (41,42). Three other homologous sequences or pseudogenes exist, but they are not coregulated and are associated with

chromosomes 3, 5, and 11 (37,43). In addition, they are much smaller than the functional X-linked HPRT gene, since interrupting, noncoding sequences are absent.

Analysis by RFLP in Lesch–Nyhan Syndrome

Assorted evidence suggests that HPRT deficiency may be genetically heterogeneous. In contrast to many genetic disorders, there is no selective advantage or ethnic association. Many mutant forms of the enzyme exist, and although a number represent single amino acid changes, the functional changes can be very diverse, ranging from changes in enzyme concentration to changes in Michaelis constants for the substrates.

The search for restriction fragment length polymorphisms in cultured cells from Lesch–Nyhan patients has been one approach to the question of genetic diversity. Subfragments of HPRT complementary DNA, representing specific exon regions of the genome, have been used to probe restriction endonuclease (BamHI, BglII, PstI, MspI)-cut DNA from 28 patients. Five patients showed HPRT loci with major deletions or rearrangements (44). Three deletion mutations showed cytogenetically normal X chromosomes. A fourth mutation showed exon duplication. A fifth mutation showed several exons with structural alterations of undetermined nature.

When messenger RNA was examined from each of the described patients (44), those with deletion mutations produced no mRNA, several normal patients showed appropriate-sized mRNA, one patient with normal DNA produced no mRNA, and the mutant with exon duplication produced a larger mRNA as expected with partial gene duplication. Each of these findings further supports the idea of genetic diversity in HPRT.

Gene Therapy

Lesch–Nyhan syndrome is one of the hereditary disorders that may be a successful candidate for therapy. A single gene abnormality appears responsible for the syndrome. Moreover, partial expression of the enzyme seems to eliminate the CNS abnormalities.

We have already described the expression of the enzyme in HPRT-deficient mouse cell lines. Cloned DNA has also been transfected into human HPRT-deficient cells. B lymphoblasts from a Lesch–Nyhan patient were infected with human HPRT cDNA using a murine retroviral vector (54). Clones integrating the HPRT cDNA were isolated and characterized by restriction fragment mapping of their genomic DNA. Enzymatic activity was restored from 4 to 23% of normal values, and many associated metabolic aberrations were nearly corrected in correspondence with the restoration of enzymatic activity.

In addition, skin fibroblasts from a Lesch–Nyhan patient, immortalized by SV40 transformation (46), have been successfully transfected with SV40 DBA vectors containing the bacterial gene coding for xanthine–guanine phosphoribosyltransferase (XGPRT). This transformation allows the cells to grow under conditions in which *de novo* purine synthesis is blocked and parent cells do not survive. The transformants appear genetically stable after 12 generations of subcloning. Thus, XGPRT appears capable of correcting the enzymatic deficiency in HPRT.

Clearly, much additional work must be pursued before one can consider the use of gene transfer as a corrective measure for Lesch–Nyhan syndrome. The above studies show that peripheral HPRT defects can be corrected, but CNS deficiencies elude treatment. However, Lesch–Nyhan disease is such a devastating disorder that the possibility of gene therapy is to be seriously considered in view of such promising preliminaries.

FRAGILE X CHROMOSOME

Clinical and genetic studies clearly show an excess of males with mental retardation, suggesting that a form of X-linked mental retardation exists. Nonspecific mental retardation became the name designated for these forms of retardation, in which mothers displayed normal intelligence and sons had a 50% probability of being affected. A puzzling aspect, however, was the extreme heterogeneity associated with nonspecific retardation. Some patients only presented with retardation, whereas others showed physical abnormalities in addition. It is now generally accepted that at least four forms of mental retardation with X-linked inheritance exist (47,48). One form, the "fragile X syndrome," is distinguished from other forms in that a fragile site is present at the distal end of the long arm of the X chromosome.

In fragile X syndrome, mental retardation is accompanied by macroorchidism and other distinct physical and neurological manifestations (48). These include increased birth weight, prominent forehead, relatively hypoplastic midface, high, arched palate, and large, often malformed ears.

The fragile X chromosome site, fra(X)(q27), was first described by Lubs in 1969 (49). Fragile chromosomal sites have several morphologically distinct features (50), the most essential being the triradial figure generated by breakage and nondisjunction at the fragile site.

A characteristic specifically associated with the fragile X site is its folate sensitivity. In media lacking folic acid and thymidine, the fragile X site is elicited in lymphocytes (50) and skin fibroblasts (51) of affected males. Expression of the site seems to depend on the absence of thymidine monophosphate during late S phase in the cell cycle. In the heterozygous female, the fragile X site also appears in those carriers showing some retardation. Expression appears age dependent, since it is often absent in the older heterozygotes (52). The fragile X site has also been demonstrated in cultured amniotic fluid cells (53) and cultured lymphocytes from fetal blood (54), suggesting a potential prenatal test for this disorder.

However, both genetic counseling and prenatal diagnosis by testing for this marker X in cultured cells are fraught with ambiguity for many reasons. First, fragile X is difficult to demonstrate in some female carriers. Second, males may have the fragile X and not be retarded (55), or vice versa. Third, there are difficulties associated with expression of fragile X in tissue culture; a lack of expression may not ensure absence of the chromosomal abnormality.

Since fragile X syndrome is not a treatable disorder, genetic screening and prenatal diagnosis are critical components to its detection. Molecular genetic approaches may provide us with viable alternatives to the screening methods described above. The linkage studies described below have already revealed critical information about the mapping of the mental retardation gene locus associated with fragile X and other closely segregating gene loci. Since the defective gene has not been identified, restriction fragment length polymorphisms of closely segregating genes may provide appropriate diagnostics.

Linkage Studies

The heritable fragile site associated with fragile X syndrome has been localized to Xq27.3 (56,57) by prophase banding (58) and scanning electron microscopy. Closely segregating with this site is the gene for glucose-6-phosphate dehydrogenase (G6PD). In human/rodent somatic cell hybrids, segregation analysis has mapped the gene coding for G6PD to Xq28 (59).

Recombinant DNA technology has provided additional linkage information. The fragile X and hemophilia B loci are very closely linked (60). Hemophilia B is caused by a functional deficiency in the coagulation factor IX. With complementary DNA for factor IX used to probe DNA from human/mouse hybrid cell lines, the gene locus for this coagulation factor has been assigned to the Xq26–27 region of the X chromosome. When a search for restriction fragment length polymorphisms was undertaken with eight endonucleases, a TaqI polymorphism was discovered. A three-generation family in which the fragile X pedigree was transmitted through the phenotypically normal grandfather was examined for segregation of the fragile X gene locus with coagulation factor IX (60). DNA from the lymphocytes of the various family members was restriction cut with TaqI and probed with coagulation factor IX cDNA. All of the affected sons and carrier daughters displayed the TaqI polymorphism, whereas the normal sons and a noncarrier daughter did not. Thus, linkage analysis suggests close association of the fragile X and coagulation factor IX genes. In addition, it has also been shown using the hybrid cell lines that the factor IX gene is distal to the HPRT gene (61).

The latter mapping was determined by characterizing a series of X-specific RFLP markers—S21, 52A, DX13, Xga, RC8, L1.28, DXYS1, HPRT, and factor IX—and using these as probes for restriction endonuclease-cut lymphocytic DNA from the families described above. By counting recombinant and nonrecombinant chromosomes, the recombination frequency was determined. This information, together with parental phase information, then permitted each of the markers to be mapped on the X chromosome (see below).

With cDNA probes to G6PD, it has further been shown by *in situ* hybridization using metaphase cells that G6PD maps distal to the fragile X site (59). Specifically, the G6PD locus is located on the Xq telomeric fragment. This observation is consistent with the segregation of the genes for deutan (62) and protan (63) colorblindness and the G6PD gene independent of factor IX. Thus, although both G6PD and factor IX genes are closely linked to the fragile X site, they flank the site and hence are not closely linked themselves.

Those genes and markers mapping around the fragile site on the long arm of the X chromosome are as follows:

xg/RC8/L1.28(centromere)DXYS1/S21/HPRT/

52A/F IX/frag X/G6PD/DX13(telomeric end)

Recently, hybridization studies using the 52A RFLP marker and DNA from human/mouse or Chinese hamster somatic cell hybrids showed that 52A is localized to Xq27/Xq28–Xqter, which is similar to factor IX (64). *In situ* hybridization has further specified the factor IX region to Xq27 (65). When families with X-linked mental retardation associated with the fragile X site were studied for TaqI polymorphisms using cDNA probes for 52A and factor IX, recombination among the 52A, factor IX, and fragile X loci was evident. Thus, although it had been previously demonstrated that the loci for 52A and factor IX were closely linked in normal families, these two loci as well as the fragile X site do not appear to be as closely linked as previously suspected. Thus, the close linkage of the fragile site with factor IX may not be preserved in many families, and factor IX linkage may be an unreliable probe for genetic counseling and prenatal diagnosis.

DOWN'S SYNDROME

Down's syndrome, first described by Langdon Down in 1866, is the single most predominant cause of mental retardation. Ten percent of mentally retarded individuals are Down's syndrome patients, with an estimated one out of 700 births resulting in an afflicted child in the United States. The majority of these children are moderately to severely retarded, and it is thus not surprising that 10% of the institutionalized mentally retarded are those with this disorder.

Over 200 physical abnormalities characterize Down's syndrome, but only a limited number are observed in any one patient. Some of these features include dwarfed stature, small rounded ears, strabismus, high cephalic index, epicanthal folds, lax ligaments, and characteristic configurations of the dermal ridges on palm and soles. The diagnosis of Down's syndrome may be difficult in newborns, but telltale indicators include hypotonia, weak or absent Moro's reflex, oblique palpebral fissures, abundant neck skin, small flattened skull, high cheekbones, protruding tongue, and broad, thick hands with single transverse palmar crease and short, inwardly curved little fingers.

Mental retardation is, of course, the prominent feature of Down's syndrome. The majority of patients have IQ scores of less than 50. In general, mental development decreases from near normal levels at the age of 1 year to about 30 in the average patient. However, the "normal" mental capacity of the infant may simply reflect our inability to assess intelligence accurately in the very young.

Despite diminished intelligence, Down's syndrome children adjust better emotionally than other mentally retarded children with comparable intelligence. Temperamentally, they are placid, cooperative, and cheerful children, although some emotional and behavioral problems may be encountered in the adolescent, particularly the institutionalized adolescent.

For most, however, the life expectancy averages 12 years. If a Down's syndrome patient lives beyond 40, early senescence develops. Other changes characteristic of Alzheimer's disease (66) also occur, suggesting an interrelationship between these two disorders.

The major cause of Down's syndrome is trisomy 21, the presence of an extra chromosome 21 as a result of nondisjunction during meiosis (67). Thus, 47 chromosomes, instead of the normal complement of 46, are present. Both maternal and paternal age appear to predispose for chromosomal nondisjunction, although the mechanism for this predisposition remains unclear.

Two other chromosomal aberrations also lead to Down's syndrome: (a) nondisjunction during any cell division following fertilization—in this case, a mosaic of both normal and trisomic cells occurs—and (b) translocation and fusion of two chromosomes, e.g., chromosomes 15 and 21. In this situation, affected patients still have 46 chromosomes, but extra chromosomal material is present. This chromosomal abnormality is inherited. Carriers are asymptomatic, although the translocation chromosome is present in both unaffected parents and offspring.

Patients with trisomic Down's syndrome show increased levels of several enzymes, including galactose-1-phosphate uridyltransferase, acid and alkaline phosphatases, glucose-6-phosphate dehydrogenase, and 5-nucleotidase. In addition, blood serotonin levels are reduced.

Several pathological abnormalities are also apparent. For example, abnormal neural development leads to a small cerebellum and brainstem and an irregular positioning of ganglion cells in layer III of the cerebral cortex. In addition, brain convolution patterns do not progress beyond those established during embryogenesis. Cardiac abnormalities, e.g., septal defects, pituitary gland abnormalities, and hypogonadism are also frequently observed.

Down's syndrome, like fragile-X-linked mental retardation, is a disorder in which the biochemical defect is unknown. Chromosome 21 is the genetic locus for a variety of genes, but those investigated so far show no apparent alterations. Since extra chromosomal material is present, it has been suggested that excesses of normal gene products mediating ontogenic events may alter CNS formation. The development of an animal model, a mouse with trisomy 16, may permit us to follow the effects of aberrations in prenatal morphogenesis (68). Several genes localized to chromosome 21 also map on mouse chromosome 16. Moreover, many features of the trisomy 16 mouse mimic the trisomy 21 human. In addition, a chimeric mouse (trisomy 16 → 2n) (67), a mosaic equivalent to the mosaic form of Down's syndrome in humans, will permit us to follow postnatal development. When the proportion of trisomic cells is high in this mosaic, the trisomic phenotype dominates. The molecular biological approaches discussed in the next sections may be particularly useful when applied to these models. Let us, therefore, examine what molecular genetic approaches have so far revealed for this disorder.

Mapping of Chromosome 21 and Linkage Studies

Chromosome 21 is the smallest of the human chromosomes and provides a good candidate for studying genetic linkages and the human diseased state. The chromosome consists of 60,000 kb or 1.6% of the haploid human genome, representing several hundred expressed genes. Only a handful of genes have been identified. These include the genes for ribosomal RNA (69), interferon receptor (IFRC) (70), cytoplasmic superoxide dismutase (SOD-1) (70), glycineamide phosphoribonucleotide synthetase (GARS) (71), aminoimidazole ribonucleotide synthetase (AIRS) (72), liver phosphofructokinase (PFKL) (72) and cystathionine β-synthetase (CBS) (73). In Down's syndrome, a normal gene product is synthesized for each, and the defect seems to be in excess production. For example, both SOD-1 (74) and GAR (75) show increased activity. For SOD-1 (74), the activity is 50% greater than normal values. However, poly(A) mRNA remains unchanged in the trisomic state.

Many loci for several genes known to be present on chromosome 21 have been mapped using chromosome-specific genomic libraries, which have been created from human DNA restriction fragments inserted into plasmid or phage vectors or somatic cell hybrids (76,77). For example, the genes responsible for the trisomic state and Down's syndrome phenotypes (78–80) have been localized to region 21q22, the distal portion of the long arm of chromosome 21; IFRC, SOD-1, PFKL, and GARS have also been localized to this region. The genes for these proteins are thus potential candidates for linkage studies.

A great deal of work has focused on copper- and zinc-dependent superoxide dismutase (81). A recombinant cDNA clone was developed for this enzyme by isolating poly(A) mRNA enriched for human SOD-1 purified from SV80 cells, a continuous cell line of human fibroblasts transformed with SV40. Double-stranded sequences were generated and inserted into the PstI site of pBR322 and cloned in *E. coli* HB101. The SOD-1 recombinant clones were selected by *in situ* hybridization with SOD-1 mRNA. Identification was verified by hybridization with mRNA, cell-free translation, immunoprecipitation, and SDS-polyacrylamide gel electrophoresis. Two clones were identified with 650-bp inserts. When used to study SOD-1 expression in human and mouse cells, these cDNA probes selected for two mRNAs containing 0.7 and 0.9 kb. Both are transcribed from the same gene on chromosome 21 as shown by Northern analysis of DNA/RNA hybrids following treatment with RNase H and by hybridization studies with chromosome 21 human/mouse somatic cell hybrids. The smaller mRNA is four times more abundant than the larger species and seems to differ in the length of the 3' untranslated region beyond the polyadenylated tail.

With these clones, the SOD-1 gene locus, representing more than 100 kb of chromosomal DNA in the 21q22 segment, was isolated and characterized by restriction mapping (82). First, several overlapping recombinants containing the SOD-1 gene were isolated from λch4A genomic libraries. Five small exons and four introns were found by nucleotide sequence and heteroduplex analysis. Only a single gene

copy, approximately 11 kb in length and 12 times the length of the larger mRNA, was present per haploid genome. In addition, four processed pseudogenes were found that do not reside on chromosome 21 based on cosegregation studies.

Restriction fragment length polymorphisms associated with trisomy 21 and SOD-1 have been evaluated (83). Human DNA isolated from cells expressing trisomy 21 were analyzed by Southern blotting using the SOD-1 cDNA probes. The restriction endonucleases EcoRI, PstI and BglII generated normal patterns consistent with the hypothesis that the encoded cellular proteins localized to 21q22 are normal but produced in excess because of the extra chromosomal material.

Transfection experiments also show a normal gene product (83). An 11-kb fragment containing the SOD-1 gene was inserted into a plasmid vector containing the bacterial gene for phosphotransferase, an enzyme inactivating the aminoglycoside antibiotic G418. Mouse L cells were transfected with the chimeric gene, and antibiotic-resistant transformants were selected. These transformants synthesized SOD-1 polypeptides with high efficiency as shown by immunoprecipitation with anti-SOD-1 antibody.

However, two recombinant clones, λA-2 and λB-1, isolated from a human fetal liver DNA library and containing the entire SOD-1 gene did show a BglII RFLP (83). When each recombinant was restriction endonuclease cut and hybridized to the SOD-1 cDNA clone, λA-2 showed 1.5-, 3.6-, and 4.1-kb fragments. In contrast, λB-1 showed only 4.1- and 5.1-kb fragments, suggesting that a mutation in the 5.1 fragment eliminated the generation of the 1.5- and 3.6-kb fragments by BglII. With samples of unrelated human DNA, it was verified that both recombinants contained the two alleles of the SOD-1 gene and that the RFLP resulted from a nucleotide alteration.

Finally, the effects of overproduction of SOD-1 genes are being assessed, since trisomy 21 cells display many phenotypic changes that may be a result of extra gene products (83). Human and mouse cells have been transformed with vectors containing the entire SOD-1 gene and are being examined for phenotypic alterations.

Clearly, as recombinant DNA probes become available for each of the other three proteins localized to 21q22, GARS, PFKL, and IFRC, similar studies can be undertaken. Perhaps each will provide us with additional information relevant to the etiology of Down's syndrome. In the section that follows, we discuss a more general use of RFLPs for studying Down's syndrome.

Nonspecific RFLPs for Studying Down's Syndrome

In cases in which the gene defect is unknown, another approach has been to search for mutations using unknown DNA markers as earlier described for fragile X-linked mental retardation. Since chromosome 21 is responsible for the defect in Down's syndrome, restriction fragment markers were generated for this chromosome.

Bacteriophage DNA from a mouse/human hybrid cell line containing only chromosome 21 was used to construct a recombinant DNA bacteriophage library (84). Recombinants were selected by their ability to hybridize with cDNA probes to the interspersed species-specific repetitive sequence in the human genome (85). By use of restriction mapping and Southern analysis with the repetitive probe, nonrepetitive restriction fragments were identified and subcloned into plasmid vectors and propagated. Twenty-nine single-copy fragments were identified from 19 recombinants, representing 1.25% of the chromosome.

Each fragment was tested as a marker for RFLPs using DNA from lymphoblastoid lines of four to six unrelated individuals and as many as 15 restriction endonucleases. DNA fragments, fractionated by agarose gel electrophoresis and supported by a nylon membrane, were hybridized to the probes and analyzed by autoradiography. If individual variations arose, Mendelian codominant inheritance was checked within the nuclear families. The results suggested that one in 100 bases represents a potential polymorphic site.

A preliminary linkage map was constructed for these markers using the Venezuelan Huntington disease family (86). The genotype of a reference pedigree (140 individuals representing 16 interrelated sibships with three to 14 children) was determined for seven DNA markers. Loci were ordered by three-point crosses following phase determination for the three markers. Two markers are located on the telomeric portion of the long arm of chromosome 21.

These markers are being used to study nondisjunction in Down's syndrome, monosomy 21, and the presence of partial diploidy. Clearly, they can also be used to study chromosome 21 translocation Down's syndrome.

In a second approach, a human chromosome 21 library was constructed by inserting EcoRI fragments of human DNA from chromosome 21 (87) into the bacteriophage vector λgtWESλB and propagating in LE392. The library generated consisted of 10,000 recombinants with inserts ranging from 2.5 to 14 kb. Since many recombinants were redundant, most but not all of chromosome 21 was represented.

Probes lacking repetitive sequences were selected (88). These probes were then tested for their ability to hybridize to total human DNA, mouse DNA, or DNA from mouse/human somatic cell hybrids containing only chromosome 21 by Southern analysis. Seven unique probes were selected, and three of these were sublocalized to specific regions on chromosome 21 based on grain distribution by in situ hybridization. Some discrepancies in specificity were apparent compared to Southern analysis. These can be ascribed to stringency during washing and hybridization, restriction fragment size of the probe, intact chromosomal morphology, and nonspecific causes during hybridization.

One specific genomic fragment, DS21D1 (89), was hybridized to EcoRI digests of total human DNA and shown to detect a 7.0-kb band. Although apparent in both normal and trisomy 21 persons, the autoradiographic signal was 50% greater in the Down's syndrome patient when averaged over several persons. Individual results were less consistent. New plasmids have been constructed, however, containing a 0.7-kb fragment of globin DNA and small fragments of DS21D1. These seem to eliminate nonspecific hybridization

and appear better quantitative markers for Down's syndrome.

CONCLUSIONS

Recombinant DNA technology applied to the four disorders we have reviewed here, phenylketonuria, Lesch–Nyhan syndrome, fragile X-linked mental retardation, and Down's syndrome, has provided invaluable information regarding the gene loci associated with these disorders, chromosomal location of the genes, linkage maps, and specific and nonspecific restriction fragment length polymorphisms to be used as markers for genetic counseling or pre- and perinatal diagnosis. In addition, where the metabolic defect is known, such as HPRT deficiency in Lesch–Nyhan syndrome or phenylalanine hydroxylase deficiency in phenylketonuria, gene therapy, involving the insertion of a functional gene into the affected tissue to correct the defect, promises to be an important medical treatment for the future.

REFERENCES

1. American Association on Mental Deficiency (1961): *A Manual on Terminology and Classification.* American Association on Mental Deficiency, Willimantic, CT.
2. American Psychiatric Association (1980): *Diagnostic and Statistical Manual of Mental Disorders,* edition 3. American Psychiatric Association, Washington.
3. Lewin, B., ed., (1983): *Genes.* John Wiley & Sons, New York.
4. Watson, J. D., Tooze, J., and Kurtz, D. T. (1983): *Recombinant DNA.* W. H. Freeman, San Francisco.
5. Southern, E. M. (1975): *J. Mol. Biol.,* 98:503–517.
6. Harper, M. E., and Saunders, G. F. (1981): *Chromosoma,* 83:431.
7. Fölling, A. (1934): *Hoppe-Seylers Z. Physiol. Chem.,* 227:169–176.
8. Dobson, J. C., Williamson, M. L., Azen, C., and Koch, R. (1977): *Pediatrics,* 60:822–827.
9. Tourian, A., and Sidbury, J. B. (1983): In: *The Metabolic Basis of Inherited Disease,* edition 5, edited by J. B. Stanbury, J. B. Wyngaarden, and D. S. Fredrickson, pp. 270–286. McGraw-Hill, New York.
10. Friedman, P. A., Kautman, S., and Kang, E. S. (1972): *Nature,* 240:157–159.
11. Woo, S. L. C., Gillam, S. S., and Woolf, L. I. (1974): *Biochem. J.,* 139:741–749.
12. Kaufman, S., and Fisher, D. B. (1970): *J. Biol. Chem.,* 245:4745–4750.
13. Robson, K. J. H., Chandra, T., McGillivray, R. T. A., and Woo, S. L. C. (1982): *Proc. Natl. Acad. Sci. U.S.A.,* 79:4701–4705.
14. Abita, J. P., Milstein, S., Chang, N., and Kaufman, S. (1976): *J. Biol. Chem.,* 251:5310–5314.
15. Tourian, A., Treiman, L., and Abe, K. (1975): *Biochemistry,* 14:4055–4060.
16. Ledley, F. D., Grenett, H. E., DiLella, A. G., Kwok, S. C. M., and Woo, S. L. C. (1985): *Science,* 228:77–79.
17. Levy, H. L. (1985): In: *Medical Genetics: Past, Present, Future,* edited by K. Berg, pp. 109–122. Alan R. Liss, New York.
18. Robson, K. J. H., Beattie, W., James, R. J., Colton, R. C. H., Morgan, F. J., et al. (1984): *Biochemistry,* 23:5671–5675.
19. Woo, S. L. C., Lidsky, A. S., Guttler, F., Chandra, T., and Robson, K. J. H. (1983): *Nature,* 306:151–155.
20. Kwok, S. C. M., Ledley, F. D., DiLella, A. G., Robson, K. J. H., and Woo, S. L. C. (1985): *Biochemistry,* 24:556–561.
21. Lidsky, A. S., Guttler, F., and Woo, S. L. C. (1985): *Lancet,* 1:549–551.

22. Woo, S. L. C., Guttler, F., Ledley, F. D., Lidsky, A., Kwok, S. C. M., DiLella, A. G., and Robson, K. J. H. (1985): In: *Medical Genetics: Past, Present, Future,* edited by K. Berg, pp. 123–135. Alan R. Liss, New York.
23. Lidsky, A. S., Robson, K. J. H., Thirumalachary, C., Barker, P. E., Ruddle, F. H. and Woo, S. L. C. (1984): *Am. J. Hum. Genet.,* 36:527–533.
24. Lesch, M., and Nyhan, W. L. (1964): *Am. J. Med.,* 36:561–570.
25. Scherzer, A. L., and Ilson, J. B. (1969): *Pediatrics,* 44:116–120.
26. Lloyd, K. G., Hornykiewicz, O., Davidson, L., Shannak, K., Farley, I., Goldstein, M., Shibuya, M., Kelley, W. N., and Fox, I. H. (1981): *N. Engl. J. Med.,* 305:1106–1111.
27. Kelley, W. N., Greene, M. L., Rosenbloom, F. M., Henderson, J. F. and Seegmiller, J. E. (1969): *Ann. Intern. Med.,* 70:155–206.
28. Holden, J. A., and Kelley, W. N. (1978): *J. Biol. Chem.,* 253: 4459–4463.
29. Kelley, W. N., and Wyngaarden, J. B. (1983): In: *The Metabolic Basis of Inherited Disease,* edited by J. B. Stanbury, J. B. Wyngaarden, and D. S. Frederickson, pp. 1115–1143. McGraw-Hill, New York.
30. Kelley, W. N., and Arnold, W. J. (1973): *Fed. Proc.,* 32:1656–1659.
31. Melton, D. W. (1981): *Cell Genet.,* 7:331–334.
32. Brennand, J., Chinault, A. C., Konecki, D. S., Melton, D. W., and Caskey, C. T. (1982): *Proc. Natl. Acad. Sci. U.S.A.,* 79:1950–1954.
33. Michelson, A. M., Markham, A. F., and Orkin, S. H. (1983): *Proc. Natl. Acad. Sci. U.S.A.,* 80:472–476.
34. Jolly, D. J., Esty, A., Bernard, H. U., and Friedmann, T. (1982): *Proc. Natl. Acad. Sci. U.S.A.,* 79:5038–5041.
35. Jolly, D. J., Okayama, H., Berg, P., Esty, A. C., Filpula, D., et al. (1983): *Proc. Natl. Acad. Sci. U.S.A.,* 80:477–481.
36. Miller, A. D., Eckner, R. J., Jolly, D. J., Friedmann, T., and Verma, I. M. (1984): *Science,* 225:630–632.
37. Melton, D. W., Konciki, D. S., Brennand, J., and Caskey, T. C. (1984): *Proc. Natl. Acad. Sci. U.S.A.,* 81:2147–2151.
38. Shapiro, S. L., Sheppard, G. L., Jr., Dreifuss, F. E., and Newcombe, D. S. (1966): *Proc. Soc. Exp. Biol. Med.,* 122:609–611.
39. Nyhan, W. L., Pesek, J., Sweetman, L., Carpenter, D. G., and Carter, C. H. (1967): *Pediatr. Res.,* 1:5–13.
40. Ricciuti, F. C., and Ruddle, F. H. (1973): *Nature,* 241:180–182.
41. Becker, M. A., Yen, R. C. K., Itkin, P., Goss, S. J., Seegmiller, J. E., et al. (1979): *Science,* 203:1016–1019.
42. McKusick, V. A. (1982): *Cytogenet. Cell. Genet.,* 32:7–23.
43. Fuscoe, J. C., Fenwick, R. G., Jr., Ledbetter, D. H., and Caskey, T. C. (1983): *Mol. Cell. Biol.,* 3:1086–1096.
44. Yang, T. P., Patel, P. I., Chinault, A. C., Stout, J. T., Jackson, L. G., et al. (1984): *Nature,* 310:412–414.
45. Willis, R. C., Jolly, D. J., Miller, A. D., Plent, M. M., Esty, A. C., et al. (1984): *J. Biol. Chem.,* 259:7842–7849.
46. Mulligan, R. C., and Berg, P. (1980): *Science,* 209:1422–1427.
47. Tariverdian, G., and Weck, B. (1982): *Hum. Genet.,* 62:95–109.
48. Turner, G., and Opitz, J. M. (1980): *Am. J. Med. Genet.,* 7:407–415.
49. Lubs, H. A. (1969): *Am. J. Hum. Genet.,* 21:231–244.
50. Sutherland, G. R. (1979): *Am. J. Hum. Genet.,* 31:125–135.
51. Fonatsch, C. (1981): *Hum. Genet.,* 59:186.
52. Jacobs, P. A., Glover, T. W., Mayer, M., Fox, P., Gerrard, J. W., et al. (1980): *Am. J. Med. Genet.,* 7:471–489.
53. Jenkins, E. C., Brown, W. T., Duncan, C. J., Brooks, J., Ben-Yishay, M., et al. (1981): *Lancet,* 2:1292.
54. Webb, G. C., Rogers, J. G., Pitt, D. B., Halliday, J., and Theobald, T. (1981): *Lancet,* 2:1231–1232.
55. Rhoads, F. A., Oglesby, A. C., Mayer, M., and Jacobs, P. A. (1982): *Am. J. Med. Genet.,* 12:205–217.
56. DeArce, M. A., and Kearns, A. (1984): *J. Med. Genet.,* 21:84–91.
57. Harrison, C. J., Jack, E. M., Allen, T. D., and Harris, R. (1983): *J. Med. Genet.,* 20:280–285.
58. Brookwell, R., and Turner, G. (1983): *Hum. Genet.,* 63:77.
59. Szabo, P., Purrello, M., Rocchi, M., Archidiacono, N., Alhadeff, B., et al. (1984): *Proc. Natl. Acad. Sci. U.S.A.,* 81:7855–7859.
60. Camerino, G., Mattei, G., Mattei, J., Jaye, M., and Mandel, J. L. (1983): *Nature,* 306:701–704.
61. Drayna, D., Davies, K., Hartley, D., Mandel, J.-L., Camerino, G., et al. (1984): *Proc. Natl. Acad. Sci. U.S.A.,* 81:2836–2839.
62. Wall, R. L., McConnel, J., Moore, D., MacPherson, C. R., and Marson, A. (1967): *Am. J. Med.,* 43:214–226.
63. Whittaker, D. L., Copeland, D. L., and Graham, J. B. (1964): *Am. J. Hum. Genet.,* 14:149–158.
64. Davies, K. E., Mattei, M. G., Mattei, J. F., Veenema, H., McGlade, S., et al. (1985): *Hum. Genet.,* 70:249–255.
65. Hartley, D. A., Davies, K. E., Drayna, D., White, R. L., and Williamson, R. (1984): *Nucleic Acids Res.,* 12:5277–5285.
66. Schweber, M. (1985): *Ann. N.Y. Acad. Sci.,* 450:233–238.
67. Lejeune, J. M., Gautier, M., and Turpin, R. (1959): *C.R. Acad. Sci.,* 248:1721–1722.
68. Epstein, C. J., Cox, D. R., and Epstein, L. B. (1985): *Ann. N.Y. Acad. Sci.,* 450:157–168.
69. Evans, H. J., Buckland, A., and Pardue, M. L. (1974): *Chromosome,* 48:405–426.
70. Tan, Y. H., Tischfield, J., and Ruddle, F. H. (1973): *J. Exp. Med.,* 137:317–330.
71. Moore, E. E., Jones, C., Kao, F.-T., and Oates, D. C. (1977): *Am. J. Hum. Genet.,* 29:389–396.
72. Patterson, D., Graw, S., and Jones, C. (1981): *Proc. Natl. Acad. Sci. U.S.A.,* 78:408–409.
73. Skovby, F., Krassikoff, N., and Franke, U. (1984): *Hum. Genet.,* 65:291–294.
74. Sinet, P. M., Allard, D., Lejeune, J., and Frezal, J. (1974): *C.R. Acad. Sci.,* 278:3267–3270.
75. Scoggin, C. H., Bleskan, J., Davison, J. N., and Patterson, D. (1980): *Clin. Res.,* 28:31A.
76. Krumleaf, R., Jeanpierre, M., and Young, B. D. (1982): *Proc. Natl. Acad. Sci. U.S.A.,* 79:2971–2975.
77. Gusella, J. F., Keys, C., Varsanyi-Breiner, A., Kao, F. T., Jones, C., et al. (1980): *Proc. Natl. Acad. Sci. U.S.A.,* 77:2829–2833.
78. Niebuhr, E. (1974): *Hum. Genet.,* 21:91–100.
79. Williams, J. D., Summit, R. L., Martens, P. R., and Kimbrell, R. A. (1975): *Am. J. Hum. Genet.,* 27:478–481.
80. Poissonier, M., St. Paul, B., Dutrillaux, B., Chassegne, M., Gruyer, M., et al. (1976): *Ann. Genet.,* 19:69–73.
81. Lieman-Hurwitz, J., Dafni, N., Lavie, V., and Groner, Y. (1982): *Proc. Natl. Acad. Sci. U.S.A.,* 79:2808–2811.
82. Levanon, D., Lieman-Hurwitz, J., Dafni, N., Wigderson, M., Sherman, L., et al. (1985): *EMBO J.,* 4:78–84.
83. Groner, Y., Lieman-Hurwitz, J., Dafni, N., Sherman, L., Levanon, D., et al., (1985): *Ann. N.Y. Acad. Sci.,* 450:133–155.
84. Gusella, J. F., Tanzi, R. E., Watkins, P. C., et al. (1985): *Ann. N.Y. Acad. Sci.,* 450:25–31.
85. Gusella, J. F., Keys, C., Varsanyi-Breiner, A., Kao, F., Jones, L., et al. (1980): *Proc. Natl. Acad. Sci. U.S.A.,* 77:2829–2833.
86. Gusella, J. F., Tanzi, R., Anderson, M. A., and Ottina, K. (1983): In: *Banbury Report 14: Recombinant DNA Applications to Human Disease,* edited by C. T. Casky and R. L. White, pp. 261–266. Cold Spring Harbor Laboratory, New York.
87. Krumlauf, R., Jeanpierre, M., and Young, B. (1982): *Proc. Natl. Acad. Sci. U.S.A.,* 79:2971–2975.
88. Benton, W. D., and Davis, R. W. (1977): *Science,* 196:180–182.
89. Devine, E. A., Brown, W. T., Houck, G. E., Fisher, S., Balàzs, I., et al. (1985): *Ann. N.Y. Acad. Sci.,* 450:85–94.

Psychopharmacology:
The Third Generation of Progress,
edited by Herbert Y. Meltzer.
Raven Press, New York © 1987.

CHAPTER 86

Psychophysiological and Pharmacological Aspects of Somnambulism and Night Terrors in Children

G. Nino-Murcia and William C. Dement

> *. . . I have seen her rise from her bed, throw her nightgown upon her, unlock her closet, take forth paper, fold it, write upon't, read it, afterwards seal it, and again return to bed; yet all this while in a most fast sleep.*
>
> *Macbeth,* Act V, scene i

Recent developments in the understanding of somnambulism and night terrors have demonstrated the important role played by changes in neurotransmitters in the manifestation and the treatment of these two disorders (1–3). The list of medications associated with the manifestation or exacerbation of these two disorders continues to grow (see Table 2). In addition, we have observed a severe negative impact on the psychological development of children and the family structure of some of our patients. Physical harm, to themselves or others, and sometimes death as a result of these two disorders have also been described (4–6). It is well known that somnambulism is more common in children than adults.

It is therefore of crucial importance that pediatricians, child psychiatrists, and other professionals involved in the treatment of children become familiar with the neurophysiological and pharmacological aspects of these two parasomnias.

SOMNAMBULISM

Clinical Manifestations

This is a disorder in which the patient suddenly sits or stands up from the sleeping position, walks about in a clumsy way, sometimes but not always avoids obstacles, mumbles or utters words that are quite often meaningless or incomprehensible, and responds to questions or statements in an irrelevant way.

Careful evaluations of these patients in sleep laboratories have demonstrated incidents of somnambulism. The patient gets out of bed, eyes open with a blank or fearful expression, and moves in a clumsy and often repetitive manner (7). Somniloquy (sleeptalking) can be observed simultaneously. The level of complexity of the motoric activity ranges from sitting up in bed or walking about the room to episodes of running and screaming. Sometimes the patient may leave the bedroom or the house while attempting to escape or avoid something. The patient is awakened with considerable difficulty only to exhibit confusion, disorientation, and complete amnesia for the episode.

Children are prone to urinate in inappropriate places, use obscene words that they would not use while awake, and frequently fall and injure themselves (8,9).

Several of our pediatric patients have come to us after fractures or major injuries produced during a somnambulistic attack. In adults, these episodes can lead to serious harm to themselves or others. For instance, Hartmann (6) reported two episodes of somnambulism, one that resulted in three deaths and another that resulted in bodily harm. The most dramatic and sad case is one of filicide: a mother, during an episode of somnambulism clearly precipitated by the use of thioridazine, stabbed her daughter to death (5).

Podolsky reported a case in which a civil engineer died after stabbing himself while in a somnambulistic episode (4). This case led Chuaqui (10) to consider somnambulism as one of the abnormalities of consciousness that can lead to suicide. Frequently, the somnambulistic patient returns to bed and continues sleeping. The patient only discovers that a somnambulistic attack occurred on being told by relatives or noticing changes in the distribution of items in the bedroom. An analysis of the cases mentioned above has reminded us of the descriptions of behavior classified as "sleep drunkenness" by other authors (11).

Sleep drunkenness is the abnormal, inappropriate behavior observed in some individuals on awakening that sometimes leads to embarrassing situations and/or harm to others with possible forensic complications (12).

A review of some of the cases of sleep drunkenness reported in the literature (11) has led us to believe that perhaps the distinction between this disorder and somnambulism is not as clear as originally thought. There appear to be many similarities between somnambulism and sleep drunkenness. In both disorders:

1. The patient has amnesia for the episode.
2. The attacks can be precipitated by external stimuli that interrupt sleep.
3. There is a personal and family history of other sleep disorders (mainly enuresis and night terrors).
4. Alcohol or drugs may play a contributory role.
5. Episodes occur from arousal during the first 2 to 3 hr after sleep onset.
6. Episodes include characteristic erratic, aimless behavior that is produced during a different level of consciousness than complete wakefulness.
7. There are similar descriptions of automatic behavior.

Both types of patients usually suffer the same emotional response of embarrassment, shame, guilt, anxiety, and perplexity after being informed of their behavior.

The only feature that appears clinically to differentiate the two disorders is that sleep drunkenness usually occurs with an arousal precipitated by external stimuli, whereas somnambulism is usually associated with a spontaneous awakening (11).

Although there are excellent reports of electroencephalographic (EEG) monitoring during somnambulistic episodes (13–16), we are not aware of any such study in patients during an episode of sleep drunkenness. It would be very helpful to determine if the EEG activity is different during somnambulism in comparison to sleep drunkenness. The latter disorder offers a difficult challenge to investigators attempting to understand it from a polysomnographic point of view.

We believe that the two disorders may have many common neurophysiological mechanisms, and perhaps the two are manifestations of arousals producing different levels of cognition.

It is important to emphasize here, however, that somnambulism can be precipitated by external stimuli such as a click, calling of the patient's name, or bringing the patient to his feet while in delta sleep (stages 3 and 4), as has been demonstrated in the sleep laboratory (7,14). Obviously, it is difficult to know the role of external stimuli in precipitating a somnambulistic episode in a patient sleeping at home.

Broughton et al. (15,17) induced somnambulistic episodes by distention of the bladder. He increased liquid intake prior to sleep onset and aroused subjects from stage 4 sleep. Based on this study, we adopted the recommendation to decrease the amount of liquid intake a few hours before the patient retires.

Broughton has explained that arousal produced by other mechanisms, such as termination of a sleep cycle and mental activity, can also trigger somnambulism (16). These observations led him to consider parasomnias as disorders of arousal (11,16). We have also wondered if an interruption in the transition between delta sleep and REM sleep plays a role in the manifestation of a sleepwalking episode.

Incidence and Family History of Somnambulism

Reports in the literature have established the incidence of sleepwalking in 1 to 15% of the population (18,19). This disorder is more common in children than in adolescents and adults. It also occurs more frequently in boys than girls. Klackenberg (20) found that the highest prevalence of somnambulism was 16.7% at 11 to 12 years of age. In his epidemiological study, Klackenberg (20) found that the frequency of sleepwalking episodes varied from once a month to once a year.

Hallstrom (21) published cases from three consecutive generations that had night terrors. He emphasized the need to consider a genetic origin in these parasomnias. On the basis of his observation that these disorders were present in three consecutive generations and in both males and females, Hallstrom (21) created the hypothesis that night terrors as a syndrome are transmitted as an autosomal dominant trait. Several authors have established the parent–child transmission of these disorders (22–26).

The genetic influence in these disorders received further confirmation with Bakwin's report (22) of the evidence of somnambulism in both monozygotic twins. He found that the concordance in monozygotic twins was six times more common than in dizygotics. The frequency of night terrors and enuresis is higher in families of children with somnambulism (15).

However, Kales et al. (23) demonstrated that the incidence of these parasomnias increases in relation to the number of affected parents: 22% when neither parent has the disorder, 45% if one was affected, and 60% when both are affected.

All of the studies mentioned above add the genetic factor to the several probable factors involved in the manifestation of these disorders.

NIGHT TERRORS

This parasomnia is characterized by a sudden arousal that could last several minutes and could be accompanied or followed by a somnambulistic episode. Like the latter, night terrors usually occur during the first third of the night, and rarely does more than one episode occur per sleep period.

TABLE 1. *Differences between night terrors and nightmares*

Night terrors	Nightmares
Also known as pavor nocturnus	Anxiety dreams
Occurs during stage 3 or 4 sleep	Occurs during REM sleep
Evident during first third of the night	Often present during the last third of the night
Could be accompanied by sleepwalking/enuresis	No major motoric activity
Severe anxiety and vocalization (screaming)	Although present, less anxiety/ vocalization
Severe autonomic discharge	Less autonomic discharge
Complete amnesia for the episode or only fragmentary recall	Vivid and detailed dream recall
Confusion if awakened	Good intellectual function at awakening
75% actual or potential injury	Minimal injury potential
Violent behavior in 55% of the patients	No violent behavior

Typically, the patient suddenly sits up in bed, screams in terror (27), exhibits stereotypic, repetitive behavior, sometimes gasps for air (28), and has severe autonomic discharge (27). This discharge is manifested by tachypnea, marked tachycardia, extrasystoles (21), flushing of the skin, diaphoresis, mydriasis (29), decreased skin resistance (16), and increased muscle tone (16). It has been said that this disorder could be one of the most terrifying experiences that occurs in man.

The patient during an episode of night terrors is unresponsive to external stimuli, confused, and disoriented if awakened. Patients have no recollection of the episode or report only fragments or brief vivid dream images or hallucinations.

The episode can be accompanied by disorganized somnambulism, making it more possible for injury to result in the patient trying to "escape." It could also be accompanied by incoherent mumbled words and/or micturition (6,29). Frequently night terrors are also associated with enuresis.

Night terrors may be confused with nightmares. Table 1 explains the main differences between these two disorders.

Several cases have been reported in which the patient's somnambulism and night terrors began during or soon after a febrile illness (31,32). The episodes were differentiated from delirium by occurrence early in the night, short duration, and persistence after the fever subsided (31).

The authors (31) explain this phenomenon as being a result of the effect of fever on sleep: fragmentation, reduction in TST, and significant decrease in stages 3 and 4. The rebound of the delta sleep could play a role in the onset of these episodes if we take into consideration Fisher's observation that longer episodes of delta sleep preceding a night terror result in a more intense episode (33).

POLYSOMNOGRAPHIC STUDIES OF SOMNAMBULISM AND NIGHT TERRORS

For several years it was postulated that parasomnias, and more specifically enuresis, were manifestations of nocturnal epilepsy (34). It was not until the Marseille group, with Gastaut's leadership, carried out several well-conducted investigations that the lack of evidence for epilepsy as the cause of the disorders was more clearly established (35–37). Even in children with diagnosed epilepsy and enuresis, there was no evidence of epileptic discharges during the enuretic event (35).

It is important here to review briefly a few well-established characteristics of normal sleep architecture before we discuss findings in patients with somnambulism or night terrors.

A normal young adult, a normal sleeper, will fall asleep in approximately 15 min and initiate the first cycle. This cycle consists of a progression through stage 1, stage 2, stages 3 and 4, then back to stage 2, and finally REM. The period of time between sleep onset and the beginning of REM is approximately 90 to 120 min. Delta sleep (stages 3 and 4) accounts for a large percentage of this first cycle, which occurs during the first third of the night.

The total amount of time spent in NREM sleep during the night is approximately 88% of the total amount of sleep in a normal adult. During childhood, the total is approximately 75%, and 80% during adolescence. In the elderly, this time in delta sleep and REM sleep is reduced in comparison with an adolescent. The fact that it is during the first third of the night that most of stages 3 and 4 occur explains why somnambulism and night terrors most commonly occur during this time. A very good summary of the normal sleep physiology has been published by Karacan and Moore (30).

As the night passes, δ sleep decreases, and simultaneously there is an increase in the duration and total amount of REM sleep. The longest period of REM sleep occurs during the last third of the night.

Gastaut et al. (17,37–39), Broughton (5,6), Tassinari et al. (36), and Jacobson et al. (7,14,44) demonstrated that night terrors and somnambulism begin in stage 3 or 4 sleep, most commonly at the end of the first cycle or the subsequent one.

These findings contradicted both the initial hypothesis

that sleepwalking was an "acting out" of a dream (40,41) and that they were epileptic phenomena (42,43). Jacobson et al. (7,14,44) demonstrated the presence of 1- to 3-Hz high-voltage activity in the EEG that persisted from 10 to 30 sec, followed by activity of lower amplitude. These authors found that if the incident persisted for more than 40 sec, there was electroencephalographic evidence of stage 2 sleep or theta, alpha, and beta frequencies. One-fourth of their patients exhibited EEGs characteristic of awakening following the incidents (7). The same authors describe the "sudden, rhythmical, high-voltage bursts of delta frequency during slow-wave sleep in all of the somnambulistics through 16 years" that they evaluated. The same pattern was not seen in their normal controls (7).

The observation that these episodes of parasomnias occur during delta sleep explains the amnesia for the episode and the absence of dream recall. Some patients relate only very simple "dream-like" episodes, but most of them deny having had a dream.

Broughton (15) demonstrated abnormalities in the visual evoked potentials of patients with these parasomnias. More specifically, he was able to demonstrate a persistence of patterns similar to the ones seen in delta sleep during the awakening following the episode. This is what Broughton (15) describes as an evoked potential "intermediate between that of slow-wave sleep and that of wakefulness." These patterns were not observed in evoked potentials after awakening from REM sleep.

Much work remains to be done to clarify why these patients with what appears to be a "tendency" for somnambulism by neurophysiological characteristics develop an episode. On the other hand, it is by now a well-known fact that somnambulism and night terrors occur with much less frequency when the patient is being observed (in a sleep laboratory or during filming for educational purposes, for instance). These clinical observations have confirmed the same findings by Gastaut et al. (17,39), Jacobson et al. (14,44), and Broughton (15,16) and pointed to the important role of psychological factors in the manifestation of these disorders.

Studies of more neurophysiological parameters in patients with these disorders are necessary. They will contribute to the understanding of the cortical and subcortical activity during the episodes. We think that evaluation of these patients with the new imaging techniques (primarily brain topographic mapping) may contribute a great deal to the clarification of this problem. We are currently performing these studies.

Our hypothesis is that these parasomnias as well as the episodes of sleep drunkenness occur during one level in a continuum of levels of consciousness between the deep sleep and wakefulness. Even though we have cited many different studies demonstrating the absence of epileptic discharges before or during episodes of night terrors or somnambulism, it is important to mention a few studies that make it necessary to include nocturnal epilepsy in any discussion of these two disorders. Fuster et al. (43) proved that 94.5% of cases with "sleep terrors during which the patient is unconscious" were associated with epileptic discharges from the parietotemporooccipital region as well as one case in which sleep terrors disappeared after excision

of a focus located in the same region. Amir et al. (45) reported that 47% of 35 of their patients showed significant interictal EEG abnormalities. Pedley and Guilleminault (46) reported six cases of unusual sleepwalking episodes that responded well to anticonvulsant medications. The main differences between Pedley's cases and the disorders usually described as somnambulism and/or night terrors are the following:

1. Their patients exhibited the bizarre behavior during the last part of the night. Patients with nonepileptic disorders (parasomnias) exhibit most of the episodes during the first third of the night. As we mentioned before, these findings are in keeping with the fact that delta sleep is more prolonged during the first third of the night.
2. Pedley's patients showed a more violent, agitated episode frequently resulting in injury (46). Most of the patients with parasomnias exhibit automatisms without the severe violent characteristics.
3. Pedley's patients presented repetitive episodes in one night. This is not a common observation in patients with parasomnias, who usually develop one episode per night.
4. There was no family history of parasomnias in Pedley's patients (46), as opposed to patients with somnambulism/night terrors.
5. The epileptic behavior may or may not be present in childhood and remain until adulthood (46). Usually the patients with parasomnias have a history of these disorders in childhood.
6. The EEG in patients with parasomnia is normal; four of the six patients described by Pedley (46) had an abnormal EEG.
7. Patients with parasomnias do not improve with anticonvulsants as Pedley's patients did.
8. Pedley's patients did not have evidence of a psychiatric component.

More cases of abnormal nocturnal automatism associated with epilepsy were reported a few years later by Guilleminault and Silvestri (47). Two of the patients with somnambulism/night terrors reported by these authors have clinical and polysomnographic evidence of sleep apnea, obstructive type. Children with these parasomnias should also be evaluated clinically and/or with a nocturnal polysomnogram to rule out sleep apnea as the precipitating factor in the manifestation of these disorders.

MEDICATIONS ASSOCIATED WITH SOMNAMBULISM AND NIGHT TERRORS

Several medications have been reported to induce or at least be associated with somnambulism and night terrors. The most dramatic association was the report of thioridazine inducing a somnambulistic episode in a 44-year-old woman who had had a history of somnambulism during adolescence (5). The episode induced by this psychotropic culminated in a filicide (the patient stabbed her daughter to death). Christianson and Perry (60) reported the presence of somnambulistic behavior associated with the use of chloral hydrate in the treatment of dermatological patients.

Lithium in combination with neuroleptics has been reported to be associated with the development of somnam-

TABLE 2. *Medications associated with somnambulism*

Thioridazine (5)
Chloral hydrate (60)
Methaqualone (55)
Methyprylon (56)
Chlorprothixene (57)
Lithium in combination with chlorpromazine, thiothixene, haloperidol, thioridazine, perphenazine, and prolixin (48)
Methaqualone in combination with diphenhydramine hydrochloride (55,61)
Desipramine in combination with chlorpromazine (59)
Doxepin (59)
Amitriptyline in combination with perphenazine (59)

bulistic behavior (49) 2 to 14 days after initiation of the treatment in 10 psychiatric patients. In these 10 cases, the episode occurred at the beginning of the night and had several of the characteristics of somnambulism previously described in this chapter.

The psychotropics used in combination with lithium, were chlorpromazine, thiothixene, haloperidol, perphenazine, prolixin, and thioridazine.

Interestingly, a decrease or discontinuation of the dose of the neuroleptic produced a disappearance of the somnambulistic episodes. Episodes only persisted in those patients who exhibited nonspecific diffuse EEG irregularity while on the medications. Two of them had drug-induced seizures. However, in four patients, the sleepwalking episodes disappeared despite the fact that they were maintained on the same dose of lithium and neuroleptics (48).

The manifestation of somnambulism in these 10 patients may be associated, according to the authors (48), with the increase in δ sleep observed as a result of lithium (50,51) or neuroleptics (52–54).

Risberg et al. (55) reported somnambulism induced by methaqualone. Other medications, including methyprylon (56), chlorprothixene (57), combinations of methaqualone and diphenhydramine hydrochloride (57), have been associated with these disorders.

Flemenbaum (58) reported that 75% of patients receiving bedtime neuroleptics and/or tricyclics developed night terrors. Unfortunately, his paper does not offer the specific medications involved.

Allen (59) reported night terrors associated with the use of doxepin and amitriptyline in combination with perphenazine and with desipramine in combination with chlorpromazine. In his cases, the utilization of benzodiazepines without discontinuation of the other medications improved the night terrors.

Therefore, if medication is prescribed (especially medications listed in Table 2), information about the history of parasomnias is necessary. This is especially important if the medication is going to be prescribed for bedtime.

NATURAL HISTORY

Kales et al. (62) evaluated 50 patients with the diagnosis of somnambulism. Out of the 50, 21 had a history of the disorder that had subsided by the time of their study, and 29 were still suffering from somnambulism. This study (62) offered many insights into the natural history of the disorder from which many clinical treatment applications could be derived.

Somnambulism that starts early in life (age of onset 5.8) (62) tends to disappear, whereas in those cases in which the age of onset was 9.9 (62), the disorder tends to persist into adulthood. In their patients in whom the somnambulism disappeared, the age of termination of the disorder was 13.8. Stress affected 80% of the patients with somnambulism at the time of the study but only 38% of those with only a history of the disorder (62).

In their patients who were still exhibiting somnambulism, 55% also had night terrors, as opposed to those with a past history of somnambulism, in whom the incidence of night terrors was only 14%. The potential for injury was higher in their patients with current evidence of somnambulism than in those with only a past history. The same was true for incidence of violent behavior.

One of the most important findings in this study by Kales et al. (62) of patients with somnambulism present after the end of adolescence was the presence of abnormalities in both the *Minnesota Multiphasic Personality Inventory* and psychiatric interviews. This was not true in their patients in whom the episodes disappeared before adulthood. Their findings illustrate the need for psychological interventions in adult patients with somnambulism. There was no major evidence of psychological disturbances in children with somnambulism. In children, the neurological component along with the genetic factors seem to be more important. The findings of Kales et al. are consistent with their hypothesis of a maturational or developmental delay in children with this disorder (62).

In another study by Kales et al. (63), adults with night terrors also had evidence of psychopathology. According to the authors, adults with night terrors inhibit the expression of aggression, and sleepwalkers showed outwardly directed expression of aggression. In both disorders these mechanisms are maladaptive.

Barabas et al. (2) found a high incidence of somnambulism in patients with Gilles de la Tourette's syndrome and created the hypothesis that sleepwalking in children with this disorder may be related to disturbed serotonin metabolism. The possible central noradrenergic hyperactivity present in Gilles de la Tourette may also play a role. The same authors (3) reported a strong association between migraine in children and somnambulism. Migraine has been associated with abnormalities in serotonin metabolism and the possible consequent disturbance in the transition between sleep stages.

Evidence of higher incidence of somnambulism, night terrors, and enuresis in patients with Gilles de la Tourette's syndrome than in children with seizures or a learning disability has been demonstrated by Barabas et al (1). These authors demonstrated that of 57 patients with Gilles de la Tourette's, 38.6% had at least one of the three: somnambulism, night terrors, or enuresis, and one patient had all three disorders.

Glaze et al. (64) described an increase in delta sleep and a decrease in REM sleep in patients with Gilles de la Tourette's. This increase in delta sleep probably explains the higher incidence of these parasomnias. The strong association between migraines and parasomnias as well as between Gilles de la Tourette's and parasomnias could give us interesting clues in the clarification of the role of neurotransmitters in the manifestation of the abnormal behavior at night. This is also true for the evidence of somnambulism and night terrors precipitated by medications such as neuroleptics and tricyclic antidepressants (see Table 2), which alter neurotransmitters in the central nervous system.

We are interested in seeing the outcome in children with parasomnias and Gilles de la Tourette when successfully treated with clonidine. We believe that clonidine as an α-adrenergic agonist could considerably reduce the severe autonomic discharge and even, perhaps, the other manifestations of the disorders. We have entertained the possibility of using clonidine even in patients with parasomnias without Gilles de la Tourette, especially those patients with severe disorders that have not responded to other modalities of treatment. The treatment is discussed below.

TREATMENT OF SOMNAMBULISM AND NIGHT TERRORS

It is very fortunate that the great majority of children with night terrors and somnambulism have only mild manifestations of the disorder and a very low frequency. Therefore, in the majority of cases, we can reassure and educate the child and the parents. By doing this, we help them discard other explanations that could generate anxiety or guilt. They are relieved to know that most children will outgrow the disorder (70).

In those patients in whom the frequency and/or the intensity of the disorder raises the possibility of psychological or especially physical harm, we should consider other measures:

1. Improvement in the patterns of sleep–wake cycle is important. In this way, we eliminate the possible role of sleep deprivation as a triggering mechanism.

2. Since Broughton (15) demonstrated that stimuli such as a full bladder could trigger an episode, we recommend a reduction in fluid intake prior to bedtime.

3. Parents should remove anything from the bedroom that could be hazardous or harmful to a child.

4. We recommend that the patient's bedroom be on the ground floor of the house. If that is not possible, the possibility of the patient easily opening windows or doors should be eliminated.

5. An assessment of a child with these disorders should include a careful review of the current medications so that modifications could be made if necessary.

6. Hypnosis has been found to be helpful in both children and adults (65–67,70).

7. A judicious psychiatric evaluation could help to decide the need for psychiatric intervention.

8. It has been demonstrated that benzodiazepines have been useful in the treatment of these disorders (68,70). A small dose of diazepam or lorazepam has been shown to eliminate the episodes or considerably reduce them. Other benzodiazepines (alprazolam, for instance) need to be explored as possibilities, especially if we consider the long half-life of diazepam and its possible interference in the daytime functioning of the child. Imipramine has also been helpful in the treatment of night terrors and somnambulism in children (69).

The use of these medications could be limited by the physician to only those times considered most "at risk" for the manifestation of the disorder (i.e., fever, stress, heavy exercise).

Physicians involved in the evaluation and treatment of these two disorders could be faced with serious legal or forensic questions as well as with difficult diagnostic puzzles.

Many challenges remain to be solved in the understanding of these disorders. With the clarification of the underlying neurophysiological mechanisms, light may be shed on the mystery of mental activity or its inhibition during sleep.

REFERENCES

1. Barabas, G., Matthews, W. S., and Ferrari, M. (1984): *Neurology (N.Y.)*, 34:815–817.
2. Barabas, G., Matthews, W. S., and Ferrari, M. (1984): *Dev. Med. Child Neurol.*, 26:457–460.
3. Barabas, G., Ferrari, M., and Matthews, W. S. (1983): *Neurology, N.Y.*, 33:948–949.
4. Podolsky, E. (1961): *Med. Sci. Law*, 1:260–265.
5. Luchins, D. J., Sherwood, P. M., Gillin, J. C., Mendelson, W. B., and Wyatt, R. J. (1978): *Am. J. Psychiatry*, 135:11.
6. Hartmann, E. (1983): *J. Nerv. Men. Dis.*, 171(8):503–505.
7. Kales, A., Jacobson, A., Paulson, M. J., Kales, J., and Walter, R. (1966): *Arch. Gen. Psychiat.*, 14:586–594.
8. Kales, A., and Kales, J. D. (1974): *N. Engl. J. Med.*, 290:487–499.
9. Kales, J. D., and Kales, A. (1975): *Int. J. Psychiatry Med.*, 6:55–56.
10. Chuaqui, C. (1975): *Can. Psychiatr. Assoc. J.*, 20:25–28.
11. Bonkalo, A. (1969): In: *5th International Meeting of Forensic Sciences*, pp. 400–409. Toronto, Canada.
12. Roffwarg, H. P. (1979): *Sleep*, 2(1):82–83.
13. Soldatos, C. R., Vela-Bueno, A., Bixler, E. O., Schweitzer, P. K., and Kales, A. (1980): *Clin. Electroencephalogr.*, 11(3):136–139.
14. Jacobson, A., and Kales, A. (1967): *Res. Publ. Assoc. Nerv. Ment. Dis.*, 45:424–455.
15. Broughton, R. J. (1968): *Science*, 159:1070–1078.
16. Broughton, R. (1982): *E.E.G. Suppl.*, 35:401–410.
17. Gastaut, H., and Broughton, R. (1965): *Recent Adv. Biol. Psychiatry*, 7:197–223.
18. Kales, J., Jacobson, A., and Kales, A. (1968): *Prog. Clin. Pathol.*, 8:63.
19. Bixler, E. O., Kales, A., Soldatos, C. R., Kales, J. D., and Healy, S. (1979): *Am. J. Psychiatry*, 136:1257–1262.
20. Klackenberg, G. (1982): *Acta Paediatr. Scand.*, 71:495–499.
21. Hallstrom, T. (1972): *Acta Pediatr. Scand.*, 48:350–352.
22. Bakwin, H. (1970): *Lancet*, 2:446.
23. Kales, A., Soldatos, C. R., Bixler, E. O., et al. (1980): *Br. J. Psychiatry*, 137:111–118.
24. Davis, E., Hayes, M., and Kirman, B. H. (1942): *Lancet*, 1:186.
25. Abe, K., and Shimakawa, M. (1966): *Psychiatr. Neurol. (Basel)*, 152:306–312.
26. Abe, K., Amatomi, M., and Oda, N. (1984): *Am. J. Psychiatry*, 141:6.
27. Fisher, C., Kahn, E., Edwards, A., and Davis, D. (1973): *J. Nerv. Ment. Dis.*, 157:75–98.
28. Kramer, M. (1979): *Psychiatr. Ann.*, 9:(7)50–68.
29. Ferris, G. (1984): *Neurol. Clin.*, 2(1):64–66.
30. Karacan, I., and Moore, C. (1985): *Annu. Rev. Psychiatry*, 4:266–293.
31. Kales, J. D., Kales, A., Soldatos, C. R., Chamberlin, K., and Martin, E. D. (1979): *Am. J. Psychiatry*, 136:1214–1215.
32. Dorus, E. (1979): *Am. J. Psychiatry*, 136:12.

33. Fisher, C., Kahn, E., Edwards, A., et al. (1974): *Psychoanal. Contemp. Sci.*, 3:317–398.
34. Pierce, C., and Lipcon, H. H. (1956): *Arch. Neurol. Psychiatr. (Clin.),* 76:310–316.
35. Saint-Laurent, J., Batini, C., Broughton, R., and Gastaut, H. (1963): *Electroencepalogr. Clin. Neurophysiol.*, 15:904.
36. Tassinari, C. A., Mancia, D., Della Bernardina, B., and Gastaut, H. (1972): *Electroencephalogr. Clin. Neurophysiol.*, 33:603–607.
37. Gastaut, H., Dongier, M., Batini, C., and Rhodes, J. (1962): *Rev. Neurol.*, 107:277–279.
38. Gastaut, H., and Broughton, R. (1963): *Percept. Motor Skills,* 17:362.
39. Gastaut, H., and Broughton, R. (1965): *Recent Adv. Biol. Psychiatry,* 7:197–223.
40. Sours, J. A., Frumkin, R., and Indermill, R. R. (1963): *Arch. Gen. Psychiatry,* 9:400.
41. Andre-Balisaux, G., and Gouse, R. (1956): *Acta Neurol. Psychiatr.,* 56:270.
42. Huber, Z. (1962): *Electroencephalogr. Clin. Neurophysiol.*, 14:577.
43. Fuster, B., Castells, C., and Etcheverry, N. (1954): *Neurology (Minneap.),* 4:531.
44. Jacobsen, A., Kales, A., Lehmann, D., and Zweizig, J. R. (1965): *Science,* 148:975–977.
45. Amir, N., Navon, P., and Silverberg-Shaler, R. (1985): *Israel J. Med. Sci.,* 21:22–26.
46. Pedley, T. A., and Guilleminault, C. (1977): *Ann. Neurol.,* 2:30–35.
47. Guilleminault, C., and Silvestri, R. (1982): In: *Sleep and Epilepsy,* edited by M. B. Sternman, M. N. Shouse, and P. Passouant, pp. 513–531. Academic Press, New York.
48. Charney, D. S., Kales, A., Soldatos, C. R., and Nelson, J. C. (1979): *Br. J. Psychiatry,* 135:418–424.
49. Gastaut, H., Batini, C., Broughton, R., Fressy, J., Roger, J., et al. (1965): In: *Le Sommeil de Nuit Normal et Pathologique,* edited by H. Fischgold, pp. 215–236. Masson, Paris.
50. Chernik, D. A., and Mendels, J. (1974): *Biol. Psychiatry,* 9:117–123.
51. Kupfer, D., Reynolds, C. F., Weiss, B. L., et al. (1974): *Arch. Gen. Psychiatry,* 30:79–84.
52. Feinberg, I., Wender, P. H., Karesko, R. L., et al. (1969): *J. Psychiatr. Res.,* 7:101–109.
53. Kaplan, J., Dawson, S., Vaughan, T., et al. (1974): *Arch. Gen. Psychiatry,* 31:62–66.
54. Jus, K., Beland, C., Jus, A., et al. (1975): *Int. Pharmacopsychiatry,* 10:58–63.
55. Risberg, A. M., Risberg, J., Elmquiest, D., et al. (1975): *Eur. J. Clin. Pharmacol.,* 8:227–231.
56. Nadel, C. (1981): *Br. J. Psychiatry,* 139:79–83.
57. Huapaya, L. (1976): *Am. J. Psychiatry,* 133:1207.
58. Flemenbaum, A. (1976): *Am. J. Psychiatry,* 133:5.
59. Allen, M. (1983): *J. Clin. Psychiatry,* 44:106–108.
60. Christianson, H., and Perry, H. (1956): *Arch. Dermatol.,* 74:232–240.
61. Huapaya, L. (1979): *Am. J. Psychiatry,* 136:7.
62. Kales, A., Soldatos, C. R., Caldwell, A. B., et al. (1980): *Arch. Gen. Psychiatry,* 37:1406–1410.
63. Kales, J. D., Kales, A., Soldatos, C. R., et al. (1980): *Arch. Gen. Psychiatry,* 37:1413–1417.
64. Glaze, D. G., Frost, J. D., and Jankovic, J. (1983): *Neurology (N.Y.),* 133:586–592.
65. Eliseo, T. S. (1975): *Clin. Hypnosis,* 17(4):272–276.
66. Clement, P. W. (1970): *J. Consult. Clin. Psychol.,* 34(1):22–26.
67. Reid, W. H., Ahmed, I., and Levie, C. A. (1981): *Am. J. Psychother.,* 35(1):27–37.
68. Reid, W. H. (1975): *Am. J. Psychother.,* 29(1):101–106.
69. Pesikoff, R. B., and Davis, P. C. (1971): *Am. J. Psychiatry,* 128:6.
70. Reid, W. H., and Gutnik, B. (1980): *Psychiatr. J. Univ. Ottawa,* 5(2):86–88.
71. Gutnik, B. D., and Reid, W. H. (1982): *Nebraska Med. J.,* 67(11):309–312.
72. Anders, T. F., and Weinstein, P. (1972): *Pediatrics,* 50(2):312–324.

Psychopharmacology:
The Third Generation of Progress,
edited by Herbert Y. Meltzer.
Raven Press, New York © 1987.

CHAPTER **87**

Neuropathology of Alzheimer's Disease and Related Dementias

Daniel P. Perl and William W. Pendlebury

In this chapter we review the neuropathologic changes seen in the brain in association with disorders characterized by progressive dementia. This follows a discussion of those changes encountered in the brain in association with normal aging. Since the list of all of the conditions that may give rise to progressive dementia is quite long, we confine our discussion to only those disease entities that are responsible for the vast majority of cases of dementia.

NORMAL AGING

With increasing age, certain changes in both the gross and microscopic appearance of the brain are noted. For the most part, these changes are variable from individual to individual and cannot be correlated to any associated significant clinical deficit.

Following the attainment of a maximum weight, at the approximate age of 18 years, the size of the human brain gradually decreases over the entire adult life-span. By age 80 years, it is estimated that the brain has lost 15% in overall weight. This loss of brain substance is encountered in both supratentorial and infratentorial structures. This decrease in brain weight is associated with the generalized atrophy of cerebral gyri as well as enlargement of the cerebral ventricles commonly encountered in the brains of elderly subjects. In a study of the relationship of total brain displacement to intracranial volume, Davis and Wright (10) showed that at the age of 55 years, the brain occupies 92% of the intracranial volume, whereas, by age 90 years, only 83% of the space within the cranial vault is taken up by the brain. This loss of brain substance is reflected in the diminished width of the cerebral cortical ribbon and enlargement of the cerebral ventricles.

Microscopically, there is evidence of loss of neurons from several regions of the brain (6). The extent of this loss is currently being assessed by computer-assisted morphometric analysis (26,35) and is not generally appreciable on routine microscopic inspection. Both neurofibrillary tangles (NFTs) and senile or neuritic plaques (NPs), lesions to be discussed in detail within the section on Alzheimer's disease, are seen in relatively small numbers in the hippocampus and neocortex from brains of nondemented individuals of advanced age (11,37). In general, there is little overlap in terms of the extent of these lesions seen in patients with advanced stages of Alzheimer's disease as compared to the normal elderly (2).

ALZHEIMER'S DISEASE AND SENILE DEMENTIA, ALZHEIMER'S TYPE

By far, the most important clinical entity responsible for progressive dementia in aging populations is Alzheimer's disease or senile dementia, Alzheimer's type. The terms Alzheimer's disease (AD) and senile dementia, Alzheimer's type (SDAT) are employed to distinguish between young and old age onset cases. More specifically, in most of the literature, AD refers to dementia with an onset prior to age 65 years, whereas SDAT refers to an onset after age 65. It should be recognized that the neuropathologic changes encountered in patients with AD and SDAT are both qualitatively and quantitatively virtually identical. Accordingly, the term AD/SDAT is employed for this discussion, recognizing that the distinction between the two terms may be an arbitrary one but is maintained until etiologic and pathogenetic mechanisms are better understood.

Gross Changes

The grossly visible changes encountered in the brains of AD/SDAT patients are nonspecific in nature; indeed, there is a considerable overlap in the appearance of the brain in AD/SDAT patients and in normal, nondemented subjects. In a study (19) of a large series of brain specimens from AD/SDAT patients, the brain weights ranged from 850 to 1,250 g with a mean value of 1,050 g. An age-matched nondemented control population had brains that, on average, weighed 100 g more than did the AD/SDAT-derived specimens; however, there was considerable overlap between the two groups. Therefore, although the AD/SDAT patients show a greater degree of cerebral atrophy when compared to the normal population, in the elderly, one cannot identify any particular brain specimen as having SDAT based on its brain weight, cortical thickness, or ventricular size.

On coronal sectioning of the cerebral hemispheres, a moderate degree of dilatation of the lateral and third ventricles is generally appreciated. This enlargement of the lateral ventricles is accompanied by a rounding of the lateral angle of the lateral ventricle. The loss of cerebral substance is related to a thinning of the cortical ribbon and likely an accompanying loss of subcortical white matter elements. Again, there is considerable overlap between the appearance of the brain with AD/SDAT and that encountered in normal aging. This concept should be kept in mind in approaching diagnostic evaluations using brain-imaging approaches. The deeper subcortical nuclei of the basal ganglia and thalamus generally retain a normal appearance.

Microscopic Changes

Autopsy studies of Alzheimer's disease have revealed a loss of neurons within several regions of the brain. This neuronal loss in the cerebral cortex is generally not detectable by routine microscopic observation and usually requires careful morphometric analysis to be appreciated (26,36). Two important subcortical regions that are characteristically depleted of neurons are the nucleus basalis of Meynert and the locus coeruleus. Studies have demonstrated that the nucleus basalis of Meynert may lose up to 90% of its normal neuronal complement, although losses of 30 to 50% are more frequently observed (39,40). Cell loss in this nucleus is of particular importance since it has recently become recognized that these neurons are the source of approximately 90% of the cholinergic input of the neocortex (25). It is postulated that the prominent loss of neocortical cholinergic activity seen in association with AD/SDAT is the result of primary cell loss in this nucleus (40). Neuronal loss in the locus coeruleus has only recently been described (5) and has not been subjected to extensive study.

The two principal neuropathologic lesions encountered in the brains of individuals with AD/SDAT are the neurofibrillary tangle (NFT) and the senile or neuritic plaque (NP). Although these had been previously observed, it was Alois Alzheimer, in 1907, who definitively described the occurrence of numerous NFTs in the brain of a 51-year-old woman who had suffered from a progressive dementing illness (1). Since that early description, there have been numerous published studies examining this cellular alteration at the light microscopic and ultrastructural levels of resolution. In cases of AD/SDAT, NFTs are widely distributed in the neocortex and are prominently found in the hippocampus and the amygdala. Other areas of involvement by NFTs include the nucleus basalis of Meynert, the claustrum, the hypothalamus, the periaqueductal nuclei, and the pontine tegmentum.

Studies have established a correlation between the density of NFTs present in the neocortex and the hippocampus and the degree of cognitive impairment displayed by the patient prior to death (2). Neurofibrillary tangles are difficult to recognize when stained with hematoxylin and eosin, and the alteration is best visualized with the use of silver impregnation stains such as the Bielschowski or Bodian techniques. With these staining methods, the NFT is seen to consist of a flame-shaped, fibrillary, strongly argyrophilic structure occupying the cytoplasm of medium- to large-sized pyramidal neurons. Neurons with a more rounded shaped perikaryon generally contain more rounded, globoid forms of NFTs.

Ultrastructurally, the NFT is composed of numerous aggregates of double-stranded twisted filaments, which are referred to as "paired helical filaments" (PHF) (20,42). The PHF are composed of two identical filaments, each measuring 10 nm in diameter, which undergo a repeated helical twist around each other with a regular periodicity of 80 nm. The PHF has been shown to be particularly insoluble in a number of harsh protein solvents and detergents, which has made biochemical characterization of its protein constituents extremely difficult (32).

The second characteristic microscopic lesion of AD/SDAT is the senile or neuritic plaque (NP). This is a relatively large structure, measuring 50 to 200 μm, that lies free within the neuropil. In cases of AD/SDAT, numerous NPs are encountered throughout the neocortex and in the hippocampus. As with the NFT, NPs are poorly visualized by hematoxylin and eosin staining, and silver impregnation methods or the fluorochrome dye thioflavin are most commonly employed to demonstrate the extent and distribution of these changes. Again, as was noted with the NFT, there is a direct correlation between the number of NPs seen in the hippocampus and neocortex and the degree of cognitive impairment seen in life (4).

Although the pathogenesis of the NP is poorly understood, the terms immature, mature, and burned-out plaques are often used in describing individual lesions based on their morphologic appearance (43). Immature NPs are composed of small collections of degenerating neurites (i.e., neuronal processes, axons, and dendrites) that, at the ultrastructural level of resolution, contain PHFs. The mature NPs contain many degenerating neurites associated with reactive astrocytes and microglial cells at the periphery of the plaque. Within the center of the structure is a stellate core of amyloid. The burned-out NPs are made up of a compact mass of amyloid surrounded by reactive astrocytes, but these lack the associated degenerating neurites. It is important to recognize that although these descriptive terms imply a developmental sequence for their formation, this concept remains speculative in nature.

Another neuropathologic lesion seen in the brains of patients with AD/SDAT is granulovacuolar degeneration (GVD). This was first described in 1911 by Simchowitz (33) and is seen almost exclusively in the neurons of the hippocampus. The cells most commonly involved by this lesion are the large pyramidal neurons of the Sommer's sector (H_1 region) of the Ammon's horn of the hippocampus. In these cells, the GVD is seen as intracytoplasmic vacuoles, each containing a dense basophilic granule. Involved neurons frequently contain clusters of these structures. The density of involvement of the hippocampus by GVD has been correlated to the degree of cognitive impairment seen prior to death (3).

Finally, an additional neuropathologic feature of AD/SDAT is the appearance of Hirano bodies. The Hirano body was first described by Hirano in 1965 (17) in the hippocampus of brains examined from natives of Guam who suffer from an endemic form of amyotrophic lateral sclerosis. The Hirano body has since been identified in most cases of AD/SDAT and has been described in association with a number of other rare neuropathologic entities and in relatively small numbers in the hippocampus of some normal elderly individuals. The Hirano body appears as a brightly eosinophilic rod-shaped structure adjacent to the pyramidal hippocampal neurons. The Hirano body has a highly regular paracrystalline filamentous ultrastructural appearance (30) and stains strongly with antibodies directed against actin (16).

It has been noted that a significant number of cases of AD/SDAT demonstrate a vascular lesion of the brain referred to as congophilic angiopathy (31). Congophilic angiopathy refers to the deposition of amyloid in the small to medium-sized arteries of the leptomeninges and the superficial cortex, particularly in the frontal and parietal regions of the brain. The white matter, deep nuclear structures, and the brainstem are characteristically spared.

These vascular changes are characterized by thickening of the vessels by eosinophilic deposits that, when stained with Congo red, show green–yellow birefringence under illumination by crossed polarized light. The amyloid deposits apparently give rise to a compromise in the integrity of the vessel walls, as spontaneous hemorrhages are common in association with this alteration (18). When hemorrhage does occur, it is frequently located in a superficial site and is commonly multifocal. These two features, namely, superficial location and multicentricity, differentiate intracerebral hemorrhage related to congophilic angiopathy from that related to systemic hypertension.

The finding of amyloid in the core of many NPs as well as within cortical blood vessels has led some investigators to suggest that amyloid may have an important pathogenetic role in AD/SDAT (15,24). However, it should be noted that congophilic angiopathy may occur as an isolated entity and in association with other neurologic disorders. Whether congophilic angiopathy and AD/SDAT represent the simultaneous occurrence of two relatively common disorders of the elderly or are linked with regard to pathogenetic mechanisms remains to be resolved with further research.

HUNTINGTON'S DISEASE

Huntington's disease represents an important cause of presenile progressive dementia. In most cases, the association of progressive dementia with a prominent movement disorder, associated personality changes, and an autosomal dominant inheritance pattern provides a clinical constellation that allows for a definitive clinical diagnosis in advance of postmortem evaluation. Gross external examination of the brain of patients with Huntington's disease reveals moderately severe generalized atrophy. Coronal sectioning of the specimen demonstrates the dramatic and characteristic loss of substance of the head of the caudate nucleus and the putamen with associated striking dilatation of the lateral ventricles.

Microscopic examination of these specimens shows profound neuronal loss in the caudate and putamen, in particular affecting the small Golgi type II neurons (7). The neuronal losses are accompanied by astrocytic proliferation and glial scarring. The cerebral cortical changes are extremely subtle, even for profoundly impaired subjects, and consist of a mild loss of deep cortical neurons and an accumulation of lipofuscin in the remaining cells (34). Senile plaques and neurofibrillary tangles are not typically encountered in the brain in Huntington's disease.

MULTIINFARCT DEMENTIA

Cerebral infarction is an extremely common disorder in the elderly. Indeed, studies have shown that the incidence of clinically apparent infarctive events involving central nervous system brain is approximately three times as high among individuals 75 years or older as among subjects less than 65 years of age (19). A postmortem study indicated that among the extreme elderly, namely, those examined at autopsy at age 85 years or more, over 30% of brain specimens show evidence of either acute or healed infarctive lesions (29). When sufficient destruction of vital cerebral structures occurs as a result of multiple cerebral infarctions, a significant degree of cognitive abilities may be lost. In such instances, the term multiinfarct dementia has been employed. Obviously, the relative mixture of cognitive loss with other superimposed neurologic signs and symptoms is extremely variable depending on the distribution and extent of the individual destructive lesions.

Based on our experience, it is estimated that 15% of all cases of dementia seen in patients over age 65 years are the result of multiple cerebral infarctions. An additional 15% of elderly demented patients represent the combined effects of SDAT with superimposed cerebral infarction. In these later cases, it is often difficult to delineate precisely the relative importance of each pathologic process in ascribing the cause of the dementia. One should realize that the relative importance of cerebral infarction as a cause of dementia in a population of elderly patients will be strongly affected by the relative incidence of poorly controlled hypertension and diabetes in that population.

In general, in cases of multiinfarct dementia, the lesions may be seen involving the cerebral cortical ribbon, the basal ganglia, and the subcortical white matter. In any individual case, one of these three sites will often predominate. The lesions are invariably multiple, bilateral, and show histologic evidence suggesting varying age. Lesions involving the cerebral cortical gray matter are most frequent in patients of this type. In these cases, the combined volume of the infarctive lesions is typically in excess of 50 μl (38). Basal ganglionic infarcts that result in dementia are virtually always bilateral, and involvement of the thalamus is extremely common. These lesions result from severe arteriosclerotic involvement of the small medial lenticulostriate perforating arteries.

A minority of multiinfarct dementia cases result from infarctive lesions involving the subcortical white matter. These lesions produce extensive demyelinization with a sparing of the overlying cerebral cortex. This entity is referred to as subacute arteriosclerotic encephalopathy or Binswanger's disease (28). These patients are frequently, but not always, hypertensive. The presence of pseudobulbar signs and motor deficits may provide important clues to distinguish these cases from AD/SDAT; however, many Binswanger's disease patients will present in a fashion that is clinically indistinguishable from this disorder.

PICK'S DISEASE

Pick's disease, a relatively rare form of progressive dementia seen in the presenile age group, has an extremely distinctive neuropathologic picture. On gross external examination, the brain demonstrates striking atrophy that is confined to the frontotemporal regions. Indeed, because of the sharp delineation between the appearance of the atrophic frontotemporal cortex and the adjacent normal-appearing parietooccipital cortex, the term lobar atrophy has been employed. The cut surface of the brain shows prominent ventricular dilatation as well as marked thinning of the involved frontotemporal and insular regions of the cerebral cortex.

Histologic examination of areas of involved cerebral cortex reveals a variable degree of neuronal loss with accompanying glial scarring. Many remaining neurons will appear, on hematoxylin and eosin staining, to be rounded and with a peripherally aligned Nissl substance. Silver impregnation stains, such as the Bielschowski technique, reveal these cells to contain prominent rounded argyrophilic Pick body inclusions, which are characteristic for the disease. These inclusions, when examined by electron microscopy, are not membrane bound and generally contain a mixture of neurofilaments, neurotubules, paired helical filaments, and other cytoplasmic components (27,30). Immunohistochemical studies have shown positive staining with polyclonal antisera directed against microtubules and neurofilaments as well as paired helical filaments (27). Some cases of Pick's disease have shown a mixture of pathologic lesions including the presence of Pick bodies as well as NFTs and NPs. However, most cases are free of AD-related neuropathologic changes, even in elderly patients. Despite the presence of these overlapping cases, Pick's disease is currently thought to be a distinct, though poorly understood, disorder.

POSTTRAUMATIC DEMENTIA (DEMENTIA PUGILISTICA)

Following the studies of Critchley (9) and of Corsellis and co-workers (8), it has become recognized that progressive dementia may ensue from the delayed effects of repeated head trauma, particularly as seen in retired boxers. This entity is referred to as posttraumatic dementia, the punch-drunk syndrome, or dementia pugilistica. Clinically, these patients show a mild to moderate degree of dementia, although it may be sufficiently severe to require institutional care. Parkinsonian features are also frequently encountered in this group of patients.

On neuropathologic examination, one sees thinning and fenestration of the septum pellucidum, depigmentation of the substantia nigra, and widespread NFT formation throughout the frontotemporal cortex. The degree of NFT formation is often quite severe and typically is seen in the absence of accompanying NPs. Electron microscopic examination of the neurofibrillary tangles of dementia pugilistica reveals an ultrastructural appearance identical to that of AD/SDAT (41). The underlying pathogenetic mechanisms leading to this poorly understood disorder are completely obscure.

CREUTZFELDT–JAKOB DISEASE

Creutzfeldt–Jakob disease, subacute spongiform encephalopathy, is an extremely rare form of progressive dementia. Following the pioneering work of Gajdusek characterizing the "slow-viral" nature of the disease kuru (12), a fatal neurodegenerative disorder seen in a restricted area among the natives of New Guinea, it was recognized that Creutzfeldt–Jakob disease represented an example of a disease seen in worldwide distribution with very similar neuropathologic features. This led to the successful transmission of a Creutzfeldt–Jakob-like disease to chimpanzees following intracerebral brain homogenate inoculation (14).

Clinically, cases of Creutzfeldt–Jakob disease often have an insidious onset of their symptoms with periods of confusion, mood disturbances, and sensory and/or motor-coordination difficulties. Within weeks to months, a progressive dementia becomes evident, frequently accompanied by myoclonus and a characteristic triphasic pattern on the electroencephalogram. The disease proceeds in a relentlessly progressive fashion with an average duration of illness until death of about 7 months. The course may be even more abrupt, and cases surviving for 3 years or more are only occasionally reported. Studies have estimated that the disease occurs with an annual incidence of approximately one case per 1 million population per year (23).

In most cases of Creutzfeldt–Jakob disease, gross examination of the brain reveals a normal appearance externally and on dissection. In cases in which there has been a longer clinical course, generalized cerebral atrophy may be found. Cases with greatly prolonged survival may demonstrate an extremely low brain weight with wide sulci and thin, firm, atrophic gyri. This latter finding is caused by a marked loss of cortical neurons with resultant glial scarring.

Microscopic examination of cases of Creutzfeldt–Jakob disease demonstrates spongiform changes, gliosis, and neuronal loss. The relative prominence of each of these three findings may vary in relation to the course of the illness. Spongiform change consists of numerous rounded vacuoles present within the tissues. This change is commonly seen within the cerebral cortex but may also be encountered in the thalamus, basal ganglia, and the molecular layer of the cerebellum. The cerebral cortical involvement is frequently patchy, with skipped areas adjacent to involved cortex. In arriving at this diagnosis, it is important to distinguish true spongiform changes from perineuronal clefts and artifacts related to immersion fixation and paraffin embedding as well as from the microcystic changes seen with nonspecific gliosis. True spongiform changes, as seen in association with Creutzfeldt–Jakob disease, are encountered within glial and neuronal processes and have distinctive features when viewed ultrastructurally (21).

Inflammatory cell infiltrates are generally not encountered in affected cases, and NFTs and NPs are rarely seen. A minority of cases (approximately 10% of cases in one series) will show the presence of amyloid plaques, similar to those seen in kuru, in the cerebellum (22). Because of the unusual resistance to inactivation of these unique infectious agents by the usual fixative agents and antiseptic procedures employed for conventional infectious agents, special precautions are required in the handling and processing of body fluids and tissues obtained from affected individuals (13).

REFERENCES

1. Alzheimer, A. (1907): *Allg. Z. Psychiatrie,* 64:146–148.
2. Ball, M. J. (1976): *Neuropathol. Appl. Neurobiol.,* 2:395–410.
3. Ball, M. J. (1977): *Acta Neuropathol. (Berl.),* 37:111–118.
4. Blessed, G., Tomlinson, B. E., and Roth, M. (1968): *Br. J. Psychiatry,* 114:797–811.
5. Bondareff, W., Mountjoy, C. Q., and Roth, M. (1982): *Neurology (N.Y.),* 32:164–168.
6. Brody, H. (1955): *J. Comp. Neurol.,* 102:511–556.
7. Bryun, G. W., Bota, A. M., and Dom, R. (1979): *Adv. Neurol.,* 23:83–93.
8. Corsellis, J. A. N., Bruton, C. J., and Freeman-Browne, D. (1973): *Psychol. Med.,* 3:270–303.
9. Critchley, M. (1957): *Br. Med. J.,* 1:357–366.
10. Davis, P. J. M., and Wright, E. A. (1977): *Neuropath. Appl. Neurobiol.,* 3:341–358.
11. Dayan, A. D. (1970): *Acta Neuropathol. (Berl.),* 16:85–94.
12. Gajdusek, D. C. (1977): *Science,* 197:943–960.
13. Gajdusek, D. C., Gibbs, C. J., Jr., Asher, D. M., Brown, P., Diwan, A., et al. (1977): *N. Engl. J. Med.,* 297:1253–1258.
14. Gibbs, C. J., Jr., Gajdusek, D. C., Asher, D. M., Alpers, M. P., Beck, E., et al. (1968): *Science,* 161:388–389.
15. Glenner, G. G. (1985): *Hum. Pathol.,* 16:433–435.
16. Goldman, J. E. (1983): *J. Neuropathol. Exp. Neurol.,* 42:146–152.
17. Hirano, A. (1965): In: *NINDB Monograph No. 2: Slow, Latent, and Temperate Virus Infections,* edited by D. C. Gajdusek and C. J. Gibbs, Jr. National Institutes of Health, Washington.
18. Ishii, N., Nishihara, Y., and Horic, A. (1984): *J. Neurol. Neurosurg. Psychiatry,* 47:1203–1210.
19. Kannel, W. B., and Wolf, P. A. (1983): In: *Vascular Disease of the Central Nervous System,* 2nd ed., edited by R. W. R. Russell. Churchill Livingstone, New York.
20. Kidd, M. (1963): *Nature,* 197:192–193.
21. Lampert, P. W., Gajdusek, D. C., and Gibbs, C. J., Jr. (1972): *Am. J. Pathol.,* 68:626–647.
22. Masters, C. L., Gajdusek, D. C., and Gibbs, C. J., Jr. (1981): *Brain,* 104:559–588.
23. Masters, C. L., Harris, J. O., Gajdusek, D. C., Gibbs, C. J., Jr., Bernoulli, C., et al. (1979): *Ann. Neurol.,* 5:177–188.
24. Masters, C. L., Multhaup, G., Simms, G., Pottgiesser, J., Martins, R. N., et al. (1985): *EMBO J.,* 4:2757–2763.
25. Mesulam, M. M., Mufson, E. J., and Levey, A. L. (1983): *J. Comp. Neurol.,* 214:170–197.
26. Mountjoy, C. Q., Roth, M., Evans, N. J. R., and Evans, H. M. (1983): *Neurobiol. Aging,* 4:1–11.
27. Munoz-Garcia, D., and Ludwin, S. K. (1984): *Ann. Neurol.,* 16:467–480.
28. Olszewski, J. (1962): *World Neurol.,* 3:359–375.
29. Peress, N. S., Kane, W. C., and Aronson, S. M. (1972): *Prog. Brain Res.,* 40:473–483.
30. Schochet, S. S., Jr., Lampert, P. W., and Lindenberg, R. (1968): *Acta Neuropathol.,* 11:330–337.
31. Scholz, W. (1938): *Z. Neurol. Psychiatry,* 162:694–715.
32. Selkoe, D. J., Ihara, Y., and Salazar, F. J. (1982): *Science,* 215:1243–1245.
33. Simchowicz, T. (1911): *Histol. Histopathol. Arb. Grosshirn.,* 4:267–444.
34. Telez-Nagel, I., Johnson, A. B., and Terry, R. D. (1973): *Adv. Neurol.,* 1:387–398.
35. Terry, R. D., and Deteresa, R. (1984): *J. Neuropathol. Exp. Neurol.,* 43:331.
36. Terry, R. D., Peck, A., Deteresa, R., and Schechter, R. (1981): *Ann. Neurol.,* 10:184–192.
37. Tomlinson, B. E., Blessed, G., and Roth, M. (1968): *J. Neurol. Sci.,* 7:331–356.
38. Tomlinson, B. E., Blessed, G., and Roth, M. (1970): *J. Neurol. Sci.,* 11:205–242.
39. Whitehouse, P. J., Price, D. L., Clark, A. W., Coyle, J. T., and DeLong, M. R. (1981): *Ann. Neurol.,* 10:122–126.
40. Whitehouse, P. J., Price, D. L., and Struble, R. G. (1983): *Science,* 215:1237–1238.
41. Wisniewski, H. M., Narang, H. K., Corsellis, J. A. N., and Terry, R. D. (1976): *J. Neuropath. Exptl. Neurol.,* 35:367.
42. Wisniewski, H. M., Narang, H. K., and Terry, R. D. (1976): *J. Neurol. Sci.,* 27:173–181.
43. Wisniewski, H. M., and Terry, R. D. (1973): In *Progress in Neuropathology,* Vol. 2., edited by H. M. Zimmerman. Grune and Stratton, New York.

Psychopharmacology:
The Third Generation of Progress,
edited by Herbert Y. Meltzer.
Raven Press, New York © 1987.

CHAPTER **88**

Cortical Neurotransmitter Chemistry in Alzheimer's Disease

Elaine K. Perry

The importance of neurotransmitters—the small molecular signals employed in rapid interneuronal communication—in normal and pathological conditions of the human brain cannot be overestimated. Almost every drug currently available to the psychiatrist or neurologist for the treatment of CNS symptoms functions either directly or indirectly by affecting specific transmitter systems. Such drugs include major and minor tranquilizers, neuroleptics, antipsychotics, a variety of antidepressants, hypnotics, anticholinergics, anticonvulsants, L-dopa, and related chemicals. No one would dispute the value of these drugs in the management of certain CNS diseases, although in many instances the precise mechanism of their action in suppressing particular clinical symptoms is unknown as is the primary nature of the disease process itself.

One group of disorders—those associated with organic or degenerative dementia—has not yet yielded to any of the pharmacologist's armamentarium. Among these disorders, Alzheimer's disease (AD) constitutes one of the greatest problems for the psychiatrist dealing with the elderly and, through its attendant social burden, for society as a whole. As yet, the only means available to alleviate the patient's suffering is through personal support and care and, in more advanced cases, through restraint via a range of tranquilizing agents. The critical need for a drug to relieve the cognitive, especially memory, impairment in the early stages and to control the broad spectrum of dementing symptoms in later stages can hardly be overemphasized.

In searching for a lesion of the brain that might be amenable to treatment, the cerebral cortex has generally been the focus of attention for research into AD. Structurally, it is the entire cortical mantle that is generally most severely affected by the presence of the microscopic hallmarks of the disease—senile plaques and neurofibrillary tangles—and chemically, the majority of abnormalities so far detected have been most prevalent in neo- and archicortical brain regions. The status of cortical neurotransmitter systems in AD is thus an area of great interest, and, thanks to a vast body of research mainly on experimental animal brains (see 20,21,28), a great deal is now known about the neuroanatomy of the various systems projecting to (ascending), from (descending), and within (intrinsic) the cerebral cortex (summarized in Table 1). It is worth noting that among the numerous systems (Table 1) so far—and no doubt more remain to be—identified, ascending input systems (such as cholinergic and noradrenergic) constitute only a small minority of cortical nerve terminals, and, by contrast, intrinsic systems such as GABA and excitatory amino acid transmitters account for a far greater proportion. Major cortical pathways with as yet unidentified transmitters include thalamocortical, transcallosal, and ipsilateral intracortical systems. Of particular interest is the observation that the majority of cortical neurons immunoreactive for such peptides as somatostatin, CCK, and substance P also contain GABA (28) and that these neurons are highly concentrated in association areas especially affected in AD.

Despite these many major advances in mapping and measuring the cellular response to cortical transmitters, knowledge regarding the physiological functions of the various pathways at the behavioral level—for example,

TABLE 1. *Cortical neurotransmitter systems*

System	Anatomy	Physiology (effect of iontophoretic application on cortical cells)
Ascending/afferent		
Cholinergic	Basal forebrain nuclei project topographically to discrete areas of entire cortex	Excitation, primarily muscarinic, in lower layers (especially pyramidal neurons); inhibition in upper layers
Noradrenergic	Projections from locus coeruleus (pons) provide diffuse and widespread innervation throughout cortex	Most cells modulated (excitation or inhibition) through effects on background spontaneous as opposed to evoked activities
Serotonergic	Projections from midbrain medial and dorsal raphe nuclei, via medial forebrain bundle, uniformly innervate entire cortex	Decreases spontaneous activity
Dopaminergic	Innervation from the ventromedial tegmental area restricted to frontal, cingulate, and entorhinal cortex	
Intrinsic and projecting/ efferent		
γ-Aminobutyric acid	Primarily associated with nonpyramidal interneurons distributed in all cortical layers and regions	Inhibition—probably the major inhibitory transmitter in the cortex
Glutamate (and aspartate)	May be associated with the majority of efferent and intrinsic excitatory projections mainly arising from cortical pyramidal neurons	Rapid and strong excitation—probably major excitatory cortical output
Somatostatin	Multipolar and bitufted nonpyramidal neurons (although pyramidal activity also reported) in most cell layers and areas (coexistence with neuropeptide Y reported)	Excitatory (and in some areas also inhibitory) effects on cortical pyramids
Vasoactive intestinal polypeptide (VIP)	Located in nonpyramidal, predominantly bipolar cells in all layers except I	Excitation
Cholecystokinin	Nonpyramidal perikarya in all layers	Excitation
Miscellaneous		
Neuropeptides	Various peptides not yet clearly located include neurotensin (may be unevenly distributed), substance P (fibers evident in frontal cortex), motilin (may be concentrated in cortex), Metenkephalin (small cells in layers II–VI), γ-MSH (fibers from hypothalamus), secretin, bombesin, CRF (intrinsic, regionally distributed)	Substance P reported to be excitatory

their role in controlling cortically governed behavior—is as yet comparatively sparse. Paradoxically, perhaps, diseases such as AD may, by virtue of the appearance of transmitter deficits associated with disturbances in specific forms of behavior, provide new clues regarding the role of particular transmitters in cerebral function.

Given the obvious need to examine cerebral and particularly cortical transmitters in AD, the investigator is currently faced with only a limited choice of means available. Ideally, the functioning of individual systems would be examined in the living brain under a variety of normal and behavioral or pharmacological test conditions, a goal that will no doubt ultimately be achieved with the emergence of more refined and clinically applicable devices for scanning or probing individual pathways in the living brain. An indirect approach that has tempted many but satisfied few is the search for marker activities reflecting cerebral abnormalities in such body fluids as lumbar CSF, blood, or urine (26). A third and by far the most extensively employed technique at present involves the measurement of transmitter activities in postmortem human brain tissue. Although this approach (see below) has undoubtedly yielded valuable information on the state of transmitters in AD (and indeed in other CNS disorders), its limitations should always be borne in mind:

1. The fact that those transmitter activities that can, by

virtue of their stability, be measured post-mortem are often relatively crude indices of transmitter function. More sensitive but unfortunately unstable indices of dynamic transmitter function such as the stimulated nerve terminal release of transmitter or receptor-induced secondary messenger responses—aspects closely related to the functioning of transmitter-governed neuronal activity in the living brain—cannot generally be examined.

2. The concern that abnormalities may, by virtue of the generally advanced stage of the disease prior to death, be secondary or indirect changes and that primary disease-related events may be obscured or even obliterated.

Despite these reservations, a growing body of evidence on the status in AD of presynaptic transmitter-related activities and of transmitter receptor binding and comparative transmitter studies in other dementing disorders merits serious consideration in relation to future basic and applied research into AD.

PRESYNAPTIC TRANSMITTER ACTIVITIES

Since the majority of biochemical studies are of necessity conducted on autopsy brain tissue, it is fortunate that a number of enzymes and transmitter, precursor, or metabolite activities, localized in individual neurons (where they are generally concentrated in varicosities or presynaptic nerve terminals) are reasonably stable post-mortem. In addition, certain transmitter synthesis, release, or uptake systems that are unstable post-mortem have been estimated in a unique collection of biopsy tissues examined by David Bowen and his colleagues (3). A summary of the numerous autopsy and biopsy studies (reviewed, 14,38,41,53) of presynaptic transmitter activities in AD is provided in Table 2.

Cholinergic

Deficits in the cholinergic system, first reported 10 years ago (4,15,43), originally aroused great interest in the pos-

TABLE 2. *Presynaptic cortical transmitter activities in Alzheimer's disease*

System	Parameter	Status in Alzheimer's disease
Cholinergic	Choline acetyltransferase	Consistently reported reduced throughout cortex
	Acetylcholinesterase	Dramatic loss histochemically; biochemically extensive loss of tetrameric (G_4) form
	High-affinity choline uptake	Decreased
	Acetylcholine synthesis	Decreased (biopsy prisms)
Noradrenergic	Norepinephrine	Moderate reductions in some areas
	3-Methoxy-4-hydroxyphenyl glycoaldehyde	Decreased/normal
	Dopamine-β-hydroxylase	Decreased/normal
Dopaminergic	Dopamine	Near normal
	Homovanillic acid	Near normal
Serotonergic	Serotonin	Moderate reductions in some areas
	5-Hydroxyindoleacetic acid	Moderate reductions in some areas
γ-Aminobutyric acid (GABA)	GABA	Normal
	Glutamate decarboxylase	Normal in biopsy (decreased in autopsy tissue)
	K^+-evoked GABA release	Normal in biopsy prisms
Glutamic (and aspartic) acid	Free amino acid	Normal
	K^+-evoked release	Normal in biopsy prisms
Somatostatin	Neuropeptide immunoreactivity	Reduced
Corticotropin-releasing factor	Neuropeptide immunoreactivity	Reduced
Substance P Met-Enkephalin Neuropeptide Y Cholecystokinin Vasoactive intestinal peptide Neurotensin Thyrotropin-releasing hormone	Neuropeptide immunoreactivity	Generally normal

sibilities of a specific transmitter involvement in AD, and the observation still stands today as the most consistent and most extensive neurochemical abnormality yet detected (6,39,46). The reduction in cerebral, particularly cortical, cholinergic markers in AD (Table 2), together with a vast body of evidence available from the effects of both cholinergic drugs and surgical or chemical lesioning of cholinergic neurons, support the now popular concept that cholinergic neurons projecting to the cortex (Table 1), which play a critical role in the memory function, degenerate in AD.

In both autopsy and biopsy tissue, the loss of, for example, choline acetyltransferase correlates well with the degree of cognitive impairment (3,44). The abnormality, which no doubt reflects the degeneration of cholinergic axons (cell bodies in the basal forebrain also degenerate as the disease advances), is apparent early in the disease process (within a year of clinical presentation), and the relationship between chemical and cognitive indices is in fact more obvious at earlier as opposed to later stages of the disease, when other transmitter deficits (see below) are apparent.

From the therapeutic viewpoint, the efficacy of potential cholinomimetic agents—and those so far tested provide only a moderate and generally clinically insignificant improvement in a proportion of patients—may depend critically on the status of cholinergic receptors and on the importance of other transmitter disturbances.

Catecholaminergic

There is little evidence of an involvement of the mesocortical dopaminergic system in AD, although this system may well play a role in the cognitive impairment of Parkinson's disease. In contrast, cortical noradrenergic markers (Table 2) are reduced in a proportion of patients, as is the population of neurons projecting to the cortex in the locus coeruleus (10,11,14,45). The clinical significance of the noradrenergic deficit in AD is still unclear, and although this system has been implicated in memory function, there is no obvious relationship between the deficit and the degree of dementia. The cortical, like the peripheral, noradrenergic system may well function in stress-related behavior, and deficits in AD may account for the rapid deterioration (usually reversible) evident in patients when, for example, their environment is suddenly altered.

Serotonergic

As with the noradrenergic system, moderate reductions in serotonergic markers (Table 2) are evident (11,14) in some patients and some brain areas, although, again, the relationship to the clinical picture is unknown. An involvement of this transmitter in some aspect of cognitive functions seems likely, although current evidence on the effects of antidepressant drugs indicates a key role for this transmitter in mood as opposed to reasoning ability (if indeed the two can be strictly separated). Indeed, those patients with serotonergic deficits may well be those who, in addition to the dementing symptoms of the disease, also suffer from depression, although this possibility has not yet been investigated.

Amino Acid Transmitters

There is as yet little evidence for an involvement of GABA or the acidic amino acid transmitters in AD, although the great importance of these systems as the major inhibitory and excitatory cortical signals prompts continued studies. The normality of free GABA or amino acid levels (Table 2) may actually be deceptive, since the former is unstable post-mortem (increasing dramatically within hours of death), and the latter may be obscured by nontransmitter general metabolic pools. The demonstration of normal glutamate decarboxylase activity and normal K^+-evoked amino acid release in biopsy tissue prisms (3,58) does, however, suggest that presynaptic terminals of these neurons may function normally at least in the cortex. Nevertheless, speculation concerning the role of excitatory amino acids in AD continues to be prompted by such provocative reports as that of De Boni and Crapper McLachlan (18) that they can induce paired helical filaments (similar to those in tangles) in cultured human neurons.

Neuropeptides

The recent discovery of a vast range of neuropeptides in the brain has naturally stimulated analyses of these in AD. So far, the only neuropeptide that has consistently been reported to be decreased in AD is somatostatin; other important intrinsic cortical peptides such as CCK and VIP are apparently unchanged (Table 2), although very recently abnormalities of CRF have also been discovered (19). The extent of the somatostatin abnormality varies according to different reports, some of which demonstrate changes in only a few brain areas and others in advanced cases only (16,23,46,54). Curiously, although somatostatin immunoreactivity is decreased, that of neuropeptide Y, with which it coexists, is apparently normal in AD, as is the level of GABA (also coexisting with somatostatin), findings that have so far defied explanation. With respect to hippocampal peptides, it will be of great interest to discover whether galanin is reduced in AD. This peptide coexists in a subpopulation of septal cholinergic neurons projecting to the hippocampus (33), and the concept that certain cortical cholinergic fibers may be differentiated on the basis of their peptide content should stimulate more refined analyses of cholinergic neuropathology in degenerative conditions such as Alzheimer's and Parkinson's diseases.

Measurement of the level (immunoreactivity) of peptides does not obviously detect changes in their turnover, a critical factor in the function of peptidergic neurons, and this aspect will no doubt be investigated in future studies using the respective messenger RNA probes. There can be no doubt that as a chemical group peptides will continue to attract attention in CNS degenerative diseases, since it is becoming progressively obvious that some, at least, function not only as hormones or neuromodulators (and even, as part of larger molecules, as actual receptors) but also as growth factors or mitogens (25).

Neuropathological Aspects

Some but not all of the transmitter abnormalities of AD described above can be related to structural changes in the brain (41,49). Thus, reductions in presynaptic components of the cholinergic, noradrenergic, and serotonergic afferent cortical fibers are most likely connected with the neuronal loss and/or shrinkage and neurofibrillary tangle formation variously seen in the respective subcortical nuclei (Meynert nucleus, locus coeruleus, and raphe systems). Accumulating evidence suggests that these subcortical neuronal abnormalities may be secondary to retrograde degeneration originating in their cortical terminations. The morphological counterparts, if any, to reductions in such neuropeptides as somatostatin and CRF, and whether these relate to the loss of cortical neurons in AD, remain to be established.

Considerable attention has been directed to the question of whether senile plaques are associated with any particular neurotransmitter system or systems (42). Neuritic processes innervating the region of the plaque (in either human or aged monkey brain) have now been shown, by immunocytochemical or histochemical techniques, to contain a variety of neurotransmitters including acetylcholine, catecholamines, and a number of neuropeptides (42). It thus seems unlikely that cortical plaque formation specifically involves any particular neuronal type, although the same may not be true of cortical tangle formation, which, with its predominance in pyramidal neurons, may primarily affect neurons containing the putative excitatory amino acid transmitters. Such a link is only speculative at present, although it might be consistent with the *in vitro* effects of these acids (see above), and indeed the whole question of the connection between the histopathological features and transmitter deficits of AD remains to be answered.

TRANSMITTER RECEPTOR BINDING

In contrast to presynaptic transmitter activities, receptors for individual transmitters are not confined to specific neurons and are generally widely distributed in the brain, not only on neurons but also, in certain instances, on cerebral blood vessels and glial cells (40). Although some receptors are situated on presynaptic nerve terminals where they govern the release of transmitter, the majority are situated postsynaptically and function to regulate, either directly or via a secondary messenger system, the membrane conductance and hence the tendency to depolarize of the target neurons. The strength of autopsy human brain receptor binding studies currently lies in the wide range of specific radiolabeled ligands now available and in the fortuitous postmortem stability of receptor ligand binding in intact brain tissue (in terms of both distribution and activity) for long periods after death. There are, however, limitations to currently available techniques that should be considered, especially where negative results are obtained in a disease condition such as AD. For example, binding to dispersed tissue membranes or to intact tissue subjected to tritium film autoradiography does not distinguish synaptic binding, which may be selectively subject to disease-related abnormalities, from nonsynaptic glial or blood vessel binding. Perhaps because of this technical restriction or the

possibility that cerebral receptors are less closely controlled than, for example, peripheral receptors, consistently detected transmitter receptor binding abnormalities (13,40) in AD (summarized in Table 3) are few in comparison to abnormalities of presynaptic transmitter activities.

Cholinergic Receptors

The majority of binding studies of cortical muscarinic sites both in isolated membrane preparations and, *in situ,* by autoradiographic localization indicate no significant abnormality in the density of total muscarinic antagonist binding sites. A few investigators have, however, reported moderate reductions, especially in archicortical areas. Research on cholinergic receptors is currently complicated by uncertainties regarding the subdivision of muscarinic receptors into agonist and antagonist subtypes. It has thus recently been reported that there is a selective reduction of the M_2 muscarinic subsite in AD, detected by carbachol displacement of muscarinic antagonist by the direct binding of the agonist oxotremorine (31). The reduction in M_2 sites is said to correlate with the loss of choline acetyltransferase (31), although, curiously, total antagonist binding has been reported to increase as this enzyme decreases (36).

If a selective M_2 loss is confirmed, then the development of specific M_2 ligands might be useful in the antemortem diagnosis of the disease using PET scanning techniques. It should, however, be noted that Cauldfield et al. (8) did not detect changes in the receptor population that was not displaced by pirenzepine (which presumably includes M_2 sites) and that our own observations (57) suggest only moderate M_2 and M_1 losses in AD (at least in the hippocampus) but not in another disease with substantial presynaptic cholinergic deficits—Parkinson's disease. Furthermore, the effects of septal or Meynert lesioning on hippocampal or neocortical muscarinic receptors are currently unclear, with some groups reporting selective M_2 losses and others only moderate losses of both M_2 and M_1 (17). All of their observations suggest caution in interpreting data on a postulated M_2 subsite in the absence of a specific ligand to detect this site.

The status of the CNS nicotinic receptor is unclear. In the cortex, a purely nicotinic-like response has not yet been observed in electrophysiological studies (29), although a receptor with mixed nicotinic and muscarinic pharmacology appears to be present (50). A major problem in neurochemical investigations of this receptor with intermediate pharmacological characteristics is the availability of suitable ligands. α-Bungarotoxin binding sites are said to be either normal or reduced in AD (Table 3), although the inability of this drug to influence the nicotinic response in CNS neurons suggests that this site may not be directly related to the nicotinic receptor. Evidence for a high-affinity nicotinic-like binding site for nicotine (9) suggests that this ligand may be a more useful tool for investigating nicotinic binding in AD. Evidence is already accumulating that the high-affinity nicotinic binding sites are reduced in AD (57). Interestingly, an endogenous factor inhibiting nicotine binding (56) in human brain may also be substantially reduced (57), raising the question of whether nicotine or a

TABLE 3. *Cortical transmitter receptor binding in Alzheimer's disease*

Receptor	Ligand	Subtype	Binding in Alzheimer's disease
Muscarinic	Quinuclidinyl benzylate (QNB) N-Methylscopolamine (NMS)		Generally normal in neocortex; moderate reductions in some limbic areas
	Pirenzepine (direct binding/QNB displacement)	M_1	Normal
	Carbachol inhibition of QNB/NMS binding	M_1 and M_2 low-affinity states	Selective loss M_2?
	Oxotremorine	M_2 high affinity	Decreased?
	cis-Dioxalane	High-affinity agonist	Normal
Nicotinic	Bungarotoxin	?	Decreased/normal
	Nicotine	?	Decreased
Serotonergic	LSD	S_1, S_2	Reduced
	Serotonin	S_1	Reduced
	Ketanserin	S_2	Reduced
Adrenergic	WB4101	α_1	Normal/increased (some areas)
	Rauwalscine	α_1	Normal
	Dihydroalprenolol	β	Normal/increased (temporal lobe)
Histamine	Pyrilamine	H_1	Normal
Dopaminergic	Spiroperidol		Normal
γ-Aminobutyric acid (GABA)	GABA		Reduced/normal
	Muscimol	A	Normal
Benzodiazepine	Diazepam/flunitrazepam		Normal
Glutamate	Glutamic acid		Normal (amygdala)/reduced
	Kainic acid		Normal
Somatostatin	Dicarba analogue/CGP, 23,996		Reduced
	Leu^8,D-Trp^{22},Tyr^{25}-Somatostatin-28		
	Tyr^{11}-Somatostatin-14		Normal
Opiate	Itorphine displacement by DAGO	μ	Normal
	Itorphine displacement by nR2266	$\kappa + \delta$	Normal
Cholecystokinin (CCK)	CCK-33		Normal
Corticotropin-releasing factor (CRF)	Tyr^0-CRF		Increased

similar agent might be worth testing in AD. Clearly, the status of the nicotinic receptor in AD merits further investigation, especially since its reduction may account for the inefficacy of certain cholinomimetic drugs tested in patients.

Serotonergic Receptors

In contrast to cholinergic and other neurotransmitter receptors, serotonergic receptor abnormalities have been consistently detected in AD (12,13,47), although the significance of these changes in terms of either clinical symptoms, pathogenesis, or possible drug effects is not yet understood. Reductions in both S_2 and to a lesser extent S_1 receptor densities are apparent (Table 3), although not in all cortical areas affected by plaques and tangles. Both receptor subtypes appear to be postsynaptic to the cortical serotonergic input: lesions of the midbrain raphe nuclei do not significantly alter the density of either in the cerebral cortex. Following lesions of the basal forebrain cholinergic neurons, the density of cortical S_2 binding sites has, in contrast, been reported to decrease (51), suggesting that a portion of S_2 receptors may exist on cholinergic terminals. The latter

observation is, however, inconsistent with the findings in human brain that in cases of Parkinson's disease in which there is a marked cholinergic deficit, S_2 binding is unaltered in the cortex (47). In AD there is no evidence for a correlation between S_2 reduction and plaques (12), although some evidence of a connection with the density of neurofibrillary tangles exists (47).

Catecholaminergic Receptors

Current evidence suggests that catecholaminergic, including α_1-, α_2-, and β-adrenergic, receptors are not affected in AD (Table 3). The normality of noradrenergic receptors in the cortex is surprising in view of the degeneration of projecting fibers from the locus coeruleus, since experimental denervation of cortical noradrenergic inputs is accompanied by changes in both α_1- and β-adrenergic receptors, which appear to be coregulated (59). The long-term pathological changes of AD are, however, likely to be distinct from those following short-term experimental lesions. One recent report (27) has indicated increased α_1- and β-adrenergic receptor binding in specific but not identical areas in AD.

Amino Acid Receptors

All except one of the reports on the GABA$_A$ receptor and its associated benzodiazepine binding site indicate normality in AD (Table 3), although the GABA$_B$ site has yet to be investigated.

The situation is less clear regarding the glutamate receptor, with one report (24), based on autoradiography, of reductions in glutamate binding in the cortex, said to reflect shrinkage of the cortical dendritic arbor, not confirmed by others (37)—at least in the amygdaloid nucleus—using isolated membranes. Glutamate receptors will no doubt continue to attract interest in AD on at least two accounts: (a) it has been suggested that during long-term potentiation, often considered to be a useful model of memory formation, the binding (particularly to the A$_1$ receptor subtype) and release of glutamate are altered (30); and (b) certain glutamate receptor subtypes bind neurotoxic molecules such as kainic acid, and the possibility that endogenous neurotoxins may act similarly in the pathogenesis of degenerative disorders such as AD arises. A key factor in the future of glutamate receptor research will be the further identification and the characterization of the various receptor subtypes.

Neuropeptide Receptors

Neuropeptide receptors are generally much less well characterized than the classical transmitter receptors. With the exception of opioid binding, the high-affinity binding of other neuropeptides has not clearly been associated with synaptic receptors and may instead affect presynaptic peptide release (25). The high-affinity binding of only a few peptides has so far been examined in AD (Table 3). Somatostatin receptor abnormalities have been reported (2), although current evidence is contradictory (Table 3), possibly reflecting the use of different ligands and in particular the problems of rapid degradation of certain of these. On the other hand, very recently an increase in CRF–receptor binding has been reported to reciprocate changes in the peptide itself (19).

COMPARISONS WITH OTHER DEGENERATIVE DEMENTIAS

Biochemical investigations of brain tissue in degenerative dementias other than AD have, with the exception of Parkinson's disease, been comparatively sparse. Examination of the cerebral cortex, as opposed to nigral–striatal pathways, in Parkinson's disease has only been carried out quite recently (5,7,22,48) and has demonstrated, in addition to cholinergic abnormalities (including increased muscarinic receptor binding), reductions in somatostatin (including the receptor) and in dopamine, norepinephrine, and serotonin, together with alterations in adrenergic receptors (Table 4). It will be of great interest to determine which, if any, of these other cortical transmitter deficits is closely associated with the cognitive impairment, usually distinct from that seen in AD although sometimes extending to severe dementia, apparent in some Parkinsonian patients.

In almost all of the other degenerative dementias so far

TABLE 4. *Cortical transmitter status in other degenerative dementias*

Disease	Cortical transmitter abnormalities
Parkinson's disease	Reductions in choline acetyltransferase (paralleled by Meynert neuron loss) correlate with the degree of dementia. Reductions in somatostatin (and its receptor) may also correlate with dementia; other changes reported include reductions in dopamine, norepinephrine, serotonin, α_2 receptors and increases in neurotensin, α_1, and β_1 receptors
Parkinsonian dementia complex of Guam	Cholinergic deficit suggested by Meynert neuron loss
Gerstmann–Straussler syndrome	Choline acetyltransferase loss
Down's syndrome	Reductions in choline acetyltransferase and norepinephrine; increased neurotensin
Progressive supranuclear palsy	Moderate choline acetyltransferase loss (?)
Alcoholic dementia	Choline acetyltransferase may be reduced in some areas
Korsakoff's psychosis	Choline acetyltransferase loss in hippocampus; neocortical cholinergic deficit also suggested by Meynert neuron loss; noradrenergic deficit indicated by CSF metabolite reductions

investigated, irrespective of the presence of Alzheimer-type pathology (for example, plaques or tangles), cholinergic abnormalities have been detected (1,34,35,52,55,60,61) either through changes in cortical biochemical marker activities or in the Meynert nucleus neuronal population (Table 4). Whether this simply reflects the current focus of attention on the cholinergic system or whether, as an end stage in a variety of pathological processes, damage to the cholinergic system invariably leads to dementia remains to be determined. It will be intriguing to learn, in the absence of cholinergic abnormalities, which other cortical transmitters, if any, are associated with the dementias of Pick's, Creutzfeldt–Jakob, and Huntington's diseases. Moreover, the psychosis of Korsakoff, which is said to involve a more specific cognitive impairment as opposed to global dementia, needs to be examined biochemically, especially in view of evidence, albeit indirect, of a noradrenergic involvement in this disorder (32).

In terms of the specificity of cortical neurochemical abnormalities in AD, it is evident that many transmitter—especially cholinergic—deficits may be apparent in other degenerative dementias with differing etiologies and pathological manifestations. This suggests that damage, by whatever means, to at least the cortical projecting cholinergic system compromises particular aspects of cognitive function;

although it remains to be established precisely which aspects, information processing related to memory is certainly a strong candidate. The only consistent transmitter-related abnormality so far detected in AD but not in other forms of dementia (such as Parkinson's and Huntington's diseases) is the decrease in serotonergic S_2 receptor binding. In view of the relatively high concentration of this receptor type in the neocortex and of the primary involvement of the cortex by plaques and tangles, it could be suggested that the S_2 receptor is situated in a critical intrinsic neuronal population affected by the disease—perhaps by the intracellular filamentous tangle deposits. Indeed, a relationship between the extent of tangle formation and decreased S_2 binding has been noted (47).

CONCLUDING REMARKS

Although current neurochemical data clearly implicating the cholinergic and possibly other transmitter systems in the dementia of Alzheimer's and perhaps other diseases are intriguing in terms of understanding the mechanisms of memory and other cognitive functions in the human brain, the ultimate goal of alleviating the suffering imposed by AD has not yet been reached. With this goal in mind, future research must continue to pursue different lines suggested by present data. From the cholinergic viewpoint, the search continues for a cholinergic agent that may be clinically effective. In this context, it will be necessary to expand further studies on cholinergic receptor status, in particular, to investigate the clinical significance of nicotinic receptor abnormalities.

With respect to the other transmitter systems, the clinical significance and possible therapeutic avenues arising from the somatostatin and CRF neuropeptide abnormalities in AD need to be pursued, as do clues regarding the involvement of various other cortical, particularly amino acid, transmitters. In fact, all of these, including the well-documented cholinergic abnormalities, can be presumed to be changes secondary to the primary disease process. At the more fundamental level, future lines of research that now need to be pursued with urgency include the following:

1. Chemical, for example, the nature of senile plaque cores and neurofibrillary tangles.
2. Epidemiological, for example, variations in the geographic distribution of the disease.
3. Genetic, for example, identification of a possible "Alzheimer gene" in familial Alzheimer's disease or Down's syndrome.
4. Molecular neurobiological, for example, detection of new protein abnormalities via corresponding messenger RNA alterations.

In summary, specific neurotransmitter deficits such as the cholinergic may well account, at least in part, for certain clinical features of AD and as such may provide a useful basis for the short-term therapeutic relief of symptoms, but, in the longer term, treatment or indeed prevention of this devastating disease is likely to emerge from more fundamental studies (such as indicated).

ACKNOWLEDGMENTS

The financial support of the Medical Research Council and Astra and the secretarial assistance of Gill Paternoster are gratefully acknowledged.

REFERENCES

1. Arendt, T., Bigl, V., Arendt, A., and Tennstedt, A. (1983): *Acta Neuropathol.,* 61:101–108.
2. Beal, M. F., Mazurek, M. F., Tran, V. T., Chattha, G., Bird, E. D., et al. (1985): *Science,* 229:289–291.
3. Bowen, D. M., and Davison, A. N. (1986): *Br. Med. Bull.,* 42:75–80.
4. Bowen, D. M., Smith, C. B., White, P., and Davison, A. N. (1976): *Brain,* 99:459–496.
5. Candy, J. M., Perry, R. H., Perry, E. K., Irving, D., Blessed, G., et al. (1983): *J. Neurol. Sci.,* 59:277–289.
6. Candy, J. M., Perry, E. K., Perry, R. H., Court, J. A., Oakley, A. E., et al. (1987): *Prog. Brain Res. (in press).*
7. Cash, R., Ruberg, M., Raisman, R., and Agid, Y. (1984): *Brain Res.,* 322:269–275.
8. Cauldfield, M. R., Straughan, D. W., Cross, A. J., Crow, T., and Birdsall, N. J. (1982): *Lancet,* 2:1277.
9. Clarke, P. B. S., Pert, C. B., and Pert, A. (1984): *Brain Res.,* 323:390–395.
10. Cross, A. J., Crow, T. J., Perry, E. K., Perry, R. H., Blessed, G., et al. (1981): *Br. Med. J.,* 282:93–94.
11. Cross, A. J., Crow, T. J., Johnson, J. A., Joseph, M. H., Perry, E. K., et al. (1983): *J. Neurol. Sci.,* 60:383–392.
12. Cross, A. J., Crow, T. J., Ferrier, I. N., Johnson, A., Bloom, S. R., et al. (1984): *J. Neurochem.,* 43:1574–1581.
13. Cross, A. J., Crow, T. J., Ferrier, I. N., and Johnson, J. A. (1986): *Neurobiol. Aging,* 7:3–8.
14. Crow, T. J., Cross, A. J., Cooper, S. J., Deakin, J. F. W., Ferrier, I. N., et al. (1984): *Neuropharmacology,* 23(12B):1561–1569.
15. Davies, P., and Maloney, A. J. F. (1976): *Lancet,* 2:1403.
16. Davies, P., Katzman, R., and Terry, R. D. (1980): *Nature,* 288:279–280.
17. De Belleroche, J., Gardner, I. M., Hamilton, M. H., and Birdsall, N. J. M. (1985): *Brain Res.,* 340:201–209.
18. De Boni, U., and Crapper McLachlan, D. R. (1985): *J. Neurol. Sci.,* 68:105–118.
19. De Souza, E. B., Whitehouse, P. J., Kuhar, M. J., Price, D. L., and Vale, W. W. (1986): *Nature,* 319:593–595.
20. Emson, P. C., and Hunt, S. P. (1984): In: *Cerebral Cortex, Vol. 2,* edited by E. G. Jones and A. Peters, pp. 145–161. Plenum Press, New York.
21. Emson, P. C., and Lindvall, O. (1986): *Br. Med. Bull.,* 42:57–62.
22. Epelbaum, J., Ruberg, M., Moyse, E., Javoy Agid, F., Dubois, B., et al. (1983): *Brain Res.,* 278:376–379.
23. Ferrier, I. N., Cross, A. J., and Johnson, J. A. (1983): *J. Neurol. Sci.,* 62:159–170.
24. Greenamyre, J. T., Penney, J. B., Young, A. B., D'Amato, C. J., Hicks, S. P., et al. (1985): *Science,* 227:1496–1499.
25. Herschman, H. R. (1986): *Trends Neurosci.,* 9:53–57.
26. Hollander, E., Mohs, R. C., and Davis, K. L. (1986): *Neurobiol. Aging,* 7:367–386.
27. Jenni-Eiermann, S., Von Hahn, H. P., Honegger, C. G., and Ulrich, J. (1984): *Gerontology,* 30:350–358.
28. Jones, E. G., and Hendry, S. H. C. (1986): *Trends Neurosci.,* 9:71–75.
29. Krnjevic, K., and Phillis, J. W. (1963): *J. Physiol. (Lond.),* 166:328–350.
30. Lynch, G., and Baudry, M. (1984): *Science,* 224:1057–1063.
31. Mash, D. C., Flynn, D. D., and Potter, L. T. (1985): *Science,* 228:1115–1117.
32. McEntee, W. J., Mair, R. G., and Langlais, P. J. (1984): *Neurology (N.Y.),* 34:648–652.

33. Melander, T., Staines, W. A., Hokfelt, T., Rakaeus, A., Eckenstein, F., et al. (1985): *Brain Res.,* 360:130–138.
34. Nakano, I., and Hirano, A. (1983): *Ann. Neurol.,* 13:87–91.
35. Nordberg, A., Larsson, C., Perdahl, E., and Winblad, B. (1982): *Drug Alcohol Depend.,* 10:333–344.
36. Nordberg, A., Larsson, C., Adolfsson, R., Alafuzoff, I., and Winblad, B. (1983): *J. Neural. Transm.,* 56:13–19.
37. Pearce, B. R., Palmer, A. M., Bowen, D. M., Wilcock, G. K., Esiri, M. M., et al. (1984): *Neurochem. Pathol.,* 2:221–232.
38. Perry, E. K. (1984): In: *Dementia: A Clinical Approach,* edited by Y. Pearce, pp. 117–134. Blackwell Scientific, Oxford.
39. Perry, E. K. (1986): *Br. Med. Bull.,* 42:63–69.
40. Perry, E. K., and Candy, J. M. (1987): In: *Receptors and Ligands in Psychiatry and Neurology,* edited by A. K. Sen and T. Lee. Cambridge University Press, Cambridge (*in press*).
41. Perry, E. K., and Perry, R. H. (1985): *Danish Med. Bull.,* 32(Suppl. 1):27–34.
42. Perry, E. K., and Perry, R. H. (1985): *Trends Neurosci.,* 8:301–303.
43. Perry, E. K., Perry, R. H., Blessed, G., and Tomlinson, B. G. (1977): *Lancet,* 1:189.
44. Perry, E. K., Tomlinson, B. E., Blessed, G., Bergmann, K., Gibson, P. H., et al. (1978): *Br. Med. J.,* 2:1457–1459.
45. Perry, E. K., Tomlinson, B. E., Blessed, G., Perry, R. H., Cross, A. J., et al. (1981): *J. Neurol. Sci.,* 51:279–287.
46. Perry, E. K., Blessed, G., Tomlinson, B. E., Perry, R. H., Crow, T. J., et al. (1981): *Neurobiol. Aging,* 2:251–256.
47. Perry, E. K., Perry, R. H., Candy, J. M., Fairbairn, A. F., Blessed, G., et al. (1984): *Neurosci. Lett.,* 51:353–357.
48. Perry, E. K., Curtis, M., Dick, D. J., Candy, J. M., et al. (1985): *J. Neurol. Neurosurg. Psychiatry,* 48:413–421.
49. Perry, R. H. (1986): *Br. Med. Bull.,* 42:34–41.
50. Phillis, J. W., and York, D. H. (1968): *Brain Res.,* 10:297–306.
51. Quirion, R., Richard, J., and Dam, T. V. (1985): *Brain Res.,* 333:345–349.
52. Robitaille, J., Wood, P. L., Etienne, P., Lal, S., Finalyson, M. H., et al. (1982): *Prog. Neurol. Psychopharmacol. Biol. Psychiatry,* 6:529–553.
53. Rossor, M., and Iversen, L. L. (1986): *Br. Med. Bull.,* 42:70–74.
54. Rossor, M. N., Emson, P. C., Mountjoy, C. G., Roth, M., and Iversen, L. L. (1980): *Neurosci. Lett.,* 20:373–377.
55. Ruberg, M., Javoy-Agid, F., Hirsh, E., Scatton, B., Heureux, R. L., et al. (1985): *Ann. Neurol.,* 18:523–529.
56. Sershen, H., Reith, M. E. A., Hashim, A., and Lajtha, A. (1984): *J. Neurosci. Res.,* 12:563–569.
57. Smith, C., Perry, E. K., Candy, J. M., Johnson, M., and Perry, R. H. (1986): *Br. J. Pharmacol.,* 88:359.
58. Smith, C. C. T., Bowen, D. M., Sims, N. R., Neary, D., and Davison, A. N. (1983): *Brain Res.,* 264:138–141.
59. Sutin, J., and Minneman, K. P. (1985): *Neuroscience,* 14:973–980.
60. Tagliavini, F., Pilleri, G., Gemignani, F., and Lechi, A. (1983): *Acta Neuropathol.,* 61:157–162.
61. Wood, P. L., Etienne, P., Lal, S., Nair, N. P. V., Finlayson, M. H., et al. (1983): *J. Neurol. Sci.,* 62:211–217.

Psychopharmacology:
The Third Generation of Progress,
edited by Herbert Y. Meltzer.
Raven Press, New York © 1987.

CHAPTER 89

In Vivo Markers in Alzheimer's Disease and Related Dementias

Neal R. Cutler

The development of *in vivo* markers for Alzheimer's disease (AD) and other dementias is important for several reasons. First and foremost among these is the ability to arrive at definitive antemortem diagnosis in AD and to develop techniques for differential diagnosis among the dementias. With the development of new therapeutic agents for the dementias, the ability of definitive diagnostic techniques is essential to ensure that the correct treatment strategy is not missed. Finally, valid and reliable inclusion and exclusion criteria for the various dementias will not only facilitate treatment but greatly enhance research efforts in an area that has been fraught with diagnostic ambiguity.

Dementias can be divided into three classifications: degenerative, vascular (or multiinfarct dementia), and other types. Degenerative dementias include Alzheimer's disease, Huntington's disease (HD), and Parkinson's disease (PD). The degenerative types of dementias are characterized by a slow, irreversible, progressive decline in mentation and personality and are usually identified after all possible etiologies for the other dementias have been excluded (22,31). Neuropathologically, there is gross atrophy of the brain, particularly of the temporal–parietal lobes, with the characteristic neurofibrillary tangles and senile plaques (22). Among the degenerative dementias, Alzheimer's disease has by far the highest incidence and has been reported to account for up to 50 to 60% of all dementias based on neuropathologic studies (22). A familial hereditary pattern has been determined for Alzheimer's disease (60).

Huntington's disease, a dementia with associated cho-

reiform movements, has an autosomal dominant hereditary pattern. The onset of HD is usually between the ages of 25 and 50. Initial clinical symptoms of choreiform movements are followed by an incipient dementia. Psychiatric symptoms, such as depression and anxiety, are also present. Neuropathologically, there is marked atrophy of the frontal lobes, caudate nuclei, and putamen. Huntington's disease represents a very small percentage of all the dementias.

Dementia associated with Parkinson's disease also accounts for a small percentage of the dementias, occurring in about 20 to 30% of PD patients. The dementia of PD usually has neuropathologic changes of the Alzheimer type. Visuospatial deficits and impairment in memory and cognition are characteristic.

Dementia of Down's syndrome (DS) also falls into the classification of degenerative dementias. Down's syndrome is a genetic disorder in which the presence of an extra portion of chromosome 21 manifests in short stature, mental retardation, premature aging, and, in 20 to 30% of cases, dementia (28,111,112). Almost all of the individuals with DS develop the neuropathologic changes of AD.

The vascular dementias, i.e., multiinfarct dementia (MID), are secondary to small vascular infarcts in the brain, which lead to gray matter loss and subsequently to dementia (55). Multiinfarct dementia accounts for approximately 17% of all the dementias (22). The dementia usually begins in the sixth or seventh decade, with gradual personality changes associated with memory and cognitive impairment. There is an abrupt step-like progression. The neuropathologic changes show local or generalized atrophy with areas of infarcted brain tissue.

Other types of dementias, such as Creutzfeldt–Jakob disease (CJD), are of the slow virus etiology. These account for a very small proportion (≈1–2%) of all dementias. Creutzfeldt–Jakob disease has a very rapid course, with dementia usually accompanied by ataxia, extrapyramidal rigidity, and myoclonus. It usually begins in the fourth or fifth decade. Approximately 10% of all CJD cases have a familial predisposition. The course is usually 8 months to 2 years. Neuropathologically, there is a widespread status spongiosus (18) throughout the brain and generalized brain atrophy (79).

CURRENT DIAGNOSTIC MEASURES

The diagnostic methodologies currently in use to assess patients with symptoms of dementia include clinical course and neurologic examination, electroencephalogram, and computerized tomographic (CT) scanning. In the majority of the degenerative dementias, diagnosis has been arrived at by exclusion of other etiologies (e.g., tumors, infections, anemias) and by clinical course and family history (31). In assessing multiinfarct dementia, the Hachinski scale (55) has been used; scores greater than 6 on this scale usually suggest the presence of MID. In addition, CT scan has been helpful in identifying multiple infarcts throughout the brain and, when combined with a Hachinski scale score greater than 6, strongly suggests MID (55,95).

Creutzfeldt–Jakob disease is diagnosed primarily by clinical course; EEG patterns provide diagnostic clues or confirmatory evidence in some cases.

Down's syndrome is unique in that it is caused by a chromosomal abnormality and invariably associated with mental retardation. The diagnosis of dementia is usually arrived at by a clinical course similar to that of AD, with behavioral problems and a progressive deterioration in general functioning (97,108,111,112).

Recently, there have been increasing research efforts to determine biologic markers for the various dementias, with a major focus on Alzheimer's disease. In these studies, comparisons of neurotransmitters, neuropeptides, amino acids, and other enzymes have been made between patients with Alzheimer's and other dementias and various controls or reference values. These studies will be reviewed in the categories of CSF and peripheral measures.

CEREBROSPINAL FLUID MEASURES

Neurotransmitters, neuropeptides, amino acids, and other potential biologic markers have been analyzed in the cerebrospinal fluid (CSF) of patients with AD. The results of these studies are summarized in Table 1 and discussed in the following sections.

Neurotransmitter Systems

Noradrenergic

Investigations of the noradrenergic system in dementia have produced mixed findings. Increased CSF levels of norepinephrine (NE) were reported by Raskind et al. (93), although Kay et al. (A. D. Kay, S. I. Rapoport, and N. R. Cutler, *unpublished data*) failed to find any differences in NE levels between AD patients and healthy controls. Differences in subject selection and procedures may explain this disparity: Raskind et al. (93) studied severely demented and agitated AD patients, whereas Kay et al. selected mildly to moderately demented AD patients who were not agitated. In addition, subjects in the Kay et al. study were at complete bedrest during the assessment and the night before, whereas patients studied by Raskind et al. (93) received only several hours of bedrest prior to lumbar puncture.

3-Methoxy-4-hydroxyphenylglycol (MHPG), a major metabolite of NE, was found in two studies to be increased in AD patients (48,93). However, four other studies reported no difference between AD patients and controls in CSF MHPG levels (A. D. Kay, S. I. Rapoport, and N. R. Cutler, *unpublished data;* 76,89,112). Dopamine-β-hydroxylase (DBH), an enzyme involved in the conversion of dopamine to NE, has been found to be decreased in two studies (83,84).

Overall, the usefulness of the noradrenergic system as a marker for AD remains to be determined in view of these inconclusive and conflicting findings.

Serotonergic

The serotonin metabolite 5-hydroxyindoleacetic acid (5-HIAA) has been found to be decreased (50,89,103), increased (106), and unchanged (7,71,113) in AD patients. Again, the only definite conclusion that can be reached is that careful selection of subjects, particularly in the patient population, is necessary to achieve reliability of results of CSF neurotransmitter studies.

Dopaminergic

The major metabolite of dopamine, homovanillic acid (HVA), has been found to be decreased in four studies of AD patients (7,50,89,103); five studies report no change in HVA (12,71,76,113,116). Methodologic limitations that may have contributed to disparities in the findings of these studies involve the inclusion of patients on medication and of agitated patients (93). Until these concerns have been addressed in carefully designed studies, the involvement of the dopaminergic system in AD will remain unclear.

Cholinergic

Enzymes and precursors that have been studied include acetylcholinesterase, butylcholinesterase, choline acetyltransferase (CAT), and choline. Several studies have found decrements in acetylcholinesterase activity in AD (4,6,103), whereas others have found no changes (4,37,104,113). It is thus not possible to determine whether acetylcholinesterase may be a specific marker for AD. Since the cholinergic system is one of the major neurotransmitter systems in AD (110), one would expect a decreased level of CAT to be found in the CSF. However, CAT activity is difficult to

TABLE 1. *Cerebrospinal fluid measures in Alzheimer's disease*

Measures	Study results		
	Increase	No change	Decrease
Noradrenergic			
Norepinephrine	Raskind et al. (93)	Kay, Rapoport, and Cutler (*unpublished data*)	
3-Methoxy-4-hydroxyphenylglycol	Gibson et al. (48)	Kay, Rapoport, and Cutler (*unpublished data*)	
	Raskind et al. (93)[a]	Mann et al. (76)	
		Palmer et al. (89)	
		Wood et al. (112)	
Dopamine-β-hydroxylase			
Serotonergic			Miyata et al. (83)
5-Hydroxyindoleacetic acid	Volicer et al. (109)[b]	Bareggi et al. (7)	Gottfries et al. (50)
		Kay et al. (70)	Palmer et al. (89)
		Wood et al. (113)	Soininen et al. (103)
Dopaminergic			
Homovanillic acid		Bowen et al. (13)	Bareggi et al. (7)
		Kay et al. (70)	Gottfries et al. (50)
		Mann et al. (76)	Palmer et al. (89)
		Wood et al. (113)	Soininen et al. (103)
		Zimmer et al. (116)	
Cholinergic			
Acetylcholinesterase		Appleyard et al. (4)	Appleyard et al. (4)
		Deutsch et al. (37)	Arendt et al. (6)
		Soininen et al. (104)	Soininen et al. (103)
		Wood et al. (113)	
Butylcholinesterase		Johnson and Domino (66)	
Choline acetyltransferase		Johnson and Domino (66)	
Choline		Growdon and Logue (51)	Yates et al. (114)
Neuropeptides			
Corticotropin-releasing factor		Nemeroff et al. (85)	May et al. (81)
			Soininen et al. (103)
Somatostatin		Thal et al. (107)	Beal et al. (8)
			Oram et al. (88)
			Serby et al. (99)
			Soininen et al. (104)
			Wood et al. (113)
Thyrotropin-releasing hormone			Oram et al. (88)
Gonadotropin-releasing hormone			Oram et al. (88)
Amino acids			
γ-Aminobutyric acid			Bareggi et al. (7)
			Enna et al. (38)
			Zimmer et al. (115)
Others			
Biopterin			Kay et al. (70)
Aluminum		Shore and Wyatt (100)	
IgA, IgD, IgE, IgG, IgM		Jonker et al. (67)	
Neuron-specific enolase	Royds et al. (96)		Cutler et al. (29)

[a] Probenecid study.
[b] Compared to Parkinson's disease patients.

assay; in the one study reviewed, no change in CAT was found (66). Butylcholinesterase has shown no change in one study (66). A clinical trial and others using cholinergic enhancing agents have not shown consistently positive results (92). Further careful studies of the enzyme CAT in CSF of patients with AD would be worthwhile.

Neuropeptide Systems

Neuropeptides that have been examined in the CSF of AD patients include corticotropin-releasing factor (CRF), somatostatin, thyrotropin-releasing hormone (TRH), and gonadotropin-releasing hormone (GRH).

Corticotropin-Releasing Factor

Two studies with carefully selected control subjects have found decreased CSF CRF levels in patients with AD dementia (81,103). Decrements in CRF levels have also been reported in postmortem brain tissue from AD patients (11). A study by Nemeroff et al. (85) found no change in AD patients compared to controls. However, this study

(85) did not use healthy controls, and the dementia population included both MID and AD patients.

Somatostatin

Somatostatin has been found to be reduced in all CSF studies (8,88,99,104,113) except one (107), which reported no change. Autopsy studies examining both somatostatin concentrations and receptor density indicate that somatostatin is deficient in AD. Recently, Beal et al. (8) found a deficiency in AD patients compared to healthy controls; however, they also found decrements in MID patients. This finding suggests that somatostatin deficiency may be secondary to brain damage per se rather than to a neurodegenerative process. Further studies are needed to compare findings in AD, MID, and in healthy controls.

Other Neuropeptides

Both thyrotropin- (88) and gonadotropin-releasing (94) hormones have been found to be decreased in AD.

Summary

The assessment of CSF concentrations of CRF and somatostatin should be pursued further. Further studies are also necessary of thyrotropin- and gonadotropin-releasing hormones in carefully selected populations of AD patients and controls.

Amino Acids

γ-Aminobutyric Acid

Three studies have reported decreased γ-aminobutyric acid (GABA) (7,38,115) in AD patients. However, GABA is very difficult to assay, and the possibility exists that the collection and assay methods used may have produced spuriously low levels. Further research in this area appears merited.

Other CSF Studies

Biopterin

Biopterin is a cofactor in the conversion of phenylalanine, tyrosine, and tryptophan hydroxylation steps leading to the production of the three neurotransmitters dopamine, NE, and serotonin (69). The CSF biopterin was found to be reduced in patients with AD and with DS (70). This finding may provide a clue as to why there have been reported similar alterations in the neurotransmitter systems in Alzheimer's disease and Down's syndrome; replication studies are called for.

Neuron-Specific Enolase

Another potential marker for Alzheimer-type dementia is neuron-specific enolase (NSE), a glycolytic enzyme that is found specifically in the neuron and has been shown to be a marker for neuronal death or neuronal production (77). Our group recently reported a deficiency in CSF NSE in 30 well-selected AD patients compared to healthy controls (29). These results may suggest a measure of neuronal degeneration in AD. Further studies are needed to support these initial findings.

Summary of CSF Studies

Of all the CSF measures studied in AD, the most consistent finding has been the deficiency in CSF somatostatin. Studies of neurotransmitter metabolites have produced mixed results and have suffered several methodologic limitations that impair their generalizability. In several cases, there were no control subjects, or controls were not healthy. Other concerns that have not been adequately addressed include diet, circadian rhythm considerations, medication-free status, and assay methodologies, as previously described (32). Cerebrospinal fluid neurotransmitter metabolite measurements still remain an area to be investigated in order to assess central nervous system responses to specific therapeutic agents.

Cerebrospinal fluid neurotransmitter metabolites and neuropeptides have not been examined carefully in the dementias associated with PD, CJD, or Pick's disease. A recent finding by Kay et al. (30; A. D. Kay, S. Kaufman, S. Milstein, and N. R. Cutler, *unpublished data;* A. D. Kay, S. I. Rapoport, and N. R. Cutler, *unpublished data*) described significant elevations of NE, 5-HIAA, HVA, and MHPG in young nondemented adults with Down's syndrome, whereas in the demented Down's syndrome subject, one finds an age-related decrement. These decreases in CSF metabolites have been found in brain metabolism with positron emission tomography (PET) scanning (97,98).

PERIPHERAL BIOCHEMICAL MEASURES

Peripheral biochemical measures have been studied in dementia of the Alzheimer's type (Table 2). Areas of investigation include monoamine oxidase (MAO) activity, the noradrenergic and the cholinergic systems, plasma proteins, plasma cortisol, growth hormone, neuron-specific enolase (NSE), and serum aluminum.

Monoamine Oxidase Activity

Platelet monoamine oxidase activity has been found to be increased in demented patients (1,3). However, increased MAO activity is also associated with normal aging (15), so the specificity of this finding as a marker for dementia is questionable.

Noradrenergic System

The noradrenergic system has been evaluated by assessing DBH. Although decrements in plasma DBH have been reported, no difference in plasma NE was found in a study comparing AD patients with healthy controls (A. D. Kay,

TABLE 2. *Peripheral biochemical measures in Alzheimer's disease*

Measures	Study results		
	Increase	No change	Decrease
Monoamine oxidase	Adolfsson et al. (1) Alexopoulos et al. (3)	Mann et al. (76)	
Noradrenergic			
Dopamine-β-hydroxylase			Miyata et al. (83)
Cholinergic			
Erythrocyte acetylcholinesterase		Markesbury et al. (78) Smith et al. (102)	Chipperfield et al. (21)
Erythrocyte choline uptake		Yates et al. (114)	
Butylcholinesterase	Smith et al. (102)		
Proteins			
IgA	Kalter and Kelly (68)	Alafuzoff et al. (2) Jonker et al. (67) Mayer et al. (82) Pentland et al. (90) Tavolata and Argentiero (106)	
IgD		Jonker et al. (67) Kalter and Kelly (68) Pentland et al. (90) Tavolata and Argentiero (106)	
IgE		Jonker et al. (67) Pentland et al. (90)	
IgG	Henschke et al. (59)	Alafuzoff et al. (2) Jonker et al. (67) Kalter and Kelly (68) Mayer et al. (82) Pentland et al. (90) Tavolata and Argentiero (106)	
IgM	Kalter and Kelly (68)	Alafuzoff et al. (2) Henschke et al. (59) Jonker et al. (67) Mayer et al. (82)	Tavolata and Argentiero (106)
Albumin		Alafuzoff et al. (2)	Behan and Feldman (9)
Others			
Plasma cortisol	Davis et al. (35)		
Growth hormone (during sleep)		Davis et al. (35)	Davis et al. (34)
Serum aluminum		Shore and Wyatt (100)	
Enolase	Cutler et al. (29)		

S. I. Rapoport, and N. R. Cutler, *unpublished data*). Assessments of the peripheral markers specific to the noradrenergic system do not support a peripheral nervous system deficit in AD as found in the central nervous system in CSF studies and on autopsy.

Cholinergic System

Studies of cholinergic measures—erythrocyte acetylcholinesterase activity, erythrocyte choline uptake, and butylcholinesterase—have been limited in number and inconclusive in results, with one report of decrease (21) and two of no change (78,102).

Other Measures

Serum immunoglobulins have also received only limited study. Overall, there have been no significant changes in these protein levels. Plasma cortisol levels have reported to be increased (35) in AD patients. Plasma growth hormone levels initially were reported to be increased (34) but were later found to be unchanged (35). No differences were seen in serum aluminum levels between AD patients and controls in one study (100). Neuron-specific enolase (NSE) was found to be increased in serum in AD patients (29). However, one cannot account for central changes in NSE based on these increases because of potential contributions of age-related changes in renal clearance, platelets, or contribution from spinal cord and other organs (29,77,96).

Summary of Peripheral Studies

The available data on peripheral biochemical measures in AD do not appear to suggest any specific relationships to the AD process. A possible exception is platelet monoamine oxidase activity. However, since this may also be an aging effect, careful examination in controlled settings is necessary to confirm any relationship to AD. Studies of peripheral markers should also be extended to include carefully defined populations of subjects with MID, CJD, and PD. The inclusion of MID patients as a comparison group, along with healthy controls, would enhance the ability to determine whether any changes observed reflect the effects of brain damage rather than a degenerative process per se.

COMPUTERIZED TOMOGRAPHY

Historically, differences between AD patients and controls have been assessed by visual inspection, then by simple measurements using planimetric methods, and finally by quantitative volumetric methods. Visual inspection is essentially determining differences by "eyeing" for changes, whereas linear and planimetric methods involve outlining the brain structures on the CT scan and making comparisons. The quantitative volumetric approach uses the computer to outline the brain structures on the CT scan image and to quantitate the measurements (24,25). Results of studies using these methods are outlined in Table 3.

Visual inspection indicated increased atrophy compared to aged-matched controls (63). Linear, planimetric, and volumetric methods have shown clear distinctions between normal aging and the changes seen in AD (25). Several studies using linear methods found increased ventricular and sulcal size (16,17,36,65). Linear, planimetric, and quantitative volumetric approaches have consistently found either increases in ventricular size or increases in ventricular brain ratios in AD patients compared to controls. One interesting finding in several studies is a consistent increase in third ventricular size in patients with mild, moderate, and severe AD (16,25,36). The statistically significant enlargement in the third ventricle may be helpful in identifying a mild form of AD and is in keeping with the suggestion

that the nucleus basalis plays a role in AD (23). Of interest also is the fact that the Creasey et al. (25) study, which included the Mattis Dementia Scale (80), showed a correlation between performance IQ score and third ventricular size, as was also seen in a study by DeLeon et al. (36). The nucleus basalis lies anterior to the third ventricle beneath the lenticular nucleus and medial to the caudate nucleus and putamen (23). Atrophy of and damage to the nucleus basalis may precede the widespread cortical atrophy and ventricular dilatation that are seen in severely demented AD patients.

There are several studies in severe AD (16,17,36,46) showing enlargement in ventricles, increased CSF volumes, and brain atrophy. Atrophy is primarily a result of loss of cortical gray matter with no change in the volume of white matter (16,17,25,46); this finding may be consistent with involvement of the association cortex in AD and with the preservation of primary sensorimotor cortex. Atrophy may also be related to the early cognitive decline in AD, whereas enlargement of the lateral ventricles appears to be related to the later cortical gray matter loss. Findings from the CT scan studies (16,17,25) are consistent with those of Hubbard and Anderson (62), who showed reduced cerebral cortical volume in AD patients under 80 years of age compared to age-matched controls. This difference was not seen in patients older than 80, whose cortical atrophy appeared to be predominantly age determined.

Only a few studies have examined MID patients using linear, planimetric, or volumetric methods. Data on this population could help to delineate differences in Alzheimer's dementia as compared to normal aging and thereby enhance the specificity of these findings. In the two MID studies reviewed, the subcortical structures, such as the lenticular and caudate nuclei and the putamen, revealed no changes from controls (33,105). It appears from CT scan studies that these structures are also not affected in AD.

TABLE 3. *Computerized tomography in Alzheimer's disease*

Investigator	Methods	Findings
Huckman et al. (63)	Visual	Increased atrophy
Jacoby and Levy (65)	Ranking, rating	Increased ventricular and sulcal size
	Linear and planimetric	Increased ventricular and sulcal size
DeLeon et al. (36)	Linear	Increased ventricular size
	Ranking	Increased third ventricle
Brinkman et al. (16)	Linear and planimetric	Increased third ventricle
		Increased ventricular brain ratio
Soininen et al. (105)	Linear	Increased ventricular and sulcal size[a]
Gado et al. (46)	Volumetric	Increased ventricular and sulcal size[b]
	Linear	No change in ventricular size
George et al. (47)	Volumetric	No change in ventricular or sulcal size
Arai et al. (5)	Volumetric	No change in ventricular or sulcal size
Dimasio et al. (33)	Linear	Increased ventricular size
Brinkman et al. (17)	Linear and planimetric	Increased ventricular brain ratio
Creasey et al. (24)	Volumetric	Increased ventricular and sulcal size
		Increased third ventricle

[a] Study included MID patients who showed less ventricular size than AD patients with more focal changes.
[b] No overlap between severe AD patients and controls.

Computerized tomographic techniques can provide quantitative estimates of the brain and its compartments in the dementia patient population. This approach permits both longitudinal and cross-sectional studies with well-defined variables. Because there is some degree of atrophy in normal aging, volumetric or quantitative methods are necessary in studies of healthy controls and AD patients.

Summary of Computerized Tomographic Studies

Volumetric CT scanning appears to be an *in vivo* marker for AD. An inherent limitation to this methodology is the need for postmortem confirmation, and we await these findings in several of the studies reviewed here. Comparison of AD to other types of dementia such as MID is also necessary.

CEREBRAL BLOOD FLOW AND POSITRON EMISSION TOMOGRAPHY

Brain-imaging methodologies such as cerebral blood flow (CBF) and positron emission tomography (PET) with various tracers such as ^{18}F-fluoro-2-deoxyglucose (^{18}FDG) and oxygen-15 (^{15}O) have been used to examine Alzheimer's disease, Huntington's disease, multiinfarct dementia,

Creutzfeldt–Jakob disease, and dementia associated with Down's syndrome.

Cerebral Blood Flow

Reduced CBF in dementia was reported as early as 1951, and subsequent studies have found consistent CBF reductions in various brain regions (Table 4). Hagberg and Ingvar (56) first attempted to relate CBF dynamics to functional aspects of the cortex and were able to demonstrate relationships between regional patterns and various cognitive abilities in AD patients. Gustafson et al. (54) showed that the cortically mediated areas were more involved in AD patients than normals and were able to confirm this finding on autopsy in several patients.

Positron Emission Tomography

With the advent of PET scanning (Table 5), Frackowiak et al. (42) examined patients with mild, moderate, and severe AD and found that the greatest reduction in early stages of the disease was in the parietal lobe, followed by the temporal, frontal, and occipital lobes. In the most severely affected patients, greatest reductions were in the frontal lobe, followed by the parietal, temporal, and occipital lobes. Farkas et al. (39) reported that in patients with AD

TABLE 4. Cerebral blood flow studies

	Subjects			
Investigator	N	Mean age (years)	Severity	Brain regions showing reduced flow[a]
Alzheimer's disease				
Freyhan et al. (43)	4	76	Descriptive	Cerebral
Lassen et al. (73)	2(?)	54	Moderate	Cerebral
Lassen et al. (74)	9	74.2	Varying	Cerebral
Hedlund et al. (58)	9	—[b]	—[b]	Frontal, temporal
Bower et al. (14)	7	—	Moderate	No reduction observed
O'Brien and Mallett (86)	6	59	—	No reduction observed
Obrist et al. (87)	10	78	Graded	Senile: temporal Presenile: temporal, parietal, occipital
Ingvar and Gustafson (64)	14	60	—	Temporal, occipital, parietal, frontal
Simard et al. (101)	14	—	Moderate–severe	Hemisphere, frontal, temporal
Gustafson and Risberg (53)	25	54 52	—	Temporal, occipital
Perez et al. (91)	10	65 63	—	Frontal, temporal, parietal
Hagberg and Ingvar (56)	57	59 56	Graded	Temporal, occipital, parietal
Grubb et al. (52)	12	33	—	Cerebral
Lavy et al. (75)	20	62	—	Hemispheric
Gustafson et al. (54)	22	66	—	Parietal, frontal
Butler et al. (19)	12	65	—	Hemispheric
Parkinson's disease				
Globus et al. (49)	14	—	—	Hemispheric

[a] All studies used ^{133}Xe except Freyhan et al. (43), Lassen et al. (75) (^{85}Kr), and Hedlund et al. (58) (^{32}P).
[b] Not mentioned.

TABLE 5. *Positron emission tomography*

	Subjects			
Investigator	N	Mean age (years)	Severity	Brain regions showing reduced metabolism
Alzheimer's disease				
Frackowiak et al. (42)[a]	13	65	Mild	Parietal > temporal > frontal > occipital
			Severe	Frontal > parietal > temporal > occipital
Farkas et al. (39)	11	73	Varying	Frontal > temporal > subcortical
Ferris et al. (40)	24	73	Varying	Temporal > frontal > parietal
Foster et al. (41)	13	59	Varying	Temporal > parietal (asymmetric focal reductions)
Friedland et al. (45)	10	65	Varying	Temporal > parietal (ratios)
Cutler et al. (25,26)	7	66	Mild–moderate	Parietal
Chase et al. (20)	17	61	Severe	Frontal, temporal, parietal
Foster et al. (41)	20	60	Mild	Parietal > temporal > occipital > frontal
			Severe	Parietal > occipital > temporal > frontal
Cutler et al. (27)	1	57	Mild	Parietal
Holman et al. (61)[b]	1	56		Posterior temporoparietal
Huntington's disease				
Kuhl et al. (72)	13	42	Varying	Caudate, putamen
	15	34	At risk	Caudate[e]
Multiinfarct dementia				
Benson et al. (10)	3	—	—	Focal and asymmetric
Creutzfeldt–Jakob disease				
Friedland et al. (44)	1[c]	54	—	Temporal lobe; hemispheric asymmetries
Down's syndrome				
Schapiro et al. (97)	2[d]	35	Severe	Parietal > temporal, frontal

[a] ^{18}F-fluoro-2-deoxyglucose (^{18}FDG) tracer except Frackowiak et al. (^{15}O).
[b] ^{123}I-3-Quinuclidinyl-4-iodobenzylate and single photon emission computerized tomography.
[c] Autopsy proven.
[d] Demented by clinical and diagnostic criteria.
[e] Six of 15 subjects.

of varying severity, the greatest metabolic reductions were in the frontal lobe, followed by the temporal and subcortical structures.

In a well-selected group of patients with moderate dementia, Foster et al. (41) and Friedland et al. (45) found temporal and parietal asymmetric reductions. Our group examined patients with mild to moderate AD and found reductions primarily in the parietal lobe (25,26) (Fig. 1). We recently examined one patient over approximately 2.5 years using serial PET scans and found that the parietal lobe was the initial area of brain reduction (27,28). Thus, overall, studies using PET scanning appear to implicate the parietal lobe as the area of brain that is most affected, or at least shows the greatest metabolic reductions, in AD (Fig. 2).

Of course, other types of dementia need to be examined to determine the specificity of this metabolic pattern. In Huntington's disease, Mazziotta et al. (72) found reduced metabolism in the caudate and putamen in symptomatic patients; 18 of 58 "at-risk" HD subjects showed caudate hypometabolism. In the one study of multiinfarct dementia using PET scanning, Benson et al. (10) found focal and asymmetric metabolic reductions. One case of Creutzfeldt–Jakob disease was examined by Friedland et al. (44), who found reductions in temporal lobe and hemispheric asymmetries. Of recent interest are studies of patients with DS by Schapiro et al. (28,97) and Schwartz et al. (98). They found age-related reductions in metabolism in nondemented DS subjects, with greater reductions in demented DS subjects than in young Down's syndrome nondemented

FIG. 1. Positron emission tomographic scans at 80 and 65 mm above the inferior orbitomeatal line (IOM) for a 65-year-old patient with a mild form of Alzheimer's disease (AD), a 49-year-old patient with a moderate form of AD, and a 73-year-old patient with a severe form of AD. rCMRglc, regional cerebral metabolic rates for glucose.

FIG. 2. A 57-year-old man with a familial form of Alzheimer's disease (AD) was evaluated at five separate evaluations with

positron emission tomographic (PET) scan at 80 mm above the inferior orbitomeatal (IOM) line. A normal 58-year-old control subject and the AD patient (**A**) in February, 1982 (**B**); October, 1982 (**C**); June, 1983 (**D**); October, 1983 (**E**); and October, 1984 (**F**). Metabolic rates for glucose (rCMRglc, in mg per 100 g per minute), decreased gradually in the parietal lobe regions, as shown by the gray areas, from metabolic rates observed in February, 1982 (**B**).

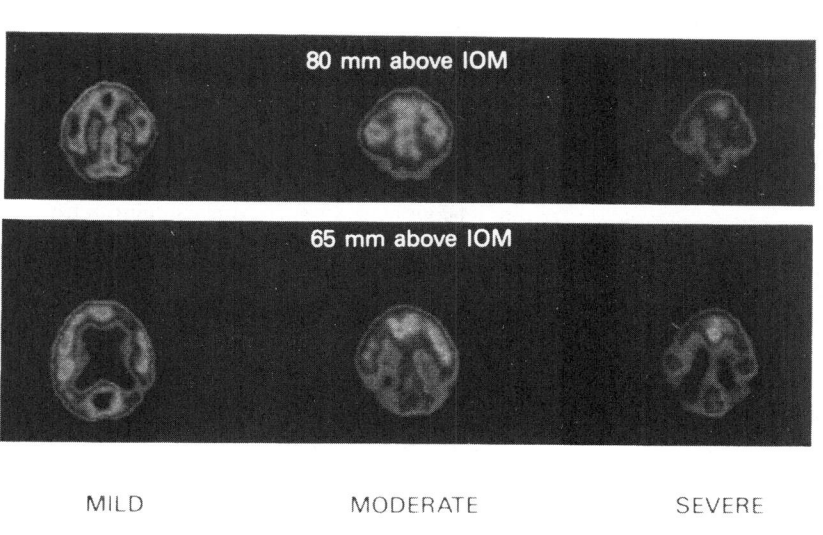

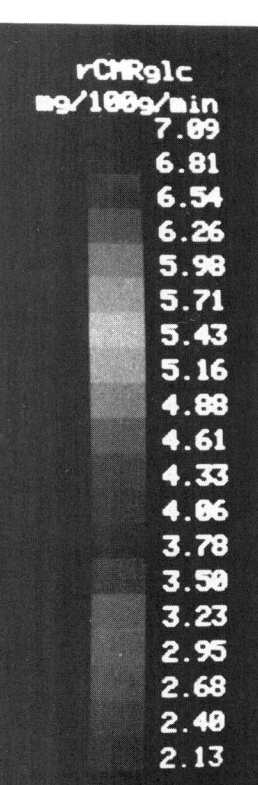

FIG. 1.

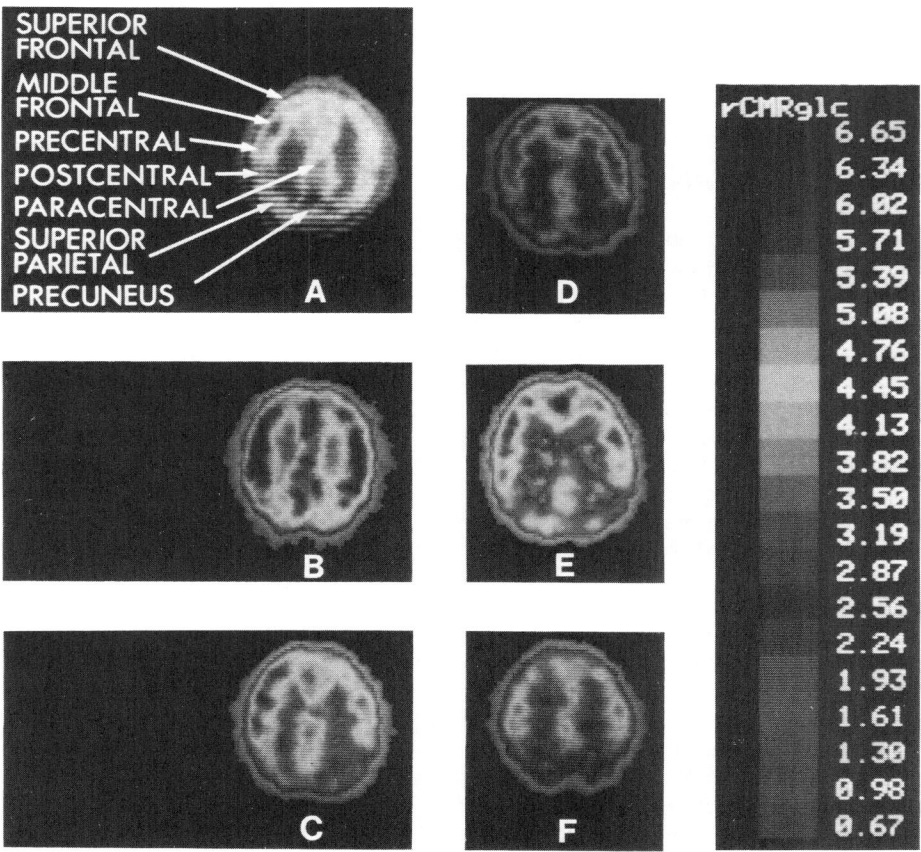

FIG. 2.

subjects (98). Further studies are needed in patients with Huntington's disease, multiinfarct dementia, Creutzfeldt–Jakob disease, and Down's syndrome to elucidate underlying mechanisms involved in these disease processes and to determine the specificity of PET methodology for the various dementias. Particularly in Huntington's disease, PET may provide a tool to determine whether striatal hypometabolism is common in asymptomatic carriers of the HD autosomal dominant gene and whether reduced metabolism is correlated with the probability that HD will develop.

Using a specific radiotracer of the cholinergic system (^{123}I-3-quinuclidinyl-4-iodobenzylate) with single photon emission computerized tomography, Holman et al. (61) found reductions in the posterior tempoparietal regions in one AD patient. Again, more studies are needed using various tracers of neurotransmitter systems to map affected brain regions and to develop identifiable "fingerprint" patterns for the various dementias.

PHARMACOLOGIC CHALLENGE

Another area that may provide useful *in vivo* markers for AD and the other dementias is the pharmacologic challenge profile. How do AD patients respond to specific pharmacologic probes as compared to patients with other dementias? Do AD patients respond differently from those with MID or CJD to arecoline (a cholinergic agonist), apomorphine (a dopaminergic agonist), or clonidine (a noradrenergic agonist)? If there are significant differences in response, could this provide a tool for differential diagnosis? Unfortunately, research in this area is almost nonexistent.

SUMMARY AND CONCLUSIONS

This review of the available data on *in vivo* markers indicates that CSF measures that may have potential utility in the differential diagnosis of dementia include reductions in levels of somatostatin and CRF. In addition, quantitative CT scanning, using volumetric methods, demonstrates third ventricular dilatation in mild, moderate, and severe Alzheimer's disease, a finding that will help discriminate between AD and the effects of normal aging. Positron emission tomography scanning may be able to assess metabolic reductions, particularly of the parietal lobe, which appears to be the cortical area of the brain that shows the earliest reductions in AD. These metabolic reductions may prove to be early markers in AD patients.

Finally, an area that has received virtually no research attention is the use of pharmacologic challenge profiles in the various dementias. Such research could be useful in developing diagnostic profiles.

The studies reviewed here present several methodologic concerns. Careful selection of control subjects, with appropriate age and health criteria, is crucial. For subjects with dementia, diagnostic criteria, age of onset, duration of illness, health status, and severity must be reported to permit assessment of the validity of results and their specificity to various types and stages of dementia and to

facilitate replication studies of potential *in vivo* markers. Autopsy confirmation is also essential to determine the specificity of the dementia and, therefore, the proposed markers. There is a need to examine carefully dementias other than the Alzheimer's type and to follow these dementias longitudinally in order to characterize their course with the *in vivo* markers.

Preliminary data from studies using radiotracers that indicate decreased uptake in the temporal–parietal lobe (such as the study with the cholinergic tracer ^{123}I-3-quinuclidinyl-4-iodobenzylate in one patient with AD) may suggest further studies to develop this tracer as a potential marker for AD.

REFERENCES

1. Adolfsson, R., Goffries, C. G., Oreland, L., Wiberg, A., and Winblad, B. (1980): *Life Sci.,* 27:1029–1034.
2. Alafuzoff, I., Adolfsson, R., Bucht, G., and Winblad, B. (1983): *J. Neurol.,* 60:465–472.
3. Alexopoulos, G. S., Lieberman, K. W., and Young, R. C. (1984): *Am. J. Psychiatry,* 141:97–99.
4. Appleyard, M. E., Smith, A. D., Wilcock, G. K., and Esiri, M. M. (1983): *Lancet,* 2:452.
5. Arai, H., Kobayashi, K., Ikeda, K., Nagao, Y., Dgihara, R., et al. (1983): *J. Neurol.,* 229:69–77.
6. Arendt, T., Bigl, V., Walther, F., and Sonntag, M. (1984): *Lancet,* 1:173.
7. Bareggi, S. R., Franceschi, M., Bonni, L., Zecca, L., and Smirne, S. (1982): *Arch. Neurol.,* 39:709.
8. Beal, M. D., Growdon, J. H., Majurek, M. D., and Martin, J. B. (1986): *Neurology (N.Y.),* 36:294–297.
9. Behan, P. O., and Feldman, R. G. (1970): *J. Am. Geriatr. Soc.,* 18:792–797.
10. Benson, D. F., Kuhl, D. E., Hawkins, R. A., Phelps, M. E., Cummings, J. L., et al. (1983): *Arch. Neurol.,* 40:711–713.
11. Bissette, G., Reynolds, G. P., Kilts, C. D., Widerlor, E., and Nemeroff, C. B. (1985): *J.A.M.A.,* 254:3067–3069.
12. Boller, F., Mizutani, T., Ryessmann, R., et al. (1980): *Ann. Neurol.,* 7:329–335.
13. Bowen, D. M., Sims, N. R., Benton, J. S., Curzon, G., Iwangoff, P., et al. (1981): *N. Engl. J. Med.,* 305:1016.
14. Bower, H. M., Andrew, J. T., and Pope, R. A. (1970): *Med. J. Aust.,* 5:209–211.
15. Bridge, T. P., Phelps, B. H., Cutler, N. R., Jeste, D. V., and Wyatt, R. J. (1984): *J. Am. Geriatr. Soc.,* 32:259–264.
16. Brinkman, S. D., Sarwar, M., Levin, H. S., and Morris, H. H. (1981): *Radiology,* 138:89–92.
17. Brinkman, S. D., and Largen, J. W., Jr. (1984): *Am. J. Psychiatry,* 141:81–83.
18. Brown, P., Cathala, F., Sadowsky, D., and Gajdusek, D. C. (1979): *Ann. Neurol.,* 6:430–437.
19. Butler, R. W., Dickinson, W. A., Katholi, C., and Halsey, J. H., Jr. (1983): *Ann. Neurol.,* 13:155–159.
20. Chase, T. N., Foster, N. L., Fedio, P., DiChiro, G., Brioks, R., et al. (1983): In: *Aging of the Brain,* edited by D. Samuel, S. Algeri, S. Gershon, V. E. Grimm, and G. Toffano, pp. 143–154. Raven Press, New York.
21. Chipperfield, B., Newman, P. M., and Moyes, I. C. A. (1981): *Lancet,* 2:199.
22. Constantidis, J. (1978): In: *Alzheimer's Disease: Senile Dementia and Related Disorders,* edited by R. Katzman, R. D. Terry, and K. L. Bick, pp. 15–25. Raven Press, New York.
23. Coyle, J. T., Price, D. L., and DeLong, M. R. (1983): *Science,* 219:1184–1190.
24. Creasey, H., Schwartz, M., Frederickson, H., Haxby, J. V., Rapoport, S. I. (1987): *Neurology,* 36:1563–1568.
25. Cutler, N. R., Duara, R., Creasey, H., Grady, C. L., Haxby, J. V., et al. (1984): *Ann. Intern. Med.,* 101:355–369.

26. Cutler, N. R., Haxby, J., Duara, R., Grady, C. L., Kay, A. D., et al. (1985): *Ann. Neurol.,* 18:298–309.
27. Cutler, N. R., Haxby, J., Duara, R., Parisi, J. E., White, J., et al. (1985): *Neurology (N.Y.),* 35:1556–1561.
28. Cutler, N. R., Heston, L. L., Davies, P., Haxby, J. V., and Schapiro, M. B. (1985): *Ann. Intern. Med.,* 103:566–578.
29. Cutler, N. R., Kay, A. D., Marangos, P. J., and Burg, C. (1986): *Arch. Neurol.,* 43:153–154.
30. Cutler, N. R., Kay, A. D., Schapiro, M. B., and Rapoport, S. I. (1984): Presented at the AMEDO Neurology Conference. Washington, D.C.
31. Cutler, N. R., and Narang, P. K. (1985): *Geriatr. Nurs.,* 6(3): 160–163.
32. Cutler, N. R., and Hodes, J. E. (1983): *Exp. Aging Res.,* 9:123–127.
33. Damasio, H., Eslinger, P., Damasio, A. R., Rizzo, M., Huang, H. K., et al. (1983): 40:715–719.
34. Davis, B. M., Levy, M. I., Rosenberg, G. S., Mathé, A., and Davis, K. L. (1982): In: *Aging, Vol. 19, Alzheimer's Disease: A Report of Progress in Research,* edited by S. Corkin, K. L. Davis, J. H. Growdon, E. Usdin, and R. J. Wurtman, pp. 55–62. Raven Press, New York.
35. Davis, B. M., Mohs, R. C., Greenwald, B. S., Mathe, A. A., Johns, J. A., et al. (1985): *J. Am. Geriatr. Soc.,* 33:741–748.
36. DeLeon, M. J., Ferris, S. H., George, A. E., Reisberg, B., Kricheff, I. I., et al. (1980): *Neurobiol. Aging,* 1:69–79.
37. Deutsch, S. I., Mohs, R. C., Levy, M. I., Rothpearl, A. B., Stocton, D., et al. (1983): *Biol. Psychiatry,* 18:1363–1373.
38. Enna, S. J., Stern, L. Z., Wastek, G. J., and Yamamura, H. I. (1977): *Arch. Neurol.,* 34:683–685.
39. Farkas, T., Ferris, S. H., Wolf, A. P., DeLeon, M. J., Christman, D. R., et al. (1982): *Am. J. Psychiatry,* 139:352–353.
40. Ferris, S. J., DeLeon, M. J., Wolf, A. P., et al. (1983): In: *Aging of the Brain,* edited by D. Samuel, S. Algeri, S. Gershon, V. E. Grimm, and G. Toffano, pp. 133–142. Raven Press, New York.
41. Foster, N. L., Chase, T. N., Fedio, P., Patronas, N. J., Brooks, R. A., et al. (1983): *Neurology (N.Y.),* 33:961–965.
42. Frackowiak, R. S. J., Pozzilli, C., Legg, N. J., DuBoulay, G. H., Marshal, J., et al. (1981): *Brain,* 104:753–778.
43. Freyhan, F. A., Woodford, R. B., and Kety, S. S. (1951): *J. Nerv. Ment. Dis.,* 113:449–456.
44. Friedland, R. P., Budinger, T. F., Koss, E., and Ober, B. A. (1985): *Neurosci. Lett.,* 53(3):235–240.
45. Friedland, R. P., Prusiner, S. B., Jugust, W. J., Budinger, T. F., and Davis, R. L. (1984): *J. Comput. Assist. Tomogr.,* 8:978–981.
46. Gado, M., Hughes, C. P., Danziger, W., Chi, D., Jost, G., et al. (1982): *Radiology,* 144:535–538.
47. George, A. E., DeLeon, M. J., Rosenbloom, S., Ferris, S. H., Gentes, C., et al. (1983): *Radiology,* 149:493–498.
48. Gibson, C. J., Logue, M., and Growdon, J. H. (1985): *Arch. Neurol.,* 42(5):489–492.
49. Globus, M., Mildworf, B., and Melamed, E. (1985): *Neurology (N.Y.),* 35:1135–1139.
50. Gottfries, C. G., Gottfries, I., and Ross, B. E. (1969): *J. Neurochem.,* 16:1341–1345.
51. Growdon, J. H., and Logue, M. (1982): In: *Aging, Vol. 19, Alzheimer's Disease: A Report of Progress in Research,* edited by S. Corkin, K. L. Davis, J. H. Growdon, E. Usdin, and R. J. Wurtman, pp. 34–43. Raven Press, New York.
52. Grubb, R. L., Jr., Raichle, M. E., Mokhtar, H., Gado, M. B., Eichling, J. O., et al. (1977): *Neurology (Minneap.),* 27:905–910.
53. Gustafson, L., and Risberg, J. (1974): *Acta Psychiatr. Scand.,* 50: 516–538.
54. Gustafson, L., Risberg, J., and Silfverskiold, P. (1981): *Adv. Biol. Psychiatry,* 6:109–116.
55. Hachinski, V. L., Iliff, L. O., Zilkha, E., et al. (1975): *Arch. Neurol.,* 32:632–637.
56. Hagberg, B., and Ingvar, D. H. (1976): *Br. J. Psychiatry,* 128: 209–222.
57. Hakim, A. M., and Mathieson, G. (1979): *Neurology (Minneap.),* 29:1209–1214.
58. Hedlund, S., Kohler, V., Nulin, G., Olsson, R., Rengstrom, O., et al. (1964): *Acta Psychiatr. Scand.,* 40:77–106.
59. Henschke, P. J., Bell, D. A., and Cape, R. D. T. (1979): *J. Clin. Exp. Gerontol.,* 1:23–37.
60. Heston, L. L., Mastri, A. R., Anderson, V. E., and White, J. (1981): *Arch. Gen. Psychiatry,* 38:1085–1090.
61. Holman, B. L., Gibson, R. E., Hill, T. C., et al. (1985): *J.A.M.A.,* 265:3063–3066.
62. Hubbard, B. M., and Anderson, J. M. (1981): *J. Neurol. Sci.,* 50: 135–145.
63. Huckman, M. S., Fox, J., and Topel, J. (1975): *Radiology,* 116: 85–92.
64. Ingvar, D. H., and Gustafson, L. (1979): *Acta Neurol. Scand.* [*Suppl.*], 46:42–73.
65. Jacoby, R. J., and Levy, R. (1980): *Br. J. Psychiatry,* 136:256–269.
66. Johnson, S., and Domino, E. F. (1971): *Clin. Chim. Acta,* 35: 421–428.
67. Jonker, C., Eikelenboom, P., and Tavenier, P. (1982): *Br. J. Psychiatry,* 140:44–49.
68. Kalter, S., and Kelly, S. (1975): *N.Y. State J. Med.,* 75:1222–1225.
69. Kaufman, S. (1963): *Proc. Natl. Acad. Sci. U.S.A.,* 50:1085–1093.
70. Kay, A. D., Milstein, S., Kaufman, S., Haxby, J., Rapoport, S. I., et al. (1987): *Neurology (N.Y.)* (*in press*).
71. Kay, A. D., Milstein, S., Kaufman, S., Rapoport, S. I., and Cutler, N. R. (1984): *Neurology (N.Y.),* 34(Suppl. 1):161.
72. Mazziotta, J. C., Phelps, M. E., Pahl, J. J., et al. (1987): *N. Engl. J. Med.,* 316:357–362.
73. Lassen, N. A., Munck, O., and Tottery, E. R. (1957): *Arch. Neurol. Psychiatry,* 77:126–133.
74. Lassen, N. A., Feinberg, I., and Lane, M. H. (1960): *J. Clin. Invest.,* 39:491–500.
75. Lavy, S., Melamed, E., Shlomo, B., Cooper, G., and Rinot, Y. (1978): *Ann. Neurol.,* 4:445–450.
76. Mann, D. M. A., Yates, P. O., and Hawkes, J. (1981): *J. Neurol. Neurosurg. Psychiatry,* 45:113–119.
77. Goodwin, F. K., Parma, A., Lanter, C., and Trams, E. (1978): *Brain Res.,* 150:117–133.
78. Markesbury, W. R., Leung, P. K., and Butterfield, D. A. (1980): *J. Neurol. Sci.,* 45:323–330.
79. Masters, C. L., and Richardson, E. P., Jr. (1978): *Brain,* 101: 333–344.
80. Mattis, S. (1976): In: *Geriatric Psychiatry: A Handbook for Psychiatrists and Primary Care Physicians,* edited by B. L. Katasut, pp. 77–122. Grune & Stratton, New York.
81. May, C., Kay, A., Hill, B., Gold, P., Chrousos, G., Rapoport, S. I., and Cutler, N. R. (1985): *Neurology (N.Y.),* 35 (Suppl. 1):91.
82. Mayer, P. P., Chughtai, M. A., and Cape, R. D. T. (1976): *Age Ageing,* 5:164–170.
83. Miyata, S., Nagata, H., Yamao, S., Nakamura, S., and Kameyama, M. (1984): *J. Neurol. Sci.,* 63:403–409.
84. Nakamura, S., Koshimura, K., Kato, T., Yamao, S., Iijima, S., et al. (1984): *Clin. Ther.,* 7:18–34.
85. Nemeroff, C. B., Widerlöv, E., Bissette, G., Walléus, H., Karlsson, I., et al. (1984): *Science,* 226:1342–1344.
86. O'Brien, M. D., and Mallett, B. L. (1979): *J. Neurol. Neurosurg. Psychiatry,* 33:497–500.
87. Obrist, W. D., Chivan, E., Cronqrist, S., and Ingvar, D. H. (1970): *Neurology (Minneap.),* 20:315–322.
88. Oram, J. J., Edwardson, J., and Millard, P. H. (1981): *Gerontology,* 27:216–223.
89. Palmer, A. M., Sims, N. R., Bowen, D. M., Neary, D., Palo, J., et al. (1984): *J. Neurol. Neurosurg. Psychiatry,* 47:481–484.
90. Pentland, B., Christie, J. E., Watson, K. C., and Yap, P. L. (1982): *Acta Psychiatr. Scand.,* 65:375–379.
91. Perez, F. I., Mathew, N. T., and Stump, D. A. (1977): *Neurologiques,* :53–62.
92. Peters, B. M., and Levin, H. S. (1979): *Ann. Neurol.,* 6:219–221.
93. Raskind, M. A., Peskind, E. R., Halter, J. B., and Jimerson, D. C. (1984): *Arch. Gen. Psychiatry,* 41:343–346.
94. Rogers, R. L., Meyer, J. S., Mortel, K. F., Mahurin, R. K., Judd, B. W. (1986): *Neurology (N.Y.),* 36:1–6.
95. Rosen, W. G., Terry, R. D., Fuld, P. A., Katzman, R., and Peck, A. (1980): *Ann. Neurol.,* 7:486–488.

96. Royds, J. A., Davies-Jones, G. A. B., Lewtas, N. A., Timperley, W. R., and Taylor, C. B. (1983): *J. Neurol. Neurosurg. Psychiatry,* 46:1031–1036.
97. Schapiro, M. B., Duara, R., Haxby, J. V., Schwartz, M., Kessler, R., et al. (1984): *Neurology (N.Y.),* 34:122.
98. Schwartz, M., Duara, R., Haxby, J., Grady, C., White, B. J., et al. (1983): *Science,* 221:781–783.
99. Serby, M., Richardson, S. B., Twente, S., Siekierski, J., Corwin, J., et al. (1984): *Neurobiol. Aging,* 5:187–189.
100. Shore, D., and Wyatt, R. J. (1983): *J. Nerv. Ment. Dis.,* 171: 553–558.
101. Simard, D., Olesen, J., Paulson, O. B., Lassen, N. A., and Skinhj, E. (1971): *Brain,* 94:273–288.
102. Smith, R. C., Ho, B. T., Hsu, L., Vrovlis, G., Claghorn, J., et al. (1982): *Life Sci.,* 30:543–546.
103. Soininen, H. I., Jolkkonen, J. T., Reinikainen, K. J., Halonen, T. O., and Riekkinen, P. J. (1984): *J. Neurol. Sci.,* 63:167–172.
104. Soininen, H., MacDonald, E., Rekonen, M., and Riekkinen, P. J. (1981): *Acta Neurol. Scand.,* 64:101–107.
105. Soininen, H., Puranen, M., and Riekkinen, P. J. (1982): *J. Neurol. Neurosurg. Psychiatry,* 45:50–54.
106. Tavolato, B., and Argentiero, V. (1980): *J. Neurol. Sci.,* 46:325–331.

107. Thal, L. J., Rosenbaum, D. M., Horowitz, S. G., Sharpless, N. S., Waltz, J. M. et al. (1983): *Neurology (N.Y.),* 33(Suppl. 2):119.
108. Thase, M. E., Liss, L., Smeltzer, D., and Maloon, J. (1982): *J. Ment. Defic. Res.,* 26:239–244.
109. Volicer, L., Greene, L., and Sinex, F. M. (1985): *Neurobiol. Aging,* 6(1):35–38.
110. Whitehouse, P. J., Price, D. L., Clark, A. W., Coyle, J. T., and Delong, M. R. (1981): *Ann. Neurol.,* 10:122–126.
111. Wisniewski, H. M., Coblentz, D. M., and Terry, R. D. (1972): *Arch. Neurol.,* 26:97–108.
112. Wisniewski, K. E., and Wisniewski, H. M. (1983): In: *Alzheimer's Disease,* edited by B. Relsberg, pp. 319–326. The Free Press, New York.
113. Wood, P. L., Etienne, P., Lal, S., Gauthier, S., Cajal, S., et al. (1982): *Life Sci.,* 31:2073–2079.
114. Yates, C. M., Blackburn, I. A., Christie, J. E., Glen, et al. (1980): In: *Biochemistry of Dementia,* edited by P. J. Roberts, pp. 185–212. John Wiley & Sons, Chichester.
115. Wilson, R. S., Fox, J. H., Huckman, M. S., Bacon, L. D., and Lobick, J. J. (1982): *Neurology (N.Y.),* 32:1054–1057.
116. Zimmer, R., Teelken, A. W., Trieling, W. B., Weber, W., Weihmayr, T., et al. (1984): *Arch. Neurol.,* 41:602–604.

Psychopharmacology:
The Third Generation of Progress,
edited by Herbert Y. Meltzer.
Raven Press, New York © 1987.

CHAPTER 90

Diagnosis and Assessment of Cognitive Dysfunctions in the Elderly

Herbert Weingartner, Robert Cohen, Trey Sunderland,
Pierre Tariot, Karen Thompson, and Paul Newhouse

Cognitive functions are not unitary but are comprised of distinct component processes. These different processes can be identified and measured. Different facets of cognitive functions can be disrupted in various neuropathologically distinct neuropsychiatric syndromes. Drug manipulations in normal subjects model the patterns of cognitive dysfunctions that are associated with neuropsychiatric syndromes (such as the amnesias, dementias, and pseudodementias) and confirm the psychobiological distinctiveness of several cognitive domains. This knowledge base can be systematically applied to the study of the complex higher mental function changes associated with aging and the dementias. Assessment approaches are presented that provide micro- and macromultivariate approaches to clinical studies of the elderly. Some of these approaches are based on clinical psychometric methods that can readily be linked to systematic clinical observational data. Other approaches make use of laboratory methods of analysis. Regardless of the type of approach that is chosen, findings will be useful when appropriate methods of scaling are used along with a means for directly comparing levels of functioning in different cognitive and noncognitive domains.

During the past decade we have seen an impressive expansion of efforts directed at understanding cognitive aspects of the aging process, the dementias, and neuropsychiatric disorders in general. During this time period, the number of studies, investigators, and patients studied has increased dramatically. Not only have clinicians been particularly active researchers in this area, but their efforts are beginning to be linked, in a systematic fashion, to the research output of neuropathologists, neuropsychologists, psychiatrists of various theoretical persuasions, neurochemists, and neuropharmacologists as well as those neuroscientists interested in cognitive science. In evaluating our most recent efforts and in directing future research, we are paying increasing attention to the multidisciplinary milieu that is necessary for understanding the psychobiological bases of thinking, learning, memory, and their pathology. It is this context that is going to allow us to begin to understand the nature of higher mental changes in the elderly.

In this chapter we outline a variety of approaches or systems that can be usefully applied to the systematic description, evaluation, and measurement (scaling) of higher mental functions in the elderly. These approaches are seen as providing diagnostic tools. Some of these approaches would serve to provide convergent confirmation and validity for systematic global observations of clinicians assessing higher mental functions in a clinical setting. A number of methods of approach may also serve to provide novel strategies for diagnosing, classifying, and evaluating cognitive treatments in the clinic. The methods and models of cognitive functioning presented here should also serve as behavioral–cognitive indices that can be systematically related to biological–neuropharmacological data, an increasingly important aspect of research in gerontology.

The structure of the chapter is as follows. We begin with a brief review of the merits of systematic evaluation of cognitive functions in the elderly and in neuropsychiatric disorders in general. In considering the usefulness of cognitive evaluations in characterizing changes in mental functions, we also consider the value of such "clinical" data for the development of viable models of how various brain systems may be involved in mediating and modulating the registration, retention, retrieval, and manipulation of information or experience. We stress the value of a continuous interplay between basic research efforts in cognitive science and systematic clinical–applied cognitive research. A variety of approaches to the study of changes in mental functioning in the elderly are then outlined. We stress that whatever cognitive methods of approach are used, such efforts must include an evaluation of the interaction between cognitive and noncognitive behaviors (such as mood or arousal). No single cognitive approach is the right approach. Potentially, many methods may be available from cognitive neuroscience, but whatever approach is chosen, it should fit clinical research needs. In some instances, a macroanalysis of higher mental functions is appropriate. In other situations, detailed analysis of highly specific types of cognitive processes is most useful (a microanalysis of cognitive functions). Many methods and strategies of approach are listed along with appropriate reference material that would provide detailed descriptions and supporting clinical research findings.

The review of methods of approach to the study of mental processes in the elderly moves from a macro- to microanalysis. Methods that would provide detailed descriptions of specific cognitive processes are based on evidence that shows how such processes can be altered selectively under different brain-state conditions. Some of these processes are described, and the types of clinical, neuropharmacological, and cognitive evidence for demonstrating the psychological distinctiveness of these domains is also presented. The cited references for each cognitive domain also contain some of the methods of evaluation that should be useful to both clinician and researcher. A similar type of analysis is provided for cognitive-like behavior in lower animals. This type of fine-grained analysis of human and lower animal cognitive processes invites comparisons and profiling of levels of functioning in different domains, an approach with important diagnostic implications. We conclude with a discussion of some of the problems that remain to be addressed and a prospectus of how future efforts can be applied most effectively to the complex problems of gerontology.

WHY EVALUATE HIGHER MENTAL FUNCTIONS IN THE ELDERLY?

Diagnosis

The clinician is confronted frequently with real or artifactual changes in higher mental functions in the elderly. Accurate characterization and interpretation of cognitive symptoms are the basis on which appropriate diagnosis can be made, which in turn defines etiology and appropriate management and intervention.

Many factors can account for the subjectively experienced and reported or clinically observed changes in mental functioning. Clinical, psychometric, and laboratory methods are available for characterizing such cognitive changes, but these methods are only now beginning to prove helpful in distinguishing the cognitive changes associated with early stages of a dementing process such as Alzheimer's disease, depression, drug effects (e.g., ethanol, benzodiazepines, or hypnotics used to induce sleep), and environmental factors (e.g., stress related to economic–socioenvironmental determinants). What makes the diagnostic problem even more complex is that any of the broad classes of determinants may have been expressed as very different types of cognitive impairments depending on individual differences in factors such as culture, intelligence, previous psychiatric histories, and concurrent familial circumstances. These types of variables must begin to be understood in terms of how they may interact with aspects of disease in altering cognition. The methods for evaluating higher mental functions can also be of greater diagnostic value if we begin to capitalize on what has been learned about the psychobiological specificity of some types of cognitive processes. This knowledge must be translated into the development of new clinical methods, which can then be applied to the diagnosis of cognitive dysfunction. Similarly, these diagnostic methods can be an important tool in characterizing changes in patients over time. It is often this ability to assess accurately the changes in mental functions over time that is the basis for accurate classification of disorders that are reflected as cognitive symptoms.

Treatment and Intervention

During the last decade we have seen the introduction of an increasing number of drug strategies for altering higher mental functions in the elderly and in cognitively impaired neuropsychiatric disorders. Several types or classes of drugs have been and continue to be tested, including antidepressants, several types of stimulants, a number of neuropeptides, cholinergic drugs, drugs that alter catecholamine activity, and nootropics (drugs whose very name implies cognitive properties). In general, the evaluation of whether any of these drugs facilitates cognitive processes in the cognitively impaired elderly has left us with no clear answers. Often findings are so ambiguous as to provide little hard data about the effectiveness or lack of cognitive responsivity of subjects to such treatments.

There are several reasons for this state of uncertainty in many current studies of drug trials that involve the evaluation of the cognitive response to such treatments. Populations studied have often been far too diagnostically or subject-characteristic heterogeneous rather than homogeneous. Cognitive measures have often been chosen almost at random as if cognition were one homogeneous function. Cognitive changes have been monitored while noncognitive changes have been ignored, thereby obscuring what aspects of patient response are specific to cognition rather than secondary responses to other aspects of their functioning. For example, activation, an antidepressant response that produces cognitive changes, must be interpreted differently from a response that alters only cognition. One recent concrete example of such interpretive confusion has involved the reports suggesting that naloxone treated memory-impaired Alzheimer's disease patients derive cognitive benefits from such treatments. It turns out that such apparent cognitive changes in these patients appear to be simply a behavioral response activation-arousal, following naloxone treatment, and reported changes in mental functioning turned out to have nothing to do with the type of cognitive dysfunctioning that is apparent in these patients (52a,62a).

Relatively few systematic findings that describe specific cognitive changes in the elderly have been applied to the design of appropriate environments for the impaired elderly. Our knowledge of the varieties of features of cognitive changes in the elderly can in fact be put to use in the design of supportive environments, including housing design, cognitive memory aids, and the structuring of support groups in the community. Design of treatment programs or environments takes into account only obvious stereotypic changes in recent memory and falls far short of our knowledge of cognitive dysfunctions that might appear in the elderly, which could be useful in the design of helpful support systems. A far more detailed and differentiated picture of cognitive changes that can occur in the elderly should and can be communicated in a meaningful manner to family members and community support groups working with the impaired elderly. Such precise information is crucial if systems are to be designed as effective instruments of support for the cognitively impaired elderly. Finally, a virtually untouched area is that of behavioral rehabilitative intervention designed around specific knowledge about the nature of cognitive changes in the elderly. This is an area that has long been found useful in working with head-injured and stroke populations but has not been explored in the elderly or in progressive dementia patients. Methods relying on selective feedback of information, forms of information presentation, and use of reinforcement strategies can be useful if we are clear about the specific nature of the cognitive changes that may be apparent in the elderly.

Neurobiological Cognitive Science

Historically, medicine has had a long tradition of using the study of "accidents of nature," diseases, in order to understand biological systems better. This has, in general,

not been the case in cognitive science. Several areas of research all concerned with the nature of cognitive processes have developed quite separate scholarly histories. The reasons for this have been detailed elsewhere (65a). It is, however, beginning to be clear that if we are to understand the psychobiology of cognitive processes, we cannot simply study unimpaired subjects in the human learning laboratory while ignoring the biology and pathology of brain function. On the other hand, extraordinarily useful tools and models have been developed within "traditional" experimental cognitive science that are ripe for translation into a form that can be used as diagnostic tools in the clinical setting. It is our conviction that those tools will provide us with extensive, sensitive, and powerful new clinical methods for defining and dissecting forms of cognitive dysfunctions.

STRATEGIES FOR CHARACTERIZING MENTAL FUNCTIONS IN THE ELDERLY: AN OVERVIEW OF A MULTISYSTEM MEASUREMENT APPROACH

When we think of mental changes that may or may not occur in the elderly, we frequently think of memory functions and nothing more. A great deal of research has shown that a measure of a patient's memory performance in an isolated context is worthless information. Characterizing mental functioning in the elderly must involve simultaneous integrated evaluation of a variety of types of cognitive functions and nominally noncognitive functions such as mood and aspects of a previous history of functioning.

Subject Characteristics

Aspects of a patient's previous history that would characterize who he is along personality–psychopathology dimensions obviously form one facet of the context for considering current mental status. A variety of psychometric tests are available for this purpose. This characterization of the subject might include not only broad aspects of psychological functioning but psychophysiological data such as responsiveness to stimuli, activation, and measures of antonomic activity.

Comparing Findings to Normative and to States of Impaired Functioning

Most clinical studies of the elderly have used normal controls as the contrast group in the evaluation of all kinds of functions. We propose that although this is an obviously logical and valuable method of approach, by itself it dramatically limits the value of such findings. Since cognitive changes are heterogeneous and are determined by many different forms of psychobiological determinants, it would be important to compare clinical cognitive findings not only with nominally unimpaired controls but also with well-defined populations of patients such as depressed subjects, or with normal control subjects treated with various types of psychoactive agents that can disrupt mental functions in variety of ways. In effect, the use of an "active placebo" group is of enormous importance in the evaluation and appreciation of changes in mental functions in the elderly.

Reliability of Measurement

Methods, procedures, and derived measures of performance may be highly reliable but nonetheless provide imprecise findings relevant to levels of mental functioning in the elderly. All clinical researchers who have explored cognitive, noncognitive, biological, and psychophysiological domains in the elderly are struck by the intrasubject variability of performance levels that are apparent in these subjects. Whether studies involve drug trials in the elderly or evaluation of functions for diagnostic purposes, it is imperative that multiple measures of performance be available per subject. Time of day, mood, factors that influence sleep, the characteristics of the examiner, and a host of internal events can affect measures of mental functioning in the elderly and can do so in a dramatic fashion. Although it is impractical, the methods used in establishing psychophysical thresholds would be the ones ideally suited to evaluating mental functions in the elderly. Multiple repeated measures within a very small group of homogeneous subjects would provide a far more valuable picture of mental functioning in the elderly than single measures of mental performance in many heterogeneously functioning subjects.

Cognitive and Noncognitive Measures

There are many aspects of higher mental functioning that should be evaluated in the elderly. Practical considerations limit what can, in fact, be measured. Perhaps most important, the approach used in evaluating cognitive functions in the elderly must be balanced. Major aspects of functioning, cognitive as well as noncognitive (social, emotional) aspects of functioning, must be appreciated at some level of detail. Recent memory function, the target area so often assessed in the elderly, is perhaps evaluated in far too great detail compared to often areas of mental functioning. This is the case because tests in this area are readily available and take little time or skill to administer. Many other aspects of cognition are often ignored because the methods of evaluation take longer to administer or require more training. Several sources provide excellent standard methods for exploring some of these domains of cognitive functioning in an orderly fashion, including sensory motor perceptual processes, language, concept formation, as well as memory. Some of the cognitive areas that may be of particular interest are defined below. Methods of approach to these distinct cognitive domains are also listed. Perhaps most important, assessment of aspects of mental functioning should be accomplished in a manner that relates the finding to those aspects of functioning that are normally not considered cognitive in nature. Motivation, sensitivity to reward, and mood are but a few of the behaviors that must

be assessed in a systematic fashion if one is to make any real sense of cognitive findings.

Patterns of Functioning

Ultimately, it would be useful to have available profiles or levels of functioning in many areas in the elderly by means of a method that is statistically reliable and valid and that meaningfully compares functioning along different dimensions in a manner easy for the clinician to interpret. Such profiles could then provide a picture of various facets of cognitive as well as noncognitive functioning. These profiles could be used in base-line descriptions of patient functioning as well as to follow changes in functioning over time or in response to drug treatment. Several methods for accomplishing such scaler profiles of assessment have been described in detail and reviewed elsewhere.

All of these approaches and issues that are important in the evaluation of mental functioning in the elderly are illustrated in summary fashion in Fig. 1.

STRATEGIES OF APPROACH: TESTS, METHODS, AND PROCEDURES

Micro- Versus Macromethods of Analysis

Systematic choices must be made about what level of detail is required and useful for characterizing aspects of mental functioning, characterizing subjects, and defining aspects of impaired functioning. The choice of approach and the precision and detail of description should be decided on the basis of how information is to be used or how it should be related to other information. The clinician or clinical researcher is faced with a staggering number of choices in terms of potentially useful methods for assessing mental functions in the elderly. Often the choice of specific instrument is based on virtually no knowledge about the procedure beyond the name of the test, which might contain the names of specific functions such as memory, perception, logic, or language. The choice of test can also be made on the basis of casual advice or visibility, but too often without a preplanned strategy of how the tests are to be used together or how test data are to fit specific research or clinical needs.

The problem of choice of methods is further complicated by the increasing use of procedures derived from experimental analysis of higher mental functions as these have emerged from the study of normal volunteers in the laboratory setting. These methods can be sensitive, powerful, and seductive but just as easily inappropriate and difficult to interpret and relate to clinical findings. Finally, the issues of time, expertise, skills at hand, and meaning of measures must all be considered in the choice of approach to the study of mental functions in the elderly.

We suggest that approaches to any cognitive domain can be broken down in the following manner with many choices of strategies serving different purposes. Based on the needs of a particular setting, it may be important to

STRATEGIES OF APPROACH FOR EXPLORING THE PSYCHOBIOLOGY OF COGNITION

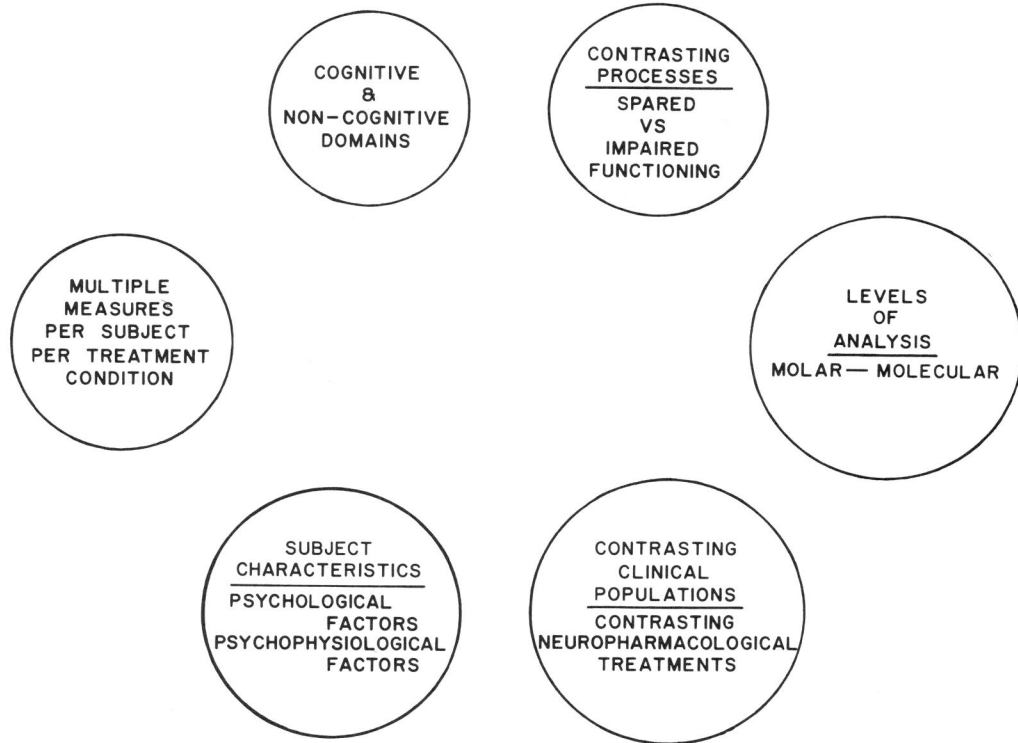

FIG. 1. Systems for exploring the psychobiology of cognition.

use well-established psychometric clinical instruments rather than more sensitive and detailed analysis using experimental methods. The interest of a clinician may be to gain a broad picture of a level of functioning (e.g., recent memory) instead of precise information about one aspect of mental activity (e.g., sustained attention). The focus of study may also be concerned with whether some types of process are intact or impaired or whether some structural aspect of intellectual functioning is affected in the elderly.

Regardless of whether one uses standard psychometric instruments or experimental laboratory methods, it is possible to dissect programmatically aspects or domains of functioning in a stepwise fashion from broad macrodescriptions to detailed definition of singular component aspects of higher mental functions. These component processes and structures may be determined by distinct psychobiological mechanisms making such a reductionistic approach to the problem of understanding details of mental functioning in the elderly of real practical clinical value. Figure 2 provides a schematic display of the sequential logic of some of these possible approaches to the study of elderly subjects. Some of the examples used involve aspects of memory, but perceptual functioning or attention or motivation could be considered using similar logic. The testing methods and procedures outlined here illustrate some of the areas that we feel require detailed analysis in the study of the elderly.

Psychometric Methods

Traditional neuropsychological test batteries assessing many types of functions are available, always with at least some normative data that can be used to compare the performance of the elderly subject. Although these methods are derived from a psychometric clinical tradition, they are often better suited for describing model group characteristics than they are effective in allowing definitive diagnostic decisions to be made about single patients. In general, these are also tests that can be administered only once and therefore are not easily suited to the study of patients in repeated-measures designs.

The historical context or tradition for the development of these tests has been of two types. In one, the attempt was to associate measures of types of higher mental functions with specific anatomically definable brain lesions. The other historical clinical tradition has been to characterize very broad aspects of mental functioning in order to allow for diagnostic classification between "functional" and "organic" disorders and among types of these disorders. Obviously, based on current knowledge about the etiology and mechanisms of forms of psychopathology, the distinction between organic and functional disorders is no more useful than 19th-century views of mind–brain distinctions within psychology are of value in the 20th century. The types of mental functions that can best be assessed in detail using

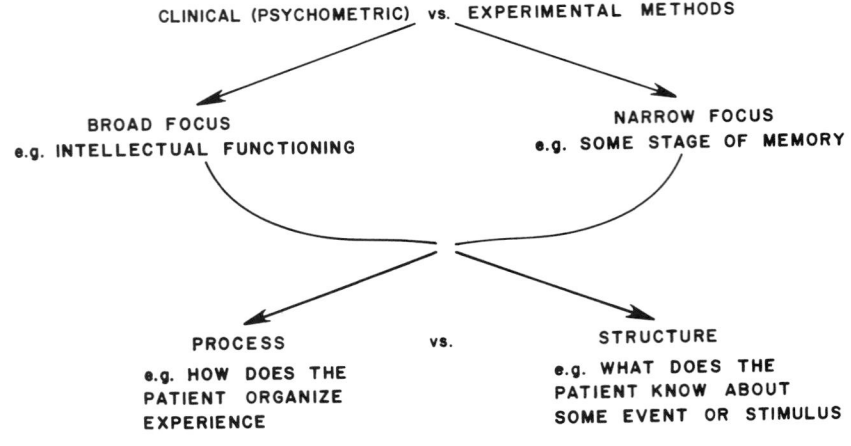

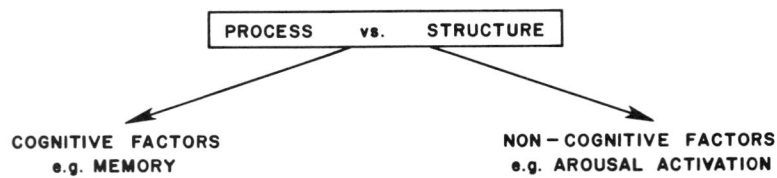

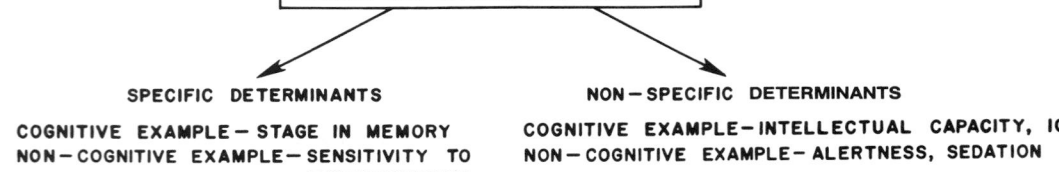

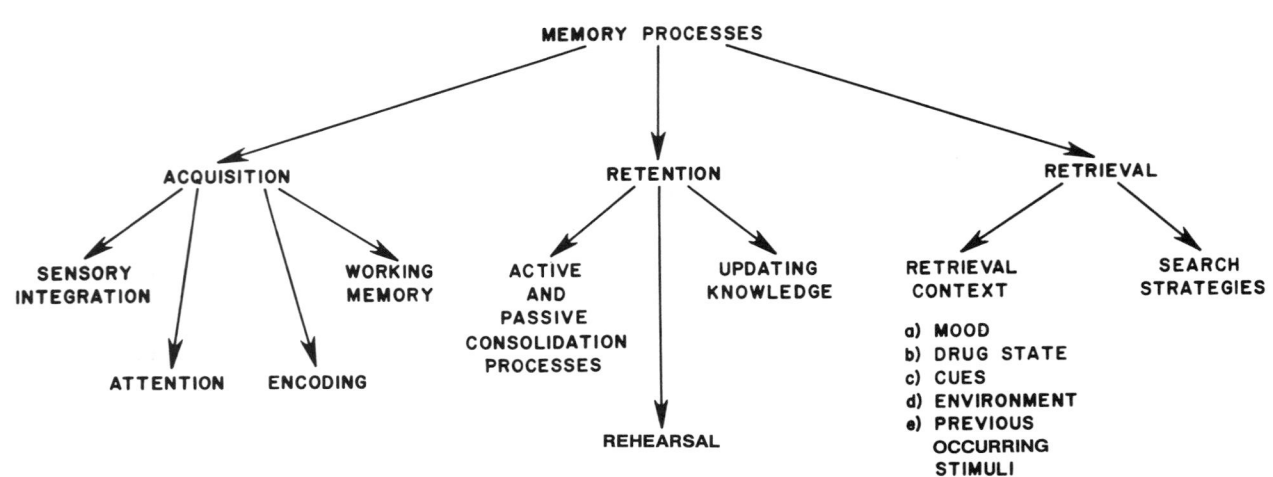

FIG. 2. Strategies for defining cognitive changes in the elderly (levels of analyses 1–3b).

(LEVELS OF ANALYSIS 3b)

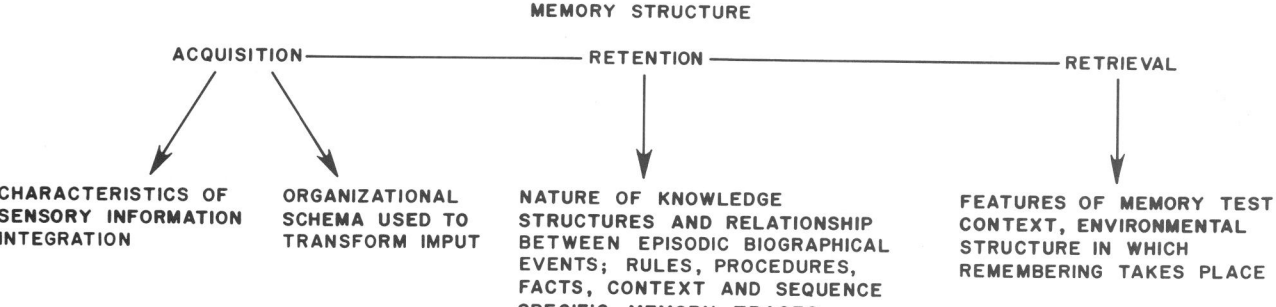

Fig. 2. *Continued.*

psychometric tools are different aspects of intelligence, memory functions, language functioning, and personality. Our inability to measure perceptual processing, thinking (e.g., concept functions, executive function, decision making), and attention accurately seriously compromises our ability to interpret other psychometric findings such as intellectual functions.

Characterizing Distinct Cognitive Processes on the Bases of Detailed Testing Using Laboratory Procedures

Possible candidates for cognitive processes that may be distinct come from several types of research. Models of memory processing in normal volunteers form a classic and obvious basis for identifying distinct cognitive processes. For example, the effects of manipulating processing conditions, stimulus material (pictures versus words), and retrieval conditions (recall versus recognition versus partial information and priming) have been used to argue for differences in some types of memory processes and representations of events in memory. Systematic clinical neuropsychological observations have also served as an important source of evidence pointing to distinctive features of memory functions (see 61 for a review of current theories about the differentiated nature of memory pathology). Animal research, too, has led to the proposal of different types of memory (48a,50a).

A number of different distinctive processes have been proposed, of which the following are the most likely to be distinguished from each other in terms of the underlying psychobiological mechanisms. Many of the distinctions among the different types of cognitive processes are apparent in a variety of clinical syndromes. Methods that can be used to assess and contrast distinct forms of cognitive processes and structures are therefore important in diagnosing accurately the determinants and presumably the etiologies of cognitive dysfunctions.

Acquisition Versus Retention Versus Retrieval Processes

Although no theory of cognition is based solely on this type of differentiation, different theories have emphasized several types of processes that may be important in each of these fundamentally different and definable "stages" of information processing.

A patient may not remember some previous event because of failures in any of these three broadly defined systems. Too often, the clinician assumes that an inability to remember an event means that it was never stored in memory. There are many clinical examples or demonstrations in which altering the retrieval conditions, such as reinstituting the context in which that event was processed, can result in successful recall. Cognitive failures associated with disturbances in mood or drug-altered states are clinical examples in which apparent memory failure may be related more to retrieval conditions than to acquisition processes. Likewise, conditions that follow successful acquisition and storage of information (retention–consolidation processes) can affect the probability that some event will be remembered. For example, a disruption of brain activity can produce a retrograde amnesia.

Attention Versus Working Memory Versus Elaborative Transformational Processes

The boundaries between attention and memory have always been unclear. Most important, attention and perhaps consciousness have represented processing systems too vague and undifferentiated to attract the programmatic interest of experimental cognitive psychologists. Nonetheless, the processes that make up these different cognitive functions are likely to involve somewhat different aspects of central nervous system activity.

A clinical example of a cognitive dysfunction related to these explanatory constructs is the heterogeneous syndrome of minimal brain dysfunction–hyperactivity–attentional disorders in children. In some instances it is possible to demonstrate alterations in attention, particularly sustained attention, as accounting for information-processing failures in subsets of these children. However, it has become increasingly clear that many of these children with "attentional dysfunctions" can successfully attend but do not transform and enrich the stimulus material in terms of their interaction with that information. Increasing evidence points to the importance of separating out these same factors in the elderly, that is, failures to attend versus impairments in elaborative encoding processes.

Short-Term Versus Long-Term Memory

This distinction is a classic dichotomy between memory processes. It has been redefined during the past decade in terms of "single memory trace" theories of information processing. Some memory theorists view this distinction as particularly useful in bridging lower animal and human learning–memory phenomena. Clinicians describing memory failure, especially those whose roots are in medicine rather than psychology, are most likely to consider this distinction useful.

Elaborate Versus Superficial Processing Operations

Distinctions between memory–learning processes are defined along a continuum in terms of the operations subjects perform at the time of information input and retrieval. Memory is successful to the degree that subjects have effectively processed input information and depends on the similarity between processing conditions and retrieval conditions.

Automatic Versus Effort-Demanding Processes

The role of capacity-demanding cognitive processes versus those that require little cognitive capacity or mental work has received increasing attention during the last decade. Some drugs and some forms of changes in brain structure and activity appear selectively to affect automatic and effort-demanding processes. As with so many other descriptive systems used to explain cognitive phenomena, initial enthusiasm yields to new questions and uncertainties (which is where matters remain at present).

Many clinical examples can be cited in support of the distinctiveness of these processes. Patients who are depressed can demonstrate selective impairments in cognition in situations that require sustained concentration and cognitive effort but are unimpaired in using processes that can be accomplished automatically, including tasks that can be quite complex. Parkinson's disease patients demonstrate a similar pattern of dysfunction. Some patients demonstrate selective impairments in automatic processing and not in effort-demanding processes. Alzheimer's, Korsakoff, and Huntington's disease patients are generally comparably impaired in both of these domains. In assessing cognitive changes in the elderly, distinguishing between levels of functioning in effort-demanding and automatic processing is therefore particularly important for both diagnosis and treatment evaluation.

Procedural Versus Declarative Memory

The distinction between learning–memory processes that are involved in knowing how to do something versus knowing that it has been done has been almost exclusively derived from clinical neuropsychological observations and not from a theory or model of normal cognitive processing. Much recent attention has been given to the distinction between these two types of learning–memory processes (14).

Some memory-impaired amnestic patients are able to learn a procedure and accurately perform that procedure at a later time without remembering the circumstances in which learning took place. This dissociation between procedural and declarative memory effects can also be seen associated with some commonly prescribed sedative drug treatments such as the benzodiazepines. Differential performance on procedural and declarative memory–learning-performance tasks can be of considerable diagnostic significance.

Episodic Versus Knowledge Memory

Some memory representations are linked to a unique context and sequence in which events have been processed. Other memories represent a knowledge base that is dissociated from the circumstances under which that information was learned. It is this knowledge that is largely the basis for encoding and organization of input (62b–d).

Impairments that result in an inability to access previously acquired knowledge are a major determinant of recent memory failure in many patients suffering senile dementia of an Alzheimer's type. The degree to which such patients are unable to bring to consciousness, or working memory, pertinent knowledge about ongoing events is linked to their inability to encode those events and therefore make them memorable. Treating unimpaired subjects with cholinergic antagonists reproduces this distinct pattern of cognitive failure. On the other hand, many memory-impaired patients exhibit marked disturbances in recent memory without any impairment in access to previously acquired knowledge in long-term memory. Several types of drug treatments in unimpaired subjects mimic this latter form of cognitive failure. These clinical and pharmacological findings provide convergent evidence that suggests that these two cognitive systems are at least partially independent and driven by different psychobiological mechanisms. Assessment of these functions is of considerable importance in establishing an appropriate diagnosis in patients or subjects presenting clinically with a disturbance in memory.

Language Versus Pattern Processing

Neuropsychological investigations have provided strong evidence for a neuroanatomic differentiation between the processing and retention of language as opposed to pattern information. This represents a historically classic area of study in neurology and neuropsychology. Findings that compare the relative effectiveness of processing (and production) of information that involves language mediation versus pattern information have been used for decades to determine the neuroanatomical systems that may account for some forms of cognitive failure.

Reward-Related Versus Reward-Independent Learning

Most studies of cognitive processes in normal subjects are designed to eliminate or at least randomize and minimize reinforcing consequences in studies of human learning. This is so despite the fact that cognitivists would acknowledge the obvious importance of reinforcement, reward, and incentive in human learning. In lower animals, learning and memory processes are almost exclusively tied to reinforcing consequences. Neuroscientists have also recently shown that brain structures and systems involved in the mediation of reward and reinforcement overlap to a considerable degree with those systems known to be important in learning and memory. The cognitive disturbances in depression and perhaps in some amnesias may well be determined by decreases in the sensitivity of the reward system.

Passive Memory Consolidation Versus Working Memory

It is apparent in psychobiological studies of memory processes in lower animals that postacquisition processing that may be involved in forming a relatively permanent trace of recent plastic representations of events may involve multiple processes including those that require active, conscious reworking and updating of information already in memory.

Context-Dependent and Context-Specific Retrieval Processes: State-Dependent Learning

The importance of retrieval context in the likelihood of successfully retrieving events from memory has been clear for some time and, in fact, increasingly has been used as a scheme to account for various types of forgetting. The link between encoding context and retrieval context has also been important in accounting for learning and memory in the unimpaired normal subject and in patients in various psychiatric and mood-altered states as well as in drug-state-dependent learning and memory.

Cognitive Processes With and Without Conscious Awareness

The role of consciousness, the subjective experience of knowing, and metacognitive operations are increasingly seen as important determinants in defining the differentiated characteristics of various types of memory processes. Are memories for events in which subjects know what they know and appreciate the circumstances in which the memories were formed the same as memories about which subjects have no awareness (35)?

Respondent (Conditioned) Learning Versus Controlled Instrumental Cognitive Processes

To the extent that patients are able to form conditioned responses and maintain a "record" of such conditioning, learning may involve different brain systems from those that are involved in "knowing" that learning has occurred and being able to encode memory for learned events. Although classical conditioning studies are rarely used in gerontological studies, we view these as providing valuable data about aspects of central nervous system functioning that are distinct from those tested by, e.g., measures of declarative, effort-demanding memory.

Evaluating Noncognitive Systems That Can Affect Cognitive Processes

Reinforcement–Reward System

This brain system (defined by self-stimulation studies of the brain) may also play an important role in the establishment of memories and in the performance of learned behaviors. Recent studies of areas of the brain that are involved in self-stimulation behavior have been useful in defining some of the chemistry and neuroanatomy of this putative reward system (36a,b). The areas of the brain and neurochemical systems that are involved in self-stimulation and reward overlap with those involved with learning and memory. This may provide confirmation of the behaviorist doctrine, i.e., that rewarded behaviors are more likely to be (remembered and) repeated. Specific components of memory–learning processes appear to be altered differentially by conditions that affect the reward system of the brain (19a). This system may have a particular role in affecting the strength of learned behaviors.

Arousal/Activation

Conditions that affect generalized brain state arousal and activation can also be seen as affecting various aspects of information processing, learning, memory, and thinking. Arousal and activation changes can alter the consolidation of memory traces (65b) and short-term and long-term memory as well as attentional strategies. The inherent vagueness of concepts such as arousal and activation has made it difficult to determine and quantify the effect that such factors have on different cognitive operations.

These modulating influences are sometimes termed "extrinsic" aspects of memory in that they do not contain the actual representation of information, the memory "trace," "engram," or "intrinsic memory" (61a), but do exert important influences on it. This behavioral concept of modulation refers to neurochemical processes that alter the function of classical neurotransmitters but do not actually conduct neuronal information across synaptic clefts. Some models of memory explicitly include nonspecific modulators. For example, the "single trace–two process" model postulates that learning involves, first, the formation of the memory trace, perhaps in the form of a reverberating neuronal circuit, and second, a nonspecific arousal that strengthens and promotes the consolidation of the trace (24a).

The multiple determinants of performance on most memory tasks add complexity to the interpretation of the effects of various types of disturbances of central nervous system function on higher mental functions. Some tasks designed to measure memory also involve factors such as sensory acuity and motor activity, which are unrelated to either intrinsic memory processes or extrinsic memory modulators. Drugs that influence these factors, however, will necessarily alter memory task performance. For example, an $ACTH_{4-9}$ peptide (Organon 2766) may enhance visual acuity and thus improve performance on visual memory tasks.

ANIMAL MODELS OF MEMORY CHANGES IN MAN

Animal modeling and research may well be of value in breaking apart aspects of cognition. If this can be done successfully, we will have available some powerful approaches for understanding and treating cognitive dysfunctions. Our success in using animal models of cognitive dysfunctions is, of course, dependent on the degree to which the model fits the clinical reality of some cognitive impairment. Simply providing an impaired memory system will not suffice.

Tests for animals must be developed that are selectively sensitive to the processes listed above, or further distinctions formulated on the basis of animal research must be proposed that can also be applied to human cognitive processes. A recent debate concerning the nature of episodic memory in animals is typical of the problems to be faced (50b,62b). The majority of individuals investigating animal learning and memory do so in the belief that although animals may be more limited in their cognitive abilities than humans, the similarities outnumber the differences. A number of recent studies support this belief. For example, if human subjects are shown a list of words and a short time later are asked to recall them, a plot of recall against serial position reveals a U-shaped function. Recall of words appearing early in the list (primacy items) or late in the list (recency items) is better than the recall of items from the middle of the list. Primacy and recency effects have now been reported in nonhuman primates, rats, and pigeons (16a,50a,68a). Furthermore, manipulations that alter the primacy and recency effects in humans produce similar effects in laboratory animals (36a).

The difference between performance on a win-shift as opposed to a win-stay strategy in a radial arm maze has been suggested to reflect a difference between automatic and effortful processing in the rat (16a), complementing the distinction made in humans by Hasher and Zacks (28). Other evidence for distinctions between cognitive processes in animals comes from lesion studies. For example, performance in passive avoidance tests, for so long the mainstay of neuropharmacological research on learning and memory in animals, appears to be dependent on processes quite different from those that are important for optimal performance in a radial arm maze (39a,50). Just what processes are tapped by the passive avoidance test remains unclear. It is, perhaps, worth noting the classic observation of Claparede, who shook hands with an amnesic patient while concealing a pin in his hand. The next day the patient was reluctant to shake hands with him but could not recall why. Would this patient's amnesia have shown up in a passive avoidance test?

REFERENCES

1. Alba, J. W., Chromiak, W., Hasher, L., and Attig, M. S. (1980): *J. Exp. Psychol. Hum. Learn. Mem.*, 6:370–378.
2. Anderson, J. R. (1976): *Language, Memory, and Thought.* Lawrence Associates, Erlbaum Hillsdale, NJ.
3. Bachrach, J., and Mintz, J. (1974): *J. Clin. Psychiatry*, 30:58–60.
4. Baddeley, A. D. (1976): *The Psychology of Memory.* Basic Books, New York.
5. Baddeley, A. D. (1982): *Psychol. Rev.*, 89:708–729.
6. Barbizet, J. (1970): *Human Memory and Its Pathology.* W. H. Freeman, San Francisco.
7. Boll, T. J. (1978): In: *Clinical Diagnosis of Mental Disorders*, edited by B. B. Wolman. New York.
8. Bower, G. H. (1970): *Cognit. Psychol.*, 1:18–45.
9. Bower, G. H. (1981): *Am. Psychol.*, 36:129–148.
10. Bradshaw, G. L., and Anderson, J. R. (1982): *J. Verb. Learn. Verb. Behav.*, 21:165–174.
11. Carr, T. H., McCauley, C., Sperber, R. D., and Parmelee, C. M. (1982): *J. Exp. Psychol. Hum. Percept. Perform.*, 8:757–777.
12. Cattell, R. B. (1963): *J. Educ. Psychol.*, 54.
13. Clifton, C., Jr., and Slowiaczek, M. L. (1981): *Mem. Cognit.*, 9:142–148.
14. Cohen, N. J., and Squire, L. R. (1980): *Science*, 210:207–210.
15. Craik, F. I. M. (1979): *Ann. Rev. Psychol.*, 30:63–102.
16. Crowder, R. G. (1982): *Acta Psychol.*, 50:291–323.
16a. Dimattia, B. V., and Kesner, R. P. (1984): *J. Exp. Psychol: Animal Behav. Proc.*, 10:557–563.
17. Drachman, D. A., and Arbit, J. (1966): *Arch. Neurol.*, 52–61.
18. Eich, J. E. (1980): *Mem. Cognit.*, 8:157–173.
19. Erickson, R. C., and Scott, M. L. (1977): *Psychol. Bull.*, 84:1130–1149.
19a. Esposito, R. V., Parker, E. S., and Weingartner, H. (1984): *Substance and Alcohol Actions and Misuse*, 5:111–119.
20. Eysenck, M. W., and Eysenck, M. C. (1979): *J. Exp. Psychol. Hum. Learn. Mem.*, 5:472–484.
21. Fisher, R. P. (1979): *Mem. Cognit.*, 7:224–231.
22. Fisher, R. P. (1981): *J. Exp. Psychol. Hum. Learn. Mem.*, 7:306–310.
23. Flexser, A. J., and Tulving, E. (1978): *Psychol. Rev.*, 85:153–171.
24. Galambos, J. A., and Rips, L. J. (1982): *J. Verb. Learn. Verb. Behav.*, 21:260–281.
24a. Gold, P. E., and McGaugh, J. L. (1975): In: *Short Term Memory*, edited by D. Deutsch, and J. L. McGaugh. Academic Press, New York.
25. Golden, C. J., Purisch, A., and Hammeke, T. A. (1979): *The Luria–Nebraska Neuropsychological Battery, a Manual for Clinical and Experimental Uses.* University of Nebraska Press, Lincoln.
26. Guilford, J. P. (1967): *Nature of Human Intelligence.* McGraw-Hill, New York.
27. Guilford, J. P., and Hoepfner, R. (1971): *The Analysis of Intelligence.* McGraw-Hill, New York.
28. Hasher, L., and Zacks, R. T. (1979): *J. Exp. Psychol. Gen.*, 108:356–388.
29. Heaton, R. R. (1976): *Clin. Psychol.*, 29:10–11.
30. Heaton, R. R., Baade, L. E., and Johnson, R. L. (1978): *Psychol. Bull.*, 85:141–162.
31. Herrmann, D. J., and Harwood, J. R. (1980): *J. Exp. Psychol. Hum. Learn. Mem.*, 6:467–478.
32. Hunt, R. R., and Einstein, G. O. (1981): *J. Verb. Learn. Verb. Behav.*, 20:497–514.
33. Hunt, R. R., and Mitchell, D. B. (1982): *J. Exp. Psychol. Learn. Mem. Cognit.*, 8:81–87.
34. Jacoby, L. L., Craik, F. I. M., and Begg, I. (1979): *J. Verb. Learn. Verb. Behav.*, 18:585–600.
35. Jacoby, L. L., and Witherspoon, D. (1982): *Can. J. Psychol.*, 36:300–324.
36. Kelly, H. P. (1964): Memory abilities: A factor analysis. *Psychol. Monogr.*
36a. Kesner, R. P. (1985): *Ann. NY Acad. Science*, 444:122–136.

36b.Kornetsky, C., Esposito, R. U. (1981): *Brain Res.*, 209:496–500.

36c.Routtenberg, A. (1979): Participation of Brain Stimulation Reward Substrates in Memory: Anatomical and Biochemical Evidence. *Federation Proceedings,* pp. 2446–2453.

37. Leight, K. A., and Ellis, H. C. (1981): *J. Verb. Learn. Verb. Behav.*, 20:251–275.

38. Lezak, M. D. (1976): *Neuropsychological Assessment.* Oxford University Press, New York.

39. Luria, A. R. (1976): *The Neuropsychology of Memory.* Halstead, Somerset, NJ.

39a.Lynch, G., and Baudry, M. (1984): *Science,* 224:1057–1063.

40. Mandler, G. (1968): In: *Verbal Behavior and General Behavior Theory,* edited by T. R. Dixon, and D. L. Horton. Prentice Hall, Englewood Cliffs, NJ.

41. Mathews, C. G. (1977): *Adult (C.A.) 15 and Older: Neuropsychological Test Battery.* C. G. Mathews, Madison, WI.

42. Mathews, C. G., Shaw, D. J., and Klove, H. (1966): *Cortex,* 2: 244–253.

43. McCloskey, M., and Santee, J. (1981): *J. Exp. Psychol. Hum. Learn. Mem.,* 7:66–71.

44. McFie, J. (1975): *Assessment of Organic Intellectual Impairment.* Academic Press, New York.

45. McGaugh, J. L., and Herz, M. J. (1972): *Memory Consolidation.* Albion, San Francisco.

46. McKoon, G., and Ratcliff, R. (1979): *J. Verb. Learn. Verb. Behav.,* 18:463–480.

47. Medin, D. L., and Smith, E. E. (1984): *Annu. Rev. Psychol.,* 35: 113–138.

48. Milner, B. (1968): *Neuropsychologia,* 6:175–179(a).

48a.Mishkin, M., and Petri, H. (1984): In: *Neuropsychology of Memory,* edited by L. R. Squire and N. Butlers, pp. 287–296. The Guilford Press, New York.

49. Norman, D. A. (1973): In: *The Physiological Basis of Memory,* edited by J. A. Deutsch. Academic Press, New York, London.

50. Olton, D. S., Gamzu, E., and Corkin, S. (1985): *Ann. N.Y. Acad. Sci.,* 444.

50a.Olton, D. S., Samuelson, R. J. (1976): *J. Exp. Psychol.: Anim. Behav. Proc.,* 2:97–116.

50b.Olton, D. S. (1984): *Behav. Brain Sci.,* 7:250–251.

51. Parsons, O. A., and Prigatano, G. P. (1978): *J. Consult. Clin. Psychol.,* 46:608–619.

52. Prigatano, G. P. (1978): *J. Clin. Psychol.,* 34:816–832.

52a.Reisberg, B., Ferris, S., Anand, R., Mir, P., Geibel, V., Deleon, M. (1983): *N. Engl. J. Med.,* 308:721–722.

53. Reitan, R. M. (1969): *Manual for the Administration of Neuropsychological Test Batteries for Adults and Children.* R. M. Reitan, Indianapolis.

54. Roediger, H. L. III, and Adelson, B. (1980): *Mem. Cognit.,* 8:65–74.

55. Russell, E. W. (1979): *J. Clin. Psychol.,* 35:611–620.

56. Salame, P., and Baddeley, A. (1982): *J. Verb. Learn. Verb. Behav.,* 21:150–164.

57. Schreiver, D. J., Goldman, H., Kleinman, K. M., Goldfader, P. R., and Snow, M. Y. (1976): *J. Nerv. Ment. Dis.,* 162:360–365.

58. Shaffer, W. O., and Laberge, D. (1979): *J. Verb. Learn. Verb. Behav.,* 18:413–426.

59. Shriffrin, R. M., and Schneider, W. (1977): *Psychol. Rev.,* 84:127–190.

60. Smith, A. (1975): *Adv. Neurol.,* 7:49–110.

61. Squire, L. R., and Butter, N. (1984): *Neuropsychology of Memory.* Guilford Press, London.

61a.Squire, L. R., and Davis, H. P. (1981): *Annu. Rev. Pharmacol. Toxicol.,* 21:323–356.

62. Squire, L. R., and Slater, P. C. (1978): *Neuropsychologia,* 16:313–322.

62a.Tariot, P., Sunderland, T., Weingartner, H., Murphy, D., Cohen, M., and Cohen, R. (1986): *Arch. Gen. Psychiatry,* 43:727–732.

62b.Tulving, E. (1983): *Elements of Episodic Memory.* Clarendon Press, Oxford.

62c.Tulving, E. (1984): *Behav. Brain Science,* 7:223–268.

62d.Tulving, E. (1985): *Amer. Psychol.,* 40:358–398.

63. Tulving, E., Schacter, D. L., and Stark, H. A. (1982): *J. Exp. Psychol. Learn. Mem. Cognit.,* 8:336–342.

64. Tulving, E., and Thomson, D. M. (1973): *Psychol. Rev.,* 80:352–373.

65. Wechlser, D. (1945): *J. Psychol.,* 19:87–93.

65a.Weingartner, H., and Parker, E. (1984): *Memory Consolidation: Psychobiology of Cognition.* Laurence Erlbaum Associates, Hillsdale, NY.

65b.Weingartner, H., Hull, B., Murphy, D. L., and Weinstein, S. (1976): *Nature,* 263:311–312.

66. Whitty, C. W. M., and Zangwill, O. L. (1977): *Amnesia.* Butterworths, London.

67. Wilson, R. S., Rosenbaum, G., Brown, G., Rourke, D., Whitman, D., et al. (1978): *J. Consult. Clin. Psychol.,* 46:1554–1555.

68. Winograd, E., and Lynn, E. S. (1979): *Mem. Cognit.,* 7:29–34.

68a.Wright, A. A., Santiago, H. C., Sands, S. F., Kendrick, D. F., and Cook, P. G. *Science,* 229:287–289.

69. Zangwill, O. L. (1969): In: *The Pathology of Memory,* edited by G. A. Talland, and N. C. Waugh, Academic Press, New York.

Psychopharmacology:
The Third Generation of Progress,
edited by Herbert Y. Meltzer.
Raven Press, New York © 1987.

CHAPTER 91

The Experimental Pharmacology of Alzheimer's Disease and Related Dementias

Richard C. Mohs and Kenneth L. Davis

STUDIES IN PATIENTS WITH ALZHEIMER'S DISEASE

Advances made during the past 10 years in our understanding of the neurochemical changes occurring in the brains of patients with Alzheimer's disease (AD) have opened an entire new era in the psychopharmacology of AD. In particular, the discovery of a dramatic and at least partially specific loss of presynaptic cholinergic markers first reported in 1976 (12,24,73) led to a tremendous increase in interest in AD on the part of psychopharmacologists. Prior to that time, AD was widely viewed as a nonspecific degenerative disease in which drugs acting on any particular neurochemical system would be unlikely to have any positive effect. The finding of the cholinergic cell loss and subsequent findings regarding other neurochemical systems have raised the possibility that specific psychopharmacologic agents might at least partially reverse the pathophysiologic and symptomatic abnormalities of this disease. As reviewed below, the most recent attempts at psychopharmacologic treatment of AD have met with only very limited success. Nevertheless, progress in the neurochemistry of AD is providing new, testable hypotheses for psychopharmacologists almost daily. This fact, together with the very substantial progress that has been made in developing new methodologies for clinical drug testing in AD patients, makes this one of the most active and exciting areas of contemporary psychopharmacology.

Methodologic Considerations

Diagnosis

During life the diagnosis of AD is a clinical one requiring both inclusion and exclusion criteria. There is no laboratory test that can be used for confirmation. Essentially, the diagnosis is given to those patients who have current symptoms and a clinical history consistent with AD and in whom other laboratory tests suggest no other condition that might be responsible for the dementia. A recent NIH concensus conference (63) developed a standard set of criteria for diagnosing AD, and, although the criteria must be operationalized for use in any particular setting, they do provide very useful guidelines for evaluating the inclusion criteria of any psychopharmacologic trial in AD. It is encouraging to note that in recent studies in which patients meeting rigorous research diagnostic criteria for AD have been followed to autopsy, over 90% of them have characteristic AD histopathology (37). Routine clinical diagnoses of AD without rigorous criteria, however, are found on follow-up to be in error as often as 30% of the time (60). Thus, careful attention to diagnosis is critical if one hopes to achieve homogeneous groups for psychopharmacologic trials.

Within the group of patients who meet rigorous clinical criteria for AD and have neuropathologic changes of AD, there will still be considerable variability in the type and extent of neurochemical abnormalities. Early patients certainly have less extensive neuronal cell loss than do later patients (20), and, although virtually all AD patients have extensive cholinergic cell loss, subgroups of patients also have a substantial loss of noradrenergic cells (22), serotonergic cells (11), and/or somatostatin-containing cells (23). Identification of patients with specific kinds and degrees of cell loss during life is currently impossible. Inevitably, clinical studies will involve patients with heterogeneous neurochemical deficits, and it is to be expected that as long as this situation persists, pharmacologic treatment approaches directed at neurotransmitter abnormalities in AD will produce heterogeneous outcomes. Progress appears to be most likely when studies are designed to investigate the clinical and neurochemical features of subgroups of patients who have a specific response to a specific agent.

Assessment

Determining whether any drug is effective in treating patients with AD has been difficult, in part, because there are no generally recognized outcome measures of improvement for AD patients. This can be contrasted with other areas of psychopharmacology where effective treatments are available. Examples include the Brief Psychiatric Rating Scale (BPRS) (72), the Hamilton Depression Rating Scale (43), and the Abnormal Involuntary Movement Scale (39), which are widely and successfully used to evaluate treatments for schizophrenia, depression, and tardive dyskinesia, respectively. Some attempts have been made to develop rating scales for Alzheimer's disease (80), but, given the importance of memory and other cognitive impairments in AD, many investigators have elected to use formal psychological tests rather than observer ratings to evaluate efficacy (84). Problems involved in using neuropsychological tests as measures of treatment efficacy include the fact that very demented patients may not be able to complete the tests, there often are no alternate forms of the tests for repeated assessments, and the tests may not be sensitive to change across a broad range of symptom severity. Our research group has recently attempted to combine some simple neuropsychological tests of memory, language, and praxis with behavioral ratings of agitation and mood disturbance to provide an overall measure of symptom severity in AD (77). This instrument, the Alzheimer's Disease Assessment Scale (ADAS), was constructed to measure all of the major clinical symptoms of AD and has high interrater and test–retest reliability; it is also sensitive to change over 12 months in a group of AD patients tested longitudinally (77).

Ideally, one would like to have demonstrated that an outcome measure used for psychopharmacologic trials is sensitive to the effects of agents generally recognized as effective. Since such assurance is impossible to obtain at present, demonstrated sensitivity to progressive increases in AD symptomatology may be the best assurance of validity presently available. However, no single scale and no uniform approach to assessment of AD patients has yet been adopted by the majority of investigators. Thus, an evaluation of studies in this area must always consider the limitations of the type of assessment procedure used. In addition, comparisons between studies are often difficult because of differences in outcome measures.

Choice of Drug and Dosage

Although the choice of drug and dosage is important in any psychopharmacologic study, investigations in patients with AD pose particular problems in this regard. Because of the rapid advances made in understanding the neurochemical abnormalities of AD, many studies have been conducted to investigate whether specific types of neuro-

transmitter enhancement will improve symptoms of AD. Since few, if any, drugs act specifically on one neurotransmitter system, and since direct measures of a drug's neurochemical effects are never available in clinical studies, the implications of any drug trial for theories about the neurochemical basis of AD symptoms must be drawn cautiously. Although it would be foolish to ignore neurochemical data when selecting drugs for trials in AD patients, no clinical trial can be viewed as more than an indirect test of a hypothesis about the relationship of neurochemistry and symptoms.

Selection of drug dosage may be more important and more difficult in AD patients than in most other study groups. Alzheimer's disease is a progressive disease, and patients undoubtedly enter clinical trials with vastly different degrees of neuronal loss. Animal studies investigating cholinomimetic drugs demonstrate that dose–response curves shift dramatically depending on the extent of cholinergic cell loss (44). Cholinergic (34) and other (1) drug effects on memory in animals are biphasic with dose, so the dose range that improves memory may be very narrow. Some evidence (2) suggests that this is also the case in humans. An implication of these findings is that in many cases it may be necessary to determine doses individually for AD patients in clinical drug trials; studies in which doses are not determined individually may fail to detect potentially important drug effects in AD patients.

Studies of Cholinergic Drugs

Two sets of facts stimulated a tremendous amount of interest in the possibility that cholinergic drugs might be useful for treating patients with AD. One, of course, was the evidence that AD is associated with a dramatic loss of cholinergic cells and that the extent of such cell loss correlates with neuropathologic and behavioral changes of AD; these results are reviewed by E. K. Perry in this volume. Second was the evidence that anticholinergic drugs such as scopolamine or atropine produce dose-related cognitive impairments (55) that, when investigated in detail, resemble the memory impairments observed in elderly people with age-related memory loss (32). It was also determined that the cholinesterase inhibitor physostigmine, but not amphetamine, could at least partially reverse the amnestic effects of scopolamine (31). Since amphetamine is a stimulant that acts primarily by increasing transmission at aminergic synapses, these data suggested quite strongly that the amnestic effects of the anticholinergics are specifically related to their effects at cholinergic synapses and are not secondary to their sedative effects. These results also suggested quite strongly that cholinomimetic drugs might improve memory in patients with a specific deficit in cholinergic transmission.

Precursors

Acetylcholine (ACh) is synthesized in cholinergic nerve terminals from two precursors, choline and acetylcoenzyme A, in a reaction catalyzed by choline acetyltransferase

(CAT) (91). The rate-limiting step in the synthesis of ACh appears to be neither the enzyme nor the availability of precursor; rather, evidence suggests that the high-affinity transport system that brings choline into the terminal is rate limiting under most conditions (81). Choline apparently cannot be synthesized *de novo* in the body, and choline for the synthesis of ACh must ultimately be derived from dietary sources, where it is usually available as phosphatidylcholine (lecithin) (91). If it were possible to increase cholinergic activity by providing additional precursor, these substances would be very valuable therapeutic agents since they can be given in large quantities with few side effects, none of which are life threatening. However, evidence on whether they can affect neurotransmission is either inconclusive or negative. Some studies have shown that in rats increasing dietary intake of choline (19) or intraperitoneal injection of choline (45) is followed by increases in ACh concentration in brain. Intraperitoneal injection of choline also increased striatal tyrosine hydroxylase activity, and the effect was blocked by atropine (86), suggesting an increase in cholinergic activity. Two oral doses of choline mimicked the effect of introperitoneal physostigmine to augment the accumulation of HVA and DOPAC in the striatum, as would be expected if both choline and physostigmine increased cholinergic transmission (65). However, not all studies have found increases in brain ACh concentrations following either dietary or intraperitoneal administration of choline (15). In addition, iontophoretic studies indicated that increases in extracellular choline did not augment the effect of physostigmine to enhance cholinergic transmission (57).

Studies investigating the effects of dietary choline supplementation in humans have found no convincing evidence that precursors have any effect on cognition. In a comprehensive review of 17 studies, Bartus et al. (2) found only one that claimed to find a substantial memory improvement (35); this finding has not been replicated. In light of the methodologic problems mentioned above, it is of interest to note that studies using sensitive outcome measures and a range of doses have not found any improvement either in AD patients (85) or in nondemented elderly people (69,70).

It has been speculated on theoretical grounds that precursors might affect memory only under very special circumstances, for example, when cholinergic neurons are firing at an increased rate or when administered over very long periods of time. The first possibility stems from studies showing that supplementary dietary choline prevents the depletion of brain ACh caused by antimuscarinic agents (87) or by electrical stimulation of cholinergic neurons (7). In normal human volunteers, a single 8-g dose of oral choline chloride slightly but significantly attenuated the amnesic effects of scopolamine (68). Lower doses that produced equivalent plasma choline levels when given over 24 hr could not produce a similar attenuation (66). Thus, even under conditions in which cholinergic transmission is enhanced, precursor supplementation has little if any effect on cognition. The possibility that long-term choline supplementation might retard degeneration of cholinergic neurons stems from the fact that cholinergic neurons are the only ones that use choline both for neurotransmitter syn-

thesis and as a membrane constituent (91). There is, however, no direct evidence to suggest that choline supplementation retards cell loss, and the one available study of long-term (1 year) administration of lecithin to AD patients found no significant effect on cognition (58).

Cholinesterase Inhibitors

The fact that precursors to acetylcholine have not shown any demonstrable effects on cognition has stimulated increased interest in both cholinesterase inhibitors and cholinergic agonists. One major difficulty encountered in testing drugs in these classes is that many of them are toxic agents that cannot be administered safely to humans. Of the cholinesterase inhibitors, only physostigmine and tetrahydroaminoacridine (THA) have been tested for their cognitive and behavioral effects in patients with AD. When given in low doses, physostigmine appears to be relatively safe, at least in people with normal cardiac functioning. It has repeatedly been demonstrated that intravenous physostigmine reverses the cognitive effects of anticholinergic drugs (31); one study (30) found that a low dose of physostigmine improved memory functioning in normal young adults, but higher doses, which have endocrine effects suggestive of a generalized stress response (26), impair memory and other cognitive functions (28). Disadvantages of physostigmine are that it has a half-life of approximately 30 min in plasma (90), and until recently it was not available in oral form.

Table 1 presents a summary of 13 studies investigating the effects of physostigmine and THA in patients with AD. Only two studies (54,83), both with small samples and one without double-blind conditions, investigated the effects of THA. A small, significant improvement of some aspect of cognition was found in both studies, but only in subgroups of patients. Five studies investigated the effects of intravenous or subcutaneous physostigmine (8,18,29,71,74). In all five studies, a range of doses was tested in each patient, and the optimal dose was determined individually. Some significant improvement in memory was found in four studies (8,18,29,74), and the fifth (71) found improved constructional praxis in three of six patients. The remaining six studies (6,16,53,67,84,88) tested the effects of oral physostigmine administered over several days. Four of these studies (6,53,67,84) found some evidence of improvement at least in a subgroup of patients. The doses most usually associated with symptomatic improvement were 2.0 and 2.5 mg every 2 hr.

No demographic factors such as age, sex, or age of onset were clear predictors of response in any study. There was, however, strong suggestive evidence that the drug only improved symptoms in a subset of patients who absorbed the drug into the CNS and in whom the drug actually enhanced central cholinergic activity. Specifically, Thal et al. (84) found that memory improvement following physostigmine was highly correlated with cholinesterase inhibition in CSF. Mohs et al. (67) found that cognitive improvement while receiving physostigmine was correlated with the percentage increase in diurnal cortisol secretion; since central cholinergic stimulation causes cortisol release

TABLE 1. *Clinical trials of cholinesterase inhibitors in patients with Alzheimer's disease*

Study	Patients	Drug and doses	Major findings
Beller et al. (6)	4M, 4F 58–83 years	Oral physostigmine 0.5, 1.0, 2.0 mg q2h	Significant increase in word recall at 2.0-mg dose
Blackwood and Christie (8)	4M, 8F 54–68 years	Physostigmine i.v. 0.75 mg	Significant improvement in recognition memory
Caltagirone et al. (16)	8 patients with onset before age 65	Oral physostigmine 1.0 mg qid	No improvement in memory or behavior
Christie et al. (18)	11 patients with onset before age 65	Physostigmine i.v. 0.25, 0.375, 0.75 mg	Significant increase in picture recognition at 0.375-mg dose
Davis and Mohs (29)	8M, 2F 50–68 years	Physostigmine i.v. 0.125, 0.25, 0.5 mg	Significant increase in recognition memory at individual best dose
Jenike et al. (53)	5M, 7F 53–89 years	Oral physostigmine 0.5–3.0 mg q2h	8 of 12 showed some evidence of improved memory
Kaye et al. (54)	10 patients 51–71 years	Oral THA 30 mg plus 60 g lecithin	Significant increase in serial learning for least demented patients
Mohs et al. (67)	8M, 4F 52–76 years	Oral physostigmine 0.5, 1.0, 1.5, 2.0 mg q2h	Cognitive improvement correlated with cortisol rise on best individual dose
Muramoto et al. (71)[a]	3M, 3F 51–63 years	Physostigmine i.v. or s.c. 0.3 to 1.0 mg	3 of 6 showed improvement in praxis
Peters and Levin (74)[a]	4M, 1F 58–79 years	Physostigmine s.c. 0.005–0.015 mg/kg plus 3.6 g lecithin	4 of 5 showed significant improvement in verbal learning
Summers et al. (83)[a]	3M, 9F 42–85 years	THA i.v. 0.25–1.5 mg/kg	Significant improvement in orientation for some patients at individual best dose
Thal et al. (84)	5M, 3F 55–78 years	Oral physostigmine 0.5–2.5 mg q2h plus lecithin 10.8 g/day	Significant increase in verbal memory at individual best dose correlated with AChE inhibition of CSF
Wettstein (88)	5M, 3F 50–70 years	Oral physostigmine 1–2 mg q2h plus lecithin 18 g/day	No improvement in praxis, language orientation, or behavior

[a] Studies not conducted under double-blind conditions.

(25), this finding suggests an association of symptom improvement with enhanced central cholinergic activity. Conversely, it appears that many patients show no effect of oral physostigmine either because they do not absorb the drug into the bloodstream or because they have such extensive cholinergic cell loss that no amount of cholinesterase inhibition can enhance cholinergic activity. Two studies of oral physostigmine found no effect on any patient. In one study (16), the 1-mg dose was clearly below the doses found effective in other studies. Why there was no effect in the study by Wettstein (88) is not clear, although it may be because the patients in this study were relatively advanced cases.

To summarize, the majority of studies investigating cholinesterase inhibitors in AD find that these drugs can improve symptoms, particularly memory, in some patients if doses are titrated individually. Even in the best cases, however, only modest and transient symptom improvements were observed. Factors that might predict a positive response to cholinesterase inhibitors are not yet established, but it appears that lack of response is often because of poor absorption of oral drug or the failure to achieve cholinergic enhancement because of extensive cell loss. The most widely studied oral drug, physostigmine, has the additional disadvantage of a short half-life, necessitating frequent administration.

Agonists

Many of the toxicity and administration problems encountered in testing cholinesterase inhibitors also apply to the agonists. Arecoline, a muscarinic agonist, has been shown to improve memory transiently when given subcutaneously to both normal young adults (82) and patients with AD (18). This drug has a short half-life and has not been given orally. It appears to have no advantage over physostigmine. Oxotremorine is a cholinergic agonist with a half-life of several hours, but the drug also is very toxic at high doses. We have administered oxotremorine to seven patients with AD in single oral doses ranging from 0.25 mg to 2.0 mg. Five of the patients experienced side effects, primarily depression and gastrointestinal upset, sufficent to warrant discontinuance of the study (27); no patient showed a measurable memory enhancement. Side effects of this sort have been reported with high doses of physostigmine (28) but appear to be particularly problematical with agonists and thus may limit their utility. One orally active cholinergic agonist, RS-86, is currently available from the Sandoz Corporation for testing. We have administered RS-86 to 12 patients with AD in oral doses ranging from 0.5 mg to 1.5 mg three times per day. Seven patients showed some improvement in cognition that was replicated when their optimal dose was readministered. Similar results have been reported by Wettstein and Spiegel (89). Although this drug clearly deserves further evaluation, it must be kept in mind that, as with oral physostigmine, even patients who improved remained quite demented, and all improvements lasted only while the drug was pharmacologically active.

Noncholinergic Drugs

As reviewed in the chapter by E. K. Perry in this volume, several noncholinergic neurochemical deficits have been identified in at least a subset of patients with AD. Whether or not pharmacotherapy aimed at reversing these other deficits will be of any benefit remains to be determined, since few studies have been conducted in this area. Of particular interest would be studies of drugs acting on the noradrenergic system, since there is good evidence that this system is involved in normal memory functioning (62), it is impaired in some AD patients (22), and, in Korsakoff patients, the α-adrenergic agonist clonidine can enhance memory (61). Methylphenidate, however, did not improve memory when given in various doses to elderly patients, some of whom probably had AD (21). Some studies have investigated the effects of dopaminergic drugs in AD patients, although the neurochemical rationale for such trials is not entirely clear. Levodopa was found to improve intellectual scores of a group of AD patients in one study (33), but others (56) have failed to confirm this result.

For a brief period of time there was interest in the possibility that opiate antagonists might be of some value in treating patients with AD. Naloxone has been shown to improve memory in rodents when given under certain conditions (51) and can reverse some effects of ischemia in man (3) and animals (49). One study (75) reported apparent dramatic improvement when naloxone was given to AD patients. A subsequent multicenter study using carefully diagnosed patients and double-blind conditions failed to find any effect of naloxone in patients with AD (9).

A variety of drugs purported to be either vasodilators and/or metabolic enhancers have been developed and tested as possible treatments for dementia. For the most part, these drugs were developed because of the view that most dementias result from inadequate blood flow to the brain or because of nonspecific metabolic deficiencies. A list of some of the drugs in these classes is presented in Table 2. As our understanding of the pathophysiology of

dementia, particularly AD, has increased, the rationale for such drugs is no longer plausible. Extensive clinical testing of many of these compounds has been conducted, although the majority of the published studies do not meet contemporary standards for diagnostic rigor or for specificity of outcome measures as described above. Previous reviews have suggested that some of these compounds may have modest beneficial effects on behavior when administered to some elderly people with poorly defined syndromes (76); however, there is no convincing evidence that any of these drugs can improve the core cognitive abnormalities of AD (92). It has been speculated that some of these drugs may have weak antidepressant or antianxiety effects in the elderly (13). Whether this is the case cannot be ascertained from available data.

STUDIES IN PATIENTS WITH MULTIINFARCT DEMENTIA

Methodologic Considerations

Many of the methodologic concerns described above regarding diagnosis, outcome measures, and choice of drug apply to studies in patients with multiinfarct dementia (MID) just as they do for studies in patients with AD. The diagnosis of MID is, if anything, even more difficult than the diagnosis of AD during life. No generally agreed-on clinical criteria for MID have been established. Although areas of cerebral infarction are sometimes visible on CT scan, they may not be evident in every case of MID (36). In addition, MID and AD frequently coexist, so evidence of MID does not rule out the possibility of AD. Clinical features and risk factors suggestive of MID have been proposed by Hachinski et al. (40) and have been partially validated with blood flow (40) and autopsy (78) data. It is likely that selection of patients with these characteristics and little evidence of other kinds of dementia may identify a relatively homogeneous group for clinical drug trials. However, few studies conducted to date have used explicit criteria to identify patients with MID, and thus it is likely that most studies including patients with MID also included other types of dementias.

The symptoms associated with MID are similar to the symptoms of AD, although, because of the different pathophysiologies of these two diseases, the longitudinal course of symptoms may be different. Psychometric tests usually do not differentiate the two conditions cross-sectionally (14). As with AD, no single instrument has been generally accepted as a measure of treatment efficacy. Given the similarity of symptoms in the two conditions, however, it seems likely that assessment instruments appropriate for AD would also be appropriate for MID.

Clinical Trials

Given the nature of the pathophysiology of MID, it is likely that drugs or other treatments acting on the vascular system could possibly be of some benefit. A number of drugs (see Table 2) have been developed as vasodilators

TABLE 2. *Vasodilators and metabolic enhancers tested for use in treating dementia*

Bencyclane
Betahistine
Cinnarizine (Mitronal®)
Cyclandelate (Cyclospasmol®)
Dihydroergotoxine mesylate (Hydergine®)
Isoxsuprine hydrochloride (Vasodilan®)
Nafronyl oxalate (Praxiline®)
Papaverine hydrochloride (Parabid®)
Pentifylline (Cosalden®)
Pyritinol plus pyridylcarbinol (Decaden®)
Xanthinol niacinate

in an attempt to increase blood flow to brain areas that have suffered ischemic damage. The theoretical rationale for drugs of this type has been questioned (41), since it may be that vasodilators actually reduce blood flow to affected areas by increasing the volume capacity of the circulatory system. In addition, since hypertension is a risk factor for MID (40,78), prevention of additional ischemic damage by control of blood pressure may be more effective in many cases than any efforts to restore lost cerebral function pharmacologically.

For many of the drugs that have been developed as vasodilators, the physiological effects are not known precisely. For some, such as papaverine (52) and dihydroergocornine (42), their effects on cerebral blood flow have been measured directly, usually via the xenon-133 inhalation technique. Although there is evidence that they can increase cerebral blood flow under some circumstances, they do not increase oxygen consumption in brain (42,52); thus, it is not clear whether these drugs have any substantial effect on neuronal activity. Clinical studies of drugs with vasoactive properties given to patients with dementia have produced mixed results, and many of the studies are difficult to interpret because they do not adequately address one or more of the methodologic problems mentioned above. Some studies have shown modest improvement in elderly patients given these drugs (5,38), but others have not (50). The latter group tends to include more studies in which objective psychometric tests rather than clinical rating scales have been used as outcome measures. One review by Yesavage et al. published in 1979 (92) concluded that drugs with mixed vasodilating and metabolic effects have generally produced more positive effects than have drugs that are primarily vasodilators. The former group includes dihydroergotoxin mesylate (Hydergine®) and nafronyl oxalate (Praxiline®). Although this generalization is still accurate as a summary of the clinical trials reported to date, there has been little further development of either the primary vasodilators or drugs with mixed effects. The rationale for using these drugs remains questionable, and the clinical evidence for their efficacy in dementia remains weak. Certainly, there is no evidence that any of these drugs is of special benefit to patients with dementia secondary to multiple cerebral infarcts.

STUDIES IN PATIENTS WITH PARKINSON'S DISEASE AND DEMENTIA

Methodologic Considerations

Parkinson's disease is primarily a movement disorder, and many early descriptions indicated that cognitive processes were unimpaired in patients with this disease (48). However, more recent investigators have observed that many parkinsonian patients evidence some cognitive impairment and that, at least in some individuals, those impairments can be quite severe (59). Since parkinsonian patients may have low motivation to perform well on cognitive tests, and because many cognitive tests require some controlled movement, it is difficult to detect subtle cognitive impairments in these patients. The problem of measuring cognitive effects of drug treatments in patients with Parkinson's disease is also difficult because of the movement disorder associated with this disease. As an obvious example, tests of praxis are very difficult to interpret in these patients. Although no satisfactory method for assessing cognitive changes completely independently of changes in motor control has been devised, it is incumbent on psychopharmacologic investigators in this area to minimize the inevitable difficulties of interpretation by including cognitive evaluation procedures that minimize the influence of motoric factors.

At present it is still not clear whether the severe dementia observed in some parkinsonian patients results from the primary brain lesions of Parkinson's disease (PD) or from concomitant Alzheimer's disease. Autopsy studies (10) indicate that a much higher than expected proportion of parkinsonian patients also have neuropathologic changes characteristic of AD. Patients with PD also have a substantial loss of cholinergic cells in the nucleus basalis (17), a lesion thought to be responsible for many of the symptoms of AD (20). Despite these neuropathologic and neurochemical similarities, there is no epidemiologic evidence to suggest that these two diseases share any common etiologic factors (46,47). Thus, the ultimate cause of dementia in PD patients remains unclear.

Clinical Trials

Several clinical studies have examined the question of whether PD patients' cognitive status changes when they are treated. Just as in normal people, anticholinergics given to PD patients cause memory impairments that are easily detectable with psychometric tests (79). Conversely, PD patients given levodopa or levodopa plus carbidopa almost invariably show improved performance on cognitive tests (4,64). The difficulty with these later studies is that it is often difficult to determine whether the improved performance represents a genuine increase in cognitive capacity or is secondary to improved motivation and movement control. Given the consistency of the finding both across studies and across cognitive tasks, it is likely that both factors play a role.

Because of the fact that cholinomimetic drugs exacerbate parkinsonian symptoms, no attempts have been made to treat the dementia of PD with drugs like physostigmine. The fact that parkinsonian dementia may be a result of even more types of cell loss than is Alzheimer-type dementia, plus the additional problems posed by trying to improve both movement and cognition, make all psychopharmacologic approaches to this condition difficult.

CONCLUSIONS

Rapid advances in our understanding of the neurochemical deficits in AD, MID, and parkinsonian dementia have opened an entire new era in the psychopharmacology of dementia. Although clinically useful treatments for most dementias are not yet available, the search for such treatments is now proceeding in a rational, scientific way. Some limited success has been achieved in trying to treat AD with cholinesterase inhibitors; additional studies in this area are warranted. Fully successful treatment of these conditions may be possible only by pharmacological agents that act on some very fundamental neurochemical defect that is responsible for the many neurotransmitter and neuromodulator abnormalities observed in demented patients.

REFERENCES

1. Altman, H. J., and Quartermain, D. (1983): *Behav. Brain Res.,* 7: 51–63.
2. Bartus, R. T., Dean, R. L., Beer, B., and Lippa, A. S. (1982): *Science,* 217:408–417.
3. Baskin, D. S., and Hosobuchi, Y. (1981): *Lancet,* 2:272–275.
4. Beardsley, J. V., and Puletti, F. (1972): *Arch. Neurol.,* 25:145–150.
5. Bell, J. A. C., and Taylor, A. R. (1967): *Br. Med. J.,* 3:525–528.
6. Beller, S. A., Overall, J. E., and Swann, A. C. (1985): *Psychopharmacology,* 87:147–151.
7. Bierkamper, G. G., and Goldberg, A. M. (1979): In: *Nutrition and the Brain,* edited by A. Barbeau, J. H. Growden, and R. J. Wurtman, pp. 243–251. Raven Press, New York.
8. Blackwood, D. H. R., and Christie, J. E. (1986): *Biol. Psychiatry,* 21:557–560.
9. Blass, J. P., Reding, M. J., Drachman, D., Mitchell, A., Glesser, G., et al. (1983): *N. Engl. J. Med.,* 309:586.
10. Boller, F., Mizutani, T., Roessmann, U., and Gambetti, P. (1980): *Ann. Neurol.,* 7:329–335.
11. Bowen, D. M., Allen, S. J., Benton, J. S., Goodhardt, M. J., Haan, E. A., et al. (1983): *J. Neurochem.,* 41:266–272.
12. Bowen, D. M., Smith, C. B., White, P., and Davison, A. N. (1976): *Brain,* 99:459–496.
13. Branconnier, R. J., and Cole, J. O. (1977): *J. Am. Geriatr. Soc.,* 25:458–562.
14. Brinkman, S. D., and Braun, P. (1984): *J. Clin. Neuropsychol.,* 6: 393–400.
15. Brunello, N., Cheney, D. L., and Costa, E. (1982): *J. Neurochem.,* 38:1160–1163.
16. Caltagirone, C., Gainotti, G., and Masullo, C. (1982): *Int. J. Neurosci.,* 16:247–249.
17. Candy, J. M., Perry, R. H., Perry, E. K., Irving, D., Blessed, G., et al. (1983): *J. Neurol. Sci.,* 54:277–289.
18. Christie, J. E., Shering, A., Ferguson, J., and Glen, A. I. M. (1981): *Br. J. Psychiatry,* 138:46–50.
19. Cohen, E. I., and Wurtman, R. J. (1976): *Science,* 191:561–562.
20. Coyle, J. T., Price, D. L., and DeLong, M. R. (1983): *Science,* 219:1184–1190.
21. Crook, T., Ferris, S., Sathananthan, G., Raskin, A., and Gershon, S. (1977): *Psychopharmacology,* 52:251–255.
22. Cross, A. J., Crow, T. J., Perry, E. K., Perry, R. H., Blessed, G., et al. (1981): *Br. Med. J.,* 2:93–94.
23. Davies, P., Katzman, R., and Terry, R. D. (1980): *Nature,* 288: 279–280.
24. Davies, P., and Maloney, A. J. F. (1976): *Lancet,* 2:1403.
25. Davis, B. M., Brown, G. M., Miller, M., Friesen, H. G., Kastin, A. J., et al. (1982): *Psychoneuroendocrinology,* 7:347–354.
26. Davis, B. M., and Davis, K. L. (1980): *Biol. Psychiatry,* 15:303–310.
27. Davis, K. L., Hollander, E., Davidson, M., Davis, B. M., Mohs, R. C., et al. (1987): *Am. J. Psychiat. (in press).*
28. Davis, K. L., Hollister, L. E., Overall, J., Johnson, A., and Train, K. (1976): *Psychopharmacology,* 51:23–27.
29. Davis, K. L., and Mohs, R. C. (1982): *Am. J. Psychiatry,* 139: 1421–1424.
30. Davis, K. L., Mohs, R. C., Tinklenberg, J. R., Hollister, L. E., Pfefferbaum, A., et al. (1978): *Science,* 201:272–274.
31. Drachman, D. A. (1977): *Neurology (Minneap.),* 27:783–790.
32. Drachman, D. A., and Leavitt, J. (1974): *Arch. Neurol.,* 30:113–121.
33. Drachman, D. A., and Stahl, S. (1975): *Lancet,* 1:809.
34. Flood, J. F., Landry, D. W., and Jarvick, M. E. (1981): *Brain Res.,* 215:177–185.
35. Fovall, P., Dysken, M. W., Lazarus, L. W., Davis, J. M., Kahn, R. L., et al. (1980): *Commun. Psychopharmacol.,* 4:141–146.
36. Fox, J. H., Kazniak, A. W., and Huckman, M. (1979): *N. Engl. J. Med.,* 300:437.
37. Fuld, P. A., Katzman, R., Davies, P., and Terry, R. D. (1982): *Ann. Neurol.,* 11:155–159.
38. Gaitz, C. M., Varner, R. V., and Overall, J. E. (1977): *Arch. Gen. Psychiatry,* 34:839–845.
39. Guy, W. (1976): *ECDEU Assessment Manual.* DHEW Publication No. (ADM) 76–338, Rockville, MD.
40. Hachinski, V. C., Hiff, L. D., Zilhka, E., Duboulay, G. H., McAllister, V. L., et al. (1975): *Arch. Neurol.,* 32:632–637.
41. Hachinski, V. C., Lassen, N. A., and Marshall, J. (1974): *Lancet,* 2:207–210.
42. Hafkenschiel, J. H., Crumpton, C. W., Moyer, J. H., and Jeffers, J. H. (1950): *J. Clin. Invest.,* 298:408–411.
43. Hamilton, M. (1960): *J. Neurol. Neurosurg. Psychiatry,* 23:56–62.
44. Haroutunian, V., Kanof, P., and Davis, K. L. (1985): *Life Sci.,* 37:945–952.
45. Haubrich, D. R., Wang, P. F. L., Clody, D. E., and Wedeking, P. W. (1975): *Life Sci.,* 17:975–980.
46. Heston, L. E., Mastri, A. R., Anderson, E., and White, J. (1981): *Arch. Gen. Psychiatry,* 38:1085–1090.
47. Heyman, A., Wilkinson, W. E., Stafford, J. A., Helms, N. J., Sigmon, A. H., et al. (1984): *Ann. Neurol.,* 15:335–341.
48. Hoehn, M. M., and Yahr, M. D. (1967): *Neurology (Minneap.),* 17:427–442.
49. Hosobuchi, Y., Baskin, D. S., and Woo, S. K. (1982): *Science,* 215:69–71.
50. Hughes, J. R., Williams, J. G., and Currier, R. D. (1976): *J. Am. Geriatr. Soc.,* 24:490–497.
51. Izuierdo, I. (1979): *Psychopharmacology,* 66:199–203.
52. Jayne, H. W., Scheinberg, P., Rich, M., and Belle, M. S. (1952): *J. Clin. Invest.,* 31:111–114.
53. Jenike, M. A., Albert, M. S., Heller, H., Gunther, J., and Goff, D. (1987): *Arch. Gen. Psychiatry (in press).*
54. Kaye, W. H., Sitaram, N., Weingartner, H., Ebert, M. H., Smallberg, S., et al. (1982): *Biol. Psychiatry,* 17:275–280.
55. Ketchum, J. S., Sidell, F. R., Crowell, E. B., Aghajanian, G. K., and Hayes, A. H. (1973): *Psychopharmacologia,* 28:121–145.
56. Kristensen, V., Olsen, M., and Theilgaard, A. (1977): *Acta Psychiatr. Scand.,* 55:41–51.
57. Krnjevick, K., and Reinhardt, W. (1980): *Science,* 206:1321–1323.
58. Levy, R., Little, A., Chuaqui, P., and Reith, M. (1983): *Lancet,* 1: 987–988.
59. Lieberman, A., Dziatolowski, M., Kupersmith, M., Serby, M., Goodgold, A., et al. (1979): *Ann. Neurol.,* 6:355–356.
60. Marsden, C. D., and Harrison, M. J. G. (1972): *Br. Med. J.,* 2: 249–252.
61. McEntee, W. J., and Mair, R. G. (1980): *Ann. Neurol.,* 7:466–470.
62. McGaugh, J. L. (1973): *Annu. Rev. Pharmacol.,* 13:229–241.
63. McKhann, G., Drachman, D., Folstein, M., Katzman, R., Price, D., et al. (1984): *Neurology (N.Y.),* 34:939–944.
64. Meier, M., and Martin, W. E. (1970): *J.A.M.A.,* 213:465–466.
65. Millington, W. R., and Wurtman, R. J. (1982): *Eur. J. Pharmacol.,* 80:431–434.
66. Mohs, R. C., and Davis, K. L. (1985): *Life Sci.,* 37:193–197.
67. Mohs, R. C., Davis, B. M., Johns, C. A., Mathe, A. A., Greenwald, B. S., et al. (1985): *Am. J. Psychiatry,* 142:28–33.
68. Mohs, R. C., Davis, K. L., and Levy, M. I. (1982): *Life Sci.,* 23: 1317–1323.
69. Mohs, R. C., Davis, K. L., Tinklenberg, J. R., and Hollister, L. E. (1980): *Neurobiol. Aging,* 1:21–25.
70. Mohs, R. C., Davis, K. L., Tinklenberg, J. R., Hollister, L. E., Yesavage, J. A., et al. (1979): *Am. J. Psychiatry,* 136:1275–1277.
71. Muramoto, O., Sugishita, M., and Ando, K. (1984): *J. Neurol. Neurosurg. Psychiatry,* 47:485–491.
72. Overall, J. E., and Gorham, D. R. (1962): *Psychol. Rep.,* 10:799–812.
73. Perry, E. K., Perry, R. H., Blessed, G., and Tomlinson, B. E. (1977): *Lancet,* 1:189.

74. Peters, B. H., and Levin, H. S. (1979): *Ann. Neurol.,* 6:219–221.
75. Reisberg, B., Ferris, S. H., Anand, R., Mir, P., Geibel, V., et al. (1983): *N. Engl. J. Med.,* 308:721–722.
76. Reisberg, B. A., Ferris, S. H., and Gershon, S. (1981): *Am. J. Psychiatry,* 138:593–600.
77. Rosen, W. G., Mohs, R. C., and Davis, K. L. (1984): *Am. J. Psychiatry,* 141:1356–1364.
78. Rosen, W. G., Terry, R. D., Fuld, P. A., Katzman, R., and Peck, A. (1979): *Ann. Neurol.,* 7:486–488.
79. Sadeh, M., Braham, J., and Modan, M. (1982): *Arch. Neurol.,* 39:666–667.
80. Shader, R. I., Harmatz, J. S., and Salzman, C. (1974): *J. Am. Geriatr. Soc.,* 22:107–113.
81. Simon, J. R., and Kuhar, M. J. (1975): *Nature,* 255:162–163.
82. Sitaram, N., Weingartner, H., and Gillin, J. C. (1978): *Science,* 201:274–276.
83. Summers, W. K., Viesselman, J. O., Marsh, G. M., and Candelora, K. (1981): *Biol. Psychiatry,* 16:145–153.
84. Thal, L. J., Fuld, P. A., Masur, D. M., and Sharpless, N. S. (1983): *Ann. Neurol.,* 13:491–496.
85. Thal, L. J., Rosen, W. G., Sharpless, N. S., and Crystal, H. A. (1981): *Neurobiol. Aging,* 2:205–208.
86. Ulus, I. H., and Wurtman, R. J. (1976): *Science,* 194:1060–1062.
87. Wecker, L., Dettbarn, W., and Schmidt, D. E. (1978): *Science,* 199:86–87.
88. Wettstein, A. (1983): *Ann. Neurol.,* 13:210–212.
89. Wettstein, A., and Spiegel, R. (1984): *Psychopharmacology,* 84:572–573.
90. Whelpton, R. (1983): *J. Chromatogr.,* 272:216–220.
91. Wurtman, R. J., Hefti, F., and Melamed, E. (1981): *Pharmacol. Rev.,* 32:315–335.
92. Yesavage, J. A., Tinklenberg, J. A., Hollister, L. E., and Berger, P. A. (1979): *Arch. Gen. Psychiatry,* 36:220–223.

Psychopharmacology:
The Third Generation of Progress,
edited by Herbert Y. Meltzer.
Raven Press, New York © 1987.

CHAPTER 92

Genetic Factors in the Etiology of Alzheimer's Disease

John C. S. Breitner

Given the enormous public health problem of Alzheimer's disease[1] (AD), the current understanding of its causes is disappointing. Epidemiologic studies (often a clue to etiology) have revealed only two firmly established risk factors for AD: advanced age and the presence of relatives affected with the disease (4,24,30,32,35,36,64). These results suggest that some interaction of aging and genetic vulnerability may ultimately predispose to the disease process of AD. Morphological, neurochemical, and pharmacologic studies (reviewed elsewhere in this volume) have suggested various mechanisms and possible causes for this process, and these are discussed briefly. The main aim of this chapter, however, is evaluation of the evidence that genetic vulnerability is a major etiologic influence in AD.

REVIEW OF ETIOLOGIC THEORIES

Although genetic theories are reserved for the bulk of this chapter, other proposed causes are reviewed here briefly. A number of plausible etiologic hypotheses for AD have prompted investigation. These include viral etiologies (including slow viruses), immunological causes, and the possible influence of toxins (either endogenous or environmental).

---

[1] This term refers throughout this chapter to the complex of presenile Alzheimer's disease and senile dementia of the Alzheimer type.

Viral Theories

The revolutionary discovery that slowly progressive neurodegenerative disorders may be caused by transmissible agents (26) has prompted speculation that the neuropathologic features of AD may be virally induced (65). Work in laboratory animals has shown that, depending on the genotype of the host and the particular strain of pathogen employed, several of the temporal and neuropathologic characteristics of AD may be seen in scrapie infection. In many host/agent combinations, the onset of clinical disease occurs near the end of the normal life-span for the animal, and the distribution of onset times is remarkably narrow (Fig. 1.), as it is also in Alzheimer's disease (see below). Scrapie-infected mice have been shown to produce typical senile plaques, neurofibrillary changes, and alterations in the blood–brain barrier suggestive of human AD (reviewed in ref. 11). A deficiency in choline acetyltransferase (ChAT) similar to that seen in AD has also been described in scrapie (43).

Such findings have prompted investigation of the transmissibility of AD to nonhuman primates. As of 1982, brain homogenates from a total of 97 AD patients had been inoculated into various animal species. Excluding 40 instances in which the inoculum was considered "suboptimal" or the period of observation was short, all of 57 experiments showed no transmission of clinical disease despite postin-

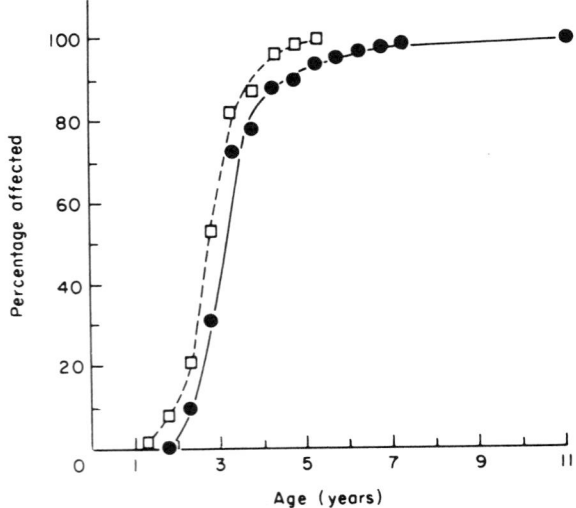

FIG. 1. The cumulative distribution of onset times for naturally occurring scrapie disease in outbred sheep. The curves apply only to those animals who are known to be "predisposed" to scrapie by virtue of the fact that they eventually developed disease. Note the similarity in shape between these curves and the distribution of onset times for AD in relatives shown in Fig. 5. Note also that the steepness of the curves produces an unexpected finding: even though the curves for males (*open squares*) and females (*closed circles*) differ only slightly in their position on the abscissa, there may be dramatic differences in age-specific cumulative incidence. Thus, at age 3 years the cumulative incidence in rams is 82%, whereas that in ewes is 30%, even though all these animals ultimately developed disease. Caution is therefore warranted when interpreting even marked differences in apparent sex-related incidence at specific ages before manifestation is largely complete. The same may apply to AD. (From Parry, ref. 53a, with permission of the editor and publishers.)

oculation observation periods exceeding by two standard deviations the mean incubation period for experimental Creutzfeldt–Jakob disease (9). Such negative results, although possibly attributable to incompatibility of agent and experimental host (27), have dampened early enthusiasm for a transmissible agent etiology (26).

Immunologic Theories

The strongest link between AD and immune function is the well-established presence of amyloid in senile plaques. Amyloid is a common finding in a number of immunologically caused illnesses (5), and immunoglobulins have been found in the amyloid of AD plaques (38). The alteration in AD of the blood–brain barrier (66) may be instrumental in deposition of immune complexes. Immunoglobulin with target specificity for neural tissue is present in the sera of some old mice and has also been found in sera of older "normal" humans and those with Alzheimer's disease (51).

Abnormality of immune function has therefore been proposed as a cause of AD. This idea has prompted investigation of immune-related HLA and complement polymorphisms in affected humans. The results of such studies (reviewed in ref. 41) are in conflict. The HLA types B_7 and C_{w3} may be unexpectedly prevalent in AD cases, and one study (62) showed the relatively rare B_7 C_{w3} haplotype in 9.1% of AD patients but only 3.6% of controls. The HLA-linked complement C4 allelic markers may also be linked to AD, and one recent study (53) showed a strong association with type C4B2. To the author's knowledge, however, no immunologic theory has yet been proposed that can account for all of the experimental observations in AD.

Toxins

Although endogenous toxins and deposition of waste products have occasionally been proposed as causes of AD, little direct evidence supports these theories. There are considerable data, however, suggesting that deposition of aluminum salts may be involved in pathogenesis (17). Intravenous administration in rabbits of soluble aluminum salts induces the formation of argyrophilic tangles resembling those seen in AD (39), although the filaments are straight rather than helical (59). Increased concentrations of aluminum have been found in AD brain tissue (16), and X-ray spectrometric methods have recently been used to demonstrate its accumulation specifically in neurofibrillary tangles (54).

Although aluminum might thus be a cause of the brain lesions of AD, its deposition may also be a passive consequence of a breakdown of normal barriers to its presence. Thus, much higher crude concentrations of aluminum are found in brains of patients with dialysis encephalopathy (2,20), but such patients do not show plaques and tangles (10) even though their brains contain aluminum concentrations sufficient to have produced tangles in experimental animals (44). Also, several case-control epidemiologic studies have investigated the possible influence of aluminum exposure on risk for AD with negative results (4,24,34). Thus, a direct etiologic role for aluminum in the pathogenesis of AD is unconfirmed.

Genetic Theories

Interest in the genetics of AD stems from pedigree studies and from the observation of familial aggregation among the pooled relatives of groups of AD index cases (probands). These two types of studies are discussed in turn.

Figure 2 typifies the results of pedigree studies of so-called familial AD. It shows the pedigree of a family with numerous cases of AD. Several points are noteworthy: (a) the disease is seen in three successive generations; (b) approximately equal numbers of males and females are affected; (c) about half of each generation eventually develops AD; but (d) presumably because of their relative youth, individuals in the fourth or fifth generation show no disease. Except for point "d," the pedigree is typical of those found in diseases caused by the operation of a simple Mendelian autosomal gene that is dominant, i.e., expressed in the heterozygote. The absence of disease in the youngest

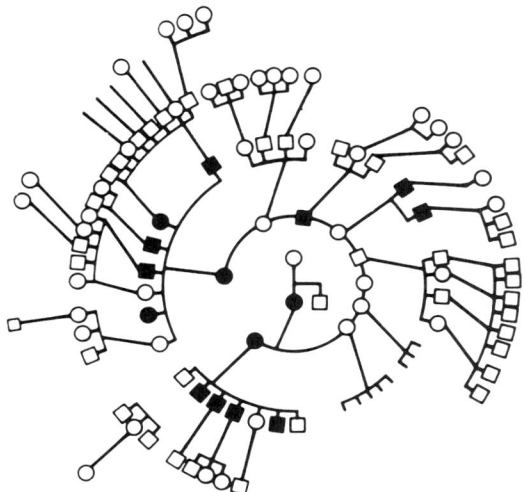

FIG. 2. Pedigree of a family where Alzheimer's disease is apparently transmitted as an autosomal dominant trait, published by Feldman et al. (21). Note transmission of disease through three generations, with roughly 50% risk among members of each generation and occurrence of disease in both males and females. Note also, however, that disease is not yet apparent in the two youngest generations. (Reproduced from Sinex and Myers, ref. 57, by permission of the authors and publishers.)

difficulties, and these are therefore addressed in some detail before the available data are reviewed.

The Issue of Diagnostic Specificity

Alzheimer's disease is only one (if admittedly the most common) among many causes of the dementia syndrome. Its definitive diagnosis requires careful clinical investigation and, ultimately, the demonstration of characteristic changes at autopsy. Before death, the presumptive diagnosis is made principally by exclusion of other specific, often focal, pathologic processes (e.g., multiple infarcts, tumor, hydrocephalus, Parkinson's disease). Although certain clinical characteristics may be typical, there are no pathognomonic signs or specific laboratory tests for AD (37).

It stands to reason that any such diagnosis of exclusion (DSM-III schizophrenia is a comparable example) may retain considerable heterogeneity in etiology and pathogenesis. This heterogeneity will have important consequences for genetic studies in pooled AD proband relatives. If AD were genetically transmitted, the "true" influence of genetic causes would be obscured by the admixture of phenocopies (index cases with a similar phenotype but lacking genetic etiology) in etiologically heterogeneous groups of index cases. To the extent that a proband population contained phenocopies, there would be a reduction in the apparent genetic predisposition among relatives.

Diagnostic specificity is thus an important precondition to the valid assessment of familial risks, and interest is growing in the identification of specific markers, including purely clinical characteristics of disease, that may identify "purer" populations of cases. For example, the recently proposed NINCDS/ADRDA consensus diagnostic criteria (45) note that the clinical diagnosis is supported by such specific features as "progressive deterioration of specific cognitive functions such as language (aphasia), motor skills (apraxia), and perception (agnosia)" as well as family history of similar disorders. Other more objective markers such as CSF cholinesterase (reviewed in ref. 37) and changes on positron emission tomography (13,25) are also under investigation.

members of the family is readily understood since, like Huntington's disease, familial polyposis coli, and a few other dominant genetic disorders, AD has its onset in later life.

Over 50 familial AD pedigrees have now been reported (52; earlier reports reviewed in ref. 22). Collectively, they suggest that, at least in some families, predisposition to AD may be transmitted as an autosomal dominant trait (46). The affected families have come to note, however, because of their rarity. They no doubt represent a biased sample of AD, and their implication for the likelihood of a genetic etiology in most AD is uncertain. Their striking feature is the early age of onset of AD, when present, generally in the 60s, 50s, or even the 40s. In population studies such early onset occurs in a small minority of AD cases (30,49). The probability of many such early onset cases in one family purely by chance is therefore small, and another explanation is required.

Since the reported pedigrees suggest the operation of an autosomal dominant AD gene, they have prompted consideration of whether such a gene may operate in AD generally. Because of its rarity and its atypical character, however, the early onset familial AD observed in selected pedigrees can yield only limited inference on possible genetic causes of AD. Broader inference becomes possible only when the disease is studied in larger samples of pooled relatives at risk, some of whom develop more typical disease. Such studies have consistently shown increased familial risks of AD in proband families, and some investigators have interpreted these risks as suggesting specific modes of genetic transmission (see below). But the interpretation of the data is complicated by a number of methodologic

The Implications of the Late Onset of AD

It is well known that the risk of AD is slight in middle age but increases rapidly thereafter, at least into the ninth decade[2] (29,30,49). Thus, any underlying genetic diathesis would likely become fully apparent only in extreme old age. Many relatives still under observation will not yet have reached such an age, and others will have died from competing causes before their genetic predisposition (if any) could be expressed (7,8,40,57). Failure to consider or adjust for this possibility must result in underestimation of the familial predisposition to AD.

---

[2] At least in one population (59a), the incidence has been shown to increase to roughly 2% per year in the early 80s. Some authors suggest that incidence falls thereafter, but the data are sparse and their implications controversial.

PREDICTED CHARACTERISTICS OF GENETICALLY CAUSED AD

What familial risks should one expect in relatives of AD probands and controls if AD were conditioned by an autosomal dominant gene? The answers to this question may be projected if certain premises are posited and their consequences considered.

If AD were in fact attributable to a dominant gene, then individuals with this gene would presumably be destined to develop the disease in late life. There should, however, be a finite probability (however small) of gene expression at any age. To avoid the ambiguity in such terms as "variable penetrance," let us require that the expression of the hypothetical AD gene must be essentially complete by extreme old age (i.e., penetrance is complete, but gene expression is age-dependent). This statement implies that the cumulative probability of gene expression in predisposed individuals must approach an asymptotic value of 1.0 at some (perhaps very late) age.[3] It cannot sensibly exceed this value. These conditions satisfy the definition of a probability distribution function (50) for gene expression. Then (excepting such anomalies as a rectangular distribution function) the age-specific probability density of gene expression would be expected to reach a maximum at some point, after which it will decline (7).

Hence, when relatives have the putative AD gene, each age x years will dictate an associated probability density $f(x)$ that the gene will be expressed (by onset of disease) in that year, and the total probability over time must be 1. Summing the age-specific probability densities up to a particular age x will yield a cumulative age-specific probability of disease expression, denoted $F(x)$, that should be reflected in the cumulative risk of disease by age x. The expected value of the cumulative incidence $I(x)$ at any age x is then equal to $F(x)$, and the curve of cumulative incidence *versus* age should approximate $F(x)$.

In reality, one does not know which individual relatives may be genetically predisposed to AD. As long as one is willing to acknowledge the existence of a dominant genetic form of AD in some cases, however, one may assume that a finite proportion of relatives must have such a genetic predisposition. This proportion will be directly related to the proportion of index cases who have genetic disease and to the population frequency of the putative gene.

In a rare dominant disorder (like Huntington's disease), the proportion of first-degree relatives (parents, sibs, children) with the gene should be 0.5 (ignoring the effects of new mutations). We may then write an expression for the age-specific cumulative probability of disease (i.e., cumulative incidence) $I(x)$ with respect to first-degree relatives as follows:

$$I(x) = 0.5 \, F(x)$$

---

[3] This means that eventually all individuals become affected. Such a statement does not, however, imply that simple addition of annual incidence rates should total 100%. Because appearance of each new case reduces the remaining number at risk (the denominator in incidence calculations), these incidence rates will increase progressively, and their total will exceed 100% substantially.

In a dominant genetic condition that is caused by a deleterious gene that is common, however, the coefficient in the above equation changes from 0.5 to a value that is larger by an amount related to the population gene frequency. The increase reflects such factors as (a) the possibility that the proband (who must bear at least one copy of the deleterious gene) may in fact be homozygous and (b) the no longer negligible risk that his mate (or, with respect to sibs, a parent from whom he did not himself acquire the gene) will also bear the gene. Such possibilities increase the probability of the gene among sibs and offspring. For example, when both parents are heterozygotes, the risk to progeny increases to three-fourths; if the proband is a homozygote, then both parents must have had the gene, and all his children will bear the gene. Formulas are available (7; J. C. S. Breitner, *unpublished results*) to describe the expected proportions of each generation of first-degree relatives who should bear the gene under the contrasting conditions that the index case does and does not himself bear the gene.

Alzheimer's disease is not rare. Therefore, if a dominant genetic form represents any substantial proportion of all AD, the population frequency of the provoking gene must be considerable. In fact, depending on diagnostic criteria employed in case ascertainment, one investigator (7) has estimated that at least three-fourths of all AD may be inherited, so that Larsson's (40) estimate that the gene frequency $q = 0.06$ appears reasonable. This gene frequency results in a prediction that 55% of the first-degree relatives of AD probands should bear the gene, and it may be shown that this proportion remains relatively stable for hypothetical gene frequencies varying between 0.03 and 0.10.

The 55% figure may be contrasted with the expected frequency of gene bearers in the general population. Since humans are diploid, the probability of an individual bearing one or two AD genes is

$$1 - (1 - q)^2$$
$$= 1 - (1 - 2q + q^2)$$
$$= 2q - q^2$$

which for small values of q is close to $2q$. Then, for example, using Larsson's estimate of gene frequency of 0.06, we would posit that 12% of the population are genetically predisposed to AD. Assuming identical age-specific gene expression in both control and proband relatives, the expected age-specific familial risks of genetically transmitted AD are then:

$$I(x) = 0.55 \, F(x) \tag{1}$$

for relatives of genetic AD probands, and

$$I(x) = 0.12 \, F(x) \tag{2}$$

for relatives of population controls.

Given the possibility of etiologic heterogeneity in cases diagnosed as having "AD," we may now examine the expected outcome when an index case series contains a proportion of nongenetic phenocopies. Because phenocopies by definition do not bear the gene, the expected incidence among their relatives is lower than that of controls (who may have it). In fact, the expected proportion of relatives with the gene closely approximates the value of the population gene frequency (7), which (because of diploidy) is roughly half the proportion with the gene in the general population. If Larsson's estimate were correct, for example, and $q = 0.06$, then the probability that relatives of phenocopies would bear one or more copies of the hypothetical gene would be about 0.06, and cumulative incidence among first-degree relatives should be

$$I(x) = 0.06\,F(x) \qquad (3)$$

If a sample of index cases in fact included two types of cases, one genetic and the other not, then the predicted age-specific cumulative incidence should be predicted by a weighted average in the two populations of relatives of equations 1 and 3. If the proportion of genetic index cases is denoted as g, then the predicted incidence $I(x)$ is

$$I(x) = [g \times 0.55\,F(x)] + [(1-g) \times 0.06\,F(x)]$$
$$= [0.55g + (0.06 - 0.06g)]F(x)$$
$$= [0.49g + 0.06]F(x). \qquad (4)$$

If, for example, the proportion of index cases with genetic disease were 0.5, then predicted cumulative incidence would be 0.30 times $F(x)$, and the asymptotic lifetime cumulative incidence of AD would be about 0.3.

REVIEW OF PREVIOUS STUDIES

Approach

The above section suggests a perspective from which to view genetic studies of AD in pooled proband families. Drawing on both pedigree data and the findings of newer studies of pooled proband relatives (see below), we may posit that a proportion of AD index cases have an autosomal dominant disorder in which gene expression is age-dependent. How closely do the data from studies to date then approximate theoretical expectations from an autosomal dominant genetic theory of etiology? If lifetime incidence in proband families is substantially below 50% but still well in excess of control values, this could suggest an admixture of phenocopies in the index cases. Can one then estimate the proportion of genetic cases from the data? If data obtained using different methods of proband ascertainment suggest the admixture of differing proportions of phenocopies, what factors might account for these differences? Are methods of diagnosis now available that appear to reduce the presence of phenocopies to low levels? How strong a case may be made presently for a dominant genetic etiology of AD?

Studies Before 1955

Early Studies

These have been reviewed by Matsuyama and Jarvik (42) and by Folstein and Powell (23). They are, for the most part, significantly flawed methodologically, so that their interpretation is difficult. Meggendorfer (47), for example, studied the families of 60 pathologically confirmed

(i.e., cerebral atrophy without evidence of vascular disease) cases of "senile dementia" and found 19 secondary cases in 16 families. At a clinical level, however, the probands included five with apparent late-onset schizophrenia that evolved into "senile dementia," another 20 cases with such "schizophrenic" symptoms as paranoia and flat affect, and six more with prominent depression and anxiety. Such symptoms, although common enough in AD, would not be expected to such a degree in a sample ascertained by modern criteria. Meggendorfer's study, in spite of its probable inclusion of conditions other than AD, suggested that 20% of cases are "familial" (cf. about one-third found typically in modern studies) and discovered one family in which the disease appeared to be "directly transmitted" through three generations. Generally similar results were reported later by Weinberger (63) and by Cresseri (18).

Sjogren's Studies

The major genetic study from the pre-1955 epoch was reported by Sjogren et al. (58). These authors studied a group of subjects including both Pick's and Alzheimer's diseases. The study was limited to presenile dementing illness, and familial risks were not examined beyond age 70. These risks were defined both in terms of simple frequencies and age-adjusted morbidity risks as estimated by the Weinberg "short method." The latter has well-known distortions, particularly in the study of late onset conditions, but the major shortcoming of the study was its failure to examine relatives over 70 years of age, prompted presumably by the view of presenile Alzheimer disease as a discrete entity apart from senile dementia. This study found a risk of disease among parents that was strikingly higher than that found among sibs, a result that is difficult to reconcile with any simple Mendelian mode of inheritance. Thus, Sjogren et al. were led to the conclusion that the most sensible explanation for the observed familial risk was some form of multifactorial inheritance. This conclusion is also difficult to justify, however, and the study is better regarded as inconclusive with respect to mode of inheritance, since the major risk period for dementing illness, ages 70 to 90, was not considered.

Studies After 1955

Larsson's Studies

In 1955, Larsson et al. (40) began a major study of "senile dementia" notable for its size (1,412 aged relatives of 377 index cases were analyzed) and its sophisticated treatment of the problem of the age-dependent manifestation of a suspected genetic diathesis toward AD.

Description. Index cases were ascertained by Roth's criteria, with age of onset ranging from 56 to 90 years (mean 74). They were selected by chart review (a few cases were available for concurrent clinical examination) from the patient populations of two large Swedish state mental hospitals, with dates of diagnosis ranging back to the first decades of this century. This method of proband ascertainment is a weakness in the study, as is the inclusion of subjects with clear evidence of multi-infarct disease as well as "senile dementia." (The authors assert, but do not demonstrate that the familial risks in these proband families were similar to those in the families of other probands without suggestion of vascular pathology.)

Disease among family members was detected by two methods: (a) "field examination," by which was meant either direct examination of living affected relatives or intensive interviewing of living relatives regarding the occurrence of disease in deceased relatives, and (b) ascertainment of disease from parish registers. The latter method would surely be expected to produce significant underestimation of incidence, since many of the deceased relatives lived at a time when "senility" was considered a natural consequence of old age. This expectation is borne out by a markedly greater incidence reported in relatives of families who were "field examined." Since the large majority of families were "field examined," however, the practical effects of this methodological difficulty are probably limited.

Larsson et al. constructed actuarial life tables (a much better approach than the Weinberg "short method") and considered risks in relatives through age 90 (which late age they justified by the large sample size—hence, the considerable number of relatives surviving to 90) as well as by the simultaneous consideration of incidence in normal population controls. They estimated the age-adjusted cumulative risk of senile dementia at 0.23 by age 90 in the first-degree relatives of probands. The risk was substantially higher, however, in sibs and children than it was among parents, a finding that is probably attributable to difficulty in the ascertainment of disease among the parents, many of whom presumably died in the late 19th or early 20th century. Incomplete ascertainment among parents, which is also suggested in several other data sets (6,35), would again lead to underestimation of true familial incidence.

Analysis. Larsson et al. suggested that senile dementia is transmitted by a simple Mendelian dominant gene, and their data enable us for the first time to examine this possibility using the methods suggested above. A recent report by Breitner et al. (7) evaluated the possible mixture of autosomal dominant disease and phenocopies in the proband sample. Based on a least-squares estimation procedure employing the gamma (multiple hit) distribution function to model the age-dependent expression of the putative AD gene, the results suggested that 52% of the Larsson probands had genetic disease. Breitner et al. noted, however, that relatively nonspecific diagnostic criteria (by modern standards) were used and suggested that at least one-quarter of these cases would not today have received a diagnosis of AD. Assuming that these other cases would not have familial disease, the proportion of "true" AD cases with a presumed genetic etiology would likely be considerably higher. Furthermore, one should not lose sight of the several probable negative biases in the incidence data themselves (see above), so that the Larsson findings appear consistent with the hypothesis that a large majority of AD (as presently diagnosed) is transmitted by a dominant genetic trait.

Åkesson's Study

Still higher estimates of familial risk were obtained by Åkesson (1), who, like Larsson, employed Roth's diagnostic criteria but used living index cases and imposed the additional diagnostic requirement that cases be continuously disoriented to time and place. This study used the Weinberg "proband method," which is known to produce significant overestimation of incidence, so the results are hard to interpret. Åkesson did, however, show markedly increased familial risks in AD as contrasted with published risk figures in a standard population. He did not propose any particular mode of inheritance.

Constantinidis's Studies

Constantinidis and associates (14,15) reviewed family history data derived primarily from hospital records (a method almost certain to produce marked underestimation of actual incidence) of cases who came to autopsy. These workers again found familial risks significantly in excess of population controls. Noting a comparable incidence in sibs and parents, these authors argued for autosomal dominant inheritance as the mechanism of increased risk. Their later work also demonstrates a noteworthy association of (a) accumulation of senile plaques and, more particularly, neurofibrillary tangles in the neocortex (as opposed to the hippocampus alone), (b) appearance of the "instrumental disorders" (aphasia, apraxia, and agnosia), and (c) familial predisposition. This work therefore extends a suggestion first made by Sjogren et al. that there exists within the Alzheimer disease–senile dementia complex a subgroup of patients who are discernible on clinical as well as neuropathologic grounds and who have a probable genetic etiology.

CURRENT STUDIES

Four major studies on the clinical genetics of AD have been reported in the present decade. Although these differ somewhat in method, all add strong support to the hypothesis that genetic factors are a major cause of AD.

The Minnesota State Hospital Studies

The best-known current work is that of Heston and colleagues (33,34), whose probands were ascertained from the neuropathology files of Minnesota state hospitals. These authors initially studied all cases dying with presenile AD over a defined time period and later added a sample of older patients who were similarly ascertained. The families were then studied by extremely careful history taking; living demented relatives received careful clinical evaluation and, in a number of cases, received later post-mortem examination; other living relatives at risk were brought in for repeated clinical assessment of possible early disease.

The results indicate that (a) there are marked differences in familial risk in early onset versus late onset probands; (b) in early onset disease (particularly where there is one affected relative), the risk to other first-degree family members increases with age and approaches 50% by age 90; (c) in all of 25 families where a secondary case has died and come to autopsy, the neuropathologic diagnosis of the relative is identical to that of the proband; (d) there is significant intrafamilial correlation in age of onset; but (e) secondary cases tend to appear at ages considerably older than the index cases.

Heston's most striking finding is the difference in apparent familial risk in early versus late onset disease. Here it must be pointed out, however, that proband ascertainment was carried out principally by autopsy diagnosis. Heston does not mention the nature or the completeness of clinical information available from the hospital records, nor does he state specifically the formal criteria employed for autopsy diagnosis. The latter point is significant, since (particularly in very old subjects) the occurrence of Alzheimer-like changes in brain is quite prevalent in "normals" (23,60). The neuropathologic features of AD, although said to be definitive, may not be entirely specific. Additional diagnostic specificity might result from a combination of clinical description and neuropathologic characterization—the approach adopted originally by Alzheimer (3) himself. Without clinical description, one may wonder particularly about the diagnostic homogeneity of the older sample. (This should presumably be less of a problem for the younger group, where plaques and tangles are probably rare except as a result of Alzheimer's dementia.)

The finding of marked familial risk in younger onset probands again suggests that a form of this disease may be transmitted by an autosomal dominant gene and that a relatively "pure" sample of such cases can be obtained when appropriate ascertainment criteria are employed. Thus, one may not have to resort to such ambiguous concepts as "variable penetrance" to account for the familial risk in AD. The intrafamilial correlation in age of onset is also important, since it suggests possible heterogeneity in the genetic predisposition to AD (55).

The Duke Collaborative Studies

Heyman et al. (35) reported results from a case sample comprising a large group of ambulatory volunteers in a comprehensive study of clinical, genetic, and epidemiologic aspects of Alzheimer's disease. Diagnostic criteria were similar to the newly proposed NINCDS standards (45), but the majority of probands showed only mild to moderate disease at ascertainment. Only patients with onset of symptoms before age 70 were studied. Family study of these probands showed greater age-specific incidence (within the age range observed) of AD among relatives than had been found in any previous investigation. The cumulative age-specific risks are shown in Fig. 3. Heston's finding of greater familial risk in early onset cases was not replicated; however, the maximum age at onset of 70 years may have precluded a meaningful comparison (Heston's early onset cases had onset before 65, and the late onset cases mostly much later.)

Because of concerns about data reliability, the Duke group did not calculate familial risks in relatives over age 75. This conservative practice may have resulted in loss of some potentially valuable data on older relatives, since recent evidence (34,56) suggests that such information can be reliably ascertained. Still, these workers found dramatic

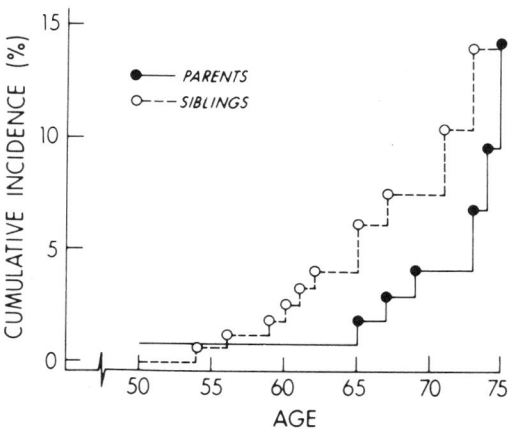

FIG. 3. Empirical cumulative incidence of AD-like illness in proband relatives through age 75, as reported by Heyman et al. (35). Probands were ascertained clinically using exacting structured diagnostic methods and criteria similar to the recent NINCDS/ADRDA criteria. Significance of the difference between risks among parents (●——●) and sibs (○---○) is not clear. The cumulative incidence by age 75, nearly 15% in both generations, is higher than had been reported in any prior study. (From Heyman et al., ref. 35, reproduced by permission of the authors and publisher.)

differences in familial risks among relatives of AD probands as contrasted with relatives of spouse controls.

The Baltimore Nursing Home Study

Further results suggesting possible genetic mechanisms were reported by Breitner and Folstein (6) from Johns Hopkins. These authors screened 3,500 Baltimore nursing home patients for AD using ascertainment criteria shown in Table 1. They found 78 eligible subjects, of whom 62

TABLE 1. *Eligibility criteria for AD probands in Baltimore nursing home study (ref. 6)*

A. Clinical criteria for AD
1. Age 50+
2. Dementia syndrome (DSM-III)
3. None of the following (exclusionary criteria):
   History of strokes or transient ischemic attacks
   Diabetes mellitus
   Hypertension (at any time) resulting in recommendation for treatment
   Alcoholism (any kind of drinking problem)
   Head trauma resulting in full loss of consciousness
   Brain tumor, epilepsy, Parkinsonism or other indication of CNS disease
   Psychiatric illness (other than present illness) requiring hospitalization

B. Other research criteria
1. Must be physically capable of participation in study
2. At least one available informant knowledgeable about subject's clinical and family history
3. Informed consent (generally from responsible relative)
4. Pedigree containing at least 2 relatives who reached age 60+

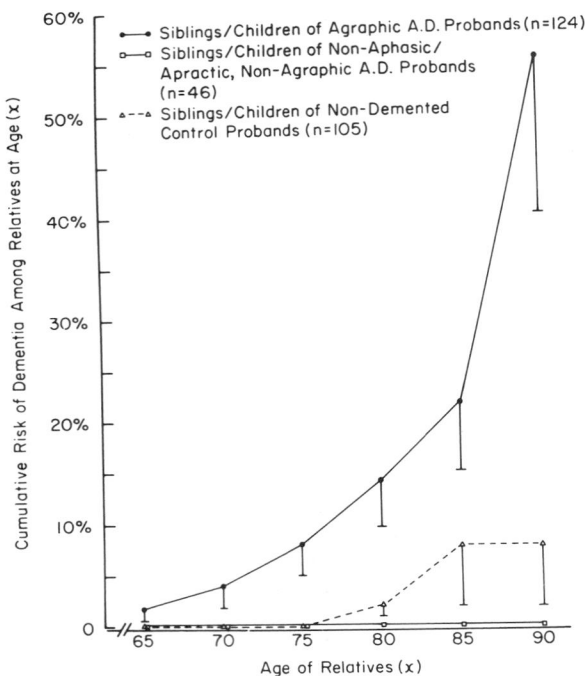

FIG. 4. Empirical cumulative incidence of AD-like illness among sibs and offspring of nursing home probands. ● —— ●, relatives of 39 language-disordered nursing home residents with AD; □ —— □, relatives of 12 residents ill 4 or more years with primary dementia but without language disorder or apraxia; △ —— △, relatives of 33 age-matched nondemented controls. (Reproduced from Breitner and Folstein, ref. 6, by permission of the publisher.)

(all white females) completed the study. A sample of 33 age- and sex-matched nursing home controls was ascertained simultaneously. The AD probands were categorized by presence of the typical middle-stage symptoms, aphasia or apraxia in addition to amnesia (*aaa;* amnesia was present in all subjects): 42 had developed such symptoms; eight had not but had been ill less than 4 years (hence, were thought still likely to develop them); and 12 had been ill over 4 years but were neither aphasic nor apractic.

Family study then revealed a marked difference in AD risks among relatives (sibs and offspring) of aphasic/apractic probands versus those ill 4 or more years but lacking these symptoms. No secondary cases were observed among the 56 relatives of the latter group, but aaa proband relatives showed cumulative risks of AD exceeding 50% by age 90 (Fig. 4). Non-demented nursing home control relatives experienced a lifetime morbid risk of 8%, which did not differ significantly from the 12% risk observed among the probands' spouses. The observed lifetime incidence of 52% (12) is consistent with the hypothesis that these probands had a relatively homogeneous autosomal dominant genetic disorder. Since 78% of the proband sample had *aaa,* the authors suggested that a majority of primary dementia cases might be genetically determined.

The New York Studies

The Baltimore findings were recently replicated in another series of clinically ascertained cases by Mohs et al. (48). Like Heyman's, these 50 subjects were mainly ambulatory volunteers for ongoing clinical studies of AD, in this case

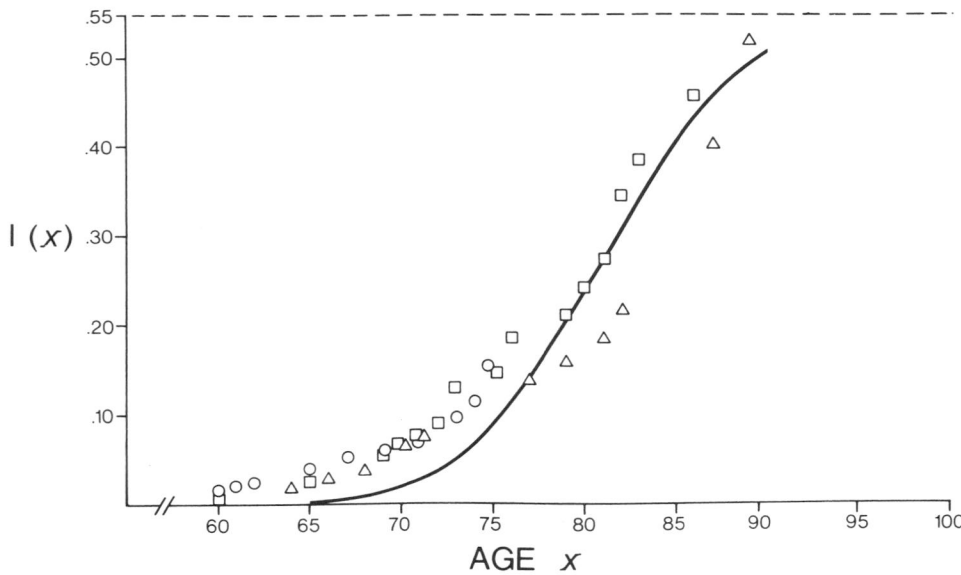

FIG. 5. Estimated cumulative incidence *I*(x) as a function of age x in first-degree relatives of the New York series (48) (□) and similar studies of Heyman et al. (35) (○; combined data from parents and sibs kindly provided for purposes of compatible presentation by Dr. A. Heyman), and the Baltimore nursing home series (6) (△). The curve shows results predicted if AD were transmitted by an autosomal dominant gene with population frequency 0.06 and age-dependent gene expression described by a normal distribution with mean 81 and standard deviation 6.12 years.

the longitudinal studies of the Alzheimer's Disease Research Center of the Mount Sinai School of Medicine and the Bronx VA Medical Center. It is noteworthy that these cases were not originally ascertained for genetic studies. Thus, it is unlikely that the cases came forward out of concern about familial risk—an important potential source of bias in family studies of clinical populations. The NINCDS diagnostic criteria were employed, with the sole additional requirement that subjects must have shown a definite progression of severity in their symptoms over the 1-year period preceding diagnosis. Age-matched (mainly spouse) controls were also studied. Family study then showed the age-specific cumulative risks to proband and control relatives indicated in Fig. 5. As in the previous study, the estimated cumulative risk by age 90 for AD relatives exceeded 50%, and that for control relatives was much lower.

Prompted in part by the findings of the Baltimore group, Mohs et al. investigated the presence of aphasia and apraxia in their AD proband sample. All but three (94%) showed some evidence of aphasia or apraxia on neuropsychological examination.

Consistency of Findings and Suggestion of Autosomal Dominant Inheritance in Several Studies

The familial risks in the two last-mentioned studies were analyzed as previously suggested to estimate the proportion of index cases possibly having a dominant genetic illness (7; R. C. Mohs, J. M. Silverman, J. C. S. Breitner, and K. L. Davis, *unpublished data*). For the Baltimore nursing home probands with *aaa* and the New York AD probands of Mohs et al., the result was identical: best fit to the empirical familial incidence data is obtained with the expression

$$I(x) = 0.55\,F(x)$$

suggesting that essentially all of the probands in both series had genetic disease. In both samples the resulting model accounts for over 97% of the total sum of squares of AD incidence with age in proband families. Thus, these two studies both suggest that AD cases ascertained clinically by modern research diagnostic criteria uniformly have familial aggregation of disease that is consistent with autosomal dominant genetic transmission. The expression of the putative predisposing gene is very late, however, with maximum probability of manifestation in the early ninth decade of life.

IMPLICATIONS AND STRATEGIES FOR FUTURE RESEARCH

Status of the Genetic Hypothesis

Although a genetic contribution to the etiology of Alzheimer's disease has long been suspected, the studies described above show a growing trend over time toward stronger suggestion of a specific genetic mechanism of disease transmission. As clinical diagnostic procedures have improved, the most recent studies have shown considerable consistency in their suggestion of strong familial aggregation

in AD. In the two studies in which cumulative incidence of disease has been estimated through age 90, it approximates 50%. This result is expected when disease transmission is through a simple Mendelian gene that is dominant in the heterozygote, i.e., the same form of transmission (with later disease expression) suggested by the well-known AD pedigrees. Moreover, these two studies suggest that such familial AD represents the large majority of AD as diagnosed by modern methods. Their findings, therefore, lend credibility to the approach to the analysis of earlier studies suggested above, which might otherwise be viewed as conjectural.

That the observed familial aggregation of AD has genetic rather than environmental causes is certainly not proven. There are many causes for familial aggregation other than genetic transmission, as evidenced by the facetious suggestion of A. Lilienfeld that attendance at medical school is transmitted in families as an autosomal dominant trait. The probability of an environmental cause is reduced, however, by several observations. (a) Despite several recent epidemiologic case-control studies exploring multiple putative risk factors, no environmental risk factor has been consistently identified. (b) In each of four studies (6,35,40,48) in which spouses of AD cases have been investigated, their risk has been indistinguishable from population controls and much lower than that of first-degree proband relatives living apart from the index cases. Spouses should logically share most environmental influences with probands. (c) Alzheimer's disease is related to Down's syndrome, a known chromosomal abnormality. Down's cases invariably develop Alzheimer-like neuropathology in middle life (67), and the incidence of Down's is increased in Alzheimer proband families (32).

Thus, in the opinion of the author, the weight of the evidence is presently against environmental and in favor of genetic causes for the observed familial aggregation of AD. Proof of genetic influences would require new and much larger twin studies or linkage studies of extensive pedigrees. Both would be extremely difficult to carry out because of the characteristic expression of AD only in late old age. With newer, molecular techniques it may be possible to overcome these difficulties by the fortunate identification of a polymorphic DNA sequence polymorphism closely linked to AD (28). Logically, one could begin the search for such linkage in the atypical large pedigrees of early-onset disease. Ultimately, one might hope to identify the gene product directly. The latter result would likely enable the subsequent study of the gene product itself, which could provide important clues to the basic mechanisms of pathogenesis of AD. Characterization of the gene product and its action might also hold out new hopes of an effective rational treatment or prevention of AD. Even a demonstration of genetic linkage might be similarly revealing if the gene were found to belong to a functionally related group controlling, say, immune function or some aspect of aging.

Additional Research Strategies

To date, there is only one published estimate of a population frequency of the putative AD gene(s) (40).

Clearly, other estimates should be made in other populations. It is quite possible that there may be important differences in gene frequency among different racial or ethnic groups. One recent study, for example, has suggested a greater than 10-fold difference in predisposition to presenile AD in Ashkenazi *versus* Sephardic Jews (61).

Even if a genetic mechanism is ultimately shown to be responsible for the familial aggregation of Alzheimer's disease, this finding would in no way invalidate the other etiologic hypotheses discussed in the beginning of this chapter. It is quite plausible, for example, that genetic makeup could influence vulnerability to slow viral infection, autoimmune disorders, or even environmental toxins.

Finally, there is the mystery of why the putative AD gene should require 80 years on average for its expression. If one could learn the mechanism for this delayed expression, one might be able to alter its timing. Because the slope of the curve of probability of gene expression versus age is quite steep, there is a real chance that an intervention capable of "pushing back" the natural history of gene expression by only a few years would relegate this gene's expression to an age beyond most people's life expectancy. A shift to the right in the curve of Fig. 5 by only 5 years could effectively prevent the large majority of cases of Alzheimer's disease.

ACKNOWLEDGMENTS

The author gratefully acknowledges helpful discussions with Drs. E. A. Murphy and M. F. Folstein. Preparation of this chapter was supported by NIH grants AG-02219 and AG-05138 and by the Medical Research Service of the Veterans Administration.

REFERENCES

1. Akesson, H. O. (1969): *Hum. Hered.*, 19:546–565.
2. Alfrey, A. C., LeGentre, G. R., and Kaehny, W. D. (1976): *N. Engl. J. Med.*, 294:184–188.
3. Alzheimer, A. (1907): *Allg. Z. Psychiatr. Ger. Med.*, 64:146–148. Translated by R. H. Wilkins and I. A. Brody, (1969): *Arch. Neurol.*, 21:109–110.
4. Amaducci, L. A., Frataglioni, L., Rocca, W. A., et al. (1986): *Neurology*, 36:922–931.
5. Behan, P. O., and Behan, W. M. H. (1979): In: *Alzheimer's Disease*, edited by A. I. M. Glen, and L. J. Whalley, pp. 33–35. Livingstone, Edinburgh, London, New York.
6. Breitner, J. C. S., and Folstein, M. F. (1984): *Psychol. Med.*, 14:63–80.
7. Breitner, J. C. S., Folstein, M. F., and Murphy, E. A. (1986): *J. Psychiatr. Res.*, 20:31–43.
8. Breitner, J. C. S., Murphy, E. A., and Folstein, M. F. (1986): *J. Psychiatr. Res.*, 20:45–55.
9. Brown, P., Salazar, A. M., Gibbs, C. J., and Gajdusek, D. C. (1982): *Ann. N.Y. Acad. Sci.*, 396:131–143.
10. Burks, J. S., Huddlestone, J., Alfrey, A. C., Norenberg, M. D., and Lewin, E. (1976): *Lancet*, 1:764–768.
11. Carp, R. I., Merz, G. S., and Wisniewski, H. M. (1984): In: *Senile Dementia: Outlook for the Future*, pp. 31–54. Alan R. Liss, New York.
12. Chase, G. A., Folstein, M. F., Breitner, J. C. S., Beaty, T. H., and Self, S. G. (1983): *Am. J. Epidemiol.*, 117:590–597.
13. Chase, T. N., Foster, N. L., Fedio, P., Brooks, R., Mansi, L., et al. (1985): *Ann. Neurol.*, 15(Suppl.):S170–S174.
14. Constantinidis, J. (1978): In: *Aging, Vol. 7: Alzheimer's Disease:*

Senile Dementia and Related Disorders, edited by R. Katzman, R. D. Terry, and K. L. Bick, pp. 15–26. Raven Press, New York.
15. Constantinidis, J., Garrone, G., and de Ajuriaguerra, J. (1962): *Encephale*, 51:301–344.
16. Crapper, D. R., Krishman, S. S., and Quittkat, S. (1976): *Brain*, 99:67–80.
17. Crapper, D. R., Karlik, S., and De Boni, U. (1978): In: *Aging, Vol. 7: Alzheimer's Disease: Senile Dementia and Related Disorders*, edited by R. Katzman, R. D. Terry, and K. L. Bick, pp. 471–486. Raven Press, New York.
18. Cresseri, A. (1948): *Boll. Soc. Ital. Biol. Sper.*, 24:200–201.
18a. Treves, T., Korezyn, A., Zilber, N., Kahana, E., Leibowitz, Y., Alter, M., and Schoenberg, B. S. (1986): *Arch. Neurol.*, 43:26–29.
19. Dickinson, A. G., Bruce, M. E., and Scott, J. R. (1983): In: *Biological Aspects of Alzheimer's Disease (Banbury Report 15)*, edited by R. Katzman, pp. 387–398. Cold Spring Harbor Laboratory Press, Cold Spring Harbor, NY.
20. Elliot, H. L., Dryburgh, F., Fell, G. B., Sabet, S., and MacDougall, A. I. (1978): *Br. Med. J.*, 1:1101–1103.
21. Feldman, R. G., Chandler, K., Levy, L., and Glaser, G. (1963): *Neurology (Minneap.)*, 13:811–820.
22. Folstein, M., Powell, D., and Breitner, J. (1983): In: *Biological Aspects of Alzheimer's Disease (Banbury Report 15)*, edited by R. Katzman, pp. 337–349. Cold Spring Harbor Laboratory Press, Cold Spring Harbor, NY.
23. Folstein, M. F., and Powell, D. (1984): *Integr. Psychiatry*, 2:163–175.
24. French, L. R., Schuman, L. M., Mortimer, J. A., Hutton, J. T., Boatman, R. A., et al. (1985): *Am. J. Epidemiol.*, 121:414–421.
25. Friedland, R. P., Budinger, T. F., Jagust, W. J., et al. (1987): In: *Positron Tomography and the Differential Diagnosis and Pathophysiology of Alzheimer's Disease*. Springer-Verlag, Heidelberg (*in press*).
26. Gibbs, C. J., and Gajdusek, D. C. (1978): In: *Aging, Vol. 7: Alzheimer's Disease: Senile Dementia and Related Disorders*, edited by R. Katzman, R. D. Terry, and K. L. Bick, pp. 559–575. Raven Press, New York.
27. Gibbs, C. J., Gajdusek, D. C., and Amyx, H. (1979): In: *Slow Transmissible Diseases of the Nervous System, Vol. 2*, edited by S. Prusiner and W. J. Hadlow, pp. 87–110. Academic Press, New York.
28. Gusella, J. F., Wexler, N. S., Conneally, P. M., Naylor, S. L., Anderson, M. A., et al. (1983): *Nature*, 306:234–238.
29. Hagnell, O., Lanke, J., Rorsman, B., and Ojusjo, L. (1981): *Neuropsychobiology*, 7:201–211.
30. Hagnell, O., Lanke, J., Rorsman, B., Ohman, R., and Ojusjo, L. (1983): *Arch. Psychiat. Nervenkr.*, 233:423–238.
31. Heston, L. L. (1979): In: *Congenital and Acquired Cognitive Disorders*, edited by R. Katzman, pp. 167–176. Raven Press, New York.
32. Heston, L. L. (1981): In: *The Epidemiology of Dementia*, edited by J. A. Mortimer and L. M. Schuman, pp. 101–114. Oxford University Press, New York.
33. Heston, L. L. (1983): In: *Biological Aspects of Alzheimer's Disease (Banbury Report 15)*, edited by R. Katzman, pp. 183–191. Cold Spring Harbor Laboratory Press, Cold Spring Harbor, NY.
34. Heston, L. L., Mastri, A. R., Anderson, V. E., and White, J. (1981): *Arch. Gen. Psychiatry*, 38:1085–1090.
35. Heyman, A., Wilkinson, W. E., Hurwitz, B. J., Schmechel, D., Sigmon, A., et al. (1983): *Ann. Neurol.*, 14:507–515.
36. Heyman, A., Wilkinson, W. E., Stafford, J. A., Helms, M. J., Sigmon, A. H., et al. (1984): *Ann. Neurol.*, 15:335–341.
37. Hollander, E., Mohs, R. C., and Davis, K. L. (1986): *Br. Med. Bull.*, 42:97–100.
38. Ishii, T., and Haga, S. (1976): *Acta Neuropathol. (Berl.)*, 36:243–249.
39. Klatzko, I., Wisniewski, H., and Streicher, E. (1965): *J. Neuropathol. Exp. Neurol.*, 24:187–199.
40. Larsson, T., Sjogren, T., and Jacobson, G. (1963): *Acta Psychiatr. Scand.*, 39(Suppl.):167.
41. Lauter, H. (1985): *Dan. Med. Bull.*, 32(Suppl. 1):1–21.
42. Matsuyama, S. S., and Jarvik, L. F. (1980): In: *Handbook of Mental Health and Aging*, edited by J. E. Birren and R. B. Sloan, pp. 134–148. Prentice-Hall, Englewood Cliffs, NJ.

43. McDermott, J. R., Fraser, H., and Dickinson, A. G. (1978): *Lancet,* 2:318–319.
44. McDermott, J. R., Ward, M. K., Smith, A. I., Parkinson, I. S., and Kerr, D. N. S. (1978): *Lancet,* 1:901–903.
45. McKhann, G., Drachman, D., Folstein, M., Katzman, R., Price, D., et al. (1984): *Neurology,* 34:939–944.
46. McKusick, V. A. (1983): *Mendelian Inheritance in Man,* 6th edition, pp. 30–31. Johns Hopkins University Press, Baltimore.
47. Meggendorfer, F. (1925): *Zentralbl. Ges. Neurol. Psychiatr.,* 40: 359.
48. Mohs, R. C., Breitner, J. C. S., Silverman, J. M., and Davis, K. L. (1987): *Arch. Gen. Psychiatry (in press).*
49. Mortimer, J. A., Schuman, L. M., and French, L. R. (1981): In: *The Epidemiology of Dementia,* edited by J. A. Mortimer and L. M. Schuman, pp. 3–23. Oxford University Press, New York.
50. Murphy, E. A. (1979): *Probability in Medicine.* Johns Hopkins University Press, Baltimore.
51. Nandy, K. (1978): In: *Aging, Vol. 7: Alzheimer's Disease: Senile Dementia and Related Disorders,* edited by R. Katzman, R. D. Terry, and K. L. Bick, pp. 555–558. Raven Press, New York.
52. Nee, L., Polinsky, R. J., Eldridge, R., Weingartner, H., Smallberg, S., et al. (1983): *Arch. Neurol.,* 40:203–208.
53. Nerl, C., Mayeux, R., and O'Neill, G. J. (1984): *Neurology (NY),* 34:310–314.
53a. Parry, H. B. (1987): In: *Scrapie Disease in Sheep,* edited by D. A. Oppenheimer. Academic Press, New York.
54. Perl, D. P., and Brody, A. R. (1980): *Science,* 208:207–209.
55. Powell, D., and Folstein, M. (1984): *J. Neurogenet.,* 1:189–197.
56. Silverman, J. M., Breitner, J. C. S., Mohs, R. C., and Davis, K. L. (1986): *Am. J. Psychiatry,* 143:1279–1282.
57. Sinex, F. M., and Myers, C. R. (1982): *Ann. N.Y. Acad. Sci.,* 396: 3–13.
58. Sjogren, T., Sjogren, H., and Lindgren, A. G. H. (1952): *Acta Psychiatr. Neurol. Scand. [Suppl.],* 82:1–152.
59. Terry, R. D., and Peña, C. (1965): *J. Neuropathol. Exp. Neurol.,* 24:200–210.
59a. Terry, R. D., and Katzman, R. (1983): *Ann. Neurol.,* 14:497–506.
60. Tomlinson, B. E. (1982): *Psychol. Med.,* 12:449–459.
61. Treves, T., Korczyn, A. D., Zilber, N., Kahana, E., Liebowitz, Y., et al. (1986): *Arch. Neurol.,* 43:26–29.
62. Walford, R. L., and Hodge, S. E. (1980): In: *Histocompatibility Testing,* edited by P. I. Terasaki, UCLA Tissue Typing Laboratory, Los Angeles.
63. Weinberger, H. L. (1926): *Arch. Ges. Neurol. Psychiatr.,* 106:666–701.
64. Whalley, L. J., Carothers, A. D., Collyer, S., DeMey, R., and Frankiewicz, A. (1982): *Br. J. Psychiatry,* 140:249–256.
65. Wisniewski, H. M. (1978): In: *Aging, Vol. 7: Alzheimer's Disease: Senile Dementia and Related Disorders,* edited by R. Katzman, R. D. Terry, and K. L. Bick, pp. 555–558. Raven Press, New York.
66. Wisniewski, H. M., and Kozlowski, P. B. (1982): *Ann. N.Y. Acad. Sci.,* 396:119–129.
67. Wisniewski, K. E., Dalton, A. J., Crapper McLachlan, D. R., Wen, G. Y., and Wisniewski, H. M. (1985): *Neurology (NY),* 35: 957–961.

Psychopharmacology:
The Third Generation of Progress,
edited by Herbert Y. Meltzer.
Raven Press, New York © 1987.

CHAPTER **93**

Dementia: Animal Models of the Cognitive Impairments Produced by Degeneration of the Basal Forebrain Cholinergic System

David S. Olton, and Gary L. Wenk

Animal models have become a critical component in the endeavor to understand the brain mechanisms involved in normal cognitive processes, the pathological bases of cognitive impairments, and the therapeutic interventions that can be used to alleviate these impairments. Their use in the study of dementia is particularly important (16,20,59, 73,78,115,116,124,166).

Because dementia is associated with different pathological changes and cognitive impairments (31,32,47), animal models are necessary to obtain detailed information to interrelate each of these different pathological and cognitive sequelae. This chapter reviews recent progress in the development of animal models of dementia. It emphasizes experiments that use behavioral tests to assess the cognitive consequences of intracranially injected neurotoxins that produce neuroanatomically and neurochemically selective neuropathological changes.

Special emphasis is placed on animal models of Alzheimer's disease for three reasons. First, this disease is having

a profound impact on society, and it promises to be a major research problem for many years (32,159).

Second, most of the relevant animal research has had Alzheimer's disease as its focus for the pathological, behavioral, and psychological dimensions of the model. One of the major sites of pathological degeneration in people with Alzheimer's disease is found in the basal forebrain cholinergic system, in the nucleus basalis of Meynert. Consequently, the experimental lesions in animals were placed in the analogous anatomical system, including the nucleus basalis magnocellularis (NBM) and the medial septal area (MSA) (25,40,41,76,99,122,137,143,162,163,177). Because some major behavioral difficulties of these patients result from a failure of memory processes (31,153), many of the behavioral tests for animals assessed memory. An impairment of memory is often the first and most consistent symptom in patients with Alzheimer's disease (34,54,80,96,159). Thus, interpretations of the behavioral impairments exhibited by animals with lesions have often used diagnostic test batteries designed to determine the extent to which the behavioral changes seen following lesions are caused by a selective impairment of memory.

Third, the cholinergic system and especially its projections to the hippocampus have been implicated in memory processes for many years (67,113,117,118,119). This body of research provides a valuable framework for developing and interpreting the more recent work reviewed here.

DEMENTIA IN HUMANS

Dementia is a progressive loss of cognitive and other higher intellectual functions. The most common cause of dementia is Alzheimer's disease, which has become a major public health problem affecting approximately 5% of Americans over the age of 65. The diagnostic criteria for Alzheimer's disease in the Diagnostic and Statistical Manual of the American Psychiatric Association (DSM-III) include the following criteria: insidious onset, relentless progression of this syndrome, and global deterioration in intellectual functioning with failures of memory (amnesia), language (aphasia), perception (agnosia), and motor skill (apraxia) (54).

The severity of the clinical symptoms associated with dementia is correlated with specific neuropathological changes (28,111,126,128). In Alzheimer's disease, the magnitude of intellectual impairment is correlated with a loss of cholinergic presynaptic markers in the cortex and hippocampus (5,6,105,168) and with the degree of pathological change in the basal forebrain (169–171), which is a major source of cholinergic innervation of the cerebral cortex and hippocampus (143,154). Neurons (1,4,57,64,93,121,127) containing monoamines, GABA (136), somatostatin (37,38,176), and other systems have also been implicated in this disease (61,95,135,179,180), but pathology in these neurons is not always found, and when present, it is not as substantial as that in cholinergic neurons (29,34,39,61,63). Thus, dementia is like many other degenerative diseases in the central nervous system. These "multisystem disorders" may involve one system more than any other throughout the course of the disease, but inevitably more than one system becomes compromised. Furthermore, the disruption of neurochemical function often appears in diverse neuroanatomical areas (67), each of which is associated with different cognitive functions. Finally, the clinical symptoms of these disorders often progress from a highly circumscribed problem to a global deterioration of many cognitive functions (54).

THE LOGIC OF ANIMAL MODELS

Determining the causal relationships among the diverse pathological and clinical symptoms of a multisystem disorder is necessary to establish the clinical–pathological correlations that are sought routinely for any disease, to understand the functional organization of different neurochemical systems as they interact with different neuroanatomical areas, and to develop therapeutic interventions to prevent or alleviate the symptoms. This type of information cannot be obtained from human patients because the invasive and experimental procedures that are necessary to obtain the required information cannot be used while patients are alive. By the time of death, the pathological and cognitive symptoms are so extensive that the information necessary for this endeavor is no longer available. Consequently, considerable effort has been put into the development of animal models that assess cognitive processes (72,134).

Existing models do not reproduce the disease itself. Instead, they generate one or more of the pathological changes associated with disease and determine the behavioral and psychological consequences of that pathology. These models assume that degeneration of a certain set of neurons will have the same functional consequences irrespective of the cause of that degeneration. Often the degeneration is produced by injecting a neurotoxin into a certain brain area to produce a lesion that has some neuroanatomical and perhaps neurochemical specificity. The behavioral effects of these injections are evaluated, and inferences are made about the cognitive processes that are spared and impaired.

Various criteria have been established to help develop and evaluate the merits of particular models. These models seek to establish a diagnostic neurological test battery for animals similar to the ones used for humans. They (a) screen for any effect of the pathology using very sensitive behavioral tests, (b) fully describe the behavioral changes produced by a given pathological change using a battery of behavioral tests to measure different abilities, and (c) infer the psychological/functional impairments responsible for the observed behavioral changes (15,16,19,20,59,73, 78,115,116,166).

NEUROTOXINS

Intracerebral injections of a neurotoxin can produce a relatively selective destruction of a particular neurochemical system in a particular neuroanatomical area (35). This approach incorporates the advantages of selective neurochemical and neuroanatomical manipulations. Systemic injections of drugs may affect a given neurochemical system, but they do so throughout the nervous system. Physical destruction of an area may produce selective neuroanatomical damage, but it often affects many neurochemical systems as well as fibers of passage.

The ideal pharmacological agent is a "magic bullet" that is specific for a given type of neurochemical substance at a given location. The extent to which a given neurotoxin attains the status of a magic bullet depends on a variety of factors. These include the selectivity of the neurotoxin for a specific neurochemical system and the functional homogeneity of the neuroanatomical area.

The pathological and biochemical changes associated with dementia have been reproduced in animals using compounds that are not neurochemically specific but are selectively toxic to neurons and do not damage axons or terminals. Three such compounds have been used extensively: kainic acid, ibotenic acid, and quinolinic acid. In addition, the ethyl choline aziridinium ion, AF64A, a putative cholinergic neurotoxin, has been tried with limited success.

Kainic Acid

Kainic acid (KA) is a conformationally restricted analog of glutamate and has potent excitatory and neurotoxic properties (33,35,82,83,108–110,114,144,149). The precise mechanism responsible for the injury to neurons is unknown. Although KA is often described as an excitotoxin, neuronal excitation alone is insufficient to explain its effects. The neurotoxic potency of KA does not correlate with its excitatory effects when compared with other conformationally restricted and synthetic glutamate analogs such as ibotenic acid, N-methyl-D-aspartate, or quisqualate (181,182).

The pyramidal cells in the CA1 and CA3 layers of the hippocampus are particularly sensitive to KA, and injections of KA at sites far away from the hippocampus can still produce degenerative changes in CA1 and CA3 (178,183). (But see ref. 23 for an effect of KA in the nucleus basalis without hippocampal damage). Thus, although KA has properties that make it a useful tool in many areas of neurobiology (83,94), its potent selectivity for CA1 and CA3 cells in the hippocampus may mean that it cannot be used to make selective lesions in other brain areas, thereby limiting its application to animal models of dementia.

Quinolinic Acid

Quinolinic acid (QA) is a potent endogenous excitotoxin that was discovered in the brain. When applied to cells in a more concentrated form, it has pathological and biochemical consequences similar to those of KA and ibotenic acid (103,125,150,158). The enzyme necessary for the synthesis of this endogenous toxin is present in rat brain, and its quantity increases with age (56,103,104). Various regions of the brain demonstrate differential sensitivity to QA. The basal forebrain cholinergic system is particularly sensitive to its neurotoxic effects, and endogenous levels are only slightly lower than those necessary to produce degeneration. Quinolinic acid is not inactivated by specific uptake or enzymatic degradation; once released, its activity is prolonged (147,150). Therefore, QA has been considered as a possible cause for abnormal neurodegeneration associated with aging and Alzheimer's disease (148).

Ibotenic Acid

Ibotenic acid (IBO) is a naturally occurring excitatory amino acid (145,146) that produces specific axon-sparing local neuronal cell loss. Lesions produced by IBO injections are more circumscribed than those produced by KA, and IBO is far less convulsive (82,109). Ibotenic acid toxicity does not depend on an intact innervation in the adult rat (82). Its excitotoxic effects are mediated by specific membrane receptors that are also activated preferentially by N-methyl-D-aspartate. Unlike KA, IBO demonstrates a pharmacological and regional selectivity and, in the immature brain, may lack the axon-sparing properties of typical excitotoxins (159).

AF64A

AF64A may be a selective cholinergic neurotoxin (50). It is an analog of choline and irreversibly inhibits sodium-dependent high-affinity choline transport into synaptosomes (138). Some of the biochemical changes associated with dementia have been reproduced by injections of AF64A into the basal forebrain and hippocampus of rats (30,51,60). However, injections of AF64A can also produce widespread lesions, killing noncholinergic neurons and axons (52,75,140,141,142).

The Lesions

The neurotoxin was injected through a cannula located in the appropriate part of the basal forebrain. The details are available in each report. These lesions produced a decrease in the activity of the rate-limiting enzyme that produces acetylcholine (161), choline acetyltransferase (CAT), in the projection area of the lesion, the frontal cortex after NBM lesions (65,76,97,99), and the hippocampus following MSA lesions (79). The CAT decrease in cortex varied from about 30% to 70% of normal. Because 20% to 30% of cortical CAT is thought to be associated with intrinsic cortical neurons (45,71), a reduction to 70% of normal indicates destruction of most of the cholinergic neurons that project to that cortical area (25). The CAT decrease in the hippocampus following MSA lesions had a similar range. Because the hippocampus has no intrinsic cholinergic neurons, these lesions may be less complete than the NBM lesions. However, any quantitative comparison is compromised by the topological projections of both the NBM and the MSA and by the need for a quantitative sampling throughout the brain. For example, following MSA lesions, CAT was reduced to a greater extent in the dorsal hippocampus than in the ventral hippocampus, and after NBM lesions, CAT was reduced more in some cortical areas than others. In any case, these lesions destroyed some but not all of the projection cells.

All measures of cholinergic activity were decreased in the appropriate projection areas. These included CAT, acetylcholinesterase, high-affinity choline uptake (HACU), acetylcholine (ACh) levels, ACh release, ACh turnover, and muscarinic receptors (3,46,65,88,124,163). Regional cerebral metabolic rate for glucose measured by the 2-deoxy-D-^{14}C-glucose technique was reduced in nine cortical areas immediately following NBM lesions (89); ^{3}H-ONB binding, however, was normal (3). Other transmitters in the projection areas have generally not been affected by these lesions (76).

BEHAVIORAL EFFECTS OF LESIONS

The behavioral effects of the lesions in the NBM and MSA are described in the sections below. Each section briefly describes an experimental testing procedure and summarizes the results obtained. The sections begin with tasks in which performance is clearly altered and end with tasks in which performance is clearly normal, with the more inconsistent results presented in the middle. Thus, a profile of the behavior of a rat with a basal forebrain lesion can be obtained by scanning the headings of each section.

This behavioral review focuses on articles published prior to 1987 describing the behavioral effects following neurotoxic lesions of the NBM in rodents. Book chapters and abstracts from meetings were not included because these did not have sufficient details about the experiments. Experiments using electrolytic lesions of the basal forebrain were not included because these lesions destroy fibers of passage at the site of the lesion so that the subsequent behavioral effects can not be attributed solely to the destruction of cell bodies in that area. Only a few experiments have tested species other than rodents so that relatively little information is available from them. In all cases, however, the data from experiments using electrolytic lesions of the NBM in rodents (42,87,88,102) or neurotoxic lesions of the NBM in marmosets (131,132) are consistent with the conclusions from the more restricted review here.

Inhibitory (Passive) Avoidance

In tests of inhibitory avoidance, the rat must inhibit a response that would normally be made in order to avoid shock. The response may be one that has a high probability because of innate predispositions (such as the tendency to avoid light and go towards the dark) or because of training.

An impairment in inhibitory avoidance is one of the most consistent behavioral consequences of lesions in the NBM. Most experiments used an apparatus composed of two compartments, one brightly lit, the other dark. The rat was placed in the lighted compartment and quickly ran into the dark compartment, where it received a shock. In single-trial training procedures, the training phase stopped here. With criterion training procedures, the rat returned to the lighted compartment (or was placed there by the experimenter), and the procedure was repeated until the rat remained in the lighted compartment for some specified period of time. The rat was removed from the apparatus and given a retention test by being replaced in the lighted compartment. Normal rats learned to remain in the lighted compartment and inhibited the tendency to return to the dark compartment.

When testing took place with at least 30 min between the training phase and the retention test, lesioned rats had a consistent impairment in inhibitory avoidance and returned to the dark compartment more quickly than controls. This result was found following bilateral (3,21,22,53,66) and unilateral (44,48) lesions of the NBM with IBO, and unilateral (58) and bilateral (86,102) lesions with KA.

When rats were tested 3 or 6 months postoperatively, without any behavioral testing in that period, lesions still produced an impairment (22,44,48). When rats were first tested in a spatial discrimination for 5 months postoperatively and then tested in inhibitory avoidance, they performed normally (21). Thus, extensive behavioral testing in some other type of task may be able to alleviate the impairment in inhibitory avoidance.

A similar impairment was found following bilateral lesions of the NBM or MSA with IBO when rats were first trained to perform a two-way active avoidance response in a shuttle box. Inhibitory avoidance was then tested by shocking the rats for going to the previously safe compartment when the warning stimulus was presented. Rats with both NBM and MSA lesions required more trials to inhibit that response than did normal rats (69).

The initial latency to enter the dark compartment (before shock was given) and the reaction to the shock were normal in all studies that reported these data. Thus, the basic sensory, motor, and motivational components of performance in the task were normal for the animals with lesions.

When the interval between the initial shock and subsequent testing was brief, mixed results were found. When the initial testing was carried out with the criterion procedure (so that each test took place immediately following a previously shocked entry into the dark compartment), some rats had a tendency to require more shocks before remaining in the lighted compartment (48), but this impairment was small; other rats had no impairments at all (44,48,86). In the single-trial acquisition procedure, a retention interval of 5 min (3) leads to a slight impairment, but not as great as that seen with longer retention intervals. As with the appetitive delayed conditional discriminations (described below), an increase in the time during which newly acquired information had to be remembered increased the magnitude of the impairment exhibited by rats with lesions.

T Maze: Discrete Trial Alternation

A rat first visited one arm of a T maze and was then given a choice between returning to that arm and going to the alternative arm. Reinforcement was given if the rat chose the arm not visited on the previous run. After that choice was made, the trial ended. The next trial was independent of the preceding trial, and again the rat had to remember which arm was first entered on that particular trial in order to choose correctly later in that trial.

An impairment in this task occurred after unilateral lesions of the NBM with QA (24), and after bilateral lesions of the NBM (69,139) or MSA (69) with IBO. One factor influencing the magnitude and duration of the impairment, which varied in these studies was the length of the delay interval within a trial. With a relatively long delay interval, which makes the task more difficult, the magnitude of the impairment relative to the choice accuracy of the controls was greater (69). Likewise, the magnitude of the impairment decreased with extended postoperative testing (69).

Delayed-Match-To-Sample

An operant chamber had two retractable levers. Each trial began with a sample phase in which one lever was extended. The rat pressed the lever, and it was retracted for a delay interval. Both levers were extended, and the rat was given reinforcement for pressing the same lever that was presented during the sample phase. Rats with bilateral lesions of the NBM with IBO had a substantial impairment in choice accuracy, especially with a long delay interval. The magnitude of this impairment decreased with postoperative testing (43).

In another experiment, 3 different compartments were available from a choice point. Each trial began with a sample phase in which the rat was forced to enter one compartment. The rat was removed from that compartment for a delay interval, and then allowed to choose among all three compartments; reinforcement was available only in the compartment entered during the sample phase. Rats with bilateral lesions of the NBM with IBO had impaired choice accuracy, especially with long delays (79).

Delayed Alternation, Continuous Trial Procedure in a T Maze

The rat first visited one of two arms in a T maze. For all subsequent trials in that session, the rat was given a choice between the two arms. Food was located only in the arm not entered in the previous trial. Thus, the optimal strategy for the rat was to go to the arm not visited on the previous trial, alternating choices between the arms. This task is the same as the discrete trial alternation procedure except that each choice determines the correct response for the succeeding choice, whereas in the discrete trial procedure, the correct choice is dependent on the first visit of that trial and not the choice in the preceding trial.

Bilateral lesions of the NBM with IBO produced a substantial impairment of choice accuracy, lowering it to the levels expected by chance (107). Unilateral lesions of the NBM with KA produced only a slight effect (23).

Radial Arm Maze: Spatial Win–Shift Discrimination with All Arms Baited

A radial arm maze has a central platform with arms extending from it like spokes on a wheel. At the beginning of each test session, one piece of food was placed at the end of each arm; the food was not replaced during the test session. Consequently, the optimal strategy for the rat was to visit each arm once and only once during a test session, using a win–shift search strategy.

Bilateral lesions of the MSA, NBM, or both MSA and NBM combined produced an impairment in choice accuracy in this task (21,42,70,81). However, choice accuracy did improve with testing and in one instance returned to normal (21).

Bilateral lesions of the NBM affected choice accuracy as a function of the interval during which the choices had to be remembered. Rats were trained preoperatively in the basic task as described above. Delays of up to 24 hr were imposed within a trial between the fourth and fifth choices on the maze. Following bilateral lesions of the NBM with IBO, choice accuracy with no delays in the trial was normal. However, choice accuracy decreased to a greater extent than normal with increasing delays (21). This impairment gradually disappeared with continued postoperative testing so that after 5 months the rats with NBM lesions had normal choice accuracy at all delay intervals (21).

These data demonstrate a consistent impairment in choice accuracy in this procedure with the radial maze and

an improvement with postoperative testing. The magnitude of the impairment was affected by the extent of preoperative and postoperative testing and the length of the delay during which information about previously visited arms had to be remembered.

Spontaneous Alternation in a T Maze

Rats visited one arm of a T maze and then chose between it and the alternative arm. No explicit reinforcement was given for either choice. Normal rats tend to choose the arm not previously visited on about 80% of the trials, presumably reflecting a tendency to explore the less recently visited area. The probability of alternation was reduced by bilateral lesions in the NBM produced by IBO (107).

Activity

Activity was measured in a variety of different types of apparatus. The rat was placed in the apparatus and allowed to move freely about it while the activity was recorded with electronic sensors or by an observer.

An increase in activity was found following bilateral lesions of the NBM with IBO (42,66,167) and bilateral lesions of the NBM with KA (86). Activity was often normal at the start of testing (3,58,167) so that the hyperactive pattern appeared most clearly with tests of long duration.

An increase in the number and duration of visits to holes drilled in the floors/walls of a compartment occurred following bilateral lesions of the NBM with IBO (42). The rats with lesions, unlike controls, showed no decrease in the tendency to visit holes during the 30-min test session (a failure of habituation). Thus, lesions of the NBM did not affect initial activity levels, but they did disrupt the usual decrease in activity during the test session (see also the discussion of hoarding in the section on Consummatory Behavior).

Water Maze

A circular tank filled with water had a platform hidden just beneath the surface of it in one quadrant. The rat was placed in the tank at different places and allowed to swim to the platform to get out of the water. Normal rats decreased the time required to get to the platform (latency) and the number of visits to quadrants without the platform (errors). The platform was then moved to a different quadrant. Normal rats showed a marked increase in latency and errors because they went to the initially correct location and spent considerable time there before going to other locations. Other rats were trained preoperatively in the task and then given a postoperative retention test two weeks following the lesions. Bilateral lesions of the NBM with IBO produced an impairment in the initial learning, increasing latency and errors. Performance was normal when the platform was moved, indicating that the rats had learned to go to the correct place in the tank (rather than detecting some cues from the platform itself). In the retention tests, rats with lesions had a slight impairment as measured by errors and latency (167).

Rats with unilateral lesions of the NBM tested 3 months after surgery had a different pattern of results. A slight impairment as measured by latency occurred during the first few days of acquisition, but it was not present thereafter. When the platform was moved to another quadrant, rats with lesions showed less of a tendency to stay in the previously correct quadrant. Swimming speed was normal (44).

Thus, NBM lesions alter behavior in the water maze, but the magnitude and characteristics of these behavioral changes may be affected by a number of variables and remain to be determined.

Two-Way (Shuttle) Active Avoidance

In two-way active avoidance, an animal must move back and forth between two compartments at the appropriate times in order to avoid shock. A warning stimulus is presented to signal the beginning of a trial. After a few seconds, a shock is given if the animal has not moved into the other box. An avoidance response is defined as moving before the shock comes on; an escape response is defined as moving after the onset of shock. An intertrial interval follows, during which the rat stays in the part of the box that had been associated with safety on the previous trial. Then the procedure is repeated, and the animal has to move back into the original compartment to avoid/escape shock. The conflict of having to return to a place in which shock was previously received in order to avoid shock during the current trial is an important characteristic of the task.

Bilateral lesions of the NBM (70,79) or the MSA (70) improved the rate at which rats reached criterion (69), a result similar to that seen following lesions of the hippocampus or septum (62). Escape responses and retention of the avoidance response 24 hr after initial learning were both normal.

Food Searching in an Open Field

In this task, food was hidden in one of 30 plastic cups in an open field 130 × 190 cm. The food was always located in the same cup, and the rat was always placed into the field at the same location. With training, normal rats learned to go directly to the cup with food and not look into other cups. Bilateral lesions of the NBM made with IBO produced a slight but durable impairment in choice accuracy in this task (107).

Serial Order (Primacy and Recency Effects) in a Radial Arm Maze

Each rat was trained to distinguish the sequential order of arms visited during a trial in a radial arm maze. The rat first visited each of the eight arms. A choice was then presented between two arms, the first and second, fourth and fifth, or seventh and eighth choices from the preceding response sequence. The arm visited earlier in the sequence was correct and had food. Normal rats exhibited a serial order effect, choosing more accurately between the first two arms (a primacy effect) and the last two arms (a recency effect) than the middle two arms.

Small lesions of the NBM made with IBO produced a selective decrement in the recency effect, impairing the ability to choose between the last two arms visited in the sequence. Large lesions of the NBM produced a decrement in both the primacy and the recency effect (77).

Temporal Discriminations

Operant procedures were developed to examine the cognitive mechanisms involved in the timing of events of relatively short duration. Three variations of this test procedure have been used with rats having bilateral lesions of the NBM and MSA produced by IBO (98,120). MSA lesions impaired performance in trials that required working memory, while NBM lesions impaired performance in trials that required divided attention.

Rats were first trained on a standard signaled FI schedule of reinforcement in which food was delivered for the first bar press after a certain interval of time from the beginning of an auditory or visual stimulus.

Peak trials tested the remembered time of reinforcement. Each peak trial began as the standard signaled FI. However, no food was provided for any bar press, and the signal continued for approximately twice as long as in the usual FI trial. Normal rats developed a symmetrical peak of responding, with the maximum rate occurring at the time when reinforcement was available in the FI schedule. The peak time was defined as the time when the maximum rate of response occurred. Lesions of the MSA produced a leftward shift of the peak time, whereas lesions of the NBM produced a rightward shift of the peak time.

The gap trials were a test of memory for the duration of a previous timed stimulus. The gap trials were the same as peak trials except that the stimulus was turned off for an interval (the gap) and then back on. Normal rats followed a stop rule with this procedure. During the gap, they stopped timing but stored the information about the duration of the stimulus prior to the gap. After the gap, they began timing again and added the duration of the stimulus prior to the gap to the duration of the stimulus after the gap. Thus, in gap trials, as compared to peak trials, normal rats had a rightward shift of the peak time by an amount equal to the gap, showing that they remembered the duration of the stimulus prior to the gap. Rats with lesions of the NBM performed normally. Those with lesions of the MSA followed a reset rule. When the stimulus was presented again after the gap, they began timing as if the stimulus prior to the gap had never occurred. Thus, the peak time was displaced to the right by an amount equal to the gap and the perceived duration of the stimulus prior to the gap (i.e., the duration of the gap corrected for the usual leftward displacement seen in peak trials).

The third procedure tested divided attention. Two stimuli were presented at the same time. Normal rats performed the task well. They timed both stimuli correctly and showed no shift of the peak time for either stimulus. Rats with

MSA lesions performed like normals. Rats with NBM lesions were able to time either stimulus when presented alone, but could not time both of them when they were presented together. When the second stimulus was presented, they stopped timing the first one, timed the second one, and then returned to the first one, showing a rightward shift of the peak time for the first stimulus by an amount equal to the usual duration of the second stimulus. Thus, the rats with NBM lesions were unable to divide attention.

Spatial Discrimination in a T Maze

The rat was given a choice between the two arms (or two sides of the stem) of a T maze. One side was correct and led to food reinforcement; the other was incorrect. In most studies, no impairment of choice accuracy occurred after lesions. The performance of rats with bilateral lesions of the NBM with IBO was impaired for only the first few days of testing (69,107); performance after unilateral lesions of the NBM with KA was normal (23). An impairment after bilateral lesions of the NBM with IBO was found in both acquisition and retention in one study (42). The rats with lesions did reach the same criterion as the controls, but they took more than twice as many trials to do so. Thus, the impairment was substantial. However, the rats in this experiment had been given several different tests of exploration prior to this discrimination, and this experience may have caused some negative transfer for the learning of this discrimination.

Bar Press Active Avoidance

A tone was presented as a warning signal. The rat had to press the bar within a short interval following the tone in order to avoid shock or press the bar after the shock had been presented in order to escape the shock. Bilateral lesions of the NBM with KA decreased the rate at which rats learned to make the avoidance response (86).

One-Way Active Avoidance

Rats were trained in a compartment that had a retractable shelf. At the beginning of a trial, the shelf was extended into the compartment. A warning signal was presented, followed by a shock. The rat could avoid the shock by jumping to the shelf when the warning stimulus was presented or escape from the shock after it had been presented by making the same response. After a brief interval, the shelf was retracted, so that the rat jumped down to the floor of the compartment, and another trial was begun.

Bilateral lesions of the NBM with IBO produced a slight impairment in the acquisition of this task (53).

Spatial Discrimination on a Radial Arm Maze: Baited and Unbaited Arms

The radial arm maze had arms extending radially from a central platform. Each of the baited arms had one pellet of food at the end of it so that the optimal strategy was to visit each of those arms once and only once during a trial. Each of the unbaited arms had no food at the end of it, so the optimal strategy was to avoid going to those arms throughout the trial.

Unilateral lesions of the NBM made with KA (24) and with IBO (106) impaired choice accuracy on both sets of arms. However, the relative magnitude of the impairments differed. Following unilateral KA lesions, choice accuracy in the baited arms was impaired to a greater extent than choice accuracy in the unbaited arms, while the opposite pattern occurred following IBO lesions.

Consummatory Behavior

Immediately after lesions of the NBM produced by almost any method, some rats exhibited a profound aphagia and adipsia. The magnitude of this syndrome varied considerably as a function of the location of the lesion, the type and amount of neurotoxin injected, and other variables that have not yet been specified. In some cases, the aphagia and adipsia lasted for only a few days and was little more than a slight exacerbation of the usual postoperative recovery following any type of surgery. In other cases, rats refused to eat or drink and had to be fed by intubation. Many rats died, and those that recovered often took up to 2 weeks to regain their normal body weight when eating laboratory chow. Aphagia and adipsia were more commonly reported by earlier studies, suggesting that current ones have found surgical parameters that can still produce effective lesions while not interfering so markedly with consummatory behaviors. Thus, the impairments of performance in many of the tasks that assess learning and memory were independent of the changes in eating and drinking.

Formal measurements of food-related behaviors in rats that had recovered from the acute aphagia and adipsia after bilateral lesions of the NBM with IBO still showed some abnormalities. Although rats with lesions ate the same amount of food as normal rats in 24 hr, they spilled more and left fewer food biscuits ungnawed, suggesting that they tended to have bouts of eating that were shorter than those of normals (42). A test of hoarding also showed abnormalities. Food was placed in an open field. Each food-deprived rat was placed in a cage next to the open field and allowed to bring the food back to the cage. Normal rats spent relatively little time in the open field, almost always carried food back to the cage when returning from the open field, and hoarded a lot of food (42). In contrast, rats with lesions spent a great deal of time in the open field, often returned to the cage without food, and hoarded less food. These results suggest that even though rats with lesions can maintain themselves on laboratory rations, they nonetheless have abnormal patterns of behavior that alter their responses to food.

Discrimination Reversal

In a typical discrimination reversal procedure, two responses are available to the animal. First, one of them is correct and produces reinforcement. Then the response–

reinforcement contingencies are reversed so that the previously correct response is incorrect, and the previously incorrect response is correct. Bilateral lesions of the NBM with IBO produced an impairment in the reversal of a spatial discrimination in the arms of a T maze (50) but not in two paths down the stem of a T maze (70). Bilateral lesions of the NBM with KA impaired the reversal of a spatial discrimination in an operant box (86).

Stone Maze (14-Choice Multiple T Maze)

The Stone maze had 14 two-choice discriminations arranged in a path from a start area to a goal where reinforcement was obtained. Combined lesions of the MSA and NBM did not alter choice accuracy in this task (81).

Sensory–Motor Coordination

When rats emerged from the anesthesia following bilateral lesions of the NBM, they sometimes exhibited psychomotor seizures. These were minimal following electrolytic lesions, varying in magnitude following IBO lesions, and severe following KA lesions (58,86). Substantial abnormalities occurred the first day after surgery. The tests included placing of forepaws to the sight or touch of an edge, orienting to a touch on the vibrissae, clasping of the forelimbs or hind limbs when lifted by the tail, rubbing of the chin, turning in an alley, and grooming (167). Although some rats continued to have occasional seizures, especially following KA lesions, all of the other signs of sensory–motor changes had disappeared 4 days after surgery (167).

Other tests showing normal coordination following bilateral lesions of the NBM with IBO include hanging on a wire, walking on an inclined screen, an elevated rod, or a plank, sensitivity to shock, latency of the initial entry into the dark compartment prior to shock in tests of inhibitory avoidance, and speed of swimming in a water maze (53,77,167).

Unilateral lesions of the NBM produced by IBO did not affect the speed of swimming in a water maze, but they did produce several asymmetries in the response to stimulation. As compared to controls, rats with NBM lesions had a greater tendency to turn towards the side of the lesion in response to a pinch of the tail, placement on an inclined grid, a light prick of a pin to the side of the body, a touch on the snout, and placement in a bowl or on a table. These differences were present 6 days after the lesion and remained throughout the subsequent 80 days of testing (44).

In summary, the unilateral lesion clearly produced an asymmetry of responding, whereas the bilateral lesion had little obvious effect several days after surgery.

INTERPRETATION

A comparison of performance on a variety of different tests is necessary to determine the reason the abnormal behavior occurred. Every test involves many psychological processes: sensation, perception, motivation, learning, memory, motor coordination, etc. Thus, an impairment of any of these processes could lead to abnormal performance. A comparison of performance in several different tasks, each of which is relatively sensitive and selective for a different psychological process, is necessary to diagnose the reason for the abnormal behavior. The logic is the same as that used in standard clinical neurological examinations for humans and when troubleshooting any defective system (117).

Rats with bilateral lesions of the NBM or MSA do not have an obvious impairment in basic sensory and motor processes. Motivation, although not yet assessed in a systematic way, appears to be normal. Although disruptions in eating and hoarding may reflect altered motivation, they may also result secondarily from changes in other processes.

The general pattern of behavioral changes seen after lesions of the basal forebrain cholinergic system with neurotoxins resembles that seen following damage to the hippocampus (62,98,113,118,120,130) and administration of anticholinergic drugs (15,18,19). Both the hippocampus and the cholinergic system have been implicated in memory, so that the similar patterns of performance suggest that a primary effect of the neurotoxic lesions is the disruption of memory. The influence of the interval during which information must be remembered (inhibitory avoidance, radial arm maze, discrete trial alternation) is an especially important part of this argument. An interaction such that the performance of the individual with the lesion relative to the performance of a control becomes worse as the delay interval increases is often taken as both necessary and sufficient to identify an amnesia. An impairment in tasks that involve a delayed conditional discrimination is striking in human amnesics and in animals with damage to temporal lobe structures. The theoretical framework used to describe the reason for this impairment has varied considerably, but considerable agreement is available concerning the empirical observations of which behaviors are impaired and spared following lesions.

The neurotoxic lesions of the basal forebrain may alter behavior in more tasks than lesions of temporal lobe structures. If such is the case, then this syndrome of behavioral changes may be more like a true dementia, with impairment in many cognitive processes, than a restricted amnesia. This conclusion is compromised by the lack of direct comparisons of performance following the different types of lesions in identical tasks, the problems of obtaining a complete lesion, and the recovery of function that may occur following neurotoxic lesions. Nonetheless, the list of tasks in which impairments have been found is striking, especially compared to the limited list of tasks in which performance is clearly unaltered by neurotoxic lesions.

In summary, rats with neurotoxic lesions of the basal forebrain certainly do not exhibit any obvious signs of apraxia or agnosia, both of which are listed as symptoms of dementia. However, they definitely have amnesia, and this appears to be more widespread than expected on the basis of many different descriptions of the amnesia syndromes (31,152,155,156). Resolution of the nature of the cognitive impairments following NBM lesions in animals and the extent to which they produce a restricted amnesic syndrome or a more global loss of cognitive function similar to that described in dementia requires experiments with more precise quantitative manipulations and analyses of extent and type of damage in the NBM and a broader battery of behavioral tests.

THERAPEUTIC INTERVENTIONS TO ALLEVIATE THE SYMPTOMS OF DEMENTIA

Because degeneration of the cholinergic system is so extensive in dementia, many experiments have attempted therapeutic interventions with compounds that alter cholinergic activity. A rationale for this approach, and the effects of compounds on normal and aged animals, is available (22). Four different strategies have been tried with animals having lesions of the basal forebrain.

The first used cholinergic precursors. Rats with basal forebrain lesions were treated with choline supplements in the diet in an attempt to increase acetylcholine production and release (18). The results of this treatment have been inconsistent.

In clinical studies with humans, choline or lecithin had no effect on cognitive scores, learning, or memory (17).

This particular approach to therapy might not be effective because the nature of the rate-limiting step for the synthesis of acetylcholine is not well known (161). Possible limiting factors include the extracellular choline concentration, the rate of choline uptake, the availability of acetylcoenzyme A, the intracellular acetylcholine concentration, and the intracellular chloride ion concentration.

A second strategy used agents that reversibly inhibit acetylcholinesterase (AChE). These agents inhibit the breakdown of acetylcholine and prolong its action in the synaptic cleft. The results of treatment in humans and rodents with physostigmine are conflicting (16,17,106,107). Therapy with anticholinesterase may have failed in humans because the number of cholinergic terminals capable of producing acetylcholine following basal forebrain lesions was probably insufficient to produce enough acetylcholine even in the presence of excess choline. The enzyme that produces acetylcholine, choline acetyltransferase, needs two substrates to produce its product: choline and acetylcoenzyme A (161). The concentration of acetylcoenzyme A is a limiting factor when the number of terminals is significantly decreased following basal forebrain injury. In addition, fewer terminals release less acetylcholine. The ability to produce significant therapeutic benefits using AChE agents is limited, therefore, by the amount of acetylcholine that can be produced. In addition, AChE inhibitors also affect peripheral enzymes and produce unpleasant side effects.

A third strategy used cholinergic agonists such as carbachol, arecoline, and pilocarpine (107). The agents do not require the presence of cholinergic terminals or acetylcholine to produce cholinergic changes following basal forebrain lesions. Agonists may improve performance in rats with basal forebrain lesions.

The fourth strategy attempted to compensate for lost neurons by transplanting embryonic cholinergic tissue (26,27,49,91). Destruction of the fimbria–fornix, the major projection pathway for cholinergic input to the hippocampus, caused behavioral impairments. When embryonic cholinergic cellular suspensions were injected into the damaged area and allowed to innervate the host tissue, significant improvement in behavioral performance followed. Impairments in rats with basal forebrain lesions were reduced with this technique.

CONCLUSIONS AND FUTURE DIRECTIONS

Intracerebrally injected neurotoxins offer an excellent neurobiological tool to produce neuroanatomically and neurochemically specific lesions. With an appropriate neurotoxin, lesions can be relatively selective for cells in a particular location and for damage to a specific neurotransmitter system. Thus, neurotoxins are capable of reproducing one or more of the pathological changes associated with diseases causing dementia.

Although excitotoxins have significantly advanced our ability to make lesions that are neuroanatomically and neurochemically specific, they still have limitations. None of the compounds described here is ideal for making lesions of selective neurotransmitter systems in the basal forebrain. Furthermore, the time course of the excitotoxic lesion is much different from that of the degenerative disorders: they take place over a few hours or days rather than many years. Furthermore, the lesions have usually been made in young adult animals, whereas dementia is primarily associated with aging in humans.

The young nervous system is capable of compensatory changes following the production of acute lesions with excitotoxins (92). These changes include compensatory sprouting as well as transsynaptic induced degeneration of noncholinergic systems (164,165). The aged brain may also be capable of sprouting (60), but much less so than is typically observed in a young brain. These factors are unlikely to affect the major conclusions drawn from previous studies, but they may affect the details of it and certainly pose interesting problems for future investigations.

More selective neurotoxins are still needed. The lesions produced by these substances are rarely complete, destroying the entire area of interest, and discrete, sparing all other neural areas. Although some have reported success with AF64A, it has not been reliable enough to merit regular use. Therefore, continued efforts to develop a specific cholinergic neurotoxin are of great importance if animal models of dementia are to continue to advance successfully.

Behavioral tasks can be used to assess the functional effects of intracerebrally injected neurotoxins. The recent emphasis on cognitive interpretations of animal behavior (72,134) has provided a conceptual framework that allows the results of experiments with animals to be integrated with those from humans. New tasks have provided additional ways to measure the functional effects of neuropathology. However, experiments with animals are not yet able to measure and analyze cognitive processes as effectively as experiments with people. Part of this discrepancy arises from a failure to conceptualize human tasks in terms sufficiently removed from the exact testing procedures so that the same type of analysis can be applied to other tests, especially ones designed for animals. However, another part is related to the lack of innovative testing with animals. Although a few new tasks have been added, and some old ones are capable of providing a great deal of useful information, new behavioral testing procedures are urgently needed to reach the goals of animal models and relate easily to the clinical procedures used to test demented patients.

More extensive behavioral testing is needed to document the parametric characteristics of the behavioral changes that follow these lesions. This review has summarized the data in terms of the presence or absence of an impairment, and sometimes indicated whether the performance recovered. Although such a simple analysis is appropriate for the initial description of the behavioral effects of these lesions, additional quantitative information is necessary to compare the effects of these lesions with those of other lesions, and evaluate the effects of therapeutic interventions. The experiments that have included extensive postoperative testing have usually found substantial recovery of performance. The experiments that have had an equivalently long postoperative recovery time, but without behavioral testing, have generally found little or no recovery of performance. These data indicate that behavioral performance can change markedly as a result of postoperative behavioral experience. This phenomenon deserves further investigation, and complicates any discussion of the behavioral effects of these lesions with a changing baseline of performance. The variables that influence the rate of recovery, and the effects of recovery on behavioral and neural function, can provide us information about the dynamic interactions of behavioral neural recovery. In order to address these and other issues, however, experiments need to provide extended postoperative testing and data analyses that provide three measures of performance: performance immediately at the start of behavioral testing, the rate of change of performance as a function of testing, and the final asymptotic level of performance at the end of testing. These quantitative parametric data will provide the means for a more accurate application of these data from animal models to issues of clinical concern.

Damage to the basal forebrain cholinergic system is capable of producing an amnesic syndrome in animals; the impairments of memory are greater than those of other cognitive processes, which is the criterion for an amnesic syndrome. Thus, among the widespread pathological changes (160,169) and cognitive impairments characteristic of dementia, a causal relationship can be established between these two: damage to the basal forebrain cholinergic system and impairments of memory.

Many issues remain to be resolved about this causal relationship. Is damage to other brain systems sufficient to produce amnesia, or is damage to the basal forebrain cholinergic system unique in this respect? What happens to the amnesic syndrome when the lesions of the basal forebrain cholinergic system are more complete or when damage extends to some of the other systems that are also involved in dementia? To what extent do lesions in the raphe (7–12,173–175) and locus coeruleus (84,85,151), either by themselves or in conjunction with lesions of the basal forebrain, influence the resulting behavioral impair-

ments? Answers to these and related questions are necessary to obtain more details about the functional interrelationships among the different neuropathologies and cognitive impairments associated with dementia and the extent to which the results with animals reflect accurately the dementia syndrome in humans.

Destruction of the basal forebrain with neurotoxins clearly produces an impairment of memory processing of some kind. Rats with these lesions have a pattern of behavioral changes indicating that basic sensory, motor, and motivational processes are intact but that the ability to remember newly acquired information for long intervals of time is disrupted.

However, the extent of this amnesia is not well documented. Amnesic syndromes are usually described in terms of memory processes that are spared and those that are impaired, yet in rats with neurotoxic lesions, few processes seem to be spared. Two issues arise from these observations. First, to what extent are the limits of the amnesia exhibited after neurotoxic lesions of the basal forebrain the same as those seen in other, clearly circumscribed amnesia syndromes? Second, to what extent do the behavioral impairments spread beyond the domain of what is usually considered an amnesic syndrome and spread into the domain of a dementia?

The basal forebrain cholinergic system has neuroanatomically discrete subdivisions and projections. Of particular importance is the distinction between the nucleus basalis and its projections to the frontal cortex and the medial septal area and its projections to the hippocampus (36,78,98,120). Behavioral testing has shown that degenerative changes in both of these systems can produce impairments of memory and of temporal discrimination. However, neurons in these two areas produce similar effects in some behavioral tasks (active avoidance, passive avoidance, radial arm maze), and divergent efforts in other tasks (temporal discriminations, serial order effects). The syndromes resulting from damage to the frontal lobes and temporal lobes in humans are distinct yet share some common elements, suggesting that the results obtained with these animal models may reflect a similar functional organization. However, an extensive and detailed analysis of the behavioral effects of selective lesions in different areas within the basal forebrain cholinergic system is necessary to provide a complete comparison of the behavioral syndromes following neuropathology limited to subcomponents of this system.

Most experiments have focused on the behavioral effects following degeneration in a single neurotransmitter system. These have provided us a great deal of information about the behavioral consequences of damage in each of these areas. However, dementia is a multisystem disorder. Thus, future animal models will need to emphasize noncholinergic pathological changes (61). Lesions should be highly specific and discrete in those transmitter systems that are affected in Alzheimer's disease. Some attempt will have to be made to follow a temporal sequence of biochemical changes in the various neurotransmitter systems. In Alzheimer's disease, the cholinergic system may begin to degenerate first (29,68), followed by changes in serotonergic (61,100), noradrenergic (121), and dopaminergic (95,179) systems. Thus, lesions might be produced in the basal forebrain cholinergic system of animals and then in the locus coeruleus, raphe system, and ventral tegmental area.

The symptoms of dementia in animals can be altered by therapeutic interventions. Some success has been obtained with compounds such as nerve growth factor (67,172), ganglioside G_{M1}, and physostigmine (78,79) and by transplants (26,27,49,91) of fetal brain tissue.

However, these interventions have not produced reliable results, and the magnitude of their effect (if any) has varied widely. Consequently, the development of an effective therapeutic or prophylactic treatment remains a high priority. Because dementia is a multisystem disorder, it may require a multimodal therapy. The changes in noncholinergic systems in Alzheimer's disease may also be responsible for components of the memory dysfunction. The performance of animals with basal forebrain lesions may be improved by providing pharmacotherapy directed at noncholinergic systems. For example, reactive synaptogenesis (2,82,90,112) may cause neuronal terminals of noncholinergic systems that coinnervate similar projection areas to increase the number and extent of their terminals to compensate for lost cholinergic inputs. The brain may attempt to recruit other compensatory processes in noncholinergic neuronal systems. Memory in animals with basal forebrain lesions may be improved by drug combinations designed to stimulate both cholinergic and noncholinergic neuronal systems.

The review in this chapter has concentrated on the effects of lesions, which is appropriate in order to understand the behavioral impairments that are likely to follow neuropathology in the cholinergic system. However, information from other techniques is important to provide information about the functioning of these systems in the normal brain. Thus, recordings from single units (101) and other electrophysiological characteristics (13,14,55,123,133) are important to obtain. Identifying the transmitter used by the neurons will have to be a major consideration as well; even though the NBM contains mostly cholinergic neurons, cells with other transmitters are present also, and these may have different electrophysiological properties.

ACKNOWLEDGMENTS

The preparation of this chapter was supported in part by funds from the U.S. Public Health Service, NIH AG05146 and NS 20471. The authors thank C. Lippa, D. Harris, and E. Kelmartin for typing the manuscript.

REFERENCES

1. Adolfsson, R., Gottfries, C. G., Roos, B. E., and Winblad, B. (1979): *Br. J. Psychiatry*, 135:216–223.
2. Akers, R. F., and Routtenberg, A. (1985): *Brain Res.*, 334:147.
3. Altman, H. J., Crosland, R. D., Jenden, D. J., and Berman, R. F. (1985): *Neurobiol. Aging*, 6:125–130.
4. Arai, H., Kosaka, K., and Iizuka, R. (1984): *J. Neurochem.*, 43: 388–393.
5. Arendt, T., Bigl, V., Tennstedt, A., and Arendt, A. (1984): *Neurosci. Lett.*, 48:81–85.
6. Arendt, T., Bigl, V., Tennstedt, A., and Arendt, A. (1985): *Neuroscience*, 14:1–14.
7. Asin, K. E., and Fibiger, H. C. (1984): *Behav. Brain Res.*, 13: 241–250.
8. Asin, K. E., and Fibiger, H. C. (1983): *Brain Res.*, 268:211–223.
9. Asin, K. E., and Wirtshafter, D. (1982): *Physiol. Behav.*, 28:89–93.
10. Asin, K. E., Wirtshafter, D., and Fibiger, H. C. (1985): *Behav. Neural Biol.*, 44:415–424.
11. Asin, K. E., Wirtshafter, D., and Kent, E. W. (1979): *Physiol. Behav.*, 23:803–806.
12. Asin, K. E., Wirtshafter, D., and Kent, E. W. (1980): *Behav. Neural Biol.*, 28:408–417.
13. Aston-Jones, G., and Bloom, F. E. (1981): *J. Neurosci.*, 1:887–900.
14. Aston-Jones, G., and Bloom, F. E. (1981): *J. Neurosci.*, 1:876–886.
15. Bartus, R. T. (1979): *Science*, 206:1086–1089.
16. Bartus, R. T., and Dean, R. (1985): In: *Normal Aging, Alzheimer's Disease and Senile Dementia*, edited by C. G. Gottfries, pp. 231–267. University of Brussels Press, Brussels.
17. Bartus, R. T., Dean, R. L., Beer, B., and Lippa, A. S. (1982): *Science*, 217:408–417.
18. Bartus, R. T., Dean, R. L., Goas, J. A., and Lippa, A. S. (1980): *Science*, 209:301–303.
19. Bartus, R. T., Dean, R. L., Pontecorvo, M. J., and Flicker, C. (1985): *Ann. N.Y. Acad. Sci.*, 444:332–358.
20. Bartus, R. T., Flicker, C., and Dean, R. L. (1983): In: *Assessment in Geriatric Psychopharmacology*, edited by T. Crook, S. Ferris, and R. Bartus, pp. 263–299. Powley Associates, New Canaan, CT.
21. Bartus, R., Flicker, C., Dean, R., Pontecorvo, M., Figueiredo, J., et al. (1985): *Pharmacol. Biochem. Behav.*, 23:125–135.
22. Bartus, R. T., Ponteconvo, M. J., Flicker, C., Dean, R. L., and Figueiredo, J. C. (1986): *Pharmacol. Biochem. Behav.*, 24:1287–1292.
23. Beninger, R. J., Jhamandas, K., Boegman, R. J., and El-Defrawy, S. R. (1986): *Pharmacol. Biochem. Behav.*, 24:1353–1360.
24. Beninger, R. J., Wirsching, B. A., Jhamandas, K., Boegman, R. J., and El-Defrawy, S. R. (1986): *Can. J. Physiol. Pharmacol.*, 64:376–382.
25. Bigl, V., Woolf, N. J., and Butcher, L. L. (1982): *Brain Res. Bull.*, 8:727–749.
26. Bjorklund, A., Gage, F. H., Stenevi, U., and Dunnett, S. B. (1983): *Acta Physiol. Scand. [Suppl.]*, 522:49–58.
27. Bjorklund, A., Gage, F. H., Schmidt, R. H., Stenevi, U., and Dunnett, S. B. (1983): *Acta Physiol. Scand. [Suppl.]*, 522:59–66.
28. Blessed, G., Tomlinson, B. E., and Roth, M. (1968): *Br. J. Psychiatry*, 11:797–783.
29. Bowen, D. M., and Davison, A. N. (1986): *Br. Med. Bull.*, 42:1–7.
30. Chrobak, J., Dettaven, D., and Walsh, T. (1985): *Neuroscience*, 14:1025–1036.
31. Corkin, S., Cohen, N. J., Sullivan, E. V., Clegg, R. A., Rosen, T. J., et al. (1985): In: *Memory Dysfunctions: An Integration of Animal and Human Research from Preclinical and Clinical Perspectives*, edited by D. S. Olton, E. Gamzu, and S. Corkin, pp. 10–40. New York Academy of Sciences, New York.
32. Corkin, S., Davis, K. L., Growdon, J. H., Usdin, E., and Wurtman, R. J. (1982): *Aging, Vol. 19 Alzheimer's Disease: A Report of Progress in Research*. Raven Press, New York.
33. Coyle, J. T. (1983): *J. Neurochem.*, 41:1–11.
34. Coyle, J. T., Price, D. L., and DeLong, M. R. (1983): *Science*, 219:1184–1190.
35. Coyle, J. T., and Schwarcz, R. (1983): In: *Handbook of Chemical Neuroanatomy*, edited by A. Bjorklund and T. Hokfelt, pp. 508–527. Elsevier, Amsterdam.
36. Crutcher, K., Kesner, R., and Novak, J. (1983): *Brain Res.*, 262: 91–93.
37. Crystal, H. A., and Davies, P. (1982): *J. Neurochem.*, 38:1781–1784.
38. Davies, P., Katzman, R., and Terry, R. D. (1980): *Nature*, 288: 279–280.

39. Davies, P., and Maloney, A. F. J. (1976): *Lancet,* 2:1403.
40. Divac, I. (1975): *Brain Res.,* 93:385–398.
41. Divac, I. (1979): *Neuroscience,* 4:455–461.
42. Dubois, B., Mayo, W., Agid, Y., LeMoal, M., and Simon, H. (1985): *Brain Res.,* 338:249–258.
43. Dunnett, S. B. (1985): *Psychopharmacology,* 87:357–363.
44. Dunnett, S. B., Toniolo, G., Fine, A., Ryan, C. N., Bjorkland, A., et al. (1985): *Neuroscience,* 16:787–797.
45. Eckenstein, F., and Thoenen, H. (1983): *Neurosci. Lett.,* 36:211–215.
46. El-Defnany, S. R., Coloma, F., Jhamandas, K., Boegman, R. J., Beninger, R. J., et al. (1985): *Neurobiol. Aging,* 6:325–330.
47. Ferry, G. (1985): *New Scientist,* 22:33–35.
48. Fine, A., Dunnett, S. B., Bjorkland, A., and Iversen, S. D. (1985): *Proc. Natl. Acad. Sci. U.S.A.,* 82:5227–5230.
49. Fine, A., Dunnett, S. B., Bjorkland, A., Clarke, D., and Iversen, S. D. (1985): *Neuroscience,* 16:769–786.
50. Fisher, A., and Hanin, I. (1980): *Life Sci.,* 27:1615–1634.
51. Fisher, A., Mantione, C. R., Abraham, D. J., and Hanin, I. (1982): *J. Pharmacol. Exp. Ther.,* 222:140–145.
52. Fisher, A., Mantione, C. R., Grauer, E., Levy, A., and Hanin, I. (1983): In: *Behavioral Models and the Analysis of Drug Action,* edited by M. Y. Spiegelstein and A. Levy, pp. 333–342. Elsevier, Amsterdam.
53. Flicker, C., Dean, R., Watkins, D. L., Fisher, S. K., and Bartus, R. T. (1983): *Pharmacol. Biochem. Behav.,* 18:973–981.
54. Folstein, M. F., and Whitehouse, P. J. (1983): *Neurobehav. Toxicol. Teratol.,* 5:631–634.
55. Foote, S. L., Aston-Jones, G., and Bloom, F. E. (1980): *Proc. Natl. Acad. Sci. U.S.A.,* 77:3033–3037.
56. Foster, A. C., Zinkand, W. C., and Schwarcz, R. (1985): *J. Neurochem.,* 44:446–454.
57. Francis, P. T., Palmer, A. M., Sims, N. R., Bowen, D. M., Davison, A. N., et al. (1985): *N. Engl. J. Med.,* 313:7–11.
58. Friedman, E., Lerer, B., and Kuster, J. (1986): *Pharmacol. Biochem. Behav.,* 19:309–312.
59. Gamzu, E. (1985): In: *Memory Dysfunctions: An Integration of Animal and Human Research from Preclinical and Clinical Perspectives,* edited by D. S. Octor, E. Gamzu, and S. Corkin, pp. 370–393. New York Academy of Sciences, New York.
60. Geddes, J. W., Monaghan, D. T., Cotman, C. W., Lott, I. T., and Wan, R. C. (1985): *Science,* 230:1179–1181.
61. Gottfries, C.-G., Adolfsson, R., Aquilonius, S. M., Carlsson, A., Eckernas, S. A., et al. (1983): *Neurobiol. Aging,* 4:261–271.
62. Gray, J. A., and McNaughton, N. (1983): *Neurosci. Biobehav. Rev.,* 7:119–188.
63. Hanin, I., Mantione, C. R., and Fisher, A. (1982): In: *Aging, Vol. 19: Alzheimer's Disease: A Report of Progress,* edited by S. Corkin, K. L. Davis, J. H. Growdon, E. Usdin, and R. J. Wurtman, pp. 267–270. Raven Press, New York.
64. Hardy, J., Adolfsson, R., Alafuzoff, I., Bucht, G., Marcusson, J., et al. (1985): *Neurochem. Int.,* 7:545–563.
65. Hartgraves, S. L., Mensah, P. L., and Kelly, P. H. (1982): *Neuroscience,* 7:2369–2376.
66. Haroutunian, V., Kanof, P., and Davis, M. D. (1985): *Life Sci,* 37:945–952.
67. Hefti, F., Dravid, A., and Hartikka, J. (1984): *Brain Res.,* 293:305–311.
68. Henke, H., and Lang, W. (1983): *Brain Res.,* 267:281–291.
69. Hepler, D. J., Olton, D. S., Wenk, G., and Coyle, J. T. (1985): *J. Neuroscience,* 5:856–873.
70. Hepler, D. J., Wenk, G. L., Cribbs, B. L., Olton, D. S., and Coyle, J. T. (1985): *Brain Res.,* 346:8–14.
71. Houser, C. R., Crawford, G. D., Salvaterra, P. M., and Vaughn, J. E. (1985): *J. Comp. Neurol.,* 234:17–34.
72. Hulse, S. H., Fowler, H., and Honig, W. K. (1978): *Cognitive Processes in Animal Behavior.* Lawrence Erlbaum Associates, Hillsdale, NJ.
73. Ingram, D. K., and Brennan, M. J. (1985): *Neurobiol. Aging,* 5:63–66.
74. Iversen, L. L. (1981): *Life Sci.,* 29:405–410.
75. Jarrard, L. E., Kant, G. J., Meyerhoff, J. L., and Levy, A. (1985): *Brain Res.* (in press).

76. Johnston, M. V., McKinney, M., and Coyle, J. T. (1983): *Exp. Brain Res.,* 43:159–172.
77. Kesner, R. T., Crutcher, K. A., and Measom, M. O. (1986): *Neurobiol. Aging,* 7:287–295.
78. Kesner, R. P., and Novak, J. M. (1982): *Science,* 218:173–174.
79. Kessler, J., Markowitsch, H. J., and Sigg, G. (1986): *Intern. J. Neuroscience,* 30:101–119.
80. Knesevich, J. W., Martin, R. L., Berg, L., and Danziger, W. (1983): *Am. J. Psychiatry,* 140:233–234.
81. Knowlton, B. J., Wenk, G., Olton, D. S., and Coyle, J. T. (1985): *Brain Res.,* 345:315–321.
82. Kohler, C., and Schwarcz, R. (1983): *Neuroscience,* 8:819–835.
83. Kohler, C., Schwarcz, R., and Fuxe, K. (1979): *Brain Res.,* 175:366–371.
84. Koob, G. F., Kelley, A. E., and Mason, S. T. (1978): *Physiol. Behav.,* 20:709–716.
85. Koob, G. F., Thatcher-Britton, K., Britton, D. R., Roberts, D. C. S., and Bloom, F. E. (1984): *Physiol. Behav.,* 3:479–485.
86. Lerer, B., Warner, J., and Friedman, E. (1986): *Behav. Neurosci.,* 99:661–667.
87. Lo Conte, G. L., Bartololini, L., Casamenti, F., Marconcini-Pepeu, I., and Pepeu, G. (1982): *Pharmacol. Biochem. Behav.,* 17:933–937.
88. Lo Conte, G. L., Casamenti, F., Bigl, V., Milaneschi, E., and Pepeu, G. (1982): *Arch. Ital. Biol.,* 120:176–188.
89. London, E. D., McKinney, M., Dam, M., Ellis, A., and Coyle, J. T. (1984): *J. Cereb. Blood Flow Metab.,* 4:381–390.
90. Lovinger, D. M., Akers, R. F., Nelson, R. B., Barnes, C. A., McNaughton, B. L., et al. (1985): *Brain Res.,* 343:137–143.
91. Low, W. C., Lewis, P. R., Bunch, S. T., Dunnett, S. B., Thomas, S. R., et al. (1982): *Nature,* 300:260–262.
92. Loy, R., and Moore, R. Y. (1977): *Exp. Neurol.,* 57:399–411.
93. Mann, J. J., Stanley, M., Neophytides, A., DeLeon, M. J., Ferris, S. H., et al. (1981): *Neurobiol. Aging,* 2:57–60.
94. McGeer, E. G., Olney, J. W., and McGeer, P. L., eds. (1978): *Kainic Acid as a Tool in Neurobiology.* Raven Press, New York.
95. McGeer, E. G. (1981): *Prog. Neuropsychopharmacol.,* 5:435–445.
96. McKhann, G., Drachman, D., Folstein, M., Katzman, R., Price, D., et al. (1984): *Neurology,* 34:939–944.
97. McKinney, M., Coyle, J. T., and Hedreen, J. C. (1983): *J. Comp. Neurol.,* 217:103–121.
98. Meck, W. H., Church, R. M., Wenk, G. L., and Olton, D. S., *J. Neuroscience* (in press).
99. Meyer, U., Wenk, H., Ott, T., and Wetzel, W. (1982): *J. Hirnforsch.,* 23:1–12.
100. Middlemiss, D. N., Palmer, A. M., Edel, N., and Bowen, D. M. (1986): *J. Neurochem.* (in press).
101. Mink, J. W., Sinnamon, H. M., and Adams, D. B. (1983): *Behav. Brain Res.,* 8:85–108.
102. Miyamoto, M., Shintani, M., Nagaoka, A., and Nagawa, Y. (1985): *Brain Res.,* 328:97–104.
103. Moroni, F., Lonbardi, G., Carla, V., and Moneti, G. (1984): *Brain Res.,* 295:352–355.
104. Moroni, F., Lombardi, G., Moneti, G., and Aldinio, C. (1984): *Neurosci. Lett.,* 47:51–55.
105. Mountjoy, C. Q., Rosor, M. N., Iversen, L. L., and Roth, M. (1984): *Brain,* 107:507–518.
106. Murray, C. L., and Fibiger, H. C. (1985): *Neuroscience,* 14:1025–1036.
107. Murray, C. L., and Fibiger, H. C. (1986): *Behav. Neurosci.,* 100:23–32.
108. Nadler, J. V., and Cuthbertson, G. J. (1980): *Brain Res.,* 195:47–56.
109. Nadler, J. V., Evenson, D. A., and Cuthbertson, G. J. (1981): *Neuroscience,* 6:2505–2517.
110. Nadler, J. V., Perry, B. W., and Cotman, C. W. (1978): *Nature,* 271:676–677.
111. Northern, B., Yates, P. O., and Davison, A. N. (1985): *J. Neurol. Psychiatry Neurosurg.* (in press).
112. Nelson, R. B., and Routtenberg, A. (1985): *Exp. Neurol.,* 89:213–224.
113. O'Keefe, J., and Nadel, L. (1978): *The Hippocampus as a Cognitive Map.* Clarendon Press, Oxford.

114. Olney, J. W., Rhee, V., and Ho, O. L. (1974): *Brain Res.*, 77: 507–512.
115. Olton, D. S. (1985): In: *Memory Dysfunctions: An Integration of Animal and Human Research from Preclinical and Clinical Perspectives*, edited by D. S. Olton, E. Gamzu, and S. Corkin, pp. 113–121. New York Academy of Sciences, New York.
116. Olton, D. S. (1983): *Neurobehav. Toxicol. Teratol.*, 5:635–640.
117. Olton, D. S. (1986): In: *Learning and Memory: A Biological View*, edited by J. L. Martinez and R. Kesner, pp. 379–397. Academic Press, New York.
118. Olton, D. S., Becker, J. T., and Handelmann, G. E. (1979): *Behav. Brain Sci.*, 2:313–365.
119. Olton, D. S., Walker, J., and Gage, F. H. (1978): *Brain Res.*, 39: 295–308.
120. Olton, D. S., Wenk, G. L., Church, R. M., and Neck, W. H. (1987): *Neuropsychologia (in press)*.
121. Palmer, A. N., Sims, N. R., Smith, C. C. T., Spillane, J. A., Esiri, M. M., et al. (1983): *J. Neurochem.*, 41:266–272.
122. Pearson, R. C. A., Gatter, K. C., Brodal, P., and Powell, T. P. S. (1983): *Brain Res.*, 259:132–136.
123. Pepeu, G. (1984): In: *Aging of the Brain and Senile Dementia: The Inventory of EEC Potentialities*, edited by D. L. Knook, G. Calderini, L. Amaducci, pp. 15–22. Eurage.
124. Pepeu, G., Casamenti, F., Bracco, L., Ladinsky, H., and Consolo, S. (1985): In: *Senile Dementia of the Alzheimer Type*, edited by J. Traber and W. H. Gispen, pp. 305–315. Springer-Verlag, Berlin, Heidelberg.
125. Perkins, M. N., and Stone, T. W. (1983): *Brain Res.*, 259:172–176.
126. Perry, E. K., Tomlinson, B. E., Blessed, G., Bergman, K., Gibson, P. H., et al. (1978): *Br. Med. J.*, 2:1457–1459.
127. Perry, E. K., Gibson, P. H., Blessed, G., Perry, R. H., and Tomlinson, B. E. (1977): *J. Neurol. Sci.*, 34:247–265.
128. Perry, E. K., and Perry, R. H. (1985): *Trends Neurosci.*, 8:301–303.
129. Price, D. L., Whitehouse, P. J., and Struble, R. G. (1986): *Trends Neurosci.*, 9:29–33.
130. Rawlins, J. N. P. (1985): *Behav. Brain Sci.*, 8:479–497, 514–528.
131. Ridley, R. M., Baker, H. F., Drewett, B., and Johnson, J. A. (1985): *Psychopharmacology*, 86:438–443.
132. Ridley, R. M., Murray, T. K., Johnson, J. A., and Baker, H. F. (1986): *Brain Res.*, 376:108–116.
133. Rogers, J., Aston-Jones, G., Dinan, T., Shaver, R., and Moss, D. E. (1983): *Soc. Neurosci. Abstr.*, 9:124.
134. Roitblatt, H. L., Bever, T. G., and Terrace, H. S. (1984): *Animal Cognition*. Lawrence Erlbaum, Hillsdale, NJ.
135. Rossor, M. N., Rehfeld, J. F., Emson, P. C., Mountjoy, C. Q., Roth, M., et al. (1985): *Ann. N.Y. Acad. Sci.*, 444:203–221.
136. Rossor, M. N., Garret, J. J., Johnson, A. L., Mountjoy, C. Q., Roth, M., et al. (1982): *Brain*, 105:313–330.
137. Rye, D. B., Wainer, B. H., Mesulam, M. M., Mufson, E. J., and Saper, C. B. (1984): *Neuroscience*, 13:627–643.
138. Rylett, B. J., and Colhoun, E. H. (1980): *J. Neurochem.*, 34:713–719.
139. Salamone, J. D., Beart, P. M., Alpert, J. E., and Iversen, S. D. (1984): *Behav. Brain Res.*, 13:63–70.
140. Sandberg, K., Hanin, I., Fisher, A., and Coyle, J. T. (1984): *Brain Res.*, 293:49–55.
141. Sandberg, K., Schnaar, R. L., McKinney, M., Hanin, I., Fisher, A., et al. (1985): *J. Neurochem.*, 44:439–445.
142. Sandberg, K., Sandberg, P. R., and Coyle, J. T. (1984): *Brain Res.*, 299:339–343.
143. Saper, C. B. (1984): *J. Comp. Neurol.*, 222:313–342.
144. Schwarcz, R., and Coyle, J. T. (1977): *Brain Res.*, 127:235–249.
145. Schwarcz, R., Hokfelt, T., Fuxe, K., and Jonsson, G. (1979): *Exp. Brain Res.*, 37:199–216.
146. Schwarcz, R., Foster, A. C., French, E. D., Whetsell, W. O., Jr., and Kohler, C. (1984): *Life Sci.*, 35:19–32.
147. Schwarcz, R., and Kohler, C. (1983): *Neurosci. Lett.*, 38:85–90.
148. Schwarcz, R., and Meldrum, B. (1985): *Lancet*, 2:140–143.
149. Schwarcz, R., Scholz, D., and Coyle, J. T. (1978): *Neuropharmacology*, 17:145–151.
150. Schwarcz, R., Wetsell, W. O., and Mangano, R. M. (1983): *Science*, 219:316–318.
151. Sessions, G. R., Kant, G. J., and Koob, G. F. (1976): *Physiol. Behav.*, 116:853–859.
152. Shacter, D. L., and Tulving, E. (1982): In: *The Expression of Knowledge*, edited by R. L. Isaacson and N. E. Spear, pp. 33–65. Plenum Press, New York.
153. Smith, C. M., and Swash, M. (1978): *Ann. Neurol.*, 3:471–473.
154. Spillane, J. A., White, P., Goodhardt, M. J., Flack, R. H. A., Bowen, D. M., et al. (1977): *Nature*, 266:558–559.
155. Squire, L. R., and Cohen, J. J. (1984): In: *Neurobiology of Learning and Memory*, edited by J. McGaugh and N. Weinberger, pp. 3–64. Guilford Press, New York.
156. Squire, L. R., and Zola-Morgan, S. (1983): In: *The Physiological Basis of Memory*, edited by J. A. Deutsch, pp. 199–268. Academic Press, New York.
157. Steiner, H. X., McBean, G. J., Kohler, C., Roberts, P. J., and Schwarcz, R. (1984): *Brain Res.*, 307:117–124.
158. Stone, T. W., and Perkins, M. N. (1981): *Eur. J. Pharmacol.*, 72: 411–412.
159. Terry, R. D., and Davies, P. (1980): *Annu. Rev. Neurosci.*, 3:77–95.
160. Tomlinson, B. E., Irving, D., and Blessed, G. (1981): *J. Neurol. Sci.*, 49:419–428.
161. Tucek, S. (1985): *J. Neurochem.*, 44:11–24.
162. Wenk, H., Bigl, V., and Meyer, U. (1980): *Brain Res. Rev.*, 2: 295–316.
163. Wenk, G. L., Cribbs, B., and McCall, L. (1984): *Exp. Brain Res.*, 56:335–340.
164. Wenk, G. L., and Engisch, K. L. (1986): *J. Neurochem.*, 47:845–850.
165. Wenk, G. L., Engisch, K. L., McCall, L. D., Mitchell, S. J., Aigner, R. L., et al. (1986): *Int. Neurochem.*, 9:557–562.
166. Wenk, G. L., and Olton, D. S., In: *Behavioral Toxicology*, edited by Z. Annau. Johns Hopkins University Press, Baltimore (in press).
167. Whishaw, I. Q., O'Connor, W. T., and Dunnett, S. B. (1985): *Behav. Brain Res.*, 17:103–115.
168. Whitehouse, P. J., Price, D. L., Clark, A. W., Coyle, J. T., and DeLong, M. R. (1981): *Ann. Neurol.*, 10:122–126.
169. Whitehouse, P. J., Price, D. L., Struble, R. G., Clark, A. W., Coyle, J. T., et al. (1982): *Science*, 215:1237–1239.
170. Whitehouse, P. J., Struble, R. G., Hedreen, J. C., Clark, A. W., and Price, D. L. (1985): In: *CRC Critical Reviews in Clinical Neurobiology*, edited by J. P. Blass, pp. 319–339. CRC Press, Boca Raton, FL.
171. Wilcock, G. K., Esiri, M. M., Bowen, D. M., and Smith, C. C. T. (1982): *J. Neurol. Sci.*, 57:407–417.
172. Will, B., and Hefti, F. (1985): *Behav. Brain Res.*, 17:17–24.
173. Wirtshafter, D., and Asin, K. E. (1982): *Physiol. Behav.*, 28:749–754.
174. Wirtshafter, D., and Asin, K. E. (1983): *Exp. Neurol.*, 79:412–421.
175. Wirtshafter, D., and Asin, K. E. (1981): *Physiol. Psychol.*, 9:263–268.
176. Wood, P. L., Eitenne, P., Gauthier, L. S., Cajal, S., and Nair, N. P. V. (1982): *Life Sci.*, 31:2073–2079.
177. Woolf, N. J., Eckenstein, F., and Butcher, L. L. (1983): *Neurosci. Lett.*, 40:98–98.
178. Wuerthele, S. M., Lovell, K. M., Jones, M. Z., and Moore, K. E. (1978): *Brain Res.*, 149:489–497.
179. Yates, C. M., Simpson, J., Gordon, A., Maloney, A. F. J., Allison, V., et al. (1983): *Brain Res.*, 200:119–126.
180. Yates, C. M., Harmar, A. J., Rose, R., Shevard, J., Sanchey de Levy, G., et al. (1983): *Brain Res.*, 258:445–452.
181. Zaczek, R., and Coyle, J. T. (1982): *Neuropharmacology*, 21:15–26.
182. Zaczek, R., Nelson, M. F., and Coyle, J. T. (1981): *Neuropharmacology*, 20:183–199.
183. Zaczek, R., Simonton, S., and Coyle, J. T. (1980): *J. Neuropathol. Exp. Neurol.*, 39:245–264.

Psychopharmacology:
The Third Generation of Progress,
edited by Herbert Y. Meltzer.
Raven Press, New York © 1987.

CHAPTER **94**

Recent Advances in the Genetics of Anxiety and Somatoform Disorders

C. Robert Cloninger

Early studies demonstrated that anxiety and somatoform disorders were relatively discrete, moderately stable over time, and showed strong familial specificity. However, many of the early studies were open to criticism because of lack of blind assessment, uniform assessment procedures, and explicit diagnostic criteria. More recently, these deficiencies have been corrected, but research and clinical practice have continued to be handicapped by approaches to clinical description and treatment that fail to integrate available neurobiological and genetic knowledge with clinical and developmental information. Nevertheless, in the past few years enough information has been accumulated to permit development of a general and testable theory of the neurobiological basis of anxiety and somatoform disorders that should facilitate future case description and research (11).

The promise of this new phase of research is that it recognizes the multidimensional nature of anxiety and that it integrates available neurobiological data with clinical and developmental information. Four types of anxiety have been distinguished and called "chronic cognitive anxiety," "chronic somatic anxiety," "panic anxiety," and "reactive dysphoria." Each of these types of anxiety can be distinguished in terms of clinical features, associated personality traits, patterns of information processing, neurophysiological and biochemical variability, and response to psychoactive drugs. Each type of anxiety has distinct genetic and environmental antecedents that have been demonstrated in recent adoption and twin studies.

In this chapter, I summarize available information about the neuropharmacology and neurophysiology of the central nervous system mechanisms that underlie the multidimensional nature of anxiety. I also integrate this with a general theory of personality and associated patterns of adaptive responses to environmental challenge. First, I present an ethological view of anxiety and the role of information processing in an organism's adaptive responses to danger and novelty. Then I summarize a general theory of personality and its role in the development of chronic anxiety, somatization, and reactive dysphoria. Predictions of this theory are compared with available neurobiological and genetic data, and recommendations are made for future research.

THE ADAPTIVE FUNCTION OF ANXIETY

Nearly all animals from lower invertebrates to man inherit a tendency to be alerted and frightened by sudden novel stimuli such as loud noises, bright lights, and unfamiliar objects (55). However, all animals have fixed limits to the amount of information they can process at any time, so significant stimuli must be filtered out from irrelevant stimuli for an organism to function successfully. If an animal reacts unselectively to all harmless stimuli, then other more significant stimuli cannot receive the intensity of response that they may require.

Responses to dangerous stimuli often have a genetically determined resistance to habituation because of the evolutionary advantage of such mechanisms for survival and

TABLE 1. *Distinguishing features of two chronic anxiety syndromes*

Characteristic feature	Type of syndrome	
	Cognitive anxiety	Somatic anxiety
Anticipation of harm from specific cues	Frequent (anticipatory worry)	Infrequent (global alarm)
Fatigability	Rapid	Slow
Muscular relaxability	Slow	Rapid
Novelty seeking	Low	High
Pain sensitivity	Low	High
Sedation threshold	High	Low

reproduction, as first noted by Darwin (25). Such resistance to habituation is seen in the genetic preparedness of man to develop avoidance responses and fear of particular stimuli such as snakes and thunderstorms (56). Anxiety-prone individuals have a greater tendency to acquire avoidance responses than normals and show a reduced tendency of some physiological responses (e.g., responses measured by galvanic skin conductance) to habituate to repeated stimuli (44,45).

The tendency to avoid novel and dangerous stimuli is an adaptive trait that benefits the survival and reproduction of an individual. However, other situations benefit from courage and fearlessness rather than fearful caution, so this can also be adaptive. Likewise, exploration of the unknown and other forms of novelty-seeking behavior may have adaptive value for the species as a whole. A tendency to form strong social attachments and to be sentimental and industrious may also have advantages in some situations, whereas tough-minded objectivity and social detachment may be advantageous in other settings. Consequently, there is wide heritable variation within a species like man in heritable tendencies to avoid harm, to explore and seek novelty, and to form social attachments (11).

Such variation is important in susceptibility to the various dimensions of anxiety. Cognitive anxiety refers to anticipatory apprehension, ruminative worrying, social anxiety and insecurity, and slow muscular relaxation (11,66,71). Susceptibility to cognitive anxiety is primarily determined by the tendency to respond intensely to aversive stimuli and hence to acquire avoidant responses to punishment, nonreward, and novelty (11). In contrast, somatic anxiety refers to generalized feelings of alarm and uneasiness associated with diverse bodily pains, distractibility, and novelty seeking (65,66). Susceptibility to somatic anxiety is primarily determined by a tendency to intense excitement in response to novel stimuli that is associated with high pain sensitivity and frequent exploratory activity. The associated features of chronic somatic anxiety and chronic cognitive anxiety are contrasted in Table 1.

Reactive dysphoria refers to acute hyperadrenergic states or recurrent states of agitated depression or dysthymia that occur in response to frustrative nonreward (11). Reactive dysphoria is associated with reward-seeking behaviors (such as overeating, grooming, and increased sexual activity) and signs of noradrenergic hyperactivity such as hypercortisolemia. Susceptibility to reactive dysphoria is primarily determined by a tendency to respond intensely to rewards

and succorance and to learn to maintain rewarded behaviors. Such reward-dependent individuals are ambitious and industrious and form strong social attachments. Susceptibility to panic attacks appears to be inherited independently of these other three forms of anxiety, as shown below.

AVOIDANCE LEARNING AND LONG-TERM SENSITIZATION

Freud (30) and Pavlov (58) noted that inborn defensive responses can be modified by experience. Each independently recognized that the ability to predict the future occurrence of dangerous situations from warning signals would be biologically adaptive. Pavlov carried out classical associative learning experiments in which neutral stimuli predicted aversive stimuli and found that animals could be conditioned so that defensive responses were elicited by previously neutral cues. Such classical conditioning involves changes primarily in the brainstem and limbic system and has been demonstrated in a wide variety of animals from lower invertebrates to man.

Aversive conditioning paradigms have been suggested as a model for acute anticipatory anxiety and acquisition of fears (27,42,67). In people with acute anticipatory anxiety, a specific premonitory signal is thought to predict the occurrence of aversive stimuli such as punishment, nonreward, or exposure to unfamiliar objects. Such anticipatory anxiety is usually transient and specific for particular situations signaled by specific premonitory cues.

However, repeated exposure to an aversive stimulus without a warning stimulus leads to long-term sensitization or chronic anxiety (42,67). The crucial difference between acute anticipatory anxiety and chronic anxiety is the presence or absence of a warning signal. When aversive events are unpredictable, safety is also unpredictable (67). Hence, in the absence of a safety signal, animals including man remain in a state of chronic anxiety.

Kandel and his associates found in sea snails that long-term sensitization led to presynaptic facilitation of the amount of neurotransmitter released at synaptic terminals of sensory neurons (42). Sensitization also led to related structural changes: the incidence and size of active zones of varicosities at presynaptic axon terminals were increased in sensitized animals (3).

The unpredictability of aversive stimuli or the unreliable recognition of warning signals can arise in either of two

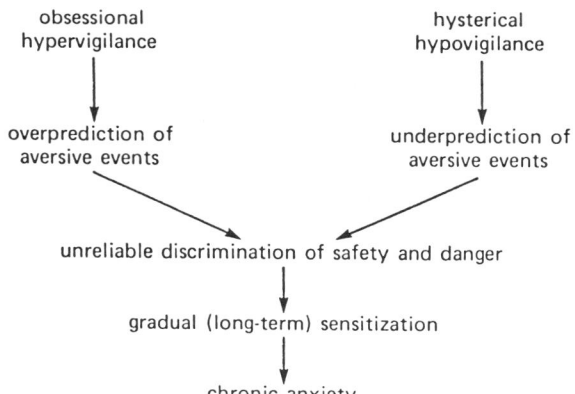

FIG. 1. Information processing and chronic anxiety.

processing style: they are hypervigilant, highly attentive to detail, fast in perceptual speed, and excel in recognizing temporal or contingent relationships (11,69).

Thus, either extreme, hypovigilance or extreme hypervigilance, leads to unreliable discrimination of safe and dangerous situations (see Fig. 1). Personality and information-processing style have an important role in susceptibility to anxiety. Histrionic and obsessional personalities simply represent the polar extremes of variation in three dimensions of personality that reflect heritable neurobiological variation in susceptibility to cognitive anxiety, somatic anxiety, and reactive dysphoria.

general ways. First, premonitory signals are not present or cannot be reliably recognized by the threatened individual. This occurs in individuals with a "histrionic" personality or information-processing style: they are hypovigilant, distractible, slow in perceptual speed, have poor attention to detail, and are poor in recognizing temporal and contingent relationships (1,7,11,12,41,49,69). Secondly, premonitory signals are ever-present or the individual remains sensitive in perceiving and predicting danger (i.e., highly vigilant) even though danger is actually rare. This occurs in individuals with an "obsessional" personality or information-

A THREE-DIMENSIONAL MODEL OF PERSONALITY VARIATION

Psychometric studies have consistently demonstrated three major dimensions of personality that are substantially heritable (29,32,50,51,72,77). However, the structure of observed phenotypic variation such as that described by Eysenck's dimensions of neuroticism–stability, introversion–extroversion, and psychoticism does not correspond well to the underlying biogenetic variation (26,50). Recently I have reviewed genetic and neurobiological studies to help define the genetic structure of these dimensions and its interaction with environmental variation in punishment, reward, and novelty (11). Here I concisely describe the

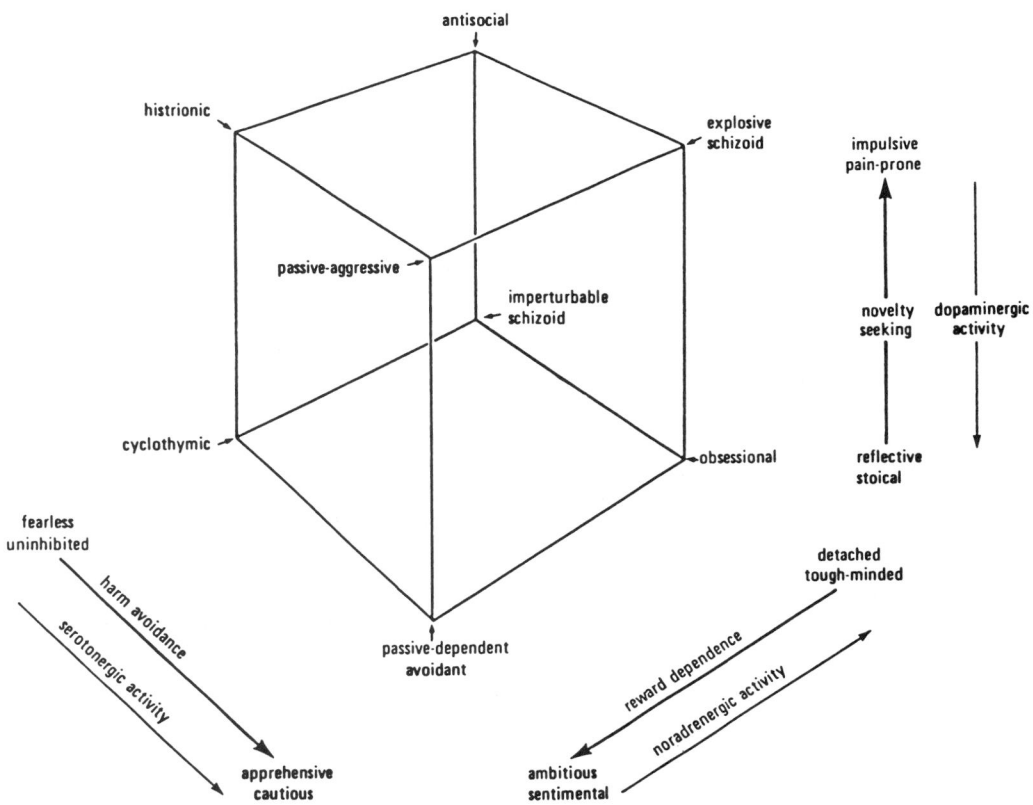

FIG. 2. Three-way interaction of personality and monoaminergic transmission.

TABLE 2. *Patterns of susceptibility to dysphoria by personality type*

Personality type[a]	Somatic anxiety	Cognitive anxiety	Reactive dysphoria
Histrionic (NhR)	++++	−	+++
Antisocial (Nhr)	+++	−	−
Passive-aggressive (NHR)	++	+	++
Explosive schizoid (NHr)	+	++	−
Passive-dependent (nHR)	−	+++	+
Obsessional (nHr)	−	++++	−
Cyclothymic (nhR)	−	−	++++
Imperturbable (nhr) schizoid	−	−	−

[a] The combination of personality traits is indicated in parentheses, novelty seeking (N or n), harm avoidance (H or h), and reward dependence (R or r), with capital letters indicating high values and lower-case letters low values.

proposed model and its predictions about the multidimensional nature of anxiety.

It is proposed that there are three genetically independent dimensions underlying variation in personality. These are called "novelty seeking," "harm avoidance," and "reward dependence." Novelty seeking is supposed to arise from a heritable tendency toward intense exhilaration and excitement in response to novel stimuli and hence a tendency toward frequent exploratory activity and pursuit of novel, potentially pleasurable activities. Reward dependence is supposed to be caused by a heritable tendency to respond intensely to reward and succorance and to learn readily to maintain rewarded behaviors. Finally, harm avoidance is supposed to be related to a heritable tendency to respond intensely to aversive stimuli and to learn readily to avoid punishment, nonreward, and novelty. Hence, harm avoidance modulates both novelty-seeking and reward-seeking behaviors that are potentially aversive or dangerous. Accordingly, environmental effects of novelty, punishment, and reward on these dimensions will not be independent, and observed phenotypic variability will be a composite of genetically independent effects and environmentally correlated variation.

Individuals who are high in novelty seeking are impulsive, quick-tempered, extravagant explorers, whereas those who are low in novelty seeking are rigid, frugal, and reflective stoics. Novelty seekers are easily bored and intolerant of monotony, preferring the thrill and exhilaration of pursuit to those of capture and consumption.

Individuals who are high in reward dependence seek rewards, including food, affection, wealth, power, fame, and other things that acquire value as rewards because of social learning. Reward-dependent individuals are described as ambitious, industrious, sentimental, and warmly affectionate, whereas reward-independent individuals are emotionally cool, tough-minded, practical, and socially detached. Reward-dependent individuals are described as moody because they need continued reward and succorance or they develop reactive dysphoria.

Individuals who are high in harm avoidance are described as fearful, cautious, apprehensive, and inhibited. They are

also easily fatigable. In contrast, individuals who are low in harm avoidance are fearless, carefree, and have little reluctance to risk personal injury. They are also highly energetic and tire only slowly.

The three-way combinations of these dimensions lead to the integrated behavior patterns summarized in Fig. 2. This is described in more detail elsewhere (11). It is important to note that these three-way combinations yield traditional personality types. It should also be noted that high novelty seeking, low harm avoidance, and high reward dependence each contribute to augmenting perceptual reactance (i.e., tendency to increase the amplitude of incoming sensory stimuli) and together define a histrionic personality pattern. Conversely, low novelty seeking, high harm avoidance, and low reward dependence each contribute to reducing perceptual reactance and together define an obsessional personality pattern.

Based on this model, specific semiquantitative predictions about patterns of susceptibility to various dysphoric states have been made (1). These are summarized in Table 2. The predictions about somatic anxiety assume it is based on high novelty seeking primarily and reduced by high harm avoidance and/or low reward dependence. The predictions about cognitive anxiety assume it is based on high harm avoidance primarily and reduced by high novelty seeking and/or high reward dependence. The predictions about reactive dysphoria assume it is based on reward dependence primarily and reduced by high harm avoidance and, to a lesser extent, high novelty seeking. In the next section, the neurobiological basis of the model and these predictions is summarized.

NEUROBIOLOGICAL BASIS OF PERSONALITY AND SUSCEPTIBILITY TO ANXIETY STATES

Central Punishment/Behavioral Inhibition System

It is postulated here that harm avoidance arises from polygenic variation in the regulation of serotonergic activity in a central behavioral inhibition system. Gray has suggested that the behavioral inhibition system functions as a comparator, checking predicted against actual events and then interrupting behavior when the unexpected is encountered (37). He suggests that this system primarily involves the limbic system, including the septohippocampal system, the Papez circuit, and the prefrontal cortex, as well as the ascending monoaminergic and cholinergic pathways that innervate these forebrain structures.

The importance of these limbic structures has been supported by recent research on benzodiazepine receptors (24). Specific high-affinity benzodiazepine receptors have been identified in the brains of all animal species phylogenetically superior to the shark. The highest densities of benzodiazepine receptors are found in cortical and limbic forebrain areas. There is an initial decrease in the number of benzodiazepine receptors in the cerebral cortex and hippocampus of rats following acute stress, and this is followed by a rebound increase that is most prominent in the hippocampus (52). Also, specific lesions of limbic structures reproduce most of the behavioral effects of benzodiazepines (24). Rats have been selectively bred for a high defecation score in a brightly lighted, unfamiliar environment, an index that is relevant to the harm avoidance dimension. Highly reactive rats have fewer benzodiazepine receptors in the hypothalamus and hippocampus than do animals selected for low defecation scores (63). The continued response to selection over many generations suggests polygenic regulation (11).

The affinity of different benzodiazepines for the receptor is highly correlated ($r = 0.78$) with their ability to reduce inhibition of behavior suppressed by contingent punishment (68). Stein has summarized extensive information showing that benzodiazepines disinhibit avoidance conditioning by GABAergic inhibition of the activity of serotonergic neurons originating in the dorsal raphe nuclei (73). Ascending serotonergic projections from the dorsal raphe nuclei to the substantia nigra inhibit nigrostriatal dopaminergic neurons and are essential for conditioned inhibition of activity by punishment and nonreward (74).

Accordingly, it is postulated that individuals high in harm avoidance have high basal levels of activity of serotonergic neurons in the behavioral inhibition system and so readily learn avoidance responses to punishment, nonreward, and novelty. In contrast, subjects who have a weak predisposition to avoid harm are supposed to be poor at avoidance learning and to have low levels of serotonergic activity in the behavioral inhibition system. This is directly supported by studies of cerebrospinal fluid (CSF) 5-hydroxyindoleacetic acid (5-HIAA), the major metabolite of serotonin. There is a strong relationship between low serotonergic turnover and impaired harm avoidance, as indicated by aggressive behavior in subjects with interpersonal problems (7,8) and by suicidal behavior in depressives (2,4). Low CSF 5-HIAA is associated with high harm avoidance as measured by low validity scores on the Marke–Nyman Personality Inventory (4). Relevant studies about biochemical variation and indices of avoidance learning are reviewed in more detail elsewhere (11).

According to the theory proposed here, susceptibility to acute anticipatory anxiety and chronic cognitive anxiety is primarily determined by variations in harm avoidance. In addition to high harm avoidance, low novelty seeking and low reward dependence contribute to a reducing perceptual reactance and obsessional information processing. Hence, susceptibility to chronic cognitive anxiety is primarily determined by high harm avoidance and to a lesser extent reduced by low novelty seeking and/or high reward dependence.

Central Incentive/Behavioral Activation System

The discovery that local brain stimulation can have reward-like properties led to studies of sites associated with self-stimulation (22). Self-stimulation at the sites of dopaminergic neurons is rapid and accompanied by marked locomotor activation, whereas many brain areas such as cortex, thalamus, and cerebellum do not support self-stimulation. Dopaminergic cell bodies in the ventral tegmentum have ascending projections to the striatum, nucleus accumbens, and frontal and limbic cortex. Available data indicate that dopaminergic pathways serve an "incentive" function to activate exploration, pursuit, and approach to rewards and environmental stimuli associated with rewards (22). Noradrenergic neurons from the locus coeruleus are supposed to be involved in reinforcement of rewarded behavior rather than the initial activation of approach or exploratory behavior.

Impulsivity and sensation-seeking behavior have been found to be associated with augmenting perceptual reactance and more intense responses to novel stimuli (53,82). Augmenting perceptual reactance is strongly correlated with high pain sensitivity and low dopaminergic activity as measured by CSF levels of homovanillic acid (HVA), the major metabolite of dopamine (36,80). However, impulsive novelty seekers may have normal conditioning to reward (39).

Accordingly, it is postulated here that low basal dopaminergic activity is associated with more intense responses to novel stimuli and hence frequent exploratory activity and novelty seeking. This is directly supported by studies of orienting responses to novel stimuli (53,82) and by studies of CSF HVA in individuals with sensation-seeking and -augmenting perceptual reactance (36,80) and in individuals with impulsive criminal behavior (47). These are reviewed in more detail elsewhere (11).

According to the theory proposed here, pain sensitivity and susceptibility to chronic somatic anxiety are primarily determined by variation in novelty seeking (11). However, low harm avoidance and high reward dependence also contribute to augmenting perceptual reactance (11) and histrionic information processing. Hence, it is predicted that susceptibility to chronic somatic anxiety is primarily determined by high novelty seeking and reduced by high harm avoidance and/or low reward dependence.

Central Reward/Behavioral Maintenance System

Noradrenergic neurons from the locus coeruleus are supposed to be involved in the maintenance of behavior by reward ("positive reinforcement") or nonpunishment ("negative reinforcement") (11). Ascending noradrenergic pathways arise from the locus coeruleus and project to limbic structures including the amygdala, septum, and hippocampus as well as the cerebral cortex. This noradrenergic system is regulated by the α_2-presynaptic receptor in a negative feedback inhibition. Electrical stimulation of the locus coeruleus of monkeys induces a state of agitated dysphoria associated with increased grooming behavior (22). A similar state is induced by reduced inhibition of the locus coeruleus from the administration of α_2-adrenergic receptor antagonists such as yohimbine and by administering β-carboline. These states of agitated dysphoria are also associated with increased plasma cortisol levels (21). Similarly, depressives show more variability in indices of basal noradrenergic output, such as plasma norepinephrine and 3-methoxy-4-hydroxyphenylglycol (MHPG), and elevated cortisol levels compared to normals (70). Clonidine, an α_2-adrenergic agonist, transiently relieves the dysphoria and decreases the cortisol to normal (70).

In contrast to these agitated dysphoric states associated with a rise in plasma cortisol and noradrenergic hyperactivity, panic attacks induced by lactate are not consistently associated with a rise in plasma cortisol and are blocked by imipramine pretreatment (D. F. Klein, *personal communication*, 1986). Panic attacks can be precipitated by lactate infusions in about 70% of patients with panic disorder but only rarely in normals or patients with other anxiety and somatoform disorders (46,59). This suggests that the mechanism for susceptibility to panic attacks is independent of these other anxiety states.

States of agitated dysphoria associated with hypercortisolemia and caused by noradrenergic hyperactivity are designated "reactive dysphoria" to distinguish them from other forms of anxiety and depression. Given the role of the noradrenergic system in the maintenance of rewarded behaviors, it is postulated here that individuals with low basal noradrenergic activity will be most sensitive to rewards and will work hard to maintain rewards. In other words, reward dependence will be associated with low basal noradrenergic activity. However, given the negative feedback relationship between the locus coeruleus and the α_2-adrenergic system, withdrawal of rewards ("frustrative nonreward") will lead to compensatory reduction of inhibition of the locus coeruleus, particularly in those with low basal noradrenergic activity. The withdrawal of rewards will be associated with increased reward-seeking behavior, but this may be inadequate in those with associated low exploratory pursuit (i.e., low novelty seeking). At the same time, the reactive increase in noradrenergic activity is supposed to lead to reactive dysphoria associated with hypercortisolemia. Serotonergic projections from the midpons also inhibit the locus coeruleus (22), so individuals with high harm avoidance (high serotonergic activity) are less likely to have marked noradrenergic hyperactivity. This is summarized in Fig. 3.

Accordingly, it is postulated here that susceptibility to reactive dysphoria will be primarily determined by high reward dependence. However, susceptibility to reactive dysphoria may be reduced by high harm avoidance and, to a lesser extent, high novelty seeking.

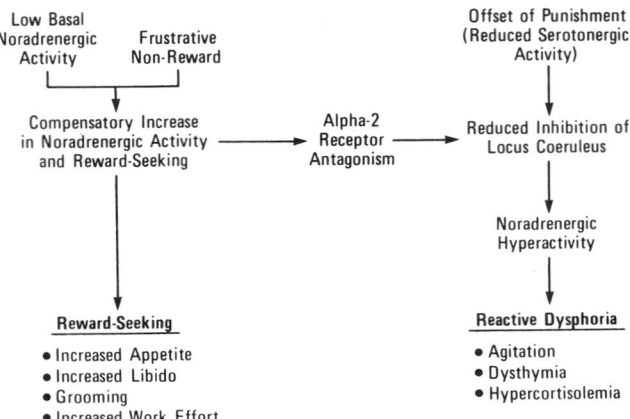

FIG. 3. Proposed mechanisms underlying "reactive dysphoria."

Susceptibility to Panic Attacks

The mechanism by which lactate infusion induces panic attacks remains uncertain. Panic attacks can be precipitated by lactate infusions in about 70% of patients with panic disorder, but only rarely in normals or patients with other anxiety or somatoform disorders (46,59). The mechanism by which lactate infusion induces panic attacks in these patients is uncertain: the direct effects of lactate suggested by Pitts and McClure have been called into doubt by later work showing that panic attacks could also be triggered by other means of inducing somatic symptoms of anxiety such as breathing in a high-CO_2 environment, strenuous exercise, or infusion of isoproterenol, which does not cross the blood–brain barrier (46).

Thus, it is possible that these different treatments trigger panic attacks by conditioned phobic responses to particular physiological signals similar to those experienced in suffocation, but not all individuals appear to be equally susceptible to acquiring such responses. Furthermore, at least some patients have the abrupt onset of spontaneous panic attacks and only subsequently develop chronic anxiety as a consequence of sensitization by recurrent unpredictable panic attacks (43). This suggests that panic attacks may involve defective regulatory mechanisms that are independent of other mechanisms of harm avoidance. Klein suggests that these mechanisms are normally involved in the regulation of responses to asphyxia or separation, events that both require a sudden outcry and appeal for help (43).

Recent PET studies indicating asymmetric blood flow (left < right) to the parahippocampal gyrus support such a role for vigilance functions in the generation of panic attacks (62) and may eventually help clarify why some patients with chronic anxiety are more susceptible to panic attacks than others.

FAMILY AND GENETIC STUDIES

Inheritance of Personality Traits

Twin and family studies indicate that measures of many personality traits and temperament factors, such as impulsivity, sociability, industry/persistence, tough-mindedness, and neuroticism, are heritable, with genetic factors accounting for 40% to 60% of overall variability on most indices in adolescence (9,26,28,31,48,60,78). Analyses of the genetic and environmental structure of Eysenck's three-dimensional model of neuroticism–stability, introversion–extraversion, and psychoticism revealed that the phenotypic structure did not correspond well with the underlying genetic structure (50). This was also shown by Eaves and Eysenck in a detailed analysis of extraversion and its components sociability and impulsivity in twins (28). Impulsivity is similar to novelty seeking as defined here, and sociability is closely related to harm avoidance. Genetic factors were largely independent between these two dimensions, as predicted by the model proposed here. Furthermore, environmental influences were highly correlated as predicted by the model here because of the joint effects of novel stimuli. A quantitative model assuming additive polygenic effects, random mating, and nonfamilial environmental effects was adequate to describe the inheritance of impulsivity and sociability. Artificial selection experiments also support polygenic effects, as noted earlier and discussed in more detail elsewhere (11).

Inheritance of Self-Reported Anxiety

As measured with the Minnesota Multiphasic Personality Inventory, the heritability of hypochondriasis and psychasthenia is low among adolescent twins (35) but is substantial in adult adopted twins (34). In a recent study of adult twins, the correlations between monozygotic cotwins who had been reared apart were significant for both hypochondriasis ($r = 0.30$) and psychasthenia ($r = 0.51$) (34). Earlier studies that had suggested that such traits were not heritable were carried out in adolescents who had seldom had time to develop chronic anxiety symptoms. This supports the developmental hypothesis described earlier in which heritable personality traits predispose to the development of chronic anxiety following long-term sensitization. Hence, genetic contributions to chronic anxiety are not apparent until adulthood in most people.

Twin and Family Studies of Chronic Anxiety Disorders

Early family history studies suggested that from 15% to 22% of first-degree relatives of probands with chronic anxiety neurosis had the same disorder (see ref. 14) compared to an estimated lifetime risk of 2% to 5% in the general population. These early studies did not distinguish panic disorder from other anxiety states as described above. Also, these early studies were open to criticism because of the lack of blind assessment, uniform assessment procedures, and explicit diagnostic criteria. An early exception to these methodological limitations was the blind study of a heterogeneous consecutive sample of same-sexed twins at the Maudsley Hospital by Slater and Shields (see ref. 10). The probandwise concordance rate for definite anxiety neurosis was 41% in 17 monozogotic twins compared to 4% of 28 dizygotic twins. These differences in concordance according

to degree of genetic relationship suggest the importance of genetic contributions to predisposition to some chronic anxiety states in adults.

The findings of Slater and Shields have been confirmed and extended by recent family and twin studies that used explicit diagnostic criteria. In the Washington University Clinic study of 500 psychiatric outpatients and their relatives, anxiety neurosis was defined as a disorder manifest by recurrent panic attacks (panic disorder) or chronic nervousness plus recurrent palpitations and/or dyspnea (other anxiety neurosis) in the absence of preexisting psychiatric disorders (14). The prevalence of a blind diagnosis of definite anxiety neurosis was 8% in 141 first-degree relatives of probands with anxiety neurosis compared to 1.9% in 1,084 first-degree relatives of probands with other diagnoses. Thus, the findings in the first-degree relatives in the Washington University Clinic Study were similar to those in the Maudsley Hospital Study, which used similar sampling and blind assessment of a heterogeneous sample.

The Washington University Clinic Study also noted that the familial aggregation of anxiety neurosis was largely accounted for by the families of probands with recurrent panic attacks complicated by agoraphobia. However, the affected relatives in these families had mostly recurrent panic attacks without agoraphobia or occasionally other mild anxiety states. This suggested the possibility that panic disorder and other anxiety disorders segregated in different families. Stated another way, not all individuals with chronic anxiety are susceptible to developing panic attacks.

Other psychiatric disorders including primary depression and alcoholism did not aggregate in families with anxiety disorders, suggesting striking diagnostic specificity (14). Similarly, among the relatives with anxiety neurosis there was no excess of depressive comorbidity, suggesting that susceptibility to anxiety neurosis and depression are not significantly correlated in most cases (11). This supports the predictions made earlier and summarized in Table 2.

Subsequently, Torgersen (75,76) carried out a twin study in Norway that also suggests that familial recurrence risks are related to severity of illness and the presence of anxiety attacks. He identified 39 monozygotic and 40 dizygotic twins with neurosis from medical records and a twin registry. The ratio of the monozygotic concordance to the dizygotic concordance increased with severity of illness in the index twin: the ratio was less than 1 for those identified from clinics and greater than 1 for those who had a psychiatric hospitalization. The less frequent male pairs were also more likely to be concordant than female pairs.

Torgersen also found that twins who had a history of panic attacks were more likely to be concordant than those without such attacks. When the probands had panic disorder, 31% of 13 monozygotic cotwins had panic attacks compared to none of 16 dizygotic cotwins (two of these did have generalized anxiety disorder as defined in DSM-III). In contrast, when the probands had generalized anxiety disorder (no panic attacks), 16% of 12 monozygotic cotwins and 10% of 20 dizygotic cotwins had the same diagnosis. Panic disorder and generalized anxiety disorder did not significantly aggregate in either the Washington University Clinic Study or the Norwegian twin study.

These results confirm that there are specific familial

factors that contribute to susceptibility to panic attacks that are not common to all types of anxiety disorder. However, patients who eventually develop recurrent panic attacks often experience other aspects of anxiety for several years prior to their first panic attack (14), so in family studies, where age and experience of relatives are variable, there is always a limited amount of aggregation of subjects with and without panic attacks. Nevertheless, the limited overlap of panic disorder and generalized anxiety disorder in families excludes the possibility that panic disorder is simply a more severe form of a single disorder. If that were true, severe (i.e., panic disorder) probands would be expected to have more relatives with the mild form (i.e., generalized anxiety disorder) than do mild probands (61).

It is still possible that the development of panic disorder requires both a specific susceptibility to panic attacks and a more severe degree of sensitization for its expression than is typical of most cases of chronic anxiety. Under this hypothesis, panic disorder probands would also tend to have greater tendency to harm avoidance and/or more threatening experiences than patients with other anxiety disorders. There is some support for this based on retrospective childhood histories of being apprehensive (14,54,64).

Several well-designed interview studies of panic disorder have been carried out in Iowa (23). The major methodological difference from other studies is that only definite cases were selected as probands, and these were compared to relatives of normal controls. This case-control design differs from the study of consecutive series of heterogeneous cases employed in the Washington University Clinic Study and the Maudsley Hospital Study. The Iowa studies have elicited somewhat higher morbid risks than the other studies despite their using strict DSM-III criteria. The morbid risk in first-degree relatives was 17.3% for definite panic disorder in panic disorder probands compared to 1.8% in relatives of normal controls. As in the other studies, other psychiatric disorders, including generalized anxiety disorder, primary unipolar depression, and alcoholism, did not aggregate with panic disorder in these families.

Harris et al. (40) further evaluated the relationship of panic disorder and agoraphobia in a family interview study in Iowa. All the agoraphobic probands had a history of recurrent panic attacks. The families of panic disorder patients had a morbidity risk of 20.5% for panic disorder and 1.9% for agoraphobia. In contrast, the families of agoraphobics had a morbidity risk of 7.7% for panic disorder and 8.6% for agoraphobia. The risks were 4.2% for each diagnosis in the control relatives. Thus, the risk of being affected with panic disorder or agoraphobia was about the same in the two groups of families, but the relatives of agoraphobics were likely to have their panic attacks complicated by agoraphobia. This suggests that agoraphobia shows familial specificity rather than being simply a nonspecific complication of severe recurrent panic attacks.

There was a high prevalence of school phobia or separation anxiety in the childhood histories of patients with panic disorder, particularly those who develop agoraphobia (33). Thus, a history of school phobia or separation anxiety may be a predictor of which panic disorder patients are most likely to develop agoraphobia. However, Roth cautions that this association has low predictive power in the general population because most school phobics do not show psychopathology as adults (64).

Because of its relative clinical homogeneity and its strong familial aggregation and specificity, many investigators have considered the possibility of Mendelian inheritance in panic disorder. Pedigree analyses have been carried out to test alternative hypotheses about the mode of inheritance of panic disorder, including polygenic models and monogenic models (23). One study showed compatibility with monogenic transmission but did not exclude alternative hypotheses (57). Later analyses took into account the sex differences in the family data that the earlier analyses had neglected (17). Both polygenic and monogenic models fit the data satisfactorily, and neither could be excluded. Hence, the results of published pedigree data do not permit discrimination of monogenic and multifactorial hypotheses.

Artificial selection experiments in animals suggest that polygenic models should be considered probable in chronic anxiety disorders in general. Nevertheless, specific clinical phenomena such as panic attacks or agoraphobia may be linked to relatively specific genetic susceptibility factors even if overall susceptibility to chronic anxiety states has a more complex multifactorial etiology. Future pedigree analyses should consider mixed models in which there is multifactorial variation in the background of each genotype at a single locus that has a large effect on particular clinical subtypes. The multifactorial background should allow for both polygenic effects and cultural inheritance or social learning. Explicit models have been developed for this purpose (15,17).

Family and Adoption Studies of Somatization

The families of patients with chronic somatic anxiety are strikingly different from those of patients with chronic cognitive anxiety. Early family studies of patients with Briquet's syndrome observed that 10% to 20% of the female first-degree relatives had the same disorder, a five- to 10-fold increase over the lifetime risk of the disorder in women in the general population (81). The male relatives of women with Briquet's syndrome also showed an increased risk of antisocial personality. Quantitative genetic analyses showed that the same familial factors predisposed to both Briquet's syndrome and antisocial personality in most cases (16). In the same families, men developed antisocial personality, whereas women developed somatization disorder when their familial predisposition was mild and antisocial personality when their predisposition was severe. These early studies were done with structured interviews and explicit behavioral criteria, but they were not blind. Recently, a blind family interview study has confirmed the familial nature of Briquet's syndrome or somatization disorder in women and also the association with antisocial personality in male and female relatives (14,38). This is consistent with the hypothesis presented earlier that both somatic anxiety and impulsivity are associated with high novelty seeking. Subjects with antisocial personality also tend to have poor avoidance learning associated with low harm avoidance. Low harm avoidance may also be characteristic of Briquet's syndrome in view of its association with frequent suicide attempts, aggressivity, and other antisocial behavior.

This familial aggregation could be caused by genetic factors, environmental influences, or both. Recently, an adoption study of somatoform disorders in Sweden has shown that the contributions of both genetic and environmental influences are substantial (6). Two relatively discrete types of somatoform disorders were distinguished in 859 Swedish women using comprehensive lifetime medical records (18). One of these disorders, called high-frequency somatization, was characterized by frequent headaches, backaches, and gastrointestinal and gynecologic complaints associated with extensive psychiatric disability. Extensive overlap with Briquet's syndrome was suggested by available psychiatric evaluations. Women who were adopted away at an early age had a fivefold increase in high-frequency somatization if their biological parents had impulsive aggressive behavior as shown by registrations for violent crimes and frequent alcohol abuse that did not require treatment compared to the adopted-away children of other parents (10% versus 2%). This is consistent with the hypothesis that this disorder is associated with a predisposition to both high novelty seeking and low harm avoidance.

The second somatoform disorder, called diversiform somatization, was characterized by less frequent but a similar range of diverse bodily pains and infrequent psychiatric treatment. Adopted-away women with diversiform somatization were more than twice as frequent (31% versus 14%) if their biological fathers had a history of nonviolent property crime in the absence of alcohol abuse or a history of early onset alcoholism complicated by criminality (6). These nonviolent property crimes were mostly petty thefts and other impulsive acts that did not involve risk of personal injury to self or others. Similarly, the subgroup of male alcoholics associated with diversiform somatization had registered behavior suggesting high novelty seeking, and this has recently been confirmed by personality tests indicating high impulsivity and sensation seeking (79). Interestingly, these subjects also had low activity of platelet monoamine oxidase, as expected in individuals predicted to have low brain monoamine turnover, since the monoamine oxidase in platelets is the predominant one in brain (MAO B, which preferentially metabolizes phenylethylamine, an amphetamine-like neurotransmitter) (19).

These findings support the hypothesis presented earlier that high novelty seeking is associated with somatic anxiety and impulsivity. When this is combined with a predisposition to low harm avoidance and poor avoidance learning, there is increased frequency of somatization and increased psychosocial disability as in the full Briquet's syndrome. A similar picture may arise when an individual with high novelty seeking but average harm avoidance begins to abuse "antianxiety" drugs such as alcohol. Such alcohol abuse artificially reduces harm avoidance and impairs avoidance learning by suppression of serotonergic activity.

Admixture analysis of quantitative scores discriminating the two types of male somatizers indicated that they were relatively discrete subtypes rather simply differing in severity of illness. The model of personality predisposition described here involves quantitative variation along three continuous dimensions. However, actual behavior involves the inter-

action of these dimensional temperament variables with qualitatively distinct environmental events. Different types of developmental experiences were observed for each type of disorder in adoptees and also often differed by the sex of the adoptee. For example, criminality, but not somatization, was associated with multiple temporary placements in childhood and other indicators of inconsistent discipline or unstable caretaking. The effect of such discrete exogenous factors on the dimensional personality variables is to produce "relatively" discrete categories with some underlying overlap but recognizable natural boundaries in terms of actual behavior.

A recent study of somatization in 807 adopted Swedish men indicated that most men with prominent somatization have features characteristic of the cognitive anxiety syndrome (20,71). Such "asthenic" male somatizers had infrequent bodily pains but recuperate slowly from minor illness and are often disabled with complaints of fatigue and weakness. Cross-fostering analyses indicated that both genetic and environmental factors contributed substantially (19). Such asthenic men had significantly fewer biological parents with criminality than did normal men or women. This indicates that high cognitive anxiety is negatively correlated with genetic antecedents of impulsivity or criminality, as expected according to the hypothesis that cognitive anxiety is associated with an extremely strong predisposition toward harm avoidance and low novelty seeking. This also indicates that genetic factors cannot be ignored in the etiology of chronic cognitive anxiety in adults.

IMPLICATIONS FOR FUTURE RESEARCH

These findings indicate that the developmental pathway to chronic anxiety states is complex, involving heritable differences between individuals in neurobiological systems that influence personality, information processing, and acquisition of adaptive responses to environmental and social circumstances. There may be relatively specific genetic susceptibility factors for particular phenomena such as panic attacks and certain types of phobic responses, but these must be considered against the multifactorial background that is involved in their development.

There is only limited information available about the relationship between personality types and the four types of anxiety states delineated here: chronic cognitive anxiety, chronic somatic anxiety, reactive dysphoria, and panic anxiety. Available information has been reviewed elsewhere (11) and is supportive, but more detailed information is needed. In particular, this should be combined with more detailed developmental information than has been customary in the past.

Progress in understanding anxiety states will be handicapped if attention is restricted to self-reported symptoms or cross-sectional signs. Measurements are needed at several levels of observation. These include (a) clinical ratings of symptoms; (b) ratings of personality traits relevant to novelty seeking, harm avoidance, and reward dependence; (c) measures of information processing including tests of neuropsychological function and performance on vigilance tasks; (d) performance in habituation and conditioning experiments for a range of incentive conditions and types of stimuli; (e) measures of neurotransmitter function and response to biochemical challenges; and (f) genetic data. Both observational and self-report information is likely to be valuable.

Longitudinal family studies offer particular promise for testing such developmental theories as that outlined here and described in more detail elsewhere (11). Family studies identify individuals at high risk who can be followed longitudinally on multiple measures. Predictions can be tested over time within individuals and also across individuals within and between families.

ACKNOWLEDGEMENTS

This work was supported in part by Research Scientist Award MH-00048 and grant MH-31302 from the National Institute of Mental Health, grant AA-03539 from the National Institute on Alcohol Abuse and Alcoholism, and a grant from the MacArthur Foundation Network on Risk and Protective Factors in Major Mental Disorders.

REFERENCES

1. Almgren, P. E., Nordgren, L., and Skantze, H. (1978): *Br. J, Psychiatry,* 132:670–673.
2. Åsberg, M., Bertilsson, L., and Martensson, B. (1984): *Adv. Biochem. Psychopharmacol.,* 39:87–97.
3. Bailey, C. H., and Chen, M. C. (1983): *Science,* 220:91–93.
4. Banki, C. M., and Arato, M. (1983): *Psychiatry Res.,* 10:253–261.
5. Bendefeldt, F., Miller, L. L., and Ludwig, A. M. (1976): *Arch. Gen. Psychiatry,* 33:1250–1254.
6. Bohman, M., Cloninger, C. R., von Knorring, A.-L., and Sigvardsson, S. (1984): *Arch. Gen. Psychiatry,* 41:872–878.
7. Brown, G. L., Goodwin, F. K., Ballenger, J. C., Goyer, P. F., and Major, L. F. (1979): *Psychiatr. Res.,* 1:131–139.
8. Brown, G. L., Ebert, M. H., Goyer, P. F., Jimerson, D. C., Klein, W. J., et al. (1982): *Am. J. Psychiatry,* 139:741–746.
9. Carey, G., Goldsmith, H. H., Tellegen, A., and Gottesman, I. I. (1978): *Behav. Genet.,* 8:299–313.
10. Carey, G., and Gottesman, I. I. (1981): In: *Anxiety: New Research and Changing Concepts,* edited by D. F. Klein and J. Rabkin, pp. 117–136. Raven Press, New York.
11. Cloninger, C. R. (1986): *Psychiatr. Develop.,* 3:167–226.
12. Cloninger, C. R. (1986): In: *Medical Basis of Psychiatry,* edited by G. Winokur and P. J. Layton. W. B. Saunders, pp. 123–151. New York, New York.
13. Cloninger, C. R., Martin, R. L., Clayton, P. J., and Guze, S. B. (1981): In: *Anxiety: New Research and Changing Concepts,* edited by D. F. Klein, and J. Rabkin, pp. 137–150. Raven Press, New York.
14. Cloninger, C. R., Martin, R. L., Guze, S. B., and Clayton, P. J. (1986): *Am. J. Psychiatry,* 143:873–878.
15. Cloninger, C. R., Rao, D. C., Rice, J., Reich, T., and Morton, N. E. (1983): *Am. J. Hum. Genet.,* 35:733–756.
16. Cloninger, C. R., Reich, T., and Guze, S. B. (1975): *Br. J. Psychiatry,* 127:11–22.
17. Cloninger, C. R., Rice, J., and Reich, T. (1979): *Am. J. Hum. Genet.,* 31:176–198.
18. Cloninger, C. R., Sigvardsson, S., von Knorring, A.-L., and Bohman, M. (1984): *Arch. Gen. Psychiatry,* 41:863–871.
19. Cloninger, C. R., von Knorring, L., and Oreland, L. (1985): *Psychiatry Res.,* 15:133–143.
20. Cloninger, C. R., von Knorring, A.-L., Sigvardsson, S., and Bohman, M. (1986): *Genetic Epidemiology,* 3:171–185.
21. Crawley, J. N., Ninan, P. T., Pickar, D., Chrousos, G. P., Linnoila, M., et al. (1985): *J. Neurosci.,* 5:477–485.
22. Crow, T. J., and Deakin, J. F. W. (1985): In: *Handbook of Psychiatry, Vol. 5: The Scientific Foundations of Psychiatry,* edited by M. Shepherd, pp. 137–182. Cambridge University Press, Cambridge.
23. Crowe, R. R. (1985): *Psychiatr. Dev.,* 2:171–186.
24. Dantzer, R. (1984): In: *Psychopharmacology of the Limbic System,* edited by M. R. Trimble and E. Zarifian, pp. 148–163. Oxford University Press, New York.
25. Darwin, C. (1873): *The Expression of the Emotions in Man and Animals.* D. Appleton & Co., New York.
26. Eaves, L., and Eysenck, H. J. (1975): *J. Pers. Soc. Psychol.,* 32:102–112.
27. Eysenck, H. J. (1979): *Behav. Brain Sci.,* 2:155–166.
28. Floderus-Myrhed, B., Pedersen, N., and Rasmuson, I. (1980): *Behav. Genet.,* 10:153–162.
29. Flynn, P. M., and McMahon, R. C. (1984): *J. Pers. Assess.,* 48:308–311.
30. Freud, S. (1964): In: *Standard Edition of the Complete Psychological Works of Sigmund Freud.* Hogarth Press, London.
31. Fulker, D. W. (1981): In: *A Model for Personality,* edited by H. J. Eysenck, pp. 88–122. Springer-Verlag, New York.
32. Gajar, A. H., and Hale, R. L. (1982): *J. Psychol.,* 112:287–293.
33. Gittelman, R., and Klein, D. F. (1984): *Psychopathology,* 17:56–65.
34. Gottesman, I. I., Bouchard, T. J., and Carey, G. (1984): Proceedings of the Fourteenth Annual Meeting of the Behavior Genetics Association, pp. 1–36. Indiana University, Bloomington.
35. Gottesman, I. I. (1962): *Eugen. Q.,* 9:223–227.
36. Gottfries, C. G., von Knorring, L., and Perris, C. (1976): *Neuropsychobiology,* 2:1–8.
37. Gray, J. A. (1983): In: *Physiological Correlates of Human Behavior. III: Individual Differences and Psychopathology,* edited by A. Gale and J. A. Edwards, pp. 31–34. Academic Press, New York.
38. Guze, S. B., Cloninger, C. R., Martin, R. L., and Clayton, P. J. (1986): *Br. J. Psychiatry,* 149:17–23.
39. Hare, R. D., and Schalling, D. (eds.) (1978): *Psychopathic Behavior: Theory and Research.* John Wiley & Sons, New York.
40. Harris, E. L., Noyes, R., Crowe, R. R., and Chaundhry, D. R. (1983): *Arch. Gen. Psychiatry,* 40:1061–1064.
41. Horowitz, M. J. (ed.) (1977): *Hysterical Personality.* Jason Aronson, New York.
42. Kandel, E. R. (1983): *Am. J. Psychiatry,* 140:1277–1293.
43. Klein, D. F. (1981): In: *Anxiety: New Research and Changing Concepts,* edited by D. F. Klein and J. Rabkin, pp. 235–264. Raven Press, New York.
44. Lader, M. (1983): In: *Physiological Correlates of Human Behavior. III: Individual Differences and Psychopathology,* edited by A. Gale and J. A. Edwards, pp. 155–169. Academic Press, New York.
45. Lader, M. H. (1969): *Br. J. Psychiatry* [*Spec. Pub.*], 3:1–215.
46. Liebowitz, M. R., Gorman, J. M., Fyer, A. J., Levitt, M., Dillon, D., et al. (1985): *Arch. Gen. Psychiatry,* 42:709–722.
47. Linnoila, M., Virkkunen, M., Scheinin, M., Nuutila, A., Rimon, R., et al. (1983): *Life Sci.,* 33:2609–2614.
48. Loehlin, J. C. (1982): *Behav. Genet.,* 12:417–428.
49. Ludwig, A. M. (1972): *Arch. Gen. Psychiatry,* 27:771–786.
50. Martin, N. G., Eaves, L. J., and Fulker, D. W. (1979): *Acta Genet. Med. Gemellol. (Roma),* 28:197–210.
51. McCrae, R. R., Costa, P. T., Jr., and Arenberg, D. (1980): *J. Gerontol.,* 35:877–883.
52. Medina, J. H., Novas, M. L., and De Robertis, E. (1983): *Eur. J. Pharmacol.,* 96:181–185.
53. Neary, R. S., and Zuckerman, M. (1976): *Psychophysiology,* 13:205–211.
54. Noyes, R., Clancy, J., Hoenk, P. R., and Slyman, D. J. (1978): *Arch. Gen. Psychiatry,* 35:173–178.
55. O'Gorman, J. G. (1983): In: *Physiological Correlates of Human Behavior, III: Individual Differences and Psychopathology,* edited by A. Gale and J. A. Edwards, pp. 45–62. Academic Press, New York.
56. Ohman, A., Eriksson, A., Fredriksson, M., Hugdahl, K., and Olofsson, C. (1974): *Biol. Psychol.,* 2:85–93.
57. Pauls, D. L., Bucher, K. D., Crowe, R. R., and Noyes, R. (1980): *Am. J. Hum. Genet.,* 31:639–644.

58. Pavlov, I. P. (1927): *Conditioned Reflexes: An Investigation of the Physiological Activity of the Cerebral Cortex,* translated and edited by G. V. Anrep. Oxford University Press, London.
59. Pitts, F. N., Jr., and McClure, J. N., Jr. (1967): *N. Engl. J. Med.,* 277:1328–1336.
60. Plomin, R. (1976): *J. Psychol.,* 94:233–235.
61. Reich, T., Cloninger, C. R., and Guze, S. B. (1975): *Br. J. Psychiatry,* 127:1–10.
62. Reiman, E. M., Raichle, M. E., Butler, F. K., Herscovitch, P., and Robins, E. (1984): *Nature,* 310:683–685.
63. Robertson, H. A., Martin, I. L., and Candy, J. M. (1978): *Eur. J. Pharmacol.,* 50:455–457.
64. Roth, M. (1984): *Psychiatr. Dev.,* 2:31–52.
65. Schalling, D. (1978): In: *Psychopathic Behavior: Approaches to Research,* edited by R. D. Hare, and D. Schalling, pp. 85–106. John Wiley & Sons, New York.
66. Schalling, D., Cronholm, B., Åsberg, M., and Espmark, S. (1973): *Acta Psychiatr. Scand.,* 49:353–368.
67. Seligman, M. E. P. (1975): *Helplessness.* W. H. Freeman, San Francisco.
68. Sepinwall, J., and Cook, L. (1980): *Fed. Proc.,* 39:3021–3031.
69. Shapiro, D. (1965): *Neurotic Styles.* Basic Books, New York.
70. Siever, L. J., and Uhde, T. W. (1984): *Biol. Psychiatry,* 19:131–156.
71. Sigvardsson, S., Bohman, M., von Knorring, A.-L., and Cloninger, C. R. (1986): *Genetic Epidemiology,* 3:153–169.
72. Sjöbring, H. (1973): *Acta Psychiatr. Scand.* [*Suppl.*], 244:1–203.
73. Stein, L. (1981): In: *Anxiety: New Research and Changing Concepts,* edited by D. F. Klein and J. Rabkin, pp. 201–214. Raven Press, New York.
74. Thiebot, M.-H., Hamon, M., and Soubrie, P. (1984): In: *Psychopharmacology of the Limbic System,* edited by M. R. Trimble and E. Zarifian, pp. 164–174. Oxford University Press, New York.
75. Torgersen, S. (1983): *Br. J. Psychiatry,* 142:126–132.
76. Torgersen, S. (1983): *Arch. Gen. Psychiatry,* 40:155–162.
77. Torgersen, S. (1980): *Arch. Gen. Psychiatry,* 37:1272–1277.
78. Vandenberg, S. G. (1962): *Am. J. Hum. Genet.,* 14:220–237.
79. von Knorring, A.-L., Bohman, M., von Knorring, L., and Oreland, L. (1985): *Acta Psychiatr. Scand.,* 72:51–58.
80. von Knorring, L., Monakhav, K., and Perris, C. (1978): *Neuropsychobiology,* 4:150–179.
81. Woerner, P. I., and Guze, S. B. (1968): *Br. J. Psychiatry,* 114:161–168.
82. Zuckerman, M. (1983): In: *Physiological Correlates of Human Behavior, Vol. 3: Individual Differences and Psychopathology,* edited by A. Gale and J. A. Edwards, pp. 99–119. Academic Press, New York.

Psychopharmacology:
The Third Generation of Progress,
edited by Herbert Y. Meltzer.
Raven Press, New York © 1987.

CHAPTER 95

Studies of the Nucleus Locus Coeruleus in Monkeys and Hypotheses for Neuropsychopharmacology

D. E. Redmond, Jr.

The nucleus locus coeruleus (LC) has been studied over the last several years with a variety of methods aimed at elucidating its functional role in humans. Data resulting from these studies have suggested a number of neurophysiological, neuropharmacological, and behavioral effects of the activity of this major central noradrenergic nucleus. This review focuses on evidence that suggests that the locus coeruleus is an essential part of the neural substrates for the emotions of anxiety and/or fear. This hypothesis has provided a basis for understanding antianxiety effects of several structurally unrelated drugs and for refining and developing strategies for studying neural mechanisms of behavior and drug actions in humans.

Whether the hypothesis itself turns out to be right or wrong may not be as important as the attempt to apply scientific principles to the study of complex human behaviors and to develop methodologies for rational and ethical human experimentation regarding these behaviors. The method builds on a base of electrophysiological and pharmacological data derived from the study of simpler organisms but largely rejects inferences attempting to interpret behaviors of these simpler organisms in the same terms used to describe the behaviors in humans. Studies in nonhuman species have been necessary to determine and refine the precision of the methods, but there is no reliance on or belief in any animal "model" of these complex behaviors. Each behavioral result merely generates a hypothesis for testing in humans, where it must ultimately stand or fall.

The nucleus locus coeruleus was chosen for study because it is the largest of the central noradrenergic nuclei, the source of over 70% of the transmitter norepinephrine (NE) in the brain, and the principal source of innervation of a number of brain regions likely to be involved in complex behaviors. Previous correlative and pharmacologic data had suggested some role for norepinephrine in the regulation of mood and behavior as well as a number of other physiologic functions. The strategy was to study the behavioral consequences of changes in the function of this nucleus induced by many different methods with different levels of specificity and selectivity but overlapping effects on NE function. Monkeys were chosen as experimental subjects because of their behavioral and social similarities with humans, which might increase the probability that their complex moods and behavioral states were analogous to human emotions. These studies led to the development of several chemical probes and hypotheses for assessing noradrenergic function in human subjects. This review indicates the current evidence supporting these hypotheses involving norepinephrine with anxiety/fear and panic states and the actions of several neuropsychopharmacologic agents.

NEUROANATOMICAL CONSIDERATIONS

The nucleus locus coeruleus consists of a compact group of a few thousand cells located bilaterally in the central gray of the isthmus on the floor of the fourth ventricle, medial to the mesencephalic tract of the trigeminal nerve. In the primate and the rat, the nucleus is compact and consists almost exclusively of a homogeneous population of norepinephrine-containing cells. Locus coeruleus neurons appear as medium-sized cells, 20 to 40 μm in diameter, with extensive dendritic arborization and axon collateralization (54,148). Axon terminals project diffusely to provide the principal noradrenergic input to the ipsilateral cerebral cortex, cingulate gyrus, hippocampus, and major projections to sensory and associational nuclei in the brainstem (superior and inferior colliculi, interpeduncular nucleus, pontine nuclei, sensory nuclei of the trigeminal nerve, and the cochlear nucleus). Massive projections to the cerebellum terminate in the molecular layer in close proximity to Purkinje cell dendrites (9,107). Noradrenergic innervation of the hypothalamus, thalamus, olfactory bulb, anterior olfactory nucleus and pyriform cortex, septal nuclei, and amygdala is shared by the LC and several smaller noradrenergic nuclei, collectively referred to as the lateral tegmental (LT) group (99). On reaching their terminal fields, LC axons collateralize to form a diffuse plexus of fine fibers regularly interspersed with varicosities (36,37,89). Fewer than 5% of NE-containing terminals in the cerebral cortex (37) and fewer than 20% of the NE terminals in the hippocampus make synaptic contact with postsynaptic elements (84). This pattern is consistent with a "global" neuromodulatory function that increases the "signal-to-noise" ratio and modulates other neurotransmitter inputs as observed neurophysiologically (166 for review) and that might be one aspect of what is variously called vigilance, anxiety, fear, or panic, depending on its intensity.

The afferents to the LC demonstrated by retrograde degeneration and horseradish peroxidase include nearly every level of the central nervous system. Projections from the forebrain include the insular cortex, the bed nucleus of the stria terminalis, magnocellular and lateral preoptic areas, the medial preoptic area, and the central nucleus of the amygdala (16,111). Afferent projections also arrive from several hypothalamic nuclei, midbrain neurons in the central gray around the dorsal raphe, the solitary tract nucleus, vestibular nucleus, the fastigial complex, reticular formation, the lateral reticular nucleus, and neurons in the marginal zone of the dorsal horn of the spinal cord. In the highly vascularized LC (and other monoamine-rich nuclei) (140), the perivascular glial sleeve found elsewhere in the brain does not prevent direct contact of capillaries on the soma and dendrites (47), making access by blood-borne substances such as hormones or systemically administered compounds more likely than in areas protected by the blood–brain barrier (96).

RECEPTOR PHARMACOLOGY OF THE LC

The compactness and homogeneity of the LC in the rat and the primate have made it possible, using single-unit electrophysiology, to characterize the pharmacology of the somatodendritic receptors that regulate this nucleus and to provide a basis for comparing specific pharmacological activation with electrical stimulation effects on behavior. Conversely, pharmacological inactivation and blockade have been compared with effects of lesions. The LC appears to receive input via receptors responsive to many different neurotransmitters. A negative feedback mechanism modulates LC neuronal firing rate via "autoreceptors" of the α_2

adrenoceptor type, responsive to NE from axon collaterals (14,15). These receptors also inhibit neuronal activity in response to low concentrations of the α_2 agonists clonidine and epinephrine (14,15), which appear to bind to somatodendritic LC receptor sites (167) and to receptors in some LC projection areas (112,154). Amphetamine, tricyclic antidepressants, and monoamine oxidase inhibitors slow the firing of LC neurons by releasing catecholamines, blocking reuptake of NE, or preventing its inactivation (46,55,63,103) at these "autoreceptors." By releasing this tonic inhibition, low doses of α_2-adrenoceptor antagonists activate impulse flow and NE release (65,95). Piperoxane (14,15), yohimbine (146), and idazoxan (137) increase net LC activity with increasing selectivity. There appear also to be postsynaptic α_2 receptors in some areas, which confound the interpretation of pharmacological effects, and most α_2 agonists and antagonists affect α_1 receptors in higher concentrations [with opposite functional effects, which were observed earlier (4,11) and are the explanation for the confusing terminology in which the most often mentioned "agonists" actually decrease the function of the affected neurotransmitter system in the doses usually employed clinically].

Locus coeruleus neurons are activated by glutamate, substance P, muscarinic acetylcholine (72,73), corticotropin-releasing factor (156), and methylxanthines (66,67) in addition to the compounds that act through α_2 receptors. The LC is also inhibited by dopamine (15), serotonin (139), glycine, γ-aminobutyric acid (GABA) (16,73), and Met-enkephalin (7), to mention the most important ones. Interactions with GABA underlie the inhibition of LC neuronal activity produced by benzodiazepines such as diazepam, chlordiazepoxide (64), and alprazolam (69). Dense concentrations of opiate receptors (109), more specifically enkephalin, endorphin, and dynorphin (6,97,98,110,162,163), are the anatomical basis for inhibition by morphine and other opioids (87) and for the specific antagonism of this effect by naloxone (2). A β-endorphin pathway from the arcuate nucleus projects through the central gray to inhibit LC impulse flow and is enhanced by morphine and blocked by naloxone (145).

The locus coeruleus is also activated by cardiovascular volume depletion and decreases in blood pressure and by increases in carbon dioxide concentration (42). Locus coeruleus activity increases during waking in comparison with slow-wave sleep or anesthesia (32,33,49). Physiologically, the locus coeruleus shows sustained responses to repeated presentations of "noxious" stimuli originating from these afferents even in anesthetized animals (17). In the awake monkey there is rapid "habituation" of locus coeruleus activity to novel nonnoxious stimuli as well as a consistent association of spontaneous LC activity with the level of "vigilance" and arousal (49,50) and clear activation in response to fear-associated stimuli (70). The efferent pathways from the locus coeruleus include target systems responsible for the physiological responses to pain and fear (see refs. 65,116), including increased blood pressure, heart rate, tremor, changes in fatty acid mobilization, and clotting tendency in the blood (of those that have been studied). In addition, pathways to and from the cerebral cortex provide the necessary feedback loops to explain the apparent influence the "meaning," "relevance," or conditioning of a stimulus may exercise on the response as well as to provide access to areas that may underlie the cognitive experience of the emotional state (or states) (113).

This neuroanatomical, biochemical, and physiological circuitry provides an outline of how the locus coeruleus (most likely in concert with other central noradrenergic nuclei) may function as a part of an alarm-relay system that modulates the disagreeable and emotional side of the response to pain as well as participating in the control of some of its physiology. Such a system is the logical one to have provided the evolutionary mechanism for elaboration of the anticipation of possible pain into the emotions generally called fear or anxiety, as theorized in different ways by Pavlov (108) and Freud (51). It may also have broader functions that subserve, or contribute to, the regulation of other physiological functions affected by fear but that also operate independently under normal conditions, such as appetite, sleep, arousal, neuroendocrine secretion, memory, attention, and learning. There is some support for this interpretation from a number of older clinical studies that have been previously reviewed (23,114,120,153) and from behavioral and pharmacological studies in rodents (35,100,126). Several contrary and alternative views have also been published based on reviews of the rodent literature or the results of specific experiments (3,12,48,86,135,136,158–160). Detailed discussion of this literature is beyond the intended scope of this chapter, which is limited to outlining the experimental evidence derived from studies of primates and to the subsequent generation and testing of hypotheses in humans.

LOCUS COERULEUS LESIONS AND ELECTRICAL STIMULATION OF LOCUS COERULEUS IN THE MONKEY

In a series of studies, electrodes or lesions were aimed at the locus coeruleus in *Macaca arctoides* (77), and concentrations of norepinephrine or its metabolite 3-methoxy-4-hydroxyphenethyleneglycol (MHPG) were measured in identified projection areas to determine the effects of activating or destroying the LC (77) on these indicators of biochemical activity. Lesions decreased MHPG concentrations compared with the same areas in normal control animals, and low-intensity electrical stimulation increased concentrations ipsilateral to the stimulating electrodes, compared either with the contralateral side or with normal unstimulated control monkeys.

Bilateral electrothermic lesions of the locus coeruleus produced unequivocal behavioral changes in seven of eight female *Macaca arctoides* studied. Emotional responses to threats were absent (143), although these monkeys would withdraw from persistent and vigorous threats and from a mildly painful stimulus. They were without apparent fear in approaching humans or dominant monkeys, maintaining eye contact more than sham-operated monkeys (78). They were also more aggressive in a social situation and moved about their cage more frequently than prior to the lesions or in comparison with sham-operated monkeys (115,121). Scratching and self-mouthing behaviors [both associated

with anxiety or mild stress (10)] decreased (114), and eating and drinking increased dramatically (123,124). Bowel motility was reduced, and the animals required regular enemas to promote defecation.

Adult male and female *M. arctoides* were studied after unilateral bipolar biphasic electrical stimulation of LC electrodes (0.2 to 1.0 mA, 0.5 msec pulse width, 10–50 Hz in 1- to 10-sec trains) (122). Stimulation of the LC in awake chair-restrained monkeys consistently induced or increased the occurrence of a group of behaviors that included yawning, chewing, scratching, startling, wringing of the hands, pulling of the hair or skin, tongue movement, grasping of the chair, struggling, self-mouthing, and self-clasping. Other physiological effects, such as pupillary dilatation, piloerection, alerting, and increases in heart rate, blood pressure, and respiratory rate were also noted (122,126). None of the behaviors occurred in exactly the same way each time, with movements to either side and with either hand in spite of unilateral stimulation. Similar responses in each monkey were obtained from stimulation of the dorsal noradrenergic bundle projections 5 mm from the locus coeruleus but not by stimulation of areas near the LC, suggesting that LC activation was necessary for the behavioral effects to occur. There were no responses suggesting that the stimulation produced pain, such as startling with stimulus onset, grimmacing, submissive facial gestures, or vocalizations. The behavioral effects were similar to those seen under circumstances in which anxiety, uncertainty, or fear may be inferred and similar to effects of some drug withdrawal states (116).

The neurochemical specificity of this electrical field stimulation was tested to determine whether the LC system was uniquely involved, since effects might have been caused by adjacent nuclei or axons incidentally activated (79,80). Piperoxane and yohimbine, administered intravenously from outside a sealed experimental chamber, both increased the identical behaviors elicited by electrical field stimulation and could not be distinguished from it or from the effects of experimentally conditioned fear by human observers scoring recorded videotapes of the behavioral effects (126). Clonidine, 10 µg/kg administered intravenously, reduced the behavioral effects of LC stimulation and also blocked and reversed the effects of piperoxane and yohimbine (116,128), as would be predicted based on the single-unit electrophysiology and pharmacology found in the rat and the effects of clonidine and piperoxane on MHPG outflow from the brain in *M. arctoides* (94). Diazepam and morphine also had similar effects in blocking the effects of electrical stimulation, piperoxane, or yohimbine (114,116,125).

In the previous experiments in chair-restrained monkeys, the restraint might have contributed to anxiety or fear as well as limited the available behavioral repertoire and made interpretation difficult. Seven monkeys, therefore, were studied one at a time with a social companion in a large cage unrestrained except by the cage, and stimulation was delivered through a long stainless steel cable or via radiotelestimulation. The lowest-intensity stimulation levels interrupted or prevented eating in food-deprived monkeys during and immediately after the stimulation without other observable effects (92). The next higher intensities, comparable to the lowest levels with behavioral effects in the chair-restraint experiments, produced an alerting response characterized by interruption of ongoing behavioral activity and visual scanning of the environment. Higher levels elicited some increases in identical behaviors seen in chair-restrained monkeys in addition to pacing, running, jumping up to a perch, and attempting to escape from the cage. As in the previous stimulation experiments, there were no responses that are usually correlated with pain (129).

Behaviors observed during opiate-antagonist-precipitated morphine withdrawal in chair-restrained *Macaca arctoides* were compared in detail with behaviors elicited by electrical field stimulation of the noradrenergic nucleus locus coeruleus (LC). Continuous LC stimulation produced a significant increase in the same behaviors found previously following pharmacological or electrical activation of the LC, without increases in general activity or distress behaviors (68). Naloxone administration in morphine-pellet-implanted monkeys increased the same behaviors as LC stimulation in a dose-dependent manner, but general activity did not increase significantly until the highest of four doses studied. Control monkeys, which had not received morphine treatment, did not exhibit significant changes in any of the behaviors following naloxone administration. Thus, behaviors associated with LC stimulation also increase during naloxone-precipitated morphine withdrawal. However, LC stimulation at the one intensity studied in this experiment produces a more specific increase in certain behaviors, whereas the most severe antagonist-precipitated morphine withdrawal appears to produce a more general behavioral activation (68).

POSSIBLE RELEVANCE TO ANXIETY OR FEAR

The preceding studies supported the hypothesis that the LC NE system is a neural substrate for alarm or fear that might be involved in pathological anxiety, panic, the effects of antianxiety drugs, and rebound withdrawal following their chronic use (113,119,122,130). Piperoxane and yohimbine, which increase LC activity and mimic the effects of electrical stimulation of the LC, had been reported to cause anxiety or fear in humans (61,76,144), whereas diazepam and morphine reduce anxiety or fear and reduce or block the behavioral effects of LC stimulation in monkeys, consistent with their reduction of the functional activity of the locus coeruleus. This interpretation was consistent with the known physiology of central noradrenergic systems and with a large body of pharmacologic and correlative data (65,114,120).

The picture of locus coeruleus function that emerges experimentally across the spectrum of its activity, from locus coeruleus lesions in the nonhuman primate to "high"-intensity electrical field stimulation, is that of an "alarm" system that filters and discriminates potentially noxious from irrelevant stimuli. High-intensity activation produces effects on nearly every major brain and autonomic function that is activated by fear, with profound effects on behavior (114). At moderate levels, locus coeruleus activity is correlated with attentiveness and vigilance to physiologically relevant stimuli (49). Progressive subnormal functioning of this system in the primate is best characterized by inattentiveness, impulsivity, carelessness, recklessness, and fearlessness (114).

Pathological anxiety might be the result of aberrations in the operation of this system at a number of points. Genetically influenced differences in catecholamine-related enzymes (101,132,164), receptor function, and neurotransmitter release mechanisms may be relevant to how active this system is in a particular individual. Changes in these same mechanisms caused by environmental exposure to strong, threatening stimuli or by chronic anxiety itself may lead to further increases in function, e.g., induction of synthetic enzyme activity or nonhomeostatic increases in receptor sensitivity or density. The further cognitive effects of learning and experience on subsequent responses may also contribute to dysfunction in some individuals who may or may not have additional biological vulnerabilities. Velley et al. (161) have noted that electrical stimulation of the locus coeruleus in rats is followed up to 4 weeks later by increased receptor binding of both α_1 and α_2 agonists and by increased behavioral effects in a "rebound" after clonidine administration. If these neurons and receptors have something to do with anxiety, these findings suggest that exposure to anxiety could have the paradoxical effect of sensitizing the individual to subsequent repeated exposures.

CLINICAL HYPOTHESES AND STUDIES

A long-range strategy was formulated for studying central noradrenergic function in human subjects. The most specific and selective pharmacologic probes available for testing in humans were tested first in monkeys, and plasma MHPG was investigated as an independent measure of noradrenergic activity that could be applied to human studies. The goal was to characterize (a) the effects of the pharmacologic probes on behavior compared with LC lesions, stimulation, or conditioned fear in monkeys, (b) effects on brain NE turnover measured directly, and (c) effects on MHPG concentrations measurable from plasma (44,45). Specific hypotheses evolved that provided explanations for empirically known pharmacological effects or predicted previously unknown ones. Some were rational and parsimonious explanations for well-established but mechanistically unexplained drug effects. These hypotheses follow, with a general indication of "confirmed" unless "not confirmed" is indicated for the clinical studies cited. A lack of citations indicates that, at present, results are not available or that the hypothesis has not been studied. Some studies are cited because their results are relevant to a hypothesis even though they might have been carried out for other reasons.

Hypotheses

1. Selective and specific α_2-adrenoceptor agonists (such as clonidine, lofexidine, guanfacine) would antagonize noradrenergically mediated functions and show similarities with opiates (118). Therefore, anti-opiate-withdrawal (13,20,21,38,57–60,74,82,134,149), antipanic (75,91), antianxiety (confirmed 75,83,85,

91,151; not confirmed in nonanxious subjects 90,150), and analgesic effects (81,142) would be postulated.

2. α_2-Adrenoceptor antagonists (yohimbine) would elicit anxiety, fear, or panic and simulate some drug withdrawal states (22,25).

3. α_2-Antagonist effects would be blocked by clondine (22), benzodiazepines (22), or opiate agonists (morphine).

4. By simultaneously disinhibiting two inhibitory systems, α_2 antagonists and opiate antagonists would have additive effects on anxiety, fear, or panic.

5. Hypercarbia (increased CO_2 concentrations) would elicit anxiety, fear, or panic (confirmed 62,165; not confirmed 157).

6. Effects of hypercarbia would be blocked by each of the inhibitory agonists [opiates, benzodiazepines (165), α_2-adrenoceptor agonists].

7. Tricyclic antidepressants and monoamine oxidase inhibitors reduce NE function as a basis for their antipanic or antianxiety effects (28,103,105,106, 138,146).

There have been a number of derivative hypotheses that have been investigated in clinical or animal studies because of the principal hypotheses. These secondary hypotheses include:

8. Morphine withdrawal increases LC unit activity in the rodent, and α_2 adrenoceptors and opiate receptors interact in regulating this activity (2,127,133,147).

9. Diazepam, chlordiazepoxide, and alprazolam reduce LC unit activity in the rat (64,69).

10. Methylxanthines such as isobutylmethylxanthine (IBMX) and caffeine, which sometimes cause anxiety or panic attacks, increase LC unit activity and MHPG turnover (52,53,67).

11. Methylxanthines would elicit anxiety or panic reversible by clonidine, benzodiazepines, or opiates (18,27).

12. Alprazolam, a very potent benzodiazepine with antipanic effects, would have antinoradrenergic actions (29,30,69).

13. Buspirone, reported to be an effective antianxiety drug, would reduce NE function (not confirmed 135,136) and have antipanic effects.

14. Benzodiazepine inverse agonists (several β-carboline compounds), reported to induce anxiety or fear (41), would increase NE activity and interact with the NE inhibitory compounds clonidine (34), morphine, and diazepam.

15. Benzodiazepine antagonists (Ro15-1788) would block the effects of the benzodiazepine agonists and facilitate effects of α_2 antagonists and drug withdrawal states associated with NE function.

16. Benzodiazepine withdrawal syndrome activates NE function (71,131) and might be reduced or prevented by clonidine or α_2 agonists.

17. Like opiate withdrawal (26), other drug withdrawal syndromes in which anxiety is a prominent feature [such as withdrawal from tricyclic antidepressants (19), alcohol (8), or nicotine (56)] might be partially noradrenergically mediated and/or ameliorated by clonidine.

18. Noradrenergic activating agents such as yohimbine might reveal differences in NE regulatory receptor function, aspects of NE turnover, or postsynaptic sensitivity between groups of subjects (categorized diagnostically) who show differential manifestations of anxiety or panic compared with their changes in NE output measures (24,25). α_2-Adrenoceptor-mediated reductions in NE function would show between-group differences (31,141).

19. Subjects who have been chronically treated with opiates, benzodiazepines, tricyclic antidepressants, monoamine oxidase inhibitors, or clonidine would show evidence of differences in NE regulatory mechanisms.

Many of the explanations or predictions referenced above have been consistent with the hypotheses linking central noradrenergic activity with anxiety, panic, or anxiety-linked drug withdrawal states. Several animal studies have not confirmed these predictions and underscored the fact that central noradrenergic neurons, even if they are essential to a brain "alarm" system that is a neural substrate for pathological or morbid anxiety or panic, are not sufficient to explain all of the clinical manifestations of these states. It should follow from this that some drugs with antianxiety properties may have their principal actions on some of these other target systems in addition to, or instead of, the NE systems. In this sense, the exceptions are important for further understanding of the "anatomy of anxiety."

The prediction that buspirone, for example, would decrease LC unit activity because of its antianxiety efficacy was not confirmed (135,136). On the contrary, buspirone seemed to increase slightly LC activity acutely, very similarly to the effects of chlorpromazine (63). This suggests that a reduction of noradrenergic function may not be involved in the effects of buspirone. It is not yet known whether or not buspirone has antipanic effects, but there are some suggestions that it might not have immediate antianxiety effects that are detectable with other antianxiety drugs that do decrease LC activity immediately. This raises the possibility that some metabolite or a secondary change must be induced in a target system before the antianxiety properties are detected. Acute LC unit activity, or several other measures of NE function, would not necessarily change.

Another compound, carbamazepine, which does have antipanic effects, also increases LC activity after acute administration (104), contrary to the simplest predictions from a noradrenergic hypothesis of anxiety. Haloperidol is an interesting neuroleptic drug because, unlike chlorpromazine, it has been shown to have antianxiety efficacy (see ref. 120). Single-dose administration, as with buspirone and carbamazepine, increases impulse activity in the LC (39). But chronic administration inactivates noradrenergic neurons (40), consistent with a noradrenergic mechanism of antianxiety action. Similar effects might be found with longer term studies of buspirone or carbamazepine. Further studies will be necessary to rule out a noradrenergic action of these compounds and to determine which other neurochemical systems might be involved in addition to or instead of the NE system.

Finally, there are a number of studies using so-called models of anxiety in rodents that appear to refute the importance of central noradrenergic function in these models. Britton et al. (12) and Koob et al. (86) have found, for example, that locus coeruleus lesions or destruction of the dorsal NE bundle does not prevent the release of punished responding by ethanol and chlordiazepoxide and appears to have other effects that could be argued to be opposite to an antianxiety one. There are problems, in my view, with the inferences drawn from these studies because of the behavioral models and because of the difficulty in interpreting the functional effects of lesions, as previously discussed in detail (126). Nonetheless, they may lead to further hypotheses for testing in humans to determine the relevance of these findings to human pathological anxiety states.

IMPLICATIONS FOR THE ANXIETY "DISORDERS"

In spite of some exceptions found so far, the neurophysiologic and biochemical changes in central noradrenergic function appear relevant to understanding and pharmacologically altering human fear, anxiety, and panic states. The identification of neural substrates for anxiety has obvious implications for treatment, not only because it would provide a rational basis for designing more effective and more specific drugs but because it would also allow the characterization of any biochemical pathophysiology of anxiety if it exists in particular groups of subjects, as some preliminary evidence suggests. Although the probes to date are still somewhat crude, there are at least some clues as to where to look. Group differences in MHPG effects of clonidine and yohimbine challenges among panic-disordered and depressed patients and controls (31) indicate dysregulation of NE activity, dysregulation of other regulatory inputs to noradrenergic neurons, or dysfunctions in α_2-adrenergic receptor–effector coupling or intracellular effector systems. By using a combination of probes with different receptors or circuits regulating noradrenergic systems, one can test some of these possibilities one by one. For example, during yohimbine challenge, can a failure of opioid inhibitory systems be demonstrated by concomitant administration of naloxone or a failure of GABA/benzodiazepine inhibition by R015-1788? The input receptor mechanisms underlying increased sensitivity of panic disorder patients to carbon dioxide challenge (165) may provide further clues.

There are also implications for future pharmacologic studies. It appears that the anxiety or panic components of several different classes of drugs, acting via independent receptor or intracellular mechanisms (1), may elicit or reduce anxiety by virtue of common effects on central noradrenergic function (2,5,93). Some new anxiolytic or anxiogenic drugs may act directly on other neural substrates of anxiety (which may include projection areas that receive input from the locus coeruleus) without altering NE impulse flow, receptor sensitivity, or turnover, but no alternative explanation has been proposed that can encompass the actions of as many different drugs as clonidine, yohimbine,

morphine, naloxone, diazepam, alprazolam, imipramine, monoamine oxidase inhibitors, β-adrenergic blockers, methylxanthines, and carbon dioxide (120).

Another concept, which continues to appear valid, is the idea that multiple receptors regulate NE activity (and its associated functions) either by shared intracellular mechanisms or by influencing the net excitatory or inhibitory forces favoring inpulse flow or transmitter release at the synapse. These parallel pathways allow morphine or benzodiazepine withdrawal to be blocked by clonidine or facilitate the effects of yohimbine with naloxone, for example. In addition to testing diagnostic or behaviorally classified differences between individuals, these multiple pathways might be utilized in several possibly beneficial ways by choosing pharmacological agents because of multiple receptor activities. Alternatively, several drugs with receptor specificity but desired combinations of effects might be used together, for example, the combination of amphetamine (46,63) with opiates (7,87) for analgesia, which decrease NE activity in an additive fashion but may conteract each other's less desirable effects mediated by other systems.

These same receptor relationships and the extensive noradrenergic neural mechanisms facilitating homeostasis and recovery of function after damage or chronic inhibition point to possible intrinsic relationships between antianxiety or antipanic activity and liability to withdrawal effects. These would vary somewhat based on the specific mechanisms by which NE function is inhibited by the compound, but it appears that potent agents for suppressing NE activity have a potential for withdrawal effects.

Partly for these reasons, the discovery of anxiolytic agents that do not suppress NE function might be advantageous. The NE system, during most of its range of function, appears to be adaptive, consistent with the familiar U-shaped performance curve associated with the effects of increasing anxiety. Suppressing or dampening this system might be the cause of mental clouding, inattention, diminished arousal, and other limiting side effects as well as contributing to possible withdrawal/rebound. Short of a molecular repair of a known and specific neuronal regulatory defect, the second-best antianxiety agent, therefore, might be a "surge limiter" that did not dampen base-line function but dampened excessive or inappropriate activation. Such an agent might also be less likely to be associated with rebound phenomena.

ACKNOWLEDGMENTS

The work cited from my laboratory was supported in part by U.S.P.H.S. grants DA02321, MH31176, MH25642, MH30929, Research Scientist Career Development Award DA-00075, Research Scientist Award MH-00643, the Harry Frank Guggenheim Foundation, the Axion Research Foundation, and the State of Connecticut. Many of my colleagues contributed significantly to studies cited as well as to the ideas expressed, including Drs. Yung H. Huang, Steven J. Grant, Dennis S. Charney, George K. Aghajanian, Robert H. Roth, George R. Heninger, James W. Maas, John H. Krystal, Mark S. Gold, Thomas Uhde, Grant N. Ko, Herbert D. Kleber, and Keith Leverenz.

REFERENCES

1. Aghajanian, G. K. (1978): *Nature,* 276:186–188.
2. Aghajanian, G. K., and Vander Maelen, C. P. (1982): *Science,* 215:1394–1396.
3. Amaral, D. G., and Sinnamon, H. M. (1977): *Prog. Neurobiol.,* 9:147–196.
4. Anden, N. E., Corrodi, H., Fuxe, K., Hokfelt, B., Hokfelt, T., et al. (1970): *Life Sci.,* 9:513–523.
5. Andrade, R., and Aghajanian, G. K. (1984): *J. Neurosci.,* 4:161–170.
6. Atweh, S. F., Murrin, L. C., and Kuhar, M. J. (1978): *Neuropharmacology,* 17:65–71.
7. Bird, S. J., and Kuhar, M. J. (1977): *Brain Res.,* 122:523–533.
8. Bjorkqvist, S. E. (1975): *Acta Psychiatr. Scand.,* 52:256–263.
9. Bloom, F. E., and Battenberg, E. L. F. (1976): *J. Histochem. Cytochem.,* 24:561–571.
10. Blurton Jones, N. G., and Trollope, J. (1968): *Primates,* 9:365–394.
11. Bolme, P., Fuxe, K., and Lidbrink, P. (1972): *Res. Commun. Chem. Pathol. Pharmacol.,* 4(3):657–697.
12. Britton, D. R., Ksir, C., Britton, K. T., Young, D., and Koob, G. F. (1984): *Physiol. Behav.,* 33:473–478.
13. Cami, J., de Torres, S., San, L., Sole, A., Guerra, D., et al. (1985): *Clin. Pharmacol. Ther.,* 38:336–341.
14. Cedarbaum, J. M., and Aghajanian, G. K. (1976): *Brain Res.,* 112:413–419.
15. Cedarbaum, J. M., and Aghajanian, G. K. (1977): *Eur. J. Pharmacol.,* 44:375–385.
16. Cedarbaum, J. M., and Aghajanian, G. K. (1978): *J. Comp. Neurol.,* 178:1–16.
17. Cedarbaum, J. M., and Aghajanian, G. K. (1978): *Life Sci.,* 23:1383–1392.
18. Charney, D. S., Galloway, M. P., and Heninger, G. R. (1984): *Life Sci.,* 35:135–144.
19. Charney, D. S., Heninger, G. R., Sternberg, D. E., and Landis, H. (1982): *Br. J. Psychiatry,* 141:377–386.
20. Charney, D. S., Sternberg, D. E., Kleber, H. D., Heninger, G. R., and Redmond, D. E., Jr. (1981): *Arch. Gen. Psychiatry,* 38:1273–1277.
21. Charney, D. S., Riordan, C. E., Kleber, H. D., Murburg, M., Braverman, P., et al. (1982): *Arch. Gen. Psychiatry,* 39:1327–1332.
22. Charney, D. S., Heninger, G. R., and Redmond, D. E., Jr. (1983): *Life Sci.,* 33:19–29.
23. Charney, D. S., and Redmond, D. E., Jr. (1983): *Neuropharmacology,* 22(12B):1531–1536.
24. Charney, D. S., Heninger, M. D., and Redmond, D. E., Jr. (1983): *N. Res. Abstr.,* NR96.
25. Charney, D. S., Heninger, G. R., and Brier, A. (1984): *Arch. Gen. Psychiatry,* 41:751–763.
26. Charney, D. S., Redmond, D. E., Jr., Galloway, M. P., Kleber, H. D., Heninger, G. R., et al. (1984): *Life Sci.,* 35:1263–1272.
27. Charney, D. S., Heninger, G. R., and Jatlow, P. I. (1985): *Arch. Gen. Psychiatry,* 42:233–243.
28. Charney, D. S., and Heninger, G. R. (1985): *Arch. Gen. Psychiatry,* 42:473–481.
29. Charney, D. S., and Heninger, G. R. (1985): *Arch. Gen. Psychiatry,* 42:458–467.
30. Charney, D. S., Brier, A., Jatlow, P. I., and Heninger, G. R. (1986): *Psychopharmacology,* 88:133–140.
31. Charney, D. S., and Heninger, G. R. (1986): *Arch. Gen. Psychiatry,* 43:1059–1065.
32. Chu, N. S., and Bloom, F. E. (1973): *Science,* 179:908–910.
33. Chu, N. S., and Bloom, F. E. (1974): *Brain Res.,* 66:1–21.
34. Crawley, J. N., Ninan, P. T., Pickar, D., Chrousos, G. P., Linnoila, M., et al. (1985): *J. Neurosci.,* 5:477–486.
35. Davis, M., Redmond, D. E., Jr., and Baraban, J. M. (1979): *Psychopharmacology,* 65:111–118.
36. Descarries, L., and Lapierre, Y. (1973): *Brain Res.,* 51:141–160.
37. Descarries, L., Watkins, K. C., and Lapierre, Y. (1977): *Brain Res.,* 133:197–222.
38. DiStefano, P. S., and Brown, O. M. (1985): *J. Pharmacol. Exp. Ther.,* 233:339–344.
39. Dinan, T. G., and Aston-Jones, G. (1984): *Brain Res.,* 307:359–362.
40. Dinan, T. G., and Aston-Jones, G. (1985): *Brain Res.,* 325:385–388.
41. Dorow, R., Horowki, R., Paschelke, G., Amin, M., and Braestrup, C. (1983): *Lancet,* 2:98–99.
42. Elam, M., Yao, T., Thoren, P., and Svensson, T. H. (1981): *Brain Res.,* 222:373–381.
43. Elam, M., Yao, T., Svensson, T. H., and Thoren, P. (1984): *Brain Res.,* 290:281–287.
44. Elsworth, J. D., Redmond, D. E., Jr., and Roth, R. H. (1982): *Brain Res.,* 235:115–124.
45. Elsworth, J. D., Roth, R. H., and Redmond, D. E., Jr. (1983): *J. Neurochem.,* 41:786–793.
46. Engberg, G., and Svensson, T. H. (1979): *Life Sci.,* 24:2245–2254.
47. Felton, D. L., and Crutcher, K. A. (1979): *Am. J. Anat.,* 155:467–482.
48. Flicker, C., and Geyer, M. A. (1982): *Brain Res. Rev.,* 4:79–103.
49. Foote, S. L., Aston-Jones, G., and Bloom, F. E. (1980): *Proc. Natl. Acad. Sci. U.S.A.,* 77:3033–3037.
50. Foote, S. L., Bloom, F. E., and Aston-Jones, G. (1983): *Physiol. Rev.,* 63:844–914.
51. Freud, S. (1936): *The Problem of Anxiety,* translated by H. A. Bunker. The Psychoanalytic Quarterly Press and W. W. Norton, New York.
52. Galloway, M. P., and Roth, R. H. (1982): *Trans. Am. Soc. Neurochem.,* 13:392.
53. Galloway, M. P., and Roth, R. H. (1983): *J. Neurochem.,* 40(1):246–251.
54. German, D. C., and Bowden, D. M. (1975): *J. Comp. Neurol.,* 161:19–29.
55. German, D. C., Sungher, M. K., Kiser, R. S., and McMillan, B. A. (1979): *Brain Res.,* 166:331–339.
56. Glassman, A. H., Jackson, W. K., Walsh, B. T., Roose, S. P., and Rosenfeld, B. (1984): *Science,* 226:864–866.
57. Gold, M. S., Redmond, D. E., Jr., and Kleber, H. D. (1978): *Lancet,* 2:929–930.
58. Gold, M. S., Redmond, D. E., Jr., and Kleber, H. D. (1978): *Lancet,* 2:599–602.
59. Gold, M. S., Pottash, A. L. C., Sweeney, D. R., Kleber, H. D., and Redmond, D. E., Jr. (1979): *Am. J. Psychiatry,* 136:7.
60. Gold, M. S., Redmond, D. E., Jr., and Kleber, H. D. (1979): *Am. J. Psychiatry,* 136(1):100–102.
61. Goldenberg, M., Snyder, C. H., and Aranow, H., Jr. (1947): *J.A.M.A.,* 135:971–976.
62. Gorman, J. M., Askanazi, J., Leibowitz, M. R., Fyer, A. J., Stein, J., et al. (1984): *Am. J. Psychiatry,* 141:857–861.
63. Graham, A. W., and Aghajanian, G. K. (1971): *Nature,* 234:100–103.
64. Grant, S. J., Huang, Y. H., and Redmond, D. E., Jr. (1980): *Life Sci.,* 27(23):2231–2236.
65. Grant, S. J., and Redmond, D. E., Jr. (1981): In: *Psychopharmacology of Clonidine,* edited by H. Lal and S. Fielding, pp. 5–27. Alan R. Liss, New York.
66. Grant, S. J., and Redmond, D. E., Jr. (1982): *J. Pharmacol. Biochem. Behav.,* 17:655–658.
67. Grant, S. J., and Redmond, D. E., Jr. (1982): *Eur. J. Pharmacol.,* 85:105–109.
68. Grant, S. J., and Redmond, D. E., Jr. (1983): *Neurosci. Abstr.,* 9:891.
69. Grant, S. J., Mayor, R., and Redmond, D. E., Jr. (1984): *Neursci. Abstr.,* 10:952.
70. Grant, S. J., and Redmond, D. E., Jr. (1984): *Exp. Neurol.,* 84:701–708.
71. Grant, S. J., Galloway, M. P., Mayor, R., Fenerty, J., Finkelstein, M., et al. (1985): *Eur. J. Pharmacol.,* 107:126–132.
72. Guyenet, P. G., and Aghajanian, G. K. (1977): *Brain Res.,* 136:178–184.
73. Guyenet, P. G., and Aghajanian, G. K. (1979): *Eur. J. Pharmacol.,* 53:319–328.
74. Hoder, E. L., Leckman, J. F., Ehrenkranz, R., Kleber, H., Cohen, D. J., et al. (1981): *N. Engl. J. Med.,* 154:1284.

75. Hoehn-Saric, R., Merchant, A. F., Keyser, M. L., and Smith, V. K. (1981): *Arch. Gen. Psychiatry,* 38:1278–1282.
76. Holmberg, G., and Gershon, S. (1961): *Psychopharmacologia,* 2: 93–106.
77. Huang, Y. H., Redmond, D. E., Jr., Snyder, D. R., and Maas, J. W. (1975): *Brain Res.,* 100:157–162.
78. Huang, Y. H., Redmond, D. E., Jr., Snyder, D. R., and Maas, J. W. (1976): *Neurosci. Abstr.,* 2:489.
79. Huang, Y. H., Redmond, D. E., Jr., Snyder, D. R., and Maas, J. W. (1977): *Brain Res. Bull.,* 2:231–234.
80. Huang, Y. H., Maas, J. W., and Redmond, D. E., Jr. (1977): *Neurosci. Abstr.,* 3:251.
81. Kleber, H. D., and Kosten, T. R. (1985): *Psychosomatics,* 26:6–8.
82. Kleber, H. D., Riordan, C. E., Rounsaville, B., Kosten, T., Charney, D., et al. (1985): *Arch. Gen. Psychiatry,* 42:391–394.
83. Ko, G. N., Elsworth, J. D., Roth, R. H., Rifkin, B. G., Leigh, H., et al. (1983): *Arch. Gen. Psychiatry,* 40:425–430.
84. Koda, L. Y., and Bloom, F. E. (1977): *Brain Res.,* 120:327–335.
85. Kolb, L. C., Blanchard, E. B., Burris, B. C., Pallmeyer, T. (1983): American Psychiatric Association, *Abstracts,* Symposium 43.
86. Koob, G. F., Thatcher-Britton, K., Britton, D. R., Roberts, D. C. S., and Bloom, F. E. (1984): *Physiol. Behav.,* 33:479–485.
87. Korf, J., Bunney, B. S., and Aghajanian, G. K. (1974): *Eur. J. Pharmacol.,* 25:165–169.
88. Lal, H., Shearman, G. R., and Ursillo, R. C. (1981): *J. Clin. Pharmacol.,* 21:16–19.
89. Lapierre, Y., Beaudet, A., Demianczuk, N., and Descarries, L. (1973): *Brain Res.,* 63:175–182.
90. Leckman, J. F., Maas, J. W., Redmond, D. E., Jr., and Heninger, G. R. (1980): *Life Sci.,* 26:2179–2185.
91. Leibowitz, M. R., Ryer, A. J., McGrath, P., and Klein, D. F. (1981): *Psychopharmacol. Bull.,* 17:122–123.
92. Leverenz, K., Redmond, D. E., Jr., and Huang, Y. H. (1978): *Neurosci. Abstr.,* 4:177.
93. Lugan, M., Lopez, E., Ramirez, R., Aguilar, H., Martinez-Olmedo, M. A., et al. (1984): *Eur. J. Pharmacol.,* 100:377–380.
94. Maas, J. W., Hattox, S. E., and Landis, D. H. (1976): *Brain Res.,* 118:167–173.
95. Maas, J. W., Hattox, S. E., Landis, D. H., and Roth, R. H. (1977): *Eur. J. Pharmacol.,* 46:228–331.
96. Medina, M. A., Giachetta, A., and Shore, P. A. (1969): *Biochem. Pharmacol.,* 18:891–901.
97. Miller, R. J., and Cuatrecasas, P. (1978): *Vitam. Horm.,* 36:297–381.
98. Miller, R. J., and Pickel, V. M. (1980): In: *Histochemistry and Cell Biology of Autonomic Neurons, SIF Cells, and Paraneurons,* edited by O. Eranko, pp. 349–359. Raven Press, New York.
99. Moore, R. Y., and Bloom, F. E. (1979): *Annu. Rev. Neurosci.,* 2: 113–168.
100. Murphy, D. L., and Redmond, D. E., Jr. (1975): In: *Catecholamines and Behavior, Vol. 2,* edited by A. J. Friedhoff, pp. 73–117. Plenum Press, New York.
101. Nies, A., Robinson, D. S., Lamborn, K. R., and Lampert, R. P. (1973): *Arch. Gen. Psychiatry,* 28:834–838.
102. Ninan, P. T., Insel, T. M., Cohen, R. M., Cook, J. M., Skolnick, P., et al. (1982): *Science,* 218:1332–1334.
103. Nyback, H., Walters, J. R., Aghajanian, G. K., and Roth, R. H. (1975): *Eur. J. Pharmacol.,* 32:302–312.
104. Olpe, H. R., and Jones, R. S. G. (1983): *Eur. J. Pharmacol.,* 91: 107–110.
105. Olpe, H. R., and Schellenberg, A. (1980): *Eur. J. Pharmacol.,* 63: 7–13.
106. Olpe, H. R., Jones, R. S. G., and Steinmann, M. W. (1983): *Experientia,* 39:242–249.
107. Olsen, L., and Fuxe, K. (1971): *Brain Res.,* 28:165–171.
108. Pavlov, I. P. (1927): *Conditioned Reflexes.* Translated by G. Anrep. Oxford University Press, New York.
109. Pert, C. B., Kuhar, M. J., and Snyder, S. H. (1975): *Life Sci.,* 16:1849–1854.
110. Pickel, V. (1982): *J. Clin. Psychiatry,* 43:13–16.
111. Pickel, V. M., Segal, M., and Bloom, F. E. (1974): *J. Comp. Neurol.,* 155:15–42.
112. Probst, A., Cortex, R., and Palacios, J. M. (1985): *Eur. J. Pharmacol.,* 106:477–488.
113. Redmond, D. E., Jr. (1977): In: *Animal Models in Psychiatry and Neurology,* edited by I. Hanin and E. Usdin, pp. 293–306. Pergamon Press, New York.
114. Redmond, D. E., Jr. (1979): In: *Phenomenology and Treatment of Anxiety,* edited by W. E. Fann, A. Pokorny, I. Karacan, and R. Williams, pp. 153–203. Spectrum Publications, New York.
115. Redmond, D. E., Jr. (1979): *Psychopharmacol. Bull.,* 15(2):26–27.
116. Redmond, D. E., Jr. (1981): In: *Psychopharmacology of Clonidine,* edited by H. Lal and S. Fielding, pp. 147–163. Alan R. Liss, New York.
117. Redmond, D. E., Jr., ed. (1982): *J. Clin. Psychiatry,* 43(6):25–29.
118. Redmond, D. E., Jr. (1982): *J. Clin. Psychiatry,* 43(6):4–8.
119. Redmond, D. E., Jr. (1982): *Trends Pharmacol. Sci.,* 3(12):477–480.
120. Redmond, D. E., Jr. (1985): In: *Anxiety and the Anxiety Disorders,* edited by A. Hussain Tuma and J. D. Maser, pp. 533–555. Lawrence Earlbaum, Hillsdale, NJ.
121. Redmond, D. E., Jr., Huang, Y. H., Snyder, D. R., Maas, J. W., and Baulu, J. (1976): *Neurosci. Abstr.,* (668):472.
122. Redmond, D. E., Jr., Huang, Y. H., Snyder, D. R., and Maas, J. W. (1976): *Brain Res.,* 116:502–510.
123. Redmond, D. E., Jr., Huang, Y. H., Snyder, D. R., Maas, J. W., and Baulu, J. (1977): *Life Sci.,* 20:1619–1628.
124. Redmond, D. E., Jr., Huang, Y. H., Baulu, J., Snyder, D. R., and Maas, J. W. (1977): In: *Anorexia Nervosa,* edited by R. Vigersky, pp. 81–96. Raven Press, New York.
125. Redmond, D. E., Jr., Gold, M. S., and Huang, Y. H. (1978): *Neurosci. Abstr.,* 4:413.
126. Redmond, D. E., Jr., and Huang, Y. H. (1979): *Life Sci.,* 25(26): 2149–2162.
127. Redmond, D. E., Jr., Roth, R. H., Hattox, S. E., Stogin, J. M., and Baulu, J. (1979): *Neurosci. Abstr.,* 5:348.
128. Redmond, D. E., Jr., and Huang, Y. H. (1982): *J. Clin. Psychiatry,* 43(6):25–29.
129. Redmond, D. E., Jr., Huang, Y. H., and Grant, S. J. (1983): *Neurosci. Abstr.* 9(Part 2):1057.
130. Redmond, D. E., Jr., and Krystal, J. H. (1984): *Annu. Rev. Neurosci.,* 7:443–478.
131. Redmond, D. E., Jr., Galloway, M. P., Grant, S. J., Fenerty, J., Mayor, R. B., et al. (1984): *Clin. Neuropharmacol.,* 7(Suppl. 1): 186–187.
132. Ross, W. B., Wetterberg, L., and Myrhed, M. (1973): *Life Sci.,* 12:529–532.
133. Roth, R. H., Elsworth, J. D., and Redmond, D. E., Jr. (1982): *J. Clin. Psychiatry,* 43(6):42–46.
134. Rounsaville, B. J., Kosten, T., and Kleber, H. (1985): *J. Nerv. Ment. Dis.,* 173:103–110.
135. Sanghera, M. K., and German, D. C. (1983): *J. Neural Transm.,* 57:267–279.
136. Sanghera, M. K., McMillen, B. A., and German, D. C. (1983): *Eur. J. Pharmacol.,* 86:107–110.
137. Scatton, B. (1982): *Life Sci.,* 31:495–504.
138. Scuvee-Moreau, J. J., and Dresse, A. E. (1979): *Eur. J. Pharmacol.,* 57:219–225.
139. Segal, M. (1979): *J. Physiol. (Lond.),* 286:401–405.
140. Shimizu, N., and Imamoto, K. (1970): *Arch. Histol. Jpn.,* 31: 329–346.
141. Siever, L. J., Uhde, T. W., Jimerson, D. C., Lake, C. R., Silberman, E. R., et al. *Am. J. Psychiatry,* 141:733–741.
142. Skingle, M., Hayes, A. G., and Tyers, M. B. (1982): *Life Sci.,* 31:1123–1132.
143. Snyder, D. R., Huang, Y. H., and Redmond, D. E., Jr. (1977): *Neurosci. Abstr.,* 3(828):261.
144. Soffer, A. (1954): *Med. Clin. North Am.,* 38:375–384.
145. Strahlendorf, H. K., Strahlendorf, J. C., and Barnes, C. D. (1980): *Brain Res.,* 191:284–288.
146. Svensson, T. H., and Usdin, T. (1978): *Science,* 202:1089–1091.
147. Swann, A. C., Charney, D. S., Elsworth, J. D., Jablons, D. M., Roth, R. H., et al. (1983): *Eur. J. Pharmacol.,* 86:167–175.

148. Swanson, L. W. (1976): *Brain Res.,* 110:39–56.
149. Uhde, T. W., Redmond, D. E., Jr., and Kleber, H. D. (1980): *Psychiatry Res.,* 2(1):37–47.
150. Uhde, T. W., Post, R. M., Siever, L. J., and Buchsbaum, M. S. (1980): *Lancet,* 2:1375.
151. Uhde, T. W., Post, R. M., Siever, L. J., Buchsbaum, M. S., Jimerson, D. C., et al. (1981): *Psychopharmacol. Bull.,* 17:125–126.
152. Uhde, T. W., Boulenger, J.-P., Siever, L. J., DuPont, R. L., and Post, R. M. (1982): *Psychopharmacol. Bull.,* 18:47–52.
153. Uhde, T. W., Boulenger, J. P., Post, R. M., Siever, L. J., Vittone, B. J., et al. (1984): *Psychopathology,* 17:8–23.
154. Unnerstall, J. R., Kopajtic, T. A., and Kuhar, M. J. (1986): *Brain Res. Rev.,* 7:69–101.
155. Valentino, R. J., and Aston-Jones, G. (1982): *Neurosci. Abstr.,* 8:228.
156. Valentino, R. J., Foote, S. L., and Aston-Jones, G. (1983): *Brain Res.,* 270:363–367.
157. Van den Hout, M. A., and Griez, E. (1984): *Br. J. Psychiatry,* 144:503–507.
158. Van der Laan, J. W., Bruinvels, J., and Cools, A. R. (1982): *Brain Res.,* 247:309–314.
159. Van Dongen, P. A. M. (1980): *Exp. Neurol.,* 67:52–78.
160. Van Dongen, P. A. M. (1981): *Prog. Neurobiol.,* 17:97–139.
161. Velley, L., Cardo, B., and Bockaert, J. (1981): *Psychopharmacology,* 74:226–231.
162. Watson, S. J., Richard, C. W. III, Ciaranello, R. D., and Barchas, J. D. (1980): *Peptides,* 1(1):23–30.
163. Watson, S. J., Khachaturian, H., Coy, D., Taylor, L., and Akil, H. (1982): *Life Sci.,* 31:1773–1776.
164. Weinshilboum, R. M., Raymond, F. A., Elveback, L. R., and Weidman, W. H. (1973): *Science,* 181:943–945.
165. Woods, S. W., Charney, D. S., Loke, J., Goodman, W. K., Redmond, D. E., Jr., et al. (1986): *Arch. Gen. Psychiatry,* 43:900–909.
166. Woodward, D. J., Moises, H. C., Waterhouse, B. D., Hoffer, B. J., and Freedman, R. (1979): *Fed. Proc.,* 38:2109–2116.
167. Young, W. S., and Kuhar, M. J. (1979): *Eur. J. Pharmacol.,* 59:317–319.

Psychopharmacology:
The Third Generation of Progress,
edited by Herbert Y. Meltzer.
Raven Press, New York © 1987.

CHAPTER **96**

The Benzodiazepine/GABA Receptor Complex and Anxiety

Daniel W. Hommer, Phil Skolnick, and Steven M. Paul

The history of the benzodiazepines as anxiolytics can be divided into two phases. The first phase began with their introduction 25 years ago and lasted until 1977. It was characterized by a nearly exponential increase in their clinical use (8) but by very little growth in our understanding of their mechanism(s) of action. The second phase began with the identification of specific receptors in the brain for benzodiazepines and has coincided with little or no increase in their clinical use but with a dramatic increase in our understanding of their CNS mechanisms of action. In this chapter we focus on the knowledge gained in the past 10 years regarding the molecular actions of the benzodiazepines and on how this information has been applied to studies of the neurobiological substrates of anxiety itself.

ANXIETY, FEAR, AND THE EFFECTS OF THE BENZODIAZEPINES

Before considering the neurobiological basis of anxiety, it is first important to have some understanding of what we mean by anxiety. Anxiety per se is neither a disease nor exclusively a symptom of disease but rather is a fundamental emotion. Most authors have considered the subjective state of anxiety to be similar to fear. From an evolutionary perspective it is easy to see the survival value of fear. Darwin (12) has characterized fear as being "preceded by astonishment, and is so far akin to it, that both lead to the senses of sight and hearing being instantly aroused. The frightened man at first stands like a statue motionless and breathless or crouches down as if instinctively to escape observation." Anxiety and fear can be considered as the cognitive and emotional concomitants of a behavioral alarm system (the so-called "flight-or-flight" response) that serves to prepare an organism to respond to impending danger. The brain mechanisms regulating fear and anxiety are likely to be present in all mammals, including humans, and to function even in the absence of clinically apparent anxiety disorder. In humans, the cerebral cortex, particularly the frontal cortex with its increased capacity for information processing, allows subtle and complex stimuli to trigger the behavioral alarm system.

ANXIOLYTICS AS PROBES OF THE NEUROBIOLOGY OF ANXIETY

The basic premise of much of the work to be reviewed here is that an understanding of neurochemical events underlying anxiety can be derived from an examination of the precise mechanisms of action of antianxiety drugs. This approach is not novel, since many of the biological theories concerning the etiology of neuropsychiatric disorders have evolved from extrapolating neurochemical data on the mode of action of psychotropic drugs. The "dopamine hypothesis of schizophrenia" and the "catecholamine theory of depression," for example, are based primarily on the accumulated preclinical and clinical data concerning the mechanisms of action of drugs that either minic or antagonize the symptoms of depression and schizophrenia, respectively (6,48). The validity of this approach depends on the specificity with which antianxiety drugs reduce the symptoms of anxiety.

Current diagnostic schemes (DSM-III; 1) describe generalized anxiety disorder as being characterized by motor tension, autonomic hyperactivity, apprehensive expectation, increased vigilance, and scanning of the environment. There is abundant evidence that benzodiazepines decrease these characteristic symptoms of anxiety in patients with generalized anxiety disorder (7,19–21,39) as well as decreasing vigilance (27), motor tension (20,30), and autonomic nervous system activity (27) in nonanxious normal volunteers. These findings support the view that the anxiety that is sensitive to benzodiazepines is not unique or confined to a specific anxiety disorder but is present, to a certain extent, in many of us. In this context, pathological anxiety can be viewed as an inappropriate or exaggerated response rather than a qualitatively unique state.

NONBENZODIAZEPINE ANXIOLYTICS

It should be noted that anxiety can be effectively decreased by a wide variety of other pharmacological agents as well as the benzodiazepines (e.g., barbiturates, propanediol carbamates, β-adrenergic blockers, and antidepressants) (7,47). However, these drugs vary in their specificity and potency, and some (e.g., the tricyclic antidepressants) are quite complex pharmacological agents with many diverse neurochemical actions (37). Benzodiazepines, on the other hand, are potent anxiolytics and at therapeutic doses (generally low microgram per kilogram doses) are devoid of the anticholinergic, antihistaminic, and α- and β-adrenolytic actions of most other psychotropic agents (19–21). Benzodiazepines are also generally regarded as being relatively ineffective antidepressant and antipsychotic agents. Thus, insofar as benzodiazepines are specific as anxiolytics, they may be useful as probes in delineating the neurobiology of anxiety.

Barbiturates (e.g., pentobarbital and phenobarbital) and subsequently the propanediol carbamates (e.g., meprobamate) were widely prescribed as anxiolytics, but because of their side effects and toxicity their use has decreased dramatically since the introduction of benzodiazepines in the early 1960s (31). Nevertheless, despite having chemically different structures, the barbiturates, propanediols, and benzodiazepines are all pharmacologically quite similar and show cross tolerance and cross dependence when chronically administered to either laboratory animals or man (7,47,56). Moreover, man's oldest and most widely used anxiolytic, ethanol, shares many pharmacological properties with the benzodiazepines and barbiturates, and all three agents can be substituted for each other in instances of tolerance and withdrawal (7). This suggests that the barbiturates, propanediol carbamates, ethanol, and benzodiazepines may share common neurochemical mechanisms of action, which may be involved in the antianxiety effects of all four agents. If a common mechanism of action for such chemically disparate drugs could be identified, it would quite likely be an important clue for understanding the pathophysiology of anxiety.

In addition to sharing anxiolytic properties, the benzodiazepines, barbiturates, propanediol carbamates, and ethanol also possess sedative and hypnotic properties. Sedation is usually the major side effect of benzodiazepine treatment, and in the clinical setting it can be difficult to separate the sedative from the anxiolytic effects of the drug. However, sedation is clearly not necessary for the antianxiety effects of the benzodiazepines, since with chronic administration, tolerance to benzodiazepine-induced sedation develops fairly rapidly, but the anxiolytic effects persist (19,20). In animals a dissociation between the sedative and the fear-reducing properties of acutely administered benzodiazepines has been demonstrated (17).

ANIMAL MODELS OF ANXIETY

In laboratory animals, benzodiazepines (as well as the other anxiolytics mentioned above) selectively attenuate the behavioral effects of three classes of environmental situations (17,18): punishment, nonreward, and novelty. Gray has proposed that these three types of environmental events activate a "behavioral inhibition system" in brain, the output of which results in an inhibition of ongoing behavior as well as an increase in arousal and attention (19). These changes are similar to the physiological and behavioral characteristics of human anxiety (1,61). Gray has also suggested that benzodiazepines and other antianxiety drugs impair activity in the behavioral inhibition system and thus "release" behavior suppressed by this system. Thus, although benzodiazepines reduce the behavioral inhibition produced by stimuli associated with punishment, they fail to alter simple escape behavior. In addition to reducing the behavioral effects of signals for punishment and nonreward, as well as for novelty itself, benzodiazepines also attenuate the accompanying autonomic and endocrine changes. The environmental situations that are sensitive to benzodiazepines in animals can usually be anthropomorphized to threats of punishment, frustration, and uncertainty.

Not surprisingly, the most widely studied behavioral action of the benzodiazepines in animals relates to their ability to reduce the behavioral inhibition produced by punishment (17). In fact, the ability of benzodiazepines to attenuate the punishment-induced suppression of behavior is a widely used screening test for uncovering the anxiolytic properties of new drugs. In one variation of this procedure, animals are deprived of food and water and then given access to a sucrose solution delivered through an electrified drinking spout from which they receive a shock every few licks. When hungry or thirsty rats are placed in this so-called "conflict" situation (i.e., a conflict between their thirst and avoidance of the shock), they generally respond by not drinking. Thus, the punishment inhibits the animal's ongoing behavior (i.e., drinking). Animals given benzodiazepines are more resistant to the ability of punishment to suppress ongoing behavior; they continue to lick despite the shocks.

The relative potencies of a large series of benodiazepines in preventing the behavioral inhibition induced by punishment in animals correlate highly with their potencies as anxiolytics in man (reviewed in ref. 46). This effect is not simply a reflection of sedation, since sedation decreases both punished and nonpunished behavior in the "conflict test" and therefore antagonizes the observed actions of benzodiazepines (17). A variety of psychotropic drugs, including stimulants, antidepressants, antipsychotics, and opiates, have been tested for their ability to prevent the behavioral inhibition induced by punishment and have been found to be devoid of "anticonflict" activity at pharmacologically relevant doses. In addition, drugs that specifically block or enhance noradrenergic, dopaminergic, cholinergic, or glycinergic neurotransmission fail to produce or alter "anticonflict" activity in animals. Other drugs, however, that show cross tolerance with the benzodiazepines, including the barbiturates, propanediol carbamates, and ethanol, also reduce the behavioral inhibition by punishment in a variety of species.

These results suggest that the mechanisms responsible for the anticonflict effect of benzodiazepines in laboratory animals may be similar, if not identical, to those responsible for their antianxiety effects in man. As we shall see, the anticonflict action of benzodiazepines has proven to be a useful model for exploring the neurobiology of anxiety. One problem, however, with using the behavioral inhibition produced by punishment as an animal model of human anxiety is whether such behavioral inhibition is a characteristic of human anxiety. Older psychodynamically oriented descriptions of anxiety contain accounts of phenomena that could be called behavioral inhibition. Freud, for example, specifically discusses the inhibitory effects of anxiety on both appetitive and sexual behavior (16). Avoidance behaviors may also constitute a form of human behavioral inhibition, and these behaviors may be included in revised editions of DSM-III.

BENZODIAZEPINE RECEPTORS

Despite their widespread clinical use, even as recently as the preceding edition of this volume the neurochemical mechanisms by which the benzodiazepines produce their anxiolytic and other behavioral effects were not known. No even tentative biochemical theory of the mechanism(s) of action of these drugs was offered. Early workers had reported a variety of neurochemical changes in brain following the administration of benzodiazepines to laboratory animals. Alterations, for example, in the turnover of a number of neurotransmitters including acetylcholine, norepinephrine, and serotonin were reported (reviewed in ref. 23), but these changes were subtle and not universally observed. Some studies even suggested that the antianxiety and muscle-relaxant effects of benzodiazepines were mediated by peripheral rather than central mechanisms. Benzodiazepines had been shown in neurophysiological experiments to potentiate the inhibitory actions of γ-aminobutyric acid (GABA), but as stated this was only one among many reported biochemical effects (24).

In 1977, two groups of investigators working independently reported the presence of saturable, high-affinity, and stereospecific recognition sites for benzodiazepines in rat brain (32,33,50). Moreover, in studying the relative affinities of a large series of benzodiazepines for these binding sites, both groups observed striking correlations between the binding affinities of various benzodiazepines in vitro and their potencies as anxiolytic agents. Similar correlations were observed between relative binding affinity and the potencies of benzodiazepines as anticonflict agents in animals (56).

Since the initial discovery of benzodiazepine receptors, literally hundreds of reports have been published further validating and extending the role of the benzodiazepine receptor in the mechanism(s) of action of these agents. It is now known that all of the major pharmacological actions of benzodiazepines are mediated through benzodiazepine receptors, since these effects can be blocked by selective benzodiazepine receptor antagonists (10,28). Benzodiazepine receptors have been demonstrated in a variety of species, including man (33), and to date no major species differences in the biochemical or pharmacological characteristics of these receptors have been demonstrated. Benzodiazepine receptors are, however, rather recent phylogenetic additions, since they are not found in invertebrates and are densest in more recently evolved brain regions.

In addition to the central benzodiazepine receptors described above, peripheral recognition sites for the benzodiazepines have also been demonstrated (3). These peripheral benzodiazepine binding sites differ from central benzodiazepine receptors in several ways; most importantly they do not appear to mediate any of the behaviorally important effects of benzodiazepine, although it is possible that these peripheral sites may represent "receptors" for heretofore unrecognized pharmacological actions of the benzodiazepines (41).

Benzodiazepines and GABA

Even prior to the discovery of benzodiazepine receptors it had been known that benzodiazepines could potentiate the inhibitory actions of GABA as measured by electrophysiological and pharmacological techniques (24). GABA is one of the most ubiquitous and important inhibitory neurotransmitters in brain and has been estimated to be present in as many as 30% of all synapses (40). Surprisingly, the initial studies of benzodiazepine receptors in brain failed to reveal any significant interaction between a number of endogenous neurotransmitters, including GABA, and the binding of radioligands to the benzodiazepine receptor. The definitive link between the benzodiazepine receptor and GABA came when Tallman and coworkers found that when GABA was added to brain membranes, the affinity of benzodiazepines for their receptor increased (56). The effects of GABA to allosterically enhance benzodiazepine receptor affinity in vivo was mimicked by GABA receptor agonists, such as muscimol, and blocked by the GABA receptor antagonist, bicucullne (56). Permeable anions such as chloride and bromide also enhance the binding of benzodiazepines to their receptor (55), suggesting the involvement of an ion channel (specifically, a chloride ion channel) in the actions of benzodiazepines. Previous electrophysiological studies had shown that GABA inhibits neuronal excitability by selectively activating membrane chloride conductance. More recent experiments involving the solubilization and purification of the benzodiazepine receptor have confirmed its close association with the GABA receptor and suggest that the binding sites for benzodiazepines and GABA exist on the same protein subunit (42). Thus, the benzodiazepine receptor may simply be a phylogenetically recent subclass of GABA receptors.

It is now generally accepted that the benzodiazepine receptor is structurally associated with the GABA receptor and, along with a chloride channel, forms a "supramolecular receptor complex" the function of which is to regulate the movement of chloride ions through neuronal membranes (36). When GABA is released into the synaptic cleft, it activates a specific postsynaptic receptor (so-called $GABA_A$ receptor),[1] causing an "opening" of the chloride channel. The negatively charged chloride ions move through the channel from the extracellular space, where they are present in high concentration, to the inside of the neuron where there is little chloride. This results in an increase in the negative charge inside the cell. The increased negative potential across the neuronal membrane hyperpolarizes the cell, making it more difficult for any excitatory synaptic input to depolarize the cell sufficiently to generate an action potential. In this way GABA produces an inhibitory effect. Benzodiazepines themselves produce little or no effect on membrane chloride conductance, but in the presence of GABA they markedly potentiate GABA-mediated increases in chloride permeability. The effect of benzodiazepines on GABA-receptor-mediated chloride conductance appears to be related to an increase in the frequency of chloride channel openings rather than an increase in chloride conductance per opening (53).

THE BENZODIAZEPINE/GABA RECEPTOR COMPLEX AS A SITE OF ACTION FOR OTHER ANXIOLYTIC DRUGS

Earlier we cited evidence that a variety of chemically dissimilar antianxiety drugs (e.g., the benzodiazepines, barbiturates, propanediol carbamates, and ethanol) shared a number of pharmacological properties including their ability to reduce anxiety-related behaviors in both laboratory animals and man (7,47). We suggested that if these agents shared a common underlying neurochemical mechanism, the latter may very likely represent an important neurobiological clue to understanding the pathophysiology of anxiety. In the initial reports describing the presence of benzodiazepine receptors in brain (50), it was also reported that most nonbenzodiazepine anxiolytics including the barbiturates failed to compete with ^{3}H-diazepam for binding to the receptor. In other words, the barbiturates, propanediol carbamates, and ethanol did not directly interact with the benzodiazepine binding or recognition site (as do the benzodiazepines), and, therefore, it was concluded that these drugs had different mechanisms of action.

The striking electrophysiological and pharmacological similarities between barbiturates and benzodiazepines as well as the ability of GABA and chloride to increase benzodiazepine receptor binding prompted a more extensive examination of the possible interaction of barbiturates with benzodiazepine receptors (36,46). Pentobarbital was found to enhance the binding of benzodiazepines to the benzodiazepine receptor in vitro. At low (i.e., sedative–hypnotic) concentrations, pentobarbital potentiated the ability of submaximal concentrations of GABA to enhance benzodiazepine receptor binding, whereas at higher (i.e., anesthetic) concentrations, barbiturates directly stimulated the binding of benzodiazepines to their receptor (46). This enhancement of benzodiazepine binding occurs through an increase in the affinity of radioligand for the receptor and, like the effects of GABA, is dependent on the presence of chloride ions (46). In addition to barbiturates, a number of other anxiolytic and anticonvulsant drugs have been reported to interact in a similar fashion with the benzodiazepine/ GABA receptor complex (ref. 47 for review).

It now appears that several classes of nonbenzodiazepine (both barbiturate and nonbarbiturate) anxiolytic, anticonvulsant as well as proconvulsant, drugs affect the benzodiazepine/$GABA_A$ receptor complex through yet another binding site. This site has been called the "picrotoxin site" since it was initially identified using this convulsant. Binding of drugs to the picrotoxin site allosterically modifies the affinity of both the benzodiazepine and the GABA receptor as well as directly affecting chloride conductance (58). In fact, recently, it has been possible to measure directly the effects of barbiturates on GABA receptor function in vitro.

Schwartz and co-workers (44) have developed a sensitive method for studying radioactive chloride transport in a subcellular brain preparation. With this method, both barbiturates and GABA have been shown to stimulate chloride uptake into resealed neuronal membranes. These effects are blocked by specific GABA receptor antagonists such as picrotoxin and bicuculline, confirming that they are mediated by a functional $GABA_A$ receptor. With the development of this method it has been possible to examine the effects of other anxiolytic drugs believed to work via the receptor complex. Significantly, ethanol, at concentrations that occur in blood during acute intoxication, increases chloride uptake in a manner quite similar to that of the barbiturates and GABA (54). From these experiments, it appears that ethanol may actually stimulate the benzodiazepine/GABA receptor complex as do pentobarbital and GABA, and at concentrations that are consistent with ethanol's antianxiety properties.

Although all of the above mentioned antianxiety drugs appear to enhance GABAergic neurotransmission by interacting with the benzodiazepine/GABA receptor complex, it is important to emphasize that there are significant differences in their precise molecular mechanisms of action. For example, benzodiazepines produce little or no effect on chloride conductance in the absence of GABA, whereas the barbiturates and ethanol can directly activate chloride conductance to produce neuronal inhibition. These differences may account for the greater toxicity and side-effect profile of barbiturates and ethanol compared with the benzodiazepines. In addition, barbiturates increase the actual

---

[1] GABA, like most neurotransmitters, interacts with more than one membrane receptor. To date, two GABA receptors have been delineated: $GABA_A$ receptors are associated with benzodiazepine receptors and chloride channels; $GABA_B$ receptors are associated with adenylate cyclase and do not appear to be modulated by benzodiazepines (15).

time of chloride channel opening rather than the frequency of openings (53). From the abundant biochemical and pharmacological data, it appears that the benzodiazepine/GABA receptor actually represents an oligomeric protein complex consisting of several subunits and containing multiple interacting binding sites for a variety of antianxiety and sedative agents. The fact that virtually all common anxiolytic drugs potentiate GABAergic neurotransmission makes this receptor complex an intriguing locus for an investigation into the brain mechanisms underlying fear and anxiety.

ANXIETY AND THE BENZODIAZEPINE/GABA RECEPTOR COMPLEX

The discovery of a specific receptor for benzodiazepines and the demonstration that this receptor complex mediates the anxiolytic actions of many antianxiety drugs raise the possibility that this complex also mediates the physiological responses underlying fear and anxiety. However, simply understanding the mechanism of action of a drug does not necessarily imply an understanding of the pathophysiological processes that are responsive to that drug. Cardiac glycosides, for example, are effective in the treatment of congestive heart failure, but their action in inhibiting Na^+,K^+-ATPase has not proven particularly useful in understanding the pathogenesis of this disorder. Nonetheless, knowing why a drug recognition site for benzodiazepines has evolved in brain, and why it is associated with a naturally occurring neurotransmitter such as GABA, may shed some light on the biological basis of anxiety and fear. One possibility, of course, is that the benzodiazepine receptor is itself subserved by an endogenous neuromodulatory substance. The benzodiazepine receptor (like the opiate receptor) may have its own endogenous ligand(s). If such a compound exists, it could theoretically mimic the benzodiazepines and reduce anxiety, or it could have an anxiogenic action.

While searching for an endogenous ligand for the benzodiazepine receptor, Braestrup and colleagues (3,4) isolated a β-carboline derivative (β-carboline-3-carboxylate ethyl ester, βCCE) that possesses an extremely high affinity for the benzodiazepine receptor. When administered to rodents, βCCE effectively antagonizes the anticonvulsant and sedative effects of the benzodiazepines (57). At first it was thought that βCCE simply blocked the effects of benzodiazepines, but later it was shown that βCCE had intrinsic pharmacological activity that was essentially opposite to that of the benzodiazepines (4). In rodents, such intrinsic actions are difficult to observe, but in primates Ninan and co-workers (35) reported marked behavioral agitation (e.g., struggling in the restraint chair, piloerection, distress vocalizations) following intravenous administration of βCCE. Significantly, the behavioral effects of βCCE in the rhesus monkey were also accompanied by increases in heart rate, blood pressure, and the stress hormones ACTH/cortisol, epinephrine, and norepinephrine. Moreover, all of the behavioral and physiologic changes produced by βCCE were blocked by pretreatment with diazepam or the selective benzodiazepine receptor antagonist Ro15-1788 (35). These data clearly

implicate the benzodiazepine receptor in mediating the "anxiogenic" effects of βCCE and argue against a nonspecific action of βCCE in producing arousal.

Although the behavioral, physiological, and endocrine effects of βCCE in subhuman primates are similar to those seen in extremely anxious patients, it is still not certain how similar the βCCE-induced syndrome is to naturally occurring fear or anxiety. Insel and co-workers (29) as well as Crawley and co-workers (9) observed that lower doses of βCCE produced highly individualistic behavioral and physiological responses in rhesus monkeys that predicted the animals' subsequent response to threatening environmental stimuli. Thus, the behavioral responses to βCCE, although varying from animal to animal, were highly characteristic of that animal and were similar to those observed under a variety of stressful or fear-provoking situations. If, for example, an animal became highly aroused and agitated when approached by a stranger, his response to βCCE administration would also be robust. Similarly, animals with low overt behavioral and physiological responses to βCCE would also be low responders to environmental stress. The fact that low, pharmacologically relevant doses of benzodiazepines completely reversed or blocked the anxiety-related behaviors produced by βCCE supports the hypothesis that this syndrome may represent a reliable pharmacological model of human fear and anxiety. Further, the α-adrenoceptor agonist clonidine, a drug shown to have anxiolytic effects in humans, also blocked the βCCE-induced syndrome, particularly the autonomic nervous system effects of βCCE (9,29). The effects of βCCE were also partially antagonized by β-adrenergic antagonists as well as serotonin antagonists (9), suggesting that full manifestation of the βCCE-induced anxiety-like syndrome requires integrity of noradrenergic and serotonergic as well as GABAergic neurotransmitter systems.

Despite the rather impressive similarities between the βCCE-induced behavioral syndrome in animals and many of the signs and symptoms of human anxiety, it is impossible to demonstrate conclusively the presence or absence of anxiety in any animal other than man. Recently, Dorow and associates (13) have administered a β-carboline derivative (FG-7142) that is closely related to βCCE to several human volunteers. The administration of FG-7142 resulted in symptoms of muscle tension, autonomic hyperactivity, and extreme apprehension. These effects were interpreted subjectively as being quite similar to anxiety and were characterized by feelings of "inner tension, excitation, and sensations of physical disturbance." The subjective effects of βCCE were accompanied by marked elevations in heart rate, blood pressure, and plasma cortisol. In one volunteer these symptoms were so severe that intravenous lormetazepam was administered, and the symptoms subsided within only a few minutes.

For obvious reasons clinical studies on the anxiogenic actions of β-carboline esters have been rather limited, but other anxiogenic compounds that work via the GABA receptor complex have also been shown to produce anxiety in man. Pentylenetetrazol, for example, is a convulsant that binds to the picrotoxin site of the benzodiazepine/GABA receptor complex (52) and has been shown to produce anxiety in humans when administered at subconvulsant doses (47). Since both the β-carboline esters and pentylenetetrazol effectively antagonize GABA-mediated chloride conductance (38,44), it appears that a decrease in GABAergic activity is associated with these drug-induced anxiety states.

More recently, Costa and his colleagues (22) have isolated, purified, and sequenced a family of peptides that compete with benzodiazepines and β-carbolines for binding to the receptor, which they have proposed as being endogenous ligands for the benzodiazepine receptor. One of these peptides (diazepam binding inhibitor or DBI) had been shown to have proconflict actions in animals (22) and to inhibit selectively the effects of GABA in electrophysiological experiments. It appears, therefore, that this peptide (or a related fragment) may function as an endogenous "anxiogenic" substance serving to attenuate GABAergic activity.

THE NEUROANATOMY OF BENZODIAZEPINE RECEPTORS AND ANXIETY

Following the demonstration of the benzodiazepine receptor in brain homogenates, an autoradiographic technique to visualize and map the distribution of benzodiazepine receptors in brain was developed (63). This technique permits tentative identification of brain regions that are targets for the benzodiazepines and may mediate their pharmacological effects. Benzodiazepine receptors are located primarily in phylogenetically recent areas of the neuroaxis such as the neocortex, particularly frontal cortex. Benzodiazepine receptors are also densely concentrated in several limbic structures. In contrast to the relatively wide distribution of benzodiazepine receptors in the forebrain, high densities of benzodiazepine receptors in the brainstem are limited to only four areas. Interestingly, three of these regions have been shown by Davis et al. (34,59) to be necessary for the ability of conditional fear to enhance the startle response in animals.

These three areas, the substantia nigra, the superior colliculus, and the ventral nucleus of the lateral lemniscus, appear to form a circuit via which central nucleus of the amygdala, another benzodiazepine-receptor-rich area, influences startle response. Since benzodiazepines selectively block the ability of fear to enhance the startle response (11), it may now be possible to examine neuroanatomical circuits that mediate specific components of fear and anxiety and to compare them with the known distribution of benzodiazepine receptors.

BENZODIAZEPINES, GABA, AND STRESS

Benzodiazepines have been commonly used for many years as pretreatment medications prior to stressful medical procedures. In addition to decreasing anxiety and fear, benzodiazepines and their receptors may play a role in the physiology and pathophysiology of stress. Recently, several laboratories have begun to examine the relationship between stress and the benzodiazepine/GABA receptor complex. Biggio and co-workers (2) were among the first to demonstrate that the benzodiazepine receptor can rapidly be altered following exposure to various stressors in rodents. More recently, Havoudjian et al. (25) have demonstrated that the effects of swim stress on the benzodiazepine/GABA receptor complex occur at the picrotoxin (barbiturate) recognition site and are manifested by an increase in the ability of permeable anions to enhance benzodiazepine binding. Functionally, these changes produce an enhancement of GABAergic receptor sensitivity, a conclusion that has recently been confirmed both biochemically and electrophysiologically in our laboratory (*unpublished observations*). Thus, immediately following stress there is a compensatory enhancement of GABA receptor sensitivity, which appears to occur directly at the postsynaptic benzodiazepine/GABA receptor complex. Consistent with this conclusion is the demonstrated increase in seizure threshold for GABA receptor antagonists such as picrotoxin and pentylenetetrazol following stress in rodents (49). It is possible that alterations in GABAergic "inhibitory tone" may serve to attenuate the physiological and perhaps cognitive components of stress.

Numerous studies in the psychiatric literature have suggested that anxiety may not simply be a symptom associated with depression but may, in fact, be essential to the development of at least some varieties of depression. The issue of whether anxiety and depression are causally related has been reviewed recently by Gray (18). Certain animal models of depression involve the administration of aversive stimuli over which the animal has no control. It has been demonstrated that it is the lack of control over aversive experiences and not the aversive events themselves that results in a behavioral syndrome characterized by failure to learn an escape task 24 hr later, reduction in aggression and social dominance, opiate-mediated stress-induced analgesia, depressed lymphocyte proliferation with increased growth of implanted tumors, decreased food intake, and ulcer formation (45). In order to see whether pharmacologically induced anxiety might be related to the development of this learned helplessness syndrome, we administered the anxiogenic β-carboline, FG-7142, to rats and tested them for deficits in learning on a subsequent shuttlebox escape task. FG-7142, like inescapable shock, produced a syndrome of learned helplessness in rats that was blocked by pretreatment with benzodiazepines or the selective benzodiazepine antagonists Ro15-1788 (14). However, these agents were ineffective in reversing the syndrome once it had developed. These data suggest that certain animal models of anxiety may be biochemically related to the learned helplessness model of depression. Whether this may be related to the vulnerability factors that determine the progression of anxiety to depression in man is unknown.

SUMMARY

The material reviewed in this chapter strongly supports a role for the GABA/benzodiazepine/chloride ionophore complex in the action of the benzodiazepines as well as other anxiolytic drugs. It appears that most, if not all, anxiolytic drugs act by increasing GABA-receptor-coupled chloride conductance. Furthermore, several anxiety-producing agents act via an opposite effect on the GABA-coupled chloride ion channel. The recent isolation of an endogenous anxiogenic peptide ligand of the benzodiazepine receptor and the demonstration of stress-induced changes in the benzodiazepine/GABA receptor complex suggest that this receptor complex may be involved in the neurochemical events underlying anxiety and fear. Obviously, much more work is required before a definite link between GABA/benzodiazepine receptor function and anxiety can be made, but at very least we now have a comprehensive and testable hypothesis of the neurobiology of anxiety.

REFERENCES

1. American Psychiatric Association. (1980): *Diagnostic and Statistical Manual of Mental Disorders,* 3rd ed. American Psychiatric Association, Washington.
2. Biggo, G. (1983): In: *Advances in Biochemical Psychopharmacology, Vol. 38,* edited by G. Biggio and E. Costa, pp. 105–119. Raven Press, New York.
3. Braestrup, C., and Squires, R. (1977): *Proc. Natl. Acad. Sci. U.S.A.,* 74:3804–3809.
4. Braestrup, C., Nielsen, M., and Olsen, C. F. (1980): *Proc. Natl. Acad. Sci. U.S.A.,* 77:2288–2292.
5. Braestrup, C., Nielsen, M., and Skovbjerg, H. (1981): In: *GABA and Benzodiazepine Receptors,* edited by E. Costa, G. DiChiara, and G. Gessa, pp. 147–155. Raven Press, New York.
6. Bunney, W. E., Jr., and Davis, J. M. (1965): *Arch. Gen. Psychiatry,* 13:483–494.
7. Cole, J. O., and Davis, J. M. (1975): In: *American Handbook of Psychiatry,* (*Second Edition*), edited by D. X. Freedman and J. E. Dyrud, pp. 247–261. Basic Books, New York.
8. Cook, L., and Davidson, A. B. (1973): In: *The Benzodiazepines,* edited by L. Levi, pp. 1–28. Raven Press, New York.
9. Crawley, J. N., Ninan, P. T., Pickar, D., Chrousos, G. P., Linnoila, M., et al. (1985): *J. Neurosci.,* 5:477–485.
10. Darragh, A., Lambe, R., Scully, M., Brick, I., O'Boyle, C., et al. (1981): *Lancet,* 2:8–10.
11. Davis, M. (1979): *Psychopharmacology (Berl.),* 61:1–7.
12. Dawrin, C. (1965): *The Expression of the Emotions in Man and Animals.* University of Chicago Press, Chicago.
13. Dorow, R., Horowski, R., Paschelke, G., Amin, M., and Braestrup, C. (1983): *Lancet,* 2:98–99.
14. Drugan, R. C., Maier, S. F., Skolnick, P., Paul, S. M., and Crawley, J. N. (1985): *Eur. J. Pharmacol.,* 113:453–457.
15. Enna, S. J., and Gallagher, J. P. (1983): *Int. Rev. Neurobiol.,* 24:181–212.
16. Freud, S. (1936): New Introductory Lectures. The Psychoanalytic Quarterly Press and W. W. Norton, New York.
17. Geller, I., and Seifter, J. (1960): *Psychopharmacologia,* 1:482–492.
18. Gray, J. A. (1982): *The Neuropsychology of Anxiety: An Enquiry into the Functions of the Septo–Hippocampal System.* Oxford University Press, New York.
19. Greenblatt, D. J., and Shader, R. I. (1974): *Benzodiazepines in Clinical Practice.* Raven Press, New York.
20. Greenblatt, D. J., Shader, R. I., and Abernethy, D. R. (1983): *N. Engl. J. Med.,* 309:354–358.
21. Greenblatt, D. J., Shader, R. I., and Abernethy, D. R. (1983): *N. Engl. J. Med.,* 309:410–416.
22. Guidotti, A., Forchetti, C. M., Corda, M. G., Konkel, D., Bennett, C. D., et al. (1983): *Proc. Natl. Acad. Sci. U.S.A.,* 80:3531–3535.
23. Haefely, W. E. (1978): In: *Psychopharmacology, A Generation of Progress,* edited by M. A. Lipton, A. DiMascio, and K. F. Killam, pp. 1359–1374. Raven Press, New York.
24. Haefely, W., Kulcsar, R., Mohler, H., Pieri, L., Polc, P., et al. (1975): *Adv. Biochem. Psychopharmacol.,* 14:131–151.
25. Havoudjian, H., Paul, S. M., and Skolnick, P. (1986): *Brain Res.,* 375:401–406.
26. Hoehn-Saric, R., Merchant, A. F., Keyser, M. C., and Smith, V. K. (1981): *Arch. Gen. Psychiatry,* 38:1278–1282.
27. Hommer, D. W., Matsuo, V., Wolkowitz, D. M., Chrousos, G. A., Weingartner, H., et al. (1986): *Arch. Gen. Psychiatry,* 43:542–551.
28. Hunkeler, W., Mohler, H., Pieri, L., Polc, P., Bonetti, E. P., et al. (1981): *Nature,* 290:514–516.
29. Insel, T. R., Ninan, P. T., Aloi, J., Jimerson, D. C., Skolnick, P., et al. (1984): *Arch. Gen. Psychiatry,* 41:741–750.
30. Linnoila, M., Erwin, C. W., Brendle, A., and Simpson, D. (1983): *J. Clin. Psychopharmacol.,* 3:88–96.
31. Mellinger, G. D., and Balter, M. B. (1983): In: *Society and Medication: Conflicting Signals for Prescribers and Patients,* edited by J. P. Morgan and D. V. Kagan, pp. 54–78. D. C. Health, Lexington, MA.
32. Mohler, H., and Okada, T. (1977): *Science,* 198:849–851.
33. Mohler, H., and Okada, T. (1978): *Life Sci.,* 22:985–996.
34. Mondlock, J. M., and Davis, M. (1985): *Neurosci. Abstr.,* 15:331.
35. Ninan, P. T., Insel, T. M., Cohen, R. M., Cook, J. M., Skolnick, P., et al. (1982): *Science,* 218:1332–1334.
36. Paul, S. M., Marangos, P. J., and Skolnick, P. (1981): *Biol. Psychiatry,* 16:213–229.
37. Paul, S. M., Janowsky, A., and Skolnick, P. (1985): In: *Psychiatry Update: The APA Annual Review, Vol. 4,* edited by R. E. Hales and A. J. Frances, pp. 37–48. APA Press, Washington, D.C.
38. Polc, P., Ropert, N., and Wright, D. M. (1981): *Brain Res.,* 217:216–220.
39. Rickels, K. (1978): *Psychopharmacology (Berl.),* 58:1–17.
40. Roberts, E., Chase, T. W., and Tower, D. B. (1976): *GABA in Nervous System Function.* Raven Press, New York.
41. Ruff, M. R., Pert, C. B., Weber, R. J., Wahl, L. M., Wahl, S. M., et al. (1985): *Science,* 229:1281–1983.
42. Schwartz, R. D., Thomas, J. W., Kempner, E. S., Skolnick, P., and Paul, S. M. (1985): *J. Neurochem.,* 45:108–115.
43. Schwartz, R. D., Jackson, J. A., Weigert, D., Skolnick, P., and Paul, S. M. (1987): *J. Neurosci. (in press).*
44. Schwartz, R. D., Skolnick, P., Seale, T. W., and Paul, S. M. (1986): In: *Advances in Biochemical Pharmacology,* edited by G. Biggio and E. Costa, pp. 33–49. Raven Press, New York.
45. Seligman, M. E. P. (1975): *Helplessness. On Depression, Development and Death.* W. H. Freeman, San Francisco.
46. Skolnick, P., Moncada, V., Barker, J. L., and Paul, S. M. (1981): *Science,* 211:1448–1450.
47. Skolnick, P., and Paul, S. M. (1982): *Int. Rev. Neurobiol.,* 23:103–140.
48. Snyder, S. H., Banerjee, S. P., and Yamamura, H. I. (1974): *Science,* 184:1243–1253.
49. Soubrie, P., Thiebot, M., Jobert, A., Montrastruc, J., Hery, F., et al. (1980): *Brain Res.,* 189:505–517.
50. Squires, R. F., and Braestrup, C. (1977): *Nature,* 266:732–734.
51. Squires, R. F., Casida, J. E., Richardson, M., and Saederup, E. (1983): *Mol. Pharmacol.,* 23:326–336.
52. Squires, R. F., Saederup, E., Crawley, J. N., Skolnick, P., Paul, S. M., et al. (1969): *J. Comp. Physiol. Psychol.,* 671:535–546.
53. Study, R. E., and Barker, J. L. (1982): *J.A.M.A.,* 247:2147–2151.
54. Suzdak, P., Schwartz, R. D., Skolnick, P., and Paul, S. M. (1986): *Proc. Natl. Acad. Sci. U.S.A.,* 83:4071–4075.
55. Tallman, J. F., Paul, S. M., Skolnick, P., and Gallager, D. W. (1980): *Science,* 207:274–281.
56. Tallman, J. D., Thomas, J., and Gallager, D. (1978): *Nature,* 274:383–395.
57. Tenen, S. S., and Hirsch, J. D. (1980): *Nature,* 288:609–610.
58. Ticku, M. K., and Maksay, G. (1983): *Life Sci.,* 33:2363–2375.
59. Tischler, M. D., and Davis, M. (1983): *Brain Res.,* 276:55–71.
60. Turski, L., Schwarz, M., Klockgether, T., and Sontas, K.-H. (1985): *Neurosci. Abstr.,* 15:1162.
61. Uhlenhuth, E. H., Balter, M. B., Mellinger, G. D., Cisin, I. H., and Clinthorne, J. (1983): *Arch. Gen. Psychiatry,* 40:1167–1173.
62. Weise, C. E., and Price, C. F. (1975): *The Benzodiazepines— Patterns of Use.* Addiction Research Foundation, Toronto.
63. Young, W. S., and Kuhar, J. J. (1979): *Nature,* 280:393–395.

Psychopharmacology:
The Third Generation of Progress,
edited by Herbert Y. Meltzer.
Raven Press, New York © 1987.

CHAPTER 97

Pharmacologic Provocation of Panic Attacks

Jack M. Gorman, Minna R. Fyer, Michael R. Liebowitz, and
Donald F. Klein

The proliferation of agents claimed capable of provoking acute panic attacks under laboratory conditions almost defies systematic categorization. Most extensively studied symptom-producing substances have been reported to induce panic in patients with panic disorder.

The prevailing strategy is to administer one or two "panicogenic" agents to susceptible patients. One goal is to establish what biochemical and physiological events occur during a panic attack. A second goal is to ascertain what other agents, administered acutely or chronically, can block the laboratory-induced panic attack. Such studies may identify clinically useful strategies for treating panics.

Finally, pharmacologic induction of panic is a method of uncovering the pathophysiology of clinical panic disorder. If a given agent has a known effect in humans and also provokes panic attacks in appropriate subjects, the assumption is often made that its specific action is etiologically involved in the generation of panic. Elaborate theories of panic disorder have evolved in this manner.

There are three difficulties with this reasoning. First, each theory fails to account for the panicogenic effects of other agents that do not affect the same neurochemical system. Second, it is possible that there are several key derangements. Third there may be many ways to affect the key derangement, making direct etiologic inferences misleading.

This review critically evaluates the work done to date with pharmacologic provocation of panic. Following Guttmacher et al. (31), the ideal panicogenic agent for laboratory studies should possess the following attributes:

1. The panic attack should combine physical symptoms of panic with a subjective sense of terror and a desire to flee. This is important because differences in the definition of panic in the literature have created confusion about the panicogenic potential of various agents.

2. The provoked attack should be judged by patients as symptomatically very similar to their own regularly occurring spontaneous attacks.

3. The induction of panic should be specific to patients with a history of spontaneous panic attacks. This may be expressed in one of two ways. Either only patients with spontaneous panic histories have attacks at all (absolute specificity) or such patients routinely panic at lower doses than other subjects (threshold specificity).

4. Drugs that block spontaneous panic attacks, such as tricyclic antidepressants (39), monamine oxidase inhibitors (38), and alprazolam (10), should also block the acute pharmacologically induced attack.

5. The effect of the agent in provoking panic should be consistent in a given patient. If a desensitization effect occurs, this should also be predictable.

6. The agent, in the panicogenic dose, should be safe for routine administration to human subjects.

7. Agents such as diazepam that do not block clinical panic (58) should not block the pharmacologically induced panic.

We will review β-adrenergic stimulants (epinephrine, isoproterenol), α-adrenergic stimulants (norepinephrine, yohimbine), cholinomimetics (methacholine, physostigmine, neostigmine, arecoline), sodium lactate, caffeine, carbon dioxide, and insulin/glucose tolerance tests.

β-ADRENERGIC STIMULANTS

Ever since William James (36) proposed that anxiety is a reaction to peripheral physical stimulation, epinephrine has been a popular tool for laboratory induction of anxiety. Epinephrine has stronger β-adrenergic than α-adrenergic stimulatory properties, producing a rise in heart rate, systolic blood pressure, and minute ventilation; peripheral vasodilation; and a decrease in diastolic blood pressure. It penetrates the blood–brain barrier poorly.

There are innumerable studies of infused epinephrine to both normal and anxious subjects. These have been reviewed elsewhere (5,44). The salient point is whether any demonstrate that epinephrine produces panic.

The answer is largely negative. Although epinephrine has never been administered to patients meeting rigorous criteria for panic disorder, Lindemann and Finesinger (50) infused "adrenalin"—a mixture of mostly epinephrine and some norepinephrine—to anxiety patients "suffering from anxiety, coming on in distinct attacks with relatively free intervals. . . ." They reported a reaction to adrenalin only in those patients whose spontaneous attacks occurred "without specific mental content." Although this description sounds like our idea of a spontaneous panic attack, the reaction to adrenalin observed by Lindemann and Finesinger (50) does not sound much like frank panic. The symptoms experienced during infusion are characterized by the authors as "self-absorption and withdrawal" (p. 365). Subsequently, Lindemann and Finesinger (51) found that patients exhibited a nonspecific response to adrenalin characterized by introspection, depression, worry, and anger but not panic. This nonspecific response to adrenalin is characteristic of the epinephrine literature.

In normal volunteers, Basowitz (1) found that each subject responded to epinephrine infusion in a way "peculiar to him in ordinary life stresses" (p. 104). Others (18,52,62) have reported that epinephrine produced an "as-if" anxiety response in both normals and psychiatric patients.

Further confounding interpretation of these results are Schacter and Singer's (72) findings that subjects given subcutaneous epinephrine were strongly influenced by cognitive expectations and environmental cues and reacted with a variety of emotions ranging from amusement to anxiety. Interestingly, this is the only study to report the accentuation of amusement as a reaction to epinephrine.

Overall, the response to epinephrine seems highly plastic, relatively nonspecific, and barely resembles panic attacks. Although unlikely, it is possible that patients with panic disorder might show a specific sensitivity to epinephrine.

Isoproterenol is a β-adrenergic agonist that, like epinephrine, does not readily permeate the blood–brain barrier. Frohlich (21) identified a group of patients with high left ventricular ejection rate, occasional systolic hypertension, often a systolic ejection murmur, and bounding arterial pulse and termed the complex "hyperdynamic β-adrenergic circulatory state." During isoproterenol infusion, these patients, but not normal controls, experienced increased cardiac awareness, exaggerated pulse response, and "emotional outbursts" that are somewhat reminiscent of panic attacks.

Subsequently, Easton and Sherman (14) described isoproterenol-induced anxiety attacks in four subjects with a history of spontaneous panic attacks. They began the infusion at 0.40 μg/min and increased the dose every 6 min until a panic attack occurred (1.7 to 2.6 μg/min). The patients' naturally occurring attacks were blocked by oral administration of propranolol (60–320 mg), and this was maintained on 4- to 24-month follow-up. Unfortunately, although the authors claim that intravenous propranolol (2 to 5 mg over 2–3 min) aborted the isoproterenol-induced attack, it was not determined whether pretreatment with propranolol blocked the isoproterenol-induced attack. In view of the poor track record of oral propranolol with panic disorder and intravenous propranolol with lactate-induced panic, it is unclear if Easton and Sherman's panics are necessarily panic disorder.

Schmidt and Elizabeth (73) first reported that intravenous isoproterenol provoked panic attacks in patients with DSM-III panic disorder but not in normals. Rainey et al. (64) have reported the largest series of isoproterenol infusions in patients with rigorously defined panic disorder. They define an acute panic attack during an infusion as an episode meeting DSM-III criteria for panic, with at least four of the 12 listed symptoms and an increase in anxiety over baseline on a 0 to 4 scale to a minimum score of 2. In 11 panic disorder patients, the rate of isoproterenol-induced panic (73%) was not significantly different from that obtained with sodium lactate infusion (91%). Both were significantly greater than placebo (36%).

The 10 normal controls had panic attacks with both lactate (30%) and isoproterenol (20%) but much less often than panic patients. Patients rated isoproterenol- and lactate-induced attacks equally similar to their spontaneously occurring attacks except that the isoproterenol attacks were described as less severe. Subsequently, these authors have reported isoproterenol infusions of 39 panic disorder patients and 18 normal controls (65). Seventy-four percent of patients and 5% of normals had isoproterenol-induced panic attacks, whereas 26% of patients and none of the controls had panic attacks with placebo infusion.

Treatment with the standard antipanic medication imipramine led to a reduction in panic to sodium lactate from 13/14 patients pre-treatment to 4/14 post-treatment and in panic to isoproterenol from 11/14 to 1/14.

It is not known whether the Rainey et al. (19,64) finding of isoproterenol-induced panic would occur repeatedly in a given patient. The high rate of placebo panic (26% to 36%) in the panic disorder patients and of sodium lactate-induced panic (30%) in the controls raises questions about whether the criteria used to define panic set too low a threshold.

The mechanism of isoproterenol-induced panic is not clear. Gorman et al. (25) and Nesse et al. (57) have reported that patients with panic disorder do not have abnormal β-adrenergic sensitivity. Nesse et al. (57) administered bolus intravenous isoproterenol (0.6 μg to 4.0 μg) to panic disorder patients and normal controls. Patients had no greater increase in anxiety over baseline compared to controls and smaller heart rate increases than controls. This was interpreted to indicate a lack of β-adrenergic hypersensitivity in panic disorder patients. Noyes et al. (58) have reported that 2 weeks of oral propranolol treatment did not lead to panic blockade.

Isoproterenol does not have direct central nervous system effects, although it may indirectly affect the central nervous system by altering blood flow to the brain. If further research indicates that isoproterenol infusion provides a good panic model, this may occur through a mechanism other than β-adrenergic stimulation, such as nonspecific stress.

α-ADRENERGIC STIMULANTS

Norepinephrine has primarily α-adrenergic stimulant properties, although it also specifically stimulates cardiac β receptors with equal potency to epinephrine. Like epinephrine and isoproterenol, it does not cross the blood–brain barrier. Most norepinephrine in peripheral blood derives from the synapses of α-adrenergic nerves.

Norepinephrine administration causes a peripheral vasoconstriction, increases in both diastolic and systolic blood pressure, and, probably because of reflex baroreceptor vagal stimulation, a drop in heart rate.

Earlier studies are inconclusive whether norepinephrine provokes panic. Frankenhauser, Jarpe, and Matell (18) compared intravenous epinephrine, norepinephrine, and placebo and found norepinephrine a much weaker anxiogen than epinephrine. Infusion of normal volunteers with an equal mixture of epinephrine and norepinephrine produced emotional reactions identical to those of epinephrine alone.

Undaunted by this lack of positive evidence, Pyke et al. (63) recently infused norepinephrine to patients with panic disorder. The protocol began with a dose of 0.25 mg/min, which was increased at 2.5-min intervals to 16 mg/min. All six subjects reportedly had typical panic attacks. Repeat norepinephrine infusion after chronic alprazolam treatment did not provoke panic.

Although this work suggests that norepinephrine may satisfy many criteria for a panic model, it is a small series that has not been replicated. All six patients reportedly panicked, but the definition of panic is sufficiently unclear that this finding remains tentative. Furthermore, no placebo control was used, and four of the six patients had discontinued benzodiazepine therapy within 4 or 5 days of the infusion. Finally, the top dose of 16 mg/min is relatively high and could conceivably be panicogenic in normals.

The experiment is interesting because norepinephrine, as expected, lowered heart rate. This suggests that tachycardia is not necessary to trigger panic, even though naturally occurring attacks are often accompanied by increased heart rate (20,43).

In recent years, a theory has repeatedly been advanced that increased central noradrenergic activity is directly related to the induction of panic. The theory derives from work on monkeys by Redmond et al. (67) showing that stimulation of the locus coeruleus, which contains most of the brain's noradrenergic neurons, causes an anxiety-like reaction. Ablation of the locus coeruleus, on the other hand, rendered the animals emotionally immune to ordinarily anxiety-provoking situations such as the introduction of a toy snake into the cage. This work has been criticized and even dismissed by Mason (53), who believes the locus coeruleus has no role in panic anxiety and merely influences the degree of arousal. He points out that serotonergic neurons are also present in the locus coeruleus.

Although Ko et al. (42) claimed to find that plasma MHPG—a metabolite of central nervous system norepi-

nephrine—rose acutely in agoraphobic subjects when confronted with their own individual phobic stimuli, more recently Woods et al. (78) found that exposure to phobic stimuli did not cause a rise in plasma MHPG. Also Ko's statistical analysis is open to criticism, since data points rather than individuals were used in the correlational analyses.

Drugs such as imipramine that block spontaneous panic appear to reduce the locus coeruleus firing rate (59,74).

Administration of an agent that acutely increases locus coeruleus discharge would be a direct test of the central noradrenergic hypothesis. Yohimbine, an α2-receptor antagonist, is such an agent. Yohimbine also easily penetrates the blood–brain barrier (55,71).

In two separate studies, Gershon et al. (24,34) administered 20 mg of oral yohimbine to a heterogeneous group of psychiatric patients. They reacted with clear-cut anxiety responses, some of which sound like panic. Ingram (35) found yohimbine a more reliable anxiogen than epinephrine. Patients with higher base-line anxiety reacted to yohimbine with the greatest amount of anxiety, suggesting that yohimbine has a specific effect on patients who experience anxiety as a prominent part of their psychiatric illness.

Charney (8) has recently given yohimbine, in a dose of 20 mg orally, to 39 patients with DSM-III panic disorder and 20 normal volunteers. Placebo, always administered the day before yohimbine, decreased anxiety in the patients. Approximately 80% of patients had an anxiety response to yohimbine. However, this high rate of response is difficult to interpret in view of the way in which it was determined. Anxiety responses were measured using a 100-mm line visual analog scale on which 0 represented no anxiety and 100 the most anxiety. An increase of at least 20 mm was considered an anxiety response to yohimbine. Rather than assessing the difference from base line in anxiety score with yohimbine, the authors chose to assess the difference in anxiety response between placebo and yohimbine. Many patients actually had a substantial decrease in anxiety with placebo. Therefore, a patient who had a large decrease with placebo and a minimal increase in anxiety with yohimbine could have been judged as an anxiety responder to yohimbine. No attempt was made to determine whether an anxiety response was an actual panic attack.

Charney et al. (10) also compared the effects of placebo and alprazolam treatment (8 to 12 weeks) on yohimbine-induced anxiety. In response to yohimbine challenge during placebo treatment, 11/14 patients experienced anxiety symptoms similar in severity to their naturally occurring panic attacks. During alprazolam treatment, only 1/14 patients reported such symptoms.

In an earlier study (7), acute pretreatment with clonidine or diazepam significantly decreased yohimbine's anxiogenic effects in normals. This finding is difficult to interpret. On the one hand, clonidine, which specifically decreases locus coeruleus firing, is known to have at least transient antipanic effects during chronic treatment of panic disorder patients (32,45). Diazepam, on the other hand, is said not to be an effective antipanic medication. Noyes et al. (58) found that although 2 weeks of treatment with diazepam decreased both the frequency and severity of panic attacks, it did not block them. M. R. Liebowitz (*personal communication*) found that pretreatment with 5 mg intravenous diazepam did not block lactate-induced panic.

Two problems seriously limit the attractiveness of yohimbine as a model of panic anxiety. First, in his original work, Gershon et al. (34) found that 3 weeks of pretreatment with imipramine worsened yohimbine-induced anxiety. Imipramine is a well-studied, well-regarded antipanic drug; any form of anxiety that gets worse after imipramine is a poor model for spontaneous panic. Charney et al. (9) have recently reported that chronic (50 to 250 mg p.o. q.d. for 8–12 weeks) imipramine treatment did not alter the anxiogenic effect of 20 mg oral yohimbine. Second, mianserin and buspirone, which like yohimbine are α_2-receptor antagonists (33,70), have not been reported to cause anxiety or exacerbate panic disorder as would be expected if the α_2-receptor is involved in the generation of panic. On the contrary, both buspirone and mianserin have anxiolytic properties (40).

It is unclear whether yohimbine provokes panic in patients with panic disorder. Also unresolved is whether yohimbine-induced anxiety is specifically related to increased noradrenergic discharge or represents a nonspecific response that can be blocked by any antianxiety agent, e.g., diazepam.

CHOLINOMIMETIC AGENTS

Although there are a number of reasons to suspect disordered parasympathetic response in patients with panic disorder, this area remains relatively neglected.

Lindemann and Finesinger (50) administered intravenous methacholine chloride (acetylmethylcholine), a predominantly muscarinic agonist, and provoked a reaction described as "panic" in a subgroup of anxious patients "who had developed definite phobias and concrete fears" (p. 363). Their description of one patient sounds very much like panic disorder; the patient had a panic attack similar to his spontaneous attacks after an injection of 15 mg methacholine but not after intravenous epinephrine or placebo.

Funkenstein et al. (22) administered intramuscular methacholine (10 mg) to 100 patients with a variety of psychiatric diagnoses and normal controls. Most of the controls have somatic symptoms but not anxiety in response to methacholine challenge. A number of patients experienced anxiety "similar to their spontaneous clinical attacks." This reaction was most common in patients with "psychoneurosis" but also occurred in subjects with a variety of other diagnoses.

In a later study, Lindemann and Finesinger (51) noted that methacholine caused a high degree of respiratory distress in anxious subjects. This is interesting in view of recent evidence linking ventilatory abnormalities to panic disorder (27; J. M. Gorman, M. R. Fyer, R. Goetz, J. Ashkenazi, J. Martinez, M. R. Liebowitz, A. J. Fyer, J. Kinney, and D. F. Klein, *unpublished data*).

Fyer et al. (A. J. Fyer, D. C. Ross, and D. F. Klein, *unpublished data*) found that the self-report of panic attacks of agoraphobics differed from those of simple or social phobics (on exposure to feared objects) in being more often characterized by the cluster of symptoms referrable to

cholinergic discharge, i.e., vomiting, urinary urgency, and urge to defecate. This finding is further evidence for a role of the cholinergic system in panic attacks. However, this may be an epiphenomenon of severity.

In normal volunteers, the administration of the cholinomimetic carbachol (Doryl®) did not induce anxiety (13).

Janowsky and Risch (37,69) have proposed that central cholinergic stimulation forms an integral part of stress responses. They reported that the centrally acting cholinesterase inhibitor physostigmine caused a nonspecific anxiety response in a number of subjects, including normals. This effect could not be mimicked by the non-centrally-acting cholinesterase inhibitor neostigmine. Atropine, but not the purely peripherally acting anticholinergic drug methscopolamine, blocked the anxiogenic effect of physostigmine.

Further supporting a role for centrally acting cholinergic stimulation in anxiety induction are studies using arecoline challenge. Arecoline produced increased anxiety in normal subjects under conditions of peripheral cholinergic blockade.

Janowsky and Risch (37,69) hypothesize that anxiety induction by central cholinergic stimulation occurs in part by activation of central sympathetic pathways. Nevertheless, it has not been demonstrated that any form of parasympathetic stimulation causes panic attacks or produces a reaction in panic disorder patients that differs from normals. The studies cited suggest that such work is worth pursuing.

CAFFEINE

It has been known for many years that caffeine makes some people nervous. The possibility that caffeine might provoke panic or have an exaggerated anxiogenic effect in anxiety patients has only recently been explored.

The neural effects of caffeine are only partially understood. Caffeine is a weak benzodiazepine receptor inhibitor (3,16). In doses of 200 to 500 mg, it can produce headaches, tremors, anxiety, and irritability (66). Acute doses of greater than 10 g can cause death (66). It remains unlikely, however, that even heavy caffeine consumers ingest sufficient amounts to make the benzodizepine antagonistic effect of routine significance.

Boulenger et al. (4) and Charney et al. (11) have argued instead that caffeine's effects on the adenosine neurotransmitter system are responsible for its anxiogenic properties. Whatever the underlying mechanism, Boulenger et al. (4) surveyed patients with panic disorder and reported that they are hypersensitive to caffeine. Thirty patients with panic disorder, 23 patients with major affective disorder, and an equal number of age- and sex-matched controls were surveyed for daily caffeine consumption (DCC) and measures of anxiety and depression. In panic disorder patients, but not in either control group, DCC was correlated with both state and trait anxiety as well as depression. Panic disorder patients reported increased sensitivity to one cup of coffee compared with controls. Depressed patients had high levels of state and trait anxiety but did not report this sensitivity. More panic patients (67%) reported having given up coffee than controls (20%).

Pursuing this, Uhde et al. (77) administered oral caffeine in doses of 240, 480, and 720 mg to 12 normal controls and found a dose-related increase in anxiety, plasma cortisol, and lactate. At the 720-mg dose, two of the 12 normals had panic attacks.

These investigators then administered 480 mg of oral caffeine to 24 panic disorder patients and 14 controls. Nine of the 24 panic patients and none of the 14 controls had panic attacks. Stringent criteria for panic were used, requiring the patient to report the experience as indistinguishable from a spontaneous panic attack. The patients all had greater increases in serum glucose, lactate, and cortisol than controls. The only variable that differentiated panicking from nonpanicking patients was an increased lactate level in panickers.

Subsequently, this group has conducted a double-blind study of alprazolam versus placebo treatment followed by caffeine challenge in 15 pairs of panic disorder patients (T. W. Uhde, *personal communication*). After treatment, on 480 mg oral caffeine challenge, 40% of the placebo and none of the alprazolam-treated group had panic attacks. Alprazolam-treated patients had serum lactate levels comparable to those usually found in normals or nonpanicking patients.

Charney et al. (11) administered oral caffeine (10 mg/kg) to patients with DSM-III panic disorder and normal volunteers. Caffeine produced more anxiety in patients than controls. Anxiety levels correlated with plasma caffeine levels in patients but not in controls. Patients reported the anxiety experienced as qualitatively similar to their spontaneous panic attacks. It is not specified whether the intensity or temporal course of the anxiety was comparable to patients' usual panic attacks.

These caffeine experiments, although interesting, create the impression that caffeine at high doses may cause panic in anyone. The study by Uhde et al. (75,76) suggests that caffeine at the 480-mg dose may provoke panic in patients with panic disorder and not normal controls (threshold specificity) and that its effect may be blocked by alprazolam. This study also raises the possibility that the panicogenic effect of caffeine may be mediated by an increase in lactate. More studies are needed to establish whether caffeine will provide a viable panic model.

SODIUM LACTATE INFUSIONS

In the last two decades sodium lactate has clearly surpassed other agents as the infusion of choice for provocation of panic in the laboratory. Hundreds of patients—most with panic disorder—and normal volunteers have undergone lactate infusion in centers around the world. The number of investigators interested in performing lactate infusion is growing steadily.

The theory behind the lactate infusion procedure stems from work begun in the 1940s by Cohen and White (12), showing that patients with "neurocirculatory asthenia" develop higher blood lactate levels than normal controls after physical exertion. They dismissed the possibility that these patients were in poor physical condition and introduced the idea that a basic defect in the capacity for aerobic metabolism was responsible for the elevated lactate levels.

Because patients with neurocirculatory asthenia sounded like panic disorder patients, Pitts and McClure (60) performed the landmark experiment demonstrating the capacity of sodium lactate infusion to provoke an acute panic attack in patients but not in normal controls.

Pitts and McClure's (60) finding has been replicated in a number of laboratories, many using double-blind, placebo-controlled technique (17,29,47,64). In the standard procedure, the subject receives a placebo infusion followed by 0.5 M racemic sodium lactate (10 cc/kg) over 20 min. Panic attacks occur in about 75% of panic disorder patients. Although there is substantial controversy about the meaning of the lactate effect, the fact that lactate infusion provokes panic in patients with panic disorder is no longer in question.

Among the agents reviewed, only lactate has been given to a large enough number of subjects under a sufficient number of varied experimental designs by different research groups to enable systematic evaluation of its suitability as a model panicogen. The abundance of data should not be assumed in any way to impart automatic validation but merely to permit the closest scrutiny.

We address the seven criteria (see above) point by point for lactate.

1. The panic attack should combine physical symptoms of panic with a subjective sense of terror and a desire to flee. The attack, therefore, should not simply be a parallel increase from a higher baseline but should be reflected in a greater increment over baseline anxiety in the panicking patient. In the work of the Klein group (47), it is explicitly stated that the criteria for calling a lactate response a panic attack go beyond simple physical symptoms and include the subjective sense of terror. Other studies, however, are not clear on this point. This is important because lactate infusion produces a number of profound physiological effects in anyone, including tachycardia, paresthesias, tremor, urinary urgency, and alkalosis. Studies like those of Rainey et al. (65), in which substantial numbers of normal volunteers are said to panic during lactate, may use measures too sensitive to these purely physical changes. Nevertheless, the literature is quite clear that patients who do panic during lactate infusion experience emotional as well as physical distress. Furthermore, Dillon et al. (D. Dillon, J. M. Gorman, M. R. Liebowitz, A. J. Fyer, and D. F. Klein, *unpublished data*) have shown that there is an incrementally greater increase in anxiety over baseline level in patients who panic to lactate than in nonpanicking patients or controls.

2. The provoked attack should be judged by patients as symptomatically very similar to their own regularly occurring spontaneous attacks. This feature has not been extensively studied, but some data indicate that lactate infusion meets this criterion.

The Acute Panic Inventory (API), a 17-item instrument measuring the severity of panic attack symptoms, was administered to panic disorder patients before and during sodium lactate infusion. At a separate time, patients were also rated on the API as if they were having a typical (for them) spontaneous panic attack, whereas normal controls rated themselves as if they were undergoing a period of very high stress. Patients who had attacks during the first half of the subsequent infusion obtained API scores very close to those of their usual panic. Patients who panicked during the second half of the infusion were somewhat lower. Patients who did not panic during the infusion obtained scores much lower than their rating of usual panic. The increment in API score from base line to infusion termination was much greater in panicking patients than in nonpanickers or normals. This indicates that patients experience lactate-induced panic as very similar to their spontaneous panic attacks and that the increase in anxiety for lactate panickers is greater than experienced by normals.

3. The induction of panic should be specific to patients with a history of spontaneous panic attacks. Here, the evidence is still incomplete. If the proper criteria for a panic attack are used, normals rarely panic during lactate infusion. Small studies have shown that social phobics (48) and obsessive–compulsives (26) are both immune to lactate panicogenesis. McGrath et al. (54) have recently reported that patients with atypical depression and a history of spontaneous panic attacks—although not meeting the full DSM-III criteria for panic disorder—experienced panic during lactate infusion. Atypical depressives without a history of panic attacks did not panic during lactate infusion. Dunner et al. (D. Dunner, *personal communication*) have found that patients with major affective disorder with concurrent panic disorder panic to lactate, whereas those with major affective disorder without concurrent panic disorder do not.

These studies suggest that lactate panicogenesis is specific to patients with a panic history. More studies are needed before the issue of specificity can be decided. Patients with generalized anxiety disorder would be of particular interest.

4. Drugs that block spontaneous panic attacks, such as tricyclic antidepressants (39), monamine oxidase inhibitors (38), and alprazolam (10), should also block the acute pharmacologically induced attack. Several similarly designed studies have tested this criterion for lactate infusion (6,38). Patients first undergo lactate infusion in the unmedicated state and are then placed on one of the usual antipanic drugs. After a sustained period of clinical remission from panic attacks, and while still on antipanic medication, the infusion is repeated. For all three types of antipanic drugs— TCAs, MAOIs, and alprazolam—the panic rate at second infusion is sharply lower. This criterion appears fulfilled by lactate infusion.

5. The effect of the agent in provoking panic should be consistent in a given patient. If the effect of the agent wanes and desensitization occurs, this should also be predictable. Bonn et al. (2), after finding that the same patient would panic repeatedly to sequential lactate infusions, attempted to use the infusion as a desensitization technique. They found that in patients suffering from "intractable anxiety," biweekly lactate infusions resulted in decreased self-rated anxiety scores. Gorman et al. (25) have also shown that a small group of patients who panicked during lactate infusion would panic again during a subsequent infusion a few days later. On the other hand, Liebowitz et al. (46) found that a group of patients who did not panic during a first infusion also did not panic a few days later during a second infusion. Although these studies used small samples, the consistency of the response to lactate in a given patient seems fairly well confirmed.

6. The agent, in the panicogenic dose, should be safe for routine administration to human subjects. There are no reports of serious adverse effects from infusion of sodium lactate. Because of the large hypertonic fluid load administered, lactate infusion is not recommended for patients with significant hypertension, congestive heart failure, or renal disease.

7. Drugs that do not block clinical panic should not block the pharmacologically induced panic.

Several attempts have been made to block acute lactate-induced panic. The addition of calcium to the lactate infusate was found to reduce the number and severity of panic attacks (60). However, early theories suggesting that lactate-induced panic is caused by hypocalcemia are now questioned. Ethylenediaminetetraacetic acid (EDTA), the powerful calcium chelator, does not produce panic attacks (61). During lactate infusion, Fyer et al. (23) have shown that ionized calcium dropped equivalently in panicking and nonpanicking patients.

Gorman et al. (25) gave intravenous propranolol (0.2 mg/kg) over 30 min immediately prior to lactate infusion to six patients who had panicked during standard lactate infusion 2 days earlier. Propranolol failed to block the repeated lactate-induced attacks in any patient. A similar finding with diazepam (5 mg i.v.) pretreatment was made by M. R. Liebowitz (*personal communication*). Liebowitz (*personal communication*) also administered intravenous clonidine (1.0 to 2.0 μg/kg) prior to lactate infusion and found that it blocked subsequent lactate panic in only four of 10 patients, all of whom had initially panicked to standard lactate infusion.

With the exception of criterion 3 (specificity), where further studies are needed, we conclude that lactate infusion provides a viable model for naturally occurring panic. Therefore, it is important to look at the biological accompaniments of lactate-induced panic.

The main biological accompaniments appear to be tachycardia and, surprisingly, hyperventilation-induced hypocapnia. One might think that metabolic alkalosis might cause hypoventilation, but that is not the case here. Increases in diastolic blood pressure, cortisol, and plasma norepinephrine are less frequently observed. Increased systolic blood pressure and plasma epinephrine and decreased blood glucose and calcium do not characterize lactate-induced panic (49). Although metabolic alkalosis is always the result of lactate infusion, this is not exaggerated in lactate panickers (28).

One limitation of the lactate model is the failure to explain adequately the pathophysiological basis of lactate-induced panic. It also remains controversial whether or not and how quickly lactate crosses the blood–brain barrier (56). A range of theories have been advanced including alkalosis, hypocalcemia, increase in NAD/NADH ratio, nonspecific factors, and increased central carbon dioxide concentration. Each of these is currently being examined.

CARBON DIOXIDE

For many years it has been assumed that hyperventilation-induced respiratory alkalosis is panicogenic. Cohen and White (12) first made the surprising observation, again in subjects dubbed "neurocirculatory asthenics," that inhalation of small amounts (4%) of carbon dioxide (CO_2) and not hyperventilation caused panic attacks.

Gorman et al. (27) reported a small series of panic disorder patients who had attacks during inhalation of 5% CO_2. Normal controls did not panic under this condition. In these patients, CO_2 also proved a somewhat more reliable panicogen than room air hyperventilation. Subsequently, Gorman et al. (J. M. Gorman, M. R. Fyer, R. Goetz, J. Ashkenazi, J. Martinez, M. R. Liebowitz, A. J. Fyer, J. Kinney, and D. F. Klein, *unpublished data*) reported preliminary data indicating that subjects who panicked to 5% CO_2 reacted with a mixture of physical and emotional symptoms similar in quality to their naturally occurring panics. Five percent CO_2 panickers have an exaggerated physiological response to CO_2 compared to normal controls and continue overbreathing after CO_2 is turned off. Social phobics and obsessive–compulsives did not panic during 5% CO_2 inhalation.

Woods et al. (79), using the Read rebreathing method, studied the effect of CO_2 on panic disorder patients and normal controls, finding that increases in anxiety occurred in both groups but were significantly greater in patients. Under strict criteria for panic (which requires fear of death, losing control, going crazy, or a desire to flee), 70% of patients panicked in contrast to 20% of matched controls. Alprazolam treatment markedly decreased CO_2-induced anxiety, with only 20% of treated patients experiencing CO_2-induced panic.

In a study of patients with panic disorder, E. Griez and M. van den Hout (*personal communication*) have shown that inhalation of a single breath of a mixture of 35% CO_2 and 65% oxygen (O_2) produces panic in patients but not in normal controls. The effect appears to be consistent for a given subject. This finding has recently been replicated in our laboratory in a small series of panic disorder patients and controls: five out of eight panic disorder patients experienced panic attacks with double-breath inhalation of 35% CO_2/65% O_2; normal controls did not.

The mechanism of the panicogenic effect of CO_2 is not understood. Elam et al. (15) have reported that CO_2 inhalation causes a dose-dependent increase in locus coeruleus discharge in rats. Gorman et al. (27) initially speculated that CO_2 may cause panic through locus coeruleus activation and subsequently that patients with panic disorder have abnormally sensitive medullary chemoreceptors. These chemoreceptors normally induce increased ventilation as arterial PCO_2 rises to hypercapnic levels but may be triggered at lower levels of CO_2 in patients with panic disorder. Interestingly, caffeine, which may provoke panic in patients with panic disorder, is known to increase the sensitivity of the medullary chemoreceptors.

Klein (41) has suggested that CO_2 chemoreceptors are linked to a specific alarm and escape mechanism sensitive to asphyxiation that is erroneously triggered in patients with panic disorder. Such a mechanism would explain the finding that many patients with panic disorder are chronic hyperventilators, that sustained hyperventilation is seen in CO_2 panickers after CO_2 is stopped, and that symptoms are consistent with the clinical symptomatology of panic.

Carr and Sheehan (6) have theorized that the primary defect in panic disorder lies in the brainstem redox-regulating system. Any challenge causing a decrease in brainstem intraneuronal pH, e.g., CO_2, stimulates the central chemoreceptors and may provoke panic in susceptible individuals. According to this theory, pyruvate infusion, which would shift the redox equation

$$\frac{[\text{lactate}]}{[\text{pyruvate}]} = K \frac{[\text{NADH}] \times [\text{H}^+]}{[\text{NAD}^+]}$$

in the opposite direction from lactate, should not be panicogenic.

These preliminary findings indicate that CO_2 may provide a good panic model, although they clearly need replication by other investigators.

MISCELLANEOUS PANICOGENS

It cannot have escaped notice that all of the agents discussed have managed to provoke panic in somebody, sometime, in someone's laboratory. The question must be raised whether there is any active agent that does not cause panic. The list is admittedly sparse. Pitts (61) reports giving panic patients infusion of the powerful calcium-chelating agent EDTA. Although patients were almost tetanic, none had panic attacks.

Uhde et al. (75) administered glucose tolerance tests to a group of panic disorder patients. A surprising number had blood glucose nadirs in the hypoglycemic range, but none reported anxiety symptoms or panic attacks. Similarly, E. Schweizer, A. Winokur, and K. Rickels, (*unpublished data*) produced significant hypoglycemia in eight of 10 patients with panic disorder during insulin tolerance tests, but no patient had a panic attack. Because hypoglycemia produces increased plasma epinephrine levels, this experiment indirectly suggests that adrenergic stimulation is inadequate to produce an attack.

Two nonpharmacologic provocations also failed to provoke panic: the mental arithmetic test (38) and the cold pressor test (30). The former has been shown to cause tachycardia, increased cortisol level, and anxiety, whereas the latter is a potent α-adrenergic stimulant that can produce significant vasoconstriction.

If the pharmacologic provocation of panic is to prove more than a nonspecific stress response, it will be necessary to document that there are agents capable of provoking profound physiological and biochemical alterations that do not routinely produce panic in panic disorder patients. In this field, a negative finding has become as valuable as a positive finding.

COMMENT

Table 1 summarizes how well each agent reviewed here satisfies our seven criteria. Lactate, caffeine, and carbon dioxide come closest to satisfying the panic model requirements. It is clear that in most cases failure to meet criteria stems more from a lack of appropriate studies rather than from an actual negative finding. Lactate comes closest to the most valid panic model primarily because it has been most extensively studied.

TABLE 1. *Criteria for panic-producing interventions*[a]

	Causes emotional and physical symptoms	Causes true panic	Specificity (absolute or threshold)	Blocked by antipanic drugs	Consistency	Safety	Not blocked by clinically ineffective agents
Anxiogenic							
Epinephrine	+	−	−	?	?	++	?
Isoproterenol	+	+	?	+	?	++	?
Norepinephrine	+	+	?	+	?	++	?
Yohimbine	+	?	?	−	?	++	−
Physostigmine	−	−	?	?	?	++	?
Arecoline	−	−	?	?	?	++	?
Methacholine	+	?	?	?	?	++	?
Caffeine	+	+	+	+	?	++	?
Lactate	++	++	++	++	++	++	+
Carbon dioxide	++	++	+	+	?	++	?
Nonanxiogenic							
EDTA	−	−	?	?	?	−	?
Glucose	−	−	?	?	?	++	?
Cold pressor	−	−	?	?	?	++	?
Mental arithmetic	−	−	?	?	?	++	?
Insulin	−	−	−	?	?	+	?

[a] ++, good positive evidence; +, preliminary positive evidence; ?, no evidence; −, negative evidence.

Pharmacologic models of panic have already made a number of contributions to our understanding of pathological anxiety. Using lactate-induced panic, several authors (38,45,65) have detected the physiological and biochemical events that occur during an acute panic attack. These include increase in heart rate and ventilation and sometimes increases in diastolic blood pressure and plasma norepinephrine. Without a laboratory model, gathering such information would depend either on accumulating sufficient subjects who happened to experience a spontaneous panic attack while in the laboratory or using ambulatory monitoring equipment that would record physiologic changes during spontaneous panic attacks. A few field studies have been carried out (20,78), but work in this area is still nascent.

Pharmacologic models have been used to debunk certain long-held beliefs about anxiety attacks, such as the idea that they are caused by hypoglycemia. The surprising findings that anxiety attacks are not accompanied by abrupt increases in plasma epinephrine or cortisol and that they cannot be blocked by acute intravenous administration of a β-adrenergic blocking agent also came from work with pharmacologic models.

It is conceivable that in the not too distant future, pharmacologically induced panic attack models will be used to screen new putative antipanic medications and to track a patient's progress through treatment. Ultimately, if one of the models meets the specificity tests, pharmacologically induced panic could even serve the clinician as a diagnostic tool.

Most problematic have been attempts to use pharmacologic models for etiologic insight. A perfect model need imply nothing about basic pathophysiology, just as the patient with coronary artery disease who becomes symptomatic during a cardiac stress test did not develop atherosclerosis because of too much exercise. At present, pharmacologic models are useful tools for studying the phenomenology of panic and the development of possible interventions. Precisely why any agent causes panic and whether understanding of these mechanisms will shed light on the basic pathology of panic disorder are as yet unknown.

ACKNOWLEDGMENTS

This work was supported in part by National Institutes of Mental Health Grants MH 33422 and MH 30906 and by Research Scientist Development Award MH 00416 (Dr. Gorman).

REFERENCES

1. Basowitz, H., Korchin, S. J., Oken, D., Goldstein, M. S., Gussach, H., et al. (1956): *A.M.A. Arch. Neurol. Psychiatry,* 76:98–106.
2. Bonn, J. A., Harrison, J., and Rees, W. L. (1971): *Br. J. Psychiatry,* 119(551):468–470.
3. Boulenger, J. P., Patel, J., and Mavango, P. J. (1982): *Neurosci. Lett.,* 30:161–166.
4. Boulenger, J. P., Uhde, T. W., Wolff, E. A. III, and Post, R. M. (1984): *Arch. Gen. Psychiatry,* 41:1067–1071.
5. Breggin, P. R. (1964): *J. Nerv. Ment. Dis.,* 139:558–568.
6. Carr, D. B., and Sheehan, D. V. (1984): *J. Clin. Psychiatry,* 45:323–330.
7. Charney, D. S., Heninger, G. R., and Redmond, D. E., Jr. (1983): *Life Sci.,* 33:19–29.
8. Charney, D. S., Heninger, G. R., and Breier, A. (1984): *Arch. Gen. Psychiatry,* 41:751–763.
9. Charney, D. S., and Heninger, G. R. (1985): *Arch. Gen. Psychiatry,* 42:473–481.
10. Charney, D. S., and Heninger, G. R. (1985): *Arch. Gen. Psychiatry,* 42:458–467.
11. Charney, D. S., Heninger, G. R., and Jatlow, P. I. (1985): *Arch. Gen. Psychiatry,* 42:233–243.
12. Cohen, M. E., and White, P. D. (1951): *Pychosom. Med.,* 13:335–357.
13. Dynes, J. B., and Todd, H. (1940): *J. Neurol. Psychiatry,* 3:1–8.

14. Easton, J. D., and Sherman, D. G. (1982): *Arch. Neurol.,* 33:689–691.
15. Elam, M., Yoa, J., Thoren, P., and Svenson, T. H. (1981): *Brain Res.,* 222:373–381.
16. File, S. E., Bond, A. J., and Lister, R. G. (1982): *Clin. Psychopharmacol.,* 2:102–106.
17. Fink, M., Taylor, M. A., and Volavka, J. (1970): *N. Engl. J. Med.,* 281:1129.
18. Frankenhaeuser, M., Jarpe, G., and Matell, G. (1961): *Acta Physiol. Scand.,* 51:175–186.
19. Freedman, R. R., Ianni, P., Ettedgui, E., Pohl, R., and Rainey, J. M. (1984): *Psychopathology,* 17(Suppl. 1):66–73.
20. Freedman, R. R., Ianni, P., Ettedgui, E., and Puthenzbath, N. (1985): *Arch. Gen. Psychiatry,* 42:244–248.
21. Frohlich, E. D., Tarazi, R. C., and Dustan, H. P. (1969): *Arch. Intern. Med.,* 123:1–7.
22. Funkenstein, D. H., Greenblatt, M., and Solomon, H. C. (1950): *Am. J. Psychiatry,* 106(11):889–901.
23. Fyer, A. J., Gorman, J. M., Liebowitz, M. R., Levitt, M., Danielson, E., et al. (1984): *Biol. Psychiatry,* 19(10):1437–1447.
24. Garfield, S., Gershon, S., Sletten, I., Sundland, D. M., and Ballon, S. (1967): *Int. J. Neuropsychiatry,* 3:426–433.
25. Gorman, J. M., Levy, G. F., Liebowitz, M. R., McGrath, P., Appleby, I., et al. (1983): *Arch. Gen. Psychiatry,* 40:1079–1082.
26. Gorman, J. M., Liebowitz, M. R., Fyer, A. J., Dillon, D. J., Davies, S. O., et al. (1983): *Am. J. Psychiatry,* 142(7):864–866.
27. Gorman, J. M., Askanazi, J., Liebowitz, M. R., Fyer, A. J. F., Stein, J., et al. (1984): *Am. J. Psychiatry,* 141(7):857–861.
28. Gorman, J. M., Cohen, B. S., Liebowitz, M. R., Fyer, A. J., Ross, D., et al. (1986): *Arch. Gen. Psychiatry,* 43:1067–1071.
29. Grosz, H. J., and Farmer, B. B. (1972): *Br. J. Psychiatry,* 120:415–418.
30. Grunhaus, L., Gloger, S., Birmacher, B., Palmer, C., and Menashe, B. (1983): *Psychiatr. Res.,* 8:171–177.
31. Guttmacher, L. B., Murphy, D. L., and Insel, T. R. (1983): *Compr. Psychiatry,* 24(4):312–326.
32. Hoehn-Saric, R., Merchant, A. F., Keyser, M. L., and Smith, V. K. (1981): *Arch. Gen. Psychiatry,* 38:1278–1282.
33. Hjorth, S., and Carlsson, A. (1982): *Eur. J. Pharmacol.,* 83:299–303.
34. Holmberg, G., and Gershon, S. (1961): *Psychopharmacology,* 2:93–106.
35. Ingram, C. G. (1962): *Clin. Pharmacol. Ther.,* 3(3):345–352.
36. James, W. (1890): *Principles of Psychology.* Holt & Co., New York.
37. Janowsky, D. S., and Risch, S. C. (1984): *Drug Dev. Res.,* 4:125–142.
38. Kelly, D., Mitchell-Heggs, N., and Shean, D. (1971): *Br. J. Psychiatry,* 119:129–141.
39. Klein, D. F. (1964): *Psychopharmacology,* 5:397–408.
40. Klein, D. F., Rabkin, J., and Gorman, J. M. (1985): In: *Anxiety and Anxiety Disorders,* edited by A. H. Tuma and J. Maser, pp. 501–532. Lawrence Erlbaum, Hillsdale, NJ.
41. Klein, D. F. (1985): Presented at the American College of Neuropsychopharmacology, Hawaii.
42. Ko, G. N., Elsworth, J. D., Roth, R. H., Riffend, B. G., Leigh, H., et al. (1983): *Arch. Gen. Psychiatry,* 40:425–430.
43. Lader, M., and Mathews, A. (1970): *J. Psychosom. Res.,* 14:377–382.
44. Lader, M. (1974): *Int. Pharmacopsychiatry,* 9:126–127.
45. Liebowitz, M. R., Fyer, A. J., McGrath, P., et al. (1981): *Psychopharmacol. Bull.,* 17:122–123.
46. Liebowitz, M. R., Gorman, J. M., and Fyer, A. J. (1984): *Am. J. Psychiatry,* 141(8):995–996.
47. Liebowitz, M. R., Fyer, A. J., Gorman, J. M., Dillon, D., Appleby, I., et al. (1984): *Arch. Gen. Psychiatry,* 41:764–770.
48. Liebowitz, M. R., Gorman, J. M., and Fyer, A. J. (1985): *Am. J. Psychiatry,* 142(8):947–949.
49. Liebowitz, M. R., Gorman, J. M., Fyer, A. J., Levitt, M., Dillon, D., et al. (1986): *Arch. Gen. Psychiatry,* 42:709–719.
50. Lindemann, E., and Finesinger, J. E. (1938): *Am. J. Psychiatry,* 95:353–370.
51. Lindemann, E., and Finesinger, J. E. (1940): *Pscyhosom. Med.,* 2:231–238.
52. Maranon, F. (1924): *Rev. Fr. Endocrinol.,* 2:301.
53. Mason, S. T., and Fibiger, H. C. (1979): *Life Sci.,* 25:2141–2147.
54. McGrath, P. J., Stewart, J. W., Harrison, W., Quitkin, F. M., and Rabkin, J. (1985): *Psychopharm. Bull.,* 21(5): 555–557.
55. Mignot, E., Laude, D., Elghozi, J., LeQuan-Bui, K. H., and Meyer, P. (1982): *Eur. J. Pharmacol.,* 83:135–138.
56. Nemato, E. M., Hoff, J. J., and Sweringhaus, J. W. (1974): *Stroke,* 5:548–553.
57. Nesse, R. M., Cameron, O. G., Crutis, G. C., McCann, D. S., and Haber-Smith, M. J. (1984): *Arch. Gen. Psychiatry,* 41:771–776.
58. Noyes, R., Jr., Anderson, D. J., Clancy, J., Crowe, R. R., Slymen, D., et al. (1984): *Arch. Gen. Psychiatry,* 41:287–292.
59. Nyback, H. V., Walter, J. R., Aghajanian, G. K., and Roth, R. H. (1975): *Eur. J. Pharmacol.,* 32:203–312.
60. Pitts, F. N., and McClure, J. N. (1967): *N. Engl. J. Med.,* 227:1329–1336.
61. Pitts, F. N., and Allen, R. E. (1979): In: *Biochemical Induction of Anxiety,* edited by W. E. Fann, I. Karacan, A. D. Pokorny, R. L. Williams, I. Karacan, and A. D. Pokorny, pp. 125–140. SP Medical & Scientific, New York.
62. Polin, W., and Goldin, S. (1961): *J. Psychiatr. Res.,* 1:50–67.
63. Pyke, R. E., and Greenberg, S. (1986): *J. Clin. Psychopharmacology,* 6(5):279–285.
64. Rainey, J. M., Jr., Pohl, R. B., Williams, M., Knitter, E., Freedman, R. R., et al. (1984): *Psychopathogy,* 17(Suppl. 1):74–82.
65. Rainey, J. M., Jr., and Noose, R. N. (1985): *Psychiatr. Clin. North Am.,* 8(1):133–144.
66. Rall, T. W. (1985): In: *The Pharmacologic Basis of Therapeutics,* edited by A. Gilman, L. Goodman, T. Rall, and A. Murad, pp. 592–608. Macmillan, New York.
67. Redmond, D. E. (1977): In: *Animal Models in Psychiatry and Neurology,* edited by I. Hanin and E. Usdin. Pergamon Press, Oxford, N.Y.
68. Rifkin, A., Klein, D. F., Dillon, D., and Levitt, M. (1981): *Am. J. Psychiatry,* 138:767.
69. Risch, S. C., Kalin, N. D., and Janowsky, D. S. (1981): *J. Clin. Psychopharm.,* 1(4):186–192.
70. Sanghera, M. K., McMillen, B. A., and German, D. C. (1983): *Eur. J. Pharm.,* 86:107–110.
71. Scatton, B., Zivkivic, B., and Dedek, J. (1980): *J. Pharm. Exp. Ther.,* 215:494–499.
72. Schacter, S., and Singer, J. E. (1969): *Psychol. Rev.,* 69:379–399.
73. Schmidt, H. S., and Elizabeth, J. I. (1982): Presented at the 37th Annual Meeting of the Society of Biological Psychiatry. Toronto, Canada.
74. Svensson, T. H., and Usdin, T. (1978): *Science,* 202:1098–1101.
75. Uhde, T. W., Vittone, B., and Post, R. M. (1984): *Am. J. Psychiatry,* 141:1461–1463.
76. Uhde, T. W., Boulenger, J. P., Jimerson, D. C., and Post, R. M. (1984): *Psychopharmacol. Bull.,* 20:426–430.
77. Uhde, T. W., Boulenger, J. P., Vittone, B., et al. (1985): In: *Proceedings of the 7th World Congress of Psychiatry.* Plenum Press, New York.
78. Woods, S. W., Charney, D. S., and Heninger, G. R. (1985): Presented at the Annual Meeting of the American Congress of Neuropsychopharmacology. Honolulu, Hawaii.
79. Woods, S. W., Charney, D. S., Lake, J., Goodman, W. K., Redmond, D. E., and Heninger, D. R. (1986): *Arch. Gen. Psychiatry,* 43(9):900–909.

Psychopharmacology:
The Third Generation of Progress,
edited by Herbert Y. Meltzer.
Raven Press, New York © 1987.

CHAPTER **98**

Introduction: Methodology in Psychopharmacology

John E. Overall

Over the past decade, much of what was previously evolving in the way of assessment and data analysis in clinical psychopharmacology has stabilized on a few instruments and standard ways of analyzing and reporting results. This is not to say that certain new issues have not come to the fore, and those will be mentioned briefly; however, it seems appropriate to mention first the conventions that have developed. These include more precise specification of patient populations from which samples are drawn, a randomized parallel-groups research design with repeated assessments, the use of a relatively few standard assessment instruments, and a uniform strategy for data analysis.

The movement toward use of specific criteria for defining psychiatric diagnoses in clinical research was well underway a decade ago, a trend initiated by the publication of *Diagnostic Criteria for Use in Psychiatric Research* (3). Generally minor modifications of the Feighner criteria produced the Research Diagnostic Criteria (RDC) of Spitzer, Endicott, and Robins (11) and the accompanying Schedule for Affective Disorders and Schizophrenia (SADS), which were developed and field tested in the NIMH Psychobiology of Depression collaborative study (5).

The emphasis on objective criteria for psychiatric diagnosis in research soon spilled over into clinical practice, as Robert Spitzer, M.D., headed up the American Psychiatric Association Task Force on Nomenclature. The revised *Diagnostic and Statistical Manual,* third edition (DSM III) (1), incorporated almost verbatim, but with some liberalization, the RDC criteria for most major psychiatric disorders. The inclusion of specific criteria enhanced the acceptability of clinical diagnosis for the definition of patient populations in clinical research.

In spite of the specified criteria for establishing a psychiatric diagnosis according to DSM III, many investigators have remained concerned about an undocumented statement that subjects in a study have met DSM III criteria for a particular diagnosis. Others have felt that DSM III diagnostic criteria may be adequate for clinical practice, but that in many areas they are overly inclusive. For example, only about two-thirds of outpatients who meet DSM III criteria for major depressive episode satisfy the more restrictive Feighner et al. research criteria. Patients within broad diagnostic categories also may differ greatly in symptom and behavior profiles, and such differences have been found relevant for treatment response.

In consideration of these issues, several different approaches have been used: restrictive research criteria have continued to be used to define patient populations (10), or broader entrance criteria have been used with careful documentation of the characteristics required for stratification of samples according to more restrictive research criteria (7). In other cases, it has been found useful to stratify broader diagnostic classifications along phenomenological or target symptom lines (6,8). Other investigators, who feel that diagnostic criteria alone provide inadequate definitions of patient samples, have emphasized the need to include minimum scores on relevant symptom rating scales among the entrance criteria (9).

During the past decade, almost all controlled clinical trials have employed random assignment of subjects between two or three treatment groups, with baseline and scheduled follow-up assessments at fixed intervals throughout the study. It is safe to say that the three-group design has become most respected in this period. It involves use of both placebo and an active reference drug as controls (e.g., 2).

Depending on the primary interest in a study, the placebo and standard drug comparisons have different purposes. If the purpose is to demonstrate that the new drug is active, it would seem that only a placebo control would be necessary. But what if no difference is found? Could it be that, for any of several reasons, the study simply was not discriminating? The presence of a standard drug with accepted therapeutic value can be a safeguard against writing off an active new drug because of a negative trial. If the standard drug cannot be discriminated from placebo, then it is reasonable to accept that the new drug probably should not be. Studies that attempt to establish equivalence of a new drug to a standard treatment use placebo to confirm that the study is discriminating. If two drugs appear about equal in efficacy, it could be because the study was poorly executed. The ability to discriminate active drug from placebo under double-blind conditions in the same study militates against that explanation.

The strategy for statistical analysis of data from parallel-groups, repeated measures designs in clinical psychopharmacology research has also assumed rather conventional form. Although the parallel-groups design appears suited for a repeated measures (split plot) analysis of variance (ANOVA), few clinical trials are completed without substantial numbers of patients dropping out along the way. Missing data pose a special problem for repeated measures ANOVA. Dropouts represent a problem in any event, and there is currently serious interest in specifying formal requirements for the proportion of study samples that must complete a trial in order for the results to be considered valid. This issue has not been resolved, however, and there are many who feel that dropouts are a realistic indication of the compliance problems in clinical practice (7). A discussion by Gail (4) concerning the distinction between pragmatic clinical trials and scientific experiments is particularly relevant here.

In the meantime, simple analysis of covariance (ANCOV) has become the statistical tool most often relied on to test the significance of difference between treatment effects at each assessment point with baseline scores entered as the covariate. Where a substantial number of dropouts has occurred, the analyses are often repeated with last available observation for dropouts carried forward to subsequent assessment points, as well as on the scores for only those patients who remain in treatment at each point. The analysis of treatment effects at the final assessment period with last available observation for each dropout carried forward, or the so-called endpoint analysis, is the single analysis that has been given most weight in evaluating the outcome of clinical trials during the past decade.

A number of special issues with regard to analysis of data from controlled clinical trials have surfaced during the period under consideration. The interpretation of results in the face of numerous dropouts has, as mentioned, been one of the most controversial. Issues related to multiple tests of significance have also received increasing attention. As described above, the repeated use of ANCOV tests for different time points is common practice; however, that is only a minor part of the problem. Often studies have involved several rating scales, each with multiple items or several composite factor scores. The probability that some portion of the multiple tests will yield apparently significant results by chance alone can be quite high. One cannot appropriately correct p values for multiple tests on different dependent measures in a simple fashion, such as dividing the alpha level by the number of tests, because of the lack of independence among them.

A solution to the multiple test problem that has gained momentum in the past few years has been specification of one or a very few primary dependent variables and the designation of one particular analysis as the critical test of the null hypothesis. The inclusion of too many different outcome measures with consequent multiplicity of significance tests has too often resulted in a checkered pattern of significant and nonsignificant findings. Thus, there has been a notable trend to select a single tried-and-true measure of treatment response and to designate a single analysis, most often the endpoint analysis, as the necessary or critical evaluation of efficacy. Any number of other measures and repeated tests of significance may then be used to explore parameters of the treatment effect, but the decision concerning efficacy depends on a specified "pivotal" analysis.

It is too relevant for the present discussion to refrain from mentioning that at this very point in drafting of this comment, the writer received a call from an industry representative who wanted advice on choosing a single primary dependent variable, from among more than a half dozen, prior to breaking the code for analysis of a study to be included in a New Drug Application (NDA). In the case of his problem, because the study involved large sample sizes, it was recommended that he include *four* of the most relevant measures in a multivariate analysis of variance (MANOVA). Where sample sizes are adequate and there is reason to believe that several variables reliably measure importantly different aspects of the treatment effect, a multivariate analysis is an excellent way to avoid the risks associated with multiple tests of significance.

Reviewing now the issues that are currently under debate as the result of problems recognized over the past decade, the treatment of dropouts looms important. A controversial proposal that has originated within the Food and Drug Administration (FDA) is that treatment comparisons should be considered valid only up to the point at which no more than 30% of the sample has dropped out of any one treatment group. Methods for combining results from multiple independent trials or multiple study sites are receiving increased attention. How to weigh a few positive studies that are embedded in a background of nonsignificant results is at issue. Methodology is being considered for adjusting final p values where interim analyses of partial results have been undertaken. The search for new and more reliable assessment instruments continues in spite of the pressure to specify in advance the critical response variable for each clinical trial. This raises the paramount issue of how to maintain flexibility that is conducive to the development of improved methodology in the face of an increasing emphasis on conventional approaches. In spite of increasing standardization, numerous recurrent problems in the design and analysis of data from clinical trials persist. These are some of the topics of concern to authors of this section on research methodology.

REFERENCES

1. American Psychiatric Association (1980): *Diagnostic and Statistical Manual*, 3rd ed. American Psychiatric Association, Washington, DC.
2. Feighner, J. P., Aden, G. C., Fabre, L. F., Rickels, K., and Smith, W. T. (1983): *JAMA*, 249:3057–3064.
3. Feighner, J. P., Robins, E., Guze, S. B., Woodruff, R. A., Winokur, G., and Munoz, R. (1972): *Arch. Gen. Psychiatry*, 26:57–63.
4. Gail, M. H. (1985): *Cancer Treat. Rep.*, 69:1107–1113.
5. Maas, J. W., Koslow, S. H., Davis, J. M., Katz, M. M., Mendels, J., Robins, E., Stokes, P. E., and Bowden, C. L. (1980): *Psychol. Med.*, 10:759–776.
6. Overall, J. E. (1984): *J. Clin. Psychiatry*, 45:85–88.
7. Overall, J. E., Donachie, N. D., and Faillace, L. A. (1987): *J. Clin. Psychiatry*, 48:51–54.
8. Overall, J. E., and Hollister, L. E. (1985): In: *Assessment of Depression*, edited by N. Sartorius and T. A. Ban. Springer-Verlag, Heidelberg.
9. Rickles, K. (1985): In: *Principles and Techniques of Human Research and Therapeutics*, edited by F. G. McMahon. Futura Publishing Company, Mount Kisco, NY.
10. Rush, A. J., Erman, M. K., Schlesser, M. A., Roffwurg, H. P., Vasavada, N., Khatami, M., Fairchild, C., and Giles, D. E. (1985): *Arch. Gen. Psychiatry*, 42:1154–1159.
11. Spitzer, R. L., Endicott, J., and Robins, E. (1978): *Arch. Gen. Psychiatry*, 35:773–782.

Psychopharmacology:
The Third Generation of Progress,
edited by Herbert Y. Meltzer.
Raven Press, New York © 1987.

CHAPTER **99**

Assessment Methods in Clinical Trials

Jerome Levine and Thomas A. Ban

Despite the explosion of knowledge and new technology during the past 10 years in the field of neuroscience, the use of clinical assessment procedures and the controlled clinical trial remains the sole final common pathway to testing (proving) the efficacy and safety of proposed therapeutic agents prior to their marketing and acceptance by the medical and scientific community. Although the rate of change in knowledge and technology about clinical assessment procedures has not paralleled that of the neurosciences, nevertheless significant changes have occurred that are now being implemented throughout the drug assessment community (academic, industrial, government, and regulatory sectors). Some of these changes relate to the design of clinical trials, to the conduct of the trials, to the documentation and analysis of the data, and to the actual data and manner in which it is being collected. This chapter will first deal with some of these changes in a non-disorder-specific fashion and then the latter part of the chapter will cover assessment instruments for anxiety, depression, and schizophrenic disorders as well as for dementia.

DESIGN ISSUES

Although the basic methodology for the design of clinical trials has not changed remarkably over the past decade, the creation of a new professional *Society for Clinical Trials* (85) and associated journal (73) and the publication of a number of textbooks (7,30,74,80,94,96,102) oriented toward the practical application of statistical principles in controlled clinical trials has done much to raise the acceptable scientific standard for such trials. A rating form useful in judging the quality of psychopharmacology clinical trials in a

systematic way (TAPS) was also developed during this period (62,94).

Unfortunately, much of the productivity has not been specific to the area of clinical trials in psychiatric disorders or psychopharmacology but rather has been general, with investigators in the areas of cardiovascular and oncologic disorders predominant. A concept that may help to "bridge" the medical and psychiatric disorders clinical trials groups is the "assessment of quality of life." Instead of looking at survival as the sole outcome endpoint, investigators in cancer and cardiovascular (110) diseases are now interested in assessing psychological functioning (mood, cognition, etc.), social and work performance, and distress caused by side effects of the treatment as other indicators of treatment utility. These outcome variables have traditionally been those used in psychiatric clinical trials.

Among the newer clinical trial texts, *Methodology of Clinical Drug Trials* by Spriet and Simon, originally written in French and recently translated into English by Edelstein and Weintraub (97), appears to be most useful for psychopharmacology investigators. A second book, also translated into English from French, *Clinical Trials* by Schwartz, Flamant, and Lellouch (91), deals extensively with a conceptual issue that is becoming increasingly important in both the design of trials and analysis of data from them. This is the concept of the "explanatory" versus "pragmatic" or management (86) trials. In the words of Schwartz et al.:

A comparative trial may be undertaken with more than one aim in view. One type of objective is both simple and well known—it is required to ascertain whether the new treatment actually possesses the favorable activity in man which laboratory studies have led us to expect. . . . In this case, the clinical trial is a direct extension of laboratory experimentation and is motivated by the same research-oriented attitude.

The other type of objective is often overlooked by scientists and is less well understood. We now wish to assess the practical value of a new treatment. . . . The trial is aimed at providing practising clinicians with a basis for decisions concerning the choice of therapy and its motivation is strictly practical in nature. . . . We shall refer to the two approaches we have outlined as "explanatory" and "pragmatic"; both approaches involve the type of comparative clinical trials which forms the main subject of this book, but the differences between them call for parallel differences in the methods adopted.

The consequences of the above statement are profound with regard to design features (e.g., homogeneous or heterogeneous sample) and analysis strategies (e.g., intent to treat or evaluable patients only) for any comparative trial. Further, at present, it appears that pragmatic or management trials are the ones considered pivotal or definitive when New Drug Applications (NDAs) are reviewed in applications for marketing a new drug in the United States. It is possible that with the further development, elucidation, and discussion of these concepts the philosophical basis of what constitutes substantial evidence and/or proof of efficacy may change.

IMPACT OF MICROCOMPUTERS

During this 10-year period (and currently) the single most important factor that has influenced the manner in which clinical trials are conducted is the introduction and widespread availability and use of the microcomputer (personal computer). This versatile tool can be used in all phases of clinical trialistics: word processing in the development of the protocol; data entry (either by patient, rater, data coordinator, data entry clerk, or directly by a laboratory instrument); and data management using a relational data base management system (which is also used in preparing data for analysis and graphic display). Descriptive and inferential statistical analysis can also be obtained from microcomputers using either specially written programs or packages of programs that were previously only available on mainframes or minicomputers such as SAS, BMDP, and SPSS. The microcomputer also has a powerful role in information dissemination (literature searches using, e.g., Medline, International Pharmaceutical Abstracts, etc.), communication with electronic mail, specialized bulletin boards, electronic on-line conferencing (e.g., PsyComNet), and actual data sharing and data transfer.

The relatively low cost of microcomputers and the development of user friendly software systems has enabled many clinical researchers to become "end users" and to carry out their own computing work directly without having to go through large data processing offices or having access to expensive mainframe computers. Because of the large number of end users it is now becoming economically feasible to develop very substantively specific software systems that can integrate a number of tasks needed by a particular field. The earliest versions of such systems were those that integrated word processing, spread sheets, data base management, and communication programs for business office applications (e.g., Framework, Symphony, etc.). In the clinical trial area a system (49) that integrates (a) data collection and data input from case report forms, (b) editing capacity, (c) file building for data selection and display (graphics), (d) statistical analysis, (e) randomization procedures, (f) a scheduler and trial management functions, and (g) an audit trial for single and multicenter (remote data entry) trials is available and actually being used as part of a large multicenter study being carried out by the National Institute of Mental Health (106). The increasing use of microcomputers and user friendly, integrated, substantively specific software systems will create a new *de facto* standard for the conduct of clinical trials within the next decade. The monitoring of clinical trials by sponsors of those trials (especially the pharmaceutical industry) has markedly increased in both quality and quantity in recent years. The kind of "quality control" that can be achieved by the combined use of on-site monitoring and microcomputer trial management support should further improve the quality of data collected in the future. It is anticipated that other technologies such as artificial intelligence (21) and, especially, so-called expert systems and decision analysis programs will be introduced and will facilitate the design, conduct, and analysis of clinical trials.

ASSESSMENT TECHNIQUE

In the clinical assessment area a distinct trend has appeared toward a more standardized way of *ascertaining* or obtaining data rather than just utilizing a uniform *recording* format. The antecedents of this trend were probably in the development of the Research Diagnostic Criteria (RDC) and the operationally defined DSM III criteria for diagnosing psychiatric disorders. Rating devices needed to be developed to capture the clinical information to tell if the criteria had been met (documented diagnosis) and whether a diagnosis could be "justified." The Diagnostic Interview Schedule (DIS) and more recently the Structured Clinical Interview for DSM III Diagnosis (SCID) have virtually provided "scripts" for how information is to be ascertained as well as recorded. The application of this type of technique in the assessment of psychopathology to establish efficacy (outcome) in clinical trials is anticipated. In an unrelated area, namely safety or side effect assessment, a completely independent development effort also resulted in an instrument (rating device) that employs a standardized or structured clinical interview organized in the way physicians conduct a "review of systems" (see below).

SIDE EFFECT ASSESSMENT

Progress in developing methods for the clinical assessment of pharmacologic treatments does not proceed at an even pace and recently little attention had been given to side effect compared to efficacy assessment. Levine and Schooler (63,64) developed and reported on a new assessment instrument named SAFTEE (Systematic Assessment for

Treatment Emergent Events) which seeks to remedy several of the shortcomings of previous instruments. Two forms of SAFTEE, General Inquiry (GI) and Systematic Inquiry (SI), are available, both of which incorporate the following features:

1. Use of a standardized inquiry procedure to elicit reports of adverse health events from patients (to reduce reporting variability).

2. Recording reports of all adverse health events, not only those suspected or prejudged to be drug related (to reduce underreporting of unanticipated events).

3. Use of a set of preferred event terms for recording (to reduce errors involved in postcoding and categorizing events).

4. Collection of comprehensive information about the onset, duration, pattern, severity, and attribution of cause in a precoded format for every reported adverse health event (to aid in interpreting the importance and significance of the event).

5. Specification of a precise time interval for the period for which adverse health events are inquired about (to better establish baseline and accurate incidence/prevalence rates).

The GI form is a subset of the inquiries of the SI, and does not include inquiries about individual body systems (e.g., Have you noticed any problems with your eyes or vision, things like swelling or irritation, blurring, double vision, poor vision, or light bothering you?) but includes general health inquiries (e.g., Have you had any physical or health problems during the past week?, etc.). Preliminary data coming from ongoing validity and reliability studies (61) indicate that using an SI technique gives rise to a greater frequency of reported adverse health events and elicits reporting of some types of events (e.g., sleep disturbance) that are rarely elicited with a GI technique. The SI: GI ratio of adverse events varies widely with the kind of event being reported. In the only study (68) so far presented comparing a group of drug-treated patients (phenelzine) to a similar group of placebo-treated patients, SAFTEE-SI treatment emergent event rates were higher for 20 of the 25 potential monoamine oxidase (MAO) side effects in the drug treated group. Thus preliminary results indicate that the SAFTEE-SI technique is likely to be a sensitive and valid approach for assessing side effects. A computer-based data entry program (15) has been developed that facilitates data display and data analysis with SAFTEE.

DOCUMENTATION AND ANALYSIS

Little systematic progress has been reported in the area of documentation and presentation of data from clinical trials over the past 10 years. However, in January 1986 the Food and Drug Administration made available a "Draft Guideline for the Format and Content of the Clinical Data Section of an Application" (107). This document, which is expected to be issued in final form by the end of 1986, gives the most explicit guidance to date on the format of clinical data presentation for an individual controlled clinical

trial issued by a regulatory agency. The document also gives guidance on the presentation of an "integrated summary" of safety information and effectiveness data covering multiple independent studies reported in a NDA. Although the document is not specific with regard to different therapeutic classes of agents, the approaches recommended are not inconsistent with the principles previously described for clinical trials in psychopharmacology (59,60,69). Various levels of specificity extending from detailed tabulations (actual observations as recorded on case report forms), through descriptive statistics (e.g., group means and standard deviations), and extending to inference testing are requested to provide a comprehensive documentation package. Whereas for some therapeutic classes of drugs the use of this type of documentation has been infrequent or unknown, the use of computer-based clinical trial data documentation systems such as BLIPS (39) has been both long-standing (40) and current (11,12) in psychopharmacologic trials.

RATING SCALES FOR THE ASSESSMENT OF PSYCHIATRIC DISORDER AND PSYCHOPATHOLOGY

The remainder of this chapter will be focused on the various devices that are primarily used to assess psychopathology or change in pathology especially during a pharmacologic intervention trial. Whereas greater progress has been seen in some areas (anxiety, pediatrics, and geriatrics) than others, this past decade has not seen the rapid expansion that was experienced in the sixties nor the cataloging and consolidation characteristic of the seventies (36). Notable, first, in the pediatric area was publication of an updated battery (105) for use with this population, and second, publication of two books specifically dealing with assessment issues in geriatric populations (19,81).

General Purpose Scales

General purpose scales are designed for the assessment of change in different psychiatric disorders and for the monitoring of change in the course of treatment.

Assessment of Change

One of the best internationally known general purpose scales is the Wittenborn Psychiatric Rating Scale (112,113). This historically important scale is translated into several languages, e.g., Czechoslovakian, French, German, Italian, Japanese, Korean, Portuguese, Swedish.

Another historically important, and currently probably more frequently used general purpose scale, also translated into several languages (e.g., Czechoslovakian, Dutch, French, German, Italian, Japanese, Russian, Spanish), is the Brief Psychiatric Rating Scale of Overall and Gorham (76). Originally designed for the assessment of change in schizophrenic patients, empirical cluster analysis revealed distinct BPRS profiles ("phenomenological types") in depressed psychiatric patients.

Monitoring Changes

There are two assessment instruments extensively used in Europe for monitoring psychopathological changes in the course of treatment: the AMDP-III and the CPRS.

AMDP stands for Association for Methodology and Documentation in Psychiatry (1,37). The third version of the system is the result of many years of methodological work in the course of which unreliable items were excluded. By employing factor analysis on the 100 psychopathological symptoms and 40 somatic signs (items) of the system, eight first-order and three second-order factors were identified. In the construction of subscales to be employed in specific diagnostic populations, the second-order factors were employed because the structure of the first-order factors was not independent of the populations studied. These second-order factors showed a stable structure during 20 days of treatment and were closely correlated to other valid and reliable scales (114).

CPRS stands for Comprehensive Psychopathological Rating Scale (2), a scale developed by a working group in collaboration with the Swedish Medical Research Council. It was constructed explicitly for the measurement of change in psychopathology with careful consideration to comprehensiveness in terms of covering a wide range of psychiatric disorders.

Rating Scales for Anxiety Disorders

For some time the measurement of anxiety was almost exclusively based on the Minnesota Multiphasic Personality Inventory (MMPI) (44) and a number of different anxiety measures derived from this scale (25). Among them probably the most extensively employed was the Taylor Scale of Manifest Anxiety (101), consisting of 50 MMPI items (chosen by agreement of raters on the basis of the content of the items), followed by the Welsh Anxiety Scale (109) and the Finney Anxiety Scales (24). Other scales employed in clinical studies were the Objective-Analytic Anxiety Battery developed at the Institute of Personality and Ability Testing by Cattell and Scheier (13) and the State-Trait Anxiety Inventory (STAI) developed by Spielberger, Gorsuch, and Lushene (93). It was Cattell and Scheier (14) who first separated "state anxiety" from "trait anxiety"; and it was in the STAI in which separate measures were given for these two aspects of anxiety. Nevertheless, measures of these two aspects of anxiety are often correlated, and it is unlikely that pure measures of "state" and "trait" anxiety can be constructed (104).

The scales reviewed are based on a unidimensional view of anxiety. Because of the recognition that there is discontinuity between normal and pathological anxiety, they are gradually being replaced by observer-rated instruments and self-reports, designed primarily to quantify levels of pathology in patients with diagnostically different anxiety disorders (103).

The most frequently employed observer-rated instruments in clinical psychopharmacological research include the Hamilton Anxiety Scale (42), the Brief Outpatient Psychopathology (29), the Physicians Questionnaire (83), and the Covi Anxiety Scale (65); and the most frequently employed self-reports include the Profile of Mood States (71), the General Health Questionnaire (34), and the Hopkins Symptom Checklist or HSCL-90 (66). Other frequently employed instruments are the Anxiety States Inventory, an observer-rated instrument, and its counterpart, the Self-Rating Anxiety Scale (117).

To answer the question whether observer-rated instruments or self-reports offer advantages in the assessment of change to psychotropic drugs, Glass, Uhlenhuth, and Kellner (33) examined a substantial number of studies in which both the Hamilton Anxiety Scale (HAS) and the Hopkins Symptom Checklist (HSCL) were employed. They found that in an overwhelming majority of studies the HAS was more sensitive than the HSCL in discriminating benzodiazepine-treated from placebo-treated patients. Further analysis of the data, however, revealed that the HSCL was about as sensitive as the HAS in discriminating drug-treated from placebo-treated patients in studies where patients in the two treatment groups reported sedation with about equal frequency.

Separation into a number of distinct illnesses within the category of anxiety disorders resulted in the construction of new scales with greater specificity for the different conditions. Included among these instruments are the three Sheehan Scales, i.e., the Sheehan Clinician Rated Anxiety Scale, the Panic and Anxiety Attack Scale, and the Marks-Sheehan Phobia Scale (92).

Rating Scales for Depressions

In a recent publication (88) the most widely used instruments for assessing depression in the different language areas and age groups were reviewed. Among the most frequently employed rating scales for the assessment of change in depressed patients are the Hamilton Rating Scale for Depression (43), the Newcastle Scale (8), the Beck Depression Inventory (4), and the Zung-Self-Rating Scale for Depression (116). The first two are completed on the basis of a clinical interview, and the latter two on the basis of self-assessment. Other frequently used scales include Kellner's Brief Depression Rating Scale (50) and Carroll's Rating Scale for Depression (9).

The most frequently employed depression scales have been translated and adapted into several languages from the original English. There are, however, a number of specially devised depression scales that are used primarily outside the English language area.

Standardized assessment instruments for depression in German include the Hamburger Depression Scale (52), the Erlanger Depression Scale (58), and the Multidimensional Mood Questionnaire (45). Among them probably the most extensively studied is the Hamburger Depression Scale, a 50-item self-rating instrument. Test-retest reliability of this scale ranges from 0.86 to 0.87, with split-half reliability of 0.90 to 0.92. Correlation with other depression scales and clinical judgments ranges from 0.72 to 0.83.

The number of depression rating scales used in French-speaking countries is steadily increasing. Some of them, e.g., the Beck-Pichot Depression Inventory, are adaptations of foreign scales (78), whereas others such as Widlocher's (111) Retardation Scale are original French assessment instruments. This carefully constructed scale is valid for the measurement of depressive retardation and sensitive for the measurement of change to treatment.

Most of the important scales used in the different language areas in the assessment of depression have been translated, standardized, and validated in Spanish by Conde and Franch (16). The one original Spanish scale, the "Test Miokinetico" of Mira Lopez (75), is useful for the evaluation of agressivity in affective disorders.

There are only a few scales for the assessment of depression in the Slavic language area. Among them the best known is the FKD, constructed by Vinar (108) in the mid-1960s. FKD stands for "quantification of depressive symptomatology for the measurement of pharmacotherapeutic effects," and the scale has been extensively employed in clinical investigations with antidepressants in Czechoslovakia. It was developed with consideration to Hamilton's depression scale and to the scale developed by Bojanovsky and Chloupkova (6) in Czechoslovakia. Other rating scales in the Slavic language areas include the scales developed by Tasher et al. (100) in Bulgaria.

There are at least two original Scandinavian depression scales, i.e., the Cronholm-Ottosson Rating Scale developed in Sweden (18) and the Bech-Rafaelsen Melancholia Scale developed in Denmark (3); and at least four original Italian depression scales, i.e., the Scale for Anxious-Depressive Symptomatology (31), the Self-Rating Scale for Depression (10), the Rome Depression Inventory (77), and the Observer-Rating Scales for the Assessment of Depression (20).

In Japan the CPRG Rating Scales of Depression are the most frequently employed (99). CPRG stands for Clinical Psychopharmacology Research Group, and the CPRG rating scales consist of three independent scales, one for use by the doctor, another by the patient, and the third by the nurse or a family member.

Assessment instruments for depression in children and adolescents were recently reviewed by Strober and Werry (98). Included among the structured interview measures are the Bellevue Index of Depression (53) and the Children's Affective Rating Scale (70); and among the self-report inventories, the Children's Depression Inventory (53), the Children's Depression Scale (56), and the Depressive Self-Rating Scale (5). Prototype of the naturalistic measures is the Peer Nomination Inventory of Depression, developed by Lefkowitz and Tesing (57).

Assessment instruments for depression in psychogeriatric patients were recently reviewed by Hovaguimian (48). Included among the scales is the Geriatric Depression Scale of Yesavage et al. (115), which includes 30 dichotomous items derived from a selection of 100 questions, and the Schwab Depression Scale, which is derived from a structured interview used in a study of mental health and aging (90). A shortened version, consisting of 10 items, was validated in a comparative study, in which the scale was found to differentiate between elderly depressives and age-matched controls. In the same study it was also shown that the scale was sensitive in depicting changes in the severity of depression from admission to discharge (32).

Rating Scales for Schizophrenias

The most frequently employed instruments in the assessment of drug-induced changes in schizophrenic patients are the ones included in the original ECDEU assessment battery (36), i.e., the Brief Psychiatric Rating Scale (BPRS) of Overall and Gorham (76) and the Nurses Observation Scale for Inpatient Evaluation of Honigfeld and Klett (47). Recently the Fischer Symptoms Checklist Neuroleptics (FSCL-NL) has been employed in some multicenter collaborative studies in Europe (26). There are indications, however, that neither the BPRS nor the FSCL-NL is an optimal instrument for the assessment of change insofar as the chronic schizophrenic population is concerned. Because of this there is a revival of interest in some of the more elaborate scales, such as the Inpatient Multidimensional Psychiatric Rating Scale of Lorr (67) and the Psychopathological Symptom Form of the AMDP-III, which consists of 100 items scored on a four-point scale (37).

Rating Scales for the Dementias

Assessment of Diagnosis

One of the frequently employed diagnostic scales for this population is the Geriatric Mental State Inventory (GMSI) developed by Copeland et al. (17) from the Mental Status Schedule of Spitzer, Fleiss, and Burdock (95). It has been shown that the GMSI can discriminate organic psychiatric syndromes from functional psychiatric disorders (27).

More specific than the GMSI are assessment instruments such as the ones specially devised by Hachinsky et al. (41) and Gustafson and Nilsson (35) for the separation of multiinfarct from primary degenerative dementia, and Alzheimer's disease from Pick's disease, respectively.

Assessment of Change

An early review of rating scales with particular usefulness in geriatric psychopharmacology was published by Salzman, Kochansky, and Shader (87). More recently Honigfeld (46) reviewed rating scales especially suitable for the assessment of "ward behavior" in psychogeriatric patients.

Frequently employed instruments in the assessment of the severity of dementia include the Mini Mental Status (28), the Brief Cognitive Rating Scale, and the Global Deterioration Scale (82); and frequently employed instruments in the assessment of institutional adjustment include the Stockton Geriatric Scale (72), the Plutchik Geriatric Rating Scale (79), the Parkside Behavior Rating Scale (22), and the Crichton Behavioral Rating Scale (84). Probably the most extensively employed assessment instrument in clinical psychopharmacological studies in psychogeriatric patients is the Sandoz Clinical Assessment Geriatric, usually referred to as the SCAG (89).

Recently the AGP System, a Manual for the Documentation of Psychopathology in Gerontopsychiatry, was published in English (38). AGP stands for Arbeitsgemeinschaft für Gerontopsychiatrie, or Association for Gerontopsychiatry, and the documentation system extends from demographic data and psychiatric history, through psychopathological symptoms and somatic signs to diagnoses.

REFERENCES

1. Angst, J., Battegay, R., Bente, D., Berner, P., Boren, W., Cornu, F., Dick, P., Englemeier, M.-P., Heimann, H., Heinrich, K., Helmchen, H., Hippius, H., Poldinger, W., Schmidlin, P., Schmitt, W., and Weiss, P. (1969): *Arzneimittelforschung,* 19:339–405.
2. Asberg, M., Perris, C., Schalling, D., and Sedvall, G. (1978): *Acta Psychiatr. Scand. (Suppl.* 271).
3. Bech, P., and Rafaelsen, O. J. (1980): *Acta Psychiatr. Scand.,* 62 (*Suppl.* 285).
4. Beck, A. T., Ward, C. H., Mendelson, J., Mock, J., and Erbaugh, J. (1968): *Arch. Gen. Psychiatry,* 4:561–571.
5. Birleson, P. (1981): *J. Child Psychol. Psychiatry,* 1:73–88.
6. Bojanowsky, J., and Chloupkova, K. (1966): *Psychiatr. Neurol.,* 151:54–61.
7. Bulpitt, C. J. (1983): *Randomised Controlled Clinical Trials.* Martinus Nijhoff Publishers, The Hague.
8. Carney, M. W. P., Roth, M., and Garside, R. F. (1965): *Br. J. Psychiatry,* 111:659–674.
9. Carroll, B. J., Feinberg, M., Smouse, P. E., Rawson, S. G., and Greden, J. F. (1981): *Br. J. Psychiatry,* 138:194–200.
10. Cassano, G. B., Castrogiovanni, P., and Rampello, E. (1986): In: *Assessment of Depression,* edited by N. Sartorius and T. A. Ban, pp. 46–54. Springer, Berlin, Heidelberg, New York.
11. Cassano, G. B., Conti, L., Massimetti, G., Fornaro, P., and Levine, J. (1982): *Pharmacopsychiatry,* 15:84–89.
12. Cassano, G. B., Conti, L., Massimetti, G., Mengali, F., Waekelin, J. S., and Levine, J. (1986): *Psychopharmacol. Bull.,* 22:52–58.
13. Cattell, R. B., and Scheier, J. H. (1960): *Handbook for the Objective-Analytic Anxiety Battery.* IPAT, Champaign, IL.
14. Cattell, R. B., and Scheier, J. H. (1961): *The Meaning and Measurement of Neuroticism and Anxiety.* Ronald Press, New York.
15. Clyde, D. J. (1986): *Psychopharmacol. Bull.,* 22:287.
16. Conde, V., and Franch, J. I. (1984): *Escalas de evaluacion comportamental para la cuantificacion de la sintomatologia psicopathologica en los trastornos angustinosos y depressivos.* Upjohn Farmaquimica, Madrid.
17. Copeland, J., Kelleher, M., Duckworth, G., and Smith, A. (1976): *Int. J. Aging Hum. Dev.,* 7:313–322.
18. Cronholm, B., and Ottosson, J. O. (1960): In: *Experimental Studies of the Mode of Action of Electroconvulsive Therapy,* edited by J. Ottosson. *Acta Psychiatr. Neurol. Scand.* 35 (*Suppl.* 145).
19. Crook, T., Ferris, S., and Bartus, R., eds. (1983): *Assessment in Geriatric Psychopharmacology.* Mark Powley Associates, New Canaan, CT.
20. Faravelli, C., Poli, E., Rosati, E., Paoli, M., and Ambronetti, A. (1982): *Riv. Psichitr.,* 17:101–105.
21. Feinberg, M. (1986): *Psychopharmacol. Bull.,* 22:311–316.
22. Fine, E. W., Lewis, D., Villa-Landa, I., and Blakemore, C. B. (1970): *Br. J. Psychiatry,* 117:157–161.
23. Fink, M., Green, A., and Bender, M. B. (1952): *Neurology,* 2: 48–56.
24. Finney, J. C. C. (1965): *Psychol. Rep.,* 17:707–713.
25. Finney, J. (1985): In: *Anxiety and the Anxiety Disorders,* edited by A. H. Tuma and J. Maser. Lawrence Erlbaum Associates, Hillsdale, NJ.
26. Fischer-Cornelssen, J. A. (1981): In: *Collegium Internationale Psychiatrie Scalarum.* Beltz Publ., Weinheim.
27. Fleiss, Y., Gurland, B., and Des Roche, P. (1976): *Int. J. Aging Hum. Dev.,* 7:323–330.
28. Folstein, M. F., Folstein, S. E., and McHugh, P. R. (1975): *J. Psychiatr. Res.,* 12:189–198.
29. Free, S. M., and Guthrie, M. B. (1969): *J. Clin. Pharmacol.,* 9: 187–194.
30. Friedman, L. M., Furberg, C. D., and DeMets, D. L. (1985): *Fundamentals of Clinical Trials.* PSG Publishing Co., Littleton, MA.
31. Gainotti, G., and Ciancheetti, C. (1968): *Riv. Patol. Nerv. Ment.,* 89:442–443.
32. Gilleard, C. J., Willmott, M., and Vaddadi, K. S. (1981): *Br. J. Psychiatry,* 138:230–235.
33. Glass, R., Uhlenhuth, E. H., and Kellner, R. (1982): Presented at Research Conference on Anxiety Disorders, Panic Attacks, and Phobias, Key Biscayne, Florida.
34. Goldberg, D. P., and Hillier, V. F. (1979): *Psychol. Med.,* 9:139–145.
35. Gustafson, L., and Nilsson, L. (1982): *Acta Psychiatr. Scand.,* 65:194–209.
36. Guy, W. (1976): *ECDEU Assessment Manual for Psychopharmacology.* DHEW Publication No. (ADM) 76-338. U.S. Department of Health, Education, and Welfare, Washington, DC.
37. Guy, W., and Ban, T. A. (1982): *The AMDP System. Manual for the Assessment and Documentation of Psychopathology.* Springer, Heidelberg.
38. Guy, W., and Ban, T. A. (1985): *The AGP System.* Springer, Heidelberg.
39. Guy, W., Bonato, R. R., Cleary, P., Yang, J., and Levine, J. (1970): *Arch. Gen. Psychiatr.,* 23:454–463.
40. Guy, W., and Cleary, P. A. (1974): In: *Psychopharmacological Agents,* edited by F. G. McMahon, pp. 53–62. Futura Publishing Company, New York.
41. Hachinsky, V. C., Iliff, L., Duboulay, G. H., et al. (1975): *Arch. Neurol.,* 32:632–637.
42. Hamilton, M. (1959): *Br. J. Med. Psychology,* 32:50–55.
43. Hamilton, M. (1960): *J. Neurol. Neurosurg. Psychiatry,* 23:56–62.
44. Hathaway, S. R., and McKinley, J. C. (1942): *The Minnesota Multiphasic Personality Inventory.* University of Minnesota Press, Minneapolis.
45. Hecheltjen, G., and Mertesdorf, F. (1973): *Gruppendynamik,* 2: 110–122.
46. Honigfeld, G. H. (1981): *Psychopharm. Bull.,* 17(4):82–95.
47. Honigfeld, G., and Klett, J. C. (1965): *J. Clin. Psychol.,* 21:65–71.
48. Hovaguimian, T. (1986): In: *Assessment of Depression,* edited by N. Sartorius, and T. A. Bann. Springer, Berlin, Heidelberg, New York.
49. International Medical Products Corporation (1986): *Clinical Research System Reference Manual.* Minneapolis.
50. Kellner, R. (1986): In: *Assessment of Depression,* edited by N. Sartorius, and T. A. Ban. Springer, Berlin, Heidelberg, New York.
51. Kendric, D. C., Gibson, A. J., and Moyers, I. C. (1979): *Brit. J. Soc. and Clin. Psychol.,* 18:240–329.
52. Kerekjarto, M. (1969): In: *Das depressive Syndrom,* edited by H. Hippius and H. Selbach. Urban and Schwarzenberg, Munich.
53. Kovacs, M., and Beck, A. T. (1977): In: *Depression in Childhood: Diagnosis, Treatment and Conceptual Models,* edited by J. G. Schultebrandt and A. Raskin. Raven Press, New York.
54. Kudo, Y. (1974): *Jpn. Med. J.,* 26:28–34.
55. Kurihara, M. (1975): *Clin. Eval.,* 3:3–17.
56. Lang, M., and Tisher, M. (1978): *The Children's Depression Scale.* The Amsterdam Council for Educational Research, Victoria.
57. Lefkowitz, M. M., and Tesing, E. P. (1980): *J. Consult. Clin. Psychol.,* 48:43–50.
58. Lehrl, S., Straub, R., and Straub, B. (1976): *Pharmakopsychiatria,* 9:247–256.
59. Levine, J. (1978): In: *Psychopharmacology: A Generation of Progress,* edited by M. A. Lipton, A. DiMascio, and K. F. Killiam, pp. 827–831. Raven Press, New York.
60. Levine, J., ed. (1979): *Coordinating Clinical Trials in Psychopharmacology: Planning, Documentation, and Analysis.* DHEW Publication No. (ADM) 79-803. U.S. Government Printing Office, Washington, DC.
61. Levine, J., Jacobson, A., Rabkin, J., and Summerfelt, A. (1986): *Controlled Clin. Trials,* 7(3):231.
62. Levine, J., and Samet, M. (1980): *Controlled Clin. Trials,* 1:177.
63. Levine, J., and Schooler, N. R. (1986): *Psychopharmacol. Bull.,* 22(2):343–381.

64. Levine, J., Schooler, N. R., and Moynihan, C. (1983): *Controlled Clin. Trials,* 4:157.
65. Lipman, R. S. (1982): *Psychopharmacol. Bull.,* 18:69–77.
66. Lipman, R. S., Covi, L., and Shapiro, A. K. (1979): *J. Affective Disord.,* 1:9–24.
67. Lorr, M., Klett, C. J., McNair, C. M., and Lasky, J. J. (1963): *Inpatient Multidimensional Psychiatric Scale.* Consulting Psychologist Press, Palo Alto.
68. Markowitz, J. S., Rabkin, J. B., Stewart, L., Quitkin, F. M., McGrath, P. J., Harrison, W., and Ocepek-Welikson, K. (1987): *Psychopharmacol. Bull.,* 23 (*in press*).
69. McGlashan, T., ed. (1973): *Documentation of Clinical Psychotropic Drug Trials.* DHEW Publication No. (HSM) 73-9038. Rockville, MD.
70. McKnew, D. J., Jr., Cytryn, L., Efron, A. M., Gershon, E. S., and Bunney, W. E. (1979): *Br. J. Psychiatry,* 134:148–152.
71. McNair, D. M., Lorr, M., and Droppleman, L. F. (1971): *Manual: Profile of Mood States.* Educational and Industrial Testing Services, San Diego.
72. Meer, B., and Baker, J. A. (1966): *J. Gerontol.,* 21:393–403.
73. Meinert, C. L., ed. (1980): *Controlled Clinical Trials.* Elsevier/North-Holland, New York.
74. Meinert, C. L. (1986): *Clinical Trials.* Oxford University Press, New York.
75. Mira Lopez, E. (1982): *Psicodiagnostica miokinetico.* Paidos, Buenos Aires.
76. Overall, J. E., and Gorham, D. R. (1962): *Psychol. Rep.,* 10:799–812.
77. Pancheri, P., and Carilli, L. (1982): *Riv. Psychiatr.,* 17:22–23.
78. Pichot, P., Piret, J., and Clyde, D. J. (1966): *Rev. Psychol. Appl.,* 16:105–115.
79. Plutchik, R., and Conte, H. (1970): *J. Am. Geriatr. Soc.,* 18:491–500.
80. Pocock, S. J. (1983): *Clinical Trials.* John Wiley & Sons, New York.
81. Raskin, A., and Jarvik, L. S. (1979): *Psychiatric Symptoms and Cognitive Loss in the Elderly.* John Wiley & Sons, New York.
82. Reisberg, B., Schneck, M. K., Ferris, S. H., et al. (1983): *Psychopharmacol. Bull.,* 19:47–50.
83. Rickels, K., and Howard, K. (1970): *Psychopharmacologia,* 17:338–344.
84. Robinson, R. A. (1961): *Gerontol. Clin.,* 3:247–257.
85. Roth, H. P. (1980): *Controlled Clin. Trials,* 1:81–82.
86. Sackett, B. L., and Gent, M. (1979): *N. Engl. J. Med.,* 301:1410–1412.
87. Salzman, C., Kochansky, J. E., and Shader, R. I. (1972): *Psychopharmacol. Bull.,* 8:3–50.
88. Sartorius, N., and Ban, T. A., eds. (1986): *Assessment of Depression.* Springer-Verlag, Berlin, New York.
89. Shader, R., Harmotz, J., and Salzman, C. (1974): *J. Am. Geriatr. Soc.,* 22:107–113.
90. Schwab, J. J., Holzner, C. E., and Warheit, G. J. (1973): *Psychosomatics,* 14:135–141.
91. Schwartz, D., Flamant, R., and Lellouch, J. (1980): *Clinical Trials* (translated by M. J. R. Healy). Academic Press, London.
92. Sheehan, D. V. (1982): *N. Engl. J. Med.,* 307:156–158.
93. Spielberger, C. D., Gorsuch, R. L., and Lushene, R. E. (1970): *Manual for the State-Trait Anxiety Inventory.* Consulting Psychologist Press, Palo Alto.
94. Spilker, B. (1984): *Guide to Clinical Studies and Developing Protocols,* pp. 191–193. Raven Press, New York.
95. Spitzer, R. L., Fleiss, J. F., and Burdock, E. I. (1964): *Compr. Psychiatry,* 5:384–395.
96. Spriet, A., and Simon, P. (1980): *Methodologie des essais cliniques des medicaments.* Les Editions de la Prospective Medicale, Paris.
97. Spriet, A., and Simon, P. (1985): *Methodology of Clinical Drug Trials* (translated by R. Edelstein and M. Weintraub). Karger Publishers, Basel.
98. Strober, M., and Werry, J. S. (1986): In: *Assessment of Depression,* edited by N. Sartorius and T. A. Ban, pp. 324–342. Springer, Berlin, Heidelberg, New York.
99. Takahashi, R. (1986): In: *Assessment of Depression,* edited by N. Sartorius and T. A. Ban, pp. 36–45. Springer, Berlin, Heidelberg, New York.
100. Tasher, T., Rogler, M., Vlakhova, V., Balabanova, V., Moldovanska, P., Kukladzhiev, B., Bakalova, S., Poncher, P., and Madzhirova, N. (1982): *Medico-biolocheskaya informacinya,* 4:30–33.
101. Taylor, J. A. (1951): *J. Exp. Psychol.,* 42:183–188.
102. Tygstrup, N., Lachin, J. M., and Juhl, E. (1982): *The Randomized Clinical Trial and Therapeutic Decisions.* Marcel Dekker, New York.
103. Uhlenhuth, E. H. (1985): In: *Anxiety and the Anxiety Disorders,* edited by A. H. Tuma and J. Maser, pp. 675–680. Lawrence Erlbaum Associates, Hillsdale, NJ.
104. Uhlenhuth, E. H., Johanson, C. E., Kilgore, K., and Kobasa, S. C. (1981): *Psychopharmacology,* 74:191–194.
105. US Department of Health and Human Services (1985): *Psychopharmacol. Bull.,* 21:713–1125.
106. US Department of Health and Human Services (1986): *Alcohol, Drug Abuse and Mental Health News,* XII(6):1 and 8.
107. U.S. Food and Drug Administration (1986): *Draft Guideline for the Format and Content of the Clinical Data Section of an Application.* Docket No. 85D-0467. Rockville, MD.
108. Vinar, O. (1966): *Act. Nerv. Super. (Praha),* 8:409–411.
109. Welsh, G. S. (1956): In: *Basic Readings on the MMPI in Psychology and Medicine,* edited by G. S. Welsh and W. G. Dahlstrom, pp. 264–281. University of Minnesota Press, Minneapolis.
110. Wenger, N. K., Mattson, M. E., Furberg, C. D., and Elinson, J., eds. (1984): *Assessment of Quality of Life.* LeJacq Publishing, USA.
111. Widlocher, D. (1981): *Psychol. Med.,* 13:53–60.
112. Wittenborn, J. R. (1950): *J. Consult. Psychol.,* 14:500–501.
113. Wittenborn, J. R. (1955): *Wittenborn Psychiatric Rating Scale Manual.* Psychological Corporation, New York.
114. Woggon, B. (1979): *Int. Pharmacopsychiatry,* 14:158–169.
115. Yesavage, J. A., Brink, T. L., Rose, T. L., et al. (1983): *J. Psychiatr. Res.,* 17:37–49.
116. Zung, W. W. K. (1965): *Arch. Gen. Psychiatry,* 12:63–70.
117. Zung, W. W. K. (1971): *Psychosomatics,* 12:371–379.

Psychopharmacology:
The Third Generation of Progress,
edited by Herbert Y. Meltzer.
Raven Press, New York © 1987.

CHAPTER **100**

Persistent Flaws in the Design and Analysis of Psychopharmacology Research

Solomon C. Goldberg

From the perspective of the past 25 years, the level of research sophistication in clinical psychopharmacology has increased substantially. Review committees for grant applications and editors of journals have justifiably become more demanding in the area of quantitative method. Psychiatrists in particular, whose training has rarely included experimental design and statistical analysis, are schooling themselves in these methodologies (5). Statisticians, epidemiologists, and quantitative psychologists have become full-time members of the research team, as opposed to the former situation of a post hoc consultation with a biostatistician after data have been collected. This is not to devalue biostatisticians; it is to criticize the practice of consulting such a person only after data have been collected. Many research enterprises today require that the biostatistical hurdle be satisfied before proceeding with the project.

With increased sophistication there is the temptation to employ the heaviest statistical artillery possible as a demonstration of one's erudition, instead of choosing a technique that is logically appropriate to the data even if this is a chi-square or *t*-test of mean differences. These and other imperfections in measurement, design, and data analysis still seem to persist. The major purpose of this chapter is to call attention to these with the hope and expectation that we will witness improvement in the next volume describing the next 10 years of progress in psychopharmacology research.

THE CASE OF THE EXCLUDED MIDDLE

It is generally recognized by most investigators that restricting the range of the variables being related results

in a lower relationship than is true in the general population from which that sample was drawn. Thus, in the general population, including infants, children, adults, and giants, one can expect to find a modest correlation between height and weight. Taller people (giants) weigh more than shorter people (infants). However, if we now restrict the range of height by doing the same correlation only on adults, the size of the correlation between height and weight will be considerably less.

A corollary of this illustration is that if our sample excluded the middle of the distribution of height by taking a sample only of newborn infants and giants, leaving out everyone else, the correlation between height and weight would be considerably higher than in the full general population. This is the case of the excluded middle. The spuriously high correlation based on the extremes of the distribution cannot validly be applied to the general population. This situation frequently occurs in clinical research where extreme groups are selected for comparison, as, for example, in comparing patients with very good vs very poor premorbid adjustment with regard to community adjustment after hospitalization. Suppose that a clinical user of this result wants to test it out in his hospital. He does a premorbid adjustment scale on all the patients coming through for a year, eventually obtains their level of community adjustment after their discharge, and finds that the correlation or variance accounted for in his sample is considerably less than what was reported in the literature on the basis of the extreme groups. Depending on his sample size, he may not even find a correlation that is significant. His disillusionment is obvious. The original investigator in the literature should not have reported results on the basis of extreme groups alone. The extreme group results are sufficient only to encourage him to do the study on the entire range of the population. Otherwise he builds up false expectations.

OMISSION OF CASES THAT EMBARRASS THE HYPOTHESIS

While strictly speaking this is considered "fudging," it is apparently done frequently enough that investigators chuckle about it. The well-known cartoon in Fig. 1 is found to be humorous because we all know people who do it. Legitimate omission of a case must be for reasons other than the outcome of the case. For example, the patient's reaction time was so slow because he was seen to doze off at the switch. The patient's plasma level of the drug was so unusual because that particular one was not analyzed in the same batch as the others. It was discovered after the case was in the study that he really did not meet the inclusion and exclusion criteria. These are legitimate.

Omitting cases that embarrass one's hypothesis is so self-evident as an abuse that it hardly seems worthy of mention. Its persistence stems partly from the recognition that everyone else is doing it. A legitimate critical question of any analysis is a review of all patients who entered the study but not the analysis.

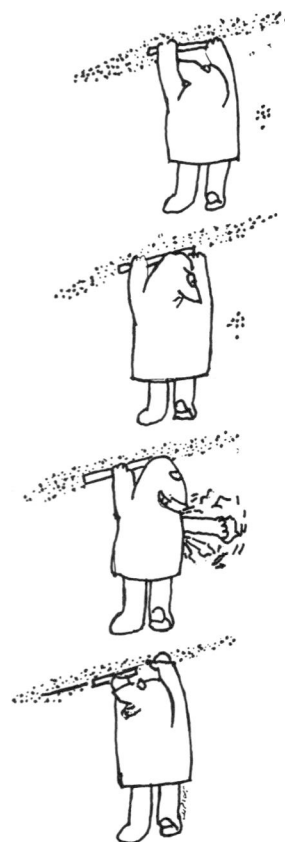

FIG. 1. Dealing with observations that do not fit the hypothesis.

OMISSION OF OUTLIERS WORKS AGAINST THE HYPOTHESIS

An opposite error is committed by those investigators who are so extremely and unduly cautious about overstating their results that they commit the type II error. For example, in testing the relationship between drug plasma level and therapeutic response, it is noted as in Figure 2 that a small number of outliers contribute heavily to the strength of the relationship. Most of the cases have blood levels between 150 and 500, and four cases are 800, 900, 1,100, and 1,500. These cautious investigators decide to omit the outlying cases because of their undue influence and then report the results on the remaining cases, which may not then reach statistical significance. They are less concerned about committing a type II error as long as they have avoided the unpardonable sin of the type I error. Moral rectitude is demonstrated as the outliers are stricken from the record.

Statistical advisors frequently have a built-in bias that the scientific investigator whom he advises errs on the side of overstating his results. Consequently, the advisor feels that he must apply a corrective by giving advice of extreme caution. He might say that these outliers are not members of the same population because of the discontinuity in the distribution. The point to be made on this issue is that outliers should not be omitted unless there is reason for omitting them other than being an outlier. First it must be decided whether the scores are realistically possible ones. If they are, they may be adjusted but never omitted. If they are not, that may be cause for omitting them.

It should be noted that the extreme scores in any distribution will always have more of an effect on the size of a relationship than less extreme scores. If both distributions are near normal, a study of 50 cases will have fewer than three cases (5%) at the extremes and these will have a greater influence on the correlation than any others. Further suppose that the outlying extreme cases appear to be unusually and discontinuously distant from the rest of the distribution so that one wishes to exercise caution in reporting the results. Here one can do so by making the scores less exaggerated before examining if the hypothesized relationship exists. This can be done in a number of ways. The first way in correlational data is to compute a rank order correlation instead of a Pearson correlation. Most computer programs such as SAS provide this option. If the Pearson correlation is due almost exclusively to the outlying case, a rank correlation would shrink greatly in size because the extreme outlying case is no longer so outlying and is simply given the next higher rank. If the rank correlation does not shrink noticeably, one is justified in retaining the Pearson correlation as is the case in Figure 2 where both the Pearson and Spearman correlations are nearly identical. Another method of adjustment might be a square root transformation. By transforming all the scores to their square roots, the blood level that was once 1,600 ng/ml now becomes 40 ng/ml. This has the effect of compressing the entire distribution.

In summary, by the very nature of scatter diagrams of two frequency distributions, the more extreme cases are far less frequent and have a greater influence on the size of

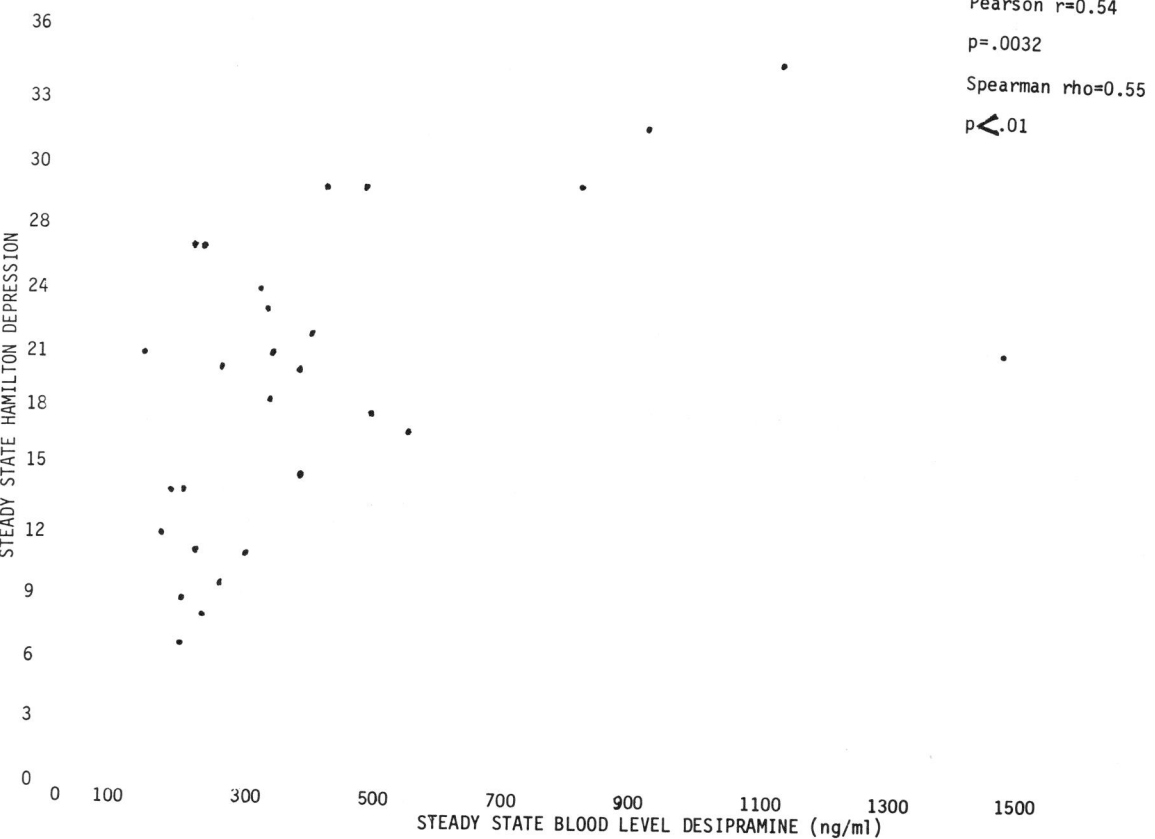

FIG. 2. Scatter diagram relating steady state Hamilton depression and steady state blood desipramine.

the relationship between the two variables. If the more extreme cases are independently judged to be legitimate, they must be retained. However, if it is suspected that the extreme cases are exaggerated, they should be adjusted by methods described above and these adjusted values should be employed in the determination of the relationship between the two variables.

DROPOUTS IN CLINICAL TRIALS

Yet another instance of omitting cases that should be included in the analysis is the practice of excluding certain kinds of dropouts in the analysis of clinical trials. Thanks to the requirements of the Food and Drug Administration, most investigators are aware of the effects of excluding dropouts when the dropout is differential by treatment. For example, in a haloperidol vs placebo study of 6 weeks duration in 50 acute schizophrenic patients, one might find that 10 patients in the placebo group had to be terminated early because of treatment failure, and 10 patients in the haloperidol group had to be terminated early and released from the hospital because of rapid remission. The remaining 15 placebo patients show more mean improvement than if the treatment failure dropouts were included, and the remaining 15 drug patients show less mean improvement than if the early remission dropouts were included. Analysis

of the 30 remaining patients who completed the full 6 weeks might not reach statistical significance because of smaller mean differences between the two groups and the reduced sample size. Yet the cruder dropout analysis of 10 treatment failures on placebo and 10 early treatment successes under drug is highly significant. Most investigators in clinical trials would now employ an endpoint analysis for all the cases, including the dropouts, and since the treatment failures would have low improvement endpoints and the treatment successes high improvement endpoints, the parametric analysis of the drug effect employing the full 50 cases would now be highly significant.

OTHER ESTIMATES OF FINAL SCORES

Endpoint analysis seems like a reasonable approach in a 6-week study since we might employ the score at, say, the end of the second week as our best available estimate of what the patient would have done by the end of the sixth week had he continued. However, one is more reluctant to employ an endpoint score of the second week in studies of longer duration, such as perhaps 26 weeks. It seems like too long a projection.

Several alternative suggestions have been made. The first is to assign the dropped patient the mean outcome score of the members of his treatment group who did not terminate early. The major virtue in this procedure is that it retains the case as part of the total sample, but it has the disadvantage of artificially reducing the variability within each treatment group, resulting perhaps in overstated significance between two groups because of spuriously low error variance.

To offset this shortcoming, some have suggested that a score be randomly selected from patients who did not drop and that this score be assigned to the dropped case. This procedure avoids the problem of artificially reducing the variability within each treatment group, and thus would result in essentially the same mean and standard deviation as the nondropped cases. The sole advantage would be in retaining the dropped case in the analysis. The greatest disadvantage is that the dropped case and its reason for being dropped would have no effect on the mean difference between the two groups.

A third procedure involves obtaining a correlation and its regression equation between the criterion of improvement and a number of pretreatment predictor variables of improvement using only the nondropped cases. Using this prediction equation, a predicted outcome score for the dropped case can be obtained. This is possibly the best approach to estimating outcome scores of early terminators, provided one can obtain a good set of predictors of outcome. To the extent that the prediction is weak, the predicted outcome scores would tend to hover about the mean outcome score of that treatment group. In this case this procedure becomes virtually equivalent to the one described earlier where dropouts are assigned the mean outcome of their treatment group.

Other investigators have argued for making subjective projections of the endpoint score according to the temporal trend up until the point of dropout. This method has obvious opportunities for experimenter bias.

Everyone legitimately finds fault with endpoint scores but eventually returns to them because the alternatives are found to be less feasible. One possible adjustment to an endpoint score that might be entertained is time in the study. This would convert an individual's improvement score to a rate of improvement per unit time. Thus an early treatment remission with marked improvement in 2 weeks should get a higher score than an early treatment remission of marked improvement in 4 weeks.

Some investigators have attempted to avoid the argument by doing two analyses, one with and one without the dropouts. If the analyses tend to agree, their confidence in the results is upheld. However, what if the analyses disagree? One is then presented with a post hoc choice that may be biased by one's hypothesis, especially if a new drug is being discovered.

DROPOUTS NOT DIFFERENTIAL BY TREATMENT

Consider another case in which the numbers of early successes and failures do not differ by treatment, there being five of each kind in each treatment group. In this instance many investigators would worry less about the effects of the dropouts on the analysis and might be content to analyze the completers only. The danger in doing so is that elimination of extreme improvement scores in both treatment groups results in an artificial reduction of the variability in each treatment group, with the result that a truly negligible difference between drug and placebo might attain statistical significance because of the artificially reduced error variance term. Here again endpoint analysis would be a corrective.

DROPOUTS FOR ADVERSE REACTIONS

Other kinds of early terminations that might be differential by treatment would be those due to adverse reactions to the drug. Suppose 10 patients terminate early under the drug condition because of adverse reactions and only two under placebo. Will it make any difference in the analysis of therapeutic outcome if it excludes these adverse reaction dropouts from the analysis? If adverse reactions are correlated with therapeutic outcome in the sense that akinesia would make a patient appear less improved, then leaving out the side effect dropouts would have the effect of overstating the mean improvement of the drug-treated group. If, however, the side effects are not correlated with therapeutic improvement, the mean of the drug group would not be affected very much by their exclusion. However, their exclusion would mean that the total sample size would be reduced by their number, making it more difficult to detect any significant difference if one exists.

Other reasons for early termination that are not differential by treatment group are moving out of town in midstudy or an intercurrent illness that prevents continuation in the study. It is highly unlikely that termination for these reasons would be associated with more or less improvement. Thus, their improvement scores are likely to scatter widely, and their exclusion probably would not have an effect on the means and standard deviations of the treatment group. However, their exclusion does mean a smaller sample size in the final analysis. Yet any particular study might suffer an odd distribution of improvement scores for people moving out of town, all clustering at one or another point in the distribution of improvement. Depending on where they cluster, they could affect the results differently. They might by their exclusion artificially inflate or deflate the variability within treatment groups or artificially increase or decrease the means of the treatment groups. Since it is impossible to predict a priori what will happen, *the wiser choice is to include in the analysis all early terminations regardless of reason by employing their endpoint or time-adjusted endpoint scores.*

Is it ever legitimate to exclude a case after it has been selected into the study? There are several reasons why this might be done. First it may be discovered after the patient is well into the study that he failed to meet some of the inclusion or exclusion criteria. He really should not have been in the study, and he should be replaced. Another instance is the patient who violates the protocol by perhaps taking another nonstudy drug that could interact with the study drug. He too should be dropped and replaced. A third instance is a bit more controversial. It asks how long the patient must be exposed to the study treatment before he is considered to have given his answer to the treatment. Obviously someone who terminates after 1 or 2 days of active treatment has not been adequately treated. How long a duration is adequate? The answer to this question is obviously arbitrary and depends on the nature of the drug, but certain conventions have been adopted. Two weeks is a common period. Thus a patient who is on the study treatment for 2 weeks and then moves out of town should be considered a legitimate case and should not be replaced.

Yet a patient might have to be dropped after only 2 days because of uncontrollable side effects. Should this patient be included in the analysis, since he has not been exposed to study treatment for 2 weeks? The imperfect solution to this problem is to include him for the purpose of side effects analysis but to exclude him from the analysis of therapeutic response. This situation would require the caution to the reader of that report if the drug is shown to be effective that the drug effectiveness applies only to those patients who did not develop early uncontrollable side effects. In other words, the drug may be effective but only for those who can tolerate the drug.

DICHOTOMIZING LOSES POWER

The widespread tendency to artificially dichotomize variables that have quantitative distributions is self-defeating. The continuous distribution of improvement on, say, the Brief Psychiatric Rating Scale (BPRS) or the Hamilton Depression Scale is frequently dichotomized into improvers and nonimprovers. The continuous distribution of postdexamethasone cortisol levels is dichotomized into positive and negative dexamethasone suppression tests (DSTs). An elaborate and lengthy interview with rich clinical material on the families of schizophrenic patients, the Camberwell Family Interview, is ultimately dichotomized into families who are high or low on expressed emotions (EE). The effect of lumping data into a dichotomy is to treat as being the same, values on a measure that may actually have different effects. Usually the investigator is hoping to find a significant relationship: between therapeutic response and perhaps drug blood level, or between escape from suppression on dexamethasone and therapeutic response, or between expressed emotion in the patient's family and clinical course and outcome in the patient. If this is their hope, they needlessly penalize themselves in dichotomizing their quantitative distributions, since doing so makes it more difficult to detect the hypothesized relationship if it exists. *The size of the correlation necessary for significance is greater if a dichotomy is employed than if the full quantitative distribution is employed.* It may be permissible and convenient for the investigator to think conceptually in terms of high and low expressed emotion or positive and negative DSTs or responders vs nonresponders, but he should not commit the error of forcing the distribution of his variables into those convenient shorthand terms.

If he is interested in improvers or responders in a depression study on the Hamilton Scale designated as a score no greater than 10, he can still inspect the scatter plots of the quantitative distributions and draw in that

cutoff score to allow him to draw appropriate conclusions. He should not confuse the question of the cutoff score, which is an arbitrary convention, with the test of significance of the relationship, which he wants to be as sensitive and as powerful as possible. If he wants to provide guidelines to clinicians with regard to a meaningful or nonmeaningful cortisol level, he can still do this by applying a number of different cutoff scores to the scatter plots of his quantitative distributions to examine what the implications are of various cutoffs. Instead of a single recommended cutoff score such as the 5 μg/dl of cortisol, the investigator might present a small range of cutoffs that might be considered. A study by Ettigi et al. (4) showed a significant relationship between therapeutic improvement and absolute cortisol level but not with the conventional dichotomized DST.

UNRELIABILITY WORKS AGAINST THE HYPOTHESIS

Reliability of measurement has received a great deal of attention in the past 20 years, so that it is extremely unusual today to find any published report that does not present reliability data on its measures. Perhaps those investigators who must deal with soft measures such as rating scales and social and psychiatric history are more keenly aware of the fallibility of their data and hence go to great pains to demonstrate some aspect of reliability. However, oftentimes investigators are less rigorous in demonstrating the reliability of their data or perhaps the sponsor of the study does not have a *requirement* of the demonstration of the reliability of the measures. In drug trials sponsored by pharmaceutical houses done by the current author, no one has *demanded* demonstration of reliability. It is too frequently assumed that since the scales such as the Hamilton or the BPRS are in the literature, and other investigators have demonstrated reliability, there is no need to do so in the study at hand. Not so. Just because reliability has been demonstrated on a scale in another study does not necessarily mean that the scale is reliable in the study currently being done unless steps are taken to insure that the measures are reliable.

The penalty for the unreliability of measures is that it attenuates whatever relationship truly exists between the variables examined. Assuming that the investigator and the sponsor have an investment in the hypothesis that there is a relationship between the variables, they are wasting their time and money by not establishing the suitable reliability of their measures.

Frequently, when reliability is demonstrated for a study, it is done for the first handful of cases but not thereafter. Data collection in clinical studies can easily go on for 2 years or more, during which time the raters can change or there may be a divergence of rating standards. Out of enlightened self-interest, reliability must be demonstrated through the full run of the study, or else risk the disconfirmation of one's hypothesis because of unreliability.

Rater training usually involves independent observation of patients, with a postinterview discussion of disagreements, so that rating standards and ground rules can be worked out for succeeding ratings. Ultimately satisfactory reliability levels are reached and then the study itself may begin. If two raters are used for every other patient or for every fifth patient, etc., to offset the possibility of a divergence of rating standards and ground rules, one should institute a postinterview discussion between the two raters concerning points of disagreement, without, however, allowing any changes in the ratings that were already made prior to the discussion. The discussion serves as a calibration for ratings that would be done in the future. It is the same kind of training procedure as before the study began. It is by this means that a high level of reliability can be maintained throughout the course of the study.

In the seemingly harder measures, such as cortisol levels, drug blood levels, ventricular size, or heart rate, data are often reported as standard errors of the mean or coefficients of variation. These are very difficult to interpret because they do not tell us whether a patient would have had the same cortisol level whether we looked at split sample A as opposed to split sample B. A reliability index such as intraclass correlation would do so. Only in rare cases is this done; for example, Saady et al. (7), showing the reliability of plasma vs serum level assays of antidepressants, demonstrated this with the intraclass correlation between split samples. Reporting a standard error of the mean or a coefficient of variation does not give this information. In the harder variables there is a great aura of objectivity compared to rating scales, and investigators do not bother to demonstrate reliability. Seemingly objective measures such as pulse, blood pressure, blood plasma levels, etc., may be less reliable than one thinks, and one's research thereby is at risk for not finding the relationship one has worked hard and long to detect. It is false economy not to take the additional effort to establish and maintain reliability of one's measures throughout the course of the study.

WANTED! REPLICATION STUDIES

The results of a single study do not make a fact. It is only when these results are confirmed by perhaps three independent investigators without other results to the contrary that the results come to be accepted as factual. However, if one attempted to compile a list of replicated facts in psychopharmacology, there would be a very short list. Part of the reason for this is that investigators tend not to give their highest priority to replicating someone else's result. They would rather discover something new on their own. This bias also obtains in priorities given to the publication of manuscripts in journals. Many journals ask their reviewers whether the manuscript presents something new or is *only* a replication of a prior finding. Obviously this policy also deters investigators from doing replication studies.

If three independent investigators, each using 20 cases, found that a neuroleptic was more effective than a placebo in acute schizophrenics, this replicated result would be far more credible than if a single investigator found the same results using 60 cases. Intuitively, independent replication of results carries more credibility than is achieved by increased sample size. If one were sponsoring a study of, say, 100 patients, would it be better to do the study in one location or to have two investigators do the study with 50 patients each? The answer must lie in favor of the replicated version of the study, because it presents the opportunity to discover that the relationship being tested in the study might apply in the one location but not in the other. Currently the credibility of any study is depicted by means of its *p* value. Most investigators are aware that with almost any size *p* value of high significance, the result presented might still be a chance finding. The *p* value is only an estimated projection of what one is likely to find if one did a replication. Instead of stopping with the *p* value of a single study why not build in a replication feature from the very beginning? This is done by collaborating with another investigator to follow essentially the same protocol. They have the opportunity to test whether their results differ from each other. If they do, they would show a failure to replicate. It is possible that each investigator might find essentially the same results each with a *p* value only at the 0.10 level, but when the two are combined, the total results reach acceptable levels of significance. If the more utopian journals in the future accepted manuscripts only if they had a replication feature built in, the literature would be cleansed of isolated sporadic findings unlikely to be replicated, and would contain documentation of ideas that failed to replicate along with those positive studies where there was positive replication.

The research world of that utopian journal would also *require* graduate students, research residents, postdoctoral research fellows, and other junior research personnel to do replication studies before embarking on anything new. The replication study is an excellent training procedure for the conduct of research, since one will want to follow the same protocol as was originally reported. Examining the failings in someone else's protocol is excellent training for designing one's own. Reports of replication studies can be very brief but would involve the incentive of publication credit, so important for junior level researchers.

CROSS VALIDATION AS MULTIVARIATE REPLICATION

A greater number of investigators are using discriminant function, multiple correlation, and regression methods in prediction of response studies. This method has been viewed with suspicion because of failures to replicate some complex multivariate results. For example, an investigator might compute a multiple correlation between five predictors and a criterion of therapeutic response. He finds the value of the multiple R (0.67) to be statistically significant ($p < 0.01$), considering the number of patients that he used and the number of predictor variables that were needed to attain this level. A common misinterpretation is to say that 45% of the outcome variance (the square of multiple R) is accounted for by the predictors. Even though multiple R tested out to be statistically significant, its face value (0.67) is known to be inflated because the prediction equation was generated on the basis of the same patients on whom it then makes predictions. This procedure capitalizes on chance factors. The true correlation between the five predictors and the outcome variable is obtained by applying the differentially weighted prediction equation developed on the original sample to a new sample of patients and correlating their predicted outcome scores with their actual outcome scores. Invariably this correlation is reduced to some extent from the one that is originally obtained in the multiple correlation. Sometimes it can reduce to near zero if there are a large number of chance predictors. The application of the old prediction equation to a new set of patients is referred to as cross validation, and if that cross validity turned out to be 0.40, then the amount of variance accounted for by the predictors would be 16% (still significant) but certainly not the original 45%.

SIZE OF THE EFFECT

With enough of a sample size one can obtain a very highly significant difference between a drug and placebo, implying that the difference between the two treatments is large. On careful inspection, the difference between the two treatments may not be as large as is implied by the significance level. Cohen (3) has suggested that, in addition to significance level, one needs to report the size of the effect. Clinicians are always asking whether the study results are perhaps statistically significant but clinically negligible. This is a good and relevant question. One way of expressing the size of an effect is in terms of the percent variance of the dependent variable accounted for by the independent variable. This can be done in any one of a variety of studies, such as (a) whether a positive DST is associated with a diagnosis of melancholia, (b) whether there is a drug-placebo difference in clinical response, or (c) whether there is a relationship between drug plasma level and cortisol level. In each of these cases one can obtain an expression of the percent variance accounted for by the independent variable. The difficulty is that these percentages are often misinterpreted. What percentage is large and what percentage is small? In the study by Hogarty, Goldberg, and Schooler (5) on the effect of maintenance medication vs placebo in the prevention of relapse in schizophrenic outpatients, some 85% of the placebo patients had relapsed by the end of 2 years, whereas the comparable figure for drug patients was about 49%. Most clinical observers agreed that this was one of the largest therapeutic effects ever to be seen in psychiatry. Yet when translated into percent of the outcome variance accounted for by the treatment, drug accounts for only 15% of the variance, a seemingly unimpressive number. Yet 15% of the variance represents an effect that knowledgeable clinical observers regard as almost revolutionary. Fleiss (4) has presented methods for deriving from any statistic an appropriate expression of percent variance accounted for. Cohen (1) has reviewed a large number of clinical studies characterizing the size of the effect, e.g., in terms of its pretreatment standard deviation units. In his review a difference in proportions of 0.30 was considered large.

Cohen regards a mean difference effect size of 0.25 standard deviation as being perhaps detectable but small. An effect size of 0.5 standard deviation was regarded as medium, whereas an effect size of one or more standard deviations was large.

One might ask whether there is a larger effect of neuroleptics on schizophrenic patients using the BPRS than there is an effect of antidepressant agents on depressed patients using the Hamilton Rating Scale. If one did a drug-placebo study in each diagnosis one could divide the mean difference of the drug and placebo by the pretreatment standard deviation on the dependent variable, and this would represent an effect size.

The concept of effect size can also be used in determining whether a treatment has a larger effect on one variable than another, as for example the effect of an antidepressant on depression and anxiety. Since the depression and anxiety variables are on different scales, they cannot be directly compared without first adjusting by means of dividing the drug-placebo difference by the pretreatment standard deviation.

SIZE OF EFFECT DESIRED IN ESTIMATING SAMPLE SIZE REQUIREMENTS

Research investigators, when soliciting statistical advice in planning a study, will need to know the number of cases in the sample that will be necessary to detect statistical significance. If the planned study is the replication of a prior study, one can look at the sample size of the prior study as a guide. Without a prior study, the projected sample size for the new study depends on the pretreatment variability on the dependent variable, e.g., BPRS, because statistical significance will require that the variability between treatments exceed the natural variability on the dependent variable prior to treatment. Often the statistical advisor will say, "If you can tell me how much of a difference between treatments you expect to get, I can calculate the number of cases you will need to detect the treatment difference of that size." Usually the investigator has little idea of the size of the difference he expects to get. He is willing to take what he can get, and this results in misunderstanding between the investigator and the statistical advisor. The guidelines offered by Cohen on more and less clinically meaningful effect sizes can be helpful. If he is seeking a drug-placebo difference, he will want at least a clinically meaningful medium effect size, which is considered approximately half a standard deviation. However, if the investigator had just discovered chlorpromazine and wanted to demonstrate that it was more effective than reserpine, the expected size of the treatment difference would be smaller than a drug-placebo difference, perhaps a quarter of the standard deviation, in which case it would require a greater sample size to detect the smaller difference as significant. Knowing the pretreatment standard deviation on the dependent variable and the desired size of the treatment difference in terms of the number of standard deviation units, one can make reasonable estimates of the number of cases necessary to detect a difference of that size. If he wants to increase his chances of finding significance, he will want to increase power with greater sample size.

The past 10 years have also witnessed greater use of power calculations in estimating sample size requirements. This is due in part to Cohen (2) on this topic. Our hypothetical investigator does not want to conclude that chlorpromazine and reserpine are equally effective only because he used too few cases. He can increase the power of his test of significance by increasing the number of cases in the sample. If he includes a placebo in the study, the number of cases necessary to detect the difference between placebo and reserpine or placebo and chlorpromazine will be substantially less than the number of cases necessary to detect the difference between reserpine and chlorpromazine. Thus he might have a larger number of cases in the active drugs than in the placebo group. It is gratifying to see that power analyses are becoming standard requirements in review committees.

NEW SCALES NEED GREATER VALIDITY

Oftentimes a clinical scale continues to be used in research because it was the first of its kind in the literature, many other investigators have used it, and one wants to compare one's own results with the prior literature. This in spite of well-recognized shortcomings of these scales. Good examples of this situation are with the Hamilton Depression Scale and the Phillips Scale of Premorbid Adjustment. Both scales have been justifiably criticized on psychometric and clinical grounds. An investigator who is sufficiently dissatisfied with the scale will either make a modification or invent a new scale. This has occurred in the area of premorbid adjustment with the Childhood Asociality Scale by Gittleman and the Goldstein Premorbid Adjustment Scale, which attempts to take into account sex differences. An investigator in schizophrenia research knowing the past literature on premorbid adjustment is obliged to include all three premorbid adjustment scales in order to make comparisons with the past literature. The investigator wishes he knew which of the three was better than the other. Since premorbid adjustment is used as a predictor of response to treatment, the investigator could find out which of the scales, if any, was a better predictor than the other. In future studies he would use the best scale, or, if they were equivalently good, he could use any one of them. While going to all this trouble, he wishes that the author of any newer scale had compared its predictive validity with the scale that he hoped to replace before making it available.

If he is dissatisfied with the Hamilton, he might invent his own depression scale. He might also demonstrate satisfactory reliability and some discriminative validity in showing that a group of known diagnostic depressions score much higher than a group of patients from a medical ward. By all rights, however, he should be required to demonstrate that his newly offered scale is *more* valid than the one that is already in common use. Otherwise, there is a needless proliferation of scales. Scale developers have typically presented reliability and validity data for their newly offered instruments, and have argued logically and clinically as to their superiority to the instruments they hope to replace, but rarely are data presented to *demonstrate* that the newly offered measure is superior in reliability and validity to the one already available.

REFERENCES

1. Cohen, J. (1962): *J. Abnorm. Soc. Psychol.,* 65:145–153.
2. Cohen, J. (1977): *Statistical Power Analysis for the Behavioral Sciences,* revised edition. Academic Press, New York.
3. Ettigi, P. E., Goldberg, S. C., Schulz, P. M., Hamer, R. M., Hayes, P. E., Narasimhachari, N., Blackard, W. G., and Friedel, R. O. (1986): (*in review*).
4. Fleiss, J. (1969): *Psychol. Bull.,* 72:273–276.
5. Goldberg, S. C., and Hamer, R. M. (1983): In: *The Handbook of Clinical Psychology. Theory, Research and Practice,* edited by C. E. Walker, pp. 75–128. Dow Jones-Irwin, Homewood, IL.
6. Hogarty, G. E., Goldberg, S. C., Schooler, N. R., and Ulrich, R. F. (1974): *Arch. Gen. Psychiatry,* 31:603–608.
7. Saady, B. J., Bloom, V. L., Narasimhachari, N., Goldberg, S. C., and Friedel, R. D. (1981): *Psychopharmacology,* 75:173–174.

Psychopharmacology:
The Third Generation of Progress,
edited by Herbert Y. Meltzer.
Raven Press, New York © 1987.

CHAPTER **101**

Adjusting p Values for Multiple Tests of Significance

John E. Overall and Howard M. Rhoades

This chapter is concerned with assigning an appropriate level of confidence to conclusions based on multiple tests of significance. The p value associated with a single test of statistical significance is an estimate of probability that the observed result has occurred by chance in the absence of any true treatment effect. When multiple tests of significance are considered, these probabilities of chance occurrence tend to be cumulative. Thus, it is generally considered appropriate to adjust the ordinary tabled p values to take into account the increased probability of chance results when multiple tests are examined.

Three somewhat different problems will be considered in this chapter, all involving the interpretation of results from multiple tests of significance. The first concerns assigning a single level of statistical significance to the combined results from several independent studies. The second concerns tests for the presence of a true treatment effect in a few positive-appearing studies that may occur in the context of several other negative or neutral studies. The final problem concerns the effect of an interim analysis on the p value for a subsequent end-of-study analysis, the interim and subsequent analysis representing multiple tests of significance on two segments of the total study sample.

The multiple tests of significance with which this chapter is concerned are tests of the same treatment effect in different samples of individuals. Each individual is represented by a single outcome observation or measurement. This chapter is not concerned with multiple tests of significance involving several measurements on the same individuals either on repeated occasions or across several different outcome measures at one point in time. The issue of adjusting p values has often been raised inappropriately with regard to the latter cases. Repeated measurements or multiple different measurements made on the same individuals pose different problems because they are not inde-

pendent. Multivariate analyses provide appropriate tests of significance for correlated measurements, but those are not the concerns of this chapter. This chapter is concerned with tests of significance for treatment effects calculated separately for a single outcome measure in several independent studies or several segments of a single study.

SIGNIFICANCE OF COMBINED RESULTS

It is often useful to be able to make a single probability statement about the significance of combined results from several independent studies. The hypothesis to which such probability statements apply concerns the presence of an average or weighted average treatment effect across all studies. It is assumed that the studies are independent and that treatment effects have been tested for statistical significance separately in the individual studies. Occasions on which the interest in a combined test occurs range from surveys of the published literature to multicenter trials following a common protocol.

Meta analysis is the popular term for statistical analysis of the results from multiple independent studies that have involved the same treatment comparisons (8). When applied to results from surveys of the published literature, the criticism of potential selective bias is a liability to be considered. Even with the best and most exhaustive summary of the literature, a bias is likely to result from the well-known tendency for negative results not to be published. Obviously, great distortion results if meta analysis is employed on only selected studies that tend to support the analyst's point of view. The concern about selective bias is not a problem when one can be confident of including all available studies, as in the case of several studies undertaken to support a New Drug Application (NDA).

The NDA is an excellent example of a situation in which meta analysis is most appropriate. Although several studies reported in an NDA concern a common treatment effect, there are usually enough differences in the patient populations or specifics of the protocols to militate against analyzing the combined data as a single stratified design. In addition, a primary interest in the significance of results from the individual studies also suggests that they should first be analyzed separately. Nevertheless, after all is said and done, one comprehensive probability statement supporting statistical significance of the combined results is relevant for the ultimate decision about drug efficacy. The procedures for obtaining a single summary probability statement concerning the presence of a treatment effect across several independent studies range from reanalyses of the combined raw data, to utilization of summary statistics, to combining of p values from previous analyses of data from the separate studies. This chapter is concerned with the latter methods.

R. A. Fisher in 1925 proposed the most widely used method for combining results from multiple independent trials in which there is reason to expect that one particular treatment should be superior to another. His own words most clearly describe the intent of this solution to the problem.

> When a number of quite independent tests of significance have been made, it sometimes happens that few or none can be claimed individually as significant, yet the aggregate gives an impression that the probabilities are on the whole lower than would often have been obtained by chance. It is sometimes desired, taking account only of these probabilities, and not of the detailed composition of the data from which they are derived, which may be of very different kinds, to obtain a single test of significance for the aggregate, based on the product of the probabilities individually observed (3).

Under the null hypothesis, p values have a uniform (rectangular) distribution over the interval 0 to 1. Minus 2 times the natural logarithm of a rectangular random variate over the interval 0 to 1 is distributed as chi-square, and independent chi-squares are additive. Thus, the sum of -2 ln p across m studies is distributed as chi-square with $2m$ degrees of freedom, where p is the one-sided p value from any appropriate test of significance for a directional hypothesis.

$$\chi^2 = -2 \sum (\ln p) \qquad [1]$$

In spite of its widespread use, Fisher's -2 ln p statistic has been criticized on what the present authors consider to be nonstatistical grounds. It is possible to construct artificial examples in which a highly positive study is combined with an equally negative study, and the resulting -2 ln p statistic is judged to be significant. However, statisticians do not generally reason from isolated extreme cases. Statistical inference is based on probability and sampling distributions, not rare cases. The question is "How likely would it be for the particular case to occur if there were no true treatment effect in the anticipated direction in any of the studies?" The answer to that question is the p value associated with the Fisher -2 ln p statistic.

The p values whose logarithms are summed to obtain the composite chi-square statistic must be one-sided p values. This is necessary because, otherwise, negative results would receive the same weight as positive results. Pertaining to a directional hypothesis, the p value associated with a negative result is greater than 0.50, and its negative logarithm is consequently smaller than that associated with a treatment effect of comparable magnitude in the expected (or positive) direction. Because the p values from the individual studies relate to a one-sided hypothesis, the probability value associated with the composite -2 ln p chi-square statistic also refers to a directional hypothesis without further modification (7).

Ordinarily, the Fisher statistic is used where there is a clear *a priori* expectation that one treatment will be superior to another and there is no interest in results to the contrary. It is possible, however, to use it for a two-sided test. One simply identifies as "positive" the direction of treatment effect that is most supported by the combined results. One-sided p values relative to that *post hoc* directional hypothesis are calculated, and -2 times their logarithms are summed to produce a composite chi-square test. The *two-sided p* value associated with this composite statistic is then twice the conventionally tabled chi-square p value for the appropriate degrees of freedom. The remainder of this section will, nevertheless, discuss results from use of the Fisher -2 ln p statistic as if an *a priori* directional expectation exists for the treatment outcomes.

The present authors have done extensive Monte Carlo evaluation of the Fisher statistic and have concluded that it will not produce significant results, beyond the specified alpha level, unless a true treatment effect in the expected direction is present in at least some of the studies, although not necessarily in all of them. If this appears to be a weak conclusion, it is no different from that strictly justified by any test of combined results; however, the -2 ln p statistic is less sensitive to a treatments $\times$ studies interaction than are most other tests. As will be explored in a later section of this chapter, the Fisher statistic is particularly sensitive to the presence of a true treatment effect in the expected direction in *any* of several studies while appropriately taking into consideration negative results that may be present. Again, it will not produce significant results with probability greater than alpha unless a true treatment effect in the expected direction is present in at least some of the studies under consideration. The Fisher statistic is concerned with a directional hypothesis and thus provides a one-sided test of significance. However, as noted, one can use it to test a two-sided hypothesis by simply doubling the p value associated with the composite chi-square statistic.

Because exact p values for tests of significance in individual studies are so readily obtainable using modern computational technology, alternative methods of combining results that start with p values should perhaps also be considered. The advantage of methods based on analysis of p values is that they are entirely general with regard to the type of data or test statistic from which the p values derive. In fact, some studies to be combined may consider a binary improve/worse outcome with a chi-square test of significance, whereas others may utilize quantitative measurements of treatment response and parametric F or t tests of significance. As long as the assumptions of the statistical models are reasonably satisfied, the results from any combination of the test statistics can be translated into p values. It is assumed, of course, that the several studies are truly independent and that all involve the same general question or treatment comparison. A word of caution is that calculations of "exact" p values may not be exact in the far tails of a statistical distribution, so it may be appropriate to replace calculated p values that are smaller than 0.001 with that value when considering the significance of combined results.

Whereas the log transformation of p values provides a chi-square test that is sensitive to the presence of a true treatment effect in *any* of several independent studies, a z-score transformation of p values provides a somewhat more conservative test of significance for the average treatment effect across the several studies. A table of areas under the unit normal distribution can be used to obtain the z-score equivalent of any p value. Again, for purposes of combining results, the p values should pertain to a directional hypothesis so that negative results are weighed appropriately. Note that z scores corresponding to $p > 0.5$ have negative signs.

The sum of the z scores for several independent studies is also a normally distributed statistic with variance equal to the number of studies entering into the sum. The statistic $z^* = \sum z/\sqrt{m}$ is thus itself a unit normal deviate, or z score, which can be referred back to the table of areas of the unit normal distribution to evaluate its probability under the null hypothesis:

$$z^* = \sum z_i/\sqrt{m} \qquad [2]$$

where z_i is the z score corresponding to the one-sided p value from a test of significance of the treatment effect in the ith study, $i = 1, 2, \ldots, m$.

Because the z scores that are summed relate to a directional hypothesis, by virtue of having been derived from one-sided p values, the z^* statistic also relates to a one-sided hypothesis. As in the case of the Fisher procedure for combining p values, it is possible to use z^* to test a two-sided hypothesis in cases where no justification exists for a directional test. One simply designates as "positive" the direction of treatment effect that is favored by the preponderance of results. The z scores corresponding to one-sided p values for that directional hypothesis are then summed to obtain z^*. The two-sided probability associated with z^* is twice the upper tail area in the unit normal distribution.

SIGNIFICANCE OF TREATMENT EFFECTS IN INDIVIDUAL STUDIES

When several investigators have independently evaluated the same drug treatments, it is not unusual for their several results to appear less than highly consistent. In some cases, a few studies may appear quite positive, whereas a majority are negative or nondiscriminating. If one examines the results from a large enough series of studies, it is almost certain that some will appear significant by chance alone unless the criterion for judging statistical significance takes the multiplicity of tests into consideration. This section is concerned with adjusting the criterion for statistical significance in individual studies to retain a conservative overall alpha level across the entire set of several independent studies.

The Bonferroni inequality provides an adjustment of required alpha level that is intuitively reasonable for judging statistical significance of individual studies (6). As noted, independent p values are randomly distributed in a uniform fashion over the interval 0 to 1 under the null hypothesis. This means that each individual p value has the same probability of falling within any specified interval near zero. Given that the p values are truly independent, the probability that any number of them will be smaller than a specified value is less than or equal to their number times the probability that *any one* will be smaller than the specified value. Let α be the desired overall alpha level, say 0.05 or 0.01. By requiring individual p values to be $p < \alpha/m$, the total probability of type I error across m studies is α, which is the sum of the probabilities of type I error for the m individual studies.

$$\sum_{m} \alpha/m = \alpha \qquad [3]$$

where α is the desired total type I error probability and α/m is the probability of type I error for each of the m independent studies under consideration. We will refer to α/m as the "simultaneous Bonferroni" criterion when it is applied uniformly to all p values under consideration without regard for the ordering of their magnitudes.

A somewhat different logic has led the present authors to view the simultaneous Bonferroni criterion as overly conservative. The p values associated with independent tests of significance have a rectangular distribution only if no true treatment effect is present. The sampling distribution for each null p value, in an ordered set from smallest to largest, is a beta distribution. Thus, one can use the incomplete beta function to define the interval within which the jth smallest observed p value in an ordered set will likely fall. It is easy to appreciate that the location and width of the interval within which the smallest observed p value can be expected to fall depend on the total number of null p values in the set. The important thing is that this applies only to p values from tests of significance in studies where no true treatment effect is present.

Suppose that a true treatment effect is present in a subset of studies, but no true treatment effect is present in the remaining $m - r$. The sampling distribution for the $m - r$ studies is known, and the Bonferroni logic applies. It does *not* apply to the p values for the studies in which a true treatment effect *is* present. It is easy to appreciate that the smallest of m null p values in an ordered set has a sampling distribution that is compressed closer to zero than does the smallest of $m - r$.

Sequential application of the Bonferroni adjustment is based on the logical assumption that rejection of the null hypothesis means that a study does not belong to the null set. That in turn redefines the sampling distributions for the remaining $m - 1$ studies. Assume that p values have been arranged in rank order from smallest to largest. The critical values for statistical significance according to the "sequential Bonferroni" procedure are as follows:

$$
\begin{array}{l}
\alpha/m \\
\alpha/(m - 1) \\
\alpha/(m - 2) \\
- \\
- \\
- \\
\alpha/(m - r)
\end{array} \qquad [4]
$$

The smallest p value in the ordered set is judged to be statistically significant if it is equal to α/m, which is the same criterion applied to all p values by the simultaneous Bonferroni procedure. If the smallest p value is judged to be statistically significant, it is assumed not to have belonged to the null set. The Bonferroni criterion for the smallest p value in the redefined null set is thus $\alpha/(m-1)$. If the smallest of the $m-1$ remaining p values is considered to be statistically significant, it is also removed from the null set. This procedure of redefining the null set is continued until the next candidate fails to reach statistical significance or until all studies have been judged to contain a true treatment effect. It is obvious that the critical values for judging statistical significance of all p values except the smallest in the original set are more liberal than the α/m applied to each p value under the simultaneous procedure.

INTERIM ANALYSES AS A MULTIPLE TEST PROBLEM

In the course of a protracted clinical trial that has originally been planned to have a sample size adequate to provide acceptable power, it sometimes becomes important to have an interim look at the data. However, interim analyses have often been discouraged because of the multiple test problem. Probability of type I error is associated with the interim analysis and again with the final analysis once the complete sample has accumulated, and those type I error probabilities are cumulative. In this section we will discuss an interim analysis strategy that maintains a conservative experiment-wide alpha level while permitting early termination if the results are already reasonably conclusive one way or the other.

This is a problem that has been of concern to several different statisticians. Most of the previously proposed solutions have been complex and have related to particular types of data and/or particular test statistics (1,4,5). A solution that is based on a similar rationale to that described herein, but which is much more conservative in its stopping rule, has been proposed by DeMets and Halperin (2). Their approach asks whether the results at an interim point are so compelling that the *most* contradictory possible result for the remainder of the originally planned sample cannot possibly change the conclusion. This, we believe, is a severely conservative approach in a field where decisions are recognized as probabilistically correct. The DeMets and Halperin solution also requires that the response variable have a restricted range in which the worst possible score and the best possible score are both clearly defined and attainable. In most practical situations, it is almost certain that subjects in one treatment group will not uniformly hit the top or bottom of a quantitative score continuum, although that is theoretically possible in the case of a binary outcome measure or a categorical rating scale. Thus, the solution that we have proposed projects the best *likely* outcome and the worst *likely* outcome for subjects not yet entered at the point of an interim analysis, not the best and worst possible results for the remainder of the sample.

The general rationale of the interim analysis proposed here is that of combining p values from a first and second test of significance (3). The first test is accomplished at an interim point with only a portion of the originally planned sample available. If the p value derived from the interim test appears significant by itself, it is considered in combination with a hypothetically worst likely outcome for the remainder of the sample in order to determine whether the combined results would still reach statistical significance. If so, the null hypothesis is rejected, and the study is terminated early with the conclusion that a true treatment effect is present.

On the other hand, if the results at the interim point appear so negative that significant results for the complete sample are highly unlikely, even if a strongly positive treatment effect were to be observed in the remainder of the study, it is only reasonable to terminate the study. In this case, the conclusion is not that no true treatment effect is present. The conclusion is that the interim results are so negative that it is highly unlikely for the remainder of the originally planned sample to change things. If a type II error is to be made, it is better to make it early and at low cost!!

Finally, if the interim results are not conclusive one way or the other, the study can be continued to its originally planned conclusion with a protected experiment-wide alpha level. The significance of the treatment effect is tested separately for the interim and remaining samples, and p values from the two analyses are combined using a statistic that resembles Fisher's $-2 \ln p$. It is necessary, however, to take the relative sample sizes for the interim and later test into consideration.

The test for significance of the treatment effect at the interim point is based on the following criterion:

$$C_1 = (\ln p_1 + \ln(0.5)) \qquad [5]$$

where C_1 is evaluated against the critical value for chi-square with 4 degrees of freedom, p_1 is a one-sided p value from the test of a directional null hypothesis at the interim point, and 0.5 is the expected value for the p_2 that would be obtained from an independent analysis of the remainder of the originally planned sample if no true treatment effect is actually present. This statistic is, thus, Fisher's method of combining p values from two independent tests of the same null hypothesis (3). In this case, the second p value is a hypothetical projection of results that might occur if the study were to be continued. If p_1 is a chance occurrence, the expected value for p_2 is 0.5. If C_1 exceeds the chi-square critical value at the desired alpha level, the presence of a true treatment effect is inferred, and the study can be terminated without entering additional subjects.

If the observed p_1 is quite large, the important question is whether a highly significant p_2 from an independent test of significance on the remainder of the originally planned sample can be expected to turn the study around. The proposed criterion for early termination due to negative results is the following:

$$C_2 = -2(\ln p_1 + \ln(\alpha/2))(1.5 - N_1/N)^{\frac{1}{2}} \qquad [6]$$

where N_1/N is the proportion of the originally planned sample that is available for the interim analysis and $p_2 = \alpha/2$ is a highly favorable projected outcome in the sample of size N_2 if the study were to be continued. The study is terminated with negative results if C_2 *fails* to exceed the critical value for chi-square with 4 degrees of freedom. It can be noted that, except for the sample size factor, $(1.5 - N_1/N)^{\frac{1}{2}}$, this statistic is also a variant of Fisher's $-2 \ln p$ for combining the results from two independent tests of significance.

If neither of the interim criteria results in termination of the study, the remaining sample of size N_2 is acquired. A test of significance for the treatment effect in the second segment of the sample produces p_2, which combined with p_1 in the following equation provides a conservative criterion for evaluating the statistical significance of the combined results:

$$C_3 = -2(\ln p_1 + \ln p_2)(0.97 + (\alpha)^{\frac{1}{2}} \cdot (N_1/N)^2) \qquad [7]$$

Again, C_3 is evaluated against the critical value for chi-square with 4 degrees of freedom.

Monte Carlo methods have been used to simulate interim analyses undertaken at various points (early, middle, or late) in a protracted clinical study involving comparison of two treatments. When no true treatment effect was present, the combined type I error for the interim analysis and the subsequent end-of-study analysis did not exceed the specified alpha level. In the absence of a true treatment effect, the interim analysis undertaken with 50% of the preplanned sample using $\alpha = 0.05$ resulted in a decision to terminate the study 67.5% of the time. Only 2.7% of these termination decisions were type I errors. The great majority thus resulted from recognition that significant results would very likely not be achieved if the study was continued.

When power of the interim procedure was compared with that of a single end-of-study analysis, a modest decrease was observed. In the presence of a true treatment effect against which the single-stage end-of-study analysis had power of 0.792, the two-stage interim analysis with 50% of total sample available had experiment-wide power of 0.749. This modest loss in power was compensated for by early termination in 41.3% of the trials. These are representative examples from a rather exhaustive evaluation of type I error and power for the two-stage interim analysis procedure that has been accomplished by the present authors. It should be noted that the interim analysis can be accomplished at any point in a study; the results from interim analysis halfway through a study are mentioned only as an example.

For a study that is initially estimated to require a total of 100 subjects divided between two treatment groups to attain power of 0.80, 10 additional subjects can be added to the total N to retain that same power as a single end-of-study analysis if an interim analysis halfway through the planned sample does not result in a decision to terminate early. Because of the substantial probability of reaching an early decision with the interim analysis, the *expected* number of subjects is actually smaller for the interim strategy. In the case cited, the interim analysis strategy will either require only 50 subjects (terminate midway) or 110 subjects (complete study) to have the same power as a single end-of-study analysis based on a total N of 100 subjects. The possible reduction in total sample is, however, not the primary motivation for proposing this approach to interim analysis. The interim analysis is proposed as an answer to

the need to know in a timely fashion how a study is likely to turn out. The saving of time is often more critical than a small probabilistic saving in number of subjects.

We believe that these results are encouraging and they might be used to recommend preplanned two-stage sampling; however, certain problems should be clearly recognized. The most salient danger concerns the possibility that knowledge of the interim results might influence the manner in which the remainder of the study is carried out if no clear decision is reached at the interim point. The p values derived from the two-stage interim analysis procedure are meaningful only if it is reasonable to assume that subjects entered before and after the interim analysis are selected and treated in the same manner.

Several drug companies have adopted the strategy of setting up "surveillance committees" to monitor the progress of studies independent of the in-house personnel or clinical investigators. The purpose is to provide a mechanism for stopping a study in which subjects are needlessly exposed to an ineffective or harmful drug, but to provide no feedback that could influence the conduct of the study if things seem to be going all right. That would seem to be a perfect environment in which to use the interim analysis strategy proposed here. The surveillance committee would have the option of terminating a study in which the results were already convincing one way or the other. If the study is not terminated early, the criterion for statistical significance would be properly adjusted to take into account the possibility that it might have been terminated. The interim analysis affords substantial probability of reaching an early decision, while it provides a conservative experiment-wide alpha level when studies are continued to their originally planned sample size.

SUMMARY

Three problems involving the interpretation of combined results from multiple tests of significance have been considered. Fisher's $-2 \ln p$ method of combining p values from tests of significance in several independent studies is the best-known test of significance for the presence of a true treatment effect in a series of several independent studies. A more conservative tests averages treatment effects, expressed as z scores, across the several studies.

Often, the results from a series of independent drug trials do not appear uniformly positive, however, and one must be concerned about the justification for accepting a few positive results in the context of several other studies that provide no evidence of a true treatment effect. An adjustment of the alpha level that is required for statistical significance is recommended. A sequential procedure that involves successively larger p values in an ordered set, beginning with the smallest, against successively less stringent criteria is described and contrasted with the more frequently used procedure of defining α/m as the critical value for evaluating the significance of each of m independent studies.

Finally, interim analyses that offer potential for early termination of a study represent another cause for concern about multiple tests of significance. Criteria for a decision to terminate at the interim point are presented together with a conservative end-of-study test, in case an interim decision is not justified. The interim and final tests together provide a conservative experiment-wide alpha level and only modest reduction in power as compared with a single end-of-study analysis.

Procedures that make use of p values from independent analyses in different studies or segments of a study sample are emphasized herein because of their wide applicability. An investigator is left free to determine the type of data and the most appropriate method of analysis. The p values that are considered in combination can derive from any appropriate tests of significance, either parametric or nonparametric. In retrospective evaluations of studies concerned with a selected research question, one is not constrained to consider only reports that contain particular types of summary statistics; most published reports contain p values for the tests of significance that have been used. Perhaps the greatest advantage of methods that make use only of p values is that they are simple to use.

REFERENCES

1. Alling, D. (1963): *J. Am. Statist. Assoc.,* 58:713–720.
2. Demets, D. L., and Halperin, M. (1982): *Controlled Clin. Trials,* 3:1–11.
3. Fisher, R. A. (1970): *Statistical Methods for Research Workers,* 14th ed. Hafner Press, New York.
4. Herrmann, N., and Szatrowski, T. H. (1985): *Controlled Clin. Trials,* 6:25–37.
5. Lan, K. K. G., Simon, R., and Halperin, M. (1982): *Commun. Statist.,* 1:107–119.
6. Miller, R. G., Jr. (1966): *Simultaneous Statistical Inference.* McGraw-Hill, New York.
7. Overall, J. E., and Rhoades, H. M. (1986): *Psychol. Bull.,* 100:121–122.
8. Strube, M. J., and Hartman, D. P. (1983): *J. Consult. Clin. Psychol.,* 51:14–27.

Psychopharmacology:
The Third Generation of Progress,
edited by Herbert Y. Meltzer.
Raven Press, New York © 1987.

CHAPTER 102

Introduction: Clinical Psychopharmacology of Affective Disorders

Gerald L. Klerman

The chapters in this section review recent advances in the clinical psychopharmacology of affective disorders.

Prominent among the advances in the past decade has been a better understanding of the complex psychopathology of affective disorders and new approaches to their diagnosis and classification. These developments are reviewed by Hirschfeld and Cross and highlight the impact of the third edition of the Diagnostic and Statistical Manual (DSM-III) of the American Psychiatric Association.

Blackwell reviews the group of new antidepressant compounds and assesses their impact on clinical therapeutics. Fink provides a reassessment of the role of ECT. Gelenberg and associates apply the newer knowledge to the treatment of depressive disorders, and similarly, Clayton and Dunner describe recent progress in the treatment of mania and bipolar disorders. Important advances have occurred in long-term treatment of affective disorders, and these are surveyed by Prien. Lastly, Weissman and associates contribute to our understanding of the relationship of psychotherapy to psychopharmacology.

The inclusion of a section on affective disorders is in itself worthy of note. The identification of affective disorders as a separate class of psychiatric conditions has only gained acceptance in the research and clinical community since the 1950s. Until the promulgation of DSM-III in 1980, official diagnostic systems, including the USAPA DSM system and the International WHO-ICD system, did not include a separate category for affective disorders. Depressions and manic states were included under either psychotic or neurotic conditions.

The separation of psychotic from neurotic conditions has been the foundation of psychiatric diagnosis for over 100 years. This classification reflects the historical origins of psychiatry in the mental hospitals, i.e., the asylums of the 18th and 19th centuries.

Until recently, the major social responsibility of psychiatry had been the identification of severely disturbed individuals (those with psychotic disorders) whose illness manifested itself in behavior that was disruptive, threatening, deviant or rendered them disabled and dependent. Almost all psychiatrists until World War I were based in mental hospitals, and the distinction between psychotic and neurotic diagnoses was often the basis for justifying legal commitment and involuntary hospitalization.

With the increasing involvement of psychiatry in community practice, general hospitals, and outpatient settings since World War II, psychiatrists have become increasingly concerned with larger and larger numbers of patients with nonpsychotic conditions. The classic concept of neuroses proved inadequate to explain their psychopathology and social dysfunction and as a guide to treatment.

The advent of effective psychopharmacologic agents further contributed to the breakdown of the psychotic–neurotic classification, particularly for depressions. The efficacy of the tricyclics and MAO inhibitors did not follow this distinction. Largely because of the pattern of clinical actions of the tricyclic antidepressants, MAO inhibitors, ECT, and lithium, it became increasingly useful clinically and valid scientifically to group together depressions, whether psychotic or neurotic, and elated states (including manic-depressive illness, cyclothymia, and hypomania) into a broad category of affective disorders. The DSM-III was the first official diagnostic nomenclature to embody this grouping, and it also appears in the proposed 10th revision of the ICD under development by the WHO.

Patients with these conditions share a common dominant presenting feature—a profound disturbance of mood, either depressed or elated. The grouping of "affective disorders" should not imply any single etiology or mode of treatment. Although genetic factors play an important role in the etiology of some of the affective disorders, particularly the bipolar disorders, no single etiology has been established. In fact, researchers, particularly those influenced by methods from epidemiology, are increasingly applying the concept of multiple risk factors, a concept that has proven useful in understanding cardiovascular illnesses and cancer. An understanding of risk factors in these disorders has contributed to interventions for control and prevention even though the etiology of these diseases is not fully established. It is hoped that a similar strategy will prove useful for psychiatric disorders in general and the affective disorders in particular.

This grouping together of the affective disorders follows the logic of classification that emerged in medicine in the late 18th and early 19th centuries. Disorders in general medicine are classified either by etiology (infectious diseases, trauma, genetic disturbances, metabolic illnesses, nutritional deficiences, etc.) or by the organ affected (cardiac disease, kidney disease, etc.). In the case of psychiatric illness, the etiologic principle remains the highest ideal. However, only a fraction of the mental disorders have had their etiologies determined. For the majority of disorders no etiology has been conclusively established. Hence, these disorders are often called "functional." Although hypotheses have been proposed for developmental, social, cultural, familial, genetic, and viral etiologies, no etiology has been established. Consequently, the diagnostic and classification systems have been based on the grouping of disorders together on the criterion of the area of behavior or mental faculty that is disturbed. The psychiatric equivalent of the "organ" becomes the mental faculty. The division of mental disorders into disorders of thinking (i.e., schizophrenia and paranoia), disorders of memory (dementia), disorders of affect (mood disorders and anxiety disorders), and disorders of behavior (eating disorders, psychosocial dysfunctions, sleep disorders, etc.) reflects this view of the morphology of the mind.

It is acknowledged that this approach to classification is far from ideal. We do not know the normal physiologic basis of mood, let alone the anatomical areas of pathology underlying clinical conditions. There is heuristic value in regarding depressive and elated syndromes as disturbances in common pathophysiology. Thus, psychiatric syndromes are logically equivalent to syndromes in medicine such as edema, jaundice, and congestive heart failure. These syndromes each have common clinical presentations and shared pathophysiological processes resulting from multiple and diverse etiologies. As with hypertension, heart failure, and jaundice, the psychiatric syndromes of depression and elation reflect such disturbances in pathophysiology.

Even with these limitations, grouping the affective disorders together has contributed to a rapid increase in scientific knowledge and improvements in clinical practice. Demonstration of the antidepressant efficacy of a range of compounds stimulates hypotheses about their mode of action, and although no definitive evidence has yet been demonstrated for abnormalities in norepinephrine or serotonin metabolism in depressions, the amine theories remain the most stimulating intellectually and the most productive heuristically.

At the clinical level, we have seen the emergence of a subspeciality of affective disorders within psychiatry. In a large number of academic and clinical settings, mood clinics, depression units, and affective disorders centers are appearing where clinical skill and knowledge can be concentrated and new research furthered. Systematic evaluation of patients using structured interviews and the newer diagnostic systems has contributed to improved care. Greater skill in psychopharmacology and in specialized psychotherapeutic techniques has resulted in reduction of hospitalization, shortened duration of illnesses, and, in some instances, reports of reduction in suicide attempts and suicide deaths.

The chapters in this section reflect these profound changes in our understanding of psychopathology and the application of knowledge for diagnostic and therapeutic purposes.

Psychopharmacology:
The Third Generation of Progress,
edited by Herbert Y. Meltzer.
Raven Press, New York © 1987.

CHAPTER **103**

Clinical Psychopathology and Diagnosis in Relation to Treatment of Affective Disorders

Robert M. A. Hirschfeld and Christine K. Cross

In the decade since the last edition of *Psychopharmacology: A Generation of Progress* was published, research devoted to clinical psychopathology and diagnosis of affective disorders has burgeoned. The classification issues raised in 1978 by Katz and Hirschfeld (50) focused on the validity and utility of the unipolar–bipolar, primary–secondary, psychotic–neurotic, and endogenous distinctions. Although closure has not been reached on these distinctions (54,88,94), recent research efforts bearing on these topics have taken a different focus, spurred by the development of the DSM-III, the new official nomenclature of the American Psychiatric Association. A distinct departure from its predecessors, the DSM-III both has facilitated research on classification and psychopathology by providing operational inclusion and exclusion criteria for diagnostic classes, which enhance diagnostic reliability, and has served as an organizing principle and stimulant for much research.

Clinical psychopathology is relevant to psychopharmacology in three respects. First, symptomatology and diagnostic classes serve as the basis for selecting subjects to participate in drug trials. Diagnostic specificity and reliability, therefore, enhance the accuracy of clinical trials and the validity of the conclusions drawn from them.

Second, clinical psychopathology and diagnosis guide clinicians in their decisions regarding specific treatments for individual patients. Again, diagnostic specificity and reliability are critical inasmuch as they increase the likelihood of effective treatment.

Finally, response to drug treatment represents an important external validator for existing and proposed diagnostic classes. That is, the demonstration that a specific symptom or cluster of symptoms is predictive of response to a certain class of drugs is an important step in establishing distinct and valid clinical entities or diagnoses. Thus, there is an iterative process whereby pharmacological response serves to clarify diagnostic classes, which, in turn, form the basis for the selection of subjects for psychopharmacological research trials.

This chapter reviews the recent advances and current status of clinical psychopathology and diagnosis of affective disorders with particular reference to their relationship to treatment. The DSM-III diagnostic categories and distinctions are described in terms of their (a) history and purpose, (b) key defining criteria, (c) clinical course, and (d) predictive ability regarding pharmacological treatment response.

Three classes of affective disorders are identified in the DSM-III: major affective disorders, subdivided into major depression and bipolar disorder; other specific affective disorders, subdivided into cyclothymic and dysthymic disorders; and atypical affective disorders, subdivided into atypical depression and atypical bipolar disorder.

A revision of the DSM-III (DSM-III-Revised) will slightly modify the current classification of affective disorders. The present organization of the chapter, however, is compatible with the anticipated changes.

MAJOR AFFECTIVE DISORDERS

Within the DSM-III, the category "major affective disorders" consists of two subcategories of disorders that are characterized by the full affective syndrome: major depressive disorder, subclassified as single episode or recurrent; and bipolar disorder, subclassified as manic, depressed, or mixed.

Major Depression

Background

In his classification of mental disorders, Kraepelin (58) applied the term manic–depressive insanity to the domain of "periodic and circular affective states." In so doing, he combined recurrent melancholia and mania as well as milder affective mood swings on the basis of their common clinical course. Leonhard (59), in 1957, proposed that manic–depressive illness be separated into two categories: bipolar disorder, characterized by both manic and depressive episodes, and monopolar (later unipolar) disorder, characterized by recurrent depression only. Leonhard suggested that these represented two distinct, separate disorders that could be differentiated clinically. Subsequent research supported the validity of Leonhard's distinction (11,73), and his classification gained rapid acceptance in the 1970s. Disorders falling within the unipolar category, however, are recognized as much more heterogeneous with regard to clinical and family history, symptomatology, course, treatment response, and presumed etiology than bipolar disorders.

The DSM-III category of major depression represents a new diagnostic category and subsumes disorders previously categorized as psychotic depression, involutional depression, psychoneurotic depressive reaction, and manic–depressive insanity. Although a sizable percentage of patients included in this category would fit Kraepelin's concept of manic-depressive illness and/or Leonhard's concept of unipolar depression, the terms are not synonymous, since major depression is much more inclusive. In addition to including single-episode as well as recurrent forms of depression, this category encompasses a proportion of cases that previously would have been termed "neurotic depression" (major depression without melancholic or psychotic features). The need to identify subtypes within the general category of major depression has been emphasized by both biological psychiatrists and psychopharmacologists, both of which view the category as too heterogeneous.

Key Diagnostic Criteria

Criteria for an episode of major depression include dysphoric mood or pervasive loss of interest or pleasure associated with such symptoms as appetite, sleep, and/or psychomotor disturbances, lethargy, feelings of worthlessness or guilt, concentration difficulties, and/or thoughts of death or suicide.

Clinical Course

Major depressions tend to be episodic with an average duration of 12 months or less. Several reports have been published by the NIMH Collaborative Study on the Psychobiology of Depression Clinical Studies investigators on the topics of recovery, relapse, and chronicity in depression (51). Overall it was found that 79% of major depressives achieved a full or partial recovery within 2 years of onset—

a figure consistent with most previous reports (56,98). This means that over 20% of patients have not recovered within 2 years, a chronicity rate of one in five. Among recovered patients, approximately 35% relapsed within 1 year. Acute onset and mildness of depressive symptomatology were factors associated with recovery, and a history of several previous episodes was associated with relapse.

Twenty-five percent of the Collaborative Study sample had "double depression," the superimposition of major depression on an underlying chronic depression (53). Identification of such patients is important in terms of assessing outcome, since full recovery from double depression—defined as remission of both acute and chronic depressive symptomatology—is much less likely than from uncomplicated major depression (39% versus 79% recovered after 2 years, respectively), and relapse of major depression is much more likely in the doubly depressed.

Treatment

Since the overall category of major depression subsumes a heterogeneous group of depressive disorders, most research directed at treatment response has focused on specific subtypes such as melancholia or psychotic major depression.

Within the general category, however, several investigators over the past 25 years have described depressive subtypes that respond preferentially to monoamine oxidase inhibitors (MAOIs). These descriptions, summarized in several recent reviews (1,27,71), each share certain features while differing in others. Overall, two general symptom complexes have been identified. In the first, depression is accompanied by severe anxiety and/or panic attacks, and in the second, depression is accompanied by atypical vegetative symptoms such as hyperphagia and hypersomnia. In addition, the importance of extreme fatigue and reactivity of mood has been emphasized. The term "atypical depression"—not to be confused with the DSM III category of atypical depression—has been applied to both symptom complexes.

Despite the purported specificity of MAOIs in the treatment of "atypical" depressions, several recent studies have reported that tricyclic antidepressants (TCAs) are equally effective in their treatment (61,72,84,89,92). In all of these studies, however, MAOIs were superior to TCAs in the treatment of depressions with prominent anxiety or panic attacks.

Melancholia

Background

The term endogenous, which denotes an innate proclivity to a disorder, was first applied to depression by Gillespie (40) in 1929 to refer to disorders unresponsive to environmental stimuli and apparently arising from internal causes. As its usage evolved, the endogenous concept took on additional components and implications (see Table 1).

The existence of an endogenous symptom cluster has been confirmed by several factor analytic investigations (64) and, more recently, by investigators using the technique

TABLE 1. *Definition and implications of the concept of endogenous depression*

A complex of symptoms including severe depressed mood, lack of reactivity, loss of interest, sleep, appetite, and psychomotor disturbances, early morning awakening, and diurnal variation of mood
Presumed biological etiology
Not precipitated by stress
Occurring primarily in those over the age of 40 with a stable, nonneurotic premorbid personality
Require somatic interventions

of cluster analysis (10,62,63). Evidence from other validation domains such as family studies, clinical course, presence of precipitating life events, and biological correlates has not been found to justify the distinctiveness of melancholia as a separate diagnostic category.

Key Diagnostic Criteria

The DSM-III subclassification of melancholia was chosen to avoid the etiologic implications of the term endogenous. Diagnosis is made strictly on the basis of manifest symptomatology without regard to etiologic assumptions. Key symptomatic criteria include pervasive loss of pleasure and lack of reactivity.

Recent evaluations of the symptoms that best distinguish melancholic from nonmelancholic depressions have consistently found lack of reactivity and psychomotor change to be the best discriminators (37,62,63,68). Ruminative thinking has also been proposed as a "distinctive" sign of melancholia (69). In addition, depressive delusions and distinct quality of depressed mood, although relatively uncommon symptoms, have also been found to be highly discriminating (37,62,63,68). On the other hand, symptoms such as sleep and appetite disturbances and loss of interest, although typical of melancholic depressions, are also frequently found in nonmelancholic depressions.

Clinical Course

Clinicians have long believed that the endogenous symptom cluster predicts a more favorable clinical course. However, most research investigations have not demonstrated this. In the Clinical Studies of the NIMH Collaborative Study of the Psychobiology of Depression, for example, no differences in recovery or relapse rates were found between melancholic and nonmelancholic major depressives.

Treatment

The response of melancholic patients to drug therapy has been widely studied, and the generally good response of such patients to TCAs has served to validate the melancholic distinction despite evidence to the contrary from other domains. Certain symptoms characteristic of melancholic depressions have consistently been reported to be predictive of a good response to TCAs. These include appetite and weight loss, early morning awakening, psychomotor retardation or agitation, and lack of reactivity (14,84). Severely melancholic patients who exhibit marked agitation and delusions have been shown to respond poorly to TCA given alone (14,83).

With regard to prophylaxis, both TCAs and lithium are reported to be effective in preventing relapse (43,47,80,90), reducing the rate of recurrence typically by some 50%. The relative efficacy of the two classes of drugs appears to be roughly comparable (90), although this is an area of some disagreement (47,80). A recent report by Prien and Kupfer (79) indicated that maintenance therapy may be safely withdrawn only after patients have been free of significant depressive symptomatology for 16 to 20 weeks.

Psychotic Depression

Background

Although in its strictest definition, the term psychotic depression refers to depressions accompanied by delusions and hallucinations, over the years the term has often been used interchangeably with endogenous depression to denote severe, incapacitating depressions presumably of a biological nature. It was not until recently that a diagnosis of psychotic depression in its most narrow sense appeared to carry with it any clinical significance.

Reports published during the 1930s and 1940s on the relationship of psychotic features to the outcome of a depressive episode concluded that the mere presence of such features was not associated with a particular outcome (48). Thus, although delusions were found to be more common among patients who failed to recover, many patients with delusions recovered completely. The introduction of ECT to treat severe depressions eliminated any doubt concerning the prognostic significance of delusions inasmuch as a good response to ECT was noted in severely depressed patients regardless of the presence of delusions.

The term schizoaffective was introduced by Kasanin (49) in 1933 to refer to patients who fit neither of Kraepelin's major psychiatric entities—dementia praecox (schizophrenia) and manic–depressive insanity. These psychotic patients presented with a mixture of schizophrenic and affective symptoms and, unlike schizophrenics, were characterized by good premorbid functioning, acute onset, and a remitting course with good recovery. Over the years, several descriptions of a similar syndrome appeared in the literature. Although they have been given various names—among them, schizophreniform psychosis, good prognosis schizophrenia, cycloid psychosis, and reactive psychosis—their key features conform to those originally delineated by Kasanin for schizoaffective (81).

In the past, schizoaffective disorder was generally studied and classified as an atypical and milder variant of schizophrenia. More recently, however, schizoaffective disorder has been conceptualized as a more severe variant of manic–depressive illness or as a hybrid or border state between affective and schizophrenic disorders (81). These changing views are reflected in the revised version of the DSM-III, the Research Diagnostic Criteria (RDC), and the International Classification of Diseases, 10th edition (ICD-10), although each system provides a slightly different treatment of schizoaffective disorder.

Key Diagnostic Criteria

Within the DSM-III, major depression may be subclassified as psychotic when delusions, hallucinations, or depressive stupor are part of the clinical picture. Psychotic features are further categorized as mood congruent or mood incongruent.

To receive a diagnosis of psychotic depression with mood-congruent features, a patient must evidence depressive stupor or delusions and/or hallucinations with mood-congruent content (e.g., themes of personal inadequacy, guilt, punishment, nihilism). A diagnosis of psychotic depression with mood-incongruent features requires a patient to have delusions and/or hallucinations that are not consistent with the depressed mood. These include delusions of persecution or control, thought broadcasting, or thought insertion.

The DSM-III-R provides a separate category for schizoaffective disorder, which it defines as a concurrent mixture of schizophrenic and affective symptoms accompanied by a 2-week period or more of hallucinations or delusions in the absence of any affective symptoms (see Table 2). The RDC and ICD-10, on the other hand, both define schizoaffective disorder simply as a concurrent mixture of schizophrenic and affective symptoms whether or not affective or schizophrenic symptoms may have occurred alone.

The DSM-III-R then defines schizoaffective disorder closer to schizophrenia. The distinction of interepisodic thought disorder has been reported to be associated with a poorer outcome, higher relapse rates, and a more deteriorating course in patients with RDC-defined schizoaffective disorder (15,46).

Psychotic depression has been found to be a remarkably stable diagnosis in that an overwhelming percentage of previous episodes of depression in psychotic patients were also psychotic (89%: 18), as are subsequent episodes (92%: 45). Moreover, even delusional content and form tend to be similar in patients across episodes (18).

Recent studies comparing symptoms, clinical history, and background characteristics of delusional (mood-congruent) and nondelusional depressives report relatively few differences. Psychotic depressives have consistently been found to display greater psychomotor disturbance (18,23,42,67) and to have more guilt (18,23,42) and greater depressed mood (16,18,23,42). No differences between the groups have been reported in vegetative symptoms (18,42), age at onset (16,18,42,67), or number of previous episodes (16,18,70), although this last finding is inconsistent (25,42,67).

As compared to mood-congruent psychotic depressives, RDC schizoaffectives have been found to have a more acute onset, less endogenous symptomatology, and more severe delusions (36). In addition, they have been reported to have an earlier age at onset (early 20s) than bipolar I patients (86)—and thus, presumably, than nonbipolar psychotic depressives—more previous episodes than psychotic depressives (36) but not bipolar I patients (86), and to have an overall lower rate of recovery (15,24) and more residual impairment (36) than psychotic depressives. These findings, however, cannot be assumed to generalize to DSM-III mood-incongruent psychotic depressives.

Clinical Course

The clinical observations of early writers concerning the similarity of long-term outcome in delusional and nondelusional depression have received recent empirical support. Coryell and Tsuang (25) compared short-term and long-term outcome in a 40-year follow-up study of predominantly untreated psychotic and nonpsychotic depressives. They found that although significantly more nonpsychotic than psychotic patients were recovered at discharge (47% versus 34%, respectively) and at the 2- to 5-year follow-up (73% versus 47%, respectively), 10- to 20-year follow-up recovery rates did not differ between the two groups (100% versus 88%, respectively). In addition, no differences were found in long-term marital, residential, or occupational outcome ratings.

In a second follow-up study, Coryell and his associates (24) compared 6-, 12-, and 24-month recovery rates in psychotic and nonpsychotic major depressives participating in the NIMH Collaborative Study on the Psychobiology of Depression. Their findings were consistent with those previously reported: although short-term (6 months) outcome was significantly poorer in psychotic depressives, recovery rates in this group increased and ultimately equaled those in the nonpsychotic group.

In a study specifically undertaken to assess the prognostic

TABLE 2. *Definitions and classification of mixed affective and schizophrenic states*

	Concurrent depressive and schizophrenic syndrome	Schizophrenic symptoms in absence of affective symptoms plus concurrent depressive and schizophrenic syndrome at another time
DSM-III-R	Mood-incongruent psychotic depression	Schizoaffective disorder
ICD-10 (proposed)	Schizoaffective disorder	Schizoaffective disorder
RDC	Schizoaffective disorder	Schizoaffective disorder

significance of mood incongruence in psychotic depression, Coryell et al. (26) compared recovery rates in psychotic depressives with mood-congruent and mood-incongruent features. At discharge, 48% of the mood-congruent and 52% of the mood-incongruent patients treated with ECT had recovered. Among untreated patients, 22% of the mood-congruent and 31% of the mood-incongruent patients had recovered at discharge. Intermediate (2–3 years) and long-term recovery rates were also comparable in the two groups (44% versus 33% and 76% versus 71%, respectively). Thus, it appears that the presence of mood-incongruent features does not predict a poorer outcome in psychotic depression.

Treatment

The validity of the concept of psychotic or delusional depression has received empirical support from several psychopharmacological studies demonstrating a differential pattern of drug response in delusional as compared to nondelusional depressives. Reports of the diminished effectiveness of TCA in the treatment of delusional depressives appeared in the literature as early as 1959 (48). However, it was not until the publication of a study by Glassman et al. (41) in 1975 that treatment response in delusional depressives became the focus of extensive investigation. Since that time several studies have documented a marked difference in TCA response rates in delusional (20–25%) as compared to nondelusional (70–80%) depressives (16,18,66,70) and a dramatic increase in recovery rates (68–95%) in delusional patients treated with a combination of TCAs and antipsychotic medication (16,18,21,66,67,93). Comparable response rates are found for psychotic depressives treated with ECT as well (16,18,48,66), a topic discussed in the chapter by M. Fink (this volume).

Bipolar Disorder

Background

The term "bipolar disorder" was originally proposed by Leonhard (59) in 1957 to refer to "manic–depressive" illnesses characterized by both manic and depressive episodes. Based on the work of several groups of investigators, the concept of bipolar disorder has broadened in recent years to include an array of variously termed subtypes with similar clinical courses, phenomenology, family histories, and treatment responses (5,6,29,30,33,35,38). These bipolar subtypes are thought to form a spectrum or continuum of disorders that, although differing in severity, are related.

Three subclasses of bipolar disorder are generally recognized: bipolar I (coded bipolar disorder in DSM-III), which includes patients with a history of depression and mania requiring hospitalization; bipolar II (coded atypical bipolar disorder in DSM-III), which includes patients with a history of depression requiring hospitalization and hypomania requiring outpatient treatment at most; and bipolar other or cyclothymia (coded cyclothymia in DSM-III), which includes patients with a history of hypomania and depression

requiring only outpatient treatment. In addition, a bipolar III or unipolar II category has been suggested by some to include patients with a history of hospitalization for depression only who have a family history of bipolar disorder.

Key Diagnostic Criteria

A diagnosis of bipolar disorder is made on the basis of clinical history: whether a patient has had or currently has mania. Key features of mania include elevated, expansive, or irritable mood accompanied by increased activity, pressure of speech, flight of ideas, grandiosity, decreased need for sleep, and/or distractibility.

In addition to distinct manic and depressive symptom pictures, bipolar disorder may present in a mixed form in which full symptom features of both mania and major depression are intermixed or alternate rapidly.

Although the same diagnostic criteria apply for both bipolar and nonbipolar major depression, the two groups have been found to differ in some aspects of symptomatology and clinical course. Two of the most frequently cited symptomatic differences between bipolar and unipolar depressives are in psychomotor activity and sleep disturbances: bipolar depressions are more often characterized by psychomotor retardation and hypersomnia, whereas unipolar depressions are more often characterized by psychomotor agitation and hyposomnia (28). However, considerable overlap exists between the two groups with respect to these variables.

Clinical Course

It has been well established that bipolar depressives typically have an earlier age at onset and are first hospitalized at a younger age (late 20s to early 30s) than unipolar depressives (early 40s) (20,28). Some 60 to 80% of cases of bipolar disorder have been estimated to begin with an episode of mania (32). In those patients whose disorder begins with an episode of depression, the interval from first depression to first manic episode has been reported to be 1 to 2 years typically (32), although it may be as long as 10 years or more (9).

The NIMH Collaborative Study investigators have found substantial differences in course of illness among subtypes of bipolar patients (52). Patients who presented with pure depression took almost twice as long to recover from their index episodes (median 25 weeks) as patients who presented with pure mania (median 13 weeks). Length of time to recovery was by far the longest, however, in patients with mixed manic and depressive features (median 79 weeks), these taking three times longer than pure depressives and six times longer than pure manics. Recovery rates at 18 months also differed among these groups, being highest in the pure manics (93%), intermediate in the pure depressives (78%), and lowest in the mixed group (68%).

In comparisons of unipolar and bipolar depressives, NIMH Collaborative Study data indicate similar rates of recovery (22). Bipolars, however, were more likely than unipolars to have multiple subsequent episodes.

A switch to bipolar disorder in patients previously diagnosed as unipolar has been reported to occur in anywhere from 4 to 18% of depressives (20). Predictors of this switch to bipolar include early age at onset of depression (25 or younger), retarded–hypersomniac and/or psychotic symptomatology, tricyclic-induced hypomania, bipolar family history, and a history of affective disorders in consecutive generations or a loaded pedigree (9).

Treatment

Bipolar disorder has been the focus of considerable psychopharmacological research, the results of which have done much to establish the validity of the concept and expand its boundaries. The efficacy of lithium in the treatment and maintenance of bipolar disorder is well documented (19,20; also see D. L. Dunner, *this volume*). Lithium has been shown to be superior to both neuroleptics and ECT in the treatment of mania (17,44) and, when used prophylactically, to reduce the frequency and duration of both manic and, to a lesser extent, depressive episodes (34,39,47,78,82). The overall response rate to lithium in bipolar disorder is approximately 80%. Factors associated with nonresponse include rapid cycling (i.e., four or more episodes per year) (31), the presence of mixed features (91), and a negative family history of bipolar disorder (65). The presence of psychotic features is not associated with treatment failure (2,3,76,77).

For a discussion of recent research on alternative drug therapies used in the treatment of bipolar disorder, see the chapter by D. L. Dunner (*this volume*).

OTHER SPECIFIC AFFECTIVE DISORDERS

The DSM-III "other specific affective disorders" include two subcategories, cyclothymia and dysthymia. Although often grouped with personality disorders in the past, cyclothymia and dysthymia were included in the affective disorders in DSM-III because of their demonstrated similarity to the major affective syndromes and because, unlike most personality disorders, they tend not to be experienced as ego-syntonic by the patient.

Cyclothymia

Background

Kraepelin (58) was among the first writers to describe cyclothymia as one of four affective temperaments. He viewed these temperaments as both subaffective forms of and substrates for the major affective disorders. Cyclothymia consisted of alternating periods of elation and depression and was associated with manic–depressive insanity. Other temperaments, according to Kraepelin, were the dysthymic or predominantly depressed, the hyperthymic or predominantly elated, and the irritable or mixed, in which elated and depressed features intermingled.

Cyclothymia has traditionally been considered relatively rare. Recent evidence has indicated, however, that cyclo-

thymia is not uncommon among psychiatric outpatients (5,6). Furthermore, in terms of its symptomatic features, family history characteristics, course, and response to treatment, cyclothymia has been shown to be more accurately considered a variant of bipolar disorder than a deviation in personality (5,6,29,33).

Key Diagnostic Criteria

For a diagnosis of cyclothymia, the DSM-III requires a 2-year history of numerous periods of depression and hypomania that do not meet the severity and/or duration criteria for major affective disorders. The presence of these biphasic patterns has been found to be critical to the differential diagnosis of cyclothymia inasmuch as a large percentage of patients with antisocial, histrionic, and borderline personalities report frequent mood swings (5).

The results of studies conducted on outpatient cyclothymics (5) and cyclothymics identified in the general population (29) indicate that the disorder is most typically characterized by brief (2 to 6 days) periods of depression and elation, which alternate irregularly. Among the more severe patients, intervening euthymic periods were rare (fewer than 10% of cases), and transitions between episodes were frequently marked by mixed, irritable mood. Although the actual figures vary between studies, "balanced" cyclothymics have been reported to make up 50 to 60% of cases, predominantly depressed another 25 to 30%, predominantly hyperthymic some 10%, and mixed or irritable the remaining 15% (5,29).

Clinical Course

The typical age of onset reported for cyclothymia is mid- to late teens (5,29). By definition, the clinical course is chronic, with as many as 35% of outpatient cases in a 3- to 4-year follow-up period reported to develop a major affective disorder (5). A high frequency of depressive episodes (12 or more per year) has been found to be associated with a chronic, nonremitting course, an earlier age at onset, and a greater likelihood of developing major depression (29).

Treatment

Lithium has been reported to be effective in attenuating mood swings and biphasic behavioral manifestations in 60% of "seriously incapacitated" cyclothymics treated in an open clinical trial, a finding consistent with reports that lithium effectively reduces subsyndromal mood swings in bipolar patients (6).

Another report on the prophylactic effect of lithium on depressive episodes only in cyclothymia put the figure much lower. Peselow and his associates (75) found that only between 25 and 30% of patients maintained on lithium remained depression-free at 1 year. However, the added finding that the interval of time between initiation of treatment and the first recurrence of depression was shorter than that between the first and second recurrences, coupled with the fact that the majority of patients completing 2 years of follow-up showed an overall reduction in number of depressive episodes, mitigates the less than striking "recovery" rates reported. Unfortunately, no other pharmacologic studies have been published in this area.

Dysthymia (Neurotic Depression)

Background

Dysthymia was originally described by Kraepelin (58) as the basic affective temperament that formed the substrate for melancholia. A newly created category in DSM-III, dysthymia subsumes many depressions previously considered to be characterologically based and thus categorized as a form of neurosis (included under "depressive neurosis") or personality disorder (included under "cyclothymia").

Despite its parenthetic name, the concept of dysthymia is not synonymous with the concept of neurotic depression in its traditional usages (see Table 3). Many depressions previously classified as "neurotic" would, within DSM-III, be classified as major depressions without melancholic or psychotic features or as atypical depressions. Thus, only a portion of "neurotic" depressions are diagnosed dysthymia in DSM-III. In turn, dysthymia includes a portion of conditions that would previously have been classified as cyclothymia. Klerman (56) has suggested that chronic depression resulting from an incompletely remitted or poorly treated major depressive episode may account for the majority of dysthymics.

Key Diagnostic Criteria

For a diagnosis of dysthymia, the DSM-III requires at least a 2-year history of continual or numerous periods of depressive symptoms characteristic of major depression but that do not meet full severity and/or duration criteria for the syndrome.

Clinical Course

By definition, dysthymia is a chronic condition. The typical age at onset varies considerably, from the early to midteens to late life (4). Dysthymic patients are at high risk for developing subsequent major depressive episodes as well as other psychiatric disorders such as alcohol and drug dependence (4,53).

Treatment

To date, only two studies provide data bearing on the issue of pharmacological treatment of dysthymia. In open clinical studies, Akiskal et al. (7) found that 45% of dysthymics show a positive response to antidepressant therapy. Kocsis et al. (57) conducted a placebo-controlled double-blind study of a group of carefully diagnosed dysthymics treated with TCA. Following a 4-week treatment period, a significantly higher percentage of drug-treated patients were found to be recovered compared to placebo-treated patients (55% vs. 14%, respectively).

TABLE 3. *Multiple usages of the term neurotic depression*

Mild depression
Nonpsychotic depression
Nonendogenous depression
Stress-precipitated or "reactive" depression
Characterological depression
Depression resulting from unresolved unconscious conflicts

DISCUSSION

In the decade since the last publication of *Psychopharmacology: A Generation of Progress,* great advances have been made in the area of clinical psychopathology and diagnosis of affective disorders in relation to psychopharmacology. A cornerstone of this progress has been the 1980 publication of the DSM-III, which codified diagnostic categories for psychiatric disorders.

The current status of the validity of the various diagnostic categories of affective disorders, however, differs considerably. The validity and pharmacological treatment implications are clearest for bipolar disorder. Moreover, increasing evidence has accumulated over the past 10 years that there exists a spectrum of bipolar disorders, including cyclothymia and bipolar II (atypical bipolar), that share common clinical and biological features, family histories, and response to drug treatment.

With regard to major depression, the category is recognized as heterogeneous. Although melancholia is generally thought to predict a good response to TCAs, research evidence has been limited and inconsistent with regard to its validity. Psychotic depression, on the other hand, has generated considerable research interest, resulting in new approaches to diagnosis and treatment of such disorders. Even greater future advances can be anticipated as the mood-congruent and mood-incongruent subtypes are examined more closely.

Several investigators have made recent attempts at further subtyping major depression. It remains for future investigators to evaluate the utility of these systems.

Klein and his associates (55,60) have proposed a classification system of major depressions that includes among its subtypes endogenomorphic depression and hysteroid dysphoria. According to Klein's schema, these depressions can be differentiated on the basis of symptoms, response to pharmacological treatment, and presumed etiology. Endogenomorphic depressions are distinguished by nonreactivity to environmental events and a pervasive inability to experience pleasure. Typical vegetative symptoms—insomnia with early morning awakening, morning worsening, and appetite loss—are also characteristic of such depressions. Klein has hypothesized that endogenomorphic depressions arise from a dysfunction of the brain's "pleasure center" and are highly responsive to TCAs.

Hysteroid dysphoria is characterized by reactive mood and extreme fatigue and is associated with atypical vegetative symptoms—hypersomnia with initial insomnia, evening worsening, and hyperphagia. It has been proposed that rejection sensitivity—extreme sensitivity to interpersonal rejection—plays a role in precipitating hysteroid dysphorias and that such depressions are responsive to MAOIs.

Winokur (96) and his associates (97) have proposed a subclassification of unipolar depressive disorders based on family psychiatric history. They describe three groups: (a) familial pure depressive disease (FPDD), in which depressed patients have a history of depression (nonbipolar) in a first-degree relative; (b) depressive spectrum disease (DSD), in which depressed patients have a history of alcoholism and/or antisocial personality in a first-degree relative (depression may be present as well); and (c) sporadic depressive disease (SDD), in which a depressed patient has a negative family history of psychiatric illness. Several characteristics including clinical history, course, and background have been reported to differentiate these groups. A positive family history (i.e., FPDD and DSD groups) has been found to be associated with a more unstable premorbid personality (12,13,95). With regard to clinical history and course, SDD patients have been found to have an age at onset averaging 8 years later than PDD and DSD, DSD patients have been found to have more previous episodes, and PDD patients have been found to have more relapses and to be more likely to develop a chronic course (95). However, no significant symptomological differences among the groups have been reported (12,13,74,95,97).

To date, little is known about dysthymia in terms of its utility as a category of affective disorders and its pharmacological implications. Akiskal (4) has proposed a classification system that subdivides dysthymia into three groups. The first is a group of late-onset primary depressives in whom dysthymia represents residual chronicity of primary major depression. A second group of dysthymics identified by Akiskal are patients in whom dysthymia is secondary to an incapacitating physical or nonaffective psychiatric disorder. Age at onset in this group is variable, and the course of the dysthymic disorder follows the course of the primary disorder. The third group of dysthymics, termed "characterological depressions" by Akiskal, are patients in whom dysthymia appears to be temperamentally or characterologically based. In this group, dysthymia has an early and insidious onset and a fluctuating course.

Akiskal further subdivides characterological depressions into "character spectrum" disorders and "subaffective dysthymic" disorders. According to his and his colleagues' research findings (7,8,87), these groups can be differentiated on the basis of personality, family history, and pharmacological variables. Thus, character spectrum disorders have dependent, histrionic, or sociopathic personalities, family histories of alcoholism, do not show TCA-induced hypomania, and are not responsive to pharmacological treatments. Subaffective dysthymias, on the other hand, evidence the classic Schneiderian depressive personality (e.g., nonassertive, brooding, pessimistic, self-critical), have family histories of affective disorders (both unipolar and bipolar), often respond to TCAs with brief hypomanic swings, and frequently demonstrate a good response to lithium or TCAs. Although future research is clearly needed to establish the validity of Akiskal's system, his subclassification of dysthymia represents a major advance in our understanding of the disorder.

In addition to the progress that has been made in specific areas of clinical diagnosis and psychopathology, the past 10 years have witnessed heightened awareness on the part of the psychiatric researcher of the importance of diagnostic rigor and external correlates in establishing the validity of subclasses of psychiatric disorders (85). This, in turn, has led to a more orderly progression of investigatory efforts. Given this and the availability of a reliable diagnostic system, even greater advances in subtyping of affective disorders for prediction of drug response can be anticipated in the next 10 years.

Specific areas that merit the attention of psychopharmacological researchers include the subclinical affective disorders cyclothymia and dysthymia. Little is known about drug treatment of either of these disorders, and dysthymia, in particular, appears to be a heterogeneous category in need of further subdivision.

Another direction for future research lies in comparison of the psychotic subtypes of affective disorders—mood congruent, mood incongruent, and schizoaffective—in terms of an analysis of effective pharmacological treatment and the clinical psychopathology that differentiates the subgroups and predicts drug response.

Finally, despite years of research, knowledge is limited concerning the prediction of response to pharmacotherapy of nonbipolar, nonpsychotic major depressions. Continued efforts to subtype these disorders are clearly needed.

REFERENCES

1. Aarons, S. F., Frances, A. J., and Mann, J. J. (1985): *Hosp. Commun. Pract.*, 36:275–282.
2. Abrams, R., and Taylor, M. A. (1976): *Am. J. Psychiatry*, 133:1445–1447.
3. Abrams, R., and Taylor, M. A. (1981): *Am. J. Psychiatry*, 138:658–661.
4. Akiskal, H. S. (1983): *Am. J. Psychiatry*, 140:11–20.
5. Akiskal, H. S., Djenderdjian, A. H., Rosenthal, R. H., and Khani, M. K. (1977): *Am. J. Psychiatry*, 134:1227–1233.
6. Akiskal, H. S., Khani, M. K., and Scott-Strauss, A. (1979): *Psychiatr. Clin. North Am.*, 2:527–554.
7. Akiskal, H. S., King, D., Rosenthal, T. L., Robinson, D., and Scott-Strauss, A. (1981): *J. Affect. Disorders*, 3:297–315.
8. Akiskal, H. S., Rosenthal, T. L., Haykal, R. F., Lemmi, H., Rosenthal, R. H., et al. (1980): *Arch. Gen. Psychiatry*, 37:777–783.
9. Akiskal, H. S., Walker, P., Puzantian, V. R., King, D., Rosenthal, T. L., et al. (1983): *J. Affect. Disorders*, 5:115–128.
10. Andreason, N. C., and Grove, W. M. (1982): *Am. J. Psychiatry*, 139:45–52.
11. Angst, J., Frey, R., Lohmeyer, B., and Zerbin-Rudin, E. (1966): *Hum. Genet.*, 55:237–254.
12. Behar, D., Winokur, G., Van Valkenburg, C., and Lowry, M. (1980): *J. Clin. Psychiatry*, 41:52–56.
13. Behar, D., Winokur, G., Van Valkenburg, C., Lowry, M., and Lachenbruck, P. A. (1981): *Neuropsychobiology*, 7:179–184.
14. Bielski, R. J., and Friedel, R. O. (1976): *Arch. Gen. Psychiatry*, 33:1479–1489.
15. Brockington, I. F., Kendell, R. E., and Wainwright, S. (1980): *Psychol. Med.*, 10:665–675.
16. Brown, R. P., Frances, A., Kocsis, J. H., and Mann, J. J. (1982): *J. Nerv. Ment. Dis.*, 170:635–637.
17. Carroll, B. J. (1979): *Arch. Gen. Psychiatry*, 36:870–878.
18. Charney, D. S., and Nelson, J. C. (1981): *Am. J. Psychiatry*, 138:328–333.
19. Clayton, P. J. (1978): *Am. J. Psychotherapy*, 32:81–92.
20. Clayton, P. J. (1981): *Comp. Psychiatry*, 22:31–43.
21. Clower, C. G. (1983): *J. Clin. Psychiatry*, 44:216–218.
22. Coryell, W., Andreasen, N. C., Endicott, J., and Keller, M. (1987): *Am. J. Psychiatry* (in press).

23. Coryell, W., Endicott, J., Keller, M., and Andreason, N. C. (1985): *J. Affect. Disorders, 9*:13–18.
24. Coryell, W., Lavori, P., Endicott, J., Keller, M., and VanEerdewegh, M. (1984): *Arch. Gen. Psychiatry, 41*:787–791.
25. Coryell, W., and Tsuang, M. T. (1982): *Arch. Gen. Psychiatry, 39*: 1181–1184.
26. Coryell, W., Tsuang, M. T., and McDaniel, J. (1982): *J. Affect. Disorders, 4*:227–236.
27. Davidson, J. R. T., Miller, R. D., Turnbull, C. D., and Sullivan, J. L. (1982): *Arch. Gen. Psychiatry, 39*:527–534.
28. Depue, R. A., and Monroe, S. M. (1978): *Psychol. Bull., 85*:1001–1029.
29. Depue, R. A., Slater, J. F., Wolfstetter-Kausch, H., Klein, D., Goplerud, E., and Farr, D. (1981): *J. Abnorm. Psychol., 90*:381–437.
30. Dunner, D. L. (1983): *Psychiatr. Dev., 1*:75–86.
31. Dunner, D. L., and Fieve, R. R. (1974): *Arch. Gen. Psychiatry, 30*:229–233.
32. Dunner, D. L., Fleiss, J. L., and Fieve, R. R. (1976): *Am. J. Psychiatry, 133*:905–908.
33. Dunner, D. L., Russek, F. D., Russek, B., and Fieve, R. R. (1982): *Comp. Psychiatry, 23*:186–189.
34. Dunner, D. L., Stallone, F., and Fieve, R. R. (1976): *Arch. Gen. Psychiatry, 33*:117–120.
35. Endicott, J., Nee, J., Andreason, N., Clayton, P., Keller, M., et al. (1985): *J. Affect. Disorders, 8*:17–28.
36. Endicott, J., and Spitzer, R. L. (1979): *Am. J. Psychiatry, 136*:52–56.
37. Feinberg, M., and Carroll, B. J. (1982): *Br. J. Psychiatry, 140*: 384–391.
38. Fieve, R. R., and Dunner, D. L. (1975): In: *The Nature and Treatment of Depression,* edited by F. Flach and S. Draghi, pp. 145–166. John Wiley & Sons, New York.
39. Fieve, R. R., Kumbaraci, T., and Dunner, D. L. (1976): *Am. J. Psychiatry, 133*:925–929.
40. Gillespie, R. D. (1929): *Guy's Hosp. Rep., 79*:306–344.
41. Glassman, A. H., Kantor, S. J., and Shostak, M. (1975): *Am. J. Psychiatry, 132*:716–719.
42. Glassman, A. H., and Roose, S. P. (1981): *Arch. Gen. Psychiatry, 38*:424–427.
43. Glen, A. T. M., Johnson, A. L., and Shepard, M. (1984): *Psychol. Med., 14*:37–50.
44. Goodwin, F. K., and Zis, A. P. (1979): *Arch. Gen. Psychiatry, 36*: 840–844.
45. Helms, P. H., and Smith, R. E. (1983): *J. Affect. Disorders, 5*:51–54.
46. Himmelhoch, J. M., Fuchs, C. Z., May, S. J., Symons, B. J., and Neil, J. F. (1981): *J. Nerv. Ment. Dis., 169*:277–282.
47. Kane, J. M., Quitkin, F. M., Rifkin, A., Ramos-Lorenzi, J., Nayak, D. D., et al. (1982): *Arch. Gen. Psychiatry, 39*:1065–1069.
48. Kantor, S. J., and Glassman, A. H. (1977): *Br. J. Psychiatry, 131*: 351–360.
49. Kasanin, J. (1933): *Am. J. Psychiatry, 13*:97–126.
50. Katz, M. M., and Hirschfeld, R. M. A. (1978): In: *Psychopharmacology: A Generation of Progress,* edited by M. A. Lipton, A. DiMascio, and K. F. Killam, pp. 1185–1195. Raven Press, New York.
51. Keller, M. B., Klerman, G. L., Lavori, P. W., Coryell, W., Endicott, J., et al. (1984): *J.A.M.A., 252*:788–792.
52. Keller, M. B., Lavori, P., Coryell, W., Andreasen, N. C., Endicott, J., et al. (1986): *JAMA, 255*:3138–3142.
53. Keller, M. B., Lavori, P. W., Endicott, J., Coryell, W., and Klerman, G. L. (1983): *Am. J. Psychiatry, 140*:689–694.
54. Kendall, R. E. (1976): *Br. J. Psychiatry, 129*:15–28.
55. Klein, D. F. (1974): *Arch. Gen. Psychiatry, 1*:447–454.
56. Klerman, G. L. (1980): In: *Comprehensive Textbook of Psychiatry,* edited by H. I. Kaplan, A. M. Freedman, and B. J. Sadock, pp. 1332–1337. William & Wilkins, Baltimore.
57. Kocsis, J. H., Frances, A., Mann, J. J., Sweeney, J., Voss, C., et al. (1985): *Psychopharmacol. Bull., 21*:698–700.
58. Kraepelin, E. (1921): *Manic-Depressive Insanity and Paranoia.* E. and S. Livingstone, Edinburgh.
59. Leonhard, K. (1957): *Aufteilung Der Endogenen Psychosen.* Akademieverlag, Berlin.
60. Liebowitz, M. R., and Klein, D. F. (1979): *Psychiatr. Clin. North Am., 2*:555–575.
61. Liebowitz, M. R., Quitkin, F. M., Stewart, J. W., McGrath, P. J., Harrison, W., et al. (1984): *Arch. Gen. Psychiatry, 41*:669–677.
62. Matussek, P., Luks, O., and Nagel, D. (1982): *Psychol. Med., 12*: 765–773.
63. Matussek, P., Soldner, M., and Nagel, D. (1981): *Br. J. Psychiatry, 138*:361–372.
64. Mendels, J., and Cochrane, C. (1968): *Am. J. Psychiatry, 124*:1–11.
65. Mendlewicz, J., Fieve, R. R., and Stallone, F. (1973): *Am. J. Psychiatry, 130*:1011–1013.
66. Minter, R. E., and Mandel, M. R. (1979): *J. Nerv. Ment. Dis., 167*:726–733.
67. Nelson, J. C., and Bowers, M. B. (1978): *Arch. Gen. Psychiatry, 35*:1321–1328.
68. Nelson, J. C., Charney, D. S., and Quinlan, D. M. (1981): *Arch. Gen. Psychiatry, 38*:555–559.
69. Nelson, J. C., and Mazure, C. (1985): *J. Affect. Disorders, 9*:41–46.
70. Nelson, W. H., Khan, A., and Orr, W. W. (1984): *J. Affect. Disorders, 6*:297–306.
71. Paykel, E. S., Parker, R. R., Rowan, P. R., Rao, B. M., and Taylor, C. N. (1983): *Psychol. Med., 13*:131–139.
72. Paykel, E. S., Rowan, P. R., Parker, R. R., and Bhat, A. V. (1982): *Arch. Gen. Psychiatry, 39*:1041–1049.
73. Perris, C. (1966): *Acta Psychiatr. Scand. [Suppl.], 194*:15–44.
74. Perris, H., Eisemann, M., Ericsson, U., Knorring, L. Von, and Perris, C. (1983): *Neuropsychobiology, 9*:103–107.
75. Peselow, E. D., Dunner, D. L., Fieve, R. R., and Loutin, A. (1981): *Comp. Psychiatry, 22*:257–264.
76. Pope, H. G., and Lipinski, J. F. (1978): *Arch. Gen. Psychiatry, 35*: 811–828.
77. Pope, H. G., Lipinski, J. F., Cohen, B. M., and Axelrod, D. T. (1980): *Am. J. Psychiatry, 137*:921–927.
78. Prien, R. F., Klett, C. J., and Caffey, E. M. (1974): *Am. J. Psychiatry, 131*:198–203.
79. Prien, R. F., and Kupfer, D. J. (1986): *Am. J. Psychiatry, 143*:18–23.
80. Prien, R. F., Kupfer, D. J., Mansky, P. A., Small, J. G., Tuason, V. B., et al. (1984): *Arch. Gen. Psychiatry, 41*:1096–1104.
81. Procci, W. R. (1976): *Arch. Gen. Psychiatry, 33*:1167–1178.
82. Quitkin, F., Rifkin, A., and Klein, D. F. (1976): *Arch. Gen. Psychiatry, 33*:337–341.
83. Rao, V. A. R., and Coppen, A. (1979): *Psychol. Med., 9*:321–325.
84. Ravaris, C. L., Robinson, D. S., Ives, J. O., Nies, A., and Bartlett, D. (1980): *Arch. Gen. Psychiatry, 37*:1075–1080.
85. Robins, E., and Guze, S. B. (1970): *Am. J. Psychiatry, 126*:107–111.
86. Rosenthal, N. E., Rosenthal, L. N., Stallone, F., Dunner, D. L., and Fieve, R. R. (1980): *Arch. Gen. Psychiatry, 37*:804–810.
87. Rosenthal, T. L., Akiskal, H. S., Scott-Strauss, A., Rosenthal, R. H., and David, M. (1981): *J. Affect. Disorders, 13*:183–192.
88. Roth, M., and Barnes, T. R. E. (1981): *Comp. Psychiatry, 22*:54–77.
89. Rowan, P. R., Paykel, E. S., and Parker, R. R. (1982): *Br. J. Psychiatry, 140*:475–483.
90. Schou, M. (1979): *Arch. Gen. Psychiatry, 36*:849–851.
91. Secunda, S. K., Katz, M. M., Swann, A., Koslow, S. H., Maas, J. W., et al. (1985): *J. Affect. Disorders, 8*:113–121.
92. Sovner, R. D. (1981): *J. Clin. Psychiatry, 42*:285–289.
93. Spiker, D. G., Weiss, J. C., Dealy, R. S., Griffin, S. J., Hanin, I., et al. (1985): *Am. J. Psychiatry, 142*:430–436.
94. van Praag, H. M. (1982): *Comp. Psychiatry, 23*:315–329.
95. Van Valkenburg, C., Lowry, M., Winokur, G., and Cadoret, R. (1977): *J. Nerv. Ment. Dis., 165*:341–347.
96. Winokur, G. (1979): *Arch. Gen. Psychiatry, 36*:47–52.
97. Winokur, G., Behar, D., Van Valkenburg, C., and Lowry, M. (1978): *J. Nerv. Ment. Dis., 166*:764–768.
98. Zis, A. P., and Goodwin, F. K. (1979): *Arch. Gen. Psychiatry, 36*: 835–839.

Psychopharmacology:
The Third Generation of Progress,
edited by Herbert Y. Meltzer.
Raven Press, New York © 1987.

CHAPTER **104**

Pharmacologic Treatment of Acute Depressive Subtypes

Andrew W. Brotman, William E. Falk, and Alan J. Gelenberg

This chapter on the drug treatment of acute depression is a guide for the research-oriented psychiatrist, with particular emphasis on efficacy data and methodological issues of pharmacologic treatments within depressive subtypes.

Although the DSM-III criteria have probably been most frequently used for diagnosis of depression by American psychiatrists since 1980, certain subtypes such as "atypical depression" are more often used to describe entities that are different from those defined by DSM-III. A useful summary of the controversies and confusion in the classification of depression can be found in a recent review article by Sinaikin (1) and in the chapter by R. M. A. Hirshfeld and C. K. Cross (*this volume*).

We have chosen to address our discussion to issues of classification and treatment in five general subtypes of depression frequently cited in the literature: (a) major depression with melancholic or endogenous features, (b) major depression without melancholia/atypical depression, (c) major depression with psychotic features, (d) bipolar depression, and (e) dysthymic disorder. We then conclude with a discussion of "treatment-resistant" depression.

GENERAL CONSIDERATIONS AND METHODOLOGIC ISSUES

Table 1 reviews the relative anticholinergic potency of the heterocyclic antidepressants, the serotonergic versus noradrenergic reuptake inhibition effect, and the efficacy of these drugs as evaluated by comparison to placebo in controlled studies and/or in comparison to a standard antidepressant (usually imipramine or amitriptyline). Al-

though these medications are consistently superior to placebo for the short-term treatment of nonpsychotic major depressive disorder, they are limited in their efficacy. The response rate from all controlled studies of imipramine averages 65% compared to a placebo response of 30% (2). Controlled trials of all heterocyclic antidepressants for various subtypes of major depression have shown an average response rate of 65 to 75% compared to a 20 to 40% placebo response rate after 1 month of treatment (3). Certain methodological features of these studies have an impact on the results, so these response rates may not match the results a clinician achieves in his or her own office. In general, the more severe the depression (excluding psychotic subtypes), the better an antidepressant will look against placebo.

Several factors must be kept in mind when one tries to interpret the response rates cited above. Virtually all of these studies are relatively short in duration (4 to 6 weeks). Most use the Hamilton rating scale for depression as the outcome measure, and the majority consider a 50% reduction in the Hamilton scale as a definition for improvement. These studies rarely provide information about duration of improvement, rates of relapse, or long-term follow-up.

This research definition of improvement may not translate into a degree of clinical improvement that a clinician or his patient would consider satisfactory: a 50% reduction in a Hamilton rating score can still leave the subject with clinically significant symptoms. By and large, few clinicians would consider an episode remitted unless the Hamilton rating score was well below 10. Further, most researchers only analyze data obtained from patients who have completed a study, and they may not report how many patients

TABLE 1. *Heterocyclic antidepressants*[a]

Name	Anticholinergic effect	Serotonin reuptake inhibition	Norepinephrine reuptake inhibition	Number of + studies vs. placebo	Number of + studies vs. imi or ami
Imipramine	++	+	++	30/44	—
Amitriptyline	+++	++	++	9/11	7/7
Desipramine	+	±	+++	3/5	6/7
Nortriptyline	+	±	++	4/4	0/0
Protriptyline	+++	±	+++	2/2	2/2
Trimipramine	++	0	±	1/1	2/2
Maprotiline	±	0	++	2/4	10/10
Doxepin	++	±	+	2/2	3/3
Trazedone	0	+	0	10/13	19/21
Amoxapine	+	+	++	3/6	15/19
Nomifensine	±	0	+++	3/3	7/8

[a] A "+" study is defined as being statistically significant in a controlled trial versus placebo or a standard TCA. Adapted from Davis (2) and Cole and Schatzberg (119).

needed to be screened for each patient entered. Dropouts are frequently not included in the analysis of efficacy, and this would most likely yield an overestimation of drug efficacy.

Drug efficacy interpretation can also be confounded by relatively brief drug trials (4 weeks or less), which may not do justice to the efficacy of the antidepressants. Quitkin's work on the duration of antidepressant drug treatment suggests that a minimum therapeutic trial should be 6 weeks, since significant improvement takes place between 4 and 6 weeks (4).

Dosage is another important concern before a conclusion can be reached about the efficacy of a drug. Many controlled studies use low to moderate dosages, which may be recommended by the *Physicians' Desk Reference* but are no longer considered adequate by most investigators. Only recently have plasma blood levels been used in studies.

Selection factors may skew the research population compared to the patients seen in practice. Most controlled studies exclude patients who have not responded to antidepressants in the past. Also, in recent years, most trials have involved mildly to moderately depressed outpatients rather than the more severely depressed inpatients. Studies rarely provide data on duration of improvement, relapse rates, or long-term follow-up.

Overall, most controlled studies of an active antidepressant versus placebo in patients with carefully diagnosed major depressive disorder, particularly with melancholic features, show that twice as many patients respond to the active drug as to placebo. However, if one takes into account patients who drop out because of side effects, it is not uncommon for half of a depressed study population not to respond to or be able to tolerate a trial of antidepressant medication.

PLASMA LEVEL MONITORING

There has been much discussion about the use of routine monitoring of plasma levels of tricyclic antidepressants with the hope that a therapeutic plasma range could be established for each medication. This would allow for precise dosing, taking into account individual variations of metabolism.

A recent American Psychiatric Association Task Force report (5) reviewed the evidence on tricyclic antidepressant blood level measurements and provided some clinical recommendations. They concluded that reliable data have been accumulated on only imipramine, nortriptyline, and, to a lesser extent, desipramine. There seems to be a linear relationship between plasma level and clinical response for imipramine and a "therapeutic window" or curvilinear relationship between plasma level and clinical response for nortriptyline. The Task Force recommended plasma level measurements for these medications only in "problem" patients who do not respond to usual oral doses or in high-risk patients who need to be treated with the lowest possible effective dose.

The Task Force did not endorse routine monitoring of plasma levels. They cautioned that even with the best-studied drugs, imipramine and nortriptyline, the data are primarily from endogenously depressed inpatient samples, and there are little data from outpatients with nonendogenous or moderate depression. Table 2 outlines usual oral dose ranges and preliminary evidence on therapeutic plasma concentrations.

There is little evidence to suggest that the newer, second-generation antidepressants have any greater efficacy than the tricyclics, although side effect profiles sometimes differ from those of tricyclics (6). Initial claims by several of the manufacturers of second-generation antidepressants about increased efficacy or faster onset of action have not been proven (3). Further, there has been no clear difference in drug efficacy or selectivity between more selective serotonin reuptake inhibitors and norepinephrine reuptake inhibitors, although this work is preliminary and under active investigation (7).

The MAO inhibitors (more fully discussed in another chapter in this book and in this chapter under atypical nonendogenous depression) are effective agents and do show efficacy for melancholic depression (8–10). As a class, the MAOIs are generally believed to be less effective than

TABLE 2. *Adult dosages and suggested therapeutic plasma level ranges for tricyclic antidepressants[a]*

Generic name	Initial dose (mg/day)	Dosage range (mg/day)	Suggested therapeutic plasma range (ng/day)
Imipramine	50	50–300	200–300[b]
Amitriptyline	50	50–300	150–250[b,c]
Desipramine	50	50–300	150–300[c]
Nortriptyline	25	30–100	50–150[c]
Protriptyline	10	50–60	70–240[c]
Maprotiline	50	50–250	—[c]
Doxepin	50	50–300	110–250[b,c]
Trazodone	50	150–400	—[c]
Amoxapine	150	50–600	—[c]
Nomifensine	100	100–300	—[c]

[a] Adapted from Cole and Schatzberg (119).
[b] Drug and metabolite.
[c] Data insufficient.

the tricyclic antidepressants in endogenous depression, but this conclusion may be biased by the fact that early studies with MAOIs used relatively low dosages (2). They may in fact be superior to TCAs in depressed patients with concomitant marked anxiety or panic symptoms. Most authorities consider the heterocyclic antidepressants the treatment of choice in endogenous depression, with the MAO inhibitors being held as second-line agents for nonresponders.

Electroconvulsive therapy (ECT) is at least as effective a treatment for melancholic depression as the antidepressants and maybe more so. At least half of patients who do not respond to heterocyclic antidepressants or MAOIs may respond to ECT (2).

Despite the limitations of pharmacotherapy and psychotherapy, the morbidity and mortality associated with major depression support the urgency of aggressive treatment. Unfortunately, recent reports suggest that only a low proportion of depressed people receive intensive treatment with either medication or electroconvulsive therapy, even among patients who are severely depressed and have a long duration of illness (11).

BIOLOGICAL TESTS AS PREDICTORS OF ANTIDEPRESSANT RESPONSE

Psychiatry's continuing search for biological markers in affective illness has been likened by Klerman to the search for the Holy Grail. Unfortunately, as of this writing, definitive biological markers continue to elude us.

Perhaps the greatest hope for a biological marker of depression was pinned on the dexamethasone suppression test (DST), which promised to open up a neuroendocrine window for clinically relevant viewing. Arana, Baldessarini, and Ornsteen conducted an extensive literature review of studies involving the DST, particularly its relevance to biological treatments of depression (12). Of 513 subjects in 18 studies, depressed patients with an initially positive DST

(i.e., nonsuppression cortisol pattern) had a treatment response rate of 81.6% versus 73.5% for those with a negative DST. When the authors focused on the eight most rigorously designed of these studies, the respective treatment response rates dropped to 75.5% and 64.4%. Both differences are significant statistically (because of the large sample sizes) but clinically modest, particularly when contrasted with the ability of clinical interviewing to predict treatment response.

These reviewers emphasize that there can be no justification for withholding vigorous antidepressant treatment from patients with initially negative DSTs. Additionally, the presence of a positive DST cannot determine the nature of biological antidepressant therapy, since some types of depression (e.g., psychotic depression, bipolar depression) may respond preferentially to other than tricyclic antidepressant drugs alone. The authors do suggest that a positive DST might weigh on the side of biological antidepressant therapy in cases in which there are some clinical suggestions of depression or where diagnostic ambiguity or concomitant illnesses may cloud the picture.

Another avenue of investigation that has consumed much time and energy concerns neurotransmitter metabolite concentrations as predictors of antidepressant response. One of the most elegant and attractive hypotheses in this area was expounded by Maas (13) in 1975. He postulated the existence of two fundamental subtypes of depression: one primarily deficient in cerebral norepinephrine, the other in serotonin. Unfortunately, a recent NIMH collaborative study failed to confirm the essence of this hypothesis (14). However, they did find that among 104 depressives, normal values for urinary norepinephrine and low values for urinary MHPG were associated with a greater incidence of drug response (imipramine and amitriptyline) in bipolar but not unipolar patients and that for unipolars (but not bipolars), low CSF levels of 5-HIAA and high urinary metanephrine concentrations were associated with a greater incidence of drug response (14). Other studies failed to find that low pretreatment urinary MHPG excretion predicted a positive response to imipramine or desipramine (15) or that depressed patients with normal or high urinary MHPG levels were more likely to improve in response to amitriptyline (16). Similarly, a study of RDC-diagnosed unipolar depressed inpatients failed to find that urinary MHPG predicted clinical response to the noradrenergic antidepressants imipramine and maprotiline, although the authors observed that most positive studies involved bipolar patients (17).

So far there have been no consistent correlations between changes in CSF MHPG concentrations and the treatment response of patients on long-term antidepressants (18). Depressed patients with low CSF concentrations of 5-HIAA, who have been reported to show an increased incidence of suicide, might be thought to respond to selective serotonin uptake inhibitors, but data so far are inconclusive (19). In fact, CSF concentrations of 5-HIAA reportedly decrease in depressed patients taking a wide variety of antidepressant drugs whether or not the depression improves (18).

Abnormal sleep patterns have also been recognized as symptoms of depression. Frank and co-workers found that patients with recurrent major depression who responded poorly to imipramine treatment tended to have a greater delay in sleep onset than imipramine responders (20). Also, slow responders to imipramine treatment and nonresponders had a lower density of REM sleep in all-night polysomnographic recordings. In addition, the investigators found that patients responsive to antidepressant treatment had higher serum cortisol concentrations during sleep.

The most frequent abnormality in major depression is a blunted thyroid-stimulating hormone (TSH) response to thyroid-releasing hormone (TRH) infusion. A Danish group reported that patients whose TRH tests fail to normalize were at a greater risk for relapse (27), and Frank et al. observed that slow responders differed from both normal responders and nonresponders by having a more robust TSH response to an infusion of TRH (19).

Ostrow and colleagues have predicted that the genetically determined rate of removal of lithium from the red blood cell via the sodium-dependent efflux pathway might ultimately be used to predict which depressed patients will respond preferentially to tricyclic or lithium treatment (22). Pharmacologic challenge tests have constituted another area of interest, with some investigators proposing that response to a stimulant might distinguish between patients more likely to respond to one versus another antidepressant drug (22).

TREATMENT OF ENDOGENOUS/ MELANCHOLIC DEPRESSION

Approximately 60% of depressed inpatients who meet DSM-III criteria for major depressive disorder have significant endogenous or melancholic symptoms (24). There is consistent evidence that the presence of melancholic symptoms predicts a positive response to tricyclic antidepressants and to electroconvulsive therapy and a more negative response to psychotherapy alone (25).

The treatment of choice for an acute episode of major depression with melancholic features and without psychosis is a trial of a tricyclic antidepressant. Bielski and Friedel's (24) review of predictors of response to tricyclic antidepressants confirms the view that these agents are most efficacious in endogenous depression compared to other subtypes of depression. Although the majority of studies have supported their conclusion (26,27), this distinction has not held up in all clinical trials (28,29). Nonetheless, Baldessarini has concluded that melancholic or endogenomorphic acute depression is the most favorable predictor of a response to antidepressants, particularly tricyclics (3).

In a recent review, Nelson and Charney (30) further broke down melancholic/endogenous depressions into two general groups: a retarded, anhedonic cluster and an agitated, delusional cluster. They concluded that the retarded cluster seems most responsive to tricyclic antidepressants and that these patients' symptoms may worsen with antipsychotic drug treatment. However, the agitated, delusional type of depression may not respond to tricyclic drugs alone but may require the concurrent use of antipsychotic agents or electroconvulsive therapy. A discussion of treatment for this latter form of depression is presented later in this chapter.

Avery and colleagues recently reviewed individual symptoms that have been correlated with a tricyclic responsiveness (32). Consistent with Nelson's observations, psychomotor retardation seems to be a consistent positive predictor, as are emotional withdrawal and loss of interest in usual activities. Although sleep and appetite disturbances are prominent in endogenous/melancholic depression, these symptoms are also found in nonendogenous depression (albeit in opposite form, i.e., hyperphagia and hypersomnia), and therefore, their predictive value of tricyclic responsiveness is equivocal (30).

Symptoms predicting a poor response to tricyclic antidepressants alone include the presence of delusions, neurotic features, hypochondriacal features, and hysterical personality traits (31). A long duration of present illness or multiple previous depressive episodes may also be poor prognostic signs (25).

MAJOR DEPRESSION WITH PSYCHOTIC FEATURES

There appear to be three viewpoints on the nature of psychotic depression, each with major treatment implications: psychotic depression is a severe form of major depressive disorder; psychotic depression is a discrete clinical entity; and psychotic depression is related to bipolar illness.

In a study of 253 patients with primary and secondary affective illness, Guze and associates found support for the severity theory (32). Psychotically depressed patients were indistinguishable from the nonpsychotic group on demographic, family history, or associated symptom variables. Since such differences would be expected if these subtypes were separate clinical entities, they concluded that major depression with psychotic features was a severe form of affective disorder.

Treatment response characteristics of psychotically depressed patients were studied by Quitkin and associates

(33). They found that such patients could be treated with tricyclic antidepressant medication alone, although higher doses and longer treatment duration were required for a successful outcome. Their results also support the severity theory of psychotic depression. Other investigators (34,35) have similarly concluded that depression with psychotic features represents a severe form of major depressive disorder.

Proponents of the view that psychotic depression is a separate clinical entity note that Guze and his associates did not determine whether the presence of psychotic features had an effect on treatment outcome or biological parameters (36). Glassman and colleagues were also critical of Quitkin's methodology, particularly the lack of a rigorous definition of psychosis (37). They further suggested that psychotic depression was usually unresponsive to tricyclic antidepressants alone but that the combination of a tricyclic plus an antipsychotic agent or the use of electroconvulsive therapy was the treatment of choice. Agreeing with this observation, Nelson and Bowers argued that tricyclic agents, used alone, could worsen the psychotic symptoms (38).

If psychotic depression is a separate entity, it would be expected to "run true" in patients and their families. Charney and Nelson found that many depressed patients who had psychotic features during their index episode had experienced very similar psychotic symptoms during previous episodes and that depressed patients without psychotic features were generally free of psychotic symptoms in previous episodes (39), findings prospectively confirmed by Helms and Smith (40). Leckman and colleagues found that a high percentage of depressed relatives of delusionally depressed probands manifest the delusional form of major depressive disorder. They concluded that their data support the contention that delusional depression is a valid if not totally discrete subtype of depression (41). In the largest prospective double-blind treatment study to date, Spiker and colleagues clearly demonstrated the superiority of amitriptyline plus perphenazine compared to the use of either agent alone. The combination provided a positive response in 78% of patients, with amitriptyline and perphenazine alone showing 41% and 19% response rates, respectively (42). The treatment outcome, course, and family history studies cited above support the view that psychotic depression is a separate entity.

In addition, biological studies have demonstrated that psychotically depressed patients have distinct characteristics compared to nonpsychotic depressives. These include significantly lower serum dopamine-β-hydroxylase activity (43), significantly lower urinary 3-methoxy-4-hydroxy phenethyleneglycol (MHPG), higher cerebrospinal fluid homovanillic acid (HVA) (44), and very high postdexamethasone cortisol levels (45).

The third alternative—that psychotic depression is related to bipolar disorder—is suggested by Weissman and colleagues, who found that the relatives of probands with psychotic depression had a sixfold higher incidence of bipolar disorder than the relatives of unipolar depressives without psychosis or than normal controls (46). Coryell also found that at 40-year follow-up, psychotically depressed patients more often developed manic symptoms than nonpsychotic patients (47). Additional support for this

thesis comes from Price and colleagues, who described six patients with psychotic depression refractory to a combination of tricyclic and antipsychotic agents: five of the six had a beneficial response when lithium carbonate was added to the treatment (48). No firm conclusions can be made from these studies, but they do suggest that psychotic depression in some individuals may be related to bipolar disorder.

From the data presented, we conclude that depression with mood-congruent psychotic features could be a heterogeneous disorder, with treatment response partially determining the subtype. Regretfully, there are no current means to predict which patients would respond to antidepressants alone. Therefore, the combination of an antipsychotic and an antidepressant, having an approximate 80% response rate, probably is the treatment of choice (35). Patients unresponsive to therapeutic dosages of the combination for 3 to 4 weeks should be given lithium augmentation, particularly if there is a family history of bipolar illness. A recent paper also reported on a case of psychotic depression unresponsive to an antidepressant, a neuroleptic, and lithium that did remit with carbamazepine (49).

Electroconvulsive therapy (ECT) provides a response rate at least as high as the combination of an antidepressant and an antipsychotic, but the relapse rate is also high, even for patients maintained on medication after remission (42). However, it remains an effective treatment for patients who fail to improve on medication and is the treatment of choice in patients clearly nonresponsive to combination treatment in the past.

Maintenance therapy for patients in remission has not been extensively studied. However, it is our experience that many patients tolerate a gradual tapering of the antipsychotic drug once full remission of their symptoms is achieved. Such short-term exposure to an antipsychotic agent would also have the benefit of diminishing the risk of tardive dyskinesia.

MAJOR DEPRESSION WITHOUT MELANCHOLIA/ATYPICAL DEPRESSION

Perhaps the most difficult part of discussing the treatment of atypical/nonmelancholic depression is arriving at a commonly accepted definition of the term. For purposes of this discussion, we equate atypical depression with nonendogenous depression along the lines described by Robinson et al. (50,51). However, other investigators have emphasized atypical neurovegetative signs such as increased sleep and increased appetite (52), the presence of marked anxiety with panic attacks (53), or the presence of an entity described as "hysteroid dysphoria" (54,55). This last subtype is characterized by histrionic personality, high activity and energy when not depressed, rejection sensitivity, and atypical depressive symptoms such as overeating, oversleeping, extreme fatigue, and mood reactivity (55). DSM-III defines atypical depression for individuals with depressive symptoms who do not meet criteria for major depression (with or without melancholia), dysthymic disorder, or adjustment disorder with depressed mood (56); it is therefore a diagnosis of exclusion and one not particularly germane to specific treatment considerations.

The view originally put forward by West and Dally in 1959 (57), that the monoamine oxidase inhibitors (MAOIs) are more effective than TCAs in nonendogenous or atypical depression, has been partially supported by the evidence over the years. However, just as some classical endogenous depressions do not respond to tricyclic antidepressants, some atypical depressions do not respond to MAO inhibitors, and efforts to define subpopulations of atypical depressives who will respond to MAOIs have not been particularly successful (58–60).

Quitkin and colleagues have recently reviewed MAOI placebo-controlled studies and have concluded that in adequate doses, these agents clearly have antidepressant effects, particularly for atypical depressives (61). In general, a dose of at least 60 to 90 mg of phenelzine, 40 mg of isocarboxazid, or 60 mg of tranylcypromine is usually required for effective antidepressive action (62).

The fact that a group of nonendogenous depressives respond to MAO inhibitors does not, however, validate the concept of a specific MAOI responsive subtype unless one can also show that these patients are resistant to tricyclic antidepressants and that endogenous depressives respond poorly to MAOIs. As discussed earlier, MAOIs have been shown effective in some studies of endogenous depression (8,59,63), and Sovner reported an open study of treatment success with TCAs in patients with atypical depressive symptoms (64). Therefore, current evidence suggests that atypical depressives and MAOI responders are a heterogeneous group (65).

Most recent pharmacological trials have compared MAO inhibitors, tricyclics, and placebo for the treatment of atypical depression. There have now been three large double-blind studies comparing tricyclics to MAOIs for patients with nonendogenous depression (8,58,64). Two of the studies, which compared amitriptyline to phenelzine (8,58), found both antidepressants to be equal in effectiveness and better than placebo. However, in both studies, patients with prominent anxiety and panic symptoms tended to respond better to MAOIs. Liebowitz et al. (60), in a preliminary report on 60 patients taking phenelzine, imipramine, or placebo, found both antidepressants superior to placebo, with phenelzine better than imipramine. However, phenelzine seemed to produce a dramatically positive and statistically significant response only in atypical depressives who also had panic attacks. In fact, atypical depressives without panic attacks or hysteroid dysphoria seemed to respond equally well to all three treatments. Two tentative conclusions that can be drawn from these studies are that MAOIs may be especially effective for nonendogenously depressed patients with panic, prominent anxiety, and/or hysteroid dysphoria, and nonendogenously depressed patients without these features may respond equally to MAOIs and TCAs or, for that matter, to placebo. This last group may not respond well to medication, with a response rate of less than 50%.

The available evidence suggests that nonendogenously depressed patients should be given a trial of a TCA or MAOI. Patients with high anxiety, panic attacks, or possibly hysteroid dysphoria may be particularly responsive to MAOIs (62,67,68). New studies with selective MAOIs may provide further clues to which subpopulation of atypical depressives respond best to a particular pharmacological intervention (69).

BIPOLAR DEPRESSION

When an individual meets criteria for major depression, with or without melancholia, it is sometimes difficult to determine whether the patient is suffering from a unipolar or bipolar disorder. That distinction is made on the basis of a history of mania or hypomania. A patient must be followed longitudinally to make the decision, because up to one-third of depressives may eventually declare themselves as bipolar (70).

Bipolar depressives, unlike unipolars, are evenly divided by sex, have an onset of illness at an earlier age, have an increased genetic loading for the disorder, and may exhibit more psychomotor retardation and hypersomnia when depressed. Further, bipolars may be more susceptible to the development of hypomania with antidepressant treatment, and they may be more likely to respond to lithium carbonate during the depressive phase of their illness (71–73).

The somatic treatment of a patient suffering from major depression in the context of a bipolar disorder is essentially the same as for unipolar depression, but with several caveats. Opinion is divided as to the risk of precipitating mania in a bipolar depressed patient following the use of antidepressants. Some investigators stress the risk of precipitating a "switch" (74,75), but others find little evidence that this is a common occurrence (76). The use of lithium carbonate along with an antidepressant has been recommended for depressed patients with bipolar disorder and with unipolar type II disorder (79,80). Lithium alone is not usually an effective treatment for most acute unipolar depressions (77,78) but may have a place in the treatment of bipolar depression.

Extein et al. recommend initial treatment with lithium alone for bipolars with depression if the patient can tolerate symptomatology for the 3 to 4 weeks it takes for lithium to alleviate an acute episode (79). However, since only half of bipolar depressives seem to respond to lithium alone (53), a tricyclic antidepressant must often be added to the treatment regimen. Other investigators feel that the combination of lithium carbonate and a TCA most effectively treats bipolar depressive disorder and suggest that lithium protects the patient against the development of a manic episode, which could be produced by the tricyclic (80,81). If the combination of lithium and a tricyclic is not successful, the tricyclic can be replaced by an MAO inhibitor, especially in "rapid cyclers" (four or more cycles of illness per year), who may not do well with tricyclic antidepressants (82). Some investigators believe that TCAs shorten cycle length and prefer to avoid them in favor of lithium alone or lithium plus MAOI.

The use of electroconvulsive therapy can also be very effective in treatment-resistant bipolar depression. Carbamazepine might be a useful antidepressant in some bipolar depressed patients (83) along with other experimental treatments that have been tried with greater or lesser degrees of success (84).

DYSTHYMIC DISORDER

Although depressive neurosis was probably the most common affective disorder to be diagnosed in DSM-II, it was "a diagnosis of theoretical unclarity and clinical confusion" (85).

The diagnosis of dysthymic disorder has replaced depressive neurosis in DSM-III (56). It does not require evidence of a precipitating event or internal conflict, nor does it necessarily occur subsequent to an identifiable loss (which is now subsumed under adjustment disorder with depressed mood). Although retaining the same code number (300.4) as depressive neurosis, dysthymic disorder is an atheoretical diagnosis requiring 2 years of fairly persistent depressed mood with the presence of at least three of 13 associated affective symptoms.

Although the nature of the association is unclear, patients with borderline, histrionic, and dependent personality disorders often have concurrent dysthymic disorder (56). In such patients, affective symptoms could be obscured clinically by the prominent and dramatic personality and behavioral characteristics. Pope and colleagues have reported that some borderline patients with a major affective disorder responded to pharmacologic interventions with an improvement in both the depressive and personality disorders (88). It is unclear at present which patients with personality disorders and minor depressions would similarly respond. There is a need for further research into the nosology of dysthymic disorder and its relationship to personality disorders.

Keller and associates have reported that 25% of patients with major depressive disorder also had a preexisting chronic minor depression (essentially synonymous with dysthymic disorder) (86,87). They emphasize that the occurrence of such a "double depression" is associated with significant differences in course, recovery rates, and cycle length compared to major depression alone. Overall, depressed patients with a preexisting dysthymia have a significantly worse outcome. Furthermore, those patients with a persistence of dysthymia after recovery from a major depressive episode have an increased likelihood to relapse into another episode of depression.

Definitive treatment recommendations for dysthymic disorder remain obscured by the heterogeneous nature of this diagnostic entity. Nonetheless, certain general treatment recommendations seem clear based on recent data. For one, dysthymia persisting after recovery from a major depressive episode requires close observation and intensive treatment (87). Although Keller does not specify the nature of this treatment, there is evidence that continuation treatment with medication as well as psychotherapy may diminish the adverse effects that premorbid neurotic traits can have on outcome (89). Weissman and colleagues have shown that psychotherapy that focuses on "the social context of the depression rather than on an exploration of intrapsychic material or past experiences" is effective in improving the outcome of depressed outpatients by reducing the amount of residual dysthymic symptoms (90).

Another clinically relevant point is that dysthymic patients without a history of major depression should be carefully evaluated for the presence of subsyndromal "endogenous"

symptoms, a waxing and waning course, and a family history of affective disorder, all of which might predict a response to antidepressant agents (90). Conversely, the presence of a precipitating event or character pathology should not preclude a trial of antidepressants. Controlled prospective treatment trials of antidepressant medication and psychotherapy for dysthymic disorder are necessary before more specific recommendations can be made.

TREATMENT-RESISTANT DEPRESSION

Significant numbers of patients do not respond to adequate therapeutic trials of antidepressants and can therefore be called "treatment resistant." The percentage of patients who fail to respond to any one trial is variably reported but usually in the neighborhood of 25 to 40% (3). Even with maximal doses of medication and blood level monitoring for adequate lengths of time (usually 4 to 6 weeks), at least 10% of patients do not improve acceptably with one or more medications.

We briefly outline several approaches that have been described for treatment resistant depressives, including the use of MAOIs, the combination of TCAs and MAOIs, adjunctive medications added to TCAs, ECT, and experimental treatments. Unfortunately, the literature is replete with open series and case reports on this topic, although rigorous research tends to be conspicuous by its absence.

There are no clear guidelines in deciding whether or when to initiate a second heterocyclic before moving to other types of treatments. However, a patient who cannot tolerate one drug should be tried on another with a different side effect profile, and a nonresponder to one type of reuptake inhibitor might be switched to another. If one or two trials of heterocyclic antidepressants are ineffective, a change to an MAO inhibitor may be indicated.

Tricyclic- and ECT-resistant conditions are frequently found in the elderly, and Georgotas et al. (91,92) have shown that MAO inhibitors can be effective in these patients. They reported on 30 patients who had all received at least two therapeutic trials of antidepressant without benefit; over a third had also failed to respond to ECT. Twenty were treated openly with phenelzine for 2 to 7 weeks, 13 of whom (65%) had a good response. The medication was well tolerated, and the authors concluded that MAO inhibitors could be effective in treatment-resistant depression in the elderly. Clinical experience suggests that MAO inhibitors can be effective in heterocyclic-resistant depressions (62). Davis, in his review of the literature, suggests a clear role for phenelzine and tranylcypromine for depressed patients (2). The latter is less well studied but has amphetamine-like properties and is an inhibitor of norepinephrine reuptake. Davis hypothesizes that tranylcypromine alone acts as a combination of amphetamine, tricyclic, and MAOI, which might explain its efficacy in treatment-resistant cases.

Until recently, the combination of MAOIs and tricyclics was thought to be dangerous. However, this combination appears safe and may be effective in some refractory patients, particularly those with severe anxiety. If the drugs are given properly, the occurrence of adverse effects is unlikely (93–97). Serious reactions seem to be caused either by overdoses, dietary indiscretion, or the use of other medications contraindicated with an MAOI. It has been suggested that 5-HT reuptake inhibitors should not be combined with MAOIs (98), and specifically, a combination of clomipramine and MAOI may be particularly dangerous (99). There is some evidence that amitriptyline, which is both a 5-HT reuptake inhibitor and a blocker of postsynaptic 5-HT receptors, may be protective against a TCA/MAOI adverse hypertensive reaction but perhaps not against the hyperthermic/hypertonic response (100). Most psychopharmacologists recommend that if the combination is to be used, one should start with low doses of the TCA and add an MAOI to the regimen several days later. Both drugs can then be increased slowly over a period of time, titrating the dose to clinical response or side effects. An MAO inhibitor can be added to a tricyclic, but the reverse should probably not be done. Although the effectiveness of the combination treatment has been reported in open studies, it has not been proven in controlled studies (101–103).

Lithium potentiation of antidepressant treatment is another approach that has received considerable attention over the last few years (104,108). DeMontigny and associates originally studied eight patients with unipolar depression who had not responded to 3 weeks of treatment with a tricyclic antidepressant. They found significant improvement, measured by the Hamilton depression scale, within 48 hr after adding lithium to the drug regimen (104). The same group had a follow-up report (105) showing that in 30 of 42 instances, depressed patients who did not respond to 3 weeks of a tricyclic antidepressant had at least a 50% improvement in their mood within 48 hr of the addition of lithium carbonate. They found that the addition of lithium to placebo was ineffective in four out of five patients.

In a related project, Henninger et al. (106) studied 15 treatment-resistant patients with major depression who had not improved with a trial of an antidepressant. In a double-blind study, they showed that the addition of lithium to a TCA produced a better response than the addition of placebo after the seventh day of treatment. They did not, however, find the beneficial effect to be as rapid as De-Montigny reported. Other research supports that lithium seems to potentiate MAO inhibitors and combination neuroleptic/TCA treatment in patients with psychotic depression (48). Most of these authors hypothesize a serotonergic basis for this synergism (107). Importantly, not all investigators have found such a robust response to the lithium adjunct approach and suggest that the response is far more variable than previously described (108).

Another approach that has received some attention is the addition of triiodothyronine (T_3) to a TCA in patients who have not had a response to the TCA alone. Several studies have shown that the addition of this thyroid hormone, in doses of 25 to 50 μg, can convert tricyclic nonresponders to responders (109,110). Interestingly, this treatment does not raise tricyclic drug levels (112) or correct subtle thyroid deficiencies (113). Its mechanism is unclear but may involve central β-receptor responsiveness to norepinephrine (114). It remains a useful intervention in patients with tricyclic treatment-resistant depression.

Other drug combinations that have occasionally been reported to be effective include the combination of a stimulant with a TCA or MAOI (95,103), the addition of L-tryptophan to TCAs or MAOIs, the addition of reserpine to a tricyclic (115), and the addition of neuroleptics, particularly in patients with delusional depression.

A number of experimental treatments have also been tried for major depression, including monoamine precursors (116), carbamazepine (117), and calcium channel blockers, among other agents. Of course, ECT remains one of the safest and most effective treatments for major depressive disorder, particularly in patients with melancholic features, and should be strongly considered if psychopharmacologic interventions fail (118).

CONCLUSION

Despite great advances in the treatment of acute depression, many patients continue to suffer because the diagnosis may not be evident, treatment may not be adequately prescribed, and, sadly, all therapeutic modalities are limited in efficacy. Most researchers agree that "depression" is a heterogeneous disorder, but the search for subtypes by studying clinical, biological, epidemiological, and treatment response variables has met with limited success. The quest for specific treatments targeted to discrete depressive subtypes will continue. Pharmacologic advances have been relatively modest since the first edition of this book was published 10 years ago, but clinicians seem to have a greater understanding of the utility of this modality for treating depression. We remain hopeful that progress will continue, skeptical of exaggerated claims of success, concerned about side effects of new medication, but aggressive in treating this common and debilitating disorder.

REFERENCES

1. Sinaikin, P. M. (1985): *J. Nerv. Ment. Dis.,* 173(4):199–211.
2. Davis, J. M. (1985): In: *Comprehensive Textbook of Psychiatry, IV,* edited by H. I. Kaplan and B. J. Sadock, pp. 1513–1536. Williams & Wilkins, Baltimore.
3. Baldessarini, R. J. (1983): *Biomedical Aspects of Depression.* APA Press, Washington.
4. Quitkin, F. M., Rabkin, J. G., Ross, D., et al. (1984): *Arch. Gen. Psychiatry,* 41:238–245.
5. APA Taskforce Report. (1985): *Am. J. Psychiatry,* 142:155–182.
6. Hollister, L. E. (1981): *Psychosomatics,* 22:872–879.
7. Nystrom, C., and Hallstron, T. (1985): *Acta Psychiatr. Scand.,* T2:6–15.
8. McGrath, P. J., Quitkin, F. M., Harrison, W., et al. (1984): *Am. J. Psychiatry,* 141:288–289.
9. Quitkin, F. M., McGrath, P., Liebowitz, M. R., et al. (1981): *J. Clin. Psychopharmacol.,* 1:70–74.
10. Giller, E., Bialos, D., Riddle, M., et al. (1982): *Psychiatr. Res.,* 6:41–48.
11. Keller, M. B., Klerman, G. L., Lavori, P. W., et al. (1982): *J.A.M.A.,* 248:1848–1855.
12. Arana, G. W., Baldessarini, R. J., and Ornsteen, M. (1985): *Arch. Gen. Psychiatry,* 42:1193–1203.
13. Maas, J. W. (1975): *Arch. Gen. Psychiatry,* 32:1357–1361.
14. Maas, J. W., Koslow, S. H., Katz, M. M., Bowden, C. L., Gibbons, R. L., et al. (1984): *Am. J. Psychiatry,* 141:1159–1171.
15. Muscettola, G., Potter, W. Z., Picker, D., and Goodwin, F. K. (1984): *Arch. Gen. Psychiatry,* 41:337–342.

16. Puzynski, S., Rode, A., Bidzinski, A., Mrozek, S., and Zaluska, M. (1984): *Acta Psychiatr. Scand.,* 69:117–120.
17. Janicak, P., Chan, C., Davis, J. M., Chang, S., Javaid, J., et al. (1985): Presented at the Fourth World Congress of Biological Psychiatry. Philadelphia, PA.
18. Charney, D. S., Menkes, D. B., and Heninger, G. R. (1981): *Arch. Gen. Psychiatry,* 38:1160–1180.
19. Asberg, M., Bertilsson, L., Thoren, P., and Traskman-Bendz, L. (1985): Presented at the Fourth World Congress of Biological Psychiatry. Philadelphia, PA.
20. Frank, E., Jarrett, D. B., Kupfer, D. J., and Grochocinski, V. J. (1984): *Psychiatr. Res.,* 13:315–324.
21. Krog-Meyer, I., Kirkegaard, C., Kijne, B., Lumholtz, B., Smith, E., et al. (1984): *Am. J. Psychiatry,* 141:945–948.
22. Ostrow, D. G., Okonek, A., Gibbons, R., Cooper, R., and Davis, J. M. (1983): *J. Clin. Psychiatry,* 44:10–13.
23. Sabelli, H. C., Fawcett, J., Javaid, J. I., and Bagri, S. (1983): *Am. J. Psychiatry,* 140:212–214.
24. Klerman, G. L. (1983): In: *Psychiatry Update, Vol II,* edited by L. Grinspoon, pp. 356–382. APA Press, Washington, D.C.
25. Bielski, R. J., and Friedel, R. O. (1976): *Arch. Gen. Psychiatry,* 33:1479–1489.
26. Paykel, E. S. (1972): *Br. J. Psychiatry,* 120:147–156.
27. Mindham, R. H. S. (1982): In: *Handbook of Affective Disorders,* edited by E. S. Paykel, pp. 231–246. Guilford Press, New York.
28. Simpson, G. M., Lee, H. L., Chuche, Z., et al. (1976): *Arch. Gen. Psychiatry,* 33:1093–1102.
29. Wittenborn, J. R., and Kiremitci, N. (1975): *Arch. Gen. Psychiatry,* 32:1172–1176.
30. Nelson, J. C., and Charney, D. S. (1981): *Am. J. Psychiatry,* 138:1–13.
31. Avery, D. H., Wilson, L. G., and Dunner, D. L. (1983): In: *Treatment of Depression: Old Controversies and New Approaches,* edited by P. J. Clayton and J. E. Barrett, pp. 193–207. Raven Press, New York.
32. Guze, S. B., Woodruff, R. A., and Clayton, P. J. (1975): *Arch. Gen. Psychiatry,* 32:1147–1150.
33. Quitkin, F., Rifkin, A., and Klein, D. F. (1978): *Am. J. Psychiatry,* 135:806–811.
34. Coryell, W., Ziegler, V. E., and Biggs, J. T. (1980): *J. Affect. Dis.,* 2:27–35.
35. Frangos, E., Athenassenas, G., Tsitourides, S., Psilolignos, P., and Katsanou, N. (1983): *J. Affect. Disorders,* 5:259–265.
36. Kantor, S. J., and Glassman, A. H. (1977): *Br. J. Psychiatry,* 131:351–360.
37. Glassman, A. H., and Roose, S. P. (1981): *Arch. Gen. Psychiatry,* 38:424–427.
38. Nelson, J. C., and Bowers, M. B. (1978): *Arch. Gen. Psychiatry,* 35:1321–1328.
39. Charney, D. S., and Nelson, J. C. (1981): *Am. J. Psychiatry,* 138:328–333.
40. Helms, P. M., and Smith, R. E. (1983): *J. Affect. Disorders,* 5:51–54.
41. Leckman, J. F., Weissman, M. M., Prusoff, B. A., Caruso, K. A., Merikangas, K. R., et al. (1984): *Arch. Gen. Psychiatry,* 41:833–888.
42. Spiker, D. G., Weiss, J. C., Dealy, R. S., Griffin, S. J., Hanin, I., et al. (1985): *Am. J. Psychiatry,* 142:430–436.
43. Meltzer, H. Y., Hyong, W. C., Carroll, B. J., and Russo, P. (1976): *Arch. Gen. Psychiatry,* 33:585–591.
44. Sweeny, D., Nelson, C., Bowers, M., Maas, J., and Heninger, G. (1978): *Lancet,* 2:100–101.
45. Schatzberg, A. F., Rothschild, A. J., Stahl, J. B., Bond, T. C., Rosenbaum, A. H., et al. (1983): *Am. J. Psychiatry,* 140:88–91.
46. Weissman, M. M., Prusoff, B. A., and Merikangas, K. R. (1984): *Am. J. Psychiatry,* 141:892–893.
47. Coryell, W., and Tsuang, M. T. (1985): *Am. J. Psychiatry,* 142:479–482.
48. Price, L. H., Conwell, Y., and Nelson, J. C. (1983): *Am. J. Psychiatry,* 140:318–322.
49. Schaffer, C. B., Mungas, D., and Rockwell, E. (1985): *J. Clin. Psychopharmacol.,* 5:233–235.
50. Robinson, D. S., Nies, A., Ravaris, C. L., et al. (1973): *Arch. Gen. Psychiatry,* 29:407–413.
51. Robinson, D. S., Nies, A., Ravaris, C. L., et al. (1978): *Arch. Gen. Psychiatry,* 35:629–635.
52. Liebowitz, M. R., Quitkin, F. M., Steward, J. W., et al. (1981): *Psychopharmacol. Bull.,* 17:159–161.
53. Tyrer, P. J. (1982): In: *Drugs and Psychiatric Practice,* edited by P. J. Tyler, pp. 227–239. Butterworths, London.
54. Klein, D. F., and Davis, J. (1968): *Diagnosis and Drug Treatment of Psychiatric Disorders.* Williams & Wilkins, Baltimore.
55. Liebowitz, M. R., and Klein, D. F. (1979): *Psychiar. Clin. North Am.,* 2:555–575.
56. American Psychiatric Association (1980): DSM III. APA Press, Washington.
57. West, E. D., and Dally, P. J. (1959): *Br. Med. J.,* 1:1491–1497.
58. Ravaris, L. L., Robinson, D. S., Ives, J. O., et al. (1980): *Arch. Gen. Psychiatry,* 37:1075–1080.
59. Giller, E., Biales, D., Riddel, M., et al. (1982): *Psychiatr. Res.,* 6:41–48.
60. Zisock, S., Braff, D. L., and Click, M. A. (1985): *J. Clin. Psychopharmacol.,* 5(3):131–140.
61. Quitkin, F. M., Rifkin, A., and Klein, D. F. (1979): *Arch. Gen. Psychiatry,* 36:749–760.
62. Pare, C. M. B. (1985): *Br. J. Psychiatry,* 146:576–584.
63. Quitkin, F. M., McGrath, P., Liebowitz, M. R., et al. (1918): *J. Clin. Psychopharmacol.,* 1:70–74.
64. Sovner, R. D. (1981): *J. Clin. Psychiatry,* 42:285–289.
65. Rowan, P. R., Paykel, E. S., Parker, R. R., et al. (1981): In: *Monoamine Oxidase Inhibitors: The State of the Art,* edited by M. B. H. Youdim and E. S. Paykel, pp. 126–139. Wiley, New York.
66. Liebowitz, M. R., Quitkin, F. M., Stewart, J. W., et al. (1984): *Arch. Gen. Psychiatry,* 41:669–677.
67. Robinson, D. S., Kayser, A., Corcella, J., et al. (1985): *Psychopharmacol. Bull.,* 21:562–567.
68. Keyser, A. K., Robinson, D. S., Nies, A., et al. (1985): *Am. J. Psychiatry,* 142(4):486–488.
69. Quitkin, F. M., Liebowitz, M. R., Stewart, J. W., et al. (1984): *Arch. Gen. Psychiatry,* 41:777–782.
70. Clayton, P. G. (1981): *Comp. Psychiatry,* 22:31–43.
71. Akiskal, H. S. (1983): In: *Psychiatry Update, Vol. II,* edited by L. Grinspoon, pp. 271–293. APA Press, Washington.
72. Kupfer, D. J., Picker, D., Himmelhoch, J. M., et al. (1975): *Arch. Gen. Psychiatry,* 32:866–871.
73. Klerman, G. L. (1983): In: *Handbook of Affective Disorders,* edited by E. S. Paykel, pp. 438–453. Guilford Press, New York.
74. Bunney, W. E. (1978): In: *Psychopharmacology: A Generation of Progress,* edited by M. A. Lipton, A. DiMascio, and K. F. Killam, pp. 1249–1259. Raven Press, New York.
75. Wehr, T. A., and Goodwin, F. K. (1979): *Arch. Gen. Psychiatry,* 36:555–559.
76. Prien, R. F. (1983): In: *Psychiatry Update, Vol. II,* edited by L. Grinspoon, pp. 303–318. APA Press, Washington.
77. Bowden, C. (1978): *Comp. Psychiatry,* 19:227–231.
78. Dunner, D. L., and Fieve, R. R. (1978): In: *Neuropsychopharmacology,* edited by P. Deniker, pp. 1109–1115. Pergamon Press, New York.
79. Extein, I., Gold, M. S., and Pottash, A. L. C. (1984): *Psychiatr. Clin. North Am.,* 7:503–517.
80. Bielski, R. J., and Friedel, R. O. (1979): *Psychiatr. Clin. North Am.,* 2:3.
81. Reid, W. H. (1984): *Treatment of the DSM-III Psychiatric Disorders,* p. 132. Brunner Mazel, New York.
82. Dunner, D. L. (1979): *Psychiatr. Clin. North Am.,* 2:661–662.
83. Okuma, T. (1983): *Psychiatr. Clin. North Am.,* 6:157–174.
84. Lerer, B. (1985): *J. Clin. Psychiatry,* 46:309–316.
85. Klerman, G. L., Endicott, J., Spitzer, R., and Hirshfeld, R. M. A. (1979): *Am. J. Psychiatry,* 136:57–61.
86. Keller, M. G., and Shapiro, R. W. (1982): *Am. J. Psychiatry,* 139:438–442.
87. Keller, M. B., Lavori, P. W., Endicott, J., Coryell, W., Klerman, G. L., et al. (1983): *Am. J. Psychiatry,* 140:689–694.
88. Pope, H. G., Jonas, J. M., Hudson, J. I., Cohen, B. M., and Gunderson, J. G. (1983): *Arch. Gen. Psychiatry,* 40:23–36.

89. Weissman, M. M., Prusoff, B. A., and Klerman, G. L. (1978): *Am. J. Psychiatry,* 135:797–800.
90. Weissman, M. M., Klerman, G. L., Prusoff, B. A., Sholomskas, D., and Padian, N. (1981): *Arch. Gen. Psychiatry,* 38:51–55.
91. Georgotas, A., Mann, J., and Friedman, E. (1981): *Biol. Psychiatry,* 16:997–1001.
92. Georgotas, A., Friedman, E., McCarthy, M., et al. (1983): *Biol. Psychiatry,* 18:195–205.
93. Shuckit, M., Robins, E., and Feighner, J. (1971): *Arch. Gen. Psychiatry,* 24:509.
94. Sethna, E. R. (1974): *Br. J. Psychiatry,* 124:265–272.
95. Georgotas, A. (1985): *Comprehensive Textbook of Psychiatry, IV.* Williams & Wilkins, New York.
96. White, K., and Simpson, G. (1981): *Clin. Psychopharmacol.,* 1:264–282.
97. Ananth, J., and Luchins, D. (1977): *Comp. Psychiatry,* 18:221–230.
98. Marley, E., and Wozniack, K. M. (1983): *Psychol. Med.,* 13:735–749.
99. Beaumont, G. (1973): *J. Intern. Med. Res.,* 1:435–437.
100. Stolz, J., and Marsden, C. A. (1982): *Eur. J. Pharmacol.,* 79:17–22.
101. Razoni, J., White, K., White, J., et al. (1983): *Arch. Gen. Psychol.,* 40:657–661.
102. Young, J. P. R., Lader, M. H., and Hughes, W. C. (1979): *Br. Med. J.,* 2:1315–1317.
103. Feighner, J. P., Herbstein, J., and Damlouju, N. (1985): *J. Clin. Psychiatry,* 46:206–209.
104. DeMontigny, C., Gronberg, E., Mayer, A., et al. (1981): *Br. J. Psychiatry,* 138:252–256.
105. DeMontigny, C., Cowinoyer, G., Marissette, R., et al. (1983): *Arch. Gen. Psychiatry,* 40:1327–1334.
106. Heninger, G. R., Gharney, D. S., and Sternberg, D. E. (1983): *Arch. Gen. Psychiatry,* 40:1335–1342.
107. Meltzer, H. Y., Lowy, M., Robertson, A., et al. (1984): *Arch. Gen. Psychiatry,* 41:391–397.
108. Lovie, A. K., and Meltzer, H. Y. (1984): *J. Clin. Psychopharmacol.,* 4(6):316–321.
109. Prange, A. J., Wilson, J. C., Rabon, A. M., et al. (1969): *Am. J. Psychiatry,* 126:457–469.
110. Earle, B. V. (1970): *Am. J. Psychiatry,* 126:1467–1469.
111. Goodwin, F. K., Pronge, A. J., Rost, R. M., et al. (1982): *Am. J. Psychiatry,* 139:34–38.
112. Garbutt, J., Malekpour, B., Brunswick, D., et al. (1979): *Am. J. Psychiatry,* 136:980–982.
113. Schwartz, G., Halaris, A., Baxter, L., et al. (1984): *Am. J. Psychiatry,* 141:1614–1616.
114. Whybrow, P. C., and Prange, A. J. (1981): *Arch. Gen. Psychiatry,* 38:106–113.
115. Ayd, F. J. (1985): *Int. Drug Ther.,* 20:5.
116. Baldessarini, R. J. (1984): *Psychopharmacol. Bull.,* 20:224–238.
117. Post, R. M., and Ehde, T. W. (1985): *Psychopharmacol. Bull.,* 21(1):10–17.
118. Weiner, R. D. (1985): *Comprehensive Textbook of Psychiatry, IV.* Williams & Wilkins, New York.
119. Cole, J. O., and Schatzberg, A. P. (1983): In: *Psychiatric Update, Vol. II,* edited by L. Grinspoon. APA Press, Washington.

Psychopharmacology:
The Third Generation of Progress,
edited by Herbert Y. Meltzer.
Raven Press, New York © 1987.

CHAPTER 105

Newer Antidepressant Drugs

Barry Blackwell

EVOLUTION, CLASSIFICATION, AND OVERVIEW

For the first 20 years of modern antidepressant drug use, the monoamine oxidase inhibitors and the tricyclic antidepressants dominated therapy, providing a relatively clear-cut classification system consistent with a single theory of drug action (the catecholamine hypothesis).

In the last decade a series of new compounds have appeared with a wide variety of chemical structures and pharmacologic profiles. The introduction of these newer compounds can be understood in a framework of dissatisfaction with earlier drugs. Following the discovery of interactions between MAO inhibitors and tyramine-containing foods, these compounds fell into relative disuse. The tricyclic antidepressants also suffered from disadvantages including their cardiac toxicity (especially in overdose), lowering of seizure thresholds, and anticholinergic activity (6).

Some authorities (70) consider iprindole to be the first of the newer compounds, although it clearly is a tricyclic

structure found subsequently to have a weak ability to block norepinephrine uptake. Other authors (15,69) have also included more recent molecular modifications of the tricyclic nucleus such as doxepin and amoxapine as newer antidepressants.

This review includes as newer antidepressants only drugs clearly differentiated from the tricyclic derivatives. Also excluded are structures whose primary action is considered sedative, such as tryptophan and alprazolam, where some antidepressant properties are alleged or still under investigation. Finally, only those compounds are included that are commercially available in the United States or Europe or are in advanced stages of the regulatory review process.

The advent of these newer drugs with their diverse structure and pharmacology has made the interpretation of clinical action increasingly complex. Explanatory models invoke at least three neurotransmitters (norepinephrine, serotonin, and dopamine) and as many different mechanisms of action. These include blockade of amine reuptake, up- or down-regulation, and blockade of receptors (15). In reality, most effective antidepressants are only partially selective and have a greater or lesser effect on more than one putative neurotransmitter or mechanism of action (66). Even drugs that have somewhat selective actions lack specificity on norepinephrine and serotonin metabolites in the cerebrospinal fluid of depressed patients (60).

Despite this heterogeneity of drug action, the consistent finding from clinical trials is that a majority of depressed patients benefit significantly compared to placebo. This suggests that their mechanism is either still unknown or that good outcome may be a final common pathway of drug action on different neurotransmitters that interact in a homeostatic manner. Such a possibility is suggested by the recently proposed "dysregulation" model (76), which explains many of the inconsistencies of the earlier and simpler catecholamine hypothesis. Even this model, however, only deals with norepinephrine, whereas the newer drugs are effective on different neurotransmitters, suggesting that dysregulation may be corrected via more than one pathway.

The earlier clinical claims for these newer compounds often reflect the deficiencies and drawbacks to existing drugs. It is hoped that each new compound will act more quickly, have fewer anticholinergic effects, be safer in overdose, and be relatively free from serious adverse effects such as alterations in cardiac function or seizure threshold. It is also hoped that these advantages can be accomplished without paying the penalty of any novel side effects.

Although there is an element of validity to some of these claims, they must be interpreted with caution. Few biological derangements are restored to normal by drugs in less than a week. Few chemically active compounds are so selective that they work at a single site or bind to only one receptor. Delayed responses, unwanted effects, and multiple actions are to be expected, especially when drugs are directed at a finely tuned and well-protected organ like the brain. Novel structures must almost inevitably incur new side effects.

The data available on new drugs are always incomplete. Final categorization of each compound awaits widespread use beyond the artificial confines of clinical trials. This includes the experience that accumulates among the victims of overdose, a tragic natural experiment in man that cannot be anticipated in animals before a new drug is released.

BUPROPRION

Structure, Pharmacology, Development, and Pharmacokinetics

Buproprion is a substituted chloropropiophenone reminiscent of anorectic drugs such as diethylproprion (51). Preclinical testing revealed mild stimulant properties and an atypical antidepressant effect. The compound has a relatively selective action on dopamine reuptake and a direct agonist action on dopamine receptors. It does not release catecholamines or produce down-regulation of post-synaptic receptors. Buproprion lacks effects on growth hormone, prolactin, and response to TRH (43) as well as any significant action on serotonergic, histaminic, or cholinergic mechanisms.

Buproprion was tested in the United States, and very little had been published until the appearance of a complete issue of the *Journal of Clinical Psychiatry* in May 1983 [Vol. 5(2)]. The FDA now considers the drug "approvable," and labeling is under negotiation.

Buproprion is rapidly absorbed with peak plasma concentrations within 2 hr (44) and has several active metabolites (69). The plasma half-life is 11 to 14 hr, and levels vary 10-fold unrelated to dosage and show a narrow therapeutic window between 75 and 100 ng/ml (61).

Clinical Effects

A majority of trials have been against amitriptyline, thus maximizing the allegedly "unique" properties of buproprion as a less sedative and mildly stimulant drug. The drug has a narrow dose range and a slower onset of action (5).

Side Effects

Buproprion has fewer anticholinergic side effects but is not free of them. There is an absence of sedation, but it has some stimulant effects including excitement, palpitations, tremor, agitation, increased motor activity, and an occasional toxic confusional state. Sedative–hypnotics may be required for insomnia or anxiety in depressed patients (13). Skin rashes and gastrointestinal disturbances (nausea and vomiting) are also reported.

One unusual side effect (3) has been an alteration in time sense, sensitivity to sensory stimuli, and vivid dreaming. These may be related to buproprion's influence on dopamine metabolism and appear more likely to occur in schizophrenic patients.

Other side effects include evidence for weight loss (33) as well as concern over the potential for amphetamine-like abuse (31,55).

Patients with sexual dysfunction on tricyclic compounds may regain normal function after switching to buproprion (27).

The incidence of seizures is estimated to be equivalent to that seen with tricyclic compounds (54).

Buproprion has produced no significant EKG or conduction changes and no alterations in pulse or blood pressure even in patients with previous postural hypotension on tricyclic drugs (24,28,29).

Overdosage

Five patients are reported (62) to have survived up to 3,000 mg without complications.

Interactions

Buproprion does not enhance the impairment of psychomotor function by alcohol or benzodiazepines (69) and has been used safely with antiarrhythmic, antihypertensive, and analgesic drugs. Patients receiving more than 600 mg daily and taking lithium appear to have an increased risk of seizures (19).

FLUOXETINE

Structure, Pharmacology, Development, and Pharmacokinetics

Fluoxetine is a substituted phenylpropylamine. The compound has highly specific actions on serotonin reuptake and relative lack of potency on norepinephrine or dopamine systems. It has a remarkable lack of affinity for receptors so that it does not produce either blockade or down-regulation in significant degrees at muscarinic, histaminic, serotonin, or noradrenergic receptors (77).

Fluoxetine appears to have been developed exclusively in the United States. Research on the compound was summarized in a special issue of the *Journal of Clinical Psychiatry* [Vol. 46(3), March 1985], and the NDA was reviewed by the FDA in October 1985, so the drug is not yet available.

Fluoxetine is slowly absorbed and metabolized (45). Peak plasma concentration occurs after 6 to 8 hr, and elimination half-life for the parent compound is 1 to 3 days, with the major metabolite (*N*-demethylfluoxetine) persisting for 7 to 15 days. Volunteers given fluoxetine showed a wide range of plasma levels and half-lives. These metabolic characteristics may create concerns about drug cumulation and variability in response.

Clinical Effects

The dosage range is 20 to 80 mg daily, and once-daily dosage (in the morning) is as effective as twice-daily administration (67). In comparison with placebo and imipramine (78), fluoxetine was not superior to placebo until the fourth week of the study, whereas imipramine (as is usual) was significantly different by weeks 2 to 3. It failed to exceed placebo in its effects on anxiety and sleep disturbance and was significantly worse than imipramine on the latter.

Similar results were obtained compared to amitriptyline, with fluoxetine showing less early benefit on anxiety and less overall benefit in sleep disturbance (14).

Side Effects

A review in patients treated for up to 2 years (82) confirmed the stimulant profile and a relative lack of anticholinergic actions. The most frequent side effects were nausea (25%), nervousness, insomnia, headache, tremor, anxiety, drowsiness, dry mouth, sweating, and diarrhea (10%). Most of these occurred early in treatment and seldom led to drug discontinuation. Weight loss may also occur. Analysis of severe side effects showed psychotic reactions including stimulant psychosis and conversion to mania.

Fluoxetine appears not to have the cardiovascular effects associated with tricyclic compounds. An analysis of electrocardiograms (25) showed a small but significant reduction in heart rate (3 beats/min) but no significant intraventricular conduction delays. Electroencephalographic studies in normals (71) show changes similar to other serotonin reuptake inhibitors and more like desipramine than other tricyclic compounds. A few seizures have been reported.

Side effects noted during long-term administration have been excessive sweating (32%) and anxiety (23%) compared to imipramine, which produced dry mouth (57%) and constipation (29%).

Overdosage

Nine patients have taken overdoses up to 3,000 mg. One patient, who also took amitriptyline, died, but the others recovered with relatively minor symptoms.

Interactions

Experiments in normal volunteers did not produce any significant changes in the metabolism of warfarin, diazepam, tolbutamide, or chlorothiazide. The concurrent administration of alcohol and fluoxetine also did not produce any evidence of additive effects (45). The combination of an MAO inhibitor and serotonin reuptake inhibitors like fluoxetine is predicted to interact on the basis of animal experiments (50).

MAPROTILINE

Structure, Pharmacology, Development, and Pharmacokinetics

Maprotiline is a modification of the basic tricyclic configuration by the addition of an ethylene bridge to the middle ring (36). The compound has a similar profile to desipramine or nortriptyline. It is relatively selective in blockade of norepinephrine uptake and inactive on serotonergic mechanisms (47), but it also has strong antihistaminic and anticholinergic properties.

Maprotiline was the first of the newer drugs. It has been marketed in other countries for over 10 years and has been available in the United States since 1981.

Maprotiline is equipotent to imipramine and has a long elimination half-life of 43 hr (81), providing a steady-state level towards the end of 1 week and permitting once-daily regimens (52). Plasma levels vary 10-fold, but there are inadequate data to correlate outcome to blood level.

Clinical Effects

An extensive review (18) concluded that maprotiline was equally effective to imipramine, amitriptyline, and doxepin. Earlier claims for a more rapid onset of action (26) have not been sustained. Concerns about its long half-life may limit its use in patients susceptible to side effects such as the elderly.

Side Effects

The principal side effects are peripheral anticholinergic manifestations in up to 30% of patients, followed by drowsiness in over 15% (69,81).

About 3% of patients develop an exanthematous skin rash, usually within 2 weeks of treatment, that is probably allergic in nature and disappears rapidly on drug cessation (26).

Of more serious concern is an increased incidence of epileptic seizures during treatment and complicating overdose (20,37). It is usual to avoid treatment in patients with a personal or family history of epilepsy and to reduce the risk of seizures by initiating treatment in low dosage and avoiding upward titration until steady state is reached.

Overdosage

In a large series of overdoses on maprotiline (40), the outcome was similar to tricyclic complications, although prolonged coma (over 72 hr) and seizures (in 36% of patients) were troublesome. Morbidity may be worsened by a long half-life and delayed excretion.

Interactions

Maprotiline produces additive effects with quinidine (85) and antagonism of neuron-blocking antihypertensive drugs including clonidine, bethanidine, and guanethidine. It does not appear to interact with β blockers (53).

MIANSERIN

Structure, Pharmacology, Development, and Pharmacokinetics

Mianserin is a tetracyclic compound of the piperazine–dibenzazepine class. It is relatively devoid of activity on reuptake mechanisms, and it blocks α_2 presynaptic, serotonin, and histamine but not muscarinic receptors (9). Quantitative EEG studies suggested its clinical utility (56).

Mianserin was synthesized in 1966 and tested as an antiallergic compound. The compound was developed in Europe from 1978 onwards. Because of the recent concerns about its toxicity, it seems unlikely that mianserin will be marketed in the United States.

The pharmacokinetics resemble those of tricyclic compounds. The half-life is from 10 to 27 hr, and the mean therapeutic plasma concentration is 50 ng/liter.

Clinical Effects

Mianserin is a sedative with a somewhat narrow dose range of 30 to 60 mg daily (79). Concerns have been expressed about a tendency to relapse during long-term maintenance therapy (75).

Side Effects

Mianserin has a sedative profile but without significant anticholinergic side effects (41).

It is devoid of effects on the cardiovascular system, including conduction, heart rate, contractability, and blood pressure (42).

A review (21) indicates that mianserin has a similar propensity to provoke seizures as tricyclic compounds. It also causes a variety of blood dyscrasias including aplastic anemia and agranulocytosis (5,6). There have been reports of arthralgia and a variety of allergic-type responses causing fever, skin rashes, and abnormal liver function.

Overdose

Mianserin appears to be unusually safe in overdose. There were no reports of convulsions, cardiac arrhythmias, or deep coma in any patient who took mianserin alone.

Interactions

A further advantage of mianserin in cardiac patients is the absence of interactions with centrally acting hypotensive drugs such as clonidine and methyldopa (22).

NOMIFENSINE

Structure, Pharmacology, Development, and Pharmacokinetics

Nomifensine is a three-ring tetrahydroisoquinoline compound (36). It is a potent reuptake inhibitor of dopamine and norepinephrine but not serotonin. It has no anticholinergic activity, is a weak α-adrenergic antagonist, and has some affinity for serotonin receptors (15).

In animals nomifensine produces amphetamine-like actions, but not in normal volunteers (70).

Nomifensine was introduced in 1977 and is now available in over 70 countries. In the United States it was released in mid-1985. Most of the U.S. studies were published in a special 1984 issue of the *Journal of Clinical Psychiatry* [Vol. 45(4), Sect. 2].

Peak plasma levels are reached within 1 to 2 hr, and elimination half-life is 2 to 4 hr (34). The electroencephalographic effects persist for up to 8 hr (72).

Clinical Effects

Nomifensine is a less sedative and more stimulating compound than other antidepressants.

The major disadvantage may be the need for twice-daily dosing and for concurrent use of sedative or hypnotic agents.

Side Effects

A major advantage is the reduced incidence of anticholinergic side effects. It also appears to produce less weight gain, less postural hypotension, and no increased incidence of epileptic seizures.

Animal work and clinical pharmacology studies (12) confirm the absence of direct cardiotoxic effects.

Nomifensine's stimulant properties and actions on dopamine metabolism incur some drawbacks. The incidence of insomnia may be increased, and reports have occurred of orofacial dyskinesia (4,8). The latter may restrict its utility in patients with Parkinson's disease.

The major drawback is the occurrence of allergic responses that are related to disturbances of immune function (1,57). These most often occur in the first weeks of treatment and are independent of dose level. The most common symptoms are a "flu-like" malaise accompanied by specific manifestations of whatever system is affected. These can include red cell hemolysis, thrombocytopenia, renal insufficiency, hepatic damage, pulmonary alveolitis (32), and a lupus-like syndrome (73).

Overdosage

The most common symptoms are drowsiness, tachycardia, and tremor. No deaths or seizures have been recorded (30).

Interactions

Single doses of nomifensine reveal no impairment of reaction time or perceptual function (35).

A case of paranoid ideation in a patient with hyperthyroidism (39) was explained on the basis that the condition is known to increase dopamine receptor sensitivity.

TRAZODONE

Structure, Pharmacology, Development, and Pharmacokinetics

Trazodone is a triazolopyridine derivative. It is a relatively selective but weak inhibitor of serotonin reuptake with sedative activity (10); it does not bind to muscarinic receptors but is active at both serotonergic and α-adrenergic receptors (64,65).

Trazodone is the first really novel nontricyclic compound. The majority of clinical research appeared in a special supplement to the *Journal of Clinical Psychopharmacology* in November 1981 prior to marketing in the United States in 1982.

Trazodone is rapidly absorbed with peak plasma levels 0.5 to 2 hr after ingestion. Despite a relatively short half-life of 6 to 11 hr, studies (83) found comparable efficacy with once-, twice-, and thrice-daily dose regimens.

Plasma levels (49) show an eightfold variation between individuals with no difference between responders and nonresponders.

Effects

Despite evidence of efficacy (17), clinicians have expressed doubts about the value of this compound based on a failure to benefit core symptoms of depression (70).

Because of its sedative profile, trazodone may be useful in patients with high anxiety or severe insomnia. It has also been studied in schizophrenic patients with depression and may produce benefit without worsening psychotic symptoms or extrapyramidal side effects (10).

Side Effects

Trazodone differs markedly from the tricyclic compounds (10,68). Anticholinergic side effects (dry mouth, blurred vision, bowel and bladder disturbance) occurred in 20% of patients on trazodone, 15% on placebo, and 51% on imipramine. Sedation was reported in 24% of trazodone patients, 12% of those on imipramine, and 6% in placebo. Trazodone also produced a variety of behavioral changes (indecision, loss of interest, forgetfulness, hostility, and fuzzy feeling or confusion), which occurred in 22% of patients compared to 11% on imipramine and 4% on placebo.

The overall incidence of seizures is low (8). Trazodone produces hypotension (69), which appears shortly after the drug is ingested and disappears after 4 to 6 hr (29).

Trazodone has no action on the conduction system of the heart but causes ventricular ectopic beats in some patients (38) and may increase cardiac irritability. Cases of priapism have been described (74), of which several required corrective surgery or suffered permanent loss of erectile function. As use increases, reports of toxic delirium, liver toxicity, skin rashes, conversion to mania, and inhibition of ejaculation have begun to appear (7,8).

Overdosage

The predominant symptom is drowsiness and rarely coma. There have been no deaths, and cardiovascular complications have not occurred (23).

Interactions

Additive effects can be anticipated with the CNS depressants including alcohol, and interactions with MAO inhibitors are predicted by an animal model (50). Trazodone has been shown to antagonize the hypotensive properties of clonidine and α-methyldopa (80) and to increase the plasma levels of phenytoin and digoxin (63,69).

VILOXAZINE

Structure, Pharmacology, Development, and Pharmacokinetics

Viloxazine is a bicyclic compound related to the β-adrenergic blocking agents.

In animal tests viloxazine possesses properties similar to both tricyclic antidepressants and amphetamine, but the mechanism of action is uncertain, and it does not interfere with amine reuptake.

Viloxazine has been available in Europe since 1975 but not in the United States. It has a half-life of 2 to 5 hr and is not therefore suitable for once-daily administration.

Clinical Effects

Viloxazine has a stimulant profile.

Side Effects

Viloxazine has a reduced frequency of anticholinergic side effects but is not devoid of them (6). The most frequent complaints are nausea, vomiting, gastrointestinal distress, and side effects of a stimulant nature (48) including weight loss (46). Migraine headaches occur even in patients with no previous history (2).

The risk of seizures appears to be significantly less than with tricyclic drugs (21).

Viloxazine is relatively free of direct cardiotoxic effects, although tachycardia and hypotension occasionally occur (58).

Overdosage

Most cases recover without serious complications, although coma and hypotension have been reported (16).

Interactions

Viloxazine might be expected to have less tendency to produce additive effects with alcohol (84). It produces increases in plasma levels of carbamazepine (59).

OTHER COMPOUNDS

There are many potential antidepressant compounds in various stages of testing around the world. In the early phases, information is often scanty and mostly available on a word-of-mouth basis between investigators. This is particularly true since pharmaceutical companies appear to have developed the strategy of discouraging early publication and speculation about their products, perhaps as a means of patent protection. Once a drug is close to regulatory approval, much of the information is then presented at a large national conference, the proceedings of which are published as a supplement to one of the (often unrefereed)

journals. Some of the articles are compilations of data by the research division of the manufacturer collected in the course of multicenter studies conducted to standard protocols.

One consequence of this practice is that the major source of published information on new compounds has often escaped critical independent scrutiny and is presented from the perspective of the developer of the drug. For this reason, clinicians should seek information on new compounds from such critical sources as the *A.M.A. Drug Evaluations,* the *Psychopharmacology Bulletin, Meyler's Side Effects of Drugs Annuals,* or recently published textbooks and independent reviews.

Some of the developmental drugs currently in various stages of investigation are listed in Table 1.

CLINICAL USE AND CHOICE AMONG NEWER COMPOUNDS

Table 2 summarizes the major characteristics of all the newer compounds that are in use today. All the drugs are more effective than placebo and equally effective with prototypic tricyclic compounds in short-term clinical trials. The only distinguishing features have been the suggestion that the effect of mianserin may wane during long-term treatment and that buproprion and fluoxetine may have slower onsets of action.

This homogeneity of outcome occurs despite differing biochemical mechanisms and behavioral profiles, which are not necessarily consistent with each other. For example, fluoxetine and trazodone are both serotonin reuptake inhibitors but differ markedly in their stimulant and sedative profiles. The primary antidepressant properties of the compounds may be separated from secondary characteristics based on different pharmacologic mechanisms just as the tricyclic antidepressants display a spectrum from the strongly sedative compound amitriptyline to the more stimulant properties of protriptyline.

At present, choice between newer compounds is based on neither differences in efficacy, alleged biochemical mechanisms, nor clinical subtypes of depression. The criteria are therefore the same as exist for the older antidepressant drugs. These are:

1. Response (or lack of it) to a particular compound in a previous episode. Except in the circumstances discussed below, there is nothing to suggest that any of the newer drugs will become a routine "first-choice" compound. They are more likely to be used after a tricyclic antidepressant has already failed or is contraindicated. Because serotonin reuptake inhibitors are especially prone to interact with MAO inhibitors, these drugs may be preferred before an MAO inhibitor is attempted. The fact that newer compounds will often remain "second-choice" treatments has important implications for the prescribing psychiatrist. Drugs used as "first-choice" agents appear to obtain better results because placebo response and spontaneous remission are attributed to them, whereas "second-choice" compounds are given more often to treatment-refractory or side-effect-sensitive individuals after failure of more traditional drugs. It is important to be aware of this built-in bias against new

TABLE 1. *Developmental antidepressant drugs*

Serotonin reuptake inhibitors
  Alaproclate
  Citalopram[a]
  Clovoxamine
  Femoxetine
  Fluvoxamine[a]
  Indalpine
  Paroxetine

Norepinephrine reuptake inhibitors
  Tandamine
  Nisoxetine
  Oxprotiline

Dopamine reuptake inhibitors
  Diclofensine

[a] Citalopram and fluvoxamine are in fairly advanced stages of clinical testing and have the potential to become available in the United States within several years.

TABLE 2. *Major characteristics of newer antidepressant drugs*

Compound	Mechanism	Clinical profile	Side effects	Overdose	Interactions	Other comments
Buproprion[a]	Dopamine reuptake inhibitor	Stimulant profile Narrow dose range Slower onset of action Adjunctive sedatives may be required Three-times-daily regimen	Less anticholinergic Stimulant actions Weight loss May aggravate schizophrenic symptoms No cardiotoxicity Some epileptogenic potential	Relatively safe (but few reports to date)	Increased seizures with lithium	Self-administered in some species
Fluoxetine[a]	Serotonin reuptake inhibitor	Stimulant profile Slow onset of action Narrow dose range Once-daily dosing Adjunctive sedatives may be required	No weight gain Not anticholinergic Noncardiotoxic Stimulant effects Headache GI disturbances	Relatively safe	Likely with MAOI	Delayed excretion
Maprotiline	Norepinephrine reuptake inhibitor	Same as imipramine	Increased seizures Skin rashes	Similar to tricyclics but exaggerated	Same as tricyclics	Long half-life
Mianserin[b]	Mixed receptor activity No affinity for uptake sites	Strongly sedative Narrow dose range Once-daily administration Possible relapse in long-term use	Not anticholinergic Noncardiotoxic Some epileptogenic potential Blood dyscrasias Immune–allergic reactions	Relatively safe	None with antihypertensive agents	
Nomifensine	Norepinephrine and dopamine reuptake inhibitor Mixed receptor activity	Stimulant profile Twice-daily dosing Adjunctive sedatives may be required Avoid in paranoid patients	Less anticholinergic Noncardiotoxic Insomnia Immune–allergic reactions Orofacial dyskinesia	Relatively safe	Enhances thyroid medications	
Trazodone	Weak serotonin reuptake inhibitor Mixed receptor activity	Sedative profile Half as potent as tricyclics May be given once daily Questionable efficacy in severe depression	Sedation Behavioral– cognitive changes Less anticholinergic Low seizure incidence Ventricular ectopic beats Priapism	Relatively safe	Antagonizes clonidine and α-methyldopa Increases levels of phenytoin and digoxin	Relatively short half-life
Viloxazine[b]	Uncertain Possible receptor activity	Stimulant profile Three-times-daily regimen Adjunctive sedatives may be required	Less anticholinergic GI disturbances Stimulant action Weight loss Migraine headaches Lower seizure risk Noncardiotoxic	Relatively safe	Increased plasma levels of carbamazepine	

[a] Not yet approved for marketing in U.S.
[b] Available in Europe, not in U.S.

compounds, since the treating psychiatrist is liable to become disillusioned when the newer drugs fail to produce results reported in clinical trials. Another bias may operate when treatment with a tricyclic compound or MAO inhibitor is abruptly terminated and withdrawal symptoms that occur are attributed to the newly prescribed drug.

2. Selection based on the desired degree of sedative or stimulant action. The degree of agitation or apathy will influence the choice between sedative agents like trazodone, mianserin, or maprotiline and compounds that have a more stimulant profile. In general, sedative antidepressants are much more widely prescribed (particularly in primary care settings), partly because they can be given at nighttime with the benefit that they alleviate insomnia and avoid the need for additional hypnotic medications. All of the newer sedative compounds can be given once daily, whereas the more stimulant compounds have shorter half-lives and require divided regimens. This means that use of the more stimulant compounds produces the double disadvantage of increased frequency of medication with the possible need for adjunctive sedative–hypnotic drugs and the risk of poorer patient compliance. This is a factor that is not well

tested within the artificial confines of a drug trial, where compliance is assured.

3. Compatibility between patient susceptibility and side effect profile of the drug. Newer drugs are particularly useful for individuals with preexisting physical conditions or idiosyncratic responses that make them susceptible to the side effects of tricyclic antidepressants or MAO inhibitors. Most of the newer compounds have been routinely tested in geriatric subpopulations and found to be relatively safe, with the same commonsense recommendations to use about half the normal adult dose and titrate upwards slowly. All of the newer drugs have been reported to lower seizure thresholds in some individuals. Since the relative risk of seizures with different antidepressants is difficult to estimate, there is no compound that can be declared unequivocally safe. There is good evidence that maprotiline poses an additional hazard. An obvious area of need is for drugs without the cardiotoxic actions of the tricyclic compounds. Although trazodone held early promise and does not cause conduction defects, there is accumulating evidence of direct myocardial actions. This leaves mianserin as the only sedative compound that has a clean cardiac profile, and with the added advantage that it does not interact with antihypertensive agents. Unfortunately, it is not available in the United States. All of the more stimulant drugs appear to be relatively noncardiotoxic. Freedom from the more common but troublesome anticholinergic and autonomic side effects of the tricyclic antidepressants is an obvious and fairly clear-cut advantage to most of the newer compounds. Absence of weight gain with the more stimulant drugs and lack of interference with sexual function are particularly valuable, although the priapism caused by trazodone is a tragic exception. Finally, with the exception of maprotiline, the newer drugs appear much safer when taken in overdose than are either the tricyclic compounds or MAO inhibitors.

4. Compatibility with concurrent medications. Knowledge about interactions is another area that waits on widespread use of a compound and its administration to individuals taking other medications. As shown in Table 2, several specific interactions have been noted once compounds have reached clinical use, including viloxazine with carbamazepine, buproprion with lithium, and nomifensine with thyroid preparations.

Within the context of the above guidelines, the newer compounds have an obvious and increasing place in psychiatric practice. New and unanticipated side effects are also inevitable either because they are less common and escaped scrutiny in clinical trials or because they masquerade as common or innocuous conditions and are sometimes mistakenly attributed to somatization. Experience with the "flu"-like symptoms that occurred early in treatment with zimelidine is a tragic example that underscores the need for the practicing psychiatrist to be continuously alert for novel or unexpected actions of new drugs.

INVESTIGATIONAL IMPLICATIONS OF NEWER COMPOUNDS

As always in new drug investigations, the major problems are avoidance of type 1 or type 2 errors with regard to efficacy and the oversight of serious or unexpected side effects.

In the last decade there have been improvements in design through the contributions of the Psychopharmacology Research Branch at NIMH and in diagnosis with application of RDC and DSM-III criteria. This enhances validity as well as the generalizability of findings from research to clinical practice. The problems of evaluating maintenance or "prophylactic" claims have been elucidated, and the newer antidepressants will have to be tested for these indications as their use increases.

The accepted efficacy of prototype antidepressants tempts investigators to shun placebo controls but opens the possibility to error, especially in small sample sizes (75). This may be compounded by failure to publish negative findings, particularly when contemporary research is strongly influenced by commercial factors.

As the number of effective drugs increases, so does the problem of recruitment of patients for study who may be unwilling to give informed consent either for placebo treatment or reversal to a prototype drug after effective short-term benefit on an investigational compound.

Unanticipated side effects can be minimized by a number of strategies including segmentation of at-risk populations (such as the elderly), longer-term studies, and postmarketing surveillance to detect problems related to overdose, drug interactions, faulty compliance, or rare side effects.

Finally, as preclinical testing becomes better able to select compounds with highly specific biochemical profiles, our improved research designs should be able to define the mechanisms that underlie therapeutic benefit and side effect susceptibility.

REFERENCES

1. Abdulgabar, A., and Mueller-Eckhardt, C. (1985): *N. Engl. J. Med.,* 313(8):469–474.
2. Barnes, T., and Greenwood, D. T. (1979): *Lancet,* 2:1368.
3. Becker, R. E., and Dufrensne, R. L. (1983): *Am. J. Psychiatry,* 139:1200–1201.
4. Black, D. A., and O'Brien, I. M. (1985): *Br. Med. J.,* 289:1272.
5. Blackwell, B. (1984): In: *Meyler's Side Effects of Drugs. Annual 8,* edited by M. N. G. Dukes, pp. 22–31. Excerpta Medica, Amsterdam.
6. Blackwell, B. (1984): In: *Meyler's Side Effects of Drugs, 10th edition,* edited by M. N. G. Dukes, pp. 24–61. Excerpta Medica, Amsterdam.
7. Blackwell, B. (1985): In: *Meyler's Side Effects of Drugs. Annual 9,* edited by M. N. G. Dukes, pp. 18–26. Excerpta Medica, Amsterdam.
8. Blackwell, B. (1986): In: *Meyler's Side Effects of Drugs. Annual 10,* edited by M. N. G. Dukes. Excerpta Medica, Amsterdam.
9. Brogden, R. N., Heel, R. C., and Speight, T. M. (1978): *Drugs,* 16:273–285.
10. Brogden, R. N., Heel, R. C., and Speight, T. M. (1981): *Drugs,* 21(6):401–429.
11. Burgess, C. D., Montgomery, S., Wadsworth, J., and Turner, P. (1979): *Postgrad. Med. J.,* 55(648):704–708.
12. Burrows, G. D., Vohra, J., Dumovic, P., Scoggins, B. A., and Davies, B. (1978): *Med. J. Aust.,* 1:341–343.
13. Chouinard, G. (1983): *J. Clin. Psychiatry,* 44:121.
14. Chouinard, G. (1985): *J. Clin. Psychiatry,* 46(3):32–37.
15. Coccaro, E. F., and Siever, L. J. (1985): *J. Clin. Pharmacol.,* 25(4): 241–260.
16. Crome, P. (1982): *Drugs,* 23:431–461.
17. Davis, J. M., and Vogel, C. (1981): *J. Clin. Psychopharmacol.,* 1(Suppl.):27S.
18. Diller, N. (1982): *Act. Neuro. Super. (Praha),* 24–28.
19. Dufresne, R. L., Weber, S., and Becker, R. (1984): *Drug Int. Clin. Pharmacol.,* 18(12):957–964.

20. Edwards, J. (1979): *Lancet,* 2:1368–1369.
21. Edwards, G. J., and Glen-Bott, M. (1984): *J. Neurol. Neurosurg. Psychiatry,* 47:960–964.
22. Elliot, H. L., Whiting, B., and Reid, J. L. (1983): *Br. J. Clin. Pharmacol.,* 15:323S–328S.
23. Faillace, L. A. (1983): *Emerg. Med.* (Suppl.)
24. Farid, F. F., Wenger, T. L., Tsai, S. Y., Singh, B. N., and Stern, W. C. (1983): *J. Clin. Psychiatry,* 44(2):170–173.
25. Fisch, C. (1985): *J. Clin. Psychiatry,* 46(Pt. 2):42–44.
26. Forrest, W. A. (1977): *J. Int. Med. Res.,* 5(Suppl. 4):116–121.
27. Gardner, E. A., and Johnston, J. A. (1985): *J. Clin. Psychopharmacol.,* 5(1):24–29.
28. Glassman, A. H. (1984): *Annu. Rev. Med.,* 35:503–511.
29. Glassman, A. H. (1984): *Psychopharmacol. Bull.,* 20:272–279.
30. Granier, R., Delaby, F., and Charbaux, C. (1982): *J. Toxicol. Med.,* 2:141–146.
31. Griffith, J. D., Carranza, J., Griffith, C., and Miller, L. L. (1983): *J. Clin. Psychiatry,* 44:206–208.
32. Ham, H., Aumiller, J., and Bohmer, R. (1985): *Lancet,* 1:1328–1329.
33. Harto-Truax, N., Stern, W. C., Miller, L. L., Sato, T. L., and Cato, A. E. (1983): *J. Clin. Psychiatry,* 44:183–186.
34. Heptner, W., Hornke, I., and Uihlein, M. (1984): *J. Clin. Psychiatry,* 45(4,Sect. 2):21.
35. Hindmarch, I., Parrott, A. C., and Stonier, P. D. (1980): *R. Soc. Med. Int. Cong. Symp.,* 25:47–54.
36. Hollister, L. E. (1981): *Psychosomatics,* 22(10):872–879.
37. Hulten, B. A., and Heath, A. (1983): *Acta Med. Scand.,* 213:275–278.
38. Janowsky, D., Curtis, G., Zisok, S., Kuhn, K., Resovsky, K., et al. (1983): *J. Clin. Psychopharmacol.,* 3(6):372–376.
39. Katona, C. (1982): *Lancet,* 2:384–385.
40. Knudsen, K., and Heath, A. (1984): *Br. Med. J.,* 288(6417):601–603.
41. Kopera, H. (1980): *Curr. Med. Res. Opin.,* 6(Suppl. 7):132–138.
42. Kopera, H., Kleinm W., and Schenk, H. (1980): *Prog. Neuropsychopharmacol.,* 4(4–5):527–535.
43. Laakmann, G., Hoffmann, N., and Hofschuster, E. (1982): *Life Sci.,* 30:1725–1732.
44. Lai, A. A., and Schroeder, D. H. (1983): *J. Clin. Psychiatry,* 44(5,Sect. 2):82–84.
45. Lemberger, L., Bergstrom, R. F., and Wolen, R. L. (1985): *J. Clin. Psychiatry,* 46(3):14–19.
46. Lennox, I. G., Ashbury, J. F. P., and Couldrick, W. G. R. (1978): *Practitioner,* 220(1315):153.
47. Lloyd, A. H. (1977): *J. Int. Med. Res.,* 5(Suppl. 4):122–138.
48. Lopes, L. J., Versiani, M., and Romildo, B. J. (1977): *Folha. Med.,* 74:75–80.
49. Mann, J. J., Georgotas, A., Newton, R., and Gershon, S. (1981): *J. Clin. Psychopharmacol.,* 1(2):75–80.
50. Marley, E., and Wozniak, K. M. (1984): *J. Psychiatr. Res.,* 18(2):191–203.
51. Mehta, N. B. (1983): *J. Clin. Psychiatry,* 44:56–59.
52. Miller, P. I., Beaumont, G., Seldrup, J., John, V., Luscombe, D. K., et al. (1977): *J. Int. Med. Res.,* 5(Suppl. 4):101–111.
53. Nemeroff, C. B., and Evans, D. L. (1983): *Biol. Psychiatry,* 18(2):237–241.
54. Peck, A. W., Stern, W. C., and Watkinson, C. (1983): *J. Clin. Psychiatry,* 44(5,Pt. 2):197–201.
55. Peck, A. W., and Hamilton, M. (1983): *J. Clin. Psychiatry,* 44(5,Pt. 2):202–205.
56. Peet, M., and Behagel, H. (1978): *Br. J. Clin. Pharmacol.,* 5:5–9.
57. Petz, R. (1985): *N. Engl. J. Med.,* 313:510–512.
58. Pinder, R. M., Brogden, R. N., Speight, T. M., and Avery, G. S. (1977): *Drugs,* 13(6):401–421.
59. Pisani, F., Narbone, M. C., Fazio, A., Crisafulli, P., Primmerano, G., et al. (1984): *Epilepsia,* 25(4):482–485.
60. Potter, W., Scheinin, M., Golden, R., Rudorfer, M. V., Cowdry, R. W., et al. (1985): *Arch. Gen. Psychiatry,* 42:1171–1177.
61. Preskorn, S. H. (1983): *J. Clin. Psychiatry,* 44(5,Pt. 2):137–139.
62. Preskorn, S. H., and Othmer, S. C. (1984): *Pharmacotherapy,* 4(1):20–34.
63. Rauch, J. L., Pavlinac, D. M., and Newman, P. E. (1984): *Am. J. Psychiatry,* 141:1472–1473.
64. Riblet, L. A., and Taylor, D. P. (1981): *J. Clin. Psychopharmacol.,* 1:17S.
65. Richelson, E. (1981): In: *Antidepressants: Neurochemical, Behavioral, and Clinical Perspectives,* edited by S. J. Enna. Raven Press, New York.
66. Richelson, E. (1982): *J. Clin. Psychiatry,* 43(11,Pt. 2):4–13.
67. Rickels, K., Smith, W. T., Glaudin, V., Amsterdam, J. M., Weise, C., et al. (1985): *J. Clin. Psychiatry,* 46(3,Pt. 2):38–41.
68. Risch, S. C., and Janowsky, D. S. (1981): *J. Clin. Psychopharmacol.,* 1:27S.
69. Robinson, D. S. (1984): *Psychopharmacol. Bull.,* 20(2):280–290.
70. Rudorfer, M. V., Golden, R. N., and Potter, W. Z. (1984): *Psych. Clin. North Am.,* 7(3):519–534.
71. Saletu, B., and Grunberger, J. (1985): *J. Clin. Psychiatry,* 46:45–52.
72. Saletu, B., Grunberger, J., Linzmayer, L., and Taeuber, K. (1982): *Int. Pharmacopsychiatry,* 17(Suppl. 1):43–72.
73. Schonhofer, P. S., and Groticke, J. (1985): *Lancet,* 2:221.
74. Sher, M., Krieger, J. N., and Juergens, S. (1983): *Am. J. Psychiatry,* 140:1362–1363.
75. Shopsin, B., Cassano, G. B., and Conti, L. (1981): In: *Antidepressants: Neurochemical, Behavioral, and Clinical Perspectives,* edited by S. J. Enna, J. Molick, and E. Richelson. Raven Press, New York.
76. Siever, L. J., and Davis, K. L. (1985): *Am. J. Psychiatry,* 142(9):1017–1031.
77. Stark, P., Fuller, R. W., and Wong, D. T. (1985): *J. Clin. Psychiatry,* 46(3):7–13.
78. Stark, P., and Hardison, C. D. (1985): *J. Clin. Psychiatry,* 46(3):53–58.
79. Van Dorth, R. M. (1983): *Acta Psychiat. Scand. (Suppl.),* 302:72–80.
80. Van Zweiten, P. A. (1977): *Pharmacology,* 15(4):331–336.
81. Wells, B. G., and Gelenberg, A. J. (1985): *Pharmacotherapy,* 1:121.
82. Wernicke, J. F. (1985): *J. Clin. Psychiatry,* 46(3):59–67.
83. Wheatley, D. (1980): *Int. Pharmacopsychiatry,* 15(4):240–246.
84. Wilson, W. H., Petrie, W. M., and Ban, T. A. (1981): *Drug Dev. Res.,* 1:223.
85. Zbiden, G., and Spichiger, H. (1983): *Arch. Toxicol.,* 51:43–51.

Psychopharmacology:
The Third Generation of Progress,
edited by Herbert Y. Meltzer.
Raven Press, New York © 1987.

CHAPTER 106

Long-Term Treatment of Affective Disorders

Robert F. Prien

Long-term treatment of affective disorders has assumed greater importance during the past decade as an increasing number of clinicians have recognized the need for considering the longitudinal nature of affective disorders in treatment and research planning. The clinical course of affective illness for many patients can best be described in terms of recurrences, remissions, and chronicity. A conservative estimate is that at least half of the individuals who have an initial episode of major depression and over 80% who have a manic episode will have one or more recurrences (3,40,52). These recurring episodes not only cause great disruption in social, familial, and career functioning but may also be fatal, as about 15 of 100 depressed persons commit suicide.

There are also growing research and therapeutic interest in the functioning between major episodes. Studies indicate that from 15 to 35% of individuals with a major affective disorder do not recover fully from any given episode (12,37,67). The incomplete recovery may represent residual chronicity resulting from inadequate treatment of the episode, a preexisting chronic disorder, or the progressive deteriorative effects of recurrences on the capacity to cope with usual life activities.

TERMINOLOGY

Purposes of Treatment

The long-term treatment of affective disorders can be classified into three categories or purposes:

1. Continuation therapy for maintaining control of an acute episode after initial subsidence of symptoms.
2. Preventive therapy for preventing or attenuating new episodes.
3. Treatment of chronicity for managing dysthymia, cyclothymia, or other long-term affective disorders.

The three categories may be blurred in clinical practice. Continuation therapy may become preventive therapy once the episode has run its course. Preventive therapy may serve the dual purpose of preventing new episodes and controlling or resolving interepisode psychopathology. Despite the potential for overlap, these categories are useful for discussing the purposes of long-term treatment and are employed with this intention.

Continuation Treatment

Affective episodes do not necessarily end with the drug-induced control of symptoms. Continued administration of the drug may be required for months after the disappearance of acute symptoms. This form of maintenance therapy is termed "continuation treatment." The use of continuation treatment is based on the assumption that antidepressant and antimanic drugs suppress manifest symptoms without immediately correcting the postulated pathophysiologic process underlying the episode.

Preventive Treatment

In this review, the term "preventive treatment" refers to the use of long-term treatment to modify the course of recurrent affective illness through reduction in the frequency and/or severity of major recurrences.

Treatment of Chronicity

The DSM-III defines two types of chronic affective disorders: dysthymic disorder and cyclothymic disorder. By definition, these disorders are long-standing (at least 2 years' duration in adults) and are characterized by persistent or intermittent affective syndromes that are not of sufficient severity or duration to satisfy the criteria for major depression or mania. Cyclothymic disorder consists of both hypomanic and depressive periods. Dysthymic disorder is characterized by depression but not hypomania.

Relapse and Recurrence

The differentiation between continuation and preventive therapies has led investigators to coin the terms "relapse" to refer to worsening of an ongoing episode and "recurrence" to represent the occurrence of a new episode.

Unipolar and Bipolar Disorders

The bipolar–unipolar distinction is employed in most preventive treatment studies and plays a vital role in understanding long-term drug treatment. Although unipolar disorder is a popular term in the therapeutic literature, it was not adopted into DSM-III because of the diversity of diagnostic criteria that have been employed in defining the disorder and the heterogeneity of conditions that it can represent. For the purposes of this report, the term unipolar disorder is limited to patients with recurrent major depression who have never had a manic episode. In DSM-III, the category of bipolar disorder describes patients who have a history of mania with or without a major depression. This disorder is sometimes referred to as bipolar I to distinguish it from bipolar II disorder (coded bipolar atypical disorder in DSM-III), which describes patients with at least one episode of major depression and a history of hypomania but not mania. Unless otherwise specified, the term bipolar disorder refers to bipolar I illness.

CONTINUATION TREATMENT

Placebo-Controlled Studies

There is evidence from several placebo-controlled studies to support the need for continuation of drug treatment following initial control of symptoms for both unipolar and bipolar disorders (15,42,51,60,61,69,73). In each study, an antidepressant or lithium was used to control acute symptoms, after which about half of the patients were switched, double blind, to a placebo and the other half continued to receive the drug. Overall, approximately 50% of the placebo-treated patients relapsed during the subsequent 6 months, compared to only about 20% of the drug-treated patients. The relapse rate with placebo was highest during the 2 months following discontinuation of medication.

Duration

To be safe, continuation therapy should be maintained for as long as the episode would be expected to last if left untreated. The problem is that when continuation treatment is effective, it may be difficult to determine when the episode is over on the basis of symptoms alone. This uncertainty may cause the clinician either to withdraw the drug prematurely, subjecting the patient to a relapse, or to prolong treatment unnecessarily.

Studies of the course of affective illness are of only limited help in estimating episode length. A longitudinal survey by Angst et al. (5) demonstrates that the duration of episodes tends to remain constant or lengthen slightly with each recurrence. These results suggest that the length of the preceding episode may serve as the lower estimate of the length of the current one. The problem with this approach is that effective drug treatment may have made the prior episode appear shorter than it was.

Work with possible biological markers of episode length such as disturbance in sleep continuity, shortened REM latency and diminished δ-phase (slow-wave) sleep activity (46,75), hypercortisolemnia (75), dexamethasone non-suppression (10,11,27), thyroid-stimulating hormone (TSH) blunting (50), and other measures of neuroendocrine secretory patterns (74,75) have provided promising leads for determining when an episode is over, but nothing that currently can be translated into clinical practice.

The only study-derived guideline for length of continuation therapy for the individual patient is provided by results from the recent Collaborative Study of Long-Term Maintenance Drug Therapy in Recurrent Affective Disorder coordinated by the National Institute of Mental Health (NIMH) (61). Results indicate that withdrawal of continuation treatment following a major depressive episode is safe only after the patient has been free of significant symptoms or has returned to his or her usual level of interepisode functioning for at least 4 months. A patient was considered to be free of significant symptoms if he or she manifested no more than minimal or transient symptoms as defined by the Global Adjustment Scale.

Continuation Treatment Following ECT

Early European trials suggest that continuation treatment with antidepressant drugs following control of acute symptoms by ECT reduces the relapse rate from approximately 50% to 15 to 20% (28,36). However, it is possible that the current relapse rate with continuation drug therapy is higher than indicated in the earlier trials. Current clinical practice tends to limit more narrowly the indications for

ECT to cases that are refractory to or are unable to tolerate antidepressant medication. Continuation treatment with ECT following successful control of acute symptoms with ECT warrants careful study.

PREVENTIVE TREATMENT

There is general agreement that certain drugs such as lithium can be effective preventive treatments. Critical issues are who should receive treatment, what treatment should be used, how long treatment should be continued, and how to maintain patient compliance.

Who Should Receive Treatment?

Numerous factors determine whether or not preventive treatment should be initiated. Among the factors to be considered are the likelihood of a recurrence in the near future, the severity and abruptness of previous episodes, the potential impact of a subsequent episode on the patient's functioning and life activities, the patient's willingness to commit himself or herself to the program, the presence of possible contraindications to treatment, and the patient's response to prior treatment regimens.

There is no fixed rule for determining who should receive preventive treatment. The factors listed above cannot be easily quantified into a formula. However, for a key factor—the likelihood of a recurrence in the near future—there is guidance from the research literature. Most clinicians who have published an opinion on the topic recommend that a patient should have at least two or three well-defined episodes requiring psychiatric intervention before he or she is treated with preventive drug therapy. Patients who have only a single attack, mild attacks, or a long interval between episodes (e.g., more than 5 years) should probably not receive long-term treatment. Possible exceptions are patients for whom a second episode would be life threatening or highly disruptive to career or family functioning or occasional patients who have an initial manic episode after age 30.

There are supportive data for administering preventive treatment after two episodes. Angst et al. (5) report that cycle length (the period between the onset of one episode and that of the next) tends to decrease with successive episodes through the first four or five episodes. The decrease in cycle length results from a shortening of the interval between episodes. After the second episode, the average cycle length drops to 20 months for bipolar patients and 22 months for unipolar patients. Assuming that the average episode lasts for 6 to 9 months, the mean interval between the second and third episodes ranges from only a year to a year and a half.

In a more recent report from a survey of over 400 patients followed for 20 years, Angst (4) indicates that patients who have two major episodes within 5 years have a 70% probability of having two or more episodes during the subsequent 5 years. Other surveys of course of affective illness (22,39) spotlight the high risk of early recurrence in patients with a history of multiple episodes.

Choice of Treatment: Unipolar Disorder

Lithium and the Antidepressants

The choice of drug for the prevention of recurrences in patients with unipolar disorder is a subject of controversy. A primary issue is the comparative efficacy of lithium and antidepressants, particularly the tricyclic antidepressants (TCAs). Six preventive studies compare lithium against an antidepressant in unipolar patients (Table 1). All the studies are in agreement that drug therapy is an effective preventive treatment for patients with unipolar disorder. However, the trials yield differing results and conclusions regarding the comparative preventive efficacy of lithium and the antidepressants. A review of the studies suggests that differences in results may be attributed in large measure to differences in design and study populations (62).

A report from the Consensus Development Conference on Mood Disorders: Pharmacologic Prevention of Recurrences convened by the NIMH and the National Institutes of Health in 1984 (52) concludes that both the TCAs and lithium are effective preventive treatments, each with advantages for certain patients. The Conference report notes that the TCAs have a logistic advantage over lithium. Because most acute unipolar depressions are treated with antidepressants rather than with lithium, continuation of the antidepressant for preventive treatment avoids the decisions and problems of when and how to switch the patient from an antidepressant to lithium. In addition, there is evidence suggesting that the TCAs are more effective than lithium in preventing severe depressive recurrences (62).

Lithium has one strong advantage over the TCAs. Lithium has potent antimanic properties, whereas the TCAs have been shown to be relatively ineffective in preventing manic recurrences and, according to some reports (48,78), may precipitate hypomania, mania, or rapid cycling in patients with latent or unrecognized bipolar disorder. The Conference report notes that 10 to 15% of patients with a diagnosis of unipolar disorder subsequently will develop a manic episode.

TABLE 1. *Trials comparing lithium and antidepressants*

Study	Lithium		Antidepressant	
	Total N	Recurrence	Total N	Recurrence
Coppen et al. (14)	12	3 (25%)	8	6 (75%)[a]
Coppen et al. (13)	15	0 (0%)	13	7 (54%)[b]
Glen et al. (26)	68	44 (65%)	54	36 (67%)[c]
Kane et al. (35)	7	2 (29%)	6	5 (83%)[d]
Prien et al. (60)	27	13 (48%)	25	12 (48%)[d]
Prien et al. (62)	31	21 (68%)	39	18 (46%)[d]
Total	160	83 (52%)	145	84 (58%)

[a] Maprotiline.
[b] Mianserin.
[c] Amitriptyline.
[d] Imipramine.

Because of the disruptive consequences of an unexpected manic episode, it is recommended that lithium therapy be given serious consideration where there is suspicion of a latent or previously undiagnosed bipolar disorder or a higher than usual risk of developing a manic episode (e.g., having a family history of bipolar disorder or a personal history of hypomania). The Conference report concludes that both lithium and the TCAs pose risks for elderly patients, who may be more vulnerable to renal complications with lithium and to urinary retention, orthostatic hypotension, and cardiac arrhythmias with the TCAs. An added disadvantage of lithium is its teratogenic effects (80), which limit its use for women of childbearing age. Earlier fears of renal failure from structural damage during lithium therapy have abated but have led to recommendations that clinicians use the lowest effective dose and monitor renal function at routine intervals (34). Comprehensive reviews of adverse reactions with lithium and the TCAs are provided by Vestergaard (77), Siris and Rifkin (71), and Blackwell (9).

Alternatives to Lithium and the TCAs

Clinicians often face the critical problem of what to use for preventive treatment when the major episode that brings the patient in for treatment is effectively controlled with a drug other than a TCA or lithium. One option is to withdraw the drug following recovery from the episode and initiate a TCA or lithium for preventive treatment. This option has several drawbacks. Taking away a drug that is producing a good response and substituting a TCA or lithium can pose logistical, ethical, and compliance problems as well as possible loss of control over symptomatology during and after the substitution. There is also the possibility that the patient may have failed to respond or had adverse reactions to prior treatment with TCAs or lithium.

The option of continuing the original drug for preventive treatment should be given serious consideration, particularly if a switch to a TCA or lithium is inappropriate for compliance, efficacy, or safety reasons. The problem is that the monoamine oxidase inhibitors (MAOIs) and newer classes of drugs have not been evaluated in controlled long-term studies of preventive efficacy. However, unless the original drug presents special risks when used on a long-term basis or has been inadequately tested for safety for long-term use, the advantages of continuing the drug seem to outweigh the disadvantages. The most cautionary statement regarding long-term use is for amoxapine because of the risk of tardive dyskinesia and extrapyramidal reactions.

A third option is to add lithium to the antidepressant regimen. There is no evidence that the combination is more effective than an antidepressant alone. However, patients who are at higher than usual risk for developing a bipolar disorder may benefit from the antimanic properties of lithium.

Role of Psychotherapy

Psychotherapies designed for the treatment of depressed patients (cognitive and interpersonal) and certain behavioral, marital, and group therapies have demonstrated efficacy in alleviating depressive symptoms. However, with the exception of an ongoing 3-year study utilizing interpersonal psychotherapy (47), none have been evaluated for long-term preventive efficacy. Short-term maintenance treatment studies suggest that psychotherapy may be beneficial in treating the mild depressive symptoms and impairment in social and interpersonal adjustment that characterize the interepisode functioning of many patients with recurrent major depressive disorders (81). There is speculation that these interepisode conditions may play a role in precipitating a subsequent episode (82).

The role of the psychological or "nonspecific psychotherapeutic" components of the clinical management of pharmacologic treatment should not be overlooked. A physician–patient interaction that provides education about the disorder and its treatment together with reassurance and encouragement serves to maintain the patient's motivation and improve compliance. The NIMH Treatment of Depression Collaborative Research Program (19) includes a clinical management condition embodying these factors in a trial evaluating psychotherapy and pharmacotherapy in acute depression. The results from this study should provide information on the effects of specific and nonspecific psychotherapeutic factors that could have implications for preventive treatment.

From a clinical standpoint, until more research information is forthcoming, psychotherapy should not be used as a substitute for pharmacotherapy for preventive treatment. Psychotherapy may be used in an adjunctive role with pharmacotherapy with the recognition that its value in this capacity has not been established.

Choice of Treatment: Bipolar Disorder (Bipolar I)

Lithium

Lithium is the recommended long-term treatment for bipolar disorder. Studies indicate that lithium is significantly superior to placebo in preventing both manic and depressive recurrences (6,16,21,59,60). With the exception of imipramine, which has been shown to be ineffective in protecting against manic attacks (60,62), no other drug has been adequately evaluated for the preventive treatment of bipolar disorder.

A major problem is what one does with the bipolar patient who does not respond to preventive treatment with lithium. However, before assuming that lithium is ineffective, the clinician should determine if the patient had an adequate serum lithium level and was complying with the medication schedule. Although some patients may respond at levels as low as 0.4 to 0.5 mEq/liter, others may require levels as high as 0.8 to 1.2 mEq/liter. An emerging recurrence at a low level in patients who can tolerate higher doses should cause one to question the adequacy of dosage.

Anticonvulsant Drugs

Carbamazepine, an anticonvulsant with a molecular structure resembling imipramine, is a promising backup treatment for lithium but has been evaluated in only three controlled double-blind trials (8,55,57), collectively involving fewer than 30 bipolar patients treated with carbamazepine. Open studies and short-term maintenance trials suggest that carbamazepine may be effective for cases not responsive to lithium (20,54,58), but this is far from an established finding. Other anticonvulsant drugs such as sodium valproate (49,63) also warrant evaluation.

Combination of Lithium and Neuroleptic

Patients who suffer severe manic recurrences while receiving lithium sometimes are treated with a neuroleptic alone or in combination with lithium. In such cases, the risk of tardive dyskinesia and other adverse effects of neuroleptic treatment is regarded as less of a danger than the highly disruptive and life-threatening consequences of repeated manic attacks. There is need for clearer definition of patients for whom this option is justifiable.

Combination of Lithium and TCA

A decade ago, the combination of lithium and a TCA was regarded as the most promising of the potential preventive treatments of bipolar disorder. The rationale for combining lithium and a TCA was that lithium would protect the patient against manic recurrences and that the TCA would protect against depressive recurrences. Two multihospital studies (62,64) indicate that the combination of lithium and imipramine provides no advantage over lithium alone.

Other Alternatives

The newer classes of antidepressants require evaluation for preventive efficacy. Some clinicians regard bupropion as the most promising of the newer drugs for preventive treatment of bipolar disorder because of its purported advantage in protecting against manic recurrences (23,84). Other experimental treatments for nonresponders to lithium include the calcium channel blocker verapamil (24,25), the serotonin precursors tryptophan and 5-hydroxytryptophan, and hypermetabolic doses of thyroid hormone (72). Two nonpharmacologic techniques, sleep advancement (or partial sleep deprivation) (79) and high-intensity light (45), subsequently may prove beneficial for selected bipolar patients who cannot tolerate medication. Light therapy may be effective for patients with seasonal affective disorders, particularly bipolar II depression (30,66).

Role of Psychotherapy

Although patients with bipolar disorder traditionally have been regarded as poor candidates for psychotherapy, there have been some promising results with combined pharmacotherapeutic–psychotherapeutic approaches. Long-term group psychotherapy or structured psychological support may enhance drug compliance and acceptance of preventive drug treatment programs (31,70). Psychotherapy may also improve social, family, and daily coping impairments that can result from frequent and severe recurrences (33).

Choices of Treatment: Bipolar II Disorder

There are only a few long-term therapeutic studies that have employed a bipolar II sample. Kane et al. (35) found lithium to be a more effective long-term treatment than imipramine or placebo in preventing depressive recurrences. Dunner et al. (18) reported no significant difference between lithium and placebo in preventing depressive recurrences but found lithium to be superior in reducing the frequency of hypomanic episodes. Peslow et al. (56), using a life table analysis to estimate probability of depressive recurrences for a 2-year period, found lithium to be more effective with bipolar II patients than with unipolar patients but reported a high recurrence rate for both groups (51% for bipolar II patients and 64% for unipolar patients).

The effectiveness of lithium in bipolar II disorder is not as well established as in bipolar I disorder, but it must still be regarded as the treatment of choice. Alternatives to lithium have not been adequately evaluated. A concern is the extent to which TCAs in bipolar II patients may precipitate hypomanic or manic episodes and how this may affect course of illness (2).

Effectiveness of Preventive Therapy in Modifying Course of Illness

Rate of Recurrence

In placebo-controlled studies of preventive therapy with unipolar patients, the average failure rates for lithium and the TCAs are 40% and 49%, respectively, compared to 75% for placebo (6,16,17,21,26,35,60,62). The average failure rate for lithium with bipolar patients is 34% compared to 81% for placebo (6,16,17,21,59,60). In most studies, failure is defined as the appearance of a major episode that requires either hospitalization or treatment with a psychopharmacologic agent other than the medication under study. Most studies range in duration from 18 to 30 months.

A caveat in interpreting failure rates from published preventive trials is that patients usually are classified as treatment failures after the first recurrence and are dropped from the study. In clinical practice, however, success or failure often is evaluated against the course of illness before treatment. Accordingly, a patient who suffers a moderately severe recurrence every 2 to 3 years may be considered a treatment success if he or she had more frequent or severe episodes before treatment.

Prevention Versus Attenuation

A prevailing issue is whether preventive drug treatments such as lithium actually prevent the occurrence of affective episodes or merely dampen the episode sufficiently to prevent a full attack. It appears that the drugs can act in both ways, depending on the individual case (7). However, Schou (68) cautions that patients who have no major recurrences during preventive treatment often have "reminders" lasting for a few days to a week when they feel as if an attack is under way. These reminders may represent recurrences that have been dampened to a very mild severity and duration.

Interepisode Functioning

A frequently overlooked issue in preventive treatment studies is the effectiveness of the treatments on functioning during episode-free periods. Outcome for preventive treatment studies is evaluated mainly in terms of incidence of major depression or mania. Clinical evaluation instruments are selected primarily for their capacity to identify and describe major episodes. The relative inattention to interepisode functioning deprives the clinician of important information regarding the effectiveness of preventive treatments. The clinician faced with the finding that two treatments are equally effective in preventing recurrences may wish to know how the treatments compared in attenuating or resolving the milder, but nonetheless disruptive, psychopathology or impairment that is often present between major episodes.

Duration of Treatment

A critical decision facing the practitioner is how long to continue preventive treatment. There is no evidence that drugs can cure recurrent affective illness. However, there is evidence that recurrences may cease spontaneously in some patients after many years of illness (5). The only way to determine whether or not a patient still requires preventive treatment is gradually to discontinue treatment and carefully follow the patient for signs of a recurrence.

Patient Compliance

A frequently neglected factor affecting the success of any program of preventive drug therapy is patient compliance. Without the cooperation of the patient and family, even the most carefully planned program is destined to fail. Surveys suggest that 25 to 50% of patients receiving long-term preventive drug treatment discontinue medication against medical advice or otherwise fail to comply with the treatment schedule (9,31,76). Many suffer recurrences as a result. Klein et al. (40), Jacobs et al. (29), and Jamison and Goodwin (32) elaborate on the reasons for noncompliance and discuss means for improving acceptance of the treatment program and adherence to the therapeutic schedule.

TREATMENT OF CHRONICITY

Dysthymic Disorder

Dysthymic disorder poses a significant public health problem. A recent survey conducted in three urban communities collected prevalence rates for DSM-III diagnoses for 9,000 randomly selected adults (65). The lifetime prevalence of dysthymia was approximately 4% for women and 2% for men. An earlier mental health survey in an urban community found that about 5% of adults suffered from chronic depression of at least 2 years' duration (83). There is significant morbidity associated with dysthymic disorder. Kovacs et al. (44), using a life table analysis in a longitudinal study of children with dysthymic disorder, report that the probability of developing an initial episode of major depression within 5 years of the onset of dysthymia is 60%. A report from the NIMH Collaborative Study of the Psychobiology of Depression (38) indicates that patients with "double depression" (a major depressive episode superimposed on a preexisting dysthymic disorder) have a significantly greater likelihood of an early recurrence than patients who have a major depressive episode without a preexisting dysthymia.

The only published controlled therapeutic study to focus exclusively on chronic depression is a 25-patient placebo-controlled trial (43) that reports that imipramine is effective in controlling both major depressive symptoms and the chronic disorder over a 6-month period.

One problem in studying the long-term treatment of dysthymic disorder is that the DSM-III classification of the disorder is too broad in scope to provide adequate guidelines for selection of patients for specific long-term treatments. One of the more promising classification systems is proposed by Akiskal (2), who differentiates chronic depression into four subtypes, two of which are reported to be responsive to pharmacologic and psychosocial treatments.

One of the treatment-responsive subtypes is an early onset "subaffective primary depression" characterized by frequent miniepisodes of depression. Patients with this disorder often have a positive family history of primary affective illness, shortened REM latency, and the potential for TCA-generated hypomania. Akiskal suggests that lithium and/or MAOIs combined with social skills training provide the most effective treatment.

A second treatment-responsive subtype is a late onset chronicity that typically occurs after age 40 in patients with no significant premorbid psychopathology who fail to recover from episodes of major depression. For treating this subtype, Akiskal recommends heterocyclic antidepressant drug treatment to attenuate vegetative and psychomotor disturbances and interpersonal or cognitive psychotherapy to reduce impairment in social adjustment and coping skills.

The subtype providing the poorest response to treatment is an early onset characterologic depression labeled "character spectrum disorder." The fourth subtype is a dysphoria secondary to a preexisting nonaffective disorder. Treatment depends on the nature of the presenting depressive symptoms and the nonaffective disorder.

Although Akiskal's subtypes require validation, they provide the basis for promising research for both short- and long-term pharmacotherapeutic and psychotherapeutic approaches. However, before research can be implemented, there must be operational definitions of the subtypes appropriate for selecting patient samples and outcome measures that are sensitive to treatment-induced changes in the symptoms characterizing the disorders.

Cyclothymic Disorder

There are little data on the treatment of cyclothymic disorder. A few open trials and anecdotal reports suggest that lithium is a useful mood stabilizer for the disorder (34,56,85), supporting arguments that cyclothymic disorder, bipolar II disorder, and bipolar I disorder should be viewed as a spectrum of related disorders of varying severity (1).

RECOMMENDATIONS AND AREAS REQUIRING RESEARCH

1. It is necessary to evaluate the preventive efficacy of drugs other than lithium in bipolar disorder and lithium and the TCAs in unipolar disorder. Carbamazepine is the most promising candidate for a carefully designed preventive trial with bipolar patients; MAOIs and bupropion are also attractive choices for long-term trials.

2. Treatment strategies should be developed for alleviating or managing dysthymic disorder. Dysthymia is a neglected disorder in the research literature despite its relatively high prevalence of 3 to 5% of the adult population. The disorder is a long-term illness that can cause significant disruption in the patient's interpersonal functioning and life activities and places the patient at relatively high risk for multiple recurrences of major depression. It should be a high-priority focus for clinical research in affective disorders during the next decade.

3. There is need for long-term (2 to 3 years) studies of psychotherapy compared to and in combination with pharmacotherapy for the prevention of relapse and recurrence of major depression. The relative contribution of each type of therapy is not clear from previous studies, primarily because no published comparative study has exceeded 36 weeks. Major goals are (a) to identify treatment-responsive subgroups and areas of functioning or psychopathology that benefit from psychotherapy alone and in combination with drugs; (b) to determine if psychotherapeutic treatments can modify impaired interepisode functioning and, if so, whether or not the modifications reduce the incidence or severity of recurrences; and (c) to determine the extent to which psychotherapeutic benefits are enduring as preventive measures.

4. It is important that preventive treatment studies focus not only on major episodes but on the often disruptive psychopathology and impairment in social functioning and coping capacity that may be present during the period between episodes. The treatment of interepisode functioning is often neglected in the study design or in the report of results, thereby omitting what could be useful information for judging the efficacy of individual treatments.

5. Attempts at identifying predictors of positive response to preventive treatment should be given high priority for research. Even with a well-studied drug such as lithium, little is known about why some patients have a complete recovery (i.e., have no further episodes) whereas other patients show only partial response (i.e., reduced frequency or severity of episodes) and still others have a poor response (i.e., no change or worsening in course of illness).

6. There should be increased efforts at identifying bio-logical markers of episode length (state-dependent markers). A valid biological or physiological state marker could serve three purposes: (a) determining when continuation drug treatment can safely be withdrawn; (b) identifying an incomplete remission that requires more aggressive treatment; and (c) detecting an emerging recurrence before appearance of clinical symptoms.

Other issues of importance are: (a) What is the minimally effective dosage range of lithium, TCAs, and other drugs for preventive treatment? (b) What is the role of maintenance ECT for patients who are refractory to medication and responsive to ECT? (c) What is the role of neuroleptics alone or in combination with lithium for patients who suffer severe breakthrough manic episodes on lithium? (d) What is the best treatment for rapid cyclers? (e) What practices can be adopted to reduce the high incidence of attrition through noncompliance in taking medication or returning for visits during long-term preventive treatment?

REFERENCES

1. Akiskal, H. S. (1983): In: *Psychiatric Update: The American Psychiatric Association Annual Review,* edited by L. Grinspoon, pp. 271–292. American Psychiatric Press, Washington.
2. Akiskal, H. S. (1985): In: *Psychiatry, Vol. 7,* edited by J. O. Cavernar, R. Michels, H. K. H. Brody, A. M. Cooper, S. D. Guze, et al., pp. 1–27. J. D. Lippincott, Philadelphia.
3. American Psychiatric Association (1980): *Diagnostic and Statistical Manual of Mental Disorders, third ed.* American Psychiatric Press, Washington.
4. Angst, J. (1981): In: *Handbook of Biological Psychiatry, Part IV,* edited by H. van Praag, M. Lader, O. J. Rafaelsen, and E. J. Sachar, pp. 225–242. Marcel Dekker, New York.
5. Angst, J., and Grof, P. (1976): In: *Lithium in Psychiatry: A Synopsis,* edited by A. Villeneuve, pp. 93–103. Les Presses de l'University Lavel, Quebec.
6. Baastrup, P. C., Poulson, J. C., Schou, M., Thomsen, K., and Amdisen, A. (1970): *Lancet,* 2:326–330.
7. Baastrup, P. C. (1980): In: *Handbook of Lithium Therapy,* edited by F. N. Johnson, pp. 26–38. MTP Press Limited, Lancaster, UK.
8. Ballenger, J. C., and Post, R. M. (1978): *Commun. Psychopharmacol.,* 2:159–175.
9. Blackwell, B. (1982): *J. Clin. Psychiatry,* 43:14–20.
10. Bowie, P. C. W., and Beaini, A. Y. (1985): *Br. J. Psychiatry,* 147:30–35.
11. Carroll, B. J. (1982): *Br. J. Psychiatry,* 140:292–304.
12. Cassano, G. B., and Maggini, C. (1983): In: *The Affective Disorders,* edited by J. M. Davis and J. W. Maas, pp. 233–242. American Psychiatric Press, Washington.
13. Coppen, A., Chose, K., and Rao, R. (1978): *Br. J. Psychiatry,* 133:206–210.
14. Coppen, A., Montgomery, S. A., Gupta, R. K., and Bailey, J. E. (1976): *Br. J. Psychiatry,* 128:479–485.
15. Coppen, A., Montgomery, S., Rao, V. A. R., Bailey, J., and Jorgensen, A. (1978): *Br. J. Psychiatry,* 133:28–33.
16. Coppen, A., Noguera, R., Bailey, J., Burns, B. H., Swani, M. S., et al. (1971): *Lancet,* 2:275–279.
17. Cundall, R. L., Brooks, P. W., and Murray, L. G. (1972): *Psychol. Med.,* 3:308–311.
18. Dunner, D. L., Stallone, F., and Fieve, R. R. (1976): *Arch. Gen. Psychiatry,* 33:117–120.
19. Elkin, I., Parloff, M. B., Hadley, S. W., and Autry, J. H. (1985): *Arch. Gen. Psychiatry,* 42:305–316.
20. Fawcett, J., and Kravitz, H. M. (1985): *J. Clin. Psychiatry,* 44:163–169.
21. Fieve, R. R., Kumbarachi, T., and Dunner, D. L. (1976): *Am. J. Psychiatry,* 133:925–929.
22. Fukuda, K., Etoh, T., Iwadate, T., and Ishii, A. (1983): *Tohoku J. Exp. Med.,* 139:299–307.

23. Gardner, E. (1983): *J. Clin. Psychiatry,* 44:163–169.
24. Giannini, A. J., Loiselle, R. H., and Price, W. A. (1985): *J. Clin. Pharmacol.,* 25:4:307–308.
25. Gitlin, M. J., and Weiss, J. (1984): *J. Clin. Psychopharmacol.,* 4: 341–343.
26. Glen, A. T. M., Johnson, A. L., and Shepard, M. (1984): *Psychol. Med.,* 14:37–50.
27. Greden, T. F., Albala, A. A., Haskett, R. F., James, N. M., Goodman, L., et al. (1980): *Biol. Psychiatry,* 15:449–458.
28. Imlah, N. W., Ryan, E., and Harrington, J. A. (1965): *J. Neuropsychopharmacol.,* 4:439–442.
29. Jacob, M., Turner, L., Kupfer, D. J., Jarrett, D. B., Buzzinotti, E., et al. (1984): *J. Affect. Disorders,* 6:181–189.
30. James, S. P., Wehr, T. A., and Sack, D. A. (1985): *Br. J. Psychiatry,* 147:424–428.
31. Jamison, K. R., and Akiskal, H. S. (1983): *Psychiatr. Clin. North Am.,* 6:175–192.
32. Jamison, K. R., and Goodwin, F. K. (1983): In: *Psychiatric Update: The American Psychiatric Association Annual Review,* edited by L. Grinspoon, pp. 319–337. American Psychiatric Press, Washington.
33. Jamison, K. R., and Goodwin, F. K. (1983): In: *Psychopharmacology and Psychotherapy,* edited by M. H. Greenhill and A. Gralnick, pp. 53–77. The Free Press, New York.
34. Jefferson, J. W., Greist, J. H., and Ackerman, D. L. (1983): *Lithium Encyclopedia for Clinical Practice.* American Psychiatric Press, Washington.
35. Kane, J. M., Quitkin, F. M., Rifkin, A., Ramos-Lorenzi, J., Nayak, D. D., and Howard, A. (1982): *Arch. Gen. Psychiatry,* 39:1065–1069.
36. Kay, D. W. K., Fahy, T., and Garside, R. F. (1970): *Br. J. Psychiatry,* 117:667–671.
37. Keller, M. B., Lavori, P. W., Rice, J., Coryell, W., and Hirschfeld, R. M. A. (1986): *Am. J. Psychiatry,* 143:24–28.
38. Keller, M. B., and Shapiro, R. W. (1982): *Am. J. Psychiatry,* 139: 438–442.
39. Keller, M. B., Shapiro, R. W., Lavori, P. W., Lewis, C. E., and Klerman, G. L. (1983): *J.A.M.A.,* 250:3299–3304.
40. Klein, D. F., Gittelman, R., Quitkin, F., and Rifkin, A. (1980): In: *Diagnosis and Drug Treatment of Psychiatric Disorders: Adults and Children.* Williams and Wilkins, Baltimore.
41. Klerman, G. L. (1978): In: *Psychopharmacology: A Generation of Progress,* edited by M. A. Lipton, A. DiMascio, and K. F. Killam, pp. 1303–1312. Raven Press, New York.
42. Klerman, G. L., DiMascio, A., and Weissman, M. M. (1974): *Am. J. Psychiatry,* 131:186–191.
43. Kocsis, J. H., Frances, A., Mann, J. J., Sweeney, J., and Voss, C. (1987): *Am. J. Psychiatry (in press).*
44. Kovacs, M., Feinberg, T. L., Crouse-Novac, M., Paulauskas, S. L., Pollock, M., et al. (1984): *Arch. Gen. Psychiatry,* 41:643–649.
45. Kripke, D. F., Risch, S. C., and Janowsky, D. (1983): *Psychiatry Res.,* 10:105–112.
46. Kupfer, D. J. (1982): In: *Biological Markers in Psychiatry and Neurology,* edited by I. Hanin and E. Usdin, pp. 387–396. Pergamon Press, New York.
47. Kupfer, D. J., and Frank, E. (1985): In: *Chronic Treatments in Neuropsychiatry,* edited by D. Kemali and G. Racagni, pp. 139–151. Raven Press, New York.
48. Kupopulos, A., Reginaldi, D., Laddomada, P., Floris, G., and Tondo, L. (1980): *Pharmakopsychiatrie,* 13:156–167.
49. Lerer, B. (1985): *J. Clin. Psychiatry,* 46:309–316.
50. Loosen, P. T., and Prange, A. J. (1982): *Am. J. Psychiatry,* 139: 405–416.
51. Mindham, R. H., Howland, C., and Shepherd, M. (1973): *Psychol. Med.,* 3:5–17.
52. NIMH/NIH Consensus Development Conference (1985): *Am. J. Psychiatry,* 142:469–476.
53. Nystrom, S. (1979): *Acta Psychiatr. Scand.,* 60:225–238.
54. Okuma, T. (1983): *Psychiatr. Clin. North Am.,* 6:157–174.
55. Okuma, T., Inanaga, K., Otsuki, S., Sarai, K., Takahashi, R., et al. (1981): *Psychopharmacology,* 73:95–96.
56. Peslow, E. D., Dunner, D. L., Fieve, R. R., and Lautin, A. (1982): *Am. J. Psychiatry,* 139:747–752.
57. Placidi, G. G., Lenzi, A., and Rampello, E. (1984): In: *Anticonvulsants in Affective Disorders,* edited by H. M. Emrich, T. Okuma, and A. A. Muller, pp. 188–197. Excerpta Medica, Amsterdam.
58. Post, R. M., Uhde, T. W., Ballenger, J. C., and Squillace, K. M. (1983): *Am. J. Psychiatry,* 140:1602–1604.
59. Prien, R. F., Caffey, E. M., and Klett, C. F. (1973): *Arch. Gen. Psychiatry,* 28:337–341.
60. Prien, R. F., Klett, C. F., and Caffey, E. M. (1973): *Arch. Gen. Psychiatry,* 29:420–425.
61. Prien, R. F., and Kupfer, D. J. (1986): *Am. J. Psychiatry,* 143:18–23.
62. Prien, R. F., Kupfer, D. J., Mansky, P. A., Small, J. G., Tuason, V. B., et al. (1984): *Arch. Gen. Psychiatry,* 41:1096–1104.
63. Puzynaki, S., and Klosiewicz, L. (1984): *J. Affect. Disorders,* 6: 115–121.
64. Quitkin, F. M., Kane, J., Rifkin, A., Ramos-Lorenzi, J. R., and Nayak, D. V. (1981): *Arch. Gen. Psychiatry,* 38:902–907.
65. Robins, L. N., Helzer, J. E., Weissman, M. M., Orvaschel, H., Gruenberg, E., et al. (1984): *Arch. Gen. Psychiatry,* 41:949–958.
66. Rosenthal, N. E., Sack, D. A., and Carpenter, C. J. (1985): *Am. J. Psychiatry,* 142:163–170.
67. Rounsaville, B. J., Sholomskas, D., and Pruskoff, B. A. (1980): *J. Affect. Disorders,* 2:73–88.
68. Schou, M. (1980): *Lithium Treatment of Manic–Depressive Illness.* S. Karger, Basel.
69. Seager, C. P., and Bird, R. L. (1962): *J. Ment. Sci.,* 108:704–707.
70. Shakir, S. A., Volkmar, F. R., and Bacon, S. (1979): *Am. J. Psychiatry,* 136:455–456.
71. Siris, S. G., and Rifkin, A. (1985): In: *Schizophrenia and Affective Disorders,* edited by A. Rifkin, pp. 117–138. John Wright, Littleton, MA.
72. Stancer, H. C., and Persad, E. (1982): *Arch. Gen. Psychiatry,* 39: 311–312.
73. Stein, M. K., Rickels, K., and Weisse, C. (1980): *Am. J. Psychiatry,* 137:370–371.
74. Targum, S. D. (1984): *Biol. Psychiatry,* 19:305–318.
75. Thase, M. E., and Kupfer, D. J. (1985): In: *Handbook of Depression: Treatment, Assessment, and Research,* edited by E. E. Beckham and W. R. Leber. Dorsey Press, Homewood, IL.
76. Van Putten, T. (1975): *Compr. Psychiatry,* 16:179–183.
77. Vestergaard, P. (1983): *Acta Psychiatr. Scand. [Suppl.]* 305:1–36.
78. Wehr, T. A., and Goodwin, F. K. (1979): *Arch. Gen. Psychiatry,* 36:555–559.
79. Wehr, T. A., Wirz-Justice, A., Goodwin, F. K., Duncan, W., and Gillan, J. C. (1979): *Science,* 206:710–713.
80. Weinstein, M. R. (1980): In: *Handbook of Lithium Therapy,* edited by N. F. Johnson, pp. 421–429. MTP Press, Lancaster, UK.
81. Weissman, M. M. (1984): In: *Psychotherapy Research,* edited by J. B. W. Williams and R. L. Spitzer, pp. 89–105. Guilford Press, New York.
82. Weissman, M. M., Kasl, S. V., and Klerman, G. L. (1976): *Am. J. Psychiatry,* 133:757–760.
83. Weissman, M. M., and Myers, J. K. (1978): *Arch. Gen. Psychiatry,* 35:1305–1311.
84. Wright, G., Galloway, L., Kim, J., Dalton, M., Miller, L., et al. (1985): *J. Clin. Psychiatry,* 46:22–25.
85. Wu, A. D. (1976): *J. Formosan Med. Assoc.,* 75:420–427.

Psychopharmacology:
The Third Generation of Progress,
edited by Herbert Y. Meltzer.
Raven Press, New York © 1987.

CHAPTER **107**

Psychotherapy and Its Relevance to the Pharmacotherapy of Major Depression: A Decade Later (1976–1985)

Myrna M. Weissman, Robin B. Jarrett, and John A. Rush

This chapter reviews the evidence for the efficacy of psychotherapy in comparison and in combination with pharmacotherapy for the treatment of major depression, surveys the progress of the past decade, and describes gaps in our understanding. For this review we include only studies that have both a pharmacotherapy and a psychotherapy condition, homogeneous samples of depressed patients (although the criteria for depression vary between studies), random assignment to treatment, and at least eight patients per treatment cell. All these studies met reasonable scientific standards, although none is completely flawless. Limitations of space preclude a detailed critique of each study. Recent reviews of psychotherapy with and without pharmacotherapy comparison conditions are available elsewhere (27,28,30,55,72–74).

THE 1976 ACNP REVIEW OF A GENERATION OF PROGRESS

When the past decade of progress in understanding the efficacy of psychotherapy in relationship to pharmacotherapy was presented by Weissman in 1976 for the last ACNP review of a generation of progress (72), the task was simple. Empirical evidence was meager, and only a few studies

were available. The 1976 review described the movement from ideologically dominated reports about the value of psychotherapy in the preceding decade, noted the lack of empirical studies, and emphasized the promises of the next decade in view of the several important clinical trials that were then under way.

That review came only 2 years after Lieberman's (41) scholarly report of the 1967 to 1974 literature on the psychotherapy of depression, which reached pessimistic conclusions about the quality of the research. It was also 1 year after Parloff and Dies (52) reviewed group psychotherapy outcome research and reached equally pessimistic conclusions about the quality of efficacy studies for depressive disorders. Among the more than 200 articles that Lieberman (41) reviewed, he found no completed controlled trials of psychotherapy that included homogeneous samples of depressed patients, used minimum scientific standards for clinical trials, and had more than 10 patients per treatment cell.

The reviews by Lieberman (41) and Parloff and Dies (52) had been preceded by the independent reviews of Cristol (17) and Luborsky et al. (46), which had noted the methodologic flaws in studies of psychotherapy. The pessimism was not about the benefits that might be achieved by the use of psychotherapy for depression but about the lack of well-designed studies. In 1974, there were no data that met reasonable scientific standards on the efficacy of psychotherapy specifically among depressed patients. Even though numerous studies had been conducted, all included diagnostically heterogeneous, inadequately defined populations and inadequately described procedures for selection and allocation to treatment.

By 1976, the design and execution of clinical trials to evaluate the efficacy of psychotherapy had improved. Although structured diagnostic interviews and specified criteria had not yet been published, several studies had begun to focus on homogeneous samples of depressed patients. There were several clinical trials examining the efficacy of psychotherapy alone, in comparison with, or in combination with a controlled condition [see Weissman (72,73) for reviews]. These were primarily pilot studies testing behavioral or cognitive approaches in small samples of depressed patients. In general, they demonstrated efficacy of the active treatment over various control groups.

At that time, only four studies included a pharmacotherapy comparison group (Table 1). Three independent maintenance trials used both pharmacotherapy and psychotherapy in the treatment of depression. These were: (a) the New Haven–Boston Collaborative Study, which examined 8 months of maintenance treatment on amitriptyline, placebo, or no pill, with or without individual interpersonal psychotherapy, in 150 partially recovered depressed women (36,76); (b) the Baltimore study, which compared 16 months of maintenance treatment on imipramine, diazepam, or placebo, with or without 4 months of group therapy, in 149 partially recovered depressed women (15); and (c) the Philadelphia study, which compared 3 months of treatment on amitriptyline or placebo, with or without marital therapy, in 196 married depressed men and women (23). This study

was considered a maintenance trial since patients were followed through to their recovery.

There was remarkable similarity in findings. All three studies showed an effect for tricyclic antidepressants. Maintenance antidepressants compared with placebo or psychotherapy were most efficacious in preventing relapse or the return of symptoms. Although some recovery of social performance occurred as a result of the reduction of symptoms, medication alone had only a limited impact on problems in living and psychosocial functioning.

All three studies showed a positive effect for psychotherapy, when compared with low contact or with medication alone, in areas related to problems in living, particularly in interpersonal relationships. The psychosocial intervention was not as effective as medication in reducing symptoms of the depressive syndrome or in preventing symptomatic relapse.

The empirical evidence that psychotherapy was effective in reducing acute depressive symptoms compared with or when combined with pharmacotherapy was only promissory. At that time, only one randomly assigned treatment trial had been completed that used cognitive therapy (CT) alone and with pharmacotherapy in acutely depressed patients (59). There were no completed studies that compared combined treatments in acutely depressed patients. The experience gained in the maintenance trials was then being applied to acute treatment trials, and several studies were under way.

The one completed acute treatment study by Rush et al. (59) included 41 acutely ill unipolar depressed outpatients randomly assigned to twice-a-week cognitive behavioral therapy compared with imipramine, up to 250 mg/day, for a maximum of 12 weeks. Both treatment groups showed statistically significant decreases in depressive symptom-

TABLE 1. *Clinical trials completed before 1976 testing the efficacy of psychotherapy in comparison or in combination with pharmacotherapy for major depression*

Treatment groups	Sample	Time (weeks)	Outcome	Investigators
CT/imip	Unipolar depressed (Feighner criteria) ($N = 41$)	12	CT showed more improvement and less attrition than imip	Rush et al. (59)
IPT/low contact with either ami, placebo, or no pill	Recovered neurotic depressives (DSM-II) ($N = 150$)	32	Ami reduced relapse rate; IPT improved social functioning in patients who did not relapse; combined treatment was additive	Klerman et al. (36)
Group therapy Imip/diaz or placebo with group or low-contact supportive psychotherapy	Moderate depressed nonpsychotic (DSM-II) ($N = 149$)	16	Imip produced more symptomatic improvement than diaz or placebo; weak effect occurred late for group therapy on perceptions of spouse, empathy, and reduction of hostility	Covi et al. (15)
Conjoint marital/marital plus ami/low contact plus ami/marital and placebo/low contact	Neurotic depressives ($N = 196$)	12	Ami reduced symptoms and had an early effect; marital improved family perception of marriage and had a late effect	Friedman (23)

atology. Cognitive therapy resulted in significantly greater improvement than did pharmacotherapy on both self-report and clinician-completed measures of depressive symptomatology. Moreover, 79% of the patients in cognitive therapy, as compared to 23% of the pharmacotherapy patients, showed marked improvement or complete remission of symptoms. The dropout rate was substantially lower in cognitive therapy. The findings of the study were controversial because of the skepticism expressed by many investigators, although not clinicians, about the positive effects of any psychological treatment over pharmacotherapy.

PROGRESS SINCE 1976

Since 1976, the situation has changed dramatically. There are many clinical trials of psychotherapy in comparison with and in combination with pharmacotherapy for major depression. Moreover, the groundwork for improving the scientific conduct of these studies has taken place. Some of the developments are those that follow.

A Catalog of Outcome Measures

In 1975, Waskow and Parloff published a catalog of outcome measures (71) suitable for measuring change in psychotherapy outcome studies. They emphasized the importance of using multiple outcome measures and noted that psychotherapy might impact on several domains, including social functioning. The main impact of their catalog was that it encouraged greater uniformity in the use of change measures and facilitated comparisons between studies.

Impact of the Therapist's Characteristics

In 1978, Parloff et al. (53) presented a review of studies on therapist variables such as experience, personality, and empathy that could affect a patient's progress and outcome in psychotherapy and should therefore be an important consideration when planning outcome. This review followed the many observations by clinicians that some therapists consistently did better than others. However, Parloff et al. (53) found only a few therapist characteristics that were promising predictors of patient progress and/or outcome in psychotherapy. According to Luborsky et al. (46), there was moderate support for the value of psychological similarities between patient and therapist and for the therapist's psychological health or sickness, with healthier therapists providing a more positive experience for the patients.

Improved Patient Specification

Between 1974 and 1979, Spitzer and associates (66) developed and published the Research Diagnostic Criteria (RDC), which made available operationally defined diagnostic criteria, and in 1980, the DSM-III was accepted as the official diagnostic criteria by the American Psychiatric Association. As the positive results from the psychophar-macologic trials began to focus attention on the importance of studying diagnostically homogeneous groups (49), more reliable methods of defining diagnoses became available and were incorporated into efficacy studies of psychotherapy.

Improved Treatment Characterization

The last decade has witnessed the use of manuals of psychotherapy in efficacy studies. These manuals specify the main procedures of the particular psychotherapy to be tested and enhance consistency among the therapists engaged in the treatment. Treatment manuals began to appear in the late 1970s. They were designed to specify the identifying characteristics of the psychotherapy, including therapeutic strategies and tactics as well as the sequence and indications for particular tactics. The tactics were operationalized by definition and illustrated by case examples. In some instances videotape examples were provided.

The behavior therapists were the first to design manuals. The behaviorists' ability to specify interventions (e.g., implosion, desensitization) with precision (although used with disorders other than depression) gave impetus to the field by providing a model to follow. The first manual was developed for cognitive therapy (CT) in 1973. The first nonbehaviorally oriented treatment manual (supportive-expressive psychoanalytically oriented psychotherapy) was developed by Luborsky (43,44) in 1976 and 1977.

The development of treatment manuals for outcome studies is now a burgeoning field. Several psychotherapies, both for depression (3,38) and for other disorders (44,68), have been developed and specified in manuals. In fact, treatment manuals are not just applicable to psychotherapy. Fawcett and Epstein at Rush Presbyterian Medical School, Chicago, have developed a comparable manual (unpublished) for the administration of antidepressant medication, which is being used in the NIMH Treatment of Depression Collaborative Research Program (21,70). There are many psychotherapies that are amenable to both specification and testing but for which manuals are not yet available. In the 1980s, manuals have become an essential feature of clinical trials, as they enhance the procedural consistency and reliability of the treatments under study.

Improved Therapist Training

Another important development in empirical studies of psychotherapy has been the use of standardized training programs based on psychotherapy manuals. The training programs developed for psychotherapy outcome studies were not designed to teach the inexperienced person how to become a therapist. Nor were they designed to teach fundamental therapeutic skills such as empathy, handling of transference, and timing. Instead, these training programs were designed to align the practices of the fully trained, experienced, and competent psychotherapist with those procedures specified in the manual (57,58,77). The development of a shared language and specified procedures in an agreed sequence was a major focus (20).

Certification criteria for psychotherapists were developed

and utilized in these training programs and were based on the goals and tasks outlined in the treatment manual. Through the viewing of videotapes of the trainees' psychotherapy sessions, several independent evaluators could determine whether the therapists had met competence criteria and could be certified to participate in the clinical trials (12,13,62).

THE FIRST NIMH COLLABORATIVE STUDY OF PSYCHOTHERAPY

These technological advances in the study of psychotherapy efficacy, many of them developed by members of the National Institute of Mental Health (NIMH) staff, together with the promising data on the efficacy of psychotherapy, led NIMH, in 1978, to begin planning and piloting the first multisite collaborative study of the treatment of depression that would include psychotherapy. Based on the models used to test the efficacy of the new psychotropic drugs in the 1960s, this study was designed to test two psychotherapies, interpersonal psychotherapy (IPT) and cognitive therapy (CT). Depressed patients were studied in three university centers simultaneously, and clinicians underwent standardized training for both psychotherapies and for the reference pharmacotherapy (imipramine) condition (21). The preliminary results of this study are discussed in the Addendum.

SUMMARY OF THE EVIDENCE

Status and Number of Studies

In 1976, there were only four clinical trials that examined the efficacy of psychotherapy in comparison or in combination with pharmacotherapy for major depression. The criteria for depression prior to specified diagnostic criteria varied. As shown in Table 2, by 1985, there were at least 14 studies, 11 completed and three in progress, and diagnostic criteria were more standardized.

Type of Treatment Studied

The most commonly studied approaches have been CT, IPT, and behavioral (39%, 28%, and 22% of the trials, respectively) (Table 3). There has been an increase in CT and IPT trials over the past decade, but the major change has been in behavioral treatments. Before 1976 there were no behavioral studies that included a pharmacotherapy cell; now there are at least four such studies. There has not

TABLE 2. *Status and number of psychotherapy studies in comparison or in combination with pharmacotherapy for major depression*

	<1976	1976–1985	Total
Completed	4	11	15
In process	—	3	3
Total	4	14	18

been a continuation of marital and family studies; only one such study has been published in the past decade. The use of combination pharmacotherapy and psychotherapy as a treatment condition has continued, and over three-quarters of the studies now include that combination. However, there has been a decrease in the use of low-contact or waiting-list control groups in psychotherapy over the past decade. There also has been a shift downward in the use of placebo controls in pharmacotherapy; only 36% of the studies in the last decade, in contrast with 75% of the studies prior to 1976, included placebo controls. This change may reflect the accumulated data from numerous placebo-controlled clinical trials on the efficacy of pharmacotherapy for the treatment of major depression. However, one might question the wisdom of this shift in view of the usefulness of the placebo-control condition to determine whether the treatments are active. It is interesting to note that insight psychodynamic therapy has been used as a comparison for behavioral or cognitive studies in only two trials despite the fact that insight psychotherapy, however defined, is the major psychological treatment in clinical practice. Data on the efficacy of insight psychodynamic therapy are still sparse. The previous trials of IPT or CT, with few exceptions, were conducted by the investigators who developed the manuals for these treatments. In the past decade, both the CT and IPT trials are being conducted at sites other than the place of their origin. These trials are most important for determining the effectiveness and the transmissibility of the respective treatments to other centers.

Duration of Treatment

Although there is a trend toward longer trials, as can be seen in Table 4, only one study goes beyond 36 weeks, the Kupfer and Frank study still in progress. A duration of 12 to 16 weeks is the most frequent treatment period, representing over 60% of the studies (Table 4), and this proportion has not changed since the previous decade. Thus, there are still sparse data on the efficacy of long-term psychotherapy for major depression. Also, there is a paucity of data on the relationship between duration of treatment and outcome or on the need for "booster sessions" for the prevention of recurrence or relapse (2).

Efficacy Studies for Major Depression

Table 5 summarizes the clinical trials for major depression that have been completed since 1976, and Table 6 the clinical trials that are currently in progress. A description of the treatment, the sample, the time period, and the outcome of each completed study is outlined in Table 5.

Psychotherapy Versus Pharmacotherapy

Three studies have data that suggest that psychotherapy may be better than pharmacotherapy for the treatment of some major depressions. The treatments represented in these studies are behavior therapy, CT, and IPT, although there is only partial evidence for CT and IPT. McLean and

TABLE 3. *Type of treatment studied in clinical trials for major depression (only studies including a pharmacotherapy condition included)*

Type of treatment studied[a]	<1975 (4)		1976–1985 (14)		Total (18)	
	N	%	N	%	N	%
CT (individual or group)	1	25	6	42	7	39
IPT	1	25	4	28	5	28
Behavioral	—	0	4	28	4	22
Marital or family	1	25	1	7	2	11
Group	—	25	—	—	1	6
Drug and psychotherapy combination	3	75	11	78	14	77
Low-contact control for psychotherapy	3	75	4	28	7	39
Placebo control for drugs	3	75	5	36	8	44
Other psychotherapy control[b]	0	0	5	36	5	28

[a] Treatments are not mutually exclusive.
[b] Control treatments include insight (N = 2); relaxation (N = 1); counseling (N = 1); group (N = 1).

Hakstian (48), in a sample of patients with primary major depression, found that behavior therapy was better than amitriptyline, which was equal to relaxation therapy and better than insight. However, the drug dose was fixed at 150 mg/day of amitriptyline, and clinical assessments were by self-report only. Blackburn et al. (9) found evidence for the efficacy of CT over pharmacotherapy, but only for patients attending the general practitioner. These patients are likely to be less chronic and less likely to have received prior treatment of any kind. Sloane et al. (65) found partial evidence for the efficacy of IPT over nortriptyline in an elderly sample at 6 weeks, primarily because the elderly did not tolerate the medications well. On the other hand, Weissman et al. (76), in a study of the treatment of acute depression, showed that IPT was equal to pharmacotherapy on symptom reduction.

Combined Treatment Versus Either Treatment Alone

Four studies have partial evidence suggesting the efficacy of combined treatment versus either pharmacotherapy or psychotherapy alone. Weissman et al. (76) found that combined treatment (IPT and amitriptyline) was additive in effect and resulted in less symptomatic failure and greater reduction of symptoms than either treatment alone. Blackburn et al. (9) found that CT plus drug was better than either treatment alone for depressed psychiatric outpatients. In the Murphy et al. (50) study, there was a trend for the efficacy of combined treatment as compared with pharmacotherapy on dropout. Dropout was highest in the pharmacotherapy alone group. Covi et al. (16) noted a trend for the clinical evaluators to find CT plus imipramine to be the most efficacious treatment, although this finding was not evident in the psychiatrists' or the patients' reports.

It is of particular note that no studies of CT in combination with pharmacotherapy have found the combination better than cognitive therapy alone. Beck et al. (5) found a trend for patients receiving CT plus amitriptyline to be doing better 1 year after treatment, although this same trend was not shown at 12 weeks (which was the end of acute treatment). Roth et al. (56) found that desipramine plus self-control therapy was better than self-control alone in speeding symptom reduction and improvement.

Two studies have shown that psychotherapy plus pharmacotherapy was equal to psychotherapy or to pharmacotherapy. Hersen et al. (25) found that all treatments, whether combined or individual, whether pharmacotherapy or social skills, were of equal efficacy. Wilson (79) also showed that behavioral techniques of various kinds plus amitriptyline were the same as behavioral techniques without pharmacotherapy at the end of 8 weeks. Patients on amitriptyline had more rapid symptom improvement initially. There was some suggestion that relaxation therapy was better than minimal therapy.

No published studies have found that psychotherapy plus pharmacotherapy produced results worse than psychotherapy alone. Three studies have shown that psychotherapy plus pharmacotherapy was equal to psychotherapy alone. The Beck et al. (5) study showed that CT plus pharmacotherapy equaled CT alone at the end of 12 weeks. Covi et al. (16) showed similar results on patient and doctor ratings

TABLE 4. *Duration of treatment phase in studies testing efficacy of psychotherapy in comparison or combined with pharmacotherapy for major depression*

Duration of trial (weeks)	<1975 (4)		1976–1985 (14)		Total (18)	
	N	%	N	%	N	%
8			1	7	1	6
10			1	7	1	6
12	2	50	6	42	8	44
16	1	25	3	21	4	22
28			1	7	1	6
32	1	25			1	6
36			1	7	1	6
176			1	7	1	6

TABLE 5. Clinical trials completed since 1976 testing the efficacy of psychotherapy in comparison or in combination with pharmacotherapy for major depression

Treatment groups	Sample	Time (weeks)	Outcome	Investigators
IPT plus ami/ami/IPT/ nonscheduled treatment	Acutely depressed (unipolar nonpsychotic) (SADS-RDC criteria) (N = 96)	16	Combined treatment additive in effect; IPT plus ami less symptomatic failure; all active treatment better than nonscheduled treatment	Weissman et al. (76)
Behavior/insight/ami/ relaxation	Primary major depression (Feighner) (N = 178)	12	B > Ami = R > I	McLean and Hakstian (48)
CT, CT + drug/drug alone	Primary major depression (RDC) (N = 64)	23	GP patients: CT, CT + drug > drug; psychiatric outpatients-CB + drug > CB > drug	Blackburn et al. (9)
Social skills + ami, social skills + placebo, insight/ psychotherapy + placebo, ami	Major depression (Feighner) (N = 125)	Weekly 12, monthly 6	Results vary; all treatments seem equal	Bellack et al. (7)
Nortrip, placebo, IPT	Hamilton of 18, major depression or dysthymia, age 60+ (RDC)	16 (only 6-wk results ready)	At 6 weeks more placebo patients dropped out; lowest in IPT	Sloane et al. (65)
CT, CT + ami	Major depression (Feighner) (N = 33)	12	Both treatments equal; CB + ami better 1 year later (trend)	Beck et al. (5)
CT, CT + nortrip, nortrip, CT + placebo	Major depression (Feighner) (N = 70)	12	All treatments equal; dropout highest in drug alone	Murphy et al. (50)
CT group + imip, CB group/traditional group	Major depression (DSM-III) (N = 70)	12	CB group = CB group + imip, traditional group	Covi et al. (16)
Task assign + ami, relaxation + ami, minimal contact + ami, task assign + placebo, relaxation + placebo, minimal contact + placebo	Unipolar; neurotic reactive depression (BPI) (N = 64)	8	More rapid improvement in drug group/no other advantage to adding ami/ less treatment sought by psychotherapy	Wilson (79)
Self-control; self-control + desip	Unipolar (RDC) (N = 26)	12	SC + drug; speeded symptom improvement	Roth et al. (56)
Doxe + CT family RX, doxe + counseling husband/wife, doxe + counseling wife alone	Married women major depression (DSM-III) (N = 27)	10	CB family less improvement than other treatment	E.M. Waring (unpublished data)

but not on the independent evaluators' ratings, where there was a trend for the combined treatment to be better. Murphy et al. (50) found that CT with nortriptyline was equal to either treatment alone.

One study by Waring et al. (E. M. Waring, L. Frelick, W. E. Keil, and D. Patton, *unpublished data*) found that family CT plus pharmacotherapy was worse than pharmacotherapy alone. They concluded that the addition of family therapy for depression during the acute phase of illness was not useful.

A review of 11 controlled studies of psychotherapy plus pharmacotherapy in the treatment of outpatients with unipolar depression, using a new statistical technique based on meta-analysis, found that the combined active treatments were appreciably more effective than placebo or minimal-contact conditions and slightly, but consistently, superior to psychotherapy alone, pharmacotherapy alone, or either of these treatments in combination with placebo (14).

Table 6 shows the three major studies currently under way. The NIMH study will provide answers on differential psychotherapy effects and the Kupfer and Frank study, on long-term treatment for recurrent depression. Preliminary results of the Hollon study (S. D. Hollon, *personal communication,* January 8, 1986) indicated that a combination

TABLE 6. *Clinical trials in progress testing the efficacy of psychotherapy in comparison or in combination with pharmacotherapy in major depression*

Treatment groups	Sample	Time (weeks)	Investigators
CT, IPT, imip + management, placebo + management	Major depression (RDC) (N = 250)	16	NIMH collaborative study
Acute treatment (IPT + imip), maintenance treatment (IPT, IPT + placebo, IPT + imip, management + imip, management + placebo)	Recurrent major depression (DSM-III) (N = 125)	Weekly 12, biweekly 8, monthly 3 years	Kupfer & Frank
CT plus drug vs. either alone	Nonbipolar major depression (DSM-III) (N = 106)	12	Hollon

of pharmacotherapy and CT was superior to pharmacotherapy alone and evidenced a nonsignificant trend relative to CT at the end of 12 weeks.

Differential Outcome by Patient Type

Information emerging from the studies conducted over the past decade will begin to answer the question about the specificity of the treatments for particular patients. Prusoff et al. (54) found that endogenous, nonsituational depressed patients responded best to the combination of drugs and psychotherapy (IPT) and worse to IPT alone, where the response was the same as in the no-treatment group. The situationally depressed patients did equally well with drugs, IPT, or the combination and better with any of these treatments than with a nonscheduled control treatment.

Blackburn et al. (9) did not find a treatment difference between endogenous and nonendogenous patients but found that psychiatric clinic patients (i.e., the more chronic or refractory patients), as compared with patients coming for treatment to a general practitioner, did best on the combination of cognitive therapy and pharmacotherapy. As noted earlier, Blackburn et al. (9) found CT alone or in combination with drugs to be slightly better than drugs alone among general-practice patients.

Kovacs (39) did not find a correlation between endogenous depression and poor response to cognitive therapy. The Blackburn et al. (9) and Kovacs (39) studies did not separate out endogenous patients who were also diagnosed as having situational depression from the patients who were diagnosed as having only endogenous depression, and neither study used RDC or DSM-III criteria for the endogenous or melancholic subtypes.

Differential Effects of Drugs and Psychotherapy

DiMascio et al. (19) found a differential effect of drugs and IPT psychotherapy. The IPT had its effect on depressed mood and on the patient's involvement in work and in other interests, whereas amitriptyline had its effect on the vegetative symptoms of depression. The effects of psychotherapy on direct measures of social functioning were found at 1-year follow-up.

Rush et al. (60) found that CT had a more pervasive and significant impact on self-concept than did imipramine and produced a greater reduction in hopelessness than did imipramine. Rush et al. (61) found that cognitive symptoms remitted before the vegetative symptoms with CT but not with imipramine.

Specificity of the Psychotherapies

Zeiss et al. (80) studied three behavioral approaches and found no differential outcome among them. Similar findings were also reported by Jarvik et al. (31) studying CT group versus psychodynamic group therapy in elderly depressed patients. However, in the studies by Bellack et al. (6) and Hersen et al. (25) comparing behavioral approaches to insight psychotherapy, the behavioral approaches were found to be somewhat more efficacious.

A partial answer to the question of specificity of treatments awaits the results of the NIMH Treatment of Depression Collaborative Research Program, in which two different psychotherapies, CT and IPT, are being compared (21). The most important features of the NIMH study are that the treatments were not developed in the centers conducting the trials; there is no ideological commitment to one or another form of treatment; and the therapists have been well trained and monitored in both treatments.

Can the Psychotherapies Be Differentiated?

DeRubeis et al. (18) undertook a study to determine whether it was possible to identify distinct and theoretically meaningful differences between two forms of therapy, CT and IPT, used in the treatment of depression. Blind ratings of videotapes enabled 12 raters to distinguish the treatments consistently in the direction of experts' predictions. Similar findings for different treatments were reported by Luborsky et al. (47), who found that independent judges were also able to distinguish three different forms of psychotherapy—cognitive–behavioral, supportive–expressive psychoanalytically oriented psychotherapy, and drug counseling. A new system for rating psychotherapies for depression to determine if they can be differentiated has been developed by

Hollon et al. (29) and will be used in the NIMH Treatment of Depression Collaborative Research Program.

Are Psychotherapy Effects Sustained?

Two separate studies (40,75) found that acutely depressed patients who had received psychotherapy alone and in combination with pharmacotherapy were doing better 1 year after treatment than those who had received only pharmacotherapy. The effects of IPT were on social functioning and were only evidenced after 16 weeks of treatment (75). Beck (4) reported follow-up results from two CT studies (10,64). In both studies, CT compared with pharmacotherapy showed greater long-term effects and prophylactic effects over the 2-year period.

The Blackburn et al. (10) study, a 2-year follow-up, included depressed patients who responded to either CT or pharmacotherapy or the combination and found significantly more relapses at 6 months in the pharmacotherapy as compared to CT alone or the combination treatment groups. The number of patients who relapsed at some point over the 2 years was also significantly higher in pharmacotherapy than in either of the treatment groups with CT. Although the findings are promising, they are still too few to draw definite conclusions about the sustained effects of psychotherapy.

CONCLUSIONS

In summary, over the last decade a number of well-designed clinical trials of the efficacy of psychotherapy have been initiated, and the pace of this research has been sustained. There has been increasing interest in understanding the elements of the therapeutic relationship or therapeutic alliance between the patient and therapist, which facilitates the application of therapeutic techniques and constructive patient change (61). There has also been increased interest in the feasibility, methodology, and policy implications of psychotherapy outcome studies (1,24,25,32–35,42,51).

The precision of the available studies, particularly the efforts to specify the treatments, the patients, and the therapists, has shown vast improvement over the past decade. There continues to be considerable interest in the efficacy of psychotherapy (particularly CT) in comparison to drugs. Research efforts to determine the specificity of which treatment for which patient are beginning to yield findings. The NIMH Treatment of Depression Collaborative Research Study, soon to be published, will yield some findings on the specificity of the treatments. Definitive conclusions must await these results.

To summarize the most recent efficacy data, there is some suggestion that psychotherapies and pharmacotherapies are approximately equivalent for the milder depressions and that the psychotherapies may even be superior. The evidence for the efficacy of the combination of pharmacotherapy and psychotherapy over either treatment alone still persists, although these findings are not as strong or as consistent in the acute treatment studies as they were in the earlier maintenance trials. There is no evidence for a negative effect of combined treatment. There is some evidence from 1- and 2-year follow-up studies for the long-term effects of psychotherapy.

FUTURE DIRECTIONS FOR RESEARCH

Although selected psychotherapies appear to reduce depressive symptoms, it is now important to identify under what conditions that effect is found or can be maximized. Especially important are studies to evaluate the comparative efficacy and indications for combined drug and psychotherapy. Studies to identify which depressed patients are most likely to respond are needed. Studies that modify the "standard" treatment are indicated to determine whether different packages are called for in different personalities or by differing histories of illness (e.g., are chronic depressions to be treated with a modified package?).

Conditions that influence treatment can be divided into two broad categories. The first category includes the relationship between the types of treatment selected and the patients' presenting cluster of problems, symptoms, and characteristics. In studying treatment–patient interactions, it may become clearer which patients respond or fail when exposed to what treatments or to which set(s) of treatments in what sequence(s).

The second category includes the variables that influence the administration or provision of treatment. In pharmacotherapy, this category corresponds to the dose-finding studies. In psychotherapy, it includes such technical questions as format of therapy presentation (individual or group; patient alone or couple), duration and frequency of treatment (biweekly versus weekly; booster sessions versus no booster sessions), and therapist training (criterion-demonstrated competency versus continued evaluation with feedback).

In beginning to examine the conditions that maximize the therapeutic effect of drugs, specific psychotherapies, or their combinations, the "effect" desired must be specified. It is likely that some treatments are more efficacious for improving acute depressive symptoms, and some may be better than others in improving social withdrawal, interpersonal problems, or cognitive distortions found in many depressed persons.

By studying the conditions that influence therapeutic effects, investigators will be confronted with the conditions associated with the treatment failures and thus can begin to study modifications of existing interventions or can design new interventions that increase the probability of a positive treatment response with maintenance across subsets of depressed patients, varied symptoms, and time.

Available data suggest that a prophylactic effect may occur. However, these data are sparse. Long-term follow-up studies are required to evaluate fully whether, when, and for whom prophylaxis is obtained with each form of psychotherapy.

Finally, it should be emphasized that all of the studies including psychotherapy described here deal with major depression and make no claims for the use of psychotherapy with psychotic depression or with bipolar disorder.

A considerable gap still remains between clinical practice and research studies. Most depressed patients, if they receive any treatment at all, and if that treatment is psychotherapy, are more likely to receive a psychodynamic psychotherapy rather than cognitive, behavioral, or interpersonal treatments. To close the gap between research and clinical practice, the next wave of clinical trials should include psychodynamic psychotherapeutic treatments. However, the studies should also include the technological advances in the specification of the treatments and the training procedures. Another method of bridging the gap between research and practice is to foster continuing education opportunities for practitioners to learn psychotherapeutic approaches whose efficacy is currently supported by empirical data from clinical trials.

ADDENDUM

Results of NIMH Collaborative Study of the Treatment of Depression

As this book was to go to press, the first results of the NIMH Collaborative Study of the Treatment of Depression were reported. Since this is the most important and largest psychotherapy–pharmacotherapy clinical trial to date, the most recent results are reported below.

In this study 250 outpatients were randomly assigned to four treatment conditions: 1) cognitive therapy, 2) interpersonal psychotherapy (IPT), 3) imipramine, and 4) a placebo clinical management. Each patient was treated for 16 weeks, and extensive efforts were made for the selection and training of psychotherapists. Outcome was assessed by a battery of scales which assess symptoms, social functioning, and cognition. One of the criteria for initial entry was a score of at least 14 on the 17-item Hamilton Rating Scale for Depression. Of the 239 patients who entered treatment, 68% completed at least 15 weeks and 12 sessions of treatment. The preliminary findings from three centers (Oklahoma City, Washington, D.C., Pittsburgh, Pennsylvania) were reported by Elkins et al. (81), Imber et al. (82), Sotsky et al. (83), and Watkins et al. (84) at the American Psychiatric Association Annual Meeting, May 13, 1986 in Washington, D.C. Overall the findings showed that all active treatments are superior to placebo in the reduction of symptoms over a 16-week period.

1. The overall degree of improvement was highly significant clinically. Over two thirds of the patients were symptom free at the end of treatment.

2. More patients in the placebo-clinical management condition dropped out or were withdrawn, twice as many as for interpersonal psychotherapy which had the lowest attrition rate.

3. At the end of 12 weeks of treatment, the two psychotherapies and imipramine were equivalent in the reduction of depressive symptoms and in overall functioning.

4. The pharmacotherapy, imipramine, had rapid initial onset of action but, by 12 weeks, the two psychotherapies had produced equivalent results.

5. Although many of the less severely depressed patients improved with all treatment conditions, including the placebo group, the more severely depressed patients in the placebo condition did poorly.

6. For the less severely depressed group there were no differences among the treatments.

7. Forty-four percent of the sample was severely depressed. The criteria of severity used was a score of 20 or more on the Hamilton Rating Scale for Depression. Patients in IPT and in the imipramine groups consistently and significantly had better scores than the placebo group on the Hamilton Rating Scale. Only one of the psychotherapies, IPT, was significantly superior to placebo for the severely depressed group. For the severely depressed group interpersonal psychotherapy did as well as imipramine.

8. Surprisingly, one of the more important predictors of patient response for IPT was the presence of an endogenous depressive symptom picture, measured by the Research Diagnostic Criteria following an interview with the Schedule for Affective Disorders and Schizophrenia (SADS). This was also true for the imipramine. However, this finding for drugs would have been expected from previous research.

ACKNOWLEDGMENTS

The NIMH Treatment of Depression Collaborative Research Program is a multisite program initiated and sponsored by the Psychosocial Treatments Research Branch, Division of Extramural Research Programs, NIMH, and is funded by cooperative agreements with six participating sites (George Washington University—MH33762; University of Pittsburgh—MH33753; University of Oklahoma—MH33760; Yale University—MH33827; Clarke Institute of Psychiatry—MH38231; and Rush Presbyterian–St. Luke's Medical Center—MH35017). The principal NIMH collaborators are Irene Elkin, Ph.D., Coordinator; John P. Docherty, M.D., Branch Chief; and Morris B. Parloff, Ph.D., Former Branch Chief. Tracie Shea, Ph.D., George Washington University, is Associate Coordinator. The Principal Investigators and Project Coordinators at the three participating research sites are: George Washington University, Stuart M. Sotsky, M.D., and David Glass, Ph.D.; University of Pittsburgh, Stanley D. Imber, Ph.D., and Paul A. Pilkonis, Ph.D; and the University of Oklahoma, John T. Watkins, Ph.D., and William Leber, Ph.D. The Principal Investigators and Project Coordinators at the three sites responsible for training therapists are: Yale University, Myrna M. Weissman, Ph.D., Eve Chevron, Ph.D., and Bruce J. Rounsaville, M.D.; Clarke Institute of Psychiatry, Brian F. Shaw, Ph.D., and T. Michael Vallis, Ph.D.; and Rush Presbyterian–St. Luke's Medical Center, Jan A. Fawcett, M.D., and Phillip Epstein, M.D. Collaborators in the data management and data analysis aspects of the program are C. James Klett, Ph.D., Joseph F. Collins, Sc.D., and Roderic Gillis (Veterans Administration Cooperative Studies Program, Perry Point, Maryland).

Appreciation is expressed to Irene Elkin, Ph.D., who commented on the initial drafts of the chapter, and to Steve Hollon, Ph.D., Aaron T. Beck, M.D., George Woody, M.D., M. Hersen, Ph.D., I. M. Blackburn, Ph.D., Neil Jacobson, Ph.D., Bruce Sloane, M.D., Lino Covi, M.D.,

Ronald S. Lipman, Ph.D., Edward M. Waring, M.D., Ellen Frank, Ph.D., and Gerald L. Klerman, M.D., who provided comments and material on their research, and to Joan Smolka for editorial assistance.

REFERENCES

1. American Psychiatric Association, APA Commission on Psychotherapies (1982): *Psychotherapy Research: Methodological and Efficacy Issues.* American Psychiatric Association, Washington.
2. Baker, A. L., and Wilson, P. H. (1985): *Behav. Ther.,* 16:335–344.
3. Beck, A. (1976): *Cognitive Therapy and the Emotional Disorders.* International Universities Press, New York.
4. Beck, A. (1985): *The Behavior Therapist,* 8:113.
5. Beck, A. T., Hollon, S. D., Young, J. E., Bedrosian, R. C., and Budenz, D. (1985): *Arch. Gen. Psychiatry,* 42:142–148.
6. Bellack, A., Hersen, M., and Himmelhoch, J. M. (1981): *Am. J. Psychiatry,* 138:1562–1567.
7. Bellack, A., Hersen, M., and Himmelhoch, J. M. (1983): *Behav. Res. Ther.,* 21:101–107.
8. Blackburn, I. M., and Bishop, S. (1983): *Br. J. Psychiatry,* 143: 609–617.
9. Blackburn, I. M., Bishop, S., Glen, A. I. M., Whalley, L. J., and Christie, J. E. (1981): *Br. J. Psychiatry,* 139:181–189.
10. Blackburn, I. M., Eunson, K. M., and Bishop, S. (1987): *Br. J. Psychiatry (in press).*
11. Blaney, P. H. (1981): In: *Behavior Therapy for Depression: Present Status and Future Directions,* edited by L. P. Rehm, pp. 1–32. Academic Press, New York.
12. Chevron, E., and Rounsaville, B. J. (1983): *Arch. Gen. Psychiatry,* 40:1129–1132.
13. Chevron, E., Rounsaville, B. J., Rothblum, E., and Weissman, M. M. (1983): *J. Nerv. Ment. Dis.,* 171:348–353.
14. Conte, H. R., Plutchik, R., Wild, K. V., and Karasu, T. B. (1986): *Arch. Gen. Psychiatry* 43:471–479.
15. Covi, L., Lipman, R. S., Derogatis, L. R., Smith, J. E., III, and Pattison, J. H. (1974): *Am. J. Psychiatry,* 131:191–198.
16. Covi, L., Lipman, R. S., Roth, D., Pattison, J. H., Smith, J. E., et al. (1987): *Am. J. Psychiatry (in press).*
17. Cristol, A. H. (1972): *Compr. Psychiatry,* 13:189–200.
18. DeRubeis, R. J., Hollon, S. D., Evans, M. O., and Bemis, K. M. (1982): *J. Consult. Clin. Psychol.,* 50:744–756.
19. DiMascio, A., Weissman, M. M., Prusoff, B. A., Neu, C., Zwilling, M., et al. (1979): *Arch. Gen. Psychiatry,* 36:1450–1456.
20. Elkin, I. (1984): In: *Psychotherapy Research: Where Are We and Where Should We Go?,* edited by J. B. W. Williams and R. L. Spitzer, pp. 150–159. Guilford Press, New York.
21. Elkin, I., Parloff, M. B., Hadley, S. W., and Autry, J. H. (1985): *Arch. Gen. Psychiatry,* 42:305–316.
22. Fiske, D. W., Hunt, H. F., Luborsky, L., Orne, M. T., Parloff, M. B., et al. (1970): *Arch. Gen. Psychiatry,* 22:22–32.
23. Friedman, A. (1975): *Arch. Gen. Psychiatry,* 32:619–637.
24. Greenspan, S. L., and Sharfstein, S. S. (1981): *Arch. Gen. Psychiatry,* 36:1213–1219.
25. Hersen, M., Bellack, A. S., Himmelhoch, J. M., and Thase, M. E. (1984): *Behav. Ther.,* 15:21–40.
26. Hine, F. R., Werman, D. S., and Simpson, D. M. (1982): *Am. J. Psychiatry,* 139:204–208.
27. Hollon, S. D. (1981): In: *Behavior Therapy for Depression: Present Status and Future Directions,* edited by L. P. Rehm, pp. 33–71. Academic Press, New York.
28. Hollon, S. D., and Beck, A. T. (1979): In: *Cognitive-Behavioral Interventions: Theory, Research and Procedures,* edited by P. C. Kendall and S. D. Hollon, pp. 153–203. Academic Press, New York.
29. Hollon, S. D., Evans, M., Waskow, I. E., and Lowery, H. A. (1984): System for rating therapies for depression. Paper presented at the Annual Meeting of the American Psychiatric Association. Washington, D.C.
30. Jarrett, R. B., and Rush, A. J. (1985): In: *Psychiatry,* edited by J. O. Cavenar, Jr., Vol. 1, pp. 1–35. J. B. Lippincott, Philadelphia.
31. Jarvik, L. F., Mintz, J., Steuer, J., and Gerner, R. (1982): *J. Am. Geriatr. Soc.,* 30:713–717.
32. Karasu, T. B. (1980): *Am. J. Psychiatry,* 137:1502–1512.
33. Karasu, T. B. (1982): *Am. J. Psychiatry,* 139:1102–1113.
34. Kazdin, A. E., and Wilson, G. T. (1978): *Arch. Gen. Psychiatry,* 35:407–416.
35. Klerman, G. L. (1987): In: *Handbook of Psychotherapy and Behavior Change,* third ed., edited by S. L. Garfield and A. S. Bergin. John Wiley & Sons, New York *(in press).*
36. Klerman, G. L., DiMascio, A., Weissman, M. M., Prusoff, B. A., and Paykel, E. S. (1974): *Am. J. Psychiatry,* 131:186–191.
37. Klerman, G. L., and Weissman, M. M. (1982): In: *Short-Term Psychotherapies for Depression,* edited by A. J. Rush, pp. 88–104. Guilford Press, New York.
38. Klerman, G. L., Weissman, M. M., Rounsaville, B. J., and Chevron, E. S. (1984): *Interpersonal Psychotherapy of Depression.* Basic Books, New York.
39. Kovacs, M. (1980): *Am. J. Psychiatry,* 137:1495–1501.
40. Kovacs, M., Rush, A. J., Beck, A. T., and Hollon, S. D. (1981): *Arch. Gen. Psychiatry,* 38:33–39.
41. Lieberman, M. (1975): *Survey and Evaluation of the Literature on Verbal Psychotherapy of Depressive Disorders.* Report prepared for the Clinical Research Branch, National Institute of Mental Health, Bethesda.
42. London, P., and Klerman, G. L. (1982): *Am. J. Psychiatry,* 139: 709–717.
43. Luborsky, L. (1976): *A General Manual for Supportive-Expressive Psychoanalytically Oriented Psychotherapy.* Unpublished; available from L. Luborsky, Hospital of the University of Pennsylvania, Philadelphia, PA 19104.
44. Luborsky, L. (1977): *Individual Treatment Manual for Supportive-Expressive Psychoanalytically Oriented Psychotherapy: Special Adaptation for Treatment of Drug Abuse.* Available from L. Luborsky, Hospital of the University of Pennsylvania, Philadelphia, PA 19104.
45. Luborsky, L. (1984): *Principles of Psychoanalytic Psychotherapy—A Manual for Supportive-Expressive Treatment.* Basic Books, New York.
46. Luborsky, L., Singer, B., and Luborsky, L. (1975): *Arch. Gen. Psychiatry,* 32:995–1008.
47. Luborsky, L., Woody, G., McLeelan, A. T., and O'Brien, C. V. (1982): *J. Consult. Clin. Psychol.,* 50:49–62.
48. McLean, P. D., and Hakstian, A. R. (1979): *J. Consult. Clin. Psychol.,* 47:818–836.
49. Morris, J. B., and Beck, A. T. (1974): *Arch. Gen. Psychiatry,* 30: 667–674.
50. Murphy, G. E., Simons, A. D., Wetzel, R. D., and Lustman, P. J. (1984): *Arch. Gen. Psychiatry,* 41:33–41.
51. Parloff, M. B. (1980): *Psychiatry,* 43:279–293.
52. Parloff, M. B., and Dies, R. R. (1975): *Int. J. Group Psychother.,* 27:281–319.
53. Parloff, M. B., Waskow, I. E., and Wolfe, B. E. (1978): In: *Handbook of Psychotherapy and Behavior Change,* second ed., edited by S. L. Garfield and A. E. Bergin, pp. 233–282. John Wiley & Sons, New York.
54. Prusoff, B. A., Weissman, M. M., Klerman, G. L., and Rounsaville, B. J. (1980): *Arch. Gen. Psychiatry,* 37:796–803.
55. Rehm, L. P., and Kornblith, S. J. (1979): In: *Progress in Behavior Modification, Vol. 7,* edited by M. Hersen, R. M. Eisler, and P. M. Miller, pp. 277–318. Academic Press, New York.
56. Roth, D., Bielski, R., Jones, M., Parker, W., and Osborn, G. (1982): *Behav. Ther.,* 13:133–144.
57. Rounsaville, B. J., Chevron, E. S., and Weissman, M. M. (1984): In: *Psychotherapy Research: Where Are We and Where Should We Go?* edited by J. B. W. Williams and R. L. Spitzer, pp. 160–172. Guilford Press, New York.
58. Rush, A. J. (1983): *Psychiatr. Clin. North Am.,* 6:105–128.
59. Rush, A. J., Beck, A. T., Kovacs, M., and Hollon, S. D. (1977): *Cognitive Ther. Res.,* 1:17–37.
60. Rush, A. J., Beck, A. T., Kovacs, M., Weissenburger, J., and Hollon, S. D. (1982): *Am. J. Psychiatry,* 139:862–866.
61. Rush, A. J., Kovacs, M., Beck, A. T., Weissenburger, J., and Hollon, S. D. (1981): *J. Affect. Disorders,* 3:221–229.
62. Shaw, B. F. (1984): In: *Psychotherapy Research: Where Are We and Where Should We Go?* edited by J. B. W. Williams and R. L. Spitzer, pp. 173–189. Guilford Press, New York.

63. Simons, A. D., Garfield, S. L., and Murphy, G. E. (1984): *Arch. Gen. Psychiatry,* 41:45–51.
64. Simons, A. D., Murphy, G. E., Levine, J. L., and Wetzel, R. D. (1986): *Arch. Gen. Psychiatry,* 43:43–48.
65. Sloane, R. B., Staples, F. R., and Schneider, L. S. (1985): In: *Clinical and Pharmacological Studies in Psychiatric Disorders: Biological Psychiatry—New Prospects,* edited by G. D. Burrows, T. R. Norman, and L. Dennerstein, pp. 344–346. John Libbey and Company, London.
66. Spitzer, R. L., Endicott, J., and Robins, E. (1978): *Arch. Gen. Psychiatry,* 35:773–782.
67. Strupp, H., and Bergin, A. E. (1969): *Int. J. Psychiatry,* 7:180–190.
68. Strupp, H., and Binder, J. (1982): *Time Limited Dynamic Psychotherapy (TLDP)—A Treatment Manual.* Center for Psychotherapy Research, Nashville.
69. Waring, E. M., and Patton, D. (1984): *Br. J. Psychiatry,* 145:641–644.
70. Waskow, I. E., Hadley, S. W., Autry, J. H., and Parloff, M. B. (1980): *NIMH Treatment of Depression Collaborative Research Program (Pilot Phase), Revised Research Plan.* Psychosocial Treatment Research Branch, National Institute of Mental Health, Rockville, MD.
71. Waskow, I. E., and Parloff, M. B., eds. (1975): *Psychotherapy Change Measures: Report of the Clinical Research Branch.* National Institute of Mental Health, U.S. Government Printing Office, Washington.
72. Weissman, M. M. (1978): In: *Psychopharmacology: A Generation of Progress,* edited by M. A. Lipton, A. DiMascio, and K. F. Killam, pp. 1313–1321. Raven Press, New York.
73. Weissman, M. M. (1979): *Arch. Gen. Psychiatry,* 36:1261–1269.
74. Weissman, M. M. (1984): *Psychotherapy Research: Where Are We and Where Should We Go?* edited by J. B. W. Williams and R. L. Spitzer, pp. 89–105. Guilford Press, New York.
75. Weissman, M. M., Klerman, G. L., Prusoff, B. A., Sholomskas, D., and Padian, N. (1981): *Arch. Gen. Psychiatry,* 38:51–55.
76. Weissman, M. M., Prusoff, B. A., DiMascio, A., Neu, C., Goklaney, M., et al. (1979): *Am. J. Psychiatry,* 136:555–558.
77. Weissman, M. M., Rounsaville, B. J., and Chevron, E. (1982): *Am. J. Psychiatry,* 139:1442–1446.
78. Whitehead, A. (1979): *Behav. Res. Ther.,* 17:495–509.
79. Wilson, P. H. (1982): *Behav. Res. Ther.,* 20:173–184.
80. Zeiss, A. M., Lewinsohn, P. M., and Munoz, R. F. (1979): *J. Consult. Clin. Psychol.,* 47:427–439.
81. Elkin, I., Shea, T., Watkins, J., and Collins, J. (1986): Comparative treatment outcome findings. Presentation of NIMH Treatment of Depression Collaborative Research Program. Annual Meeting of the American Psychiatric Association. Washington, D.C.
82. Imber, W., Pilkonis, P., Sotsky, S., and Elkin, I. (1986): Differential treatment effects. Presentation of NIMH Treatment of Depression Collaborative Research Program. Annual Meeting of the American Psychiatric Association, Washington, D.C.
83. Sotsky, S., Glass, D., Shea, T., and Pilkonis, P. (1986): Patient predictors of treatment response. Presentation of NIMH Treatment of Depression Collaborative Research Program. Annual Meeting of the American Psychiatric Association, Washington, D.C.
84. Watkins, J., Leber, W., Imber, S., and Collins, J. (1986): Temporal course of symptomatic change. Presentation of NIMH Treatment of Depression Collaborative Research Program. Annual Meeting of the American Psychiatric Association, Washington, D.C.

Psychopharmacology:
The Third Generation of Progress,
edited by Herbert Y. Meltzer.
Raven Press, New York © 1987.

CHAPTER **108**

Convulsive Therapy in Affective Disorders: A Decade of Understanding and Acceptance

Max Fink

Convulsive therapy is a complex, technical, and labor-intensive treatment in psychiatry that, after more than a half century of use, still arouses emotional as well as scientific debate. Despite the controversies, our continuing failure to find effective and safe therapies for the major psychoses and the increasing recognition of "therapy-resistant syndromes" have led many therapists and their patients to reexamine this long-established therapy. Greater usage of ECT in the past decade has also been encouraged by improved methods of administration, understanding of the relative efficacy and safety of different electrode placements and different electric currents, and answers to the vexing question, "Is a seizure really necessary for therapeutic efficacy?" The publication of guidelines for ECT practice that optimize the safety and the efficacy of the treatments has also been encouraging. The indications for ECT and predictors of good outcome have been clarified, and interest has increased in theories of its antidepressant action. In this review, studies of the past decade that most affected our practice and theory are highlighted.

RECENT HISTORY

Our interest in convulsive therapy was rekindled by the politicization of medicine, especially by public demands and legislative fiats to stop the use of what were considered "intrusive" treatments in psychiatry. These demands came to a head early in the 1970s when the California legislature sought to stop the use of psychoactive drugs, leucotomy, and convulsive therapy in the belief that these treatments were being abused by physicians acting as agents of the state against the best interests of the individual. The attacks on drug therapies were deflected by a consensus among psychiatrists and legislators that these treatments were

essential to patient care. The attack on leucotomy led to the formation of a Presidential Commission to assess the treatment. The Commission found leucotomy to have merit, that it was rarely used, and that further research and even greater clinical use were warranted (47). Despite these recommendations, public pressure against its use has been so great that leucotomy has virtually been abandoned.

The impact of public attitudes on convulsive therapy was unexpected. To defend against complaints that the treatments were dangerous and abused, psychiatric associations established commissions to assess efficacy and usage (7,53,58). The surveys found convulsive therapy to be widely used in patients with depressive disorders, with less acceptance of its use in other types of illness. British surveyors actually visited 100 treatment centers and found many units to function poorly, with poor equipment, poor facilities, and poorly trained staff. Their report led to a public outcry (24) and to many modifications of practice (52). The publication of guidelines for therapy in the APA report, as well as new texts, provided bases for clinicians and administrators to reintroduce ECT in their practices and institutions with assurance that they could meet standards for indications and practice (1,7,25,30). Public pressure continued, however, culminating most recently in the NIH-sponsored Consensus Conference on Electroconvulsive Therapy. This assessment again found the treatment to be singularly effective, and although it noted the controversial nature of the public argument, it encouraged further usage and research to improve the treatment's safety (21).

USAGE

Among fears expressed by antipsychiatrists was that ECT was used disproportionately among those least able to protect themselves—women, the poor, the disadvantaged, and the minorities. But surveys found the opposite to be true—few patients were offered ECT in city, state, or federally supported hospitals, institutions where such disadvantaged populations receive most of their medical care; indeed, convulsive therapy was largely reserved for patients in private and university hospitals, and principally among patients from the middle and upper classes (7,8,25). This disparity is seen within one institution, where usage was much greater among private pay patients than among those supported by public funds (10). Within the state of California, political pressures clearly affected the usage of ECT so that it continues to be used in the independent academic and private hospitals but not in public hospitals (38).

The APA survey (7) estimated that 100,000 patients were treated with ECT annually in the nation, for a usage of about 4.4 patients per 10,000 population. This estimate was based on reports by practitioners responding to a survey. A 1985 NIH estimate, extrapolated from national hospital reporting statistics, found usage to be about half the earlier estimate (69). Estimates of usage rates in other countries include 7.0 patients per 10,000 population in Denmark in 1972; 5.6/10,000 in Great Britain in 1980; and 10.4/10,000 in Ireland in 1982 (25,42). But usage is less in France, The Netherlands, Switzerland, and Germany and probably higher in India and other Third World nations, but actual data are lacking.

Usage is dependent on clinical indications and the psychopathology of patients but also varies according to a complex calculus of staff attitude and training, cost of personnel, supplies, and equipment, and institutional and community arrangements for cost reimbursement. Although social and economic factors clearly influence all aspects of psychiatric practice, they become compelling in convulsive therapy because of the labor intensity and technical complexity of present treatment practices and because adverse community attitudes have so influenced the teaching and practice of this complex therapy.

INDICATIONS FOR USE

In a treatment that has been available for more than five decades, it is not unexpected that our present appreciation of its indications differs from its role in earlier decades. Our appreciation has been changing rapidly since the assessments of the mid-1970s. Indeed, one of the unexpected consequences of the NIH Consensus Conference was the positive response to the use of ECT in patients with delusional depression, schizoaffective disorders, schizophrenia, and mania in addition to the established usage in patients with major depressive disorders and melancholia (21,59,60,70).

We still teach, and in some jurisdictions this teaching is rooted in law, that patients must have "adequate" trials of all other treatments before they are subjected to ECT. Thus, the primary subject for the use of ECT is the depressed patient unresponsive to adequate trials of drug or psychotherapy. In such cases, the efficacy of ECT remains high, often recorded as 80 to 90% of trials. Indeed, in patients with major depressive disorders, convulsive

therapy is as effective or more effective than sham ECT, placebo, tricyclic drugs, or monoamine oxidase inhibitors (25). This is particularly true among the elderly, especially those with greater degrees of vegetative dysfunction and melancholia, who are clearly responsive (DSM-III 296.2, 296.3, 296.5, 296.6, 296.8; each with .x3).

Depressed patients with delusions fare poorly with antidepressant drugs alone, and in such patients the initial use of ECT is a consideration (9,63). Among delusional depressed patients, we can identify improvement rates of 30% for tricyclic drugs, 50% for antipsychotic drugs, 65 to 70% for their combination, and 85 to 90% for ECT (39). Although we lack direct evidence from prospective studies (which have not been done), the reasonable therapist can conclude that ECT may be an initial treatment in patients with severe delusional depression, particularly if they are middle-aged or elderly and describe thoughts of worthlessness, guilt, or somatic concern (DSM-III 296.24, 296.34, 296.54, 296.64, 296.84).

For patients who have a compelling suicidal drive, especially if inanition is a feature of their condition, convulsive therapy is a primary intervention. This is true for patients who are severely agitated, requiring physical restraint or complex polypharmacy. There is also an indication, based on less data, for the use of ECT in schizoaffective patients, especially among patients in whom trials with other therapies have failed (DSM-III 295.7, 295.74).

The separation of depressed patients into subpopulations of unipolar or bipolar disorders is not useful in predicting the response to convulsive therapy. Bipolar patients in the manic phase are as responsive to convulsive therapy as in the depressive phase. We lack evidence, however, from comparative studies of the relative efficacy and safety of convulsive therapy compared with lithium or an antipsychotic drug or lithium combined with an antipsychotic drug or carbamazepine alone (60). Lacking such direct evidence, we are compelled to consider the clinical reports that encourage our belief that convulsive therapy is effective in manic states, particularly for patients with the more severe varieties of manic delirium and in patients who are so excited as to require restraints, high doses of sedative drugs, or polypharmacy for management. Indeed, the adverse effects that are so clearly defined in the treatment of mania with lithium and antipsychotic drugs are less apparent in manic patients treated with ECT alone and compel our consideration of ECT as an effective therapy (DSM-III 296.6, 296.4, 296.7; also .x4).

Confusional syndromes are not an infrequent manifestation of a severe depressive disorder, leading to descriptions of cases with "pseudodementia" or "reversible dementia." When such patients have been treated with ECT, the recovery to familial integrity has often been dramatic (6,18,19,44).

Because of the risks of teratogenicity of drug therapies during pregnancy, consideration has been given to the use of convulsive therapy for its efficacy and relative safety in patients with severe affective disorders. Clinical data support convulsive therapy in patients with bipolar or schizophreniform disorders during pregnancy and for the schizophreniform and affective disorders seen during the postpartum period (DSM-III 269.xx; 295.4x) (48,57).

In young patients it is often difficult to determine whether the first illness is a manifestation of an affective or a schizophrenic disorder. In mixed populations of schizophrenics, most patients respond poorly to any intervention, including convulsive therapy (59). But studies find a subgroup (DSM-III 295.2), chiefly those with catatonic and affective symptoms, that responds rapidly to ECT (17,33,68). For patients who have been ill for less than 2 years, ECT is as effective as antipsychotic drugs. The ease of use of drug therapies, however, leads to their initial selection in almost all patients. In patients with psychoses of long duration, there seems to be as little to be gained from ECT as from drug therapies. In severely ill patients who have failed to respond to drug and psychotherapies alone, however, there are reports that ECT combined with antipsychotic drugs has been effective in reducing the more severe aspects of the illness; indeed, one recent optimistic report finds an unusually high recovery rate for patients treated with ECT and thiothixene after they have failed courses of thiothixene alone (31) (DSM-III 295.3, 295.9).

RISKS AND THEIR MANAGEMENT

Perhaps the decade's most important contributions to treatment practice have been the routine acceptance of seizure monitoring and the understanding of the contributions of electrode placement and current type to the efficacy and safety of the treatments. Modern seizure inductions are done with ultrashort barbiturate anesthesia, muscle relaxation using succinylcholine, and continuous ventilation with oxygen. The use of succinylcholine, however, provides an opportunity for the therapist to misjudge seizure duration and to assume a satisfactory seizure has occurred when, in fact, it has not. The 1980 British survey of practice found that fully one-third of treatment units were unable to determine whether their patients had a fit or not, and therapeutic efficacy was severely compromised (53). Indeed, much of the reluctance of British psychiatrists to use ECT may have resulted from their awareness that the treatments were less effective than expected, clearly the direct result of abysmal clinical practices. Seizure duration monitoring is now routinely accomplished by observations of a fit in a limb in which the action of succinylcholine has been blocked by an inflated blood pressure cuff or by direct measurement of EEG seizure length using a paper recorder or an auditory monitor or by measurement of the seizure-induced tachycardia (28,41).

Ever since the mid-1950s, when unmodified seizure inductions were replaced by the routine use of anesthesia and oxygenation, the mortality of the treatments has been reduced to rates less than those of anesthesia alone. With seizure monitoring now an accepted part of practice, other complications are reduced to levels that suggest that these inductions are safer than psychotropic drug therapies alone, especially in patients with cardiovascular disorders, which increase the risks of drug therapies. Electroconvulsive therapy is often the treatment of choice in pregnancy, and it has been safely administered to medically ill and compromised patients and to the elderly (23,32,55,56).

The principal risk of convulsive therapy remains the patient's complaints of cognitive impairment. Impairment is usually described for the period of the illness and the events associated with the treatments, but there are some patients who continue to express losses of retrograde memories earlier than the period of the illness (43). Cognitive impairment results, in part, from the path of electric currents and the type or amount of electric energy used. Since cognitive impairment is less with unilateral electrode placement than with bilateral (36), present practice recommends unilateral electrode placement over the nondominant hemisphere for all patients except the most suicidal or most severely ill (2) or those with mania (62). But not all seizures are therapeutically the same. Seizures induced with bilateral placement seem to be more effective than those induced through unilateral placement, so that bilateral treatments are recommended in the most severely ill and in those who have not responded within five to six treatments (5,45,54). There are some observers, however, who contend that treatments through unilateral electrode placements, when properly done, are equally effective to those in which bilateral electrode placements have been used (36,64).

A similar difference in cognitive effects and efficacy exists in comparisons of inductions using brief pulse and sine-wave stimuli: brief pulse currents elicit less cognitive impairment but have less efficacy (43). The use of threshold currents is associated with less cognitive impairment as well as less efficacy, so that threshold currents are no longer recommended for clinical purposes. Modern brief-pulse current instruments induce seizures with apparently equivalent efficacy and less effects on cognition than sine-wave currents, and brief-pulse current instruments are now favored both in the United States and Great Britain for routine use.

Studies of serum prolactin levels during seizures find associations with the intensity of the currents and with electrode placement. Greater amounts of prolactin are released into the serum with both higher-intensity currents and bilateral electrode placements, suggesting that the release of peptides from hypothalamic pituitary centers may have some influence on the therapeutic course (3,4,12,50,65–67).

One aspect of the treatment that has been thoroughly studied is the importance of a seizure in the therapeutic process. Many in Britain (presumably because they could not determine whether a patient had indeed had a therapeutic seizure) believed that a seizure was not necessary for clinical success. Numerous clinical trials comparing the efficacy of seizures in ECT with sham treatments were undertaken (37,49). The most recent reports of the Leicestershire and Nottingham studies conclude that there is a distinct therapeutic advantage for treatments with seizures compared to sham treatments, both in patients with depression and in those with schizophrenia (16,17,33).

Although questions were raised about the relative efficacy of electrical and chemically induced seizures, no recent studies have been undertaken. The clinical data from inductions with pentylenetetrazol (Metrazol®) and flurothyl (Indoklon®) show that such inductions are clearly effective, as effective as electrical inductions, but the ease of administration of electric inductions compels their general clinical use.

Many patients with severe medical illnesses are referred for ECT, and the management of high-risk patients has become a matter of considerable interest (19,23,56). Monitoring of blood pressure, heart rate, and electrocardiogram is now routine in the very ill, and pretreatment amelioration of blood gas, metabolic, and hematologic abnormalities is expected. Most clinically indicated medications are given before or during ECT without compromising the patient. For example, there is a transient increase in blood pressure accompanying each seizure, and in hypertensive patients, the elevations may be quite high. It is common practice to administer prophylactic nitroglycerin or propranolol before each induction. Reports that some antiarrhythmic drugs, such as lidocaine, markedly raise seizure thresholds and interfere with ECT efficacy suggest that such agents not be used (35).

Unfortunately, few studies of drug interactions and ECT have been undertaken. Since there is no evidence that the concurrent use of tricyclic antidepressants or monoamine oxidase inhibitors augments the efficacy of ECT, and because these may have unwanted cardiovascular effects, antidepressant drugs are rarely combined with ECT. For antipsychotic drugs, however, greater efficacy has been reported when they have been combined with ECT, and it is not unusual to treat patients, particularly those with mania and schizophrenia, with this combination (1,25). Lithium use during ECT is associated with severe cognitive effects, and the combination is generally avoided (61).

Major affective illnesses are recurrent disorders, and continued or maintenance treatment is a feature of their care, whether the primary treatment is with medications or with ECT. Little attention has been paid to this problem, however, and our present practice of maintaining patients on a tricyclic antidepressant, a monoamine oxidase inhibitor, lithium, or even biweekly or monthly seizures remains unchanged from our experience of earlier decades.

PREDICTORS OF RESPONSE

Convulsive therapy is indicated in severely ill, affectively disturbed patients, and much of our knowledge of predictors of good outcome comes from the experience of earlier decades. Those with high scores on the Hamilton depression scale are usually responsive to ECT, with higher scores generally associated with greater degrees of improvement. Prominent vegetative features presage a good prognosis, as does agitation, cognitive impairment, or severe withdrawal. Older patients generally respond rapidly, and age is not an impediment to treatment.

Tests of neuroendocrine dysregulation are a focus of recent interest. The TSH response to TRH, dexamethasone suppression of serum cortisol, and growth hormone response to apomorphine and to insulin have each been examined for their predictive value (20). In general, dysregulation is prominent in our patients, and the abnormal neuroendocrine tests normalize with successful treatment (27). We have been unable to define a pattern of dysregulation that predicts either good or poor outcome with treatment, and although some recent studies find the failure of tests to normalize to be associated with early relapse, others are not so assured (11).

Interest was once shown in neurophysiologic and neuropsychologic predictors of outcome, but such studies are clearly out of fashion now, and little has been added to the reviews published earlier. But with the development of inexpensive methods for multilead real-time EEG analysis, our interest has once again been quickened into the characteristics of the seizure, the postseizure period of electrical silence, and the changes in the interseizure records as indicators of a therapeutic seizure and as predictors of outcome. Indeed, one study team has focused attention on the postseizure period of isoelectric EEG activity and has proposed that treatments with isoflurane anesthesia may be associated with antidepressant response. Isoflurane is a unique anesthetic in producing extended periods of isoelectric EEG activity at standard anesthetic dosages (40).

MECHANISM OF ANTIDEPRESSANT ACTION

The essential ingredient for an antidepressant effect in convulsive therapy remains the repeated induction of bilateral grand mal seizures, two to five times weekly, for seven to twelve seizures. To explain the antidepressant effect, it is logical to search for biochemical changes in the brain that may follow repeated seizures. But seizures involve massive electrical and biochemical discharges in brain tissues, activation of the autonomic nervous system, release of secretions of endocrine glands, and, unless there is neuromuscular blockade, tonic and clonic convulsions of body muscles. These activities cause so many changes in biochemistry and physiology of the body that there is no dearth of demonstrable effects. Our difficulty lies not in demonstrating changes but in differentiating those that may be central to antidepressant activity and those that may be clearly secondary.

Many of the problems that beset psychopharmacologic research also affect ECT research: variability among patients, limitations on experimentation in humans, inaccessibility of brain tissues to direct examination, anxieties engendered by such simple procedures as cerebrospinal fluid examinations, and the cost of any procedure that delays treatment. These limitations compel studies in animals, but alas, these have been of little help to our understanding of the ECT process. What progress has been made has come from human research precisely because the conditions under study, the affective and psychotic disorders, have no duplicate in animal species or animal tissues.

Indeed, where suggestions from animal studies have been examined in patients, they usually fail of replication. Studies of CSF do not find relationships between catecholamine metabolites and seizures; and studies of naloxone fail to find connections between opioid receptors and the ECT process (26,27,34,51). Perhaps the single compelling observation from animal studies that has been replicated in man is the observation that ECS increases dopaminergic activity in centrencephalic regions. The conclusion that patients with parkinsonism may be helped by ECT was verified, clarifying the role of this neurohumor in parkinsonism (13–15,46).

Two threads are now being studied to explain the antidepressant efficacy of ECT. One focuses on the neurohumoral mechanisms that have been used to explain the action of antidepressant drugs. In this formulation, the acute release of norepinephrine and dopamine and the increase in the turnover of norepinephrine in the brain that occur during ECS are emphasized. Receptor sensitivity is also increased during ECS. Sensitivity to agents mimicking the actions of brain monoamines is increased such that postsynaptic responses mediated by serotonin, dopamine, and norepinephrine are enhanced. These biochemical changes are seen as reversing the pathophysiology of the depressive disorder (22).

The other view focuses on the signs of neuroendocrine dysregulation that are so prominent in patients with affective disorders and that normalize during the recovery process. In this view, hypothalamic dysfunction (probably hypofunction) is postulated as central to endogenous depressive disorders. The antidepressant activity of convulsive therapy is seen to result from its stimulation of hypothalamic–pituitary centers, releasing natural substances, probably peptides, which modify mood, vegetative symptoms, and behavior associated with mood disturbances (26,27,29).

The theory takes into account observations that the grand mal seizure, with its centrencephalic features and release of brain substances, is essential to a treatment response. It claims nothing from the induction process or the peripheral manifestations. It recognizes that convulsive therapy is particularly effective in relieving melancholic features in patients with a prominence of vegetative symptoms. And it takes advantage of the observations that seizures release peptides from the central nervous system and that some peptides are behaviorally active.

The continued use of convulsive therapy compels our interest in improved treatment efficacy and in alternate treatments that may be more effective. Recent descriptions of electroacupuncture convulsive therapy from China and of isoflurane narcosis therapy from Vienna are encouraging. Hormones with behavioral effects derived from centrencephalic brain regions provide tools for the study of affective disorders. And the more widespread awareness that convulsive therapy is still a most effective and safe therapy and its greater acceptance by psychiatrists may encourage scientists to develop new theories of the antidepressant activity of seizures and to increase our understanding of the interaction of brain functions and behavior.

ACKNOWLEDGMENT

This work was aided in part by grants from the International Association for Psychiatric Research, Inc., St. James, New York 11780.

REFERENCES

1. Abrams, R., and Essman, W. B., eds. (1982): *Electroconvulsive Therapy. Biological Foundations and Clinical Applications.* Spectrum Publications, New York.
2. Abrams, R., and Fink, M. (1984): *J. Affec. Disorders,* 7:245–247.
3. Abrams, R., and Swartz, C. M. (1985): *Convuls. Ther.,* 1:38–42.
4. Abrams, R., and Swartz, C. M. (1985): *Convuls. Ther.,* 1:115–119.
5. Abrams, R., Taylor, M. A., Faber, R., Ts'o, T. O., Williams, R. A. et al. (1983): *Am. J. Psychiatry,* 140:463–465.
6. Allen, R. M. (1982): *Biol. Psychiatry,* 17:1435–1443.
7. American Psychiatric Association (1978): *Electroconvulsive Therapy. Task Force Report 14.* American Psychiatric Association, Washington.
8. Asnis, G. M., Fink, M., and Saferstein, S. (1978): *Am. J. Psychiatry,* 135:479–482.
9. Avery, D., and Lubrano, A. (1979): *Am. J. Psychiatry,* 136:559–562.
10. Bailine, S. H., and Rau, J. H. (1981): *Compr. Psychiatry,* 22:274–281.
11. Baldessarini, R., and Arana, G. W. (1985): *J. Clin. Psychiatry,* 42:25–29.
12. Balldin, J. (1982): *Acta Psychiatr. Scand.,* 65:365–369.
13. Balldin, J., Granerus, A. K., Linstedt, G., Modigh, K., and Walinder, J. (1981): *J. Neural. Transm.,* 52:199–211.
14. Balldin, J., Granerus, A. K., Lindstedt, G., Modigh, K., and Walinder, J. (1982): *Psychopharmacology,* 76:371–376.
15. Baruch, P., Jouvent, R., Vindreau, C., Drouillon, C., Widlocher, D., et al. (1985): *World Cong. Biol. Psychiatry Abstr.,* 1985:425.2.
16. Brandon, S., Cowley, P., McDonald, C., Neville, P., Palmer, R., et al. (1984): *Br. Med. J.,* 288:22–25.
17. Brandon, S., Cowley, P., McDonald, C., Neville, P., Palmer, R., et al. (1985): *Br. J. Psychiatry,* 146:177–183.
18. Bulbena, A., and Berrios, G. E. (1986): *Br. J. Psychiatry,* 148:87–94.
19. Burke, W. J., Rutherford, J. L., Zorumski, C. F., and Reich, T. (1985): *Compr. Psychiatry,* 26:480–486.
20. Christie, J. E., Whalley, L. J., Brown, N. S., and Dick, H. (1982): *Br. J. Psychiatry,* 140:268–273.
21. Consensus Conference (1985): *J.A.M.A.,* 254:103–108.
22. Costain, D. W., Cowen, P. J., Gelder, M. G., and Grahame-Smith, D. G. (1982): *Lancet,* 1:400–404.
23. Dec, G. W., Jr., Stern, T. A., and Welch, C. (1985): *J.A.M.A.,* 253:2525–2529.
24. Editor (1981): *Lancet,* 2:1207–1208.
25. Fink, M. (1979): *Convulsive Therapy: Theory and Practice.* Raven Press, New York.
26. Fink, M. (1984): In: *Neurobiology of Manic Depressive Illness,* edited by R. M. Post and J. C. Ballenger, pp. 721–730. Williams & Wilkins, Baltimore.
27. Fink, M. (1984): *Adv. Biochem. Psychopharmacol.,* 39:345–357.
28. Fink, M., and Johnson, L. (1982): *Arch. Gen. Psychiatry,* 39:1189–1191.
29. Fink, M., and Ottosson, J.-O. (1980): *Psychiatry Res.,* 2:49–61.
30. Fraser, M. (1982): *ECT: A Clinical Guide.* John Wiley & Sons, Chichester.
31. Friedel, R. O. (1985): *World Cong. Biol. Psychiatry Abstr.,* 1985:532.6.
32. Gerring, J. P., and Shields, H. M. (1982): *J. Clin. Psychiatry,* 43:140–143.
33. Gregory, S., Shawcross, C. R., and Gill, D. (1985): *Br. J. Psychiatry,* 146:520–524.
34. Haskett, R. F., Zis, A. P., and Albala, A. A. (1985): *Biol. Psychiatry,* 20:623–633.
35. Hood, D. D., and Mecca, R. S. (1983): *Anesthesiology,* 58:379–381.
36. Horne, R. L., Pettinati, H. M., Sugerman, A. A., and Varga, E. (1985): *Arch. Gen. Psychiatry,* 42:1087–1092.
37. Kiloh, L. G. (1985): *Psychiatr. Dev.,* 3:205–218.
38. Kramer, B. A. (1985): *Am. J. Psychiatry,* 142:1190–1192.
39. Kroessler, D. (1985): *Convul. Ther.,* 1:173–182.
40. Langer, G., Neumark, J., Koinig, G., Graf, M., Aschauer, H., et al. (1985): *Neuropsychobiology,* 14:118–120.
41. Larson, G., Swartz, C., and Abrams, R. (1984): *Am. J. Psychiatry,* 141:1269–1271.
42. Latey, R. H., and Fahy, T. J. (1985): *Br. J. Psychiatry,* 147:438–439.
43. Malitz, S., and Sackeim, H., eds. (1986): *Electroconvulsive Therapy: Clinical and Basic Research Issues.* New York Academy of Sciences, New York.
44. McAllister, T. W., and Price, T. R. (1982): *Am. J. Psychiatry,* 139:626–629.
45. McAllister, T. W., Price, T. R. P., and Ferrell, R. B. (1985): *J. Clin. Psychiatry,* 46:430–431.
46. Modigh, K., Balldin, J., Eden, S., Granerus, A. K., and Walinder, J. (1981): *Acta Psychiatr. Scand. [Suppl.],* 290:91–99.
47. National Commission for the Protection of Human Subjects of Biomedical and Behavioral Research (1977): *Report and Recommendations.* DHEW Publication (OS)77-0001, Washington.

48. Nurnberg, H. G., and Prudic, J. (1984): *Hosp. Commun. Psychiatry,* 35:67–71.
49. Palmer, R. L. (1981): *Electroconvulsive Therapy: An Appraisal.* Oxford University Press, New York.
50. Papakostas, Y., Stefanis, C., Sinouri, A., Trikkas, G., Papadimitriou, G., et al. (1984): *Am. J. Psychiatry,* 141:1623–1624.
51. Papakostas, Y. G., Stefanis, C. S., Markianos, M., and Papadimitriou, G. N. (1985): *Biol. Psychiatry,* 20:1326–1327.
52. Pippard, J. (1986): *Convuls. Ther.,* 2:62–64.
53. Pippard, J., and Ellam, L. (1981): *Electroconvulsive Treatment in Great Britain, 1980.* Gaskell, London.
54. Price, T. R. (1981): *N. Engl. J. Med.,* 304:53.
55. Regestein, Q. R., and Lind, L. J. (1980): *Compr. Psychiatry,* 21:288–291.
56. Regestein, Q. R., and Reich, P. (1985): *Convuls. Ther.,* 1:101–114.
57. Repke, J. T., and Berger, N. G. (1984): *Obstet. Gynecol.,* 63:39S–41S.
58. Royal College of Psychiatrists (1977): *Br. J. Psychiatry,* 131:261–271.
59. Small, J. G. (1985): *Convuls. Ther.,* 1:263–270.
60. Small, J. G. (1985): *Convuls. Ther.,* 1:271–276.
61. Small, J. G., Kellams, J. J., Milstein, V., and Small, I. F. (1980): *Biol. Psychiatry,* 15:103–112.
62. Small, J. G., Small, I. F., Milstein, V., Kellams, J. J., and Klapper, M. H. (1985): *Biol. Psychiatry,* 20:125–134.
63. Spiker, D. G., Weiss, J. C., Dealy, R. S., Griffin, S. J., Hanin, I., et al. (1985): *Am. J. Psychiatry,* 142:430–436.
64. Strömgren, L. S. (1984): *Acta Psychiatr. Scand.,* 69:484–490.
65. Swartz, C. M. (1985): *Convuls. Ther.,* 1:81–88.
66. Swartz, C. M. (1985): *Convuls. Ther.,* 1:252–257.
67. Swartz, C., and Abrams, R. (1984): *Br. J. Psychiatry,* 144:643–645.
68. Taylor, P., and Fleminger, J. J. (1980): *Lancet,* 1:1380–1382.
69. Thompson, J. W. (1985): In: *Proceedings, Consensus Development Conference on Electroconvulsive Therapy,* pp. 32–36. OMAR, Washington.
70. Van Valkenburg, C., and Clayton, P. J. (1985): *Biol. Psychiatry,* 20:699–700.

Psychopharmacology:
The Third Generation of Progress,
edited by Herbert Y. Meltzer.
Raven Press, New York © 1987.

CHAPTER 109

Drug Treatment of Bipolar Disorder

David L. Dunner and Paula J. Clayton

The most crucial issue in treating mania is recognizing it. In that regard, the most innovative feature of the treatment of bipolar affective disorders in recent years has been the clarification of the criteria for diagnosis of these conditions. The use of the DSM-III has enabled greater attention to the diagnosis of bipolar illnesses, specifically mania, compared with previous diagnostic systems. This change came about in large measure because of the efficacy of lithium salts in bipolar affective disorder, particularly for maintenance therapy of recurrent attacks of bipolar illness. It thus became important for American psychiatrists to diagnose bipolar illness, which up to the mid-1970s they had had difficulty recognizing because of different formulations.

The change from DSM-II to DSM-III was largely a change in philosophy from an intuitive-based diagnosis to a symptom-based diagnosis. Major results of the adoption of DSM-III include a widening of the concept of bipolar affective disorder and a narrowing of the concept of schizophrenia. Psychosis and even the presence of Schneiderian first-rank symptoms no longer automatically result in a diagnosis of schizophrenia.

The system allows the clinician to code a bipolar disorder as mixed, manic, or depressive and to indicate whether the manic episode is nonpsychotic, psychotic with mood-congruent features, or psychotic with mood-incongruent features. This third category is similar to what some American and European researchers call schizoaffective mania. In a study of definitions of mania, the concordance rate between RDC schizoaffective mania and DSM-III mood incongruent psychotic mania was 0.75 (5). Most researchers agree that schizoaffective mania should be considered a manic syndrome for treatment purposes (9). Some even claim the outcome is the same, whereas others report it to be better than schizophrenia but not as good as bipolar (4,32).

It is clear that a high percentage of patients with acute mania will have psychotic symptoms. Approximately 20 to 40% of patients will evidence Schneiderian first-rank symptoms during their acute manic episode (1,39). These symptoms, although not necessarily mood-congruent, occur in the presence of other manic symptoms and should not dissuade the clinician from making the diagnosis of mania. The treatment of psychotic mania, however, may present problems. A review of studies of treatment of "schizoaffective manic" patients suggests that lithium treatment is effective but not as rapidly effective as in less psychotic manic patients (22). The use of lithium combined with antipsychotic drugs is often warranted for this complication of manic illness. However, complications of combined therapy suggest the need for alternate treatment strategies.

Similarly, most patients with classic mania are no longer admitted to hospitals except for their first attack. This is because of the positive clinical effects of lithium carbonate maintenance therapy in both manic and depressive phases of the illness. Thus, bipolar patients most frequently seen today have first episodes of mania or are relapsing because they are either noncompliant with lithium treatment or have complications of their clinical picture such as concomitant use of alcohol or hallucinogenic or other street drugs. The typical manic patient has by and large disappeared from the large metropolitan hospital setting to be replaced by patients whose relapses tend to be recurrent and somewhat refractory to maintenance therapy. New approaches to stabilize such patients need to be found. Furthermore, in studying lithium maintenance therapy, it has been found that a group of patients do not respond well to lithium.

These so-called frequent-failing patients have been found to be rapidly cycling, and alternate treatments for their care are essential.

In this chapter we discuss recent developments in the treatment of bipolar disorder, both acute mania and depression. The rationale for development of alternative therapies to lithium carbonate in acute mania is discussed.

TREATMENT OF ACUTE MANIA

Lithium

Historically, treatment of acute mania has included hospitalization, restraints, exercise, physical treatment (wet sheet packs, electroconvulsive therapy), and sedation. The introduction of antipsychotic medication in the 1950s was a major advance in treatment of acute mania, and these agents remained the treatment of choice until replaced by lithium carbonate in the 1960s and early 1970s. The efficacy of lithium treatment for acute mania was established through placebo-controlled trials as well as comparative trials against antipsychotic medication (13,14,35). In summary, lithium has been found to be clearly more effective than placebo in the treatment of acute mania in trials conducted over 2-week periods. Lithium has been shown to be at least as effective as antipsychotic medication (usually controlled with chlorpromazine) for the treatment of acute mania, again in relatively brief trials. It takes several days to achieve a therapeutic blood lithium concentration, and the antipsychotic medications tend to be sedating early in treatment. Thus, common clinical practice since the 1970s has been to treat the acutely manic patient with a combination of lithium and antipsychotic medication.

Although combined treatment is usually safe and effective, there have been occasional but unpredictable complications regarding this type of management. For example, some patients treated with lithium in combination with neuroleptics have been reported to experience lithium toxicity (10). Some manics can be treated with neuroleptics alone; however, the occurrence of a rare but at times fatal syndrome (neuroleptic malignant syndrome) during treatment with neuroleptics has been reported with increasing frequency (27). Furthermore, repeated use of potent neuroleptics for brief periods of time (as one might treat a relapsing manic patient) has resulted in some bipolar patients developing tardive dyskinesia.

Not all acutely manic patients show a prompt therapeutic response to lithium. Some patients seem refractory to treatment, and some patients are unsuited for lithium treatment secondary to medical problems. All of the above-mentioned problems have resulted in attempts to find new and alternative treatments for acute mania. Research and recent developments are useful in defining which manic patient should be treated with what medication. As noted above, several studies showed that lithium was efficacious in the treatment of acute mania when used alone. Whereas most of these studies were of 2 or 3 weeks' duration, one study continued treatment for 5 weeks, and some additional patients responded (46). Furthermore, data from a VA–NIMH collaborative project suggested that hospitalized manic patients who were not too psychotic, aggressive, or noncompliant were best treated with lithium as compared with chlorpromazine (36). (There was similar efficacy for the two treatments but fewer side effects with lithium.) In contrast, the more psychotic, aggressive, and noncompliant patient showed greater improvement with chlorpromazine than with lithium. (There were more dropouts in the lithium-treated group.) The fact that lithium can be given only orally (not intramuscularly) also limits its use to the more compliant patient.

A clinical problem frequently encountered is the manic patient who does not seem to respond promptly to treatment. Clinicians have become concerned about the need to shorten duration of hospitalization, and in many communities hospital stays of only 2 weeks are common for treatment of acutely manic patients. If the patient is not responding by day 10, there may be concern that treatment is not working fast enough or possibly that lithium is not an appropriate medication.

Past research is helpful in the above situation. The natural history of untreated mania is described as a 6-month illness in about 50% of patients (49). It is likely that some patients who are not responding to treatment at the end of 2 weeks will respond with longer duration of treatment. In the Takahashi et al. (46) study, three patients who had not responded by 3 weeks responded during an additional 2 weeks of therapy. Thus, there may be no need for concern about inappropriate diagnosis if patients do not respond in what today is considered a very prompt manner.

Lithium is measured in the serum, and doses are usually determined by serum concentration. However, lithium works intracellularly. The erythrocyte has been used as an index of lithium intracellular concentration (19,40). Some patients who have seemingly adequate serum concentrations of lithium have low erythrocyte concentrations. Thus, one factor in the failure of many patients to respond in a timely manner to treatment with lithium alone may be related to inadequate tissue levels of lithium. Some laboratories measure lithium erythrocyte:plasma ratios, and we have found this test to be clinically useful in instances in which the patient is not responding at usual lithium serum concentrations. In case of low erythocyte:plasma ratios, the dose of lithium can be increased, and the red blood cell:plasma ratio (and clinical condition of the patient) monitored. The patients should be monitored for side effects of lithium but can be treated at higher than usual plasma lithium concentrations if the erythrocyte:plasma ratio is monitored.

In summary, treatment of the acutely manic patient who is at the mild end of the severity spectrum and who is compliant could consist of psychosocial structure, exercise, hypnotics for regulation of sleep, and lithium carbonate alone.

Lithium with Neuroleptics

The more psychotic and/or noncompliant patient is difficult to treat with lithium alone. Such patients are commonly treated with neuroleptics alone, with lithium combined with neuroleptics, or with neuroleptics alone with lithium added later. As noted above, however, there may be a developing controversy regarding the use of neuroleptics in such patients.

In 1974, Cohen and Cohen (10) described four patients who developed neurotoxicity during combined treatment of lithium and haloperidol. These cases resulted in confusion among clinicians, since that combination of medication was in wide clinical use. If the combination was by itself toxic, it would seem logical that multiple instances of neurotoxicity would have been evident. Although the use of that particular combination of medication has been considered safe after extensive review of clinical experience, sporadic case reports of neurotoxicity with combined neuroleptic–lithium treatment have persisted. These reports have included a variety of neuroleptics in addition to haloperidol.

Lithium toxicity is usually characterized by symptoms of ataxia, confusion, hyperactive reflexes, chorea, slurred speech, and, at times, coma. Spring and Frankel (45) reviewed several cases of lithium toxicity occurring in the presence of neuroleptics. They suggested that some of these cases may have represented instances of simple lithium toxicity. However, other cases may have represented instances of the neuroleptic malignant syndrome. The neuroleptic malignant syndrome has recently been reviewed by Levenson (27). It is described as an uncommon but potentially fatal reaction occurring during treatment with neuroleptics, being characterized by muscular rigidity, fever, autonomic dysfunction, and altered consciousness. Several laboratory abnormalities are noted during this syndrome, and they include leukocytosis and elevated serum creatinine phosphokinase. This clinical syndrome can result in death or permanent neurotoxic damage. Neuroleptic malignant syndrome is somewhat different clinically from pure and uncomplicated lithium toxicity. The etiology of neuroleptic malignant syndrome is unknown. Its occurrence may explain some isolated instances of lithium in combination with neuroleptics producing a toxic state as noted above by Spring and Frankel (45). Alternative explanations for the syndrome of neurotoxicity during combined treatment may also be pertinent. For example, patients treated with neuroleptics in combination with lithium are often dehydrated and oversedated, and the dehydration associated with this combination may result in lithium toxicity itself. Furthermore, mania in its severe form has been known to include symptoms of confusion, fever, and even death. Thus, severe untreated mania may itself present as a neurotoxic syndrome and possibly have long-term neurological sequelae. Fortunately, the syndromes of neurotoxicity occurring with lithium, neuroleptic malignant syndrome, and confusional mania with fever are each rare occurrences. The rarity of these conditions, however, makes it difficult to determine the relationship of neuroleptics in the picture of lithium toxicity in such cases and makes research on this problem extremely difficult.

Tardive dyskinesia is another recently described side effect of chronic administration of neuroleptic medication. One theory explaining this syndrome is that the blockade of postsynaptic dopamine receptors during chronic neuroleptic treatment results in an increased production of dopamine by the presynaptic neuron as well as postsynaptic

supersensitivity. When the neuroleptic is stopped, the results of either or both of these chemical effects are to produce a dopamine excess manifested particularly by abnormal dyskinetic movements. Schizophrenic patients are frequently treated with neuroleptics chronically, often over the course of their lifetime. However, bipolar patients often experience pulse treatments of neuroleptics, i.e., are treated with neuroleptics during periods of mania, and the neuroleptics are stopped during periods of remission or periods of postmanic depression. Thus, the course of use of neuroleptics in patients with bipolar affective disorder is one of high doses separated by drug-free periods. This is exactly the model that would lead to cases of tardive dyskinesia. In the past, neuroleptics commonly used to treat mania were of a less potent variety (usually chlorpromazine or thioridazine), but in the past 10 years there has been an increasing clinical usage of the more potent neuroleptics (haloperidol and thiothixine). Frequently, clinicians have used these neuroleptics at relatively high doses, i.e., chlorpromazine-equivalent units of 4 g or more. Although the change from less potent to more potent neuroleptic use is related to fewer acute side effects during treatment with more potent neuroleptics, the rate of tardive dyskinesia among bipolar patients may actually be increased.

In summary, the treatment of the very agitated psychotic patient has recently included the use of potent neuroleptic agents in combination with lithium; however, the reports of severe side effects associated with the use of neuroleptics raise the issue of caution needing to be exercised in the treatment of such patients. Therefore, alternative treatments for acute mania have been studied. These treatments include carbamazepine, benzodiazepines, and other medications. One additional problem with lithium therapy has been the concern about nephritis associated with lithium toxicity. This concern was raised in the mid-1970s, when biopsy tissue from patients who had histories of lithium toxicity showed a chronic nephritis (6,23,37). It has been well known that lithium has a variety of renal effects including a mild polyuria, which occurs subclinically in most patients, as well as inability to concentrate urine (nephrogenic diabetes insipidus) (38). The latter can be a clinical problem in about 5% of chronic lithium-treated patients. The issue of chronic renal disease secondary to long-term lithium usage created a controversy regarding whether lithium, which needed to be administered chronically in order to effect maintenance therapy for recurrent bipolar disorder, was indeed safe on a long-term basis. This question seemingly has been resolved with recommendations that the least effective dose of lithium be used and that the lithium be given in a single daily dosage. However, all of these concerns—both toxicity of lithium itself and difficulties in the combination of lithium with neuroleptics—have created a situation in which the development of alternative therapies for acute mania is relevant to clinical practice. These alternative therapies have not been studied as extensively as lithium in acute mania, and the rarity of untreated mania in modern research facilities makes it unlikely that extensive research can provide the definitive data necessary to demonstrate clearly the efficacy of these agents. Many of these treatments have recently been summarized by Lerer (26).

ALTERNATIVE TREATMENTS FOR ACUTE MANIA

Carbamazepine

Carbamazepine is an anticonvulsant that is particularly useful in patients with temporal lobe epilepsy. Japanese investigators were the first to report the use of this compound in patients with mania. Takezaki and Honaoka (47) reported some improvement in six of 10 manic patients using carbamazepine. Okuma et al. (30), who studied the drug in acute mania and also for its maintenance effects, found carbamazepine to be effective in 13 of 33 acutely manic patients and somewhat effective in a further six subjects. However, in most of the cases treated by Okuma et al. (30), carbamazepine was not used alone but was used in conjunction with other treatments for mania including lithium and neuroleptics. Okuma et al. (31), in a study of manic patients assigned randomly to carbamazepine or chlorpromazine, found that carbamazepine improved symptoms in 70% of patients and chlorpromazine in 60%. The improvement was noted early in the course of treatment, suggesting that the efficacy may have been related to sedative effects. Ballenger and Post (2,3) also have studied carbamazepine in mania in a design using carbamazepine switching with placebo in the same patient. They noted a marked-to-moderate improvement in manic symptoms during carbamazepine treatment as compared with placebo treatment in five of nine subjects.

Although carbamazepine has a different side effect picture than lithium, the drug has a number of gastrointestinal side effects, and doses should be increased slowly in order to minimize the gastrointestinal disturbances. Blood dyscrasias have also been reported as side effects of carbamazepine (24). Furthermore, blood levels of carbamazepine should be obtained, since the drug at high blood levels produces a toxicity. Cases of neurotoxicity associated with the combined use of lithium and carbamazepine have also been reported (41). Finally, carbamazepine may be of benefit for maintenance therapy, particularly of rapidly cycling bipolar patients (33).

Carbamazepine remains the best-studied treatment for mania other than lithium. It is widely used clinically and should be considered the first option to lithium treatment in the lithium-nonresponsive manic patient.

Clonidine

Clonidine is an α-adrenergic agonist that is centrally active. The use of clonidine in acute mania was reported initially in 1980 and subsequently in a few isolated case reports. Zubenko et al. (50) recently reported three patients whose acute mania was treated with the administration of clonidine on an open basis. One patient was possibly treated with a combination of clonidine, carbamazepine, and lithium. A second patient seemed to have a prompt response to initiation of clonidine and a relapse when clonidine was discontinued. This patient again showed a prompt response when clonidine was reinstituted. The response was described to occur within 48 hr of treatment with clonidine. Zubenko et al. (50) considered these open

data to be of interest and suggested the need for double-blind trials. Hypotension is an important side effect of clonidine.

Lorazepam

Modell and co-workers (28) have recently reported the treatment of four patients with acute mania using the combination of lithium and a benzodiazepine, lorazepam. Three of the patients were described as having psychotic symptoms for 5 to 7 days prior to treatment. Lorazepam, at doses of 2 to 4 mg every 2 hr on an as-needed basis in order to achieve sedation was combined with lithium carbonate. One patient required 30 mg a day, two 20 mg a day, and one was treated with about 10 mg a day of lorazepam. Side effects of this treatment included mild ataxia, and there was no benzodiazepine withdrawal syndrome when lorazepam was discontinued. High doses of lorazepam were continued for the initial week of treatment, and then lorazepam was tapered. Although only mild side effects were reported by Modell (28), a patient of ours became apneic after a single oral dose of 2 mg of lorazepam (S. Cohen, *personal communication*).

Clonazepam

Clonazepam is an anticonvulsant benzodiazepine derivative that has been tried in manic patients in a randomly assigned crossover design. Chouinard et al. (8) tested clonazepam against lithium in 12 manic subjects (haloperidol was available on an as-needed basis for severe agitation). Doses of clonazepam ranged from 4 to 16 mg per day, and results indicated that clonazepam was found to be significantly more effective than lithium over a 10-day trial. Clonazepam was reported to be highly sedative, and patients required less p.r.n. haloperidol during clonazepam than during lithium treatment. However, it should be pointed out that a 10-day trial of lithium carbonate is generally considered too brief a time period for an adequate lithium effect to occur. Nonetheless, these results suggest that clonazepam may be of use early in the course of treatment as an alternative to neuroleptic treatment.

Verapamil

Verapamil is a calcium agonist that was first reported useful for the treatment of an acutely manic patient in 1982 by Dubovsky et al. (11). This group also reported a double-blind placebo-controlled crossover trial in three patients, and the authors report that verapamil may be of use in about 70% of unselected manic patients (12). Antimanic effects have been noted by other investigators (21). Verapamil is one of a type of medication—calcium channel-blocking agents—that has been found to be useful for treatment of hypertension and arrhythmias.

Valproic Acid

Valproic acid is a GABAergic drug that has anticonvulsant effects. This medication has been tested in a few bipolar patients by Emrich and colleagues (17), who noted that the compound may be effective in mania and also had some effects in rapidly cycling patients, i.e., maintenance effects. The maintenance effects were noted when patients were given valproic acid in combination with lithium.

L-Tryptophan

L-Tryptophan is an amino acid precurser of serotonin. This compound was administered to depressed patients as a means of testing the "biogenic amine" theory of depression. (Brain serotonin levels are theorized to be low in depressed patients, who might respond clinically to elevation in brain serotonin effected by administration of L-tryptophan.) Administration of L-tryptophan to acutely manic patients has shown clinical efficacy in some but not all studies (7,29,34). Doses of up to 12 mg/day were used. One advantage of L-tryptophan over other medication is the lack of side effects with its use.

Electroconvulsive Therapy

Although electroconvulsive therapy (ECT) is usually considered a treatment for depression, Small et al. (44) have recently reported that manic patients failed to respond to unilateral ECT but ultimately responded to bilateral ECT. This observation was noted in a prospective comparison of ECT against lithium in acute manics and represents an incidental finding. The small number of cases (six) warrants caution in interpreting results. However, ECT might be considered an effective alternative to medication for the treatment of acute manic patients. Small (42) notes that ECT is as effective as lithium in the treatment of acute mania. However, ECT should not be administered concomitantly with lithium, since neurotoxicity may occur in such instances (43).

SUMMARY

Lithium carbonate is an established treatment for acute mania. Clinically, acutely manic patients are usually treated with a combination of lithium and potent antipsychotic medications. However, this combination of medication has been reported to yield severe neurological side effects, albeit on rare occasions. Alternative treatments to lithium for acute mania have been less well studied for safety and efficacy. Also, it is unclear if some of these treatments are "antimanic" or purely sedative in nature. Thus, benzodiazepines are highly sedative: is their use in manic patients a mere replacement of the barbiturates of the past?

The following recommendations seem warranted by data currently available. First, lithium alone should be considered as the initial treatment of choice for the first-episode manic patient. If the patient refuses oral medication and/or is very psychotic, intramuscular medication should be used. Either benzodiazepines or neuroleptic treatment appears justified, the choice of drug being predicated on factors unique to the patient. However, the patient treated with lithium and neuroleptics may be at increased risk for side effects and should be closely monitored. Electroconvulsive

treatment can be an effective alternative to pharmacotherapy.

TREATMENT OF "SECONDARY MANIA"

Diagnostic criteria developed at Washington University in St. Louis preceded DSM-III. These criteria categorized psychiatric patients as having "primary" and "secondary" illnesses dependent on a prior history of a defined psychiatric (or medical) disorder preceding current symptoms (in the case of secondary illness) or lack thereof (in the case of primary illness). Thus, mania occurring in a patient who had no prior psychiatric history was termed a "primary" affective disorder. Mania occurring in an alcoholic patient would be termed "secondary."

Krauthammer and Klerman (25) described five broad illness categories that can present with a manic syndrome as a complication. For example, treatment with corticosteroids, systemic lupus erythematosis, and some cases of viral encephalitis may present with a manic-like psychiatric syndrome. Although DSM-III does not utilize the primary-secondary distinction, treatment of secondary mania is a common clinical problem. As noted in the introduction of this chapter, hospitalized manic patients frequently are those who have complicated histories.

It is beyond the scope of this chapter to discuss treatment of every type of secondary mania. However, the following principles of treatment may be of use. If the mania is secondary to a medication, the medication should be discontinued or its dosage reduced. Often the mania will respond to this simple manipulation. If the mania occurs in an active alcoholic, care should be taken to avoid neuroleptics (which may decrease the seizure threshold in a patient who might undergo alcohol withdrawal). Furthermore, treatment of both disorders is imperative. Indeed, most cases of secondary mania involve treatment of two conditions—mania and the preexisting disorder. As a general rule, treatment prescribed for either condition should not worsen the other.

TREATMENT OF DEPRESSIVE DISORDER OF BIPOLAR ILLNESS

Studies of the natural history of mania reveal that mania is often a triphasic illness. There is commonly a premanic depression, a rapid "switch" into the manic condition, and a slower transition into a postmanic depressive phase. Some bipolar patients experience only the premanic or postmanic depression as characteristic for their cycles. Each manic episode with its associated depression can be considered a "cycle." A small percentage of bipolars (about 5–10%) will not experience any depression—so-called "unipolar manics."

Studies of lithium maintenance therapy using the life table method of analysis and excluding rapid cyclers suggest that a bipolar patient, once euthymic, has a decreased probability of relapse if lithium treated as compared to placebo or no treatment (18). However, lithium-treated patients can and do experience relapse during maintenance therapy. The rate of failure during lithium treatment seems to be biphasic. For the first 6 months of lithium treatment (beginning when the patient is euthymic), the failure rate is about five times greater than over the ensuing 3-year period.

We have interpreted these data to make several clinical suggestions. The patient who is experiencing his first manic episode should be treated with lithium through the post-manic depression and continued on lithium for 6 additional months. Lithium therapy can then be terminated and the patient advised to return for treatment promptly should hypomanic symptoms or depressive symptoms recur. (The latter may represent the premanic depressive phase of the next cycle.) The above is predicated on natural history data, since some patients will not experience a second cycle, and it seems unnecessary to apply maintenance therapy to first-cycle patients. The 6-month period of continued lithium treatment after the patient has recovered from the postmanic depression is based on data showing this period to be the highest for relapse (18).

Treatment of depression of bipolar patients is dependent on which phase of the cycle one is treating. The premanic depression is of variable duration. (The authors have treated patients whose premanic depression lasted for 2 years.) Also, some patients who present for treatment of their first depressive episode may be bipolar and in a premanic depressive phase. A patient should not be considered "unipolar" until he has experienced a 6-month period of euthymia after recovery from the first depressive episode.

If the patient is a known bipolar and is presenting for treatment of what appears to be a premanic depression, the clinician should be concerned that the course of such a premanic depression probably is to switch into mania, and this switch process may be hastened by treatment with tricyclic antidepressants or some of the more recently introduced antidepressants. [Bupropion may be the exception here, since preliminary data suggest an absence of "switches" into mania/hypomania during use of bupropion in clinical treatment of depressed patients (20).] Treatment of this depression might include restarting lithium (in order to begin maintenance therapy) along with cautious use of antidepressants. The clinician should advise the patient and family about the possibility of a switch into mania and have the patient monitor sleep and other symptoms.

If the patient is presenting for treatment of an initial depressive episode, the clinician should consider the possibility that the patient is a "latent bipolar" who may be in a premanic depressive phase of the cycle. A switch into mania occurs in about 5% of first-episode depressives (13). Factors that may suggest that the patient may be a "latent bipolar" include a family history of bipolar illness and/or a personal history of cyclothymia.

Treatment of the postmanic depressive phase depends in part on severity of symptoms. About half of bipolar patients experience their postmanic depression as a period of tiredness, fatigue, mild oversleeping, and diminished concentration. Such patients may not require any pharmacotherapy for their (mild) depression other than lithium. In other patients, the depression may be severe and require treatment with pharmacotherapy or ECT.

Pharmacotherapy of the postmanic depressive phase may be difficult. This depression is frequently characterized by oversleeping and severe psychomotor retardation. Antidepressants that are more activating may be of particular benefit in contrast to the more sedating antidepressants. However, individual patients may respond uniquely to one particular agent, and this should be taken into account in planning treatment.

In general, treatment of any depressive episode should consist of education of the patient, assessment for the presence of other (medical) causes, and a tailoring of the treatment to the patient. The choice of pharmacotherapy, psychotherapy (such as cognitive therapy), or the combination of treatments is dependent on a number of factors. Other "treatments" that may be useful include regular structure of the patient's activities, exercise, and light therapy.

TREATMENT OF RAPID CYCLERS

Rapid cyclers are patients who experience four or more episodes of affective illness per year (16). Such patients do not respond well to lithium, although there is some improvement in their course with lithium treatment. We have suggested that rapidly cycling patients may respond well to a combination of lithium and antipsychotic drugs and the avoidance of antidepressants. [Tricyclic antidepressants have been noted to increase rapid cycling in some bipolar patients (48).] In addition, some rapid cyclers have been reported to have elevated levels of thyroid antibodies, suggesting that they may have an underlying history of thyroiditis that somehow interacts with their bipolar illness to create the rapid cycling. In such cases, the addition of thyroid hormone, even in euthyroid patients, may be of benefit. Carbamazepine alone or in combination with lithium has also been advocated by some as useful for the treatment of rapid cyclers. In general, we would recommend a trial of lithium alone, then possibly the addition of small doses of less potent antipsychotic medication to the patient's course. Tricyclic antidepressants should be avoided. If the patient does not seem to respond, then other medication such as carbamazepine may be added to the regimen.

CONCLUSION

For the most part, the introduction of lithium salts for the treatment of acute mania has proven to be a safe and efficacious treatment and is clinically accepted. Development of alternative treatments has been partially compromised by the success of lithium, since many patients who used to relapse and require rehospitalization are now stabilized as outpatients with lithium maintenance therapy. However, it is important that alternative treatments for acute mania be developed and their safety and efficacy demonstrated.

REFERENCES

1. Abrams, R., and Taylor, M. A. (1976): *Am. J. Psychiatry,* 133: 1445–1447.
2. Ballenger, J. C., and Post, R. M. (1978): *Commun. Psychopharmacol.,* 2:159–175.

3. Ballenger, J. C., and Post, R. M. (1980): *Am. J. Psychiatry*, 137:782–790.
4. Brockington, I. F., Wainwright, S., and Kendell, R. E. (1980): *Psychol. Med.*, 10:73–83.
5. Brockington, I. F., Hillier, V. F., Francis, A. F., Helzer, J. E., and Wainright, S. (1983): *Am. J. Psychiatry*, 140:435–439.
6. Bucht, G., and Wahlin, A. (1980): *Acta Med. Scand.*, 207:309–314.
7. Chambers, C. A., and Naylor, G. J. (1978): *Br. J. Psychiatry*, 132:555–559.
8. Chouinard, G., Young, S. N., and Annable, L. (1983): *Biol. Psychiatry*, 18:451–466.
9. Clayton, P. J. (1982): *J. Nerv. Ment. Dis.*, 170:646–650.
10. Cohen, W. J., and Cohen, N. H. (1974): *J.A.M.A.*, 230:1283–1288.
11. Dubovsky, S. L., Franks, R. D., Lifschitz, M. L., and Coen, P. (1982): *Am. J. Psychiatry*, 139:502–504.
12. Dubovsky, S. L., Franks, R. D., and Schrier, D. (1985): *Biol. Psychiatry*, 20:1009–1014.
13. Dunner, D. L. (1983): In: *Psychiatry Update, Vol. II*, edited by L. Grinspoon, pp. 293–303. American Psychiatric Press, Washington.
14. Dunner, D. L., and Fieve, R. R. (1978): In: *Neuropsychopharmacology*, edited by P. Deniker, C. Radouco-Thomas, and A. Villeneuve, pp. 1109–1115. Pergamon Press, New York.
15. Dunner, D. L., Fleiss, J. L., and Fieve, R. R. (1976): *Am. J. Psychiatry*, 133:905–908.
16. Dunner, D. L., Patrick, V., and Fieve, R. R. (1977): *Compr. Psychiatry*, 18:561–566.
17. Emrich, H. M., Zerssen, D., Kissling, W., and Moeller, H. J. (1981): *Am. J. Psychiatry*, 138:256.
18. Fleiss, J. L., Prien, R. F., Dunner, D. L., and Fieve, R. R. (1978): *Compr. Psychiatry*, 19:355–362.
19. Frazer, A., Mendels, J., Secunda, S. K., and Bianchi, C. P. (1973): *J. Psychiatr. Res.*, 10:1–8.
20. Gardner, E. A. (1983): *J. Clin. Psychiatry*, 44:157–162.
21. Giannini, H., House, W. L., Loiselle, R. H., Giannini, M. D., and Price, W. (1984): *Am. J. Psychiatry*, 141:1602–1603.
22. Goodnick, P. J., and Meltzer, H. Y. (1984): *Schizophrenia Bull.*, 10:30–48.
23. Hestbech, J., Hansen, H. E., Amdisen, A., and Olsen, S. (1977): *Kidney Int.*, 12:205–213.
24. Joffe, R. T., Post, R. M., Roy-Byrne, P. P., and Uhde, T. W. (1985): *Am. J. Psychiatry*, 142:1196–1199.
25. Krauthammer, C., and Klerman, G. (1978): *Arch. Gen. Psychiatry*, 35:1333–1339.
26. Lerer, B. (1985): *J. Clin. Psychiatry*, 46:309–316.
27. Levenson, J. L. (1985): *Am. J. Psychiatry*, 142:1137–1145.
28. Modell, J. G., Lenox, R. H., and Weiner, S. (1985): *J. Clin. Psychopharmacol.*, 5:109–113.
29. Murphy, D. L., Baker, M., Goodwin, F. K., Miller, F. K., Kotin, J., et al. (1974): *Psychopharmacologia*, 34:11–20.
30. Okuma, T., Kishimoto, A., Inoue, K., Matsumoto, H., Ogura, A., et al. (1973): *Folia Psychiatr. Neurol. (Jpn.)*, 27:281–297.
31. Okuma, T., Inanaga, K., Otsuki, S., Sarai, K., Takahashi, R., et al. (1979): *Psychopharmacology*, 66:211–217.
32. Pi, E. H., and Surawicz, F. G. (1982): *J. Clin. Psychiatry*, 43:235–236.
33. Post, R. M., Ballenger, J. C., Uhde, T. W., and Bunney, W. E., Jr. (1984): In: *Neurobiology of Mood Disorders*, edited by R. M. Post and J. C. Ballenger, pp. 777–816. Williams & Wilkins, Baltimore.
34. Prange, A. J., Wilson, I. C., Lynn, C. W., Alltop, L. B., and Stikeleather, R. A. (1974): *Arch. Gen. Psychiatry*, 30:56–62.
35. Prien, R. F. (1979): In: *Lithium: Controversies and Unresolved Issues*, edited by T. B. Cooper, S. Gershon, N. S. Kline, and M. Schou, pp. 3–29. Excerpta Medica, Amsterdam.
36. Prien, R. F., Klett, C. J., and Caffey, E. M. (1972): *Arch. Gen. Psychiatry*, 26:146–153.
37. Rafaelsen, O. H., Bolwig, T. G., Lagefoged, J., and Brun, C. (1979): In: *Lithium: Controversies and Unresolved Issues*, edited by T. B. Cooper, S. Gershon, N. S. Kline, and M. Schou, pp. 578–583. Excerpta Medica, Amsterdam.
38. Ramsey, T. A., and Cox, M. (1982): *Am. J. Psychiatry*, 139:443–449.
39. Rosenthal, N. E., Rosenthal, L. N., Stallone, F., Dunner, D. L., and Fieve, R. R. (1980): *Arch. Gen. Psychiatry*, 37:804–810.
40. Schreiner, H. C., Dunner, D. L., Meltzer, H. L., and Fieve, R. R. (1979): *Biol. Psychiatry*, 14:207–213.
41. Shukla, S., Goodwin, C. D., Long, L. E. B., and Miller, M. G. (1984): *Am. J. Psychiatry*, 141:1604–1606.
42. Small, J. G. (1985): *Convuls. Ther.*, 1:271–276.
43. Small, J. G., Kellams, J. J., Milstein, V., and Small, I. F. (1980): *Biol. Psychiatry*, 15:103–112.
44. Small, J. G., Small, I. F., Milstein, V., Kellams, J. J., and Klapper, M. H. (1985): *Biol. Psychiatry*, 20:125–134.
45. Spring, G., and Frankel, M. (1981): *Am. J. Psychiatry*, 138:810–821.
46. Takahashi, R., Sakuma, A., Itoh, K., Kurihara, M., Saito, M., and Watanabe, M. (1975): *Arch. Gen. Psychiatry*, 32:1310–1318.
47. Takezaki, H., and Honaoka, M. (1971): *Seishin Shinkeigaku Zasshi*, 48(13):173–183.
48. Wehr, T. A., and Goodwin, F. K. (1979): *Arch. Gen. Psychiatry*, 36:555–559.
49. Winokur, G., Clayton, P. J., and Reich, T. (1969): *Manic-Depressive Illness*. C. V. Mosby, St. Louis.
50. Zubenko, G. S., Cohen, B. M., Lipinski, J. F., and Jonas, J. M. (1984): *Am. J. Psychiatry*, 141:1617–1618.

Psychopharmacology:
The Third Generation of Progress,
edited by Herbert Y. Meltzer.
Raven Press, New York © 1987.

CHAPTER **110**

Introduction: Schizophrenia

John M. Kane

Advances over the past decade in the diagnosis and assessment of schizophrenia have involved increasing attention to the reliability and validity of diagnostic criteria in conjunction with greater appreciation of the potential heterogeneity of the syndrome and its clinical manifestations.

New structured diagnostic interviews have been developed that provide more comprehensive documentation of both positive and negative signs and symptoms. In addition, the recognition that a longitudinal approach to diagnosis is required in schizophrenia has been reinforced.

Although many hypotheses relating to heterogeneity in etiology, treatment response, and course are not new, they are being tested with greater degrees of methodological sophistication from a broader array of perspectives, some of which (e.g., new techniques in brain imaging) have emerged over the past decade.

The extent to which clinical phenomena are in and of themselves useful for identifying meaningful subtypes within the schizophrenic syndrome remains controversial; however, the establishment of diagnostic or selection criteria in a systematic and replicable fashion for inclusion in all studies relating to any aspect of schizophrenia (etiology, pathophysiology, or treatment response) remains critical to advances in the field.

As both Andreasen and Carpenter point out, there are no pathognomonic signs of schizophrenia, and various psychopathologic domains associated with the illness may be only loosely linked, with enormous variability between subjects and within subjects over time. In addition, the fact that there is such a degree of heterogeneity in onset, pattern of illness, long-term outcome, and a variety of genetic and biologic factors has placed renewed emphasis on predictors of drug response to identify subgroups that may not require or may not benefit from short- or long-term neuroleptic treatment. At present, these efforts have not led to major successes, and recent 2- to 3-year follow-up studies of first-episode schizophrenics admitted to hospital suggest that the overwhelming majority experience a recurrence. At the same time, much longer-term follow-up studies suggest that some patients experience considerable improvement with aging. The long-term outcome studies also point out discrete patterns of illness, with some individuals experiencing an insidious onset and poor outcome whereas others may have an acute onset associated with either very good response or very poor response to treatment.

The impact of currently available forms of treatment (e.g., neuroleptics) on the long-term course of the illness and ultimate outcome is difficult to assess given the naturalistic nature of these outcome studies, whereas the data are quite compelling with regard to the overall positive impact of neuroleptic treatment in those controlled trials lasting 1 or 2 years following an index episode.

Although neuroleptics remain the most effective pharmacologic treatment in schizophrenia, other classes of medication and electroconvulsive therapy may also be helpful in some subgroups, as reviewed by Rifkin and Siris; however, means to identify these subgroups a priori remain unavailable. A major continuing problem in schizophrenia research is the identification of subgroups within a larger population. For example, we assume that all marketed neuroleptics are equally efficacious, yet we also note that some patients may do better on one drug than another. Comparisons between drugs within the neuroleptic class are based on overall response rates (which are comparable), but this does not indicate potential differences between patients in response to one drug versus another. The kinds of research strategies necessary to delineate subtypes based on pharmacologic response require careful longitudinal assessment with appropriate controls, particularly with regard to the passage of time. If a patient fails to respond to a first treatment but responds to a subsequent treatment, this may simply reflect additional time on medication, and a control group receiving the original treatment for the additional interval is necessary to draw meaningful conclusions. The issue of dose equivalence also remains a critical problem in comparing different compounds. Dose equivalencies have been estimated based on clinical trials that utilize a range of doses. However, conversion ratios appropriate at one end of the dosage spectrum may not be applicable at the other extreme.

Despite the clinical efficacy of neuroleptics, there is an array of signs and symptoms labeled as "negative" or "deficit state" that do not respond in a parallel fashion with more positive symptoms such as delusions, hallucinations, and thought disorder. However, these symptoms may also vary in response to neuroleptics depending on which phase of illness the patient is in. During an acute exacerbation, even symptoms that may be considered negative (e.g., psychomotor retardation, withdrawal) can be shown to benefit from neuroleptics, whereas during the maintenance phase following recovery from an episode, neuroleptics may increase psychomotor retardation, emotional withdrawal, and blunted affect, perhaps through the neurologic side effects we label as parkinsonism. Negative symptoms must also be differentiated from depression and demoralization; therefore, several strategies may be necessary to validate the nature of these symptoms in specific patients. The extent to which positive and negative symptom clusters represent different pathophysiologic processes remains to be established, as does the extent to which the presence or absence of specific symptoms is associated with different phases of the illness in a specific individual.

Clearly, neuroleptics have not succeeded in overcoming many of the psychosocial and vocational limitations that we associate with schizophrenia, regardless of their etiology. In addition, a variety of environmental, familial, personality, and nonsomatic treatment factors may play important roles in determining the level of functioning achieved by patients with this illness; therefore, neuroleptic effects must be viewed in this context. Schooler and Hogarty discuss these issues.

A further concern with currently available neuroleptics is their propensity to produce neurologic side effects, particularly tardive dyskinesia (TD). Prevalence estimates suggest that this condition is present in over 20% of chronically institutionalized neuroleptic-treated patients. The incidence of tardive dyskinesia appears to be 3 to 4% per year of neuroleptic exposure. Though the majority of cases are not severe, the occurrence of severe and disabling cases of TD has been a major impetus for both the development of safer antipsychotic compounds and the development of alternative strategies to reduce cumulative neuroleptic exposure.

As Tamminga and Gerlach discuss, there have been considerable efforts over the past decade to identify and determine the clinical effects of a variety of "novel" or "atypical" antipsychotic compounds. To some extent this research has grown out of the further elucidation of the basic anatomy and physiology of dopamine systems in brain, but it has also been stimulated by the limitations of traditional neuroleptics in spectrum of activity and propensity to produce adverse effects, particularly tardive dyskinesia. Further study of dopaminergic systems within the brain has identified multiple dopamine receptors for which different antipsychotic drugs display varying degrees of selectivity. In addition, specific neuroleptic drugs have different effects in cholinergic, serotonergic, and noradrenergic systems and, in all likelihood, a variety of other neurotransmitter or neuromodulator systems as well. Though the atypical drugs produce relatively few extrapyramidal side effects, it remains to be determined whether they provide a substantially reduced risk of tardive dyskinesia. Ultimately the test of this possibility will require carefully controlled clinical trials. Tamminga and Gerlach review experience to date with several atypical compounds.

During the past decade we have witnessed a "second generation" of long-term clinical trials in schizophrenia. As Kane and Lieberman point out, these studies have benefited from advances in methodology and statistical analysis as well as including a more comprehensive array of assessment techniques, examining not only rates of psychotic relapse and rehospitalization but also subjective well-being, psychopathology outside of the psychotic range, psychosocial and vocational adjustment, and family interactions. In addition, increasing attention has been given to identifying and quantifying a variety of adverse effects. Although to some extent the gains in this area have involved extensions of previous observations, more sophisticated testing of specific hypotheses, and increasingly comprehensive assessment of risks and benefits, we should not lose sight of the enormous advantage that incremental improvements in treatment can provide when applied to large numbers of patients. In addition, further exploration and understanding of the heterogeneity in outcome with both acute and long-term pharmacotherapy should provide important clues to a better understanding of schizophrenia in general.

Psychopharmacology:
The Third Generation of Progress,
edited by Herbert Y. Meltzer.
Raven Press, New York © 1987.

CHAPTER 111

Schizophrenia: Diagnosis and Assessment

Nancy C. Andreasen

Our present decade is likely to be one of reassessment and growth in our understanding of the concept of schizophrenia. Psychiatry at present seems to have a divided mind about this illness. One group looks on it with pessimism, with regard to both our ability to understand it and our ability to treat it. Others view the puzzle of schizophrenia as a tantalizing challenge. For them, the complexity of schizophrenia is its fascination. The problems involved in understanding schizophrenia are the fundamental and archetypal ones that psychiatry must face. If we understand and solve this illness, the remainder of our tasks are likely to be relatively easy.

DIAGNOSTIC ISSUES

Part of the puzzle of schizophrenia is the definition of what this disorder is. Since it was originally defined by Kraepelin and Bleuler at the turn of the century (12,34), our understanding of it has evolved and shifted. Diagnostic controversies can be summarized by four major questions: What are the boundaries of the concept? What are the characteristic symptoms that define this concept? How much emphasis should be given to course and longitudinal factors in defining the concept? Is the disorder homogeneous or heterogeneous and, if heterogeneous, how should it be subdivided or subtyped?

Boundary Issues

Most clinicians and investigators can agree on a concept of "core" or "nuclear" schizophrenia. Although its presenting symptoms may vary and its longitudinal course may fluctuate, this form of the disorder is severe, incapacitating, and characterized by at least some deterioration in functioning or personality that is relatively persistent. Controversy arises, however, when people begin to discuss the related disorders that may or may not circle around this nucleus. The most serious debate involves two disorders that may possibly be related: schizoaffective disorder and schizotypal personality.

The concept of schizophrenia proposed by Kraepelin, referred to by him as dementia praecox, is very similar to what we now call nuclear or core schizophrenia. Since his original definition of dementia praecox, however, the concept has steadily broadened. Kraepelin's definition linked the disorder to a deteriorating course, whereas Bleuler's emphasized the importance of cross-sectional symptoms. Further, Bleuler stressed symptoms as fundamental that are on a spectrum with normality: associative loosening, autistic thinking, ambivalence in thoughts and emotions, and abnormalities of affect. Since these symptoms could be present in relatively mild form, and since Bleuler deemphasized florid or psychotic symptoms such as delusions or hallucinations, the concept of schizophrenia expanded to include latent or nonpsychotic forms. When Kasanin introduced the concept of schizoaffective disorder, mixed affective and psychotic syndromes were also brought into the schizophrenia spectrum (29).

During the late 1960s and early 1970s, the results of the International Pilot Study of Schizophrenia and the U.S./U.K. Study led to a major reassessment of the boundaries of the concept of schizophrenia (18,55). These two cross-national studies made it clear that, at least in the United States, the concept of schizophrenia may have expanded so far that its limits were stretched to the breaking point. At the very least, the United States was out of step with the rest of the world. Armed with this recognition, American nosologists began to reassess and redefine. The result was a slimming of the concept in the DSM-III classification—

if not to its early Kraepelinian trimness, then at least to a proportion that seemed lean and functional. The DSM-III has shed both schizoaffective disorder and latent or nonpsychotic forms from the core concept in addition to requiring some evidence for chronicity (6 months duration) and evidence for deterioration in functioning (22).

This narrowing occurred because clinicians and researchers were concerned that the concept of schizophrenia had become "too soft." The selection of treatment and the conduct of research had become impaired. More recently, some have begun to wonder if the pendulum has swung too far. It is perhaps now time to reassess the implications, both pro and con, of the narrowing of the concept of schizophrenia.

Schizoaffective Disorder

Clinicians have recognized for many years that some patients with schizophrenia also have affective symptoms such as depression, especially relatively early in the illness. Early work indicated, in fact, that the presence of affective symptoms was a good prognostic sign, particularly when tied to other important indicators such as acute onset, good premorbid adjustment, and family history of affective disorder. When lithium became widely available as a treatment for mania, it was only natural that conscientious and caring clinicians would also attempt to use it as a treatment for schizoaffective disorder. When many patients with schizoaffective disorder were found to respond well to lithium, the whole concept of schizoaffective disorder was reevaluated through a broad range of data-based research.

This research has now been summarized in a large number of review articles (17,19,43,54). Many of these are flawed, however, by the fact that they pool many different definitions of schizoaffective disorder—some of them emphasizing acuteness of onset, others response to treatment, and others mixed phenomenology. Brockington and others have summarized the many different criteria that have been applied to define schizoaffective disorder (14).

In general, most of the recent studies and summaries have concluded either that schizoaffective disorder is a variant of affective disorder or that it represents some type of syndrome that is intermediate between affective disorder and schizophrenia. The emphasis varies depending on the external validator used. Those explored most commonly include family history, response to treatment, and outcome. In a recent review, Coryell concludes that most of the 17 studies that look at outcome find that schizoaffectives do less well than patients with pure affective disorder but better than patients with schizophrenia (19). Studies of treatment response appear to indicate that patients with schizoaffective disorder are less likely to respond to lithium alone but do respond relatively well to combinations of lithium and antipsychotics and that they show an overall better response than patients with pure schizophrenia (43). The family history studies indicate that patients with schizoaffective disorder have higher rates of schizophrenia in their families than do patients with pure affective disorder, but they also have higher rates of affective disorder in their families than do patients with pure schizophrenia. Family

studies do seem to indicate, however, that schizoaffectives with manic features (schizobipolars or schizomanics) may be much more closely allied to the affective disorders than are schizoaffectives who manifest only depression (17,46).

Most of these findings can be explained by the assumption that the current definitions of schizoaffective disorder probably identify a mixture of atypical patients with schizophrenia and with affective disorder. As research progresses further, we may be more successful in identifying the best criteria for classifying these atypical patients. At the present time, the term schizoaffective disorder, as it is usually used, probably refers to a "mixed bag."

In this context, the boundary between schizophrenia and affective disorders must remain flexible, depending on whether the goal is research or patient care. A narrow definition of schizophrenia, as manifested by DSM-III, is well suited to patient care, since it minimizes the chance that a patient who might respond well to lithium or ECT will be denied such treatment because of being prematurely diagnosed as having an illness (schizophrenia) that does not usually call for such treatment. For research purposes, a narrow definition allows for minimum contamination of schizophrenic cohorts by patients with affective disorder, although it may produce contamination of samples of patients with affective disorder by including some patients who in fact have schizophrenia. Although this might seem a desirable situation for investigators interested in studying schizophrenia, since it identifies a relatively pure sample of schizophrenics, it may be inappropriate for some types of studies. In particular, genetic and family studies might benefit from a broader concept of schizophrenia, since studies of diagnostic concordance among twins or in individual patients over time could be subject to falsely elevated estimates of discordance if further research supports that the full range of pathology in schizophrenia is in fact broader.

Schizotypal Personality

The concept of schizoaffective disorder requires that we consider the bounds of schizophrenia with respect to affective symptoms, whereas the concept of schizotypal personality asks that we consider the bounds of schizophrenia with respect to severity.

In the preneuroleptic era, mild nonpsychotic forms of schizophrenia were gradually added to the concept under a variety of different names: latent, pseudoneurotic, and simple schizophrenia. It was frequently observed that these patients did not respond particularly well to psychotherapy. When neuroleptics became available, they did not seem particularly efficacious either. As the risk of tardive dyskinesia became more apparent, pressure mounted to narrow the concept of schizophrenia in order to prevent the excessive or inappropriate use of neuroleptics. The impetus to narrow the concept of schizophrenia in terms of severity thus also arose for a psychopharmacologic reason—in this instance, to prevent a particular somatic treatment rather than to suggest a specific one.

Although this narrowing has been important because of its implications for treatment, more recent genetic and family data suggest that the boundaries may have been set too narrow. From an etiologic or pathophysiologic perspective, schizophrenia may exist as a spectrum of disorders including milder personality disorders (33). Differences in genetic loading or the exposure to other etiologic factors may simply lead to a milder schizophrenic syndrome in some individuals.

There are a number of studies that examine schizoid or schizotypal traits in twins, adopted offspring, or the first-degree relatives of schizophrenic probands. In a reanalysis of the Danish adoption study of schizophrenia, Kendler and colleagues found that schizotypal personality occurred in 10.5% of the biologic relatives of schizophrenics, none of the adopted relatives, and none of the control relatives (30,31). In addition, biologic relatives of adoptees with schizophrenia were at higher risk for schizotypal personality than were relatives of adoptees without schizophrenic psychoses (14.3% versus 0%). An increased incidence of schizotypal personality in the first-degree relatives of family members has also been reported (31).

Schizotypal features are also linked phenomenologically to schizophrenia. In fact, five of the eight criteria for schizotypal personality in DSM-III are nearly identical to the criteria for prodromal schizophrenia.

The possible etiologic link between schizotypal traits and schizophrenia certainly merits further research using a variety of paradigms, including genetics, neurochemistry, and brain imaging. The clinical importance of these findings is, however, relatively limited. It is certainly not appropriate to consider all schizotypal patients as preschizophrenic, since most do not eventually develop schizophrenia. There is a dearth of treatment studies of schizotypal traits, but the risk of tardive dyskinesia does imply that the clinician should not treat the schizotypal personality with the same eagerness that is used to try antidepressants on dysthymic patients.

Characteristic Symptoms

Debate swirls around the issue of the defining features of schizophrenia because this disorder is complex in its clinical presentation. Whereas affective disorders are characterized by a clear disorder in mood or affect and dementia has memory impairment as its hallmark, schizophrenia lacks a single defining feature.

In an attempt to simplify the concept, clinicians and researchers have sought a pathognomonic feature. Bleulerian "thought disorder" held this position of preeminence for many years. It is now clear that this was a misleading oversimplification; thought disorder occurs in mania and depression and is even observed in normal individuals (2,3,7). A similar position of preeminence was given for a time to Schneiderian first-rank symptoms, but it is now clear that these cannot be regarded as pathognomonic either (15,37).

We must confront squarely the fact that, at our present level of understanding, schizophrenia is characterized by a multiplicity of symptoms that reflect a broad range of cognitive dysfunctions. Patients with schizophrenia suffer from abnormalities in perception, attention, communica-

tion, volition, affective modulation, cognition, and motor function. We refer to these abnormalities as hallucinations, delusions, thought disorder, avolition, affective blunting, catatonia, etc. Although these abnormalities, signs, and symptoms occur in the broad range of patients suffering from schizophrenia and characterize it as a disease, no single patient manifests all of these symptoms at a given time or even during the entire course of his illness. In fact, a given patient may have only one or two, such as delusions combined with inattentiveness, although this is relatively uncommon if patients are followed over a period of time.

Thus, the clinical picture that is referred to as schizophrenia can be quite diverse when it is observed over a broad range of patients. This illness has many defining features, none of which is pathognomonic. Stated conceptually, the definition of schizophrenia is polythetic rather than monothetic: it is defined by a characteristic clustering of a variety of symptoms, no single one of which is specific to the disorder. (The affective disorders, by contrast, are monothetic, since they have the single defining feature of a disorder in mood.)

More recently, the emphasis has shifted from "pathognomonic symptoms" to signs and symptoms that are simply clinically useful. In order to meet the criterion of clinical utility, signs and symptoms must fulfill three requirements: adequate reliability, adequate base rate, and potential validity. Reliability refers to the ability of two observers to agree on the presence or absence (and sometimes the severity) of a particular sign or symptom. It is axiomatic that if features of an illness cannot be evaluated reliably, they will not be useful diagnostically, not to mention suitable measures for research. Base rate refers to the frequency with which a sign or symptom occurs; a symptom may be quite important when it occurs but may occur very infrequently and therefore be of little value either clinically or in research. Validity refers to the capacity to make useful predictions, such as response to treatment.

During the past several decades, considerable progress has been made in identifying and defining the signs and symptoms of schizophrenia in order to satisfy these three criteria. Early efforts focused on symptoms that promised better reliability, such as delusions and hallucinations or, particularly, Schneiderian first-rank symptoms (37). As these were shown to have good reliability and usually an adequate base rate, work continued on other more difficult symptoms such as affective blunting or thought disorder (1–7). Delusions and hallucinations by their very nature are discontinuous from normal function and can relatively easily be rated as present or absent. On the other hand, other symptoms of schizophrenia, such as affective blunting or difficulties in communicating in language, are not so clearly discontinuous and are therefore more difficult to define and to rate reliably. During recent years, however, considerable progress has been made in this area, and reliable definitions are now available for the broad range of the signs and symptoms of schizophrenia (26,38; M. Moscarelli, C. Maffei, and C. Cazzullo, *personal communication*).

In an effort to bring some coherence to the broad range of schizophrenic symptoms, during recent years investigators have begun to group them into two major groups: positive or florid symptoms and negative or defect symptoms (5,6,8–10). As a group, positive symptoms tend to represent an abnormality, distortion, or exaggeration of a normal function and include a variety of delusions and hallucinations and abnormalities in language and behavior. Negative symptoms, on the other hand, represent a diminution or loss of function and include such features as poverty of speech and content of speech (alogia), affective blunting, asociality-anhedonia, and avolition. Some evidence suggests that positive symptoms may occur more frequently during the early stages of schizophrenia, whereas negative symptoms are more prominent during the later phases. Further, once they occur, negative symptoms tend to persist (41,42). There is also some evidence suggesting that negative symptoms respond less well to treatment with neuroleptics than do positive symptoms (28,53). This latter point is a matter of some controversy, however, and is likely to be a topic of research during the next few years.

Subtypes of Schizophrenia

Given the breadth and diversity of the symptoms that characterize schizophrenia, it is only natural to wonder whether this disorder is truly heterogeneous or whether it is a related group of disorders. Identifying possible subtypes is of great importance both in the search for underlying pathophysiology and etiology and in the search for predictors of treatment response. If a diverse group of disorders is pooled together in studies of biological correlates or of treatment response, important findings may be lost because fundamental differences have been averaged out. Only a broad spread of variance is left behind as a clue to suggest the possibility of heterogeneity. Because so many studies of schizophrenia do display a large variance across a diversity of measures in schizophrenic samples, many investigators suspect that schizophrenia may indeed be a cluster of heterogeneous disorders that share the characteristics of psychotic features and a relatively poor outcome.

Traditional Subtypes

Both Kraepelin and Bleuler subdivided schizophrenia into several different groups, and modern nosology follows their example. In fact, the current standard approach to subtyping schizophrenia codified in the American Psychiatric Association's *Diagnostic and Statistical Manual* is nearly identical to the subtypes recommended by Kraepelin and Bleuler. The paranoid subtype is characterized by well-organized delusions with relatively preserved affect and very little formal thought disorder. The disorganized (hebephrenic) subtype is characterized by fragmented delusions and hallucinations as well as prominent formal thought disorder and flat or inappropriate affect. Patients whose clinical picture is dominated by catatonic motor symptoms (stupor, negativism, rigidity, excitement, or posturing) are subtyped as catatonic. Patients who display some mixture of these symptoms and do not easily fall into any of these three categories are classified as undifferentiated.

The main purpose of subtyping is to improve predictive

validity. To the clinician, subtypes hold out the promise of refinement in treatment selection and prediction of outcome. To the researcher, the delineation of more homogeneous subtypes promises faster progress in identifying etiological factors. Since these promises remain largely unfulfilled, traditional approaches to subtyping schizophrenia must be considered inadequate. A few studies suggest some differences between these subtypes and age of onset, family history, long-term outcome, and a variety of biological parameters, but most of these studies are plagued by problems in replication and lack of specificity (32,44,50).

Alternative Strategies

Dissatisfaction with traditional subtypes has led some investigators to propose alternate strategies. One that appears to hold promise is the use of outcome variables to generate new classes of subtypes (56). In this approach, cross-sectional phenomenology is not treated as the identifying feature of the class, and instead some important clinical or biological measures such as response to treatment or evidence of structural brain abnormality are used as the principle by which subtypes are defined. For example, Weinberger et al. subdivided a sample of schizophrenic patients into those with prominent ventricular enlargement and those without evidence of structural brain abnormality (53). These two groups were then examined in terms of their response to treatment, showing that patients with prominent ventricular enlargement are less likely to respond to treatment with neuroleptics. An alternate strategy is to use response to treatment as the independent variable, identifying those patients who respond well to neuroleptics and then examining the various defining features of this group, such as signs and symptoms, cognitive functioning, etc. Although this approach is promising, it has been used only infrequently to date. Further, this approach is only as good as the variables selected to define the new classes.

Another alternative approach for subtyping schizophrenia involves the use of positive and negative symptoms to identify separate diagnostic classes (5,6,20). This approach has clear heuristic and theoretical appeal, since it unites phenomenology, pharmacology, and pathophysiology into a single comprehensive hypothesis, originally proposed by Crow (20). According to this model, negative symptoms are associated with poor premorbid functioning, cognitive impairment, evidence of structural brain abnormality (e.g., enlarged ventricles on CT scan), poor response to treatment, and an underlying pathophysiology and etiology characterized by neuronal loss. Positive symptoms, on the other hand, respond well to treatment and occur in the context of normal cognitive function and generally good premorbid adjustment; their underlying pathophysiology and etiology are hypothesized to be related to hyperdopaminergic transmission, perhaps in the limbic system.

Some evidence supports this distinction. Positive symptoms tend to respond relatively well to neuroleptics, whose major mechanism of action is blockade of dopamine transmission (28). Other drugs that enhance dopamine transmission, such as the amphetamines, are likely to exacerbate positive symptoms (11). On the other hand, patients with prominent negative symptoms or evidence of ventricular enlargement tend to respond less well to neuroleptic therapy (53). Several studies have also shown that patients with prominent negative symptoms tend to have evidence of cognitive impairment and a higher rate of structural brain abnormalities (5,6,27,45). A few studies also suggest that negative symptoms may be associated with dopamine deficiency rather than dopamine overactivity (16,35,36).

Some studies of this model have failed to confirm it, however (40). The model has problems (as in fact do all approaches to subtyping) in dealing with longitudinal aspects of schizophrenia, since in any individual patient the symptoms may vary widely from one time to another. The concept of negative symptoms has also been criticized, since these may result from a variety of sources such as the effects of institutionalization, neuroleptic side effects, demoralization, and depression. Further, negative symptoms may sometimes be secondary side effects of positive symptoms (e.g., the paranoid patient who avoids social activity because of suspiciousness and fear), a fact that makes neuroleptic effects on negative and positive symptoms difficult to interpret.

Course and Outcome

The current narrow definition of schizophrenia embodied in DSM-III represents a return to Kraepelinian principles in that it stresses longitudinal features in addition to cross-sectional ones. The DSM-III definition succeeded in dramatically narrowing the concept of schizophrenia by adding in two longitudinal characteristics: a 6-month duration of symptoms and evidence for some deterioration from the previous level of functioning.

The requirement that the concept of schizophrenia involve evidence of both chronicity and deterioration has inevitably aroused some controversy. The work of Manfred Bleuler is often cited as evidence that many patients with schizophrenia may have a relatively good outcome (13). There are few large studies examining long-term outcome for schizophrenia using criteria comparable to DSM-III. The "Iowa 500" is one of the better studies of this type (52). Two hundred consecutive admissions for schizophrenia were retrospectively diagnosed as schizophrenic using criteria that required 6 months of symptoms and an absence of symptoms of affective disorder. At follow-up 30 years later, 20% were completely asymptomatic, 25% had moderate symptoms, and 55% had severe symptoms. At the present time, it therefore seems reasonable to suggest that even when there is some evidence of chronicity, as many as one in five patients with schizophrenia will have a relatively good outcome, and many will avoid the severe deterioration considered by some to be a hallmark of the disease.

ASSESSMENT

Methods for assessing schizophrenia will vary depending on whether the goal is to make a clinical diagnosis or to collect data for research. At a minimum, clinical evaluation must include an overview of current and past symptoms.

Sampling Problems in Research

As the above discussion suggests, one of the basic questions that the researcher must ask himself is: Which schizophrenia am I studying? Depending on his goals, he may wish to have a broad sample or a narrow one. For example, an investigator interested in phenomenologic research may choose to explore a specific subgroup, such as those patients with prominent negative symptoms, with the goal of comparing pharmacologic intervention versus social skills training versus a combined approach. An investigator interested in exploring the neurochemical mechanisms that underlie symptoms and response to treatment might wish to choose a neuroleptic highly selective for D2 receptors and to examine the effects of this medication on a broad range of patients with both positive and negative symptoms in order to explore whether dopamine blockade selectively diminishes positive symptoms. Investigators interested in genetic mechanisms will probably wish to include the entire schizophrenia spectrum in their sample in order to determine whether an illness such as schizotypal personality is in fact a subclinical variant of classic schizophrenia.

Although the sample selected may vary depending on the hypothesis to be explored, it is incumbent on researchers to describe their sample as clearly, accurately, and precisely as possible so that subsequent investigators can replicate their work or make intelligent and accurate comparisons across a variety of studies. Careful description of samples is always important in research, but it is especially important in the case of schizophrenia, given the conceptual blurring that marks current discussions of this disorder. One center will describe its sample as "chronic," meaning that the patients had been ill for more than 6 months, even though the patients function as outpatients most of the time. In another center, the term "chronic" is used to refer to patients who are chronically institutionalized. Diagnostic subtypes, such as paranoid or undifferentiated, are typically used with similar imprecision. Consequently, investigators will do best to resort to more quantitative descriptions of their samples and describe them in terms of duration of illness (dated from the time of first hospitalization), age of onset, total duration of hospitalization during the patient's lifetime, inpatient versus outpatient status, etc. These quantitative measures are likely to give a much more detailed and accurate indication of chronicity, severity, etc.

Instruments Available

Many different kinds of instruments are available for assessing patients suffering from schizophrenia. These include interviews, standardized diagnostic criteria, and rating scales. Although investigators will pick and choose among these various assessment procedures, depending on their goals, a few axiomatic principles should shape this selection. First, in most centers "chart diagnoses" are not usually sufficient to make a diagnosis for the purposes of research, even in the post-DSM-III era. Patients entered into research protocols with a specific diagnosis such as schizophrenia should be evaluated by the investigators with some type of standardized clinical interview and diagnosed according to some prespecified criteria. Second, in most ongoing or long-term projects, assessment instruments should be selected in order to document the broad range of symptoms that characterize schizophrenia; just making a diagnosis will not be sufficient over the long run, since (as the above overview has shown) the boundaries of our diagnostic concepts are likely to continue to shift over time; data should be collected so that, when the "standard" diagnostic criteria change (as they inevitably will), the investigator can redefine his sample accordingly. Third, for a complex illness such as schizophrenia, evaluations should be done by clinicians or by other individuals who have had extensive training and patient contact; the symptoms of schizophrenia can be evaluated reliably, but good reliability cannot be achieved by inexperienced or untrained raters; subtle judgments concerning affective flattening or thought disorder require a broad clinical background before judgments as to presence or absence or degree of severity can be made wisely and accurately.

Structured Interviews and Diagnostic Criteria

Many different structured interviews are now available for studies designed to assess schizophrenia. Each of these has its inherent strengths and weaknesses.

The Present State Examination (PSE) was developed by Wing and others, originally for use in the International Pilot Study of Schizophrenia (55). It is the prototype of structured interviews and has good reliability and other psychometric properties. The time set is the past month, and direct interview with the patient is the primary source of information. Diagnoses are made by a computer program (CATEGO). This interview does not offer direct comparability with DSM-III, and it does not provide any detailed longitudinal information such as duration of illness, lifetime duration of hospitalization, etc. It cannot be used to make lifetime diagnoses or to document lifetime symptoms.

The Schedule for Affective Disorders and Schizophrenia (SADS) has both a current and a lifetime version (23). Interviewers are encouraged to collect information from all sources available (e.g., family members, medical records). Its coverage includes a broad range of symptoms, such as delusions, hallucinations, depressive symptoms, manic symptoms, and anxiety. It has well-documented reliability. It does not cover negative symptoms or cognitive symptoms such as problems with memory or attention.

The Diagnostic Interview Schedule (DIS) was developed as an epidemiologic field instrument in order to make DSM-III diagnoses in large population surveys (25). Its coverage of schizophrenia is relatively rudimentary. It was designed for use by nonclinicians and relies primarily on direct interview data.

The Structured Clinical Review for DSM-III (SCID) was also designed to make DSM-III diagnoses (49). It exists in different forms, which emphasize different clusters of symptoms depending on the sample to be studied. The version of the SCID appropriate for research in schizophrenia is the SCID-P, designed for use with patients suffering from psychosis. The SCID is primarily a diagnostic instrument and does not provide detailed coverage of a broad range of symptoms.

The Comprehensive Assessment of Symptoms and History (CASH) was designed primarily to evaluate patients suffering from major psychoses such as schizophrenia and affective disorders (10). It provides broad coverage of symptoms, including both positive and negative symptoms, information about premorbid adjustment, past history and course, and indices of cognitive impairment. It has both a current and a past section. The interviewer is encouraged to use information from all sources available.

Four different sets of diagnostic criteria are currently in use.

The St. Louis or Washington University Criteria were the first diagnostic criteria to be developed (24). The criteria for schizophrenia are relatively narrow, and they mix indices of social function with longitudinal features and phenomenology (i.e., the criteria include such things as marital status, age of onset, and types of symptoms present). Although they are probably no longer state of the art, they continue to be widely used.

The Research Diagnostic Criteria (RDC) offer a relatively broad definition of schizophrenia in that the duration criterion is only 2 weeks (49). Investigators who wish to use a narrower criterion can change the diagnostic threshold by lengthening the duration, however. Except for the duration criterion, the RDC definition of schizophrenia is quite similar to DSM-III. The RDC were written as diagnostic criteria to accompany the SADS interview.

The DSM-III and DSM-IIIR are probably now the most widely used criteria in the United States, and many non-American investigators have begun to use them as well (22). Their definition of schizophrenia includes both longitudinal and cross-sectional features and is relatively narrow.

Rating Scales

Although the above structured interviews and diagnostic criteria will be used to make diagnoses and to identify a broad range of symptoms in patients, rating scales will usually be used in order to measure change in clinical status over time. Rating scales are particularly appropriate in psychopharmacologic research. Many are available for research with schizophrenic patients.

The Brief Psychiatric Rating Scale (BPRS) is the prototype rating scale for use in psychopharmacologic research (39). In its most widely used form, it includes 12 factors originally developed through factor analysis. These factors include such symptoms as conceptual disorganization, blunted affect, emotional withdrawal, distorted thinking, depressed mood, and psychic anxiety.

The Scale for the Assessment of Thought, Language, and Communication (TLC) was developed in order to find a detailed means for evaluating formal thought disorder in schizophrenia (2,3). It contains scales for rating 18 different types of thought disorder. It is used for studies that focus on this particular variable or as a supplement to interviews that lack adequate coverage of thought disorder, such as the SADS.

The Affect Rating Scale was developed as a companion to the TLC in order to provide a reliable method for evaluating abnormalities in affect (4). It relies heavily on clinical observation, using indices of affective flattening such as poor eye contact, lack of vocal inflections, or failure to smile when prompted.

The Scale for Emotional Blunting (SEB) is another scale developed to rate abnormalities in affect (1). These abnormalities are divided into three broad groups: affect, behavior, and thought content.

The Scale for the Assessment of Negative Symptoms (SANS) was developed in order to provide a comprehensive method for evaluating negative symptoms (5,6,8). It covers five negative symptoms: alogia, affective blunting, avolition-apathy, anhedonia–asociality, and attentional impairment. It includes both scale scores and global ratings.

The Scale for the Assessment of Positive Symptoms (SAPS) is designed as a companion to the SANS (5,6,9). Together, these two scales cover most of the phenomenology of schizophrenia. The SAPS provides detailed ratings for types of hallucinations, types of delusions, bizarre behavior, and positive formal thought disorder.

The SADS-C is a short version of the SADS designed for longitudinal evaluation of patients with repeated interviews. Various forms are available that focus on particular sets of symptoms (e.g., depression, psychosis).

In psychopharmacologic research, clinicians are typically seeking scales that are sensitive to change over time. Ratings are most frequently done at weekly interviews, although they may occur more often in some studies. The BPRS is perhaps the most widely used instrument in psychopharmacologic research because of its sensitivity to change. The SANS and SAPS are newer instruments that also appear to have good sensitivity in measuring change.

ACKNOWLEDGMENTS

This research was supported in part by NIMH Grant MH31593, a Scottish Rite Schizophrenia Research Grant, the Nellie Ball Trust Fund, and Grant RR59 from the General Clinical Research Centers Program, Division of Research Resources, NIH.

REFERENCES

1. Abrams, R., and Taylor, M. A. (1976): *Am. J. Psychiatry,* 135:226–229.
2. Andreasen, N. C. (1979): *Arch. Gen. Psychiatry,* 36:1315–1320.
3. Andreasen, N. C. (1979): *Arch. Gen. Psychiatry,* 36:1325–1330.
4. Andreasen, N. C. (1979): *Am. J. Psychiatry,* 136:944–947.
5. Andreasen, N. C. (1982): *Arch. Gen. Psychiatry,* 39:784–788.
6. Andreasen, N. C. (1982): *Arch. Gen. Psychiatry,* 39:789–794.
7. Andreasen, N. C., Hoffman, R. E., and Grove, W. M. (1985): In: *Controversies in Schizophrenia: Changes and Constancies,* edited by M. V. Seeman and M. Menuck, pp. 97–120. Macmillan, New York.
8. Andreasen, N. C. (1983): *The Scale for the Assessment of Negative Symptoms (SANS).* The University of Iowa, Iowa City.
9. Andreasen, N. C. (1984): *The Scale for the Assessment of Positive Symptoms (SAPS).* The University of Iowa, Iowa City.
10. Andreasen, N. C. (1985): *Comprehensive Assessment of Symptoms and History (CASH).* The University of Iowa, Iowa City.
11. Angrist, B., Rotrosen, J., and Gershon, S. (1980): *Psychopharmacology,* 11:1–3.
12. Bleuler, E. (1950): *Dementia Praecox or the Group of Schizophrenias,* translated by J. Zinkin. International Universities Press, New York.
13. Bleuler, M. (1978): *The Schizophrenic Disorders: Long-term Patient and Family Studies,* translated by S. M. Clements. Yale University Press, New Haven.
14. Brockington, I. F., Wainwright, S., and Kendell, R. E. (1979): *Psychol. Med.,* 9:91–99.
15. Carpenter, W. T., and Strauss, J. S. (1973): *Arch. Gen. Psychiatry,* 27:847–852.
16. Chouinard, G., and Jones, B. D. (1978): *Lancet,* 2:99–100.
17. Clayton, P. (1984): *J. Nerv. Ment. Dis.,* 170:646–650.
18. Cooper, J. E., Kendell, R. E., and Gurland, B. J. (1972): *Psychiatric Diagnosis in New York and London: Maudsley Monograph No. 20.* Oxford University Press, London.
19. Coryell, W. H. (1986): In: *The Medical Basis of Psychiatry,* edited by G. Winokur and P. Clayton, pp. 102–104. W. B. Saunders Co., Philadelphia.
20. Crow, T. J. (1980): *Br. J. Med.,* 280:66–68.
21. Creese, I., Burt, D. R., and Snyder, S. H. (1976): *Science,* 182:481–483.
22. Diagnostics Committee, American Psychiatric Association (1980): *Diagnostic and Statistical Manual (DSM-III).* American Psychiatric Association, Washington.
23. Endicott, J., and Spitzer, R. L. (1978): *Arch. Gen. Psychiatry,* 35:837–844.
24. Feighner, J. P., Robins, E., and Guze, S. B. (1972): *Arch. Gen. Psychiatry,* 26:57–63.
25. Helzer, J. E., Robins, L. M., McEvoy, L. T., Spitznagel, E. L., Stoltzman, R. K., et al. (1985): *Arch. Gen. Psychiatry,* 42:657–666.
26. Humbert, M., Salvador, L., Segui, J., Obiols, J., and Obiols, J. E. (1986): *Rev. Depto. Psiq. Univ. Barcelona,* 13:28–36.
27. Johnstone, E. C., Crow, T. J., and Frith, C. D. (1976): *Lancet,* 2:924–926.
28. Johnstone, E. C., Crow, T. J., Frith, C. D., Carney, M. W., and Price, J. S. (1978): *Lancet,* 1:848–851.
29. Kasanin, J. (1933): *Am. J. Psychiatry,* 90:97–126.
30. Kendler, K. S., and Gruenberg, A. M. (1982): *Am. J. Psychiatry,* 139:1185–1186.
31. Kendler, K. S., Masterson, C., Ungaro, R., and Davis, K. (1984): *Am. J. Psychiatry,* 141:424–427.
32. Kendler, K. S., and Tsuang, M. T. (1981): *Schizophrenia Bull.,* 7:594–619.
33. Kety, S. S., Rosenthal, D., Wender, P. H., and Schulsinger, F. (1971): *Am. J. Psychiatry,* 128:302–306.
34. Kraepelin, E. (1919): *Dementia Praecox and Paraphrenia,* translated by R. M. Barclay. E. & S. Livingstone, Edinburgh.
35. Lecrubier, Y., Puech, A. J., Simon, P., and Widlocher, D. (1980): *Psychol. Med.,* 12:2431–2441.
36. Mackay, A. V. P. (1980): *Br. J. Psychiatry,* 137:279–283.
37. Mellor, C. S. (1970): *Br. J. Psychiatry,* 117:15–23.
38. Ohta, T., Okazaki, Y., and Anzai, N. (1984): *Jpn. J. Psychiatry,* 13:999–1010.
39. Overall, J. E., and Gorham, D. R. (1962): *Psychol. Rep.,* 10:799–812.
40. Owens, D. G. C., Johnstone, E. C., Crow, T. J., Frith, C. D., Jagoe, J. R., et al. (1985): *Psychol. Med.,* 15:43–54.
41. Pfohl, B., and Winokur, G. (1982): *Br. J. Psychiatry,* 141:567–572.
42. Pfohl, B., and Winokur, J. (1983): *J. Nerv. Ment. Dis.,* 171:296–300.
43. Pope, H. G., and Lipinski, J. S. (1978): *Arch. Gen. Psychiatry,* 35:811–828.

44. Potkin, S. G., Cannon, H. E., and Murphy, D. L. (1978): *N. Engl. J. Med.*, 298:61–66.

45. Rieder, R. O., Donnelly, E. F., and Herdt, J. R. (1979): *Psychiatr. Res.*, 1:108.

46. Rosenthal, M. E., Rosenthal, L. N., and Stallone, F. (1980): *Arch. Gen. Psychiatry*, 37:804–810.

47. Seeman, P., Lee, T., Chang-Wong, M., and Wong, K. (1976): *Nature*, 261:717–719.

48. Spitzer, R. L., Endicott, J., and Robins, E. (1985): *Research Diagnostic Criteria (RDC) for a Selected Group of Functional Disorders* (second edition). Biometric Research, New York State Psychiatric Institute, New York.

49. Spitzer, R. L., and Williams, J. B. W. (1985): *Structured Clinical Interview for DSM-III-Patient Version (SCID-P)*. Biometric Research, New York State Psychiatric Institute.

50. Tsuang, M. T., and Winokur, G. (1974): *Arch. Gen. Psychiatry*, 31:43–47.

51. Tsuang, M. T. (1979): *Arch. Gen. Psychiatry*, 36:633–634.

52. Tsuang, M. T., Woolson, R. F., and Fleming, J. A. (1979): *Arch. Gen. Psychiatry*, 36:1295–1301.

53. Weinberger, D. R., Bigelow, L. B., Kleinman, J. E., Klein, S. T., Rosenblatt, J. E., et al. (1980): *Arch. Gen. Psychiatry*, 37:11–13.

54. Welner, A., Croughan, J. L., and Robins, E. (1974): *Arch. Gen. Psychiatry*, 31:628–637.

55. Wing, J. K., Cooper, J. E., and Sartorius, N. (1974): *The Measurement and Classification of Psychiatric Symptoms*. Cambridge University Press, Cambridge.

56. Wyatt, R. J., Potkin, S. G., and Kleinman, J. E. (1981): *J. Nerv. Ment. Dis.*, 169:100–112.

Psychopharmacology:
The Third Generation of Progress,
edited by Herbert Y. Meltzer.
Raven Press, New York © 1987.

CHAPTER 112

Drug Treatment of Acute Schizophrenia

Arthur Rifkin and Samuel Siris

Our ability to treat schizophrenia is one of the major achievements of psychopharmacology. Prior to the introduction of chlorpromazine, the first neuroleptic, the usual course of an acute episode of schizophrenia was to last several months, with many patients not reaching remission for years if at all. Today, with the routine use of neuroleptics, the great majority of such episodes remit or markedly improve within 6 weeks. The picture is hardly rosy, however. Despite this great achievement in reducing symptoms during an acute episode, many patients have residual symptoms, and relapse remains a risk.

STANDARD TREATMENT WITH NEUROLEPTICS

The overall efficacy of neuroleptics compared to placebo is one of the most thoroughly researched questions in psychopharmacology (36). Neuroleptic treatment is indicated in every patient with acute schizophrenia unless there are compelling contraindications (e.g., a clearly established history of lack of response during past episodes or one of severe adverse reactions).

Choice of Neuroleptic

Despite a wide variety of different chemicals, there are no convincing data that any neuroleptic is more effective than any other, either in global terms of reducing psychotic symptoms or in being more effective for a particular symptom (with the exception of promazine, which early on was shown to be less effective than chlorpromazine) (13,37). The research showing the equivalence of neurolep-tics is based on group data; i.e., there are no persistent trends demonstrating that a group of patients given one drug does better than a comparison group given another. Such data cannot rule out the possibility that there are individuals within these groups who respond better to one drug than another. This has led clinicians to consider using a different neuroleptic if the first is ineffective and to the commendable practice of using the neuroleptic that had been effective during a previous episode for treatment of a relapse.

The equivalence in clinical efficacy applies only partially to adverse reactions. Although the range of adverse reactions is the same, there are distinct quantitative differences. These differences roughly correlate with a division of neuroleptics into two categories: less potent ones, such as chlorpromazine, chlorprothixene, thioridazine, and mesoridazine, and all the others, which can be called high-potency drugs. The less potent drugs are more sedating, have more anticholinergic adverse reactions, and produce more postural hypotension but less intense extrapyramidal side effects. Thus, the choice of neuroleptic depends on which adverse reactions are more bothersome or dangerous. In general, we recommend that the high-potency drugs be used. Except for the extrapyramidal side effects, which usually can be handled adequately by antiparkinson agents, they are better tolerated.

The greater sedation of the lower-potency drugs is sometimes considered an advantage in the patient who is agitated and has difficulty sleeping. This has not been apparent from the many studies showing low- and high-potency neuroleptics to be equally efficacious in treating agitation or hyperarousal. These symptoms are seen usually early during the acute episode. If a low-potency drug is used because of its alleged superiority in treating agitation, it would then be necessary to switch to a high-potency one if the sedation became bothersome, which it usually does. In the absence of evidence that one drug is better than another in treating agitation, we prefer to use a high-potency agent. Rapid relief of symptoms of behavioral dyscontrol probably depends on sedation more than any specific antipsychotic action of a neuroleptic, although this is far from certain. Using a low potency neuroleptic to achieve control often leads to difficulty with postural hypotension. Our recommendation is to use as treatment of agitation and violent behavior sedatives such as barbiturates or benzodiazepines, parenterally or orally depending on the speed of action desired and the cooperativeness of the patient. If this does not help sufficiently, neuroleptics should be used. Delaying the use of neuroleptics for several days has the advantage of permitting a more extensive diagnostic evaluation, which is especially useful in newly admitted inpatients who are not well known to the treating psychiatrist.

Dose

Despite the overwhelming evidence that neuroleptics are superior to placebo in the treatment of acute schizophrenia when given in a dose of at least 400 mg/day of chlorpromazine or its equivalent, there are relatively few studies comparing different doses. This literature has been reviewed recently (62). We suggest that there is no value in using doses higher than standard (400 to 1,200 mg/day in chlorpromazine units); i.e., "rapid neuroleptization" has not proven helpful.

It is interesting and puzzling to find in reviewing the studies that not only are higher doses not more effective, but also they do not appear to cause more adverse reactions. This appears inconsistent with clinical experience, but it points out a difficulty faced by the clinician in choosing dosage: neuroleptics are very safe, and the usual guideline available with most drugs, the appearance of side effects, is often not useful with neuroleptics. The dosages that can be given without significant adverse reactions seem astounding, but this is a fact that the clinician must be aware of. Despite lack of data justifying the use of higher doses, there has been a trend in recent years to escalate dosage.

Since the dose with which a patient is discharged usually determines the dose that will be used for long-term outpatient treatment, and the long-term adverse reaction of tardive dyskinesia may be related to dose (31), the lower end of usual dosage should be used in most patients, e.g., 10 to 20 mg/day of haloperidol.

Compliance is always a worry even if the patient is hospitalized. If there is any doubt, the oral dose should be given in liquid form. In the case of fluctuating compliance or cooperativeness, a long-acting depot preparation can be used.

Duration of Treatment Before Changing Treatment

How long should the usual dosage of a neuroleptic be continued in the face of inadequate response? Unfortunately, there are very few data concerning this important question. A study by Quitkin et al. (56) comparing megadosage of

fluphenazine, 1,200 mg/day, to standard dose, 30 mg/day, sheds some light. Subjects were chosen who had not responded to 6 weeks of standard treatment, which meant 30 mg/day of fluphenazine. They then received experimental treatment for an additional 6 weeks. Surprisingly, about 60% of those continued on the lower dose of 30 mg/day responded, a better rate than achieved by the megadose. Among other conclusions, this suggests that 6 weeks is an inadequate period to judge nonresponse. Yet it is difficult to continue a treatment that has not been effective within 4 to 6 weeks. We recommend that at least 4 weeks be allowed at a steady standard dose before a change be considered.

Since there is no evidence that within the usual standard dose range of 400 to 1,200 mg/day of chlorpromazine, or its equivalent, one dose is better than another, there is no reason to continue a dose that causes bothersome adverse reactions if the dose is above the minimum. If it is at the minimum, another drug may be tried. If a patient has responded well previously, it is best to use the same drug and dose. (The role of blood levels is discussed elsewhere in this volume.)

Managing Adverse Reactions

Sedation

There is no antidote for sedation. The best response is to reduce the dose and/or switch to a high-potency neuroleptic. Sedation is not a dramatic side effect, and the patient may stop complaining about it although it is bothersome and limits functioning.

Extrapyramidal Side Effects

These are the most common troublesome adverse reactions. They range from dramatic dystonias to symptoms difficult to distinguish from psychopathology. These are dealt with in detail elsewhere in this volume. Here we discuss only briefly some of the practical problems in the diagnosis and treatment of extrapyramidal side effects (EPS). The most difficult problems in the diagnoses of EPS concern the differentiation of akathisia from agitation and anxiety, and akinesia from depression or residual symptoms of schizophrenia. It is best to accept the uncomfortable fact that we lack good clinical tools to distinguish the adverse reaction from the symptom of psychopathology and realize that we must test the diagnosis if the distinction is important. If the patient is not receiving an antiparkinson agent, it can be given. If the symptom in question remits, the diagnosis is made. But antiparkinson drugs are not completely effective. In the absence of a response, the only sure way to make the correct diagnosis is to discontinue the neuroleptic for several weeks. During an acute episode, this strategy is not practical but is more relevant for long-term maintenance treatment, when an interruption of several weeks is less dangerous. If during acute treatment the differentiation is difficult, it is best to lower the dose, use antiparkinson agents, and, if those are ineffective, to try a different neuroleptic. In such an instance, this may be one of the uncommon indications for a low-potency neuroleptic, since it is less likely to cause EPS.

Should antiparkinson drugs be used prophylactically? This is a controversial question. The evidence has been reviewed (58). The advantages are to spare the patient frightening and painful symptoms, to forestall antipathy toward drug treatment, and to avoid akinesia and akathisia that can mimic symptoms of psychopathology and lead to mistaken diagnoses and treatments. The disadvantages are to add to the anticholinergic burden and to use a drug that might not be necessary. Opinion is divided in the field, but in our view, there is more to gain than to lose by using antiparkinson drugs prophylactically. If anticholinergic side effects are troublesome, the anticholinergic antiparkinson drug may be replaced with amantadine, which is not anticholinergic. There is no evidence that any one antiparkinson drug is superior to the others.

Agranulocytosis and Leukopenia

These two conditions should be differentiated. Agranulocytosis is usually an abrupt and complete loss of granulocytes. Leukopenia is a different condition; the leukocyte count falls slowly and usually stabilizes above 3,000, and this is not generally associated with symptoms.

Anticholinergic Adverse Reactions

These side effects consist of blurred vision, dry mouth, constipation, and delayed micturition. These symptoms are usually annoying but not serious. However, at times they can cause serious problems such as fecal impaction and urinary retention. Even when not serious, they are very bothersome and deserve attention and treatment. A seemingly unimportant symptom like dry mouth can be a cause of noncompliance with its major consequences.

The treatment for most anticholinergic adverse reactions is to provide cholinergic stimulation with neostigmine, 15 to 30 mg p.o. t.i.d., or bethanecol, 25 mg p.o. b.i.d. to q.i.d. Cholinergic drugs are less helpful for blurred vision. Even when these are given as ophthalmic drops, the effective concentration is reached only briefly, and there is the danger of causing considerable miosis, which could reduce vision. For blurred vision, the best treatment is reading glasses. Before further drugs are used to treat anticholinergic side effects, the dose of the neuroleptic should be kept at its minimum, and switching to another neuroleptic should be considered, especially if the original one is a low-potency drug that is more likely to cause anticholinergic adverse reactions.

Constipation should be treated initially with mild laxatives with progression to stronger ones if necessary. It is far easier to deal with constipation before it becomes an impaction.

Other Adverse Reactions

Postural hypotension occurs more frequently with the low-potency neuroleptics and is more serious with advancing age. In the elderly this is probably the most serious common adverse reaction because it can cause falls and fractures. Especially in the elderly, sitting and standing blood pressure readings should be done regularly. A drop of 20 mm Hg of systolic pressure and 10 mm Hg of diastolic is probably more than should be tolerated. The best guide is the patient's symptoms, such as dizziness and unsteadiness, although serious falls, particularly in the elderly, may occur even in the absence of these symptoms. The presence of postural hypotension prior to drug treatment may be a predictor of subsequent orthostatic problems after the drug is started.

The relationship of dose to postural hypotension has not been established, but, if clinically possible, the dose should be lowered if postural hypotension occurs; or the clinician may switch from a low- to a high-potency neuroleptic. The risk of postural hypotension would be an indication to begin treatment with a high- rather than a low-potency neuroleptic. The patient should be educated to the need not to stand abruptly from a recumbent position and, when standing, to have a source of support for the first few minutes, should dizziness occur. Such advice may be difficult for a patient with acute schizophrenia to follow, and close nursing attention is required. Surgical hose may be a means to reduce postural hypotension.

DRUG TREATMENT OF POSTPSYCHOTIC DEPRESSION

The diagnosis of depression associated with schizophrenia is difficult because there are at present no reliable clinical means of differentiating several conditions that can present with similar symptoms (63). These include depressive symptoms as an integral part of the disorder, as in schizoaffective disorder, or "depression" as a late development in schizophrenia itself, which does not require any additional diagnosis, "depression" as an understandable situational response to the disorder and the demoralizing effect it has on the patient's life, or "depression" as an adverse reaction to the neuroleptic, such as akinesia. The most pressing clinical question is how to treat depressive symptoms that emerge or, perhaps, were unnoticed because of other more dramatic symptoms.

Most studies of an antidepressant in combination with a neuroleptic have not demonstrated any advantage for the combination, but the patients were not selected because they had concomitant depression (65). Two studies of patients selected for depressive symptoms among those with schizophrenia found the combination superior (55,60). Siris et al. (64) found imipramine superior to placebo as adjunctive medication to fluphenazine decanoate. Johnson reached contrary results (28). He compared nortriptyline to placebo as adjunctive drugs to a depot neuroleptic. He found no signifiant difference between the two groups in the outcome of depressive symptoms but did find more side effects in those given nortriptyline. However, the dose of nortriptyline used was higher than is usually used to treat depression, and no blood levels were done to determine if the "therapeutic window" had been exceeded. In another negative study, Waehrens and Gerlach (70) found no benefit in a double-blind trial of maprotiline plus a neuroleptic compared to the neuroleptic alone in patients described as having schizophrenia and "emotional withdrawal." Interpretation of these data is difficult because the diagnostic criteria were not given and the dose of maprotiline may not have been adequate.

The double-blind, controlled studies of monoamine oxidase inhibitors in the treatment of schizophrenia have been reviewed by Siris et al. (65) and Brenner and Shopsin (3). The results are not impressive, but, again, the samples did not include patients selected for depressive symptoms.

Patients with schizophrenia with a premorbid history of childhood asociality, i.e., patients who have never had a period of good social adjustment and who as children were often picked on, may develop more psychotic symptoms when an antidepressant is added to their neuroleptic (15). Patients with schizophrenia with marked agitation may also be poor risks for adjunctive antidepressants according to several anecdotal reports (65).

We conclude from the available data that a tricyclic antidepressant should be added to the continuing neuroleptic regimen of a patient with schizophrenia who develops a depression-like syndrome following the remission of the psychosis. Before doing this, the possibility of akinesia masquerading as depression should be considered by treating with full dosage of an antiparkinson drug. This is not a completely effective method of detecting akinesia, but it is helpful. Patients given the combination of an antidepressant and a neuroleptic should be monitored closely for adverse reactions, since they interfere with each other's metabolism, and the blood levels of both can rise.

NONSTANDARD TREATMENT OF ACUTE SCHIZOPHRENIA

When the preceding treatments have not been effective, the clinician is faced with a difficult decision. Some other treatment should be tried, but there are insufficient data from systematic studies to determine which treatments should be tried and in which order. In this section we review the evidence for several drugs that are being used for this indication.

Lithium

Biederman et al. (2) found the combination of lithium and haloperidol superior to haloperidol alone in newly admitted patients—not a sample selected for unresponsiveness to neuroleptic treatment. Small et al. (66) showed that adding lithium to a neuroleptic in chronic patients hospitalized for a long time diminished symptoms. Yet Shopsin et al. (59) found lithium not helpful in a study comparing chlorpromazine to lithium (each drug used separately) in newly admitted patients not demonstrated refractory to standard treatment. Overall, we find sufficient evidence for a trial of lithium if standard treatment has been ineffective—even in the absence of affective symptoms—with a low level of certainty that it will work.

Propranolol

Four controlled studies have compared propranolol with a neuroleptic to a neuroleptic alone. Three of the studies showed statistically significant improvement for adjunctive propranolol using doses from 400 to 2,000 mg/day (39,46,53,71).

Since Peet et al. (49) found that propranolol raised the blood levels of chlorpromazine, its sulfoxide, prolactin, and the total neuroleptic level (as measured by the radioreceptor assay), the results indicating that chlorpromazine plus propranolol was superior to the neuroleptic alone could be interpreted as resulting from an elevation of the blood levels of the neuroleptic. This is doubtful since the dose or blood level of a neuroleptic has not been found to be a predictor of response.

Three studies have examined the effect of propranolol given alone to patients with schizophrenia. King et al. (35), using patients with chronic schizophrenia, found no difference between propranolol and placebo. Yorkston et al. (72) found no difference between propranolol, 670 mg/day, and chlorpromazine, 300 mg/day, in 46 newly admitted patients. However, it is puzzling that only 39% of those treated with chlorpromazine improved during the 3-month trial. Perhaps the dose of chlorpromazine was too low, or this group of patients was atypical.

Peet et al. (48) compared chlorpromazine, 400 mg/day, and propranolol, 640 mg/day, to placebo for 3 months following removal from neuroleptic treatment in subjects with chronic schizophrenia. They found no difference in improvement between the groups. This study is also difficult to interpret. During the 1-month washout from the neuroleptic, no patient worsened, an unexpected finding. And it is puzzling that chlorpromazine was not more effective than placebo. Perhaps these patients were extremely refractory to treatment, which would make them a poor sample choice with whom to test the efficacy of propranolol.

What conclusions can we draw from this review of the studies of propranolol in schizophrenia? The studies using it as an adjunctive drug to a neuroleptic are encouraging; those using it alone are not. Yet two of the three latter studies are difficult to interpret. The studies differ in their samples: some are chosen for being refractory to treatment, some are newly admitted patients, and some are chronic patients whose degree of remission is partial. There is also a large range in the dose used. Although the data are insufficient for any definitive conclusion, we judge that there is enough evidence to make a trial of high-dose propranolol indicated for patients who are unresponsive to an adequate course of neuroleptic drugs. It is difficult to know what dose to use. This leaves the clinician with a wide choice of dose. The literature, as reviewed here and in a large number of anecdotal reports, shows that doses have ranged from 400 mg/day to almost 2,000 mg/day. Our procedure is to aim at a final dose of about 1,000 mg/day, if tolerated, and wait at least 2 months to assess benefits.

Benzodiazepines

Studies of benzodiazepines in schizophrenia have been either negative (22–25,32,42) or slightly encouraging (27,33,40,41).

Anecdotal reports are encouraging about the use of high-dosage (200–400 mg/day) diazepam (1,47). There is insufficient evidence to support the routine use of high-dose benzodiazepines in patients with schizophrenia who do not respond to other treatments. Yet it should be considered when all else has been ineffective.

Clonazepam, a benzodiazepine marketed as an anticonvulsant, was tested in nine patients with chronic schizophrenia as an adjunct to a neuroleptic. Under double-blind conditions they were given placebo clonazepam for 2 weeks before and after treatment with clonazepam for 32 days, the last 14 of which were for tapering. Clonazepam appeared to have no effect on symptoms (32). There are anecdotal reports of clonazepam's effectiveness in mania and schizoaffective disorder (21,69).

High-Dose Neuroleptic Treatment

Prien and Cole (53) compared 2,000 to 300 mg/day of chlorpromazine. They found that younger patients hospitalized for a shorter period did better on the higher dose. A similar study using trifluoperazine, 80 versus 15 mg/day, reached the same conclusion (54).

Clark et al. (11) compared 600 mg/day of chlorpromazine to 150 to 300 mg/day and found the higher dose better. Gardos et al. (18) found 40 mg/day of thiothixene better than 10 mg/day. Brotman et al. (7) showed 60 mg/day of butaperazine superior to 15 to 30 mg/day. On the contrary, Carseallen et al. (9) found that 100 mg/day of trifluoperazine was no different from 10 mg/day; however, both groups showed a poor response, indicating a sample unresponsive to neuroleptic medication. By present-day standards the lower dose used in many of these studies would be considered too low, and these studies may not reflect the best comparison of "high dose to standard dose."

A comparison of haloperidol, 100 mg/day, to chlorpromazine, 600 mg/day, in 18 patients was done by McGreadie et al. (44). On a rating scale of symptoms, the patients treated with haloperidol did better, although this was not seen in measures of global improvement.

Anecdotal reports supported the use of very high doses of fluphenazine (16,17,19,38). Three double-blind studies compared megadosages of fluphenazine, 800 to 1,200 mg/day, to standard doses, 30 to 60 mg/day (14,26,50). Each study reported superiority for the megadose, although there were no reports that the improvement was sufficient to allow the patient to be discharged. These patients had all been treated extensively before the trial with standard doses of neuroleptics.

Quitkin et al. (56) did a study (described previously) of megadosage in patients with schizophrenia who were newly admitted and had not responded to 6 weeks of standard treatment. No one had been hospitalized for longer than 2 months. They compared two doses of fluphenazine: 1,200 to 39 mg/day. Overall, the patients receiving the lower dose did better. They had an improvement rate of 60%. This study indicates not only that it is questionable that megadosage is superior in such patients but also that 6 weeks of standard dosage is an insufficient time to judge a patient as refractory.

There is enough evidence to support the use of megadosage in treatment-refractory patients to make it worth a trial without high hopes.

Electroconvulsive Therapy

Brill et al. (4) compared ECT to simulated ECT in 67 patients with schizophrenia. They found no difference between groups. May (43) compared ECT to treatment with a neuroleptic, psychotherapy, or ward milieu therapy alone. Treatment with the neuroleptic with or without psychotherapy was better than milieu treatment or psychotherapy alone to a statistically significant extent; ECT was intermediate.

Childers (10) studied four treatments: ECT, fluphenazine (20 mg/day), chlorpromazine (1,000 mg/day), and chlorpromazine with ECT. Siris et al. (61) analyzed these data further and found the combination of ECT with chlorpromazine superior to either drug ($p < 0.05$) but not superior to ECT alone.

Taylor and Fleminger (68), using 20 patients who had received neuroleptics for at least 2 weeks, compared ECT to simulated ECT. Those getting real ECT did better ($p = 0.004$). The other published studies are difficult to interpret because they involved very chronic patients whose likelihood of improvement was low.

The most clinically relevant question is the value of ECT in patients who have not responded to an adequate trial of neuroleptic treatment, since it is not likely that ECT will be considered as the first treatment. There are no controlled studies of this question. An anecdotal report by Ries et al. (57) is encouraging. They describe nine patients with schizoaffective disorder who did well on ECT after not responding to drug treatment. Whether the response in schizophrenia would be similar is not known, and one anecdotal report is not much to go on. Yet, in the patient who has not responded to other treatments, there seems to be enough evidence for ECT to justify a trial in this very serious disorder. Clinicians who gave many patients with schizophrenia ECT during the years before the introduction of reserpine and chlorpromazine favored giving a large number (20) to prevent relapse even if improvement occurred earlier.

Methadone

There is the intriguing possibility that methadone may be an antipsychotic drug (20,34,45,51).

In a double-blind controlled study, Brizer et al. (5) compared methadone to placebo as adjunctive drugs to a neuroleptic in seven patients who had chronic paranoid schizophrenia and had not responded to long trials of adequate doses of various neuroleptics. Despite methodological limitations and sparse analyses, this study does suggest that methadone may be effective in patients with schizophrenia refractory to neuroleptics. The six patients who were withdrawn from methadone did not have any difficulty stopping the drug and on follow-up have not shown drug-seeking behavior. Giving an addicting drug to patients with schizophrenia is not an easy decision. Before using methadone as routine treatment for neuroleptic-resistant patients, there should be much more research on its efficacy and safety. Yet in patients suffering severely from schizophrenia who have not responded to other treatments, methadone might be considered.

TREATMENT OF SCHIZOAFFECTIVE DISORDER

There is a paucity of good studies of this disorder, perhaps at least in part because of the controversy about the criteria to be used in its diagnosis.

Prien et al. (52), in a large 18-hospital collaborative study of 83 patients, compared lithium and chlorpromazine in a 3-week trial. The dose of chlorpromazine varied widely from 200 to 3,000 mg/day. There was little difference between the treatments. The sample was divided into "highly active" and "mildly active," although all patients required hospitalization. In the "highly active" group there were no differences between the treatments.

Brockington et al. (6) studied a small number of patients with schizoaffective disorder–excited (11 completers), comparing lithium to chlorpromazine, and found no difference. In another comparison of lithium and chlorpromazine, Johnson et al. (29,30) found that lithium was less effective.

The conclusion from these few studies seems to be that chlorpromazine is at least equal and probably superior to lithium in excited patients with schizoaffective disorder. There have been even fewer studies of the combination of a neuroleptic plus lithium. Biederman et al. (2), in a study described previously, found that haloperidol plus lithium was superior to haloperidol alone in newly admitted patients, whom they sorted into several groups between "pure" mania and "pure" schizophrenia. In each group, excluding the "pure" extremes, which were not studied, the combination was superior.

In a small study, Carman et al. (8) studied five patients who had been stabilized for 8 weeks on a neuroleptic and then, under double-blind conditions, had lithium or its placebo added. During the lithium period, excitement was reduced further.

Those studies that suggest that the combination of lithium and neuroleptic is superior to the neuroleptic alone have not described any cases of neurotoxicity, an adverse reaction that has been of concern with the combination (12,67). Yet it is our judgment that the treatment of choice for excited schizoaffective disorder is the same as outlined for acute schizophrenia. Since the results of treatment are usually excellent for the acute episode, there seems little reason to run the possible additional risk of neurotoxicity from the combination with lithium.

GENERAL CONCLUSION

Overall, drug treatment of acute schizophrenia is the pride and despair of psychiatry. Usually patients respond to treatment using standard doses of a neuroleptic. This is a tremendous advance and the greatest achievement of modern psychiatry. Unfortunately, if the patient does not respond to this first treatment, there is shockingly little research on what should be done. There remain many patients whose recovery from an acute attack takes a long time or never occurs at all. These patients are a serious challenge and deserve much further research focusing on alternative treatment strategies.

ACKNOWLEDGMENT

Research for this chapter was partially supported by grant MH 34309 from the National Institute of Mental Health.

REFERENCES

1. Beckmann, H., and Haas, S. (1980): *Psychopharmacology*, 71:79–82.
2. Biederman, J., Lerner, Y., and Belmaker, R. H. (1979): *Arch. Gen. Psychiatry*, 36:327–333.
3. Brenner, R., and Shopsin, B. (1980): *Biol. Psychiatry*, 15:633–647.
4. Brill, N. Q., Crumpton, E., and Eiduson, S. (1959): *A.M.A. Arch. Neurol. Psychiatry*, 81:627–635.
5. Brizer, P. A., Hartman, N., and Sweeney, J. (1985): *Am. J. Psychiatry*, 142:1106–1107.
6. Brockington, I. F., Kendell, R. E., and Kellett, J. M. (1978): *Br. J. Psychiatry*, 133:162–168.
7. Brotman, R. K., Muzekari, L. N., and Shanken, P. M. (1969): *Curr. Ther. Res.*, 11:5–8.
8. Carman, J. S., Bigelow, L. B., and Wyatt, R. J. (1981): *J. Clin. Psychiatry*, 42:124–128.
9. Carseallen, H. B., Rochman, H., and Lovegrove, T. D. (1968): *Can. Psychiatr. Assoc. J.*, 13:459–461.
10. Childers, R. T. (1964): *Am. J. Psychiatry*, 120:1010–1011.
11. Clark, M. L., Ramsey, H. R., Ragland, R. E., Rahhal, D. K., Serufetinides, E. A., et al. (1970): *Psychopharmacologia*, 18:260–270.
12. Cohen, W. J., and Cohen, N. H. (1974): *J.A.M.A.*, 230:1283–1287.
13. Davis, J. M. (1976): *Psychiatr. Ann.*, 6:71–106.
14. DeBuck, R. P. (1972): In: *Proceedings of the Eighth Congress of the Collegium Internationale Neuro-Psychopharmacologium*. Excerpta Medica, Copenhagen.
15. Fink, M., Pollack, M., and Klein, D. F. (1964): *Neuropsychopharmacology*, 3:370–372.
16. Fouks, L. (1967): In: *Neuropsychopharmacology*, edited by H. Brill, J. O. Cole, P. Deniker, H. Hippius, and P. S. Bradley, pp. 1152–1155. Excerpta Medica, Amsterdam.
17. Fouks, L., Perivier, R., Lerno, J., and Gilbert, M. M. E. (1966): *Ann. Med. Psychol. (Paris)*, 124:698.
18. Gardos, G., Orzack, M. H., Finn, G., and Cole, J. O. (1975): *Dis. Nerv. Syst.*, 35:55–58.
19. Gayral, L., and Lambert, P. (1967): In: *Neuropsychopharmacology*, edited by H. Brill, J. O. Cole, P. Deniker, H. Hippius, and P. S. Bradley, pp. 1128–1134. Excerpta Medica, Amsterdam.
20. Gold, M. S., Donabediam, R. K., and Dillard, M. (1977): *Lancet*, 2:398–399.
21. Greenspan, D., and Levine, D. (1985): *Am. J. Psychiatry*, 142:774–775.
22. Gundlach, R., Engelhardt, D. M., and Hankoff, L. (1966): *Psychopharmacologia*, 9:81–82.
23. Holden, J. M. C., and Holden, U. P. (1970): *Psychosomatics*, 11:551–561.
24. Holden, J. M. C., Itil, T. M., and Keskiner, A. (1968): *Compr. Psychiatry*, 9:633–643.
25. Hollister, L. E., Bennett, J. J., and Kimbell, I., Jr. (1963): *Dis. Nerv. Syst.*, 24:746–750.
26. Itil, T., and Keskiner, A. (1970): *Dis. Nerv. Syst.*, 31:37–42.
27. Jimmerson, D. C., vanKammen, D. P., and Post, R. M. (1982): *Am. J. Psychiatry*, 139:489–491.
28. Johnson, D. A. W. (1981): *Br. J. Psychiatry*, 139:89–101.
29. Johnson, G., Gershon, S., and Burdock, E. I. (1971): *Br. J. Psychiatry*, 119:267–276.
30. Johnson, G., Gershon, S., and Hekimian, L. J. (1968): *Compr. Psychiatry*, 9:563–573.
31. Kane, J. M., Rifkin, A., Woerner, M., Reardon, G., Sarantakos, S., et al. (1983): *Arch. Gen. Psychiatry*, 40:893–896.
32. Karson, C. N., Weinberger, D. R., and Bigelow, L. (1982): *Am. J. Psychiatry*, 139:1627–1628.

33. Kellner, R., Wilson, R. M., and Muldauer, M. D. (1975): *Arch. Gen. Psychiatry,* 32:1246–1254.

34. Khantzian, E. J., Mack, J. E., and Schatzberg, A. F. (1974): *Am. J. Psychiatry,* 131:160–164.

35. King, D. J., Turkson, S. N. A., and Leddle, J. (1980): *Br. J. Psychiatry,* 137:458–468.

36. Klein, D. F., and Davis, J. M. (1969): *Diagnosis of Drug Treatment of Psychiatric Disorders.* Williams & Wilkins, Baltimore.

37. Klerman, G. L. (1973): *Drug Ther.,* 3:94–106.

38. Lambert, P. A., Charriot, G., Delaunay, J., and Marcon, G. (1965): *Ann. Med. Psychol. (Paris),* 123:823.

39. Lindstrom, L., and Persson, E. (1980): *Br. J. Psychiatry,* 137:126–130.

40. Lingjaerde, O. (1982): *Acta Psychiatr. Scand.,* 65:339–354.

41. Lingjaerde, O., Engstrand, E., and Ellingsen, P. (1979): *Curr. Ther. Res.,* 26:505–514.

42. Maculans, G. A. (1964): *Dis. Nerv. Syst.,* 25:164–168.

43. May, P. R. (1968): *Treatment of Schizophrenia.* Science House, New York.

44. McGreadie, R. B., and MacDonald, I. M. (1977): *Br. J. Psychiatry,* 131:310–316.

45. McKenna, G. J. (1982): *Ann. N.Y. Acad. Sci.,* 398:44–55.

46. Myers, D. H., Campbell, L., and Cocks, N. M. (1981): *Br. J. Psychiatry,* 139:118–121.

47. Nestoros, J. N., Nair, N. P. V., and Pulman, J. R. (1983): *Psychopharmacology,* 81:42–47.

48. Peet, M., Bethell, M. S., and Coates, A. (1982): *Br. J. Psychiatry,* 139:105–111.

49. Peet, M., Middlemiss, D. N., and Yates, R. A. (1981): *Br. J. Psychiatry,* 138:112–117.

50. Polvan, N., Vagcioglu, V., Itil, T., and Fink, M. (1968): In: *Proceedings of the Sixth Congress of the Collegium Internationale Neuropsychopharmacologium.* Excerpta Medica, Amsterdam.

51. Powell, D. (1973): *Arch. Gen. Psychiatry,* 28:586–594.

52. Prien, R. F., Caffey, E. M., and Klett, C. J. (1972): *Arch. Gen. Psychiatry,* 27:182–189.

53. Prien, R. F., and Cole, J. O. (1968): *Arch. Gen. Psychiatry,* 18:482–495.

54. Prien, R. F., Levine, J., and Cole, J. O. (1969): *Am. J. Psychiatry,* 126:305–313.

55. Prusoff, B. A., Williams, D. H., and Weissman, M. M. (1979): *Arch. Gen. Psychiatry,* 36:569–575.

56. Quitkin, F., Rifkin, A., and Klein, D. F. (1975): *Arch. Gen. Psychiatry,* 32:1276–1281.

57. Ries, R. K., Wilson, L., and Bokan, J. A. (1981): *Compr. Psychiatry,* 22:167–173.

58. Rifkin, A., Quitkin, F., Kane, J., Struve, F., and Klein, D. F. (1978): *Arch. Gen. Psychiatry,* 35:483–489.

59. Shopsin, B., Kim, S. S., and Gershon, S. (1971): *Br. J. Psychiatry,* 119:435–440.

60. Singh, A. N., Saxena, B., and Nelson, H. L. (1978): *Curr. Ther. Res.,* 23:485–501.

61. Siris, S. G., Glassman, A. H., and Stetner, F. (1982): In: *Electroconvulsive Therapies: Biological Foundations and Clinical Applications,* edited by W. B. Essman and R. Abrams, pp. 91–111. Spectrum Publications, New York.

62. Siris, S. G., and Rifkin, A. (1983): In: *Schizophrenia and Affective Disorders: Biology and Treatment,* edited by A. Rifkin, p. 245. John Wright–PSG, Boston.

63. Siris, S. G., and Rifkin, A. (1983): In: *Schizophrenia and Affective Disorders: Biology and Treatment,* edited by A. Rifkin, p. 281. John Wright–PSG, Boston.

64. Siris, S. G., Rifkin, A., and Reardon, G. T. (1985): *Psychopharmacol. Bull.,* 21:114–116.

65. Siris, S. G., vanKammen, D. P., and Docherty, J. P. (1978): *Arch. Gen. Psychiatry,* 35:1368–1377.

66. Small, J. G., Kellams, J. J., and Milstein, V. (1975): *Am. J. Psychiatry,* 132:1315–1317.

67. Spring, G. K. (1979): *J. Clin. Psychiatry,* 40:135–138.

68. Taylor, P., and Fleminger, J. J. (1980): *Lancet,* 1:1380–1383.

69. Victor, B. S., Link, N. A., Binder, R. L., and Bell, I. R. (1984): *Am. J. Psychiatry,* 141:1111–1112.

70. Waehrens, J., and Gerlach, J. (1980): *Acta Psychiatr. Scand.,* 61:438–444.

71. Yorkston, N. J., Zaki, S. A., and Pitcher, D. R. (1977): *Lancet,* 2:575–578.

72. Yorkston, N. J., Zaki, S. A., and Weller, M. P. (1981): *Acta Psychiatr. Scand.,* 63:13–27.

Psychopharmacology:
The Third Generation of Progress,
edited by Herbert Y. Meltzer.
Raven Press, New York © 1987.

CHAPTER **113**

Maintenance Pharmacotherapy in Schizophrenia

John M. Kane and Jeffrey A. Lieberman

Maintenance antipsychotic drug treatment has proven to be of enormous value in preventing psychotic relapse and rehospitalization in patients with schizophrenia. Numerous double-blind placebo-controlled clinical trials support this conclusion and have been the subject of several review articles (13,14,22).

NEW RESEARCH

In the last decade we have seen the initiation of much more sophisticated long-term clinical trials, which have focused not only on relapse and rehospitalization but on a variety of other factors relevant to assessing the overall benefits and risks of maintenance drug treatment. Several issues have determined the types of studies conducted in recent years: first of all, the frequent occurrence of adverse effects, particularly tardive dyskinesia (36) with an estimated incidence of 3 to 4% per year of neuroleptic exposure (41); second, the relative lack of substantial improvement in "deficit" or residual symptoms and signs with continued impairment in psychosocial and vocational adjustment in many patients; third, the considerable variability in clinical course among patients and the potential influence of other therapeutic, environmental, and personality variables on outcome; and last, increasingly sophisticated methodologic and data analytic strategies that have been developed and applied in the design and interpretation of long-term clinical trials.

The present chapter focuses on the results of published pharmacologic treatment trials of at least 9 months' duration. Table 1 summarizes results of double-blind comparisons of either active drug versus placebo, two different active drugs, or active drug given in different forms (e.g., oral versus depot injection) or in different dosages or dosage ranges.

HETEROGENEITY OF OUTCOME

It is clear that there is enormous variability in relapse rates reported in these studies. Even among patients receiving guaranteed medication delivery (i.e., depot injections), relapse rates vary from 0 to 40% at the end of 1 year. Relapse rates after the same interval among those patients receiving placebo ranged from 30% to 86%. One difficulty in comparing relapse rates across studies, however, is that not all of these reports have presented cumulative relapse rates or "life table analyses," which allow for appropriate handling of patients with incomplete data (e.g., those who drop out or are discontinued from the trial because of adverse effects). The life table analysis allows for the frequent incomplete periods of observation occurring in long-term clinical trials. When cumulative relapse curves are presented, then data from different studies can be contrasted even though investigators may have utilized different assessment intervals, conducted trials for different lengths of time, or experienced different drop out rates.

METHODOLOGIC FACTORS

There are a variety of other factors that may play a role in producing the variability in outcome between different studies, and these factors are important to consider not only in the design and interpretation of clinical trials but

TABLE 1. *Maintenance pharmacotherapy in schizophrenia*

Author	N	Age (mean or range)	Sex	Prior episodes	Time since discharge (weeks)	Level of remission	Duration	Outcome (relapse)		Dropout
Trochinsky et al. (56)	43	40–50	63% Female	2–3	2–4 years	No halluc. del. or obvious thought disorder; required 300 mg CPZ	1 year	Drug PBO	4% 63%	?
Engelhardt et al. (17–19)	446	18–44	?	?	?	?	48 months	CPZ 1 yr 15%, 4 yr 20% PBO 1 yr 30%, 4 yr 31%		36% in 18 months
Leff and Wing (45)	35	16–55	?	?	6–12	Preadmission level	12 months	Drug PBO	35% 80%	14%
Hirsch et al. (26)	81	43	36% Female	70%	50% 52	?	9 months	FD PBO	8% 66%	9%
Crawford and Forrest (11)	31	20–65	71% Female	?	?	?	10 months	Stel FD	40% 14.3%	7%
Hogarty et al. (27)	374	34	58% Female	60% two or more	?	?	24 months	Drug 12 months 31%, 24 mos 48% PBO 12 months 68%, 24 mos 80%		8%
Chien (9)	47	43	57% Female	Former long-term inpatients	?	?	12 months	FE[a] FE[b] PBO	12% 37% 86%	?
Rifkin et al. (54)	73	23	32% Female	1.9	Mean 26	Remitted or stable plateau	12 months	FD + oral PBO	5% 75%	11%
Kelly et al. (43)	60	42	66% Female	?	?	?	9 months	Fluph dec Flupen dec	10% 10%	2%
Falloon et al. (20)	44	17–60 (mean 39)	55% Female	2 or more 80%	0	?	12 months	Pimozide FD	24% 40%	12%
Quitkin et al. (53)	56	26	44% Female	2.7	Mean 64	Remitted or stable plateau	12 months	Pen FD	7% 10%	20%
Hogarty et al. (29)	105	34	54% Female	4.6	0	?	24 months	Oral 2 years 65% 12–24 months 42% FD 2 years 40% 12–24 months 8%		13%
McGreadie et al. (51)	35	50	All male	?	?	"Well controlled"	9 months	Pimozide FD	19% 17%	3%
Schooler et al. (55)	214	29	41% Female	2 or more	0	?	12 months	FHCL FD	38% 46%	25%
Cheung (8)	30	40	60% Female	1.6	3–5 years	Fully remitted 3–5 years	18 months	Antipsychotic Benzodiazepine	13% 62%	7%
Kane et al. (35)	28	22	50% Female	1	Mean 17	Remitted	1 year	Drug PBO	0% 41%	35%
McCreadie et al. (51)	28	55	All male	?	Inpatients	"Well controlled"	10 months	Pimozide FD	15% 7%	25%
Odejide and Aderounmu (52)	70	?	?	2 or more	?	Well for at least 12 months	12 months	FD PBO	19% 56%	25%
Kane et al. (37)	126	29	37% Female	3.2	Mean 64	Remitted or stable plateau	12 months	Low-dose FD Intermed. dose Std. dose FD	56% 24% 14%	10%
Marder et al. (47)	50	36	All male	?	Mean 23 months	Stable	1 year	Low-dose FD 1 year 22% 2 years 44% Std. dose FD 1 year 20% 2 years 31%		14%
Crow et al. (12)	120	26	38% Female	1	1 month	Able to be discharged	2 years	Drugs PBO	58% 70%	11%

[a] Doctor-regulated interval.
[b] Patient-regulated interval.

also in making judgments of the clinical applicability of alternative maintenance strategies to specific patients.

Generalizability

The extent to which results from a particular study can be generalized to the larger population of patients suffering from the same illness is a critical consideration. Given the established efficacy of neuroleptic medication and the appropriate increase in emphasis on informed consent over the past decade, we must recognize the fact that many patients may choose not to participate in clinical trials (particularly if placebo is a possible treatment), and many clinicians and/or investigators may explicitly or implicitly exclude certain patients. Reports of clinical trials have varied in the extent to which information is presented on the "screening" and selection process producing the actual participants. Interestingly, two (30,55) of the studies with relatively high relapse rates on "guaranteed" medication had the highest percentage entering the trial of those individuals screened. Since there may be lack of uniformity in the definition or selection of "eligible" patients, it is difficult to make comparisons on this issue. Clearly, details with regard to patient selection, diagnostic criteria, and demographic and treatment history characteristics (as well as other variables), which might influence outcome, are important in determining the generalizability of results from a specific clinical trial.

Diagnostic Criteria

With the introduction of the Feighner criteria, the Research Diagnostic Criteria, and the DSM-III, there have been improvements in the reliability of diagnostic criteria; however, it is difficult to determine the impact of utilizing these criteria on outcome in clinical trials, since it is not possible to determine the procedures employed in those studies that did not involve specific inclusion and exclusion criteria.

Level and Duration of Remission

Those patients who have fully recovered from any psychotic signs and symptoms may have a different degree of vulnerability to relapse following drug withdrawal than those patients who continue to be symptomatic (referring more specifically to positive symptoms, e.g., delusions, hallucinations, thought disorder). In addition, it is possible that the risk of psychotic relapse is greatest immediately following recovery (or partial recovery) from a psychotic exacerbation compared to some months later, particularly for patients undergoing medication discontinuation (or substantial dosage reduction) but even for patients continuing on stable doses of medication. Few reports have fully described the level and/or length of remission at study entry, but the available data do suggest that this may be an important factor. Those studies that involved patients recently discharged from a brief hospitalization tend to report higher relapse rates than studies involving patients who have been stable and out of the hospital for many months.

This interpretation, however, should not be taken to mean that there is a steadily declining risk of relapse with time in remission, suggesting that for those patients in remission for many months or several years the risk of medication discontinuation is minimal. This does not appear to be the case. The Cheung (8) study involved patients who had been in remission for 3 to 5 years, and 62% of the subjects withdrawn from neuroleptics relapsed within 18 months. A similar finding was reported by Hogarty et al. (28) in an uncontrolled neuroleptic discontinuation involving patients who had been in good remission for at least 2 years, among whom 65% relapsed within 1 year. Dencker et al. (15) and Johnson (34) have also reported equivalent results in uncontrolled discontinuation studies.

Definition of Relapse

There has been enormous variation in the outcome criteria utilized in long-term maintenance trials. Most frequently "relapse" or "rehospitalization" have been employed as major outcome measures. Neither of these is an objective, reproducible, or reliable measure. Many factors influence rehospitalization rates besides level of psychopathology, and the determination of relapse has frequently been a subjective clinical judgment that may be influenced by a variety of patient, physician, and family factors. Some studies in recent years have attempted to utilize more objective and reproducible relapse criteria such as predefined changes on specific psychotic items on a rating scale; however, such strategies may not be sensitive to other important factors that might influence clinical judgment. Whatever methods are used to categorize outcome, attempts to make criteria objective, reliable, and reproducible will help to foster generalizability and meaningful comparison between studies employing different treatment strategies.

Compliance and the Role of Depot Injections

Noncompliance in medication taking has always been a major problem in the long-term treatment of schizophrenia. Denial, lack of insight, social stigma, adverse effects, and lack of information regarding benefits and risks remain frequent problems for patients with schizophrenia. Noncompliance, by its very nature, has been a difficult phenomenon to study; however, even in the context of controlled clinical trials (where noncompliant patients are probably underrepresented), there is a great deal of evidence that noncompliance in medication taking is a frequent event. The introduction of long-acting injectable medications produced considerable optimism in overcoming this problem; however, a series of controlled trials (54,55) involving double-blind random assignment to oral versus injectable neuroleptics did not confirm the considerable advantages for depot drugs suggested by the initial "mirror image" studies.

There are problems, however, in interpreting these results. First of all, patients engaged in these studies had to agree to participate in a research protocol and to receive both oral and injectable medication, one of which was placebo. Secondly, given recent results on substantial dosage reduction in maintenance treatment (to be discussed subsequently), it is likely that patients participating in these trials and receiving active oral medication may have had considerable leeway for partial noncompliance without precipitating a relapse. Thirdly, we suggest that noncompliance, particularly among patients initially cooperative enough to participate in a long-term clinical trial, is a gradually developing phenomenon. Unless patients are specifically selected on the basis of past noncompliance, it is likely that this behavior will develop gradually over time. In addition, when a patient in complete or relative remission discontinues medication, the consequential psychotic relapse may not occur for several months (the modal period from available data appears to be 3–7 months). These factors suggest that in a general population of outpatients with schizophrenia (not selected specifically for noncompliance), a controlled clinical trial lasting well beyond 1 year would be necessary to demonstrate the real value of guaranteed medication delivery. This conclusion is supported by the results of the only such trial, which lasted 2 years (30). In this study the relapse rate on oral medication during the second year was 42% in comparison to 8% on depot injectable medication. (This difference failed to reach statistical significance because of inadequate sample size.)

Kane and Borenstein (39) reviewed the problem of sample size and study duration in the context of guaranteed medication versus oral medication and carried out Monte Carlo analyses suggesting that 100 patients per group followed for 2 years would only provide minimally adequate power (0.71) to detect a clinically important difference given the time frame involved in the development and consequences of noncompliance.

This highlights the importance of adequate sample size as well as study duration in addressing a variety of important clinical questions. This issue becomes even more critical in attempting to determine the interaction and relative influence of multiple treatment strategies within the same trial.

Guaranteed medication delivery has played an important role in most of the major maintenance treatment studies in recent years because it enables the investigator to be certain that relapse occurring in the context of long-term pharmacotherapy is not caused by noncompliance, and, therefore, the impact of other patient, treatment, or environmental factors can be considered and explored. In addition, the use of long-acting injectable medication has been favored in the controlled trials of dosage reduction for the same reason, as well as the investigator's ability to titrate dosage more carefully within a specific range and to overcome some individual variation in absorption and first-pass metabolism.

At the same time, however, many clinicians have refrained from utilizing long-acting injectable drugs because of concern regarding adverse effects. Some reports in the literature had encouraged these concerns, particularly with regard to acute extrapyramidal side effects and tardive dyskinesia. With regard to the former, it is our impression that higher than necessary doses of long-acting injectable drugs were utilized in some early trials, leading to a higher than necessary incidence of akinesia, akathisia, and other extrapyramidal side effects. With regard to tardive dyskinesia, a few reports in the literature (36) had suggested that fluphenazine decanoate might be associated with a higher incidence of tardive dyskinesia than other neuroleptic drugs; however, since this drug is not subject to the substantial rates of noncompliance seen in oral medication taking, it is likely that any such association, if it did occur, is an epiphenomenon of actual increased neuroleptic exposure rather than exposure to a particular drug.

DRUG DOSAGE IN LONG-TERM TREATMENT

Initially, the major focus in maintenance treatment studies was the efficacy of neuroleptic drugs in preventing relapse. In recent years the focus has shifted towards improving the benefit-to-risk ratio of long-term pharmacotherapy. In this context, several studies conducted in the past decade have focused on alternative strategies to reduce cumulative neuroleptic exposure and to identify minimum effective dosages for long-term treatment (38). (Strategies involving intermittent or targeted pharmacotherapy are discussed subsequently.)

Caffey et al. (5) conducted the first controlled dosage reduction study in hospitalized inpatients and demonstrated that those patients whose dosage was reduced to three-sevenths of their original dosage experienced a 15% relapse rate within 4 months as compared to 45% for those patients receiving placebo and 5% for those continuing on their original dose.

Goldstein et al. (23) studied the efficacy of two dose levels of fluphenazine enanthate with and without crisis-oriented family therapy in 104 recently discharged schizophrenic patients. These predominantly first-episode (69%) patients were randomly assigned to fluphenazine enanthate 25 mg or 6.25 mg i.m. every 2 weeks and were studied for 6 weeks following hospital discharge. Relapse was defined as the need to alter medication substantially or to rehospitalize the patient. Only 10% relapsed within the 6 weeks following discharge, but 24% of those in the low-dose/no-therapy condition relapsed as compared to none of the high-dose/therapy. The low-dose/therapy and the high-dose/no-therapy groups had relapse rates of 9% and 10%, respectively. Although this study involved a relatively brief period of controlled treatment, it is a classic study in suggesting the potential additive effects of neuroleptics and such psychotherapeutic strategies as crisis-oriented family therapy.

Kane et al. (37,40) have reported results from a 1-year random assignment study of different dosage ranges of fluphenazine decanoate (12.5–50 mg every 2 weeks as compared to 1.25–5.0 mg every 2 weeks) involving stable outpatient schizophrenics. At the end of 1 year, the cumulative relapse rate (utilizing objective criteria on psychotic items of the BPRS) on low dose was 56% compared to 14% for the standard dose. An intermediate dose (2.5–10.0 mg every other week) was also studied and produced a cumulative relapse rate of 24% (42). Despite the significantly higher relapse rate among the patients receiving the low-dose treatment, most of the patients who did relapse were restabilized with temporary dosage increase and without requiring rehospitalization. In addition, significantly fewer early signs of tardive dyskinesia were observed in these patients, and they were performing better on some measures of psychosocial adjustment than the patients treated with standard dose.

Interestingly, the patients receiving the very low doses manifested less evidence of emotional withdrawal, blunted affect, tension, and psychomotor retardation. These differences were statistically significant in group comparisons of rating scale data but were not of such magnitude as to be obvious in individual patients. These findings, however, emphasize the potential importance of ongoing parkinsonian side effects, even during the maintenance phase of treatment, and highlight the complexity of assessing so-called negative symptoms.

Marder et al. (47,48) studied 66 male veteran outpatients randomly assigned, double-blind, to 5 mg or 25 mg of fluphenazine decanoate administered every 2 weeks. Patients were followed for 2 years and were maintained on the assigned fixed dose of 5 or 25 mg as long as they did well. The investigators defined three levels of unfavorable outcome that would lead to a dosage change. When patients experienced an increase of 3 or more points on BPRS cluster scores for thought disturbance or paranoia, they were considered to have had a "psychotic exacerbation." (These were relatively mild and seldom led to rehospitalization, but the clinician was allowed to increase the dose up to 10 or 50 mg for the respective groups.) When patients could not be adequately controlled within this range, they were considered to have had a "relapse." The third level of outcome was rehospitalization. The results from this study highlight the importance of a long-term perspective. At the end of 1 year, the "exacerbation" rate was almost identical in the two treatment groups (35% on 5 mg and 43% on 25 mg); however, during the second year the two doses produced different rates of exacerbation. Sixty-nine percent experienced an exacerbation on 5 mg as compared to only 36% on 25 mg. When the clinician has the flexibility to double the dose and the outcome of "relapse" is considered, the two treatments produced similar results after 2 years: 44% relapsed on the lower dose and 31% on the higher dose (a nonsignificant difference). Relapse rates at 1 year were 22% with the lower dose range and 20% with the higher.

Results from both of these studies suggest that dosage reduction can lead to a diminution in adverse effects and improvement in some subjective and objective measures of well-being; however, the risk of psychotic exacerbation increases, and patients must be observed carefully with a readiness to increase medication when necessary and usually on a temporary basis. This highlights the importance of viewing this approach as a strategy within the context of flexible, observant clinical management. In addition, there may be patients for whom dosage reduction is not feasible based on past attempts or potential dire consequences of psychotic relapse (e.g., history of serious suicide attempts or dangerousness).

Hogarty (31) has reported preliminary results from a study comparing a standard dose of fluphenazine decanoate (average 20 mg every 2 weeks) and a low dose (averaging 4 mg every 2 weeks) representing 20% of the standard. At 1 year, five of 20 patients (25%) assigned to the standard dose and five of 22 (23%) assigned to the low dose relapsed.

ALTERNATIVE STRATEGIES

The rationale for maintenance treatment is based on the assumption that pharmacotherapy is necessary to prevent an increase in or reemergence of psychotic signs and symptoms. The relative benefits of maintenance treatment in general, or alternative strategies in particular, undoubtedly vary from patient to patient but may also vary depending on the stage of the illness for a given individual. Results from long-term naturalistic follow-up studies emphasize the heterogeneity of outcome in this illness, with some patients experiencing a chronic deteriorating course while others experience a much more benign outcome after 10 or 20 years. We have relatively little information on the impact of drug treatment on the very-long-term outcome of schizophrenia despite the very dramatic benefits of neuroleptics over the course of several years as demonstrated in controlled trials.

Identifying true drug effect is also complicated by variability in symptom patterns and drug responsiveness even among patients presenting with similar symptoms. The extent to which maintenance pharmacotherapy is truly prophylactic in terms of preventing a new episode as compared to suppressing continuously present symptomatology may also vary from patient to patient, and if this distinction could be made it would clearly be useful in establishing the appropriate treatment strategy.

The possibility that some patients may not require continuous medication has fostered research on "intermittent" or "targeted" strategies, which go well beyond earlier studies of "drug holidays" in suggesting that some patients may do very well completely off of neuroleptics for substantial periods of time and that a full-blown relapse can be prevented by detecting early or prodromal signs of exacerbation and reinstituting medication at that point.

The strategy is an outgrowth of observations by Herz and Melville (24) and others that many patients experience characteristic signs or symptoms during the early stages of relapse and that knowledge of this pattern obtained from the patient, family, and previous treatment sources may facilitate early recognition and treatment. In addition, the strategy assumes that lengthy interruptions in drug administration may minimize the risks of adverse effects. This is clearly the case for many adverse effects (e.g., parkinsonian, cognitive, and neuroendocrine); however, the impact of this strategy on the incidence of tardive dyskinesia has not been established.

Herz et al. (25) and Carpenter et al. (6,7) have demonstrated the feasibility of targeted treatment; however, we must await the results of Schooler and Keith's ongoing NIMH multicenter study to allow a direct comparison of continuous low dose versus intermittent strategies. Both of these pharmacotherapy strategies are clinically limited, however, to settings that allow close clinical monitoring as well as to patients and/or families who can recognize and respond appropriately to early signs of relapse.

FUTURE DIRECTIONS

Ideally, we would like to be able to predict which patients are best suited for a particular strategy based on their propensity to relapse within a relatively short time without medication. The work of Lieberman et al. (46) utilizing response to methylphenidate infusions as a potential predictor may prove useful in this regard and is a logical extension of earlier work by Janowsky et al. (32,33) and Angrist et al. (1,2). Lieberman's results suggest that those patients experiencing a transient exacerbation of psychotic signs and symptoms following 0.5 mg/kg of methylphenidate given intravenously will relapse sooner (following neuroleptic discontinuation) than patients not responding to methylphenidate in that fashion. This strategy does not necessarily identify patients who can be maintained medication-free indefinitely; however, in our experience this remains a very small subgroup.

We have found (35) that even among patients recovering from an acute-onset first schizophrenic episode, a statistically significant drug effect is apparent in preventing relapse during the subsequent year (40% relapsing on placebo, none on drug), and as these patients are followed for longer intervals, the overwhelming majority experience recurrence of psychosis when untreated.

Crow et al. (12) reported a less striking drug effect after 2 years in a population of first-episode patients: 58% relapsed on active medication as compared to 70% on placebo. However, these results also suggest that most patients will have a recurrence within 2 to 3 years following their first episode of schizophrenia.

The lack of a more dramatic drug effect in the Crow et al. study is surprising. There are several potentially important differences between these studies. Kane et al. included only acute onset patients, whereas in the Crow et al. study, a large proportion of the trial participants had lengthy insidious onsets, and these investigators reported a significant relationship between length of time ill prior to initiation of neuroleptic treatment and poorer outcome. In addition, Crow et al. randomized patients to drug or placebo after a month out of hospital, and patients were seen monthly for the first 6 months and then every 6 weeks by nonresearch clinicians. In the Kane et al. study, patients were in stable remission for an average of 17 weeks prior to randomization and were seen every 2 weeks by research psychiatrists throughout the trial.

Although it has been difficult to identify patients who can be withdrawn from neuroleptics indefinitely, there remains a substantial subgroup of patients who relapse despite ongoing pharmacotherapy. It is difficult, however, in such cases to presume that medication is without any effect in that relapse may be even more frequent or more severe without drug treatment. We are not aware of any studies that have specifically focused on alternative treatment strategies for patients who experience psychotic relapse despite continuous pharmacotherapy. There have been some studies suggesting that the measurement of blood levels and/or prolactin may be useful in identifying patients at risk for relapse despite continued neuroleptic treatment; however, we have insufficient data at present on which to base clinical guidelines (3,4,44).

Although a variety of medications have been utilized in the treatment of schizophrenic patients who do not respond acutely to neuroleptics, there are few data on such drugs as carbamazepine, lithium, propranolol, benzodiazepines, or electroconvulsive therapy in long-term treatment either alone or in conjunction with neuroleptics. In fact, the potential value of switching neuroleptic or neuroleptic class has not been studied adequately. Data are also needed on adjunctive use of various pharmacologic agents to treat specific symptoms or symptom patterns (e.g., dysphoria, depression, negative symptoms) in the maintenance phase of treatment. This is not to ignore the potential importance of personality, psychosocial, environmental, and other factors in amplifying or limiting response to somatic treatments, and these interactions are discussed elsewhere in this volume.

A question has also arisen as to whether neuroleptics may have a negative impact on the course of schizophrenia over the long term. The suggestion (10) that neuroleptics might produce a "supersensitivity psychosis" implies that following neuroleptic treatment the risk of relapse is increased by an increased sensitivity of dopamine receptors in relevant brain areas. This could be manifested clinically by more rapid relapse following drug discontinuation than would have occurred without maintenance drug treatment or by the need for increasing dosages of neuroleptics to maintain the same level of remission. There are insufficient data to allow firm conclusions in this area, and there are enormous methodologic problems in adequately testing this hypothesis. At the same time, it is also necessary to consider the fact that some patients with schizophrenia have a deteriorating course despite or without neuroleptic treatment rather than as a consequence of such treatment. In addition, the lack of, or delay in, pharmacologic treatment may have a negative impact on subsequent course even if medication is ultimately utilized as suggested by the classic study of May et al. (49). This phenomenon may be mediated biologically and/or psychologically, and further work would be necessary to consider potential mechanisms.

Although advances in maintenance treatment over the past decade have largely involved extensions of previous observations, more sophisticated testing of specific hypotheses, and increasingly comprehensive assessment of risks and benefits, we should not lose sight of the enormous advantages that incremental improvements in treatment can provide when applied to large numbers of patients. Further exploration and understanding of the heterogeneity of long-term pharmacotherapy outcome in schizophrenia should provide important clues to a better understanding of schizophrenia in general.

ACKNOWLEDGMENTS

This research was supported in part by NIMH grants 31776, 32369, 38880, and 00537.

REFERENCES

1. Angrist, B., Rotrosen, J., and Gershon, S. L. (1980): *Psychopharmacology,* 67:31–38.
2. Angrist, B., Pesselow, E., Rubenstein, M., Wolkin, A., and Rotrosen, J. (1985): *Psychopharmacology,* 85:277–283.

3. Brown, W. A., and Laughren, T. P. (1981): *Am. J. Psychiatry,* 183:237–239.
4. Brown, W. A., Laughren, T., Chisholm, E., and Williams, B. W. (1982): *Arch. Gen. Psychiatry,* 39:998–1000.
5. Caffey, E. M., Jr., Diamond, L. S., Frank, T. V., Grasberger, J. C., Herman, L., et al. (1964): *J. Chron. Dis.,* 17:347–358.
6. Carpenter, W. T., Stephens, J. H., Rey, A. C., Hanlon, T. E., and Heinrichs, D. W. (1982): *Psychopharmacol. Bull.,* 18:21–23.
7. Carpenter, W. T., and Heinrichs, D. W. (1984): In: *Drug Maintenance Strategies in Schizophrenia,* edited by J. Kane, pp. 82–89. American Psychiatric Press, Washington.
8. Cheung, H. K. (1981): *Br. J. Psychiatry,* 138:490–494.
9. Chien, C.-P. (1975): In: *Drugs in Combination with Other Therapies,* edited by M. Greenblatt, pp. 13–29. Grune & Stratton, New York.
10. Chouinard, G., and Jones, B. (1980): *Am. J. Psychiatry,* 137:16–21.
11. Crawford, R., and Forrest, A. (1974): *Br. J. Psychiatry,* 124:385–391.
12. Crow, T. J., MacMillan, J. F., Johnson, A. L., and Johnstone, E. C. (1986): *Br. J. Psychiatry,* 148:120–127.
13. Davis, J. M. (1975): *Am. J. Psychiatry,* 132:1237–1245.
14. Davis, J. M., Schaffer, C. B., Killian, G. A., Kinard, C., and Chan, C. (1980): *Schizophrenia Bull.,* 6:70–87.
15. Dencker, S. J., Lepp, M., and Malm, U. (1980): *Acta Psychiatr. Scand. [Suppl.],* 279:64–76.
16. Engelhardt, D. M., Freedman, N., Glick, B. S., Hankoff, L. D., Mann, D., et al. (1960): *J.A.M.A.,* 173:147–149.
17. Engelhardt, D. M., Rosen, B., Freedman, N., Mann, D., and Margolis, R. (1963): *J.A.M.A.,* 186:981–983.
18. Engelhardt, D. M., Freedman, M., Rosen, B., Mann, D., and Margolis, R. (1964): *Arch. Gen. Psychiatry,* 11:162–169.
19. Engelhardt, D. M., Rosen, B., Freedman, N., and Margolis, R. (1967): *Arch. Gen. Psychiatry,* 16:98–101.
20. Falloon, I. R. H., Watts, D. C., and Shepherd, M. (1978): *Psychol. Med.,* 8:59–70.
21. Falloon, I. R. H., Boyd, J. L., McGill, C. W., Razani, J., Moss, H. B., et al. (1982): *N. Engl. J. Med.,* 306:1347–1440.
22. Gittelman-Klein, R., and Klein, D. F. (1968): *Psychopharmacology—A Review of Progress 1957–1967,* edited by D. H. Efron, pp. 1119–1153. Government Printing Office, Washington.
23. Goldstein, M. J., Rodnick, E. H., Evans, J. R., May, P. R. A., and Steinberg, M. R. (1978): *Arch. Gen. Psychiatry,* 35:1169–1177.
24. Herz, M. I., and Melville, C. (1980): *Am. J. Psychiatry,* 137:801–805.
25. Herz, M. I., Szymanski, H. V., and Simon, J. C. (1982): *Am. J. Psychiatry,* 139:918–922.
26. Hirsch, S. R., Gaind, R., Rohde, P. D., Stevens, B. C., and Wing, J. K. (1973): *Br. Med. J.,* 1:633–637.
27. Hogarty, G. E., Goldberg, S. C., and Collaborative Study Group (1974): *Arch. Gen. Psychiatry,* 28:54–64.
28. Hogarty, G. E., Ulrich, R. F., Mussare, F., and Aristigueta, N. (1976): *Dis. Nerv. Syst.,* 37:494–500.
29. Hogarty, G. E., Goldberg, S. C., Schooler, N. R., and Ulrich, R. F. (1979): *Arch. Gen. Psychiatry,* 31:603–608.
30. Hogarty, G. E., Schooler, N. R., Ulrich, R. F., Mussare, F., Ferro, P., et al. (1979): *Arch. Gen. Psychiatry,* 36:1283–1294.
31. Hogarty, G. E. (1984): *J. Clin. Psychiatry,* 45(5):36–42.
32. Janowsky, D. S., El-Yousef, K., Davis, J. M., and Sekerke, J. (1973): *Arch. Gen. Psychiatry,* 28:185–191.
33. Janowsky, D. S., and Davis, J. M. (1976): *Arch. Gen. Psychiatry,* 33:304–308.
34. Johnson, D. A. W. (1979): *Br. J. Psychiatry,* 135:524–530.
35. Kane, J. M., Rifkin, A., Quitkin, F., Nayak, D. V., and Ramos-Lorenzi, J. R. (1982): *Arch. Gen. Psychiatry,* 39:70–73.
36. Kane, J. M., and Smith, J. M. (1982): *Arch. Gen. Psychiatry,* 39:473–481.
37. Kane, J. M., Rifkin, A., Woerner, M., Reardon, G., Sarantakos, S., et al. (1983): *Arch. Gen. Psychiatry,* 40:893–896.
38. Kane, J. M., ed. (1984): *Drug Maintenance Strategies in Schizophrenia.* American Psychiatric Press, Washington.
39. Kane, J. M., and Borenstein, M. (1985): *Psychopharmacol. Bull.,* 21:23–27.
40. Kane, J. M., Rifkin, A., Woerner, M., Reardon, G., Kreisman, D., et al. (1985): *Psychopharmacol. Bull.,* 21:533–537.
41. Kane, J. M., Woerner, M., Borenstein, M., Wegner, J., and Lieberman, J. (1986): *Psychopharmacol. Bull.,* 22:254–258.
42. Kane, J. M., Woerner, M., and Sarantakos, S. (1986): *J. Clin. Psychiatry,* 47(5):30–33.
43. Kelly, H. B., Freeman, H. L., Banning, B., and Schiff, A. A. (1977): *Int. Pharmacopsychiatry,* 12:54–64.
44. Laughren, T. P., Brown, W. A., and Williams, B. W. (1979): *Am. J. Psychiatry,* 136:108–110.
45. Leff, J. P., and Wing, J. K. (1971): *Br. Med. J.,* 3:559–604.
46. Lieberman, J. A., Kane, J. M., Gadaleta, D., Brenner, R., Lesser, M. S., et al. (1984): *Am. J. Psychiatry,* 141:633–638.
47. Marder, S. R., Van Putten, T., Mintz, J., McKenzie, J., Lebelle, M., et al. (1984): *Arch. Gen. Psychiatry,* 41:1025–1029.
48. Marder, S. R., Van Putten, T., Mintz, J., Lebell, M., McKenzie, J., et al. (1987): *Arch. Gen. Psychiatry (in press).*
49. May, P. R. A., Tuma, A. H., Yale, C., Potepan, P., and Dixon, W. J. (1976): *Arch. Gen. Psychiatry,* 33:481–506.
50. McCreadie, R. G., Dingwall, J. M., Wiles, D. H., and Heykants, J. J. P. (1980): *Br. J. Psychiatry,* 137:510–517.
51. McCreadie, R., Mackie, M., Morrison, D., and Kidd, J. (1982): *Br. J. Psychiatry,* 140:280–286.
52. Odejide, O. A., and Aderounmu, A. F. (1982): *J. Clin. Psychiatry,* 43(5):195–196.
53. Quitkin, F., Rifkin, A., Kane, J. M., Ramos-Lorenzi, J. R., and Klein, D. F. (1978): *Arch. Gen. Psychiatry,* 35:889–892.
54. Rifkin, A., Quitkin, F., Rabiner, C. J., and Klein, D. F. (1977): *Arch. Gen. Psychiatry,* 34:43–47.
55. Schooler, N. R., Levine, J., Severe, J. B., Brauzer, B., DiMascio, A., et al. (1980): *Arch. Gen. Psychiatry,* 37:16–24.
56. Troshinsky, C. H., Aaronson, H. G., and Stone, R. K. (1962): *Penn. Psychiatry Q.,* 2:11–15.

Psychopharmacology:
The Third Generation of Progress,
edited by Herbert Y. Meltzer.
Raven Press, New York © 1987.

CHAPTER **114**

Medication and Psychosocial Strategies in the Treatment of Schizophrenia

Nina R. Schooler and Gerard E. Hogarty

The past decade of research contains an interesting and, at times, quite different focus from earlier work regarding the effects of pharmacotherapy and psychosocial interventions administered to schizophrenic persons—a direction influenced by studies in the neurosciences and environmental psychology as well as by such political concerns as deinstitutionalization, insurance limitations, and decreased funding for community mental health services. This is the third review on this general topic to appear in volumes reflecting progress in psychopharmacology research (29,33) and in some ways has the least material to cover. If it were narrowed to studies that are diagnostically precise, involve random assignment to treatment, and are experimentally complete (i.e., include experimental variation of both the drug and psychosocial treatments), then very little of this recent history would be included. Only two studies have appeared in this decade that meet these criteria (14,20). Therefore, we shall loosen our criteria to include studies of psychosocial treatment:

1. That are limited to patients diagnosed as schizophrenic or in which schizophrenic patient subgroups can be distinguished.
2. In which an experimental psychosocial treatment is compared to a control or second psychosocial treatment.
3. In which assignment to treatment is random.

Thus, the review includes a number of studies that do not control drug treatment experimentally. Attention is not directed to studies of pharmacologic treatment that do not address psychosocial treatments directly, because this work is well reviewed elsewhere in this volume. Our goal is to review recent history and attempt a formulation that reflects both the state of the art and the seeds for future research.

IDENTIFIED THEMES OF THE PAST DECADE

The character of some research on psychosocial treatment during the past decade, and particularly the early part of the decade, has been captured by Klein (24), who distinguishes between psychosocial treatment of schizophrenia and psychosocial help for people with schizophrenia. The design of many treatments was based largely on common sense approaches—providing assistance in areas of obvious need, be that social, environmental, or personal (14,19), or on the extension of established psychotherapeutic approaches to schizophrenia (31).

A series of investigations completed since 1981 has studied psychosocial treatments for schizophrenia based on specific hypotheses regarding the nature of the illness, most frequently a stress/diathesis model (2,8,17,25,26,39). Characteristically, the investigators have frequently been the architects of the treatments being studied. Much of this work rejects former ideas about the role of the family in the pathogenesis of the illness, which resulted in therapeutic prescriptions for distancing patients and families. These treatment models seek an informed relationship with families.

HISTORICAL CONTEXT

Immediately before 1975, we and our colleagues, in the first two-factor, placebo-controlled (but atheoretical) study of an antipsychotic drug (chlorpromazine) and psychosocial treatment, provided evidence for the prophylactic effect of maintenance chemotherapy (48% relapse in 2 years), the limitations of placebo alone or a psychosocial treatment administered in the absence of medication (80% relapse), as well as a delayed effect of combined psychosocial therapy and medication in forestalling schizophrenic relapse (19). Exponential relapse rates for medication (3.6% per month) and placebo (10.4% per month) suggested that the magnitude of the prophylactic effect was considerably greater than cumulative relapse rates might indicate (21).

Regarding adjustment, a disordinal interaction indicated a superiority of combined treatment and a deleterious effect of psychosocial treatment when administered in the absence of medication (18). Later, we provided evidence that the characteristics of patients interacted with psychosocial treatment such that less insightful, cognitively disorganized, and withdrawn patients did poorly on a high-expectation psychosocial treatment, whereas better integrated patients improved (13). Criticism of this study focused on the possibility that noncompliance with medication might have contributed to the relatively high relapse rate on medication and thus might have mitigated the effect of combined psychosocial treatment as well. Further, criticism concerning the effects of treatment on adjustment focused on our restriction of the analysis of adjustment to long-term survivors.

A subsequent study addressed the compliance question by a comparison of fluphenazine decanoate and hydrochloride (or their placebos) administered in the randomized context of psychosocial treatment. First-year relapse showed no significant difference between routes of administration (35% and 40% relapse, respectively). However, no patient relapsed in the second year while receiving the combination of fluphenazine decanoate and social therapy (20). A series of other studies comparing oral and depot fluphenazine yielded similar 1-year outcomes (32,35), as did a study comparing oral pimozide to fluphenazine decanoate (10).

Although these studies were consistent in their inability to detect differences between medication regimens guaranteeing compliance (depot administration) and those allowing noncompliance (oral administration), the extent of the influence of medication noncompliance on the course of schizophrenic illness is still being questioned (23). It is clear though that relapse does occur under guaranteed medication (depot administration), varies depending on length of time since an index episode, and may be as high as 40% in the first year following discharge. Noncompliance, per se, is not a sufficient explanation for schizophrenic relapse. This renewed recognition that relapse occurs under guaranteed medication served as a further spur to development of psychosocial treatments to be administered in conjunction with medication.

METHODOLOGIC CONSIDERATIONS

An ideal study should be diagnostically specific to schizophrenia, have experimental control of both medication and psychosocial treatment, use randomization or another method to insure comparability of groups, and include blind evaluation or other techniques to insure unbiased assessment of treatment effects. Few studies in the literature of the past decade satisfy these criteria. In this section we describe, briefly, appropriate standards for each of these methodologic criteria and in the subsequent descriptions identify studies that come reasonably close to meeting them.

The "complete" study design is one in which there are experimental and control conditions for both medication and the psychosocial treatment so that independent, additive, and interactive effects of the two treatment modalities can be assessed (33). A design frequently used to assess psychosocial treatment is one that does not control drug treatment experimentally. In such studies, drug treatment may become an outcome or dependent variable, as in a study of length of hospital stay (16) or behavioral family therapy (6). However, in these designs it is unclear whether outcomes are a direct effect of the psychosocial treatment or are mediated by changes in drug treatment.

A further concern is that of power to detect differences. It is a common observation that negative studies are less likely to be fully analyzed and published and that small studies may have insufficient power to detect differences of moderate size that may be of substantial clinical relevance.

A second issue is the diagnosis of patients studied. In principle, our focus is on patients diagnosed as schizophrenia or its variants (schizophreniform, schizoaffective) according to operational clinical criteria such as those of the American Psychiatric Association, the World Health Organization, or other specified criteria (36,40). The literature of the past decade on drug treatment is quite consistent in its reliance on such criteria, but much of the literature on psychosocial treatments that would be relevant often includes multiple diagnoses without operational criteria. Since it is difficult to assess the relevance of such work to treatment research in schizophrenia, we have excluded studies unless schizophrenic patients are distinguished from other diagnoses in data analysis.

Randomization of patients to treatment conditions is an obvious control to insure lack of bias. Even when assignment is randomized, if treatment is not blind (usually the case for psychosocial treatments), it is possible clinician bias could play a role in determining patient assignment. In situations in which double-blind conditions cannot be maintained, independent blind assessment of outcome is advisable. This may be especially difficult because of the added financial burden and because patients are less cooperative with assessors who are unknown to them. Self-ratings, ratings by family members, and more "objective" measures such as task performance, resource utilization, and hospitalization provide useful and potentially less biased measures of outcome than nonblind clinician ratings, although some of these may be less relevant outcomes for psychosocial treatment.

Another issue in the measurement of outcome is whether what is being measured is a variable of genuine clinical value or simply an indicator that the experimental condition has been appropriately manipulated. For example, plasma concentration of an antipsychotic drug may be a more sensitive measure of dosage administered than the prescribed dose, but it is not the clinical outcome measure of interest in a study comparing two dosages of a drug. Similarly, differences in duration of eye contact between two forms of social skills training may indicate that the therapies adhere to their theoretical models but are not a measure of the therapy's efficacy. Thus, it is necessary to include in treatment research, particularly research that looks at both drug and psychosocial treatment effects, outcome measures that assess the hypothesized effects of the treatments under study but that are not simply reflections of the experimental manipulations.

Finally, research designs concerned with the relationship of the effects of pharmacologic and psychosocial treatments are faced with an inherent difficulty. Psychotherapy research regards the maintenance of gains well after the end of therapy as a major source of validation that the therapy is successful. Psychopharmacologic treatment efficacy, especially long-term efficacy in schizophrenia, is frequently established through discontinuation or withdrawal study designs. Thus, assessment of outcome at the conclusion of treatment exposure is the design strategy favored by pharmacologic researchers, whereas follow-up studies are often considered more definitive by psychosocial treatment researchers. Clearly, the optimal design is one that maintains an experimental drug treatment throughout a follow-up period for the psychosocial treatment. In this way, at the end of the total study period, each treatment modality will be assessed under the conditions most relevant to it.

Because we are interested in the interaction and relationship of drug and psychosocial treatments from the perspective of psychopharmacology research, our mandate has been to explore the psychotherapy literature from this perspective. We are distressed to find that psychotherapy researchers do not take proper account of drug treatment as a mediating and influential determinant of outcome. It is probably true that a psychotherapy reviewer would find our pharmacologic literature equally lacking.

EXPERIMENTAL STUDIES OF PSYCHOSOCIAL TREATMENT

In this section we review studies of specific psychosocial treatments: individual psychotherapy, social skills training, group psychotherapy, and family treatment. We have excluded a series of studies that manipulate environments such as comparisons of hospitalization to community care, ward milieus, length of hospital stay, day hospitals, or foster care. Although such system approaches are of substantial interest in the overall treatment of schizophrenic patients, they are beyond the scope of this review.

Individually Oriented Treatment

Only one study of insight-oriented psychotherapy has appeared in the past decade that meets our minimum criteria for inclusion—specific diagnosis of schizophrenia, prospective and random assignment to treatment. Stanton, Gunderson, and their colleagues (15,37) compared expressive insight-oriented (EIO) psychotherapy provided three times a week to a reality adaptive supportive (RAS) psychotherapy in which patients were seen once a week. The EIO fostered a "detailed exploration of the patients' inner experience and relations with others . . . to increase insight . . . an understanding of the fact of his illness, its nature

and its implication" (p. 537). The RAS focused on problems in the current living situation of the patient with the goal of identifying solutions or improving future coping strategies. Therapists emphasized the biological origins of the illness and the need for long-term pharmacologic treatment and were active in topic selection and advice giving. Patients were recruited from three hospitals in the Boston area: a private psychoanalytically oriented facility, a university-affiliated mental health center, and a Veterans Administration hospital. Treatment, provided by 81 experienced therapists, was initiated during hospitalization and continued for up to 2 years following discharge. One hundred sixty-four recently hospitalized patients who met International Pilot Study for Schizophrenia criteria and had functioned out of hospital for at least 4 months in the past 2 years were included. Fifty percent were experiencing a first hospitalization; about 68% were male. Only 58% ($N = 95$) completed the 6-month period, defined as minimum treatment exposure, and only 31% completed 2 years of treatment. Dropout rates differed by hospital (the analytically oriented hospital had a lower dropout rate than the others). Analysis of outcome was restricted to patients who completed 6 months of treatment, and the most sweeping test of hypotheses to the 50 patients still in treatment after 24 months.

Medication administration was not controlled, and only two statistical comparisons of drug treatment are reported. There were no differences between the groups in number of days on antipsychotic drugs. This was counter to the prediction that less drug would be needed under EIO. The RAS patients spent more days on lithium, significantly more in the second year. Days on medication is a crude measure of need for medication that obscures possible dosage differences.

Counter to hypotheses, the RAS group showed significantly better outcome: fewer job changes, less time dependent on family, a larger share of household responsibilities, and fewer days in hospitalization during the first year. The authors report a "nonsignificant advantage" for EIO in cognitive functioning and a moderate effect on ego functioning. No differences in interpersonal relationships or signs and symptoms of schizophrenia were found. Unfortunately, there is no control for psychotherapy in the form of a medication-treated group with minimal psychotherapeutic support. The high attrition rate further restricts interpretation of the findings. However, the high attrition rate itself may be the clearest outcome. Neither RAS nor EIO was sufficiently attractive to a majority of the 164 patients who initially accepted them to stay the 2-year course.

A study conducted by us was designed to investigate the role of individual social therapy and injectable neuroleptic in preventing relapse through enhanced compliance and provision of enriched social support (20). Newly discharged patients ($N = 105$) were randomly assigned to either injectable depot fluphenazine or oral fluphenazine and high or low social therapy. Thus, the study included experimental control of both drug and psychosocial treatment. Social therapy focused on solution of personal/environmental problems impinging on instrumental role performance as well as on reduction of social isolation and resolution of a wide range of reality-based problems. Treatment continued until relapse or up to 2 years. There were no significant main effects of either treatment on relapse over the 2 years of the study, but a trend for reduced relapse among patients treated with depot fluphenazine and high social therapy. In fact, no patient treated with the combination relapsed after 8 months. This suggests that patients who were stabilized on medication were able to benefit from the resource provided by the social therapy. The relapse rates for other groups were more constant over time. However, prediction of which patients would relapse receiving high social therapy was not possible.

Social and Life Skills Training

Interest in improving the social skills of schizophrenic patients stems from obvious patient deficits and also from experimental psychological studies of the ability to change behavior through carefully designed reinforcement paradigms. More research effort has been directed to the relative effectiveness of components of behavioral training than to assessment of efficacy. From the extensive literature, we identified only four studies that were restricted to patients diagnosed as schizophrenic or analyzed outcome separately for schizophrenic patients.

Eisler et al. (5) randomly assigned 24 schizophrenic and 24 nonpsychotic male inpatients to social skills training, social skills training plus modeling, and a control condition of behavioral rehearsal. Six sessions were conducted during a 5-day period. Patients in both social skills groups improved more on measures of social skills, speech loudness, and duration than the control group, but for schizophrenic patients the addition of modeling provided a significant advantage over social skills training alone, suggesting that the schizophrenic patients required the additional cues provided by modeling. This difference was not seen for the nonpsychotic patients.

Brown and Munford (3) compared "life skills" training (including behavioral rehearsal, modeling, and homework) to "traditional VA rehabilitation programming" (20 hr a week for 7 weeks) in 28 chronic schizophrenic male inpatients. At the end of treatment, patients in the experimental group improved significantly in a Life Skills Inventory that assessed skills in areas of health, finance, communication, and use of community resources. Depression, as measured by the Hamilton Depression Rating Scale (nonblind), and a self-rating of relapse probability also improved. Neither of these studies provides any information about drug treatment. Further, the duration and/or maintenance of gains are not reported.

Wallace and Liberman (39) reported results of a study comparing social skills training (SST) to holistic health therapy (HHT) in 28 hospitalized male schizophrenic inpatients who lived on a ward that functioned as a token economy. Inclusion was restricted to patients who had lived with a relative rated high in "expressed emotion" immediately prior to hospitalization and relative remission from florid psychotic symptoms. This study, reviewed here because of the inpatient population and experimental treatment, is also linked to a series of investigations of family

treatment and social skills in outpatients that derive from the literature on expressed emotion (EE). Patients received "optimal doses" of neuroleptic medication (mean 350 mg/day chlorpromazine equivalence) with no differences between the two treatment groups. The HHT focused on coping with stressors by increasing physical and psychological well-being and included activities such as yoga, jogging, meditation, and group discussions on stress. The SST focused on interpersonal problem solving designed to improve "receiving, processing, and sending" communication skills. Treatment in both groups was intensive—up to 6 hr a day for 9 weeks. In addition, both groups participated in weekly family therapy sessions reflecting the differing approaches: in the SST group, a behavioral therapy emphasizing communication and problem solving; in the HHT group, education, coping, and insight into family dynamics.

Acquisition of the skills emphasized in SST (but not specific measures relevant to the HHT condition) and more general outcome in terms of psychopathology, relapse up to 24 months post-discharge, and family ratings of patients were assessed. Compared to HHT patients, patients in the SST group improved significantly in a social skills test similar to the SST sessions both immediately following the 9-week treatment and at a 9-month post-discharge follow-up. Other measures derived from a social interaction task supported this sustained improvement. Further, after 9 months, relatives rated SST patients as less negative or obstreperous and showing less psychopathology than HHT patients. Both groups improved over time in self-rated symptoms and psychopathology, but there were no differences between the groups. Relapse or rehospitalization rates were not different, although the direction of effect in these measures favored the SST group. The difficulty in interpreting the results of this study derives from the complexity of the "treatment package" delivered to patients, the inadequate power to detect effects both because of the very small sample and the very large number of comparisons made, and the absence of either control of drug treatment following discharge or information about it.

Bellack and his colleagues (2) investigated SST in the context of a 12-week, day hospital (DH) program for chronically ill schizophrenic patients. Both men and women were included, but gender differences are not reported. Neuroleptic medication was administered to all patients "in accord with current clinical practice." Sixty-four patients were randomly assigned to either DH ($N = 20$) or DH and one of two procedurally different social skills training approaches ($N = 49$) for 3 hr per week of training in basic skills helpful in establishing a social network and reducing interpersonal stress. Evaluations of outcome were conducted both at the end of the 12-week treatment period and 6 months later. The authors analyzed pre–post differences separately for the SST and DH groups after 12 weeks and found significant improvement for both groups in symptoms (ratings made blind to treatment group assignment), in patient self-ratings only for the DH group, and in specific measures of social skills only for the SST groups. No statistical comparisons between DH and SST are presented. There were no differences in rehospitalization rates during a 12-month follow-up period. At a 6-month assessment, a comparison of change from posttreatment to 6 months showed significant improvement in the SST group compared to DH alone in patient self-ratings and psychiatric symptoms but not specific social skills measures. However, attrition was substantial—only 35% of DH patients and 45% of the SST group were assessed at 6 months. With such a low follow-up rate, the question of biases in the group assessed is raised, particularly if there were differences in who was followed between the treatment groups. For example, since patients who are rehospitalized may be easier to locate, were such patients overrepresented in the control group?

With two exceptions—the Bellack study reviewed here and a study of family therapy and SST by one of us (G.E.H.) to be reviewed in the section on family therapy—the knowledge about SST for schizophrenia is based on studies conducted with male inpatients, primarily chronically hospitalized. To some degree this is because much of the work was carried out at VA hospitals, but even studies conducted in other hospital settings have been restricted to men. Whether results would be different for women is moot. Treatment studies of schizophrenia that included women and report gender effects suggest that there are differences both for antipsychotic drugs (12) and for psychosocial treatments (13). The studies we have reviewed indicate that SST leads to measurable changes in the specifically targeted behaviors such as eye contact and assertiveness and that these changes do reflect more substantial clinical outcome. How enduring that outcome is and its relationship to drug treatment remain largely unexplored.

Group Therapy

After reviewing the available literature on group therapy in schizophrenia in 1980, Mosher and Keith (30) concluded that a suitably controlled study was needed comparing group therapy to individual psychotherapy, with patient groups maintained and withdrawn from neuroleptic drugs. Neither that study nor any other that incorporates control conditions for both group therapy and drug treatment has been conducted. The only relevant study to appear that meets our criteria for review is a well-described trial conducted by Malm (28).

Eighty newly hospitalized schizophrenic patients who had signs and symptoms of autism, ego disturbance, and thought process disturbances were randomly assigned either to depot fluphenazine and a standard 3-month social skills training program or to an experimental program in which a year of communication-oriented group therapy was added to the standard package. Group therapy, designed to "increase ego awareness, verbal and emotional communication and to alleviate symptoms," was provided by experienced nurse clinicians without formal psychotherapy training.

On average, patients received about 10 mg weekly of fluphenazine decanoate in the first year. This was reduced to about 6 mg weekly in the second year. No information is provided about frequency of injections, but there were no dosage differences between the two groups.

Outcome was assessed for the 68 patients (34 in each group) who completed the 2-year study including 11 who had not had a full year of group therapy, a very conservative

data analytic strategy. Nevertheless, the experimental group showed significantly greater improvement in measures of emotional communication, anhedonia, free time activities, and "entry into the social field." When patients were further divided into more and less psychotic, the more psychotic patients in group therapy had more days out of hospital than the control group; among the less psychotic patients, the rate of remission was higher in the therapy group. However, there were no overall differences in course of illness between the two treatment groups. This is an important study incorporating some attractive design features. Assessment of outcome after a follow-up period for the group therapy during which patients were maintained on antipsychotic medication allows determination of the persistence of the effects. A number of therapists provided treatment so that the results cannot be linked to a particular therapist. Further, since all patients were maintained on fluphenazine decanoate and there were no dosage differences between treatment groups, the additive effects of group therapy to drug treatment are quite convincing.

Family Treatment

Perhaps the most striking characteristic of psychosocial treatment research during the past decade has been a renewed interest in treatment that involves families. In the first of these studies and the only one to include experimental variation of drug treatment, Goldstein and his colleagues (14) compared a brief 6-week crisis-oriented family therapy to no therapy in acutely ill schizophrenic patients, both men and women, discharged after brief (14-day) hospitalization. Patients were also randomized to either a fixed standard (25 mg) or low (6.25 mg) dose of fluphenazine enanthate every 2 weeks during the 6-week study. Therapy focused on acknowledgment of the illness, identification of possible precipitating and future stressors, and development of coping strategies. These still acutely ill patients were highly vulnerable to relapse; 10% relapsed during the 6-week period. The relapse rate was highest (24%) in the group that received low dose and no therapy. The group receiving standard dose and therapy experienced no relapses, and the remaining two groups (standard dose with no therapy or low dose with therapy) experienced the overall 10% rate. These results suggest an additive effect of drug and family therapy.

The same ordering of treatment groups persisted for 6 months with no relapses in the group receiving standard dose and therapy rising to 48% in the low-dose, no-therapy group. Effects on symptomatology are more complex and involve disordinal effects of dosage, therapy, sex, and premorbid functioning. However, a consistent positive benefit of family therapy both for men and women was found for withdrawal symptoms after 6 weeks. This benefit of family therapy persists after 6 months primarily in patients who received the higher dose. The 6-month outcome reflects a follow-up period during which treatment was not controlled. Virtually all effects of dosage on symptoms were dependent on sex. Men showed greater residual symptoms on high than low dose, and the reverse was true for women. Thus, if the study had included men only, or the data had not been examined for gender effects, very different conclusions would have been drawn.

Glick and his colleagues (11) randomly assigned newly hospitalized patients with schizophrenia ($N = 80$) or major affective disorders ($N = 64$) to a brief inpatient family intervention (IFI) or routine hospital care. Schizophrenic patients were further divided into groups with high and low prehospital functioning. Experimental subjects received at least six, but on average nine family sessions during a 5-week hospital stay. Treatment focused on acceptance and understanding of the illness, identification and management of stressors, and the need for continuing posthospital treatment. These goals are similar to those of Goldstein and his colleagues, and although Goldstein's patients were outpatients, their hospital stay was so short that patients in the two studies seem to be at a similar point in their illness. Medication was "balanced" between the two groups. The IFI group had a higher proportion of women than men, but no comparisons of outcome by sex are provided. Design of the study included assessment of outcome at discharge, 6-, and 18-month follow-up. Results have been reported for three-quarters of the sample through the 6-month follow-up on two global measures. Schizophrenic patients who showed higher levels of functioning prior to hospitalization showed significant benefit from IFI both at discharge and 6 months later. There were no treatment effects for the poorly functioning schizophrenic patients or for the affective disorder patients. The benefit of therapy solely for better-functioning patients is congruent with our own earlier results (13) and with other studies in the literature but not with the family treatment studies we review below.

Four more recent studies of family therapy have been stimulated by the concept of expressed emotion (EE) mentioned earlier in this review (22). Evidence from a number of sources suggests that the stimulation of cultural expectations in developed countries, the stress of developmental and other life experiences, and some "affects" associated with family life may represent natural environmental stressors, stimuli that could precipitate or exacerbate psychosis in vulnerable patients. Affects expressed by a family member toward a schizophrenic patient during a standardized interview focused on information about events and activities in the home as well as attitudes and feelings provide the measure of EE. High EE is characterized by criticism, hostility, and/or overinvolvement with the patient. Low EE is defined by an absence (or less than a threshold value) of the rated affective characteristics. A series of naturalistic studies has found that high familial EE at the time a patient is hospitalized with a schizophrenic illness is predictive of subsequent relapse. In several of these studies, the concurrent use of medication lessened the impact of high EE, especially when face-to-face contact with family members was reduced. In a focal study, Vaughn and Leff (38) reported 9-month relapse rates of 13% in patients from low-EE families contrasted to 51% in patients from high-EE families. However, within the high-EE group, patients who were maintained on medication and had less than 35 hr a week of face-to-face contact with their families relapsed at a rate comparable to the low-EE group (15%). Relapse rose to 92% for patients from high-EE homes who

experienced neither of these protective factors, an impressive finding.

These findings have been replicated in several studies, but in the largest attempted replication by one of us (G.E.H.) a main effect of EE was not observed (17). In this study, relapse was accounted for by medication (68% of those discontinued versus 34% of those maintained) and number of prior hospitalizations. The EE status was predictive of relapse for subsamples of the population, primarily for young men living in parental homes. Sex and age appear confounded with EE; young never-married men are more likely to live in high-EE homes, and older never-married women in low-EE homes.

Recently, four studies have used differing strategies of family treatment to approach families selected for high-EE status.

Leff and his colleagues (26) randomly assigned 24 schizophrenic patients from high-EE families to either a 9-month social intervention package or a control condition of routine outpatient care. Social intervention included education provided in the home, a relatives' group that focused on problems and included low-EE families, and a variable number of family sessions conducted in the home. An equal number of men and women were in the two treatment groups, but no analyses of sex differences are reported. Virtually all patients received long-acting injectable neuroleptics and are described as compliant. Treatment goals were to reduce EE and thereby lower relapse rates and improve patient functioning. Families in the social intervention group showed a significant reduction in the "critical comments" aspect of EE, suggesting that the intervention met its objective. Further, relapse in the experimental group was 9% in the 9-month period compared to 50% in the control group. In a 2-year follow-up of these patients restricted to those who remained on medication (27), 78% of the control group had relapsed compared to 20% in the experimental group. However, if the entire experimental group was considered, 50% had a poor outcome—relapse or suicide.

A study by Falloon and associates (8) included 36 schizophrenic outpatients at high risk for relapse either because of high EE or other environmental stressors. Patients were treated with "optimal" doses of antipsychotic medication and randomly assigned to receive either home-based behavioral family therapy (BFT), including education about the illness and training in communication skills and problem solving, or clinic-based, individual, supportive psychotherapy. After a 9-month treatment period, only one patient in the experimental group relapsed compared to eight in the control group. Significantly greater reductions in measures of symptom and burden and improvement in social functioning were found in the BFT group compared to the individual psychotherapy. Since medication was not experimentally controlled, both compliance with medication and drug dosage were examined as dependent variables. Compliance ratings were not different in the family and individually treated groups. Drug dosage tended to be lower in the BFT group; 245 mg of CPZ per day or equivalent compared to 338 mg/day for individually treated cases. There has been speculation that the mechanism of psychosocial treatment effects is through insuring compliance or higher levels of neuroleptic treatment. Although this study cannot provide evidence regarding independent effects of drug treatment, the family therapy effect goes beyond insurance of compliance or adequate dose and in fact suggests that dose reduction may be possible. In a 2-year uncontrolled follow-up (9), the advantage to the BFT patients persisted: 15 of the 18 controls experienced an episode of "florid" schizophrenia compared to two of the 18 BFT patients. Family treatment continued during this time at a supportive level, and some patients assigned to the individual treatment group were offered some family therapy sessions.

Nine-month analyses of an ongoing 2-year study of group therapy for high-EE families and patients have been reported by Kottgen and her colleagues (25). Three groups are compared: a high-EE group receiving therapy ($N = 16$) and two control groups—a high-EE group ($N = 14$) and a low-EE group ($N = 20$) that did not. First-episode patients were diagnosed as showing nuclear symptoms of schizophrenia with the Present State Examination (40). It appears that most of the therapy was conducted following discharge. No information is provided on drug treatment. Patients and families were seen in separated groups. The goals of treatment included resolution of painful situations using examples from everyday life, reduction of prejudice and negative expectations, exploration of the origins of critical and hostile overinvolvement, reduction of stress and isolation through mutual support, encouragement of autonomy, and provision of information about the illness and medication. Nine-month outcome showed no significant differences among the three groups: 33% relapsed in the experimental group compared to 53% in the combined control groups. Although inspired by the EE concept, the therapeutic goals and techniques of this group are different from those of the other investigators, emphasizing review of prior painful experiences and development of insight, which seems at odds with a goal of reducing high affect.

Most recently, one of us (G.E.H.) and colleagues have reported 1-year results of a study comparing family psychoeducation, social skills training, and their combination to maintenance antipsychotic medication in a 2-year outpatient study (17). Patients were diagnosed according to Research Diagnostic Criteria (RDC; 36) during hospitalization and assessed for EE status. High-EE patients were randomly assigned to one of two ongoing studies: the family treatment–social skills study and a maintenance drug dosage study. Patients in the psychosocial treatment study were further randomized to one of three conditions: family treatment ($N = 22$), social skills training ($N = 23$), or their combination ($N = 23$). All these patients received maintenance medication, in most cases injectable fluphenazine decanoate. Patients randomized to the drug dosage study were further randomized to maintenance with standard or reduced dosage. The standard dosage group ($N = 35$) in the dosage study also served as a "drug-alone" control group for the psychosocial treatment study. This novel strategy was designed to minimize the problem of "extra" attention that may be associated with control groups in psychosocial treatment studies that are of necessity

nonblind. Approximately half of the patients in the drug-alone control group were female, but only 25% of patients in the three psychosocial treatment groups, because more women refused to participate in the psychosocial treatment study.

The goals of both family treatment and social skills training were reduction of conflict and EE in the home: in the former by providing information about the illness and its management in individual family sessions; in the latter by increasing patient social competence in individual therapy sessions by changing behaviors believed to elicit high EE, particularly criticism, from families. Instruction, modeling, rehearsal, role play, and homework were used in SST.

Among patients who received either of the psychosocial treatments alone, relapse was approximately 20%, compared to those who received both (no relapse in the first year) or maintenance medication alone (41%). These differences are statistically significant and support an additive effect of the two psychosocial treatments. When analysis was restricted to patients compliant with medication, a significant effect of family treatment and the additive effects of both treatments were still seen. Neither dosage nor gender differences among treatment groups have been reported yet.

Three of the family treatment studies carried out with patients from high-EE families assessed changes in EE during the course of treatment and related this change to outcome. Leff and his colleagues (27) report that if EE or face-to-face contact was reduced, only one of seven patients relapsed in 2 years. Unfortunately, the interview to assess change was conducted at relapse (if that occurred during the 9-month period), thus continuing the confounding of the rating of EE with the symptomatic state of the patient. Hogarty et al. (17) provide the most detailed analysis of change in EE and its relationship to relapse. Family treatment was associated with a higher rate of reduction in EE (39%) compared to SST and controls (25%). However, regardless of treatment, there was no relapse in households that changed to low-EE status. Finally, Kottgen et al. (25) found that 70% of relatives change from high to low EE over an 18-month period. In contrast, relatives initially rated as low are stable over time. These data suggest a complex relationship between the patient's symptomatic state and EE.

On balance, results of studies of family treatment suggest that a wide range of approaches—behavioral, group, educational—are useful in long-term treatment of schizophrenia. Whether modification of the family emotional climate is the mechanism of action is unclear both because of problems in assessment and because all the studies, with the exception of Goldstein's and Glick's work, were restricted to families largely defined by high EE status. If these family approaches are successful with families not preselected for high EE status, some other mechanism must account for the effect.

DISCUSSION

Perhaps our most striking conclusion is that we have identified only two studies that incorporated full experimental controls both for drug and a psychosocial treatment in schizophrenia during the decade under review: Goldstein and his colleagues' two-factor study of family therapy and two dosages of fluphenazine enanthate (14) and our own study of sociotherapy and oral versus injectable fluphenazine (20). In neither study was the experimental control for drug treatment a "no-drug" group. In one study the difference was between oral and injectable medication, and in the other between two dose levels of the same drug. In both studies there are interactive as well as additive effects of medication and psychosocial treatment. Further, in both studies there are differences in treatment outcome for men and women, suggesting, as we have noted, the importance both of inclusion of men and women in studies of treatment in schizophrenia and the obvious corollary of analyzing data so as to evaluate rather than ignore possible sex differences in treatment outcome.

Although there have been few studies that had the capacity to assess the interaction of drug and psychosocial treatment during this past decade, important information to guide such studies in future has been accumulating. First, a number of the more recent studies provide evidence of medication compliance through use of parenteral administration, plasma assays, or careful pill counts in both the psychosocial experimental and control groups. In such studies it is possible to conclude that the effect of a psychosocial treatment is not "just" enhancement of compliance. Thus, these studies demonstrate a specific effect of psychosocial treatment beyond encouragement of medication adherence. For outpatients, differences in adjustment often appear to reflect differential relapse rates. Development of data analytic methods that disentangle relapse and adjustment represents both a conceptual and a methodologic challenge. If data from all patients are included, the adjustment generally mirrors relapse. Exclusion of relapsing patients restricts generalizability, particularly if one treatment has a very high relapse rate. For inpatient and short-term outpatient studies, benefits of psychosocial treatment seem to be stronger for better-functioning patients who have the psychological resources to benefit from the treatments.

Second, we now have cumulative development of information about two psychosocial treatments—social skills training and family therapy. Previously, few studies of psychosocial treatments systematically evaluated similar variables or treatments, so that integrating results across studies was difficult. Many of the studies of family therapy and social skills training include common elements: education about the illness, a focus on communication and other skills, and an emphasis on reality-based issues rather than insight and understanding. These studies are also more explicit about treatment procedures than an earlier generation was. Although none of them can boast formal treatment manuals, the studies by Hogarty and his colleagues (1) and Falloon and his colleagues (7) have resulted in volumes that provide an approximation of manuals for therapy. Both groups have explicit training methods, making the replication of these treatments in other studies and the transfer to clinical practice possible.

Where do we go from here? We can identify three broad areas that should be addressed. Two of these are within the purview of psychosocial treatment researchers. The first is the isolation of the specific elements of effective psychosocial therapies that make them effective. The second is the development of therapies to meet the needs of patients not served by available treatments. For example, the family treatment approaches described above are restricted to patients living with or involved with a high-EE family. The extension of these strategies to patients who live in low-EE families or have become isolated from their families represents a significant challenge.

The third research area is the study of drug and psychosocial treatments in studies that are capable of examining both additive and interactive effects of drug and psychosocial treatments. The National Institute of Mental Health has recently instituted such a study under the direction of one of us (N.R.S.) and Samuel J. Keith in collaboration with investigators at five hospitals (34). The drug treatment component compares standard antipsychotic drug maintenance treatment with two strategies for dosage reduction hypothesized to reduce risk of developing tardive dyskinesia. One group (standard dosage) receives fluphenazine decanoate in dosages between 12.5 and 50 mg biweekly. A second group (continuous low dose) receives between 2.5 and 10 mg biweekly. The third group (targeted) receives the injection vehicle only. Patients in all groups are administered open-label fluphenazine at the first signs of impending relapse. Studies employing both of these strategies are reviewed elsewhere in this volume.

Patients and their families also participate in one of two treatment approaches designed to improve social functioning and to buffer the increased risk for relapse incurred by reducing medication. The design of these treatments grows out of the studies reviewed above in the section on family treatment. Both treatment groups participate in an initial workshop designed to provide education about the illness, stress and its management, communications, and problem-solving skills modeled after the Survival Skills Workshop developed by Anderson and one of us (G.E.H.) (1) as well as monthly family group meetings. The elements represent the Supportive Family Management condition. In addition, patients and families in the Applied Family Management group participate in individual family sessions conducted in the home, modeled after the behavioral family therapy developed by Falloon and his colleagues (7). Although the elements of the psychosocial treatments were developed originally with the paradigm of EE in mind, this study tests their potential applicability to a wider range of families by including families without regard to EE status. This study represents a significant advance in research on treatment efficacy for schizophrenia. First, it is the first study begun in almost a decade that will be able to examine both additive and interactive effects of psychosocial and drug treatments for schizophrenia. Second, it builds directly on positive results of a generation of studies in both psychosocial and psychopharmacologic treatments.

There are many questions regarding the relationship of drug and existing psychosocial treatments that need to be addressed. The studies of social skills training we have reviewed show substantial evidence of efficacy, but we have little information on whether drug treatment (dosage?) enhances or restricts acquisition and retention. If the principles of the family interventions described can be extended to nonfamily groups and environments in which schizophrenic patients live and work, then these strategies will require assessment in relation to drug treatment.

Finally, we can expect both advances and consolidation of our understanding of the neurobiological basis of schizophrenic disorders in the coming years. Attention to these characteristics in both the development of psychosocial treatments and the matching of specific psychosocial treatment elements to specific neurobiological deficits may be possible in the next decade.

REFERENCES

1. Anderson, C. M., Reiss, D. J., and Hogarty, G. E. (1986): *Schizophrenia in the Family.* Guilford Press, New York.
2. Bellack, A. S., Turner, S. M., Hersen, M., and Luber, R. F. (1984): *Hosp. Commun. Psychiatry,* 35:1023–1028.
3. Brown, M. A., and Munford, A. M. (1983): *J. Nerv. Ment. Dis.,* 171:466–470.
4. Carpenter, W. T., Jr., Strauss, J. S., and Bartko, J. J. (1973): *Science,* 182:1275–1278.
5. Eisler, R. M., Blanchard, E. B., Fitts, H., and Williams, J. G. (1978): *Behav. Mod.,* 2:147–172.
6. Falloon, I. R. H. (1985): *Family Management of Schizophrenia.* Johns Hopkins University Press, Baltimore.
7. Falloon, I. R. H., Boyd, J. L., and McGill, C. W. (1984): *Family Care of Schizophrenia: A Problem Solving Treatment for Mental Illness.* Guilford Press, New York.
8. Falloon, I. R. H., Boyd, J. L., McGill, C. W., Razani, J., Moss, H. B., et al. (1982): *N. Engl. J. Med.,* 306:1437–1440.
9. Falloon, I. R. H., Boyd, J. L., McGill, C. W., Williamson, M., Razani, J., et al. (1985): *Arch. Gen. Psychiatry,* 42:887–896.
10. Falloon, I. R. H., Watt, D. C., and Shepherd, M. (1978): *Psychol. Med.,* 8:59–70.
11. Glick, I. D., Clarkin, J. F., Spencer, J. H., Haas, G. L., Lewis, A. B., et al. (1985): *Arch. Gen. Psychiatry,* 42:882–886.
12. Goldberg, S. C., Schooler, N. R., Davidson, E. M., and Kayce, M. (1966): *Psychopharmacologia,* 9:31–47.
13. Goldberg, S. C., Schooler, N. R., Hogarty, G. E., and Roper, M. (1977): *Arch. Gen. Psychiatry,* 34:171–184.
14. Goldstein, M. J., Rodnick, E. H., Evans, J. R., May, P. R. A., and Steinberg, M. R. (1978): *Arch. Gen. Psychiatry,* 35:1169–1177.
15. Gunderson, J. G., Frank, A. F., Katz, H. M., Vannicelli, M. L., Frosch, J. P., et al. (1984): *Schizophrenia Bull.,* 10:564–584.
16. Hargreaves, W. A., Glick, I. D., Drues, J., Showstack, J. A., and Feigenbaum, E. (1977): *Arch. Gen. Psychiatry,* 34:305–311.
17. Hogarty, G. E., Anderson, C. M., Reiss, D. J., Kornblith, S. J., Greenwald, D. P., et al. (1986): *Arch. Gen. Psychiatry,* 43:633–642.
18. Hogarty, G. E., Goldberg, S. C., and Schooler, N. R. (1974): *Arch. Gen. Psychiatry,* 31:609–618.
19. Hogarty, G. E., Goldberg, S. C., Schooler, N. R., and Ulrich, R. F. (1974): *Arch. Gen. Psychiatry,* 31:603–608.
20. Hogarty, G. E., Schooler, N. R., Ulrich, R., Mussare, F., and Herron, E. (1979): *Arch. Gen. Psychiatry,* 36:1283–1294.
21. Hogarty, G. E., and Ulrich, R. F. (1976): *Arch. Gen. Psychiatry,* 33:297–301.
22. Hooley, J. M. (1985): *Clin. Psychol. Rev.,* 5:119–139.
23. Kane, J. M., and Borenstein, M. (1985): *Psychopharmacol. Bull.,* 21:23–27.
24. Klein, D. F. (1980): *Schizophrenia Bull.,* 6:122–130.
25. Kottgen, C., Sonnichsen, I., Mollenhauer, K., and Jurth, R. (1984): *Int. J. Fam. Psychiatry,* 5:84–94.
26. Leff, J., Kuipers, L., Berkowitz, R., Eberlein-Vries, R., and Sturgeon, D. (1982): *Br. J. Psychiatry,* 141:121–134.
27. Leff, J., Kuipers, L., Berkowitz, R., and Sturgeon, D. (1985): *Br. J. Psychiatry,* 146:594–600.
28. Malm, U. (1982): *Acta Psychiatr. Scand. [Suppl.],* 297:1–65.
29. May, P. R. A. (1967): In: *Psychopharmacology: A Review of Progress 1957–1967,* edited by D. H. Efron, pp. 1155–1176. Government Printing Office, Washington.
30. Mosher, L. J., and Keith, S. J. (1980): *Schizophrenia Bull.,* 6:10–41.
31. Paul, G. L., and Lentz, R. J. (1977): *Psychosocial Treatment of Chronic Mental Patients.* Harvard University Press, Cambridge.
32. Rifkin, A., Quitkin, F., Rabiner, C. J., and Klein, D. F. (1977): *Arch. Gen. Psychiatry,* 34:43–47.
33. Schooler, N. R. (1978): In: *Psychopharmacology: A Generation of Progress,* edited by M. A. Lipton, A. DiMascio, and K. F. Killam, pp. 1155–1168. Raven Press, New York.
34. Schooler, N. R., and Keith, S. J. (1983): *Treatment Strategies in Schizophrenia Study Protocol.* National Institute of Mental Health, Rockville, MD.
35. Schooler, N. R., Levine, J., Severe, J. B., Brauzer, B., DiMascio, A., et al. (1980): *Arch. Gen. Psychiatry,* 37:16–24.
36. Spitzer, R. L., Endicott, J., and Robins, E. (1978): *Research Diagnostic Criteria for a Selected Group of Functional Disorders,* third ed. New York State Psychiatric Institute, New York.
37. Stanton, A. H., Gunderson, J. G., Knapp, P. H., Frank, A. F., Vannicelli, M. L., et al. (1984): *Schizophrenia Bull.,* 10:520–551.
38. Vaughn, C. E., and Leff, J. P. (1976): *Br. J. Psychiatry,* 129:125–137.
39. Wallace, C. J., and Liberman, R. P. (1985): *Psychiatry Res.,* 15:239–247.
40. Wing, J. K., Cooper, J. E., and Sartorius, N. (1974): *The Measurement and Classification of Psychiatric Symptoms.* Cambridge University Press, London.

Psychopharmacology:
The Third Generation of Progress,
edited by Herbert Y. Meltzer.
Raven Press, New York © 1987.

CHAPTER **115**

The Phenomenology and Course of Schizophrenia: Treatment Implications

William T. Carpenter, Jr.

In the first edition of this volume, May and Goldberg (52) reviewed research relevant to predicting the schizophrenic patient's response to pharmacotherapy. They noted a number of factors of prognostic significance in schizophrenia such as premorbid adjustment. These factors interact with drug response, and maximum drug/placebo differences are observed in the prognostic mid-range. A number of seemingly discrete factors may relate to patient response to the antipsychotic neuroleptic drugs (e.g., females have a larger drug/placebo response difference), but these factors seem continuous (e.g., males also have a robust drug/ placebo response difference), and between-subject variability is great. Also, although not subjected to extensive empirical research, it is evident from clinical observation that within-subject variability of drug response occurs over time. Similar problems mitigate progress in defining pharmacodynamics or pharmacokinetic predictors of drug response. May and Goldberg were able to summarize that "there are probably two subgroups who perhaps should not receive drugs. The first is a subgroup who do well in the community without drugs, and the second a subgroup who do poorly in general and are not helped further by drugs. The trouble is that at present we have no certain way to identify either group." Although those who do well without drugs remain to be identified, interesting recent work suggests that endocrine, pharmacologic, radiologic, and phenomenologic tools may define individuals most vulnerable to relapse or most likely to be drug resistant.

Brown and Laughren (3) report data suggesting that serum prolactin levels during antipsychotic drug therapy sometimes fail to demonstrate the elevation expected from postsynaptic dopamine blockade. These cases appear more vulnerable to early relapse. Lieberman and colleagues (48,49)

report an inverse correlation between symptom exacerbation with a methylphenyldate challenge and time to relapse. These initiatives suggest a dopaminergic/symptom interaction germane to pharmacotherapy. Van Putten and May (76) report that neuroleptic-induced dysphoria predicts poor therapeutic response to antipsychotic drugs in patients hospitalized for treatment of a psychotic episode. Weinberger (78) has reported that patients with high ventricle-to-brain ratios measured on CT scan are poor drug responders, and Crow (18) uses poor drug response as a defining characteristic of type II schizophrenia. Long-term low-dose strategies also suggest some difference in prophylaxis between very low dose and standard dose, suggesting that it may still prove possible to define the minimal drug blood concentration associated with treatment response, but no guidelines are now available. Despite promising initiatives during the past 10 years, we do not presently have tools that can be applied with confidence to the prediction of treatment response of the individual patient.

The situation is comparable when addressing the question of differential pharmacotherapy in schizophrenia. Extensive efforts to ascertain therapeutic differences among the antipsychotic neuroleptic drugs has led to the conclusion that principal differences reside in side effect profiles. Direct therapeutic effects are quite similar across compounds despite occasional interesting hypotheses to the contrary (27). May and Goldberg (52) conclude that "The association of patient subtypes with response to different neuroleptics cannot be considered sufficiently established to be theoretically or practically useful." Little subsequent work in this area has been reported, and there is no basis for present revision of this conclusion. There is, however, considerable interest in the possibility that atypical neuroleptics now being studied will be substantially safer than presently approved compounds.

Another area receiving increasing attention concerns subgroups of the schizophrenia syndrome that may be responsive to psychotherapeutic drugs other than neuroleptic antipsychotic medication. This area has been recently reviewed by Donaldson and colleagues (20). Although some patients appear responsive to alternative drugs, no success in defining these subgroups has yet been achieved.

The intense study of differential drug effects, predictors of drug response, and treatment-specific subtypes of schizophrenia, which waxed in the 1960s and 1970s, has waned in the 1980s. This effort has given way to a reexamination of the disease manifestations and course characteristics associated with the clinical syndrome of schizophrenia, a recognition of the heterogeneity of the syndrome, and the study of integrated treatment approaches. From these considerations emanate more complex strategies for clinical therapeutics, with emphasis on phase of illness, individual differences, and empirical observation of each patient's response dispositions.

Ideally, the treatment of schizophrenia is based on an appreciation of the phenomenology and course of illness in each individual patient. This includes ascertainment of those descriptive features germane to an accurate differential diagnosis as the first step in treatment planning. The clinician must go far beyond these descriptive factors, however, in determining optimal treatment for each patient. The nature of the course of illness, the phase in its development, the particular constellation of symptoms, the personality in whom they are manifest, and the interaction of the illness with psychological and social milieu must all be considered in determining an appropriate treatment strategy. It is important, therefore, to appreciate the richness and variability of phenomena emanating through the schizophrenia process and to understand the interactions of these phenomena over time in shaping the course and ultimate outcome of the illness.

Schizophrenia may be conceptualized as a clinical syndrome (24,56) within the context of a developmental, interactive medical model (7,8,72), and both the syndromal status and the medical model (21) have implications for treatment. It is through knowledge of the behavior and subjective experience of an individual, interpreted in the context of a scientifically valid medical model, that the specificity of treatment decisions can be articulated and treatment-relevant subgroups identified. The discussion to follow thus provides overviews of phenomenology, course, the medical model, and clinical syndrome as a general background to treatment considerations.

PHENOMENOLOGY

Jaspers (35) brought the philosophic tradition of phenomenology into the action-oriented arena of medicine. Psychiatric phenomenology refers to description, classification, and understanding of the subjective experiences of illness. These are the data most germane to the care and study of patients with schizophrenia and from which we appreciate the form, content, and circumstances of psycho-pathologic expression. An understanding of this material is shaped by consideration of the individual's life story and expanded through the use of correlational techniques of medical sciences, which elucidate underlying mechanisms by examining their coexistence and cause-and-effect relationships (56). The phenomenology associated with schizophrenia is rich and varied. The content of inner experiences is extensively determined by the person's personality, culture, and interactions with the environment. This is meaningfully (as distinguished from causally) (35) related to the individual and his/her personal history.

The form (e.g., somatic hallucination) rather than content of subjective experience seems to derive more directly from illness and, as such, plays a critical role in differential diagnosis and the assessment of treatment effects. It is not yet clear how many distinct psychopathologic processes are associated with the schizophrenia syndrome. An atomistic approach would consider each form as distinct. Hallucinatory phenomena in each sense modality would be distinguished from each other and from each form of disordered thought process, and so forth. For convenience in organizing data, and because psychometric and conceptual approaches to the data suggest that some forms cluster together, it has been useful to describe the manifestation of schizophrenia under three general headings: positive symptoms, negative symptoms, and social manifestations (61). Motor aberrations comprise an informative fourth category (25,41,47).

Positive, or expressive, symptomatology refers to those psychopathologic processes that appear to be exaggerations or disinhibitions of normal processes. Hallucinations, delusions, pressured speech, and excessive or painful affect would be examples of positive symptoms. The most blatant manifestations of schizophrenia that demarcate the psychotic process are positive symptoms. As such, they have been the focus of diagnostic and treatment considerations. They have often been thought to provide an adequate definition of nuclear schizophrenia, with implications of a deteriorating process and poor prognosis (42,63). However, it has been established that within the psychotic classes of illness, positive symptomatology has only modest prognostic implication (9,16,31,39,69). Differentiating the prognoses in schizophrenia from those of other psychoses requires an ascertainment of developmental history, pattern and course of illness, and psychopathologic features other than positive symptoms (e.g., prepsychotic asociality) (4,53,62,67,70,71,74).

Negative symptoms may be conceptualized as the absence or diminution of ordinary functions (61,62). Absence of social drive, lack of sense of purpose, diminished curiosity and spontaneity, and restricted or blunted emotional arousal are examples. Since negative symptoms may emanate from a variety of causes (e.g., drug side effects, depression), it is useful to define schizophrenic deficit symptomatology as those negative symptoms that are present as enduring traits and do not appear to be secondary to other conditions (13). Such symptoms account for much of the long-term impairment observed in patients with schizophrenia, and deficit processes are central to prognosis.

Social symptomatology is a more ambiguous area where observed psychopathology is revealed through its impact on social role performance (e.g., occupational impairment, social withdrawal). Such symptoms may emanate from both positive and negative psychopathologic processes. For example, social withdrawal may be a consequence of either paranoid ideation or lack of social drive. It may be a consequence of illness, in the sense that social engagement skills and gratifications are curbed because of the presence of chronic illness, or this type of symptomatology may relate more directly to distinct psychopathologic processes. The response of others to a person chronically burdened with a stigmatizing illness also determines manifestations in this area of symptomatology and behavior. Treatment considerations largely derive from presumptions regarding proximal causation. For example, social withdrawal in floridly psychotic patients vulnerable to social overstimulation may be a coping device reactive to the psychotic process. In such a case, pharmacotherapy of the psychosis may simultaneously reduce social dysfunction. This is not the case, however, when social withdrawal is based on a deficit in social drive.

Motor symptomatology (1,25,41,47,50) in schizophrenia includes a wide variety of alterations observable in a clinical neurological examination. Manifestations such as posturing, stiffness, facial grimacing, and dyskinesia, among others, may be secondary to drug side effects. However, preneuroleptic descriptions of schizophrenia make it clear that a similar variety of motor manifestations was observed in patients prior to pharmacotherapy, and catatonia was viewed by Kraepelin as a subtype of schizophrenia (41). Presently, motor symptomatology is particularly (68) important as a potential guide to anatomic localization and may prove important in ascertaining the relationship between early risk factors (e.g., birth and pregnancy complications) and brain structural alterations in schizophrenia.

Conceptualizing psychopathologic manifestations of schizophrenia in these separate domains is useful in clarifying the objectives of treatment and in assessing the limitations of each treatment approach (6). Until recently, pharmacotherapeutic strategies were evaluated exclusively with respect to impact on positive symptoms or on negative symptoms solely in the context of active psychotic processes (14). As a consequence, few empirical data are available in the literature on the long-term drug effects on negative or deficit symptomatology or on social or motor symptomatology. Taxonomic criteria have shifted from an almost exclusive focus on positive symptoms to an emphasis on deficit symptoms. This shift has important implications for pharmacologic treatment strategies, since diagnosis is now based less on those illness attributes most likely to be treatment responsive and more on longitudinal psychopathologic processes for which robust treatment effects are not presently available.

COURSE

The view of the course of illness in schizophrenia has undergone considerable revision in recent years. Both Kraeplin (41) and Bleuler (1), early in this century, observed a downhill course and poor outcome in the majority of patients with dementia preacox, the group of schizophrenias. However, both of these pioneers observed cases of good improvement and recovery and recognized that course was not progressive throughout life in a substantial proportion of cases. Many workers felt that certain constellations of psychotic symptoms indicated the presence of a psychotic illness with deteriorating course and poor outcome (42,63). It is now clear that various psychopathologic domains in schizophrenia are only loosely linked and that a longitudinal view of each domain is necessary to achieve a robust prediction of course and outcome (2,54,64,70). Past social functioning is a good predictor of future social functioning but a poor predictor of future positive symptoms status. Exacerbation of illness requiring hospitalization is predicted by the extent to which hospital treatment has been necessary in the past but is not predicted by prior occupational or social functioning. A past pattern of positive symptoms would be a good predictor of a future pattern of positive symptoms (80) but a poor predictor of deficit symptomatology.

Contributing to the recognition of the diversity of psychopathologic development within the individual patient is the observation that the individual tends to progress to maximum symptom manifestation within the first 5 to 10 years of illness (2,17). However, the phenomenon of late improvement has now been described by several workers, suggesting that even chronically impaired cases may show areas of improvement associated with aging (2,17,29,30,34). Another consideration is the typology of course per se. From the vantage of the European long-term follow-up of schizophrenic patients, several discrete patterns of illness can be characterized, with meaningful implications for treatment (17). Some patients gradually proceed into psychosis from a long-standing background of poor development and negative symptomatology and may never manifest full recovery. Others become abruptly psychotic without displaying evidence of prior morbidity. They show rapid response to treatment and good recovery, sometimes without subsequent positive symptom episodes. Others with a similarly rapid onset run a devastating course of illness. This diversity of pattern belies the hope of viewing schizophrenia, as presently defined, as a disease entity wherein patients have extensive similarity with respect to the nature of onset, symptom manifestation, treatment response, course, and presumed cerebral pathology.

Finally, it has become clear that the syndrome of schizophrenia is associated with considerable variability in ultimate outcome, including, on the one hand, substantial numbers of patients who manifest severe deterioration over time and, on the other, cases who show remarkable improvement and relatively modest illness-related impairment in the long term.

SCHIZOPHRENIA IN THE CONTEXT OF THE MEDICAL MODEL

Engel (21) has criticized reductionistic approaches in medicine and calls particular attention to the limitation of the biomedical model in defining the range of relevant information for the study of disease and care of patients. This criticism can aptly be applied to schizophrenic illnesses. There have been a number of competing models put forward within the context of medical practice. They have attempted to develop an understanding of schizophrenia at one level of explanation (e.g., biological, psychological, or social) by excluding from consideration data not readily incorporated within the scope of the dominant theory. A broader medical model appears more scientifically valid, and Engel has articulated the implications of general systems theory in biology for conceptualizing illness within the medical framework (21). This biopsychosocial medical model incorporates a range of data that would otherwise require multiple models and does so in an integrative framework that assumes that perturbations at any level of organization have effects within other levels. For example, a treatment intervention initiated at the subcellular level (e.g., neuroleptic drug action at neuronal synapses) will have influences throughout higher levels of organization (e.g., nervous system, subjective experience, social functioning), just as a treatment initiated at the social level (e.g., family intervention) can be expected to modify subordinate levels such as the patient's subjective experience and functioning attributes of the nervous system.

There are several implications of the biopsychosocial model for the care and study of patients with schizophrenia. First, operating concepts must integrate biological, psychological, and social data. Second, treatment interventions will not be conceptualized solely at the level of initiation, thus expanding the range of observation relevant to ascertaining treatment mechanisms and effects. Third, although treatments may be distinguished by the operations of initiation, as psychotherapy is distinguished from pharmacotherapy, the effect of treatment at each functional level is a matter for empirical investigation. This model discourages the a priori assumption that treatments initiated at different levels (or based on different theories of illness) are dissimilar in their functional consequences.

A developmental view within this medical framework enables the integration of a number of early risk factors documented in schizophrenia (e.g., prenatal and birth complications, genetic factors, winter birth) with developmental processes leading to vulnerability to illness (15). A stress diathesis hypothesis has been put forward to illuminate the influence of environmental stress on the occurrence of manifest illness (60,66). This hypothesis separates factors associated with etiology of illness from factors that determine the probability and timing of manifest illness.

CLINICAL SYNDROME

The fact that there is heterogeneity within schizophrenia with regard to onset, symptom manifestation, pattern of course, and ultimate outcome argues against schizophrenia, as presently defined, being a single disease entity. The presence of multiple risk factors, some of which appear unrelated, further strengthens the view that schizophrenia is a heterogeneous syndrome comprising multiple disease entities. Some would argue that a disease entity cannot be confirmed in the absence of specific tissue pathology (56). It is sufficient for the present purposes merely to argue that there is little basis for presuming that any current definition of schizophrenia results in a cohort of patients with uniformity of etiology, pathogenesis, illness manifestation, course,

treatment response, or cerebral pathology. If syndromal status is accepted for diagnostic purposes, it is evident that treatment of the individual case becomes highly dependent on specific manifestations rather than on diagnostic classification per se.

PRELIMINARY CONCLUSIONS

The following conclusions relevant to treatment derive from the above considerations:

1. Schizophrenia is a clinical syndrome with diverse etiology, pathogenesis, symptom manifestation, course, and outcome. The age of onset and impact of illness vary tremendously from patient to patient.
2. Only first-order approximations of treatment requirements emerge from differential diagnoses. A broad phenomenologic perspective of the individual case is necessary for implementing treatment.
3. The general systems-based medical model implies a necessity to consider treatment intervention as being initiated at different levels of the functioning organism. Within this model, treatment strategies are derived in an integrated framework, and the various treatment modalities are not prejudged as alternatives or mutually exclusive.
4. Because the domains of psychopathology within the schizophrenia syndrome are only modestly correlated, a robust treatment effect in one domain may not be beneficial in others. Because the nature of the illness shifts over time within the individual patient, optimal treatment for one phase of illness may be inappropriate in another.
5. Most definitions of schizophrenia skew the illness toward chronicity, with long-standing functional impairment. Most treatment research has been based on short-term paradigms. We do not presently have a comprehensive data-based framework for understanding the long-range therapeutics of schizophrenia.

Presently popular restrictive diagnostic criteria for schizophrenia create many cases that fall into poorly defined, equivocal diagnostic classes (e.g., DSM-III psychoses not elsewhere classified) or widen the boundaries of the affective disorders to create a large and unwieldy class. Many of these cases will be treated with antipsychotic drugs. The following discussion of treatment is sufficiently broad to include those psychoses requiring pharmacotherapy usually reserved for schizophrenia.

TREATMENT IMPLICATIONS

Despite the fact that the effectiveness of neuroleptic drugs in schizophrenia has led to a biochemical hypothesis of illness (5,57,65,66), pharmacotherapy has continued to be based entirely on empirical evidence of effectiveness. The antipsychotic drugs have a demonstrable effect on positive symptom expressions in most, but not all, psychotic patients (57). In addition to acute management and therapeutic considerations, the long-term use of these medications stabilizes the clinical picture and decreases the rate of psychotic exacerbation (28).

In the presence of acute and florid psychotic symptoms,

a broad range of psychopathologic responsivity is observed, including improvement in negative symptoms. However, during periods of clinical stability, it has not yet been demonstrated that antipsychotic drugs are therapeutically efficacious for the deficit syndrome or for long-standing social or motor symptomatology. These considerations reveal that the greatest benefit-to-risk profile is seen in the context of florid positive symptoms and in circumstances in which frequent psychotic exacerbation can be anticipated.

A differential diagnosis is particularly relevant in identifying patients with chronic exacerbating illnesses where long-term pharmacotherapy with antipsychotic drugs is warranted. These cases are to be distinguished from those in classes of illness for which effective alternative pharmacotherapy is available (e.g., lithium prophylaxis in bipolar affective disorder) and from those that are not highly vulnerable to recurrent exacerbations (e.g., single episode patients and late phase patients no longer manifesting an episodic course). In such instances, pharmacotherapeutic strategies can be based on the course of illness data. For example, on the basis of long-term follow-up studies of Bleuler (1) and Ciompi (17), it appears that about 25 to 30% of schizophrenic cases have a good premorbid development followed by an acute onset of psychosis and remission of the illness. Most cases proceed to subsequent episodes that are not always followed by good recovery. However, about 10% prove to have only the single episode. These patients will not benefit from long-term prophylactic antipsychotic drugs. Hence, this subgroup of patients merits only short-term antipsychotic drug therapy (19) with follow-up over time off medication and pharmacotherapeutic intervention at first signs of a second episode (12). Efforts to define this population in clinical practice can be based on descriptive factors (e.g., premorbid development, catatonic and affective features admixed with psychosis, quality of recovery).

Another instance of course consideration is based on Bleuler's observation that aging has a tranquilizing effect on illness (1). About half of the patients progress to relatively stable "end states" with moderate to severe illness. However, the course is less punctuated by psychotic exacerbations, and aging reduces the need for the calming effects of drugs. Also, the patient may be more able to relate to others and show improvement in role functioning. During this phase, the risks associated with antipsychotic drugs are increased, and benefits are reduced. Hence, drug reduction or drug elimination strategies are recommended for these patients during this phase of illness.

The presumption that different pathologic mechanisms are involved in the various disease manifestations comprising the schizophrenia syndrome suggests a therapeutic role for drugs other than antipsychotic neuroleptics. Although this area has received only preliminary exploration, the clinician dealing with a patient who is unresponsive to antipsychotic medication or in whom the risks of such medication are considerable may wish to evaluate the short-term efficacy of other psychoactive drugs in the context of individualized treatment. Based on phenomenologic and course assessment, patients displaying symptoms similar to behavioral dyscontrol phenomena having a putative ictal basis may merit a trial with antiseizure medication (20,58). Patients with

affective instability, a family history of affective disorder, and important components of depression or mania in the presenting picture may merit a trial with lithium (20). Patients with emerging tardive dyskinesia who appear to require neuroleptic drugs for clinical stability may merit a trial with clonidine or benzodiazepine therapy as a possible alternative to the neuroleptic (26,40,77,79,81). Admittedly, in each of these instances, evidence of efficacy is scant, and the guidelines are not confirmed. However, where the risk of neuroleptic treatment outweighs benefit, using an alternative medication in brief empirical trials with selected cases is justified even if only a small proportion of patients prove responsive. Considering the heterogeneity of schizophrenia, this is an especially appropriate strategy. Pertinent information on the use of clinical manifestations to guide the clinician in drug selection has recently been reviewed (20).

The relatively high risk of tardive dyskinesia associated with long-term administration of antipsychotic drugs has prompted innovative drug reduction strategies in neuroleptic-responsive patients. Recent controlled clinical trials support the hypothesis that drug benefits can be achieved despite a substantial reduction in medication administration. Continuous low-dose strategies and symptom-targeted intermittent pharmacotherapy appear to achieve results approximating those of continuous standard dose therapy in a substantial proportion of patients with schizophrenia (12,32,33,37,38,46,51,59). Known risk for tardive dyskinesia (36,73) and hypothesized risk for the deficit syndrome with long-term antipsychotic drug use (50) provide a basis for the clinician to attempt drug reduction strategies in pharmacotherapeutic management. Although such an approach appears suitable for a majority of schizophrenic patients, especially appropriate candidates would include patients who are beginning to manifest evidence of dyskinesia and patients with infrequent, gradual, or nonsevere relapse patterns. The use of long-term antipsychotic medication for prophylactic purposes may not be warranted in single-episode patients prior to evidence of the presence of a relapsing illness (19), and targeting the administration of drugs to the appearance of prodromal symptoms can safeguard those who do proceed to a relapse. Similarly, patients become more vulnerable to dyskinesia and less vulnerable to recurrent florid psychotic exacerbations as they age; hence, a shift in the benefit-to-risk ratio gradually takes place over time.

The circumstances under which pharmacotherapy is undertaken should contribute to the determination of an appropriate strategy. Although biochemical effects of the drugs are initiated at the subcellular level, the process of pharmacotherapy is initiated in the context of the doctor/patient relationship. Some patients, for example, have a history of noncompliance to medication, and alternative strategies based on patient attitude may be necessary. Also, alternative drugs, low-dose regimens, and targeted early intervention strategies may prove helpful in patients who refuse continuous neuroleptic antipsychotic drugs because of unpleasant side effects.

The clinician also considers factors extraneous to the illness in making pharmacotherapeutic decisions. For example, patients vulnerable to relapse who live in highly emotion-arousing circumstances may show considerable benefit with prophylactic medication. Conversely, patients who live in low-arousal circumstances may not require the same degree of prophylactic protection from drugs (43,44) and may find their quality of life and functioning capabilities enhanced off medication (55,75).

Some typologic distinctions within the schizophrenia syndrome have apparent treatment implications. The type I and type II distinction put forward by Crow (18) and the related concept of deficit and nondeficit schizophrenia (15,50) may define patients who differ with respect to treatment responsivity. Although these concepts may not go beyond indicating that poor-prognosis patients are not as treatment responsive as good-prognosis patients, Leff and Wing (45) believe that maximum drug benefits are achieved in the midprognosis range. Evans and colleagues (22) have provided preliminary evidence that good-prognosis, nonparanoid patients have a brisker therapeutic response and reach a higher level of adjustment from a treatment strategy that does not initially rely on neuroleptic medication, whereas poor-prognosis patients and paranoid patients require early treatment with antipsychotic drugs. The use of clinical data defining treatment-relevant subgroups in planning an individual's pharmacotherapy has been detailed elsewhere (11).

With regard to the integration of treatment, the general systems concept and the stress diathesis hypothesis point toward the likelihood of diverse treatment interventions taking place simultaneously at several levels of initiation. This concept has recently been reinforced by the results of clinical trials indicating additive or synergistic interactions between interpersonal and pharmacotherapeutic strategies. A review of this literature has been published recently (23), and a large-scale NIMH multicenter collaboration comparing three drug administration strategies within the context of two interpersonal strategies promises new information on the integration of treatments and on the identification of treatment-relevant subgroups (N. Schooler and S. Keith, *unpublished data*, 1983).

FUTURE DEVELOPMENTS

The past 10 years has been a period of consolidation in the pharmacotherapy of schizophrenia. The polemics of drug versus psychotherapy in the treatment of schizophrenia have unequivocally given way to the acceptance of pharmacotherapy and the development of strategies for integrating interpersonal and pharmacologic treatments. The limitations and risks of antipsychotic drug therapy have been elucidated; the use of these drugs has been sharply curtailed in disorders other than schizophrenia; and safer strategies for the drug therapy of schizophrenia have been introduced.

The development of effective new drugs for schizophrenia has been difficult. The number of dopamine-blocking neuroleptic drugs on the market has multiplied, but they appear to share a common mode of therapeutic action and differ principally in side-effect profiles. Atypical neuroleptics with more specific sites of action are currently being evaluated and appear promising for preventing extrapyramidal side effects. Psychoactive drugs effective in such disorders as depression, mania, epilepsy, hypertension, and anxiety may prove useful in selected cases but do not represent a breakthrough in the treatment of schizophrenia. New strategies aimed at reducing the risks of antipsychotic drugs while maintaining benefits have been favorably reported; however, no effective treatment for the chronic patient unresponsive to neuroleptic drugs has been successfully developed.

Substantial progress is anticipated in the prediction of pharmacotherapeutic responsiveness. Methods for subdividing the schizophrenia syndrome can be implemented and the treatment-related merits of various subdivisions assessed. Also, previously unaddressed attributes of illness, such as enduring deficit symptoms, are becoming the object of therapeutic initiatives. The relationship of risk factors to therapeutic response will be scrutinized, working on the assumption that risk factors may define different pathogenic processes. Pedigree loading for schizophrenia and related processes, the excess in winter births and in birth and pregnancy complications, a variety of developmental deviations, and familial communication deviancy and affective style illustrate markers of interest in risk paradigms and merit investigation to determine therapeutic relevance.

Tools associated with clinical neurology, neuropsychology, and brain imaging will increasingly be employed to identify subtypes of schizophrenia associated with structural brain changes, alterations in information processing, and clinical neurologic signs. Preliminary evidence already associates structural brain changes with diminished treatment responsivity (78). Putative biologic markers will be examined for their potential in predicting treatment response. Some, such as diminished prolactin response to neuroleptic drugs and symptom increase on methylphenidate challenge, already appear promising in identifying patients with heightened vulnerability to relapse (3,49). Similarly, information-processing tasks and environmental assessment tools will be increasingly used to subdivide schizophrenia into meaningful treatment response categories.

The material reviewed above encourages a shift in the concept of psychopathology in schizophrenia. Implications for future work include, first, recognition that domains of psychopathology in schizophrenia may be only weakly related or orthogonal. Present thinking defines deficit psychopathology as distinct from positive symptoms. Whereas the latter symptoms have guided clinical investigations of pharmacotherapy and provide the basis for a neuropsychopharmacologic-derived dopamine hypothesis of schizophrenia, the former symptoms may represent the core psychopathology of schizophrenia as defined by Kraepelin and Bleuler. The deficit domain contributes most heavily to the long-term burden of illness. As such, it merits special scrutiny in the next generation of research in schizophrenia.

Second, it is now evident that disturbed perception, thought, and emotion underlying disruptive subjective experiences and referred to as psychotic aberrations are not pathognomonic of a diagnostic class. Psychotic symptoms and antipsychotic drug reactivity do not adhere to specific nosologic boundaries of classes of psychotic illnesses. The study of the etiology, pathogenesis, and therapeutics of psychosis may be hampered by presumptions of the distinctiveness of psychosis per se. The psychobiology of psychosis and the relevance of drug-induced psychosis as models for illness may best be applied to psychosis generically rather than schizophrenia specifically. Development of models, exploration of psychobiology and therapeutics, and the study of risk factors as illness specific may focus on core features of illness (e.g., deficit syndrome) that may be more informative in defining putative disease entities.

Third, the observed stabilization and, at times, improved condition of chronic patients as they age raise issues of different pharmacologic effects associated with age. Research on special therapeutic requirements and special risks (e.g., dyskinesia, sedation) in elderly patients will no doubt provide important new information of clinical relevance to the rapidly growing numbers of elderly patients with schizophrenia. The fact that course of illness alters with the aging process may provide a clue to pathophysiology, as surely must be the case with the age of onset of schizophrenia. Neither of these age-related phenomena has yet been explained.

TWO CAVEATS

In chronic illness, longitudinal designs are necessary to assess adequately the impact of the illness over time. In schizophrenia, a variety of pressures, opportunities, and misconceptions have led to an emphasis on acute paradigms in treatment research. Evidence from pre- and postneuroleptic comparisons and from the European long-term follow-up studies suggests that the decisive short-term effects of pharmacotherapy are not generally translated into a long-term impact on outcome of illness. We are not presently knowledgeable with respect to the long-term interaction between antipsychotic medication and the deficit syndrome in schizophrenia. It is important to provide a suitably broad and extended framework for the study of the illness, including the assessment of treatment effects on the core psychopathology in addition to assessments of those psychopathologic domains most likely to reflect treatment responsivity. There is the corollary need to distinguish long-standing deficits from transitory negative symptoms. The literature is already confounded with a diversity of opinion as to whether neuroleptics are an effective treatment of negative symptoms. In spite of this, it seems quite evident that such symptoms improve in the context of effective treatment of florid psychotic episodes, although the deficit syndrome is not effectively treated by neuroleptic drugs in the long term.

The second caveat has to do with the centrality of the clinical relationship to all treatment approaches. Too often, the intimate involvement of clinician with patient is avoided, with the belief that brief ascertainment of certain conspicuous symptoms is sufficient to guide diagnosis and treatment. In opposing circumstances, an intimate involvement is implemented over time but is dominated by theoretical presentiments as to the etiology and treatment of the illness (8,10). Because most patients with schizophrenia often have difficulty in sharing a sense of purpose, maintaining insight into the nature of their illness, and persevering in treatment, it is imperative that the continuity of a clinical relationship

with a familiar professional be the backbone of treatment. In this context, the phenomenologic evaluation can be assured, thus permitting the initiation of multiple treatments, the integration of treatments, and the shifting of treatment tactics as circumstances and psychopathology change over time. Also operating within this context are the therapeutic effects of a structuring and supportive relationship, an identification process that enhances coping skills and reduces idiosyncratic responsiveness by fostering a consensually validated reality orientation.

The above approach should be viewed in contrast to theoretically driven, intensive psychotherapy on the one hand and minimal clinical engagement in exploring the course of illness on the other. The biopsychosocial medical model provides a framework for the integration of various treatment approaches as well as for the cooperative involvement of various professionals who participate in the care of any given patient. The centrality of the principal clinical relationship within this framework cannot be overstated.

REFERENCES

1. Bleuler, E. (1950): In: *Dementia Praecox or the Group of Schizophrenias,* translated by J. Zinken. International Universities Press, New York.
2. Bleuler, M. (1978): In: *The Schizophrenic Disorders: Long-term Patient and Family Studies,* translated by S. M. Clemens. Yale University Press, New Haven, London.
3. Brown, W. A., and Laughren, T. (1981): *Am. J. Psychiatry,* 138: 237–239.
4. Cannon-Spoor, H. E., Potkin, S. G., and Wyatt, R. J. (1982): *Schizophrenia Bull.,* 8:470–484.
5. Carlsson, A., and Lindqvist, M. (1963): *Acta Pharmacol. Toxicol.,* 20:140–144.
6. Carpenter, W. T. (1980): In: *Presentations and Sessions of the V.A. Advisory Conference on Chronic Schizophrenia, Harpers Ferry, West Va., 1979,* edited by D. F. Baxter and T. Melnechuk. Raven Press, New York.
7. Carpenter, W. T. (1983): *Schizophrenia Bull.,* 9:9–10.
8. Carpenter, W. T. (1984): *Strecker Monograph Series. The 21st Institute of Pennsylvania Hospital Award Lecture.* Philadelphia.
9. Carpenter, W. T., Bartko, J. J., Strauss, J. S., and Hawk, A. B. (1978): *Am. J. Psychiatry,* 135:940–945.
10. Carpenter, W. T., and Heinrichs, D. W. (1980): In: *Psychotherapy of Schizophrenia. Current Status and New Directions,* edited by J. S. Strauss, S. Fleck, M. Bowers, I. Levine, T. W. Downey, et al. Plenum Press, New York.
11. Carpenter, W. T., and Heinrichs, D. W. (1981): *J. Nerv. Ment. Dis.,* 169:113–119.
12. Carpenter, W. T., and Heinrichs, D. W. (1983): *Schizophrenia Bull.,* 9:533–542.
13. Carpenter, W. T., Heinrichs, D. W., and Alphs, L. D. (1985): *Schizophrenia Bull.,* 11:440–452.
14. Carpenter, W. T., Heinrichs, D. W., and Hanlon, T. E. (1981): *Am. J. Psychiatry,* 138:465–471.
15. Carpenter, W. T., Heinrichs, D. W., and Wagman, A. M. I. (1985): In: *Controversies in Schizophrenia,* edited by M. Alpert. Guilford Press, New York.
16. Carpenter, W. T., Strauss, J. S. and Bellak, L., eds. (1979): *Disorders of the Schizophrenic Syndrome.* Basic Books, New York.
17. Ciompi, L. (1980): *Br. J. Psychiatry,* 136:413–420.
18. Crow, T. J. (1985): *Schizophrenia Bull.,* 11:471–486.
19. Davis, J. M. (1975): *Am. J. Psychiatry,* 132:1237–1245.
20. Donaldson, S. R., Gelenberg, A. J., and Baldessarini, R. J. (1983): *Schizophrenia Bull.,* 9:504–527.
21. Engel, G. (1977): *Science,* 196:129–136.
22. Evans, J. R., Goldstein, M. J., and Rodnick, E. H. (1973): *Arch. Gen. Psychiatry,* 28:666–672.

23. Faloon, I. R. H., and Liberman, R. P. (1983): *Schizophrenia Bull.,* 9:543–554.

24. Feinstein, A. R. (1974): *Clinical Judgment.* Robert E. Krieger, Huntington, NY.

25. Fish, F. J. (1962): *Schizophrenia.* John Wright & Sons, Bristol.

26. Freedman, R., Kirch, D., Bell, J., Adler, L. E., Pecevich, M., et al. (1982): *Acta Psychiatr. Scand.,* 65:35–45.

27. Gould, R. J., Murphy, K. M. M., Reynolds, I. J., and Snyder, S. H. (1983): *Proc. Natl. Acad. Sci. U.S.A.,* 80:5122–5125.

28. Haracz, J. L. (1982): *Schizophrenia Bull.,* 2:438–459.

29. Harding, C. M., Brooks, G. W., Askihaga, T., Strauss, J. S., and Breier, A. (1987): *Am. J. Psychiatry,* (in press).

30. Harding, C. M., Brooks, G. W., Askihaga, T., Strauss, J. S., and Breier, A. (1987): *Am. J. Psychiatry,* (in press).

31. Hawk, A. B., Carpenter, W. T., and Strauss, J. S. (1975): *Arch. Gen. Psychiatry,* 32:343–347.

32. Herz, M. I. (1984): In: *Drug Maintenance Strategies in Schizophrenia,* edited by J. M. Kane. American Psychiatric Press, Washington.

33. Hogarty, G. E. (1985): Paper presented at American College of Neuropsychopharmacology Annual Meeting. Maui, Hawaii.

34. Huber, G., Gross, G., and Scheuttler, R. (1979): *Schizophrenie. Eine Verlaufs- und Sozial-Psychiatristhe Langreistudie.* Springer-Verlag, Berlin, Heidelberg, New York.

35. Jaspers, K. (1963): *General Psychopathology (1923),* translated by J. Hoenig and M. Hamilton. Manchester University Press, Manchester.

36. Jeste, D. V., and Wyatt, R. J. (1982): *Understanding and Treating Tardive Dyskinesia.* Guilford Press, New York.

37. Kane, J. M. (1983): *Schizophrenia Bull.,* 9:528–541.

38. Kane, J. M. (1984): *Drug Maintenance Strategies in Schizophrenia.* American Psychiatric Association, Washington.

39. Kendell, R. E., Brockington, I. F., and Leff, J. P. (1979): *Arch. Gen. Psychiatry,* 36:25–31.

40. Klein, E., Bental, E., Lerer, B., and Balmaker, R. H. (1984): *Arch. Gen. Psychiatry,* 41:165–170.

41. Kraepelin, E. (1971): *Dementia Praecox and Paraphrenia,* translated by R. M. Barclay. Robert R. Krieger, Huntington, New York.

42. Langfeldt, G. (1937): *The Prognosis of Schizophrenia and the Factors Influencing the Course of the Disease.* E. Munksgaard, Copenhagen.

43. Leff, J. P., Kuipers, L., Berkowitz, R., Eberlein-Vries, R., and Sturgeon, D. (1982): *Br. J. Psychiatry,* 141:121–134.

44. Leff, J. P., and Vaughn, C. E. (1981): *Br. J. Psychiatry,* 139:102–104.

45. Leff, J. P., and Wing, J. K. (1971): *Br. Med. J.,* 2:599–604.

46. Lehmann, H., Wilson, W. H., and Deutsch, M. (1983): *Compr. Psychiatry,* 24:293–303.

47. Leonhard, K. (1979): In: *The Classification of Endogenous Psychoses,* translated by R. Berman, edited by E. Robins. Halstead Press, New York.

48. Lieberman, J., Kane, J., Gadaleta, D., Brenner, R., Lesser, M., et al. (1984): *Am. J. Psychiatry,* 141:633–638.

49. Lieberman, J., Kane, J., Gadaleta, D., Ramos-Lorenzi, J., Bergmann, K., et al. (1985): *Psychopharmacol. Bull.,* 21:123–129.

50. Manschreck, T. C. (1983): *Prog. Exp. Person. Res.,* 12:53–96.

51. Marder, S. R., Van Putten, T., Mintz, J., Lebell, M., McKenzie, J., et al. (1984): In: *Drug Maintenance Strategies in Schizophrenia,* edited by J. M. Kane. American Psychiatric Press, Washington.

52. May, P. R. A., and Goldberg, S. C. (1978): *Psychopharmacology:* *A Generation of Progress,* edited by M. A. Lipton, A. DiMascio, and K. F. Killam, pp. 1139–1154. Raven Press, New York.

53. McGlashan, T. H. (1984): *Arch. Gen. Psychiatry,* 41:585–601.

54. McGlashan, T. H. (1986): *Arch. Gen. Psychiatry,* 41:167–176.

55. McGlashan, T. H., and Carpenter, W. T. (1976): *Am. J. Psychiatry,* 133:14–19.

56. McHugh, P. R., and Slavney, P. R. (1983): *The Perspectives of Psychiatry.* The Johns Hopkins University Press, Baltimore.

57. Meltzer, H. Y., and Stahl, S. M. (1976): *Schizophrenia Bull.,* 2: 19–76.

58. Monroe, R. R. (1970): *Episodic Behavioral Disorders: Psychodynamic and Neuropsychiatric Analyses.* Harvard University Press, Cambridge.

59. Rifkin, A., and Kane, J. M. (1984): In: *Drug Maintenance Strategies in Schizophrenia,* edited by J. M. Kane. American Psychiatric Press, Washington.

60. Rosenthal, D., Goldberg, I., Jacobsen, B., Wender, P. H., Kety, S. S., et al. (1974): *Psychiatry,* 37:521–539.

61. *Schizophrenia Bulletin* (1970): *Issue No. 11, Winter, 1974.* Superintendent of Documents, Washington.

62. *Schizophrenia Bulletin* (1982): *Volume 8, No. 3, 1982.* Superintendent of Documents, Washington.

63. Schneider, K. (1959): *Clinical Psychopathology,* translated by M. W. Hamilton. Grune & Stratton, New York.

64. Schwartz, C. C., Myers, J. K., and Astrachan, B. M. (1976): *Arch. Gen. Psychiatry,* 32:1221–1227.

65. Snyder, S. H. (1981): *Am. J. Psychiatry,* 138:460–464.

66. Spring, B., and Zubin, J. (1977): In: *Primary Prevention in Psychopathology, Vol. 1: The Issues,* edited by G. W. Albee and J. M. Joffe. University Press of New England,

67. Stephens, J. H. (1970): *Semin. Psychiatry,* 2:464–485.

68. Stevens, J. R. (1982): In: *Schizophrenia as a Brain Disease,* edited by F. A. Henn, and H. A. Nasrallah. Oxford University Press, New York.

69. Strauss, J. S., and Carpenter, W. T. (1974): *Arch. Gen. Psychiatry,* 31:37–42.

70. Strauss, J. S., and Carpenter, W. T. (1977): *Arch. Gen. Psychiatry,* 34:159–163.

71. Strauss, J. S., and Carpenter, W. T. (1979): In: *Disorders of the Schizophrenic Syndrome,* edited by L. Bellak. Basic Books, New York.

72. Strauss, J. S., and Carpenter, W. T. (1981): In: *Schizophrenia,* edited by S. M. Woods. Plenum Press, New York.

73. Task Force on Late Neurological Effects of Antipsychotic Drugs (1980): *Am. J. Psychiatry,* 137:1163–1172.

74. Vaillant, G. (1962): *J. Nerv. Ment. Dis.,* 135:534–543.

75. Van Putten, T. (1974): *Arch. Gen. Psychiatry,* 31:67–72.

76. Van Putten, T., and May, P. R. A. (1978): *Arch. Gen. Psychiatry,* 35:477–480.

77. Von Kammen, D. P., Peters, J., Rosen, J., Fields, R., Rogol, A., et al. (1985): Clonidine and Schizophrenia. Behavioral and biochemical evaluations. Poster Session at the ACNP Meeting. Maui, Hawaii.

78. Weinberger, D. R. (1984): In: *Guidelines for Use of Psychotropic Drugs,* edited by P. E. Garfinkel. Spectrum, New York.

79. Wolkowitz, O. M., Pickar, D., Doran, A. R., Breier, A., Tarell, J., et al. (1987): *Am. J. Psychiatry* (in press).

80. World Health Organization (1978): *Report of the International Pilot Study of Schizophrenia, Vol. 2.* WHO Press, Geneva.

81. Zemlan, F. P., Hirschowitz, J., Sautter, F. J., and Garver, D. L. (1984): *Br. J. Psychiatry,* 144:65–69.

Psychopharmacology:
The Third Generation of Progress,
edited by Herbert Y. Meltzer.
Raven Press, New York © 1987.

CHAPTER 116

New Neuroleptics and Experimental Antipsychotics in Schizophrenia

Carol A. Tamminga and Jes Gerlach

Advances in the pharmacology of schizophrenia may contribute to an understanding of the brain mechanisms involved in the disorder as well as indicate agents for improved therapeutics. A reproducible response of a psychotic symptom to a pharmacologically selective drug could implicate a particular transmitter system in the pathophysiology of psychosis, localize a psychosis-related area of brain, or suggest a novel therapeutic approach to the illness. Three decades ago, the discovery of the potent antipsychotic action of neuroleptic drugs focused scientific inquiry on the nature and function of dopamine (DA) systems in mammalian brain. Although this research has yet to serve as a direct pathway to an improved understanding of schizophrenia, it has launched a broadly productive area of neuropsychiatric inquiry. Not only have the basic anatomy and physiology of DA systems in brain been explicated but also multiple types and locations of DA receptors have been discovered, the heterogeneity of dopaminergic pathways described, and unusual clinical actions of some neuroleptics identified, thus providing greater opportunity for targeted symptomatic improvement in psychosis. In addition to studying central DA-containing neural systems in schizophrenia, investigators have begun to examine the role of other specific neurotransmitters and probes in psychosis, describing their functions in brain and their clinical action. In addition to these classical transmitters, new neurotransmitters and modulators are being studied, especially the multitude of peptides thought to influence CNS neural functions, only a few of which have been evaluated in any detail in schizophrenia.

The concept that schizophrenia is a single disease entity with one etiology, one mechanism, and a single optimal treatment has been increasingly questioned. Observations drawn from pharmacologic studies of schizophrenia support the hypothesis that schizophrenia may be pathophysiologically heterogeneous and have multiple, sometimes multiple and coincident, neural mechanisms. Drugs that modify psychosis might be symptom specific or symptom complex specific, not disease specific; and drug effects on different symptom clusters might be additive in schizophrenia. An example would be the hypothesis that the positive symptom state in schizophrenia is different in mechanism, biology, and pharmacology from the deficit state (24,37): where positive symptoms are described as episodic, often accompanying the onset of schizophrenia, the deficit state is said to be persistent and may intensify or extend with progression of the illness. Deficit state has been associated with organicity (77), structural brain changes (151), resistance to neuroleptic treatment, and a family history of severe schizophrenia (23); positive-symptom schizophrenia lacks these characteristics; it is productive, episodic, and presumably functional. Dopamine agonists appear to worsen positive symptoms (6) while they may improve negative symptoms; DA antagonists are reported to do the opposite (7). Whereas all of these speculations need yet to be rigorously established, at least the suggestion of multiple subtypes of schizophrenia, with multiple pharmacologies of the syndrome, is strongly argued by these kinds of observations. Analysis of drug effects on specific symptoms and symptom clusters in schizophrenia will continue to provide data to evaluate this hypothesis.

ATYPICAL NEUROLEPTICS: SPECIFIC RECEPTOR AFFINITY PROFILES

In the past decade, a series of interesting developments have begun in the pharmacology of schizophrenia. Traditional neuroleptics have been modified along two parameters: the development of increasingly selective antidopaminergic drugs (e.g., sulpiride) and diminution of the antidopaminergic component of neuroleptic drugs together with an increase of antiserotonergic and antinoradrenergic potency (e.g., clozapine). These two types of antipsychotic medication have been united under the term "atypical neuroleptics," and both are well established in clinical psychiatry in Europe and Asia. They are characterized by potent antipsychotic effects and a relatively low level of extrapyramidal side effects.

Neuroleptics block multiple amine receptors in the brain (75). Some neuroleptics are highly D_2 receptor selective, whereas others are more "broad spectrum," affecting multiple kinds of receptors. Figure 1 shows a selection of clinically used antipsychotics classified according to receptor affinity, beginning with the D_2-selective drug sulpiride and proceeding to the "broad-spectrum," nonselective drug clozapine. Pimozide and haloperidol follow sulpiride in their D_2 selectivity. Haloperidol affects serotonin and α_1 receptors more than sulpiride and pimozide, which may influence the therapeutic effect profile of this drug compared to the two others. It can be seen that perphenazine, compared to haloperidol, blocks histamine receptors, which

also may contribute to the antipsychotic effect. However, the implications of this changing receptor affinity profile may become more evident when the pure DA-selective drugs (like sulpiride) are compared with DA-nonselective drugs (like clozapine), which have marked antiserotonergic and antinoradrenergic effects. Both types of drugs possess antipsychotic properties, but their effect on mental functions may be different in salient respects. It will be a task for the future to define more specifically the behavioral and antipsychotic effects that relate to the varying receptor affinities of antipsychotic drugs.

Although it is difficult to associate receptor affinity profiles with psychic effects of neuroleptics, it is far easier to relate these receptor affinities to the side effects of these drugs. The DA-selective antipsychotic drugs have few autonomic and sedating actions, but they induce extrapyramidal motor symptoms; the DA-nonselective drugs produce the opposite side-effect profile.

Another potentially important characteristic of the receptor affinity profiles of neuroleptic drugs should be noted: antipsychotics influence D_1 and D_2 receptors to different degrees (Fig. 1). Most neuroleptics, including the substituted benzamides (e.g., sulpiride), butyrophenones (e.g., haloperidol), and the diphenylbutylpiperidines (e.g., pimozide)

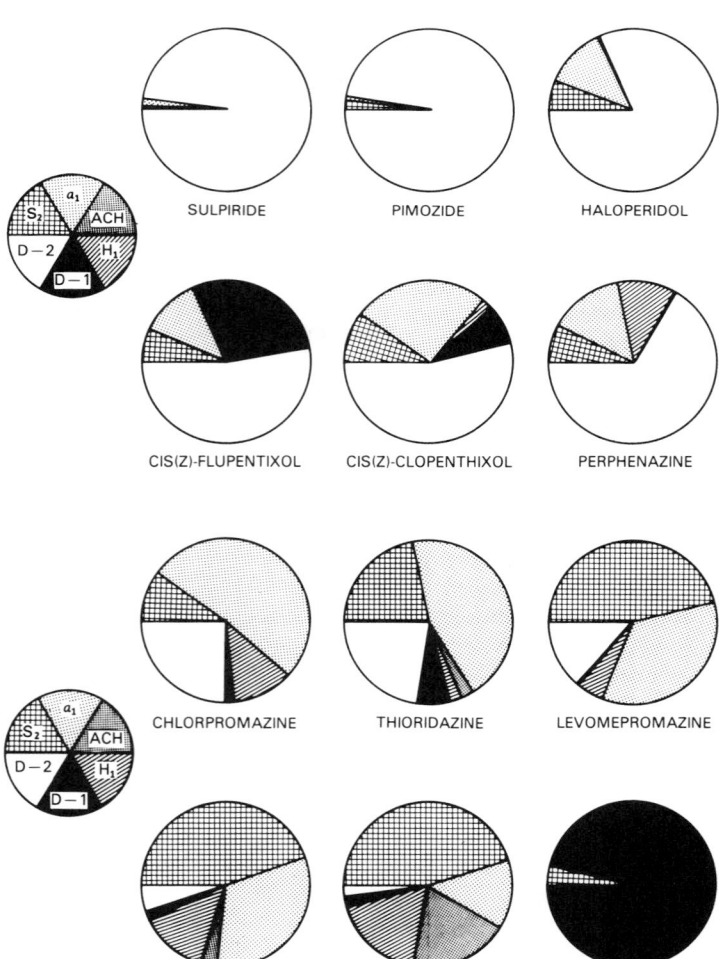

FIG. 1. A selection of neuroleptic drugs classified according to receptor affinity profile (*pie charts*). D_1, D_2, ACH (acetylcholine), α_1-adrenergic, and S-2 (serotonin) receptor affinities were determined from receptor binding experiments with ^{3}H-pifluthixol, ^{3}H-spiroperidol, ^{3}H-PrBCM, ^{3}H-prazosin, and ^{3}H-spiroperidol, respectively. H_1 receptor affinity was determined from inhibition of histamine-induced contractions of guinea pig ileum *in vitro* (76).

have little effect on D_1 receptors. Phenothiazines (e.g., chlorpromazine) have a weak D_1-blocking action, whereas thioxanthenes (e.g., flupenthixol) have a more pronounced effect. SCH 23390, the last drug in Fig. 1, is a pure D_1 antagonist that is available for animal experimentation only. The clinical implications of the varying D_1–D_2 potency are, however, far from clarified (see below). Figure 1 clearly illustrates the pharmacologic characteristics of the two groups of atypical neuroleptics: the DA-selective drugs represented by sulpiride and the DA-nonselective drugs represented by clozapine. In the next two sections, we discuss the pharmacological and clinical properties of these two groups of drugs compared to traditional neuroleptics.

Dopamine Receptor-Selective Neuroleptics

The DA receptor-selective antipsychotics are neuroleptics that unite a traditional antipsychotic effect with a low level of autonomic and sedating side effects. The antidopaminergic action of these drugs provides for an antipsychotic effect, whereas the lack of anticholinergic and antinoradrenergic actions results in few autonomic and cardiovascular side effects. Furthermore, the putative selectivity of some of the compounds for the D_2 receptor may result in relatively few extrapyramidal side effects.

Sulpiride

Sulpiride is the oldest and clinically most established member of the substituted benzamides. The main pharmacological characteristics of this drug are the following:

1. Sulpiride binds to a subgroup of D_2 receptors that are sodium dependent (79) and are preferentially located on the presynaptic membrane (141).
2. Sulpiride increases brain DA turnover in DA terminal areas as demonstrated by an elevated concentration of homovanillic acid (HVA) in the brains of rodents (118) and humans (69).
3. Sulpiride in very high doses induces no or atypical catalepsy. At relatively low doses, it inhibits apomorphine-

induced locomotion, whereas at higher doses it counteracts apomorphine-induced stereotypy (79,108) (Fig. 2). Traditional neuroleptics like haloperidol produce all three behaviors at the same dose level. Sulpiride has even been shown to aggravate amphetamine-induced stereotypy (114).
4. With long-term treatment, sulpiride induces no increase in D_2 receptors in the experimental animal but a significant increase in D_1 receptors, in contrast to traditional neuroleptics like haloperidol, which elevate the D_2 but not D_1 receptors (80).

In clinical double-blind studies, sulpiride (800–2,300 mg/day) has been shown to have an antipsychotic effect in chronic schizophrenic patients not significantly different from that of chlorpromazine (17), haloperidol (111), and trifluoperazine (43). The potential advantages of this drug appear to be relatively few extrapyramidal side effects and, in small to moderate doses, an antiautistic and antidepressant effect (45,105).

In a recent double-blind study, 20 chronic, severely ill schizophrenic patients were treated with sulpiride and haloperidol in a crossover design (two 12-week periods) (55). The median dose of sulpiride was 2,000 mg/day (range 800–3,200) and of haloperidol 12 mg/day (range 6–24). As in other studies, sulpiride proved to have an antipsychotic effect not significantly different from that of haloperidol, and the symptom response profiles were similar for the two drugs. However, in spite of the high doses of sulpiride, parkinsonism and akathisia occurred less frequently during the first 4 weeks of the sulpiride period compared with the corresponding haloperidol period. These differences disappeared during the remaining part of the study, in which five sulpiride patients and 10 haloperidol patients received biperiden. Cardiovascular side effects were equally rare for both drugs.

In another study, sulpiride was used in lower doses (800 mg/day) and compared with chlorpromazine (400 mg/day) in young and more acute schizophrenic patients (68). In this study, sulpiride resulted in a more rapid improvement than chlorpromazine. After 1 to 2 weeks, patients treated with sulpiride had a significantly lower global psychosis morbidity score than those treated with chlorpromazine;

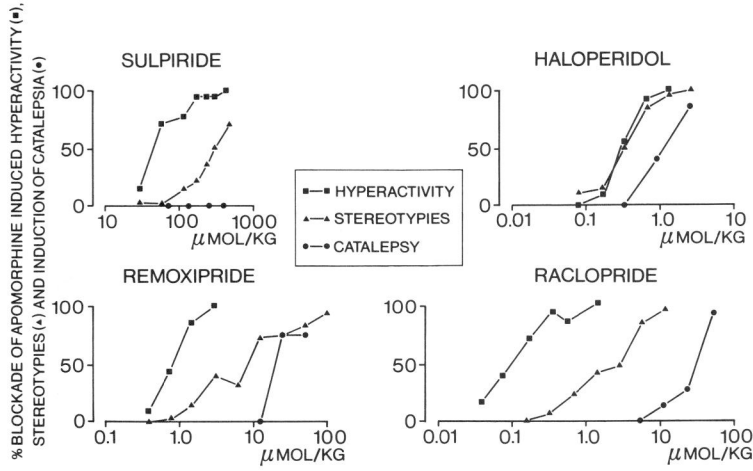

FIG. 2. The potency of sulpiride, remoxipride, haloperidol, and raclopride in blocking apomorphine-induced locomotion and stereotypies and to induce catalepsy in rats (18,37). The compounds were injected i.p. 60 min prior to apomorphine (1 mg/kg s.c.). The results on catalepsy are based on the peak time effect of each compound in the bar test.

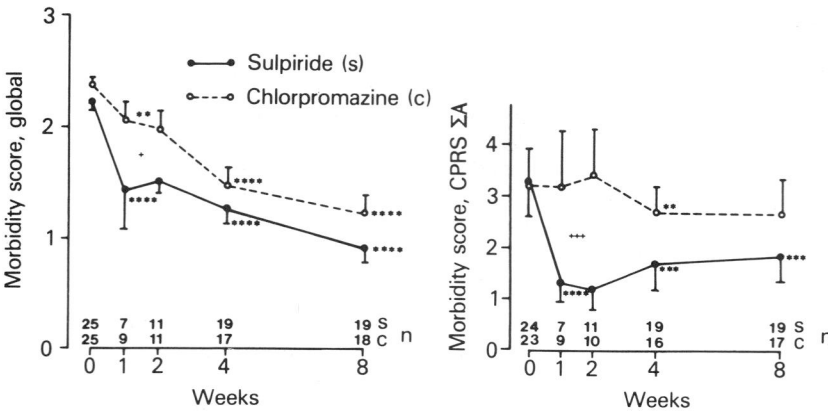

FIG. 3. Global evaluation of schizophrenic symptomatology and autism in schizophrenic patients treated with sulpiride and chlorpromazine (27). Autism comprises the following five items: inability to feel, lassitude, emotional withdrawal, reduced speech, slowness of movements. Data indicate means ± SE. Rating scores of 1 and 2 were pooled in the statistical analysis. Figures below indicate numbers of patients in the two groups. Comparison with pretreatment scores: $^{**}p < 0.025$; $^{***}p < 0.01$; $^{****}p < 0.001$. Comparison between groups: $^{+}p < 0.05$; $^{+++}p < 0.001$.

however, after 4 and 8 weeks, there were no significant differences between the two drugs (Fig. 3).

The authors have examined the concentrations of HVA in cerebrospinal fluid and found them increased to the same degree during sulpiride treatment as during chlorpromazine (69). This indicates that the central DA receptor blockade effect of sulpiride was comparable to that of chlorpromazine. Other studies also suggest that sulpiride given in low doses (100–300 mg/day) may be an appropriate treatment for slightly depressed patients including endogenous depression (15), but more controlled studies are warranted in this area.

It has been claimed that sulpiride should be less liable to induce tardive dyskinesia (TD) than traditional neuroleptics. This assertion has been based on the following observations: sulpiride induces no or weak DA supersensitivity with chronic administration (80); sulpiride suppresses TD in monkeys without subsequent TD rebound aggravation (in contrast to traditional neuroleptics) (67); uncontrolled observations worldwide indicate that only six patients have developed TD during sulpiride treatment (3). However, TD may not be a DA supersensitivity phenomenon (53) nor a rebound aggravation phenomenon (54), and uncontrolled observations (mainly comprising patients treated with sulpiride in relatively small doses) are not useful for a judgment of the TD-inducing effect of sulpiride (in high antipsychotic doses). Furthermore, sulpiride can suppress TD in humans to the same degree as other antidopaminergic drugs (25). Therefore, the claim that sulpiride fails to induce TD has to be reevaluated. In fact, there are good reasons for doing so because (a) the selective action of sulpiride on a subgroup of D_2 receptors may be an advantage in light of the new hypothesis that TD is caused by a blockade of a subgroup of DA receptors related to the striatofugal GABA-mediated projections (53,66); (b) the D_1 receptor increase during prolonged sulpiride treatment may protect against TD development (80); and (c) if non-DA mechanisms are involved in the pathogenesis of TD—and this may well be the case (140)—then DA-selective drugs such as sulpiride should represent an additional advantage compared to less-specific neuroleptics. Therefore, the potential of sulpiride to induce reversible and irreversible TD deserves to be more carefully evaluated in long-term comparative clinical trials with observation of the immediate

withdrawal aggravation and the more persisting level of dyskinesias.

Other Substituted Benzamides

In the search for new selective D_2 antagonists, a series of novel substituted benzamides has been developed (106). Remoxipride and raclopride are two interesting members of this series. They share some of the behavioral effects of sulpiride but have the advantage of being more potent and causing less prolactin increase. Remoxipride [S-3-bromo-N-(1-ethyl-2-pyrrolidinyl)methyl-2,6-dimethoxybenzamide hydrochloride monohydrate] is a selective D_2 receptor blocker with preferential action in mesolimbic areas and substantia nigra (107). It displaces ^{3}H-spiperone in vivo in limbic and in ventral tegmental structures but not in striatal tissue at doses that selectively block apomorphine-induced hyperactivity. Blockade of ^{3}H-spiperone in striatum was observed only at high doses, which produce catalepsy (Fig. 2). Moreover, remoxipride, like sulpiride, causes a low maximal DA receptor binding displacement in striatum compared to other DA terminal areas. Even at high doses, neither drug displaced striatal ^{3}H-spiperone more than 40 to 50% in contrast to the 80 to 90% displacement by chlorpromazine and haloperidol (66).

Raclopride [(−)-(S)-3,5-dichloro-N-(1-ethyl-2-pyrrolidinyl)methyl-6-methoxysalicylamide tartrate] is characterized by the same clear separation between doses producing catalepsy and inhibition of stereotypy and locomotion induced by apomorphine (Fig. 2), but raclopride penetrates readily into the brain tissue and binds with high affinity to D_2 receptors in DA-rich areas including the striatum (107). This observation suggests that the atypical behavioral profile of the substituted benzamides cannot be explained only by a special regional distribution pattern of the drugs into the brain but more likely by the existence of different populations of D_2 receptors within striatum as well as in extrastriatal regions.

Remoxipride has been tested in four pilot studies (29,91,95,101), which all showed the drug (90–1,200 mg/day) to have an antipsychotic effect comparable to traditional neuroleptics. Side effects include slight parkinsonism and akathisia, sedation, fatigue, and headache. Only very few autonomic side effects have been observed. Prolactin is elevated by remoxipride, but to a lesser degree than by sulpiride.

Raclopride has been tested in healthy volunteers (Astra Lakemedel, *personal communication*). One developed acute dystonia after 4 mg b.i.d. for 2 days, and akathisia was seen in most subjects at 4 to 8 mg/day. No parkinsonism and no autonomic or cardiovascular reactions occurred. Thus, raclopride appears to be the first "low-dose" benzamide comparable in motor side effects to haloperidol. The question is whether it may have therapeutic advantages or may induce less parkinsonism than haloperidol.

Broad-Spectrum Dopamine-Receptor Neuroleptics

Clozapine

Clozapine [8-chloro-11-(4-methyl-1-piperazinyl)-5H-dibenzo(*b,e*)(1,4)diazepine] belongs to the chemical class of dibenzodiazepines, which also includes powerful traditional neuroleptics such as loxapine and clothapine. The main pharmacological characteristics of this drug are as follows:

1. Clozapine binds to several types of receptors, especially serotonin (S_2), α_1-adrenergic, and histaminergic (H_1) receptors (75). D_1 and D_2 receptors are affected to a lesser degree (Fig. 1), and the binding to DA receptors appears to be looser than that for other neuroleptics (70).

2. In small doses, clozapine decreases DA release in the brain of rodents (63), and in moderate doses (225 mg/day), it causes a decrease in HVA in cerebrospinal fluid of schizophrenic patients (61). Higher doses of clozapine increase DA turnover in experimental animals as well as in the human patient (119).

3. Clozapine is not cataleptogenic. It inhibits the locomotion but not the stereotypies induced by apomorphine (97,128). Like sulpiride, it may even potentiate amphetamine-induced stereotypy (113).

4. With chronic treatment in the experimental animal, clozapine produced no increase in D_2 receptor number or affinity, but, like sulpiride, it may increase D_1 receptors (80).

Early trials clearly demonstrated that the antipsychotic effect of clozapine was at least equal to, and often greater than, comparable effects with other high-dose neuroleptics such as chlorpromazine (50), levomepromazine (9), and thioridazine (65).

Another study from that time demonstrates the special symptom reduction profile of clozapine compared to that of haloperidol (57). Twenty schizophrenic patients were treated in a crossover design with clozapine (100–800 mg/day, mean 200) and haloperidol (3–32 mg/day, mean 10) in periods of 82 days preceded by long drug-free periods (7–71 days, until relapse). The therapeutic effect of clozapine and haloperidol is shown in Fig. 4. It can be seen that clozapine caused a highly significant reduction not only in the productive schizophrenic symptoms but in anxiety and tension as well. In addition, significant effects were noted on the negative symptoms of emotional withdrawal and blunted affect. Haloperidol also reduced the intensity of the schizophrenic core symptoms significantly, but not anxiety and tension. A comparison between clozapine and haloperidol showed that clozapine was significantly superior with regard to the effect on somatic concern, anxiety,

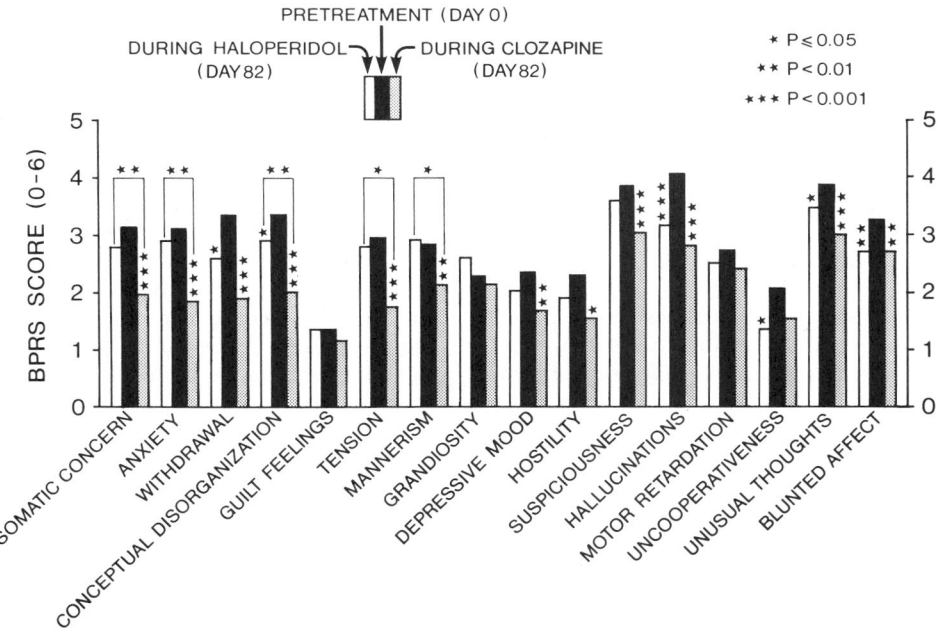

FIG. 4. Mean BPRS scores before and following treatment with clozapine and haloperidol (56). The significance signs above the bars indicate the difference between ratings at day 0 and day 82. In five items a significant difference was found between clozapine and haloperidol.

conceptual disorganization, tension, and mannerism. The therapeutic advantage of clozapine was most pronounced in the more severely disturbed patients who, in addition to their schizophrenic symptoms, suffered from anxiety, tension, and psychomotor restlessness. This particular therapeutic effect profile of clozapine is entirely consistent with the results of a subsequent study in the United States (122).

The difference between the antipsychotic effect profiles of clozapine and haloperidol might, at least partly, be related to different side effects of the two drugs. In severe cases of schizophrenia, clozapine brings about an often desirable relaxation and sedation, whereas haloperidol may instead cause restlessness, often associated with anxiety and tension, symptoms that can only partly be reversed by antiparkinsonian drugs. These differential clinical effects probably represent a correlate to the differential affinity of the two drugs to brain receptors (Fig. 1) and their different effects on dopaminergic neurotransmission (60).

In the recommended dose level (up to 600 mg/day), clozapine does not induce extrapyramidal side effects, although some slowing of movements and reduced facial expression may be seen related to the sedative effect (9,50,57,65,122). Even more interesting is the finding of an antitremor effect of clozapine not only in parkinsonian tremor (Parkinson's disease and neuroleptic-induced parkinsonism) but also in essential tremor (12.5–75 mg/day) (109,145). This and the sedative effect make, in some cases, the combination of clozapine and a traditional neuroleptic such as haloperidol a particularly beneficial antipsychotic treatment.

Clozapine may prove to be an interesting drug in relation to tardive dyskinesia, both with respect to the treatment and prevention of the syndrome. In high doses (400–900 mg/day), clozapine can dampen the TD symptoms moderately (124), but in general, because of the side effects of clozapine (see below), such high-dose treatment cannot be recommended for elderly TD patients. However, in a subgroup of severely psychotic patients suffering from severe atypical tardive dyskinesia associated with productive psychotic symptoms, bizarre behavior, and possibly some form of brain damage, clozapine in relatively high doses (600–900 mg/day) may lead to improvement of all symptoms, especially if traditional neuroleptics like haloperidol have resulted in insufficient effect or maybe even an aggravation of the psychomotor disturbances (103; *unpublished observations*).

In low doses (50–250 mg/day), clozapine has no significant dyskinesia-suppressing effect (59). In these cases, however, a spontaneous recovery of the syndrome may be predicted to occur during the treatment, because clozapine in such doses may not induce or aggravate the primary pathophysiological mechanisms underlying TD.

The question of whether clozapine may produce the primary pathophysiological alterations underlying TD is not completely clarified, but available evidence indicates that clozapine may well be least likely to induce tardive dyskinesia of all available antipsychotics. The drug has weak D_1 and D_2 receptor-blocking effects, and in low doses, it may have no such effect at all. In cebus monkeys with dyskinesias, clozapine does not induce symptom suppression or withdrawal aggravation as classical neuroleptics do (67).

Uncontrolled clinical observations and follow-up studies (110) also suggest that clozapine does not induce tardive dyskinesia. Only one case of the disorder developing during clozapine treatment has been reported (40).

Clozapine, however, strongly influences cardiovascular and autonomic functions. It may cause a fall in orthostatic blood pressure (especially in the initial treatment phase) and sinus tachycardia. In the above mentioned clinical trial with clozapine and haloperidol (57), it was found that three patients collapsed during the first day of treatment with clozapine, 100 mg b.i.d., and for the material as a whole the cardiac frequency rose from 88 ± 15 beats/min (day 0) to 112 ± 19 (day 40) and 108 ± 15 (day 82) during clozapine treatment, whereas no changes were seen during haloperidol treatment. The electrocardiogram showed a sinus tachycardia, a corresponding shortening of the PQ interval, and a flattening (in 7%, an inversion) of the T waves. These ECG changes diminished slightly during the period of treatment and disappeared following the discontinuation of clozapine.

Since the introduction of increased hematologic surveillance and tightly restricted utilization following eight deaths in Finland from agranulocytosis, there has been a drastic decrease in the number of cases of bone marrow suppression, from 0.38% to 0.06%, and a decrease in mortality in those clozapine-treated patients who develop agranulocytosis from 42% to 19% (88). For comparison, the incidence of agranulocytosis caused by phenothiazines is stated to be 0.1 to 1.0%, and the mortality in these cases of agranulocytoses to be 11 to 38% (5,116). It remains unclear whether the risk is significantly presented by other neuroleptics, and further data from carefully monitored patients are necessary.

Other Dopamine-Nonselective Atypical Neuroleptics

Fluperlapine and BW 234 U are two interesting drugs belonging to the group of atypical neuroleptics. Fluperlapine [3-fluoro-6-(4-methylpiperazinyl)-11H-dibenz-(*b,e*)-azepine] is a result of the search for new clozapine-like neuroleptics. It is a dibenzazepine derivative chemically and pharmacologically related to clozapine (44). It has the same weak affinity for D_1 and D_2 receptors and a strong affinity for serotonin receptors. However, in contrast to clozapine, it causes no α_1 blockade but facilitates noradrenergic neurotransmission through presynaptic mechanisms. BW 234 U {*cis*-9-[3-(3,4-dimethyl-1-piperazinyl)propyl]carbazole dihydrochloride} has no or minimal affinity for DA, noradrenergic, serotonergic, histaminergic, and muscarinic receptors but counteracts apomorphine-induced aggression and locomotion without producing catalepsy or sedation (49).

Both fluperlapine (152) and BW 234 U (30) have been tested clinically and have shown antipsychotic properties and only weak EPS-inducing effects. Unfortunately, like clozapine, both drugs have demonstrated the potential for inducing granulocytopenia. Therefore, further clinical research with these drugs has been stopped. Nevertheless, from a theoretical and research point of view, they both represent an interesting step forward in the direction of non-DA antipsychotics.

Amperozide is another DA-nonselective drug that has reached phase II evaluation. This drug exhibits a new atypical pharmacological profile that is characterized by a weak D_2-blocking effect in limbic areas but at the same time an enhanced release of presynaptic DA without causing a general increase in DA turnover (33). Like other atypical neuroleptics, it causes no catalepsy and no antagonism against apomorphine stereotypy but inhibition of locomotion and conditioned behavior. Like fluperlapine, it facilitates noradrenergic neurotransmission and has a strong serotonin antagonistic and, in higher doses, agonistic effect. Amperozide has been found to have a unique antiaggressive effect in animals without sedation (in contrast to other neuroleptics), and it causes an anxiolytic and antistress effect corresponding to the effect of diazepam (33). In healthy volunteers, amperozide (30–40 mg/day) has caused tinnitus, dizziness, and some T-wave flattening in electrocardiograms (Ferrosan, Malmö, *personal communication*). The drug is now under clinical evaluation in schizophrenia.

Uncommon Antidopaminergic Drugs

Based on findings from early experiments with chlorpromazine (21), it has been widely accepted that classical neuroleptics act to reduce psychosis by their blockade of the DA receptor (126). But DA receptor blockade as a technique for antipsychotic action has been less than completely effective clinically and is related to serious acute and chronic drug side effects. Thus, the strategy has been pursued of developing new antipsychotic compounds by directing antagonists at various alternative sites in the dopaminergic system. Furthermore, extensive detail has accumulated to help characterize central DA neuronal systems. This has provided information to develop new antidopaminergic strategies: much about the anatomy (4,38), biochemistry (12,18), and physiology (28,146) of brain DA systems as well as details of diverse receptor subtypes (32,84), heterogeneity of the projection tracts (11,130), and multiplicity of modulatory transmitters related to DA-containing neurons have been described. These pieces of information have provided the nidus for various novel pharmacologic approaches to the treatment of schizophrenia.

Reserpine is one of the earliest antipsychotic compounds, reputed to have been used in folk medicine for its tranquilizing effect even prior to its chemical identification (71). Its action in brain is mediated by the depletion of catecholamines from nerve terminals, thus reducing availability of DA in the synapse; its administration is accompanied by hypotension and clinical depression as the most limiting side effects at the high daily doses required for antipsychotic action. Despite this, the drug is still used today for its antidyskinetic effects in special circumstances. α-Methyl-*para*-tyrosine (AMPT), which acts presynaptically on dopaminergic neurons, has mild antipsychotic effects in schizophrenia, presumably mediated by inhibition of the rate-limiting synthetic enzyme for DA, tyrosine hydroxylase, thereby reducing DA availability in the synapse (125). The administration of AMPT alone has not been effective in treating schizophrenia (62); however, the drug reportedly potentiates the antipsychotic effect of thioridazine when coadministered (22,31). Whether this activity of AMPT could be practically applied in the treatment of schizophrenia has been partially explored but became irrelevant

because of its renal side effects (99). These observations have lent support to the hypothesis that symptoms of schizophrenia improve in response to a decrease in DA-mediated neural transmission.

An opportunity whose potential for antipsychotic treatment has yet to be explored lies in the differential stimulation of the dopamine receptor subtypes D_1 and D_2 (84). At this time, data derived from biochemical, binding, and behavioral experiments do not yet present a consistent functional picture of the D_1 and the D_2 receptors, suggesting that the current categorization may be to some extent incomplete. The D_1 receptor has been defined as the DA-sensitive membrane recognition site positively linked to adenylate cyclase, and the D_2 site as the one that either lacks or is negatively coupled to adenylate cyclase (83,84). It is assumed that subcategories of each of the subtypes exist. Results of functional studies of the D_1 and D_2 receptors suggest that the two receptors may often interact, sometimes reciprocally and other times cooperatively. The state of receptor sensitization (i.e., normosensitive versus supersensitive) also appears to determine the resultant action of specific D_1 and D_2 probes. For example, in superfused striatal slices, cyclic AMP efflux was stimulated by a D_1 agonist (SKF 38393) and antagonized by a D_2 agonist (LY141865) (129). In another experiment, a D_1 agonist inhibited a D_2-agonist-stimulated decrease in DA turnover in striatum (117). However, in the reserpinized rat, both D_1 and D_2 agonists were required for full restoration of normal motor activity (61). But in rotational models, either a D_1 or D_2 agonist could stimulate turning (64,83,120). In addition, blockade of D_1 as well as of D_2 receptors produces catalepsy and stereotypy antagonism in rodents (115) and parkinsonism with dystonia in monkeys (56), but in rodents the effect of D_2 receptor blockers (but not of D_1 blockers) can be antagonized by anticholinergics, benzodiazepines, and GABA agonists. Much future work is required for the mere explication of the multiple types of DA receptors, and even more to study in detail their functional interactions in mammalian behaviors.

A novel DA receptor strategy, whose functional application in schizophrenia is more developed than the D_1/D_2 receptor dichotomy, is the utilization of DA autoreceptor agonists. Among the multiple types of DA receptors postulated to exist in mammalian brain is the DA-sensitive autoreceptor located on the cell body and terminal areas of certain DA-containing neurons (1); stimulation of this receptor reduces DA synthesis and release (85), inhibits DA-neuronal firing (147), and diminishes DA-mediated animal behaviors (20). Because of the high ligand affinity of the autoreceptor compared with the postsynaptic receptor, it can be differentially stimulated with low doses of DA agonist. Thus, selective stimulation of presynaptic DA receptors in the schizophrenic patient has been pursued for its potential antipsychotic effect. Results from early trials of apomorphine in schizophrenia carried out to test this hypothesis (34,135) were reminiscent of reports from the early 1900s of the tranquilizing effects of apomorphine (42); they showed a reduction in psychotic symptoms lasting a short time. Some (35,81) but not all (48,94) subsequent attempts to replicate this work have been positive. Those studies failing entirely to observe an antipsychotic effect with apomorphine generally used low doses of apomorphine. The other studies suggest a variable mental status response, sometimes including psychosis reduction. The variability in patient response to apomorphine remains unexplained: whereas some individuals have a significant decrease in psychosis, others fail to change at all, and an occasional patient worsens. Whether this response is a state or trait phenomenon and whether it is stable within a single individual and/or has a kinetic explanation remain unanswered. Biochemical analysis of plasma and CSF after apomorphine administration has demonstrated transient reductions in DA metabolites, supporting the proposed DA autoreceptor mechanism of drug effect. Clinical studies utilizing nonapomorphine DA agonists to reduce psychosis, chiefly ergots, have been uniformly negative (16,102,134). Although unexplained, this may be accounted for by the other transmitter actions of these compounds. N-Propyl-norapomorphine (NPA), an N-propyl analog of apomorphine, has antipsychotic effects acutely, but repeated administration produces tolerance to this effect (132). To what extent these theoretically interesting findings can be applied to the actual treatment of schizophrenia needs to be answered.

The use of DA agonist stimulation in the treatment of schizophrenia, directed toward the postsynaptic receptor, although generally found to stimulate psychotic symptoms (8), may actually treat a subset of psychotic symptoms, the deficit state symptoms of schizophrenia (58,76). Both anecdotal and controlled-study data support the idea that L-DOPA or other agonists such as bromocriptine may improve deficit symptoms in schizophrenia. However, the full development of this idea will depend on additional testing in subpopulations of schizophrenics.

OTHER TRANSMITTER SYSTEM DRUGS

Two other CNS monoamine transmitter systems, serotonin and norepinephrine, have been considered at one time or another to be pivotal to the pathophysiology of schizophrenia (73,153). There is renewed interest in the strategy of manipulating the serotonin system in schizophrenia for therapeutic response with the report that fenfluramine, a drug that releases and depletes serotonin, improves symptoms of autism, a disease whose symptoms can parallel some of those found in schizophrenia (52). Although several initial studies of fenfluramine in schizophrenia indicate that it has no antipsychotic or antiautistic effects (26,127), studies with direct-acting serotonin receptor antagonists appear more promising. The idea that serotonin receptor antagonists may be therapeutically useful in schizophrenia is supported by several observations: clozapine has unusually potent serotonin antagonist activity, which might explain some component of its antipsychotic action, and there have been promising early reports of the antipsychotic action of selective serotonin antagonists (26). This question remains to be explored further.

Norepinephrine (NE)-containing neurons may be abnormal in schizophrenia as evidenced by a deficit of the amine in cerebrospinal fluid from schizophrenic patients (90). An explanation of this abnormality has been elusive, in part because the pharmacology of schizophrenia does not support a potent involvement of NE in the symptoms of psychosis. Not only do noradrenergic agonists (a tricyclic or amphetamine) fail to improve symptoms of schizophrenia, but they often exacerbate the condition. Moreover, propranolol, as detailed in the next paragraph, has been hypothesized to improve psychosis with high-dose administration. Presumably, the CSF deficit in NE in schizophrenia could be spurious; it could be a compensatory neural change associated with schizophrenia or a long-lived neuroleptic side effect.

Propranolol, as a β-adrenergic receptor blocker, has therapeutic indications in the treatment of heart disease, hypertension, and headache. Based on its pharmacologic action, the drug has been tested in schizophrenia in a number of European studies (10,154) and, later, in clinical trials in the United States (51,121), which initially suggested some psychosis improvement. However, reports from controlled clinical trials carried out as a follow-up of the initial observations are rare. But among a group of the best studies, no more than half of the patients sustained an antipsychotic response of even a mild degree to high doses of propranolol. There was no consistency as to the type of symptomatic improvement in psychosis from study to study. Nor was the symptom response reported of the magnitude as that which commonly occurs with DA receptor blockers.

The other traditional brain neurotransmitter systems that have been studied in schizophrenia are γ-aminobutyric acid (GABA) and acetylcholine. Pharmacologic manipulation of CNS cholinergic activity fails to alter psychotic symptoms or to improve the disease. GABA is a ubiquitous neurotransmitter in brain, subserving not only long tracts but local neuronal networks as well (87,148). Its general function as an inhibitory transmitter has led to the concept, proposed by Roberts (112), that a generalized GABA-mediated neuronal network in the mammalian central nervous system preserves organized cognitive, affective, and behavioral activities by selective disinhibition. Thus, augmenting GABA-mediated neural inhibition should theoretically improve schizophrenia. Also, evidence suggests that GABA interacts with the nigral DA-containing neurons, albeit in a complex fashion (149), to inhibit electrical activity in DA-containing neurons. Thus, GABA agonism was proposed as a mechanism for reducing DA system activity and improving psychosis. When GABAmimetics were actually tested in schizophrenia, however, they failed to improve psychosis. Indeed, they do not have any consistent action on psychosis. The direct-acting agonist muscimol, instead of being antipsychotic, is psychotomimetic in schizophrenia, mimicking the action it has in normals (131). Other GABAmimetics, such as γ-acetylenic GABA and THIP, while producing variable mental status changes do not alleviate psychosis. Two others, γ-vinyl GABA and progabide, appear to have no effect on mental status at all in schizophrenia (140). Clinical evidence supports the generalization that GABAmimetic drugs do not alter psychotic symptoms in schizophrenia by modifying GABA-mediated neurotransmission.

PEPTIDERGIC DRUGS

The discovery and identification of peptides that behave as transmitters in the brain have opened a new chapter in CNS pharmacology. The discovery that a number of peptides are also colocalized with traditional neurotransmitters and with each other has prompted speculation that peptides may also be transmission modulators. Thus, not only do many different peptidergic transmitters exist in brain, but they may behave in multiple ways as well. The identification, localization, and basic biochemistry of the peptide-mediated neurons has preceded much of an appreciation of their functional roles. Thus, where clinical application of many of these peptides has taken place, it has preceded a full understanding of their function in mammalian brain. Also, any clinical application has been difficult because of methodologic difficulties, especially their CNS tissue penetrability and their rapid degradation by plasma and tissue peptidases.

One family of peptide neurotransmitters in brain, the opiates, is characterized by their ability to bind to the opiate receptors. Manipulation of the opiate subsystems with agonists and antagonists, monitored by functional measures of these systems, has been actively studied in schizophrenia. The CSF levels of an opiate-like endorphin (other than β-endorphin or enkephalin) have been reported elevated in acute unmedicated schizophrenic subjects and subsequently normalized in those same subjects following neuroleptic-induced psychosis remission (96,138). β-Endorphin itself has been reported to be elevated in acutely psychotic schizophrenics (41). With these pieces of evidence used to hypothesize opiate system excess in schizophrenia, naloxone, an opiate antagonist, was administered to symptomatic schizophrenic volunteers. Although no therapeutic effect was initially demonstrated, subsequent studies reported a naloxone-induced improvement, but only in isolated psychotic symptoms such as hallucinations (47,93,150); other investigators failed to find any such therapeutic effects (78,89,144). Overall, naloxone appears to have little consistent action in psychosis.

Curiously, although some investigators found rationale enough to diminish central endorphin system action with an opiate receptor-blocking drug, others found reason to stimulate those same opiate systems with agonists. β-endorphin was administered to schizophrenic subjects in an uncontrolled clinical trial, with striking symptomatic improvement reported, in some cases a prolonged effect (86). This report led to a vigorous search for antipsychotic actions of opiate agonists. The met-enkephalin analog FK 33-824 was tested and reported lacking in antipsychotic efficacy (81). Subsequent studies with β-endorphin have failed to confirm any antipsychotic activity of this peptide (13).

In addition to the opiate peptidergic system, nonopiate peptides have been studied for their antipsychotic efficacy. The β-lipotropin (β-LPH) fragment γ-endorphin and its destyrosine derivative des-tyrosine-γ-endorphin (DTγE, β-LPH$_{62-77}$) alter active avoidance learning in rats in a fashion similar to neuroleptics (39); thus, DTγE was tested in schizophrenic subjects for active antipsychotic effects. Initial trials (46,142,143) found antipsychotic effects of DTγE in select subgroups of schizophrenic subjects, but later investigators were unable to reproduce the original results in other patients (136). Work has begun in testing another endorphin derivative, desenkephalin-γ-endorphin (DEγE), believed to be the active antipsychotic metabolite of DTγE in man and suggested to have the same antipsychotic activity (143). No replicable demonstration of the antipsychotic activity of this family of drugs has yet been accomplished.

Cholecystokinin octapeptide (CCK-8), another nonopiate peptidergic transmitter, has received considerable attention as an antipsychotic drug. Two features of its distribution in brain suggest a potential involvement in schizophrenia: (a) its cortical localization (14) and (b) its colocalization with DA in certain of the mesencephalic DA-containing neurons, particularly in the A10 region (72). Even before its physiologic or behavioral actions had been characterized, it was tested for antipsychotic efficacy in schizophrenic patients (104). This early study reported CCK-8 to be a rather potent antipsychotic drug. Thus, preclinical and additional clinical studies commenced to address questions of efficacy and mechanism. Although preclinical studies even now continue to support more strongly the rationale for CCK-8 efficacy in schizophrenia (36), the subsequent controlled clinical experiments have been uniformly negative (74,98,133). Not only psychosis but also other centrally mediated functions such as visual evoked potential and involuntary movements in the patients fail to change with CCK-8. The peptide also fails to alter parkinsonian symptoms in severely affected Parkinson's disease patients (19). On the other hand, in animal model and in vitro experiments, CCK-8 modulates the release of DA from nerve terminals (100); it modifies prolactin secretion, but not through the dopaminergic system (137); it may also interact with dopaminergic transmission postsynaptically at the DA receptor or membrane effector system. These central actions of CCK-8 occur in rats when the peptide is administered intraventricularly or directly into tissue. Even though behavioral, electrophysiologic, and biochemical changes in neural function are reported with systemic CCK-8 administration, at least some of these changes can be attributed to stimulation of vagal afferent fibers. An explanation of the negative clinical results of CCK-8 in the treatment of schizophrenia that is consistent with the promising preclinical data is that CCK-8 fails to enter the mammalian brain with systemic administration. Neither systemic administration of radiolabeled CCK-8 in monkeys with CSF analysis (unpublished observation) nor in vivo receptor occupancy tests in rats provides evidence to support the claim that systemically administered CCK-8 enters the brain (27). Thus, the hypothesis that CCK-8 will improve psychosis in schizophrenia has not yet been effectively tested because of drug delivery problems.

Any number of other neurally active peptides that have already been identified are of interest in schizophrenia based on their localization in brain, their apparent interaction with DA neural systems, and their behavioral actions. These include such peptides as neurotensin, corticotropin-releasing factor, somatostatin, and substance P, among others. In summary, the area of peptide pharmacology in schizophrenia is probably one of the most exciting and rapidly changing areas of current research. Although the mechanisms required to modify central peptidergic systems in humans have not yet been clearly defined, the demand for data from clinical application and the clinical enthusiasm for new pharmacologic directions fuels both basic and applied research. Currently, little work in the therapeutic application of clinical peptide pharmacology has been positive, but this area of developing basic neurobiology is bound to afford significant gains in clinical applicability in the future. In addition, one might anticipate that a reduction in the proposed heterogeneity of schizophrenia by defining pathophysiologically homogeneous groups might allow some of these treatments to emerge as effective in particular disease subtypes.

Overall, the development of new and novel antipsychotic compounds has depended on advances in the design of known neuroleptics or on the application of putative antipsychotic strategies derived from preclinical studies. Neither of these approaches has identified fully effective therapies directed at the core pathophysiology of schizophrenia. However, technical advances in the field may provide new opportunities. Recently, new technologies have allowed visualization of the living human brain with positron emission tomography using labeled deoxyglucose or selective receptor ligands. Findings from these investigations promise to reveal a new level of understanding about localization of function, perhaps of symptoms, in the schizophrenic brain. Pharmacologic approaches derived from PET studies might provide a basis for more potent and specific antischizophrenic treatments. Traditionally, antipsychotic treatments, regardless of the transmitter system targeted, have modified synaptic transmission. The rapid rate of developments in the field of molecular genetics suggests that, shortly, pharmacology in psychiatry may be moved to the level of the gene and the gene product. Modification of enzyme production, receptor synthesis, or membrane regeneration carried out by modifying gene translation or posttranslational processing could conceivably modify centrally mediated behaviors in man in a powerful and specific manner. The diversity of new and potential pharmacologic approaches becoming available and the sophisticated technologies for studying human brain pathophysiology may contribute to conceptually new approaches to the treatment of schizophrenia.

REFERENCES

1. Aghajanian, C. K., and Bunney, B. S. (1973): In: *Frontiers in Catecholamine Research,* edited by E. Usdin and S. Snyder, pp. 643–645. Pergamon Press, New York.
2. Aghajanian, C. K., and Haigler, H. J. (1974): *Adv. Biochem. Psychopharmacol.,* 10:167–177.
3. Alberts, J. L., Francois, F., and Josserand, F. (1985): *Semin. Hop. Paris,* 61:1351–1357.
4. Anden, N. E., Carlsson, A., Dahlstrom, A., Fuxe, K., Hillarp, N. A., et al. (1964): *Life Sci.,* 3:523–530.
5. Anderman, B., and Griffith, R. W. (1977): *Eur. J. Clin. Pharmacol.,* 11:193–198.
6. Angrist, B. M., and Gershon, S. (1970): *Biol. Psychiatry,* 2:95–107.
7. Angrist, B. M., Rotrosen, J., and Gershon, S. (1982): *Psychopharmacologia,* 72:17–19.
8. Angrist, B. M., Sathananthan, G., and Gershon, S. (1973): *Psychopharmacologia,* 31:1–12.
9. Angst, J., Haenicke, U., Padrutt, A., et al. (1971): *Pharmakopsychiatrie,* 4:192–200.
10. Atsmon, A. (1976): *Adv. Clin. Pharmacol.,* 12:86–90.
11. Bannon, M. J., Reinhard, J. F., Bunney, B. S., and Roth, R. H. (1982): *Nature,* 296:444–446.
12. Bannon, M. J., Wolf, M. E., and Roth, R. H. (1983): *Eur. J. Pharmacol.,* 91:119–125.
13. Barchas, J. D., Berger, P. A., Watson, S. J., Akil, H., and Hao Li, C. (1980): In: *Neural Peptides and Neuronal Communication,* edited by E. Costa and M. Trabucchi, pp. 447–453. Raven Press, New York.
14. Beinfeld, M. D., Meyer, D. K., Eskay, R. L., Jensen, R. T., and Brownstein, M. J. (1981): *Brain Res.,* 212:51–57.
15. Benkert, O., and Holsboer, F. (1984): *Acta Psychiatr. Scand.,* 69(Suppl. 311):42–48.
16. Brambilla, F., Scarone, S., and Pugnetti, L. (1983): *Psychiatr. Res.,* 8:159–169.
17. Bratfos, O., and Haug, J. O. (1979): *Acta Psychiatr. Scand.,* 135:164–173.
18. Brownstein, M. J. (1979): In: *Dopaminergic Ergot Derivatives and Motor Functions,* edited by K. Fuxe and D. B. Calne, pp. 33–43. Pergamon Press, New York.
19. Bruno, G., Ruggeri, S., Chase, T. N., Bakker, K., and Tamminga, C. A. (1985): *Clin. Neuropharmacol.,* 8:266–270.
20. Carlsson, A. (1975): In: *The Basal Ganglia,* edited by M. D. Yahr, pp. 137–141. Raven Press, New York.
21. Carlsson, A., and Lindquist (1963): *Acta Pharmacol. Toxicol.,* 20:140.
22. Carlsson, A., Roos, B. E., Walinder, J., and Skott, A. (1973): *J. Neural Transm.,* 34:125–132.
23. Carpenter, W. T., Heinrichs, D. W., and Alphs, L. D. (1985): *Schizophrenia Bull.,* 11:440–453.
24. Carpenter, W. T., Heinrichs, D. W., and Wagman, A. M. I. (1987): *Arch. Gen. Psychiatry (in press).*
25. Casey, D. E., Gerlach, J., and Simmelsgaard, H. (1979): *Psychopharmacology,* 66:73–77.
26. Ceulemans, D. L. S., Gelders, Y. G., Hoppenbrouwers, J. A., Reyntjens, J. M., and Janssen, P. A. J. (1985): *Psychopharmacology,* 85:329–332.
27. Chase, T. N., Barone, P., Bruno, G., Cohen, S. L., Juncos, J., et al. (1985): In: *Neuronal Cholecystokinin,* edited by J. N. Crawley and J. J. Vanderhaegen, pp. 553–561. New York Academy of Sciences, New York.
28. Chiodo, L. A., and Bunney, B. S. (1983): *J. Neurosci.,* 3:1607–1619.
29. Chouinard, G. (1987): *Psychopharmacology (in press).*
30. Chouinard, G., and Annable, L. (1984): *Psychopharmacology,* 84:282–284.
31. Chouinard, G., Pinard, G., Serrano, M., and Tetreault, L. (1973): *Curr. Ther. Res.,* 15:473–482.
32. Christensen, A. V., Arnt, J., and Svendsen, O. (1985): In: *Dyskinesia: Research and Treatment,* edited by D. E. Casey, T. N. Chase, A. V. Christensen, and J. Gerlach, pp. 182–190. Springer-Verlag, Heidelberg.
33. Christensen, E., Bjork, A., and Gustavsson, B. (1985): *Acta Physiol. Scand.,* 124(Suppl. 542):281.
34. Corsini, G. U., Del Zompo, M., Manconi, S., Cianchetti, C., Magoni, A., et al. (1977): *Adv. Biochem. Psychopharmacol.,* 16:645–649.
35. Corsini, G. U., Piccardi, M. P., Bocchetta, A., Bernardi, F., and Del Zompo, M. (1981): In: *Apomorphine and Other Dopaminomimetics, Vol. 2: Clinical Pharmacology,* edited by G. U. Corsini and G. L. Gessa, pp. 13–24. Raven Press, New York.
36. Crawley, J. N., and Vanderhaegen, J. J., eds. (1985): *Neuronal Cholecystokinin.* New York Academy of Sciences, New York.
37. Crow, T. J. (1980): *Br. Med. J.,* 280:66–68.
38. Dahlstrom, A., and Fuxe, K. (1964): *Acta Physiol. Scand. [Suppl.],* 232:1–55.
39. De Wied, D., Kovacs, G. L., and Bohus, B. (1978): *Eur. J. Pharmacol.,* 49:427–438.
40. Doepp, S., and Buddeberg, C. (1975): *Nervenarzt,* 46:589–590.
41. Domschke, W., Dickschas, A., and Mitznegg, P. (1979): *Lancet,* 1:1024.

42. Douglas, C. J. (1900): *Mercks Arch.,* 11:212–213.
43. Edwards, J. G., Alexander, J. R., Alexander, M. S., Gordon, A., and Zutchi, T. (1980): *Br. J. Psychiatry,* 137:522–529.
44. Eichenberger, E. (1984): *Arzneim. Forsch. Drug Res.,* 34:110–114.
45. Elizur, A., and Davison, S. (1975): *Curr. Ther. Res.,* 18:578–584.
46. Emrich, H. W. (1980): *Pharmakopsychiatr. Neuropsychopharmakol.,* 13:290–298.
47. Emrich, H. W., Cording, C., and Piree, S. (1977): *Neuropsychopharmakology,* 10:265–270.
48. Ferrier, E. C., Johnstone, E. C., and Crow, T. J. (1984): *Br. J. Psychiatry,* 144:341–348.
49. Ferris, et al. (1982): *J. Pharm. Pharmacol.,* 34:388–390.
50. Fisher-Cornelssen, K., Ferner, U., and Steiner, H. (1974): *Arzneim. Forsch.,* 24:1006–1007.
51. Gardos, G., Cole, J., Volicer, L., Orzack, M. H., and Oliff, A. C. (1973): *Curr. Ther. Res.,* 15:314–323.
52. Geller, E., Ritvo, E. R., Freeman, B. J., and Yuwiler, A. (1982): *N. Engl. J. Med.,* 307:165–168.
53. Gerlach, J. (1985): In: *Dyskinesia. Research and Treatment,* edited by D. E. Casey, T. N. Chase, A. V. Christensen, and J. Gerlach, pp. 98–103. Springer-Verlag, Berlin, Heidelberg, New York.
54. Gerlach, J., Ahlfors, U. G., Dencker, S. J., Gravem, A., Gunby, B., et al. (1987): *Psychopharmacology* (in press).
55. Gerlach, J., Behnke, K., Heltberg, J., Munk-Andersen, E., and Nielsen, H. (1985): *Br. J. Psychiatry,* 147:283–288.
56. Gerlach, J., Kistrup, K., and Korsgaard, S. (1987): In: *Selectivity of Psychotropic Drug Action,* edited by S. Dahl, L. Gram, S. Poal, and W. Potter. Springer-Verlag, Berlin.
57. Gerlach, J., Koppellnis, P., Helweg, E., and Monrad, A. (1974): *Acta Psychiatr. Scand.,* 50:410–424.
58. Gerlach, J., and Luhdorf, K. (1975): *Psychopharmacologia,* 44:105–110.
59. Gerlach, J., and Simmelsgaard, H. (1978): *Psychopharmacology,* 59:105–112.
60. Gerlach, J., Thorsen, K., and Fog, R. (1975): *Psychopharmacologia,* 40:341–350.
61. Gershanik, O., Heikkila, R. E., and DuVoisin, R. C. (1983): *Neurology (N.Y.),* 33:1489–1492.
62. Gershon, S., Heikimian, L., Floyd, A., and Hollister, L. (1967): *Psychopharmacologia,* 11:189–194.
63. Gianutsos, G., and Moore, K. E. (1977): *Res. Commun. Chem. Pathol. Pharmacol.,* 17:29–39.
64. Gower, A. J., and Marriott, A. S. (1982): *Br. J. Pharmacol.,* 77:185–194.
65. Gross, H., Langner, E., and Pfolz, H. (1970): *Arzneim. Forsch.,* 24:987–989.
66. Gunne, L.-M., Haggstrom, J.-E., and Sjoquist, B. (1984): *Nature,* 309:347–351.
67. Haggstrom, J.-E. (1984): *Acta Psychiatr. Scand.,* 69(Suppl. 311):103–108.
68. Harnryd, C., Bjerkenstedt, L., Bjork, K., Gullberg, B., Oxenstierna, G., et al. (1984): *Acta Psychiatr. Scand.,* 69(Suppl. 311):7–30.
69. Harnryd, C., Bjerkenstedt, L., Gullberg, B., Oxenstierna, G., Sedvall, G., et al. (1984): *Acta Psychiatr. Scand.,* 69(Suppl. 311):75–92.
70. Hartvig, P., Eckernas, S. A., Lindstrom, L., Ekblom, B., Bondesson, U., et al. (1987): *Psychopharmacology* (in press).
71. Himwich, H. E. (1967): In: *Comprehensive Textbook of Psychiatry,* edited by A. M. Freedman and H. I. Kaplan, pp. 67–77. Williams & Wilkins, Baltimore.
72. Hokfelt, T., Rehfeld, L., Skirboll, B., Ivemark, M., Goldstein, M., et al. (1980): *Nature,* 285:476–478.
73. Holden, J., Itil, T., Keskiner, A., and Gannon, P. (1971): *J. Clin. Pharmacol.,* 11:220–226.
74. Hommer, D. W., Pickar, D., Roy, A., Ninan, P., Boronow, J., et al. (1984): *Arch. Gen. Psychiatry,* 41:617–622.
75. Hyttel, J., Larsen, J. J., Christensen, A. V., and Arnt, J. (1985): In: *Dyskinesia: Research and Treatment,* edited by D. E. Casey, T. N. Chase, A. V. Christensen, and J. Gerlach, pp. 9–18. Springer-Verlag, Berlin, Heidelberg, New York.
76. Inanaga, K., Nakazawa, Y., Inoue, K., Tachibana, H., Oshima, M., et al. (1975): *Folia Psychiatr. Neurol. Jpn.,* 29:123–143.
77. Ingvar, D. H., and Franzen, G. (1974): *Acta Psychiatr. Scand.,* 50:425–462.
78. Janowsky, D. S., Segal, D. S., and Bloom, F. (1977): *Am. J. Psychiatry,* 134:926–927.
79. Jenner, P., and Marsden, C. D. (1984): *Acta Psychiatr. Scand.,* 69(Suppl. 311):109–123.
80. Jenner, P., Rupniak, N. M. J., and Marsden, D. C. (1985): In: *Dyskinesia: Research and Treatment,* edited by D. E. Casey, T. N. Chase, A. V. Christensen, and J. Gerlach, pp. 174–181. Springer-Verlag, Berlin, Heidelberg, New York.
81. Jeste, D. V., Zalcman, S., Weinberger, D. R., Cutler, N. R., Bigelow, L. B., et al. (1983): *Prog. Neuropsychopharmacol. Biol. Psychiatry,* 7(1):83–88.
82. Jorgensen, A., Fog, R., and Veilis, B. (1979): *Lancet,* 1:935.
83. Kebabian, J. W. (1978): *Life Sci.,* 23:479–484.
84. Kebabian, J. W., and Calne, D. B. (1979): *Nature,* 277:93–96.
85. Kehr, W., Carlsson, A., Lindquist, M., Magnusson, T., and Atack, C. (1972): *J. Pharm. Pharmacol.,* 24:744–747.
86. Kline, N. S., Hao Li, C., Lehmann, H. E., Lajtha, A., Laski, E., et al. (1977): *Arch. Gen. Psychiatry,* 34:1111–1113.
87. Krogsgaard-Larsen, P., Scheel-Kruger, J., and Kofod, H. (1979): *GABA-Neurotransmitters: Pharmacochemical, Biochemical, and Pharmacologic Aspect.* Munksgaard, Copenhagen.
88. Krupp, P., and Monka, C. (1982): Situation Report, March 31, 1982. Sandoz Document, April 26, 1982. Sandoz, Basel, Switzerland.
89. Kurland, A. A., McCabe, O., Hanlon, T. E., and Sullivan, D. (1977): *Am. J. Psychiatry,* 134:1408–1410.
90. Lake, C. R., Sternberg, D. E., van Kammen, D. P., Ballenger, J. C., Ziegler, M. G., et al. (1980): *Science,* 207:331–333.
91. Laursen, A. L., and Gerlach, J. (1986): *Acta Psychiatr. Scand.,* 73:17–21.
92. Lee, T., and Tang, S. W. (1984): *Psychiatr. Res.,* 12:277–285.
93. Lehmann, H., Vasavan Nair, N. P., and Kline, N. S. (1979): *Am. J. Psychiatry,* 136:762–766.
94. Levy, M. I., Davis, B. M., Mohs, R. C., Kendler, K. S., Mathe, A. A., et al. (1984): *Arch. Gen. Psychiatry,* 41:520–524.
95. Lindstrom, L., Besev, G., Stening, G., and Widerlov, E. (1985): *Psychopharmacology,* 86:241–243.
96. Lindstrom, L. H., Widerlov, E., Gunne, L. M., Wahlstrom, A., and Terenius, L. (1978): *Acta Psychiatr. Scand.,* 57:153–164.
97. Ljungberg, T., and Ungerstedt, U. (1979): *Psychopharmacology,* 60:303–307.
98. Lotstra, F., Verbanck, P., Mendelewicz, J., and Vanderhaegen, J. J. (1984): *Biol. Psychiatry,* 6:877–882.
99. Magelund, G., Gerlach, J., and Casey, D. E. (1979): *Acta Psychiatr. Scand.,* 60:185–189.
100. Markstein, R., and Hokfelt, T. (1984): *J. Neurosci.,* 4:570–575.
101. McCreadie, R. G., Morrison, D., Eccleston, D., Gall, R. G., Loudon, J., et al. (1985): *Acta Psychiatr. Scand.,* 72:139–143.
102. Meltzer, H. Y. (1980): *Schizophrenia Bull.,* 6:456–475.
103. Meltzer, H. Y., and Luchins, D. J. (1984): *J. Clin. Psychopharmacol.,* 4:286–287.
104. Moroji, T., Watanabe, N., Aoki, N., and Itoh, S. (1982): *Arch. Gen. Psychiatry,* 39:485–486.
105. Niskanen, P., Tamminen, T., and Viukari, M. (1975): *Curr. Ther. Res.,* 17:281–284.
106. Ogren, S. O., Hall, H., Kohler, C., Magnusson, O., de Paulis, T., et al. (1987): (in press).
107. Ogren, S. O., Hall, H., Kohler, C., Magnusson, O., Lindbom, L.-O., et al. (1983): *Eur. J. Pharmacol.,* 102:459–474.
108. Ogren, S. O., Hall, H., Kohler, C., Magnusson, O., and Sjostrand, S.-E. (1987): *Psychopharmacology* (in press).
109. Pakkenberg, H., and Pakkenberg, B. (1986): *Acta Neurol. Scand.,* 73:295–297.
110. Povlsen, U. J., Noring, U., Fog, R., and Gerlach, J. (1985): *Acta Psychiatr. Scand.,* 71:176–185.
111. Rao, V. A. R., Bailey, J., Kirkin, A., and Coppen, A. (1980): *Psychopharmacology,* 80:73–77.
112. Roberts, E. (1976): In: *GABA in Nervous System Function,* edited by T. N. Chase and D. B. Tower, pp. 515–540. Raven Press, New York.
113. Robertson, A., and MacDonald, C. (1984): *Pharmacol. Biochem. Behav.,* 21:97–101.

114. Robertson, A., and MacDonald, C. (1985): *Eur. J. Pharmacol.,* 109:81–89.
115. Rosengarten, H., Schweitzer, J. W., and Friedhoff, A. J. (1983): *Life Sci.,* 33:2479–2482.
116. Rudenko, G. M., and Lepakhin, V. K. (1979): In: *Side Effects of Drugs, Annual 3,* pp. 50–53. Excerpta Medica, Amsterdam.
117. Saller, C. F., and Salama, A. I. (1985): *Eur. J. Pharmacol.,* 109: 297.
118. Scatton, B., Bischoff, S., Dedek, J., and Korf, J. (1977): *Eur. J. Pharmacol.,* 44:287–292.
119. Sedvall, G., Bjerkenstedt, L., Lindstrom, L., and Wode-Helgodt, B. (1986): *Life Sci.,* 23:425–430.
120. Setler, P. E., Sarau, H. M., Zirkle, C. L., and Saunders, H. L. (1978): *Eur. J. Pharmacol.,* 50:419–430.
121. Shopsin, B., Hirsch, J., and Gershon, S. (1975): *Biol. Psychiatry,* 10:105–107.
122. Shopsin, B., Klein, H., Aaronsom, M., and Collora, M. (1979): *Arch. Gen. Psychiatry,* 36:657–664.
123. Simpson, G. M., and Cooper, T. A. (1978): *Am. J. Psychiatry,* 135:99–100.
124. Simpson, G. M., Lee, J. H., and Shrivastava, R. K. (1978): *Psychopharmacology,* 56:75–80.
125. Sjoerdsma, A. (1966): *Pharmacol. Rev.,* 18:673–684.
126. Snyder, S. H. (1972): *Arch. Gen. Psychiatry,* 27:169–179.
127. Stahl, S. M., Uhr, S. B., and Berger, P. A. (1985): *Biol. Psychiatry,* 20:1098–1102.
128. Stille, G., Lauener, H., and Eichenberg, E. (1971): *Farmaco Ed. Prat.,* 26:603–625.
129. Stoof, J. F., and Kebabian, J. W. (1981): *Nature,* 294:366–368.
130. Tam, S.-Y., and Roth, R. H. (1985): *Biochem. Pharmacol.,* 34: 1595–1598.
131. Tamminga, C. A., Crayton, J. C., and Chase, T. N. (1978): *Am. J. Psychiatry,* 135:746–748.
132. Tamminga, C. A., Gotts, M. D., Thaker, G. K., Alphs, L. D., and Foster, N. L. (1986): *Arch. Gen. Psychiatry,* 43:398–402.
133. Tamminga, C. A., Littman, R. L., Alphs, L. D., Chase, T. N., Thaker, G. K., et al. (1986): *Psychopharmacology,* 88:387–391.
134. Tamminga, C. A., and Schaffer, M. H. (1979): *Psychopharmacology,* 66:239–242.
135. Tamminga, C. A., Schaffer, M. H., Smith, R. C., and Davis, J. M. (1978): *Science,* 200:567–568.
136. Tamminga, C. A., Tighe, P. J., Chase, T. N., DeFraites, E. G., and Schaffer, M. H. (1981): *Arch. Gen. Psychiatry,* 38:167–168.
137. Tanimoto, K., Tamminga, C. A., and Chase, T. N. (1985): *Neurosci. Abstr.* 11:1298.
138. Terenius, L., Wahlstrom, A., Lindstrom, L., and Widerlov, E. (1976): *Neurosci. Lett.,* 3:157–162.
139. Thaker, G. K., Tamminga, C. A., Alphs, L. D., Lafferman, J., Ferraro, T. et al. (1987): *Arch. Gen. Psychiatry (in press).*
140. Ungerstedt, U., Herrera-Marschitz, M., Stahle, L., Tossman, U., and Zetterstrom, T. (1985): In: *Dyskinesia: Research and Treatment,* edited by D. E. Casey, T. N. Chase, A. V. Christensen, and J. Gerlach, pp. 19–30. Springer-Verlag, Berlin, Heidelberg, New York.
141. Verhoeven, W., Van Praag, H. M., and Van Ree, J. M. (1979): *Arch. Gen. Psychiatry,* 36:294–298.
142. Verhoeven, W. M., Van Ree, J. M., de Wied, D., and Van Praag, H. M. (1981): *Arch. Gen. Psychiatry,* 38:1182–1183.
143. Volavka, J., Mallya, A., Baig, S., and Perez-Cruet, J. (1977): *Science,* 196:1227–1228.
144. Von Zander, K. J., and Ruther, E. (1978): *Arzneim. Forsch.,* 28: 1495–1496.
145. Walters, J. R., Bunney, B. S., and Roth, R. H. (1975): *Adv. Neurol.,* 9:273–284.
146. Walters, J. R., Bunney, B. S., and Roth, R. H. (1975): *Adv. Neurol.,* 9:273–284.
147. Walters, J. R., and Chase, T. N. (1977): In: *Neurotransmitter Function: Basic and Clinical Aspects,* edited by W. S. Fields, pp. 193–211. Stratton Intercontinental, New York.
148. Walters, J. R., and Lakoski, J. M. (1978): *Eur. J. Pharmacol.,* 47:469–472.
149. Watson, S. J., Berger, P. A., Akil, H., Mills, M. J., and Barchas, J. D. (1978): *Science,* 201:73–75.
150. Weinberger, D. R., Jeste, D. V., Teychenne, P. F., and Wyatt, R. J. (1985): In: *Schizophrenia Paranoia and Schizophreniform Disorders of Late Life,* edited by N. Miller and G. Cohen. Guilford Press, New York.
151. Woggon, B., Heinrich, K., Kufferle, B., Muller-Oerlinghausen, B., Polding, W., et al. (1984): *Arzneim. Forsch. Drug Res.,* 34: 122–125.
152. Wyatt, R. J., Gillin, J. C., Kaplan, J., Stillman, R., Mandel, L., et al. (1974): In: *Serotonin—New Vistas,* edited by D. Costa, G. L. Gessa, and M. Sandler, pp. 299–314. Raven Press, New York.
153. Yorkston, N. J., Zaki, S. A., Pitcher, D. R., Grizelier, J. H., Hollander, D., et al. (1977): *Lancet,* 1:575–578.

Psychopharmacology:
The Third Generation of Progress,
edited by Herbert Y. Meltzer.
Raven Press, New York © 1987.

CHAPTER 117

Treatment of Anxiety in the Elderly

Richard I. Shader, John S. Kennedy, and David J. Greenblatt

Although the differentiation among stress responses, fear, and anxiety is of general theoretical and practical value, this distinction is particularly important for the elderly. At a practical level, phenomenological distinctions among these states are meaningful because their etiology and specific management are likely different. As concepts they are highly interrelated semantically; unfortunately, the essential aspects of what they share and how they differ remain somewhat obscure. When an elderly woman living alone in a disadvantaged neighborhood on a fixed income has fallen several times, does not want to leave her room, and complains of tension and trouble falling asleep, is this fear, stress, or anxiety, or some combination of any two or all three?

CONCEPTS

Stress itself is not an affective state. In our view, stress can be best understood as an adaptation to environmental or internal demands that exceed an individual's capacities or resources. Study of particular stressors and their consequences may have utility in understanding the elderly. In our experience, certain variables (e.g., an increase in rent or other costs, the illness of a pet, the loss of teeth) may have more significance for the elderly than for younger groups. It is not at all clear why not all individuals exposed to seemingly comparable troubles reveal stress and why not all individuals reveal stress in the same way. The concept of stress as it relates to the elderly is reviewed more extensively elsewhere (41,59).

Many current definitions conceptualize the differences between fear and anxiety states as being recognizable by any of three elements:

1. The presence or absence of a consensually determined threat to homeostasis;
2. The extent to which the observed or felt reactions are proportionate to the threat; and
3. The potential adaptiveness of the response defined in terms of survival value.

Definitions using this framework are fraught with difficulty because they are subjective. As an example of the difficulty associated with these definitions, it is said that the elderly commonly "freeze," a behavior hypothesized to be a result of actual quantitative somatic losses or losses in the qualitative aspects of certain functions such as speed of action (i.e., those which would make successful fight or flight impossible) (26). Such persons show acquiescence or compliance on demand (10). Faced with a "frozen" nursing home patient who has been recently transferred to the home, it is not unlikely that some observers would view this behavior as an appropriate adaptation. Others might see "freezing" behavior as less adaptive than becoming difficult to manage or regressed.

In our view, some degree of fear is a primary and adaptive affective response to any threatening situation characterized by conflict, unfamiliarity, and/or anticipation of pain. Fear, like worry, is a self-limited emotion occurring under certain conditions and has survival value. Fear may become so intense and temporarily disabling that intervention or treatment may be indicated. Fear should dissipate as soon as conditions move from threat to safety. With fear, the memory of the threatening experience is integrated in a reality- and time-based fashion; this allows the individual to mobilize coping skills and behaviors that permit conscious choice to avoid similar experiences in the future, thereby promoting the capacity for the mastery of such situations.

TABLE 1. *Symptoms/syndromes that may be seen on first presentation in the elderly*

Somatization	Abdominal upset or
Hypochondriasis	gastrointestinal complaints
Fatigue	Motor restlessness
Vague aches and pains	Initial or sleep onset insomnia
Headaches	Phobic symptoms
Tachycardia	

Anxiety is the descriptor that applies when the fear-like affective response persists over excessively long periods or occurs without a known time-related stimulus. Anxiety may be persistent, leading to a sense of being constantly "uptight" or nervous, or it can be situational or have an attack-like course. Fear and anxiety can be difficult to differentiate in the elderly. Because physical illnesses associated with anxiety symptoms are common in the elderly, consideration of use of the term anxiety should invite particular caution in this age group. Only when a patient's symptoms appear after careful investigation to have no cause, when the pattern meets criteria for an "endogenous" anxiety state such as panic disorder, or when response to the fear-provoking stressor seems irrational, excessive, unremitting, or unwarranted, is it considered appropriate to label the patient's complaint as an anxiety disorder. Anxiety disorders appearing for the first time in an older person are uncommon; often such symptoms reflect stress or fear or some underlying autonomic nervous system dysregulation coming from hypoxia, thyroid dysfunction, or some other disorder. Perhaps most commonly, anxiety in older persons is a manifestation of a depressive disorder.

Anxiety in younger individuals is classically described as consisting of an anxious or apprehensive mood; intrusive ideation such as thoughts, fears, images, impulses, or dreams; trouble concentrating or altered feelings such as depersonalization or derealization; physiological signs and symptoms such as dyspnea, choking or smothering sensations, tachycardia, palpitations, muscle tension, trembling or shaking; and behaviors such as withdrawal, avoidance, agitation, or difficulty with decision making. Such behaviors and symptoms are often more obscurely delineated and organized into the presenting problems listed in Table 1. Table 1 highlights one of the difficulties in the evaluation of anxiety in the elderly—namely, physical illnesses often can coexist with or obscure anxiety symptoms.

EPIDEMIOLOGY, PREVALENCE, AND INCIDENCE AND ASSESSMENT ISSUES

There have been no prospective incidence studies of anxiety states in the elderly. The meager relevant literature is best summarized in Blazer's statement that " 'neuroses' (anxiety states and dysthymic disorders) probably decrease in incidence with increasing age" (3). As we have suggested, clinical wisdom suggests that *de novo* development of true anxiety states is uncommon or rare in the aged. Among disorders arising *de novo*, adjustment disorder with anxious mood [a *Diagnostic and Statistical Manual of Mental Disorders,* 3rd edition (DSM-III) diagnosis] is suggested to be most common (40), followed by simple phobias (58). Conditions that rarely develop *de novo* in the elderly are suggested to include panic disorder (40) and obsessive-compulsive disorder (43).

Certain problems regularly obscure the assessment of anxiety in the elderly. For example, symptom-based rating scales commonly include somatic complaints; hence, overestimates of dysfunction are common. Another problem with such scales is that the clusters or factors derived are not necessarily translatable into diagnostic entities. Indeed, Blazer (2) has suggested that symptom checklists are probably of less value in the elderly than in other age groups. The elderly may demonstrate a differential response to structured questionnaires compared to unstructured interviews and have a propensity for endorsing somatic items more frequently while denying the presence of associated or underlying affects.

One study of urban and rural adults (773 males and 1,338 females) over age 55 found, using the trait portion of the Speilberger State-Trait Inventory, that anxiety symptoms had a prevalence of 17.1 and 21.5% in males and females, respectively (24). Another, employing SCL-90 self-ratings in patients (79 males and 99 females) over age 60 on a geriatric medical inpatients unit compared to adult psychiatric inpatients (100 males and 101 females) under age 60, noted that 13% of the elderly patients had moderate to high anxiety scores: 50% of the younger patients reported moderate to high levels of anxiety as defined by this scale (34). A frequently cited prevalence study is by Bergmann (1), who evaluated each of 300 randomly sampled elderly individuals between ages 60 and 80 for psychiatric, medical, and cognitive problems. Anxiety states were defined to include anxiety neurotics and anxiety-prone personalities; obsessional or hysterical personalities were excluded. In retrospectively determining the age of initial onset for these problems, Bergmann found that the prevalence of late onset neurosis, defined as onset after age 60, was 8.6%. Chronic neurosis, defined as onset before age 60 but with persistence, had a prevalence of 10%. The finding of an approximately 20% prevalence of anxiety neurosis and anxiety-prone personality is at odds with data from most other prevalence studies, where mild to moderate neurosis has generally been reported in the range of 5 to 10% (51). It is possible that the inclusion of the so-called anxiety-prone personality accounts at least in part for some of this discrepancy. It should be noted that difficulties with retrospectively constructed diagnoses and presumably also ages of onset and with using a single interview in the absence of use of all available information have been pointed out by Leckman and co-workers (32). In their case-control family study of lifetime diagnoses, data derived from a single interview approximated diagnoses made on all available information for simple phobias, but this did not hold for panic disorder or generalized anxiety. More recently, preliminary results of the U.S. Epidemiological Catchment Area (ECA) program have been published (58). The ECA data suggest that the total prevalence of all disorders, including, among others, dementia, depression, and anxiety, for persons over age 65 is 10.8%. Given the lack of consensus among the various attempts at determining the incidence and prevalence of anxiety disorders among the elderly, further research clearly is needed. To be truly helpful, such research should try to differentiate among the symptom pictures of stress, anxiety, and fear. The ECA study's rates for agoraphobia and panic states deserve comment in this regard. Clinical experience suggests, as in our opening clinical example, that not infrequently elderly persons become housebound because of falls. They report concern about being jostled by crowds or slipping. They may not acknowledge that their fears may be excessive (perhaps even qualifying as anxiety), because such an admission is not seen as a socially desirable response; also their fears may not be excessive—a fear of falling in some elderly may be quite appropriate, since they can lead to severe injury and sometimes to death.

It follows that it may be difficult to make the *de novo* diagnosis of agoraphobia in the elderly, particularly when there has been an associated fall or even a pattern of neighborhood muggings. Agoraphobia not linked to panic attacks is uncommon in the young but not uncommon in the elderly. The ECA data on panic disorder are of interest because of a putative dramatic drop in prevalence for this disorder after age 65. It would be useful to know the nature of the relationships among fears of leaving the house or falling, the actual occurrence of falls and victimization in the elderly, and agoraphobia with and without panic attacks. Such data might assist in the development of a more useful taxonomy of fear states and anxiety states in the elderly. In summary, it is likely that the prevalence of anxiety states in the elderly ranges between 5 and 10% and that relative to younger ages there may be a modest decrease in prevalence because of a decreased incidence (37). Further research is needed to assess the clinical impression that in the elderly acute severe anxiety is relatively infrequent whereas low-grade chronic anxiety is more common.

ANXIETY AND DELIRIUM AND STRESS

Medical and drug-related etiologies for anxiety symptoms are particularly common in the elderly. These are numerous and reviewed elsewhere (23,27). For many of the drugs typically cited in such reviews, it is likely that the induced anxiety symptoms either are a direct effect on the autonomic nervous system or are the manifestations of subclinical drug-induced delirium (i.e., delirium in which fluctuating orientation is not readily apparent).

Anxiety and delirium are distinct phenomena which in the elderly can merge at times and present difficulty in clinical differentiation. Essential features, however, for the diagnosis of delirium are inattention and acutely fluctuating orientation. When autonomic nervous system overactivity is involved, tachycardia, tremor, dilated pupils, and increased perspiration are frequently seen. Delirium, which may occur in 30 to 50% of the hospitalized elderly at some time during their hospitalization, is linked with high mortality rates, longer lengths of stay for nonmedical reasons, anguish for families, and increased risk for a diagnosis of dementia and referral to a chronic care facility (33). There is suggestive evidence from the literature that even in younger adults, anxiety symptoms may at times of situational stress be the presenting manifestations of subclinical

drug toxicity, which may under the circumstances of sustained psychosocial stress evolve into a delirium (53). The frequent precipitation of delirium in the elderly by psychosocial stressors is a regularly observed phenomena (28). Eisdorfer (10) has reported that stress can manifest itself in the elderly by antidiuretic hormone (ADH) hypersecretion leading to hyponatremia and an anxiety-like clinical picture. Electrolyte replacement therapy is critically important. The pertinence of this example is that even the presence of an identifiable psychosocial stressor should never militate against a thorough search for other rectifiable etiologies.

ANXIETY AND AGITATION

Agitation is an observable behavioral state characterized by fidgetiness, inability to sit still, hand wringing, nail biting, pawing, and such. It can be present in a range of psychiatric disorders including anxiety states, depression, hypomania, mania, schizophrenia, and delirium or dementia.

EVALUATION OF *DE NOVO* ANXIETY STATES AND ANXIETY SIGNS

Since *de novo* anxiety states are thought to be infrequent in the elderly, routine inquiry should include elucidation of the frequency of use of caffeine, hypnotics, and alcohol. Total caffeine use by older persons may be lower relative to younger persons (56), but pharmacodynamic sensitivity to the drug may be increased (25). Hypnotic use by the elderly is very prevalent (35), usually prescribed by nonpsychiatrists, and, with the emergence of shorter-acting drugs, it is likely that unrecognized withdrawal will increasingly evidence itself as anxiety. Alcohol use by the elderly is also underrecognized and understudied. Its use is often linked to loneliness and social isolation. It may be used to mask anxiety, and abstinence may present with anxiety. Evaluation of all elderly patients should include an inquiry of both the patient and a family member or friend about these drugs as well as about the use of over-the-counter and other prescribed drugs.

ANXIETY, FEAR, AND ABUSE

The exact prevalence of abuse of the elderly is unknown. Its existence has led to rising social concern about its occurrence, and numerous publications have addressed the issue (39). Perhaps the most common form is neglectful abuse involving a range of errors of omission and commission on the part of caretakers (29). According to one study of 22 cases, anxiety was the most common psychological manifestation of abuse (39). Abuse should be considered in the evaluation of any older person presenting with anxiety who is reliant on caretakers. Again, what is appropriately called fear and what is anxiety is not clear.

ANXIETY, FEAR, AND VICTIMIZATION

Little research has evaluated the long-term effects of crime on the elderly. One study of worries about the future in the elderly noted that 11 and 44 of 58 individuals had been assaulted and robbed, respectively, in the 6 months preceding the study (52). The concern that was most related to actual life events was the fear of being assaulted. A report of four cases that examined the effects of burglary and vandalism on the health of older people noted that one died within 1 month of being at home during a burglary, one went from being relatively high-functioning and independent to requiring permanent dependent care in a nursing home, and the remaining two required extended hospital care (5). Since it is possible that one could find similar cases of younger patients, any differential sensitivity in the elderly to such stressors is not established. Documenting the ramifications of assault on the elderly may lead to a better understanding of the issues by the public and to a better understanding of how to help with the consequences of this type of trauma in the elderly.

PSYCHOPHYSIOLOGIC MEASURES AND BIOLOGICAL TESTS IN THE AGED

There have been several reviews of this area in recent years (9,36). These reviews demonstrate that the major focus of research has been on the differentiation between younger and older subjects' psychophysiologic responses to experimentally induced stress and has been directed at attempting to relate observed differences in physiology to behavior. There has been little work directed specifically at differentiation of psychophysiologic states in nonanxious elderly as compared to elderly with anxiety disorders. Lader (31) has noted in young anxious individuals as compared to young nonanxious that the psychophysiologic variables, blood pressure, heart rate, muscle blood flow, muscle tone, tremor, and galvanic skin response (GSR)-measured sweat gland activity, are increased, finger blood flow is decreased, and the electroencephalogram (EEG) demonstrates little change in activity or the response is usually one of overattention. A lack of habituation to a monotonously repeated stimulus is also evidenced in the anxious subject but not in the nonanxious.

Electromyogram (EMG)-measured muscle tension is increased in the anxious aged (9). Heart rate and blood pressure demonstrate less variability in the elderly compared to the young. In older males as compared to older females and younger adults, free fatty acids have been shown to increase during learning of a simple verbal test; they have been shown not to rise after pretreatment with propranolol (11). The GSR is the most consistent measure of anxiety (?fear) across all ages, and the proportionate response from baseline levels increases with age in men more than in women. These findings suggest that overarousal responses to stress may be causally related to a diminished capacity to learn in the elderly. A recent study using relaxation training to improve memory lends some support to this hypothesis (60).

PRINCIPLES OF TREATMENT

Decisions concerning treatment arise from the background of a careful evaluation of the patient as an individual within the context of his or her biopsychosocial framework. Successful treatment of anxiety disorders in the elderly often involves the family and social agencies, psychosocial therapies, and the judicious use of medication. Because successful treatment may require the coordination of multiple modalities of treatment, the involvement of a multidisciplinary team is sometimes of paramount importance.

DISORDER CLASSIFICATION AND SPECIFICITY OF TREATMENT

With respect to DSM-III classification, Adjustment Disorders typically require environmental interventions and a supportive therapeutic relationship. The role of medication is not well defined, but many authors suggest that for mild anxiety it is not initially indicated (44,47). Treatment of simple phobias and social phobias is suggested to best involve behavioral approaches (47). Medications may have a limited role (46). For persistent mild and, more consensually, for moderate to severe anxiety, medication is viewed as useful (38,44,47,50). For chronic anxiety, agoraphobia with panic attacks, and panic states, it is likely that principles of treatment for younger patients are equally valid in the elderly. It is readily apparent that most of what is known about the relationship between diagnostic classification and treatment is at best anecdotal in the elderly. As such, other approaches deserve comment.

One study reported that using a radiotransmitter trigger that signaled an Emergency Response Center (prearranged responders) significantly reduced anxiety in homebound elderly (S. Sherwood, *personal communication*); obviously, this and similar strategies should receive further evaluation. A randomized, controlled trial of surveillance health visitation to the elderly by employed visitors was undertaken in rural and urban settings (57). At the end of 2 years, service utilization was noted to be increased, but there was no evidence of significant improvement beyond baseline in anxiety and depression as evaluated by questionnaires.

There have been two studies of relaxation training in the elderly and its relationship to memory improvement during stress, one an uncontrolled study of list learning (61) and the other a controlled study of visual and mnemonic learning (60). Both concluded that relaxation training significantly reduced performance anxiety and significantly improved learning. Another placebo-controlled study examined and found efficacy for β-blockers in the reduction of stress (?fear, ?anxiety), using a similar learning paradigm (11). No study has directly compared β-blockers to relaxation treatments in reducing performance concerns in the elderly.

BENZODIAZEPINES

At the present time, benzodiazepines are still the most frequently used drugs when pharmacotherapy is indicated to treat anxiety symptoms in the elderly.

Their usage should involve an understanding of the pharmacokinetic and pharmacodynamic characteristics applicable to this age group (a more detailed discussion of the pharmacokinetics of benzodiazepines appears elsewhere in this volume). They are as follows:

1. Rate of absorption and volume of distribution (determined largely by lipid solubility) after single oral doses are the major determinants of onset and duration of clinical activity.

2. During multiple dose or chronic therapy, the rate and extent of accumulation are determined by half-life and clearance of the particular benzodiazepine.

3. Benzodiazepines may be classified according to rate of clearance, as reflected by elimination half-life.

   a. Ultrashort half-life benzodiazepines with elimination half-lives of less than 5 hr do not accumulate. Drugs of this category (such as brotizolam, midazolam, and triazolam) are administered to elderly patients but almost always as hypnotics rather than as anxiolytics.

   b. Short and intermediate half-life benzodiazepines have elimination half-lives of 5 to 24 hr. Limited drug accumulation occurs, and accumulation of active metabolites is not significant. Age has little effect on drug clearance for those members of this group metabolized by conjugation (e.g., oxazepam). However, oxidatively metabolized agents (e.g., diazepam) have impaired clearance, resulting in an increased potential for accumulation in the elderly.

   c. Long half-life benzodiazepines have elimination half-lives greater than 24 hr, frequently have active metabolites, and both parent drug and metabolite(s) may accumulate during chronic therapy. Clearance is not uncommonly impaired in the elderly.

4. Pharmacokinetic differences between the young and elderly may in part explain clinical impressions of enhanced drug effect in the elderly. However, other factors, perhaps at central nervous system benzodiazepine receptor sites, may also be important in understanding differences in drug effect between young and elderly populations.

Table 2 summarizes the pharmacokinetic features of four benzodiazepines that have received considerable study in the elderly: alprazolam, diazepam, lorazepam, and oxazepam (14,15,17,18,20–22,45). Diazepam and lorazepam were introduced in generic form in 1985.

Because cost considerations may promote the use of other generically available drugs in the elderly, chlordiazepoxide deserves mention even though it is not an extensively used drug at present. Shader and colleagues (49) studied the effect of age on chlordiazepoxide pharmacokinetics using a single oral dose. Under the assumption of 100% systemic availability, chlordiazepoxide clearance was significantly reduced in the elderly, resulting in prolongation of elimination half-life from 10.1 hr in young male subjects to 18.2 hr in elderly males. Impaired formation of the major active metabolite, desmethylchlordiazepoxide, was also documented in the elderly subjects. This finding has been confirmed using an intravenous dose (42). Among elderly female subjects, no data are available.

In general, these observations can be extended to all other benzodiazepines metabolized by pathways other than direct conjugation (glucuronide formation). In short-term or single-dose usage in volunteers or general hospital patients, the elderly as compared to younger groups (at comparable dosages) develop higher blood levels or have an increased frequency of unwanted sedation with other benzodiazepines such as clorazepate (48,49), flurazepam (16,19), nitrazepam (4,13) and temazepam (8,54)—the latter three are primarily used as hypnotics. In one long-term usage study of flurazepam and nitrazepam (12–15 months and in some cases up to 15 years), blood levels were "substantially higher than those . . . in younger individuals," effectiveness and patient satisfaction were maintained, and there was apparent clinical tolerance to unwanted sedation, confusion, and motor unsteadiness (55).

It must be emphasized that the elderly are a heterogeneous group; hence, individualized dosage considerations are always appropriate. It must also be noted that because most kinetic research is carried out in volunteer populations, the relationship between these findings and the desired goal of reduction in anxiety in the elderly is not firmly established.

TABLE 2. *Summary of changes with aging in pharmacokinetic parameters of four benzodiazepine antianxiety agents*

Drug	Metabolism pathway	Significant active metabolites	Relative lipid solubility	GI absorption Δ/age		Relative protein binding Δ/age	Volume of distribution Δ/age	Clearance Δ/age	Approximate values of elimination half-life (hr)	
									Young adult	Elderly
Oxazepam	Hepatic conjugation	None	1 (least)	Intermediate & slow	Slower & erratic	2 No Δ	No Δ	No Δ (M > F)	9	9
Lorazepam	Hepatic conjugation	None	2	Intermediate	Slight ↓	3 ↓	No Δ	No Δ	14	16
Alprazolam (triazolo-benzo-diazepine)	Hepatic oxidation	None	3	Intermediate	Slight ↑ in females (F)	1 No Δ	↓	(↓ M > F)	10	17 (↑ M > F)
Diazepam	Hepatic oxidation	N-Desmethyl-diazepam	4 (most)	Rapid	Slight ↓	4 ↓	(↑ M < F)	↓	40	85 (↑ M > F)

We could locate only four trials published since the last American College of Neuropsychopharmacology volume that examined the effects of benzodiazepines on anxiety in non-brain-impaired elderly. Because of the paucity of such reports, each trial will be described in brief. A 1982 report examined 220 elderly outpatients mostly with a primary diagnosis of anxiety neurosis ($N = 201$) (30). Conducted as a multicenter, randomized, double-blind trial, 108 patients received oxazepam (initial dose 30 mg, with a range to 60 mg) and 112 patients received placebo. Mean age was 67.5, and the 19 patients not diagnosed as anxiety neurosis suffered from adjustment reaction of adult life with anxiety ($N = 7$) or anxiety reaction with depression ($N = 12$). Two-thirds of the group had concomitant chronic medical illnesses (e.g., cardiorespiratory illnesses), and 73% were receiving other medications. Eighty-three percent completed the 4-week trial. Relevant to anxiety reduction, statistically significant differences in favor of oxazepam were found on the anxious mood, tension, and insomnia items of the Hamilton Anxiety Scale, on the anxiety, trouble concentrating, phobia-obsession, insomnia, ruminations, and hypochondriasis variables of the Physician's Target Symptom Scale, and the obsessive-compulsive factor of the Hopkins Symptom Checklist (a trend was noted for the anxiety factor, $p = 0.089$). The anxiolytic value of oxazepam could be demonstrated even in the presence of a reasonably clear placebo response.

A 1984 report examined alprazolam (0.25–1.5 mg) versus placebo in geriatric outpatients or nursing home residents over age 60 (mean age 69 years) suffering from "clinical anxiety" or "anxiety associated with depression" (6). Eighty-three patients (alprazolam, $N = 40$; placebo, $N = 43$) completed the 4-week trial. Hamilton Anxiety Scale total scores showed significant improvement with alprazolam as compared to placebo, and individual item decrements were comparable to those in the oxazepam study already reviewed. Significant differences in favor of alprazolam were also noted on a Physician's Global Impressions rating and on a Target Symptoms scale.

In the third article, a 1985 report comparing brotizolam (0.25 mg) and nitrazepam (0.50 mg) in a randomized, double-blind, crossover trial, daytime anxiolytic properties were noted, even though the primary purpose of the trial focused on the hypnotic properties of these drugs (12). There were 20 patients in the trial, all over age 64 with a mean age of 69.3 years. All had "primitive sleep problems, but were without psychiatric symptoms." There was no placebo. However, based on "post" versus "pre" scores, both drugs reduced the time taken to fall asleep and the number of nighttime arousals. On the Mood Adjective Checklist of Nowlis, both drugs reduced daytime anxiety and increased enthusiasm, concentration, and vigor. In light of the placebo response in the first two reports, however, these results are at best suggestive.

A fourth article is mentioned merely for completeness. This report describes 671 anxious patients treated with bromazepam or lorazepam in a double-blind, multicenter trial, again with no placebo (7). Although 24 bromazepam and 19 lorazepam patients were over age 65, results were not presented separately for this elderly cohort. In this group of reports, the primary unwanted effect was excessive drowsiness or somnolence. In none was the frequency of this effect excessive, however.

BUSPIRONE

Marketed while these volumes were going to press, data on buspirone in the elderly are insufficient to draw conclusions. An open study on 12 elderly patients (5 males, 7 females), ages 66 to 80 (mean 72.4), with generalized anxiety disorder suggests that dosages between 5 and 30 mg per day in divided doses produced significant anxiety reduction over the 28-day trial (D. S. Robinson, *personal communication*).

β-BLOCKERS

Since fear and situational anxiety are common in the elderly, it seems probable that β-blockers would have a useful role in this age group. However, we could find no trials to support this usage.

ANTIDEPRESSANTS (INCLUDING MONOAMINE OXIDASE INHIBITORS) AND NEUROLEPTICS

These groups of drugs, although used extensively by clinicians in older populations with symptoms of anxiety, have not been the focus of carefully controlled trials. They also have been helpful in elderly patients showing anxiety symptoms accompanying depression and/or psychosis. However, we could find no studies in the last decade supporting their use in anxiety states *per se* in the elderly.

ACKNOWLEDGMENTS

This work was supported in part by USPHS Grant 2-R01-MH-34223 (Drs. Shader and Greenblatt) and by the Alberta Heritage Foundation for Medical Research Clinical Fellowship 004325 (Dr. Kennedy).

REFERENCES

1. Bergmann, K. (1971): In: *Recent Developments in Psychogeriatrics: A Symposium,* edited by D. W. K. Kay and A. Walk, pp. 39–50. Headley Brothers, Ashford, Kent.
2. Blazer, D. (1980): *J. Am. Geriatr. Soc.,* 28:52–58.
3. Blazer, D. (1983): In: *Psychiatry Update, Vol. II,* edited by L. Grinspoon, pp. 87–95. American Psychiatric Press, Washington, DC.
4. Castleden, C. M., George, C. F., Marcer, D., and Hallett, C. (1977): *Br. Med. J.,* 1:10–12.
5. Coakley, D., and Woodford-Williams, E. (1979): *Lancet,* 2:1066–1067.
6. Cohn, J. B. (1984): *Curr. Ther. Res.,* 35:100–112.
7. Cordingley, G. J., Dean, B. C., and Hallett, C. (1985): *Curr. Med. Res. Opin.,* 9:505–510.
8. Divoll, M., Greenblatt, D. J., Harmatz, J. S., and Shader, R. I. (1981): *J. Pharm. Sci.,* 70:1104–1107.
9. Eisdorfer, C. (1978): In: *Aging: The Process and the People,* edited by G. Usdin and C. K. Hofling, pp. 96–128. Brunner/Mazel, New York.

10. Eisdorfer, C. (1979): In: *Phenomenology and Treatment of Anxiety,* edited by W. E. Fann, I. Karacan, A. D. Pokorny, and R. L. Williams, pp. 43–49. SP Medical and Scientific Books, New York.

11. Eisdorfer, C., Nowlin, J., and Wilkie, F. (1970): *Science,* 170: 1320–1327.

12. Ferrara, N., Valentini, P., Sestito, M., DePrisco, F., Veniero, A. M., Canonico, V., Breglio, R., and Rengo, F. (1985): *Curr. Ther. Res.,* 37:295–308.

13. Greenblatt, D. J., and Allen, M. D. (1978): *Br. J. Clin. Pharmacol.,* 5:407–413.

14. Greenblatt, D. J., Allen, M. D., Harmatz, J. S., and Shader, R. I. (1980): *Clin. Pharmacol. Ther.,* 27:301–312.

15. Greenblatt, D. J., Allen, M. D., Locniskar, A., Harmatz, J. S., and Shader, R. I. (1979): *Clin. Pharmacol. Ther.,* 26:103–113.

16. Greenblatt, D. J., Allen, M. D., and Shader, R. I. (1977): *Clin. Pharmacol. Ther.,* 21:355–361.

17. Greenblatt, D. J., Arendt, R. M., Abernethy, D. R., Giles, H. G., Sellers, E. M., and Shader, R. I. (1983): *Br. J. Anaesthes.,* 55:985–989.

18. Greenblatt, D. J., Divoll, M., and Abernethy, D. R. (1983): *Arch. Gen. Psychiatry,* 40:287–292.

19. Greenblatt, D. J., Divoll, M., Harmatz, J. S., MacLaughlin, D. S., and Shader, R. I. (1981): *Clin. Pharmacol. Ther.,* 30:475–486.

20. Greenblatt, D. J., Divoll, M., Harmatz, J. S., and Shader, R. I. (1980): *J. Pharmacol. Exp. Ther.,* 215:86–91.

21. Greenblatt, D. J., and Shader, R. I. (1985): In: *The Benzodiazepines: Current Standards for Medical Practice,* edited by D. E. Smith and D. R. Wesson, pp. 43–58. MTP Press, Boston.

22. Greenblatt, D. J., Shader, R. I., Franke, K., MacLaughlin, D. S., Harmatz, J. S., Allen, M. D., Werner, A., and Woo, E. (1979): *J. Pharm. Sci.,* 68:57–63.

23. Hall, R. C. W., Levenson, A. J., and LeCann, A. F. (1981): In: *Aging, Vol. 14: Neuropsychiatric Manifestations of Physical Disease in the Elderly,* edited by A. J. Levenson and R. C. W. Hall, pp. 133–149. Raven Press, New York.

24. Himmelfarb, S., and Murrell, S. A. (1984): *J. Psychol.,* 116:159–167.

25. Isso, J. L., Ghosal, A., Kwong, T., Freeman, R. B., and Jaenike, J. R. (1983): *Am. J. Cardiol.,* 52:769–773.

26. Jarvik, L. S. (1980): In: Symposium, Department of Psychiatry, University of Arizona, November 1977, pp. 29–43, Roche Laboratories, Nutley, NJ.

27. Johnson, D. A. W. (1981): *Drugs,* 22:57–69.

28. Kennedy, A. (1959): *Gerontol. Clin.,* 1:71–82.

29. Kimsey, L. R., Tarbox, A. R., and Bragg, D. F. (1981): *J. Am. Geriatr. Soc.,* 29:465–472.

30. Koepke, H. H., Gold, R. L., Linden, M. E., Lion, J. R., and Rickels, K. (1982): *Psychosomatics,* 23:641–645.

31. Lader, M. (1983): *J. Clin. Psychol.,* 44:5–10.

32. Leckman, J. F., Sholomskas, D., Thompson, W. D., Belanger, A., and Weissman, M. M. (1982): *Arch. Gen. Psychiatry,* 39:879–883.

33. Lipowski, Z. J. (1983): *Am. J. Psychiatry,* 140:1003–1005.

34. Magni, G., and Diego, D. L. (1984): *Psychol. Rep.,* 55:607–612.

35. Mellinger, G. D., and Balter, M. B. (1981): In: *Epidemiological Impact of Psychotropic Drugs,* edited by G. Tognoni, C. Bellantyono, and M. Lader, pp. 117–135. Elsevier/North-Holland Biomedical Press, Amsterdam.

36. Michalewski, J. H., Thompson, L. W., and Patterson, J. V. (1979): In: *Psychiatric Symptoms and Cognitive Loss in the Elderly: Evaluation and Assessment Techniques,* edited by A. Raskin and L. F. Jarvik, pp. 73–124. Hemisphere Publishing Corp., Washington, DC.

37. Murphy, J. M., Sobol, A. M., Neff, R. K., Olivier, D. C., and Leighton, A. H. (1984): *Arch. Gen. Psychiatry,* 41:990–997.

38. Nobel, K. (1979): In: *Geriatric Psychopharmacology,* edited by K. Nandy, pp. 105–116. Elsevier/North-Holland, New York.

39. O'Malley, T. A., O'Malley, H. C., Everett, D. E., and Sarson, D. (1984): *J. Am. Geriatr. Soc.,* 32:362–369.

40. Pfeiffer, E. (1983): In: *Psychiatry Update, Vol. II,* edited by L. Grinspoon, pp. 140–161. American Psychiatric Press, Washington, DC.

41. Renner, V. J., and Birren, J. E. (1980): In: *Handbook of Mental Health and Aging,* edited by J. E. Birren and R. B. Sloane, pp. 310–336. Prentice-Hall, Englewood Cliffs, NJ.

42. Roberts, R. K., Wilkinson, G. R., Branch, R. A., and Schenker, S. (1978): *Gastroenterology,* 75:479–485.

43. Roth, M. (1975): *Psychiatr. Ann.,* 6:417–445.

44. Salzman, C. (1984): In: *Clinical Geriatric Psychopharmacology,* edited by C. Salzman, pp. 132–148. McGraw-Hill, New York.

45. Salzman, C., Shader, R. I., Greenblatt, D. J., and Harmatz, J. S. (1983): *Arch. Gen. Psychiatry,* 40:293–297.

46. Shader, R. I., and Greenblatt, D. J. (1982): *J. Clin. Psychiatry,* 43:8–16.

47. Shader, R. I., and Greenblatt, D. J. (1986): In: *American Handbook of Psychiatry,* Vol. 8, edited by P. A. Berger and H. K. H. Brodie, pp. 597–619. Basik Books, Inc., New York.

48. Shader, R. I., Greenblatt, D. J., Ciraulo, D. A., Divoll, M., Harmatz, J. S., and Georgotas, A. (1981): *Psychopharmacology,* 75:193–197.

49. Shader, R. I., Greenblatt, D. J., Harmatz, J. S., Franke, K., and Koch-Weser, J. (1977): *J. Clin. Pharmacol.,* 17:709–718.

50. Shamoian, C. A. (1983): *Med. Clin. North Am.,* 67:361–378.

51. Simon, A. (1980): In: *Handbook of Mental Health and Aging,* edited by J. E. Birren and R. B. Sloane, pp. 653–670. Prentice-Hall, Englewood Cliffs, NJ.

52. Stein, S., Linn, M. W., Slater, E., and Stein, E. (1984): *J. Am. Geriatr. Soc.,* 32:431–434.

53. Stillner, V., Popkin, M. K., and Pierce, C. (1978): *Am. J. Psychiatry,* 135:855–856.

54. Swift, C. G., Haythorne, J. M., Clarke, P., and Stevenson, I. H. (1981): *Br. J. Clin. Pharmacol.,* 11:413–414.

55. Swift, C. G., Swift, M. R., Hamley, J., Stevenson, I. H., and Crooks, J. (1984): *Age Ageing,* 13:335–343.

56. Vener, A. M., Krupka, L. R., and Climo, J. J. (1979): *J. Am. Geriatr. Soc.,* 27:83–90.

57. Vetter, N. J., Jones, D. A., and Victor, C. R. (1984): *Br. Med. J.,* 288:369–372.

58. Weissman, M. M., Meyers, J. K., Tischler, G. L., Holzer, C. E., Leaf, P. J., Orvaschel, H., and Brody, J. A. (1985): *Acta Psychiatr. Scand.,* 71:366–379.

59. Wilkie, F. L., Eisdorfer, C., and Staud, J. (1982): *Psychiatr. Clin. North Am.,* 5:131–143.

60. Yesavage, J. A. (1984): *Am. J. Psychiatry,* 141:778–781.

61. Yesavage, J. A., Rose, T. L., and Spiegel, D. (1982): *Exp. Aging Res.,* 8:195–198.

Psychopharmacology:
The Third Generation of Progress,
edited by Herbert Y. Meltzer.
Raven Press, New York © 1987.

CHAPTER **118**

Antidepressant Drug Treatment in the Elderly

Daniel A. Plotkin, Sylvia C. Gerson, and Lissy F. Jarvik

Depression is one of the most common psychiatric disorders afflicting the elderly. Reported prevalence rates range from 2% to 18% (9,13,54,80,97) and estimates are even higher in patients with physical disorders (68), particularly stroke (116). Ever since the discovery of the mood-elevating properties of monoamine oxidase inhibitors and imipramine in the 1950s, antidepressant drugs have been a major method of treatment for depression. However, relatively little information has been systematically collected on the efficacy and safety of these compounds in the elderly. Persons over 65 years of age have frequently been excluded from treatment outcome research, due in part to difficulties in recruiting physically healthy, medication-free older subjects and in part to concern over the potentially dangerous side effects of these drugs (94,143).

Due to the growing interest in aging, there have recently been a number of double-blind, controlled studies dealing specifically with drug treatment of unipolar depression in the elderly (43). A systematic literature survey of controlled double-blind studies through 1985 yielded 22 clinical trials (plus one in 1986) of tricyclic and tetracyclic antidepressants, trazodone, nomifensine, and some newer experimental compounds such as bupropion, and fluoxetine (Table 1). More recent controlled and uncontrolled trials of antidepressants that have come to our attention (including lithium and monoamine oxidase inhibitors) are also discussed in this review. We relied heavily on computerized literature searches for our survey, and over and over it was clear how inadequate they are. We hope that omissions will be drawn to our attention, and we would like to stress to our readers the importance of including key words (like depression and

elderly) in titles of further publications so that computers will register them appropriately.

EFFICACY IN THE ELDERLY

Treatment of depression in the elderly is generally assumed to be fraught with multiple difficulties. Further, it has been assumed that depressed elderly individuals are more "refractory" to pharmacologic or psychologic treatment approaches than are younger adults. Although there is evidence that some elderly depressed patients ultimately have a poor outcome [e.g., those with ventricular enlargement on computerized tomographic (CT) head scan (64,65) or delusions and severe initial disease (19,95)], there is a deplorable lack of data. Instead, we have opinions by leading experts, sometimes diametrically opposed. For example: "there is convincing evidence that affective illness in the aged . . . tends to be more chronic, more severe, and more treatment-resistant than it is in younger patients" (61, p. 26) versus "there is no evidence that these drugs [antidepressants] are less effective" in the elderly (21, p. 36) and the conclusion that elderly patients may be incorrectly or prematurely labeled as "treatment-resistant" (47).

Convincing data are lacking. For example, a retrospective chart review of endogenously depressed inpatients (24 over and 16 under the age of 50 years) treated with imipramine, amitriptyline, or desipramine concluded that older depressed patients were significantly more likely (8 of 24) to demonstrate response failure than younger depressed patients (1 of 16), when matched for depressive subtypes and severity

TABLE 1. *Double-blind studies of antidepressant drug treatment in older patients*

Authors & year	Drugs	Dose (mg/day)	Weeks of treatment	Age (years)	Sex (% women)	Baseline N[a]	Percent dropout[b]	Outcome: mean % improvement on HAM-D[c]
Lakshmanan et al., 1986 (86)[d]	Doxepin	10–20	3	70–83	36[e]	29	17[e]	52[e]
	Placebo				62[e]	(total)		22[e]
Feighner & Cohn, 1985 (35)	Doxepin	50–200	6	61–90	52	79	61[e]	36[e]
	Fluoxetine	20–80			63	78	47[e]	35[e]
Assalian et al., 1985 (8)	Trimipramine	75–150	4	$\bar{x}=59^e$	45[e]	25	24[e]	64[j]
	Doxepin	75–150			27[e]	(total)	(total)	48[j]
Weissman et al., 1984 (144)	Alprazolam[f]	0.5–1.9[g]	6	60–85	76	25	44[e]	63[e]
	Imipramine[f]	25–102.5[g]			(total)	(total)	(total)	66[e]
	Placebo[f]							60[e]
Jansen & Siegfried, 1984 (67)	Nomifensine[h]	100[l]	4	65+	75	25	8[e]	51[j]
	Placebo			$\bar{x}=75$	(total)	25	8–20[e,i]	9[j]
Lipsey et al., 1984 (89)[d,k]	Nortriptyline	20–100	4–6	$\bar{x}=61^e$	36[e]	39	35[e]	Insufficient data presented
	Placebo				35[e]	(total)	32[e]	
Cohn et al., 1984 (24)	Imipramine	75–200	4	60+	62[e]	21	14[e]	50[j]
	Nomifensine[h]	75–200		$\bar{x}=66^e$	52[e]	21	5[e]	46[j]
	Placebo				76[e]	21	14[e]	23[j]
Merideth et al., 1984 (93)	Imipramine	50–200	5	60+	73[e]	22	36[e]	57[j]
	Nomifensine[h]	50–200		$\bar{x}=69^e$	70[e]	20	20[e]	56[j]
	Placebo				79[e]	19	47[e]	25[j]
Gwirtsman et al., 1983 (55)	Doxepin	25–129[g]	6	55+	8[e]	25	28[e]	44[j]
	Maprotiline	25–144[g]		$\bar{x}=64$	(total)	24	17[e]	60[j]
Branconnier et al., 1983 (16)	Bupropion-450	300–450	5	55–80	56[e]	18	21[e]	51[j,m]
	Bupropion-150	150[l]			(total)	18	(total)	44[j,m]
	Imipramine	25–150				18		51[j,m]
	Placebo					9		22[j,m]
Kane et al., 1983 (74)	Bupropion-450	300–450	4	55–77	70	51	25[e]	42[e]
	Bupropion-150	150[l]			(total)	(total)	(total)	41[e]
	Imipramine	75–200						52[e]
	Placebo							38[e]
Jarvik et al., 1982 (69)	Doxepin	25–225	26	55–81	72	12	40[n]	52
	Imipramine	25–250			(total)	10	67[n]	50
	Placebo					10	100[n]	19
Scardigli & Jans, 1982 (122)[d]	Mianserin	30–60	4	51–88	36[o]	29	17[e]	78[e]
	Nomifensine[h]	75–150			(total)	29	14[e]	54[e]
	Trazodone	202–405[o]				29	38[e]	61[e]
Goldstein et al., 1982 (48)[d,p]	Amitriptyline	75–150	4	64–88	56[e]	9	(Not	40[j]
	Nomifensine[h]	75–150			57[e]	7	given)	31[j]
Branconnier et al., 1982 (15)[q]	Amitriptyline	75–150	4–5	60–85	59[q]	25	16[e]	46[j]
	Mianserin	30–60			(total)	25	(total)	47[j]
	Placebo					25		35[j]
Gerner et al., 1980 (42)	Imipramine	50–200	4	60–90	62	21	57[e]	68[j]
	Trazodone	100–400			(total)	19	37[e]	56[j]
	Placebo					20	35[e]	16[j]
Nugent 1979 (102)[d,r]	Amitriptyline	75–150	4	60–89	100	25	0	74[e]
	Viloxazine	150–300			(total)	23	9[e]	69[e]
Olsen et al., 1978 (103)	Gerovital-H3	week 1: 100 × 3 weeks 2–4: 200 × 3	4	48–77	52 (total)	11	0	49[e]
	Placebo					12	0	33[e]
Brodie et al., 1975 (17)[d]	Fluphenazine/ nortriptyline	1.5/30[l]	4	65+ $\bar{x}=73^e$	(Not given)	32	0	Insufficient data. Hard to interpret
	Promazine	150[l]				32	6[e]	
Zung et al., 1974 (154)	Gerovital-H3	week 1: 100 × 3 weeks 2–4: 200 × 3	4	60–79	(Not given)	36 (total)	17[e] (total)	19[e,s]
	Imipramine	25–86						19[e,s]
	Placebo							9[e,s]

TABLE 1. (*Continued*)

Authors & year	Drugs	Dose (mg/day)	Weeks of treatment	Age (years)	Sex (% women)	Baseline N^a	Percent dropout[b]	Outcome: mean % improvement on HAM-D[c]
Beber 1971 (10)[d]	Perphenazine/ amitriptyline Chlordiazepoxide hydrochloride	2/10–8/40 10–40	4 + 4 crossover	68–90	87[e] (total)	63 (total)	3[e] (total)	Insufficient data. Rating measures hard to interpret
Kernohan et al., 1967 (81)[d,t]	Nortriptyline Placebo	25–100	12	$\bar{x} = 70^e$	61[e] (total)	46[e] 46[e]	9[e] (total)	Insufficient data. Rating measures hard to interpret
Chesrow et al., 1964 (23)[d]	Nortriptyline Placebo	75[l]	About 7 months 1–2 months	34–87 $\bar{x} = 60$	31[e] (total)	65 (total)	6[e] (total)	Insufficient data. Rating measures hard to interpret

[a] Number of patients enrolled in study.

[b] Dropouts were reported according to a variety of criteria. Our attempts to present them in a uniform manner resulted in recalculation of some published data. The percent dropouts reported here represent the total number of patients who dropped out for any reason divided by the total number of patients who started the study. Some published reports were ambiguous, and we may have erred in our interpretation. Inquiries should be directed to the authors of individual articles. We hope the data from this table will at least give a general idea of the attrition rates.

[c] HAM-D, Hamilton Depression Rating Scale.

[d] Does not specify limitation to major affective disorder or equivalent.

[e] Calculated from published data.

[f] All patients in this study were receiving weekly Interpersonal Therapy (IPT) in addition to drug.

[g] Mean maximum dose.

[h] Nomifensine has been withdrawn from the market.

[i] Two different numbers are given for final sample size (depressed patients receiving placebo).

[j] Estimated from published figure.

[k] Poststroke depression. Half of the patients had major depression.

[l] Fixed dose.

[m] Outcomes reported for 4 weeks instead of 5 weeks of treatment.

[n] Protocol provided for reassignment to another drug by nonblind clinical pharmacologist. If patients assigned to another drug are not included as dropouts, the rates become doxepin 20%, imipramine 50%, and placebo 30% (calculated from raw data).

[o] As reported by authors. Unclear how dose reached with 50 mg unit dose. Data for sex given as of 14 days ($N = 75$).

[p] Study patients divided into two groups (endogenous and reactive depression) for each drug. Only data for endogenous groups are reported here.

[q] Patients had documented cognitive impairment. Data for sex reported as of 28 days ($N = 63$).

[r] "Use of a benzodiazepine was permitted."

[s] Hamilton Depression Scale not used; psychiatric rating scale used was Depression Status Inventory (DSI).

[t] "Majority of patients in both groups received other types of medication, including tranquilizers."

(18). However, this finding alone cannot support the assertion that older patients are less likely than younger ones to *respond* to tricyclic antidepressants (TCAs)—only that older patients are more likely to show response failure. Indeed, one might conclude from the same data that age had no effect on the rate of remission, since a good response was seen in 12 of the 24 older patients compared to 8 of the 16 younger patients. Only 4 patients in the older group (17%) had a partial response, however, compared to 7 of the younger ones (44%); thus, age may influence partial response.

DISTRIBUTION OF OUTCOMES

In Hamilton's (57) report of melancholic patients (average age middle to late forties) who were treated with imipramine or phenelzine, he noted that outcomes clearly distinguished between drug responders and nonresponders. There were but a few in the intermediate gray zone of slightly improved, and Hamilton suggested that others attempt replication of this bimodal distribution. One double-blind placebo-controlled study comparing imipramine and doxepin (69) also reported a distinctly bimodal distribution of outcomes, this time in older patients (mean age 67 years); half of the patients treated with active drug went into remission, but most of the others (41% of the total sample) were still depressed enough at the end of the study to meet admission criteria according to both psychiatric evaluation and Hamilton Depression Rating Scale (HAM-D) score. Further data are needed to verify this bimodal distribution, which has important clinical relevance in terms of duration of drug treatment in non-responders.

EARLY RESPONSE

In the previously cited study of imipramine and doxepin in geriatric patients (69), symptomatic improvement occurred after only one week, although full response, if it occurred at all, sometimes took as long as five weeks. An early response to antidepressant drug treatment in the elderly has also been observed by others (19,40,55,86, 103,106,119,144).

Early response is in keeping with the statement of Winokur (145) that in the general adult population the most common antidepressant drug response is "immediate . . . in terms of one week." Winokur cites the findings of Braithwaite and colleagues (14) and Ziegler and associates (153) to support his impression. By contrast, Quitkin and colleagues (110) concluded from their pattern analysis, carried out for three studies of antidepressant drug efficacy (four drugs) in a mixed group of mild to moderately depressed adult (not elderly) outpatients, that "true" drug responders differ from "nonspecific" responders in that they respond *after* two weeks of drug treatment. The issue of response time needs to be resolved. It is especially important for the elderly, who could benefit from not having to endure prolonged administration of drugs that will prove ineffective and have the potential for serious side effects.

ADVERSE SIDE EFFECTS

The adverse side effects of antidepressant drugs are described elsewhere in *this volume*. Despite the commonly held belief that adverse effects of antidepressant drugs are particularly common and problematic in the elderly, few studies have directly addressed that issue. Instead, pharmacologic findings are extrapolated to the elderly (113, 130). The side effects profile does generally dictate the clinical choice of antidepressant drug in the elderly patient. Anticholinergic properties cause bothersome symptoms in younger adults but the consequences, such as acute confusional state, may be intolerable in the elderly. Even so relatively benign a side effect as dry mouth may preclude the wearing of artificial dentures; constipation may lead to fecal impaction, and acute glaucoma may be precipitated in the presence of a narrow occludable chamber angle. Good data on the incidence of these side effects in the elderly are notable for their absence. Data gathered on normal elderly (20) cannot be applied directly to patients with major depressive disorders.

Cardiovascular effects are of great concern in the depressed elderly, given the prevalence of concomitant cardiovascular disease in this population. The most common serious cardiovascular adverse effect is orthostatic hypotension (45), which can lead to falls and injuries. Nortriptyline (NT) (117) and doxepin (100) have been reported to cause less orthostasis than imipramine. Another report, however, noted significant orthostatic hypotension in elderly patients on nortriptyline (112). Pretreatment orthostatic hypotension has been an inconsistent and unreliable predictor of drug induced orthostasis, and so has drug dosage.

Theoretically, the antiarrhythmic effects of the tricyclics should have clinical usefulness (12,44). And yet, surprisingly little information has become available during the past decade.

Electrocardiographic studies of TCAs in elderly patients have yielded contradictory results. There is one report (75) of prolonged intraventricular conduction times in seven patients treated with imipramine while others (58) failed to find an effect on mean conduction time in 21 patients on imipramine, or prolongation of conduction time in 12 patients on nortriptyline (112). However, in the latter two studies, new conduction abnormalities did develop in some patients (e.g., one patient on imipramine developed a first-degree heart block and three patients developed intraventricular conduction disturbances). Clearly, it would be advantageous to be able to correlate the development of conduction disturbances with some known parameter, and recent work suggests that EKG changes correlate with hydroxylated metabolites of TCA rather than the parent compound (85,123,148,150).

Studies using radionuclide angiography in depressed cardiac patients indicate that neither imipramine nor doxepin have the anticipated serious depressant effect on the mechanical function of the heart (46,141).

In conclusion, our information on side effects in the elderly is inadequate for the tricyclics (the most studied compounds) as well as other antidepressant drugs.

A POSSIBLE PREDICTOR OF TREATMENT RESPONSE

Several avenues have been explored to predict clinical response in the elderly, so far without consistent results. They include clinical and demographic characteristics (111,118), neuroendocrine parameters [dexamethasone suppression test (147)], biochemical measures [urinary 3-methoxy-4-hydroxyphenylglycol (MHPG) (36), platelet monoamine oxidase (MAO) levels (39,40)], radiologic measures [quantitative CT scan of the head (64,65)], and stimulant challenge [methylphenidate test (131)]; although there have been encouraging leads, none have revealed clear-cut predictors, and approach to treatment remains on a trial-and-error basis. One of the first questions to be answered is which agent to use. Since available data do not indicate differential efficacy, traditional clinical wisdom dictates that drug selection be based on the side-effects profiles (41,121). Important considerations include anticholinergic properties, effects on cardiac conduction, and orthostatic hypotension.

The measurement of pretreatment systolic orthostatic hypotension in one study (70) predicted remission in geriatric (mean age 66 years, range 55–81 years) patients treated with doxepin or imipramine with high sensitivity and specificity. Patients with pretreatment systolic orthostatic hypotension (PSOP) of 12 mm Hg or more tended to go into remission (92%), whereas those with a drop of 10 mm Hg or less rarely did (18%). Another study (124) supports the predictive value of PSOP in unipolar depressed elderly outpatients (mean age 64 years, range 60–82 years) who were treated with a 16-week course of nortriptyline.

The patients with a PSOP ≥ 10 mm Hg had a 2.5 times greater improvement than those with a PSOP of <10 mm Hg.

PLASMA ANTIDEPRESSANT LEVELS AND DAILY DOSES OF TCAs

The numerous studies on antidepressant plasma levels that emerged in the 1970s were essentially restricted to the TCAs and yielded contradictory results. A thoughtful review published in 1983 concluded that efforts to relate plasma levels to therapeutic outcome were, in general, disappointing (127). We focus here on findings specifically concerning the elderly, and most information is available for amitriptyline, imipramine, desipramine, and nortriptyline (4), with the greatest consensus for nortriptyline. Unanswered questions include (a) Do the elderly require smaller doses to achieve therapeutic plasma levels? and (b) Do they respond to lower plasma levels?

Although data are generally lacking for the elderly, clinical experience indicates that they tend to require lower doses than do younger patients. Age-related changes in distribution (decreased plasma protein, increased body fat), metabolism (decreased hepatic hydroxylation and demethylation), and elimination (decreased glomerular filtration rate), result in increased plasma levels for prolonged duration (although increased alpha-glycoprotein levels may have the opposite effect). There is evidence (101,108) that indeed, elderly patients achieve higher plasma levels for a given dose of imipramine or amitriptyline than do younger patients, and there may be a sex difference (108). The findings for secondary amine TCAs are less clear. In a study of imipramine and amitriptyline (83), a significant correlation was found between age and concentration of tertiary amine TCAs but not between age and the demethylated metabolites of the parent compounds (i.e., secondary amine TCAs). It has also been reported (29,30) that a mean "therapeutic" level of nortriptyline (NT) of 104 ng/ml was achieved with relatively low daily doses (mean 50 mg) in the elderly, while another group (129), noted that mean steady-state plasma and red blood cell NT levels were similar in elderly compared to younger patients, on the same dosage schedule (50 mg t.i.d). Others too (152) reported no effect of age on amitriptyline (AMI) or NT plasma levels, although patients as young as 40 years were included (mean age: AMI 50 years, NT 51 years). In a study of desipramine (99), only a weak and non-significant correlation between age and TCA steady state plasma levels was observed. Similarly, another publication (28) reported that desipramine plasma levels per milligram dose were the same for seven elderly depressed women (age range 69–92 years) as for a group of younger patients (open trial). A review of desipramine (66) concluded that recent studies do not suggest a buildup of desipramine or its metabolites in healthy geriatric patients.

With regard to hydroxylated metabolites, increased steady state concentrations of 2-hydroxydesipramine were reported (82) in elderly compared to younger patients, and so were increased ratios of 10-hydroxynortriptyline (10-OH-NT, the pharmacologically active metabolite of NT) to NT with age (11,149). In the latter study, plasma NT concentrations did not differ significantly between age groups (mean ages 20.7 and 73.5 years). However, the steady state plasma concentration of unconjugated 10-OH-NT was considerably higher in older than in younger adults. It should be noted that there was considerable interindividual variability in the ratio of plasma 10-OH-NT to plasma NT in all age groups, although the ratio within individuals was stable. Even without considering hydroxylated metabolites, great interindividual variability in plasma levels seems to be the rule rather than the exception (14,22,38,152).

An additional source of variability in the dose/plasma level relationship is suggested by a recent case report (34) indicating that steady state desipramine serum levels in a 65-year-old man fit a nonlinear rather than linear pharmacokinetic model. The authors propose that saturation of hepatic metabolic processes (leading to large increases in serum concentrations from small increases in dosage) may account for this observation, and they advise caution in using serum concentrations to predict daily dosage. There are other reports, however, of success in predicting steady state levels of desipramine (6) and NT (30) from single dose parameters.

Since the elderly frequently take multiple medications, the clinician must constantly watch for drugs (e.g., neuroleptics) that increase plasma levels of antidepressants (50,98), or induce hepatic enzymes (e.g., barbiturates) and lead to decreased plasma antidepressant levels (107).

With regard to the relationship of clinical response to antidepressant plasma levels in elderly patients, the data are conflicting. In an open study of desipramine (28), five of the seven patients showed a clinical response to a dose of 25 mg b.i.d., and only one of the five had a steady state plasma level greater than 34 ng/ml. In another study (99), mean desipramine plasma levels of responders (post-treatment HAM-D score of ≤ 11) were higher than those of nonresponders in elderly depressed patients (age range 60–81 years, $N = 20$). Thirty-one younger melancholic patients (mean age 40 years) met similar criteria and underwent similar treatment. The same threshold for response (115 ng/ml) was identified in both groups; however, examination of the data set reveals that one of the six elderly initial responders had a blood level of 502 ng/ml, with the next highest level being 223 ng/ml, whereas for another it was 50 ng/ml. This observation seems to be at variance with the authors' conclusion that low desipramine levels are not effective in elderly melancholic patients. When the dose was increased, there were five additional responders. Were the higher plasma levels needed for therapeutic response or was it due to longer duration of treatment? The authors note that of five non-responders whose plasma desipramine levels were above 115 ng/ml, none responded even after 4 to 9 additional weeks of treatment, arguing against the second explanation above. However, in a study of doxepin and imipramine (69), in which the protocol allowed for adjustment of dose in accordance with clinical indication, the maximum dose rarely exceeded 75 mg/day for the majority of remitters. These data do not support the practice of increasing the dose for patients who fail to show improvement within one or two weeks; however, since plasma drug levels were not available, it is impossible to know whether the remitters had "therapeutic" levels. A recent double-blind, placebo-controlled study of low-dose doxepin treatment (10–20 mg daily) in depressed geriatric rehabilitation patients suggests that such doses are effective without achieving plasma levels greater than 20 ng/ml, at least in a group of patients not selected according to *Diagnostic and Statistical Manual of Mental Disorders,* 3rd edition (DSM-III) criteria for major depressive episode (86).

Another protocol that allowed for dosage adjustment on clinical grounds was an open trial using doxepin to treat elderly depressed nursing home residents (38). In that study, responders had a higher mean daily dose (185 mg) and higher plasma levels (mean 127 ng/ml) than did non-responders (80 mg and 49 ng/ml, respectively). According to at least one study (129), the upper limit of the "therapeutic window" of nortriptyline was similar for younger and older patients (approximately 140 ng/ml). A recent study (5) of 79 younger unipolar depressed outpatients (mean age 42 ± 13 years for women and 40 ± 12 years for men) failed to show correlation between clinical response and plasma concentrations of desipramine and/or 2-hydroxydesipramine. Another recent study (83) in younger patients failed to show correlation between clinical response and plasma levels of amitriptyline, imipramine, nortriptyline, and desipramine. One must be cautious, however, in extrapolating these findings to the elderly. Information from dose prediction studies cannot be applied to the elderly without specific data for them, and such data are still sparse.

OTHER DRUGS USED TO TREAT DEPRESSION IN THE ELDERLY

Benzodiazepines

There is little evidence that the benzodiazepines have a specific antidepressant action, although they are sometimes helpful for the anxiety or insomnia that may accompany depression, particularly in the early phase of treatment with an antidepressant agent when the full effect has not yet occurred. The only benzodiazepine for which there is some evidence of an antidepressant effect is alprazolam, which is purported to have an antianxiety action at low daily dosages and an antidepressant action at higher dosages, although this has not been studied in elderly patients. There is one published double-blind controlled study comparing alprazolam, imipramine, and placebo (144), although all patients received psychotherapy in conjunction with pharmacotherapy, and the antidepressant effect of different dosages of alprazolam was not specifically examined (see Table 1).

The benzodiazepines do lack the adverse cardiovascular actions that are a problem with heterocyclic antidepressant medications (51); and, indeed, there is one report (88) of a case of successful treatment of depression with alprazolam in a patient with cardiac disease for whom the usual antidepressant agents were deemed inadvisable.

Monoamine Oxidase Inhibitors

Although monoamine oxidase inhibitors (MAOIs) are thought to be effective in "atypical" depression (with prom-

inent anxiety symptoms) and in "refractory" depression (both of which occur in the elderly), and although the side effects of the more commonly used TCAs (particularly central and peripheral anticholinergic effects) provide ample motivation to test alternative antidepressants, MAOIs have not been studied well in the elderly depressed population. Hypotension and hypertensive crises following ingestion of foods containing tyramine have been the major deterrents. Theoretically, the MAOIs ought to be especially effective in the elderly depressed patient because MAO has been shown to increase with age (2,114,115). Platelet MAO is thought to correlate with MAO type B in brain (37), although the correlation has recently been challenged (151). Since MAO breaks down biogenic amines, a clinical depression could ensue secondary to diminished neurotransmitter(s) (90). While the precise mechanism of antidepressant action of MAOIs remains in question (92), there is evidence that the antidepressant action indeed occurs by inhibition of MAO (140). MAOIs could be particularly effective for depressive symptoms associated with dementia of the Alzheimer type (DAT), since in some DAT patients the reduction in MAO exceeds that found in normal aging (49). This inference has some support from open clinical trials (7,72), although there are no definitive published studies. There have also been encouraging preliminary results in treating elderly depressed, nondemented patients (39,115,118), including successful treatment of tricyclic-nonresponders (39,118). A question remains as to why some patients who show adequate (>80%) inhibition of MAO do not respond to treatment, and one study suggests that age at onset of the depressive illness may provide the answer (2). In that study, patients with onset of depression before age 55 had lower MAO activity than did controls or patients with later onset. One might speculate that the patients with low initial MAO levels represent a subtype unlikely to respond to MAOIs. Clearly, further research is needed.

Lithium Salts

In the United States, lithium salts have traditionally been used in the treatment and prophylaxis of bipolar disease. As the general patient population ages, clinical observations on the safety and efficacy of lithium in the elderly have been accumulating, but placebo-controlled, double-blind studies are lacking. Uncontrolled studies indicate that lithium is effective in elderly patients (1,60,61,71,96,126), and that poor response correlates with neurologic illness ("dementiform" illness or "extrapyramidal dysfunction") rather than age, age at onset of disease, duration of affective symptoms, or presence of other medical illness (61).

The literature on adverse effects of lithium in the elderly is sparse. Uncontrolled studies suggest that lithium toxicity depends upon pre-existing neurologic disease (26,62,73,125), as well as lithium plasma levels (139). Although such studies provide only indirect evidence that lithium is safe and effective in lower doses in neurologically normal elderly bipolar patients, more recent reports add support. Thus, it was reported (1) that there were no significant differences in affective morbidity over a one-year period among three groups of elderly patients randomly assigned to different lithium ranges (0.45–0.59 mM/liter, 0.60–0.79 mM/liter, ≥0.80 mM/liter; total $N = 22$). However, tremor and thyroid dysfunction (elevated TSH level) were significantly reduced in patients maintained at lithium levels below 0.8 mM/liter. In another study (53), where 78 inpatients were partitioned into three groups according to age (≤45 years, 46–64 years, ≥65 years), the ratio of dose/kg body weight to plasma level declined by 36% from the youngest to the oldest group, and a lower daily dose of lithium was sufficient to produce "therapeutic" serum levels (0.61–0.70 ± 0.15 mM/liter) in the older patients. Fifty years of age was the threshold for the need to lower the daily lithium dose.

In summary, it appears that elderly patients are capable of responding to lithium therapy (albeit they may require lower daily doses and/or lower serum lithium levels), and that such therapy should not be withheld on the basis of age alone. Instead, other factors, such as pre-existing renal, thyroid, or neurologic disease, should be determinants.

There have been recent reports (32,33,59) of the efficacy of lithium added to an antidepressant drug for unipolar nonresponders. This effect would appear to apply to elderly as well as younger patients, but double-blind controlled studies have not been reported for the geriatric population. One report (85) cites five elderly patients who responded only after lithium carbonate was added to a single antidepressant. It also appears that the order of drug administration can be reversed, i.e., an antidepressant can be added to ongoing lithium treatment with resultant robust response (104,109).

Stimulants

Psychostimulants (methylphenidate, dextroamphetamine) as antidepressant agents have been investigated for over 40 years, with the general consensus that they are not true antidepressants and do not have a primary effect on mood; however, few controlled double-blind studies have been performed. A recent double-blind study (91) in young adult patients with "mild depression" failed to show benefit of methylphenidate compared to placebo, and an earlier double-blind study which included 61 elderly patients (mean age 71 years) also failed to show superiority of methylphenidate over placebo (87). Nonetheless, open trials in elderly patients suggest that there may still be a place for psychostimulants in particular subtypes of elderly depressed patients. Thus, methylphenidate has been reported useful (63) as an adjunct to psychotherapy (54 "depressed" outpatients, 50–70 years of age), and stimulants were deemed beneficial for medically ill depressed elderly patients who were not candidates for conventional antidepressant agents (78,79).

Neuroleptics

Although neuroleptics are still used, either alone or in combination with antidepressants in elderly depressed patients, there are a paucity of data on outcome. An early double-blind study compared thioridazine to imipramine in 92 patients with "mixed symptoms of anxiety and depression," 24 of them between 51 and 70 years of age,

and found the drugs approximately equal in efficacy, although results were not given separately for age groups (138).

COMBINED TREATMENTS

There have been two reports on the use of a TCA in combination with a neuroleptic to treat anxiety/depression in patients over age 70 years. One study (17) combined fluphenazine with NT and compared this to a neuroleptic alone (promazine). Another study (10) evaluated the combination of perphenazine and amitriptyline to chlordiazepoxide. Unfortunately, neither the ratings nor data were adequately explained, and the results are difficult to evaluate. Recently, a more carefully controlled, double-blind study of delusional depression demonstrated the superiority of amitriptyline plus perphenazine over either agent alone, but elderly patients were excluded from the study (132).

Lithium-antidepressant combination treatment is discussed above. Data on other drug combinations (e.g. thyroid, estrogens) remain to be accumulated for the elderly.

Even though this volume is devoted to progress in psychopharmacology, other treatment modalities deserve at least a brief mention. They include ECT which appears to be reasonably safe in the elderly, lacking the cardiovascular, anticholinergic and other side effects of so many of the antidepressant drugs (27,31,77,120). The effect of ECT on memory, however, remains controversial as does the use of unilateral as opposed to bilateral treatments (3,52,133). Data for the elderly are notably scarce, although anecdotal evidence supports its use, especially for those who are severely depressed and refractory to drug treatment (particularly when there is a prior history of successful treatment with ECT).

Psychotherapy also can be successful in the treatment of older depressed patients, especially outpatients (134,146). As in the case of psychopharmacology, the elderly have usually been, and still are excluded from psychotherapy outcome studies. The few exceptions provide valuable data on cognitive, behavioral, supportive-expressive psychodynamic, and cognitive-behavioral psychotherapy (136,137). Even though combined use of drugs and psychotherapy would theoretically seem to be the soundest approach (76), data for the elderly are practically nonexisting [for one notable exception see (142)]. More data are certainly needed.

MAINTENANCE TREATMENT FOR DEPRESSION IN THE ELDERLY

Data are virtually absent from the literature. Anecdotally, and in one report (25), relapse is common, especially when treatment lasts less than a year, but a firm database needs to be accumulated before any conclusions can be drawn.

SPECIAL TREATMENT CONSIDERATIONS IN ELDERLY DEPRESSED PATIENTS

Space does not allow for discussion of the special issues which need to be considered in the elderly. The reader is referred instead to existing reviews (34,56,87). They range from phenomenologic [e.g. memory loss (105), guilt (128), somatic complaints (135)] and pathophysiologic (e.g., disease, drug-disease, and drug-drug interactions) to coexistence of depression with stroke, dementia, Parkinson and other diseases.

CONCLUSION

In our attempt to gather the facts concerning pharmacologic treatment of depression in geriatric patients, we found support for our claim that "more data are needed." We found only 23 double-blind controlled studies in the 22-year period between 1964 and 1986, and half of them included only 50 individuals or fewer. However, since nearly two-thirds of them appeared in the last five years, it is likely that future studies will continue the trend. The TCAs and trazodone remain the standard treatments for depression in the elderly, although MAOIs and lithium salts appear to be gaining acceptance. We expect that some of the methodological problems (including non-standard diagnostic criteria) that make the available data difficult to evaluate will be overcome in the course of the next decade. Finally, we anticipate that more effective treatments will be developed. Currently, response rates are disappointingly low, ranging around 50 to 60%, so that there is ample room for improvement.

ACKNOWLEDGMENTS

This work was supported in part by National Institute of Mental Health research grants MH31357, MH36205, MH40059, and the Veterans Administration. The opinions expressed are those of the authors and not necessarily those of the Veterans Administration.

REFERENCES

1. Abou-Saleh, M. T., and Coppen, A. (1983): *Br. J. Psychiatry,* 143:527–528.
2. Alexopoulos, G. S., Lieberman, K. W., Young, R. C., and Shamoian, C. A. (1984): *Am. J. Psychiatry,* 141:1276–1278.
3. Alexopoulos, G. S., Young, R. C., and Shamoian, C. A. (1984): *Biol. Psychiatry,* 19(5):783–787.
4. APA Task Force on the Use of Laboratory Tests in Psychiatry (1985): *Am. J. Psychiatry,* 142:155–162.
5. Amsterdam, J. D., Brunswick, D. J., Potter, L., Winokur, A., and Rickels, K. (1985): *Arch. Gen. Psychiatry,* 42:361–364.
6. Antal, E. J., Lawson, I. R., Alderson, L. M., Chapron, D. J., and Kramer, P. A. (1982): *J. Clin. Psychopharmacol.,* 2:193–198.
7. Ashford, J. W., and Ford, C. V. (1979): *Am. J. Psychiatry,* 136:1466–1467.
8. Assalian, P., Rosengarten, M. D., and Phillips, R. (1985): *J. Clin. Psychiatry,* 46:90–94.
9. Ban, T. (1984): *J. Clin. Psychiatry,* 45(3, Sec. 2):18–23.
10. Beber, C. R. (1971): *J. Fla. Med. Assoc.,* 58:35–38.
11. Bertilsson, L., Mellström, B., and Sjöqvist, F. (1979): *Life Sciences,* 25:1285–1292.
12. Bigger, J. T., Giardina, E. G. V., Perel, J. M., Kantor, S. J., and Glassman, A. H. (1977): *N. Engl. J. Med.* 296:206–208.
13. Blazer, D., and Williams, C. D. (1980): *Am. J. Psychiatry,* 137:439–444.
14. Braithwaite, R. A., Goulding, R., Theano, G., Bailey, J., and Coppen, A. (1972): *Lancet,* 2:1297–1300.
15. Branconnier, R. J., Cole, J. O., Ghazvinian, S., and Rosenthal, S. (1982): In: *Typical and Atypical Antidepressants: Clinical Practice,* edited by E. Costa and G. Racagni, pp. 195–212. Raven Press, New York.
16. Branconnier, R. J., Cole, J. O., Ghazvinian, S., Spera, K. F., Oxenkrug, G. F., and Bass, J. L. (1983): *J. Clin. Psychiatry,* 44:130–133.
17. Brodie, N. H., McGhie, R. L., O'Hara, H., Valle-Jones, J. C., and Schiff, A. A. (1975): *Practitioner,* 215:660–664.
18. Brown, R. P., Sweeney, J., Frances, A., Kocsis, J. H., and Loutsch, E. (1983): *J. Clin. Psychopharmacol.,* 3:176–178.
19. Brown, R. P., Kocsis, J. H., Glick, I. D., and Dhar, A. K. (1984): *J. Clin. Psychopharmacol.,* 4:311–315.
20. Burns, M., Moskowitz, H., and Jaffe, J. (1986): *J. Clin. Psychiatry,* 47:252–254.
21. Busse, E., and Simpson, D. (1983): *J. Clin. Psychiatry,* 44(5, Sec. 2):35–39.
22. Carr, A. C., and Hobson, R. P. (1977): *Br. Med. J.,* 2:1151.
23. Chesrow, E. J., Kaplitz, S. E., Breme, J. T., Sabatini, R., Vetra, H., and Marquardt, G. H. (1964): *J. Am. Geriatr. Soc.,* 12:271–277.
24. Cohn, J. B., Varga, L., and Lyford, A. (1984): *J. Clin. Psychiatry,* 45(4, Sec. 2):68–72.
25. Cook, B. L., Helms, P. M., Smith, R. E., and Tsai, M. (1986): *J. Affective Disord.,* 10:91–94.
26. Corcoran, A. C., Taylor, R. D., and Page, I. H. (1949): *JAMA,* 139:685–688.
27. Crowe, R. R. (1984): *N. Eng. J. Med.,* 311(3):163–167.
28. Cutler, N. R., Zavadil, A. P., Eisdorfer, C., Ross, R. J., and Potter, W. Z. (1981): *Am. J. Psychiatry,* 138:1235–1237.
29. Dawling, S., Crome, P., Braithwaite, R. A., and Lewis, R. R. (1980): *Eur. J. Clin. Pharmacol.,* 18:147–150.
30. Dawling, S., Crome, P., Heyer, E. J., and Lewis, R. R. (1981): *Br. J. Psychiatry,* 139:413–416.
31. Dec, G. W. Jr., Stern, T. A., and Welch, C. (1985): *JAMA,* 253(17):2525–2529.
32. de Montigny, C., Cournoyer, G., Morissette, R., Langlois, R., and Caillé, G. (1983): *Arch. Gen. Psychiatry,* 40:1327–1334.
33. de Montigny, C., Elie, R., and Caillé, G. (1985): *Am. J. Psychiatry,* 142:220–223.
34. Dugas, J. E., and Bishop, D. S. (1985): *J. Clin. Psychopharmacol.,* 5:43–45.
35. Feighner, J. P., and Cohn, J. B. (1985): *J. Clin. Psychiatry,* 46(3, Sec. 2):20–25.
36. Filser, J. G., Muller, W. E., and Beckmann, H. (1986): *Br. J. Psychiatry,* 148:95–97.
37. Fowler, C. J., Tipton, K. F., MacKay, A. V. P., and Youdim, M. B. H. (1982): *Neuroscience,* 7:1577–1594.
38. Friedel, R. O. (1980): In: *Psychopathology in the Aged,* edited by J. O. Cole and J. E. Barrett, pp. 157–163. Raven Press, New York.
39. Georgotas, A., Friedman, E., McCarthy, M., Mann, J., Krakowski, M., Siegel, R., and Ferris, S. (1982): *Biol. Psychiatry,* 18:195–205.
40. Georgotas, A., Kim, O. M., Hapworth, W., Bow, A. D., and Friedman, E. (1983): *Psychopharmacol. Bull.,* 19:662–665.
41. Gerner, R. H. (1985): *J. Affective Disord.,* 1(suppl.):S23–S31.
42. Gerner, R., Estabrook, W., Steuer, J., and Jarvik, L. (1980): *J. Clin. Psychiatry,* 41:216–220.
43. Gerson, S. C., Jarvik, L. F., and Mintz, J. (1987): In: *Perspectives in Psychopharmacology,* edited by J. D. Barchas and W. E. Bunney, Jr. A. J. Liss, New York (in press).
44. Giardina, E. G. V., Bigger, J. T., Glassman, A. H., Perel, J. M., and Kantor, S. J. (1979): *Circulation,* 60:1045–1052.
45. Glassman, A. H., and Bigger, J. T. (1981): *Arch. Gen. Psychiatry,* 38:815–820.
46. Glassman, A. H., Johnson, L. L., Giardina, E. G. V., Walsh, B. T., Roose, S. P., Cooper, T. B., and Bigger, J. T., Jr. (1983): *JAMA,* 250:1997–2001.
47. Goff, D. C., and Jenike, M. A. (1986): *J. Am. Geriatr. Soc.,* 34:63–70.
48. Goldstein, S. E., Birnbom, F., and Laliberte, R. (1982): *J. Clin. Psychiatry,* 43:287–289.
49. Gottfries, C-G., Adolfsson, R., Aquilonius, S-M., Carlsson, A.,

Eckernas, S-A., Nordberg, A., Oreland, L., Svennerholm, L., Wieberg, A., and Winblad, B. (1983): *Neurobiol. Aging,* 4:261–271.

50. Gram, L. F., and Overø, K. F. (1972): *Br. Med. J.,* 1:463–465.
51. Greenblatt, D. J., and Shader, R. I. (1972): *N. Engl. J. Med.,* 291:1239–1243.
52. Gregory, S., Shawcross, C. R., and Gill, D. (1985): *Br. J. Psychiatry* 146:520–524.
53. Greil, W., Stoltzenburg, M. C., Mairhofer, M. L., and Haag, M. (1985): *J. Affective Disord.,* 9:1–4.
54. Gurland, B. J., and Cross, P. S. (1982): *Psychiatr. Clin. North Am.,* 5:11–26.
55. Gwirtsman, H. E., Ahles, S., Halaris, A., DeMet, E., and Hill, M. A. (1983): *J. Clin. Psychiatry,* 44:449–453.
56. Halaris, A. (1986): *Int. J. Psychiatry Med.,* 16(1):1–19.
57. Hamilton, M. (1982): *Br. J. Psychiatry,* 140:223–230.
58. Hayes, R. L., Gerner, R. H., Fairbanks, L., and Moran, M. (1983): *J. Clin. Psychiat.,* 44:180–183.
59. Heninger, G. R., Charney, D. S., and Sternberg, D. E. (1983): *Arch. Gen. Psychiatry.* 40:1335–1342.
60. Hewick, D. S., Newbury, P., Hopwood, S., Naylor, G., and Moody, J. (1977): *Br. J. Clin. Pharmacol.* 4:201–205.
61. Himmelhoch, J. M., Neil, J. F., May, S. J., Fuchs, C. Z., and Licata, S. M. (1980): *Am. J. Psychiatry,* 137:941–945.
62. Himmelhoch, J. M., Auchenbach, R., and Fuchs, C. Z. (1982): *J. Clin. Psychiatry,* 43(Sec. 2):26–32.
63. Jacobson, A. (1958): *Psychiatr. Q.,* 32:474–485.
64. Jacoby, R. J., Levy, R., and Bird, J. M. (1981): *Br. J. Psychiatry,* 139:288–292.
65. Jacoby, R. J., Dolan, R. J., Levy, R., and Baldy, R. (1983): *Br. J. Psychiatry,* 143:124–127.
66. Janowsky, D. S., and Byerley, B. (1984): *J. Clin. Psychiatry,* 45(10, Sec. 2):3–7.
67. Jansen, W., and Siegfried, K. (1984): *J. Clin. Psychiatry,* 45(4, Sec. 2):63–67.
68. Jarvik, L. F., and Perl, M. (1981): Neuropsychiatric Manifestations of Physical Disease in the Elderly, In: *Aging,* Vol. 14, edited by A. J. Levenson and R. C. W. Hall, pp. 1–15. Raven Press, New York.
69. Jarvik, L. F., Mintz, J., Steuer, J., and Gerner, R. (1982): *J. Am. Geriatr. Soc.,* 30:713–717.
70. Jarvik, L. F., Read, S. L., Mintz, J., and Neshkes, R. E. (1983): *J. Clin. Psychopharmacol.,* 3:368–372.
71. Jefferson, J. W. (1983): *Compr. Psychiatry,* 24:166–178.
72. Jenike, M. A. (1985): *Am. J. Psychiatry,* 142:763–764.
73. Johnson, G., Maccario, M., Gershon, S., and Korein, J. (1970): *J. Nerv. Ment. Dis.,* 151:273–289.
74. Kane, J. M., Cole, K., Sarantakos, S., Howard, A., and Borenstein, M. (1983): *J. Clin. Psychiatry,* 44(5, Sec. 2):134–136.
75. Kantor, S. J., Bigger, J., Glassman, A. H., MacKen, D. L., and Perel, J. M. (1975): *JAMA,* 231:1364–1366.
76. Karasu, T. B. (1982): *Am. J. Psychiatry,* 139(9):1102–1113.
77. Karlinski, H., and Shulman, K. (1984): *J. Am. Geriatr. Soc.,* 32:183–186.
78. Katon, W., and Raskind, M. (1980): *Am. J. Psychiatry,* 137:963–965.
79. Kaufmann, M. W., Murray, G. B., and Cassem, N. H. (1982): *Psychosomatics,* 23:817–819.
80. Kay, W. K., and Bergmann, K. (1980): In: *Handbook of Mental Health and Aging,* edited by J. E. Birren and R. B. Sloane, pp. 34–56. Prentice-Hall, Englewood Cliffs, New Jersey.
81. Kernohan, W. J., Chambers, J. L., Wilson, W. T., and Daugherty, J. F. (1967): *J. Am. Geriatr. Soc.,* 15:196–202.
82. Kitanaka, I., Zavadil, A. P., Cutler, N. R., and Potter, W. Z. (1981): *Clin. Pharmacol. Ther.,* 29:258.
83. Kocsis, J. H., Hanin, I., Bowden, C., and Brunswick, D. (1986): *Br. J. Psychiatry,* 148:52–57.
84. Kushnir, S. L. (1986): *Am. J. Psychiatry,* 143:3–4.
85. Kutcher, S. P., Reid, K., Dubbin, J. D., and Shulman, K. I. (1986): *Br. J. Psychiatry,* 148:676–679.
86. Lakshmanan, M., Mion, L. C., and Frengley, J. D. (1986): *J. Am. Geriatr. Soc.,* 34:421–426.
87. Landman, M. E., Preisig, R., and Perlman, M. (1958): *J. Med. Soc. NJ,* 55:55–58.

88. Levy, A. B., Davis, J., and Bidder, T. G. (1984): *J. Clin. Psychiatry,* 45:480–481.
89. Lipsey, J. R., Robinson, R. G., Pearlson, G. D., Rao, K., and Price, T. P. (1984): *Lancet,* 1:297–300.
90. Maas, J. W. (1975): *Arch. Gen. Psychiatry,* 32:1357–1361.
91. Mattes, J. A. (1985): *J. Clin. Psychiatry,* 46:525–527.
92. Mendis, N., Pare, C. M. B., Sandler, M., Glover, V., and Stern, G. M. (1981): *Psychopharmacology,* 73:87–90.
93. Merideth, C. H., Feighner, J. P., and Hendrickson, G. (1984): *J. Clin. Psychiatry,* 45(4, Sec. 2):73–77.
94. Mintz, J., Steuer, J., and Jarvik, L. F. (1981): *J. Consult. Clin. Psychol.,* 49:542–548.
95. Murphy, E. (1983): *Br. J. Psychiatry,* 142:111–119.
96. Murray, N., Hopwood, S., Balfour, D. J. K., Ogston, S., and Hewick, D. S. (1983): *Psychol. Med.,* 13:53–60.
97. Murrell, S. A., Himmelfarb, S., and Wright, K. (1983): *Am. J. Epidemiol.,* 117:173–185.
98. Nelson, J. C., and Jatlow, P. I. (1980): *Am. J. Psychiatry,* 137:1232–1234.
99. Nelson, J. C., Jatlow, P. I., and Mazure, C. (1985): *J. Clin. Psychopharmacol.,* 5:217–220.
100. Neshkes, R., Gerner, R., Jarvik, L. F., Mintz, J., Joseph, J., Linde, S., Aldrich, J., Connolly, M. E., Rosen, R., and Hill, M. (1985): *J. Clin. Psychopharmacol.,* 5:102–106.
101. Nies, A., Robinson, D. S., Friedman, M. J., Green, R., Cooper, T. B., Ravaris, C. L., and Ives, J. O. (1977): *Am. J. Psychiatry,* 134:790–793.
102. Nugent, D. (1979): *Clinical Trials Journals,* 16:13–16.
103. Olsen, E. J., Bank, L., and Jarvik, L. F. (1978): *J. Gerontol.,* 33:514–520.
104. Pande, A. D., and Max, P. (1985): *Am. J. Psychiatry,* 142:1228–1229.
105. Plotkin, D. A., Mintz, J., and Jarvik, L. F. (1985): *Am. J. Psychiatry,* 142:1103–1105.
106. Post, F., and Shulman, K. (1985): In: *Recent Advances in Psychogeriatrics,* edited by T. Arie, pp. 119–140. Churchill Livingstone, London.
107. Preskorn, S. H. (1986): *J. Clin. Psychiatry,* 47(Suppl.):24–30.
108. Preskorn, S. H., and Mac, D. S. (1985): *J. Clin. Psychiatry,* 46:276–277.
109. Price, L. H., Charney, D. S., and Heninger, G. R. (1985): *Am. J. Psychiatry,* 142:619–623.
110. Quitkin, F. M., Rabkin, J. G., Ross, D., and McGrath, P. J. (1984): *Arch. Gen. Psychiatry,* 41:238–245.
111. Rabins, P. V., Merchant, A., and Nestadt, G. (1984): *Br. J. Psychiatry,* 144:488–492.
112. Reed, L., Smith, R. C., Schoolar, J. C., Hu, R., Doddamane, E., Leelavathi, E., Mann, E., and Lippman, L. (1980): *Am. J. Psychiatry,* 137:986–989.
113. Richelson, E. (1982): *J. Clin. Psych.,* 43:4–11.
114. Robinson, D. S. (1975): *Fed. Proc.,* 34:103–107.
115. Robinson, D. S., Davis, J. M., Nies, A., Ravaris, C. L., and Sylvester, D. (1971): *Arch. Gen. Psychiatry,* 24:536–539.
116. Robinson, R. G., Starr, L. B., and Price, T. R. (1984): *Br. J. Psychiatry,* 144:256–262.
117. Roose, S. P., Glassman, A. H., Siris, S., Walsh, T., Bruno, R. L., and Wright, L. B. (1981): *J. Clin. Psychopharmacol.,* 1:316–321.
118. Roose, S. P., Glassman, A. H., Walsh, B. T., and Woodring, S. (1986): *Am. J. Psychiatry,* 143:345–348.
119. Rothblum, E. D., Sholomskas, A. J., Berry, C., and Prusoff, B. A. (1982): *J. Am. Geriatr. Soc.,* 30:694–699.
120. Salzman, C. (1982): *Psychiatr. Clin. North. Am.,* 5:191–197.
121. Salzman, C. (1985): *Annu. Rev. Med.,* 36:217–228.
122. Scardigli, G., and Jans, G. (1982): In: *Typical and Atypical Antidepressants: Clinical Practice,* edited by E. Costa and G. Racagni, pp. 229–237. Raven Press, New York.
123. Schneider, L. S. (1986): *N. Engl. J. Med.,* 314:15.
124. Schneider, L. S., Sloane, R. B., Staples, F. R., and Bender, M. (1986): *J. Clin. Psychopharmacol.,* 6:172–176.
125. Shopsin, B., Johnson, G., and Gershon, S. (1970): *Int. Pharmacopsychiatry,* 5:170–182.
126. Shulman, K., and Post, F. (1980): *Br. J. Psychiatry,* 136:26–32.
127. Simpson, G. M., Pi, E. H., and White, K. (1983): *J. Clin. Psychiatry,* 44(5, Sec. 2):27–34.

128. Small, G. W., Komanduri, R., Gitlin, M., and Jarvik, L. F. (1987): *International Journal of Geriatric Psychiatry*, 1:121–126.

129. Smith, R. C., Reed, K., and Leelavathi, D. E. (1980): *Psychopharmacol. Bull.*, 16:54–57.

130. Snyder, S. H., and Yamamura, H. I. (1977): *Arch. Gen. Psychiatry*, 34:236–239.

131. Spar, J. A., and LaRue, A. (1985): *J. Clin. Psychiatry*, 46:466–469.

132. Spiker, D. G., Weiss, J. C., Dealy, R. S., Griffin, S. J., Hanin, I., Neil, J. F., Perel, J., Rossi, A. J., and Soloff, P. H. (1985): *Am. J. Psychiatry*, 142:430–436.

133. Squire, L. R. (1982): In: *Electroconvulsive Therapy*, edited by W. B. Essman and R. Abrams, pp. 169–186. Spectrum Publications, Inc., Jamaica, New York.

134. Steuer, J. (1982): *Psychiatr. Clin. North Am.*, 5:199–213.

135. Steuer, J., Bank, L., Olsen, E. J., and Jarvik, L. F. (1980): *J. Geront.*, 35(5):683–688.

136. Steuer, J., Mintz, J., Hammen, C. L., Hill, M., Jarvik, L. F., McCarley, T., Motoike, P., and Rosen, R. (1984): *J. Consult. Clin. Psychol.*, 52:180–189.

137. Thompson, L., and Gallagher, D. (1984): *Advances of Behavioral Research Therapy*, 6:127–139.

138. Thompson, W. (1972): *Practitioner*, 209:95–98.

139. van der Velde, C. D. (1971): *Am. J. Psychiatry*, 127:1075–1077.

140. van Praag, H. M. (1983): *Neuropharmacology*, 22:433–440.

141. Veith, R. C., Raskind, M. A., Caldwell, J. H., Barnes, R. F., Gumbrecht, G., and Ritchie, J. L. (1982): *N. Engl. J. Med.* 306:954–959.

142. Weissman, M. (1987): UCLA Intensive Course in Geriatric Medicine (No. 616) Syllabus, pp. 21–29.

143. Weissman, M., and Myers, J. (1979): *J. Geriatr. Psychiatry.* 12:187–201.

144. Weissman, M. M., Prusoff, B. A., Sholomskas, A. J., and Berry, C. (1984): In: *Biological Psychiatry: Recent Studies,* edited by G. D. Burrows, T. R. Norman and K. P. Maguire, pp. 167–174. John Libbey, London.

145. Winokur, G. (1980): *Biol. Psychiatry*, 15:599–611.

146. Yesavage, J. A., and Karasu, T. B. (1982): *Am. J. Psychother.*, 36:41–55.

147. Young, R. C., Alexopoulos, G. S., Manley, M. W., Shamoian, C. A., Dhar, A. K., and Kutt, H. (1984): In: *Frontiers in Biochemical and Pharmacological Research in Depression,* edited by E. Usdin, M. Åsberg, L. Bertilsson and F. Sjöqvist, pp. 207–211. Raven Press, New York.

148. Young, R. C., Alexopoulos, G. S., Shamoian, C. A., Dhar, A. K., and Kutt, H. (1984): *Am. J. Psychiatry*, 141:432–433.

149. Young, R. C., Alexopoulos, G. S., Shamoian, C. A., Manley, M. W., Dhar, A. K., and Kutt, H. (1984): *Clin. Pharmacol. Ther.*, 35:540–544.

150. Young, R. C., Alexopoulos, G. S., Shamoian, C. A., Kent, E., Dhar, A. K., and Kutt, H. (1985): *Am. J. Psychiatry*, 142:866–868.

151. Young, W. F., Jr., Laws, E. R., Jr., Sharbrough, F. W., and Weinshilboum, R. M. (1986): *Arch. Gen. Psychiatry*, 43:604–609.

152. Ziegler, V. E., and Biggs, J. T. (1977): *JAMA*, 238:2167–2169.

153. Ziegler, V. E., Clayton, P. J., and Biggs, J. T. (1977): *Arch. Gen. Psychiatry*, 34:607–612.

154. Zung, W. W. K., Gianturco, D., Pfeiffer, E., Wang, H. S., Whanger, A., Bridge, P., and Potkin, S. J. (1974): *Psychosomatics*, 15:127–131.

Psychopharmacology:
The Third Generation of Progress,
edited by Herbert Y. Meltzer.
Raven Press, New York © 1987.

CHAPTER **119**

Treatment of Sleep Disorders in the Elderly

Thomas H. Crook, David J. Kupfer, Carolyn C. Hoch,
and Charles F. Reynolds, III

Sleep disturbances represent a major clinical problem among elderly individuals, with 25 to 40% of persons over 65 years of age complaining of disturbed sleep (37,41,78). Sleep disturbances are almost always multiply determined by age-dependent changes in sleep (amount, composition, and circadian distribution), concurrent medical/neuropsychiatric disorders and their treatments, and psychosocial/environmental changes (67,68). Given this complex background, the widespread prescription and use of hypnotics in this age group for symptomatic relief of sleep disturbances warrants reevaluation. This chapter considers psychobiological research findings related to the effects of age on the pattern and structure of sleep, specific sleep disorders that are prevalent in the elderly, diagnostic approaches, and treatment.

ALTERATIONS IN PATTERN AND STRUCTURE OF SLEEP

Comparative studies of elderly individuals and younger adults have shown relatively little difference over an adult's lifetime in total amount of sleep across a 24-hr period (46,52,78). However, there are alterations in sleep pattern and structure that occur with advancing age which contribute to the sleep-related complaints of spending more time in bed, having difficulty with falling asleep, staying asleep, and feeling sleepy or needing frequent naps during the day (52).

The natural periodicity of circadian rhythms apparently changes with age (33,52). In an environment free of time cues, healthy elderly individuals have been found to show a shorter circadian period, with an associated phase advance of body temperature rhythm (82). Circadian rhythm disturbances are manifested by the redistribution of sleep across the 24-hr day. Many persons find themselves retiring earlier and earlier at night as they become older, reflecting a phase advance of their sleep period. Some elderly persons even develop multiple, shorter sleep-wake periods over a 24-hr period or a polyphasic sleep-wake cycle resembling that of infants (52).

Another salient feature of sleep in later life is daytime napping. In a sample of normal 50- to 60-year olds, 75% reported some daytime napping (80). When given a chance to do so, both healthy elderly and those with complaints of disturbed sleep fell asleep faster during the day than did healthy younger controls (8). Whether or not the individual takes a regular nap, a midafternoon bout of sleepiness appears to be nearly universal (8). The question arises: Are daytime naps simply a reflection of fundamental changes in circadian rhythm, or are they a compensatory response to disturbed nocturnal sleep? There is some evidence that daytime sleepiness is at least partially compensatory, since napping and drowsiness are more frequent in individuals with fragmented nocturnal sleep (8,11). In addition to these biological factors, social factors may enforce and reinforce napping behavior in the elderly, such as boredom, custom, and socioeconomic pressures (47).

Electrophysiologic studies of sleep structure have also revealed clear changes with advancing age. It is well documented that a dramatic reduction in the amplitude of delta activity in the sleep electroencephalogram (EEG) and a sharp decrease in those sleep segments that are characterized by a high arousal threshold occur (52,53,61,67,70). Corresponding to these EEG changes, older people often report frequent nocturnal awakenings, and in systematic studies of auditory threshold they have been shown to be more susceptible to external stimuli during sleep (50).

Changes in rapid eye movement (REM) sleep have also been widely reported, though there has been some disagreement as to the extent and nature of the changes. One reported difference is in the distribution of REM sleep through the night. REM sleep appears to be reasonably uniform in elderly persons, whereas in young normals a greater proportion of REM sleep occurs in the second half of the night (29,67,70). Several investigators have also reported that REM periods are shorter among older persons, especially in the second half of the night (40,61,80,81). Reduction of REM sleep periods is particularly marked in extreme old age (35,52,84) and in individuals suffering from Alzheimer's disease (31,62). The shortening of REM periods in these groups is of clinical interest because of the hypothesized significance of REM sleep in maintaining perception and memory functions (52,62). Finally, altered REM sleep distribution and increased percentage of REM sleep occur in elderly depressives (28,71).

Questions exist as to whether sleep changes with age differ in males and females. In general, physicians receive far fewer sleep-related complaints from men than from women, especially postmenopausal women, and hypnotic drugs are prescribed much less frequently for men than for women (54). In laboratory research as well, women tend to express a lower level of satisfaction with their sleep (18,77) than do men. However, several objective studies suggest that older men actually have more disturbed nocturnal sleep than do women and nap more frequently during the day (80,81). In a study of the healthy elderly, aged men showed diminished sleep continuity compared with aged women, reflecting on increased difficulty maintaining sleep, particularly in the last 2 hr of the sleep period (70). Also, the amount of slow-wave sleep (stages 3 and 4) was lower among men than among women (70).

SLEEP DISORDERS IN THE ELDERLY

In addition to sleep changes associated with the normal aging process are sleep disorders related to specific etiological factors. These factors will be considered individually (Table 1).

TABLE 1. *Etiology of sleep disorders in elderly*

Age-dependent changes in sleep
Transient situational disorders
Poor sleep habits
Pain and chronic illnesses
Dementias
Affective disorders
Sleep-disordered breathing
Drugs
Periodic leg jerks

Transient Situational Disorders

Persons with sleep disorders resulting from transient situational factors are generally considered to be those who have slept normally prior to a clearly stressful event, such as the death of a loved one, and who develop insomnia that lasts less than 3 weeks (3,17). The goal of treatment in such cases is generally to provide the patient with much-needed rest and to prevent a temporary problem from becoming chronic. Pharmacotherapy may be useful in such cases, as discussed in the treatment section (17,22,67).

Sleep Habits

Common correlates of sleep disorders are those associated with poor sleep hygiene such as irregular sleep-wake schedule, excessive environmental temperature or noise, or evening use of alcohol, nicotine, or caffeinated beverages. Adverse conditioning factors such as obsessive worry about sleep or use of the sleep setting for activities not conducive to sleep may also impair sleep (28,67,68).

Medical Disorders

Approximately two-thirds of individuals over 65 have one or more chronic medical disorders. Chronic pain contributes significantly to sleep changes; for example, pain may awaken the person as arthritic joints stiffen during the inactivity of sleep, or as angina signals coronary artery vasoconstriction at the onset of REM sleep (28,30,58). In chronic obstructive pulmonary disease, oxygen saturation may produce inadequate ventilatory changes during sleep. Hence, the individual's frequent arousals may be a physiologically adaptive response to improved ventilation (28,86). Epigastric pain that causes awakening can result from reflux of gastric acid into the esophagus or from the increase in gastric acid secretion that is associated with exacerbation of peptic and duodenal ulceration during periods of REM sleep (39). Fluid accumulation in the lungs of elderly individuals who have congestive heart failure may produce difficult breathing and sleeplessness. Benign prostatic enlargement, prostatic disease, diabetes mellitus, and urethritis (the latter especially in elderly women) may produce nocturnal awakening (30).

Dementias

Diminished sleep efficiency, impaired sleep maintenance, decreased REM sleep percentage, increased waking, and fragmentation of sleep stages have been observed in elderly demented patients (16,61,62,71). Nighttime wakefulness, wandering, and confusion are major problems that often lead to excessive sedation, falls, and other accidents (68).

Affective Disorders

Disturbances in sleep continuity, taking longer to fall asleep, difficulty in maintaining sleep during the night, and early morning awakening are part of the constellation of depressive symptoms at all ages (47). These sleep changes also occur, to a lesser extent, during normal aging itself. There are, however, other predictable sleep abnormalities in depression: (a) diminished slow-wave sleep with a shift of electroencephalogram (EEG) delta activity from the first to the second non-rapid eye movement (NREM) sleep period; (b) an abbreviated first NREM sleep period (shortened REM latency) leading to more rapid appearance of the first REM sleep; and (c) altered intranight temporal distribution of REM sleep with increased REM sleep time and REM activity earlier in the night (53,66,71). Thus, the effects of age and depression combine to produce pronounced sleep disturbances in the elderly.

Sleep Disordered Breathing

During the past 10 years it has become increasingly clear that sleep-related respiratory disorders are prevalent among the elderly. Between 25 and 40% of elderly persons in the general population are reported to experience such disorders (2,5,6,9,12,43,51,65,77,79), and sleep apnea is reported to be the most frequent cause of disordered sleep among persons over 65 years of age seen at sleep disorders clinics (51). It has been argued that sleep apnea may account for a substantial number of deaths among the elderly (44). Finally, a higher proportion of sleep apnea appears to occur in elderly Alzheimer patients than in healthy elderly (31,69,74,75).

In elderly patients, both central and obstructive sleep apnea are of concern. In the latter condition, a pharyngeal obstruction blocks airflow and may cause profound anoxia and a reflex sympathetic response marked by increased systemic and pulmonary blood pressure, tensing of the pharyngeal muscles allowing airflow to resume, and compensatory hyperventilation (45,47,63,64). Such episodes may continue throughout the night, although the patient may simply report excessive daytime sleepiness and may be unaware of frequent awakenings and periods of breathing cessation.

In contrast to obstructive apnea, central sleep apnea is marked by periods in which central nervous system mechanisms for initiating respiration fail and movement of the diaphragm and intercostal muscles ceases (48). As in the case of obstructive sleep apnea, periods of breathing cessation may occur throughout the course of the night without the patient's awareness.

Most elderly patients with sleep apnea show signs of both central and obstructive apnea (1,45). An apneic episode may begin with central respiratory failure, leading to airway collapse when breathing resumes, or, alternatively, episodes of both obstructive and central apnea may occur in the same patient over the course of the night. In both cases, the term "mixed apnea" is applied.

Medications

Stimulants, depressants, and other drugs may trigger or exacerbate sleep disturbances. The elderly are particularly at risk because chronic illnesses—hence medication usage—

increase with age. Age-dependent changes in pharmacokinetics, especially in the distribution, metabolism, and excretion of drugs, tend to interfere with the sleep-wake cycle in elderly (30,32).

Sleep is also disturbed by alcohol, caffeine, or nicotine. Although alcohol is initially a depressant and may have hypnotic effects, it soon fragments sleep and contributes to disturbed, restless sleep.

Periodic Leg Movements

Periodic movements during sleep (PMS), or nocturnal myoclonus, have been reported in 10 to 20% of persons with disordered sleep (12) and 44% of persons over 65 years of age (1). The periodic movements are highly stereotyped leg twitches recurring every 20 to 40 sec and lasting for epochs of 5 min to 2 hr during NREM sleep; these episodes alternate with periods of normal sleep. It is often a bed partner who reports these movements, since the individuals themselves are seldom aware of their own leg movements and typically complain only of fragmented and unrefreshing sleep. Persons with PMS also sleep for a shorter period, 100 min less on average, than do others (1,38).

CLINICAL EVALUATION

The aims of clinical evaluation are to identify, first, the type of sleep disturbance and its duration, and second, its probable etiology. Sources of diagnostic information include (a) interviews with the elderly individual and bed partner; (b) a sleep-wake diary kept for at least 14 days in order to establish the distribution and amount of sleep during the 24-hr day; (c) physical and neuropsychiatric examination; and (d) clinical evaluation to explore sleep habits, adverse conditioning factors, medication use, and indicators of sleep apnea or nocturnal myoclonus (67).

The patient should be referred to a sleep disorders specialist or clinical polysomnographer if the clinical evaluation indicates any of the following:

Sleep apnea syndrome, suggested by heavy snoring and excessive daytime sleepiness, particularly in men and postmenopausal women;

Nocturnal myoclonus, suggested by complaints of restless legs, kicking, or bed sheets in disarray every morning;

Snoring and excessive daytime sleepiness, particularly in men;

Narcolepsy-cataplexy, suggested by a history of sudden, irresistible daytime sleep attacks and emotion-triggered loss of muscle tone with usual onset prior to age 30;

Sleep phase irregularity with advancement of major sleep period or fragmented sleep-wake scheduling.

TREATMENT

Nonpharmacologic Treatment

It is necessary to "strengthen" the sleep-wake cycle and to combat the age-related tendency to develop several brief sleep episodes in a 24-hr period. Elderly individuals and their families need to know that some sleep disturbances may be unavoidable. It is not that less sleep is needed, but that the ability to sleep in a consolidated fashion seems to diminish with age (7,28,30,68).

It has been recommended that emphasis be placed on the use of stimulus controls and promotion of sleep hygiene practices such as urging elderly individuals to go to bed at a consistent time each night, to get up at the same time each morning, and to eliminate or at least reduce napping. Similarly, it has been advocated that the bedroom should be maintained as a stimulus and avoided for nonsleep activities, such as watching television or obsessing about sleep. In addition, attention should be given to omitting alcohol and caffeine and having a comfortable bed and comfortable surroundings, as well as timing of meals, activities, and medications (28,30,67,68).

Pharmacologic Treatment

Hypnotics may be appropriate in the management of transient sleep disturbance for persistent psychophysiologic insomnia (sleep loss from negative conditioning or somatized tension factors), or in persistent insomnia associated with nonpsychotic psychiatric disorders. Additional factors to consider in prescribing hypnotics for elderly persons are age-related changes in metabolism, effects on sleep apnea, effects on daytime alertness and performance, and other concurrent medications that might potentiate sedative effects. Contraindications for prescribing hypnotics for the elderly include heavy snoring, tendency to abuse drugs, lung, kidney, or liver disease, risk for injury at work, and suicidal risk (67).

If it is determined that hypnotic drugs are indicated for the elderly person, it is advisable to establish the lowest effective dose, tell the patient when to take the medication, monitor daytime sequelae, follow the patient regularly, limit use to less than 20 doses per month for not more than three months (19,22), and, finally, encourage the patient to increase reliance on the nonpharmacologic treatment measures (4).

Some of the frequently prescribed hypnotic drugs for treatment of disordered sleep in elderly are chloral derivatives, benzodiazepines, L-tryptophan, and barbiturates.

Chloral Derivatives

Oldest among available prescription hypnotics, and least studied in the past decade, are the chloral derivatives, particularly chloral hydrate. After centuries of use, these drugs remain reasonable choices for short-term therapy in elderly patients because of an onset of action of generally less than 30 min, minimal interactive effects with other drugs, and a half-life in the range of 8 hr (19,22). On the negative side, chloral derivatives may be associated with gastrointestinal disturbances, and may diminish in efficacy with long-term use (19,22).

Benzodiazepines

The benzodiazepines are the hypnotic drugs most widely used in the United States and are also commonly prescribed in the elderly (19,22). Although all benzodiazepines are likely to have hypnotic properties, the three commonly prescribed compounds are flurazepam, temazepam, and triazolam. These compounds will be described individually.

Flurazepam. After its introduction in 1970, flurazepam was for many years the only benzodiazepine marketed specifically as a hypnotic in the United States. The drug is a complicated combination of short-acting and long-acting compounds. The major active metabolite of flurazepam, desalkylflurazepam, accumulates in the blood and is eliminated very slowly, particularly in elderly patients (21). The half-life of the drug is over 45 hrs in young adults, and significant levels of desalklylflurazepam may be found in the blood of elderly patients many days or even weeks after a single dose (22).

Because of receptor adaptation, hypnotic effects of flurazepam do not precisely mirror desalkylflurazepam blood levels, but as the drug accumulates, daytime sedation and impaired psychomotor performance may be seen in elderly patients (10,21). Falls and other accidents appear to be more frequent with flurazepam and other long-acting benzodiazepines than with placebo or shorter-acting hypnotics, even several days after discontinuation (42,60). An advantage of the slow elimination of flurazepam is that rebound insomnia is rarely seen (49). In general, flurazepam may be least appropriate when the elderly patient's daytime alertness is very important and most appropriate when the patient reports both insomnia and daytime anxiety (49).

Temazepam. Temazepam is a conjugated benzodiazepine with a mean half-life of approximately 13 to 14 hr in healthy young males and a longer half-life among elderly patients because of slower clearance (14).

A frequently noted problem with temazepam has been its reported slow rate of absorption resulting in minimal impact on sleep latency (76), although this criticism is being challenged (72). Apparently, the rate of absorption is significantly increased with a soft gelatin capsule rather than with the hard capsule used in the United States (57).

In view of the half-life of temazepam, it is not surprising that in multiple doses the drug accumulates less than flurazepam and more than triazolam (57). Severe withdrawal effects are not often reported, but tapering of dosage at the termination of therapy is suggested to minimize this possibility.

Triazolam. The short-acting benzodiazepine triazolam became available in the United States early in 1983. The elimination half-life of the drug is in the range of 1.5 to 5 hr, with a mean of 2 to 3 hr. Because of the drug's short half-life, sleep may worsen in the later hours of the night. For this reason, triazolam is sometimes seen as more suitable for younger adult insomniacs whose main problem is falling asleep than for older persons who tend to awaken throughout the night and in the early morning.

Age-related differences in clearance time have been documented and are believed to be explained by reduced hepatic oxidizing capacity in the elderly, and possibly by a reduction in hepatic blood flow (23,24,83). Since older persons clear the drug more slowly and are more likely to have unpredicated negative responses to medication, an initial dose of 0.125 mg may be advisable, whereas in younger adults an appropriate initial dose may be 0.25 or 0.50 mg.

The short half-life of triazolam means that there is unlikely to be much daytime carry-over. Most studies report that vigilance and performance are unimpaired the day after triazolam is taken (10,56), and triazolam has even been reported to improve alertness or decrease daytime drowsiness (10).

The most frequent criticisms of triazolam and other short-acting benzodiazepines are daytime anxiety during administration and rebound insomnia after the drug has been discontinued (36). As with temazepam, withdrawal from triazolam should be accomplished through gradual tapering to minimize the occurrence of rebound insomnia (20).

L-Tryptophan

The amnio acid L-tryptophan is a serotonin precursor and is regarded by advocates as a "natural sedative" without the drawbacks of hypnotic drugs (25–27,34,55,73). Little is known of the effects of the compound in the elderly, but in view of the limitations of standard hypnotics, careful clinical studies with L-tryptophan in elderly insomniacs would appear worthwhile. The compound is rapidly metabolized and cleared by the body, but has been reported to improve sleep after short-term use is terminated (73). Why this would be the case is not clear, and even the immediate effects of L-tryptophan are not fully understood (85). In general, multiple studies suggest that L-tryptophan at doses of 1 to 5 g reduces sleep latency and waking time, at least in the early hours of the night (27).

Barbiturate and "Nonbarbiturate" Hypnotics

The barbiturates and so-called "nonbarbiturate" hypnotics—glutethimide, ethchlorvynol, methprylon, and methaqualone—distort normal sleep physiology, have a high potential for dependence, induce hepatic microsomal enzymes, and are extremely dangerous in overdose (22). These drugs would very rarely, if ever, be indicated for elderly patients.

A DECADE OF PROGRESS

During the past decade, significant advances have been made in sleep research in general and research on the treatment of sleep disorders in the elderly in particular. When Miles and Dement (52) reviewed the literature of the 1960s and 1970s on the treatment of sleep disorders in the elderly, they found striking gaps. For example, they found only one sleep laboratory study using subjects over the age of 65. Studies typically had no evaluation of daytime carry-over effects, no performance or alertness measures, and often no control group. By contrast, studies of drug efficacy in the 1980s have been much more thorough and carefully controlled and have often included elderly subjects. Moreover, an increasing sophistication in polygraphic and physiological recording techniques has enabled researchers to gather more precise information on the effects of hypnotics in normal and patient populations.

Attention in sleep research has also shifted to interactions of variables affecting sleep rather than isolated examinations of individual factors. For example, studies have focused on the interaction of hypnotics and respiratory difficulties and on the combined impact of sleep apnea and periodic movements in sleep. Investigations that consider the interplay of multiple variables in determining sleep difficulties and response to treatment are clearly required in dealing with an issue as complex as the nature and treatment of sleep disorders in the elderly.

FUTURE RESEARCH: TOWARD AN IDEAL HYPNOTIC

Clearly, research during the past two decades has led to very substantial improvements in the treatment of sleep disorders, and multiple pharmacologic options are now available to the clinician. Although the benzodiazepines, in particular, offer very clear advantages over the drugs of previous decades (particularly the barbiturates and "nonbarbiturate" sedative hypnotics), they are also clearly not ideal. A consensus appears to exist on the characteristics of an ideal hypnotic for the elderly (13,15,22,32,59), and these may be outlined as follows:

Induces sleep promptly after administration
Maintains sleep for an adequate period without undesired awakenings
Promotes a sleep state identical to undrugged or "natural" sleep
Leaves the individual feeling refreshed and well rested on awakening
Does not cause undesired daytime sedation or drowsiness
Causes no impairment of coordination and psychomotor function
Does not lose efficacy when taken repeatedly (for a number of consecutive nights or on a chronic basis)
Does not accumulate in the body during chronic usage
Does not lead to dependence
Is not harmful if an overdose is taken
Does not cause "rebound insomnia" when suddenly discontinued
Does not exacerbate sleep apnea or other conditions contributing to disturbed sleep
Causes no undesired reactions, such as cardiovascular or gastrointestinal distress
Does not cause enzyme induction or participate in other clinically important drug interactions
Is inexpensive

A goal of sleep research in the coming decade will be the development of compounds that approximate this ideal. Such drugs would be of inestimable value to individuals suffering from sleep disorders in the large and rapidly expanding elderly population.

REFERENCES

1. Ancoli-Israel, S., Kripke, D. F., Mason, W., and Kaplan, O. J. (1985): *J. Gerontol.,* 40:419–425.
2. Ancoli-Israel, S., Kripke, D. F., Mason, W., and Messin, S. (1981): *Sleep,* 4:349–358.
3. Association of Sleep Disorders Center (1979): *Diagnostic Classification of Sleep and Arousal Disorders,* 1st ed. *Sleep,* 2:1–131.
4. Association of Sleep Disorders Center (1982): *Project Sleep Educational Program.* Upjohn, Kalamazoo, MI.
5. Block, A. J. (1980): *Heart Lung,* 9:1011–1024.
6. Block, A. J., Wynne, J. W., and Boysen, P. G. (1980): *Am. J. Med.,* 69:75–79.
7. Bootzin, R. R., and Nicassio, P. (1978): In: *Progress in Behavior Modification,* edited by M. Hersen, R. Eisler, and P. Miller. Academic Press, New York.
8. Carskadon, M. A., Brown, E. D., and Dement, W. C. (1982): *Neurobiol. Aging,* 3:321–327.
9. Carskadon, M., and Dement, W. (1981): *J. Gerontol.,* 36:420–423.
10. Carskadon, M. A., Seidel, W. F., Greenblatt, D. J., and Dement, W. C. (1982): *Sleep,* 5:361–371.
11. Carskadon, M., van den Hoed, J., and Dement, W. (1980): *J. Geriatr. Psychiatry,* 13:135–151.
12. Coleman, R. M., Miles, L. E., Guilleminault, C. C., Zarcone, V. P., van den Hoed, J., and Dement, W. C. (1981): *J. Am. Geriatr. Soc.,* 29:289–296.
13. Dement, W. C. (1983): Paper presented for National Institute of Mental Health Consensus Development Conference on Drugs and Insomnia, November.
14. Divoll, M., Greenblatt, D. J., Harmatz, J. S., and Shader, R. I. (1981): *J. Pharm. Sci.,* 70:1104–1107.
15. Drugs and Insomnia (1983): National Institute of Mental Health Consensus Development Conference Summary, 4(10). Washington, DC.
16. Feinberg, I., Koresko, R. L., and Heller, N. (1967): *J. Psychiatr. Res.,* 5:107–144.
17. Freedman, D. X., Derryberry, J. S., Federman, D. D., et al. (1984): *JAMA,* 251:2410–2414.
18. Gerber, M., Ancoli-Israel, S., Mason, W. J., and Kripke, D. F. (1985): *Sleep Res.,* 14:106.
19. Greenblatt, D. J. (1981): In: *Physicians Handbook on Psychotherapeutic Drug Use in the Aged,* edited by T. Crook and G. Cohen, pp. 58–65. Mark Powley Associates, New Canaan, CT.
20. Greenblatt, D. J., Divoll, M., Abernethy, D. R., Locniskar, A., and Shader, R. I. (1983): *Pharmacology,* 27(Suppl.)2:70–75.
21. Greenblatt, D. J., Divoll, M., Harmatz, J. S., McLaughlin, D. S., and Shader, R. I. (1981): *Clin. Pharmacol. Ther.,* 30:475–486.
22. Greenblatt, D. J., and Prien, R. F. (1984): In: *Physicians' Guide to the Recognition and Treatment of Sleep Disorders in the Elderly,* edited by D. J. Kupfer and T. Crook, pp. 33–43. Mark Powley Associates, New Canaan, CT.
23. Greenblatt, D. J., and Shader, R. I. (1980): *Arzneim. Forsh.,* 30:886–890.
24. Guilleminault, C., and Silvestri, R. (1982): *Neurobiol. Aging,* 3:379–386.
25. Hartmann, E. (1965): Presented to the Association for the Psychophysiological Study of Sleep, Washington, DC, March.
26. Hartmann, E. (1968): In: *Proceedings of the Fourth World Congress of Psychiatry, Part 4,* edited by J. J. Lopez-Ibor, pp. 3100–3102. Excerpta Medica Foundation, New York.
27. Hartmann, E. (1977): *Am. J. Psychiatry,* 134:366–370.
28. Hauri, P., ed. (1982): *The Sleep Disorders.* Upjohn, Kalamazoo, MI.
29. Hayashi, Y., and Endo, S. (1982): *Sleep,* 5:277–283.
30. Hoch, C. C., and Reynolds, C. F. (1986): *Geriatric Nurs.,* 7:24–27.
31. Hoch, C. C., Reynolds, C. F., Kupfer, D. J., Houck, P. R., Berman, S. R., and Stack, J. A. (1986): *J. Clin. Psychiatry,* 47:499–503.
32. Hollister, L. E. (1977): *Geriatrics,* 32:71–73.
33. Ingram, D. K., London, E. D., and Reynolds, M. A. (1982): *Neurobiol. Aging,* 3:287–297.
34. Jouvet, M., and Renalt, J. (1966): *C. R. Soc. Biol. (Paris),* 160:1461–1465.
35. Kahn, E., and Fisher, C. (1969): *J. Nerv. Ment. Dis.,* 148:474–494.
36. Kales, A. (1983): Presented at the National Institute of Mental Health Consensus Development Conference on Drugs and Insomnia: The Use of Medications to Promote Sleep, Washington, DC.
37. Kales, A., Bixler, E. O., Leo, L. A., Healy, S., and Slye, E. (1974): *Sleep Res.,* 3:139.
38. Kales, A., Bixler, E. O., Soldatas, C. R., Vela-Bueno, A., Caldwell, A. B., and Cadieux, R. J. (1982): *Psychosomatics,* 23:589–600.
39. Kales, A., and Kales, J. D. (1974): *N. Engl. J. Med.,* 290:487–499.
40. Kales, A., Wilson, T., Kales, J. D., Jacobson, A., Paulson, M. J., Kollar, E., and Walter, R. D. (1967): *J. Am. Geriatr. Soc.,* 15:405–414.
41. Karacen, I., Thornby, M., Anch, M., Holzer, C., Warheit, G., Schwab, J., and Williams, R. L. (1976): *Soc. Sci. Med.,* 10:239–244.
42. Kramer, M., and Schoen, L. S. (1984): *J. Clin. Psychiatry,* 45:176–177.
43. Krieger, J., Megnin, P., and Kurtz, D. (1980): *Rev. EEG Neurophysiol.,* 10:177–185.
44. Kripke, D. F., and Ancoli-Israel, S. (1983): In: *Sleep/Wake Disorders: Natural History, Epidemiology, and Long-Term Evolution,* edited by C. Guilleminault and E. Lugaresi. Raven Press, New York.
45. Kripke, D. F., Ancoli-Israel, S., and Okudaira, N. (1982): *Neurobiol. Aging,* 3:329–336.
46. Kripke, D. F., Simons, R. N., Garfinkel, L., and Hammond, E. C. (1979): *Arch. Gen. Psychiatry,* 37:103–116.
47. Kupfer, D. J., and Reynolds, C. F. (1983): *Psychiatr. Dev.,* 4:367–386.
48. Kupfer, D. J., and Reynolds, C. F. (1983): *Hosp. Pract.,* 18:101–119.
49. Lamy, P. P. (1984): *Am. Fam. Phys.,* 30:187–191.
50. Lukas, J. S. (1975): *J. Acoust. Soc. Am.,* 58:1232–1242.
51. McGinty, D., Littner, M., Beahm, E., Ruiz-Primo, E., Young, E., and Sowers, J. (1982): *Neurobiol. Aging,* 3:337–350.
52. Miles, L. E., and Dement, W. C. (1980): *Sleep,* 3:119–220.
53. Miller, N. E., and Bartus, R. T. (1982): *Neurobiol. Aging,* 3:283–286.
54. Morgan, K. (1983): *Arch. Gerontol. Geriatr.,* 2:181–199.
55. Mouret, J., Bobillier, P., and Jouvet, M. (1967): *C. R. Soc. Biol. (Paris),* 161:1600–1603.
56. Nicholson, A. N., and Stone, B. M. (1980): *Br. J. Clin. Pharmacol.,* 9:187–194.
57. Ochs, H. R., Greenblatt, D. J., and Heuer, H. (1984): *J. Clin. Pharmacol.,* 24:58–64.
58. Orem, J., and Baines, C. D., eds. (1981): *Physiology in Sleep.* Academic Press, New York.
59. Oswald, I. (1984): *Psychopharmacology (Suppl.),* 1:84–90.
60. Oswald, I., Adam, K., Borrow, S., and Idzikowski, C. (1979): In: *Pharmacology of the States of Alertness,* edited by P. Passouant and I. Oswald, pp. 51–63. Pergamon Press, Oxford.
61. Prinz, P. N., and Halter, J. B. (1983): In: *Sleep Disorders: Basic and Clinical Research,* edited by M. Chase and E. D. Weitzman, pp. 463–487. SP Medical and Scientific Books, New York.
62. Prinz, P. N., Vitaliano, P. P., Vitiello, M. V., Bokan, J., Raskind, M., Peskind, E., and Gerber, C. (1982): *Neurobiol. Aging,* 3:361–370.
63. Remmers, G. E., Anch, A. M., and deGroot, W. J. (1980): In: *Clinics in Chest Medicine, Vol. 1,* edited by M. H. Williams, pp. 57–71. W. B. Saunders, Philadelphia.
64. Remmers, J. (1984): *Rev. Respir. Dis.,* 130:153–155.
65. Reynolds, C. F., Coble, P. A., Black, R. S., Holzer, B., Carroll, R., and Kupfer, D. J. (1980): *J. Am. Geriatr. Soc.,* 28:164–170.
66. Reynolds, C. F., and Kupfer, D. J. (1987): In: *Mental Health Aspects of Physical Disease in Old Age,* edited by N. Miller and G. Cohen. Guilford Press, New York (*in press*).
67. Reynolds, C., Kupfer, D. J., Hoch, C. C., and Sewitch, D. E. (1985): *J. Clin. Psychiatry,* 46:9–12.

68. Reynolds, C. F., Kupfer, D. J., and Sewitch, D. E. (1984): *Hosp. Community Psychiatry,* 35:779–781.
69. Reynolds, C. F., Kupfer, D. J., Taska, L. S., Hoch, C. C., Sewitch, D. E., Restifo, K., Spiker, D. G., Zimmer, B., Marin, R. S., Nelson, J., Martin, D., and Morycz, R. (1985): *J. Clin. Psychiatry,* 46:257–261.
70. Reynolds, C. F., Kupfer, D. J., Taska, L. S., Hoch, C. C., Sewitch, D. E., and Spiker, D. G. (1985): *Sleep,* 8:20–29.
71. Reynolds, C. F., Kupfer, D. J., Taska, L. S., Hoch, C. C., Spiker, D. G., Sewitch, D. E., Zimmer, B., Marin, R. S., Nelson, J. P., Martin, D., and Morycz, R. (1985): *Biol. Psychiatry,* 20:431–442.
72. Roehrs, T., Lamphere, J., Paxton, C., Wittig, R., Zorick, F., and Roth, T. (1984): *Br. J. Clin. Pharmacol.,* 17:691–696.
73. Schneider-Helmert, D. (1981): *Int. Pharmacopsychiatry,* 16:162–173.
74. Smallwood, R. G., Vitiello, M. V., Giblin, E. G., and Prinz, P. (1983): *Sleep,* 6:16–22.
75. Smirne, S., Franceschi, M., Bareggi, S. R., Comi, G., Mariani, E., and Mastrangelo, M. (1980): In: *Sleep, Sleep Research,* 5th European Congress, edited by W. P. Koella, pp. 442–444. S. Karger, Basel.
76. Soldatas, C. R. (1983): Presented at the Consensus Development Conference on Drugs and Insomnia: The Use of Medications to Promote Sleep.
77. Spiegel, R., ed. (1981): *Sleep and Sleeplessness in Advanced Age.* SP Medical and Scientific Books, New York.
78. Tune, G. S. (1969): *Br. J. Med. Psychol.,* 42:75–80.
79. Webb, P. (1974): *J. Appl. Psychol.,* 37:899–903.
80. Webb, W. B. (1982): *Neurobiol. Aging,* 3:311–319.
81. Webb, W. B. (1983): In: *Sleep Disorders: Basic and Clinical Research,* edited by M. Chase and E. D. Weitzman, pp. 489–501. SP Medical and Scientific Books, New York.
82. Weitzman, E. D., Moline, M. L., Czeisler, C. A., and Zimmerman, J. C. (1982): *Neurobiol. Aging,* 3:299–309.
83. Wilkinson, G. R., and Shand, D. G. (1975): *Clin. Pharmacol. Ther.,* 18:377–390.
84. Williams, R. L., Karacen, I., and Hursch, C. J., eds. (1974): *EEG of Human Sleep: Clinical Applications.* John Wiley and Sons, New York.
85. Wurtman, R. J., and Fernstrom, J. D. (1976): *Biochem. Pharmacol.,* 25:1691–1696.
86. Wynne, J. W. (1978): *Johns Hopkins Med. J.,* 143:3–7.

Psychopharmacology:
The Third Generation of Progress,
edited by Herbert Y. Meltzer.
Raven Press, New York © 1987.

CHAPTER 120

Treatment of Agitation in the Elderly

Carl Salzman

Among the most distressing manifestations of old age are the restlessness, agitation, and uncontrolled, socially inappropriate behavior that sometimes accompany various forms of stress or illness. At times, agitation is a consequence of organically impaired central nervous system function, as in dementia; at other times, such as following a loss, it resembles the protest and rage of an infant who has been separated from nurturing parents. Agitation, restlessness, and assaultiveness are also common components of psychosis and depression of later life (20,56,62,87,111), and it is not unusual to observe older agitated people who are suffering from various degress of dementia, loss, and psychosis simultaneously. Regardless of its manifestations or etiology, however, agitation may be a more serious management problem than the stresses that caused it. At these times, medication is usually indicated.

Drugs are frequently used to control agitation in older people. Neuroleptic drugs, the class of compounds most widely used to control agitation, are the third most frequently used class of drugs in skilled nursing facilities (67). In one nursing home survey, chlorpromazine was the most prescribed drug and thioridazine the third most prescribed drug (112). Thioridazine was also the third most frequently prescribed drug (15% of all patients) in a widely cited survey of Veterans Administration hospital treatment of elderly patients with organic brain syndrome (84).

STUDIES OF CLINICAL EFFECT OF NEUROLEPTICS IN THE CONTROL OF AGITATION

Although a variety of nonneuroleptic psychotropic drugs, including benzodiazepines, β-blockers, and reserpine, has also been employed to control agitation in the elderly, neuroleptics continue to be the drugs most frequently prescribed for the control of agitation (6,8,12,32,35,41, 46,67,69,84,87,93–95,97,99,100–103,116–120,128,135).

Studies Prior to 1976

The preponderance of clinical information regarding the effect of neuroleptics for controlling agitation in elderly patients prior to 1976 is derived from uncontrolled studies published in the two decades following the introduction of neuroleptics. Thirty-one published reports of over 3,000 patients of mixed diagnoses appeared in the literature between 1955 and 1976 (Table 1). These early reports included observations of patients with a variety of different diagnoses, different neuroleptics in varying doses, nonspecific and usually nonquantitative outcome criteria, and a variable duration of clinical observation. These uncontrolled clinical reports as a group demonstrate an overall therapeutic response rate of "good to excellent" results in approximately 60 to 70% of elderly patients with a wide variety of organic and emotional disorders. Nevertheless, since age, severity of illness, specificity of diagnosis, and dosage vary from study to study, no conclusions can be drawn regarding differential efficacy or toxicity among the various neuroleptics that were studied.

Twenty-three controlled studies comparing neuroleptics with either placebo or another active compound were also published prior to 1976 (Table 2). Although these studies attempted to bring an increased measure of scientific rigor by comparing neuroleptics with a placebo or a comparison drug, the results of these studies, like the uncontrolled reports, must be viewed with considerable caution. The symptoms of patients included in these studies were quite diverse, and diagnostic criteria were rarely specified. Most of these studies, however, did use standardized outcome measures (rating scales) and adequate length of treatment. As a group, these studies demonstrated the superiority of neuroleptic over placebo in the control of restlessness,

TABLE 1. *Neuroleptic treatment of agitation in the elderly: uncontrolled studies prior to 1976*

Drug (ref.)	N	Age (years)	Dose[a] (mg)	Results
Trifluoperazine (19)	12	60–74	4–10	8/12 no better or worse because of EPS[b]
Thioridazine (2)	14	74	75	Good control of agitation; few EPS
Thioridazine (53)	69	65–88	100	Marked reduction in confusion and agitation
Thioridazine (65)	37	65+	20–200	75% of patients "benefited"
Thioridazine (38)	56	74.9	47–90	44/56 good or excellent response
Thioridazine (23)	40	81.7	66–95	26/40 excellent or good behavioral control
Thioridazine (74)	27	80.4	75	All patients showed decreased agitation and restlessness
Thioridazine (134)	64	72	75	90% had good response
Thioridazine (116)	47	79	20–300	21/47 marked response: reduced agitation, restlessness, hostility
Thioridazine (89)	49	80	50	43/49 had reduced hostility, agitation, combativeness
Thioridazine (9)	98	66.6	200	68/98 showed good improvement; restlessness, "abnormal behavior pattern" reduced
Chlorpromazine (82)	200	65+	200–300	79% of patients had decreased aggression, restlessness, hostility; 55% of psychotic patients improved "significantly"
Chlorpromazine (135)	1,000	65+	150–200	Marked improvement in agitation, excited, hostile patients
Chlorpromazine (73)	677	65+	Not given	70% favorable response
Chlorpromazine (66)	26	60–90	150	12/26 marked or moderate improvement of severe behavioral problems
Chlorpromazine (52)	79	Not given	75	43/79 showed "significant" improvement
Chlorpromazine (105)	60	60–84	12–48	51/60 good to excellent response
Chlorpromazine (125)	22	72–93	30–75	20/22 good to excellent response
Trifluoperazine (135)	24	60–81	12	6/24 improved
Trifluoperazine (83)	7	60+	30	"Significant number" improved
Trifluoperazine (49)	27	71	4–8	Apathetic patients: showed no improvement, many side effects, especially EPS
Trifluoperazine (71)	100	31–79	9	63% of patients improved
Haloperidol (42)	10	Not given	0.4–0.6	Moderate or marked improvement in 6/10 patients
Haloperidol (68)	331	16–76	8.1	
Haloperidol (128)	18	74.8	0.5–2.0	10/18 good or excellent response
Mesoridazine (44)	43	80.7	45	31/43 much improved; less aggression, agitation
Mesoridazine (43)	25	55–88	75	16/25 showed reduced agitation; 10/25 had reduced hostility
Thiothixene (7)	26	Not given	9.2; 12	Better therapeutic results with low doses and highly motivated hospital nursing staff
Perphenazine (21)	Not given	Not given	64	Good behavioral control
Prochlorperazine (108)	50	60–88	20	Good symptom relief in 85%
Prochlorperazine (106)	70	60–94	15–40	Overall effectiveness of 77%

[a] Dose expressed in mean daily dose, when given; otherwise, dose range used.
[b] EPS, Extrapyramidal symptoms.

tension, and agitation. There was no consistent advantage of any one neuroleptic over another in those studies of direct comparison between drugs, although neuroleptics as a class of compounds were superior to other compounds such as benzodiazepines, steroids, and reserpine (1,24,28,63, 69,91,126). Two of the 23 studies did not find neuroleptics helpful and, in fact, reported deterioration of patients on these medications (91,126).

Studies During 1976–86

Fourteen reports of neuroleptics used to control agitation in the elderly were published in the decade from 1976 to 1986 (Table 3). More than 500 patients were studied, and, as a group, these studies demonstrated that neuroleptics were more therapeutic than placebo; there were no therapeutic differences among neuroleptics. As noted in a recent

TABLE 2. *Neuroleptic treatment of agitation in the elderly: controlled studies prior to 1976[a]*

Drug (ref.)	N	Diagnosis (mean age, years)	Dose[b] (mg)	Duration	Ratings	Results
Thioridazine, PBO (59)	40	Schizophrenia (63)	75–500	5 weeks	Multidimension rating	Thioridazine caused marked improvement in agitation and socialization. Mild EPS
Thioridazine, diazepam (63)	56	Organic brain syndrome (72.5)	T:38.9 DZ:9	4 weeks	Ham Anx, NOSIE	Thioridazine better than diazepam for anxiety; diazepam better than thioridazine for agitation, insomnia and depression
Thioridazine, diazepam (24)	56	"Senile" (NAG)	T:79 DZ:12	4 weeks	Ham Anx, NOSIE	Drugs equal for anxiety, agitation, and tension; thioridazine better than diazepam for behavioral improvement
Thioridazine, chlorpromazine (3)	151	Organic brain syndrome (72)	T:70 CPZ:78	12 weeks		Drugs equal on behavioral ratings
Thioridazine, thiothixene (61)	40	Chronic brain syndrome (NAG)	Not given	Not given	BPRS, video	Thioridazine more calming, thiothixene more stimulating
Thioridazine, haloperidol (130)	60	Psychotic (72.6)	T:113 H:2	12 weeks	BPRS, NOSIE, mental status	Drugs equal for treatment of excitement, irritability, hostility, and suspiciousness
Haloperidol, PBO (122)	18	Organic brain syndrome (71.6)	1–4.5	18 weeks	Global ratings	Haloperidol much better than placebo in reducing overactivity, restlessness, and tension. EPS common with haloperidol
Chlorpromazine, PBO (104)	46	Dementia and chronic schizophrenia (72.5)	150–225	8 weeks	Clinical ratings	Chlorpromazine superior to PBO in reducing psychotic symptoms
Chlorpromazine, pentylene, tetrazol, reserpine, PBO (91)	80	Chronic brain syndrome (24)	Not given	6 weeks	Fergus-Falls	Chlorpromazine patients deteriorated faster than PBO patients
Chlorpromazine, reserpine-pipradol (1)	80	Paranoid (79)	CPZ:75	8 weeks	Not given	No difference between drug and PBO
Chlorpromazine, PBO (11)	53	Dementia (76.5)	CPZ: 137.5	3 weeks	Not given	Chlorpromazine superior for agitation
Acetophenazine, PBO (48)	27	Organic brain syndrome (61)	60	3–8 weeks	Ward behavior	Acetophenazine much superior to PBO for improved behavior and assaultiveness
Acetophenazine, imipramine, trifluoperazine (51)	251	Chronic schizophrenia and organic brain syndrome (66)	A:20–126 IMI:25–150 TFP:2–12	24 weeks	NOSIE, IMPS	Acetophenazine and trifluoperazine equally effective in reducing motor disturbance, psychosis, thinking disorder; acetophenazine better than trifluoperazine in decreasing irritability and improving social competence
Thioridazine, diazepam (28)	59	Organic brain syndrome (80)	T:33 DZ:7.2	4 weeks	Ham Anx, NOSIE	Thioridazine superior to diazepam on all ratings
Thioridazine, haloperidol, chlorpromazine (13)	30	No dx given (80.5)	T:25–100 H:0.5–2 CPZ:25–100	9 days	Blood pressure ratings	All drugs statistically equal on BP. CPZ and thioridazine caused large decrease in blood pressure
Thioridazine, amitriptyline, fluoxymesterone, meprobamate, tybamate (69)	38	Mixed diagnosis (72)	T:75–150	8–10 weeks	Verdun, BPRS	Thioridazine better than all other drugs for irritability and excitement
Thioridazine, fluoxymesterone, nicotinic acid, PBO (70)	120	Mixed (NAG)	T:75–100	12 weeks	Verdun, BPRS	BPRS total score improved only on combination of thioridazine and fluoxymesterone; thioridazine alone best only for blunted affect

TABLE 2. (Continued)

Drug (ref.)	N	Diagnosis (mean age, years)	Dose[b] (mg)	Duration	Ratings	Results
Thioridazine, halo-peridol, chlor-promazine, oxa-zenam, tybamate (126)	37	Restless elderly (73)	T:50–150 H:4.5 CPZ:50–150 Ox:20–30 Tyb:700–950	36 weeks	Not given	No drug helpful. Oxazepam least but haloperidol worst; thioridazine and chlorpromazine produced least deterioration
Haloperidol, thiorida-zine (112)	46	Senile psychosis (76.5)	H:2 T:106.7	6 weeks	BPRS, global rating, NOSIE	Drugs equal in efficacy
Acetophenazine, phenobarbital (133)	76	Anxiety, tension; no dx (60s–70s)	A:80	Not given	Not given	Drugs equally effective, but only $\frac{1}{3}$ of patients had a response
Acetophenazine, chlorpromazine, PBO (107)	45	Paranoid schizo-phrenia (73)	A:41–80 CPZ:52–100	8 weeks	Paranoia rating scale	Both drugs effective in reducing paranoia; acetophenazine better for delusions and bizarre posture
Acetophenazine, PBO (26)	80	Mixed dx (NAG)	20	6 months	Personal audit	Excellent or good results in 85% by clinical observation and 93% by psychological tests
Trifluoperazine, PBO (49)	27	Chronic brain syndrome (71)	71	8 weeks	Multiple adjective checklist; clinical observation	Drug not effective; caused EPS

[a] Abbreviations: Ham Anx, Hamilton Anxiety Scale; NOSIE, Nurses Observation Scale for Inpatient Evaluation; BPRS, Brief Psychiatric Rating Scale; IMPS, Inpatient Multidimensional Psychiatric Scale; PBO, placebo; Fergus-Falls, Fergus Falls Geriatric Rating Scale; Verdun, Verdun Target Rating Scale; NAG, no age given; EPS, Extrapyramidal Symptoms Scale.
[b] Dose expressed in mean daily dose, when given; otherwise, dose range used.

review of some of these studies, however (50), the research methodology employed was often insufficiently rigorous to permit valid scientific conclusions. Two of the studies, one of haloperidol (132) and one of molindone (77), were conducted without any control or comparison group, although rating scales and an adequate study period were employed in both. These studies offered little more than a clinical impression that both drugs in the prescribed doses were helpful in reducing psychotic symptoms. Two other studies compared a neuroleptic with ongoing doctor's choice treatment. In the first (86), fluphenazine enanthate was more therapeutic for paranoid hostility than doctor's choice medication but caused more psychomotor depression and retardation. In the second of these studies, thiothixene given to elderly schizophrenic patients was not associated with any therapeutic improvement at doses of 75 to 90 mg a day and offered no advantage over doctor's choice medication (75).

In a well-designed multihospital study, Stotsky (121) compared the effect of thioridazine with placebo or diazepam in four separate populations comprising 610 demented, nonpsychotic patients whose mean ages ranged from 72 to 81. Thioridazine was given in doses of 10 to 200 mg versus placebo or diazepam in daily doses of 2 to 40 mg. The study was conducted over a 4-week period and outcome criteria included the Nurses Observation Scale for Inpatient Evaluation (NOSIE) and Hamilton Anxiety Rating Scales. At the end of 4 weeks, thioridazine was associated with significantly greater improvement compared to placebo on all eight symptoms and factors of the Hamilton Anxiety

Scale. Thioridazine was also superior to diazepam, although the differences between the two active drugs were less striking than the difference between thioridazine and placebo.

Two other well-designed studies from the same period compared thioridazine to haloperidol for the control of agitation in the elderly. In the first study, Cowley (29) compared the effect of thioridazine (mean daily dose 153 mg) to that of haloperidol (mean daily dose 2.1 mg) in 40 demented inpatients age 65 years or over. In the second study, Rosen (92) examined the difference between thioridazine (mean daily dose, 58 mg) and haloperidol (mean daily dose, 1.3 mg) in 56 outpatients with mixed diagnoses who had a mean age of 69 years. The Brief Psychiatric Rating Scale (BPRS) was used in both studies to measure outcome criteria. Both of these studies concluded that the drugs were therapeutically equivalent, although Cowley found greater therapeutic improvement with thioridazine on some of the subscales of the BPRS, whereas Rosen found a significantly larger increase in Wechsler Memory Scale scores of patients treated with haloperidol. The differences favoring thioridazine in the first study and haloperidol in the second may reflect the difference between the thioridazine/haloperidol dosage ratio in the first study of 75:1 versus 50:1 in the second study, as well as the differences in patient diagnosis and hospital status.

In a third study published in the past decade, thioridazine was also compared to loxapine in 53 demented patients over the age of 65 years (10). In this 8-week study utilizing standard rating scale outcome measures, a mean daily dose

TABLE 3. *Neuroleptic treatment of agitation in the elderly: controlled trials since 1976*

Drug (ref.)	N	Diagnosis (mean age, years)	Dose[a] (mg)	Duration	Ratings	Results
Thioridazine, diazepam, PBO (121)	60	Demented nonpsychotic (76.4)	T:10–200 D:20–40	4 weeks	NOSIE, HAM	Thioridazine better than diazepam on all behavioral ratings; drugs equal in sedation
Thioridazine, haloperidol (29)	40	Demented (65+)	T:153 H:2.1	4 weeks	BPRS	Drugs equal in efficacy
Thioridazine, loxapine (10)	53	Demented (65+)	T:62.5 L:10.5	8 weeks	BPRS, SCAG, CGI, NOSIE	Drugs equal on all scales, both drugs better than PBO. Most patients showed only modest improvement. Loxapine more sedating and more EPS; thioridazine more hypotension
Thioridazine, haloperidol (92)	56	Mixed dx; out pts. (69)	T:58 H:1.3	6 weeks	BPRS, Wechsler memory, Katz adjustment	Drugs equal in therapeutic efficacy and social adjustment
Thioridazine, fluphenazine (18)	30	Chronic schizophrenia (67)	T:84–285 F:1.5–5	6 weeks	CGI, BPRS, EPS	Drugs equal in therapeutic efficacy. Fluphenazine produced rigidity. Thioridazine strong in producing hypotension, weight gain and prolonging the QT interval
Haloperidol, chlormethiazole (124)	87	Demented or psychotic (65+)	H:2.5 C:576	10 weeks	Stockton ADL ratings	Haloperidol better in reducing aggression, confusion and depression. Haloperidol less sedating
Haloperidol, clopenthixol (45)	47	Demented (80.6)	H:0.5 Cl:5	8 weeks	Crichton, CGI, Gottfries	Neither drug affected cognition; haloperidol caused more behavioral deterioration
Haloperidol decanoate, no control (131)	11	Chronic psychotic (24)	1 i.m. q 4 weeks	5 months	BPRS	Equal efficacy to oral haloperidol
Loxapine, haloperidol (81)	64	Demented (72.5)	L:21.9 H:4.6	8 weeks	CGI, SCAG, BPRS, NOSIE	Both drugs equal improvement on all scales; both better than PBO. Haloperidol caused more sedation, retardation, and orthostatic hypotension. Drugs equal in producing EPS
Fluphenazine enanthate, doctor's choice (86)	26	Paranoid (71.5)	5 mg q 2 weeks	6 weeks	CGI, BPRS	Fluphenazine enanthate better than doctor's choice in paranoid hostility; caused more depression and retardation
Molindone, no control (79)	28	Mixed dx; 50% demented (72.7)	85.8	8 weeks	BPRS, CGI	Reduced psychotic symptoms; few side effects
Thiothixene, doctor's choice (75)	11	Schizophrenia (69.9)	75–90	7–8 months	BPRS	No improvement with thiothixene
Thiothixene, PBO (85)	42	Organic brain syndrome (75.5)	15	4 weeks	BPRS, NOSIE	Thiothixene and PBO equal on all ratings
Melperone, no control (38)	14	Organic brain syndrome (75.2)	91	4 weeks	SCAG, CGI	12/14 better effect than prior neuroleptics (not specified)
Melperone, PBO (34)	20	Mixed dx; nonpsychotic (76)	5–10	3 weeks	Paranoid belligerence scale	Melperone added to prestudy neuroleptic; combination significantly decreased ratings of belligerence.

Abbreviations: SCAG, Sandoz Clinical Assessment, Geriatric; CGI, Clinical Global Index; ADL, Activities of Daily Living; NOSIE, Nurses Observation Scale for Inpatient Evaluation; HAM, Hamilton Anxiety Scale; BPRS, Brief Psychiatric Rating Scale; EPS, Extrapyramidal Symptoms Scale; Crichton, Crichton Geriatric Rating Scale; Gottfries, Gottfries-Cronholm Geriatric Rating Scale.

[a] Dose expressed in mean daily dose, when given; otherwise, dose range used.

of 62.5 mg of thioridazine was compared with a mean daily dose of 10.5 mg of loxapine. Both drugs were better than placebo but were therapeutically equal to each other, although most patients showed only modest improvement in symptoms of behavioral excitement. Loxapine produced more extrapyramidal symptoms, and thioridazine was associated with greater hypotension. Surprisingly, however, loxapine was the more sedating of the two drugs.

In two European studies, haloperidol was compared to chlormethiozole, a nonneuroleptic sedative, in 87 demented or psychotic patients over the age of 65 (124) and was compared to chlopenthixol in 47 demented elderly patients (mean age 78.1 years) (45). In the first of these studies, haloperidol was clearly superior in reducing aggression, confusion, and depression. In the second study, neither drug was noted to improve cognitive function, and haloperidol was associated with a worsening of behavior. Haloperidol was also compared to loxapine in 64 demented inpatients having a mean age of 72.5 (81). Utilizing average daily doses of 21.9 mg for loxapine versus 4.6 mg of haloperidol for 8 weeks, investigators found both drugs to be therapeutically equivalent. Both drugs also produced an equivalent frequency and intensity of extrapyramidal symptoms; but haloperidol, surprisingly, was associated with more sedation, and also with orthostatic hypotension.

In a controlled study of thiothixene versus placebo in 42 patients with organic brain syndrome (etiology not specified) having a mean age of 75.5, 15 mg per day of thiothixene was not superior to placebo on BPRS and NOSIE outcome criteria (85). Two studies, one open (38) and one placebo-controlled (34) of a new butyrophenone, melperone, demonstrated its effectiveness in controlling psychosis, aggression, and paranoid belligerence in elderly psychiatric patients (mean age 75.2 years and 76 years, respectively).

Taken together, these studies, despite their methodological deficiencies, support the previous conclusions that neuroleptic drugs are therapeutically useful in the control of agitation, restlessness, and hostility in elderly patients with a variety of diagnoses. No therapeutic differences among neuroleptics can be inferred. It should be noted, however, that the therapeutic effect of neuroleptics was modest; and in two studies of thiothixene, the neuroleptic was superior neither to placebo nor to ongoing doctor's choice medication. In a third study, haloperidol caused frank behavioral deterioration.

When these reports of the past decade are taken together with the earlier reports of neuroleptic control of agitated behavior in elderly patients, three conclusions are justified, despite methodology that would not be acceptable according to current research criteria:

1. Neuroleptics have consistent and reliable therapeutic effect in controlling agitation for elderly patients who are demented, psychotic, or both.

2. The overall therapeutic efficacy of these drugs is modest rather than striking. For some patients, in fact, these drugs are not more therapeutic than placebo, and may even contribute to a worsening of behavior.

3. No single neuroleptic, or class of neuroleptics, seems to offer any advantage as a treatment for agitation.

PHARMACOLOGY OF NEUROLEPTICS IN THE ELDERLY

Several assumptions have been made regarding the pharmacology of neuroleptic drugs, with respect to both pharmacokinetics and pharmacodynamics. All of these assumptions are based on the general observation that drug effects observed in younger patients are likely to be exaggerated in the elderly (17,90,96,98). For example, absorption of neuroleptics, which is slow in young adults, is assumed to be even slower in the elderly. Second, neuroleptic binding to serum albumin is assumed to be decreased in the elderly, as has been found with tricyclic antidepressants. Third, volume of distribution of neuroleptics is assumed to increase with age following the same pattern as the benzodiazepines. Last, hepatic metabolism and clearance of neuroleptics are assumed to be delayed and less efficient in elderly patients, as is the case for both benzodiazepines and cyclic antidepressants (64,98).

Actual data concerning the effect of age on neuroleptic pharmacokinetics are sparse. An increase in elimination half-life associated with age with thioridazine has been reported (5). The effect of age on steady-state plasma concentration of neuroleptics has produced conflicting conclusions (27). A relationship between the plasma concentration of thioridazine and metabolites and age could not be demonstrated in one study (78), in contrast to two other studies (5,27) in which a significant positive correlation between age and plasma level of thioridazine and metabolites in schizophrenic populations was observed. Adding to the confusion, Forsman and Ohman were unable to demonstrate any significant correlation between age and plasma haloperidol concentration in one study (40), but did find a positive correlation in a second, pilot study (39).

Pharmacodynamic responsiveness to neuroleptic medication, like pharmacokinetic parameters, has been assumed to alter with age. As a consequence of age-related reductions in neurotransmitter function, it has been inferred that the older central nervous system may be increasingly sensitive to neuroleptic drugs (37,98). Thus, reductions in dopamine neurotransmission in the nigrostriatal tract of the aged central nervous system theoretically predispose the older patient to an increased likelihood of developing extrapyramidal symptoms from neuroleptic-induced dopamine blockade. Observations of increased extrapyramidal side effects with neuroleptics in the elderly (109) support the inference that decreased nigrostriatal dopamine may be responsible for the increase in these drug effects (47,101,115,118). Similarly, age-related reductions in central baroreceptors (98) should predispose the older patient to an increased sensitivity to neuroleptic-induced orthostatic hypotension. This increased sensitivity is reflected in an increased incidence of hypotension with neuroleptics (14). Reduced acetylcholine transmission associated with advanced age has also been linked to marked increase in anticholinergic toxicity and delirium in elderly neuroleptic recipients (98,101,127).

Thus, although direct research evidence is lacking, clinical observations suggest that the elderly person is likely to be more sensitive to both therapeutic and toxic effects of neuroleptic drugs as a result of age-related alterations in pharmacodynamic drug sensitivity, as well as in pharmacokinetic drug disposition.

SIDE EFFECTS OF NEUROLEPTICS IN THE ELDERLY

Clinical observations have suggested that the older patient is especially sensitive to sedation (11,32,46,47,56, 67,73,87,93,94,100–103), orthostatic hypotension (14), and the development of abnormal involuntary movements (47,109). The development of side effects, or the increased predisposition to developing side effects, may also depend on the health of the central nervous system of the older patient as well as on pharmacodynamic and pharmacokinetic factors. Increased drug sensitivity, especially to the development of abnormal involuntary movements, is more likely in older patients with central nervous system pathology (47,101,109).

Neuroleptic drugs differ from one another in the frequency and intensity of the side effects that they produce. It has been assumed that the differences observed in young adults are likewise true for the elderly. For instance, in younger patients, low-potency neuroleptics such as chlorpromazine and thioridazine are associated with clinically significant sedation and orthostatic hypotension but with relatively less intense extrapyramidal symptoms. High-potency neuroleptics such as haloperidol and fluphenazine tend to produce relatively less sedation and orthostatic hypotension, but are extremely potent inducers of extrapyramidal symptoms. Clinical observation suggests that, controlling for dose, these relationships between type of neuroleptic and side effects are true for older patients as well (56,67,99,100). For example, in one study of older patients, as would be predicted, chlorpromazine and thioridazine caused larger decreases in blood pressure than haloperidol (13). Some studies, however, have reported that elderly patients respond differently from younger patients. Haloperidol caused more

orthostatic hypotension and sedation than loxapine in one study (87) and loxapine was more sedating than thioridazine in another (10).

Although data regarding these acute neuroleptic side effects and age are relatively sparse, there is a large body of evidence that strongly demonstrates a relationship between age and an increased incidence and severity of tardive dyskinesia. Crane, reviewing information on 279 patients, noted that the highest incidence of dyskinesia occurred between ages 50 and 70 (30,31). Tepper (123) reviewed 44 epidemiologic studies concerning tardive dyskinesia. Fifteen of these studies directly addressed the effect of age and risk of developing tardive dyskinesia. In 9 of the 15, tardive dyskinesia was clearly associated with neuroleptic use, and the severity of the symptoms was correlated with advanced age, as was the prevalence. Smith and Baldessarini (113) pooled published data on over 4,000 patients studied up until 1980. Five hundred and six patients had documented tardive dyskinesia, with a progressive increase in the incidence of dyskinesias up to, but not beyond, age 70. They concluded that advanced age up to 70 is associated with an increased risk of incidence and severity of tardive dyskinesia, which levels off after the age of 70. Kane (60) noted that 13 of the 20 studies of tardive dyskinesia found a statistically significant association between the increase in age and the prevalence of tardive dyskinesia. Jeste and Wyatt (57) summarized 10 studies with 783 patients and found that the prevalence of tardive dyskinesia was almost three times higher in patients over the age of 40 than under the age of 40; reviews by the American Psychiatric Association Task Force on Tardive Dyskinesia (4), by Casey (22), and Jenike (54) reached similar conclusions.

Taken together, the many literature reviews of earlier research as well as more recent reports (summarized in Table 4) demonstrate an increase in both the incidence of tardive dyskinesia as well as its severity with age.

In contrast to the above-mentioned side effects, there are no data to suggest that the elderly are more likely than younger adults to develop the following side effects: ob-

TABLE 4. *Association of age and tardive dyskinesia*

Author	N	Age (years)	Results
Smith et al. (1978) (114)	377	60	Overall prevalence: 62%; prevalence of moderate and severe tardive dyskinesia (t.d.): 30%; significant linear relationship between age and t.d. for females, curvilinear for males (decreased prevalence after age 70)
Bourgeois et al. (1980) (15)	270	81.8	25% had t.d.; incidence of t.d. was 2.35 times greater in those who took neuroleptics
Johnson et al. (1982) (58)	66	57+	56% prevalence in patients 45+; increased incidence and severity in older patients; incidence does not correlate with duration of treatment
Mukherjee et al. (1982) (77)	153	48.4	No prevalence rate given for elderly patients (overall prevalence: 45.8); age significantly correlated with prevalence and severity of t.d.
Lieberman et al. (1984) (72)	79	85.5	Prevalence of t.d. in neuroleptic-treated elderly was 16.5% as compared with institutionalized elderly who did not receive neuroleptics (4.8%) and nontreated elderly in the country (1.2%)
Chacko et al. (1985) (25)	87	67	30/64 patients taking neuroleptics had t.d. (47%)

structive jaundice, agranulocytosis, weight gain, skin rashes, grand mal seizures, and neuroleptic malignant syndrome. Furthermore, neuroleptic malignant syndrome is more common among young patients than old patients (76).

NONNEUROLEPTIC TREATMENT OF AGITATION IN THE ELDERLY

During the early years of the neuroleptic era, when the efficacy of these drugs for controlling agitation was still uncertain, a variety of nonneuroleptic drugs such as meprobamate (16), reserpine alone (110), or reserpine combined with a central nervous system stimulant such as methylphenidate or amphetamine (36), were considered effective in controlling overactive, aggressive, and hostile elderly patients. According to uncontrolled clinical observations, these drugs were often helpful in reducing agitation.

Benzodiazepines have also been used in attempts to quiet disruptive behavior of the elderly. As noted earlier, diazepam was compared in three separate studies with thioridazine (see Table 2). Diazepam was found to have some mild calming properties but was not as therapeutically effective for behavioral control as was thioridazine. Oxazepam was studied utilizing doses of up to 200 mg per day with an additional 50 mg given at bedtime as needed. The author reported considerable reduction in psychomotor agitation and aggressiveness with this treatment, although research data were not provided (33).

The most promising nonneuroleptic treatment of agitation in the elderly has been the use of β-blockers. These drugs have been observed to control agitation and violence in young adult patients, as well as in mentally retarded children (88,136). In a recent case report, three patients aged 54, 71, and 86 years, all with a diagnosis of primary degenerative dementia and severe destructive, aggressive, and disorganized behavior, responded well to propranolol, 60 mg per day, despite prior failure with neuroleptics (55). These three cases as well as the report by Yudofsky (136) have been cited (55,80) as evidence supporting the use of propranolol for agitation secondary to dementia in the elderly. There have been no double-blind controlled studies of propranolol or other β-blockers for the treatment of agitation, however, and although clinical use of these agents is increasing, additional clinical reports are lacking.

SUMMARY

Reversible medical factors as well as social, environmental, or psychological stress such as a death in the family or moving to unfamiliar surroundings may contribute to agitation in elderly patients. Before any medication is prescribed for agitated behavior, therefore, it is essential to perform a comprehensive medical, psychiatric, and psychosocial evaluation.

If the elderly patient's symptoms of agitation, restlessness, assaultiveness, aggression, or violence are severe enough to disrupt normal functioning, then medication should be employed. The literature and research studies reviewed and cited, both prior to 1976 and since that time, support the judicious use of neuroleptics for behavioral control. No neuroleptic is especially effective for behavioral control; therefore, selection of a drug rests on differential toxicity among drugs rather than on differential therapeutic efficacy. Older patients are more sensitive to sedation, orthostatic hypotension, anticholinergic symptoms, and the development of abnormal involuntary movements including tardive dyskinesia. The studies as a group also suggest that adequate behavioral control may be achieved with doses substantially lower than those used with younger adult patients. Treatment of agitation with propranolol seems promising on the basis of a few published case histories and slowly growing clinical experience, but further research is necessary.

Despite the wide use of neuroleptics for the control of behavior, and their positive effect reported in the literature, considerable pharmacodynamic and pharmacokinetic research is desirable to refine neuroleptic treatment in the future.

REFERENCES

1. Abse, W., and Dahlstrom, W. G. (1960): *JAMA*, 174:2036–2042.
2. Ahmed, A. (1968): *J. Am. Geriatr. Soc.*, 16:945–947.
3. Altman, H., Mehta, D., and Evenson, R. C. (1973): *J. Am. Geriatr. Soc.*, 21:241–248.
4. American Psychiatric Association (1980): *Tardive Dyskinesia Task Force*, pp. 25–27. American Psychiatric Association, Washington, DC.
5. Axelsson, R. (1977): *Curr. Ther. Res.*, 21:587–600.
6. Ayd, F. J. (1961): *J. Am. Geriatr. Soc.*, 8:909–914.
7. Ban, T. A. (1978): *Psychopharmacology of Thiothixene*, p. 156. Raven Press, New York.
8. Ban, T. A. (1980): *Psychopharmacology for the Aged*, pp. 62–72. Karger, Basel.
9. Barksdale, B. (1971): *Curr. Ther. Res.*, 13:359–363.
10. Barnes, R., Veith, R., Okimoti, J., Raskind, M., and Oumbrecht, G. (1982): *Am. J. Psychiatry*, 139:1170–1174.
11. Barton, R., and Hurst, L. (1966): *Br. J. Psychiatry*, 112:989–990.
12. Bercel, N. A. (1961): *Am. Pract. Digest. Treat.*, 12:44–48.
13. Birkett, D. P., and Boltuch, B. (1972): *J. Am. Geriatr. Soc.*, 20:403–406.
14. Blumenthal, M. D., and Davie, J. W. (1980): *Am. J. Psychiatry*, 137:203–206.
15. Bourgeois, M., Bouilh, P., Tignot, S., and Yesavage, J. (1980): *J. Nerv. Ment. Dis.*, 168:177–178.
16. Bower, W. H. (1957): *Ann. NY Acad. Sci.*, 67:801–809.
17. Braithwaite, R. (1982): In: *Psychopharmacology of Old Age*, edited by D. Wheatley, pp. 46–54. Oxford University Press, New York.
18. Branchey, M. H., Lee, J. H., Arun, R., and Simpson, F. M. (1978): *JAMA*, 239:1860–1862.
19. Brooks, G. W., and MacDonald, M. G. (1961): *Am. J. Psychiatry*, 117:932–933.
20. Burnside, I. M. (1980): In: *Handbook of Mental Health and Aging*, edited by J. E. Birren and R. B. Sloane, pp. 719–744. Prentice-Hall, Englewood Cliffs, NJ.
21. Busse, E. W. (1960): *Geriatrics*, 15:673.
22. Casey, D. E. (1985): In: *Chronic Treatments in Neuropsychiatry*, edited by D. Kemali and G. Racagui, pp. 15–24. Raven Press, New York.
23. Cavero, C. V. (1966): *J. Am. Geriatr. Soc.*, 14:617–622.
24. Cervera, A. A. (1974): *Psychiatr. Digest*, 35:15–21.
25. Chacko, R. C., Root, L., Marmion, J., Molinari, V., and Adams, G. L. (1985): *J. Clin. Psychiatry*, 46:55–57.
26. Chesrow, E. J., and Kaplitz, S. E. (1963): *J. Am. Geriatr. Soc.*, 11:445–448.
27. Cooper, T. B., and Robinson, D. S. (1981): In: *Age and the Pharmacology of Psychoactive Drugs*, edited by A. Raskin, D. S. Robinson, and J. Levine, pp. 181–192. Elsevier, New York.

28. Covington, J. S. (1975): *South. Med. J.,* 68:719–724.
29. Cowley, L. M., and Glen, R. S. (1979): *J. Clin. Psychiatry,* 40:411–419.
30. Crane, G. E. (1968): *Am. J. Psychiatry,* 124:40–48.
31. Crane, G. E., and Smeets, R. A. (1974): *Arch. Gen. Psychiatry,* 30:341–343.
32. Dawson-Butterworth, K. (1970): *J. Am. Geriatr. Soc.,* 18:97–114.
33. Deberdt, R. (1978): *Acta Psychiatr. Scand. (Suppl.),* 274:104–110.
34. DeCuyper, H., van Praag, H. M., and Verstraeten, D. (1985): *Neuropsychobiology,* 13:1–6.
35. DiMasco, A., and Goldberg, H. L. (1975): *Hosp. Physician,* 11:35–39.
36. Fergueson, J. T., and Funderburk, W. H. (1956): *JAMA,* 160:279–283.
37. Finch, C. E. (1977): In: *Handbook of the Biology of Aging,* edited by C. E. Finch and L. Hayflick, pp. 262–280. Van Nostrand, New York.
38. Fisher, R., Blair, M., Shedletsky, R., Lundell, A., and Napoliello, M. (1983): *Can. J. Psychiatry,* 28:193–196.
39. Forsman, A., and Ohman, R. (1974): In: *Pharmacodynamics and Pharmacokinetics,* edited by G. Sedvall, B. Uvnes, and Y. Zotterman, pp. 359–366. Pergamon Press, Oxford.
40. Forsman, A., and Ohman, R. (1976): *Curr. Ther. Res.,* 20:319–336.
41. Fraiberg, P. L. (1972): *Dis. Nerv. Syst.,* 33:178–182.
42. Gerle, B., Petersson, B., and Widmark, M. (1961): *Svenska Lak Tidn.,* 58:415–418.
43. Goldstein, B. J., and Dippy, W. E. (1967): *Curr. Ther. Res.,* 9:256–260.
44. Goldstein, S. E. (1974): *Curr. Ther. Res.,* 16:316–323.
45. Gotestam, K. G., Ljunghell, S., and Olsson, B. (1981): *Acta Psychiatr. Scand. (Suppl.),* 294:46–53.
46. Hader, M. (1965): *J. Mt. Sinai Hosp.,* 32:622–633.
47. Hamilton, L. D. (1966): *Geriatrics,* 21:131–138.
48. Hamilton, L. D., and Bennett, J. L. (1962): *Geriatrics,* 17:596–601.
49. Hamilton, L. D., and Bennett, J. L. (1962): *J. Am. Geriatr. Soc.,* 10:140–147.
50. Helms, P. M. (1985): *J. Am. Geriatr. Soc.,* 33:206–209.
51. Honigfeld, G., and Newall, P. N. (1965): *Dis. Nerv. Syst.,* 26:427–429.
52. Howell, T. H., Harth, J. A. D., and Dutuch, M. (1954): *Practitioner,* 173:172–173.
53. Jackson, E. B. (1961): *Am. J. Psychiatry,* 118:543–544.
54. Jenike, M. A. (1983): *J. Am. Geriatr. Soc.,* 31:71–73.
55. Jenike, M. A. (1983): *Geriatrics,* 38:29–31.
56. Jenike, M. A. (1985): *Handbook of Geriatric Psychopharmacology,* pp. 17–38. PSG Publishing, Littletown.
57. Jeste, D. V., and Wyatt, R. J. (1982): *Understanding and Treating Tardive Dyskinesia,* pp. 32–34, 96–98. Guilford Press, New York.
58. Johnson, G. F. S., Hunt, E. G., and Rey, J. M. (1982): *Arch. Gen. Psychiatry,* 39:486.
59. Judah, L., Murphee, D., and Seager, L. (1959): *Am. J. Psychiatry,* 115:1118–1119.
60. Kane, J. M., and Smith, J. M. (1982): *Arch. Gen. Psychiatry,* 39:473–481.
61. Katz, M. M., and Itil, T. M. (1974): *Arch. Gen. Psychiatry,* 31:204–210.
62. Kay, D. A. K., and Roth, M. (1961): *J. Ment. Sci.,* 107:619–626.
63. Kirven, L. E., and Montero, E. F. (1973): *J. Am. Geriatr. Soc.,* 21:546–551.
64. Klotz, U., Avant, G. R., Hoyumpa, A., Schenker, S., and Wilkinson, G. R. (1975): *J. Clin. Invest.,* 55:347–359.
65. Kral, V. A. (1961): *Can. Med. Assoc. J.,* 84:152–154.
66. Kurland, A. A. (1955): *Dis. Nerv. Syst.,* 16:336–369.
67. Lamy, P. P. (1980): *Prescribing for the Elderly,* pp. 501–592. PSG Company, Littleton.
68. Lapolla, A., and Nash, L. R. (1966): *Int. J. Neuropsychiatry,* 2:129–134.
69. Lehmann, H. E., and Ban, T. A. (1967): *Laval Med.,* 38:588–595.
70. Lehmann, H. E., and Ban, T. A. (1974): *Psychopharmacol. Bull.,* 1:75–76.
71. Lesse, S. (1962): *Am. J. Psychiatry,* 118:934–935.
72. Lieberman, J., Kane, J. M., Woerner, M., and Weinhold, P. (1984): *Psychopharmacol. Bull.,* 20:22–26.
73. Lifshitz, K., and Kline, N. S. (1963): In: *Clinical Principles and Drugs in the Aging,* edited by J. T. Freeman, pp. 421–457. Charles C Thomas, Springfield, IL.
74. Maurer, A. S. (1973): *J. Am. Geriatr. Soc.,* 21:226–228.
75. Mohler, G. (1976): *Curr. Ther. Res.,* 12:377–385.
76. Mueller, P. S. (1985): *Psychosomatics,* 26:654–668.
77. Mukherjee, S., Rosen, A. M., Cardenas, C., Varia, V., and Olarte, S. (1982): *Arch. Gen. Psychiatry,* 39:466–469.
78. Muusze, R. G., and Vanderheeren, F. A. J. (1977): *Eur. J. Clin. Pharmacol.,* 11:141–147.
79. Peper, M. (1985): *J. Clin. Psychiatry,* 46:26–29.
80. Petrie, W. M., and Ban, T. A. (1981): *Lancet,* 1:324.
81. Petrie, W. M., Ban, T. A., Baney, S., Fujimzi, M., Guy, W., Raghet, M., Wilson, W. H., and Schaffer, J. D. (1982): *J. Clin. Psychopharmacol.,* 2:122–128.
82. Pollack, B. (1986): *Geriatrics,* 11:253–259.
83. Post, F. (1962): *Gerontol. Clin.,* 4:137.
84. Prien, R. F., and Caffe, E. M., Jr. (1977): *Compr. Psychiatry,* 18:551–560.
85. Rada, R. T., and Kellner, R. (1976): *J. Am. Geriatr. Soc.,* 24:105–107.
86. Raskind, M., Alvarez, C., and Herlin, R. N. (1979): *J. Am. Geriatr. Soc.,* 27:459–463.
87. Raskind, M., and Eisdorfer, C. (1976): In: *Drug Treatment of Mental Disorders,* edited by L. L. Simpson, pp. 237–266. Raven Press, New York.
88. Ratey, J. J., Morrill, R., and Oxenkrug, G. (1983): *Am. J. Psychiatry,* 140:1356–1357.
89. Reedy, W. J. (1967): *J. Am. Geriatr. Soc.,* 15:587–592.
90. Ritschel, W. A. (1983): In: *Pharmacologic Aspects of Aging,* edited by L. A. Pagliano and A. M. Pagliano, pp. 219–256. C. V. Mosby, St. Louis.
91. Robinson, D. B. (1969): *Arch. Gen. Psychiatry,* 25:41–46.
92. Rosen, H. J. (1979): *J. Clin. Psychiatry,* 40:24–31.
93. Salzman, C. (1979): *Geriatrics,* 34:87–90.
94. Salzman, C. (1982): *Am. J. Psychiatry,* 139:67–74.
95. Salzman, C. (1982): *Hosp. Community Psychiatry,* 33:133–136.
96. Salzman, C. (1982): *Psychiatr. Clin. North Am.,* 5:181–190.
97. Salzman, C. (1982): In: *Health and Disease in Old Age,* edited by J. W. Rowe and R. W. Besdine, pp. 115–136. Little Brown, Boston.
98. Salzman, C. (1984): *Clinical Geriatric Psychopharmacology,* pp. 18–31. McGraw-Hill, New York.
99. Salzman, C. (1985): *Annu. Rev. Med.,* 36:217–228.
100. Salzman, C., Hoffman, S. A., and Schoonover, S. C. (1983): In: *Practitioner's Guide to Psychoactive Drugs,* edited by E. L. Bassuk, S. C. Schoonover, and A. Gelenberg. Plenum Press, New York.
101. Salzman, C., Shader, R. I., and Pearlman, M. S. (1970): In: *Psychotropic Drug Side Effects,* edited by R. I. Shader and A. DiMascio, pp. 261–279. Williams and Wilkins, Baltimore.
102. Salzman, C., Shader, R. I., and van der Kolk, B. A. (1975): In: *Manual of Psychiatric Therapeutics,* edited by R. I. Shader, pp. 171–184. Little Brown, Boston.
103. Salzman, C., Shader, R. I., and van der Kolk, B. A. (1976): *NY State J. Med.,* 76:71–77.
104. Seager, C. P. (1955): *Br. Med. J.,* 1:882–884.
105. Settel, E. (1956): *Gen. Pract.,* 12:74–76.
106. Settel, E. (1957): *J. Am. Geriatr. Soc.,* 5:827–831.
107. Sheppard, C., Bhattacharyya, A., DiGiacomo, M., and Merlis, S. (1964): *J. Am. Geriatr. Soc.,* 12:884–888.
108. Shubin, H., and Sherson, J. (1959): *J. Am. Geriatr. Soc.,* 7:405.
109. Siede, H., and Muller, H. F. (1967): *J. Am. Geriatr. Soc.,* 15:517–522.
110. Silverman, M., Parker, J. B., and Busse, E. W. (1959): *NC Med. J.,* 20:428–432.
111. Sloane, R. B. (1978): *Cont. Educat.,* 11:42–47.
112. Smith, G. R., Taylor, C. W., and Linkous, P. (1974): *Psychosomatics,* 15:134–138.
113. Smith, J. M., and Baldessarini, R. J. (1980): *Arch. Gen. Psychiatry,* 37:1368–1373.

114. Smith, J. M., Oswald, O. L., Kucharski, T., and Waterman, L. J. (1978): *Psychopharmacology,* 58:207–211.
115. Solomon, K. (1980): In: *Haloperidol Update 1958–1986,* edited by F. J. Ayd, Jr., pp. 155–173. Ayd Medical Communications, Baltimore.
116. Spencer, T. (1969): *Md. State Med. J.,* 18:73–76.
117. Steinhart, M. J. (1974): *NY State J. Med.,* 74:976–978.
118. Stotsky, B. A. (1972): In: *Butyrophenones in Psychiatry,* edited by A. DiMascio and R. I. Shader, pp. 71–86. Raven Press, New York.
119. Stotsky, B. A. (1973): In: *Psychopharmacology and Aging,* edited by C. Eisdorfer and W. E. Fann, pp. 193–202. Plenum Press, New York.
120. Stotsky, B. A. (1975): In: *Aging, Vol 2: Genesis and Treatment of Psychological Disorders in the Elderly,* edited by S. Gershon and A. Raskin, pp. 239–258. Raven Press, New York.
121. Stotsky, B. A. (1984): *Clin. Ther.,* 6:546–559.
122. Sugerman, A. A., Williams, H., and Adlerstein, A. M. (1964): *Am. J. Psychiatry,* 120:1190–1192.
123. Tepper, S. J., and Haas, J. F. (1979): *J. Clin. Psychiatry,* 40:508–516.
124. Ter Haar, H. W. (1977): *Age and Aging,* 6(*Suppl.*):73–82.
125. Terman, L. A. (1955): *Geriatrics,* 10:520–522.
126. Tewfik, G. I., Jain, V. K., Harcup, M., and Magowan, S. (1970): *Gerontol. Clin.,* 12:351–359.
127. Thompson, T. L. H., Morgan, M. G., and Nies, A. S. (1983): *N. Engl. J. Med.,* 308:194–199.
128. Tobin, J. M., Brosseau, E. R., and Lorenz, A. A. (1970): *Geriatrics,* 25:119–122.
129. Toennissen, L. M., Casey, D. E., and McFarland, B. H. (1985): *Arch. Gen. Psychiatry,* 42:278–284.
130. Tsuang, M. M., Min, L. L., Stotsky, B. A., and Cole, J. O. (1971): *J. Am. Geriatr. Soc.,* 19:593–600.
131. U.S. Senate Special Committee on Aging (1975): *Drugs in Nursing Homes.* U.S. Government Printing Office, Washington, DC.
132. Viukari, M., Salo, H., Lamminsiva, U., and Gordin, A. (1982): *Acta Psychiatr. Scand.,* 65:301–308.
133. Wellborn, W. S. (1961): *Psychosomatics,* 2:450–455.
134. Wilson, J. D., and Mathis, F. (1968): *J. Arkansas Med. Soc.,* 65:210–213.
135. Wolff, K. (1963): *Geriatric Psychiatry,* pp. 78–86. Charles C Thomas, Springfield, IL.
136. Yudofsky, S. (1981): *Am. J. Psychiatry,* 138:218–230.

Psychopharmacology:
The Third Generation of Progress,
edited by Herbert Y. Meltzer.
Raven Press, New York © 1987.

CHAPTER 121

Differential Diagnosis and Assessment of Anxiety: Recent Developments

Abby J. Fyer, Salvatore Mannuzza, and Jean Endicott

The conceptual direction of anxiety research over the past 30 years has been toward ever increasing specificity. The 1952 *Diagnostic and Statistical Manual of Mental Disorders* (DSM-I) contained only three anxiety disorder categories (3). Implicit in its nosology were the beliefs that (a) anxiety existed on a continuum from normal to pathological without intervening qualitative distinction, and (b) etiology and symptoms of anxiety disorders were determined by intrapsychic conflict or developmental deficit.

Empirical research during the 1960s repeatedly questioned these assumptions. Klein (66) observed that imipramine successfully blocked panic attacks but not generalized anxiety. Pitts and McClure (104) demonstrated that intravenous sodium lactate precipitated panic in patients whose illness was characterized by these attacks but not in normal controls. Marks (87) delineated four groups of phobia patients who differed in age of onset, symptomatology, course, and treatment outcome. Wolpe (145), Marks (87), and others demonstrated that specific symptomatically based behavioral treatments were effective in many phobic patients.

By the early 1970s, diagnostic criteria incorporating the implications of these findings were routinely used by several research groups. Published in 1972, the Feighner criteria (40) operationalized definitions of anxiety neuroses, phobic, and obsessive compulsive disorders. Several years later the Research Diagnostic Criteria (RDC) (118) split anxiety neuroses into panic and generalized anxiety disorders and included four subtypes of phobic disorder (agoraphobia, simple, social, mixed).

The *Diagnostic and Statistical Manual of Mental Disorders,* 3rd edition, (DSM-III) (5) adopted the central tenets of this nosology with three further conceptual modifications. Agoraphobia was given status as a separate disorder. Though it remained in the general category of phobic disorders, it was split into two subtypes depending on presence or absence of panic attacks. Simple and social phobia were also made separate disorders allowing for the possibility of differential etiology. Posttraumatic stress disorder was added.

The past decade has seen a geometric progression in the volume of research on anxiety disorders. These are "second generation studies" applying, criticizing, and refining the criteria created by the RDC and DSM-III. One result of this abundance of work has been to make clear the benefits of increased specificity in diagnosis and measurement. Reliability of diagnosis of anxiety disorders, facilitated by the introduction of operationalized criteria and detailed anxiety interview schedules, has been considerably improved. This enables productive cross-center comparison of outcome in natural history and family studies. Discrimination between anxiety and depressive disorders has also improved, though their relationship remains controversial.

Measures assessing treatment outcome now focus on frequency and intensity of specific types of anxiety (e.g., number of panic attacks, time spent in compulsive rituals, numbers and kinds of social interactions) rather than total scores or percent change in mean overall anxiety scores. Newer methods give precise information about the patient's condition and improve the comparison of treatments with respect to specific symptoms.

This chapter reviews the progress of the new nosology and its impact on assessment procedures. The first section, Diagnosis, reviews the DSM-III anxiety disorder criteria, the revisions of these criteria recommended in the revised draft DSM-III-R (6), and current controversies related to diagnostic definitions. Available validity and reliability data on DSM-III anxiety disorders are summarized. New interview schedules for anxiety disorder diagnosis, recent studies on heterogeneity within diagnostic categories, and relationship of anxiety to depression are also discussed. The second section, Psychological Assessment, reviews the anxiety measurement instruments most frequently employed. The significance of new scales is indicated.

DIAGNOSIS

Panic and Generalized Anxiety Disorders

The qualitative distinction between panic and generalized anxiety has achieved significant face validity in the United States and is part of the DSM-III. However, many investigators outside the United States, as well as some within the United States, consider panic a more severe form of generalized anxiety (64,133). Data addressing this issue are discussed in this section.

The separation of panic and generalized anxiety was based in part on the observation that imipramine blocked spontaneous panic but not anticipatory anxiety or avoidance in agoraphobics with panic attacks (67). Previously panic had been considered merely a more severe form of generalized anxiety. However, a drug response in which the severe but not the mild form of a disorder is effectively treated is virtually unknown. An example would be a severe pneumococcal pneumonia that responded better to penicillin than did a milder case caused by the same bacteria. On the other hand, even severe pneumococcal pneumonia responds to penicillin, whereas colds (a milder but etiologically distinct disorder) do not.

Family data further contest the continuum hypothesis. If panic disorder (PD) were a severe form of generalized anxiety disorder (GAD), then one would expect GAD to be more common in relatives of PD patients than in relatives of normal controls. Family studies have found equal or less GAD in relatives of PD patients as compared to normals (26,31). Torgersen's (131) twin study indicated a genetic factor in PD but did not show greater concordance for monozygotic (MZ) vs dizygotic (DZ) twins for GAD and PD, as would be expected if GAD were a milder form.

The quantitative model also suggests that panic occurs following a buildup of generalized anxiety. However, in retrospective life history studies the great majority of panic patients report onset of generalized anxiety *after* rather than before onset of panic attacks (18,134). Uhde et al. (134) also reported a group of male panic patients who meet all disorder criteria except for generalized anxiety between attacks. Preliminary data from biological studies also support a distinction between panic and generalized anxiety (27,70,78,100,137; M. R. Liebowitz, *personal communication*).

A further question is the significance of proposed distinctions among types of panic with respect to the existence of and relationship to precipitants. The DSM-III definition of panic disorder requires panic attacks that are "not precipitated only by exposure to a circumscribed phobic stimulus." The draft DSM-III-R (6) requires unexpected panic attacks, which are defined as those "1) not occurring immediately before or upon exposure to a situation that almost always causes anxiety, and 2) not triggered by situations in which the individual was the focus of other's attention." Attacks precipitated by known organic factors are excluded in both documents.

Barlow (11) uses the term "cued" attacks to describe panic attacks triggered by a stimulus of which the subject may or may not be aware and has hypothesized that apparently unexpected attacks are actually "cued," but that the individual himself is unaware of the triggering event. However, his group (14) found some distinction in that uncued panics were significantly more frequently associated with symptoms of dizziness and fear of loss of control.

In the SADS-Lifetime Anxiety Version (SADS-LA) (44), our group has defined three categories of panic: spontaneous, situationally predisposed, and stimulus-bound. Spontaneous attacks are unexpected. Situationally predisposed is used to describe panic attacks that occur frequently, but not always, in particular situations. The occurrence of an attack in any particular instance remains unpredictable. Stimulus-bound attacks occur only in anticipation of or on exposure to a stimulus (phobic situation) that always causes anxiety for the individual.

Imipramine has been shown to block spontaneous and situationally predisposed attacks in panic and agoraphobic patients, but not stimulus-bound attacks of specific simple and social phobics (147). Data from our group (in agreement with Barlow) also support a phenomenological distinction between spontaneous and stimulus-bound panic. Agoraphobics with panic have significantly more severe and frequent feelings of faintness, dizziness, and fears of doom or dying during panic than do patients with specific phobias (A. J. Fyer et al., *unpublished data*).

The term panic attack is currently used to describe a variety of discrete episodes of intense anxiety. The data discussed here suggest the possibility of qualitative distinction between types of intense anxiety. Further research should clarify these distinctions and determine their significance for diagnosis and treatment.

Diagnostic Criteria for Panic Disorder

Panic disorder is defined in the DSM-III in terms of frequency of panic attacks over a specified period. The Feighner (40) and Research Diagnostic Criteria (118) require six panic attacks in a 6-week period. DSM-III (5) requires only three attacks in 3 weeks. Individuals with lower frequencies are given a diagnosis of generalized anxiety disorder or atypical anxiety disorder. However, recent findings suggest that even the DSM-III's lowered threshold may be inappropriately restrictive.

Torgersen (131) reported that inclusion of GAD patients

with a history of infrequent panic in the panic disorder group resulted in MZ twins having 5 times greater concordance for anxiety disorders with panic attacks than DZ twins. When these infrequent panickers were placed in GAD category, there was only a slight excess of MZ concordance for panic disorder. Norton et al. (99) found that untreated individuals with a lifetime history of occasional panic had similar panic attack symptomology, anxiety rating scale responses, and family histories of psychiatric illness to panic disorder patients. Pharmacologic treatment studies of "atypical" depression indicate that patients with a lifetime history of infrequent panic attacks have similar responses to those who have met the disorder frequency criteria (81). Both groups may differ from nonpanicking depressive patients.

In clinical settings one often sees individuals who do not meet current frequency criteria but in all other ways resemble "true" panic disorder patients (58,99,110). Barlow (14), however, found that the majority of 60 anxiety patients studied had had unexpected (spontaneous) panic attacks regardless of primary diagnosis. Only the frequency criterion prevented many patients with other primary anxiety disorder diagnoses (e.g., obsessive-compulsive disorder, GAD) from being given an additional panic disorder diagnosis.

The draft DSM-III-R has recommended a lowering of the panic frequency criterion so that a disorder diagnosis can be given if an individual has had (a) three attacks in a 3-week period or (b) three attacks in his or her lifetime, *and* "one or more of the attacks has been followed by a period of at least one month of persistent fear of having another attack" (6). The impact of this redefinition remains to be seen. It is conceivable that some patients have occasional true panics but do not develop persistent fear. The significance of panic attack frequency is an area for further investigation.

Subtypes of Panic Disorder

The working draft of the DSM-III-R (6) describes three subtypes of panic disorder, depending on the degree of secondary phobic anxiety and/or avoidance. Panic disorder without phobic avoidance includes patients with panic attacks and no avoidance. The existence of these patients has been documented by several research groups (11,134). Panic disorder with extensive phobic avoidance includes patients who were previously categorized under agoraphobia with panic attacks. Individuals who have some phobic anxiety and/or avoidance but do not meet criteria for the extensive category are given the residual label of panic disorder with limited phobic avoidance. Initial work with these categories indicates poor reliability for the distinction between limited and extensive avoidance. The current DSM-III-R committee recommendation is for two categories; panic disorder uncomplicated by phobic avoidance and panic disorder with agoraphobia (PDA). PDA is graded mild, moderate, or severe according to the degree of phobic avoidance (or endurance with intense anxiety) (R. L. Spitzer, *personal communication*).

Diagnostic Criteria for GAD

GAD is the residual anxiety category in DSM-III. GAD was created to provide for patients who had significant pathological anxiety but not other specific symptoms (i.e., panic, phobias, obsessions, or compulsions). The DSM-III criteria for GAD include 1 month of persistent anxiety, three anxiety symptoms, and exclusion of another psychiatric disorder as a cause. Empirical work in the past few years has led to considerable modification in the original criteria. Patients who met DSM-III GAD appeared to be a heterogeneous group. Some had or continued to have panic but did not meet disorder criteria. In one comorbidity study, 80% of GAD patients had a coexisting anxiety disorder diagnosis (11). Confusion also arose as to how to classify other anxiety disorder patients who had significant generalized anxiety not related to their diagnosis (e.g., a man with a cat phobia who complained of constant excessive worry about his job and family, insomnia, muscle tension, and throat tightness, all of which were unrelated to actual or possible contact with the phobic situation, i.e., cats).

The draft DSM-III-R requires excessive or unrealistic worry about two or more life circumstances, six associated anxiety symptoms (from a list of 18), and a duration of at least 6 months. In addition GAD is no longer considered the anxiety residual category. Simultaneous diagnosis of both GAD and another anxiety disorder is made provided the focus of the generalized anxiety is unrelated to the other disorder (e.g., worry about panic attacks in panic disorder, contamination in obsessive-compulsive disorder). Simultaneous diagnosis of GAD and a psychotic disorder is prohibited if the anxiety disorder has occurred only in the presence of the psychotic disorder. Overlap of GAD and mood disorders is discussed in the section Relationship of Panic Disorder and GAD to Depression.

The original GAD 4-week duration criterion was chosen somewhat arbitrarily and overlaps with the criteria for adjustment reaction. Clinical research samples have normally included patients with longer duration (6 months to many years) (8,59,110). However, a recent study suggests that pure GAD is relatively transient and cases of long duration are rare. Breslau and Davis (19) found that the rate of DSM-III GAD decreased fivefold if duration criterion was increased from 1 month to 6 months. However, most individuals who had 6 months duration also met criteria for DSM-III major depression. In view of these data it may be premature to exclude individuals who are ill less than 6 months.

Validity of Panic Disorder and GAD

Findings of descriptive, biological, family, and genetic studies carried out in the last decade support the diagnostic validity of panic disorder. The small amount of existing longitudinal data is inconclusive as to the relationship between panic disorder, depression, and other anxiety disorders. Results of descriptive and biological studies indicate considerable heterogeneity in GAD as well as overlap with other disorders. A heritable contribution to etiology has not been found for GAD.

Family and twin studies. Family and twin data provide strong support for the diagnostic validity of panic disorder and its distinction from GAD (22,26,31). Consistent family patterns have not been found in GAD. The only applicable twin study does not indicate a hereditary contribution to GAD (131). This literature is reviewed in detail in Chapter 94, *this volume.*

Descriptive studies. Five comparative studies of descriptive aspects of panic disorder and GAD in clinical samples have been reported (8,13,58,110,132). Developmental differences were identified in two of three studies that addressed this issue. In Torgersen's sample (132) a history of chronic anxiety in childhood was significantly more frequent in panic disorder (132), whereas loss of a parent before age 16 was significantly more frequent in GAD. Raskin (110) found no diagnostic differences in childhood separations/losses. However, her panic patients had a significantly higher rate of environmental disruptions during childhood. Hoehn-Saric (58) found no childhood differences at all. Age of onset differentiated the two diagnoses in only one (8) of the three studies in which it was reported (8,58,110). Significantly more somatic autonomic symptoms were reported by PD than GAD patients in three studies (8,13,58).

These distinctions seem fairly robust, since they were found in spite of relatively small sample sizes and, in some cases, inclusion in GAD samples of patients with history of panic attacks or disorder.

Longitudinal studies. Very few follow-up or retrospective life history studies have been reported. Existing data indicate that the life history of panic patients frequently includes other symptomatology. Most frequent are other anxiety syndromes, depression, and alcohol abuse. Findings are suggestive but as yet inconclusive with respect to the relationship of panic to GAD and depression. Generalized anxiety occurred in most panic patients and usually followed onset of panic attacks. Depression was episodic and could occur before or after panic onset. In almost all cases, panic attacks preceded the onset of agoraphobia.

Cloninger et al. (26) conducted a 5-year prospective follow-up of anxiety patients. Of 32 patients who had follow-up diagnosis of panic disorder, 60% had panic disorder alone or with another disorder at original interview, 20% had another anxiety diagnosis, and the rest either depression or alcoholism.

Patients who received panic diagnoses at both occasions frequently gave a lifetime history of other anxiety symptoms: 84% had simple phobias, 78% social phobias, 16% had agoraphobia, and 22% mild obsessions and compulsions. All cases of agoraphobia and most obsessions and compulsions (5/7) followed the onset of panic attacks.

Uhde et al. (134) conducted a retrospective life history study of 38 patients with panic attacks. Eighty-four percent (32/38) had associated generalized anxiety and agoraphobia. Ninety-four percent of those who developed generalized anxiety and 97% of those who became agoraphobic did so after the onset of panic attacks. These investigators noted a small group of patients (6/38), all male, who met all DSM-III and RDC criteria except for that of "between panic nervousness." This group tended to have short episodes of stress-precipitated illness and no history of psychiatric treatment.

Breier et al. (18) conducted a retrospective life history study of 54 agoraphobia with panic and 6 panic disorder patients. Depression (70%), childhood separation disorder (18%), obsessive compulsive disorder (17%), and alcoholism (17%) were the most common additional diagnoses. Eighty percent of subjects at some time also met all except exclusion criteria for DSM-III GAD. Anticipatory anxiety (worry about panic) was distinguished from GAD. Ninety-three percent of subjects reported this symptom.

Agoraphobia followed onset of panic in 98% of cases. Approximately one-third (18/48) of GAD and depression (18/42) episodes occurred prior to or overlapping with onset of panic attacks. The remaining two-thirds followed and were temporally distinct from onset of panic disorder. In this sample, course of panic disorder, agoraphobia, generalized and anticipatory anxiety were chronic and unremitting. Mean episode duration in months was panic 85 ($\pm$13), agoraphobia 112 ($\pm$15), anticipatory anxiety 110 ($\pm$14), and GAD 77 ($\pm$15).

Relationship of Panic Disorder and GAD to Depression

The DSM-III excludes diagnosis of panic or generalized anxiety disorders in presence of major depressive disorder (MDD). This convention is contradicted by recent family study data. Leckman et al. (73) found that rates of anxiety disorders and depression were higher in relatives of probands who had MDD plus an anxiety disorder than in relatives of probands who had MDD only. This difference existed even if anxiety symptoms occurred only during an episode of MDD.

Further analyses indicated that the excess relative risk for MDD or anxiety disorder was accounted for by probands who had MDD and either panic disorder or GAD. Relatives of probands with MDD + PD had higher rates of MDD, PD, and GAD than relatives of normals and MDD only probands. Relatives of MDD + GAD probands had higher risks of only GAD and MDD. MDD + agoraphobia (AG) in the proband did not confer higher risk for PD, AG, or GAD in relatives than MDD only. However, this last finding cannot as yet be generalized, as (in contrast to most clinical samples) a large number of agoraphobics in this sample reported no panic attacks.

In accordance with these data, the draft DSM-III-R has modified the exclusion criteria for PD so that diagnosis of PD can be made even in the presence of MDD. Concurrent diagnosis of GAD and MDD can be made only if GAD has also occurred at times other than during a major depression (R. L. Spitzer, *personal communication*). This latter restriction is inconsistent with the data of Leckman et al. cited above. It was felt that since GAD symptoms (unlike panic attacks) are a usual part of MDD, a separate diagnosis of GAD was not merited unless the anxiety also occurred independently. In addition, since previous family and twin study data do not indicate that GAD is familial, the significance of excess GAD in the relatives of individuals who have both anxiety and depressive disorders is less clear than in the case of panic disorder.

Phobic Disorders

The DSM-III describes three phobic disorders: agoraphobia, social phobia, and simple phobia.

Agoraphobia

Agoraphobia has been well described in the literature for over 100 years. However, its classification remains controversial. Early case reports focused on avoidance behavior and placed agoraphobia in the category of phobic disorders. Learning and psychoanalytic theories adopted this approach. The observation that imipramine blocked spontaneous panics but had no immediate effect on anticipatory anxiety or avoidance in agoraphobics led to the conceptualization of agoraphobia as a complication of recurrent spontaneous panic (67). In this view, patients fear and/or avoid situations in which they are afraid they would not be able to function, escape, and/or get help if they had a panic attack. The DSM-III divides agoraphobia into two categories: agoraphobia with and without panic attacks.

Agoraphobia with panic attacks. Several studies indicate that the large majority of patients with agoraphobia with panic report panic attacks antecedent to the development of avoidant behavior and anticipatory anxiety (18,36,134). Patients with agoraphobia with panic are also indistinguishable from panic disorder patients with respect to age of onset, sex ratio, rates of MDD (130), sodium lactate vulnerability (77), and response of panic attacks to imipramine and phenelzine (113,147).

Preliminary family study results also confirm a relationship between the two diagnoses. Harris et al. (54) found significantly higher rates of panic disorder in first-degree relatives of panic disorder and agoraphobia with panic attack probands than in relatives of controls. However, though overall prevalence of anxiety disorder was equal, the two types of families were not indistinguishable. Panic disorder rates were higher in relatives of panic disorder probands than in relatives of agoraphobics. Agoraphobia was significantly more prevalent in relatives of agoraphobics than in relatives of normal controls. Relatives of panic disorder patients did not differ from those of normal controls with regard to agoraphobia. These data may indicate either a partial genetic overlay or difference in severity. However, sample size is small and firm conclusions must await replication.

In contrast, descriptive studies support a diagnostic distinction between agoraphobia with panic and specific phobic disorders (simple and social phobias) (7, 14, 69, 78, 87, 95, 148; A. J. Fyer et al., *unpublished data*).

Agoraphobia without panic attacks. Two out of three recent studies using DSM-III or RDC criteria found no incidence of agoraphobia without panic in clinic populations (18,36). The third reported that 20% of agoraphobics give no history of panic attacks (130). In contrast, the New Haven Epidemiological Catchment Area site (141,142) found the rate of agoraphobia with a lifetime absence of panic disorder ever was 2.9/100 as compared to 0.3/100 rate of agoraphobia with panic and 0.9/100 rate of panic without agoraphobia. Of the 144 individuals who had agoraphobia without panic disorder, 67 (47%) were found to have some panic-like symptoms which were below threshold for DSM-III panic disorder criteria (e.g., less than three in 3 weeks, or attacks only when confronted with phobic stimuli). One-third of the remaining 77 had MDD. Eliminating these groups left a population rate of "pure" agoraphobia without panic of 1/100.

One explanation for the discrepancy between the epidemiologic and clinical samples may be variation in interview methodology and definition of agoraphobia. Patient samples were diagnosed by clinicians using semistructured interview schedules and DSM-III criteria. Epidemiological catchment area (ECA) data were collected by lay interviewers using the DIS (111). The central feature of the DSM-III definition of agoraphobia is fear and consequent avoidance of places "from which escape might be difficult or help not available in case of sudden incapacitation." Avoidance and/or fear must be severe enough that one's life is progressively constricted. The Diagnosis Interview Schedule (DIS) definition of DSM-III agoraphobia has a slightly different focus and a lower threshold of severity. It requires unreasonable fear of only one of six possible agoraphobic situations (going out of the home, crowds, being alone, bridges, tunnels, or public transportation). The reason for the fear(s) is not addressed.

Therefore, the DIS definition can include individuals whose fears are *not* centered around availability of help or escape if suddenly incapacitated. The DIS severity criterion requires only that the subject has told a doctor or other professional about the phobia, taken medication for it, or found it to interfere "a lot" with his or her life.

Since the ECA data are based in part on retrospective life history, another explanation may be that some subjects who deny a history of panic attacks have forgotten infrequent panic or limited symptom attacks which occurred at the start of their illness. It is also possible that agoraphobics with panic are disproportionately overrepresented in clinic samples because of the added distress of panic attacks, though it seems unlikely that this would account for all of the observed difference.

In the draft DSM-III-R, agoraphobia without panic attacks was replaced by agoraphobia with limited symptom attacks. The data described above indicate that this change, though correct for many cases, may be premature. In the interest of a conservative approach to nosology, the current recommendation of the DSM-III-R committee is reestablishment of the more general agoraphobia without a history of panic attacks category, while awaiting clarification of the epidemiological data (R. L. Spitzer, *personal communication*).

Social Phobia

The core feature of social phobia is fear of humiliation or embarrassment while performing an activity observed by others. Anxiety is experienced on anticipation of or actual exposure to situations that involve doing things in front of other people. Social phobia was first described by Marks and Gelder (88) in 1966. The original definition included both performance anxiety (e.g., public speaking) and more diffuse social anxiety (e.g., dating, parties, casual social interaction). Patients with both discrete and pervasive illness were included in the category.

In contrast, the DSM-III states that "usually one fear only" is present. It has been suggested that patients with more pervasive illness be included under avoidant personality disorder (52). There are no comparative validity data concerning either social phobic patients with single vs multiple fears or the relationship of social phobia and avoidant personality disorder. Existing clinical studies indicate that multiple performance and/or diffuse social fears commonly occur (7,49,76,87). The draft DSM-III-R has adopted a conservative approach. Patients with single and multiple fears are included in social phobia. Diagnosis of avoidant personality and social phobia can be given simultaneously. Only individuals whose social phobic stimulus is related to obsessions or sexual dysfunction are excluded. Panic disorder patients often avoid social situations because they fear embarrassment were they to panic in front of others. An example would be a fear of visiting friends because the need to "flee" if a panic attack occurred might lead to abrupt awkward departures. An individual may also avoid performance situations because he is afraid if he has a panic attack while there, he will be embarrassed by his subsequent inability to function adequately.

Liebowitz (79) has suggested that patients with this history be classified as "secondary" social phobics. "Primary" social phobics fear only those situations in which they are observed by others. However, panic patients with secondary social phobia will fear any situation in which they might panic.

Whether panic patients with secondary social phobia are in any way more like social phobics than other panic patients is not known.

Validity studies of social phobia. There are very few validity data on social phobia. Two consecutive series are consistent with respect to clinical and demographic characteristics of these patients (7,87). On average as compared to agoraphobics, social phobia patients have an earlier and more gradual onset, are more often male, less often married, and have a more affluent socioeconomic background. Preliminary studies suggest that social phobic anxiety is not decreased by tricyclic antidepressants, but may respond well to monoamine oxidase (MAO) inhibitors or β-blockers (49,76).

Vulnerability to panic when given intravenous sodium lactate has also been demonstrated to be significantly less in social phobia patients than in those with panic disorder or agoraphobia with panic (78).

Social phobics as a group are also distinguished from simple phobics by age at onset, sex distribution, generalized anxiety, increased galvanic skin response fluctuation, and response to systematic desensitization (87). Data on direct pharmacologic comparisons of simple and social phobia patients are not available. Family studies of social phobia as compared to normals or other anxiety disorders have not been reported.

Simple Phobia

Simple phobia is the residual phobic disorder in DSM-III. It is defined as persistent irrational or excessive fear and/or avoidance of a particular object or situation that is not associated with agoraphobia, social phobia, or obsessive-compulsive disorder.

A second issue concerns the necessity of avoidance for the diagnosis. Certain individuals have persistent irrational fear(s) of a situation(s), but because of life circumstances (job security, a spouse or child's needs), they will expose themselves to it. The draft DSM-III-R allows the diagnosis in such cases, provided the individual reports persistent discomfort (endurance with intense anxiety) when exposed to the phobic stimulus.

A related unresolved issue is the threshold for a "case" of simple phobia. Here a conflict of interest may exist between clinicians and researchers. The clinician hopes to identify individuals who require treatment. The researcher tries to establish criteria which best facilitate etiological investigation. The draft DSM-III-R simple phobia diagnosis requires "fear or avoidant behavior (that) causes marked distress or interferes with social or occupational functioning."

Twin and family data suggest that what is transmitted (if anything) in simple phobias is a proneness to irrational fear of certain situations rather than impairment or avoidance (21,22). Diagnostic criteria that include impairment and avoidance may obscure findings if used to identify cases in genetic studies.

Most simple phobics experience intense anxiety when forced to confront the phobic object. The physiological relationship of this intense anxiety (stimulus-bound panic) to spontaneous or situationally predisposed panic attacks and "normal" fear is not known.

Subtypes of simple phobia. There are several lines of evidence suggesting heterogeneity within the group of simple phobics. However, at present there are insufficient data to establish any one subtype as a separate diagnosis. The most clearly differentiated group are blood-injury-needle phobics. Marks first noted the association between fainting and this type of phobia (87). Several recent case reports document bradycardia, hypotension and vasovagal fainting in this group (29,32,103). Patients appeared to respond to behavioral treatment as do other simple phobics. Further controlled studies are necessary before separating this group from the remainder of simple phobics.

Animal phobias appear to have a uniformly early age of onset and chronic course (1,87). Neither is true for other types of simple phobias (e.g., fears of storms, driving, heights, etc.). Marks and Gelder considered animal phobias a separate diagnostic group (88).

Studies of onset of simple phobias also indicate diversity. Trauma related to phobic object, parental teaching or modeling, and stressful life events have been causative agents in varying numbers of cases. A considerable number of individuals also report no known precipitant (102,116).

Validity studies of simple phobia. Preliminary results from the Epidemiological Catchment Area studies indicate that simple phobia is one of the most common psychiatric disorders in the population (112). In contrast, these patients comprise only a small fraction of anxiety disorders seen in clinical settings (11). Perhaps for this reason, relatively few systematic validity studies have been conducted.

Simple phobias are distinguished from agoraphobia by

clinical psychopathology, lower spontaneous GSR fluctuation (69), greater improvement with desensitization (95), and nonresponse to imipramine (147). Marks also found that one type of simple phobia, i.e., animal phobias, had an earlier age of onset and lower overt anxiety levels than agoraphobia or social phobia (87). There are fewer data concerning the relationship of simple and social phobias. Marks (87) reported a higher female/male ratio among simple than among social phobics. There are no drug treatment, follow-up, or family studies comparing simple and social phobias.

Obsessive-Compulsive Disorder

The definition of obsessive-compulsive disorder (OCD) has been the most stable among the anxiety disorder diagnoses. However, recent research has provoked new questions and reraised old ones.

The DSM-III requires that obsessions and compulsions are regarded by the patient as senseless and are resisted or ignored whenever possible. Stern and Cobb (122) in a study of 45 obsessive-compulsives found that 46% of patients reported little or no resistance to their rituals at the time of assessment. Similarly, Rachman and Hodgson (108) reported that only 14% of 83 subjects resisted rituals all the time. Walker (139) also found resistance in less than 100% of patients. Reflecting these findings, the draft DSM-III-R eliminates resistance from the definition of compulsions. Initial resistance to obsessions or neutralization of them with some other thought or object is retained.

Though necessary for clinical purposes, the use of an impairment criterion may obscure significant findings in a research setting. Carey and Gottesman (22) found an 88% concordance rate for obsessive-compulsive features in MZ twins as compared to 47% for DZ twins. The term features was used to describe symptoms that met DSM-III criteria except that they did not "interfere with social or role function and were not a significant source of distress." Concordance rates based only on symptoms that met disorder criteria were not significantly different for MZ and DZ pairs.

A further issue concerning definition is raised by recent ECA findings. Lifetime population rates of OCD were found to be between 2 and 3% (112). This is strikingly higher than suggested by the less than 1% rates seen in clinical populations. The differences between treated and untreated cases remain to be studied. However, it is possible that results will significantly alter current definitions of the disorder.

Relationship of OCD to Anxiety and Depressive Disorders

Insel (63) and others have argued that OCD would be more appropriately classified with the affective disorders or in its own category than with anxiety disorders. One type of OCD patient, those with primary obsessional slowness, frequently do not report anxiety either in normal course or when prevented from carrying out rituals (63,105). In addition many other obsessive-compulsive patients do not report anxiety or nervousness as a major complaint. Instead self-criticism for wasteful and senseless behavior, decreased function, and depression are the common presenting complaints.

Lifetime history of major depressive disorder has been reported as high as 50% in patients with OCD (47,143). Obsessional symptoms are common in depressive disorders. Even when not depressed, OCD patients exhibit other common affective symptoms, including low self-esteem, guilt, and indecisiveness. However, the two disorders have different ages of onset and sex incidence ratios.

OCD patients have similar shortened rapid eye movement (REM) latency (62) and blunted growth hormone response to clonidine (115) to those seen in depressed samples. However, these findings remain to be replicated.

Data from clomiprimine (CMI) treatment studies are controversial concerning the relationship between OCD and depression. Two of the four reported studies (109,129) have found no relationship between pretreatment depressive symptomatology and effect of CMI on obsessions and compulsions. Two others (90,93) reported that high pretreatment depression was correlated with good response of OCD symptoms to CMI. Additional support for etiologic distinction between OCD and affective disorder comes from two studies correlating CMI metabolite blood levels with changes in OCD and depressive symptomatology (123,128). These data suggest the existence of different mechanisms responsible for CMI's antidepressant and antiobsessive-compulsive effects.

An interesting link between OCD and depression is suggested by the work of Rachman's group. Comparing nonclinical subjects and OCD patients, these investigators (125) found that most normals had obsessional thoughts similar in form and content to those experienced by patients. Abnormal obsessions were more difficult to dismiss as well as being more strongly resisted, more frequent, and more vivid. However, when dysphoric mood was induced in nonclinical subjects, it took them longer to dismiss intrusive thoughts than when euthymic or euphoric.

Controversy exists as to the relationship between OCD and other anxiety disorders. OCD patients frequently report anxiety with onset of obsessions, contact with contaminants, or prevention of rituals. Foa (42,43) and Mavissakalian (92) have noted that avoidance of "contaminants" has a similar function to social phobic avoidance of parties or the agoraphobic's avoidance of crowded stores. In the patient's eye, it prevents the onslaught of anxiety. However, Insel (63) has pointed out that in contrast to phobics, OCD patients remain perpetually uncertain as to the efficacy of their avoidance.

Approach to stimuli that evoke rituals has also been shown to produce similar physiological response (increased heart rate and skin conductance) to that seen when phobics are confronted with phobic object (65). Obsessional symptoms are frequently reported in patients with other anxiety disorders (26,62). Investigators have differed as to the extent these are complications of OCD or representative of additional anxiety disorder (63).

Another area of interest is the relationship between OCD and tic disorders suggested by recent family study data (100a).

Subtypes of Obsessive-Compulsive Disorder

Several attempts to subdivide OCD patients have been made. Lewis (74) suggested a division between obsessional patients and those with compulsive urges and rituals. However, studies suggest that in clinical populations most patients have both types of symptoms (63,106,108,143). Roughly 25% of patients have obsessions only, and very few (5 to 6%) have only compulsions.

Barlow and Beck (12) found that behavioral therapy produced more favorable outcome in subjects with both obsessions and compulsions than in those with only obsessions. In contrast, two follow-up studies have found the absence of compulsions to be a favorable prognostic sign (2,83).

Content of obsessions and compulsions has also been used as a basis for subtyping. Three series have found washers or cleaners (i.e., individuals who ritually wash or clean to prevent contamination) to make up 50% of the clinical population (63,108,122). Checkers (individuals who obsessionally doubt and repeatedly check to ward off the doubt) were the next most frequent group. Insel (63) and Rachman and Hodgson (108) found that among washers females greatly exceeded males, whereas there were equal numbers of men and women in other subgroups. Rachman and Hodgson also found that most cleaners had a sudden onset (24/32), whereas among checkers a gradual onset was the rule (21/29).

Primary obsessional slowness was also reported in a minority of patients in all three series. This subtype of OCD is characterized by exceedingly slow ritualized carrying out of activities of daily living (e.g., washing, dressing, showering). Typically, rituals are not associated with anxiety.

Posttraumatic Stress Disorder

The concept of PTSD has face validity, but there are few controlled studies that address the empirical validity of the diagnosis and even fewer that specifically test the DSM-III criteria. There remains considerable controversy about the definition of this disorder.

The DSM-III requires that the precipitating event in PTSD be "outside of range of usual human experience." This criterion is retained in the draft DSM-III-R. There is evidence that a PTSD-like syndrome can occur following more usual life traumas (e.g., bereavement) (61). However, further studies characterizing the types of usual stress that can precipitate a PTSD-like syndrome and the syndrome itself are needed before criterion alteration is merited.

Several subtypes of PTSD—acute (onset within 6 months of trauma, duration up to 6 months), delayed (onset at least 6 months after trauma), and chronic (duration of symptoms more than 6 months)—are described in DSM-III. The deletion of the delayed subtype has been suggested, since (a) difficulties often arise in ascertaining whether delayed onset symptoms are truly attributable to the original stress, and (b) minor symptoms often occur between the trauma and diagnosis of delayed onset PTSD (i.e., onset is not *really* delayed (135).

Numerous case reports of delayed onset have appeared in the literature (10,51). Systematic clinical and epidemiologic data are not yet reported. The draft DSM-III-R has eliminated the subtyping of PTSD. The revised diagnostic criteria for PTSD do not require that symptoms begin within any prescribed period following the trauma. However, in the case that delayed onset occurs (more than 6 months after the trauma), it is specified as part of the diagnosis.

Validity Studies of PTSD

Two studies have reported a high prevalence (75–84%) of concurrent psychiatric diagnoses in PTSD patients (51,114). The most common disorders found were depression, other anxiety disorders, and alcohol or substance abuse. A third retrospective life history study found a similar pattern (33).

Preliminary results of the one reported family study of PTSD showed patterns of prevalence of psychiatric disorder in first-degree relatives to be more similar to those of GAD patients than to those of depressive patients (33). Alcohol and drug abuse (60%), depression (20%), generalized anxiety disorders (14%), and antisocial personality (11%) were most commonly found.

Using an experimental approach, Blanchard et al. (16) reported that heart rate response to audiotape of combat sounds successfully differentiated normals from PTSD patients in 95.5% of cases. Systolic blood pressure and forehead electromyographic response also differed between groups.

Reliability of Diagnosis of Anxiety Disorders

Though operationalized diagnostic criteria were introduced during the 1970s, reliability of anxiety disorder diagnosis was inconsistent until the last several years. The major factors contributing to this were probably (a) lack of structured interview schedules that included items applicable to anxiety disorder criteria; (b) the small numbers of anxiety patients included in most samples; (c) lack of rater familiarity with anxiety patients; and (d) difficulty discriminating between anxiety and depression.

The recent revival of interest in anxiety disorder research has led to development of several new interview schedules which include items providing DSM-III and/or RDC anxiety disorder diagnoses. These instruments are the Diagnosis Interview Schedule (DIS) (111), the Anxiety Disorders Interview Schedule (ADIS) (36), the Structured Clinical Interview for DSM-III (SCID) (119), and the Schedule for Affective Disorders and Schizophrenia—Lifetime Anxiety Version (SADS-LA) (44). Use of these schedules has greatly improved reliability.

In this section we will briefly describe the new anxiety interview schedules and review current reliability data.

Diagnostic Interview Schedule

The DIS (111) was developed for use in the Epidemiological Catchment Area studies. It is a completely structured interview schedule designed to be administered by lay interviewers. The DIS provides focused psychiatric diagnostic evaluation in 45 to 60 min. Computerized diagnostic output from the DIS is available using RDC, Feighner, and DSM-III criteria. Since it is a completely structured schedule, the DIS does not allow for clinician input. If a subject misinterprets a question, there is little or no leeway for connection. The specific questions and structure are much more crucial than in semistructured clinician-administered schedules.

Robins et al. (111) compared lay-interviewer DIS diagnosis to diagnosis by a psychiatrist who used the DIS followed by an open clinical question session. Kappas for agreement between lay interviewer and psychiatrist on DSM-III anxiety disorders in a clinic patient population were panic disorder .40, agoraphobia .67, simple phobia .47, and obsessive-compulsive disorder .60. GAD and PTSD were not included. Helzer et al. (56) reported kappas and Y statistic (coefficient of colligation) (146) for a similar comparison using subjects from a general population sample. Low base rates alone can lead to low kappa values regardless of level of reliability (20,28). The Y statistic is less sensitive to base rates and therefore useful in general population samples where cases may be rare events. Unweighted kappas and Y statistic agreement between lay and psychiatrist diagnosis of DSM-III anxiety disorders were as follows (kappas listed first followed by Y in parentheses): agoraphobia .46 (.63), social phobia .40 (.61), simple phobia .31 (.46), panic disorder .42 (.63), and OCD .12 (.40). Two significant systematic biases were noted. Lay interviewers overdiagnosed OCD and underdiagnosed major depression.

In a third study, Anthony et al. (9) from the Baltimore ECA site compared DIS lay interviewer diagnoses to psychiatrist DSM-III diagnosis in clinical interview. Kappas for the three anxiety disorders included were phobic disorders .24, panic disorder −.02, and OCD .05. Factors cited as contributing to diagnostic disagreement were incomplete criteria coverage, overinclusive questions in DIS, unclear criteria for past vs current disorder, insufficient information, and the heavy reliance of the DIS on symptom report (as compared to clinician judgment about symptom report).

The kappa values cited in the DIS studies are lower than those reported below by investigators using the ADIS and SADS-LA. However, the cases are not directly comparable. The DIS data are derived from test-retest studies of comparative diagnoses by two different types of interviewers and interviews (lay interviewer DIS vs clinician interview or clinician DIS + clinical questions). These answer the question of how closely lay interviewer DIS diagnosis approximates clinician diagnosis. Data for DIS lay interviewer vs lay interviewer comparisons are not available. The ADIS and SADS-LA data report formal test-retest reliability of two clinicians of similar expertise using the same instrument.

Additional discrepancies between DIS and clinical diagnosis may arise in part from the structured format of the DIS. A semistructured format allows the interviewer to probe for clarification if need arises. In contrast, structured format may lead to difficulty in making certain kinds of distinctions. For example, confusion may arise when psychiatric and lay uses of a term differ (e.g., panic attack vs severe anxiety or the definition of alcohol abuse). Another

source of error is the case in which a similar behavior pattern can result from one of several subjective causes (e.g., avoidance of social situations might be due to social phobic fears of humiliation or anhedonia and social withdrawal in depression).

Anxiety Diagnosis Interview Schedule

The ADIS (36) was developed by Barlow and colleagues at the Center for Anxiety and Stress (Albany, NY). It is a semistructured clinician-administered interview schedule that provides current DSM-III anxiety diagnoses as well as clinical history of presenting problem, detailed information about structural and cognitive influences on anxiety, anxiety and depressive symptom description, and Hamilton Anxiety and Depression scale scores.

DiNardo et al. (36) reported initial results on reliability between two independent interviews (test-retest reliability) using the ADIS to evaluate 60 sequential subjects at an anxiety research clinic. Barlow recently reported on an augmented sample of 125 patients (11). Agreement was defined as exact agreement on primary diagnosis. Kappas for DSM-III anxiety diagnoses were as follows: panic disorder .65, agoraphobia with panic attacks .85, simple phobia .55, social phobia .90, OCD .82, and GAD .57. All except simple phobia and GAD are well within acceptable range. Disagreements about GAD involved decisions about its presence or absence in context of other anxiety disorders (e.g., When does general anxiety in a panic patient merit a separate GAD diagnosis?). This problem is addressed by the draft DSM-III-R revisions.

Difficulties in diagnosis of simple phobia were reported to concern decisions about degree of impairment that met case threshold. Too few PTSD patients were seen for stable kappas to be calculated.

Structured Clinical Interview for DSM-III

The SCID (119) provides current and lifetime DSM-III diagnoses periodically updated to conform to DSM-III revisions. It was developed to provide an instrument that fits easily into most clinical contexts but also gives reliable and accurate diagnosis. The SCID is clinician-administered and takes from 30 to 75 min, depending on the subject's degree of psychopathology. An important feature of the SCID is its initial overview section. The interviewer first allows the subject to present a full picture of the problem and its impact on his life before going into the structured interview. Age of onset and some descriptive material are included (e.g., treatment, types of phobic fears). Reliability studies of the SCID are currently ongoing.

Schedule for Affective Disorders and Schizophrenia— Lifetime Anxiety Version

Our group has developed the SADS-LA (44), which provides DSM-III, draft DSM-III-R, and RDC anxiety diagnoses as well as detailed assessment of lifetime anxiety symptoms and overall psychiatric evaluation.

The standard SADS Lifetime Version (SADS-L) (117) provides information about lifetime symptoms, including, if applicable, the current episode. The SADS-LA is a modification of the SADS-L and was designed specifically for use in studies requiring detailed lifetime information on anxiety disorders, symptoms, and traits.

In addition to the items included in the SADS-L, the SADS-LA includes (a) Items providing more detailed descriptive information about anxiety symptoms (e.g., panic attack response to different treatments, chronological development of symptoms in PTSD, quantitative assessment of obsessive-compulsive symptoms). An extensive section has been added on fears (e.g., fear of heights, public speaking, performing), their age at onset, treatment history, precipitants, course, severity, effect on behavior, etc. (b) Sections on anxiety symptoms that do not quite meet criteria for currently recognized symptoms or disorders (e.g., "near panic" attacks, avoidant tendencies, "near" Generalized Anxiety Disorder). (c) DSM-III and draft DSM-III-R criteria as well as RDC criteria for anxiety and affective disorders. (d) Sections on the following DSM-III disorders (which do not appear in RDC): Separation Anxiety Disorder, Tourette Syndrome, PTSD, and Adjustment Disorder with Anxious Mood. (e) Sections on the depressive subtypes, Major Depression with Melancholia and Atypical Depression (81). (f) A section on Demoralization secondary to an anxiety disorder.

In addition to the above supplemental items and sections, the SADS-LA also includes several procedural modifications which distinguish it from the SADS-L: (a) The appropriate hierarchies are used for the DSM-III and RDC diagnoses of anxiety and affective disorders. However, the form also provides for recording these syndromes *whenever present,* regardless of the rules of the diagnostic hierarchies. (b) A Life Chart of the history of psychiatric symptoms and disorders is prepared for each subject. The Life Chart is a visual representation of the subject's lifetime history of psychiatric disorders and symptoms. (c) A summary section including items on the overlap of disorders and symptoms is filled out by the rater at the end of the Anxiety Disorders Section. Though the SADS-LA was developed as a whole clinical interview, including assessment of anxiety disorders as well as any other psychiatric disorder, it is possible to extract the Anxiety Section and use it either (a) in conjunction with another semistructured interview, or (b) as a supplement to a general clinical psychiatric interview.

Results of initial expert test-retest reliability trials (i.e., two independent interviews) are shown in Table 1. Subjects were current and past patients at our anxiety and depression research clinics. In most cases, both interviews were done on the same day; however, several patients were reinterviewed as much as several weeks later. The kappa values, except for simple phobia, are well within the acceptable range and are similar to those obtained by Barlow's (11) group. In our case, low reliability of simple phobia was also due to disagreements as to what degree of impairment was needed to meet case threshold. Too few patients with PTSD, agoraphobia without panic, and GAD have been completed to allow calculation of stable kappas for these disorders.

TABLE 1. *SADS-LA test-retest reliability kappas[a]*

DSM-III Diagnosis	Rater 1 vs rater 2		Raters 1 or 2 vs 3	
	N[b]	Kappa[c]	N[b]	Kappa[c]
Panic disorder	8	1.00	7	.72
Agoraphobia with panic attacks	5	.84	10	.86
Simple phobia	2	.00	4	.15
Social phobia	3	.76	8	.87
Obsessive-compulsive disorder	2	1.00	3	1.00
Separation anxiety disorder	2	1.00	0	—

[a] Each column is the result of 15 pairs of interviews, i.e., 15 subjects each interviewed on two separate occasions.
[b] N = Total number of cases diagnosed by *either* rater.
[c] Each column of kappas reflects 30 *different* subjects.

PSYCHOLOGICAL ASSESSMENT

Measures of anxiety vary widely in their format and coverage. Older methods tend to be quite general, whereas newer procedures focus on the more specific symptoms, syndromes, and associated features of anxiety disorders.

Self-monitoring procedures involve the ongoing recording of target behaviors or recording at preset or random intervals. Since events are recorded soon after they occur, forgetting and distorted recall are minimized (127). However, a major difficulty is that behavior is influenced by self-observation (98). These procedures primarily are employed to assess behavioral interventions, and are less frequently used in drug trials.

Self-rating questionnaires and checklists include general (71) and specific (86) fear inventories, measures of trait (38) and state anxiety (138), and scales of general psychopathology (34,35). Most of these instruments are brief and easily scored, and are thus well suited for some drug trials. However, they are not without shortcomings. Finney (41) has criticized self-report measures for their "transparency" and inclusion of "obvious items," which are easily faked. Many do not contain items descriptive of specific target behaviors. Also, the use of undefined scale points in certain instruments is susceptible to rater variance in interpretation. Even in the detection of pre- and posttreatment changes *within* subjects, ceiling, floor, and restricted range effects can camouflage real differences (as can the failure to cover symptoms of interest).

Clinical ratings are available in the form of brief, general scales (53,82,148) and in more comprehensive and focused semistructured interviews (36,37,44,111,119,144). Provided that clinicians receive adequate training, these instruments are less susceptible to errors of rater variance and interpretation. Also, semistructured schedules often provide diagnoses in one or more systems of classification. However, clinical rating instruments are often not used, since experienced personnel are needed for their administration and they usually require from 45 min to 3 hr to complete.

Behavioral measures tend to focus on the effects of anxiety on avoidance or performance, and are sometimes referred to as measures of "motoric anxiety" (15). The most frequently used procedures in this class, the behavioral avoidance tests (BATs), employ some measure of escape or avoidance (68,84,97). The main problems with BATs are the influence of demand characteristics (96) and the lack of transfer to nonexperimental, *in vivo* settings (75).

A number of *personality inventories* have been developed (23,39,55). Factor analytic studies of early measures have revealed general factors that correlate highly with several diverse scales (41). These studies raise the question of what is being measured (general maladjustment? emotionality?). In addition, the separation of anxiety and depression has been a perennial problem, with most studies showing a high association between the two dimensions. Factor analyses that have yielded independent factors for "anxiety" and depression typically have shown high loadings of phobic avoidance, rather than general anxiety, on the anxiety dimension (37). In their review of treatment studies of patients with Phobic Disorder, Agras and Jacob (1) found that personality inventories, compared to other measures, were least sensitive in discriminating treatment groups and in showing pre-post changes.

The development of rating scales in psychiatric research has followed a trend from the more general measures of overall severity and global symptomatology to the more specific. This tendency has paralleled changes in the U.S. classification system that also reflect increased specificity. The inclusion of diagnostic criteria and a multiaxial system in DSM-III and the splitting of Anxiety Neurosis (DSM-II) into Panic and Generalized Anxiety Disorders are examples.

The assessment of the features of currently recognized, specific anxiety disorders is reviewed in the following sections. Emphasis is on the most widely employed and most promising measures.

Phobic Disorders

Agoraphobia

The most frequently used self-rating scale for the assessment of agoraphobia is the Fear Questionnaire (89). The FQ is a 17-item scale that yields a "total phobia" score, three subscores (agoraphobia, blood-injury phobia, social phobia), a global phobic distress rating, and an "anxiety-depression" score.

Chambless et al. (25) criticized the FQ for including few items on agoraphobia and for not distinguishing between accompanied and unaccompanied avoidance. They developed the Mobility Inventory for Agoraphobia (MI), a 26-item self-rating questionnaire that does not have these limitations. The MI discriminated between patients with social phobia and agoraphobia. Also, in support of the value of separate measures of accompanied and unaccompanied avoidance: (a) only moderate correlations were found between these scores (.44 and .67 for two samples of patients with agoraphobia); (b) unaccompanied scores significantly exceeded accompanied scores on most items for patients, but not for normal controls (25).

Chambless and colleagues (24) also developed the Agoraphobic Cognitions Questionnaire to evaluate thoughts of negative consequences to anxiety and the Body Sensations Questionnaire to measure the severity of being frightened by autonomic arousal. Unlike other scales, these questionnaires provide information on the cognitive aspects of agoraphobia. Also, good internal consistency, test-retest reliability, concurrent and discriminant validity, and sensitivity to changes with treatment have been demonstrated for these measures (24).

Behavioral measures also are used frequently in the assessment of agoraphobia (101). Procedures such as the "structured walk" provide standardized measures which are comparable across subjects. However, only one dimension, distance, is represented. For many patients with agoraphobia, this dimension might not accurately reflect the severity of their condition.

Accurate representation and measurement are particularly important when the concepts, concordance and synchrony, are considered. Concordance refers to a high correlation between two or more areas of measurement (behavioral, cognitive, and physiological). Synchrony refers to high covariance of measures over time. It has been suggested that *de*synchrony during treatment and *dis*cordance following treatment predict relapse in patients with panic disorder (101). Adequate assessment in all response systems is needed to support or refute these findings.

Social Phobia

Among the most frequently used measures of social fears are the Social Avoidance and Distress Scale (140), the Fear of Negative Evaluation Scale (140), and the Willoughby Personality Schedule (79). Also, some general scales, such as the Fear Questionnaire (89) and the Hopkins Symptom Check List (35), include social phobia subscales.

Leary (72) has criticized most self-report measures for confounding social anxiousness with social avoidance. Some individuals are highly anxious in social situations yet show no avoidance. Others avoid social situations for reasons unrelated to anxiousness. Leary developed a social anxiousness scale that was specifically designed to measure self-reported distress. High internal consistency, test-retest reliability, and construct and criterion validity were demonstrated (72).

One criticism of Leary's scale is that the reason for the individual's subjective distress is not assessed. A person might become anxious in social situations because of fears associated with humiliation or embarrassment, because of fears of having a panic attack, or for some other reason. Few items in Leary's scale provide this information (e.g., "When I speak in front of the others, I worry about making a fool out of myself.").

Simple Phobia

Fear and avoidance of nearly every imaginable phobic stimulus have been studied (e.g., dogs, cats, spiders, blood, snakes, heights, elevators, needles, storms, escalators, rats, knives, and darkness). A review of the literature is beyond the scope of this article. The reader is referred to Sturgis and Scott (124), Taylor and Agras (126), and Agras and Jacob (1).

Leary's comments on social anxiety scales are also true for measures of simple phobias. It is important not to confound fear with avoidance, and vice versa. However, it is also important to assess both facets of phobic disorder.

Concluding Comment on Phobia Scales

The Marks-Sheehan Phobia Scale (MSPS) deserves special mention. The MSPS is one of several scales being used in the Cross-National Collaborative Panic Study sponsored by the Upjohn Company. It includes several items on miscellaneous phobias (e.g., fear of eating, drinking, or writing in public, feeling trapped or caught in closed spaces), an item on the furthest distance the subject can travel alone, and a global item (0–10) on degree of distress or impairment. Each situation is rated on a fear scale (0–10) and an avoidance scale (0–4).

The MSPS appears to provide a wealth of important information. Future investigations are needed to assess the psychometric characteristics and clinical utility of the instrument.

Obsessive-Compulsive Disorder

One of the most widely used scales to assess OCD symptoms and traits is the Leyton Obsessional Inventory (LOI) (30). However, despite its popularity and adequate psychometric properties, the LOI does not include items for horrific obsessions and handwashing compulsions.

The Maudsley Obsessional/Compulsive Inventory (MOC) (57) is a 30-item self-rating scale. It has good test-retest reliability and external validity, and is also sensitive to treatment effects (108). However, the MOC does not include obsessional ruminations.

Steketee and Foa (120) recently developed the Cues for Urges to Ritualize Inventory to assess internal and external cues and expected consequences, and the Thought Inventory to assess the specific consequences feared by the patient with OCD. Future investigations are needed to determine the psychometric properties and clinical sensitivity of these measures.

For most of these inventories, it is difficult to determine whether the patient is obsessional/compulsive, or has obsessions/compulsions. This is true even for instruments that purport to measure both symptoms and traits. For example, "symptom" items on the Sandler-Hazari Obsessionality Inventory (108) include "I dislike making hurried decisions," and "I often have to check up to see whether I have closed a door or switched off a light." Neither of these statements necessarily reflects the ego-alien nature of obsessions and compulsions.

Self-monitoring procedures and behavioral measures (107) are rarely used to study patients with OCD. Some recent studies (121) have used daily measures of time spent in rituals.

Posttraumatic Stress Disorder

Most investigators have used currently existing schedules to assess PTSD, or have modified existing measures, or have developed instruments patterned to their needs. For example, Malloy et al. (85) used the Fear Thermometer, a self-rating scale, to study PTSD in combat veterans. They also employed a behavioral avoidance measure in which subjects viewed neutral and combat videotapes, and pressed a stop button "if the scene becomes upsetting." Veronen and Kilpatrick (136) modified the Fear Survey Schedule to study PTSD in rape victims.

A neglected scale in the assessment of stress response syndromes is the Impact of Event Scale (IES) (60). The IES is a self-rating questionnaire in which items such as "My feelings about it were kind of numb," and "I stayed away from reminders of it" are rated on a frequency scale. With few exceptions (e.g., exaggerated startle response), symptoms of DSM-III PTSD are represented. High internal consistency, test-retest reliability, and sensitivity to clinical improvement have been demonstrated (60). Investigators in the field of rape, combat, and other trauma syndromes should consider using the IES. However, scales with content specific to the stress, the flashbacks, etc. are needed.

Panic Disorder

One instrument that was specifically designed to measure the severity of symptoms that typically occur during a panic attack is the Acute Panic Inventory (API). The API was originally developed at Hillside Hospital and later used (in modified form) in a series of studies at the New York State Psychiatric Institute. The inventory includes severity ratings (1–4) for 17 panic attack symptoms and 15 multiple-choice questions on the frequency, situational occurrence, and severity of panic attacks, spontaneous panic attacks, and derealization/depersonalization.

Liebowitz et al. (77) reported that the API differentiated panic disorder patients experiencing an acute, lactate-induced panic attack from panic disorder patients and normal control subjects who did not panic during infusion. These investigators also found that lactate-induced and naturally occurring attacks in patients with panic disorder were phenomenologically similar, as indexed by the API. Fyer et al. (*unpublished data*) reported that several items on the API discriminated between the panic attacks of patients with agoraphobia and specific phobias. Dillon et al. (35a) found that the API differentiated the panic attacks of patients with panic disorder from stress reactions in normal control subjects. These studies suggest that the API possesses high discriminant validity and is keenly sensitive to panic (versus other forms of) anxiety.

The Sheehan Panic Attack and Anticipatory Anxiety Scale (currently being used in the Upjohn Company Cross-National Collaborative Panic Study) includes items on panic attacks, minor (or limited symptom) attacks, and anticipatory anxiety. Panic attacks are defined as a sudden surge of intense discomfort or fear accompanied by at least three of 14 characteristic symptoms. In minor attacks, only one or two associated symptoms are experienced and subjective discomfort (dread or apprehension) may or may not be present. Spontaneous and situational panic attacks are rated separately. Items are included for coding the number (past week, past month), average duration (minutes), and average intensity (0–10) of panic and minor attacks, and episodes of anticipatory anxiety. Daily diaries are used (self-monitoring) to assure that accurate data are obtained.

Self-rating scales such as the SCL-90 (34) include items that presumably identify panic attacks (Item 72—"Spells of terror or panic"). Also, most semistructured interviews include a section on Panic Disorder. For example, the lifetime anxiety version of the Schedule for Affective Disorders and Schizophrenia (44) has an extensive section on panic attacks, their characteristics, frequency, and effect on functioning.

It is important to define precisely what is considered a "panic attack" for purposes of replication and comparability across studies. For example, the Mobility Index defines panic attack as "a high level of anxiety accompanied by strong body reactions with the temporary loss of the ability to plan, think, or reason and the intense desire to escape or flee the situation" (25). This definition does not entirely conform to official nomenclature; certain key aspects (e.g., sudden onset) are not included, whereas others (e.g., "loss of the ability to plan") are added. It is not known how these differences may cause inconsistent findings across studies.

Generalized Anxiety Disorder

DSM-III GAD is defined in terms of symptoms of motor tension (e.g., muscle aches), autonomic hyperactivity (e.g., palpitations), apprehensive expectation (e.g., rumination), and vigilance and scanning (e.g., hyperattentiveness resulting in distractability).

There are no standardized scales specifically designed to assess GAD, although scales of general psychopathology include most GAD symptoms. A major problem with using general scales to assess GAD is that differential diagnostic distinctions cannot be made. For example, were palpitations limited to panic attacks, or were they experienced intermittently, throughout the day? Did "spells of terror" occur spontaneously, or only when the patient was confronted with a phobic stimulus? Was distractability limited to periods of depression? In summary, general scales might prove useful as an index of severity of anxiety symptoms but should not be relied on as diagnostic measures.

The measurement of the symptoms of nonspecific anxiety (e.g., nonphobic, nonpanic, non-OCD) apart from depressive symptoms has always presented a problem. The lack of specificity of the symptoms may reflect a lack of specificity of the disorder, as noted in an earlier section.

CONCLUDING REMARK

During the last 5 years, several scales have been introduced to separate cognitive and behavioral aspects of mental disorders. Examples include Leary's (72) measure of social anxiousness in social phobia, Steketee and Foa's (120) Cues for Urges to Ritualize Inventory and Thought Inventory in OCD, and Chambless and co-workers' (24) Agoraphobic Cognitions Questionnaire and Body Sensations Questionnaire in agoraphobia.

This trend toward increasing specificity reflects progress in our understanding of mental disorders: From naturalistic observations of unfamiliar phenomena, to the design of controlled experiments to study these phenomena. From Anxiety Neurosis in DSM-III, to GAD plus three subtypes of PD proposed for DSM-III-R (6). From the global questions that are asked during the introduction of a mental status exam, to the more focused questions asked as the interview progresses. These are other examples of a general-to-specific trend. In each, advances in knowledge lead to increased specificity, which results in further advances in knowledge, and so on. Information obtained by reliable and valid assessment tools ultimately will benefit the patient by identifying the most appropriate treatment strategies.

ACKNOWLEDGMENTS

This work was supported in part by National Institute of Mental Health grants MH 34292 and MH 30906. The authors thank Peggy Ray for her editorial assistance.

REFERENCES

1. Agras, W. S., and Jacob, R. G. (1981): In: *Phobia: Psychological and Pharmacological Treatment*, edited by M. Mavissakalian and D. H. Barlow, pp. 35–62. Guilford Press, New York.
2. Akhtar, S., Wig, N. H., Pershod, D., and Verma, J. K. (1975): *Br. J. Psychiatry*, 127:342–348.
3. American Psychiatric Association, Committee on Nomenclature and Statistics (1952): *Diagnostic and Statistical Manual of Mental Disorders*. American Psychiatric Association, Washington, DC.
4. American Psychiatric Association, Committee on Nomenclature and Statistics (1968): *Diagnostic and Statistical Manual of Mental Disorders*, 2nd ed. American Psychiatric Association, Washington, DC.
5. American Psychiatric Association, Committee on Nomenclature and Statistics (1980): *Diagnostic and Statistical Manual of Mental Disorders*, 3rd ed. American Psychiatric Association, Washington, DC.
6. American Psychiatric Association, Work Group to Revise DSM-III (1985): *DSM-III-R in Development (10/5/85)*. American Psychiatric Association, Washington, DC.
7. Amies, P. L., Gelder, M. G., and Shaw, P. M. (1983): *Br. J. Psychiatry*, 142:174–179.
8. Anderson, D., Noyes, R., Jr., and Crowe, R. R. (1984): *Am. J. Psychiatry*, 142:572–575.
9. Anthony, J. C., Folstein, M., Romanoski, A. J., Von Korff, M. R., Nestadt, G. R., Chahal, R., Merchant, A., Brown, C. H., Shapiro, S., Kramer, M., and Gruenberg, E. M. (1985): *Arch. Gen. Psychiatry*, 42:667–675.
10. Atkinson, R. M., Henderson, R. G., Sparr, L. F., and Deale, S. (1982): *Am. J. Psychiatry*, 139:1118–1121.
11. Barlow, D. H. (1985): In: *Anxiety and the Anxiety Disorders*, edited by A. H. Tuma and J. D. Maser, pp. 479–500. Lawrence Erlbaum Associates, Hillsdale, NJ.
12. Barlow, D. H., and Beck, J. G. (1984): In: *Psychotherapy Research*, edited by J. B. Williams and R. L. Spitzer, pp. 19–69. Guilford Press, New York.
13. Barlow, D. H., Cohen, A. S., Waddell, M. T., Vermilyea, J., Klosko, J. S., Blanchard, E. B., and DiNardo, P. A. (1984): *Behav. Ther.*, 15:431–449.

14. Barlow, D. H., Vermilyea, J., Blanchard, E. B., Vermilyea, B., DiNardo, P. A., and Cerny, J. A. (1985): *J. Abnorm. Psychol.,* 94:320–328.
15. Bellack, A. S., and Lombardo, T. W. (1984): In: *Behavioral Theories and Treatment of Anxiety,* edited by S. M. Turner, pp. 51–90. Plenum Press, New York.
16. Blanchard, E. B., Kolb, L. C., Pallmeyer, T. P., and Gerardi, R. J. (1982): *Psychiatr. Q.,* 54:220–229.
17. Breier, A. W., Charney, D. S., and Heninger, G. R. (1985): *Am. J. Psychiatry,* 142:787–797.
18. Breier, A., Charney, D. S., and Heninger, G. R. (1986): *Arch. Gen. Psychiatry,* 43(11):1029–1036.
19. Breslau, N., and Davis, G. C. (1985): *Psychiatry Res.,* 15:231–238.
20. Carey, G., and Gottesman, I. I. (1978): *Arch. Gen. Psychiatry,* 35:1454–1459.
21. Carey, G., and Gottesman, I. I. (1981): In: *What Is a Case: The Problem of Definition in Psychiatric Community Surveys,* edited by J. K. Wing, P. Bebbington, and L. Robins, pp. 29–41. Grant McIntyre, London.
22. Carey, G., and Gottesman, I. I. (1981): In: *Anxiety: New Research and Changing Concepts,* edited by D. F. Klein and J. G. Rabkin, pp. 117–136. Raven Press, New York.
23. Cattell, R. B., Eber, H. W., and Tatsuoka, M. M. (1970): *Handbook for the Sixteen Personality Factor Questionnaire.* Institute for Personality and Ability Testing, Champaign, IL.
24. Chambless, D. L., Caputo, C. G., Bright, P., and Gallagher, R. (1984): *J. Consult. Clin. Psychol.,* 52:1090–1097.
25. Chambless, D. L., Caputo, C. G., Jasin, S. E., Gracely, E. J., and Williams, C. (1985): *Behav. Res. Ther.,* 23:35–44.
26. Cloninger, C. R., Martin, R. L., Clayton, P., and Guze S. B. (1981): In: *Anxiety: New Research and Changing Concepts,* edited by D. F. Klein and J. G. Rabkin, pp. 137–154. Raven Press, New York.
27. Cohen, A. S., Barlow, D. H., and Blanchard, E. B. (1985): *J. Abnorm. Psychol.,* 94:96–101.
28. Cohen, J. (1960): *Educ. Psychol. Measurement,* 20:37–46.
29. Connolly, J., Hallam, R. S., and Marks, I. M. (1976): *Behav. Ther.,* 7:8–13.
30. Cooper, J. (1970): *Psychol. Med.,* 1:48–64.
31. Crowe, R. R., Noyes, R., Jr., Pauls, D. L., and Slyman, D. (1983): *Arch. Gen. Psychiatry,* 40:1065–1069.
32. Curtis, G. C., and Thyer, B. A. (1983): *Am. J. Psychiatry,* 140:771.
33. Davidson, J., Swartz, M., Storck, M., Krishnan, R. R., and Hammett, E. (1985): *Am. J. Psychiatry,* 142:90–93.
34. Derogatis, L. R., Lipman, R. S., and Covi, L. (1973): *Psychopharmacol. Bull.,* 9:13–28.
35. Derogatis, L. R., Lipman, R. S., Rickels, K., Uhlenhuth, E. H., and Covi, L. (1974): In: *Psychological Measurements in Psychopharmacology,* edited by P. Pichot and R. Olivier-Martin, pp. 79–110. S. Karger, New York.
35a.Dillon, D. J., Gorman, J. M., Liebowitz, M. R., Feyer, A. J., and Klein, D. F. (1987): *Psychiatry Research (in press).*
36. DiNardo, P. A., O'Brien, G. T., Barlow, D. H., Waddell, M. T., and Blanchard, E. B. (1983): *Arch. Gen. Psychiatry,* 40:1070–1074.
37. Endicott, J., Spitzer, R. L., and Fleiss, J. L. (1975): *Compr. Psychiatry,* 16:285–301.
38. Endler, N. S., and Okada, M. (1975): *J. Consult. Clin. Psychol.,* 43:319–329.
39. Eysenck, H. J., and Eysenck, S. B. G. (1975): *Manual of the Eysenck Personality Questionnaire.* Hodder and Stoughton, London.
40. Feighner, J. P., Robins, E., Guze, S. B., Woodruff, R. A., Jr., Winokur, G., and Munoz, R. (1972): *Arch. Gen. Psychiatry,* 26:57–63.
41. Finney, J. C. (1985): In: *Anxiety and the Anxiety Disorders,* edited by A. H. Tuma and J. D. Maser, pp. 645–673. Lawrence Erlbaum Associates, Hillsdale, NJ.
42. Foa, E. B., and Kozak, M. J. (1985): In: *Anxiety and the Anxiety Disorders,* edited by A. H. Tuma and J. D. Maser, pp. 421–452. Lawrence Erlbaum Associates, Hillsdale, NJ.
43. Foa, E. B., Steketee, G., and Young, M. C. (1984): *Clin. Psychol. Rev.,* 4:431–457.

44. Fyer, A. J., Endicott, J., Mannuzza, S., and Klein, D. F. (1985): *Schedule for Affective Disorders and Schizophrenia—Lifetime Version* (modified for the Study of Anxiety Disorders). Anxiety Disorders Clinic, New York State Psychiatric Institute, New York.
45. Gittelman, R., and Klein, D. F. (1984): *Psychopathology,* 17(Suppl. 1):56–65.
46. Gittelson, N. (1966): *Br. J. Psychiatry,* 112:705–708.
47. Goodwin, D., Guze, S., and Robins, E. (1969): *Arch. Gen. Psychiatry,* 20:182–187.
48. Gorman, J. M., Levy, G. F., Liebowitz, M. R., McGrath, P., Appleby, I., Dillon, D. J., Davies, S. O., and Klein, D. F. (1983): *Arch. Gen. Psychiatry,* 40:1079–1082.
49. Gorman, J. M., Liebowitz, M. R., Fyer, A. J., Campeas, R., and Klein, C. F. (1985): *J. Clin. Psychopharmacol.* 5:298–301.
50. Gorman, J. M., Liebowitz, M. R., Fyer, A. J., Dillon, D., Davies, S. O., Stein, J., and Klein, D. F. (1985): *Am. J. Psychiatry,* 142:864–866.
51. Green, B. L., Lindy, J. D., and Grace, M. C. (1985): *J. Nerv. Ment. Dis.,* 173:406–411.
52. Greenberg, D., and Stravynski, A. (1983): *Br. J. Psychiatry,* 143:526.
53. Hamilton, M. (1959): *Br. J. Med. Psychol.,* 32:50–55.
54. Harris, E. L., Noyes, R., and Crowe, R. R. (1983): *Arch. Gen. Psychiatry,* 40:1065–1069.
55. Hathaway, S. R., and McKinley, J. C. (1942): *The Minnesota Multiphasic Personality Schedule.* University of Minnesota Press, Minneapolis.
56. Helzer, J. E., Robins, L. N., McEvoy, L. T., Spitznagel, E. L., Stoltzman, R. K., Farmer, A., and Brockington, I. F. (1985): *Arch. Gen. Psychiatry,* 42:657–666.
57. Hodgson, R. J., and Rachman, S. (1977): *Behav. Res. Ther.,* 15:389–395.
58. Hoehn-Saric, R. (1982): *Psychopharm. Bull.,* 18:104–108.
59. Hoehn-Saric, R., and McLeod, D. R. (1985): *Psychiatr. Clin. North Am.,* 8:73–88.
60. Horowitz, M., Wilner, N., and Alvarez, W. (1979): *Psychosom. Med.,* 41:209–218.
61. Horowitz, M. J., Wilner, N., Kaltreider, N., and Alvarez, M. A. (1980): *Arch. Gen. Psychiatry,* 37:85–92.
62. Insel, T. R., Gillin, J. C., Moore, A., Mendelson, W. B., Loewenstein, R. J., and Murphy, D. L. (1982): *Arch. Gen. Psychiatry,* 39:1372–1377.
63. Insel, T. R., Zahn, T., and Murphy, D. L. (1985): In: *Anxiety and the Anxiety Disorders,* edited by A. H. Tuma and J. D. Maser, pp. 577–590. Lawrence Erlbaum Associates, Hillsdale, NJ.
64. Jablensky, A. (1985): In: *Anxiety and the Anxiety Disorders,* edited by A. H. Tuma and J. D. Maser, pp. 735–758. Lawrence Erlbaum Associates, Hillsdale, NJ.
65. Kelly, D. (1980): *Anxiety and Emotions: Physiological Basis and Treatment.* Charles C Thomas, Springfield, IL.
66. Klein, D. F. (1964): *Psychopharmacology,* 5:397–408.
67. Klein, D. F. (1981): In: *Anxiety: New Research and Changing Concepts,* edited by D. F. Klein and J. G. Rabkin, pp. 235–263. Raven Press, New York.
68. Kroll, H. W. (1975): *J. Behav. Ther. Exp. Psychiatry,* 6:325–326.
69. Lader, M. H. (1967): *J. Psychosom. Res.,* 11:271–281.
70. Lader, M. H., and Mathews, A. (1970): *J. Psychosom. Res.,* 14:377–382.
71. Lang, P. J., and Lazovik, A. D. (1963): *J. Abnorm. Soc. Psychol.,* 66:519–525.
72. Leary, M. R. (1983): *J. Pers. Assess.,* 47:66–75.
73. Leckman, J. R., Merikangas, K. R., Pauls, D. L., Prusoff, B. A., and Weissman, M. M. (1983): *Am. J. Psychiatry,* 140:880–882.
74. Lewis, A. J. (1936): *Proc. R. Soc. Med.,* 29:325–336.
75. Lick, J. R., and Unger, T. (1975): *J. Consult. Clin. Psychol.,* 43:864–866.
76. Liebowitz, M. R., Fyer, A. J., Gorman, A. J., Campeas, R., and Levin, A. (1986): *J. Clin. Psychopharmacol.,* 6:93–98.
77. Liebowitz, M. R., Fyer, A. J., Gorman, J. M., Dillon, D., Appleby, I. L., Levy, G., Anderson, S., Levitt, M., Palij, M., and Davies, S. O. (1984): *Arch. Gen. Psychiatry,* 41:764–770.
78. Liebowitz, M. R., Fyer, A. J., Gorman, J. M., Dillon, D., Davies, S., and Stein, J. M. (1985): *Am. J. Psychiatry,* 142:947–950.

79. Liebowitz, M. R., Gorman, J. M., Fyer, A. J., and Klein, D. F. (1985): *Arch. Gen. Psychiatry*, 42:729–736.
80. Liebowitz, M. R., Gorman, J. M., Fyer, A. J., Levitt, M., Dillon, D., Levy, G., Appleby, I. L., Anderson, S., Palij, M., and Davies, S. O. (1985): *Arch. Gen. Psychiatry*, 42:709–719.
81. Liebowitz, M. R., Quitkin, F. M., Stewart, J. W., McGrath, P. J., Harrison, W., Rabkin, J. G., Tricamo, E., Markowitz, J. S., and Klein, D. F. (1984): *J. Clin. Psychiatry*, 45(7 Pt.2):22–25.
82. Lipman, R. S. (1982): *Psychopharmacol. Bull.*, 18:69–77.
83. Lo, W. H. (1967): *Br. J. Psychiatry*, 113:823–832.
84. Mac, R., and Fazio, A. F. (1972): *Behav. Res. Ther.*, 10:283–285.
85. Malloy, P. F., Fairbank, J. A., and Keane, T. M. (1983): *J. Consult. Clin. Psychol.*, 51:488–494.
86. Mandler, G., and Sarason, S. B. (1952): A study of anxiety and learning. *J. Abnorm. Soc. Psychol.*, 47:166–173.
87. Marks, I. M. (1969): *Fears and Phobias*. Academic Press, New York.
88. Marks, I. M., and Gelder, M. G. (1966): *Am. J. Psychiatry*, 123:218–221.
89. Marks, I. M., and Mathews, A. M. (1979): *Behav. Res. Ther.*, 17:263–267.
90. Marks, I. M., Stern, R. S., Mawrson, D., Cobb, J., and McDonald, R. (1980): *Br. J. Psychiatry*, 136:1–25.
91. Mavissakalian, M. (1979): *J. Behav. Assess.*, 1:271–279.
92. Mavissakalian, M., and Barlow, D. H. (1981): In: *Phobia: Psychological and Pharmacological Treatment*, edited by M. Mavissakalian and D. H. Barlow, pp. 1–33. Guilford Press, New York.
93. Mavissakalian, M., and Michelson, L. (1983): *J. Nerv. Ment. Dis.*, 171:301–306.
94. Mellman, T. A., and Davis G. C. (1985): *J. Clin. Psychiatry*, 46:379–382.
95. Michelson, L., and Mavissakalian, M. (1983): *Behav. Res. Ther.*, 21:695–698.
96. Miller, B. V., and Bernstein, D. A. (1972): *J. Abnorm. Psychol.*, 80:206–210.
97. Miller, B. V., and Levis, D. J. (1971): *Behav. Res. Ther.*, 9:17–21.
98. Nelson, R. O., Lipinski, D. P., and Black, J. L. (1975): *Behav. Ther.*, 6:337–349.
99. Norton, G. R., Harrison, B., Hauch, J., and Rhodes, L. (1985): *J. Abnorm. Psychol.*, 94:216–221.
100. Noyes, R., Jr., Anderson, D. J., Clancy, J., Crowe, R. R., Slymen, D. J., Ghoneim, M. M., and Hinrichs, J. V. (1984): *Arch. Gen. Psychiatry*, 41:287–292.
100a. Pauls, D. L., Towbin, K. E., Leckman, J. F., Zahner, G. E. P., and Cohen, D. J. (1986): *Arch. Gen. Psychiatry*, 43:1180–1182.
101. O'Brien, G. T., and Barlow, D. H. (1984): In: *Behavioral Theories and Treatment of Anxiety*, edited by S. M. Turner, pp. 143–186. Plenum Press, New York.
102. Ost, L. G., and Hugdahl, K. (1981): *Behav. Res. Ther.*, 19:439–447.
103. Ost, L. G., Sterner, U., and Lindahl, I. L. (1984): *Behav. Res. Ther.*, 22:109–117.
104. Pitts, F. N., and McClure, J. N. (1967): *N. Engl. J. Med.*, 22:1329–1336.
105. Rachman, S. J. (1974): *Behav. Res. Ther.*, 11:463–471.
106. Rachman, S. J. (1985): In: *Obsessive-Compulsive Disorder: Psychological and Pharmacological Treatment*, edited by M. Mavissakalian, S. M. Turner, and L. Michelson, pp. 1–47. Plenum Press, New York.
107. Rachman, S., Cobb, J., Grey, S., MacDonald, B., Mawson, D., Sartory, G., and Stern, R. (1979): *Behav. Res. Ther.*, 17:467–478.
108. Rachman, S. J., and Hodgson, R. J. (1980): *Obsessions and Compulsions*. Prentice-Hall, Englewood Cliffs, NJ.
109. Rappaport, J., and Ismond, D. R. (1982): *J. Am. Acad. Child Psychiatry*, 21:543–548.
110. Raskin, M., Peeke, H. V. S., Dickman, W., and Pinsker, H. (1982): *Arch. Gen. Psychiatry*, 39:687–689.
111. Robins, L. N., Helzer, J. E., Croughen, J., and Ratcliff, K. S. (1981): *Arch. Gen. Psychiatry*, 38:381–389.
112. Robins, L. N., Helzer, J. E., Weissman, M. M., Orvaschel, H., Gruenberg, E., Burke, J. D., and Regier, D. A. (1984): *Arch. Gen. Psychiatry*, 41:949–958.

113. Sheehan, D. V., Ballenger, J., and Jacobsen, G. (1980): *Arch. Gen. Psychiatry*, 37:51–59.
114. Sierles, F. S., Chen, J.-J., McFarland, R. E., and Taylor, M. D. (1983): *Am. J. Psychiatry*, 140:1177–1179.
115. Siever, L. J., Insel, T. R., Jimerson, D. C., Lake, C. R., Udhe, T. W., Aloi, J., and Murphy, D. L. (1983): *Br. J. Psychiatry*, 142:184–187.
116. Snaith, R. P. (1968): *Br. J. Psychiatry*, 114:673–697.
117. Spitzer, R. L., and Endicott, J. (1979): *Schedule for Schizophrenic and Affective Disorders—Lifetime Version*, 3rd ed. Research Assessment and Training Unit, New York State Psychiatric Institute, New York.
118. Spitzer, R. L., Endicott, J., and Robins, E. (1978): *Arch. Gen. Psychiatry*, 35:773–782.
119. Spitzer, R. L., and Williams, J. B. W. (1985): *Structured Clinical Interview for DSM-III*. Biometrics Research Department, New York State Psychiatric Institute, New York, February.
120. Steketee, G., and Foa, E. B. (1985): In: *Clinical Handbook of Psychological Disorders*, edited by D. H. Barlow, pp. 69–144. Guilford Press, New York.
121. Steketee, G., Foa, E. B., and Grayson, J. B. (1982): *Arch. Gen. Psychiatry*, 39:1365–1371.
122. Stern, R. S., and Cobb, J. P. (1978): *Br. J. Psychiatry*, 132:233–239.
123. Stern, R. S., Marks, I. M., Mawson, D., and Lusconbe, D. K. (1980): *Br. J. Psychiatry*, 136:161–166.
124. Sturgis, E. T., and Scott, R. (1984): In: *Behavioral Theories and Treatment of Anxiety*, edited by S. M. Turner, pp. 91–141. Plenum Press, New York.
125. Sutherland, G., Newman, B., and Rachman, S. (1982): *Br. J. Med. Psychol.*, 55:127–128.
126. Taylor, C. B., and Agras, S. (1981): In: *Behavioral Assessment of Adult Disorders*, edited by D. H. Barlow, pp. 181–208. Guilford Press, New York.
127. Tellegen, A. (1985): In: *Anxiety and the Anxiety Disorders*, edited by A. H. Tuma and J. D. Maser, pp. 681–706. Lawrence Erlbaum Associates, Hillsdale, NJ.
128. Thoren, P., Asberg, M., Bertilsson, L., Mellstrom, B., Syogvista, F., and Trashman, L. (1980): *Arch. Gen. Psychiatry*, 37:1289–1294.
129. Thoren, P., Asberg, M., Cronholm, B., Jornested, L., and Trashman, L. (1980): *Arch. Gen. Psychiatry*, 37:1281–1285.
130. Thyer, B. A., Himle, J., Curtis, G. C., Cameron, O. G., and Nesse, R. M. (1985): *Compr. Psychiatry*, 26:208–214.
131. Torgersen, S. (1983): *Arch. Gen. Psychiatry*, 40:1085–1089.
132. Torgersen, S. (1986): *Arch. Gen. Psychiatry*, 143:630–632.
133. Tyrer, P. (1984): *Br. J. Psychiatry*, 144:78–83.
134. Uhde, T. W., Boulenger, J. P., Roye-Byrne, P. P., Geraci, M. F., Vittone, B. J., and Post, R. M. (1985): *Prog. Neuropsychopharmacol. Biol. Psychiatry*, 9:39–51.
135. Van Putten, T., and Yager, J. (1984): *Arch. Gen. Psychiatry*, 41:411–413.
136. Veronen, L. J., and Kilpatrick, D. G. (1980): *Behav. Modif.*, 4:383–396.
137. Waddell, M. G., Barlow, D. H., and O'Brien, G. T. (1984): *Behav. Res. Ther.*, 22:393–402.
138. Walk, R. D. (1956): *J. Abnorm. Soc. Psychol.*, 22:171–178.
139. Walker, V. J. (1973): *Br. J. Psychiatry*, 123:675–680.
140. Watson, D., and Friend, R. (1969): *J. Consult. Clin. Psychol.*, 33:448–457.
141. Weissman, M. M. (1985): In: *Anxiety and the Anxiety Disorders*, edited by A. H. Tuma and J. D. Maser, pp. 275–296. Lawrence Erlbaum Associates, Hillsdale, NJ.
142. Weissman, M. M., Leaf, P. J., Holzer, C. E., and Merikangas, K. R. (1985): *Psychopharmacol. Bull.*, 21:539–572.
143. Welner, A., Reich, T., Robins, I., Fishman, R., and Van Doren, T. (1976): *Compr. Psychiatry*, 17:527–539.
144. Wing, J. K., Cooper, J. E., and Sartorius, N. (1974): *Measurement and Classification of Psychiatric Symptoms*. Cambridge University Press, New York.
145. Wolpe, J. (1958): *Psychotherapy and Reciprocal Inhibition*. Stanford University Press, Stanford.
146. Yule, G. U. (1912): *J. R. Stat. Soc.*, 75:581–642.
147. Zitrin, C. M., Klein, D. F., Woerner, M. G., and Ross, D. C. (1983): *Arch. Gen. Psychiatry*, 40:125–138.
148. Zung, W. W. K. (1971): *Psychosomatics*, 12:371–378.

Psychopharmacology:
The Third Generation of Progress,
edited by Herbert Y. Meltzer.
Raven Press, New York © 1987.

CHAPTER **122**

Current Pharmacotherapy of Anxiety and Panic

Karl Rickels and Edward E. Schweizer

With the introduction of meprobamate in 1955 and subsequently the first benzodiazepines in the early 1960s, the pharmacotherapy of anxiety emerged from a half-century-long reliance on barbiturates and a much longer prehistory of self-medication with herbal preparations, opiates, bromides, and alcohol. Progress since then has been notable not just for specific advances in pharmacotherapy, but also for the way in which these advances, in turn, have altered our core ideas about the diagnosis and pathophysiology of anxiety and other mental disorders. In a sense, clinical psychopharmacology has become the improvisational laboratory of biological psychiatry, giving rise to diagnostic and etiologic insights for subsequent refinement and testing. The successful use of antidepressants for the treatment of certain anxiety disorders is an example. Beginning with Klein's 1964 observations on the effects of imipramine (54), the efficacy of antidepressants in subtypes of anxiety forced, somewhat grudgingly, a reconceptualization of the nosology of anxiety disorders (55). The benzodiazepine receptor hypothesis of anxiety (44) is another example of an etiologic theory derived from leads provided by pharmacotherapy.

In a more general sense, the advent of psychopharmacology is itself largely responsible for the emergence of the descriptive, operational nosology enshrined in the *Diagnostic and Statistical Manual of Mental Disorders,* 3rd edition (DSM-III). The introduction of new drugs required some demonstration of safety and efficacy. Quantification of improvement was difficult for patients suffering only from "intrapsychic conflict" or *"praecox gefuehl."* Various rating scales, such as the venerable Hamilton Depression and Anxiety scales, proved more useful. This empirical trend, represented by increasing reliance on objective symptom scales, resulted in wider and wider acceptance of operational definitions of psychiatric syndromes (51).

Our diagnostic conceptions of anxiety have been among the most profoundly altered by this change in the psychiatric *Weltanschauung.* We can now confidently assert that much pathological anxiety is inadequately explained by the concept of neurosis with its implication of intrapsychic conflict and threatening libidinal or aggressive drives. We can also be confident that anxiety has a neurobiologic substrate, and that this substrate can be decisively affected by anxiolytic drugs. (This is not to deny that other cognitive or behavioral techniques might also have an equal effect on the biologic substrate.) This chapter will highlight some of what is new in the increasingly heterogeneous field of anxiety pharmacotherapy. Due to considerations of space, the main emphasis will be on treatment of generalized anxiety (GAD) and panic (PD).

DIAGNOSIS AND PREVALENCE OF ANXIETY DISORDERS

An anxiety diagnosis is the most frequent psychiatric diagnosis made in America. A recently conducted National Institute of Mental Health (NIMH) Catchment Area Household Survey (129), which involved almost 10,000 persons, estimated that 8.3% of the adult U.S. population suffered from anxiety disorders during the past 6 months. The next most frequent diagnoses were alcohol and drug abuse (6.4%) and depression (6.0%), followed by schizophrenia (1.0%). These rates are in rough agreement with those obtained in an earlier 1979 National Household Survey conducted by Balter and associates (74,147), who found the following diagnostic frequencies for the past year: agoraphobia-panic disorder (1.2%), other phobic disorders (2.3%), generalized anxiety disorder (6.4%), and depressive disorders (5.1%). Lifetime prevalence of DSM-III anxiety diagnoses, including simple phobias and obsessive-compulsive disorder, but excluding transient and situational anxiety conditions, appears to be approximately 13 to 15%.

It is worth noting that alcoholism, the second most prevalent diagnosis, also appears to have significant comorbidity with anxiety. Structured interviews of alcoholics (148) have demonstrated premorbid anxiety disorders in more than 20%. Conversely, as many as 20 to 25% of such anxiety disorders as social phobia (3,137) have been found to be associated with alcohol dependence. In addition, the frequently reported association of alcoholism and affective illness seems, on genetic grounds, to stem in large measure from the previously unrecognized contribution of coexisting anxiety disorder (75).

Despite the prevalence and the often intense distress, disability, and unremitting nature of anxiety (82), adequate professional evaluation and treatment is the exception rather than the rule. Recent surveys (129) have found that fewer than one-quarter of patients suffering anxiety disorders received any professional evaluation or treatment for it. When they did, nonpsychiatric medical personnel often provided the treatments. Another survey (147) found that among patients categorized as GAD, only 27% were receiving antianxiety medication. This tends to confirm the suspicion that alcohol and other nonprescribed drugs may still be the mainstay of treatment for a dishearteningly large percentage of patients suffering with anxiety. Any discussion of the present or future direction of anxiety pharmacotherapy must take account of this gap between treatment theory and actual practice. Parenthetically, there is no evidence to suggest that these anxious patients had eschewed pharmacotherapy in favor of intensive attempts at symptom reduction through dynamic, behavioral, or cognitive treatments, as effective as these often are.

Since the last volume in this series appeared, the treatment of anxiety has begun to move beyond almost exclusive reliance on benzodiazepines, though they are still considered the pharmacologic treatment of choice for most anxiety conditions. The hue and cry in the past decade over benzodiazepine overuse and misuse (57) has served its purpose in awakening consumer and clinician alike to the physical dependence liability of these drugs. In retrospect, the alarm was perhaps overstated in that the self-reinforcing properties of benzodiazepines in humans are much less than they are for other drugs of abuse (45). Epidemiological confirmation of this has come from recent surveys (74,147) suggesting that patients prescribed benzodiazepines actually consume them much less frequently and at lower doses than had previously been thought.

Another change since the last volume is the increasing attention paid to the issue of careful differential diagnosis.

It is an article of faith in medicine that making a proper diagnosis carries with it implications, not only about general prognosis, but about choice of treatment. In the field of psychiatry we hope we are beyond the stage, though perhaps not by much, where we lob medication in the general direction of a patient's symptom cluster and hope we hit something. A good illustration of this evolving refinement in diagnosis is the subtyping of anxiety disorders that has taken place as DSM-III has supplanted DSM-I and DSM-II (142).

Starting with the all-inclusive heterogeneity of anxiety neurosis, phobic anxiety was initially split off in recognition of the differential responsiveness of this subset of the neurosis to behavioral interventions (flooding, in vivo exposure, etc.). The phobic subgroup was further subdivided when generalized phobic symptoms were found to require different treatments, and to have different histories, than simple phobias. The usefulness of antidepressants in another subgroup of anxiety neurotics, as was mentioned above, resulted in detachment of an agoraphobic-panic group. In this way, generalized anxiety disorder (GAD), as it is called today, has been successively restricted in its definition, to the point that it is much less common than before to see GAD "in pure culture."

If the proposed increase in the duration requirement for GAD from 1 to 6 months is included in the final version of DSM-III-R (140), it will further restrict GAD and will further reduce both its heterogeneity and its prevalence. Although current diagnostic trends appear to represent an advance in an understanding of anxiety disorders, we would question the elaboration of too many anxiety diagnosis subcategories, unless they can be validated by differential treatment response, and unless they help to better differentiate GAD from depression. The implications that diagnosis has for treatment, and vice versa, is an important current theme in anxiety research and clinical practice, but one that requires much more study.

TREATMENT OF GENERALIZED ANXIETY

Depending on its definition, anxiety is considered a normal emotion, a frequently fluctuating symptom, a syndrome, or a diagnostic illness. As a mild symptom, it may stimulate productive thinking, motivate entrepreneurial activity, and be the driving force behind many accomplishments. As a debilitating syndrome or illness, it may reduce a productive, intelligent person to an emotional wreck, unable to function adequately. Anxiety may be primary or secondary; acute, intermittent, or chronic; and mild, moderate, or severe. Anxiety can be operationally defined in terms of scores on a variety of rating scales, as well as according to various diagnostic schemata.

Nonpsychotic anxiety at the time of the DSM-II was mainly diagnosed as "anxiety neurosis," which also included "panic attacks" and which was often given the qualifier "with or without significant concomitant depression." Thus, for almost 20 years anxious patients in clinical studies included those suffering from generalized anxiety as well as those suffering from various degrees of panic disorders and often also dysthymic disorders. The following diagnostic categories respond favorably to anxiolytics: generalized anxiety disorder, atypical anxiety disorder, panic disorder, posttraumatic stress disorder, adjustment disorder with anxious mood, somatization disorder, and the many anxiety conditions not diagnosable by DSM-III because of either symptom severity or duration of illness restrictions (93,95).

Clinicians learned swiftly that anxiolytics were not nearly as effective in anxiety associated with schizophrenia or borderline personality, in agitation associated with chronic brain syndrome, and in the phobic or obsessive-compulsive disorders. Many social phobias, while frequently improving with behavior therapy or with imipramine and monoamine oxidase inhibitors (MAOIs), do, however, also respond at least to some degree to treatment with anxiolytics. Clinicians also have learned that symptoms of anxiety may frequently mimic physical disease, and it is therefore most important to rule out the large number of physical illnesses that can present with anxiety-like complaints before fully considering a diagnosis of an anxiety disorder (4). Psychiatric conditions other than anxiety may also masquerade as anxiety complaints, rendering diagnosis and treatment considerations more complicated.

Benzodiazepines

The efficacy of the benzodiazepines in the symptomatic treatment of nonpsychotic anxiety has been well established. Hundreds of studies, many of them conducted under stringent double-blind conditions, have consistently shown that the benzodiazepines produce significantly more improvement than placebo in many of the somatic and emotional manifestations of anxiety (33,58,91). In fact, comparing the clinical efficacy of the benzodiazepines with that of the barbiturates, meprobamate, and placebo, one finds again and again the same rank order of efficacy, with benzodiazepines producing the most and placebo the least amount of improvement (17,60,91). Yet not every patient, by far, improves with benzodiazepines, and moderate to marked improvement is obtained in only about 65 to 75% of those treated with benzodiazepines. In addition, as Rickels' research group demonstrated years ago, even patients reporting moderate improvement, representing about 40% of patients treated with benzodiazepines, do not nearly achieve their "normative" preanxious baseline (91). Recent reviews summarizing the current status of benzodiazepine treatment have been provided by Greenblatt, Shader, and Abernethy (35) and Beckmann and Haas (11).

Eight benzodiazepines are presently available in the United States as anxiolytics. Five of them have long half-lives and include chlordiazepoxide, the first benzodiazepine introduced into medicine; diazepam, the most frequently prescribed benzodiazepine; and clorazepate, prazepam, and halazepam, pharmacologically inactive prodrugs of the major active metabolite of diazepam, namely, desmethyldiazepam. The remaining three benzodiazepines have short to intermediately long half-lives. Two of them, oxazepam and lorazepam, have no active metabolites, and the recently introduced triazolo-benzodiazepine, alprazolam, has several active but clinically insignificant metabolites. In equipotent dosages, alprazolam appears to be less sedating than other benzodiazepines (2,21,105), and, most interestingly, it also has been reported to possess antidepressant properties (25,107).

No consistent data have ever been provided in the literature that benzodiazepines differ significantly from each other in general global anxiolytic efficacy. All benzodiazepine derivatives have similar pharmacological properties. They reduce anxiety and tension, cause sedation and sleep, and possess varying degrees of anticonvulsant and muscle relaxant properties. They also are helpful in depressive symptoms secondary to anxiety. The most common side effects arise from their central nervous system depressant effects. Sedative side effects are commonly seen in early phases of treatment and are usually dose-related. Interestingly, although some tolerance to the sedative effects of the benzodiazepines develops initially, this usually is not true for the anxiolytic effect (35,41,66). When such CNS effects as drowsiness, impairment of intellectual functioning, reduced motor coordination, and impairment of short-term memory and recall complicate treatment (46,72,152), these symptoms usually occur early in treatment and, similar to sedation, decrease or disappear with time because of adaptation or tolerance, or after dosage adjustment. Patients are therefore warned to exercise caution when driving or using heavy machinery should they feel drowsy.

As with any type of sedative drug, the addition of other sedating substances such as antihistamines, many of which are available over the counter, and particularly alcohol, may lead to increased sedation. Although the combination of alcohol in small quantities, i.e., one or two drinks, with a normal dose of benzodiazepines (e.g., 5–10 mg per day of diazepam) does not produce much of a problem, the overuse of either or both may produce serious consequences. In fact, benzodiazepines are extremely safe drugs, and unless combined with alcohol or other CNS depressant drugs taken in excessive dosages, BZ overdosing is not lethal (93). Benzodiazepines, just like other medications, although not associated with birth defect formation (120,136), should be used sparingly, if at all, during pregnancy, and particularly during the first trimester. Some of the literature related to toxicity and drug overuse has recently been reviewed (93).

Despite overall comparability, small but clinically relevant differences in benzodiazepine pharmacology do exist. The most lipophilic of the benzodiazepines, diazepam, for example, produces a more immediate effect than the more water-soluble benzodiazepine, oxazepam; and of two desmethyldiazepam prodrugs, clorazepate has a rather swift onset of action whereas prazepam does not. Thus, the pattern of absorption and distribution determines acute drug effects, whereas the pattern of elimination becomes important during chronic therapy.

Since oxazepam and lorazepam have no active metabolites but are directly glucuronized into inactive compounds, it is suggested that these drugs are preferable in the management of the elderly or persons with serious liver impairment (34,43). Yet long-acting benzodiazepines with active metabolites can also be used quite effectively in these indications by prescribing them in smaller than usual dosages and by increasing the time intervals between dosing. Thus, anxiety can be appropriately managed even in the elderly with both short- and long-half-life benzodiazepines (8).

The clinical significance of drug interactions between benzodiazepines with and without active metabolites and such medications as cimetidine, propranolol, and oral contraceptives is still far from established, as patients and physicians easily adjust treatment regimen to cope with increased or impaired drug clearance (1,13). Length of benzodiazepine plasma half-life may be relevant in determining the time course of return of symptoms after the benzodiazepine is abruptly discontinued (99). One may expect that the shorter the half-life, the sooner the original symptoms may return, and the longer the half-life, the longer it will take for the original symptoms to reappear (22,87). Half-life may also play a role in determining the incidence and intensity of rebound anxiety and/or withdrawal reactions when a benzodiazepine, prescribed in therapeutic doses, is stopped abruptly after months of therapy (26,145).

Finally, antidepressant properties other than those secondary to antianxiety effects have not generally been attributed to the benzodiazepines (122). In fact, alprazolam, a triazolo-benzodiazepine with an intermediately long half-life, has been the first benzodiazepine for which clear antidepressant properties have been demonstrated (25,107).

Predictors of Treatment Response

Research conducted over many years has shown that nonpsychotic anxious patients respond best to short-term anxiolytic therapy if they suffer from high levels of emotional and somatic symptoms of anxiety and from low levels of depression and interpersonal problems (90,106). Alprazolam may represent an exception to the above. One of the strongest and most significant predictors of benzodiazepine treatment outcome is initial response during the first week of therapy (24). In fact, if a patient does not respond within a few weeks, the physician would be wise to reassess his earlier diagnosis. He may have overlooked a depression or missed a personality problem. Finally, if a patient fails to improve and if a reassessment of the diagnosis confirms the original anxiety diagnosis, one may consider measuring benzodiazepine plasma levels. Plasma levels of benzodiazepines correlate strongly with daily dosage (99). Determination of benzodiazepine plasma levels may help the physician if compliance appears to be a problem. It may also help to identify the occasional fast or slow drug metabolizers (i.e., patients with excessive side effects on low dosages or unimproved patients with a lack of side effects on high daily dosages). Other predictors of positive response to anxiolytic therapy are no prior anxiolytic therapy or good response to such, expectations of receiving anxiolytic drugs, presence of precipitating stress, positive physician attitudes toward drug use, and physician empathy and emotional support (91).

Acute vs Chronic Benzodiazepine Therapy

Many anxious patients improve simply with the passage of time and/or with support provided by a variety of sources, not necessarily a psychiatrist. The addition of a benzodiazepine may, however, make even a short anxiety episode more bearable. Short-term therapy should be the rule rather than the exception when benzodiazepines are prescribed. Rickels et al. (100) have reported that 50% of chronically anxious patients treated for 6 weeks with diazepam remained symptom-free when blindly switched to 8 weeks of placebo. A similar level of maintained improvement was observed after only 4 weeks of benzodiazepine therapy in nonchronically anxious patients (95).

In those patients for whom prolonged therapy is considered advisable, it is important to be aware that maximum improvement with benzodiazepines is usually obtained within the first 6 weeks of treatment, and, as a rule, no significant additional improvement occurs after that time (98). One may speculate that state anxiety is more susceptible to anxiolytic drug therapy than trait anxiety. At the same time, tolerance to the anxiolytic effect of the benzodiazepine does not seem to be a significant problem even with long-term therapy (32,41,66,100,101).

Patients treated chronically with benzodiazepines should be regularly evaluated by a caring and understanding physician, kept on the lowest but not ineffective daily dosage, and provided enough emotional support so that they may at regular intervals attempt to get along without medication for limited or even extended periods of time. Such a treatment approach will prevent the development in most instances of physical dependence and will also assure that a patient does not continue on medication simply to counteract withdrawal experiences or even only mild symptoms of rebound anxiety. Since anxiety frequently waxes and wanes, p.r.n. dosing or intermittent use should be considered whenever possible. When patients are treated with any type of drug for prolonged periods of time, the benefit/risk ratio has to be assessed and should clearly favor treatment benefits.

A variety of nondrug therapies ranging from simple support to analytic psychotherapy should also be considered as treatment options by patient and physician, either alone or in combination with benzodiazepine therapy (7).

The fact that relapse rates in chronically anxious patients were found at 1-year follow-up to range from 69% (102) to 80% (97) still does *not* support the use of uninterrupted, continuous benzodiazepine therapy for these patients, but it does stress the need many chronically anxious patients have for prolonged, albeit, if possible, intermittent therapy, i.e., each therapy lasting only a few weeks, to be interrupted by months or at least weeks without therapy. In general, patients suffering from panic disorder may need longer benzodiazepine therapy than patients suffering from GAD. This same intermittent treatment approach should, whenever possible, also be employed if benzodiazepines are given chronically for nonpsychiatric conditions (23,150). *Continuous uninterrupted* benzodiazepine therapy for months and years, even when prescribed in therapeutic dosages, seems to represent an inappropriate treatment approach for most anxious patients.

Low Dose Dependence with Benzodiazepines

It has been demonstrated for a long time that physical dependence to benzodiazepines can be produced with excessive dosages given for a prolonged period of time (42). More recently, it has become clear that even in low therapeutic dosages, benzodiazepines, when prescribed for prolonged periods of time, may produce physical dependence, as evidenced by the appearance of withdrawal symptoms after abrupt drug discontinuation (68,85,100, 124,144,151). The time course of withdrawal symptoms has been clearly defined in that symptoms of withdrawal occur within a few days of abrupt drug discontinuation, peak within 5 to 7 days, and then slowly decrease with time. Some mild rebound anxiety may already be present in a few patients treated for only 4 to 6 weeks (26). These rebound symptoms generally last for only a few days. In contrast, return of original symptomatology occurs more gradually; it is frequently noticeable only 1 to 2 weeks after discontinuation of treatment; its symptoms are similar to those the patient had originally; and they do not decrease with time (92). Short-half-life benzodiazepines seem to cause earlier and more marked withdrawal than long-half-life benzodiazepines (116,145), but the incidence of patients experiencing withdrawal does not seem to differ between the two groups of benzodiazepines (116).

In a prospective study of maintenance diazepam therapy, Rickels et al. (100) showed that 43% of patients who had been taking a benzodiazepine for a year or longer suffered from clear-cut withdrawal responses, and another 14% from transient responses or anxiety rebound. More recently, in patients who visited a benzodiazepine withdrawal clinic after having taken benzodiazepines for many years, the incidence of definite withdrawal was found to be 68% (102). Thus, what Winokur et al. (151) reported in the first placebo-controlled case report published is still true, namely, that even severe withdrawal responses can be abated temporarily by a single dose of a benzodiazepine, and that patients abruptly withdrawn will lose their withdrawal symptoms with time. Withdrawal symptoms are usually less marked when patients are being gradually discontinued from benzodiazepine therapy, a procedure now considered to be the treatment of choice; yet, even during gradual withdrawal, patients frequently experience disturbing withdrawal symptoms, which, while of a milder nature, may last for prolonged periods of time. Therefore, some patients prefer to withdraw "cold turkey," thus assuring that the withdrawal period will most likely be over within several weeks. There also are a significant number of long-term users who are simply not able to fully withdraw from their benzodiazepines. We observed that the longer a patient was on a low-dose benzodiazepine and the more chronic his or her emotional problems were, including characterological ones, the more difficulty such patient had in his or her attempt to withdraw from a benzodiazepine (102). Sometimes authors blame long-lasting psychiatric symptoms occurring after the discontinuation of a long-term chronic benzodiazepine therapy as having been caused either by the benzodiazepine or by its discontinuation. In most instances these symptoms, however, probably rather represent an emergence of old or new symptoms related to the patient's loss of benzodiazepine support.

Withdrawal responses to abrupt discontinuation of pharmacological therapy are not unique to benzodiazepines, but have also been reported for tricyclic antidepressants (14), for low-potency neuroleptics (16), and for such anti-

hypertensive drugs as propranolol, clonidine, and methyl-dopa, to mention only a few (28,69,88). In most, but not all, cases benzodiazepine withdrawal reactions can be treated by tapering off drug intake slowly, usually by one-eighth to one-fourth the daily dose every 1 to 2 weeks (138,151).

In real life, however, most patients tend to take benzodiazepines only for short periods of time or to use them on an "as needed" basis. If benzodiazepines are taken for a prolonged period of time, they usually are discontinued slowly. Therefore, the actual incidence of withdrawal experiences observed with benzodiazepines in the general practice of medicine may be rather small indeed (68).

Antihistamines, Neuroleptics, β-Blockers, and Clonidine

Antihistamines such as hydroxyzine possess some anxiolytic properties; however, this is usually seen only in doses so high that marked sedation occurs (109). Nevertheless, drugs such as hydroxyzine do have limited usefulness in the treatment of anxiety in addiction-prone personalities, alcoholics, or patients for whom benzodiazepines are not effective. Other antihistamines, such as diphenhydramine and doxylamine, are helpful over-the-counter sleep aids, although less effective than benzodiazepines (112).

Neuroleptics in low daily dosages have been claimed to possess anxiolytic properties. These claims have never been fully substantiated, and the evidence to date points, at most, to an intermediate efficacy between benzodiazepines and placebo (96,108,111,114,117,118,123). Since neuroleptics also possess troublesome side effects, including the potential to cause tardive dyskinesia, their use should be restricted to those anxious patients not responding to other medications, to patients whose anxiety is secondary to such diagnoses as borderline personality or schizophrenia, and to elderly patients who suffer primarily from agitation rather than anxiety (76).

β-Blockers, primarily propranolol, have been advocated in the treatment of schizophrenia, alcoholism, lithium tremor, stage fright, and anxiety (to mention only a few suggested indications), based on the perhaps oversimplified reasoning that anxiety bears some relation to overactivity of the sympathetic nervous system. Although β-blockers decrease somatic manifestations of anxiety such as palpitations, tremors, and sweaty palms, they do not affect the emotional components of anxiety. They may also produce sedation and, in certain individuals, extremely low pulse rate, leading to faintness and dizziness—some of the very symptoms they are prescribed to treat. β-blockers apparently work primarily by blocking peripheral rather than central β-adrenergic neurons. In 1979 Cole et al. (18) intensively reviewed the use of β-blockers in anxiety, and concluded that the evidence in their favor was rather minimal in the daily dosages used, which actually may have been insufficient.

Since that time, several further studies have also concluded that β-blockers, while possibly having some effect in selected patients (e.g., those suffering from stage fright; 12,38), are generally not as effective as benzodiazepines in the treatment of anxiety (36,49,80). Interestingly, Hallstrom and colleagues (36) found that the combination of diazepam and propranolol produced more positive results than diazepam alone. This would suggest more an adjunctive than a primary therapeutic role for β-blockers in the treatment of generalized anxiety.

Clonidine is a relatively selective α₂-agonist for an inhibitory autoreceptor that modulates central noradrenergic function (146). The use of clonidine as an antianxiety agent appears, at least in part, to have been that rare example, a canny clinical application of a biologic model derived from animal research. The locus ceruleus model suggests noradrenergic overactivity as a substrate for anxiety (89). Initial clinical application was to the treatment of opiate withdrawal (30), where anxiety is a well-known and prominent feature. The successful use of clonidine in moderating opiate withdrawal symptoms has led to speculation about an anxiolytic role for clonidine. To date, only one pilot study of nine patients (40) has assessed the effect of clonidine in generalized anxiety. The anxiolytic effect was modest, and most patients clearly preferred their previous benzodiazepine.

Antidepressants

The lack of treatment research on DSM-III-defined GAD is felt most keenly when it comes to the use of antidepressants. Despite their efficacy, benzodiazepines do possess liabilities that make the availability of alternative treatments desirable. Sedation, memory and performance effects, interaction with alcohol, selected unresponsiveness, and dependence and withdrawal are among the major drawbacks. Demonstration of direct anxiolytic benefit from antidepressant treatment would provide a useful treatment option that might avoid some of these drawbacks.

Evidence concerning the effectiveness of antidepressants in the treatment of generalized anxiety not associated with panic, phobic, obsessive-compulsive, or depressive symptoms is sparse. Findings of possible relevance are based on studies that antedate DSM-III and thereby antedate not only our current definition of GAD, but also the current emphasis on thorough documentation of diagnosis which DSM-III has promoted. Studies using samples of "mixed anxiety-depression" patients or mixed neurotics (20,47, 53,103,110,113,128) leave unanswered the question of the extent to which any effectiveness found for antidepressants is due simply to their relieving anxiety only because they relieve depression.

The most convincing evidence for the anxiolytic effect of imipramine comes from a large collaborative study in which imipramine, chlordiazepoxide, and placebo were compared for their antianxiety properties (48). Imipramine clearly showed significantly more antianxiety properties than chlordiazepoxide. Controlled studies on more restrictively diagnosed GAD populations are currently underway to confirm or refute any specific anxiolytic role for antidepressants when prescribed to nondepressed GAD patients.

To our knowledge, there are no controlled studies of the use of MAOIs or third-generation antidepressants in GAD. Again, there are uncontrolled pre-DSM-III studies on mixed anxious-depressed-phobic populations that make direct generalized anxiety benefit difficult to disentangle. It is hoped that GAD will, in the near future, be the focus of more well-designed research, since differential treatment response might help subtype this "residual" diagnosis. For now, the use of antidepressants in GAD should probably be reserved for patients in whom the liability of benzodiazepine use has been shown to be unacceptable (though the use of antidepressants is not without possibly greater risks). Antidepressants might also have some utility in patients with inadequate therapeutic response to benzodiazepines and possibly in those requiring long-term treatment.

Buspirone

The search for effective and safe nonbenzodiazepine anxiolytics has been going on for many years (94). Recently, buspirone has become of particular interest, as it is the first nonbenzodiazepine anxiolytic for which a New Drug Application has been filed in the United States, and it is already marketed in West Germany (119).

Buspirone, an azaspiro-decane-dione, was developed in the early 1970s. It has a chemical structure different from other anxiolytics, antidepressants, and neuroleptics. Buspirone does not bind to the benzodiazepine receptor and does not seem to influence γ-aminobutyric acid (GABA), at least directly. The buspirone development program conducted in the United States demonstrated that buspirone was equally effective as diazepam and clorazepate, and significantly more effective than placebo in treating symptoms of GAD for 4-week periods. Drug-placebo differences already were present after 1 week of treatment (86).

Most controlled studies conducted with buspirone showed a slightly, but insignificantly, slower onset of action during the first week of treatment for buspirone than for diazepam; none of these differences, however, reached statistical significance. In a more recently conducted 7-day study comparing two dosage levels of buspirone with placebo and with 15 to 20 mg of diazepam in a small group of patients, the authors again observed a slight but nonsignificant advantage for diazepam after 1 week of treatment, possibly related to the fact that many patients also had significant degrees of insomnia as part of their anxiety syndrome (Rickels, Lucki, and Giesecke, *unpublished data*). In the same study, diazepam produced more sedation than either buspirone or placebo. Since buspirone is a nonsedating compound, one would not expect the drug to be effective within the first several days of treatment.

Besides producing improvement comparable to the benzodiazepines, buspirone produced significantly less sedation. Furthermore, based on animal, normal volunteer, and patient research, buspirone produced fewer detrimental effects in psychomotor functions than benzodiazepines (59,77), did not seem to interact with alcohol (70), and seemed to lack the potential to be abused or to cause physical dependence (19,104).

Rickels et al. (119) also observed that diazepam, as compared to buspirone, was slightly more effective in alleviating somatic symptoms of anxiety, whereas buspirone was slightly more effective than diazepam in relieving symptoms of anger and hostility. Finally, in a prospective 6-month study conducted with anxious patients comparing clorazepate with buspirone, no tolerance to either drug developed, and when placebo was abruptly substituted for either drug under double-blind conditions after 6 months of treatment, clorazepate, but not buspirone, caused rebound anxiety and/or withdrawal symptoms (104).

One may conclude that buspirone, the first nonbenzodiazepine developed for the treatment of generalized anxiety disorder, represents an important addition to the physician's armamentarium for the treatment of anxious patients. Although lack of sedation will clearly be beneficial for some patients, it may be a hindrance in the treatment of others. Lack of physical dependence is certainly a plus, particularly for patients in need of chronic treatment. For those patients, however, who are in need of only a limited treatment period, this finding may be of little relevance. Slow onset of action, which would possibly prevent its p.r.n. use, may represent a disadvantage. As with any new compound that is novel in its structure, only extensive clinical experience will fully delineate buspirone's spectrum of action in terms of speed of therapeutic onset, diagnostic indications favorable to its use, and the final adverse effect pattern, a pattern that can only be established after years of therapeutic use.

TREATMENT OF PANIC DISORDER

Evaluating current treatments for panic disorder is easier in some ways than it is for generalized anxiety. The target population is more homogeneous, and because formal diagnostic recognition came only in 1980, much of the research is on populations defined in currently accepted terms. In reviewing treatment studies, one caveat that emerged is that perhaps too little attention has been paid, when it comes to analyzing treatment effects, to confounding clinical variables such as the presence or absence of agoraphobia.

Tricyclic Antidepressants

Klein's initial pilot study (54) demonstrating a role for imipramine in panic disorder has been confirmed by several controlled studies. In some, imipramine has been compared to placebo or to behavioral therapies (67,153,154). In others it has been compared to benzodiazepines (73) or to MAOIs (132). Patients studied suffered varying degrees of phobic avoidance. No uncomplicated panic disorder subgroups were delineated for study. Significant antipanic benefit from imipramine was demonstrated in all studies but one (67). This latter study by Marks demonstrated a nonsignificant trend in improvement for imipramine over placebo (74% much improved versus 55%), though on closer examination the placebo group appears to have been receiving active behavioral treatment. Also, 11% of enrolled patients had failed a previous antidepressant trial. A reanalysis of Marks' data, using a more limited number of outcome indices, did indicate a significant imipramine effect (A. Raskin, *personal communication*).

The efficacy of antidepressants in *uncomplicated* panic disorder has only been demonstrated in non-placebo-controlled studies (27,29,79) of clomipramine and imipramine. Clomipramine has also shown significant benefit in a large

($N = 480$) uncontrolled study of anxiety associated with agoraphobia or social phobia (10). This finding has been confirmed (84) in a double-blind study that found clomipramine to have significant benefit in panic disorder also associated with agoraphobia and social phobia.

Besides clomipramine and imipramine, there are, to our knowledge, no controlled or blinded studies of other non-MAOI antidepressants in panic disorder. Anecdotal reports suggest antipanic efficacy for other antidepressants, such as desipramine (37,63,79), trazodone, and maprotiline (130), though there have been reports that amoxapine (131) and bupropion (134) may have no antipanic properties.

Though the efficacy of imipramine in panic disorder with or without phobic avoidance appears to be fairly well established, the generalizability of this finding to other antidepressants remains to be demonstrated. This should be an important avenue of future research, since antidepressants appear to offer a distinct alternative to alprazolam for the treatment of panic disorder. They pose no dependence liability, though withdrawal symptoms are occasionally elicited on abrupt discontinuation. In addition, the lack of dietary prohibitions also recommends them over the MAOIs. Side effects of imipramine, though, limit its effectiveness and acceptance in over one-third of patients in some studies (67,71). Desipramine would likely be a comparably effective drug whose significantly lower anticholinergic properties might make it much better tolerated. The confirmation, by controlled studies, of antipanic properties for other antidepressants would be welcome.

MAO Inhibitors

The fact that MAOIs have survived the vicissitudes of their first 25 years of use is testimony, by itself, to their often remarkable efficacy. Initial favorable uncontrolled clinical studies of MAOIs (5,52,121,149) included patients with a remarkable heterogeneity of anxious and depressive symptoms and syndromes. More restrictive studies on more typical or classic depressions yielded less than encouraging results and led to calls for abandoning MAOI use altogether.

Kelly's large 1970 retrospective study (50) of over 200 phobically anxious and agoraphobic patients showed such striking benefit from MAOIs that it provided the impetus for the first controlled studies in anxiety disorders (65,139,143). These studies confirmed the value of MAOIs in the treatment of mixed agoraphobic, phobically anxious, and socially phobic patients. Prior to 1980, MAOI research was almost exclusively confined to England or the Commonwealth, while research on tricyclics for panic anxiety states was, under the influence of Donald Klein, largely confined to the United States. This has changed since the publication in 1980 of Sheehan's study (132) comparing phenelzine to imipramine and placebo. This study was the first to report the effect of an MAOI on a DSM-III-defined PD population. It demonstrated strong antipanic properties for both drugs, with a trend favoring phenelzine. Since then there have been studies (133) confirming the benefit of MAOIs in PD and phobic anxiety.

There have been no controlled studies we are aware of on MAOIs other than phenelzine for the treatment of PD.

Anecdotally (125), both tranylcypromine and isocarboxazid have been reported to be effective. Given that phenelzine may be the single most efficacious antipanic agent currently available, the paucity of MAOI research is unfortunate. This is especially true in this case, since it is unusual for a psychiatric disorder to be so responsive to three drugs (phenelzine, imipramine, and alprazolam) with such different chemical structures and mechanisms of action. Differential treatment response might help to identify more specific PD subtypes, and might provide pathophysiologic clues.

Benzodiazepines

The use of benzodiazepines in PD represents, as Samuel Johnson once said of second marriages, the triumph of hope over experience. Historically, as we have mentioned, the delineation of PD stemmed from recognition of the differential sensitivity of its core crescendo episodes of anxiety to antidepressants. To turn around and discover a treatment affinity between benzodiazepines and PD might partially undermine our confidence in the validity of the diagnostic discrimination of GAD and PD.

But what is the evidence, if any, of a role for benzodiazepines in PD? To answer this it is useful to divide the benzodiazepines into those of low potency (diazepam, chlordiazepoxide, clorazepate) and those of high potency (alprazolam, lorazepam). Questions of current research interest are, Is there any effect by low-potency benzodiazepines on panic attacks themselves? Is there significantly greater specific antipanic efficacy by high-potency benzodiazepines, and if so, is that efficacy unique to the triazolo ring (of alprazolam)?

Taking up the question of low-potency benzodiazepines first: Pre-DSM-III studies (115) found significant antipanic effects from diazepam in patients high on rating scale panic dimensions. What percent would actually have met DSM-III diagnostic criteria, though, is uncertain. Only two controlled studies we know of have assessed the benefit of low-potency benzodiazepines in PD with agoraphobia, and both have methodologic drawbacks. McNair and Kahn (73) compared chlordiazepoxide to imipramine in 26 patients in an 8-week double-blind trial. A composite panic score showed significantly greater improvement for imipramine over chlordiazepoxide, but this only emerged from the composite score, and significance was not achieved until the final week. Individual self- or physician-rated clusters from HSCL panic anxiety, POMS tension-anxiety, and agoraphobia did not significantly favor imipramine. There was no placebo group and no comment by the authors as to the degree of benefit over time due to chlordiazepoxide. It should be noted that the mean maximum daily doses for each drug were perhaps low (chlordiazepoxide 55 mg, imipramine 132 mg). Noyes et al. (81) studied 21 patients in a 2-week double-blind crossover comparison of diazepam (median dose 30 mg) to propranolol (median dose 240 mg) also in PD and agoraphobia. They reported moderate to marked improvement in panic symptoms that was not just limited to generalized or anticipatory anxiety. Blockade of actual panic attacks was effective enough that seven patients

"remarked spontaneously that they 'felt better than they had in years.' "

Antipanic effects (of low-potency benzodiazepines) have certainly not been well enough documented to merit their inclusion as front-line drugs. They show some promise, though, and it is perhaps premature to be overconfident or overly neat in the diagnostic inferences one draws based on the presumption of their total inefficacy.

Turning to high-potency benzodiazepines, the evidence for specific antipanic effects is much more solid and convincing. This is especially true for alprazolam, the triazolo derivative first marketed in 1981 (for GAD). Since then, alprazolam has been the subject of several controlled studies (6,15,133,135), numbering over 700 patients, that have demonstrated its remarkable antipanic effects in patients with or without agoraphobia. Its efficacy is well trumpeted and well known, as is testified to by its rapid rise in prescription use. In light of its benefit-risk ratio, and its generally minimal and well-tolerated side effects, it rightfully occupies a central position among current antipanic treatments. The major drawback, especially at recommended doses of 6 to 10 mg per day, is its potential, similar to other benzodiazepines, to cause physical dependence and withdrawal symptoms after discontinuation from long-term therapy. Pretreatment informed consent regarding the issue of dependence is becoming as essential to clinical practice as it is to inform patients considered for treatment with neuroleptics about the risk of tardive dyskinesia.

A pilot investigation (9) suggests that clonazepam, the high-potency, nontriazolo benzodiazepine marketed as an antiepileptic, may have antipanic properties comparable to alprazolam. If these preliminary findings are confirmed, it would corroborate antipanic effects we have observed for lorazepam, especially in patients suffering panic disorder uncomplicated by agoraphobia (126).

To the extent that benzodiazepines have antipanic effects, one must call into question as overdrawn the distinction between panic attacks as "spontaneous" sui generis events discrete from generalized anxiety (115). Antipanic effects might result from any adequate general anxiolysis, though the example of alprazolam suggests that this may require 40 to 100 mg of diazepam or its equivalent. The utility of traditional benzodiazepines in PD remains an open question requiring further controlled research.

β-Blockers and Clonidine

The use of β-adrenergic blocking agents for the treatment of panic provides, as it did for generalized anxiety, belated confirmation of the James-Lange theory of emotion (61), but in doing so damns it with faint praise. Only two studies to date (78,81) have tested the efficacy of propranolol in PD, and results provide little support for an antipanic effect. Propranolol also does not appear to block lactate-induced panic (31). Corroborating this, we have observed that patients treated by their internist with β-blockers, either empirically or for MVP, not infrequently apply to our clinic for anxiety treatment while reporting no significant anxiolytic effect from their cardiac drug. One unconfirmed and uncontrolled exception is a report by Heiser and

DeFrancisco (39) that six of nine patients achieved marked blockade of their panic attacks on a relatively low dose of propranolol (mean 42 mg per day). In general, though, β-blockers have not been found to significantly control panic attacks, despite partial amelioration of peripheral adrenergic symptoms. In light of this it is of interest to note that hypoglycemic stimulation of peripheral adrenergic symptoms, in PD patients by i.v. insulin, conversely, does not reliably elicit panic (127). These two observations suggest caution in any overexclusive focus on adrenergic symptoms as the sole significant manifestations of panic. In conclusion, β-blocking drugs, on the basis of current evidence, would appear to have, at most, a minor or adjunctive role in the treatment of panic disorder.

Four studies (56,64,142,146) that we are aware of have tested clonidine in panic anxiety. The small N of 35 makes any conclusions tentative, but what evidence there is provides moderate support for a possible antipanic and antianxiety effect. The effect appears to be acute (<1 week onset), and may be correlated with reduced noradrenergic indices such as 3-methoxy-4-hydroxyphenylglycol (MHPG). Limitations on the utility of clonidine may be its side effects (significant hypotension, sedation, and fatigue) and the possibility that for some patients tolerance may eventually develop to the antipanic effects (64). For the time being, and before well-controlled clinical trials prove or disprove these early findings, clonidine use should probably be reserved for carefully selected treatment-resistant PD patients.

General Comments

Overall, the treatment of PD represents one of the most gratifying success stories of psychopharmacology. Intensely distressing attacks of panic anxiety, often associated with disabling phobic symptoms, have been demonstrated to respond remarkably to at least three chemically distinct classes of agents. This success in the acute treatment of panic disorder raises as many clinical issues as it resolves. By way of example, little research has been addressed to the question of how the presence or absence of phobic avoidant or hypochondriacal and somatic symptoms affects choice of drug or treatment outcome. Indeed, little is known about the long-term natural history of PD, how treatment might alter its course, or even what constitutes adequate maintenance treatment.

Questions have even been raised as to whether the antipanic effects of tricyclic antidepressants (TCAs) and MAOI might actually be antidepressant effects. After all, genetic (141), course of illness (62), and neuroendocrine (127) studies suggest syndromic overlap of PD and major depression. With regard to this issue, research has provided preliminary evidence (73,132,153,154) favoring antipanic effects being independent of antidepressant effects, though there are dissenting voices (67). The evidence cited to support this contention is of several kinds. First, degree of baseline depression is generally not predictive of antipanic response (50,143,153,154). Second, mean antipanic doses of TCA/MAOI are often lower than for MDD, and antipanic effects often manifest earlier (131). Third, anecdotal evidence

is cited suggesting that some patients with concurrent MDD and PD will have an antipanic response to a tricyclic which is dissociated from any antidepressant response (83). We have also clinically observed patients remit in their panic after treatment with alprazolam, but subsequently develop a major depression (while still on the drug) without recurrence of their panic. Antidepressants, though, often improve not just focal panic symptoms, but also associated phobias and depression (73,84). On this basis, it has been suggested (67) that antidepressants in panic may be generally "patholytic."

SUMMARY AND CONCLUSION

In summary, the pharmacotherapy of anxiety in the past decade can best be characterized as being in transition. We have moved beyond almost exclusive reliance on benzodiazepines, but they remain the most widely used, safe, and effective anxiolytics. Even more effective and safe anxiolysis is likely to emerge from current research on such issues as low dose dependence, drug self-reinforcing properties, the nature and management of withdrawal, acute vs maintenance treatment, etc.

The last decade has also witnessed confirmation of a role for both tricyclic and MAOI antidepressants in PD. On the other hand, β-blockers have not lived up to their promise, whereas agents such as clonidine remain of largely research interest.

On the horizon are indications that antidepressants may have a role in GAD, whereas traditional benzodiazepines may have been prematurely written off as having no antipanic properties. If these suggestions are confirmed by clinical testing, they may partly undermine the discrete distinction between panic and GAD. Also on the horizon is buspirone, a nonbenzodiazepine anxiolytic which may be the harbinger of a whole new class of novel anxiolytics. It promises to be a substantive alternative to the benzodiazepines.

Additionally, it may do what past anxiolytics have always done—shed new light on the diagnosis and pathophysiology of anxiety itself.

ACKNOWLEDGMENT

This research was supported in part by USPHS research grant MH-08957.

REFERENCES

1. Abernethy, D. R., Greenblatt, D. J., Ochs, H. R., and Shader, R. I. (1984): *Curr. Med. Res. Opin.,* 8(*Suppl.* 4):80.
2. Aden, G. C., and Thein, S. G. (1980): *J. Clin. Psychiatry,* 41: 245–248.
3. Aimes, P. L., Gelden, M. G., and Shaw, P. M. (1983): *Br. J. Psychiatry,* 142:174–179.
4. Altesman, R. I., and Cole, J. O. (1983): *J. Clin. Psychiatry,* 44(8, Sec. 2):12–18.
5. Arnot, R. (1960): *Dis. Nerv. Syst.,* 11:448.
6. Ballenger, J. C. (1985): IVth World Congress of Biological Psychiatry, Philadelphia.
7. Balmer, R., Battegay, R., and von Marschall, R. (1981): *Int. Pharmacopsychiatry,* 16:221–234.

8. Bandera, R., Bollini, P., and Garrattini, S. (1984): *Curr. Med. Res. Opin.,* 8(*Suppl.* 4):94.
9. Beaudry, P., Fontaine, R., Mercier, P., and Chouinard, G. (1985): Presented at The Society for Biological Psychiatry, Dallas.
10. Beaumont, G. (1977): *J. Int. Med. Res.,* 5(*Suppl.* 5):116–123.
11. Beckmann, H., and Haas, S. (1984): *Nervenarzt,* 55:111–121.
12. Brantigan, C. O., Brantigan, T. A., and Joseph, N. (1982): *Am. J. Med.,* 72:88–94.
13. Breckenridge, A. (1983): In: *The Benzodiazepines: From Molecular Biology to Clinical Practice,* edited by E. Costa, pp. 237–246. Raven Press, New York.
14. Charney, D. S., Heninger, G. R., Sternberg, D. E., and Landis, H. (1982): *Br. J. Psychiatry,* 141:377–386.
15. Chouinard, G., Annable, L., Fontaine, R., and Solyom, L. (1982): *Psychopharmacology,* 77:229–233.
16. Chouinard, G., Bradwejn, J., Annable, L., Ross, B. D., and Ross-Chouinard, A. (1984): *J. Clin. Psychiatry,* 45:500–502.
17. Cohen, J., Gomez, E., Hoell, N. L., Kotin, J., Rickman, E. E., and Ruessler, R. L. (1976): *Curr. Ther. Res.,* 20:184–193.
18. Cole, J. O., Altesman, R. I., and Weingarten, C. H. (1979): *McLean Hosp. J.,* 4:40–67.
19. Cole, J. O., Orzack, M. H., Beake, B., Bird, M., and Bar-tal, Y. (1982): *J. Clin. Psychiatry,* 43(12, Sec. 2):69–74.
20. Conti, L., and Pinder, R. M. (1979): *J. Int. Med. Res.,* 7:285–289.
21. Dawson, G. W., Jue, S. G., and Brogden, R. N. (1984): *Drugs,* 27:132–147.
22. de Figueiredo, R., Franchini, A., Martinho, A., and Hindmarch, I. (1981): *Int. Pharmacopsychiatry,* 16:57–65.
23. Dowling, J. T. (1980): *Drugs,* 19:437–442.
24. Downing, R. W., and Rickels, K. (1987): *Acta Psychiatr. Scand.,* 72:522–528.
25. Feighner, J. P., Aden, G. C., Fabre, L. R., Rickels, K., and Smith, W. T. (1983): *JAMA,* 249:3057–3064.
26. Fontaine, R., Chouinard, G., and Annable, L. (1984): *Am. J. Psychiatry,* 141:848–852.
27. Garakani, H., Zitrin, C. M., and Klein, D. F. (1984): *Am. J. Psychiatry,* 141:446–448.
28. Garbus, S. B., Weber, M. A., Priest, R. T., Brewer, D. D., and Hubbell, F. A. (1979): *J. Clin. Pharmacol.,* 19:476–486.
29. Gloger, S., Grunhaus, L., Birmacher, B., and Troudart, T. (1981): *Am. J. Psychiatry,* 138:1215–1217.
30. Gold, M. S., Redmond, D. E., and Kleber, H. D. (1978): *Lancet,* 1:929–930.
31. Gorman, J. M., Levy, G. F., and Liebowitz, M. R. (1983): *Arch. Gen. Psychiatry,* 40:1079–1082.
32. Greenblatt, D. J., Laughren, T. P., Aleen, M. D., Harmatz, J. S., and Shader, R. I. (1981): *Br. J. Clin. Pharmacol.,* 11:35–40.
33. Greenblatt, D. J., and Shader, R. I. (1974): *Benzodiazepines in Clinical Practice.* Raven Press, New York.
34. Greenblatt, D. J., and Shader, R. I. (1980): *Drug Res.,* 30:886–890.
35. Greenblatt, D. J., Shader, R. I., and Abernethy, D. R. (1983): *N. Engl. J. Med.,* 309:354–358,410–416.
36. Hallstrom, C., Treasaden, I., Guy Edwards, J., and Lader, M. (1981): *Br. J. Psychiatry,* 139:417–421.
37. Hamlin, C., and Gold, M. S. (1984): In: *Advances in Psychopharmacology,* edited by M. S. Gold, R. B. Lydiard, and J. S. Carman, pp. 225–275. CRC Press, Inc., Boca Raton.
38. Hartley, L. R., Ungapen, S., Davie, I., and Spencer, D. J. (1983): *Br. J. Psychiatry,* 142:512–517.
39. Heiser, J. F., and DeFrancisco, D. (1976): *Am. J. Psychiatry,* 133:1389–1394.
40. Hoehn-Saric, R., Merchant, A. F., Keyser, M. L., and Smith, V. K. (1981): *Arch. Gen. Psychiatry,* 38:1278–1282.
41. Hollister, L. E., Conley, F. K., Britt, R. H., and Suer, L. (1981): *JAMA,* 246:1568–1570.
42. Hollister, L. E., Motzenbecker, F. P., and Degan, R. O. (1961): *Psychopharmacologia,* 2:63–68.
43. Hoyumpa, A. M. (1978): *South. Med. J.,* 7:23–28.
44. Insel, T. R., Ninan, P. T., Aloi, J., Jimerson, D. C., Skolnick, P., and Paul, S. M. (1984): *Arch. Gen. Psychiatry,* 41:741–750.
45. Johanson, C. E., and Uhlenhuth, E. H. (1980): *Psychopharmacology,* 71:269–273.
46. Johnson, L. C., and Chernik, D. A. (1982): *Psychopharmacology,* 76:101–113.
47. Johnstone, E. C., Cunningham-Owens, D. E., Frith, C. D., McPherson, K., Dowie, C., Riley, G., and Gold, H. (1980): *Psychol. Med.,* 10:321–328.
48. Kahn, R. J., McNair, D. M., Lipman, R. S., Covi, L., Rickels, K., Downing, R., Fisher, S., and Frankenthaler, L. M. (1986): *Arch. Gen. Psychiatry,* 43:79–85.
49. Kelly, D. (1985): *Stress Med.* 1:143–152.
50. Kelly, D., Guirguis, W., Frommer, E., Mitchell-Heggs, N., and Sargant, W. (1970): *Br. J. Psychiatry,* 116:387–398.
51. Kendell, R. E. (1982): *Arch. Gen. Psychiatry,* 39:1334–1339.
52. King, A. (1962): *Med. J. Aust.,* 1:879–883.
53. Kleber, R. J. (1979): *J. Clin. Psychiatry,* 40:165–170.
54. Klein, D. F. (1964): *Psychopharmacologia,* 5:397–408.
55. Klein, D. F. (1981): In: *Anxiety: New Research and Changing Concepts,* edited by D. F. Klein and J. Rabkin, pp. 235–262. Raven Press, New York.
56. Ko, G. N., Elsworth, J. D., Roth, R. H., Rifkin, B. G., Leigh, H., and Redmond, D. E. (1983): *Arch. Gen. Psychiatry,* 40:425–430.
57. Lader, M. (1978): *Neuroscience,* 3:159–165.
58. Lader, M. (1980): *Drug Res.,* 30:910–913.
59. Lader, M. (1982): *J. Clin. Psychiatry,* 43(12, Sec. 2):62–67.
60. Lader, M. H., Bond, A. J., and James, D. C. (1974): *Psychol. Med.,* 4:381–387.
61. Lange, C. G., and James, W. (1922): *The Emotions.* Williams and Wilkins, Baltimore.
62. Leckman, J. F., Weissman, M. M., Merikangas, K. R., Pauls, D. L., and Prusoff, B. A. (1983): *Arch. Gen. Psychiatry,* 40:1055–1060.
63. Liebowitz, M. R., Fyer, A. J., Gorman, J. M., Dillon, D., Appleby, I. L., Levy, G., Anderson, S., Levitt, M., Palij, M., Davies, S. O., and Klein, D. F. (1984): *Arch. Gen. Psychiatry,* 13:764–770.
64. Liebowitz, M. R., Fyer, A. J., McGrath, P., and Klein, D. F. (1981): *Psychopharmacol. Bull.,* 17:122–123.
65. Lipsedge, J. S., Hattoff, J., and Huggins, P. (1973): *Psychopharmacologia,* 32:67–80.
66. Lucki, I., Rickels, K., and Geller, A. M. (1985): *Psychopharmacol. Bull.,* 21:93–96.
67. Marks, I. M., Gray, S., Cohen, D., Hill, R., Mawson, D., Ramm, E., and Stern, R. S. (1983): *Arch. Gen. Psychiatry,* 40:153–162.
68. Marks, J. (1983): *J. Psychoactive Drugs,* 15:137–149.
69. Martin, P. R., Ebert, M. H., Gordon, E. K., Weingartner, H., and Kopin, I. J. (1984): *Psychopharmacology,* 84:58–63.
70. Mattila, M. J., Aranko, K., and Seppala, T. (1982): *J. Clin. Psychiatry,* 43(12, Sec. 2):56–60.
71. Mavissakalian, M., and Perel, J. (1985): *Am. J. Psychiatry,* 142:1032–1036.
72. McNair, D. M. (1973): *Arch. Gen. Psychiatry,* 29:611–617.
73. McNair, D. M., and Kahn, R. J. (1981): In: *Anxiety: New Research and Changing Concepts,* edited by D. F. Klein and J. Rabkin, pp. 69–79. Raven Press, New York.
74. Mellinger, G. D., and Balter, M. B. (1981): In: *Epidemiological Impact of Psychotropic Drugs,* edited by G. Tognoni, C. Bellantuono, and M. Lader, pp. 117–135. Elsevier-North Holland, New York.
75. Merikangas, K. R., Leckman, J. F., Prusoff, B. A., Pauls, D. L., and Weissman, M. M. (1985): *Arch. Gen. Psychiatry,* 42:367–372.
76. Morris, R., and Rickels, K. (1984): *Curr. Ther. Res.,* 35:519–531.
77. Moskowitz, H. (1982): *J. Clin. Psychiatry,* 43(12, Sec. 2):45–55.
78. Munjack, D. J., Rebal, R., Shaner, R., Staples, F., Braun, R., and Leonard, M. (1984): *Compr. Psychiatry,* 26:80–89.
79. Muskin, P. R., and Fyer, A. J. (1981): *J. Clin. Psychopharmacol.,* 1:81–90.
80. Noyes, R., Jr. (1982): *Psychosomatics,* 23:155–170.
81. Noyes, R., Anderson, D. J., Clancy, J., Crowe, R. R., Slymen, D. J., Ghoneim, M. M., and Hinrichs, J. V. (1984): *Arch. Gen. Psychiatry,* 41:287–292.
82. Noyes, R., Clancy, J., Hoenk, P. R., and Slymen, D. J. (1980): *Arch. Gen. Psychiatry,* 37:173–178.
83. Nurnberg, H. G., and Coccaro, E. F. (1982): *Am. J. Psychiatry,* 139:1060–1062.
84. Pecknold, J. C., McClure, D. J., Appeltauer, L., Allan, T., and Wrzesinski, L. (1982): *Br. J. Psychiatry,* 140:484–490.

85. Petursson, H., and Lader, M. H. (1981): *Br. Med. J.,* 283:643–645.
86. Pitts, F. N., ed. (1982): *J. Clin. Psychiatry,* 43(12, Sec. 2).
87. Ponciano, E., Relvas, J., and Mendes, F. (1981): *R. Soc. Med. Int. Cong. Symp. Ser.,* 43:125–131.
88. Rangno, R. E., and Langlois, S. (1982): *Br. J. Clin. Pharmacol.,* 13S:345–351.
89. Redmond, D. E. (1977): In: *Animal Models in Psychiatry and Neurology,* edited by I. Hamin and E. Usdin, pp. 116–139. Pergamon Press, Oxford.
90. Rickels, K. (1968): In: *Non-Specific Factors in Drug Therapy,* edited by K. Rickels, pp. 3–26. Charles C Thomas, Springfield, IL.
91. Rickels, K. (1978): *Psychopharmacology,* 58:1–17.
92. Rickels, K. (1980): In: *Benzodiazepines 1980: Current Update; Psychosomatics,* 21(Suppl.):15–20.
93. Rickels, K. (1981): *Br. J. Clin. Pharmacol.,* 11S:71–83.
94. Rickels, K. (1983): *J. Clin. Psychiatry,* 44:38–43.
95. Rickels, K. (1985): In: *Drug Treatment of Neurotic Disorders— Focus on Alprazolam,* edited by M. H. Lader and H. C. Davies, pp. 84–93. Churchill Livingstone, Edinburgh.
96. Rickels, K., Case, W. G., Csanalosi, I., Pereira-Ogan, J., Sandler, K. R., and Schless, A. P. (1978): *Curr. Ther. Res.,* 23:111–120.
97. Rickels, K., Case, W. G., and Diamond, L. (1980): *Int. Pharmacopsychiatry,* 15:186–192.
98. Rickels, K., Case, W. G., and Downing, R. W. (1982): *Psychopharmacol. Bull.,* 18:38–41.
99. Rickels, K., Case, W. G., Downing, R. W., Dixon, R., and Fridman, R. (1984): *Pharmacopsychiatry,* 17:44–49.
100. Rickels, K., Case, W. G., Downing, R. W., and Winokur, A. (1983): *JAMA,* 250:767–771.
101. Rickels, K., Case, W. G., Downing, R. W., and Winokur, A. (1985): In: *Chronic Treatments in Neuropsychiatry,* edited by D. Kemali and G. Racagni, pp. 193–204. Raven Press, New York.
102. Rickels, K., Case, G. W., Winokur, A., and Swenson, C. (1984): *Psychopharmacol. Bull.,* 20:608–615.
103. Rickels, K., Csanalosi, I., Chung, H. R., Case, W. G., Pereira-Ogan, J. A., and Downing, R. W. (1974): *Am. J. Psychiatry,* 131:25–30.
104. Rickels, K., Csanalosi, I., Chung, H., Case, W. G., and Schweizer, E. E. (May 1985): Presented at the Annual Meeting of the American Psychiatric Association, Dallas, TX.
105. Rickels, K., Csanalosi, I., Greisman, P., Cohen, D., Werblowsky, J., Russ, H. A., and Harris, H. (1983): *Am. J. Psychiatry,* 140:82–85.
106. Rickels, K., Downing, R., and Winokur, A. (1978): In: *Handbook of Psychopharmacology,* edited by L. L. Iversen and S. D. Iversen, p. 13. Plenum, New York.
107. Rickels, K., Feighner, J. P., and Smith, W. T. (1985): *Arch. Gen. Psychiatry,* 42:134–141.
108. Rickels, K., Gingrich, R. L., Csanalosi, I., Werblowsky, J., Schless, A., Sandler, K., and Rosenfeld, H. (1981): *Curr. Ther. Res.,* 29:156–164.
109. Rickels, K., Gordon, P. E., Zamostien, B. B., Case, W., Hutchison, J., and Chung, H. (1970): *Compr. Psychiatry,* 11:457–474.
110. Rickels, K., Hesbacher, P., and Downing, R. W. (1970): *Dis. Nerv. Syst.,* 31:468–475.
111. Rickels, K., Hutchison, J., Morris, R. J., Csanalosi, I., Parsia, K., and Pereira-Ogan, J. A. (1972): *Curr. Ther. Res.,* 14:1–9.
112. Rickels, K., Morris, R. J., Newman, H., Rosenfeld, H., Schiller, H., and Weinstock, R. (1983): *J. Clin. Pharmacol.,* 23:235–242.
113. Rickels, K., Perloff, M., Stepansky, W., Dion, H. S., Case, W. G., and Sapra, R. K. (1969): *Psychopharmacologia,* 15:265–279.
114. Rickels, K., Raab, E., Gordon, P. E., Laquer, K. G., DeSilverio, R. V., and Hesbacher, P. (1968): *Psychopharmacologia,* 12:181–192.
115. Rickels, K., and Schweizer, E. E. (1986): *Psychopharmacol. Bull.,* 22:93–99.
116. Rickels, K., Case, W. G., Schweizer, E. E., Swenson, C., and Fridman, R. B. (1986): *Psychopharmacol. Bull.,* 22:407–415.
117. Rickels, K., Weise, C. C., Clark, E. L., Jenkins, B. W., Rose, C. K., Rosenfeld, H., and Gordon, P. E. (1974): *Br. J. Psychiatry,* 125:79–87.

118. Rickels, K., Weise, C. C., Whalen, E. M., Csanalosi, I., Jenkins, B. W., and Stepansky, W. (1971): *J. Clin. Pharmacol.,* 11:440–449.
119. Rickels, K., Wiseman, K., Norstad, N., Singer, M., Stoltz, D., Brown, A., and Danton, J. (1982): *J. Clin. Psychiatry,* 43(12, Sec. 2):81–86.
120. Rosenberg, L., Mitchell, A. A., Parsells, J. L., Pashayan, H., Louike, C., and Shapiro, S. (1983): *N. Engl. J. Med.,* 309:1282–1285.
121. Sargant, W. (1962): *J. Neurophysiol.,* 3(Suppl. 1):96–103.
122. Schatzberg, A. F., and Cole, J. O. (1978): *Arch. Gen. Psychiatry,* 35:1359–1365.
123. Schless, A., Weise, C. C., Sandler, K., and Rickels, K. (1978): *Prog. Neuropsychopharmacol. Biol. Psychiatry,* 2:191–196.
124. Schoepf, J. (1983): *Pharmacopsychiatria,* 16:1–8.
125. Schweizer, E., and Rickels, K. (1986): *Am. J. Psychiatry,* 143:1590–1592.
126. Schweizer, E., Fox, I., Clary, C., and Rickels, K. (1987): (submitted).
127. Schweizer, E., Winokur, A., and Rickels, K. (1986): *Am. J. Psychiatry,* 143:654–655.
128. Shamas, E. (1977): *Dis. Nerv. Syst.,* 38:201–207.
129. Shapiro, S., Skinner, E. A., Kessler, L. G., Von Kroff, M., and German, P. S. (1984): *Arch. Gen. Psychiatry,* 41:971–982.
130. Sheehan, D. V. (1982): *Drug Ther.,* 12:179–193.
131. Sheehan, D. V. (1985): *Psychiatr. Clin. North Am.,* 8:49–62.
132. Sheehan, D. V., Ballenger, J., and Jacobsen, G. (1980): *Arch. Gen. Psychiatry,* 37:51–59.
133. Sheehan, D. V., Claycomb, J. B., and Surman, O. S. (1984): Presented at the Annual Meeting of the American Psychiatric Association, Los Angeles.
134. Sheehan, D. V., Davidson, J., and Manschreck, T. C. (1983): *J. Clin. Psychopharmacol.,* 3:23–31.
135. Sheehan, D. V., Uzogara, E., and Coleman, J. H. (1982): Presented at the Annual Meeting of the American Psychiatric Association, Toronto.
136. Shiono, P. H., and Mills, J. L. (1984): *N. Engl. J. Med.,* 311:919–920.
137. Smail, P., Stockwell, T., Canter, S., and Hodgson, R. (1984): *Br. J. Psychiatry,* 144:53–57.
138. Smith, D. E. (1979): Newsletter, California Society for the Treatment of Alcoholism and Other Drug Dependencies, 6:1–3.
139. Solyom, L., Heseltine, G. F. D., and McClure, D. J. (1973): *Can. Psychiatry Assoc. J.,* 18:25–31.
140. Spitzer, R. L. (1985): Draft: DSM III-R in Development. American Psychiatric Association, Chicago.
141. Torgersen, S. (1983): *Arch. Gen. Psychiatry,* 40:1085–1089.
142. Tyrer, P. (1984): *Br. J. Psychiatry,* 144:78–83.
143. Tyrer, P., Candy, J., and Kelly, D. (1973): *Psychopharmacology,* 32:237–254.
144. Tyrer, P., Owen, R., and Dawling, S. (1983): *Lancet,* 1402–1406.
145. Tyrer, P., Rutherford, D., and Huggett, T. (1981): *Lancet,* 1:520–522.
146. Uhde, T. H., Siever, L. J., and Post, R. M. (1984): In: *Neurobiology of Mood Disorders,* edited by R. M. Post and J. C. Ballenger, pp. 554–571. Williams and Wilkins, Baltimore.
147. Uhlenhuth, B. H., Balter, M. B., Mellinger, G. D., Cisin, I. H., and Clinthorne, J. (1983): *Arch. Gen. Psychiatry,* 40:1167–1173.
148. Weiss, K. J., and Rosenberg, D. J. (1985): *J. Clin. Psychiatry,* 46:3–6.
149. West, E. D., and Dally, P. J. (1959): *Br. Med. J.,* 1:1491.
150. Wheatley, D. (1980): *Prog. Neuropsychopharmacol. Biol. Psychiatry,* 4:537–544.
151. Winokur, A., Rickels, K., Greenblatt, D. J., Snyder, P. J., and Schatz, N. J. (1980): *Arch. Gen. Psychiatry,* 37:101–105.
152. Wittenborn, J. R. (1979): *Br. J. Clin. Pharmacol.,* 7(Suppl. 1):61S–67S.
153. Zitrin, C. M., Klein, D. F., and Woerner, M. G. (1980): *Arch. Gen. Psychiatry,* 37:63–72.
154. Zitrin, C. M., Klein, D. F., Woerner, M. G., and Ross, D. C. (1983): *Arch. Gen. Psychiatry,* 40:125–138.

Psychopharmacology:
The Third Generation of Progress,
edited by Herbert Y. Meltzer.
Raven Press, New York © 1987.

CHAPTER 123

Psychopharmacologic Approaches to Obsessive-Compulsive Disorder

Thomas R. Insel and Joseph Zohar

Obsessive-compulsive disorder (OCD) traditionally has been considered a treatment-refractory syndrome. Although patients with this disorder may display many of the classic psychodynamic principles of defense and symptom formation, psychodynamic treatments have generally not been effective in reducing obsessions or compulsions (50). Behavioral approaches have proven more successful for the reduction of compulsive rituals, but the cognitive symptoms, the obsessions, may not be as responsive to behavior therapy (54). The outlook with pharmacologic treatments, until recently, was summed up by Salzman and Thaler (60) in their review of the pre-1978 literature: "With regard to drugs . . . there is neither convincing nor suggestive evidence that more can be accomplished than the relief of some anxiety—at a cost that often outweighs the potential benefits" (p. 295).

In the past 5 years, controlled studies of the use of medications for OCD have provided convincing evidence that a psychopharmacologic treatment can help many of these patients. Although the disorder is classified as an anxiety disorder, few data support the use of classic anxiolytics for these patients (31). Most case reports and nearly all controlled studies have focused on the antidepressants. In this chapter we review the evidence that one antidepressant, clomipramine, appears to decrease obsessions and compulsions; we then discuss whether or not these effects are antidepressant or truly antiobsessional; and finally, we consider the implications that so far only one antidepressant of those studied appears significantly effective. The distinctive psychopharmacologic features of this particular compound may ultimately provide a clue to the neurobiology of this syndrome.

CLINICAL FEATURES

Obsessive-compulsive disorder presents in several forms (23). The most common syndrome involves obsessions with contamination ("germ phobia") accompanied by ritualistic washing. Other patients, preoccupied with a feeling that they have done something wrong, have to check repetitively that they have not left the gas on or hit someone while driving. Sometimes obsessional doubt will be manifest as a need for symmetry, with hours spent checking that the books on the shelf are lined up "just right." Some patients present with intrusive, reprehensible thoughts or impulses not accompanied by rituals. As many as one-third of adult obsessive-compulsives describe symptoms beginning in childhood, often before puberty (14).

The prevalence of OCD in the general population, although traditionally thought to be 0.05% (76), has been reported to be more than 2.0% in the recent NIMH-sponsored Epidemiologic Catchment Area (ECA) Survey (58). This surprisingly high prevalence might reflect a problem in the diagnostic criteria, as the ECA survey did not require interference with functioning for a diagnosis of OCD. It should also be noted that many patients with OCD are very secretive about their symptoms and do not seek help until they develop complications, the most common complication being depression (19). In one study, for instance, the average interval between onset of obsessional symptoms and first visit to a therapist was 7.5 years (51).

Although this syndrome has recently been grouped with the anxiety disorders, anxiety may be a secondary rather than a primary feature of the clinical picture. Obsessionals often manifest discrete phobias with avoidant behavior, but the inescapable and internal quality of these "fears" is quite different from that described by true phobics (31). When there is an external, phobic stimulus for an obsession (such as "dirt" or "cancer germs" or "radiation"), the source is usually invisible and ubiquitous, in contrast to the discrete stimulus for a simple phobia. Likewise, panic attacks have not been noted with great frequency in OCD (31, although also see 8). Pharmacologic challenge with agents that provoke panic attacks or anxiety such as d-lactate (20) or yohimbine (D. Charney, *personal communication*) have failed to induce an increase in either anxiety or obsessions in patients with OCD. These results run counter to psychodynamic or behavioral formulations of obsessions as anxiety-reducing mechanisms. In fact, recent psychobiological data support more of a link with depression, rather than the traditional view of the obsessional syndrome as an anxiety disorder.

INTERACTION WITH DEPRESSION

Before the twentieth century, OCD was known as religious melancholy (41), or even as melancholy itself (22). In modern times, phenomenologic studies have demonstrated not only that obsessions are common in primary affective illness, but that depression is the most common complication of OCD (19,73) as well. Moreover, the ECA survey (58), like earlier studies (18,37), found significant overlap between "obsessive-compulsive disorder" and major depressive disorder.

As biological markers have been proposed as specific for primary depression, a number of recent studies have examined some of these same markers in OCD (28). Several (6,10,26), but not all (38,46), reports have described nonsuppression of the dexamethasone suppression test in OCD patients. Sleep electroencephalographic (EEG) abnormalities, including shortened rapid eye movement (REM) latency and decreased stage 4 sleep, have been demonstrated even in nondepressed patients with OCD (25). Reduced [³H]imipramine binding in the platelets of OCD patients has been reported in one (75) but was not evident in another study (27). And a blunted growth hormone response to clonidine, well documented in depressives (63), has also been reported in a small cohort of OCD patients (62).

On the other hand, the natural courses of these two illnesses are different. OCD is usually chronic, in contrast to primary depression, which tends to be episodic (9). The age of onset for OCD patients is young compared to primary depression, and the male/female ratio is different between these two disorders (lower for depression). At least one biological marker, platelet serotonin (5-HT) uptake, appears to be normal in OCD (27,75) yet is abnormal in most studies of major depressive disorder (45). Conversely, Shagass and co-workers (61) have reported an abnormal pattern in the middle latency waves of the somatosensory averaged evoked response (AER) that appears specifically in OCD and not in other psychiatric disorders, including depression. Therefore, it appears that though there are both clinical and biological similarities between the two syndromes, there are also significant differences that emerge from a careful comparison of OCD and affective illness.

This complicated relationship needs to be kept in mind when reviewing the pharmacologic treatment of OCD.

CLOMIPRAMINE TREATMENT FOR OBSESSIVE-COMPULSIVE DISORDER

Various medications have been given to OCD patients (2,29). The most promising developments, however, have been with the tricyclic antidepressant clomipramine (Anafranil, Ciba-Geigy). This drug is still not marketed in the United States but is widely used elsewhere. As early as 1968, Reynghe de Voxrie reported that clomipramine reduced the obsessional symptoms in 10 of his 15 depressed patients (57). During the 1970s a series of confirmatory but uncontrolled studies from England and Canada extended this initial observation for other patients with primary OCD (1,4,55).

More recently a group of carefully controlled double-blind studies using clomipramine have been published (Table 1) (3,15,30,40,47,68,74). These controlled studies show that clomipramine is more effective than placebo in reducing OCD symptomatology. Patients with rituals, as well as those with pure obsessions, appear to respond equally well to the drug. Combining the data from all the studies in Table 1, of 106 OCD patients treated with clomipramine, approximately two-thirds improved significantly, as measured by blind clinical ratings of their obsessive-compulsive symptoms. It is not always clear, however, how many of these patients were entirely free of their obsessions or compulsions following treatment. In the study by Insel et al. (30) the mean improvement on ratings of obsessions was only 34%, without any patient showing a complete response (four subsequently showed a full remission). The Flament et al. (15) study found two of 19 children to be symptom free at the end of 5 weeks on

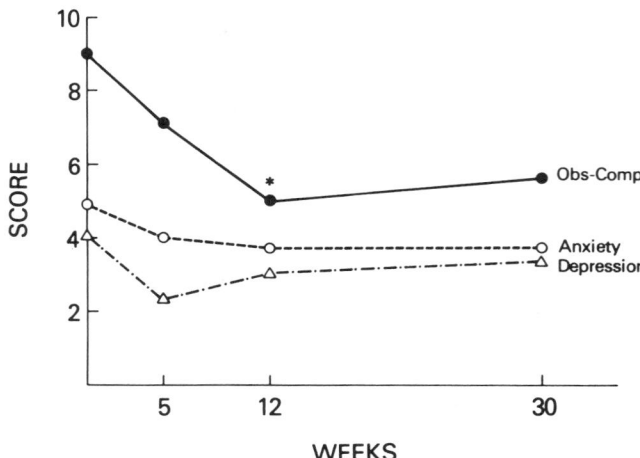

FIG. 1. Six OCD patients (fulfilling *Diagnostic and Statistical Manual-III* diagnostic criteria) were followed for 30 weeks on clomipramine (dose range: 150–300 mg/day). NIMH global rating (1–15 scale) of symptom severity shows maximal decrease ($p < 0.05$) in obsessive-compulsive symptoms at week 12.

TABLE 1. *Double-blind studies of clomipramine in obsessive-compulsive disorder*[a]

Ref.	No.	Design	Improvement in obsess Sx
68	35 (I)	Parallel CMI (150 mg) vs NOR (150 mg) vs PLAC	CMI > PLAC (5 weeks); NOR not >PLAC
40	40 (I then O)	Parallel CMI (183 mg) vs PLAC 4 weeks, then behav Rx	CMI > PLAC (4-week self rating only); CMI + behav Rx > PLAC + behav Rx (depressed subgroup only)
47	14	Crossover; CMI (75 mg) vs PLAC	CMI > PLAC (4 weeks)
3	20 (I + O)	Parallel; CMI (133 mg) vs AMI (197 mg)	CMI not AMI improved from baseline (4 weeks)
30	13 (I + O)	Crossover; CMI (236 mg) vs CLG (28 mg); PLAC control	CMI > CLG (4 + 6 weeks); PLAC ineffective
74	19 O	CMI (275 mg) vs IMI (265 mg)	CMI ≥ IMI (6 weeks)
	then 16 O	Parallel	CMI > IMI (12 weeks)
15	19 (I + O)	Crossover; CMI (141 mg) vs PLAC	CMI > PLAC (5 + 5 weeks) (childhood OCD)

[a] Abbreviations: I, inpatients; O, outpatients; CMI, clomipramine; NOR, nortriptyline; PLAC, placebo; AMI, amitriptyline; CLG, clorgyline; IMI, imipramine.

clomipramine, although the overall group improvement was again approximately 35%.

In contrast to depression, a relatively long period of time was needed in most studies for clomipramine to appear significantly effective. Volavka et al. (74) found clomipramine's reduction of obsessional symptomatology exceeded imipramine's effects only at 12 weeks of treatment. Marks et al. (40) pointed out that it took 10 weeks for clomipramine to reach its maximum response. Thoren et al. stated that "amelioration with clomipramine is a relatively slow process and it is not until the fifth week that the differences between treatments (clomipramine, placebo, nortriptyline) are clear cut" (68). Our experience is in line with these observations. As can be seen from Fig. 1, in six patients followed for 30 weeks on clomipramine, global ratings (0–15 scale) of symptom severity showed maximal decreases in obsessive-compulsive symptoms only after 12 weeks of treatment. Note that in this group, depression and anxiety scores are relatively low at baseline and show little change with treatment.

ANTIDEPRESSANT OR ANTIOBSESSIONAL?

Do these results with clomipramine reflect a specific antiobsessional effect or is the drug simply an effective antidepressant for a group of patients who frequently become depressed? Data from several different approaches to this question have provided somewhat conflicting answers. Marks et al. (39,40) attempted to answer this question by separating the OCD patients into most and least depressed subgroups based on depression ratings prior to treatment. A beneficial effect for clomipramine emerged only in the most depressed subgroup, suggesting an antidepressant but not a specific antiobsessional effect. Unfortunately, this study included behavior therapy, which may be more effective in nondepressed obsessionals, and thus may have obscured a medication effect in this subgroup. Mavissakalian and Michelson (42) in a small sample of eight OCD patients also reported improvement only in their depressed subgroup.

Only three of their patients received clomipramine, however; the remaining five received imipramine. In a subsequent extension of this study including seven additional subjects treated with clomipramine, Mavissakalian et al. (43) found *identical* decreases in obsessional symptoms between the most and least depressed subgroups.

Following the strategy of Marks et al., Insel and co-workers also compared most and least depressed OCD patients (30), but found equivalent responses of obsessional symptoms to clomipramine. In a single case studied with repeated blind trials of clomipramine following both high and low baseline depression ratings, these same investigators found robust and equal decreases in obsessional ratings (24). Thoren et al. (68) also found no significant statistical difference between pretreatment severity of depressive symptomatology (as measured by the Montgomery and Asberg scale) in 12 OCD patients who responded to clomipramine and 10 OCD patients who did not respond to clomipramine. They concluded that "The anti-obsessional effect of clomipramine is not confined only to patients who also have a manifest depression." Similarly, Montgomery (47), in his study of 19 OCD patients treated with clomipramine, found no significant change in depression (as measured by Montgomery and Asberg Depression Rating Scale) compared with placebo treatment, but significant improvement in obsessional symptoms. Ananth et al. (3) also reported that "There was no relationship between the improvement in depression and decrease in obsessive symptoms in 9 patients who were treated with clomipramine." Recently both Volavka et al. (74) and Flament et al. (15) also reported that the effect of clomipramine on OCD symptomatology was independent of the initial severity of depression.

It seems, therefore, that high depression ratings are not a prerequisite for an antiobsessional response to clomipramine. In this regard OCD resembles other nonaffective disorders such as panic disorder, bulimia, enuresis, migraine, and chronic pain syndrome, in which tricyclics are found to be effective also in the absence of initial (either primary or secondary) depression (49). What is curious about OCD and clomipramine is the lack of evidence that other antidepressants are effective.

OTHER ANTIDEPRESSANTS

The antiobsessional effect of clomipramine has been compared to nortriptyline (68), amitriptyline (3), clorgyline (30), imipramine (74), zimelidine (27), and desipramine (27) in controlled studies that were carried out in order to evaluate other antidepressants for antiobsessional effects. Clomipramine was found to be clearly more effective than the monoamine oxidase (MAO) inhibitor clorgyline in a crossover, double-blind, placebo-controlled study that involved 13 OCD patients (30). Thoren et al. (68) reported that the effects of nortriptyline were intermediate between placebo and clomipramine and not significantly different from either. Volavka et al. (74) reported clomipramine to be more effective than imipramine in its antiobsessional properties at 12 but not at 6 weeks of treatment. The lack of a placebo control and differences in the baseline severity and symptom clusters between the drug groups hamper the interpretation of these results.

Experience with electroconvulsive therapy (ECT), while limited, has not been particularly promising in OCD. Several authorities have discouraged the use of ECT for these patients (21,59,66) even while recognizing the efficacy of this treatment for depression. Mellman and Gorman (44) described an excellent response to ECT in a *nondepressed* 60-year-old obsessional. This report, however, appears to be an exception. Guttmacher (*unpublished manuscript*) recently reviewed eight well-diagnosed cases of OCD treated with ECT and found four to have both antiobsessional and antidepressant responses. The improvement in obsessions required a prolonged series of treatments which in one case was associated with subjective memory impairment and in two others was transient. In three other patients, ECT was followed by improvement in depressive but not obsessional symptoms.

The evidence thus is accumulating that clomipramine might be more effective than other antidepressant treatments for reducing obsessional symptomatology. Table 2 summarizes data from a series of double-blind trials in OCD patients performed over the past 5 years by our group (27, 30, *unpublished data*). These results suggest that desipramine, clorgyline, and zimelidine, all excellent antidepressants, are generally not useful to patients with OCD. Clearly more studies comparing clomipramine to other tricyclics are needed.

As might be expected with such a chronic and treatment-refractory condition, there have been case reports documenting antiobsessional responses to a wide range of psychotropic drugs. These reports include tranylcypromine (33,34), phenelzine (5,32), clonidine (36), alprazolam (67,70), trazodone (7,53), and lithium (65). Of particular interest, Rasmussen (56) and others (11,65) reported that the addition of lithium could increase the antiobsessional effect of a tricyclic antidepressant. This effect had been previously documented for treatment of refractory depressed patients by de Montigny (48). Further studies with lithium are needed. In the United States, where clomipramine is not available, it would be useful to know whether lithium might augment the effects of other tricyclics.

CLOMIPRAMINE AND THE SEROTONIN HYPOTHESIS

If clomipramine is more effective than other tricyclics in OCD, is there some neurochemical effect of clomipramine that might be relevant to the pathophysiology of OCD? Clomipramine is distinguished from other tricyclics by its high potency for inhibiting serotonin reuptake. This observation has led to the so-called "serotonin hypothesis" of OCD. Evidence supporting a role for clomipramine's effects on serotonin as mediating the drug's antiobsessional effects is as follows: (a) The plasma level of clomipramine (which selectively blocks serotonin reuptake), but not the plasma level of its primary metabolite, desmethylclomipramine (which blocks both serotonin and norepinephrine reuptake), correlates significantly with a reduction in obsessive-compulsive symptoms (30,64). (b) There is a significant correlation between the drug-induced reduction of OCD symptoms and the reduction in the cerebrospinal fluid (CSF) serotonin metabolite 5-hydroxyindoleacetic acid (5-HIAA) (69) and platelet serotonin (15). (c) Preclinical evidence suggests that the addition of lithium to chronic tricyclic administration (clinically associated with an increased an-

TABLE 2. *Change in CPRS-measured obsessional symptoms*[a]

Drug	Total no.	Moderately improved	Slightly improved	No change	Worse
		Change Score ≥3	(2–1)	(0)	(<0)
Clomipramine	25	13	10	1	1
Clorgyline	11	0	7	1	3
Desipramine	14	2	4	4	4
Zimelidine	5	1	1	1	2
Placebo	16	0	4	5	7

[a] CPRS indicates Comprehensive Psychiatric Scale—Obsessive-Compulsive Subscale (68) (8 items rated 0–3). Data are taken from a series of double-blind trials in both inpatients and outpatients with primary OCD. Change is calculated by subtracting baseline score from score at either 5 or 6 weeks of treatment.

tiobsessional effect) induces an increase in serotonergic electrophysiologic activity (48). (d) In an uncontrolled trial, the serotonin precursor L-tryptophan was reported to reduce obsessional symptoms (78).

Following the line of this hypothesis, one might expect that other potent serotonergic reuptake blockers would have antiobsessional properties as well. Initial reports have been mixed. Although most studies with zimelidine (17,35,52) and fluoxetine (16,71) have been promising, the effects in some cases (71) have been subtle. One placebo-controlled double-blind study (27) could not demonstrate that zimelidine was more effective than desipramine and found both less effective than clomipramine for reducing OCD symptoms. This study, while limited to only five patients on zimelidine, was notable because CSF measures of serotonin turnover were roughly equal in the zimelidine and clomipramine groups. It appeared, therefore, that changes in serotonergic function may be necessary, but were not sufficient, for an antiobsessional response in this small group treated with zimelidine.

Although serotonin has been implicated in the mediation of aggression, anxiety, and social dominance in animal studies (72), there is no compelling evidence for a serotonergic abnormality as etiologic in OCD. Yaryura-Tobias reported reduced whole blood serotonin in OCD patients (77), but more recent studies focusing on serotonin platelet uptake have failed (27,75) to find an abnormality. Platelet [^{3}H]imipramine binding was reduced in one (75) but not another (27) cohort of OCD patients. Using a different approach, oral administration of the 5 HT-lb agonist m-chlorophenylpiperazine (m-CPP), which has very limited behavioral effects in normal volunteers, appears in preliminary studies to profoundly increase obsessional symptoms in patients with OCD (80).

Whether clomipramine's antiobsessional effects are mediated via the serotonergic system is a separate question that deserves further study. Although it is tempting to associate the drug's potency for reducing obsessional symptoms with its potency for blocking serotonin reuptake, several other actions of clomipramine, such as its potent uncoupling effects on oxidative phosphorylation (79), its distinct potency for Ca^{2+} channel blockade (author's *unpublished data*), and its actions on the opiate system (12,13) may be equally important.

CONCLUSION

In the last decade new therapeutic approaches to OCD have increased scientific interest in a disorder that has long been considered to be chronic and resistant to treatment. Behavioral treatments have repeatedly been shown to reduce compulsive behaviors. Drug treatment may augment behavioral therapy (1) although an increased effectiveness for such a combined approach is still not proven. Patients who do not have avoidant behavior or rituals amenable to behavior therapy are certainly excellent candidates for medication. Depression should not be considered a prerequisite for using medication in an OCD patient. Clomipramine is currently the drug treatment of choice with antiobsessional effects apparently independent of antidepressant

effects. More information is needed about the long-term pharmacologic management of the patient with OCD. Since this syndrome is more chronic than depression, studies in the next few years will need to focus on duration of treatment and long-term outcome.

Obsessive-compulsive disorder offers the psychopharmacologist a unique opportunity. Here is a syndrome that appears refractory to most psychotropics, with, thus far, response being clearly demonstrated to the tricyclic clomipramine and, to some extent, to newer, serotonin-selective antidepressants. The careful unraveling of those features that distinguish antiobsessional compounds from structurally related but ineffective agents may reveal a mechanism of action. Ultimately, such a mechanism could implicate a particular neurochemical system in the pathophysiology of this disorder.

REFERENCES

1. Amin, M. M., Ban, T. A., and Pecknold, J. C. (1977): *J. Int. Med. Res.,* 5:33–37.
2. Ananth, J. (1976): *Psychosomatics,* 17:180–184.
3. Ananth, J., Pecknold, J. C., van der Steen, N., and Engelsmann, F. (1981): *Prog. Neuropsychopharmacol. Biol. Psychiatry,* 5:257–264.
4. Ananth, J., Solyom, L., Bryntwick, S., and Krischnappa, U. (1979): *Am. J. Psychiatry,* 136:700–701.
5. Annesley, P. T. (1969): *Br. J. Psychiatry,* 115:748.
6. Asberg, M., Thoren, P., and Bertilsson, L. (1982): *Psychopharmacol. Bull.,* 18:13–21.
7. Baxter, L. R. (1985): *J. Nerv. Ment. Dis.,* 173:432–433.
8. Boyd, J. H., Burke, J. D., Gruenberg, E., Holzer, C. E., Rae, D. S., George, L. K., Karno, M., Stoltzman, R., McEvoy, L., and Nestadt, G. (1984): *Arch. Gen. Psychiatry,* 41:983–989.
9. Coryell, W. (1981): *J. Nerv. Ment. Dis.,* 169:220–224.
10. Cottraux, J. A., Bouvard, M., Claustrat, B., and Juenet, C. (1984): *Psychiatry Res.,* 13:157–165.
11. Eisenberg, J., and Asnis, G. (1985): *Am. J. Psychiatry,* 142:663.
12. Eschalier, A., Montastrus, J. L., Devoize, J. L., Rigal, G., Gaillard-Plaza, G., and Pechadre, J. C. (1981): *Eur. J. Pharmacol.,* 74:1–7.
13. Eschalier, A., Rigal, F., Devoize, J. L., Trolese, J. F., and Grillon, C. (1983): *Eur. J. Pharmacol.,* 91:505–507.
14. Flament, M., and Rapoport, J. (1984): In: *New Findings in Obsessive-Compulsive Disorder,* edited by T. R. Insel, pp. 24–43. American Psychiatric Press, Washington, DC.
15. Flament, M. F., Rapoport, J. L., Berg, C. J., Sceery, W., Kilts, C., Mellstrom, B., and Linnoila, M. (1985): *Arch. Gen. Psychiatry,* 42:977–986.
16. Fontaine, R., and Chouinard, G. (1985): *Am. J. Psychiatry,* 142: 989.
17. Fontaine, R., Chouinard, G., and Iny, L. (1985): *Curr. Ther. Res.,* 37:326–332.
18. Gittleson, N. (1966): *Br. J. Psychiatry,* 112:883–887.
19. Goodwin, D., Guze, S., and Robins, E. (1969): *Arch. Gen. Psychiatry,* 20:182–187.
20. Gorman, J. M., Liebowitz, M. R., Fyer, A. J., Dillon, D., Davies, S. O., Stein, J., and Klein, D. F. (1985): *Am. J. Psychiatry,* 142: 864–866.
21. Grimshaw, L. (1965): *Br. J. Psychiatry,* 111:1051–1056.
22. Hunter, R., and MacAlpine, I. (1963): *Three Hundred Years of Psychiatry.* Oxford University Press, London.
23. Insel, T. R. (1984): In: *New Findings in Obsessive-Compulsive Disorder,* edited by T. R. Insel, pp. 2–22. American Psychiatric Press, Washington, DC.
24. Insel, T. R., Alterman, I., and Murphy, D. L. (1982): *Psychopharmacol. Bull.,* 18:315–319.
25. Insel, T. R., Gillin, J. C., Moore, A., Loewenstein, R., Murphy, D. L., and Mendelson, W. (1982): *Arch. Gen. Psychiatry,* 39: 1372–1377.

26. Insel, T. R., Kalin, N. H., Guttmacher, L. B., Cohen, R. M., and Murphy, D. L. (1982): *Psychiatry Res.,* 6:153–158.
27. Insel, T. R., Mueller, E. A., Alterman, I., Linnoila, M., and Murphy, D. L. (1985): *Biol. Psychiatry,* 20:1174–1188.
28. Insel, T. R., Mueller, E. A., Gillin, J. C., Siever, L. J., and Murphy, D. L. (1984): *J. Psychiatry Res.,* 18:407–425.
29. Insel, T. R., and Murphy, D. L. (1981): *J. Clin. Psychopharmacol.,* 1:304–311.
30. Insel, T. R., Murphy, D. L., Cohen, R. M., Alterman, I., Linnoila, M., and Kilts, C. (1983): *Arch. Gen. Psychiatry,* 40:605–612.
31. Insel, T. R., Zahn, T., and Murphy, D. L. (1985): In: *Anxiety and the Anxiety Disorders,* edited by H. Tuma and J. Masur, pp. 577–589. Lawrence Erlbaum, Englewood Cliffs, NJ.
32. Jain, V. K., Swinson, R. P., and Thomas, J. E. (1970): *Br. J. Psychiatry,* 127:237–238.
33. Jenike, M. A. (1981): *Am. J. Psychiatry,* 138:1249–1250.
34. Jenike, M. A., Surman, O. S., Cassem, N. H., Zusky, P., and Anderson, W. H. (1983): *J. Clin. Psychiatry,* 4:131–132.
35. Kahn, R. S., Westenberg, H. G. M., and Jolles, J. (1984): *Acta Psychiatr. Scand.,* 69:259–261.
36. Knesevich, J. W. (1982): *Am. J. Psychiatry,* 139:364–365.
37. Lewis, A. J. (1936): *Proc. R. Soc. Med.,* 29:325–336.
38. Lieberman, J. A., Kane, J. M., Sarantakos, S., Cole, K., Houvard, A., Borenstein, M., Novacenko, H., and Puig-Antich, J. (1985): *Am. J. Psychiatry,* 142:747–751.
39. Marks, I. M. (1983): *Br. J. Psychiatry,* 143:338–347.
40. Marks, I. M., Stern, R., Mawson, D., Cobb, J., and McDonald, R. (1980): *Br. J. Psychiatry,* 136:1–25.
41. Maudsley, H. (1895): *The Pathology of the Mind.* Macmillan, London.
42. Mavissakalian, M., and Michelson, L. (1983): *J. Nerv. Ment. Dis.,* 171:301–306.
43. Mavissakalian, M., Turner, S., Michelson, L., and Jacob, R. (1985): *Am. J. Psychiatry,* 142:572–576.
44. Mellman, L. A., and Gorman, J. M. (1984): *Am. J. Psychiatry,* 141:596–597.
45. Meltzer, H. H., Arora, R. C., and Song, P. (1982): In: *Biological Markers in Psychiatry and Neurology,* edited by E. Usdin and E. Costa. Pergamon Press, New York.
46. Monterio, W., Marks, I. M., Noshiruani, H., and Checkley, S. (1986): *Br. J. Psychiatry,* 148:326–329.
47. Montgomery, S. A. (1980): *Pharm. Med.,* 1:189–192.
48. Montigny, C. de, and Cournoyer, G. (1987): In: *Treating Resistant Depression,* edited by J. Zohar and R. H. Belmaker. Pergamon Press, New York (*in press*).
49. Murphy, D. L., Siever, L. J., and Insel, T. R. (1985): *Prog. Neuropsychopharmacol. Biol. Psychiatry,* 9:3–13.
50. Nemiah, J. (1984): In: *New Findings in Obsessive-Compulsive Disorder,* edited by T. R. Insel, pp. xi–xii. American Psychiatric Press, Washington, DC.
51. Pollitt, J. (1957): *Br. Med. J.,* 1:194–197.
52. Prasad, A. (1984): *Pharmacopsychiatry,* 17:61–62.
53. Prasad, A. (1985): *Pharmacol. Biochem. Behav.,* 22:347–348.
54. Rachman, S. (1983): In: *Failures in Behavior Therapy,* edited by E. B. Foa and P. M. G. Emmelkamp, pp. 35–58. Wiley Press, New York.
55. Rack, P. H. (1977): *J. Int. Med. Res.,* 5:81–96.
56. Rasmussen, S. A. (1984): *Am. J. Psychiatry,* 141:1283–1285.
57. Renynghe de Voxrie, G. V. (1968): *Acta Neurol. Belg.,* 68:787–792.
58. Robins, L. N., Helzer, Y. E., Weissman, M. M., Orvaschel, H., Gruenberg, E., Burke, J. D., and Regier, D. A. (1984): *Arch. Gen. Psychiatry,* 41:949–967.
59. Roth, M. (1965): *Practitioner,* 194:613–620.
60. Salzman, L., and Thaler, F. H. (1981): *Am. J. Psychiatry,* 138:286–296.
61. Shagass, C., Roemer, R. A., Straumanis, J. J., and Josiassen, R. C. (1984): *Biol. Psychiatry,* 19:1507–1524.
62. Siever, L. J., Insel, T. R., Jimerson, D. L., Lake, C. R., Uhde, T. W., Aloi, J., and Murphy, D. L. (1983): *Br. J. Psychiatry,* 142:184–187.
63. Siever, L. J., and Uhde, T. W. (1984): *Biol. Psychiatry,* 19:131–156.
64. Stern, R. S., Marks, I. M., and Wright, J. (1980): *Postgrad. Med. J.,* 56:134–139.
65. Stern, T. A., and Jenike, M. A. (1983): *Psychosomatics,* 24:673–674.
66. Sternberg, M. (1974): In: *Obsessional States,* edited by H. R. Beech, pp. 291–307. Methuen, London.
67. Tesar, G. E., and Jenike, M. A. (1984): *Am. J. Psychiatry,* 141:689–690.
68. Thoren, P., Asberg, M., Bertilsson, L., Mellstrom, B., Sjoqvist, F., and Traskman, L. (1980): *Arch. Gen. Psychiatry,* 37:1289–1294.
69. Thoren, P., Asberg, M., Cronholm, B., Jornestedt, L., and Traskman, L. (1980): *Arch. Gen. Psychiatry,* 37:1281–1285.
70. Tollefson, G. (1985): *J. Clin. Psychopharmacol.,* 5:39–42.
71. Turner, S., Jacob, R., Beidel, D. C., and Himmelhach, J. (1985): *J. Clin. Psychopharmacol.,* 5:207–212.
72. Valzelli, L. (1984): *Prog. Neuropsychopharmacol. Biol. Psychiatry,* 8:311–325.
73. Vaughan, M. (1976): *Br. J. Psychiatry,* 129:36–39.
74. Volavka, J., Neziroglu, F., and Yaryura-Tobias, J. A. (1985): *Psychiatry Res.,* 14:83–91.
75. Weizman, A., Carmi, M., Hermesh, H., Shahar, A., Apter, A., Tyano, S., and Rehavi, M. (1986): *Am. J. Psychiatry,* 143:335–339.
76. Woodruff, R., and Pitts, F. (1969): *Am. J. Psychiatry,* 120:1075–1080.
77. Yaryura-Tobias, J. A., Bebirian, R. J., Neziroglu, F. A., and Bhagavan, H. N. (1977): *Res. Commun. Psychol. Psychiatry Behav.,* 2:279–286.
78. Yaryura-Tobias, J. A., and Bhagavan, H. N. (1977): *Am. J. Psychiatry,* 234:1298–1299.
79. Zilberstein, D., and Dwyer, D. M. (1984): *Science,* 226:977–979.
80. Zohar J., Mueller, E. A., Insel, T. R., Zohar-Kodouch, R., and Murphy, D. L. (1987): *Arch. Gen. Psychiatry* (*in press*).

Psychopharmacology:
The Third Generation of Progress,
edited by Herbert Y. Meltzer.
Raven Press, New York © 1987.

CHAPTER 124

Pediatric Psychopharmacology: The Last Decade

Judith L. Rapoport

This greatly expanded section on pediatric psychopharmacology reflects the many changes since the 1978 publication of *A Generation of Progress.* There has been an explosion in rating and diagnostic scales, new areas of major interest, some implications for diagnosis, and areas of research expansion. In a separate section, more basic studies are reviewed having specific relevance to childhood disorders. This provides an overview of the section on clinical studies, and current, more general issues in pediatric psychopharmacology.

METHODOLOGY

In the last decade, pediatric psychopharmacology has come into its own with the first two major textbooks of pediatric psychopharmacology (30,31). The December 1985 special issue of *Psychopharmacology Bulletin* devoted to Rating Scales and Methodology for Pediatric Psychopharmacological studies, edited by Rapoport and Conners (24), the first revision since the 1976 ECDEU Assessment Manual for Psychopharmacology, is greatly expanded in scope. The 1976 *Bulletin* contained pediatric scales primarily for ward ratings of psychotic, hyperactive, and aggressive behaviors. There are now scales for rating hyperactivity in adolescents and adults, and the ratings for autistic and stereotyped behaviors have been made clearer to differentiate these behaviors from adverse drug effects. In addition to the new level of sophistication in assessments, there is a greatly broadened range of assessments. This is reflected in the new sections on structured interviews for children, social skills, cognitive measures, compliance, and side effect measures in children. In addition, depression, anxiety, Tourette's syndrome, and obsessive compulsive disorder are included.

Finally, side effects are covered in greater depth with inclusion of systematic ratings of abnormal involuntary movements.

From the variety of scales one realizes that stimulant drug studies have become a virtual cottage industry, with rating scales sensitive to drug effects on peer and family interaction, behavioral change in adolescents, and more subtle cognitive effects including effects on new learning.

There is a new sizable section on childhood depression, although the lack of clearly demonstrated efficacy of antidepressants for depressed pediatric populations remains puzzling (see below). Finally, there is a greatly expanded repertoire of rating methods for eating behaviors, reflecting the recent interest in drug treatment of anorexia and bulimia.

DSM-III-R AND PEDIATRIC PSYCHOPHARMACOLOGY

Diagnostically, as Gittelman, Spitzer, and Cantwell (12) had stressed, it was hoped that drug responsivity of pediatric groups would contribute to the validity of diagnostic categories. *Diagnostic and Statistical Manual of Mental Disorders,* 3rd edition (DSM-III) brought major changes to the U.S. diagnostic system, but particularly important were the addition of numerous subgroups, and new entities in the pediatric area, during a time when pediatric psychopharmacology was expanding dramatically.

The most important changes were the descriptive, operational definition of syndromes, urging the use of multiple diagnosis, the multiaxial approach, that included placing specific developmental disabilities on a separate axis (axis II). Within axis I (behavioral syndromes), the most notable changes from DSM-II were the clear separation of Pervasive Developmental Disorders from Schizophrenic disorders, the subtyping of Conduct Disorders and renaming "Hyperkinetic Reaction" as Attention Deficit Disorder. Several anxiety disorders were specifically placed in the childhood category, and the Eating Disorders section was expanded.

Studies using psychopharmacologic agents in pediatric groups have implications for DSM-III; therapeutic efficacy can indicate continuity with adult conditions and support the validity (or lack) of diagnostic distinctions. Conversely, new distinctions in DSM-III might lead to "cleaner" therapeutic drug trials. At the time of this writing (1985), there are only relatively few methodologically sound, relevant studies; these are reviewed by diagnostic category.

"Externalizing Disorders": Attention Deficit Disorder, Conduct Disorder, and Oppositional Disorder

A major diagnostic question for the externalizing disorders group is the continuity/discontinuity between conduct disorder and attention deficit disorder. Certainly there is some reason to think that stimulants might be useful both for conduct disorders and for hyperactivity, supporting continuity between the two. A few studies have addressed this point.

Early studies with stimulants took place in a training school for delinquent boys (6), and recently a more careful examination of mixed cases, the rule in most clinics, indicates decrease in both restless/inattentive and aggressive behaviors with stimulant drug treatment in such cases (2). However, a key question remains: Do "pure" conduct disordered children respond to stimulants?

The only attempt to address this question to date is that of Taylor et al. (26). This study of 38 boys with presenting problems of serious conduct disorder indicated that methylphenidate (maximum 30 mg/day) for 3 weeks, compared to placebo, decreased restless/inattentive behavior most conspicuously, and the decrease in antisocial behavior was less impressive.

However, some (e.g., teacher-rated) measures of defiance were significantly reduced even though parent reports did not indicate such changes. The study supports some diagnostic validation of "ADD" by stimulants, but several problems in interpretation of these data remain. First, defiant behaviors are typically less frequent than restlessness and inattention and the short time period (3 weeks) may have been insufficient for adequate rating of change. More important, the mixed cases seen in Taylor's study may not be the ones most instructive to treat; the study remaining is of stimulant drug response of severely conduct-disordered children who are not motorically restless and who do not differ from age-matched controls in attentional tasks. The response or lack of response of this rare but instructive group would be of particular interest.

The use of stimulants in adults giving childhood histories of hyperactivity is of particular practical concern; Wender (29) has pioneered the use of stimulants for an often ignored and untreated adult patient group. However, only one study has addressed the specificity of this response, that is, whether the adults with childhood history have a *different* response to stimulant than does an adult group

with similar current problems but *without* a childhood history of hyperactivity. Mattes et al. (17) carried out such a comparison study in which 26 adults with ADDH-RT were compared with 35 "hyperactive" adults without childhood history using a maximum of 30 mg of methylphenidate for 3 weeks, twice a day with a counter-balanced double-blind placebo control.

The results were disappointing. No overall benefit of methylphenidate was evident regardless of childhood history. Approximately 25% of the sample did seem to gain some benefit, but no clear-cut predictors of drug response were identified. Most notably the history of childhood hyperactivity had no prediction for response.

This is an important study; it questions the usefulness of stimulant drug treatment in at least a large group of "likely" adult subjects, and casts doubt upon the stimulant drug response as validating the particular diagnostic group (ADD-RT) as had been hoped.

Childhood ADD *without* hyperactivity is a controversial category. Some have found such groups quite heterogeneous, and not continuous clinically with hyperactivity (16,18). However, a study waiting to be undertaken is a stimulant drug trial of children with academic failure who receive such a diagnosis. If a (rare) subgroup of, for example, "learning-disabled" children are handicapped primarily or exclusively by inattention, then such a trial would be particularly worthwhile.

Whereas stimulant drugs have generally proved disappointing in the treatment of learning disabilities and academic failure (8), a useful study would be of stimulant drug treatment of children with academic failure in whom careful diagnostic educational testing indicated *only* inattention as the basis for educational lag. Such a group would most probably have failure of classroom performance but be found to read on grade level with individual testing. Individual case reports are suggestive (25), and although such a group might be difficult to identify, successful treatment of a subgroup of attention-disordered children would indicate continuity with at least one variety of ADD with childhood hyperactivity. At this writing, however, Attention Deficit Disorder without hyperactivity will probably be dropped from DSM-III-R (revised) because of the rarity of use and questionable status discussed above.

Finally, an important review by Aman (1) reminds us of the lack of efficacy of stimulants in autistic and retarded populations. Although there is work to be done in this area (dose-response relationship, more homogeneous populations), it does seem that at least *some* populations of children manifesting behavioral overactivity will not respond to stimulants and even worsen. In a broad sense, then, stimulant drug studies have contributed to conceptual validation.

Childhood Depressive Disorder

There has been dramatic increase in interest in childhood depression with important studies on biological validation of this syndrome (20,21), suggesting continuity with adult disorder. However, the status of antidepressant treatment for this disorder remains ambiguous. To date, there is no unequivocal evidence of a drug-placebo difference in response to antidepressants in prepubertal depressed children or depressed adolescents. The first well-controlled study of Puig-Antich et al. (22) did not find such a difference, owing, perhaps, to the sizable improvement (68%) in the placebo-treated group. In spite of this lack of drug-placebo difference, the significant correlation with plasma tricyclic concentration and clinical improvement indicated that concentrations over 150 mg/ml were differentially effective. Since then, other studies have suggested that children may be safely treated with tricyclics and that plasma concentrations between 125 and 225 mg/ml of imipramine are best for maximal clinical improvement (19,28). However, only the study of Kashani et al. (15) has showed superiority to placebo in a controlled trial. Kashani et al. treated nine prepubertal depressed children (mean age 10.8 years) by random assignment to 4 weeks of amitriptyline (maximum dose 1.5 mg/kg/day) or placebo, following which the children received 4 weeks of the alternate treatment. There was a trend ($p = 0.08$) for drug treatment to be superior. However, the relatively low doses of drug, and crossover design (which permits maximum "guess" about drug phase), antidepressants (TCAs) are only indicated after other supportive measures, including extended placebo trial, have failed.

A number of interesting diagnostic approaches might be tried if antidepressant treatment were efficacious. For example, for mixed conduct disordered-depressed adolescents, a trial of TCAs with *delayed* drug action that improved both mood and conduct disorder would suggest underlying depression as primary to the conduct disorder. However, even in adolescent populations diagnosed as major depressive disorder, significant differential effects of TCAs compared with placebo are lacking (23).

In summary, whereas the DSM-III diagnosis of major depressive disorder seems valid for children at least above the age of 7, the contribution of pediatric psychopharmacology to this validation has been ambiguous. Further details are given by Ambrosini (Chapter 129, *this volume*).

Childhood Obsessive-Compulsive Disorder

A recent series of studies has investigated the treatment of obsessive-compulsive disorder with the tricyclic antidepressant clomipramine (Anafranil, Ciba Geigy), which is not yet available in the United States although widely prescribed in Europe, Canada, and South America. At least one-third of adult obsessives had the onset of their disorder in childhood, but only one study has specifically addressed the pharmacological treatment of children and adolescents. Flament et al. (7), using a double-blind, crossover design, found that clomipramine (mean dose 140 ± 30 mg) at the end of 5 weeks was superior to placebo. In this study, the presence of depression did not predict the antiobsessional effect of the drug, indicating the independence of the obsessive-compulsive disorder and its amelioration from depression. This provides strong evidence and continuity between the childhood-onset and adult-onset disorder. The mechanism for clomipramine effect remains unclear. Insel et al. (14) found another, generally effective antidepressant, clorgyline, to be clinically ineffective for obsessions, and a recent study by Insel (*personal communication*) has demonstrated the superiority of clomipramine over desmeth-

ylimipramine for a small group of adult obsessional patients, as has also been found with adolescents (Leonard, *personal communication*).

The failure of this disorder to generally respond well to antianxiety agents is one of several arguments against placing the disorder within the anxiety disorders section of DSM-III. It is intriguing to speculate that at least the childhood onset obsessives are those who later may develop secondary depressive or anxiety symptomatology but who initially have quite a separate "pure" condition. The family history of the adolescent group studied at NIH also indicated *discontinuity* from depressive disorder, although these data are beyond the scope of this review.

Childhood Anxiety Disorders

Since the landmark study of Gittelman and Klein (9) demonstrating a significant benefit from 6 weeks treatment with imipramine (mean dose 159 mg/day) compared to placebo for 45 school-phobic children, there has been little additional work. One study, that of Berney et al. (3), found clomipramine (40–75 mg/day) to be ineffective, but the low doses of the latter study make interpretation difficult.

The response of adult agoraphobics to imipramine suggests continuity between childhood separation anxiety and adult agoraphobia. Family studies indicate that childhood separation anxiety is linked specifically to adult panic disorder rather than to parental generalized anxiety (27). However, the presence of previous or current separation anxiety in adult patients with panic disorder does not predict the response to imipramine (10).

The use of antianxiety agents in childhood conditions is unexplored. The specificity of tricyclic treatment has not been established; for example, no trial of imipramine for childhood generalized anxiety disorder has been reported. Similarly, the use of other agents (e.g., diazepam or alprazolam) for childhood separation anxiety has also not been studied systematically. This will be the major new thrust of research in the next decade for pediatric psychopharmacology. The evidence that both imipramine and monoamine oxidase inhibitors are superior to the benzodiazepines in the treatment of adult panic attacks and agoraphobia has lent support to a biological basis for these disorders; such support is already present from genetic studies and lactate stimulation of attacks. The application of this notion to nosology of childhood anxiety disorders remains one of the most intriguing problems in our field. A circular problem exists at present: Pediatric patients do not fit readily into the present DSM-III subgroups, often presenting with some feature of separation anxiety, phobia, and/or generalized anxiety. Drug studies rely on careful patient definition. Until clarifying family and follow-up studies are carried out, drug trials in this area remain a bootstrap operation.

Specific Developmental Disorders (Axis II)

DSM-III separated specific childhood developmental disorders on a separate axis, in part to ensure that they be noted in addition to the axis I disorders—the major behavioral syndromes. There have been a few interesting trials of drug treatment in this area: specifically, piracetam, a substance structurally related to γ-aminobutyric acid (GABA) and vasopressin (DDAVP). Piracetam (4,13) and DDAVP (5) have shown some mild beneficial effect in laboratory measures similar to that found with methylphenidate by Gittelman et al. (11).

Recently piracetam has been studied in neuropsychological paradigms in several populations, but most frequently in dyslexic groups. A total of 12 double-blind trials with dyslexic boys indicates improvement in verbal learning, single-word reading, short-term memory, or reading rate. The status of this drug is still uncertain in the United States, but it is likely to prompt more studies with learning-disabled children. It is still too soon to see whether this agent will reveal subgroups of responsive children that might break down along the usual subgrouping of dyslexics (e.g., language-disordered vs those with visual motor dysfunction).

About one-third of dyslexic children make gains (compared to none of most studies' control groups). Whether these findings are clinically meaningful is unclear, but as learning-disabled populations are so massive, there is great impetus for continued pharmacologic research.

In summary, DSM-III has provided clearer diagnostic guidelines for pediatric drug trials and has greatly facilitated communication among clinicians. However, further validation of new subgroups is yet to come.

NEW DIRECTIONS

As indicated in the section on diagnosis, there is interesting new work in the area of anxiety disorders, obsessive-compulsive disorder, and learning disorders and still some interest in the pharmacological treatment of depression (see Chapter 129, *this volume*). At this time, it is most clear that clinical treatment of obsessive adolescents is being modified to include pharmacological treatment. Whether behavior modification will have an equal place with clomipramine for pediatric patients remains to be seen. It may be that family management and problems with therapeutic alliance will place behavioral treatment at a disadvantage for pediatric subjects, but a comparative study with this group has yet to be undertaken.

There has not yet been sufficient new work on drug treatment of anxiety disorders in childhood to warrant a separate chapter. However, as this goes to press, a number of double-blind trials have been initiated using alprazolam for treatment of separation anxiety and generalized anxiety disorder in childhood, and a new study comparing behavior modification with imipramine in the treatment of separation anxiety disorder is being launched. As noted, the lack of diagnostic validation of subgrouping of childhood anxiety disorders is a stumbling block. Whether psychopharmacological trials will help clarify this is unclear. As panic attacks are extremely rare in childhood and adolescence, the major diagnostic issue will be between separation anxiety and GAD.

SUMMARY

The greatly expanded sections of this volume devoted to childhood conditions testify to the importance of this area. There are still conspicuously weak areas. There is little reliable data about childhood anxiety disorders or developmental disabilities, and extremely few studies specifically with adolescent populations. Studies with these groups have great practical and theoretical importance for our field. It is hoped that the next edition of this volume will remedy this lack.

REFERENCES

1. Aman, M. (1982): *J. Autism Dev. Disord.,* 12:385–398.
2. Amery, B. R., Minichiello, M., and Brown, G. (1984): *J. Am. Acad. Child Psychiatry,* 23:291–294.
3. Berney, T., Kolvin, I., Bhate, S., Garside, R., Jeans, J., Kay, B., and Scarth, L. (1981): *Br. J. Psychiatry,* 138:110–118.
4. Conners, C. K., Blouin, A., Winglee, M., Lougee, L., O'Donnell, D., and Smith, A. (1984): *Psychopharmacol. Bull.,* 20:667–673.
5. Eisenberg, J., Chazan-Gologorsky, S., Hattab, J., and Belmaker, R. H. (1984): *Biol. Psychiatry,* 19:1137–1141.
6. Eisenberg, L., Lachman, R., Molling, P., Lockner, A., Mizelle, J., and Conners, C. K. (1963): *Am. J. Orthopsychiatry,* 33:431–447.
7. Flament, M., Rapoport, J. L., Berg, C. J., and Kilts, C. (1985): *Arch. Gen. Psychiatry,* 21:150–152.
8. Gadow, K. D. (1983): *J. Learn. Dis.,* 16:290–299.
9. Gittelman, R., and Klein, D. F. (1973): *J. Nerv. Ment. Dis.,* 156:199–215.
10. Gittelman, R., and Klein, D. F. (1984): *Psychopathology,* 17(*Suppl.* 1):56–65.
11. Gittelman, R., Klein, D., and Feingold, I. (1983): *J. Child Psychol. Psychiatry,* 24:193–212.
12. Gittelman, R., Spitzer, R., and Cantwell, D. (1978): In: *Pediatric Psychopharmacology: The Use of Behavior Modifying Drugs in Children,* edited by J. Werry, pp. 136–170. Brunner/Mazel, New York.
13. Helfgott, E., Rudel, S. R., and Krieger, J. (1984): *Psychopharmacol. Bull.,* 20:688–690.
14. Insel, T., Murphy, R., Cohen, R., et al. (1983): *Arch. Gen. Psychiatry,* 40:605–621.
15. Kashani, J., Shekim, W., and Reid, J. (1984): *J. Am. Acad. Child Psychiatry,* 23:348–351.
16. Leahey, B., Schaughnecy, E., Strauss, C., and Frame, C. (1984): *J. Am. Acad. Child Psychiatry,* 23:302–309.
17. Mattes, J., Boswell, L., and Oliver, H. (1984): *Arch. Gen. Psychiatry,* 41:1059–1063.
18. Maurer, R., and Stewart, M. (1980): *J. Clin. Psychiatry,* 417:232–233.
19. Preskorn, S., Weller, E., and Weller, R. (1982): *J. Clin. Psychiatry,* 43:450–453.
20. Puig-Antich, J. (1986): In: *Depression in Young People: Development and Clinical Perspectives,* edited by M. Rutter, C. Izard, and P. Read, pp. 341–382. Guilford Press, New York.
21. Puig-Antich, J., Blau, S., Marx, N., et al. (1978): *J. Am. Acad. Child Psychiatry,* 17:695–707.
22. Puig-Antich, J., Perel, J., Luptakin, W., et al. (1979): *J. Am. Acad. Child Psychiatry,* 18:616–627.
23. Puig-Antich, J., Perel, J., Luptakin, W., Chambers, W., Tabrizi, M., King, J., Goetz, R., Johnson, R., and Stiller, R. (1987): *Arch. Gen. Psychol.,* 44:81–92.
24. Rapoport, J., and Conners, C. K., eds. (1985): *Psychopharmacol. Bull.,* 21:713–1124.
25. Schmidt, K., Solanto, M., Sanchez, M., Vargas, P., and Wein, S. (1984): *J. Clin. Psychopharmacol.,* 4:100–103.
26. Taylor, E., Schachar, R., Wieselberg, M., and Thorley, G. (1987): *J. Child Psychol. Psychiatry* (in press).
27. Weissman, M., Myers, J., Leckman, J., et al. (1982): Talk presented on Anxiety Disorders, Key Biscayne.
28. Weller, E., Weller, R., Preskorn, S., and Glotzbach, R. (1982): *Am. J. Psychiatry,* 139:506–509.
29. Wender, P., Reimherr, F., and Wood, D. (1981): *Arch. Gen. Psychiatry,* 38:449–456.
30. Werry, J. (1978): In: *Pediatric Psychopharmacology: The Use of Behavior Modifying Drugs in Children.* Brunner/Mazel, New York.
31. Wiener, J. M. (1977): In: *Psychopharmacology in Childhood and Adolescence.* Basic Books, New York.

Psychopharmacology:
The Third Generation of Progress,
edited by Herbert Y. Meltzer.
Raven Press, New York © 1987.

CHAPTER **125**

Pharmacotherapy of Childhood Hyperactivity: An Update

Rachel Gittelman Klein

The efficacy of various pharmacological interventions for the management of hyperactive children[1] has been established for well over a decade. As is the case in other pharmacotherapy research, recent scientific investigations have progressed to more refined issues of drug effect. Since the overall clinical efficacy of stimulants is no longer an issue, attention has turned to the identification of more subtle treatment effects, such as drug effects on mother/child and teacher/child interaction, clinical significance of stimulant effects, optimal dosage, and the relationship between plasma level and clinical action. Because no single treatment is completely effective, much hope has been placed in the addition of other types of interventions with pharmacotherapy. The study of combination treatments has been actively pursued in recent years.

This decade has seen a beginning interest in determining whether the psychostimulants that are so effective in childhood are appropriate in adolescence, and whether treatment in childhood has a positive effect on long-term outcome.

The deleterious effects of pharmacotherapy are a continuing concern. Two possible major deleterious consequences of stimulant treatment have been raised: one, the possibility of state-dependent effects on learning and memory; two, interference with the growth process.

A few new compounds have been used in hyperactive children with encouraging results, these include bupropion, monoamine oxidase (MAO) inhibitors, and clonidine; other compounds have not proved promising.

This chapter summarizes recent evidence concerning the above clinical issues in the pharmacotherapy of childhood hyperactivity. Several detailed reviews have appeared recently (30,44,57) that provide literature surveys through the early 1980s. Therefore, this chapter will be limited to new advances, mostly those since 1980, with earlier studies included whenever the sense of the discussion demands it.

NEW EFFECTS OF OLD TREATMENTS: THE PSYCHOSTIMULANTS

Social Behavior

It had been believed by some that the cost of reducing the symptoms of hyperactivity included, in part, impaired social functioning, taking the forms of abulia and lack of spontaneity. Contrary to expectation, hyperactive children showed increases in positive social behavior in school while on 0.6 mg/kg of methylphenidate, as compared to a lower dose, 0.3 mg/kg, and to placebo (78).

A group of studies (4,5,7,41) has reported on the interaction between hyperactive children and their mothers

---

[1] The terms hyperactive and hyperactivity are used to refer to the diagnosis of Attention Deficit Disorder with Hyperactivity (ADDH).

while the children received placebo or methylphenidate (Table 1). The results have been consistent in indicating that methylphenidate treatment of the child enhances co-operation between mother and child, reduces the mother's intrusive behavior, increases the mother's positive responses to the child, and increases compliance to maternal commands. These effects are more marked with higher doses; moreover, in reports by Barkley et al. (6,7), positive changes in the mother's behavior toward the treated child were apparent only when the child received the higher of the doses investigated (0.7 and 1 mg/kg/day). A further study, in kindergarten-age children, whose control group was too small to permit a test of methylphenidate ($N = 3$), failed to find significant positive changes in the mother's behavior among drug-treated children ($N = 8$) compared with controls (18). A study of teacher interactions with treated and untreated hyperactive children has also found that, when hyperactive children are treated with methylphenidate,

TABLE 1. *Studies of methylphenidate effects on interaction between hyperactive children, their mothers, and teachers[a]*

Authors	N	Dose	Results
Mother/child studies			
Humphries et al. (41)[b]	26	Mean, 12.5 mg	Mothers Decrease directions Increase praise Decrease criticism Children Increase directions Increase praise Decrease criticism
Barkley and Cunningham (4,5)[b]	20	Mode, 10 mg	Mothers Decrease directions Decrease negative behavior Increase rate of no response Increase responses to child's approach Increase facilitation of play Children Increase compliance Increase attention to mother's commands
Cohen et al. (18)	21	4 groups 1) Cognitive behavior modification (N = 6) 2) Methylphenidate (N = 8), 10–30 mg/day 3) 1 & 2 combined (N = 4) 4) No treatment (N = 3)	No group differences in mother/child interactions
Barkley et al. (7)[b]	54	0.3 mg/kg/day 1.0 mg/kg/day	Mothers Decrease directions Decrease negative behavior (only at 1.0 mg/kg) Children Increase compliance Decrease off-task behavior (at both doses)
Barkley et al. (6)[b]	60	0.6 mg/kg/day 1.4 mg/kg/day	Mothers Interact less (at higher dose only; no difference between high and low dose) Direct less (at higher dose only) Control less (at both doses) Attend more (at both doses) Children Comply better (at higher dose only; high dose superior to low dose)
Teacher/child study			
Whalen et al. (76,77)[b]	22	Mean a.m. dose 12.3 mg	Teachers Decrease controlling behavior Decrease intensity of interaction Decrease calling child's name No change in ordinary (noncontrol) interactions Children Initiate fewer contacts with teachers

[a] Studies listed in chronological order.
[b] Placebo-controlled, crossover studies.

teachers are less controlling, less disciplining, and have less intense interactions with the children (76,77).

The well-executed studies indicate that the medication status of hyperactive children has a positive impact on their social behavior and on the responses they elicit from adults. The latter effect has been shown to be clinically significant since teachers' behavior toward the medicated hyperactive children became indistinguishable from their behavior toward normal students.

Clinical Significance of Drug Effects

Although the statistical superiority of the stimulants over placebo in the management of hyperactive children is incontrovertible, some have raised questions as to the clinical significance of the beneficial effects induced by active treatments (40,44). In order to assess the magnitude of clinical effect, the behavior of stimulant-treated children has been contrasted to that of normal children. Several small studies have reported that off-task behavior in the classroom was normalized with methylphenidate (49,54,55). The medication was also found to normalize many behaviors of hyperactive children in experimental classrooms (74,75). Controlled naturalistic studies of treated hyperactive children as well have reported normalization of motor activity (56) and of classroom behaviors such as noncompliance and interference (2). However, in a study that included multiple aspects of classroom behavior, hyperactive children on relatively high doses of methylphenidate continued to differ significantly from their normal classmates on a few behavioral measures (2). Therefore, methylphenidate appears to normalize much, but not all, of the problematic behavior of hyperactive children, even at seemingly adequate dosages.

Stimulant Effects on Acquisition of Academic Skills

Until now, few have disagreed with the notion that stimulant medications do not ameliorate deficient complex cognitive processes or the acquisition of academic skills. Some have condemned the use of these treatments because of this single failure (31). Only one study (22) has investigated the effect of methylphenidate on the academic performance of hyperactive children in a design that remedied the failings of previous studies. Significant improvement with methylphenidate was noted on arithmetic and language tasks; in some instances, it was functionally meaningful. The results raise doubts about the firmly held opinion regarding the lack of stimulant effects on classroom learning and performance.

DOSAGE

As is the case for all pharmacotherapy, one cannot speak of drug effects without considering dosage. What constitutes optimal psychostimulant dosage for the treatment of hyperactive children has been controversial. It has been claimed that optimal dose levels for clinically significant behavioral improvement have the unfortunate consequence of impairing cognitive performance, whereas lower doses enhance learning but lead to less satisfactory behavioral changes. In a study of visual memory, 0.3 mg/kg had a superior effect than 1.0 mg/kg on visual memory and matching tasks, whereas the higher dose had a more favorable effect on classroom behavior (12,66). Further attempts to document dissociation between the psychostimulant effects on cognition and behavior have not been successful (3,16,20,26,54,58,59,65,71) (see Table 2). The

TABLE 2. *Effects of methylphenidate dosage in hyperactive children*[a]

Authors	Drug	N	Doses	Measures	Results
Sprague and Sleator (66)	Methyl/placebo	20	0.3 mg/kg 1.0 mg/kg	Visual memory	0.3 mg/kg better than placebo and 1.0 mg/kg 1.0 mg/kg no different from placebo
				Teacher ratings	0.3 mg/kg and 1.0 mg/kg better than placebo 1.0 mg/kg better than 0.3 mg/kg
Brown and Sleator (12)[b]	Methyl/placebo	11	0.3 mg/kg 1.0 mg/kg	MFFT[c]	Errors 0.3 mg/kg better than placebo and 1.0 mg/kg 1.0 mg/kg no different from placebo Latency Unaffected by 0.3 and 1.0 mg/kg
Charles et al. (16)	Methyl	42	0.2 mg/kg 0.4 mg/kg[d] (N = 11) 0.6 mg/kg[d] (N = 20) 0.8 mg/kg[c] (N = 11)	Children's checking task; teacher ratings Parent ratings	Linear positive relationship between dosage and improvement on cognitive and behavioral measures

TABLE 2. (*Continued*)

Authors	Drug	N	Doses	Measures	Results

Walker (71)	Methyl/placebo	18	0.3 mg/kg
			0.7 mg/kg
				Visual memory	Error rate
					  0.3 mg/kg no different from placebo
					  0.7 mg/kg better than placebo and 0.3 mg/kg
					Response rate
					  0.3 mg/kg and 0.7 mg/kg better than placebo
					  0.3 mg/kg better than placebo
					  0.7 mg/kg no different from placebo and 0.3 mg/kg

Gan and Cantwell (26)[d]	Methyl/placebo	20	0.3 mg/kg
			0.5 mg/kg
			1.0 mg/kg
				Visual learning task	Errors (acquisition)
					  0.3 mg/kg better than placebo
					  0.5 and 1.0 mg/kg no different from placebo, from each other, and from 0.3 mg/kg
					Errors (retention)
					  0.3 mg/kg better than placebo
					  No drug better than placebo
					  0.5 and 1.0 mg/kg no different from placebo, from each other, and from 0.3 mg/kg

Solanto and Conners (65)	Methyl/placebo	10	0.3 mg/kg 0.6 mg/kg 1.0 mg/kg	Reaction time Seat movements Errors of commission	Reaction time and seat movements Drug reduced both. No dose differences Linear positive relationship between dosage and reduction in number of errors

Peeke et al. (53)	Methyl/placebo	9	10 mg (0.25–0.3 mg/kg)
			21 mg (0.5–0.6 mg/kg)
				Verbal tasks	Recognition
					  10 mg better than placebo
					  21 mg no different from placebo and from 10 mg
					Immediate recall
					  10 and 21 mg no different, both better than placebo
					Delayed recall
					  10 mg better than 21 mg and placebo
					  21 mg no different from placebo
					Recognition of errors
					  10 mg better than placebo
					  21 mg no different from 10 mg and from placebo

Ballinger et al. (3)	Methyl/placebo	9	0.3 mg/kg 0.64 mg/kg	Verbal tasks Reading	Linear positive relationship between dosage and improvement No significant drug effect ($p < 0.10$)
Pelham et al. (54)	Methyl/placebo	29	0.15 mg/kg 0.3 mg/kg 0.6 mg/kg	Arithmetic Reading Spelling	Peak positive effect at 0.3 mg/kg No decrement with 0.6 mg/kg Significant positive effect at 0.6 mg/kg only Trend for 0.6 mg better than placebo

TABLE 2. (*Continued*)

Authors	Drug	N	Doses	Measures	Results
Rapport et al. (58,59)	Methyl/placebo	12	5 mg (0.22 mg/kg) 10 mg (0.43 mg/kg) 15 mg (0.65 mg/kg)	Classroom observations: On task Negative behaviors Visual learning task Continuous performance Classroom observations: Off task Classroom performance Teacher ratings	Linear positive relationship between dosage and improvement in off task and negative behaviors Linear positive relationship between dosage and improvement on cognitive, academic, and behavioral measures

[a] Studies listed in chronological order.
[b] Same study as Sprague and Sleator (66).
[c] MFFT, Matching Familiar Figures Test.
[d] N who reached each dose (progressive dosage increase in total sample).
[e] Interpretation complicated by having separate placebo conditions for each dose, so that each dose is compared to a different "no drug" performance level.

hypothesis that optimal clinical efficacy is feasible only at the cost of impaired learning ability has not been corroborated. However, little investigation of the higher dose range (1.0 mg/kg/day and above) has been undertaken. The issue of dose-related cognitive effects is complicated by the fact that not all cognitive tasks are similarly affected by stimulants, and at the same dosage (53). However, this observation is very different from the claim that some aspects of learning are actually impaired by treatment.

RELATIONSHIP BETWEEN PLASMA LEVELS OF PSYCHOSTIMULANTS AND BEHAVIORAL IMPROVEMENT

Several groups have investigated the relationship between plasma level of psychostimulants (79) and clinical response. So far, one (80) has found a significant positive relationship between level of drug and clinical outcome, others have not (10,37). A very small pilot reports an inverse relationship between plasma levels and errors on rote learning tasks (45). Large intraindividual variance in plasma levels at constant oral doses have been noted (37). Unless a given dose produces consistent plasma levels in any one child, it is unlikely that they will turn out to be a meaningful pharmacological measure. However, the positive report precludes ruling out any significance to plasma levels.

EFFICACY OF COMBINED PHARMACOTHERAPY AND PSYCHOTHERAPY

Because of the very different clinical focus of pharmacological and psychotherapeutic approaches, the reasonable expectation has been held that by combining them, clear advantage would accrue in the management of hyperactive children. A large clinical report of combined treatments

suggests that it may be the case (62). Systematic investigations of this premise have been conducted by combining methylphenidate with behavior modification (32,52,54,81), parent training in behavior management (25), and cognitive training (1,13,14,17).

In a partial sample of the largest study to date of the effect of methylphenidate alone compared to methylphenidate combined with an active behavior modification program in school and at home (N = 61) (32), children who received the combination did not differ from those who received methylphenidate alone on direct measures of classroom disruptive behavior, and on teacher ratings. In the expanded, complete sample (N = 86), the combination treatment group was rated significantly better by teachers than the group on methylphenidate alone. However, the direct classroom observations did not corroborate the teachers' evaluations (44a). Another study of behavior modification combined with low doses of methylphenidate failed to indicate accrued improvement during behavioral treatment (81). Unexpectedly and curiously, children who had received behavior modification worsened when this ineffective intervention ceased.

In a study that compared methylphenidate treatment alone to methylphenidate combined with parent training, no significant advantage was obtained from the added intervention of parent training to the medication (25).

Cognitive training, a more recent form of behavioral management, was devised in the face of disappointing results regarding the often weak effects of behavioral managements, and their lack of generalized efficacy across settings and over time in children with various behavior disorders. Cognitive training aims to modify children's careless, disorganized, impulsive responses, by teaching reflective, thoughtful approaches to mental problems and social situations. Cognitive training in kindergarten hyperactive boys was compared to methylphenidate and to the combination of the two treatments, as well as to no

TABLE 3. *Studies of stimulant medication combined with other interventions in hyperactive children[a]*

Authors	N	Treatments	Results
Bugental et al. (14)	36	Naturalistic groups 1) Methylphenidate (dosage unspecified) 2) No medication Assigned to either 1) Cognitive training 2) Social reinforcement	No advantage for combination treatment on cognitive measures and teacher ratings
Wolraich et al. (81)	20	Crossover Methylphenidate (0.3 mg/kg) Placebo With and without behavioral treatment	No advantage for combination treatment over medication alone
Brown (11)	120	Naturalistic treatment groups 1) Methylphenidate or dextroamphetamine (dosage unspecified) 2) No medication Assigned to 3 groups 1) Modeling (cognitive training) 2) Instruction 3) No intervention	No advantage for combination treatment over medication alone (no behavioral measures included)
Gittelman-Klein et al. (32)	61	3 groups 1) Methylphenidate (mean 38 mg/day) 2) Behavior therapy 3) 1 and 2 combined	Teacher ratings and classroom observations No advantage for combination treatment over medication alone on teacher ratings, on classroom observations or disruptive behavior, and on academic performance Combination treatment better than methylphenidate for observed classroom minor motor movements, and for global teacher improvement
Firestone et al. (25)	43	3 groups 1) Methylphenidate alone (22 mg/day) 2) Methylphenidate (or dextroamphetamine) + parent training 3) Placebo + parent training	No advantage for combination treatment over medication alone on academic and behavioral measures
Cohen et al. (17)	24	4 groups 1) Methylphenidate (10–30 mg/day) (N = 8) 2) Cognitive training (N = 6) 3) 1 and 2 combined (N = 6) 4) Untreated (N = 4)	No treatment differences across 4 groups, on cognitive and behavioral measures, so no advantage for combination treatment over medication alone
Pelham et al. (54)		Crossover Methylphenidate 0.15, 0.3, and 0.6 mg/kg (0.25–0.29 mg/day) Placebo With and without behavior therapy to enhance academic performance and reduce negative behaviors in class	No advantage for combination treatment over medication alone
Brown et al. (13)	40	3 groups 1) Methylphenidate 0.3 mg/kg (5–15 mg/day) 2) Cognitive training 3) 1 and 2 combined	No between-group analyses reported. Examination of data indicates no advantage for combination treatment on numerous cognitive and behavioral measures
Abikoff and Gittelman (1)	50	3 groups 1) Psychostimulants (methylphenidate equivalent, ca. 45 mg/day) 2) Psychostimulants[b] + cognitive training 3) Psychostimulants + attention control	No advantage for combination treatment over drug alone on numerous behavioral, cognitive, and academic measures

[a] Studies listed in chronological order.

[b] Only contrasts between stimulants alone and the combination of stimulants with training are summarized. [All studies except Cohen et al. (17) found stimulant treatment superior to other treatments used singly.]

treatment. No difference across these four conditions was obtained. However, the study is flawed by the small number of subjects in each group, thereby limiting the likelihood of detecting treatment differences (17).

A study of methylphenidate, cognitive training, and their combination failed to provide direct treatment comparisons (13); only within-group analyses are presented, but the descriptive statistics clearly reveal a lack of superiority for the combination over drug alone.

A larger study in school-aged children investigated whether an extensive period of cognitive training would enhance academic performance and behavioral improvement in hyperactive children on maintenance stimulant treatment (1). Children who received cognitive training in combination with methylphenidate showed no superiority on the multiple academic measures obtained when compared to children who remained on methylphenidate alone, and to children who received the combination of an attention control and methylphenidate. Similar negative results were obtained on all behavioral ratings tapping adjustment at home and in school. Not a single trend in favor of cognitive training was obtained, but some potential negative treatment effects were discovered. Children who received cognitive training were significantly slower in their performance, leading to significantly worse Performance IQs.

Many other reports have appeared concerning the relative efficacy of stimulants alone versus stimulants with behavioral treatment. However, these are case studies, or they involve very brief treatment periods (such as 2 days) so that their contribution to our understanding of the potential advantages of combining interventions is very limited (for a review see ref. 1).

Table 3 summarizes studies of stimulants alone and stimulants compared with other modalities.

PSYCHOSTIMULANTS IN ADOLESCENTS

In spite of the long-standing observation that many hyperactive children remain symptomatic through adolescence, and in spite of the huge literature supporting the use of psychostimulants in childhood, very little has been done to investigate the usefulness of stimulant treatment in adolescents. To some extent, the lack of clarity in the diagnosis of adolescents probably has limited the undertaking of treatment studies in this age group. A recent report documents the feasibility of identifying the syndrome in those above the age of 16 (34). Only one small study has examined the effects of methylphenidate in youngsters aged 13 to 18. They received placebo and methylphenidate in low (mean 15 mg/day) and higher (mean 31 mg/day) doses, for 1 week each in random order. Parent and teacher scales indicated significant advantage for the two drug conditions over the placebo; in addition, the higher doses were superior to the low doses of methylphenidate on a measure obtained from parents and teachers (70). A problem of this study is the fact that almost two-thirds of the adolescents were on methylphenidate at the time of referral to the study. Some self-selection for drug responders may have occurred, since the patients had chosen to remain on medication. However,

the short length of treatment was likely to minimize drug effects, since these become more salient as exposure to medication continues. In spite of these limitations, the study is consistent with the expectation that stimulants are effective in adolescents with the diagnosis of ADDH.

LONG-TERM EFFECTS OF STIMULANTS

An important clinical question is whether successful treatment in childhood leads to better ultimate outcome, as the children had several years of improved adjustment. In 1975, Weiss and co-workers (73) compared children who had been treated with methylphenidate to children who had received no medication, and to those who had been treated with chlorpromazine. In early adolescence, the children did not differ on multiple measures of outcomes. However, the original length of treatment was variable, and most children had not received long-term methylphenidate.

A subsequent report on the same children (39) selected only those who had received at least 3 years of continuous methylphenidate treatment during elementary school age. These youngsters were reevaluated in adulthood and compared to hyperactive children who had not received stimulants because the medications were not then in use; therefore, the different treatment groups do not reflect different diagnostic practices. The formerly untreated hyperactive patients were significantly worse than those treated. For instance, the latter had less psychiatric treatment and fewer car accidents; more led independent lives; more were attending school; they had a more positive view of their childhood and tended to have less aggression than the untreated group. They were rated also as having better social skills and rated themselves as having better self-esteem than the previously untreated hyperactive children. Two items favored the untreated groups: they had held their last job for a longer period of time, and fewer of them reported concentration problems. This study is encouraging in its observation that early stimulant treatment may have some ultimate advantage. Its limitation comes from the fact that the treated group followed up consists of 20 children from an original 25 who had received 3 years methylphenidate; moreover, these 25 came from a cohort of over 100 children and whether they are representative of the original diagnosed group is unclear.

Loney et al. (47) also found that exposure to stimulants in childhood (6 months or more) was positively associated with better parent ratings, less police contact for alcohol and drug use, and less drunken driving, in early adolescence. In another report, Loney postulated that drug treatment was not likely to be influential in diminishing long-term symptomatology, since childhood aggression, which is not believed to be ameliorated by stimulant treatment, rather than childhood hyperactivity, was the critical antecedent in the later development of psychiatric problems (48). The pathogenic model of outcome that views early hyperactivity as unimportant in the evolution of later psychiatric disorders was not corroborated in a recent follow-up study (35), which found that conduct disorders in adolescence occurred almost exclusively among youngsters who retained the ADDH. If these findings are valid, the long-term use of medication, when it is effective, could be construed as important in modifying the natural history of the disorder.

A related study (15) examined children 4 years after methylphenidate had been initiated, comparing those who had remained on medication for extended time to those who had not. Length of treatment was not associated with a superior outcome, whether behavioral or scholastic.

Interpretation of all these data is complicated by the fact that exposure to medication is self-selected. Attempts to understand the long-term effects of stimulant treatment will provide only suggestive evidence, since they must rely on naturalistic groups whose treatment fate is not under experimental control.

From the mixed results, it does not follow that long-term treatment has a questionable place in the management of hyperactive children. Clinical observation from diverse sources supports the expectation that stimulant treatments are effective over long spans; but, even in the context of such long-term efficacy, ultimate outcome may not be appreciably affected.

DELETERIOUS EFFECTS OF PSYCHOSTIMULANTS

Decrements in Growth

The observation by Safer et al. (61) of significant decrement in growth velocity in children treated for extended periods of time with psychostimulant has led to multiple investigations yielding markedly contradictory results (60). The extreme variability in dosage used across studies has confused the picture, since some negative studies used only low doses. A prospective study of children treated for up to 3 years failed to find an effect by methylphenidate (up to 0.77 mg/kg/day dosages) on predicted adult stature (43). Another recent prospective study of hyperactive children treated with methylphenidate for up to 4 years at higher doses (average 40 mg/day) found a significant decrease in height percentile, cumulative dosage being significantly associated with the decrease (51). The same children were followed up into late adolescence and were not found to be shorter than controls (29). Similar results were obtained in a smaller study that identified 20 hyperactive children treated with methylphenidate for at least 3 years (39). As young adults, the previously treated hyperactive children did not differ in height from hyperactive children who had not been treated with stimulants and from normals.

The weight of the evidence seems to be that methylphenidate has significant effects on growth velocity in childhood, but the growth spurt compensates for the earlier effects, and eventual height is not compromised. These observations were made in instances where treatment had been interrupted during adolescence. It is not known whether the same pattern would occur if treatment were sustained throughout adolescence.

State-Dependent Learning

The report of state-dependent effects on children treated with stimulant (69) generated much concern, since stimulant treatment is protracted in most, occurring during a devel-

opment period requiring the acquisition of important skills. One study replicated the earlier report of state-dependent effects of methylphenidate (63), but several others have failed to do so (8,67,68,72). In a large study of learning-disabled children who had received tutoring while being treated with high doses of methylphenidate or a placebo, no evidence for state-dependent learning was found (33).

NEW TREATMENTS

The newness of an intervention is a relative phenomenon; here, it refers to compounds that emerged subsequent to the standard treatments (dextroamphetamine and methylphenidate). Two other stimulant drugs were introduced in the early 1970s (magnesium pemoline and caffeine), but they were not fully investigated until the late 1970s and early 1980s.

Caffeine

A total of 146 children with hyperactivity or other unspecified behavior problems have been included in nine studies of the clinical efficacy of caffeine (19,24,27,36,38). The clinical results with caffeine are, on the whole, negative. The only positive clinical effect was reported in a study using whole versus decaffeinated coffee (38). In one study (28), low doses of caffeine (159 mg) combined with a low dose of methylphenidate (10 mg) led to significantly greater improvement than did higher doses of caffeine (309 mg) alone, the drug alone, or the drug combined with a high dose of caffeine. The finding is weakened by the fact that only six children participated in this crossover study that included seven experimental conditions. However, high caffeine doses have been found to lead to increased restlessness in normal children (23). Since this effect has never been reported with dextroamphetamine or methylphenidate, the findings with caffeine represent a special clinical pattern that has theoretical interest. They suggest that motor and attentional systems may respond independently, and that the action of stimulants may not consist of a primary enhancement of vigilance that, in turn and only secondarily, leads to reduction in motor activity.

Magnesium Pemoline

The early reports of effectiveness of magnesium pemoline have been documented in a trial comparing the drug (dosage ±60 mg/day) to methylphenidate (±22 mg/d) and to placebo (21). The magnitude of clinical impact does not seem quite as great as that obtained with the other stimulants, and the time of onset is somewhat delayed. The distinctive characteristic of pemoline is its longer clinical action, making it potentially useful for children with severe rebound effect from methylphenidate or dextroamphetamine, and for children unable to take multiple daily doses. However, the longer activity is not consistent across children and cannot be relied on.

Monoamine Oxidase Inhibitors

Monoamine oxidase inhibitors have been investigated because they affect the dopamine, serotonin, and norepinephrine neurotransmitter systems, believed to be the mediating mechanisms for the therapeutic efficacy of established stimulants. Small groups of children received clorgyline (average 12 mg/day), a selective MAO-A inhibitor, or tranylcypromine sulfate (average 10 mg/day), a MAO-(A + B) inhibitor (82). Significant behavioral improvement was obtained to a degree equivalent to dextroamphetamine. Together with results from studies of compounds with selective acute neurotransmitter alterations, the results with the MAOIs argue for a model of drug action in ADDH that involves multiple neurochemical systems. Interestingly, the clinical drug effects ceased immediately on withdrawal of the MAOIs, whereas alterations in norepinephrine metabolism continued for 2 weeks thereafter. These findings are interpreted as revealing a dissociation between the clinical effectiveness of the drug and changes in norepinephrine.

Bupropion

Because of previously reported beneficial effects with antidepressant medications (tricyclics) in hyperactive children, a trial of bupropion was undertaken by Simeon and colleagues (64). Of 17 patients, 12 (70%) had moderate to marked clinical efficacy on doses from 50 to 150 mg/day (mean 130 mg/day). Confusingly, the teacher rated the children as better when they were substituted to a placebo following the bupropion trial. No controlled trial of bupropion has appeared.

Clonidine

One clinical trial of clonidine in 10 hyperactive children reported significant improvement on parent and teacher ratings with doses of 4 to 5 µg/kg/day administered q.i.d. (42). Treatment may not have been blind, since all children were on clonidine after 2 weeks into the trial. However, the marked deterioration in several children upon placebo substitution documents the efficacy of clonidine. Because of the markedly different neuropharmacological profile of clonidine compared with the psychostimulants, its clinical efficacy in ADDH is of considerable interest.

FAILED TREATMENTS

Based on the dopamine hypothesis of attention deficit disorder with hyperactivity, several dopamine agonists have been investigated in open clinical trials. Neither piribidal (9) nor amantadine (50) nor L-dopa (46) was found to have clinical action.

SUMMARY

Clinical research in the treatment of hyperactive children has moved from global efficacy studies to the identification of more refined treatment effects. The study of social behavior and interaction has yielded consistent positive findings. Treated children are more sociable; mothers and teachers relate to them more positively, in a less directive,

intense, and controlling fashion. Similarly, multiple aspects, but not all, of hyperactive children's behavior are normalized with methylphenidate.

Several fields of inquiry have yielded negative results. The notion that there is a dosage-related dissociation of stimulant effects on learning and behavior has not been substantiated. Plasma levels of methylphenidate mostly have been unrelated to clinical effect, but the issue remains open. The additional use of various forms of psychotherapies (behavioral treatment, parent training, cognitive therapy) with stimulants has not resulted in superior outcomes than medication alone.

Only a small, brief study of methylphenidate in adolescents has appeared supporting the expectation that stimulants are effective in this age group.

The long-term impact of early stimulant treatment remains controversial. Two reports have found some advantages in the outcome of previously treated hyperactive children compared to controls. At the same time, early treatment cannot be construed as preventing later dysfunction altogether. Extended stimulant treatment appears to be associated with a reduction in growth velocity, the latter being a function of cumulative dosage. However, the eventual height of those treated in childhood does not appear affected.

Based on various theories of drug efficacy, several new compounds have been investigated in small trials. The MAO inhibitors have been reported to be as effective as psychostimulants. In clinical trials, bupropion and clonidine have also been reported effective. Other compounds selected because of their dopaminergic activity (piribidal, L-dopa, amantadine) have not yielded encouraging results. Because of several negative studies, caffeine has ceased to be a potentially interesting compound.

Recent investigations have placed the role of stimulants in hyperactive children on a firmer basis. The effectiveness of these compounds is broad, influencing important cognitive and interpersonal relationships; several of the suspected costs have not been documented.

REFERENCES

1. Abikoff, H., and Gittelman, R. (1985): *Arch. Gen. Psychiatry*, 42: 953–961.
2. Abikoff, H., and Gittelman, R. (1985): *J. Abnorm. Child Psychol.*, 13:33–44.
3. Ballinger, C. T., Varley, C. K., and Nolen, P. A. (1984): *Am. J. Psychiatry*, 141:1590–1593.
4. Barkley, R. A., and Cunningham, C. E. (1979): *Arch. Gen. Psychiatry*, 36:201–208.
5. Barkley, R. A., and Cunningham, C. E. (1980): In: *Treatment of Hyperactive and Learning Disordered Children*, edited by R. M. Knights and D. J. Bakker, pp. 219–236. University Park Press, Baltimore.
6. Barkley, R. A., Karlsson, J., Pollard, S., and Murphy, J. V. (1985): *J. Child Psychol. Psychiatry*, 26:705–715.
7. Barkley, R. A., Karlsson, J., Strzelecki, E., and Murphy, J. V. (1984): *J. Consult. Clin. Psychol.*, 52:750–758.
8. Becker-Mattes, A., Mattes, J. A., Abikoff, H., and Brandt, L. (1985): *Am. J. Psychiatry*, 142:455–459.
9. Brown, G. L., Ebert, M. H., and Mikkelsen, E. J. (1979): Presented at the annual meeting of the American Academy of Child Psychiatry, Chicago.
10. Brown, G. L., Hunt, R. D., Ebert, M. H., Bunney, W. E., Jr., and Kopin, I. J. (1979): *Psychopharmacology*, 62:133–140.
11. Brown, R. T. (1980): *J. Learn. Disabil.*, 13:249–254.

12. Brown, R. T., and Sleator, E. K. (1979): *Pediatrics,* 64:408–410.
13. Brown, R. T., Wynne, M. E., and Medenis, R. (1985): *J. Abnorm. Child Psychol.,* 13:69–87.
14. Bugental, D. B., Whalen, C. K., and Henker, B. (1977): *Child Dev.,* 48:874–884.
15. Charles, L., and Schain, R. (1981): *J. Abnorm. Child Psychol.,* 9: 495–505.
16. Charles, L., Schain, R., and Zelniker, T. (1981): *J. Dev. Behav. Pediatr.,* 2:78–81.
17. Cohen, N. J., Sullivan, J., Minde, K., Novak, C., and Helwig, C. (1981): *J. Abnorm. Child Psychol.,* 9:43–54.
18. Cohen, N. J., Sullivan, J., Minde, K., Novak, C., and Keens, S. (1983): *Child Psychiatry Hum. Dev.,* 13:213–244.
19. Conners, C. K. (1975): In: *Recent Advances in Child Psychopharmacology,* edited by R. Gittelman-Klein, pp. 136–147. Human Sciences Press, New York.
20. Conners, C. K., and Solanto, M. V. (1984): In: *Attention Deficit Disorder: Diagnostic, Cognitive and Therapeutic Understanding,* edited by L. N. Bloomingdale, pp. 191–204. Spectrum Publications, New York.
21. Conners, C. K., and Taylor, E., (1980): *Arch. Gen. Psychiat.,* 37: 922–930.
22. Douglas, V. I., Barr, R. G., O'Neill, M. E., and Britton, B. G. (1986): *J. Child Psychol. Psychiatry,* 27:191–211.
23. Elkins, R. N., Rapoport, J. L., Zahn, T. P., Buchsbaum, M. S., Weingartner, H., Kopin, I. J., Langer, D., and Johnson, C. (1981): *Am. J. Psychiatry,* 138:178–183.
24. Firestone, P., Davey, J., Goodman, J. T., and Peters, S. (1978): *J. Am. Acad. Child Psychiatry,* 17:445–456.
25. Firestone, P., Kelly, M. J., Goodman, J. T., and Davey, J. (1981): *J. Am. Acad. Child Psychiatry,* 20:135–147.
26. Gan, J., and Cantwell, D. P. (1982): *J. Am. Acad. Child Psychiatry,* 21:237–242.
27. Garfinkel, B., Webster, C., and Sloman, L. (1975): *Am. J. Psychiatry,* 132:723–728.
28. Garfinkel, B. D., Webster, C. D., and Sloman, L. (1981): *Can. J. Psychiatry,* 26:395–401.
29. Gittelman, R. (1982): Presented at the annual meeting of the American College of Neuropsychopharmacology, Puerto Rico.
30. Gittelman, R. (1983): In: *Stimulants: Neurochemical, Behavioral, and Clinical Perspectives,* edited by I. Creese, pp. 205–226. Raven Press, New York.
31. Gittelman, R. (1983): In: *Developmental Neuropsychiatry,* edited by M. Rutter, pp. 437–449. Guilford Press, New York.
32. Gittelman, R., Abikoff, H., Pollack, E., Klein, D. F., Katz, S., and Mattes, J. A. (1980): In: *Hyperactive Children: The Social Ecology of Identification and Treatment,* edited by C. K. Whalen and B. Henker, pp. 221–243. Academic Press, New York.
33. Gittelman, R., Klein, D. F., and Feingold, I. (1983): *J. Child Psychol. Psychiatry,* 24:193–212.
34. Gittelman, R., and Mannuzza, S. (1985): *Psychopharmacol. Bull.* (Special feature: ADDH and Mental Retardation), 21:237–242.
35. Gittelman, R., Mannuzza, S., Shenker, R., and Bonagura, N. (1985): *Arch. Gen. Psychiatry,* 42:937–947.
36. Gross, M. (1975): *Psychosomatics,* 58:423–431.
37. Gualtieri, C. T., Wargin, W., Kanoy, R., Patrick, K., Shen, C. D., Youngblood, W., Mueller, R. A., and Breese, G. R. (1982): *J. Am. Acad. Child Psychiatry,* 21:19–26.
38. Harvey, D. H. P., and Marsh, R. W. (1978): *Dev. Med. Child Neurol.,* 20:81–86.
39. Hechtman, L., Weiss, G., and Perlman, T. (1984): *J. Am. Acad. Child Psychiatry,* 23:261–269.
40. Henker, B., Whalen, C. K., and Collins, B. E. (1979): *J. Abnorm. Child Psychol.,* 7:1–13.
41. Humphries, T., Kinsbourne, M., and Swanson, J. (1978): *J. Child Psychol. Psychiatry.,* 19:13–22.
42. Hunt, R. D., Minderaa, R. B., and Cohen, D. J. (1985): *J. Am. Acad. Child Psychiatry,* 24:617–629.
43. Kalachnik, J. E., Sprague, R. L., Sleator, E. K., Cohen, M. N., and Ullman, R. K. (1982): *Dev. Med. Child Neurol.,* 24:586–595.
44. Klein, D. F., Gittelman, R., Quitkin, F., and Rifkin, A. (1980): *Diagnosis and Drug Treatment of Psychiatric Disorders: Adults and Children.* Williams & Wilkins, Baltimore.
44a. Klein, R. G. (1986): Presented at the annual meeting of the American College of Neuropsychopharmacology, December, Washington, D.C.

45. Kupietz, S. S., Winsberg, B. G., and Sverd, J. (1982): *J. Am. Acad. Child Psychiatry,* 21:27–30.
46. Langer, D., Rapoport, J., Brown, L., Ebert, M., and Bunney, W. (1982): *J. Am. Acad. Child Psychiatry,* 21:10–19.
47. Loney, J., Kramer, J., and Kosier, T. (1981): Presented at the annual meeting of the American Psychological Association, Los Angeles.
48. Loney, J., Kramer, J., and Milich, R. S. (1981): In: *Psychosocial Aspects of Drug Treatment for Hyperactivity,* edited by K. D. Gadow and J. Loney, pp. 381–415. Westview Press, Boulder, CO.
49. Loney, J., Weissenburger, F. E., Woolson, R. F., and Lichty, E. C. (1979): *J. Abnorm. Child Psychiatry,* 7:133–143.
50. Mattes, J. A. (1980): *Psychopharmacol. Bull.,* 16:67–69.
51. Mattes, J. A., and Gittelman, R. (1983): *Arch. Gen. Psychiatry,* 40:317–321.
52. O'Leary, S. G., and Pelham, W. E. (1978): *Pediatrics,* 61:211–217.
53. Peeke, S., Halliday, R., Callaway, E., Rael, R., and Reus, V. (1984): *J. Clin. Psychopharmacol.,* 4:82–88.
54. Pelham, W. E., Bender, M. E., Caddell, J., Booth, S., and Moorer, S. H. (1985): *Arch. Gen. Psychiatry,* 42:948–952.
55. Pelham, W. E., Schnedler, R. W., Bologna, N. C., and Contreras, J. A. (1980): *J. Appl. Behav. Anal.,* 13:221–236.
56. Porrino, L. J., Rapoport, J. L., Behar, D., Ismond, M. A., and Bunney, M. D., Jr. (1983): *Arch. Gen. Psychiatry,* 40:688–693.
57. Rapoport, J. L. (1983): In: *Developmental Neuropsychiatry,* edited by M. Rutter, pp. 385–403. Guilford Press, New York.
58. Rapport, M. D., DuPaul, G. J., Stoner, G., and Jones, J. T. (1986): *J. Consult. Clin. Psychol.,* 54:334–341.
59. Rapport, M. D., Stoner, G., DuPaul, J., Birmingham, B. K., and Tucker, S. (1985): *J. Abnorm. Child Psychol.,* 13:227–244.
60. Roche, A. F., Lipman, R. S., Overall, J. E., and Hung, W. (1979): *Pediatrics,* 63:647–650.
61. Safer, D., Allen, R. P., and Barr, E. (1972): *N. Engl. J. Med.,* 287: 217–220.
62. Satterfield, J. H., Satterfield, B. T., and Cantwell, D. P. (1981): *Behav. Pediatr.,* 98:650–655.
63. Shea, V. T. (1982): *Psychopharmacology,* 78:226–270.
64. Simeon, J. G., Furgeson, H. B., Knott, V., Rochon, R., and Fleet, J. V. W. (1985): Presented at the annual meeting of the American College of Neuropsychopharmacology, Maui, Hawaii.
65. Solanto, M. V., and Conners, C. K. (1982): *Psychophysiology,* 19: 658–667.
66. Sprague, R. L., and Sleator, E. K. (1977): *Science,* 198:1274–1276.
67. Steinhausen, H.-C., and Kreuzer, E.-M. (1981): *Psychopharmacology,* 74:389–390.
68. Stephens, R. S., Pelham, W. E., and Skinner, R. (1984): *J. Consult. Clin. Psychol.,* 52:104–113.
69. Swanson, J., and Kinsbourne, M. (1976): *Science,* 192:1354–1357.
70. Varley, C. K. (1983): *J. Am. Acad. Child Psychiatry,* 22:351–354.
71. Walker, M. A. (1982): In: *Drugs and Mental Retardation,* edited by S. E. Breuning and A. D. Poling, pp. 235–266. Charles C Thomas, Springfield, IL.
72. Weingartner, H., Langer, D., Grice, J., and Rapoport, J. L. (1982): *Psychiatr. Res.,* 6:21–29.
73. Weiss, G., Kruger, E., Danielson, U., and Elman, M. (1975): *Can. Med. Assoc. J.,* 112:159–165.
74. Whalen, C. K., Collins, B. E., Henker, B., Alkus, S. R., Adams, D., and Stapp, J. (1978): *J. Pediatr. Psychol.,* 4:177–187.
75. Whalen, C. K., Henker, B., Collins, B. E., Finck, D., and Dotemoto, S. (1979): *J. Appl. Behav. Anal.,* 12:65–81.
76. Whalen, C. K., Henker, B., and Dotemoto, S. (1980): *Science,* 208:1280–1282.
77. Whalen, C. K., Henker, B., and Dotemoto, S. (1981): *Child Dev.,* 52:1005–1014.
78. Whalen, C. K., Henker, B., Swanson, J. M., Granger, D., Kliewer, W., and Spencer, J. (1987): *J. Consult. Clin. Psychol.* (in press).
79. Winsberg, B. G., Hungund, B. L., and Perel, J. M. (1980): *Psychopharmacol. Bull.,* 16:69–71.
80. Winsberg, B. G., Kupietz, S. S., Sverd, J., Hungund, B. L., and Young, N. (1982): *Psychopharmacology,* 76:329–332.
81. Wolraich, M., Drummond, T., Salomon, M., O'Brien, M., and Sivage, C. (1978): *J. Abnorm. Psychol.,* 6:149–161.
82. Zametkin, A., Rapoport, J. L., Murphy, D. L., Linnoila, M., Karoum, F., Potter, W. Z., and Ismond, D. (1985): *Arch. Gen. Psychiatry,* 42:969–973.

Psychopharmacology:
The Third Generation of Progress,
edited by Herbert Y. Meltzer.
Raven Press, New York © 1987.

CHAPTER **126**

Drug Treatment of Infantile Autism: The Past Decade

Magda Campbell

SUMMARY OF PROGRESS MADE BETWEEN 1960 AND 1978

Since 1960, when psychopharmacology in this population began in a systematic fashion, the most visible progress has been made in the past decade. In the 1960s Fish (31) and associates worked intensively on developing rating scales appropriate for this population and sensitive to change due to drug administration. Fish also made the important, and still valid, clinical observation that autistic children respond poorly to the low-potency neuroleptics and develop sedation on low doses, whereas on high-potency neuroleptics decrease of symptoms without sedation can be obtained (32,33). In a series of pilot studies, a variety of psychoactive drugs were explored; these were reviewed by Campbell et al. (12). The groundwork for future research was established and was based on very careful clinical diagnosis.

In the decade following Fish's historical chapter on methodology concerning autistic children, a modest progress has been made in this area of psychopharmacology, and it was summarized in the predecessor of this volume (5). Serious attempts were made to use larger and diagnostically homogeneous patient samples and to assess drug effect under rigorous conditions (20). In order to promote communication with other investigators, rating scales developed by the Psychopharmacology Research Branch of the National Institute of Mental Health (NIMH) (50) were used, employing multiple raters under different rating conditions. The emphasis was on improving methodology (5).

GOALS FOR THE PAST DECADE

The goals were discussed in the previous volume (5). The problems involved diagnosis, classification, subgroups of autistic children with differential response to drugs, study design and treatment evaluation, and rating conditions. Most drugs that were evaluated prior to 1978 seemed to be of limited value, or ineffective, in this population based on short-term studies. This was thought to be due partly to the fact that most autistic children function on a retarded level, and cognition was not positively affected by drug. However, no attempts were made to study cognition, learning, or performance in a systematic way.

AREAS OF PROGRESS

Diagnosis

With the advent of the *Diagnostic and Statistical Manual of Mental Disorders,* 3rd edition (DSM-III) (28), it was made possible for investigators to use diagnostic and other criteria that were clearly spelled out and that were used in the entire country. Infantile autism entered the official nomenclature of the American Psychiatric Association. Similar diagnostic criteria were the Definition of Autism of the National Society for Autistic Children, forwarded by Ritvo and Freeman (53). Thus communication between investigators was made possible or facilitated.

Demographic Characteristics

In order to define responders to a drug, it is necessary to define the patient sample by a variety of parameters. The Children's Personal Data Inventory (CPDI), which is part of the Early Clinical Drug Evaluation Unit (ECDEU) Pediatric Packet (38), was supplemented by a Template (4,6). This Template consists of 156 items related to family history of mental illness and pre- and perinatal history of the patient; its use is described elsewhere (16). The Research Obstetrical Scale (ROS) by Sameroff et al. (58) has been also used in clinical trials and differentiated autistic children from other diagnostic categories (37). Reports now define their patients not only by chronological age, but also by IQ and socio-economic status (SES). With one exception (47), studies reviewed here include diagnostically homogeneous patient samples. Patient's status (inpatient vs outpatient) is specified.

Indications

As a group, in children with symptoms of hyperactivity, aggressiveness, stereotypies, and withdrawal, neuroleptics, specifically haloperidol, are indicated. It has been demonstrated in more than one controlled and well-designed study that these symptoms significantly decrease, both statistically and clinically, with administration of haloperidol, both when given on a short-term (1,8,9,21,26) and on a long-term (7,19) basis. However, there are individuals with this symptom profile who fail to respond to such drugs. In exclusively hypoactive and anergic autistic children, this class of drug is not indicated, since the response is usually poor and sedation develops invariably at very low doses; therefore, in some studies hypoactivity is listed among exclusion criteria.

No clear-cut indications have been established yet for such drugs as fenfluramine or naltrexone.

Treatment Evaluation

Design

Much attention has been given to this issue, and, as shown in Table 1, in most studies the basic requirements of a good clinical trial were met: certainly an improvement over the previous decade.

Crossover vs parallel or combination of intensive and extensive design. In a rare and chronic clinical condition, such as infantile autism, to employ an intensive or within-individual design (42) seems to be a reasonable approach. Intensive and extensive design (60) were combined in four major studies (1,8,9,21,26). However, because of the problems of drug washout and carryover (24,25,44), comparative or parallel design may be preferable to crossover or intensive design; these issues were recently reviewed elsewhere (14).

Duration of treatment. Clearly it is important to differentiate short-term efficacy of a drug from its long-term efficacy. In the past it was shown that in a young child, when a lengthy crossover design is employed (14–21 weeks, mean 18.6 weeks), it is impossible to differentiate the effect of drug from the effect of time or maturation (20), an issue raised by Fish many years ago (31). In systematic studies of haloperidol, this issue was addressed and the duration of short-term studies was 14 weeks (1,8,9,21), whereas the length of long-term studies was a minimum of 6 months (7,19,49).

Assessments

Rating scales and other assessment instruments are presented in a recent update (51) of the Special Issue on Pharmacotherapy in Children (50).

Behavioral. No single behavioral scale is yet being used in autistic children across studies. This is in contrast to the universal use of the rating scales of Conners developed for hyperactive children. However, some progress has been made here, too. With the development and publication of the ECDEU Pediatric Packet, the first 28 items of the Childrens Psychiatric Rating Scale (CPRS) and the Clinical Global Impressions (CGI) have been consistently used by one research unit; the former was used in 175 children, and the latter in 182 (17). Both reflected change due to drug treatment. The Parent Teacher Questionnaire (PTQ) was also used in a large number of patients (total $N = 79$) and was appropriate when employed by either teachers or parents (1,2,20). The Nurse's Global Impressions (NGI) was used in 70 children and was also sensitive to changes due to drug (8,20). On the other hand, the Children's Behavior Inventory (CBI), a standardized developmental scale (3,39), was not sensitive to reflect change due to drug (8,20).

The Ritvo-Freeman Real Life Rating Scale for Autism (34) was used in a multicenter study involving a total of 150 autistic children and adolescents (55). Data are published only on 81 subjects (2,43,54–56).

The Timed Behavior Rating Scale was developed specifically for autistic children; it was sensitive to reflect decreases of stereotypies due to haloperidol administration in an ABA design (26).

Other scales developed for autistic children but not yet used in drug studies are commented on elsewhere (17). In order to maximize objectivity, electronic devices were used to measure stereotypies and motor activity in an automated laboratory (1,9,17). These measures, and the use of videotapes, are discussed by Campbell and Palij (17) and Meiselas et al. (46).

Cognitive. A major step forward is the attempt to measure not only behavioral effects of drugs in this population, but also their effects on cognition, in general. The same assessments may not be appropriate for short- and for long-term studies, and practice effect is to be taken into consideration. In the case of short-term trials, learning or performance tasks are appropriate, whereas in long-term studies, intelligence tests may be utilized (17). Table 2 details some of the features of drug trials in which cognitive and learning measures were administered to autistic subjects.

Untoward effects. A greater concern in regard to short-term untoward effects (e.g., excessive sedation, adverse effect on cognitive functions, behavioral toxicity) and long-term untoward effects of drugs (abnormal involuntary movements associated with neuroleptic administration, effect of drugs on height, weight, and IQ) in children is reflected in an extensive discussion on measures of side effects in a book by Campbell et al. (14) and in a review article (18).

Biochemical Abnormalities Underlying the Behavioral and Cognitive Deviancies and Their Relationship to Choice of Drug Treatment

There are serious and unresolved methodological problems involved in studies of biochemical markers in autistic patients. The patient samples are invariably small, and the age ranges are wide. Recent studies confirm that serotonin and catecholamine (63) abnormalities exist in subgroups of autistics and that they may be related to various behavioral and cognitive abnormalities (64,65). More recent work suggests abnormal level or activity of endogenous opiates, again, only in subgroups of these patients (36,62). The rationale of administering fenfluramine and naltrexone (or naloxone) was an attempt to correct simultaneously the behavioral and the underlying biochemical abnormalities with a psychopharmacological agent. As with other pharmacological agents, these approaches, or attempts, in humans may be less successful than in laboratory animals.

Clinical Drug Trials: Therapeutic and Untoward Effects (Short- and Long-Term Efficacy and Safety)

An overview of clinical trials is presented in Table 1.

In the past decade it was clearly demonstrated in carefully designed and double-blind studies that haloperidol, a potent antidopaminergic drug, is an effective therapeutic agent for many autistic children when given in an enriched psychosocial environment. This finding is important both clinically and theoretically, since there is a suggestion that a subgroup of autistic children show evidence of excess dopaminergic activity (65). Administration of conservative doses to inpatients, ages 2 to 7 years, was associated with statistically and clinically significant changes, including decreases of stereotypies, hyperactivity, and negativism (1,8,26), and facilitation of learning in the laboratory (1,8). Furthermore, no untoward effects were observed at these doses, when haloperidol was individually regulated and given up to 3 months, cumulatively. This drug remained therapeutically effective when administered up to $4\frac{1}{2}$ years and helped many autistic children to remain with their families and/or in educational programs (7,19,21), and it had no adverse effects on IQ (29).

However, when haloperidol was administered cumulatively for longer than 3 to 12 months, 22% of autistic children developed tardive or withdrawal dyskinesias, in a study employing a prospective design (15,49). The movements involved mainly the areas of mouth, jaws, and tongue; their duration ranged from 16 days up to 9 months. It was difficult at times to differentiate withdrawal dyskinesias from stereotypies, which were suppressed by drug and reemerged upon discontinuation of haloperidol, particularly in the area of mouth, jaws, and tongue (46).

Because of the association of abnormal involuntary movements with haloperidol, as well as with other neuroleptic agents, other types of drugs should be considered for the treatment of this population.

Ritvo and associates (35) explored and subsequently studied fenfluramine in a crossover, double-blind, placebo-controlled study involving a large number of autistic subjects who participated in a multicenter study (2,43,45,54–56). The data were published recently, involving 81 subjects, aged 33 months to 24 years, all of whom were outpatients (55). About 33% of patients showed marked improvement of behavior, which was associated with increases of IQs, but not in all studies (2,45). Furthermore, Leventhal (45) found no clinical response to fenfluramine in 16 autistic children. Only a few side effects were reported: loss of weight and transient sedation. Volkmar et al. (61) reported deterioration of behavior in two autistic children, with irritability, fearfulness, agitation, and disrupted sleep.

Fenfluramine is a potent antiserotonergic drug (59); Ritvo explored this agent because about one-third of autistic children have hyperserotonemia (11,57), which is thought to be associated with severe behavioral abnormalities and severe intellectual subnormality (11,64,65). Fenfluramine administration was associated with marked decrease of serotonin in the multicenter study (55); however, the responders were subjects who had low baseline serotonin levels, and, as a group, they had higher IQs than the nonresponders (55,56).

In an open pilot study involving 10 autistic children aged 3 to 5.75 years, the results suggested that the most marked improvements were rated in four children who had low IQs (10). Decreases of irritability, temper tantrums, aggressiveness, self-mutilation, and hyperactivity, and improved sleep pattern as well as increased relatedness were among therapeutic changes observed; however, in some children the positive changes were transient. Unlike in the study of Ritvo et al. (55), a flexible dosage schedule was employed; optimal doses of fenfluramine ranged from 1.1 to 1.8 mg/kg/day, mean, 1.413 mg/kg/day (10). The most common untoward effects were transient weight loss, drowsiness, and uncontrollable irritability.

Preliminary data analyses of a small sample of autistic children who completed their study, and who represent part of a large, ongoing double-blind study of fenfluramine, employing a parallel groups design, suggest much weaker therapeutic effects with fenfluramine (22). Based on a small number of children, there is also a suggestion that fenfluramine may have adverse effects on discrimination learning in the laboratory.

Kalat (41) and Panksepp (48) forwarded the hypothesis that the neurochemical basis of infantile autism is abnormalities of the endogenous opioid system, and that administration of an opiate antagonist, such as naloxone or naltrexone, should yield decreases of behavioral and other associated abnormalities (48). This hypothesis is based on animal studies conducted by Panksepp (48) and supported by two studies involving autistic subjects and controls (36,62). This was the rationale for exploring naltrexone, a potent opiate antagonist with long-lasting effects and relatively free of side effects.

TABLE 1. Survey of publications[a]

Drug	Ref.	Age (range) of subjects (years)	Sample	Dosage (range) mg/day	mg/kg/day	Design	Measures	Drug effect
Haloperidol	8	2.6–7.2	Homogeneous; N = 40 inpatients	0.5–4 (mean = 1.65)	Mean = 0.07–0.15	Double-blind, placebo-controlled, random assignment to 4 groups in a factorial design (drug vs behavior therapy and the combination of both)	CPRS, CGI, NGI, CBI; ratings of video-taped sessions (task-appropriate behavior); cognitive battery; language acquisition; DOTES, TESS, side effect checklist	Decreases of stereotypies and withdrawal; facilitation of language acquisition; no effect on cognitive battery
Haloperidol	26	2.1–7.0	Homogeneous; N = 10 inpatients		Mean = 1.65–1.90	Double-blind, placebo-controlled, random assignment; within-subjects reversal design	Interval recording scale of 8 categories of maladaptive behaviors; DOTES, TESS, side effect checklist	Decreases of stereotypies and withdrawal
Haloperidol	1	2.33–6.92	Homogeneous; N = 40 inpatients	0.5–3.0 (mean = 1.11)	0.019–0.217 (mean = 0.05)	Double-blind, placebo-controlled, random assignment to one of the 2 treatment sequences: HPH or PHP (crossover)	CPRS, CGI, PTQ, DOTES, TESS, side effect checklist, AIMS, ADS; videotaping	Decrease in stereotypies, withdrawal, abnormal object relationships, hyperactivity, fidgetiness, negativism, angry and labile affect[b]
Haloperidol	47	3–16	Heterogeneous; N = 87 (34 autistics)	0.75–6.75		Double-blind, placebo-controlled, random assignment; cross-over		
Pimozide	47	3–16	Heterogeneous; 34 autistics (total N = 87)	1–4		Double-blind and placebo-controlled comparison with haloperidol; random assignment; crossover; multicenter study; no washout at switching		
Megadoses of vitamin B6 (pyridoxine)	52	4–19	Heterogeneous; N = 16 outpatients	75–3,000	2.4–94.3	Double-blind, placebo-controlled, random assignment; cross-over (BABAB)	TSCL	Decreases in global symptom ratings
Fenfluramine	35	3–5/4	Homogeneous; N = 3 outpatients	40		Double-blind, placebo-controlled; no randomization; crossover (ABA); 4 months	Ward Symptom Rating Scale; EPEC; serial IQ testing	Decreases in symptoms; increases in IQ

1228

Drug	Ref	Age	Sample	Dose (mg)	Dose (mg/kg)	Design	Measures	Effects
Fenfluramine	54	3–18	Homogeneous; N = 14 outpatients		1.5	Double-blind, placebo-controlled; no randomization; crossover; 7.5 months	Ritvo-Freeman Real Life Rating Scale for Autism; Alpern-Boll Developmental Profile; serial IQ testing; parent interviews; family daily diaries; weekly weights	Decreases in stereotypies, restlessness, and withdrawal; improvements in language, and sleep pattern; increases IQ
Fenfluramine	56	2½–18	Homogeneous; N = 14 outpatients		1.5	As above, in ref. 54; 17.5 months	As above, in ref. 54	Decreases in stereotypies, hyperactivity, and withdrawal; increases in communication and in cognitive functioning (IQ)
Fenfluramine	2	5–13	Homogeneous; N = 9 outpatients		1.5	As above, in ref. 54; 7.5 months	Ritvo-Freeman Real Life Rating Scale for Autism; serial IQ testing; Conners PTQ	Decreases in hyperactivity, distractibility, and stereotypies
Fenfluramine	55	33 months–24 years	Homogeneous; N = 81 outpatients		1.5	As above, in ref. 54; 7.5 months		33% "strong clinical improvement"; 52% "some improvement"; and 15% "absolutely no changes"
Fenfluramine	45	3–12	Homogeneous; N = 16		1.5	As above, in ref. 54; 7.5 months	As in ref. 54	No effect
Fenfluramine	10		Homogeneous; N = 10 inpatients	15–30	1.093–1.787	Placebo baseline followed by 4–8 weeks of drug	CPRS, CGI, AIMS, ADS, side effect checklist	Stimulating and tranquilizing effects: increased relatedness, decreases in irritability, aggressiveness, self-mutilation, and hyperactivity; improved sleep pattern
Naltrexone	23	3.75–6.42	Homogeneous; N = 5 inpatients		0.5–2.0	Open acute dose range tolerance study design	CPRS, CGI, PTQ, NGI, cognitive battery, side effect checklist, AIMS, ADS	Tranquilizing (decreases of aggressiveness directed against self and others and hyperactivity) and stimulating (decreases of withdrawal, increases of language production and more responsive affect)

[a] Abbreviations: ADS, Abbreviated Dyskinesia Scale; AIMS, Abnormal Involuntary Movement Scale; CBI, Children's Behavior Inventory; CGI, Clinical Global Impressions; CPRS, Children's Psychiatric Rating Scale; DOTES, Dosage Record and Treatment Emergent Symptoms Scale; EPEC, Evaluation and Prescription for Exceptional Children; NGI, Nurse's Global Impressions; PTQ, Parent Teacher Questionnaire; TESS, Treatment Emergent Symptoms Scale; TSCL, Target Symptom Checklist.

[b] In the laboratory, facilitation of discrimination learning is seen without affect on stereotypies or motor activity.

TABLE 2. *Cognitive and learning measures in clinical drug trials*[a]

Measure	Duration of study	Subjects		Ref.
		Ages in years	Sample size	
Cognitive battery (based on items from Gesell Developmental Schedules, WPPSI[b], and Stanford-Binet)	1) 12 weeks 2) 14–21 weeks	2.6–7.2 2.25–7.17	40 30	8 20
Language acquisition	12 weeks	2.6–7.2	40	8
Discrimination learning (auditory and visual stimuli)	1) 14 weeks 2) 14 weeks	2.33–6.92 3.17–7.5	40 42	1 22
Serial IQ testing (Merrill-Palmer Preschool Performance, Cattell or Stanford-Binet Scales, age-appropriate Wechsler Scale)	1) 7.5 months (Note: IQ measured once every month) 2) Same as 1. above 3) Same as 1. above	3–18 5–13 3–12	14 9 16	54 2 45
IQ and/or DQ testing (Gesell Developmental Schedules, age-appropriate Wechsler Scale, Stanford-Binet)	9 months–3.8 years (mean 3.0 years) (Note: IQ measured twice: on baseline and after 9 months–3.8 years)	3.3–8.11	15	29

[a] Adapted from ref. 17.
[b] WPPSI, Wechsler Preschool and Primary Scale of Intelligence.

Naltrexone HCl was administered to 5 autistic boys, ages 3.75 to 6.42 years, whose intellectual functioning ranged from mildly to profoundly retarded. Their symptoms included withdrawal, hyperactivity, stereotypies, aggressiveness against self or others, and irritability. An open acute dose range tolerance design was employed; naltrexone was given in ascending doses, once a week only. The doses were 0.5, 1.0, and 2.0 mg/kg/day. Three of the 5 children were responders; decreases of withdrawal, hyperactivity, aggressiveness against self and others, and increases of language production and responsiveness of affect were rated (23). Mild sedation of short duration was the only side effect; all laboratory studies, including liver enzymes and electrocardiogram remained unchanged. These encouraging findings warrant further studies.

Comparison and Interaction of Pharmacotherapy and Psychosocial Treatments

Only a small number of autistic children will lead independent lives as adults (13); none of the currently available treatments will yield dramatic changes (13,27). Acquisition of normal language and speech by the age of 5 or 6 years seems to be the single and most important predictor for outcome (30). In view of these findings, it is important to compare drug treatment to another quantifiable treatment, behavior modification, and if both are effective, to determine whether the combination of both is more effective than either treatment modality alone. This was the purpose of a double-blind, placebo-controlled study in 40 hospitalized autistic children, aged 2.6 to 7.2 years (8). Here, haloperidol was compared to behavior therapy focusing on language acquisition. Only the combination of both treatments increased significantly the acquisition of words and was superior to the other treatments in this factorial design, where children were randomly assigned to one of the four treatment groups. The purpose of drug therapy should be to make the autistic child more amenable to other treatment modalities; as pointed out by Irwin (40) the only lasting effect of drug administration is due to conjoint psychosocial treatment. The findings of the above study are important, and if replicated they have far-reaching implications.

ACKNOWLEDGMENTS

This work was supported in part by NIMH Grants MH-32212 and MH-40177, by a grant from the Stallone Fund for Autism Research, and by Social and Behavioral Sciences Research Grant No. 12-108 from the March of Dimes Birth Defects Foundation.

REFERENCES

1. Anderson, L. T., Campbell, M., Grega, D. M., Perry, R., Small, A. M., and Green, W. H. (1984): *Am. J. Psychiatry,* 141:1195–1202.
2. August, G. J., Raz, N., and Baird, T. D. (1985): *J. Autism Dev. Disord.,* 15:97–107.
3. Burdock, E. I., and Hardesty, A. S. (1967): In: *Psychopathology of Mental Development,* edited by J. Zubin and J. A. Jervis. Grune and Stratton, New York.
4. Campbell, M. (1977): *Psychopharmacol. Bull.,* 13(2):30–33.
5. Campbell, M. (1978): In: *Psychopharmacology: A Generation of Progress,* edited by M. A. Lipton, A. DiMascio, and K. F. Killam, pp. 1451–1461. Raven Press, New York.
6. Campbell, M. (1978): In: *Proceedings of the Third International Symposium on Psychopharmacology,* edited by H. C. B. Denber, pp. 63–92. Raven Press, New York.
7. Campbell, M., Anderson, L. T., Cohen, I. L., Perry, R., Small, A. M., Green, W. H., Anderson, L., and McCandless, W. H. J. (1982): *Psychopharmacol. Bull.,* 18(1):110–112.

8. Campbell, M., Anderson, L. T., Meier, M., Cohen, I. L., Small, A. M., Samit, C., and Sachar, E. J. (1978): *J. Am. Acad. Child Psychiatry,* 17:640–655.

9. Campbell, M., Anderson, L. T., Small, A. M., Perry, R., Green, W. H., and Caplan, R. (1982): *J. Autism Dev. Disord.,* 12:167–175.

10. Campbell, M., Deutsch, S. I., Perry, R., Wolsky, B. B., and Palij, M. (1986): *Psychopharmacol. Bull.,* 22:141–147.

11. Campbell, M., Friedman, E., Green, W. H., Collins, P. J., Small, A. M., and Breuer, H. (1975): *Int. Pharmacopsychiatry,* 10:213–221.

12. Campbell, M., Geller, B., and Cohen, I. L. (1977): *J. Pediatr. Psychol.,* 2:153–161.

13. Campbell, M., and Green, W. H. (1985): In: *Comprehensive Textbook of Psychiatry,* 4th ed., Vol. 2, edited by H. I. Kaplan and B. J. Sadock, pp. 1672–1683. Williams & Wilkins, Baltimore.

14. Campbell, M., Green, W. H., and Deutsch, S. I. (1985): *Child and Adolescent Psychopharmacology.* Sage Publications, Beverly Hills & London.

15. Campbell, M., Grega, D. M., Green, W. H., and Bennett, W. G. (1983): *Clin. Neuropharmacol.,* 6:207–222.

16. Campbell, M., and Palij, M. (1985): *Psychopharmacol. Bull.,* 21(4):719–733.

17. Campbell, M., and Palij, M. (1985): *Psychopharmacol. Bull.,* 21(4):1047–1053.

18. Campbell, M., and Palij, M. (1985): *Psychopharmacol. Bull.,* 21(4):1063–1082.

19. Campbell, M., Perry, R., Bennett, W. G., Small, A. M., Green, W. H., Grega, D. M., Schwartz, V., and Anderson, L. (1983): *Psychopharmacol. Bull.,* 19(1):80–82.

20. Campbell, M., Small, A. S., Hollander, C. S., Korein, J., Cohen, I. L., Kalmijn, M., and Ferris, S. J. (1978): *J. Autism Child. Schizophr.,* 8:371–381.

21. Campbell, M., Small, A. M., Palij, M., Perry, R., Meiselas, K., and Shell, J. (1987) (in press).

22. Campbell, M., Small, A. M., Palij, M., Perry, R., and Polonsky, B. B. (1987): *Psychopharmacol. Bull.,* 23(1):123–127.

23. Campbell, M., Sokol, M. S., Small, A. M., Palij, M., Perry, R., Nobler, M., Addrizzo, D. (1986): *Am. Acad. Child and Adolescent Psychiatry,* 2:34.

24. Chassan, J. B. (1979): *Research Design in Clinical Psychology and Psychiatry,* 2nd ed. Irvington Publishers, New York.

25. Cochran, W. G., and Cox, G. M. (1957): *Experimental Designs,* 2nd ed. John Wiley, New York.

26. Cohen, I. L., Campbell, M., Posner, D., Small, A. M., Triebel, D., and Anderson, L. T. (1980): *J. Am. Acad. Child Psychiatry,* 19:665–677.

27. DeMyer, M. K. (1981): *Schizophr. Bull.,* 7:388–451.

28. *Diagnostic and Statistical Manual of Mental Disorders (DSM-III),* 3rd ed. (1980): American Psychiatric Association, Washington, DC.

29. Die Trill, M. L., Wolsky, B. B., Shell, J., Green, W. H., Perry, R., and Campbell, M. (1984): Presented at the 31st Annual Meeting of the American Academy of Child Psychiatry, Toronto, October 10–14.

30. Eisenberg, L. (1956): *Am. J. Psychiatry,* 112:607–612.

31. Fish, B. (1968): In: *Psychopharmacology, A Review of Progress, 1957–1967,* edited by D. H. Efron, J. O. Cole, J. Levine, and J. R. Wittenborn, pp. 989–1001. Public Health Service Publication No. 1836, U.S. Government Printing Office, Washington, DC.

32. Fish, B. (1970): *Psychopharmacol. Bull.,* 6:12–15.

33. Fish, B., Shapiro, T., and Campbell, M. (1966): *Am. J. Psychiatry,* 123:32–39.

34. Freeman, B. J., Ritvo, E. R., Yokota, A., and Ritvo, A. (1986): *J. Am. Acad. Child Psychiatry,* 25:130–136.

35. Geller, E., Ritvo, E. R., Freeman, B. J., and Yuwiler, H. (1982): *N. Engl. J. Med.,* 307:165–169.

36. Gillberg, C., Terenius, L., and Lonnerholm, G. (1985): *Arch. Gen. Psychiatry,* 42:780–783.

37. Green, W. H., Campbell, M., Hardesty, A. S., Grega, D. M., Padron-Gayol, M., Shell, J., and Erlenmeyer-Kimling, L. (1984): *J. Am. Acad. Child Psychiatry,* 23:399–409.

38. Guy, W. (1976): *ECDEU Assessment Manual for Psychopharmacology* (revised). Department of Health, Education and Welfare Publication No. (ADM) 76-338, Rockville, MD.

39. Hardesty, A. S., and Burdock, E. I. (1979): *Psychopharmacol. Bull.,* 15:14–21.

40. Irwin, S. (1968): *Am. J. Psychiatry (Suppl.),* 124:1–19.

41. Kalat, J. W. (1978): *J. Autism Child Schizophr.,* 8:477–479.

42. Kazdin, A. E. (1982): *Single-Case Research Designs.* Oxford University Press, New York.

43. Klykylo, W. M., Feldis, D., O'Grady, D., Ross, D. L., and Halloran, C. (1985): *J. Autism Dev. Disord.,* 15:417–423.

44. Laska, E., Meisner, M., and Kushner, H. B. (1983): *Biometrics,* 39:1087–1091.

45. Leventhal, B. L. (1985): Presented at the 25th NCDEU Annual (Anniversary) Meeting, Key Biscayne, Florida, May 1–4.

46. Meiselas, K., Peselow, E. D., Die Trill, M. L., Deutsch, S. I., Perry, R., Cicero, S. D., and Campbell, M. (1984): Presented at the 31st Annual Meeting of the American Academy of Child Psychiatry, Toronto, October 10–14.

47. Naruse, H., Nagahata, M., Nakane, Y., Shirahashi, K., Takesada, M., and Yamazaki, K. (1982): *Acta Paedopsychiatr.,* 48:173–184.

48. Panksepp, J., Sahley, T. L. (1987): In: *Neurobiological Issues in Autism,* edited by E. Schopler and G. B. Mesibov, pp. 357–372. Plenum Press, New York.

49. Perry, R., Campbell, M., Green, W. H., Small, A. M., Die Trill, M. L., Meiselas, K., Golden, R. R., and Deutsch, S. I. (1985): *Psychopharmacol. Bull.,* 21:140–143.

50. *Psychopharmacol. Bull.* (1973): Special Issue: *Pharmacotherapy of Children.*

51. *Psychopharmacol. Bull.* (1985): Special Feature: *Rating Scales and Assessment Instruments for Use in Pediatric Psychopharmacology Research.* Vol. 21, No. 4.

52. Rimland, B., Callaway, E., and Dreyfus, P. (1978): *Am. J. Psychiatry,* 135:472–475.

53. Ritvo, E. R., and Freeman, B. J. (1978): *J. Am. Acad. Child Psychiatry,* 17:565–575.

54. Ritvo, E. R., Freeman, B. J., Geller, E., and Yuwiler, A. (1983): *J. Am. Acad. Child Psychiatry,* 22:549–558.

55. Ritvo, E. R., Freeman, B. J., Yuwiler, A., Geller, E., Schroth, P., Yokota, A., Mason-Brothers, A., August, G. J., Klykylo, W., Leventhal, B., Lewis, K., Piggott, L., Realmuto, G., Stubbs, E. G., and Umansky, R. (1986): *Psychopharmacol. Bull.,* 22:133–140.

56. Ritvo, E. R., Freeman, B. J., Yuwiler, A., Geller, E., Yokota, A., Schroth, P., and Novak, P. (1984): *J. Pediatr.,* 105:823–829.

57. Ritvo, E. R., Yuwiler, A., Geller, E., Ornitz, E. M., Saeger, K., and Plotkin, S. (1970): *Arch. Gen. Psychiatry,* 23:566–572.

58. Sameroff, A. J., Seifer, R., and Zax, M. (1982): *Early Development of Children at Risk for Emotional Disorder.* Monographs of the Society for Research in Child Development, 47(7, Serial No. 199), pp. 1–82.

59. Schuster, C. R., Lewis, M., and Seiden, L. S. (1986): *Psychopharmacol. Bull.,* 22(1):148–151.

60. Turner, D. A., Purchatzke, G., Gift, T., Farmer, C., and Uhlenhuth, E. H. (1974): In: *Principles and Techniques of Human Research and Therapeutics, Vol. 8,* edited by J. Levine, B. C. Schiele, and W. J. R. Taylor, pp. 105–118. Futura Publishing Co., Mt. Kisco, New York.

61. Volkmar, F. R., Paul, R., Cohen, D. J., and Schaywitz, B. A. (1983): *N. Engl. J. Med.,* 309:187.

62. Weizman, R., Weizman, A., Tyano, S., Székely, G., Weissman, B. A., and Sarne, Y. (1984): *Psychopharmacology,* 82:368–370.

63. Young, J. G., Cohen, D. J., Brown, S.-L., and Caparulo, B. K. (1978): *J. Am. Acad. Child Psychiatry,* 17:671–678.

64. Young, J. G., Kavanagh, M. E., Anderson, G. M., Shaywitz, B. A., and Cohen, D. J. (1982): *J. Autism Dev. Disord.,* 12:147–165.

65. Young, J. G., Ludman, W. L., and Knott, P. J. (1986): In: *Biological Psychiatry 1985,* edited by C. Shagass, R. C. Josiassen, W. H. Bridger, K. J. Weiss, D. Stoff, and G. M. Simpson, pp. 1495–1497. Elsevier Science Publishing Co., New York.

Psychopharmacology:
The Third Generation of Progress,
edited by Herbert Y. Meltzer.
Raven Press, New York © 1987.

CHAPTER **127**

Toward a Movement Control Perspective of Tardive Dyskinesia

Robert L. Sprague and Karl M. Newell

Most writers on the history of tardive dyskinesia cite a German paper by Schönecker (33) as the beginning of the study of tardive dyskinesia in 1957 (4,19). If one considers only populations of the mentally retarded, as is the focus of this paper, the history of investigation of the topic is even more recent (38). In 1975, some 18 years after the first report, Paulson et al. (29) reported a clinical study classifying the kinds of abnormal movements leading to tardive dyskinesia in an institutional population of mentally retarded people. Surprisingly, there were no other reports of research with the mentally retarded until Gualtieri and colleagues (13,14) wrote about it in the early 1980s. Once an interest became expressed in this area, several articles were published in the 1980s, which are reviewed by Kalachnik (21).

CLINICAL MANIFESTATION

Mentally Retarded Populations

Although there are books that describe the abnormal involuntary movements of tardive dyskinesia in the psychiatric populations (4,19), there are relatively few such descriptions of these abnormal movements in mentally retarded people. Therefore one of the more thorough descriptions will be quoted at length:

(a) in the facial area, grimacing, tics, and brow arching, (b) in the ocular area, bursts of blinking and fine tremor or twitching of the eyelids or periorbital area, (c) in the oral area, lip smacking, puckering, sucking, chewing, lateral jaw movement, lower lip thrusting, and cheek puffing, (d) in the lingual area, tongue thrusting, pushing the tongue

against the cheek, lower lip producing a noticeable bulge, and worm-like (athetoid) and jerking (myokymic) movements of the tongue inside the mouth, (e) in the head, neck, and truncal areas, shoulder torsion or rotation, a thrusting or circulatory movement of the pelvic area (axial hyperkinesia), and snapping the head back (retrocollis) or to the side (torticollis), (f) in the upper limb area, jerking as well as rhythmic serpentine writhing movements and (g) in the lower limb area, toe movement, foot tapping, and ankle flexion. A myriad of other possible manifestations such as gait disturbances, restless legs, diaphragmatic (throat) movements, head nodding, ballistic movements (i.e. sudden, fast, large swinging movements of the arms and legs), and rubbing the thighs or caressing the face and hair are mentioned as well. Some of the more colorful, though nonfunctional, terms for the movements listed above are the "anteater sign" or "flycatcher syndrome" for tongue thrusting, the "bon-bon sign" for tongue in cheek, and "piano playing movements" for twisting, spreading, and flexion-extension of the fingers (ref. 21, p. 135).

What is important in this context is an attempt to establish a basis for distinguishing between the abnormal involuntary movements of tardive dyskinesia in populations of mentally retarded people and similar rhythmic movements of stereotypy also seen, particularly, in institutionalized populations of mentally retarded individuals. Although the distinction between these two disorders has great implications for theory and major implications for clinical treatment, there is surprisingly little written on the topic. One of the themes of this chapter is an attempt to lay some conceptual framework for distinguishing between these two major classes of abnormal movement, particularly in populations of developmentally disabled individuals, although the differential diagnostic problem is not exclusive to this population.

It is not very clearly explicated in the literature, but the general assumption is that tardive dyskinetic movements are associated with the use and withdrawal of neuroleptic medication (22) and stereotypic movements with the deprivation of stimulation in institutional settings and the presence of role models that encourage the development of such odd movements, as reviewed by Lewis and Baumeister (26). What is implicit in this thinking is that tardive dyskinesia is attributable to some type of lesion in the central nervous system, probably neurochemical, whereas stereotyped activity is a learned behavior pattern that is highly repetitive and attributable to learning in unique situations of deprived stimulation. To repeat, this is all highly speculative because there have been no empirical attempts to clarify the differences between these two serious disorders.

Illustrative Case

One of the authors of this paper (R.L.S.), in conversation with the researchers of stereotyped movement disorders of the mentally retarded, was urged to write the case history of a foster infant his family raised. About 15 years ago the author and his wife were foster parents as certified by a state agency until numerous difficulties resulted in ending the foster care relationship (37). One of the babies placed in the home was an infant girl, the daughter of a teenager who had one previous child and who reportedly attempted to abort the pregnancy that resulted in this infant girl. The mother refused to have any prenatal care, and it was reported to us that her brother had to take her forcibly to the hospital for the delivery of this baby. As could be inferred from such a history, the pregnancy and delivery had more than its share of traumas, so it is not surprising that the baby was born with a convulsive disorder and mild microcephaly. After about 2 years and numerous problems with the child, a neurological consultation was sought and obtained at a large metropolitan children's hospital where it was decided to hospitalize the child for a few days. Because the hospital was some distance from the home of the foster parents, it was not possible to visit the infant regularly. At the time of the hospitalization, the infant walked—ran is a more apt description—and was especially adept at climbing with careless abandonment on furniture, drapes, stairwells, etc. Before leaving the child in the hospital, the foster parents suggested to the nurse that it might be useful to place a transparent plastic bubble top over the crib to ensure that the child stayed in the crib in the strange environment. The nurse rejected the foster parents' suggestion out of hand, but when the child climbed out of the crib and ran after them and joined the foster parents in the hall as they were leaving, the nurse reconsidered the suggestion.

Upon returning to the hospital to pick up the child about 5 days later, the foster father was amazed to see that not only had the plastic bubble been placed on top of the crib but a blanket had been tied around the sides of the crib to prevent the child from seeing out. As Lewis and Baumeister (26) so aptly discuss, a "cage" stereotypy had developed in those few days. Other than overactivity and climbing, the foster parents had not noticed any body rocking by the child prior to the hospitalization. But after a few days of severely reduced visual stimulation in a strange setting, the child had developed a full-blown body-rocking stereotypy. The child rocked in the middle of the hospital crib with her body swinging back and forth at a typical rate of about one per second. This case history is included in this chapter because there is practically no historical information or case material available in the literature as to how stereotypic patterns develop in children. One case history does not particularly prove anything, but it may illustrate the susceptibility of a child with presumed damage to the central nervous system to develop quite rapidly severe stereotyped movement patterns.

Distinguishing Tardive Dyskinesia from Stereotypy

It is quite clear that the observable movement patterns of individuals with stereotyped movements and individuals with tardive dyskinesia may be quite similar, if not identical. Thus a serious problem of differential diagnosis may be presented to the clinician in this situation. At recently sponsored National Institute of Mental Health workshops on the topic of psychopharmacology in the mentally retarded (31,32), it was the consensus of the experts in attendance that usually stereotyped behavior could be distinguished from tardive dyskinesia by close attention to the total movement pattern and to the context in which it was observed. For example, it was speculated that the stereotyped behavior usually involved larger segments of the body in a highly ritualistic, repetitive movement. Perhaps just as important, it was speculated that there were certain patterns of movement very typical of stereotypy but less typical of tardive dyskinesia. Some of these patterns of movement are head rocking, body rocking, and repetitive complex patterns of hand movements, often in front of the face, such as flipping fingers before the eyes, patting the head a certain number of times, then rubbing the nose and finally waving the hand before the eyes. It seems that tardive dyskinetic movements typically involve smaller segments of the body in patterns of motions that are less complex than those previously identified with institutionalized mentally retarded individuals.

ASSESSMENT OF ABNORMAL MOVEMENT PATTERNS

Rating Scale Methodology

Some form of rating scale assessment is the most popular assessment technique used to evaluate the abnormal voluntary movements associated with tardive dyskinesia (10). Kalachnik (21) has reviewed the six rating scales available in the literature that have been used to assess tardive dyskinesia. These are (a) AIMS (Abnormal Involuntary Movements Scale) (18), which is probably the most prevalent scale, although it may not be the most widely used scale with the mentally retarded; (b) DIS-Co (Dyskinesia Identification System–Coldwater) (40), which is being rather widely used with mentally retarded populations; (c) TDRS (Tardive Dyskinesia Rating Scale) and the Abbreviated

Simpson/Rockland Abbreviated Dyskinesia Scale (34); (d) TRIMS (Texas Research Institute of Mental Sciences) (35); and (e) WES (Withdrawal Emergent Symptom Checklist) (9). Although there are no empirical data on how often each of these scales is used in people with developmental disabilities, it is our impression that there are only two used very frequently (AIMS and DIS-Co), whereas the other three scales are used infrequently or almost not at all.

Psychometric Properties

It is most unfortunate that, although psychometric theory has been available for at least 85 years to assess the adequacy of instruments designed to evaluate the behavior of people, ranging from intelligence to psychiatric symptoms, this body of theory and empirical knowledge has hardly been acknowledged by scholars developing rating scales for tardive dyskinesia. As has been discussed previously (41), with the exception of DIS-Co, most of the other scales, at best, give small sample data on test/retest reliability and/ or some information on interrater agreement, with almost no attention to other important characteristics such as stability over time, validity with external measures, and the whole subarea of quality of the item as it contributes to an overall score. Several professional societies have issued pamphlets for a number of years listing principles that should be used to evaluate such rating scale assessments. The most recent bulletin—the fifth in this series of booklets—was issued by a group of three professional societies in 1985 (3). In a recent article, Sprague and Kalachnik (39) surveyed the 180 principles enunciated in the *Standards,* and 21 were identified as directly applying to the area of tardive dyskinesia. Even a cursory review of the literature on rating scales will show that most of the scale developers are either unaware of, or ignore, suggestions for rating scale construction as outlined in the *Standards.*

In contrast to this trend of ignoring psychometric theory, a revision of DIS-Co was undertaken, using six quality-of-item indicators as criteria for the revision and using statistical weights as the basic empirical data for the revision (41). This revision started with a pool of 34 items and, using a large sample of institutionalized mentally retarded people, reduced the redundancy and noncontributing items to 15. The elimination of items was based on the quality-of-item indicators, which resulted in a more sensitive rating scale that was obviously shorter and much easier to use.

Thus, since a revision of the scale improved the instrument, the question immediately arose whether this system (21) can be used effectively to teach personnel to rate abnormal movements. If a scale is only effective in the hands of a small body of experts, its usefulness as an applied technique in a large number of clinical settings is highly dubious (21). Surprisingly, there are only a very few studies that have even attempted to investigate on a very small scale whether a rating scale can be taught to other individuals (43). Recently, however, a study has been completed with reasonably large samples for both the DIS-Co ($N = 201$) and the revision, DISCUS ($N = 95$).

Using deviation from the criterion score as the primary metric, it was clearly shown that, although personnel from an institutional setting initially overrate abnormal movements as assessed by videotape, after 8 hr of training the tendency to overrate is either greatly reduced or eliminated (in fact, there is a tendency to underrate), and the generalization to live patients from the clinical setting of the raters is exceptionally good (39). For example, on the revised scale (DISCUS) the mean deviation score from criterion on pretest examination with videotape was 4.65, whereas the mean deviation criterion score on live patients was 0.08, which is a highly significantly statistical reduction in the amount of deviation from criterion. Just as important, the variance of the ratings of the trainees around the criterion score was also reduced. The next finding, which may come as a surprise to some people, is that there was no difference in the trainability as measured, again, by deviation from criterion score in different discipline groups of trainees, including these four groups: nurses, licensed practical nurses, physicians, and others consisting of psychologists, special educators, etc. Thus, it would seem that using psychometric theory as a foundation for a program of developing a rating scale and evaluating the scale following psychometric principles is a most useful procedure, and the procedure has led to the development of a rating scale instrument that is reliable (40), trainable (39), and has considerable validity (22).

Problems Remaining

This progress with rating scale technology must not, however, be taken as a satisfactory conclusion to the diagnostic problems, because there are many other issues still unresolved in tardive dyskinesia assessment for practical applications (16) and in research support for this area (15). Some of these issues involve differential diagnosis of patterns of abnormal movements as displayed in different disorders such as stereotypic movement and tardive dyskinesia. Ultimately, a series of assessment technologies should be developed that would permit reliable, accurate differential diagnosis not only of tardive dyskinesia and stereotypy, but also of other important conditions resulting in repetitive abnormal movements, such as parkinsonism, pseudoparkinsonism associated with beginning treatment with neuroleptic medications, Huntington's chorea, etc. In order to develop such reliable and sensitive diagnostic instruments, the authors firmly believe that a sound conceptual basis needs to be laid to guide researchers in the development of these techniques. Unfortunately, the clinical assessment of abnormal involuntary movements as revealed by rating scale techniques has not utilized theory and empirical knowledge in the disciplines that have sought understanding of coordination and control in human movement. Whatever diagnostic procedures eventually develop must take into consideration the dynamics of abnormal human movement, which involve some basic considerations of moving the mass of biological tissue in space as linked by joints and propelled by coordinated muscle contractions. This obvious point is often forgotten in the concepts underlying the development of diagnostic tests. A conceptual framework is particularly important in the mid-1980s, because a number of exciting technological advances have been made that allow very precise quantification of the movements of body parts and that promise exact specification of movements and their patterns. But before this new technology can be effectively utilized, a conceptual framework should be developed. This leads to a discussion of the movement control characteristics implicit in any understanding of abnormal movement patterns.

MOVEMENT CONTROL CHARACTERISTICS

Basic Considerations

Natural observation of abnormal movements leads intuitively to the categorization of behaviors such as body rocking, hand waving, head banging, facial grimacing, tongue thrusting, and so on. The natural categorization of abnormal movements has been operationalized by the development of rating scales and the standardization of DIS-Co, as previously described. Rating scales attempt to define a formal system for the nominal categorization of movements. The rating scale categorization of abnormal movements provides a useful approach to identifying disorders and the basis for the development of movement disorder screening tests that can be administered by personnel in a number of clinical settings. However, rating scales do not provide any insight into the movement control characteristics of the disorder, and the observer categorization approach is probably not the most sensitive technique for discriminating among various pathological conditions.

It would seem that only a dynamic (kinematic and kinetic) analysis of the movement sequence will open the window to an understanding of the motor control properties of abnormal movements. Kinematics is that branch of dynamics which relates to the dimensions of length and time and their various derivatives such as velocity and acceleration. Kinetics is that branch of dynamics which relates to mass, force, and time and their various derivatives. A particular need with respect to tardive dyskinesia is an understanding of how these dynamic properties of movement may differ in persons on and withdrawn from neuroleptic medication, and how these movement properties differ from those of institutionalized stereotypic movements together with those of "normal" movement control.

In a recent article, one of us (28) has elaborated on work in perception (7,20) and action (24,25), to suggest that the topological properties of the relative motion of limbs and torso may be taken to reflect coordination, whereas the scaling characteristics of a given set of relative motions may be taken as an index of control. Topological kinematic properties are those which remain invariant in the face of transformations in absolute scale of movement parameters due to speed or effort changes and may be utilized to characterize what is often referred to as the form of the movement sequence (27,28). Arguably, it is perception of the topological properties of movement that specifies the categorization of actions, such as those conducted in rating scales. Even in postural activities, which may be viewed as the attempt to maintain a stable body configuration with respect to the environment, there is still relative motion of each body link (17). Thus, in both posture and movement, topological properties of the kinematics reflect the form of the action. Skill is the optimal configuration of coordination

and control for the individual, given the constraints at hand in the organism-environment interaction.

Given the operational framework for coordination, control, and skill briefly described above, it is apparent that there have been very few investigations of the pattern of coordination of the abnormal stereotypic movements. Where kinematic analysis has been conducted, it has primarily been limited to an examination of the frequency characteristics of a single biomechanical degree of freedom movement in the act of body rocking (26,30,44). The few studies of the frequency components of stereotypic behavior have been interpreted as supportive of a centralist account of motor control (26,44), after the central pattern generator concept (8,12).

In the balance of this section we lay out some of the key motor control issues to be resolved regarding tardive dyskinesia and develop briefly the significance of these issues for a theoretical account of these drug-induced movement disorders. It is anticipated that the development of a link between the motor control and tardive dyskinesia literatures may enable the latter to go beyond the traditional descriptive characterization of behavioral acts to a more principled account of the dynamic properties of the abnormal movements evident in tardive dyskinesia. It is proposed that only this latter approach can open the door to the development of a psychopharmacological theory of tardive dyskinesia that is consistent with the biophysical principles of movement disorders.

The unnatural properties of stereotypic movement disorders relate primarily to (a) their "involuntary" nature, which has been discussed above, and (b) their atypical movement properties, in contrast to movements viewed as reflective of "normal" action patterns. In the remainder of this chapter we focus on the description of the motor control properties of stereotypic movements. The goal is to provide an outline of ways to develop a movement control perspective of the abnormal movements displayed by people with tardive dyskinesia.

DEGREES OF FREEDOM AND ABNORMAL MOVEMENTS

A fundamental problem for the motor system is regulation of the many organismic degrees of freedom (6,42). Variables are free to vary at all levels of biological analysis, and it is the coordination of this regulatory process that is a central question in action theory. At a behavioral biomechanical level of analysis, Bernstein (6) has estimated that there must be in excess of 100 degrees of freedom that necessitate coordination and control. It is also the case that the number of free variables requiring constraint typically increases the more micro the level of analysis. Thus, for example, if the system regulates muscles, approximately 700 degrees of freedom would require constraint, whereas tens of thousands of degrees of freedom would require constraint in a motor system regulating motor units.

Observation of the movements that are characteristic of tardive dyskinesia suggests that many of these abnormal acts involve coordination and control of only a few degrees of freedom at the behavioral level. For example, there is often only one anatomical segment involved in the abnormal action, and the stereotypic movement sequence takes place around a single axis of motion. Many of the instances of tongue thrusting, arm movements, and foot tapping reflect repetitive movements of a single degree of freedom. Furthermore, where more than a single degree of freedom is involved in stereotypic movement, the activities often reflect the symmetrical activity of body parts on either side of the body midline, a constraint that in and of itself probably reduces the degrees of freedom to be regulated.

The above set of observations does not, of course, reflect all the activities characteristic of tardive dyskinesia. The important point being advanced, however, is that in many instances the stereotypic movements reflect the coordination and control of only a few biomechanical degrees of freedom. The rhythmic characteristics displayed within these simple movements contain, however, interesting cyclical properties of amplitude, period, and phase.

It is clear that the activities reflective of tardive dyskinesia need a formal analysis from a degrees of freedom perspective. Several immediate questions need to be addressed. First, how many degrees of freedom are being coordinated and controlled in each repetitive activity? Second, is there any systematic change from a degrees of freedom perspective in the development of abnormal movements with progressive states of tardive dyskinesia? Third, how does drug withdrawal interact with the coordination process in patients with tardive dyskinesia? Fourth, is there a systematic directional order from a cephalocaudal or proximal-distal perspective to the development of tardive dyskinesia as is often claimed with the development of "normal" fundamental movement patterns (11).

Bernstein (6) viewed skill as the mastery of redundant degrees of freedom. In voluntary movement, the individual typically "relaxes the ban" in the coordination of the degrees of freedom, as is reflected by the transition of jerky movements to the smooth coordinated movement of the skilled performer. A degrees of freedom analysis of tardive dyskinesia could reveal some of the basic motor control properties of the abnormal stereotypic movements.

Rhythmic Properties of Stereotypic Movements

Rhythmic phenomena are common at macro- and microlevels of biological systems. For example, they are evident in the daily rhythm of life, the movement patterns of animal locomotion, and at the microlevel of neuronal networks. Viewed in this light, the rhythmical qualities of stereotypic movement disorders are at first glance not atypical. Indeed, some of the action patterns identified with the disorder of tardive dyskinesia are sometimes produced voluntarily by individuals viewed as normal. For example, certain whole body stereotypies of institutionalized patients may match a movement segment performed by a dancer. Thus, the display of rhythmic movement behavior is not in and of itself an aberrant phenomenon.

There have been a few analyses of the frequency characteristics of stereotypic movements, particularly in the act of body rocking (26,30,44). These studies have shown that intraindividual rates of rocking are stable over considerable periods of time. Alpert et al. (2) have also provided an indication that shifts in the frequency component of finger movement tremor may occur with the application of neuroleptic medication (chlorpromazine), perhaps due to changes in dopamine receptor sensitivity (1). A few movement-recording techniques have been utilized with patients exhibiting tardive dyskinesia (10), but no systematic relationships regarding movement properties have emerged that may be contrasted with the rhythmical properties of normal motor behavior or other categories of stereotypic movement. In summary, there is at present very little useful data regarding the rhythmical properties of tardive dyskinesia.

There is considerable evidence from repetitive "normal" movement tasks that subjects naturally gravitate to a preferred frequency of movement that is consistent with biophysical principles of optimization in terms of the efficiency of motion (36). Efficiency is defined by the ratio of mechanical work done to energy expended. An understanding of the frequency characteristics of tardive dyskinesia and other abnormal stereotypic movement disorders would open the door to an efficiency analysis of the stereotypic movement disorders. This kind of approach to dyskinetic patients would also provide the basis to examine the influence of neuroleptic drugs on the efficiency of motion and the specific hypothesis of Alpert et al. (2) that drugs change the frequency characteristics of movement. Observation suggests that tardive dyskinetic patients are, in effect, "skilled" at producing the various categories of stereotypic movements, in that they appear to be less exhausted or more accustomed to their actions than "normal" people may be when attempting to mimic the same action patterns. That is, tardive dyskinesia patients may be producing the optimal movement pattern for the constraints at hand.

TOWARD A MOVEMENT CONTROL THEORY OF TARDIVE DYSKINESIA

A fuller understanding of the biodynamics of stereotypic movement disorders would provide a stronger platform from which to develop theories of movement disorders. The extant theoretical positions of stereotypic movements (5,26) follow in the main the theories of normal motor behavior that have developed around the central versus peripheral debate for motor control (23). The focus of this polemic has shifted in recent years from an either/or debate to a matter of emphasis of the respective positions. The central pattern generator literature has clearly indicated that timing properties of various biological systems are intrinsic to the system in that they do not necessitate an external stimulus to initiate or sustain rhythmic behavior (8). Traditional feedback concepts have been relegated to the secondary role of modifying centrally generated action patterns.

No matter what position one takes on the central versus peripheral debate for movement control, one is locked into some form of representation accounting for the order and regularity displayed in human action. Recently, Kugler et al. (24,25) have argued for a contrasting account of action theory in which symbolic representations are set aside (for the moment) as the principled account of movement in favor of a stronger examination of the response dynamics. Drawing on the principles of self-organization in biological systems through thermodynamics and the information perspective of ecological psychology, Kugler and colleagues propose that the order in biological and physiological processes is primarily owing to dynamics, and that the constraints that arise, both anatomical and functional, serve only to channel and guide dynamics. It is not that actions are caused by constraints; it is, rather, that some actions are excluded by them (see ref. 24, p. 9). This perspective requires a fuller understanding of the constraints on action (28), given that the patterns of coordination that arise are emergent properties.

The coordinative structure theory of Kugler et al. (24,25) provides a principled basis for which to understand the dynamics that are evident in abnormal stereotypic movements. The examination of this theoretical perspective requires, as was argued previously, the measurement of the response dynamics rather than the mere nominal categorization of the behaviors. This orientation also has implications for clinical practice and the development of more sophisticated diagnostic procedures than check-list categorization. In summary, it appears that recent developments in motor control provide a strong theoretical and empirical basis to reexamine tardive dyskinesia and the stereotypic movements which are all too common in institutionalized residents.

ACKNOWLEDGMENT

This paper was supported in part by PHS grant MH 32206 awarded to Robert L. Sprague.

REFERENCES

1. Alpert, M., Diamond, R., and Friedhoff, A. J. (1982): *Psychopharmacol. Bull.,* 18:90–92.
2. Alpert, M., Diamond, F., Weisenfreund, J., Taleporos, E., and Friedhoff, A. J. (1978): *Br. J. Psychiatry,* 133:169–175.
3. American Educational Research Association, et al. (1985): *Standards for Educational and Psychological Testing.* American Psychological Association, Washington, DC.
4. American Psychiatric Association (1979): *Tardive Dyskinesia.* American Psychiatric Association, Washington, DC.
5. Berkson, G. (1983): *Am. J. Ment. Defic.,* 88:239–246.
6. Bernstein, N. (1967): *The Coordination and Regulation of Movements.* Pergamon, London.
7. Cutting, J. E., and Proffitt, D. R. (1982): *Cognitive Psychol.,* 14:211–246.
8. Delcomyn, F. (1980): *Science,* 210:492–498.
9. Englehardt, D. M. (1974): *Withdrawal Emergent Symptoms (WES) Checklist.* Department of Psychiatry, Downstate Medical Center, New York.
10. Gardos, G., Cole, J. O., and La Brie, R. L. (1977): *Arch. Gen. Psychiatry,* 34:1206–1212.
11. Gesell, A. (1929): *Psychol. Rev.,* 36:307–319.
12. Grillner, S. (1985): *Science,* 228:143–149.
13. Gualtieri, C. T., Barnhill, J., McGimsey, J., and Schell, D. (1980): *J. Am. Acad. Child Psychiatry,* 19:419–450.
14. Gualtieri, C. T., and Hawk, B. (1980): *Appl. Res. Ment. Retard.,* 1:55–69.
15. Gualtieri, C. T., and Keppel, J. M. (1985): *Psychopharmacol. Bull.,* 21:304–309.
16. Gualtieri, C. T., and Sprague, R. L. (1984): *Psychopharmacol. Bull.,* 20:346–348.
17. Gurfinkel, V. S., Kots, Y. M., Paltsev, E. I., and Feldman, A. G. (1971): In: *Models of the Structural-Functional Organization of Certain Biological Systems,* edited by I. M. Gelfand, V. S. Gurfinkel, S. V. Fomin, and M. L. Tsetlin, pp. 382–395. MIT Press, Cambridge.
18. Guy, W., ed. (1976): *ECDEU Assessment Manual for Psychopharmacology.* U.S. Government Printing Office, Washington, DC.
19. Jeste, D. V., and Wyatt, R. J. (1982): *Understanding and Treating Tardive Dyskinesia.* Guilford Press, New York.
20. Johansson, G., von Hofsten, C., and Jansson, G. (1980): *Annu. Rev. Psychol.,* 31:27–63.
21. Kalachnik, J. E. (1985): In: *Advances in Learning and Behavior Disabilities,* edited by K. D. Gadow, pp. 133–180. JAI Press, Greenwich, CT.
22. Kalachnik, J. E., Harder, S. R., Kidd-Nielson, P., Errickson, E., Doebler, M., and Sprague, R. L. (1984): *Psychopharmacol. Bull.,* 20:27–32.
23. Kelso, J. A. S., and Stelmach, G. E. (1976): In: *Motor Control: Issues and Trends,* edited by G. E. Stelmach, pp. 1–40. Academic Press, New York.
24. Kugler, P. N., Kelso, J. A. S., and Turvey, M. T. (1980): In: *Tutorials in Motor Behavior,* edited by G. E. Stelmach and J. Requin, pp. 3–47. North-Holland, Amsterdam.
25. Kugler, P. N., Kelso, J. A. S., and Turvey, M. T. (1982): In: *The Development of Movement Control and Coordination,* edited by J. A. S. Kelso and J. E. Clark, pp. 5–78. Wiley, New York.
26. Lewis, M. H., and Baumeister, A. A. (1982): In: *International Review of Research in Mental Retardation, Vol. 11,* edited by N. R. Ellis, pp. 123–161. Academic Press, New York.
27. McGinnis, P. M., and Newell, K. M. (1982): *Hum. Movement Sci.,* 1:289–305.
28. Newell, K. M. (1985): In: *Differing Perspectives in Motor Control,* edited by D. Goodman, I. Franks, and R. Wilberg, pp. 295–317. North-Holland, Amsterdam.
29. Paulson, G. W., Rizvi, C. A., and Crane, G. E. (1975): *Clin. Pediatr.,* 14:953–955.
30. Pohl, P. (1977): *Dev. Med. Child Neurol.,* 19:811–817.
31. Reatig, N., and Raskin, A. (1985): *Psychopharmacol. Bull.,* 21:167–168.
32. Reatig, N., and Schooler, N. (1983): NIMH workshop, Washington, DC.
33. Schönecker, M. (1957): *Nervenarzt,* 28:35–36.
34. Simpson, G. M., Lee, J. H., Zoubok, B., and Gardos, G. (1979): *Psychopharmacology,* 64:171–179.
35. Smith, R. C., Allen, R., Gordon, J., and Wolff, J. (1983): *Psychopharmacol. Bull.,* 19:266–276.
36. Sparrow, W. A. (1983): *J. Motor Behav.,* 15:237–261.
37. Sprague, R. L. (1976): In: *Learning Disability/Minimal Brain Dysfunction Syndrome,* edited by R. P. Anderson and C. G. Halcomb, pp. 94–125. Charles C Thomas, Springfield, IL.
38. Sprague, R. L. (1982): Paper presented at the annual meeting of the American Academy of Child Psychiatry, Washington, DC.
39. Sprague, R. L., and Kalachnik, J. E. (1985): Paper presented at the annual meeting of the American College of Neuropsychopharmacology, Maui, HA.
40. Sprague, R. L., Kalachnik, J. E., Breuning, S. E., Davis, V. J., Ullmann, R. K., Cullari, S., Davidson, N. A., Ferguson, D. G., and Hoffner, B. A. (1984): *Psychopharmacol. Bull.,* 20:328–338.
41. Sprague, R. L., White, D. M., Ullmann, R., and Kalachnik, J. E. (1984): *Psychopharmacol. Bull.,* 20:339–345.
42. Turvey, M. T. (1977): In: *Perceiving Acting and Knowing,* edited by R. Shaw and J. Bransford. Lawrence Erlbaum Associates, Hillside, NJ.
43. Whall, A. L., Engle, V., Edwards, A., Bobel, L., and Haberland, C. (1983): *Nurs. Res.,* 32:151–156.
44. Wolff, P. H. (1968): *Can. Psychol.,* 9:474–484.

Psychopharmacology:
The Third Generation of Progress,
edited by Herbert Y. Meltzer.
Raven Press, New York © 1987.

CHAPTER 128

Tic Disorders

James F. Leckman, John T. Walkup, Mark A. Riddle, Kenneth E. Towbin, and Donald J. Cohen

Tic disorders constitute a family of related disorders of childhood onset which display a broad range of clinical manifestations and severity. The most severe tic disorder is usually designated as Gilles de la Tourette's syndrome (TS). TS is a rare, familial neuropsychiatric disorder of unknown etiology that is characterized by waxing and waning multiform motor and phonic tics and a range of complex and intriguing behavioral symptoms (15,57,97). It is typically a lifelong disorder that can be disabling.

Scientific interest in tic disorders has increased dramatically over the past decade (14). Presently, intense research efforts show promise of identifying specific genetic and nongenetic factors of etiological significance. Although these causative factors are doubtless mediated by central neurochemical mechanisms, the identification of the neuroanatomic substrates and particular pathophysiological mechanisms involved in tic disorders has been an elusive goal. Central dopaminergic systems localized in the striatum and in the mesolimbic areas remain a major focus of research interest. Expanding knowledge of the complexity of these systems and their intimate association with other neurotransmitter and neuromodulator systems, however, has made a unitary dopaminergic hypothesis increasingly untenable. More complex pathophysiologic hypotheses have been advanced, based largely on drug efficacy studies in which nondopaminergic agents have been reported to worsen or improve symptoms. Interactions between various central neurochemical systems have been posited to account for the putative clinical effects of centrally active agents. A

central cholinergic-dopaminergic imbalance has been proposed to account for the effects of cholinergic and anticholinergic agents (105). Alternatively, "interactions" between central noradrenergic and dopaminergic systems have been advanced to account for the beneficial effects of clonidine in some TS patients (19,58). Other recent data have implicated endogenous opioid systems (42a). Although these hypotheses have been heuristically useful in directing basic (10) and clinical investigations (56,58,62,72,111), little can be said with certainty concerning the pathophysiology of TS or other tic disorders.

This review examines recent advances in the understanding of tic disorders, focusing on the natural history of the disorder and prevailing etiological and pathophysiological hypotheses, with the aim of identifying promising areas for future clinical investigation.

NATURAL HISTORY

The natural history of TS is a complex and partially age-dependent set of phenomena. Attentional problems and difficulties with motoric hyperactivity and impulse control frequently precede the emergence of frank motor and phonic tics in young children (46). Motor tics typically appear well before phonic tics. The motor tics usually show a rostral-caudal progression, so that tics involving the face and head regularly precede those involving the extremities and trunk (46,97). Simple motor tics are rapid meaningless muscular events, such as eye blinking, grimacing, and shoulder jerks. The complex motor movements are slower and more "purposive" in appearance. Often they involve repetitive grooming behaviors, but can be any movement the body can produce, including touching, clapping, throwing, hopping, as well as bending, writhing, and sudden "dystonic" postures. A small proportion of patients develop self-abusive, complex motor tics of biting or hitting. Simple phonic tics are linguistically meaningless noises or sounds, such as sniffing, throat clearing, hissing, or barking. Complex phonic tics are multiform and can involve the sudden ejaculation of inappropriate words or phrases. Sudden alterations in the pitch, volume, and/or rhythm of speech, and echolalia can occur.

Obsessive-compulsive symptoms are present in a substantial proportion of cases (74,76,81,116). Onset is typically during adolescence. Compulsive rituals usually precede obsessional thoughts. Infrequently the obsessive-compulsive symptoms completely overshadow the tic symptoms.

Other salient features of the natural history of TS include the moment-to-moment, situation-dependent variation in the frequency of symptoms; tic related sensory phenomena; the "volutionary" suppression of symptoms for brief periods; the waxing and waning of symptoms over weeks to months; and the emergence of a more stable repertoire of symptoms in adulthood.

GENETIC FACTORS

Arguably the most significant advances in the understanding of tic disorders during the past decade have not come from neuropharmacologic studies, but rather have followed family-genetic and twin studies which suggest that hereditary factors are involved in the vertical transmission of tic disorders in some families. Segregation of risk within these families is consistent with an autosomal dominant mode of genetic transmission (22,26,50,80a). These results, taken with recent advances in molecular genetics and the identification of high-density families in Canada (55) and Oregon, have led to intensive efforts to locate the putative gene responsible for TS using genetic linkage techniques.

"Genetic linkage" refers to the tendency of two pieces of adjacent genetic material (usually genes) to segregate together across generations in a single family. Recently developed recombinant DNA techniques have produced many new markers suitable for linkage studies throughout the genome (49). These markers can be used to follow the inheritance (segregation) of pieces of DNA in a family and to assess its cosegregation with the putative TS gene.

Genetic linkage studies, therefore, require an extensive diagnostic evaluation of all family members in order to discriminate affected from unaffected individuals. Family study and twin data support the notion that chronic multiple tics (CMT) are a more prevalent but less severe manifestation of the same underlying genetic predisposition as TS (80,85). The identification of alternative phenotypes in affected pedigrees in addition to TS and CMT remains a critically important area of research. The relationship between TS and attention deficit disorder (ADD) is controversial, with some studies suggesting that ADD is etiologically related to TS (21), whereas other reports are more consistent with the hypothesis that ADD is a comorbid condition and that the high prevalence of ADD in TS clinic populations may result from an ascertainment bias (79).

Increased rates of obsessive-compulsive symptoms in TS patients (1,74,76,81,116), and the finding that approximately 20% of the adult first-degree relatives of TS probands display prominent obsessive-compulsive symptoms (76,81), has led to the provocative hypothesis that some forms of obsessive-compulsive disorder (OCD) may be alternate phenotypic expressions of the TS gene (80a,81). If confirmed, this finding would have a major impact on genetic linkage studies by expanding the range of phenotypic expression associated with the TS gene. It would also have considerable heuristic value for future metabolic and pharmacologic studies of OCD.

Should genetic linkage studies be successful and culminate in the location of the gene, a new era in tic disorder research would commence. Molecular genetic strategies would be used to isolate and clone the relevant DNA material so that the abnormal gene product could be identified. Subsequent studies would be expected to lead to an understanding of the functional significance of the putative gene product, its neuroanatomic localization, and its role in the pathophysiology of the disorder (49). Improved diagnostic procedures would be expected to follow from these discoveries, and children at risk for the disorder could be identified. Preventative strategies and more rational and potentially curative treatments could emerge (65).

NONGENETIC FACTORS

Twin studies, in addition to supporting the presence of hereditary factors in the transmission of TS, indicate that nongenetic factors are also important in the expression of TS and related tic disorders (31,85). In a recent twin study, Price et al. (85) reported that among 30 monozygotic (MZ) twin pairs, 53% were fully concordant for TS. Another 23% of these pairs were partially concordant, with the cotwin displaying milder tic symptoms. The remaining 23% were fully discordant, with the cotwin displaying neither TS nor tics. If TS is etiologically homogeneous, these data indicate that the same genetic predisposition may be associated with a broad range of phenotypic expression and other (nongenetic) factors are responsible for this variability of expression.

The study of nongenetic risk and protective factors is an emerging area of research. A number of potentially important risk factors have been identified for TS and related disorders. The frequency and magnitude of pre- and postnatal factors have not been fully documented in tic disorder families. Pasmanick and Kawi (78), in evaluating the hospital records of children with tics, found that mothers of children with tics were 1.5 times more likely to have experienced a complication during pregnancy than the mothers of children without tics. In a recent reexamination of the TS twin data reported by Price et al. (85), all of the index twins with TS had a lower birth weight than their unaffected cotwins, again suggesting the potential importance of prenatal factors (64a).

Clinical experience and pilot epidemiologic studies of TS indicate that periods of increased anxiety and emotional stress regularly produce exacerbations of TS symptoms (46,106). We have further speculated that stress and heightened anxiety may also play a role in the expression of the disorder among vulnerable individuals (60).

A third environmental factor that has been linked to the emergence of tic symptoms is exposure to stimulant medications (26,29,38,39,53,66,84). This is a complicated and controversial issue. In a recent examination of the question, Price et al. (85) assessed information concerning 34 cases (16 twins and 18 nontwins) of stimulant exposure prior to the age of 18 years who had or who later developed TS. Only 27% of these cases reported a clear association between stimulant exposure and tic onset. Among the MZ twin pairs, three pairs were concordant for stimulant exposure and all were concordant for TS. Six other MZ pairs were discordant for stimulant exposure. In each case, the unexposed cotwin also developed TS, although their age of onset was on average 12 months later. The broad range of response argues against there being a simple one-to-one relationship between stimulant exposure and the appearance of tics (29,88).

PATHOPHYSIOLOGICAL MECHANISMS

Dopaminergic Mechanisms

Several neurochemical systems have been implicated in the pathogenesis of tic disorders. The most compelling data concern central dopaminergic mechanisms. These data include reports from three independent laboratories of lowered baseline and postprobenicid cerebrospinal fluid (CSF) homovanillic acid (HVA) levels in TS patients compared to available contrast groups (11,17,18,47,103); the suppression of tics by dopaminergic blocking agents, such as haloperidol, fluphenazine, pimozide, and penfluridol in a majority of TS patients (21,37,90,96–100); the suppression of tics by α-methyl-p-tyrosine, an inhibitor of dopamine synthesis (109); the emergence of TS-like syndromes following the withdrawal of neuroleptics in a small number of cases (51,52); and the exacerbation of tic behaviors following exposure to agents which may increase central dopaminergic activity such as L-dopa, amphetamine, methylphenidate, and pemoline (25,28,36–38,66,84,86). Several investigators have postulated that hypersensitive postsynaptic dopaminergic receptors may account for this body of metabolic and pharmacological data (11,17,18). This hypothesis, in turn, has lead Friedhoff and coworkers (35) to give gradually increasing amounts of L-dopa in an attempt to down-regulate the hypersensitive dopamine receptors.

Other investigators have used rank order correlations of neuroleptic efficacy in TS versus the effect of neuroleptics on a number of *in vitro* tests of dopamine receptor functioning to hypothesize that the agents that either inhibit the presynaptic release of dopamine or specifically block D-2 dopaminergic receptors would be particularly effective in the suppression of tic symptoms (104). Preliminary evidence suggests there may be a reduction of TS symptoms following low doses of dopamine receptor agonists, such as apomorphine, which presumably act via presynaptic dopaminergic receptors and produce a net reduction in activity

in those dopaminergic systems with autoreceptors (30). Trials of specific dopamine autoreceptor agonists, as they become available, will be of theoretical and practical interest. Similarly, ongoing European experience with substituted benzamides that selectively block D-2 dopaminergic receptors, including tiapride and sulpiride, show considerable promise in the treatment of TS (91). Preliminary studies with RO22-1319, a water-soluble pyrroloisoquinoline derivative with selective D-2 dopaminergic-blocking activity, are also encouraging (112). Additional clinical trials are needed to confirm these optimistic results.

Although the preponderance of these data supports the view that central dopaminergic mechanisms are involved in the pathophysiology of tic disorders, it is important to keep in mind that the reported effects are partial. Dopamine receptor blocking agents suppress tics, they do not eliminate them. There is also a significant minority of patients who do not respond to these agents. With few exceptions, most of the clinical trials involve small numbers of patients treated over relatively brief periods of time without adequate controls. The effect of stimulant medications in exacerbating tic behaviors is even more problematic, with recent surveys indicating that there are many patients who have had long-term exposure to these agents without experiencing significant difficulty (28,86). Taken together these data suggest that the observed dysfunction in dopaminergic systems may not be the primary pathophysiologic mechanism in all tic disorder patients. The hypothesis that abnormalities in central dopaminergic systems predispose genetically vulnerable individuals to a more severe expression of the disorder may be an attractive alternative (60). This interactive model might account for the variable phenotypic expression of the TS trait, as observed in the study of MZ twins and first-degree relatives, and open the door to prospective longitudinal studies that focus in part on those events which can affect the development of central dopaminergic systems. Such events would include pre- and postnatal exposure to specific pharmacologic agents, e.g., antiemetics and CNS stimulants, as well as the documentation of pre- and postnatal stresses that may be associated with endogenous processes that activate central dopaminergic systems.

Another model that tic disorders are etiologically heterogeneous, with dopaminergic mechanisms having a more central role in some but not all forms of the disorder, also merits attention. Reports suggesting that a positive response to haloperidol is associated with a positive family history of tics and TS are consistent with this view (75,87). A third hypothesis, that abnormalities in central dopaminergic activity associated with tic disorders are a frequent, but not universal, result of tic behaviors, is untenable based on the available pharmacologic data.

Noradrenergic Mechanisms

Evidence of noradrenergic involvement in the pathophysiology of TS is based largely on the reported beneficial effects of clonidine, an imidazoline derivative with specific α_2-adrenergic receptor agonist activity (7,8,19,61). Other data include reduced levels of urinary 3-methoxy-4-hydroxyphenylethylene glycol (MHPG) excretion in TS patients (2,108) and reduced clonidine-stimulated growth hormone release (59). More complex hypotheses involving noradrenergic-dopaminergic and noradrenergic-serotonergic-dopaminergic interactions have also been proposed (60), based on altered plasma HVA levels after chronic clonidine treatment (62,64), increased plasma HVA levels after acute withdrawal from clonidine (64), and the concordance of clonidine and haloperidol in a double crossover study of these agents (7). The effectiveness of clonidine in TS is controversial, with some investigators reporting promising results (7,8,19,61) that have not been replicated by other investigators (98). The waxing and waning course of the syndrome and the relatively high rate of placebo response further caution against an overly optimistic appraisal of the available data on the magnitude and time course of the clonidine response [a 35% reduction in symptoms over a 12-week period (61)] and emphasize the need for additional controlled clinical trials.

Although MHPG is a major metabolite of norepinephrine in the brain, the relationship between urinary MHPG excretion and central adrenergic neuronal activity remains unclear (68). Reports that CSF MHPG levels appear to be normal, with the exception of an occasional patient with elevated CSF MHPG levels (18,103), cast doubt on the heuristic value of the urinary MHPG data *per se*. The reported changes in plasma HVA after chronic clonidine have not consistently been observed (62,64), and the increase in plasma HVA following acute clonidine withdrawal is likely due to increased sympathetic activity in the periphery rather than any dramatic change in central dopaminergic activity (64).

The B_{max} and K_D of [^{3}H]yohimbine binding to α_2-receptors on platelets have been reported as normal in TS patients compared to controls (101). Subsequent changes in specific binding parameters during clonidine treatment did not parallel the course of clinical improvement, suggesting that other mechanisms may be responsible for the efficacy of clonidine in TS. Many other aspects of peripheral catecholaminergic metabolism have been evaluated in TS and are largely inconclusive (27,95).

The finding of elevated salivary amylase excretion in TS patients versus a contrast group of ADD children is suggestive of the involvement of β-adrenergic receptors in the pathophysiology of TS (19,94). However, a controlled clinical trial found no difference in treatment response to varying doses of propranolol compared to placebo (107).

Heuristically, the hypothesis that noradrenergic mechanisms are involved in the pathophysiology of TS has been generative of basic research. Efforts have intensified to explore the functional interrelationship of the noradrenergic locus ceruleus and the nigrostriatal and mesolimbic systems.

Serotonergic Mechanisms

There is insufficient evidence to support a hypothesis of direct serotonergic involvement in the pathogenesis of TS. Medications that act by increasing or decreasing serotonergic activity do not consistently alter TS symptoms (12,24, 41,48,70,110,114,115). Similarly, studies of CSF 5-hydroxy-indoleacetic acid (5-HIAA), the principal central metabolite

of serotonin, have reported a range of low and normal levels in TS patients compared to contrast groups (11,17,18,103). In addition, whole blood tryptophan, but not whole blood serotonin, levels were found to be significantly lower in TS patients compared to normal controls (59). Serotonergic projections from the dorsal raphe have been suggested as the link between central noradrenergic and dopaminergic mechanisms (10).

Cholinergic Mechanisms

Dysfunction of cholinergic systems in the pathophysiology of TS has been postulated on the basis of the effects of cholinergic and anticholinergic agents on tic symptoms (3,4,32,72,82,83), increased RBC choline concentrations in TS patients compared to controls (43), and reduced choline uptake into cultured fibroblasts (88). Elevated levels of RBC choline concentration have also been reported in affected and unaffected first-degree relatives of TS probands (20). A more complex hypothesis of a dopaminergic-cholinergic imbalance has also been proposed in which there is heightened dopaminergic activity as well as diminished cholinergic activity, as in other movement disorders affecting the basal ganglia (105).

Evidence supporting a central role of cholinergic mechanisms in the pathophysiology of TS is not convincing. Intravenous physostigmine, a selective and potent inhibitor of acetylcholinesterase, has been reported by some investigators to decrease acutely motor and phonic tics (105). Other investigators have reported that intramuscular physostigmine aggravates motor tics and can block the beneficial effects of scopolamine, a muscarinic blocking agent (111). These agents also are associated with appreciable side effects, which were not adequately controlled for in these studies.

Clinical trials with choline, lecithin, and deanol have been disappointing overall (3,4,32,72,82,83). Although precursor loading with choline and lecithin appears to increase brain acetylcholine levels, evidence does not indicate that the synaptic release of acetylcholine is increased by this maneuver (69). The recent report of Singer and co-workers of normal levels of CSF acetylcholinesterase and butyrylcholinesterase in TS compared to normal controls also argues against a primary defect in brain cholinergic systems (102). However, if central dopaminergic mechanisms are involved in the pathophysiology of tic disorders, as appears likely, secondary alterations in cholinergic activity could be expected, given their close interrelationship.

GABAergic Mechanisms

The benzodiazepine clonazepam has been reported to be effective in the treatment of TS (41,48,70). Clonazepam, however, has significant effects on serotonergic systems. Other benzodiazepines, including diazepam (23), have not been reported to diminish TS symptoms. In a recent open trial, progabide, a direct γ-aminobutyric acid (GABA) agonist, was effective in reducing tics in two of four patients with TS (73). Taken together, these clinical findings suggest that GABAergic systems warrant further evaluation in TS patients. However, a primary defect in GABAergic mechanisms is unlikely, given the data of van Woert and colleagues, who did not find a significant difference in CSF GABA or whole blood GABA between 15 TS patients and a group of controls (113).

Endogenous Opioid Mechanisms

Endogenous opioid peptides appear to play a role in the control of human motor functions and in the pathophysiology of abnormal movement disorders (9). Endogenous opioid mechanisms have been proposed in TS based on neuropathological and neuropharmacological data. Haber and coworkers (42a) have reported low levels of postmortem immunoreactivity to dynorphin in the basal ganglia in a single case study. If this provocative finding can be confirmed, a very promising area of investigation will rapidly emerge. The available neuropharmacological data is less promising as naloxone, an opioid receptor antagonist, which does not have consistent effects in patients with TS (5,92,93).

Other Pathophysiological Mechanisms

Two recent case reports described dramatic symptomatic improvement in patients with TS following treatment with nifedipine, a *calcium channel blocker* (6,40). Decreased calcium influx at presynaptic neurons could lead to decreased neurotransmitter release, which, in turn, could result in symptom reduction. Current understanding of calcium channels and calcium channel blockers, although preliminary, suggests that these drugs may have a role in the treatment of TS. This view is also supported by evidence that pimozide and penfluridol are potent calcium channel antagonists (42).

Several other medications, which have multiple or unknown mechanisms of actions, have been tried in TS patients. In general, *tricyclic antidepressants* exacerbate TS symptoms, although a few positive responses have been reported (12,33,34). *Carbamazepine* has been reported to increase and to decrease tics (67,77). Marked acute exacerbation, followed by symptom reduction, has been reported following *lithium carbonate* therapy (29,71). One TS patient reportedly improved following administration of *prednisolone* (54).

The theoretical implications of these disparate findings *vis à vis* the major pathophysiological mechanisms in TS are unclear.

PROMISING DIRECTIONS FOR CLINICAL RESEARCH

Phenomenology and Clinimetrics

Assessment methodologies are critical to clinical research. They are indispensable in genetic-family studies as well as drug trials. Only recently have reliable measures been established to permit valid across-patient comparisons in TS (45,63,96). Further refinement of these instruments is crucial to continued progress. Special attention needs to be focused on the assessment of milder syndromes to document better the progression of the syndrome and to establish the range of phenotypic expression. Efforts to characterize and document the ADD and obsessive-compulsive symptoms in TS patients are also needed.

Genetics

Molecular genetic strategies have considerable promise in TS research; however, major obstacles remain. Genetic linkage studies require the precise identification of "affected" individuals in order to trace the segregation of known genetic markers and the putative TS gene. Barring a fortuitous discovery of the sort recently reported by Comings et al (22a), efforts to locate the TS gene are likely to require the careful testing of hundreds of chromosomal markers. Location of the "gene" will permit improved diagnostic techniques and facilitate the identification of at-risk individuals in affected pedigrees. This last step is crucial in the study of nongenetic risk and protective factors that appear to mediate the expression of the TS gene. The location of the putative gene is also only the first step in acquiring a thoroughgoing knowledge of the pathogenesis of TS by cloning the gene and determining the functional significance of the abnormal gene product.

Pharmacological Strategies

Since the efficacy of haloperidol in reducing dramatically the frequency and intensity of tics was demonstrated two decades ago, other medications, including clonidine and pimozide, have become an integral part of the treatment of patients with TS. Unfortunately, each of these three drugs has limitations. The usefulness of haloperidol is limited by frequent side effects of sedation, cognitive blunting, and weight gain. The risk of persistent tardive dyskinesia in TS patients already afflicted with one movement disorder is particularly troubling (39). Pimozide, which has the same spectrum of potential side effects as haloperidol, also has been associated with cardiac-related deaths and carcinogenesis in animals. Clonidine, although free of serious side effects when used in low doses, regularly sedates a small proportion of subjects and is not as effective in controlling tics as the dopaminergic blocking agents. Given these limitations, a continuing search for safer and more effective medications is needed.

Areas of particular promise include the development and testing of more specific dopaminergic agents such as tiapride and RO22-1319. The exploratory use of newly developed centrally active pharmaceuticals may be warranted in severe and refractory patients. The optimistic reports of calcium channel blocking agents being effective in TS should be pursued in controlled clinical trials.

Metabolic Studies

The relative inaccessibility of the CNS for *in vivo* study is a clear obstacle to direct pathophysiologic studies. The complexity of the neurochemical systems being studied and the impossibility of frequent sampling seriously limit the potential value of CSF studies. Postmortem brain specimens are needed for additional neuropathologic studies and precise biochemical studies of specific brain regions. Development of peripheral strategies for studying central catecholamine metabolism, such as the debrisoquin technique (89), may provide a means to study CNS metabolism during periods of waxing and waning symptoms, before and after medication trials, as well as in the study of other factors associated with the natural history of tic disorders.

Imaging Studies

Although no specific neuropathological abnormalities have been documented and no structural abnormalities have been observed on computerized tomography (CT) scan (44), the full potential of the emerging positron emission tomography (PET) and molecular resonance imaging (MRI) technologies has not been realized in the study of tic disorders (13).

CONCLUSION

TS has been described as a model neuropsychiatric disorder of childhood onset. As the factors involved in the pathogenesis of tic disorders more clearly emerge over the next decades, we can anticipate the unfolding of a complex and intriguing story of "gene-environment" interactions set against the backdrop of the ongoing development and maturation of brain neurochemical systems (60).

Major advances in the understanding of the ontogeny of brain neurochemical systems and the mechanisms by which environmental and psychological factors influence the course of neuronal development are needed before some of the most fascinating questions posed by the natural history of TS and related disorders can be answered. Why do tic disorders emerge and progress during a particular period of CNS development? What accounts for the appearance of specific symptoms, their moment-to-moment fluctuation, their waxing and waning course, and their disappearance? What governs the emergence of self-destructive behaviors or the obsessive-compulsive symptoms? Why do some patients report premonitory sensations that suddenly enter their consciousness as irrational and often irresistible urges? The pursuit of the etiological and pathophysiological mechanisms responsible for these phenomena will lead basic and clinical researchers to the frontier between the mind and the body.

ACKNOWLEDGMENTS

This work was supported by NIMH grants MH18268 and MH30929, NICHHD grant HD03008, NINCDS grant NS16648, NIH grant RR00125, the John Merck Fund, the MacArthur Foundation, the Tourette Syndrome Association, and the Gateposts Foundation. The authors also wish to acknowledge the contributions of Drs. D. L. Pauls, G. M. Anderson, and R. A. Price, and Ms. S. Ort and Ms. M. Hardin to this work.

REFERENCES

1. Abuzzahab, F. S., and Anderson, F. O. (1973): *Minn. Med.,* 56:492.
2. Ang, L., Borison, R., Dysken, M., and Davis, J. M. (1982): In: *Gilles de la Tourette Syndrome, Advances in Neurology, Vol. 35,* edited by A. J. Friedhoff and T. N. Chase, pp. 171–175. Raven Press, New York.
3. Barbeau, A. (1978): *Can. J. Neurol. Sci.,* 5:157–160.
4. Barbeau, A. (1980): *N. Engl. J. Med.,* 302:1310–1311.
5. Berecz, J. M., Dysken, M. W., and Davis, J. M. (1979): *Neurology,* 29:1316–1317.
6. Berg, R. (1985): *Acta Psychiatr. Scand.,* 72:400–401.
7. Borison, R. L., Ang, L., Hamilton, W. J., Diamond, B. I., and David, J. M. (1983): *Brain Res. Bull.,* 11:205–208.
8. Bruun, R. D. (1984): *J. Am. Acad. Child Psychiatry,* 23:126–133.
9. Buck, S. H., and Yamamura, H. I. (1982): In: *Gilles de la Tourette Syndrome, Advances in Neurology, Vol. 35,* edited by A. J. Friedhoff and T. N. Chase, pp. 121–132. Raven Press, New York.
10. Bunney, B. S., and DeRiemer, S. (1982): In: *Gilles de la Tourette Syndrome, Advances in Neurology, Vol. 35,* edited by A. J. Friedhoff and T. N. Chase, pp. 99–104. Raven Press, New York.
11. Butler, I. J., Koslow, S. H., Siefert, W. E., Capriolo, R. M., and Singer, H. S. (1979): *Ann. Neurol.,* 6:37–39.
12. Caine, E. D., Polinsky, R. J., Ebert, M. H., Rapoport, J. L., and Mikkelsen, E. J. (1977): *Ann. Neurol.,* 5:305–306.
13. Chase, T. M., Foster, N. L., Fedro, P., Brooks, R., Mansi, L., Kessler, R., and DiChiro, G. (1984): *Ann. Neurol.,* 15(Suppl. S17).
14. Cohen, D. J., and Leckman, J. F. (1984): *J. Am. Acad. Child Psychiatry,* 23:123–125.
15. Cohen, D. J., Leckman, J. F., and Shaywitz, B. A. (1984): In: *Diagnosis and Treatment in Pediatric Psychiatry,* edited by D. Shaffer, A. A. Ehrhardt, and L. Greenhill, pp. 3–28. MacMillan Free Press, New York.
16. Cohen, D. J., Ort, S., Caruso, K. A., Anderson, G. M., Hunt, R. D., Shaywitz, B. A., Kremenitzer, M., and Leckman, J. F. (1987): *J. Am. Acad. Child Psychiatry,* 26:65–68.
17. Cohen, D. J., Shaywitz, B. A., Caparulo, B., Young, J. G., and Bowers, M. B. (1978): *Arch. Gen. Psychiatry,* 35:245–250.
18. Cohen, D. J., Shaywitz, B. A., Young, J. G., Carbonari, C. M., Nathanson, J. A., Lieberman, D., Bowers, M. B., and Maas, J. W. (1979): *J. Am. Acad. Child Psychiatry,* 18:320–341.
19. Cohen, D. J., Young, J. G., Nathanson, J. A., and Shaywitz, B. A. (1979): *Lancet,* 2:551–553.
20. Comings, D. E., Brenda, T. G., Avelino, E., Kopp, U., and Hanin, I. (1982): In: *Gilles de la Tourette Syndrome, Advances in Neurology, Vol. 35,* edited by A. J. Friedhoff and T. N. Chase, pp. 255–258. Raven Press, New York.
21. Comings, D. E., and Comings, B. G. (1984): *J. Am. Acad. Child Psychiatry,* 23:138–146.
22. Comings, D. E., Comings, B. G., Devor, E. J., and Cloninger, D. R. (1984): *Am. J. Hum. Genet.,* 36:586–600.
22a. Comings, D. E., Comings, B. G., Diez, G. et al. (1986): Evidence of the Tourette gene is at 18q22 I. Seventh Int. Cong. Hum. Genet. Berlin; part II: 620 (abstr.).
23. Connell, P. H., Corbett, J. A., Horne, D. J., and Mathews, A. M. (1976): *Br. J. Psychiatry,* 113:375–381.
24. Crosley, C. J. (1979): *Ann. Neurol.,* 5:596–597.
25. Denkla, M. D., Bemporad, J. R., and MacKay, M. C. (1976): *JAMA,* 235:1349–1351.
26. Devor, E. J. (1984): *Am. J. Hum. Genet.,* 36:704–709.
27. Eldridge, R., Sweet, R., Lake, C. R., Ziegler, M., and Shapiro, A. K. (1977): *Neurology,* 27:115–124.
28. Erenberg, G., Cruse, R. P., and Rothner, A. D. (1985): *Neurology,* 35:1346–1348.
29. Erikson, H. M., Goggin, J. E., and Messiha, F. S. (1977): *Adv. Med. Biol.,* 90:197–205.
30. Feinberg, M., and Carroll, B. J. (1970): *Arch. Gen. Psychiatry,* 36:979–985.
31. Fernando, S. J. M. (1967): *Br. J. Psychiatry,* 113:607–617.
32. Finney, J. W., Christophersen, E. R., and Ziegler, D. K. (1981): *Lancet,* 2:989.
33. Fras, I. (1978): *NY State J. Med.,* 78:1230–1232.
34. Fras, I., and Karlavage, J. (1977): *Am. J. Psychiatry,* 134:195–197.
35. Friedhoff, A. J. (1982): In: *Gilles de la Tourette Syndrome, Advances in Neurology, Vol. 35,* edited by A. J. Friedhoff and T. N. Chase, pp. 133–140. Raven Press, New York.

36. Goetz, C. G., Tanner, C. M., and Klawans, H. L. (1984): *Arch. Neurol.*, 41:271–272.
37. Golden, G. S. (1974): *Dev. Med. Child Neurol.*, 16:76–78.
38. Golden, G. S. (1977): *Ann. Neurol.*, 2:69–70.
39. Golden, G. S. (1985): *Pediatr. Neurol.*, 1:192–194.
40. Goldstein, J. A. (1984): *J. Clin. Psychiatry*, 45:360.
41. Gonce, M., and Barbeau, A. (1977): *Can. J. Neurol. Sci.*, 4:279–283.
42. Gould, R. J., Murphy, K. M. M., Reynolds, I. J., and Snyder, S. H. (1983): *Proc. Natl. Acad. Sci. USA*, 80:5122–5125.
42a. Haber, S. N., Kowall, N. W., Vonsattel, J. P., Bird, E. D., and Richardson, E. P. (1986): *J. Neurological Sciences*, 75:225–241.
43. Hanin, I., Merikangas, J. R., Merikangas, K. R., and Kopp, U. (1979): *N. Engl. J. Med.*, 301:661–662.
44. Harcherik, D. F., Cohen, D. J., Paul, R., Ort, S., Shaywitz, B. A., Volkmar, F. R., Rothman, S., and Leckman, J. F. (1985): *Am. J. Psychiatry*, 142:731–734.
45. Harcherik, D. F., Leckman, J. F., Detlor, J., and Cohen, D. J. (1984): *J. Am. Acad. Child Psychiatry*, 23:153–160.
46. Jagger, R. L., Prusoff, B. A., Cohen, D. J., Kidd, K. K., Carbonari, C. M., and John, K. (1982): *Schizophr. Bull.*, 8:267–278.
47. Johansson, B., and Roos, B. (1974): *Eur. Neurol.*, 1137–1145.
48. Kaim, B. (1983): *Brain Res. Bull.*, 11:213–214.
49. Kidd, K. K. (1985): In: *Genetic Aspects of Human Behavior*, edited by T. Sakai and T. Tsuboi, pp. 235–246. Igaku-shoin Ltd., Tokyo.
50. Kidd, K. K., and Pauls, D. L. (1982): In: *Gilles de la Tourette Syndrome, Advances in Neurology, Vol. 35*, edited by A. J. Friedhoff and T. N. Chase, pp. 243–249. Raven Press, New York.
51. Klawans, H. D., Falk, D. A., Nausieda, P. A., and Weiner, W. J. (1978): *Neurology*, 28:1064–1065.
52. Klawans, H. D., Nausieda, P. A., Goetz, C. L., Tanner, C. M., and Weiner, W. J. (1982): In: *Gilles de la Tourette Syndrome, Advances in Neurology, Vol. 35*, edited by A. J. Friedhoff and T. N. Chase, pp. 415–418. Raven Press, New York.
53. Klempel, K. (1974): *S. Afr. Med. J.*, 48:1379–1380.
54. Kondo, K., and Kabasawa, T. (1978): *Ann. Neurol.*, 4:387.
55. Kurland, R., Behr, J., Medved, L., Shoulson, I., Pauls, D. L., Kidd, J. R., and Kidd, K. K. (1985): *Neurology*, 35:176(s).
56. Leckman, J. F., Anderson, G. M., Cohen, D. J., Ort, D. I., Harcherik, D. F., Hoder, E. L., and Shaywitz, B. A. (1984): *Life Sci.*, 35:2497–2503.
57. Leckman, J. F., and Cohen, D. J. (1987): In: *Tourette Syndrome and Tic Disorders: Clinical Understanding and Treatment*, edited by D. J. Cohen, R. D. Bruun, and J. F. Leckman. John Wiley and Sons, New York (*in press*).
58. Leckman, J. F., Cohen, D. J., Detlor, J., Young, J. G., Harcherik, D., and Shaywitz, B. A. (1982): In: *Gilles de la Tourette Syndrome, Advances in Neurology, Vol. 35*, edited by A. J. Friedhoff and T. N. Chase, pp. 391–401. Raven Press, New York.
59. Leckman, J. F., Cohen, D. J., Gertner, J. M., Ort, S., and Harcherik, D. (1984): *J. Am. Acad. Child Psychiatry*, 23:174–181.
60. Leckman, J. F., Cohen, D. J., Price, R. A., Riddle, M. A., Minderaa, R. B., Anderson, G. M., and Pauls, D. L. (1986): In: *Movement Disorders*, edited by N. S. Shah and A. G. Donald, pp. 257–272. Plenum Medical Book Company, New York.
61. Leckman, J. F., Detlor, J., Harcherik, D., Ort, S., and Cohen, D. J. (1985): *Neurology*, 35:343–351.
62. Leckman, J. F., Detlor, J., Harcherik, D. F., Young, J. G., Anderson, G. M., Shaywitz, B. A., and Cohen, D. J. (1983): *J. Am. Acad. Child Psychiatry*, 22:433–440.
63. Leckman, J. F., Ort, S. I., Towbin, K. E., and Cohen, D. J. (1987): In: *Tourette Syndrome and Tic Disorders: Clinical Understanding and Treatment*, edited by D. J. Cohen, R. D. Bruun, and J. F. Leckman. John Wiley and Sons, New York (*in press*).
64. Leckman, J. F., Ort, S., Cohen, D. J., Caruso, K. A., Anderson, G. M., and Riddle, M. A. (1986): *Arch. Gen. Psychiatry*, 43:1168–1176.
64a. Leckman, J. F., Price, R. A., Walkup, J. T., Ort, S., Pauls, P. L., Cohen, D. J. (1987): *Arch. Gen. Psychiatry*, 44:100.
65. Leckman, J. F., Weissman, M. M., Pauls, D. L., and Kidd, K. K. (1987): *Br. J. Psychiatry* (*in press*).
66. Lowe, T. L., Cohen, D. J., Detlor, J., Kremenitzer, M. W., and Shaywitz, B. A. (1982): *JAMA*, 247:1731–1739.
67. Lutz, E. G. (1977): *Am. J. Psychiatry*, 134:99–100.

68. Maas, J. W., and Leckman, J. F. (1983): In: *MHPG: Basic Mechanisms and Psychopathology*, edited by J. W. Maas, pp. 33–43. Academic Press, New York.
69. McIntosh, F. C. (1981): In: *Basic Neurochemistry*, edited by G. F. Siegel, R. W. Albers, B. W. Agranoff, and R. Katzman, pp. 183–204. Little, Brown, Boston.
70. Merikangas, J. R., Merikangas, K. R., Kopp, U., and Hanin, I. (1985): *Acta Psychiatr. Scand.*, 72:395–399.
71. Messiha, F. S., Erickson, J., and Goggin, J. E. (1976): *Res. Commun. Chem. Pathol. Pharmacol.*, 15:609–612.
72. Moldofsky, H., and Sandor, P. (1983): *Am. J. Psychiatry*, 140:1627–1629.
73. Mondrup, K., Dupont, E., and Braindgaard, H. (1985): *Acta Neurol. Scand.*, 72:341–343.
74. Montgomery, M. A., Clayton, P. J., and Friedhoff, A. J. (1982): In: *Gilles de la Tourette Syndrome, Advances in Neurology, Vol. 35*, edited by A. J. Friedhoff and T. N. Chase, pp. 335–339. Raven Press, New York.
75. Nee, L. E., Caine, E. D., Polinsky, R. J., Eldridge, R., and Ebert, M. H. (1980): *Ann. Neurol.*, 7:41–49.
76. Nee, L. E., Polinsky, R. J., and Ebert, M. H. (1982): In: *Gilles de la Tourette Syndrome, Advances in Neurology, Vol. 35*, edited by A. J. Friedhoff and T. N. Chase, pp. 291–295. Raven Press, New York.
77. Neglia, J. P., Glaze, D. G., and Zion, T. E. (1984): *Pediatrics*, 73:841–844.
78. Pasamanick, B., and Kawi, A. (1956): *Pediatrics*, 48:596–601.
79. Pauls, D. L., Hurst, C., Kruger, S. D., Leckman, J. F., Kidd, K. K., and Cohen, D. J. (1986): *Arch. Gen. Psychiatry*, 43:1177–1179.
80. Pauls, D. L., Kruger, S. D., Leckman, J. F., Cohen, D. J., and Kidd, K. K. (1984): *J. Am. Acad. Child Psychiatry*, 23:134–137.
80a. Pauls, D. L., and Leckman, J. F. (1986): *N. Eng. J. Med.*, 35:993–996.
81. Pauls, D. L., Towbin, K. E., Leckman, J. F., Zahner, G. E. P., and Cohen, D. J. (1986): *Arch. Gen. Psychiatry*, 43:1180–1182.
82. Pinta, E. R. (1977): *Dis. Nerv. Syst.*, 38:214–215.
83. Polinsky, R. J., Ebert, M. H., Caine, E. D., Ludlow, C., and Bassick, C. J. (1980): *N. Engl. J. Med.*, 302:1310.
84. Pollack, M. A., Cohen, N. L., and Friedhoff, A. J. (1977): *Arch. Neurol.*, 34:630–632.
85. Price, R. A., Kidd, K. K., Cohen, D. J., Pauls, D. L., and Leckman, J. F. (1985): *Arch. Gen. Psychiatry*, 42:815–820.
86. Price, R. A., Leckman, J. F., Pauls, D. L., Cohen, D. J., and Kidd, K. K. (1986): *Neurology*, 36:232–237.
87. Price, R. A., Pauls, D. L., Kruger, S. D., and Caine, E. D. (1984): *Am. J. Hum. Genet.*, 36:178.
88. Rickland, D., Breakfield, X., and Roth, R. (1980): Program and Abstracts of the Third International Symposium on Dystonia, Vancouver, Canada.
89. Riddle, M. A., Shaywitz, B. A., Leckman, J. F., Anderson, G. M., Shaywitz, S. E., Hardin, M. T., Ort, S. I., and Cohen, D. J. (1986): *Life Sci.*, 38:1041–1048.
90. Ross, M. S., and Moldofsky, H. (1978): *Am. J. Psychiatry*, 135:585–587.
91. Rothenberger, A. (1984): *Z. Kinder Jugend Psychiat.*, 12:284–301.
92. Sandyk, R. (1985): *Life Sci.*, 37:1655–1663.
93. Sandyk, R. (1985): *Ann. Neurol.*, 18:367–368.
94. Selinger, D., Cohen, D. J., Ort, S., Anderson, G. M., Caruso, K. A., and Leckman, J. F. (1984): *J. Am. Acad. Child Psychiatry*, 23:392–398.
95. Shapiro, A. K., Baron, M., Shapiro, E., and Levitt, M. (1984): *Arch. Neurol.*, 41:282–285.
96. Shapiro, A. K., and Shapiro, E. (1984): *J. Am. Acad. Child Psychiatry*, 23:161–173.
97. Shapiro, A. K., Shapiro, E. S., Bruun, R. D., and Sweet, R. D., eds. (1978): *Gilles de la Tourette Syndrome*. Raven Press, New York.
98. Shapiro, A. K., Shapiro, E., and Eisenkraft, G. J. (1983): *Arch. Gen. Psychiatry*, 40:1235–1240.
99. Shapiro, A. K., Shapiro, E., and Eisenkraft, G. J. (1983): *Am. J. Psychiatry*, 140:1183–1186.
100. Shapiro, A. K., Shapiro, E., and Eisenkraft, G. J. (1983): *Compr. Psychiatry*, 24:327–331.
101. Silverstein, F., Smith, C. B., and Johnston, M. V. (1984): *Dev. Med. Child Neurol.*, 27:793–799.

102. Singer, H. S., Oshida, L., and Coyle, J. T. (1984): *Arch. Neurol.,* 41:756–757.
103. Singer, J. S., Tune, L. E., Butler, I. J., Zaczck, R., and Coyle, J. T. (1982): In: *Gilles de la Tourette Syndrome, Advances in Neurology, Vol. 35,* edited by A. J. Friedhoff and T. N. Chase, pp. 177–183. Raven Press, New York.
104. Stahl, S. M., and Berger, P. A. (1981): *Am. J. Psychiatry,* 138: 240–242.
105. Stahl, S. M., and Berger, P. A. (1982): In: *Gilles de la Tourette Syndrome, Advances in Neurology, Vol. 35,* edited by A. J. Friedhoff and T. N. Chase, pp. 141–150. Raven Press, New York.
106. Surwillo, W. W., Shafii, M., and Barrett, C. L. (1978): *J. Nerv. Ment. Dis.,* 166:812–816.
107. Sverd, J., Cohen, S., and Camp, J. A. (1983): *J. Autism Dev. Disord.,* 13:207–213.
108. Sweeney, R. D., Pikar, D., Redmond, D. E., and Maas, J. (1978): *Lancet,* 1:872.

109. Sweet, R. D., Bruun, R. D., Shapiro, A. K., and Shapiro, E. (1976): *Arch. Gen. Psychiatry,* 31:857–861.
110. Sweet, R. D., Bruun, R. D., Shapiro, A. K., and Shapiro, E. (1976): In: *Clinical Neuropharmacology, Vol. 1,* edited by H. L. Klawans, pp. 81–105. Raven Press, New York.
111. Tanner, C. M., Goetz, C. G., and Klawans, H. L. (1982): *Neurology,* 32:1315–1317.
112. Uhr, S. B., Berger, P. A., Pruitt, B., and Stahl, S. M. (1985): *N. Engl. J. Med.,* 311:989.
113. van Woert, M. H., Rosenbaum, D., and Enna, J. J. (1982): In: *Gilles de la Tourette Syndrome,* edited by A. J. Friedhoff and T. N. Chase, pp. 369–376. Raven Press, New York.
114. van Woert, M. H., Yip, L. C., and Balis, M. E. (1977): *N. Engl. J. Med.,* 296:210–212.
115. Yaryura-Tobias, J. A. (1975): *Am. J. Psychiatry,* 132:1221.
116. Yaryura-Tobias, J. A. (1981): *Orthomolec. Psychiatry,* 10:263–268.

Psychopharmacology:
The Third Generation of Progress,
edited by Herbert Y. Meltzer.
Raven Press, New York © 1987.

CHAPTER **129**

Pharmacotherapy in Child and Adolescent Major Depressive Disorder

Paul J. Ambrosini

Recognition of affective disorders in children and adolescents is gaining wider prominence in the last two decades. Prior conceptualizations that youngsters could not exhibit a major depression or only revealed depression in masked form (1) are losing sway (2,3). This shift has coincided with the experience that both Research Diagnostic Criteria (RDC) and *Diagnostic and Statistical Manual of Mental Disorders,* 3rd edition (DSM-III) criteria are applicable for diagnosing childhood and adolescent affective disorders (4,5). The application of standard diagnostic criteria has led not only to identification of samples of prepubertal and adolescent children with depressive disorders but also to identification of several phenomenological subtypes, such as endogenous, nonendogenous (6), psychotic (7), dysthymic (8), and bipolar (9). By reliably identifying these youngsters with affective disorders, researchers are now mapping various characteristic parameters of this syndrome, which helps validate both the syndrome's existence and its continuity with adult affective disorders. Numerous reports are available on the epidemiology, symptomatology, family history, outcome, psychosocial characteristics, and biological correlates of childhood and adolescent affective disorders (10). Furthermore, there is a growing body of data on the use of pharmacotherapy in major depressive disorder (MDD).

This area of pediatric psychopharmacology is gaining wider visibility as a viable treatment modality; however, the quality of the clinical literature available to date varies considerably. It is heavily weighted toward open and poorly designed investigations with only a handful of well-designed placebo-controlled studies. Although there are some findings suggesting efficacy for antidepressant treatment of childhood and adolescent affective disorders and correlations of response with plasma tricyclic antidepressant (TCA) levels, there currently is no study that has shown that tricyclics

are superior to placebo. Further placebo-controlled, random-assignment, double-blind studies are essential in order to delineate the guidelines for judicious use of antidepressants in depressed youngsters.

The aim of this chapter is to review the last decade's progress in the pharmacotherapy of childhood and adolescent major depressive disorder and to prepare the reader to properly evaluate future trends. Advances in this field were spurred by progress in diagnostic nosology and measurement, proper attention to pharmacotherapy research design, and advances in pediatric pharmacokinetics of tricyclic antidepressants. These topics will be incorporated into this review to adequately present both the advances in this last decade and the areas available for advancement in the coming period of progress.

DIAGNOSTIC AND MEASUREMENT CONSIDERATIONS

The use of psychotropic medication in pediatric psychiatry implies an attempt to ameliorate the dysfunction of a disorder with medication. The psychopharmacologist's goal, therefore, is to identify the "right" drug for a specific disorder. The discovery of the ability of lithium to quell the polarity swings in bipolar disorder is the classic example of this approach in psychiatry. Such pharmacological specificity has clear diagnostic significance in validating a syndrome. However, this has not been the case in pediatric psychopharmacology. For example, the antipsychotics do not affect the syndrome of pervasive developmental disorder (childhood psychoses), but are used primarily for their general ability to reduce motoric activity (11). Nor are stimulants necessarily specific for the syndrome of attention deficit disorder (ADD), since they lessen motoric activity in normal children (12) and their efficacy in adults with residual ADD is also being questioned (13). It is common practice in pediatric psychopharmacology, therefore, to prescribe psychotropics in a symptom-specific manner, since clinical experience has not yet identified syndrome-specific drugs.

In the last decade, however, progress in pharmacotherapy of child and adolescent major depressive disorder has occurred because of the commitment to the concept of using pharmacotherapeutic response as one means of validating the existence of the syndrome in youngsters. A corollary of this concept is that antidepressants should be used in those children meeting the criteria for the syndrome of MDD and not indiscriminately in those merely having the symptom of depression. Only in this last decade has a more systematic nosological framework been established to diagnose the syndrome of MDD in children and adolescents.

Weinberg et al. (14) initially proposed modifying the Feighner criteria (15) for diagnosing adult MDD for use in children. He prospectively identified a group of depressed youngsters and followed their response to antidepressants. Pearce (16) noted that the symptoms of the depressive disorder clustered together. Puig-Antich et al. (6) used unmodified RDC to diagnose and treat a prepubertal major depressive group. DSM-III subsequently specified that the same essential symptom profile should be used to diagnose childhood major depression as was used in adults. There are significant overlaps in the Weinberg, RDC, and DSM-III criteria for MDD (2). The RDC and the DSM-III essentially cover the same symptom profiles, except that the RDC require one more symptom than the DSM-III criteria for making a definitive diagnosis. A perusal of the Weinberg criteria reveals that several symptom groups kept distinct by RDC or DSM-III (e.g., loss of interest and decreased concentration, guilt and suicidal ideation) were combined by this group. Therefore, although each criteria set is appropriate to use in pharmacotherapy studies of depressed youngsters, all three will identify different depressive subsets (17,18). Unresolved diagnostic issues remain. Those of particular importance are, What are the lower limits of the diagnostic threshold for disorder in children, and Is the syndrome of MDD continuous across ages? Biologic validation studies of child and adolescent MDD may clarify this area (10).

Concomitant with the establishment of specific diagnostic criteria, several interview schedules were devised that permitted a reliable methodology for diagnosing children both among multiple raters in a single setting and among geographically distinct research groups. The Interview Schedule for Children (ISC) was published by Kovacs in 1977 (19), followed by the childhood version of the Schedule for Affective Disorders and Schizophrenia, the Kiddie-SADS (K-SADS) compiled by Puig-Antich and Chambers (20). Each instrument is a semistructured interview conducted individually with the parent and child which, systematically assesses the symptom clusters required to make DSM-III or RDC diagnoses. Structured epidemiological interview schedules are also available, the Diagnostic Interview for Children and Adolescents (DICA) developed by Herjanic and Welner (21) and the Diagnostic Interview

Schedule for Children (DISC), constructed by Costello (22). These latter two instruments are particularly suited for epidemiological studies, since they can be reliably administered by lay interviewers. An epidemiological version of the K-SADS is also in use (23).

Coinciding with the development of the ISC, K-SADS, DICA, and DISC was the standardization for use in the pediatric population of traditional depression rating scales used in adult affective disorder research. Poznanski et al. (24) modified the Hamilton depression rating scale, and she has published psychometric data on the 18-item Children's Depression Rating Scale (CDRS). The following depression severity criteria are established: 17–29 normal, 30–35 borderline, 36–45 mild, 46–55 moderate, 56+ severe. In a similar fashion, Kovacs (25) adapted the Beck Depression Inventory (BDI) for use with children. Although this instrument, the Children's Depression Inventory (CDI), is widely used and appears to segregate out among a cohort of psychiatrically referred youngsters those with significant depressive symptomatology (26), specific severity criteria cutoffs for this 27-item scale have not yet been published. This work is ongoing (S. Paulauskas, *personal communication*). As with the CDRS, the CDI is primarily used in children. The BDI has been shown to be directly applicable in the adolescent population (27) using the following severity cutoff points: 0–9 normal, 10–15 mild, 16–19 moderate, 20–29 moderate-severe, 30–63 severe. The Bellevue Index of Depression (BID), a 40-item severity scale based on the Weinberg criteria, has also been used in several studies (28). Kazdin and Petti (29) systematically reviewed most scales and interview measures used in child and adolescent depression.

The use of the CDRS, CDI, and BDI has given the pediatric psychopharmacologist simple, easy-to-administer rating scales to measure both baseline depression severity and response to medication. It must be emphasized, nonetheless, that these instruments do not diagnose an episode of MDD. They measure the severity of depressive symptoms. Approximately 20% of adolescents scoring above 16 on the BDI were not clinically diagnosed as depressed by DSM-III criteria (27). Similarly, with a shortened 13-item version of the CDI, only 75% of children with high scores were clinically diagnosed as having the depressive syndrome using DSM criteria (30).

From this discussion, it is also apparent that response criteria must be established prior to implementing a pharmacotherapy protocol. Since the CDRS and CDI do not identify syndromatic state, an alternative approach used by Puig-Antich has been to repeat the K-SADS interview and identify responders and nonresponders in a dichotomous fashion or by summing the ordinal scoring assigned to each symptom of the depressive syndrome (depression subscale score) generated by this interview. Such a methodology allows for assessment of both syndromal remission and severity improvement.

Most pharmacotherapy studies of depressed youngsters during this last decade have also used an endpoint analysis time frame to assess drug response. This entails identifying improvement status at the end of the protocol. An endpoint analysis may not be the best method applied to identify drug effects, as Quitkin et al. (31) have noted in their analysis of adult depressive pharmacotherapy trials. Pattern analysis over the 4 to 6 weeks of treatment with weekly or biweekly ratings may identify true drug responding individuals (i.e., those with delayed and persistent improvement). Pattern analysis would necessitate a repeat measures design using the CDRS, CDI, or K-SADS. The practice effect of such a procedure has not been clearly delineated, particularly in the prepubertal population.

PHENOMENOLOGICAL AND CLINICAL CONSIDERATIONS

An assessment of a pharmacological treatment response must also consider phenomenological and clinical characteristics of the depressive disorder in the young. The importance of this perspective is apparent from recent advances in pharmacotherapy of adult affective disorder, which show the specific response or lack of response of most subtypes to particular drug regimens (32,33). Although most of the major depressive subtypes are identified in children and adolescents, there appears to be more phenotypic homogeneity in the prepubertal depressive groups, since it is uncommon to identify an atypical or bipolar depressed child. Epidemiological studies of hospitalized adult bipolars (34,35) seem to confirm this clinical observation by noting that the most common age of onset of bipolar depressive illness is the late teens and early 20s. Although the onset of bipolar illness in prepuberty is rare, Joyce (35) noted that among 10 adults with their first episode before 15, 70% had an initial depression.

Spontaneous improvement of the depressive disorder is also a confounding variable to consider in any treatment outcome study. It is reported that prepubertal and adolescent major depressive disorder from its onset lasts approximately 30 weeks (8,36). Though the time frame from onset of illness to study entry cannot be controlled, this variable should be considered as a covariate in any analysis. These issues take on greater significance, since at least 20% of depressed youngsters no longer meet criteria for the depressive syndrome on repeated assessment in 2 weeks. These phenomenological constraints and the epidemiological fact of an approximately 2% prevalence rate for MDD in the general prepubertal population (37), and 5 to 13% rate in the adolescent population (38), have made it technically difficult to conduct a large-scale psychopharmacology study in the depressed young.

The issue of an inpatient versus an outpatient study group does not appear to be as important a study variable reflecting severity of illness as is the case in the adult population. This is particularly so in the prepubertal group, since the criteria for hospital admission frequently reflect family and psychosocial factors impinging on continuity of care. Clearly, an inpatient study will have greater control over medication compliance, so outpatient studies should routinely include plasma drug level monitoring.

Finally, the issue of segregating the prepubertal and adolescent population for study has heuristic value. Prepubertal MDD has phenomenological differences from its adult counterpart. For example, 38% of psychotic prepubertal depressives generally have dysphoric auditory hallu-cinations, whereas the psychotically depressed adult is more commonly deluded (7,39). This may reflect the influence of cognitive development on psychopathic phenomenology. A shift from prepuberty to adolescence also is significant, given reports of sex hormones either inducing depressive states (40) or improving depressed mood (41).

METHODOLOGICAL CONSIDERATIONS: THE DRUG PROTOCOL

Once an agent is found effective in an open trial it must be tested against placebo or the standard drug or class of drugs which themselves are superior to placebo. The parameters of such protocols should include a double-blind, placebo-controlled design with random assignment to each treatment cell. Sample size must be sufficient to provide adequate statistical power. Dose, duration of the treatment, and plasma drug level should be controlled and monitored. An understanding of pediatric pharmacokinetics is also necessary, since the metabolism, drug distribution, half-life, and protein-binding characteristics of antidepressants in the young require different dosing practices from those used in adults (42). This is particularly so with the tricyclic antidepressants imipramine, desipramine (43), and nortriptyline (44). Only in the last decade are more such methodologically sound studies entering into common practice in pediatric psychopharmacology.

Following an assessment of drug benefit during the active phase of illness, continuation and prophylaxis studies are indicated. A continuation study can answer the question of how long an individual should remain on medication once recovery has occurred. A prophylaxis study can assess the benefits of long-term maintenance medication in preventing recurrence. This is of particular importance in affective disorders, which are episodic illnesses in both adults (45) and children (46). Since the methodological tools to begin assessing the efficacy of antidepressants in child and adolescent MDD have been in place only in the last decade, studies completed to date are those conducted during active illness. Very preliminary evidence is available on continuation treatment (47), but prophylaxis studies are not available.

STATE OF PHARMACOTHERAPY PROGRESS

Tricyclic antidepressants have been used in pediatric psychopharmacology for the last two decades to ameliorate symptoms of enuresis (48), school phobia (49), and hyperactivity (50). Their efficacy in these disorders does not suggest that youngsters exhibiting these syndromes are depressed. It is more likely that TCAs have multiple pharmacological effects (51). However, this experience with TCAs in children and adolescents has shown that these agents can be safely administered to the pediatric age group.

The use of TCAs in depressed children began in the 1960s, yet the majority of this published work is flawed because of poor methodological design. Heterogeneous samples of children with anxious, behavioral, or psychotic features were treated; few reports delineated the diagnostic or recovery criteria; and dose and duration of medication treatment were inadequate or not specified. This body of work therefore describes the treatment of the symptom of depression and not necessarily the depressive syndrome. Petti systematically reviewed this earlier work (52).

An often-quoted article by Weinberg et al. (14) heralded the beginning of a more systematic methodological approach to pharmacotherapy in youngsters with MDD. The importance of this study is not necessarily in its treatment outcome findings. Even though 18 of the 19 children in the depressed treatment group demonstrated a definite improvement on 25 mg of amitriptyline daily, this was an open design in which the investigators did not control the treatment phase or standardize the time when outcome (recovery) was assessed. The significance of this work is that criteria were first established to diagnose depressive disorder in children, the Weinberg criteria. Since the mid-1970s more rigorously designed studies have been appearing. Although only a small array of treatment trials are available, a foundation of knowledge now exists to guide the next wave of investigations.

Numerous single case reports of TCA efficacy or preliminary findings followed by publication of a final report are available. Those studies presented here are the final reports that include sufficient data to assess study design, sample size, diagnostic and response criteria, length of treatment, dosage, and plasma level parameters. The major studies that meet these criteria are listed in Table 1.

Three studies are open-medication trials with a total sample size of $N = 62$ (range 8–34), whereas four are a double-blind design with a total sample size of $N = 73$ (range 6–38). Of the seven reports, Puig-Antich's group (6,53,54) studied the majority of both the cases treated openly (42/62) and those treated blindly (38/73). Petti et al. (55) used a small double-blind sample size of 6, which made statistical analysis invalid, whereas Kashani et al. (56) used a sample of 9, which had weak power. The medications used included imipramine (IMI) and amitriptyline (AMI). None of the double-blind studies found TCAs

superior to placebo, although they were considered effective in the open trials.

All studies listed in Table 1 used either RDC, DSM-III, or Weinberg diagnostic criteria with the CDRS, CDI, or BID to identify depressed youngsters. Kramer et al. (57), however, used specified scores from a psychiatric depression rating scale and also scaled scores of psychometric tests. Response criteria in each study included either repeat K-SADS assessment and its depression subscale score, or the CDI, CDRS, or BID. Kramer's group repeated their original diagnostic battery. All studies defined response in an end-point analysis that generally was after 4 to 6 weeks of pharmacotherapy. However, Preskorn et al. (58) initially identified responders at 3 weeks, adjusted medication, and reassessed recovery at 6 weeks.

Several other studies are available that were not listed in Table 1. The work by Geller et al. using nortriptyline (NT) in an open design is of particular note. This group reported efficacy in prepubertal depressives whose NT plasma levels were maintained in a similar "therapeutic window" range as has been found in studies of NT in adult depressives (47,59). However, these published studies are not clear in defining response criteria, nor was the time to response necessarily standardized. The strength of this group's work lies in their investigations of the pharmacokinetic parameters of NT in the pediatric population (44,60,61) and its cardiotoxicity (62).

A study completed but not yet reported by S. H. Preskorn, E. B. Weller, et al. (*personal communication*) appears particularly interesting. This is a double-blind, placebo-controlled investigation of over 30 prepubertal inpatients diagnosed depressed by the DICA and DSM-III criteria. Response measures included the CDI, CDRS, and a global assessment scale completed after 6 weeks of IMI. Medication was administered at 100 mg/day up to 5 mg/kg to maintain plasma levels of tricyclics between 150 and 250 ng/ml. Preliminary analyses revealed a slight trend for medication superiority over placebo. However, when subjects were

TABLE 1. *Pharmacotherapy studies in child and adolescent major depression[a]*

Author	Design	Criteria Dx.	Criteria Resp.	Age	N	Drug and dose	Length (weeks)	Resp. TCA	Resp. PL	Plasma level resp. range
Puig-Antich (6)	Open	RDC	RDC	Prepub. 6–12	8	IMI 5 mg/kg	6–8	6/8		
Kramer (57)	DB	Rating scale[b]	Rating scale[b]	Adol. 13–17	20	AMI 200 mg	6	8/10	6/10	
Preskorn (58)	Open	DSM DICA	CDI CDRS	Prepub. 7–12	20	IMI 50–5 mg/kg	3–6	12/16 12/20		125–225 ng/ml
Petti (55)	DB	Weinberg BID CDI	BID CDI	Prepub. 6–12	6	IMI 5 mg/kg	6	2/3	0/3	
Kashani (56)	DB crossover	DSM BID	DSM BID	Prepub. 9–12	9	AMI 1.5 mg/kg	4–8	3/5– 3/4[b]	1/4– 1/2[b]	
Puig-Antich (53)	DB	RDC	RDC subscales	Prepub. 7–12	38	IMI 5 mg/kg	5	9/16	15/22	>150 ng/ml
Ryan (54)	Open	RDC	RDC	Adol. 10–17	34	IMI 5 mg/kg	6	15/34		Not correlated

[a] Abbreviations: IMI, imipramine; AMI, amitriptyline; DB, double-blind; PL, placebo.
[b] See text.

segregated according to their dexamethasone suppression test (DST) status, DST nonsuppressors were noted to respond preferentially to IMI whereas DST suppressors did not follow this pattern.

Two other reports using maprotoline (63) or mianserin (64) are available. An open study by Minuto and Gallo (63) investigated a diagnostically heterogeneous sample where only 7 of 20 youngsters had depressive diagnoses. The second report by Dugas et al. (64) was an open study in prepubertal and adolescent depressives, and it suggests efficacy after 1, 2, 4 and 10 weeks of treatment. However, 30 of the 110 subjects are not accounted for, study entry was based solely on a history of depressed mood for 4 weeks and a CDRS score greater than 30, and the length of treatment and time to response assessment were not standardized.

PREPUBERTAL MAJOR DEPRESSION

The prepubertal studies include the works by Puig-Antich et al. (6,53), Preskorn et al. (58), Petti and Law (55), and Kashani et al. (56). All groups used either IMI up to 5 mg/kg/day or AMI at 1.5 mg/kg/day. However, only Puig-Antich and Preskorn meaningfully employed plasma IMI levels to assess dose-response relationships. Although Petti and Law's report is well designed and double-blind, with only three subjects in each treatment cell, it is impossible to generalize on their findings. Furthermore, medication was only maintained for 3 weeks; thereafter it was tapered and discontinued during the sixth week of treatment. A conservative interpretation of this work reveals that two of three drug-treated subjects had better than a moderate improvement, whereas none of the three placebo-treated subjects improved sufficiently to not require open IMI treatment.

Preskorn et al. (58) studied 20 prepubertal youngsters in an open fashion over 6 weeks. The first 3 weeks of treatment were at a fixed dose of 75 mg of IMI followed by altered dosage in the nonresponders. After 3 weeks there was a 20% (4/20) response rate in which four of the five responders had a total TCA (IMI + DMI) plasma level of 125 to 225 ng/ml. During the remaining 3 weeks, four nonresponders were lost to follow-up; 12 of 16 children finally recovered at 6 weeks; and 11 of the 12 had total plasma TCA in the "therapeutic range." These authors noted a significant correlation of response with both total TCA plasma level and with plasma DMI levels. There was a 92% (11/12) response rate within this window but only a 25% (1/4) response outside these guidelines. However, the choice of these TCA ranges may be premature, since only four subjects had total plasma TCA levels above 250 ng/ml. Furthermore, identifying a therapeutic window after 3 weeks may allow insufficient time to test whether IMI is effective at "nontherapeutic" levels (65). Conservative estimates of the overall response in this study range from 60 to 75%, depending on whether lost cases are included as nonresponders. Furthermore, because the response criteria were the CDI, CDRS, and a clinical global impression scale, it is unclear how many children recovered from the depressive syndrome.

The fixed-dose, double-blind, crossover study conducted by Kashani et al. (56) involved nine prepubertal depressives. Amitriptyline was administered up to 1.5 mg/kg/day. Each treatment phase lasted 4 weeks and it was immediately followed by the alternate treatment regimen. Subjects were diagnosed clinically by DSM-III criteria and given the BID. Response criterion was a BID score less than 20. The drug group was noted to have a greater decrease in their BID scores than when treated with placebo ($p < 0.09$). During the first phase three of five children responded to AMI, whereas only one of four responded to placebo. In phase two, three of four subjects responded to AMI and one of two to placebo. These authors noted no significant carryover effect between phases and therefore classified six of nine subjects as AMI responders and two of nine as placebo responders. One child was a nonresponder to both placebo and AMI.

This study is well-designed, but its small sample size makes it difficult to generalize the findings. Furthermore, there was only a trend for the depressed youngsters to have improved BID scores, whereas no comments were made about remission of the depressive syndrome. Plasma levels of AMT were not monitored, so it is also unclear whether therapeutic levels of AMI or its metabolite, nortriptyline, persisted during the placebo phase.

The study by Puig-Antich et al. (53) is the most extensive double-blind, placebo-controlled protocol available. It evolved from initial pilot observations that six of eight prepubertal major depressed children responded to imipramine after 6 to 8 weeks of treatment (6). The final report studied 38 youngsters, 16 treated with IMI up to 5 mg/kg/day and 22 with placebo. An endpoint analysis of response completed after 5 weeks of treatment included remission of the depressive syndrome, change in a depression subscale score, and a global assessment scale, all ascertained by a repeat K-SADS interview. Response rates were not significantly different between the placebo (68%, 15/22) and IMI (56%, 9/16) group.

In a second analysis of predictors of clinical response to IMI, these investigators included 15 additional cases treated openly, with 15 of the 16 children randomly assigned to active drug. Total plasma TCA level (IMI + DMI) positively correlated with predicting response of the depressive syndrome ($p < 0.003$). There was no evidence of response inhibition at high plasma levels as noted by Preskorn. Response was less likely in the psychotic subtype, although neither endogeneity nor the presence of separation anxiety predicted response. The clinical response rate in those children with maintenance plasma levels above the median value (214 ng/ml) was 87% (13/15), whereas only 47% (7/15) below this cutoff improved. A *post hoc* total plasma level cutoff of 150 ng/ml correctly identified 85% of the responders. An intriguing finding was that children with low total plasma TCA level had a worse outcome compared to the placebo treatment group. The explanation for this finding is unclear.

Few methodological flaws can be found in this study. Therefore the fact that IMI is not superior to placebo is a robust finding. That no difference existed between active and inactive treatment clearly bears on the 68% placebo response, which was quite high compared to the depressed adult placebo response rate of approximately 40% (66). Yet the inactivity of placebo has been questioned and briefly reviewed by Puig-Antich et al. (39). Finally, length of episode at entry into the study and phenomenological characteristics of this depressive cohort also may account for the negative findings. The responders in this study may have been in the recuperative phase of their disorder. Only a placebo washout would minimize this subset. Secondly, it still remains to be elucidated whether prepubertal major depressives identified with uniform diagnostic criteria also are biologically similar. Clearly, as reviewed earlier, the lack of more refined subtyping of prepubertal MDD at this stage of our knowledge implies that, although we can identify phenomenologically homogeneous samples, we cannot be sure that they represent biologically distinct groups.

ADOLESCENT MAJOR DEPRESSION

Kramer et al. (57) completed the only random-assignment, double-blind, placebo-controlled treatment study of 20 adolescents. Subjects were inpatients and diagnosed via predefined criteria. The same diagnostic battery was then employed to assess recovery. Ten youngsters randomly received 200 mg/day of amitriptyline (AMT) or placebo. An endpoint response analysis was reported after 6 weeks of treatment. Plasma levels were not followed. Although all the response measures revealed statistically significant improvement, there was no difference between active and placebo groups. Eighty percent (8/10) of the AMT group improved to either a moderate or maximal level, whereas 60% (6/10) of the placebo cohort improved to the same degree.

Several factors may have impinged on these negative findings. Boys predominated in the placebo group whereas girls predominated in the AMI group. In a retrospective reassessment mentioned by the authors, three placebo subjects would have been excluded. Finally, plasma levels were not available. This study makes clear the necessity of adhering to one's diagnostic criteria set and the power available from plasma blood sampling in order to maximize our understanding of pharmacotherapy efficacy in the young.

The remaining adolescent study reported by Ryan et al. (54) is a well-designed open protocol in 34 primarily outpatient adolescents. Diagnosis was made with the K-SADS and RDC criteria. IMI was titrated up to 5 mg/kg/day with plasma level monitoring. An endpoint analysis was completed after 6 weeks of medication. Response criteria included remission of the depressive syndrome and changes on depression subscale scores, both identified with repeat K-SADS interview. Overall, 44% (15/34) of subjects responded, yet clinical response was not correlated with plasma tricyclic level as was found in prepuberty. Variables that were noted to predict a negative response included female sex, higher plasma IMI level, and a pretreatment diagnosis of separation anxiety. There was no substantiation in this adolescent group, as was shown in prepuberty, that the psychotic subtype was less likely to respond to medication. However, the number of psychotic youngsters was low in this adolescent study.

Overall this is a well-designed study whose main drawback is its open methodology. Nevertheless, the negative findings with this methodology contrast to the open studies in prepubertal depressives, which uniformly reported a benefit from pharmacotherapy. The significant finding of this report, therefore, is a suggestion that adolescent MDD may be a distinctly different syndrome to treat pharmacologically. Ryan et al. hypothesize that this lack of response pattern could represent a negative influence of increased estrogen during adolescent development. This hypothesis was further supported by the facts of an increasing prevalence of depression in adolescence (38), the side effect of depression induced by birth control pills (40), and findings of lower antidepressant response rates in younger adults compared to the older populations (39).

SUMMARY OF PHARMACOTHERAPY STUDIES

The works reviewed here have been collated in Table 2 to reveal the overall rate of the efficacy of pharmacotherapy in prepubertal and adolescent MDD. Where there remained a question of lost cases or only mild response, the final outcome was computed conservatively by considering these subjects as nonresponders. In the one crossover design study, results from the first stage were used to minimize any carryover effects. The summary figures reported, therefore, are rough estimates of recovery rates. In prepuberty, of 52 children on active medication 62% improved, whereas 55% of 29 children recovered on placebo. Overall, approximately 60% of prepubertal depressives improved in 4 to 6 weeks regardless of their medication status. In the adolescent group the figures are similar but slightly lower. Of 44 adolescents treated with active medication, 52% recovered, whereas 60% of 10 adolescents improved on placebo. Overall, approximately 55% of adolescent depressives responded within 4 to 6 weeks regardless of their medication regimen.

These compiled figures clearly reflect the fact that no double-blind, placebo-controlled study found tricyclics to be superior to placebo. However, these figures also hide the fact that a new body of knowledge is emerging from this work completed over the last decade. The primary considerations are the following:

TABLE 2. TCA versus placebo: percent response[a]

	N	Pre-pubertal +	Pre-pubertal −	N	Adolescent +	Adolescent −
TCA	(52)	62	38	(44)	52	48
Placebo	(29)	55	45	(10)	60	40
Total	(81)	59	41	(54)	54	46

[a] Data obtained from refs. 53–58.

1. Prepubertal major depression may exhibit a distinct pharmacological response pattern in contrast with adolescent depressives because of the lack of plasma level correlations with response in teenagers.

2. Pharmacotherapy response was similar in the endogenous and nonendogenous subtypes, but it was less likely in the psychotic depressed prepubertal child.

3. DST nonsuppression in prepubertal depressed inpatients may predict a favorable response to imipramine.

4. A minimum total plasma TCA level of 150 ng/ml should be attained when treating prepubertal depressives with IMI or DMI.

AREA FOR FUTURE PROGRESS

The work during this last decade in pediatric psychopharmacology of children and adolescents with MDD has identified the need for placebo-controlled efficacy studies. These investigations must include strict adherence to proper methodological design, including a placebo washout and monitoring of plasma drug levels. The inclusion of scales assessing family environment and family life stresses may also be useful as predictors of response (67) because of the youngster's greater dependence on the family system. Continuation studies are also clearly needed. Investigations with other classes of antidepressants, such as lithium, monoamine oxidase inhibitors, minor tranquilizers, and the newer generation of antidepressants, may help isolate which agents or treatment combinations have benefit in youngsters.

Many theoretical issues remain in our understanding of child and adolescent MDD. Its continuities and discontinuities with adult affective disorders are only slowly being sorted and analyzed. Naturalistic outcome in epidemiological studies is clarifying the morbidity of the disorder and therefore the true need for any pharmacological intervention. Biological studies in high-risk families and family history investigations may aid in finding biogenetic subtypes. The confluence of these investigative strategies all focusing on the syndrome of MDD in the young will be invaluable in guiding psychopharmacologists through the next decade of progress.

ADDENDUM

Following the publisher's deadline for this text, Geller et al. (68) reported preliminary results of an open nortriptyline (NT) trial in 22 prepubertal outpatient depressives six to twelve years old. Diagnoses were made with the K-SADS and depressed subjects recruited into the study if their CDRS score was at least 40. Pharmacotherapy began after a two week drug free interval if the CDRS remained above 35. Treatment lasted six weeks with oral NT doses ranging from 20 to 50 mg/d; 14 of 22 subjects improved (64%). Responders had significantly higher mean steady state plasma NT levels; all subjects with NT levels greater than 60 ng/ml improved. Although maximal clinical response appeared in a plasma NT range from 60 to 100 ng/ml, this study was not designed to assess the efficacy of higher plasma NT levels. It should be noted that although most subjects in this study were endogenously depressed at baseline, it was unclear how many youngsters remained syndromatically depressed when pharmacotherapy began. The response rate reported in this study corresponds with the pharmacotherapy data just reviewed.

REFERENCES

1. Cytryn, L., and McKnew, D. J. (1972): *Am. J. Psychiatry,* 129: 149–155.
2. Cytryn, L., McKnew, D. H., and Bunney, W. E. (1980): *Am. J. Psychiatry,* 137:22–25.
3. Carlson, G. A., and Cantwell, D. P. (1980): *Am. J. Psychiatry,* 137:445–449.
4. Robbins, D., Alessi, N., Cook, S. C., et al. (1982): *J. Am. Acad. Child Psychiatry,* 21:251–255.
5. Puig-Antich, J. (1982): *J. Am. Acad. Child Psychiatry,* 21:291–293.
6. Puig-Antich, J., Blau, S., Marx, N., et al. (1978): *J. Am. Acad. Child Psychiatry,* 17:695–707.
7. Chambers, W. J., Puig-Antich, J., Tabrizi, M., et al. (1982): *Arch. Gen. Psychiatry,* 39:921–928.
8. Kovacs, M., Feinberg, T. L., Crouse-Novak, M. A., et al. (1984): *Arch. Gen. Psychiatry,* 41:229–237.
9. Strober, M., and Carlson, G. (1982): *Arch. Gen. Psychiatry,* 39: 549–555.
10. Cantwell, D. (1985): *Psychiatr. Clin. North Am.,* 4:779–792.
11. Winsberg, B. G., and Yepes, L. E. (1978): In: *Pediatric Psychopharmacology,* edited by J. S. Werry, pp. 234–273. Brunner/Mazel, New York.
12. Rapoport, J. L., Buchsbaum, M. S., Weingartner, H., et al. (1980): *Arch. Gen. Psychiatry,* 37:933–943.
13. Mattes, J. A., Boswell, C., Oliver, H., et al. (1984): *Arch. Gen. Psychiatry,* 41:1059–1063.
14. Weinberg, W. A., Rutman, A., Sullivan, L., et al. (1973): *J. Pediatrics,* 83:1065–1072.
15. Feighner, J. P., Robins, E., Guze, S. B., et al. (1972): *Arch. Gen. Psychiatry,* 26:57–61.
16. Pearce, J. (1977): *J. Child Psychol. Psychiatry,* 18:79–82.
17. Carlson, G. A., and Cantwell, D. (1982): *J. Am. Acad. Child Psychiatry,* 21:247–250.
18. Poznanski, E., Mokros, H., Grossman, J., et al. (1985): *Am. J. Psychiatry,* 142:1168–1173.
19. Kovacs, M. (1978): *Interview Schedule for Children* (ISC), 10th revision. University of Pittsburgh, Pittsburgh, PA.
20. Puig-Antich, J., and Chambers, W. J. (1978): *Schedule for Affective Disorders and Schizophrenia for School Age Children,* 2nd draft. N.Y. State Psychiatric Institute, New York.
21. Orvaschel, H. (1985): *Psychopharmacol. Bull.,* 21:737–745.
22. Costello, A. J., Edelbrock, C., Kalas, R., et al. (1982): *Diagnostic Interview Schedule for Children* (DISC). Western Psychiatric Institute & Clinic, Pittsburgh, PA.
23. Orvaschel, H., Puig-Antich, J., Chambers, W., et al. (1982): *J. Am. Acad. Child Psychiatry,* 4:392–397.
24. Poznanski, E. O., Grossman, J. A., Buchsbaum, Y., et al. (1984): *J. Am. Acad. Child Psychiatry,* 23:191–197.
25. Kovacs, M. (1980–81): *Acta Paedopsychiatr.,* 46:305–315.
26. Kovacs, M. (1985): *Psychopharmacol. Bull.,* 21:995–998.
27. Strober, M., Green, J., and Carlson, G. (1981): *J. Consult. Clin. Psychol.,* 49:482–483.
28. Petti, T. A. (1978): *J. Am. Acad. Child Psychol.,* 17:49–59.
29. Kazdin, A. E., and Petti, T. A. (1982): *J. Child Psychol. Psychiatry,* 23:437–457.
30. Carlson, G., and Cantwell, D. P. (1980): *J. Child Psychol. Psychiatry,* 21:19–25.
31. Quitkin, F., Rabkin, J., Ross, D., et al. (1984): *Arch. Gen. Psychiatry,* 41:782–786.
32. Spiker, D. G., Weiss, J. D., and Dealy, R. S. (1985): *Am. J. Psychiatry,* 142:430–436.
33. Liebowitz, M. R., Klein, D. F., Quitkin, F. M., et al. (1984): In: *Neurobiology of Mood Disorders,* edited by R. M. Post and J. C. Ballenger, pp. 107–120. Williams & Wilkins, Baltimore.

34. Loranger, A. W., and Levine, P. M. (1978): *Arch. Gen. Psychiatry,* 35:1345–1348.
35. Joyce, P. R. (1984): *Psychol. Med.,* 14:145–149.
36. Strober, M. (1985): *Psychiatr. Ann.,* 15:375–378.
37. Kashani, J. H., McGee, R. O., Clarkson, S. E., et al. (1983): *Arch. Gen. Psychiatry,* 40:1217–1223.
38. Cohen, P., Velez, C. N., and Garcia, M. (1985): Presented at American Academy of Child Psychiatry, San Antonio, October 26.
39. Puig-Antich, J., Ryan, N. D., and Rabinovich, H. (1985): In: *Diagnosis and Psychopharmacology of Childhood and Adolescent Disorders,* edited by J. M. Weiner, pp. 149–178. John Wiley, New York.
40. Herzberg, B. N., Johnson, A. L., and Brown, D. (1970): *Br. Med. J.,* 4:142–145.
41. Klaiber, E. L., Broverman, D. M., Vogel, W., et al. (1979): *Arch. Gen. Psychiatry,* 36:550–554.
42. Rave, E., and Wilson, J. T. (1983): In: *Handbook of Clinical Pharmacokinetics,* edited by M. Gibaldi and L. Prescott, pp. 142–168. Adis Health Science Press, New York.
43. Perel, J. M. (1974): In: *Report of Chairman. Ad Hoc Committee on Tricyclic Antidepressant Cardiotoxicity,* edited by O. S. Robinson, F.D.A., pp. 1–4. Washington, DC.
44. Geller, B., Cooper, T. A., Chestnut, E., et al. (1984): *J. Clin. Psychopharmacol.,* 4:265–269.
45. Keller, M. B., Shapiro, R. W., Lavori, P. W., et al. (1982): *Arch. Gen. Psychiatry,* 39:911–915.
46. Kovacs, M., Feinberg, T. L., Crous-Novak, M. A., et al. (1984): *Arch. Gen. Psychiatry,* 41:643–649.
47. Geller, B., Perel, J., Knitter, E. F., et al. (1983): *Psychopharmacol. Bull.,* 19:62–64.
48. Shaffer, D., and Ambrosini, P. J. (1985): In: *Diagnosis and Psychopharmacology of Childhood and Adolescent Disorders,* edited by J. M. Weiner, pp. 305–331. John Wiley & Sons, New York.
49. Gittelman-Klein, R., and Klein, D. F. (1971): *Arch. Gen. Psychiatry,* 25:204–207.
50. Donnelly, M., Zametkin, A. J., Rapoport, J. L., et al. (1986): *Clin. Pharmacol. Ther.,* 39:72–81.
51. Rapoport, J., and Mikkelson, E. J. (1978): In: *Pediatric Psycho-pharmacology,* edited by J. S. Werry, pp. 208–233. Brunner/Mazel, New York.
52. Petti, T. A. (1983): Imipramine in the treatment of depressed children. In: *Affective Disorders in Childhood and Adolescence: An Update,* edited by D. P. Cantwell and G. A. Carlson, pp. 375–415. SP Medical & Scientific Books, New York.
53. Puig-Antich, J., Perel, J. M., Lupatkin, W., et al. (1987): *Arch. Gen. Psychiatry,* 44:81.
54. Ryan, N., Puig-Antich, J., Rabinovich, H., et al. (1985): *Acta Psychiatr. Scand.,* 72(Suppl. 320):48.
55. Petti, T., and Law, W. (1982): *J. Clin. Psychopharmacol.,* 2:107–110.
56. Kashani, J., Shekim, W. O., and Reid, J. C. (1984): *J. Am. Acad. Child Psychiatry,* 23:348–351.
57. Kramar, A. D., and Feiguine, R. J. (1981): *J. Am. Acad. Child Psychiatry,* 20:636–644.
58. Preskorn, S. H., Weller, E. B., Weller, R. A., et al. (1982): *J. Clin. Psychiatry,* 43:450–453.
59. Geller, B., Cooper, T. A., Farooki, Z. Q., et al. (1985): *Am. J. Psychiatry,* 142:336–338.
60. Geller, B., Cooper, T. B., Chestnut, E. C., et al. (1985): *J. Clin. Psychopharmacol.,* 5:154–158.
61. Geller, B., Cooper, T., and Chestnut, E. (1985): *J. Clin. Psychopharmacol.,* 5:213–216.
62. Geller, B., Farooki, Q., Cooper, T. B., et al. (1985): *Am. J. Psychiatry,* 142:1095–1097.
63. Minuti, E., and Gallo, V. (1982): *Adv. Biochem. Psychopharmacol.,* 32:223–227.
64. Dugas, M., Mouren, M. C., Halfon, O., et al. (1985): *Acta Psychiatr. Scand.,* 72:48–53.
65. Quitkin, F. M., Rabkin, J. G., and Ross, D. (1984): *Arch. Gen. Psychiatry,* 41:238–245.
66. Klein, D. F., Gittelman, R., Quitkin, F., et al. (1980): *Diagnosis and Drug Treatment of Psychiatric Disorders: Adults and Children,* pp. 268–408. Williams & Wilkins, Baltimore.
67. Werry, J. S. (1978): In: *Pediatric Psychopharmacology,* edited by J. S. Werry, pp. 29–78. Brunner/Mazel, New York.
68. Geller, B., Cooper, T. B., Chestnut E. C., et al. (1986): *Amer. J. Psych.,* 143:1283–1286.

Psychopharmacology:
The Third Generation of Progress,
edited by Herbert Y. Meltzer.
Raven Press, New York © 1987.

CHAPTER **130**

Basic Biological Overview of the Eating Disorders

Katherine A. Halmi, Sigurd Ackerman, James Gibbs, and Gerard Smith

Research in the neuropsychopharmacology of the eating disorders has burgeoned in the past decade. There was no section on eating disorders in the previous *Generation of Progress* volume. However, in the past decade, the increased need to develop clinical treatment programs for anorexia nervosa and bulimia syndrome patients and the recognition of the usefulness of pharmacological methods in the treatment of these disorders spurred further research. This section focuses on investigations in anorexia nervosa, bulimia syndrome, and obesity. Definitions for the first two conditions are given in Table 1. It should be noted that an anorexia nervosa patient who also binges and purges has two diagnoses: anorexia nervosa and bulimia syndrome. Emphasis on studying neurotransmitter and opioid metabolism in anorexia nervosa and the bulimia syndrome has occurred with the recognition that many of the signs and symptoms of these disorders are significantly affected by the function of various neurotransmitters. The physiological changes that occur before, during, and after a bulimic episode and the physiological changes that maintain bulimic and starvation behavior are not known. The mechanisms by which antidepressants are effective in reducing binge eating episodes are not known. These questions will be studied in the next generation.

The recent progress in basic research relevant to eating disorders can be characterized as the movement away from analysis of eating syndromes produced by brain lesions to the analysis of specific neurochemical mechanisms of specific aspects of the control of eating. A field dominated by the ventral–medial hypothalamic syndrome and the lateral hypothalamic syndrome is now dominated by the specific effects of monoamines and peptides at specific locations in the brain or peripheral nervous system. For example, norepinephrine in the paraventricular nucleus may be considered a specific probe for initiating eating, and gut peptides administered peripherally are probes for the termination of eating.

A major conceptual shift has been to accept the idea that the meal is the functional unit of eating behavior. Basic research on the control of initiation, on the maintenance and positive reinforcing effect of food, and on the termination of eating have immediate relevance to eating disorder patients in which the same kind of behavioral eating information can be obtained in the same form. This should make it much easier to exploit concepts and results obtained in animal work for the analysis of the eating disorders.

THE PHYSIOLOGY OF EATING

The successful psychological and physiological analysis of eating a meal is necessary for understanding the eating disorders and for the development of effective therapies—nutritional, psychological, and pharmacological. To analyze eating is to analyze the psychobiological mechanisms that determine the form of the meal, because the meal is the functional unit of eating behavior (118). Since the newborn infant eats meals without requiring instruction from her or his caretaker, the mechanisms for the initiation, maintenance, and termination of a meal must be "hard-wired." As the child develops and matures, the physiological mech-

TABLE 1. *DSM-III-R criteria*

Eating disorders
  Anorexia nervosa
  A. Intense fear of becoming obese, which does not diminish as weight loss progresses.
  B. Disturbance in the way in which one's body weight, size, or shape is experienced, e.g., claiming to "feel fat" even when emaciated; belief that one area of the body is "too fat" even when obviously underweight.
  C. Refusal to maintain body weight over a minimal normal weight for age and height, e.g., weight loss leading to maintenance of body weight 15% below expected; failure to make expected weight gain during period of growth, leading to body weight 15% below expected.
  D. In females, absence of at least three consecutive menstrual cycles when otherwise expected to occur (primary or secondary amenorrhea).
  Bulimia nervosa
  A. Recurrent episodes of binge eating (rapid consumption of a large amount of food in a discrete period of time, usually less than 2 hr).
  B. During the eating binges there is fear of not being able to stop eating.
  C. The individual regularly engages in either self-induced vomiting, use of laxatives, or rigorous dieting or fasting in order to counteract the effects of the binge eating.
  D. A minimum average of two binge-eating episodes per week for at least 3 months.

Eating disorders NEC
  Examples:
  1. An individual of normal weight who does not have binge eating episodes but frequently engages in self-induced vomiting for fear of gaining weight.
  2. All of the features of anorexia nervosa in a female except for absence of menses.
  3. All of the features of bulimia nervosa except for the frequency or duration of binge-eating episodes.

anisms are supplemented and enriched by learned or conditioned mechanisms. Although it is commonly assumed that eating in the adult is primarily under the control of these learned mechanisms, there is little experimental evidence for this view. In fact, the relative contribution of congenital or unconditioned mechanisms and of learned mechanisms for the control of meal size and frequency is an empirical question of great importance. Given the lack of relevant data on this point, we briefly review neural and hormonal mechanisms that are currently considered as putative controls for normal eating. We emphasize "putative" because none of these mechanisms has been demonstrated to be a natural component of the physiological structure of a meal.

The psychobiological mechanisms thought to be involved in distortions of eating associated with stress (see J. E. Morley, *this volume*), restraint, externality, and depression have not been sufficiently delineated to merit discussion at this time. A discussion of the other clinically relevant area of acquired preferences and aversions for food is beyond the scope of this chapter.

Meal Initiation: Hunger

Gastric Contractions

In 1912, Walter Cannon published a paper entitled "An Explanation of Hunger" (9). In this study, Cannon reported a good temporal correlation in one human subject between periods of increased gastric motility (recorded via an inflated gastric balloon) and the subjective sense of hunger; it may have been significant for the results that this subject was coached by Cannon to recognize and respond to hunger sensations. Based on the temporal correlation he found, Cannon referred to these periods of increased motility as "hunger contractions." Using similar techniques, Carlson apparently confirmed these results in a large number of subjects (10). It seemed that solid experimental evidence in support of a traditional speculation about the necessary stimulus for hunger had been produced. But the evidence was less solid than it seemed. Christensen (14) did not observe the correlation in a study of young men. The correlation was never present in subjects when motility was measured by a small telemetering capsule instead of by a large balloon (111) or when subjects were not coached in advance to associate hunger with increased gastric motility (138). The fact that gastrectomized patients clearly experienced hunger (60) was also not consistent with Cannon's "explanation of hunger." The contractions do not make a significant contribution to the initiation of eating.

Glucoprivation and the Glucostatic Hypothesis

Another theory to account for the beginning of meals explained eating in terms of changes in cellular metabolism. The initial event was thought to be a decrease in levels of circulating glucose or, alternatively, a decrease in the glucose utilization by cells (glucoprivation); such a decrease was postulated to occur as a result of a period of nonfeeding. Thus, the initiation of a meal was seen as a response to a metabolic deficit that accrued between meals. Mayer called this the glucostatic hypothesis to emphasize the pivotal role of glucose utilization. The glucostatic hypothesis had intuitive appeal: we eat in response to a need, and that need is a deficit in the availability of a prime fuel, glucose, for cellular use.

The glucostatic hypothesis was supported by numerous experiments in animals in which meal size increased after the administration of insulin to produce hypoglycemia, which led indirectly to glucoprivation, or after the administration of 2-deoxy-D-glucose (2-DG), which produced direct intracellular blockade of glucose utilization [for details, see review by Smith (132)]. Both insulin hypoglycemia and 2-DG also increased meal size in humans and, furthermore, produced self-reports of increased hunger (128,140). Thus, significant hypoglycemia and/or intracellular glucoprivation are sufficient signals for the initiation of a meal in animals and humans. But most meals do not begin in the context of this metabolic emergency (130), and for that reason the glucostatic hypothesis has not been considered to be relevant to the initiation of meals under the usual circumstances of *ad libidum* feeding.

Three experimental observations appeared recently, however, that revived interest in a modified form of the glucostatic hypothesis. The first observation was that if rats treated with 2-DG were not given food until after glucose utilization had returned to normal, the rats still initiated a meal (105). This observation was important because it dissociated the effect of 2-DG on meal initiation from the acute metabolic responses to intracellular glucoprivation. Thus, a meal could be initiated as the result of an episode of glucoprivation that occurred hours before—an apparent demonstration of a "metabolic memory." Since none of the previous animal or human experiments had searched for this kind of delayed relationship, this reopened the possibility that this type of glucostatic mechanism could be initiating meals without the simultaneous appearance of other neuroendocrine responses to glucoprivation.

The other two observations concerned the occurrence of a decrease in blood glucose shortly before the initiation of a meal in rats with constant access to food (8,88). These decreases in glucose were small (approximately 10%), and they were revealed by constant monitoring of glucose during experiments that lasted hours. These decreases are not sufficient to produce hypoglycemia, and, on the basis of current knowledge, they would not decrease cellular glucose utilization in any tissue. Thus, the decrease in blood glucose appears to function as a signal for initiating eating in the absence of the concurrent metabolic need that was postulated in the original glucostatic hypothesis. The best evidence that this decrease in blood glucose causes the initiation of eating and is not simply correlated with the onset of eating is that infusions of exogenous glucose sufficient to shorten the duration of the fall in blood glucose prevented the initiation of a meal. Thus, this new glucostatic hypothesis postulates that a small decrease of blood glucose has informational value for the eating system that is not directly related to a current metabolic need. This new possibility should receive extensive testing in normal animals and humans and in patients with eating disorders.

Neurochemistry

There is compelling pharmacological evidence that a noradrenergic α_2 receptor-mediated action in the paraventricular nucleus of the hypothalamus initiates eating in sated rats (39,80). This mechanism is modulated by circulating corticosterone (81) and has a circadian rhythm of sensitivity, being most sensitive in the early hours of the dark phase (73).

Neuropeptide Y, a peptide that is colocalized in some peripheral noradrenergic neurons, has also recently been demonstrated to initiate eating after microinjection into a variety of hypothalamic sites including the paraventricular nucleus (15,84,136; see J. E. Morley, *this volume*). Chronic injections of neuropeptide Y or of norepinephrine into the paraventricular nucleus produce chronic hyperphagia and increased body weight.

Although this noradrenergic mechanism is established beyond reasonable doubt, and the eating response to neuropeptide Y is a robust phenomenon, the relevance of these paraventricular synaptic events to the initiation of spontaneous eating remains to be demonstrated.

Opioid peptides can also initiate eating under certain conditions. These pharmacological effects are reviewed by J. E. Morley (*this volume*).

Learned Cues

Rats can learn to initiate eating to external stimuli previously associated with food (41,123,150). Food-associated cues are associated with increased dopaminergic turnover in the hypothalamus (129), and their potency for initiating a meal is increased by food deprivation, decreased by peripheral administration of cholecystokinin, and not changed by peripheral cholinergic blockade (123,151,152). This new work suggests that the pharmacological analysis of meals initiated by learned cues in humans would be interesting and may yield new therapeutic approaches to patients with eating disorders.

Meal Maintenance: Pleasure and Reward

The positive reinforcing or rewarding effects of food stimuli sustain eating once a meal has been initiated. These rewarding effects are innate, e.g., sweet taste, or they are acquired, e.g., chili pepper (119). Wise (153) suggested that central dopamine mechanisms mediate the rewarding effects of food just as they mediate the rewarding effects of intracranial self-stimulation and of the self-administration of psychoactive drugs. The experimental basis for Wise's suggestion was that the dopamine antagonist pimozide inhibited the rewarding effect of food (153). This was supported by evidence of increased turnover of hypothalamic dopamine during feeding (53,54).

Sclafani and his colleagues extended this hypothesis to the reward of sweet fluids by demonstrating that pimozide decreased the intake of a saccharin–glucose solution in a fashion similar to the decrease produced by dilution of the sweet fluid (126,157,158). The use of sweet solutions to analyze the dopamine hypothesis of food reward has the advantage that good stimulus control is provided by the tight linkage between the concentration of sugar solutions and their reward value as measured by preference or palatability tests (19,112). Since this linkage is tightest during sham feeding of sucrose solutions because sham feeding minimizes the postingestive inhibitory effect of sugar solutions, Geary and Smith (30) tested the effect of pimozide on the sham intake of sucrose solutions (5–40%). Pimozide inhibited sham feeding rate, and the temporal pattern of decreases in sham feeding rate after pimozide were similar to those produced by decreasing the concentration of sucrose sham-fed. Schneider et al. (124) have observed a similar result with other specific D_2 receptor antagonists such as sultoperide and sulpiride.

This pharmacological evidence has been supported by the observation that dopaminergic turnover in the hypothalamus increases as a direct function of the concentration of sucrose that was sham fed for 9 min prior to decapitation (4). This effect appeared to be limited to the hypothalamus because it was not observed in other dopaminergic terminal fields such as the accumbens, olfactory tubercle, caudate, amygdala, or frontal cortex.

These data support Wise's hypothesis, but they do not prove it, because it is not clear that the increased hypothalamic dopamine turnover is reflecting the rewarding effect of sham-fed sucrose rather than some other aspect of sensory or motor processing. And the pharmacological evidence can be criticized on the same grounds: it is extremely difficult to rule out some motor disability as being responsible for the inhibitory effect of the D_2 antagonists. With these reservations in mind, however, it is clear that Wise's hypothesis is of significant heuristic value for investigating the possibility that the normal rewarding effect of food is disturbed in patients with eating disorders (see J. E. Morley, *this volume,* for the possibility that endogenous opioids are also involved in food reward).

Meal Termination: Satiety

Where Does Food Act to Produce Satiety?

Since we experience satiety before large amounts of food can be digested and absorbed, ingested food must produce the necessary signals at one or more sites along the surface of the upper gastrointestinal tract. In order to determine whether these powerful signals arise from oral, gastric, or intestinal sites—or from all three—simple surgical techniques have been tested in animals. When chronic cannulas or catheters are placed in the esophagus or stomach so that they can be temporarily opened during a test to allow drainage and recovery of an ingested food (sham feeding), all species overeat (20,34,61,62,160). These observations demonstrate that food stimuli in the mouth are not sufficient to exert a normal satiety reaction. Meal termination cannot totally be controlled by past experience and the learning associated with the taste and texture of food. Furthermore, if these results, obtained in several animal species under a variety of conditions, have any relevance to human feeding, meal termination is not primarily controlled by the scheduling of meals enforced by social customs.

The results of this kind of behavioral testing in animals can be more dramatic and more interesting: when total recovery of an ingested liquid food is achieved in sham feeding of rhesus monkeys, satiety is absent (see Fig. 1). These results mean that the accumulation of food in the stomach and/or the entry of food into the intestine are necessary for satiety.

We investigated this problem further by asking whether food infused directly into the small intestine would reduce sham feeding in rhesus monkeys. Small amounts of intestinal food produced a highly significant dose-related suppression of sham feeding (34). Similar results have been obtained in rats (85,117). These findings were important on several counts. First, they established the potency of food in the small intestine for inhibiting food intake. Second, intestinal food did not require the presence of gastric distention to inhibit sham feeding, since gastric distention cannot occur when gastric cannulas are open for sham feeding. Third, intestinal food not only inhibited food intake, but it elicited the other behaviors normally seen in animals when a meal ends: grooming, exploration, and apparent sleep. This was good evidence that natural satiety, not discomfort or some other artifact, had occurred.

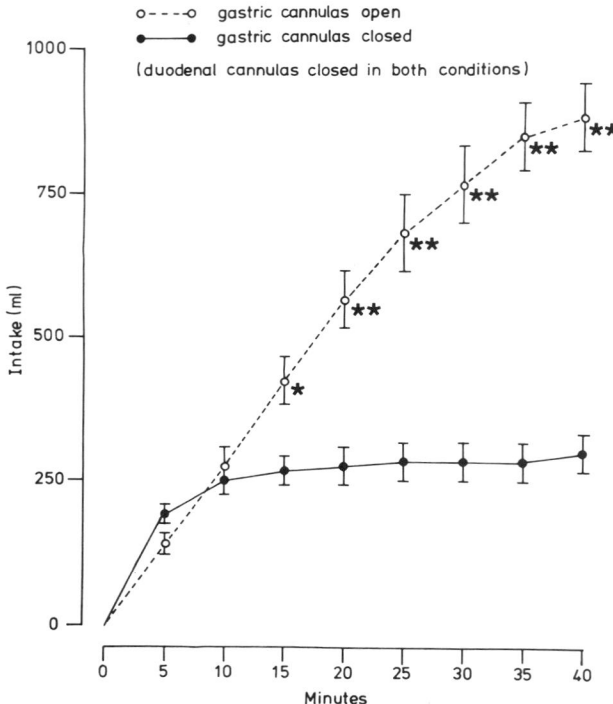

FIG. 1. When no food accumulates in the stomach or small intestine, satiety disappears. The figure shows the mean cumulative liquid food intakes (mean ± S.E.M., milliliters) by four rhesus monkeys during tests under two different conditions: on days when gastric fistulas were closed (*filled circles*) and all ingested food remained within the gastrointestinal tract; and on days when gastric fistulas were open (*open circles*). All tests were carried out after overnight food deprivation. Under both conditions, food was smelled, tasted, and swallowed normally, but when fistulas were open, and no food remained in the gut, feeding was continuous. Liquid food was a high-carbohydrate preparation with a density of 1 kcal/ml. *$p < 0.05$; **$p < 0.01$, statistical differences from results when cannulas were closed. (Reprinted by permission from Gibbs et al., ref. 34.)

It is of special interest to note that an early instance of human sham feeding (the result of a chronic fistula following a traumatic penetrating wound of the upper intestine) has been recorded. In this report, the victim's physician noted: ". . . It is not easy to imagine the intense hunger and greed with which the patient consumed colossal amounts of food . . . without reaching the feeling of satiation . . ." (6). The experimental studies and the clinical case converge to indicate that the intestine (or possibly an early postabsorptive event) plays an important role in ending meals.

Is the role of the intestine a necessary component of satiety? This question has been experimentally addressed by artificially preventing the normally rapid initial emptying of ingested food from stomach into intestine. This can be achieved by using a noose device (74) or an inflatable cuff (21) at the pylorus to inhibit gastric emptying temporarily. Whatever the technique, the results are the same: rats do not overeat when food is restricted to the stomach. They display normal satiety. Thus, the stomach, as well as the intestine, is the source of at least one satiety signal.

How Does Food Act to Produce Satiety?

It is widely thought that afferent fibers of the abdominal vagus provide the primary avenue of satiety traffic produced by food in the stomach. But we found that vagotomized rats in which ingested food was limited to the stomach by a pyloric noose were no different from similar sham-operated rats in the amount of food they ate at a test meal (75). Thus, gastric satiety did not require vagal innervation of the stomach or of the abdomen. Koopmans (72) extended this finding. Using an inbred strain, he transplanted an extra stomach from donor rats into recipient rats. The transplanted stomach opened into the small intestine of each recipient rat, but passage of experimentally injected food into the intestine during a test could be prevented by the use of a pyloric noose. Injections of food into the transplanted stomach had a strikingly accurate satiety effect even though the transplanted stomach had no extrinsic neural connections.

These results suggested that the gastric satiety signal might be hormonal. Since gastrin, the classic gastric peptide, had no effect on food intake even in huge doses (86), we turned our attention to bombesin, a recently discovered peptide. Bombesin, or a peptide closely resembling bombesin, is present in large amounts in the gastrointestinal tract, and at particularly high concentrations in the stomach. Systemic injections of bombesin produced a potent and dose-related inhibition of normal feeding (33) and a similar effect on sham feeding, and it elicited the natural behavioral sequence of satiety in rats (93). Recently, bombesin was shown to reduce food intake significantly at a test meal in normal-weight human volunteers (102). Obese subjects have not been tested yet.

In a parallel effort, we attempted to decipher the code for intestinal satiety. Once again, hormones appear important. Cholecystokinin (CCK) is an intestinal peptide that is released into blood in proportion to the amount of food that enters the duodenum. Cholecystokinin has several established gut functions such as contraction of the gallbladder, decrease of gastric emptying, and stimulation of pancreatic enzyme secretion. Systemic injections of CCK produce potent dose-related suppressions of feeding in a wide variety of animals, including rhesus monkeys. Like food in the intestine, CCK elicits a sequential display of satiety-related behaviors. (For review of the satiety actions of CCK in experimental animals, see ref. 35.) Finally, in humans, intravenous infusion of CCK reduces food intake at a test meal in lean (71,135) and obese (113) subjects. Whether the chronic administration of CCK will reduce body weight in obese humans is not known, but CCK did produce weight loss in genetically obese rats when it was administered over a 3-week period (7).

How Do Gut Signals Reach the Brain?

In no case is the mechanism of action of a putative satiety signal understood. It has been assumed that CCK must first act somewhere in the periphery because it is unlikely to cross the blood–brain barrier to have a direct central effect. Consistent with this assumption, Moran and McHugh (100) obtained evidence to support their suggestion that the satiety action of CCK is indirect, depending on its well-known inhibition of gastric emptying. What is clear is that the satiety action of systemically administered exogenous CCK is critically dependent on the integrity of the abdominal vagus nerve and specifically on its gastric branches (131). Furthermore, the vagal afferent fibers are the ones necessary for CCK's satiety function (133). It is possible that central processing of the CCK satiety signal carried to the brain over vagal afferents may also involve the synaptic action of neuronally released CCK in the paraventricular nucleus. The evidence for this suggestion is that bilateral lesions of the paraventricular nucleus block the satiety effect of peripherally administered CCK (17), microinjection of CCK into the nucleus inhibits food intake (25), and microinjection of CCK antagonists, such as proglumide or benzotript, increases food intake (137).

One can see that clear distinctions between these two putative signals are emerging: they have different anatomical sites of origin, they are blocked by different neural lesions, and they must consequently have different mechanisms of action.

Pancreatic glucagon (29,139,142), pancreatic insulin (106), and somatostatin (84,87) are three other candidates for

TABLE 2. Characteristics of five putative satiety signals

Peptide	Inhibition of feeding	Inhibition of sham feeding	Means of blockade	Interaction with	Effect in human
Cholecystokinin	Yes	Yes	Gastric vagotomy	Pregastric food Gastric load Exogenous BBS	Yes
Bombesin	Yes	Yes	Visceral disconnection	Exogenous CCK	Yes
Pancreatic glucagon	Yes	No	Hepatic vagotomy Glucagon antibody		Yes
Somatostatin	Yes	—	Subdiaphragmatic vagotomy	?[a]	?
Pancreatic insulin	Yes	Yes	—	?	?

[a] ? indicates that the relevant data are not currently available.

satiety signals. These gastrointestinal peptides are also released by ingested food, and they show interesting similarities to, and differences from, CCK and bombesin (Table 2). The characteristics of these five peptides listed in Table 2 strongly suggest that the seeming unitary state we experience regularly after meals may actually be the complex summation of a mosaic of neuroendocrine messages, each of which responds to different features of ingested food, each with a different mediating mechanism to allow privileged entry into brain tissue, and each interacting in intricate ways with other members of the group. Further research will determine whether this suggestion has merit. Further research will no doubt reveal other candidate signals and should also tell us whether a functional excess or deficit of one of these peptide messages plays a role in the psychopathology of the eating disorders.

WEIGHT AND APPETITE CHANGES IN DEPRESSION

Many investigators have considered the possibility that disturbances in mood may be an intrinsic feature of appetite disorders such as anorexia nervosa and bulimia nervosa (see ref. 48 for a recent review). It is clear, however, that a disturbance of appetite is a cardinal feature of depressive disorders. There is a large body of data available about the epidemiology, phenomenology, associated neurobiological findings, and pharmacologic interventions that bear on the links between disturbances of mood and appetite, which may ultimately contribute to our understanding of appetite regulation per se.

Disturbances in appetite are reported by 77% to 90% of all depressed patients (12,18,97,110,156), although the diagnostic criteria for depression vary among studies. Among depressed patients with symptoms of appetite disturbance, about four out of five will have a decrease in appetite and one out of five an increase (12,52,97,110,156), a relationship that appears to be constant across cultures (97).

Why some depressed patients have an increased appetite and others a decreased appetite remains an unresolved question. Hyperphagia tends to be overrepresented in less severe depressions, in women (12,77,110), in patients with a history of mania or hypomania (12), and in younger patients (12,110). Interestingly, the NIMH Collaborative Depression Study found that increased appetite as a feature of depression tends to be associated with greater hostility, greater interpersonal sensitivity, and decreased libido but did not distinguish well among any of the Research Diagnostic Criteria subtypes of depression (12).

Hyperphagia is often associated with hypersomnia in depressed patients, an association that has been characterized as atypical. However, more recent studies have suggested that this association may be quite typical of some forms of depression, such as seasonal affective disorder (121), which appears to occur nearly always as a bipolar disorder.

On the other hand, for patients with unipolar depression, appetite disturbance per se may have singular significance as a predictor of risk for depression among their relatives. In a study of 133 probands and 810 relatives by Leckman et al. (78), the occurrence of appetite disturbance (direction unspecified) and guilt during a depressive episode in a proband confers twice the risk for depression among the relatives studied compared to the absence of these symptoms. Appetite disturbance, among all symptoms, is the single symptom that confers the greatest risk for depression among the relatives. In this study, appetite disturbance was dissociated from other "biological" signs such as sleep disturbance and loss of interest in sex, in that the occurrence of these signs carried with them no increased risk for depression among the relatives. These data led to the conclusion that "the neurochemical and neurophysiological mechanisms that regulate appetite may be closely linked to some forms of depression" (78).

Depressed patients treated with tricyclic antidepressants (TCAs) and/or monoamine oxidase inhibitors (MAOIs) frequently gain weight in the course of recovery (2,110). There is increasing evidence that the weight changes are attributable to pharmacologic effects of the drugs that are independent of their antidepressant effects. First, patients treated with TCAs report a carbohydrate craving (109), which is not observed otherwise. Second, the effects of TCAs in weight can be dissociated from their effects on appetite and the course of depression. For example, in a short-term study comparing the response to amitriptyline with the response to placebo, amitriptyline was associated with increased weight, but the weight gain did not correlate with either increased appetite or recovery from depression (77).

Third, TCAs can produce weight gain in persons who are not acutely depressed. Two separate studies show that weight gain is associated with TCA treatment in patients who are on maintenance therapy after recovery from their depression. Paykel et al. (109) studied 51 women who had been successfully treated with amitriptyline. During a 6-month follow-up period, they were randomized to amitriptyline (100–150 mg/day), placebo, or no drug. The patients treated with amitriptyline had significant weight gain, whereas patients in the other two groups did not. There were no group differences in depression ratings. Carbohydrate craving was related to drug dose, but weight gain was not. In a similar study by Berken et al. (3), 40 depressed outpatients were treated for 6 months with imipramine, nortriptyline, or amitriptyline. There was an approximately linear increase in weight over the 6-month period, i.e., including the period after recovery from depression. In this study the weight gain was dose related.

Tricyclics and MAOIs may, therefore, have selective effects on appetite and weight that are not related to their antidepressant effects. Additional support for this view comes from the observation that two second-generation antidepressant drugs, bupropion and zimelidine, have not been found to produce weight gain during recovery from depression in either short-term or long-term use (1,16,40). In fact, zimelidine treatment may be associated with weight loss (1).

The pharmacologic actions that account for these appetitive and weight changes are uncertain. The antidepressants that produce hyperphagia [the TCAs, MAOIs, and, among the newer agents, mianserin (50)] are also those that increase available presynaptic or synaptic norepinephrine. It is possible that they act on norepinephrine-sensitive pathways related to the regulation of food intake. This view can be supported by data from animal studies. Leibowitz et al. (79) have shown that injection of TCAs into the hypothalamic paraventricular nucleus elicits eating in sated rats. This effect can be blocked either by antagonizing postsynaptic α-adrenergic receptors or by inhibiting local norepinephrine synthesis. These observations would also be consistent with the finding in humans that weight gain is not associated with treatment with zimelidine (a serotonin uptake inhibitor) or bupropion (which probably down-regulates postsynaptic norepinephrine α-receptors).

Against the body of evidence connecting TCA and MAOI use with weight gain, a study by Harris et al. (51) shows that these antidepressants can also be associated with weight loss as well as weight gain. In this short-term study using a variety of TCAs and MAOIs, weight and appetite changes were frequent findings, but the direction of the changes was dependent on the starting weight. Thus, patients had increased appetite and weight gain if they had lost weight initially in the course of their depression but had a decrease in appetite and weight loss if they had gained weight prior to treatment. These findings were independent of the drug used for treatment.

The effects of lithium on weight gain are well known (70,143) but not well understood. Weight gain averaging 10 kg during lithium prophylaxis (i.e., during euthymia) occurs in as many of two-thirds of patients (143). Here, weight gain tends to occur in persons who are overweight at the start of treatment (rather than underweight) and is more often associated with increased thirst rather than with increased appetite (143). This observation raises the possibility that the weight gain is attributable to excess ingestion of high-caloric liquids.

Other investigators have shown that the lithium-induced weight gain may result from its effects on intermediary metabolism. There is both an "insulin-like" effect of lithium, i.e., an increase in glucose tolerance (141), as well as an increase in serum insulin in some patients (96), although the serum insulin level does not correlate well with weight or weight gain.

Lithium may affect lipid metabolism by promoting the use of glucose and inhibiting the use of glycerides in the synthesis of triglycerides (76).

Overall, these studies show that disturbances of appetite and weight in affective disorders are common but variable in character and that by and large the variability cannot yet be explained.

Drugs used to treat disorders of mood regulation can also affect appetite and/or weight but apparently do so in ways that are unrelated, or only indirectly related, to their effects on mood.

HYPOTHALAMIC FUNCTION

Satiety and Taste in Eating Disorders

Eating behavior and weight changes in anorexia nervosa and the bulimia syndrome provide a good suspicion for differences in the detection of satiety. All of these patients wish to lose weight; however, the outcome of their dieting endeavors varies considerably. There are anorexia nervosa patients who maintain their underweight condition exclusively by restricting food intake. Other anorexia nervosa patients do not have this control and alternate severe food restriction with binge eating. Bulimia syndrome patients may have weight fluctuations that are large but are within 10% of normal weight range. In these patients, food restriction alternates with binge eating, or constant binge eating is present with purging behaviors. For some reason these patients are not successful in reaching and maintaining an underweight condition. It is reasonable to hypothesize that physiological changes occur with the dieting endeavors and influence hunger and satiety through a variety of mechanisms resulting in a variety of disturbed eating behavior patterns.

Serotonin enhances satiety and norepinephrine reduces satiety in the paraventricular and medial hypothalamic regions (56). During food deprivation there is a decrease of α-adrenergic receptor binding in the paraventricular nucleus (PVN). This could mean an increase in release of PVN norepinephrine (NE), resulting in receptor down-regulation and an inhibition of satiety. Increased α-adrenergic receptor binding is present in the lateral hypothalamus during food deprivation. This could mean a suppression of NE release here and a receptor proliferation or up-regulation to facilitate increased hunger (63). Impairment in the regulation of receptor sites could account for differences in satiety among normal-weight bulimics, underweight anorectics, and underweight anorectics with bulimia. Hypothalamic centers that mediate feeding and satiety also mediate reward and aversion. β-Endorphin, morphine, and long-acting enkephalin analogs all induce feeding when injected into the PVN (55). Dopaminergic systems are necessary for self-administrative behaviors and could be a major link in the role of food as a reinforcer. Dopamine blockers, such as pimozide, can decrease intravenous self-injection, self-stimulation, or feeding (36). Bulimia could be considered a self-administrative or stimulation behavior. Many bulimics have an urge to binge, alleviate tension or anxiety by binging, and are unable to stop their binging behavior.

One study using a test meal paradigm to examine differences in detection of hunger and satiety in patients with anorexia nervosa and the bulimia syndrome found both quantitative and qualitative differences in the eating disorder patients compared with control subjects. Over the course of a meal prior to treatment, anorectic restrictors showed a greater change compared with anorectic bulimics and in both hunger ratings and fullness ratings. After reaching a normal weight, anorectic restrictors showed much less change in these ratings. At a normal weight status, both groups of patients and controls took in the same amount of liquid meal; however, the anorectic restrictors had significantly less change in their fullness ratings over the course of the meal compared to the anorectic bulimics and controls. After treatment, the anorectic restrictors behaved like restrained eaters in that they ended a meal when they were still hungry and not satiated (108).

There was also a qualitative change in the hunger and satiety ratings over treatment and between groups. In the control subjects and in the emaciated anorectic restrictors, the hunger and satiety curves were inversely proportioned;

however, in the anorectic bulimics there was a rapid rebound of hunger. After weight restoration, the anorectic restrictors showed a marked disturbance in hunger and fullness curves. This was an unexpected finding. Their curves were no longer reciprocal as in normal controls, but at some points these patients could not distinguish between fullness and hunger, a phenomenon noted consistently in the anorectic bulimic patients (108). The hunger–fullness curves showed distinct differences between the anorectic patients and controls, indicating a marked disturbance in the way anorectic patients experience hunger and satiety. The continued development of a valid test meal paradigm would allow the specific testing of various neurotransmitter agonists and antagonists relevant to satiety and hunger mechanisms on the detection of satiety in anorexia nervosa and the bulimia syndrome.

The various patterns of eating behavior such as severe restriction of calorie-dense foods and/or binge eating of high-fat and high-sugar foods lead to the suspicion that there may be differences in taste preferences in the eating disorder patients. The hypothalamus may be involved in conditioning mechanisms of taste. Lateral hypothalamic cells alter their firing rate in response to the taste of a palatable food and fire with a background rate that is correlated with food deprivation (120). Lateral hypothalamic cells can fire during operant bar-press responses to obtain food and fire discriminately to food cues (104). Specific neurotransmitter systems can trigger specific appetites. For example, norepinephrine-induced feeding is preferential for carbohydrates. Morphine-treated rats tend to select fatty foods, and naloxone shifts food choice away from fats (83,94).

Two studies have examined taste preferences for sweetness and fatness in eating disorder patients. In both studies the increasing concentration of both sweetness and fatness was detected accurately by both eating disorder patient groups and normal controls with no significant differences. However, both studies show significant differences in the preferences for sucrose and lipid mixtures among all groups. The first study showed that anorexia nervosa patients had a preference for much lower lipid concentration compared with normal college students and obese adults. In this study, obese subjects had a very high preference for high-lipid-containing solution and had an optimal preference for a very low sucrose concentration (23). In a second study comparing taste preferences of anorectic restrictors, anorectic bulimics, and normal-weight bulimics, the bulimic patients gave the greatest pleasantness scores and showed an enhanced liking for intensely sweet and high-fat-containing solutions. Exclusive dieting (restrictor) anorectics consistently rated all sucrose and fat stimuli as more unpleasant than did the bulimics or anorectics with bulimia. These differences were not substantially altered by weight gain during treatment. Taste preferences to sugar and fat appear to be linked to eating patterns that define the eating disorder groups and thus may provide a psychobiological marker of a psychiatric diagnosis (49). Specific pharmacological interventions to treat bulimic behavior may well affect taste preference. Treatment outcome could well be predicted by taste preferences in the eating disorder patients.

Temperature Regulation

In 1970, Wakeling and Russell (145) proposed that a primary defective temperature regulation in anorexia nervosa was linked with the feeding disorder characteristic of the illness. They found an abnormally high rise in central body temperature to be necessary for a peripheral vasodilatation response to occur, and when it did occur it was delayed and developed abnormally slowly. In response to a standard meal, the central body temperature of the patients rose significantly, whereas in control subjects it remained constant. After refeeding, there was still evidence of the same disorder of temperature regulation, although it was not as marked as in the malnourished state. Another study (26) found peripheral blood flow to be 50 to 60% lower in anorectic patients compared with normal controls, and this marked difference was maintained after a heat load. These investigators suggested that a heat-conserving selective peripheral vasoconstriction was present in the anorectic patient.

However, a study of thermoregulatory sweating showed a lower threshold for sweating and vasodilatation in patients with anorexia nervosa. The onset of thermosweating occurred at a lower core and mean skin temperature in the patients with anorexia compared with controls (89). After ingestion of a meal, the patients had a significant increase in core temperature and a significant rise in peripheral blood flow, but the control subjects had no change in core temperature and no change in peripheral blood flow. The authors suggest that the finding of vasodilatation and sweating may be a contributory factor to the abnormally low core temperature of the anorectic patients and may explain their common complaints relating to feelings of warmth in their hands and feet after meals. These investigators showed that the peripheral vessels in anorectic patients are unusually reactive to cold. In a water immersion study, the anorectic patients preferred temperatures that were significantly higher than those of control subjects, and these abnormally high preference responses persisted after a substantial weight gain had occurred (91). Elevation in deep body temperature produced a shift in preference towards a lower stimulus temperature in the control group, but in the patients who preferred the high stimulus temperature, hyperthermia produced little change in their thermal preference. The authors proposed that an elevation in the set point temperature for thermal regulation was present in some patients with anorexia nervosa (90).

Endocrinology

A source of controversy concerning the endocrine abnormalities present in anorexia nervosa is whether these aberrations are merely reflecting a malnourished condition or whether they reflect a primary hypothalamic impairment. Of the many endocrine investigations conducted on anorexia nervosa patients, the majority indicate endocrine abnormalities to be directly related to the malnourished condition. However, there is impressive indirect evidence that the nutritional state cannot explain the extent of endocrine aberrations. This evidence suggests an additional primary hypothalamic impairment.

Hypothalamic–Pituitary–Ovarian Axis

Amenorrhea occurs in many patients with anorexia nervosa before the weight loss has occurred (18). After treatment, the return of normal menstrual cycles lags behind the return to a normal body weight (127). Resumption of menses in treated normal-weight anorectic patients is associated with marked psychological improvement (24). Early investigations showed that urinary excretion of estrogen was diminished in emaciated anorectics (95). Both urinary excretion and plasma levels of gonadotropins are decreased in anorexia nervosa (103).

Another study showed only 22% of the variance in LH levels to be accounted for by the degree of weight loss or percentage below ideal body weight (5). Weiner (149) points out that if 78% of the variance in LH levels must be accounted for by factors other than weight loss, then there can be no simple relationship among weight loss, LH levels, and amenorrhea. In this excellent article, Weiner also pointed out that the amenorrheic runners in a study (125) had increased LH levels compared to exercising women who retained their menses. Weiner suggests that evidence against a direct relationship between weight and gonadotropin levels is that women who lose weight but do not develop anorexia nervosa and have secondary amenorrhea can have normal LH levels. Age-inappropriate gonadotropin secretion patterns are present in some patients who have full recovery of body weight to a normal range but still have the persistence of symptoms of anorexia nervosa or bulimia (64).

Further evidence indicating that the amenorrhea in anorexia is not simply related to weight status is found in the feedback studies (146). The positive feedback release of LH to estrogen stimulus was absent in nine of 12 weight-restored patients, indicating that the hypothalamus was not able to respond normally to the estrogen. A similar phenomenon was seen when chlomiphene was tested in weight-restored anorectics. The second LH peak after chlomiphene administration was not present. This suggests a hypothalamic defect that is not related to the patient's nutritional status. Persistent exposure of anorectic women to gonadotropin-releasing hormone (GnRH) produces the same changes in the pituitary FSH and LH response that occur with restoration of weight (103). This is further indication of a hypothalamic impairment. Although a recent study (116) has shown that normal women, when starved to 10% below normal body weight, can assume prepubertal LH patterns, this does not mean that the age-inappropriate LH secretion pattern seen in anorexia is caused solely by weight loss. The studies discussed above give ample evidence that many factors influence the secretion of LH, and it is certainly plausible that weight loss is not the sole factor initiating amenorrhea in anorexia nervosa.

Maintenance of some of the behavioral signs and symptoms of anorexia may be mediated via catechol estrogens, which are disproportionally increased in emaciated anorectic women. There is a shift of estradiol metabolism from 16α hydroxylation to 2 hydroxylation (159). Catechol estrogens have the potential of interacting with both catecholamine-mediated and estrogen-mediated systems in the central nervous system.

Hypothalamic–Pituitary–Thyroid Axis

The changes in thyroid function such as low serum triiodothyronine (T_3) and a normal thyrotropin (TSH) reserve are present in emaciated states and are not peculiar to anorexia nervosa (13,99,101,144). The TSH responses to TRH in anorexia nervosa patients tend to be delayed in about 70% of the cases studied (11,38,144). In most of these studies there was an abnormal growth hormone response to TRH. Likewise, most bulimic patients show an abnormal growth hormone response to TRH. In one of these studies bulimia syndrome patients responded normally to TRH with a prompt rise in TSH serum level (98), and in another study eight of 10 bulimic patients showed a blunted TSH response (43). In the anorectic patients, the thyroid metabolism appears to reflect the metabolic state associated with the emaciation; however, in the bulimic patients there are too few studies with too few numbers and contradictory results so that no interpretation is possible.

Hypothalamic–Pituitary–Adrenocortical Axis

The reduced metabolic rate of cortisol and the incomplete suppression of ACTH and cortisol levels by dexamethasone in malnourished anorectic patients are also seen in protein–calorie malnutrition (147,148). A recent study has shown the increased adrenocortical activity to be caused by increased secretion of corticotropin-releasing factor (CRF) from the hypothalamus (69) and found elevated cerebrospinal fluid levels of CRF in underweight patients with anorexia nervosa. Both the level of CSF CRF and pituitary-adrenal function return to normal with weight recovery.

Dexamethasone nonsuppression was present in about one-half to two-thirds of normal-weight bulimia syndrome patients tested in two studies (59,98). Nonsuppression was not associated with the degree of depression, body weight, or severity of abnormal eating-related behaviors. More complete and extensive cortisol secretion studies are needed in bulimia syndrome patients.

Growth Hormone

Growth hormone (GH) is elevated in basal measurements in about one-third of malnourished anorectic patients (28). Although this increase in serum growth hormone is also found in protein–calorie malnutrition (122), the mechanism may be different for the increase in anorexia nervosa. Severe protein deprivation is necessary and is associated with a drop in serum alanine and albumin (115) when serum growth hormone is elevated in protein–calorie malnutrition. Serum alanine and albumin levels are normal in anorexia nervosa (44). In pharmacological perturbation studies, a decreased response of GH to L-dopa and apomorphine has been observed even after weight recovery (47). This suggests that there may be a specific abnormality in dopaminergic regulation of growth hormone secretion in anorexia nervosa. The adenohypophysis of an anorexia nervosa patient who was emaciated at the time of death was examined with a battery of differential stains and immunocytochemically (45). The ACTH, GH, TSH, and prolactin cells stained with the same intensity as those in normal control pituitaries. The gonadotrophs stained for LH with immunostaining much more faintly in the anorectic pituitaries than in normal glands. These findings reflect a selective pituitary deficiency in the emaciated state of anorexia nervosa.

NEUROTRANSMITTER STUDIES

The first studies of neurotransmitters in anorexia nervosa were those measuring urinary methylhydroxyphenoglycol (MHPG), which was decreased in all studies in emaciated anorectics and increased with weight recovery (42,46). Studies of neurotransmitter metabolites in the CSF are difficult to interpret. In one study opioid activity was increased in the emaciated state and returned to normal with weight recovery (66), and in another study β-endorphin immunoreactivity was normal in underweight anorectics (31). GABA CSF levels were normal in emaciated anorectics, and CSF HVA, 5-HIAA, and tyrosine levels were decreased in the emaciated anorectic state and returned to normal with weight recovery in two studies (32,67). Another study showed a reversal of the normal CSF/plasma ratio of arginine vasopressin in emaciated anorectics (38). This ratio corrected with weight gain. A decreased plasma NE and increased platelet α_2-adrenergic receptor density in malnourished anorectics suggest an inverse relationship between NE output and α_2-adrenergic receptor activity (92). The unusual finding of lower plasma and CSF levels of NE and MHPG in patients with long-term weight maintenance raises the question of whether anorectics have a trait-related disturbance of NE metabolism (69). These observations could be related to continued peculiar eating habits and continued anorectic symptoms such as anxiety over weight gain and overactivity. Since CRF is disinhibited by low CNS NE, one would expect to find elevated serum cortisol levels in these patients or dexamethasone resistance. Unfortunately, these measures were not reported in the above study.

After probenecid administration, weight-recovered anorectic restricting patients had a higher concentration of 5-HIAA than weight-recovered bulimic patients (66). These alterations in serotonin metabolism may be a trait-related phenomenon or may be a reflection of the different eating behavior patterns in the two groups of anorectic patients.

Impaired growth hormone response to L-dopa (47) and impaired prolactin response to chlorpromazine (107) with decreased CSF HVA suggest a disturbance in dopamine regulation, possibly at the postsynaptic receptor site. It needs to be determined whether the changes found in norepinephrine, dopamine, and serotonin neurotransmitter functions merely reflect nutritional disturbances or represent a biological trait identifying the eating disorder patients.

GENETIC MECHANISMS IN THE EATING DISORDERS

A comparison of monozygotic versus dizygotic twins for concordance rate of anorexia nervosa was done in 30 female twin pairs in a study (58). Nine of 16 monozygotic and one of 14 dizygotic pairs were concordant for anorexia nervosa. These numbers certainly suggest a genetic component to this disorder. Because of the relatively low prevalence rate of this disorder, it has not been possible to do comparisons of twins reared together with those reared apart for concordance rates. The study of genetic markers and examination of the adopted-away offspring of an anorectic individual have not been used to study genetic factors in anorexia nervosa.

REFERENCES

1. Aberg, A., and Holmberg, G. (1979): *Acta Psychiatr. Scand.*, 59: 45–58.
2. Arenillas, L. (1964): *Lancet*, 1:432–433.
3. Berken, G. H., Weinstein, D. O., and Stern, W. (1984): *J. Affect. Disorders*, 7:133–138.
4. Bourbonais, K., Jerome, C., Simansky, K. J., and Smith, G. P. (1983): *Soc. Neurosci. Abstr.*, 9:193.
5. Brown, G. M. (1977): In: *Anorexia Nervosa*, edited by R. A. Vigersky, pp. 123–125. Raven Press, New York.
6. Busch, W. (1858): *Arch. Patol. Anat. Physiol. Klin. Med.*, 14: 140–186.
7. Campbell, R. G., and Smith, G. P. (1983): *Soc. Neurosci. Abstr.*, 9:902.
8. Campfield, L. A., Brandon, P., and Smith, F. J. (1985): *Brain Res. Bull.*, 14:605–616.
9. Cannon, W. B., and Washburn, A. L. (1912): *Am. J. Physiol.*, 29:441–454.
10. Carlson, A. J. (1913): *Am. J. Physiol.*, 31:175–192.
11. Casper, R. C., and Frohman, L. A. (1982): *Psychoneuroendocrine*, 7:59–68.
12. Casper, R. C., Redmond, D. E., Katz, M. M., Schaffer, C. B., Davis, J. M., et al. (1985): *Arch. Gen. Psychiatry*, 42:1098–1104.
13. Chopra, I. A. (1975): *J. Clin. Endocrinol. Metab.*, 40:221–227.
14. Christensen, O. (1931): *Acta Med. Scand.* [*Suppl.*], 37:170.
15. Clark, J. T., Kalra, P. S., Crowley, W. R., and Kalra, S. P. (1986): *Endocrinology*, 115:427–429.
16. Coppen, A., Rama Rao, V. A., Swode, C., and Wood, R. (1979): *Psychopharmacology*, 63:199–202.
17. Crawley, J. N., and Kiss, J. Z. (1985): *Ann. N.Y. Acad. Sci.*, 448: 586–588.
18. Dally, P. (1969): *Anorexia Nervosa*. Heinemann, London.
19. Davis, J. D. (1973): *Physiol. Behav.*, 11:39–45.
20. Davis, J. D., and Campbell, C. S. (1973): *J. Comp. Physiol. Psychol.*, 83:379–387.
21. Deutsch, J. A., Young, W. G., and Kalogeris, T. J. (1978): *Science*, 201:165–167.
22. Dorfman, D. B., Schwartz, D., and Hoebel, B. G. (1986): *Brain Behav. Rev.*, 82:200–221.
23. Drewnowski, A., Greenwood, M. R. C., Halmi, K. A., Gibbs, J., and Duberstein, P. (1984): *Fed. Proc.*, 43:475.
24. Falk, J. R., and Halmi, K. A. (1982): *J. Biol. Psychol.*, 17:799–806.
25. Faris, P. L., and Olney, J. W. (1985): *Soc. Neurosci. Abstr.*, 11: 39.
26. Freyschuss, U. (1978): 67:225–228.
27. Gander, D. R. (1965): *Lancet*, 1:107–109.

28. Garfinkel, P., Brown, G. M., Stanser, H. C., and Moldofsky, H. (1975): *Arch. Gen. Psychiatry,* 32:739–744.
29. Geary, N., and Smith, G. P. (1982): *Physiol. Behav.,* 28:313–322.
30. Geary, N., and Smith, G. P. (1985): *Pharmacol. Biochem. Behav.,* 22:787–790.
31. Gerner, R. H., and Sharp, B. (1982): *Brain Res.,* 237:244–247.
32. Gerner, R. H., Cohen, D. J., Fairbanks, L., Anderson, G. M., Young, J. G., et al. (1984): *Am. J. Psychiatry,* 141:1441–1444.
33. Gibbs, J., Fauser, D. J., Rowe, E. A., Rolls, B. J., Rolls, E. T., et al. (1979): *Nature,* 282:208–210.
34. Gibbs, J., Madison, S. P., and Rolls, E. T. (1981): *J. Comp. Physiol. Psychol.,* 95:1003–1015.
35. Gibbs, J., and Smith, G. P. (1984): In: *Frontiers in Neuroendocrinology,* edited by L. Martini, and W. F. Ganong, pp. 223–245. Raven Press, New York.
36. Glimcher, P., and Margolin, D. (1986): *Brain Res.,* 266:348–352.
37. Gold, M. S. (1981): *Int. J. Psychiatry Med.,* 10:51–57.
38. Gold, P. W., Kaye, W., Robertson, G. L., and Ebert, M. (1983): *N. Engl. J. Med.,* 308:1117–1123.
39. Goldman, C. K., Marino, L., and Leibowitz, S. F. (1985): *Eur. J. Pharmacol.,* 53:69–81.
40. Gottfries, C. G. (1981): *Acta Psychiatr. Scand. [Suppl.],* 210(63): 353–356.
41. Grant, D. P., and Milgram, N. W. (1973): *Can. J. Psychol.,* 27: 305–316.
42. Gross, H. A., Lake, C. R., Ebert, M. H., Ziegler, M. G., and Kopin, I. J. (1979): *J. Clin. Endocrinol. Metab.,* 49:805–809.
43. Gwirtsman, H. E. (1983): *Am. J. Psychiatry,* 140:559–563.
44. Halmi, K. A. and Stegink, L. D. (1987): *J. Parental and Enteral Nutr. (in press).*
45. Halmi, K. A. (1976): In: *Hormones, Behavior and Psychopathology,* edited by E. J. Sachar, pp. 285–289. Raven Press, New York.
46. Halmi, K. A., Dekirmenjian, H., Davis, J. M., Casper, R., and Goldberg, S. (1978): *Arch. Gen. Psychiatry,* 35:458–460.
47. Halmi, K. A., and Sherman, B. S. (1979): In: *Biological Psychiatry Today,* edited by J. Obiols and E. Ballus, pp. 609–614. Elsevier/North-Holland Biomedical Press, Amsterdam.
48. Halmi, K. A. (1985): *Int. J. Eat. Disorders,* 4(4a):663–676.
49. Halmi, K. A., Drewnowski, A., Pierce, B., Gibbs, J., and Smith, G. P. (1985): *APA Syllabus and Proceedings,* p. 81. American Psychiatric Association, Washington.
50. Harris, B., and Harper, M. (1980): *Lancet,* 1:493.
51. Harris, B., Young, J., and Hughes, B. (1984): *Br. J. Psychiatry,* 145:645–648.
52. Harris, B., Young, J., and Hughes, B. (1984): *J. Affect. Disorders,* 6:331–339.
53. Heffner, T. G., Hartman, J. A., and Seiden, L. S. (1986): *Science,* 208:1168–1170.
54. Heffner, T. G., Vosmer, G., and Seiden, L. S. (1984): *Pharmacol. Biochem. Behav.,* 20:947–949.
55. Hoebel, B. (1979): *Fed. Proc.,* 38:2454–2461.
56. Hoebel, B. (1984): In: *Eating and Its Disorders,* edited by E. Stellar and A. Stunkard, pp. 15–38. Raven Press, New York.
57. Hoebel, B. G. (1985): *Brain Res. Bull.,* 14:525–528.
58. Holland, A. J., Hall, A., Murray, R., Russell, G. F. M., and Crisp, A. H. (1984): *Br. J. Psychiatry,* 145:414–419.
59. Hudson, J. I., Pope, H. G., Jonas, J. M., Laffer, P. S., Hudson, M. S., et al. (1983): *Psychiatr. Res.,* 8:111–117.
60. Inglefinger, F. J. (1944): *N. Engl. J. Med.,* 231:321–327.
61. James, W. T. (1963): *Psychol. Rep.,* 12:31–39.
62. Janowitz, H. D., and Grossman, M. I. (1949): *Am. J. Physiol.,* 159:143–148.
63. Jhanwar-Uniyal, M., Fleischer, F., and Levine, B. E. (1982): *Abstr. Soc. Neurosci.,* 8:711.
64. Katz, J. L. (1978): *Psychosom. Med.,* 40:549–567.
65. Kaye, W. H., Pickar, D., Naber, D., and Ebert, M. H. (1982): *Am. J. Psychiatry,* 139:643–645.
66. Kaye, W. H., Ebert, M. H., Gwirtsman, H. E., and Weiss, S. R. (1984): *Am. J. Psychiatry,* 141:1598–1601.
67. Kaye, W., Ebert, M. H., Raliegh, M., and Lake, R. (1984): *Arch. Gen. Psychiatry,* 41:350–355.
68. Kaye, W., Gwirtsman, H., George, D. T., Ebert, M., Jimerson, D., et al. (1984): In: *ANCP,* Abstract 105.
69. Kaye, W. H., Jimerson, D. C., Lake, C. R., and Ebert, M. H. (1985): *Psychiatr. Res.,* 14:333–342.
70. Kerry, R. F., Leibling, L. I., and Owen, G. (1970): *Acta Psychiatr. Scand.,* 46:238–243.
71. Kissileff, H. R., Pi-Sunyer, F. X., Thornton, J., and Smith, G. P. (1981): *Am. J. Clin. Nutr.,* 34:154–160.
72. Koopmans, H. S. (1981): In: *The Body Weight Regulatory System: Normal and Disturbed Mechanisms,* edited by L. A. Cioffi, W. P. T. James, and T. B. van Itallie. Raven Press, New York.
73. Kraeuchi, K., Wiry-Justice, A., Suetterlin-Willener, R., and Ferr, H. (1985): *IRCS Med. Sci.,* 13:561.
74. Kraly, F. S., and Smith, G. P. (1978): *Physiol. Behav.,* 21:405–408.
75. Kraly, F. S., and Gibbs, J. (1980): *Physiol. Behav.,* 24:1007–1010.
76. Krulik, R., Janko, L., and Cerny, M. (1971): *Acta Univ. Carol.,* 12:533–540.
77. Kupfer, D. J., Coble, P. A., and Rubinstein, D. (1979): *Psychosom. Med.,* 41(7):535–544.
78. Leckman, J. F., Caruso, K. A., Prusoff, B. A., Weissman, M. M., Merikangas, K. R., et al. (1984): *Arch. Gen. Psychiatry,* 41:839–844.
79. Leibowitz, S. F., Arcomano, A., and Hammer, N. J. (1978): *Prog. Neuropsychopharmacol.,* 2:349–358.
80. Leibowitz, S. F. (1980): In: *The Handbook of the Hypothalamus, Vol. 3, Part A, Behavioral Studies of the Hypothalamus,* edited by P. J. Morgane and J. Panksepp, pp. 299–437. Marcel Dekker, New York.
81. Leibowitz, S. F., Roland, C. R., Hor, L., and Squillari, V. (1984): *Physiol. Behav.,* 32:857–864.
82. Levine, A. S., and Morley, J. E. (1982): *Pharmacol. Biochem. Behav.,* 16:897–902.
83. Leibowitz, S. V. (1982): *Handbook Hypothalamus,* 3:299–437.
84. Levine, A. S., and Morley, J. E. (1984): *Peptides,* 5:1025–1030.
85. Liebling, D. S., Eisner, J. D., Gibbs, J., and Smith, G. P. (1975): *Comp. Physiol. Psychol.,* 89:955–965.
86. Lorenz, D. N., Kreielsheimer, G., and Smith, G. P. (1979): *Physiol. Behav.,* 23:1065–1072.
87. Lotter, E. C., Krinsky, R., McKay, J. M., Treneer, C. M., Porte, D., Jr., et al. (1981): *J. Comp. Physiol. Psychol.,* 95:278–287.
88. Louis-Sylvestre, J., and LeMegnen, J. (1980): *Neurosci. Biobehav. Rev.,* 4:13–15.
89. Luck, P., and Wakeling, A. (1980): *Br. Med. J.,* 281:906–908.
90. Luck, P., and Wakeling, A. (1980): *Clin. Sci.,* 62:677–682.
91. Luck, P., and Wakeling, A. (1981): *Clin. Sci.,* 61:559–567.
92. Luck, P., Mikbailidis, D. P., and Dashwood, M. R. (1983): *J. Clin. Endocrinol. Metab.,* 57:911–914.
93. Martin, C. F., and Gibbs, J. (1980): *Peptides,* 1:131–134.
94. Marx-Kaufman, R., and Kamarek, R. B. (1981): *Psychopharmacology,* 74:321–324.
95. McCullagh, E. P., and Tupper, W. R. (1940): *Ann. Intern. Med.,* 14:817–838.
96. Mellerup, E. T., Gronlund Thomsen, H., Bjorum, N., and Rafaelsen, O. J. (1972): *Acta Psychiatr. Scand.,* 48:332–336.
97. Mezzich, J. E., and Raab, E. S. (1980): *Arch. Gen. Psychiatry,* 37:818–823.
98. Mitchell, J. E., and Bantele, J. P. (1983): *Biol. Psychiatry,* 18: 355–365.
99. Miyai, K. (1975): *J. Endocrinol. Metab.,* 40:334.
100. Moran, T. H., and McHugh, P. R. (1982): *Am. J. Physiol.,* 242: R491–R497.
101. Moschang, T. (1975): *J. Endocrinol. Metab.,* 40:470–473.
102. Muurahainen, N. E., Kissileff, H. R., Thornton, J., and Pi-Sunyer, F. X. (1983): *Soc. Neurosci. Abstr.,* 9:183.
103. Nillius, S. J., and Wide, L. (1979): *Uppsala J. Med. Sci.,* 80:21–35.
104. Nishino, H. (1982): In: *The Neural Basis of Feeding and Reward,* edited by B. G. Hoebel and D. Novin, pp. 355–372. Haer Institute, Brunswick, ME.
105. Nonavinakere, V. K., and Ritter, R. C. (1983): *Appetite,* 4:177–185.
106. Oetting, R. L., and VanderWeele, D. A. (1985): *Physiol. Behav.,* 34:557–562.

107. Owen, W. P., Halmi, K. A., Lasley, E., and Stokes, P. (1983): *Psychopharmacol. Bull.,* 19:578–581.
108. Owen, W. P., Halmi, K. A., Gibbs, J., and Smith, G. P. (1985): *J. Psychiatr. Res.,* 19:279–284.
109. Paykel, E. S., Mueller, P. S., and La Vergne, P. M. (1973): *Br. J. Psychiatry,* 123:501–507.
110. Paykel, E. S. (1977): *J. Psychosom. Res.,* 21:401–407.
111. Penick, S. B., Smith, G. P., Wieneke, K., Jr., and Hinkle, L. E., Jr. (1963): *Am. J. Physiol.,* 205:421–426.
112. Pfaffman, C. (1982): In: *The Physiological Mechanisms of Motivation,* edited by D. W. Pfaff, pp. 61–79. Springer-Verlag, New York.
113. Pi-Sunyer, X., Kissileff, H. R., Thornton, J., and Smith, G. P. (1982): *Physiol. Behav.,* 29:627–630.
114. Pimstone, B. L., Barbezat, G., Hanson, J. D., and Murray, P. (1968): *Am. J. Clin. Nutr.,* 20:482–491.
115. Pimstone, B. (1973): *J. Clin. Endocrinol. Metab.,* 36:779–783.
116. Pirke, K. M. (1983): *Int. J. Eat. Disorders,* 2:151–158.
117. Reidelberger, R. D., Kalogeris, T. J., Leung, P. M. B., and Mendel, V. E. (1983): *Am. J. Physiol.,* 244:R872–R881.
118. Richter, C. (1922): *Comp. Psychol. Monogr.,* 1:2.
119. Rozin, P., and Schiller, D. (1980): *Motivat. Emotion,* 4:77–101.
120. Rolls, E. T. (1982): In: *The Neural Basis of Feeding and Reward,* edited by B. G. Hoebel and D. Novin, pp. 323–339. Haer Institute, Brunswick, ME.
121. Rosenthal, N. E., Sack, D. A., Gillin, J. C., Lewy, A. J., Goodwin, F. K., et al. (1984): *Arch. Gen. Psychiatry,* 41:72–80.
122. Samuel, A. M., and Deshpande, U. R. (1972): *J. Clin. Endocrinol. Metab.,* 35:863–867.
123. Schallert, T., Pendergrass, M., and Farrar, S. B. (1982): *Appetite,* 3:81–90.
124. Schneider, L. H., Gibbs, J., and Smith, G. P. (1986): *Peptides,* 7:135–140.
125. Schwartz, B. (1981): *Am. J. Obstet. Gynecol.,* 141:662–670.
126. Sclafani, A., Aravich, P. F., and Xenakis, S. (1982): In: *The Neural Basis of Feeding and Reward,* edited by B. G. Hoebel and D. Novin, pp. 507–515. Haer Institute, Brunswick, ME.
127. Sherman, B. M., and Halmi, K. A. (1977): In: *Anorexia Nervosa,* edited by R. A. Vigersky, pp. 211–214. Raven Press, New York.
128. Silverstone, J. T., and Besser, M. (1971): *Postgrad. Med. J.,* 47:427–429.
129. Simansky, K. J., Bourbonais, K. A., and Smith, G. P. (1985): *Pharmacol. Biochem. Behav.,* 23:253–258.
130. Smith, G. P., Gibbs, J., Strohmayer, A. J., and Stokes, P. E. (1972): *Am. J. Physiol.,* 222:77–81.
131. Smith, G. P., Jerome, C., Cushin, B. J., Eterno, R., and Simansky, K. J. (1981): *Science,* 213:1036–1037.
132. Smith, G. P. (1984): In: *Behavioral Neuroendocrinology,* edited by C. Nemeroff and A. Dunn, pp. 463–495. Spectrum Publications, New York.
133. Smith, G. P., Jerome, C., and Norgren, R. (1985): *Am. J. Physiol.,* 249:R638–R641.
134. Smith, S. R., Bledsoe, T., and Chetri, M. K. (1975): *J. Clin. Endocrinol. Metab.,* 40:43–52.
135. Stacher, G., Steinringer, H., Schmierer, G., Schneider, C., and Winklehner, S. (1982): *Peptides,* 3:133–136.
136. Stanley, B. G., Chin, A. S., and Leibowitz, S. F. (1985): *Brain Res. Bull.,* 14:521–525.
137. Stuckey, J., Gibbs, J., and Smith, G. P. (1987): *Peptides (in press).*
138. Stunkard, A. J., and Fox S. (1971): *Psychosom. Med.,* 33:123–134.
139. Stunkard, A. J., Van Itallie, T. B., and Reis, B. B. (1955): *Proc. Soc. Exp. Biol. Med.,* 89:258.
140. Thompson, D. A., and Campbell, R. G. (1977): *Science,* 198:1065–1068.
141. Van der Velde, C. D., and Gordon, M. W. (1969): *Arch. Gen. Psychiatry,* 21:478–485.
142. VanderWeele, D. A., Geiselman, P. J., and Novin, D. (1979): *Physiol. Behav.,* 23:155–158.
143. Vendsborg, P. B., Bech, P., and Rafaelsen, O. J. (1976): *Acta Psychiatr. Scand.,* 53:139–147.
144. Vigersky, R. (1976): *J. Clin. Endocrinol. Metab.,* 43:893–900.
145. Wakeling, A., and Russell, G. F. M. (1970): *Psychol. Med.,* 1:30–39.
146. Wakeling, A. (1976): *Psychol. Med.,* 6:371–388.
147. Walsh, B. T., Katz, J., Levin, J., Kream, J., Fukushima, D., et al. (1978): *Psychosom. Med.,* 40:499–506.
148. Walsh, B. T., Katz, J., Levin, J., Kream, J., Fukushima, D., et al. (1981): *J. Clin. Endocrinol. Metab.,* 53:203–205.
149. Weiner, H. (1983): *Int. J. Eat. Disorders,* 2:109–116.
150. Weingarten, H. P. (1983): *Science,* 220:431–433.
151. Weingarten, H. P. (1984): *Appetite,* 5:147–158.
152. Weingarten, H. P. (1984): *Physiol. Behav.,* 32:403–408.
153. Wise, R. A., Spindler, J., deWit, H., and Gerber, G. J. (1978): *Science,* 201:262–264.

Psychopharmacology:
The Third Generation of Progress,
edited by Herbert Y. Meltzer.
Raven Press, New York © 1987.

CHAPTER 131

Behavioral Pharmacology for Eating and Drinking

John E. Morley

Over the past decade it has become clear that numerous pharmacological agents are capable of modulating ingestive behaviors in animals and in humans. Based on pharmacological studies, the regulation of feeding can be divided into a peripheral satiety system and a central feeding system. We have previously suggested that the activation of feeding is dependent on the interaction of a number of neurotransmitters within the central nervous system arranged in a cascade system similar to the complement fixation system or that responsible for blood clotting (42). This clearly represents a gross oversimplification of the complexities of appetite regulation. It is now recognized that at least two central feeding systems are present, i.e., an opioid–dopaminergic system responsible for causing the organism to choose foods that are highly palatable or have a high fat content and a second system that leads to the selection of carbohydrate-rich foods and that appears to involve the activation of neuropeptide Y (Fig. 1). Similarly, the regulation of drinking involves multiple neurotransmitter and hormonal inputs. Nutrient selection also appears to play a role in drinking behavior, as some pharmacological stimuli cause a craving for salt and water, e.g., angiotensin II, whereas others appear to produce a pure thirst, e.g., carbachol.

PEPTIDES AS MODULATORS OF FOOD INTAKE IN HUMANS

In 1924 it was demonstrated by Barbour that peripherally administered insulin stimulated feeding in undernourished diabetic, malnourished, and normal children (7). This phenomenon is well recognized by clinicians today when they are forced to put obese type II diabetics onto insulin.

In these unfortunate individuals, insulin leads to hyperphagia and further weight gain, much to the chagrin of their physicians. A conundrum yet to be fully resolved is that in baboons central administration of insulin leads to a decrease in food intake (76). It is possible that this effect of insulin is secondary to its pharmacological ability to activate insulin growth factor (IGF) receptors, as IGF has been demonstrated to be a potent anorexic agent after cerebroventricular injection in the rat (70). The only other peptide that has been shown to stimulate feeding in any species after peripheral administration is motilin. Motilin increases feeding in starved rats, possibly secondary to its salutatory effect on gastric emptying (18). The role of motilin in the disturbed gastric motility seen in anorexia nervosa is worthy of investigation.

The majority of peptides released during a meal appear to be predominantly involved in the termination of the meal. Knoll (25) has isolated and partially purified two glycoproteins, satietin I and II, from human serum that are potent anorectic agents. Many studies have demonstrated that a variety of gastrointestinal hormones will decrease food intake after administration in pharmacological doses. Whether these peptides play a physiological role in the regulation of food intake is currently the subject of much debate. However, a number of them have been demonstrated to decrease food intake over a single meal in humans. The best studied of these is cholecystokinin (CCK), which decreases food intake in doses just below those necessary to produce nausea in lean and obese subjects (58). The effect on food intake can be divorced from its inhibitory effect on gastric emptying, and it has been shown to decrease food intake in at least some human subjects who have had a vagotomy (63). These data suggest that the effects of CCK in humans are, as is the case in the dog

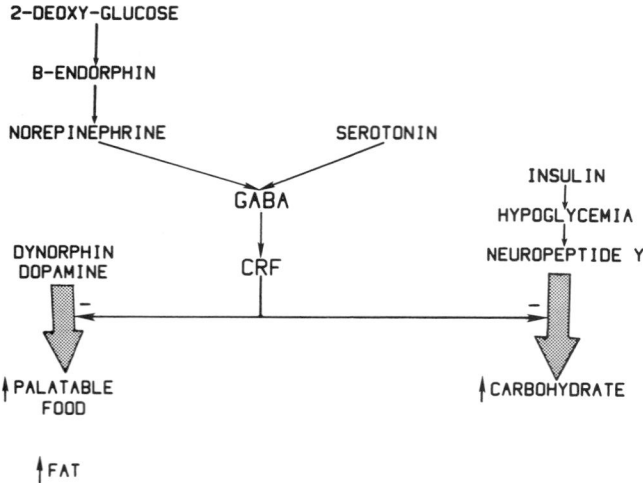

FIG. 1. Cascade system of neurotransmitters involved in central appetite regulation. GABA, γ-aminobutyric acid; GRF, corticotropin-releasing factor.

(36), independent of the vagus. Glucagon (64) and bombesin (54) also decrease food intake in humans.

Calcitonin is a potent anorectic agent in rats and is released following meals (16). It appears to produce its effect by inhibiting calcium uptake into the hypothalamus (34). Studies in humans have demonstrated that calcitonin can decrease weight in doses that do not produce nausea (50).

OPIOIDS AS MODULATORS OF FEEDING AND BODY WEIGHT

Since the original report by Holtzman (24) that the opioid antagonist naloxone decreases feeding, a vast body of literature has confirmed a role for endogenous opioids in the modulation of feeding (49). Studies in the Siberian tiger have suggested that opioids may play a central role in the recognition of which foods are safe to eat, and thus opioid blockade was shown to lead to neophobia (9). This is in keeping with the data suggesting a major role of opioids in the choice of highly palatable food (*vide infra*). Although opioid feeding systems appear to be involved in numerous species, there are some species such as the Chinese hamster and the raccoon that feed perfectly normally and yet appear to lack an opioid feeding system (8,56). Further, with advancing age, there appears to be a decrease in the effectiveness of the opioid feeding system, which may provide a partial explanation for the anorexia associated with advancing age (20).

In the rat numerous pharmacological studies have established a role for the κ opioid system in the initiation of feeding (48). Dynorphin, the endogenous κ-receptor ligand, is a potent stimulator of feeding following central administration (44), and its levels in the central nervous system fluctuate with the nutritional state of the animal (43). The major site of action of dynorphin appears to be within the paraventricular nucleus (21). Other studies have demon-

strated that there are, in fact, multiple opioid-sensitive feeding sites within the central nervous system (21,75), and pharmacological studies have suggested that more than one opioid receptor may play a role in feeding behaviors (32).

Naloxone has been demonstrated to decrease food intake in humans over a single meal in normal and obese individuals (3,14,73), in a patient with hypothalamic hyperphagia (46), and in response to 2-deoxyglucose administration (72). Of particular interest is the fact that naloxone decreases food intake without altering the individual's perception of hunger (72,73). Similarly, the κ agonist butorphanol tartrate increases food intake in normal humans without producing any effect on appetite as measured by a satiety analog scale (53). Nalmefene, a long-acting opioid antagonist, has been shown to decrease food intake for up to 24 hr (10).

Despite these encouraging short-term results, studies with the long-acting oral preparation naltrexone have turned out to be disappointing. Atkinson (4) showed only a small effect of naltrexone on enhancing weight loss in obese women. Mitchell et al. (41) could demonstrate no advantage of naltrexone over placebo using high doses of naltrexone. This trial was discontinued prematurely because of an unacceptable rate of abnormal liver function tests. As animal studies have demonstrated an increased sensitivity of diabetics to naloxone (35), we also studied the effect of naltrexone on weight loss in obese patients with type II diabetes mellitus. Again the results were negative.

A careful reevaluation of the animal and human literature makes these results somewhat less surprising. Opiate addiction is clearly associated with weight loss in animals and in humans. When we studied patients on methadone maintenance, we found that the majority of them were below 100% of ideal body weight despite marked hyperphagia (69). Animal studies suggest that morphine administration decreases weight gain, most probably by a direct effect on lipolysis (38,57), and passive immunization with β-endorphin leads to weight gain (40). In keeping with this hypothesis is the recent report that nalorphine, a mixed opiate agonist/antagonist, is a potent long-term anorectic agent in obese subjects (6).

In summary, it appears that opioids, and in particular the κ agonist dynorphin, are important but not essential neurotransmitters involved in the initiation of feeding. However, in the long term, it appears that the peripheral effects of opiates on lipolysis play a more crucial role in the regulation of body weight than does the central effect on feeding.

NEUROPEPTIDE Y: A POTENT OREXIGENIC SUBSTANCE

Recent studies have shown that central administration of neuropeptide Y (NPY) produces a potent increase in food intake (13,66). In our studies we showed that the effect of NPY is independent of norepinephrine's effect on food intake (37). In view of the fact that many NPY fibers terminate in the paraventricular nucleus (23), it is not surprising that direct injections into this nucleus more potently increase feeding than do intraventricular injections (51,66).

We also investigated the effects of repeated injections of the closely related peptide, peptide YY, and found that tolerance to its effects did not develop (51). The animals showed marked weight gain, though much of this was caused by gut fill. Similar findings have been reported by Stanley et al. (67) using chronic injections of NPY. Of particular interest is the ability of NPY to continue to increase feeding in the face of marked stomach distention. This shows that central factors can override satiety signals from the gut.

In view of the potent orexigenic effect of NPY, it has been suggested that it may play a role in the pathogenesis of bulimia and that a suitable trivial name for NPY would be bulimin.

NEUROPHARMACOLOGY OF NUTRIENT SELECTION

There is now increasing evidence that different neurotransmitters produce their increase in food intake by preferentially increasing a specific dietary macronutrient. Thus, NPY produces a highly specific increase in carbohydrate intake (51). This is more selective than the effect of norepinephrine, which predominantly increases carbohydrate but also increases fat (32; *unpublished observations*). Serotonin and its agonists have been reported specifically to decrease carbohydrate intake (11). However, a recent study by Blundell and Hill (12) suggested that while sparing protein they reduce fat as well as carbohydrate intake.

Studies by Marks-Kaufman and her colleagues have shown that opioid agonists and antagonists specifically modulate fat intake. We have recently confirmed this preference of the opioid system to modulate fatty foods (22), and in our studies in humans using the opioid antagonist nalmafene, we again saw a specific decrease in fat intake (10). However, other studies (2) have suggested that the primary effect of the opioid system is to modulate the intake of highly palatable foods. This formulation would be compatible with the preferential effect on fatty foods, which are usually perceived as being highly palatable.

STRESS-INDUCED EATING

Feeding responses to stress in humans are variable, with 46% increasing eating when stressed and 48% decreasing food intake (77). Studies in rats using the tail-pinch model of stress-induced eating have provided clear evidence that this form of feeding involves activation of the endogenous opioid system (39,45). Other studies have suggested that this form of eating also involves activation of the dopaminergic system (48). Activation of the dopaminergic system appears to result predominantly in chewing, whereas the opioid system appears to be related to ingestive behavior.

Evidence is accumulating to suggest that stress-induced undereating is mediated by release of corticotropin-releasing factor (CRF); CRF is a potent inhibitor of feeding after central administration (47). The anorectic effect of CRF is produced by local injection into the paraventricular nucleus. Corticotropin-releasing factor inhibits norepinephrine-in-duced feeding, and it appears that CRF may be the substance that norepinephrine inhibits to produce its feeding effect. In view of the known activation of the hypothalamic–pituitary–adrenal axis in patients with anorexia nervosa, it has been suggested that CRF may play a role in the pathophysiology of anorexia nervosa.

THE NEUROPHARMACOLOGY OF DRINKING

Since the original evidence in the early 1900s by Andre Meyer and Hugo Wettendorf that alterations in body water correlated directly with thirst, it has become clear that there are two major pathways capable of stimulating thirst (60). Thus, combining of stimuli to both osmotic and volumic thirst results in drinking equivalent to the sum of water intakes provoked by either stimulus by itself.

Angiotensin II stimulates water and salt intake, most probably by a direct effect on the subfornical organ (17,60). Further, all stimuli that produce extracellular hypovolemia also activate the renin–angiotensin system. Angiotensin II does not appear to be the only effector of thirst secondary to hypovolemia, as anephric animals, who do not have a renin–angiotensin system, still drink following hypotension (60), and a combination of angiotensin II and hypovolemia acts synergistically to produce drinking (5). In view of the ease with which angiotensin-induced drinking is blocked by multiple manipulations, it seems to represent a relatively minor physiological stimulus of drinking (60).

A number of monoamines have been shown to modulate drinking (Table 1). Thus, β-adrenergic agonists such as isoproterenol increase drinking, whereas α-adrenergic agonists, e.g., metaraminol and clonidine, decrease drinking (29,30). The effect of isoproterenol on drinking is blocked by the angiotensin II antagonist saralasin, suggesting that it produces drinking by activation of the renin–angiotensin system (59). Norepinephrine within the paraventricular nucleus decreases feeding at doses lower than those required to increase feeding (30). Norepinephrine is a potent antidipsogenic, decreasing drinking produced by carbachol, angiotensin II, hypertonic saline, and polyethyleneglycol (31,60). Depletion of central catecholamines with 6-hydroxydopamine produces a reduction in the dipsogenic response to angiotensin, and intrahypothalamic phentolamine blocks the drinking response to angiotensin II. Serontonin increases drinking after both peripheral injection and direct injection into the paraventricular nucleus (31).

TABLE 1. *Pharmacological agents that modulate drinking*

Increase drinking	Decrease drinking
Hypertonic saline	α-Adrenergic agonists, e.g.,
Angiotensin II	metaraminol, clonidine,
β-Adrenergic agonists, e.g.,	norepinephrine
isoproterenol	β-Adrenergic antagonists,
Carbachol	e.g., propranolol
Serotonin	Dopamine antagonists
Histamine	Antihistamines
Neurotensin	Substance P
Prostaglandins	Atrionatriuretic factor
	Prostaglandins

Carbachol increases drinking after water deprivation (31). This effect is specific for water and does not cause an increase in saline intake. Histamine is another potent dipsogenic whose effectiveness is decreased 50% by β blockers (19,31). Dopamine antagonists in low doses are potent inhibitors of drinking, though the specificity of this effect is in some doubt (31,60).

Other neurotransmitters have also been demonstrated to alter water intake. These include neuropeptide Y (13,37,66), neurotensin (65), and the prostaglandins (33), which all increase drinking. The role of the opioids in modulating fluid intake is of interest in that there is evidence for opioids both stimulating and inhibiting water intake. Numerous studies have shown that the opioid antagonist naloxone decreases drinking (61) and that enkephalins and endorphins attenuate both angiotensin-II- and hypertonic saline-induced drinking through naloxone-sensitive mechanisms (68). However, central administration of a μ-selective agent increases water intake at low doses, whereas there is some evidence that dynorphin, despite producing a diuresis and increasing feeding, both factors that should increase drinking, does, in fact, inhibit fluid intake (B. A. Gosnell et al., *unpublished observations*). Thus, it appears that μ-receptor agonists are dipsogenic, whereas κ agonists are antidipsogenic. There is some evidence favoring a more specific role for opioids in the regulation of salt appetite than in drinking per se (35). Substance P stimulates water intake in pigeons but inhibits it in rats (74). Since substance P inhibits the renin–angiotensin system, its effect on drinking may be secondary to this effect. Recently atrionatriuretic factor, which produces a potent salt diuresis, has been shown to be antidipsogenic (55).

The original experiments by Richter in 1936 demonstrated that adrenalectomy produced a specific salt appetite. Subsequent studies have clearly delineated that the renin–angiotensin–aldosterone system is the major determinant of salt appetite (17). Fluharty and Epstein (15) have provided evidence that mineralocorticoids and angiotensin act synergistically to produce the appetite for the taste of salt. Other hormonal systems also appear to play a role in salt

appetite, as both hypothyroidism and estrogen administration lead to salt craving (17).

As already pointed out, ingested food represents a stimulus for drinking. Kraly (27) has strongly argued that one of the neurotransmitter mediators of drinking is histamine. Histamine is released from endocrine-like nonmast cells of the gastric mucosa during a meal, and histamine antagonists decrease the drinking associated with starvation-induced feeding (26). The vagus appears to play an important role as the neuronal mediator of the drinking response associated with eating (26). Accumulating evidence, although favoring histamine as an important mediator of meal-induced drinking, does suggest that multiple sequential interactions of neurotransmitters and hormonal controls are involved in the regulation of this process.

In view of the complex interactions involved in the regulation of drinking and salt ingestion, it is useful to display the available information in a diagrammatic form (Fig. 2). It should be stressed that this diagrammatic approach represents only a crude approximation to reality, and many further experiments will be necessary before a rigorous model can be assembled. The model suggests that there are four major stimuli to the activation of the desire to drink: S1, hypovolemia; S2, osmotic; S3, food ingestion; and S4, motivational factors. It is suggested that there is a final common pathway (F) for the activation of drinking by S1, S2, and S3 and that F can be inhibited by an inhibitory system involving α-adrenergic agonists and the κ opioids (28). Salt ingestion is seen as being secondary to activation of the angiotensin system acting in concert with hormonal factors such as the mineralocorticoids and estrogens. The higher cortical factors (S4) are given a special position in this schema, allowing them to override the other mechanisms.

THIRST DISORDERS

In view of the essentiality of drinking to survival of the organism, it is not surprising that disorders leading to

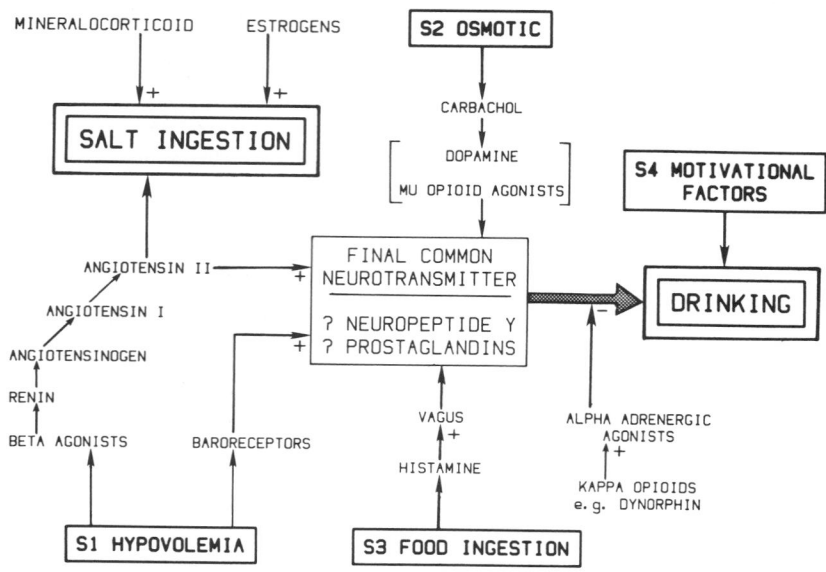

FIG. 2. Multiple factors involved in the initiation of drinking. See text for details.

adipsia are extremely rare. Tumors and other lesions involving the anterior wall of the third ventricle can lead to hypodipsia and impaired release of vasopressin (11). In addition, it has been demonstrated that elderly individuals fail to drink sufficient fluid and suffer periods of dehydration. This would explain the higher prevalence of dehydration associated with infections in the elderly.

Appropriate polydipsia can be present in a number of conditions associated with excessive renal water loss and occasionally in patients with extreme hyperreninemia (1). In both these situations, the brain is responding appropriately to circulating signals concerning the body's state of hydration. Of more interest is the condition of primary polydipsia in which the desire to drink persists in the absence of known physiological stimuli. In rare cases, primary polydipsia is secondary to a cerebral lesion. Mostly, however, it is psychogenic and is especially common in postmenopausal women suffering from chronic or acute psychosis. It appears that either clonidine or naloxone may be useful in the therapy of psychogenic polydipsia. Finally, in patients with polydipsia, hyperkalemia and hypercalcemia need to be excluded. Both of these disturbances potently stimulate prostaglandin synthesis, suggesting this neurotransmitter as a potential mediator of this form of polydipsia.

REFERENCES

1. Anderson, B., and Lundgren, M. (1982): *Annu. Rev. Med.*, 33:231–239.
2. Apfelbaum, M., and Madenoff, A. (1981): *Pharmacol. Biochem. Behav.*, 15:89–91.
3. Atkinson, R. L. (1982): *J. Clin. Endocrinol. Metab.*, 55:196–198.
4. Atkinson, R. L. (1983): *Abstr. 4th Int. Cong. Obesity*, 30A:81.
5. Atkinson, R., Kaesermann, H. P., Lambelet, J., Peters, G., and Peters-Haefeli, L. (1979): *J. Physiol. (Lond.)*, 291:61–73.
6. Balkanyi, I., Mohair, L., and Balkanyi, L. (1985): *Abstr. Cong. Hung. Pharmacol. Soc.*, 4:8.
7. Barbour, O. (1924): *Arch. Pediatr.*, 41:707–711.
8. Billington, C. J., Morley, J. E., Levine, A. S., and Gerritsen, G. C. (1984): *Am. J. Physiol.*, 267:R405–411.
9. Billington, C. J., Morley, J. E., Levine, A. S., Wright, F., and Seal, U. S. (1985): *Physiol. Behav.*, 36:641–663.
10. Billington, C. J., Shafer, R. B., and Morley, J. E. (1985): *Endocrinology*, 116:946A.
11. Blundell, J. E. (1976): In: *Serotonin in Health and Disease*, edited by W. B. Emson, pp. 403–450. Spectrum, New York.
12. Blundell, J. E., and Hill, A. S. (1985): In: *Abstracts, Disorders of Eating Behavior: A Psychoneuroendocrine Approach*, p. 106. University of Paira, Paira.
13. Clark, J. J., Kalra, P. S., Crowley, W. R., and Kalra, S. P. (1984): *Endocrinology*, 115:427–429.
14. Cohen, M. R., Cohen, R. M., Pickard, D., and Murphy, D. L. (1985): *Psychosom. Med.*, 47:132–138.
15. Fluharty, S. J., and Epstein, A. N. (1983): *Behav. Neurosci.*, 97:746–758.
16. Freed, W. J., Perlow, M. J., and Wyatt, R. D. (1979): *Science*, 206:850–852.
17. Fregly, M. J., and Rowland, N. E. (1985): *Am. J. Physiol.*, 248:R1–11.
18. Gartwaite, T. L. (1985): *Peptides*, 6:41–44.
19. Gerald, M. C., and Maukel, R. F. (1972): *Br. J. Pharmacol.*, 44:462–471.
20. Gosnell, B. A., Levine, A. S., and Morley, J. E. (1983): *Life Sci.*, 32:2793–2799.
21. Gosnell, B. A., Morley, J. E., and Levine, A. S. (1986): *Brain Res.*, 369:177–184,
22. Gosnell, B. A., Romsos, D. R., Morley, J. E., and Levine, A. S. (1985): *Behav. Neurosci.*, 99:1181–1191.
23. Gray, T. S., and Morley, J. E. (1986): *Life Sci.*, 38:389–401.
24. Holtzman, S. G. (1974): *J. Pharmacol. Exp. Ther.*, 189:51–60.
25. Knoll, J. (1985): In: *Endocoids*, edited by H. Lal, F. La Bella, and J. Lane, pp. 512–522. Alan R. Liss, New York.
26. Kraly, F. S. (1983): *Nature*, 302:65–66.
27. Kraly, F. S. (1984): *Psychol. Rev.*, 91:478–490.
28. Kraly, F. S., Gibbs, J., and Smith, G. P. (1975): *Nature*, 258:226–228.
29. Lehr, D., Mallow, J., and Krukowski, M. (1967): *J. Pharmacol. Exp. Ther.*, 158:150–163.
30. Leibowitz, S. F. (1978): *Pharmacol. Biochem. Behav.*, 8:163–175.
31. Leibowitz, S. F. (1980): In: *Handbook of the Hypothalamus, Vol. 3*, edited by P. J. Morgane and J. Panksepp, pp. 299–437. Raven Press, New York.
32. Leibowitz, S. F., Weiss, G. F., Yee, F., and Tretter, J. B. (1985): *Brain Res.*, 14:561–567.
33. Leksell, L. G. (1976): *Acta Physiol. Scand.*, 98:85–93.
34. Levine, A. S., and Morley, J. E. (1981): *Brain Res.*, 222:187–191.
35. Levine, A. S., Murray, S. S., Kneip, J., Grace, M., and Morley, J. E. (1982): *Physiol. Behav.*, 28:23–25.
36. Levine, A. S., Sievert, C. E., Morley, J. E., Gosnell, B. A., and Silvis, S. E. (1984): *Peptides*, 5:675–678.
37. Levine, A. S., and Morley, J. E. (1984): *Peptides*, 5:1025–1030.
38. Levine, A. S., Grace, M., Billington, C., Gosnell, D. M., et al. (1985): *Proc. Soc. Neurosci.*, 15:241.
39. Lowy, M. T., Maickel, R. P., and Yim, G. K. W. (1980): *Life Sci.*, 26:2113–2118.
40. McLaughlin, C. L., and Baile, C. A. (1985): *Physiol. Behav.*, 35:365–370.
41. Mitchell, J. E., Morley, J. E., and Hatsukami, D. (1984): In: *The Neural and Metabolic Bases of Feeding*, p. 69. University of California Press, Davis.
42. Morley, J. E. (1980): *Life Sci.*, 27:355–368.
43. Morley, J. E., Elson, M. K., Levine, A. S., and Shafer, R. B. (1982): *Peptides*, 3:901–906.
44. Morley, J. E., and Levine, A. S. (1981): *Life Sci.*, 29:901–1903.
45. Morley, J. E., and Levine, A. S. (1980): *Science*, 209:1259–1261.
46. Morley, J. E., and Levine, A. S. (1982): *Am. J. Clin. Nutr.*, 35:757–761.
47. Morley, J. E., and Levine, A. S. (1982): *Life Sci.*, 31:1459–1464.
48. Morley, J. E., Levine, A. S., and Rowland, N. (1983): *Life Sci.*, 32:2169–2182.
49. Morley, J. E., Levine, A. S., Yim, G. K. W., and Lowy, M. T. (1983): *Neurosci. Biobehav. Rev.*, 7:281–305.
50. Morley, J. E., Gosnell, B. A., Krahn, D. D., Mitchell, J. E., and Levine, A. S. (1985): *Psychopharmacol. Bull.*, 21:400–405.
51. Morley, J. E., Levine, A. S., Gosnell, B. A., and Krahn, D. D. (1985): *Brain Res. Bull.*, 14:511–519.
52. Morley, J. E., Levine, A. S., Kneip, J., Grace, M., Zeugner, H., et al. (1985): *Eur. J. Pharmacol.*, 112:17–25.
53. Morley, J. E., Parker, S., and Levine, A. S. (1985): *Am. J. Clin. Nutr.*, 42:1175–1178.
54. Muurahainen, N. E., Kissileff, M. R., Thomston, J., and Pi-Sunyer, F. X. (1983): *Soc. Neurosci. Abstr.*, 9:183.
55. Nakamura, M., Katsuura, G., Nakoo, K., and Imura, H. (1985): *Neurosci. Lett.*, 58:1–6.
56. Nizielski, S. E., Morley, J. E., Gosnell, B. A., Seal, U. S., and Levine, A. S. (1985): *Physiol. Behav.*, 36:171–176.
57. Ottaviani, R., Mastropaolo, J. P., and Riley, A. L. (1985): *Proc. Soc. Neurosci.*, 15:1059.
58. Pi-Sunyer, F. X., Kisseleff, H. R., Thornton, J., and Smith, G. P. (1982): *Physiol. Behav.*, 29:629–630.
59. Ramsay, D. J. (1978): *Fed. Proc.*, 37:2689–2693.
60. Rowland, N. (1980): In: *Analysis of Motivational Processes*, edited by F. M. Toates and T. R. Halliday, pp. 39–59. Academic Press, London.
61. Rowland, N. (1982): *Pharmacol. Biochem. Behav.*, 16:87–91.
62. Ruggy, J., and Fisher, A. E. (1974): *Nature*, 250:733–735.
63. Shaw, M. J., Hughes, J. J., Morley, J. E., Levine, A. S., Silvis, S. E., et al. (1985): *Ann. N.Y. Acad. Sci.*, 448:640–641.
64. Schulman, J. C., Carelton, J. L., Whitney, G., and Whitehorn, J. C. (1957): *J. Appl. Physiol.*, 11:419–421.
65. Stanley, B. G., Hoebel, B. G., and Leibowitz, S. F. (1983): *Peptides*, 4:493–500.

66. Stanley, B. G., and Leibowitz, S. F. (1984): *Life Sci.,* 33:2635–2642.

67. Stanley, B. G., Kyrkouli, S. E., Lampert, S., and Leibowitz, S. F. (1985): *Proc. Soc. Neurosci.,* 15:162.

68. Summy-Long, J. Y., Keil, L. C., Deen, K., Rosella, L., and Severs, W. B. (1981): *J. Pharmacol. Exp. Ther.,* 217:619–629.

69. Tallman, J. R., Willenbring, M., Carlson, G., Boorales, M., Krahn, D. D., et al. (1984): *Fed. Proc.,* 63:1058.

70. Tannebaum, G. S., Guyda, H. J., and Posner, B. I. (1983): *Science,* 220:777–779.

71. Thompson, D. A., Welle, S. L., Lilivavat, U., Penicaud, L., and Campbell, R. G. (1983): *Life Sci.,* 31:847–852.

72. Thompson, D. A., Welle, S. L., Lilivavat, U., Penicaud, L., and Campbell, R. G. (1983): *Life Sci.,* 31:847–852.

73. Trenchard, E., and Silverstone, T. (1983): *Appetite,* 4:43–50.

74. Uemura, H., Okawara, Y., and Kabayashi, H. (1985): *Neuroendocrinol. Lett.,* 7:175–184.

75. Woods, J. C., and Leibowitz, S. F. (1985): *Pharmacol. Biochem. Behav.,* 23:431–438.

76. Woods, S. C., West, D. B., Stein, L. J., McKay, L. D., Lotter, E. C., et al. (1981): *Diabetologia,* 20:305–313.

77. Willenbring, M. L., Levine, A. S., and Morley, J. E. (1986): *Int. J. Eating Disorders,* 5:855–864.

78. Wilson, K. M., Rowland, N., and Fregly, M. J. (1984): *Appetite,* 5:31–38.

Psychopharmacology:
The Third Generation of Progress,
edited by Herbert Y. Meltzer.
Raven Press, New York © 1987.

CHAPTER **132**

Psychopharmacology of Anorexia Nervosa

James E. Mitchell

The current interest in drug therapies for anorexia nervosa has resulted from several lines of reasoning. First, anorexia nervosa is a condition that is not easily treated (42), and the development of new, improved therapies is much in order. Second, patients with anorexia nervosa frequently demonstrate symptoms that, on a theoretical basis, might be responsive to psychotropic drugs, such as depression (9,16). Third, our growing knowledge of the underlying basic mechanisms that control appetite and feeding has suggested possible approaches to the manipulation of food intake in patients with anorexia nervosa (32). However, none of the drug therapies that have been used have proven therapeutic for all of the major symptoms of this disorder, although certain pharmacologic strategies appear to benefit certain patients in certain ways. Therefore, drug therapy for anorexia nervosa currently should be viewed as adjunctive.

ANTIPSYCHOTIC THERAPY

There are theoretical reasons to consider the use of antipsychotics in anorexia nervosa, since there is considerable evidence that dopamine is involved in the biology of feeding (30). Barry and Klawans (4) in 1976 proposed that increased activity at dopamine receptors might be responsible for many of the symptoms of anorexia nervosa. However, the role of dopamine in feeding is complex, and recent studies in animals suggest that dopamine has variable effects depending on location and dosage (30).

The first pharmacological trial using neuroleptics in anorexia nervosa was reported in 1958 by Dally et al. (13), who described the use of chlorpromazine in 11 patients in dosages to a maximum of 1,000 mg a day (average dose of 600 mg) combined with insulin as an appetite stimulant (60–80 units a day). In 1960 (14) and in 1966 (15), these authors summarized their treatment experience with an expanded series of 48 patients. The authors compared the outcome of these patients to the outcome of historical controls, consisting of 48 patients who had been treated in their facility over the preceding 20 years who had not received chlorpromazine. Treatment outcome data showed that the patients treated with chlorpromazine plus insulin gained weight more rapidly and were discharged from the hospital more quickly than the historical controls; however, at follow-up there were no significant differences between the two groups.

Crisp and Roberts (12) in 1962 reported on the use of chlorpromazine without insulin in the treatment of a male anorexia nervosa patient, and Crisp subsequently reported a series of 21 anorexia nervosa patients, many of whom received chlorpromazine as part of treatment (11). A few other reports or uncontrolled trials have appeared describing the use of antipsychotics to treat anorexia nervosa (22,39). Subsequently, two controlled trials have been reported. Vandereycken and Pierloot in 1982 reported a trial of pimozide in 18 female inpatients with anorexia nervosa who were also receiving a uniform contingency management program (49). After a base-line period of 7 to 10 days, the behavioral therapy program was supplemented by a double-blind crossover treatment consisting of two periods of 3 weeks when subjects received either pimozide, 4 or 6 mg, or placebo. Eight patients were initiated on pimozide and 10 on placebo. Analysis showed that the direct effect of pimozide tended to be significantly greater ($p = 0.067$) than that of placebo. No evidence was obtained of any differences in response between the 4- and 6-mg dosage.

Vandereycken subsequently reported a double-blind placebo-controlled crossover trial using sulpiride, another dopamine antagonist, in 18 patients receiving the same therapeutic program described in the 1982 study (50). After a base-line period of 1 week, patients were assigned to 3-week periods of either sulpiride, in a dosage of 300 to 400 mg a day, or placebo. Crossover analysis failed to establish any statistically significant direct effects of sulpiride either on mean daily weight change or on the behavioral or attitudinal variables used in the study; however, weight gain was greatest while receiving sulpiride in 13 of the 18 patients.

Taken together, the available studies have not proven antipsychotic drugs to be superior to placebo or to be an effective therapy for most patients with the disorder. This conclusion is tempered by the fact that the controlled studies reported to date have generally been small and of short duration and have used the neuroleptic as an adjunctive therapy to an established treatment program. It is certainly possible that certain patients, particularly those with severe agitation, may benefit from neuroleptic therapy. However, existing data do not support the use of these compounds on a routine basis in this population.

CYPROHEPTADINE

Serotonin is known to play an important role in food intake (30,32). Augmentation of serotonergic transmission in the medial hypothalamus induces satiety responses in animals, and suppression of serotonergic transmission can stimulate appetite. Cyproheptadine, a potent serotonin and histamine antagonist, has been used for some time to stimulate appetite in patient populations other than anorexia nervosa (6,46). Benady (5) in 1970 reported the use of cyproheptadine to treat a 12-year-old female with anorexia nervosa and suggested that cyproheptadine might be useful in helping patients with anorexia nervosa gain weight, and Silverstone and Schuyler reported a small outpatient trial of the medication in 1972, again suggesting a therapeutic advantage for the drug (43).

In 1977, Vigersky and Loriaux (51) reported a double-blind placebo-controlled trial of cyproheptadine in patients with anorexia nervosa. Thirteen patients were treated with active drug (12 mg/day) and 11 with placebo for a total of 8 weeks. There were no significant outcome differences between the two groups. Goldberg et al. (17) in 1979 reported a double-blind placebo-controlled multicenter trial that incorporated four treatment combinations: cyproheptadine plus behavior therapy, cyproheptadine plus no behavior therapy, placebo plus behavior therapy, placebo plus no behavior therapy. Subjects were treated with cyproheptadine at dosages ranging from 12 to 32 mg. The overall difference between drug and placebo groups in terms of weight gain was small and nonsignificant (drug, 5.11 kg; placebo, 4.32 kg). However, a *post-hoc* analysis suggested that the drug might be most effective in those individuals with more severe forms of the disorder.

Halmi et al. (21) subsequently completed a multicenter trial in 72 patients comparing high-dose cyproheptadine to both amitriptyline and placebo. The daily dosage of medication was increased to a maximum of 32 mg of cyproheptadine, 160 mg of amitriptyline, or placebo at the discretion of the treating physician. Patients taking cyproheptadine and amitriptyline attained their target weights an average of 10.5 days earlier than patients taking placebo. The authors found an unexpected differential drug effect on the bulimic subgroup of the anorectic patients: cyproheptadine

significantly increased treatment efficiency in nonbulimic patients and significantly impaired treatment efficiency in bulimic patients when compared with amitriptyline and placebo. The authors concluded that cyproheptadine was useful for increasing the rate of weight gain and reducing depressive symptoms in nonbulimic anorectics and that amitriptyline may also increase weight gain in anorectics but that the side effects of that drug were more problematic.

Taken together, the available studies suggest that there is a role for high-dose cyproheptadine in the treatment of anorexia nervosa in nonbulimic patients. The drug appears to be relatively free of side effects, the most common side effect being sedation. It must be remembered that the drug was used in these studies in combination with established, structured inpatient treatment programs.

ANTIDEPRESSANTS

The relationship between anorexia nervosa and affective disorders is complex and currently a matter of debate. Some researchers have suggested a close relationship between these two disorders based on clinical similarities, pharmacological response similarities, and family history studies, some of which have suggested familial relatedness (24). Other authors have argued against this close relationship (1).

Several case reports and reports of series of patients have suggested a role for antidepressants in the treatment of anorexia nervosa (24,34,35,37,38,52). The report by Hudson et al. (24) in 1985 reviews much of this literature and adds a series of nine patients, several of whom received more than one agent during the course of treatment. This report suggested that antidepressants can indeed help patients with anorexia nervosa but that many anorexia nervosa patients tolerate these medications poorly, and most are very sensitive to their anticholinergic side effects.

Only three controlled trials using antidepressants in anorexia nervosa have been reported. One is the study of Halmi et al. (21) discussed previously. Lacey and Crisp (28) in 1980 reported a placebo-controlled double-blind trial in 13 inpatients who were treated for 10 to 11 weeks with chlomipramine, 50 mg a day ($N = 6$), or placebo ($N = 7$). The authors found no significant advantage for active drug over placebo. However, the dosage selected for this trial, although a rational starting point for an initial controlled trial in this population, in retrospect may have been too low. Recently Biederman et al. (7) reported a double-blind placebo-controlled trial of amitriptyline in a series of 25 patients, 11 assigned to active drug and 14 to placebo. There were no significant differences on the main outcome variables between drug and placebo patients. The mean dose attained in week 5 was 115 mg per day with a mean end-point serum level of 140.0 ± 95.1 ng/ml (amitriptyline plus nortriptyline). No significant association was established between serum level and outcome.

These studies suggest that despite the presence of depressive symptoms in many patients with anorexia nervosa, these medications should not be used on a routine basis. Most authors have commented on the problems with side effects, particularly anticholinergic side effects, in this population, suggesting that researchers planning trials in this patient group should consider using low-anticholinergic agents at higher dosages in order to maximize the likelihood of demonstrating a drug effect. Another issue concerns acute treatment versus maintenance. It is possible although untested that an important use for these drugs might be found after acute weight recovery, when patients are more likely to tolerate the side effects.

LITHIUM CARBONATE

A few case reports of patients with anorexia nervosa who were successfully treated with lithium suggest that this compound might be useful for some anorectic patients (3,44). Gross et al. (20) in 1981 reported the first controlled evaluation in an inpatient trial of 16 subjects who were also being treated with a behavior modification program. Serum levels were maintained between 0.9 and 1.4 mEq/liter, and subjects were treated for a total of 28 days. The lithium-treated group had gained more weight at week 3 and week 4 relative to the placebo-treated group. Although encouraging, the sample sizes were small, and the study was of brief duration. However, clinicians must bear in mind that lithium is a potentially highly toxic drug in this population. Patients in the Gross et al. study were inpatients who were closely monitored for signs of toxicity. Careful attention to fluid, electrolyte, and cardiac status would be requisite for using lithium in these patients.

OTHER TREATMENTS

The endogenous opioid system has been shown to play an important role in hypothalamic control of appetite and eating (32). Moore et al. (36) in 1981 attempted to modulate this system in order to evaluate the effects on eating in anorexia nervosa patients. Subjects received 3.2 to 6.4 mg a day of naloxone intravenously by continuous infusion for several days and were found to have a significantly greater weight gain during the period of naloxone infusion. Unfortunately, the design of this study makes interpretation of the results difficult. Also, there is considerable evidence in both human and infrahuman species suggesting that endogenous opioids stimulate feeding (33) and that the administration of opioid antagonists usually suppresses feeding in humans (2,45,48), a finding opposite to the results of the Moore et al. study.

Johanson and Knorr reported the treatment of nine individuals with anorexia nervosa using L-dopa for periods up to 4 months (25,26). This therapeutic strategy was based on their assessment of behavioral and cognitive similarities—such as rigid, obsessive–compulsive, stereotyped behaviors—between patients with anorexia nervosa and patients with parkinsonism. The maximum dosage of L-dopa ranged from 1.0 to 3.0 g per day. The authors concluded that five of the nine patients treated with L-dopa responded well without evidence of adverse effects.

Because of the commonly reported observation that marijuana stimulates appetite in many individuals, Gross et al. (19) undertook a controlled trial of Δ^9-tetrahydrocannabinol. The protocol was 4 weeks in duration and double-blind crossover in design, with 11 females participating. Medication was given 90 min before meals, with the dosage of Δ^9-THC gradually increasing from a total daily dosage of 7.5 mg to 30 mg. Diazepam was given as an active control in increasing dosages from 3.0 to 15 mg daily. There was no advantage for the Δ^9-THC, and three patients experienced severe dysphoric reactions consisting of paranoid ideation and feelings of loss of control.

Patients with anorexia nervosa frequently have delayed gastric emptying (41), which contributes to the frequent complaints of bloating and abdominal pain reported during refeeding. Several authors have reported that emptying time can be improved in patients with anorexia nervosa by the administration of drugs that promote gastric emptying, such as metoclopramide (29,31) and domperidone (41). However, metoclopramide may be associated with depression and, because of its central as well as peripheral dopamine-blocking properties, may cause tardive dyskinesia.

Several other agents have been mentioned in isolated case reports or series. Zinc is known to be an important element in processes related to taste perception, and zinc deficiency can present with impaired taste and anorexia (23). A case of a patient with anorexia nervosa who responded to zinc supplementation has recently appeared (8), but controlled studies have not been reported. A case report of a patient who responded to the adrenergic blocker phenoxybenzamine has been published (40). Cases have also been reported involving treatment with glycerol (10) (in an attempt to provide a source of glucose and assist repletion of carbohydrate stores), nandrolone (47) (an anabolic steroid), and ACTH and cortisone (18), therapeutic approaches that are no longer tenable given our current knowledge of the effects of these compounds.

CONCLUSIONS

The history of pharmacological treatment for anorexia nervosa underscores quite clearly the need for placebo-controlled double-blind trials before therapies can be accepted. The progress of the literature in this area has been from positive and enthusiastic single case reports to controlled trials with generally negative or equivocal results.

A major limiting factor in the antidepressant trials appears to have been the high level of intolerance to these medications by anorexia nervosa patients and the use of highly anticholinergic drugs. The work with cyproheptadine looks particularly promising, the results suggesting that nonbulimic (restrictor) anorectics may benefit from this medication, which is reasonably well tolerated by most patients. The results with lithium are also promising; however, this is a difficult drug to use in this group, and careful monitoring is required. The use of agents to stimulate gastric emptying appears to be useful for patients who are bothered by postprandial distress early in the course of treatment.

Although there are many interesting leads and directions, much of the research of greatest promise has yet to be translated into human studies. As with many areas of neurobiology, much progress has been made in the last two decades unraveling the biology of appetite and eating. These findings offer many interesting opportunities better to understand and better to treat humans with eating disorders.

REFERENCES

1. Altshuler, K. Z., and Weiner, M. F. (1985): *Am. J. Psychiatry,* 142:328–332.
2. Atkinson, R. L. (1982): *J. Clin. Endocrinol. Metab.,* 55:196–198.
3. Barcai, A. (1977): *Acta Psychiatr. Scand.,* 55:97–101.
4. Barry, V. C., and Klawans, H. L. (1976): *J. Neural Transm.,* 38:107–122.
5. Benady, D. R. (1970): *Br. J. Psychiatry,* 117:681–682.
6. Bergen, S. S. (1964): *Am. J. Dis. Child.,* 108:270–273.
7. Biederman, J., Herzog, D. A., Rivinus, T. M., Harper, G. P., Ferber, R. A., et al. (1985): *J. Clin. Psychopharmacol.,* 5:10–16.
8. Bryce-Smith, D., and Simpson, R. I. D. (1984): *Lancet,* 2:350.
9. Cantwell, D. P., Sturzenberger, S., Burroughs, J., Salkin, B., and Green, J. K. (1977): *Arch. Gen. Psychiatry,* 34:1087–1093.
10. Caplin, H., Ginsburg, J., and Beaconsfield, P. (1973): *Lancet,* 1:319.
11. Crisp, A. H. (1965): *Br. J. Psychiatry,* 112:505–512.
12. Crisp, A. H., and Roberts, F. J. (1962): *Postgrad. Med. J.,* 38:350–353.
13. Dally, P. J., Oppenheim, G. B., and Sargant, W. (1958): *Br. Med. J.,* 2:633–634.
14. Dally, P. J., and Sargant, W. (1960): *Br. Med. J.,* 1:1770–1773.
15. Dally, P., and Sargant, W. (1966): *Br. Med. J.,* 2:793–795.
16. Eckert, E. D., Goldberg, S. C., Halmi, K. A., Casper, R. C., and Davis, J. M. (1982): *Psychol. Med.,* 12:115–122.
17. Goldberg, S. C., Halmi, K. A., Eckert, E. D., Casper, R. C., and Davis, J. M. (1979): *Br. J. Psychiatry,* 134:67–70.
18. Greenblatt, R. B., Barfield, W. M. E., and Clarks, S. L. (1951): *J. Med. Assoc. Georgia,* 40:229–301.
19. Gross, H., Ebert, M., Faden, V. B., Goldberg, S. C., Kaye, W. H., et al. (1983): *J. Clin. Psychopharmacol.,* 3:165–171.
20. Gross, H. A., Ebert, M. H., Faden, V. B., Goldberg, S. C., Nee, L. E., et al. (1981): *J. Clin. Psychopharmacol.,* 1:376–381.
21. Halmi, K. A., Eckert, E., LaDu, T., and Cohen, J. (1986): *Arch. Gen. Psychiatry,* 43:177–181.
22. Hoes, M. (1980): *J. Orthomol. Psychiatry,* 9:48–51.
23. Horrobin, D. F., and Cunnane, S. C. (1980): *Med. Hypotheses,* 6:277–296.
24. Hudson, J. I., Pope, G. P., Jonas, J. M., and Yurgelun-Todd, D. (1985): *J. Clin. Psychopharmacol.,* 5:17–23.
25. Johanson, A. J., and Knorr, N. J. (1974): *Lancet,* 2:591.
26. Johanson, A. J., and Knorr, N. J. (1977): In: *Anorexia Nervosa,* edited by R. A. Vigersky, pp. 363–372. Raven Press, New York.
27. Kendler, K. S. (1978): *Am. J. Psychiatry,* 135:1107–1108.
28. Lacey, J. H., and Crisp, A. H. (1980): *Postgrad. Med. J.,* 56:79–85.
29. Lebwohl, P. (1980): *Am. J. Gastroenterol.,* 74:127–132.
30. Leibowitz, S. F. (1980): *Handbook of the Hypothalamus.* Raven Press, New York.
31. Moldofsky, H., Jeuniewic, N., and Garfinkel, P. E. (1977): In: *Anorexia Nervosa,* edited by R. A. Vigersky, pp. 373–375. Raven Press, New York.
32. Morley, J. E. (1980): *Life Sci.,* 27:355–368.
33. Morley, J. E., Levine, A. S., and Yim, G. K. (1983): *Neurosci. Biobehav. Rev.,* 7:281–305.
34. Mills, I. H. (1976): *Lancet,* 2:687.
35. Moore, D. C. (1977): *Am. J. Psychiatry,* 134:1303–1304.
36. Moore, R., Mills, I. H., and Forster, A. (1981): *J. R. Soc. Med.,* 74:129–131.
37. Needleman, H. L., and Waber, D. (1976): *Lancet,* 2:580.
38. Needleman, H. L., and Waber, D. (1977): In: *Anorexia Nervosa,* edited by R. A. Vigersky, pp. 357–362. Raven Press, New York.
39. Plantley, F. (1977): *Lancet,* 1:1105.
40. Redmond, D. E., Swann, A., and Heninger, G. R. (1976): *Lancet,* 2:307.
41. Russell, D. M., Freedman, M. L., Feiglin, D. H. I., Jeejeebhoy, K. N., Swinson, R. P., et al. (1983): *Am. J. Psychiatry,* 140:1235–1236.
42. Steinhausen, H.-C., and Glanville, K. (1983): *Psychol. Med.,* 13:239–249.
43. Silverstone, T., and Schuyler, D. (1975): *Psychopharmacologia,* 40:335–340.
44. Stein, G. S., Hartshorn, S., Jones, J., and Steinberg, D. (1982): *Br. J. Psychiatry,* 140:526–528.
45. Sternbach, H. A., Annitto, W., Pottash, A. L. C., and Gold, M. (1982): *Lancet,* 1:388–389.
46. Stiel, J. N., Liddle, G. W., and Lacy, W. W. (1970): *Metabolism,* 19:192–200.
47. Tec, L. (1974): *J.A.M.A.,* 229:1423.
48. Trenchard, E., and Silverstone, T. (1983): *Appetite J. Intake Res.,* 4:43–40.
49. Vandereycken, W., and Pierloot, R. (1982): *Acta Psychiatr. Scand.,* 66:445–450.
50. Vandereycken, W. (1984): *Br. J. Psychiatry,* 144:288–292.
51. Vigersky, R. A., and Loriaux, D. L. (1977): In: *Anorexia Nervosa,* edited by R. A. Vigersky, pp. 346–356. Raven Press, New York.
52. White, J. H., and Schnaultz, N. L. (1977): *Dis. Nerv. Syst.,* 38:567–571.

Psychopharmacology:
The Third Generation of Progress,
edited by Herbert Y. Meltzer.
Raven Press, New York © 1987.

CHAPTER **133**

Psychopharmacology of Bulimia

B. Timothy Walsh

Bulimia is an eating disorder whose salient characteristic is episodic binge eating. Patients with bulimia are aware that the behavior is abnormal but feel that they are unable to control their eating during a binge. Most patients with bulimia attempt to avoid weight gain by inducing vomiting after binges, by abusing laxatives or diuretics, or by severely restricting their diets between binges. Bulimia can occur at both ends of the weight spectrum; about half of patients hospitalized for anorexia nervosa also binge eat, so they can be considered to have both anorexia nervosa and bulimia (3,7). Conversely, a fraction of overweight patients also engages in binge-eating behavior (8,44). However, the majority of patients who present to clinics requesting treatment for bulimia are of normal body weight (28). In such patients, the frequency of binges ranges from a few times a month to five or more episodes a day, and the average amount of food consumed per binge is of the order of 2500 calories.

Although this pattern of eating was described in antiquity, bulimia attracted little medical attention until the late 1970s. Since that time, there has been a flurry of popular and professional interest in this syndrome. However, we have few accurate estimates of its frequency in the population. Surveys of selected populations, typically college students, suggest that loosely defined "binge eating" is a common occurrence. When more restrictive criteria are applied, such as a minimum binge frequency of once a week and the routine use of purging, estimates of the frequency of bulimia drop considerably but are still in the range of 1 to 5% of young women, a disturbingly high prevalence (4,11,13,33,36).

In normal-weight individuals, bulimia appears to be generally well tolerated physically. The disturbances most frequently noted are fluid and electrolyte abnormalities related to recurrent vomiting and/or laxative and diuretic abuse (26). These metabolic derangements can produce physical symptoms and are occasionally of sufficient severity to require acute medical intervention. Gastric dilatation

and rupture, which are life-threatening complications, have rarely been reported (5,25). Patients who induce vomiting may develop significant dental disease, probably related to the effects of stomach acid on the teeth, and painless, benign salivary gland enlargement (12,24,45). Women with bulimia also appear to have a higher than expected frequency of menstrual disturbance.

Pharmacological approaches to the treatment of bulimia have been based on two conceptual models of this syndrome: one model posits that bulimia is related to a seizure disorder and implies that anticonvulsant medication may be a useful form of treatment; the other, more recent, model suggests that bulimia is in some way related to affective illness and that antidepressant medication may be of use.

ANTICONVULSANT TREATMENT OF BULIMIA

The model of bulimia as a seizure equivalent was developed by Rau and Green between 1974 and 1979 (9,10,37,38). These authors were struck by several clinical similarities between binge eating and seizures. The episodes of binging were described by patients as being episodic, ego-dystonic, and uncontrollable and were sometimes preceded by an altered state of consciousness that could be likened to an aura. Green and Rau obtained EEGs on a series of 59 patients with binge eating and noted abnormalities in 64%. They therefore proposed that "compulsive eaters have a primary neurological disorder similar to epilepsy" (37, p. 228). On the basis of this formulation, they openly treated a total of 47 patients with the antiepileptic drug phenytoin and described impressive symptom relief in 27 (57%). The most frequently observed EEG abnormality was the occurrence of 14- and 6-per-sec spikes, and 21 (78%) of the 27 patients with this abnormality responded to phenytoin treatment.

There has only been one controlled trial of significant size of phenytoin in binge eating. In 1977, Wermuth et al.

(50) described the results of a double-blind study of crossover design examining the effectiveness of phenytoin in the treatment of 20 patients. The patient population was more heterogeneous with respect to body weight than those in more recent pharmacological studies; at entry, nine patients were overweight, and one had anorexia nervosa. The patients were also less severely ill; the mean binge frequency was 3.7/week before treatment compared to binge frequencies of approximately 10/week in more recent studies. Ten patients were randomized to begin treatment with phenytoin (300 mg daily), and there was a significant decline over 6 weeks in binge frequency in this group. However, contrary to predictions based on a seizure model, the binge frequency in this group did not increase when the medication was switched to placebo. In the group that received placebo first, there was no change in binge frequency during the first 6 weeks, but the patients did improve when they received phenytoin in the second phase. Overall, there was no significant difference between placebo treatment and phenytoin treatment, and only one patient ceased binging entirely.

The authors obtained EEGs on all patients prior to the study and found abnormalities in only three patients. Furthermore, there was no relationship between clinical response and either the presence of pretreatment EEG abnormalities or plasma phenytoin level. This study provides no support for the hypothesis of Rau and Green that patients with binge eating have a neurological disorder similar to epilepsy: EEG abnormalities were infrequent, and the clinical response to phenytoin was not consistent with predictions based on a seizure model. The results suggest that impressive clinical response to phenytoin is not common but do not exclude the possibility that some patients respond favorably to such treatment. Unfortunately, there have been no further controlled studies of phenytoin in bulimia.

One other controlled study may be pertinent to the seizure model of bulimia. Kaplan et al. (22) have reported on their experience with the anticonvulsant carbamazepine in the treatment of six patients with bulimia. Patients were treated in 6-week intervals with placebo and carbamazepine in a placebo–carbamazepine–placebo or carbamazepine–placebo–carbamazepine double-blind design. Although five of the six patients had no more than an equivocal response to carbamazepine, one patient had no response to placebo, improved dramatically on carbamazepine, and relapsed when she switched back to placebo. Carbamazepine is widely used in the treatment of seizure disorders but has a chemical structure similar to that of the tricyclic antidepressants and has been shown to be effective in the treatment of bipolar affective illness (35). Therefore, the response of the patient of Kaplan et al. to treatment with carbamazepine is as consistent with an association between bulimia and affective illness as with an association between bulimia and seizure disorder. In addition, although small in size, their study suggests that impressive response of bulimia to carbamazepine therapy is uncommon.

ANTIDEPRESSANT TREATMENT OF BULIMIA

The clinical feature of bulimia that has prompted most pharmacological trials in the 1980s is that of mood distur-

bance. There is broad agreement among clinicians treating patients with bulimia that, compared with their peers, such patients have increased frequencies of depression and of anxiety (6,49). In addition, several studies have documented that patients with bulimia are prone to develop not merely depressed mood but full depressive syndromes (14,17,48). There is far less agreement about whether the association between bulimia and mood disturbance suggests that bulimia is an unusual form of depression or whether the mood disturbance is "secondary" to the eating disorder. Reports are inconsistent concerning the frequency of mood disturbance among the relatives of patients with bulimia and about the prevalence and the significance of biological findings characteristic of major depressive illness, such as increased adrenal activity and short REM latencies. In short, although there is good evidence of an association between bulimia and mood disturbance, the nature of that relationship is uncertain.

Although the relationship between mood disturbance and bulimia has been, and remains, unclear, the presence of depression prompted clinicians to treat patients with bulimia with antidepressant medication. A single case report appeared in 1978 and was followed in 1982 by reports of two series of patients openly treated with tricyclic antidepressants (TCAs) and monoamine oxidase inhibitors (MAOIs) (30,40,46). Since that time, reports of the treatment of over 200 patients with bulimia have appeared in the literature, and the majority of these have described successful outcome (2,15,16,18,23,27,32,34,41–43,47). The vast majority of these reports concern women with bulimia who are of normal body weight. The medications suggested to be effective have ranged from TCAs and MAOIs to the newest antidepressant medications and have also included lithium carbonate. Five double-blind, placebo-controlled trials have been reported.

The first controlled study examined mianserin and was flawed by the probable inclusion of patients who were only mildly ill and by the use of only a modest dose of drug (60 mg/day) (42). Both placebo- and mianserin-treated patients improved on several symptom measures, but the number of days per week the subjects reported binging did not change in either group.

Three of the five controlled studies have examined tricyclic antidepressants. Pope et al. (31) and Hughes et al. (18) studied imipramine (200 mg/day) and desipramine (200 mg/day), respectively, and found that both were more effective than placebo in reducing the mean number of binges per week. Mitchell and Groat (27) studied amitriptyline (150 mg/day) and, although they used a design very similar to that of the other two TCA studies, found no difference between drug and placebo in the effect on eating behavior. The most striking difference between the study of Mitchell and Groat and the other two TCA studies was that Mitchell and Groat's placebo group improved substantially, whereas the placebo groups in the other two TCA studies did not. In all three studies, the patients treated with active medication improved to a similar degree, attaining on the average about a 75% reduction in binge frequency.

One controlled study has examined the treatment of patients with bulimia with MAOIs. Walsh et al. (47) found that the MAOI phenelzine (60 mg/day) was superior to placebo in reduction of the number of binges per week and in the fraction of patients whose binge eating had ceased entirely at the termination of the study.

Thus, three of five double-blind, placebo-controlled trials have found evidence of antidepressant drug superiority over placebo in the treatment of patients of normal body weight with bulimia. These studies provide persuasive evidence of the short-term efficacy of antidepressant medication in this syndrome. However, a number of questions remain unanswered. Probably the most intriguing question is why antidepressant medication is useful in the treatment of bulimia. In fact, its utility in this syndrome seems paradoxical in light of reports that antidepressant medication sometimes leads to increased weight and sugar craving (29).

As noted, one of the features of bulimia that prompted psychiatrists to treat this syndrome with antidepressants was the presence of mood disturbance. However, two of the placebo-controlled studies have found that the pretreatment presence of mood disturbance had little bearing on treatment response. Hughes et al. (18) excluded patients with current major depression from their study and, nonetheless, found a significant drug/placebo difference. Walsh et al. (47) stratified their sample at randomization into depressed and nondepressed groups and found a significant drug/placebo difference in both groups. Thus, it appears that some nondepressed patients with bulimia derive benefit from treatment with antidepressant medication.

One attractive hypothesis to account for this result is related to anxiety. Among patients with bulimia, feelings of anxiety or tension are probably the most frequent precipitants of binge eating (1,19). In addition to their antidepressant efficacy, both TCAs and MAOIs have significant anxiolytic properties (20,21,39). Thus, in some bulimic patients, antidepressants may be of therapeutic value because they relieve anxiety and hence remove one of the precipitants of binge eating. Unfortunately, although this hypothesis is heuristically appealing, no studies have addressed this proposal experimentally.

A second question is whether MAOIs are superior to TCAs in the treatment of patients with bulimia. The MAOIs have long been believed to be particularly effective in the treatment of patients with atypical depression characterized by a high degree of anxiety as well as depression and sometimes by overeating. The mixture of anxiety and depression noted in many patients with bulimia bears some resemblance to "atypical" depression and suggests that MAOIs might be especially useful in bulimia. Because of differences in patient populations and in experimental designs, it is difficult to compare the controlled trials of TCAs to that of the MAOI phenelzine. Nonetheless, MAOIs do not appear to be dramatically more effective than TCAs. On the other hand, it is clear that there are bulimic patients who fail to respond to TCAs who do respond to MAOIs. Therefore, although there are suggestions that MAOIs may be superior to TCAs in bulimia, the difference, if it exists, appears to be modest and may be detected only by a study directly comparing a MAOI to a TCA in a large patient population.

In clinical terms, one of the major unanswered questions about drug treatment for bulimia is the long-term outcome of such therapy. All of the double-blind controlled trials have been short-term, none lasting more than 10 weeks, and long-term outcome data are extremely limited. Preliminary reports suggest that although relapse on drugs does occur, it is not typical, but that discontinuation of medication after short-term treatment may be frequently followed by relapse. It is currently unknown whether a longer course of treatment, lasting 6 months, for example, leads to sustained remission of bulimia or if the eating disorder is likely to return upon cessation of medication.

A second important clinical question is how treatment with medication compares to other forms of treatment for bulimia such as group or cognitive/behavioral therapy. We do not know if one form of treatment is superior, if there are some patients who respond best to a specific form of therapy, or if medication should ideally be combined with other forms of therapy. None of the pharmacological studies have carefully reported the number of bulimic patients who refuse to take medication or the problem of drug compliance and dropouts. Side effects such as hypotension, dizziness, and headaches can be a problem. Patients who have completed a phenelzine trial also agreed to follow the "MAOI diet." Thus, a biased bulimia population participated in the drug studies, and results cannot be generalized to the entire bulimia population.

In short, the last decade has witnessed the development of potentially useful pharmacological treatments for bulimia. However, the delineation of the precise role of pharmacology in the treatment of this eating disorder requires much additional investigation.

ACKNOWLEDGMENTS

This work was supported, in part, by NIMH grants (MH-38355 and MH-00383), by the Parke-Davis Division of the Warner Lambert Company, and by Communities Foundation of Texas, Inc.

REFERENCES

1. Abraham, S. F., and Beumont, P. J. V. (1982): *Psychol. Med.,* 12:625–635.
2. Brotman, A., Herzog, D. B., and Woods, S. W. (1984): *J. Clin. Psychiatry,* 45:7–9.
3. Casper, R. C., Eckert, E. D., Halmi, K. A., Goldberg, S. C., and Davis, J. M. (1980): *Arch. Gen. Psychiatry,* 37:1030–1035.
4. Cooper, P. J., Waterman, G. C., and Fairburn, C. (1984): *Br. J. Clin. Psychol.,* 23:45–52.
5. Devitt, P. G., and Stamp, G. W. H. (1983): *Gut,* 24:678–679.
6. Fairburn, C. G., and Cooper, P. J. (1984): *Br. J. Psychiatry,* 144:238–246.
7. Garfinkel, P. E., Moldofsky, H., and Garner, D. M. (1980): *Arch. Gen. Psychiatry,* 37:1036–1040.
8. Gormally, J., Black, S., Daston, S., and Rardin, D. (1982): *Addict. Behav.,* 7:47–55.
9. Green, R. S., and Rau, J. H. (1974): *Am. J. Psychiatry,* 131:428–432.
10. Green, R. S., and Rau, J. H. (1977): In: *Anorexia Nervosa,* edited by R. A. Vigersky, pp. 377–382. Raven Press, New York.
11. Halmi, K., Falk, R. J., and Schwartz, E. (1981): *Psychol. Med.,* 11:697–706.
12. Harrison, J. L., George, L. A., Cheatham, J. L., and Zinn, J. (1985): *Gen. Dent.,* 33:65–68.
13. Hart, K. J., and Ollendick, T. H. (1985): *Am. J. Psychiatry,* 142:851–854.
14. Herzog, D. B. (1984): *Am. J. Psychiatry,* 141:1594–1597.

15. Horne, R. L. (1985): Bupropion in the treatment of bulimia. Presented at the 138th Annual Meeting of the American Psychiatric Association, Dallas, Texas.
16. Hsu, L. K. G. (1984): *Am. J. Psychiatry,* 141:1260–1262.
17. Hudson, J. I., Pope, H. G., Jonas, J. M., and Yurgelun-Todd, D. (1983): *Psychiatry Res.,* 9:345–354.
18. Hughes, P. L., Wells, L. A., Cunningham, C. J., Ilstrup, D. M. (1986): *Arch. Gen. Psychiatry,* 43:182–186.
19. Johnson, C., and Larson, R. (1982): *Psychosom. Med.,* 44:341–351.
20. Johnstone, E. C., Cunningham-Owens, D. G., Frith, C. D., McPherson, K., Dowie, C., et al. (1980): *Psychol. Med.,* 10:321–328.
21. Kahn, R. J., McNair, D. M., Covi, L., Dowing, R. W., Fisher, S., et al. (1981): *Psychopharmacol. Bull.,* 17(3):97–100.
22. Kaplan, A. S., Garfinkel, P. E., Darby, P. L., and Garner, D. M. (1983): *Am. J. Psychiatry,* 140:1225–1226.
23. Kennedy, S. H., Piran, N., and Garfinkel, P. E. (1985): *J. Clin. Psychopharmacol.,* 5:279–285.
24. Levin, P. A., Falko, J. M., Dixon, K., Gallup, E. M., and Saunders, W. (1980): *Ann. Intern. Med.,* 93:827–829.
25. Matikainen, M. (1979): *Am. J. Surg.,* 138:451–452.
26. Mitchell, J. E., Pyle, R. L., Eckert, E. D., Hatsukami, D., and Lentz, R. (1983): *Psychol. Med.,* 13:273–278.
27. Mitchell, J. E., and Groat, R. (1984): *J. Clin. Psychopharmacol.,* 4:186–193.
28. Mitchell, J. E., Hatsukami, D., Eckert, E. D., and Pyle, R. L. (1985): *Am. J. Psychiatry,* 142:482–485.
29. Paykel, E. S., Mueller, P. S., and De La Vergue (1973): *Br. J. Psychiatry,* 123:501–507.
30. Pope, H. G., and Hudson, I. (1982): *Psychopharmacology,* 78:176–179.
31. Pope, H. G., Hudson, J. I., Jonas, J. M., and Yurgelun-Todd, D. (1983): *Am. J. Psychiatry,* 140:554–558.
32. Pope, H. G., Hudson, J. I., and Jonas, J. M. (1983): *J. Clin. Psychopharmacol.,* 3:274–281.
33. Pope, H. G., Hudson, J. I., and Yurgelun-Todd, D. (1984): *Am. J. Psychiatry,* 141:292–294.
34. Pope, H. G., Herridge, P. L., Hudson, J. I., Fontaine, R., and Yurgelun-Todd, D. (1985): Treatment of bulimia with nomifensine. Presented at the 138th Annual Meeting of the American Psychiatric Association, Dallas, Texas.
35. Post, R. M., and Uhde, T. W. (1985): *Psychopharmacol. Bull.,* 21(1):10–17.
36. Pyle, R. L., Mitchell, J. E., Eckert, E. D., Halvorson, P. A., Neuma, P. A., et al. (1983): *Int. J. Eating Disorders,* 2:75–85.
37. Rau, J. H., and Green, R. S. (1975): *Compr. Psychiatry,* 16:223–231.
38. Rau, J. H., Struve, F. A., and Green, R. S. (1979): *Clin. Electroencephalogr.,* 10:180–189.
39. Ravaris, C. L., Nies, A., Robinson, D. S., Ives, J. O., Lamborn, K. R., et al. (1979): *Arch. Gen. Psychiatry,* 33:749–760.
40. Rich, C. L. (1978): *J.A.M.A.,* 239:2688–2689.
41. Roy-Byrne, P., Gwirtsman, H., Edelstein, C. K., Yager, J., and Gerner, R. H. (1983): *J. Clin. Psychopharmacol.,* 3:60–61.
42. Sabine, E. J., Yonace, A., Farrington, A. J., Barratt, K. H., and Wakeling, A. (1983): *Br. J. Clin. Pharmacol.,* 15:195S–202S.
43. Shader, R. I., and Greenblatt, D. J. (1982): *J. Clin. Psychopharmacol.,* 2:233–234.
44. Stunkard, A. J. (1959): *Psychiatr. Q.,* 33:284–295.
45. Walsh, B. T., Croft, C. B., and Katz, J. L. (1981–1982): *Int. J. Psychiatry Med.,* 11:255–262.
46. Walsh, B. T., Stewart, J. W., Wright, L., Harrison, W., Roose, S. P., et al. (1982): *Am. J. Psychiatry,* 139:1629–1630.
47. Walsh, B. T., Stewart, J. W., Roose, S. P., Gladis, M., and Glassman, A. H. (1984): *Arch. Gen. Psychiatry,* 41:1105–1109.
48. Walsh, B. T., Roose, S. P., Glassman, A. H., Gladis, M., and Sadik, C. (1985): *Psychosom. Med.,* 47:123–131.
49. Weiss, S. R., and Ebert, M. U. (1983): *Psychosom. Med.,* 45:293–303.
50. Wermuth, B. M., Davis, K. L., Hollister, L. E., and Stunkard, A. J. (1977): *Am. J. Psychiatry,* 134:1249–1253.

Psychopharmacology:
The Third Generation of Progress,
edited by Herbert Y. Meltzer.
Raven Press, New York © 1987.

CHAPTER 134

The Pharmacotherapy of Obesity

Louis Lasagna

CRITICISMS OF ANOREXIANT DRUGS

There is a widespread belief that appetite suppressants are not significantly useful in the treatment of obesity. Academicians tend to teach that such drugs are only trivially effective, rapidly induce tolerance to their effects, are frequently abused and lead to addiction, and often produce intolerable side effects (4).

In fact, none of these clichés is true, and it may be helpful, as background, to examine the basis for their existence. To begin with, most physicians are not interested in treating obesity and are not particularly good at it. There is often a presumption that if fat people only had moral fiber and simply restrained their piggish appetites, obesity would not exist. For many physicians, obesity becomes a medical condition only when it complicates "real" illness such as hypertension, coronary artery disease, congestive heart failure, diabetes mellitus, or sleep apnea. The fact that obesity can not only cause emotional distress but predisposes to diabetes, hypertension, cancer, gallbladder disease, varicose veins, orthopedic problems, etc., is not sufficiently appreciated by the medical profession. Nor does it help that when physicians try to manage obesity they often fail and thus get negatively reinforced.

A second factor is a report the FDA made a number of years ago (7) that rather mindlessly lumped together 39 controlled trials of anorexiants in the FDA files, ignoring dosage, duration, patient mix, protocol differences, dropouts, etc., and then compared the weight loss on pooled active treatments with that on placebo. Twenty of these studies had lasted 4 weeks, 18 lasted 8 weeks, and only one study had lasted for a year. The conclusion was that the difference between active drugs and placebo was trivial when these treatments were added to dietary restriction.

A third factor is the frequently encountered difficulty that people have in distinguishing "medical addiction" from "recreational" drug use. It is uncontested that certain stimulants (amphetamines most notoriously) have been abused and have been popular as "street drugs." The fact is that most illicit drug users have not become addicts because appetite suppressants were prescribed properly for them by physicians. Furthermore, physicians tend to lump all appetite suppressants together, although the track record in regard to abuse varies dramatically from drug to drug.

A fourth factor is the seamy image of the unscrupulous "fat doctor," whose office is a front for doling out "feel good" pills. Such doctors, sad to say, do exist, but there are also legitimate bariatricians who prescribe drugs wisely and ethically as part of an effective weight reduction regimen.

A final factor is the knowledge that antiobesity drugs can cause harm. In large dosages, amphetamines, for example, can produce a toxic psychosis. Although this is true, it is no more relevant to the proper use of appetite suppressants than the knowledge of cocaine's ability to produce a paranoid psychosis is relevant to the proper use of cocaine as a topical anesthetic. The old drug dinitrophenol, which inhibited energy-rich phosphate bond transfer and increased metabolic rate and oxygen consumption, on the other hand, is no longer used because the side effects from its clinical use were deemed excessive and intolerable.

THE AVAILABLE AGENTS

Prescription Drugs

There are many prescription drugs on the market for the treatment of obesity (see Table 1). Although most of these are stimulants, one, fenfluramine, is a sedative.

TABLE 1. *Popular prescription anorectic drugs*

Generic name	Brand name*	Recommended dose in package insert
Amphetamine (racemic)		5 to 30 mg daily
Dextroamphetamine	Dexedrine®	5 to 10 mg t.i.d. or 10 to 15 mg in extended release form daily
Methamphetamine	Desoxyn®	5 mg t.i.d. or 10 to 15 mg extended release form daily
Amphetamine plus dextroamphetamine resin complex	Biphetamine®	12.5 to 20 mg daily
Benzphetamine	Didrex®	25 to 150 mg daily
Diethylpropion	Tenuate®, Tepanil®	25 mg t.i.d. ± one midevening dose
Fenfluramine	Pondimin®	20 to 40 mg t.i.d.
Mazindol	Sanorex®	1 to 3 mg daily
Phendimetrazine	Plegine®	35 mg b.i.d. or t.i.d.
Phenmetrazine	Preludin®	75 mg daily in extended release form
Phentermine HCL	Adipex®	18.75 to 37.5 mg daily
	Fastin®	30 mg daily
Phentermine Resin	Ionamin®	15 to 30 mg daily

* Some of these drugs are sold generically or by other brand names.

Over-the-Counter Drugs

In recent years, phenylpropanolamine (PPA) has become popular as an over-the-counter (OTC) appetite suppressant. Phenylpropanolamine is an old drug and has been used OTC for decades as an ingredient of cough/cold remedies. It has a remarkably benign track record in regard to this usage. More recently, the FDA asked an advisory committee to review the evidence on PPA as a weight-reducing agent, and the agency was advised that the drug was safe and effective and that its efficacy was statistically difficult to distinguish from standard prescription anorexiants.

Most of the clinical data available for scrutiny in fact deal with PPA/caffeine combinations, but because the animal data are convincing in regard to PPA's effect on food intake and weight, and because in one controlled clinical trial PPA with caffeine was not significantly more effective than PPA alone, the prevailing FDA regulatory philosophy was to allow marketing of both kinds of products. More recently, caffeine has been withdrawn from OTC PPA appetite suppressant products because of the suspicion that the combination was more toxic than PPA alone.

MECHANISM OF ACTION

In theory, weight loss can be achieved in the following ways: (a) decreased food intake, (b) decreased food absorption, and (c) increased metabolism.

Since most appetite suppressants are stimulants, mechanism c has been difficult to rule out as a contributory factor. There is not much support for mechanism b. This leaves mechanism a as the most popular mode of action.

Food intake may be decreased by a depressant effect on appetite and hunger, so that the seeking out of food is diminished, or by allowing satiety to be more readily achieved, i.e., causing a feeling of fullness or satisfaction of hunger after less food intake than would ordinarily be required. Older neurophysiologic experiments in animals supported the existence of both kinds of centers, i.e., "appetite" and "satiety" centers. More recently, however, research has moved away from this simpler focus, and current thinking emphasizes the great complexity of the central and peripheral processes involved in controlling food intake (2,8,9). Anorectic drug research has dealt extensively with the role of neurotransmitters in feeding, with the catecholamines and serotonin receiving the lion's share of attention. Interesting and unpredictable differences have been seen. For instance, despite the apparent chemical similarity of fenfluramine and amphetamines, fenfluramine is less like amphetamine than is mazindol, which is structurally quite different.

Although not readily studied in animals, it has been postulated that the effects of stimulant anorexiants on mood may also play a role in controlling appetite in humans. It is a fact that drugs like amphetamine can elevate mood, and it is also true that depression is often encountered in the early stages of weight control regimens as food intake is decreased. Hence, it is not possible to exclude a useful contribution of stimulant anorexiants via their euphoriant effects.

In experimental animals one can see a rebound hyperphagia when appetite suppressants are discontinued; whether such rebound occurs clinically is less clear.

THE AVAILABLE CLINICAL DATA ON SAFETY AND EFFICACY

Safety

In clinical doses, the stimulant anorexiants are similar in their side effect profile. These drugs tend to produce such adverse effects as insomnia, dysphoria, excitement, agitation, dizziness, tremor, headache, dry mouth, unpleasant taste, impotence, hallucinations, confusion, assaultiveness, panic states, hypertension, palpitations, and tachycardia. With fenfluramine, side effects include drowsiness, vivid dreams, and diarrhea. Phenylpropanolamine has been reported to produce severe hypertension, stroke, and CNS disturbances. Most of the reported PPA cases, which are few in number, have followed the ingestion of overdoses or of combinations of drugs.

There is one troublesome syndrome seen occasionally in patients on amphetamines. Typically, a young woman who has been obese most of her life loses weight and becomes lively and active on drug treatment. If amphetamine is eventually stopped, there is a rebound ballooning up of weight plus a picture of lethargy and depression that is difficult to treat.

Efficacy

There are not many comparative trials available for analysis, and it would be difficult to make a persuasive case for one anorexiant drug being better than another on average. Although comparisons of PPA and prescription anorexiants have generally failed to show statistically significant differences, the trends in such data usually favor the prescription drugs. There is no evidence that tolerance to the anorexiant effects is less likely with one drug than another.

A RATIONAL APPROACH TO THE USE OF ANOREXIANTS

The Need for Multimodal Programs

Most obese patients have to resign themselves to a life of partial deprivation. Since dietary restriction and restraint must be a part of any successful regimen, behavior modification training is also helpful in developing good eating habits. The behavior therapy of obesity includes such techniques as self-monitoring, stimulus control, control of the act of eating (such as slowing down the rate of eating and taking smaller bites), contingency contracting, self-reinforcement, cognitive restructuring, nutrition education, and a social support system (10).

Because the achievement of weight loss tends to cause a decrease in metabolic rate, exercise programs are usually advisable, since this metabolic decrease can be at least partially counteracted by such exercise. Exercise advice should be neither stereotyped nor excessive; the personal preference of the patient for exercise style needs to be listened to and used as the foundation for the exercise program.

If a nondrug obesity program encompassing the above components achieves the desired weight loss, clearly no adjuvant drug therapy is necessary. For most significantly obese patients, however, a drug will need to be added if satisfactory weight loss is to be achieved.

Dosage Schedule Considerations

Attention to dosage regimen may be as important a determinant of success or failure as the choice of drug. For instance, many obese patients are not "large breakfast" eaters and have their big meal of the day in the evening. It is therefore not sensible to prescribe dosage three times daily, before breakfast, lunch, and dinner, for such patients. Giving the initial dose to such patients before lunch makes more sense. Likewise, since drugs need time to be absorbed, reach the site of action, and produce their effect, an hour before the time of desired peak effect is a reasonable time for the ingestion of drug. A range of 30 to 90 min before desired peak effect probably will accommodate the needs of most patients. Since most of the drugs are central nervous system stimulants, the taking of drug late in the day may interfere with sleep. Because of this, the time of the evening meal and of bedtime may have to be modified, as well as the timing of the last dose.

It is not necessary for all obese patients to take appetite suppressants continually. There are individuals who will want to achieve short-term weight loss, such as for a wedding or an audition. Holiday times, such as Thanksgiving and Christmas, pose serious threats to the waistline because of the overeating that occurs at family celebrations. On the other hand, long-term trials indicate that complete tolerance to the effects of appetite suppressants is by no means the rule (1,3,5). Effective doses of appetite suppressants allow many patients to keep weight off for many months (or even indefinitely), although there is considerable variability from person to person.

There is some confusion about the definition of tolerance to an appetite suppressant. On any weight control regimen, the rate of weight loss is greatest early in treatment, and there is an inevitable plateauing of body weight. In a double-blind controlled trial of effective drug against placebo (added to diet, exercise, etc.), the patients on placebo will lose weight for a time but begin to gain weight after a few weeks. The average weight of the patients on active drugs will continue to drop, plateau later, and then stay fairly level. This prevention of weight gain is an extremely important phenomenon and is a measure of maintained efficacy and should not be misinterpreted as tolerance.

A combination of fenfluramine and a stimulant anorexiant may be a useful regimen in some patients, since clinical trials with such a combination indicate that weight loss can be achieved with half doses of each drug taken together that is equivalent to that with full doses of either drug alone. Such a combination is associated with fewer side effects because of the different pharmacodynamics of fenfluramine and stimulant anorexiants.

Special Considerations in the Treatment of Obesity

Other medical conditions may pose serious problems for the management of the obese. Surgery is associated with higher morbidity and mortality not only in the morbidly obese but in the moderately obese as well. Hence, if surgery is elective, an attempt at weight loss should be made before the operation.

In the case of diabetes mellitus or hypertension, there is good evidence that the achievement of weight loss will have a beneficial effect on these underlying diseases. At least in mild cases of these disorders, weight loss may obviate the need for any specific antidiabetic or antihypertensive treatment. Even if weight control alone does not suffice to control blood sugar or blood pressure, it may diminish the dosage requirements of antidiabetic or antihypertensive drugs.

For patients with coronary artery disease or congestive heart failure, there is a clear mechanical benefit if weight loss is achieved, with a diminished work load for the cardiovascular system.

Preventing orthopedic troubles such as low back pain and arthritis of the weight-bearing joints is a good reason for weight control programs in the obese. Even when orthopedic problems already exist, the achievement of weight loss may be a significant factor in rehabilitation.

OTHER DRUGS IN THE TREATMENT OF OBESITY

A variety of other drugs have been proposed for the management of obesity (4). Some, such as human chorionic gonadotrophin, "starch blockers," or bulking agents, seem simply not to work very well. Others, such as digitalis and diuretics, seem irrational. Thyroid preparations will certainly induce hypermetabolism (and weight loss) if taken in sufficiently high doses, but their use has (perhaps unfairly) a bad reputation because of the serious toxicity seen from the use of "diet pills" that contained thyroid hormone, digitalis, and diuretics.

CONCLUSION

Drugs are not the answer to obesity but, as part of a multimodal approach, can have effects that range from mild to profound over the short term as well as the long term. Physicians should stop mouthing unscientific clichés about anorexiants and take seriously the challenge of obesity, which is a serious national health problem (6). There are relatively few medical entities for which preventive measures have been shown to work. Obesity, however, is one medical problem where the achievement of the therapeutic goal has both therapeutic and preventive benefits.

A short-term approach to the control of obesity is not sensible for most overweight patients. Weight that is lost is often promptly put back on by the obese. The role that anorectic drugs should play for a given patient should be determined by mutual decision of the patient and the physician. For some patients, drugs will not be necessary or will not work. For others, intermittent use of the drugs may be a wise choice. Others may require the drugs for the long term. Although we do not know the implications of continuous long-term anorectic drug use, it is not evident that whatever long-term risks are associated with these drugs are greater than the long-term risks of untreated obesity.

REFERENCES

1. Allen, G. S. (1975): *J. Int. Med. Res.,* 3:40–44.
2. Blundell, J. E. (1980): In: *Obesity,* edited by A. J. Stunkard, pp. 182–207. W. B. Saunders, Philadelphia.
3. Bolding, O. T. (1974): *Curr. Ther. Res.,* 16:40–48.
4. Lasagna, L. (1980): In: *Obesity,* edited by A. J. Stunkard, pp. 292–299. W. B. Saunders, Philadelphia.
5. McKay, R. H. G. (1973): *Curr. Med. Res. Opin.,* 1:489–493.
6. NIH Consensus Development Conference (1985): *Ann. Intern. Med.,* 103:147–151.
7. Prout, T. E. (1980): In: *Controversies in Therapeutics,* edited by L. Lasagna, pp. 184–189. W. B. Saunders, Philadelphia.
8. Smith, G. P. (1983): *Lancet,* 2:88–89.
9. Sullivan, A. C., and Green, R. K. (1985): *Fed. Proc.,* 44:135–144.
10. Tan, T.-L., Handford, H. A., and Soldatos, C. R. (1984): *Rational Drug Ther.,* 18(2).

Psychopharmacology:
The Third Generation of Progress,
edited by Herbert Y. Meltzer.
Raven Press, New York © 1987.

CHAPTER 135

Drug Delivery Systems: Applicability to Neuropsychopharmacology

Louis Lemberger, Sigmund Schildcrout, and George Cuff

The treatment of patients with neuropsychiatric diseases is indeed complex. Although many useful, potent therapeutic agents may be available, difficulty in treatment stems from the unresponsiveness, uncooperativeness, or varying degrees of unreliability and noncompliance of patients suffering from severe neurologic or psychiatric diseases. Thus patients with Parkinson's disease, stroke, or other neuropsychiatric afflictions in which hand-mouth coordination and gastrointestinal reflexes are incapacitated present a special problem in drug delivery. In addition, certain diseases presenting with psychotic behavior manifested by irrationality may result in an unwillingness of patients to take medications. Moreover, at times aggressive behavior of patients directed toward nursing staff instructed to administer drugs makes the conventional methods of drug administration impractical. Therefore, a great need exists in neuropsychiatric disorders for unique delivery systems to facilitate the administration of drugs to patients to assure the drug's distribution to its site of action. The main goal of drug delivery is to get the drug to the site of action in optimal concentration to produce the desired pharmacologic effects without producing unacceptable adverse or undesirable effects. Therefore, the various processes of absorption, distribution, metabolism, and excretion play a major role. Once the drug enters the central compartment and distributes to its site of action, several processes are involved in getting it to the site of action and having its effect terminated. The major barrier to absorption or passage of a drug through various systems and conveying it to its site of action is the biomembrane or the cellular membrane. Many processes may be involved when drugs pass through this membrane, and it is important to consider these in developing drug-delivery systems to allow drugs to enter the systemic circulation and distribute to their specific sites of action.

When oral medication can be taken, controlled or sustained-release preparations may increase the duration of the absorptive phase of the drug and thus extend its duration of activity. Therefore, a controlled-release drug preparation may be a valuable adjunct to conventional dosage therapy.

A need also exists for long-acting preparations of injectable drugs, administered by the intramuscular or subcutaneous routes. Such preparations are useful for the administration of antipsychotic drugs. These are given intramuscularly, and are formulated as either insoluble salts, e.g., fluphenazine decanoate, or as solutions in oil. These formulations insure a slow "payout" of drug and assure sufficient plasma and brain concentrations to control the abnormal behavior.

Recently the concept of transdermal administration of medications has been popularized and shown to be of some value in the treatment of certain cardiovascular diseases and motion sickness. This technology may also be of future value in the area of neuropsychopharmacology.

An important drug-delivery system, utilized in research as well as in the prevention and therapy of diseases or conditions, is implantable drug preparations. This concept may employ technology that combines drugs with materials such as silastic or biodegradable matrices. An example of a research usage is the utilization and implantation of morphine pellets in animals. This enables the researcher to produce morphine-dependent animals that can be used to study addiction and intolerance development. From a therapeutic standpoint, usage of this concept is exemplified by the potential benefits derived from implanting Naltrexone, a narcotic antagonist in subcutaneous tissue. This drug-delivery system has been used in an attempt to prevent addiction in highly susceptible populations.

A totally new, clinically useful area involving unique drug-delivery systems is that of infusion pumps employed to administer drugs by either the subcutaneous or intravenous route. The prototype example of this is the insulin infusion pump. Application of this technology has made inroads in the area of neuropsychopharmacology, where drugs such as L-dopa and lisurgide have been given intravenously to control the "on-off" symptoms associated with Parkinson's disease and to assure continuous therapeutic concentrations of the drugs. Implantable pumps have also demonstrated utility in the area of analgesia for the control of severe pain. Studies have shown that individuals using a self-injection apparatus and thus having control over the delivery and dosing regimen of their own pain medication are capable of controlling their pain quite adequately. Thus, drugs such as morphine and other analgesics have been administered by this route.

In addition to the classical neurotransmitters (e.g., norepinephrine, serotonin, dopamine, acetylcholine, etc.), a whole series of neuropeptides have been identified that also are responsible for modulating neuronal function and that can serve as neurotransmitters or cotransmitters. As our understanding and knowledge regarding these new neurotransmitters increase, the need for systemic administration of these novel compounds becomes important. Studying these agents in a clinical research protocol would have limitations because the neuropeptides are not reliably absorbed after oral administration; therefore, preparations have been developed that might facilitate uniform absorption. It appears that some limited success may be achieved in facilitating the transport of these compounds across membranes by administering them via the intranasal route. Two clinical examples of this approach have been with the use of Pitressin (vasopressin) and insulin. This route has also been considered for the administration of enkephalin analogs. Clearly, as new discoveries are made in the area of the pharmacology of the neuropeptides and as their utility is demonstrated in a variety of neuropsychopharmacologic diseases, the intranasal route of administration may be very important and may be accepted similarly to the intranasal use of Pitressin in individuals who have liver cirrhosis, esophageal varices, and elevated portal pressure.

The importance of unique delivery systems can be further underscored based on their use in research studies and their potential adaptability in the therapeutic arena. The pharmaceutical development of various formulations designed to take advantage of very active drugs that may have only limited oral absorption, or of drugs with unique chemical properties that limit their therapeutic utility when given in the usual manner, may be overcome by the use of novel techniques. For example, drugs that have very poor absorption may have their absorption enhanced by allowing the drug to stay in a specific area of the intestinal tract for an optimum period. Likewise, drugs that are rapidly metabolized by the liver and, therefore, have very short durations of activity may have their durations of activity increased either by reformulation in a controlled release preparation, or by possibly using an alternate route, such as a transdermal administration. This latter technique may cause the drug to escape metabolism in the liver or intestinal tract and, therefore, could salvage a drug that would ordinarily be discarded.

SPECIFIC ROUTES AND TECHNIQUES

Oral Route

Oral Immediate Release

The oral route of administration is that which is most widely utilized. This route is most acceptable and when appropriate is the ideal route. The usual type of formulations are capsules and tablets, and these provide an immediate-release form. The solid formulation undergoes disintegration, then dissolution, and the drug can then be absorbed in the appropriate portion of the GI tract. However, in some instances a drug does not provide the necessary pharmacologic response when given in an immediate release preparation, and thus a controlled release formulation is required or desired.

Oral Controlled Release

Rationale.

The dosing regimen for tablets or capsular products may be up to three to four times daily, as illustrated in Fig. 1. With this schedule it is possible for a given dose both to elicit side effects (from the peak plasma level) and to be subtherapeutic (in the period immediately preceding the next dose). Moreover, it is not uncommon for patients to be noncompliant and to miss a dose in the course of normal daily activity. Similar issues must be considered when dealing with sustained-release preparations (Fig. 2). The rationale for oral controlled release medication would thus be (a) minimize patient compliance problems associated with less frequent dosing; (b) minimize side effects by avoiding blood level peaks; (c) enhance therapeutics via more constant blood levels and protection against trough blood levels; (d) produce efficient drug utilization by the body.

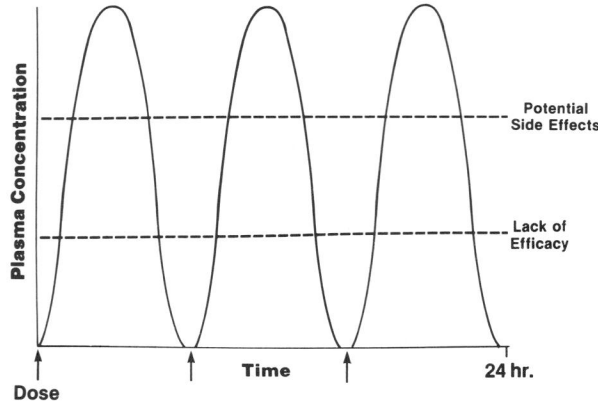

FIG. 1. Illustration of plasma vs time profile for a conventional oral product.

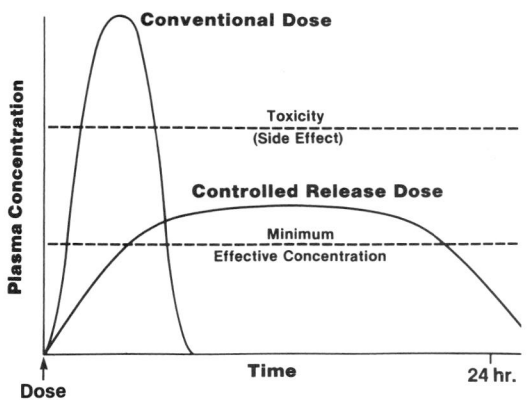

FIG. 2. Comparison of conventional and controlled-release formulations.

General description of concepts.

Some of the concepts that have been used to achieve oral controlled release are illustrated in Fig. 3. The type A system contains drug in an insoluble matrix with release by diffusion (e.g., refs. 1, 2). The type B system contains drug in a soluble core, coated with a soluble/insoluble polymer combination (e.g., refs. 3, 4); the soluble polymer dissolves, creating channels through which the drug can diffuse. In the case of a hydrophilic gum containing matrix, type C, the drug may be released by processes of both diffusion and erosion (5,6). The osmotic pump, type D, is surrounded by a semipermeable membrane that permits water to enter at a controlled rate; the drug solution exits through the laser-drilled hole (7). Additional mechanisms

include the use of erodible coatings, pH-sensitive polymers, and various combinations.

The choice of an oral sustained release system is usually made by the pharmaceutical scientist after careful review of the physical and chemical properties of the drug.

Influence of gastrointestinal transit.

There are several criteria that should be met for oral sustained release to be considered a logical therapeutic alternative. Bianchi and Graziani using X-ray methods determined that the transit time of oral dosage form from mouth to cecum was 3 to 8+ hours (8). Davis and co-workers, using scintigraphic methods, found that tablets and pellets took about 5 to 6 hr to reach the large intestine (9,10). Thus, in the extreme, a drug with a short pharmacological half-life and a duodenal absorption window would be a poor candidate for once-a-day oral therapy.

A logical scheme for justifying the development of a once-a-day dosage form is illustrated in the case of metoprolol (11–16). Metoprolol is completely absorbed after oral administration with an elimination half–life of 3 hr (11). By means of intubation methods, drug was infused directly into the stomach, duodenum, and jejunum (12), jejunum and ileum (13), and colon (14) of humans. These studies concluded that the drug is absorbed from all segments of the gastrointestinal tract except the stomach. The rate of absorption from the jejunum was additionally determined to be unaffected by bile salts and other endogenous secretions (15). Further, the *in vivo* release, absorption of drug, and systemic availability were not influenced by food, when drug was administered via Oros osmotic pump over a 32-hr period (16). All these factors lead to a legitimate rationale for the ongoing clinical trials for metoprolol via the osmotic pump.

Clinical use.

The clinical use of oral controlled release concepts is extensive and a thorough listing is beyond the scope of this writing (see, e.g., ref. 17, for a selected summary through the mid-1970s). One of the more widely investigated drugs for oral sustained release therapy is theophylline. Some examples of studies that have been conducted in support of once-a-day therapy include the establishment of *in vitro/ in vivo* correlations for hydrophilic gum formulations (18), and comparison of inter- and intrasubject variation for sustained release tablet and pellet product (19).

Clomipramine clinical studies have been conducted comparing a once daily schedule of sustained release preparation with similar dosage of three times daily conventional formulation. The two formulations showed similar therapeutics and tolerability in depressed patients (20). Moreover, they were shown to exhibit similar therapeutics and slightly better tolerability in phobic and obsessional patients (21).

Parenteral Route

Usual i.v., i.m., or s.c.

Parenteral administration is the injection of drugs under or through the skin or mucous membrane. A parenteral

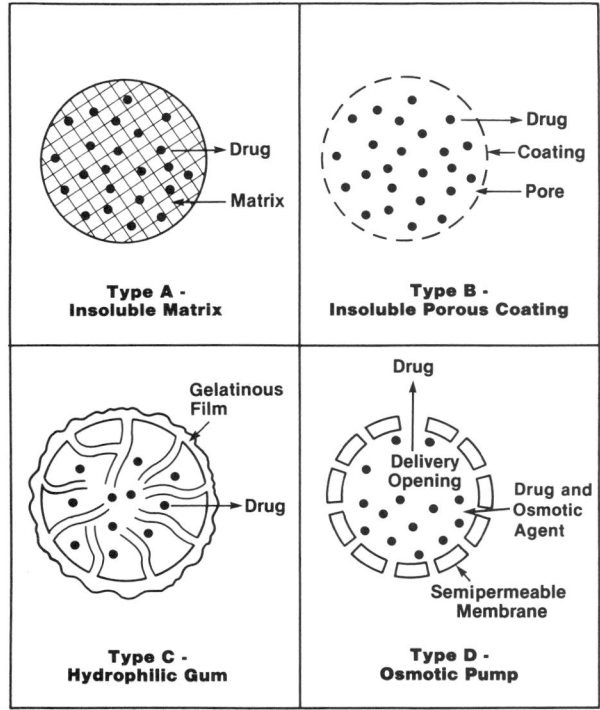

FIG. 3. Concepts for oral controlled-release formulations.

route of administering a drug is used when desired effects from a drug cannot be achieved by simpler routes of dosing. Some indications for choosing a parenteral route are (a) for drugs not absorbed orally; (b) for drugs not stable in the gastric tract; (c) when a rapid onset of action is required; (d) to obtain and maintain precisely controlled blood levels of a drug; (e) patients who are unconscious, uncontrollable, vomiting, or experiencing convulsions; (f) fluid or electrolyte imbalance; (g) hyperalimentation; (h) to achieve a local effect such as a spinal block. The most widely used parenteral routes are intravenous (i.v.), intramuscular (i.m.), and subcutaneous (s.c.). Most parenteral techniques fall into one of these three broad classes.

All parenteral dosage forms should be sterile and pyrogen free. In general, i.v. dosage forms should not contain particulates, although oil-in-water emulsions may be used for hyperalimentation. Other exceptions are noted in the use of microspheres in localizing drugs to specific target organs (22) for treatment of disease. The i.v. route affords the advantage of achieving immediate blood levels of drug and thus a rapid pharmacological activity. This is particularly important in the management of certain emergency situations such as life-threatening cardiac arrhythmias or status epilepticus.

When drugs are to be administered i.v. an aqueous (isotonic) vehicle is preferable. Some agents, such as diazepam, are not sufficiently soluble in aqueous media to be formulated without the use of a cosolvent. Diazepam i.v. may be indicated for emergencies such as status epilepticus, even though the vehicle contains 40% propylene glycol, which could be cardiotoxic if given too rapidly as an intravenous injection (23,24). For neuroleptic drugs, the i.v. route is usually not necessary, except when used during surgery as an adjunct to other analgesics or in such cases as treatment of intractable hiccups (25). Although i.v. administration guarantees the delivery of a drug into the blood as rapidly as possible, it entails acceptance of certain risks, including thrombosis or infection at the site of injection and toxic side effects resulting from too rapid injection rate.

The i.m. and s.c. routes have a slower onset of action than the i.v. route, but generally offer a safer means to administer drugs parenterally. These routes are more popular and convenient for the patient and physician. The i.m. route is preferred over the s.c. route when a more rapid absorption is required. There are a variety of muscle sites available, but the gluteal muscle is often preferred because of its ability to tolerate large volumes of fluid. The most rapid absorption is reported to occur via the deltoid muscle (26), although the volume injected must be restricted to less than 2 ml. Drugs to be administered by the i.m. or s.c. route may be formulated in nonaqueous media and may be formulated as suspensions. The rate of absorption from the i.m. route is more rapid than that from the s.c. route; however, the s.c. route offers more rapid and predictable absorption than the oral route. Some of the factors that affect the rates of drug absorption from the i.m. and s.c. routes include (a) the solubility of the drug in the surrounding fluid; (b) vascularity at the injection site; (c) partition coefficient of the drug or its lipid solubility; (d) vehicle components; (e) particle size if the drug is present as a

suspension; (f) stability of the drug in the injection site; and (g) physiological state of the patient.

The i.m. and s.c. routes do have certain liabilities. Neither route should be used in patients with severe cardiac failure or in cardiovascular collapse, as absorption would be unpredictable. The main risks of i.m. administration are (a) accidental injection into a vein or artery; (b) injection into a nerve; and (c) pain or inflammation at the injection site. Potential adverse effects of s.c. administration include pain and inflammation at the injection site and infection.

One of the primary indications for the i.m. route of administration of neuroleptic agents is in the management of acutely psychotic individuals. Often such individuals resist taking oral medication or may be aggressive and violent. To achieve rapid control of the patient, the i.m. route is both effective and humane. Virtually all major tranquilizers are supplied in an i.m. preparation. The i.m. route also is used for depot injections to provide prolonged blood levels of neuroleptics.

Depot Injectables

A depot injection is one that provides a localized reservoir that gradually releases drug for absorption. Those drugs best suited for depot forms have short half-lives and are very potent, since the total drug required for several weeks of therapy must be supplied in one dosage form. This last problem is often made easier to handle, since the total amount of drug given in a depot is often significantly less than that required for a comparable effect when given orally (27). Depot dosage forms are especially advantageous with psychiatric patients, who may be noncompliant. Patients known to rapidly metabolize oral chlorpromazine have responded to depot fluphenazine (28). Also, since a depot injection is administered in a clinical setting and may last for 2 to 6 weeks, the risk of accidental or intentional overdose is greatly reduced. In the hospital setting, considerable time and effort on the part of the nurses and staff are directed at getting patients to take drugs, administering them, and maintaining an appropriate inventory with records. This burden can be greatly relieved by the use of depot dosage forms. The depot antipsychotic dosage forms are indicated for those who make up the "revolving door" population of hospitals in that they increase the length of time such individuals may be able to live outside a hospital (29). Depot antipsychotic medications should not be administered to a patient unless that patient has been demonstrated to be responsive to a trial of the medication when given orally. If the patient fails to respond, the oral dosage form offers greater flexibility and ease of reducing or stopping the medication so that a different drug could be tried. If a patient exhibits allergy, neuroleptic malignant syndrome, or other toxicity, the results may be fatal when the depot dosage form is administered, since there is no way to reduce the blood levels of the drug for such extended periods (30). Because depots initially release drug slowly, it may take 1 to 2 days to achieve a therapeutic blood level. Clinically this can result in fewer side effects or reduced toxicity of the drug. For example, flupenthixol decanoate has fewer extrapyramidal side effects and less sedation than the dihydrochloride or free base (31,32).

The premise in developing depot injectables entails gradual absorption of drug from a specific site. A number of biological factors affect absorption from depots, but the properties of the drug and dosage form are more amenable to manipulation by the pharmaceutical chemist. The driving force for absorption is the drug concentration (or activity) in the biological fluids at the site of injection. By controlling the drug concentration in the biological fluids at the depot site, the rate of absorption may be controlled. Thus, the most rapidly absorbed dosage form is an aqueous solution. Exceptions to this occur if the drug in solution precipitates at the injection site. This is a common method of decreasing the rate of drug absorption (33–35). For example, sodium phenytoin precipitates in aqueous solution at a pH less than 11.7 (pH of a saturated solution), and 1 g dissolves in about 66 ml water (36). Following i.m. injection the acidic form of phenytoin precipitates in the lower pH of the muscle (37,38). Chlordiazepoxide HCl has an aqueous solubility of 165 mg/ml at room temperature, the free base solubility is 2 mg/ml, and the pKa is 4.76 (39). The i.m. formulation of the hydrochloride contains 20% propylene glycol and has a pH of 3.0. At physiological pH in muscle tissue, precipitation of the free base is thought to occur. Drug precipitation from an injectable solution may occur even when a depot is not desired, causing decreased bioavailability and pain at the site of injection. When the depot forms particulate drug in the muscle, absorption is controlled by the solubility and dissolution rate of the drug. Thus, the particle size (40) has been shown to be proportional to the absorption of drugs. The crystalline form of a drug can significantly affect solubility, and many drugs exhibit polymorphism. A classical example (41) of dissolution rate control by controlling crystallinity and particle size is that of insulin zinc suspensions U.S.P. Prompt insulin zinc suspension is an amorphous zinc complex. Extended insulin zinc suspension is a crystalline zinc complex. The prompt insulin zinc suspension acts more quickly because the amorphous form dissolves more rapidly than the crystalline form and because the amorphous material uses a smaller particle size than the crystalline preparation.

The use of an oil vehicle in which the drug is dissolved is also helpful in controlling drug release. The most widely used oils are corn oil, cottonseed oil, peanut oil, sesame oil, almond oil, and castor oil (42). Sesame oil is used most often because it is generally the most stable. The drug must partition from the oil phase to the surrounding biological fluid. The slow release from oils is a result of the large oil/water partition coefficient, since most neuroleptics tend to be very lipid-soluble compounds. Drugs having small partition coefficients or very poor lipid solubility are not suitable for this dosage form. Some of the factors influencing the absorption of a drug from an oil vehicle are (a) the extent to which the depot remains in one area or spreads to others; (b) absorption of the vehicle (43); and (c) the viscosity of the vehicle. These factors can be controlled to some extent by the judicious choice of oils and by adding a viscosity enhancer to the oil. Gelling agents like aluminum monostearate (44,45) both increase viscosity, thus decreasing molecular diffusion rates, and localize the depot so that the surface area is reduced and

better controlled. The apparent partition coefficient (K) is the crucial factor in the success of this approach and is a function of the drug and the oil system used. The value of K can be changed by using poorly water-soluble salts or prodrug derivatives that are very oil-soluble. Fluphenazine enanthate (heptanoic acid ester) as a solution in sesame oil provides a therapeutic effect lasting for 1 to 3 weeks (46). The enanthate ester undergoes cleavage so that only free fluphenazine crosses the blood-brain barrier (47). Similar results were seen with fluphenazine decanoate. Most reports describe more side effects with the enanthate than with the decanoate ester (48,49), which is more often used. In using megadoses (10 times or more than standard doses) the enanthate has been reported to be more effective than the decanoate (50). Side effects that developed over the 4- to 8-year period using the enanthate were not significant, although not all criteria for tardive dyskinesia could be defined because the severity of schizophrenia prevented a sufficient drug-free period for evaluation. Four of the fourteen patients involved in this study developed orange-sized masses bilaterally (1–2 cm thick) in the buttocks, but there was no correlation with the total dose and volume of oil given.

Infusion Pumps

Infusion pumps have been used for some time in hospitals when a very accurate and precisely controlled rate of administration is needed. Such pumps have tended to be fairly large, heavy, and bulky. In recent years portable infusion pumps for ambulatory patients have been developed to deliver variable or constant rate infusions. These devices may be designed to be worn externally or to be surgically implanted.

External infusion pumps have been used in prolonged treatment of patients requiring chemotherapy, insulin infusion in diabetics, and for the relief of pain. Such pumps avoid the need for multiple injections and provide much better control of drug blood levels than multiple injections. These pumps do have certain potential problems, including slippage of the needle, irritation or infection at the site of the injection pump, failure due to clogged lines, leaking or kinking of the cannula, susceptibility to external trauma, and patient compliance.

Topical Route

Transdermal

Physical features of the skin.

The skin is one of the largest and most accessible organs of the body. It separates the external environment from the underlying blood circulation and serves as a barrier against physical, chemical, and microbial attack. The skin plays principal roles in homeostasis, the regulation of blood pressure and body temperature (51).

History and rationale.

Until recent times the skin has been generally regarded as impermeable (52). However, the application of topical medications traces its origin to the plasters and ointments of the ancient Greeks (53,54). Perhaps the history of modern transdermal delivery systems dates back to 1879 when Murrell first described the use of nitroglycerine (55).

The rationale for transdermal delivery systems for systemic therapy, as contrasted to oral administration, normally includes (a) elimination of the vagaries of gastrointestinal absorption such as pH, food, and transit time; (b) avoidance of the first-pass effect of the liver; (c) providing constant and continuous administration; (d) possible elimination of pulsed-entry-associated side effects; (e) utilization of drugs with short half-lives; (f) simple termination of therapy in mid-dose by removal of the device; (g) limitation to potent drugs (56,57).

General description of devices.

There are currently three principal designs of transdermal delivery systems (Fig. 4). Each system is bounded on one face by a peel strip, which is removed at the time of intended administration to permit the device to be adhered to the appropriate body surface; the other face is bounded by a backing that is impermeable to the drug and protects the product from the external environment. The simplest system in design is type A, which contains a disk of drug in appropriate diffusion matrix and an annular adhesive ring. Next in complexity (to the pharmaceutical manufacturer) is type B, in which the diffusion matrix must additionally be formulated to achieve adhesive properties. Type C systems are a variation of type B, but further engineered with a rate-controlling membrane, to set a maximum limit to release of drug from the device.

Although current interest in transdermal delivery is for systemic indications (see discussion which follows), it has also been shown that some drugs can penetrate to deep tissue in both humans and dogs (58).

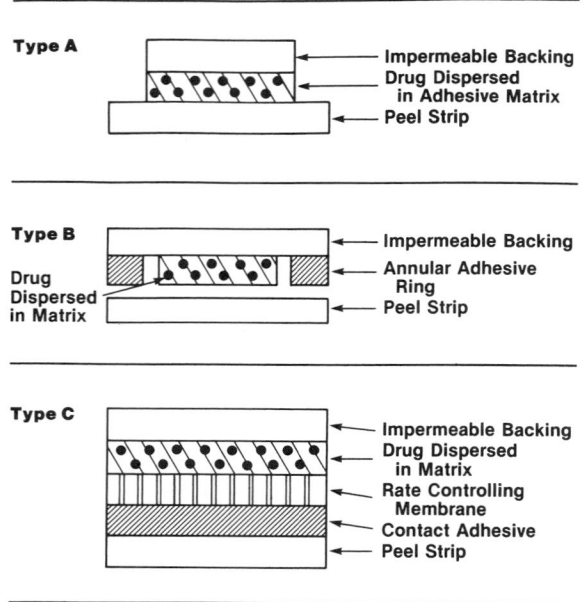

FIG. 4. Components of transdermal therapeutic systems.

Clinical use.

Scopolamine and nitroglycerine. The first drug to be introduced in a transdermal therapeutic system (TTS) was scopolamine (type C of Fig. 4). Scopolamine has a pharmacokinetic half-life of less than 1 hr and had occasionally been used intramuscularly to prevent motion sickness at sea. Pharmacological effects have been shown to correlate with urinary excretion; side effects of dry mouth, drowsiness, and tachycardia are common following intramuscular administration. A TTS-scopolamine patch has been developed for application behind the ear over a 3-day period (59). This patch has been shown to be clinically effective (60), with the most common side effect being dry mouth. It is interesting to note that q.i.d. intramuscular administration at 0.2 mg per dose results in a total 3-day dosage of 3.2 mg; by contrast, the TTS-scopolamine patch delivers 0.5 of the contained 1.5 mg over this period of time.

In late 1981, three transdermal devices were approved by the Food and Drug Administration for administration of nitroglycerine. Following oral administration, nitroglycerine undergoes extensive first-pass metabolism, has a 3-min elimination half-life, a high apparent volume of distribution of approximately 3 liters/kg, and a high plasma clearance of approximately 0.7 liters/min/kg (61). Consequently, sublingual nitroglycerine tablets, which promptly relieve the pain associated with anginal attacks, provide minimal duration of action or prophylactic protection; further, nitroglycerine ointments, which have to be applied several times a day, are regarded as inconvenient, messy, and poorly reproducible (62). In a recent clinical study, Chu et al. (62) compared the nitroglycerine plasma concentrations for 1×/day TTS-nitroglycerine system and 3×/day ointment application. The normalized areas under the curves were determined to be not statistically different. Transdermal nitroglycerine patches have been shown to improve performance and hemodynamic function during treadmill exercise tests (63,64); however, there may be some attenuation with continued use (63), suggesting that tolerance may develop to its pharmacologic action.

Other drugs. In addition to the transdermal delivery systems already discussed for nitroglycerine (1-day delivery) and scopolamine (3-day delivery), there are also published reports on transdermal forms of estradiol and clonidine (53). The clonidine patch is particularly interesting, as it is designed to deliver up to 0.3 mg/day for 1 week (65).

Iontophoresis

The conventional transdermal therapeutic systems rely on passive diffusion to deliver drugs through the skin. However, for molecules that are charged (either naturally, or in the particular limited pH ranges), it has been shown that greatly enhanced transport can be achieved by the application of low-level direct current, a process known as iontophoresis. Iontophoresis has been used to treat hyperhidrosis (66) and to deliver topical anesthetics (67), antiviral agents (68), and antiinflammatory drugs (69). In pigs, the animals whose skins are thought to be closest to humans, there has been a report of iontophoretic insulin delivery evidencing transport by both a reduction in blood glucose and increase in serum insulin levels (70). Considering the high molecular weight of insulin, this may have positive implications for neuropeptides that would otherwise be deactivated via the oral route.

Implants

Rationale.

The ideal drug delivery system would sense a physiological need and deliver the therapeutic agent via a feedback mechanism, as per the concept of glucose-sensor-actuated insulin pumps (71). Lacking the sophistication of elaborately fail-safe-controlled feedback mechanisms, the next best alternative would be a continuous intravenous infusion at a predetermined basal rate. However, with the risks, medical supervision, and hospitalization requirements of the continuous intravenous route, a practical alternative might thus become the subcutaneously implanted control delivery matrix.

An effective subcutaneous drug delivery system would have to fulfill many of the following requirements for the duration of treatment: (a) facilitate and maximize patient compliance; (b) release drug at a controlled rate while reducing side effects; (c) not require major surgery for implantation; (d) free of potential medical complications; (e) minimal risk of misuse or unauthorized termination; (f) readily retrievable by medical personnel (72).

Historical.

The modern era of the use of polymeric materials to control drug delivery probably owes its origin to a chance observation by Folkman and Long in the early 1960s: that silicone polymers absorb certain dyes from solution and release them reversibly. This finding was followed by studies involving the use of implanted silicone capsules for prolonged administration of cardioregulatory agents (73) and anesthetics (74). In 1966 Dziuk and Cook reported on the permeability of silicone polymers to a variety of steroids. They also determined that implanted melangestrol-acetate-containing silicone capsules would inhibit fertility in cattle (75). These results were confirmed by Kincl and co-workers (76), who further determined that silicones were considerably more permeable to steroids than other polymers.

Consideration of bioerodible polymers for surgical implant was stimulated by Kulkarni and co-workers in 1966 (77). They reported that polylactic acid (PLA) appeared to be a suitable material for surgical implantation, as it undergoes hydrolytic deesterification to lactic acid, a normal product of muscle metabolism. Histological studies demonstrated that PLA was nontoxic and nonreactive to tissue. Some of the early animal experiments involving polylactic acid as a drug delivery composite involved systems for narcotic antagonists (78) and anticancer agents (79).

Considerations for use.

The usual indication for an implanted drug delivery system is the treatment of a chronic condition. Major therapeutic concerns must include some assurance against the possibility of dose dumping. Depending on the mechanism of drug release, an additional consideration would be the time to achieve steady state. Further, the release rate may tend to decrease with time due to both depletion of drug and fibrotic tissue encapsulation, and this must be taken into account, since the desired therapeutic effect would be diminished.

Biological compatibility is another subject of major concern. The acute phase of the inflammatory reaction leads to the formation of an exudate and fibrous network at the affected site. Vascular and lymphatic systems are activated and may generate an immune response. Further, leaching out of additives can cause toxic reactions. Biological compatibility with soft tissues, ease of fabrication, and excellent mechanical properties have made silicone-based materials the most widely used in implants. However, silicones require surgical removal, whereas the polylactic acid series can be bioerodible and biodegradable.

Applications.

As mentioned previously, the silicones have been the most widely used materials in drug delivery implants. Early applications were in contraceptive steroid administration to women (80,81), where the contraceptive effectiveness was found to be dependent on the dose administered. Other agents delivered from silicone implants include antiinflammatory drugs to rats (82) and antineoplastic agents to hamsters (83).

Another material that appears to exhibit acceptable biocompatibility properties for implant purposes is ethylene/vinyl acetate (EVA). The subcutaneous implantation of insulin-containing EVA disks to diabetic rats has been shown to produce normoglycemic blood levels within 1 day with the effects lasting nearly 1 month (84). After the insulin appeared to have stopped being released from the disks, as indicated by return to the hyperglycemic state, new disks were implanted; the blood levels were then found to return to the normoglycemic state.

Implantable drug delivery matrices have also been used to induce diseased states in animals. An example of this is the implantation of deoxycorticosterone acetate-releasing silicone pellets in rats to develop an animal model for hypertension (85). Similarly, to study narcotic addiction, morphine sulfate-releasing silicone pellets have been implanted in rats (86).

A drug delivery device that has been used for continuous controlled delivery to laboratory animals is the subcutaneously implanted osmotic pump. The literature on the use of this device is immense; some drugs that have been administered include insulin (87), morphine sulfate (88), haloperidol (89), and dopamine (90).

Copolymers of lactic and glycolic acid have been used to produce naltrexone-releasing beads for narcotic antagonism studies. In both monkeys and mice, *in vitro* and *in vivo* release profiles were determined to be very similar (91). Narcotic antagonist activity for these biodegradable beads was found to persist for more than 1 month.

Lactic/glycolic copolymer beads containing naltrexone have also been studied clinically by implantation in humans

(92). The results demonstrated that opiate effects could be successfully blocked for up to 1 month if therapeutic drug levels were maintained. However, varying degrees of tissue inflammation were noted in most of the subjects, raising the question about the feasibility of this approach with the present vehicle system.

Intranasal

The nasal cavity is the area between the floor of the cranium and the roof of the mouth, extending anteriorly to the nostrils and posteriorly to the pharynx. The primary physiological function of the nasal cavity is to modify the inhaled air by removing particulates and by controlling the temperature and humidity of the air. The physical features responsible for modifying the air cause considerable resistance to the airflow as well as an intimate contact between the airstream and the mucosal surfaces. The highly vascular nasal mucosa offers an opportunity for rapid absorption of compounds that may be degraded in the GI tract, undergo extensive presystemic hepatic metabolism, or not be absorbed when taken orally. The nasal mucosa has very little capacity for metabolism of drugs (93). The nasal circulatory and mucociliary systems are important features for removal of materials from the nasal cavity, and anything that influences their behavior can markedly affect drug absorption. For example, a vasoconstrictive agent may reduce absorption simply by reducing the local blood flow. Irritating agents may evoke excessive secretion of mucus and remove a drug before absorption is complete.

Drugs are usually administered intranasally as drops or as a spray. Hardy et al. utilized gamma scintigraphy to assess coverage of nasal mucosa and clearance of ^{99}Tc-labeled human serum albumin when administered as a drop or a spray (94). They found that one drop spread more extensively than the spray and that three drops covered most of the wall of the nasal cavity. The more intimate contact of drops with the nasal cavity suggests more complete absorption than from a spray. Y. W. Chien and S. F. Chang have reviewed the development of nasal dosage forms (95).

Certain drugs are effectively absorbed when administered intranasally as a powder. For example, cocaine has been reported to provide a slightly more rapid peak plasma level when administered intranasally as crystals rather than a solution (96). Further, the mean elimination half-life of cocaine was greater when given intranasally than orally. This may be because the vasoconstrictive action of cocaine on the nasal vasculature results in prolonged absorption and is consistent with the finding that cocaine was present on nasal mucosa 3 hr after application in humans (97,98).

Insulin

Insulin currently is administered to diabetics by injection. The discomfort, local reactions, and inconvenience experienced by many make an alternative route attractive. Recently Hirai et al. reported that mixtures of insulin and a surfactant (sodium glycocholate, saponin, or polyoxy-

ethylene-9-laurylether) could be given intranasally to dogs and resulted in elevated serum insulin levels (99). Other researchers (100,101) have reported that an intranasally administered insulin-bile salt aerosol provided reproducible kinetics, with the peak insulin level seen in 10 to 15 min. The efficiency of intranasal insulin dosing was found to be a fraction of that obtained after i.v. administration. The authors note that a local nasal irritation, manifested as a burning sensation, occurred with the bile salts. Yakosuka et al. in 1977 described the nasal absorption of insulin in 18 healthy adults (102). They found the use of 1% sodium glycocholate caused a greater reduction in glucose levels within 15 min of intranasal administration. The peak blood levels of insulin when given intranasally were almost as rapid as when given i.v. and more rapid than when given subcutaneously.

Peptides and Neuropeptides

In general, peptides are not effective when taken orally, making the intranasal route an attractive alternative. One example is vasopressin or antidiuretic hormone (ADH), used as intranasal lysine vasopressin in treating diabetes insipidus. A snuff powder form has been used but has the potential for local, systemic, and pulmonary allergic reactions (103). Intranasal lysine vasopressin has practically eliminated these side effects. Luteinizing hormone-releasing hormone (LHRH) is suitable for treatment of cryptorchidism (104), even though only 1.5% of the administered dose is absorbed. Surprisingly, absorption of LHRH is not affected by common colds and rhinitis. LHRH analogs such as Nafarelin acetate have been investigated for contraception (105). Absorption was enhanced by using a concentrated solution and the relative bioavailability was found to be 10%. Anovulation was achieved in women after once daily dosing, thus providing a convenient and effective method of contraception. In patients with cortisol deficiencies, corticotropin (ACTH) prolonged release formulations cannot be used for long-term therapy because they alter normal adrenal function and can cause adrenal atrophy. However, ACTH administered intranasally may prevent the adrenal cortex atrophy seen with constant blood levels of ACTH. ACTH and related peptides are known to enhance motivational and attentional processes and may affect memory and retrieval processes (106,107). Various neuropeptides, such as endorphins, enkephalins, substance P, somatostatin, neurotensin, and cholecystokinin, have been suggested as having roles in mental illness (106,108,109), although these are not understood. However, any therapeutic applications of such agents will require absorption from some delivery system, and the nasal route may become a very important part of such treatment.

Miscellaneous

A variety of other drug-delivery systems and routes of administration exist, but none currently represent a primary mode of treatment for neuropsychiatric illness. These include suppositories, sublingual or buccal dosage forms, inhalation methods, prodrugs, liposomes, microcapsules, and microspheres.

Suppositories

Suppositories may be administered into the rectum, vagina, or urethra. Generally the rectal route is used when systemic drug absorption is desired. A suppository may be used to avoid the first-pass effect of the liver or for drugs unstable in the stomach or small intestine. This route is indicated when a patient is nauseated or vomiting, unconscious, having an asthmatic attack, or having other illnesses where there is difficulty in swallowing or a likelihood of choking. The choice of vehicle can alter rate and extent of absorption, and it must be nonirritating. A discussion of vehicles commonly used is given by Hersey (110).

Sublingual and Buccal

The sublingual and buccal administration of drugs like nitroglycerin or methyltestosterone provides rapid drug absorption, avoids the first-pass effect with the liver, and circumvents the possibility of degradation in the stomach or small intestine. The highly vascular mucosa in the mouth has no stratum corneum, thus most drugs have a high degree of permeability across the oral mucosa. The drug is absorbed through the sublingual or buccal vasculature and carried through the jugular vein to the superior vena cava and directly into the heart and arterial circulation. Patients should be instructed, after a sublingual or buccal tablet has been placed in position, to minimize eating, drinking, chewing, smoking, and swallowing saliva until the tablet is completely dissolved.

Inhalation

The inhalation route takes advantage of the permeability, surface area, and vascularity of the lung tissue, which results in rapid absorption. Inhalation also avoids the first-pass liver effect. Most agents are presented as gases, mists, aerosols, or very fine particles. Delivery of particulates such as cromolyn sodium is complicated by problems associated with particle size control and efficiency of delivery, since much of the drug is lost in the mouth and trachea prior to reaching the lungs (111). This route is very effective for treating asthma with β-agonists and steroids. The pulmonary tissue has a highly developed cytochrome p-450 system and is capable of phase I oxidations as well as phase II conjugation reactions, such as glucuronidation and sulfation (111). Although this route is not used therapeutically in neuropsychopharmacology, it is important as a route of administration for drugs of abuse including cannabis, nicotine, and volatile solvents.

Prodrugs

Prodrugs are chemical derivatives of drugs that regenerate the free drug *in vivo*. Prodrugs may be more stable, more efficiently absorbed, formulated into controlled-release products, or less susceptible to metabolism than the active drug. Prodrugs have been used extensively in injectable depot dosage forms. An example previously discussed is fluphenazine enanthate. This approach may have considerable potential in neuropsychopharmacology in that it provides a means to allow drugs to cross the blood-brain barrier. An example of systems described by N. Bodor (112) entails the conversion of the charged quaternary pyridinium salt of N-methylpyridinium-2-carbaldoxime (2-PAM) into the corresponding dihydropyridine, which as a tertiary amine would easily penetrate the lipoidal blood-brain barrier. Subsequent oxidation regenerated the active 2-PAM. This approach allowed 13 times more pro-2-PAM than 2-PAM to cross the blood-brain barrier.

Liposomes

Liposomes are spherical vesicles made of a thin lipid membrane enclosing an aqueous system or multiple concentric lipid membranes enclosing multiple concentric aqueous spaces. The aqueous space contains the drug of interest. The size varies from about 0.2 to 20 μm. Liposomes containing thyrotropin releasing hormone (TRH) have been reported to deliver TRH across the blood-brain barrier of rabbits (113). However, only 0.44% of the injected dose was taken up by the brain. The barriers to obtaining a sufficient efficiency of brain uptake by liposomes are considerable. However, if these problems are resolved, the ability to deliver peptides and hormones to the CNS could be very important in neuropsychopharmacology.

Microcapsules and Microspheres

Microcapsules or microspheres are utilized to deliver drugs by many different routes. Systems have been developed to deliver peptides, steroids (114), and other drugs for prolonged periods as injectable depots of microparticulates suspended in a vehicle. The release of a drug may be by diffusion through a polymer membrane or as a result of erosion of a matrix material. The polymers used must be biodegradable and biocompatible and may be synthetic or of natural origin. Numerous systems have been researched for delivery of microsphere systems to specific organs (115). Most of this work has been directed toward treatment of various tumors, with relatively little use of microspheres in the treatment of neuropsychiatric illnesses.

SUMMARY AND CONCLUSIONS

Implementation of the technology developed in the pharmaceutic field of drug-delivery systems will be beneficial to the treatment of neuropsychiatric disorders. Changes in our concept of drugs, such as the development of drugs that are peptides and our desire to produce continuous pharmacologic effects without variability in blood concentrations, have created a need to utilize this new technology. This should result in more predictable clinical effects, better patient compliance, and advances in the treatment of certain disease states.

REFERENCES

1. Schwartz, J. B., Simonelli, A. P., and Higuchi, W. I. (1968): *J. Pharm. Sci.,* 57:278–282.
2. Goodhart, F. W., McCoy, R. H., and Ninger, F. C. (1974): *J. Pharm. Sci.,* 63:1748–51.
3. Coletta, V., and Rubin, H. (1964): *J. Pharm. Sci.,* 53:953–955.
4. Wood, J. H., and Syarto, J. (1964): *J. Pharm. Sci.,* 53:877–881.
5. Lapidus, H., and Lordi, N. G. (1966): *J. Pharm. Sci.,* 55:840–843.
6. Huber, H. E., Dale, L. B., and Christenson, G. L. (1966): *J. Pharm. Sci.,* 55:974–976.
7. Theeuwes, F. (1975): *J. Pharm. Sci.,* 64:1987–1991.
8. Bianchi, L., and Graziani, C. (1984): *Curr. Therap. Res.,* 36:797–809.
9. Davis, S. S. (1983): In: *Topics in Pharmaceutical Sciences,* edited by D. D. Breimer, p. 205–214. Elsevier, Amsterdam.
10. Davis, S. S., Hardy, J. G., Taylor, M. J., Whalley, D. R., and Wilson, C. G. (1984): *Int. J. Pharmaceutics,* 21:167–177.
11. Regardh, C. G., and Johnsson, G. (1980): *Clin. Pharmacokinet.,* 5:557–569.
12. Jobin, G., Cortot, A., Godbillon, J., Duval, M., Schoeller, J., Hirtz, J., and Bernier, J. (1985): *Br. J. Clin. Pharmacol.,* 19:97S–105S.
13. Vidon, N., Evard, D., Godbillon, J., Rongier, M., Duval, M., Schoeller, J., Bernier, J., and Hirtz, J. (1985): *Br. J. Clin. Pharmacol.,* 19:107S–112S.
14. Godbillon, J., Evard, D., Vidon, N., Duval, M., Schoeller, J., Bernier, J., and Hirtz, J. (1985): *Br. J. Clin. Pharmacol.,* 19:113S–118S.
15. Evard, D., Vidon, N., Godbillon, J., Bovet, M., Duval, M., Schoeller, J., Bernier, J., and Hirtz, J. (1985): *Br. J. Clin. Pharmacol.,* 19:119S–125S.
16. Lecaillon, J. B., Massias, P., Schoeller, J., and Hbadie, E. (1985): *Br. J. Clin. Pharmacol.,* 19:245S–249S.
17. Ballard, B. E. (1978): In: *Sustained and Controlled Release Drug Delivery Systems,* edited by J. R. Robinson, pp. 1–70. Marcel Dekker, New York.
18. Nakano, M., Ohmori, N., Ogata, A., Sugimoto, K., Tobino, Y., Iwaoku, R., and Juni, K. (1983): *J. Pharm. Sci.,* 72:378–380.
19. Pollack, G. M., Baswell, B., Szefler, S. J., and Shen, D. D. (1984): *Int. J. Pharmaceutics,* 21:3–16.
20. Bloom, A. J., Hevest, H. P., Krypsin-Exner, K., and Van der Poel, F. W. (1983): *Ther. Vinschau.,* 40:805–809.
21. Paula, A. J. M., Oggero, U., and Vale, R. D. C. (1982): *J. Bras. Psiquiatria,* 31:63.
22. Tomlinson, E., Burger, J. J., Schoonderwoerd, E. M. A., and McVie, J. G. (1984): In: *Microspheres and Drug Therapy,* edited by S. S. Davis, J. G. McVie, and E. Tomlinson, pp. 75–89. Elsevier, Amsterdam.
23. Ginn, P. D. (1975): In: *Applied Therapeutics for Clinical Pharmacists,* edited by M. A. Koda-Kimble, L. Young, and B. Katcher, p. 592. Applied Therapeutics, San Francisco.
24. *Physician's Desk Reference* (1984): B. Huff, managing editor, p. 1671.
25. *Physician's Desk Reference* (1984): B. Huff, managing editor, pp. 1896–1899.
26. Duma, R., and Akers, M. (1984): In: *Pharmaceutical Dosage Forms: Parenteral Medications, Vol. 1,* edited by K. H. Vis, L. Lochman, and H. Lieberman, pp. 13–45. Marcel Dekker, New York.
27. Lee, V., and Robinson, J. (1978): In: *Sustained and Controlled Release Drug Delivery Systems,* edited by J. Robinson, pp. 123–210. Marcel Dekker, New York.
28. Adamson, L., Curry, S. H., Bridges, P. K., Firestone, A. F., Lavin, N. I., Lewis, D. M., Watson, R. D., Xavier, C. M., and Anderson, J. A. (1973): *Dis. Nerv. Syst.,* 34:181–191.
29. Denham, J., and Adam, L. (1971): *Acta Psychiatr. Scand.,* 47:420.
30. Gold, D. (1984): *Hosp. Formul.,* 19:153–176.
31. Nielson, I., Pedersen, V., Nymark, M., Franck, K., Boeck, V., Fjalland, B., and Christensen, A. (1973): *Acta Pharmacol. Toxicol.,* 33:353–362.
32. Christensen, A., and Nielsen, I. (1974): *Psychopharmacologia,* 34:119–126.
33. Ritschel, W. (1973): In: *Drug Design,* edited by E. Ariens, *Vol. 4,* pp. 75–92. Academic Press, New York.
34. Thompson, R. (1960): *Parenteral Drug Assoc. Bull.,* 14:6–17.
35. Schroeder, H., and DeLuca, P. (1974): *Parenteral Drug Assoc. Bull.,* 28:1–14.
36. *Merck Index,* 10th ed., p. 7210. Merck and Company, Rahway, New Jersey.
37. Wilensky, A. (1973): *Neurology,* 23:318–324.
38. Serrano, E., Roye, D., Hammer, R., and Wilder, J. (1973): *Neurology,* 23:311–317.
39. MacDonald, A. (1972): In: *Analytical Profiles of Drug Substances,* edited by K. Florey, *Vol. 1,* pp. 25, 26, 45. Academic Press, New York.
40. Buckwalter, F., and Dickson, H. (1958): *J. Am. Pharm. Assoc./Sci. Ed.,* 47:661–666.
41. Haleblian, J., and McCrone, W. (1969): *J. Pharm. Sci.,* 58:911–929.
42. Boylan, J., and Fites, Alan (1979): In: *Modern Pharmaceutics,* edited by G. Banker and C. Rhodes, pp. 429–478. Marcel Dekker, New York.
43. Deanesly, R., and Parkes, A. (1933): *J. Physiol. (Lond.),* 78:155–160.
44. Romansky, M., and Rittman, G. (1944): *Science,* 100:196–198.
45. Thompson, R., and Hecht, R. (1959): *Am. J. Clin. Nutr.,* 7:311–317.
46. Daniels, T., and Jorgensen, E. (1977): In: *Textbook of Organic Medicinal and Pharmaceutical Chemistry,* 7th ed., edited by C. Wilson, O. Giswald, and R. Doerge, p. 389. J. B. Lippincott, Philadelphia.
47. Ebert, A. G., and Hess, S. M. (1965): *J. Pharmacol. Exp. Ther.,* 148:412–421.
48. Christodoulidis, H., and Frangos, H. (1975): *Curr. Ther. Res.,* 18:193–198.
49. Davis, J., Janicak, P., Linden, R., Maloney, J., and Pavkovic, I. (1983): In: *Neuroleptics: Neurochemical, Behavioral, and Clinical Perspectives,* edited by J. Coyle and S. Enna, pp. 15–64. Raven Press, New York.
50. Dencker, S., Enoksson, P., Johansson, R., Lundin, L., and Malm, U. (1981): *Acta Psychiatr. Scand.,* 63:1–12.
51. Chien, Y. W. (1982): *Novel Drug Delivery Systems,* Chapter 5, pp. 149–217. Marcel Dekker, New York.
52. Scheuplein, R. J., and Bronaugh, R. L. (1983): In: *Biochemistry and Physiology of the Skin,* edited by L. A. Goldsmith, pp. 1255–1295. Oxford University Press, New York.
53. Shaw, J. E., and Mitchell, C. (1983/84): *J. Toxicol. Cutan. Ocular Toxicol.,* 2:249–266.
54. Kligman, A. M. (1984): *Am. Heart J.,* 108:200–206.
55. Murrell, W. (1879): *Lancet,* 1:80,113,151,225. In: Thompson, R. H., *Angiology,* 34:23, 1983.
56. Shaw, J. E., Chandrasekaran, S. K., and Taskovich, L. (1975): *Pharmaceutical J.,* Sept. 27, p. 325–328.
57. Chandrasekaran, S. K., Benson, H., and Urquhart, J. (1978): In: *Sustained and Controlled Release Delivery Systems,* edited by J. R. Robinson, Chapter 7, pp. 557–593. Marcel Dekker, New York.
58. Rabinowitz, J. L., and Baker, D. (1984): *J. Clin. Pharmacol.,* 24:532–539.
59. Shaw, J., and Urquhart, J. (1980): *Trends Pharmacol. Sci.,* April, pp. 208–211.
60. Shaw, J. E., Bayne, W., and Schmitt, L. (1976): *Clin. Pharmacol. Ther.,* 19:115.
61. Karim, A. (1983): *Angiology,* 34:11–22.
62. Chu, L., Gale, R. M., Schmitt, L. G., and Shaw, J. E. (1984): *Angiology,* 35:545–552.
63. Hollenberg, M. (1984): *Am. Heart J.,* 108:223.
64. Thompson, R. H. (1983): *Angiology,* 34:23–31.
65. Shaw, J. E. (1984): *Am. Heart J.,* 10:217–223.
66. Grice, K. (1980): *Physiotherapy,* 66:43–44.
67. Gangarosa, L. P. (1981): *Methods Find. Exp. Clin. Pharmacol,* 3:83–93.
68. Hill, J. M., Gangarosa, L. P., and Park, N. H. (1977): *Ann. NY Acad. Sci.,* 22:604–612.

69. Bertolucci, L. E. (1982): *J. Orthop. Sports Phys. Therapy*, 4:103–108.
70. Stephen, R. L., Petelenz, T. J., and Jacobsen, S. C. (1984): *Biomed. Biochim. Acta*, 43:553–558.
71. Soegijoko, S., Selam, J. L., Ferrand, D., Mirouze, J., Pham, T. C., Pistoulet, B., and Renaud, F. (1982): *Horm. Metab. Res. (Suppl.)*, Ser. 12:165.
72. Chien, Y. W. (1982): *Novel Drug Delivery Systems*, pp. 311–412. Marcel Dekker, New York.
73. Folkman, J., and Long, D. M. (1964): *Ann. NY Acad. Sci.*, 111:857–868.
74. Folkman, J., Winsey, S., and Moghul, T. (1968): *Anesthesiology*, 29:410–418.
75. Dziuk, P. J., and Cook, B. (1966): *Endocrinology*, 78:208–211.
76. Kincl, F. A., Benagiano, G., and Anges, I. (1968): *Steroids*, 11:673–680.
77. Kulkarni, R. K., Pani, K., Neuman, C., and Leonard, F. (1966): Technical Report 6608, Walter Reed Army Medical Center, Washington, DC.
78. Woodland, J. H. R., and Yoltes, S. (1973): *J. Med. Chem.*, 16:897–901.
79. Yolles, S., Leofe, T. D., and Meyer, F. J. (1975): *J. Pharm. Sci.*, 64:115–116.
80. Croxatto, H., Diaz, S., Vera, R., Etchart, M., and Atria, P. (1969): *Am. J. Obstet. Gynecol.*, 105:1135–1138.
81. Tatum, H. J., Coutinho, E. M., Filho, J. A., and Santanna, R. S. (1969): *Am. J. Obstet. Gynecol.*, 105:1139–1143.
82. Jones, R. C., and Datko, L. J. (1977): *Agents Actions*, 7:555–562.
83. Long, D. M., Sehgal, L. R., DeRios, M. E., Rios, M. V., Szanto, P. B., and Forrest, R. (1973): *Rev. Surg.*, 30:229–240.
84. Creque, H. M., Langer, R., and Folkman, J. (1980): *Diabetes*, 29:37–40.
85. Chien, Y. W., Lambert, H. J., and Rozek, L. F. (1976): In: *Controlled Release Polymeric Formulations*, edited by D. Paul and F. Harris, ACS Symposium Series No. 33, American Chemical Society, pp. 72–86.
86. McGinity, J. W., and Mehta, C. S. (1978): *Pharmacol. Biochem. Behav.*, 9:705–708.
87. Harshfield, D. L., and Griffey, M. A. (1979): *Fed. Proc.*, 38:878.
88. Lange, D. G., Fujimoto, J. M., and Roerig, S. C. (1979): *Pharmacologist*, 21:228.
89. Login, I. S., Nagy, I., and MacLeod, R. M. (1979): *Physiologist*, 22:72.
90. Moore, R. H. (1979): *Fed. Proc.*, 38:858.
91. Wise, D. L., Schwope, A. D., Harrigan, S. E., McCarthy, D. A., and Howes, J. F. (1978): In: *Polymeric Delivery Systems*, edited by R. J. Kostelnik, p. 75. Midland Macromolecular Monographs. Gordon and Breach, New York.
92. Chiang, C. N., Kishimoto, A., Barnett, G., and Hollister, L. E. (1985): *Psychopharmacol. Bull.*, 21:672–675.
93. Parr, G. (1983): *Pharm. Int.*, 4:202–205.
94. Hardy, J., Lee, S., and Wilson, C. (1985): *J. Pharm. Pharmacol.*, 37:294–297.
95. Chien, Y. W., and Chang, S. F. (1985): In: *Transnasal Systemic Medications*, edited by Y. W. Chien, pp. 1–100. Elsevier Science Publishers, Amsterdam.
96. Wilkinson, P. K., Dyke, C. V., Jatlow, P., Barash, P., and Byck, R. (1980): *Clin. Pharmacol. Ther.*, 27:386–394.
97. Byck, R., Jattow, P., Barash, P., and Dyke, C. V. (1976): In: *Cocaine and Other Stimulants*, edited by E. H. Ellinwood and M. M. Kilbey, pp. 629–646. Plenum Press, New York.
98. Dyke, C., Barash, P. G., Jatow, P., and Byck, R. (1976): *Science*, 195:859–861.
99. Harai, S., Ikenaga, T., and Matsuzawa, T. (1978): *Diabetes*, 27:296–299.
100. Moses, G., Gordon, M., Carey, C., and Flier, J. S. (1983): *Diabetes*, 32:1040–1047.
101. Flier, S., Moses, A. C., Gordon, G. S., and Silver, R. S. (1985): In: *Transnasal Systemic Medications*, edited by Y. W. Chien, pp. 217–226. Elsevier Science Publishers, Amsterdam.
102. Yokosuka, T., Omori, Y., Hirata, Y., and Hirai, S. (1977): *J. Jpn. Diab. Soc.*, 20:146–152.
103. Gambertoglio, J. G., and Mangini, R. J. (1978): In: *Applied Therapeutics for Clinical Pharmacists*, 2nd ed., edited by M. Koda-Kimble, B. Katcher, and L. Young, p. 374. Applied Therapeutics, San Francisco.
104. Sandow, J., and Petri, W. (1985): In: *Transnasal Systemic Medications*, edited by Y. Chien, pp. 183–199. Elsevier Science Publishers, Amsterdam.
105. Vickery, B. H., Anik, S., Chaplin, M., and Henzl, M. (1985): In: *Transnasal Systemic Medications*, edited by Y. W. Chien, pp. 201–215. Elsevier Science Publishers, Amsterdam.
106. DeWied, D. (1982): *Eur. J. Clin. Invest.*, 12:281–284.
107. Pigache, R. M., and Rigter, H. (1981): *Front. Horm. Res.*, 8:193–207.
108. Manchanda, R., and Hirsch, S. (1982): *Int. Pharmacopsychiatry*, 17:147–152.
109. Tamminga, C. (1983): In: *Neuroleptics: Neurochemical, Behavioral and Clinical Perspectives*, edited by J. Coyle and S. Enna, pp. 281–295. Raven Press, New York.
110. Hersey, J. (1979): In: *Modern Pharmaceutics*, edited by G. Banker and C. Rhodes, pp. 565–589. Marcel Dekker, New York.
111. Juliano, R. L. (1984): *Pharmac. Ther.*, 24:355–365.
112. Bodor, N. (1977): In: *Design of Biopharmaceutical Properties Through Prodrugs and Analogs*, edited by E. Roche, pp. 98–135. American Pharmaceutical Association Academy of Pharmaceutical Sciences, Washington, D.C.
113. Postmes, J. and Coengracht, J. (1983): *J. Drug Res.*, 8(9) 2051–2053.
114. Lim, F. (1984): In: *Biomedical Applications of Microencapsulation*, CRC Press.
115. Davis, S. S., Illum, L., McVie, J., and Tomlinson, E. (1984): *Microspheres and Drug Therapy*, Elsevier, Amsterdam.

Psychopharmacology:
The Third Generation of Progress,
edited by Herbert Y. Meltzer.
Raven Press, New York © 1987.

CHAPTER 136

Monoamine Oxidase Inhibiting Drugs: Pharmacologic and Therapeutic Issues

Donald S. Robinson and Neil M. Kurtz

Over the past decade monoamine oxidase inhibitors (MAOIs) have gained widespread acceptance as effective alternatives to the more widely prescribed tricyclic antidepressants. In addition, more recent studies have established the therapeutic efficacy of MAOIs in a broad spectrum of psychiatric disorders, often with unique clinical effects. MAOIs are generally accepted as one of the most effective therapies for panic disorders (83). Their clinical utility in the management of eating disorders (92,93), obsessive-compulsive disorders (32), social phobias (42), attention deficit disorder (95), and chronic pain (17) has been reported. Also of interest is the apparent superiority of MAOIs compared to tricyclic antidepressants in relieving anxiety and panic symptoms associated with depressive illness (36,44,75). The efficacy of this antidepressant drug class in these heterogeneous psychiatric disorders suggests that MAOIs possess either novel antidepressant activity or separate anxiolytic effects. This has led to the further suggestion that MAOIs possess more than a single pharmacologic mechanism of action, accounting for their apparent broad therapeutic spectrum. This issue is addressed further in the discussion of electrophysiological and neurochemical effects.

Issues unresolved 10 years ago regarding this antidepressant drug class have been further elucidated in the ensuing period (78). The largely unstudied pharmacokinetics of MAOIs have been investigated extensively in humans in the case of phenelzine (72) and to a lesser extent for tranylcypromine (5,85). Guidelines for maintenance treatment with an MAOI are being developed in long-term, placebo-controlled studies (74). The two active subtypes of the enzyme, MAO$_A$ and MAO$_B$, have been extensively characterized. Several enzyme inhibitors with relative subtype specificity are under development and being evaluated

clinically (4,69). Promising preliminary results have been reported for several investigational drugs which are thought to be reversible inhibitors of MAO (18,59). These may offer the advantage of equivalent efficacy with a lesser potential for troublesome side effects or toxicity.

Additional experience has been gained with the combined use of MAOIs with other psychotropic drugs, including tricyclic antidepressants, trazodone, lithium, monoamine precursors, and other psychoactive agents. Growing experience over the past decade supports the cautious use of the MAOIs, phenelzine, or isocarboxazid in particular, in combination with other antidepressants and stimulant drugs for the treatment of refractory patients (27).

Finally, MAOIs have been shown to be efficacious in many different diagnostic subgroups of depression. Both endogenous and nonendogenous forms of major depression can be effectively treated with MAOIs (52,66,89). These agents have been shown to be useful in atypical depression associated with hysteroid features (36,44), prominent somatic anxiety or panic symptoms (75), and minor depressive disorder (75,79). Therapeutic indications for MAOIs in treating depression are reviewed in Chapter 104, *this volume.*

MECHANISM OF ACTION

The profound effects on monoamine systems of antidepressant drugs introduced in the late 1950s led to development of the catecholamine hypothesis of affective disorders, which postulated a deficiency in adrenergic neuronal transmission (11,65,80). A serotonin deficiency state in depressive illness has also been proposed (15).

It became quickly evident that there was a temporal dissociation between the delayed onset of therapeutic effect and the more immediate pharmacologic effect of tricyclic antidepressants to inhibit monoamine uptake. Chronic studies using radiolabeled receptor binding techniques in animals documented additional pharmacological effects with a gradual onset, including the development of α_2- and β-adrenergic receptor subsensitivity, a characteristic of nearly all effective therapies for depression.

Neurochemical Studies

Determinations of the effects of MAOIs on brain neurotransmitter concentrations have revealed marked differences between the acute and chronic effects of these agents on norepinephrine, serotonin, and dopamine (13,71). Peak increases in tissue concentrations of these monoamines usually occurred within the first 7 days of treatment, with levels then gradually declining with continuing administration over a 6-week period of study, even though the degree of MAO inhibition was maintained. These observations lent further support to the growing belief that secondary adaptive changes in neuronal systems play an integral, and possibly pivotal, role in antidepressant drug action. In the case of MAOIs, the degree of enzyme inhibition as well as the intraneuronal transmitter concentration changes observed during the first weeks of treatment were not proportional with the biologic or clinical effects of these agents.

It was also interesting in these studies that brain serotonin concentrations were elevated more rapidly and to a greater extent than were the two catecholamines, norepinephrine and dopamine, although with continued administration, levels of all three amines tended to return toward baseline. The prominent effect of MAOI treatment on brain serotonin raises the possibility that this neurotransmitter may play a more pivotal role than other neurotransmitter systems in the treatment of depressive and anxiety disorders.

Neuronal receptor binding studies under conditions of chronic treatment have shown that both tricyclic and MAOI antidepressant drugs reduce the apparent concentration of serotonin binding sites (down-regulation) (29,64). Although the MAO$_A$-selective inhibitor clorgyline shares this property with the clinically available nonselective inhibitors, the MAO$_B$ inhibitor deprenyl, which seemingly lacks antidepressant efficacy, does not affect serotonin binding in brain tissue. Current evidence is substantial that a compensatory decrease in cortical 5-HT$_2$ receptors (as measured by [^{3}H]ketanserin or [^{3}H]spiperone binding) may be a prerequisite for therapeutic activity of most antidepressants (3). Following discontinuation of repeated administration of nialamide, cortical serotonin concentrations have been shown to return to baseline gradually over a several-day period, whereas even longer is required for down-regulation of 5-HT$_2$ receptor binding sites in brain to normalize (24). These dynamic changes in serotonin function evidenced by delayed gradual changes in neurotransmitter levels and receptor binding, which are secondary to MAOI therapy, may in part contribute to the so-called therapeutic lag as well as the carryover effects of MAOIs, which in some cases require a drug-free interval after stopping treatment.

Additional evidence for a functional role for serotonin down-regulation in the pharmacology of MAOIs is provided by behavioral studies. Pretreatment with drugs of this class can attenuate the "serotonin syndrome" in rats induced by the serotonin agonist 5-methoxy-N,N-dimethyltryptamine (47). In general, tricyclic antidepressants lack this property. Presumably, this effect of MAOI pretreatment can be explained in part by a decrease in the number of [^{3}H]serotonin receptor-binding sites in brainstem and/or spinal cord. Interestingly, pretreatment with phenelzine enhances the quipazine-induced head shake response in rats, which assesses 5-HT$_2$ receptor function (48), in a manner similar to clinically effective and novel anxiolytic agents (F. Yocca, *personal communication*). This finding lends credence to the claim that MAOIs affect central serotonin systems and may share properties common to anxiolytic drugs.

Electrophysiological Studies

Measurement of neuronal electrophysiological activity has provided a rather different perspective into the mechanism of action of MAOIs. Receptor binding studies have the limitation that they provide little information concerning the functional activity of intact *in vivo* neuronal systems. Electrophysiology provides a useful measure of the functional effect of such neuronal adaptive changes, which is critical to an understanding of the therapeutic activity of antidepressant drugs. Evidence suggests that chronic MAOI administration enhances the efficacy of serotonergic neurotransmission (9). The time course of this electrophysiological effect is temporally consistent with the onset of therapeutic effects of MAOIs.

Within the first 2 weeks of MAOI administration, there is a decrease in neuronal firing patterns for both the noradrenergic and serotonergic systems as mediated by α_2, β, and serotonin auto- and postsynaptic receptors. Adrenergic transmission mediated by α_2 and β sites remains depressed throughout ongoing treatment, but the situation is different for serotonergic systems. After 2 weeks of chronic treatment the serotonin presynaptic autoreceptor remains functionally depressed; however, the postsynaptic neuron not only recovers from the acutely depressed baseline firing pattern but exhibits evidence of enhanced responsiveness. These electrophysiological effects on adrenergic and serotonergic systems are apparently common to all antidepressant treatments so far studied, including tricyclics (8,22,60,81), electroconvulsive therapy (ECT) (20), misanserin (7), iprindol (19), and zimelidine (21).

Complementing these studies is a recent report of differential effects of an MAOI and tricyclic antidepressant on the serotonin presynaptic autoreceptor (61). Chronic nialamide treatment, but not chlorimipramine treatment, abolished autoreceptor activity and significantly augmented the efflux of [^{3}H]serotonin *in vitro* from superfused hypothalamic slices. Taken together with the electrophysiologic data, these findings suggest that the therapeutic activity of MAOIs may in some way be linked to adaptive changes in either pre- or postsynaptic serotonergic systems.

MAO Subtype and Neurotransmitters

In 1968 Johnston described two forms of MAO on the basis of a bimodal pattern of inhibition of tyramine deamination found with clorgyline. This led to the designation of two enzyme subtypes, MAO_A and MAO_B (34). Since then, a considerable literature has developed showing varying amounts of MAO_A and MAO_B activity in several tissues of interest such as brain, kidney, liver, intestine, and platelets. These enzyme subtypes have in addition been characterized by differences in monoamine substrate specificity, electrophoretic mobility of radiolabeled subunits (1), and, most recently, by immunological (23) and chromatographic techniques (24). However, attempts to purify, sequence, and delineate their primary structure have been unsuccessful.

Although no substrate is completely specific for one or the other form of MAO, certain substrates are highly selective (28). To be regarded as selective for MAO_A, substrates must have a high ratio for the following:

$$\frac{K_m(MAO_B)}{K_m(MAO_A)} \quad \text{and} \quad \frac{V_{max}(MAO_A)}{V_{max}(MAO_B)}$$

Serotonin appears to meet this criterion. Substrates with low values for these ratios, such as phenylethylamine, are selective for MAO_B. However, it is apparent that metabolism of a given substrate is concentration dependent so that enzyme specificity is only relative and not absolute. Furthermore, sufficiently high monoamine concentrations *in vivo* may be encountered in some brain regions so that oxidation may occur by the nonpreferred form of the enzyme. Substrate specificity should therefore be viewed as a continuum rather than as discrete enzyme activities (28).

There are large species differences in the ratio of A and B forms (30,56). Rat brain is thought to contain nearly equivalent proportions of MAO_A (55%) and MAO_B (45%). Hamster brain, on the other hand, has been found to contain 95% MAO_A activity. Human brain is now believed to contain a preponderance of MAO_B (70–75%) activity, and that of other nonhuman primates, such as the rhesus monkey, may have even higher proportions of MAO_B activity. However, this does not provide insight into regional brain differences in MAO subtype, which are still open to question. In the rat MAO_A is thought to be localized predominantly intraneuronally, whereas MAO_B has been found extraneuronally and also in high concentrations in serotonin-rich areas (40). In humans, however, the two subtypes may be found both intra- and extraneuronally (62).

With specific MAO_A inhibitors intracellular concentrations of norepinephrine and serotonin are most affected. When the nonspecific MAOIs are examined, in addition to norepinephrine, serotonin, and dopamine, levels of other amines whose concentrations are normally quite low, i.e., tryptamine, phenylethylamine, and epinephrine, also increase. The high concentrations of these amines in vesicles and cytoplasm may produce feedback inhibition of monoamine synthetic pathways. This effect, most clearly established for noradrenergic systems, results in decreased turnover, which contributes to altered metabolite production (45).

A direct consequence of acute MAO inhibition with either a specific MAO_A inhibitor, such as clorgyline, or a nonspecific inhibitor, such as phenelzine, is reduction of the noradrenergic metabolites 3-methoxy,4-hydroxy-phenylglycol (MHPG), 3,4-dihydroxyphenylglycol (DOPEG), and vanillylmandellic acid (VMA), and an increase in normetanephrine (46,55,73). A comparable effect on noradrenergic metabolite patterns is not seen with MAO_B-specific inhibitors (2,55).

The data in humans concerning serotonin metabolites are less clear. Two studies have shown that high-dose clorgyline treatment produces a relatively small decrement in 5-hydroxyindoleacetic acid (5-HIAA) CSF or urine concentration compared to the pronounced effect on MHPG (46,55). Major and co-workers (49) found CSF 5-HIAA to be significantly reduced in depressed patients treated with either clorgyline or pargyline, suggesting that in humans serotonin may not be a selective substrate for MAO_A and that MAO_B may also contribute significantly to its metabolism. These findings are in contrast to *in vitro* and *in vivo* animal experiments which indicate that serotonin is a preferred substrate for MAO_A (1,54). In this regard the anatomical localization of MAO_B in serotonin-rich brain regions is an important finding (40). In the same study Major and co-workers found that homovanillic acid (HVA), the principal acidic metabolite of dopamine, was also significantly reduced by 4 weeks of treatment with either clorgyline or pargyline, with the latter producing the greater decline (49). Murphy and co-workers (57) showed that CSF HVA was only slightly decreased even with high clorgyline doses (30 mg/day). Taken together, these data suggest that dopamine is a substrate for both MAO_A and MAO_B, but may be a preferred substrate for the B-form in humans (55). Findings of this type have led to investigations of the clinical potential of MAO_B inhibitors such as *l*-deprenyl in the treatment of Parkinson's disease (38).

INVESTIGATIONAL SELECTIVE AND REVERSIBLE MAO-INHIBITING DRUGS

Consistent with this renewed interest in MAOIs, the past 10 years have seen a number of new agents in this drug class being developed for clinical use. Much of the work has focused on developing selective MAO_A or nonselective reversible inhibitors for the treatment of depressive illness (88,91). Promising examples of these are amiflamine, moclobemide, and sercloremine (69). The latter two drugs show preliminary clinical evidence of efficacy in the treatment of depressive illness (18,59). There is reason to think that a reversible inhibitor of monoamine metabolism may protect against some of the troublesome side effects associated with nonreversible inhibitors. Of particular interest is evidence that suggests that the reversible inhibitors may not potentiate tyramine-induced pressor effects, thereby diminishing the risk of a hypertensive crisis and obviating the need for dietary restrictions.

A particularly innovative approach is the new MAOI, MDL72145 (96). This is a prodrug that crosses the blood-brain barrier where it is selectively taken up by neurons and decarboxylated to a specific, irreversible MAO_B inhibitor. It is possible that the use of the prodrug mechanism may obviate some of the troubling side effects attributable to MAO inhibition in the periphery, e.g., intestine and liver. This could also substantially reduce the risk of hypertensive crisis and might allow for easing dietary restrictions necessitated by MAOI therapy.

PHARMACOKINETICS AND METABOLISM OF MAOIs

Relatively little was known about the metabolic degradation and clinical pharmacokinetics of MAOIs until recent years. Studies have shown that the irreversible enzyme inhibitors used in clinical practice, i.e., tranylcypromine, phenelzine, and isocarboxazid, are substrates for MAO. By forming irreversible covalent bonds to the active site of the enzyme, these drugs functions as "suicide" enzyme inhibitors (63,86). This process could account in part for the brief plasma elimination half-life $t_{\frac{1}{2}\alpha}$ of MAOIs, as has been reported following single doses of phenelzine (14,72). Since MAOIs act as substrates for the enzyme MAO, long-term administration could impair their own metabolism, resulting in nonlinear pharmacokinetics and a potential for drug accumulation. In this regard plasma concentrations of phenelzine have been reported to increase progressively in depressed patients over the first several weeks of treatment (76).

Acetylation has been proposed as a major metabolic pathway for the degradation of hydrazine MAOIs, such as phenelzine and isocarboxazid. It has received extensive study in humans because of the possibility that dose relates to acetylator phenotype (25,33). More recent studies have failed to confirm an association between acetylator status and clinical effects of phenelzine (16,51,78).

Extremely limited data are available on the metabolic fate of phenelzine, isocarboxazid, and tranylcypromine in either animals or humans. Preliminary studies suggested that phenelzine primarily undergoes oxidation rather than acetylation as the major degradative pathway in humans (12,58). Using site-specific, stable isotope-labeled phenelzine, Robinson and co-workers (72) investigated the metabolism of phenelzine in both normal subjects and chronically treated patients. This mass fragmentographic technique proved particularly useful because several of phenelzine's probable metabolites, such as phenylacetic acid, and parahydroxyphenylacetic acid, are also normally present in urine from endogenous sources. Study findings suggest that phenelzine is rapidly converted to phenylacetic acid and its ring-hydroxylated metabolite rather than to any acetylated metabolites. No detectable levels of phenelzine acetate were found in plasma or urine samples. It was concluded that acetylation is not a metabolic route for phenelzine and acetylator phenotype does not relate to the clinical dose.

More limited information is available on the pharmacokinetics of tranylcypromine and isocarboxazid. Simpson and co-workers report that following a single 10-mg challenge dose of tranylcypromine, peak plasma levels occurred at 1 to 2 hr, with a plasma elimination $t_{\frac{1}{2}\alpha}$ under 2 hr (85). Significant platelet MAO inhibition persisted for at least 1

week following this single dose. Two other studies also report a very short $t_{\frac{1}{2}\alpha}$ for tranylcypromine (5,94). In a study to assess the biologic half-life of tranylcypromine, Bieck and Antonin (6) estimated the pharmacodynamic $t_{\frac{1}{2}}$ to be of the order of several days. This conclusion was based on persisting sensitivity to tyramine infusion for several days after discontinuation of 4 weeks of tranylcypromine treatment. One subject maintained tyramine supersensitivity for several weeks following discontinuation.

These human pharmacokinetic studies consistently find MAOIs to be cleared very rapidly from plasma while biologic effects persist for much longer periods. Studies suggest that the pharmacokinetics and pharmacodynamics of MAOIs are unique, as would be predicted for a drug of the suicide enzyme inhibitor class. Further investigation is required to more fully characterize the complex pharmacokinetics and pharmacodynamics of MAOIs in humans.

SIDE EFFECTS AND TOXICITY OF MAO-INHIBITING DRUGS

The reemergence of MAOIs into fairly widespread clinical use over the past decade was a result of both more conclusive evidence of their therapeutic efficacy and of accumulated safety experience about this drug class. An overriding concern has been the potential liability for hypertensive crisis, often a medical emergency. Fortunately, with modest dietary restriction in a reliable patient, the risk of this untoward event seems to be very low in the experience of most investigators. Review of the safety data from two centers, involving more than 100 patients each, shows that the incidence of severe hypertensive reactions in patients receiving MAOIs is less than 1% (67: D. S. Robinson and A. Kayser, *unpublished data*).

On the other hand, it has become apparent that MAOIs have certain troublesome side effects, which often lead to drug intolerance by the patient and discontinuation despite a favorable therapeutic response. Studies conducted in recent years probably provide more accurate assessments of the true incidence of side effects with MAOIs because of the trend to use higher doses which are in the recognized therapeutic range. There seems to be consensus that the most clinically significant side effects are symptomatic orthostatic hypotension, excessive weight gain associated with hyperphagia, sexual dysfunction, hypomania (usually in bipolar patients), insomnia, and bipedal edema (67,68,74). The MAOIs appear to have no important direct cardiac effects; the postural hypotension and slight showing of heart rate appear to be manifestations of decreased sympathetic tone (77). A decrease in circulating levels of plasma norepinephrine is a concomitant of MAOI therapy (73).

Other less common or troublesome MAOI side effects which have been reported include myoclonic jerks, often more related to sleep onset (41), and induction of pyridoxine deficiency with phenelzine treatment (31).

As more long-term studies are being done to assess the value of maintenance antidepressant treatment, the adverse experience with chronic MAOI use is emerging. Such data are pertinent because of the trend to treat depressive episodes for at least 6 to 12 months or longer. In a study of maintenance treatment with phenelzine for up to 2 years, interim findings indicate that of 79 patients treated for an index episode of depression, 20 patients (25%) ultimately discontinued, primarily for reasons of side effects (74). This is especially noteworthy because 65 of the 79 patients (82%) had experienced an initial favorable therapeutic response to phenelzine, and most were strongly motivated to remain on MAOI therapy. Of the 20 discontinuing patients, four were in acute treatment (up to 2 months) and 16 had reached the continuation or maintenance treatment phases of the study. Excessive weight gain was experienced by 10 of these patients, followed in decreasing order of frequency by bipedal edema, hypomania, orthostatic hypotension, insomnia, and sexual dysfunction. No withdrawal symptoms were encountered in any of the patients terminating from either acute or long-term phenelzine treatment.

In a small sample of 14 patients on long-term phenelzine treatment, Evans and co-workers (26) noted that 10 of the patients had side effects that emerged after 2 months of therapy. These patients, in order of frequency, experienced weight gain with increased appetite, edema resistant to diuretics, muscle symptoms, paresthesias responsive to pyridoxine, and anorgasmia. Long-term adverse experience has not been reported for tranylcypromine or isocarboxazid.

With the growing utilization of MAOIs in clinical practice it is predictable that drug overdoses will be encountered in increasing numbers. Fortunately, documented deaths due to MAOIs have been infrequent. A toxic syndrome characterized by altered mental status, hyperpyrexia, and hyperreflexia is seen that may progress to metabolic acidosis, seizures, and cardiovascular collapse. As for most drugs, treatment of MAOI overdose is primarily nonspecific and supportive, and should include measures to reduce or retard further drug absorption. A case report has recently described a patient who ingested at least 1,000 mg of phenelzine, resulting in coma, acidosis, and temperature elevations up to 41°C. The patient responded rapidly to intravenous dantrolene administration, which has been used successfully in the treatment of malignant hyperthermia and neuroleptic malignant syndrome (35). It is postulated that this reversal of malignant hyperthermia syndrome by dantrolene is mediated by its inhibitory action on the release of sarcoplasmic calcium ions.

UNIQUE AND NONAPPROVED CLINICAL APPLICATIONS OF MAOIs

The apparent broad spectrum of action of MAOIs, encompassing both depressive and anxiety disorders, has led to their evaluation in other conditions that may have an affective component and that lack effective treatments. It would appear that MAOIs have important therapeutic actions in addition to their intrinsic antidepressant efficacy. These include specific antianxiety properties useful in the treatment of both mood and anxiety-related disorders.

Some of the more important and interesting of these newer clinical applications of MAOIs will be discussed.

Depression

Like much of the earlier psychopharmacologic literature, MAOI research was hampered by lack of properly controlled studies employing rigorous experimental design (70). Another important recent advance has been the use of operationalized diagnostic criteria and interview techniques combined with more sophisticated rating scales. These developments have allowed clinical drug actions to be more precisely defined, and in the case of the MAOIs their therapeutic efficacy in a wide variety of depressive disorders is evident.

MAOIs do not appear to have selectivity in treating various subtypes of depression. Recent well-controlled studies support the efficacy of the nonselective MAOIs and the specific MAO_A inhibitor clorgyline in more severely, "endogenously" depressed patients, with therapeutic benefit equivalent to that of the tricyclic antidepressants (66,75). Deprenyl may also be effective as an antidepressant, but only at higher dosages where MAO_B specificity may be lost (50,53). Current evidence would hold that inhibition of MAO_A activity is essential to the treatment of severe depression (55).

Major depression appears to be a heterogeneous disorder with variously defined overlapping subgroups characterized by anxiety, phobic, and histrionic symptoms and "atypical" features such as prominent somatic complaints, excessive fatigue and hypersomnia, reversed diurnal variation, etc. Studies of patients with nonendogenous and atypical forms of depression suggest that MAOIs may be more effective than the tricyclics class (36,43,66,75).

Much of the investigation of this last patient category has been performed by the group at Columbia. A recent controlled trial comparing phenelzine (60–90 mg/day), imipramine (200–300 mg/day), and placebo in atypical depression found the MAOI superior to placebo and tricyclic therapy (44). Of interest was the additional finding that patients with a history of panic attacks responded particularly well to phenelzine. This is consistent with findings in a study by Robinson and co-workers (75). Phenelzine (60 mg/day) was compared to amitriptyline (150 mg/day) in a double-blind trial involving 169 outpatients with primary depression. Although the overall efficacy of the two drugs was nearly equivalent, depressed patients with panic attacks, phobic avoidance, or prominent somatic symptoms responded significantly better and more rapidly to phenelzine. Depressed patients reporting panic symptoms were also less likely to discontinue phenelzine treatment than amitriptyline treatment (75).

Therefore, evidence suggests that the MAOI and tricyclic classes of antidepressants are equally effective in treating severe or melancholic major depression. The former appears to be superior to tricyclics in a number of subgroups of depression with more atypical features and may be the preferred drugs in selected patients. On balance, the findings of these more recent comparative studies in depression support the notion that MAOIs may have intrinsic anxiolytic properties in addition to an antidepressant effect.

Panic Disorder

There is growing evidence that MAOIs are the most efficacious treatment currently available for panic disorder. In a definitive, controlled clinical trial, Sheehan and co-workers found both active drugs, phenelzine (45 mg/day) and imipramine (150 mg/day), superior to placebo in a large sample of patients diagnosed as panic disorder by *Diagnostic and Statistical Manual of Mental Disorders,* 3rd edition (DSM-III) criteria (83). In this study there was a trend for phenelzine to be superior to imipramine. In a subsequent study, Sheehan compared higher doses of phenelzine to imipramine and alprazolam, a triazolobenzodiazepine reported to have antipanic properties (84). Again, phenelzine appeared to be the superior treatment, particularly with regard to measures of disability or avoidance behavior. It has been suggested that the advantage of phenelzine lies in its ability not only to block the panic attacks, but also to reduce the accompanying anticipatory anxiety and phobic avoidance (42).

There may be a genetic as well as a clinical linkage between panic disorder and depression (10,39,82). Phenelzine is effective in treating patients with panic symptoms, even in the absence of depressive symptomatology. This suggests that the mechanism of action of MAOIs in relieving distress in panic disorder is not necessarily the same as that in treating depression.

Phobic Avoidance

As noted above, MAOIs may be particularly helpful in treating phobic-avoidance behavior associated with both mood and anxiety disorders. Controlled trials have indicated phenelzine to be as efficacious as behavior therapy and superior to placebo in treating mixed agoraphobic social phobia (87,90). Liebowitz and co-workers recently reported an open study that indicates that phenelzine, independent of any antidepressant properties, may be particularly effective in the treatment of social phobias as defined by DSM-III criteria (42). Additional studies are needed to define the role of MAOIs in treating these frequently disabling avoidance behaviors.

Attention Deficit Disorder

Rapaport and co-workers (95) recently reported a provocative finding suggesting that MAOI therapy may be highly effective in treating children with attention deficit disorder characterized by hyperactivity. It was found that children had an immediate and unequivocal response to several different MAOIs, including phenelzine, tranylcypromine, and clorgyline. The rapid response suggests a separate mechanism of action than that mediating antidepressant effects. These investigators go on to report that in their extensive experience, MAOIs are the first agents to

parallel the effects of dextroamphetamine so closely that treating physicians could not distinguish between them. This success of the MAOIs is in contrast to the unsatisfactory results obtained with other agents, including tricyclic antidepressants, mianserin, and L-dopa. If these promising results are confirmed, it could have important implications in understanding and treating attention deficit disorder.

Other Clinical Indications

Preliminary evidence of efficacy for MAOIs in the treatment of bulimia and chronic pain associated with depression has been shown in double-blind, placebo-controlled trials. Open trials in obsessive-compulsive disorder have also shown promising therapeutic effects for MAOIs.

In a preliminary report, Walsh and co-workers found that 56% (5/9) of the bulimia patients treated with phenelzine stopped bingeing entirely while the remaining four patients experienced at least a 50% reduction in bingeing (93). This contrasted sharply with placebo therapy, which failed to show significant antibingeing activity. Preliminary evidence of efficacy in this disorder has also been shown with isocarboxazid (37).

Davidson and co-workers reported that phenelzine was superior to both placebo and impramine in the treatment of patients with chronic pain associated with depression (17). In a retrospective analysis of their data, these investigators report that the presence of atypical vegetative symptoms, including increases in appetite, weight, and libido, correlated with analgesic response to phenelzine.

In a small open trial of eight patients, Jenike and co-workers reported rapid and sustained response in four of the patients treated with either phenelzine or tranylcypromine (32). It is of interest that all of the responders but none of the nonresponders had phobic anxiety and/or panic attacks as part of their overall symptom picture. These investigators suggest that these results, although promising, should be replicated in controlled trials. It is particularly interesting that serotonin has been implicated as playing a central role in the physiology or pharmacology of these disorders. Consistent with this, another class of antidepressant agent, the serotonin reuptake blocking drugs, are currently being extensively evaluated as treatment for some of these disorders. More work will be needed to define the role of MAOIs and other antidepressants in the treatment of chronic pain, eating disorders, and obsessive-compulsive disorder and their relationships, if any, to serotonergic systems.

REFERENCES

1. Achee, F. M., Gabay, S., and Tipton, K. F. (1977): *Prog. Neurobiol.,* 8:325–348.
2. Alken, R. G., Palfreyman, M. G., Brown, M. J., Davies, D. S., Lewis, P. J. and Schecter, P. J. (1984): *Proc. Br. Pharmacol. Soc.,* 615–616.
3. Andree, T. H., Mikuni, M., and Meltzer, H. Y. (1984): *Psychopharmacol. Bull.,* 20:349–353.
4. Ask, A. L., Fagervall, I., and Ross, S. B. (1983): *Naunyn Schmiedebergs Arch. Pharmacol.,* 324:79–87.

5. Bailey, E., and Barrow, E. J. (1980): *J. Chromatogr.*, 183:25–31.
6. Bieck, P. R., and Antonin, K. H. (1982): *Eur. J. Clin. Pharmacol.*, 22:301–308.
7. Blackshear, M. A., and Sanders-Bush, E. (1982): *J. Pharmacol. Exp. Ther.*, 221:303–308.
8. Blier, P., and deMontigny, C. (1980): *Naunyn Schmiedebergs Arch. Pharmacol.*, 314:123–128.
9. Blier, P., and deMontigny, C. (1985): *Neuroscience*, 16:949–955.
10. Breier, A., Charney, D. S., and Heninger, G. R. (1984): *Arch. Gen. Psychiatry*, 411:1129–1135.
11. Bunney, W. E., and Davis, J. M. (1965): *Arch. Gen. Psychiatry*, 13:483–494.
12. Caddy, B., Stead, A. H., and Johnstone, E. C. (1978): *Br. J. Clin. Pharmacol.* 6:185–188.
13. Campbell, I. C., Robinson, D. S., Lovenberg, W., and Murphy, D. L. (1979): *J. Neurochem.*, 32:49–55.
14. Cooper, T. B., Robinson, D. S., and Nies, A. (1978): *Commun. Psychopharmacol.*, 2:505–512.
15. Coppen, A. (1967): *Br. J. Psychiatry*, 113:1237–1264.
16. Davidson, J., McLeod, M. N., and Blum, M. R. (1978): *Am. J. Psychiatry*, 135:467–469.
17. Davidson, J., and Raft, D. (1985): *Arch. Gen. Psychiatry*, 42:635–636.
18. Delini-Stula, A., Fischbach, R., Bures, E., and Poldinger, W. (1985): *Drug Dev. Res.* 6:371–384.
19. deMontigny, C. (1984): *Mod. Probl. Pharmacopsychiatry*, 18:102–116.
20. deMontigny, C. (1984): *J. Pharmacol. Exp. Ther.*, 228:230–234.
21. deMontigny, C., Blier, P., Caille, G., and Konassi, E., (1981): *Acta Psychiatr. Scand.*, 63(Suppl. 290):79–90.
22. deMontigny, C., Blier, P., and Chaput, Y. (1984): *Neuropharmacology*, 23:1511–1520.
23. Denny, R. M., Fritz, R. R., Patel, N. T., and Abell, S. W. (1982): *Science*, 215:1400–1403.
24. Denny, R. M., Fritz, R. R., Patel, N. T., Widen, S. G., and Abell, C. W. (1983): *Mol. Pharmacol.*, 24:60–68.
25. Evans, D. A. P., Davison, K., and Pratt, R. T. C. (1965): *Clin. Pharmacol. Ther.*, 6:430–435.
26. Evans, D. K., Davidson, J., and Raft, D. (1982): *J. Clin. Psychopharmacol.*, 2:208–210.
27. Feighner, J. P., Herbstein, J., and Damlouji, N. (1985): *J. Clin. Psychiatry*, 46:206–209.
28. Fowler, C. J., and Tipton, K. F. (1984): *J. Pharm. Pharmacol.*, 36:1112–1115.
29. Frazer, A., and Lucki, I. (1982): In: *Typical and Atypical Molecular Mechanisms*, edited by E. Costa and C. Racagni, pp. 69–90. Raven Press, New York.
30. Garrick, N. A., and Murphy, D. L. (1980): *Psychopharmacology*, 72:27–33.
31. Gelenberg, A. J. (1984): *Biol. Therap. Psychiatry*, 7:39.
32. Jenike, M. A., Surman, O. S., Cassem, N. H., Zusky, P., and Anderson, W. H. (1983): *J. Clin. Psychiatry*, 44:131–132.
33. Johnstone, E. C., and Marsh, W. (1973): *Lancet*, 1:567–570.
34. Johnstone, J. P. (1968): *Biochem. Pharmacol.*, 17:1285–1297.
35. Kaplan, R. F., Feinglass, N. G., Webster, W., and Mudra, S. (1986): *JAMA*, 225:642–644.
36. Kayser, A., Robinson, D. S., Nies, A., and Howard, D. (1985): *Am. J. Psychiatry*, 142:486–488.
37. Kennedy, S. H., Piran, N., and Garfinkel, P. E. (1985): *J. Clin. Psychopharmacol.*, 5:279–285.
38. Knoll, J. (1983): *Acta Neurol. Scand.*, (Suppl. 95):57–80.
39. Leckman, J. F., Merikangas, K. P., Pauls, D. L., Prusoff, B. A., and Weissman, M. M. (1983): *Am. J. Psychiatry*, 140:880–882.
40. Levitt, P., Pintar, J. E., and Breakfield, X. O. (1982): *Proc. Natl. Acad. Sci. USA*, 79:6385–6389.
41. Lieberman, J. A., Kane, J. M., and Reife, R. (1985): *J. Clin. Psychopharmacol.*, 5:221–228.
42. Liebowitz, M. R., Fyer, A. J., Gorman, J. M., Campeas, R., and Levin, A. (1986): *J. Clin. Psychopharmacol.*, 6:93–97.
43. Liebowitz, M. R., and Klein, D. F. (1979): In: *Affective Disorders*, edited by H. S. Akiskal, pp. 555–575. W. B. Saunders, Philadelphia.
44. Liebowitz, M. R., Quitkin, F. M., Stewart, J. W., McGrath, P. J., Harrison, W., Rabkin, J., Tricamo, E., Markowitz, J. S., and Klein, D. F. (1985): *Psychopharmacol. Bull.*, 21:558–561.
45. Lin, R. C., Neff, N. H., Ngar, S. H., and Costa, E. (1969): *Life Sci.* 8:1077–1984.
46. Linnoila, M., Karoum, F., and Potter, W. Z. (1982): *Arch. Gen. Psychiatry*, 39:513–516.
47. Lucki, I., and Frazer, A. (1982): *Psychopharmacology*, 77:205–211.
48. Lucki, I., Nobler, M. S., and Frazer, A. (1984): *J. Pharmacol. Exp. Ther.*, 63:328–341.
49. Major, L. F., Murphy, D. L., Lipper, S., and Gordon, E. (1979): *Neurochemistry*, 32:229–231.
50. Mann, J. J., Frances, A., Kaplan, R. D., Kocsis, J., Peselow, E. D., and Gershon, S. (1982): *J. Clin. Psychopharmacol.*, 2:54–57.
51. Marshall, E. F., Mountjoy, C. Q., Campbell, I. C., Garside, R. F., Lietch, I. M., and Roth, M. (1978): *Br. J. Clin. Pharmacol.*, 6:247–254.
52. McGrath, P. J., Quitkin, F. M., Harrison, W., and Stewart, J. W. (1984): *Am. J. Psychiatry*, 14:288–289.
53. Mendlewicz, J., and Youdim, B. H. (1983): *Br. J. Psychiatry*, 142:508–511.
54. Murphy, D. L. (1978): *Biochem. Pharmacol.*, 26:921–930.
55. Murphy, D. L., Cohen, R. M., Garrick, N. A., Siever, L. J., and Campbell, I. C. (1984): In: *Neurobiology of Mood Disorders*, edited by R. M. Post and J. C. Ballenger, pp. 710–720. William and Wilkins, Baltimore.
56. Murphy, D. L., Garrick, N. A., Aulakh, C. S., and Cohen, R. M. (1984): *J. Clin. Psychiatry*, 45:37–43.
57. Murphy, D. L., Lipper, S., and Campbell, I. C. (1979): *Monoamine Oxidase: Structure, Function and Altered Functions*, edited by T. P. Singer, R. W. VonKroff, and D. L. Murphy, pp. 457–475. Academic Press, New York.
58. Narasimhachari, N., and Friedel, R. O. (1980): *Res. Commun. Psychol. Psychiatry Behav.*, 5:185–197.
59. Norman, T. R., Ames, D., Burrows, G. D., and Davies, B. (1985): *J. Affective Disord.*, 8:29–35.
60. Nyback, H. V., Walter, J. R., Aghajanian, G. K., and Roth, R. H. (1975): *Eur. J. Pharmacol.*, 32:302–312.
61. Offord, S. J., and Warwick, R. O. (1985): *Pharmacologist*, 27:264.
62. Oreland, L., Arai, Y., Stenstrom, A., and Fowler, C. J. (1983): In: *Monoamine Oxidase and Its Selective Inhibitors*, edited by H. Beckmann and P. Riederer, pp. 246–254. S. Karger, Basel.
63. Paech, C., Salach, J. I., and Singer, T. P. (1979): In: *Monoamine Oxidase: Structure, Function and Altered Functions*, edited by T. P. Singer, R. W. VonKroff, and D. L. Murphy, pp. 39–50. Academic Press, New York.
64. Peroutka, S. J., and Snyder, S. H. (1980): *Science*, 210:88–90.
65. Prange, A. J. (1965): *Dis. Nerv. Syst.*, 25:217–221.
66. Quitkin, F., Rifkin, A., and Klein, D. F. (1979): *Arch. Gen. Psychiatry*, 36:749–760.
67. Rabkin, J., Quitkin, F., Harrison, W., Tricamo, E., and McGrath, P. (1984): *J. Clin. Psychopharmacol.*, 4:270–278.
68. Ravaris, C. L., Robinson, D. S., Ives, J. O., Nies, A., and Bartlett, D. (1980): *Arch. Gen. Psychiatry*, 37:1075–1080.
69. Riederer, P., Jellinger, J., and Seeman, D. (1984): In: *Monoamine Oxidase and Disease*, edited by K. F. Tipton, P. Dostert, and M. Strolin Benedetti, pp. 403–415. Academic Press, London.
70. Robinson, D. S. (1986): *Psychopharmacol. Bull.*, 1;12–16.
71. Robinson, D. S., Campbell, I. C., Walker, M., Statham, N. J., Lovenberg, W., and Murphy, D. L. (1979): *Neuropharmacology*, 18:771–776.
72. Robinson, D. S., Cooper, T. B., Jindal, S. R., Corcella, J., and Lutz, T. (1985): *J. Clin. Psychopharmacol.*, 5:333–337.
73. Robinson, D. S., Johnson, G. A., Nies, A., Corcella, J., Cooper, T. B., Albright, D., and Howard, D. (1983): *J. Clin. Psychopharmacol.*, 3:282–287.
74. Robinson, D. S., Kayser, A., Bennett, B., Devereaux, E., Lerfald, S., Albright, D., Laux, D., and Corcella, J. (1986): *Psychopharmacology Bull.*, 22:553–557.
75. Robinson, D. S., Kayser, A., Corcella, J., Laux, D., Yingling, K., and Howard, D. (1985): *Psychopharmacol. Bull.*, 21:562–567.
76. Robinson, D. S., Nies, A., Corcella, J., and Cooper, T. B. (1982): *Psychopharmacol. Bull.*, 17:154–157.
77. Robinson, D. S., Nies, A., Corcella, J., Cooper, T. B., Spencer, C., and Keefover, R. (1982): *J. Clin. Psychiatry*, 43:8–15.

78. Robinson, D. S., Nies, A., Ravaris, C. L., Ives, J. O., and Bartlett, D. (1978): In: *Psychopharmacology: A Generation of Progress,* edited by M. A. Lipton, A. DiMascio, and K. F. Killam, pp. 961–973. Raven Press, New York.

79. Rowan, P., Paykel, E. S., Parker, R. R., and West, E. (1980): *Neuropharmacology,* 19:1223–1225.

80. Schildkraut, J. J. (1965): *Am. J. Psychiatry,* 122:505–518.

81. Sheard, M. H., Solvick, A., and Aghajanian, G. K. (1972): *Brain Res.,* 43:690–694.

82. Sheehan, D. V. (1984): *J. Clin. Psychiatry,* 45:29–36.

83. Sheehan, D. V., Ballenger, J., and Jacoban, G. (1980): *Arch. Gen. Psychiatry,* 37:51–59.

84. Sheehan, D. V., Barry, J., Claycomb, M. D., Surman, O. S., Gelles, L., Gallo, J., and LeGros, B. S. (1984): Presented at the 137th Annual Meeting of the American Psychiatric Association, May 8, 1984.

85. Simpson, G. M. Frederickson, E., Palmer, R., Pi, E., Sloane, B., and White, J. (1985): *Biol. Psychiatry,* 20:680–684.

86. Sjoerdsma, A. (1981): *Clin. Pharmacol. Ther.,* 30:3–22.

87. Solyom, C., Solyom, L., LaPierre, Y., Pecknold, J., and Morton, L. (1981): *Biol. Psychiatry,* 16:239–247.

88. Tipton, K. F., Dostert, P., and Strolin Benedetti, M., ed. (1984): *Monoamine Oxidase and Disease: Prospects for Therapy with Reversible Inhibitors.* Academic Press, London.

89. Tyrer, P. (1976): *Br. J. Psychiatry,* 128:354–360.

90. Tyrer, P., Candy, J., and Kelly, D. (1973): *Psychopharmacologia,* 32:237–254.

91. Waldmeir, P. C., Tipton, K. F., Bernasconi, R., Felner, A. E., Bauman, L., and Maitre, L. (1985): *Eur. J. Pharmacol.,* 107:79–89.

92. Walsh, B. T., Roose, S. P., Glassman, A. H., Gladis, M., and Sadik, C. (1985): *Psychosom. Med.,* 47:123–131.

93. Walsh, B. T., Stewart, J. W., Roose, S. P., Gladis, M., and Glassman, A. H. (1984): *Arch. Gen. Psychiatry,* 41:1105–1109.

94. Youdim, M. B. H., Aronson, J. K., Blau, K., Green, A. R., and Grahame-Smith, D. G. (1979): *Psychol. Med.,* 9:377–382.

95. Zametkin, A., Rapoport, J. L., Murphy, D. L., Linnoila, M., and Ismod, D. (1985): *Arch. Gen. Psychiatry,* 42:962–977.

96. Zreika, M., McDonald, I. A., Bey, P., and Palfreyman, M. G. (1984): *J. Neurochem.,* 43:448–454.

Psychopharmacology:
The Third Generation of Progress,
edited by Herbert Y. Meltzer.
Raven Press, New York © 1987.

CHAPTER **137**

Medications in the Treatment of Sleep Disorders

Wallace B. Mendelson

When evaluating problems related to sleep, it is useful to view the complaints of insomnia or hypersomnolence as symptoms of a variety of discrete disorders. Before we examine the available pharmacologic treatments—which are the subject of this review—it might be well to briefly survey the classification of sleep disorders. Perhaps the most widely accepted classification system was developed by the Association of Sleep Disorders Centers (3) and appears in its nosology and with some modifications in the proposed *Diagnostic and Statistical Manual of Mental Disorders,* 3rd edition, revised draft (DSM-III-R) (26). There are four main categories:

1. DIMS: Disorders of initiating and maintaining sleep (insomnia)
2. DOES: Disorders of excessive somnolence (hypersomnia)
3. Disorders of the sleep-wake cycle (circadian rhythm disorders)
4. Dysfunctions associated with sleep, sleep stages, or partial arousals (parasomnias)

Each of these categories is composed of a number of individual disorders. It should be noted that the same condition, e.g., sleep apnea or nocturnal myoclonus, may appear in more than one category, reflecting the belief that it may result in both insomnia (DIMS) and hypersomnia (DOES). We will examine here some of the major disorders, with emphasis on pharmacologic approaches to their management.

PERSISTENT PSYCHOPHYSIOLOGICAL DIMS

In this disorder one gets a sense that the patient is trying so hard to sleep that the anxiety related to sleeping actually becomes the cause of the insomnia. A classical history—which usually only comes out after several interviews—is that at some time in the past the patient experienced an emotional upset that might reasonably be expected to disturb sleep, e.g., a romantic setback. During this period of initial sleep loss, the patient seems to focus on the sleep-related aspects of his situation. After awhile, when the distress over the original trauma has finally healed, the sleep disturbance remains. The key element in the history is that the patient can sleep when he is not trying. Hence he may describe falling asleep while watching television in the living room, yet be unable to sleep when he gets up and goes into the bedroom. Paradoxically, such a patient will often sleep well in the laboratory. It has been speculated that this is because he has given himself permission to sleep, i.e., he has decided that it will be impossible to sleep in this situation and hence will not try. Since he does not then experience anxiety about whether he will sleep, he is able to do so.

Another aspect of this disturbance is that there may be a conditioned quality to the insomnia. It has been suggested that the bedroom becomes associated in the patient's mind with the uncomfortable sensation of being unable to sleep. Such a patient will often comment that he sleeps better when away from home.

Psychophysiologic insomnia may be helped by nonpharmacologic as well as pharmacologic means. Probably the first step is to have the patient keep a sleep diary, which not only documents the starting condition, but also seems to give him a sense of having more control over his poor sleep; somehow it seems less mysterious when it is measurable. One useful approach is the technique of "stimulus control" (8), the essence of which is to remove from the bedroom all behaviors incompatible with sleep—including worrying about sleep. In essence, the patient is told that the bedroom should be reserved exclusively for sleep. If he finds himself engaged in any other activity—including lying in bed unable to sleep—he should get up and go into another room, and return only when he feels ready to sleep. Other approaches include various relaxation techniques such as biofeedback and progressive relaxation (9,13) and behavioral self-management (20), which emphasize the active role of the patient and the relation of the nighttime distress to daytime life (38). Pharmacotherapy may also be of benefit as an adjunctive treatment, and will be considered at the end of the next section.

SUBJECTIVE DIMS COMPLAINT WITHOUT OBJECTIVE FINDINGS

The hallmark of this disorder is that the distress seems disproportionate to the polygraphically measured sleep, which is usually only mildly disturbed. Such patients are, then, seemingly poor judges of their sleep as measured by the polygraph. It has been speculated that the distress derives either from some disturbance in the ability to perceive the state of consciousness, or some disability in the process of generalizing from the immediate experience to one's habitual status (40).

The patient with subjective DIMS has a somewhat different experience in the laboratory than the patient with persistent psychophysiologic DIMS. In the latter case, sleep in the laboratory is usually relatively good. Whether it is or not, however, the patient in that case tends to be a good judge of how the sleep was. In contrast, the patient with subjective DIMS will describe a poor night, when in fact polygraphic measures showed relatively little disturbance. One promising approach for this disorder is the sleep restriction technique (55). In summary, the patient keeps a careful diary of his hours in bed, and of how many hours he believes that he slept during that period. His time in bed is then restricted to the number of hours he has been sleeping, and is gradually lengthened. The principle is that in the restricted hours now available his sleep will become more efficient.

HYPNOTICS

There are no firm guidelines available on the pharmacotherapy of these chronic conditions; a useful summary of current thinking may be found in the paper resulting from the National Institute of Mental Health consensus conference on Drugs and Insomnia (44). In general, many persons feel that it is appropriate to use hypnotics for treatment of "transient" and "short-term" insomnia, which may last for a few days, or up to a few weeks, respectively. Examples of transient insomnia may be that due to hospitalization for elective surgery, whereas short-term insomnia might be due to an acute personal loss. In contrast, the use of hypnotics for the chronic insomnias such as we have presented here (persistent psychophysiological DIMS or subjective DIMS without objective findings) is less clear. Most laboratory efficacy studies of nightly administration (which have usually been less specific about the nature of the chronic insomnia) have only been carried out to approximately 1 month's duration, so the benefits beyond this point are not well documented. [One study of nitrazepam in normal volunteers did suggest some modest benefits over 10 weeks (1).] It has not been established whether occasional use is beneficial in the long term. Virtually no laboratory studies have been done on this, presumably because the methodologic difficulties are so great. Speaking as a clinician—with no systematic data available—this author finds hypnotics useful as adjunctive therapy while engaging in nonpharmacologic techniques. In this approach, a prescription is written with enough medication for two or three doses a week. In essence, one tells the reluctant patient, who is searching for a pharmacologic answer, "Work with me. While you are learning these techniques, you will never go more than three nights without a good night's sleep." For patients who are not engaged in therapy, one's judgment should be used as to whether to give hypnotics for occasional use. It is clearly important to make a "therapeutic contract" with the patient, explaining that there is little evidence that nightly use is of benefit in the long term, and creating an understanding that future requests for increased quantities of hypnotics will not be honored.

The choice of which hypnotic to prescribe involves many factors, including desired rate of onset and duration of effect, the medical status of the patient, presence of other medications, types of side effects that might be most easily tolerated, and likelihood of overdose. The benzodiazepines are particularly useful as outpatient medications, due to relatively low toxicity when taken alone in overdose, and lack of hepatic enzyme induction. Since these compounds are available with greatly differing half-lives, it is possible to choose an agent tailored to the patient's complaint of difficulty falling asleep or awakenings during the night. If daytime anxiety is also a concern, then the long-acting benzodiazepines (i.e., half-lives of 24 hr or more) may be particularly suitable. They might be less appropriate in a situation when maximum daytime alertness is desired.

Before prescribing a hypnotic, it is also well to consider the complications arising from their use. Certainly among these is the possibility that the patient may become reliant upon them. One study seems to suggest that 4 years after starting a benzodiazepine, 15 to 20% of patients may still be taking it (17,19). Although the potential for abuse differs across pharmacologic classes, there is some suggestion that reliance on recommended doses of hypnotics is as likely to occur with benzodiazepines as with barbiturates (18). Another area of concern is the possible appearance of daytime residual effects. The long-acting benzodiazepines in particular may alter alertness and ability to perform a variety of tasks, without the patient's awareness of impairment (38). On the other hand, there has been one report of daytime anxiety following use of a short-acting benzodiazepine (41), and this issue needs to be explored more thoroughly. Other areas of concern include interactions with alcohol. It should be remembered that if a patient is taking a long-acting benzodiazepine at bedtime, he will have active drug in his bloodstream when he takes a drink during the following evening. Use of hypnotics in the elderly also presents special problems. Due to a combination of altered body content (increased percentage of adipose tissue), changes in rate of clearance of some (but not all) hypnotics, and possible changes in nervous system sensitivity, they are more likely to develop side effects (39). For these reasons it is particularly desirable to try nonpharmacologic alternatives in elderly patients. It is also important to consider the possibility of sleep apnea syndrome before prescribing hypnotics. Although benzodiazepines have relatively modest respiratory depressant qualities compared to other classes of hypnotics, there is some tentative evidence that they may greatly enhance respiratory difficulties in patients with sleep apnea (39). Aspects of history that may lead one to suspect sleep apnea will be discussed in the next section.

SLEEP APNEA SYNDROMES

Sleep apnea syndromes are traditionally divided into obstructive and central forms, which in general (with many exceptions) are associated with excessive daytime sleepiness and insomnia, respectively. The archetypal patient with obstructive apnea is middle-aged and male, often overweight and often hypertensive. It was originally thought that this disorder resulted from a relatively straightforward problem of collapse of the pharynx as a result of hypotonia during sleep. More recently, emphasis on the frequently mixed nature of apneic events, and recognition of the very complex actions of the upper airway musculature during respiration, suggest that there may be a much more complex etiology. This presumably involves an interaction of nervous system dysregulation with the anatomic problem of a narrowed airway (40).

Obstructive sleep apnea may lead to a sense of having slept poorly, daytime sleepiness, medical problems such as pulmonary and systemic hypertension, and psychiatric symptoms including poor concentration, irritability, difficulty with memory, and depressive symptoms, Although the physiology is poorly understood, it may also be associated with impotence. (Indeed screening tests for sleep apnea performed during nocturnal penile tumescence studies for evaluation of impotence are often positive, an issue that needs further study.) Some patients may also experience hypnagogic hallucinations and automatic behavior (29), symptoms usually associated with narcolepsy.

Central apnea tends to increase in frequency with age. Several studies suggest that some degree of sleep apnea may be found in 44 to 67% of elderly persons in general (2,6,14,35,53); among the elderly who do complain of poor sleep, as many as 87% may be found to have such disorders as sleep apnea, nocturnal myoclonus, or narcolepsy (24). The etiology is poorly understood, but appears to involve a periodic failure of the nervous system to stimulate respiratory activity by the diaphragm and accessory muscles of respiration. A history of loud snoring, which is very common with obstructive apnea, is less often seen in central apnea.

Treatments for obstructive sleep apnea range from very conservative steps involving weight loss and sleeping position, to pharmacological approaches, to surgery on the upper airway (40). Weight loss of 20 kg or more may be of some benefit to some patients, and there is some evidence that it is more beneficial to those with apneas in both rapid eye movement (REM) and non-REM sleep (31). It is common experience that snoring is less likely when one sleeps on the side instead of the back; using this observation, Cartright (15) has shown a reduction in apneas in patients sleeping on the side. The difference in respiration in the two positions was greatest in those who were less heavy.

TRICYCLIC ANTIDEPRESSANTS

In the early 1970s, several case reports suggested that tricyclic antidepressants might be useful in sleep apnea. Since protriptyline is much less sedating than most tricyclics, it seemed an appropriate agent for clinical trials, and indeed several studies have confirmed its usefulness (12,16,28,54). The mechanism of action is not certain. It seems to decrease the frequency of disordered breathing events in non-REM sleep (54), and may help in patients whose apneas are largely confined to non-REM sleep (16). In REM sleep, some studies have suggested that its benefits are due merely to shortening the duration (54), whereas others indicate that it actually reduces the number of disordered breathing events and degree of oxygen desaturation in REM sleep (28). On the other hand, benefits of protriptyline are limited. One study, for instance, found that only 7 of 14 patients could be managed by protriptyline alone (16). Side effects that should be considered include anticholinergic symptoms such as dry mouth or urinary hesitancy, and alterations in cardiac conduction and possibly contractility. The latter is of particular concern, since these patients may already be more likely to experience arrhythmias.

MEDROXYPROGESTERONE ACETATE

Progesterone, which has respiratory stimulant properties, had been reported to reduce P_aCO_2 in normal volunteers and patients with obesity-hypoventilation syndrome (52,57). It seemed reasonable, then, to determine its benefits in sleep apnea syndrome. The results have shown at best modest improvement. Orr et al. (45), for instance, found no change in frequency and duration of apneas; there was some improvement in daytime somnolence and P_aO_2, which may have been related to improved cardiac status. Other studies reported no improvement in the group as a whole, although about half had reduced sleepiness and number of apneas (56), no change except for a reduction in maximum duration of apneas (6), or improved daytime blood gases with no major changes in respiratory status during sleep (25).

The mechanism of action of progesterone *vis à vis* respiration is unclear. It has been suggested that it stimulates the muscles of the upper airway as well as the diaphragm and intercostals (56). Another interesting speculation is that its respiratory stimulant effects are a nonspecific consequence of its thermogenic properties. Side effects include alopecia and decreased libido. One patient in the study of Strohl et al. (56) had a substantial increase in apneas; it has been speculated that this could be due to relatively greater stimulation of the diaphragm and intercostals relative to the musculature of the upper airway such as the genioglossus.

There is clearly a need, then, for better pharmacologic treatments for sleep apnea syndrome. There has been some tentative evidence that L-tryptophan might have benefits in sleep apnea (50). It may be particularly useful in those patients in whom the disordered breathing events are primarily in non-REM sleep, or in whom they are of equal severity in non-REM and REM sleep. One promising avenue of basic research might be to examine drugs that are "inverse agonists" of benzodiazepines, i.e., that bind to the receptor complex yet have opposite pharmacologic properties compared to traditional hypnotics. Another might be to examine the effects of drugs that alter body temperature on respiration during sleep.

There are also a variety of other approaches to obstructive sleep apnea, which are beyond the scope of the present paper (40). These include the use of low flow oxygen during sleep (the benefits of which appear to be relatively limited), continuous positive air pressure, and surgical interventions including uvulopalatopharyngoplasty or chronic tracheostomy.

Treatments available for central sleep apnea are relatively limited. In practice protriptyline is often used, although there are few systematic data on this. The carbonic anhydrase inhibitor acetazolamide has been reported to reduce apnea-associated awakenings and rate of apneas with improved daytime wakefulness in the short term, but results at 1 year followup were mixed. Another approach is diaphragm pacing, although at present this is available at relatively few medical centers. Patients with central alveolar hyperventilation syndrome have been maintained for as long as 10 years using this technique (33), and certainly its use with central sleep apnea will be of great interest.

NOCTURNAL MYOCLONUS AND RESTLESS LEGS SYNDROME

Like sleep apnea, nocturnal myoclonus appears in the Association of Sleep Disorders Centers nosology as a cause of both insomnia and excessive daytime sleepiness. This disorder involves periodic clonic movements of the legs during sleep, resulting in brief arousals. Current criteria for diagnosis are that there are at least three episodes during the night during each of which at least 30 such movements occur. Inside each of these episodes movements occur periodically, usually every 20 to 40 sec.

Myoclonic movements also occur in asymptomatic persons. In one study, 6% of asymptomatic subjects met the formal diagnosis of nocturnal myoclonus and another 5% had some movements (4). Myoclonic movements are also found in patients with many other sleep disorders, including narcolepsy and sleep apnea (23). This seems to raise the possibility that although nocturnal myoclonus may be an entity in its own right, it may also be a consequence of sleep disturbance due to other causes. The hallmark of this disorder is that the patient is usually unaware of it, complaining only of poor sleep or daytime sleepiness. Thus it is useful when taking a history to ask the patient's bed partner if he/she is aware of any clonic leg movements. It may also be useful to ask the patient if the bedcovers are very disturbed in the morning, or whether the bed remains relatively neat.

In contrast to nocturnal myoclonus, patients with restless legs syndrome are very much aware of a difficulty with their legs—they complain of a hard-to-describe discomfort that is worst at rest, and is relieved by movement. Because of this discomfort they find it very difficult to lie still and go to sleep. Restless legs syndrome tends to occur in patients with nocturnal myoclonus. It often occurs in uremia, and has been estimated to be found in 5 to 20% of dialysis patients (48). It has also been reported in 15% of surgical outpatients (10).

Patients with nocturnal myoclonus are not found to have epileptiform activity on standard clinical electroencephalograms, and most traditional antiepileptic medications are not of benefit. Perhaps the most widely accepted treatment is the use of clonazepam, often given in doses of 0.5 to 1.5 mg. Results have been variable. In a study of 15 patients at Stanford University, the patients' reports were mixed, with clear success in only a few cases (22). Oshtory and Vijayan (46) described two patients treated successfully. Coleman (21) found that only one of three patients had clear improvement in polygraphic measures of movements. The major side effect is daytime sleepiness. Some physicians prescribe short-acting benzodiazepines and believe that there is benefit. This awaits confirmation by a systemic study. Baclofen has been found to decrease waking time and movement-induced sleep fragmentation, but may actually increase the number of movements (30). It should also be noted that nocturnal myoclonus has been thought to be a side effect of treatment with tricyclic antidepressants, and to occur during hypnotic withdrawal. Coleman (21), reviewing the histories of 53 patients, however, did not find it to be associated with one particular class of medications.

NARCOLEPSY

Narcolepsy is a disorder of excessive sleepiness in combination with a series of secondary symptoms. The sleepiness often takes the form of sleep attacks, episodes of a seemingly irresistible need to sleep, usually lasting about 15 min or less, from which the patient often awakens feeling at least briefly refreshed. The key to the history of sleep attacks would seem to be the inappropriateness of the timing of the events; the actual total sleep of the narcoleptic over 24 hr may not be much greater than that of normals. Another major symptom is cataplexy. This is characterized by brief (often less than a minute) loss of muscle tone, occurring in association with the expression of emotion. The resulting weakness may be mild, causing no more than a need to briefly sit down, or may be a major event resulting in collapse. In general the patient retains consciousness during these episodes, although during longer ones visual hallucinatory experiences may occur. Other secondary symptoms include sleep paralysis—a sensation of being unable to move just as one is going to sleep or waking up—and hypnogogic or hypnopompic hallucinations, vivid dreamlike experiences that occur at those times. They may also have episodes of what clinically may appear to be automatic behavior, which is associated with brief microsleep episodes. Somewhat paradoxically, perhaps, they may complain of disturbed nocturnal sleep, with frequent awakenings and a sense of not having been refreshed.

A critical observation in understanding the pathophysiology of narcolepsy was the report of REM sleep occurring in the first few minutes of sleep (49). This may occur in as many as 44% of patients during nocturnal sleep (43). In clinical practice, an evaluation is usually done of both nocturnal sleep and a multiple sleep latency test consisting of four daytime naps; a diagnosis is made when two of these five possible sleep onsets involve REM onset sleep. Forty-nine percent may also exhibit significant numbers of myoclonic leg movements, and 9% may have significant sleep apnea (43).

The biochemical alterations that underlie the observed pathophysiology of narcolepsy have been the subject of intensive study. Work with narcoleptic dogs suggests that they have a defect in dopamine utilization and/or turnover (37), as well as elevated numbers of acetylcholine receptors in the brainstem (7). The latter may imply cholinergic hypersensitivity. There are also data suggesting that the observed temperature minima in narcoleptic patients occur about an hour after sleep onset, compared to 4 to 5 hr after sleep onset in controls (42). How intimately this circadian phase advance of temperature is linked to the REM onset sleep is not yet certain. Recent evidence also suggests that almost all patients with narcolepsy may have the major histocompatibility complex antigen HLA DR2, compared with 21.5% of controls (36). This would seem to link the disorder to the short arm of chromosome 6, and represents a major step forward in understanding its genetic basis.

Stimulants and Tricyclic Antidepressants

The traditional pharmacotherapy for narcolepsy is determined by the target symptoms. For treatment of sleep attacks, stimulants such as dextroamphetamine (29), methylphenidate, or pemoline are often used. This author prefers pemoline because of its somewhat longer half-life of 12 hr, and because of the clinical impression that it may have less euphoriant qualities. The major side effect of concern is overstimulation resulting in poorer nocturnal sleep. For this reason, doses should be given in the morning, and a second dose, if needed, should be administered no later than noon. Although early clinical reports suggested that tolerance to dextroamphetamine does not develop during

a 6-month trial (47), many physicians have the impression that this is indeed a major difficulty. For this reason it may be wise to have a drug holiday 1 day a week. If tolerance does develop, it is best to withdraw the medication slowly—after carefully cautioning the patient that he may experience severe rebound sleepiness—and begin treatment again with low doses.

For the symptom of cataplexy, the tricyclic antidepressants are often used. Perhaps the most widely administered compound has been imipramine, usually in doses of 50 to 100 mg. Such doses are obviously less than those used to treat major depressions. The timing of benefits is also somewhat different than in the treatment of depression, insofar as amelioration of cataplexy may often occur after 1 or 2 days in narcolepsy. Other tricyclics may also be useful; some clinicians employ protriptyline, taking advantage of its stimulant properties. Clomipramine has been reported to effectively prevent secondary symptoms for periods of 10 to 21 months (29,51).

Other Pharmacologic Agents

Patients with intractable narcolepsy have also been treated with the monoamine oxidase inhibitor phenelzine for periods as long as 1 year (58), with improvement in both secondary symptoms as well as subjective daytime sleepiness. The many side effects, including hypotension, edema, and impaired sexual functioning, make monoamine oxidase inhibitors less desirable, however, except in cases unresponsive to traditional treatments. Other compounds have been reported to benefit daytime sleepiness in case studies or small patient groups, including L-dopa (32), methysergide (59), and propranolol (34). A case report with L-tryptophan suggested that REM periods tended more often to follow non-REM periods when the patient was on drug (60). Amantadine, which may have some amphetamine-like properties, has been thought to be not beneficial (27).

Although the pharmacologic treatment of narcolepsy is vital, it is important to bear in mind the nonpharmacologic management as well. Narcolepsy is a very debilitating illness. One study comparing its psychosocial consequences with that of epilepsy showed that the narcoleptics had higher frequencies of disease-attributed problems at work, poorer driving records, greater problems in planning recreation, and other problems (11). These persons also have often done less well in their personal and professional lives than they might have, with inevitable loss of self-esteem. For these reasons, supportive counseling is very important. It is also very useful for these patients to plan brief daytime naps into their schedules, as these seem to offer at least temporary increases in daytime wakefulness.

SUMMARY AND CONCLUSIONS

From the brief descriptions of these major disorders several general thoughts emerge. The first is that disturbed sleep is a symptom that may result from various discrete, diagnosable, and treatable conditions. The same diagnostic reasoning that is used in other areas of medicine is, then, very applicable when evaluating a complaint of poor sleep. The second point is that in several cases, including nocturnal myoclonus and sleep apnea, the same pathophysiology may result in complaints of either insomnia or daytime sleepiness, the latter presumably appearing as the nocturnal sleep becomes more disturbed. In some sense, then, myoclonus and apnea have a common feature. In both cases sleep is interrupted by aberrant physiologic disturbances that cause many brief awakenings, greatly compromising sleep continuity. Thus, although some symptomatology may occur as a direct consequence of the altered physiology (e.g., the repeated arterial oxygen desaturations in sleep apnea), other symptoms may result from the fragmentation of sleep itself.

Another interesting theme is that myoclonic symptoms may appear in several contexts, either as a possible free-standing entity, or possibly as a nonspecific consequence of sleep disturbance due to other disorders such as narcolepsy. In cases where it appears in the context of another disorder, the appropriate approach is to treat the primary disorder. One situation that is particularly clinically irksome is when some myoclonic movements appear in a patient with disordered breathing events, even though they may fall short of a formal diagnosis of sleep apnea syndrome. The problem here is that drugs that might be useful for myoclonus are often respiratory suppressants to some degree, and hence should only be used with great caution in such patients.

It should also be noticed that tricyclic antidepressants are mentioned in several different sections of this review—including those on psychophysiologic insomnia, sleep apnea, and narcolepsy—and are also used in other conditions such as nocturnal enuresis. It is not clear why tricyclics are so beneficial in a variety of situations. The experience with sleep apnea suggests that it is not merely a matter of their REM sleep suppressant properties (as there is at least some evidence that protriptyline is beneficial in non-REM sleep apnea as well). Similarly, the different dosage and time course of response in narcolepsy seem to imply that the mechanism of action may be different in the various disorders. The significance of the utility of these agents in many conditions will remain one of the intriguing questions for the years ahead.

The discussion of subjective insomnia without objective findings raises another interesting topic: the recognition that the subjective experience of being asleep is a somewhat different process than the act of being asleep in terms of electroencephalogram (EEG)-defined sleep stages. It may be that one aspect of the pathophysiology of this disorder is a dissociation between the normal relationship of the experience of sleep and the usual EEG markers of sleep. This raises the interesting possibility that hypnotics—the agents that seem to bring some relief to this condition—may work not only by altering EEG-defined sleep stages themselves, but also by changing the subjective experience of the state of consciousness associated with that stage (W. Mendelson et al., *submitted for publication*).

Finally, it should be noticed that although there are useful pharmacologic approaches to each of these disorders, the administration of medication is only one aspect of their management. In most cases it is equally important to institute appropriate behavioral steps (e.g., taking naps in narcolepsy), to help the patient understand what is happening to him, and to help instill a sense that he is more in control of his condition than he may have at first believed.

REFERENCES

1. Adam, K., Adamson, L., Brezinova, L., Hunter, W. M., and Oswald, I. (1976): *Br. Med. J.,* 1:1558–1560.
2. Anconi-Israel, S., Kripke, D. F., Mason, W., et al. (1981): *Sleep,* 4:349–358.
3. Association of Sleep Disorder Center (1979): *Sleep,* 2:1–137.
4. Bixler, E. O., Kales, A., Vela-Bueno, Jacoby, A., Scarone, J. A., and Soldatos, C. R. (1982): *Res. Commun. Chem. Pathol. Pharmacol.,* 36:129–140.
5. Block, A. J., Boysen, P. G., Wynne, J. W., et al. (1979): *N. Engl. J. Med.,* 300:513–517.
6. Block, A. J., Wynne, J. W., Boysen, P. G., Lindsey, S., Martin, C., and Cantor, B. (1981): *Am. J. Med.,* 70:510.
7. Boehme, R. E., Baker, T. L., Mefford, I. N., Barchas, J. D., and Dement, W. C. (1984): *Life Sci.,* 34:1825–1828.
8. Bootzin, R. R. (1977): In: *Behavioral Self-Management,* edited by R. B. Stuart, pp. 176–195. Brunner/Mazel, New York.
9. Borkovek, T. C., and Fowles, D. C. (1973): *J. Abnorm. Psychol.,* 82:153–158.
10. Braude, W., and Barnes, T. (1982): *Br. Med. J.,* 284:510.
11. Broughton, R. J., Guberman, A., and Roberts, J. (1984): *Epilepsia,* 25:423–433.
12. Brownell, L. G., West, P., Sweatman, P., Acres, J. C., and Kryger, M. H. (1982): *N. Engl. J. Med.,* 307:1037–1042.
13. Budzynski, T. H. (1973): *Semin. Psychiatry,* 5:537–547.
14. Carskadon, M. A., and Dement, W. C. (1981): *J. Gerontol.,* 36: 420–423.
15. Cartright, R. D. (1984): *Sleep,* 7:110–114.
16. Clark, R. W., Schmidt, H. S., Schaal, S. F., Boudoulas, H., and Schuller, D. E. (1979): *Neurology,* 29:1287–1292.
17. Clift, A. D. (1975): In: *Sleep Disturbance and Hypnotic Drug Dependence,* edited by A. D. Clift, pp. 97–105. Excerpta Medica, Amsterdam.
18. Clift, A. D. (1975): In: *Sleep Disturbance and Hypnotic Drug Dependence,* edited by A. D. Clift, pp. 107–153. Excerpta Medica, Amsterdam.
19. Clift, A. D. (1975): In: *Sleep Disturbance and Hypnotic Drug Dependence,* edited by A. D. Clift, pp. 155–177. Excerpta Medica, Amsterdam.
20. Coates, T. J., and Thoresen, C. E. (1977): *How to Sleep Better.* Prentice-Hall, Englewood Cliffs, NJ.
21. Coleman, R. M. (1979): Ph.D. Thesis, Yeshiva University. University Microfilm, Ann Arbor, MI.
22. Coleman, R. M. (1982): In: *Sleeping and Waking Disorders: Indications and Techniques,* edited by R. Guilleminault, pp. 265–295. Addison Wesley, California.
23. Coleman, R. M., Pollak, C. P., and Weitzman, E. D. (1980): *Ann. Neurol.,* 8:416–421.
24. Dement, W. C. (1980): Presentation to Project Sleep.
25. Dolly, F. R., and Block, A. J. (1983): *Chest,* 84:394–398.
26. DSM IIIR (1985): *Psychiatr. News,* 9–10.
27. Ersmark, B., and Lidvall, H. (1973): *Psychopharmacologia,* 28: 308.
28. Fletcher, E., Lavoi, M., Zenner, G., Malitz, W., and Nickeson, D. (1984): *Am. Rev. Respir. Dis. (Suppl.),* 129:A59.
29. Guilleminault, C., Carskadon, M. A., and Dement, W. C. (1974): *Arch. Neurol.,* 30:90–93.
30. Guilleminault, C., and Flagg, W. (1984): *Ann. Neurol.,* 15:234–239.
31. Guilleminault, C., van den Hoed, J., and Mitler, M. M. (1978): *Sleep Apnea Syndromes.* Alan R. Liss, New York.
32. Gunne, L. M., Lidvall, H. F., and Widen, L. (1971): *Psychopharmacologia,* 19:204–206.
33. Hambrecht, F. T. (1980): *Ann. Biomed. Eng.,* 8:333–338.
34. Kales, A., Soldatos, C. R., Cadieux, R., Bixler, E. O., Tan, T. L., and Scharf, M. B. (1979): *Ann. Int. Med.,* 91:741–742.

35. Krieger, J., Mangin, P., and Kurtz, D. (1980); *Rev. EEG Neurophysiol.,* 10:177–185.
36. Langdon, N., Welsch, K. I., van Dam, M., Vaughn, R. W., and Parkes, D. (1984): *Lancet,* 2:1178–1180.
37. Mefford, I. N., Baker, T. L., Boehme, R., Foutz, A. S., and Ciaranello, R. D. (1983): *Science,* 22:632–669.
38. Mendelson, W. B., ed. (1980): *The Use and Misuse of Sleeping Pills.* Plenum, New York.
39. Mendelson, W. B. (1985): In: *American Psychiatric Assoc. Psychiatry Update, Vol. IV,* edited by R. E. Hales and A. J. Frances, pp. 379–394. American Psychiatric Press, Washington, DC.
40. Mendelson, W. B. (1987): In: *Human Sleep: Research and Clinical Care.* Plenum, New York (*in press*).
41. Morgan, K., and Oswald, I. (1982): *Br. Med. J.,* 284:942.
42. Mosko, S. S., Holowach, J. B., and Sassin, J. F. (1983): *Sleep,* 6: 137–146.
43. Mosko, S. S., Shampain, D. S., and Sassin, J. F. (1984): *Sleep,* 7: 115–125.
44. National Institute of Mental Health (1984): *Conn. Med.,* 48:373–378.
45. Orr, W. C., Imes, N. K., and Martin, R. J. (1979): *Arch. Intern. Med.,* 139:109–111.
46. Oshtory, M., and Vijayan, N. (1980): *Arch. Neurol.,* 37:119–120.
47. Parkes, J. D., and Fenton, G. W. (1973): *J. Neurol. Neurosurg.,* 36:1076–1081.
48. Read, D. J., Feest, T. G., and Nassim, M. A. (1981): *Br. Med. J.,* 283:885–886.
49. Rechtschaffen, A., Wolpert, E. A., Dement, W. C., Mitchell, S. A., and Fisher, C. (1963): *Electroencephalogr. Clin. Neurophysiol.,* 15:599–609.
50. Schmidt, H. S. (1983): *Bull. Eur. Physiopathol.,* 19:625–629.
51. Shapiro, W. R. (1975): *Arch. Neurol.,* 32:653–656.
52. Skatrud, J. B., Dempsey, J. A., Iber, C., and Berssenbrugge, A. (1981): *Am. Rev. Respir. Dis.,* 124:260–268.
53. Smallwood, R. F., Vitiello, M. V., Giblin, E. C., et al. (1983): *Sleep,* 6:16–22.
54. Smith, P. L., Haponik, E. F., Allen, R. P., and Bleecker, E. R. (1983): *Am. Rev. Respir. Dis.,* 127:8–13.
55. Spielman, A. J., Saskin, P., and Thorpy, M. J. (1984): *Sleep Res.,* 13:167.
56. Strohl, K. P., Hensley, M. J., Saunders, N. A., Scharf, S. M., and Brown, R. (1981): *JAMA,* 245:1230–1232.
57. Sutton, F. D., Zwillich, C. W., Creagh, C. E., Peirson, D. J., and Weil, J. V. (1975): *Ann. Intern. Med.,* 83:476–479.
58. Wyatt, R. J., Fram, D. H., Buchbinder, R., and Snyder, F. (1971): *N. Engl. J. Med.,* 285:987–991.
59. Wyler, A. R., Wilkus, R. J., and Troupin, A. S. (1975): *Arch. Neurol.,* 32:265–268.
60. Zarcone, V., Gulevich, G., and Greenberg, S. (1968): *Psychophysiology,* 5:236–237.

Psychopharmacology:
The Third Generation of Progress,
edited by Herbert Y. Meltzer.
Raven Press, New York © 1987.

CHAPTER **138**

A Model Psychopharmacology Curriculum for Psychiatric Residents

Ira D. Glick, David S. Janowsky, Carl Salzman, and Richard I. Shader

After a number of years of discussion and planning by the Committee on Education and Training of the American College of Neuropsychopharmacology (ACNP) an *ad hoc* committee, consisting of the authors of this chapter, was appointed to develop and produce a model psychopharmacology curriculum for use in psychiatric residency programs. Supported in part by a National Institute of Mental Health (NIMH) grant (No. 83M055989510D), the curriculum was reviewed by the parent committee and by the ACNP Council and subsequently distributed in 1985 to psychiatric residency programs. What follows is the essence of the curriculum. It has been shortened, largely through the omission of examples rather than through any omission of concepts.

OBJECTIVES

Designed to provide a basis for planning and teaching basic and clinical psychopharmacology in a psychiatric residency, this model curriculum originated from the following assumptions:

- The teaching of psychopharmacology at the residency level is underrepresented both in numbers of programs providing adequate content and in the time allotted
- There is great variance in the effectiveness of such teaching, even when there is appropriate representation

- There is a need to assure adequate, science-based knowledge and skills among psychiatric residents
- Resources for designing such educational programs are not uniformly distributed nationally

These impressions originated from requests to the ACNP by the American Psychiatric Association (APA) and the American Association of Directors of Psychiatric Residency Training (AADPRT), data developed by the NIMH, and numerous teachers of psychopharmacology who asked for a structured curriculum and teaching aids.

OVERVIEW

This teaching package assumes that there is not only psychopharmacologic "theory and practice" to be taught but also underlying principles to be learned. Psychiatric residents learn in different ways, at different speeds, and in very different settings, and repetition of appropriate concepts and data at various steps in the residency is necessary for the integration and consolidation of this information base. Case-based learning is essential. The involvement of senior supervisors, who can be models for the integration of psychopharmacology into the total treatment planning for care, is also important.

We believe that the terminal objectives of a clinical psychopharmacology program should be to impart the ability to

- Integrate psychodynamic-psychosocial and psychobiol-ogic-psychopharmacologic aspects of a given patient's care
- Use psychotropic drugs safely
- Know when and when *not* to use psychotropic drugs
- Understand the limitations of psychotropic usage and their dangers and pitfalls
- Possess reasonable theoretical models to understand the biologic mechanisms underlying the use of psychotropic drugs

We have not included *enabling objectives* (i.e., what should be learned in each year), because they are too dependent on local program conditions (e.g., whether residents start psychiatry on inpatient or outpatient rotations or in emergency room settings, or the sequencing of other curricula).

We have also not included material on the legal, regulatory, and ethical aspects of psychopharmacologic prescribing practices. For example, programs should include material on the rights of physicians in emergency clinical situations (suicidal or assaultive patients) and the rights of patients to refuse treatment.

WHAT AND HOW TO TEACH

Obviously, each program needs to develop its own style for teaching psychopharmacology, based on its resources, expertise, and available clinical arenas. The following are suggestions for developing an optimal teaching curriculum and program. We have *not* delineated "priorities versus the ideal." Therefore, although each program will have to decide that question, we would emphasize that didactic lectures and the Journal Club conference have been the "irreducible minimum" as opposed to the fullest program possible in the best of all worlds.

The question of which learning groups should be interdisciplinary must be considered, since many beginning residents are "ashamed" to reveal their rudimentary knowledge in psychopharmacology in front of, for example, ward nurses and other personnel. A survey of the content and formats of what we consider the "better" programs that include psychopharmacology teaching is found in Appendix A of the full monograph. Interested readers should consult the monograph, which is available from the Secretariat of the ACNP, Box 1823, Station B, Vanderbilt University, Nashville, TN 37235.

Didactic Program

A Psychopharmacology Lecture Series (to cover the basic and the sophisticated use of psychotropic drugs)

Development, advantages/disadvantages, and integration with other formats. We view the didactic curriculum as being taught at three different levels—a "crash course" (taught in the PG I year or in the summer of the PG II year), a basic course, and an advanced course with components taught sequentially during the 4 years of training. In addition, formal didactic teaching of psychopharmacology should be provided within the larger context of the teaching of neurobiology and biological psychiatry.

We strongly believe that programs should include a series of introductory psychopharmacology lectures—i.e., the "crash course"—for the beginning resident as part of the core curriculum. Careful attention must be paid to these lectures, since they may form the basis for the developing psychiatrist's future clinical practice.

Although up-to-date scientific knowledge may be imparted to trainees during a series of lectures, it is important to emphasize that for resident training, didactics may not be as directly useful as small group and individual supervision and case-conference methods of teaching. Nevertheless, formal didactic teaching often stimulates interest in psychopharmacology and broadens intellectual and clinical perspectives in the treatment of psychiatric patients. It is important to allow a question-and-answer format during and/or after a specific didactic lecture to help consolidate learning.

A didactic lecture series is obviously a useful way of conveying information. Issues of lack of "absorption" and "retention" of lecture material suggest that, whenever possible, lectures be accompanied by relevant, clinically oriented (or otherwise appropriate) journal articles and textbook reading assignments. Time should be allotted in each lecture for resident and lecturer dialogue, either after each subtopic or at the end of the lecture. In a 1-hr lecture, at least 15 min should be devoted to discussion.

Because of ever-increasing demands on both trainee and faculty time, one program has begun to develop a videotape library of lectures in basic and clinical psychopharmacology. These tapes are available for residents who, because of clinical duties, miss the scheduled times; other uses are possible. However, the passive experiences of listening and/or watching audio and video tapes are not optimal for learning. Interaction with experts and the opportunity to ask questions about exceptions to the rule are essential.

In the next two sections, we present a list of General Issues and Concepts and Specific Topics that may be helpful in developing a didactic lecture series. Suggested introductory themes are delineated. Both the "issues" and the "topics" also are appropriate for consideration in the more mentorial and supervisory forms of teaching psychopharmacology, such as in psychopharmacology case conferences or psychopharmacology rounds.

In addition to the utilization of the above-mentioned outlines as guides to the content of didactic lectures, such outlines may be helpful in preparing a series of slides for utilization in didactic lectures. Slide sets to accompany most lecture topics are being developed and should soon be available for a nominal charge from the ACNP.

Appendix B in the full monograph presents model lecture outlines, which were readily available to us and which may be useful in organizing a lecture series for residents. The lecture outlines included are intended to be representative and are not "model" outlines in the sense of being considered without flaw. It is hoped that they offer useful guidelines for the preparation of similar outlines. Contributors were Leo Hollister, M.D., Sidney Zisook, M.D., Lewis Judd, M.D., J. Hampton Atkinson, M.D., David Braff, M.D., Marc Schuckit, M.D., Gary Tollefson, M.D., Sheldon Preskorn, M.D., Carl Salzman, M.D., James Kocsis, M.D., Rachel Gittelman, Ph.D., Richard Shader, M.D., Charles Rich, M.D., David Janowsky, M.D., and Max Fink, M.D.

General issues and concepts. The following are suggested general issues and concepts that are worth covering in specific clinical psychopharmacology lectures about a given drug or class of drugs. The level of the course (i.e., "basic" or "advanced") should determine which of the following to include:

- Proposed mechanisms of action of drug
- Basic pharmacologic issues (pharmacokinetic issues, physiologic effects, etc.)
- Diagnostic issues (overlap between efficacies, delineation of syndromes, etc.)
- Efficacy of drugs in related or complementary classes versus each other and versus placebo
- Age-related issues (child, geriatric, etc.)
- Drug dosages; timing of dosages
- Specific indications (specific use of drugs: differential efficacies between drugs)
- Uses of drugs in nonpsychiatric settings
- Uses across diagnoses (specificity issues)
- General principles of drug use (models of administration, timing of dosages, use of blood levels, predictors of effect, etc.)
- Drug-drug interactions (psychotropic-psychotropic; medical-psychotropic; recreational-psychotropic)
- Drug-combination therapies
- Side effects (CNS, metabolic, cardiovascular, dermatologic, peripheral autonomic, electrocardiographic effects)
- Medical and laboratory workup needed to use a given drug
- Drug withdrawal effects
- Overdose signs, effects, and treatment
- Addiction-habituation-dependency potential
- Contraindications
- Uses of blood levels
- Issues of acute, continuation, and maintenance phase psychopharmacology
- Strategies for the treatment-resistant patient

Specific topics. The following is a series of lecture topics of importance in constructing a didactic psychopharmacology series. We recognize that the list is long and the topics may not seem to be of parallel importance, but we leave the job of tailoring the topics to local program coordinators.

Topics 1–9 are most appropriate for the first-year resident who needs to rapidly master the use of psychotropic agents. Such lectures may occur within the context of a "crash course" offered in a resident's first year of psychiatry training. A crash course covers issues of diagnosis [i.e., *Diagnostic and Statistical Manual of Mental Disorders,* 3rd edition (DSM-III)] and treatment with antipsychotics and antidepressants—emphasizing indications, contraindications, and dose regimens including routes of administration and side effects. It may be useful to repeat such lectures in greater depth in the second half of the PG II year, after the beginning resident has had a greater amount of integrated clinical experience. In general, these topics are presented in order of how they could be presented over the course of the residency.

1. General principles
   - Dose-response relationships
   - Blood levels
   - Evaluation of effects
   - Placebo effects
   - Pharmacokinetics
2. Biologic hypotheses (genetic, biochemical, electrolyte, circadian) relating to the etiology of the following diagnoses:
   - Affective disorders
   - Schizophrenic disorders
   - Anxiety, phobic, and panic disorders
   - Attention deficit disorders
   - Childhood psychoses
   - Dementias
   - Other
3. Antipsychotic Drugs
   - Neuroleptic
   - Antiparkinsonian agents used with antipsychotics
4. Antidepressants
   - Tricyclic antidepressants
   - Monoamine oxidase inhibitors
   - Newer antidepressants
   - Psychostimulants
   - Lithium
   - Unconventional antidepressants
5. Antimanic agents and mood normalizers
   - Lithium
   - Carbamazepine
   - Sodium valproate
   - Antipsychotic drugs
   - Others
6. Antianxiety agents
   - Sedative and hypnotic drugs
   - Benzodiazepines
   - Others (e.g., buspirone, tricyclics, monoamine oxidase inhibitors, hydroxyzine)
7. Child psychopharmacology
   - General management considerations
   - Indications by diagnosis
   - Indications by presenting symptoms
8. Liaison consultation psychopharmacology
   - Uses of psychotropic drugs in the medically ill
   - Medical drug-induced psychopathology
   - Drug-drug interactions
   - Drug side effects in the medically ill patient
9. Geriatric psychopharmacology
   - Uses of psychotropic drugs in the medically ill
   - Medical drug-induced psychopathology
   - Drug-drug interactions
   - Drug side effects in the medically ill patient
   - Differential pharmacology
10. Treatment of resistant depression and mania
11. Treatment of resistant schizophrenia
12. Treatment of resistant anxiety, panic disorder, and agoraphobia
13. Exotic uses of psychotropic drugs
14. Drug treatment of sleep disorders
15. Precursor loading therapies in schizophrenia and depression
   - Choline

- L-dopa
- Phenylalanine
- Tryptophan
- 5-Hydroxytryptophan

16. Substance abuse and recreational uses of drugs
    - Opiates
    - Sedative hypnotics
    - Stimulants
    - Marijuana
17. Alcohol
    - Disease concept
    - Alcohol misuse
    - Habituation
    - Toleration
    - Dependence
    - Withdrawal
    - Treatment
    - Etiology
18. Drug treatment of personality disorders
    - Antisocial disorder
    - Obsessive-compulsive disorder
    - Depressive personality disorder
    - Borderline personality disorder
    - Schizoid personality disorder
    - Other (i.e., the violent personality)
19. The interface for psychopharmacology with other modalities such as psychotherapy, electroconvulsive therapy, etc.
20. Psychotropic drug-drug interactions
21. The "sociopsychology" of psychopharmacology
22. When to stop, withhold, or not start drugs (issues of why to use drugs, why to change doses, why to continue medications)
23. The sociology of medicine giving (influence of social status, age, and site of treatment on drug treatment)
24. The education of patients (in drug effects, drug compliance, and drug side effects)
25. Working with patient resistance to, or overuse of, drugs
26. Roles, settings, and sociology of psychotropic drug uses and abuse
27. Electroconvulsive therapy (ECT)
28. Research approaches in psychopharmacology (instruments, design, etc.)

Development of a Literature Review Seminar (Journal Club) and Outside Guest Lecturer Series

We also recommend an integrated literature review seminar (or Journal Club) and guest lecturer series for all 3 years of residency training in which the literature read is directly related to the lecture presented.

An important aspect of any Journal Club, which should occur at least once a month, is the development of the critical ability to read and critique scientific articles. In one program, "good" and "bad" articles on psychopharmacology subjects are presented in a monthly Journal Club meeting. Residents critique the "good" and "bad" articles and then, in turn, are critiqued on their critique by a senior psychopharmacologist. Residents should be encouraged to ask "controversial" questions and question assumptions underlying the presentations.

Development of a Formal Case Conference

Case conferences should be offered in all 3 years of psychiatric residency training. Patients are selected because of difficulties in their treatment, particular features in their clinical presentations, or because they illustrate a particular aspect of psychopharmacology. The patient is presented and interviewed with a focus on at least these perspectives:

- Diagnosis and differential diagnosis
- Review of prior psychopharmacologic treatment
- Current reasoning for use of medications
- Selection of drug and dose and/or ECT
- Integration of the case from psychotherapeutic and psychopharmacologic perspectives

Basic pharmacology principles can be discussed as related to actual patient care, and specific psychopharmacology principles can be developed. Side effects of long-term treatment can also be discussed; followup conferences are often useful after a 3-month hiatus.

Continuous Clinical Psychopharmacology Case Conferences Focusing on the Integration of Psychotherapy and Psychopharmacology

Another didactic technique is the use of a continuous longitudinal clinical psychopharmacology case conference, approximately twice monthly, which illustrates the need for psychopharmacologic interventions and for other psychotherapies. Alternatively, cases can be seen for only a few sessions. Videotapes or live interviews can be utilized to focus on the psychotherapy-psychopharmacology interface.

Development of Individual or Small Group Supervision

Use of Small Group, Clinical, Mentorial Teaching by Psychopharmacology Experts Using Selected Case Material

Modeled after individual or small group psychotherapy supervision, the discussion may focus on the effects of role and setting on the trainee or on the tendency to treat patients entirely by diagnosis, socioeconomic status, and location of treatment. For example, a resident whose first exposure to psychiatry is on a busy inpatient unit may naturally develop a "give drugs first" attitude. Similarly, an "antidrug" attitude may be inherent in the outpatient setting.

In supervision with beginning trainees, the focus most commonly is on inpatient treatment. Residents should meet with psychopharmacologists (meaning a senior psychopharmacologist or a clinical psychiatrist with some special expertise in psychopharmacology) at least weekly and review individual patient treatment problems, especially illustrating the use of drug classes from a drug treatment point of view. Supervision should be either on an individual (one-on-one) or a very small group (maximum three to four trainees) basis once a week to allow for maximum informality and is envisioned as the time during which the beginning trainee can ask very simple questions without fear or embarrassment. It is also a time that the trainee(s) and supervisor can *see patients together,* review treatment records, discuss philosophical decisions to use or not use drugs, and read psychopharmacology literature together if so desired.

Advanced supervision should include the use of psychotropic drugs in outpatient settings (especially if the program has a psychopharmacology clinic), general hospitals, community programs, schools, nursing homes, etc. Advanced supervision includes discussion of mechanisms of drug actions, pharmacokinetics, and research data as well as basic treatment principles. Supervision using this mode should be to some extent category-based, for example, pharmacokinetics of antipsychotic agents.

ECT can also be taught as part of the psychopharmacology curriculum. The most effective form of teaching is during the actual administration of ECT, emphasizing learning through practice and observation.

Supervision by Senior Residents (i.e., PGY IIIs and IVs) of Junior Residents In Situ in Such Settings as Drug Clinics, Inpatient Units, and Emergency Rooms

A considerable amount of psychopharmacology teaching can occur in the context of direct clinical care, with junior residents learning from more senior residents or "frontline" faculty, as in medical and surgical rotations. When possible, a senior resident, selected as a chief resident in psychopharmacology, supervises the teaching of psychopharmacology within the context of patient care. In centers with many trainees, the chief resident, supervised by the senior psychopharmacology faculty, may conduct psychopharmacology consultation rounds with first and second year residents on their assigned units, specifically reviewing all cases, as in the medical/surgical residency model.

Development of Psychopharmacology Units

It may be helpful to develop specific psychopharmacology treatment units as subcomponents of outpatient psychiatry rotations and/or liaison-consultation units. A drawback to the "drug specialty clinic" concept is that it may fragment resident thinking into a nonintegrative view of the patient.

Utilization of Reading Lists

Introduction to the relevant psychopharmacologic literature is important in the training of residents in psychopharmacology. Appendix C in the full monograph gives references that may be helpful. We believe these articles, and the derivatives obtained from their bibliographies, should only be given selectively (because of time considerations) to residents, although a program of comprehensive reading is an alternative.

With respect to the literature list, we have elected not to discriminate the value of articles. We feel such annotations might generate undue controversy. Generally, a reading list may be derived from the following journals, as well as from

looking up specific drugs in *Index Medicus* and similar reference sources. Furthermore, the *Psychopharmacology Bulletin* offers periodic lists of articles under specific pharmacologic topics, categorized in the *Index Medicus* format.

A list of both classic articles and seminal new references can be compiled by the Coordinator of each local program on an ongoing basis.

Use of Psychopharmacology-Psychobiology Journals and Newsletters

Journals

("C" means mostly clinical emphasis, "B" means mostly basic)

- *Journal of Clinical Psychopharmacology*   C

This journal has a strong clinical focus, publishing articles, reviews, letters, and case reports dealing almost exclusively with the clinical use of psychotropic drugs.

- *American Journal of Psychiatry*   C

This journal publishes a number of psychopharmacologic articles. Especially timely and relevant are the brief reports and the clinical and research reports.

- *Acta Psychiatrica Scandinavica*   C

Frequently publishes clinically oriented psychopharmacologic reports.

- *Archives of General Psychiatry*   C & B

This journal often has psychopharmacologically oriented reports. Generally, it is relatively research oriented and less practically oriented.

- *Journal of Clinical Psychiatry*   C

General psychiatry clinical journal which publishes a variety of reviews and articles on the use of drugs, as well as on other issues in general psychiatry.

- *British Journal of Psychiatry*   C

This journal occasionally has good, drug-oriented articles.

- *Biologic Psychiatry*   B

A basic science psychiatry journal with occasional articles on the use of drugs. More often than not, articles are about drug mechanisms and modes of action.

- *Psychopharmacology*   B

A basic psychopharmacology journal with infrequent, clinically oriented articles.

- *Psychopharmacology Bulletin*   C & B

A journal that frequently publishes brief abstracts and proceedings of meetings such as the ACNP. A good way to get a rapid overview of the "news" of important psychopharmacology meetings.

Newsletters

- *The International Drug Therapy Newsletter*
- *Biologic Therapies in Psychiatry*

Representative Basic Psychopharmacology Books

Since new texts appear regularly, the interested reader should consult with colleagues, read journal book reviews, or contact the ACNP.

Development of a Psychiatric Neurobiology Lecture Series

In some programs, it may be useful to provide a series of lectures and didactic seminars on the most up-to-date thinking on the current neurobiologic concepts underlying psychiatry and psychopharmacology. This specific course can occur concurrently with a clinical psychobiology seminar and lecture series, or as part of this series. An integrative approach might be, for example, to precede (or follow) a lecture on antipsychotic drugs by a lecture on the neurobiology of schizophrenia. Representative topics of such a series could include the following:

- Basic neurobiologic principles (i.e., synaptic mechanisms, available neurotransmitters, anatomy of neurobiologic function, etc.)
- Major neurotransmitters and neuromodulators in psychiatry
- Receptor mechanisms
- Neurobiologic hypotheses of affective disorders
    Adrenergic hypothesis
    Cholinergic hypothesis
    Serotonin hypothesis
    Endorphin hypothesis
    Electrolyte hypothesis
    Circadian hypothesis
    Other hypotheses
- Neurobiologic hypotheses of schizophrenia
    Endorphin hypothesis
    Dopamine hypothesis
    Norepinephrine hypothesis
    Transmethylation hypothesis
    GABA (γ-aminobutyric acid) hypothesis
    Other hypotheses
- Anxiety disorders
    GABAergic hypothesis
    Noradrenergic hypothesis
- Neurobiologic hypothesis of other psychiatric disorders
- Other newly noted neurotransmitters, neuromodulators, and other chemical hypotheses

It is suggested that the above series consider supporting evidence from at least the following perspectives:

- Animal neurochemical data and models
- Animal pharmacologic data
- Human neurochemical data
- Human clinical pharmacologic data

HOW TO EVALUATE

Both to understand whether a given clinical psychopharmacology program is achieving its teaching goals (see section II) and to point out areas of weakness in individual trainees, several standardized techniques are available to evaluate trainee competence before and after curriculum exposure.

An optimal evaluation of a clinical psychopharmacology program should consist of a pre- and posteducation formal examination, a pre- and posteducation review of the trainees' charting patterns, and ongoing written evaluation by psychopharmacology supervisors. Another possibility is that resident knowledge and skills can be evaluated during a "mock boards" type of clinical examination at least three times during the residency.

Formal Examination

We strongly believe a pre- and posttest exam is valuable. An example is Nelson, J. C., *Psychiatry: Pre Test Self-Assessment and Review,* 2nd edition, New York: McGraw-Hill, 1982. Questions can also be taken from the psychopharmacology component of the PRITE exam or the American Psychiatric Association PKSAP Exam (psychopharmacology component; selected questions from other sections).

Of course we (or any group of experts) would not agree with all the answers. Rather the questions are used as an evaluation instrument and as a springboard for learning.

Charting Patterns

A trainee should be taught how to keep systematic, concise psychopharmacology records during training so that this skill can be taken into practice. A global rating form to evaluate this function can be developed on a pre- and post-basis.

The educational basis for this evaluative exercise is that psychiatrists often seem loath to maintain written records. Presumably the feeling is that the confidential relationship with the patient will be jeopardized. Although the thoughts, behaviors, fantasies, and other psychological phenomena of patients might pertain to confidences that might be embarrassing to patients if generally revealed, information about the drugs they are taking, when they are being taken, how much has been ordered and over what periods of time, and, some would argue, when there has been departure from the usual conservative practices of *the Physician's Desk Reference* (PDR), should be well documented. Such information does not violate confidences and provides a continuing rationale for the "medical" aspects of care. In our present litigious era, the psychiatrist who does not maintain such records is put at great risk for a legal action, and at great disadvantage in defending against anything that may develop.

Supervisor's Evaluation

We feel the best method to evaluate a trainee's ability to apply to clinical practice what is learned in didactic and other formal sessions is an evaluation by a psychopharmacology supervisor. Evaluation should be done at least yearly or every 6 months, presumably by a new psychopharmacology supervisor each year. The scale could be the one illustrated in the Appendix.

Trainee Evaluation of the Program

Needless to say, trainee evaluations and feedback are mandatory and necessary for a viable program.

HOW TO INTEGRATE PSYCHOPHARMACOLOGY INTO AN ONGOING RESIDENCY CURRICULUM ("THE POLITICS")

To make this curriculum work, both national and local steps must be taken. Some may ask why we included the national-level steps in a model curriculum. This is done so that local directors of psychopharmacological training can be aware of both the issues and the recommendations that have been, or will be, made to various groups involved with psychiatric education, and that underlie this curricula (see Appendix E in the full monograph).

National Level

Consult the full monograph for this section.

Local Level

- For each program, one individual should be identified as "Coordinator" or "Director" of Psychopharmacology Training. This individual should have a broad orientation and a strong committment to clinical psychopharmacology and be an integral part of the particular department's residency education committee.
- For programs without a faculty member with special expertise in psychopharmacology, a psychopharmacology expert should be identified in the region to consult with the local person in charge of organizing the psychopharmacology curriculum.
- Each residency program should (ideally) have a Psychopharmacology Subcommittee which meets regularly, at least monthly, and has liaison with the Curriculum Committee. Here, "critical mass" is important.
- We recommend that the person identified as Director or Coordinator of Psychopharmacology Training make a very strong attempt to obtain the support of the Chairman and the Director of Residency Training.
- Each program should have available relevant readings on reserve in the library concerning the interface of psychopharmacology and psychotherapy.
- Programs of moderate to large size should have a "Chief Resident" in psychopharmacology (although some believe that having such "specialists" at the Chief Resident level is counterproductive).
- A monthly faculty seminar, serving as an update in psychopharmacology, is strongly recommended.
- An alternative technique for integrating a psychopharmacology program into an existing residency program is

to build psychopharmacology into the existing residency structure. In such a setting, the individual designated in charge of psychopharmacology teaching would be a regular member of the residency education committee. However, we feel that in most programs it is important for psychopharmacology to be represented as a specific content area, with some system of advocacy, because of its tendency to be "swallowed up" and diluted in the usual curriculum committees, especially those with an antidrug bias.

In any case, before instituting any changes, we would suggest taking the model curriculum to a joint faculty-resident committee and encouraging the faculty and students to study the curriculum first, and then adapt it to the local ecology.

- A major goal of the development of a clinical psychopharmacology program should be to develop faculty and residents who have an integrated approach to the drug and psychosocial treatment of the patient. Too often, such approaches are represented by different individuals with divergent biases, so that the resident cannot speak comprehensively to a single supervisor about his or her patients. Obviously, such divergent foci and biases are difficult to overcome.

- As to child psychopharmacology, it is important that general psychiatry residencies provide training via didactic lectures and individual supervision for residents rotating through child psychiatry. Emphasis of such lectures should be on the drug treatment of childhood disorders as well as on liaison psychopharmacology. A specific series of psychopharmacology lectures when a resident is rotating through a child program, as well as psychopharmacology supervision, may be indicated using the above-described techniques. Similar programs may be useful for child psychiatric fellows.

CLINICAL PSYCHOPHARMACOLOGY: RELATIONSHIP OF RESEARCH TO TEACHING

The relationship of clinical psychopharmacology teaching and psychobiologic-psychopharmacologic research is important to define. Obviously, research underlies the major clinical psychopharmacologic practices utilized. However, it is important to note that psychopharmacologic research and the teaching of clinical psychopharmacology are not synonymous. A program may have excellent basic or clinical psychopharmacologic researchers who are either poor teachers or uninterested in teaching clinical psychopharmacology. Furthermore, one does not necessarily need to be a "front line" researcher in psychopharmacology to effectively teach the art of psychopharmacology. In many ways, we feel that psychiatrists interested in understanding clinical psychopharmacology and in teaching it in a practical sense, as well as from a theoretical perspective, are the key to developing a viable psychopharmacology program.

PSYCHOPHARMACOLOGY CURRICULA: THE PAST AND THE FUTURE

A previous review by the NIMH has documented that there was relatively limited formal teaching of psychopharmacology in the 1960s and 1970s. The previous volumes in this series did not explicitly consider the teaching of psychopharmacology. A review of two decades of the NIMH Career Teacher Program revealed very few recipients with a primary commitment to the teaching of psychopharmacology. We view this curriculum as a start; it will be modified by us and by those who use it over the next decades of progress.

As to the future, we predict more of the same (i.e., there will be a continuous explosion of new data that will need to be taught). Of even greater importance will be the need to teach how to rapidly integrate psychopharmacology into modern multimodal psychiatric treatment plans. Furthermore, we speculate that psychopharmacology will be even more of an integral part of the subject matter of both general medicine and pharmacology. Although we now see increasing numbers of young psychiatrists interested in psychopharmacology, our prediction, unfortunately, is that there will continue to be a shortage of those interested in and capable of teaching this material.

ACKNOWLEDGMENTS

We are indebted to O. Ray, Ph.D., S. Fisher, Ph.D., A. Abraham, M.D., H. Pincus, M.D., C. Bowden, M.D., L. Baxter, M.D., L. Hollister, M.D., R. Nemiroff, M.D., C. O'Brien, M.D., Ph.D., D. Dunner, M.D., D. Gallant, M.D., J. Lomax, M.D., and R. Brunstetter, M.D., for help in the development of this curriculum and for support in part from the National Institute of Mental Health (No. 83M055989501D).

APPENDIX

Resident Performance Rating for Psychopharmacology

(From the Department of Psychiatry of the Tufts University School of Medicine and the New England Medical Center)

Name of Resident _____

Period Covered _____

Name of Rater _____

Role of Rater and Context of Evaluation _____

Number of Hours Per Week With Resident _____

Please rate this resident in the areas listed below and indicate your level of certainty regarding your evaluation.

Please note that *average means that the resident performs as you would expect a resident at this level to perform. Thus, only a few residents would be expected to have higher or lower ratings than "Pass."*

	Outstanding	High Pass (above average)	Pass (average)	Low Pass (below average)	Unacceptable	Not Applicable	Level of Certainty High	Average	Low
1) Knowledge of neurobiological theories related to use of psychotropic drugs									
2) Degree of sophistication in differential diagnosis related to use of psychotropic drugs									
3) Knowledge of clinical indications and contraindications for use of the major classes of psychotropic drugs									
4) Knowledge of side effects and complications of major classes of psychotropic drugs									

5) Degree of sophistication in use _____
of psychotropic agents
(awareness of kinetic factors,
avoidance of polypharmacy)

6) Knowledge of special factors _____
regarding use of psychotropic
agents in geriatric and medically
ill patients

7) Degree of understanding of _____
interaction between pharmacologic
and psychosocial factors in
patient care

GENERAL COMMENTS (Use other side)

Psychopharmacology:
The Third Generation of Progress,
edited by Herbert Y. Meltzer.
Raven Press, New York © 1987.

CHAPTER **139**

Monitoring of Plasma Drug Concentrations in Clinical Psychopharmacology

Sally Guthrie, Elizabeth A. Lane, and Markku Linnoila

In the early 1970s, when adequate assay methods were available at only a few centers, clinical psychopharmacology was at the forefront of clinical pharmacology and biological psychiatry. Psychotropic drugs were used as probes to investigate the complexities of pharmacokinetics of compounds with a high first-pass metabolism, and the tremendous interindividual variability in their kinetics was established. This discovery led to pressure to apply plasma concentration measurements to the clinical practice of psychiatry, and to the commercialization of these measurements. Most of the ensuing studies replicated previous results, using new drugs, but providing no improvement or innovation in study design. In the meantime, an explosion of knowledge was taking place in the neurosciences, and this became a very attractive area for young biological psychiatrists. The field of clinical psychopharmacology lost some of its scientific momentum as a result of this shift in emphasis.

The application of recent advances in analytical techniques, a better understanding of the kinetics of active drug metabolites, and the use of precise diagnostic systems in psychiatry should lead to improved experimental design and renewed interest in the field of clinical psychopharmacology. Below we describe and compare the various analytical methods used for psychotropic drug assays, with particular emphasis on differences in the lower limit of detection and specificity. In the following section we review pharmacokinetics with respect to the relationship of dose rate to drug and metabolite plasma concentrations, the

prediction of dose rates, and the relationship of concentrations in plasma and at the site of action. We then discuss factors affecting study design, such as diagnosis, severity of illness, drug regimen, and minimum durations of pretreatment washout and active drug treatment. All of the foregoing topics have an important impact on the last section, in which studies investigating the relationship between plasma psychotropic drug concentrations and treatment response are reviewed.

ANALYTICAL METHODS

Analytical methods that may be considered for monitoring of psychotropic drugs include gas chromatography (GC), high-performance liquid chromatography (HPLC), radioimmunoassay (RIA), and radioreceptor assay (RRA). Regardless of the technique, for a method to be clinically useful it has to achieve high selectivity, accuracy, and precision, and a low detection limit.

Selectivity of a method is particularly important for this class of drugs, because they are extensively metabolized and produce active and inactive metabolites that accumulate in the body. These have to be separated from each other for a meaningful interpretation of plasma concentration measurements. High-potency antipsychotic drugs are present in plasma in low concentrations, and the criterion of a low enough limit of detection (<1 ng) has not been met until recently. As more potent anxiolytic agents have been produced, the limit of detection for benzodiazepines has also had to be improved (<1 ng). Most antidepressants accumulate to concentrations greater than 100 ng/ml during chronic dosing, but much lower limits of detection (1–5 ng) have become necessary in order to utilize single-dose kinetics to predict dose rate and to quantify metabolites. Accuracy (the closeness of the assay result to the true concentration) and precision (the closeness of replicate assay results to each other) have to be established for each assay in each laboratory.

Gas Chromatography

GC is a highly selective technique whereby chemicals, at high temperatures, are first separated by differential partitioning between a mobile gas phase and a stationary liquid phase and then measured by a detector depending on specific chemical reactions.

The flame ionization detector (FID) is the least sensitive and least selective of the detectors. A number of GC-FID methods for measurement of antidepressants to a lower limit of 10 to 50 ng have been published (137). These are adequate for the monitoring of the secondary and tertiary amines during steady state and for forensic applications.

An electron capture (EC) detector is more selective than an FID. Its selectivity depends on the presence of an electronegative group in the molecule. GC-EC has been an excellent method for the analysis of many benzodiazepines because of the presence of at least one halogen or nitro group in the molecules. Depending on the benzodiazepine, the limit of detection varies between 0.05 to 5 ng, which is adequate for monitoring levels after a single dose (49).

Benzodiazepines containing a 3-hydroxy group, such as oxazepam, temazepam, and lorazepam, are unstable under GC conditions, and sensitivity and reproducibility are improved by silylation of the hydroxyl group.

Detection limits of 0.5 to 10 ng apply to the use of GC with a nitrogen-phosphorus detector (NPD) for the analysis of tricyclic antidepressants. Since the NPD has high selectivity for nitrogen and phosphorus atoms, it has a broad application in the analysis of psychoactive drugs, including many secondary and tertiary amine antidepressants.

Mass spectrometric (MS) detection is commonly interfaced with gas chromatographic separation. A mass spectrometer is the most specific of the GC detectors and acts as a second separation technique. The other detectors (FID, EC, NPD) do not discriminate between similar chemical substances such as metabolites that elute from the GC at the same time, but a mass selective detector can be used to measure a mass that arises only from the chemical of interest, even in the presence of other substances that coelute. GC-MS methods for antidepressants have about the same detection limit as GC-NPD methods, whether electron impact (EI) or chemical ionization (CI) has been used in the massspectrometer. However, CI results in less fragmentation than EI and may have better selectivity, especially when closely related metabolites yield identical smaller fragments. GC-MS with chemical ionization optimized for negative ions has been reported to have a 10-times lower limit of detection than does optimization for positive ions when applied to benzodiazepines (49).

Liquid Chromatography

LC is similar to GC in that chemicals are first separated by either differential partitioning between a mobile liquid phase and a stationary phase or adsorption to the stationary phase and then measured by a detector depending on specific physicochemical properties. A major difference from GC is the temperature at which the chromatography is carried out. LC is usually performed at or a little above ambient temperature, whereas GC is run at high temperatures in order to volatilize the analyte. Therefore, LC can be applied to substances that are unstable at high temperatures or do not volatilize (42). A second difference from GC is the ease of chromatographic separation of amines and hydroxylated compounds by LC without derivatization. Therefore, the quantification of a drug and various metabolites may be more directly accomplished by LC than by GC. For example, measurement of imipramine and its metabolites (hydroxyimipramine, desipramine, and hydroxydesipramine) can be accomplished by a single step extraction and separation by LC with fluorescence detection (186). In contrast, analysis by GC usually requires a three-step extraction and derivatization of the secondary amine and the hydroxyl groups in order to achieve satisfactory chromatographic separation of the four chemicals. In a recent review (137) there were nineteen references to LC analysis of hydroxylated antidepressants but only four to GC methods.

The most widely used method of detection following LC is absorption spectroscopy. Most psychoactive drugs can be detected by this means, and the limit of detection is satisfactory for plasma concentration monitoring for most antidepressants (1–10 ng), some neuroleptics (10 ng) (43), and some benzodiazepines (approximately 10 ng). A number of substances present in plasma also absorb the low wavelengths used for detection, so a chromatographic system that separates the drug and its metabolites from such substances must be found. Greater selectivity for certain drugs can be achieved by using a fluorescence detector. Fluorescence detection is as good as absorbance for imipramine, but the detection limit for hydroxyimipramine is approximately 10 times lower. In contrast, fluorescence detection is much less sensitive for clomipramine and its metabolites.

Electrochemical detectors have had limited application to the analysis of antidepressants and their metabolites. However, adequately low limits of detection for the antipsychotics haloperidol (0.1 ng) (90), chlorpromazine (0.5 ng), and trimeprazine (0.25 ng) (116) have been accomplished by LC with electrochemical detection. The assays for haloperidol and an LC-absorbance method for perphenazine also allow simultaneous determination of the metabolites: reduced haloperidol (0.5 ng) (90) and dealkylated perphenazine (1.5 ng) (100).

Thin Layer Chromatography

TLC has been used to separate compounds quantified by densitometry. In general, this method is rarely capable of detecting the concentrations present after single doses and is suitable only for some secondary and tertiary amines during steady state dosing (45,50,71,136,139,177).

Radioimmunoassay

RIA is particularly attractive because it can theoretically work on unextracted, small volume samples and measure amounts as low as 50 pg of the substance of interest. However, since psychoactive drugs are small molecules and produce significant quantities of metabolites, which have structures similar to the parent drug, RIAs frequently lack the selectivity necessary for therapeutic monitoring. To improve selectivity a more elaborate sample preparation involving extraction, derivatization, and separation has been applied to an RIA that detects haloperidol and its main metabolite, reduced haloperidol (29,60,168). Both haloperidol and its metabolite are measured, with results comparable to those obtained by LC with electrochemical detection. With these complex modifications the RIAs tend to lose their advantage of simplicity over the chromatographic methods, although they may retain the advantage of a lower limit of detection (RIA, 50 pg; HPLC-EC, 500 pg; GC, 250 ng for haloperidol). Another approach to resolving the problem of poor selectivity of the RIA is to produce and screen a large number of antibodies. This is a very time-consuming process but has been successful in the case of trifluoperazine (75). An RIA using an optimal antibody provided measures of 24-hr AUC of trifluoperazine similar to those obtained by GC-MS (120–122).

RIAs for fluphenazine have significant cross-reactivity with metabolites (98% for 8-hydroxyfluphenazine and 57% for 7-hydroxyfluphenazine) (197) and have not been compared with the more selective GC-MS, GC-NPD, or TLC assays (46,117). Similarly, an RIA reported for chlorpromazine has 10 to 20% cross-reactivity with each of the metabolites hydroxylated in the 7 or 8 positions (86).

Monoclonal antibody techniques have not yet been used to produce RIAs for psychotropic drugs. Theoretically, they hold a promise of great selectivity for this application and can thus remedy the biggest single weakness of the RIAs used so far.

Radioreceptor Assay

The radioreceptor assay for neuroleptics is the least specific of any of the methods described here, because it does not detect a specific chemical structure but an averaged sum of all chemicals present that bind to receptors in rat or bovine brain membranes. The radioreceptor assay was originally described by Creese and Snyder (41) and presented as a measure of the total amount of dopamine-2 receptor-blocking activity in a sample, and, by inference, the total amount of neuroleptic activity in patient plasma. That is, the assay measures active metabolites as well as the parent drug and corrects for their relative potencies. It was claimed that the radioreceptor assay could be applied to all neuroleptics and that results for different drugs and different subjects could be compared directly.

The limit of detection of the assay is relatively high. It is sufficient to measure steady state activity after usual doses of haloperidol (7 ng/ml), chlorpromazine (26 ng/ml), thioridazine (280 ng/ml), and fluphenazine (3.6 ng/ml) in most patients. Concentrations of drugs at the low end of the observed ranges will not be detected. Intraassay and interassay coefficients of variation are high (20 and 30%, respectively) (98). The relationships between measures of plasma concentrations of various neuroleptics and their metabolites and the results of the radioreceptor assay have been reviewed recently (89).

Major criticisms of the original claims for the radioreceptor assay have focused on the inappropriateness of direct comparison of results for different neuroleptics (42) and the observation that variability in concentrations of plasma proteins, especially α_1-acid glycoprotein, causes inaccuracies in results (89,112). The effect of α_1-acid glycoprotein concentrations depends on the relative affinities of the test drug and probe ([^{3}H]spiroperidol) to α_1-acid glycoprotein concentration in the sample in which nonspecific binding is determined. Qualitatively, the effect of a higher concentration of α_1-acid glycoprotein in the test sample than in

TABLE 1. *Comparison of analytical methods[a]*

	Specificity	Detection limit[b]	Speed	Low cost
Radioimmunoassay	++	++++	++++	++++
Radioreceptorassay	+	+++	+++	++++
Gas chromatography				
FID	+++	+++	++	++
EC	++++	++++	+	++
NPD	++++	++++	++	++
MS (CI/EI)	+++++	++++	++	+
High pressure liquid chromatography				
Absorbance	++	+++	++	++
Fluorescence	++++	++++	++	++
EC	++++	++++	++	++

[a] Abbreviations: FID, flame ionization detector; EC, electron capture; NPD, nitrogen-phosphorus detector; MS, mass spectrometry; CI, chemical ionization; EI, electron impact.
[b] Detection limit: ++++ 0.5–10 ng, +++ 10–50 ng.

the calibration samples results in an apparently higher drug concentration if the affinity of the test drug to α_1-acid glycoprotein is less than or equal to the affinity of the probe. Conversely, an apparently lower drug concentration is expected if the affinity of the test drug to α_1-acid glycoprotein is greater than the affinity of the probe.

Until the factors that affect the results of the radioreceptor assay are understood and controlled, one cannot expect to apply it successfully to studies of concentrations effective for treatment or to the simple decision of how to adjust a patient's dose.

A radioreceptor assay for benzodiazepines has been reported (80,178). It measures the inhibition of the specific binding of diazepam to synaptosomal membranes. Similarly, a radioreceptor assay for tricyclic antidepressants has been proposed, based on specific binding to a muscarinic cholinergic receptor (81).

The radioreceptor assay with the greatest promise for therapeutic drug monitoring is the one for neuroleptics. This analytical approach could be useful in drug development to screen plasma samples for the presence of unknown active metabolites. Theoretically, the radioreceptor assay for neuroleptics could be improved by using a ligand which, unlike spiroperidol, would not have a high affinity to receptor sites other than the dopamine-2 receptors and would have a low affinity for α_1-acid glycoprotein. Certain substituted benzamides may fulfill these theoretical requirements (57). (See Table 1 on page 1325.)

When faced with selection of an analytical method to use in drug monitoring or in an experiment to determine the therapeutic range of a drug, preference should be given to a method that is specific. The second necessary characteristic of the assay method is that its lower limit of detection is low enough for the purpose intended. Accuracy and precision depend on sensitivity of the method and vary among laboratories and individual chemists, but can only be meaningful variables for a specific assay.

PHARMACOKINETICS

Drug and Metabolite Concentrations

Clearance Concepts

Drug plasma concentrations in clinical psychopharmacology are often obtained during steady-state dosing. The dose rate and concentration are related by clearance, so that a higher dose rate results in a proportionately higher average concentration. This relationship depends on there being no saturation of elimination pathways at the concentrations usually encountered, as is the case for most psychotropic drugs. There have been some indications, however, that there may be exceptions to this rule even at therapeutic dose rates, e.g., doxepin (84), imipramine, and desipramine (20,51). Furthermore, after an overdose, the elimination of amitriptyline appears to be saturated and, thus, nonlinear (141). Autoinduction of chlorpromazine and diazepam metabolism leading to an increased clearance occurs in certain individuals during chronic dosing (2,70,85).

A number of psychoactive drugs have active metabolites; e.g., imipramine dosing results in significant concentrations of desipramine and hydroxydesipramine; diazepam dosing results in significant concentrations of N-desmethyldiazepam. At steady state, the concentrations of a parent drug ($C_{ss,p}$) and metabolites ($C_{ss,m}$) are related by their clearances: $C_{ss,m}/C_{ss,p} = Cl_{p-m}/Cl_m$ where Cl_{p-m} is the clearance of the parent drug to this particular metabolite, and Cl_m is the elimination clearance of the metabolite. Also the dose rate (Ro) of the parent drug is related to the metabolite concentration by clearances: $C_{ss,m} = Ro fm_{p-m}/Cl_m$, where fm_{p-m} is the fraction of the parent drug metabolized to this particular metabolite and may be thought of as a ratio of clearances, namely Cl_{p-m}/Cl_p where Cl_p is the total clearance of the drug. Therefore, a higher dose rate of parent drug results in a proportionately higher concentration of a metabolite (147).

These simple equations apply to the simplest example of a metabolite formed from the parent drug by one metabolic pathway. A number of metabolites of psychoactive drugs may be formed by multiple metabolic steps via other metabolites. For example, hydroxydesipramine may be formed from imipramine via either desipramine or hydroxyimipramine. Although the equations that take these steps into consideration are more complex, the net relationship of the dose rate of a parent drug to the steady-state concentration of a metabolite is still a simple proportionality, provided none of the intermediate metabolic steps is saturated at the usual dosing rates (102).

Usually the relationship of a dose rate and steady-state concentration of a drug and metabolites is the same regardless of the drug's extraction ratio across the liver or gastrointestinal tract. Extraction ratio is the fraction of the dose that is metabolized during a single pass across a particular organ. Thus that fraction of the dose never appears in the systemic circulation as the parent drug. If the metabolite extraction ratio is small ($E_m < 0.01$), then the fraction of the dose transformed into the metabolite and the fraction of the dose leaving the liver as the metabolite are equal. However, if the metabolite extraction ratio is large ($E_m > 0.1$), then the fraction of the dose transformed into the metabolite is greater than the fraction of the dose that escapes the liver as the metabolite, and it is the latter fraction that affects the steady-state concentration of the metabolite (99). This distinction should be made, for example, when relating the steady-state concentration of desipramine ($E =$ approximately 0.6) (169) to the dose rate of imipramine.

Many metabolites are formed in the liver but eliminated by renal excretion, e.g., hydroxydesipramine and hydroxydesipramine glucuronide. Therefore, the decrease in the renal function seen in most older patients can affect metabolite concentration even if it does not affect the parent drug concentration. For example, the concentration of hydroxydesipramine depends on the dose rate of desipramine (Ro), the fraction of desipramine metabolized to hydroxydesipramine (fm_{p-m}), and the clearance of hydroxydesipramine by conjugation and renal excretion (Cl_m). In older patients, with decreased hydroxydesipramine renal clearance, the concentration of hydroxydesipramine is increased (88,150). This also results in an increase in the ratio of metabolite to parent drug concentration. The explanation for the increased hydroxydesipramine concentration is, however, complicated. The fraction of hydroxydesipramine excreted unchanged is small, and an age-related decrease in renal clearance of hydroxydesipramine is not, as such, sufficient to explain the size of the increase in metabolite concentration. Hydroxydesipramine glucuronide is probably hydrolyzed in the body (e.g., via enterohepatic recirculation) to hydroxydesipramine. When this phenomenon is combined with decreased renal clearance of the glucuronide, then the magnitude of the age-related elevation of hydroxydesipramine concentrations can be explained by the decrease in renal function. Psychoactive drugs with conjugated metabolites that are eliminated by renal excretion but are also subject to enterohepatic recirculation are tricyclic antidepressants, phenothiazines, thioxanthenes, and certain benzodiazepines. The reduced metabolite of haloperidol (hydroxyhaloperidol) can be reoxidized to haloperidol in the liver (91), but the fraction excreted in the urine is currently unknown.

Sampling Time at Steady State

Often, when concentrations of drugs and their metabolites are measured during steady state a single blood sample is collected just prior to the next dose. This concentration is usually treated as if it represented the average steady state. However, it may be far from the average steady-state concentration, depending on the absorption rate constant, the elimination half-life of the drug in an individual patient, and the dosing interval.

A general view of acceptable sampling times at steady state has been presented by Rowland and Unadkat (166). For a drug that is absorbed rapidly and dosed at an interval equal to the population half-life, they described a range of sampling times at which the concentration would be within 20% of the average steady-state concentration in individuals in whom the half-life ranged between 0.33 and 3 times the population average. A sample collected at any time during the dosing interval was acceptable in an individual in whom the elimination half-life was 3 times the average. However, in an individual in whom the elimination half-life was 0.33 of the average, the sampling time should be approximately at the middle of the dosing interval. In this latter individual, the concentration in a sample collected at the end of the dosing interval would be less than one-half the average steady-state concentration.

Many psychoactive drugs have long half-lives (approximately 12 hr) and are dosed once or twice daily. Desipramine, for example, had an average elimination half-life of 20 hr in one study (range 10.3–38.4 hr) (169). In the case of desipramine dosed every 12 hr, sampling at the end of the dosing interval would underestimate the average steady-state concentration in those patients in whom the half-life is close to or less than 12 hr. Of 30 subjects in the above study, six (20%) fell into that category. In the case of desipramine dosed once daily, the concentration obtained at the end of a dosing interval would underestimate the average steady-state concentration by more than 20% in

approximately 75% of subjects. In the case of lithium, Perry et al. (143) found that 18 subjects had half-lives ranging from 9.5 to 22.5 hr. If lithium were administered every 12 hr and the concentration measured immediately prior to the next dose, consistent with the recommendation of Amidsen (3), the C_{ss} would be significantly underestimated in only one subject (6%) of the sample. No similar evaluation has been made for metabolite concentrations. However, the error in estimating the average steady-state concentration of a metabolite from the concentration at the end of a dosing interval should be no greater than the error in the parent drug concentration, because the apparent elimination half-life of the metabolite must be equal to or greater than that of the parent drug, due to the fact that the metabolite is biotransformed from the parent compound.

Plasma Concentration and Concentration at the Site of Action

Protein Binding

The plasma concentration of a drug measured in most assays is the sum of the concentrations unbound and bound to plasma proteins. Since it is axiomatic that it is the steady-state concentration of the unbound drug that is the driving force for drug distribution throughout the body, including the site of action, it would be more useful to monitor the concentrations of unbound drugs and metabolites. Also, it is the unbound drug which is eliminated from the body. However, estimation of unbound concentrations is indirect, time-consuming, and subject to methodological errors such as pH and temperature effects.

The main plasma proteins to which psychoactive drugs are bound are albumin, α_1-acid glycoprotein (orosomucoid), and lipoproteins. Albumin concentrations do not vary much within an individual, but the concentration of albumin and binding to albumin may be significantly decreased in patients with liver or kidney diseases. For these patients the clearance of a drug may also be decreased so that total drug concentration ($C_{ss,p}$) tends to be decreased by decreased plasma protein binding (increased free fraction, f_p) but this trend is counteracted by a decreased clearance of the unbound drug (Cl'_p): $C_{ss,p} = Ro/(f_p Cl'_p)$. Therefore, measurement of unbound drug concentration is necessary for a rational use of drug concentration monitoring in therapeutic management of such patients. Since α_1-acid glycoprotein is an acute phase reactant, its concentrations may be significantly increased in individuals with inflammatory conditions or acute illnesses. For example, concentrations of α_1-acid glycoprotein have been reported to increase from normal values of 70 mg/100 ml to 160 mg/100 ml after a myocardial infarction. Many basic drugs bind to this protein with high affinity so that this amount of change in α_1-acid glycoprotein concentration can increase the total concentration of a drug significantly. Concentrations of α_1-acid glycoprotein that were 78% higher than in controls (166 vs 93 mg/100 ml) resulted in 61% higher total plasma concentrations of the basic drug, lidocaine (4.81 vs 2.99 μg/ml) but no significant difference in the concentration of unbound lidocaine (0.94 vs 1.00 μg/ml) (12). Similar behavior is expected of the basic psychoactive drugs such as tricyclic antidepressants, for which variability of plasma protein binding in normal volunteers is related to differences in concentrations of α_1-acid glycoprotein, apolipoprotein B, and complement $C3_c$, but not albumin (95). Concentrations bound to α_1-acid glycoprotein may be increased by age (47), anticonvulsant drug therapy (162), uremia (69), liver and other cancers (36,183,195), minor infections such as common cold (94), or trauma (53), or decreased by chronic hepatitis (77). A statistically significant decrease in the free fraction of chlorpromazine has been reported in Crohn's disease (0.93% vs 1.63%) and rheumatoid arthritis (1.08% vs 1.63%) (146), associated with an increase in α_1-acid glycoprotein concentration from 69 mg/100 ml in controls to 165 mg/100 ml in patients with Crohn's disease and 149 mg/100 ml in patients with arthritis. Albumin concentrations were lower in both disease groups than in control subjects. There have been two reports of small, statistically significant, though clinically insignificant, increases in the concentration of α_1-acid glycoprotein in physically healthy patients treated with imipramine (33) and amitriptyline (13). An increase in the absolute amount of α_1-acid glycoprotein is not the only mechanism of plasma protein binding interaction: phenobarbital treatment has been shown to increase the affinity of binding of desipramine to α_1-acid glycoprotein in rats (26). Other drugs, such as diazepam, bind to both albumin and α_1-acid glycoprotein, and variability in the concentrations of both of these plasma proteins contributes significantly to interindividual variability in the bound concentration of diazepam (163).

When the relative concentrations of metabolite and parent drug are considered, it cannot be assumed that the protein binding of each species is equal. The concentrations should be corrected for any difference in plasma protein binding before speculation on the relative contribution of each to a pharmacologic effect. That is, $C'_{ss,m}/C'_{ss,p} = fp_m C_{ss,m}/fp_p C_{ss,p}$, where C'_{ss} represents the unbound steady state concentration and fp represents the fraction in plasma that is not bound. For example, the free fractions of imipramine and desipramine are very similar to each other, so the ratio of unbound concentrations is approximately equal to the ratio of total concentrations. However, the free fractions of nortriptyline ($fp = 0.05$) and hydroxynortriptyline ($fp = 0.35$) are very different, so that the ratio of the unbound concentration of hydroxynortriptyline to nortriptyline is three to four times greater than the ratio of the total concentrations (23,25) (Table 2).

The clinical significance of this lies in the efforts to evaluate the relative contribution of metabolites to the therapeutic effect, which have been largely unsuccessful to date. For example, the relative concentrations of hydroxy nortriptyline and nortriptyline to be compared with relative pharmacological potency data should be the unbound concentrations rather than the total concentrations in plasma, i.e., a ratio of 9 not 2. Similarly, the plasma protein binding of thioridazine and its metabolites differ from each other (Table 2). Because the total concentrations of many active metabolites in plasma are currently measured, there is a need to know the plasma protein binding of these metabolites so that their contribution to pharmacological effects can be more realistically evaluated. These data are currently lacking for most psychotropic drugs.

The measurement of plasma concentrations of bound and unbound drug has been discussed above as if the total concentration were measured by the analytical method. This is true for most of the methods currently used, and the measurement of total drug concentrations has not been shown to be affected by the concentrations of plasma proteins. The exception is the radioreceptor assay, which is very significantly affected by the variability in the concentrations of plasma proteins in the sample, as discussed in the analytical section (89,112). This difference between the response of the radioreceptor assay to plasma protein concentrations and that of other analytical methods must contribute to the different results obtained when the radioreceptor assay is compared with results from other analytical methods.

Cerebrospinal Fluid Concentrations

Since the site of action of psychoactive drugs is the CNS, the question of the relationship of plasma drug concentration to the concentration in the CNS has arisen. Theoretically, the CNS drug concentration interacting with the "receptor,"

TABLE 2. *Plasma protein binding of two psychoactive drugs and their active metabolites*

	$f_p(\%)$[a]	CSF/plasma conc (%)	Plasma total	Conc (ng/ml) unbound
Amitriptyline			120 (1)[b]	7 (1)
Hydroxyamitriptyline			30 (0.25)	5 (0.7)
Nortriptyline	5	3.7–5.2	60 (0.5)	4.5 (0.6)
		5.9–14.2		
Hydroxynortriptyline	35	5.1–5.8	130 (1.1)	42 (6)
Refs.	23, 25		14	14
Thioridazine	2.6		(1)	(1)
Mesoridazine	13.4		(1.18)	(6.1)
Sulforidazine	10.4		(0.41)	(1.6)
Refs.	15		9	

[a] f_p, Free fraction in plasma.
[b] Normalized to amitriptyline concentration.

the concentration unbound at the receptor site, and should be equal to the concentration in cerebrospinal fluid (CSF) at steady state. At steady state the concentrations of a drug and its metabolites in the CSF should be equal to the concentrations of the respective chemicals in plasma not bound to plasma proteins. This assumes that the chemicals enter and leave the CNS by passive diffusion only, that they are not actively transported into or out of the CNS, and, in the case of metabolites, that these are not formed in the CNS. There is not a great deal of data available for comparison of CSF to plasma concentrations. The reported CSF concentrations of nortriptyline and desipramine are approximately equal to unbound concentrations in plasma (17,23,148,169). The CSF concentration of imipramine has been reported to be about one-third the unbound concentration in plasma (149). However, the unbound fraction in plasma reported by these investigators was about three times greater than that reported by others (0.31 compared with 0.14, 0.04, and 0.08) (23,67,145,152), so it is unclear whether the CSF concentration of imipramine is less than or equal to the unbound plasma concentration. Whereas the CSF and unbound plasma concentrations of nortriptyline and desipramine appear to be equal, the CSF concentration of the hydroxylated metabolite of nortriptyline appears to be less than the unbound plasma concentration (Table 2). This implies that there is an active transport of hydroxynortriptyline out of the CNS and is consistent with a finding of hydroxydesipramine renal clearance greater than creatinine clearance, implying active renal excretion of this hydroxylated tricyclic antidepressant (169). Similarly, the CSF concentration of lithium, which does not bind to plasma proteins, is reported to be only 40% of the plasma concentration at steady state (11), and lithium is known to be a substrate of active transport systems.

The ratio of CSF to plasma concentrations of chlorpromazine at steady state (2) is approximately equal to the unbound fraction of chlorpromazine in plasma (44,145), indicating that the CSF concentration is equal to unbound concentration in plasma. The ratio of CSF to plasma concentrations of haloperidol (4.3%) (155) is about half the unbound fraction of haloperidol in plasma (8–12%) (61,165). The CSF and plasma results (155) were obtained using an RIA shown to overestimate plasma haloperidol concentration (167,168), therefore, the CSF to plasma ratio may be underestimated.

In comparing CSF and unbound plasma concentrations of any drug, it is presumed that steady state has been reached at both sampling sites. Steady state of plasma concentrations is easily confirmed by daily sampling. However, it has not been established that steady-state CSF concentrations are achieved at the same time.

PLASMA CONCENTRATION-RESPONSE RELATIONSHIPS FOR PSYCHOTROPIC DRUGS

Diagnostic Considerations

A prerequisite for finding meaningful relationships between plasma concentrations of a psychotropic drug and a favorable therapeutic outcome is a diagnostic uniformity of the patient population. A good example of this is that the ranges of "therapeutic" plasma concentrations, which have been defined for the tricyclic antidepressants imipramine and nortriptyline, are valid only in patients with "endogenous" depression (105).

Severity of Illness

Probably the single greatest advance in biological psychiatry during the past 15 years has been the accumulation of a data base that permits rational dosing of psychotropic drugs. At the same time, this success has hampered investigations into "therapeutic" plasma concentrations of these drugs. This is because an increasing proportion of patients receives adequate treatment from practitioners in the community. Thus, a disproportionate number of genuine treatment nonresponders reach the tertiary care facilities, which are typically involved in the studies on plasma concentration-treatment outcome relationships. By definition, it is impossible to find meaningful relationships between plasma concentrations and treatment outcomes of a drug associated with a favorable treatment outcome by studying treatment nonresponders (8).

The opposite situation may be true in outpatient treatment programs, where responses to nonspecific interventions (in drug research often described as "placebo" responses), can make the finding of "therapeutic" plasma concentration ranges impossible. These response biases, nonresponsiveness, and responsiveness to interventions other than psychotropic drugs, have greatly contributed to the confusion concerning "therapeutic" plasma concentrations of many psychotropic drugs (8).

Duration of Current Episode and Cycle Length

Major affective disorders and schizoprenia are chronic conditions with a fluctuating severity of symptoms. Affective disorders in particular are often characterized by periods of a total freedom from symptoms and a cycle length typical of each patient. Thus, "spontaneous" remissions can be expected, particularly in patients with a relatively short cycle length. A longitudinal perspective of a patient's illness is necessary for a comprehensive interpretation of characteristics of an individual treatment response.

In general, patients whose current episode of depression has lasted in excess of 6 months, despite apparently adequate treatment, and patients with a rapid-cycling illness should not be included in studies concerning plasma concentration-treatment response relationships. Chronically institutionalized schizophrenics are not appropriate subjects to be used in studies on neuroleptics, because this population contains a disproportionately large number of patients with drug treatment nonresponsive defect states (194).

Choice of Dosing Regimen

As a result of the well-known very large interindividual variability in pharmacokinetics of psychotropic drugs, fixed dose studies usually produce enough scatter of plasma concentrations for investigation of correlations between plasma concentrations and response. When specific hypotheses concerning "therapeutic" plasma concentrations are tested, a fixed plasma concentration design can be used. In such an experiment groups of patients are brought to predetermined plasma concentrations and response rates are compared across groups (92). A flexible dose design, which leaves the selection of doses to the clinician responsible for treatment, has to be discouraged. It may lead to the administration of higher doses to treatment-resistant patients and, therefore, skewed results.

Duration of Treatment

Duration of treatment in trials of antidepressants and neuroleptics should be a minimum of 6 weeks. A significant number of depressed patients respond to treatment between weeks 3 and 6 (153), and certain biochemical changes associated with the antipsychotic action of neuroleptics appear only after 5 to 6 weeks of treatment (147). For anxiolytic benzodiazepines used to treat mental disorders with primary anxiety symptoms, shorter trials are probably adequate. The length of such trials may be determined in part by the pharmacokinetic characteristics of the anxiolytic and, when appropriate, its active metabolites. A full treatment response to antidepressants in anxious patients takes up to 6 weeks to appear (106). In some obsessive-compulsive patients, responses to clomipramine treatment have been observed to appear after 10 weeks on the drug (184).

Duration of Pretreatment Washout

Optimally, only patients who have not been previously exposed to psychotropic drugs would be studied. In practice, however, many patients included in studies have to have their previous drug treatment discontinued. Biochemical and certain behavioral changes, directly related to psychotropic drug treatments, can be found up to 4 weeks after discontinuing the administration of a drug (35,147). Washout periods required for biochemical studies are, however, impractical in most clinical settings. Thus, the length of the pretreatment washout period is primarily determined by the pharmacokinetic characteristics and the mechanism of action of the previous drug treatment. Two-week washout periods are usually adequate in symptomatic patients for studies on plasma concentration-therapeutic response relationships. The clear exceptions to this rule are patients treated previously with monoamine oxidase inhibitors or lithium.

Maintenance Treatments

Studies concerning appropriate plasma concentrations for the maintenance of remission should include data on previous cycle length in relapsing patients with affective disorders. In schizophrenics, data should be collected on patterns of interaction and their changes over time in the patient's family, because these can significantly alter the length of the symptom-free period even in patients who comply with medication (101).

Antidepressants

Amitriptyline

Whether or not amitriptyline plasma concentration can be correlated with treatment response is still obscure. In many of the studies the placebo washout or drug-free period was either nonexistent or lasted less than 1 week, confounding the results by including potential placebo responders and baseline ratings contaminated by withdrawal symptoms from previous drug treatments (24,25,37,39,40,103,130, 191,201). Furthermore, several studies that lasted less than 4 weeks on a fixed dose of active drug may have missed subjects responding at a later time point (37,96,97,119,191).

Ten of the studies in the literature report no correlation between amitriptyline or amitriptyline + nortriptyline concentrations and therapeutic response (25,37,40,103,119,130, 160,161,164,191). Five of six studies conducted on outpatients (37,160,161,164,191,201) do not show any such relationship. Two of these studies (37,164) used a variable dose of amitriptyline. Liisberg et al. (103) excluded patients who were candidates for electroconvulsive treatment. These patients often are good candidates for a favorable therapeutic response to tricyclics. Thus, the study is biased against finding any relationships. Breyer-Pfaff et al. (25) found no correlation between treatment response and plasma concentrations of 10-hydroxynortriptyline, nortriptyline, or amitriptyline, although they found that amitriptyline plus nortriptyline in the range between 95 and 200 ng/ml was associated with the greatest amount of improvement. Moyes et al. (130) found no correlation between response and amitriptyline or amitriptyline + nortriptyline concentration, but they did find improvement associated with an amitriptyline concentration of 50 to 100 ng/ml and a combined plasma amitriptyline + nortriptyline level of 75 to 150 ng/ml.

Seven other studies (24,39,96,97,126,191,201) found either a linear or a curvilinear relationship between amitriptyline + nortriptyline concentrations and a favorable therapeutic response. Vandel et al. (191) associated improvement with a combined amitriptyline + nortriptyline plasma concentration of 60 to 180 ng/ml, but they used neuroleptics in combination with amitriptyline. Kupfer et al. (97) associated improvement in an inpatient group with a combined amitriptyline + nortriptyline plasma concentration of >200 ng/ml. Ziegler et al. (201) found that improvement was associated with a combined plasma concentration of >95 ng/ml. Montgomery et al. (126) found positive correlations (albeit weak: $r = 0.3$–0.4) between the percent improvement of symptoms on the Comprehensive Psychiatric Rating Scale and plasma concentrations of nortriptyline and combined amitriptyline + nortriptyline. Braithwaite et al. (24) found that improvement was associated with a combined amitriptyline + nortriptyline plasma concentration of 80 to 200 ng/ml.

Although differing thresholds for therapeutic response are probably due to different experimental designs, diagnostic groups, and methods of assay, the fact remains that very little consensus has been reached regarding optimal plasma concentrations of amitriptyline and its metabolites for the treatment of depression.

Clomipramine

Of the six studies investigating clomipramine plasma concentrations and treatment response, three report a correlation of desmethylclomipramine concentration with response (27,48,190), whereas one (154) found a correlation of clomipramine plasma concentration with response. The other two studies (107,130) found no correlation between either desmethylclomipramine or clomipramine concentrations and a favorable treatment response.

"Therapeutic" ranges for either desmethylclomipramine or clomipramine have been reported by two groups. Reisby et al. (154) observed that a clomipramine plasma concentration greater than 90 to 110 ng/ml was associated with an optimal treatment outcome. Della Corte et al. (48) reported that most responders had desmethylclomipramine concentrations in the range of 240 to 700 ng/ml. Only three of six studies used a drug-free observation or placebo period of at least 1 week (107,154,190). Studies were performed on patient groups with varying diagnoses, including "endogenous" depression (27), "neurotic" depression (107), or a combination of both (154,190). No studies were conducted in "endogenously" depressed patients employing both a study length of at least 4 weeks and an adequate placebo washout period. Consequently, it is difficult to draw any conclusions about correlations between clomipramine concentrations and effect, and in fact, much of the antidepressant effect of clomipramine may be due to desmethylclomipramine, which, at steady state, is present in higher concentrations than the parent compound.

Desipramine

Eleven studies appear in the literature exploring the relationship between desipramine concentrations and antidepressant response (1,4,5,30,63,87,132–134,175,185). Three studies were conducted for a period exceeding 3 weeks of fixed-dose drug treatment and contained some provision for excluding placebo responders (87,175,185). Of these, Khalid et al. (87) found a correlation between improvement in Hamilton Depression Rating Scale scores and desipramine plasma concentrations after 4 weeks of treatment, whereas Simpson et al. (175) and Stewart et al. (185) found none. Several investigators (5,132) have searched for a relationship between 2-hydroxydesipramine or combined 2-hydroxydesipramine + desipramine concentrations and treatment outcome, but none has yet been found. In summary, the best-designed inpatient study has reported no correlation between desipramine concentration and therapeutic response (175).

Doxepin

Few investigators have studied the relationship between doxepin plasma concentration and treatment response (30,62,107,193). Diagnostically different study populations were used in most of these studies. Brunswick et al. (30) found no correlation between doxepin or desmethyldoxepin + doxepin concentrations and treatment response in patients with "endogenous" depression. Plasma concentrations of desmethyldoxepin + doxepin ranged between 44 and 771 ng/ml. Although the responders tended to have higher plasma concentrations than the nonresponders, there was no statistically significant difference in plasma concentrations between the two groups. In a variable dose study where the dose was titrated upwards weekly, Ward et al. (193) found that favorable responses were more likely in patients within the plasma concentration range of 125 to 250 ng/ml of doxepin + desmethyldoxepin. Friedel and Raskin (62) studied depressed nursing home patients older than 60 years, using a variable dose protocol. They found that a positive treatment outcome was associated with a plasma doxepin + desmethyldoxepin concentration of ≥110 ng/ml. Linnoila et al. (107) studied a group of "neurotic" depressives and found significantly higher combined plasma doxepin + desmethyldoxepin concentrations in the group of responders. However, their patients responded at much lower plasma concentrations than endogenous depressives (30). In summary, a doxepin plasma concentration range associated with a favorable therapeutic outcome in depression has not been defined.

Imipramine

The plasma concentration-response relationship for imipramine has been explored for both depressed and agoraphobic patients. Although most studies are somewhat less than optimal in design, the consensus of opinion in four (68,138,176,192) of the five (131) studies utilizing "endogenously" depressed inpatients is that there is a correlation between a favorable therapeutic response and combined imipramine + desipramine plasma concentration. Concentrations in excess of 220 ng/ml are associated with a favorable treatment outcome in two of these studies (68,176). It is noteworthy that no relationship has been found between plasma imipramine + desipramine concentrations and the treatment outcome in "neurotic" depression.

Mianserin

Montgomery et al. (125,127) reported a poorer response in subjects with plasma mianserin concentrations above 70 ng/ml. Their study contained 50 patients, 26 with "endogenous" and 24 with "reactive" depressions. Of the patients achieving plasma concentrations > 70 ng/ml, only one had been diagnosed as having a "reactive" depression. In the group of patients diagnosed as "endogenous" depressives, there was a negative correlation between the plasma concentration of mianserin and amelioration of Hamilton Depression Rating Scale scores (r = −0.48), higher concentrations being associated with poorer responses. Perry et al. (142) found a correlation between the improvement in Hamilton Depression Rating Scale scores and plasma mianserin concentration following 3 weeks of treatment. Although the correlation was fairly strong (r = 0.69), the number of patients was small (N = 10) and the mean reduction in depression rating scores was similar for both mianserin- and placebo-treated patients (18.4 and 18.8, respectively). Thus, although no therapeutic range can be defined based on these studies, the Montgomery et al. study suggests that an upper limit for favorable therapeutic responses may exist.

Nortriptyline

Nortriptyline has been extensively studied by six different groups, who have published a total of nine reports (6,7,31,32,76,92,109,124,200). Of these studies, three have found either a linear (200) or a curvilinear (7,92) correlation between nortriptyline plasma concentration and response. Many of these reports have attempted to establish a "therapeutic" concentration range. The lower limit of this proposed range has been reported to be 50 ng/ml (7,92,200), whereas the upper limit varies from 140 to 200 ng/ml (6,7,92,124,200). Most of these studies have deficiencies, such as a short treatment period, treatment with drugs capable of interacting with nortriptyline, or inadequate pretreatment drug-free periods. Nevertheless, the weight of evidence, based on the well-controlled inpatient studies, favors the existence of a therapeutic range for plasma concentrations of nortriptyline in the treatment of "endogenous" depression.

Protriptyline

The protriptyline plasma concentration-response relationship has been studied by two groups (19,192). Protriptyline is difficult to study because it has a long half-life (approximately 78 hr) (128), consequently it takes 2 weeks to reach a steady-state plasma concentration on the average, and much longer in some patients. Whyte et al. (196) noted that only 19 of 28 of their patients had reached steady state after $3\frac{1}{2}$ weeks of fixed-dose treatment. They still reported a relationship between plasma concentrations and treatment response with the optimum plasma levels between 132 to 248 ng/ml. Biggs and Ziegler (19) found that after 3 weeks of fixed-dose treatment 3 of 21 patients had not yet attained steady state. They found a correlation between treatment response and plasma concentration, with a significantly better response rate in subjects with plasma concentrations exceeding 70 ng/ml. The plasma concentrations in this study were generally lower than those in the study by Whyte et al. (196). Consequently, the authors' inability to find an upper limit of a "therapeutic" plasma concentration range does not contradict the results of Whyte et al. (196).

In summary, the evidence for a plasma concentration-response relationship for antidepressants is strongest for nortriptyline and imipramine, but it pertains only to patients with "endogenous" depression. Glassman et al. (68) reported an 84% response rate for such patients, whose plasma imipramine concentrations were greater than 200 ng/ml, and Kragh-Sorensen (92) reported a recovery rate of 100% for patients whose nortriptyline plasma concentrations ranged between 80 and 150 ng/ml.

Maintenance Treatment

Studies relating plasma concentration to long-term prophylactic response to antidepressants are not numerous. Two reports (38,64) investigated amitriptyline, one nortriptyline (93), and the last (108) a variety of antidepressants, including clomipramine, maprotiline, amitriptyline, and imipramine. All investigators found that prophylactic antidepressant therapy for periods ranging between 3 and 26 months was more effective in prevention of relapse than placebo. Kragh-Sorensen et al. (93) found that depressive relapses were related to low nortriptyline plasma concentrations (<72 ng/ml). Studies using amitriptyline found that those patients who had the lowest plasma concentrations tended to relapse (38,64). Loo et al. (108) found that, in general, for all the tricyclic antidepressants used in their study, a plasma concentration ranging between 70 and 250 ng/ml was associated with successful long-term maintenance treatment. The consensus seems to be that maintenance treatment is necessary for prophylaxis against further depressive episodes, and that the effective prophylactic plasma concentrations are similar to those used for the treatment of an acute episode.

Lithium

In contrast to most other psychotropic agents, there is a well-accepted therapeutic plasma concentration range for lithium. The lower (0.4–0.6 mEq/liter) and upper (1.2 mEq/liter) limits are determined by therapeutic response and toxicity, respectively (135,174,187). The optimal steady-state plasma concentration ranges vary with respect to the duration of treatment. For acute antimania therapy, plasma levels of 0.8 to 1.4 mEq/liter have been found to be effective (151). Hullin et al. (78,79) have shown that a plasma concentration of at least 0.4 mEq/liter is an adequate maintenance concentration in 80% of bipolar patients receiving lithium as a prophylactic treatment.

Anxiolytics

Chlordiazepoxide

There is only one report in the literature on the plasma concentration-effect relationship for steady-state chlordiazepoxide (104). Anxious subjects were recruited by newspaper advertisements and those having Hamilton Anxiety Rating Scale scores greater than 12 were included in the study. The subjects received chlordiazepoxide or placebo according to a double-blind, crossover design. At 1 week, plasma chlordiazepoxide concentration did not correlate with the reduction of anxiety symptoms. Concentrations of two metabolites (desmethylchlordiazepoxide and demoxepam) correlated with decreases in anxiety and somatic symptomatology. However, 7 days is not a sufficient time for desmethylchlordiazepoxide to reach steady state.

Desmethyldiazepam

The hypnotic effect of desmethyldiazepam has been investigated by an Italian group (188,189). In one study nine anxious-depressed inpatients received desmethyldiazepam and nortriptyline (189). The quality and quantity of sleep was assessed by both the patients and the nursing staff. Blood was drawn at 5 and 10 days following commencement of the desmethyldiazepam treatment. Pharmacokinetic parameters were determined following the final desmethyldiazepam dose on day 10. The mean half-life of desmethyldiazepam was found to be 51 hr (range 26–86 hr). Some patients were not yet at steady state when blood was sampled. The maximum hypnotic effect was noted after the first dose and it did not correlate with the plasma concentration. Another study (188) was conducted with 45 inpatients suffering from primary "anxiety neurosis" and insomnia. Patients were randomized to placebo, 10 or 20 mg desmethyldiazepam, or 200 mg amylobarbitone. Again, no correlation was found between clinical ratings of hypnotic efficacy and plasma concentrations.

Diazepam

More reports concerning the relationship between plasma concentrations and antianxiety effect have been published for diazepam than for all the other anxiolytics combined (18,22,45,59,83,85,159). Three of these studies report no correlation between plasma concentrations and therapeutic response (22,59,85). Four other studies report some relationship between plasma diazepam concentrations and the antianxiety response. Dasberg et al. (45) treated a group of 14 anxious inpatients with 20 mg/day of diazepam for a period of 5 days. They found a weak ($r = 0.51$, $p < 0.05$) correlation between plasma diazepam concentrations at 5 days and a decrease in a combined score of three major anxiety symptoms in each patient. Desmethyldiazepam concentration, although it had not yet reached steady state, was correlated with improvement in gastrointestinal complaints ($r = 0.66$, $p < 0.05$). Robin et al. (159) studied outpatients with persistent anxiety states. They administered placebo, clorazepate, and diazepam using a double-blind, crossover design. Each treatment lasted 2 weeks. Although a lack of data points precluded a formal statistical analysis, they reported the indication of a negative correlation in the individual patients between symptom rating scores and plasma desmethyldiazepam concentration. There was no washout period between treatment blocks, consequently desmethyldiazepam was present in the placebo treatment period, which confounded the findings. Johnstone et al. (83) administered diazepam, amitriptyline, diazepam + amitriptyline, or placebo in a double-blind study to 240 neurotic outpatients. All patients, including those receiving placebo, showed improvement. The change in Spielberger Rating Scores over 4 weeks was positively correlated with the plasma diazepam concentration ($p < 0.05$, r not reported).

Anxiety may be even more difficult to quantify than depression or psychosis because of marked fluctuations in the severity of symptoms over relatively short periods of time. The issues are further complicated when the sample contains patients with high scores on various anxiety rating scales but rigorous diagnostic criteria are not applied. Including patients with, for example, agoraphobia and generalized anxiety disorder without differentiating the two groups can only be expected to add to the existing confusion. Generally, anxiety states do not require hospitalization, and consequently most studies have been conducted on an outpatient basis, making compliance difficult to monitor. Also, most of these studies have not been optimally designed. Few provide a placebo observation period, and exclusion criteria have, in most cases, not eliminated subjects who might be abusing alcohol or other recreational drugs that might interact with the anxiolytics. According to the current literature, there is no robust correlation between anxiolytic plasma concentrations and treatment response. There is, however, an emerging literature suggestive of superior long-term efficacy of traditional antidepressants, both monoamine oxidase inhibitors and tricyclics, over the conventional benzodiazepines in the treatment of various anxiety disorders (106). Presently very little is known concerning plasma concentration-therapeutic efficacy relationships for antidepressants in the treatment of anxiety (83,113).

Neuroleptics

Butaperazine

Two reports by Garver et al. (34,65) have found a curvilinear relationship between butaperazine plasma and red blood cell concentrations and treatment response in hospitalized schizophrenics. The red blood cell concentrations of butaperazine fit a quadratic polynomial model relating concentration to change in symptom scores better than plasma concentrations. The authors have hypothesized that red blood cell concentrations may parallel free plasma concentrations, and thus be a better index of the concentration of the drug at central receptor sites.

Chlorpromazine

Studies relating chlorpromazine concentration to effect are complex because at least two active metabolites (7-hydroxychlorpromazine and nor-l-chlorpromazine) are formed. Meltzer et al. (118) reported no correlation between the improvement in Brief Psychiatric Rating Scale scores and chlorpromazine "equivalents," as measured by NRRA, in 21 schizophrenic patients. All other published studies employed GC assays. Rivera-Calimlim et al. have reported a correlation between chlorpromazine plasma concentrations and response in acute schizophrenics, especially improvement in thought disorder and paranoid delusions (157,158). They proposed a threshold of 30 ng/ml in one study (156) and a "therapeutic" range of 50 to 300 ng/ml (158) in a later study. Wode Helgodt et al. (199) found that a threshold plasma concentration of 40 ng/ml was necessary for a favorable therapeutic effect. The concentrations of chlorpromazine metabolites have also been related to treatment outcome by various groups. Phillipson et al. (144) reported that 7-hydroxychlorpromazine was correlated with an improvement in both "perceptual disorder" and a group of symptoms associated with schizophrenia. Sakalis et al. (172) found no correlation between plasma chlorpromazine concentration and response, nor did they find any correlation between the ratio of chlorpromazine + 7-hydroxychlorpromazine to chlorpromazine sulfoxide and micrographia (used as a measure of subclinical hypokinesia) (171). However, four groups (10,170,173,198) have found significantly higher ratios of the therapeutically inactive chlorpromazine sulfoxide to chlorpromazine in nonresponders, and one study reports a higher 7-hydroxychlorpromazine to chlorpromazine ratio in responders (110). Few studies have used a fixed-dose design (171,172,198,199).

Fluphenazine

In two studies neuroleptic activity in plasma was measured using an NRRA. In one study (74), patients more likely to respond had "concentrations" > 2.2 ng/ml, and in the other (82), patients who relapsed had "concentrations" < 2.2 ng/ml. These can be compared with two studies in which fluphenazine concentrations were measured with gas chromatography. In one of these (55), no correlation between plasma concentration and clinical improvement was observed. Plasma concentrations ranged from 0.1 to 1.8 ng/ml after 7 days of treatment. In the other, Dysken et al. (52) found a significant curvilinear relationship between treatment response and plasma concentrations during oral dosing and proposed a "therapeutic" range of 0.2 to 2.8 ng/ml. The majority of patients in both of these studies improved. However, the three patients with plasma concentrations in excess of 2.8 ng/ml were nonresponders in the study of Dysken et al. (52), whereas in the other study (55) no patient had a plasma concentration above 1.8 ng/ml.

Haloperidol

In the last 5 years, at least 11 articles describing the plasma concentration-response relationship for haloperidol have appeared in the literature (21,54,56,66,111,114, 123,129,179,181,182). Eight of these studies report either a curvilinear relationship or have defined a therapeutic range (56,66,111,114,123,179,181,182). Haloperidol is an almost ideal drug to use in this kind of research because it has only one known active metabolite, reduced haloperidol (28). Smith et al. (179,181,182) have consistently found a significant curvilinear relationship between haloperidol plasma or red blood cell concentrations and response in well-designed inpatient studies. Their findings have been replicated by most other groups (66,114,123). A "therapeutic" concentration range for treating acute relapses in chronic schizophrenics from approximately 3 to 17 ng/ml is found by the majority of investigators (56,66, 111,114,179,182), although Miller et al. (123) found a higher range of 10 to 40 ng/ml.

Perphenazine

Hansen et al. have explored plasma concentration-response relationships in two studies (72,73). In both trials acutely psychotic, schizophrenic, or paranoid patients received a stable, individually adjusted, daily oral dose of perphenazine over a 5-week period. Although Hansen et al. did not find a correlation between plasma levels measured with GC and antipsychotic response, they proposed a "therapeutic" range between 0.8 and 1.2 ng/ml to provide maximal efficacy and a low risk for extrapyramidal side effects.

Thioridazine

Three different groups have used three different assay methods to determine plasma concentrations of thioridazine and its major metabolites in an effort to relate these to therapeutic response. Bergling et al. (16) used a fluorometric assay to measure thioridazine concentrations in plasma drawn at three different time points after dosing. When these three concentrations were averaged and compared to response, no correlation was found. Papadopoulos et al. (140) used GC to measure thioridazine, two of its active metabolites, mesoridazine and sulforidazine, and one inactive metabolite, thioridazine sulfoxide, in plasma from 16 elderly psychotic inpatients with varying diagnoses. Those with better control of symptoms had sulforidazine concentrations in excess of >0.13 ug/ml. This group also used the NRRA assay and found that patients with values more than 214 "units" exhibited better control of symptoms. Smith et al. (180) found no correlations between plasma or red blood cell thioridazine or mesoridazine concentrations measured with GC and efficacy in chronic schizophrenics.

Thus, the plasma concentration-treatment response data are too inconsistent to guide in choosing the optimal thioridazine dose rate in the treatment of schizophrenia.

Thiothixene

Bergling et al. (16) studied 21 patients with schizophrenic or paranoid syndromes and found no correlation between thiothixene plasma concentrations and response. However, Mavroidis et al. (115) observed a significant curvilinear relationship and proposed a possible "therapeutic" range extending from 2 to 15 ng/ml. Inspection of the data reveals that most of the subjects improving 40% or better on the New Haven Schizophrenic Index had plasma levels below the proposed therapeutic threshold.

Of the neuroleptic drugs, haloperidol is the only one for which there appears to be some consensus of opinion. However, the "therapeutic" range between 3 and 17 ng/ml is not yet firmly established. The difficulty of defining strict plasma-concentration response relationships for neuroleptics is due in part to the heterogeneity of the schizophrenic syndrome, difficulties in quantifying the antipsychotic response, and the fact that adequate assay methodology is still quite demanding.

TABLE 3. *Therapeutic plasma concentration ranges*

Drug	Indication	Therapeutic range	Refs.
Imipramine	"Endogenous" depression	(imi- + desipramine) >220 ng/ml >240 ng/ml	68 176
Nortriptyline	"Endogenous" depression	<175 ng/ml 50–139 ng/ml <200 ng/ml 50–150 ng/ml	6 7 200 124 92
Lithium	Mania	0.4–1.2 mEq/liter	Multiple authors (see text)
Haloperidol	Acute exacerbation of schizophrenia	3–17 ng/ml	179, 182 114 56 111 66
		10–40 ng/ml	123

In summary, except for lithium, whose therapeutic plasma concentration range in the maintenance treatment of bipolar affective disorders is well established, imipramine and nortriptyline in "endogenous" depression, and haloperidol in acute exacerbations of schizophrenia, current knowledge concerning therapeutic plasma concentrations of psychotropic drugs is still rudimentary (Table 3). This is largely because of the difficulty of designing and conducting the necessary experiments and represents a general failure to take advantage of the latest advances in clinical pharmacology in psychiatry. The problems are often compounded by inadequate characterization of patients and their living environment in outpatient studies. There is reason for optimism, however, because many of the flaws in past experimental designs are known and they can be avoided in future studies.

REFERENCES

1. Aberg-Wistedt, A., Jostell, K.-G., Ross, S. B., and Westerlund, D. (1981): *Psychopharmacology*, 74:297–305.
2. Alfredsson, G., Wode-Helgodt, B., and Sedvall, G. (1976): *Psychopharmacology*, 48:123–131.
3. Amdisen, A. (1983): In: *Handbook of Clinical Pharmacokinetics*, edited by M. Gibaldi and L. Prescott, pp. 109–131. ADIS Health Science Press, Balgowlah.
4. Amin, M. M., Cooper, R., Khalid, R., and Lehmann, H. E. (1978): *Psychopharmacol. Bull.*, 14:45–46.
5. Amsterdam, J. D., Brunswick, D. J., Potter, L., Winokur, A., and Rickels, K. (1985): *Arch. Gen. Psychiatry*, 42:361–364.
6. Asberg, M. (1973): *Clin. Pharmacol. Ther.*, 16:215–229.
7. Asberg, M., Cronholm, B., Sjoqvist, F., and Tuck, D. (1971): *Br. Med. J.*, 3:331–334.
8. Asberg, M., and Sjoqvist, F. (1978): *Commun. Psychopharmacol.*, 2:381–391.
9. Axelsson, R., and Martensson, E. (1977): *Curr. Ther. Res.*, 20: 561–586.
10. Axelsson, S., Jonsson, S., and Nordgren, L. (1975): *Arch. Psychiatr. Nervenkr.*, 221:167–170.
11. Baldessarini, R. J. (1980): In: *The Pharmacological Basis of Therapeutics*, edited by A. G. Gilman, L. S. Goodman, and A. Gilman, p. 432. MacMillan Publishing Co., New York.
12. Barchowsky, A., Shand, D. G., Stargel, W. W., Wagner, D. G. S., and Routledge, P. A. (1982): *Br. J. Clin. Pharmacol.*, 13:411–415.
13. Baumann, P., Tinguely, D., and Schopf, J. (1982): *Br. J. Clin. Pharmacol.*, 14:102–103.
14. Baumann, P., Tinguely, D., Schopf, J., Koef, L., Perey, M., Michel, L., Balant, A., and Dick, B. (1981): In: *Clinical Pharmacology in Psychiatry*, edited by E. Usdin, S. G. Dahl, P. Kragh-Sorensen, F. Sjoqvist, and P. L. Morselli, pp. 227–237. Macmillan Press, London.
15. Belpaire, F. M., Vanderheeren, F. A. J., and Bogaert, M. G. (1975): *Arzneimittelforsch.*, 25:1969–1971.
16. Bergling, R., Mjorndal, T., Oreland, L., Rapp, W., and Wold, S. (1975): *J. Clin. Pharmacol.*, 15:178–186.
17. Bertilsson, L., Mellstrom, B., and Sjoqvist, F. (1979): *Life Sci.*, 25:1285–1292.
18. Bianchi, G. N., Fennessy, M. R., Phillips, J., and Everitt, B. S. (1974): *Psychopharmacologia*, 35:113–122.
19. Biggs, J. T., and Ziegler, V. E. (1977): *Clin. Pharmacol. Ther.*, 22:269–273.
20. Bjerre, M., Gram, L. F., Kragh-Sorensen, P., Kristensen, C. B., Pedersen, O. L., Moller, M., and Thayssen, P. (1981): *Psychopharmacology*, 75:354–357.
21. Bjorndal, N., Bjerre, M., Gerlach, J., Kristjansen, P., Magelund, G., Oestrich, I. H., and Waehrens, J. (1980): *Psychopharmacology*, 67:17–23.
22. Bond, A. J., Hailey, D. M., and Lader, M. H. (1977): *Br. J. Clin. Pharmacol.*, 4:51–56.
23. Borga, O., Azarnoff, D. L., Forschell, G. P., and Sjoqvist, F. (1969): *Biochem. Pharmacol.*, 18:2135–2143.
24. Braithwaite, R. A., Goulding, R., Theano, G., Bailey, J., and Coppen, A. (1972): *Lancet*, 1:1297–1300.
25. Breyer-Pfaff, U., Gaertner, H. J., Kreuter, F., Scharek, G., Brinkschulte, M., and Wiatr, R. (1982): *Psychopharmacology*, 76:240–244.
26. Brinkschulte, M., and Breyer-Pfaff, U. (1982): *Biochem. Pharmacol.*, 31:1749–1754.
27. Broadhurst, A. D., James, H. D., Della Corte, L., and Heeley, A. F. (1977): *Postgrad. Med. J.*, 53(Suppl. 4):139–145.
28. Brown, W. A., and Silver, M. A. (1985): *J. Clin. Psychopharmacol.*, 5:143–147.
29. Browning, J. L., Harrington, C. A., and Davis, C. M. (1985): *J. Immunol.*, 6:45–66.
30. Brunswick, D. J., Amsterdam, J. D., Potter, L., Caroff, S., and Rickels, K. (1983): *Acta Psychiatr. Scand.*, 67:371–377.
31. Burrows, G. D., Davies, B., and Scoggins, B. A. (1972): *Lancet*, 2:619–623.

32. Burrows, G., Scoggins, B. A., and Davis, B. (1974): In: *Classification and Prediction of Outcome in Depression, Symposium Medicum Hoechst,* edited by Angst, pp. 173–179. Schuttauer Verlag, Stuttgart.

33. Carroll, B. J., Mukhopadhyay, S., and Feinberg, M. (1981): In: *Clinical Pharmacology in Psychiatry: Neuroleptic and Antidepressant Research,* edited by E. Udsin, S. G. Dahl, L. F. Gram, and O. Lingjaerde, pp. 19–25. Macmillan, London.

34. Casper, R., Garver, D. L., Dekirmenjian, H., Chang, S., and Davis, J. M. (1980): *Arch. Gen. Psychiatry,* 37:301–305.

35. Charney, D. S., Heninger, G. R., Sternberg, D. E., and Landis, H. (1982): *Br. J. Psychiatry,* 141:377–386.

36. Chio, L.-F., and Oon, C.-J. (1979): *Cancer,* 43:596–604.

37. Click, M. A., and Zisook, S. (1982): *J. Clin. Psychiatry,* 43:369–371.

38. Coppen, A., Ghose, K., Montgomery, S., Rama Rao, V. A., Bailey, J., and Jorgensen, A. (1978): *Br. J. Psychiatry,* 133:28–33.

39. Corona, G. L., Fenoglio, L., Pinelli, P., and Zerbi, F. (1977): *Pharmakopsychiatrie,* 10:299–308.

40. Corona, G. L., Zerbi, F., Pinelli, P., Fenoglio, L., Frattini, P., Cucchi, M. L., and Santagostino, G. (1980): *Commun. Psychopharmacol.,* 4:309–316.

41. Creese, I., and Snyder, S. H. (1977): *Nature,* 270:180–182.

42. Curry, S. H. (1985): *J. Clin. Psychopharmacol.,* 5:263–271.

43. Curry, S. H., Brown, E. A., Hu, O. Y.-P., and Perrin, J. (1982): *J. Chromatogr.,* 231:361–376.

44. Curry, S. H., Davis, J. M., Janowsky, D. S., and Marshall, J. H. L. (1970): *Arch. Gen. Psychiatry,* 22:209–215.

45. Dasberg, H. H., van der Klein, E., Guelen, P. J. R., and van Praag, H. M. (1974): *Clin. Pharmacol. Ther.,* 15:473–483.

46. Davis, C. M., and Fenimore, D. C. (1983): *J. Chromatogr.,* 272:157–165.

47. Davis, D., Grossman, S. H., Kitchell, B. B., Shand, D. G., and Routledge, P. A. (1980): *Clin. Res.,* 28:234A.

48. Della Corte, L., Broadhurst, A. D., Sgaragli, G. P., Filippini, S., Heeley, A. F., James, H. D., Faravelli, C., and Pazzagli, A. (1979): *Br. J. Psychiatry,* 134:390–400.

49. DeSilva, J. A. F. (1982): In: *Pharmacology of Benzodiazepines,* edited by E. Usdin, P. Skolnick, J. F. Tallman, D. Greenblatt, and S. M. Paul, pp. 239–256. Verlag Chemie, Florida.

50. DeSilva, J. A. F., Bekersky, I., and Puglisi, C. V. (1974): *J. Pharm. Sci.,* 63:1837–1841.

51. Dugas, E. J., and Bishop, D. S. (1985): *J. Clin. Psychopharmacol.,* 5:43–45.

52. Dysken, M. W., Javaid, J. I., Chang, S. S., Schaffer, C., Shahid, A., and Davis, J. M. (1981): *Psychopharmacology,* 73:205–210.

53. Edwards, D. J., Lalka, D., Cerra, F., and Slaughter, R. L. (1982): *Clin. Pharmacol. Ther.,* 31:62–67.

54. Ereshefsky, L., Davis, C. M., Harrington, C. A., Jann, M. W., Browning, J. L., Saklad, S. R., and Burch, N. R. (1984): *J. Clin. Psychopharmacol.,* 4:138–142.

55. Escobar, J. I., Barron, A., and Kiriakos, R. (1983): *J. Clin. Psychopharmacol.,* 3:359–362.

56. Extein, I., Angusthy, K. A., Gold, M. S., Pottash, A. L. C., Martin, D., and Potter, W. Z. (1982): *Psychopharmacol. Bull.,* 18:156–158.

57. Farde, L., Hall, H., Ehrin, E., and Sedvall, G. (1986): *Science,* 231:258–261.

58. Fischbach, R. (1979): *Arzneimittelforsch.,* 29:352–355.

59. Fontaine, R., Annable, L., Chouinard, G., and Ogilvie, R. I. (1983): *J. Clin. Psychopharmacol.,* 3:80–87.

60. Forsman, A., Martensson, E., Nyberg, G., and Ohman, R. (1974): *Arch. Pharmacol.,* 286:113–124.

61. Forsman, A., and Ohman, R. (1976): In: *Antipsychotic Drugs: Pharmacodynamics and Pharmacokinetics,* edited by G. Sedvall, B. Uvnas, and Y. Zotterman, pp. 359–365. Pergamon Press, New York.

62. Friedel, R. O., and Raskin, M. A. (1975): In: *Sinequan: A Monograph of Recent Clinical Studies,* edited by J. A. Mendels, pp. 51–53. Excerpta Medica, Amsterdam.

63. Friedel, R. O., Veith, R. C., Bloom, V., and Bielski, R. J. (1979): *Commun. Psychopharmacol.,* 3:81–87.

64. Furlong, F. W., Sellers, E. M., and Kapur, B. M. (1977): *Can. Psychiatr. Assoc. J.,* 22:275–284.

65. Garver, D. L., Dekirmenjian, H., Davis, J. M., Casper, R., and Ericksen, S. (1977): *Am. J. Psychiatry,* 134:304–307.

66. Garver, D. L., Hirschowitz, J., Glicksteen, G. A., Kanter, D. R., and Mavroidis, M. L. (1984): *J. Clin. Psychopharmacol.,* 4:133–137.

67. Glassman, A. H., Hurwic, M. J., and Perel, J. M. (1973): *Am. J. Psychiatry,* 130:1367–1369.

68. Glassman, A. H., Perel, J. M., Shostak, M., Kantor, S. J., and Fleiss, J. L. (1977): *Arch. Gen. Psychiatry,* 34:197–204.

69. Grossman, S. H., Davis, D., Kitchell, B. B., Shand, D. G., and Routledge, P. A. (1982): *Clin. Pharmacol. Ther.,* 31:350–357.

70. Guentert, T. W. (1984): *Clin. Pharmacokinet.,* 9:203–210.

71. Haefelfinger, P. (1978): *J. Chromatogr.,* 145:445–451.

72. Hansen, L. B., and Larsen, N.-E. (1985): *Psychopharmacology,* 87:16–19.

73. Hansen, L. B., Larsen, N.-E., and Gulmann, N. (1982): *Psychopharmacology,* 78:112–115.

74. Harris, P. Q., Friedman, M. J., Cohen, B. M., and Cooper, T. B. (1982): *Biol. Psychiatry,* 17:1123–1130.

75. Hawes, E. M., Aravagiri, M., Dulos, R. A., Rauw, G. A., and Stonkus, M. D. (1983): *Prog. Neuropsychopharmacol. Biol. Psychiatry,* 7:709–714.

76. Hollister, L. E., Pfefferbaum, A., and Davis, K. L. (1980): *Am. J. Psychiatry,* 137:485–486.

77. Huet, P. M., Arsene, D., and Richer, G. (1981): *Clin. Pharmacol. Ther.,* 29:252–253.

78. Hullin, R. P. (1979): In: *Lithium: Controversies and Unresolved Issues,* edited by T. B. Cooper, S. Gershon, N. S. Kline, and M. Schou, pp. 333–334. Excerpta Medica, Amsterdam.

79. Hullin, R. P. (1980): In: *Handbook of Lithium Therapy,* edited by F. N. Johnson, pp. 243–247. University Park Press, Baltimore.

80. Hunt, P., Husson, J.-M., and Raynaud, J.-P. (1979): *J. Pharm. Pharmacol.,* 31:448–451.

81. Innis, R. B., Tune, L., Rock, R., Depaulo, R., U'Prichard, D. C., and Snyder, S. H. (1979): *Eur. J. Pharmacol.,* 58:473–477.

82. Johnstone, E. C., Bourne, R. C., Cotes, P. M., Crow, T. J., Ferrier, I. N., Owen, F., and Robinson, J. D. (1980): In: *Drug Concentrations in Neuropsychiatry,* Ciba Foundation Symposium 74, pp. 99–114. Excerpta Medica, Amsterdam.

83. Johnstone, E. C., Bourne, R. C., Crow, T. J., Frith, C. D., Gamble, S., Lofthouse, R., Owen, F., Owens, D. G. C., Robinson, J., and Stevens, M. (1981): *Psychopharmacology,* 72:233–240.

84. Joyce, P. R., and Sharman, J. R. (1985): *Clin. Pharmacokinet.,* 10:365–370.

85. Kanto, J., Iisalo, E., Lehtinen, V., and Salminen, J. (1974): *Psychopharmacologia,* 36:123–131.

86. Kawashima, K., Dixon, R., and Spector, S. (1975): *Eur. J. Pharmacol.,* 32:195–202.

87. Khalid, R., Amin, M. M., and Ban, T. A. (1978): *Psychopharmacol. Bull.,* 14:43–44.

88. Kitanaka, I., Ross, R. J., Cutler, N. R., Zavadil, A. P., and Potter, W. Z. (1982): *Clin. Pharmacol. Ther.,* 31:51–55.

89. Ko, G. N., Korpi, E. R., and Linnoila, M. (1985): *J. Clin. Psychopharmacol.,* 5:253–262.

90. Korpi, E. R., Phelps, B. H., Granger, H., Chang, W.-H., Linnoila, M., Meek, J. L., and Wyatt, R. J. (1983): *Clin. Chem.,* 29:624–628.

91. Korpi, E. R., and Wyatt, R. J. (1984): *Psychopharmacology,* 83:34–37.

92. Kragh-Sorensen, P., Hansen, C. E., Baastrup, P. C., and Hvidberg, E. F. (1976): *Psychopharmacologia,* 45:305–312.

93. Kragh-Sorensen, P., Hansen, C. E., Larsen, N.-E., Naestoft, J., and Hvidberg, E. F. (1974): *Psychol. Med.,* 4:174–180.

94. Kragh-Sorensen, P., and Larsen, N.-E. (1980): *Clin. Pharmacol. Ther.,* 28:796–803.

95. Kristensen, C. B. (1983): *Clin. Pharmacol. Ther.,* 34:689–694.

96. Kupfer, D. J., Hanin, I., Grau, T., and Coble, P. (1977): *Clin. Pharmacol. Ther.,* 22:904–911.

97. Kupfer, D. J., Hanin, I., Spiker, D., Neil, J., Coble, P., Grau, T., and Nevar, C. (1978): *Commun. Psychopharmacol.,* 2:441–450.

98. Lader, S. R. (1980): *J. Immunoassay,* 1:57–75.

99. Lane, E. A., and Levy, R. H. (1985): *J. Pharmacokinet. Biopharm.*, 13:373–386.
100. Larsson, M., and Forsman, A. (1983): *Ther. Drug. Monit.*, 5: 225–228.
101. Leff, J. P., and Wing, J. K. (1971): *Br. Med. J.*, 3:599–604.
102. Levy, G. (1964): *J. Pharm. Sci.*, 53:342–343.
103. Liisberg, P., Mose, H., Amdisen, A., Jorgensen, A., and Petersen, H. E. H. (1978): *Acta Psychiatr. Scand.*, 57:426–435.
104. Lin, K., and Friedel, R. O. (1979): *Am. J. Psychiatry*, 136:18–23.
105. Linnoila, M. (1981): In: *Prevention and Treatment of Depression*, edited by T. A. Ban, R. Gonzales, A. S. Jablonsky, N. A. Sartorius, and F. E. Vartanian, pp. 219–232. University Park Press, Baltimore.
106. Linnoila, M. (1984): In: *Guidelines for the Use of Psychotropic Drugs*, edited by H. C. Stancer, P. E. Garginker, and V. Rakoff, pp. 329–339. SP Medical and Scientific Books, New York.
107. Linnoila, M., Seppala, T., Mattila, M. J., Vihko, R., Pakarinen, A., and Skinner, J. T. (1980): *Arch. Gen. Psychiatry*, 37:1295–1299.
108. Loo, H., Benyacoub, A. K., Rovei, V., Altamura, C. A., Vadrot, M., and Morselli, P. L. (1980): *Br. J. Psychiatry*, 137:444–451.
109. Lyle, W. H., Braithwaite, R. A., Brooks, P. W., Cuthill, J. M., Early, D. F., Goulding, R., Leggett, W. P., Pearson, I. B., Silverman, G., Snaith, R. P., and Strang, G. E. (1974): *Postgrad. Med. J.*, 50:282–287.
110. MacKay, A. V. P., Healey, A. F., and Baker, J. (1974): *Br. J. Clin. Pharmacol.*, 1:425–430.
111. Magliozzi, J. R., Hollister, L. E., Arnold, K. V., and Earle, G. M. (1981): *Am. J. Psychiatry*, 138:365–367.
112. Mailman, R. B., Dettaven, D. L., Halpern, E. A., and Lewis, M. H. (1984): *Life Sci.*, 34:1057–1064.
113. Mavissakalian, M., Perel, J. M., and Michelson, L. (1984): *J. Clin. Psychopharmacol.*, 4:36–40.
114. Mavroidis, M. L., Kanter, D. R., Hirschowitz, J., and Garver, D. L. (1983): *Psychopharmacology*, 81:354–356.
115. Mavroidis, M. L., Kanter, D. R., Hirschowitz, J., and Garver, D. L. (1984): *J. Clin. Psychopharmacol.*, 4:155–157.
116. McKay, G., Geddes, J., Cooper, M. J., and Gurnsey, T. S. (1983): *Prog. Neuropsychopharmacol. Biol. Psychiatry*, 7:703–707.
117. McKay, G., Hall, H., Edom, R., Hawes, E. M., and Midha, K. K. (1983): *Biomed. Mass Spectrom.*, 10:550–555.
118. Meltzer, H. Y., Busch, D. A., and Fang, V. S. (1983): *Psychiatry Res.*, 9:271–283.
119. Mendlewicz, J., Linkowski, P., and Rees, J. A. (1980): *Br. J. Psychiatry*, 136:154–160.
120. Midha, K. K., Hawes, E. M., Korchinski, E. D., Hubbard, J. W., McKay, G., Cooper, J. K., and Roscoe, R. M. H. (1984): *Biopharm. Drug Dispos.*, 5:25–32.
121. Midha, K. K., Hubbard, J. W., Cooper, J. K., Hawes, E. M., Fournier, S., and Yeung, P. (1981): *Br. J. Clin. Pharmacol.*, 12: 189–193.
122. Midha, K. K., Roscoe, R. M. H., Hall, K., Hawes, E. M., Cooper, J. K., McKay, G., and Shetty, H. U. (1982): *Biomed. Mass Spectrom.*, 9:186–190.
123. Miller, D. D., Hershey, L. A., Duffy, J. P., Abernathy, D. R., and Greenblatt, D. J. (1984): *J. Clin. Psychopharmacol.*, 4:305–310.
124. Montgomery, S., Braithwaite, R., Dawling, S., and McAuley, R. (1978): *Clin. Pharmacol. Ther.*, 23:309–314.
125. Montgomery, S. A., McAuley, R., and Montgomery, D. B. (1978): *Br. J. Clin. Pharmacol.*, 5:71s–76s.
126. Montgomery, S. A., McAuley, R., Rani, S. J., Montgomery, D. B., Braithwaite, R., and Dawling, S. (1979): *Br. Med. J.*, 1: 230–231.
127. Montgomery, S. A., Montgomery, D. B., McAuley, R., and Rani, S. J. (1978): *Acta Psychiatr. Belg.*, 78:798–812.
128. Moody, J. P., Whyte, S. F., Macdonald, A. J., and Naylor, G. J. (1977): *Eur. J. Clin. Pharmacol.*, 11:51–56.
129. Morselli, P. L., Zarifian, E., Cuche, H., Bianchetti, G., Cotterau, M. J., and Deniker, P. (1980): *Adv. Biochem. Psychopharmacol.*, 24:529–536.
130. Moyes, I. C. A., Ray, R. L., and Moyes, R. B. (1980): *Postgrad. Med. J.*, 56(Suppl. 1):127–129.
131. Muscettola, G., Goodwin, F. K., Potter, W. Z., Claeys, M. M., and Markey, S. P. (1978): *Arch. Gen. Psychiatry*, 35:621–625.
132. Nelson, J. C., Bock, J. L., and Jatlow, P. I. (1983): *Clin. Pharmacol. Ther.*, 33:183–189.
133. Nelson, J. C., Jatlow, P. I., Bock, J., Quinlan, D. M., and Bowers, M. B. (1982): *Arch. Gen. Psychiatry*, 39:1055–1061.
134. Nelson, J. C., Jatlow, P. I., and Mazure, C. (1985): *J. Clin. Psychopharmacol.*, 5:217–220.
135. Noack, C. H., and Trautner, E. M. (1951): *Med. J. Aust.*, 38: 219–222.
136. Norman, T. R., and Burrows, G. D. (1981): In: *Psychotropic Drugs, Plasma Concentration and Clinical Response*, edited by G. D. Burrows and T. R. Norman, pp. 83–138. Marcel Dekker, New York.
137. Norman, T. R., and Maguire, K. P. (1985): *J. Chromatogr.*, 340: 173–197.
138. Olivier-Martin, R., Marzin, D., Buschsenschutz, E., Pichot, P., and Boissier, J. (1975): *Psychopharmacologia*, 41:187–195.
139. Overo, K. F. (1980): *Acta Psychiatr. Scand. (Suppl.)*, 279:92–103.
140. Papadopoulos, A. S., Chand, T. G., Crammer, J. L., and Lader, S. (1980): *Br. J. Psychiatry*, 136:591–596.
141. Pedersen, O. L., Gram, L. F., Kristensen, C. B., Moller, M., Thayssen, P., Bjerre, M., Kragh-Sorensen, P., Klitgaard, N. A., Sindrup, E., Hole, P., and Brinklov, M. (1982): *Eur. J. Clin. Pharmacol.*, 23:513–521.
142. Perry, G. F., Fitzsimmons, B., Shapiro, L., and Irwin, P. (1978): *Br. J. Clin. Pharmacol.*, 5:35s–41s.
143. Perry, P. J., Alexander, B., Prince, R. A., and Dunner, F. J. (1984): *J. Clin. Psychopharmacol.*, 4:242–246.
144. Phillipson, O. T., McKeown, J. M., Baker, J., and Healey, A. F. (1977): *Br. J. Psychiatry*, 131:172–184.
145. Piafsky, K. M., and Borga, O. (1977): *Clin. Pharmacol. Ther.*, 22:545–549.
146. Piafsky, K. M., Borga, O., Odar-Cederlof, I., Johansson, C., and Sjoqvist, F. (1978): *N. Engl. J. Med.*, 299:1435–1439.
147. Pickar, D., Labarca, R., Linnoila, M., Roy, A., Hommer, D., Everett, D., and Paul, S. (1984): *Science*, 225:954–956.
148. Potter, W. Z., Calil, H. M., Sutfin, T. A., Zavadil, A. P., Jusko, W. J., Rapoport, J., and Goodwin, F. K. (1982): *Clin. Pharmacol. Ther.*, 31:393–401.
149. Potter, W. Z., Muscettola, G., and Goodwin, F. K. (1979): *Psychopharmacology*, 63:187–192.
150. Potter, W. Z., Rudorfer, M. V., and Lane, E. A. (1984): In: *Frontiers in Biochemical and Pharmacological Research in Depression*, edited by E. Usdin, M. Asberg, L. Bertilsson, and F. Sjoqvist, pp. 373–390. Raven Press, New York.
151. Prien, R. F., Caffey, E. M., and Klett, C. J. (1972): *Br. J. Psychiatry*, 120:409–414.
152. Pruitt, A. W., and Dayton, P. G. (1971): *Eur. J. Clin. Pharmacol.*, 4:59–62.
153. Quitkin, F. M., Rabkin, J. G., Ross, D., and McGrath, P. J. (1984): *Arch. Gen. Psychiatry*, 41:238–245.
154. Reisby, N., Gram, L. F., Bech, P., Sihm, F., Krautwald, O., Elley, J., Ortmann, J., and Christiansen, J. (1979): *Commun. Psychopharmacol.*, 3:341–351.
155. Rimon, R., Averbuch, I., Rozick, P., Fijman-Davilovich, L., Kara, T., Dasberg, H., Ebstein, R. P., and Belmaker, R. H. (1981): *Psychopharmacology*, 73:197–199.
156. Rivera-Calimlim, L., Castaneda, L., and Lasagna, L. (1973): *Clin. Pharmacol. Ther.*, 14:978–986.
157. Rivera-Calimlim, L., Gift, T., Nasrallah, H. A., Wyatt, R. J., and Lasagna, L. (1978): *Commun. Psychopharmacol.*, 2:215–222.
158. Rivera-Calimlim, L., Nasrallah, H., Strauss, J., and Lasagna, L. (1976): *Am. J. Psychiatry*, 133:646–652.
159. Robin, A., Curry, S. H., and Whelpton, R. (1974): *Psychol. Med.*, 4:388–392.
160. Robinson, D. S., Cooper, T. B., Howard, D., Corcella, J., and Albright, D. (1985): *J. Clin. Psychopharmacol.*, 5:83–88.
161. Robinson, D. S., Cooper, T. B., Ravaris, C. L., Ives, J. O., Nies,

A., Bartlett, D., and Lamborn, K. R. (1979): *Psychopharmacology,* 63:223–231.

162. Routledge, P. A., Stargel, W. W., Finn, A. L., Barchowsky, A., and Shand, D. (1981): *Br. J. Clin. Pharmacol.,* 12:663–666.

163. Routledge, P. A., Stargel, W. W., Kitchell, B. B., Barchowsky, A., and Shand, D. G. (1981): *Br. J. Clin. Pharmacol.,* 11:245–250.

164. Rowan, P. R., Paykel, E. S., Marks, V., Mould, G., and Bhat, A. (1984): *Neuropsychobiology,* 12:9–15.

165. Rowell, F. J., Hui, S. M., Fairbairn, A. F., and Eccleston, D. (1981): *Br. J. Clin. Pharmacol.,* 11:377–382.

166. Rowland, M., and Unadkat, J. D. (1981): *Br. J. Clin. Pharmacol.,* 12:687–689.

167. Rubin, R. T., Forsman, A., Heykants, J., and Ohman, R. (1980): *Arch. Gen. Psychiatry,* 37:1069–1074.

168. Rubin, R. T., Tower, B. B., Hayes, S. E., and Poland, R. E. (1982): *Methods Enzymol.,* 84:532–542.

169. Rudorfer, M. V., Lane, E. A., Chang, W.-H., Zhang, M., and Potter, W. Z. (1984): *Br. J. Clin. Pharmacol.,* 17:433–440.

170. Sakalis, G., Chan, T. L., Gershon, S., and Park, S. (1973): *Psychopharmacologia,* 32:279–284.

171. Sakalis, G., Chan, T. L., Sathananthan, G., Schooler, N., Goldberg, S., and Gershon, S. (1977): *Commun. Psychopharmacol.,* 1:157–166.

172. Sakalis, G., Curry, S. H., Mould, G. P., and Lader, M. H. (1972): *Clin. Pharmacol. Ther.,* 13:931–946.

173. Sakurai, Y., Takahashi, R., Nakahara, T., and Ikenaga, H. (1980): *Arch. Gen. Psychiatry,* 37:1057–1062.

174. Schou, M., Baastrup, P. C., Grof, P., Weis, P., and Angst, J. (1970): *Br. J. Psychiatry,* 116:615–619.

175. Simpson, G. M., Pi, E. H., Abdelmalek, E., Boyd, J. L., Carroll, R. S., Cooper, T. B., and Miller, A. (1983): *Psychopharmacology,* 80:240–242.

176. Simpson, G. M., White, K. L., Boyd, J. L., Cooper, T. B., Halaris, A., Wilson, I. C., Raman, E. J., and Ruther, E. (1982): *Am. J. Psychiatry,* 139:358–360.

177. Sistovaris, N., Dagrosa, E. E., and Keller, A. (1983): *J. Chromatogr.,* 277:273–281.

178. Skolnick, P., Goodwin, F. K., and Paul, S. M. (1979): *Arch. Gen. Psychiatry,* 36:78–80.

179. Smith, R. C., Baumgartner, R., Misra, C. H., Mauldin, M., Shvartsburd, A., Ho, B. T., and DeJohn, C. (1984): *Arch. Gen. Psychiatry,* 41:1044–1049.

180. Smith, R. C., Baumgartner, R., Ravichandran, G. K., Shvartsburd,

A., Schoolar, J. C., Allen, P., and Johnson, R. (1984): *Psychiatry Res.,* 12:287–296.

181. Smith, R. C., Baumgartner, R., Shvartsburd, A., Ravichandran, G. K., Vroulis, G., and Maudlin, M. (1985): *Psychopharmacology,* 85:449–455.

182. Smith, R. C., Vroulis, G., Shvartsburd, A., Allen, R., Lewis, N., Schoolar, J. C., Chojnacki, M., and Johnson, R. (1982): *Am. J. Psychiatry,* 139:1054–1056.

183. Snyder, S., and Ashwell, G. (1971): *Clin. Chim. Acta,* 34:449–455.

184. Stern, R. S., Marks, I. M., Mawson, D., and Luscombe, D. K. (1980): *Br. J. Psychiatry,* 136:161–166.

185. Stewart, J. W., Quitkin, F., and Fyer, A. (1980): *Psychopharmacol. Bull.,* 16:52–54.

186. Sutfin, T. A., and Jusko, W. J. (1979): *J. Pharm. Sci.,* 68:703–705.

187. Talbott, J. H. (1950): *Arch. Intern. Med.,* 85:1–10.

188. Tansella, M., Siciliani, O., Burti, L., Schiavon, M., Tansella, C. Z., Gerna, M., Tognoni, G., and Morselli, P. L. (1975): *Psychopharmacologia,* 41:81–85.

189. Tognoni, G., Gomeni, R., DeMaio, D., Alberti, G. G., Franciosi, P., and Scieghi, G. (1975): *Br. J. Clin. Pharmacol.,* 2:227–232.

190. Traskman, L., Asberg, M., Bertilsson, L., Cronholm, B., Mellstrom, B., Neckers, L. M., Sjoqvist, F., Thoren, P., and Tybring, G. (1979): *Clin. Pharmacol. Ther.,* 26:600–610.

191. Vandel, S., Vandel, B., Sandoz, M., Allers, G., Bechtel, P., and Volmat, R. (1978): *Eur. J. Clin. Pharmacol.,* 14:185–190.

192. Walter, C. J. S. (1971): *Proc. Soc. Med.,* 64:282–285.

193. Ward, N. G., Bloom, V., Wilson, L., Raskind, M., and Raisys, V. A. (1982): *J. Clin. Psychopharmacol.,* 2:126–128.

194. Weinberger, D. R., Torrey, E. F., Neophytides, A. N., and Wyatt, R. J. (1979): *Arch. Gen. Psychiatry,* 36:735–739.

195. Weiss, J. F., Morantz, R. A., Bradley, W. P., and Chretien, P. B. (1979): *Cancer Res.,* 39:542–544.

196. Whyte, S. F., Macdonald, A. J., Naylor, G. J., and Moody, J. P. (1976): *Br. J. Psychiatry,* 128:384–390.

197. Wiles, D. H., and Franklin, M. (1978): *Br. J. Clin. Pharmacol.,* 5:265–268.

198. Wiles, D. H., Kolakowska, T., McNeilly, A. S., Mandelbrote, B. M., and Gelder, M. G. (1976): *Psychol. Med.,* 6:407–415.

199. Wode-Helgodt, B., Borg, S., Fyro, B., and Sedvall, G. (1978): *Acta Psychiatr. Scand.,* 58:149–173.

200. Ziegler, V. E., Clayton, P. J., Taylor, J. R., Co, B. T., and Biggs, J. T. (1976): *Clin. Pharmacol. Ther.,* 20:458–463.

201. Ziegler, V. E., Co, B. T., Taylor, J. R., Clayton, P. J., and Biggs, J. T. (1976): *Clin. Pharmacol. Ther.,* 19:795–801.

Psychopharmacology:
The Third Generation of Progress,
edited by Herbert Y. Meltzer.
Raven Press, New York © 1987.

CHAPTER **140**

Introduction: Pharmacokinetics in Clinical Psychiatry and Psychopharmacology

David J. Greenblatt and Richard I. Shader

A major thrust of this decade's "Generation of Progress" is an overview of progress that the discipline of clinical psychopharmacology has made in understanding individual variations in the response to psychotropic drugs. During this last decade, considerable effort and attention has focused on the role of pharmacokinetic factors in accounting for this individual variability. The chapters in the present section review selected advances in this important area of basic and clinical science.

Pharmacokinetics utilizes mathematical models to account for the time course in changes of drug concentrations in body fluids and tissues. To study pharmacokinetics of psychotropic drugs in experimental or clinical models, sensitive and specific methods must be available for repeated measurement of the drug in question, and/or its pertinent metabolites, in a body fluid or tissue. Progress in our knowledge of psychopharmacokinetics made during the last decade would not have been possible without the technological advances in analytical chemistry that allowed the necessary quantitative measurements. Areas of particular importance included chromatographic column separation technology [for example, microparticular high-performance liquid chromatography (HPLC) columns and capillary gas chromatography (GC) columns], as well as detection technology (such as electrochemical detectors for HPLC and improved nitrogen-phosphorous detection systems for GC). New analytical methods have also been developed. These include the radioreceptor assays, the enzyme-multiplied immunoassays, and new radioimmunoassay techniques. Along with each new methodologic development inevitably comes questions and problems regarding assay sensitivity, specificity, and replicability. The increasing use of plasma concentration determinations in clinical psychiatry likewise raises general issues of reliability and quality control in commercial laboratories. Appropriate application and interpretation of analytical methodologies are issues that are of concern to all of our section authors.

The application of pharmacokinetic models lies at the core of psychopharmacokinetics. All of our authors are individuals with extensive experience and expertise in the use and interpretation of these pharmacokinetic techniques. Even more important, each chapter deals critically with the limitations and drawbacks of pharmacokinetic methodologies, thereby emphasizing not only what the discipline has taught us, but also how we might be misled into pitfalls of interpretation. Furthermore, the authors attempt to put pharmacokinetic data into proper clinical focus, and emphasize how the data may be of use to scientists and clinicians in understanding individual variations in response to psychotropic drugs.

Readers need not have a working knowledge of the mathematically sophisticated fine points of clinical pharmacokinetics to assimilate the chapters in this section. However, authors have assumed a knowledge of some basic concepts of pharmacokinetics, such as volume of distribution, elimination half-life, clearance, drug accumulation, and the use of serum drug concentrations for therapeutic monitoring. Detailed review of these concepts can be found elsewhere (1–5). It is our hope that readers will take away from this section a balanced and realistic understanding of the contributions of pharmacokinetics to clinical psychiatry and psychopharmacology.

REFERENCES

1. Gibaldi, M. (1984): *Biopharmaceutics and Clinical Pharmacokinetics.* Lea and Febiger, Philadelphia.
2. Gibaldi, M., and Perrier, D. (1975): *Pharmacokinetics.* Marcel Dekker, New York.
3. Greenblatt, D. J., and Shader, R. I. (1985): *Pharmacokinetics in Clinical Practice.* W. B. Saunders, Philadelphia.
4. Rowland, M., and Tozer, T. N. (1980): *Clinical Pharmacokinetics: Concepts and Applications.* Lea and Febiger, Philadelphia.
5. Wagner, J. G. (1975): *Fundamentals of Clinical Pharmacokinetics.* Drug Intelligence Publications, Illinois.

Psychopharmacology:
The Third Generation of Progress,
edited by Herbert Y. Meltzer.
Raven Press, New York © 1987.

CHAPTER 141

The Search for Correlations Between Neuroleptic Plasma Levels and Clinical Outcome: A Critical Review

Kamal K. Midha, Edward M. Hawes, John W. Hubbard,
Elarien D. Korchinski, and Gordon McKay

In 1978 May and Van Putten (62) published a critical review of the literature entitled "Plasma Levels of Chlorpromazine in Schizophrenia." They pointed out a number of experimental conditions essential to the generation of useful information: (a) a sensitive and reliable drug assay; (b) an adequate number of patients entered in the study; (c) careful selection of patients to ensure a diagnostically homogeneous and treatment-responsive group; (d) the use of fixed dosages to ensure that plasma levels remain independent of clinical impression and improvement; (e) the use of randomized double-blind conditions when more than one dosage level is used; (f) a fixed and adequate length of treatment, since the "sustained dosage" concentration of a drug may determine the *speed* of recovery, rather than the *amount* of change that is possible; (g) avoidance of contamination from other treatments, such as lithium carbonate, electroshock therapy, or other antipsychotic drugs; (h) avoidance of contamination by age effects or sex differences; (i) avoidance of contamination by previous drug taking by allowing the longest "washout period" that is ethically feasible; (j) the necessity to avoid overreliance on coefficients of correlation between "steady-state" blood levels and determinants of clinical outcome, either of which can be confounded by a variety of factors; and (k) use of appropriate statistical methods in the analysis of data.

The task of reviewing literature on neuroleptic drugs is made very difficult by the fact that, even today, all too many researchers leave themselves open to the kind of common-sense criticisms leveled by May and Van Putten. There are so many variables and points of contention involved that one simply cannot report experimental conclusions without consideration of the experimental design and methodology. In this chapter, we shall not attempt a comprehensive survey of the literature; we shall focus on some important trends, developments, and controversies in antipsychotic drug monitoring research over the past decade.

The search has continued for correlations between the concentrations of neuroleptic drugs in plasma, serum, or red blood cells and therapeutic response or side effects. Clinical pharmacokinetic data have accumulated for drugs such as chlorpromazine, thioridazine, and haloperidol, which give relatively high plasma concentrations, and some data have also emerged on drugs that are harder to analyze, such as fluphenazine, perphenazine, and flupenthixol. There appears to be a consensus emerging on a "therapeutic window" of sorts for haloperidol, but the phenothiazine and thioxanthene-type neuroleptics have continued to present a challenge. That a sizeable proportion of recent publication on neuroleptic drug research has concerned haloperidol, is attributable to the belief that the butyrophenones are much less complicated in their metabolism and disposition than are phenothiazines or thioxanthenes (see 86 for a review on haloperidol). For example, Moller and co-workers (70) stated that "haloperidol is an especially good model for the elucidation of these issues of clinical and theoretical relevance because, in contrast to most other neuroleptics, it has no therapeutically active metabolites." Indeed, it was held initially that the first step in the metabolism of haloperidol was oxidative dealkylation, which broke the "backbone" of the drug and yielded only inactive metabolites (6,24). Subsequently, it was shown that the keto group of haloperidol can be reduced to a hydroxy group to give the metabolite now known as "reduced haloperidol" (25).

Reduced haloperidol has a similar lipid solubility to the parent drug (46) and can be found at postmortem in "high concentrations" in the brain tissues of patients who have been medicated with haloperidol (44). Korpi and co-workers (44) also referred to unpublished data on the presence of reduced haloperidol in the plasma of 35 schizophrenic patients treated chronically with haloperidol (0.4 mg/kg, p.o.). Concentrations of reduced haloperidol were said to range from 6 to 300% of the corresponding concentrations of the parent drug. Two published abstracts (7,34) also make reference to the presence of reduced haloperidol in plasma of patients medicated with haloperidol. A more detailed report (21) describes the reduced haloperidol to haloperidol ratios in the plasma of five hospitalized schizophrenic patients chosen for their "poor initial response to therapy or their need for high doses of haloperidol." Four of these patients, who were judged by Clinical Global Impression (CGI) Scale not to have responded to high-dose haloperidol, were found to have plasma levels of reduced haloperidol higher than those of the parent drug. Thus, some individuals appear to produce relatively high plasma concentrations of reduced haloperidol, which these limited data suggest may be associated with a poor therapeutic response to haloperidol (7,21,34).

The implication that reduced haloperidol is not an active neuroleptic is supported by experiments in which this metabolite was applied directly to rat brain neurons from multibarrel micropipettes (42). Reduced haloperidol showed no evidence of neuroleptic-like antagonist activity in either dopaminergic or noradrenergic systems. Thus, it seems that earlier reports attributing possible psychoactivity to reduced haloperidol (25) may have been confounded by the oxidation of the metabolite to haloperidol in vivo. Haloperidol was found in the plasma, liver, and brain tissues of rats injected intraperitoneally with synthetic reduced haloperidol (47). Whether or not interconversion between haloperidol and reduced haloperidol occurs in humans is yet unknown, but it does appear that the metabolism and disposition of haloperidol are more complicated than first thought. Certainly one must exercise caution in the interpretation of data from experiments that take no account of reduced haloperidol.

Lack of knowledge about the role played by reduced haloperidol is probably only one of several reasons why studies trying to establish useful relationships between haloperidol concentrations and therapeutic outcome have yielded variable results. Other reasons include (a) the use of different analytical methods, some of which are usually specific for the parent drug [high-performance liquid chromatography (HPLC), gas-liquid chromatography (GLC)], whereas other methods [radioimmunoassay (RIA), radioreceptor assay (RRA)] often are not; (b) the measurements of drug (and sometimes metabolites) in different tissues (plasma, serum, red cells); (c) the use of different methods to assess therapeutic outcome; and (d) inadequacies in study design that lead to ambivalent or inconclusive results (62). Thus, haloperidol must now be included in the controversy on neuroleptic drugs: what to measure, how to measure, where to measure, when to measure, with what measures of outcome to relate.

THE ANALYTICAL METHOD (HOW TO MEASURE, WHAT TO MEASURE)

In the 1970s, several publications suggested that there may be a relationship between clinical improvement in some schizophrenic patients medicated with chlorpromazine and plasma levels of its active 7-hydroxy metabolite (55,76,82–84). Other workers (17,43,108) were unable to confirm these findings, and it was suggested (11) that technical difficulties in the measurement of the unstable phenolic metabolite needed further investigation. These studies (reviewed in 11) emphasized the need to take into consideration the contribution of active metabolites and the need for the development of reliable and robust analytical methods for them.

Radioreceptor assay is a new biological technique that has been developed and applied over the past decade (14). This method depends on the ability of neuroleptic drugs and their active metabolites to bind to dopamine receptors (13,97). The neuroleptic drug and dopamine-blocking metabolites compete with tritiated spiroperidol (or tritiated haloperidol) for dopamine D-2 binding sites on preparations of membranes from rat striatum (14). Inactive metabolites that do not interact with dopamine receptors do not bind and are not measured. The RRA does not measure concentrations per se, but has been posited to estimate the overall "neuroleptic activity" in plasma, which is often expressed in "chlorpromazine equivalents" (i.e., the concentration of chlorpromazine that would reduce the binding of tritiated spiroperidol to the dopamine receptors to the same extent as the drug under study).

Theoretically, all neuroleptic drugs, given at therapeutic doses, should produce similar levels of plasma "neuroleptic activity" in terms of chlorpromazine equivalents. This does seem to be the case; however, there are two notable exceptions (97). After administration of intramuscular fluphenazine decanoate, plasma chlorpromazine equivalents were much lower (2–25 ng/ml) than after administration of (presumably oral) fluphenazine hydrochloride (60–230 ng/ml), which is in the normal range. The reason for this discrepancy is unknown. By contrast, thioridazine (350–1,700 ng/ml) and mesoridazine (2,207–2,433 ng/ml) gave extraordinarily high chlorpromazine equivalent values (97). Other investigators have also observed high RRA values for thioridazine (10,37,50,54,101,103). Mailman and co-workers (58) subsequently reported that the normal displacement of tritiated spiroperidol from striatal membranes by thioridazine is altered in the presence of sera. The magnitude of this effect differs with serum from different individuals, making it difficult to control. Moreover, these workers (57) found that sera from drug-free healthy subjects caused a marked inhibition of spiroperidol binding, the extent of which varied with different striatal membranes, whether prepared from rat or cow brains. These data suggest that RRA, in its present form, is inappropriate for the estimation of thioridazine or mesoridazine, and that the use of RRA in the estimation of other neuroleptic drugs cannot be approached in a cavalier manner.

Theoretically, since RRA measures the total dopamine D-2 receptor blocking activity of drug and metabolites in the plasma or serum, the RRA values should reflect dopamine D-2 receptor blocking activity in the brain, provided that the more polar dopamine D-2 blocking metabolites are able to penetrate the blood-brain barrier. Therefore, RRA values should correlate especially with measures of the positive symptoms (15) of schizophrenia (hallucinations, delusions, thought disorder) which are responsive to dopamine-blocking drugs. Several reports (8,10,49,80,81,102,103) suggest that plasma or serum RRA values do tend to correlate with measures of positive symptoms such as change in Brief Psychiatric Rating Scale (BPRS) psychosis factor scores; however, it is not possible to reach a consensus because experimental designs vary so much between studies.

By its very nature, the RRA is responsive to all drugs and metabolites that have dopamine D-2 receptor blocking activity. This has encouraged some researchers to include a multitude of different neuroleptic drugs in the same study (29,49,102,103) and even to include patients medicated with more than one neuroleptic (49,103). In most cases, no fixed dose was used, and in some studies (49,81), the dose was titrated according to response. Furthermore, in two of the studies (102,103), there was apparently no attempt to measure C_{min} RRA values or to demonstrate that steady states existed. In our view, RRA has the promise of becoming a tool very useful to the practicing psychiatrist, but it would be a pity if its potential were to be abrogated through misuse before the ground rules are established.

Since the tissues used in RRA are preparations of striatal or caudate membranes, it is logical that there should be some correlation between plasma or serum RRA values and extrapyramidal side effects, which are mediated through blockade of dopamine receptors in the basal ganglia. Aoba and co-workers (2) conducted a study in 41 patients [27 schizophrenics diagnosed by *Diagnostic and Statistical Manual of Mental Disorders,* 3rd edition (DSM-III) and 14 patients with organic mental disorders] who were dosed orally with haloperidol for a period of 6 weeks before plasma samples were harvested for analysis by RRA (details given). They found a significant difference in plasma RRA values between patients with and without signs of parkinsonism. They suggested that parkinsonism symptoms, induced by haloperidol, occur simply in a plasma-neuroleptic-level-dependent manner. By contrast, they could detect no significant differences in plasma RRA values among three age groupings of the patients in the study (<45 years, $N = 15$; 45–60 years, $N = 10$; >60 years, $N = 16$).

That RRA is posited to reflect overall "neuroleptic activity" in plasma or serum rests on the dual hypotheses that schizophrenia is entirely a matter of dopamine receptors, and that calf caudate or rat striatal receptors possess similar characteristics to whatever nonstriatal receptors are involved in schizophrenia. The RRA certainly does not take into account that most classic neuroleptic drugs also interact with noradrenergic and serotonergic receptors (75) or that transmitters other than dopamine also may be involved in the disease process (15,31,98). The use of classic neuroleptic drugs to palliate the symptoms of schizophrenia

likely involves interference with noradrenergic, dopaminergic, and serotonergic receptors in cortical and mesolimbic areas and also the unwanted blockade of dopaminergic receptors in the basal ganglia. Nakahara and co-workers (71) developed separate RRAs to enable them to estimate the antinoradrenergic and antiserotonergic components of neuroleptic activity. They applied their new methods, in combination with the antidopaminergic RRA, to examine the serum of schizophrenic patients on long-term medication with chlorpromazine. They found that the spectrum of serum antinoradrenergic, antiserotonergic, and antidopaminergic activities varied among patients receiving the same dose of chlorpromazine. This is probably related to the wide intersubject variation in the metabolism of chlorpromazine and to the fact that each metabolite has different activities at the three types of receptor (9). Hence, we believe that the RRA for antidopaminergic activity should be referred to as such, at least until there is clarification of the role of other receptor systems in the disease process.

Lindenmayer and co-workers (53) used RRA to examine the sera of 24 refractory schizophrenics who were each under medication with one of five neuroleptic drugs. The authors concluded that the majority of their patients had more than adequate serum levels of neuroleptic drug and went on to discuss other possible reasons for their refractoriness. This study illustrates a useful practical application for RRA, although the authors commented that individualized methods to measure concentrations of specific neuroleptic drugs need to be used in conjunction with RRA, in order to address some of the questions posed by their data.

A few studies have been carried out in which RRA has been compared with other analytical methods. Smith and co-workers (93) studied 27 schizophrenic or schizoaffective patients treated with several fixed doses of haloperidol. They investigated relationships between decrease in BPRS psychosis factor scores and plasma level data measured by RRA and gas-liquid chromatography with nitrogen-phosphorus detection (GLC-NPD). It was concluded that steady-state plasma levels of haloperidol, determined by GLC-NPD, were better predictors of decrease in BPRS psychosis factor scores than plasma RRA values. In a similar study, Miller and co-workers (68) compared RRA and GLC-NPD methods in the analysis of serum samples drawn from 21 acute schizophrenic inpatients treated with haloperidol. Unfortunately, the RRA proved to be too insensitive to be useful in the study. The authors attributed the problem to their use of freeze-dried caudate, rather than fresh caudate which was used by Creese and Snyder (14).

Silverstone and co-workers (89) were unable to find any relationship between clinical outcome and plasma measurements by either RRA or RIA in a study in which the effectiveness of pimozide and haloperidol was compared in 22 acute schizophrenics. There were, however, a number of serious flaws in the experimental design: (a) 1 week free of oral antipsychotic or 4 weeks free of long-acting depot drug are inadequate "washout" periods; (b) there was apparently no blind; and (c) administration of intramuscular chlorpromazine was allowed when "the clinical situation demanded urgent parenteral administration of antipsychotic drug."

Korpi and co-workers (45) examined serum and plasma samples harvested from 32 chronic schizophrenics who were on constant oral haloperidol treatment (0.3–1.3 mg/kg/day). RRA tended to give higher values (nanograms per milliliter haloperidol equivalents) than the direct measurement of haloperidol (nanograms per milliliter) concentrations by HPLC. It is a moot point whether or not it is appropriate to compare RRA values and HPLC measurements directly, but the authors calculated a coefficient of correlation as 0.68 (Table 4, ref. 45). The authors speculated that the RRA values might have been elevated by interaction of reduced haloperidol, and calculated a correlation of 0.73 for the total haloperidol plus reduced haloperidol measured by HPLC, versus haloperidol equivalents measured by RRA. Unfortunately, the correlation between reduced haloperidol levels and RRA values was almost as good (0.61). Furthermore, we note that in the former correlation ($r = 0.73$), the y-intercept in the x/y correlation was 20-fold greater than the slope, whereas in the latter ($r = 0.61$), the y-intercept was 34 times greater than the slope. This suggests that the RRA values may have been inflated through nonspecific binding (see 57). In this context it is also worth noting that the RRA (45) was based on rat *or* bovine caudate membranes.

In contrast to RRA values, RIA measurements consistently *underestimated* haloperidol levels measured by HPLC ($r = 0.62$). RIA is a competitive binding assay (like RRA) and can also be subject to interference from nonspecific binding and unwanted cross reactions with metabolites. Korpi and co-workers (45) carried out the RIA measurements on extracts of the patient samples similar to those employed in their HPLC method. The authors suggested a number of possible reasons why the RIA measurements underestimated those by HPLC, but in our view, a most plausible explanation is that the standard curves for the RIAs were prepared from "unextracted haloperidol solutions, whereas the samples were extracted." In our experience, we have found that standard curves for "extraction RIAs" must be generated via the same type of procedure used in the test samples.

The foregoing discussion demonstrates that measurement of haloperidol by RRA is not as simple as sometimes supposed. The study by Korpi et al. (45) illustrates the value of comparing different types of methods of analysis with appropriate attention to detail. It is also clear that it is necessary to have robust analytical methods available to permit study of key metabolites of antipsychotic drugs, if there is to be understanding of the molecular basis of antidopaminergic activity in RRA or neuroleptic activity in therapeutic outcome.

CHOICE OF TISSUES (WHERE TO MEASURE)

Over the past decade, the debate has continued on whether it is desirable to measure drug concentrations in plasma, serum, red cells, or whole blood. It has become quite fashionable to measure drug concentrations in red cells, since it was suggested that concentrations in the red cell fraction may be a better reflection of brain levels than are plasma or serum levels (26,27).

Drug analysis in whole blood or red cells requires even more care than in plasma or serum because red cells contain reactive oxidation-reduction systems that can cause artifacts in analysis (18,19,23). Furthermore, there have been suggestions that metabolic sulfoxidation of phenothiazine antipsychotics occurs in red cells (69,100), although Kaul and co-workers (39) suspected that this phenomenon was an artifact, and questioned "the ability of an assay method to accurately determine chlorpromazine in red cells and/or blood." Subsequently it was shown that the sulfoxidation of chlorpromazine in whole blood is almost entirely due to the use of alkaline extraction methods in the analysis (64). After incubation of chlorpromazine with human whole blood under simulated "physiological" conditions *in vitro,* only a very small amount (1%) was found as sulfoxide when the red cell fraction was extracted by a method that did not require the red cells to come into contact with alkali (30).

In 1980 it was reported (12) that the N-oxide metabolite was present in the plasma of patients medicated with chlorpromazine. Although there is some dispute whether or not chlorpromazine N-oxide is pharmacologically active as such (48), or after metabolic conversion back to the parent drug (52), the realization of its presence in blood has important consequences for the analyst. On addition of alkali to whole blood, chlorpromazine N-oxide is rapidly reduced to chlorpromazine, a portion of which undergoes oxidation to chlorpromazine sulfoxide (64). Even in plasma, chlorpromazine N-oxide can be reduced to chlorpromazine when strong alkalis like sodium hydroxide interact with plasma proteins to generate reducing equivalents *in situ* (32). This can lead to spurious elevation of plasma chlorpromazine concentrations (by as much as 340%) when the use of strong alkali is combined with a lengthy extraction procedure.

Apparently chlorpromazine N-oxide does not penetrate into the red cells to any great extent (about 4%; ref. 30). Consequently, there should be minimal interference from N-oxide breakdown during analysis of red cells, provided they are separated from plasma. The plasma fraction can then be analyzed by a method that avoids the use of sodium hydroxide (32). However, the facile sulfoxidation of chlorpromazine suggests that the use of any alkali may be unwise in the extraction of phenothiazines from red blood cells (30,64).

Smith and co-workers (94) carried out a fixed-dose study on thioridazine in 26 patients with a diagnosis of schizophrenia ($N = 22$) or schizoaffective disorder ($N = 4$). The patients were randomly assigned to receive fixed-dose treatment with 150, 250, 650, or 750 mg thioridazine per day. Patients known to be nonresponsive to neuroleptic drugs were excluded from the study. The authors stated that almost all the patients included in the study improved sufficiently to be discharged from the hospital. Nevertheless, no relationship was found between steady-state levels of thioridazine and/or mesoridazine in plasma or red cells and clinical response, judged by improvement in total BPRS or BPRS psychosis factor scores. The authors discussed possible reasons for the apparent lack of relationships between clinical response and plasma or red cells measures, including a frank admission that there were problems in the precise measurement of mesoridazine by their GLC-

NPD method. Details of the analytical method (88) show it to be an adaptation of the GLC-NPD procedure for butaperazine, developed by Javaid and co-workers (35). This method calls for the addition of sodium hydroxide to the plasma or resuspended red cells, before extraction with a mixture of isopropanol (10%) in heptane. Unfortunately, there are no data on the stability of thioridazine (or butaperazine) and their metabolites under these conditions, although the observed interconversions between chlorpromazine and metabolites under similar conditions (32,64) show that there is cause for concern. That there were problems with unwanted oxidation-reduction reactions is evidenced by the inclusion of small quantities of the reducing agent sodium diethylthiocarbamate in the organic extraction solvent (35) and by the addition of the antioxidant sodium metabisulfite to the separated plasma and red cells fractions before committing the samples to the freezer to await analysis (88). It is possible that these precautions may have been sufficient to prevent spurious oxidation reactions from occurring in alkalinized red cell material, but carefully designed and executed experiments will be required if the question is to be answered.

Certainly any future studies on clinical pharmacokinetics of thioridazine should include measurement of the side chain sulfone metabolite (sulforidazine), which appears to be even more actively antidopaminergic than either the parent drug or mesoridazine, the side chain sulfoxide metabolite (40,73). Indeed, Lewis and co-workers (51) have pointed out that the clinical effects of thioridazine appear to depend in large measure on the biotransformation of the parent drug into biologically active metabolites, as indicated in earlier studies by Axelsson and Martensson (3,4).

IS THERE A "THERAPEUTIC WINDOW" FOR NEUROLEPTICS?

A therapeutic window, in simple terms, is a range of concentrations of drug, usually measured in plasma or serum, that is associated with a good therapeutic outcome. Plasma levels outside the window are either too low to ensure good therapeutic efficacy or high enough to induce toxic effects. In the case of drugs like the phenothiazine antipsychotics, which undergo extensive metabolism, it may be necessary to take into account the contribution of active metabolites to the therapeutic response and side effects. The use of conventional chromatographic or immunoassay techniques to measure parent drug (and important metabolites) could lead to the revelation of optimum therapeutic ranges for antipsychotics, but each drug would have to be dealt with separately. Radioreceptor assay, however, is a method that has the capacity to furnish information about levels of total antidopaminergic activity in the plasma, because RRA is based on the binding of all antidopaminergic ligands. Thus, RRA measurements ideally have the potential to reveal a universal therapeutic window for neuroleptics, if such a thing exists. Cohen and co-workers (10) reported a strong correlation ($r = 0.91$, $p < 0.01$) between plasma RRA values and change in BPRS, 2 weeks after commencement of fixed-dose medication with thioridazine, in a group of eight patients with manic-depressive psychosis (five males and three females). Thus, although this study design can be criticized on a number of counts (small number of patients, mixed diagnostic types, inclusion of males and females, spurious RRA values for thioridazine), four important points emerge. First, whatever the RRA values mean in absolute terms, they do at least take into account the activities of all antidopaminergic metabolites in the plasma. Second, the patients were drug free for 1 month before the study and none had ever received depot neuroleptic. Furthermore, the patients were observed for a 3-day period, without medication, to decrease the likelihood that any subject included in the study would have a spontaneous remission. These measures were presumably sufficient to ensure minimization of contamination from previous drug treatments, thereby increasing the chance of significant change in BPRS scores, after 2 weeks of treatment with the drug. Third, the encouraging results of this pilot study underscore the observation (5) that neuroleptic drugs are *antipsychotic* rather than antischizophrenic or antimanic. Fourth, the *rate* of improvement seemed to be related to the plasma RRA values. Those patients with the highest values improved most rapidly; those with intermediate values improved more slowly, and patients with the lowest RRA values did poorly or relapsed.

Van Putten and co-workers (104) discussed the rate of improvement in the context of timing and the therapeutic window concept (when to measure). They conducted a study in 47 newly admitted schizophrenic patients who were randomly assigned to receive fixed doses of 5, 10, or 20 mg of haloperidol over a period of 4 weeks. After this, the dose could be increased in poorly responding patients for another 4 weeks of treatment. Before entering the study, the patients were observed in a drug-free state, and no patient was allowed to participate if there was spontaneous improvement. Clinical improvement was measured by BPRS, NOSIE, and CGI, and plasma haloperidol was measured by RIA. After 1 week of treatment, curvilinear relationships emerged between plasma haloperidol levels and percent improvement on the BPRS psychosis factor, total BPRS scores, and CGI. There was also a suggestion of a therapeutic window between 5 and 16 ng haloperidol per milliliter plasma, although the authors cautioned that there were only two patients with plasma levels above the upper limit, and both these individuals were wracked with side effects.

By the second week of treatment, there was no relationship between plasma haloperidol and any measure of change in clinical outcome. The reasons for this appeared to be that by the second week, some patients with plasma haloperidol levels below 5 ng/ml had started to improve, whereas others with plasma levels above 16 ng/ml also did well. The authors suggested that high plasma levels may not be psychotoxic unless the patient experiences disabling side effects. The second period of 4 weeks of treatment with higher doses of haloperidol (up to 30 mg) did not lead to further improvement (BPRS) but to an increase (worsening) in BPRS depression ratings. Treatment-resistant EPS (notably akathisia) was better related to treatment failure at higher doses, and the authors suggested that treatment-resistant akathisia may be a more powerful determinant of outcome than plasma levels of haloperidol.

Other workers have reported similar evidence of a therapeutic window for haloperidol levels in plasma: Smith et al. (92), 6.5 to 16.5 ng/ml at 24 days; Mavroidis et al. (59), 4 to 11 ng/ml at 14 days; and Magliozzi et al. (56), 8 to 18 ng/ml at 3 to 12 weeks. Potkin and co-workers (77) reported a similar therapeutic range (4 to 22 ng/ml) in a cohort of Chinese schizophrenics. None of these correlations is very strong: The percentage of variance accounted for ranges from only 8% (77) to 43% (59). The difficulties involved in achieving a reasonable balance between statistical rigor and common-sense interpretation of clinical observation are well illustrated in a series of letters (41,105) and replies (90,91) published in the *Archives of General Psychiatry.* In the course of these discussions, Smith (90) briefly reviewed the studies pertinent to haloperidol (56,59,77,92,104), presenting the data in convenient table form. Certainly, to our knowledge, there is only a single report (22) of a patient in whom the initial antipsychotic effect of haloperidol was lost and then regained as plasma levels went above (27.5 ng/ml) and then were brought back into the therapeutic window (10 ng/ml).

In a preliminary report, Smith and co-workers (96) suggested that red blood cell haloperidol levels may be a better predictor of clinical response, as judged by change in total BPRS, than plasma haloperidol levels. However, in a more recent study (95), no significant differences emerged in relationships between plasma or red cell haloperidol levels and clinical response measured by change in BPRS psychosis factor scores. The ranges associated with optimal clinical response were reported to be 6.5 to 16.5 ng/ml plasma and 2.2 to 6.8 ng/ml red cells. On the other hand, Neborsky and co-workers (72) and Garver and colleagues (28) suggested that plasma to red cell haloperidol *ratios* might predict the likely outcome of haloperidol treatment. Both groups of workers reported that high plasma to red cell ratios on the seventh day of treatment were highly correlated with measures of clinical improvement, although by day 14, correlation was no longer evident in the one study (28) that was continued for 2 weeks. In earlier work, Shvartsburd and colleagues (87) had reported red cell to plasma haloperidol ratios (0.39 ± 0.04) similar to those calculated by Garver and co-workers (28) (0.41 ± 0.09), who used the same GLC method (87). By contrast, Neborsky and co-workers (72) used an analytical method (74) that requires adjustment of the biological material to pH 12 followed by solvent extraction before measurement of haloperidol by RIA. This procedure yielded red cell to plasma haloperidol ratios of 0.63 to 1.10, approximately double those determined by Shvartsburd (87) and Garver (28). This leads one to suspect that the use of strong alkali in contact with red cell material may have compromised the subsequent analysis of the extracts by RIA (72). Note that the GLC method (87) allows for the extraction of resuspended red cells without the use of alkali. Certainly the measurement of haloperidol (and reduced haloperidol) in red cells requires further investigation.

It is also worthy to note that after administration of haloperidol, serum or plasma RRA values have so far given disappointingly poor correlations with measures of clinical outcome (68,89,92,93) and with chromatographic (45,68, 92,93) or immunoassay (45) methods. Tang and co-workers (99) used RRA to measure levels of antidopaminergic activity in a cohort of male schizophrenic patients who were randomly assigned to receive fixed doses of either haloperidol or chlorpromazine over a period of 25 days. Plasma samples were obtained twice weekly and subjected to equilibrium dialysis so that total and free "neuroleptic activity" could be measured by RRA. The total BPRS was administered twice in the first week and once a week thereafter.

Of the 19 patients who completed the trial, 11 were on haloperidol and eight were on chlorpromazine. No correlation was detected between decrease in BPRS scores and RRA values when all 19 patients were considered together. This led the authors to conclude that the RRA "did not detect a narrow therapeutic window for neuroleptic drugs." Such a conclusion is based on the premise that RRA ought to be equally effective or reliable for all neuroleptic drugs. In fact, the lack of correlation among the 19 subjects was due to lack of correlation between change in BPRS scores and RRA values in plasma from 11 patients treated with haloperidol. When the data from the eight patients treated with chlorpromazine were considered separately, remarkably good linear correlations emerged between decrease in BPRS scores (1–25 days) and both plasma total ($r = -0.7$, $p < 0.03$) and plasma free ($r = -0.8$, $p < 0.02$) RRA values. These results certainly bear out the conclusion of Korpi and colleagues (45) that "further exploration is needed before radioreceptor assay can be approved for general use."

Relatively few publications on chlorpromazine have appeared in the early 1980s compared with the plethora of studies that were carried out over the previous decade and that have been surveyed in several reviews (11,16,38, 62,78,85). In one of the most rigorously controlled studies on any antipsychotic drug, Wode-Helgodt and colleagues (109) carried out a multiple of fixed-dose, placebo-"double dummy" controlled double-blind study in 44 patients (18 men, 26 women) who were voluntarily admitted to hospital for the duration of the study. The patients were selected for the presence of psychotic symptoms (thought disorder, delusions, or auditory hallucinations) rather than for a diagnosis of schizophrenia *per se,* because of the uncertainty of diagnosis in acute psychosis at the first admission. After a drug-free period of 1 month, followed by a period on placebo (1–7 days), the patients were randomly assigned to receive 200, 400, or 600 mg chlorpromazine per day, in roughly equal proportions of men and women. Psychotherapeutic outcome was monitored during the placebo period and after treatment for 2 and 4 weeks with chlorpromazine by means of the Comprehensive Psychopathological Rating Scale (CPRS). Samples of blood and CSF were harvested at these same time points. Chlorpromazine was measured by a gas-liquid chromatography-mass spectrometric (GLC-MS) method (1).

The results showed a startling difference in outcome between men and women. After 2 weeks of treatment, there were very modest correlations between CPRS measures and chlorpromazine in CSF ($r = -0.54$) and plasma ($r = -0.34$) among the women. There were no such correlations evident among the men. After 4 weeks of treatment, the women improved significantly more than the men, although the correlations with CSF and plasma chlorpromazine were poorer. The authors pointed out that the women tended to have higher plasma chlorpromazine levels than the men, possibly due to lower body weights (and therefore the fixed absolute dosages tended to give higher doses in milligrams per kilogram body weight in the women). In fact, the women seemed to improve equally well on all three doses studied after both 2 and 4 weeks of treatment. Only those men on the highest dose appeared to improve significantly, although by 4 weeks, all doses were related to significant decreases in the morbidity scores.

Once again, these data raise the difficult question of the relationship between dose (and plasma level) and the *time* required for the full effect of the therapeutic response to become evident. Furthermore, as the patient begins to improve with time at sustained dosage, he or she acquires an enhanced ability to interact with psychosocial factors (109), a point that has also been raised by May and colleagues (63). In other words, the drug treatment cannot be divorced from nondrug factors that affect outcome. In this context, it is interesting to note that measures of EPS at 4 weeks were significantly related to both plasma and CSF chlorpromazine levels and in both men and women (109). One would not expect EPS to be modified by nondrug treatments. There is also the possibility that the profile of metabolites may have undergone significant change after 4 weeks continuous treatment with the drug and that metabolites contribute significantly to the onset of EPS.

The study by Wode-Helgodt and colleagues (109) suggested that chlorpromazine levels greater than 40 ng/ml plasma or 1 ng/ml CSF were associated with marked clinical improvement, although many studies carried out in the 1970s failed to show anything of practical value that could be achieved by measurement of plasma levels of chlorpromazine (for a review, see 16). Rivera-Calimlim and co-workers (79) suggested that optimal plasma levels of chlorpromazine were between 30 and 150 ng/ml, on the basis of a retrospective study in psychotic patients. By contrast, Van Putten and colleagues (106) concluded that improvement occurred over a range of 3 to 72 ng/ml after the administration of a fixed dose of chlorpromazine (6.6 mg/kg/day, e.g., 450 mg/day for a 67.5-kg person) for 28 days, in 48 newly admitted (or readmitted) schizophrenic patients (sex unspecified). The authors state that when clinically permissible, a 2- to 10-day washout period was allowed, although most of the patients were believed not to have taken medication "recently." Clinical outcome was measured before and after treatment by means of the BPRS (blind rater) and plasma chlorpromazine levels were measured by GLC-MS. A "responder" was defined as a patient whose total BPRS score had changed by six or more by the 28th day.

That Van Putten and co-workers (106) found no correlation between plasma chlorpromazine and clinical improvement at 28 days is consistent with the lack of correlation observed by Wode-Helgodt and co-workers (109) after 4 weeks of treatment with chlorpromazine. Although there are differences between the two studies (rating scales, probability of heterogeneity of subjects, use of placebo), there are also similarities (fixed doses, similar number of subjects, all subjects hospitalized, same duration of study, blind raters, GLC-MS method). In fact, the apparent lack of concordance about the plasma levels of chlorpromazine associated with good clinical outcome is likely more attributable to the radically different methods of treatment of data than to any other reason. Wode-Helgodt and co-

workers (109) used Fisher's exact test to arrive at the conclusions that "the results indicated marked clinical improvement with chlorpromazine concentrations above 1 ng/ml in CSF and 40 ng/ml in plasma" after 2 weeks of treatment. Van Putten and co-workers (106), on the other hand, chose to define a "responder" as a patient whose total BPRS score changed by six or more by the end of the 4-week study period. Although this method may seem arbitrary at first sight, it does reflect the way clinicians tend to categorize the patients in practice. After 4 weeks of treatment, half the patients were judged to be "responders" and the other half "nonresponders," yet the plasma chlorpromazine concentrations in the "nonresponders" were spread over almost exactly the same range of concentrations found in the "responders." Scrutiny of the information presented by Wode-Helgodt and colleagues (109) suggests that the same trend may be present in their data. After 2 weeks, there appears to be about the same number of good responders with plasma concentrations less than 40 ng/ml as there are with chlorpromazine levels greater than 40 ng/ml. Clearly, it would be little more than an academic nicety to think of raising the dose in a patient who was responding well to treatment but happened to have a plasma concentration lower than a number generated from a mere statistical test.

There is also the question of the *time* required for clinical improvement to become apparent in response to a given steady-state plasma level of the drug. Van Putten and co-workers (106) increased the dose in 11 of their "nonresponders." Four of these patients improved, although their plasma concentrations all remained below 72 ng/ml, and in one case actually appeared to be lower, despite the increase in dose. It must be emphasized that no attempt was made to prove that steady states existed either before or after the dosage increment, but one wonders if these patients might have improved eventually merely if they had been given more time to respond to the lower dosage regimen. It certainly appears that "time to respond" is a significant confounding variable in the search for correlations between plasma levels and therapeutic response.

Studies with the more potent piperazine-type phenothiazine drug, fluphenazine, are even more difficult to carry out because plasma concentrations are often subnanogram. The most sensitive assay methods for fluphenazine to date are by RIA (66,107) and GLC-MS (65).

There have been only two fixed-dose studies of oral fluphenazine in psychotic patients. Dysken and co-workers (20) conducted a study in 29 newly admitted, floridly psychotic schizophrenic or schizoaffective patients who were held medication free for 1 week before the study began. The patients were assigned to receive a dose of 5, 10, or 20 mg fluphenazine hydrochloride, although the dosing procedure was neither randomized nor blind. Plasma fluphenazine was measured by a GLC-NPD method which is reliable down to 0.5 ng/ml. This is barely adequate for the assay of fluphenazine, because even after 2 weeks on fixed dose, 12 of 29 subjects apparently had plasma fluphenazine concentrations of less than 0.5 ng/ml.

Clinical outcome was assessed by the serial New Haven Schizophrenic Index (NHSI). The authors noted that there was marked variability in the clinical response over the range of plasma levels found, stating that it was possible to fit a quadratic regression line (curvilinear relationship) on the data with a level of probability of less than 0.02 (correlation coefficient not stated). On the basis of these data, Dysken and colleagues guardedly suggested a therapeutic window from 0.2 to 2.8 ng/ml plasma fluphenazine, pointing out that the upper and lower limits of the window were each defined by only three subjects. (Three nonresponders had plasma levels less than 0.2 ng/ml and three nonresponders had plasma levels greater than 2.8 ng/ml.)

An interesting point of similarity between the fluphenazine study of Dysken and co-workers (20) and the chlorpromazine study of Van Putten, May, and Jenden (106) is that both experimental protocols allowed for the dose to be adjusted at the end of the fixed dose period. At the end of the 2-week period of fixed-dose fluphenazine, the physician was permitted to adjust the dose upwards or downwards or to continue the same level of medication. (It is not stated how many physicians were involved or whether they were privy to the plasma level data. One would assume *not*, because it would take several days for the plasma samples to be analyzed.) The physicians (20) chose to maintain the same dosage regimen in 12 patients (mean percentage change in NHSI score 57.7 ± 9.7 SEM), whereas the dosage was increased in 15 patients (mean percentage change in NHSI score 24.5 ± 9.4 SEM). Two patients were dropped from the study at this stage. Dysken and colleagues pointed out that in no case was there a reduction in dosage in order to improve clinical response.

Scrutiny of the data reported by Dysken and co-workers (see Fig. 3 in ref. 20) reveals another interesting similarity with the chlorpromazine study (106). Following the "practitioner-friendly" technique of Van Putten and colleagues, we assigned an arbitrary cutoff point of 50% change in NHSI to distinguish "adequate responders" from "inadequate responders." Within Dysken's therapeutic window of 0.2 to 2.8 ng/ml, there appear to be an equal number of adequate responders and inadequate responders (12 of each). One would surmise that these "adequate responders" correspond to the 12 patients in whom the physicians chose to maintain the initial dose. The physicians would likely have come to this decision with or without plasma level data. It is in deciding what to do about the "inadequate responder" that the clinician might find plasma level data helpful. If the therapeutic window concept for antipsychotic drugs has any validity, the course of action to be taken should be defined by its upper and lower limits. Appropriate adjustment of dosage should be made only for those "inadequate responders" whose plasma levels fall outside the window. No adjustment at all is required for the (majority) inadequate responders whose plasma levels fall within the window. This brings us back to the importance of considering the *rate* of improvement, a point discussed in Dysken's article (20).

Mavroidis and co-workers (60,61) carried out a study in 19 schizophrenic patients in an attempt to define more precisely the therapeutic window for oral fluphenazine proposed by Dysken and co-workers. The patients were actively psychotic and were readmitted to the hospital for the duration of the study. Each patient was randomly assigned to receive 2.5, 5, or 10 mg fluphenazine b.i.d. over a period of 2 weeks. Clinical improvement was monitored

by means of the NHSI, the system employed by Dysken and co-workers. Raters were blind to the plasma concentration data, but it is not stated whether they were also blind to dose. Plasma samples were harvested at days 7 and 14 (and also at day 12 where possible) in order to evaluate the steady state. NHSI ratings were taken at baseline and on days 7, 12, and 14.

There was a significant curvilinear relationship between clinical improvement at 2 weeks and the mean plasma levels ($r = 0.47$, $p < 0.05$). The therapeutic range was defined as the portion of the regression line associated with an improvement of at least 45% on the NHSI. The optimum therapeutic range, defined by this criterion, appeared to occur in the range 0.13 to 0.70 ng/ml. Patients with fluphenazine plasma levels within this range showed a mean improvement of $59\% \pm 6.27$ (SEM), whereas patients with higher plasma levels showed a mean improvement of $34\% \pm 5.73$ (SEM).

There are two important criticisms of this study. First, neither report (60,61) makes any mention of any washout or observation period. Secondly, the GLC-NPD analytical method employed (36) is just not sensitive enough to define plasma levels below 0.5 ng/ml. The coefficient of variation at 0.2 ng/ml is reported to be 20% (which means the fluphenazine peak is hard to distinguish from background noise).

Examination of the curvilinear relationship (see Fig. 1 in ref. 61) reveals that the ends of the curve slope upwards, quite unlike the familiar inverted "U" shape. Furthermore, if one applies the arbitrary 50% improvement criterion to distinguish "adequate responders" (more than 50% improvement) from "inadequate responders" (less than 50% improvement), one finds that there are two "adequate responders" well outside the upper limit of the proposed therapeutic range of 0.13 to 0.7 ng/ml. Nevertheless, the plasma levels of these two patients are within the therapeutic range proposed by Dysken and co-workers (20). In fact, if the wider therapeutic range of 0.1 or 0.2 to 2.8 ng/ml is applied to the data of Mavroidis and co-workers (60,61), once again one finds that the patients are almost equally divided among "adequate responders" and "inadequate responders."

Thus, although there is some evidence for the applicability of the therapeutic window concept to neuroleptic drugs, it must be admitted that plasma concentration-response correlations rarely account for more than 25% of the variance. Some of the remaining variance factors can be identified, but they are very difficult to cope with experimentally. The psychoses, characterized as they are by disordered thought and loss of contact with reality, are disorders of an intensely personal nature that emphasize the individuality of the patient. Nondrug variance factors are, therefore, highly individualized because they involve psychosocial interactions, intentional or unintentional. Some patients respond to antipsychotic drugs quickly, so that the best drug-related correlations have all been found within 1 or 2 weeks of starting drug treatment. However, as these patients became more amenable to psychosocial therapy, the nondrug variance factors assume a greater role and correlations are lost. Other patients respond more slowly to a given dose of neuroleptic, and it is in these individuals that a plasma concentration measurement, taken after 1 or 2 weeks of treatment, may be helpful. This can assist the practitioner in deciding whether or not it is necessary to adjust the dose up or down to bring the plasma concentration within the putative therapeutic range.

Mavroidis and colleagues (60) have proposed such a strategy for fluphenazine, in which they suggest starting the patient on an average dose (5 mg b.i.d.), supplemented, if necessary, by a nonantipsychotic sedative to control agitation, until the patient has time to show his or her response to the regimen. Division of the daily dose makes sense from the kinetic point of view. Itoh and co-workers (33) have indicated that steady state tends to be achieved more quickly with a divided daily dose schedule than with a single daily dose regimen. There are always peaks and valleys in plasma concentrations within a steady state, but there was significantly less variation in plasma levels during the day when the dose was divided (33). Dysken and co-workers (20) defined single-dose plasma concentration-time profiles by taking frequent blood samples during the day after the administration of 20 mg fluphenazine to nine patients. Mean plasma levels peaked at 6.0 ng/ml, which is double the upper limit of the putative therapeutic range (2.8 ng/ml). By contrast, after the administration of single oral doses of 5 mg fluphenazine hydrochloride to six healthy volunteers, the highest C_{max} value reached in any individual was approximately 1.0 ng/ml, whereas the mean C_{max} value was 0.56 ng/ml (67). Even peak values remained within the putative therapeutic range for fluphenazine after a single 5-mg dose. Thus, the dose and dosage interval are *both* important criteria that determine the length of time to reach steady state, the level of the steady state, and the variation in plasma concentration within the steady state. Dosage regimens of 5 mg q.i.d., 10 mg b.i.d., and 20 mg H.S. all provide for the ingestion of 20 mg of drug per day, but the pharmacokinetics of each regimen are different. The clinical consequences of high peak plasma concentrations following the administration of the dose are largely unknown. Therefore, more research is needed on the effects of dosing schedules on the within-day variation in steady-state levels of antipsychotic drugs and their major metabolites. In seeking relationships between steady-state levels and therapeutic outcome, most authors take pains to justify clinical and methodological aspects of their study designs, but few venture to discuss the pharmacokinetic implications of the type of dosage regimen.

In summary, the question of whether there is a "therapeutic window for neuroleptic drugs" has not been answered definitively as yet. There may be ranges of plasma concentrations associated with optimum antipsychotic action, but these will have to be defined separately for each drug. There is evidence that some nonresponders may do better when their plasma drug levels are lowered. The conventional practice of raising the dose of antipsychotic drug in poor responders may be inappropriate in some patients. Over the next decade, experience in the use of putative therapeutic ranges of plasma concentrations should clarify their general validity and usefulness in clinical practice. The development of sensitive and reliable methods for the assessment of clinical outcome and of good analytical methods that can be applied routinely would be of great value.

CONCLUSIONS

Some important trends and developments can be identified, which have emerged since the review of May and Van Putten (62).

There have been improvements in the sensitivity and reliability of analytical methods for parent antipsychotics, although metabolite analysis still presents some challenges. The concept of RRA has been applied to neuroleptic drugs, but there are still some technical difficulties that remain to be solved before its application can be considered universal. Newer techniques, such as the combination of specific receptor-labeling ligands with positron emission tomography, have begun to be applied to studies on the pharmacodynamics of neuroleptics in brains of living patients.

There appears to have been a greater awareness of the need for the careful selection of patients, judging by the widespread use of rigorous diagnostic criteria such as DSM-III. There is also a recognition that neuroleptic drugs are primarily antipsychotic rather than antischizophrenic; some researchers have sought to correlate the positive symptoms of schizophrenia with plasma concentration data.

The importance of considering the *rate* of improvement, rather than the amount of change that is possible, has been borne out in several studies. The best correlations between clinical outcome and plasma level data have typically been observed 2 weeks after commencement of drug therapy, although the correlations rarely account for more than approximately 25% of the variance, even when data on plasma levels of active metabolites are also considered.

The length of the "washout" period continues to be a contentious issue. Evidence is beginning to emerge that following withdrawal of antipsychotic, dopamine receptors in the brain remain blocked for a substantial time after plasma concentrations have declined. These preliminary findings confirm the view that the "washout" period should be the longest period that is ethically feasible. Firm data on the rates of disappearance of neuroleptic drugs from the central nervous system should become available in the foreseeable future.

Despite all the methodological and technical difficulties, there are encouraging signs that it may be possible to define "therapeutic ranges" of plasma concentrations of neuroleptic drugs. More research is needed on intersubject variation in rate of improvement in response to sustained fixed dose therapy.

ACKNOWLEDGMENTS

The authors gratefully acknowledge the Medical Research Council of Canada for Program Grant PG-34. We thank Drs. P. R. A. May and S. R. Marder of U.C.L.A. and Brentwood VA, California, for helpful discussions during preparation of the manuscript.

REFERENCES

1. Alfredsson, G. B., Wode-Helgodt, B., and Sedval, G. (1976): *Psychopharmacology,* 48:123–131.
2. Aoba, A., Katika, Y., Yamaguchi, N., Shida, M., Tsuneizumi,

T., Shibata, N., Kenichi, K., and Hasegawa, K. (1985): *J. Gerontol.*, 40:303–308.

3. Axelsson, R., and Martensson, E. (1978): *Curr. Ther. Res. Clin. Exp.*, 24:232–242.

4. Axelsson, R., and Martensson, E. (1980): *Curr. Ther. Res. Clin. Exp.*, 28:463–489.

5. Baldessarini, R. J. (1977): *Chemotherapy in Psychiatry.* Harvard University Press, Cambridge.

6. Braun, G. A., Poos, G. I., and Soudijn, W. (1967): *Eur. J. Pharmacol.*, 1:58–62.

7. Browning, J. L., Harrington, C. A., Burch, N. R., and Davis, C. M. (1982): *Fed. Proc.*, 41:1635.

8. Cahil, H. M., Avery, D. H., Hollister, L. E., Creese, I., and Snyder, S. H. (1979): *Psychiatry Res.*, 1:39–44.

9. Cohen, B. M., Herschel, M., and Aoba, A. (1979): *Psychiatry Res.*, 1:199–208.

10. Cohen, B. M., Lipinski, J. F., Pope, G. H., Harris, P. Q., and Altesman, R. I. (1980): *Psychopharmacology*, 70:191–193.

11. Cooper, T. B. (1978): *Clin. Pharmacokinet.*, 3:14–38.

12. Craig, J. C., Gruenke, L. D., Hitzeman, B. A., Holaday, J., and Loh, H. H. (1980): In: *Phenothiazines and Structurally Related Drugs*, edited by E. Usdin, H. Eckert, and I. S. Forrest, pp. 129–132. Elsevier/North Holland, New York.

13. Creese, I., Burt, D. R., and Snyder, S. H. (1976): *Science*, 192:481–483.

14. Creese, I., and Snyder, S. H. (1977): *Nature*, 270:180–182.

15. Crow, T. J. (1980): *Br. Med. J.*, 280:66–68.

16. Curry, S. H. (1981): In: *Plasma Levels of Psychotropic Drugs and Clinical Response*, edited by G. D. Burrows and T. Norman, pp. 243–286. Marcel Dekker, New York.

17. Curry, S. H., and Evans, S. (1975): *Psychopharmacol. Commun.*, 1:481–490.

18. Diepold, C., Eyer, P., Kampffmeyer, H., and Reinhardt, K. (1982): *Adv. Exp. Med. Biol.*, 136B:1173–1181.

19. Dolle, B., Topner, W., and Neuman, H. G. (1980): *Xenobiotica*, 10:527–536.

20. Dysken, M. W., Javaid, J. I., Chang, S. S., Schafer, C., Shahid, A., and Davis, J. M. (1981): *Psychopharmacology*, 73:205–210.

21. Ereshefsky, L., Davis, C. M., Harrington, C. A., Jann, M. W., Browning, J. L., Saklad, S. R., and Burch, N. R. (1984): *J. Clin. Psychopharmacol.*, 4:138–142.

22. Extein, I., Pottash, A. L. C., and Gold, M. S. (1983): *Lancet*, 1:1048–1049.

23. Eyer, P., and Lierheimer, E. (1980): *Xenobiotica*, 10:517–526.

24. Forsman, A., Folsch, G., Larsson, M., and Ohman, R. (1977): *Curr. Ther. Res.*, 21:606–617.

25. Forsman, A., and Larsson, M. (1978): *Curr. Ther. Res.*, 24:567–568.

26. Garver, D. L., Davis, J. M., Dekirmenjian, H., Jones, F. D., Casper, R., and Haraszti, J. (1976): *Arch. Gen. Psychiatry*, 33:862–866.

27. Garver, D. L., Dekirmenjian, H., Davis, J. M., Caspar, R., and Ericksen, S. (1977): *Am. J. Psychiatry*, 134:304–307.

28. Garver, D. L., Hirschowitz, J., Glicksteen, G. A., Kanter, D. R., and Mavroidis, M. J. (1984): *J. Clin. Psychopharmacol.*, 4:133–137.

29. Harris, P. Q., Brown, S. J., Friedman, M. J., and Bacopoulos, N. G. (1984): *Biol. Psychiatry*, 19:849–860.

30. Hawes, E. M., Hubbard, J. W., Martin, M., McKay, G., Yeung, P. K. F., and Midha, K. K. (1986): *Ther. Drug Monit.*, 8:37–41.

31. Hornykiewicz, O. (1982): *Nature*, 299:484–486.

32. Hubbard, J. W., Cooper, J. K., Hawes, E. M., Jenden, D. J., May, P. R. A., Martin, M., Van Putten, T., and Midha, K. K. (1985): *Ther. Drug Monit.*, 7:222–228.

33. Itoh, H., Yagi, G., Tateyama, M., Fujii, Y., Iwamura, K., and Ichikawa, H. (1984): *Prog. Neuropsychopharmacol. Biol. Psychiatry*, 8:51–62.

34. Jann, M. W., Ereshefsky, L., Saklad, S. R., Richards, A., and Davis, C. M. (1984): *Drug Intell. Clin. Pharm.*, 18:507.

35. Javaid, J. I., Dekirmenjian, H., Liskevych, U., and Davis, J. M. (1979): *J. Chromatogr. Sci.*, 17:666–670.

36. Javaid, J. I., Dekirmenjian, H., Liskevych, U., Lin, R.-L., and Davis, J. L. (1981): *J. Chromatogr. Sci.*, 19:439–443.

37. Javaid, J. I., Linden, R. D., and David, J. J. (1982): *Psychopharmacol. Bull.*, 18:227–228.

38. Kane, J., Rifkin, A., Quitkin, F., and Klein, D. (1976): In: *Progress in Psychiatric Drug Treatment*, edited by D. Klein and R. Gittelman Klein, pp. 399–408. Brunner-Mazel, New York.

39. Kaul, P. N., Chopde, C. T., and Clark, M. L. (1980): In: *Phenothiazines and Structurally Related Drugs*, edited by E. Usdin, H. Eckert, and I. S. Forrest, pp. 159–162. Elsevier/North-Holland, New York.

40. Kilts, C. D., Knight, D. L., Mailman, R. B., Widerlov, E., and Breese, G. R. (1984): *J. Pharmacol. Exp. Ther.*, 231:334–342.

41. Kirch, D. G., Bigelow, L. B., and Wyatt, R. J. (1985): *Arch. Gen. Psychiatry*, 42:838–839.

42. Kirch, D. G., Palmer, M. R., Egan, M., and Freedman, R. (1985): *Neuropharmacology*, 24:375–379.

43. Kolakowska, T., Wiles, D. H., Gelder, M. G., and McNeilly, A. S. (1976): *Psychopharmacology*, 49:101–107.

44. Korpi, E. R., Kleinman, J. E., Costakos, D. T., Linnoila, M., and Wyatt, R. J. (1984): *Psychiatry Res.*, 11:259–269.

45. Korpi, E. R., Ko, G. N., Phelps, B. H., and Wyatt, R. J. (1984): *J. Clin. Psychopharmacol.*, 4:332–335.

46. Korpi, E. R., Phelps, B. H., Granger, H., Chang, W.-H., Linnoila, M., Meek, J. L., and Wyatt, R. J. (1983): *Clin. Chem.*, 29:624–628.

47. Korpi, E. R., and Wyatt, R. J. (1984): *Psychopharmacology*, 83:34–37.

48. Krieglstein, J., Rieger, H., and Schutz, H. (1979): *Eur. J. Pharmacol.*, 56:363–370.

49. Kucharski, L. T., Alexander, P., Tune, L., and Coyle, J. (1984): *Psychopharmacology*, 82:194–198.

50. Lai, A. A., Fleck, R. J., Patzke, J. V., Glueck, B. G., Shaskan, E. G., and Rosenberg, B. J. (1982): *Ther. Drug Monit.*, 4:89–93.

51. Lewis, M. H., Mobilio, J. N., Rissmiller, D. J., and Mailman, R. B. (1984): *J. Am. Osteopath. Assoc.*, 84:124–128.

52. Lewis, M. H., Widerlov, E., Knight, D. L., Kilts, C. D., and Mailman, R. B. (1983): *J. Pharmacol. Exp. Ther.*, 225:539–545.

53. Lindenmayer, J. P., Smith, D., and Katz, I. (1984): *J. Clin. Psychiatry*, 45:117–119.

54. Linnoila, M., Rosenblatt, J. E., Jeske, D., Potter, W. Z., and Wyatt, R. J. (1982): *Acta Pharmacol. Toxicol.*, 50:25–29.

55. MacKay, A. V. P., Healey, A. F., and Baker, J. (1974): *Br. J. Clin. Pharmacol.*, 1:425–430.

56. Magliozzi, J. R., Hollister, L. E., Arnold, K. V., and Earle, G. M. (1981): *Am. J. Psychiatry*, 138:365–367.

57. Mailman, R. B., De Haven, D. L., Halpern, E. A., and Lewis, M. H. (1984): *Life Sci.*, 34:1057–1064.

58. Mailman, R. B., Pierce, J. P., Crofton, K. M., Petitto, J., De Haven, D. L., Kilts, C. D., and Lewis, M. H. (1984): *Biol. Psychiatry*, 19:833–847.

59. Mavroidis, M. L., Kanter, D. R., Hirschowitz, J., and Garver, D. L. (1983): *Psychopharmacology*, 81:354–356.

60. Mavroidis, M. L., Kanter, D. R., Hirschowitz, J., and Garver, D. L. (1984): *J. Clin. Psychiatry*, 45:370–373.

61. Mavroidis, M. L., Kanter, D. R., Hirschowitz, J., and Garver, D. L. (1984): *Psychopharmacol. Bull.*, 20:168–170.

62. May, P. R. A., and Van Putten, T. (1978): *Arch. Gen. Psychiatry*, 35:1081–1087.

63. May, P. R. A., Van Putten, T., Jenden, D. J., Yale, C., and Dixon, W. J. (1981): *Arch. Gen. Psychiatry*, 38:202–207.

64. McKay, G., Cooper, J. K., Hawes, E. M., Hubbard, J. W., Martin, M., and Midha, K. K. (1985): *Ther. Drug Monit.*, 7:472–477.

65. McKay, G., Hall, K., Edom, R., Hawes, E. M., and Midha, K. K. (1983): *Biomed. Mass Spectrom.*, 10:550–555.

66. Midha, K. K., Cooper, J. K., and Hubbard, J. W. (1980): *Commun. Psychopharmacol.*, 4:107–114.

67. Midha, K. K., McKay, G., Korchinski, E. D., Hawes, E. M., and Hall, K. (1983): *Eur. J. Clin. Pharmacol.*, 25:709–711.

68. Miller, D. O., Hershey, L. A., Duffy, J. P., Abernethy, D. R., and Greenblatt, D. J. (1984): *J. Clin. Psychopharmacol.*, 4:305–310.

69. Minder, R., Schetzer, G., and Bickel, M. H. (1971): *Naunyn Schmiedebergs Arch. Pharmacol.*, 268:334–347.

70. Moller, H.-J., Kissling, W., Lang, C., Doerr, C., Pirke, K.-M., and Von Zerssen, D. (1982): *Am. J. Psychiatry*, 139:1571–1575.

71. Nakahara, T., Hirano, M., Uchimura, H., Saito, M., Kim, J. S.,

Matsumoto, T., Yokoo, H., Shimomura, M., and Mukai, A. (1983): *Psychopharmacology,* 79:266–270.

72. Neborsky, R. J., Janowski, D. S., Perel, J. M., Munson, E., and Deprey, D. (1984): *J. Clin. Psychiatry,* 45:10–13.

73. Niedzwiecki, D. M., Mailman, R. B., and Cubeddu, L. X. (1984): *J. Pharmacol. Exp. Ther.,* 228:636–639.

74. Pajerski, J., Stiller, R., Perel, J. M., and Nathan, R. S. (1982): *Fed. Proc.,* 41:1065.

75. Petroutka, S. J., and Snyder, S. H. (1980): *Am. J. Psychiatry,* 137:1518–1522.

76. Phillipson, O. T., McKeown, J. M., Baker, J., and Healey, A. F. (1977): *Br. J. Psychiatry,* 131:172–184.

77. Potkin, S. G., Shen, Y., Dongfeng, Z., Pardes, H., Shu, L., Phelps, B., and Poland, R. (1985): *Psychopharmacol. Bull.,* 21:59–61.

78. Rivera-Calimlim, L., and Hershey, L. (1984): *Annu. Rev. Pharmacol. Toxicol.,* 24:361–386.

79. Rivera-Calimlim, L., Nasrallah, L., Strauss, J., and Lasagna, L. (1976): *Am. J. Psychiatry,* 133:646–652.

80. Rosenblatt, J. E., Pary, R. J., and Bigelow, L. B. (1980): *Am. J. Psychiatry,* 133:646–652.

81. Rosenblatt, J. E., Pert, C. B., Colison, J., Van Kammen, D. P., Scott, R. J., and Bunney, W. E., Jr. (1979): *Commun. Psychopharmacol.,* 3:153–158.

82. Sakalis, G., Chan, T. L., Gerhson, S., and Park, S. (1973): *Psychopharmacologia,* 32:279–284.

83. Sakalis, G., Chan, T. L., Sathananthan, G., Schooler, N., Goldberg, S., and Gershon, S. (1977): *Commun. Psychopharmacol.,* 1:157–166.

84. Sakalis, G., Curry, S. H., Mould, G. P., and Lader, M. H. (1972): *Clin. Pharmacol. Ther.,* 13:931–946.

85. Sedvall, G. (1981): In: *Clinical Pharmacology in Psychiatry,* edited by E. Usdin, pp. 243–249. Elsevier, New York.

86. Settle, E. C., and Ayd, F. J., Jr. (1983): *J. Clin. Psychiatry,* 44:440–448.

87. Shvartsburd, A., Dekirmenjian, H., Chang, S., and Davis, J. M. (1983): *J. Clin. Psychopharmacol.,* 3:7–12.

88. Shvartsburd, A., Nwokeafor, V., and Smith, R. C. (1984): *Psychopharmacology,* 82:55–61.

89. Silverstone, T., Cookson, J., Ball, R., Chin, C. N., Jacobs, D., Lader, S., and Gould, S. (1984): *J. Psychiatr. Res.,* 18:255–258.

90. Smith, R. C. (1985): *Arch. Gen. Psychiatry,* 42:835–838.

91. Smith, R. C. (1985): *Arch. Gen. Psychiatry,* 42:839–840.

92. Smith, R. C., Baumgartner, R., Burd, A., Ravichandran, G. K., and Maudlin, M. (1985): *Psychopharmacol. Bull.,* 21:52–58.

93. Smith, R. C., Baumgartner, R., Misra, C. H., Mauldin, M., Shvartsburd, A., Ho, B. T., and De John, C. (1984): *Arch. Gen. Psychiatry,* 41:1044–1049.

94. Smith, R. C., Baumgartner, R., Ravichandran, G. K., Shvartsburd, A., Schoolar, J. C., Allen, P., and Johnson, R. (1984): *Psychiatry Res.,* 12:287–296.

95. Smith, R. C., Baumgartner, R., Shvartsburd, A., Ravichandran, G. K., Vroulis, G., and Maudlin, M. (1985): *Psychopharmacology,* 85:449–456.

96. Smith, R. C., Vroulis, G., Shvartsburd, A., Lewis, A. R., Schoolar, J. C., Chojnacki, M., and Johnson, R. (1982): *Am. J. Psychiatry,* 139:1054–1056.

97. Snyder, S. H. (1981): *Am. J. Psychiatry,* 138:460–464.

98. Snyder, S. H. (1982): *Lancet,* 2:970–974.

99. Tang, S. W., Glaister, J., Davidson, L., Toth, R., Jeffries, J. J., and Seeman, P. (1984): *Psychiatry Res.,* 13:285–293.

100. Traficante, L. J., Sakalis, G., Siekierski, J., Rotrosen, J., and Gershon, S. (1979): *Life Sci.,* 24:337–345.

101. Tune, L. E., and Coyle, J. T. (1982): *Ther. Drug Monit.,* 4:59–62.

102. Tune, L. E., Creese, I., De Paulo, J. R., Slavney, P. R., Coyle, J. T., and Snyder, S. H. (1980): *Am. J. Psychiatry,* 137:187–190.

103. Tune, L. E., Creese, I., De Paulo, J. R., Slavney, P. R., and Snyder, S. H. (1981): *J. Nerv. Ment. Dis.,* 169:60–63.

104. Van Putten, T., Marder, S. R., May, P. R. A., Poland, R. E., and O'Brien, R. P. (1985): *Psychopharmacol. Bull.,* 21:69–72.

105. Van Putten, T., Marder, S. R., and Mintz, J. (1985): *Arch. Gen. Psychiatry,* 42:835.

106. Van Putten, T., May, P. R. A., and Jenden, D. J. (1981): *Psychol. Med.,* 11:729–734.

107. Wiles, D. H., and Franklin, M. (1978): *Br. J. Clin. Pharmacol.,* 5:265–268.

108. Wiles, D. H., Kolakowska, T., McNeilly, A. S., Mandelbrote, B. M., and Gelder, M. G. (1976): *Physiol. Med.,* 6:407–415.

109. Wode-Helgodt, B., Borg, S., Fryo, B., and Sedvall, G. (1978): *Acta Psychiatr. Scand.,* 58:149–173.

Psychopharmacology:
The Third Generation of Progress,
edited by Herbert Y. Meltzer.
Raven Press, New York © 1987.

CHAPTER **142**

Pharmacokinetics of Antidepressants

Matthew V. Rudorfer and William Z. Potter

During the last 15 years the effort to describe relationships between antidepressant concentrations and clinical response has been paralleled by pharmacokinetic studies of these compounds both in healthy volunteers and in patients. The focus on human studies is an important one since, as is being demonstrated in studies of new antidepressant compounds, pharmacokinetic behavior in animals does not predict whether parent drug or (potentially) active metabolites will predominate under clinical conditions of chronic treatment. Test doses of model compounds in humans are also being assessed as a possible means of predicting an individual's metabolism of a variety of antidepressants and thereby anticipating problems that might arise from differential pharmacokinetics. What emerges is more an appreciation of the principles determining concentration of drugs that are subject to multiple metabolic pathways than simple generalizable tests. Knowledge of these principles currently provides the greatest help in anticipating whether a drug is likely to produce effects consistent with a single compound interacting with a single receptor. In what follows, we will use examples from recent investigations to highlight those pharmacokinetic principles most relevant to understanding the biochemical and therapeutic actions of antidepressants in humans.

First, we note that extensive interindividual variability in the pharmacokinetics of antidepressants, especially classic tricyclic compounds, is so generally recognized that numerous clinical laboratories determine plasma concentrations for the purpose of therapeutic monitoring. It is still not clear, however, that knowledge of plasma concentrations is always clinically useful. The status of the therapeutic utility of such measures has been extensively reviewed (and

is critically discussed in *this volume*). Therefore, we will only focus on aspects of the relationship(s) between concentration and effect that demonstrate the pharmacodynamic consequences of complex pharmacokinetics.

BASIS OF METABOLISM

New antidepressants, such as tricyclic compounds, are highly lipophilic and therefore subject to multiple biotransformation steps yielding polar metabolites that can be readily excreted in the urine. The major site of this drug metabolism is the liver, where tricyclic antidepressants (TCAs), for instance, undergo mainly demethylation and hydroxylation, followed by glucuronide conjugation (44). The oxidative reactions are usually the rate-limiting ones and are subject to stimulation or blockade by exogenous agents as well as having their primary activity determined by an individual's genetic makeup. A useful concept is that of intrinsic clearance, which refers to the ability of the liver to remove a drug by all pathways in the absence of any blood flow limitations. *In vivo,* in addition to the intrinsic clearance, the physiologic context of drug presentation to the liver, including factors such as hepatic blood flow and binding of drug to blood proteins and to tissues, influences the actual rate of antidepressant metabolism (136).

MAJOR METABOLIC PATHWAYS

At least for the TCAs, of the two major oxidative pathways (Fig. 1), demethylation and hydroxylation, the latter appears to more closely approximate a functional

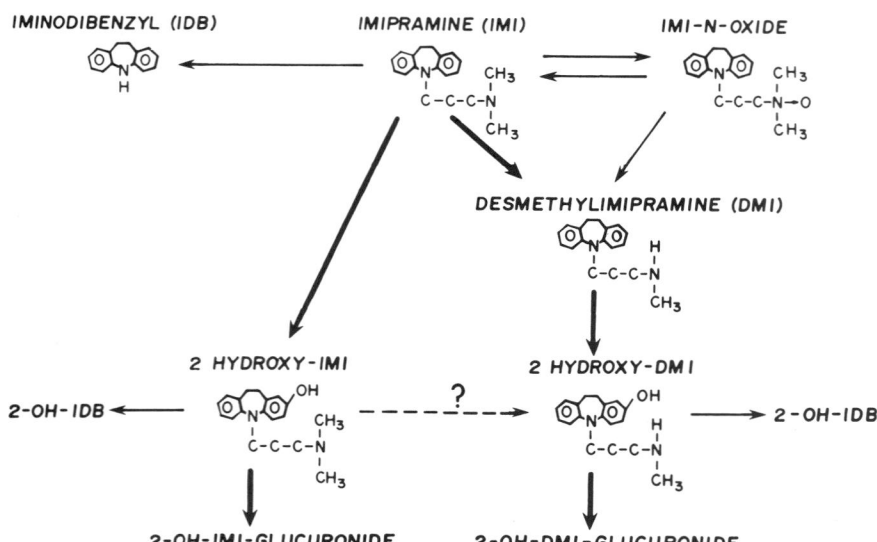

IMINODIBENZYL (IDB)   IMIPRAMINE (IMI)   IMI-N-OXIDE

DESMETHYLIMIPRAMINE (DMI)

2 HYDROXY-IMI   2 HYDROXY-DMI

2-OH-IDB ←   ? - - - - - →   → 2-OH-IDB

2-OH-IMI-GLUCURONIDE   2-OH-DMI-GLUCURONIDE

FIG. 1. Metabolic pathways of the prototypical tricyclic antidepressant, imipramine, in humans.

"rate-limiting" step (since it is needed prior to conjugation and to produce sufficient polarity to permit renal excretion). First-pass metabolism results from the extremely high affinity for hepatic microsomal cytochrome P450 as drug flows through the liver via the portal vein to the hepatic vein prior to entering the systemic circulation. This is much greater following oral or (in animals) intraperitoneal administration compared with intravenous (IV) infusion or intramuscular injection (86). Consequently, bioavailability is maximal with intravenous administration, as calculated from the ratio of the area under the plasma concentration versus time curves (AUCs) following oral and IV presentation of the same dose, respectively, assuming complete absorption of the former (27). First-pass metabolism of several TCAs has been quantitated in humans, including nortriptyline (approximately 30–50%; refs. 3, 8, 49), amitriptyline (30–69%; ref. 22), and imipramine (23–71%; refs. 48, 86). The most extensive first-pass metabolism has been reported for doxepin, averaging 70% (133) with a range of 55 to 87% (143). Similarly variable and extensive first-pass metabolism can be expected to occur with newer antidepressants. As for the metabolic route(s) that are ultimately most important for nontricyclics, these will, of course, be compound-specific (113). For instance, in the case of the new antidepressant bupropion, reduction of the intact parent aminoketone to an amino alcohol appears to be important (70).

The relative contributions of various pathways have been thoroughly worked out for the TCAs, as mentioned before, with hydroxylation assuming special prominence. Thus, for imipramine (27), the major metabolites are 2-OH-desipramine (free plus conjugated, 40%), 2-OH-imipramine (25%), and 2-OH-iminodibenzyl 2-OH-IDB (15%). Conjugated plus unconjugated OH-nortriptyline accounts for 55% of an oral dose of amitriptyline (131). Similarly, the 10-hydroxy metabolite in urine represents 49% (2) or 43% (80), and 2-OH-desipramine an average of 38% (99), of an oral dose of nortriptyline or desipramine, respectively.

PHARMACODYNAMIC CONSEQUENCES OF ACTIVE METABOLITES

Metabolism by hydroxylation can have important functional pharmacodynamic consequences, since unconjugated hydroxy metabolites are present in blood and brain in concentrations that can exceed that of the parent compound, especially in the case of OH-nortriptyline. The data base profiling the similar biologic spectrum of activity of hydroxy metabolites of TCAs and the relative amounts found in animal and human tissue is now extensive and has been reviewed elsewhere (97). Only in the case of nortriptyline, however, has the hydroxy metabolite been proposed to be other than additive; the possibility that high levels of OH-nortriptyline may in some way block or reverse the antidepressant action of nortriptyline and thereby account for the relatively low upper therapeutic level of nortriptyline is under investigation in Scandinavia. As has been shown for both nortriptyline and desipramine, the concentration of hydroxy metabolite at steady state is highly correlated with that of the parent compound (97). Thus, a concentration of 150 ng/ml of nortriptyline is likely to be associated with an OH-nortriptyline concentration in excess of 200 ng/ml. It should be appreciated, however, that to date no one has shown that OH-nortriptyline by itself has adverse or depressogenic effects.

The other major metabolic pathway for TCAs is side chain demethylation (Fig. 1), which in the case of converting a tertiary to a secondary amine TCA produces active metabolites. These are now generally appreciated to be more potent norepinephrine uptake inhibitors than the tertiary amine TCAs, which are more potent inhibitors of serotonin uptake. Again, however, as discussed elsewhere in detail, the pharmacokinetics are such that following administration of a tertiary amine TCA (amitriptyline, imipramine, or clomipramine) there will always be high enough concentrations of the secondary amine to produce extensive norepinephrine uptake inhibition (12). Thus, no

TCAs can be considered to be selective serotonin uptake inhibitors following chronic oral administration.

PHARMACOKINETIC RELATIONSHIPS OF PARENT DRUG AND METABOLITES

Interestingly, there is no correlation between plasma concentration of parent drug and demethylated metabolite for imipramine (31) or clomipramine (74), despite significant correlations between parent TCA and hydroxy metabolites, consistent with even greater variability in demethylation than in hydroxylation. Bock et al. (14) find a modest but significant ($r = 0.53$) correlation between the sum of parent (amitriptyline) + demethylated metabolite (nortriptyline) concentrations and the total of all unconjugated hydroxy metabolites in amitriptyline-treated patients. Different controlling factors in hepatic P450-dependent metabolism appear to be involved in oxidative demethylation and hydroxylation, since there is no correlation between the plasma clearance of amitriptyline by demethylation and the extent of hydroxylation as measured by the urinary ratio of parent drug to hydroxy metabolite after single dose debrisoquine (79); the use of debrisoquine as a metabolic marker in pharmacogenetic studies will be discussed below.

Not only are demethylated TCAs hydroxylated, but also recent *in vitro* studies demonstrate demethylation of hydroxy metabolites of TCAs, including conversion of 10-OH-amitriptyline to 10-OH-nortriptyline (B. Mellstrom and L. Bertilsson, *personal communication*) and 2-OH-imipramine to 2-OH-desipramine (Fig. 1; T. Monks and J. R. Gillette, *personal communication*). Thus ultimate plasma levels of active drug forms depend on multiple pathways of formation and clearance. Secondary amine TCAs such as desipramine and nortriptyline can also be further demethylated, although didesmethylated metabolites of TCAs are not considered clinically important (100), since only small amounts are recovered in urine following administration of imipramine (27) or nortriptyline (2).

Finally, TCA metabolic pathways may not all be unidirectional. *In vitro* one can achieve methylation of several secondary amine tricyclics by *N*-methyl-transferase present in rabbit lung (32,88). In one clinical report (89), 15% of a group of patients treated with therapeutic doses of desipramine had measurable amounts of the tertiary amine compound imipramine in their blood, presumably resulting from direct methylation of the desipramine. A case report of a fatal nortriptyline overdose (2 g) also provides evidence of methylation, since approximately 12 hr after ingestion there was 51 ng/ml of amitriptyline as well as 886 ng/ml of nortriptyline in plasma (118); no amitriptyline was assayed in plasma from two patients with less serious nortriptyline overdoses. However, one large survey of routine plasma level monitoring failed to identify secondary amine TCAs in samples from patients receiving therapeutic doses of tertiary amine tricyclics (75).

POSSIBLE NONLINEAR PHARMACOKINETICS

Of course, overdose and therapeutic situations are not necessarily comparable, and at very high drug concentra-

tions, usual (first-order kinetics) metabolic pathways may be saturated (47). This has been suggested to occur even in the case of demethylation, such that the ratio of imipramine to desipramine in the brain after imipramine overdose was disproportionately high (23), although preferential saturation of hydroxylation of imipramine could equally well explain the finding (Fig. 1). In more than 60% of imipramine or amitriptyline overdoses, plasma parent TCA to demethylated metabolite concentration ratios are twice those observed under normal therapeutic steady-state conditions (10,119), then progressively decline with time as tertiary amine levels fall and secondary amine concentrations remain the same (126) or rise (47). Gram and associates (47) identified imipramine-*N*-oxide in the plasma of patients early after imipramine overdose but not in any patients taking therapeutic doses; they also found hydroxylation to be saturable even in the latter group. Possible saturation of hydroxylation has also been reported after high doses of desipramine (25,35). Despite apparent saturation of a particular metabolic pathway, elimination half-life ($t_\frac{1}{2}$) can be within normal limits for parent tricyclic and demethylated and hydroxylated metabolites after overdose (47) or chronic megadosing (19), though prolonged elevation of TCA plasma concentrations following overdose has been reported (69,125,126). Slowed, albeit first-order TCA and OH-TCA elimination after amitriptyline overdose in one patient was apparently related to hepatotoxicity (69). Patients in renal failure also have relatively normal elimination half-lives of parent drug and nonconjugated metabolites; excretion of polar glucuronide, however, is dramatically reduced (72).

Since none of the above studies provide direct data on the total fraction of TCAs metabolized over different pathways under conditions of high doses or overdoses, it is impossible to conclude definitively that there is selective saturation of a particular pathway. Nonetheless, the data do show nonlinear kinetics such that above a certain dose biologically active forms will accumulate disproportionately; thus, one cannot simply keep increasing doses of TCAs in nonresponders without a significant risk of a rather sudden transition to truly toxic plasma concentrations. Similarly, following an overdose, one cannot always count on the usual elimination half-life and must be prepared for prolonged (several days) periods of risk.

CLASSIC PHARMACOKINETIC PARAMETERS UNDER CONDITIONS OF LINEARITY

The "usual" pharmacokinetics of TCAs have been mostly based on single-dose studies with patients and healthy volunteers. In at least half of the subjects, a two-compartment open model (42) best fits the disposition data, with other individuals' data more consistent with a single central compartment (1,31,38,39). Plasma protein binding is typically 90% for tricyclics, with free fraction of 6% for nortriptyline (16), 11% for imipramine (68,84), and 14% for desipramine (84). Plasma free fraction of TCAs is approximately equal to CSF drug concentration (84) and shows less than 100% interindividual variability (68); this is small in comparison to other kinetic parameters such as clearance, suggesting that plasma protein binding is not the prime

TABLE 1. *Elimination half-lives of tricyclic antidepressants after a single dose*

TCA	$t_\frac{1}{2}$ (hr)		
	Mean	Range	Refs.
Imipramine	7.6	4.0–17.6	86
	8.6	6.0–11.2	46
	11.7	8.0–14.0	48
	12	7–22	20
	28.4	18.5–34.0	101
Desipramine	17.1	12.5–24.7	1[a]
	20	12–30	101
	18.2	10.3–31.8	115[b]
Amitriptyline	24.1	20.3–30.8	110[c]
	36.1	31.0–46.6	141
Nortriptyline	26.8	18.2–35.0	1[a]
	28.2	22.0–39.4	110[c]
	33.3	17.8–57.8	46
	46.4	21.5–88.1	17
Doxepin	16.8	8.2–24.5	144
	17.9	10.9–47.3	133
Protriptyline	74.3	53.6–91.7	143
	78.4	54.6–124.0	83
Clomipramine	24.7	20.1–39.6	85
Dothiepin	25	17–42	77

[a] Same subjects; [b] Caucasian subjects; [c] same subjects.

TABLE 3. *Plasma clearance of tricyclic antidepressants after an oral dose*

TCA	Clearance (liters/hr)		
	Mean	Range	Refs.
Imipramine	79.0	39.5–172.4	101
	138.6	85.8–227.4	46[c]
	151.2	54.6–212.4	48
	184.8[a]	64.8–300.0	86
Desipramine	123.0	54.2–221.0	115[b]
	130.2[a]	70.0–202.3[a]	1[d]
	130.2[a]	81.2–156.1[a]	31
Amitriptyline	96.0	48.6–140.4	110[e]
	148.2	58.2–204.6	141
Nortriptyline	30.0	15.0–44.4	110[e]
	53.9[a]	29.4–100.1[a]	1[d]
	62.4[a]	38.4–85.2	46[c]
Doxepin	65.1[a]	54.6–75.6[a]	133
	266.7[a]	107.8–557.2[a]	143
Protriptyline	11.9[a]	7.7–19.6[a]	142
	14.9[a]	7.5–22.8[a]	83
Clomipramine	64.2	35.4–119.4	85
Dothiepin	144.9[a]	44.8–353.5[a]	77

[a] Corrected for 70 kg body wt; [b] Caucasian subjects; [c] same subjects; [d] same subjects; [e] same subjects.

locus of interindividual TCA kinetic variability. Clearance rates and $t_\frac{1}{2}$ of nortriptyline (1) or desipramine (101) do not differ in single versus multiple dose paradigms within a given individual (see Tables 1 and 3), consistent with the long-term stability of steady-state TCA plasma concentrations in patients maintained on a constant dose (68,101), and suggesting lack of autoregulation of TCAs of their own metabolism or saturation of pathways at usual clinical doses at least with these compounds. Interpretation of a 15% fall in TCA and OH-TCA plasma levels between weeks 3 and 6 of chronic amitriptyline dosing in one outpatient study (36) is complicated by methodological

TABLE 2. *Elimination half-lives of "second generation" antidepressants after a single dose*

Drug	$t_\frac{1}{2}$ (hr)		
	Mean	Range	Refs.
Maprotiline	43	27–58	108
Amoxapine	8		52
Nomifensine	1.7	1.6–1.8	56
	3.9	3.4–4.9	132
Trazodone	6.3		138
	13.9		61
Mianserin	21.6	10.7–40.8	57
Bupropion	11.9	10.7–13.8	38
	18.8		94
	9.8	3.9–23.1	70
Zimelidine	5.1	4.3–6.0	55
Citalopram	33	23.0–75	67

problems, including non-steady-state sampling times. Slow clearance of nortriptyline in most of the patients in one study (17) was felt to differ from kinetics in normals, but most investigators have found similar antidepressant pharmacokinetics in depressives and healthy volunteers (57,76,114).

Half-lives of TCAs derived from such studies are summarized in Table 1. These relatively long half-lives permit the practice of single daily (bedtime) doses. Chronopharmacological studies indicate a lack of a circadian effect on single-dose kinetics of nortriptyline or amitriptyline in volunteers (87). Similarly, patient studies comparing nortriptyline (145), desipramine (141), or maprotiline given thrice daily versus once at night find no differences in steady-state plasma concentrations for any drug. The now withdrawn "second generation" antidepressant nomifensine, with a $t_\frac{1}{2}$ of only 2 to 4 hr (18) (Table 2), on the other hand, must be given at least three times a day. The tables of half-lives show why a general rule emerges that there is a wide variation in elimination rates of antidepressants. These observations also provide much of the impetus to identify the determining factor(s) in each individual that would predict the behavior of most if not all such drugs.

GENETIC BASIS OF PHARMACOKINETIC VARIATION

Perhaps the factor that is most invoked to form the basis for pharmacokinetic predictions is the genetic component for interindividual variability in hepatic metabolism. In what remains the landmark work in this area, 39 healthy middle-aged twin pairs in separate Swedish households were administered low doses of nortriptyline for 8 days (4). Among those not taking other medication, there was virtually no intrapair difference in steady-state concentrations for the monozygotic twins, whereas four of the 11 such dizygotic twinships showed significant intrapair differences. As recalculated by Potter et al. (96), intrinsic clearance varied as much as 3.35 liters/min within dizygotic twinships but not more than 1.08 liters/min between monozygotic twins. Concomitant use of other drugs eliminated the high concordance in nortriptyline steady-state concentrations within identical twin pairs, indicating the role of environmental as well as genetic factors (5), the former to be discussed later in this chapter.

Within individuals, degree of variability in metabolism of two or more TCAs may indicate regulation by common genetic and environmental factors (5). For example, metabolism of the secondary amines nortriptyline and desipramine is closely related; although absolute plasma clearance of desipramine is twice as rapid as that of nortriptyline (1), the two drugs' clearance values are highly correlated ($r = 0.90$). In contrast, clearance of nortriptyline is only weakly correlated with that of imipramine (46); single-dose kinetics of protriptyline also fail to correlate with those of doxepin in healthy volunteers (143). Looking at two tertiary amines, amitriptyline and clomipramine, in a crossover study, Mellström et al. (81) found a 0.87 correlation between steady-state levels of the parent drugs and a 0.77 correlation for the respective desmethyl metabolites. The tetracyclic compound maprotiline, which is metabolized similarly to conventional TCAs (see below and Tables 2 and 4), correlated with imipramine in terms of single-dose kinetic parameters (58).

The metabolic pathway of hepatic acetylation, long believed responsible for monoamine oxidase inhibitor (MAOI) disposition (135), is also under polymorphic genetic control, the gene for slow acetylation being autosomally recessive. Despite early suggestions that acetylation status might predict MAOI responsiveness, controlled studies do not support this idea (111). Recent data challenge the assumption of MAOI acetylation. Robinson and co-workers (109), using isotope-labeled phenelzine, identified oxidation as the major biotransformation pathway of this MAOI; most of the administered drug was recovered as aromatic acid derivatives, with no acetylphenelzine detected.

PHARMACOGENETIC PROBES

A current approach to the genetics of TCA breakdown involves comparison of tricyclic kinetics with that of marker drugs that undergo metabolism of known inheritance patterns. Clearance of antipyrine, under polymorphic genetic control, occurs via several pathways and shows modest correlation with imipramine, but not nortriptyline, clearance (13,46), possibly because demethylation is more important for the former TCA. With regard to psychotropic medications, antipyrine clearance is most closely correlated with that of benzodiazepines, including the triazolobenzodiazepine compound alprazolam (51), with putative antidepressant properties. Drugs metabolized primarily by hydroxylation demonstrate the closest relationship to tricyclic disposition. Single-dose $t_{\frac{1}{2}}$ of oxyphenylbutazone (53) parallels steady-state plasma concentrations of nortriptyline or desipramine. Similarly, phenylbutazone has been used as a marker of TCA clearance; Perel et al. (93) observed a positive correlation (magnitude unreported) between phenylbutazone $t_{\frac{1}{2}}$ and later steady-state concentration of imipramine + desipramine in the same depressed individuals.

More recently much attention has focused on the antihypertensive compound debrisoquine (63). Deficient hydroxylation of debrisoquine, commonly defined as a high ratio of debrisoquine to 4-hydroxy debrisoquine in an 8-hr urine sample after a single dose, is inherited as a single autosomal recessive trait (78) and varies widely across populations, including 9% of British Caucasians (104) and >30% of Orientals (60). This is relevant to the observation that TCA level outliers appear to belong to a different population from the rest (54), such as the 5% of a mixed group of patients treated with desipramine who exhibited unusually low hydroxy metabolite concentrations (98).

An association between debrisoquine and TCA metabolism has been suggested by studies showing significant correlations between debrisoquine hydroxylation and E-hydroxylation clearance of nortriptyline (80) and between debrisoquine hydroxylation and desipramine steady-state concentration (11). In another study in 18 volunteers, a high correlation between the urinary ratios of desipramine/OH-desipramine and debrisoquine/OH-debrisoquine was found; in addition, formation rates of hydroxylated metabolites of desipramine and debrisoquine were highly correlated in a study using liver microsomal preparations from 10 patient biopsies (127). Both of the clinical studies were carried out on groups selected to include at least 20% of slow hydroxylators of debrisoquine. In a randomly selected population that by chance did not include slow hydroxylators, we were unable to document a relationship between debrisoquine hydroxylation and total or hydroxylation clearance of single dose desipramine in Caucasian as well as Chinese volunteers (116). Despite the fact that none of the subjects were slow hydroxylators of debrisoquine, we

TABLE 4. *Plasma clearance of "second generation" antidepressants after an oral dose*

Drug	Clearance (liters/hr)		Refs.
	Mean	Range	
Maprotiline	41.1	5.5–20.0[a]	6
Amoxapine	250.0		Unpublished[b]
Nomifensine	78.9	63.1–89.7	132
Trazodone	8.9		Unpublished[c]
Mianserin	36.4[a]	23.1–56.7[a]	57
	68.6[a]	32.9–122.5[a]	76
	148.7[a]	136.9–155.8[a]	38
	90.3[a]		94
Bupropion	204.7	116.0–362.0	70
Zimelidine	120.0	86.4–177.6	55
Citalopram	25.8	16.8–38.4	67

[a] Corrected for 70 kg body weight; [b]Lederle Laboratories, data on file; [c]Mead Johnson & Co., Product Monograph, 1982.

found clear interethnic differences in desipramine clearance (115), suggesting that pathways other than hydroxylation were of major importance. One such pathway, that of demethylation, has also been shown to lack correlation with debrisoquine hydroxylation in the case of amitriptyline (79).

As noted elsewhere (63), the urinary metabolic ratio does not necessarily reflect drug metabolizing ability. Moreover, even as a pharmacogenetic probe, urinary metabolic ratios are limited, since they can only identify the small (when present) presumably homozygous genotype of slow metabolizers and have no ability to distinguish between homozygous and heterozygous rapid metabolizers (128).

Since extensive population studies on the metabolism of antidepressants are not available, one must be very circumspect in the interpretation of correlative studies based on the inclusion of a few outliers. Certainly, it is likely that persons identified as very slow hydroxylators of debrisoquine will be unusually slow metabolizers of those antidepressants most dependent on metabolism by hydroxylation. But even among the bulk of subjects who are rapid metabolizers, one can demonstrate a seven-fold range of clearance of a TCA and hence a high likelihood that many individuals will fall outside of a therapeutic range on a standard dose. From a practical point of view, simply obtaining a plasma level of antidepressant at the earliest sign of unexpected side effects would provide more specific and relevant information. The general principle that emerges is that, despite overall similarities in metabolic pathways, specific drugs are subject to specific metabolic processes that limit the application of pharmacokinetic phenotyping compounds. If one really wants to know the pharmacokinetic behavior of a certain drug in a person, a test dose of that particular drug must be administered to the individual in question.

TEST DOSES OF ANTIDEPRESSANTS FOR PHARMACOKINETIC PREDICTION

This approach for antidepressants was pioneered by Alexanderson (1), who found correlations near unity between clearance after a single dose and steady-state concentration (C_{ss}) on chronic administration for both nortriptyline and desipramine. Numerous investigators have extended and in some cases streamlined for clinical use the inverse relationship expressed in this simple equation: C_{ss} = AUC × maintenance dose/dosing interval × loading dose (86,101).

Employment of a single concentration measurement at a fixed time point—generally 24–48 hr after loading dose administration—is a simpler procedure for patient dosing but dependent on the degree to which such a level reflects actual AUC (12). Clinically acceptable results have been reported for a number of TCAs (17,20,21,26,30,77, 83,101,120).

The specific nomograms that have been derived for each of the studied compounds can be found in the studies referred to above. The general principle to remember is that single-dose pharmacokinetic predictions work well for antidepressants and can usually be simplified to one or two blood drawings. In our experience, this is mostly of use in

a research setting to carry out studies in which we want to control the plasma concentration (28,112). To date, there have been no convincing demonstrations that use of a test dose significantly accelerates or improves the frequency of therapeutic response.

ENVIRONMENTAL FACTORS THAT INFLUENCE PHARMACOKINETICS

Age

In this final section we consider factors other than the genetically determined intrinsic clearance that influence antidepressant pharmacokinetics. It is reasonable to postulate alterations in antidepressant metabolism as a function of aging. Conclusions, however, are limited by the difficulty in factoring out other confounding variables (96). A comparison between young and elderly male volunteers following a single dose of amitriptyline (121) illustrates the problem: Clearance was nonsignificantly lower (10%) in the older subjects, attributable to the expected decrease in liver weight and hepatic blood flow. Mean $t_{\frac{1}{2}}$, however, was considerably (34%) elevated in the elderly, based not only on the reduction in clearance (Cl), but also on an observed increase in volume of distribution (V); each of these factors can independently affect $t_{\frac{1}{2}}$, which equals 0.693 V/Cl. Changes in V may relate to alterations in body composition with age or to variation in plasma protein binding. Sometimes, however, particularly in the elderly, concomitant somatic disease does affect the concentration of plasma proteins. For instance, increases in α_1-acid glycoprotein with inflammation or malignancy result in decreased free fraction and increased total steady-state concentrations of antidepressants. Nonetheless, as noted elsewhere, clearance and the unbound pharmacologically active drug concentration, and therefore drug effect, will not change (96). In another study, clearance was slower and $t_{\frac{1}{2}}$ prolonged after a single dose of nortriptyline in elderly depressed inpatients (30), although the presence of significant medical illness and concomitant polypharmacy limited interpretations from this study. In contrast, psychiatrically healthy individuals, most of them relatives of patients known to achieve unusually high plasma nortriptyline steady-state concentrations, showed no age effect on nortriptyline kinetics (9). Other studies in naturalistic patient settings have yielded mixed results. These are reviewed in detail elsewhere (117) and summarized in Table 5. As a general rule, although there may be effects of age per se on antidepressant metabolism, these are modest and do not by themselves justify an assumption that elderly patients require lower doses.

Although specific data are even sparser than in the elderly, drug metabolism at the other extreme of the life cycle—infancy and childhood—is also frequently different from that in adults. Findings are reviewed elsewhere (106), and if any single principle emerges it would involve an apparent ability of children to demethylate tertiary amine TCAs more rapidly than adults. In any event, doses in children should be at least as high as in adults on a milligram per kilogram basis.

TABLE 5. *Age effects on tricyclic antidepressant steady-state plasma concentrations in depressed patients*

Drug	Effect of increased age on plasma concentration	Refs.
Imipramine	Increased	91
	Increased (in males)	50
Desipramine	Increased	91
	Unchanged	101
	Unchanged	28, 29
	Unchanged	90
Amitriptyline	Increased	91
	Unchanged	140
	Unchanged	73
	Increased	103
Nortriptyline	Unchanged	140
	Increased	68
	Unchanged	139
	Unchanged (children and adolescents)	41
Doxepin	Unchanged	40
Clomipramine	Increased	130
	Increased	62

Renal Function

Perhaps of greater relevance is the role of renal function in antidepressant elimination. It has long been recognized that lithium does not undergo metabolism but is nearly completely excreted through the kidneys. Thus the normal decline in glomerular filtration rate with age causes up to a 60% decrease in lithium renal clearance, with lengthening of $t_{\frac{1}{2}}$ up to 36 hr in the elderly versus 24 hr in middle-aged adults (105). Whereas unchanged TCAs are not subject to renal excretion, their metabolites are. It was originally shown by Alexanderson and Borga (2) that the renal clearance of hydroxynortriptyline was over 100 ml/min. A similarly high urinary clearance has been shown for unconjugated hydroxydesipramine (65), with a decrease in truly elderly depressed patients with an average age of over 80 years ($r = -0.73$ between age and 2-OH-desipramine renal clearance) accompanied by an increase in the plasma OH-desipramine/desipramine ratio. This is interpreted to mean that the rate of desipramine hydroxylation was not altered, since desipramine plasma concentrations were the same in the elderly as in younger populations (28). Even without truly elderly subjects (115), our Chinese and Caucasian volunteers demonstrated after single-dose desipramine a significant reduction in renal clearance of OH-desipramine with increasing age (99). A weaker but still significant association has been noted between age and plasma OH-nortriptyline/nortriptyline ratio in patients treated with nortriptyline or amitriptyline (95,124,139), despite unchanged levels of the unmetabolized drug. In some populations with different age ranges, a higher hydroxy metabolite ratio in the elderly cannot be shown (47). From among 45 desipramine-treated patients with a nearly four-fold age range (15), there was only a trend toward higher relative levels of hydroxy metabolite with increasing age. We would still suggest that in truly elderly patients therapeutic and/or toxic actions mediated by TCA hydroxy metabolites may be exaggerated unless allowances are made in dosing (42).

Sex

No general principle with regard to effects of sex on antidepressants can be identified. Most studies that have specifically compared male and female plasma concentrations of nortriptyline (4,9,30), amitriptyline and/or nortriptyline (140) [including after overdose (119)], imipramine (43,47), or desipramine (15) have not found a significant difference. The sole exception involves a report of higher imipramine concentrations in older males as compared to younger females (50); this could, of course, have been an age effect. More recently, prolonged $t_{\frac{1}{2}}$ and reduced clearance in advanced age for alprazolam (51) were observed only in men.

Race

On the assumption that races are likely to manifest a wide range of genetic differences, effects on drug metabolism are to be expected. Most reports of antidepressant use, however, do not account for the race of subjects under study. Ziegler and Biggs (140) found 50% higher steady-state plasma nortriptyline concentrations in black patients compared to whites (although this difference was small compared to the seven-fold overall variation in nortriptyline concentrations); in another group of patients treated with amitriptyline, there was a smaller racial difference which was not significant. Earlier studies reported a more rapid response to TCA and phenothiazine therapy in blacks (92) and more improvement on imipramine at 1 week (107). These older works presumably all reflected slower rates of TCA metabolism in black patients, but their interpretation is limited by their failure to assay TCA plasma concentrations and by diagnostic heterogeneity in treatment groups. Following amitriptyline overdose, blacks developed plasma total TCA levels adjusted for amount ingested twice that of whites (119), with a nonsignificantly higher amitriptyline/nortriptyline concentration ratio.

Anecdotal reports have long described the need for lower routine doses of TCAs in Asian as opposed to Western countries, suggesting racially based pharmacokinetic differences. In the only English language report we are aware of documenting TCA plasma concentrations in Asian patients, Yamashita and Asano (137) did not find elevated plasma levels in their uncontrolled sample and proposed that pharmacodynamic or psychosocial factors might explain the efficacy of low doses. However, healthy Asian volunteers had higher plasma drug concentrations for 24 hr after a single dose of clomipramine than their native British counterparts (7,71).

Extending these investigations, we traced the fate of a single oral dose of desipramine over 5 days in healthy

Chinese and Caucasian volunteers (115). Total desipramine clearance was significantly slower in the Chinese (mean of 73.5 liters/hr compared with 123 liters/hr for the Caucasians), with a trimodal distribution including a minority of outliers in each group (29% Chinese, slow clearance; 25% Caucasians, rapid clearance). Surprisingly, there were no significant interethnic differences in specific hydroxylation clearance. A similar increase in bioavailability of single-dose nortriptyline has been observed in Japanese volunteers (64).

Smoking

Tobacco smoke contains both inducers and inhibitors of drug oxidizing enzymes. The net effect, that of stimulation of drug metabolism, probably occurs in organs, e.g., lung, other than liver. There is contradictory evidence of a significant impact of smoking on TCA metabolism, with evidence for lower (62,73,93) or unchanged (4,140) steady-state TCA concentrations. The reasons for this discrepancy in the literature are unclear. Careful prospective documentation of tobacco use by subjects in antidepressant studies should help clarify this issue and judge its practical importance.

Alcohol

Chronic heavy drinking, defined as daily consumption of alcoholic beverages containing at least 200 g of absolute ethanol, can induce the metabolism of drugs handled by the hepatic cytochrome P450 enzyme system (59). At least one study supports possible relevance for antidepressants. This involved 11 depressed alcoholic men who had an intrinsic clearance of imipramine 2.5-fold higher than that of controls matched for smoking status (24), resulting in lower steady-state concentrations not only of imipramine but also of 2-OH-imipramine, desipramine, and 2-OH-desipramine in the alcohol-dependent group. In contrast, *acute* alcohol loading can impair TCA clearance. Pretreatment with ethanol caused an increase in total TCA concentration (in brain and blood, respectively) of approximately 200% (mainly in parent drug) following single-dose amitriptyline administration in both rats (102) and humans (33). These effects are still modest in comparison to interindividual differences in metabolism and are relatively easy to control. Acute alcohol did not produce significant changes in clearance of single-dose bupropion in male healthy volunteers (94).

Drug Interactions

Depressed patients often are prescribed multiple medications, many of which can alter antidepressant kinetics. For instance, barbiturates are among the most potent nonspecific inducers of hepatic microsomal metabolism, resulting in lower steady-state concentrations of concurrent TCAs (4,83,130). Interestingly, and fortunately, the benzodiazepines do not share this effect on TCA metabolism (83,123). Autoinduction of hepatic oxidizing enzymes, not

described for TCAs, occurs with carbamazepine (37) and—in rats and mice—bupropion (122).

Perhaps more dramatic than induction of metabolism is blockade resulting from competition for the same degradative enzymes, with resultant reduction in TCA clearance and elevation of tricyclic plasma concentrations. Such a clinically significant interaction has been observed particularly, in a dose-dependent fashion, with a variety of antipsychotic drugs (45); this effect—more pronounced in tertiary than secondary amine TCAs—is reduced by introduction of the tricyclic first (66). Although competitive inhibition of hepatic metabolism appears responsible for this neuroleptic-antidepressant interaction, other actions of neuroleptics, including reduction in hepatic blood flow (45) or competition for nonmetabolizing hepatic binding sites, may contribute to this effect. Decreased hepatic blood flow due to reduced cardiac output and competition for microsomal oxidizing enzymes apparently accounts for the elevation of maprotiline steady-state concentrations induced by addition of the β-blocker propranolol (129); similar interactions would be expected with the older tricyclics as well.

Decreased TCA hydroxylation with resultant reduction in clearance has been observed as well for the central stimulant methylphenidate (134)—although a negative report has appeared (34)—and the histamine H_2-receptor antagonist, cimetidine (82). Pharmacokinetic interactions of antidepressants with other drugs have been reported. These include oral contraceptives, anticonvulsants, and anticoagulants. Insufficient data are available to make generalizations for these specific classes. Available studies have been recently reviewed (117).

SUMMARY OF RELEVANT PRINCIPLES

Three principles related to pharmacokinetics emerge from the research literature as clearly relevant to understanding antidepressant action both from research and clinical points of view. With antidepressants one should expect the following:

1. Large interindividual variability in plasma concentration as a function of genetically determined metabolic capacity
2. A high probability of biologically active metabolites that may be relevant to therapeutic and toxic effects
3. Considerable specificity of metabolic profiles for most compounds even within an individual; i.e., that pharmacokinetic predictions across drugs have limited precision

Thus, in the foreseeable future, with *in vivo* studies of antidepressant action one should quantitate all biologically active forms to control pharmacokinetic sources of variance. Ideally this would be free drug concentration, but in practice total concentration provides a generally accurate relative measure. Although individuals can be screened for membership in a subgroup of approximately 5% of Caucasians who are unusually slow hydroxylators of a variety of antidepressants and antihypertensives, such tests do not obviate the need for specific measures of a specific drug in situations in which knowledge of relative amounts of active forms is desired. Single test doses of a specific compound, however, provide accurate predictions of ultimate steady-state concentrations of parent compound, even with one or two blood samples drawn 24 to 36 hr later, given a sensitive enough method. With some drugs such predictions may also hold for active metabolites, although the approach is not generally established. When one considers the practical limitations to giving a test dose and obtaining immediate reliable results, it would still be necessary to evaluate actual steady-state concentrations if knowledge of this is wanted.

As reviewed in *this volume,* knowledge of pharmacokinetic variance explains only a modest fraction of variations in clinical or chronic biochemical effects. We would emphasize, however, that our models for relating drug concentration to effect are based primarily on acute *in vivo* and *in vitro* studies and may not always apply to chronic effects on interacting neurotransmitter systems which themselves have been shown to undergo gradual drug-induced changes. Progress in our understanding of how to analyze chronic drug effects may reveal that even twofold or less differences in drug concentration will have important pharmacodynamic consequences. Since control of pharmacokinetic variance is now relatively simple as well as feasible, we strongly recommend that investigators apply the straightforward principles summarized in this chapter in anticipation of such advances, in an effort to analyze effects as well as to identify those individuals in whom absent or unexpected effects are clearly the consequences of being at either extreme of drug metabolizing ability.

REFERENCES

1. Alexanderson, B. (1972): *Eur. J. Clin. Pharmacol.,* 5:1–10.
2. Alexanderson, B., and Borga, O. (1973): *Eur. J. Clin. Pharmacol.,* 5:174–180.
3. Alexanderson, B., Borga, O., and Alvan, G. (1973): *Eur. J. Clin. Pharmacol.,* 5:181–185.
4. Alexanderson, B., Price Evans, D. A., and Sjoqvist, F. (1969): *Br. Med. J.,* 4:764–768.
5. Alexanderson, B., and Sjoqvist, F. (1971): *Ann. NY Acad. Sci.,* 179:739–751.
6. Alkalay, D., Wagner, W. E., Jr., Carlsen, S., Khemani, L., Volk, J., Bartlett, M. F., and LeSher, A. (1980): *Clin. Pharmacol. Ther.,* 27:679–703.
7. Allen, J. J., Rack, P. H., and Vaddadi, K. S. (1977): *Postgrad. Med. J.,* 53(Suppl. 4):79–86.
8. Alvan, G., Borga, O., Lind, M., Palmer, L., and Siwers, B. (1977): *Eur. J. Clin. Pharmacol.,* 11:219–224.
9. Alvan, G., Price Evans, D. A., and Sjoqvist, F. (1971): *J. Med. Genet.,* 8:129–135.
10. Bailey, D. N., Van Dyke, C., Langou, R. A., and Jatlow, P. I. (1978): *Am. J. Psychiatry,* 135:1325–1328.
11. Bertilsson, L., and Aberg-Wistedt, A. (1983): *Br. J. Clin. Pharmacol.,* 5:388–390.
12. Bertilsson, L., Asberg, M., and Thoren, P. (1974): *Eur. J. Clin. Pharmacol.,* 7:365–368.
13. Bertilsson, L., Eichelbaum, M., Mellstrom, B., Sawe, J., Schulz, H.-U., and Sjoqvist, F. (1980): *Life Sci.,* 27:1673–1677.
14. Bock, J. L., Giller, E., Gray, S., and Jatlow, P. (1982): *Clin. Pharmacol. Ther.,* 31:609–616.
15. Bock, J. L., Nelson, J. C., Gray, S., and Jatlow, P. I. (1983): *Clin. Pharmacol. Ther.,* 33:322–328.
16. Borga, O., Azarnoff, D. L., Plym-Forshell, G., and Sjoqvist, F. (1969): *Biochem. Pharmacol.,* 18:2135–2143.
17. Braithwaite, R. A., Montgomery, S., and Dawling, S. (1978): *Clin. Pharmacol. Ther.,* 23:303–308.
18. Brogden, R. N., Heel, R. C., Speight, T. M., and Avery, G. S. (1979): *Drugs,* 18:1–24.
19. Brown, G. M., Stancer, H. C., Moldofsky, H., Harman, J., Murphy, J. T., and Gupta, R. N. (1978): *Arch. Gen. Psychiatry,* 35:1261–1264.
20. Brunswick, D. J., Amsterdam, J. D., Mendels, J., and Stern, S. L. (1979): *Clin. Pharmacol. Ther.,* 25:605–610.
21. Brunswick, D. J., Amsterdam, J. D., Schless, A., Rothbart, M., Sandler, K., and Mendels, J. (1980): *J. Clin. Psychiatry,* 41:337–340.
22. Burch, J. E., and Hullin, R. P. (1981): *Psychopharmacology,* 74:35–42.
23. Christiansen, J., and Gram, L. F. (1973): *J. Pharm. Pharmacol.,* 25:604–608.
24. Ciraulo, D. A., Alderson, L. M., Chapron, D. J., Jaffe, J. H., Subbarao, B., and Kramer, P. A. (1982): *J. Clin. Psychopharmacol.,* 2:2–7.
25. Cooke, R. G., Warsh, J. J., Stancer, H. C., Reed, K. L., and Persad, E. (1984): *Clin. Pharmacol. Ther.,* 36:343–349.
26. Cooper, T. B., and Simpson, G. M. (1978): *Am. J. Psychiatry,* 135:333–335.
27. Crammer, J. L., Scott, B., and Rolfe, B. (1969): *Psychopharmacologia,* 15:207–225.
28. Cutler, N. R., Zavadil, A. P., III, Eisdorfer, C., Ross, R. J., and Potter, W. Z. (1981): *Am. J. Psychiatry,* 138:1235–1237.
29. Cutler, N. R., Zavadil, A. P., III, Linnoila, M., Scheinin, M., Rudorfer, M. V., and Potter, W. Z. (1984): *Biol. Psychiatry,* 19:549–556.
30. Dawling, S., Crome, P., and Braithwaite, R. (1980): *Clin. Pharmacokinet.,* 5:394–401.
31. DeVane, C. L., Savett, M., and Jusko, W. J. (1981): *Eur. J. Clin. Pharmacol.,* 19:61–64.
32. Dingell, J. V., and Sanders, E. (1966): *Biochem. Pharmacol.,* 15:599–605.
33. Dorian, P., Sellers, E. M., Warsh, J. J., Reed, K. L., Hamilton, C., and Fan, T. (1982): *Clin. Pharmacol. Ther.,* 31:219.
34. Drimmer, E. J., Gitlin, M. J., and Gwirtsman, H. E. (1983): *Am. J. Psychiatry,* 140:241–242.
35. Dugas, J. E., and Bishop, D. S. (1985): *J. Clin. Psychopharmacol.,* 5:43–45.
36. Edelbroek, P. M., Zitman, F. G., Schreuder, J. N., Rooymans, H. G. M., and de Wolff, F. A. (1984): *Clin. Pharmacol. Ther.,* 35:467–473.
37. Eichelbaum, M., Erbom, K., Bertilsson, L., Ringberger, V., and Rane, A. (1975): *Eur. J. Clin. Pharmacol.,* 8:337–341.
38. Findlay, J. W. A., Van Wyck Fleet, J., Smith, P. G., Butz, R. F., Hinton, M. L., Blum, M. R., and Schroeder, D. H. (1981): *Eur. J. Clin. Pharmacol.,* 21:127–135.
39. Fredricson Overo, K., Gram, L. F., and Hansen, V. (1975): *Eur. J. Clin. Pharmacol.,* 8:343–347.
40. Friedel, R. O. (1980): In: *Psychopathology in the Aged,* edited by J. O. Cole and J. E. Barrett. Raven Press, New York.
41. Geller, B., Cooper, T. B., and Chestnut, E. C. (1985): *J. Clin. Psychopharmacol.,* 5:213–216.
42. Gibaldi, M., and Perrier, D. (1982): *Pharmacokinetics,* 2nd ed. pp. 45–111. Marcel Dekker, New York.
43. Glassman, A. H., Perel, J. M., Shostak, M., Kantor, S. J., and Fleiss, J. L. (1977): *Arch. Gen. Psychiatry,* 34:197–204.
44. Gram, L. F. (1974): *Dan. Med. Bull.,* 21:218–231.
45. Gram, L. F. (1977): *Dan. Med. Bull.,* 24:81–89.
46. Gram, L. F., Andreasen, P. B., Fredricson Overo, K., and Christiansen, J. (1976): *Psychopharmacology,* 50:21–27.
47. Gram, L. F., Bjerre, M., Kragh-Sorensen, P., Kvinesdai, B., Molin, J., Pedersen, O. L., and Reisby, N. (1983): *Clin. Pharmacol. Ther.,* 33:335–342.
48. Gram, L. F., and Christiansen, J. (1975): *Clin. Pharmacol. Ther.,* 17:555–563.
49. Gram, L. F., and Fredricson Overo, K. (1975): *Clin. Pharmacol. Ther.,* 18:305–314.
50. Gram, L. F., Sondergaard, I., Christiansen, J., Petersen, G. O., Bech, P., Reisby, N., Ibsen, I., Ortmann, J., Nagy, A., Dencker, S. J., Jacobsen, O., and Krautwald, O. (1977): *Psychopharmacology,* 54:255–261.
51. Greenblatt, D. J., Divoll, M., Abernethy, D. R., Moschitto, L. J.,

Smith, R. B., and Shader, R. I. (1983): *Arch. Gen. Psychiatry,* 40:287–290.

52. Greenblatt, E. N., Hardy, R. A., Jr., and Kelly, R. G. (1978): *Pharmacol. Biochem. Prop. Drug Sub.,* 2:1–19.

53. Hammer, W., Martens, S., and Sjoqvist, F. (1969): *Clin. Pharmacol. Ther.,* 10:44–49.

54. Hammer, W., and Sjoqvist, F. (1967): *Life Sci.,* 6:1895–1903.

55. Heel, R. C., Morley, P. A., Brogden, R. N., Carmine, A. A., Speight, T. M., and Avery, G. S. (1982): *Drugs,* 24:169–206.

56. Heptner, W., Badian, M. J., Baudner, S., Christ, O. E., Fraser, H. M., Rupp, W., Weimer, K. E., and Wissmann, H. (1977): *Br. J. Clin. Pharmacol.,* 4(Suppl. 2):123S–127S.

57. Hrdina, P. D., Lapierre, Y. D., McIntosh, B., and Oyewumi, L. K. (1983): *Clin. Pharmacol. Ther.,* 33:757–762.

58. Hrdina, P. D., Rovei, V., Henry, J. F., Hervy, M. P., Gomeni, R., Forette, F., and Morselli, P. L. (1980): *Psychopharmacology,* 70:29–34.

59. Iber, F. L. (1977): *Clin. Pharmacol. Ther.,* 22:735–742.

60. Inaba, T., Otton, S. V., and Kalow, W. (1981): *Clin. Pharmacol. Ther.,* 33:394–399.

61. Jauch, Von R., Kopitar, Z., Prox, A., and Zimmer, A. (1976): *Arzneimittelforsch.,* 26:2084–2089.

62. John, V. A., Luscombe, D. K., and Kemp, H. (1980): *J. Int. Med. Res.,* 8(Suppl. 3):88–95.

63. Kalow, W. (1982): *Can. J. Physiol. Pharmacol.,* 60:1–12.

64. Kishimoto, A., and Hollister, L. E. (1984): *J. Clin. Psychopharmacol.,* 4:171–172.

65. Kitanaka, I., Ross, R. J., Cutler, N. R., Zavadil, A. P., III, and Potter, W. Z. (1982): *Clin. Pharmacol. Ther.,* 31:51–55.

66. Kragh-Sorensen, P., Borga, O., Garle, M., Hansen, L. B., Hansen, C. E., Hvidberg, E. F., Larsen, N.-E., and Sjoqvist, F. (1977): *Eur. J. Clin. Pharmacol.,* 11:479–483.

67. Kragh-Sorensen, P., Fredricson Overo, K., Lindegaard Pederson, O., Jensen, K., and Parnas, W. (1981): *Acta Pharmacol. Toxicol.,* 48:53–60.

68. Kragh-Sorensen, P., and Larsen, N.-E. (1980): *Clin. Pharmacol. Ther.,* 28:796–803.

69. Kuhn, W. F., Jones, D. R., Lippmann, S. B., Embry, C. K., Williams, W. M., Manshadi, M. S., and Hurst, H. E. (1984): *J. Clin. Psychopharmacol.,* 4:158–160.

70. Laizure, S. C., DeVane, C. L., Stewart, J. T., Dommisse, C. S., and Lai, A. A. (1985): *Clin. Pharmacol. Ther.,* 38:586–589.

71. Lewis, P., Vaddadi, K. S., Rack, P. H., and Allen, J. J. (1980): *Postgrad. Med. J.,* 56(Suppl. 1):46–49.

72. Lieberman, J. A., Cooper, T. B., Suckow, R. F., Steinberg, H., Borenstein, M., Brenner, R., and Kane, J. M. (1985): *Clin. Pharmacol. Ther.,* 37:301–307.

73. Linnoila, M., George, L., Guthrie, S., and Leventhal, B. (1981): *Am. J. Psychiatry,* 138:841–842.

74. Linnoila, M., Insel, T., Kilts, C., Potter, W. Z., and Murphy, D. L. (1982): *Clin. Pharmacol. Ther.,* 32:208–211.

75. Lydiard, R. B., Martin, D., Gold, M. S., and Pottash, A. L. C. (1985): *J. Clin. Psychopharmacol.,* 5:60.

76. Maguire, K. P., Norman, T. R., Burrows, G. D., and Scoggins, B. A. (1982): *Eur. J. Clin. Pharmacol.,* 21:517–520.

77. Maguire, K. P., Norman, T. R., McIntyre, I., and Burrows, G. D. (1983): *Clin. Pharmacokinet.,* 8:179–185.

78. Mahgoub, A., Idle, J. R., Dring, L. G., Lancaster, R., and Smith, R. L. (1977): *Lancet,* 2:584–586.

79. Mellstrom, B., Bertilsson, L., Lou, Y.-C., Sawe, J., and Sjoqvist, F. (1983): *Clin. Pharmacol. Ther.,* 34:516–520.

80. Mellstrom, B., Bertilsson, L., Sawe, J., Schulz, H.-U., and Sjoqvist, F. (1981): *Clin. Pharmacol. Ther.,* 30:189–193.

81. Mellstrom, B., Bertilsson, L., Traskman, L., Rollins, D., Asberg, M., and Sjoqvist, F. (1979): *Pharmacology,* 19:282–287.

82. Miller, D. D., and Macklin, M. (1984): *Am. J. Psychiatry,* 141:153.

83. Moody, J. P., Whyte, S. F., MacDonald, A. J., and Naylor, G. J. (1977): *Eur. J. Clin. Pharmacol.,* 11:51–56.

84. Muscettola, G., Goodwin, F. K., Potter, W. Z., Claeys, M. M., and Markey, S. P. (1978): *Arch. Gen. Psychiatry,* 35:621–625.

85. Nagy, A. (1977): *J. Pharm. Pharmacol.,* 29:104–107.

86. Nagy, A., and Johansson, R. (1975): *Naunyn Schmiedebergs Arch. Pharmacol.,* 290:145–160.

87. Nakano, S., and Hollister, L. E. (1983): *Clin. Pharmacol. Ther.,* 33:453–459.

88. Narasimhachari, N., and Lin, R.-L. (1976): *Psychopharmacol. Commun.,* 2:27–38.

89. Narasimhachari, N., Saady, J. J., Joseph, A., Ettigi, P., and Friedel, R. O. (1982): *J. Clin. Psychopharmacol.,* 2:413–416.

90. Nelson, J. C., Jatlow, P. I., and Mazure, C. (1985): *J. Clin. Psychopharmacol.,* 5:217–220.

91. Nies, A., Robinson, D. S., Friedman, M. J., Green, R., Cooper, T. B., Ravaris, C. L., and Ives, J. O. (1977): *Am. J. Psychiatry,* 134:790–793.

92. Overall, J. E., Hollister, L. E., Kimbell, I., Jr., and Shelton, J. (1969): *Arch. Gen. Psychiatry,* 21:89–94.

93. Perel, J. M., Shostak, M., Gann, E., Kantor, S. J., and Glassman, A. H. (1976): In: *Pharmacokinetics of Psychoactive Drugs,* edited by L. A. Gottschalk and S. Merlis, pp. 229–241. Spectrum Press, New York.

94. Posner, J., Bye, A., Jeal, S., Peck, A. W., and Whiteman, P. (1984): *Eur. J. Clin. Pharmacol.,* 26:627–630.

95. Pottash, A. L. C., Martin, D. M., Extein, I., Mas, F., Jarvis, A. H., Zirk, R. G., and Gold, M. S. (1983): *Soc. Neurosci. Abstr.,* 9:428.

96. Potter, W. Z., Bertilsson, L., and Sjoqvist, F. (1981): In: *Handbook of Biological Psychiatry: Part VI, Practical Applications of Psychotropic Drugs and Other Biological Treatments,* edited by H. M. van Praag, O. Rafaelson, M. Lader, and E. Sachar, pp. 71–134. Marcel Dekker, New York.

97. Potter, W. Z., and Calil, H. M. (1981): In: *Clinical Pharmacology in Psychiatry,* edited by E. Usdin, pp. 311–324. Elsevier, New York.

98. Potter, W. Z., Calil, H. M., Sutfin, T. A., Zavadil, A. P., III, Jusko, W. J., Rapoport, J., and Goodwin, F. K. (1982): *Clin. Pharmacol. Ther.,* 31:393–401.

99. Potter, W. Z., Lane, E. A., and Rudorfer, M. V. (1983): In: *Clinical Pharmacology in Psychiatry: Bridging the Experimental-Therapeutic Gap,* edited by L. F. Gram, E. Usdin, S. G. Dahl, P. Kragh-Sorensen, F. Sjoqvist, and P. Morselli, pp. 203–216. Macmillan Press, London.

100. Potter, W. Z., and Linnoila, M. (1984): In: *Neurobiology of Mood Disorders,* edited by R. M. Post and J. C. Ballenger, pp. 698–709. Williams and Wilkins, Baltimore.

101. Potter, W. Z., Zavadil, A. P., III, Kopin, I. J., and Goodwin, F. K. (1980): *Arch. Gen. Psychiatry,* 37:314–320.

102. Preskorn, S. H., and Hughes, C. W. (1983): *Psychopharmacology,* 80:217–220.

103. Preskorn, S. H., and Mac, D. S. (1985): *J. Clin. Psychiatry,* 46:276–277.

104. Price Evans, D. A., Mahgoub, A., Sloan, T. P., Idle, J. R., and Smith, R. L. (1980): *J. Med. Genet.,* 17:102–105.

105. Prien, R. F. (1981): In: *Age and the Pharmacology of Psychoactive Drugs,* edited by A. Raskin, D. S. Robinson, and J. Levine, pp. 163–169. Elsevier, New York.

106. Rapoport, J. L., and Potter, W. Z. (1981): In: *Age and the Pharmacology of Psychoactive Drugs,* edited by A. Raskin, D. S. Robinson, and J. Levine, pp. 105–123. Elsevier, New York.

107. Raskin, A., and Crook, T. H. (1975): *Arch. Gen. Psychiatry,* 32:643–649.

108. Riess, W., Dubey, L., Funfgeld, E. W., Imhof, P., Hurzeler, H., Matussek, N., Rajagopalan, T. G., Raschdorf, F., and Schmid, K. (1975): *J. Int. Med. Res.,* 3(Suppl. 2):16–41.

109. Robinson, D. S., Cooper, T. B., Jindal, S. P., Corcella, J., and Lutz, T. (1985): *J. Clin. Psychopharmacol.,* 5:333–337.

110. Rollins, D. E., Alvan, G., Bertilsson, L., Gillette, J. R., Mellstrom, B., Sjoqvist, F., and Traskman, L. (1980): *Clin. Pharmacol. Ther.,* 28:121–129.

111. Rose, S. (1982): *J. Clin. Psychopharmacol.,* 2:161–164.

112. Ross, R. J., Zavadil, A. P., III, Calil, H. M., Linnoila, M., Kitanaka, I., Blombery, P., Kopin, I. J., and Potter, W. Z. (1983): *Clin. Pharmacol. Ther.,* 33:429–437.

113. Rudorfer, M. V., Golden, R. N., and Potter, W. Z. (1984): In: *Clinical Psychopharmacology,* edited by C. R. Lake. *Psychiatr. Clin. North Am.,* 7:519–534.

114. Rudorfer, M. V., Karoum, F., Ross, R. J., Potter, W. Z., and Linnoila, M. (1985): *Clin. Pharmacol. Ther.,* 37:66–71.

115. Rudorfer, M. V., Lane, E. A., Chang, W.-H., Zhang, M., and Potter, W. Z. (1984): *Br. J. Clin. Pharmacol.,* 17:433–440.
116. Rudorfer, M. V., Lane, E. A., and Potter, W. Z. (1985): *J. Clin. Psychopharmacol.,* 5:89–92.
117. Rudorfer, M. V., and Potter, W. Z. (1985): In: *Pharmacotherapy of Affective Disorders: Theory and Practice,* edited by W. G. Dewhurst and G. B. Baker, pp. 382–448. Croom Helm, London.
118. Rudorfer, M. V., and Robins, E. (1981): *Am. J. Psychiatry,* 138: 982–983.
119. Rudorfer, M. V., and Robins, E. (1982): *J. Clin. Psychiatry,* 43: 457–460.
120. Rudorfer, M. V., and Young, R. C. (1980): *Commun. Psychopharmacol.,* 4:185–188.
121. Schulz, P., Turner-Tamiyasu, K., Smith, G., Giacomini, K. M., and Blaschke, T. F. (1983): *Clin. Pharmacol. Ther.,* 33:360–366.
122. Shroeder, D. H. (1983): *J. Clin. Psychiatry,* 44(Sec. 2):79–81.
123. Silverman, G., and Braithwaite, R. A. (1973): *Br. Med. J.,* 3:18–20.
124. Sjoqvist, F. (1981): In: *Age and the Pharmacology of Psychoactive Drugs,* edited by A. Raskin, D. S. Robinson, and J. Levine, pp. 195–204. Elsevier, New York.
125. Spiker, D. G., and Biggs, J. T. (1976): *JAMA,* 236:1711–1712.
126. Spiker, D. G., Weiss, A. N., Chang, S. S., Ruwitch, J. F., Jr., and Biggs, J. T. (1975): *Clin. Pharmacol. Ther.,* 18:539–546.
127. Spina, E., Birgersson, C., von Bahr, C., Ericsson, O., Mellstrom, B., Steiner, E., and Sjoqvist, F. (1984): *Clin. Pharmacol. Ther.,* 36:677–682.
128. Steiner, E., Iselius, L., Alvan, G., Lindsten, J., and Sjoqvist, F. (1985): *Clin. Pharmacol. Ther.,* 38:394–401.
129. Tollefson, G., and Lesar, T. (1984): *Am. J. Psychiatry,* 141:148–149.
130. Traskman, L., Asberg, M., Bertilsson, L., Cronholm, B., Mellstrom, B., Neckers, L. M., Sjoqvist, F., Thoren, P., and Tybring, G. (1979): *Clin. Pharmacol. Ther.,* 26:600–610.
131. Vandel, B., Vandel, S., Allers, G., Bechtel, P., and Volmat, R. (1979): *Psychopharmacology,* 65:187–190.
132. Vereczkey, L., Bianchetti, G., Garattini, S., and Morselli, P. L. (1975): *Psychopharmacologia,* 45:225–227.
133. Virtanen, R., Scheinin, M., and Iisalo, E. (1980): *Acta Pharmacol. Toxicol.,* 47:371–376.
134. Wharton, R. N., Perel, J. M., Dayton, P. G., and Malitz, S. (1971): *Am. J. Psychiatry,* 127:1619–1625.
135. Whitford, G. M. (1978): *Int. Pharmacopsychiatry,* 13:126–132.
136. Wilkinson, G. R., and Shand, D. G. (1975): *Clin. Pharmacol. Ther.,* 18:377–390.
137. Yamashita, I., and Asano, Y. (1979): *Psychopharmacol. Bull.,* 15:40–41.
138. Yamato, C., Takahashi, T., and Fujita, T. (1976): *Xenobiotica,* 6:295–306.
139. Young, R. C., Alexopoulos, G. S., Shamoian, C. A., Manley, M. W., Dhar, A. K., and Kutt, H. (1984): *Clin. Pharmacol. Ther.,* 35:540–544.
140. Ziegler, V. E., and Biggs, J. T. (1977): *JAMA,* 238:2167–2169.
141. Ziegler, V. E., Biggs, J. T., Ardekani, A. B., and Rosen, S. H. (1978): *J. Clin. Pharmacol.,* 18:462–467.
142. Ziegler, V. E., Biggs, J. T., Rosen, S. H., Meyer, D. A., and Preskorn, S. H. (1978): *J. Clin. Psychiatry,* 39:660–663.
143. Ziegler, V. E., Biggs, J. T., Wylie, L. T., Coryell, W. H., Hanifl, K. M., Hawf, D. J., and Rosen, S. H. (1978): *Clin. Pharmacol. Ther.,* 23:580–584.
144. Ziegler, V. E., Biggs, J. T., Wylie, L. T., Rosen, S. H., Hawf, D. J., and Coryell, W. H. (1978): *Clin. Pharmacol. Ther.,* 23: 573–579.
145. Ziegler, V. E., Knesevich, J. W., Wylie, L. T., and Biggs, J. T. (1977): *Arch. Gen. Psychiatry,* 34:613–615.

Psychopharmacology:
The Third Generation of Progress,
edited by Herbert Y. Meltzer.
Raven Press, New York © 1987.

CHAPTER **143**

Pharmacokinetics of Lithium

Thomas B. Cooper

Lithium was found to be effective in the treatment of manic-depressive disorders in the late 1940s but was not approved by the Food and Drug Administration (FDA) for the treatment of manic episodes in the United States until 1970, and for maintenance therapy in manic-depressive illness patients with a history of mania in 1974. The use of lithium for these indications is now well established and widespread throughout the Western world. Schou (115) compared data from lithium clinics in Denmark, Sweden, Norway, Great Britain, Canada, and the United States and estimated that one to two individuals per thousand of the population in these countries are being treated with lithium. Reifman and Wyatt (106) estimate that the economic impact of the introduction of lithium on mental health costs in the United States over the 10-year period 1970–1980, using the conservative assumption of a 60% response rate, points to a saving of $2.8 billion in medical costs and $1.28 billion in increased productivity. Thus, use of this simple element in psychiatric care has resulted in savings of approximately $400 million yearly in the United States!

Knowledge of the pharmacokinetics of a drug or medication after it has been ingested is of paramount interest in rational therapy in any branch of medicine. However, it has been slow to assume an importance in psychiatry due in part to the technical difficulties in measuring the low quantities of drug present in the various body fluids. Of equal importance is the fact that many of these compounds produce numerous psychoactive metabolites that further complicate interpretation of such data.

Lithium, a drug with low therapeutic index, has the ideal advantage of being an active therapeutic agent that is not metabolized and is easily quantified. Information on the absorption, distribution, and excretion of lithium could therefore be used as a paradigm of what was desirable in other branches of biological psychiatry. Lithium was first used in the treatment of manic-depressive illness without plasma lithium monitoring. Because of this low therapeutic index, Cade (17) stated in his original article:

It is therefore of utmost importance that when a patient is on maximum doses he should be seen each day and the nursing staff should be instructed to look for early signs of saturation.

Talbot (135) in a followup study of the use of lithium as a salt substitute measured plasma-lithium concentration and observed that toxicity did not occur in patients with blood levels less than 1.0 mEq/liter. Noack and Trautner (86) reported similar findings in the treatment of manic-depressive illness where blood levels of lithium were monitored. By the late 1950s, monitoring of blood lithium was recommended as a routine (113). Thus lithium was one of the earliest psychotropic drugs in which plasma level monitoring was both necessary and feasible.

Lithium was introduced as a treatment for manic-depressive illness at a most fortunate time. Chemical methods for determination of electrolyte concentrations had just undergone a major change with the introduction of commercially available, relatively inexpensive flame photometers. Flame instrumentation involving atomic absorption became generally available in the early 1960s, and even more recently the exquisitely sensitive flameless atomic absorption spectrophotometers (AAS) have been introduced (24,26). Microanalysis methodology requiring 25 to 50 μl plasma has been described (2,32,113,118), and accurate quantitation using as little as 1 μl plasma with flameless atomic absorption spectrophotometry is possible (46). Good laboratory practice results in coefficients of variation below 2% within and 4% between assay. Better than this can be achieved if the assay is carefully standardized each day. Jefferson (66) reported that quality control data for a representative month in their laboratory demonstrated a coefficient of variation at 0.65 mEq/liter of 2% with a ±2 standard deviation range of 0.62 to 0.68 mEq/liter. One often finds statements in the literature suggesting that a coefficient of variation of 10% or greater is to be expected in clinical laboratories for such assays. Clearly this is not acceptable practice using current modern analytical instrumentation.

PHARMACOKINETIC PROPERTIES OF LITHIUM

Lithium is readily absorbed when administered *per os,* which is the only route used in humans. Although a number of lithium salts have been used for the preparation of lithium tablets or capsules, there are no significant qualitative differences between these formulations.

Lithium is rapidly absorbed, and therefore the serum lithium concentration shows steep rises during the first hours after intake (Fig. 1). These rises often coincide with initial side effects, e.g., gastrointestinal irritation, a dazed feeling, and muscular weakness. But there is some evidence that the side effects that occur in chronic treatment, such as hand tremor, polyuria, polydypsia, and weight gain, may be related to these concentration peaks (114).

The rapid absorption and the resultant high peak concentration have led to attempts to develop a slow or sustained release preparation (Fig. 1). In the United States at the present time there are two such formulations in which the lithium salt is embedded in a matrix so that the release of lithium ion occurs over protracted periods of time. With these preparations it is also possible, even in patients who eliminate lithium rapidly, to divide the dosage into two instead of three or even four daily doses, thus increasing the compliance rate. Schou (114) also points out that an additional advantage of the sustained release preparation is that when a patient has attempted suicide by taking an overdose of lithium, aspiration and gastric lavage are much more likely to be successful if the patient has ingested the sustained or slow release preparation.

Distribution

As stated previously, lithium is an ideal model for pharmacokinetics, in that the ion is not bound to plasma or tissue proteins. It passes from the systemic circulation into the tissues and a dynamic equilibrium is established between plasma and cells. In steady state, therefore, the plasma lithium concentration is an indicator of the total lithium content and may be used to monitor treatment. Bergner (9) has shown that the total body lithium content can be predicted from the serum curve. The volume of distribution for lithium is about the same as that of total body water, but in equilibrium there are differences in a variety of tissue plasma concentration gradients. In the liver, the lithium concentration is lower than the concentration in the extracellular fluid. In other tissues, such as muscle, bone, and thyroid, it is two to four times higher (114). The concentration in the brain is of the same order of magnitude as that in extracellular fluid, i.e., <50% of the plasma concentration. There are no apparent differences between lithium concentration in various brain regions (11,109,137).

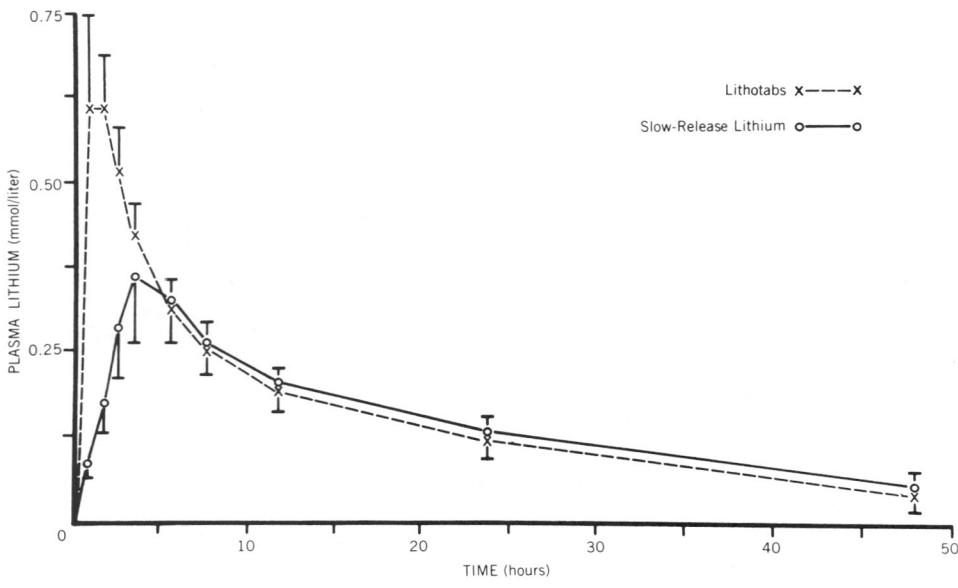

FIG. 1. Single-dose plasma lithium profiles obtained in 11 volunteer subjects after ingesting a standard release formulation (Lithotabs) and a slow release formulation. Time points show mean ±1 standard deviation. (From ref. 33.)

Elimination

Lithium is not metabolized and therefore excretion is of the unchanged ion. Very little is lost in feces and its elimination depends primarily on the renal lithium clearance (104,136). We have found in our own work that more than 95% of lithium is excreted via this route (33) and under normal circumstances renal clearance is independent of the serum concentration, and accordingly there is a direct proportionality between the maintenance dose and the serum concentration.

Lithium is filtered freely through the glomerulus, and approximately 80% of the filtered load is absorbed with sodium and water in the proximal tubules. The remaining 20% passes to the distal parts of the nephron where essentially no lithium is absorbed, and therefore this portion is excreted in the urine. In normal adults the lithium clearance ranges from 10 to 40 ml/min with a modest decrease with age (138).

PATIENT MONITORING

Blood Collection

Blood samples are collected in plain dry tubes or tubes containing an anticoagulant using either a syringe or vacuum tube system. The use of lithium heparin as an anticoagulant or any anticoagulant containing lithium obviously must be avoided. Normal, good clinical technique should be observed in the collection of any blood sample to avoid hemolysis. However, a slight degree of hemolysis has no clinically significant effect on the determination of lithium in plasma. In a recent publication, Hisayasu et al. (63) deliberately hemolyzed blood samples to the point where a 3% change in hematocrit (ca 8% hemolysis) was effected and showed that plasma lithium levels were not changed to any level of clinical significance.

Time of Blood Sampling

When lithium therapy is initiated, serum samples should be drawn once or twice weekly until clinical condition and serum levels are stable. Because of the well-demonstrated fluctuation in lithium levels between a dosing interval, it is necessary to standardize blood sampling times. Amdisen (4–6) has made a major contribution in describing in detail the requirements and necessity for the standard 12-hr lithium level. Samples are usually drawn in the morning 12 hr after the last dose. The 12-hr sampling interval is essential for correct interpretation of the serum level because therapeutic ranges were developed from data using this time interval. Amdisen, however, is careful to point out that selection of this time point is arbitrary and does not reflect the average plasma concentration during a single dose interval (7). Samples drawn shortly after ingestion of lithium would reflect the absorption peak and give results considerably higher than samples taken 12 hr postdose (Fig. 1). A rough estimate of 0.3 mEq/liter above the 12-hr steady state level for each 300 mg tablet ingested gives an idea of the fluctuations observed. Thus a patient on a dosage regimen of 900 mg b.i.d. with a 12-hr steady-state level of 0.5 mEq/liter would have a peak level (2–3 hr postdose) of approximately 1.4 mEq/liter (0.5 + 0.9). An example of the clinical problems caused by this type of error has been reported by Jefferson and Greist (69). The frequency of blood level monitoring depends on the patient's response, whether frequent dosage changes are made, and the presence of factors that interfere with the elimination of lithium: administration of thiazide diuretics, reduction of salt intake, development of kidney damage, dehydration brought about by a variety of illnesses, etc. Since the pharmacokinetic data indicate that it would take at least 4 to 7 days, with an average of 5 days, for most patients to achieve steady state after initial medication, serum levels need not be obtained more frequently than this when stabilizing a dose unless there is concern for toxicity. Dosage adjustment based on serum levels prior to reaching steady state can be misleading and dangerous unless interpreted with a firm understanding of the pharmacokinetics of this ion. Well-stabilized patients on maintenance therapy may only require monitoring every 1 to 3 months (4). Age differences are important in clinical management, with advancing age bringing a likelihood of cardiovascular and renal disease as renal lithium clearance decreases. Consequently elderly patients often need lower doses to achieve comparable blood levels (105). Increased susceptibility of side effects in the elderly may require more than two divided doses per day or the use of a slow release form of lithium (45,65,144).

Plasma Level Interpretation

Despite the fact that efforts to absolutely correlate serum levels with clinical response have been unsuccessful, therapeutic ranges have been proposed. Grof (57) placed the minimum effective level for treatment for acute mania between 0.8 and 1.0 mEq/liter, with a maximum between 1.4 and 1.5 mEq/liter. The study of Prien et al. (102) demonstrated no therapeutic advantage in maintaining blood levels above the 1.4 mEq/liter level. Patients treated with higher lithium doses showed no greater improvement but ran a higher risk in terms of side effects (102,131). Because of interindividual differences in response, it is better to start at lower recommended levels and increase as necessary. For maintenance therapy, somewhat lower serum concentrations are usually required, with a minimum between 0.6 and 0.8 mEq/liter. Schou (113) in very early studies recommended plasma lithium levels between 0.8 and 1.2 mEq/liter. Some older patients do well on even lower maintenance levels (114). The lower dosage (contrasted to blood level) required by the elderly may be attributed to the fact that in the elderly renal clearance of lithium is diminished, and plasma levels are therefore higher. Recent prospective studies were unable to demonstrate significant differences in relapse rate when patients were maintained at three different plasma level ranges: <0.49, 0.5 to 0.69, and >0.7 mEq/liter (74). In a followup report these same patients were followed for an additional year, during which time the plasma level range was adjusted downward to 0.25 to 0.39, 0.4 to 0.59, and 0.6 to 1.0 mEq/

liter. A relapse rate of 51.5% was found among the patients monitored with plasma lithium levels of <0.4 mEq/liter, whereas there was no significant difference between the higher groups (64). These data give support to the experience of many clinicians: Maintenance lithium levels of 0.8 to 1.2 mEq/liter may well be unnecessarily high for many medium- to low-risk patients during prophylactic treatment. These observations need further validation in controlled studies, but there is no *a priori* reason to assume that long-term prophylactic treatment requires the same plasma lithium concentration as is required for its antimanic effects. Severe toxic effects occur most often at serum levels above 2.5 mEq/liter. When levels reach 3.0 mEq/liter or higher, hemodialysis or peritoneal dialysis treatment is necessary to prevent severe and possibly irreversible complications. Concentrations above 3.5 mEq/liter are considered life-threatening (59).

The ability to define a therapeutic range rests on the correlation between dose of the drug, level of clinical response, and clinical deterioration caused by manifest toxic effects of the drug (a curvilinear relationship). This concept, in turn, permits one to separate toxicity occurring above the upper limit of the therapeutic range from side effects that occur below this upper limit. These side effects, although unwanted, may well be part of a treatment regimen in which cessation of treatment is not necessary; on the other hand, they do permit one to investigate effects within the therapeutic range. This latter concept is of importance, since there are serious neurological effects that do occur in therapy within the "therapeutic range." It should be stressed that these are quite rare and, in many cases, can be attributed to other factors (e.g., tremors severe enough to making writing or working impossible) seen with the use of lithium and high doses of tricyclic antidepressant or with antipsychotic agents. Lithium side effects have been succinctly reviewed by Mielke (84).

APPLICATION OF PHARMACOKINETICS

The pharmacokinetic approach to the use of lithium has enabled one to investigate dosage predictions, optimize dosage regimens, and examine the pharmacokinetics of possible drug interactions, intracellular lithium levels, and urinary excretion.

The lithium ion is the ideal drug for pharmacokinetic analysis. It is water soluble, rapidly absorbed, and excreted quantitatively via the kidneys in first-order kinetics. Lithium can be accurately quantified in body fluids and tissues after a single oral dose; it has no metabolic products; and there is a generally accepted therapeutic range of serum levels.

The renal clearance of lithium has been shown to be independent of serum concentration (139) and is strongly correlated with steady-state lithium concentration (117). Schou et al. (117) developed a formula for predicting the maintenance dose required to keep the "average" serum lithium level at steady state within the therapeutic range. The "average" lithium is 20 to 30% higher than the standard 12-hr standard serum level described earlier. These investigators observed that clearance of lithium is remarkably constant, with little day-to-day or month-to-month

variation. Sedvall et al. (118) made the additional observation that there was a stronger correlation between the steady-state lithium level ($r = 0.87$) and the products of lithium clearance and body weight.

Renal clearance studies have also been used by Norman et al. (87) and Tyrer et al. (140) where creatinine clearance data calculated from serum creatinine were used to predict optimal dosage.

The now classic single-dose, multiple blood sample pharmacokinetic approach has been used by several investigators working with lithium. The data from such experiments are fitted by a variety of model-dependent and model-independent procedures utilizing techniques from simple planimetry to extremely complex iterative curve-fitting procedures designed to fit data with a variety of mathematical functions. The parameters derived from such studies can be and have been used to examine the effects of drug regimen and type of formulations on the fluctuation in the serum lithium level during a single dosing interval, bioavailability, etc. (4,10,18). In addition, Bergner et al. (10), Amdisen (4), Poust et al. (100), Tyrer et al. (140), Fava et al. (48), Gengo et al. (54), Chang et al. (20–22), and Ereshevsky and Jann (47) all confirm the observation that steady-state plasma lithium levels can be predicted from the pharmacokinetic dose curve with acceptable accuracy.

In our own laboratory, while investigating the pharmacokinetics of lithium and other psychotropic drugs, we observed that after a single dose the level obtained 24 hr postdose was highly correlated with the steady-state level obtained when patients were placed on a fixed dose regimen. In our first study of lithium in 17 patients given a single oral loading dose of 600 mg lithium with bloods collected at 24 hr, then receiving 1,800 mg lithium/day on a t.i.d. regimen, a correlation ($r = 0.97$) was obtained between the 24-hr level and the steady state (25). Using this regression equation, we prepared a table of ranges of 24-hr values and the dosages associated with the ranges. These ranges were set conservatively low at the extremes of dosage, because they were calculated by extrapolation of the line of best fit. The table was then "fine tuned" by examining all of our available data obtained from patients on dosages other than 600 mg t.i.d., i.e., data in addition to those which determined the regression equation. Our general policy has been that if any bias is to be present in the tables, then it should be toward recommending a dosage that might be slightly lower rather than one that might result in toxicity. In a 2-year followup study of our original technique, we found that the table did not require alteration (27). Chang et al. (21), in a carefully controlled study using a minor modification of our procedure, were able to show marked advantages to using the prediction method. Other investigators have published confirmation of the validity of this procedure (21,48,54,119,140), and we have published data on a pharmacokinetic study of three lithium formulations and the calculated relationship between the 24-hr level and steady state and confirmed the original observation (30). Recently Slattery et al. (126), Devane et al. (40), and Gram et al. (55) all have demonstrated, on theoretical grounds, that such a strong correlation is to be expected in drugs with linear pharmacokinetic properties.

Several attempts have been made to refine the procedure.

Chang et al. (20) have used a 25-hr postdose time point and a larger dose, the latter presumably to increase accuracy of the lithium measure. The reason for the selection of a 25-hr rather than a 24-hr time point is obscure. Perry et al. (96) have shown that accuracy and prediction can be improved by using different equations to predict discrete ranges, and in their hands this procedure did indeed increase the accuracy of prediction (93). Such a finding could in turn be anticipated from the theoretical analysis of Slattery et al. (126), Devane et al. (40), and Gram et al. (55).

Perry et al. (92) also explored a two-point method using 12- and 36-hr serum levels after a test dose adjusted for weight and age. In this method the authors were able to predict 20 of 22 steady-state serum levels to within 0.1 mEq/liter. Another variation on the original procedure has been the use of the one-point prediction as a repeated procedure using two test doses and two accompanying serum levels. Marr et al. (83) were able to predict target serum levels to within 0.1 mEq/liter in five of six psychiatric inpatients. Amdisen (6) has outlined a procedure for basing maintenance dosage on three daily 12-hr serum lithium levels following a week of low-dose lithium. The method clearly is one of the safest procedures available, but does necessitate three separate blood samples collected after treatment with low doses of lithium, which would seem to make the procedure too cumbersome. This latter observation is particularly pertinent when one considers that a large majority of patients achieve steady state within 5 to 7 days of commencing treatment on a fixed dose regimen. Therefore blood collected after 3 days of treatment, i.e., before the morning dose on day 4, will approximate 87% of steady state in the majority of patients, and from this dosage adjustments can be readily made.

Mathematical models have been used by Zetin et al. (150), Gaillot et al. (51), Swartz (133), Swartz and Wilcox (134), and Dugas and Feeney (42). These procedures involved the determination of population pharmacokinetic parameters and applying these in a straightforward computer simulation to blood samples collected after loading dose or after multiple doses obtained from chart review. Acceptable predictions are reported.

The single-point procedure has been confirmed in many studies for lithium and also for several other medications in use in psychiatry and elsewhere (13,15,29,38,76, 81,99,149). In carefully controlled studies high correlations have always been found. A number of studies in the literature state that the latter is not the case, i.e. that a high correlation between these two variables (24-hr point and steady state) does not exist—despite three theoretical articles demonstrating that such high correlations are to be expected. Close inspection of these data indicates that one has to suspect laboratory error or gross misinterpretation of the actual theoretical basis for the procedure (16,31,37), i.e., the 24-hr level is highly correlated with steady state only when all patients are administered the same fixed dose.

Fava et al. (48) found that 29 of 30 patients (96%) were within therapeutic range of 0.6 to 1.2 mEq/liter; the outlier patient had a lithium of 1.33 mEq/liter. These authors, while enthusiastic about the accuracy of prediction, temper their observations by suggesting that in contrast to the data

of Chang et al. (21) this procedure did not shorten hospital stay or time to achieve steady state. Examination of the experimental design indicates that in both groups blood levels were obtained three times per week during this study. This strict protocol would clearly militate against finding any temporal differences in the prediction technique versus clinician's choice. Indeed, if blood level monitoring is to be performed three times per week, there seems to be no value in attempting dosage prediction.

The article by Pallidino et al. (89) found a very low correlation between the 24-hr blood level following a 600-mg dose of lithium and the steady-state level at fixed dosage. These authors state that their analytical method had a systematic bias of +0.11 mEq/liter serum, demonstrated when lithium free serum was run as an unknown. Despite this, their data were not corrected for this bias, which clearly has major impact on the 24-hr measure where levels of <0.5 mEq/liter are obtained (all patients were predicted to require 600 mg/day using the uncorrected data). Not surprisingly, only eight of 17 patients achieved the therapeutic range of 0.6 to 1.2 mEq/liter and five of these eight had <0.7 mEq/liter. If one corrects the 24-hr level by subtracting the systematic error of 0.11 mEq/liter, then the predicted dosages range from 600 to 1,800 mg/day. Recalculation of these steady-state data using the revised dosage prediction showed 16 of 17 patients would have achieved steady-state levels within the therapeutic range; the single outlier would have had a blood level of 0.59 mEq/liter. Nevertheless there are sufficient technical problems associated with these procedures to have formed major obstacles to widespread use. This reviewer must again reemphasize that any procedure utilizing laboratory measures is meant as an aid to the clinician and cannot be substituted for good clinical common sense. Patients at the extreme of dosage requirements, i.e., where dosage predictions are extraordinarily high or low, can be quickly identified, and such patients clearly warrant careful monitoring. This is an advantage that has been emphasized by this author and colleagues utilizing the technique. Obviously one should not embark on giving a patient 3,600 mg/day on the basis of a single blood level! One would, however, be forewarned that this patient could have a potential treatment problem. Similarly, the prediction of 300 mg/day or less would also very clearly alert the careful physician to potential clinical problems.

CLINICAL RELEVANCE OF OTHER CELL AND BODY FLUID MEASURES

Erythrocytes

In the 1970s there were a number of promising reports that the lithium transport characteristics of circulating erythrocytes may be useful in predicting response and for identifying subgroups of patients. The previous review by Cooper and Simpson (28) devoted considerable time to a critical discussion of this topic. Subsequent reports have given little support to these hypotheses. In the late 1970s an important step was made when an *in vitro* test to predict the *in vivo* erythrocyte concentration was developed by

Pandey and Davis (90). This procedure allowed screening of large numbers of patients of various diagnostic categories and normal volunteers. The *in vitro* ratio was found to be highly correlated with the *in vivo* ratio ($r > 0.9$). Application of this procedure by a large number of investigators has resulted in the conclusion that the lithium ratio has no diagnostic value, and no consistent relationship between the lithium ratio and clinical efficiency has been demonstrated (19,56). Recently Garver et al. (52) evaluated 141 consecutively admitted patients using the *in vitro* procedure and found that lithium response could be identified with high sensitivity but low specificity when examining the extreme modes of the distribution of this ratio. The procedure, however, was less efficacious than *Diagnostic and Statistical Manual of Mental Disorders,* 3rd edition (DSM-III) diagnoses in detecting lithium responders (61 vs 85%). The erythrocyte/plasma ratio has been recommended as a marker for compliance (19,53). The erythrocyte concentration does not show the wide fluctuations of plasma lithium during a single dosing interval and is useful in detecting non-compliance (12).

Investigation of this ratio has contributed to our basic understanding of the lithium countertransport system and other membrane transport mechanisms. Diamond et al. (41) have suggested the delay in onset of action of lithium may be directly related to the inhibition of the countertransport system, which these authors have demonstrated to be a slow process.

Saliva

The possibility of using salivary lithium for monitoring dosage has been investigated quite extensively during the past 15 years. Shopsin et al. (122) suggested that this saliva measure may be substituted for plasma lithium level monitoring. Such a technique has obvious appeal in that this body fluid is easily obtained and involves a noninvasive collection procedure. The quantitation of lithium in saliva is readily accomplished because the salivary concentration is approximately 2 to 3 times that of plasma. The sample requires centrifugation to remove particulate matter but is then processed essentially as plasma or serum, although additional care must be taken to ensure that the electrolyte concentration of the mixture is comparable to that of the standards used. Unfortunately, the individual patient saliva to plasma ratio shows considerable interindividual variation, and there is controversy over the interindividual stability of this ratio (58,101,123,145). Thus intraindividual variation means that before saliva monitoring can be substituted for plasma or serum level monitoring, this ratio must be determined for each patient (36). Marked intraindividual variation would render the measure useless! A review of this topic is to be found in the chapter by Sims (123). Recently Selinger et al. (120) reported a new method for the determination of salivary lithium concentrations in which saliva secretion was maximally stimulated by citric acid and pure parotid saliva analyzed for lithium content. Extremely high correlations between saliva lithium and plasma lithium were obtained ($r = 0.98$). These authors have subsequently investigated the effect of anticholinergic drugs on the saliva-plasma lithium measure, and again

found that there was a high correlation with little difference between the two groups of patients (121). However, a recent report by Richardson and King (110) tested the feasibility of this procedure in an underdeveloped country where plasma level monitoring was not possible. Their conclusion was that the correlation obtained "in the field" was not good enough to render the method clinically useful. Despite more than 50 publications on this topic, saliva monitoring is very rarely used in general clinical practice.

Spinal Fluid

Lithium is easily measured in spinal fluid, but the test has little clinical utility even in monitoring toxicity. The cerebrospinal fluid (CSF) plasma-lithium ratio is 0.5 or less and does not seem to correlate with diagnosis or therapeutic response and is not readily altered by hemodialysis (148). A study in which plasma, erythrocyte, and CSF lithium concentrations were measured concurrently yielded interesting results in that the erythrocyte and CSF concentrations showed slower rises and falls than did the plasma concentration. From such data one might predict that a closer correlation between CSF and erythrocyte concentrations would be expected. That this failed to occur, together with the fact that the erythrocyte lithium proved significantly higher than CSF lithium, supports the hypothesis that transfer of lithium into and out of the CSF and erythrocytes takes place by a different mechanism (148). In fact, considerable experimentation (43,44) has now established several mechanisms of transport by the erythrocyte membrane, whereas more scanty data (60,103) on lithium transport to and from CSF suggests that this occurs primarily by bulk flow and simple diffusion. Other work has shown that in animals the CSF has no advantage over serum lithium as a predictor of brain lithium concentration, whereas CSF lithium in humans has also failed to predict therapeutic effect (109,146).

Tears and Sweat

Tear and sweat measures have been reported, and it has been suggested by one group (14) that lithium could be monitored via tear analysis, but questioned by another (73). Sweat has been implicated in extensive lithium loss during heavy exercise or heat exposure, resulting in lower plasma lithium levels (71,85). Neither of these measures has much clinical utility, and the possibility of routine use of such esoteric measures seems highly unlikely.

Urine

During steady state the amount of lithium excreted per 24 hr is essentially equal to the daily dose (90% or greater). However, during the 24-hr interval the amount of lithium excreted per unit time (excretion rate) varies considerably. This is because the excretion rate is proportional to the plasma concentration, which can show a threefold variation during a single dosing interval. The resulting lithium concentration may in practice be regarded as unpredictable and of no value in the monitoring of lithium treatment, even when one can be sure of complete sample collection. However, in the case of suspected impaired renal function it may be useful to document the plasma lithium clearance rate. Urine lithium can be measured relatively simply but does require more preparation than does plasma. However, as this measure has little practical clinical relevance, the reader interested in further technical details on measurement is referred to the detailed article by Amdisen (3).

TOXICITY

Pharmacokinetic Mechanisms

Lithium has a low therapeutic index, and therefore modest increases in plasma lithium move a patient from the therapeutic range into potential toxicity. The causes and underlying mechanisms of lithium toxicity essentially can be dichotomized, namely, deliberate intake of a large dose with suicidal intent, or reduction in renal lithium clearance with concomitant increase in plasma and tissue concentrations if this change is not followed by appropriate reduction in dosage. Obviously the deliberate ingestion of an overdose of this medication will cause toxicity, and, without adequate treatment, death. Schou (114) has suggested that there is an additional safety factor in prescribing slow release lithium preparations, in that such patients, if treated promptly, may still have considerable quantities of unabsorbed medication, which can be removed by gastric lavage.

Renal mechanisms involved in toxicity in the patient without kidney disease are closely tied to the sodium balance, and hence pharmacokinetic changes result if this balance is disturbed (59). Sodium deficiency can lead to a reduction in lithium clearance (138). The mechanisms involved are as follows: In electrolyte balance sodium and lithium are primarily reabsorbed from the proximal tubules; sodium but not lithium can be reabsorbed from the distal tubules. In extreme sodium deficiency, however, lithium may also be reabsorbed from the distal segments of the tubules. In a modest sodium deficit the reabsorption of sodium in the distal tubules maintains sodium balance and lithium toxicity is avoided. In more pronounced sodium deficiency the reabsorption of lithium becomes more pronounced and the plasma level increases. When the plasma concentration reaches a certain lithium level, lithium inhibition of the aldosterone-stimulated reabsorption of sodium in the distal tubule segments becomes such that sodium deficiency is further increased. This in turn leads to a further decrease in lithium clearance, with a resulting increase in plasma lithium. Thus a vicious cycle is in place, which without intervention will certainly lead to toxicity. It follows that any increase in the 12-hr steady-state lithium without concomitant change in dosage must be thoroughly investigated to ascertain that this process is not underway and that a toxicity may be pending that requires appropriate treatment.

Long-Term Changes in Renal Function

In human studies a significant decrease in concentrating capacity is a common finding and occurs relatively early in treatment and remains significantly reduced thereafter (116,142,143). Thomsen (138) has postulated an unexplained but direct effect of lithium on glomerular filtration rate (GFR). Until recently GFR had not been demonstrated to be affected by long-term lithium treatment, but Lokkeggard et al. (80), in a study of 153 manic-depressive patients treated with lithium for at least 5 years, with a mean of 10 years' treatment, did demonstrate a modest decrease in GFR. However, it required 17 years of treatment before the regression line crossed the lower 95% confidence interval of the control population. These investigators emphasize that very few of their patients developed markedly decreased GFR.

There exists some controversy over the advisability of divided or single-dose regimens of lithium and renal toxicity. It has been suggested that a large single dose of lithium will cause more dose-related side effects, and thus a divided dose regimen will avoid this problem. Conversely, it has been suggested that kidney damage caused by lithium may be minimized by giving a large single dose daily, thus allowing a quiescent low-lithium period for repair mechanisms to operate (98). Vestergaard et al. (142), Vestergaard and Thomsen (143), and Perry et al. (95) have shown that once a day dosing resulted in less diminution in concentrating capacity, which may give additional support for such a strategy. Schou et al. (116) investigated this problem in a collaborative study between two clinical research institutes. One of these utilized a slow release preparation given twice per day, the other used a standard release preparation given at bedtime. In both hospitals many patients developed polyuria. Neither regimen differentially affected glomerular filtration rate or proximal tube reabsorption, but distal tube reabsorption of water and polyuria were less pronounced in the single-dose regimen patients. While conceding the finding, one of these groups quite properly points out that a controlled study in a single research clinic to rule out patient and environmental differences is essential before the above evidence can be regarded as conclusive. The study of Plenge et al. (98) attempted this, but the treatment groups were not randomly assigned (116). Such an important observation obviously needs confirmation, but, if proven, will clearly require that we rethink our current dosing regimens.

DRUG INTERACTIONS

Diuretics

It is well established that thiazide diuretics decrease renal lithium clearance and increase serum lithium levels (97). Himmelhoch et al. (62) anticipated a 40% increase in serum lithium levels in patients given 500 mg chlorothiazide daily (or its equivalent) and therefore decreased lithium dose by 40% to maintain the same levels. These diuretics have been used to treat lithium-induced nephrogenic diabetes insipidus (49) and may be of some value when combined with lithium in treating patients who require large doses of lithium to reach therapeutic lithium concentrations (61). Other classes of diuretics have been less thoroughly studied, and one cannot generalize to all clinical situations. Available data in normal volunteers suggest that the potassium-sparing diuretics may increase serum lithium levels. Loop diuretics do not cause lithium retention (72), and osmotic diuretics, carbonic anhydrase inhibitors, and xanthine diuretics may actually increase lithium excretion (67,139). Given the above, one should anticipate interactions between lithium and diuretics, and appropriate increased frequency of monitoring is indicated (70).

Amiloride

Vasopressin-resistant diabetes insipidus is a common side effect of lithium treatment. Amiloride, a potassium-sparing diuretic that acts on the cortical collecting tubule, antagonizes the inhibition brought about by lithium on vasopressin-induced water transport (75). In a detailed study, Battle et al. (8) demonstrated amiloride could be used to provide specific therapy for polyuria associated with long-term lithium treatment.

Theophylline

Theophylline has been reported to increase renal clearance of lithium (139) and reduce plasma lithium levels by as much as 30% (94). It follows, therefore, that increased frequency of monitoring is mandatory when theophylline is added to treatment or when theophylline administration is discontinued; the former may result in loss of efficacy, the latter, toxicity.

Neuroleptic and Antidepressant Drugs

Animal studies have demonstrated that lithium delays gastric emptying and impairs absorption of chlorpromazine (111). It has been unequivocally demonstrated that chlorpromazine and other neuroleptic drugs undergo extensive first-pass metabolism, with a major proportion of this metabolism taking place in the gut wall (34,35). It follows that any delay in gastric emptying would allow additional time for metabolism to occur, thus reducing availability of the drug to the systemic circulation. Rivera-Calimlim et al. (112) have confirmed this observation in humans, demonstrating a marked decrease in availability of chlorpromazine (ca 50%) when single-dose pharmacokinetic profiles were obtained in normal volunteers given chlorpromazine or chlorpromazine plus lithium in random crossover design. Phenothiazine drugs have been shown to increase intracellular content of lithium. This is brought about by an increase in the influx of lithium into the erythrocyte, with resulting increase in the erythrocyte/plasma ratio (91). This effect appears to be relatively specific for the phenothiazines, with no changes obtained for haloperidol, tricyclic antidepressants, or the monoamine oxidase inhibitor phenelzine (91). The observation that tricyclic antidepressants do not change the erythrocyte plasma/lithium ratio is apparently contradicted by the data of Ostrow et al. (88), who claim a 25% increase in the *in vitro* ratio test at comparable lithium concentrations. Lingjaerde et al. (78) and DeMontigny et al. (39) report synergism in clinical action with the tricyclic antidepressant plus lithium combination but did not examine kinetic changes. Westiuk et al. (147)

claim that the combination of lithium plus haloperidol lowers the erythrocyte/plasma ratio and cite the work of Zimmer et al. (151,152) demonstrating membrane fluidity changes caused by haloperidol as supportive of their findings.

The phenothiazine data are not controversial; i.e., it is generally accepted that intracellular lithium content is increased, and this pharmacokinetic interaction has been suggested, but not proven, as an explanation of neurotoxicities reported with the combination of lithium and neuroleptic drug (1,125–128,130).

One of the most frequently quoted drug interactions with lithium is that of haloperidol, first reported by Cohen and Cohen (23). This observation was particularly disturbing in that irreversible neurological damage occurred in the four subjects comprising this report. The evidence for compatibility or lack of compatibility of this particular combination has been extensively and critically reviewed (68,141), and although additional toxicities have been reported since the first report, to this reviewer's knowledge, only one has been irreversible (129). A pharmacokinetic explanation of these haloperidol-lithium neurotoxicities cannot be supported by published data. Increased intracellular lithium or increased intracellular haloperidol has not been demonstrated in carefully controlled studies. Indeed, the data of Westiuk may indicate that there is a decrease in intracellular lithium in a subgroup of patients (bipolar manic-depressive) when this combination is used (147).

Antiinflammatory Drugs

Indomethacin (50,105,107), diclofenac (108), and phenylbutazone (124) have been demonstrated to cause clinically significant decreases in renal clearance of lithium. Aspirin does not cause these changes (107). A reduction in dosage and careful plasma lithium monitoring are indicated for patients placed on these medications. There are few or no data for the newer nonsteroidal antiinflammatory agents, but again additional precautions should be observed until adequate information is available.

CONCLUSION

Knowledge of the pharmacokinetics of lithium has enabled us to define therapeutic and toxic ranges in humans. Prediction of individual dosage requirements from a single challenge dose of medication has proven possible, and noncompliance can be readily detected by examination of the erythrocyte/plasma ratio. The application of pharmacokinetic principles in combination with sound clinical common sense and experience has permitted interpretation of difficult clinical problems. The pharmacokinetic profiles obtained from various lithium formulations have made it possible to adjust dosage regimens to suit individual patient needs. In addition, these same principles have allowed us to place the treatment of lithium toxicity on a firm theoretical and practical basis. Current efforts appear to be exploring the lowest possible lithium level that needs to be maintained to protect patients from recurrence of their illness. Work cited in this review suggests that it may be necessary to rethink current dosing strategies in light of the findings of Schou et al. (116).

The author wishes to bring to the attention of the reader the availability of a Lithium Information Center at the University of Wisconsin, Department of Psychiatry. Run by Drs. Greist and Jefferson, this valuable library is available to all research investigators. The cost is modest and it is truly the source for lithium research bibliographies.

REFERENCES

1. Alevizos, B. (1979): *Br. J. Psychiatry*, 135:482.
2. Amdisen, A. (1967): *Scand. J. Clin. Lab. Invest.*, 20:104–108.
3. Amdisen, A. (1975): In: *Lithium Research and Therapy*, edited by F. N. Johnson, pp. 181–185. Academic Press, New York.
4. Amdisen, A. (1977): *Clin. Pharmacokinet.*, 2:73–92.
5. Amdisen, A. (1978): *J. Anal. Toxicol.*, 2:193–202.
6. Amdisen, A. (1980): In: *Handbook of Lithium Therapy*, edited by F. N. Johnson, pp. 179–195. MTP Press, Lancaster, England.
7. Amdisen, A. (1985): In: *Therapeutic Drug Monitoring*, edited by B. Widdop, pp. 301–331. Churchill Livingstone, Edinburgh.
8. Battle, D. C., von Riotte, A. B., Gaviria-Moises, M., and Grupp, M. (1985): *N. Engl. J. Med.*, 312:408–414.
9. Bergner, P.-E. E. (1977): *Bull. Math. Biol.*, 39:167–178.
10. Bergner, P.-E. E., Berniker, K., Cooper, T. B., Gradijan, J. R., and Simpson, G. M. (1973): *Br. J. Pharmacol.*, 49:328–339.
11. Bond, P. A. (1978): In: *Lithium in Medical Practice*, edited by F. N. Johnson and S. Johnson, pp. 215–223. University Park Press, Baltimore.
12. Bone, S., Roose, S. P., Dunner, D. L., and Fieve, R. R. (1981): *J. Clin. Psychopharmacol.*, 1:390–391.
13. Braithwaite, R., Montgomery, S., and Dawling, S. (1978): *Clin. Pharmacol. Ther.*, 23:303–308.
14. Brenner, R., Cooper, T. B., Yablonski, M. E., Lieberman, J. A., Lesser, M., Siris, S. G., and Rifkin, A. E. (1982): *Am. J. Psychiatry*, 139:678–679.
15. Brunswick, D. J., Amsterdam, J. D., Mendels, J., and Stern, S. L. (1979): *Clin. Pharmacol. Ther.*, 25:605–610.
16. Brunswick, D. J., and Cooper, T. B. (1983): *J. Clin. Psychopharmacol.*, 3:57.
17. Cade, J. F. J. (1949): *Med. J. Aust.*, 2:349–352.
18. Caldwell, H. C., Westlake, W. J., Connor, S. M., and Flanagan, T. (1971): *J. Clin. Pharmacol.*, 11:349–356.
19. Carroll, B. J. (1979): *Arch. Gen. Psychiatry*, 36:870–878.
20. Chang, S. S., Dysken, M. W., Pandey, G. N., and Davis, J. M. (1981): Presented at APA Annual Meeting, New Orleans.
21. Chang, S. S., Pandey, G. N., Casper, R. C., Kinard, C. O., and Davis, J. M. (1979): In: *Lithium: Controversies and Unresolved Issues*, edited by T. B. Cooper, S. Gershon, N. S. Kline, and M. Schou, pp. 419–426. Excerpta Medica, Amsterdam.
22. Chang, S. S., Pandey, G. N., Dysken, M., Schaffer, C., and Davis, J. M. (1979): *Clin. Pharmacol. Ther.*, 25:217.
23. Cohen, W. J., and Cohen, N. H. (1974): *JAMA*, 230:1283–1287.
24. Cooper, T. B. (1980): In: *Handbook of Lithium Therapy*, edited by F. N. Johnson, pp. 169–178. MTP Press, Lancaster, England.
25. Cooper, T. B., Bergner, P.-E. E., and Simpson, G. M. (1973): *Am. J. Psychiatry*, 130:601–603.
26. Cooper, T. B., and Carroll, B. J. (1981): *J. Clin. Psychopharmacol.*, 1:53–58.
27. Cooper, T. B., and Simpson, G. M. (1976): *Am. J. Psychiatry*, 133:440–443.
28. Cooper, T. B., and Simpson, G. M. (1978): In: *Psychopharmacology: A Generation of Progress*, edited by M. A. Lipton, A. DiMascio, and K. F. Killam, pp. 923–931. Raven Press, New York.
29. Cooper, T. B., and Simpson, G. M. (1978): *Am. J. Psychiatry*, 135:333–335.
30. Cooper, T. B., and Simpson, G. M. (1979): In: *Lithium: Controversies and Unresolved Issues*, edited by T. B. Cooper, S. Gershon, N. S. Kline, and M. Schou, pp. 346–353. Excerpta Medica, Amsterdam.
31. Cooper, T. B., and Simpson, G. M. (1982): *Am. J. Psychiatry*, 139:969.
32. Cooper, T. B., Simpson, G. M., and Allen, D. (1974): *At. Absorpt. Newsl.*, 13:119–120.
33. Cooper, T. B., Simpson, G. M., Lee, J. H., and Bergner, P.-E. E. (1978): *Am. J. Psychiatry*, 135:917–922.
34. Curry, S. H., D'Mello, A., and Mould, G. P. (1971): *Br. J. Pharmacol.*, 42:403–411.
35. Dahl, S. G., and Standjord, R. E. (1977): *Clin. Pharmacol. Ther.*, 21:437–448.
36. Danhof, M., and Breimer, D. D. (1978): *Clin. Pharmacokinet.*, 3:39–57.
37. Davis, R. A., Taylor, M. A., and Abrams, R. (1978): *Biol. Psychiatry*, 13:595–599.
38. Dawling, S., Crome, P., Braithwaite, R. A., and Lewis, R. R. (1980): *Eur. J. Clin. Pharmacol.*, 18:147–150.
39. DeMontigny, C., Grunberg, F., Mayer, A., and Deschenes, J.-P. (1981): *Br. J. Psychiatry*, 138:252–256.
40. DeVane, C. L., Wolin, R. E., and Jusko, W. J. (1979): *Commun. Psychopharmacol.*, 3:353–357.
41. Diamond, J. M., Ehrlich, B. E., and Freedman, J. C. (1982): *N. Engl. J. Med.*, 307:1646.
42. Dugas, J. E., and Feeney, A. M. (1983): *Clin. Pharmacokinet.*, 2:249–252.
43. Duhm, J., and Becker, B. F. (1977): *Pflugers Arch.*, 367:211–219.
44. Duhm, J., Eisenried, F., Becker, B. F., and Greil, W. (1976): *Pflugers Arch.*, 364:147–155.
45. Dunner, D. L., Roose, S. P., and Bones, S. (1979): In: *Lithium: Controversies and Unresolved Issues*, edited by T. B. Cooper, S. Gershon, N. S. Kline, and M. Schou, pp. 427–431. Excerpta Medica, Amsterdam.
46. Ehrlich, B. E., and Diamond, J. M. (1978): *Biochim. Biophys. Acta*, 543:264–268.
47. Ereshefsky, L., and Jann, M. W. (1983): In: *Applied Clinical Pharmacokinetics*, edited by D. Mungall, pp. 245–270. Raven Press, New York.
48. Fava, G. A., Molnar, G., Block, B., Lee, J. S., and Perini, G. I. (1984): *Am. J. Psychiatry*, 141:812–813.
49. Forrest, J. N., Cohen, A. D., Torretti, J., Himmelhoch, J. M., and Epstein, F. H. (1974): *J. Clin. Invest.*, 53:1115–1123.
50. Frolich, J. C., Leftwich, R., Ragheb, M., Oates, J. A., Riemann, I., and Buchanan, D. (1979): *Br. Med. J.*, 1:1115–1116.
51. Gaillot, J., Steimer, J.-L., Mallet, A. J., Thebault, J. J., and Bieder, A. (1979): *J. Pharmacokinet. Biopharm.*, 7:579–628.
52. Garver, D. L., Hitzemann, R., and Hirschowitz, J. (1984): *Arch. Gen. Psychiatry*, 41:497–505.
53. Gengo, F., Frazer, A., Ramsey, T. A., and Mendels, J. (1980): *Comp. Psychiatry*, 21:276–280.
54. Gengo, F., Timko, J., D'Antonio, J., Ramsey, A., Frazer, A., and Mendels, J. (1980): *J. Clin. Psychiatry*, 41:319–321.
55. Gram, L. F., Bech, P., Reisby, N., and Jorgensen, O. S. (1981): In: *Clinical Pharmacology in Psychiatry*, edited by E. Usdin, pp. 155–171. Elsevier, New York.
56. Greil, W., Becker, B. F., and Duhm, J. (1979): In: *Lithium: Controversies and Unresolved Issues*, edited by T. B. Cooper, S. Gershon, N. S. Kline, and M. Schou, pp. 209–217. Excerpta Medica, Amsterdam.
57. Grof, P. (1979): *Arch. Gen. Psychiatry*, 36:891–893.
58. Groth, U., Prellwitz, W., and Jahnchen, E. (1974): *Clin. Pharmacol. Ther.*, 16:490–498.
59. Hansen, H. E., and Amdisen, A. (1978): *Q. J. Med.*, 186:123–144.
60. Hesketh, J., and Glen, I. (1978): *Biochem. Pharmacol.*, 27:813–814.
61. Himmelhoch, J. M., Forrest, J., Neil, J. F., and Detre, T. P. (1977): *Am. J. Psychiatry*, 134:149–152.
62. Himmelhoch, J. M., Poust, R. I., Mallinger, A. G., Hanin, I., and Neil, J. F. (1977): *Clin. Pharmacol. Ther.*, 22:225–227.
63. Hisayasu, G. H., Cohen, J. L., and Nelson, R. W. (1977): *Clin. Chem.*, 23:41–45.
64. Hullin, R. P. (1980): In: *Handbook of Lithium Therapy*, edited by F. N. Johnson, pp. 243–247. MTP Press, Lancaster, England.
65. Jefferson, J. W. (1983): *Compr. Psychiatry*, 24:166–178.
66. Jefferson, J. W. (1984): In: *Handbook of Psychiatric Diagnostic Procedures*, edited by R. C. W. Beresford and T. P. Beresford, pp. 161–181. Spectrum, New York.
67. Jefferson, J. W., and Greist, J. H. (1979): In: *Psychopharmacology Update: New and Neglected Areas*, edited by J. M. Davis and D. Greenblatt, pp. 81–104. Grune and Stratton, New York.

68. Jefferson, J. W., and Greist, J. H. (1980): In: *Haloperidol Update: 1958-1980*, edited by F. J. Ayd, pp. 73-82. Ayd Medical Communications, Baltimore.

69. Jefferson, J. W., and Greist, J. H. (1981): *Am. J. Psychiatry*, 138:93-94.

70. Jefferson, J. W., Greist, J. H., and Baudhuin, M. (1981): *J. Clin. Psychopharmacol.*, 1:124-134.

71. Jefferson, J. W., Greist, J. H., Clagnaz, P. J., Eischens, R. R., Marten, W. C., and Evenson, M. A. (1982): *Am. J. Psychiatry*, 139:1593-1595.

72. Jefferson, J. W., and Kalin, N. H. (1979): *JAMA*, 241:1134-1136.

73. Jefferson, J. W., Kaufman, P., and Ackerman, D. (1984): *J. Clin. Psychiatry*, 45:304-305.

74. Jerram, T. C., and McDonald, R. (1978): In: *Lithium in Medical Practice*, edited by F. N. Johnson and S. Johnson, pp. 407-413. MTP Press, Lancaster, England.

75. Kosten, T. R., and Forrest, J. N. (1982): *Clin. Res.*, 30:540A (Abstr.).

76. Koup, J. R., Sack, C. M., Smith, A. L., and Gibaldi, M. (1979): *Clin. Pharmacokinet.*, 4:460-469.

77. Lehmann, W. D., Bahr, U., and Schulten, H. R. (1978): *Biomed. Mass Spectrom.*, 5:536-539.

78. Lingjaerde, O., Edlund, A. H., Gormsen, C. A., Gottfries, C. G., Haugstad, A., Hermann, I. L., Hollnagel, P., Makimattila, A., Rasmussen, K. E., Remvig, J., and Robak, O. H. (1974): *Acta Psychiatr. Scand.*, 50:233-242.

79. Lloyd, J. R., and Field, F. H. (1981): *Biomed. Mass Spectrom.*, 8:19-24.

80. Lokkegaard, H., Andersen, N. F., Henriksen, E., Bartels, P. D., Brahm, M., Baastrup, P. C., Jorgensen, H. E., Larsen, M., Munck, O., Rasmussen, K., and Schroder, H. (1985): *Acta Psychiatr. Scand.*, 71:347-355.

81. Madakasira, S., Preskorn, S. H., Weller, R., and Pardo, M. (1982): *J. Clin. Psychopharm.*, 2:136-139.

82. Maessen, F. J. M. J. (1980): In: *Handbook of Lithium Therapy*, edited by F. N. Johnson, pp. 169-178. MTP Press, Lancaster, England.

83. Marr, M. A., Djuric, P. E., Ritschel, W. A., and Garver, D. L. (1983): *Clin. Pharmacokinet.*, 2:243-248.

84. Mielke, D. H. (1976): In: *Depression: Behavioral, Biochemical, Diagnostic and Treatment Concepts*, edited by D. M. Gallant and G. M. Simpson, pp. 273-308. Spectrum, New York.

85. Miller, E. B., Pain, R. W., and Skripal, P. J. (1978): *Br. J. Psychiatry*, 133:477-478.

86. Noack, C. H., and Trautner, E. M. (1951): *Med. J. Aust.*, 38:219-222.

87. Norman, K. P., Cerrone, K. L., and Reus, V. I. (1982): *Am. J. Psychiatry*, 139:1625-1626.

88. Ostrow, D. G., Southam, A. S., and Davis, J. M. (1980): *Biol. Psychiatry*, 15:723-739.

89. Palladino, A., Longenecker, R. G., and Lesko, L. J. (1983): *J. Clin. Psychiatry*, 44:7-9.

90. Pandey, G. N., and Davis, J. M. (1979): In: *Lithium: Controversies and Unresolved Issues*, edited by T. B. Cooper, S. Gershon, N. S. Kline, and M. Schou, pp. 346-353. Excerpta Medica, Amsterdam.

91. Pandey, G. N., Goel, I., and Davis, J. M. (1979): *Clin. Pharmacol. Ther.*, 26:96-102.

92. Perry, P. J., Alexander, B., Dunner, F. J., Schoenwald, R. D., Pfohl, B., and Miller, D. (1982): *J. Clin. Psychopharm.*, 2:114-118.

93. Perry, P. J., Alexander, B., Prince, R. A., and Dunner, F. J. (1984): *J. Clin. Psychopharmacol.*, 4:242-246.

94. Perry, P. J., Calloway, R. A., Cook, B. L., and Smith, R. E. (1984): *Acta Psychiatr. Scand.*, 69:528-537.

95. Perry, P. J., Dunner, F. J., Hahn, R. L., Tsuang, M. T., and Berg, M. J. (1981): *Acta Psychiatr. Scand.*, 64:281-294.

96. Perry, P. J., Prince, R. A., Alexander, B., and Dunner, F. J. (1983): *J. Clin. Psychopharmacol.*, 3:13-17.

97. Peterson, C., Hvidt, S., Thomsen, K., and Schou, M. (1974): *Br. J. Psychiatry*, 3:143-145.

98. Plenge, P., Mellerup, E. T., Bolwig, T. G., Brun, C., Hetmar, O., Ladefoged, J., Larsen, S., and Rafaelsen, O. J. (1982): *Acta Psychiatr. Scand.*, 66:121-128.

99. Potter, W. Z., Zavadil, A. P., and Goodwin, F. K. (1978): *Psychopharmacol. Bull.*, 14:29-32.

100. Poust, R. I., Mallinger, A. G., Mallinger, J., Himmelhoch, J. M., and Hanin, I. (1976): *Psychopharmacol. Comm.*, 2:91-103.

101. Preskorn, S. H., Abernethy, D. R., and McKnelly, W. V., Jr. (1978): *J. Clin. Psychiatry*, 39:756-758.

102. Prien, R. F., Caffey, E. M., and Klett, C. J. (1972): *Br. J. Psychiatry*, 120:409-414.

103. Prockop, L. D., and Marcus, D. J. (1972): *Life Sci.*, 11:859-868.

104. Radomski, J. L., Fuyat, H. N., Nelson, A. A., and Smith, P. K. (1950): *J. Pharmacol. Exp. Ther.*, 100:429-444.

105. Ragheb, M., Ban, T. A., Buchanan, D., and Frolich, J. C. (1980): *J. Clin. Psychiatry*, 41:397-398.

106. Reifman, A., and Wyatt, R. J. (1980): *Arch. Gen. Psychiatry*, 37:385-388.

107. Reimann, I. W., Diener, U., and Frolich, J. C. (1983): *Arch. Gen. Psychiatry*, 40:283-286.

108. Reimann, I. W., and Frolich, J. C. (1981): *Clin. Pharmacol. Ther.*, 30:348-352.

109. Rey, A. C., Jimerson, D. C., and Post, R. M. (1979): *Commun. Psychopharmacol.*, 3:267-278.

110. Richardson, R. E., and King, J. R. (1984): *Biol. Psychiatry*, 19:1129-1132.

111. Rivera-Calimlim, L. (1976): *Psychopharmacol. Commun.*, 2:263-272.

112. Rivera-Calimlim, L., Kerzner, B., and Karch, F. E. (1978): *Clin. Pharmacol. Ther.*, 23:451-455.

113. Schou, M. (1958): *Acta Pharmacol. Toxicol.*, 15:70-84.

114. Schou, M. (1978): In: *Principles of Psychopharmacology*, 2nd ed., edited by W. G. Clark and J. del Guidice, Chapter 17. Academic Press, New York.

115. Schou, M. (1982): *Pharmacopsychiatrica*, 15:128.

116. Schou, M., Amdisen, A., Thompsen, K., Vestergaard, P., Hetmar, O., Mellerup, E. T., Plenge, P., and Rafaelsen, O. J. (1982): *Psychopharmacology*, 77:387-390.

117. Schou, M., Baastrup, P. C., Grof, P., Weis, P., and Angst, J. (1970): *Br. J. Psychiatry*, 116:615-619.

118. Sedvall, G., Petterson, U., and Fyro, B. (1970): *Pharmacol. Clin.*, 2:231-235.

119. Seifert, R., Bremkamp, H., and Junge, C. (1975): *Psychopharmacologia*, 43:285-286.

120. Selinger, D., Hailer, A. W., Nurnberger, J. I., Simmons, S., and Gershon, E. S. (1982): *Biol. Psychiatry*, 17:99-102.

121. Selinger, D., Simmons, S., Hailer, A. W., Nurnberger, J. I., and Gershon, E. S. (1982): *Biol. Psychiatry*, 17:1145-1155.

122. Shopsin, B., Gershon, S., and Pinckney, L. (1969): *Int. Pharmacopsychiatry*, 2:148-169.

123. Sims, A. (1980): In: *Handbook of Lithium Therapy*, edited by F. N. Johnson, pp. 200-204. MTP Press, Lancaster, England.

124. Singer, L., Imbs, J. L., Danion, J. M., Schmidt, M., and Sebban, M. (1978): 11th CINP Congress, Vienna, Abstracts, p. 272.

125. Singh, S. V. (1982): *Lancet*, 2:278.

126. Slattery, J. T., Gibaldi, M., and Koup, J. R. (1980): *Clin. Pharmacokinet.*, 5:377-385.

127. Spring, G. K. (1979): *J. Clin. Psychiatry*, 40:135-138.

128. Spring, G. K., Abrams, R., and Taylor, M. A. (1979): *Am. J. Psychiatry*, 136:1099-1100.

129. Spring, G., and Frankel, M. (1981): *Am. J. Psychiatry*, 138:818-821.

130. Spring, G. K., and Gould, D. J. (1978): Presented at the American Psychiatric Association Annual Meeting, p. 29. Syllabus and Scientific Proceedings.

131. Spring, G., Schweid, D., Gray, C., Steinberg, J., and Horwitz, M. (1970): *Am. J. Psychiatry*, 126:1306-1310.

132. Stafford, D. T., and Saharovici (1974): *Spectrochim. Acta*, 29B:277-281.

133. Swartz, C. M. (1983): *Comput. Psychiatry Psychol.*, 5:13-17.

134. Swartz, C. M., and Wilcox, J. (1984): *Arch. Gen. Psychiatry*, 41:1154-1158.

135. Talbott, J. H. (1950): *Arch. Intern. Med.*, 85:1-10.

136. Talso, P. J., and Clarke, R. W. (1968): *Am. J. Physiol.*, 215:823-827.

137. Terhaag, B., Scherber, A., Schaps, P., and Winkler, H. (1978): *Int. J. Clin. Pharmacol. Biopharmacol.*, 16:333-335.

138. Thomsen, K. (1978): *Dan. Med. Bull.*, 25:106-115.

139. Thomsen, K., and Schou, M. (1968): *Am. J. Physiol.,* 215:823–827.
140. Tyrer, S. P., Grof, P., Kalvar, M., and Shopsin, B. (1981): *Neuropsychobiology,* 7:152–158.
141. Tyrer, S. P., and Shopsin, B. (1980): In: *Handbook of Lithium Therapy,* edited by F. N. Johnson, pp. 289–309. MTP Press, Lancaster, England.
142. Vestergaard, P., Amdisen, A., Hansen, H. E., and Schou, M. (1979): *Acta Psychiatr. Scand.,* 60:504–520.
143. Vestergaard, P., and Thomsen, K. (1981): *Psychopharmacology,* 72:203–204.
144. Vinar, O., and Vinarova, E. (1978): *Acta Nerv. Super. (Praha),* 20:91–92.
145. Vlaar, H., Bleeker, J. A. C., and Schalken, H. F. A. (1979): *Acta Psychiatr. Scand.,* 60:423–426.

146. Watanabe, S., Taguchi, K., Ebara, T., Iguchi, K., and Otsuki, S. (1973): *Folia Psychiatr. Neurol. Jpn.,* 27:299–303.
147. Werstiuk, E. S., Grof, P., Rotstein, E., and Werner, L. (1983): *Prog. Neuropsychopharmacol. Biol. Psychiatry,* 7:831–834.
148. White, K., Cohen, J., Boyd, J., and Nelson, R. (1979): *Int. Pharmacopsychiatry,* 14:185–189.
149. Wilkens, J. H., Neuenkirchen, H., Sybrecht, G. W., and Oellerich, M. (1984): *Eur. J. Clin. Pharmacol.,* 26:491–498.
150. Zetin, M., Garber, D., and Cramer, M. (1983): *J. Clin. Psychiatry,* 44:144–145.
151. Zimmer, G., Gross, W., Mehler, U., and Dorn-Zachertz, D. (1980): *Arzneimittelforsch.,* 30:221–228.
152. Zimmer, G., and Schulze, P. (1981): *Arzneimittelforsch.,* 31:1389–1392.

Psychopharmacology:
The Third Generation of Progress,
edited by Herbert Y. Meltzer.
Raven Press, New York © 1987.

CHAPTER **144**

Pharmacokinetics of Antianxiety Agents

David J. Greenblatt and Richard I. Shader

Despite an ongoing trend toward more cautious and conservative prescribing of psychotropic drugs, benzodiazepine anxiolytics and hypnotics continue to be extensively prescribed and utilized drugs (65,91,92). Seven benzodiazepines appeared among the 100 most commonly dispensed drugs by American retail pharmacies in 1985 (Table 1). Continuing review and evaluation of the pharmacologic properties of benzodiazepine derivatives is appropriate and necessary for scientists aiming to understand the mechanisms of action of psychotropic drugs, as well as for patients and clinicians who must evaluate the realistic risks and benefits of psychotropic drug therapy.

PHARMACOKINETIC COMPONENTS OF ANXIOLYTIC AND HYPNOTIC DRUG ACTION

Benzodiazepine derivatives differ considerably among themselves in milligram potency. These differences probably reflect at least in part a differential quantitative affinity for the receptor site mediating pharmacologic action (96). Clinical doses of some benzodiazepines (for example, triazolam, clonazepam, and flunitrazepam) generally fall in the range of less than 2 mg, whereas for others (such as chlordiazepoxide, oxazepam, flurazepam, and halazepam) clinical doses often exceed 20 mg. Despite these large quantitative variations in intrinsic potency, qualitative differences among benzodiazepine derivatives in the character of clinical action are difficult to demonstrate. After appropriate adjustment of dosage to account for differences in potency, all benzodiazepines appear to share anxiolytic, sedative-hypnotic, and anticonvulsant effects in ascending order of dose and brain concentration. Likewise, it is not easy to find consistent scientific evidence to validate the primary (FDA-approved) clinical indications for some ben-

zodiazepines as anxiolytics, some as hypnotics, some as anticonvulsants, and others primarily as preoperative medications. Nonetheless, clinical differences do exist among benzodiazepines in the time course of onset, intensity, and duration of clinical activity, both following single doses, and during multiple dosage. Many of these differences can be accounted for by specific pharmacokinetic properties. This chapter reviews the physicochemical and pharmacokinetic properties of benzodiazepines, and the relation of these to their clinical actions (16,32,34,49,50,64,66,69,83). Also discussed are methodologic problems that can complicate the interpretation of pharmacokinetic data, and the relation of these data to pharmacodynamic action. Since "anxiolytic" and "hypnotic" benzodiazepines are actually indistinguishable in their primary pharmacologic actions, the two categories will be considered together.

PHYSICOCHEMICAL PROPERTIES OF BENZODIAZEPINES

Lipid Solubility

All benzodiazepine derivatives are weak organic bases. Some of these drugs, such as chlordiazepoxide, flurazepam, and midazolam, form water-soluble salts at acidic pH. In the case of midazolam, this property has been widely publicized, and has led midazolam to be termed "the first water-soluble benzodiazepine" (82). In any case, once buffered to physiologic pH as would occur *in vivo,* all benzodiazepines become moderately to highly lipid-soluble substances. Two methods used for *in vitro* quantitation of benzodiazepine lipophilicity are (a) the partitioning of drugs between an aqueous buffer at physiologic pH and an organic solvent (usually octanol), and (b) the evaluation of

TABLE 1. *Benzodiazepines appearing among the 100 drugs most commonly dispensed by American retail pharmacies[a]*

Drug	1985 rank	1984 rank
Diazepam	5	4
Alprazolam	20	32
Lorazepam	23	23
Flurazepam	38	29
Clorazepate	41	36
Triazolam	42	73
Temazepam	58	50

[a] Source: *American Druggist,* February, 1986.

TABLE 2. *Relative lipid solubility of benzodiazepines*

Drug	HPLC retention index[a]
Midazolam	1.54
Camazepam	1.36
Quazepam	1.22
Flurazepam	1.10
Diazepam	1.00
Desmethyldiazepam	0.79
Chlorodesmethyldiazepam	0.74
1-Hydroxymethyl midazolam	0.71
Brotizolam	0.67
Triazolam	0.64
4-Hydroxymidazolam	0.59
Desalkylflurazepam	0.56
Alprazolam	0.54
Temazepam	0.54
Lorazepam	0.48
Oxazepam	0.45
Clobazam	0.40
Estazolam	0.39
Flurazepam aldehyde	0.38
Flunitrazepam	0.31
Nitrazepam	0.29
Desmethylclobazam	0.29
Clonazepam	0.28
Desmethylflunitrazepam	0.25
Bromazepam	0.24
Lormetazepam	0.22
Hydroxyethyl flurazepam	0.20
Ro-15-1788	0.15

[a] Higher values indicate greater lipid solubility (all numbers are relative to diazepam). See ref. 11 for description of method.

retention on a reverse-phase high-pressure liquid chromatographic (HPLC) system (10,11,45,98). Using either of these approaches, there are considerable differences among benzodiazepines in their characteristics of lipid solubility (Table 2). These variations, in turn, may alter some of their pharmacokinetic properties, including the rate of absorption from the gastrointestinal tract, the extent of distribution *in vivo,* and possibly also the rate of onset of activity following single doses (45).

Plasma Protein Binding

Benzodiazepine derivatives as a group of compounds also are extensively bound to serum or plasma protein (114). The extent of binding varies considerably among drugs, ranging from a free fraction of less than 2% in the case of diazepam, up to 30% or more in the case of alprazolam (95). For all benzodiazepines studied to date, free fraction is independent of total plasma concentration over a wide range of total concentrations (95) (Fig. 1).

The clinical importance of benzodiazepine plasma protein binding has been subject to considerable misinterpretation. Knowing the extent of binding of a specific benzodiazepine

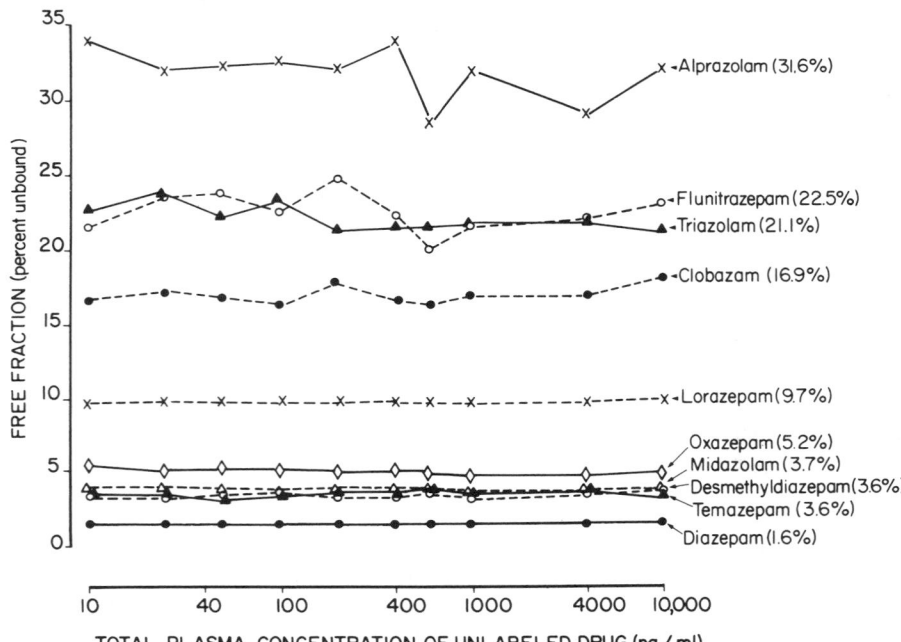

FIG. 1. Relationship of benzodiazepine free fraction in normal human plasma (*y*-axis) versus the total plasma drug concentration (*x*-axis). There are wide differences among the various benzodiazepines in the extent of protein binding (free fraction). Diazepam is most extensively bound (mean free fraction, 1.6%), whereas alprazolam is the least extensively bound (mean free fraction, 31.6%). Other benzodiazepines fall in between these extremes. However, for each benzodiazepine tested, free fraction in plasma was independent of total plasma concentration up to concentrations of 10,000 ng/ml. See ref. 95 for further explanation.

is of importance in *interpreting* pharmacokinetic data based on total plasma concentrations, particularly in the study of physiologic conditions or disease states [such as renal insufficiency (60,101), severe burns (88,89), and possibly old age] which may lead to alterations in protein binding (56,62,63). On the other hand, protein binding of benzodiazepines has no direct influence on clinical activity (62).

The primary binding protein for benzodiazepines appears to be albumin, although variations in serum albumin concentration account for only a small fraction of individual variability in the extent of protein binding. There is some evidence to suggest that the triazolobenzodiazepine triazolam binds to some degree to α_1-acid glycoprotein (85).

ONSET OF ACTION AFTER SINGLE INTRAVENOUS OR ORAL DOSES

The brain is the principal pharmacologic site of benzodiazepine activity. Pharmacodynamic effects are necessarily mediated by interaction with one or more functional molecular recognition sites located in brain tissue, which are widely assumed to correspond to the specific benzodiazepine binding site reported to be present in brain tissue of animals and humans (96,118,121). The extent of benzodiazepine uptake into brain must be an important determinant of the amount of drug available to interact with the receptor. The extent of entry of benzodiazepines into brain tissue is a process governed mainly by passive diffusion. Variations in lipid solubility explain a significant portion of the variability among the benzodiazepines in partitioning between brain and systemic plasma, that is, the extent of their uptake into brain tissue relative to any given unbound plasma concentration (43). Similar relationships may exist when benzodiazepine uptake into other tissues is examined, whether in experimental studies (31,75,123) or in human autopsy studies (30). Thus, benzodiazepine availability to the target tissue occurs as a result of passive diffusion, and the amount present in brain is proportional to the unbound drug concentration in plasma.

Not only is the extent of benzodiazepine uptake into brain determined by predictable physicochemical properties, but the rate of uptake and equilibrium is very rapid. The rapidity of this equilibrium has been demonstrated in a number of studies directed at quantitation of (a) actual measurement of the relative time course of benzodiazepine concentrations in brain and plasma following single doses in animals (29,73); (b) the entry of drug and subsequent equilibration with the cerebrospinal fluid (11,61,108); (c) the rapidity of onset of pharmacodynamic activity when measured by objective techniques such as the appearance of characteristic electroencephalographic activity (11) or alterations in saccadic eye movement velocity (122). Some studies suggest that although the onset of activity of all benzodiazepines is rapid following single intravenous injections, the small variability in time of onset of action may be explained by differences in their lipophilicity (122). Thus benzodiazepine equilibration between systemic plasma and brain tissue is rapid.

When benzodiazepines are given by extravascular routes of administration, such as by mouth or by intramuscular injection, the rate of absorption from the gastrointestinal tract or the site of injection appears to be the rate-limiting step in onset of clinical activity (45,50,90). Those benzodiazepines that are rapidly absorbed from the gastrointestinal tract have a prompt onset of clinical action, whereas those that are slowly absorbed have a much slower onset of action. Diazepam, desmethyldiazepam (formed from its precursor clorazepate), flurazepam (leading to its aldehyde and hydroxyethyl metabolites), and midazolam are the most rapidly absorbed benzodiazepines, generally reaching peak concentrations in blood within 1 hr after dosage (24,117). In the treatment of insomnia, rapid onset of action after oral dosage is a desirable objective for the treatment of sleep onset insomnia. During treatment of anxiety, the benefits of rapid onset of action are less well defined. Many patients experience the rapid onset of drug effects due to rapidly absorbed benzodiazepines as therapeutically beneficial, whereas others perceive the very same effects unfavorably, sensing some degree of drowsiness, loss of control, muscle relaxation, or feeling "spaced out." Whether favorable or unfavorable, these perceptions reflect the identical pharmacokinetic property of rapid drug absorption. How this is experienced by a given patient depends on his or her expectations, prior drug experience, and specific reason for drug administration.

Slowly absorbed benzodiazepines such as oxazepam, temazepam, and prazepam likewise must be evaluated in light of the specific clinical situation and the sensitivity of the individual patient. This type of drug might be of benefit for anxious patients wishing to avoid the prompt onset of central effects following each dose. Prazepam (117) or slow-release diazepam (Valrelease) (70,86), for example, is a reasonable choice for highly drug-sensitive individuals who feel excessively drowsy or "spaced out" after taking rapidly absorbed benzodiazepines.

All else being equal, benzodiazepine absorption will probably be more rapid when taken on an empty stomach than when given along with or just after food, since the drug must be delivered to the proximal small bowel before it can be absorbed into the systemic circulation (22,41). Absorption will also be slowed if a drug is given together with an aluminum-containing antacid such as Maalox (41).

FACTORS DETERMINING THE DURATION OF PHARMACODYNAMIC ACTION

The duration of clinical action of benzodiazepines is of considerable importance. For example, if a hypnotic agent has sedative actions that persist longer than the patient wishes to stay asleep, the sedation during the waking hours may be unfavorable, and is often termed "hangover." On the other hand, hypnotic drug effects that are too short in duration may lead to early morning awakening. Analogous scenarios are possible in other clinical situations, as when benzodiazepines are used for the treatment of anxiety, for preoperative sedation, or for the treatment of acute seizure disorders.

Clinical activity of benzodiazepines following single doses may be terminated by at least three mechanisms. Two of these mechanisms are pharmacokinetic, whereas the third

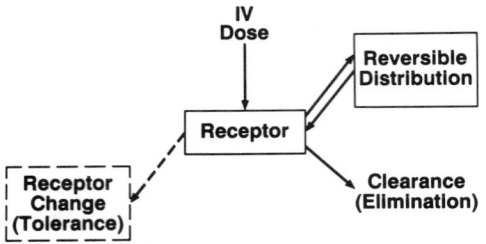

FIG. 2. Schematic representation of possible mechanisms by which benzodiazepine action may be terminated. It is assumed that following a rapid intravenous dose of a benzodiazepine derivative, the drug has rapid access to the receptor site in brain. Thereafter, drug action may be terminated by one or more of several mechanisms. Acute adaptation or tolerance (**lower left**) describes a change in intrinsic receptor sensitivity, such that any given drug concentration at the receptor elicits a reduced pharmacologic effect. This mechanism is important for all benzodiazepines. Drug action may also be terminated if the drug disappears from the receptor site due to pharmacokinetic mechanisms. The first possibility is reversible distribution (**upper right**), in which the drug distributes from the central compartment to peripheral storage sites, consisting mainly of adipose tissue, skeletal muscle, and liver. The drug may also be removed by irreversible clearance or elimination, in which the substance is biotransformed by the liver.

involves a functional change in the pharmacologic receptor mediating drug action (Fig. 2). In pharmacokinetic terms, benzodiazepine action may be terminated if the drug disappears from its receptor site. This may occur by reversible drug distribution, in which the drug egresses from its site of action in the brain and diffuses to peripheral storage sites, principally adipose tissue, skeletal muscle, and liver. A second pharmacokinetic mechanism is irreversible biotransformation or clearance, in which the drug disappears from the receptor site due to hepatic metabolism. The

receptor or molecular mechanism for termination of drug action is independent of the above two pharmacokinetic events, and is often called "acute tolerance" or "acute adaptation." Acute tolerance operationally describes the observation that receptors become less sensitive to drug effects as the duration of exposure to the drug becomes longer. Although the drug may have a constant concentration in blood, in whole brain, and at the receptor site, its pharmacodynamic effects are reduced because the receptor's intrinsic sensitivity to the drug decreases.

Acute tolerance contributes at least partly to the termination of action of essentially all benzodiazepines (28). These compounds are notorious for their capacity to produce adaptation or tolerance to a number of central actions. The precise molecular mechanisms are not fully understood, but many studies demonstrate tolerance to benzodiazepines following chronic dosage, as well as acute tolerance following single doses (17,28,68,111,120). It is likely that tolerance develops to different central actions of benzodiazepines at different rates, and that for any given central effect, different benzodiazepines may show different rates of inducing tolerance (27,28). Tolerance phenomena complicate attempts to relate benzodiazepine plasma concentrations to clinical effect, and indicate that duration of drug exposure must clearly be considered in studies of this type.

Pharmacokinetic contributions to termination of drug action can be quite different among the various benzodiazepines. Current data suggest that distribution rather than clearance is the most important pharmacokinetic terminator of action of benzodiazepines after single doses (11). Because all of these drugs are lipophilic substances, their plasma concentration profile following single doses—particularly single, rapid, intravenous injections—has a biphasic profile (Fig. 3). The initial rapid and precipitous phase of drug disappearance from plasma is attributed to drug distribution from the central compartment (including brain) to peripheral compartments. The extent of peripheral distribution

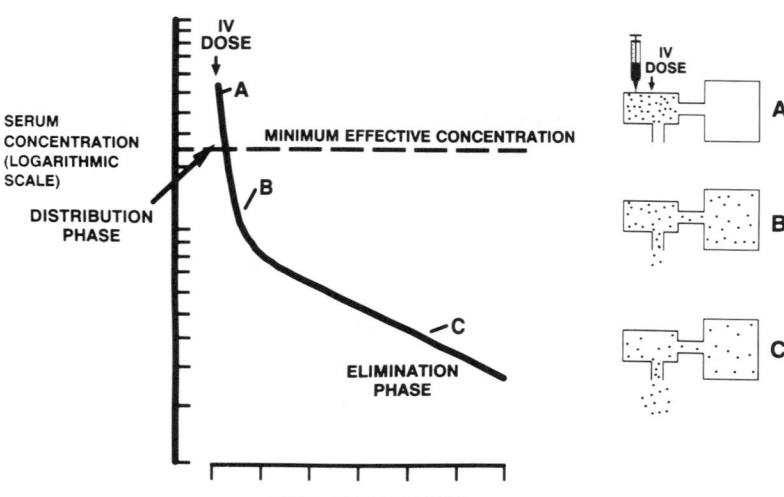

FIG. 3. Schematic representation of serum drug concentrations following an intravenous dose of a lipophilic substance, such as a benzodiazepine derivative, whose pharmacokinetic properties are consistent with a two-compartment model. On the **right** are diagrams representing phases of drug distribution, corresponding to the points on the serum concentration curve. Immediately after an intravenous dose (point A), drug concentrations in serum, and at the receptor site, are high, since the entire dose is confined within the central compartment. Between points A and B, there is a considerable decrement in drug concentrations in the central compartment (serum and brain), due mainly to distribution from central to peripheral compartments (point B), with only a small amount of drug removed by biotransformation. Assuming a minimal effective drug concentration as shown on the **left** of the slide, the decrement in concentrations due to the distribution phase may actually be responsible for terminating drug action. After distribution equilibrium is attained, drug disappearance from serum and from the receptor site enters a slower phase, which is governed mainly by biotransformation and elimination (point C).

(as determined by volume of distribution) increases as benzodiazepines become increasingly lipophilic (11,44). For highly lipid-soluble benzodiazepines such as diazepam and midazolam, the initial distribution phase following a single intravenous dose may actually cause a five- to 10-fold decline in plasma concentrations over the first 30 min to 3 hr after dosage, as the drug egresses from the "central compartment" into peripheral tissues. This phase of drug distribution can lead to termination of clinical effects, depending on which pharmacodynamic variable is under evaluation and how it is being quantitated. The drug's apparent elimination half-life represents a much slower phase that is determinable only after the distribution phase is complete (33). It is not surprising, therefore, that elimination half-life of benzodiazepines is not necessarily related to the time course of effects following single doses. Drugs with long half-lives may actually have very short durations

of action after single doses because of their very extensive distribution. Conversely, drugs that are relatively less lipophilic and have smaller volumes of distribution may have longer durations of action after single doses. In only a few cases does elimination or clearance contribute to terminating drug action in the first few hours after dosage. Midazolam is the most important example of such a drug (37). Midazolam has not only a high degree of lipophilicity and a large volume of distribution *in vivo,* but also a very high metabolic clearance and short half-life (Table 3). Thus, for midazolam, both clearance and distribution contribute to terminating drug action.

The dependence of single-dose pharmacodynamic action on drug distribution as opposed to elimination half-life explains why some clinical "paradoxes" are not really paradoxical. Comparable intravenous doses of diazepam and lorazepam, for example, may have very different

TABLE 3. *Pharmacokinetic summary of benzodiazepines*

Administered drug	Most common indication	Initial biotransformation pathway	Substances present in blood[a] (with usual range of elimination half-life, hr)	Representative references
Diazepam	Anxiolytic	Oxidation	Diazepam (20–70) Desmethyldiazepam (36–96) Oxazepam* Temazepam*	2, 4, 24, 25, 40, 87
Clorazepate[b]	Anxiolytic	Oxidation	Desmethyldiazepam (36–96)	105, 106, 115, 116
Prazepam[b]	Anxiolytic	Oxidation	Desmethyldiazepam (36–96)	7, 105
Oxazolam[b]	Anxiolytic	Oxidation	Desmethyldiazepam (36–96)	105
Halazepam	Anxiolytic	Oxidation	Halazepam* Desmethyldiazepam (36–96)	18, 58
Alprazolam	Anxiolytic	Oxidation	Alprazolam (8–15)	3, 48, 120
Lorazepam	Anxiolytic	Conjugation	Lorazepam (10–20)	1, 2, 5, 9, 32, 42, 53, 67, 97
Oxazepam	Anxiolytic	Conjugation	Oxazepam (5–15)	5, 32, 52, 104
Bromazepam	Anxiolytic	Oxidation	Bromazepam (20–30)	69, 83
Clobazam	Anxiolytic	Oxidation	Clobazam (20–30) Desmethylclobazam	54, 55, 103
Flurazepam	Hypnotic	Oxidation	Desalkylflurazepam (36–120) Hydroxyethyl flurazepam (1–4) Flurazepam aldehyde Flurazepam*	21, 26, 51, 76
Temazepam	Hypnotic	Conjugation	Temazepam (8–20)	23, 35, 76, 100, 119
Lormetazepam	Hypnotic	Conjugation	Lormetazepam (8–20)	74
Triazolam	Hypnotic	Oxidation	Triazolam (1.5–5)	3, 47, 76, 119
Brotizolam	Hypnotic	Oxidation	Brotizolam (4–7)	59, 113
Nitrazepam	Hypnotic	Nitroreduction	Nitrazepam (20–30)	38, 76, 80
Flunitrazepam	Hypnotic; perioperative	Oxidation; nitroreduction	Flunitrazepam (10–40) Desmethylflunitrazepam	15, 76, 81
Quazepam	Hypnotic	Oxidation	Quazepam (15–35) Oxoquazepam (25–35) Desalkylflurazepam (36–120)	71, 72
Estazolam	Hypnotic	Oxidation	Estazolam (20–30)	6
Midazolam	Perioperative; hypnotic	Oxidation	Midazolam (1–4) 1-Hydroxymethyl midazolam* 4-Hydroxy midazolam*	8, 12, 37, 82, 109
Clonazepam	Antiseizure	Nitroreduction	Clonazepam (30–60)	69, 83

[a] Asterisk (*) indicates compounds present in quantitatively minor amounts, and/or those that have reduced pharmacologic activity.

[b] Clorazepate, prazepam, and oxazolam all serve as desmethyldiazepam precursors.

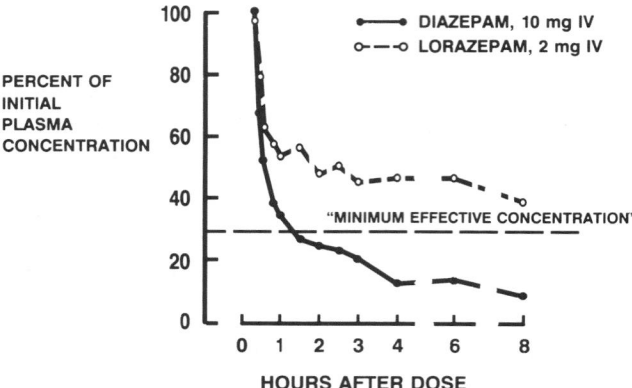

FIG. 4. A pharmacokinetic study in a healthy volunteer who received a single 10-mg intravenous dose of diazepam on one occasion and a single 2-mg intravenous dose of lorazepam on another occasion. Plasma concentrations for the first 8 hr after dosage are depicted as the fraction of the initial plasma concentration. It is further assumed that the drug's clinical activity will be evident as long as the plasma concentration remains equal to or higher than 30% of the initial plasma level. Because diazepam has a very large volume of distribution, plasma concentrations fall below the minimum effective level between 1 and 2 hr after dosage, leading to an apparent termination of drug action. In the case of lorazepam, having a smaller pharmacokinetic volume of distribution, plasma concentrations remain above the minimum effective level for a full 8 hr after dosage. Although lorazepam has a shorter elimination half-life than diazepam, the duration of action of lorazepam following a single intravenous dose may considerably exceed that of diazepam, because the extent of peripheral distribution of lorazepam is much smaller.

durations of action (Fig. 4). All else being equal, lorazepam will have a longer duration of action after a single dose than will a clinically comparable dose of diazepam (20,46). This occurs even though the elimination half-life of lorazepam is much shorter than that of diazepam.

ACCUMULATION OF BENZODIAZEPINES DURING MULTIPLE DOSAGE

The extent of benzodiazepine accumulation during repeated dosage depends in large part on the drug's elimination half-life in relation to the interval between doses (56,63). Benzodiazepines with long values of elimination half-life will accumulate extensively and slowly during repeated dosage at intervals of 24 hr or less (4,13,25,51,55,93,112). When treatment is terminated they will also disappear from the body at an equally slow rate (13,25,51,55,112,115). Benzodiazepines with short values of elimination half-life will accumulate minimally during repeated dosage and will reach the steady-state condition shortly after initiation of therapy (42,100,112). Short half-life benzodiazepines likewise disappear rapidly after termination of multiple-dose treatment (Table 3).

Both pharmacokinetic profiles have advantages and disadvantages. For long half-life benzodiazepines, possible cumulative sedative and performance-impairing effects may

develop over time during repeated dosage (19). The increasing drug concentrations in brain may theoretically produce correspondingly increased central nervous system depression, possibly leading to daytime drowsiness, sedation, or impairment of psychomotor or intellectual performance. Although this has been demonstrated with several long half-life benzodiazepines, particularly during the treatment of insomnia, the degree of central depression is not directly proportional to their concentration in blood. Despite the continuously increasing drug concentrations in blood and at the receptor site, central depression does not increase in parallel because of tolerance to the nonspecific depressant effects of the drug (13,77,112). Drowsiness, sedation, or impairment of performance may occur during the initial days or weeks of treatment, but these effects tend to abate over time despite continued administration of the same dose and continued drug accumulation (99). Thus adaptation at least partially offsets the tendency of accumulating benzodiazepines to produce cumulative sedative effects. After termination of treatment, long half-life benzodiazepines disappear from the body as slowly as they accumulated. This pattern of slow washout after termination of treatment may be beneficial, since "uncovering" of the receptor occurs at a similarly slow rate, thereby minimizing the likelihood of rapid recurrence of symptomatology and/or the development of withdrawal symptoms after treatment is terminated (13,78,79).

In contrast, the relative nonaccumulation of short half-life benzodiazepines during multiple dosage probably minimizes the likelihood of daytime sedative or performance-impairing effects. Patients may in fact experience increased alertness or even anxiety during the daytime (94). After termination of treatment, the rapid disappearance of the drug from blood and brain rapidly uncovers the receptor and increases the likelihood that recurrence of symptoms or drug withdrawal will be of rapid onset (78,79,93). Thus short half-life benzodiazepines must be tapered rather than abruptly discontinued at the termination of treatment.

BENZODIAZEPINE OXIDATION VERSUS CONJUGATION

The two major pathways for most currently available benzodiazepines involve hepatic biotransformation by one of two principal mechanisms: oxidation or conjugation. Only a few drugs are transformed by a third mechanism, nitroreduction (Table 3). Oxidative pathways produce relatively minor molecular modifications that may yield active pharmacologic intermediates (63). The two most common oxidative transformations are aliphatic hydroxylation and N-dealkylation, and many benzodiazepines are biotransformed by one of these pathways. The second principal biotransformation pathway of benzodiazepines is hepatic conjugation to glucuronic acid (63). Oxazepam, lorazepam, temazepam, and lormetazepam are metabolized by this mechanism. Unlike many products of oxidative biotransformation, glucuronide conjugates are pharmacologically inactive and are excreted in the urine as such.

Oxidation is termed a "susceptible" pathway, since oxidative activity can be impaired by a number of influences, including old age (47,48,72,116), liver disease such as cirrhosis or hepatitis (99), and coadministration of metabolic inhibitors such as cimetidine or estrogens (2,3,26,84,102). Conjugation, on the other hand, is a "nonsusceptible" pathway, since the same factors that can profoundly impair benzodiazepine oxidation may have little or no effect on conjugation (2,5,35,36,84,102,107).

These pharmacokinetic differences have led some to conclude that benzodiazepines transformed by conjugation may be "preferable" for the treatment of the elderly patient, those with liver disease, or those also receiving inhibitors such as cimetidine. Oxidized benzodiazepines, on the other hand, may be "potentially hazardous" in the same group of patients. This argument has sound theoretical rationale, but at present is only incompletely supported by clinical findings.

During multiple dosage with a benzodiazepine (or any other drug), its steady-state concentration (C_{ss}) in serum or plasma will be determined as follows:

$$C_{ss} = \frac{\text{Dosing Rate}}{\text{Clearance}}$$

At any given dosing rate, C_{ss} will increase if some factor intervenes to impair the drug's total metabolic clearance (63). However, the resulting increase in C_{ss} is not necessarily clinically important. Because benzodiazepines have an inherently large therapeutic index, an increase in C_{ss} in a given patient does not necessarily increase clinical effects or precipitate toxicity. In one study, multiple dosage with diazepam in cirrhotic patients led to higher steady-state levels compared to healthy controls; these higher levels were correlated with an increased perception of sedative effects (99). In this particular case, the impaired clearance of diazepam in cirrhotic patients appears to be of clinical importance, and the dosing rate of diazepam should be lower in cirrhotics relative to comparable patients with normal liver function. A second pharmacokinetic interaction whose clinical importance has been evaluated is the diazepam-cimetidine interaction (39). Coadministration of diazepam to cimetidine-treated patients caused increased steady-state concentrations of diazepam and desmethyldiazepam, but there were minimal alterations in therapeutic effects, and no appearance of potentially toxic drug effects. Thus the clinical importance of altered benzodiazepine clearance in disease states or from drug interactions cannot be assumed until established in controlled clinical trials.

THE IMPORTANCE OF BENZODIAZEPINE METABOLITES

Many benzodiazepines are biotransformed into pharmacologically active metabolites, which in turn appear in the systemic circulation in unconjugated and therefore potentially clinical important form (Table 3). This inevitably raises the question of which metabolites contribute to clinical activity, and the relative contribution of each metabolite to the activity of the parent compound. Unfortunately, this question usually does not have a simple or straightforward answer, since the ultimate clinical effect of such metabolic products depends on a composite of several factors, which must be evaluated collectively. The first of these is the quantitative extent to which a specific metabolite is formed. Some metabolites, such as the 4-hydroxy derivative of midazolam, appear in quantitatively small amounts relative to the parent compound or to other metabolic products (12). In other cases, as with the desmethyl products of diazepam or of clobazam, metabolite concentrations are similar to or higher than those of the parent drug. Sometimes it is the *parent drug* concentrations that are quantitatively small relative to the metabolites; this is the case, for example, with flurazepam, plasma concentrations of which are much lower than those of the aldehyde, hydroxyethyl, and desalkyl products (21). The second determinant of metabolite activity is the extent to which it reaches brain tissue. This, in turn, is related to its lipid solubility and its binding to serum or plasma protein. Increasing lipophilicity is associated with increased uptake into brain tissue. Reduced protein is associated with an increased fraction of the total plasma concentration available for diffusion out of the vascular system into peripheral tissues, including brain. Brain uptake of specific benzodiazepines can be measured in experimental models, based on the ratio of the brain concentration divided by the unbound plasma

TABLE 4. *Evaluating possible clinical importance of benzodiazepine metabolites*

	Quantitative importance	Lipophilicity (HPLC Index)[a]	Brain/free plasma ratio[b]	Receptor K_i[c]
I. Diazepam and desmethyldiazepam				
Parent drug: diazepam	+	1.00	26.1	9.6
Metabolite: desmethyldiazepam	+	0.79	22.8	5.6
II. Clobazam and desmethylclobazam				
Parent drug: clobazam	+	0.40	6.0	222.5
Metabolite: desmethylclobazam	++	0.29	8.0	2,843.0

[a] Higher numbers indicate greater lipid solubility (see Table 2). Data kindly provided by Dr. Rainer M. Arendt.

[b] Based on data from ref. 43.

[c] Based on *in vitro* affinity using GABA-free membranes. Data kindly provided by Dr. Steven M. Paul.

concentration at equilibrium. Finally, the contribution of a metabolite to overall clinical outcome depends also on its "intrinsic" activity, usually measured by its affinity for the benzodiazepine receptor *in vitro*.

How the above factors should be combined or weighted is not established. However, an intuitive approach may yield a reasonable estimate as to whether a particular metabolite is of importance. As one example, consider diazepam (DZ) and its metabolite, desmethyldiazepam (DMDZ). During multiple-dose therapy with DZ, steady-state plasma concentrations of DMDZ equal or slightly exceed those of DZ, indicating quantitative importance (14,25,57,110). DMDZ lipophilicity is close to that of DZ, and the brain/unbound plasma concentration ratio for the two compounds is similar. Finally, the affinity of DMDZ for the benzodiazepine receptor actually exceeds that of DZ (Table 4). Taken collectively, these data indicate that DMDZ most probably does contribute to overall clinical activity during chronic therapy with DZ. As a contrasting example, consider clobazam (CBZ), and its metabolite desmethylclobazam (DMCBZ). During chronic treatment with CBZ, DMCBZ is of quantitative importance, with steady-state DMCBZ concentrations exceeding those of CBZ by twofold or more (55,103). Furthermore, the brain/unbound plasma ratios for CBZ and DMCBZ are similar. However, the affinity of DMCBZ for the benzodiazepine receptor is more than 10-fold lower than that of CBZ (Table 4), making it unlikely that DMCBZ adds an important component to the overall clinical action of CBZ.

ACKNOWLEDGMENTS

We are grateful for the collaboration and assistance of D. R. Abernethy, H. R. Ochs, R. M. Arendt, J. M. Scavone, H. Friedman, M. K. Divoll, J. S. Harmatz, L. G. Miller, and A. Locniskar. This work was supported in part by grants MH-34223 and AG-00106 from the United States Public Health Service.

REFERENCES

1. Abernethy, D. R., Greenblatt, D. J., Ameer, B., and Shader, R. I. (1985): *J. Pharmacol. Exp. Ther.,* 234:345–349.
2. Abernethy, D. R., Greenblatt, D. J., Divoll, M., Ameer, B., and Shader, R. I. (1983): *J. Pharmacol. Exp. Ther.,* 224:508–513.
3. Abernethy, D. R., Greenblatt, D. J., Divoll, M., Moschitto, L. J., Harmatz, J. S., and Shader, R. I. (1983): *Psychopharmacology,* 80:275–278.
4. Abernethy, D. R., Greenblatt, D. J., Divoll, M., and Shader, R. I. (1983): *J. Clin. Pharmacol.,* 23:369–376.
5. Abernethy, D. R., Greenblatt, D. J., Ochs, H. R., Weyers, D., Divoll, M., Harmatz, J. S., and Shader, R. I. (1983): *Clin. Pharmacol. Ther.,* 33:628–632.
6. Allen, M. D., Greenblatt, D. J., and Arnold, J. D. (1979): *Psychopharmacology,* 66:267–274.
7. Allen, M. D., Greenblatt, D. J., Harmatz, J. S., and Shader, R. I. (1980): *Clin. Pharmacol. Ther.,* 28:196–202.
8. Allonen, H., Ziegler, G., and Klotz, U. (1981): *Clin. Pharmacol. Ther.,* 30:653–661.
9. Ameer, B., and Greenblatt, D. J. (1981): *Drugs,* 21:161–200.
10. Arendt, R. M., and Greenblatt, D. J. (1984): *J. Pharm. Pharmacol.,* 36:400–401.
11. Arendt, R. M., Greenblatt, D. J., deJong, R. H., Bonin, J. D., Abernethy, D. R., Ehrenberg, B. L., Giles, H. G., Sellers, E. M., and Shader, R. I. (1983): *J. Pharmacol. Exp. Ther.,* 227:95–106.
12. Arendt, R. M., Greenblatt, D. J., and Garland, W. A. (1984): *Pharmacology,* 29:158–164.
13. Bliwise, D., Seidel, W., Greenblatt, D. J., and Dement, W. (1984): *Am. J. Psychiatry,* 141:191–195.
14. Bowden, C. L., and Fisher, J. G. (1980): *South. Med. J.,* 73: 1581–1584.
15. Boxenbaum, H. G., Posmanter, H. N., Macasieb, T., Geitner, K. A., Weinfeld, R. E., Moore, J. D., Darragh, A., O'Kelly, D. A., Weissman, L., and Kaplan, S. A. (1978): *J. Pharmacokin. Biopharm.,* 6:283–293.
16. Breimer, D. D. (1979): *Br. J. Clin. Pharmacol.,* 8(Suppl.):7s–13s.
17. Breimer, D. D., Jochemsen, R., Kamphuisen, H. A. C., Nicholson, A. N., Spencer, M. B., and Stone, B. M. (1985): *Br. J. Clin. Pharmacol.,* 19:807–815.
18. Chung, M., Hilbert, J. M., Gural, R. P., Radwanski, E., Symchowicz, S., and Zampaglione, N. (1984): *Clin. Pharmacol. Ther.,* 35:838–842.
19. Church, M. W., and Johnson, L. C. (1979): *Psychopharmacology,* 61:309–316.
20. Conner, J. T., Katz, R. L., Bellville, J. W., Graham, C., Pagano, R., and Dorey, F. (1978): *J. Clin. Pharmacol.,* 18:285–292.
21. Cooper, S. F., Drolet, D., and Dugal, R. (1984): *Biopharm. Drug. Dispos.,* 5:127–139.
22. Divoll, M., Greenblatt, D. J., Ciraulo, D. A., Puri, S. K., Ho, I., and Shader, R. I. (1982): *J. Clin. Pharmacol.,* 22:69–73.
23. Divoll, M., Greenblatt, D. J., Harmatz, J. S., and Shader, R. I. (1981): *J. Pharm. Sci.,* 70:1104–1107.
24. Divoll, M., Greenblatt, D. J., Ochs, H. R., and Shader, R. I. (1983): *Anesth. Analges.,* 62:1–8.
25. Eatman, F. B., Colburn, W. A., Boxenbaum, H. G., Posmanter, H. N., Weinfeld, R. E., Ronfeld, R., Weissman, L., Moore, J. D., Gibaldi, M., and Kaplan, S. A. (1977): *J. Pharmacokinet. Biopharm.,* 5:481–494.
26. Eckert, M., Ziegler, W. H., Cano, J. P., Bovey, F., Amrein, R., Coassolo, P. H., Schalch, E., and Burckhardt, J. (1983): *Drugs Exp. Clin. Res.,* 9:77–99.
27. Ellinwood, E. H., Heatherly, D. G., Nikaido, A. M., Bjornsson, T. D., and Kilts, C. (1985): *Psychopharmacology,* 86:392–399.
28. File, S. E. (1985): *Neurosci. Biobehav. Rev.,* 9:113–121.
29. Friedman, H., Abernethy, D. R., Greenblatt, D. J., and Shader, R. I. (1986): *Psychopharmacology,* 88:267–270.
30. Friedman, H., Ochs, H. R., Greenblatt, D. J., and Shader, R. I. (1985): *J. Clin. Pharmacol.,* 25:613–615.
31. Friedman, H. L., Scavone, J. M., Greenblatt, D. J., and Shader, R. I. (1985): *Pharmacology,* 27:207.
32. Greenblatt, D. J. (1981): *Clin. Pharmacokinet.,* 6:88–105.
33. Greenblatt, D. J. (1985): *Annu. Rev. Med.,* 36:421–427.
34. Greenblatt, D. J., Abernethy, D. R., Divoll, M., Harmatz, J. S., and Shader, R. I. (1983): *J. Clin. Psychopharmacol.,* 3:129–132.
35. Greenblatt, D. J., Abernethy, D. R., Divoll, M., Locniskar, A., Harmatz, J. S., and Shader, R. I. (1984): *J. Pharm. Sci.,* 73:399–401.
36. Greenblatt, D. J., Abernethy, D. R., Koepke, H. H., and Shader, R. I. (1984): *J. Clin. Pharmacol.,* 24:187–193.
37. Greenblatt, D. J., Abernethy, D. R., Locniskar, A., Harmatz, J. S., Limjuco, R. A., and Shader, R. I. (1984): *Anesthesiology,* 61:27–35.
38. Greenblatt, D. J., Abernethy, D. R., Locniskar, A., Ochs, H. R., Harmatz, J. S., and Shader, R. I. (1985): *Clin. Pharmacol. Ther.,* 38:697–703.
39. Greenblatt, D. J., Abernethy, D. R., Morse, D. S., Harmatz, J. S., and Shader, R. I. (1984): *N. Engl. J. Med.,* 310:1639–1643.
40. Greenblatt, D. J., Allen, M. D., Harmatz, J. S., and Shader, R. I. (1980): *Clin. Pharmacol. Ther.,* 27:301–312.
41. Greenblatt, D. J., Allen, M. D., MacLaughlin, D. S., Harmatz, J. S., and Shader, R. I. (1978): *Clin. Pharmacol. Ther.,* 24:600–609.
42. Greenblatt, D. J., Allen, M. D., MacLaughlin, D. S., Huffman, D. H., Harmatz, J. S., and Shader, R. I. (1979): *J. Pharmacokin. Biopharm.,* 7:159–179.
43. Greenblatt, D. J., and Arendt, R. M. (1985): *Pharmacologist,* 27: 207.
44. Greenblatt, D. J., Arendt, R. M., Abernethy, D. R., Giles, H. G., Sellers, E. M., and Shader, R. I. (1983): *Br. J. Anaesthes.,* 55: 985–989.

45. Greenblatt, D. J., Arendt, R. M., and Shader, R. I. (1984): In: *Sleep, Benzodiazepines, and Performance,* edited by I. Hindmarch, H. Ott, and T. Roth, pp. 92–97. Springer-Verlag, Berlin.

46. Greenblatt, D. J., and Divoll, M. (1983): In: *Status Epilepticus: Mechanisms of Brain Damage and Treatment (Advances in Neurology, Vol. 34),* edited by A. V. Delgado-Escueta, C. G. Wasterlain, D. M. Treiman, and R. J. Porter, pp. 487–491. Raven Press, New York.

47. Greenblatt, D. J., Divoll, M., Abernethy, D. R., Moschitto, L. J., Smith, R. B., and Shader, R. I. (1983): *Br. J. Clin. Pharmacol.,* 15:303–309.

48. Greenblatt, D. J., Divoll, M., Abernethy, D. R., Moschitto, L. J., Smith, R. B., and Shader, R. I. (1983): *Arch. Gen. Psychiatry,* 40:287–290.

49. Greenblatt, D. J., Divoll, M., Abernethy, D. R., Ochs, H. R., and Shader, R. I. (1983): *Drug Metab. Rev.,* 14:251–292.

50. Greenblatt, D. J., Divoll, M., Abernethy, D. R., Ochs, H. R., and Shader, R. I. (1983): *Clin. Pharmacokinet.,* 8:233–253.

51. Greenblatt, D. J., Divoll, M., Harmatz, J. S., MacLaughlin, D. S., and Shader, R. I. (1981): *Clin. Pharmacol. Ther.,* 30:475–486.

52. Greenblatt, D. J., Divoll, M., Harmatz, J. S., and Shader, R. I. (1980): *J. Pharmacol. Exp. Ther.,* 215:86–91.

53. Greenblatt, D. J., Divoll, M., Harmatz, J. S., and Shader, R. I. (1982): *J. Pharm. Sci.,* 71:248–252.

54. Greenblatt, D. J., Divoll, M., Puri, S. K., Ho, I., Zinny, M. A., and Shader, R. I. (1981): *Br. J. Clin. Pharmacol.,* 12:631–636.

55. Greenblatt, D. J., Divoll, M., Puri, S. K., Ho, I., Zinny, M. A., and Shader, R. I. (1983): *Clin. Pharmacokinet.,* 8:83–94.

56. Greenblatt, D. J., and Koch-Weser, J. (1975): *N. Engl. J. Med.,* 293:702–705.

57. Greenblatt, D. J., Laughren, T. P., Allen, M. D., Harmatz, J. S., and Shader, R. I. (1981): *Br. J. Clin. Pharmacol.,* 11:35–40.

58. Greenblatt, D. J., Locniskar, A., and Shader, R. I. (1983): *Psychopharmacology,* 80:178–180.

59. Greenblatt, D. J., Locniskar, A., and Shader, R. I. (1983): *Sleep,* 6:72–76.

60. Greenblatt, D. J., Murray, T. G., Audet, P. R., Locniskar, A., Koepke, H. H., and Walker, B. R. (1983): *Nephron.,* 34:234–238.

61. Greenblatt, D. J., Ochs, H. R., and Lloyd, B. L. (1980): *Psychopharmacology,* 70:89–93.

62. Greenblatt, D. J., Sellers, E. M., and Koch-Weser, J. (1982): *J. Clin. Pharmacol.,* 22:259–263.

63. Greenblatt, D. J., and Shader, R. I. (1985): *Pharmacokinetics in Clinical Practice.* W. B. Saunders, Philadelphia.

64. Greenblatt, D. J., and Shader, R. I. (1985): In: *The Benzodiazepines: Current Standards for Medical Practice,* edited by D. E. Smith and D. R. Wesson, pp. 43–58. MTP Press, Lancaster, England.

65. Greenblatt, D. J., Shader, R. I., and Abernethy, D. R. (1983): *N. Engl. J. Med.,* 309:354–358,410–416.

66. Greenblatt, D. J., Shader, R. I., Abernethy, D. R., Ochs, H. R., Divoll, M., and Sellers, E. M. (1982): In: *Pharmacology of Benzodiazepines,* edited by E. Usdin, P. Skolnick, J. F. Tallman, D. Greenblatt, and S. M. Paul, pp. 257–269. Macmillan Press, London.

67. Greenblatt, D. J., Shader, R. I., Franke, K., MacLaughlin, D. S., Harmatz, J. S., Allen, M. D., Werner, A., and Woo, E. (1979): *J. Pharm. Sci.,* 68:57–63.

68. Greenblatt, D. J., Shader, R. I., Harmatz, J. S., and Georgotas, A. (1979): *Psychopharmacology,* 66:289–290.

69. Guentert, T. W. (1984): *Prog. Drug Metab.,* 8:241–386.

70. Gustafson, J. H., Weissman, L., Weinfeld, R. E., Holazo, A. A., Khoo, K.-O., and Kaplan, S. A. (1981): *J. Pharmacokinet. Biopharm.,* 9:679–691.

71. Hilbert, J. M., Chung, M., Maier, G., Gural, R., Symchowicz, S., and Zampaglione, N. (1984): *Clin. Pharmacol. Ther.,* 36:99–104.

72. Hilbert, J. M., Chung, M., Radwanski, E., Gural, R., Symchowicz, S., and Zampaglione, N. (1984): *Clin. Pharmacol. Ther.,* 36:566–569.

73. Hironaka, T., Fuchino, K., and Fujii, T. (1984): *J. Pharmacol. Exp. Ther.,* 229:809–815.

74. Hümpel, M., Nieuweboer, B., Milius, W., Hanke, H., and Wendt, H. (1980): *Clin. Pharmacol. Ther.,* 28:673–679.

75. Igari, Y., Sugiyama, Y., Sawada, Y., et al. (1982): *Drug Metab. Dispos.,* 10:676–679.

76. Jochemsen, R., van Boxtel, C. J., Hermans, J., and Breimer, D. D. (1983): *Clin. Pharmacol. Ther.,* 34:42–47.

77. Johnson, L. C., and Chernik, D. A. (1982): *Psychopharmacology,* 76:101–113.

78. Kales, A., and Kales, J. D. (1983): *J. Clin. Psychopharmacol.,* 3:140–150.

79. Kales, A., Soldatos, C. R., Bixler, E. O., and Kales, J. D. (1983): *Pharmacology,* 26:121–137.

80. Kangas, L., and Breimer, D. D. (1981): *Clin. Pharmacokinet.,* 6:346–366.

81. Kangas, L., Kanto, J., and Pakkanen, A. (1982): *Int. J. Clin. Pharmacol. Ther. Toxicol.,* 20:585–588.

82. Kanto, J. H. (1985): *Pharmacotherapy,* 5:138–154.

83. Klotz, U., Kangas, L., and Kanto, J. (1980): *Prog. Pharmacol.,* 3(3):1–72.

84. Klotz, U., and Reimann, I. (1980): *Eur. J. Clin. Pharmacol.,* 18:517–520.

85. Kroboth, P. D., Smith, R. B., Sorkin, M. I., Silver, M. R., Rault, R., Garry, M., and Juhl, R. P. (1984): *Clin. Pharmacol. Ther.,* 36:379–383.

86. Locniskar, A., Greenblatt, D. J., Zinny, M. A., Harmatz, J. S., and Shader, R. I. (1984): *J. Clin. Pharmacol.,* 24:255–263.

87. Mandelli, M., Tognoni, G., and Garattini, S. (1978): *Clin. Pharmacokinet.,* 3:72–91.

88. Martyn, J. A. J., Abernethy, D. R., and Greenblatt, D. J. (1984): *Clin. Pharmacol. Ther.,* 35:535–539.

89. Martyn, J. A. J., Greenblatt, D. J., and Quinby, W. C. (1983): *Anesthes. Analges.,* 62:293–297.

90. Mattila, M. J., Mattila, M., and Tuomainen, P. (1985): *Med. Biol.,* 63:21–27.

91. Mellinger, G. D., Balter, M. B., and Uhlenhuth, E. H. (1984): *JAMA* 251:375–379.

92. Mellinger, G. D., Balter, M. B., and Uhlenhuth, E. H. (1985): *Arch. Gen. Psychiatry,* 42:225–232.

93. Mitler, M. M., Seidel, W. F., van den Hoed, J., Greenblatt, D. J., and Dement, W. C. (1984): *J. Clin. Psychopharmacol.,* 4:2–13.

94. Morgan, K., and Oswald, I. (1984): *Br. Med. J.,* 284:942.

95. Moschitto, L. J., and Greenblatt, D. J. (1983): *J. Pharm. Pharmacol.,* 35:179–180.

96. Müller, W. E. (1981): *Pharmacology,* 22:153–161.

97. Nielsen-Kudsk, F., Jensen, T. S., Magnussen, I., Jakobsen, P., Jensen, P. B., Mondrup, K., and Peterson, T. (1983): *Acta Pharmacol. Toxicol.,* 52:121–127.

98. Ochs, H. R., Greenblatt, D. J., Abernethy, D. R., Arendt, R. M., Gerloff, J., Eichelkraut, W., and Hahn, N. (1985): *J. Pharm. Pharmacol.,* 37:428–431.

99. Ochs, H. R., Greenblatt, D. J., Eckardt, B., Harmatz, J. S., and Shader, R. I. (1983): *Clin. Pharmacol. Ther.,* 33:471–476.

100. Ochs, H. R., Greenblatt, D. J., and Heuer, H. (1984): *J. Clin. Pharmacol.,* 24:58–64.

101. Ochs, H. R., Greenblatt, D. J., Kaschell, H. J., Klehr, U., Divoll, M., and Abernethy, D. R. (1981): *Br. J. Clin. Pharmacol.,* 12:829–832.

102. Ochs, H. R., Greenblatt, D. J., and Knüchel, M. (1983): *Br. J. Clin. Pharmacol.,* 16:743–746.

103. Ochs, H. R., Greenblatt, D. J., Lüttkenhorst, M., and Verburg-Ochs, B. (1984): *Eur. J. Clin. Pharmacol.,* 26:499–503.

104. Ochs, H. R., Greenblatt, D. J., and Otten, H. (1981): *Klin. Wochenschr.,* 59:899–903.

105. Ochs, H. R., Greenblatt, D. J., Verburg-Ochs, B., and Locniskar, A. (1984): *J. Clin. Pharmacol.,* 24:446–451.

106. Ochs, H. R., Steinhaus, E., Locniskar, A., Knüchel, M., and Greenblatt, D. J. (1982): *Klin. Wochenschr.,* 60:411–415.

107. Patwardhan, R. V., Yarborough, G. W., Desmond, P. V., Johnson, R. F., Schenker, S., and Speeg, K. V. (1980): *Gastroenterology,* 79:912–916.

108. Ramsay, R. E., Hammond, E. J., Perchalski, R. J., and Wilder, B. J. (1979): *Arch. Neurol.,* 36:535–539.

109. Reves, J. G., Fragen, R. H., Vinik, H. R., and Greenblatt, D. J. (1985): *Anesthesiology,* 62:310–324.

110. Rickels, K., Case, W. G., Downing, R. W., Dixon, R., and Fridman, R. (1984): *Pharmacopsychiatry,* 17:44–49.

111. Rosenberg, H. C., and Chiu, T. H. (1985): *Neurosci. Biobehav. Rev.,* 9:123–131.

112. Salzman, C., Shader, R. I., Greenblatt, D. J., and Harmatz, J. S. (1983): *Arch. Gen. Psychiatry,* 40:293–297.

113. Scavone, J. M., Greenblatt, D. J., Harmatz, J. S., and Shader, R. I. (1986): *Br. J. Clin. Pharmacol.,* 21:197–204.

114. Sellers, E. M., Naranjo, C. A., Khouw, V., and Greenblatt, D. J. (1982): In: *Pharmacology of Benzodiazepines,* edited by E. Usdin, P. Skolnick, J. F. Tallman, D. J. Greenblatt, and S. M. Paul, pp. 271–284. Macmillan Press, London.

115. Shader, R. I., Ciraulo, D. A., Greenblatt, D. J., and Harmatz, J. S. (1982): *Clin. Pharmacol. Ther.,* 31:180–183.

116. Shader, R. I., Greenblatt, D. J., Ciraulo, D. A., Divoll, M., Harmatz, J. S., and Georgotas, A. (1981): *Psychopharmacology,* 75:193–197.

117. Shader, R. I., Pary, R. J., Harmatz, J. S., Allison, S., Locniskar, A., and Greenblatt, D. J. (1984): *J. Clin. Psychiatry,* 45:411–413.

118. Skolnick, P., and Paul, S. M. (1982): *Int. Rev. Neurobiol.,* 23:103–140.

119. Smith, R. B., Divoll, M., Gillespie, W. R., and Greenblatt, D. J. (1983): *J. Clin. Psychopharmacol.,* 3:172–176.

120. Smith, R. B., Kroboth, P. D., Vanderlugt, J. T., Phillips, J. P., and Juhl, R. P. (1984): *Psychopharmacology,* 84:452–456.

121. Tallman, J. F., Paul, S. M., Skolnick, P., and Gallager, D. W. (1980): *Science,* 207:274–281.

122. Tedeschi, G., Smith, A. T., Dhillon, S., and Richens, A. (1983): *Br. J. Clin. Pharmacol.,* 15:103–107.

123. van der Kleijn, E. (1969): *Arch. Int. Pharmacodyn.,* 178:193–215.

Psychopharmacology:
The Third Generation of Progress,
edited by Herbert Y. Meltzer.
Raven Press, New York © 1987.

CHAPTER **145**

Pharmacokinetics and Actions of Methylphenidate

Kennerly S. Patrick, Robert A. Mueller, C. Thomas Gualtieri, and George R. Breese

The central stimulant methylphenidate (MPH, Ritalin), is the drug of choice in the management of symptoms of attentional deficit disorder with hyperactivity (ADD-H). MPH can produce a variety of responses in children with ADD-H symptoms. At similar doses of MPH, exaggerated, variable, or insufficient behavioral changes can be observed. Although such findings may indicate diagnostic subgroups, individual differences in absorption and disposition of MPH could also explain the variability in drug response. Accordingly, the pharmacokinetics of MPH and selected MPH metabolites have recently been evaluated in children undergoing therapy. This work was complemented by preclinical studies of the distribution and pharmacological activity of MPH and metabolites. It is possible that a better understanding of the pharmacokinetics and pharmacodynamics of MPH will permit an improvement in the quality of pharmacotherapy for these children, analogous to the improvement presently being realized in the management of epilepsy through monitoring of anticonvulsant blood levels (63).

In the present chapter, the pharmacokinetics of MPH are summarized, the available analytical techniques for measuring MPH are presented, and the relevance of the MPH pharmacokinetics to drug effect is discussed.

CHEMISTRY

MPH [methyl phenyl-2-(2′-piperidyl)acetate] is a secondary amine containing a methyl ester and possessing two chiral centers that give rise to four optical isomers: *d-threo, l-threo, d-erythro,* and *l-erythro.* Synthesis of MPH yields an 80:20 *dl*-erythro:*dl* = threo mixture (90). Only the *threo* racemate produces the desired central stimulant action, whereas the *erythro* racemate contributes to hypertensive side effects and exhibits lethality in rats comparable to that of the *threo* racemate (84). The current pharmaceutical products contain only the *threo* racemate. The *d-threo* enantiomer of MPH possesses the 2R:2′R absolute stereochemistry (Fig. 1) (74). This enantiomer is believed to be responsible for the therapeutic activity of the racemic drug, though data to support this position are limited (48,56).

Intramolecular hydrogen bonding of MPH (64,90) may account for its being a weaker base than the structurally related amphetamines (48). At physiologic pH, approximately 7% of MPH is present as the lipid-diffusible free base. This fraction is sufficiently high to permit rapid extraction and accumulation in highly perfused tissues (55,57).

The stability of MPH in aqueous solution at 80°C was observed to be greatest at pH 2.86 (79). At pH 7.0 and 37°C in Sorensen's phosphate buffer, 50% of MPH is hydrolyzed in 25 hr, at 7.4 and 7.6 the $t_{\frac{1}{2}}$ is reduced to 11 and 6.3 hr, respectively (20), demonstrating the extreme dependence of the rate of hydrolysis on pH. At room temperature in pooled human plasma, MPH is comparatively stable, with a $t_{\frac{1}{2}}$ of 42.8 hr. The hydrolysis $t_{\frac{1}{2}}$ decreases to 5.68 hr at 37°C (89). Deesterification of MPH occurs rapidly in mouse liver or kidney homogenates, but is slow in brain tissue (62). Such data clearly indicate the need to cool biological samples after collection to minimize hydrolysis. Further, storage with ethylenediaminetetraacetic acid may reduce the rate of hydrolysis (41).

Since MPH is a basic drug, plasma protein binding

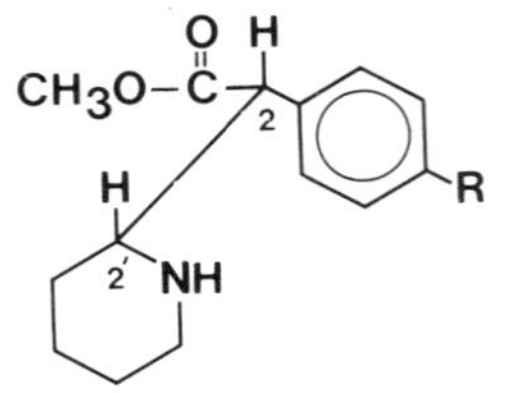

FIG. 1. d-threo-[2R:2R']-MPH.

would be expected to be associated with α-acid glycoprotein and lipoprotein fractions, not primarily with albumin, which generally binds acidic drugs (9). However, binding of MPH to 4% albumin in pH 7.4 buffer (25) is comparable to binding to whole plasma, 12 and 15%, respectively (41,93). The large free fraction of MPH should facilitate metabolism and tissue extraction, perhaps contributing to the short plasma elimination $t_{\frac{1}{2}}$ of MPH (89).

METABOLISM

Although early studies examining the metabolism of MPH in rats (8) and guinea pigs (78) postulated extensive drug biotransformation, only the deesterified product, ritalinic acid, was identified (Fig. 2). After oral administration of radiolabeled MPH to humans, approximately 70 to 80% of the radioactivity is excreted in urine in 24 hr, primarily as ritalinic acid (25,67) and 6-oxoritalinic acid (7). Thin layer chromatographic analysis of human plasma samples collected 2 hr following administration of labeled MPH indicates that >75% of the total radioactivity is ritalinic acid, whereas compounds appearing to be p-hydroxyritalinic acid and 6-oxoritalinic acid comprise approximately 1 and 2% of the activity, respectively. In rat, unlike human or dog, an appreciable amount of MPH metabolites is eliminated in feces (25). As with amphetamine (81), rats generate substantially more p-hydroxylated metabolites of MPH than do humans. Accordingly, rats excrete in urine p-hydroxy-MPH (15%), p-hydroxyritalinic acid (20%), and its glucuronide (10%) after an i.p. dose of MPH (25).

Lactam formation rather than para-hydroxylation is the predominant oxidative route of metabolism in the dog. After oral MPH, Egger et al. (23) determined that 6-oxoritalinic acid and its glucuronide accounted for 47% of the urinary excretion products in this species. Dogs were found to further metabolize 6-oxo-MPH enantioselectively to 5-hydroxy-6-oxo-MPH (1%), its glucuronide (12%), and the corresponding ritalinic acid conjugate (4%). Several minor metabolites were also identified, including 4-hydroxy-6-oxo-MPH glucuronide, N-carbamyl-MPH, N-carbamyl-ritalinic acid, and p-hydroxy-6-oxoritalinic acid taurine amide.

ROLE OF METABOLITES IN THE PHARMACOLOGY OF METHYLPHENIDATE

Metabolic hydroxylation of such structurally diverse psychotropic agents as chlorpromazine (46), diazepam (2), and amphetamine (13) yields centrally active derivatives that may contribute to the pharmacology of the parent compounds in humans. The detection of p-hydroxy-MPH as the principal metabolite in rat brain and its hydrolytic product as a urinary metabolite in humans (25) prompted speculation that the hydroxy ester may represent a clinically significant metabolite of MPH (20,41). Although this metabolite was believed to diffuse into the CNS more readily

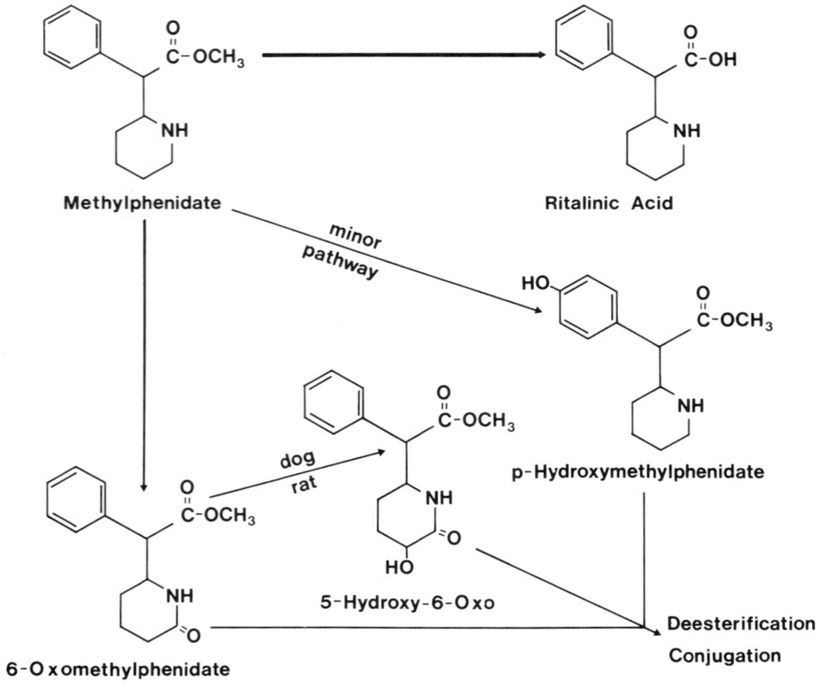

FIG. 2. Metabolic pathway for MPH.

Methylphenidate

Ritalinic Acid

minor pathway

p-Hydroxymethylphenidate

dog rat

5-Hydroxy-6-Oxo

6-Oxomethylphenidate

Deesterification
Conjugation

than the parent drug (20,41,93), this view has been discounted (60). A role for *p*-hydroxy-MPH in the pharmacology of MPH is appealing in view of the very low concentration of MPH in plasma after therapeutic doses. Since typical doses of amphetamine result in significantly higher plasma concentrations than for MPH (77), the latter drug is either a very potent stimulant or is converted to an active metabolite. Adding to the initial interest in *p*-hydroxy-MPH, the metabolite was believed to be a serotonin agonist (93). An early evaluation of locomotor-inducing activity of this metabolite indicated relatively low potency. However, the administered substance contained only 30% of the pharmaceutically relevant *threo* racemate (25). Patrick et al. (59) subsequently synthesized pure *dl-threo-p*-hydroxy-MPH, and the locomotor-inducing activity after intracerebroventricular administration was found to be nearly twice that of the parent compound (Fig. 3).

As attractive as this role for an active metabolite was, the notion was dispelled when highly specific and sensitive analytical methods were brought to bear on the question. Using a deuterated variant of *p*-hydroxy-MPH as an internal standard for gas chromatography-mass spectrometry (GC-MS) quantitation, the metabolite is not detected in plasma samples from human subjects administered MPH, and in contrast to an earlier report (25), is detected only in trace amounts relative to the parent drug in the brain of rats administered MPH. However, microgram per gram quantities of *p*-hydroxy-MPH are detected in rat liver (57) and low nanogram per milliliter concentrations in human urine (58).

Faraj et al. (25) speculated that metabolically formed *p*-hydroxy-MPH may be optically active due to enantioselective hydroxylation of the racemic drug. Recent studies in our laboratory have demonstrated stereoselective *p*-hydroxylation of MPH in rats. On administration of the separate enantiomers of MPH, only the levo compound yields appreciable free *p*-hydroxy-MPH (56). By analogy, a greater fraction of a dose of *l*-amphetamine is excreted as the *p*-hydroxy metabolite in human and rat than is excreted after a dose of *d*-amphetamine (22).

The concentration-time profile of the principal metabolite of MPH, ritalinic acid, has been studied extensively (25,89,93). However, plasma concentration has little clinical significance, since this amino acid is pharmacologically inactive (78), even after intracerebroventricular administration (59). The 6-oxo-MPH metabolite likewise produces little or no pharmacological effect (25). In conclusion, it appears that the pharmacological actions of MPH in humans can be attributed solely to the parent compound.

ANALYTICAL METHODS FOR METHYLPHENIDATE DETERMINATIONS

The low clinical blood concentration of MPH (2–20 ng/ml) is below that of most psychotherapeutic agents and requires sensitive analytical methodology for therapeutic drug monitoring. Initial attempts to quantify circulating concentrations of MPH utilized gas chromatography (GC) with flame ionization (71,91) or electron capture detection (21,39,66). These procedures require large volumes of blood (4–10 ml) and/or lack an internal standard. Recent methods involving GC-nitrogen phosphorus detection provide the requisite sensitivity to measure MPH levels of 2 ng/ml. Whereas the method of Hungund et al. (40) requires several solvent extractions, Potts et al. (65) described a procedure that incorporates a solid phase extraction to simplify sample preparation. High-performance liquid chromatographic procedures do not offer the necessary sensitivity to be useful for clinical MPH samples (54,82).

More practical methods for measuring MPH from biological samples involve GC-MS. The inherent molecular specificity of this approach provides chromatograms exhibiting little or no background. Because the piperidine ring fragment of MPH dominates its EI mass spectrum (Fig. 4), with no other fragment of appreciable relative abundance, selected ion monitoring (SIM) of this high-yield fragment provides an exceptionally strong ion current for high sensitivity. Milberg and co-workers (49) first applied GC-MS-SIM to the analysis of underivatized MPH. This approach requires a large plasma volume (5 ml) and an internal standard is not included. Further, quantitation is variable due to thermal decomposition of the underivatized drug during chromatography (27).

In subsequent GC-MS studies (14,28,40), MPH has been

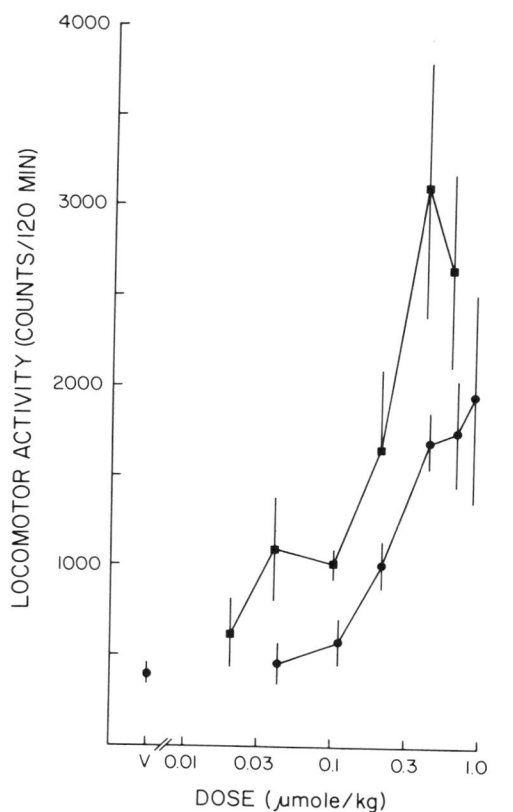

FIG. 3. Effects of MPH (●) and *p*-hydroxy-MPH (■) on the locomotor activity of rats. The locomotor response to the vehicle is indicated by V. Symbols represent the mean of three to six separate determinations, and vertical lines represent 1 SEM. (Adapted from ref. 59.)

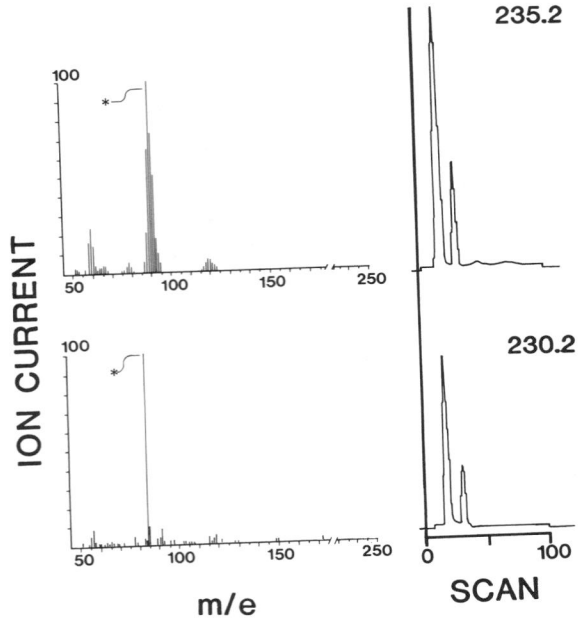

FIG. 4. Electron impact mass spectra of MPH·HCl (**lower left**) and internal standard, deuterated MPH·HCl (**upper left**). The indicated (*) ions represent the [²H₀] and [²H₅] piperidyl fragments, respectively. These are monitored from a spiked plasma extract as the *N*-pentafluoropropionyl derivatives (230.2 and 235.2 *m/e⁻*) in the ion chromatograms to the **right**. The later-eluting peaks are derived from the corresponding *p*-hydroxy compounds. Abscissa time scale: 2 sec per scan number.

acylated prior to chromatography to increase volatility and diminish thermal lability. This permits analysis of only 1 to 2 ml of plasma. In most procedures, ethylphenidate (ritalinic acid ethyl ester) serves as the internal standard. A disadvantage in this approach is the frequent overlap of the MPH and internal standard peaks, as observed by Hungund et al. (40) and by our laboratory. Also, the internal standard cannot efficiently control for hydrolysis of MPH, because the rate of hydrolysis of the ethyl ester is considerably slower than that of MPH (64).

A GC-MS-chemical ionization (CI) assay utilizing methane as the carrier and reagent gas has been developed (42). The base peaks of MPH and ethylphenidate are not monitored because, again, chromatographic peak overlap occurs. This difficulty is circumvented by monitoring the separate masses of the protonated molecular ions. In so doing, some potential sensitivity is lost, since these ions do not generate the strongest ion currents. Furthermore, the EI mode offers operational advantages over CI.

Patrick and co-workers (58) developed a GC-MS-EI method for the simultaneous determination of MPH and *p*-hydroxy-MPH (59) from biological samples using the deuterated variants as internal standards to circumvent the chromatographic problems associated with the ethylphenidate standard. Use of these deuterated standards improves overall assay performance (58). The mass spectra of deuterated MPH (Fig. 4) demonstrate the extensive incorporation of deuterium atoms into the piperidine ring, with

most combinations of deuterons and protons appearing in appreciable abundance. The pentadeutero form is the most abundant variant for both standards, representing approximately 25% of the total of each deuterated mixture. The remaining 75% of each contributes to the analysis in a carrier capacity. Accordingly, the corresponding pentadeuterated derivatized piperidyl fragment ions are chosen for SIM of the internal standards. The contribution of trace amounts of the [²H₀] species from the internal standards to the ion current of the unknowns is exceedingly small. Samples are derivatized with pentafluoropropionic anhydride rather than trifluoroacetic anhydride, since the additional mass imparted to the adducts permits SIM at a higher mass (235 A.M.U.) to provide cleaner ion chromatograms (Fig. 4).

METHYLPHENIDATE PHARMACOKINETICS

Evaluation of pharmacokinetic parameters for MPH obtained by various laboratories is summarized in Table 1. Although the number of investigations is small, these data appear sufficiently consistent to allow general conclusions. The available MPH attains peak plasma concentrations in approximately 1 to 2 hr. Investigators describe that peak concentrations are highly variable. MPH is rapidly distributed to tissues and is eliminated rapidly with a $t_{\frac{1}{2}}$ between 2 and 2.5 hr. These characteristics of MPH elimination necessitate twice daily dosing to maintain therapeutic drug concentrations during school hours in children being treated for ADD-H.

Several studies have demonstrated a linear plasma concentration-dose relationship for the kinetics of MPH (31,77,94). Gualtieri et al. (31) report dose proportionality for oral administration of 0.15 and 0.3 mg/kg MPH to 16 adults and 27 children with ADD-H. Mean 1-hr serum concentration for MPH in adults and children who received 0.3 mg/kg is 11.1 and 13.2 ng/ml, respectively, indicating that age has little effect on the pharmacokinetics of MPH.

Although early work suggested that MPH is absorbed completely (25), recent studies utilizing more specific techniques reevaluated the bioavailability of MPH. Wargin et al. (89) found bioavailability of MPH to be 19% in rat and 22% in the monkey. Chan et al. (15) administered MPH intravenously to children with ADD-H and compared results with oral administration in order to evaluate the bioavailability. In these studies, the fraction reaching the systemic circulation was calculated to be 11 to 53%. After i.v. administration, MPH rapidly distributes, followed by monoexponential decline, and exhibits a mean steady-state volume of distribution of 5.95 liters/kg. The calculated mean clearance of 2.3 liters/kg/hr is greater than liver blood flow, suggesting multiple sites of metabolism.

MPH has been recommended to be taken before meals, because food was believed to interfere with the absorption (52). However, two studies have recently demonstrated that the pharmacokinetics of MPH is not adversely affected by coadministration with food. At two doses in a small but rigorously controlled study (*N* = 6), Gualtieri et al. (31) report that 1-, 2-, and 3-hr serum concentrations of MPH were not significantly different between the fasting state

TABLE 1. *Summary of mean pharmacokinetic parameters of MPH[a]*

References	Dose, route	Number of subjects	Age (years)	$t_{\frac{1}{2}}$ (hr)	CL (liters/kg/hr)[b]	t_{max} (hr)	C_{max} (ng/ml)
Hungund et al. (41)	10–20 mg, p.o.	4	7–11	2.56	5.47		
Chan et al. (14)	10–20 mg, i.v.	6	7–14	2.02	2.33		
Shaywitz et al. (77)	0.34–0.65 mg/kg, p.o.	12–14	7–12	2.53		1.9–2.5	11.2–20.2
Wargin et al. (89)	0.3 mg/kg, p.o.	5	7–12	2.43	10.2	1.5	10.8
	0.3 mg/kg, p.o.	10	21–40	2.14	10.5	2.1	7.8
	0.15 mg/kg, p.o.	5	21–40	2.05	10.5	2.2	3.5
Chan et al. (15)	0.25–0.65 mg/kg, p.o.	5	7–12	2.14		1.0	34.7

[a] Abbreviations: t_{max}, time of peak concentration; C_{max}, peak concentration; Cl, clearance; $t_{\frac{1}{2}}$, half-life.
[b] Oral studies based on 100% availability.

and *post cibum*. Chan and co-workers (15) explored the effect of food on bioavailability in a group of seven boys, applying a more thorough pharmacokinetic analysis. Results indicate that if any differences do exist, food may actually accelerate absorption of MPH. Time to peak plasma concentration in the oral fasted state was 1.6 ± 0.42 hr, but occurred at 1.0 ± 0.35 hr when administered with breakfast. Perhaps the food increases the retention of the drug in the upper small intestines, where absorption is expected to be most rapid. The elimination $t_{\frac{1}{2}}$ values after i.v. MPH in the fasted state, oral administration in the fasted state, or oral administration with breakfast were 2.04 ± 0.42, 2.10 ± 0.36, and 2.14 ± 0.32 hr, respectively. The bioavailability for fasted versus fed conditions is 27.9 ± 11.5% and 31.4 ± 15.9%. The considerable variability in plasma concentrations observed between and within individuals (31,76) may reflect day-to-day variability in presystemic metabolism.

The bioavailability of MPH in a sustained-release formulation (Ritalin-SR) has not been directly evaluated. A pharmacokinetic study relating a single 20-mg sustained-release tablet to a b.i.d. schedule for the 10-mg immediate-release MPH tablet in pediatric patients was conducted (17) through analysis of urine concentrations of the principal metabolite, ritalinic acid (67). The extent of absorption for the two formulations was concluded to be equivalent. However, in view of the recent studies demonstrating that a major portion of an oral dose of MPH is metabolized to ritalinic acid before reaching the systemic circulation in humans (15,89), this indicates that monitoring urinary elimination of ritalinic acid may not reflect the extent of MPH absorbed intact. Further, it is well documented that the systemic availability of drugs may be dependent on the dosage formulation (5,68,76). Thus, more direct analytical procedures will need to be applied to the pharmacokinetics of the sustained-release product before any conclusions can be made concerning the bioavailability of this MPH formulation.

TISSUE DISTRIBUTION

Since the therapeutic effects of MPH depend on its access to brain, several studies evaluated the distribution of MPH concentrations in brain and other tissues. Within 1 to 5 min after i.v. administration, a brain/serum MPH ratio of 7 to 8 is achieved (28,57). This rapid accumulation of MPH in brain is consistent with its rapid effects when administered i.v. for treatment of hiccups (50). Whereas Gal et al. (28) found a parallel decay of MPH from brain and blood, Patrick et al. (57) found brain levels of MPH fell somewhat more rapidly than serum concentrations. After oral administration, a similar accumulation in brain relative to serum is noted (Fig. 5). However, brain variability is considerably greater after oral dosing, suggesting a source of variability in clinical response. Like amphetamine (19), MPH accumulates in highly perfused tissues (Table 2) and appears to occur primarily by physicochemical extraction into environments more lipid than the general circulation (55,85). Radioisotopic studies have evaluated the regional distribution of MPH within the CNS. After intracerebro-

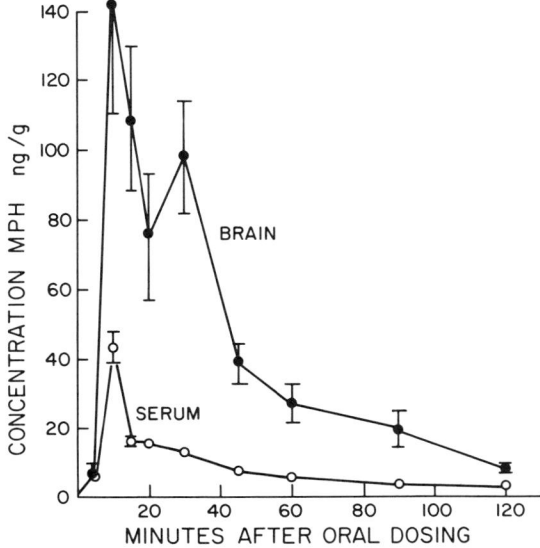

FIG. 5. MPH concentration in serum (○) and brain (●) after oral administration of 1 mg/kg. Each value represents the mean ± SE (vertical bars unless too small to illustrate) of at least four rats. (From ref. 57.)

TABLE 2. *Tissue distribution of MPH and p-hydroxy-MPH in rat*

Tissue	MPH	p-Hydroxy-MPH	Conjugated p-hydroxy-MPH
	μg/g	μg/g	μg/g
Serum	1.5 ± 0.12	0.02 ± 0.01	—
Red cell fraction	1.8 ± 0.3	0.02 ± 0.002	—
Brain	18.0 ± 2.7	0.02 ± 0.003	—
Kidney	33.7 ± 2.4	1.9 ± 0.3	—
Liver	5.0 ± 0.4	1.3 ± 0.2	13.7 ± 2.5
Lung	26.9 ± 2.9	0.2 ± 0.06	—
Heart	7.2 ± 0.6	0.2 ± 0.01	—

Rats were administered 20 mg/kg of MPH i.p. and sacrificed after 30 min. Each value represents the mean ± SE of five animals. —, Values not determined. (From ref. 57).

ventricular administration of MPH to rabbits, an uneven distribution between brain regions is observed (75). However, this may be an artifact of route of administration, since i.p. or i.v. administration to rats does not produce significant regional differences in the distribution of MPH (73). Similarly, *d*-amphetamine is homogeneously distributed throughout rat brain (19).

SITE OF ACTION

Stimulant effects of both MPH and *d*-amphetamine appear to depend prominently on an indirect action on dopaminergic neurons (11,12,51). However, it has been suggested that the effects of MPH differ from those of *d*-amphetamine because MPH is more easily antagonized by reserpine pretreatment (16,70). A further difference is that *d*-amphetamine decreases brain dihydroxyphenylacetic acid whereas MPH increases the concentration of this metabolite (11). These results are compatible with the thesis that *d*-amphetamine increases release of dopamine, whereas MPH acts by inhibiting dopamine uptake (16,51,69).

Schweri et al. (72) report the presence of saturable, stereoselective, and sodium-dependent binding sites of [³H]MPH in synaptosomal membranes from striatal tissue. The highest density of MPH binding is found in areas with a high density of dopamine terminals (43,72,86). A good correlation is found between the ability of compounds to reduce the extent of binding of MPH and their ability to antagonize dopamine uptake and to produce motor stimulation (72). Since lesions to dopamine-containing neurons reduce binding of MPH, binding is presumed to be associated with a presynaptic dopamine transport complex (43). *d*-Amphetamine has also been found to bind to striatum, brainstem, and hypothalamus (34,61). In contrast to binding of MPH, binding of *d*-amphetamine is not dependent on sodium and does not correlate with the locomotor action of compounds that displace specific binding of *d*-amphetamine (61). MPH only weakly inhibits binding of *d*-amphetamine to hypothalamic membranes (72), which is enhanced by glucose administration (1). Binding studies in the hypothalamus are consistent with the lesser anorectic

effect of MPH compared to *d*-amphetamine (38). These reports provide evidence that the binding sites for MPH and amphetamine are discrete entities.

PHARMACOKINETICS AND THERAPEUTIC ACTIONS OF METHYLPHENIDATE

Although the improvement of symptoms of ADD-H with MPH is considered by many to be diagnostic of this syndrome, a difficulty with this interpretation is that pharmacokinetics has not been considered in those patients who did not respond favorably to this stimulant therapy. The interindividual variability in the pharmacokinetics of MPH is consistent with the possibility that insufficient levels of the drug in the systemic circulation might account for a negative therapeutic outcome. Further, although MPH is not considered a dangerous medication, it does have a "silent" toxicity in the form of negative cognitive and affective effects (83). The therapeutic index for such toxic effects is very low. Thus, it was reasonable to pursue the idea that blood level analysis might improve clinical management and diminish the occurrence of "silent" toxicity. Using multiple response measures including standardized rating scales, direct behavioral observations, neuroendocrine and cardiovascular measures, neuropsychological tests, and blood levels, the relationships of the pharmacokinetics to physiological and therapeutic responses induced by MPH were correlated. The most relevant finding is that the concentration of MPH in children with ADD-H who do not have a favorable therapeutic response did not differ from those who received an advantage from this therapy (30). In a given individual, serum concentration is variable on a day-to-day basis. This variability does not appear related to the clinical variability that occurs in children with ADD-H who take the medication on a daily basis.

Table 3 shows correlations between MPH blood levels and the different response measures taken. Along the pharmacokinetic time profile of the drug, occasional associations of dose can be demonstrated with certain measures, such as the neuroendocrine response. Neither 1-hr serum levels nor any other pharmacokinetic parameter correlates

TABLE 3. *Correlations of methylphenidate serum levels and response measures (hyperactive children, acute effects study)*

Dependent measure	Dose = 0.3 mg/kg		Dose = 0.6 mg/kg		Dependent measure	Dose = 0.3 mg/kg		Dose = 0.6 mg/kg	
	n	r	n	r		n	r	n	r
Conners parent rating scale					4	10	−0.384	13	−0.169
Total score	49	−0.104	39	−0.080	5	17	0.039	11	0.110
Hyperactivity items	39	−0.136	37	0.012	6	12	0.199	12	−0.203
Distractibility items	39	−0.049	36	−0.065	9	11	0.375	10	0.055
Conners teacher rating scale					10	27	0.088	26	−0.144
					12	14	0.596	10	−0.161
Total score	26	−0.237	23	0.319	13	23	0.050	20	0.091
Hyperactivity items	23	−0.220	21	0.027	14	13	−0.604[a]	10	0.315
Distractibility items			20	0.324	15	17	−0.037	16	−0.308
Pulse rate	31	0.311	33	0.370[a]	16	5	−0.224	8	0.027
Systolic blood pressure	31	0.395[a]	33	0.178	17	25	−0.244	22	−0.132
Diastolic blood pressure	29	0.479[a]	32	0.248	18	5	−0.302	10	0.438
Growth hormone	39	0.318	40	0.207	19	7	0.310	5	−0.112
Prolactin	33	−0.062	34	0.291	20	6	−0.153	7	−0.286
Thyroid-stimulating hormone	14	−0.361	14	−0.148	21	25	−0.162	23	−0.101
					22	22	−0.027	18	0.029
Continuous performance task					23	5	0.758		
					24	4	−0.965		
Correct responses	36	0.109	37	−0.043	25	6	−0.251	10	0.489
False alarms	34	−0.215	36	−0.210	Behavioral observations by teacher				
Actometer	33	−0.061	34	−0.194	1	3	−0.715		
Matching familiar figures					2	12	0.078	8	−0.267
Latency	28	−0.139	28	0.104	3	9	−0.005	6	−0.041
Errors	27	−0.344	26	−0.309	4	3	0.931	3	0.321
Routh activity room					5	5	0.652	6	−0.082
Quadrant entries	38	0.133	35	0.317	6	4	−0.146		
Toy changes	38	0.004	38	0.128	7	11	0.148	11	0.381
Behavioral observations by research assistant					8	13	0.045	11	0.399
3	11	−0.300	14	−0.224	9	12	−0.039	11	−0.204

[a] Significant at *p* = 0.05 level.
(From ref. 30.)

with any of the host of measures employed to measure drug response in hyperactive children. In the within-subjects analyses, changes in plasma growth hormone and prolactin follow a pattern that reflects the pharmacokinetic profile of the drug. In Fig. 6 blood levels are plotted relative to the occurrence of side effects. It is apparent that differences occur among the groups with respect to blood levels. Toxic effects are more likely to occur in the high dose (0.6 mg/kg) condition, but once the dose effect is partialled out of the regression, there is no portion of variance attributable to blood level. However, MPH serum level does not distinguish between drug "responders" and "nonresponders." Likewise, the serum level is not correlated with the severity of toxic effects, and does not correlate with other dependent measures.

Results of other studies are at variance with these conclusions. Kupietz et al. (47) associated plasma MPH and learning errors in five ADD-H children. However, the regression analysis appears not to have tested the relative impact of time (along the curve) or dose on the variance

in learning scores. The study by Shaywitz et al. (77) correlated improvement on the Conners Teacher Rating Scale with plasma MPH drawn at different times after administration of drug in different children, and in many cases the drug was actually administered by the parent before the child came to the clinic. In neither study was an attempt made to factor out the effects of dose on clinical response. The clinically essential question is not whether blood levels correlate with response, but whether any additional variance in response is attributable to blood levels once the variance in response attributable to dose is excluded. That is, will blood levels predict any more about the patient's clinical response than will dose? In a third study (93) associating MPH concentrations with response, no additional variance in response was explained by blood levels after the effects of dose were removed. Thus, on the basis of the research described herein, it is concluded that blood MPH levels are not statistically related to clinical response, nor are they likely to prove clinically helpful until this lack of correlation is understood.

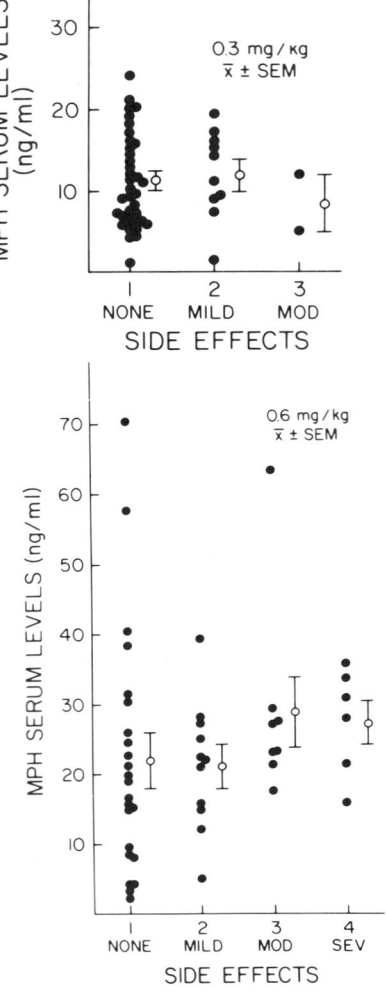

FIG. 6. MPH serum levels and side effects in hyperactive children at 0.3 and 0.6 mg/kg doses.

FUTURE DIRECTIONS

Meaningful blood MPH-therapeutic response correlations may depend on a knowledge of the enantiomeric disposition of the circulating drug (45,92). The significance of inter-individual differences in enantioselective metabolism of other drugs administered in the racemic form is apparent from studies of propranolol (6,80), verapamil (24,87), and warfarin (37,53). Accordingly, the individual response to racemic MPH therapy may depend on individual differences in stereochemically dependent pharmacokinetics. Since most of an oral dose of MPH is metabolized by hydrolysis before reaching the systemic circulation (15,89), and enzymes that govern the hydrolysis of esters structurally similar to MPH exhibit stereoselectivity (36), it is possible that systemically available MPH is differentially enriched in one or the other stereoisomer to account for variability in response. The importance of stereochemistry to stimulant drug activity is apparent for the individual enantiomers of amphetamine. Each has been reported to be more efficacious for different subpopulations of ADD-H children (3,10), to produce different profiles of side effects (3,10,44), and to exhibit unique pharmacokinetics (29,88).

It is well established that the stereochemistry about the MPH structure is pharmacologically important (26,48). Recently, in the only defined *in vivo* evaluation of the separate enantiomers of MPH, *d*-MPH was found to be much more active than the *l*-isomer in inducing locomotor activity in rats (56). Further, enantioselective metabolism was evident. The individual enantiomers of MPH could even produce differences in *direction* rather than *degree* of certain pharmacological effects, as observed with the differential pharmacology of the enantiomers of the dopaminergic agents 3-(3-hydroxyphenyl)-*N-n*-propylpiperdine (4) and *p*-fluorococaine (18,35).

Thus, it is possible that the individual therapeutic response to racemic MPH may in part depend on the enantiomeric disposition of circulating MPH, i.e., responders may metabolize MPH with enantioselectivity differing from nonresponders, thereby producing a different profile of effects. Future MPH studies should utilize chiral chromatographic methods (56) designed to correlate enantiomeric drug levels with therapeutic and toxic responses.

ACKNOWLEDGMENTS

Research from this laboratory was supported by USPHS grants MH-36294, HD-03110, and HD-10570.

REFERENCES

1. Angel, I., Hauger, R. L., Luu, M. D., Giblin, B., Skolnick, P., and Paul, S. M. (1985): *Proc. Natl. Acad. Sci. USA,* 82:6320–6324.
2. Arnold, E. (1975): *Acta Pharmacol. Toxicol.,* 36:335–352.
3. Arnold, L. E., Hvestis, R. D., Smeltzer, D. J., Scheib, J., Wemmer, D., and Colner, G. (1972): *Arch. Gen. Psychiatry,* 33:292–300.
4. Arnt, J., Bogeso, K. P., Christensen, A. V., Hyttel, J., Larsen, J. J., and Svendsen, O. (1983): *Psychopharmacology,* 81:199–207.
5. Barr, W. H. (1969): *Drug Inform. Bull.,* 3:27–45.
6. Barrett, A. M., and Cullum, V. A. (1968): *Br. J. Pharmacol.,* 34:43–55.
7. Bartlett, M. F., and Egger, H. P. (1972): *Fed. Proc.,* 31:537.
8. Bernhard, K., Buhler, V., and Bickel, M. H. (1959): *Helv. Chim. Acta,* 42:802–807.
9. Borga, O., Piafsky, K. M., and Nilsen, O. G. (1977): *Clin. Pharmacol. Ther.,* 22:539–544.
10. Bradley, C. (1950): *Pediatrics,* 5:24–36.
11. Braestrup, C. (1977): *J. Pharm. Pharmacol.,* 29:463–470.
12. Breese, G. R., Cooper, B. R., and Hollister, A. S. (1975): *Psychopharmacologia,* 44:5–10.
13. Brodie, B. B., Cho, A. K., and Gessa, G. L. (1970): In: *Amphetamines and Related Compounds,* edited by E. Costa and S. Garattini, pp. 217–230. Raven Press, New York.
14. Chan, Y. M., Soldin, S. J., Swanson, J. M., Deber, C. M., Thiessen, J. J., and Macleod, S. (1980): *Clin. Biochem.,* 13:266–272.
15. Chan, Y. M., Swanson, J. M., Soldin, S. S., Thiessen, J. J., Macleod, S. M., and Logan, W. (1983): *Pediatrics,* 72:56–59.
16. Chuich, C. C., and Moore, K. E. (1975): *J. Pharmacol. Exp. Ther.,* 193:559–563.
17. Ciba-Geigy Corp. (1980): New Drug Application 18029.
18. Clarke, R. L., Daum, S. J., Gambino, A. J., Aceto, M. D., Pearl, J., Levitt, M., Cumiskey, W. R., and Bogado, E. F. (1973): *J. Med. Chem.,* 16:1260–1267.
19. Danielson, T. J., and Boulton, A. A. (1976): *Eur. J. Pharmacol.,* 37:257–264.
20. Dayton, P. G., Perel, J. M., Israili, Z. H., Faraj, B. A., Rodewig, K., Black, N., and Goldberg, L. I. (1975): In: *Clinical Pharmacology of Psychoactive Drugs,* pp. 183–202. Alcoholism and Drug Addiction Foundation, Toronto.
21. Delbee, F. T., and Debackere, M. (1975): *J. Chromatogr.,* 106:412–417.

22. Dring, L. G., Smith, R. L., and Williams, R. T. (1970): *Biochem. J.,* 116:425–435.
23. Egger, H., Bartlett, F., Dreyfuss, R., and Karliner, J. (1981): *Drug Metab. Dispos.,* 9:415–423.
24. Eichelbaum, M., Mikus, G., and Vogelgesang, B. (1984): *Br. J. Clin. Pharmacol.,* 17:453–458.
25. Faraj, B. A., Israili, Z. H., Perel, J. M., Jenkins, M. L., Holtzman, S. G., Cucinell, S. A., and Dayton, P. G. (1974): *J. Pharmacol. Exp. Ther.,* 191:535–547.
26. Ferris, R. M., Tang, F. L. M., and Maxwell, R. A. (1972): *J. Pharmacol. Exp. Ther.,* 181:407–416.
27. Flamm, B. L., and Gal, J. (1975): *Biomed. Mass Spectrom.,* 2: 281–283.
28. Gal, J., Hodshon, B. J., Pintauro, C., Flamm, B. L., and Cho, A. K. (1977): *J. Pharm. Sci.,* 66:866–969.
29. Goldstein, M., and Anagnoste, B. (1965): *Biochim. Biophys. Acta,* 107:168–170.
30. Gualtieri, C. T., Hicks, R. E., Patrick, K., Schroeder, S. R., and Breese, G. R. (1984): *Ther. Drug Monit.,* 6:379–392.
31. Gualtieri, C. T., Kanoy, R., Hawk, B., Koriath, U., Schroeder, S., Youngblood, W., Breese, G. R., and Prange, A. J. (1981): *Psychoneuroendocrinology,* 6:331–339.
32. Gualtieri, C. T., Wargin, W., Kanoy, R., Patrick, K., Shen, D., Youngblood, W., Mueller, R. A., and Breese, G. R. (1982): *J. Am. Acad. Child Psychiatry,* 21:19–26.
33. Gualtieri, C. T., Wargin, W., Kanoy, R., Youngblood, W., and Breese, G. R. (1982): *Res. Commun. Psychol. Psychiatry Behav.,* 7:381–384.
34. Hauger, R., Hulihan-Giblin, B., Skolnick, P., and Paul, S. M. (1984): *Life Sci.,* 34:771–782.
35. Heikkila, R. E., Manzino, L., and Cabbat, F. C. (1981): *Subst. Alcohol Actions Misuse,* 2:115–121.
36. Hein, G. E., and Niemann, C. (1962): *J. Am. Chem. Soc.,* 84: 4487–4494.
37. Hignite, C., Vetrecht, J., Tschanz, C., and Azarnoff, D. (1980): *Clin. Pharmacol. Ther.,* 28:99–105.
38. Hollister, A. S., Ervin, G. N., Cooper, B. R., and Breese, G. R. (1975): *Neuropharmacology,* 14:715–723.
39. Huffman, R., Blake, J. W., Ray, R., Noonan, J., and Murdick, P. W. (1974): *J. Chromatogr. Sci.,* 12:382–384.
40. Hungund, B. L., Hanna, M., and Winsberg, B. G. (1978): *Commun. Psychopharmacol.,* 2:203–208.
41. Hungund, B. L., Perel, J. M., Hurwic, M. J., Sverd, J., and Winsberg, B. G. (1979): *Br. J. Clin. Pharmacol.,* 8:571–576.
42. Iden, C. R., and Hungund, B. L. (1979): *Biomed. Mass Spectrom.,* 6:422–425.
43. Janowsky, A., Schweri, M. M., Berger, P., Long, R., Skolnick, P., and Paul, S. M. (1985): *Eur. J. Pharmacol.,* 108:187–191.
44. Janowsky, D. S., and Davis, J. M. (1976): *Arch. Gen. Psychiatry,* 33:304–308.
45. Jenner, P., and Testa, B. (1973): *Drug Metab. Rev.,* 2:117–184.
46. Kleinman, J. E., Llewellyn, B., Bigelow, A. R., Rogol, A., Weinberger, D. R., Nasrallah, A., Wyatt, R. J., and Gillin, C. (1980): In: *Phenothiazines and Structurally Related Drugs: Basic and Clinical Studies,* edited by E. Usdin, H. Eckert, and I. S. Forrest, pp. 275–278. Elsevier North Holland, New York.
47. Kupietz, S. S., Winsberg, B. G., and Sverd, J. (1982): *J. Am. Assoc. Child Psychiatry,* 21:27–30.
48. Maxwell, R. A., Chaplin, E., Batmanglidj Eckhardt, S., Soares, J. R., and Hite, G. (1970): *J. Pharmacol. Exp. Ther.,* 173:158–165.
49. Millberg, R. M., Rinehart, K. L., Sprague, R. L., and Sleator, E. K. (1975): *Biomed. Mass Spectrom.,* 2:2–8.
50. Nathan, M. D., Leshner, R. T., and Keller, A. P. (1980): *Laryngoscope,* 90:1612–1618.
51. Nielsen, J. A., Chapin, D. S., and Moore, K. E. (1983): *Life Sci.,* 33:1899–1907.
52. Oettinger, L. (1976): *South. Med. J.,* 69:161–163.
53. O'Reilly, R. A. (1974): *Clin. Pharmacol. Ther.,* 16:348–354.
54. Padmanabian, G. R., Fogel, J., Mollica, J. A., O'Connor, J. M., and Strusz, R. (1980): *J. Liquid Chromatogr.,* 3:1079–1085.
55. Pardridge, W. M., and Connor, J. D. (1972): *Experientia,* 29:302–304.
56. Patrick, K. S., Caldwell, R. W., Davis, K. R., Mueller, R. A., and Breese, G. R. (1986): *Fed. Proc.,* 46:933.
57. Patrick, K. S., Ellington, K. R., and Breese, G. R. (1984): *J. Pharmacol. Exp. Ther.,* 231:61–65.
58. Patrick, K. S., Ellington, K. E., Breese, G. R., and Kilts, C. D. (1985): *J. Chromatogr. Biomed. Appl.,* 343:329–338.
59. Patrick, K. S., Kilts, C. D., and Breese, G. R. (1981): *J. Med. Chem.,* 24:1237–1240.
60. Patrick, K. S., Kilts, C., and Breese, G. (1982): *J. Label. Compounds Radiopharm.,* 9:485–490.
61. Paul, S. M., Hulihan-Giblin, B., and Skolnick, P. (1982): *Science,* 218:487–490.
62. Perel, J. M., and Black, N. (1970): *Fed. Proc.,* 29:345.
63. Pippenger, C. E., Penry, J. K., and Cutt, H. (1978): *Antiepileptic Drugs: Quantitative Analysis and Interpretation.* Raven Press, New York.
64. Portoghese, P. S., and Malspeis, L. (1961): *J. Pharm. Sci.,* 50:494–501.
65. Potts, B. D., Martin, C. A., and Vore, M. (1984): *Clin. Chem.,* 30:1374–1377.
66. Ray, R. S., Noonan, J. S., Murdick, P. W., and Tharp, V. L. (1972): *Am. J. Vet. Res.,* 33:27–31.
67. Redalieu, E., Bartlett, M. F., Waldes, L. M., Darrow, W. R., Egger, H., and Wagner, W. E. (1982): *Drug Metab. Dispos.,* 10: 708–709.
68. Riegelman, S., and Rowland, M. (1973): *J. Pharmacokinet. Biopharm.,* 1:419–434.
69. Ross, S. B. (1979): *Life Sci.,* 24:159–168.
70. Scheel-Kruger, J. (1971): *Eur. J. Pharmacol.,* 14:47–59.
71. Schubert, B. (1970): *Acta Chem. Scand.,* 24:433–438.
72. Schweri, M. M., Skolnick, P., Rafferty, M. F., Rice, K. C., Janowsky, A. J., and Paul, S. M. (1985): *J. Neurochem.,* 45:1062–1070.
73. Segal, J. L., Cunningham, R. F., Dayton, P. G., and Israili, Z. H. (1976): *Drug Metab. Dispos.,* 4:140–146.
74. Shafiee, A., and Hite, G. (1969): *J. Med. Chem.,* 12:266–270.
75. Shah, N. S., Powell, D. A., and Shan, A. B. (1983): *Prog. Neuropsychopharmacol. Biol. Psychiatry,* 7:101–106.
76. Shand, D. G., Rangno, R. E., and Evans, G. H. (1972): *Pharmacology,* 8:344–352.
77. Shaywitz, S. E., Hunt, R. D., Jatlow, P., Cohen, D. J., Young, J. G., Pierce, R. N., Anderson, G. M., and Shaywitz, B. A. (1982): *Pediatrics,* 69:688–694.
78. Sheppard, H., Tsien, W. H., Rodegker, W., and Plummer, A. J. (1960): *Toxicol. Appl. Pharmacol.,* 2:352–362.
79. Siegel, S., Lackman, L., and Malspeis, L. (1959): *J. Am. Pharm. Assoc.,* 48:431–439.
80. Silber, B., and Riegelman, S. (1980): *J. Pharmacol. Exp. Ther.,* 215:643–648.
81. Smith, R. L., and Dring, L. G. (1970): In: *Amphetamines and Related Compounds,* edited by E. Costa and S. Garattini, pp. 121–139. Raven Press, New York.
82. Soldin, S. J., Chan, Y. M., Hill, B. M., and Swanson, J. M. (1979): *Clin. Chem.,* 25:401–404.
83. Sprague, R. L., and Sleator, E. K. (1977): *Science,* 198:1274–1276.
84. Szporny, L., and Gorog, P. (1961): *Biochem. Pharmacol.,* 8:263–268.
85. Thoenen, H., Hurlimann, A., and Haefely, W. (1968): *J. Pharm. Pharmacol.,* 20:1–11.
86. Unis, A. S., Dawson, T. M., Gehlert, D. R., and Wamsley, J. K. (1985): *Eur. J. Pharmacol.,* 113:155–157.
87. Vogelgesang, B., Echizen, H., Schmidt, E., and Eichelbaum, M. (1984): *Br. J. Clin. Pharmacol.,* 18:733–740.
88. Wan, S. H., Martin, S. B., and Azernoff, D. L. (1978): *Clin. Pharmacol. Ther.,* 23:585–590.
89. Wargin, W., Patrick, K., Kilts, C., Gualtieri, C. T., Ellington, K., Mueller, R. A., Kraemer, G., and Breese, G. R. (1983): *J. Pharmacol. Exp. Ther.,* 226:382–386.
90. Wiesz, I., and Dudas, A. (1960): *Monatshefte Fuer Chemie.,* 91: 840–849.
91. Wells, R., Hammond, K. B., and Rodgerson, D. O. (1974): *Clin. Chem.,* 20:440–443.
92. Williams, K., and Lee, E. (1985): *Drugs,* 30:333–335.
93. Winsberg, B. G., Hungund, B. L., and Perel, J. M. (1980): *Psychopharmacol. Bull.,* 16:69–71.
94. Winsberg, B. G., Kupietz, S. S., Sverd, J., Hungund, B. L., and Young, N. L. (1982): *Psychopharmacology,* 76:329–332.

Psychopharmacology:
The Third Generation of Progress,
edited by Herbert Y. Meltzer.
Raven Press, New York © 1987.

CHAPTER 146

Pharmacokinetics of Psychotropic Drugs in Selected Patient Populations

E. M. Sellers and R. Bendayan

Theoretically, pharmacokinetic changes in some patient populations may be sufficiently large to require routine dosage adjustment. Kinetic changes have been ascribed to age, diseases (e.g., hepatic, renal), smoking, ethanol use, drug interactions, and drug abuse and dependence. However, many scientific and practical problems undermine the reliability and usefulness of many such studies, for example: small numbers of subjects; extremely variable and poorly described clinical conditions; failure to adequately identify, characterize, and/or control for diet, weight, body composition, drug consumption, concurrent medications, status of hepatic and renal function, and racial and genetic background. Failure to recognize the confounding effects of age, smoking, ethanol consumption, drug use, and decreasing renal function limits many studies.

A variety of pharmacokinetic methodologic problems are prominent. The term clearance is used synonymously with half-life in some early studies; the rationale or method for curve-fitting procedures is poorly described; blood samples have often been taken for a short duration after administration of the drug; oral administration of drugs has been associated with the implicit assumption of complete systemic bioavailability; metabolites are infrequently measured; no calculations of total body clearance are made or even possible; and most studies involve single dose administration (14). Despite the understandable difficulties in trying to identify and/or control these and other variables, their presence frequently casts the interpretation of results into doubt and precludes statements about the general applicability of the results. Hence conclusions are qualitative and lack both mechanistic implication and predictive value in populations and individual patients.

Ideally, kinetic studies should include determination of oral and systemic clearance, renal clearance, and metabolite kinetics. The extent to which single dose data are predictive of the multiple dose therapeutic setting should be determined (14). Studies of three different dose rates are needed. Since so many psychotropic drugs undergo considerable hepatic extraction, and thus bioavailability (F) is variable and low, it is not reasonable to assume that F is unchanged in clearance calculations for psychotropic drugs.

Kinetic data are usually analyzed using statistics that assume a normal (Gaussian) data distribution. Careful data inspection often indicates nonnormal data distribution, and nonparametric data handling is often needed. The assumption of normal distribution focuses attention on group mean changes rather than the mechanistically interesting outlier. Genetic sources of variation have usually been suspected by such deviant results. Even in "healthy normal volunteers," four- to sixfold variations in half-life and clearance are common (38). However, identification of the sources of variation requires establishment of strict basal conditions and subject selection. Conversely, such large variability decreases the likelihood that changes in a single variable detected in a strictly controlled study, e.g., renal function, will be generalizable to a less selected population.

Finally, a significant kinetic change obviously says nothing about the clinical importance of such a change. Several studies suggest that pharmacokinetic changes of apparent importance (e.g., cimetidine-diazepam interaction) may be of little clinical importance (8). Studies to establish clinical importance are essential.

The objectives of this chapter are to discuss how the pharmacokinetics of psychotropic drugs are influenced by hepatic and renal disease, smoking, ethanol consumption, and drug abuse.

HEPATIC DISEASE

The liver is the major organ for the biotransformation and elimination of psychotropic drugs; hence hepatic dys-

function may result in drug accumulation and alteration of pharmacologic effect. Drug pharmacokinetic changes in hepatic disease have been extensively reviewed (43, 45, 46; Table 1). The type and severity of liver dysfunction, concomitant disease, concurrent factors affecting biotransformation (e.g., age, sex, nutritional status), the kinetic characteristics of the drug (e.g., high or low hepatic extraction ratio), and concurrent drug therapy may all be important. Some of these factors can also modify pharmacodynamics.

Hepatic drug biotransformation occurs by three principal mechanisms: mixed function oxidase enzymatic oxidation,

TABLE 1. *Pharmacokinetic parameters of psychotropic drugs in hepatic disease*

Drug	Dose and route of administration	Hepatic disease	N	Plasma clearance	V_d	$t_{\frac{1}{2}}B$ (hr)
Barbiturates						
Phenobarbital	0.85–2.55 mg/kg (duodenal intubation)	Cirrhosis	6	—	—	130 ± 15*
		Acute viral hepatitis	8	—	—	104 (60–127)
			(6)	—	—	(86.0 ± 3.0)
Pentobarbital	200 mg (p.o.)	Infective hepatitis	5	—	—	13.4 ± 1.5
		Alcoholic fatty liver	5	—	—	13.2 ± 2.0
		Cirrhosis	5	—	—	14.4 ± 1.2*
		Malignancy	5	—	—	17.7 ± 1.1*
			(5)	—	—	(12.7 ± 1.2)
Hexobarbital	2.97–7.32 mg/kg (i.v. infusion)	Acute hepatitis	13	1.94 ± 0.85* ml/kg/min	1.1 ± 0.4ª liters/kg	8.17 ± 3.1*
			(14)	(3.57 ± 0.83 ml/kg/min)	(1.1 ± 0.12 liters/kg)	(4.4 ± 1.2)
Hexobarbital	3.1–14.6 mg/kg (i.v. infusion)	Cirrhosis				
		Compensated	8	1.9 ± 0.7* ml/kg/min	1.14 ± 0.26ª liters/kg	8.48 ± 2.9*
		Uncompensated	22	1.3 ± 0.5* ml/kg/min	1.57 ± 0.64 liters/kg	16.95 ± 7.5*
			(22)	(3.3 ± 1.0 ml/kg/min)	(1.25 ± 0.24 liters/kg)	(5.66 ± 1.83)
Amylobarbital	3.2 mg/kg (i.v.)	Chronic liver disease				
		Albumin <3.5 g%	5	41.0 ± 5.1* ml/min	39.4 ± 6.6*	
		Albumin >3.5 g%	5	118.9 ± 12.5 ml/min	17.7 ± 1.9	
			(10)	(92.0 ± 7.0 ml/min)	—	(21.1 ± 1.2)
Other hypnotics						
Meprobamate		Chronic liver disease	9	—	—	24.3 ± 4.4*
						(12.6 ± 2.6)
Chlormethiazole	192 mg (p.o. & i.v.)	Alcoholic cirrhosis	8	12.8 ± 1.7* ml/kg/min	—	8.7 ± 1.4
			(6)	(18.1 ± 1.2 ml/kg/min)	—	(6.6 ± 1.0)
Benzodiazepines						
Chlordiazepoxide	0.6 mg/kg (i.v.)	Alcoholic cirrhosis	8	7.7 ± 2.1* ml/min	0.48 ± 0.14*ª liters/kg	62.7 ± 27.3*
			(8)	(15.3 ± 4.4 ml/min)	(0.33 ± 0.06 liters/kg)	(23.8 ± 11.6)
	0.6 mg/kg (i.v.)	Acute viral hepatitis	5	6.1 ± 4.3* ml/min	0.4 ± 0.2*ª liters/kg	91.0 ± 99.5*
			(5)	(18.1 ± 7.1 ml/min)	(0.3 ± 0.03 liters/kg)	(11.1 ± 2.7)

TABLE 1. (*Continued*)

Drug	Dose and route of administration	Hepatic disease	N	Plasma clearance	V_d	$t_{\frac{1}{2}}B$ (hr)
Chlordiazepoxide	50 mg (i.v.)	Cirrhosis	11	0.19 ± .03* ml/kg/min	0.34 ± 0.02[a] liters/kg	34.9 ± 8.7
			(14)	0.54 ± 0.13 ml/kg/min	(0.38 ± 0.04 liters/kg)	(10.0 ± 0.9)
Diazepam	0.1 mg/kg (i.v.)	Alcoholic cirrhosis	9	13.8 ± 2.4 ml/min	1.74 ± 0.21*[a] liters/kg	105.6 ± 15.2*
			(5)	(26.6 ± 4.1 ml/min)	(1.13 ± 0.28 liters/kg)	(46.6 ± 14.2)
	10 mg (p.o.)	Acute viral hepatitis	8 (6)	— —	— —	74.5 ± 27.5* (32.7 ± 8.9)
	0.1 mg/kg (i.v.) or	Chronic active hepatitis	(4)	—	—	59.7 ± 23.0
	10 mg (p.o.)		(6)			(32.7 ± 8.9)
		Chronic Liver Disease				
Diazepam	0.3 ± 0.39 mg/kg (i.v.)	Ascites	7	0.09 ± 0.022* ml/kg/min	0.59 ± 0.11[c] liters/kg	77.4 ± 4.3*
	0.3 ± 0.03 mg/kg (i.v.)	No ascites	10	0.178 ± 0.033 ml/kg/min	0.69 ± 0.14 liters/kg	48.7 ± 12.1
	0.4 ± 0.07 mg/kg (i.v.)		(5)	(0.243 ± 0.050 (ml/kg/min)	(0.98 ± 0.18 liters/kg)	(43 ± 3.2)
Diazepam	10 mg (i.v.)	Cirrhosis	9	17.1 (7.4–24.2) ml/min	2.86 (0.89[a]– 8.04) liters/kg	164* (28.6–517.2)
			(4)	[35.0 (17.7–53.6) ml/min]	[1.16 (0.54–1.57) liters/kg]	[32.1 (14.3–61.2)]
Diazepam	0.1 mg/kg (i.v.)	Cirrhosis	6			111.9 ± 21.7*
		Fibrosis	5			83.9 ± 14.7
			(13)			46.6 ± 14.2
Desmethyldiazepam	20 mg (p.o.)	Cirrhosis	4	4.6 ± 1.1* ml/min	0.63 ± 0.12 liters/kg	108.2 ± 40.3*
			(4)	(11.3 ± 3.1 ml/min)	(0.64 ± 0.17 liters/kg)	(50.9 ± 6.2)
Lorazepam	2 mg (i.v.)	Cirrhosis	13	0.81 ± 0.48 ml/kg/min	2.01 ± 0.82*[b] liters/kg	31.9 ± 9.6*
		Acute viral hepatitis	9	0.74 ± 0.34 ml/kg/min	1.52 ± 0.61 liters/kg	25 ± 6.4
			(11)	(0.75 ± 0.23 ml/kg/min)	(1.28 ± 0.34 liters/kg)	(22.1 ± 5.4)
Oxazepam	45 mg (p.o.)	Cirrhosis	6	155.5 ± 31.5 ml/min	60.9 ± 9.5 liters[b]	5.8 ± 0.5
			(8)	(136.0 ± 17.5 ml/min)	(61.2 ± 4.6 liters)	(5.6 ± 0.3)

N, Number of subjects; V_d, volume of distribution; [a]V_d at steady state; [b]V_d during the elimination phase B (two-compartment models); [c]V_d of one-compartment model; $t_{\frac{1}{2}}B$, elimination half-life; ( ), values for the control group of subjects; * indicates statistical significance.

conjugation between the drug and an endogenous substrate such as glucuronic acid, and nonmicrosomal enzymatic action, e.g., acetylation. Drug elimination by the liver depends on the hepatic blood flow, the intrinsic ability ("intrinsic clearance") of the liver to metabolize the drug, and the extent of the drug binding to plasma proteins. The relative importance of these differs according to the efficiency of the liver in extracting the drug. For highly extracted drugs (intrinsic clearance ≫ hepatic blood flow), hepatic clearance is sensitive to changes in liver blood flow, but much less so to alterations in protein binding or intrinsic

hepatic drug metabolizing activity. In contrast, for drugs that are poorly extracted by the liver (intrinsic clearance ≪ hepatic blood flow), drug hepatic clearance largely reflects the intrinsic clearance and a change in either binding or drug metabolizing activity will affect total drug clearance (44). In liver disease, blood flow and drug metabolizing activity may be altered. In acute inflammatory liver disease, the major alteration is a hepatocellular dysfunction, whereas in cirrhosis the major abnormalities are a reduction in hepatic blood flow and the presence of portosystemic shunting. In liver disease, a decrease in hepatic blood flow will lead to a decrease in the hepatic clearance of highly extracted drug (e.g., tricyclic antidepressant), with a consequent large increase in the drug's systemic bioavailability. For poorly extracted drugs (e.g., benzodiazepines, barbiturates), a decrease in the hepatic intrinsic clearance will lead to a decrease of the hepatic clearance of the drug.

Protein synthesis is often decreased in liver disease and drug binding to plasma proteins may decrease. Two mechanisms are responsible for changes in drug binding in liver disease. Decreases in protein concentration predictably decrease binding capacity. Decreases in serum albumin will be accompanied by a proportionate decrease in binding (3,16,33). Increases in AGP or globulin concentrations with inflammation can increase binding capacity for selected drugs. Even in the absence of changes in protein concentration, the binding of drugs to plasma protein can be altered by changes in the affinity of drug and binding site. Binding can be decreased by competition with endogenous substances or increased by cooperative effects modifying albumin conformation, e.g., fatty acids (3,15,28). Increases in free fraction in hepatic disease have been reported for amobarbital, diazepam, meperidine, morphine, phenytoin, and thiopental (3,16,33). The importance of these changes depends in large part on the volume of distribution of the drug and the absence of other effects. Most psychotropic drugs have a large volume of distribution. In general, a decrease in affinity results in loss of drug from the plasma compartment, a fall in total drug concentration (D_T), an increase in free fraction, but little change in free drug (D_F) concentration ($D_F = \alpha \cdot D_T$). Since free drug concentration is relatively unchanged, no alteration in drug effect is detectable. On the other hand, kinetic calculations under conditions of changed binding and serum drug concentration interpretation are fraught with error (9,33).

Specific Drugs

Barbiturates

Significant reductions in the plasma clearance of hexobarbital occur in patients with cirrhosis and acute hepatitis (5,47). Half-life increases particularly in patients with decompensated cirrhosis (47), and amobarbital clearance is reduced in patients with chronic liver disease and low serum albumin concentrations. Serum amobarbital binding to plasma is reduced if the serum albumin is less than 3.5 g/dl. In contrast, phenobarbital, which is excreted to some extent by the kidney, shows only slight prolongation of the elimination half-life in patients with cirrhosis and acute viral hepatitis (1). Chronic dosing studies are not available.

Benzodiazepines

Most benzodiazepines are extensively metabolized by the liver. The clearance of benzodiazepines eliminated primarily by oxidation pathways of liver biotransformation is typically decreased by one-half to one-third in patients with liver disease, but the pharmacokinetics of the derivatives metabolized by conjugation, e.g., oxazepam and lorazepam, are not altered. For example, important reductions in plasma

clearances of diazepam (15) and chlordiazepoxide (29), along with significant prolongations of their elimination half-lives, are found in cirrhosis and acute viral hepatitis. Kinetics of desmethyldiazepam are similarly altered. Oxazepam pharmacokinetic parameters are not altered in patients with hepatic disease (37). In patients with cirrhosis, the elimination half-life of lorazepam is slightly elevated, but the plasma clearance of the drug is not altered. The slight increase in the elimination half-life can be explained by the increase in the volume of distribution (17).

Antidepressants and Antipsychotic Drugs

The major route of antidepressant and antipsychotic drug metabolism is oxidation by the hepatic microsomal mixed-function oxidase enzymes. Since these drugs typically undergo important first-pass metabolism when administered orally, their bioavailability is expected to increase importantly in the presence of hepatic dysfunction. Surprisingly very few data are available. The oral clearance of the femoxetine is reduced in patients with cirrhosis and the area under the plasma concentration-time curve increased (11). These results imply an increase in the drug's bioavailability with subsequent accumulation of the drug.

Other Drugs

Kinetic studies done with nonpsychotropic drugs in patients with cirrhosis and hepatitis suggest that important changes in bioavailability and intrinsic clearance of psychotropic drugs should occur. Opiates (e.g., morphine, methadone, heroin, meperidine), amitriptyline, L-dopa, phencyclidine, and peptides all fall into this category. No specific studies have been done to test this prediction.

SMOKERS AND SMOKING

Numerous studies and reviews document altered disposition of drugs in "heavy" cigarette smokers (13,35,42). Increased clearance (e.g., diazepam, lorazepam, N-desmethyldiazepam, oxazepam), lowered plasma drug concentrations (e.g., clomipramine, imipramine), and decreased urinary excretion (e.g., pentazocine, nicotine) are postulated to have occurred through induction of hepatic microsomal oxidizing enzymes, resulting in enhanced biotransformation. However, other drugs biotransformed through identical steps are unaffected (e.g., nortriptyline).

In contrast, insignificant changes in the kinetics of drugs that undergo conjugation reactions (e.g., glucuronidation of oxazepam, lorazepam) or nonmicrosomal metabolism are typical.

When heavy smoking affects clearance, twofold increases in mean oral clearance may occur [e.g., N-desmethyldiazepam: smokers, 0.044 liters/kg/hr, nonsmokers, 0.016 liters/kg/hr (23); and oxazepam (25)]. In contrast, when diazepam, lorazepam, and midazolam are given intravenously (24), no significant differences in mean systemic clearance are found. These data emphasize the difference between oral clearance and systemic clearance. Only chronic oral dosing studies can establish the steady-state kinetic and clinical consequences of the smoking effect. The relative lack of effect on total clearance suggests that decreases in sensitivity to drugs in heavy smokers may not be due to kinetic changes. There is evidence that heavy smoking is associated with a lesser degree of sedation, in particular for diazepam and chlordiazepoxide (4) and N-desmethyldiazepam (23). The therapeutic importance of this is unknown.

Although interpretation of most studies is consistent with enzyme induction, no graded response with respect to intensity of tobacco exposure is readily apparent. There are a number of reasons for this. For example, smoking history and the methods used to determine smoke constituent exposure are often inadequate (35).

ETHANOL

Acute and chronic ethanol ingestion alters the pharmacodynamics and disposition of psychotropic drugs (Tables 2 and 3). In most cases pharmacodynamic interaction appears to be more important than any concurrent pharmacokinetic interaction. The mechanisms of kinetic interactions and effects on drug metabolism have been reviewed (19,21,32,34,36).

A major flaw in most clinical patient studies is a relative lack of knowledge of the alcohol use history. The technologic power brought to bear on most pharmacokinetic studies stands in contrast to the lack of attention to obtaining reliable, valid, precise, stable, and objectively corroborated information on acute and chronic alcohol consumption (cf. tobacco). A "time-line follow-back" interview technique can be reliable and valid by objective indicators and collaterals, and in various alcoholic populations and in test-retest situations. Simple quantity-frequency methods of estimating alcohol consumption fail to characterize the pattern of alcohol consumption. Although good-quality data can be obtained using a time-line follow-back technique, either for a lifetime, for a month, or for up to a year, such an inquiry should be coupled to other measures to establish convergent validity of the characterization of the drinking history: for example, breath or urine alcohol.

Presystemic Hepatic First-Pass Drug Interaction

Theoretically, drugs with high bioavailability and low hepatic clearance may be expected to be less susceptible to the presystemic effects of prior administration of ethanol than drugs with low bioavailability and high hepatic extraction (45). Studies in the isolated perfused rat liver indicate that ethanol affects the initial rapid uptake phase into the liver and inhibits subsequent biotransformation of propranolol, a high-extraction drug, to its metabolites (7). Such studies suggest that the timing of the presentation of ethanol could be important to the type and extent of pharmacokinetic interaction (7,19,32,34). The hypothesis that high-extraction drugs are particularly susceptible to ethanol effects has been tested with amitriptyline, chlormethiazole, propoxyphene, and zimelidine. During the early absorptive phase, there is a marked relative increase in free amitriptyline concentration when ethanol has been administered 1 hr before. Such marked increases in amitriptyline concentrations associated with marked clinical pharmacodynamic interactions suggest that for this drug both pharmacokinetic and pharmacodynamic interactions are important.

However, even "low-extraction" drugs can demonstrate susceptibility to a presystemic absorptive phase interaction with ethanol. Ethanol, for example, causes a 96% relative increase in diazepam concentration 18 min after intravenous administration, and a 100% increase 15 min after oral diazepam administration compared with a diazepam-alone condition. Studies of the mechanism of pharmacodynamic interactions should therefore include numerous drug concentration measurements during the absorptive phase.

Specific Drugs

Three sequences of drug administration are relevant: (a) concurrent acute ingestion of single doses of ethanol and the psychotropic; (b) chronic ethanol abuse plus a single dose of a psychotropic drug in intoxicated and recently abstinent chronic alcoholics; and (c) chronic therapeutic use of a psychotropic drug plus an acute single dose of ethanol. All other clinical situations are variants on these three patterns (Tables 2 and 3).

Acute Ethanol Administration

Acute administration of ethanol to laboratory animals or incubation of microsomal preparations with ethanol (50 mM) inhibits the mixed-function oxidase enzymes. In the human, the clearance of various benzodiazepines that undergo oxidative biotransformation, chloral hydrate, and phenytoin decreases, and plasma elimination half-life of amitriptyline, chlordiazepoxide, diazepam, desmethyldiazepam, meprobamate, pentobarbital, and zimelidine is increased by acute ethanol administration. Such inhibition occurs with blood alcohol concentrations as low as 800 mg/liter. In general, as long as ethanol is present, inhibition continues. This results in an approximately 30% average increase in peak and area under the curve (AUC) plasma concentrations of psychotropic drugs administered orally, e.g., diazepam, chlordiazepoxide, and clobazam. Concurrent with inhibition of biotransformation and decrease in free drug clearance of parent compound, production of active metabolites is decreased. Ethanol has a lesser effect on drugs that are conjugated (e.g., lorazepam, oxazepam) (Table 2).

For those drugs susceptible to acute ethanol inhibition, the extent and nature of the pharmacokinetic interaction after coadministration can be importantly affected by the order of ethanol and drug administration. For example, administration of diazepam prior to the ingestion of alcohol results in relatively little effect of ethanol on diazepam pharmacokinetics (19,32). This is largely due to the absence of a presystemic hepatic first-pass drug interaction.

For a number of other drugs, e.g., methadone, methaqualone, and chlorpromazine, less convincing changes have been reported after acute ethanol.

TABLE 2. *Pharmacokinetic interactions of acute ethanol ingestion and psychotropic drugs administration[a]*

Drug (route of administration)	Effect of ethanol on drug pharmacokinetics
Barbiturates	
Pentobarbital (p.o.)	Increased $t_{\frac{1}{2}}$ (100%)
Amobarbital no alterations (p.o.)	
Other hypnotics	
Meprobamate (p.o.)	Increased $t_{\frac{1}{2}}$ (1–500%)
Glutethimide (p.o.)	Reduction of glutethimide plasma and urine concentrations
Chloral hydrate (p.o.)	Increased plasma concentration of trichlorethanol
Chlormethiazole (p.o.)	Reduction of chlormethiazole oral Cl (50%)
	Increased chlormethiazole bioavailability; $t_{\frac{1}{2}}$ unchanged
Benzodiazepines	
Chlordiazepoxide (p.o.)	Increased chlordiazepoxide plasma concentration
Chlordiazepoxide (i.v.)	Decreased total and unbound Cl of chlordiazepoxide (37%); increased $t_{\frac{1}{2}}$ (66%)
	Increased plasma concentration of N-desmethylchlordiazepoxide
Clobazam (p.o.)	Increased clobazam plasma concentration and AUC; Cl decreased (66%)
Diazepam (p.o.)	Increased initial diazepam concentrations
Diazepam (p.o.)	No alterations
Diazepam (p.o.)	Increased AUC of diazepam
Diazepam (p.o.)	Increased diazepam concentration at 90 min
Diazepam (p.o.)	Increased peak diazepam concentration
Diazepam (p.o.)	Decreased peak concentration, unchanged AUC
Diazepam (p.o.)	Increased diazepam concentration at 60 and 90 min
Diazepam (i.v.)	Increased diazepam AUC for total and unbound drug
Lorazepam (i.v.)	Reduced lorazepam (Cl 18%)
Oxazepam (p.o.)	Delayed absorption; unchanged disposition
Oxazepam (p.o.)	Unchanged disposition
Triazolam (p.o.)	Increased triazolam AUC
	Decreased triazolam total Cl (15%)
Antipsychotics	
Chlorpromazine (p.o.)	Reduced urine concentrations of chlorpromazine metabolites
Antidepressants	
Amitriptyline (p.o.)	Increased amitriptyline AUC; metabolite increased
Zimelidine (p.o.)	Norzimelidine production decreased (46%)

[a] Abbreviations: $t_{\frac{1}{2}}$, elimination half-life; Cl, clearance; AUC, area under the drug concentration-time curve.

A number of studies fail to detect kinetic changes after acute ethanol, e.g., buspirone, diazepam, fluoxetine, lithium, trazodone, triazolam, and zimelidine. The impact of trial design and other factors on the results is important but beyond the scope of this chapter.

Chronic Ethanol Administration

Chronic administration of ethanol to rats and humans causes proliferation of the smooth endoplasmic reticulum and an increase in microsomal protein content and cytochrome P-450 and results in an augmentation in drug-metabolizing ability of the microsomes *in vitro*. Ethanol is a much less potent inducer in rats than phenobarbital. In the human, the biotransformation and free clearance of oxidatively metabolized benzodiazepines, barbiturates, meprobamate, and phenytoin is increased. Since concurrent liver disease may alter plasma albumin concentration or be associated with impaired drug metabolism, measurement of free drug clearance may be necessary (Table 3).

In considering the effects of chronic ethanol administration, it is important to distinguish those studies of intoxicated chronic alcoholics from those of recently abstinent chronic alcoholics. Acutely intoxicated chronic alcoholics show a prolonged half-life of orally administered chlordiazepoxide compared to normal volunteers. These observations may reflect an impaired metabolic conversion of chlordiazepoxide to its desmethyl metabolite. Inconclusive or contradictory results probably reflect an offsetting combination of actions,

TABLE 3. *Pharmacokinetic interactions of chronic ethanol ingestion and psychotropic drugs administration[a]*

Drug (route of administration)	Effect of ethanol on drug pharmacokinetics
CNS depressants	
Pentobarbital (p.o.)	Decreased $t_{\frac{1}{2}}$ (25%)
Meprobamate (p.o.)	Decreased $t_{\frac{1}{2}}$ (50%)
Phenytoin	Decreased $t_{\frac{1}{2}}$ (40%)
	Cl increased (50%)
Benzodiazepines	
Chlordiazepoxide (p.o.)	Decreased plasma concentrations of chlordiazepoxide and desmethylchlordiazepoxide
Chlordiazepoxide (p.o.)	Decreased chlordiazepoxide AUC (p.o.)
Chlordiazepoxide (p.o.)	Increased $t_{\frac{1}{2}}$
Diazepam (i.v.)	Decreased AUC up to 24 hr
Diazepam (i.v.)	$t_{\frac{1}{2}}$ shorter on day 1 than after withdrawal; Cl and V_d unchanged
Antidepressants	
Imipramine	Decreased concentrations of imipramine and 2-hydroxy-imipramine decreased bioavailability (?)

[a] Abbreviations: $t_{\frac{1}{2}}$, elimination half-life; Cl, clearance; AUC, area under the drug concentration-time curve.

e.g., ethanol inhibition plus induction of biotransformation, as well as the difficulty of studying a transient ethanol effect in the presence of a drug with long half-life and low hepatic clearance.

In recently abstinent chronic alcoholics, the peak and area under the curve (AUC) for diazepam are lower, but the terminal elimination rate is no different after oral diazepam than in control subjects. Whether these results are due to a decrease in serum albumin with an increase in the volume of diazepam distribution, decreases in bioavailability, or increased biotransformation is not known. A comparable study in chronic alcoholics given intravenous diazepam also showed decreased peak diazepam and AUC up to 12 hr postdose and lower desmethyldiazepam levels, suggesting an increased initial volume of distribution.

The ability of chronic ethanol administration to induce metabolizing enzymes is the best available explanation of the observed decrease in chlordiazepoxide and diazepam blood levels; however, confirmatory evidence for this is needed, as are studies of the effect of chronic ethanol administration on the disposition of psychotropic drugs that are predominantly conjugated.

The clinical consequence of an increased drug clearance is that the average steady-state drug level will be lower. However, since the relationship of psychotropic drug concentration to effect is usually not established, the clinical importance of such changes is unknown. The clinical implication of increased clearance of CNS depressants is further confused, because there is cross tolerance between ethanol and such drugs, suggesting that chronic ethanol ingestion might not only decrease blood levels but also decrease central nervous system sensitivity to the drugs.

Chronic Psychotropic Drug Use and Single Doses of Ethanol

This pattern of study most closely simulates the usual circumstances of coingestion of the two drugs and is least studied. Theoretically, kinetic changes in psychotropic drug disposition may only be small because of their typically large volume of distribution. In addition, the relatively rapid elimination of ethanol compared to the long half-life of many psychotropic drugs makes it less likely that an important kinetic interaction will occur.

RENAL DISEASE

Renal elimination of drugs depends on the drug concentration in blood, the extent of protein binding, glomerular filtration rate, and tubular secretion and reabsorption (14,44). Although disease can affect these processes differentially, in practice this has not been shown to be of kinetic importance. Creatinine clearance provides a sufficient indicator of overall renal function. Since most psychotropic drugs are primarily metabolized by the liver, changes in their kinetics are not expected in renal disease. However, the elimination of the more water-soluble metabolites of these agents can be altered, and if they are pharmacologically active, unexpected therapeutic toxic effects may occur.

Finally, hepatic conjugation is reduced in uremic rats and humans, and there may well be altered drug metabolism in renal dysfunction (38) (Table 4).

Calculation of renal clearance requires knowledge of the free drug concentration. Since renal disease can profoundly affect protein binding of drugs, kinetic studies must include this. They rarely do. Renal failure is associated with decreases in binding (increased free fraction) for alprazolam, amobarbital, chlordiazepoxide, clobazam, diazepam, flurazepam, lorazepam, N-desmethyldiazepam, oxazepam, pentobarbital, and phenytoin. The effects of chronic renal failure on binding of basic drugs are more complex, since the binding proteins are often different than for acidic drugs, e.g., AGP and lipoproteins. In general, binding of basic drugs is not affected in renal failure.

Single-dose kinetic studies in normal subjects can establish the extent of renal excretion of a drug. Since changes in renal drug clearance and creatinine clearance are usually closely related, the estimation of creatinine clearance allows dosage adjustments for drugs that are primarily eliminated by the kidney (2). Specific studies in patients with renal disease become confirmatory.

Specific Drugs

Barbiturates

The metabolic clearance, elimination half-life, and volume of distribution of single doses of pentobarbital are unchanged in uremic patients (28). Pentobarbital protein binding is significantly reduced in uremic patients even when serum albumin concentration is normal. This suggests the presence of an endogenous inhibitor or inhibitors of binding, which decrease binding affinity (26). Since phenobarbital relies on the kidneys for approximately 30% of its excretion, slight kinetic changes are expected (2). This drug can be hemodialyzed and should be readministered after dialysis (2). Barbital is the only barbiturate that is primarily eliminated by the kidney; hence, important accumulation occurs in patients with end-stage renal failure even with hemodialysis. However, since the kinetic data are so sparse, drug dose should be adjusted in individual patients on the basis of serum drug concentrations and pharmacologic response.

Benzodiazepines

The high serum protein binding, large volume of distribution, and lipid solubility of benzodiazepines have kinetic implications in renal disease. First, their high volume of distribution and low free drug serum concentrations result in low dialysance. Second, changes in binding may importantly change total drug concentration (9).

Dosage adjustment of oxazepam in patients with renal insufficiency seems unnecessary on kinetic grounds. Single doses of oxazepam show an increase in the elimination half-life and the oral clearance of total drug in patients with chronic renal failure (20). Although the percent of oxazepam unbound increases, the intrinsic clearance of unbound drug and the free serum concentration is unchanged.

TABLE 4. *Pharmacokinetic parameters of psychotropic drugs in renal disease*

Drug	Dose and route of administration	Severity of renal insufficiency	N	Systemic clearance	Renal clearance	V_d	$t_{\frac{1}{2}}B$ (hr)
Barbiturates Pentobarbital	100 mg (p.o.)	HD	9	2.0 ± 0.6 liters/hr	—	58 ± 24 liters[b]	21.3 ± 8.7
			(11)	(1.6 ± 0.4 liters/hr)	—	(62 ± 25 liters)	(26.5 ± 9.5)
Benzodiazepines Lorazepam	2.5 mg (p.o.)	CRF $Cl_{cr} < 2$ ml/min	7				11.3 ± 0.6
		HD	7				9.4 ± 1.0
			(6)				(11.1 ± 0.9)
Oxazepam	30 mg (p.o.)	CRF $Cl_{cr} = 13 ± 2$ ml/kg/hr	4	170 ± 7* ml/kg/hr	0.61 ± 0.22 ml/kg/hr	5.8 ± 2.3*[a] liters/kg	25 ± 4*
		HD	4	120 ± 2 ml/kg/hr	—	3.4 ± 0.3*[a] liters/kg	33 ± 3*
			(13)	(90 ± 6) ml/kg/hr	(0.52 ± .07) ml/kg/hr	(1.0 ± 0.1) liters/kg	(10 ± 1)
Triazolam	0.5 mg (p.o.)	HD (7) CAPD (4)	11	5.5 (1.5–31.2) ml/kg/min	—	—	2.3 (1.4–5.7)
			(11)	[3.50 (1.41–8.58) ml/kg/min]			[2.6 (1.68–5.17)]
Tricyclic antidepressants Nortriptyline	75 mg (p.o.)	HD	5				26.3
		CRF	10				29.5
			(8)				(24.8)

N, Number of subjects; V_d, volume of distribution; [a]V_d at steady state; [b]V_d of one-compartment model; $t_{\frac{1}{2}}B$, elimination half-life; HD, hemodialyzed patients; CRF, chronic renal failure; * indicates statistical significance; ( ), values for the control group of subjects; CAPD, continuous ambulatory peritoneal dialysis; Cl_{cr}, creatinine clearance.

The plasma elimination half-life of lorazepam is not altered in chronic renal failure patients on hemodialysis, but plasma lorazepam glucuronide is higher (40). The accumulation of lorazepam glucuronide may not be clinically important as long as deconjugation does not occur, since this metabolite is inactive. In the only steady-state study, lorazepam serum concentration and half-life were significantly prolonged in two patients in chronic renal failure (22).

Single-dose triazolam oral clearance and elimination half-life are unaltered in end-stage renal insufficiency (18).

Antipsychotic Drugs

Studies on the effect of renal disease on the kinetics of antipsychotic drugs are not available. A report of toxic psychosis occurring in four patients receiving chlorpromazine, along with the theoretical distant effects of renal failure on hepatic extraction and metabolism of high-extraction drugs, suggests studies of such drugs are needed.

Antidepressants

Single-dose pharmacokinetics of nortriptyline and its two major metabolites (conjugated and unconjugated 10-hy-droxynortriptyline) have been evaluated in chronic renal failure and hemodialysis patients. Nortriptyline pharmacokinetics were not altered. In the hemodialyzed patients, however, concentrations of conjugated 10-hydroxynortrip-tyline were elevated, suggesting decreased elimination (6). Serum concentrations of amitriptyline, desipramine, imipramine, nortriptyline, and their metabolites, under steady-state conditions in patients with chronic renal failure undergoing hemodialysis, are not changed (20). Levels of conjugated hydroxylated metabolites are markedly elevated. Some data suggest that tricyclic antidepressant glucuronides may have some pharmacologic effect.

CHRONIC DRUG ABUSE

The use of single or multiple drugs in high doses over long periods of time would be expected to modify the kinetics of numerous psychotropic drugs. Ethanol, barbiturates, glutethimide, and smoking are all known enzyme inducers during chronic use. Drug abusers frequently combine the use of CNS depressants. Probably because proper studies in this free-spirited population are so difficult, none have been reported. Autoinduction has been shown with secobarbital. Unpublished single case studies suggest that the disposition of some psychoactive drugs in this population can be markedly changed. For example, secobarbital $t_{\frac{1}{2}} =$

6 hr; phenytoin $t_{\frac{1}{2}}$ = 3 hr; high total methadone plasma concentrations associated with high AGP; very low amitriptyline levels but higher nortriptyline.

CONCLUSION

From this survey of the changes in kinetics of psychotropic drugs, certain predictions can be made about the effects of liver disease, ethanol use, smoking, and renal disease on psychotropic drug kinetics. In severe liver disease, drug oxidation will be impaired but conjugation unaffected. Acute ethanol inhibits oxidation and relatively spares glucuronidation and acetylation. Chronic ethanol and heavy smoking result in enzyme induction and increase drug clearance. In chronic renal disease relatively minor effects are found, since most psychotropic drugs are metabolized by the liver. Despite persuasive overall data to support these generalizations, the data for individual drugs and selected clinical situations are sparse and often methodologically seriously flawed.

In this chapter hepatic and renal disease have been regarded as stable phenomena. They are not. Hence knowledge of average changes in kinetics is not very useful in a particular patient and clinical circumstance. The available information only provides a general understanding and data base available for decision making. The clinician is therefore forced to monitor drug concentrations and clinical responses in each patient.

In general, the overall quality of kinetic studies (with some notable exceptions) with psychotropic drugs is relatively poor compared to the methodologic standards of the pharmacokinetics discipline.

Obviously, kinetic changes say little about the therapeutic importance of the changes. It is surprising that so few studies have attempted to relate the altered kinetics to clinical effects. Such studies are urgently needed. Drugs that undergo substantial hepatic extraction are prime candidates to be associated with clinically important changes in the selected populations discussed in this chapter. Many unstudied psychotropic drugs are within this group.

Conversely, psychotropic drugs that are inactivated in the liver by conjugation and have high systemic bioavailability will not be affected by ethanol, smoking, drug abuse, liver disease, or inhibitors of drug metabolism. Such drugs will also have less variable kinetics and in the long term will be the preferred psychotropic drugs in therapeutic use. Preclinical studies should take this into consideration in the identification of new clinical leads.

ACKNOWLEDGMENTS

We thank our colleagues with whom we have collaborated and Ms. Donna Campbell and Ms. Karen Cauch-Bontje for their assistance in preparing this chapter.

NOTE

A complete bibliography is available on request to the authors.

REFERENCES

1. Alvin, J., McHorse, T., Hoyumpa, A., Bush, M. T., and Schenker, S. (1975): *J. Pharm. Exp. Ther.*, 192:224–235.
2. Bennett, W. J., Aronoff, G. R., Morrison, G., Golper, T. A., Pulliam, J., Wolfson, M., and Singer, I. (1983): *Am. J. Kidney Dis.*, 3:155–193.
3. Blaschke, T. F. (1977): *Clin. Pharmacokinet.*, 2:32–44.
4. Boston Collaborative Drug Surveillance Program (1973): *N. Engl. J. Med.*, 288:277–280.
5. Breimer, D. D., Zilly, W., and Richter, E. (1975): *Clin. Pharmacol. Ther.*, 18:433–440.
6. Dawling, S., Lynn, K., Rosser, R., and Braithwaite, R. (1982): *Clin. Pharmacol. Ther.*, 32:322–329.
7. Dorian, P., Sellers, E. M., Carruthers, G., Hamilton, C., and Fan, T. (1982): *Clin. Pharmacol. Ther.*, 31:219.
8. Greenblatt, D. J., Abernethy, D. R., Morse, D. S., Harmatz, J. S., and Shader, R. I. (1984): *N. Engl. J. Med.*, 310:1639–1643.
9. Greenblatt, D. J., Sellers, E. M., and Koch-Weser, J. (1982): *J. Clin. Pharmacol.*, 22:259–263.
10. Grossman, S. H., Davis, D., Kitchell, B. B., Shand, D. G., and Routledge, P. A. (1982): *Clin. Pharmacol. Ther.*, 31:350–357.
11. Hansen, B. A., Mengele, H., Keiding, S., and Lund, J. (1984): *Acta Pharmacol. Toxicol.*, 55:386–389.
12. Hoyumpa, A. M., Jr., Desmond, P. V., Roberts, R. K., Nichols, S., Johnson, R. F., and Schenker, S. (1980): *J. Lab. Clin. Med.*, 95:310–321.
13. Jusko, W. J. (1978): *J. Pharmacokinet. Biopharm.*, 6:7–39.
14. Jusko, W. J. (1980): In: *Applied Pharmacokinetics, Principles of Therapeutic Drug Monitoring*, edited by W. E. Evans, J. J. Schentag, and W. J. Jusko, pp. 639–680. Applied Therapeutics, San Francisco.
15. Klotz, U., Avant, G. R., Hoyumpa, A., Schenker, S., and Wilkinson, G. R. (1975): *J. Clin. Invest.*, 55:347–359.
16. Koch-Weser, J., and Sellers, E. M. (1976): *N. Engl. J. Med.*, 294: 311–316, 526–531.
17. Kraus, J. W., Desmond, P. V., Marshall, J. P., Johnson, R. F., Schenker, S., and Wilkinson, G. R. (1978): *Clin. Pharmacol. Ther.*, 24:411–419.
18. Kroboth, P. D., Smith, R. B., Silver, M. R., Rault, R., Sorkin, M. I., Puschett, J. B., and Juhl, R. P. (1985): *Br. J. Clin. Pharmacol.*, 19:839–842.
19. Lane, E. A., Guthrie, S., and Linnoila, M. (1985): *Clin. Pharmacokinet.*, 10:228–247.
20. Lieberman, J. A., Cooper, T. B., Suckow, R. F., Steinberg, H., Borenstein, M., Brenner, R., and Kane, J. M. (1985): *Clin. Pharmacol. Ther.*, 37:301–307.
21. Linnoila, M., Mattila, M. J., and Kitchell, B. S. (1979): *Drugs*, 18: 299–311.
22. Murray, T. G., Chiang, S. T., Koepke, H. H., and Walker, B. R. (1981): *Clin. Pharmacol. Ther.*, 30:805–809.
23. Norman, T. R., Fulton, A., Burrows, G. D., and Maguire, K. P. (1981): *Eur. J. Clin. Pharmacol.*, 21:229–233.
24. Ochs, H. R., Greenblatt, D. J., and Knuchel, M. (1985): *Chest*, 87:223–226.
25. Ochs, H. R., Greenblatt, D. J., and Otten, H. (1981): *Klin. Wochenschr.*, 59:899–903.
26. Odar-Cederlof, I. (1986): In: *Drug Protein Binding*, edited by M. M. Reidenberg and S. Erill, pp. 175–187. Praeger Press, New York.
27. Reidenberg, M. M., and Erill, S., eds. (1986): *Drug Protein Binding*. Praeger Press, New York.
28. Reidenberg, M. M., Lowenthal, D. T., Briggs, W., and Gasparo, M. (1976): *Clin. Pharmacol. Ther.*, 20:67–71.
29. Roberts, R. K., Wilkinson, G. R., Branch, R. A., and Schenker, S. (1978): *Gastroenterology*, 75:479–485.
30. Rowland, M., and Tozer, T. N., eds. (1980): *Clinical Pharmacokinetics: Concepts and Applications*. Lea and Febiger, Philadelphia.
31. Sellers, E. M. (1979): In: *Metabolic Effects of Alcohol*, edited by P. Avogaro, C. R. Sirtori, and E. Tremoli, pp. 113–138. Elsevier/North Holland Biomedical Press, Amsterdam.
32. Sellers, E. M. (1984): *Psychopharmacol. Bull.*, 20:497–499.
33. Sellers, E. M. (1986): In: *Drug Protein Binding*, edited by M. M. Reidenberg and S. Erill, pp. 257–273. Praeger Press, New York.

34. Sellers, E. M., and Busto, U. (1982): *J. Clin. Psychopharmacol.,* 2:249–262.
35. Sellers, E. M., Frecker, R. C., and Romach, M. K. (1983): *Drug Metab. Rev.,* 14:225–250.
36. Sellers, E. M., and Holloway, M. R. (1978): *Clin. Pharmacokinet.,* 3:440–452.
37. Shull, H. J., Wilkinson, G. R., Johnson, R., and Schenker, S. (1976): *Ann. Intern. Med.,* 84:420–425.
38. Verbeeck, R. K. (1982): *Drug Metab. Dispos.,* 10:87–89.
39. Verbeeck, R. K., Tjandramaga, T. B., De Schepper, P. J., and Verberckmoes, R. (1981): *Br. J. Clin. Pharmacol.,* 12:749–751.
40. Verbeeck, R. K., Tjandramaga, T. B., Verberckmoes, R., and De Schepper, P. J. (1976): *Br. J. Clin. Pharmacol.,* 3:1033–1039.
41. Vesell, E. S., and Penno, M. B. (1983): *Clin. Pharmacokinet.,* 8: 378–409.
42. Vestal, R. E., and Wood, A. J. (1980): *Clin. Pharmacokinet.,* 5: 309–319.
43. Wilkinson, G. R., and Schenker, S. (1976): *Biochem. Pharmacol.,* 25:2675–2681.
44. Wilkinson, G. R., and Shand, D. G. (1975): *Clin. Pharmacol. Ther.,* 18:377–390.
45. Williams, R. L. (1983): *N. Engl. J. Med.,* 309:1616–1622.
46. Williams, R. L., and Mamelok, R. D. (1980): *Clin. Pharmacokinet.,* 5:528–547.
47. Zilly, W., Breimer, D. D., and Richter, E. (1978): *Clin. Pharmacol. Ther.,* 23:525–534.

Psychopharmacology:
The Third Generation of Progress,
edited by Herbert Y. Meltzer.
Raven Press, New York © 1987.

CHAPTER **147**

Introduction: Side Effects

Richard Jed Wyatt

This book summarizes the dramatic advances in psychopharmacology that have taken place during the last 30 years. Although modern psychopharmacology has profoundly decreased suffering in our patients, this progress has not been made without discomfort, toxicity, and, at times, death. It is almost axiomatic that no prevention or intervention in medicine occurs without some human cost. Being severely ill is risky business, and even the most charmed magic bullet leaves its trace (10). Nevertheless, it is up to the physician to know the risks involved, to be alert to adverse effects, and to weigh the advantages of treatment against his oath to "do no harm."

Until this century, medical knowledge had not evolved sufficiently to provide effective treatment for most illnesses. The physician could offer little more than comfort and hope. Physicians were obliged by the Hippocratic tradition not to alarm their patients but to convey the appearance of resolution regardless of the difficulties (3). By the late nineteenth century, Tolstoy complained, "What tormented Ivan Ilych most was the deception, that lie, which for some reason they all accepted, that he was not dying but was simply ill" (9, p. 137). All this changed dramatically, however, with the introduction of modern medicine. The quick progress of medicine and the related sciences in this century has made the social interaction between patient and physician very complex. Physician and patient have suddenly become shared decision makers; Hippocrates' admonition to protect the patient from knowledge is no longer possible or advisable. Nevertheless, because of the patient's fear and unwillingness to cope with reality, some denial of knowledge must necessarily exist. When we go as patients to the physician, our main concern is not for knowledge but for healing and restoration to our original selves. Unfortunately, though, no matter how effective the treatment, the health or imagined health of our youth rarely fully returns following a serious illness.

The physician must not collude with the patient by witholding information that may be frightening but helpful to the treatment process. In order for effective collaboration to be established, the physician must know the boundaries of his science and art, educate his patient about them, and go into battle against the illness with the patient as an ally. For both physician and patient, determining a reasonable balance between assault on the disease and assault on the body can be extremely difficult.

The following six chapters describe some of these difficulties as they are manifest in the side effects, complications, and adverse effects of powerful medical tools. Often these effects are so mild that they cannot be differentiated from normal variations in life. On other occasions, however, they seem as frightening as the disorders the medications treat. Perhaps most discomforting for physician and patient alike is that the hazards of the diseases and the hazards of their treatments, in most cases, cannot be measured on the same scale; they are calibrated differently and do not relate to each other in a linear mode.

How can lithium's blunting of life be weighed against the erasure of suicidal thoughts or against the destruction left in the wake of a manic hurricane? Similarly, how can the neuroleptic's blunting of affect be balanced against its dissolution of satanic schizophrenic delusions? How can we assess the relative value of terminating hallucinations commanding a patient to jump from a bridge against the potential of tardive dyskinesia's motoric distortions or the lethal potential of the neuroleptic malignant syndrome?

In evaluating the relative risk of developing adverse treatment effects, one must be able to make comparisons with patients not receiving the treatment. Since adverse effects are almost always qualitatively similar to signs and symptoms encountered on occasion in the absence of medications, it is important to know the percentage of patients who would develop the effects if they had never been medicated. For example, tardive dyskinesia-like movements were described in psychiatric patients many years before the introduction of neuroleptic medication. In 1919 Emil Kraepelin wrote:

Some of them resemble movements of expression, wrinkling of the forehead, distortion of the corners of the mouth, irregular movements of the tongue and lips, twisting of the eyes, opening them wide and shutting them tight, in short, those movements which we bring together under the name of making faces or *grimacing;* they remind one of the corresponding disorder of choreic patients. . . .Connected with these are further, smacking and clicking with the tongue, sudden sighing, sniffing, laughing and clearing throat. But besides, we observe specially in the lip muscles, fine lightning-like or rhythmical twitchings, which in no way bear the stamp of voluntary movements. . . .Several patients continually carried out peculiar sprawling, irregular, choreiform, outspreading movements, which I think can best be characterised by the expression 'athetoid ataxia' (8, p. 83).

Spontaneously occurring tardive dyskinesia-like movements are present in up to 6% of chronically hospitalized psychiatric patients who have never been on neuroleptic medication (4,11).

An evaluation of the risk of neuroleptic-induced tardive dyskinesia must compare patients with spontaneously developing dyskinesias to the total group developing tardive dyskinesia-like movements. When this comparison is performed, the risk of developing neuroleptic-induced persistent tardive dyskinesia (about 13%) is found to be approximately twice as great as developing tardive dyskinesia-like movements if no neuroleptic were used. The incidence of crippling tardive dyskinesia is not known, but it appears to be far less than 5% of the patients who are given chronic neuroleptic medications.

When possible, risks such as those just cited are best presented numerically so that arithmetic comparisons can be made and physicians and their patients can make informed judgments. Physicians need to be expert technicians at balancing the odds, interpreting them for their patients, and using their art to read the subtle clues of the sometimes frightened and impaired patient.

There is perhaps even more important information that is often not presented to the psychiatric patient. What is the course of the symptoms and illness in patients not treated in a prescribed manner? Often the morbidity or mortality can only be surmised. Some data, however, are available. In a recent study in our research setting (7) we had many more serious assaultive events over a 6-week period when patients were off medications than when medicated. Similarly, in a well-controlled prospective study, Johnson et al. (6) followed schizophrenic patients who discontinued their neuroleptic medications after a lengthy period of stability as well as a group who remained on their medications. In the group who discontinued their medications, there was not only the expected higher number of relapses, but also, increased antisocial behavior and self-injury.

The patient, his family, and society need to consider the potential of suicide in any decision to take or not take psychotropic medications. In both schizophrenia and the affective disorders, the lifetime risk of suicide is about 15%. The mortality and treatment benefits in severe affective disorders are better recognized than for schizophrenia. The best available and admittedly limited data suggest that lithium treatment has decreased the successful suicide rate in patients with bipolar affective disorder from about 15% to almost zero (2). This statement must not be construed as an invitation for complacency.

It is natural that we want to provide the least toxic treatments possible for our patients, and harm to any patient is cause for concern and study. But when placed in perspective, we may be doing quite well. The relative number of patients with serious psychotropic medication-related adverse effects is small. This is especially true when we consider the things to which people voluntarily subject themselves. For example, the toll from cigarettes and alcohol is greater than from psychotropic medications. The average male smoker will lose 2,250 days of his life from smoking. Smoking cigars will cause 330 days of lost life and smoking a pipe 220 days of lost life. The alcoholic may lose 12 to 15 years of his life. Being 30 pounds overweight will cause an average of 1,300 days of lost life. And these facts do not begin to take into consideration the profound qualitative disturbance produced. Yet these are situations over which one can exert at least some control.

Not wearing seat belts (only one of seven people regularly uses seat belts despite considerable education and a number of state laws requiring their use), riding motor bikes without helmets, or living on the San Andreas fault are potentially more lethal than the taking of prescribed psychotropic medications. Deaths from taking neuroleptics or antidepressants are comparatively rare and most of those from antidepressants are from fatal overdoses. Thus, given the risks individuals knowingly court every day or compared with the illnesses treated with the psychotropic medications, these drugs are relatively safe.

Further, not only are the psychotropic medications relatively safe, but their side effects, when viewed from a long-range perspective, have proved to be important to the advance of medicine. One might argue that because of the wealth of new knowledge gained simply from drug side effects, these medications have produced greater good than harm.

The sedation of benzodiazepines is used in the management of presurgical patients. Lithium's ability to increase the white blood cell count has been advantageous for patients with depleted white blood cell counts. The tricyclic antidepressants are being used as antiarrhythmic agents (Glassman, *this volume*). Chlorpromazine ointment has recently been shown to promote healing in diffuse cutaneous leishmaniasis, a condition resistant to other treatments (4). Even the thalidomide disaster was turned into something positive: a treatment for leprosy or Hansen's disease.

Despite the bewildering contradictions of our modern life, the physician, through the tradition of the Hippocratic Oath, has been charged "to do no harm." More specifically, the Hippocratic Oath says:

I will apply dietetic measures for the benefit of the sick according to my ability and judgement; I will keep them from harm and injustice (1).

When "do no harm" is taken out of context, however, it is a starkly paralyzing phrase that is not the intent of the Hippocratic Oath. One cannot practice medicine without sometimes inflicting hurt. The only approach that can be taken is to do the greatest amount of good while doing the least amount of harm. Each decision is an artful balance.

REFERENCES

1. Edelstein, L. (1943): *The Hippocratic Oath: Text, Translation and Interpretation.* Johns Hopkins Press, Baltimore.

2. Goodwin, F. K., and Jamison, K. R. (1988): *Manic-Depressive Illness.* Oxford University Press (*in press*).
3. Gregory, J. (1817): *Lectures on the Duties and Qualifications of a Physician.* M. Carey & Son, Philadelphia.
4. Henriksen, T. H., and Lende, S. (1983): *Lancet,* 1:126.
5. Jeste, D. V., and Wyatt, R. J. (1982): *Understanding and Treating Tardive Dyskinesia.* Guilford Press, New York.
6. Johnson, D. A. W., Pasterski, G., Ludlow, J. M., Street, K., and Taylor, R. D. W. (1983): *Acta Psychiatr. Scand.,* 67:339–352.
7. Karson, C. N., and Bigelow, L. B. (1986): *Journal of Nervous and Mental Disorders* (*in press*).
8. Kraepelin, E. (1919): *Dementia Praecox and Paraphrenia,* R. M. Barclay and G. M. Roberston, trans. Robert E. Krieger, Huntington, NY (reprinted 1971).
9. Tolstoy, L. (1982): "The Death of Ivan Ilych." In: *The Death of Ivan Ilych and Other Stories,* pp. 95–157. New American Library, New York.
10. Wyatt, R. J. (1985): In: *Comprehensive Textbook of Psychiatry/ IV,* No. 2, edited by H. I. Kaplan and B. J. Sadock, pp. 2016–2027. Williams and Wilkins, Baltimore.
11. Wyatt, R. J., and Jeste, D. V. (1984): *Psychiatr. News,* January, p. 2.

Psychopharmacology:
The Third Generation of Progress,
edited by Herbert Y. Meltzer.
Raven Press, New York © 1987.

CHAPTER **148**

Tardive Dyskinesia

Daniel E. Casey

Tardive dyskinesia (TD) is a syndrome of involuntary hyperkinetic abnormal movements that occur in predisposed individuals during or following the cessation of long-term neuroleptic drug therapy. The increasing concern about this syndrome has led to a reconsideration of the proper indications for these highly efficacious and widely used drugs. In addition, TD has focused substantial research into the mechanisms of current drug treatments and stimulated the pursuit of new antipsychotic agents that are free of troublesome side effects.

TD has a relatively brief history. The first description of this syndrome was by Schönecker (87) in 1957 in German, followed by a second description in French in 1959 (88). The next report was the first English language publication from a Danish group in 1960 (96). Until Faurbye et al. in 1964 (35) offered the term "tardive dyskinesia," it was variably described as the "bucco-linguo-masticatory syndrome" and "terminal extrapyramidal insufficiency syndrome." From then until the early 1970s the debate gradually evolved from whether TD actually existed to the epidemiological aspects of this syndrome. In the past decade there has been an explosion of research in all areas of TD.

CLINICAL DESCRIPTION

TD is characterized by involuntary, repetitive, purposeless hyperkinetic movements. The original descriptions emphasized orofacial signs: chewing, tongue protrusion and vermicular movements, lip smacking, puckering, and pursing,

as well as rapid eye blinking and blepharospasm. TD can also affect the upper and lower limbs with choreoathetosis. Occasionally the hands and fingers move in a repetitious pattern that resembles playing an invisible piano or guitar. Axial symptoms of forward and backward pelvic thrusting or discontinuous rotatory hip motions may also develop. Rarely, breathing or swallowing dyskinesias produce irregular respiratory rates or grunting noises (14).

Though atypical forms of TD have been recognized for many years (30), recent interest has focused on these less characteristic presentations. Tardive dystonia occurs more often in younger patients and is predominated by sustained abnormal positions with torticollis, blepharospasm, grimacing, and truncal torsion (10). Tardive akathisia is persisting restlessness (3). Like tardive dystonia, this syndrome can also occur by itself, but both are more often accompanied by typical TD movements. It is unclear if these different symptoms represent distinct pathophysiological mechanisms or are better explained as symptom clusters that reflect the breadth of the TD syndrome. Early reports of TD in children noted that axial dystonic features predominated over orofacial signs, but later evaluations suggested that the syndrome in children was more similar to than different from the adult presentations (12,47).

TERMINOLOGY

The temporal aspects of TD have been specifically characterized (40). Covert dyskinesia is unmasked when neuroleptic drugs are reduced or discontinued. Withdrawal dyskinesia appears under similar treatment conditions, but disappears spontaneously in 6 to 12 weeks. Overt dyskinesia is present during neuroleptic treatment. Defining persisting TD as irreversible after 6 or 12 months is arbitrary and too narrowly conceptualizes the long-term outcome. Some TD improves or resolves over many years (26). The most plausible explanation of these different outcomes is that TD occurs along a continuum of reversible to irreversible dysfunction, but specific pathophysiological mechanisms have not been identified.

A separate approach establishes research diagnostic criteria that have been widely accepted (86). Three prerequisites are (a) at least 3 months of cumulative neuroleptic exposure; (b) at least moderate abnormal involuntary movements in one or more body areas or mild movements in two or more body areas; and (c) the absence of other conditions that produce involuntary hyperkinetic dyskinesias. Commonly used scales are the Abnormal Involuntary Movements Scale (AIMS), the Dyskinesia Rating Scale, and the St. Hans Scale (41,51,89). After these three criteria are met, drug treatment status and temporal aspects determine the different TD categories of probable, masked probable, transient, withdrawal, persisting, and masked persisting TD. However, the caution applies that a particular point on a rating scale does not constitute a diagnosis. Rating scales are for descriptive and quantitative purposes. Diagnoses require in-depth analyses of epidemiological, etiological, and temporal aspects of symptoms.

DIFFERENTIAL DIAGNOSIS

Idiopathic (Spontaneous) Dyskinesias

The controversy surrounding the role of abnormal movements in psychosis is not new. Kraepelin and Bleuler debated the existence and meaning of choreiform dyskinesias as they set the foundation for our current concepts of dementia praecox (schizophrenia). Kraepelin believed that abnormal movements were an integral part of the biological basis of schizophrenia:

Some of these movements correspond exactly to the movements of expression: wrinkling of the eyebrow, distortion of the mouth, rolling the eyes, and those other facial movements which are characterized as grimacing. These movements remind one of choreic movements and are quite independent of ideas and feelings. There may be associated with them smacking of the lips, clucking the tongue, sudden grunting, sniffing, and coughing. Furthermore, in the lips we observe very rapid rhythmical movements. More often there exists a peculiar choreiform movement of the mouth which may be described as athetoid ataxia (72).

By tying together some of these seemingly unrelated signs, Kraepelin may have grouped heterogeneous disorders of idiopathic, postinfectious, traumatic, or hereditary neurodegenerative origin.

Bleuler took an opposing view about the meaning of chorea in schizophrenia:

The expressive gestures are also modified. Every conceivable stilted gesture occurs. . . . Grimaces of all kinds, peculiar

ways of shrugging the shoulders, extraordinary movements of the tongue and lips, finger play, sudden involuntary gestures—all of these peculiarities are the reasons why some authors have spoken of choreic or tetanic movements in catatonia, quite mistakenly though.

Choreal, athetotic, and tetanic phenomena are entirely different from the motor symptoms which accompany schizophrenia. The confinement of the movements to specific groups of muscles can be much better explained on a psychic than on an anatomic basis (8).

Is it possible to reconcile these seemingly disparate perspectives? Were Kraepelin and Bleuler seeing the same signs and symptoms, or were they making fundamentally different observations about disorders of movement in schizophrenia? An unequivocal answer to the question is impossible. However, the most parsimonious explanation centers around issues of definition of terms and theoretical framework. Both these astute clinicians observed similar signs of "grimacing" and "irregular (extraordinary) movements of the tongue and lips," but adopted polar positions when interpreting these phenomena. Resolving this apparent conflict is possible by proposing that Kraepelin may have overinclusively combined diverse and unrelated signs within a biological framework, whereas Bleuler offered an overly strict psychological explanation for abnormal movements.

Stereotypies and mannerisms of psychosis, as well as other idiopathic dyskinesias, are part of a differential diagnosis of movement disorders. Syndromes termed spontaneous orofacial dyskinesia and blepharospasm-oromandibular dystonia syndrome or Meige syndrome (54) must be distinguished from other focal and segmental dystonias. Tourette's syndrome is a disorder of involuntary tics and vocalizations; it starts in childhood and continues with a waxing and waning course through adult life. Simple persisting tics in an isolated muscle group are another consideration. Dental problems can also cause orofacial movements (14).

Neuroleptic Acute Extrapyramidal Syndromes

Acute dystonia occurs most often during the first few days of neuroleptic treatment, whereas drug-induced parkinsonism (tremor, rigidity, and bradykinesia) usually develops after several days of drug therapy. Akathisia, a subjective feeling of restlessness that may have motor manifestations of an inability to sit still and continuous motions of the trunk, can be misdiagnosed as a psychotic exacerbation or as TD. The rabbit syndrome is rapid rhythmical twitching in the lips and perioral area which improves with anticholinergic agents (14). Coexisting TD and acute extrapyramidal syndromes (EPS) are infrequently written about, though these dyskinesias simultaneously occur in 20 to 30% of TD patients receiving neuroleptics (82).

A syndrome phenomenologically similar but pharmacologically opposite to TD is occasionally described as paradoxical TD or initial hyperkinesia (21,43,74). It may be a distinct acute EPS syndrome because it often reverses with anticholinergics or quickly resolves when neuroleptics are discontinued. Increased cholinergic or antidopaminergic influences aggravate the symptoms. Alternatively, this syndrome may be a subtype of TD. It probably occurs more often than is recognized, as many pharmacological studies of TD note that a few patients have responses that are opposite or paradoxical to the main predicted treatment effect. This emphasizes the point that different pathophysiological mechanisms may be expressed clinically by similar symptoms, such as hyperkinetic dyskinesias.

Other Drug-Induced Dyskinesias

Many other drugs can produce movement disorders that must be differentiated from TD. Anticholinergics and antihistaminics rarely cause dyskinesias after prolonged use. Chorea, as well as stereotyped behavior, can occur with chronic amphetamine abuse. Several anticonvulsants, oral contraceptives, chloroquine, and other antimalarial drugs can also evoke reversible orofacial and limb dyskinesias (2,14,59).

Hereditary and Systemic Illnesses Associated with Dyskinesia

The hereditary neurodegenerative syndromes of Huntington's disease and Wilson's disease (hepatolenticular degeneration) may initially present with signs that resemble TD and/or psychosis, but are usually distinguishable by clinical signs, laboratory tests, and family history. Endocrinopathies of hyperthyroidism and hypoparathyroidism, and other syndromes such as chorea in pregnancy (chorea gravidarum), systemic lupus erythematosis, Henoch-Schönlein's purpura, and encephalitis can all be associated with hyperkinetic dyskinesias (14).

EPIDEMIOLOGY

Prevalence

The prevalence of TD greatly varies from 0.5 to 100% (2,6,20,61). This wide range undoubtedly reflects many variables, including different populations at risk, characteristics of past and present treatment, and criteria for diagnosis. Conservative estimates of average TD prevalence rates are 15 to 20%, but may exceed 70% in high-risk populations, such as the elderly. Spontaneous dyskinesia (SD) rates average 5% (2,20,59,61).

Although most studies show TD prevalence rates are higher than SD rates, a few do not. This has led some to question whether TD exists. A recent study that initially reported no significant difference between prevalence of TD (67%) and SD (53%) in chronically psychotic schizophrenics (77) did show a significant drug effect when the data were reanalyzed with age-matched groups (32).

TD prevalence rates have steadily increased by approximately 1% per year over the past two decades (20,59,61). However, SD rates have also increased at about 1% per year. The difference between the two rates has remained relatively stable at approximately 15% when similar patient groups were compared at the same time. When TD rates were low, SD rates were low, as in the 1960s, and when TD rates were high, SD rates were high, as in the early 1980s. This suggests that greater awareness and vigilance may have increased the reported rates of all abnormal movements. Both TD and SD were probably underdiagnosed 20 years ago, and are overdiagnosed currently (20).

SD and TD may be associated. They can be phenomenologically similar and share risk factors of increasing age and female sex (25). Perhaps a preexisting vulnerability interacts with additional elements, such as disease (schizophrenia, etc.), drugs (neuroleptics, etc.), and environment (toxins, etc.) to convert a covert predisposition to clinically overt symptoms (20). This hypothesis could account for the findings of a naturally occurring 5% SD base rate and an uncorrected 20% TD rate, yielding a corrected net neuroleptic drug contribution of 15% (2,20,61).

The large majority of prevalence rates are cross-sectional analyses that identify the number of existing cases at a specified time. They do not reflect the important but complex influence of some existing cases resolving and some new cases developing. For example, the TD prevalence rate decreased from 31 to 27% over 1 year (5), but the true change in TD prevalence is clouded by an increase in neuroleptic dosage—a factor known to suppress TD. A separate 3-year follow-up study (4) reported a TD prevalence increase from 39 to 47%, which included 22 new and 14 resolved cases, where the average drug dose also increased. Picking single points and not accounting for treatment status may lead to considerably different conclusions regarding TD prevalence.

Criteria for defining a case of TD markedly influence prevalence rates. When the mildest symptoms are included, prevalence can be 70%, whereas severe symptom rates are 2.5% (2). When minimal symptom criteria were used to assess elderly retarded patients, prevalence rates of TD and SD were 100 and 85%, respectively (6). Case definition criteria also affect idiopathic orofacial SD rates in monkeys. The prevalence averaged 5% for mild symptoms, which is remarkably similar to SD rates in patients (2,25,61) and ranged from 24.4 to 0.4% (20). The highest rate occurred when the least restrictive criteria (minimal symptoms) were applied to the oldest monkeys, whereas the lowest rate occurred when the strictest criteria (severe symptoms) were applied to the youngest animals.

RISK FACTORS

Age/Gender

TD frequency and severity increase with age. Pooled data from nine studies showed TD in approximately 10% of patients under 40 years old and a steady increase in prevalence to over 50% in patients 60 years or older (90). TD usually occurs more often in females (1.68:1) (61).

Neuroleptic Dose/Duration of Treatment

The relationship between TD and parameters of drug exposure (i.e., total, average, or peak dose; duration of treatment) is obscure. Most studies looking at long treatment durations failed to find an association between drug intake and TD (2,61,95). The few investigations showing a positive correlation evaluated short treatment periods of 3 years or less (31,95). Methodological issues may partly explain these conflicting findings, since several studies required minimum treatment durations of many years, and some did not control for age. A recent study addressing these points in a fixed age group (average 65 years) showed the largest increase in the 50% TD prevalence occurred in the first 3 years of treatment. There was no significant difference in TD in those patients treated between 5 and 25 years (95). These data confirm both the short- and long-term treatment literature and suggest that, at least in older patients, there is a period of maximum vulnerability to TD which is best described by a sigmoid dose-response curve.

In contrast, a prospective TD study in younger patients (average age 28 years) shows a steady annual incidence of 3 to 4% of new cases (64). These data imply there is a linear rather than sigmoid relationship to risk. The varying results in these two studies may be due to the large age difference and/or prevalence vs incidence measures. Prevalence rates will level off over time if the number of resolving cases is similar to the number of developing cases that arise from a steady annual incidence rate. Also, the period of greatest TD risk may vary with age. Neither study has teased apart the very complex interaction of concomitantly increasing age and treatment duration.

Only prospective studies of drug blood levels and TD that control dosing parameters will be able to sort out issues of cause and effect. One cross-sectional study found neuroleptic blood levels were higher in TD than in non-TD patients, but this association was not observed in additional studies with either oral or depot neuroleptics (33,55).

Neuroleptic Drug Type

Conflicting findings across several studies do not clarify whether one drug, chemical class, or milligram potency characteristic correlates with increased risk of TD. None of these hypotheses is supported by adequate data (13). The suggestion that depot neuroleptics are associated with higher rates of TD may be severely confounded by parameters of prior treatment, forced compliance, and different rates and amounts of drug delivery. Drug receptor site specificity for limbic rather than striatal dopamine (DA) receptors has been proposed (9), but this claim could not be replicated (81).

It is also unclear if atypical neuroleptics, such as clozapine, whose antipsychotic effect may not be mediated through DA receptor blockade, will be less likely to produce TD. Unfortunately, the necessary prospective comparative data with typical neuroleptics do not exist. Another purported atypical neuroleptic is sulpiride, a substituted benzamide drug commonly used in Europe. The low EPS rate (and speculated low TD liability) may be explained on the basis of relatively low brain drug levels, since sulpiride poorly penetrates the blood-brain barrier. The cautious interpretation is that any neuroleptic drug that suppresses TD, which sulpiride does (24), may have the capacity to produce TD.

Though the hypotheses about relationships between different types of DA receptors, neuronal pathways, and pharmacological effects in various dyskinesias are intriguing, they are insufficiently tested to guide clinical practice. However, the proposals about unique mechanisms of drug action are so attractive and potentially useful that they undoubtedly will and should be exploited in future research. Regarding TD, the commercially available neuroleptic drugs appear to be more similar than different, and it is not possible to implicate one drug or class as more or less liable to produce this syndrome.

Trial Periods Without Neuroleptics

Discontinuing neuroleptics as a drug holiday has the advantages of reducing drug exposure and unmasking covert dyskinesia, but exposes the patient to a risk of psychotic relapse. One retrospective study and a review of this topic associated frequent drug holidays with higher rates of irreversible TD (57,60). Other investigations show that many patients successfully tolerate drug-free periods or are maintained on lower daily neuroleptic doses and TD may improve (4,26). Overall, there are far too few data to adequately address the role of interrupted vs continuous drug therapy in either the causation or the outcome of TD. Reducing the neuroleptic dose to the lowest effective level or discontinuing the drug for as long as possible continues to be the most rational approach.

Anticholinergic Drugs/EPS

There is no consensus about the etiological role of anticholinergic agents in TD; correlational data exist both for and against such an association (2,61). Anticholinergic drugs may temporarily aggravate existing TD, but symptoms return to baseline when these drugs are discontinued (2,21,40,43).

Acute EPS have been hypothesized as a TD risk factor (31). A prospective TD study shows parkinsonian side effects significantly correlate to the early (less than 1 year of drug treatment) onset of TD, but EPS are not associated with TD onset after 2 or more years of neuroleptics (64). Identifying the relationship between acute EPS and the later evolution of TD will be difficult because acute EPS are influenced by patient parameters such as age and sex, factors of drug type and dose, and the widely divergent treatment and prophylactic practices with anti-EPS drugs (66). Since anticholinergic drugs are used to treat EPS, the retrospective associations of anticholinergics with TD may be indirect measures of EPS and TD vulnerability.

Psychiatric Diagnosis

Several reports note that affective disorders may be a risk factor for TD (16,63,75). Management strategies of concomitant lithium and intermittent high dose short-term neuroleptic treatment may contribute to these differences. It is not known if schizophrenia is a risk or protective factor for TD, but it is clear that TD can occur in anyone who receives neuroleptic drugs but who has never been psychotic.

Organic Brain Factors

Early reports identified organic brain disease, lobotomy, and electroconvulsive therapy (ECT) as predisposing factors to TD, but subsequent reviews questioned these associations (2,61). Studies with computerized tomography (CT) have conflicting findings about TD and brain pathology (34,65). Possible explanations for these differences include subtypes of TD, lack of age-matched controls, and confounding effects of current drug treatment that masks TD via drug-induced parkinsonism. Though associations between brain disease and TD are difficult to define, there is face validity to the rationale that existing deficits enhance the expression of other dysfunctions. For example, the SD prevalence is significantly greater for patients with than without organic mental disorders (25).

ETIOLOGY

There is no direct evidence of CNS alterations to explain TD. Rather, current concepts must rely on indirect data and the statistical argument that dyskinesias are more common in neuroleptic-treated than untreated patients.

Attempts to identify the structural pathology of TD used several approaches. Radiological investigations with CT scans do not consistently show significant differences between TD and non-TD patients. Whereas one light microscopic study noted higher rates of nigral degeneration and gliosis in TD patients (28), another suggested that these findings may be nonspecific and reflect age-related changes (52). Brains from rodents exposed to neuroleptics for several months at standard or high doses also show either cell loss or no change (76).

The mode of action of neuroleptic drugs is central to any theory of TD. The motor system effects of these drugs are presumably due to DA receptor blockade in the nigro-striatal basal ganglia system. Most neuroleptics block to varying degrees both DA receptor subtypes D-1 (adenylate cyclase-linked) and D-2 (non-adenylate cyclase-linked) (53,73). Some drugs have a relatively equal effect on D-1 and D-2, whereas others are nearly exclusive D-2 receptor blockers. This implies that the antipsychotic and dyskinetic mechanisms are mediated by the effect in common on D-2 receptors. However, the as yet unknown role of D-1 may be elucidated when pure D-1 drugs are available for testing in the clinic.

Though the research focus has been on DA receptor mechanisms because these most closely correlate with clinical effects, it is essential to emphasize that the vast majority of neuroleptic drugs also affect several neurotransmitter systems, including serotonin, norepinephrine, acetylcholine, and histamine (53,73). The contributions of these other systems to both the desired antipsychotic effect and undesired side effects over the short, intermediate, and long term are inadequately studied.

Theories of TD

DA receptor hypersensitivity is the most widely accepted explanation of TD. The strongest support for DA involve-ment comes from clinical observations. DA antagonists cause and usually suppress TD, whereas DA agonists increase symptoms. A secondary influence on DA effects involves the reciprocal cholinergic system. However, there are several aspects of TD that do not support the DA hypersensitivity theory.

Receptor-binding studies of human postmortem CNS comparing schizophrenic patients with and without TD find no significant differences in either the D-1 or D-2 receptors (32). These data must be considered with the concern that at the time of death, drug status may be unknown, and the findings could reflect treatment conditions rather than TD.

Biochemical data from the clinic also do not support DA dysfunction as the explanation of TD. When comparing TD and non-TD patients, prolactin and growth hormone show no differences, whereas CSF plasma and urinary homovanillic acid changes are inconsistent (56,65,92).

With no direct evidence in patients, much of what is believed about the pathogenesis and pathophysiology of TD derives from animal models. Rodents show increased behavioral responses to DA agonists following DA antagonist treatment of a single dose, a few days, several weeks, and 1 year (27,29,67,85,94). Biochemical changes of increased D-2 receptor numbers in treated animals correlate with behavioral changes in most (11) but not all (98) studies. These occur in all rodents, and are reversible within days to weeks of discontinuing neuroleptics. Several of these observations are not compatible with essential clinical aspects of TD: symptoms without agonist provocation, individual vulnerability, late onset, coexisting TD and acute EPS, and potentially irreversible course.

Spontaneous chewing in rodents has been more recently proposed as a model of TD. These behaviors increase with neuroleptic treatment and age (83,98), but may not correlate with changes in DA receptor numbers (98). Reversibility is unclear; one study noted prompt resolution with discontinuing neuroleptics or giving antiparkinson drugs (83), but another noted persistence for at least 2½ months after neuroleptics were stopped (98).

Other models include CNS destruction. Unilateral lesioning of the basal ganglia with 6-hydroxydopamine is followed by DA agonist-induced abnormal rotational behavior (97). Cortical ablation and neuroleptic exposure increase spontaneous chewing (45).

Interestingly, concomitant lithium and neuroleptics block behavioral and biochemical DA hypersensitivity in rodents (68,79). Specificity of this preventive effect (Is it seen with other drugs?) and how it applies to TD is unknown.

The cebus monkey model of TD has several strengths: the symptoms are identical to those in patients, occur in only some monkeys, require long-term neuroleptic treatment, respond to the same drug therapy, coexist with acute EPS, and have a reversible/irreversible course (15,48,71). Monkeys also show increased behavioral responses to DA agonists following antagonist treatment (19). DA turnover was significantly decreased in the caudate and substantia nigra in the TD monkeys 2 months after neuroleptics were discontinued (49), though no DA receptor characterizations were done to compare and contrast with human findings. There were also changes in GABA with decreased glutamic acid decarboxylase, the γ-aminobutyric acid (GABA) synthesizing enzyme, in the substantia nigra, medial globus pallidus, and subthalamic nucleus. Most importantly, these DA and GABA results were specific to dyskinetic monkeys; there were no significant differences between untreated and treated but non-TD monkeys (49,50).

These and other data about GABA effects in rodents provide the basis for a GABA deficiency theory of TD (36,84). However, clinical studies with GABA agonists in TD do not show uniform benefits from these compounds.

With the notable exception of TD in monkeys, animal models of TD are more appropriately characterized as general paradigms of acute and chronic neuroleptic treatment. Though the purported rodent models of TD are almost uniformly accepted, they are limited by many findings that are inconsistent with TD. Much of the data could be used to argue that the observed changes in DA function underlie the desirable therapeutic antipsychotic effect rather than the undesirable TD effect (19,85).

A noradrenergic dysfunction theory of TD has also been proposed (56). This derives in part from data showing significantly greater dopamine β-hydroxylase activity in TD patients than in those without TD. CSF norepinephrine was also significantly correlated with severity of TD (65). As further support for this theory, it is noted that drugs that improve or aggravate TD affect both DA and norepinephrine.

In summary, little evidence has been developed to identify the basis of TD. Human studies and animal models have been a rich but incomplete source of data about the effects of neuroleptic treatment. Though DA dysfunction is widely believed to underlie TD, it may be necessary but not sufficient to explain this complex disorder. In the presence of conflicting findings and the absence of direct data, it is best to keep an open mind about the pathogenesis and pathophysiology of TD.

TREATMENT

Treating TD is a difficult challenge. No drugs are both safe and effective over extended treatment periods. The long list of agents used for TD attests to their general ineffectiveness.

Dopamine

Reducing DA function is the most effective way of suppressing TD. Neuroleptics consistently mask TD. Decreasing presynaptic DA activity via depletion or false transmission with reserpine, tetrabenazine, α-methyl-para-tyrosine, or α-methyl-dopa has produced variable effects ranging from nearly complete suppression to minimal change (2,58). Though reserpine has only rarely been associated with causing TD, it and the other drugs that decrease amine function should be used cautiously because they may be reproducing similar neurochemical alterations (decreased DA neurotransmission) implicated in the etiology of TD. Possibly the degree of suppression is related to the degree of eventual aggravation or persistence of TD (17).

The theoretically attractive approach of treating TD by desensitizing hypersensitive DA receptors with DA agonists has been unsuccessful. The reported benefit with levodopa (1) was not replicated in subsequent trials. Direct receptor stimulation with agonists also did not significantly affect TD (22,42).

Acetylcholine

Anticholinergic drugs usually aggravate or uncover existing TD (2,18,39,42,58). Infrequently anticholinergics reduce rather than worsen symptoms, as described above in paradoxical dyskinesia (21,43,74). A review of anticholinergic drugs in 14 TD studies with 177 patients noted an improvement rate of 7.3% (58).

Augmenting a relatively underfunctioning cholinergic system is a logical approach to treating TD. Physostigmine, an acetylcholine esterase inhibitor, often decreased TD, but occasionally produced no change or aggravated symptoms. Some of these inconsistent effects may be due to TD subtypes or complicating effects of physostigmine, such as sedation, nausea, and vomiting. Cholinergic precursor loading with deanol, choline, or lecithin was initially encouraging, but much less successful in subsequent reports (18,42,58). In 68 studies with 379 TD patients, cholinergic drugs improved 47% of the patients in open studies and 30% in double-blind trials (58).

GABA

The GABA-inhibiting effect on DA neurons provides the rationale that increasing GABA influences might successfully treat TD. Inhibiting the catalytic enzyme GABA-transaminase with γ-acetylenic GABA, γ-vinyl-GABA, or sodium valproate led to variable decreases in TD (23,42,70). This effect was most evident in older patients taking concomitant neuroleptic drugs and who had drug-induced parkinsonism (23,42,70). Direct GABA receptor stimulation with the agonist muscimol decreased TD (93), but another GABA agonist, tetrahydroisoxazolopyridinol (THIP), had no significant effect (69). Baclofen, a structural analog of GABA with unclear effects on GABA mechanisms, also had a variable and generally ineffective influence on TD (18,44,58).

Benzodiazepines, which also may enhance GABA function, have either reduced or aggravated TD. Clonazepam was as effective as phenobarbital in reducing TD, which raises questions about whether the antihyperkinetic effects of benzodiazepines occur through specific mechanisms or nonspecific sedative effects (18,58). In a review of 19 studies with GABA agents involving 204 patients with TD, 58% improved in open studies and 43% improved in double-blind evaluations (58).

Other

Studies with serotonergic agonists of tryptophan and 5-hydroxytryptophan and the antagonist cyproheptadine yielded mixed results (18,58). The initial studies with lithium were encouraging, but later double-blind evaluations showed limited benefit. In 10 studies with 90 TD patients receiving lithium, only 27% improved (58). The β receptor antagonist propranolol has shown either suppression or no benefit (58,78), and a preliminary report about clonidine, an α-adrenergic agonist, noted TD decreased in two patients (18,58). Studies with neuropeptides in TD included a synthetic met-enkephalin, morphine, naloxone, des-tyrosine-γ-endorphin, and vasopressin, but all showed minimal or no benefit (7,18,42). Many other drugs used to treat TD produced inconsistent results, or evaluated too few patients to draw conclusions. These include estrogen, pyridoxine, fusaric acid, manganese, phenytoin, hydergine, papaverine, and several others (18,58).

LONG-TERM OUTCOME

The underlying fear that continued drug treatment will inevitably worsen symptoms has led to admonitions against using neuroleptics in patients with TD. However, the reversible course of TD, even in some patients continuing drug therapy, has been regularly noted since the initial publications identifying this syndrome (87,88,96).

Improvement across studies varies widely from 0 to 92% (17). This wide range undoubtedly reflects multiple factors of patient variables (age, sex, and psychiatric diagnosis), treatment parameters (drug dose and cumulative exposure), and temporal aspects (duration of treatment and psychosis). Age is most consistently correlated with a favorable outcome of TD. Younger patients are more likely to improve, whereas older patients are less likely to do so (17,90,91). However, this trend does not exclude symptom resolution in any age group, as some elderly patients have TD improve over 5 to 8 years. Duration of follow-up and degree of improvement are positively associated (26). There are insufficient data to clarify whether sex or diagnosis correlates with TD outcome.

Discontinuing neuroleptic drugs leads to stable or gradually improving TD (26,37,80,87,95,99). The few studies addressing TD outcome when neuroleptics are continued also show that symptoms may stabilize or improve over many years, though they can increase in a minority of patients (4,17,26,38,91,96). Interrupted treatment may be related to higher rates of irreversible TD (57,60).

Duration of TD and treatment are probably important factors in outcome. Early detection has been associated with TD reversibility (46,80). Also, longer duration of treatment and higher cumulative doses correlated with less likelihood of TD reversibility (62), implying that continued treatment may retard the rate of improvement that would occur without neuroleptic exposure.

CONCLUSIONS

Patients receiving prolonged neuroleptic treatment have significantly higher rates of hyperkinetic dyskinesias than non-drug-treated patients. Though the mechanisms are unknown, this may occur by neuroleptic treatment converting a covert, underlying predisposition to overt clinical symptoms. Risk factors include increased age, female sex, and probably affective disorders. Recent studies show pa-

rameters of drug exposure are related to TD. Other possible risk factors of acute EPS, anticholinergic treatment, and brain damage require further study. There is no direct evidence to characterize the pathogenetic or pathophysiological basis of TD. Animal models in monkeys and rodents have been valuable but incomplete sources of knowledge about acute and chronic neuroleptic treatment. In a final explanation of TD, DA, noradrenergic, or GABA dysfunction may be necessary but not sufficient to account for this complex syndrome. The large number of different drug treatment trials attests to the conclusion that none is proven to be both safe and effective for TD. Favorable long-term outcome correlates with younger age, early detection, lesser drug exposure, and increasing length of follow-up. With so much unknown about TD, it is appropriate to retain an open view on all aspects of this syndrome. The current and future direction of intensely pursued research is to produce antipsychotic drugs that are more efficacious and free of troublesome side effects—particularly TD.

ACKNOWLEDGMENTS

This project was supported in part by funds from the Veterans Administration Research Merit Review Programs and NIMH Grant MH-36657. Marian Karr prepared the typescript.

REFERENCES

1. Alpert, M., and Friedhoff, A. (1980): In: *Tardive Dyskinesia—Clinical and Basic Research,* edited by R. Smith, W. Fann, and R. Davis, pp. 471–473. Spectrum, New York.
2. Baldessarini, R. J., Cole, J. O., Davis, J. M., Gardos, G., Preskorn, S. H., Simpson, G. M., and Tarsy, D. (1980): *Tardive Dyskinesia: A Task Force Report.* American Psychiatric Press, Washington, DC.
3. Barnes, T. R. E., and Braude, W. M. (1985): *Arch. Gen. Psychiatry,* 42:874–878.
4. Barnes, T. R. E., Kidger, T., and Gore, S. M. (1983): *Psychol. Med.,* 13:71–81.
5. Barron, E. T., and McCreadie, R. G. (1983): *Br. J. Psychiatry,* 143:423–424.
6. Bicknell, D. J., and Blowers, A. J. (1980): *Br. J. Psychiatry,* 136:315–316.
7. Bjørndal, N., Casey, D. E., and Gerlach, J. (1980): *Psychopharmacology,* 69:133–136.
8. Bleuler, E. (1950): *Dementia Praecox or the Group of Schizophrenias,* p. 191. International Universities Press, New York.
9. Borison, R. L., Fields, J. Z., and Diamond, B. I. (1981): *Neuropharmacology,* 20:1321–1322.
10. Burke, R. E., Fahn, S., Jankovic, J., Marsden, C. D., Lang, A. E., Gollomp, S., and Ilson, J. (1982): *Neurology,* 32:1335–1346.
11. Burt, D. R., Creese, I., and Snyder, S. H. (1977): *Science,* 196:326–328.
12. Campbell, M., Grega, D. M., Green, W. H., and Bennett, W. G. (1983): *Clin. Neuropharmacol.,* 6:207–222.
13. Carpenter, W. T., Casey, D. E., Cole, J. O., Davis, J. M., Kane, J. M., and Tamminga, C. A. (1984): *Arch. Gen. Psychiatry,* 41:415–416.
14. Casey, D. E. (1981): *Acta. Psychiatr. Scand. (Suppl. 291),* 63:71–87.
15. Casey, D. E. (1984): *Psychopharmacol. Bull.,* 20:376–379.
16. Casey, D. E. (1984): In: *Tardive Dyskinesia and Affective Disorders,* edited by D. E. Casey and G. Gardos, pp. 1–20. American Psychiatric Press, Washington, DC.
17. Casey, D. E. (1985): In: *Dyskinesia: Research and Treatment,*

edited by D. E. Casey, T. Chase, A. V. Christensen, and J. Gerlach, pp. 88–96. Springer, Berlin.

18. Casey, D. E. (1985): In: *Dyskinesia: Research and Treatment,* edited by D. E. Casey, T. Chase, A. V. Christensen, and J. Gerlach, pp. 137–142. Springer, Berlin.

19. Casey, D. E. (1985): In: *Dyskinesia: Research and Treatment,* edited by D. E. Casey, T. Chase, A. V. Christensen, and J. Gerlach, pp. 211–216. Springer, Berlin.

20. Casey, D. E. (1985): *J. Clin. Psychiatry,* 46(Sect. 2):42–47.

21. Casey, D. E., and Denney, D. (1977): *Psychopharmacology,* 54:1–8.

22. Casey, D. E., Gerlach, J., and Bjørndal, N. (1982): *Psychopharmacology,* 78:89–92.

23. Casey, D. E., Gerlach, J., and Magelund, G. (1980): *Arch. Gen. Psychiatry,* 37:1376–1379.

24. Casey, D. E., Gerlach, J., and Simmelsgaard, H. (1979): *Psychopharmacology,* 66:73–77.

25. Casey, D. E., and Hansen, T. E. (1984): In: *Neuropsychiatric Movement Disorders,* edited by D. Jeste and R. J. Wyatt, pp. 69–84. American Psychiatric Press, Washington, DC.

26. Casey, D. E., Povlsen, U. J., Meidahl, B., and Gerlach, J. (1986): *Psychopharmacol. Bull.,* 22:250–253.

27. Christensen, A. V., Fjalland, B., and Møller Nielsen, I. (1976): *Psychopharmacology,* 48:1–6.

28. Christensen, E., Møller, J. E., and Faurbye, A. (1970): *Acta Psychiatr. Scand.,* 46:14–23.

29. Clow, A., Jenner, P., and Marsden, C. D. (1979): *Eur. J. Pharmacol.,* 57:365–375.

30. Crane, G. E. (1973): *Br. J. Psychiatry,* 122:395–405.

31. Crane, G. E., and Smeets, R. A. (1974): *Arch. Gen. Psychiatry,* 30:341–343.

32. Crow, T. J., Cross, A. J., Johnstone, E. C., Owen, F., Owens, D. G. C., and Waddington, J. L. (1982): *J. Clin. Psychopharmacol.,* 2:336–340.

33. Fairbairn, A. F., Rowell, F. J., Hui, S. M., Hassanyeh, F., Robinson, A. J., and Eccleston, D. (1983): *Br. J. Psychiatry,* 142:579–583.

34. Famuyiwa, O. O., Eccleston, D., Donaldson, A. D., and Garside, R. F. E. (1979): *Br. J. Psychiatry,* 135:500–504.

35. Faurbye, A., Rasch, P. J., Peterson, P. B., Brandborg, G., and Pakkenberg, H. (1964): *Acta Psychiatr. Scand.,* 40:10–27.

36. Fibiger, H. C., and Lloyd, K. G. (1984): *TINS,* 7:462–464.

37. Gardos, G., and Cole, J. O. (1980): *Am. J. Psychiatry,* 137:776–781.

38. Gardos, G., Cole, J. O., Perenyi, A., and Casey, D. E. (1985): In: *Chronic Treatments In Neuropsychiatry,* edited by D. Kemali and G. Racagni, pp. 37–42. Raven Press, New York.

39. Gardos, G., Cole, J. O., Rapkin, R. M., LaBrie, R. A., Baquelod, E., Moore, P., Sovner, R., and Doyle, J. (1984): *Arch. Gen. Psychiatry,* 41:1030–1035.

40. Gardos, G., Cole, J. O., and Tarsy, D. (1978): *Am. J. Psychiatry,* 135:1321–1324.

41. Gerlach, J. (1979): *Dan. Med. Bull.,* 26:209–245.

42. Gerlach, J., Casey, D. E., and Korsgaard, S. (1986): In: *Movement Disorders,* edited by N. S. Shah and A. G. Donald, pp. 119–147. Plenum, New York.

43. Gerlach, J., Reisby, N., and Randrup, A. (1974): *Psychopharmacologia,* 34:21–35.

44. Gerlach, J., Rye, T., and Kristjansen, P. (1978): *Psychopharmacology,* 56:145–151.

45. Glassman, R. B., and Glassman, H. N. (1980): *Psychopharmacology,* 69:19–25.

46. Glazer, W. M., Moore, D. C., Schooler, N. R., Brenner, L. M., and Morgenstern, H. (1984): *Arch. Gen. Psychiatry,* 41:623–627.

47. Gualtieri, C. T., Quade, D., Hicks, R. E., Mayo, J. P., and Schroeder, S. R. (1984): *Am. J. Psychiatry,* 141:20–23.

48. Gunne, L. M., and Barany, S. (1976): *Psychopharmacology,* 50:237–240.

49. Gunne, L. M., and Häggström, J. E. (1985): In: *Dyskinesia: Research and Treatment,* edited by D. E. Casey, T. Chase, A. V. Christensen, and J. Gerlach, pp. 191–193. Springer, Berlin.

50. Gunne, L. M., Häggström, J. E., and Sjöquist, B. (1984): *Nature,* 309:347–349.

51. Guy, W. (1976): In: *ECDEU Assessment Manual for Psychophar-macology,* pp. 534–537. US Government Printing Office, Washington, DC.

52. Hunter, R., Blackwood, W., and Smith, M. C. (1968): *J. Neurol. Sci.,* 7:263–273.

53. Hyttel, J., Larsen, J. J., Christensen, A. V., and Arnt, J. (1985): In: *Dyskinesia: Research and Treatment,* edited by D. E. Casey, T. N. Chase, A. V. Christensen, and J. Gerlach, pp. 9–18. Springer, Berlin.

54. Jankovic, J., and Ford, J. (1983): *Ann. Neurol.,* 13:402–411.

55. Jeste, D. V., DeLisi, L. E., Zalcman, S., Wise, D., Phelps, B., Rosenblatt, J., Potkin, S., Bridge, P., and Wyatt, R. J. (1981): *Psychiatry Res.,* 4:327–334.

56. Jeste, D. V., Lohr, J. B., Kaufmann, C. A., and Wyatt, R. J. (1986): In: *Tardive Dyskinesia and Neuroleptics: From Dogma to Reason,* edited by D. E. Casey and G. Gardos, pp. 16–32. American Psychiatric Press, Washington, DC.

57. Jeste, D. V., Potkin, S. G., Sinha, S., Feder, S., and Wyatt, R. J. (1979): *Arch. Gen. Psychiatry,* 36:585–590.

58. Jeste, D. V., and Wyatt, R. J. (1982): *Arch. Gen. Psychiatry,* 39:803–816.

59. Jeste, D. V., and Wyatt, R. J. (1982): *Understanding and Treating Tardive Dyskinesia.* Guilford Press, New York.

60. Jeste, D. V., and Wyatt, R. J. (1985): *J. Clin. Psychiatry,* 46(Sect. 2):14–18.

61. Kane, J. M., and Smith, J. M. (1982): *Arch. Gen. Psychiatry,* 39:473–481.

62. Kane, J. M., Woerner, M., Sarantakos, S., Kinon, B., and Lieberman, J. (1986): In: *Tardive Dyskinesia and Neuroleptics: From Dogma to Reason,* edited by D. E. Casey and G. Gardos, pp. 100–107. American Psychiatric Press, Washington, DC.

63. Kane, J. M., Woerner, M., Weinhold, P., Kinon, B., Lieberman, J., and Borenstein, M. (1984): In: *Tardive Dyskinesia and Affective Disorders,* edited by G. Gardos and D. E. Casey, pp. 22–28. American Psychiatric Press, Washington, DC.

64. Kane, J. M., Woerner, M., Weinhold, P., Wegner, J., Kinon, B., and Borenstein, M. (1984): *Psychopharmacol. Bull.,* 20:387–389.

65. Kaufmann, C. A., Jeste, D. V., and Shelton, R. C. (1986): *Biol. Psychiatry,* 21:799–812.

66. Keepers, G. A., Clappison, V. J., and Casey, D. E. (1983): *Arch. Gen. Psychiatry,* 40:1113–1117.

67. Klawans, H. L., and Rubovits, R. (1972): *J. Neural. Transm.,* 33:235–246.

68. Klawans, H. L., Weiner, W. J., and Nausieda, P. A. (1977): *Prog. Neuropsychopharmacol.,* 1:53–60.

69. Korsgaard, S., Casey, D. E., and Gerlach, J. (1982): *Arch. Gen. Psychiatry,* 39:1017–1021.

70. Korsgaard, S., Casey, D. E., and Gerlach, J. (1983): *Psychiatry Res.,* 8:261–269.

71. Kovacic, B., and Domino, E. F. (1982): *J. Clin. Psychopharmacol.,* 2:305–307.

72. Kraepelin, E. (1907): *Clinical Psychiatry.* Macmillan, New York.

73. Leysen, J. (1981): In: *Clinical Pharmacology in Psychiatry,* edited by E. Usdin, S. Dahl, L. Gram, and O. Lingjaerde, pp. 35–62. Macmillan Publishers Ltd., London.

74. Moore, D. C., and Bowers, M. B. (1980): *Am. J. Psychiatry,* 137:1202–1205.

75. Mukherjee, S., Rosen, A. M., Caracci, G., and Shukla, S. (1986): *Arch. Gen. Psychiatry,* 43:342–346.

76. Nielsen, E. B., and Lyon, M. (1978): *Psychopharmacology,* 59:85–89.

77. Owens, D. G. C., Johnstone, E. C., Crow, T. J., and Frith, C. D. (1982): *Arch. Gen. Psychiatry,* 39:452–461.

78. Perenyi, A., and Farkas, A. (1983): *Biol. Psychiatry,* 18:391–394.

79. Pert, A., Rosenblatt, J. E., and Sivit, C. (1978): *Science,* 201:171–173.

80. Quitkin, F., Rifkin, A., Gochfeld, L., and Klein, D. F. (1977): *Am. J. Psychiatry,* 134:84–87.

81. Reynolds, G. P., Cowey, L., Rossor, M. N., and Iversen, L. L. (1982): *Lancet,* 2:499.

82. Richardson, M. A., and Craig, T. J. (1982): *Am. J. Psychiatry,* 139:341–343.

83. Rupniak, N. M. J., Jenner, P., and Marsden, C. D. (1983): *Psychopharmacology,* 79:226–230.

84. Scheel-Kruger, J., and Arnt, J. (1985): In: *Dyskinesia: Research and Treatment,* edited by D. E. Casey, T. Chase, A. V. Christensen, and J. Gerlach, pp. 19–30. Springer, Berlin.

85. Schelkunov, E. L. (1967): *Nature,* 214:1210–1212.

86. Schooler, N. R., and Kane, J. (1982): *Arch. Gen. Psychiatry,* 39:486–487.

87. Schönecker, M. (1957): *Nervenarzt,* 28:35.

88. Sigwald, J., Bouttier, D., and Raymondeaud, C. (1959): *Rev. Neurol.,* 100:751–755.

89. Simpson, G. M., Lee, J. H., Zuobok, B., and Gardos, G. (1979): *Psychopharmacology,* 64:171–179.

90. Smith, J. M., and Baldessarini, R. J. (1980): *Arch. Gen. Psychiatry,* 37:1368–1373.

91. Smith, J. M., Burke, M. P., and Moon, C. O. (1981): *Psychopharmacol. Bull.,* 17:120–121.

92. Stahl, S. M., Faull, K. F., Barchas, J. D., and Berger, P. A. (1985): *Arch. Neurol.,* 42:166–169.

93. Tamminga, C. A., Crayton, J. W., and Chase, T. N. (1979): *Arch. Gen. Psychiatry,* 36:595–598.

94. Tarsy, D., and Baldessarini, R. J. (1973): *Nature,* 245:262–263.

95. Toenniessen, L. M., Casey, D. E., and McFarland, B. H. (1985): *Arch. Gen. Psychiatry,* 42:278–284.

96. Uhrbrand, L., and Faurbye, A. (1960): *Psychopharmacologia,* 1:408–418.

97. Ungerstedt, U. (1971): *Acta Physiol. Scand (Suppl.),* 367:1–48.

98. Waddington, J. L., Cross, A. J., Gamble, S. J., and Bourne, R. D. (1983): *Science,* 220:530–532.

99. Yagi, G., Ogita, K., Ohtsuka, N., Itoh, H., and Miura, S. (1976): *Keio J. Med.,* 27–35.

Psychopharmacology:
The Third Generation of Progress,
edited by Herbert Y. Meltzer.
Raven Press, New York © 1987.

CHAPTER 149

Neuroleptic Malignant Syndrome

Charles A. Kaufmann and Richard Jed Wyatt

Neuroleptic malignant syndrome (NMS) is a life-threatening complication of neuroleptic treatment characterized by fever, rigidity, altered consciousness, and autonomic instability (41). It is the most serious of a range of "catatonic reactions" to high-potency antipsychotic drugs, which also include akinesia (127), withdrawal, negativism, posturing, and waxy flexibility (58).

INCIDENCE

NMS, although relatively rare, is being recognized with increasing frequency: only 60 cases had been described in the world literature by 1980 (25); that number has nearly doubled in the past 5 years (91). The increase in case reports is not surprising: in their original description of the syndrome, Delay and Deniker (41) estimated the incidence among patients treated with haloperidol as 0.5 to 1.0%; Pope has recently arrived at a similar estimate (cited in 33). Nonetheless, NMS is far less frequent than other neuroleptic-induced neurologic syndromes, occurring in 15 to 50% of patients (132).

Men appear to be more susceptible than women (relative risk 2:1) (25,89). Younger patients are more often affected; >80% of patients are <40 years old (25), and the youngest reported patient was 12 years old (59).

Haloperidol has been the neuroleptic most frequently implicated in NMS (89). This may in part reflect the fact that haloperidol and thioridazine are the two most prescribed neuroleptics. It may also reflect the facts that high-potency neuroleptics are often prescribed at greater relative doses than low-potency neuroleptics, or that these agents are used to treat medically ill and acutely agitated patients who might otherwise be predisposed to NMS (91, vide infra). Nonetheless, it is worth noting that the relative frequency of NMS (case reports/million drug mentions) with different neuroleptics is highly correlated with their ability to antagonize dopamine (D-2) receptors in striatum (data based on ref. 89, 131, and the National Disease and Therapeutic Index 1979–1984, IMS America, Ltd.) (Fig. 1). Other drugs that have been implicated in NMS include chlorpromazine (108), fluphenazine (3,105), loxapine (47), thioridazine (74), thiothixene (101), and trifluoperazine (121).

NMS has been described with oral, intramuscular, and intravenous routes of administration (92). Although neuroleptics alone have been implicated, 23% of patients were also receiving anticholinergics (158), 15% lithium, and 4% tricyclic antidepressants (89).

CLINICAL FEATURES

NMS begins with neurological signs (rigidity, akinesia, dyskinesia) (41) which invariably precede or accompany the onset of fever (up to 42°C). Rare cases suggest fever may occur in the absence of rigidity (67,107), but concurrent medical conditions (sedative-hypnotic withdrawal and possible delirium tremens) complicate their interpretation. Signs of autonomic dysfunction (tachycardia, labile hypertension, diaphoresis, pallor) are common and may also precede the appearance of fever (12,161). Changes in mental status (from mild obtundation through stupor and coma) occur in 70% of patients. "Signs in the lungs", originally described by Delay and Deniker (41) and occurring in 30% of patients, are conceivably related to a primary toxic effect of neuroleptics, but are more likely secondary phenomena, the late results of pulmonary embolus due to prolonged immobilization or of aspiration pneumonia due to dysphagia.

NMS usually appears within 2 weeks of initiating neuroleptic treatment or increasing dose (in 47/52 cases in one

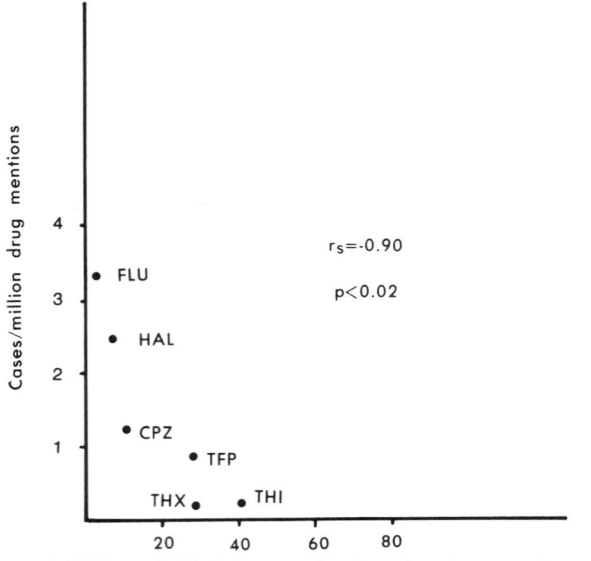

FIG. 1. Association between neuroleptic malignant syndrome and dopamine-2 receptor antagonism. The relative incidence of NMS with different neuroleptics was determined based on the number of cases reported in the literature (89) and on the frequency with which such drugs were prescribed (National Disease and Therapeutic Index, 1979–1984). These data were then compared with the relative ability of these neuroleptics (IC_{50}) to inhibit *in vitro* binding of the radiolabeled antagonist [³H]spiperone to dopamine-2 receptors in rat striatum (131). A strong inverse correlation was found between relative incidence and IC_{50} values (alternatively, a direct correlation between relative incidence and equilibrium association constants, K_A). FLU, fluphenazine; HAL, haloperidoc; CPZ, chlorpromazine; TFP, trifluoperazine; THX, thiothixene; THI, thioridazine.

series) (89). However, it may also occur following months of stable-dose treatment. Episodes evolve over 24 to 72 hr and last 5 to 10 days following oral medications and 2 to 3 times as long after depot medications.

Anecdotal reports describe NMS as more common in patients with preexisting neurologic dysfunction (41,72,105), although a survey of the world literature (25) found a history of organic brain syndrome in only 18% of patients.

Other authors suggest that schizophrenic patients may be at higher risk for NMS. Although this might relate to an underlying instability in autonomic and temperature regulation, especially among younger patients, as originally described in the preneuroleptic era (20), it could also reflect their greater exposure to neuroleptic medication. NMS has also been described in patients with depression, mania, amphetamine psychosis (29), sedative-hypnotic withdrawal (67), Huntington's disease (21), Parkinson's disease (150), and during anesthetic preinduction (109).

LABORATORY FINDINGS

A variety of laboratory abnormalities have been described in NMS; these are probably not diagnostic. Leukocytosis (15,000–30,000) with a shift to the left appears in 40% of

patients (89). Elevated creatine phosphokinase (CPK) (muscle isoenzyme) (up to 15,400) (108) also appears in approximately 40% of patients (89), may be an early marker of the disorder, and probably results from myonecrosis (105) or calcium flux (vide infra).

Liver enzymes [serum glutamic oxaloacetic transaminase (SGOT)], lactate dehydrogenase (LDH), alkaline phosphatase) may also be elevated (80,94), and may result from acute fatty changes in liver produced by high fever. Electroencephalographic abnormalities, primarily generalized slowing, are an inconstant feature.

DIFFERENTIAL DIAGNOSIS

The occurrence of fever and rigidity in patients on psychotropic medication presents a complex problem in differential diagnosis. NMS must be distinguished from other causes of the catatonic syndrome (57), including infectious [viral encephalitis, rickettsial encephalitis (36,139), encephalitis lethargica (41), tetanus], collagen vascular (polymyositis), and metabolic (hyperparathyroidism) disorders. Patients with thyrotoxicosis may also present with fever, tremors, and autonomic dysfunction.

Akinetic mutism and central hyperthermia, disorders resulting from a variety of CNS lesions, may also resemble NMS. Similarly, an akinetic crisis with rigidity and autonomic dysfunction may complicate the withdrawal of L-dopa or amantadine from patients with Parkinson's disease (31,136).

Patients on neuroleptics may develop marked hyperthermia with heat stroke. Here elevation in ambient temperature, strenuous activity (96,135), and peripheral anticholinergic effects (especially of low-potency neuroleptics) combine to raise core temperature. In NMS, unlike heat stroke, rigidity precedes or accompanies the fever.

Patients on neuroleptics may also be susceptible to malignant hyperthermia (MH), a potentially fatal genetic myopathy, which, like NMS, is associated with fever, rigidity, and autonomic dysfunction. MH has been most commonly linked to the use of inhaled anesthetics, depolarizing muscle relaxants, and local anesthetics (18). However, it can also appear in response to phenothiazines, tricyclic antidepressants, monoamine oxidase inhibitors (42,69), and stress. Although MH may be overrepresented among psychiatric patients (51) and may bear a marked similarity to NMS, the two disorders may be distinguished (vide infra), for example on the basis of family history and *in vitro* muscle contractile properties.

Patients on combined neuroleptic-lithium therapy are at risk to develop not only NMS but also lithium neurotoxicity (143). The latter condition, characterized by delirium, seizures, and EEG abnormalities, is felt to resemble intoxication with lithium alone and to result from enhanced intracellular lithium transport by phenothiazines like thioridazine (117). It is not accompanied by fever, which appears late, if at all, in simple lithium intoxication (129). Such lithium toxicity can be contrasted with an NMS in patients on lithium and high-potency neuroleptics, in which both extrapyramidal symptoms and fever appear and in which lithium is felt to potentiate neuroleptic toxicity (95) rather than the converse. NMS in the setting of combined lithium-neuroleptic treatment may not be associated with EEG abnormalities (1) or elevated intracellular (erythrocyte) lithium levels (117). Neurotoxicity from combined lithium-neuroleptic therapy may be associated with a disastrous outcome (34), perhaps accounting for the widespread attention it has received. It should be noted, however, that the combination has been used extensively (9,71,137), with fewer than 10 cases of the full NMS reported (120).

Lastly, NMS may be difficult to distinguish from acute lethal catatonia, a (possibly familial) disorder associated with extreme hyperactivity, followed by fever, rigidity, and acrocyanosis. Both disorders may be conceptualized as hypothalamic "crises" superimposed on (iatrogenic or psychogenic) catatonic reactions (52,147). Although acute lethal catatonia was first described in the preneuroleptic era (145), affected patients were often medicated with anticholinergics (hyoscine, scopolamine—the sedatives then available), prior to the onset of fever, undoubtedly complicating the clinical picture and interfering with evaporative heat loss.

Both NMS and lethal catatonia may temporarily respond to barbiturates; sodium amobarbital interviews may therefore not differentiate between them. The two conditions may be distinguishable on clinical grounds: patients with NMS, despite frequently being mute, appear cooperative (156). At one time, differentiating NMS from lethal catatonia appeared critical (72,119); the former disorder was precipitated by neuroleptics; the latter life-threatening disorder required their use. Today, such distinctions may be less critical with the availability of therapeutic agents (for example, potent benzodiazepines) that appear to ameliorate both conditions.

PATHOETIOLOGY

NMS at the Organ Level: Disordered Thermogenesis

NMS may be distinguished from other neuroleptic-induced catatonic syndromes (58) by the presence of fever.

Hyperthermia may result from excess heat production (through shivering or mobilization of calorigenic energy reserves), inappropriate heat conservation (through increased peripheral vasomotor tone), impaired evaporative heat loss (through diminished sweating), or alterations in hypothalamic temperature control centers which couple (warm and cold) thermosensors to appropriate effectors in order to maintain core temperature (14) (Fig. 2).

Increased heat production has been implicated in NMS, through both shivering and nonshivering thermogenesis. Furthermore, enhanced muscle activity (rigidity, tremor), characteristic of NMS, may be divided into that occurring on a peripheral or central basis.

Similarities between NMS and MH, a myopathy, suggest muscle pathology in the former. Both disorders are associated with increased CPK (105). Moreover, neuroleptics like chlorpromazine may induce contractures in isolated frog skeletal muscle (although only at high concentrations) (5) and affect the contractile response of muscle from control subjects (26) and patients with MH (128). Similarly, muscle obtained from patients who have recovered from NMS may show 10-fold greater sensitivity to fluphenazine-induced contractions (27).

However, there are also differences between the two disorders. MH is by and large a genetic disorder (primarily autosomal dominant), although sporadic cases do occur; NMS appears to be sporadic. Elevations in CPK appear between episodes in MH patients (and their first-degree relatives (79), but not in NMS patients (76). MH patients may have abnormal amounts of phosphorylase A and characteristic muscle morphology; NMS patients do not (19,21,148). Muscle from patients with MH is sensitive to contractions produced by caffeine or caffeine and halothane; that of patients with NMS may only be sensitive to halothane alone (27,148). Curare (108), pancuronium bromide (138), and diazepam (108,138) do not produce muscle relaxation in MH but do so in NMS (73). Lastly, patients with MH have subsequently received neuroleptics without incident (17,69), whereas patients with NMS have subsequently tolerated depolarizing muscle relaxants like succi-

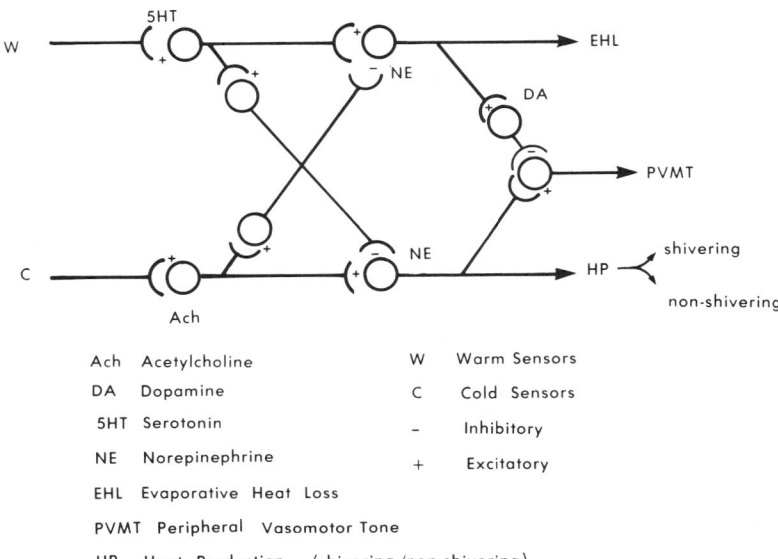

Ach Acetylcholine
DA   Dopamine
5HT Serotonin
NE   Norepinephrine
EHL Evaporative Heat Loss
PVMT Peripheral Vasomotor Tone
HP   Heat Production (shivering/non-shivering)

W Warm Sensors
C Cold Sensors
− Inhibitory
+ Excitatory

FIG. 2. Neuronal model of mammalian thermoregulation. Warm and cold thermosensors are coupled to appropriate effectors in order to maintain core temperature: dopamine appears to play an important role in such coupling. Hyperthermia may result from excess heat production (↑HP), inappropriate heat conservation (↑PVMT), impaired heat loss (↓EHL), or altered coupling between sensors and effectors. (Adapted from ref. 38.)

nylcholine (94). Thus, central mechanisms (for example, blockade of striatal dopamine receptors—vide infra) probably play a major role in the rigidity and shivering thermogenesis of NMS.

Nonshivering thermogenesis may also play a role in the hyperthermia of NMS. Muscle flaccidity induced by curare only partly reverses the elevated temperature (108). Such increase in metabolic rate is mediated by the sympathetic nervous system, which may also be responsible for the tachycardia and hypertension seen in the syndrome. Of note, elevated levels of plasma and urinary norepinephrine and epinephrine have been seen in NMS (48), and one patient with NMS was successfully treated with propranolol (R. B. Schiffer in ref. 89). Also of note, circulating catecholamine levels may also be increased during episodes of MH in an experimental porcine model (70), suggesting that MH, too, may be a systemic disorder and not merely a myopathy.

Inappropriate heat conservation in NMS is suggested by pallor in the face of increased core temperature. Whereas neuroleptics might exert peripheral anticholinergic effects and interfere with evaporative heat loss through sweating, NMS is most often caused by high-potency neuroleptics with fewer anticholinergic effects and is often accompanied by profuse sweating (80), implying intact cholinergic sudomotor effectors.

Possible alterations in hypothalamic temperature control will be considered in the discussion of dopamine blockade which follows.

NMS at the Cellular Level: Dopamine Blockade

The lack of consistent findings at autopsy in muscle, basal ganglia, and hypothalamus of patients with NMS (108) suggests an abnormality at a more microscopic level. There is ample evidence that diminished dopamine neurotransmission may be of prime pathogenic significance in NMS. NMS is often associated with high-potency neuroleptics which are potent dopamine-receptor blockers (77, 131, and Fig. 1), but, as noted above, have other effects. However, NMS has also been reported in association with drugs that inhibit dopamine synthesis (α-methylparatyrosine) or interfere with dopamine storage (tetrabenazine) (21), drugs that have no direct effects on muscle contraction or on peripheral cholinergic tone. Furthermore, NMS has been described following discontinuation of dopamine agonists (L-dopa, amantadine) (76,150) in patients with Parkinson's disease (patients who are known to have a loss of nigrostriatal and hypothalamic dopaminergic neurons) (46) and following discontinuation of amphetamine and institution of neuroleptics in patients with narcolepsy (29) (chronic dopamine agonist treatment possibly inducing postsynaptic dopamine receptor subsensitivity and potentiation of neuroleptic blockade).

Marked elevations in CSF dopamine metabolites (homovanillic acid, HVA; dihydroxyphenylacetic acid, DOPAC) have been described in NMS and are consistent with postsynaptic blockade. Compare Tollefson and Garvey's (149) concentration of DOPAC (26.7 pmol/ml) with the maximum values we found with similar techniques in 36

unmedicated (6.04 pmol/ml) and 9 neuroleptic-medicated (6.65 pmol/ml) schizophrenic patients (C. A. Kaufmann, unpublished observation). It should be noted, however, that other studies of CSF metabolites in NMS have not replicated the elevation in HVA (65,153).

Dopamine blockade may influence NMS at any of several levels. Dopamine may have an inhibitory effect at the neuromuscular junction (16); dopamine blockade might therefore be associated with direct neuromyal facilitation. Dopamine blockade in nigrostriatal pathways may also contribute to rigidity. Diencephalospinal dopamine projections ordinarily inhibit thoracolumbar sympathetic outflow (93); their blockade may account for increased sympathetic tone and nonshivering thermogenesis in NMS.

Lastly, dopamine blockade may have a direct effect on hypothalamic thermoregulatory centers. Dopaminergic neurons appear to modulate peripheral vasomotor tone, an important effector in heat conservation (14). Direct application of dopamine or apomorphine (a dopamine agonist) in preoptic/anterior hypothalamus of cats or rats results in decreased peripheral vasomotor tone, increased tail skin temperature, enhanced heat exchange, and diminished core temperature (38,83). Other direct and indirect dopamine agonists such as L-dopa (160), bromocriptine (125), amantadine (37,40), and D-amphetamine (160) likewise produce a fall in core temperature. This effect appears to be mediated by D-1 (adenylate cyclase facilatory) dopamine receptors (38) and may be blocked by parenteral or intrahypothalamic pimozide (a dopamine antagonist). In the face of a heat load, neuroleptics elicit an undesirable increase in peripheral vasomotor tone, minimal increase in tail skin temperature, and rise in core temperature (38,39). Similar mechanisms might account for pallor, despite hyperthermia, and an inability to handle the heat load of shivering and nonshivering thermogenesis in NMS. Of interest, patients with Parkinson's disease (who have sustained a loss of hypothalamic dopaminergic neurons) show impaired heat loss through vasodilation (46).

Dopamine blockade may also account for the reported occurrence of NMS in patients on combined lithium and neuroleptic treatment. Lithium is known to enhance the extrapyramidal symptoms of neuroleptic treatment (99). Chronic lithium treatment alone may prevent apomorphine-induced stereotypy (49) and locomotor hyperactivity (154), suggesting that lithium may itself antagonize striatal dopamine receptors; lithium may also inhibit striatal dopamine synthesis, augmenting this receptor blockade (54).

In considering alterations in dopamine neurotransmission in NMS we must remember that dopamine projections do not exist in isolation but in dynamic balance with other neurotransmitter systems. Alterations in dopamine tone may result from or result in alterations in these other systems, possibly with pathogenic consequences. Thus, the nigrostriatal system contains not only dopaminergic, but cholinergic, GABAergic, and possibly other neurons (Fig. 3). Dopamine blockade may result in increased acetylcholine turnover in striatum (144) as well as decreased γ-aminobutyric acid (GABA) turnover in substantia nigra (86). Intranigral administration of muscimol, a GABA-A (postsynaptic) receptor agonist (140), protects against haloperidol-induced catalepsy, whereas benzodiazepines (like diazepam),

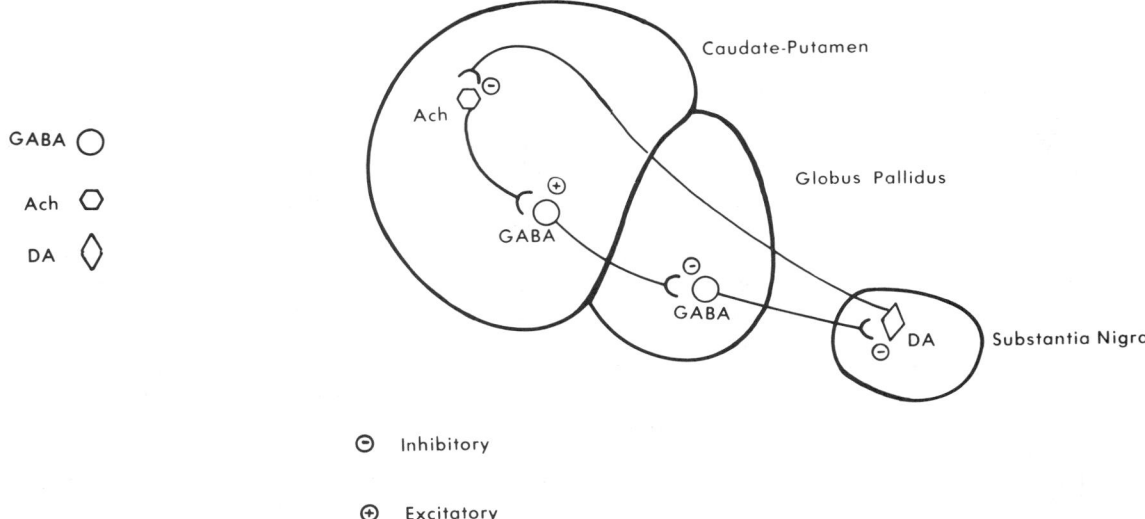

GABA ○

Ach ⬡

DA ◇

⊖ Inhibitory

⊕ Excitatory

FIG. 3. Chemical neuroanatomy of the basal ganglia. Dopaminergic neurons exist in dynamic balance with other neurons, including cholinergic and GABAergic neurons. Alterations in dopamine tone may result from or result in alterations in these other systems. (Adapted from ref. 104.)

which act at receptors allosterically linked to GABA receptors (140) and facilitate GABAergic transmission (98), reverse haloperidol-induced increases in dopamine turnover (82). These considerations suggest a potential therapeutic role for benzodiazepines (or anticholinergics) in the treatment of rigidity associated with NMS (vide infra).

Likewise, GABAergic neurons may have a role in hypothalamic thermoregulation. Whereas intracerebroventricular GABA itself appears to have little effect on thermoregulation, muscimol (possibly more readily entering brain) lowers peripheral vasomotor tone (like dopamine) (14), again suggesting a role for GABA-agonists/benzodiazepines in the treatment of NMS.

NMS at the Molecular Level: Calcium and Cyclic AMP

Nonetheless, dopamine blockade does not provide a fully adequate explanation for NMS. All neuroleptics antagonize dopamine receptors, yet NMS is relatively uncommon. NMS may appear even at low neuroleptic doses (41), months after treatment is instituted. It may persist long after neuroleptics are withdrawn, even after urinary drug metabolites are no longer detectable (149). Patients with NMS do not invariably develop a recurrence when rechallenged with the offending drug (21,89,105). Thus, dopamine blockade may be a necessary, but not sufficient, condition for NMS. Certain states may facilitate the appearance of NMS, for example, dehydration (80), prolonged agitation (157), previous dopamine agonist treatment (29), or concurrent lithium therapy (143). Moreover, NMS bears considerable similarity to other syndromes—MH and acute lethal catatonia—which, while distinct, might share some pathogenic mechanisms. Once again, the inadequacy of dopamine blockade as an explanation suggests a lesion at

a more microscopic molecular level of stimulus-response coupling, downstream to the dopamine receptor.

Cyclic AMP and calcium constitute dual systems of intracellular messengers coupling stimulus to response (122). Several steps in the coupling process can be identified for both systems: (a) recognition of an external signal by a cell surface receptor and coupling to a transducing element; (b) transduction of this signal within the membrane into a new intracellular signal; (c) intracellular reception of this new signal by specific receptor proteins; (d) modulation of cell proteins by the signal receptor and their consequent response; and (e) termination of the signal to limit its temporal domain.

In dopamine neurons (for example, in striatum or hypothalamus), specific receptors (on which we have focused) recognize synaptic dopamine, are coupled within the plasma membrane by GTP-binding coupling protein (G/F protein) (28) to adenylate cyclase, which transduces the signal by catalyzing the formation of intracellular cyclic AMP. Cyclic AMP in turn binds to specific cyclic AMP receptor proteins activating protein kinases and changing cell function. The cyclic AMP signal is terminated by phosphodiesterases. Although the cyclic AMP system just described predominates, a calcium information transfer system also operates and may modulate the cyclic AMP system. Thus, calcium enters the cell through specific channels, binds within the cell to a calcium-receptor protein, calmodulin (30), which in turn may activate either adenylate cyclase (if membrane bound) or phosphodiesterase (if cytosolic). Likewise, the cyclic AMP system may modulate the calcium system (i.e., they are "synarchic" messengers).

In muscle, the calcium system predominates. Calcium is taken up by the cell via voltage-independent and voltage-dependent channels, sequestered in the sarcoplasmic reticulum, and rapidly released in response to depolarization. It diffuses to a receptor protein, troponin-C, which changes conformation, allowing heavy meromyosin to interact with actin and produce muscle contraction (118). The calcium signal is terminated by a variety of pump-reuptake mechanisms in plasma membrane, sarcoplasmic reticulum, and mitochondria. Once again, cyclic AMP may modulate this system. For example, cyclic AMP may alter the behavior of voltage-dependent calcium channels in the plasma membrane (116), may cause increased calcium release from the sarcoplasmic reticulum (84), and may increase efflux of calcium from the mitochondria (15).

These two interacting systems are obviously complicated, but a full consideration of both may ultimately provide both a necessary and a sufficient explanation for NMS and related conditions, as well as potentially novel therapeutic interventions.

In NMS alterations in the two pathways may account for many of the observed features. Consider the idealized hypothalamic dopamine neuron shown in Fig. 4. Intracellular calcium levels are in part determined by a Na^+/Ca^{2+} exchange mechanism (10): increases in extracellular sodium are associated with decreases in intracellular calcium. Likewise, decreases in extracellular calcium may be associated with decreases in intracellular calcium. We might expect such decreased intracellular calcium to inactivate membrane-bound calmodulin, in turn inactivating adenylate cyclase and ultimately preventing heat loss through diminished peripheral vasomotor tone. In fact, third ventricle concentrations of both sodium and calcium appear to affect temperature regulation. As expected, increased sodium produces hyperthermia (113). Likewise, lower calcium concentrations are associated with greater core temperature elevations (and smaller tail temperature elevations) with exercise in both rats (61) and macaque monkeys (112). Increases in serum (and ventricular) sodium accompany dehydration, perhaps accounting for its association with NMS (77, but see 155). Moreover, cerebrospinal fluid calcium, reflecting ventricular and brain extracellular fluid calcium (78), may fall during acute psychotic agitation (24), perhaps accounting for the described association between prolonged agitation and NMS, as well as providing a mechanism for the hyperthermia accompanying acute lethal catatonia (similar mechanisms in striatal dopamine neurons might also account for the rigidity seen in acute lethal catatonia).

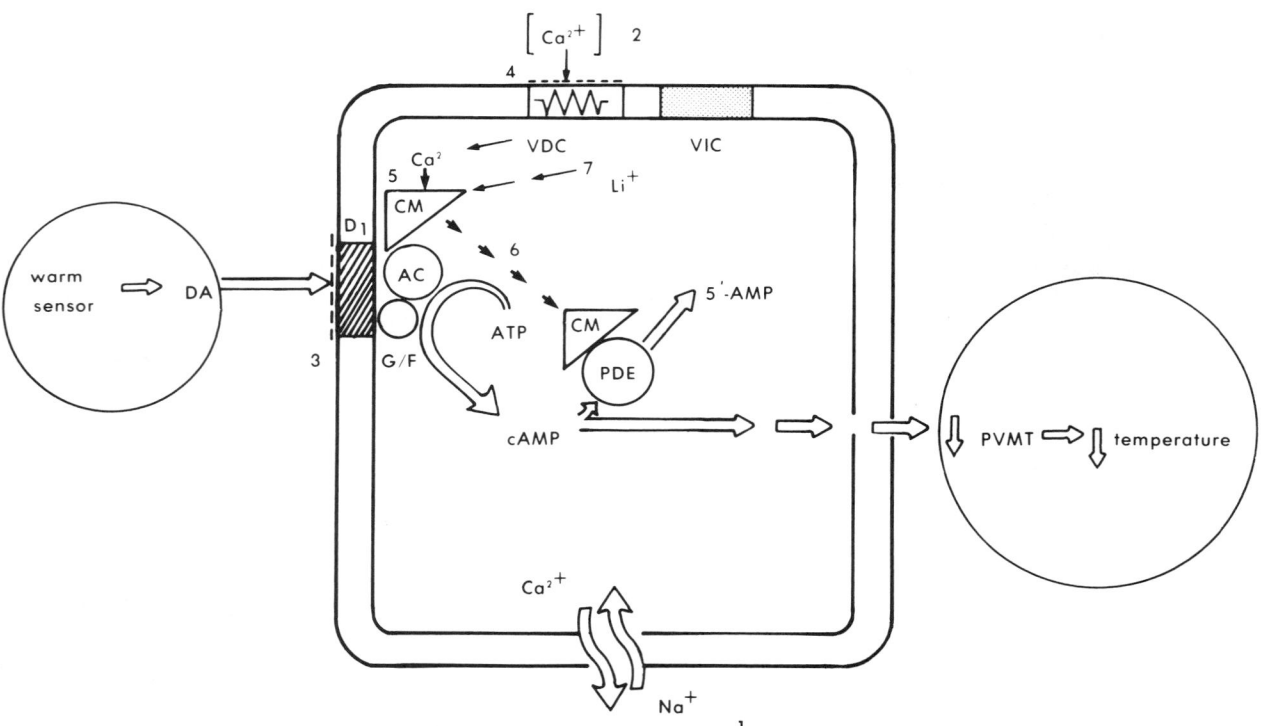

FIG. 4. An idealized hypothalamic dopamine neuron. Calcium and cyclic AMP (cAMP) represent interdependent intracellular messengers coupling stimulus (from thermosensors) to response (peripheral vasomotor tone). Intracellular calcium concentrations may vary [1] inversely with extracellular sodium concentrations and [2] directly with extracellular calcium concentrations. Alterations in calcium concentration might be expected to affect coupling via calmodulin (CM) and adenylate cyclase (AC). Neuroleptics may affect AC directly through [3] dopamine (DA) receptor antagonism. Neuroleptics may also affect intracellular calcium by blocking voltage-dependent calcium channels (VDC) [4]. Furthermore, acute neuroleptic treatment [5] may inhibit AC indirectly, by interfering with calmodulin binding to membrane. Similarly, chronic dopamine agonist treatment [6] may induce translocation of calmodulin from membrane to cytosol, also inhibiting AC and activating phosphodiesterase (PDE), thereby lowering cAMP. Finally, lithium may inhibit AC [7], perhaps by interference with calcium binding to calmodulin. These alterations may ultimately prevent heat loss through diminished peripheral vasomotor tone (PVMT). VIC, Voltage-independent calcium channel; G/F, GTP-binding coupling protein.

Neuroleptics may also influence calcium influx. In addition to blocking dopamine receptors, diphenylbutylpiperidine neuroleptics (like pimozide) may block voltage-dependent (verapamil-sensitive) calcium channels (63). Furthermore, acute neuroleptic treatment may interfere with calmodulin binding to membrane, inhibiting adenylate cyclase. In muscle, neuroleptics like chlorpromazine may inhibit calcium reuptake by the sarcoplasmic reticulum (5).

Chronic dopamine (D-1) agonist treatment also induces translocation of calmodulin from membrane to cytosol, inhibiting adenylate cyclase, activating phosphodiesterase, and lowering cyclic AMP (75,106). Once again, hypothalamic dopamine neurons might become subsensitive with impairment in peripheral heat exchange and increased susceptibility to NMS.

Lithium may also inhibit dopamine-sensitive adenylate cyclase (146) (perhaps through interference with calmodulin, as hydrated lithium is approximately the same size as calcium), possibly explaining its association with NMS.

Malignant hyperthermia may also be associated with alterations in adenylate cyclase; here the enzyme may be (pharmacogenetically) more sensitive (159). Increased levels of cyclic AMP in muscle would be expected to produce increased calcium release from sarcoplasmic reticulum and an increased contractile response, as has been seen when muscle fibers from patients with MH are exposed to the phosphodiesterase inhibitor, caffeine (55).

These theoretical considerations have practical implications for treatment. Two drugs affecting calcium metabolism, nifedipine and verapamil, have been used recently with some success in NMS (114,126), while a third drug, calcitonin, has been studied extensively in a patient with rapid cycling periodic psychosis associated with spontaneous rigidity and fever (perhaps a recurrent form fruste of acute lethal catatonia) (22). In the latter patient, episodes of agitation and hyperthermia were accompanied by relative elevations in serum calcium (which is inversely proportional to CSF calcium) (24) and marked elevations in CPK (not surprising, as increased extracellular calcium may be associated with CPK leakage from skeletal muscle) (141). In prior studies, calcitonin had resulted in a rise in CSF calcium, a fall in serum calcium (24), and normalization of CPK in patients with previous elevations (23). The patient with periodic psychosis responded to a therapeutic trial of calcitonin with prompt defervescence (within 2 hr vs 40 hr for untreated episodes). Several mechanisms might have been involved: a rise in CSF calcium (restoring dopamine-mediated thermoregulation), a fall in serum calcium (reducing sarcoplasmic calcium and contractile response), or an increase in calcium sequestration by mitochondria (similarly decreasing muscle contraction) (123). This provocative study highlights our ignorance of the role played by calcium metabolism in neuroleptic-induced catatonic reactions (45) and suggests that consideration be given to calcitonin as a treatment for neuroleptic-induced rigidity and fever.

TREATMENT

The cornerstone of treatment of NMS is prompt discontinuation of psychotropic medications. Temporary discontinuation of neuroleptics should be considered whenever the course of treatment with such agents becomes unexpectedly adverse. Such discontinuation may not result in immediate improvement, even in those patients who eventually recover fully, because of the long elimination half-life of neuroleptics (58,156). Although discontinuation of all medication remains the most prudent therapeutic approach, NMS resulting from combined lithium-neuroleptic treatment has been treated by merely reducing the dose of lithium along with stopping the neuroleptic (32).

Supportive treatment, including temperature reduction with cooling blankets and antipyretics and restoration of fluid and electrolyte balance, should be aggressively pursued. Evidence of intercurrent infections should be sought. Artificial ventilation may be required (11). If myoglobinuria and acute renal failure appear imminent, diuresis with intravenous fluids and appropriate diuretics and alkalinization of the urine may minimize damage (87). Although dialysis may be useful in the treatment of associated renal failure, it probably does not otherwise favorably influence the course of NMS, as neuroleptics are tightly bound to serum proteins.

Several treatments have been suggested to reverse the symptoms of NMS, including nonspecific somatic approaches (such as electroconvulsive therapy, ECT) and specific pharmacologic interventions. ECT has reportedly led to improvement in NMS, possibly by increasing dopamine (81) or GABA (52) turnover. However, in other studies, ECT has failed to demonstrate such improvement (119) and has been associated with cardiac arrest and permanent neurological damage (124), arguing against the use of such nonspecific treatment.

The development of specific pharmacologic approaches to NMS has paralleled the evolution of specific theoretical formulations. Given the successful use of the muscle relaxant, dantrolene, in MH (88), and the similarity between MH and NMS, several trials of dantrolene (and other muscle relaxants like pridinolum mesylate) (60) have been reported in NMS. Dantrolene appears to interfere with excitation-contraction coupling, perhaps by decreasing the amount of calcium released from the sarcoplasmic reticulum (152) (although central effects, for example on GABA metabolism, may also be important) (52). Although dantrolene alone (35,62,64,100) or in combination with bromocriptine (65) has generally had a favorable effect, especially when administered early in the course of the syndrome (85,130) and in oral doses between 4 and 10 mg/kg/day (13,65), some improvement may have been coincidental with the simultaneous discontinuation of neuroleptics. Moreover, as we have seen, skeletal muscle excitation-contraction coupling may not be of prime pathogenic significance in NMS. These theoretical considerations, along with practical concern over potential serious hepatotoxicity with dantrolene (especially with prolonged use), limit the value of this drug in the pharmacotherapy of NMS.

Noradrenergic antagonists such as propranolol, which diminish the autonomic hyperactivity associated with NMS (89), may play an ancillary role in therapy.

Other treatment approaches have attempted to reverse the dopamine receptor blockage associated with NMS: either directly (with drugs affecting dopamine turnover) or indirectly (with drugs affecting acetylcholine and GABA turnover). Drugs directly affecting dopamine have included L-dopa (a dopamine precursor) (90), amantadine (a drug enhancing synaptic dopamine) (4,56,58,102), and bromocriptine (a postsynaptic dopamine agonist) (43,110,111,161), and have generally been effective.

Anticholinergic medications have had both favorable (59,72,80) and unfavorable (156) effects. Unfortunately, high doses (for example, trihexyphenidyl 20 mg i.m./day) may need to be used (72), possibly contributing to alterations in mental status and in evaporative heat loss. Anticholinergics have been specifically described as ineffective in reversing NMS associated with combined lithium and neuroleptic therapy (151), and may not influence the mortality rate of NMS (25).

Benzodiazepines, drugs that enhance GABA-A (postsynaptic) receptor binding (140) in striatum (and possibly hypothalamus), appear to have greatest promise as therapeutic agents in NMS (53). They have been effective even in cases in which dopamine agonists and anticholinergics have not worked (92). They appear to be well tolerated, even in high doses (68). Moreover, in addition to reversing symptoms of NMS, they may be of some benefit in treating underlying psychotic symptoms, especially if adequate doses are used (115), perhaps by increasing mesolimbic GABAergic transmission (97). In particular, catatonic symptoms, such as mannerisms and posturing, may respond to high-dose diazepam (mean dose 100 mg p.o./day) (115). This is of practical importance, as acute lethal catatonia, often difficult to distinguish from NMS, is felt to require continued antipsychotic treatment; benzodiazepines, unlike neuroleptics, may have a favorable effect in both conditions.

As noted, benzodiazepines have a large volume of distribution, requiring a substantial bolus of drug on initiating treatment. Small doses of diazepam (for example, 5 mg p.o. q.i.d.) may be of little value (111), as opposed to larger doses (for example, 10–20 mg i.v. followed by 10 mg p.o. q.i.d.) (92,103). More potent benzodiazepines (for example, lorazepam 2 mg i.v. followed by 2 mg p.o. q. 12 hr), which are more tightly bound to benzodiazepine receptors than diazepam (142), may be of particular value. Significant doses may be necessary and effects may be cumulative.

Also as noted, neuroleptics, especially depot preparations, have a long elimination half-life; treatment with any of the aforementioned drugs (dopaminergic, anticholinergic, GABAergic) may therefore need to be continued for several days to prevent a recurrence of symptoms. Finally, it is clear that further research is needed into drugs (like calcitonin) which more directly affect the molecular lesion in NMS.

PROGNOSIS

Approximately 20% of patients diagnosed as suffering from NMS have died (25,91) within 3 to 30 days of the onset of symptoms from such complications as cardiovascular collapse, respiratory failure [due to tachypneic hypoventilation (7), pulmonary embolus (124), or aspiration pneumonia], and renal failure [due to rhabdomyolysis and myoglobinuria (44)]. Nonfatal complications have also

included *Escherichia coli* fasciitis (134). Patients on depot neuroleptics may be at greater morbid risk ($p = 0.066$; Fisher exact test) perhaps because of longer exposure to the offending drug (25).

However, in those patients who survive, recovery is usually complete. Six patients have been left with permanent neurologic sequelae, five in whom NMS followed combined lithium and neuroleptic therapy. Cohen and Cohen (34) described four patients left with dementia, dyskinesia, and cerebellar dysfunction following combined treatment. High doses of haloperidol were given despite near toxic levels of lithium, undoubtedly contributing to the poor outcome (8). Frankel and Spring (50) described one patient left with dyskinesia and cerebellar dysfunction again following combined treatment. Of note, persistent dementia, choreoathetosis, and cerebellar dysfunction may follow toxicity due to lithium alone (6,66).

Eiser et al. (44) described one patient who was left with dysarthria and dysphagia following haloperidol alone; his deficits were felt to be due to a diffuse neuropathy that resulted from prolonged hyperpyrexia.

Maintenance treatment of the patient surviving NMS and requiring neuroleptics remains controversial. Nonetheless, there is anecdotal evidence suggesting that low-potency neuroleptics may be well tolerated, especially if they are pharmacologically distinct from the offending drug (2,133).

ACKNOWLEDGMENTS

The authors wish to thank Stanley N. Caroff, M.D., for reviewing the manuscript and Gail A. Miller for its preparation.

REFERENCES

1. Abrams, R., and Taylor, M. A. (1979): *Am. J. Psychiatry,* 136:336–337.
2. Aizenberg, D., Shalev, A., and Munitz, H. (1985): *Br. J. Psychiatry,* 146:317–318.
3. Allan, R., and White, H. D. (1972): *Br. Med. J.,* 1:221–222.
4. Amdurski, S., Radwan, M., Levi, A., and Elizur, A. (1983): *Curr. Ther. Res.,* 33:225–259.
5. Andersson, K.-E. (1972): *Acta Physiol. Scand.,* 85:532–546.
6. Apte, S. N., and Langston, J. W. (1983): *Ann. Neurol.,* 13:453–455.
7. Auzepy, P., Poivet, D., and Nitenberg, G. (1977): *Nouv. Presse Med.,* 6:1236.
8. Ayd, F. J. (1975): *Int. Drug Ther. Newsletter,* 10:29–36.
9. Baestrup, P. G., Hollnagel, P., Sorenson, R., and Schou, M. (1976): *JAMA,* 236:2645–2646.
10. Baker, P. F. (1976): In: *SEB Symposium XXX: Calcium in Biological Systems,* edited by C. J. Duncan, pp. 67–88. Cambridge University Press, New York.
11. Bates, I., and Courtenay-Evans, R. J. (1984): *Br. Med. J.,* 288:1913.
12. Bernstein, R. A. (1979): *Psychosomatics,* 20:840–846.
13. Bismuth, C., de Rohan-Chabot, P., Goulon, M., and Raphael, J. C. (1984): *Acta Neurol. Scand. (Suppl.),* 100:193–198.
14. Bligh, J. (1979): *Neuroscience,* 4:1213–1236.
15. Borle, A. (1974): *J. Membr. Biol.,* 16:221–228.
16. Bowman, W. C., and Raper, C. (1967): *Ann. NY Acad. Sci.,* 139:741–753.
17. Britt, B. A. (1971): *Anesth. Analg.,* 50:1107–1111.
18. Britt, B. A. (1979): *Fed. Proc.,* 38:44–48.

19. Britt, B. A., and Kalow, W. (1970): *Can. Anesth. Soc. J.,* 17: 293–315.
20. Buck, C. W., Carscallen, H. B., and Hobbs, G. E. (1950): *Arch. Neurol. Psychiatry,* 64:828–842.
21. Burke, R. E., Fahn, S., Mayeux, R., Weinberg, H., Louis, K., and Willner, J. H. (1981): *Neurology,* 31:1022–1026.
22. Carman, J. S., and Wyatt, R. J. (1977): *Lancet,* 2:1124–1125.
23. Carman, J. S., and Wyatt, R. J. (1978): Presented at the 131st Annual Meeting, American Psychiatric Association, Atlanta.
24. Carman, J. S., and Wyatt, R. J. (1979): *Biol. Psychiatry,* 14:295–336.
25. Caroff, S. (1980): *J. Clin. Psychiatry,* 41:79–83.
26. Caroff, S., Rosenberg, H., and Gerber, J. C. (1983): *J. Clin. Psychopharmacol.,* 3:120–121.
27. Caroff, S., Rosenberg, H., and Gerber, J. C. (1983): *Lancet,* 1: 244.
28. Cassel, D., and Selinger, Z. (1977): *Proc. Natl. Acad. Sci. USA,* 74:3307.
29. Chayasirisobohn, S., Cullis, P., and Veeramasuneni, R. R. (1983): *Hosp. Community Psychiatry,* 34:548–550.
30. Cheung, W. Y. (1980): *Science,* 207:19–27.
31. Clough, C. G. (1983): *Br. Med. J.,* 287:128–129.
32. Coffey, C. E., and Ross, D. R. (1980): *Am. J. Psychiatry,* 137: 736–737.
33. Cohen, B. M., Baldessarini, R. J., Pope, H. G., Jr., and Lipinski, J. F., Jr. (1985): *N. Engl. J. Med.,* 313:1293.
34. Cohen, W. J., and Cohen, N. H. (1974): *JAMA,* 230:1283–1287.
35. Coons, D. J., Hillman, F. J., and Marshall, R. W. (1982): *Am. J. Psychiatry,* 139:944–945.
36. Cope, R. V., and Gregg, E. M. (1983): *Br. Med. J.,* 286:1938.
37. Cox, B. (1979): In: *Body Temperature,* edited by P. Lomax and E. Schonbaum, pp. 231–255. Marcel Dekker, New York.
38. Cox, B., Kerwin, R., and Lee, T. F. (1978): *J. Physiol. (Lond.),* 282:471–483.
39. Cox, B., and Lee, T. F. (1977): *Br. J. Pharmacol.,* 61:83–86.
40. Davies, J. A., and Redfern, P. H. (1973): *J. Pharm. Pharmacol.,* 25:705–707.
41. Delay, J., and Deniker, P. (1968): In: *Handbook of Clinical Neurology,* edited by P. J. Viken and G. W. Bruyn, pp. 248–266. North Holland, Amsterdam.
42. Denborough, M. A. (1980): *Pharmacol. Ther.,* 9:357–365.
43. Dhib-Jalbut, S., Hesselbrock, R., Brott, T., and Silbergeld, D. (1983): *JAMA,* 250:484–485.
44. Eiser, A. R., Neff, M. S., and Slifkin, R. F. (1982): *Arch. Intern. Med.,* 142:601–603.
45. El-Defrawi, M. H., and Craig, T. J. (1984): *Compr. Psychiatry,* 25:539–545.
46. Elliott, K., Cote, L. J., and Frewin, D. B. (1974): *Neurology,* 24: 857–862.
47. Ewart, A. L., Kloek, J., Wells, B., and Phelps, S. (1983): *J. Clin. Psychiatry,* 44:37–38.
48. Feibel, J. H., and Schiffer, R. B. (1981): *Am. J. Psychiatry,* 138: 1115–1116.
49. Flemenbaum, A. (1977): *Biol. Psychiatry,* 12:563–572.
50. Frankel, M. H., and Spring, G. K. (1982): *Am. J. Psychiatry,* 139:537–538.
51. Franks, R. D., Aoueille, B., Mahowald, M. C., and Masson, N. (1982): *Am. J. Psychiatry,* 139:1065–1066.
52. Fricchione, G. L. (1985): *Biol. Psychiatry,* 20:304–313.
53. Fricchione, G. L., Cassem, N. H., Hooberman, D., and Hobson, D. (1983): *J. Clin. Psychopharmacol.,* 3:338–342.
54. Friedman, E., and Gershon, S. (1973): *Nature,* 243:520–521.
55. Gallant, E. M., and Ahern, C. P. (1983): *Mayo Clin. Proc.,* 58: 758–763.
56. Gangadhar, B. N., Desai, N. G., and Channabasavanna, S. M. (1984): *J. Clin. Psychiatry,* 45:526.
57. Gelenberg, A. J. (1976): *Lancet,* 1:1339–1341.
58. Gelenberg, A. J., and Mandel, M. R. (1977): *Arch. Gen. Psychiatry,* 34:947–950.
59. Geller, B., and Greydanus, D. E. (1979): *J. Clin. Psychiatry,* 40: 102–103.
60. Giordani, L., Amore, M., Montanari, A., Berlinzani, L., and Gentili, C. (1985): *Am. J. Psychiatry,* 142:389–390.
61. Gisolfi, C. V., Wilson, N. C., Myers, R. D., and Phillips, M. I. (1976): *Brain Res.,* 101:160–164.
62. Goekoop, J. G., and Carbaat, P. A. T. (1982): *Lancet,* 2:49–50.
63. Gould, R. J., Murphy, K. M. M., Reynolds, I. J., and Snyder, S. H. (1983): *Proc. Natl. Acad. Sci. USA,* 80:5122–5125.
64. Goulon, M., de Rohan-Chabot, P., Elkharrat, D., Gajdos, P., Bismuth, C., and Conso, F. (1983): *Neurology,* 33:516–518.
65. Granato, J. E., Stern, B. J., Ringel, A., Karim, A. H., Krumholz, A., Coyle, J., and Adler, S. (1983): *Ann. Neurol.,* 14:89–90.
66. Green, J. B. (1984): *Ann. Neurol.,* 15:111.
67. Greenblatt, D. J., Gross, P. L., Harris, J., Shader, R. I., and Ciraulo, D. A. (1978): *J. Clin. Psychiatry,* 39:673–675.
68. Greenblatt, D. J., and Shader, R. I. (1978): In: *Psychopharmacology: A Generation of Progress,* edited by M. A. Lipton, A. DiMascio, and K. F. Killam, pp. 1381–1390. Raven Press, New York.
69. Gronert, G. A. (1980): *Anesthesiology,* 53:395–423.
70. Gronert, G. A., Milde, J. H., and Theye, R. A. (1977): *Anesthesiology,* 47:411–415.
71. Growe, G. A., Crayton, J. W., Klass, D. B., Evans, H., and Strizich, M. (1979): *Am. J. Psychiatry,* 136:454–455.
72. Grunhaus, L., Sancovici, S., and Rimon, R. (1979): *J. Clin. Psychiatry,* 40:99–100.
73. Guze, B. H., and Baxter, L. R., Jr. (1985): *N. Engl. J. Med.,* 313: 163–166.
74. Haberman, M. L. (1978): *Arch. Intern. Med.,* 138:800–801.
75. Hanbauer, I., and Costa, E. (1982): In: *Calcium and Cell Function,* edited by W. Y. Cheung, pp. 253–272. Academic Press, New York.
76. Henderson, V. W., and Wooten, G. F. (1981): *Neurology,* 31: 132–137.
77. Hermesh, H., Huberman, M., Radvan, H., and Kott, E. (1984): *J. Nerv. Ment. Dis.,* 172:692–695.
78. Hunter, G., and Smith, H. V. (1960): *Nature,* 186:161.
79. Isaacs, H. (1970): *Br. J. Anesth.,* 42:1077–1084.
80. Itoh, H., Ohtsuka, N., Ogita, K., Yagi, G., Miura, S., and Koga, Y. (1977): *Folia Psychiatr. Neurol. Jpn.,* 31:559–576.
81. Jessee, S. S., and Anderson, G. F. (1983): *J. Clin. Psychiatry,* 44: 186–188.
82. Keller, H. H., Schaffner, R., and Haefely, W. (1976): *Naunyn Schmiedebergs Arch. Pharmacol.,* 294:1–7.
83. Kennedy, M. S., and Burks, T. F. (1974): *Neuropharmacology,* 13:119–128.
84. Kentera, D., and Varagic, V. (1975): *Br. J. Pharmacol.,* 54:375–381.
85. Khan, A., Jaffe, J. H., Nelson, W. H., and Morrison, B. (1985): *J. Clin. Psychiatry,* 46:244–246.
86. Kim, J. S., and Hassler, R. (1975): *Brain Res.,* 88:150–153.
87. Knochel, J. P. (1974): *Arch. Intern. Med.,* 133:841–864.
88. Kolb, M. E., Horne, M. L., and Martz, R. (1982): *Anesthesiology,* 56:254–262.
89. Kurlan, R., Hamill, R., and Shoulson, I. (1984): *Clin. Neuropharmacol.,* 7:109–120.
90. Kurlan, R., and Shoulson, I. (1983): *Neurology,* 33:162.
91. Levenson, J. L. (1985): *Am. J. Psychiatry,* 142:1137–1145.
92. Lew, T.-Y., and Tollefson, G. (1983): *Biol. Psychiatry,* 18:1441–1446.
93. Lindvall, O., Bjorklund, A., and Skagerberg, G. (1983): *Ann. Neurol.,* 14:255–260.
94. Lotstra, F., Linkowski, P., and Medlewicz, J. (1983): *Biol. Psychiatry,* 18:243–247.
95. Loudon, J. B., and Waring, H. (1976): *Lancet,* 2:1088.
96. Mann, S. C., and Boger, W. P. (1978): *Am. J. Psychiatry,* 135: 1097–1100.
97. Mao, C. C., and Costa, E. (1978): In: *Psychopharmacology: A Generation of Progress,* edited by M. A. Lipton, A. DiMascio, and K. F. Killam, pp. 307–318. Raven Press, New York.
98. Mao, C. C., Guidotti, A., and Costa, E. (1975): *Naunyn Schmiedebergs Arch. Pharmacol.,* 289:369–378.
99. Marhold, J., Zimanova, M., and Lachman, M. (1974): *Act. Nerv. Super. (Praha),* 16:199–200.
100. May, D. C., Morris, S. W., Stewart, R. M., Fenton, B. J., and Gaffney, F. A. (1983): *Ann. Intern. Med.,* 98:183–184.
101. McAllister, R. G., Jr. (1978): *Arch. Intern. Med.,* 138:1154–1156.

102. McCarron, M. M., Boettger, M. L., and Peck, J. J. (1982): *J. Clin. Psychiatry,* 43:381–382.
103. McEvoy, J. P., and Lohr, J. B. (1984): *Am. J. Psychiatry,* 141: 284–285.
104. McGeer, P. L., Eccles, J. C., and McGeer, E. G. (1978): *Molecular Neurobiology of the Mammalian Brain.* Plenum Press, New York.
105. Meltzer, H. Y. (1973): *Psychopharmacologia,* 29:337–346.
106. Memo, M., Lovenberg, W., and Hanbauer, I. (1982): *Proc. Natl. Acad. Sci. USA,* 79:4456–4460.
107. Misiaszek, J. J., and Potter, R. L. (1985): *Psychosomatics,* 26: 62–66.
108. Morris, H. H., McCormick, W. F., and Reinarz, J. A. (1980): *Arch. Neurol.,* 37:462–463.
109. Moyes, D. (1973): *Br. J. Anesth.,* 45:1163–1164.
110. Mueller, P. S. (1985): *Psychosomatics,* 26:654–662.
111. Mueller, P. S., Vester, J. W., and Fermaglich, J. (1983): *JAMA,* 249:386–388.
112. Myers, R. D., Gisolfi, C. V., and Mora, F. (1977): *Nature,* 266: 178–179.
113. Myers, R. D., and Veale, W. L. (1970): *Science,* 170:95–97.
114. Nesemann, M. E., Michels, J. T., and Pollei, S. R. (1984): *Wis. Med. J.,* 83:12–14.
115. Nestoros, J. N., Nair, N. P. V., Pulman, J. R., Schwartz, G., and Bloom, D. (1983): *Psychopharmacology,* 81:42–47.
116. Oota, I., and Nagai, T. (1977): *Jpn. J. Physiol.,* 27:195–213.
117. Pandey, G. N., Goel, I., and Davis, J. M. (1979): *Clin. Pharmacol. Ther.,* 26:96–102.
118. Potter, J. D., Johnson, J. D., and Dedman, J. R. (1977): In: *Ca²⁺ Binding Proteins and Ca²⁺ Function,* edited by R. H. Wasserman, R. A. Corradino, E. Carofoli, and R. H. Kretsinger, pp. 239–247. Elsevier, New York.
119. Powers, P., Douglass, R., and Waziri, R. (1976): *Dis. Nerv. System,* 37:359–361.
120. Prakash, R., Kelwala, S., and Ban, T. A. (1982): *Compr. Psychiatry,* 23:567–571.
121. Preston, J. (1959): *Am. Pract. Digest. Treat.,* 10:627.
122. Rasmussen, H. (1981): *Calcium and cAMP as Synarchic Messengers.* John Wiley & Sons, New York.
123. Rasmussen, H., and Pechet, M. (1972): In: *Pharmacology of the Endocrine System and Related Drugs,* edited by H. Rasmussen, p. 237. Oxford University Press, New York.
124. Regestein, G., Alpert, J., and Reich, P. (1977): *JAMA,* 238:618–620.
125. Reid, J. L. (1975): In: *Advances in Neurology,* edited by D. B. Calne, T. N. Chase, and A. Barbeau, pp. 73–80. Raven Press, New York.
126. Reis, J., Felten, P., Rumbach, L., and Collard, M. (1983): *Rev. Neurol. (Paris),* 139:595–596.
127. Rifkin, A., Quitkin, F., and Klein, D. F. (1975): *Arch. Gen. Psychiatry,* 32:672–674.
128. Rosenberg, H. (1977): *Anesth. Analg.,* 3:466.
129. Schou, M., Amdisen, A., and Trap-Jensen, J. (1968): *Am. J. Psychiatry,* 125:520–527.
130. Scott, J. (1984): *Br. J. Psychiatry,* 144:98.
131. Seeman, P. (1980): *Pharmacol. Rev.,* 32:229–313.
132. Shader, R. I., and DiMascio, A. (1970): *Psychotropic Drug Side Effects.* Williams & Wilkins, Baltimore.
133. Shalev, A., Hermesh, H., Aizenberg, D., and Munitz, H. (1985): *N. Engl. J. Med.,* 313:1292–1293.
134. Sherman, C. B., Hashimoto, F., and Davidson, E. J. (1983): *JAMA,* 250:361.
135. Shibolet, S., Coll, R., Gilat, T., and Sohar, E. (1967): *Q. J. Med.,* 36:525–547.
136. Simpson, D. M., and Davis, G. C. (1984): *Am. J. Psychiatry,* 141:796–797.
137. Small, J. G., Kellams, J. J., Milstein, V., and Moore, J. (1975): *Am. J. Psychiatry,* 132:1315–1317.
138. Smego, R. A., and Durack, D. T. (1982): *Arch. Intern. Med.,* 142:1183–1185.
139. Smith, J. A., III, and Carter, J. H. (1984): *Am. J. Psychiatry,* 141:609.
140. Snyder, S. H. (1984): *Science,* 224:22–31.
141. Soybel, D., Morgan, J., and Cohen, L. (1978): *Res. Commun. Chem. Pathol. Pharmacol.,* 20:317.
142. Spirt, N. M., Bautz, G., Zanko, M., Horst, W. D., and O'Brien, R. A. (1981): *Soc. Neurosci. Abstr.,* 7:865.
143. Spring, G., and Frankel, M. (1981): *Am. J. Psychiatry,* 138:818–821.
144. Stadler, H., Lloyd, K. G., Gadea-Ciria, M., and Bartholini, G. (1973): *Brain Res.,* 55:476–480.
145. Stauder, H. K. (1934): *Arch. Psychiatr. Nervenkr.,* 121:614–634.
146. Stefanini, E., Longoni, R., Fadda, F., Spano, P. F., and Gessa, G. L. (1978): *J. Neurochem.,* 30:257–258.
147. Stoudemire, A., and Luther, J. S. (1984): *Int. J. Psychiatry Med.,* 14:57–63.
148. Tollefson, G. (1982): *J. Clin. Psychopharmacol.,* 2:266–270.
149. Tollefson, G. D., and Garvey, M. J. (1984): *J. Clin. Psychopharmacol.,* 4:150–153.
150. Toru, M., Matsuda, O., Makiguchi, K., and Sugano, K. (1981): *J. Nerv. Ment. Dis.,* 169:324–327.
151. Tyrer, P., Alexander, M. S., Regan, A., and Lee, I. (1980): *Br. J. Psychiatry,* 136:191–194.
152. Van Winkle, W. B. (1976): *Science,* 193:1130–1131.
153. Verhoeven, W. M., Elderson, A., and Westenberg, H. G. (1985): *Biol. Psychiatry,* 20:680–684.
154. Verimer, T., Goodale, D. B., Long, J. P., and Flynn, J. R. (1980): *J. Pharm. Pharmacol.,* 32:665–666.
155. Wedzicha, J. A., and Hoffbrand, B. I. (1984): *Lancet,* 1:963.
156. Weinberger, D. R., and Kelly, M. J. (1977): *J. Nerv. Ment. Dis.,* 165:263–268.
157. West, P. A., and Meltzer, H. Y. (1979): *Am. J. Psychiatry,* 136: 963–966.
158. Westlake, R. J., and Rastegar, A. (1973): *JAMA,* 225:1250.
159. Willner, J. H., Cerri, C., and Wood, D. S. (1982): In: *Disorders of the Motor Unit,* edited by D. L. Schotland, pp. 423–440. John Wiley & Sons, New York.
160. Yehuda, S., and Wurtman, R. J. (1972): *Nature,* 240:477–478.
161. Zubenko, G., and Pope, H. G., Jr. (1983): *Am. J. Psychiatry,* 140:1619–1620.

Psychopharmacology:
The Third Generation of Progress,
edited by Herbert Y. Meltzer.
Raven Press, New York © 1987.

CHAPTER **150**

Serious Nonextrapyramidal Adverse Effects of Neuroleptics: Sudden Death, Agranulocytosis, and Hepatotoxicity

Douglas F. Levinson and George M. Simpson

Neuroleptics have been demonstrated or alleged to be responsible for a number of grave adverse effects unrelated to the extrapyramidal system. This chapter will review the literature on three areas of concern. The first is the long-standing question about whether neuroleptics may be responsible for some cases of sudden death in psychiatric patients. The second is the well-documented risk of agranulocytosis due to clozapine, an atypical antipsychotic that is investigational in the United States and is in widespread use elsewhere in the world, and the much smaller risk associated with other antipsychotics. The third is the risk of hepatocellular damage during neuroleptic therapy.

CAN NEUROLEPTICS CAUSE SUDDEN DEATH?

Neuroleptic drugs were widely introduced to psychiatric hospitals during the mid to late 1950s. During the late 1950s and early 1960s case reports began appearing in the literature suggesting that some sudden or unexpected deaths among psychiatric patients might be related to the prescription of phenothiazines (26). Although a number of pathophysiological mechanisms were proposed, no clear relationship between neuroleptics and sudden death could be established. Questions continued to arise about individual cases. In 1980, similar questions were raised by the U.S. Food and Drug Administration (FDA) concerning haloperidol, and the issue was reviewed at a meeting of the FDA Psychopharmacologic Drug Advisory Committee. Again, no clear conclusions could be reached (25). The American Psychiatric Association (APA) then commissioned an expert panel to review the issue, for a report to be completed in

1986 (39). Once again, no clear relationship could be established. Nevertheless, because of the importance of this issue, and the controversy surrounding it, the questions and evidence will be reviewed here.

A series of early case reports (1963–1966) was reviewed by Leetsma and Koenig (26). These reports included 58 patients, of whom 24 were observed to collapse suddenly, 21 were found dead or dying, 9 died "unexpectedly," and 4 died under other unusual circumstances. All but 6 were under the age of 55. The reports varied greatly in completeness of medical information and in the nature of the clinical pictures. The authors concluded that at least some of these deaths may have been directly related to neuroleptic effects, and that attention should be focused on two probable mechanisms for neuroleptic-related sudden death: (a) aspiration with asphyxia, and (b) cardiovascular collapse related to (i) arrhythmia and/or (ii) hypotension.

Such hypotheses have proven difficult to confirm or refute. At the outset, there are major problems related to the definitions of sudden, unexplained, and unexpected death. This has been thoroughly reviewed in the APA report (39). A number of distinctions must be made. For example, there are well-known adverse effects of neuroleptics that can contribute ultimately to a patient's death. For example, severe and persistent parkinsonism can lead to physical immobilization and subsequent complications such as pulmonary embolus, dehydration and electrolyte disturbances, and myoglobinuria (27). Such patients may die "suddenly," but thorough medical evaluation would show that the death was due to "expectable" results of known pathophysiological mechanisms that had been present and observable for some time before the death. A question exists as to how many of the reported cases in this area are of this type, as opposed to cases where an undetermined pathophysiological mechanism might suddenly bring about a death that could not otherwise have been expected or explained.

There are numerous definitions of sudden, unexpected death in the literature. For example, one of the leading medical studies (23) defined sudden death as death within 24 hr of onset of symptoms. Ungvari (44) proposed the following definition for consideration of the neuroleptic issue: "an apparently healthy person's death occurring literally instantaneously or within 1 hour of the onset of symptoms, excluding suicide, homicide and accident." The APA report (39) adopted the following criteria: death discovered in less than 24 hr after symptom onset, in a healthy patient with no preexisting illness on usual doses of psychotropics, with a negative autopsy (unable to explain the cause of death), and with complete medical data available for analysis.

Clearly, if neuroleptics did contribute to sudden death, such an effect would not be limited to such previously healthy cases, but these criteria may be useful in identifying cases that are informative for isolation of a specific role for the drug. Only 35 cases meeting this definition were published between 1957 and 1980, of whom 20 were found dead, 8 showed evidence of cardiovascular collapse, 7 had seizures, and 3 had difficulty breathing just before death. They were taking a variety of neuroleptic drugs, generally proportional to the range of drugs in clinical use (39). By definition, there were no positive autopsy findings.

The fact that such a small number of relevant cases can be identified raises the question of whether any significant excess of sudden and unexplained deaths exists among neuroleptic-treated psychiatric patients. Several studies have attempted to examine this on a large scale. Brill and Patton (6) found that for all inpatients in New York state psychiatric hospitals, age-corrected death rates were identical for the years 1955 and 1960 (before and after the introduction of neuroleptics). Craig and Lin (10) compared mortality rates in psychiatric inpatients in Norway between 1926 and 1941, in Michigan between 1950 and 1954, and in New York State between 1969 and 1977; they also obtained rates for the general population in each location during the same era. The mortality rates for the general population were similar across locations, with higher rates for psychiatric inpatients in each case (40.4–70.7/1000/year, vs 12.3–17.3/1000/year). The postneuroleptic New York mortality rates were lower than the rates for the two preneuroleptic samples, but similar to the Michigan rates. Tsuang and Simpson (43) also reported an increased mortality rate for schizophrenic patients. All of these studies considered rates for death by all causes. They suggest that, if neuroleptic-treated patients have any increase in sudden death, it is rare enough not to affect the overall mortality rate measurably.

Two other studies examined incidence of sudden death specifically. Swett and Shader (42) found two sudden deaths among 1,932 consecutive psychiatric admissions to six U.S. and Finnish hospitals (1968–1974). One patient with preexisting left ventricular disease died "suddenly" after a 16-day period during which her blood urea nitrogen (BUN) had risen from 30 to 60 mg/dl (normal below 25 mg/dl), and her potassium decreased from 4.6 to 3.3 mEq/liter

(normal 3.5–5.5 mEq/liter) as of 5 days before death (the last testing); she was receiving a potassium-wasting diuretic, potassium, and 2 mg haloperidol daily. Cardiac and electrolyte disorders seem more likely than haloperidol to have contributed to this death. The second death occurred suddenly in a 23-year-old man receiving 10 mg haloperidol and four antiseizure medications (diazepam, phenytoin, primidone, and ethosuximide) daily. This rate of sudden death is similar to the rate of one or two per thousand per year suggested by Richardson, Groupner, and Richardson (36) as likely to occur on a cardiac basis alone (although the lack of full one-year follow-up in the Swett and Shader study makes the two rates not entirely comparable). A second study reported 21 sudden and unexpected deaths among 31,960 admissions at Shanghai Psychiatric Hospital between 1970 and 1979, again roughly comparable to one or two per thousand per year (although, again, the exact observation period per subject is not known) (M. Y. Zhang and T. S. Zhou, unpublished, cited in ref. 39). Thus, no excess of sudden death among psychiatric patients has been found.

If neuroleptics contribute to death or sudden death in individual patients, this must occur rarely enough to be nondetectable in these epidemiologic studies. One possible mechanism involves the cardiac repolarization abnormalities that can occur during phenothiazine treatment. This was initially reported for thioridazine by Kelly, Fay, and Laverty (22), who attributed two fatalities to the effect. Cardiovascular effects of neuroleptics have been recently reviewed by Risch, Groom, and Janowsky (37). On the electrocardiogram (ECG), abnormal T-waves, U-waves, increased Q-T interval, and depressed S-T segment may be seen, although it should be noted that as many as 29% of placebo-treated controls may also show ECG abnormalities, usually T-wave changes (16). Changes are clearly most common with thioridazine. Axelsson and Aspenstrom (4) reported that most patients with thioridazine plasma levels found by them to be therapeutic (>1 µM/liter) had T-wave changes, and that intraindividual changes in thioridazine level were correlated with grade of T-wave change up to an individual plateau level. No clinically deleterious effects, and no other ECG effects, were seen. Elderly patients may be particularly at risk for ECG effects; in a crossover study of elderly patients, thioridazine was far more likely than fluphenazine to cause both T-wave and QT abnormalities (5). It would thus be a reasonable precaution to obtain periodic ECGs during periods of dosage increase and stabilization in phenothiazine-treated patients with preexisting cardiac disease, and particularly those with repolarization abnormalities, because of the possible risk of induction of ventricular arrhythmia (15). Special caution is advised in the use of thioridazine and other low-potency phenothiazines in patients with preexisting cardiac disease.

Other mechanisms of death have been proposed. Cancro and Wilder (7) reported a patient with a near-fatal episode of fainting with head trauma, probably directly related to severe hypotension, after 8 days of chlorpromazine therapy. Apparently, such events are uncommon. Brauchitsch and May (45) studied 35 cases of asphyxiation and aspiration deaths among psychiatric inpatients. Patients were generally regressed, and most had concurrent neurological disorders.

There were both neuroleptic-treated and untreated patients, and no direct relationship to drugs could be found. Two of the patients had "peculiar manneristic stereotype movements involving the tongue, lips and cheeks" (19, p. 131); the drug status of these patients is not given, but it has since become apparent that dystonic and dyskinetic symptoms involving the pharynx and larynx may present a risk of aspiration and asphyxiation (13). Fatal heat stroke has been attributed to the anticholinergic and thermoregulatory effects of neuroleptics (46). We have recently reported that in all cases of death from "neuroleptic malignant syndrome" in the reports reviewed, morbidity could be attributed to medical complications related to neuroleptic-induced rigidity or circumstances surrounding the treatment of these complications, rather than to a directly malignant effect of the drugs themselves (27).

There is currently insufficient evidence to support a conclusion that antipsychotic drugs directly cause sudden death. Certainly there is no evidence that any measurable number of patients die because of neuroleptics, and there is some evidence that mortality among psychiatric patients has decreased since the introduction of neuroleptics. There may be individual cases in which there is a causal relationship. Possible examples of such cases should be reported in full, and prior to publication these reports should be subjected to critical examination of the completeness of medical information and the soundness of causal inferences. We believe that there is a relationship between serious morbidity and mortality—but typically neither sudden nor unexplained death—and the occurrence of severe and persistent drug-induced rigidity or hypotension. These are most likely when high doses are used and when adverse effects are not systematically monitored. The current trend toward use of lower doses of neuroleptics, except in patients with well-documented treatment-resistant illness, may reduce the incidence of such adverse outcomes.

NEUROLEPTIC-INDUCED AGRANULOCYTOSIS

Chlorpromazine-induced agranulocytosis was first reported in 1954 (29), only 2 years after the introduction of the drug. Other phenothiazines were subsequently implicated, including thioridazine, promazine, mepazine, methtrimeprazine, and others. Pisciotta and associates have reviewed these cases at intervals (31,33); thioridazine-associated cases were reviewed by Ferguson, Hodges, and Bogner (12). By 1965, 138 cases had been reported in patients treated with phenothiazines alone, and 283 with phenothiazines plus other drugs, making these agents the leading cause of agranulocytosis in adults (31). This literature will be reviewed briefly here, followed by a discussion of agranulocytosis associated with clozapine.

Early data demonstrated that large doses of chlorpromazine were associated with a measurable decline in granulocytes, apparently peaking at 3 months (30). Pisciotta (31) reported that of 6,200 psychiatric patients treated with phenothiazines who were systematically monitored, 2,000 (1:3) developed "transient, moderate leukopenia," whereas 5 (1:1,240) developed agranulocytosis. Litvak and Kaelbing (28) reported that of 5,993 inpatients on psychotropic drugs (most but not all phenothiazines) who received weekly complete blood counts (CBCs), 41 on phenothiazines alone and 9 on phenothiazines plus other drugs developed total white blood counts (WBCs) below $3,700/mm^3$ (1:120), 5 had WBC below 2,000 (1:1,200), and 3 had clinical agranulocytosis with infection (1:2,000). At the time of these studies, high doses of low-potency phenothiazines were the major form of antipsychotic therapy.

Reports of antipsychotic-related agranulocytosis have since become less frequent, presumably because the high-potency and nonphenothiazine agents (which appear to be less likely to cause the problem) are used more often, and high doses of the low-potency phenothiazines are used less often. It should also be noted that many of the early cases occurred in large institutions with heterogeneous patients and variable levels of care. For example, of 16 deaths reported in Maryland hospitals from 1956 to 1966, 11 had serious concurrent medical illnesses (30). Further, in the series of Litvak and Kaelbing (28), in addition to 50 cases of leukopenia associated with phenothiazines (including all 3 deaths), there were 26 cases considered related to other causes and 30 that occurred in the absence of drug treatment or any other apparent cause. Therefore, it is quite possible that some cases with other or unknown causes have been attributed to phenothiazines in the literature.

Pisciotta has presented data to provide the best explanation to date for this phenomenon. Bone marrow cells from patients who had recovered from chlorpromazine-induced agranulocytosis showed inhibition of mitosis in the presence of chlorpromazine (34). Cells from such patients were subsequently found to have a reduction in the incorporation of tritiated thymidine, suggesting a defect in the final stage of DNA synthesis; patients sensitive to other drugs lacked the defect, and other pathways could not be implicated (32). It was therefore hypothesized that phenothiazine-sensitive patients may have a defect in DNA synthesis that is normally benign, but that predisposes to complete cessation of granulocyte production in the presence of phenothiazine for a sufficient period of time (32).

Phenothiazine-induced agranulocytosis usually appears between 10 and 90 days after initiation of the offending drug, although a few cases with later onset have been seen (31). Daily and total doses have been quite variable, although higher doses are apparently associated with a higher incidence of leukopenia. Plasma levels have not been available. As discussed above, it is often clinically silent. Recovery generally occurs over 1 to 3 weeks; deaths occur in a minority of cases. No specific therapy has been found. It has been suggested that older females and whites are more vulnerable (30). Rechallenge with the offending drug produces recurrence; it is usually possible to switch to a chemically unrelated drug, usually a nonphenothiazine, but an unusual case has been reported in which multiple subsequent trials of various antipsychotic drugs from different classes produced leukopenia that remitted on discontinuation of each drug (3). It has been repeatedly suggested (and we agree) that frequent WBC measurements are of little value, as they identify primarily silent, benign leukopenia. Even where routine surveillance has been attempted, clinically significant agranulocytosis has usually been identified only after symptoms of infection have occurred

(28,31). In patients on low-potency phenothiazines in particular, signs of infection early in therapy should be followed immediately by a WBC examination.

Currently, the drug of greatest concern worldwide is clozapine, a novel antipsychotic that can cause agranulocytosis. This drug, of the dibenzazepine class, has been considered of theoretical and clinical importance because of its apparent differences from other available antipsychotics. Specifically, it has weak or absent effects in some of the standard animal models for dopaminergic blockade, such as inhibition of amphetamine-induced stereotypies and induction of catalepsy (20), although striatal single-neuron electrophysiological effects have been reported in some studies (35), and prominent anticholinergic effects are also seen. It does not cause parkinsonism. It is generally considered to have a low potential for causing tardive dyskinesia (TD), although Simpson et al. reported short-term amelioration of TD after initiation of clozapine, with recurrence of movements after discontinuation of drug (40). This suggests that striatal DA blockade may have occurred and thus that long-term exacerbation of TD might occur. Despite these inconsistencies, interest in clozapine has continued because of the compelling problems of reducing the incidence of TD, treating patients with special sensitivity to developing extrapyramidal symptoms, and treating psychosis in TD patients. Furthermore, clinical reports have found clozapine to be an antipsychotic that is at least as effective as other drugs, and that may be more effective in at least some treatment-resistant patients (24,41).

In the summer of 1975, an unusual number of cases of agranulocytosis were noted in Finnish patients receiving clozapine. Subsequent survey of all Finnish hospitals revealed that in at most 2,800 patients receiving clozapine, 16 (1:175) cases of granulocytopenia (defined as WBC < 3,200/mm^3) occurred, including 13 (1:215) cases of agranulocytosis (no or few peripheral granulocytes) and 8 (1:350) related deaths secondary to infection (2). In 13 of the 16 cases, clozapine was the only drug being administered. The dyscrasia occurred during the first 3 months of treatment, and recovery occurred over 1 to 2 weeks after discontinuation of drug; the pattern was similar to that reported for chlorpromazine, suggesting an effect on DNA synthesis rather than immediate, allergic cellular destruction. Deaths occurred in patients who continued to receive the drug after signs of infection (2). Many features of this epidemic were puzzling, such as the fact that some clinics had multiple cases and others none, despite prescription of similar dosages from the same batches of drug. Nevertheless, the association with clozapine appeared clear.

Between 1977 and 1984, 85 cases of agranulocytosis were reported to the manufacturer; 36 were fatal. In U.S. trials, incidence has been calculated as the proportion of total patients treated, and of cases "at risk" (receiving 6 weeks of treatment or more) who developed total WBC of less than 1,500. As of February, 1984, there had been 2 cases out of 429 total cases (4.66 per 1000) and 203 cases at risk (9.85 per 1000). As of April, 1986, there had been 3 cases out of 627 total (4.78 per 1000) and 379 at risk (7.91 per 1000); the U.S. manufacturer therefore currently estimates a risk of approximately 1 case per 100 treated for over 6 weeks (Dr. G. Honigfeld, Sandoz Research Institute, personal communication. None of these cases was fatal. Thus, although careful monitoring may reduce mortality, a significant proportion of patients do develop clinical agranulocytosis.

Clozapine has been marketed in 36 countries. Premarket testing had begun in the United States at the time of the Finnish epidemic. The occurrence of the non-fatal agranulocytosis in an American patient led to suspension of trials by the FDA in 1977. The company also restricted use of the drug worldwide to treatment-resistant patients and those with TD. A number of related drugs have been developed, but as yet none have been shown to have a profile of adverse effects preferable to clozapine. Because of the advantages cited above, clozapine has continued to be viewed as a potentially useful drug by psychopharmacologists. Clozapine has recently again been approved for investigational use in the United States to determine its value for patients with TD and also for patients poorly responsive to other antipsychotic treatment. It is likely that testing of clozapine will proceed, and that in the future clozapine and/or clozapine-like drugs may become available for marketing in the United States, at least for specific indications. Current studies are likely to produce clearer guidelines for monitoring WBC counts and for appropriate response to low counts. Current Sandoz protocols in the United States call for maximum clozapine dosage of 900 mg/day, with CBC pretreatment and every 7 days throughout treatment, with discontinuation of treatment for any total WBC < 4,000/mm^3, or total granulocytes (polys plus bands) < 1,500.

HEPATOTOXICITY OF NEUROLEPTICS

Jaundice and liver function abnormalities were reported during chlorpromazine (CPZ) therapy 30 years ago (9). CPZ has since become a model for drug-induced cholestatic hepatitis. Yet the mechanism is still unclear, as is the relationship of reactions to CPZ and to other antipsychotics. Although there have been few new data on this issue in recent years, it deserves review because of the frequency of clinical questions concerning hepatic effects of antipsychotics.

CPZ is by far the most common antipsychotic to be associated with hepatic effects. For example, the Danish Board of Adverse Reactions to Drugs analyzed 572 cases of hepatotoxicity between 1968 and 1978 (11). Of these, the 93 reactions to psychotropics were second only to the 144 associated with halothane; CPZ was the psychotropic in 54 of the cases. The incidence of CPZ-related jaundice can be estimated from the eight large series giving such figures reviewed by Ishak and Irey (19): of a total of 12,210 treated patients, 149 (1.2%) developed clinical jaundice. Closely monitored series of patients have shown an incidence of elevated liver enzymes ranging from 22 to 50% (19).

As is true for many other adverse effects, CPZ may be most frequently implicated because it has been the most frequently prescribed antipsychotic, particularly during the first decade of antipsychotic use when newly discovered adverse effects received the closest attention. Thus, laboratory models of phenothiazine-induced hepatic changes have also involved CPZ, as it has reliable effects and clear-cut clinical relevance. Jaundice has also been associated with promazine, prochlorperazine, mepazine, perphenazine, trifluoperazine, thioridazine, and fluphenazine, suggesting that any phenothiazine may produce some degree of risk (19). This suggestion is supported by Jones et al. (21), who examined spontaneous drug-related hepatitis reports to the FDA and found that all phenothiazine subclasses (aliphatic, piperidine, piperazine) were implicated. They also used computerized Medicaid records from two states to demonstrate that phenothiazine-treated patients had a significantly higher number of hepatitis-related diagnoses than patients not on such treatment, with no difference among the drug subclasses. (There was no excess of hepatitis in patients over 50, which may be due to lower doses often used in this group, to absence of drug abuse-related hepatitis found in younger psychotic patients, or to other unknown factors.)

Cases associated with haloperidol have also been reported (14). No cases associated with thioxanthene derivatives were identified in a computer-assisted literature search.

In the Danish survey cited above, CPZ-related liver disease was primarily cholestatic in 80% and primarily cytotoxic in 20% of cases with sufficient data, based on the pattern of liver enzyme abnormalities. About 10% developed chronic disease, of the biliary cirrhotic type. There were 5 deaths reported in the 54 cases, and 9 cases of severe liver impairment (11).

Ishak and Irey (19) conducted one of the most complete pathological studies in phenothiazine-related armed forces cases (1954–1969). Of 96 alleged cases, 36 were felt to be confirmed after careful study. The 36 patients on CPZ had received a mean of 2.78 g, over a mean of 15.3 days prior to symptoms. Two-thirds of their cases had a systemic prodrome for 2 to 14 days prior to jaundice, including symptoms such as GI complaints and fever with chills, malaise, fatigue, and muscle aches. Liver enzymes (serum glutamic-oxaloacetic transaminase, SGOT, and/or serum glutamic-pyruvic transaminase, SGPT) were typically between 50 and 300 Karmen units; most patients had peripheral eosinophilia. The pathological findings were typical of studies involving these drugs: cholestasis was found in the canaliculi, hepatocytes, and Kupffer cells, usually centrilobular or central and midzonal; however, some degree of inflammation and focal necrosis was also seen in most cases, as well as sinusoidal eosinophilia. Most patients recovered within 8 weeks, but some took 12 to 78 weeks to normalize lab values. In four cases, chronic biliary cirrhosis resulted (9–11% incidence in this and the Danish series).

There is still mixed evidence concerning the mechanism in such cases. The time course, low incidence, eosinophilia, and occasional occurrence after a single dose of drug all point to an immunologic mechanism such as the hypersensitivity reaction. The much higher incidence of liver enzyme abnormalities in CPZ-treated patients suggests cytotoxic effects as well. Numerous authors have suggested that both mechanisms may be involved in cases of clinically significant cholestasis (38). CPZ may form free radicals within the liver that directly inhibit Na^+K^+-ATPase, impairing bile salt-independent biliary flow (bile salt excretion) (38). This

may occur to some degree in many or most patients, leading to frequent silent elevations of liver enzymes. This conclusion is supported by a report that 5 of 20 CPZ-treated patients, and 0 of 25 placebo-treated patients, had subtle and clinically silent changes on liver biopsy read by an experienced pathologist as suggesting cholestatic processes (18). It has been suggested that these cytotoxic effects may lead to membrane alterations and thus to hypersensitivity reactions in certain susceptible patients, although susceptibility could also be due to idiosyncrasy of free radical formation and damage or to independent hypersensitivity effects (38). Reactions to other phenothiazines have shown pathology similar to that caused by CPZ; two well-described cases associated with haloperidol also showed evidence of hypersensitivity reaction with predominantly cholestatic and some cellular damage (14).

It must be emphasized that in the individual case, it can be difficult to determine whether liver disease is related to antipsychotic drugs. Ishak and Irey were able to confirm only 36 of 94 cases (19). Hollister and Hall reported that over half of 45 psychiatric inpatients had nonspecific abnormalities on liver biopsy whether or not they had received drugs, with CPZ only apparently contributing to the specific cholestatic changes described above (18). Viral hepatitis, extrahepatic biliary disease of all types, cholestasis due to other drugs (such as tetracycline), and liver abnormalities related to alcohol or substance abuse may all be confused with drug effects, particularly in the typical case where only blood values are available, rather than biopsy material.

Clinically, the following conclusions appear to be warranted. It would be prudent to assess liver functions before and during the first 1 to 2 weeks of therapy with phenothiazines (and particularly the low-potency agents). Significant reactions may occur at any point and are more likely to be identified during investigation of symptoms (jaundice or the prodrome of fever, GI or systemic symptoms) rather than with blood tests at any arbitrary time point. It is not known whether routine testing would be useful with nonphenothiazine antipsychotics. The appropriate response to mild and clinically silent liver enzyme elevations is often unclear. Particularly where other drugs or substances could be at fault, great care should be taken not to force premature discontinuation of an otherwise beneficial antipsychotic. When clinically insignificant abnormalities occur, or have been reported in the past, continued monitoring on the drug may be appropriate in some cases to determine whether continued therapy is possible. Any overt symptoms or signs that could be related to hepatic disease should be fully evaluated in any patient receiving antipsychotic drugs, and these drugs should be discontinued if it is believed that they are causal. Definitive diagnosis is only possible when biopsy findings of typical drug-related cholestasis can be correlated with the clinical course. Affected patients must be monitored until laboratory values are entirely normal, to identify cases with chronic cirrhosis. There is no documented treatment for drug-induced cholestasis, except for supportive therapy.

No definitive guidelines can be given for future antipsychotic treatment. Hollister (17) reported that 70% of phenothiazine-induced jaundice patients had recurrence of liver abnormalities after rechallenge with low doses, yet some were able to resume CPZ therapy; four of Ishak and Irey's cases received other phenothiazines without apparent harm, but cases of cross sensitivity have been reported (19). Because there are now multiple classes of antipsychotic drugs, a switch is usually made to a different (and non-phenothiazine) class, both after clinical jaundice and after mild enzyme elevations; there are no data to determine how often such switches are in fact necessary. Although a conservative approach may protect some patients from overt hepatic damage, it must be emphasized again that many patients are denied potentially beneficial drugs because of previous poorly documented reports of "elevated liver enzymes" coincidental with administration of a particular drug. Suspicion of drug-induced changes should be followed by careful documentation of alternative diagnoses and, in questionable cases, continuation or rechallenge with the drug with the patient's consent. Liver disease may be less common with the thioxanthene and butyrophenone derivatives.

Finally, there is often a question about administering antipsychotics to patients with known liver disease. The major interaction in these cases is simply that impaired liver function will tend to produce greatly elevated plasma and tissue levels of these drugs (1), which are excreted largely by the liver. For patients with preexisting noncholestatic disease, the incidence of significant liver reactions even with phenothiazine derivatives is still low. Such reactions are due to mechanisms unrelated to the concurrent disease, so that no increased risk of drug-induced liver injury should be expected if doses are adjusted appropriately. Nevertheless, it would be wise to avoid phenothiazine derivatives, to minimize the likelihood of even minor or transient further compromise of function. Patients with cholestatic diseases should be given only nonphenothiazine antipsychotics. Liver enzymes should be monitored during the first 2 months of antipsychotic therapy in all patients with preexisting liver disease.

ACKNOWLEDGMENTS

Julie Holub and Mary Maisey assisted in the preparation of this chapter.

REFERENCES

1. Alexander, G. J., Machiz, S., and Alexander, R. B. (1972): *Adv. Exp. Med. Biol.,* 27:151–160.
2. Amsler, H. A., Teerenhovi, L., Barth, E., Harjula, K., and Vuopio, P. (1977): *Acta Psychiatr. Scand.,* 56:241–248.
3. Ananth, J. V., Valles, J. V., and Whitelaw, J. P. (1973): *Am. J. Psychiatry,* 130:100–102.
4. Axelsson, R., and Aspenstrom, G. (1982): *J. Clin. Psychiatry,* 43:332–335.
5. Branchey, M. H., Lee, J. H., Amin, R., and Simpson, G. M. (1978): *JAMA,* 239:1860.
6. Brill, H., and Patton, R. E. (1962): *Am. J. Psychiatry,* 119:20–35.
7. Cancro, R., and Wilder, R. (1970): *Am. J. Psychiatry,* 127:368–371.
8. Claghorn, J. L., Abuzzahab, F. S., Wang, R., Larson, C., Gelenberg, A. J., Klerman, G. L., Tuason, V., and Steinbook, R. (1983): *Psychopharmacol. Bull.,* 19:138–140.
9. Cohen, I. M., and Archer, J. D. (1958): *JAMA,* 159:99–101.
10. Craig, T. J., and Lin, S. P. (1981): *Arch. Gen. Psychiatry,* 38:935–938.
11. Dossing, M., and Andreasen, B. (1982): *Scand. J. Gastroenterol.,* 17:205–211.
12. Ferguson, R. L., Hodges, G. R., and Bogner, P. J. (1977): *South. Med. J.,* 70:110–111.
13. Flaherty, J. A., and Lahmeyer, H. W. (1978): *Am. J. Psychiatry,* 135:1414–1415.
14. Fuller, C. M., Yassinger, S., Donlon, P., Imperato, T. J., and Ruebner, B. (1977): *West. J. Med.,* 127:515–518.
15. Giles, T. O., and Modlin, R. K. (1968): *JAMA,* 205:108–110.
16. Holden, M., and Itil, T. (1977): In: *Stress and Heart,* edited by D. Wheatley, pp. 87–119. Raven Press, New York.
17. Hollister, L. E. (1957): *Am. J. Med.,* 23:870–879.
18. Hollister, L. E., and Hall, R. A. (1966): *Am. J. Psychiatry,* 123:211–212.
19. Ishak, K. G., and Irey, N. S. (1972): *Arch. Pathol.,* 93:283–304.
20. Jenner, P., and Marsden, C. D. (1983): In: *Psychopharmacology—Part I: Preclinical Psychopharmacology,* edited by D. G. Grahame-Smith and P. J. Cowen, pp. 180–217. Excerpta Medica, Oxford.
21. Jones, J. K., Van de Carr, S. W., Zimmerman, H., and Leroy, A. (1983): *Psychopharmacol. Bull.,* 19:24–27.
22. Kelly, H. G., Fay, J. E., and Laverty, S. G. (1963): *Can. Med. Assoc. J.,* 89:546–554.
23. Kuller, L., Lilienfeld, A., and Fisher, R. (1966): *Medicine,* 46:341–361.
24. Lapierre, Y. D., Ghadirian, A., St.-Laurent, J., and Chaudhry, R. P. (1980): *Curr. Ther. Res.,* 27:391–400.
25. Leber, P. (1981): *Psychopharmacol. Bull.,* 17:6–9.
26. Leestma, J. E., and Koenig, K. L. (1968): *Arch. Gen. Psychiatry,* 18:137–148.
27. Levinson, D. F., and Simpson, G. S. (1986): *Arch. Gen. Psychiatry,* 43:839–848.
28. Litvak, R., and Kaelbling, R. (1971): *Arch. Gen. Psychiatry,* 24:265–267.
29. Lomas, J. (1954): *Br. Med. J.,* 2:358–359.
30. Mandel, A., and Gross, M. (1968): *Dis. Nerv. Syst.,* 29:32–36.
31. Pisciotta, A. V. (1969): *JAMA,* 208:1862–1868.
32. Pisciotta, A. V. (1971): *J. Lab. Clin. Med.,* 78:435–448.
33. Pisciotta, A. V. (1982): *Haematologica,* 67:292–318.
34. Pisciotta, A. V., Westring, D. W., and DePrey, C. (1967): *J. Lab. Clin. Med.,* 70:229–235.
35. Rebec, G. V., Bashore, T. R., Zimmerman, K. S., and Alloway, K. D. (1979): *Pharmacol. Biochem. Behav.,* 11:529–538.
36. Richardson, H., Groupner, K. I., and Richardson, M. E. (1966): *JAMA,* 194:254–260.
37. Risch, S. C., Groom, G. P., and Janowsky, D. S. (1982): *J. Clin. Psychiatry,* 43:16–31.
38. Sherlock, S. (1979): *Gut,* 20:634–648.
39. Simpson, G. M., Jefferson, J., Davis, J., and Perez-Cruet, J. (1987): *Report of the APA Task Force on Sudden Death (in press).*
40. Simpson, G. M., Lee, J. H., and Shrivastava, R. K. (1978): *Psychopharmacology,* 56:75–80.
41. Simpson, G. M., and Varger, E. (1974): *Curr. Ther. Res.,* 16:679–686.
42. Swett, C. P., and Shader, R. I. (1977): *Dis. Nerv. System,* 38:69–72.
43. Tsuang, M. T., and Simpson, J. C. (1985): *Arch. Gen. Psychiatry,* 42:98–103.
44. Ungvari, G. (1980): *Pharmakopsychiatrie,* 13:29–33.
45. Von Brauchitsch, H., and May, W. (1968): *Arch. Gen. Psychiatry,* 18:129–136.
46. Zelman, S., and Guillan, R. (1970): *Am. J. Psychiatry,* 126:787–790.

Psychopharmacology:
The Third Generation of Progress,
edited by Herbert Y. Meltzer.
Raven Press, New York © 1987.

CHAPTER **151**

Cardiovascular Effects of Tricyclic Antidepressants

Alexander H. Glassman, Steven P. Roose, Elsa-Grace V. Giardina, and J. Thomas Bigger, Jr.

Shortly after tricyclic antidepressants (TCAs) were introduced it was noted that people who took fatal overdoses of TCAs most frequently died from heart block and/or arrhythmias (58). This observation led to the concern that in vulnerable patients these drugs might produce similar complications at the lower plasma concentrations used for antidepressant treatment.

In the early 1960s, two large epidemiological studies attempted to assess the relationship between TCA drugs and cardiovascular death rate. The Boston Collaborative Drug Surveillance Program (4) reported that among 4,074 hospitalized patients with a diagnosis of "cardiovascular disease," 80 were taking TCAs. There was no difference between cardiovascular patients taking TCAs and those not taking TCAs with regard to the frequency of arrhythmias, heart block, shock, syncopy, hypertension, and cardiac failure during hospitalization. The Aberdeen General Hospital's group, however, found the opposite result (11,28,29). Of 864 patients who received amitriptyline, 119 had a diagnosis of cardiac disease. An identical number of nondepressed patients who matched the TCA cases for age, gender, cardiac diagnosis, and length of hospital stay were selected as controls. The overall mortality rate in both the index cases and controls was high (19 and 12%, respectively) but not significantly different. The rate of sudden unexpected death, however, was significantly higher in the amitriptyline-treated cases (86%).

Since a number of studies have established that there is an increased incidence of cardiovascular deaths in depressed patients *per se,* it is possible that the high mortality rate associated with depressive illness, rather than the amitriptyline, accounted for the difference in mortality between cases and controls in the Aberdeen study (1). Nonetheless, the contradictory results in these two epidemiological studies are indicative of the complexity of the cardiovascular effects of the TCAs. Only after 25 years have we gradually acquired an accurate understanding of the cardiac effects of the TCAs. This chapter will review these effects in the following order: (a) orthostatic hypotension, (b) conduction, (c) contractility, (d) rhythm, and (e) overdose. A brief review of normal cardiac electrophysiology has been published previously (19).

ORTHOSTATIC HYPOTENSION

One of the most frequent and potentially serious side effects of TCA treatment is orthostatic hypotension. Fractures, lacerations, myocardial infarctions, and sudden deaths have all been reported (20,31).

By far the most studied drug in this context is imipramine. An early study by Muller et al. (31) observed "moderate to severe" postural hypotension in 24% of 82 depressed patients treated with imipramine. The patients were split into two groups: half with a mean age of 70, all of whom had some cardiovascular disease, and half with a mean age of 39, all free from cardiovascular disease. Most of the untoward reactions attributed to orthostatic hypotension occurred in the older group. We have examined the effects of imipramine on blood pressure in 120 patients in a retrospective study, and 44 patients in a prospective study (20). In the retrospective study, the average age was 56 and the dose of drug was 261 mg. In nine (8%) of the 120 patients who started imipramine, orthostatic hypotension necessitated the discontinuation of drug.

In the prospective study, 44 depressed patients with an

average age of 59 were treated with therapeutic plasma levels of imipramine. One minute after standing, the average fall in systolic blood pressure was 26 mm Hg, which represented a statistically significant increase ($p < 0.001$) as compared to the predrug orthostatic drop. An important clinical characteristic of this on-drug orthostatic fall was that there was no tendency for patients to accommodate to the effect of the drug over a 4-week period of observation.

The data available on the orthostatic effect of other TCAs are not as complete, but the works of Nelson et al. (32), Hayes et al. (22), Kopera (26), and our own group (44) strongly imply that this orthostatic effect exists for amitriptyline and desmethylimipramine as well. It is interesting that for over a decade doxepin has been marketed as the safest tricyclic in patients with cardiovascular disease, even though very little is known concerning doxepin's potential to cause orthostatic hypotension. A recent study suggests that doxepin may cause less orthostatic hypotension. Since a mean dose of only 76 mg of doxepin was given, however, and blood pressure measured only weekly, the conclusions reasonably drawn from this study are very limited (33).

Nortriptyline is the only TCA presently marketed that is significantly different in its orthostatic effect. Freyschuss et al. (13) reported that the orthostatic effect of nortriptyline in 40 healthy and relatively young (mean age 44) depressed patients was negligible. In a study of 20 patients with a mean age of 42 and no cardiovascular illness, Vohra et al. (55) and Thayssen et al. (51) have also reported that there were no postural systolic drops with nortriptyline.

We have examined the effects of nortriptyline on blood pressure in 33 patients in a retrospective study and 15 patients in a prospective study. In the retrospective study, the mean age of the group was 67, mean daily dose of nortriptyline 85 mg, and mean plasma concentration 98 ng/ml (43). None of the 33 patients developed orthostatic hypotension. In the prospective study, we compared the orthostatic effect of nortriptyline in 15 patients with an average age of 59, and compared the results to the orthostatic effect of imipramine in a comparable group of patients (45). The average orthostatic drop on nortriptyline was 13 mm Hg, which is significantly less than the 26 mm Hg orthostatic drop in the patients on imipramine. Furthermore, we treated eight patients with both imipramine and nortriptyline, thereby allowing a comparison of the differential orthostatic effect of the two drugs, using the patient as his own control. In this group, which includes a number of patients who developed severe orthostatic drops on imipramine, nortriptyline caused significantly less orthostatic hypotension. In fact, the patients who were forced to stop their imipramine because they repeatedly fell or passed out when standing showed no significant symptoms of orthostatic hypotension when switched to nortriptyline.

Thus, in medically healthy, depressed patients, treated with TCAs, orthostatic hypotension is the most frequent serious cardiovascular side effect. This problem is best documented for imipramine, which induced intolerable orthostatic hypotension in approximately 8% of the patients with melancholia, and all available data would conclude that the same is probably true of desmethylimipramine and amitriptyline as well. Nortriptyline, however, clearly causes less orthostatic hypotension than the other TCAs and generally can be used when the other drugs cannot be tolerated because of this side effect.

Both the rate of orthostatic hypotension induced by imipramine and the magnitude of difference between imipramine and nortriptyline increase dramatically when one starts treating depressed patients with cardiac disease. We have now treated 25 depressed patients with preexisting congestive heart failure with imipramine and the rate of drug-induced orthostatic hypotension was approximately 50% (21,41). In 21 patients with preexisting congestive failure treated with therapeutic plasma concentrations of nortriptyline, however, only one patient (4.8%) developed orthostatic hypotension (42). Furthermore, 19 of the 21 nortriptyline-treated patients had, at some previous time, a trial of imipramine, and eight of 19 fell down while on imipramine. Thus, even in depressed patients with congestive heart failure, nortriptyline can most often be used safely when imipramine is discontinued because of orthostatic hypotension.

The mechanism by which TCAs induce orthostatic hypotension is unclear. Interestingly, a significant risk factor for the development of orthostatic hypotension with imipramine may be the diagnosis of depression itself. Giardina et al. (18) have reported that in 22 nondepressed cardiac patients with some degree of congestive heart failure (mean ejection fraction 33% by radionuclide angiography), treated with imipramine for arrhythmia control, only one patient (4%) discontinued medication because of orthostatic hypotension. This compares to the rate of approximately 50% of patients developing intolerable orthostatic hypotension in our depressed patients with a similar degree of left ventricular impairment who were treated with comparable plasma concentrations of imipramine (21,41). Thus, it would seem that when treated with imipramine, patients with heart disease and melancholia are at significantly greater risk to develop orthostatic hypotension than patients with heart disease alone (chi-square = 8.98, $p < 0.005$).

EFFECTS OF THERAPEUTIC DOSES OF TCAs ON CONDUCTION

In one of the first cardiovascular studies to incorporate plasma level measurements, Vohra et al. (55) examined the effect of drug on the electrocardiogram (ECG) in 32 patients treated with nortriptyline or doxepin. The data showed a significant drug-related increase in the PR interval for patients treated with nortriptyline but not for those treated with doxepin. The mean nortriptyline level, however, was 186 ng/ml and the doxepin level was not reported, thereby raising the concern that the drug effect on the ECG may have been evaluated when the drugs were not at comparable plasma concentrations.

In a subsequent effort to clarify the apparent difference in conduction effect between nortriptyline and doxepin, Burrows et al. (7) crossed over 12 depressed patients using 150 mg/day doses for each drug. They found that nortriptyline significantly increased conduction in four of the 12 patients, whereas doxepin did not. The plasma concentration of nortriptyline in the four patients who developed significant increases, however, ranged from two to five times the usual therapeutic level of nortriptyline, whereas the average plasma concentration of doxepin was relatively low (52 ng/ml). Little can be concluded from this study with respect to possible intrinsic differences in the cardiac effects between these two drugs.

Further studies of the ECG effects of nortriptyline within the "therapeutic window" (50–150 ng/ml) were conducted by Freyschuss et al. (13) and Ziegler et al. (60). These studies are comparable in that they both included relatively young depressed patients essentially free from cardiovascular disease. Among the total of 57 patients, only two developed modest ECG changes while on nortriptyline. Thus, the studies to date indicate that in middle-aged, depressed patients, free from serious cardiovascular disease, therapeutic plasma levels of nortriptyline are unlikely to increase significantly either the PR or QRS measurements. Significant changes in these measurements, however, do occur more often at plasma concentrations of drug only slightly higher than the upper limit of the therapeutic window.

Vohra was the first to attempt to identify more precisely where TCAs exert their influence on conduction. An increased PR interval could be the result of either AH (AV nodal) or HV (intraventricular) prolongation. His bundle electrocardiography is a technique by which the components of AV conduction can be isolated and evaluated separately. Vohra et al. (54) performed these measures in 12 patients prior to and while taking nortriptyline. They found that the AH interval was unaffected, but a prolongation of the HV interval occurred in one of eight patients with plasma concentrations less than 200 ng/ml and in all four patients with plasma concentrations above 200 ng/ml. That the TCAs exert their major effect on the HV interval has subsequently been supported by the electrophysiological studies of Weld and Bigger (56) and Rawling and Fozzard (40).

With respect to the more widely used TCAs, we have studied the ECG effects of therapeutic plasma concentrations of imipramine (mean level 282 ng/ml) in 44 depressed patients, and found that the drug regularly produced significant increases in the PR, QRS, and QT$_c$ measurements (25). Despite amitriptyline's being the most frequently prescribed TCA in the United States, few systematically collected data are available on its ECG effects at presumed therapeutic plasma concentrations. The data that are available suggest that, like imipramine, amitriptyline prolongs cardiac conduction and in overdose it seems to be at least as cardiotoxic as the other TCAs (6,34,37,59). The limited information available, however, does not allow specific comparisons between amitriptyline and other TCAs.

Summarizing the literature, one can conclude that TCA drugs at, or just above, therapeutic plasma concentrations, frequently prolong PR and QRS intervals, and that they exert their major action on intraventricular (HV) conduction. In depressed patients with normal cardiac conduction as reflected by a normal pretreatment ECG, it is important to realize that the moderate increases in either the PR or QRS caused by TCA drugs are not, by themselves, clinically significant.

The propensity of TCAs to reduce conduction velocity raises the question of whether patients with preexisting cardiac conduction disease would be at increased risk to develop AV block when treated with a tricyclic. This concern is supported by the frequency of AV block after TCA overdose, and by well-documented case reports of patients with preexisting bundle branch block who developed 2 to 1 AV block when treated with imipramine (24). We have recently completed a prospective study of 41 depressed patients with 1° AV block and/or bundle branch block compared to 151 patients with normal pretreatment ECGs. Both groups were treated with therapeutic plasma concentrations of imipramine or nortriptyline (43). The rate of 2 to 1 AV block was significantly higher (9%) in patients with preexisting bundle branch block, as compared to the rate (0.7%) in patients with normal pretreatment ECGs ($p < 0.05$ by Fisher's exact test). In fact, the one patient with a normal pretreatment ECG who developed 2 to 1 AV block on tricyclic had an abnormal His Purkinje conduction apparent only by catheterization.

EFFECTS ON MECHANICAL FUNCTION OF THE HEART

Until recently, it has been widely assumed that the TCAs adversely affect left ventricular function (LVF). A number of early studies looking at nortriptyline, amitriptyline, and imipramine found evidence of TCA-induced impairment of LVF (5,38,50). The method used to assess LVF, however, was the systolic time interval, a measurement that is dependent, in part, on the QRS duration. Since QRS prolongation is a characteristic effect of the TCAs, there exists the possibility that the effect of TCAs on the systolic time interval in these early studies was due to their effects on conduction, not on LVF. This possibility was supported when studies using an alternate measure of LVF, specifically the echocardiogram, failed to demonstrate TCA impairment of LVF (16).

The introduction of radionuclide angiography provided a more reliable means of assessing TCA effect on LVF. Using this methodology, Veith et al. (53) evaluated the effect of imipramine and doxepin in 17 depressed patients and found no evidence that either drug impaired LVF. This study used, however, only relatively low doses of drug and included few patients with ejection fractions below 40%.

Subsequently, we reported radionuclide data on a series of 15 depressed patients with moderate to severe impairment of LVF (mean ejection fraction, 33%), treated at therapeutic plasma concentrations of imipramine (21). Though imipramine had no deleterious effect on any measure of LVF, as previously discussed, it produced intolerable orthostatic hypotension in approximately 50% of patients. We have replicated this finding in a second series of 10 depressed patients with heart failure (mean pretreatment ejection fraction, 31%) who also had no change in any measure of LVF when treated with therapeutic plasma concentrations of imipramine (41). As before, however, 50% of these patients developed intolerable orthostatic hypotension.

In contrast, we have recently completed a study in which we administered therapeutic plasma concentrations of nortriptyline to depressed patients with preexisting impaired

LVF, and measured the effect on blood pressure and LVF (42). Twenty-one patients with a mean age of 68 ± 9 years and a mean pretreatment ejection fraction of 33% were treated with therapeutic plasma concentrations (mean level 107 ng/ml of nortriptyline). Nortriptyline did not cause any deleterious effect on LVF, and induced intolerable orthostatic hypotension in only one of 21 patients. Thus, nortriptyline would seem to be a relatively safe drug in the treatment of depressed patients with congestive heart failure, provided there is no preexisting conduction disease.

ANTIARRHYTHMIC EFFECTS OF TRICYCLICS

Because TCAs can cause severe arrhythmias in overdose, it had been widely held that their use was contraindicated in patients with preexisting arrhythmias (58). It is not necessarily true, however, that a drug will produce the same cardiovascular effect at a therapeutic plasma concentration as it does when at a toxic level. This has proved to be the case for the tricyclic drugs. Over the past 10 years, it has been established that at plasma concentrations approximating therapeutic levels for treatment of depression, these drugs have powerful antiarrhythmic activity that is of significant clinical importance (2,14,17). The antiarrhythmic effect of imipramine was first noted in two depressed patients with ventricular premature depolarizations (VPDs) treated in a clinical outcome study of depression (2). This observation was confirmed in a second series of 11 depressed patients with VPDs, 10 of whom subsequently had 90% VPD suppression at imipramine plasma concentrations ranging from 100 to 302 ng/ml (17). The possibility was raised whether the VPD activity itself, and its subsequent suppression by imipramine, was intrinsically related to the presence of affective disorder. This possibility was subsequently disproved by a study of Giardina et al. (15) in which 17 of 22 cardiac patients with VPDs, but without depression, had more than 75% VPD suppression after imipramine treatment. In this study, imipramine was not only effective in suppressing the total number of VPDs, but of particular importance from the cardiologist's perspective, imipramine was also potent against the complex features. Significant reductions occurred in the frequency of bigeminy ($85 \pm 45\%$), pairs ($89 \pm 30\%$), and ventricular tachycardia ($99 \pm 2\%$).

Preliminary results indicate that nortriptyline is similar to imipramine with respect to antiarrhythmic activity against VPDs, including the complex features (14). It is not clear to what extent other TCAs share imipramine's and nortriptyline's antiarrhythmic activity, though it is likely that many have this property to some extent (39).

The observation that imipramine has a major effect on the initial inward sodium current of the Purkinje fiber (43,45), together with the data from the His bundle studies that demonstrate that TCAs depress conduction velocity (26), gives the TCAs an electrophysiological profile that is characteristic of type 1 antiarrhythmic compounds such as quinidine and procainamide. This electrophysiological profile also extends to desmethylimipramine and the hydroxy metabolites (30,57). In fact, 2-hydroxyimipramine is equipotent to imipramine with respect to slowing conduction

velocity in isolated Purkinje fibers and suppressing ouabain-induced arrhythmias (43,45). These data support the view that the TCAs exert their antiarrhythmic effect, at least in part, by direct action on the heart, although a central mechanism, or the possibility of a combination of direct cardiac and central effects, cannot be ruled out.

In summary, imipramine and nortriptyline, and probably to some extent other TCAs as well, have significant antiarrhythmic activity against VPDs. These drugs share electrophysiological properties characteristic of type 1 antiarrhythmic compounds (23) and, presently, are being used in cardiac patients free from depression for the exclusive purpose of arrhythmia control.

OVERDOSE

The importance of issues involving the cardiovascular effects of TCAs in overdose stems from both the frequency with which tricyclic overdoses occur and the frequency with which those overdoses result in a cardiovascular death. TCA drugs are now the third most common cause of drug-related death, trailing only alcohol-drug combinations and heroin (12). Although it is well known that TCAs can be fatal in overdose, the mechanism by which this occurs, and the most appropriate therapeutic interventions, are far less clear. This lacuna in our knowledge results, in large part, from the difficulty in collecting, systematically studying, and controlling treatment in a reasonable number of overdose cases.

It is clear that all of the standard tricyclics, including doxepin, can be fatal in overdose, and the same is true for the newer nontricyclics, maprotyline and amoxapine. The signs and symptoms frequently seen in TCA overdose include slurred speech, confusion, coma, tachycardia, hypotension, respiratory distress, conduction delays, and seizures. In a recent series of 32 *fatal* TCA ingestions, 14 patients died en route to the hospital, nine were alive on arrival but already had major symptoms, and the remaining nine arrived without major symptoms (10). Subsequently these nine patients developed major symptomatology within 2 hr of arriving, and all deaths from the direct toxicity of the drug occurred within the first 24 hr.

A major clinical problem in TCA overdose is determining when a patient is no longer in danger. Earlier reports had suggested that TCA overdose could produce late sudden fatalities (9). Most of these "late" deaths, however, actually involved patients who died from complication of severe symptoms that had presented earlier and were not actually sudden "late" deaths *de novo* (46,48). It would seem probable that many TCA overdoses have been hospitalized unnecessarily and/or for unnecessarily long periods because of this concern. It appears that if, after 6 hr, a patient has not developed any major symptomatology (depressed level of consciousness, hypotension, depressed respiration, seizures, conduction block, or arrhythmia), it is very unlikely he or she will.

The one principle in TCA overdose about which there is no dispute is that there should be aggressive treatment directed toward removal of drug from the body (8). The contents of the stomach should be removed in any suspected

TCA overdose. Once absorption has occurred, neither hemodialysis, charcoal hemoperfusion, nor peritoneal dialysis has met with much success in reducing drug load. Recently, Swartz and Sherman (49) reported evidence that a slurry of activated charcoal given repeatedly through a nasogastric tube following an initial emptying of the stomach greatly accelerates tricyclic elimination. This would appear to be the result of a large enterohepatic circulation of tricyclic that is interrupted by the repeated charcoal. They suggest that this method would be preferable to aspiration near the ampulla of Vater because it will not produce significant electrolyte abnormalities. This technique would seem encouraging but has been subjected to limited study in actual cases of overdose.

The cardiovascular effects of acute TCA overdose most frequently seen are tachycardia and hypotension. Both occur in over 50% of cases. The hypotension is, at least partially, related to a relative volume depletion. Complete correction of the hypotension, however, does not entirely correct the tachycardia. Recent radionuclide studies have shown that at therapeutic plasma concentrations, TCAs do not impair LVF (21,53). In fact, catheterization studies have shown that in moderately severe overdose, function is not impaired (52). Data, however, are not available from overdose cases that fail to survive. Recently, N. L. Benowitz (personal communication) has described two cases of fatal TCA overdose in which ventricular pacing produced regular ventricular depolarization but minimal cardiac output. This would suggest that at very high concentrations, TCAs might directly impair the myocardium. The most characteristic and serious sequelae of overdose involve disturbances in conduction and repolarization. These are manifested clinically by AV block, intraventricular conduction defects, and prolongation of the QT_c interval.

Heart block and ventricular arrhythmias are regularly a part of fatal overdoses. Malignant ventricular arrhythmias are uncommon in most TCA overdoses (27), but they are likely to be seen in severe cases. Faced with a patient who has taken a TCA overdose and is having ventricular arrhythmias, the emergency room physician might consider treating these arrhythmias with quinidine or other similar antiarrhythmic drugs. Only if the physician realizes that the TCAs themselves are type 1 antiarrhythmic drugs, does the danger of this procedure become apparent. Although systematic studies are not yet available, it would seem most reasonable to treat TCA overdoses that develop arrhythmias as one would quinidine overdoses, i.e., with hypertonic sodium bicarbonate and pacing (35,36). This therapeutic regimen should significantly increase the percentage of patients surviving TCA overdose, or, at least, insure that the treatment will not unintentionally exacerbate the presenting problem.

The literature emphasizes that seizures and arrhythmias are associated with plasma level of TCAs above 1,000 ng/ml (47). Recently, Boehnert and Lovejoy (3) have suggested that QRS duration might be a better predictor of these sequelae than serum levels. They noted that in their series of 49 TCA overdoses, seizures occurred only in cases with a QRS duration above 0.10 sec, and ventricular arrhythmia was seen with a QRS greater than 0.16 sec. Thus, for acute ingestions, the ECG may provide a reliable measure of increased risk with TCA overdose. How well a QRS of less than 0.10 predicts ultimate safety, however, or how long after ingestion the ECG must be followed, remains to be established more firmly.

REFERENCES

1. Avery, D., and Winokur, G. (1976): *Arch. Gen. Psychiatry,* 33: 1029–1037.
2. Bigger, J. T., Jr., Giardina, E. G. V., Perel, J. M., Kantor, S. J., and Glassman, A. H. (1977): *N. Engl. J. Med.,* 296:206–208.
3. Boehnert, M. T., and Lovejoy, F. H., Jr. (1985): *N. Engl. J. Med.,* 313:474–479.
4. Boston Collaborative Drug Surveillance Program (1972): *Lancet,* 1:529–531.
5. Burckhardt, D., Raeder, E., Muller, V., Imhof, P., and Neubauer, H. (1978): *JAMA,* 239:213–216.
6. Burgess, C. D., Turner, P., and Wadsworth, J. (1978): *Br. J. Clin. Pharmacol.,* 5:21s–28s.
7. Burrows, G. D., Vohra, J., Dumovic, P., Maguire, K., Scoggins, B. A., and Davies, B. (1977): *Prog. Neuropsychopharmacol.,* 1: 329–334.
8. Callaham, M. (1979): *JACEP,* 8:413–425.
9. Callaham, M. (1982): *West. J. Med.,* 137:425–429.
10. Callaham, M., and Kassel, D. (1985): *Ann. Emerg. Med.,* 14:1–9.
11. Coull, D. C., Crooks, J., Dingwall-Fordyce, I., Scott, A. M., and Weir, R. D. (1970): *Lancet,* 2:590–591.
12. Department of Health, Education and Welfare (1978): *Facts of Life and Death.* Publication No. (PHS) 79-1222:39–47.
13. Freyschuss, U., Sjoqvist, F., Tuck, D., and Asberg, M. (1970): *Pharmacol. Clin.,* 2:68–71.
14. Giardina, E. G. V., Barnard, T., Johnson, L., Saroff, A. L., Bigger, J. T., Jr., and Louie, M. (1986): *J. Am. Coll. Cardiol.,* 7:1363–1369.
15. Giardina, E. G. V., and Bigger, J. T., Jr. (1982): *Am. J. Cardiol.,* 50:172–179.
16. Giardina, E. G. V., Bigger, J. T., Jr., and Glassman, A. H. (1982): *Clin. Pharmacol. Ther.,* 31:230.
17. Giardina, E. G., Bigger, J. T., Jr., Glassman, A. H., Perel, J. M., and Kantor, S. J. (1979): *Circulation,* 60:1045–1052.
18. Giardina, E. G. V., Johnson, L. L., Vita, J., Bigger, J. T., Jr., and Brem, R. F. (1985): *Am. Heart J.,* 109:992–998.
19. Glassman, A. H., and Bigger, J. T., Jr. (1981): *Arch. Gen. Psychiatry,* 38:815–820.
20. Glassman, A. H., Bigger, J. T., Jr., Giardina, E. V., Kantor, S. J., Perel, J. M., and Davies, M. (1979): *Lancet,* 1:468–471.
21. Glassman, A. H., Johnson, L. L., Giardina, E. G. V., Walsh, B. T., Roose, S. P., Cooper, T. B., and Bigger, J. T., Jr. (1983): *JAMA,* 250:1997–2001.
22. Hayes, J. R., Born, G. F., and Rosenbaum, A. H. (1977): *Mayo Clin. Proc.,* 52:509–512.
23. Hoffman, B. F., and Bigger, J. T., Jr. (1971): In: *Drill's Pharmacology in Medicine,* 4th ed., edited by J. R. DiPalma, pp. 824–852. McGraw-Hill, New York.
24. Kantor, S. J., Bigger, J. T., Jr., Glassman, A. H., Macken, D. L., and Perel, J. M. (1975): *JAMA,* 231:1364–1366.
25. Kantor, S. J., Glassman, A. H., Bigger, J. T., Jr., Perel, J. M., and Giardina, E. V. (1978): *Am. J. Psychiatry,* 135:534–538.
26. Kopera, H. (1978): *Br. J. Clin. Pharmacol.,* 5:29s–34s.
27. Langou, R. A., Van Dyke, C., Tahan, S. R., and Cohen, L. S. (1980): *Am. Heart J.,* 100:458–464.
28. Moir, D. C., Cornwell, W. B., Dingwall-Fordyce, I., Crooks, J., O'Malley, K., Turnbull, M. J., and Weir, R. D. (1972): *Lancet,* 2: 561–564.
29. Moir, D. C., Dingwall-Fordyce, I., and Weir, R. D. (1973): *Eur. J. Clin. Pharmacol.,* 6:98–101.
30. Muir, W. W., Strauch, S. M., and Schaal, S. F. (1982): *J. Cardiovasc. Pharmacol.,* 4:82–90.
31. Muller, O. F., Goodman, N., and Bellet, S. (1961): *Clin. Pharmacol. Ther.,* 2:300–307.
32. Nelson, J. C., Jatlow, P. I., Bock, J., Quinlan, D. M., and Bowers, M. B., Jr. (1982): *Arch. Gen. Psychiatry,* 39:1055–1061.

33. Neshkes, R. E., Gerner, R., Jarvik, L. F., Mintz, J., Joseph, J., Linde, S., Aldrich, J., Conolly, M. E., Rosen, R., and Hill, M. (1985): *J. Clin. Psychopharmacol.*, 5:102–106.

34. Peet, M., Tienari, P., and Jaskari, M. O. (1977): *Pharmakopsychiatr. Neuropsychopharmakol.*, 10:309–312.

35. Pentel, P., and Benowitz, N. (1984): *J. Pharmacol. Exp. Ther.*, 230:12–19.

36. Pentel, P. R., Goldsmith, S. R., Salerno, D. M., Nasraway, S. A., and Plummer, D. W. (1986): *Am. J. Cardiol.*, 57:878–880.

37. Petit, J. M., Spiker, D. G., Ruwitch, J. F., Ziegler, V. E., Weiss, A. N., and Biggs, J. T. (1977): *Clin. Pharmacol. Ther.*, 21:47–51.

38. Raeder, E. A., Burckhardt, D., Neubauer, H., Walter, R., and Gastpar, M. (1978): *Br. Med. J.*, 2:666–667.

39. Raeder, E. A., Zinsli, M., and Burckhardt, D. (1979): *Br. Med. J.*, 2:102.

40. Rawling, D. A., and Fozzard, H. A. (1979): *J. Pharmacol. Exp. Ther.*, 209:371–375.

41. Roose, S. P., Glassman, A. H., Giardina, E. G. V., Johnson, L. L., Walsh, B. T., and Bigger, J. T., Jr. (1987): *J. Clin. Psychopharm.* (in press).

42. Roose, S. P., Glassman, A. H., Giardina, E. G. V., Johnson, L. L., Walsh, B. T., Woodring, S., and Bigger, J. T., Jr. (1986): *JAMA*, 256:3253–3257.

43. Roose, S. P., Glassman, A. H., Giardina, E. G. V., Walsh, B. T., Woodring, S., and Bigger, J. T., Jr. (1987): *Arch. Gen. Psychiatry*, 44:273–275.

44. Roose, S. P., Glassman, A. H., Siris, S. G., and Bruno, R. L. (1980): Presented at American Psychiatric Association, San Francisco.

45. Roose, S. P., Glassman, A. H., Siris, S. G., Walsh, B. T., Bruno, R. L., and Wright, L. B. (1981): *J. Clin. Psychopharmacol.*, 1: 316–319.

46. Sedal, L., Korman, M. G., Williams, P. O., and Mushin, G. (1972): *Med. J. Aust.*, 2:74–79.

47. Spiker, D. G., Weiss, A. N., Chang, S. S., Ruwitch, J. F., and Biggs, J. T. (1975): *Clin. Pharmacol. Ther.*, 18:539–546.

48. Sunshine, P., and Yaffe, S. J. (1963): *Am. J. Dis. Child.*, 106:501–506.

49. Swartz, C. M., and Sherman, A. (1984): *J. Clin. Psychopharmacol.*, 4:336–340.

50. Taylor, D. J., and Braithwaite, R. A. (1978): *Br. Heart J.*, 40: 1005–1009.

51. Thayssen, P., Bjerre, M., Kragh-Sorensen, P., Moller, M., Petersen, O. L., Kristensen, C. B., and Gram, L. F. (1981): *Psychopharmacology*, 74:360–364.

52. Thorstrand, C. (1974): *Acta Med. Scand.*, 195:505–514.

53. Veith, R. C., Raskind, M. A., Caldwell, J. H., Barnes, R. F., Gumbrecht, G., and Ritchie, J. L. (1982): *N. Engl. J. Med.*, 306: 954–959.

54. Vohra, J., Burrows, G. D., Hunt, D., and Sloman, G. (1975): *Eur. J. Cardiol.*, 3:219–227.

55. Vohra, J., Burrows, G. D., and Sloman, G. (1975): *Aust. NZ J. Med.*, 5:7–11.

56. Weld, F. M., and Bigger, J. T., Jr. (1980): *Circ. Res.*, 46:167–175.

57. Wilkerson, R. D. (1978): *J. Pharmacol. Exp. Ther.*, 205:666–674.

58. Williams, R. B., Jr., and Sherter, C. (1971): *Ann. Intern. Med.*, 74:395–398.

59. Ziegler, V. E., Co, B. T., and Biggs, J. T. (1977): *Dis. Nerv. Syst.*, 38:697–699.

60. Ziegler, V. E., Co, B. T., and Biggs, J. T. (1977): *Am. J. Psychiatry*, 134:441–443.

Psychopharmacology:
The Third Generation of Progress,
edited by Herbert Y. Meltzer.
Raven Press, New York © 1987.

CHAPTER **152**

Renal and Other Controversial Adverse Effects of Lithium

Erling T. Mellerup, Per Plenge, and Ole J. Rafaelsen

For almost 40 years lithium has been established as a psychotropic agent with antimanic properties. Even more important, it has been generally accepted and widely used as a prophylactic treatment against affective episodes for more than 20 years. In the last 10 years, however, there has been widespread concern regarding the adverse effects of lithium treatment, especially the renal side effects.

During all these years numerous experimental and clinical studies have addressed most aspects of lithium biology and pharmacology. It is obvious, however, that despite the extensive research it is still unknown how lithium exerts its psychotropic effects. The same is also true for other psychopharmacological medications, although for some of them, e.g., neuroleptics and benzodiazepines, the research has concentrated on specific receptors that seem to be of central importance. In contrast, lithium has more effects than most other drugs, and it has been impossible to single out any of these that are decisively related to its relapse-preventing action. This situation is probably attributable to the fact that lithium on a molecular level interferes with sodium, potassium, magnesium, and calcium at many functional macromolecules, thereby producing numerous biochemical effects, which then are integrated into the physiological and behavioral effects of lithium.

Besides the studies of basic mechanisms involved in the action of lithium, much work has been done in the fields of lithium administration and lithium side effects. Because lithium therapy is mainly prophylactic, the administration period is very long, extending from years to the rest of the patient's life. This means that even minor side effects may grow into major problems, possibly leading to discontinuation of lithium treatment. In a study by Bech and co-workers (5), side effects were the main reason for discontinuation of lithium treatment more often than insufficient effect on mood stabilization.

Lithium therapy of manic-depressive patients is accompanied by many different effects, among which only the relapse-preventive effect is wanted. Most of the other effects are completely unnoticed by the patients, although many of these biochemical effects form the basis for the disturbing and inconvenient side effects. Some of the most common side effects are renal impairment, tremor, weight gain, gastrointestinal symptoms, and thyroid hyperplasia, but many others have been described (73). The mechanisms behind these side effects are largely unknown, although suggestions and hypotheses exist that may be more substantiated than hypotheses about the psychotropic effect.

Irrespective of the mechanisms, it has been necessary to design lithium treatment procedures that take these side effects into consideration. Adjunctive treatment is used to counteract the tremor, where β-blockers like propranolol are given. To compensate for the hypothyroidism, thyroxine is used, and thiazide diuretics (20) and amiloride (4) may be used to reduce excessive urine output. Weight gain can be controlled by slimming diets. Otherwise side effects are avoided by reducing the lithium intake.

A reduction in lithium dosage has primarily been advocated by those concerned about the renal side effects, and the reduction can take place in two ways. Either the amount of lithium in each dose is reduced and the number of doses remains unchanged, or the amount of lithium in a single dose is unchanged or increased, but the number of doses is reduced. The difference between these two treatment strategies is in principle the same as the difference between a treatment regimen with two or three daily doses of lithium and a once-daily dose regimen. There are controversies about how severe and extensive the renal side effects are, and about whether the two different treatment schedules affect the kidneys differently.

RENAL DISTURBANCES

The polyuria-polydipsia syndrome is the most common and most investigated side effect in lithium-treated patients, occurring in about 60%. It has been recognized from the start of lithium use, and was considered a purely functional and thus reversible side effect. In 1977, however, it was found that a small number of lithium-treated patients—all having suffered episodes of lithium intoxication—showed various morphological changes in their kidneys (17,18). These reports caused considerable concern among psychiatrists, as well as patients and led to numerous studies of kidney function in lithium-treated patients. The methods used to assess the lithium effects have been pathological-anatomical investigations of kidney biopsies, analysis of urine osmolality, serum creatinine, clearances of various substances, glomerular filtration rate, and measurement of urine volume.

Structural Changes

The biopsy studies vary with respect to the selection of patients and controls and also with respect to the variables analyzed. Generally, more lesions will be found in patients with a history of lithium intoxication, severe polyuria, or signs of reduced kidney function (3,17,18). When unselected lithium-treated patients are studied, the proportion with pathological renal changes is reduced to about 10% (10,25,56).

The types of renal lesions noticed by different workers are also important in determining the incidence of pathological changes. In the previously mentioned studies, the lesions found were interstitial fibrosis, tubular atrophy, and glomerular sclerosis; however, when less severe lesions, directly related to primary biochemical effects of lithium, are added to this list more patients will be included in the pathological group. Thus Walker and his co-workers (76) noted, among other changes, accumulation of glycogen granules in the cells of the distal tubules and collecting ducts, and this change could be found in all lithium-treated patients, including some who had received lithium for 5 days only. This finding is in agreement with the lithium-induced increase in glycogen synthesis known from other cell types (39). If the glycogen accumulation and the associated changes in carbohydrate metabolism form the biochemical basis for the more pronounced structural and functional changes, these changes should be present in all lithium-treated patients. The fact that only some of the patients show such side effects indicates that other mechanisms are involved in the formation of lesions or that regenerative processes may occur in varying degrees in individual patients.

Pathological renal changes similar to those seen in lithium-treated patients have been observed in lithium-treated animals, using toxic (59,81) as well as low doses of lithium (15,28,51).

Changes in Tubular Function

The functional kidney changes in lithium-treated patients have been studied much more than the structural changes. The most common finding has been a decreased tubular function with respect to water-conserving ability. Almost all studies have found that lithium reduced urine-concentrating ability after a period of thirst or administration of antidiuretic hormone or both.

The maximum urine osmolality measured in lithium patients may be compared with the usual control groups or with manic-depressive patients not treated with lithium. When no control group is available the patient's urine-concentrating ability may be compared with the normal range, where the cutoff point usually is chosen as 800 mOsm/kg H_2O. The mean values for the lithium-treated patients have been below this value in most studies (13,19,24,25,65,72,74,77). The proportion of patients with a maximum urine osmolality below 800 mOsm/kg H_2O varies in the different studies between 30 and 90%. In the reports of Coppen and co-workers (13) and Hullin and co-workers (21), the maximum urine osmolality in the lithium-treated patients was not significantly lower than in the control groups of psychiatric patients not on lithium, but all groups were below the threshold of 800 mOsm/kg H_2O. In other studies the maximum urine osmolality in the lithium-treated patients was lower than in the manic-depressive control group, and this group was lower than the normal control group (72,74). These studies indicate that the reduced urine-concentrating ability in the lithium-treated patients may be attributed in part to other factors associated with affective illness.

Some studies also found that the urine osmolality decreased with increasing total intake of lithium (32,77), with duration of treatment (13,19a,24,25,72,78), and serum lithium level (65,72).

Urine volume and urine osmolality are normally not correlated, as the effect on urine volume of fluid intake, salt intake, and glomerular filtration may be more important than the maximal urine-concentrating ability. With a pathological or drug-induced decrease in urine-concentrating ability, however, it is obvious that urine volume will increase. Accordingly, some studies have reported that urine volume and urine osmolality are correlated in lithium-treated patients (8,10,13,78).

Changes in Glomerular Function

Glomerular filtration rate has been studied by analysis of the clearance of various substances, mostly creatinine and a chelate of 51Cr with ethylene diamine tetraacetic acid (51Cr-EDTA). The glomerular function in lithium-treated patients is much less affected than the tubular function; and, in particular, the number of patients with reduced filtration rate is low compared with the number of patients showing reduced concentration ability. In one study none of the patients had glomerular filtration rates below normal (14); however, the mean treatment time for these patients was only about 3 years. In two studies where the mean treatment periods were 7 and 8 years, 10% of the patients had a decrease in glomerular filtration rate, although no correlation between filtration rate and duration of lithium treatment was found (19,25). In patients who had a mean treatment time of 10 years, 19% showed a glomerular filtration rate below the 95% confidence limits of the control group, and there was a significant negative correlation between filtration rate and time on lithium (32). Bendz (7) reviewed a large number of these studies and concluded that the reduction in glomerular filtration rate probably is secondary to the reduction in tubular function.

The Mechanism

The exact cellular mechanisms producing the functional and structural changes in the kidney remain to be clarified, but some experimental studies have demonstrated lithium effects that may be pertinent with respect to the functional changes. First, lithium inhibits the effect of vasopressin in the kidney, partly by direct inhibition of the hormone-stimulated activity of the adenylate cyclase (11,16). Second, lithium may decrease concentrating ability because of effects on plasma and kidney urea concentration. It is known that low concentrations of urea generally reduce urinary concentrating ability (47). Urea enhances urinary concentration by the creation in the kidney of a steep corticopapillary gradient of urea that osmotically extracts water into the medullary interstitium (22,29). In lithium-treated rats this corticopapillary gradient of urea is greatly reduced because of a decrease in plasma urea concentration (11). As plasma urea in lithium-treated patients (36) is reduced to the same degree as in lithium-treated rats, the proposed mechanism may come into play, hereby explaining the vasopressin-resistant polyuria.

The structural changes may not be explained by these lithium effects, but as lithium has numerous other effects, particularly on energy metabolism, it may be possible that, for example, the glycogen accumulation in the tubular cells (76) is a parallel phenomenon not directly related to the lithium effects of water handling in the kidneys.

Treatment Schedule

Although the precise mechanisms that produce the renal changes still remain to be clarified, it has been suggested that the peak lithium concentration might be a risk factor after lithium intake. The arguments for his idea were based on knowledge of the toxic effects of lithium, which may start to appear at serum lithium concentrations around 2 mmol/liter. Accordingly, it has been concluded that high peak concentrations of lithium should be avoided, and this could be accomplished by giving multiple doses of slow-release lithium preparations.

Although it is true that high lithium concentrations in the body produce toxic effects, it may not be true that side effects can be avoided by giving two or three daily doses. The price paid for a treatment procedure that avoids high peak concentration is that the minimum lithium concentration in the body will be relatively high. Patients who

receive two or three daily doses may obtain very moderate peak lithium concentrations, but they may never obtain lower concentrations than the 12-hr post-absorption value, at which time they take a further lithium dose. Patients who receive one daily lithium dose may reach higher peak concentrations (30), but they may also obtain very low minimum lithium concentrations; more important, they will have low serum lithium concentrations for many hours each day.

The difference between one daily dose of lithium and multiple doses has been studied especially with regard to lithium-induced polyuria. In an animal study two groups of rats received the same amount of lithium each day. One group was injected intraperitoneally once a day, leading to very high serum lithium peak concentrations, but also very low concentrations before the next injection. The other group received lithium in the food, leading to relatively constant serum concentrations between 0.6 and 0.9 mmol/liter. After 15 days of treatment, polyuria became much more pronounced in the lithium-fed rats than in the lithium-injected rats, and this difference persisted throughout the study. After 5 months of treatment, kidney morphology was studied, and it was found that structural changes, such as fibrosis and tubular atrophy, were more severe in the rats with constant serum lithium than in rats with both high and low serum lithium concentrations (51).

In some clinical studies patients receiving one daily dose of lithium were compared with patients receiving two or three daily doses. Each of these studies showed that one daily dose was associated with significantly lower diuresis (19,32,50,61). In one of these studies renal biopsies showed that 5% of the one daily dose patients had sclerotic glomeruli, fibrosis, or atrophic tubuli, whereas 13% of the multiple-dose patients had these changes (19b,50).

Thus all these studies indicate that renal function was less affected in organisms receiving lithium once a day compared with more frequent intake. As the one daily administration was associated with higher peak serum concentrations of lithium, the advantage of this treatment regimen may be related to the long periods each day with very low lithium concentrations. In other words, low diuresis may be correlated with low serum lithium minimum concentrations.

This hypothesis was tested in a study of 65 lithium-treated patients in whom serum lithium concentrations were determined over a 24-hr period in which urine collection also took place. Multiple linear regression was performed with urine volume as the independent variable and lithium dose, peak serum lithium concentration, 12-hr serum lithium, minimum serum lithium, length of treatment, and age of patients as the dependent variables. Only minimum serum lithium and urine volume showed a significant positive correlation, whereas the peak concentration of lithium correlated poorly to urine volume (35).

The importance of a low minimum serum lithium concentration may be that regenerative processes in the kidney are very lithium sensitive, and thus preferentially occur in periods with low lithium concentrations. Another explanation may be that some lithium-induced metabolic changes return to normal in periods with low lithium concentrations, but become permanent without these periods. Such persistent metabolic changes may then form the basis for progressive pathological changes.

OTHER SIDE EFFECTS

Tremor is another common side effect seen in approximately 40% of lithium-treated patients. The mechanism that produces the tremor is unknown; it may be caused by lithium interaction with other cations important for nerve and muscle cell excitability, or it may be because of lithium effects on, e.g., peripheral or central β-adrenergic receptors. The tremor can be reduced by administration of propranolol or other β-blocking drugs (26). In the first days of lithium treatment most patients may have an exaggerated physiological tremor that declines after 1 to 2 weeks (55). The tremor seen in long-term lithium-treated patients may be similar to a physiological tremor (23), or it may be more like a parkinsonian tremor because it has also been reported that the peak tremor frequency is decreased in some of these patients (64).

The relationship between tremor and lithium has been studied by Persson (45). He found that high doses and high concentrations of lithium were associated with tremor, but also a dose-independent steep gradient in the serum lithium concentration after intake was positively correlated with tremor. In agreement with these findings, it has been found that slow-release lithium preparations can reduce the tremor (34). It has also been suggested to give a lower dose of lithium in the morning in order to reduce the gradient of serum lithium, thereby reducing the tremor during the day (60). In our clinic the morning dose of lithium was discontinued, and only one dose, taken just before bedtime, was given. In this way the steep gradient in serum lithium occurred during sleep, and no new gradient occurred in the daytime. As tremor normally is absent during sleep (23) or does not interfere with sleep as such, it seems of minor importance—in this respect—that one daily dose of lithium gives rise to a steeper gradient in serum lithium than divided doses. Another factor that also may contribute to a reduction in tremor is that the once daily evening dose should be less than the sum of divided doses to produce the same 12-hr serum lithium concentration. This is because of the lower lithium clearance during sleep (30).

Thus by giving lithium in one daily dose in the evening, it seems possible to reduce the inconveniences of tremor occurring in relation to the temporarily elevated serum lithium. Whether this treatment regimen also is able to influence the shift in peak tremor frequency seen after long-term lithium therapy has not been studied.

Weight gain is a relatively common side effect seen in approximately 30% of lithium-treated patients. The percentage of patients with weight gain, however, varies considerably from study to study. Values from 4% (68) to 60% of the patients (71) are reported, probably reflecting demographic variability in diet and body weight.

The weight gain in lithium-treated patients has been regarded as an adjustment to the weight these patients might have reached had they not been ill (27). Such patients, however, do not deviate with respect to prelithium body weight compared with normal controls; furthermore postlithium body weight in relation to ideal weight is

increased more in these patients than in control persons (38,46). The weight gain is not a combined effect of lithium and affective disease, since lithium-treated rats increase their body weight above control animals (6,42,48,52).

The mechanism producing the lithium-induced weight gain is unknown, but several explanations have been suggested. The weight gain may simply be a result of a lithium-induced increase in appetite leading to a higher food intake (42); or the increased thirst of the polyuria may be satisfied by beverages rich in calories (71). In addition to these indirect lithium effects, it is also known that lithium influences energy metabolism in numerous ways. Glucose transport is increased by lithium (12); various enzymes involved in glycogen synthesis and glycolysis are influenced by lithium (39); and glucose tolerance and insulin secretion are also influenced by lithium (33,69). Recently blood glucose was found to be slightly elevated in euthymic lithium-treated patients (37).

All these metabolic effects possibly occur in all lithium-treated patients, but only the susceptible patients, e.g., those with high numbers of fat cells, develop a weight gain (70). Renal disturbances, tremor, and weight gain are probably the most common side effects associated with lithium treatment, but numerous other side effects are known.

Gastrointestinal discomfort with nausea and abdominal pain are side effects clearly related to the intake of lithium (45). The immediacy of these side effects can be reduced by the use of slow release tablets, but the symptoms may appear later after the intake (1).

During the early years of lithium treatment it was observed that lithium influenced the thyroid gland (62). The lithium effects may vary from subtle changes in biochemical variables to goiter or hypothyroidism; cases with hyperthyroidism have also been reported (2,40,63).

In a number of patients cutaneous reactions to lithium treatment have been reported. Lithium may aggravate the disease in patients suffering from psoriasis, but the disease may also develop for the first time subsequent to lithium therapy. Acne and several other dermatoses may also appear after the start of lithium treatment (57).

Electrocardiogram (ECG) changes with T-wave depression can occur during lithium treatment (67). Although such changes are considered benign and reversible, there have been some reports of serious sinus bradycardia associated with lithium therapy (41,43,80).

All these side effects are disturbing to the patients, whereas other types of side effects are not noticed by the patient, and are revealed only by laboratory analyses. They are of concern to the psychiatrist, however, because of possible potential risk. Among such side effects are the leukocytosis and lymphopenia often reported in lithium-treated patients (44,67,75) and the accumulation of calcium and phosphate in the body during lithium treatment (53).

None of these other side effects have been studied with respect to differences between several daily doses or one daily dose of lithium. It could be expected that the gastrointestinal symptoms would be particularly disturbing when all the lithium is taken in a single dose; however, it seems that the discomfort, if noticed by the patient at all, is not strong enough to disturb the sleep.

CONCLUSION AND SUMMARY

Administration of lithium will always be followed by numerous biochemical changes that can be measured as enzyme inhibition or activation or as changes in concentration of various metabolites and electrolytes. The number and intensity of the biochemical changes will increase with increasing amounts of lithium in the body. Homeostatic mechanisms may counteract the lithium-induced changes, however, and biochemical deviations can often be more pronounced during periods with changing lithium concentrations than during periods with relatively constant lithium concentrations (48,49).

The side effects as well as the psychotropic effects are probably integrated phenomena, each depending on several direct lithium effects, on the status of the metabolic machinery, and on the quality of the homeostatic mechanisms. Regenerative or repair processes may also be important because they may counteract slowly accumulating pathological changes caused by the daily effects of lithium on the biochemistry of sensitive cells. The individual biological factors may explain why the various side effects are not seen in all lithium treated patients, and also why the side effects may vary in the course of lithium treatment.

In patients with severe side effects, secondary treatment can be used for a few of the side effects, but the most important treatment is to reduce the lithium dose. Normally, this is accomplished by reducing the amount of lithium in each dose. This procedure may, however, increase the number of relapses (54,66,79). We have recommended an alternative strategy viz to reduce lithium intake to one daily dose at bedtime.

Experimental and clinical studies indicate that one daily dose is associated with lower diuresis and fewer renal changes than two or three daily doses. The explanation for this finding may be that the very low lithium concentration for many hours each day allows regenerative processes to occur to a higher degree than in those patients who, with two or three doses of lithium, never have serum lithium concentrations lower than the 12-hr value.

Whether other side effects or the psychotropic effect of lithium depends on the number of daily doses has not been thoroughly studied. It is noteworthy that, despite the many years of lithium maintenance or prophylactic use, three pertinent questions remain unanswered. First, we do not know when the minimum threshold of lithium concentration should be reached in order to produce the psychotropic effect. Second, it is not known how long the lithium concentration should remain at this threshold. Third, it is not known how often this threshold should be reached.

The answer to the first question probably varies from patient to patient. Some may avoid relapses with relatively low lithium concentrations. Others may need lithium concentrations above the tolerable level, and accordingly such patients will be nonresponders. The second and third questions cannot be answered, but at least it is known that the necessary prophylactic concentration does not have to be kept constant, since the patients receiving one daily dose have serum lithium concentrations below this value for many hours each day.

The various lithium treatment schedules applied by researchers and clinicians have given new insight into the advantages and disadvantages of continuous or discontinuous administration of a psychopharmacologically active drug, and thus helped to produce a general understanding of these problems, which are also encountered in antibiotic therapy (9) and evidently are important for the understanding of the impact of alcoholism on the liver (31). Lithium has proved to be an interesting research tool, and results obtained will help to open new vistas of pharmacokinetics and pharmacodynamics of general importance in psychopharmacology as well as in other therapeutic fields.

REFERENCES

1. Amdisen, A. (1975): In: *Lithium Research and Therapy,* edited by F. N. Johnson, pp. 197–210. Academic Press, London.
2. Amdisen, A., and Andersen, C. J. (1982): *Pharmacopsychiatria,* 15:149–155.
3. Aurell, M., Svalander, C., Wallin, L., and Alling, C. (1981): *Kidney Int.,* 20:663–670.
4. Battle, D. C., von Riotte, A. B., Gaviria, M., and Grupp, M. (1985): *N. Engl. J. Med.,* 312:408–414.
5. Bech, P., Vendsborg, P., and Rafaelsen, O. J. (1976): *Acta Psychiatr. Scand.,* 53:70–81.
6. Bellwinkel, S., Schafer, A., Minne, H., and Ziegler, R. (1975): *Int. Pharmacopsychiatry,* 10:9–16.
7. Bendz, H. (1983): *Acta Psychiatr. Scand.,* 68:303–324.
8. Bendz, H., Andersch, S., and Aurell, M. (1983): *Acta Psychiatr. Scand.,* 68:325–334.
9. Bennett, W. M., Plamp, C. E., Gilbert, D. N., Parker, R. A., and Porter, G. A. (1979): *J. Infect. Dis.,* 140:576–580.
10. Bucht, G., and Wahlin, A. (1980): *Acta Med. Scand.,* 207:309–314.
11. Christensen, S., Kusano, E., Yusufi, A. N. K., Murayama, N., and Dousa, T. P. (1985): *J. Clin. Invest.,* 75:1869–1879.
12. Clausen, T. (1968): *Biochim. Biophys. Acta,* 150:66–72.
13. Coppen, A., Bishop, M. E., Bailey, J. E., Cattell, W. R., and Price, R. G. (1980): *Acta Psychiatr. Scand.,* 62:343–355.
14. Donker, A. J. M., Prins, E., Meijer, S., Sluiter, W. J., van Berkestijn, J. W. B. M., and Dols, L. C. W. (1979): *Clin. Nephrol.,* 12:254–262.
15. Evan, A. P., and Ollerich, D. A. (1972): *Am. J. Anat.,* 134:97–106.
16. Forrest, J. N., Jr., Cohen, A. D., Torretti, J., Himmelhoch, J. M., and Epstein, F. H. (1974): *J. Clin. Invest.,* 53:1115–1123.
17. Hansen, H. E., Hestbech, J., Olsen, S., and Amdisen, A. (1977): *Proc. Eur. Dial. Transplant. Assoc.,* 14:518–527.
18. Hestbech, J., Hansen, H. E., Amdisen, A., and Olsen, S. (1977): *Kidney Int.,* 12:205–213.
19. Hetmar, O., Bolwig, T. G., Brun, C., Ladefoged, J., Larsen, S., and Rafaelsen, O. J. (1986): *Acta Psychiatr. Scand.,* 73:574–581.
19a. Hetmar, O., Clemmesen, L., Ladefoged, J., Larsen, S., and Rafaelsen, O. J. (1987): *Acta Psychiatr. Scand. (in press).*
19b. Hetmar, O., Brun, C., Clemmesen, L., Ladefoged, J., Larsen, S., and Rafaelsen, O. J. (1987): *Acta Psychiatr. Scand. (in press).*
20. Himmelhoch, J. M., Forrest, J., Neil, J. F., and Detre, T. P. (1977): *Am. J. Psychiatry,* 134:149–152.
21. Hullin, R. P., Coley, V. P., Birch, N. J., Thomas, T. H., and Morgan, D. B. (1979): *Br. Med. J.,* 1:1457–1459.
22. Jamison, R. L., and Oliver, R. E. (1982): *Am. J. Med.,* 72:308–321.
23. Jankovic, J., and Fahn, S. (1980): *Ann. Intern. Med.,* 93:460–465.
24. Johnson, G. F. S., Hunt, G. E., Duggin, G. G., Horvath, J. S., and Tiller, D. J. (1984): *J. Affective Disord.,* 6:249–263.
25. Jørgensen, F., Larsen, S., Spanager, B., Clausen, E., Tangø, M., Brinch, E., and Brun, C. (1984): *Acta Psychiatr. Scand.,* 70:455–462.
26. Kellet, J. M., Metcalfe, M., Bailey, J., and Coppen, A. J. (1975): *J. Neurol. Neurosurg. Psychiatry,* 38:719–721.
27. Kerry, R. J., Liebling, L. I., and Owen, G. (1970): *Acta Psychiatr. Scand.,* 46:238–243.

28. Kling, M. A., Fox, J. G., Johnston, S. M., Tolkoff-Rubin, N. E., Rubin, R. H., and Colvin, R. B. (1984): *Lab. Invest.,* 50:526–535.
29. Kokko, J. P., and Rector, F. C., Jr. (1972): *Kidney Int.,* 2:214–223.
30. Lauritsen, B. J., Mellerup, E. T., Plenge, P., Rasmussen, S., Vestergaard, P., and Schou, M. (1981): *Acta Psychiatr. Scand.,* 64:314–319.
31. Lelbach, W. K. (1974): In: *Recent Advances in Alcohol and Drug Problems, Vol. 1,* edited by R. J. Gibbins, Y. Israel, H. Kalant, R. E. Popham, W. Smidt, and R. G. Smart, pp. 142–145. John Wiley and Son, New York.
32. Løkkegaard, H., Andersen, N. F., Henriksen, E., Barteis, P. D., Brahm, M., Baastrup, P. C., Jørgensen, H. E., Larsen, M., Munck, O., Rasmussen, K., and Schrøder, H. (1985): *Acta Psychiatr. Scand.,* 71:347–355.
33. Malaisse, W. J., Mailaisse-Lagae, F., and Brisson, G. (1971): *Horm. Metab. Res.,* 3:65–70.
34. Matussek, N., and Hessling, P. V. (1971): *Nervenarzt,* 42:376–378.
35. Mellerup, E. T., Dam, H., Plenge, P., Widding, A., and Rafaelsen, O. J. (1985): *Psychiatry Res.,* 14:309–313.
36. Mellerup, E. T., Dam, H., Wildschiødtz, G., and Rafaelsen, O. J. (1979): *Acta Psychiatr. Scand.,* 60:177–184.
37. Mellerup, E. T., Dam, H., Wildschiødtz, G., and Rafaelsen, O. J. (1983): *J. Affective Disord.,* 5:341–347.
38. Mellerup, E. T., Grønlund Thomsen, H., Bjørum, N., and Rafaelsen, O. J. (1972): *Acta Psychiatr. Scand.,* 48:332–336.
39. Mellerup, E. T., and Rafaelsen, O. J. (1975): In: *Lithium Research and Therapy,* edited by F. N. Johnson, pp. 381–388. Academic Press, London.
40. Mellerup, E. T., Vendsborg, P. B., and Rafaelsen, O. J. (1982): In: *Psychiatry and Endocrinology,* edited by P. J. V. Beumont and G. D. Burrows, pp. 305–324. Elsevier Biomedical Press, Amsterdam.
41. Montalescot, G., Levy, Y., and Yes Hatt, P. (1984): *Int. J. Cardiology,* 5:94–96.
42. Opitz, K., and Schafer, G. (1976): *Int. Pharmacopsychiatry,* 11:197–205.
43. Palileo, E. V., Coelho, A., Westveer, D., Dhingra, R., and Rosen, K. M. (1983): *Am. Heart J.,* 106:1443.
44. Perez-Cruet, J., Dancey, J. T., and Waite, J. (1978): In: *Lithium in Medical Practice,* edited by F. N. Johnson, pp. 271–277.
45. Persson, G. (1977): *Acta Psychiatr. Scand.,* 55:208–213.
46. Peselow, E. D., Dunner, D. L., Fieve, R. R., and Lautin, A. (1980): *J. Affective Disord.,* 2:303–310.
47. Pitts, R. F. (1969): In: *Physiology of the Kidney and Body Fluids,* pp. 94–128. Yearbook Medical Publishers Inc., Chicago.
48. Plenge, P. (1978): *Psychopharmacology,* 58:317–322.
49. Plenge, P. (1982): *Psychopharmacology,* 77:348–355.
50. Plenge, P., Mellerup, E. T., Bolwig, T. G., Brun, C., Hetmar, O., Ladefoged, J., Larsen, S., and Rafaelsen, O. J. (1982): *Acta Psychiatr. Scand.,* 66:121–128.
51. Plenge, P., Mellerup, E. T., and Nørgaard, T. (1981): *Acta Psychiatr. Scand.,* 63:303–313.
52. Plenge, P. K., Mellerup, E. T., and Rafaelsen, O. J. (1973): *Int. Pharmacopsychiatry,* 8:234–238.
53. Plenge, P., and Rafaelsen, O. J. (1982): *Acta Psychiatr. Scand.,* 66:361–373.
54. Prien, R. F., and Caffey, E. M. (1976): *Am. J. Psychiatry,* 133:567–570.
55. Pullinger, S., and Tyrer, P. (1983): *Br. J. Psychiatry,* 143:40–41.
56. Rafaelsen, O. J., Bolwig, T. G., Ladefoged, J., and Brun, C. (1979): *Excerpta Medica,* 578–583, series 478.
57. Sarantidis, D., and Waters, B. (1983): *Br. J. Psychiatry,* 143:42–50.
58. Sashidharan, S. P., and McGuire, R. J. (1983): *Acta Psychiatr. Scand.,* 68:126–133.
59. Schou, M. (1958): *Acta Pharmacol. Toxicol.,* 15:70–84.
60. Schou, M. (1974): *Nervenartz,* 45:408–413.
61. Schou, M., Amdisen, A., Thomsen, K., Vestergaard, P., Hetmar, O., Mellerup, E. T., Plenge, P., and Rafaelsen, O. J. (1982): *Psychopharmacology,* 77:387–390.
62. Schou, M., Amdisen, A., Eskjaer Jensen, S., and Olsen, T. (1968): *Br. Med. J.,* 3:710–713.
63. Smigan, L., Wahlin, A., Jacobsson, L., and von Knorring, L. (1984): *Neuropsychobiology,* 11:39–43.
64. Tyrer, P., Lee, I., and Trotter, C. (1981): *Br. J. Psychiatry,* 139:59–61.
65. Tyrer, S. P., Schacht, R. G., McCarthy, J., Menard, K. N., Leong, S., and Shopsin, B. (1983): *Psychol. Med.,* 13:61–69.
66. Tyrer, S. P., Shopsin, B., and Aronson, M. (1983): *Br. J. Psychiatry,* 142:427.
67. Vacaflor, L. (1975): In: *Lithium Research and Therapy,* edited by F. N. Johnson, pp. 211–225. Academic Press, London.
68. Vecchio, M. del, Maj, M., and Kemali, D. (1980): In: *The Prediction of Lithium Response,* edited by A. H. Dufour, D. Pringuey, and T. Milech, pp. 75–82. Marseille.
69. Vendsborg, P. B. (1979): *Acta Psychiatr. Scand.,* 59:306–316.
70. Vendsborg, P. B., Bach-Mortensen, N., and Rafaelsen, O. J. (1976): *Acta Psychiatr. Scand.,* 53:355–359.
71. Vendsborg, P. B., Bech, P., and Rafaelsen, O. J. (1976): *Acta Psychiatr. Scand.,* 53:139–147.
72. Vestergaard, P., and Amdisen, A. (1981): *Acta Psychiatr. Scand.,* 63:333–345.
73. Vestergaard, P. (1983): *Acta Psychiatr. Scand.,* 67(Suppl. 305):33.
74. Wahlin, A., Bucht, G., von Knorring, L., and Smigan, L. (1980): *Int. Pharmacopsychiatry,* 15:253–259.
75. Wahlin, A., von Knorring, L., and Roos, G. (1984): *Neuropsychobiology,* 11:243–246.
76. Walker, R. G., Dowling, J. P., Alcorn, D., Ryan, G. B., and Kincaid-Smith, P. (1983): *Pathology,* 15:403–411.
77. Waller, D. G., Guy Edwards, J., Naik, R., and Polak, A. (1984): *Q. J. Med.,* 211:369–379.
78. Wallin, L., Alling, C., and Aurell, M. (1982): *Clin. Nephrol.,* 18:23–28.
79. Waters, B., Lapierre, Y., and Gagnon, A. (1982): *Biol. Psychiatry,* 17:1323–1329.
80. Weintraub, M., Hes, H. P., Rotmensch, H. H., Soferman, G., and Liron, M. (1983): *Isr. J. Med. Sci.,* 19:353–355.
81. Yavorskii, A. N., Goryanov, O. A., Rychko, A. V., and Samoilov, N. N. (1976): *Bull. Exp. Biol. Med.,* 82:1780–1782.

Psychopharmacology:
The Third Generation of Progress,
edited by Herbert Y. Meltzer.
Raven Press, New York © 1987.

CHAPTER **153**

Cognitive Impairment and Benzodiazepines

Joy L. Taylor and Jared R. Tinklenberg

The most common side effect of the benzodiazepines is excessive CNS depression, which is subjectively reported as drowsiness, dizziness, fatigue, light-headedness, and incoordination (29,70). These symptoms of benzodiazepine-induced CNS depression are frequently associated with the objective indications of memory deficits and impairments in performance. This chapter provides an update on what is known about the cognitive side effects of the benzodiazepines.

COGNITIVE SIDE EFFECTS ASSOCIATED WITH THE INITIAL ADMINISTRATION OF BENZODIAZEPINES

In clinically effective oral doses, the initial administration of benzodiazepines generally induces a wide array of cognitive impairments. The various benzodiazepines in common clinical practice appear to have qualitatively similar effects on memory and performance (28,47,57). The main quantitative differences are in the onset and duration of effects.

Effects of Benzodiazepines on Learning and Memory

One of the most pronounced cognitive effects of the benzodiazepines is impaired ability to learn new information. Acquisition of both verbal and visual information can be impaired (2,15,17,19,20,22–25,34,38,42,47,49,57,58, 67,71,73,77–79,85,92) by as much as 66% (35). This reduction in ability to learn is most marked in the first hour or two after drug ingestion for diazepam and in the third or fourth hour for lorazepam (15). The time required for recovery from this impairment depends on the specific benzodiazepine, the dose, and the sensitivity of the cognitive testing, but can be as long as 6 hr (20). It should be noted that since patients may not be aware that their memory is impaired (35), they should be explicitly warned of this possibility.

The benzodiazepines usually do not impair retrieval of already-learned information (47,49,85), especially if it is well-learned. For example, retrieval of knowledge about semantic categories, such as naming various kinds of fruits, is not appreciably altered (7,20,57). In some instances, the benzodiazepines can enhance recall of information learned immediately before drug administration (20,34,57,58,86). Characteristically in these studies, a word list is presented and immediate recall is tested. A benzodiazepine is then administered and new word lists are presented. Before recovery from the benzodiazepine, delayed recall of the predrug list is tested. Benzodiazepine-treated subjects show superior delayed recall of the predrug list, compared to placebo-treated subjects. This "retrograde facilitation" of recall seems to result from reduced interference between the predrug and postdrug information, which results from reduced learning of the postdrug information (34). In other words, the benzodiazepines reduce the acquisition of new postdrug words that would otherwise interfere with recall of the words learned before drug ingestion. Retrograde facilitation of memory is dose related, such that larger doses produce greater facilitation (20).

Benzodiazepines do not appreciably reduce the accuracy of recalling very recently presented items (37,58), i.e., the benzodiazepines do not impair accuracy of retrieving verbal information from short-term memory (7,47,58). The benzodiazepines, however, may reduce the speed of retrieval somewhat and may slow the rate at which information is manipulated in short-term memory (87). An overly simplified conclusion of these results is that the benzodiazepines slow short-term memory "working memory" procedures without substantially diminishing memory capacity.

Effects of Benzodiazepines on Performance

Laboratory Tests

Therapeutic doses of benzodiazepines frequently slow performance of repetitive, self-paced tasks (36,92). Benzodiazepines do not usually affect accuracy of performance, at least when the task is relatively simple. The DSST (Digit Symbol Substitution Task), one of the more sensitive complex psychomotor tasks, can show benzodiazepine-induced deficits in doses as low as 5 mg diazepam (31) or 1 mg lorazepam (15,31,48), and for time periods as long as 12 hr after 15 mg flurazepam (3). Other clerical-type tasks, such as letter cancellation and arithmetic calculation tasks, are of intermediate sensitivity, but performance on them can be impaired in the range of diazepam 10 mg (30,31,37,59,82) or lorazepam 2.5 mg (15,16). Reaction time (RT) tasks, which may be either purely reflexive (i.e., "simple RT") or may require a decision (i.e., "choice RT"), are among the less sensitive of the common laboratory psychomotor measures (24,36,92), although reaction time slowing can occur at higher doses, such as triazolam 0.5 mg (85). Benzodiazepines can also slow performance on tests of spatial ability, such as those requiring mental manipulations of geometric forms (21,89).

Benzodiazepines have been shown to impair both sustained attention (vigilance) (31) and divided attention in many (43,84,90,93) but not all (37,43) laboratory studies. Decrements in attention have been found in doses as low as 2.5 mg diazepam (31). We have argued elsewhere (90) that many benzodiazepine effects on complex cognitive functions might be parsimoniously explained in terms of nonspecific effects such as impaired attention. In any event, these findings clearly indicate that benzodiazepines can exert a variety of deleterious effects on performance in laboratory settings. The next section addresses studies closer to real life.

Driving Studies

Studies generally find that benzodiazepines in the range of 10 mg diazepam impair driving performance (44,63,82). In a well-done simulator study of young military drivers treated with diazepam, subjects drove faster, neglected instructions to turn, and caused more collisions (44). They did not show any reliable changes in the ability to stay on the road. The results of two other studies, in contrast, were more remarkable for decreased ability to stay on course as well as decision errors. No changes in driving speed were observed. One study (63) involved driving instructors for the police academy who were tested on a straight, level highway at night for 1 hr. The other study (82) involved students who were tested on two tasks that have been found to correlate with accident rates of city bus drivers. It should be noted that some driving simulator studies have not shown consistent benzodiazepine impairment (13,45), perhaps because of insensitive methodology (83). Taken together, however, these results suggest that many drivers who take a single dose of diazepam for the first time will be at increased risk for accidents. In highway driving, the risk may be an increased tendency to stray out of the lane of travel. In more congested situations, the risk may be an impaired ability to select rapidly the correct action. Clinicians are obligated to warn their patients about the increased hazards of driving while taking benzodiazepines, even after single doses.

It should be noted that these benzodiazepine-induced objective changes in performance are congruent with the most commonly reported subjective side effects of benzodiazepines, namely drowsiness, dizziness, light-headedness, and incoordination (29).

Dose-Response Relationships, and Onset and Duration of Effects

Although the benzodiazepines as a group produce qualitatively similar cognitive impairments (28,47,57), they vary a great deal in terms of time course of effects, particularly with respect to duration of effects. Benzodiazepines are commonly subgrouped as "short-acting" versus "long-acting," because of differences in metabolism and elimination half-lives. In the case of the benzodiazepines, however, the terms short- versus long-acting belie the duration of clinical action. Given clinically comparable doses, drugs with shorter plasma half-lives can induce longer-lasting impairments than those with longer half-lives. For example, lorazepam, a "short-acting" benzodiazepine with a half-life of 12 to 20 hr produces longer-lasting effects than diazepam, a "long-acting" benzodiazepine with a half-life of 35 to 50 hr (1,82). Duration of effects may be more a function of the relative lipophilicity of the benzodiazepines, with lorazepam, e.g., being relatively less lipophilic than diazepam and exerting more prolonged effects (27).

After oral administration, benzodiazepines exert their peak effects within 1 to 3 hr. The duration of effects ranges between 3 and 24 hr, depending on the drug as previously mentioned and the dose. More specific details of the time courses subsequent to oral ingestion of various benzodiazepines are described as follows.

Diazepam exerts its peak effects between 0.5 and 1 hr after ingestion (20,21). Recovery time for a 0.1-mg/kg dose, the equivalent of 7 mg for a 150-lb person, is approximately 3.5 hr (20). As noted above, recovery times are dose-related; recovery times for a 15-mg dose range between 5 hr (20) and 15 hr (4). These findings indicate that a single administration (one night) of 10 mg diazepam can be safely used as a hypnotic by individuals who do not show unusual sensitivity to CNS depressants (60).

In oral doses, lorazepam has a later onset and a longer duration of cognitive side effects in comparison with diazepam. Lorazepam exerts its peak effects between 3 and 4 hr after ingestion (15). Recovery times have not been systematically determined for various dose levels, but one study suggests that one should allow 12 or even 24 hr for complete recovery from 2.5 mg lorazepam (82). A 1-mg dose is probably at the threshold for producing impairments, given that one study found a trend for memory to be impaired at 3 hr postdrug (78) and another found memory to be reliably impaired at this time (15). Lorazepam, in doses of 2 mg and higher, has been observed to produce the most prolonged cognitive impairments in comparison to other benzodiazepines, with impairments persisting throughout the day following evening administration (77,82). At the higher dose levels, intense and striking amnesia has been reported in some individuals (49,77).

There is scant information available concerning the onset of side effects of triazolam and flurazepam. This paucity is not surprising, because these benzodiazepines are primarily marketed as hypnotics. Triazolam 0.5 mg does produce significant impairments of memory and psychomotor performance between 1.5 and 7 hr after ingestion (85,86). Recovery from effects of 0.5 mg triazolam appears to take 7 hr (86) to 11 hr (61). Thus, most studies (33,66,74,85,86) but not all (61,91) indicate that 0.5 mg triazolam should be safe for administration as a hypnotic. In comparison with triazolam 0.5 mg, flurazepam 15 mg has a smaller likelihood of producing "hangover effects," whereas 30 mg has a greater likelihood of producing persistent, sedative daytime effects (36).

COGNITIVE SIDE EFFECTS ASSOCIATED WITH THE REPEATED ADMINISTRATION OF BENZODIAZEPINES

As noted above, in clinically effective doses, the initial administration of benzodiazepines usually induces a wide array of cognitive impairments. These impairments have been observed in patients as well as in normal volunteers (23,43,76). With repeated administration, these impairments usually become less pronounced, but not always (43). Tolerance to benzodiazepine cognitive impairments develops even when there is progressive accumulation of benzodiazepines in the blood. The greatest increase in tolerance occurs between the first and second drug administrations (18). A range of schedules of benzodiazepine administration is associated with tolerance. Tolerance to cognitive side effects has been shown when benzodiazepines are taken several times a day, on a daily basis (1,24), or as infrequently as once a week (18). Tolerance develops regardless of whether the benzodiazepine has a short or long elimination half-life (22). At present, it is unclear whether complex cognitive functions, such as learning, develop tolerance to benzodiazepine effects more quickly or more slowly than simple cognitive functions. In any event, after repetitive benzodiazepine treatment has been stopped, all benzodiazepine cognitive effects subside, usually within a few days (22,24).

There are a few clinical situations where the repeated administration of benzodiazepines does not result in diminishing cognitive side effects. The most common one is where the patient increases the dose of benzodiazepine or takes additional CNS-sedative medication, alcohol, or other psychotropic drugs.

Benzodiazepines are often administered to insomniac patients for the purpose of maintaining next-day performance that otherwise would be impaired by lack of sleep. There is no evidence, however, that benzodiazepines consistently maintain next-day performance even when sleep is subjectively improved (11,36,56). Instead, especially after the first few nights of treatment, there may be next-day

cognitive impairment (56), of which subjects are sometimes unaware (56,64). Some studies indicate that these initial carryover impairments of daytime performance do not persist (11,32,56), and most indicate that there is no buildup of impairments (75,85), even though blood concentrations of benzodiazepines may increase. There may be exceptions to this generalization. With chronic bedtime benzodiazepine administration, older insomniac patients may show more persistent and perhaps even progressive performance deficits (64). There may be some cumulative adverse effects of flurazepam on certain psychomotor tasks (11).

The mechanism(s) of the tolerance associated with the repetitive administration of benzodiazepines has not been convincingly established. Most speculations focus on decreases in the number or sensitivity of benzodiazepine receptor sites in the central nervous system during long-term treatment (12,72). Alterations in drug metabolism are not marked enough to provide a convincing explanation (14,39). Neither the intensity nor the duration of the initial cognitive effects of benzodiazepines nor the subsequent development of tolerance is consistently explained by the pharmacokinetics of the benzodiazepines. Despite the suggestions of some advertisements for "short-acting" benzodiazepines, blood concentrations of benzodiazepines do not precisely reflect benzodiazepine-induced performance decrements (56).

INDIVIDUAL VARIABILITY IN SENSITIVITY TO COGNITIVE SIDE EFFECTS

There is considerable between-individual variability in the cognitive responses to the same schedule of repetitive administration of benzodiazepines. Some patients initially show marked cognitive impairments to which tolerance develops only slowly; other patients with the same body weight show little vulnerability and little change with continued benzodiazepine administration. The limited available evidence, however, indicates that a given individual who responds to benzodiazepine with impairment on one occasion will usually show, on subsequent trials, progressively diminishing impairment. Interestingly, patients who show considerable drug-induced impairments on certain tasks do not necessarily show great impairment on others (18). It has been observed, though, that those individuals who are most sensitive to the hypnotic effect of benzodiazepines tend to be the same individuals who experience more marked cognitive side effects (11,73). Reports of sleepiness may thus provide some indication of cognitive impairment. It should be noted that subjective reports are often not very sensitive to benzodiazepine effects on cognition. Simple clinical questioning can often lead to an underestimation of benzodiazepine-induced deficits.

Increased Sensitivity of the Elderly to Benzodiazepine Side Effects

In the 1970s clinical reports from the Boston Collaborative Drug Surveillance Program indicated that the elderly were more likely to experience excessive sedation from diazepam (5) and flurazepam (26) than were younger individuals. A recent epidemiologic study (40) and two placebo-controlled studies (69,88) confirm the earlier retrospective reports. The epidemiologic study found that individuals over the age of 70 who experienced a fall during a hospital stay were 3.7 times more likely to have been prescribed flurazepam, a trend that was not seen in younger patients. Although this finding does not establish a causal relationship between flurazepam use and performance impairment, it is provocative. The two controlled studies compared benzodiazepine-induced impairments in young and older subjects who were matched for gender and body size. These studies found that diazepam produced greater and more prolonged cognitive impairments in the elderly subjects. Remarkably, elderly individuals were impaired by a dose as low as 2.5 mg (69). This dose has seldom, if ever, produced detectable impairments in younger individuals.

The increased sensitivity of the elderly to benzodiazepines may be partially accounted for by age-related differences in pharmacokinetics (62). The oxidative processes of demethylation and hydroxylation are generally slower in the elderly. Diazepam and chlordiazepoxide are metabolized by oxidation, and reduced plasma clearance of these drugs has been found in the elderly in most but not all studies (88). Pharmacokinetic differences between young and old, however, are not the sole factor in explaining the increased vulnerability of older individuals to the side effects of the benzodiazepines. As noted elsewhere in this section, increased plasma levels of benzodiazepines do not necessarily mean greater performance deficits. Precisely controlled studies of nitrazepam (10) and temazepam (88) have found age differences in benzodiazepine sensitivity even though clearance of these benzodiazepines appears to be unchanged in the elderly (88). (Nitrazepam and temazepam do not undergo oxidation, but are metabolized via reduction of the nitro group and glucuronide conjugation, respectively.)

Other possible mechanisms for increased sensitivity in the elderly are age-related changes in the permeability of the blood-brain barrier to benzodiazepines, increases in the number and/or affinity of benzodiazepine receptors, reductions in the concentration of naturally occurring benzodiazepine-like receptor ligands, and/or impairment of homeostatic mechanisms in the central nervous system (88). Animal research yields some support for age-related changes in the permeability of the brain to benzodiazepines; the other possibilities are areas of active investigation (9).

In conclusion, although arguments can be made for using preferentially the "short-acting," conjugated benzodiazepines (e.g., lorazepam, triazolam, temazepam) in the elderly, most performance studies indicate they are not significantly safer for use in the elderly than the "long-acting," oxidated benzodiazepines (e.g., diazepam, chlordiazepoxide, and flurazepam). The clinical use of benzodiazepines in older individuals should focus on lower initial doses, explicit discussion of the risk of greater drug sensitivity with elderly patients and their caregivers, and close monitoring of clinical response.

BENZODIAZEPINES IN COMBINATION WITH OTHER PSYCHOACTIVE DRUGS

Alcohol and caffeine are the two psychoactive drugs most likely to be taken concurrently with benzodiazepines.

It has long been established that the combination of alcohol and benzodiazepines causes greater cognitive impairment than either drug ingested alone. Quite recently, it has been determined that caffeine counteracts some benzodiazepine effects. Performance and pharmacologic studies of these drug combinations are reviewed below.

Most performance studies of the benzodiazepine-alcohol combination have involved relatively low concentrations of alcohol, e.g., blood alcohol of less than 0.08 mg/dl and relatively low benzodiazepine dosages, in the range of 5 to 10 mg diazepam or 1 mg lorazepam. At these drug levels, benzodiazepines and alcohol taken separately may have no effect on performance or may even enhance it (54), whereas the combination of the two drugs impairs virtually all measures of performance (44–46,48). These findings suggest that the concurrent use of benzodiazepines and alcohol should be avoided or approached cautiously, even at low doses (83).

Studies of the benzodiazepine-alcohol combination in general reveal a weak pharmacologic interaction between the two drugs (80). Since acute alcohol consumption impairs drug oxidizing capacity in many individuals (6), benzodiazepines that are metabolized by oxidation (e.g., diazepam and flurazepam) show elevated plasma levels when alcohol is consumed concurrently (41,51). Inhibition of oxidation, however, is apparently just one mechanism involved in the interaction between benzodiazepines and alcohol (54). Other possible mechanisms are altered binding of benzodiazepines to plasma proteins (81) and enhanced binding of benzodiazepines to receptors in the brain (8).

Three studies have looked at the effects of caffeine, alone and in combination with benzodiazepines. The caffeine levels that were studied ranged between 75 and 500 mg, which is the equivalent of 0.75 to 5 cups of coffee in humans. The benzodiazepines studied were 10 to 20 mg diazepam (50,55) and 2.5 mg lorazepam (16). In these studies caffeine was found to counteract partially some of the psychomotor impairments produced by benzodiazepines. Caffeine did not diminish benzodiazepine-induced memory impairments (16,50). Of particular clinical significance is the finding that higher levels of caffeine counteracted the anxiolytic effects of the benzodiazepines (14,55). These results suggest that drinking 1 or 2 cups of coffee about 1 hr before the time of the peak effects produced by a benzodiazepine might be useful for counteracting some of the unwanted effects of benzodiazepines. Drinking coffee, however, might also reduce the therapeutic effects of benzodiazepines.

There is a pharmacologic interaction between caffeine and diazepam, such that plasma levels of diazepam may be slightly reduced when caffeine is ingested concurrently with diazepam (19). This reduction, however, does not precisely correspond to objective changes in performance. The basic mechanisms involved in benzodiazepine-caffeine interactions are areas of active investigation (52,53,65,68), but the mechanisms are unclear at this time.

SUMMARY

There is convincing laboratory and clinical evidence that benzodiazepines are frequently associated with cognitive deficits and other impairments in human performance. These deficits are often more pronounced in older individuals. The magnitude and duration of these side effects are not precisely correlated with the plasma half-life of the benzodiazepine. These impairments usually decrease with repetitive administration. The clinician is obligated to instruct patients regarding these side effects, especially how they may adversely affect driving and other daily activities.

REFERENCES

1. Aranko, K., Mattila, M. J., and Seppala, T. (1983): *Br. J. Pharmacol.,* 15:545–552.
2. Block, R. I., and Berchou, R. (1984): *Pharmacol. Biochem. Behav.,* 20:233–241.
3. Bond, A. J., and Lader, M. H. (1973): *Psychopharmacologia,* 32:223–235.
4. Borland, R. G., and Nicholson, A. N. (1977): *Br. J. Clin. Pharmacol.,* 4:86–89.
5. Boston Collaborative Drug Surveillance Program (1973): *N. Engl. J. Med.,* 288:277–280.
6. Breckenridge, A. (1983): In: *The Benzodiazepines: From Molecular Biology to Clinical Practice,* edited by E. Costa, pp. 237–246. Raven Press, New York.
7. Brown, J., Brown, M. W., and Bowes, J. B. (1983): *Neuropsychologia,* 21:501–512.
8. Burch, T., and Ticku, M. (1980): *Eur. J. Pharmacol.,* 67:325–326.
9. Burchinsky, S. G. (1984): *Exp. Gerontol.,* 19:227–239.
10. Castleden, C. M., George, C. F., Marcer, D., and Hallett, C. (1977): *Br. Med. J.,* 1:10–12.
11. Church, M. W., and Johnson, L. C. (1979): *Psychopharmacology,* 61:309–316.
12. Crawley, J. N., Marangos, P. J., Stivers, J., and Goodwin, F. K. (1982): *Neuropharmacology,* 21:85–89.
13. Durrman, I., and Norrman, B. (1975): *Psychopharmacologia,* 40:279–284.
14. File, S. E. (1981): *Psychopharmacology,* 73:240–245.
15. File, S. E., and Bond, A. J. (1979): *Psychopharmacology,* 66:309–313.
16. File, S. E., Bond, A. J., and Lister, R. G. (1982): *J. Clin. Psychopharmacol.,* 2:102–106.
17. File, S. E., and Lister, R. G. (1982): *Br. J. Clin. Pharmacol.,* 14:545–550.
18. File, S. E., and Lister, R. G. (1983): *Br. J. Clin. Pharmacol.,* 16:645–650.
19. Ghoneim, M. M., Hinrichs, J. V., Chiang, C. K., and Loke, W. H. (1986): *J. Clin. Psychopharmacol.,* 6:75–80.
20. Ghoneim, M. M., Hinrichs, J. V., and Mewaldt, S. P. (1984): *Psychopharmacology,* 82:291–295.
21. Ghoneim, M. M., Hinrichs, J. V., and Mewaldt, S. P. (1984): *Psychopharmacology,* 82:296–300.
22. Ghoneim, M. M., Hinrichs, J. V., and Mewaldt, S. P. (1986): *Clin. Pharmacol. Ther.,* 39:491–500.
23. Ghoneim, M. M., Hinrichs, J. V., Noyes, R., and Anderson, D. J. (1984): *Neuropsychobiology,* 11:229–235.
24. Ghoneim, M. M., Mewaldt, S. P., Berie, J. L., and Hinrichs, J. V. (1981): *Psychopharmacology,* 73:147–151.
25. Ghoneim, M. M., Mewaldt, S. P., and Hinrichs, J. V. (1984): *Pharmacol. Biochem. Behav.,* 21:231–236.
26. Greenblatt, D. J., Allen, M. D., and Shader, R. I. (1977): *Clin. Pharmacol. Ther.,* 21:355–361.
27. Greenblatt, D. J., and Divoll, M. (1983): *Adv. Neurol.,* 34:487–491.
28. Greenblatt, D. J., Shader, R. I., and Abernethy, D. R. (1983): *N. Engl. J. Med.,* 309:354–358, 410–416.
29. Greenblatt, D. J., Shader, R. I., Divoll, M., and Harmatz, J. S. (1984): *J. Clin. Psychiatry,* 45:192–195.
30. Haffner, J. F. W., Morland, J., Setekleiv, J., Stromseather, C. E., Danielsen, A., Frivik, P. T., and Dybing, F. (1973): *Acta Pharmacol. Toxicol.,* 32:161–178.
31. Hart, J., Hill, H. M., Bye, C. E., Wilkenson, R. T., and Peck, A. W. (1976): *Br. J. Clin. Pharmacol.,* 3:289–298.
32. Hindmarch, I. (1977): *Acta Psychiatr. Scand.,* 56:373–381.
33. Hindmarch, I., and Clyde, C. A. (1980): *Arzneimittelforsch.,* 30:1163–1166.
34. Hinrichs, J. V., Ghoneim, M. M., and Mewaldt, S. P. (1984): *Psychopharmacology,* 84:158–162.
35. Hinrichs, J. V., Mewaldt, S. P., Ghoneim, M. M., and Berie, J. L. (1982): *Pharmacol. Biochem. Behav.,* 17:165–170.
36. Johnson, L. C., and Chernik, D. A. (1982): *Psychopharmacology,* 76:101–113.
37. Jones, D. M., Lewis, M. J., and Spriggs, T. L. B. (1978): *Br. J. Clin. Pharmacol.,* 6:333–337.
38. Kleinknecht, R. A., and Donaldson, D. (1975): *J. Nerv. Ment. Dis.,* 161:399–411.
39. Klotz, U., and Reimann, I. (1981): *Eur. J. Clin. Pharmacol.,* 21:161–163.
40. Kramer, M., and Schoen, L. S. (1984): *J. Clin. Psychiatry,* 45:176–177.
41. Laisi, U., Linnoila, M., Seppala, T., Himberg, J.-J., and Mattila, M. J. (1979): *Eur. J. Clin. Pharmacol.,* 16:263–270.
42. Liljequist, R., Linnoila, M., and Mattila, M. J. (1978): *Eur. J. Clin. Pharmacol.,* 13:339–343.
43. Linnoila, M., Erwin, C. W., Brendle, A., and Simpson, D. (1983): *J. Clin. Psychopharmacol.,* 3:88–96.
44. Linnoila, M., and Hakkinen, S. (1974): *Clin. Pharmacol. Ther.,* 15:368–373.
45. Linnoila, M., and Mattila, M. J. (1973): *Eur. J. Clin. Pharmacol.,* 5:186–194.
46. Linnoila, M., Saario, I., and Maki, M. (1974): *Eur. J. Clin. Pharmacol.,* 7:337–342.
47. Lister, R. G. (1985): *Neurosci. Biobehav. Rev.,* 9:87–94.
48. Lister, R. G., and File, S. E. (1983): *J. Clin. Psychopharmacol.,* 3:66–71.
49. Lister, R. G., and File, S. E. (1984): *Psychopharmacology,* 83:183–187.
50. Loke, W. H., Hinrichs, J. V., and Ghoneim, M. M. (1985): *Psychopharmacology,* 87:344–350.
51. MacLeod, S. M., Giles, H. G., Patzalek, G., Thiessen, J. J., and Sellers, E. M. (1977): *Eur. J. Clin. Pharmacol.,* 11:345–349.
52. Marangos, P., Martino, A., Paul, S., and Skolnick, P. (1981): *Psychopharmacology,* 72:269–274.
53. Marangos, P., Paul, S., Parma, A., Goodwin, F., Syapin, P., and Skolnick, P. (1979): *Life Sci.,* 24:851–858.
54. Mattila, M. J. (1984): *Br. J. Clin. Pharmacol.,* 18:21S–26S.
55. Mattila, M. J., and Nuotto, E. (1983): *Med. Biol.,* 61:337–343.
56. Mendelson, W. B., Weingartner, H., Greenblatt, D. J., Garnett, D., and Gillin, J. C. (1982): *Sleep,* 5:350–360.
57. Mewaldt, S. P., Ghoneim, M. M., and Hinrichs, J. V. (1986): *Psychopharmacology,* 88:165–171.
58. Mewaldt, S. P., Hinrichs, J. V., and Ghoneim, M. M. (1983): *Mem. Cognition,* 11:557–564.
59. Morland, J., Setekleiv, J., Haffner, J. F. W., Stromsaether, C. E., Danielsen, A., and Holstwethe, G. (1974): *Acta Pharmacol. Toxicol.,* 34:5–15.
60. Nicholson, A. N. (1981): *Br. J. Clin. Pharmacol.,* 11:61S–69S.
61. Nicholson, A. N., and Stone, B. M. (1980): *Br. J. Clin. Pharmacol.,* 9:187–194.
62. Ochs, H. R., Greenblatt, D. G., Divoll, M., Abernethy, D., Feyeraben, H., and Dengler, H. J. (1981): *Pharmacology,* 23:24–30.
63. O'Hanlon, J. F., Haak, T. W., Blaauw, G. J., and Riemersma, J. B. J. (1982): *Science,* 217:79–81.
64. Oswald, I., Adam, K., Borrow, S., and Idzikowski, C. (1979): *Adv. Biosci.,* 21:51–65.
65. Paul, S., and Skolnick, P. (1981): In: *Anxiety: New Research and Changing Vistas,* edited by D. Klein and J. Rabkin, pp. 215–234. Raven Press, New York.
66. Peabody, C. A., Thiemann, S., Thompson, J. M., Miller, T. P., Taylor, J. L., Petersen, R. C., and Tinklenberg, J. R. (1985): *Curr. Ther. Res.,* 37:822–829.
67. Petersen, R. C., and Ghoneim, M. M. (1980): *Prog. Neuropsychopharmacol.,* 4:81–89.
68. Polc, P., Bonetti, E. P., Pieri, L., Cumin, R., Angioi, R. M., Mohler, H., and Haefely, W. E. (1981): *Life Sci.,* 28:2265–2275.
69. Pomara, N., Stanley, B., Block, R., Berchou, R. C., Stanley, M., Greenblatt, D. J., Newton, R. E., and Gershon, S. (1985): *J. Clin. Psychiatry,* 46:185–187.

70. Rickels, K., Downing, R. W., Case, G. W., Csanalosi, I., Chung, H., Winokur, A., and Gingrich, R. L., Jr. (1985): *J. Clin. Psychiatry,* 46:470–474.
71. Roehrs, T., Zorick, F. J., Sicklesteel, J. M., Wittig, R. M., Hartse, K. M., and Roth, T. (1983): *J. Clin. Psychopharmacol.,* 3:310–313.
72. Rosenberg, H. C., and Chiu, T. H. (1981): *Eur. J. Pharmacol.,* 70:453–460.
73. Roth, T., Hartse, K. M., Saab, P. G., Piccione, P. M., and Kramer, M. (1980): *Psychopharmacology,* 70:231–237.
74. Roth, T., Kramer, M., and Lutz, T. (1977): *Drugs Exp. Clin. Res.,* 1:279–286.
75. Saario, I., and Linnoila, M. (1976): *Acta Pharmacol. Toxicol.,* 38:382–392.
76. Saario, I., Linnoila, M., and Mattila, M. J. (1976): *Br. J. Clin. Pharmacol.,* 3:843–848.
77. Scharf, M. B., and Jacoby, J. A. (1982): *Clin. Pharmacol. Ther.,* 31:175–179.
78. Scharf, M. B., Khosla, N., Brocker, N., and Goff, P. (1984): *J. Clin. Psychiatry,* 45:51–53.
79. Scharf, M. B., Khosla, N., Lysaght, R., Brocker, N., and Moran, J. (1983): *J. Clin. Psychiatry,* 44:362–364.
80. Sellers, E. M., and Busto, U. (1982): *J. Clin. Pharmacol.,* 22:249–262.
81. Sellers, E. M., Naranjo, C. A., Giles, H. G., Frecker, R. C., and Beeching, M. (1980): *Clin. Pharmacol. Ther.,* 28:638–645.
82. Seppala, T., Korttila, K., Hakkinen, S., and Linnoila, M. (1976): *Br. J. Clin. Pharmacol.,* 3:831–841.
83. Seppala, T., Linnoila, M., and Mattila, M. J. (1979): *Drugs,* 17:389–408.
84. Seppala, T., Palva, E., Mattila, M. J., Korttila, K., and Shrotriya, R. C. (1980): *Psychopharmacology,* 69:209–218.
85. Spinweber, C. L., and Johnson, L. C. (1982): *Psychopharmacology,* 76:5–12.
86. Spinweber, C. L., Johnson, L. C., and Webb, S. C. (1985): *Sleep Res.,* 14:60.
87. Subhan, Z., and Hindmarch, I. (1984): *Neuropsychobiology,* 12:244–248.
88. Swift, C. G., and Stevenson, I. H. (1983): In: *The Benzodiazepines: From Molecular Biology to Clinical Practice,* edited by E. Costa, pp. 225–236. Raven Press, New York.
89. Taylor, J., Hunt, E., and Coggan, P. (1987): *Psychopharmacology* (*in press*).
90. Tinklenberg, J. R., and Taylor, J. L. (1984): In: *The Neuropsychology of Memory,* edited by L. R. Squire and N. Butters, pp. 213–223. Guilford Press, New York.
91. Veldkamp, W., Straw, R. N., Metzler, C. M., and Demissianos, H. V. (1974): *J. Clin. Pharmacol.,* 14:102–111.
92. Wittenborn, J. R. (1979): *Br. J. Clin. Pharmacol.,* 7:61S–67S.
93. Wolkowitz, O. M., and Tinklenberg, J. R. (1985): *Psychopharmacology,* 85:221–223.

Psychopharmacology:
The Third Generation of Progress,
edited by Herbert Y. Meltzer.
Raven Press, New York © 1987.

CHAPTER **154**

Introduction: Effects of Psychotropic Drugs on Major Functions in Normal Humans and Infrahuman Species

E. H. Uhlenhuth

This section exists because of the widespread conviction that studies of the effects of psychotropic drugs on normal behavior, especially in humans, can provide important information about behavior, its disturbances, and especially their amelioration. Advocates of this approach maintain that the absence of pathology significantly simplifies the experimental situation and thereby facilitates reliable interpretation of the data. Detractors maintain that information obtained from the study of normals cannot be generalized reliably to pathological behavior. The recently demonstrated similarity between the effects of stimulants on patients with attention deficit disorder and on normal controls (see Chapter 156) do not support this view. Whatever the merits on each side of the controversy, the advocates of studies in normals have generated copious data with heuristic value for understanding behavior and its deviations and often with practical implications for therapeutics, particularly in the realm of adverse effects.

The past decade witnessed a substantial increase in sophistication about the multiple factors that require consideration for precise investigations of the behavioral effects of drugs. Ellinwood and Nikaido (Chapter 155), for example, lay out six functional areas that influence perceptual-neuromotor assessment. Harvey (Chapter 158) points out that behavioral measurement of associative learning requires clear differentiation from sensory and motoric factors. Judd and Squire (Chapter 156) address the role of the particular cognitive task as it reflects specific, and presumably different, aspects of cognition, such as performance accuracy versus time or information storage versus retrieval. They also point toward electrophysiological correlates of behavior as means of further specifying cognitive functions.

The authors represented in this section also concern themselves with pharmacologic factors in the behavioral effects of drugs. Judd's group, for instance, addresses the differences observed between acute and chronic dosing with some compounds. The main thrust of the report by Ellinwood and Nikaido is to surmount the oversimplification

of drug plasma levels as an explanation for the quantitative changes in the pharmacodynamic effects of psychotropic drugs over time after administration. Thus the field is clearly advancing in terms of identifying, describing, and accounting for the complex set of parameters that are relevant to the relationship between the neurochemical and the behavioral effects of psychotropic drugs.

Although it is always difficult to separate "methodologic" from "substantive" advances, an interesting trend becomes apparent as one views the set of chapters in this section from the latter perspective. Some authors have found the data of their area much more coherent in terms of neurotransmitter system concepts than others. Eichelman (Chapter 68) especially finds evidence from pharmacologic probes to suggest clearly that the noradrenergic, dopaminergic, and cholinergic systems enhance aggressive behavior, while the serotonergic and GABAergic systems suppress it. Pedersen and Prange (Chapter 157), too, find rather consistent evidence that dopaminergic drugs and certain central hormones stimulate sexual behavior, whereas serotonergic drugs and opioids suppress it. In this case, however, the evidence for enhancement by β-adrenergic drugs and suppression by α-adrenergic drugs is less clear.

Judd and Squire, in contrast, find little association between cognitive function and the effects of drugs on specific neurotransmitter systems, with the possible exception of inhibiting effects of opioids and facilitating effects of opioid antagonists. Harvey, indeed, makes a special point of emphasizing the lack of correlation between the effects of drugs on associative learning, measured in a tightly controlled paradigm, and their effects on neurotransmitter systems.

These differences among authors in organizing their material, of course, may arise from a variety of sources, including personal interests and styles. But from this observer's distance, the behaviors addressed in this section seem to arrange themselves according to the cognitive complexity that they require. Thus aggressive and sexual behaviors, especially with the emphasis here on data from infrahuman species, probably depend less on cognitive modulation and more on the mobilization of energy or arousal. Behaviors reflecting primarily perceptual-neuro-motor function may occupy an intermediate position. Finally, behaviors reflecting cognition, including memory and especially associative learning, by definition depend largely on these highly complex functions.

This line of thinking suggests that neurotransmitter system concepts, at least in their present rather global form, may be especially applicable to understanding behavior that depends more on "affect" than on cognition. Currently the available knowledge of neuroanatomical systems (Chapters 155, 158) and neurophysiology (Chapter 156) may be more useful in understanding behaviors with a large cognitive component. As Pedersen and Prange suggest (Chapter 157), more complete comprehension of all the functions addressed here and their therapeutic manipulation will develop from further studies of the behavioral effects of drugs on specific neurotransmitters in specific neuroanatomical locations.

In the context of this discussion, it may seem regrettable that this section includes no chapter describing the effects of psychotropic drugs on mood in normal humans and the attendant implications about neurotransmitter systems involved. Chapters devoted specifically to drug effects on mood also are conspicuously absent from earlier volumes in this series, even though motor and cognitive functions, including memory, are well represented in every volume.

Our consultants judged the new material dealing with mood as insufficient for useful review at this time. The interested reader, however, can find mention of the mood-altering effects of stimulants (see Chapter 166) and sedatives (see Chapter 165) elsewhere in this book, together with references to the authors' publications. Other major contributors to the recent literature on drugs and mood include J. O. Cole's group on antianxiety agents (1), C. E. Johanson's group on stimulants and sedatives (2), and L. L. Judd's group on lithium (3).

This volume is the first of this series to feature full chapters on the effects of psychotropic agents on aggressive, sexual, and maternal behaviors. Hopefully, the data on drug effects on mood will be ready for comprehensive review and synthesis in time for the next volume in this series.

REFERENCES

1. Cole, J. O., Orzack, M. H., Blake, B., Bird, M., and Bar-Tal, Y. (1982): *J. Clin. Psychiatry,* 43:69–74.
2. DeWit, H., Uhlenhuth, E. H., and Johanson, C. E. (1986): *Drug Alcohol Depend.,* 16:341–360.
3. Judd, L. L. (1979): *Arch. Gen. Psychiatry,* 36:860–865.

Psychopharmacology:
The Third Generation of Progress,
edited by Herbert Y. Meltzer.
Raven Press, New York © 1987.

CHAPTER **155**

Perceptual–Neuromotor Pharmacodynamics of Psychotropic Drugs

E. H. Ellinwood, Jr. and A. M. Nikaido

In recent years there has been a growing recognition of the importance of elucidating the mechanisms that mediate the impairment of perceptual–neuromotor performance by psychotropic drugs, especially in terms of describing the pharmacokinetic–pharmacodynamic relationship. The rationale underlying this area of research is based on important clinical concerns, including the development of ways to increase the ratio of therapeutic to toxic side effects and the potential contribution of psychotropic medications to the serious impairment of work-related, driving, and other types of performance, which may result in accidental injury.

Our exploration of this area addresses several important questions: (a) the types of perceptual–neuromotor functioning that can reliably be measured; (b) the development of sensitive and reliable tasks for use in a dynamically changing drug environment; (c) the magnitude and duration of impairment; and (d) the nature of rate-limiting processes associated with the time course of drug effects. The following discussion highlights the relationship between the pharmacokinetics and pharmacodynamics of benzodiazepine-induced perceptual–neuromotor impairment.

PERCEPTUAL–NEUROMOTOR TASKS AS BEHAVIORAL CORRELATES OF CNS FUNCTIONS

As Broadbent (11) has pointed out, human performance involves numerous subfunctions and cannot be treated as a unit, particularly when we are attempting to understand how drugs affect behavior. Considerable research has been directed toward determining the nature of tasks and related CNS processes that are sensitive or insensitive to various classes of drugs. Kleinknecht and Donaldson (52) classified 40 to 50 tasks used in studies on the diazepam effect into broader categories, including reflex speed, psychomotor performance, attention and vigilance, decision making, and learning and memory. In a more recent correlational and factor analytic study of cognitive and perceptual motor tasks used with sedative-anxiolytics, the main factor, psychomotor performance speed, accounted for 30% of the total variance (98). The second and third factors were related to accuracy and concentration and personality qualities involving extraversion. In their investigation of anxiolytics, antidepressants, antihypoxidotic, and nootropic drugs, Grunberger and Saletu (40) concluded that quantitative measures of psychomotor impairment could be used to describe time and dose–efficacy relationships and thus provide important data on pharmacodynamic properties.

There are a number of extensive reviews of the literature on the psychomotor and cognitive effects of psychotropic drugs, and the interested reader is referred to these reports (16,17,44,49,63,96). Johnson and Chernik (49) and Wittenborn (96) concluded that speed of performance was a common denominator of tasks most sensitive to the benzodiazepines, barbiturates, and other sedative–hypnotics; the insensitive tasks involved established faculties or were not time dependent. Relatively fewer experimental studies have examined the effect on perceptual–neuromotor skills of drugs with anticholinergic, antihistaminic, or antidopaminergic properties, such as antidepressant and neuroleptic medications (38,60,67,73,78,88).

COMPONENTS OF PERCEPTUAL–NEUROMOTOR ASSESSMENT

Complex Neuromotor Tasks

At the very minimum, the selection of tasks for a perceptual–neuromotor task battery should consider the following components of drug-induced behavioral toxicity: (a) information sampling and sequential processing (81,87), (b) attention-arousal mechanisms, for example, concentrated versus divided attention (69), (c) neuromotor and psychomotor performance (27,28), (d) motivation, (e) judgment, including risk taking (11,19), and (f) cognitive processes that involve learning, memory and higher cortical functions (L. L. Judd, L. R. Squires, N. Butters, D. P. Salmon, and K. A. Paller, *this volume*). Although the complexity of evaluating each of these effects in a dynamically changing drug environment can easily become overwhelming, one needs to be aware of these processes when designing experiments.

Several methodological considerations are important in the choice of tasks. First, there is the need to sample a spectrum of perceptual, cognitive, and neuromotor capacities. Second, tasks to be used for repeated testing should show substantial concentration–effect relationships at given times in postdrug testing. Third, each measure must demonstrate inter- and intrasubject stability across and within test sessions for the predrug and placebo conditions (57).

An approach that is productive in delineating the specific CNS faculties affected by a drug is the fractionization of the multiple components involved in a single complex task (D. Heatherly, A. M. Nikaido, E. H. Ellinwood, Jr., and D. Dubow, *unpublished work*). Furthermore, computerization of a task allows for a more refined analysis of the differential contribution of individual components to performance and magnifies the power of the task. For example, in a recent unpublished study examining the effects of three benzodiazepines, Heatherly et al. factored out measures of both the motor and learning components of a computerized version of the digit–symbol substitution test (DSST) in the same way that the symbol-copying effect can be removed from scores of the paper-and-pencil DSST. Figure 1 illustrates the differential pharmacologic effect offset rates for the learning versus performance phases of the DSST.

Simple Neuromotor Tasks

The establishment of a stable base-line performance level during training is an important prerequisite for the use of complex tasks. Thus, another consideration in the development of a battery is the inclusion of tasks that evaluate neuromotor performance without major learning or mental concentration involvement (27), such as transducer–computer assessment of rapid alternation movements (finger tapping), ataxia, and various components of saccadic and smooth pursuit eye tracking. These tasks assess simple posturomotor coordination and automatic eye-tracking capabilities that are not necessarily related to intellectual, motivational, or attentional processes. Consequently, they are ideal for testing a broader population range, including patients, and are robust and sensitive in assessing alcohol intoxication even under roadside conditions (14).

Smith et al. (86) have described a very efficient microprocessor-based system for assessing saccade velocity, duration, and reaction time. Saccadic eye movements are sensitive not only to psychotropic drugs, such as the benzodiazepines, carbamazepine, phenytoin, valproate, papaveretum, and methadone, but also to tolerance effects despite a relatively long duration of impairment following a single dose (39). This task is sufficiently sensitive and reliable to be used to describe the onset characteristics and duration of effects for various benzodiazepines (90). Although smooth pursuit eye movement is also sensitive to drug effects at higher doses, the signal-to-noise ratio measure for this task (59) is not as reliable or sensitive at lower concentrations (27). Another important test in the practical application of psychomotor testing is dynamic visual acuity, which is correlated with the incidence of auto accidents and laterality of the defect (12,13). More recently, this task has been described as being sensitive to antihistamine impairment (8).

Because of its simplicity, the evaluation of ataxia with a microprocessor-controlled sway table has been recommended as a reliable method of assessing the degree of recovery after anesthesia and for monitoring drug side effects (27,54). Postural ataxia is well established as a sensitive index of impairment for psychotropic drugs, including alcohol (37), barbiturates (27,54), marijuana (55), and benzodiazepines (36,54). In fact, interesting differences between alcohol- and benzodiazepine-induced sway indicate different loci for the two types of drug perturbation. Alcohol increased ataxia in the anterior–posterior direction, which is completely compensated for by visual stabilization; similar types of behavior are observed in patients with atrophy of the anterior lobe of the spinocerebellum (25). In contrast, benzodiazepines (54) and lesions of the flocculonodular lobe of the cerebellum (vestibulocerebellum) (66) were associated with lateral sway with eyes open and virtually no visual stabilization. These comparisons suggest that the benzodiazepine effect on sway may be mediated by multiple benzodiazepine interactions in the vestibulocerebellum, including input to the Purkinje cell at the molecular neuronal level and at the Purkinje cell outflow to the vestibular nucleus of Dieter (41).

Neuromotor tasks, including the rhomberg, eye–hand coordination, slow pursuit tracking, and saccadic eye velocity, are hypothesized to involve cerebellar and brainstem circuitry associated with neuromodulators, such as the benzodiazepines. These measures differ from cognitive tasks such as memory encoding, which probably reflect greater contribution from the hippocampus and cortex. Comparing the two types of tasks can facilitate an evaluation of the hypothesis that benzodiazepine action is based on differential affinities to receptor subtypes in certain CNS regions (26). Variations in receptor kinetics and adaptation in different brain areas may also be related to differences in acute tolerance observed for neuromotor versus cognitive tasks (31).

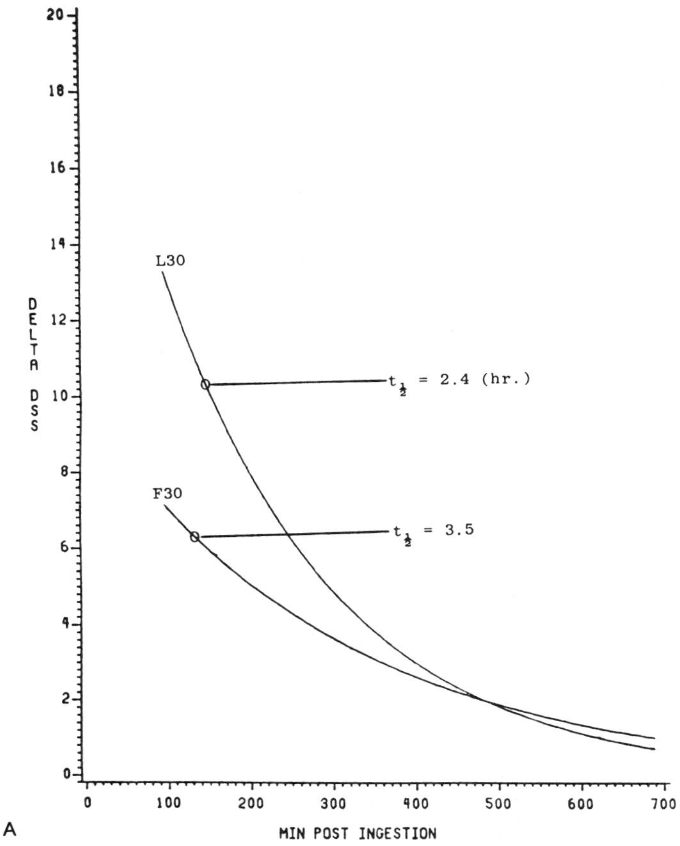

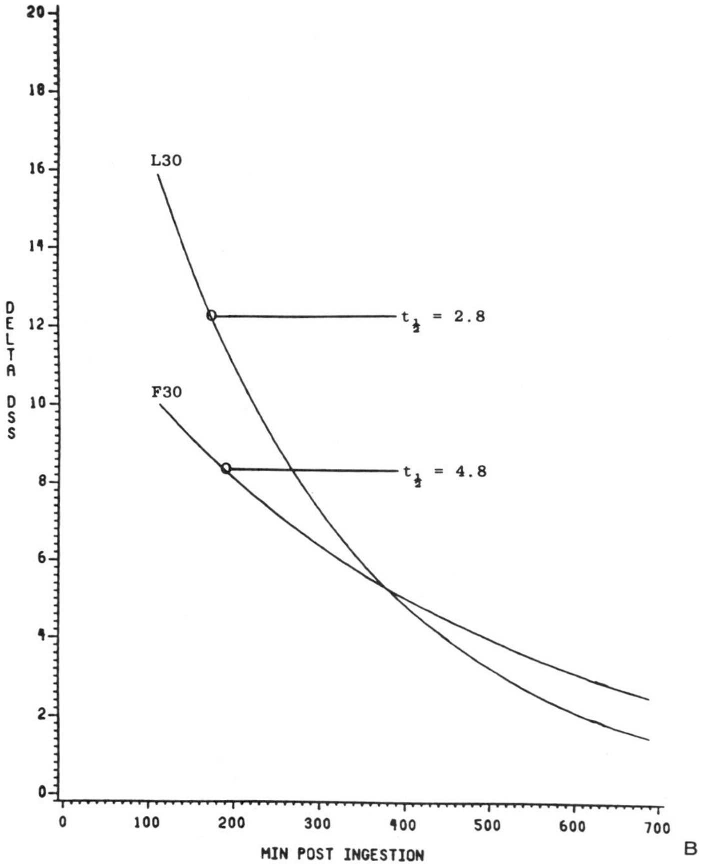

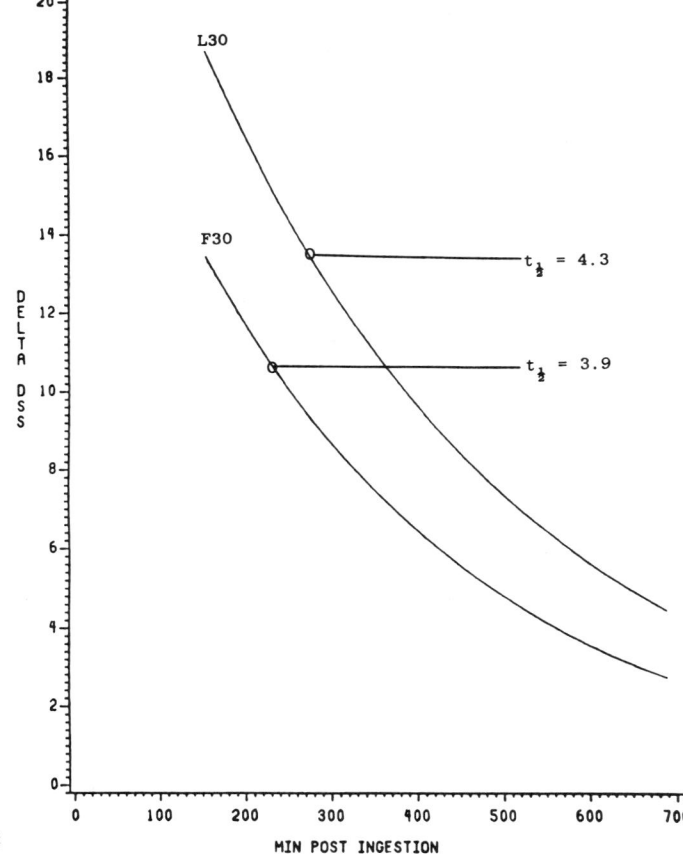

FIG. 1. Predicted drug effect offset curves for the DSST after single oral doses of diazepam (**A**), alprazolam (**B**), and lorazepam (**C**). The curves were determined by nonlinear regression fits of the pooled DSST performance scores. The first 30 trials (F30) represent the learning encoding phase, and the last 30 (L30) represent the psychomotor performance speed component. DSS = number of correct responses divided by mean reaction time. Delta score is defined as the unit changes from the predrug base line. Note that diazepam and alprazolam rates of recovery from peak impairment were slower for F30 than L30, but offset rates were similar for lorazepam.

THE PHARMACOKINETIC–PHARMACODYNAMIC RELATIONSHIP

Discrepancies between pharmacokinetic and pharmacodynamic profiles frequently have been reported following single doses of psychotropic drugs, for example, the marked acute tolerance of many sedative–anxiolytics (29,56,84,97). Such data dramatically demonstrate that a large source of unexplained variance needs to be investigated systematically. In addition, the rapidly expanding knowledge base on the kinetic events at the drug biophase level emphasizes the importance of receptor adaptation or receptor–ligand kinetics, including desensitization and the receptor synthesis-degradation life cycle (71), to pharmacodynamic models of acute and chronic drug action. Partially successful attempts have been undertaken to incorporate estimated receptor dissociation rates into pharmacokinetic–pharmacodynamic models (30,48). The perception of the biophase based on *in vitro* equilibrium kinetics is being replaced by mathematical models of kinetics of agonist-induced processing of receptors under initial to steady-state conditions (5,95). The analogously restrictive definition of pharmacodynamics as a constant relationship between drug concentration and effect or as time independent is also being reconsidered (45).

Since many perceptual–neuromotor measures possess reasonable linearity, robustness, and sensitivity, these objective tasks provide a more logical choice for the investigation of pharmacodynamic mechanisms in contrast to "noisy" or insensitive and less reliable therapeutic variables (45) such as global, subjective measures of anxiety or depression. Clinically, CNS adaptation to drug perturbation may play a more important role in producing therapeutic changes than the direct drug effect (e.g., adrenergic receptor adaptation following chronic tricyclic antidepressant treatment) (91) and therefore needs to be explicated further.

As indicated above, mathematical models that specify precisely the nature of the relationship between drug concentration and impairment across time could be valuable in explaining important pharmacologic phenomena such as acute and chronic tolerance, tachyphylaxis, and sensitization. By incorporating the pharmacokinetic parameters into the pharmacodynamic model, an examination of the variance unaccounted for by drug concentration may reveal other salient mechanisms. Presently, the detailed characterization of the rate-limiting pharmacodynamic processes is not possible; therefore, utilization of hybrid rate constants and descriptive offset rates that "summarize" the interactive effects of mechanisms is necessary. One example is the following pharmacokinetic–pharmacodynamic model that expresses the behavioral effect in terms of serum concentration and a hybrid rate constant (31):

$$E = FF \times P + A_0 \times e^{(-K_{ATC} \times t)} \qquad (1)$$

where E is the performance score, P is serum drug concentration (ng/ml), FF is the free fraction for the drug, t the time after drug ingestion in hours, K_{ATC} the hybrid acute tolerance rate constant, and A_0 the coefficient for the K_{ATC} term. Because of the differential contribution of various preequilibrium pharmacokinetic factors to the absorption onset and plateau performance phases, the model was restricted to the examination of the offset period, extending

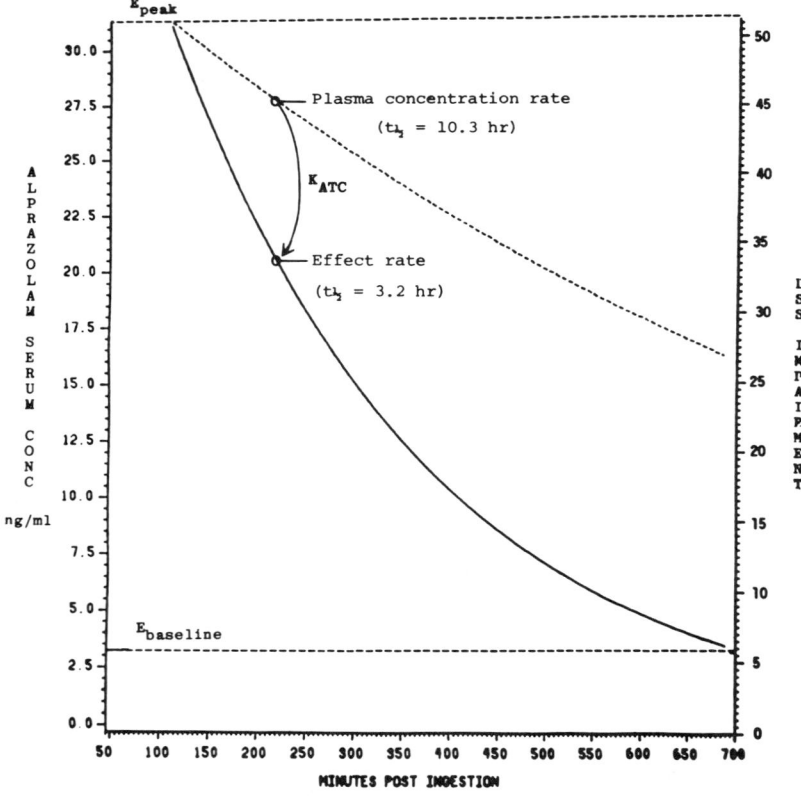

FIG. 2. A descriptive pharmacokinetic–pharmacodynamic model for the effect of alprazolam on DSST performance. The predicted segmented drug concentration and effect curves are based on single exponential models determined by nonlinear fits of the pooled data for serum concentration and performance, respectively. E_{peak} is maximum impairment; $E_{baseline}$ is predrug performance score plus 10% of E_{peak}; plasma concentration rate is drug concentration offset rate from E_{peak} to $E_{baseline}$; effect rate is performance effect offset rate from E_{peak} to $E_{baseline}$; K_{ATC} is hybrid exponential rate constant that best relates the offset rates of drug effect and concentration.

from the final impairment peak to the return of performance to base-line levels (see segmented curves in Fig. 2). K_{ATC} and A_0 were determined by performing nonlinear regression analyses on all pooled scores for drug concentration and performance. The degree of acute tolerance is expressed by the hybrid exponential rate constant (K_{ATC}) that best relates the pharmacokinetic to behavioral impairment offset rates.

Another method of describing the entire onset, plateau, and offset phases of the drug effect is the hysteresis or phase-plot curve, which relates drug concentration to performance across time. Figure 3 illustrates the leading and lagging relationships between the pharmacokinetic and impairment time courses for diazepam and lorazepam, respectively, during the impairment onset phase. Alprazolam

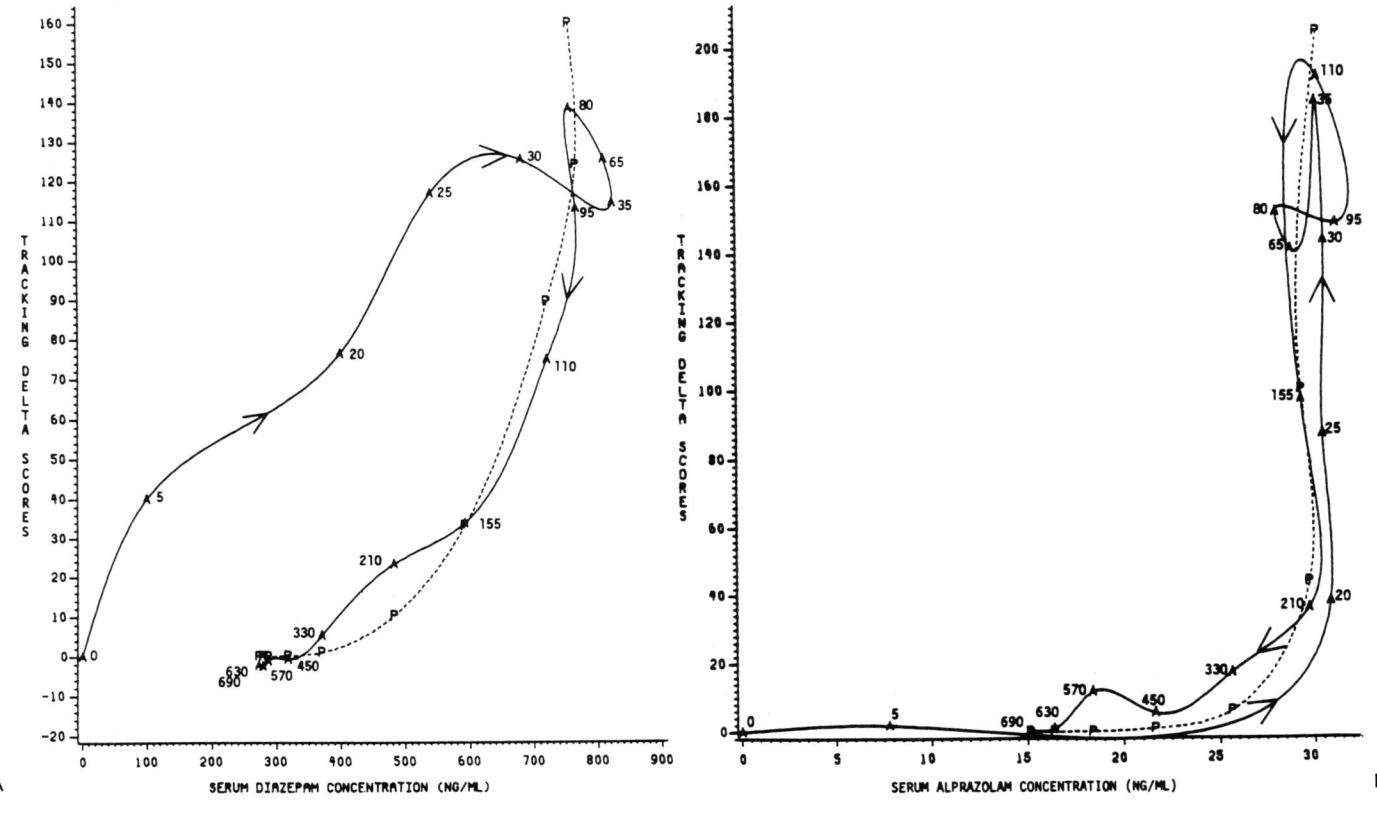

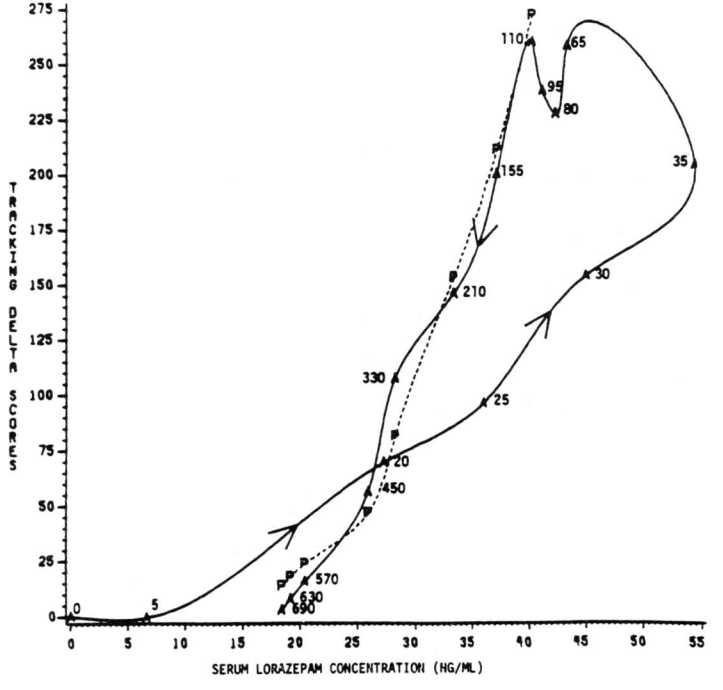

FIG. 3. Hysteresis curves of subcritical tracking performance versus drug serum concentration for diazepam (**A**), alprazolam (**B**), and lorazepam (**C**). Delta score is defined as unit change from the predrug level. Points represent the means of actual (A) and predicted (P) scores for consecutive testing time periods. Predicted values are based on the K_{ATC} model. *Arrows* denote the sequence of the testing times. [Curves previously appeared in Ellinwood et al. (31)].

had a highly unusual profile; the onset and offset of the drug effect occurred while drug levels were invariant (31). At the present stage of scientific development, however, caution must be exercised in the interpretation of comparisons between the pharmacokinetic and drug effect offset rates across different segments of the pharmacokinetic profile as well as comparisons between tasks.

Drug effect half-life ($t_{\frac{1}{2}}$) represents the time required for one-half of the impairment effect to dissipate for exponential functions; an efficacy rate would be calculated for drugs with zero-order offset profiles. Based on data from Ellinwood et al. (31), the drug effect $t_{\frac{1}{2}}$ ranged from 3 to 4 hr for the DSST and was highly similar for three benzodiazepines with varying pharmacokinetic properties (Table 1). Recent unpublished studies found similar DSST half-lives of 3 to 4 hr for two additional drugs, quazepam and triazolam, with very different pharmacokinetic and receptor binding characteristics. The theoretical implication is that the rate-limiting process (3 to 4 hr) for DSST impairment is relatively independent of the differential pharmacokinetic and receptor kinetic properties of these drugs.

Independent receptor mechanisms, such as benzodiazepine ligand–receptor complex degradation half-life (7), need to be considered as potential rate-limiting processes. In this regard, recent studies in neuron cultures (7) provide evidence of fast (3.8-hr) and slow (32-hr) benzodiazepine receptor degradation half-lives. The faster degradation rate is compatible with the DSST drug effect half-lives of the above drugs and with the hypothesis of a receptor rate-limiting process that is common across benzodiazepines.

On the other hand, Table 1 indicates that the coordination (tracking) task demonstrated dramatic differences when comparing the very rapid drug effect $t_{\frac{1}{2}}$ for diazepam and alprazolam to the much longer $t_{\frac{1}{2}}$ for lorazepam. Similar differences were noted for the coordination-performance component of the DSST (L30PW). Kaplan and Jack (51) proposed that the more prolonged effect of lorazepam is a function of relative binding affinity. However, our data do not support the affinity hypothesis, since alprazolam and lorazepam have very similar binding affinities and pharmacokinetic half-lives (10), but alprazolam produced a much shorter duration of coordination impairment than lorazepam (31). In general, the drug effect $t_{\frac{1}{2}}$ of the coordination task is much shorter than for the DSST, which is more dependent on learning and memory processes (Fig. 4).

One hypothetical explanation for the differences in drug effect $t_{\frac{1}{2}}$ observed for the two types of tasks may be the differential CNS distributions of heterogeneous benzodiazepine receptors, that is, greater concentrations of BZ_1 and peripheral receptors in the cerebellum and brainstem and of central and BZ_2 receptors in the hippocampus and cortex (1,26,61). Differential affinities for the peripheral and central receptors have been determined for a number of benzodiazepines, and very fast dissociation rates have been observed for the peripheral and BZ_1 receptors (26,83,92). Drugs specific for the peripheral receptor, such as Ro 5-4864, have been reported to have CNS effects, including increasing the firing rate in neurons of the substantia nigra reticulata and inducing seizures (94).

Another hypothesis is that the differential binding ratios of heterogeneous receptors in the cerebellum and brainstem may mediate the very-fast-tracking drug effect offset rates of diazepam and alprazolam. Ex vivo binding studies have shown that diazepam has a dissociation rate that is approximately nine times that of lorazepam (48). In addition, the structure of lorazepam, triazolam, and clonazepam includes a chloride ion in the ortho position of the "C" ring. This type of structure has been related to the high receptor affinity of these benzodiazepines and may account in part for the finding that neither lorazepam nor triazolam shows the fast drug effect offset profile for the coordination task (31; E. H. Ellinwood et al., unpublished results).

In the previous discussion, the potential biophase mechanisms were highlighted to demonstrate that humans may represent the ideal subjects for studies designed to explore pharmacokinetic–pharmacodynamic models of perceptual–neuromotor effects. A different perspective is gained from comparing the various components of performance on a task battery across drugs as opposed to examining only one or two dependent measures, which are usually the extent of the capacity of experimentation with lower animals. The same argument is also evident in the capacity to fractionate various components of a single task, as discussed earlier.

As a final but important comment, our models, involving the K_{ATC} and drug effect $t_{\frac{1}{2}}$, have used an approach that differs from other pharmacokinetic–pharmacodynamic modeling techniques (20,21,45,46) to determine the potential contribution of receptor kinetics and other mechanisms. First, whereas other models encompass the entire drug effect time course, we have focused on the effect offset phase, during which the receptor dissociation rate is hypothesized to be the rate-limiting mechanism. In contrast, receptor association and dissociation, as well as complicated

TABLE 1. *Pharmacokinetic and pharmacodynamic half-lives[a] determined by a pooled nonlinear fitting procedure Pharmacodynamic half-lives*

Task[b]	Diazepam (20 mg)	Alprazolam (2.0 mg)	Lorazepam (4.0 mg)
TRACKING	0.67	0.76	2.31
DSSOVRPW	3.30	3.15	4.33
DSSF30PW	3.48	4.85	3.87
DSSL30PW	2.36	2.83	4.28

Pharmacokinetic half-lives

Time[c] (min)	Diazepam (20 mg)	Alprazolam (2.0 mg)	Lorazepam (4.0 mg)
Total $t_{1/2\beta}$	33.3	14.5	15.7
Segmented $t_{1/2\beta}$			
80–690	7.6		
110–690		10.3	9.3
155–690			9.8

[a] Half-lives are expressed in hours.
[b] Performance scores were calculated as delta scores, that is, unit changes from the predrug level.
[c] Time describes the time interval used to determine the pharmacokinetic half-lives.

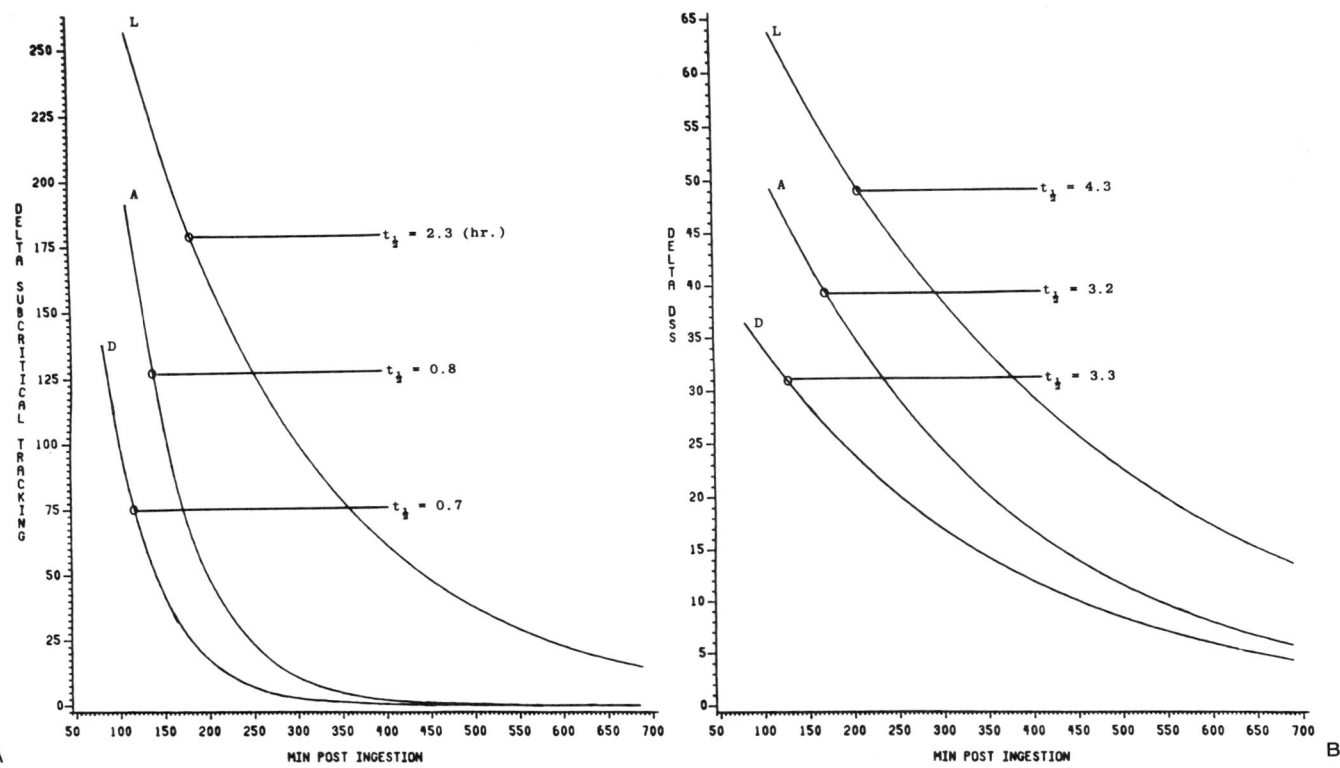

FIG. 4. Predicted drug effect offset curves on the tracking (**A**) and DSST (**B**) tasks for lorazepam (L), alprazolam (A), and diazepam (D). (See Fig. 1 for further explanation.)

absorption–distribution pharmacokinetic rates, determine the onset of the effect. Second, other pharmacodynamic models are estimated by using the pharmacokinetic parameters; however, the pharmacokinetic rate constants may be similar to and consequently mask the pharmacodynamic rate constants (see discussion on ultrashort drugs). Thus, we calculated the drug effect $t_\frac{1}{2}$ based only on performance data and then related the drug effect (pharmacodynamic) $t_\frac{1}{2}$ to the pharmacokinetic $t_\frac{1}{2}$. The resulting marked similarities across benzodiazepines in the drug effect $t_\frac{1}{2}$ for certain cognitive tasks and the variable ultrafast $t_\frac{1}{2}$ for other coordination tasks imply that the role of pharmacokinetic constants in the pharmacodynamic model needs to be reconsidered. Our results demonstrate that the comparison of the drug effect between diverse tasks and between drugs with differing pharmacokinetic properties may be used to determine the nature of benzodiazepine pharmacodynamic mechanisms.

Short Pharmacokinetic Half-Life Drugs

The correlation between drug plasma concentration and effect has generally been considerably higher for benzodiazepines with ultrashort pharmacokinetic half-lives (24,50) than for drugs with longer distribution–elimination phases (28,29). For midazolam with a $t_{\frac{1}{2}\alpha}$ of 6 to 15 min and $t_{\frac{1}{2}\beta}$ of 1.7 to 4 hr (79), plasma levels were strongly associated with psychomotor impairment ($r = 0.68$–0.92) (50) and reaction time ($r = 0.78$, $p < 0.001$) (24). Baktir et al. (3) also found parallel offsets for triazolam plasma levels and

complex tasks such as the DSST. The data support, but do not prove unequivocally, that pharmacokinetics is the main causal driving force for the drug effect.

An equally plausible and parsimonious explanation, however, is that the pharmacokinetic $t_{\frac{1}{2}\beta}$ of 2 to 4 hr for short-acting benzodiazepines corresponds closely to the kinetics of the pharmacodynamic rate-limiting mechanism. A good illustration of this hypothesis is the case of tetra-hydrocannabinol (THC), an abused psychotropic drug with an ultrashort $t_{\frac{1}{2}\alpha}$ of less than 1 hr. Previous data show that tracking errors under conditions of divided attention had a fast pharmacologic effect half-life of 0.8 hr and a linear correlation of 0.87 with higher plasma levels (5.0–28 ng/ml) of the fast initial distribution phase, whereas critical tracking (breakpoint) with an effect half-life of 5 hr did not correlate with the full range of plasma levels but did demonstrate a significant sigmoid relationship for very low plasma values (0.4–4 ng/ml) in the distribution phase (4). As mentioned earlier, however, correlations calculated for different pharmacokinetic parameters should be interpreted with caution.

Others have described parallel decay rates following peak impairment and plasma THC levels (18,75). During the later offset phase, the counterclockwise hysteresis indicates a consistent and substantial phase delay in psychological measures (subjective rating) when the entire onset–offset period is considered (18,47,76). Cocchetto et al. (18) found a consistent zero-order decay constant for subjective rating, which returned to base line in approximately 150 min. In this case, the pharmacodynamic offset (a) was linear, (b) showed no acute tolerance, and (c) had a fast offset rate that lagged behind plasma levels. Similarly, chronic THC use did not display substantial tolerance effects (58).

Given the lack of acute and chronic tolerance, THC levels above 10 ng/ml could be considered as a legal indicator of intoxication. However, considerable testing of dose–response relationships in light and heavy users would be required, since levels of 2 to 7 ng/ml have been reported in heavy users up to 32 hr after the last self-reported use of THC (15). In summary, for several drugs the very rapid distribution half-life is followed by a considerably slower time-dependent pharmacodynamic profile (45); yet, because of the relative approximation of the pharmacokinetic and drug effect offset rates, there is a greater correspondence between plasma and performance measures for drugs with short pharmacokinetic half-lives than for those with longer half-lives.

Drug Interaction and Chronic Tolerance

The study of drug interaction, including the facilitating effects of some drugs as well as chronic and cross tolerance, may also provide important clues concerning the nature of the pharmacodynamic mechanisms independent of pharmacokinetic properties. Caffeine and theophylline have been shown to antagonize the diazepam effects on conflict avoidance tasks and muscle relaxation in animals (77) and on perceptual–neuromotor performance in humans (34,42,64,65); both drugs have a lower affinity for the benzodiazepine receptor and higher affinity for the adenosine receptor (9,93). On the other hand, enprophylline (a novel methylxanthine without adenosine receptor blocking properties) failed to antagonize the CNS effects of diazepam, suggesting that adenosine receptor blockade may be an important mechanism for methylxanthine–benzodiazepine antagonism (72). The specificity of the antagonizing effect of caffeine for the benzodiazepines is further indicated by the finding that doses of caffeine as high as 500 mg/kg did not affect ethanol-induced psychomotor impairment (69,74). These interactions are significant, since ethanol and substances containing methylxanthines, such as coffee and tea, are utilized by many individuals in combination with benzodiazepines.

The nature of chronic and cross tolerance poses a complex and intriguing challenge for understanding pharmacodynamic tolerance mechanisms. Patients who were chronic benzodiazepine users showed no psychomotor performance deficits yet reported significantly greater feelings of tranquilization than drug-free controls (62). In addition, the diazepam plasma concentrations necessary to induce anesthesia were significantly higher when patients, ranging in age from 20 to 80 years, chronically ingested alcohol or sedatives (22). These results are clinically important, since high concentrations of ethanol (3 to 3.5 mg/ml) and diazepam (2.5 to 3.5 ng/ml) may be on board simultaneously in chronic abusers without producing toxic effects, indicating tremendous capacity for chronic tolerance (82).

Cross tolerance to diazepam did not occur in young healthy subjects on as many psychomotor tasks as for lorazepam after a 7-day treatment period with lorazepam (2). Moskowitz and Smiley (70) also found that diazepam-induced deficits on driving-related skills persisted after 8 days of chronic buspirone administration. Both the presence and absence of chronic tolerance have been described as well in elderly normal and patient populations for different benzodiazepines (22,68,89). Various mechanisms have been proposed to explain chronic tolerance, namely, a reduction of benzodiazepine binding sites (23,80), competitive binding to receptors by active metabolites (32,43), and changes in drug metabolism (33,53). However, none of these hypotheses fully explains all aspects of this phenomenon.

CONCLUSIONS

A current issue receiving considerable national attention is the mortality and morbidity associated with accidents facilitated by drug impairment, for example, falls reported by the elderly and occupational and vehicular accidents. Although the data are quite sparse, epidemiological studies clearly suggest that psychotropic drugs, including the individual or combined use of alcohol and benzodiazepines, are significantly related to the occurrence of traffic accidents (6,35,85). In light of these statistics, an important question concerns the development of valid and reliable procedures for assessing the degree of drug-induced impairment. Previous research with psychotropic drugs has strongly demonstrated that drug plasma levels are insufficiently correlated with perceptual–neuromotor impairment and would be an inadequate criterion for defining the condition of driving under the influence of drugs other than alcohol.

Therefore, an important application of perceptual–neuromotor testing is the evaluation of the behavioral effects of psychotropic drugs, especially sedative–anxiolytics, in a variety of clinical situations, including (a) testing for street readiness following outpatient anesthesia, (b) monitoring drug side effects during chronic use of psychotropic medications in vulnerable populations such as the aged, (c) testing for interactive side effects when two or more drugs with possible mutual potentiation are administered, and (d) development of impairment testing for legal purposes. The advantages of these tasks are their simplicity and ability to measure specific components of the overall driving task. We have also emphasized that perceptual–neuromotor tests can provide insights into the nature of pharmacodynamic rate-limiting processes that contribute to the effect offset rate. In conclusion, although the relationship of laboratory assessment to performance in actual driving and other dangerous situations has never been adequately evaluated, the further development and application of perceptual–neuromotor testing in clinical settings are important to insure the safer utilization of psychotropic drugs.

REFERENCES

1. Anholt, R. R. H., Murphy, K. N. M., Mack, G. E., and Snyder, S. H. (1984): *J. Neurosci.*, 4:593–603.
2. Aranko, K., Mattila, M. J., and Seppala, T. (1983): *Br. J. Clin. Pharmacol.*, 15:545–552.
3. Baktir, G., Fisch, H. U., Huguenin, P., and Bircher, J. (1983): *Clin. Pharmacol. Ther.*, 34:195–201.

4. Barnett, G., Licko, V., and Thompson, T. (1985): *Psychopharmacology,* 85:51–56.

5. Beck, J. S., and Goren, H. J. (1983): *J. Recept. Res.,* 3:561–577.

6. Bo, O., Haffner, J. F. W., Langard, O., Trumpy, J. H., Bredesen, J. E., et al. (1975): In: *Alcohol, Drugs, and Traffic Safety,* edited by S. Israelstam and S. Lambert.

7. Borden, L. A., Czajkowski, C., Chan, C. Y., and Farb, D. H. (1984): *Science,* 226:857–860.

8. Borland, R. G., and Nicholson, A. N. (1984): *Br. J. Clin. Pharmacol.,* 18:69S–72S.

9. Boulenger, J., Patel, J., and Marangos, P. J. (1982): *Neurosci. Lett.,* 30:161–166.

10. Braestrup, C., and Nielsen, M. (1983): In: *Handbook of Psychopharmacology: Biochemical Studies,* edited by L. L. Iversen, S. D. Iversen, and S. H. Snyder, pp. 285–384. Plenum Press, New York.

11. Broadbent, D. E. (1984): *Br. J. Clin. Pharmacol.,* 18:5S–9S.

12. Burg, A. (1968): *Visual Test Scores and Driving Record: Additional Findings, Vol. 2.* Dept. of Engineering, University of California, Los Angeles.

13. Burg, A. (1974): *Visual Degradation in Relationship of Specific Accident Types.* Institute of Transportation and Traffic Engineering, School of Engineering and Applied Science, University of California, Los Angeles.

14. Burns, M., Kayne, P., Studdard, R., and Tharp, V. (1982): *J. Forensic Sci.,* 22:315.

15. Chesher, G. B., and Starmer, G. A. (1983): *Cannabis and Human Performance Skills. N.S.W. Drug and Alcohol Authority Research Report Series B.*

16. Clayton, A. B. (1976): *Hum. Factors,* 18:241–252.

17. Coccaro, E. F., and Siever, L. J. (1985): *J. Clin. Pharmacol.,* 25:241–260.

18. Cocchetto, D. M., Owens, S. M., Perez-Reyes, M., Diguiseppi, S., and Miller, L. (1981): *Psychopharmacology,* 75:158–164.

19. Cohen, J. M. (1966): *A New Introduction to Psychology.* Allen and Unwin, London.

20. Colburn, W. A. (1981): *J. Pharmacokinet. Biopharmacol.,* 9:367–388.

21. Colburn, W. A., and Brazzell, R. K. (1985): In: *Opioid Analgesics in the Management of Clinical Pain,* edited by K. M. Foley and C. Inturrisi, pp. 425–438. Raven Press, New York.

22. Cook, P. J., Flanagan, R., and James, I. M. (1984): *Br. Med. J.,* 289:351–353.

23. Crawley, J. N., Marangos, P. J., Stivers, J., and Goodwin, F. K. (1982): *Neuropharmacology,* 21:85–89.

24. Crevoisier, C., Ziegler, W. H., Eckert, N., and Heizmann, H. (1983): *Br. J. Clin. Pharmacol.,* 16:51S–61S.

25. Diener, H. C., Dichgans, J., Bacher, M., and Gompf, B. (1984): *Electroencephalogr. Clin. Neurophysiol.,* 57:134–142.

26. Dubnick, B., Lippa, A. S., Klepner, C. A., Coupet, J., Greenblatt, E. N., et al. (1983): *Pharmacol. Biochem. Behav.,* 13:311–318.

27. Ellinwood, E. H., Jr., Linnoila, M., Angle, H. V., Moore, J. W., Jr., Skinner, J. T. III, et al. (1981): *Psychopharmacology,* 73:350–354.

28. Ellinwood, E. H., Jr., Linnoila, M., Easler, M., and Molter, D. (1981): *Clin. Pharmacol. Ther.,* 30:534–538.

29. Ellinwood, E. H., Jr., Linnoila, M., Easler, M. E., and Molter, D. W. (1983): *Psychopharmacologia (Berl.),* 79:137–141.

30. Ellinwood, E. H., Jr., Nikaido, A., and Heatherly, D. (1984): *Psychopharmacology,* 83:297–298.

31. Ellinwood, E. H., Jr., Heatherly, D. G., Nikaido, A. M., Bjornsson, T. D., and Kilts, C. (1985): *Psychopharmacology,* 86:392–399.

32. Elsass, P., Hendel, J., Hvidberg, E. F., Hansen, T., Gymoese, E., et al. (1980): *Psychopharmacology,* 70:307–312.

33. File, S. E. (1981): *Psychopharmacology,* 73:240–245.

34. File, S. E., Bond, A. J., and Lister, R. (1982): *J. Clin. Psychopharmacol.,* 2:102–106.

35. Garriott, J. C., DiMaio, V. J. M., Zumwalt, R. E., and Petty, C. S. (1977): *J. Forensic Sci.,* 22:383–389.

36. Ghoneim, M. M., Hinrichs, J. V., and Mewaldt, S. P. (1984): *Psychopharmacology,* 82:291–295.

37. Goldberg, L. (1966): *Psychosom. Med.,* 28:570–595.

38. Goode, D. J., Manning, A. A., Middleton, J. F., and Williams, B. (1981): *Psychiatr. Res.,* 5:247–255.

39. Griffiths, A. N., Marshall, R. W., and Richens, A. (1984): *Br. J. Clin. Pharmacol.,* 18:73S–82S.

40. Grunberger, J., and Saletu, B. (1980): *Prog. Neuropsychopharmacol.,* 4:417–434.

41. Haefely, W., Polc, P., Pieri, L., Schaffner, R., and Laurent, J.-P. (1983): In: *Benzodiazepines: From Molecular Biology to Clinical Practice,* edited by E. Costa, pp. 21–65. Raven Press, New York.

42. Henauer, S. A., Hollister, L. E., Gillespie, H. K., and Moore, F. (1983): *Eur. J. Clin. Pharmacol.,* 24:743–747.

43. Hendel, J., Elsass, P., Sorenson, K. H., Moller, I. W., Hvidberg, E. F., et al. (1980): *Psychopharmacology,* 70:303–305.

44. Hindmarch, I. (1980): *Br. J. Clin. Pharmacol.,* 10:189–209.

45. Holford, N. H., and Sheiner, L. B. (1981): *Crit. Rev. Bioeng.,* 5:273–322.

46. Holford, N. H., and Sheiner, L. B. (1982): *Pharmacol. Ther.,* 16:143–166.

47. Hollister, L. E., Gillespie, H. K., Ohlsson, A., Lindgren, J. E., Wahlen, A., et al. (1981): *J. Clin. Pharmacol.,* 21:1971S–1977S.

48. Jack, M. L., Colburn, W. A., Spirt, N. M., Bautz, G., Zanki, M., et al. (1983): *Prog. Neuropsychopharmacol. Biol. Psychiatry,* 7:5–6.

49. Johnson, L. C., and Chernik, D. A. (1982): *Psychopharmacology,* 76:101–113.

50. Kanto, J., and Allonen, H. (1983): *Int. J. Clin. Pharmacol. Ther. Toxicol.,* 21:460–463.

51. Kaplan, S. A., and Jack, M. L. (1983): In: *Benzodiazepines: From Molecular Biology to Clinical Practice,* edited by E. Costa, pp. 173–199. Raven Press, New York.

52. Kleinknecht, R. A., and Donaldson, D. (1975): *J. Nerv. Ment. Dis.,* 161:399–411.

53. Klotz, U., and Reimann, I. (1981): *Eur. J. Clin. Pharmacol.,* 21:161–163.

54. Korttila, K., Ghoneim, M. M., Jacobs, L., and Lakes, R. S. (1981): *Anesthesiology,* 55:625–630.

55. Kvolseth, T. O. (1977): *Percept. Mot. Skills,* 45:935–939.

56. Lader, M. (1979): In: *Sleep Research,* edited by R. G. Priest, A. Pletscher, and J. Ward, pp. 99–108. MTP Press, Lancaster.

57. Lehmann, H. E., and Knight, D. A. (1961): *Rev. Can. Biol.,* 20:525–536.

58. Lindgren, J.-E., Agurell, S., Hollister, L. E., and Gillespie, H. K. (1981): *Psychopharmacology,* 74:208–212.

59. Lindsey, T. Z., Holzman, P. S., Haberman, S., and Ysaillo, N. J. (1978): *J. Abnorm. Psychol.,* 87:491–496.

60. Linnoila, M., Johnson, J., Dubyoski, K., Buchsbaum, M. S., Schneinin, M., et al. (1984): *Br. J. Clin. Pharmacol.,* 18:109S–120S.

61. Lo, M. M. S., Trifelleti, R. R., and Snyder, S. H. (1982): In: *Pharmacology of the Benzodiazepines,* edited by E. Usdin, pp. 165–173. Macmillan, New York.

62. Lucki, I., Rickels, M. D., and Geller, A. M. (1985): *Psychopharmacol. Bull.,* 21:93–96.

63. Mattila, M. J. (1984): *Br. J. Clin. Pharmacol.,* 18:21S–26S.

64. Mattila, M. J., and Nuotto, E. (1984): *Med. Biol.,* 61:337–343.

65. Mattila, M. J., Palva, E., and Savolainen, K. (1982): *Med. Biol.,* 60:121–123.

66. Mauritz, K. H., Dichgans, J., and Hufschmidt, A. (1979): *Brain,* 102:461–482.

67. Meyer, F. P., Neubuser, G., Weimeister, O., and Walther, H. (1983): *Int. J. Clin. Pharmacol. Ther. Toxicol.,* 21:192–196.

68. Morgan, K. (1984): *Psychopharmacology [Suppl.],* 1:79–83.

69. Moskowitz, H. (1984): *Br. J. Clin. Pharmacol.,* 18:51S–61S.

70. Moskowitz, H., and Smiley, A. (1982): *J. Clin. Psychiatry,* 43:45–55.

71. Motulsky, H. J., Mahan, L. C., and Incel, P. A. (1985): *Trends Pharmacol. Sci.,* 6:317–319.

72. Niemand, D., Martinell, S., Arvidsson, S., Svedmyr, N., and Ekstrom-Jodal, B. (1984): *Lancet,* 1:463–464.

73. Nuotto, E. (1983): *Eur. J. Clin. Pharmacol.,* 24:603–609.

74. Nuotto, E., Mattila, M. J., Seppala, T., and Konno, K. (1982): *Clin. Pharmacol. Ther.,* 31:68–76.

75. Ohlsson, A., Lindgren, J.-E., Wahlen, A., Agurell, S., Hollister, L. E., et al. (1980): *Clin. Pharmacol. Ther.,* 28:409–416.

76. Perez-Reyes, M., DiGuiseepi, S., Davis, K., Schindler, V. H., and Cook, C. E. (1982): *Clin. Pharmacol. Ther.,* 31:617–624.

77. Polc, P., Bonetti, E. P., Pieri, L., Cumin, R., Angioi, R. M., et al. (1981): *Life Sci.,* 28:2265–2275.

78. Raskin, A., Friedman, A. S., and DiMascio, A. (1983): *Psychopharmacol. Bull.,* 19:649–652.

79. Reeves, J. G., Fragen, R. J., Vinik, H. R., and Greenblatt, D. J. (1985): *Anesthesiology,* 62:310–324.
80. Rosenberg, H. C., and Chiu, T. H. (1981): *Eur. J. Pharmacol.,* 70:453–460.
81. Sanders, A. F. (1981): In: *Machine Pacing and Occupational Stress,* edited by G. Salvendy and M. J. Smith, pp. 57–64. Taylor and Francis, London.
82. Schmidt, G., and Bosche, J. (1981): In: *Proceedings of 8th International Conference on Alcohol, Drugs and Traffic Safety, Vol. III,* edited by L. Goldberg, pp. 984–995. Almqvist and Wiksell, Stockholm.
83. Schoemaker, H., Boles, R. G., Horst, W. D., and Yamamura, H. I. (1983): *J. Pharmacol. Exp. Ther.,* 225:61–69.
84. Sellers, E. M., Naranjo, C. A., Giles, H. G., Frecker, R. C., and Beeching, M. (1980): *Clin. Pharmacol. Ther.,* 28:638–645.
85. Skegg, D. C. G. (1979): *Br. Med. J.,* 1:917–919.
86. Smith, A. T., Bittencourt, P. R. M., Lloyd, D. S. L., and Richens, A. (1981): *J. Biomed. Eng.,* 3:39–43.
87. Sternberg, S. (1969): In: *Attention and Performance II,* edited by W. G. Koster, pp. 276–315. North-Holland, Amsterdam.
88. Swift, C. G., Haythorne, J. M., Clarke, P., and Stevenson, I. H. (1981): *Acta Psychiatr. Scand.,* 290:425–432.
89. Swift, C. G., Swift, M. R., Hamley, J., Stevenson, I. H., and Crooks, J. (1984): *Age Ageing,* 13:335–343.
90. Tedeschi, G., Smith, A. T., Dhillon, S., and Richens, A. (1983): *Br. J. Clin. Pharmacol.,* 15:103–107.
91. Tyrer, P., and Marsden, C. (1985): *Trends Neurosci.,* 8:427–431.
92. Wang, J. K. T., Taniguchi, T., and Spector, S. (1984): *Mol. Pharmacol.,* 25:349–351.
93. Weir, R. L., and Hruska, R. E. (1983): *Arch. Int. Pharmacodyn.,* 265:42–48.
94. Weissman, B. A., Cott, J., Jackson, J. A., Bolger, G. T., Weber, K. H., et al. (1985): *J. Neurochem.,* 44:1494–1499.
95. Wiley, H. S., and Cunningham, D. D. (1981): *Cell,* 25:435–440.
96. Wittenborn, J. R. (1979): *Br. J. Clin. Pharmacol.,* 7:61S–67S.
97. Ziegler, G., Ludwig, L., and Klotz, U. (1983): *Pharmacopsychiatry,* 16:71–76.
98. Zimmermann-Tansella, C. Z. (1984): *Percept. Mot. Skills,* 58:803–810.

Psychopharmacology:
The Third Generation of Progress,
edited by Herbert Y. Meltzer.
Raven Press, New York © 1987.

CHAPTER **156**

Effects of Psychotropic Drugs on Cognition and Memory in Normal Humans and Animals

Lewis L. Judd, Larry R. Squire, Nelson Butters, David P. Salmon, and Ken A. Paller

The vast majority of studies of psychoactive drug effects on cognition have been conducted in psychiatric patients. Although these investigations have made valuable contributions, there are limits to what can be learned from such studies. In mentally disordered patients, it is difficult to know whether drug effects result from the preexisting mental state, the effects of the drug on that state, or by direct action on the cognitive behavior under study. There are methodological advantages to studying the effects of psychoactive drugs in cognitively intact normal subjects. It is these studies, together with supporting studies in experimental animals, which are the focus of this chapter. The following classes of psychoactive drugs are covered: lithium, antidepressants, neuroleptics, psychostimulants, and opiate agonists and antagonists.

LITHIUM

There have been consistent reports that therapeutic serum levels of lithium affect cognition in normal subjects. Schou et al. (142,143) reported themselves on lithium to be less responsive to the environment and less able to concentrate and memorize. Later controlled studies confirmed small but consistent impairments of mental functioning from lithium. Normal subjects were self-rated as less clear mentally, less alert, and less efficient, and some subjects exhibited poorer school performance on lithium (148). Lithium also slowed choice reaction time, which was attributed to a slowing of information processing (102). Normals manifested small decreases in mean IQ scores, deficits in the Trail Making Test (Part A) of the Halstead-Reitan Neuropsychological Battery, the Digit Symbol Substitution Test (DSST) of the Wechsler Adult Intelligence Scale (WAIS), and the Minnesota Clerical Test after 2 weeks of lithium treatment. These authors concluded that lithium appeared to slow the rate of performance, but did not impair response accuracy (79,80).

In another report, subjects felt cognitively impaired on lithium and scored lower on a memory test (84). Similarly, lithium did not affect immediate (2 hr) free recall, but did impair memory 14 days later. Lithium also subtly impaired performance on the initial component of a learning task (91). In an uncontrolled study, lithium slowed performance on the Porteus Maze Test and the choice reaction time test (173). In a follow-up to their original study, Judd (81) suggested that lithium-induced slowing of psychomotor performance is due to a central slowing of information processing. They also found several measures of memory to be normal after 2 weeks of lithium, but psychomotor performance was impaired on tests requiring speed (154). More recently Weingartner et al. have reported that normals on lithium produced more errors of commission in recalling previous events, but errors of omission were not affected. These authors suggested that lithium specifically disrupts memory retrieval (167–170). The above observations, based on objective cognitive measures, have been supported indirectly by electrophysiological studies in which lithium slowed the EEG (55,148), altered event-related brain potentials (ERPs), and delayed nerve conduction velocity (6).

In summary, lithium often induces subjective feelings of cognitive slowing together with decreased ability to learn, concentrate and memorize. In addition, controlled studies have consistently described small but consistent performance decrements on various cognitive tests, including memory tests. The available data suggest that the slowing of performance is likely to be secondary to a slowing in rate of central information processing.

Lithium in Animals

Studies of lithium's effect on animal behavior have primarily focused on stereotypy, locomotor behavior, and classical conditioning. A few studies have attempted to explore lithium's influence on learning and memory. Johnson (77,78) reported that lithium decreased exploratory behavior of rats and impaired one-trial passive avoidance learning. He suggested that lithium reduces the influence of environmental stimuli secondary to disrupting central sensory processing. This hypothesis is consistent with the data from studies of normal human subjects (79,80,100). However, criticisms of this animal work have cited methodological problems such as different routes of drug administration across studies, different drug doses, species differences, and absence of appropriate controls (149,150). Thus, there is little agreement at this time about the type, the magnitude, or the specificity of lithium's effects on learning and memory in animals.

THE ANTIDEPRESSANTS

The effects of administration of antidepressant drugs on the cognitive functions of healthy human volunteers have been the focus of a number of investigations over the last decade (161). The most interesting studies have been those in which the tricyclic antidepressants were administered in the chronic dose regimens required for therapeutic efficacy in the clinical situation. A therapeutic dose schedule of imipramine (200 mg/day for 4 weeks) impaired performance on the Porteus Maze and on the Trail Making Test (Part B), but performance on a paired-associate learning task was actually enhanced by the drug (82). Amitriptyline (75 mg/day for 14 days) increased the mistakes made in classifying visual and auditory stimuli in a choice reaction time task, but reaction time itself was not affected (146). In another study (99), 14 days of amitriptyline decreased performance levels in paired-associate learning.

Single-dose studies of amitriptyline have reported decreased performance on the DSST, an arithmetic test (21), and an information-processing task (104). However, two other studies report unimpaired performance on simple cognitive tests from single doses of amitriptyline (35,118). Amitriptyline's most pronounced effects on normals are in immediate memory, where a deficit has been observed in three of four studies after single doses of the drug (20,121,122,166). Linnoila et al. also observed a decrement in a free recall task from an acute dose of the drug (103). Normal subjects when administered a total of 150 mg of imipramine over an 8-hr period were impaired in both the DSST and time estimation accuracy (176).

A thorough evaluation of the acute administration of amitriptyline on memory was conducted by Branconnier et al. (14), in which no effects on iconic and incidental memory or on memory scanning were found. However, amitriptyline did impair free recall and recall after the semantic, but not the phonemic, cues. Because the pattern of memory deficits associated with amitriptyline and imipramine was considered to be similar to that induced by scopolamine, Branconnier et al. suggested that their findings may be due to anticholinergic effects of the tricyclics. Support for this cholinergic hypothesis of memory impairment was also found when these (13) and other investigators (166) were unable to demonstrate memory deficits with trazodone, an antidepressant without central anticholinergic properties.

Two weeks' administration of the tricyclic nortriptyline (30 mg/day on days 1–7; 75 mg/day on days 8–14) impaired backward, but not forward, recall in a digit span test and increased the number of mistakes in a paired associate learning task (96). However, another study using a single dose (25 mg) of nortriptyline found no impairment on the DSST, the Digit Span, an arithmetic test, and memory function (20). Other studies have failed to demonstrate significant cognitive effects from the tricyclics chlorimipramine (96) and desmethylimipramine (104,134).

Additional studies of the cognitive effects of nontricyclic antidepressants have resulted in negative results with the following drugs: maprotiline (100), mianserin (99), clovoxamine (137), fluvoxamine (138), bupropion (61,121,122), nomifensine (120,176), zimelidine (103–105,169,170), and tranylcypromine (56).

In summary, several of the tricyclic antidepressants, notably imipramine and amitriptyline, produce measurable cognitive impairment in normal subjects following acute or chronic administration. However, there is a suggestion in some studies that certain aspects of cognition may be improved during chronic treatment, implying a potential differential effect in a chronic versus an acute regimen. Nontricyclic compounds, in contrast, appear to have little or no effect on normal cognition, although the sparsity of systematic studies requires further research before such a conclusion is warranted.

Antidepressants in Animals

Thompson (161) demonstrated that imipramine (2.5, 5, 10, and 20 mg/kg) administered to pigeons increased, in a dose-dependent manner, the number of errors on a complex discrimination task. Amitriptyline impaired the performance of rats on a staircase maze task (23) and delayed extinction of a runway response (40). Imipramine, amitriptyline, desimipramine, and mianserin disrupted rats' performance of a shuttle box conditioned avoidance response (64,139,159). However, desimipramine (107) failed to influence resistance to extinction, nor was imipramine shown to affect the memory of rats in a one-trial appetitive learning task (94). In contrast, zimelidine was found to improve the memory of mice on a passive avoidance task (1). Thus, depending on the drug or the task, antidepressants have been reported to produce decrements, to enhance, or to have no effects on learning and memory in animals.

THE NEUROLEPTICS

The few systematic studies of neuroleptic effects on normal human memory and cognition reported during the last decade have found little change in cognitive functioning from the antipsychotic medications. For example, no effect was observed in digit span, paired-associate learning, and retention after either a single dose (25 mg) or 2-weeks administration (30 mg/day for week 1, 60 mg/day for week 2) of chlorpromazine (97,98). Thioridazine administered for 2 weeks (30 mg/day for week 1, 60 mg/day for week 2) also had no effect on digit span or paired-associate learning. However, single doses of thioridazine (50 mg) have been reported to both enhance (158) and impair (160) performance on the DSST.

The small number of studies examining the influence of neuroleptic drugs on cognitive processes of normals precludes any general conclusions. Only two of the most widely used neuroleptics, chlorpromazine and thioridazine, have been systematically examined to date, and no consistent effects on cognition have emerged. It appears that neuroleptics may have only mild effects on the learning and memory processes of healthy subjects, but further research is necessary employing a wider variety of antipsychotic agents administered under standard therapeutic regimens.

Neuroleptics in Animals

Very few studies have been reported assessing the effects of neuroleptic drugs on the cognitive processes of animals. Bartus (7) administered haloperidol (0.006–0.05 mg/kg) to rhesus monkeys in a delayed response task, and only the higher doses of the drug resulted in a decrement in performance at all delays. In contrast to Bartus' negative findings, other investigators have reported the following detrimental or facilitating consequences from neuroleptics: impaired memory in rats from haloperidol (116); impaired memory of passive shock avoidance in rats from haloperidol, chlorpromazine, and clozapine (45); and enhanced passive avoidance learning in chicks after haloperidol (37).

The majority of investigations of the behavioral effects of neuroleptic drugs in animals have employed active avoidance tasks, which have proven to be sensitive to the neuroleptics. A number of studies have reported a decrease in active avoidance responses, without affecting the rodent's ability to perform escape responses, from the following drugs: haloperidol, clozapine, thioridazine, pimozide, flu-

phenazine, perphenazine, and other neuroleptics (12,36,85,119,139,159,165). For example, when the neuroleptic drug phenfluridol (2–8 mg/kg) was administered to rats for 10 days while they were performing a lever-press conditioned avoidance task, the number of avoidance responses they made decreased over the first 4 days of treatment and then stabilized at lower levels (93).

Although it is possible to interpret these deficits in active avoidance performance as a breakdown in the associations between environmental stimuli and events, a recent explanation (175) suggests that the neuroleptics produce their behavioral effects by changing the subjective value of reinforcers (i.e., the anhedonia hypothesis). In any event, given the inconsistencies in the results and the differences in species, drugs, and dosages across studies, general conclusions concerning the relationship between neuroleptics and cognition seem premature at this time.

THE PSYCHOSTIMULANTS

This section focuses on the cognitive effects of amphetamine (usually dextroamphetamine), methylphenidate, caffeine, and cocaine. Other chapters discuss stimulant effects on mood (31) and associative conditioning (66).

Psychostimulants can produce subjective effects such as improved concentration, increased energy and motivation, heightened confidence, decreased boredom, and clearer thinking. Nevertheless, the classic review of Weiss and Laties (171) suggests that the primary effect of low to moderate doses of psychostimulants is to promote alertness and counteract fatigue. Facilitated intellectual performance under the influence of stimulants was attributed largely to antifatigue effects. Recent work has explored the effects of stimulants with a broader range of tasks.

Amphetamine

The facilitatory effects of amphetamine on vigilance and tasks requiring quickness have long been recognized. Amphetamine generally improves performance on tasks of sustained attention, such as letter cancellation, signal detection, and arithmetic (62,171). In other tasks of intellectual function, such as paired-associate learning, amphetamine has been reported to facilitate (70,172), to impair (19), or not to affect (90) performance. However, indirect drug effects (e.g., delayed sleep onset) were not always recognized (152).

Among the more recent studies, those of Rapoport, Weingartner, and colleagues (124,125,167) are notable for demonstrating similar cognitive effects of amphetamine in both normal and attention deficit disorder (ADD) children, contradicting the view that the calming effect is unique to ADD. Both ADD and normal children improved in tests of free recall, cued recall, and vigilance. Since memory improvements did not correlate significantly with vigilance, reaction time, or mood changes, the authors rejected the idea that memory facilitation was mediated by improvements in attention.

Not all studies have consistently noted improvements in performance from amphetamine. For example, in one study normal subjects improved on the performance portion of an IQ test, while not improving on tests of recall (38). In a study of twins, amphetamine impaired performance on an arithmetic test did not change digit span (34). In a complex reaction-time task, phentermine (an amphetamine derivative) had no effect on stimulus evaluation, slowed response selection, and speeded response execution (51).

Methylphenidate

In ADD patients, this drug can improve performance on tasks of focused attention and memory (54,123,127, 157,164). One study showed improved paired-associate learning in ADD children, with a nonsignificant trend toward impairment in control children (156). Also, methylphenidate in children with ADD apparently disrupted performance in the Wisconsin card-sort test, which requires shifting attention between different cognitive sets (39).

In healthy adults, the lower of two doses of methylphenidate facilitated the learning of Chinese characters under difficult conditions (92). In contrast, a high intravenous dose of methylphenidate impaired memory, probably due to disrupted attention during learning (173). Methylphenidate can also improve vigilance (2,33). In some studies, ERPs supplemented behavioral measures of cognition. For example, methylphenidate attenuated a fatigue-induced vigilance decrement in a visual detection task, while also influencing a late positive ERP component (P300) in a manner that implicated improved efficiency of stimulus evaluation (88,111,155). In other experiments using complexity manipulations in a choice reaction-time task, ERP changes suggested that methylphenidate improved response-related processing rather than stimulus evaluation (21,115). These opposite conclusions may reflect the differing cognitive requirements of the tasks used. In any case, the results support the idea that stimulants do more than simply improve alertness.

Caffeine

This drug, a methylxanthine, has pharmacological properties different from the other psychostimulants (15), although its effects on performance are similar in many respects (141,171). Caffeine-related improvements have been found in vigilance, letter cancellation, and divided attention tasks (8,28,114). Caffeine was found to increase the decay rate of the orientation-specific, chromatic aftereffect of McCullough (3,147). In the embedded figures task, caffeine impaired performance when the task was novel, but later facilitated performance (17). In contrast to the findings with amphetamine and methylphenidate, caffeine usually had no effect on memory (8,28,106,126). Segregating subjects on the basis of personality showed that performance on tests of verbal abilities was impaired by caffeine in introverted subjects but improved in extroverted subjects (57,128,129). These personality types are thought to have basic differences in baseline arousal (43).

Cocaine

Since Freud's early observations on cocaine (50) there have been few studies of the psychological effects of this drug, and fewer still with systematic experimental manipulations (47,48). One study deserves mention because it bears on the issue of whether stimulants affect stimulus- or response-related processes. In an auditory discrimination task, alterations in ERPs suggested that stimulus evaluation resources had been reduced due to distracting autonomic and subjective effects (69). Cocaine can also disrupt learning of a fixed sequence of key press responses (48). In another study, cocaine speeded reaction time in sleep-deprived subjects but not in rested subjects (49).

Psychostimulants in Animals

An important recent finding is that the well-known facilitatory effect of posttraining amphetamine on retention (112) is due to drug effects on the peripheral nervous system (108,109). Amphetamine facilitates retention by its actions on the adrenal gland, and epinephrine released by the adrenal gland can modulate memory—perhaps by altering the experience of stress, which ordinarily accompanies learning in these paradigms. Thus, memory facilitation may be based on an interaction between the stimulant dose and the animal's arousal state (58,59,67,68).

There are several reports of facilitated learning in animals given amphetamine: attenuated forgetting of a spatial task in rats (140), accelerated relearning of object discrimination in mice (153), better visual discrimination in mice (25), and better left-right discrimination in goldfish (136). Methylphenidate facilitated active avoidance and water maze performance in rats (87) and enhanced acquisition of serial discrimination reversals in rats, but impaired acquisition at high doses (63). In rats, caffeine facilitated maze performance in one case (135) and disrupted it in another (23).

Studies using a wide variety of paradigms have reported learning deficits with amphetamine: in monkeys (9,130,163), in rats (11,18,41,86,89,117,144), and in pigeons (151). In addition, caffeine, methylphenidate, and amphetamine impaired spatial alternation in dogs (131). However, it was suggested that some of the stimulant-induced deficits may have been secondary to motor perseveration.

Summary

Psychostimulants can clearly influence human performance by counteracting fatigue and improving vigilance. Many recent reports have explored these effects using constructs like arousal and alertness. On the other hand, better explanations might require considering arousal as a multidimensional factor, not a single parameter that varies only quantitatively (44). Nonetheless, it has been useful to suppose that stimulant effects on performance depend on whether a dose-dependent increment in arousal will approach or surpass an optimal arousal level. Further, changes in arousal might indirectly influence many other cognitive processes. Alternatively, stimulants may directly influence cognition independently of arousal effects. Studies using

ERPs and tasks that discriminate between stimulus- and response-related processing have suggested that stimulants may act more selectively than would be predicted by a simple arousal hypothesis. Finally, it has been suggested that a fundamental effect of stimulants is to facilitate overlearned or automatic cognitive operations (e.g., perseveration), while impairing performance that requires the development of new strategies or the flexible use of old ones (16,132,145).

THE OPIATE AGONISTS AND ANTAGONISTS

Recently, there has been increasing interest in the possibility that opioid peptides might modulate learning and memory in both humans and animals. Some of this work has involved the systematic manipulation of CNS opioid peptide systems by exogenous opiate agonist and antagonist drugs, and it is these studies which will be reviewed here.

For many years anecdotal reports have appeared in the literature describing an opiate-mediated impairment of mental concentration and cognition in humans (76). However, few studies have methodically attempted to investigate the effects of opiates and their antagonists on cognition in normal subjects. In one report a single dose of the opiate antagonist naltrexone improved performance on a task requiring continuous sustained attention (60). In contrast (101), another report found a naloxone-reversible improvement in performance and recall of serial learning after codeine administration. Other investigators (46) reported naloxone produced feelings of mental slowness and incompetence but did not affect performance on several cognitive tasks. Wolkowitz and Tinklenberg (177) found naloxone caused no memory or psychomotor performance decrements in normals. However, other workers (29,30) have reported disruption of memory when naloxone is administered at doses much higher than are needed to reverse the usual opiate effects (2 or 4 mg/kg i.v.). Investigation of naloxone's ability to block cognitive performance decrements from other drugs has yielded inconsistent results. For example, naloxone attenuated ethanol-induced cognitive impairment (42), but had no effect on diazepam-related performance decrements (177). It is therefore difficult to summarize the cognitive effects of opiate agonists and antagonists in normals. Nevertheless, there are indications that at high doses (e.g., 2–4 mg/kg) naloxone may disrupt learning and memory, but the effects of opiates on these functions remain unclear. Finally, it is of interest that two recent studies in normal subjects have described a systematic alteration in the ERP indices of selective attention (N100) following administration of opiate agonists and antagonists. In these studies naloxone enhanced selective attention (4), and methadone produced a decrement (83), suggesting a specific role for the CNS opioid peptides in the capacity for selective attention in humans.

Opiate Agonists and Antagonists in Animals

The possibility that the opioid peptide systems are involved in learning and memory has generated a number of studies in animals. Until recently, few generalizations could

be drawn from this research, and the literature was characterized by replication failures, conflicting reports, and controversy. This circumstance is undoubtedly due to the enormous complexity of the area and also to inconsistencies in methodology between the studies (e.g., different experimental learning paradigms, issues of dose and timing of drug administration, genetic factors, and species differences).

The literature has been especially confusing in studies on the effects of opiate agonists on learning and memory. For example, Mondadori et al. (113) found posttrial administration of morphine facilitated learning and memory of a one-trial passive avoidance test, but only when the drug was administered at medium (40 mg/kg) or relatively high (100 mg/kg) doses. At other doses, morphine was either ineffective or had the opposite effect by impairing memory retention (27,113). Beatty (10) observed no effect of morphine on retention of spatial memory. Similarly, Rodgers et al. (133) reported no morphine (0.5–5.0 mg/kg) effect on hot-plate avoidance when administered posttrial, nor was there an effect on memory at retesting 48 to 72 hr later. Jacobs et al. (75) found postconditioning administration of morphine did not significantly alter memory retention of a previously acquired taste aversion. All of these authors concluded that their findings were inconsistent with an involvement of opioid peptides in memory processes.

However, other groups have reported that opiates disrupted learning and memory. In one study, both morphine and heroin impaired long-term memory of discrimination learning when the drugs were administered before and after training (24). Subsequent studies by Castellano (26) demonstrated a dose-dependent effect of morphine, given prior to training, on memory of pattern discrimination. When administered after training, morphine disrupted memory for passive avoidance learning in a dose-dependent way (>1.0 mg/kg). Izquierdo (72) reported that posttraining administration of subanalgesic doses of opiates produced retrograde amnesia, which was reversed by naloxone. Mauk et al. (110) found morphine abolished an undertrained, but not an overtrained, classically conditioned eyeblink response, and this effect was also immediately reversed by naloxone. These authors concluded that the opioid peptides can affect memory in certain learning paradigms, especially when performance depends on conditioned fear.

Studies using opiate antagonists, such as naloxone, have resulted in more consistent agreement and convergence of findings. Despite some reports to the contrary (10,133), the weight of evidence in the literature suggests that naloxone can enhance memory. Izquierdo and Graudenz (74) observed that posttraining administration of naloxone facilitated memory retention and postulated that this effect was due to a central release of dopaminergic and β-adrenergic mechanisms. This same group (22) also found that naloxone reversed the retrograde amnesia caused by electroconvulsive shock (ECS). Gallagher et al. (53) reported that posttraining administration of both naloxone and dyphenorphine significantly improved spatial memory; the effect was attenuated when drugs were administered 2 hr after learning. This report is significant for showing that the facilitatory effects of antagonists on memory can be found in appetitively motivated tasks. In another study (52), pretraining administration of naloxone improved acquisition but not retention, whereas posttraining administration of naloxone did appear to improve retention. These authors hypothesized that opioid peptide effects on memory were mediated through CNS catecholaminergic systems.

Using a different research strategy, Liang et al. (95) found that naloxone reversed the impaired retention of learned avoidance by subseizure electrical stimulation of the amygdaloid area. In a related study (32), subseizure stimulation of the dentate gyrus impaired spatial memory, which could be prevented by naloxone pretreatment. Finally, naloxone administered during the posttraining period of a step down-inhibitory avoidance task produced memory facilitation, but naloxone had no effect on performance when administered before training (73). Based on these findings with naloxone, each of the previous authors hypothesized time- and dose-dependent effects of opioid peptides on memory consolidation. Some have postulated direct involvement of opioid peptides in memory processes, whereas others suggest that the observed effects are secondary to influences on various CNS neurotransmitter systems. Of particular interest in this regard is recent work linking opioid peptides to central cholinergic mechanisms (5,71), which in turn has stimulated clinical trials of naloxone in Alzheimer's disease.

In summary, the literature supports the conclusion that opioid peptides affect learning and memory, either directly or indirectly. Studies involving naloxone are the most consistent, and they suggest that naloxone has memory-enhancing properties that are time and dose dependent and observable across a range of tasks. There is also evidence, although not all studies support this idea, that the administration of opiate antagonists after learning and during memory consolidation improves retention. Less consistency exists at this time in studies with opiate agonists, which seem to be virtually evenly divided between investigations reporting memory disruption, memory enhancement, and no effect.

CONCLUSION

There is little doubt that all classes of psychoactive agents produce both generalized and specific effects on learning and memory.

As the reader will note, it is very difficult to summarize the effects of multiple classes of psychotropic drugs, some with CNS stimulant and others with CNS depressant properties, on behaviors as complex and as difficult to define and quantify as cognition and memory. As a result, the literature and research in this very important area of investigation can be conflictual, characterized by replication failures, and inconclusive. In part, this is also due to a failure to develop a more standardized methodology for assessing cognitive and memory processes in both animals and humans. In addition, as in other areas of psychopharmacology, the differential effects of dose and timing on the exquisitely sensitive and complex behaviors of cognition compound the problem. The authors made the decision to present the data in the literature as it is and have not attempted to force a synthesis or an integration where it was not possible.

On the other hand, when a generalized confluence of findings emerged, these commonalities were highlighted and emphasized. More specifically, lithium, despite some studies to the contrary, generally produced a slowing of cognitive performance, which was felt to be due to an influence on central processing capacities. The stimulants, in general, facilitated specific components of thinking behavior by enhancing vigilance and counteracting fatigue. The opiate antagonists appeared to influence and enhance memory consolidation. The other drugs covered in this chapter appeared to produce sufficiently disparate effects on learning and memory to preclude any generalizations at this point in time.

There appear to be distinct methodological advantages in studying cognitive effects in intact, normal humans and animals. This field of scientific endeavor, which combines the methods of classical psychopharmacology with cognitive and experimental psychology, will provide in the future important probes into the understanding of the biology of cognition. Even though a number of important studies have been already reported, it remains a wide open area of scientific inquiry where there are still far more questions than potential answers.

REFERENCES

1. Altman, H. J., Nordy, D. A., and Ogren, S. O. (1984): *Psychopharmacology*, 84:496–502.
2. Aman, M. G., Vamos, M., and Werry, J. S. (1984): *Aust. NZ J. Psychiatry*, 18:86–88.
3. Amure, B. O. (1979): *J. Physiol.*, 195:32P.
4. Arnsten, A. F. T., Segal, D. S., Neville, H. J., Hillyard, S. A., Janowsky, D. S., Judd, L. L., and Bloom, F. E. (1983): *Nature*, 304:725–727.
5. Baratti, C. M., Introni, I. B., and Huggens, P. (1984): *Behav. Neurol. Biol.*, 40:155–169.
6. Barratt, E. S., Russell, G., Creson, D. and Tupin, J. (1970): *Diseases of the Nervous System*, 31:335–337.
7. Bartus, R. (1978): *Pharmac. Biochem. Behav.*, 9:353–357.
8. Battig, K., Buzzi, R., Martin, J. R., and Feierabend, J. M. (1984): *Experientia*, 40:1218–1223.
9. Bauer, R. H., and Fuster, J. M. (1978): *Pharmacol. Biochem. Behav.*, 8:243–249.
10. Beatty, W. W. (1983): *Pharmacol. Biochem. Behav.*, 19:397–401.
11. Beatty, W. W., Bierley, R. A., and Boyd, J. (1984): *Behav. Neural Biol.*, 42:169–176.
12. Bloss, J. L., and Singer, G. H. (1978): *Psychopharmacology*, 57:295–302.
13. Branconnier, R. J., and Cole, J. O. (1981): *J. Clin. Psychopharmacol.*, 1:825–855.
14. Branconnier, R. J., DeVitt, D. R., Cole, J. O., and Spera, K. F. (1982): *Neurobiology of Aging*, 3:55–59.
15. Breese, G. (1987): In *Psychopharmacology: The Third Generation of Progress*, edited by H. Y. Melzer, pp. 1387–1396. Raven Press, New York.
16. Broverman, D. M., Klaiber, E. L., Kobayashi, Y., and Vogel, W. (1968): *Psychol. Rev.*, 75:23–50.
17. Broverman, D. M., and Casagrande, E. (1982): *Psychopharmacology*, 78:252–255.
18. Buresova, O., and Bures, J. (1982): *Psychopharmacology*, 77:268–271.
19. Burns, J. T., House, R. F., Fensch, F. C., and Miller, J. G. (1967): *Science*, 155:849–851.

20. Bye, C., Clubley, M., and Peck, A. W. (1978): *Br. J. Clin. Pharmac.*, 6:155–161.
21. Callaway, E. (1983): *Psychophysiology*, 20:359–370.
22. Carrasco, M. A., Dias, R. D., and Izquierdo, I. (1982): *Beh. Neurol. Biol.*, 34:352–357.
23. Cassone, M. C., and Molinengo, L. (1981): *Life Sci.*, 29:1983–1988.
24. Castellano, C. (1975): *Psychopharmacologia*, 42:235–242.
25. Castellano, C. (1979): *Psychopharmacology*, 62:35–40.
26. Castellano, C. (1980): *Psychopharmacology*, 67:235–239.
27. Classen, W., and Mandadori, C. (1984): *Experientia*, 15:405–406.
28. Clubley, M., Bye, C. E., Henson, T. A., Peck, A. W., and Riddington, C. J. (1979): *Br. J. Clin. Pharmacol.*, 7:157–163.
29. Cohen, M. R., Cohen, R. M., Pickar, D., Weingartner, H., and Murphy, D. L. (1982): *Arch. Gen. Psychiat.*, 40:613–619.
30. Cohen, R. M., Cohen, M. R., Weingartner, H., Pickar, D., and Murphy, D. L. (1983): *Psychiatry Research*, 8:127–136.
31. Cole, J. O., and Bird, M. (1987): In: *Psychopharmacology: The Third Generation of Progress*, edited by H. Y. Meltzer. Raven Press, New York (*in press*).
32. Collier, T. J., and Routtenberg, A. (1984): *Brain. Res.*, 310:384–392.
33. Coons, H. W., Peloquin, L. J., Klorman, R., Bauer, L. O., Ryan, R. M., Perlmutter, R. A., and Salzman, L. F. (1981): *Electroencephalogr. Clin. Neurophysiol.*, 51:373–387.
34. Crabbe, J. C., Jarvik, L. F., Liston, E. H., and Jenden, D. J. (1983): *Acta Genet. Med. Gemellol.*, 32:139–149.
35. Crome, P., and Newmann, B. (1978): *J. Int. Med. Res.*, 6:430–434.
36. Davidson, A. B. and Weidley, E. (1976): *Life Sci.*, 18:1279–1284.
37. Davis, J. L., and Cherkin, A. (1979): *Psychopharmacology*, 63:269–272.
38. Drachman, D. A. (1977): *Neurology*, 27:783–790.
39. Dyme, I. Z., Sahakian, B. J., Golinko, B. E., and Rabe, E. F. (1982): *Prog. Neuropsychopharmacol. Biol. Psychiatry*, 6:269–273.
40. Egan, J., Earley, C. J., and Leonard, B. E. (1979): *Psychopharmacology*, 61:143–147.
41. Evenden, J. L., and Robbins, T. W. (1983): *Psychopharmacology*, 80:67–73.
42. Ewing, J. A., Mills, K. C., Bisgrove, E. Z., and McManus, K. (1984): *Adv. Alcohol Subst. Abuse*, 3:47–59.
43. Eysenck, H. J. (1967): *The Biological Basis of Personality*, edited by Thomas. Springfield, Ill.
44. Eysenck, M. W., and Folkard, S. (1980): *J. Exp. Psychol. Gen.*, 109:32–41.
45. Fernandez-Tome, M. P., Sanchez-Blazquez, P., and Rio, J. (1979): *Psychopharmacology*, 61:43–47.
46. File, S. E., and Silverstone, T. (1981): *Psychopharmacology*, 74(4):353–354.
47. Fischman, M. (1987): In: *Psychopharmacology: The Third Generation of Progress*, edited by H. Y. Meltzer, pp. 1543–1554. Raven Press, New York.
48. Fischman, M. W. (1984): *Natl. Inst. Drug Abuse Res. Monogr. Ser.*, 50:72–91.
49. Fischman, M. W., and Schuster, C. R. (1980): *Psychopharmacology*, 72:1–8.
50. Freud, S. (1974): *Cocaine Papers*, edited by R. Byck. New American Library, New York.
51. Frowein, H. W. (1981): *Acta Psychologica*, 47:105–115.
52. Fulginiti, S., and Cancela, L. M. (1983): *Psychopharmacology*, 9:45–48.
53. Gallagher, M., King, R. A., and Young, N. B. (1983): *Science*, 221:975–976.
54. Gan, J., and Cantwell, D. P. (1982): *J. Am. Acad. Child Psychiatry*, 21:237–242.
55. Gartside, I. B., Lippold, O. C. J., and Meldrum, B. S. (1966): *Electroenceph. Clin. Neurophysiol.*, 20:382–390.
56. Gentil, V., Alevizos, B., Felix-Gentil, M., and Lader, M. (1978): *Br. J. Clin. Pharmac.*, 5:536–538.
57. Gilliland, K. (1980): *J. Res. Personal.*, 14:482–492.
58. Gold, P. E., and McGaugh, J. L. (1975): In: *Short-Term Memory*, edited by D. Deutsch, and J. A. Deutsch, pp. 355–378. Academic Press, New York.
59. Gold, P. E., and van Buskirk, R. (1978): *Behav. Biol.*, 24:168–184.
60. Gritz, E. R., Shiffman, S. M., Jarvik, M. E., Schlesinger, J., and Charuvastra, V. C. (1976): *Clin. Pharmacol. Therap.*, 19:773–776.
61. Hamilton, M. J., Bush, M., Smith, P., and Peck, A. W. (1982): *Br. J. Clin. Pharmac.*, 14:791–797.
62. Hamilton, M. J., Smith, P. R., and Peck, A. W. (1983): *Br. J. Clin. Pharm.*, 15:367–374.
63. Handley, G. W., and Calhoun, W. H. (1978): *Psychopharmacology*, 57:115–117.
64. Hano, J., Vetulani, J., Sansone, M., and Oliverio, A. (1981): *Psychopharmacology*, 73:265–268.
65. Hartmann, E., Orzack, M. H., and Branconnier, R. (1977): *Psychopharmacology*, 53:185–189.
66. Harvey, J. A. (1987): In: *Psychopharmacology: The Third Generation of Progress*, edited by H. Y. Meltzer, pp. 1485–1492. Raven Press, New York.
67. Haycock, J. W., van Buskirk, R., and Gold, P. E. (1977): *Psychopharmacology* 54:21–24.
68. Hellman, P. A., Crider, A., and Solomon, P. R. (1983): *Behav. Neurosci.*, 97:1017–1021.
69. Herning, R. I., Jones, R. T., Hooker, W. D., and Tulunay, F. C. (1985): *Psychopharmacology*, 87:178–185.
70. Hurst, P. M., Radlow, R., Chubb, N. C., and Bagley, S. K. (1969): *Am. J. Psychology*, 82:307–319.
71. Introni, I. B., and Baratti, C. M. (1985): *Behav. Neurol. Biol.*, 41:152–163.
72. Izquierdo, I. (1982): *Braz. J. Med. Biol. Res.*, 15:119–134.
73. Izquierdo, I., and Dias, R. D. (1985): *Psychoneuroendocrinology*, 10:165–172.
74. Izquierdo, I., and Graudenz, M. (1980): *Psychopharmacology*, 67:265–268.
75. Jacobs, M. J., Zellner, D. A., LoLordo, V. M., and Biley, A. L. (1981): *Pharmacol. Biochem. Behav.*, 14:779–785.
76. Jaffe, J. H., and Martin, W. R. (1980): In: *Pharmacological Basis of Therapeutics*, 6th edition, edited by A. G. Gilman, L. S. Goodman, and A. Gilman, pp. 494–534. Macmillan, New York.
77. Johnson, F. N. (1979): In: *Lithium: Controversies and Unresolved Issues*, edited by T. B. Cooper, S. Gershon, N. S. Kline, and M. Schou, pp. 945–951. Excerpta Medica, Amsterdam.
78. Johnson, F. N.: In: *Lithium Research and Therapy*, edited by F. N. Johnson, pp. 339–350. Academic Press, London.
79. Judd, L. L., Hubbard, B., Janowsky, D. S., Huey, L. Y., and Attewell, P. A. (1977): *Arch. Gen. Psychiat.*, 34:346–351.
80. Judd, L. L., Hubbard, B., Janowsky, D. S., Huey, L. Y., and Takahashi, K. I. (1977): *Arch. Gen. Psychiat.*, 34:355–357.
81. Judd, L. L. (1979): *Arch. Gen. Psychiat.*, 36:860–865.
82. Judd, L. L., Rausch, J. L., Janowsky, D. S., and Huey, L. Y. (1981): Effect of imipramine on cognition in normals. Paper presented at the annual meeting of the American Psychiatric Association, New Orleans.
83. Judd, L. L., Segal, D. S., Budnick, B., McAdams, L. A., Risch, S. C., Janowsky, D. S., and Hillyard, S. A. (1987): *Psychopharmacol. Bull. (in press)*.
84. Karniol, I. G., Dalton, J., and Lader, M. H. (1978): *Psychopharmacology*, 57:289–294.
85. Kazdova, E., and Dlabac, A. (1975): *Activ. Nerv. Sup.*, 17:284–285.
86. Kesner, R. P., Bierley, R. A., and Pebbles, P. (1981): *Pharmacol. Biochem. Behav.*, 15:673–676.
87. Kinney, L., and Vorhees, C. V. (1979): *Pharmacol. Biochem. Behav.*, 10:437–439.
88. Klorman, R., Bauer, L. O., Coons, H. W., Lewis, J. L., Peloquin, J., Perlmutter, R. A., Ryan, R. M., Salzman, L. F., and Strauss, J. (1984): *Psychopharmacol. Bull.*, 20:3–9.
89. Koek, W., and Smangen, J. L. (1984): *Psychopharmacology*, 83:346–350.
90. Kornetsky, C. (1958): *J. Pharmacol.*, 123:216–219.
91. Korpf, D., and Muller-Oerlinghausen, B. (1979): *Acta Psychiat. Scan.*, 59:97–124.

92. Kupietz, S. S., Richardson, E., Gadow, K. D., and Winsberg, B. G. (1980): *Psychopharmacology,* 69:69–72.

93. Kuribara, H., and Tadokoro, S. (1976): *Japan J. Pharmacol.,* 26:693–702.

94. Lalonde, R., and Vikis-Freibergs, V. (1985): *Pharmac. Biochem. Behav.,* 22:377–382.

95. Liang, K. C., Messing, R. B., and McGaugh, J. L. (1983): *Brain Res.,* 271:41–49.

96. Liljequist, R., Linnoila, M., and Mattila, M. J. (1974): *Psychopharmacologia,* 39:181–186.

97. Liljequist, R., Linnoila, M., Mattila, M. J., Saario, J., and Seppala, T. (1975): *Psychopharmacologia,* 44:205–208.

98. Liljequist, R., Linnoila, M., and Mattila, M. J. (1978): *Europ. J. Clin. Pharmacol.,* 13:339–343.

99. Liljequist, R., Seppala, T., and Mattila, M. J. (1978): *Br. J. Clin. Pharmac.,* 5:149–153.

100. Liljequist, R., Mattila, M. J., and Linnoila, M. (1981): *Acta Pharmacol. et Toxicol,* 48:190–192.

101. Liljequist, R. (1981): *Eur. J. Clin. Pharmacol.,* 20:99–107.

102. Linnoila, M., Saario, I., and Maki, M. (1974): *Europ. J. Clin. Pharmacol.,* 7:337–342.

103. Linnoila, M., Johnson, J., Dubyoski, T., Ross, R., Buchsbaum, M., Potter, W., and Weingartner, H. (1983): *Acta Psychiatr. Scand. Suppl. 308,* 68:175–181.

104. Linnoila, M., Johnson, J., Dubyoski, K., Buchsbaum, M. S., Schneinin, M., and Kilts, C. (1984): *Br. J. Clin. Pharamac.,* 18:1095–1205.

105. Linnoila, M., Dubyoski, K. V., Rawlings, R. R., Rudorfer, M. V., and Eckardt, M. J. (1985): *J. Clin. Psychopharmac.,* 5:148–153.

106. Loke, W. H., Hinrichs, J. V., and Ghoneim, M. M. (1985): *Psychopharmacology,* 87:344–350.

107. Lucki, I., and Frazer, A. (1985): *Psychopharmacology,* 85:253–259.

108. Martinez, J. L., Jenson, R. A., Messing, R. B., Vasquez, B. J., Soumireu-Mourat, B., Geddes, D., Liang, K. C., and McGaugh, J. L. (1980): *Brain Res.,* 182:157–166.

109. Martinez, J. L., Vasquez, B. J., Rigter, H., Messing, R. B., Jensen, R. A., Liang, K. C., and McGaugh, J. L. (1980): *Brain Res.,* 195:433–443.

110. Mauk, M. D., Warren, J. T., and Thompson, R. F. (1982): *Science,* 216:434–436.

111. McCarthy, G., and Donchin, E. (1981): *Science,* 211:77–80.

112. McGaugh, J. L. (1973): *Ann. Rev. Pharmacol.,* 13:229–241.

113. Mondadori, C., and Wasser, P. D. (1979): *Psychopharmacology,* 63:297–300.

114. Moskowitz, H., and Burns, M. (1981): In: *Alcohol, Drugs, and Traffic Safety,* Vol. III, edited by L. Goldberg, pp. 969–983. Almquist and Wiksell International, Stockholm.

115. Naylor, H., Halliday, R., and Callaway, E. (1985): *Psychopharmacology,* 86:90–95.

116. Oades, R. D. (1981): *Biological Psychology,* 12:77–85.

117. Oades, R., Taghqouti, K., Simon, H., and Le Moal, M. (1985): *Psychopharmacology,* 85:123–128.

118. Ogura, C., Kishimoto, A., Mizukawa, R., Kunimoto, N., Hazama, H., Ryoke, K., Takeda, A., Honma, H., and Kawalara, K. (1983): *Neuropsychobiology,* 10:103–107.

119. Oka, M., Kamei, C., and Shimizu, M. (1977): *Japan J. Pharmacol.,* 27:807–815.

120. Parrott, A. C., Hindmarch, I., and Stonier, P. D. (1982): *Eur. J. Clin. Pharmacol.,* 23:309–313.

121. Peck, A., and Hamilton, M. (1983): *J. Clin. Psychiat.,* 44:202–205.

122. Peck, A. W., Bye, C. E., Clubley, M., Henson, T., and Riddington, C. (1979): *Br. J. Clin. Pharmac.,* 7:469–478.

123. Peeke, S., Halliday, R., Callaway, E., Prael, R., and Reus, V. (1984): *J. Clin. Psychopharmacol.,* 4:82–88.

124. Rapoport, J. L., Buchsbaum, M. S., Weingartner, H., Zahn, T. P., Ludlow, C., and Mikkelsen, E. J. (1980): *Arch. Gen. Psychiat.,* 37:933–943.

125. Rapoport, J. L., Buchsbaum, M. S., Zahn, T. P., Weingartner, H., Ludlow, C., and Mikkelsen, E. J. (1978): *Science,* 199:560–563.

126. Rapoport, J. L., Jensvold, M., Elkins, R., Buchsbaum, M. S., Weingartner, H., Ludlow, C., Zahn, T. P., Berg, C. J., and Neims, A. H. (1981): *J. Nerv. Ment. Dis.,* 169:726–732.

127. Rapport, M. D., Stoner, G., Dupaul, G. J., Birmingham, B. K., and Tucker, S. (1985): *J. Abnorm. Child Psychol.,* 13:227–243.

128. Revelle, W., Amaral, P., and Turriff, S. (1976): *Science,* 192:149–150.

129. Revelle, W., Humphreys, M. S., Simon, L., and Gilliland, K. (1980): *J. Exp. Psychol. Gen.,* 109:1–31.

130. Ridley, R. M., Baker, H. F., and Weight, M. L. (1980): *Psychopharmacology,* 67:241–244.

131. Risner, M. E., and Jones, B. E. (1979): *Psychopharmacology,* 63:137–141.

132. Robbins, T. W., and Sahakian, B. J. (1979): *Neuropharmacology,* 18:931–950.

133. Rodgers, R. J., Randall, J., and Pittock, F. (1985): *Neuropharmacology,* 324:333–336.

134. Ross, R. J., Smallberg, S., and Weingartner, H. (1984): *Psychiat. Res.,* 12:89–97.

135. Roussinov, K. S., and Yonkov, D. I. (1976): *Acta Physiol. Pharmacol. Bulg.,* 2:61–68.

136. Sahagian, D. E., and Ingle, D. J. (1977): *Science,* 198:67–69.

137. Saletu, B., Grunberger, J., and Rajna, P. (1983): *Br. J. Clin. Pharmac.,* 15:3695s–3845s.

138. Saletu, B., Grunberger, J., Rajna, P., and Karobath, M. (1980): *J. Neural Transm.* 49:63–86.

139. Sanger, D. J. (1985): *Pharmac. Biochem. Behav.,* 23:591–593.

140. Sara, S. J., and Deweer, B. (1982): *Behav. Neural Biol.,* 36:146–160.

141. Sawyer, D. A., Julia, H. L., and Turin, A. C. (1982): *J. Behav. Med.,* 5:415–439.

142. Schou, M. (1966): *J. Psychiat. Res.,* 6:67–95.

143. Schou, M., Amdisen, A., and Thomsen, K. (1968): In: *D. E. Psychiatria Progrediente, Volume II,* edited by P. Baudes, E. Peterova, and V. Sedivec. Zapadoveski Nakladatelstvi, Plzen, Czechoslavakia.

144. Schrot, J., and Thomas, J. R. (1983): *Pharmacol. Biochem. Behav.,* 18:529–534.

145. Segal, D. S., and Janowsky, D. S. (1978): In: *Psychopharmacology, A Generation of Progress,* edited by M. A. Lipton, A. DiMascio, and K. F. Killam, pp. 1113–1123. Raven Press, New York.

146. Seppala, T. (1977): *Annals Clin. Res.,* 9:66–72.

147. Shute, C. C. (1978): *J. Physiol.,* 278:47P.

148. Small, J. G., Milstein, A., Perez, H. D., Small, I. F., and Moore, D. F. (1972): *Biological Psychiatry,* 5(1):65–77.

149. Smith, D. F. (1977): *Pharmakopsychiat.,* 10:79–88.

150. Smith, D. F. (1979): In: *Lithium: Controversies and Unresolved Issues,* edited by T. B. Cooper, S. Gershon, N. S. Kline, and M. Schou, pp. 936–944. Excerpta Medica, Amsterdam.

151. Spetch, M. L., and Treit, D. (1984): *Pharmac. Biochem. Behav.,* 21:663–666.

152. Spiegel, R. (1979): In: *Pharmacology of the States of Awareness,* edited by P. Passouant and I. Oswald, pp. 189–201. Pergamon Press, Oxford.

153. Squire, L. R. (1979): *Brain Res.,* 177:401–406.

154. Squire, L. R., Judd, L. L., Janowsky, D. S., and Huey, L. Y. (1980): *Am. J. Psychiat.,* 137:1042–1046.

155. Strauss, J., Lewis, J. L., Klorman, R., Peloquin, L. J., Perlmutter, R. A., and Salzman, L. F. (1984): *Psychophysiology,* 21:609–621.

156. Swanson, J. M., and Kinsbourne, M. (1976): *Science,* 192:1354–1357.

157. Swanson, J. M., Sandman, C. A., Deutsch, C., and Baren, M. (1983): *Pediatrics,* 72:49–55.

158. Szabadi, E., Bradshaw, C. M., and Gaszner, P. (1980): *Psychopharmacology,* 68:125–134.

159. Taboada, M. E., Sonto, M., Hawkins, H., and Monti, J. M. (1979): *Psychopharmacology,* 62:83–88.

160. Theofilopolous, N., Szabadi, E., and Bradshaw, C. M. (1984): *Br. J. Clin. Pharmac.,* 18:135–144.

161. Thompson, D. M. (1976): *Pharmac. Biochem. Behav.,* 4:671–677.

162. Thompson, P. J., and Trimble, M. R. (1982): *Psychological Medicine,* 12:539–548.
163. Thompson, D. M., and Moerschbaecher, J. M. (1984): *Pharmacol. Biochem. Behav.,* 20:601–607.
164. Thurston, C. M., and Sobol, M. P. (1979): *J. Abnormal Child Psychology,* 7:471–481.
165. Usuda, S., Nishikori, K., Noshiro, O., and Maeno, H. (1981): *Psychopharmacology,* 73:103–109.
166. Warrington, S. J., Ankier, S. I., and Turner, P. (1984): *Br. J. Clin. Pharmac.,* 18:549–557.
167. Weingartner, H., Rapoport, J. L., Buchsbaum, M. S., Bunney, W. E., Jr., Ebert, M. H., Mikkelsen, E. J., and Caine, E. D. (1980): *J. Abnorm. Psychol.,* 89:25–37.
168. Weingartner, H., Buchsbaum, M. S., and Linnoila, M. (1983): *Life Sci.,* 33:2159–2163.
169. Weingartner, H., Rudorfer, M. V., Buchsbaum, M. S., and Linnoila, M. (1983): *Science,* 221:472–474.
170. Weingartner, H., Rudorfer, M. V., and Linnoila, M. (1985): *Psychopharmacology,* 86(4):472–474.
171. Weiss, B., and Laties, V. G. (1962): *Pharm. Rev.,* 14:1–36.
172. Weitzner, M. (1965): *J. Psychol.,* 60:71–79.
173. Wetzel, C. D., Squire, L. R., and Janowsky, D. S. (1981): *Behavioral and Neural Biology,* 31:413–424.
174. White, K., Bohart, R., Whipple, K., and Royd, J. (1979): *Int. Pharmacopsychiat.,* 14:176–183.
175. Wise, R. A. (1982): *Behavioral and Brain Sciences,* 5:39–87.
176. Wittenborn, J. R., Flaherty, C. F., McGough, W. E., Bossange, K. A., and Nash, R. J. (1976): *Psychopharmacology,* 51:85–90.
177. Wolkowitz, D. M., and Tinklenberg, J. R. (1985): *Psychopharmacology,* 85(2):221–223.

Psychopharmacology:
The Third Generation of Progress,
edited by Herbert Y. Meltzer.
Raven Press, New York © 1987.

CHAPTER **157**

Effects of Drugs and Neuropeptides on Sexual and Maternal Behavior in Mammals

Cort A. Pedersen and Arthur J. Prange, Jr.

Reproductive behaviors include sexual behavior and maternal behavior. These behaviors have multiple determinants. Both the prenatal stress and the perinatal gonadal steroid environment experienced by neonates influence sexual differentiation of later reproductive behaviors (20,70). In adult animals, gonadal steroids directly control reproductive behaviors (13,20,53). However, male sexual behavior and maternal behavior are also shaped by experience (34,53). In this chapter, we do not review investigation in these important areas. Rather, we review studies in mammals of the effects on reproductive behaviors of neuropeptides or drugs that alter classical neurotransmitter systems. We discuss steroid and experiential factors only to the degree necessary to understand the experimental conditions under which drugs and neuropeptides have been tested.

DESCRIPTION AND QUANTIFICATION OF BEHAVIOR

We briefly discuss quantification of sexual and maternal behavior in the rat because most studies of drug and neuropeptide effects on these behaviors have been conducted in this species.

Female Sexual Behavior

Female sexual behavior includes proceptive behaviors, which stimulate sexual advances from males, and receptive behaviors, which facilitate attempts by males to copulate. Sexually receptive female rats respond to mounting by males by adopting a lordosis posture, which affords access to the vagina. Most studies of drug and neuropeptide effects on female sexual behavior in rats have focused on the lordosis response. Meyerson et al. (34) have described this behavior and its quantification; Pfaff and Modianos (46) have reviewed its neural control.

Large doses of estrogen alone or small doses of estrogen followed by progesterone 1 to 6 hr prior to behavioral testing produce high rates of proceptive behavior and lordosis in ovariectomized female rats. Facilitating effects of substances on lordosis have generally been tested in ovariectomized rats treated with low doses of estrogen that by themselves do not produce high rates of lordosis. Inhibitory effects of substances on lordosis have generally been tested in ovariectomized rats treated with large doses of estrogen or with estrogen and progesterone. Reviews of the role of ovarian steroids in female sexual behavior are available (13,20).

Male Sexual Behavior

The intact, sexually experienced male rat initiates copulation shortly after discovering a sexually receptive female. The male repeatedly mounts the female from behind. During a mount the male grasps the flanks of the female with his forelegs and displays rapid pelvic thrusting. If he achieves intromission, he quickly dismounts by jumping backward. Almost immediately he remounts. After a number of intromissions, the male ejaculates. The ejaculation is accompanied by prolonged and intense grasping of the flanks of the female and a slower dismount followed by licking of his genitals. After a period of recovery, the male resumes mounting and intromitting until he ejaculates again. Several dimensions of this sequence of events have been measured by investigators to quantify the effects of treatments.

Most studies have utilized intact males, although some work has been done with castrate, testosterone-treated males. Treatments often affect different parameters of male sexual behavior in experienced versus inexperienced males, vigorous versus sluggish copulators, or, in castrate males, in those receiving optimal versus suboptimal testosterone replacement. Hart and Leedy (26) have described the neural basis of male sexual behavior; Meyerson et al. (34) have reviewed the issues that pertain to the measurement of male sexual behavior.

Maternal Behavior

Maternal behavior is composed of a number of coordinated component behaviors that result in the cleaning, warming, feeding, and protection of young animals until they are able to take care of themselves. Detailed descriptions of maternal behavior in mammalian species have been provided by Rheingold (50). Most investigators determine the presence or absence of one or a few of the component behaviors to determine if maternal behavior is present, assuming that the components of maternal behavior tend to occur as a unit so that if one component is present the others are as well. Some investigators, however, record the presence or absence of several components of maternal behavior. Some investigators also measure the intensity of component behaviors rather than only their presence or absence.

The rapid onset of maternal behavior that occurs postpartum in rats depends on the rising estrogen and falling progesterone levels that occur during the last few days of gestation. Treatment of naive, nulliparous female rats on a schedule that mimics the ovarian steroid changes that occur in late gestation markedly shortens the latency of onset of maternal behavior. Shortly after parturition, the maintenance of maternal behavior becomes independent of ovarian steroids. Once postpartum rats acquire some mothering experience, maternal behavioral responses to pups reemerge rapidly even after long periods of separation from pups. Current knowledge of the role of ovarian steroids and experience in the expression of maternal behavior is well summarized by Rosenblatt et al. (53).

The effects of some drug or neuropeptide treatments on maternal behavior have been tested in parturient or lactating animals, and other treatments have been tested in ovarian steroid-treated nulliparous animals. Some treatments have been addressed to the onset of maternal behavior and some to established maternal behavior, its maintenance or its reemergence; few treatments have been addressed to both. Because the mechanisms of onset appear to differ in some ways from the mechanisms of maintenance or reemergence

of maternal behavior (53), the effects of drug or neuropeptide treatments may differ between these phases of maternal response.

EFFECTS OF DRUGS ON SEXUAL AND MATERNAL BEHAVIOR

Serotonin-Active Drugs

Sexual Behavior

Peripheral administration of a variety of monoamine oxidase inhibitors (MAOIs) diminished both lordosis and mounting behavior (34,60). Doses of MAOIs sufficient to block sexual behavior increased brain serotonin (5-HT) levels more than other monoamine levels (34). Peripheral administration of the 5-HT precursor 5-HTP, 5-HT agonists, the 5-HT releaser fenfluramine, or 5-HT reuptake blockers inhibited male and female sexual behavior (34,60). Depletion of 5-HT by administration of the tryptophan hydroxylase inhibitor para-chlorophenylalanine (PCPA) increased copulatory behavior (34,60). Peripheral administration of 5-HT antagonists increased both lordosis and mounting (34). Implants of the serotonergic antagonists methysergide or cianserin into the preoptic–anterior hypothalamic area, posterior hypothalamus, medial forebrain bundle, corticomedial amygdala, or dorsal hippocampus or infusion of methysergide into the medial preoptic area (MPOA) or arcuate–ventromedial area of the hypothalamus (ARC–VMH) increased lordosis, whereas infusion of 5-HT into the MPOA or ARC–VMH suppressed lordosis (14,21,34). Destruction of ascending axons from serotonergic neurons in the midbrain with local application of the specific neurotoxin 5,7-dihydroxytryptamine (5,7-DHT) either moderately increased proceptive and receptive behavior or had no effect on female sexual behavior (34). Intrahypothalamic injection of 5,7-DHT increased lordosis (27). Thus, in the rat, there is considerable experimental agreement that treatments that increase central 5-HT neurotransmission inhibit whereas treatments that decrease central 5-HT neurotransmission facilitate sexual behavior.

The role of 5-HT in sexual behavior in other species is less clear. Although fenfluramine inhibited lordosis, administration of PCPA and methysergide had no effect or inhibited lordosis in guinea pigs (14,34). Intracerebroventricular (i.c.v.) infusion of the 5-HT agonist quipazine inhibited lordosis in guinea pigs when given after but not before the onset of sexual receptivity (20). para-Chlorophenylalanine treatment in rhesus monkeys has been reported by different investigators to restore proceptivity after adrenalectomy (19) or to decrease sexual receptivity (7). Administration of 5-HTP decreased proceptive behavior, and chlorimipramine treatment, which decreases 5-HT reuptake, decreased proceptive and receptive behavior in rhesus monkeys (19).

The effect on sexual behavior in the rat of peripheral administration of 5-HT agonists such as lysergic acid diethylamide (LSD) varied with dose. High doses decreased whereas lower doses enhanced both female and male copulatory behavior (34). Low doses are thought to stimulate preferentially autoreceptors and thereby decrease transmission in 5-HT synapses, whereas high doses mimic high rates of neurotransmission by preferentially stimulating postsynaptic receptors (34). The effects of 5-HT on lordosis appear to be progesterone dependent. Higher doses of 5-HTP and other agonists were more effective in inhibiting lordosis in rats treated with estrogen and progesterone than in rats treated with estrogen alone (34). Moreover, lordosis-enhancing effects of low doses of LSD were increased by progesterone treatment (34). It has been hypothesized that progesterone enhances sexual behavior by increasing presynaptic 5-HT activity (34).

Maternal Behavior

Chlorimipramine, which blocks reuptake of 5-HT, had no effect on maternal behavior in rats treated throughout gestation or lactation (10). Administration of 5-HT increased the latency to kill pups but did not decrease the high incidence of infanticide in olfactory bulbectomized mice (38).

Catecholamine-Active Drugs

Sexual Behavior

Two observations—that amphetamine, a potent releaser of catecholamines, suppressed lordosis and that α-methyl-para-tyrosine, an inhibitor of catecholamine synthesis, increased lordosis but decreased mounting—stimulated investigations into the role of catecholamines in sexual behavior (34). Peripheral administration of dopamine (DA) agonists or precursors to rats inhibited lordosis at higher doses and facilitated at lower doses. Meyerson et al. (34) argued that lower doses of DA agonists facilitated lordosis by selectively affecting presynaptic autoreceptors, thereby decreasing DA neurotransmission. Low doses of the DA agonist bromocriptine increased proceptive behavior in female rhesus monkeys (19). In rats, DA antagonists facilitated lordosis (the immobile component of female sexual behavior) but inhibited proceptive behavior (the mobile component) (34). Dopamine antagonists did not increase lordosis in guinea pigs (34). Infusion of DA agonists into the MPOA or ARC–VMH facilitated lordosis in rats, whereas infusion of antagonists into these brain sites inhibited lordosis (36). The difference in effects on lordosis of peripheral versus intrahypothalamic administration of DA agonists and antagonists suggests that peripheral drug effects may be mediated primarily at extrahypothalamic brain sites such as the basal ganglia.

In contrast to their effects on lordosis, L-dopa and DA agonists such as apomorphine, lisuride, and pergolide increased mounting behavior (34,60). Dopamine antagonists such as pimozide or haloperidol decreased male sexual behavior and blocked many of the facilitating effects of apomorphine or L-dopa (80). Dopamine neurotransmission appears to play an important role in penile erection and ejaculation independent of its facilitating role in copulatory behavior. Drugs that stimulate DA receptors (amantadine, L-dopa, amphetamine, apomorphine) produced repeated

erections followed by ejaculation in male rats housed alone or with other males (60).

The effects on sexual behavior of drugs that alter norepinephrine (NE) neurotransmission are difficult to fit into a clear mechanistic scheme. Peripheral administration of α-adrenergic agonists inhibited, whereas β-adrenergic agonists facilitated, male sexual behavior in rats (14). Clonidine, an α_2 agonist, inhibited lordosis but decreased the latency to mount while decreasing frequency of mounts in rats (34). However, clonidine facilitated lordosis in guinea pigs, apparently by acting at postsynaptic α-adrenergic receptors (20). Infusion of the β-adrenergic agonist isoproterenol or NE or epinephrine into the MPOA or ARC–VMH facilitated lordosis, whereas infusions of the α-adrenergic agonist methoxamine inhibited lordosis (14). Peripheral administration of α-adrenergic antagonists inhibited lordosis; on male copulatory behavior they were either facilitative (yohimbine) or without effect (phenoxybenzamine) (12,34). β-Adrenergic antagonists facilitated lordosis but inhibited male copulatory behavior (34). Ward et al. [as cited by Meyerson et al. (34)] reported that implantation of the β-adrenergic antagonist LB-46 into hypothalamic sites increased lordosis, whereas the α-adrenergic antagonist phentolamine had no effect. In contrast, Foreman and Moss [as cited by Crowley and Zemlan (14)] observed that infusion of phentolamine and phenoxybenzamine into the MPOA or ARC–VMH enhanced lordosis, whereas infusions of the β antagonist propranolol decreased lordosis. The β blocker oxprenolol increased copulatory behavior in male rhesus monkeys (19).

Treatments that alter NE levels in the brain affect sexual behavior in differing ways. Lesioning of the ventral noradrenergic bundle with 6-hydroxydopamine (6-OHDA) inhibited lordosis but had no effect on proceptive behavior in rats (34). Infusions of 6-OHDA into the spinal subarachnoid space suppressed female receptivity and proceptivity as well as some parameters of male mounting behavior in rats, suggesting that descending NE pathways mediate sexual behavior (24). Suppression of NE synthesis with dopamine β-hydroxylase inhibitors decreased lordosis in guinea pigs but increased frequency of mounts in rats (20,32,34). Chronic administration of phenylethylamine derivatives, which selectively increase the NE content of the MPOA, increased male-to-male mounting (59). Administration of the NE precursor dihydrophenylserine in rats pretreated with pargyline and the decarboxylase inhibitor MK486 inhibited male copulatory behavior (34).

Maternal Behavior

Administration of DA agonists produced no deficits of onset or maintenance of maternal behavior in rats but decreased maternal aggression and other components of maternal behavior in hamsters (53,55). Dopamine antagonists, however, inhibited maternal behavior. Chlorpromazine treatment in lactating rats diminished contact with dispersed pups and nest-building behavior (22). Haloperidol inhibited in a dose-related manner both the onset and the reemergence of several components of maternal behavior in ovarian steroid-treated (43) and postpartum rats (23). Haloperidol inhibited pup retrieval more than food-seeking behavior, suggesting a specific effect on maternal motivation (23). Apomorphine reinstated pup retrieval in rats treated with haloperidol.

Amphetamine administration in lactating rats inhibited maternal behavior over a dose range that increased locomotor behavior (47). Low doses of amphetamine in vervet monkey mothers eliminated initiation of physical and visual contact with their infants (58). Chronic administration of imipramine, which decreases reuptake of NE, diminished "overall" maternal behavior in lactating rats (10).

Administration of 6-OHDA prior to impregnation, resulting in 50% or greater NE and DA depletion in the brain, decreased latency to retrieve and increased aggression in postpartum rats (67). However, i.c.v. administration of 6-OHDA 2 days prepartum, resulting in a 30% or greater depletion of brain NE, produced marked deficits in nursing and nest-building behavior in rats. The same treatment 4 days postpartum had no deleterious effect on the maintenance of maternal behavior (14). In rats treated with 6-OHDA and desmethyimipramine (to spare NE neurons), a 30% or greater depletion of brain DA was associated with prolonged crouching in the nursing posture but with no other changes in maternal behavior (48). Amphetamine effects on maternal behavior were the same in these animals as in controls receiving no 6-OHDA, suggesting that amphetamine effects may be mediated primarily by NE (48).

Acetylcholine-Active Drugs

Sexual Behavior

Lordosis was decreased 30 min after, but increased 3 hr after, peripheral administration of muscarinic agonists (34). Because the inhibitory effects of muscarinic agonists were increased by MAOIs and reversed by *para*-chlorophenylalanine (PCPA) but not by α-methyl-*para*-tyrosine, it was concluded that 5-HT but not catecholamines mediated muscarinic inhibition of lordosis (34). Hypophysectomy prevented the delayed effects of muscarinic agonists, suggesting that facilitation of lordosis may have resulted from release of adrenal progestins (34). Peripheral administration of the muscarinic antagonist atropine inhibited male copulatory behavior (34). Peripheral administration of nicotine has been reported to increase lordosis and either to facilitate or inhibit male sexual behavior (34). Implantation or infusion of carbachol or atropine into hypothalamic and limbic sites increased lordosis (34,52).

Maternal Behavior

Infusion of atropine i.c.v. had a dose-related inhibitory effect on the onset of maternal behavior in ovarian steroid-treated nulliparous rats; the nicotinic antagonist hexamethonium was ineffective (44). Over the same dose range, atropine had no effect on the reemergence of maternal behavior in experienced rat mothers separated from pups for 24 hr.

γ-Aminobutyric Acid-Active Drugs

Sexual Behavior

Infusion of the γ-aminobutyric acid (GABA) receptor blocker picrotoxin into the substantia nigra inhibited the high rates of lordosis that occur with bilateral lesions of the septum (30). Intranigral infusion of hydrazinopropionic acid, which inhibits GABA transamination, or the GABA agonist muscimol in sham-lesioned rats facilitated lordosis.

Maternal Behavior

Compared to virgin rats, lactating rat mothers display less immobility in response to startling stimuli, consume larger quantities of food, and behave more aggressively towards conspecific animals (25). Drugs that decrease GABA neurotransmission (e.g., caffeine, pentylenetetrazol) significantly decreased food intake and aggression and increased startle-elicited immobility in rat mothers (25).

EFFECTS OF NEUROPEPTIDES ON SEXUAL AND MATERNAL BEHAVIOR

Gonadotropin-Releasing Hormone

Sexual Behavior

Moss and McCann and Pfaff first reported that s.c. administration of a single dose of gonadotropin-releasing hormone (GnRH) increased lordosis in female rats [as cited by Meyerson et al. (34)]. Subcutaneous administration of GnRH also decreased latencies to mount, intromit, and ejaculate in male rats (60). Infusion of GnRH into the MPOA, the ARC–VMH, the mesencephalic central gray (MCG), or the spinal subarachnoid space proved effective in facilitating lordosis (14,36,51,56). Infusion of 5-HT, methoxamine, propranolol, or haloperidol into the MPOA or ARC–VMH blocked the lordosis-facilitating effects of GnRH (14,36). Infusion of GnRH i.c.v. increased or maintained high rates of mounting in genitally anesthetized male rats (60).

Studies of analogs of GnRH have revealed little correlation between potencies in facilitating or blocking gonadotropin release and effects on sexual behavior (36,56,74). The terminal five-amino-acid sequence of GnRH is particularly important for the lordosis-facilitating effect of this decapeptide (17).

Opioid Peptides

Sexual Behavior

Opioids inhibit female and male sexual behavior. Peripheral administration of morphine decreased receptivity in female hamsters (39) and decreased copulatory behavior in male rats (14,60). Methadone inhibited sexual behavior in male hamsters (37). Intrathecal morphine inhibited lordosis in female rats and increased the number of intromissions before ejaculation in male rats (71). Infusion i.c.v. of morphine, β-endorphin, or enkephalin analogs inhibited male and female sexual behavior in rats (34,60,72). Infusion of β-endorphin into the MCG inhibited lordosis, but Met-enkephalin had no effect (61).

Peripheral administration of opioid antagonists (naloxone or naltrexone) decreased latencies to mount, intromit, and ejaculate and decreased the number of mounts or intromissions prior to ejaculation in rats (14,60) but failed to facilitate lordosis in rats or hamsters (40,72). Naltrexone administration did not facilitate male sexual behavior in hamsters (37). Intrathecal administration of naloxone did facilitate lordosis and decrease the number of intromissions before ejaculation in rats (71). Infusion of naloxone into the MCG also increased lordosis, possibly by blocking β-endorphin inhibition of GnRH release (61). Naloxone inhibited other parameters of male sexual behavior in rats, e.g., prolonging the latency to intromit after an ejaculation and decreasing the number of penile flips in tests of penile reflexes (55). The inhibitory effect of naltrexone on sexual behavior in male talapoin monkeys (31) raises questions about the comparative role of opioids in male sexual behavior in rodents and primates.

Maternal Behavior

Peripheral administration of morphine inhibited both the onset and maintenance of maternal behavior in rats (8). Implants or infusions of morphine into the preoptic area but not the ventromedial area of the hypothalamus also blocked maternal behavior (54). Endogenous opioids have not been tested. In rats given naltrexone pellets the day before delivery or treated with naloxone at the beginning of labor, both placentophagia and cleaning of pups of birth membranes, umbilical cords, and birth fluids were significantly decreased (28).

Prolactin

Sexual Behavior

Most investigators have reported deficits in male and female sexual behavior in rodents during chronic hyperprolactinemia produced by intrahypothalamic implants of estradiol, subcutaneous placement of capsules containing diethylstilbestrol, or ectopic placement of pituitary grafts (4,6,16,36,65). Deficits in male sexual behavior persisted long after removal of diethylstilbestrol capsules and normalization of prolactin (PRL) and testosterone levels (6). However, decreased latencies to mount and intromit have also been observed shortly after transplantation of pituitary grafts (60). Treatment with the DA agonist bromocriptine for 2 weeks reversed deficits in sexual behavior produced by ectopic placement of pituitary grafts (16). Administration of the peripheral DA antagonist domperidone, which increased PRL secretion, decreased (4) or had no effect (60) on male sexual behavior but did increase lordosis (65). Subcutaneous and i.c.v. administration of PRL b.i.d. for

15 days had no effect on male copulatory behavior in rats (60). Infusion of PRL i.c.v. decreased, whereas infusion into the MCG increased, lordosis in rats (20,36).

Maternal Behavior

Early reports that PRL administration facilitates the onset of maternal behavior in rats have not been confirmed (9,53), though peripheral and intrahypothalamic administration of PRL in mice increased retrieval and licking of pups as well as nest building (9). Dopamine agonists that block PRL release did not inhibit the onset or maintenance of maternal behavior (9,53). However, PRL administration reversed the inhibition produced by hypophysectomy of the onset of maternal behavior in ovarian steroid-treated rats (9). Daily treatment with domperidone, which increased PRL secretion, decreased latency of onset of maternal behavior in male rats, whereas suppression of PRL release with bromocriptine had no effect (66).

Adrenocorticotropin, ACTH Fragments, and α-Melanocyte-Stimulating Hormone

Sexual Behavior

In female rats, peripheral administration of ACTH or ACTH$_{1-24}$ increased both progesterone levels and lordosis (14,15). Adrenalectomy abolished both effects. Infusion of ACTH$_{1-24}$ i.c.v. increased lordosis in rabbits but decreased or had no effect on lordosis in rats (5,69). Peripheral administration of ACTH fragments in rats treated with estrogen and progesterone increased lordosis in animals with low pretreatment receptivity and decreased lordosis in animals with high pretreatment receptivity (73). ACTH$_{4-10}$ and ACTH$_{4-9}$ (which have little effect on adrenal steroidogenesis) as well as α-MSH were as potent or more so than ACTH or ACTH$_{1-24}$ in their effects on lordosis (18,68,73). Infusion of ACTH$_{4-10}$ i.c.v. increased (69) or had no significant effect (33) on lordosis in rats. Central administration of ACTH$_{4-10}$ in rabbits also had no effect on lordosis (57). Intracerebroventricular administration of α-MSH in rats increased lordosis (69).

In isolated male rats, intracerebroventricular administration of ACTH$_{1-24}$ and related peptides such as α-MSH induced repeated penile erections, ejaculations, and copulatory movements. Under heterosexual testing conditions, administration of these peptides decreased ejaculation latencies and number of mounts and intromissions prior to ejaculation but failed to increase the percentage of sexually sluggish males that copulated (60). Administration of ACTH$_{4-10}$ decreased copulation (60).

Oxytocin and Arginine Vasopressin

Sexual Behavior

Intracerebroventricular infusion of oxytocin (OXY) increased lordosis in rats (2,11), whereas i.c.v. infusion of arginine vasopressin (AVP) has been reported either to inhibit (64) or to facilitate (11) lordosis. Central administration of OXY decreased the latency to ejaculate and the latency to intromit after ejaculation in male rats (3).

Maternal Behavior

Vaginal stimulation, a well-established releaser of OXY, induced maternal behavior in goats and sheep (45). However, intravenous administration of OXY was ineffective in facilitating attachment to newborns in goats or maintaining high levels of maternal response during the third week of lactation in rats (45). Some investigators observed a high incidence of maternal behavior in rats shortly after i.c.v. infusion of OXY and AVP, but other investigators observed no effect (41,42,45). Central administration of OXY antiserum or OXY antagonists inhibited the onset of maternal behavior in ovarian steroid-treated rats (45). Intracerebroventricular infusion of OXY in experienced rat mothers produced a more rapid reemergence of maternal behavior (45). Subcutaneous administration of OXY decreased pup killing and increased maternal behavior in nulliparous wild mice (29).

Corticotropin-Releasing Hormone

Sexual Behavior

Infusion of ovine corticotropin-releasing hormone (CRH) into the ARC–VMH or MCG potently inhibited lordosis and increased active rejection of male rats by females (62). These effects may have been mediated by release of β-endorphin (62).

Maternal Behavior

Intracerebroventricular infusion of ovine CRH significantly inhibited the onset and maintenance of maternal behavior in ovarian steroid-treated nulliparous rats (49). Infusion of CRH also increased pup killing in rats naive to pups but produced no pup killing in experienced rat mothers (49).

CONCLUDING REMARKS

The foregoing review is of only limited value in understanding reproductive behavior in humans. It acknowledges the importance of experience and of the gonadal steroid environment but by intention omits them from consideration. Consideration is limited to the influences of drugs and neuropeptides that affect brain transmitter systems. Studies of such influences have been performed mainly in rats. Although brain neurotransmitter systems in the rat are generally regarded as apt models for cognate systems in the human, this consensus about neurochemical similarities does not establish behavioral correspondence between the two species. The degree to which rat reproductive behavior is a model for human reproductive behavior remains a moot question.

An additional limitation follows as an instance of the broader problem stated above. Human reproductive behavior includes paternal behavior, but in no species has paternal behavior been studied according to the variables that are the focus of this discussion. The rat does not exhibit such behavior. Studies of the neurotransmitter and the neuropeptide bases of paternal behavior in mammalian species in which parenting by the father is important for survival of the offspring would be of great interest.

The studies reviewed have almost always employed the administration of substances in the periphery. Although this practice may have clinical relevance, it has limited utility for revealing the behavioral role of various neurotransmitters in discrete brain regions. The behavioral effects of peripheral administration of a drug or a neuropeptide may simply result from peripheral effects plus the algebraic sum of effects, possibly of opposite sign, in various brain areas. Administration of substances to specific brain sites will be required to elucidate the behavioral role of various neurotransmitters within discrete regions of the brain.

In future work it will be important to compare the interactions among the various neurotransmitters, among the various neuropeptides, and between neurotransmitters and neuropeptides in the regulation of reproductive behaviors within discrete brain regions. Some brain regions, e.g., the medial preoptic area (MPOA) (26,45,46), appear to play a central role in male and female sexual behavior as well as in maternal behavior. It will be of interest to determine how sexual differentiation or varying sex steroid conditions alter the function of neurotransmitter or neuropeptide systems in such brain regions. Such studies will allow us to understand better the neuroendocrine hierarchy of control of reproductive behaviors.

REFERENCES

1. Ahlenius, S., and Larsson, K. (1984): *Eur. J. Pharmacol.*, 99:279–286.
2. Arletti, R., and Bertolini, A. (1985): *Neuropeptides*, 6:247–253.
3. Arletti, R., Bazzani, M., Castelli, M., and Bertolini, A. (1985): *Horm. Behav.*, 19:14–20.
4. Bailey, D. J., and Herbert, J. (1982): *Neuroendocrinology*, 35:186–193.
5. Baldwin, D. M., Haun, C. K., and Sawyer, C. H. (1974): *Brain Res.*, 80:291–301.
6. Bartke, A., Doherty, P. C., Steger, R. W., Morgan, W. W., Amador, A. G., et al. (1984): *Neuroendocrinology*, 39:126–135.
7. Boelkins, R. C. (1973): In: *Serotonin and Behavior*, edited by Barchas and Usdin, pp. 357–364. Academic Press, New York.
8. Bridges, R. S., and Grimm, C. T. (1982): *Science*, 218:166–168.
9. Bridges, R. S., Loundes, D. D., DiBase, R., and Tate-Ostroff, B. A. (1985): In: *Prolactin: Basic and Clinical Correlates*, edited by R. M. MacLeod, M. O. Thorner, and U. Scapagnini, pp. 591–599. Liviana Press, Padova.
10. Broitman, S. T., and Donoso, A. O. (1978): *Psychopharmacology*, 56:93–101.
11. Caldwell, J. D., Pedersen, C. A., and Prange, A. J., Jr. (1986): *Neuropeptides*, 7:175–189.
12. Clark, J. T., Smith, E. R., and Davidson, J. M. (1984): *Science*, 225:847–849.
13. Clemens, L. G., and Weaver, D. R. (1985): In: *Handbook of*

Behavioral Neurobiology, 7: Reproduction, edited by N. Adler, D. Pfaff, and R. W. Goy, pp. 183–227. Plenum Press, New York.
14. Crowley, W. R., and Zemlan, F. P. (1981): In: *Neuroendocrinology of Reproduction,* edited by N. T. Adler, pp. 451–484. Plenum Press, New York.
15. De Catanzaro, D., Gray, D. S., and Gorzalka, B. B. (1981): *Physiol. Behav.,* 26:207–213.
16. Doherty, P. C., Bartke, A., and Smith, M. S. (1981): *Horm. Behav.,* 15:436–450.
17. Dudley, C. A., Vale, W., Rivier, J., and Moss, R. L. (1983): *Neuroendocrinology,* 36:486–488.
18. Everard, D., Wilson, C. A., and Thody, A. J. (1977): *J. Endocrinol.,* 73:32.
19. Everitt, B. J. (1979): *Ciba Found. Symp.,* 329–358.
20. Feder, H. H. (1984): *Annu. Rev. Psychol.,* 35:165–200.
21. Franck, J. E., and Ward, I. L. (1981): *Neuroendocrinology,* 32:50–56.
22. Frankova, S. (1977): *Psychopharmacology,* 53:83–87.
23. Giordano, A. L., Johnson, A. E., and Rosenblatt, J. S. (1985): In: *Abstracts: Conference on Reproductive Behavior,* p. 50.
24. Hansen, S., and Ross, S. B. (1983): *Brain Res.,* 268:285–290.
25. Hansen, S., Ferreira, A., and Selart, M. E. (1985): *Psychopharmacology,* 86:344–347.
26. Hart, B. L., and Leedy, M. G. (1985): In: *Handbook of Behavioral Neurobiology, 7: Reproduction,* edited by N. Adler, D. Pfaff, and R. W. Goy, pp. 373–422. Plenum Press, New York.
27. Luine, V. N., Frankfurt, M., Rainbow, T. C., Biegon, A., and Azmitia, E. (1983): *Brain Res.,* 264:344–348.
28. Mayer, A. R., Faris, P. L., Komisaruk, B. R., and Rosenblatt, J. S. (1985): *Pharmacol. Biochem. Behav.,* 22:1035–1044.
29. McCarthy, M. M., Bare, J. E., and vomSaal, F. S. (1986): *Physiol. Behav.,* 36:17–24.
30. McGinnis, M. Y., Gordon, J. H., and Gorski, R. A. (1980): *Brain Res.,* 184:179–191.
31. Meller, R. E., Kerverne, E. B., and Herbert, J. (1980): *Pharmacol. Biochem. Behav.,* 13:663–672.
32. Melman, A., Fersel, J., and Weinstein, P. (1984): *J. Urol.,* 132:804–808.
33. Meyerson, B. J., and Bohus, B. (1976): *Pharmacol. Biochem. Behav.,* 5:539–545.
34. Meyerson, B. J., Malmnäs, C. O., and Everitt, B. J. (1985): In: *Handbook of Behavioral Neurobiology, 7: Reproduction,* edited by N. Adler, D. Pfaff, and R. W. Goy, pp. 495–536. Plenum Press, New York.
35. Morali, G., and Larsson, K. (1984): *Pharmacol. Biochem. Behav.,* 20:185–187.
36. Moss, R. L., and Dudley, C. A. (1982): In: *Behavior and the Menstrual Cycle,* edited by R. C. Freedman, pp. 65–76. Marcel Dekker, New York.
37. Murphy, M. R. (1981): *Pharmacol. Biochem. Behav.,* 14:561–567.
38. Neckers, L. M., Zarrow, M. X., Myers, M. M., and Denenberg, V. H. (1975): *Pharmacol. Biochem. Behav.,* 3:545–550.
39. Ostrowski, N. L., Stapleton, J. M., Noble, R. G., and Reid, L. D. (1979): *Pharmacol. Biochem. Behav.,* 11:673–681.
40. Ostrowski, N. L., Noble, R. G., and Reid, L. D. (1981): *Pharmacol. Biochem. Behav.,* 14:881–888.
41. Pedersen, C. A., and Prange, A. J., Jr. (1979): *Proc. Natl. Acad. Sci. U.S.A.,* 76(12):6661–6665.
42. Pedersen, C. A., Ascher, J. A., Monroe, Y. L., and Prange, A. J., Jr. (1982): *Science,* 216:648–651.
43. Pedersen, C. A., Caldwell, J. D., and Prange, A. J., Jr. (1984): In: *Abstracts: Conference on Reproductive Behavior,* p. 60.
44. Pedersen, C. A., Caldwell, J. D., Brooks, P. J., and Prange, A. J., Jr. (1985): *Soc. Neurosci. Abstr.,* p. 1293.
45. Pedersen, C. A., and Prange, A. J., Jr. (1985): *Pharmacol. Ther.,* 28:287–302.
46. Pfaff, D., and Modianos, D. (1985): In: *Handbook of Behavioral Neurobiology, 7: Reproduction,* edited by N. Adler, D. Pfaff, and R. W. Goy, pp. 423–493. Plenum Press, New York.
47. Piccirillo, M., Alpert, J. E., Cohen, D. J., and Shaywitz, B. A. (1980): *Psychopharmacology,* 70:195–199.
48. Piccirillo, M., Alpert, J. E., Cohen, D. J., and Shaywitz, B. A. (1980): *Pharmacol. Biochem. Behav.,* 13:391–395.
49. Prange, A. J., Jr., Caldwell, J. D., Brooks, P. J., and Pedersen, C. A. (1985): *Soc. Neurosci. Abstr.,* p. 619.
50. Rheingold, H. L. (1963): *Maternal Behavior in Mammals.* John Wiley & Sons, New York.
51. Riskind, P., and Moss, R. L. (1983): *Brain Res. Bull.,* 11:481–485.
52. Rodgers, C. H., and Law, O. T. (1968): *Physiol. Behav.,* 3:241–246.
53. Rosenblatt, J. S., Mayer, A. D., and Siegel, H. I. (1985): In: *Handbook of Behavioral Neurobiology, 7: Reproduction,* edited by N. Adler, D. Pfaff, and R. W. Goy, pp. 229–298. Plenum Press, New York.
54. Rubin, B. S., and Bridges, R. S. (1984): *Brain Res.,* 307:91–97.
55. Sachs, B. D., Valcourt, R. J., and Flagg, H. C. (1981): *Pharmacol. Biochem. Behav.,* 14:251–253.
56. Sakuma, Y., and Pfaff, D. W. (1983): *Neuroendocrinology,* 36:218–224.
57. Sawyer, C. H., Baldwin, D. M., and Haun, C. K. (1975): In: *Sexual Behavior: Pharmacology and Biochemistry,* edited by Sandler and G. Gessa, pp. 259–267. Raven Press, New York.
58. Schiørring, E., and Hecht, A. (1979): *Psychopharmacology,* 64:219–224.
59. Segal, M., Shohami, E., and Jacobowitz, D. M. (1984): *Pharmacol. Biochem. Behav.,* 20:133–135.
60. Serra, G., and Gessa, G. L. (1984): In: *Psychoneuroendocrine Dysfunction,* edited by N. S. Shah and A. G. Donald, pp. 141–155. Plenum Press, New York, London.
61. Sirinathsinghji, D. J. S., Whittington, P. E., Audsley, A., and Fraser, H. M. (1983): *Nature,* 301:62–64.
62. Sirinathsinghji, D. J. S., Rees, L. H., Rivier, J., and Vale, W. (1983): *Nature,* 305:232–235.
63. Sirinathsinghji, D. J. S. (1983): *Physiol. Behav.,* 31:717–723.
64. Sodersten, P., Henning, M., Melin, P., and Ludin, S. (1983): *Nature,* 301:608–610.
65. Sodersten, P., Hansen, S., and Eneroth, P. (1983): *J. Endocrinol.,* 99:181–187.
66. Sodersten, P., and Eneroth, P. (1984): *J. Endocrinol.,* 102:115–119.
67. Sorenson, C. A., and Gordon, M. (1975): *Pharmacol. Biochem. Behav.,* 3:331–335.
68. Thody, A. J., Wilson, C. A., and Everard, D. (1979): *Physiol. Behav.,* 22:447–450.
69. Thody, A. J., Wilson, C. A., and Everard, D. (1981): *Psychopharmacology,* 74:153–156.
70. Ward, I. L., and Ward, O. B. (1985): In: *Handbook of Behavioral Neurobiology, 7: Reproduction,* edited by N. Adler, D. Pfaff, and R. W. Goy, pp. 77–98. Plenum Press, New York.
71. Wiesenfeld-Hallin, Z., and Sodersten, P. (1984): *Nature,* 309:257–258.
72. Wiesner, J. B., and Moss, R. L. (1984): *Life Sci.,* 34:1455–1462.
73. Wilson, C. A., Thody, A. J., and Everard, D. M. (1979): *Horm. Behav.,* 13:293–300.
74. Zadina, J. E., Kastin, A. J., Fabre, L. A., and Coy, D. H. (1981): *Pharmacol. Biochem. Behav.,* 15:961–964.

Psychopharmacology:
The Third Generation of Progress,
edited by Herbert Y. Meltzer.
Raven Press, New York © 1987.

CHAPTER **158**

Effects of Drugs on Associative Learning

John A. Harvey

It is an interesting historical fact that behavioral pharmacology has focused primarily on the ability of drugs to affect performance rather than learning. According to Laties (29), the first experimental study of drug action on behavior appeared in 1908 and was based on experiments carried out by I. V. Zavadskii in Pavlov's laboratory. These studies employed previously trained dogs to examine the effects of alcohol, morphine, cocaine, and caffeine on the conditioned salivary reflex (29). Indeed, subsequent studies in Russia and elsewhere continued to use Pavlovian conditioning to examine the effects of drugs on the performance of previously acquired responses rather than on learning as measured by the acquisition of new responses. This is especially surprising since, as noted below, Pavlovian conditioning provides the most elegant and precise set of procedures for determining the effects of drugs on learning (12,14,16,24,41). Moreover, Pavlovian conditioning as such did not become a widely used method in behavioral pharmacology. Instead, the principle of pairing a conditioned stimulus (CS) with an unconditioned stimulus (UCS) was used either as part of a transfer design or combined with instrumental and operant procedures as in the conditioned emotional response, the conditioned avoidance response, or Sidman avoidance (see refs. 12,14).

Although instrumental (31) and operant (40) procedures were used occasionally to examine drug effects on the performance of maintained behaviors, the pioneering studies of Dews beginning in 1955 (7) set the stage for a technology and paradigm that were to become the predominant force in behavioral pharmacology. Consequently, the most systematic and elegant data available of drug effects on behavior have come from operant studies in which behaviors are maintained by a variety of events under various schedules of reinforcement. The continued emphasis on the effects of drugs on performance thus stems, at least in part, from the spectacular success of a behavioral analysis that emphasized performance characteristics and distrusted any inferred processes including learning. This emphasis has

further been reinforced by the difficulty of using operant methods for a systematic analysis of drug actions on learning, as indicated below (see also 12,14,41). It is not surprising, therefore, to note that although drugs have been reported to affect performance by altering the ability of stimuli to control behavior (8,28), few behavioral pharmacologists have been willing to deal directly with the possible consequences of such changes in stimulus properties on associative or cognitive processes. However, the continued emphasis on performance factors in behavioral pharmacology becomes quite puzzling when one considers that the salient therapeutic actions of most psychopharmacological agents are on sensory processing of stimuli and associative processes, not motor acts.

Although operant methods per se have not been used to examine drug effects on learning, many experimenters have assumed that such effects could be measured by observing the acquisition of conditioned avoidance responses in the shuttle box. However, with but rare exceptions, attempts to examine the effects of drugs on learning have often employed inadequate response systems, methodologies, and control procedures to allow for an unambiguous interpretation of drug effect on acquisition. Consequently, premature and contradictory interpretations have been provided by various investigators for identical effects of drugs. For example, the enhanced acquisition of the conditioned avoidance response produced by LSD has variously been attributed to an increase in learning (5), pseudoconditioning (23), and motivational factors (2). Therefore, in some cases this meant that a drug effect would be either erroneously attributed to learning when the results were actually caused by changes in performance factors or erroneously dismissed as a result of effects on the ability of the animals to initiate responses. Others have avoided the problem entirely by simply measuring retention of a response after a period of time. In short, in order to study drug effects on learning, one requires a procedure and paradigm at least as precise as the operant methods used to study drug effects on performance. This means that the procedure must allow an unambiguous assessment of learning in control animals and methods that can differentiate the effects of drugs on sensory, associative, and motoric factors (12). Pavlovian conditioning of the nictitating membrane reflex of the rabbit has been demonstrated to meet these criteria (14,16).

THE NICTITATING MEMBRANE REFLEX

It is widely recognized that Pavlovian conditioning is a powerful paradigm for examining the biological bases of learning (12,14,16,24,41). In particular, Pavlovian conditioning of the nictitating membrane reflex in the rabbit has provided an excellent experimental model for examining both the incremental and decremental effects of drugs on associative learning in a mammal (12,14,16,39). For example, a great deal is known about the anatomy and physiology of this corneal–sixth nerve reflex. Unconditioned stimuli such as tactile stimulation of the cornea or electrical stimulation of the skin just lateral to the eye activate trigeminal inputs to the pars oralis, from which second-order trigeminal neurons project to retractor bulbi motoneurons in the accessory abducens nucleus either directly or indirectly via the reticular formation (20). Activation of the accessory abducens nucleus leads to contraction of the retractor bulbi muscle via the sixth nerve, which in turn pulls the eye back into the orbit, and the force of this mechanical action squeezes the nictitating membrane out over the cornea. Extension of the nictitating membrane has been shown to be caused solely by retraction of the eyeball (32,33).

Auditory stimuli are reflexly subliminal in that they do not elicit an overt retraction of the eyeball and the correlated extension of the nictitating membrane, but they do produce small but detectable increases in neuronal activity within the unconditioned reflex arc (1). Thus, prior to conditioning, an auditory stimulus can produce heterosynaptic reflex facilitation as measured by an increased amplitude of the unconditioned response (UCR) of membrane extension when a tone precedes the UCS (15,19,41). It should be noted that heterosynaptic reflex facilitation provides a measurement of the unconditioned excitatory properties of the tone that is to be used as a CS in conditioning. During the paired presentations of a tone CS with a UCS, the tone becomes supraliminal and capable of eliciting conditioned responses (CRs) of nictitating membrane extension. Given these anatomical details, one advantage of this conditioning model becomes obvious, since both the CR and the UCR are mediated by the same final common pathway involving the accessory abducens nucleus and sixth nerve (21).

ASSOCIATIVE AND NONASSOCIATIVE EFFECTS OF DRUGS

The second and more important advantage of this corneal–sixth nerve reflex is that it is able to provide an unambiguous measure of associative learning in control rabbits; i.e., the acquisition of CRs occurs only during the explicit pairings of CS and UCS (14). As noted above, prior

to conditioning, auditory (as well as visual) CSs do not evoke extensions of the nictitating membrane. In addition, the base-line rate of membrane extension is low (less than 2%), and the explicitly unpaired presentations of tone, light, and shock stimuli never produce any significant increase in either base-line responding or responding to tone and light CSs in control animals (14). Because control animals demonstrate the virtual absence of nonassociative responding and hence the absence of sensitization, pseudoconditioning, or alterations in base-line rate of responding, their acquisition of CRs during paired presentations of CSs and UCS can be attributed unambiguously to associative learning.

In many conditioning situations, CR acquisition by controls can be shown to be a mixture of both nonassociative and associative processes, so that it becomes difficult or impossible to tease these factors apart when examining the effects of drugs on learning. For example, many experimenters have reported that both d-lysergic acid diethylamide (LSD) and d-amphetamine increase the acquisition of conditioned avoidance responses in the shuttle box during the paired presentations of the tone CS and shock UCS (Table 1), but as a rule a control for nonassociative responding (i.e., the use of explicitly unpaired presentations of the tone and shock stimuli) has not been employed. When such controls were employed (11,22,23), it was found that vehicle-injected animals demonstrated levels of nonassociative responding of 9% and that both LSD and d-amphetamine significantly increased these levels of nonassociative responding to 18 and 26%, respectively (Table 1). It was concluded, therefore, that the increased acquisition produced by d-amphetamine and LSD was not through

TABLE 1. *Drug effects on nonassociative processes*

Drug and dose (μmole/kg)	Percentage conditioned responses[a]	
	Paired CS–UCS	Unpaired CS/UCS
Shuttle box avoidance procedure		
Vehicle	47[b]	9
d-amphetamine (10.8)	85[b]	26[b]
LSD (0.174)	68[b]	18[b]
Pavlovian conditioning of nictitating membrane reflex		
Vehicle	57	2
d-amphetamine (10.0)	59	2
LSD (0.030)	74[b]	5
DOM (3.0)	76[b]	11[b]

[a] Data for the shuttle box avoidance procedure obtained from references 11, 22, and 23, and for the conditioned nictitating membrane reflex from references 13 and 17. All data are for responding to a tone CS when the tone CS was paired with a shock UCS or when these two stimuli were unpaired. Abbreviations as in Table 2.
[b] Significantly different from vehicle control value ($p < 0.01$).

learning but rather through the occurrence of pseudoconditioning (11,23,24).

However, the difficulty of such conclusions is illustrated by the data obtained with Pavlovian conditioning of the nictitating membrane reflex (Table 1). As indicated above, control animals demonstrate low levels of nonassociative responding during the explicitly unpaired presentations of CS and UCS (2%), which is not affected by either d-amphetamine (2%) or LSD (5%) (Table 1). Under these conditions, the absence of any effect of d-amphetamine on associative learning becomes more apparent. However, it is also clear that LSD does increase associative learning.

Because of the low levels of nonassociative responding demonstrated by control rabbits, the nictitating membrane reflex is also quite sensitive for detecting changes in sensitization or pseudoconditioning. For example, the hallucinogen DOM (2,5-dimethoxy-4-methylamphetamine) was also found to increase significantly the acquisition of CRs during Pavlovian conditioning of the nictitating membrane reflex (Table 1). However, DOM also produced a significant increase in nonassociative responding over that of vehicle controls (Table 1). Moreover, this increased responding produced by DOM (11%) was found to reflect an increase in responding to the tone stimulus from 6.7 to 17.8% across the 10 days of unpaired presentations of CS and UCS (17). Thus, the effects of DOM on CR acquisition did not occur solely through a change in associative learning but may have also reflected pseudoconditioning.

The data presented in Table 1 illustrate just one of the methodological problems that arises in the use of operant and instrumental procedures to examine the acquisition of learned behaviors. It is not surprising, therefore, that many investigators either distrusted any studies purporting to measure drug effects on learning or focused on the examination of memory, the persistence of a learned behavior.

LOCALIZING THE EFFECTS OF DRUGS ON ASSOCIATIVE LEARNING

Tables 2 and 3 present a summary of experiments that have examined the effects of drugs on CR acquisition using Pavlovian conditioning of the nictitating membrane reflex. With the exception of the studies with pentylenetetrazol (10), pimozide (15), chlordiazepoxide (6), and harmaline (42), which did not employ unpaired presentations of CS and UCS as a control for nonassociative responding, increases or decreases in CR acquisition produced by the remaining drugs listed in Table 2 could be attributed to an effect on associative learning. Table 3 presents a list of drugs that had no effect on acquisition.

Once it had been determined that a drug was altering associative learning, it was possible to examine further the behavioral processes being affected. For example, one obvious manner by which a drug might increase or decrease the rate of learning would be through a direct effect on the unconditioned reflex itself. Such an effect of a drug is impossible to determine in procedures employing the conditioned avoidance response because the escape response to shock is not an unconditioned response but a learned response. Moreover, there is no consistent final common

pathway for either the avoidance or escape response. Thus, changes in the unconditioned aversiveness of the shock or in the ability of the animal to make a response cannot directly be determined within the context of the shuttle box. It should be noted that if a decrease in the rate of CR acquisition in the shuttle box occurs when there is also a sign of sedation, one cannot conclude that the drug is having no effect on associative learning. Rather, this again simply indicates that the response system and/or paradigm being employed are inappropriate for determining an effect on learning. In contrast, such determinations are easily carried out for the nictitating membrane reflex.

On the basis of experiments using a range of intensities of either the air puff or shock UCS, it has been uniformly reported that changes in associative learning produced by the drugs listed in Table 2 could not be attributed to an effect on the threshold of the UCS for elicitation of UCRs or on the amplitude of the elicited UCR. Since both the unconditioned and conditioned extensions of the nictitating membrane are mediated by the same final common pathway and result from activation of the same effector system, the absence of any effect on the unconditioned reflex would indicate that the drug had also not affected the motoric expression of the CR to the tone CS (see also 16,19,39). This latter conclusion has been supported by the findings that the retarded acquisition of CRs produced by morphine (36), scopolamine (18), and haloperidol (J. A. Harvey and I. Cormezano, *unpublished data*) could still be detected after animals had been withdrawn from drug and then returned to the conditioning situation 5 days later, indicating that the drugs were not retarding CR acquisition through an effect on performance factors per se.

Another mechanism by which a drug might affect learning is by altering the excitatory properties of the tone CS. It is remarkable that every drug that has been found to enhance or retard the rate of associative learning also increases or decreases the conditioned excitatory properties of the tone CS (Table 4). To determine the effects of drugs on the excitatory properties of a CS, animals were first trained until they achieved asymptotic levels of conditioned responding to a tone CS. The animals were then injected with drug or vehicle, and the intensity of the tone CS was varied to obtain a measure of the percentage of CRs elicited across a range of CS intensities. For control animals, the overall percentage of CRs decreased with decreasing intensity of the tone. However, drugs that enhanced or retarded CR acquisition produced a comparable increase or decrease, respectively, in the percentage of CRs as compared with vehicle controls. Table 4 compares these effects of drugs as the percentage change during acquisition and the percentage change during maintenance when CS intensity was varied. These two measures are highly correlated ($r = 0.985$), indicating that there is also a good association between the degree to which a drug enhances or retards learning and the degree to which it increases or decreases the ability of a tone CS to elicit CRs. A similar relationship has been found by correlating the rate of CR acquisition with the change in the intensity threshold of the CS for eliciting CRs (39).

The close correspondence between the effects of drugs on the excitatory properties of a conditioned tone stimulus

TABLE 2. *Effects of drugs on CR acquisition*[a]

Drugs and route of injection[h]	ED50 (μmole/kg)[b]	References
Increased acquisition		
LSD i.v.	0.003	17
DOM i.v.	0.250	17
Pentylenetetrazol s.c.	181.0[c]	10
Decreased acquisition		
Haloperidol i.v.	1.52	J. A. Harvey and I. Gormezano (*unpublished data*)
Pimozide i.v.	>0.66	15
Chlordiazepoxide i.p.	<40.0[d]	6
Harmaline i.v.	<46.7[e]	42
Scopolamine i.v.	0.195	18
Atropine s.c.	23.0[c]	9
Morphine i.v.	4.19; 18.5[f]	36, 38
Ethylketocyclazocine i.v.	0.56[f]	38
U-50-488H i.v.	0.84[f]	38
N-Allylnormetazocine i.v.	8.98[f]	C. V. Schindler and J. A. Harvey (*unpublished data*)
Phencyclidine i.v.	1.07[f]	C. V. Schindler and J. A. Harvey (*unpublished data*)
Pentazocine i.v.	49.1[f]	C. V. Schindler and J. A. Harvey (*unpublished data*)
L-PIA s.c.	3.67	44; L. Winsky and J. A. Harvey (*unpublished data*)

[a] All of the studies cited used classical conditioning of the rabbit's nictitating membrane response. Unless otherwise noted, the offset of an 800-msec tone or light CS occurred simultaneously with the onset of a 100-msec shock UCS. There were 30 tone–shock and 30 light–shock pairings on each of 10 consecutive daily conditioning sessions.

[b] ED50 values calculated as the dose of drug producing a half-maximal increase or decrease in CR acquisition based on the overall percentage of CRs during acquisition, the number of trials required to achieve a criterion of 10 consecutive CRs, or the percentage of animals achieving criterion. Where only one dose of drug was employed, the value given indicates whether the ED50 would be less than (<) or greater than (>) the indicated dose.

[c] For acquisition, the offset of a 750-msec tone CS occurred simultaneously with the onset of a 300-msec shock UCS. There were 32 or 33 tone–shock pairings on each of eight or nine consecutive daily sessions.

[d] For acquisition, a 50-msec shock UCS overlapped the last 50 msec of a 350-msec tone CS. There were 60 tone–shock pairings on each of four consecutive daily sessions.

[e] For acquisition, a 350-msec tone CS was paired with a 100-msec UCS consisting of an air puff directed at the cornea. The UCS onset occurred 260 msec after CS onset. There were 100 tone–air puff pairings on each of four consecutive daily sessions.

[f] For acquisition, the offset of a 400-msec tone CS occurred simultaneously with the onset of a 100-msec shock UCS. There were 40 tone–shock pairings on each of five consecutive daily sessions.

[g] Effects of d-amphetamine were modality specific with no effect on CR acquisition to the tone CS but a significant enhancement in acquisition to the light CS with an ED50 of 1.2 μmole/kg.

[h] Abbreviations: BOL, d-2-bromolysergic acid diethylamide; DOM, 2,5-dimethoxy-4-methylamphetamine; LSD, d-lysergic acid diethylamide; PIA, N^6-(phenylisopropyl)adenosine (L-PIA and D-PIA are the R and S forms, respectively, in absolute configuration); U-50-488H, trans-(±)-3,4,dichloro-N-methyl-N-[2-(1-pyrrolidinyl)cyclohexyl]benzeneacetamide.

TABLE 3. *Drugs with no effect on CR acquisition[a]*

Drugs and route of injection	Highest dose tested (μmole/kg)	References
BOL	0.300	17
Lisuride i.v.	0.300	J. A. Harvey and I. Gormezano (*unpublished data*)
Atropine methylnitrate s.c.	49.1[c]	9
Methscopolamine i.v.	3.8	18
Naloxone i.v.	27.5	37
d-Amphetamine i.v.	30.0[g]	17
Caffeine s.c.	300.0	45
Theophylline s.c.	200.0	45
D-PIA s.c.	10.0	L. Winsky and J. A. Harvey (*unpublished data*)
Rolipram s.c.	3.0	L. Winsky and J. A. Harvey (*unpublished data*)

[a] See Table 2 for abbreviations and footnotes.

and learning suggested that drugs might also alter the excitatory properties of auditory stimuli prior to learning. The effects of drugs on the unconditioned excitatory properties of a tone were determined by measuring changes in reflex facilitation. Both haloperidol and scopolamine not only retarded associative learning (Table 2) but also produced a large and significant decrease in the unconditioned excitatory properties of an auditory stimulus. Thus, prior to any conditioning, the duration and amplitude of reflex facilitation produced by a tone were significantly reduced by haloperidol (15) and scopolamine (19). Taken together, these findings suggested that all drugs examined so far (Tables 2 and 3) increased or decreased the rate of associative learning by increasing or decreasing both the unconditioned and conditioned excitatory properties of the tone CS (15,19).

THE RETICULAR FORMATION AS THE SITE OF DRUG ACTION ON LEARNING

The summary presented in Table 2 indicates that a wide variety of drugs can enhance or retard CR acquisition. The list of those that have been demonstrated to alter associative learning includes drugs that have been classified as a hallucinogen (LSD), neuroleptic (haloperidol), muscarinic blocking agent (atropine and scopolamine), opioid (morphine), and adenosine analog (L-PIA). Moreover, these drugs are presumed to produce their effects through a variety of transmitter systems. Such an outcome suggests that learning involves a large number of neural systems employing many different transmitters so that the effect of

TABLE 4. *Effects of drugs on CR acquisition and maintenance[a]*

Drugs	Dose (μmole/kg)	Percentage change from control	
		Acquisition[a]	Maintenance[a]
LSD	0.030	+57[b]	+56[b]
Haloperidol	0.665	−31[b]	−30[b]
Scopolamine	0.95	−77[b]	−71[b]
Morphine	59.8	−65[b]	−85[b]
Ethylketocyclazocine	1.26	−70[b]	−82[b]
U-50-488H	2.15	−69[b]	−71[b]
L-PIA	5.0	−74[b]	−66[b]
Naloxone	2.7	+3	+8
Caffeine	300.0	+2	+2
Theophylline	200.0	+4	+3

[a] For acquisition, drug effects are based on average percentage of CRs across all days of training. For maintenance, drug effects are based on average percentage of CRs during testing across a range of CS intensities. See text for details. Footnotes, abbreviations, and routes of injection as in Table 2. $r = 0.985$ for correlation between drug effect on acquisition and maintenance.

[b] Significantly different from vehicle control ($p < 0.05$).

a drug on any particular transmitter in widely separated portions of the brain could modify associative learning.

However, since all of the drugs so far examined produce their effects on learning through a common mechanism, i.e., on the excitatory properties of the CS, one would assume that some common functional system must be mediating the actions of all of these drugs. This latter possibility is strongly supported by a number of electrophysiological studies dealing with the effects of drugs on the reticular formation. These studies have indicated that a variety of drugs with different presumed mechanisms of action act on the reticular formation to enhance or block the unconditioned and conditioned excitatory effects of auditory stimuli as measured by changes in both behavioral and EEG arousal thresholds (3,27). For example, in agreement with the data in Table 4, neuroleptics (25,26) and muscarinic blocking agents (30,35,43) blocked both behavioral and EEG arousal to a tone, whereas LSD had exactly the opposite effect (4,25,34). In addition, Bradley (3) and Killam and Killam (27) suggested that drugs may affect learning by altering the excitatory effects of a CS on these reticular formation neurons.

These conclusions suggest that the multisynaptic portion of the corneal–sixth nerve reflex that involves the reticular formation (20) provides a point at which drugs could modify the excitatory/arousal effects of the CS on reticular neurons. If such neurons receive inputs from both the auditory system and cornea (20), then the drug would also be altering the interaction of CS and UCS, thereby producing the observed changes in heterosynaptic reflex facilitation and associative learning (19). In agreement with previous suggestions that heterosynaptic reflex facilitation represents the plastic changes responsible for learning (24,41), it has been found that the effect of a drug on the ability of a tone to facilitate the nictitating membrane reflex provides a good prediction of the effects the drug will have on subsequent associative learning (15,19).

The results obtained with Pavlovian conditioning of the nictitating membrane response and the earlier electrophysiological studies described above provide a common basis for the effects of drugs on associative learning. By increasing or decreasing the unconditioned excitatory or arousal properties of a tone that is to be used as a CS, a drug would increase or decrease the ability of that tone CS to enter into associative learning. Similarly, to the extent that the drug would increase or decrease the conditioned excitatory properties of the tone CS, then it would be expected to increase or decrease the ability of the CS to elicit CRs once learning had occurred.

SUMMARY

This review has attempted to indicate how the use of reflexive behaviors in general, and of Pavlovian conditioning in particular, provides one with the opportunity to determine the anatomical systems on which drugs act to produce changes in learning and performance. The challenge for coming research is to map out the precise pathways and synaptic transmitters employed for both the conditioned and unconditioned reflexes and to identify the points at which they converge on the final common pathway. Such an approach would provide the unique opportunity to describe the effects of drugs on learning in terms of both anatomical loci and neurochemical mechanisms. This, in turn, may provide clues to the neurochemical basis of learning and memory for simple reflexes and by extension for more complex cognitive processes.

ACKNOWLEDGMENTS

I thank Dr. Victor G. Laties for calling my attention to several of the historical references used in this chapter. Supported by United States Public Health Service Grant MH16841.

REFERENCES

1. Berthier, N. E., and Moore, J. W. (1983): *Brain Res.*, 258:201–210.
2. Bignami, G. (1972): *Psychopharmacologia*, 25:146–151.
3. Bradley, P. B. (1958): In: *Reticular Formation of the Brain*, edited by H. H. Jasper, L. D. Proctor, S. S. Knighton, W. C. Noshay, and R. T. Costello, pp. 123–149. Little, Brown, Boston.
4. Bradley, P. B., and Key, B. J. (1958): *Electroencephalogr. Clin. Neurophysiol.*, 10:97–110.
5. Bridger, W. H. (1975): In: *Neurobiological Mechanisms of Adaptation and Behavior*, edited by A. J. Mandell, pp. 287–298. Raven Press, New York.
6. Chisholm, D. C., Couch, J. V., and Moore, J. W. (1971): *Psychonom. Sci.*, 23:203–204.
7. Dews, P. B. (1955): *J. Pharmacol. Exp. Ther.*, 113:393–401.
8. Dews, P. B. (1955): *J. Pharmacol. Exp. Ther.*, 115:380–389.
9. Downs, D., Cardozo, C., Schneiderman, N., Yehle, A. L., VanDercar, D. H., et al. (1972): *Psychopharmacologia*, 23:319–333.
10. Elliott, R., and Schneiderman, N. (1968): *Psychopharmacologia*, 12:133–141.
11. Evangelista, A. M., and Izquierdo, I. (1971): *Psychopharmacologia*, 20:42–47.
12. Gormezano, I., and Harvey, J. A. (1978): In: *Psychopharmacology of Hallucinogens*, edited by R. Stillman and R. Willette, pp. 207–219. Pergamon Press, New York.
13. Gormezano, I., and Harvey, J. A. (1980): *J. Comp. Physiol. Psychol.*, 94:641–649.
14. Gormezano, I., Kehoe, E. J., and Marshall, B. S. (1983): In: *Progress in Psychobiology and Physiological Psychology*, edited by J. M. Sprague and A. N. Epstein, pp. 197–275. Academic Press, New York.
15. Harvey, J. A., and Gormezano, I. (1981): *J. Pharmacol. Exp. Ther.*, 218:712–719.
16. Harvey, J. A., and Gormezano, I. (1986): In: *Advances in Behavioral Pharmacology*, edited by N. A. Krasnegor and T. Thompson, pp. 115–132. Erlbaum Press, New York.
17. Harvey, J. A., Gormezano, I., and Cool, V. A. (1982): *J. Pharmacol. Exp. Ther.*, 221:289–294.
18. Harvey, J. A., Gormezano, I., and Cool-Hauser, V. A. (1983): *J. Pharmacol. Exp. Ther.*, 225:42–49.
19. Harvey, J. A., Gormezano, I., and Cool-Hauser, V. A. (1985): *J. Neurosci.*, 5:596–602.
20. Harvey, J. A., Land, T., and McMaster, S. E. (1984): *Brain Res.*, 301:307–321.
21. Harvey, J. A., Marek, G. J., Johannsen, A. M., McMaster, S. E., Land, T., et al. (1983): *Soc. Neurosci. Abstr.*, 9:330.
22. Izquierdo, I. (1974): *Psychopharmacologia*, 35:189–193.
23. Izquierdo, I. (1975): *Behav. Biol.*, 15:193–205.
24. Kandell, E. R. (1979): *Harvey Lect.*, 73:19–92.
25. Key, B. J. (1961): *Psychopharmacologia*, 2:352–363.
26. Key, B. J., and Bradley, P. B. (1960): *Psychopharmacologia*, 1:450–462.

27. Killam, K. F., and Killam, E. K. (1958): In: *Reticular Formation of the Brain,* edited by H. H. Jasper, L. D. Proctor, S. S. Knighton, W. C. Noshay, and R. T. Costello, pp. 111–222. Little, Brown, Boston.

28. Laties, V. G. (1975): *Fed. Proc.,* 34:1880–1888.

29. Laties, V. G. (1979): *J. Exp. Anal. Behav.,* 32:463–472.

30. Lindsley, D. F., Carpenter, R. S., Killam, E. K., and Killam, K. F. (1968): *Electroencephalogr. Clin. Neurophysiol.,* 24:497–513.

31. Macht, D. I., and Mora, C. F. (1921): *J. Pharmacol. Exp. Ther.,* 16:219–235.

32. Marek, G. J., McMaster, S. E., Gormezano, I., and Harvey, J. A. (1984): *Brain Res.,* 299:215–229.

33. Prince, J. H. (1964): *The Rabbit in Eye Research.* Charles C Thomas, Springfield, IL.

34. Purpura, D. P. (1956): *Arch. Neurol. Psychiatry,* 75:122–131.

35. Sadowski, B., and Longo, V. G. (1962): *Electroencephalogr. Clin. Neurophysiol.,* 14:465–476.

36. Schindler, C. W., Gormezano, I., and Harvey, J. A. (1983): *J. Pharmacol. Exp. Ther.,* 227:639–643.

37. Schindler, C. W., Gormezano, I., and Harvey, J. A. (1984): *Psychopharmacology,* 83:114–121.

38. Schindler, C. W., Gormezano, I., and Harvey, J. A. (1985): *Fed. Proc.,* 44:1723.

39. Schindler, C. W., Gormezano, I., and Harvey, J. A. (1985): In: *Behavioral Pharmacology: The Current Status,* edited by L. S. Seiden and R. Balster, pp. 55–71. Alan R. Liss, New York.

40. Skinner, B. F., and Heron, W. T. (1937): *Psychol. Rec.,* 1:340–346.

41. Thompson, R. F., Berger, T., Cegavske, C., Patterson, M. M., Roemer, R., et al. (1976): *Am. Psychol.,* 31:209–227.

42. Turker, K. S., and Miles, T. S. (1984): *Brain Res. Bull.,* 13:229–233.

43. White, R. P., and Boyajy, L. D. (1960): *Arch. Int. Pharmacodyn.,* 127:260–273.

44. Winsky, L., Gormezano, I., and Harvey, J. A. (1984): *Soc. Neurosci. Abstr.,* 10:793.

45. Winsky, L., Gormezano, I., and Harvey, J. A. (1985): *Soc. Neurosci. Abstr.,* 11:874.

Psychopharmacology:
The Third Generation of Progress,
edited by Herbert Y. Meltzer.
Raven Press, New York © 1987.

CHAPTER **159**

Nonpharmacological Factors Determining the Behavioral Effects of Drugs

James E. Barrett

One of the distinguishing characteristics of the field of behavioral pharmacology has been the emphasis on the identification and analysis of behavioral variables that determine the effects of drugs. This emphasis stems to a large extent from the fact that many individuals conducting early research in this field were initially trained in experimental psychology and approached the analysis of drug action from that perspective. The period in the mid-1950s, in which major advances were made in the discovery and use of psychotherapeutic drugs, coincided with a period during which significant progress also occurred in the experimental analysis of behavior. Research in operant conditioning, using procedures originally developed by Skinner (35) and significantly elaborated by Ferster and Skinner (19), yielded valuable methods for establishing, controlling, and analyzing behavior. These methods, together with an accompanying theoretical approach, helped shape as well as direct much of the research in behavioral pharmacology.

Few experiments have so forcefully and elegantly illustrated the important contribution of behavioral variables to the effects of drugs as did the original studies by Dews (16,17). These well-known experiments, demonstrating that the behavioral effects of pentobarbital and amphetamine depended on the manner in which behavior was controlled by its consequences (i.e., the schedule of reinforcement), have been widely regarded as providing a major impetus for establishing behavioral pharmacology as an independent discipline. Since those initial experiments, behavioral pharmacology has developed in several different directions. As occurs in many fields that undergo expansion and progress, objectives and directions in behavioral pharmacology have

become somewhat diffuse. In many cases, the emphasis on the analysis of behavioral variables and drug effects has shifted to one that uses behavior primarily as an assay system comparable to that of an isolated organ or tissue preparation. Further, since behavioral pharmacology has become a discipline more or less independent of its predecessors, it can form and has formed new alliances with other fields that also represent synthetic approaches. Although the discipline currently embraces a wide variety of individuals with diverse backgrounds and objectives, it would appear that behavioral pharmacology involves the predominant use of behavior, both conditioned and unconditioned, as a basis for the analysis of drug action. This chapter reviews relatively recent progress in the traditional area of behavioral pharmacology that has focused on behavioral variables that influence the effects of drugs.

BEHAVIORAL CONSEQUENCES AS DETERMINANTS OF DRUG EFFECTS

Schedule-Controlled Response Rate

The use of schedule-controlled behavior, in which selected responses are differentiated, developed, and maintained by consequent events, has been an integral part of research in behavioral pharmacology. Schedules of reinforcement have provided the degree of experimental control necessary for establishing objective, stable, and reproducible behavioral performances that can be manipulated over a range broad enough to allow meaningful investigation of the interactions between drugs and behavior. Initial analyses of the effects of drugs on different rates and patterns of responding maintained under various schedules helped identify the important contribution of schedule-controlled response rate to the effects produced by certain drugs (24). Under a wide range of circumstances there is an inverse relationship between the effects of a drug and the rate of responding that occurs under nondrug conditions. Experiments that have manipulated response rate and isolated relevant variables that contribute to rate of responding, such as reinforcement frequency, have repeatedly confirmed the importance of response rate in determining the effects of various drugs, particularly the psychomotor stimulants (18,32,33). Response rate has also been a valuable keystone in isolating and revealing other determinants of the behavioral effects of drugs.

Type of Reinforcer

One area in which the use of schedule-controlled response rate has permitted the identification of a variable capable of influencing drug effects has been that of the role of the type of maintaining event. When comparable rates of responding are maintained under similar fixed-interval schedules by different events (e.g., food, electric shock presentation, or by the termination of a stimulus correlated with shock), a number of drugs will produce effects that depend on the event (4–6,30). For instance, chlordiazepoxide, ethanol, and pentobarbital, as well as many serotonin antagonists, increase behavior maintained by food but only decrease responding maintained by electric shock. Drugs from other classes, however, such as morphine (25) and the serotonin agonist quipazine (5), generally only increase performances maintained by shock at doses that decrease food-maintained responding. The psychomotor stimulants, amphetamines and cocaine, as well as dopamine agonists (piribedil and apomorphine), increase behavior maintained by either type of consequence, whereas most dopamine antagonists (e.g., chlorpromazine and haloperidol) typically only decrease responding under these conditions (5). Differential or selective drug effects occur when response rates maintained by different events are comparable (Fig. 1), thereby reducing the possibility that these effects might be related to differences in control rate of responding. Additionally, though, when control response rates maintained by different events under fixed-interval schedules have been manipulated over a wide range, effects were still related to the type of event (2).

Drug effects on punished or suppressed responding can also depend on the type of maintaining event. For example, except under certain conditions (described below), d-amphetamine decreases punished behavior maintained by food. However, when punished responding is studied using the termination of a stimulus correlated with shock as the maintaining event, d-amphetamine produces large increases in punished behavior (26). Similarly, pentobarbital has been shown to produce increases in punished responding suppressed by shock at doses that did not increase punished responding reduced by the presentation of a stimulus correlated with a timeout period during which food was unavailable (13). Since the type of reinforcing or punishing event can be an important factor in determining drug

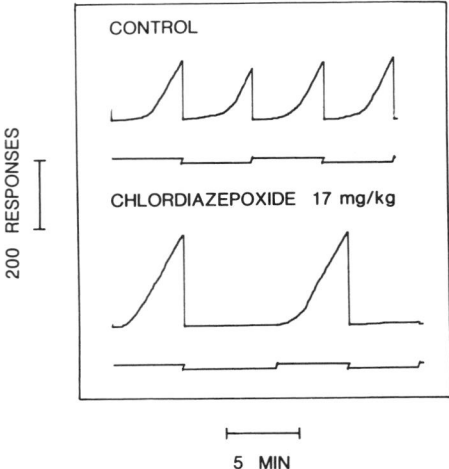

FIG. 1. Comparable control rates of responding maintained under fixed-interval schedules by food or electric shock presentation (squirrel monkey). The line beneath each cumulative record was offset during the shock-presentation component, which was correlated with a pair of white lights; the food-presentation component was correlated with red stimulus lights. If a response did not occur after 6 min in either component, the schedule components automatically alternated. A 1-min timeout period separated the two components. Chlordiazepoxide (17.0 mg/kg) markedly increased responding maintained by food but eliminated responding during the shock-presentation component. (Adapted from ref. 9.)

effects, it would appear that the processes of reinforcement and punishment are not unitary behavioral phenomena. Drugs can reveal or clarify subtle aspects of the way behavior is controlled by its consequences that, otherwise, are difficult to detect.

Drugs that produce one effect depending on the type of maintaining event presented under fixed-interval schedules may produce different effects under fixed-ratio schedules. For instance, although pentobarbital, ethanol, and chlordiazepoxide differentially affect responding maintained by food or stimulus-shock termination under fixed-interval schedules, performances maintained by these events under fixed-ratio schedules are affected similarly (22). However, the comparable effects obtained with d-amphetamine under fixed-interval schedules with different maintaining events do not always occur under fixed-ratio schedules (6,21,23), although this issue warrants some clarification (28). Thus, as with many variables, there are some conditions under which the type of event matters substantially and other conditions under which it matters little. Selective drug effects that depend on the type of event and on the schedule that maintains responding do, however, provide strong additional bases for emphasizing the crucial importance of behavioral variables as determinants of drug effects. The degree of control exerted by these variables is often quite dramatic, occurring within very short time periods, as shown in Fig. 1, and even simultaneously, as when chlordiazepoxide decreases or completely eliminates responding on one lever that produces shock while enhancing responding maintained simultaneously by food on a second lever (Fig. 2).

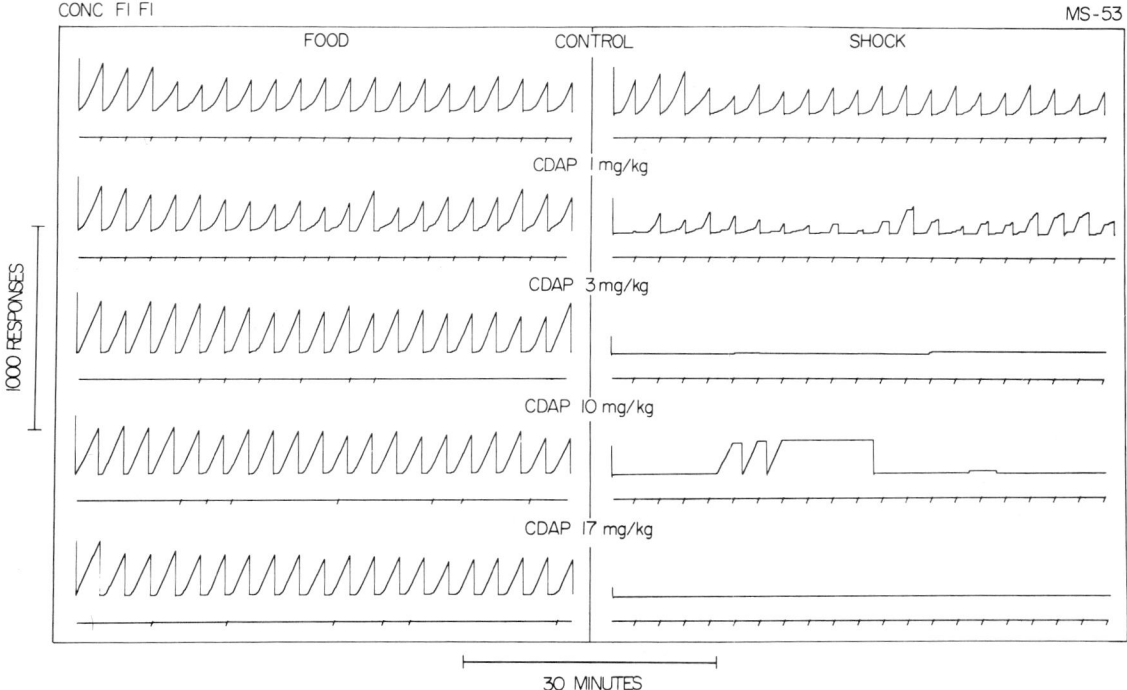

FIG. 2. Effects of chlordiazepoxide on responding simultaneously maintained on different levers by a concurrent fixed-interval schedule of food or shock presentation (squirrel monkey). The pens reset to baseline after the occurrence of each event. Records are from one session and were recorded simultaneously. Note that increasing doses of chlordiazepoxide decreased responding on the lever that produced shock, while at the same time, responding on the lever that produced food was increased.

Although the basis for differential drug effects that depend on the type of consequent event remains to be more thoroughly explored, it is evident that, under conditions when all else appears equal, the effects of certain drugs can be directly related to the type of consequence maintaining behavior. There is a considerable degree of order in these effects, as indicated in Fig. 3, which summarizes the effects of amphetamines, minor tranquilizers (e.g., chlordiazepoxide, pentobarbital), and opioids on reinforced and punished behavior maintained under fixed-interval schedules by food or escape from shock. The arrows beside each drug class indicate whether any dose of these compounds increases responding; if the drug does not produce increases across the entire dose range the arrow points in the downward direction. The top two quadrants show that amphetamines increase rates of responding maintained by either event, whereas the effects of minor tranquilizers and opioids, although different from each other, both depend on the event that maintains responding. The bottom two quadrants show that when behavior maintained by either event is punished, effects of amphetamines depend on the maintaining event; however, with punished responding, neither the effects of minor tranquilizers nor those of the opioids depend on the maintaining event. Furthermore, the effects of amphetamines, but not minor tranquilizers or opioids, on responding maintained by the presentation of food depend on whether responding is punished (compare upper and lower left-most panels). In contrast, the effects of minor tranquilizers and opioids, but not amphetamines, on behavior maintained by the termination of electric shock depend on whether responding is punished (compare upper and lower right-most panels). Perhaps the most interesting feature of this figure is the fact that the diagonal quadrants show remarkable symmetry (solid arrows) and asymmetry (broken arrows), respectively, as indicated in the center. That is, the effects of the compounds on behavior reinforced by food (top left) are identical to those obtained with punished responding maintained by shock escape (lower right). Precisely the opposite relation holds for behavior maintained by escape from shock and punished behavior maintained by food. This figure, though somewhat oversim-

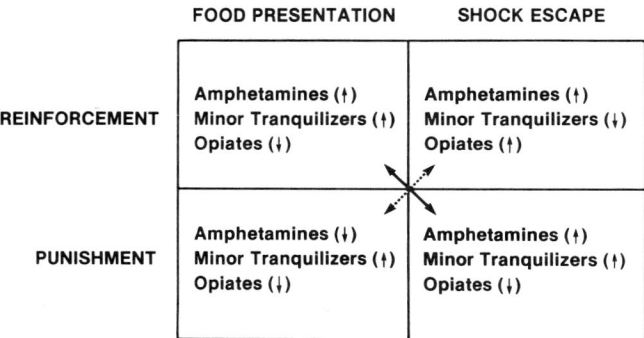

FIG. 3. Effects of amphetamines, minor tranquilizers, and opiates under fixed-interval schedules of food presentation or termination of a stimulus correlated with shock (shock escape) under conditions of reinforcement and punishment. See text for details.

plified because these effects are also subject to other influences (e.g., the schedule, as well as other variables described below), not only conveys a remarkable degree of order in what could be viewed as a diverse array of effects, but also delineates and captures the importance of behavioral variables in the expression of drug effects.

Environmental Context

The schedule-controlled rate of responding and type of reinforcing event are two nonpharmacological variables that appear to influence drug action fairly directly; response rate is evident from ongoing behavior and the maintaining event is a salient and recurring consequence of responding. In some cases, however, drug effects on behavior under one condition can depend on behavioral consequences occurring under a different condition that, although temporally removed, is still part of the more immediate environmental context. As such, the particular behavior under study may not change, except when a drug is administered, thereby revealing an indirect effect or latent interaction between the different conditions controlling behavior. For example, the typical rate-decreasing effects of d-amphetamine on punished food-maintained responding, maintained in one component of a multiple schedule, are reversed if animals are exposed to a shock-avoidance schedule in a separate, distinct component (29). Similarly, the effects of ethanol on responding maintained by food under a fixed-interval schedule can be altered markedly by manipulating the value of a fixed-ratio schedule occurring in a different component (7). Similar effects have been reported with chlorpromazine in unpublished studies by Waller (summarized in ref. 27). Modification of the effects of drugs on these behaviors occurred even though baseline performances during the unchanged portion of the schedule did not differ across conditions. Interactions of this type are striking because the qualitative effects of a drug on behavior (i.e., whether the drug will predominantly increase or decrease responding) can change even though the characteristics of that behavior appear unaffected by modifications in contingencies, consequences, or stimulus conditions (42) during the alternate component of the schedule.

HISTORICAL AND EXPERIENTIAL INFLUENCES

Behavioral History

Those determinants of the behavioral effects of drugs described in the previous sections—response rate, event type, and environmental context—are all part of the relatively immediate environment. However, other conditions that have occurred previously, but that are no longer part of the current environment, can also profoundly influence drug action. These factors comprise the behavioral history of the organism. Perhaps the earliest demonstration of the influence of prior experience on drug effects was reported by Terrace (38), who found that chlorpromazine and imipramine had different effects on discrimination perfor-

mances of pigeons depending on whether training initially occurred under an "errorless" procedure or under a procedure where responses ("errors") were allowed to occur to a stimulus in the presence of which food was not delivered (S⁻). These drugs increased responses to S⁻ when the discrimination was trained with errors but did not do so if training occurred under the errorless procedure.

More recently, several studies have shown that the typical rate-decreasing effects of d-amphetamine on punished responding can be reversed if monkeys are exposed to a shock-postponement schedule (1,3). Figure 4 shows the effects of d-amphetamine on punished responding of squirrel monkeys before and after training under an avoidance schedule in which responding postponed electric shocks. Prior to avoidance training, responding was unaffected or decreased by d-amphetamine (left panel), whereas following exposure to the avoidance schedule, d-amphetamine produced large increases in punished responding. Rate-increasing effects of d-amphetamine on punished behavior occurred even though the rate and patterning of punished responding after exposure to the avoidance schedule were identical to that maintained before avoidance training.

In an effort to delineate some of the variables that might contribute to the modification of amphetamine's effects on punished responding after an avoidance history, a "yoked" experimental procedure was employed to evaluate the role of the shock contingency in these effects (9). After first determining dose-response curves for d-amphetamine under a punishment procedure with food-maintained responding,

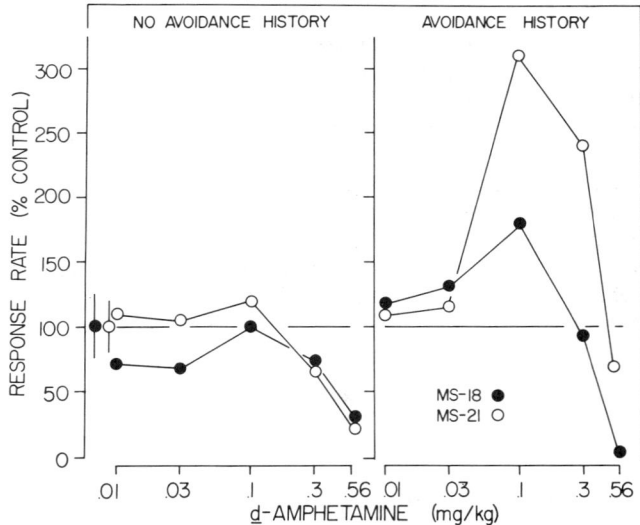

FIG. 4. Modification of the effects of d-amphetamine on punished behavior of squirrel monkeys by behavioral history. Responding maintained by a 5-min fixed-interval schedule of food presentation was punished by delivery of a 7-mA electric shock that followed every 30th response within each interval. Panel on the **left** shows the effects of d-amphetamine on punished responding prior to training under an avoidance or shock-postponement schedule. Panel on the **right** shows effects of d-amphetamine on punished responding after the same monkeys (MS-18 and MS-21) were exposed to an avoidance schedule for approximately 2 weeks. (Adapted from ref. 3.)

some monkeys were then trained under an avoidance schedule where responding postponed the scheduled presentation of shocks. Other monkeys were "yoked" to the avoidance animals and received the same frequency and temporal pattern of shocks that were delivered to the avoidance monkeys when those animals failed to respond. In the case of the yoked subjects, however, shocks were unavoidable and were delivered independently of responding. When dose-response curves were redetermined under the punishment procedure, after exposure to the shock-avoidance or response-independent shock schedules, d-amphetamine produced increases only in responding of animals trained under the avoidance schedule (Fig. 5). Thus, exposure to shock alone was not sufficient to produce a change in the effects of d-amphetamine on punished responding. Figure 5 also shows the effects of d-amphetamine on response duration, a variable analyzed to determine whether the avoidance history altered certain topographical features of the response. However, as indicated in Fig. 5, response duration effects were largely unchanged after exposure to the avoidance schedule. This study appears to eliminate the possibility that the reversal of the effects of d-amphetamine on punished behavior was due to a modification of the response itself or to a general, nonspecific effect of "stress" produced by shocks, regardless of how those shocks were delivered. Response-independent shocks may produce other effects which, under different experimental circumstances, could be important in modifying drug effects. However, the specific contingencies and behavior engendered under the avoidance schedule appear to be responsible for reversing the effects of amphetamine on punished responding.

A number of other studies have also demonstrated the importance of behavioral history under different procedures and with different drugs (9). For instance, exposure of monkeys to a schedule where performances were maintained by response-produced shock reversed the rate-decreasing effects of morphine on avoidance responding (8). As in previous studies, these effects of morphine on responding under the avoidance schedule occurred without alteration of the initial baseline performances. Similarly, the effects of chlordiazepoxide on responding maintained by electric shock were reversed by interpolated training under a punishment schedule (9). In all these cases, including those described for d-amphetamine, the alteration in the qualitative effects of the drugs was not transient but appeared to last indefinitely unless the animals were exposed to another condition.

The role of behavioral history has also been studied in experiments in which animals were exposed to certain schedules of reinforcement and then drug effects were evaluated after this history. In one experiment, the effects of d-amphetamine were studied on lever pressing by rats maintained under a fixed-interval schedule of food delivery (41). Prior to training under the fixed-interval schedule, different groups of rats were exposed to either a fixed-ratio 40 response schedule, which engendered high response rates, or to a schedule where low response rates were maintained due to the requirement of an 11-sec pause between successive responses for food to be delivered. The effects of d-amphetamine on fixed-interval responding differed depending on prior schedule history; responding was decreased in animals with the fixed-ratio history, whereas responding was increased in rats trained previously under

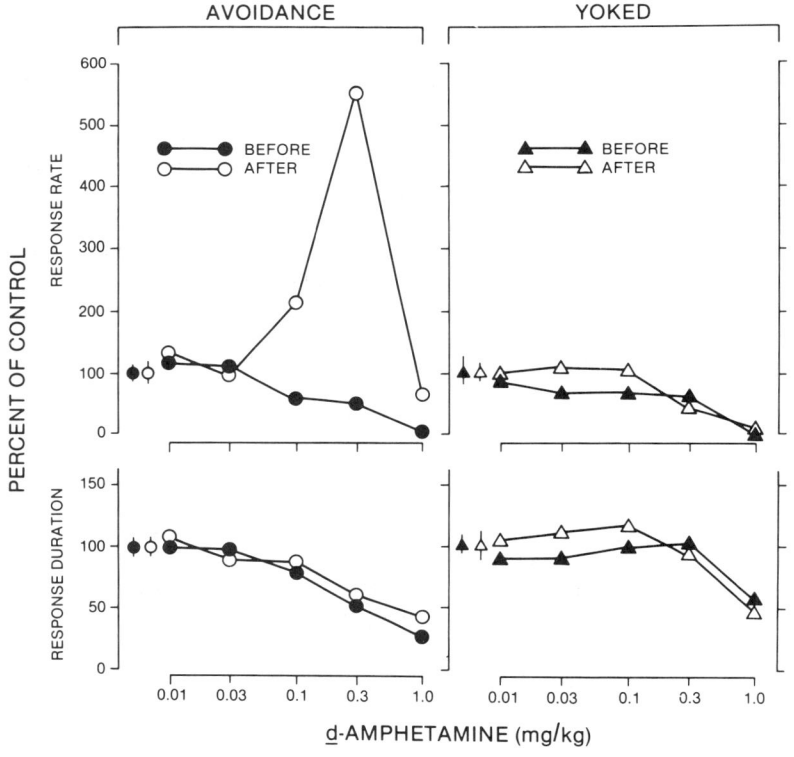

FIG. 5. Effects of d-amphetamine on punished responding of squirrel monkeys before and after exposure to either an avoidance schedule (**left** panels) or a yoked procedure in which the animal received the same frequency and temporal distribution of shocks as did the avoidance monkey (**right** panels). **Top** portion shows data for response rates, which, before exposure to the avoidance or yoked schedule, were 0.038 and 0.024 responses per second for the avoidance and yoked animals, respectively. **Bottom** panels show effects of d-amphetamine on response durations, which, before avoidance or yoked-avoidance training, were 1.12 and 0.252 sec per response for the avoidance and yoked animals, respectively; response duration did not change for the yoked animal but decreased to nearly half for the animal exposed to the avoidance schedule. (Adapted from ref. 9.)

the schedule with the pause requirement. Although there was a clear effect of history, this effect was also apparent in baseline response rate performances. Compared to rats trained initially under the schedule that engendered low response rates, rats that were given fixed-ratio experience showed higher rates of responding under the fixed-interval schedule; drug effects were consistent with a tendency for *d*-amphetamine to increase relatively lower rates of responding and decrease higher response rates.

In a study with a similar design, pigeons were first trained under a variable-interval schedule, following which they responded under either a fixed-ratio or differential-reinforcement-of-low-rate schedule (31). Dose-response curves were determined for methadone under the variable-interval schedule before and after exposure to these schedules. Methadone produced greater decreases in pigeons with the history of low-rate responding, even though the control rates of responding in the different groups did not differ. Further, pigeons with the low-rate history developed tolerance to the rate-decreasing effects of methadone more rapidly and completely than did animals trained under the fixed-ratio schedule. Thus, behavioral history can not only influence the acute effects of drugs, but can also affect the course of tolerance. Further use of selected schedules that engender different specific types of behavioral performances may help identify the salient features of prior experience that contribute to the modification of drug effects.

Taken together, these several studies provide ample support for the importance of behavioral history as a significant factor in determining the effects of drugs. Such studies imply that the effects of drugs on the behaving organism are modifiable over an extremely wide range and that behavioral experience initiates a cascade of effects which then produce differential sensitivity to the effects of drugs.

Pharmacological History

Experience with certain drugs has been known for some time to influence subsequent drug effects. Chronic exposure to one compound frequently produces tolerance to that compound and cross-tolerance to compounds with similar pharmacological activity. Repeated administration of drugs can also enhance the response to certain agents, as when chronic haloperidol produces "supersensitivity" to apomorphine. Recent experiments focusing on the behavioral effects of drugs have also demonstrated similar shifts, as well as alterations, in dose-response functions that were a function of pharmacological experience (20). Unlike traditional findings with drug tolerance, however, these changes in drug effects occurred under conditions where the drug was administered infrequently. Furthermore, experience with one drug produced changes in the behavioral effects of a drug from a different class. These results are shown in Fig. 6, which depicts the effects of pentobarbital on punished responding of squirrel monkeys maintained under a stimulus-shock termination schedule. If monkeys previously received morphine when responding under this schedule, with the dose-response curve determined by twice-weekly administration of morphine (0.01–1.0 mg/kg), the admin-

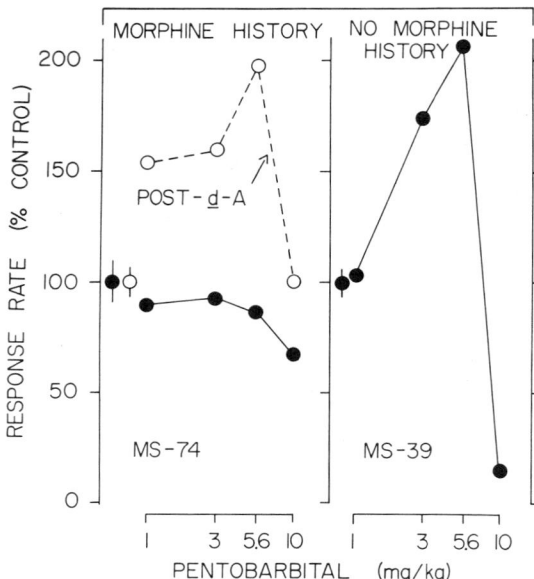

FIG. 6. Effects of pentobarbital on punished behavior of squirrel monkeys with (**left**) and without (**right**) a history of morphine administration. Note that pentobarbital did not increase punished behavior in animals that had previously received acute injections of morphine. However, after *d*-amphetamine, pentobarbital increased responding. (Adapted from ref. 20.)

istration of pentobarbital decreased responding. If, however, pentobarbital was studied first, and there was no prior administration of morphine, pentobarbital produced large increases in response rates. Thus, initial exposure to morphine appeared to prevent or markedly attenuate the rate-increasing effects of pentobarbital. The blockade of the rate-increasing effects of pentobarbital by morphine can, however, be reversed by the administration of *d*-amphetamine. If *d*-amphetamine, which consistently increases responding under these conditions, is subsequently administered to monkeys that first received morphine, the experience with amphetamine overrides the initial effects of morphine such that pentobarbital will produce increases in responding (the dashed curve in Fig. 6 shows pentobarbital's effects after exposure to *d*-amphetamine).

Although all of these effects occur under conditions where drugs are not administered chronically, chronic administration can also reveal different drug effects that depend on how behavior is controlled by its consequences. For example, as described above, *d*-amphetamine generally increases responding under fixed-interval schedules regardless of the type of maintaining event. However, under conditions where performances of squirrel monkeys were maintained by food, by electric shock presentation, or by escape from a stimulus correlated with shock, chronic administration of *d*-amphetamine produced tolerance only in performances under the food and escape schedules (11). Further, in this same study, doses of *d*-amphetamine that initially increased responding maintained by shock produced decreases after chronic administration was discontinued. Both acute and chronic exposure to drugs can produce lasting influences that, again, illuminate the importance of behavioral variables.

Many questions remain about the specific factors responsible for the effects of prior pharmacological experience on the subsequent behavioral effects of drugs. It is not yet known whether mere exposure to these compounds is sufficient to modify drug activity or whether that experience must occur under the specific experimental contingencies of the experiment. A number of studies, described in the following section, suggest that direct changes in the consequences of behavior produced by the drug can dramatically alter the effects of that drug when administered later. If drug-produced changes are responsible for these effects, the studies summarized in this section suggest that behavioral consequences produced by one drug can also influence the effects obtained with other drugs even when those drugs are from pharmacologically distinct classes. Thus, behavioral variables can produce effects that allow the actions of drugs to cross pharmacological boundaries. Regardless of the eventual clarification of these issues, it is apparent that experience with certain drugs can significantly attenuate or preclude the behavioral actions of certain compounds; in other instances drug experience can produce effects that would not otherwise occur.

Drug-Behavior Interaction History

Drug administration often produces direct behavioral effects that may alter the balance of factors that have played an important part in establishing and maintaining behavior. In some cases, it appears that the effects produced by a drug on one occasion can rather dramatically modify the subsequent effects of that drug and, as indicated above, perhaps other drugs as well. For example, Smith and McKearney (37) reported that the first administration of 1.0 mg/kg d-amphetamine markedly increased response rates of pigeons under a schedule in which food was delivered only when a 30-sec pause occurred between responses. The rate increases not only eliminated the extended pauses, but also substantially decreased reinforcement frequency. On the second through fourth injections, there was a marked, progressive diminution of the initial drug effect, even though successive injections were separated by several days. Subsequently, when the pause requirement was removed during drug sessions, increases in responding produced by d-amphetamine occurred consistently on injection. This study demonstrated that the initial effects of a drug can be modified by the specific changes that occur in behavioral consequences when that drug is administered. Unanswered by this study are several questions that focus on issues related to pharmacological tolerance. Although these are tolerance-like phenomena, i.e., there is a progressive decline in the effects of the drug, these effects do not fulfill other defining characteristics of tolerance. For example, the dose-effect curve is not shifted to the right, but only depressed. Studies of this nature do, however, generate additional questions concerning behavioral tolerance (14,15) by demonstrating that progressive changes in the behavioral effects of drugs can occur under conditions where pharmacological tolerance may not be present.

Related experiments using different procedures have also demonstrated marked interactions between behavioral consequences produced by a drug and changes in the subsequent actions of that drug. For example, Smith, Branch, and McKearney (36) studied the effects of d-amphetamine in squirrel monkeys trained under two different procedures in which responses adjusted the intensity of a continuous electric shock. Under one procedure responses decreased shock intensity which, in the absence of responding, increased automatically (escape). Under the second procedure, responses produced food but also increased shock intensity that, otherwise, periodically decreased (punishment). d-Amphetamine increased responding maintained under the escape schedule but not under the punishment schedule. However, if the monkeys first received amphetamine under the punishment schedule, increases did not occur when the drug was then administered under the escape schedule. Mere exposure to the punishment schedule, without d-amphetamine, did not prevent the increases in escape responding produced by d-amphetamine. The combination of the drug plus exposure to the punishment schedule blocked the typical rate-increasing effects of amphetamine on escape responding.

A similar drug-behavior interaction history was found to reverse the usual rate-decreasing effects of morphine on punished responding of squirrel monkeys (10). In this

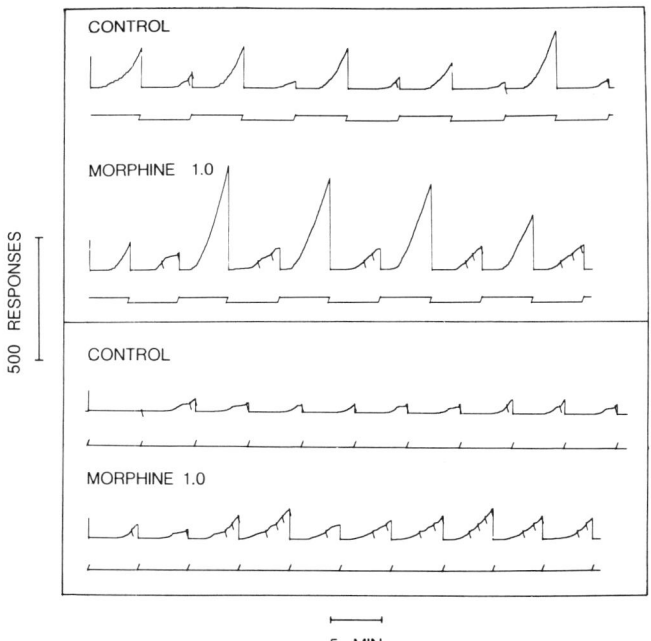

FIG. 7. Top two records show effects of morphine on responding of squirrel monkeys maintained under a multiple schedule of stimulus-shock termination with punishment in one component (pen beneath record offset). Shocks are indicated by diagonal slashes. Morphine increased responding in both components under the multiple schedule. Morphine also increased punished responding when studied alone (**lower two records**). Increases in punished responding with morphine were due to the administration of morphine under the multiple schedule. (Adapted from ref. 10.)

experiment, morphine was first studied on punished and unpunished responding maintained during different components of a multiple schedule. In both components of the schedule, responding under a fixed-interval schedule terminated visual stimuli correlated with shock delivery. During one of the components, responding was also punished by the presentation of shock following each thirtieth response. When morphine was administered, large increases in punished responding occurred; these effects persisted even when morphine was studied later on punished responding alone (Fig. 7). Since these effects on punished responding differed from those found previously (20), the possible contributing factors were analyzed systematically. The effects of morphine were studied on punished behavior alone, before and after exposure to the multiple schedule, and were then studied when the multiple schedule was in effect. Morphine did not increase punished responding when studied before or after exposure to the multiple schedule in which responding was not punished in one component. However, morphine increased punished responding when administered under the multiple schedule, and, as before, these effects persisted even when punished responding was later studied alone. This study indicated that both the environmental context and the effects of the drug under that situation can markedly alter the effects that drug has on behavior. Furthermore, these altered effects persisted even when the critical initial, precipitating influences were removed.

In these studies the effects of different drugs were shown to depend on the combination of the drug and the specific consequences of behavior produced by the drug. Drug-induced changes in the manner in which behavior was controlled by those consequences altered the subsequent actions of that drug and, apparently, other drugs as well. These findings provide additional testimony to the potentially overwhelming significance that behavioral factors can exert in determining the effects of drugs on behavior.

SIGNIFICANCE AND ORIGIN OF BEHAVIORAL INFLUENCES ON DRUG ACTION

Research and theory in behavioral pharmacology have attempted to identify general behavioral variables influencing the effects of drugs and to impose order on the cumulative results of the past 30 years of experimentation. There has been a long-term emphasis on, and a recent renewed interest in, the analysis of behavioral mechanisms of drug action (12,34,39,40). Some of these efforts have attempted to account for the behavioral effects of drugs by analyzing whether drugs produce effects comparable to those obtained when the variables controlling behavior are manipulated. Presumably, if manipulations of these variables produce effects comparable to those produced by a drug, then it could be argued that the drug was exerting its effect by modifying the control of behavior by this variable. However appealing this notion may be, there has not yet been sufficient research to allow adequate evaluation of the merits or feasibility of this approach. There are also enormous difficulties involved. Although our knowledge about

behavior and behavioral processes is still emerging, we currently do know enough about behavior and the behavioral effects of drugs to appreciate the fact that analyses of whether drugs produce effects similar to those found when variables such as delay of reinforcement or reinforcement magnitude are manipulated would be extraordinarily complex. Complexity itself should not be a deterrent. However, manipulation of most controlling variables typically degrades or decreases behavioral measures such as response rate, in contrast to many drug effects, which frequently increase these measures. Additionally, when such manipulations do produce effects, they are relatively small compared to those obtained when a drug is administered. Differences of this type between behavioral manipulations and drug effects are difficult to reconcile and do not strongly endorse the pursuit of behavioral mechanisms that focus on controlling relations of this type. Finally, even if one were to obtain drug effects that were comparable to those, for example, of changing the magnitude of reinforcement, there is no assurance that such effects are functionally equivalent in other respects. Different manipulations can produce similar effects but not share a common mechanism.

Behavior is unquestionably the result of controlling relations, or contingencies, both past and present, but it is unlikely that a drug changes behavior either by mimicking or altering those controlling variables or their functional properties. As indicated some time ago by Kelleher and Morse (24), drugs affect the behavior of the individual, not the controlling relations. It is more a matter of how behavior *is* and *has been* controlled that is critical. Controlling variables are important because they have generated the current behavior, not because they are modified by the actions of a drug. Behavior with a complex history differs in many ways from behavior without such a history. There may be differences in the control of behavior by relevant stimuli or even in the dimensions of the response. Furthermore, even though the controlling relations may appear similar, behavior with a particular history may not only be differentially sensitive to drugs but also to other behavioral interventions. Research in behavioral pharmacology has reemphasized the importance of certain variables that require novel approaches to the analysis of behavior and the behavioral determinants of drug action. Unlike many physiological systems, behavior has not yet been characterized well enough to understand and appreciate the multiple interrelationships and dimensions involved. Whether on the basis of further research these yield behavioral mechanisms of drug action is secondary to arriving at a more complete understanding of behavioral factors involved in drug effects.

SUMMARY

Research in behavioral pharmacology has, without doubt, demonstrated repeatedly and emphatically that the effects of a large number of drugs are sensitive to and, in some cases, dependent on behavioral factors. Behavior is the product of complex interactions between circumstances that occurred previously, but which no longer exist, those that currently exist but are temporally remote, and the more immediate surrounding conditions. Ongoing behavior is dynamic and, unlike systems that tend to be relatively static, embodies the combined influences, both past and present, that can exert powerful control over drug effects. It has often been argued that, because behavioral pharmacology performs research on intact behaving organisms ("whole animal research"), little can be learned about the mechanisms by which drugs exert their effects. This restrictive view, which appears to regard drug action as relatively fixed, recognizes the complexity of behavior but does not adequately acknowledge the myriad orderly and reproducible effects, as well as the dramatic changes in drug effects, that can be obtained when significant behavioral variables are manipulated. Because behavioral variables are so critical in determining the effects of drugs, an understanding of those variables is as fundamental to drug action as is the understanding of traditional pharmacological mechanisms. Fruitful, productive, and innovative research is being conducted in molecular pharmacology that will undoubtedly greatly expand our understanding of basic drug-receptor interactions, neuromodulation, and other fundamental pharmacological mechanisms of drug action. Apparently, however, these mechanisms can be modified or overridden by numerous behavioral variables. An understanding of how the basic molecular mechanisms are behaviorally driven, together with a better understanding of critical behavioral variables, should greatly expand our knowledge of the dynamic interactions between behavioral and pharmacological mechanisms of drug action.

ACKNOWLEDGMENTS

This work was supported in part by PHS Grant DA-02873 from the National Institute on Drug Abuse. I thank Myra J. Zimmerman for assistance in the preparation of the manuscript. Drs. N. A. Ator, J. L. Katz, M. A. Nader, and J. M. Witkin provided helpful comments on the manuscript.

REFERENCES

1. Bacotti, A. V., and McKearney, J. W. (1979): *J. Pharmacol. Exp. Ther.*, 211:80–85.
2. Barrett, J. E. (1976): *J. Pharmacol. Exp. Ther.*, 196:605–615.
3. Barrett, J. E. (1977): *Science*, 198:67–69.
4. Barrett, J. E. (1985): In: *Behavioral Pharmacology: The Current Status*, edited by L. S. Seiden and R. L. Balster, pp. 7–22. Alan R. Liss, New York.
5. Barrett, J. E. (1985): In: *Handbook of Squirrel Monkey Research*, edited by L. A. Rosenblum and C. L. Coe, pp. 315–348. Plenum Publishing Corp., New York.
6. Barrett, J. E., and Katz, J. L. (1981): In: *Advances in Behavioral Pharmacology, Vol. 3*, edited by T. Thompson, P. B. Dews, and W. A. McKim, pp. 119–168. Academic Press, New York.
7. Barrett, J. E., and Stanley, J. A. (1980): *J. Exp. Anal. Behav.*, 34:185–198.
8. Barrett, J. E., and Stanley, J. A. (1983): *Psychopharmacology*, 81:107–110.
9. Barrett, J. E., and Witkin, J. M. (1986): In: *Behavioral Analysis of Drug Dependence*, edited by S. R. Goldberg and I. Stolerman, pp. 195–223. Academic Press, New York.
10. Brady, L. S., and Barrett, J. E. (1986): *J. Exp. Anal. Behav.*, 45:221–228.
11. Branch, M. N. (1979): *J. Pharmacol. Exp. Ther.*, 210:354–360.
12. Branch, M. N. (1984): *J. Exp. Anal. Behav.*, 42:511–522.
13. Branch, M. N., Nicholson, G., and Dworkin, S. I. (1977): *J. Exp. Anal. Behav.*, 28:285–293.
14. Corfield-Sumner, P. K., and Stolerman, I. P. (1978): In: *Contemporary Research in Behavioral Pharmacology*, edited by D. E. Blackman and D. J. Sanger, pp. 391–448. Plenum Press, New York.
15. Demelweek, C., and Goudie, A. J. (1983): *Psychopharmacology*, 80:287–307.
16. Dews, P. B. (1955): *J. Pharmacol. Exp. Ther.*, 113:393–401.
17. Dews, P. B. (1958): *J. Pharmacol. Exp. Ther.*, 122:137–147.
18. Dews, P. B., and Wenger, G. R. (1977): In: *Advances in Behavioral Pharmacology, Vol. 1*, edited by T. Thompson and P. B. Dews, pp. 167–227. Academic Press, New York.
19. Ferster, C. B., and Skinner, B. F. (1957): *Schedules of Reinforcement.* Appleton-Century-Crofts, New York.
20. Glowa, J. R., and Barrett, J. E. (1983): *Science*, 220:333–335.
21. Johanson, C. E. (1978): *J. Pharmacol. Exp. Ther.*, 204:118–129.
22. Katz, J. L., and Barrett, J. E. (1978): *Psychopharmacology*, 56:153–155.
23. Katz, J. L., and Barrett, J. E. (1978): *Pharmacol. Biochem. Behav.*, 8:35–39.
24. Kelleher, R. T., and Morse, W. H. (1968): *Ergeb. Physiol. Chem. Exp. Pharmakol.*, 60:1–56.
25. McKearney, J. W. (1974): *J. Pharmacol. Exp. Ther.*, 190:141–153.
26. McKearney, J. W. (1976): *J. Exp. Anal. Behav.*, 26:281–287.
27. McKearney, J. W. (1979): In: *Advances in Behavioral Pharmacology, Vol. 2*, edited by T. Thompson and P. B. Dews, pp. 39–64. Academic Press, New York.
28. McKearney, J. W. (1980): *Psychopharmacology*, 70:35–39.
29. McKearney, J. W., and Barrett, J. E. (1975): *Psychopharmacologia*, 41:23–26.
30. Morse, W. H., McKearney, J. W., and Kelleher, R. T. (1977): In: *Handbook of Psychopharmacology, Vol. 7*, edited by L. L. Iversen, S. D. Iversen, and S. H. Snyder, pp. 151–180. Plenum Press, New York.
31. Nader, M. A., and Thompson, T. (1987): *J. Exp. Anal. Behav. (in press).*
32. Robbins, T. W. (1982): In: *Theory of Psychopharmacology*, edited by S. J. Cooper, pp. 1–63. Academic Press, New York.
33. Sanger, D. J., and Blackman, D. E. (1976): *Pharmacol. Biochem. Behav.*, 4:73–83.
34. Sidman, M. (1959): *Psychopharmacologia*, 1:1–19.
35. Skinner, B. F. (1938): *Behavior of Organisms.* Appleton-Century-Crofts, New York.
36. Smith, J. B., Branch, M. N., and McKearney, J. W. (1978): *J. Pharmacol. Exp. Ther.*, 207:159–164.
37. Smith, J. B., and McKearney, J. W. (1977): *Psychopharmacology*, 53:151–157.
38. Terrace, H. S. (1963): *Science*, 140:318–319.
39. Thompson, T. (1984): In: *Advances in Behavioral Pharmacology, Vol. 4*, edited by T. Thompson, P. B. Dews, and J. E. Barrett, pp. 1–45. Academic Press, New York.
40. Thompson, T., and Schuster, C. R. (1968): *Behavioral Pharmacology.* Prentice-Hall, Englewood Cliffs, NJ.
41. Urbain, C., Poling, A., Millam, J., and Thompson, T. (1978): *J. Exp. Anal. Behav.*, 29:385–392.
42. Witkin, J. M. (1986): *J. Exp. Anal. Behav.*, 45:195–205.

Psychopharmacology:
The Third Generation of Progress,
edited by Herbert Y. Meltzer.
Raven Press, New York © 1987.

CHAPTER **160**

Environmental and Cultural Factors in the Behavioral Action of Drugs

John L. Falk and David A. Feingold

The last 30 years have seen increased attention given to the contribution that environmental conditions can make to the behavioral action of drugs. A tradition of behavioral analysis under controlled laboratory conditions has produced a technology and a body of knowledge that relates the rules governing the occurrence of certain consequences of an act to the future patterns of occurrence of that act (40). The behavior patterns generated by these "schedules of reinforcement" have functioned as invaluable baseline conditions for analyzing the effects of drugs on behavior. But the environmentally arranged contingencies of reinforcement have effects on the stream of behavior that are more profound than just the passive production of a baseline upon which drugs then reveal their characteristics. Rather, the behavioral effects of drugs are determined not only by their intrinsic pharmacologic properties, but also by environmental contexts within which they act.

Both behavior analysis and anthropology have, within their own disciplines, attempted to make explicit the notion of "environmental context" and to use it to clarify the complex interactions that constitute their realms of study. Within behavior analysis, the study of schedules of reinforcement and the way in which they determine a host of behavioral dynamic effects, as well as unexpected behavioral and physiologic phenomena, has begun to map how profound the influence of the environment can be on the behavioral effects of drugs. Anthropologists study environmental contexts as cultural factors which are determinants of such things as how drugs are taken, under what circumstances, in what amounts, and for what purposes. In behavior analysis, environmental contexts were shown to be important determinants of the major effects of drugs: whether a particular dose stimulates or depresses behavioral output, whether the drug functions as a positive reinforcer or an aversive event, or whether or not functional tolerance is present (e.g., 50). Anthropologists are interested in how drug-determined physiological states, acting within a cultural context, can then be further defined and evaluated as perhaps religious, recreational, or dangerous outcomes.

Although behavior analysis as practiced in laboratory settings, and anthropology with its emphasis on natural settings, might seem to have little in common, there is nonetheless an overriding mutual interest in how the physical, social, and economic environment determines the phenomena that are their subject matters. For our present purposes, we wish to consider how these disciplines can illuminate drug effects, drug-seeking, and drug-taking, with an eye to broadening the ultimate context within which studies in psychopharmacology are viewed.

SUBSTANCE, SET, AND SETTING: INTRINSIC AND INTERACTIONAL EFFECTS

Increased recognition has been given to the importance of analyzing the behavioral action of a drug as a cluster of interactions among the pharmacological substance, the individual set of the organism, and the environmental setting. Yet, at present, with respect to resultant behaviors, it is unclear just which components and interactions of the substance-set-setting cluster produce intrinsically specific outputs, and which might evoke or permit considerable malleability in drug-induced behavior. Understandably, many researchers are most interested in explicating whatever might be the intrinsic specificities of drug action before considering complex interactions. In what sense do drugs have intrinsically specific sensory discriminative dimensions, reinforcing properties, or focused behavioral paths, such as triggering integrated attack, sexual, or ingestive acts? To what extent can substance-set-setting interactions alter or completely transform the behavioral outcomes of drug action? Systematic studies of such questions are recent, but a provisional picture is beginning to take shape.

Intrinsic Response to Drugs and to Environmental Contingencies of Reinforcement

The complex specific receptor systems now known to be present in the brain lend credence to the notion that a host of psychoactive drugs produce their characteristic effects through specific, intrinsic pharmacological actions. These effects are physiological, but include behaviors such as convulsions, sleep, and food and fluid ingestion. Long-term environmental arrangements also can result in specific rates and patterns of behavioral output owing to the intrinsic relations that exist between the environmentally determined contingencies of reinforcement and the resultant patterns of behavior (40). The complex and enduring patterns of behavior that flow on the one hand from the intrinsic actions of drugs, and on the other hand from intrinsic actions of reinforcement contingencies, are qualitatively different. The first consists mainly of unconditioned behaviors, whereas the second is composed of a learned operant unit response that is emitted in a characteristic pattern primarily determined by the particular environmental contingency currently in effect.

Interaction of Intrinsic Responses: Production of Quantitative and Qualitative Changes in Drug Response

Interactions between the two kinds of intrinsic determinants of behavior have received extensive laboratory study. Drugs, as one might expect, affect the behavior patterns produced by schedules of reinforcement. The quantitative details of how this occurs made it evident that even in the simplified and highly controlled context of the laboratory many of the initial notions of the behavioral effects of classes of drugs had to be amended. For example, a particular dose of pentobarbital when administered to an animal trained on a multiple fixed-ratio 50, fixed-interval 15-min schedule[1] increased the fixed-ratio rate of behavior

but decreased the rate produced by the fixed-interval component (24). This study and a host of ensuing experiments made it clear, for example, that drugs could no longer be simply classified as stimulants or depressants of behavior. In Dews' (24) study, a particular dose of pentobarbital in the same organism with respect to the same reinforcer at proximal points in time functioned as a stimulant or a depressant depending on what component schedule of reinforcement was brought to bear. Hence when even intrinsic determinants interact, the behavioral outcomes, while quite lawful, produce effects that make it impossible to characterize a drug's behavioral action independently of the contingency of reinforcement controlling behavior.

Schedules of reinforcement can determine not only how drugs affect the quantitative aspects of behavioral output such as response rate; they also can affect the qualitative properties of drugs as reflected by the kind of control they exert over behavior. For example, many studies have analyzed the powerful reinforcing effects of cocaine in animals and humans (43). Nevertheless, monkeys self-administering cocaine intravenously in accordance with a variable-interval schedule[2] will simultaneously work on a second lever where a fixed-interval schedule produces 1-min periods of time-out from the opportunity to continue with the cocaine self-administration schedule (77). This result is counterintuitive if one believes that when positive reinforcers are being actively approached they should not be simultaneously escaped. But given the explicit environmental option, quite clearly they can be.

Another sort of motivational duality can be unmasked for nicotine (42). It is intravenously self-administered by monkeys on a fixed-interval 5-min schedule, indicating its efficacy as a reinforcer. But similar doses effectively punished[3] lever-pressing in a fixed-ratio 30 food schedule. As Goldberg and Spealman (42) state: "Thus, under different conditions, nicotine was found to have pronounced effects either as a punisher or as reinforcer. These findings are important because they emphasize that the behavioral effects of nicotine are neither immutable nor predictable solely on the basis of the drug's inherent pharmacological qualities."

Prior Experience with One Kind of Environmental Contingency Can Alter Drug Response to a Different Contingency

Current schedules of reinforcement, then, can change and even completely transform the effects of drugs on

---

[1] In a multiple schedule, reinforcement is programmed by two or more schedules of reinforcement which occur in random sequence with each schedule accompanied by a particular stimulus during the time it is in effect. In a fixed-ratio schedule, reinforcement is scheduled to occur upon the completion of a fixed number of responses since the last reinforced response. In a fixed-interval schedule, reinforcement is scheduled to occur following the first response after a given interval

of time has elapsed since the last reinforced response. In the example given, reinforcement occurs after every fiftieth response in the fixed-ratio 50 component of the multiple schedule, and after the first response that occurs 15 min after the last reinforced response in the fixed-interval 15-min component.

[2] In a variable-interval schedule, reinforcement is scheduled to occur following the first response after a random interval of time has elapsed since the last reinforced response. The given mean of the intervals lies between two assigned values.

[3] In a punishment procedure, an event that occurs contingent upon some response decreases the probability of that response occurring under similar circumstances.

behavior. However, until recently, it was not evident that prior experience with a behavior schedule can change the characteristic way in which a particular drug affects a current schedule of reinforcement. Stated another way, the "set" of the individual can be radically altered by experience with a reinforcement contingency so that a drug affects a current schedule performance in a manner quite differently from how it affects an individual without such an interpolated experience (62). For example, a simple, undrugged history of responding under a shock-avoidance schedule[4] reversed the usual effects of d-amphetamine when the drug was administered weeks later in connection with a punishment schedule in which responding reinforced by food presentation is suppressed by response-produced electric shock[5] (7). For morphine, the dose-effect relation on a shock-avoidance schedule was reversed by a prior history of response-produced shock; for chlordiazepoxide it was reversed for response-produced shock by a history of punished responding (8). Thus, environmental factors in the form of behavior schedules, both those in the remote past that change the individual's "set" and those currently in effect, can quantitatively and qualitatively influence the behavioral effects of drugs.

Environmental Factors Determining the Development of Drug Tolerance

Classical pharmacology assumed that a phenomenon such as the acquisition of tolerance to a drug was a function of repeated drug administration altering the individual's "set" owing to the metabolic or CNS physiological changes that were intrinsic effects of the drug-exposure history. Recent investigations have changed this view by presenting evidence that the presence of tolerance is strongly related to crucial environmental variables: (a) whether the test for drug tolerance is performed in the same environment in which the agent was previously administered, and (b) whether the criterion behavioral measure used to assess tolerance has been performed under the influence of the course of repeated drug administrations given prior to the test for tolerance. The contingent nature of drug tolerance alluded to in (a) above is illustrated by the following experiment (75). Rats injected with morphine daily and then tested for analgesia following the fourth injection in the same environment showed much less analgesia (i.e., they were morphine tolerant) than animals given the same course of daily morphine injections but receiving the fourth-day analgesia test in a different environment. The arrangement described in (b) was used in an early experiment by Carlton and Wolgin (13). Food-deprived rats injected with amphetamine daily for 8 days prior to consuming a daily meal became tolerant to the anorectic effect of the drug after the fourth day of drug administration. Another group got the same course of injections but received them after the daily meal, rather than before. When this second group was then switched to the procedure used for the first group to assess their response to amphetamine, they gave no evidence of tolerance to the drug. Despite the same daily exposure to the drug, they too took 4 days to become tolerant under the new procedure. That is, they responded to amphetamine as if they were drug naive. Clearly, for behavioral tolerance to a drug to develop, the behavior must occur in the daily portion of the induction phase during which the organism is in the drugged state.

THE ENVIRONMENT AS A CRUCIAL CATALYZER IN DRUG RESPONSE

Thus far, the discussion has been centered on how intrinsic responses to drugs and to environmental contingencies interact to produce current and long-term changes in the organism's response to drugs. But the environment can affect responses to drugs in ways that do not work directly through contingencies of reinforcement. Two prototypical experiments illustrate how a seemingly small change in environmental circumstances can (a) radically alter a drug's dose-effect relation, or (b) induce behavioral changes that can precipitate, among other effects, massive increases in drug intake.

The Dose-Response Relation

The LD_{50} point for amphetamine sulfate in mice was reduced by approximately 50% when animals were confined in jars with a small floor area after injection compared to larger area jars. But the LD_{50} dose difference was almost 10 times lower when mice were simply caged with a few other mice, rather than singly, after injection (16,17,56). Thus, even a dose-effect relation for lethality, which would not seem to be a strong candidate for modulation by the environment, can be nevertheless shifted radically by relatively benign and noninvasive environmental factors.

Excessive Behavior Induction and Drug-Taking

The imposition of another kind of simple environmental constraint can induce a variety of exaggerated behaviors, including overindulgence in drugs. Briefly, about 25 years ago it was observed that rats reduced to 80% of their normal body weights and allowed to obtain a small pellet of food on a variable-interval 1-min schedule for approximately 3 hr each day drank approximately 10 times as much water compared to a control condition in which they were given the same total amount of food all at once and water intake was recorded for a similar 3-hr period (32,33). Although such animals are never water deprived, nor do the environmental conditions impose any water balance derangement, they continue their food-schedule-induced polydipsia during each daily session for months on end. During the remainder of each 24-hr cycle they were housed in individual home cages with free access to water, but little was ingested. If animals exposed to such a schedule-induced polydipsia procedure are given their usual session

---

[4] In an avoidance schedule, a response postpones for a period of time the occurrence of an aversive event.

[5] Using schedules such as fixed-interval or variable-interval, it has been shown that responding can be maintained by the response-produced presentation of electric shock.

amount of food all at once as a single ration, then the water intake for that session falls to normal, control amounts; when returned to their home cages they do not ingest unusual amounts of water. Clearly, they are not under any physiological constraint to drink unusual amounts of fluid. Unlike drinking that is produced by water depletion or by an NaCl load, this polydipsia is largely unaffected by intubating even a large load of water into the stomach before a session. Neither does it depend on the intermittent eating of a dry food pellet; appropriate liquid food portions engender water overdrinking as well. The overdrinking, then, is a behavioral phenomenon and is not attributable to metabolic need.

Experimental analysis has revealed that schedule-induced polydipsia, as well as several other excessive adjunctive behaviors, is (a) a bitonic function of the rate at which food pellets are delivered, and (b) an inverse function of body weight as determined by the degree of food deprivation. Thus, sessions with small interpellet times (a few seconds) and large times (5 or 10 min) do not induce overdrinking; but as time is increased beyond a few seconds, drinking increases up to a maximum point, whereas longer interpellet times produce proportional decreases in drinking. Food deprivation is a necessary, but not a sufficient, condition; the degree of overdrinking in daily sessions decreases progressively over a several-day period if body weight is allowed to increase beyond approximately 95% of normal.

If schedule-induced polydipsia in rats were an isolated phenomenon it would hardly be of systematic importance. However, not only are a variety of excessive behaviors induced as adjuncts to the delivery of scheduled reinforcers, but a broad range of species reveal these exaggerated behaviors. Intermittent food delivery can generate not only polydipsia, but also severe attack behavior in pigeons and in squirrel monkeys (for reviews of these and further studies described, see refs. 34 and 35). Further, attack behavior, like polydipsia in rats, Java macaque, and rhesus monkeys, is a bitonic function of interfood time, and a direct function of deprivation-produced decreases in body weight. Schedule-induced exaggeration of several kinds of general activities occurs in animals and humans. For example, scheduled access to monetary gain, gambling opportunities, or maze-solving induced greatly increased locomotor activities and body movements in humans compared to unscheduled conditions. Studies on humans usually do not employ deprivation and scheduled access to food as the inducing condition. Besides hyperactivity, humans have shown schedule-induced increases in fluid intake, eating, grooming, and smoking (e.g., 18).

A variety of schedule-induced excessive behaviors can occur given the appropriate environmental generating conditions. In general terms, deprivation of a valued commodity or activity does not in itself produce excessive adjunctive behavior. It is deprivation in conjunction with the temporal constraint of episodic delivery of limited portions of a valued commodity in one domain that induces excessive behavior in relation to commodities in some other domains. Schedule-induced chronic excessive intake has been demonstrated for a number of drugs taken orally: alcohol (37), pentobarbital (64), phenobarbital (81), nicotine (74), morphine (57), etonitazene (63,65), amphetamine (73), phen-

cyclidine (14), chlordiazepoxide (72), and midazolam (38). Intermittent food delivery schedules were used to induce chronic overindulgence of these drug solutions. For some of these drugs, physical dependence was demonstrated to have developed (alcohol, phenobarbital, midazolam). Not just oral drug overindulgence occurs. Similar schedules also induce animals to intravenously self-administer excessive heroin, methadone, cannabis, and nicotine (66,76,80).

Since schedule-induction conditions can produce chronic and excessive oral drug-taking in animals in preference to water, or even to some glucose solutions (71,82), it is possible that these conditions are similar to ones catalyzing drug overindulgence in humans. For humans too, when life's crucial commodities are in short supply and available only on intermittent, marginal schedules, such as may occur in an impoverished, inner-city environment, drugs can become all-powerful in reinforcing efficacy. Further, such an environment fails to foster the acquisitions of skills important for attaining the conventional crucial commodities, ensuring that marginality becomes endemic. Again, in accordance with the aforementioned bitonic functional relation, excessive drug-taking would not be expected under too attenuated a rate of commodity attainment (destitution), but rather would be characteristic of intermediate rates.

Also, it is not just economically and educationally inadequate environments that constitute generating conditions for drug abuse and other excesses. An attenuated social reinforcement matrix, which nevertheless sets high standards for achievement, may constitute quite adequate schedule-induced drug-taking conditions. If this is coupled with an affluence providing easy access to expensive drugs, it could result in a lack of engagement with conventional schedules of reinforcement and an excessive engagement with drugs, the taking of which is further sustained by an alternative socially reinforcing matrix of drug-culture denizens. This is possibly the context generating drug abuse among affluent youth.

Finally, drug abuse also seems overrepresented in groups that work on schedules of reinforcement with intermediate intermittency rates characteristic of occupations where problematic consequentiality is continually faced. Goffman (41) has described this diverse set of occupations as being located "where the action is." They include market speculators, prospectors, high-construction workers, test pilots, a variety of hustling jobs such as commission salesmen and promoters, performing jobs such as politicians, actors, sports performers, and a variety of small-time criminals who must continually engage in street-wise action to "make it." The rather continuous facing of events with possible critical importance at an intermediate reinforcement rate is a life situation that seems to generate adjunctive behavior excesses such as drug abuse.

DRUGS AS CULTURAL ARTIFACTS

The use of psychopharmacological agents is virtually a panhuman trait. In fact, there is some evidence that even nonhuman animal species in the wild seek out certain plants that contain potentially psychoactive drugs (26). Alcohol, the drug with widest geographical and historical distribution, was discovered and rediscovered untold times in the history of the human race. "Only Pacific Islanders and the indigenes of most of North America failed to discover the manufacture of alcoholic beverages on their own" (61, p. 2).

As far as we know, there is no society in the world that does not make use of some psychoactive substance. However, there is also no society we know of that permits unrestricted use of the full range of drugs available by all members of the society. Drugs are cultural artifacts (60), or more precisely, the processes that define drugs and delineate consumption behaviors are culturally mediated. Therefore, both the primary inducements toward and constraints on drug consumption are cultural. These are the determinants of the societal, situational, environmental, and scene and/or subcultural appropriateness of drug-using behaviors.

For well over a century, evidence has accumulated of significant cultural variation in patterns of drug use and in responses to specific drugs. Testimony before the Royal Opium Commission and published debate in Britain in the 1890s, for example, puzzled over the fact that the same opium that was widely used in India without noticeable harm produced widespread addiction in China.

Even earlier, *The Jesuit Relations* commented extensively on the perceived differences in alcohol use patterns between Indians and non-Indians in North America, and often accounted for these in what today we would see as cultural terms (21).

Turkey and Iran are both Moslem societies that have produced opium commercially for over a century. The Persians consumed significant quantities of opium; the Turks never did.

More recently, there has been increased interest in examining the relationships between drug effects and social situations. It has been noted that "there is strong evidence attesting to the powerful impact of social environments, relations, and structures upon physiology—and, as an intervening variable, upon drug effects" (6, p. 80). They develop a concept of "sociopharmacology" stressing three issues: the effects of social situations on drug responses, the effects of drugs on social situations, and the interaction between the two. The emphasis, however, is on microsocial processes, rather than on larger cultural ones. It may be useful, therefore, to supplement the sociopharmacological agenda with a formulation of what might be called "cultural pharmacology."

Culture, in the sense used here, refers to hierarchically structured sets of rules, by which humans endow experience with meaning. Such rules may be seen as of two types: definitional (parametric) and strategic. The former operate to define and delimit events and categories. These are the rules that tell us what "game" is being played; they allow us to differentiate a chess match from the Super Bowl, a striptease from a church service, an Akha pig sacrifice from simply eating pork, or the American Association for the Advancement of Science from the Independent Order of Odd Fellows. However, although these rules define the game being played, they don't define how to play it well. Whether playing chess or "copping" heroin, there are strategic rules of effective social performance. Not all rules are equally powerful, and not all players equally adept. Similarly, in social encounters, definitions of the situation are problematic and emergent from a process of negotiation and renegotiation. Cultural rules set the parameters of this process. These rules must be learned, and, therefore, are susceptible to investigation—whether they concern learning to drink in France (5), drunken comportment in the United States (59), the rituals of heroin among urban American heroin addicts (4), the behavioral rules for heroin sales in Hawaii (12), or drug dealing in California (2).

The contributions of cultural anthropology to the understanding of the behavioral actions of drugs essentially entail three elements: a comparative perspective, an ethnographic methodology, and an interpretive theoretical paradigm. Obviously, not every study embodies all three: Anthropological studies have been carried out in our own society (e.g., 3,68,78,83); many studies do not limit themselves to ethnographic methods, narrowly construed (e.g., 11,15,70,85); and a number of anthropologists have been ecological, rather than interpretive, in their theoretical orientation (e.g., 9,11). Nevertheless, these elements are those that most clearly characterize the anthropological research agenda.

CULTURAL PATTERNING OF DRUG EFFECTS

In the public mind (and sometimes in other academic fields), anthropology is often viewed as the disciplinary repository of obscure knowledge of esoteric practices in societies very remote from our own. Yet, from the very inception of the discipline, cultural (or social) anthropology has taken as its aim not merely the acquisition of ethnological trivia, but rather the elucidation of sociocultural processes. To this end, it has emphasized cross-cultural comparison to test theories derived from the experience of Western societies and what has come to be known as "controlled comparison."

Ruth Bunzel (10), in her ground-breaking paper on the role of alcoholism in two Central American cultures, presented the initial attempt at controlled comparison between very similar cultures that differed markedly in their patterns of alcohol use.

Much of the anthropological literature on drugs and alcohol has been concerned with the traditional use of psychoactive substances, particularly hallucinogens, in a religious ritual context. La Barre (54) and Aberle (1) produced classic studies of the peyote religion among Native Americans of the Southwest. Numerous other studies have explored the use of *ayahuasca* and other hallucinogens among the native peoples of the Amazon region (25,45,52). Wilbert (89) has drawn attention to the magicoreligious use of tobacco among the Indians of South America. In Africa, Fernandez (39) described the use of *Tabernanthe iboga* by two cults among the Fang of Gabon. Various *Datura* preparations are also used in trance possession ceremonies in different African societies. Such uses of drugs represent only a portion of the repertoire of induction techniques used by communicants among peoples for whom trance and/or hallucination are sacrillized and, therefore, highly valued experiences. Nondrug techniques include chanting, drumming, repetitive dance movements, induced hyperventilation, and meditation exercises, among others.

It is also true that whereas trance possession may be deemed necessary for specialists such as spirit mediums or shamans in many societies, these same societies frequently see trance behavior in nonspecialists as potentially dangerous to both the individual experiencing it and those around him or her. Feingold's research among the Akha of the Thai-Burma frontier has shown that whereas Spirit Mediums (*nipa*), who make contact with the spirit world through trance, are utilized as one vehicle for the culturally appropriate diagnoses of disease, the trance experience itself is viewed as highly undesirable. Although other types of religious practitioners, such as Spirit Doctors (*Pima*), are accorded high status and respect, the Spirit Medium is often a female of relatively low status and the object of considerable ambivalence. This accords with similar patterns that have been reported for other regions (e.g., 58).

The cultural patterning of hallucinatory experience, whether induced by drug or nondrug means, is clear from the ethnographic record (26,30). Individuals belonging to cultures in which hallucinogens have been traditional vehicles for religious experience "enter a drug experience with certain expectations about the content and form of drug-induced visionary experience: this is especially so when specific beliefs are held and the individual's experience is programmed by a skillful shaman or priest" (26, p. 402).

CULTURAL FACTORS AFFECTING USE AND ABUSE

It is evident that such processes are not limited to non-Western societies. By now, the role of hallucinogens in European witchcraft is widely recognized (45). For earlier periods, the ritual use of psychotropic botanicals in the Old World can be demonstrated for periods from 7,000 to 8,000 years ago, with some indications of still more ancient use of some substances (55). Such uses of hallucinogens have been related by La Barre and others to theories of the shamanic origins of religion (55). It must be noted, however, that these theories have not won universal acceptance among anthropologists and archaeologists, particularly as they pertain to relations between cultural complexes found in the New World and the Old. Nevertheless, the antiquity of the use of psychotropics is clearly indicated, even if the details of their introduction await further clarification.

The comparative perspective of anthropology, both across cultures and across time, has not been limited to the study of alcohol and hallucinogens. Ground-breaking studies on the use of cannabis, sponsored by both the National Institute of Mental Health (NIMH) and NIDA, have been conducted in Jamaica (19,20,29,69,70), Greece (79), Colombia (67), and Costa Rica (15). These studies, focusing on chronic cannabis user populations, have called into question many of the assertions that have been made regarding the long-term effects of cannabis. Although these studies have been conducted in diverse cultural and social settings, by different researchers, utilizing a variety of interdisciplinary approaches, there has been a remarkable coherence to their findings. The "stepping-stone hypothesis"

finds little support in any of these studies, and the universality of the so-called "amotivational syndrome" is clearly refuted (15,20). In sum, the cross-cultural studies of chronic cannabis use have shown little evidence of long-term effects as compared to nonusers. In Costa Rica, for example, in which the chronic smokers had "smoked an average of nearly ten marihuana cigarettes (2.0 gm of material or exposure to 24–70 mg of THC) per day for a minimum of ten years (mean 16.9 years) prior to the beginning" of the project (15, p.11), the conclusion of the $2\frac{1}{2}$-year project was that "if chronic marihuana use leads, in the long run, to deleterious effects, these must be subtle indeed" (15, p. 207).

Not surprisingly, many of these results have proved politically unpalatable to policy-makers. Nevertheless, collectively they represent major landmarks in long-term study of chronic cannabis use, the data and conclusions of which must be confronted by any serious investigator in this field.

Although many of the cross-cultural studies of marijuana (see above), opiates (e.g., 85–88), and alcohol (31,46,47) have been interdisciplinary, combining anthropological, biomedical, and psychological techniques, it is the ethnographic component that has set anthropological studies apart.

Ethnography focuses on the contexted investigation of naturally occurring situations. The emphasis is on intensive, rather than extensive, methods, the careful control over analogy, and the use of "natural experiments." Ethnography should not be equated with simply any form of open-ended interview or "hanging out." Instead, it should aim at what Clifford Geertz has called "thick description," which is context-rich and situationally grounded. Unlike questionnaire research (which may be used to supplement ethnography), the emphasis is on what people do, not simply what they say they do. This requires extended periods of observation, in natural environments, and for most purposes, control of the local language. Participant observation requires the skills of the field biologist, rather than the laboratory biochemist. Both have important contributions to make; each has limitations.

All experiments are based on analogy to an external world. Laboratory conditions allow excellent control over variables, but inferior control of analogy. Ethnography allows outstanding control over analogy, if less precise control over variables. However, since the consumption of drugs by humans is a social activity, *par excellence,* this analogical control is vital to any real understanding of drug-seeking and drug-using behaviors.

We have noted before that anthropological studies of drugs have been characterized by an interpretive theoretical paradigm. Anthropology seeks to understand the processes by which humans endow experience with meaning. Physiological states are endowed with meaning, which, in turn, influences those states. It is clear, for example, that expectations play an important role in human experiences with psychotropic substances, both on a societal and an individual level (22,36,53,59,90). Opium has very different meanings for Akha, Yao, or Hmong in the hills of Thailand than for De Quincey or Cocteau, for example. In consequence, there is relatively little similarity in their experience of the drug or natural performance under its influence.

The cultural factors that influence drug consumption in any society are diverse. Most commonly, consumption is limited by sex, age, role, and condition of life. For example, among the Akha of North Thailand, Laos and Burma, "recreational" opium smoking is socially restricted to adult males, as is the drinking of alcohol. Women and children of both sexes are sometimes given opium for illness, though not generally by pipe. Moreover, although some adult women will smoke, most often introduced to the practice by their husbands, they are few compared to men, and the amount of opium each consumes is significantly less than that consumed by their male counterparts. In contrast to opium and alcohol, tobacco is allowed to both women and children of both sexes as soon as they show any desire to smoke.

Similarly, social roles delineate consumption patterns, in that types and amounts of drug use that are appropriate to occupants of certain social roles are not appropriate to others. For example, among a number of different societies, the use of certain drugs is restricted to ritual specialists (45). In addition, in many groups particular roles carry with them restrictions on consumption that do not apply to other members of the society (e.g., airplane pilots in the United States).

In addition to illness necessitating or precluding the consumption of a particular drug, other conditions of life can influence drug-using behaviors. Ritual purity or impurity may prescribe or proscribe the use of particular substances. It is also obvious that social class membership can encourage the consumption of some drugs, while discouraging the use of others. Through the centuries, many hierarchically organized societies have had sumptuary laws that limited use or consumption of certain goods to members of a particular class (when Robin Hood was poaching the King's deer he was violating a sumptuary law, as was anyone, other than the Emperor, who placed a five-toed dragon on his house in late traditional China). Less formal social rules also operate. Class-based drug choices are functions of what might be called "style rules" as well as of economics; solvent abuse, to cite an obvious case, is rarely found among upper-class adults.

Macrocultural factors influence the availability and cost of drugs, and hence influence consumption patterns. Westermeyer (84), in an important article, demonstrates "the pro-heroin effects of anti-opium laws in Asia." Similarly, the net result of marijuana suppression campaigns in Mexico has been to move American users from relatively low THC Mexican marijuana to higher THC Colombian- and Californian-grown product.

The cultural patterning of time, setting, and occasion also influences drug use. In many societies (including our own) there are periods of licensed intoxication (e.g., Mardi Gras, Carnival, New Year's Eve), during which behavior that might otherwise be denigrated or punished is allowed or even encouraged. Abstinence is also enforced during certain periods either through taboo or the milder dictates of etiquette. Physical location and social setting have profound effects on both quantity of drugs consumed and subjective experiences of their effects. The pub in Britain, the kat room in Yemen, the opium den in nineteenth-century China, and the New York heroin "shooting gallery"

all have their protocols that operate on the amounts, timing, and co-occurrence of the drugs used.

Consumption factors that are influenced by cultural rules include the following: dosage, drug interactions, and the antecedent biological state of the user. Cultural rules play a large role in determining dosage both because of the use of culturally defined measures for dispensing drugs and because of cultural definitions of appropriate levels of consumption (23,28,44,47,49,51,91). Drug interactions occur because of appropriateness rules regarding what substances are consumed together. For example, Akha opium smokers smoke raw opium which has been mixed with opium ash and white powder packaged as Chinese medicine which turns out to be powdered aspirin. The mixture is moistened, most usually with tea. At an opium-smoking session, tobacco and tea are invariable accompaniments to opium. In China in the early part of the century, opium was often mixed with strychnine. Fermented tea, chewed in northern Thailand and Shan States for at least 500 years, is mixed with a variety of other substances as flavor enhancers.

Antecedent biological states of users are influenced by such factors as fasting, sleep deprivation, trance practice, feasting, etc. These, in turn, clearly impact on drug effects, and constitute important environmental factors in the assessment of drug actions.

REFERENCES

1. Aberle, D. F. (1966): *The Peyote Religion Among the Navaho.* Aldine, Chicago.
2. Adler, P. A. (1985): *Wheeling and Dealing.* Columbia University Press, New York.
3. Agar, M. (1973): *Ripping and Running.* Seminar Press, New York.
4. Agar, H. M. (1977): In: *Drugs, Rituals and Altered States of Consciousness,* edited by B. M. DuToit, pp. 137–148. A. A. Balkema, Rotterdam.
5. Anderson, B. G. (1979): In: *Beliefs, Behaviors, and Alcoholic Beverages,* edited by M. Marshall, pp. 429–432. University of Michigan Press, Ann Arbor.
6. Barchas, P. R., and Barchas, J. D. (1977): In: *Psychopharmacology,* edited by J. D. Barchas, P. A. Berger, R. D. Ciaranello, and G. R. Elliott, pp. 81–87. Oxford University Press, New York.
7. Barrett, J. E. (1977): *Science,* 198:67–69.
8. Barrett, J. E., and Witkin, J. M. (1986): In: *Behavioral Analysis of Drug Dependence,* edited by S. R. Goldberg and I. Stolerman, pp. 195–223. Academic Press, New York.
9. Bolton, R. (1973): *Ethnology,* 12:257–277.
10. Bunzel, R. (1940): *Psychiatry,* 3:361–387.
11. Burchard, R. E. (1975): In: *Cannabis and Culture,* edited by V. Rubin, pp. 463–484. Aldine, Chicago.
12. Carlson, K. A. (1977): In: *Drugs, Rituals and Altered States of Consciousness,* edited by B. M. DuToit, pp. 191–205. A. A. Balkema, Rotterdam.
13. Carlton, P. L., and Wolgin, D. L. (1971): *Physiol. Behav.,* 7:221–223.
14. Carroll, M. E., and Meisch, R. A. (1980): *J. Pharmacol. Exp. Ther.,* 215:339–346.
15. Carter, W. E., ed. (1980): *Cannabis in Costa Rica.* Institute for the Study of Human Issues, Philadelphia.
16. Chance, M. R. A. (1946): *J. Pharmacol. Exp. Ther.,* 87:214–219.
17. Chance, M. R. A. (1947): *J. Pharmacol. Exp. Ther.,* 89:289–296.
18. Cherek, D. R. (1982): *Pharmacol. Biochem. Behav.,* 17:523–527.
19. Comitas, L. (1975): In: *Cannabis and Culture,* edited by V. Rubin, pp. 119–132. Aldine, Chicago.
20. Comitas, L. (1976): *Ann. NY Acad Sci. USA,* 282:24–32.

21. Dailey, R. C. (1979): In: *Beliefs, Behaviors and Alcoholic Beverages,* edited by M. Marshall, pp. 116–127. University of Michigan Press, Ann Arbor.
22. Davis, W. (1985): *The Serpent and the Rainbow.* Simon and Schuster, New York.
23. Dennis, P. A. (1979): In: *Beliefs, Behaviors, and Alcoholic Beverages,* edited by M. Marshall, pp. 54–64. University of Michigan Press, Ann Arbor.
24. Dews, P. B. (1955): *J. Pharmacol. Exp. Ther.,* 113:393–401.
25. Dobkin de Rios, M. (1973): In: *Hallucinogens and Shamanism,* edited by M. J. Harner, pp. 67–85. Oxford University Press, New York.
26. Dobkin de Rios, M. (1975): In: *Cannabis and Culture,* edited by V. Rubin, pp. 401–416. Aldine, Chicago.
27. Dobkin de Rios, M. (1977): In: *Drugs, Rituals and Altered States of Consciousness,* edited by B. M. DuToit, pp. 237–249. A. A. Balkema, Rotterdam.
28. Doughty, P. L. (1979): In: *Beliefs, Behaviors, and Alcoholic Beverages,* edited by M. Marshall, pp. 64–81. University of Michigan Press, Ann Arbor.
29. Dreher, M. R. (1982): *Working Men and Ganja.* Institute for the Study of Human Issues, Philadelphia.
30. DuToit, B. M. (1977): *Drugs, Rituals and Altered States of Consciousness.* A. A. Balkema, Rotterdam.
31. Everette, M. W., Waddell, J. O., and Health, D. R., eds. (1970): *Cross-Cultural Approaches to the Study of Alcohol: An Interdisciplinary Perspective.* World Anthropology Series. Mouton, The Hague.
32. Falk, J. L. (1961): *Science,* 133:195–196.
33. Falk, J. L. (1969): *Ann. NY Acad. Sci. USA,* 157:569–593.
34. Falk, J. L. (1971): *Physiol. Behav.,* 6:577–588.
35. Falk, J. L. (1981): In: *Behavior in Excess,* edited by S. J. Mulé, pp. 313–337. Free Press, New York.
36. Falk, J. L. (1983): *Pharmacol. Biochem. Behav.,* 19:385–391.
37. Falk, J. L., Samson, H. H., and Winger, G. (1972): *Science,* 177:811–813.
38. Falk, J. L., and Tang, M. (1985): *Drug Alcohol Depend.,* 15:151–163.
39. Fernandez, J. W. (1972): In: *Flesh of the Gods,* edited by P. T. Furst, pp. 237–260. Praeger Publishers, New York.
40. Ferster, C. B., and Skinner, B. F. (1957): *Schedules of Reinforcement.* Appleton-Century-Crofts, New York.
41. Goffman, E. (1967): *Interaction Ritual.* Anchor, Garden City, NY.
42. Goldberg, S. R., and Spealman, R. D. (1982): *Fed. Proc.,* 41:216–220.
43. Grabowski, J., ed. (1984): *Cocaine: Pharmacology, Effects, and Treatment of Abuse (NIDA Res. Monogr. 50).* US Government Printing Office, Washington, DC.
44. Harding, W. M., and Zinberg, N. E. (1977): In: *Drugs, Rituals, and Altered States of Consciousness,* edited by B. M. DuToit, pp. 111–133. A. A. Balkema, Rotterdam.
45. Harner, M. J., ed. (1973): *Hallucinogens and Shamanism.* Oxford University Press, New York.
46. Heath, D. B. (1974): *J. Alcoholism Related Addict.,* 10:24–42.
47. Heath, D. B. (1975): In: *Research Advances in Alcohol and Drug Problems, Vol. 2,* edited by R. J. Gibbins, Y. Israel, H. Kalant, R. E. Popham, W. Schmidt, and R. G. Smart, pp. 1–92. John Wiley & Sons, New York.
48. Honigmann, J. J. (1979): In: *Beliefs, Behaviors, and Alcoholic Beverages,* edited by M. Marshall, pp. 30–35. University of Michigan Press, Ann Arbor.
49. Honigmann, J. J. (1979): In: *Beliefs, Behaviors, and Alcoholic Beverages,* edited by M. Marshall, pp. 414–428. University of Michigan Press, Ann Arbor.
50. Kelleher, R. T., and Morse, W. H. (1968): *Ergeb. Physiol. Biol. Chem. Exp. Pharmacol.,* 60:1–56.
51. Keller, M. (1979): In: *Beliefs, Behaviors, and Alcoholic Beverages,* edited by M. Marshall, pp. 404–414. University of Michigan Press, Ann Arbor.
52. Kensinger, K. M. (1973): In: *Hallucinogens and Shamanism,* edited by M. Harner, pp. 9–14. Oxford University Press, New York.
53. Kornetsky, C. (1976): *Pharmacology: Drugs Affecting Behavior.* John Wiley and Sons, New York.
54. La Barre, W. (1938): *The Peyote Cult.* Yale University Publications in Anthropology, No. 19, New Haven, Connecticut.
55. La Barre, W. (1972): In: *Flesh of the Gods,* edited by P. T. Furst, pp. 261–278. Praeger Publishers, New York.
56. Lasagna, L., and McCann, W. P. (1957): *Science,* 125:1241–1242.
57. Leander, J. D., McMillan, D. E., and Harris, L. S. (1975): *J. Pharmacol. Exp. Ther.,* 195:279–287.
58. Lewis, I. M. (1971): *Ecstatic Religion.* Penguin Books, Baltimore.
59. MacAndrew, C., and Edgerton, R. B. (1969): *Drunken Comportment: A Social Explanation.* Aldine, Chicago.
60. Mandelbaum, D. G. (1965): *Current Anthropology.,* 6:281–293.
61. Marshall, M., ed. (1979): *Beliefs, Behaviors, and Alcoholic Beverages.* University of Michigan Press, Ann Arbor.
62. McKearney, J. W. (1979): In: *Advances in Behavioral Pharmacology, Vol. 2,* edited by T. Thompson and P. B. Dews, pp. 39–64. Academic Press, New York.
63. McMillan, D. E., and Leander, J. D. (1976): *Pharmacol. Biochem. Behav.,* 4:137–141.
64. Meisch, R. A. (1969): *Psychon. Sci.,* 16:16–17.
65. Meisch, R. A., and Stark, L. J. (1977): *Pharmacol. Biochem. Behav.,* 7:195–203.
66. Oei, T. P. S., Singer, G., and Jefferys, D. (1980): *Psychopharmacology,* 67:171–176.
67. Partridge, W. L. (1975): In: *Cannabis and Culture,* edited by V. Rubin, pp. 147–172. Aldine, Chicago.
68. Preble, E., and Casey, J. J. (1969): *Int. J. Addict.,* 4:1–24.
69. Rubin, V. (1975): In: *Cannabis and Culture,* edited by V. Rubin, pp. 257–266. Aldine, Chicago.
70. Rubin, V., and Comitas, L., eds. (1975): *Ganja in Jamaica.* Mouton, The Hague.
71. Samson, H. H., and Falk, J. L. (1974): *J. Pharmacol. Exp. Ther.,* 190:365–376.
72. Sanger, D. J. (1977): *Pharmacol. Biochem. Behav.,* 7:1–6.
73. Sanger, D. J. (1977): *Psychopharmacology,* 54:273–276.
74. Sanger, D. J. (1978): *Pharmacol. Biochem. Behav.,* 8:343–346.
75. Siegel, S. (1975): *J. Comp. Physiol. Psychol.,* 89:498–506.
76. Smith, L. A., and Lang, W. J. (1980): *Pharmacol. Biochem. Behav.,* 13:215–220.
77. Spealman, R. D. (1979): *Science,* 204:1231–1233.
78. Spradley, J. P. (1970): *You Owe Yourself a Drunk: Ethnography of Urban Nomads.* Little, Brown, Boston.
79. Stefanis, C., Liakos, A., and Boulougouris, J. C. (1976): *Ann. NY Acad. Sci. USA,* 282:58–63.
80. Takahashi, R. N., and Singer, G. (1980): *Pharmacol. Biochem. Behav.,* 13:877–881.
81. Tang, M., Ahrendsen, K., and Falk, J. L. (1981): *Pharmacol. Biochem. Behav.,* 14:405–408.
82. Tang, M., and Falk, J. L. (1977): *Pharmacol. Biochem. Behav.,* 7:471–474.
83. Weppner, R. S. (1973): *J. Soc. Appl. Anthropol.,* 22:111–121.
84. Westermeyer, J. (1976): *Arch. Gen. Psychiatry,* 33:1135–1139.
85. Westermeyer, J. (1982): *Poppies, Pipes, and People: Opium and Its Use in Laos.* University of California Press, Berkeley.
86. Westermeyer, J., and Peng, G. (1977): *J. Nerv. Ment. Dis.,* 164:346–350.
87. Westermeyer, J., and Peng, G. (1977): *J. Nerv. Ment. Dis.,* 164:351–354.
88. Westermeyer, J., and Peng, G. (1978): *Br. J. Addict.,* 73:181–187.
89. Wilbert, J. (1975): In: *Cannabis and Culture,* edited by V. Rubin, pp. 439–461. Aldine, Chicago.
90. Wilson, G. T. (1981): In: *Advances in Substance Abuse: Behavioral and Biological Research, Vol. 2,* edited by N. Mello, pp. 1–40. JAI Press, Greenwich, CT.
91. Yamamura, B. (1979): In: *Beliefs, Behaviors, and Alcoholic Beverages,* edited by M. Marshall, pp. 270–277. University of Michigan Press, Ann Arbor.

Psychopharmacology:
The Third Generation of Progress,
edited by Herbert Y. Meltzer.
Raven Press, New York © 1987.

CHAPTER **161**

Alcoholism and Drug Abuse: An Overview

Nancy K. Mello and Roland R. Griffiths

Substance abuse disorders are the most prevalent of all psychiatric disorders in this country according to a 1984 survey of metropolitan areas organized by the National Institute of Mental Health (NIMH). Alcohol abuse and alcohol dependence ranked first of all psychiatric disorders in lifetime prevalence rates, followed by phobias, major depressive disorders, and drug abuse and dependence (8). In 6-month prevalence rates, alcohol abuse and alcohol dependence ranked first among psychiatric disorders in men aged 18 to 64 and fourth in women aged 18 to 24. Drug abuse and/or dependence was the second most common psychiatric disorder among men and women aged 18 to 24. These data are striking testimony to the current public health impact of substance abuse disorders in relation to phobias, depression, schizophrenia, and other psychiatric disorders (7,8).

The escalating social and economic costs of alcoholism and drug abuse parallel the prevalence of substance abuse disorders. In 1984, the National Institute on Drug Abuse (NIDA) estimated that the annual cost of drug abuse is about $100 billion (3). Of this figure, perhaps $10 to $16 billion is accounted for by expenditures for health care, general welfare, law enforcement, and loss of job productivity. The costs of criminal drug trafficking may account for $70 to $80 billion dollars each year. In 1975, the total economic costs of alcoholism, including health care, loss of productivity, accidents, and crime were estimated at $42.75 billion (1). Over the ensuing 10 years, this figure, adjusted for inflation, may approach $80 billion. Thus, a conservative estimate of the total annual economic cost of alcoholism and drug abuse combined could exceed $160 billion. Such estimates of economic costs are useful to dramatize the societal impact of substance abuse disorders, but dollars alone cannot convey the human costs involved—these are incalculable.

Through biomedical and behavioral research, there have been many advances in our understanding of alcohol and drug abuse disorders. The 15 chapters in this section summarize some recent research on substance abuse problems. They describe current knowledge about the behavioral and biological effects of alcohol and other drugs. The determinants of risk for and the medical consequences of alcohol and drug abuse are examined. Recent advances in the treatment of alcohol and drug dependence are also described with a critical appraisal of the advantages and limitations of new pharmacotherapies. It has not been possible to cover the entire spectrum of substance-abuse-related research in this section. Rather, an attempt has been made to review selectively research on drugs of particular concern today and to emphasize some of the areas where there has been significant progress in research.

TRENDS IN SUBSTANCE ABUSE PROBLEMS

The chapters in this section illustrate that substance use and abuse can take many forms. The spectrum of drug abuse problems continually changes, and trends in particular drug use patterns are often evanescent, almost faddish. The past two decades have witnessed a shift from hallucinogens (LSD, mescaline) during the 1960s to abuse of heroin and marijuana in the early 1970s, followed by introduction of another hallucinogen, phencyclidine (PCP), during the late 1970s (R. L. Balster, *this volume*). The recent increase in cocaine abuse is reminiscent of the cocaine epidemic at the turn of the century (6; M. Fischman, *this volume*). Drug Abuse Warning Network (DAWN) mentions of cocaine increased by 55% between 1979–80 and 1981–82 (2). But in the mid 1980s, there appears to be a gradual decline in marijuana use by young adults (J. H. Mendelson, *this volume*). However, the lifetime prevalence of marijuana use among adults over 26 is estimated at about 23% (2). The abuse of anxiolytic and sedative drugs also appears to be declining according to survey and DAWN report data (R. R. Griffiths and C. A. Sannerud, *this volume*). Heroin abuse ranked second in DAWN mentions between 1979–

80 and 1981–82, and emergency ward mentions involving heroin increased by 48% during this period (2). After a period of relative quiescence, PCP reemerged as the fifth most frequently reported drug in hospital emergency room admissions during 1984.

Other recent entries into the kaleidoscope of abused drugs are synthetic analogs of PCP, stimulants, and opioids. Although alteration in the molecular structure of a drug is beyond the capacity of the average drug abuser, some illicit drug suppliers, sophisticated in chemistry, have developed so-called "designer drugs," which involve minor variations in chemical structures of regulated compounds (thus evading legal regulatory control). These drug analogs may have major toxic consequences because of increased potency and/or increased concentrations of toxic contaminants. MDMA or "ecstasy" is one well-publicized entry into the designer drug market (R. A. Glennon, *this volume*). The specter of a proliferation of "designer drugs" portends an ominous future for eclectic drug abusers.

Despite intensive antismoking campaigns orchestrated by the federal Department of Health and Human Services (DHHS) and private organizations, tobacco smoking remains one of the most prevalent forms of drug use in this country. In 1982, an estimated 55 million smokers purchased 623 billion cigarettes (R. Jones, *this volume*). A gradual shift in public attitudes about the acceptability of smoking has paralleled accumulating evidence of the adverse medical consequences of smoking. Moreover, recent research on the pharmacology of nicotine has led many to conclude that nicotine is a "prototypic" drug of abuse (R. Jones, *this volume*).

In this country, the majority of people drink alcohol and use alcohol responsibly. However, alcohol abuse and alcoholism are increasingly visible problems, rivaled only by heart disease and cancer in public health impact (N. K. Mello, *this volume*). Surveys estimate that approximately 10 million people are alcoholic or have serious drinking problems. But the social stigma associated with alcoholism has always led to denial of the problem and underreporting. Inconsistencies in criteria for alcohol abuse and spontaneous remission of alcohol problems further complicate the counting process (5).

POLYDRUG ABUSE: SOME IMPLICATIONS

Most chapters in this section focus on a single drug or drug class, i.e., alcohol, sedative anxiolytics, cocaine, marijuana, opioids, phencyclidine, and tobacco. But there is increasing evidence that substance abuse often involves the use of several drugs, concurrently or simultaneously. Alcoholics may also abuse tobacco, tranquilizers, opioids, depressants, and caffeine (N. K. Mello, *this volume*). Similarly, opioid addicts may also abuse alcohol, benzodiazepines, cocaine, marijuana, and other available drugs (M. J. Kreek, *this volume;* R. R. Griffiths and C. A. Sannerud, *this volume*). Marijuana is often used with alcohol and tobacco (J. H. Mendelson, *this volume*). Historically, multiple drug use may have been more common than is usually recognized—the combined use of wine and opium (laudanum) was not unusual in Victorian times (5).

But an increased awareness of the prevalence of polydrug abuse today challenges many traditional concepts about the origins of substance abuse and further complicates analysis of these disorders. One potentially salutary effect of a polydrug abuse perspective is that examination of similarities in drug use patterns and their behavioral consequences becomes almost mandatory. There is a possibility that various forms of drug abuse may have common characteristics that transcend the pharmacological distinctions between drugs. If the concept of substance abuse facilitates identification of meaningful commonalties among abused drugs, this should help to evaluate and perhaps alleviate the inevitable substance abuse problems of tomorrow.

SOME MEDICAL CONSEQUENCES OF ALCOHOL AND DRUG ABUSE

The adverse medical consequences of drug abuse are emphasized throughout this section. The most prevalent type of medical disorder is often associated with the route of drug administration. For example, smoking tobacco, marijuana, and cocaine all are associated with compromised pulmonary function (R. Jones, M. Fischman, J. H. Mendelson, *this volume*). Intravenous use of cocaine and opioids enhances risk of a variety of infectious diseases ranging from viral hepatitis to bacterial or fungal endocarditis to acquired immunodeficiency disorder (AIDS) (M. Fischman, M. J. Kreek, *this volume*). By January 1986, 16,458 AIDS cases had been reported by the Center for Disease Control, and 17% of these were intravenous drug users. Intravenous drug users accounted for 56% of all females with documented AIDS (4). Alcohol abuse is associated with liver disease, gallbladder and pancreatic disease, gastric disorders, pulmonary disease, and cardiovascular disorders (N. K. Mello, *this volume*). The combined use of alcohol, cocaine, and heroin can enhance risk of toxic effects of each drug used independently (M. J. Kreek, *this volume*).

The potential hazards of drug abuse may be altered by changes in the route of drug administration. For example, overdose deaths from cocaine appear to reflect increased use of intravenous cocaine and of free-base cocaine smoking (M. Fischman, *this volume*). The use of chewing tobacco instead of smoking tobacco has less deleterious effects on pulmonary function, but it appears to increase the risk for oral cancer (R. Jones, *this volume*).

Alcohol and opioids each may have profound adverse effects on reproductive function in both men and women (M. J. Kreek, N. K. Mello, *this volume*). Marijuana also disrupts pituitary–gonadal hormones essential for reproduction in females and decreases sperm count and motility in males (J. H. Mendelson, *this volume*). Alcohol, opioids, marijuana, and tobacco all have been shown to have adverse effects on fetal growth and development (N. K. Mello, M. J. Kreek, J. H. Mendelson, R. Jones, *this volume*).

The adverse effects of abused drugs on brain function and behavior can be as toxic as effects on organ systems. Phencyclidine, a dissociative anesthetic, can produce a toxic psychosis similar to schizophreniform disorders

(R. L. Balster, *this volume*). The transient mood elevation associated with cocaine intoxication is rapidly replaced by a profound dysphoria characterized by anxiety, depression, and fatigue (M. Fischman, M. J. Kreek, *this volume*). Alcohol and heroin intoxication also may be associated with depression and anxiety after an initial positive change in mood (N. K. Mello, *this volume*). Recent longitudinal studies show that depression is often a consequence of alcohol dependence, not an antecedent (N. K. Mello, *this volume*). Although the physical dependence-inducing capacity of benzodiazepines has been recognized for some time, recently it has been shown that normal therapeutic doses of these widely prescribed drugs also produce physical dependence after prolonged treatment (R. R. Griffiths and C. A. Sannerud, *this volume*).

RISK FOR SUBSTANCE ABUSE DISORDERS

It is very difficult to define the parameters of enhanced risk for substance abuse disorders. The diversity of drug abusers and the ever-changing array of abused drugs and drug combinations present many obstacles to a search for simple origins. The importance of peer pressure in initial drug experimentation is well recognized, but the factors that maintain or sustain an ongoing pattern of drug abuse are less clearly understood.

Like other substance use disorders, alcoholism has long eluded the best efforts of scientists to identify the factors that mitigate for risk, remission, and relapse. But recent research strongly implicates genetic factors in contributing to the risk for alcohol problems (M. A. Schuckit, *this volume*). Systematic analyses of the behavioral and biological correlates of a family history of alcoholism are under way. Identification of reliable predictors could eventually clarify the biological mechanisms that underlie enhanced risk for alcohol problems (M. A. Schuckit, *this volume*). To date, biological risk factors for other substance use disorders have not been systematically explored.

RESEARCH STRATEGIES FOR ANALYSIS OF ALCOHOL AND DRUG ABUSE

Clinical studies of illicit drugs of abuse have always been limited by constraints associated with the reliability of information provided by the street drug user and the illegality of the drug use behavior. During the past decade there have been significant advances in clinical research on drug abuse problems. It is now well recognized that it is essential to study drug effects during a period of drug intoxication in well-controlled clinical studies rather than to rely on recalled impressions. As valid data about drug abuse are acquired and street lore is relegated to the realm of questionable anecdote, the opportunity for understanding drug abuse disorders is increased immeasurably. Effective strategies for treatment and eventually for prevention depend critically on systematic clinical research on alcohol and drug abuse problems.

One recurrent theme that emerges from these reviews is the concordance between data obtained from clinical studies and from basic studies in animal models. Twenty years of research has consistently demonstrated that drugs that are abused by man are usually self-administered by laboratory animals (R. L. Balster, R. R. Griffiths and C. A. Sannerud, M. Fischman, C. Johanson, W. L. Woolverton, and C. Schuster, N. K. Mello, J. H. Woods and G. Winger, *this volume*). Alcohol, cocaine, opioids, phencyclidine, barbiturates, benzodiazepines, amphetamines, and nicotine are just a few examples of drugs abused by man and self-administered in animal models. The availability of a reliable and valid animal model of drug self-administration has a number of practical and heuristic implications. The model permits the prediction of potential liability for abuse of new drugs and analysis of many of the possible behavioral and medical consequences of human drug abuse. For example, the toxic consequences of cocaine abuse were completely predictable from behavioral pharmacological studies of cocaine self-administration by animals (M. Fischman, *this volume*). A primate model of alcohol self-administration developed disruptions of reproductive function like those seen in alcoholic women (N. K. Mello, *this volume*). Phencyclidine, opioids, barbiturates, and benzodiazepines are also self-administered by experimental animals, and these models have been particularly useful for examining withdrawal signs under spontaneous and antagonist-precipitated withdrawal conditions (R. L. Balster, J. H. Woods and G. Winger, R. R. Griffiths and C. A. Sannerud, *this volume*). The value of animal models for investigating the pharmacological and behavioral mechanisms underlying drug dependence has been repeatedly demonstrated (C. Johanson, W. L. Woolverton, and C. Schuster, *this volume*).

Animal models can also provide a sensitive behavioral assay of drug similarities and differences and can be used to categorize new drugs on the basis of their discriminative effects. The unique profile of PCP intoxication described by PCP abusers is paralleled by basic studies of drug discrimination in animals, which show that PCP effects are discriminable from those of many other psychotropic drugs (R. L. Balster, *this volume*). Furthermore, the disarmingly simple, yet powerful drug discrimination methodologies have recently shown their utility in providing useful and unique functional information about structure–activity relationships and drug receptor systems. Such contributions to understanding of basic pharmacological mechanisms of action of abused drugs are well illustrated in the reviews of PCP (R. L. Balster, K. M. Johnson, *this volume*), MDA-like hallucinogens and stimulants (R. A. Glennon, *this volume*), and opioids (J. H. Woods and G. Winger, *this volume*). For example, recent studies have shown that a behavioral analysis of drug discriminative and reinforcing effects can differentiate between μ and κ opioid agonists. The exciting implications of this approach to analysis of opioid agonists, mixed agonists, and mixed agonist–antagonists is more fully discussed in the review of opioids, receptors, and abuse liability (J. H. Woods and G. Winger, *this volume*).

Another important new application of animal models of drug self-administration is in the prediction and evaluation of new pharmacotherapies for drug abuse (C. Johanson, W. L. Woolverton, and C. Schuster, *this volume*). In addition to the value of these drug self-administration models for assessing abuse liability, evaluation of the effects of a treatment drug on self-administration of an abused drug can provide an indication of its clinical treatment efficacy (C. Johanson, W. L. Woolverton, and C. Schuster, *this volume*). Potentially adverse interactions between treatment drugs and other abused drugs can be evaluated in such animal models before exploratory clinical trials.

The increasing prevalence of multiple drug use and abuse poses new challenges for all aspects of research on drug abuse (M. J. Kreek, *this volume*). Treatment of alcohol and drug abuse is greatly complicated by polydrug abuse problems, and judicious selection of pharmacotherapies has become even more difficult (M. J. Kreek, J. Jaffe, *this volume*). Yet systematic clinical studies have already shown that some drugs modify the effects and use patterns of other drugs, often in ways not entirely predictable from the pharmacology of each compound. An improved understanding of multiple drug interactions will be an important dimension of substance abuse research during the next decade. Development of animal models of polydrug abuse is another obvious and valuable extension of basic behavioral pharmacological research. The escalating prevalence of substance abuse disorders in comparison to other psychiatric disorders (8) provides a renewed impetus for a continuing commitment to scientific research and for allocation of federal resources for research that are commensurate with the magnitude of the problem.

ACKNOWLEDGMENTS

Preparation of this review was supported by Grants DA 02519, DA 00101, DA 01147, DA 03889, and DA 03890 from the National Institute on Drug Abuse (NIDA) and by Grants AA 04368 and AA 06252 from the National Institute on Alcohol Abuse and Alcoholism (NIAAA).

REFERENCES

1. Alcohol and Health (1981): *Fourth Special Report to the U.S. Congress, DHHS Publ. No. (ADM) 81-1080.* U.S. Government Printing Office, Washington.
2. Clayton, R. (1984): In: *Drug Abuse and Drug Abuse Research, DHHS Triennial Reports to Congress,* pp. 13–34. U.S. Government Printing Office, Washington.
3. Department of Health and Human Services (1984): *Drug Abuse and Drug Abuse Research, DHHS Triennial Reports to Congress.* U.S. Government Printing Office, Washington.
4. Fauci, A. F. (1985): *Ann. Intern. Med.,* 102:800–813.
5. Mendelson, J. H., and Mello, N. K. (1985): *Alcohol: Use and Abuse in America.* Little, Brown, Boston.
6. Musto, D. F. (1973): *The American Disease: Origins of Narcotic Control.* Yale University Press, New Haven, London.
7. Myers, J. K., Weissman, M. M., Tischler, G. L., Holzer, C. E., Leaf, P. J., et al. (1984): *Arch. Gen. Psychiatry,* 41:959–967.
8. Robins, L. N., Helzer, J. D., Weissman, M. M., Orvaschel, H., Gruenberg, E., et al. (1984): *Arch. Gen. Psychiatry,* 41:949–958.

Psychopharmacology:
The Third Generation of Progress,
edited by Herbert Y. Meltzer.
Raven Press, New York © 1987.

CHAPTER 162

Alcohol Abuse and Alcoholism: 1978–1987

Nancy K. Mello

Since the last ACNP review of research on alcoholism and alcohol effects on behavior in 1978 (21), there have been a number of advances in our understanding of alcohol problems and the medical consequences of alcohol abuse. This review describes some recent studies of the extent of alcohol problems as well as new information about the adverse health consequences of alcohol abuse. The relationship between alcoholism and other forms of substance use and abuse are also examined. Recent developments in the treatment of alcoholism are reviewed by J. Jaffe elsewhere in this volume. The effects of alcohol on aggression, memory, mood, performance, sexuality, sleep, and sociability were described in a previous ACNP review (21).

ALCOHOLISM AND ALCOHOL ABUSE DEFINED

Research on alcoholism has always been complicated by ambiguities in the definition of alcoholism and controversy over whether or not alcoholism is a disease (29). In 1980, the American Psychiatric Association revised its diagnostic criteria for alcohol abuse and alcoholism to facilitate early recognition of alcohol problems (5). The revised APA criteria (DSM-III) emphasize a pathological drinking pattern and evidence of social or occupational impairment. Alcohol abuse is inferred if these disturbances have persisted for "at least one month." Alcoholism is distinguished from alcohol abuse by tolerance and physical dependence. Tolerance is defined as the "need for markedly increased amounts of alcohol to achieve the desired effect, or a markedly diminished effect with regular use of the same amount." Dependence is defined as "the development of alcohol withdrawal (e.g., morning shakes and malaise relieved by drinking) after cessation of or reduction in drinking" (5).

The DSM-III diagnostic criteria for alcoholism, the end stage of alcohol abuse, are relatively specific because the pharmacological criteria of tolerance and physical dependence (withdrawal) are clearly defined. Diagnostic criteria for alcohol abuse are more ambiguous, but one advantage of the new DSM-III criteria is that cultural criteria are not used as the basis for diagnosis. Also noteworthy is that the frequency-of-intoxication criteria used in DSM-II have been replaced by a more realistic duration-of-drinking criteria. But it is obvious that episodic drinking for 1 month has no intrinsic advantage over episodic drinking once each month in establishing an unequivocal diagnosis of alcohol abuse (29). Conspicuously absent from the DSM-III criteria are ill-defined constructs such as "craving" and "loss of control." These constructs once were offered as simplistic explanations for alcoholism but have not survived the empirical test of scientific scrutiny (29).

THE EXTENT OF ALCOHOL PROBLEMS TODAY

Alcoholism is rivaled only by heart disease and cancer as a major public health problem. It has been estimated that alcohol-abuse-related expenses account for about 12% of the nation's total expenditures for health (1). The economic costs in terms of lost productivity, accidents, crime, and health care expenditures were estimated at $42.75 billion in 1975 (2).

Accurate estimates of the number of persons who are alcoholic or have serious drinking problems have always been limited by imprecise standards for what constitutes a drinking problem. The stigma usually associated with alcoholism has led to denial by the patient, the family, and the physician. Moreover, alcoholism fluctuates in severity as do other chronic diseases such as diabetes or arthritis. However, it has been estimated that 9% of adult men and

5% of adult women are at risk for the development of alcoholism or alcohol abuse (2).

In 1984, the first reports of the National Institute of Mental Health (NIMH) collaborative studies on the prevalence of psychiatric disorders showed that alcohol abuse and dependence are currently one of the most common forms of psychiatric disorders (33,40). In lifetime prevalence rates, alcohol abuse and alcohol dependence ranked first of all psychiatric disorders, followed by phobias, major depressive episodes, and drug abuse and dependence (40). In the 6-month prevalence rates, alcohol abuse and alcohol dependence ranked first among psychiatric disorders in men aged 18 to 64. In men over 65, alcohol abuse and alcohol dependence ranked third after severe cognitive impairment and phobias. In women, rates of alcohol abuse and dependence for 6-month and lifetime prevalence were significantly lower than in men, but alcohol abuse and dependence were the fourth most common psychiatric disorders for young women aged 18 to 24. The prevalence of alcohol abuse among women has prompted increased concern over the effects of substance use on women's health (39). The NIMH data, based on a survey of 10,000 persons, are probably the most accurate estimates of the prevalence of alcohol abuse and dependence yet available (33,40).

ANTECEDENTS OF ALCOHOL PROBLEMS

Anyone can develop a serious drinking problem, and alcohol abuse can take many forms. Efforts to identify significant predisposing factors and to predict who is at greatest risk for alcoholism have been disappointing. Research has not yet identified any biological, psychological, or social/cultural variable that uniformly predicts alcohol abuse or alcoholism (22). But there is increasing evidence that children of alcoholics are at high risk for the development of alcohol problems, and data concerning the biology of risk for alcoholism are reviewed by M. A. Schuckit in this volume. However, many people develop alcohol problems independently of a family history of alcoholism, and the great diversity of developmental and social experiences suggests that no one factor can "explain" or predict why some people develop drinking problems and others do not.

It was once believed that depressive illness was a frequent antecedent of alcoholism, and antidepressants were often prescribed for the treatment of alcoholism. Improved definitions of alcoholism and of depression have shown that although these disorders may coexist, alcoholism is not necessarily a symptom of depression. A recent analysis of over 10,000 first admissions for alcoholism treatment showed that only 1.5% were diagnosed as suffering from an affective disorder (28). In 1983, results from a prospective longitudinal study showed that alcoholism may develop first, and depression may be a consequence of problem drinking rather than the obverse (47). A sample of professional school graduates was studied for up to 20 years, and it was shown that the development of depression before problem drinking was far less common than severe depression following chronic alcoholism or alcohol abuse (47). There is also little firm evidence to support the notion that

drinking problems develop as a consequence of a reactive depression to a major loss or stressful experience. Some people drink in an effort to ameliorate stress, tension, or sadness, whereas others do not. It is increasingly recognized that alcohol is not an effective antidepressant and may actually increase despondency at high doses (22).

Alcohol abuse is a complex behavioral disorder determined by many interrelated factors. Attempts to unravel the origins of alcohol problems may prove to be less productive than attempts to understand how abusive drinking patterns are maintained. Behavioral science research suggests that it may be meaningful to try to identify factors that determine an ongoing pattern of alcohol abuse, abstinence, and relapse. Drinking behavior is maintained by its consequences. Although these consequences are complex and varied, analysis of the functional relationship between particular consequences and drinking episodes offers an approach to understanding how alcohol abuse is maintained (see ref. 22 for review).

ALCOHOLISM AND THE PREVALENCE OF MEDICAL DISORDERS

It is well known that chronic alcohol abuse and alcohol dependence are associated with a variety of medical disorders and that gastrointestinal disorders, especially liver disease, can be directly related to alcohol toxicity (3,19,43). Pancreatic dysfunction, a variety of malabsorption syndromes, and alcoholic cardiomyopathy also are commonly observed in alcohol abusers. Tobacco smoking appears to be an important factor contributing to pulmonary disease among alcoholic men. There is also an association among smoking, heavy drinking, and increased risk for cancer of the mouth and larynx (3). Alcohol has many adverse effects on male reproductive function (9). However, systematic attention to the effects of alcohol on female reproductive function and possible implications for normal fetal growth and development have attracted scientific attention only recently. Current research on alcohol effects on reproductive function in women is discussed in a later section of this chapter.

Studies of the medical concomitants of alcoholism and alcohol abuse traditionally have relied on patients with compromised social and economic resources treated in city, state, or federally supported facilities. Recent surveys of medical disorders in over 10,000 first admissions for alcoholism treatment to proprietary hospitals have documented the medical concomitants of alcoholism in middle-income people (28,31). Men comprised 76% of the sample, and women accounted for 24%. The age range was from 15 to 85 years, but the majority of patients were between 35 and 59. Twenty percent of the men and 14% of the women were over 60 years old at first admission. Over 70% of the patients had a significant medical problem other than alcoholism. Liver disease, gallbladder and pancreatic disease, and pulmonary disease (bronchitis, emphysema, and asthma) were the most prevalent disorders based on International Classification of Diseases (ICDA-8) diagnoses. Hypertensive disease was present in 15% of the males and 7% of the females. The high prevalence of medical disorders among middle-class patients suggests that inpatient treatment for alcoholism should be undertaken where serious medical illnesses can be concurrently treated (28).

Balancing these adverse consequences of alcohol abuse on health, there is some evidence that moderate alcohol use (three or more drinks per day) may be associated with a lower rate of nonfatal myocardial infarction and sudden cardiac death (17). There is also evidence that moderate alcohol use may protect against premature (before age 50) cardiovascular disease in women (41). The precise mechanism of this apparent protective effect of alcohol is unknown (17). However, three or more drinks per day was associated with higher systolic and diastolic blood pressure in both men and women compared to alcohol abstainers and people who drank two or fewer drinks each day (17), and alcoholism has been implicated as a risk factor in stroke (46). Clinical studies of alcoholics reveal a diverse pattern of cardiac dysfunctions (38), and basic studies of the cardiovascular effects of alcohol also suggest that alcohol abuse may increase risk for cardiomyopathy (see refs. 4, 42 for review). But the beneficial or harmful effects of alcohol may differ for particular cardiovascular conditions, and the precise determinants of "risk" are poorly understood (17).

ALCOHOL EFFECTS ON BRAIN FUNCTION

Chronic alcohol abuse is associated with a variety of deficits of brain function including disorders of memory, attention, cognitive processes, and sleep (see refs. 21, 34 for review). Some of these disorders are accentuated during alcohol withdrawal and then appear to be reversible during sobriety. Repeated alcohol intoxication combined with nutritional deficiencies may lead to permanent brain dysfunction such as Wernicke's disease and Korsakoff's psychosis, which are characterized by profound impairment of memory and deranged thinking processes. The degree of impairment appears to covary with the duration and severity of alcoholism.

The mechanisms by which alcohol disrupts CNS processes during intoxication and permanently impairs brain function in some alcoholics are poorly understood. Although some disorders have been shown to be associated with discrete CNS lesions, as in the case of Wernicke–Korsakoff psychoses, a more diffuse deterioration of brain tissue has also been observed. The development of new imaging techniques now permits the noninvasive quantitative measurement of radioactivity concentrations in human brain tissue and are useful for diagnostic localization and functional analysis of a variety of CNS disorders (35). There is evidence that alcoholics may have ventricular enlargement, widening of the sulci, and diffuse cortical atrophy (51), but the relationship to drinking history has been difficult to establish. In some instances, CT scan abnormalities were found to be reversible (7), and it appears that the radiological appearance of the brain may change during abstinence. Recent studies of magnetic resonance imaging of the brain in alcoholic patients 24 hr after cessation of drinking showed that brain water was significantly higher during acute alcohol withdrawal than after 7 to 21 days of abstinence (44). Consequently, it is possible that apparent ventricular dilatation and widening of the sulci in some alcoholics reflect transient changes in brain water rather than loss of neural tissue. A number of methodological problems limit clear interpretation of the relationships between duration of alcoholism and neuropsychological and structural impairments. It is usually impossible to determine the premorbid state and to identify contributing factors other than alcoholism.

ALCOHOL EFFECTS ON REPRODUCTIVE FUNCTION

There is considerable evidence that alcohol has adverse effects on male reproductive function. Impotence, testicular atrophy, gynecomastia, and loss of sexual interest are often associated with chronic alcoholism (9). Acute and chronic alcohol intoxication significantly suppressed plasma testosterone levels in both alcohol-dependent and normal men and in animal models (9). Alcohol appears to inhibit testosterone biosynthesis in the testes through several converging mechanisms, and the contribution of acetylaldehyde or changes in NAD-to-NADH ratios in the testes remains to be clarified (9).

In contrast to the extensive literature on alcohol effects on male reproductive function, there has been surprisingly little attention to the effects of alcohol on reproductive function in women (8,49). In 1975, there was one clinical report that chronic alcohol intoxication disrupted ovarian function (32), and in 1980, a more extensive study of 31 alcoholic women was described (15). These clinical reports indicate that alcoholism in women is associated with several disorders of reproductive function including anovulation, luteal phase dysfunction, and amenorrhea (15,32). In 1984, the first data on drinking and female reproductive dysfunction from a representative national sample were reported (52). A stratified household sample of 917 women showed a strong association between alcohol consumption and a variety of menstrual disorders including dysmenorrhea, heavy menstrual flow, and premenstrual discomfort. The incidence of these disorders increased with usual drinking levels. Women who consumed six or more drinks per day at least five times a week had elevated rates of gynecological surgery (other than hysterectomy) and obstetric disorders. These are the first data to provide evidence that drinking and reproductive dysfunction are related in the general (nonclinical) population (52).

The pathogenesis of reproductive disorders associated with alcohol use and abuse is poorly understood. In alcoholic women, it has been difficult to determine the relative contribution of alcohol-associated liver disease, malnutrition, and the direct toxic effects of alcohol (15). Malnutrition associated with profound weight loss or hepatic dysfunction can disrupt menstrual cycle regularity. Clear evaluation of the effects of chronic alcoholism on reproductive function requires development of an experimental animal model in which nutritional factors and intercurrent illness can be controlled. In 1983, a model of alcoholism in the female Macaque monkey was developed using operant behavioral techniques (24). Monkeys that self-administered high doses of alcohol (2.9 to 4.4 g/kg/day) for 3 to 6½ months developed amenorrhea, atrophy of the uterus, decreased ovarian mass, and suppressed luteinizing hormone (LH) levels. The pathological picture in the alcohol-dependent Macaque monkey was consistent with that in alcoholic women. Decreased ovarian mass and an absence of corpora lutea have also been observed in alcoholic women at autopsy. Since there was no laboratory or pathological evidence of liver disease and food self-administration remained stable or increased during the period of alcohol self-administration, it appeared that alcohol toxicity accounted for the observed disruptions of menstrual cycle regularity (24).

It is not yet known if the toxic effects of chronic alcohol dependence occur primarily at the level of the hypothalamus, the pituitary, or the ovary or if alcohol simultaneously disrupts each component of the hypothalamic–pituitary–gonadal axis (8,9,49). Studies of the effects of a single acute dose of alcohol on pituitary and gonadal hormones in normal human females and in female rhesus monkeys have not shown an alcohol-induced suppression of pituitary gonadotropins or ovarian steroid hormones (20,23,30,48). These findings in females are somewhat surprising, since acute alcohol administration does significantly suppress testosterone levels in human males (9). New strategies for assessing the sites of alcohol toxicity include the use of provocative tests of hypothalamic and pituitary function such as stimulation with naloxone, an opioid antagonist, and synthetic luteinizing hormone-releasing hormone (LHRH). These provocative tests are commonly used in clinical endocrinology for the evaluation of reproductive dysfunction (37,53). Systematic studies of the acute and chronic effects of alcohol on hypothalamic–pituitary function when pituitary hormones are exogenously stimulated should eventually yield a clearer picture of the sites of alcohol's disruptive effects on reproductive function.

ALCOHOL EFFECTS ON FETAL GROWTH AND DEVELOPMENT

The disruptive effects of alcohol on menstrual cycle function are accompanied by infertility and increased risk for spontaneous abortion (13,18). Yet, women who are chronic alcohol abusers do become pregnant, and their children may be afflicted with physical congenital anomalies, abnormal brain function, and pre- and postnatal retardation of growth and development. Behavioral disorders range from hyperactivity to mental retardation. Since alcohol diffuses freely across the placental barrier, the fetus is exposed to the same effective dose of alcohol as the mother. In the 1983 Special Report to Congress on Alcohol and Health, it was estimated that the overall prevalence of alcohol-related fetal malformations and developmental anomalies was one to three per 1,000 births (3).

In 1981, the Surgeon General issued an Advisory to inform women of the risk of drinking during pregnancy (11). Warnings against drinking during pregnancy have been traced to Aristotle, repeated in the Bible, and reaffirmed in clinical observations during the 19th and early 20th centuries (45,50). Yet, despite the sanction of history, the 1973 report of a fetal alcohol syndrome (FAS), i.e., a specific pattern of dysmorphologies and growth retardation in the children of alcoholic women (16), was met with

considerable skepticism. Controversy over the extent to which alcohol is a specific teratogen was based on the fact that FAS mothers often used other drugs, were malnourished, and had inadequate medical care during pregnancy. Any of these alone or in combination with alcohol could lead to birth defects, and similar patterns of malformation could occur independently of alcohol abuse. Specific attribution of birth defects to alcohol required conditions in which malnutrition and polydrug use could be controlled, a situation impossible to achieve in pregnant women.

Recently, a number of animal models of alcoholism have been developed to address these issues (see refs. 36, 45 for review). The weight of current evidence suggests that alcohol is a teratogen in several species studied under controlled laboratory conditions. For example, in a primate model, alcohol (2.5 to 4.1 g/kg) was administered by gavage once a week from 40 days post-conception to delivery (6,10). These alcohol doses produced average blood alcohol levels between 240 and 256 mg/dl and 338 to 415 mg/dl, respectively, within 2 hr after alcohol administration (6). This regimen resulted in one spontaneous abortion and three live births. Infants were followed for 6 months and compared with age- and sex-matched controls. Prenatal exposure to the highest alcohol dose, 4.1 g/kg, resulted in neurologic, developmental, and facial anomalies similar to those seen in human FAS infants. Behavioral examinations showed profound retardation, and neuropathological examination revealed cerebral asymmetry, minimal cortical organization, and hydrocephalus *ex vacuo*. Of two surviving infants exposed to 2.5 g/kg of alcohol prenatally, the female had no developmental or neuropathological abnormalities, whereas the male was hyperkinetic and showed evidence of developmental retardation and brain abnormality (6).

The alcohol-exposed Macaque infants differed from human FAS infants in two respects: (a) all were abnormally large at birth, whereas low birth weight is common in humans; (b) none showed malformations of heart, kidney, or other organs often seen in human FAS infants. The absence of organ malformations is probably related to the fact that alcohol administration to the mother did not begin until the end of the organogenic period. Factors accounting for the size of the infants are unclear, but the weekly alcohol exposure is different from the daily drinking pattern of alcoholic women, and nutritional status during pregnancy was probably better in the Macaque mothers than in many alcoholic women (6).

Within the next decade, evidence from well-controlled animal studies should further confirm (or refute) the hypothesis that alcohol is a specific teratogen. Although it seems likely that alcohol, in sufficient doses, is teratogenic, the extent to which the human fetal alcohol syndrome is specific to alcohol remains unresolved. Increasing clinical evidence suggests that other drugs are also fetotoxic and that drug abuse during pregnancy can result in a profile of low birth weight, delayed development, and brain malformations similar to those reported for alcohol abuse (see J. H. Mendelson, *this volume*). Also unresolved is the range of alcohol doses and the duration of drinking likely to produce adverse consequences for the fetus. Such information is important because most women (60%) of child-bearing age use some alcohol (3) and confirmation of pregnancy often does not occur until midway into the first trimester.

ALCOHOL AND POLYDRUG ABUSE

Many of the adverse medical consequences of alcohol abuse and alcoholism may be increased by the concurrent use of other substances. The medical consequences of polydrug use are reviewed by M. J. Kreek elsewhere in this volume. The behavioral effects of interactions between alcohol and other abused drugs are poorly understood, but there is compelling evidence that alcohol has a direct effect on concurrent tobacco smoking. Anecdotal observations that alcohol intoxication and smoking covary have been confirmed under laboratory conditions (12). Smoking by alcoholic men was measured when alcohol or a nonalcohol vehicle control solution was available. Subjects could consume one drink every 30 min or a total of 12 drinks over 6 hr. Subjects could smoke their preferred brand of cigarettes, but all cigarettes were cut to an equal length. Alcohol availability was consistently associated with an increase in cigarette smoking in comparison to control sessions when no alcohol was available. Measures of the number of cigarette puffs and butt weight indicated that increased smoking during drinking was not due to smoking less of each cigarette (12). These findings in alcoholic men have been confirmed (14) and extended to social drinkers (27). When social drinkers were given unrestricted access to alcohol over several days, there was a striking covariation between alcohol consumption and cigarette smoking (27).

The mechanisms by which alcohol influences tobacco use are unknown, but drug-related effects on smoking are not unique to alcohol. Opiate agonists, heroin and methadone, as well as an opioid mixed agonist–antagonist, buprenorphine, and certain stimulants have also been shown to be associated with increased cigarette smoking during intoxication (see ref. 25 for review). Since these drugs have a broad spectrum of actions, it is difficult to construct a plausible hypothesis concerning specific pharmacological effects on cigarette smoking. In contrast to tobacco, alcohol did not increase or decrease marijuana smoking by young men (26).

Multiple drug use appears to be an increasingly common pattern, and the way in which drugs interact to modulate use patterns is an important area for further study. Traditionally, alcoholism and other forms of drug abuse have been studied as if these were discrete disorders that exist in relative isolation from each other, but this separatist approach is not tenable on empirical or theoretical grounds. Alcoholics may also abuse tobacco, tranquilizers, depressants, and caffeine, just as opiate addicts may also abuse alcohol, cocaine, marijuana, and other available drugs (see M. J. Kreek, *this volume*). It is unlikely that future drug abuse problems will be adequately defined by the exclusive use of a single agent. The concept of substance abuse implies that there may be similarities between addictive disorders that transcend the specific pharmacological properties of abused drugs. Identification of the critical similarities and differences between the behavioral consequences of drugs from different pharmacological classes promises to be a productive research strategy. An improved synthesis of existing information about alcohol and drug abuse should reveal the extent to which there are common processes in the development and maintenance of substance abuse patterns.

ACKNOWLEDGMENTS

Preparation of this review was supported in part by Grant DA 00101 from the National Institute on Drug Abuse and Grants AA 04368 and AA 06252 from the National Institute on Alcohol Abuse and Alcoholism, ADAMHA.

REFERENCES

1. *Alcohol and Health* (1978): Third Special Report to the U.S. Congress, DHEW Publ. No. (ADM) 79-832. U.S. Government Printing Office, Washington.
2. *Alcohol and Health* (1981): Fourth Special Report to the U.S. Congress, DHHS Publ. No. (ADM) 81-1080. U.S. Government Printing Office, Washington.
3. *Alcohol and Health* (1984): Fifth Special Report to the U.S. Congress, DHHS Publ. No. (ADM) 84-1291. U.S. Government Printing Office, Washington.
4. Altura, B. M., and Altura, B. T. (1982): *Fed. Proc.*, 41:2447–2451.
5. American Psychiatric Association Task Force on Nomenclature and Statistics (1980): *Diagnostic and Statistical Manual of Mental Disorders*, third edition. American Psychiatric Association, Washington.
6. Bowden, D. M., Weathersbee, P. S., Clarren, S. K., Fahrenbruch, C. E., Goodlin, B. L., et al. (1983): *Am. J. Primatol.*, 14:143–157.
7. Carlen, P. L., and Wilkinson, D. A. (1980): *Acta. Psychiatr. Scand.* [*Suppl.*], 286:103–118.
8. Cicero, T. J. (1980): In: *Advances in Substance Abuse, Behavioral and Biological Research, Vol. 1,* edited by N. K. Mello, pp. 1201–1254. JAI Press, Greenwich, CT.
9. Cicero, T. J. (1982): *Alcoholism Clin. Exp. Res.*, 6:207–215.
10. Clarren, S. K., and Bowden, D. M. (1982): *J. Pediatr.*, 101:819–824.
11. Food and Drug Administration, Surgeon General's Advisory on Alcohol and Pregnancy. (1981): *FDA Drug Bull.*, 11:9–10.
12. Griffiths, R. R., Bigelow, G. E., and Liebson, I. (1976): *J. Exp. Anal. Behav.*, 25(3):279–292.
13. Harlap, S., and Shiono, P. H. (1980): *Lancet*, 2:173–176.
14. Henningfield, J. E., Chait, L. D., and Griffiths, R. R. (1984): *Psychopharmacology*, 82:1–5.
15. Hugues, J. N., Cofte, T., Perret, G., Jayle, M. S., Sebaoun, J., et al. (1980): *Clin. Endocrinol.*, 12:543–551.
16. Jones, K. L., Smith, D. W., Ulleland, C. N., and Streissguth, A. P. (1973): *Lancet*, 1:1267–1271.
17. Klatsky, A. L., Friedman, G. D., and Siegelaub, A. B. (1979): *Alcoholism Clin. Exp. Res.*, 3(1):33–39.
18. Kline, J., Stein, Z., and Shrout, P. (1980): *Lancet*, 2:176–180.
19. Korsten, M. A., and Lieber, C. S. (1985): In: *The Diagnosis and Treatment of Alcoholism*, second edition, edited by J. H. Mendelson and N. K. Mello, pp. 21–64. McGraw-Hill, New York.
20. McNamee, B., Grant, J., Ratcliffe, J., Ratcliffe, W., and Oliver, J. (1979): *Br. J. Addict.*, 74:316–317.
21. Mello, N. K. (1978): In: *Psychopharmacology: A Generation of Progress*, edited by M. A. Lipton, A. DiMascio, and K. F. Killam, pp. 1619–1637. Raven Press, New York.
22. Mello, N. K. (1983): In: *The Pathogenesis of Alcoholism, Biological Factors, Vol. 7*, edited by B. Kissin and H. Begleiter, pp. 133–198. Plenum Press, New York.
23. Mello, N. K., Bree, M. P., Ellingboe, J., Mendelson, J. H., and Harvey, K. L. (1984): *Pharmacol. Biochem. Behav.*, 120:293–299.
24. Mello, N. K., Bree, M. P., Mendelson, J. H., Ellingboe, J., King, N. W., et al. (1983): *Science*, 221:677–679.

25. Mello, N. K., and Mendelson, J. H. (1986): In: *Strategies for Research on the Interactions of Drugs of Abuse,* edited by M. C. Braude and H. M. Ginzburg, pp. 154–180. U.S. Government Printing Office, Washington, DC.

26. Mello, N. K., Mendelson, J. H., Kuehnle, J. C., and Sellers, M. (1978): *J. Pharmacol. Exp. Ther.,* 207(3):922–935.

27. Mello, N. K., Mendelson, J. H., Sellers, M. L., and Kuehnle, J. C. (1980): *Clin. Pharmacol. Ther.,* 27(2):202–209.

28. Mendelson, J. H., Babor, T. F., Mello, N. K., and Pratt, H. (1986): *J. Stud. Alcohol,* 47(5):361–366.

29. Mendelson, J. H., and Mello, N. K. (1985): In: *The Diagnosis and Treatment of Alcoholism,* second edition, edited by J. H. Mendelson and N. K. Mello, pp. 1–20. McGraw-Hill, New York.

30. Mendelson, J. H., Mello, N. K., and Ellingboe, J. (1981): *J. Pharmacol. Ther.,* 218:23–26.

31. Mendelson, J. H., Miller, D., Mello, N. K., Pratt, H., and Schmitz, R. (1982): *Alcoholism Clin. Exp. Res.,* 67:377–383.

32. Moskovic, S. (1975): *Srpski Arhiv za Celokupno Lekarstvo,* 103(9):751–758.

33. Myers, J. K., Weissman, M. M., Tischler, G. L., Holzer, C. E., Leaf, P. J., et al. (1984): *Arch. Gen. Psychiatry,* 41:959–967.

34. Parsons, O. A., Butters, N., and Nathan, P., eds. (1987): *Neuropsychology of Alcoholism: Implications for Diagnosis and Treatment.* Guilford Press, New York (*in press*).

35. Phelps, M. E., Mazziotta, J. C., and Huang, S.-E. (1982): *J. Cereb. Blood Flow Metab.,* 2:113–162.

36. Randall, C. L., and Noble, E. (1980): In: *Advances in Substance Abuse, Behavioral and Biological Research, Vol. 1,* edited by N. K. Mello, pp. 201–254. JAI Press, Greenwich, CT.

37. Rebar, R. W. (1978): In: *Reproductive Endocrinology: Physiology, Pathophysiology and Clinical Management,* edited by S. S. C. Yen and R. B. Jaffe, pp. 469–518. W. B. Saunders, Philadelphia.

38. Regan, T. J., and Ettinger, P. O. (1979): *Alcoholism Clin. Exp. Res.,* 3(1):40–45.

39. *Report of the Public Health Service Task Force on Women's Health Issues* (1985): Public Health Report 100:73-106. U.S. Government Printing Office, Washington.

40. Robins, L. N., Helzer, J. E., Weissman, M. M., Orvaschel, H., Gruenberg, E., et al. (1984): *Arch. Gen. Psychiatry,* 41(10):949–958.

41. Rosenberg, L., Sloane, D., Shapiro, S., Kaufman, D., Miettinen, O., et al. (1981): *Am. J. Public Health,* 71:82–85.

42. Rubin, E. (1982): *Fed. Proc.,* 41:2460–2464.

43. Seixas, F. A., Williams, K., and Eggleston, S., eds. (1975): *Ann. N.Y. Acad. Sci.,* 252:1–339.

44. Smith, M. A., Chick, J., Kean, D. M., Douglas, H. B., Singer, A., et al. (1985): *Lancet,* 1:1273–1274.

45. Streissguth, A. F., Landesman-Dwyer, S., Martin, J. C., and Smith, D. W. (1980): *Science,* 209:353–361.

46. Taylor, J. R., Combs-Orme, T., Anderson, D., Taylor, D. A., and Koppenol, C. (1984): *Alcoholism Clin. Exp. Res.,* 8(3):283–286.

47. Vaillant, G. E. (1983): *The Natural History of Alcoholism.* Harvard University Press, Cambridge.

48. Välimäki, M., Härkönen, M., and Ylikahri, R. (1983): *Alcoholism Clin. Exp. Res.,* 7:289–293.

49. Van Thiel, D. H., and Gavaler, J. S. (1982): *Alcoholism Clin. Exp. Res.,* 6:179–185.

50. Warner, R. H., and Rosett, H. L. (1975): *J. Stud. Alcohol,* 36(11):1395–1420.

51. Wilkinson, D. A. (1982): *Alcoholism Clin. Exp. Res.,* 6:31–45.

52. Wilsnack, S. D., Klassen, A. D., and Wilsnack, R. W. (1984): *Alcoholism Clin. Exp. Res.,* 8:451–458.

53. Yen, S. S. C., Quigley, M. E., Reid, R. L., Ropert, J. F., and Cetel, N. S. (1985): *Am. J. Obstet. Gynecol.,* 152:485–493.

Psychopharmacology:
The Third Generation of Progress,
edited by Herbert Y. Meltzer.
Raven Press, New York © 1987.

CHAPTER **163**

Biochemical Pharmacology of Alcohol

Boris Tabakoff and Paula L. Hoffman

Much work has, in the past, been directed at examining alcohol (ethanol)-induced peripheral organ damage, especially damage to the liver. Although these problems still attract significant attention, some of the emphasis in alcohol research has shifted to a detailed examination of the mechanisms by which alcohol produces its acute intoxicating or sedative effects; how tolerance, physical dependence, and brain damage develop; and to studies of the biochemical basis of the reinforcing effects of ethanol and for excessive intake of this drug. This chapter attempts to highlight the research advances that have been made toward answering these questions during the last decade.

ALCOHOL: A DRUG WITHOUT A RECEPTOR

In 1901, Meyer proposed that ethanol produces its physiological effects (i.e., intoxication, sedation) through perturbation of neuronal membrane lipids (1). This "membrane hypothesis" of the actions of ethanol has been widely accepted. However, only during the past several years have sensitive physicochemical techniques, including electron paramagnetic resonance (EPR) and fluorescence polarization, provided convincing evidence that physiologically attainable concentrations of ethanol (25–100 mM) significantly increase the "fluidity" of cell membrane lipids. Furthermore, it has been found that these changes in membrane fluidity can be correlated with ethanol-induced sedation (2–4). One crucial study involved lines of mice that had been selectively bred for differential sensitivity to the hypnotic effect of ethanol. By use of EPR techniques, neuronal cell membranes obtained from the more sensitive mice ("LS" mice) were also found to be more sensitive to the lipid-fluidizing effect of ethanol added *in vitro,* compared to membranes from the less sensitive animals ("SS" mice) (5). These results appear to support the postulate that ethanol produces some of its physiological effects via a relatively nonspecific effect on membrane lipid structure. However, other research has indicated significant specificity of the effects of ethanol at the molecular level. For example, the effects of ethanol on fluidity of neuronal membranes obtained from the selectively bred lines of mice discussed above were reexamined using fluorescence polarization as well as EPR (6). No differences between the lines were observed by use of fluorescence polarization, in contrast to the EPR results (6). Since the fluorescent probe monitors a different membrane region than the EPR probe (6), these results suggested that the primary site affected by genetic selection—i.e., the site that influences the hypnotic response to ethanol—is probably localized within a restricted area of the neuronal membrane (6).

Neuronal cell membranes are heterogeneous mixtures of lipids and proteins, and areas of differential sensitivity to ethanol within the membrane may result from the presence of "microdomains" of particular composition. Gangliosides as well as phospholipids and cholesterol are major components of neuronal membranes and may contribute to determining the sensitivity of a membrane to ethanol. Gangliosides were very recently found to enhance significantly the "fluidizing" effect of ethanol when they were added to model phospholipid bilayers (7).

The evidence (see ref. 8) that specific regions within neuronal membranes can show selective sensitivity to ethanol suggested that various membrane-bound proteins, which are dependent on their immediately surrounding lipids for optimal activity (e.g., ref. 9), should also differ in sensitivity to ethanol. Since neuronal membrane proteins—i.e., receptors, ionophores, and enzymes—represent the functional moieties of the neuronal membranes, their responses to ethanol would contribute to the specific collage of neuropharmacological effects produced by ethanol. As an example, certain membrane-bound ionophores that control ion flux and, therefore, neurotransmitter release and neuronal excitability appear to be quite sensitive to ethanol. "Fast-phase" calcium uptake into synaptosomes, a process specifically associated with neurotransmitter release, was significantly inhibited by 25 mM ethanol (10). Phosphatidylinositol breakdown, which is believed to mediate intracellular calcium mobilization, also was reported to be inhibited by relatively low concentrations of ethanol in cerebral cortex (12), and the combination of these effects could severely perturb neurotransmitter release. In support of a role of CNS calcium flux in the physiological response to ethanol, intraventricular administration of calcium ions or a calcium ionophore to mice was shown to enhance the hypnotic effect of ethanol (13).

Not only are particular classes of membrane-bound proteins sensitive to low concentrations of ethanol, but selective effects of ethanol on particular areas of neuronal membranes also appear to result in a high degree of selectivity with respect to actions on proteins, even among closely related proteins in various cell membranes in brain (Table 1). This specificity could be a result of both neural membrane heterogeneity (i.e., different lipid microenvironments) and the membrane characteristics of different cells or organelles. For instance, the two forms of monoamine oxidase (MAO), MAO-A and MAO-B, are closely related functionally and structurally (14), but ethanol selectively inhibits the B form of MAO in human platelet and brain (15).

Another membrane-bound neuronal enzyme that repeatedly has been found to be affected by ethanol *in vitro,* as well as by chronic ethanol ingestion, is Na^+,K^+-ATPase (see ref. 16). This enzyme appears to exist in two forms with differing affinity for the inhibitor ouabain (17). Very recent studies suggest that the form of the enzyme that is localized to neuronal membranes (17), rather than glial membranes, is selectively sensitive to the effects of ethanol (18,18a).

A third membrane-bound enzyme, adenylate cyclase, also has been studied in detail. This enzyme is coupled to various neurotransmitter receptors in the CNS and plays a role in synaptic transmission. Receptor–adenylate cyclase systems, in general, consist of three membrane-bound proteins: the receptor, a guanine-nucleotide-dependent coupling protein ("G"), and the catalytic unit of adenylate cyclase (see ref. 19). Ethanol activates adenylate cyclase activity in brain (20–22), and in the presence of guanine nucleotides, low, physiologically attainable concentrations of ethanol significantly increase activity (20–22). A critical distinction has been noted, however, in the actions of ethanol on dopamine-sensitive adenylate cyclase in striatum compared to norepinephrine-sensitive adenylate cyclase in cerebral cortex (20–24). In striatum, ethanol has a single site of action, i.e., on the interaction of G and the enzyme (20). In contrast, in cerebral cortex, ethanol has multiple sites of action in the receptor–adenylate cyclase complex (22–24). That is, even though certain of ethanol's actions on adenylate cyclase may be mediated by effects on membrane "fluidity" (20–24), the resulting effects on protein-protein interactions are rather specific and depend on the anatomical source of the neuronal membranes.

Another receptor–effector coupling system that is affected by ethanol in a particularly specific manner is the GABA-benzodiazepine (BDZ) receptor–chloride channel complex (see ref. 16). Ethanol, *in vitro,* has little effect on GABA or BDZ binding to their receptors. More recently, however, ethanol, at low concentrations, was shown to inhibit the binding to brain membranes of *tert*-butylbicyclophosphorothionate (TBPS), a ligand believed to interact with a

---

TABLE 1. *Evidence for specificity of the CNS effects of ethanol*

System	Specificity	Reference
Receptors and receptor–effector coupling		
A. GABA–BDZ–barbiturate receptor–chloride ionophore	Ethanol affects binding of ligand associating with chloride ionophore only	25, 26
B. Catecholamine receptor–adenylate cyclase	Ethanol primarily affects G_s function, but actions depend on anatomical source of complex	20–24
C. Receptor-mediated polyphosphoinositide (PI) breakdown	Ethanol affects muscarinic cholinergic, but not α_1-adrenergic receptor-stimulated PI breakdown	11
D. Opiate receptor binding	Ethanol preferentially inhibits ligand binding to δ as compared to μ receptors; κ receptors are resistant to ethanol	27, 28
Membrane-bound enzymes		
A. Monoamine oxidase (MAO)	Ethanol selectively inhibits MAO-B activity	15
B. Na^+,K^+-ATPase	The activity of the neuronally localized form of the enzyme is more sensitive to ethanol	18, 18a

membrane site closely associated with the chloride channel (25,26). The fact that ethanol affects only one component of the oligomeric GABA–BDZ receptor–chloride channel complex again indicates the specificity of action of ethanol. Particularly in this receptor–effector system, and also in the adenylate cyclase systems where ethanol primarily affects the activity of G (20–24), it is possible that ethanol may interact directly with hydrophobic areas of the membrane-bound proteins in addition to interacting with membrane lipids.

A further example of the selectivity of action of ethanol is evident in the influence of ethanol on ligand binding to opiate receptors in brain (27,28). There are a number of subtypes of opiate receptor, which differ in their affinity for various opiates and opioid peptides (29). The δ opiate receptor, with high affinity for enkephalin, is particularly sensitive to ethanol (which decreases receptor affinity for ligand), whereas the κ receptor subtype is very resistant to the effect of ethanol (29a).

The specificity of the neurochemical responses to ethanol suggests that, even though there is no distinct CNS "receptor" for ethanol as there are for other psychotropic drugs, ethanol may interact selectively with particular "receptive" regions of proteins or cell membranes, leading to defined physiological effects. Although ethanol affects the activity of a large number of neurotransmitter and neuromodulator systems (see ref. 16), each system displays a specific and circumscribed response to ethanol. Therefore, the "membrane hypothesis" of ethanol's action may be correct conceptually, but it must include a recognition of the selectivity of biochemical responses to ethanol.

BIOCHEMICAL PHARMACOLOGY OF TOLERANCE AND PHYSICAL DEPENDENCE

Chronic ingestion of ethanol leads to the development of functional (cellular) tolerance and physical dependence, presumably as a result of adaptive changes in response to the initial effects of ethanol (see ref. 30). In attempting to delineate the neurochemical changes associated with adaptation to ethanol, it is natural to investigate the systems that are initially affected by ethanol. In terms of the "membrane hypothesis" for the action of ethanol, one would postulate that cell membranes, which ethanol initially "fluidizes," would become more "rigid" and resistant to the fluidizing effect of ethanol. Such a change would be consistent with the presence of ethanol tolerance, and, in the absence of ethanol, membrane malfunction could contribute to the generation of withdrawal symptoms. In fact, synaptosomal membranes from ethanol-tolerant animals did show increased base-line "order" in the absence of ethanol and resistance to the disordering effect of ethanol *in vitro* (3,31).

However, a number of unresolved issues compromise attempts to relate changes in bulk membrane lipid properties to tolerance or physical dependence. First, in spite of a significant amount of work, no consistent biochemical basis for the alteration in neuronal membrane properties—e.g., changes in phospholipid or cholesterol composition—has emerged (see ref. 16). Measurements of total lipid composition may not be sensitive enough to detect significant changes, since it seems likely that only particular lipid regions within the neuronal membrane may be altered after chronic ethanol ingestion (see above). Another issue is that tolerance to different effects of ethanol develops at different rates (30), and a single change in membrane properties cannot easily account for this differential development of tolerance. Furthermore, ethanol tolerance has recently been shown to be complex, involving "environment-independent" and "environment-dependent," or conditioned, aspects (30) in both animals and humans. For instance, repeated exposure to the same test environment, or mental rehearsal of the task to be performed, facilitated tolerance development in humans (32). It seems simplistic to suggest that a single change in bulk membrane lipid properties can account for these diverse consequences.

The problem of evaluating the neurochemical basis of ethanol tolerance has, on the other hand, been most profitably approached by ascertaining the influence of certain neurochemical systems on the development of tolerance. With the use of specific neurotoxins (6-hydroxydopamine; 5,7-dihydroxytryptamine), it has been demonstrated that brain noradrenergic and serotonergic systems play important roles in the development of ethanol tolerance. In mice, partial destruction of noradrenergic systems completely blocked the development of both environment-dependent and environment-independent tolerance (33,34), and depletion of serotonin delayed the development of environment-dependent tolerance (34). In rats, destruction of a specific serotonergic pathway in brain also delayed the development of ethanol tolerance (35), and combined destruction of noradrenergic and serotonergic neurons completely blocked tolerance development (35).

These studies not only revealed the importance of particular neurochemical systems for the development of different forms of ethanol tolerance but also provided information about the basis of the adaptive response to ethanol. The results showed that the simple presence of ethanol in an individual is not sufficient to produce functional ethanol tolerance. The other prerequisite is optimal activity of certain neuronal pathways in the CNS. In addition, these experiments demonstrated that the development of ethanol tolerance could be blocked without interfering with the development of physical dependence (33). This dissociation of tolerance and physical dependence provided evidence contrary to earlier theories of tolerance and physical dependence that postulated a unitary neurochemical basis for these phenomena.

Ethanol tolerance in mice and rats is also influenced by a naturally occurring neuropeptide, arginine vasopressin (36,37). This peptide, which is a mammalian antidiuretic hormone, and which has also been implicated in learning and memory (38), was shown to maintain tolerance in mice or rats that had been rendered tolerant to ethanol, even in the absence of further ethanol ingestion (36,37). Very recent evidence suggests that antagonists of vasopressin can facilitate the loss of tolerance, implicating the endogenous hormone in the maintenance or expression of tolerance (37a). Similarly, rats (Brattleboro strain) that lack endogenous vasopressin were reported not to develop ethanol tolerance (39). The action of vasopressin on tolerance is, however, dependent on the presence of intact noradrenergic and/or serotonergic systems in brain (37,40). It has been known for some time that ethanol affects vasopressin secretion from the neurohypophysis in both animals and humans (41), and it appears that circulating vasopressin levels in humans are increased after chronic ethanol ingestion (41). Further examination of the action of ethanol on vasopressin-containing neuronal networks in brain is, of course, critical for elucidating the contribution of this neuropeptide to the development and maintenance of ethanol tolerance.

In contrast to the results that have been obtained on the neuropharmacology of ethanol tolerance, less progress has been made in determining neurochemical systems that are responsible for physical dependence or the symptoms of ethanol withdrawal. Although much interest has focused on the GABA–benzodiazepine systems, there is currently little evidence for their role in physical dependence on ethanol (16). The most consistent neurochemical changes associated with physical dependence appear to be an increase in muscarinic cholinergic receptors and alterations in the function of noradrenergic systems in brain following chronic ethanol ingestion. The increase in muscarinic cholinergic receptors in animals consuming ethanol occurs primarily in cerebral cortex and hippocampus (12,42,43), and the number of receptors reverts to normal at the time that overt withdrawal symptoms (i.e., seizures, etc.) have dissipated (42). Recently, the changes in muscarinic cholinergic receptor number have been found to be associated with alterations in receptor-mediated stimulation of phosphatidylinositol turnover (11), which is believed to couple the receptors to calcium mobilization (44).

Norepinephrine turnover in the CNS has consistently been found to be increased during chronic ethanol ingestion by animals and humans (16,45,46), and the properties of brain β-adrenergic receptors also change during chronic ethanol ingestion (47). These changes persist throughout the early part (up to 3 days) of the withdrawal period (45,47). It has also been shown that the changes in β-adrenergic receptor properties are associated with alterations in receptor-stimulated adenylate cyclase activity (48). Certain of these aberrations in the function of brain noradrenergic systems may be responsible for the sleep disturbances (e.g., REM rebound, insomnia) that are characteristic of ethanol withdrawal (49).

Much evidence has accumulated to indicate that genetic factors contribute to individual sensitivity to ethanol and to the development of alcoholism in certain individuals (50,51). Further indicators of the role that genetics plays in ethanol-related events have been derived from studies with lines of mice that have been selectively bred for differential sensitivity to ethanol withdrawal. These mice are designated withdrawal-seizure prone (WSP) and withdrawal-seizure resistant (WSR) and have been shown to differ in their sensitivity only to ethanol withdrawal seizures and not to other drugs that produce generalized seizures (52). Not only does this selection indicate a genetic basis for susceptibility to the development of ethanol withdrawal seizures, but it also provides a model in which to investigate further the biochemical factors associated with physical dependence on ethanol. These animals have already been used to demonstrate that differences in the physical properties of brain membrane lipids are not associated with differential sensitivity to ethanol withdrawal (53). On the other hand, there appear to be specific differences in brain proteins between the two lines of mice (54). These differences may well be related to the differing susceptibilities to ethanol withdrawal seizures. With respect to the genetics of tolerance, it has been shown that various inbred strains of rats and mice develop tolerance to ethanol at different rates and to differing degrees (55,56). The heterogeneous stock developed from these animals (57) can, in the future, be used as a basis for development of selected lines with differential characteristics of ethanol tolerance and will allow for additional detailed investigation of the biochemical basis of tolerance.

ETHANOL AS A REINFORCER: WHAT IS THE BASIS FOR EXCESSIVE ETHANOL INTAKE?

A genetic approach has also proved valuable for investigating the reinforcing effects of ethanol. It is generally assumed that ethanol is ingested for its pharmacological effects and that certain of these effects are reinforcing and will maintain ethanol consumption. However, although ethanol self-administration has been demonstrated in animals under some conditions, it has been difficult to develop a suitable, consistent model for voluntary ethanol ingestion (58). Recently, selective breeding has been used to develop lines of rats that differ significantly in their ethanol-drinking behavior. These lines include the AA (alcohol-preferring) and ANA (alcohol-avoiding) rats (59) as well as the P (preferring) and NP (nonpreferring) lines of rats (60). The AA and P rats prefer to drink a 10% ethanol solution in a free-choice situation with food and water available, whereas ANA and NP rats avoid alcohol under these circumstances. The preferring rats will also bar-press for ethanol reward (61). The generation of these lines of rats indicates that there may be a genetic basis for ethanol "preference" or for a predilection to ingest ethanol [this is not simply a matter of taste preference, since P rats will self-administer ethanol intragastrically (62)]. P rats will also consume sufficient ethanol to display signs of physical dependence (61). These P and NP animals have already provided initial data on the biochemical characteristics that may be related to ethanol intake or to the reinforcing properties of ethanol. Differences in brain amine levels (particularly in serotonin levels) and in physiological responses to ethanol have been characterized in the different lines of rats (63,64).

The neurochemical systems that mediate ethanol reinforcement have, to date, not been identified clearly, in part because of difficulties in demonstrating the reinforcing properties of ethanol in certain model systems (65,66). Noradrenergic and dopaminergic systems have been considered, based on their role in the expression of the rewarding properties of other drugs (67,68). Endogenous opioid systems have also been suggested to modulate ethanol-induced reinforcement, since, in at least one study, naltrexone interfered with ethanol self-administration (69). The most intriguing results to date, however, have implicated serotonergic neuronal systems in modulation of ethanol ingestion. Zimelidine, a blocker of serotonin uptake, was reported to reduce ethanol intake, apparently by increasing the availability of serotonin at the synapse. In animal studies, rats that were injected daily with zimelidine showed reduced ethanol ingestion in a free-choice situation in which the animals could choose water or increasing concentrations of ethanol (70). Furthermore, zimelidine reduced ethanol intake by humans who were heavy drinkers (71). In 13 subjects, zimelidine increased days of abstinence and decreased the daily number of drinks consumed. It was suggested that zimelidine modified ethanol intake by affecting a central neuronal mechanism that controls drinking of alcohol (71). Serotonergic systems mediate the intake of a number of rewarding substances (72), and increasing serotonin at central synapses may provide a promising approach for controlling ethanol ingestion. The use of serotonergic drugs in the lines of rats with differing ethanol "preference" may generate additional evidence for the importance of serotonergic systems in ethanol-induced reinforcement.

SUMMARY AND CONCLUSIONS

Significant progress has been made over the last several years toward elucidating the biochemical pharmacology of ethanol. Even though ethanol does not interact with a CNS "receptor" in the classical sense, specific molecular sites of action have been identified for this drug. These sites of action include particular areas of lipids ("microdomains") within neuronal membranes and/or hydrophobic ("receptive") regions of membrane-bound proteins. Advances have also been made in elucidating the neurochemistry of functional ethanol tolerance, and certain neuronal systems involved in development or expression of tolerance have been identified: these include neurons containing norepinephrine, serotonin, and the neuropeptide vasopressin. The development of selected lines of animals with differential intensity of ethanol withdrawal symptoms promises to provide further information on the neurochemistry of physical dependence on ethanol.

Similarly, the most promising approach to understanding the basis for voluntary ethanol ingestion is the genetic approach; lines of animals have been developed with differing propensities to drink alcohol. These animals should provide a powerful tool for elucidating the neurochemistry of ethanol preference and the reinforcing properties of ethanol. Initial studies in animals and in humans suggest that serotonergic systems may be important modulators of ethanol intake. Overall, the use of new techniques, in particular genetic approaches to study various aspects of the actions of ethanol, promises even more substantial progress in the near future.

REFERENCES

1. Meyer, H. H. (1901): *Arch. Exp. Pathol. Pharmacol.*, 46:338–346.
2. Harris, R. A., and Schroeder, F. (1981): *Mol. Pharmacol.*, 20:128–137.
3. Chin, J. H., and Goldstein, D. B. (1976): *Science*, 196:684–685.
4. Chin, J. H., and Goldstein, D. B. (1977): *Mol. Pharmacol.*, 13:435–441.
5. Goldstein, D. B., Chin, J. H., and Lyon, R. C. (1982): *Proc. Natl. Acad. Sci. U.S.A.*, 79:4231–4233.
6. Perlman, B. J., and Goldstein, D. B. (1984): *Mol. Pharmacol.*, 26:547–552.
7. Harris, R. A., Groh, G. I., Baxter, D. M., and Hitzemann, R. J. (1984): *Mol. Pharmacol.*, 25:410–417.
8. Chin, J. H., and Goldstein, D. B. (1981): *Mol. Pharmacol.*, 19:425–431.
9. Farias, R. N., Bloj, B., Morero, R. D., Sineriz, F., and Trucco, R. E. (1975): *Biochim. Biophys. Acta*, 415:231–251.
10. Leslie, S. W., Barr, E., Chandler, C., and Farrar, R. P. (1983): *J. Pharmacol. Exp. Ther.*, 225:571–575.
11. Hoffman, P. L., Moses, F., Luthin, G. R., and Tabakoff, B. (1986): *Mol. Pharmacol.*, 30:13–18.
12. Smith, T. L. (1983): *Neuropharmacology*, 22:661–663.
13. Harris, R. A. (1979): *Pharmacol. Biochem. Behav.*, 10:527–534.
14. Jain, M. (1977): *Life Sci.*, 20:1925–1977.
15. Tabakoff, B., Lee, J. M., De Leon-Jones, F., and Hoffman, P. L. (1985): *Psychopharmacology*, 87:152–156.
16. Hoffman, P. L., and Tabakoff, B. (1985): In: *Alcohol and the Brain: Chronic Effects*, edited by R. E. Tarter and D. H. van Thiel, pp. 19–68. Plenum Press, New York.
17. Sweadner, K. J. (1979): *J. Biol. Chem.*, 254:6060–6067.
18. Marks, M. J., Smolen, A., and Collins, A. C. (1984): *Alcohol Clin. Exp. Res.*, 8:390–396.
18a. Nhamburo, P. T., Salafsky, B. P., Tabakoff, B., and Hoffman, P. L. (1987): *Biochem. Pharmacol.* (in press).
19. Stadel, J. M., deLean, A., and Lefkowitz, R. J. (1982): *Adv. Enzymol.*, 53:1–43.
20. Luthin, G. R., and Tabakoff, B. (1984): *J. Pharmacol. Exp. Ther.*, 228:579–587.
21. Rabin, R. A., and Molinoff, P. B. (1981): *J. Pharmacol. Exp. Ther.*, 216:129–134.
22. Saito, T., Lee, J. M., and Tabakoff, B. (1985): *J. Neurochem.*, 44:1037–1044.
23. Rabin, R. A., and Molinoff, P. B. (1983): *J. Pharmacol. Exp. Ther.*, 227:551–556.
24. Tabakoff, B., Luthin, G. R., Saito, T., and Lee, J. M. (1984): *Psychopharmacol. Bull.*, 20:481–484.
25. Thyagarajan, R., and Ticku, M. K. (1985): *Brain Res. Bull.*, 15:343–345.
26. Liljequist, S., Culp, S., and Tabakoff, B. (1986): *Life Sci.*, 38:1931–1939.
27. Tabakoff, B., and Hoffman, P. L. (1983): *Life Sci.*, 32:192–204.
28. Hiller, J. M., Angel, L. M., and Simon, E. J. (1981): *Science*, 214:468–469.
29. Pfeiffer, A., and Herz, A. (1982): *Mol. Pharmacol.*, 21:266–271.
29a. Khatami, S., Salafsky, B., Shibuya, T., and Hoffman, P. L. (1987): *Neuropharmacol.* (in press).
30. Tabakoff, B., Melchior, C. L., and Hoffman, P. L. (1982): *Alcoholism Clin. Exp. Res.*, 6:252–259.
31. Harris, R. A., Baxter, D. M., Mitchell, M. A., and Hitzemann, R. J. (1984): *Mol. Pharmacol.*, 25:401–409.
32. Annear, W. C., and Vogel-Sprott, M. (1985): *Psychopharmacology*, 87:90–93.
33. Tabakoff, B., and Ritzmann, R. F. (1977): *J. Pharmacol. Exp. Ther.*, 203:319–331.
34. Melchior, C. L., and Tabakoff, B. (1981): *J. Pharmacol. Exp. Ther.*, 219:275–280.
35. Khanna, J. M., Kalant, H., Le, A. D., and LeBlanc, A. E. (1981): *Prog. Neuropsychopharmacol. Biol. Psychol.*, 5:459–465.
36. Hoffman, P. L., Ritzmann, R. F., Walter, R., and Tabakoff, B. (1978): *Nature*, 276:614–616.
37. Le, A. D., Kalant, H., and Khanna, J. M. (1982): *Eur. J. Pharmacol.*, 80:337–345.
37a. Szabó, G., Ishizawa, H., Tabakoff, B., and Hoffman, P. L. (1987): *Alcoholism: Clin. Exp. Res.* (in press).
38. Van Wimersma Greidanus, T. B., van Ree, J. M., and de Wied, D. (1983): *Pharmacol. Ther.*, 20:437–458.
39. Pittman, Q. J., Rogers, J., and Bloom, F. E. (1982): *Regul. Peptides*, 4:33–41.
40. Hoffman, P. L., Melchior, C. L., and Tabakoff, B. (1983): *Life Sci.*, 32:1065–1071.

41. Beard, J. D., and Sargent, W. Q. (1979): In: *Biochemistry and Pharmacology of Ethanol, Vol. 2,* edited by E. Majchrowicz and E. P. Noble, pp. 3–16. Plenum Press, New York.
42. Tabakoff, B., Munoz-Marcus, M., and Fields, J. Z. (1979): *Life Sci.,* 25:2173–2180.
43. Rabin, R. A., Wolfe, B. B., Dibner, M. D., Zahniser, N. R., Melchior, C. L., et al. (1980): *J. Pharmacol. Exp. Ther.,* 213:491–496.
44. Berridge, M. J., and Irvine, R. F. (1984): *Nature,* 312:315–321.
45. Borg, S., Czarneka, A., Kvande, H., Mossberg, D., and Sedvall, G. (1983): *Alcoholism Clin. Exp. Res.,* 7:411–415.
46. Pohorecky, L. A. (1982): *J. Pharmacol. Exp. Ther.,* 223:348–354.
47. Banerjee, S. V., Sharma, V. K., and Khanna, J. M. (1978): *Nature,* 276:407–409.
48. French, S. W., Palmer, D. S., Narod, N. E., Reid, P. E., and Ramey, C. W. (1975): *J. Pharmacol. Exp. Ther.,* 194:319–326.
49. Lester, B. K., Rundell, O. H., Cowden, L. C., and Williams, H. L. (1973): In: *Alcohol Intoxication and Withdrawal Experimental Studies,* edited by M. M. Gross, pp. 261–279. Plenum Press, New York.
50. Propping, P. (1977): *Hum. Genet.,* 35:309–334.
51. Bohman, M. (1978): *Arch. Gen. Psychiatry,* 35:269–276.
52. McSwigan, J. D., Crabbe, J. C., and Young, E. R. (1984): *Life Sci.,* 35:2119–2126.
53. Harris, R. A., Crabbe, J. C., and McSwigan, J. D. (1984): *Life Sci.,* 35:2601–2608.
54. Goldman, D., and Crabbe, J. (1986): *Prog. Neuropsychopharmacol. Biol. Psych.,* 10:177–189.
55. Tabakoff, B., Ritzmann, R. F., Raju, T. S., and Deitrich, R. A. (1980): *Alcohol Clin. Exp. Res.,* 4:294–297.
56. Tabakoff, B., and Culp, S. G. (1984): *Alcohol Clin. Exp. Res.,* 8:495–499.
57. McClearn, G. E. (1967): In: *Behavior—Genetic Analysis,* edited by J. Hirsch, pp. 307–321. McGraw-Hill, New York.
58. Cicero, T. J. (1980): In: *Alcohol Tolerance and Dependence,* edited by H. Rigter and J. C. Crabbe, Jr., pp. 1–51. Elsevier/North-Holland, Amsterdam.
59. Eriksson, K. (1968): *Science,* 159:739–741.
60. Lumeng, L., Hawkins, T. D., and Li, T.-K. (1977): In: *Alcohol and Aldehyde Metabolizing Systems, Vol. 3,* edited by R. G. Thurman, J. R. Williamson, H. R. Drott, and B. Chance, pp. 537–544. Academic Press, New York.
61. Li, T.-K., Lumeng, L., McBride, W. T., and Waller, M. B. (1981): In: *NIAAA Research Monograph 6,* pp. 171–191. U.S. Government Printing Office, Washington.
62. Waller, M. B., McBride, W. J., Gatto, G. J., Lumeng, L., and Li, T.-K. (1984): *Science,* 225:78–80.
63. Lumeng, L., Waller, M. B., McBride, W. J., and Li, T.-K. (1982): *Pharmacol. Biochem. Behav.,* 16:125–130.
64. Kakihana, R., and Butte, J. C. (1980): In: *Animal Models in Alcohol Research,* edited by K. Eriksson, J. D. Sinclair, and K. Kiianmaa, pp. 21–33. Academic Press, New York.
65. Asin, K. E., Wirtshafter, D., and Tabakoff, B. (1985): *Pharmacol. Biochem. Behav.,* 22:169–173.
66. Numan, R. (1981): *Pharmacol. Biochem. Behav.,* 15:101–108.
67. Wise, R., and Routtenberg, A. (1983): In: *Biology of Alcoholism, Vol. 7,* edited by B. Kissin and H. Begleiter, pp. 77–105. Academic Press, New York.
68. Fibiger, H.-C. (1978): *Annu. Rev. Pharmacol. Toxicol.,* 18:37–56.
69. Altshuler, H. L., Phillips, P. E., and Feinhandler, D. A. (1980): *Life Sci.,* 26:679–688.
70. Rockman, G. E., Amit, Z., Carr, G., Brown, Z. W., and Ogren, S.-O. (1979): *Arch. Int. Pharmacodyn. Ther.,* 241:245–259.
71. Naranjo, C. A., Sellers, E. M., Roach, C. A., Woodley, D. V., Sanchez-Craig, M., et al. (1984): *Clin. Pharmacol. Ther.,* 35:374–381.
72. Rockman, G. E., Amit, Z., Bourque, C., Brown, Z. E., and Ogren, S.-O. (1980): *Arch. Int. Pharmacodyn. Ther.,* 244:123–129.

Psychopharmacology:
The Third Generation of Progress,
edited by Herbert Y. Meltzer.
Raven Press, New York © 1987.

CHAPTER **164**

Biology of Risk for Alcoholism

Marc A. Schuckit

This chapter reviews biological factors that might contribute to the risk for alcoholism. The effort to identify trait markers of a predisposition towards this disorder is based on the premise that alcoholism is genetically influenced. The usual study approach focuses on populations at elevated risk as determined by the presence of an alcoholic biological parent (68).

Before reviewing relevant studies, it is important to recognize several methodological issues. First, the focus of most investigations has been on alcoholism, not on possible genetic contributors to the decision to drink nor those that might influence the development of more temporary alcohol-related life problems in the late teens to early 20s (10,19,75). Second, although the definition of alcoholism used in different investigations has varied, most studies have centered on persistent heavy drinking with associated pervasive alcohol-related life problems, which in turn indicate a high likelihood of a continuation of such difficulties in the future (63,67,68). Third, in order to maximize the chances of identifying a genetic predisposition if it exists, the subjects of research have usually been relatives of severe primary alcoholics, i.e., individuals for whom alcoholism developed in the absence of any preexisting psychiatric disorder (67,68). This avoids the distractions imposed by combining together samples with genetic vulnerabilities to diverse problems such as the antisocial personality disorder, bipolar major affective disorder, and so on.

A fourth methodological consideration involves the sex of the subjects. Sons of relatively severe alcoholics are usually studied in order to maximize the chance that genetic factors will be identified. This reflects the fact that on follow-up men can be expected to show higher rates of expression of an alcoholism vulnerability if it exists (11,72). A second advantage to the study of males is the possibility that results from an alcohol challenge could vary with the

phase of the menstrual cycle or consumption of contraceptive pills, problems that could jeopardize study results if women were used (36). Most research has also been limited to sons of alcoholic fathers, not mothers, to minimize the possible impact of a fetal alcohol syndrome.

Finally, in most recent investigations, groups of sons of alcoholics are identified prior to the onset of alcoholism and studied cross-sectionally with the hope that the same population can be followed up to observe the correlation between identified markers and the future development of the disorder. Some studies have chosen prepubertal boys in order to observe them before exposure to ethanol, but these run the risk of missing markers that are only apparent after puberty or following exposure to modest drinking (1,2,47). Other investigations have selected older subjects, usually in their late teens to early or mid-20s, populations that give investigators the opposite pattern of assets and liabilities.

The comments offered in the following sections begin with a brief review of the data supporting the conclusion that alcoholism is genetically influenced and then progress to two different methodological approaches to identifying factors associated with the vulnerability. The chapter concludes with a summary and recommendations for future research.

DATA SUPPORTING GENETIC FACTORS IN ALCOHOLISM

The conclusion that alcoholism is genetically influenced is supported by family, twin, and adoption studies in humans. Family investigations have revealed a fourfold increased risk for this disorder in sons and daughters of alcoholics without clear evidence of a heightened vulnerability towards other major primary psychiatric diseases (16,69). However, demonstrating the familial nature of a disorder does not directly support the contribution of genetic influences.

Twin research attempts to evaluate the relative contribution of genetics and environment by comparing the rate of alcoholism in identical twins of alcoholics with the rate for fraternal twins. Although members of a twin pair share similar childhood environments no matter what type of twinship is involved, identical twins have 100% of their genes in common, but fraternal twins share only 50% (60). As a result, if the future development of alcoholism is related to childhood environmental events, the rate of similarity (or concordance) for alcoholism within a twin pair should be similar for the two types of twins. However, if genetic factors are also important, the level of concordance should be significantly higher within the identical twins. Most studies to date have revealed a significantly higher level of concordance for identical than fraternal twins, with conclusions varying with the population studied and the methodology invoked (37,48).

The third type of study evaluates the risk for alcoholism in biological children of alcoholics who were raised separately from their biological parents (i.e., adoption-type studies). Whether approached through a half-sibling methodology or actual adoption records, these investigations have revealed a three- to fourfold higher risk for alcoholism in adopted-out sons of alcoholics; although the findings are a bit more controversial, there is a similar heightened risk for adopted-out daughters as well (4,5,7–9,13,23–29,76). After controlling for the impact of an alcoholic biological parent, being reared by an alcoholic appears to add little, if anything, to the risk (28,76).

Human research is also presently under way in an attempt to identify potentially important subgroups among primary alcoholics. For example, one preliminary series of studies has named at least two subtypes. The first is more likely to be seen in males and is closely allied with criminality (male-limited type), whereas the second is equally likely to be seen in both sexes and appears to be more responsive to environmental factors (milieu-limited type) (14). Although the findings are preliminary, they highlight the fact that not all alcoholics are likely to have been equally sensitive to genetic influences.

Animal studies have also contributed to our understanding of how biological factors might influence the decision to drink, the level of central nervous system (CNS) sensitivity to the effects of ethanol, and the voluntary intake of enough alcohol to cause intoxication (17,41,45). At least one recently developed animal model is evaluating biological factors that interact with reinforcing properties of ethanol to yield oral intake to the point of intoxication, tolerance, and physical dependence (41).

This panoply of studies indicates that there is extensive evidence supporting the importance of genetic influences in the development of alcoholism. Most researchers have concluded that this is a polygenic and multifactorial problem in which genetically influenced biological factors contribute significantly to the risk for developing alcoholism through interactions with environmental events (11,12,75). Until new research methods are produced, there is enough evidence supporting genetic factors to justify the search for biological markers of a risk for developing this disorder. These studies are carried out through comparisons of alcoholics and controls and through observations of populations at high risk for the future development of alcoholism.

COMPARISONS OF ALCOHOLICS AND CONTROLS

The easiest way to begin to search for biological markers associated with alcoholism is to compare alcoholics with controls, an approach with both liabilities and assets. Evaluations of alcoholics have the advantages of large numbers of potential people for study and the fact that almost all subjects definitely have the disorder. On the other hand, many differences between alcoholics and controls are the result of years of heavy drinking and the associated life-style (i.e., they are markers of the state of the illness—state markers) and, thus, tell us little about biological factors related to the actual vulnerability towards alcoholism (68). For example, many changes on personality tests, hormonal abnormalities, neurological deficits, and deteriorations in liver functioning are caused by alcohol or associated trauma and nutritional deficiencies and, although useful in diagnosing alcoholism, do not relate to an actual predisposition (63). On the other hand, some characteristics of alcoholics do not revert to normal with abstinence or involve systems that were unlikely to have been affected by heavy drinking. These findings could be worth further evaluation as possible biological markers of the predisposition towards alcoholism. They include the qualitative evaluation of some enzyme systems, differential vulnerabilities to developing adverse consequences of heavy drinking, some neurophysiological parameters, and some blood antigens.

Isoenzyme Patterns

The isoenzyme patterns of the two major enzymes involved in human ethanol degradation, alcohol dehydrogenase (ADH) and aldehyde dehydrogenase (ALDH), are genetically controlled (6,39,40,94). Thus, the ethanol elimination rate for an individual appears to be genetically influenced, as does the postdrinking level of the psychoactive first breakdown product of ethanol, acetaldehyde (6,94). Alcohol dehydrogenase controls the first step in the degradation of beverage alcohol, and the isoenzyme pattern of this protein is dictated by a minimum of three gene loci, each with possible alleles, and each producing one or more polypeptide chains (6,39). As a result, there are up to 15 bands of human ADH with unique biochemical profiles of optimal temperature, Michaelis constant (K_m), substrate specificity, and sensitivity to inhibitors such as disulfiram. Although the pattern of these isoenzymes normally changes with age, and their quantity is affected by environmental factors, the actual pattern the enzyme forms is a genetically controlled phenomenon present before alcoholism develops. To date, the usefulness of the ADH isoenzyme patterns has been limited by the need for liver tissue for evaluation, although recent developments in analyses of hair root and lymphocyte proteins offer the opportunity for progress in the future (22,31,32). Despite the potential importance of ADH as a trait marker for an alcoholism predisposition, there are few significant ADH isoenzyme pattern differences between alcoholics and controls.

The second enzyme of importance, ALDH, is responsible for the metabolism of aldehydes in diverse body areas (30,40,51). There are four or more isoenzymes of ALDH in human liver cytosol and mitochondria, each with different biochemical properties (30). At least one isoenzyme, the low-K_m mitochondrial form, varies markedly among different ethnic groups and is missing in 30% to 50% of Orientals (31,32). In the absence of this isoenzyme form, acetaldehyde levels are significantly elevated after drinking, with a subsequent syndrome of facial flushing, palpitations, and nausea that resembles a mild ethanol–disulfiram reaction. It is not surprising that Orientals missing this enzyme are less likely than their coevals to drink, less likely to drink heavily, and appear to have a lower rate of alcoholism (22,84). However, although developing high levels of acetaldehyde after drinking appears to be associated with a decreased risk for alcoholism in some ethnic groups, other populations might also produce higher acetaldehyde but have high levels of alcoholism, e.g., American Indians (70,96). This underscores the manner in which a biological factor could influence the development of alcoholism but is unlikely to predestine a high or low risk. It is probably the interaction between biological and environmental factors that determines the final clinical outcome.

Factors That Influence the Problem Pattern in Alcoholics

Another approach to the search for biological vulnerabilities towards alcoholism takes advantage of the fact that not all alcoholics develop the same profile of problems. Thus, it is conceivable that for some individuals the biological predisposition may translate as an enhanced vulnerability towards one problem or towards another. Supporting this contention, studies of twins have revealed a higher level of similarity or concordance for alcoholic psychoses and for alcoholic cirrhosis within identical alcoholic twins than within fraternal alcoholic twins (34). In a similar fashion, it has also been demonstrated that a genetically controlled deficiency in the enzyme transketolase may be closely linked with the vulnerability of only some alcoholics to develop Wernicke–Korsakoff's syndrome (3). It is conceivable that there are a series of biological vulnerabilities increasing the chances of being identified as an alcoholic, with different factors operating in different families.

Results of Some Other Comparisons of Alcoholics and Controls

A number of blood proteins unlikely to be "caused" by alcoholism have been reported to be "abnormal" in alcoholics. These include the brain protein Pt 1 Durarte (15), a possible linkage in repulsion between the D gene of the Rh system and alcoholism, as well as a linkage between alcoholism and the SS phenotype for complement C3 (33). Each of these potential markers requires further evaluation in populations at high alcoholism risk.

Finally, it should be noted that most of the work reported below takes advantage of nonreversible differences between alcoholics and controls. These include several neurophysiological attributes such as the brain waves of the event-related potentials (ERPs) and the differential pattern of slow and fast waves on the background cortical EEGs (1,52,53). Another potential trait marker being tested in high-risk groups is monoamine oxidase (MAO), an enzyme important in the degradation of brain neurotransmitters. Platelet MAO activity appears to be low in alcoholics, and although it is not clear whether it returns to normal with long-term abstinence (56,81,83), MAO may serve as trait marker for a predisposition towards alcoholism.

In summary, comparisons of alcoholics and controls can help identify potential trait markers of a vulnerability towards alcoholism. This occurs by identifying biological traits that do not return to normal with abstinence and outlining differences from controls that are unlikely to have been caused by years of heavy drinking or associated problems. Results to date include interesting leads on several enzyme systems, some blood proteins, and at least two types of brain waves.

STUDIES OF POPULATIONS AT HIGH RISK FOR ALCOHOLISM

Methodological Considerations

The goal of these studies is to identify markers associated with a predisposition towards alcoholism (i.e., trait markers) (67,68). These should be relatively easily measured properties that are present before the illness develops and that can be observed during remission from active problems. The markers might be fortuitous, indirectly associated with a predisposition, perhaps because the genes influencing the marker are located on the same chromosome and relatively close to the genes influencing the development of alcoholism (68). On the other hand, it is possible that the trait markers observed are actually directly involved in the mechanisms that mediate the alcoholism risk.

There are at least three possible approaches to studies of populations at high risk for the future development of alcoholism. First, and most potentially potent, are studies of children of alcoholics adopted out and reared by non-alcoholic parents. These people are then followed with repeated evaluations over time to observe potential differences from controls and the way that these markers actually associate with the later development of alcoholism. Unfortunately, detailed evaluations of adopted-away children of alcoholics are expensive and difficult to carry out. Only two such cohort investigations of offspring adopted out are now in progress, one using children born between 1924 and 1927 in Copenhagen (28,35,89) and the second using records from two adoption agencies in Iowa (7–9).

A second approach is to study intensively multiple generations of a limited number of families of alcoholics, searching for markers that are present in alcoholic relatives but are not seen in nonalcoholic relatives. Such investigations have the asset of giving useful information about the probable pattern of inheritance of alcoholism. However, these studies carry the expensive and time-consuming liability of requiring personal interviews and testing of multiple generations of families as well as the need to interpret results while controlling for the effects of prior drinking patterns, age, and so on. As a result, such investigations can rarely gather data from more than a limited number of families. Therefore, this type of study is probably best reserved for use after preliminary data have indicated those markers that are most appropriate for further investigation. One study of multiple generations in families of alcoholics is now in progress in Quebec (C. Radouce Thomas, *personal communication*).

Third, most work with populations at high risk for alcoholism have utilized cohorts or groups of normal individuals identified because of their date of birth, their educational institution, or through their use of public resources or contact with police agencies. A Danish cohort of 9,000 complication-free full-term births (some of whom have an alcoholic parent) gathered from 1951 to 1961 is presently being evaluated (20,21,52,82). In a different approach, the recent investigations of populations at elevated risk for alcoholism begun in the United States evaluate biological sons of alcoholics who were identified at various ages and then followed over time.

The attributes of work with populations at high risk for the future development of alcoholism have been discussed extensively elsewhere (67). In short, these studies are relatively costly but pave the way for more efficient research in the future; the investigations cannot isolate the mode of inheritance of a marker (this is best done through studies of multiple members of multiple generations of a limited number of families) but can indicate the best markers to look for; the studies address unique populations of limited generalizability, but robust markers from this group can then be applied to larger groups once acceptable study methods have been developed. The prospective study of cohorts at high risk offers unique advantages not found in other study methods but must be viewed as only one important part of research aimed at identifying markers of a predisposition towards alcoholism.

Some Findings from Studies of High-Risk Cohorts

Most of the information on potential biological markers of a predisposition towards alcoholism has come from the cross-sectional evaluation of cohorts of sons of alcoholics who are compared to sons of nonalcoholics (67,68). This section briefly outlines some of those findings.

A Decreased Intensity of Reaction to Ethanol

The series of studies carried out in our own laboratory since 1978 has documented a decreased intensity of reaction to modest doses of ethanol in sons of alcoholics (family history positive or FHP men). The subjects have been students and nonacademic staff at a university who were identified through a mailed questionnaire. This instrument, taking approximately 20 min to complete, identified demography, alcohol/drug/tobacco use histories, personal histories of medical and psychiatric disorders, and family histories of psychiatric illness and alcoholism. After excluding all men who had major medical or psychiatric illness or who had already fulfilled criteria for alcoholism or drug abuse, the remaining individuals who were drinkers and FHPs were selected for study. Each higher-risk man was matched with a family history negative (FHN) subject on age, sex, race, religion, educational level, drinking history, drug use history, and smoking history. In most studies, FHPs and FHNs were individually brought to the laboratory on three occasions, where they received, in random order, placebo, 0.75 ml/kg of ethanol (about three drinks), and 1.1 ml/kg of ethanol administered as a 20% solution in a sugar-free carbonated beverage drunk over 10 min.

In both our own laboratory as well as two additional investigations carried out elsewhere, the two family groups expressed similar expectations of how they would feel after three drinks, developed identical blood alcohol concentrations (BACs) after drinking, and exhibited similar reactions during the placebo session. However, following active alcoholic beverages, the FHP men rated themselves significantly less intoxicated than the FHNs (44,50,59,64,66). The family history group differences were most marked following the low-dose ethanol challenge. At the same time as reporting less intense feelings of intoxication, the FHPs also demonstrated less decrement in cognitive and psychomotor performance associated with ethanol and showed less change in two hormones known to be affected by drinking, cortisol and prolactin (65,77). Thus, one of the more consistent findings coming out of studies of populations at high risk for alcoholism is their significantly less intense subjective feelings of intoxication after drinking, a finding that correlates with some physiological and cognitive/psychomotor reports.

The relationship between the less intense feelings of intoxication and the future development of alcoholism will be established through follow-up of subjects over the next 10 to 15 years. Research is also needed to establish the possible biological mechanisms controlling the decreased intensity of reaction to ethanol and then to demonstrate any level of genetic control. Hypothetically, however, it is possible that a decreased intensity of reaction to low doses of alcohol along with a "more usual" intense intoxication following high ethanol loads could place an individual at a disadvantage in a heavy-drinking society. Most young men and women may "learn" how to drink by occasionally overimbibing but then take advantage of their experiences to recognize how to stop drinking before intense levels of intoxication occur. Thus, a relative insensitivity to effects of modest doses of ethanol could impair an individual's ability to learn to stop drinking at blood levels where control of behavior is still likely. This would not be necessary or sufficient to cause alcoholism but is an example of how possible biological factors might interact with environment to produce a level of alcoholism risk.

Some Possible Electrophysiological Markers

Event-related potentials (ERPs) are computer-averaged brain waves measuring electrophysiological reactions to stimuli. One part of the ERP, the positive wave occurring at approximately 300 msec after a stimulus (the P300), occurs in normal individuals after they experience an anticipated but rare event (53). The P300 is thought to correlate with a person's ability to attend selectively to an anticipated stimulus. Following up on observations of a persistent dampened amplitude of P300s in alcoholics, Begleiter and colleagues have documented a similar deficiency in preadolescent sons of alcoholics (1,53). Possible differences from controls on other aspects of the ERPs have also been reported (18,57). Theoretically, a decreased ability to attend to a stimulus might make it more difficult to discriminate effects of modest ethanol doses or might be associated with other deficits in cognition or in interpersonal functioning that might directly increase the alcoholism risk.

In other work, alcoholics have been shown to demonstrate relatively lower levels of slow waves (i.e., α waves) on background cortical EEGs before ethanol and/or to be more likely to increase the amount of this wave after an ethanol challenge (20,21,44,52,93). Following up on this finding, studies have revealed a similar EEG pattern in sons of alcoholics. It is possible that ethanol has different reinforcing properties in individuals at high risk for alcoholism, perhaps "correcting" for a lower level of α activity and thus producing more feelings of relaxation (61,79).

In summary, to follow up on studies of alcoholics and controls and focus on electrophysiological characteristics that do not appear to return to normal with abstinence, two possible trait markers for alcoholism have been studied in sons of alcoholics. Future investigations must look at the correlation between these findings and the actual development of alcoholism. They will also need to explore the interrelationship between these two factors and other potential markers of a predisposition towards alcoholism, including the apparent decreased intensity of reaction to ethanol in sons of alcoholics.

Possible Persistent Cognitive or Psychomotor Impairment

Studies of young sons of alcoholics identified through their association with juvenile authorities have revealed possible defects on cognitive tests. Compared to sons of nonalcoholics, within these groups the FHPs tended to demonstrate decreased verbal IQs, decreased auditory word-span performance, lower levels of reading comprehension, an increased number of errors on the Category Test of the Halstad–Reitan battery, as well as problems with constructional praxis and abstract problem solving (21,38,55,87,88). Although these findings are impressive, other studies question their generalizability. For instance, in our own studies of university students and nonacademic staff, no base-line differences on cognitive and psychomotor tests were observed for FHPs and FHNs (64,66,67). Of course, it may be that some sons of alcoholics do have a higher risk for cognitive impairment but that these individuals would be the least likely to attain entrance into a university or a steady job in early adulthood. However, using another approach, studies of large general cohorts that were followed over time have found few correlations between apparent cognitive decrements during childhood and the later development of alcoholism (90,92).

Another interesting finding is the observation of an association between the risk for alcoholism and signs of hyperactivity during childhood (26) as well as the demonstration of increased impulsiveness within some high-risk groups (38,43,44,85). On the other hand, childhood hyperactivity can reflect nonspecific stressors such as living with an alcoholic parent and might be temporary and distinct from a true hyperactive child syndrome or attention deficit disorder (78). A number of studies following cohorts over time have not demonstrated a close association between impulsivity or a full-blown hyperactive child syndrome and the actual future development of alcoholism, and in our own laboratory, FHPs were no more likely to have demonstrated hyperactivity in childhood or to show more signs of impulsivity on the Minnesota Multiphasic Personality Inventory (MMPI) than FHNs (55,86,90–92).

In summary, for some men there may be an association between cognitive and psychomotor test impairment and/or signs of hyperactivity in childhood and the future development of alcoholism. However, these are not seen in moderately functional sons of alcoholics (such as those identified as workers or students at a university) and are not strong enough to be identified in general population prospective cohort studies of initially healthy populations.

Possible Personality Profiles and the Future Development of Alcoholism

Alcoholics are likely to show "abnormalities" on a variety of personality tests (63,71). However, many of these results could reflect the actions of ethanol as well as the mood swings and life crises inherent in a life-style of heavy ethanol intake. As a result, most personality test abnormalities tend to return towards normal with abstinence. In addition, some of the traits that do remain after cessation of drinking may reflect primary diagnoses such as antisocial personality disorder and not alcoholism per se (58,63).

Thus, it is not surprising that there are few impressive differences from controls for personality attributes of young men at high risk for the future development of alcoholism. Although a personality profile of increased risk-taking and impulsivity divorced from hyperactivity may be noted for some offspring of alcoholics (42,54), the results for FHPs are usually still within "normal" range. Also, in our laboratory, the comparisons of FHP and FHN college students have revealed no significant differences for scores on neuroticism, extraversion, state anxiety, locus of control, or on an indirect measure of personality, the portable Rod and Frame Test (46,54,61,62,73). However, no definitive answers are available because of limitations in the number of pairs studied thus far, the fact that an absence of a significant difference between groups is sometimes difficult to prove, and trends from some other studies (85), all of which justify further work in this area.

Some Possible Biochemical Markers

As alluded to above, it is probable that alcoholics demonstrate lower platelet MAO activity levels than controls. A similar, although nonsignificant, trend has been observed in sons of alcoholics (56,81), with parallel findings for dopamine-β-hydroxylase (DBH) levels (80,81). Definitive conclusions are jeopardized by the absence of statistical significance for these findings as well as debate about the best measurement methodology.

A similar controversy exists regarding the levels of the first breakdown product of ethanol, acetaldehyde. Although most investigators agree that, at least temporarily, the levels of this highly active compound are significantly higher in the blood of alcoholics after drinking than in controls, there is much debate about whether the finding generalizes to sons of alcoholics as well. Several investigations in our own laboratory as well as trends reported from two other groups reveal a possible important elevation in postdrinking acetaldehyde levels in blood and breath of sons of alcoholics. However, these levels are either adulterated with spuriously produced acetaldehyde or so low as to tax the limit of accuracy of the measurement methodology (74,95,96). It is likely that a final answer must await the development of new, more sensitive and specific acetaldehyde measurement procedures.

A SYNTHESIS AND CONCLUSION

There have been great advances in the study of biological markers of a predisposition towards alcoholism in the last decade. It is now generally accepted that alcoholism is a genetically influenced disorder, a conclusion that has stimulated the search for biological markers of a predisposition.

This chapter has described a number of methodologies that have been used in this search. Comparisons of alcoholics and controls have revealed several potentially important blood protein markers and have identified neurophysiological measures that have been applied to studies of populations at high risk. Reflecting the methodological considerations discussed above, most activity in the search for biological markers has centered on studies of young men at high risk for the future development of alcoholism as determined by the presence of a severely alcoholic first-degree family member. The results have revealed a number of factors that appear to correlate with risk but that will require further investigation in order to determine their actual correlation with future problems, find biological mechanisms controlling the observations, and reveal the genetic mechanisms underlying their expression.

Among the more prominent findings to date is a behavioral observation documenting a decreased intensity of reaction to a modest ethanol challenge in sons of alcoholics compared to controls. This might make it more difficult for subjects at high risk to determine when they are becoming drunk at drug blood levels at which they still have enough self-control to stop drinking. This is an example of a possible genetically influenced factor that might contribute to the risk for alcoholism but does not predestine any individual to become an alcoholic. Other prominent and potentially interesting findings are the de-

creased amplitude of the P300 wave of the ERP as well as the possible differences between FHPs and FHNs on the pattern of brain waves of the background cortical EEG.

These results show that studies of populations at high risk for alcoholism can be carried out successfully. In the future, investigations would be strengthened if the small number of laboratories engaged in this work would standardize criteria for defining alcoholism and follow similar procedures for base-line testing as well as for administering ethanol and observing test results. It may also be appropriate in the near future to apply some of the more prominent differences between FHPs and FHNs to studies of multiple generations of families of alcoholics. It will also be important to try to increase the number of studies of the characteristics of children of alcoholics who were adopted out near birth and raised without knowledge of their biological parent's problems. Finally, to be maximally effective, the series of studies discussed in this chapter should follow up tested groups to determine the combinations of background variables and test results that best predict the development of alcoholism.

ACKNOWLEDGMENTS

This work was supported by USPHS grant AA05562-03, the Research Service of the Veterans Administration, and the Joan B. Kroc Foundation.

REFERENCES

1. Begleiter, H., Porjesz, B., Bihari, B., and Kissin, B. (1984): *Science*, 227:1493–1496.
2. Behar, D., Berg, C. J., and Rapoport, J. L. (1983): *Alcohol Clin. Exp. Res.*, 7:404–410.
3. Blass, J. P., and Gibson, G. E. (1977): *N. Engl. J. Med.*, 297:1367–1370.
4. Bohman, M. (1978): *Arch. Gen. Psychiatry*, 35:269–276.
5. Bohman, M., Sigvardsson, S., and Cloninger, C. R. (1981): *Arch. Gen. Psychiatry*, 38:965–969.
6. Bosron, W. F., and Li, T. K. (1981): *Semin. Liver Dis.*, 1:179–188.
7. Cadoret, R. J., Cain, C. A., and Grove, W. M. (1980): *Arch. Gen. Psychiatry*, 37:561–563.
8. Cadoret, R. J., and Gath, A. (1978): *Br. J. Psychiatry*, 132:252–258.
9. Cadoret, R. J., O'Gorman, T. W., Troughton, E., and Heywood, E. (1985): *Arch. Gen. Psychiatry*, 42:161–167.
10. Cahalan, D., and Cisin, I. H. (1968): *Q. J. Stud. Alcohol*, 29:130–151.
11. Cloninger, C. R., Christiansen, K. O., Reich, T., and Gottesman, I. I. (1978): *Arch. Gen. Psychiatry*, 35:941–951.
12. Cloninger, C. R., Riech, T., and Yokoyama, S. (1983): *Psychiatry Dev.*, 3:225–246.
13. Cloninger, C. R., Bohman, M., and Sigvardsson, S. (1981): *Arch. Gen. Psychiatry*, 36:861–868.
14. Cloninger, C. R., Bohman, M., Sigvardsson, S., and von Knorring, A.-L. (1984): In: *Recent Developments in Alcoholism*, edited by M. Galanter, pp. 37–51. Plenum Press, New York.
15. Comings, D. E. (1979): *Nature*, 277:28–32.
16. Cotton, N. S. (1979): *J. Stud. Alcohol*, 40:89–116.
17. Deitrich, R. A. (1984): *Alcohol Clin. Exp. Res.*, 8:487–490.
18. Elmasian, R., Neville, H., Woods, D., Schuckit, M. A., and Bloom, F. (1982): *Proc. Natl. Acad. Sci. U.S.A.*, 79:7900–7903.
19. Fillmore, K. M., and Midanik, L. (1984): *J. Stud. Alcohol*, 45:228–236.

20. Gabrielli, W. F., Mednick, S. A., Volavka, J., Pollock, V. E., Schulsinger, F., et al. (1982): *Psychophysiology,* 19:404–407.
21. Gabrielli, W. F., and Mednick, S. A. (1983): *J. Nerv. Ment. Dis.,* 171:444–447.
22. Goedde, H. W., Agarwal, D. P., and Harada, S. (1980): *Enzyme,* 25:281–286.
23. Goodwin, D. W. (1979): *Arch. Gen. Psychiatry,* 36:57–61.
24. Goodwin, D. W. (1985): *Arch. Gen. Psychiatry,* 42:171–174.
25. Goodwin, D. W., Schulsinger, F., Hermansen, L., Guze, S. B., and Winokur, G. (1973): *Arch. Gen. Psychiatry,* 28:238–242.
26. Goodwin, D. W., Schulsinger, F., Hermansen, L., Guze, S. B., and Winokur, G. (1975): *J. Nerv. Ment. Dis.,* 160:349–353.
27. Goodwin, D. W., Schulsinger, F., Knop, J., Mednick, S., and Guze, S. B. (1977): *Arch. Gen. Psychiatry,* 34:751–755.
28. Goodwin, D. W., Schulsinger, F., Moller, N., Hermansen, L., Winokur, G., et al. (1974): *Arch. Gen. Psychiatry,* 31:164–169.
29. Goodwin, D. W., Schulsinger, F., Moller, N., Mednick, S., and Guze, S. (1977): *Arch. Gen. Psychiatry,* 34:1005–1009.
30. Greenfield, N. J., and Pietruszko, R. (1977): *Biochim. Biophys. Acta,* 483:35–45.
31. Harada, S., Agarwal, D. P., Goedde, H. W., and Ishikawa, B. (1983): *Pharmacol. Biochem. Behav.,* 18:151–153.
32. Harada, S., Misawa, S., Agarwal, D. P., and Goedde, H. W. (1980): *Am. J. Hum. Genet.,* 32:8–15.
33. Hill, S. Y., Goodwin, D. W., Cadoret, R., Osterland, C. K., and Doner, S. M. (1980): *J. Stud. Alcohol,* 36:981.
34. Hrubec, Z., and Omenn, G. S. (1981): *Alcohol Clin. Exp. Res.,* 5: 207–214.
35. Jacobsen, B., and Schulsinger, F. (1981): In: *Prospective Longitudinal Research: An Empirical Basis for the Primary Prevention of Psychosocial Disorders,* edited by S. A. Mednick and A. E. Baert, pp. 225–230. Oxford University Press, Oxford.
36. Jones, B. M., and Jones, M. K. (1976): In: *Alcoholism Problems in Women and Children,* edited by M. Greenblatt and M. A. Schuckit, pp. 103–136. Grune & Stratton, New York.
37. Kaij, L. (1960): *Studies on the Etiology and Sequels of Abuse of Alcohol.* Department of Psychiatry, University of Lund, Lund.
38. Knop, J., Goodwin, D., Teasdale, T. W., Mikkelsen, U., and Schulsinger, F. (1984): In: *Longitudinal Research in Alcoholism,* edited by D. W. Goodwin, D. Teilmann Van Dusen, and S. A. Mednick, pp. 107–122. Kluwer-Nijhoff Publishing, Boston.
39. Li, T. K. (1981): *Alcohol Clin. Exp. Res.,* 5:451–459.
40. Li, T. K. (1977): In: *Enzymology of Human Alcohol Metabolism,* edited by A. Meister, pp. 19–56. John Wiley & Sons, New York.
41. Li, T. K. (1986): Animal studies in the genetics of alcoholism. *Alcohol Clin. Exp. Res.,* 9:475–492.
42. MacAndrew, C. (1979): *Addict. Behav.,* 4:11–20.
43. McCord, J. (1981): *J. Stud. Alcohol,* 42:739–748.
44. Mednick, S. A. (1983): Subjects at risk for alcoholism. Presented at the 14th Medical and Scientific Conference of National Alcoholism Focus, Houston, Texas.
45. Meisch, R. (1982): *Br. J. Psychiatry,* 141:113–120.
46. Morrison, C., and Schuckit, M. A. (1983): *J. Clin. Psychiatry,* 44: 306–307.
47. Mukherjee, A. B., Ghayourmanesh, S., Fisher, A., Ghazanfari, A., Martin, P., et al. (1983): In: *Abstracts of Contributed Papers, XV International Congress of Genetics. Part I.,* p. 75. Oxford and IBH Publishing, New Delhi.
48. Murray, R. M., Clifford, C., Gurling, H. M. D., Topham, A., Clow, A., et al. (1983): *Psychiatr. Dev.,* 2:179–192.
49. Murray, R. M., Clifford, C. A., and Gurling, H. M. D. (1983): In: *Recent Developments in Alcoholism,* edited by M. Galanter, pp. 25–48. Plenum Press, New York.
50. O'Malley, S. S., and Maisto, S. A. (1985): The effects of family drinking history on responses to alcohol: Expectancies and reactions to intoxication. *J. Stud. Alcohol,* 46:289–297.
51. Pietruszko, R., Theorell, H., and de Zalenski, C. (1972): *Arch. Biochem. Biophys.,* 153:279–293.
52. Pollock, V. E., Volavka, J., and Goodwin, D. W. (1983): *Arch. Gen. Psychiatry,* 40:857–861.
53. Porjesz, B., and Begleiter, H. (1983): In: *The Pathogenesis of Alcoholism,* edited by B. Kissin and H. Begleiter, pp. 415–483. Plenum Press, New York.
54. Saunders, G. R., and Schuckit, M. A. (1981): *J. Nerv. Ment. Dis.,* 168:456–458.
55. Schaeffer, K. W., Parsons, O. A., and Yohman, J. R. (1984): *Alcohol Clin. Exp. Res.,* 8:347–358.
56. Scher, K. J. (1983): *Arch. Gen. Psychiatry,* 40:466.
57. Schmidt, A. L., and Neville, H. J. (1985): *Alcohol,* 2:529–533.
58. Schuckit, M. A. (1973): *J. Stud. Alcohol,* 34:157–164.
59. Schuckit, M. A. (1980): *J. Stud. Alcohol,* 41:242–249.
60. Schuckit, M. A. (1983): *Am. J. Psychiatry,* 104:439–443.
61. Schuckit, M. A. (1982): *J. Clin. Psychiatry,* 43:238–239.
62. Schuckit, M. A. (1983): *Am. J. Psychiatry,* 40:1223–1224.
63. Schuckit, M. A. (1984): *Drug and Alcohol Abuse: A Clinical Guide to Diagnosis and Treatment,* 2nd edition, pp. 44–82. Plenum Press, New York.
64. Schuckit, M. A. (1984): *Arch. Gen. Psychiatry,* 41:879–884.
65. Schuckit, M. A. (1984): *J. Clin. Psychiatry,* 45:374–379.
66. Schuckit, M. A. (1985): *Arch. Gen. Psychiatry,* 42:375–379.
67. Schuckit, M. A. (1985): *Psychiatr. Dev.,* 3:31–63.
68. Schuckit, M. A. (1985): In: *Psychiatry,* Vol. 3, edited by R. Michaels, pp. 1–19. J. P. Lippincott, Philadelphia.
69. Schuckit, M. A. (1986): *Am. J. Psychiatry,* 143:140–147.
70. Schuckit, M. A., and Duby, J. (1982): *J. Clin. Psychiatry,* 43:415–418.
71. Schuckit, M. A., and Haglund, R. M. J. (1982): In: *Alcoholism: Development, Consequences, and Interventions,* edited by N. Estes and E. Heinemann, pp. 16–31. C. V. Mosby, St. Louis.
72. Schuckit, M. A., and Morrisey, E. R. (1979): *Am. J. Psychiatry,* 136:611–617.
73. Schuckit, M. A., and Penn, N. E. (1985): *Am. J. Drug Alc. Abuse,* 2:113–118.
74. Schuckit, M. A., and Rayses, V. (1979): *Science,* 203:54–55.
75. Schuckit, M. A., and von Wartburg, J. P. (1988): *Prog. Neuropsychopharm. Biol. Psychiatry,* 10:191–199.
76. Schuckit, M. A., Goodwin, D. A., and Winokur, G. A. (1972): *Am. J. Psychiatry,* 128:1132.
77. Schuckit, M. A., Parker, D. C., and Rossman, L. R. (1983): *Biol. Psychiatry,* 18:1153–1159.
78. Schuckit, M. A., Petrich, J., and Chiles, J. (1978): *J. Nerv. Ment. Dis.,* 166:79–87.
79. Schuckit, M. A., Engstron, D., Alpert, R., and Duby, J. (1981): *J. Stud. Alcohol,* 42:918–924.
80. Schuckit, M. A., O'Connor, D. T., Duby, J., Vega, R., and Moss, M. (1981): *Biol. Psychiatry,* 16:1067–1075.
81. Schuckit, M. A., Shaskan, E., and Duby, J. (1982): *Arch. Gen. Psychiatry,* 39:137–140.
82. Schulsinger, F. (1972): *Psychophysiology,* 1:190–206.
83. Sullivan, J. L., Cavenar, J. O., Maltbie, A. A., Lister, P., and Zung, W. W. K. (1979): *Biol. Psychiatry,* 14:385.
84. Suwaki, J., and Ohara, H. (1985): *J. Stud. Alcohol,* 46:196–198.
85. Tarter, R. E., and Alterman, A. (1985): *J. Stud. Alc.,* 46:329–356.
86. Tarter, R. E., Hegedus, A. M., and Gavaler, J. S. (1985): *J. Stud. Alcohol,* 46:259–261.
87. Tarter, R. E., Hegedus, A. M., Goldstein, G., Shelly, C., and Alterman, A. (1984): *Alcohol Clin. Exp. Res.,* 8:216–222.
88. Tarter, R., Hill, S., Jacob, T., Hegedus, A., and Winsten, K. J. (1984): *J. Stud. Alc.,* 45:1–9.
89. Utne, H. E., Hensen, F. V., Winkler, K., and Schulsinger, F. (1977): *J. Stud. Alcohol,* 38:1219–1223.
90. Vaillant, G. E. (1984): In: *Psychiatry Update,* edited by L. Grinspoon, pp. 311–319. American Psychiatric Press, Washington.
91. Vaillant, G. E., and Milofsky, E. S. (1982): *Arch. Gen. Psychiatry,* 39:127–133.
92. Vaillant, G. E., and Milofsky, E. S. (1982): *Am. Psychol.,* 37:494–502.
93. Volovka, J., Pollock, V., Gabrielli, W. F., and Mednick, S. A. (1985): In: *Currents in Alcoholism, Vol. VIII,* edited by M. Galanter, pp. 116–123. Grune & Stratton, New York.
94. von Wartburg, J. P. (1980): *Acta Psychiatr. Scand. [Suppl.],* 268: 179–188.
95. Ward, K., Weir, D. G., McCrodden, J. M., and Tipton, K. F. (1983): *IRCS Med. Sci.,* 11:950.
96. Zeiner, A. R., Girardot, J. M., Nichols, N., and Jones-Saumty, D. (1984): *Clin. Exper. Res.,* 8:129.

Psychopharmacology:
The Third Generation of Progress,
edited by Herbert Y. Meltzer.
Raven Press, New York © 1987.

CHAPTER **165**

Abuse of and Dependence on Benzodiazepines and Other Anxiolytic/Sedative Drugs

Roland R. Griffiths and Christine A. Sannerud

The anxiolytic/sedative drugs are among the most widely prescribed of all compounds. Therapeutically, these compounds are used predominantly in the management of anxiety, insomnia, muscle rigidity and spasticity, and convulsions. The purpose of this review is to summarize recent information on the extent of medical and nonmedical use, the reinforcing effects, and the physical dependence-producing effects of these compounds. Space limitations preclude discussion of a range of other adverse effects that are relevant to a comprehensive assessment of abuse liability (26). Such effects, which have been discussed elsewhere (12,13,21,26), include psychomotor impairment, interactions with ethanol, anterograde amnesia, impaired awareness of degree of drug effect, other psychiatric/behavioral disturbances, and drug-associated mortality. Because the benzodiazepine compounds have largely replaced the barbiturate and nonbarbiturate anxiolytic/sedatives as therapeutic agents, the primary emphasis of this review is on benzodiazepines.

EXTENT OF MEDICAL USE

After introduction of benzodiazepine compounds in the early 1960s, use of these compounds as sedatives and anxiolytics in the United States, as reflected in number of prescriptions, steadily increased through 1975 to peak levels of approximately 100 million prescriptions per year. Subsequently, benzodiazepine prescriptions decreased monotonically to approximately 65 million prescriptions in 1981 and then leveled off (3,18). With the increased use of benzodiazepines, use of nonbenzodiazepine sedatives and anxiolytics (e.g., barbiturates and meprobamate) decreased markedly (4,18). Since most anxiolytics are benzodiazepines, trends in anxiolytic prescriptions (Fig. 1) have been similar to those of benzodiazepines. The recent trend of decreasing anxiolytic prescription is probably attributable to a decreased rate of refilling prescriptions, with little change in prescription size or proportion of the population receiving prescriptions each year (M. B. Balter, *this volume*). This tendency toward conservative anxiolytic use is probably attributable to a substantial recent increase in negative attitudes of patients toward use of these compounds (11). The trend toward conservative use of benzodiazepines since the mid-1970s has occurred in some, but not all, West and North European countries (5,46).

Despite recent decreases in anxiolytic use, the high prevalence of use is striking. Household survey data for the United States in 1979 and 1981 showed that 11 to 13% of the adult population has taken an anxiolytic one or more times during the last year, and 2.3 to 2.5% of the population has taken anxiolytics on a daily basis for 4 months or longer (2,48). The latter daily use rate is relevant to estimating the population at risk for development of therapeutic dose physical dependence. Both the past year and daily use rates in the United States are only intermediate in comparison to European countries, in which past-year prevalence rates as high as 18% and daily use rates (≥ 4 months) as high as 7.2% have been reported in a cross-national survey (2).

Although prevalence of anxiolytic use is high, the available evidence suggests that these anxiolytic drugs are generally

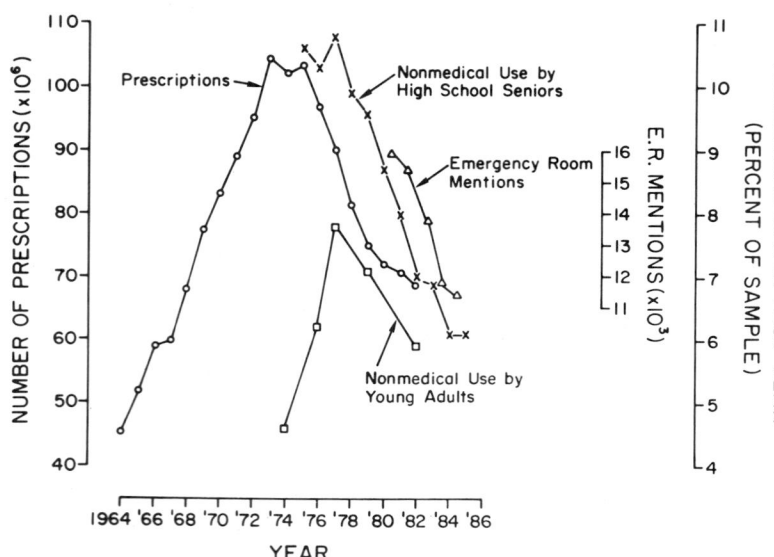

FIG. 1. Trends in use and abuse of anxiolytics in the United States. Data on the number of prescriptions (in millions) were derived from the National Prescription Audit, IMS America Inc., and were organized courtesy of M. B. Balter. Data on the percentages of high school seniors and young adults reporting nonmedical use during the past year were from ongoing national surveys (38,50). Data on the number of emergency room mentions (in thousands) for the five major anxiolytics, were supplied by NIDA and were derived from a panel of consistently reporting emergency rooms in the DAWN system (see text for details).

being used appropriately, and possibly even conservatively, within the broad context of the health care system (46,48,61,80). Some inappropriate prescribing of anxiolytics, however, cannot be entirely ruled out (63,72,73). In any case, given the concerns associated with development of physical dependence, there is an increasing clinical consensus that chronic maintenance of patients on anxiolytics is not desirable and that patients so maintained should be regularly evaluated for termination of the medication (30,32,55,63,64).

EXTENT OF NONMEDICAL USE

There are numerous documented case reports involving the nonmedical use of benzodiazepine, barbiturate, and other anxiolytic/sedative drugs. It is clear from such reports and various surveys that benzodiazepines and other sedatives are sometimes used nonmedically for their psychoactive effects (i.e., to get high) and that they are bought and sold illicitly. Clearly, accurate estimates of the extent of nonmedical use are critical to an understanding of the magnitude and trends of the drug abuse problem with these compounds. As with estimates of medical use, there have been several rigorously conducted national surveys in the United States that have provided such information.

One survey, which has been conducted annually since 1975, has provided information about the nonmedical use of drugs among high school seniors (37,38). A second national survey, which has been conducted six times over an 11-year period (1972–1982), has provided information about the nonmedical use of drugs among persons living in households (50). In 1982, the two surveys showed that 14 to 15% of high school seniors and young adults (18–25 years) reported past nonmedical use of anxiolytics, whereas 15 to 19% of these groups reported past nonmedical use of sedatives (e.g., barbiturates and methaqualone). In both surveys, these lifetime prevalence rates were generally below those for other major drug classes except for heroin and opioid analgesics: alcohol (93–95%), tobacco cigarettes (70–

77%), marijuana (59–64%), stimulants (18–28%), cocaine (16–28%), and hallucinogens (15–21%). With regard to recent trends, both surveys showed that the nonmedical use of anxiolytics has been decreasing since 1977 (Fig. 1). With the sedatives, the high school survey showed monotonic decreases from 1981 to 1985, but the less current household survey (most recent survey in 1982) failed to show this decrease.

Another source of national data about the nonmedical use of drugs is the DAWN system, which is sponsored by the National Institute on Drug Abuse (NIDA). Part of this system involves structured reports from emergency rooms of nonmedical drug use. Although the reliability of DAWN reports has been questioned (74,75), the system provides unique information that supplements the national survey data. Five-year trend data for the period ending with the second quarter of 1985 show a monotonically decreasing number of emergency room mentions for the major anxiolytics (Fig. 1: total mentions for diazepam, chlordiazepoxide, clorazepate, lorazepam, and meprobamate) and sedatives (barbiturate and nonbarbiturate). These data were supplied courtesy of A. Blanken of NIDA and were derived from a panel of consistently reporting emergency rooms. These 5-year trend data from the DAWN system are generally consistent with the results of the two national surveys discussed previously and suggest that the incidence of drug abuse problems with anxiolytic and sedative drugs in the United States has been decreasing in recent years.

Although the national surveys and the DAWN system provide valuable information about large segments of the population, they provide relatively little information about extent and patterns of anxiolytic abuse within the illicit drug culture. Regrettably, information of this type is sparse. At present, the best information is provided by clinical observations of professionals working with drug abuse patients and by rather limited surveys of drug use at drug abuse treatment clinics. Clinical observations suggest that, in the illicit drug culture, anxiolytic/sedatives are most frequently used by polydrug abusers (51,67,77). Benzodiazepines, in particular, are frequently, though not exclusively, abused in combination with other drugs rather than as a primary drug of abuse (41,67). A recurring clinical observation, which has been supported by several surveys, has been the relatively high rate of abuse of diazepam by methadone maintenance patients (7,10,40,42,68,78,81,82). In one survey 65 to 70% of the 224 patients at two geographically separate methadone clinics had positive urinalysis tests during a single month (68). These patients reported using relatively high doses of diazepam in abusive (i.e., nontherapeutic) patterns to "boost" the effects they obtained from their methadone. A related double-blind clinical pharmacology study showed that diazepam does indeed enhance some subjective and physiological opioid effects in methadone maintenance patients while concurrently producing sedative-like subjective effects (59).

Although anxiolytic abuse clearly represents a significant problem in some methadone maintenance clinics, there is substantial variability across clinics, even within the same geographical region (10,67). Such variability may reflect unknown differences in clinic policies (e.g., discharging patients who show unauthorized drug use), differences in local illicit availability of drug, and/or differences in preferences for the drug related to sociological factors associated with the particular clinic population (10). Thus, at present a valid estimate of such anxiolytic abuse among methadone maintainance patients is unknown, nor is it clear whether the pattern of abuse among these patients is typical of the much larger population of opioid abusers not in methadone treatment.

REINFORCING EFFECTS

Reinforcing efficacy of a drug refers to the relative effectiveness in maintaining behavior on which delivery of the drug is dependent. Reinforcing properties are a defining characteristic of abused drugs.

Reinforcing Effects in Animals

Drug self-administration procedures in laboratory animals permit assessment of the relative efficacy with which different drugs maintain drug self-administration. The validity of this approach for providing information relevant to human drug abuse is supported by the good correspondence between those drugs that are self-administered by laboratory animals and those that are self-administered and abused by humans or produce profiles suggesting abuse liability in human experiments (23,25).

Numerous experimental studies with rats and nonhuman primates have examined self-administration of a variety of anxiolytic/sedatives via the intravenous, oral, and intragastric routes (22,26,83). These studies show that the benzodiazepines are less efficacious as reinforcers than barbiturates with intermediate half-lives (pentobarbital, amobarbital, secobarbital) and psychomotor stimulants such as cocaine. Among the benzodiazepines, triazolam and midazolam, which are rapidly eliminated in man, maintain higher levels of self-injection than a variety of other benzodiazepines that are slowly eliminated in man (26,27). Triazolam and midazolam do not, however, maintain the high consistent levels of self-injection maintained by the barbiturates with intermediate half-lives. It is not clear whether the difference in self-administration between the rapidly and slowly eliminated benzodiazepines indicates that the rapidly eliminated compounds are more efficacious reinforcers than other benzodiazepines.

Reinforcing Effects and Subjective "Liking" in Humans

The best-validated human experimental approach for providing information about the abuse liability of drugs is to utilize placebo-controlled, double-blind methodologies to characterize subjective effects and/or behavioral reinforcing properties in subjects with histories of drug abuse (24). With this experimental approach, the abuse liability of a drug is inferred from the ability of a drug (a) to serve as a reinforcer (i.e., increase the probability of behavior that results in its administration) and/or (b) to produce pleasant subjective effects, sometimes called "euphoria" or "liking." Reinforcing effects can be assessed by using various drug self-administration procedures, whereas pleasant ("euphoric") subjective effects can be assessed by using various scale or item-based questionnaires.

Using placebo-controlled, double-blind designs, 14 experiments in subjects with histories of drug abuse have demonstrated that benzodiazepines produce reinforcing effects (i.e., maintain self-administration) and/or produce subjective effects indicating some liability for abuse (24). These results have been obtained with a variety of different benzodiazepines (diazepam, triazolam, oxazepam, prazepam, halazepam, lorazepam, and chlordiazepoxide), representing compounds with different pharmacokinetic profiles (fast versus slow onset of effects; fast versus slow elimination) and compounds used for different clinical indications (anxiolytic and hypnotic). No study that examined a reasonable range of doses failed to demonstrate such reinforcing/subjective effects of benzodiazepines.

In eight studies that compared the reinforcing/subjective effects of a benzodiazepine (diazepam, chlordiazepoxide, or triazolam) with those of pentobarbital, the barbiturate has generally been shown to have the greater liability for abuse (24). These results are consistent with the animal drug self-administration results discussed previously.

Several studies that compared the reinforcing/subjective effects of different benzodiazepines indicate there are meaningful differences among these compounds. Specifically, lorazepam appears to produce reinforcing/subjective effects similar to those of diazepam, whereas oxazepam, halazepam, and chlordiazepoxide may have less liability for abuse than diazepam (24). The most thoroughly characterized comparison was that between diazepam and oxazepam (28,29). When these drugs were compared over a wide range of doses (10–160 mg diazepam; 30–480 mg oxazepam), several types of data suggested that diazepam had a greater liability for abuse. Compared with oxazepam, diazepam produced greater liking and euphoria and was judged to be of greater monetary street value. The subjective effects of diazepam were categorized as being similar to those of barbiturates more frequently than were those of oxazepam. Diazepam was associated with a more rapid onset of effect than was oxazepam, and this rapid onset was repeatedly cited by subjects in written comments as being a desirable feature of the drug effect. Finally, behavioral choice tests showed that diazepam was a more efficacious reinforcer than oxazepam.

The overall conclusion from these studies, that diazepam has a greater liability for abuse than oxazepam, was confirmed in subsequent analyses of epidemiological drug abuse data from the United States and from Sweden (6,29). After adjustment for differences in rates of use, it was shown that diazepam abuse uniformly exceeded oxazepam abuse on various epidemiological measures of drug abuse (e.g., prescription forgeries, theft and loss reports, Drug Enforcement Administration illicit cases, emergency room mentions involving illicitly obtained drug). This effect was not an artifact of unequal rates of prescribing and occurred when data were calculated to exclude Valium®, the original and most widely known brand of diazepam.

The difference in reinforcing/subjective effects among benzodiazepines is analogous to differences in reinforcing/subjective effects among barbiturates. Phenobarbital has been shown to produce relatively less liking and euphoria than pentobarbital and secobarbital (19,77). This observation is consistent with the clinical observation that, relative to these other barbiturates, phenobarbital has an extremely low incidence of abuse characterized by drug-seeking behavior (19).

PHYSICAL DEPENDENCE

Physical dependence is manifested by biochemical, physiological and/or behavioral disruptions that occur on termination of chronic drug administration. Physical dependence is not a defining characteristic of an abused drug; there are drugs that produce physical dependence without eliciting drug-seeking behavior (e.g., cyclazocine, nalorphine), and there are drugs thought not to produce physical dependence that do produce substantial drug-seeking behavior (e.g., cocaine, amphetamine) (26). Among the sedative/anxiolytics, phenobarbital is an example of a drug that is fully capable of producing physical dependence, although there is an extremely low incidence of abuse characterized by drug-seeking behavior (19). Although not a defining characteristic of abuse liability, physical dependence may contribute to the abuse liability of a drug in two ways: (a) as an adverse effect of drug use that is revealed on discontinuation of drug use and (b) as a potential mechanism by which the reinforcing effects of a drug may be enhanced.

Physical Dependence in Animals

Physical dependence on anxiolytic/sedative drugs has been extensively studied in laboratory animals using three general approaches: (a) substitution tests in which the ability of the test drug to suppress withdrawal signs of animals physically dependent on another drug is assessed;

(b) spontaneous withdrawal tests in which withdrawal signs are assessed when administration of test drug is abruptly terminated after a period of chronic administration; (c) precipitated withdrawal tests in which a benzodiazepine-like test drug is given chronically and withdrawal signs are assessed after administration of a benzodiazepine antagonist.

Studies in mice, rats, dogs, cats, and monkeys have clearly shown that withdrawal severity is an increasing function of dose and duration of administration of barbiturate and benzodiazepine drugs (19,44,54,65). Among the most severe signs of anxiolytic/sedative withdrawal are delirium and grand mal convulsion. In an elegant series of studies with barbiturates, Okomoto (54) demonstrated that withdrawal severity is also an inverse function of the rate of drug elimination. To date, no such relationship has been clearly demonstrated in spontaneous withdrawal studies with various benzodiazepines (26,80). In fact, substitution, spontaneous, and precipitated withdrawal studies in laboratory animals to date have not provided convincing data differentiating among benzodiazepines with respect to withdrawal severity.

It is of interest that studies of precipitated benzodiazepine withdrawal have revealed a remarkable degree of adaptive sensitivity of the central nervous system to benzodiazepine administration. Precipitated benzodiazepine withdrawal signs have been observed in baboons and cats after chronic treatment with relatively low doses (0.25–0.5 mg/kg) of diazepam or flurazepam and after only 1 to 3 days of exposure to higher benzodiazepine doses (44,65).

Studies comparing the physical dependence-producing properties of benzodiazepines and barbiturates in laboratory animals have provided only a limited basis for differentiating between these classes. Benzodiazepines have generally been shown to suppress barbiturate withdrawal signs in drug substitution procedures (19,80,83). However, several substitution studies suggest that cross dependence between barbiturates and benzodiazepines may be weak or incomplete (26,47), and one study, which used the rigorous "chronically equivalent" dosing procedure, concluded that a benzodiazepine (chlordiazepoxide) produced less severe withdrawal than a barbiturate (phenobarbital) (9).

Physical Dependence in Humans

Repeated use of anxiolytic/sedative drugs by humans can result in physical dependence. The signs and symptoms associated with termination of chronic dosing of these compounds include anxiety, insomnia, agitation, anorexia, tremor, muscle twitching, nausea/vomiting, hypersensitivity to sensory stimuli and other perceptual disturbances, depersonalization, hallucination, delirium, grand mal convulsions, and occasionally death (19,35,45,66). The more severe of the signs and symptoms are generally observed only following prolonged exposure to high doses.

Physical Dependence Following High Daily Doses

The withdrawal syndrome following termination of intermediate-duration barbiturates (pentobarbital, secobarbital, and amobarbital) and alcohol has been carefully characterized in a series of nonblind experiments in subjects with and without histories of drug abuse (19,20,35). Following a progressive decrease in signs of intoxication over 6 to 15 hr, patients show increasing minor withdrawal signs and symptoms, which may be followed after 24 hr or more by grand mal convulsions, auditory or visual hallucinations, and delirium. With barbiturates, withdrawal severity is an increasing function of dose. The proportion of subjects showing grand mal seizures after prolonged administration of high-dose (0.9–2.2 g/day), intermediate-dose (0.6–0.8 g/day), or low-dose (0.4 g/day) pentobarbital or secobarbital was 78%, 13%, and 0%, respectively. The proportion of subjects showing minor withdrawal effects at these same dose levels was 100%, 61%, and 6%, respectively. Severe withdrawal reactions (i.e., seizures and psychoses) following abrupt discontinuation of high doses of various nonbarbiturate sedatives, including meprobamate, glutethimide, ethinamate, ethchlorvynol, and methyprylon, have also been reported (15).

Experimental characterization of the high-dose benzodiazepine withdrawal syndrome has been somewhat less complete. In a classic study, Hollister (34) abruptly switched 11 psychiatric patients to placebo after 2 to 6 months of receiving high daily doses of chlordiazepoxide (300–600 mg/day, 8–20 times the usual therapeutic dose). Withdrawal signs, which occurred in 10 of the 11 patients, appeared between 2 and 8 days after drug termination and included depression, aggravation of psychoses, agitation, insomnia, loss of appetite, and nausea; two patients had grand mal convulsions on days 7 and 8.

Subsequent studies and clinical observation have confirmed and extended these findings to other benzodiazepines (33,56). One such assessment was made in a group of 10 patients who had used high doses of diazepam for 3 to 14 years (49). The daily dose taken 6 months prior to abrupt nonblind drug termination ranged between 60 and 120 mg/day; none had used other drugs during this period. A withdrawal syndrome lasting up to 6 weeks occurred in all 10 subjects on termination of drug dosing. Although there were no convulsions, alcohol- or barbiturate-like delirium occurred in four subjects during the first 10 days of withdrawal; minor withdrawal signs and symptoms, which occurred throughout a 6-week period in almost all subjects, included anxiety, insomnia, agitation, anorexia, tremor, muscle twitching, and a variety of perceptual changes such as paresthesias and hypersensitivity to light and noise.

As with the laboratory animal data on physical dependence, the available human data provide only a limited basis for differentiating between barbiturates and benzodiazepines. Most of the signs and symptoms that have been described in experimental studies of pentobarbital and secobarbital withdrawal have also been noted in studies or case reports of benzodiazepine withdrawal. A major difference has been that benzodiazepine withdrawal has been associated with a considerably lower frequency of severe signs such as seizures and delirium. It should be noted, however, that all of the high-dose benzodiazepine studies and reports have involved benzodiazepines that are slowly eliminated or have active metabolites that are slowly eliminated. Thus, at present, it is not clear whether the differences in withdrawal severity between drugs like pentobarbital (which is relatively rapidly eliminated) and diazepam (which is relatively slowly eliminated) represent inherent pharmacodynamic differences or whether they simply reflect pharmacokinetic differences (31).

Benzodiazepine Physical Dependence Following Therapeutic Doses

In addition to producing physical dependence after chronic high doses, it is now clear that benzodiazepines can also produce physical dependence after prolonged treatment at normal therapeutic doses (43,55,66,79,80). The profile, intensity, and time course of signs and symptoms that emerge on termination of drug administration have permitted differentiation of true pharmacological withdrawal from a simple reemergence of preexisting anxiety or insomnia. Although the most severe withdrawal signs (seizures and delirium) are generally absent in therapeutic dose dependence, a variety of disturbing signs and symptoms remain, including anxiety, insomnia, irritability, tremor, muscle twitching, headache, gastrointestinal disturbance, depersonalization, and a wide variety of perceptual changes such as paresthesias and hypersensitivity to light and noise (66). Because many more therapeutic dose withdrawal studies have focused on benzodiazepines than on barbiturates, it is not clear whether the profiles of subtle withdrawal signs and symptoms differ between these drug classes. It is known that barbiturate withdrawal can be associated with a variety of subtle perceptual changes (14,20), which are possibly similar to those described during benzodiazepine withdrawal.

Speed of onset of withdrawal after abrupt cessation of benzodiazepines varies from 1 to 10 days (55). Estimates of the duration of the therapeutic dose withdrawal syndrome have been extremely variable. Although clinical investigators have often estimated its duration to be 4 weeks or less (as short as 5 days) (55), there are an increasing number of clinical reports describing protracted withdrawal syndromes lasting 6 months or longer (1,30). The proportion of long-term users that are at risk for withdrawal effects is difficult to estimate because withdrawal studies have often involved self-selected patients who have previously had difficulty withdrawing from medication (55,57). However, in studies of relatively unselected patient groups, the proportion of patients experiencing withdrawal after long-term benzodiazepine use has been as high as 45%, even when drug has been withdrawn incrementally (70,71). The minimum duration of benzodiazepine treatment necessary to produce significant therapeutic dose dependence is controversial. It has been estimated to be as short as 4 to 6 weeks (17,53,58) and as long as 8 months (62). If rebound insomnia (a significant worsening of sleep after treatment with hypnotic drugs) is taken as a measure of drug withdrawal, therapeutic dose dependence has occasionally been demonstrated after only 2 weeks of drug administration (8,39).

Withdrawal severity and latency to onset of withdrawal may differ between benzodiazepines. Benzodiazepine compounds that are relatively rapidly eliminated (e.g., lorazepam, triazolam) tend to have shorter latencies to withdrawal onset than relatively slowly eliminated compounds or compounds with slowly eliminated metabolites (e.g., diazepam, flurazepam) (26,69,71), although there is considerable overlap in these distributions. There is some evidence that the probability and intensity of withdrawal effects are greater with rapidly eliminated than with slowly eliminated compounds (17,76), and this certainly seems to be the case if rebound insomnia is taken as a measure of withdrawal for hypnotic benzodiazepines (39).

By analogy to what is known about barbiturate dependence, it has been hypothesized that benzodiazepine withdrawal severity should be an inverse function of the rate at which drug leaves the brain (31). Although an inverse relationship between benzodiazepine plasma level and withdrawal intensity or probability of withdrawal symptoms was shown in one study (71), other studies failed to confirm this relationship (1,52,60,70), thus leaving the validity of this pharmacokinetic hypothesis in some doubt. The best-controlled experimental study that seems to support the hypothesis is one by Tyrer (69,71), who showed that in self-referred patient groups undergoing abrupt benzodiazepine detoxification, the severity of early withdrawal symptoms and the dropout rate were higher with the quickly eliminated lorazepam than with diazepam, which has a slowly eliminated metabolite. However, another recent withdrawal study (16) has shown that lorazepam also produced greater rebound anxiety and a higher dropout rate than bromazepam. Since both lorazepam and bromazepam have similar metabolic half-lives (both about 12 hr) with no significant accumulation of active metabolite (36), this study suggests that there may be intrinsic differences in the ability of benzodiazepines to produce physical dependence independent of pharmacokinetic factors. Taken together, these studies also suggest that lorazepam physical dependence may be more problematic than that with other benzodiazepines. This conclusion is consistent with the observations of Kemper (41), who reviewed a large number of cases of benzodiazepine abuse and concluded that lorazepam withdrawal is particularly severe.

SUMMARY

Benzodiazepines, which are among the most safe, effective, and widely prescribed of all psychotropic compounds, have largely replaced barbiturates as anxiolytics, sedatives, and hypnotics over the last two decades. The nonmedical use (i.e., abuse) of barbiturates and benzodiazepines has tended to decrease in recent years. Clinical observation suggests that in the illicit drug culture these drugs are most frequently used by polydrug abusers. Benzodiazepines tend to be abused in combination with other drugs; diazepam–opioid combinations seem to be a particular problem in this regard. Experiments in laboratory animals have shown that benzodiazepines have reinforcing properties; however, they are clearly less efficacious as reinforcers than barbiturates with intermediate half-lives such as pentobarbital or psychomotor stimulant compounds such as cocaine. Analogous studies in humans have confirmed that the reinforcing/subjective effects of benzodiazepines are less than those of pentobarbital. In addition, human studies suggest that the reinforcing/subjective effects of lorazepam are similar to those of diazepam and that the reinforcing/subjective effects of diazepam are greater than those of other benzodiazepines including oxazepam. Studies in laboratory animals and humans have shown that abrupt termination of high chronic doses of barbiturates and benzodiazepines can produce a severe withdrawal syndrome, which may include delirium

and grand mal convulsions. Some limited animal and human data suggest that high doses of barbiturates may produce a more severe withdrawal syndrome than high doses of benzodiazepines. It is now clear that benzodiazepines also can produce a withdrawal syndrome after prolonged treatment with normal therapeutic doses. The area of benzodiazepine therapeutic dose dependence has received considerable scientific and public attention because of both known and unknown potential problems associated with physical dependence and because of the large population potentially at risk—more than 2% of the U.S. adult population. Such withdrawal occurs in a significant proportion of long-term benzodiazepine users, and there is some evidence that lorazepam produces more withdrawal problems than other anxiolytic benzodiazepines. Although additional research will be required to address adequately the risk/benefit ratio of long-term benzodiazepine use, there is an increasing clinical consensus that chronic maintenance of patients on anxiolytics is not desirable and that patients so maintained should be regularly evaluated for termination of medication.

ACKNOWLEDGMENTS

Preparation of this paper was supported, in part, by National Institute on Drug Abuse grants R01 DA01147 and R01 DA03889.

REFERENCES

1. Ashton, H. (1984): *Br. Med. J.*, 288:1135–1140.
2. Balter, M. B., Manheimer, D. I., Mellinger, G. D., and Uhlenhuth, E. H. (1984): *Curr. Med. Res. Opin.*, 8:5.
3. Baum, C., Forbes, M. B., and Kennedy, D. L. (1984): Poster presentation at the American Psychological Association Annual Convention, Toronto, Canada.
4. Baum, C., Kennedy, D. L., Forbes, M. B., and Jones, J. K. (1982): *Drug Utilization in the U.S.—1981. Third Annual Review.* Food and Drug Administration, Washington.
5. Bergman, U., and Dahlstrom, M. (1986): In: *Drug Treatment of Neurotic Disorders: Focus on Alprazolam*, edited by M. H. Lader and H. C. Davies, pp. 43–52. Churchill Livingstone, Edinburgh.
6. Bergman, U., and Griffiths, R. R. (1986): *Drug Alcohol Depend*, 16:293–301.
7. Bigelow, G., Stitzer, M., Lawrence, C., Krasnegor, N., D'Lugoff, B., et al. (1980): *Int. J. Addict.*, 15:427–437.
8. Bixler, E. O., Kales, J. D., Kales, A., Jacoby, J. A., and Soldatos, C. R. (1985): *J. Clin. Pharmacol.*, 25:115–124.
9. Boisse, N. R., Ryan, G. P., Guarino, J. J., and Gay, M. H. (1981): *Pharmacologist*, 23:192.
10. Budd, R. D., Walkin, E., Jain, N. C., and Sneath, T. C. (1979): *Am. J. Drug Alcohol Abuse*, 6:511–514.
11. Clinthorne, J. K., Cisin, I. H., Balter, M. B., Mellinger, G. D., and Uhlenhuth, E. H. (1986): *Arch. Gen. Psychiatry*, 43: 527–532.
12. Cole, J. O., Haskell, D. S., and Orzack, M. H. (1981): *McLean Hosp. J.*, 6:46–74.
13. Edwards, J. G. (1981): *Drugs*, 22:495–514.
14. Epstein, R. S. (1980): *Am. J. Psychiatry*, 137:107–108.
15. Essig, C. F. (1966): *J.A.M.A.*, 196:714–717.
16. Fontaine, R., Annable, L., Beaudry, P., Mercier, P., and Chouinard, G. (1985): *Psychopharmacol. Bull.*, 21:91–92.
17. Fontaine, R., Chominard, G., and Annable, L. (1984): *Am. J. Psychiatry*, 141:848–852.
18. Food and Drug Administration (1981): *Benzodiazepines: Extent of Use, Misuse, and Abuse.* Drug Use Analysis Branch, Division Drug Experience, FDA, Washington.
19. Fraser, H. F., and Jasinski, D. R. (1977): In: *Handbook of*

Experimental Pharmacology, Vol. 45, edited by W. R. Martin, pp. 589–612. Springer-Verlag, New York.

20. Fraser, H. F., Wikler, A., Essig, C. F., and Isbell, H. (1958): *J.A.M.A.,* 166:126–129.

21. Greenblatt, D. J., Shader, R. I., and Abernethy, D. R. (1983): *N. Engl. J. Med.,* 309:410–416.

22. Griffiths, R. R., and Ator, N. A. (1981): In: *Benzodiazepines,* edited by J. Ludford and S. Szara, pp. 22–36. National Institute on Drug Abuse Monograph No. 33, DHHS Publication No. ADM 81-1052, U.S. Government Printing Office, Washington.

23. Griffiths, R. R., and Balster, R. L. (1979): *Clin. Pharmacol. Ther.,* 25:611–617.

24. Griffiths, R. R., and Roache, J. D. (1985): In: *The Benzodiazepines: Current Standards for Medical Practice,* edited by D. E. Smith and D. R. Wesson, pp. 209–225. MTP Press, Lancaster.

25. Griffiths, R. R., Bigelow, G. E., and Henningfield, J. E. (1980): In: *Advances in Substance Abuse: Behavioral and Biological Research,* edited by N. K. Mello, pp. 1–90. JAI Press, Greenwich, CT.

26. Griffiths, R. R., Lamb, R. J., Ator, N. A., Roache, J. D., and Brady, J. V. (1985): *Neurosci. Biobehav. Rev.,* 9:133–151.

27. Griffiths, R. R., Lukas, S. E., Bradford, L. D., Brady, J. V., and Snell, J. D. (1981): *Psychopharmacology (Berl.),* 75:101–109.

28. Griffiths, R. R., McLeod, D. R., Bigelow, G. E., Liebson, I. A., and Roache, J. D. (1984): *Psychopharmacology (Berl.),* 84:147–154.

29. Griffiths, R. R., McLeod, D. R., Bigelow, G. E., Liebson, I. A., Roache, J. D., et al. (1984): *J. Pharmacol. Exp. Ther.,* 229:501–508.

30. Higgitt, A. C., Lader, M. H., and Fonagy, P. (1985): *Br. Med. J.,* 291:688–690.

31. Hollister, L. E. (1981): *Psychiatr. Ann.,* 11:26–31.

32. Hollister, L. E. (1985): In: *The Benzodiazepines: Current Standards for Medical Practice,* edited by D. E. Smith and D. R. Wesson, pp. 87–96. MTP Press, Lancaster.

33. Hollister, L. E., Bennett, J. L., Kimbell, I., Savage, C., and Overall, J. E. (1963): *Dis. Nerv. Syst.,* 24:746–750.

34. Hollister, L. E., Motzenbecker, F. P., and Degan, R. O. (1961): *Psychopharmacologia,* 2:63–68.

35. Isbell, H., Altschul, S., Kornetsky, C. H., Eisenman, A. J., Flanary, H. G. et al. (1950): *A.M.A. Arch. Neurol. Psychiatry,* 64:1–28.

36. Jochemsen, R., and Breimer, D. D. (1984): *Curr. Med. Res. Opin.,* 8:60–79.

37. Johnston, L. D., O'Malley, P. M., and Bachman, J. G. (1984): *Drugs and American High School Students, 1975–1983.* DHHS Publication No. (ADM) 85-1374, U. S. Government Printing Office, Washington.

38. Johnston, L., O'Malley, P., and Bachman, J. G. (1985): *Use of Licit and Illicit Drugs by America's High School Students, 1975–1984.* DHHS Publication No. (ADM) 85-1394, U.S. Government Printing Office, Washington.

39. Kales, A., Soldatos, C. R., and Vela-Bueno, A. (1985): In: *The Benzodiazepines: Current Standards for Medical Practice,* edited by D. E. Smith and D. R. Wesson, pp. 121–147. MTP Press, Lancaster.

40. Kaul, B., and Davidow, B. (1981): *Am. J. Drug Alcohol Abuse,* 8:17–25.

41. Kemper, N., Poser, W., and Poser, S. (1980): *Deut. Med. Wochenschr.,* 105:1707–1712.

42. Kleber, H. D., and Gold, M. S. (1978): *Ann. N.Y. Acad. Sci.,* 311:81–98.

43. Lader, M., and Petursson, H. (1984): In: *Antianxiety Agents,* edited by G. D. Burrows, T. R. Norman, and B. Davies, pp. 127–141. Elsevier, Amsterdam.

44. Lukas, S. E., and Griffiths, R. R. (1984): *Eur. J. Pharmacol.,* 100:163–171.

45. Marks, J. (1978): *The Benzodiazepines—Use, Overuse, Misuse, Abuse.* University Park Press, Baltimore.

46. Marks, J. (1985): In: *The Benzodiazepines: Current Standards of Medical Practice,* edited by D. E. Smith and D. R. Wesson, pp. 67–86. MTP Press, Lancaster.

47. Martin, W. R., McNicholas, L. F., and Cherian, S. (1982): *Life Sci.,* 31:721–730.

48. Mellinger, G. D., Balter, M. B., and Uhlenhuth, E. H. (1984): *J.A.M.A.,* 251:375–379.

49. Mellor, C. S., and Jain, V. K. (1982): *Can. Med. Assoc. J.,* 127:1093–1096.

50. Miller, J. D., Cisin, I. H., Gardner-Keaton, H., Harrel, A. V., Wirtz, P. W., et al. (1983): *National Survey on Drug Abuse: Main Findings 1982.* DHHS Publication No. (ADM) 83-1263, U.S. Government Printing Office, Washington.

51. Mitchelson, M., Davidson, J., Hawks, D., Hitchens, L., and Malone, S. (1970): *Lancet,* 1:606–607.

52. Mitler, M. M., Seidel, W. F., Van Den Hoed, J., Greenblatt, D. J., and Dement, W. C. (1984): *J. Clin. Psychopharmacol.,* 4:2–13.

53. Murphy, S. M., Owen, R. T., and Tyrer, P. J. (1984): *Lancet,* 2:1389.

54. Okamoto, M. (1984): In: *Mechanisms of Tolerance and Dependence,* edited by C. W. Sharp, pp. 333-347. NIDA Research Monograph No. 54, DHHS publication number (ADM) 84-1300, U.S. Government Printing Office, Washington.

55. Owen, R. T., and Tyrer, P. (1983): *Drugs,* 25:385–398.

56. Petursson, H., and Lader, M. H. (1981): *Br. J. Addict.,* 76:133–145.

57. Petursson, H., and Lader, M. H. (1981): *Br. Med. J.,* 283:643–645.

58. Power, K. G., Jerrom, D. W. A., Simpson, R. J., and Mitchell, M. (1985): *Br. Med. J.,* 290:1246–1248.

59. Preston, K. L., Griffiths, R. R., Stitzer, M. L., Bigelow, G. E., and Liebson, I. A. (1984): *Clin. Pharmacol. Ther.,* 36:534–541.

60. Rhodes, P. J., and Rhodes, R. S. (1984): *Clin. Toxicol.,* 22:371–385.

61. Rickels, K. (1981): *Br. J. Clin. Pharmacol.,* 11:71S–83S.

62. Rickels, K., Case, G. W., Downing, R. W., and Winokur, A. (1983): *J.A.M.A.,* 250:767–771.

63. Rickels, K., Case, G. W., Winokur, A., and Swenson, C. (1984): *Psychopharmacol. Bull.,* 20:608–615.

64. Rickels, K., Case, G. W., Downing, R. W., and Winokur, A. (1985): In: *Chronic Treatments in Neuropsychiatry,* edited by D. Kemali and G. Racagni, pp. 193–204. Raven Press, New York.

65. Rosenberg, H., and Chiu, T. H. (1985): *Neurosci. Biobehav. Rev.,* 9:123–131.

66. Schopf, J. (1983): *Pharmacopsychiatria,* 16:1–8.

67. Smith, D., and Marks, J. (1985): In: *The Benzodiazepines: Current Standards for Medical Practice,* edited by D. E. Smith and D. R. Wesson, pp. 179–199. MTP Press, Lancaster.

68. Stitzer, M. L., Griffiths, R. R., McLellan, A. T., Grabowski, J., and Hawthorne, J. W. (1981): *Drug Alcohol Depend,* 8:189–199.

69. Tyrer, P. J., and Seivewright, N. (1984): *Postgrad. Med. J.,* 60:41–46.

70. Tyrer, P. J., Owens, R., and Dawling, S. (1983): *Lancet,* 1:1402–1406.

71. Tyrer, P. J., Rutherford, D., and Huggett, T. (1981): *Lancet,* 1:520–522.

72. Uhlenhuth, E. H., Balter, M. B., Mellinger, G. D., Cisin, I. H., and Clinthorne, J. (1983): *Arch. Gen. Psychiatry,* 40:1167–1173.

73. Uhlenhuth, E. H., Balter, M. B., Mellinger, G. D., Cisin, I. H., and Clinthorne, J. (1984): *Curr. Med. Res. Opin.,* 8:37–47.

74. Ungerleider, J. T., Lundberg, G. E., Sunshine, I., and Walberg, C. B. (1980): *Arch. Gen. Psychiatry,* 37:106–109.

75. Ungerleider, J. T., Lunberg, G. E., Sunshine, I., and Walberg, C. B. (1980): *J. Anal. Toxicol.,* 4:269–271.

76. Walters, L., and Nel, P. (1981): *South Afr. Med. J.,* 24:115–116.

77. Wesson, D. R., and Smith, D. E. (1977): *Barbiturates: Their Use, Misuse, and Abuse.* Human Sciences Press, New York.

78. Wiersum, J. (1974): *J.A.M.A.,* 227:79.

79. Winokur, A., Rickels, K., Greenblatt, D. J., Snyder, P. J., and Schatz, N. J. (1980): *Arch. Gen. Psychiatry,* 37:101–105.

80. Woods, J. H., Katz, J. L., and Winger, G. (1983): In: *Eighth Review of Psychoactive Substances for International Control.* WHO, Geneva, Switzerland.

81. Woody, G. E., Mintz, J., O'Hare, K., O'Brien, C. P., Greenstein, R. A., et al. (1975): *J. Psychedel. Drugs,* 7:373–379.

82. Woody, G. E., O'Brien, C. P., and Greenstein, R. (1975): *Int. J. Addict.,* 10:843–848.

83. Yanagita, T. (1981): In: *Psychotropic Agents Part II: Anxiolytics, Gerontopsychopharmacological Agents, and Psychomotor Stimulants,* edited by F. Hoffmeister and G. Stille, pp. 395–406. Springer-Verlag, New York.

Psychopharmacology:
The Third Generation of Progress,
edited by Herbert Y. Meltzer.
Raven Press, New York © 1987.

CHAPTER **166**

Cocaine and the Amphetamines

Marian W. Fischman

The past decade has seen an enormous upsurge in the use of cocaine, which persists despite severe penalties associated with its possession and sale. Such an increase in psychomotor stimulant use presents a serious public health problem, and much clinical and basic research has been carried out to investigate the effects of these drugs. This chapter describes the behavioral pharmacology of amphetamine and cocaine, reviewing research from the past 10 years but drawing on earlier work when appropriate. A brief description of the current cocaine use epidemic and its relation to earlier amphetamine epidemics is followed by a discussion of animal laboratory research with amphetamine and cocaine. The available methods for studying psychotropic drugs in animals are important tools for the evaluation of a drug's abuse liability and dependence potential. Much of what we have learned about the clinical toxicity of cocaine and amphetamine could have been predicted from the animal laboratory results. In addition, research on the behavioral pharmacology of these drugs in humans both extends and provides generality for the conclusions to be drawn from the laboratory research. By necessity, this chapter is a selective review of cocaine and amphetamine; the papers referenced serve only as examples of the available literature. During the past 10 years a number of extensively detailed reviews and books have been published (55,59,83,90,122), which achieve comprehensive coverage of the literature.

Amphetamine and cocaine, very different in their pharmacological development, share the properties of central nervous system stimulant activity and substantial abuse liability. Cocaine is a naturally occurring local anesthetic, isolated from the plant *Erythroxylon coca* in 1860 (55). It enjoyed almost immediate popularity, praised by such notables as Sigmund Freud (1884, translated in ref. 18), who accurately described its central effects and suggested that this "magical drug" could cure neurasthenia, depressed mood, and alcohol and morphine addiction. Clearly, the early popularity of cocaine can be attributed as much to its mood-altering properties as to any therapeutic local anesthetic properties. It was not long before concern about its toxic dependence-producing properties was also publicized, and the passage of the Harrison Narcotic Act of 1914 effectively limited availability of this drug. Amphetamine, on the other hand, was first synthesized in 1887 (20) as part of a program on the manufacture of aliphatic amines, although its use as a bronchial dilator did not take hold until the early 1930s. The CNS stimulant properties of the amphetamines were described in 1933 (5), and reports of abuse soon followed. They rapidly replaced cocaine in "street" use since they were cheaper, more readily available, and had a longer duration of action (9). The optimism with which the amphetamines were greeted was, however, followed by a condemnation, which paralleled the cyclic pattern of acceptance seen with cocaine.

These two drugs share a range of effects, most of which are related to their sympathomimetic properties. Amphetamine and cocaine increase concentrations of both dopaminergic and noradrenergic transmitters at the neuronal synapse, cocaine by blocking reuptake and amphetamine by both augmenting release and blocking reuptake (143). These effects are discussed in detail elsewhere in this volume (see L. S. Seiden, *this volume*).

CLINICAL UTILITY

Cocaine is, as stated above, a local anesthetic, and although it has largely been replaced by synthetics (e.g., procaine, lidocaine), it is still used in surgery of the upper respiratory tract because of its unique (to the local anesthetics) vasoconstriction properties.

Stimulant drugs are frequently indicated for the treatment of narcolepsy, obesity, and childhood hyperactivity (9). Although patients with narcolepsy require large doses of amphetamine for prolonged periods of time, tolerance does not seem to develop to the therapeutic effects of the drug, since patients can be maintained at a fixed dose (87). The use of amphetamines in the treatment of hyperkinetic behavioral disorders in children, however, remains controversial. Those promoting their use point to their potential benefits and advocate care in limiting treatment dose and duration (9). Although the major therapeutic utility of amphetamine is in the short-term treatment of obesity (85), considerable evidence exists for a rapid development of tolerance to the anorectic effects of this drug. Therefore, these drugs should only be given for 4 to 6 weeks and, if needed for longer-term treatment, should be administered intermittently with drug-free periods interspersed (9). Amphetamine therapy has also been attempted with little success in the treatment of Parkinson's disease (102), and both amphetamine and cocaine have been suggested for the treatment of depression, although little evidence exists to support their efficacy (81,109).

Despite endorsement for the treatment of a range of ailments, the therapeutic utility of these drugs is, at best, limited. Their abuse liability and dependence potential should therefore be weighed against this minimal therapeutic utility in evaluating the toxic consequences of these drugs.

GENERAL EFFECTS

Humans given single moderate doses of cocaine and amphetamine generally show a decrease in food intake and fatigue and an increase in activity, talkativeness, and reports of euphoria and general well-being. At higher doses, repetitive motor activity (stereotyped behavior) is often seen, and with further increases in dose, convulsions, hyperthermia, coma, and death can ensue.

The primary physiological parameters measured after cocaine and amphetamine administration have been cardiovascular functions. These drugs cause dose-related increases in heart rate and blood pressure (48,131). Intravenous cocaine (4–32 mg) has not been shown to have any effect on the electrocardiogram (48) or on respiratory rate and body temperature (10–25 mg; 111). Oral cocaine (30–200 mg/day) given in divided doses does not affect pulse, temperature, blood pressure, or respiration (108). As with amphetamine (110), these oral doses do have a suppressive effect on both rapid eye movement (REM) sleep and total sleep.

Although early research (77) reported that cocaine increased α frequency and amplitude and β activity 20 min after injection, Herning and his colleagues (61) recently reported that intravenous and oral cocaine in humans appears to increase β activity but not α, perhaps because subjects in the latter study were engaged in a demanding task. Unlike other stimulants, however, it also decreased the amplitude of the P300 component of an auditory evoked response recorded while subjects were attending to a demanding task (77).

The effects of cocaine and amphetamine in most non-human species parallel those seen in humans. At lower doses, animals are active and alert, showing increases in responding maintained by other reinforcers but often decreasing food intake. Higher doses produce species-specific stereotyped behavior patterns, and further increases in dose are followed, as in humans, by convulsions, hyperthermia, coma, and death (72).

EPIDEMIOLOGY

The amphetamines and cocaine do not have concurrent abuse histories, although they share many characteristics, and experienced stimulant users are unable to discriminate them when administered intravenously (48). In fact, it appears that, at least over the past 40 to 50 years, they have alternated in popularity. Reports of amphetamine abuse began to appear in the early 1940s, with the first widespread outbreak reported in Japan in the early 1950s (17). The amphetamine epidemic peaked in the United States in the middle 1960s, and it was estimated that in 1969 13.5% of college students had used amphetamines at least once (9). A survey of amphetamine use in 1976 (1) found that the largest group of users was the 18- to 25-year-old group, with a lifetime prevalence of use of almost 17%. There was evidence of a general decline in amphetamine use in the population by 1978 (97), which contrasts with data on cocaine use trends during that period.

Reports from a range of sources suggest that we are currently in the midst of an epidemic of cocaine use and abuse, exacerbated by extraordinary levels of cocaine availability. The evidence for this comes from estimates of prevalence of use (83), clinician reports of increases in those seeking treatment (50,53), emergency room reports of cases in which cocaine was involved (26), and use by high school students (99).

The number of people who report having used cocaine increased dramatically from 5.4 million in 1974 to 21.6 million in 1982 (3), and data from the National Survey on Drug Abuse (2) as well as a survey of the nation's high school seniors (76) indicate a low prevalence and comparative stability in cocaine use between 1972 and 1976 followed by dramatic increases in prevalence from 1976 to 1979 (from 13% to 27.5%), with a leveling off of prevalence between 1979 and 1982. However, the increase in current use is reflected in data from an ongoing survey of high school seniors, which obtained the highest rate ever of cocaine use (17%) for this population during 1985 (75).

The impressive reinforcing properties of cocaine are well known (e.g., ref. 71). If more than 22 million people have used it at least once, given the fact that this drug is such an efficacious reinforcer, it is likely that many will use it again. As was recently suggested (26), if only 10% are at risk, and half or even a quarter of those get into trouble, we can expect 550,000 people to be having serious cocaine abuse problems. The 450,000 telephone calls to a toll-free "cocaine hot-line" telephone number offering free advice and referral sources to cocaine abusers during the first 18 months of its existence lend credence to this estimate (53). The toxicity of this drug does not depend on a "dangerous" route of administration. Data collected from callers to the "cocaine hot-line" (53) found that 61% of those requesting help were primarily intranasal users, whereas 21% were free-basing, and 18% used intravenously. This reflects other reports that serious cocaine toxicity is common after all three routes of administration (e.g., refs. 49,127). The current concern about the severe public health problem posed by cocaine use in this country is justified in light of reports such as these. The temporal abuse patterns of cocaine and amphetamine appear quite similar. The predominant pattern of uncontrolled amphetamine use was the discreet "run," with few periods of mild daily use (84), and this development of periods of high-intensity prolonged use has also been reported for cocaine users seeking treatment (52).

The 1984 National Survey on Drug Abuse profiled the cocaine user as an occasional user, combining cocaine most frequently with marijuana, nicotine cigarettes, or alcohol. The demographic profile of cocaine use among young adults depicts a white college-educated male residing in a large metropolitan area, predominantly in the northeast or western portions of the United States. In addition, although the risk pattern for most drugs of abuse increases sharply through the teens, with rates declining rapidly at age 18 (78), cocaine appears to be the only illicit drug that shows continuing increases in the risk of initiation through age 24. The subgroup appearing most vulnerable to use appears to be the 18- to 25-year-old group (99), although clinical reports do not single out this group in reports of the drug's toxicity (53).

ABUSE LIABILITY AND DEPENDENCE POTENTIAL

Self-Administration

The laboratory self-administration model has provided abundant evidence that cocaine and amphetamine are potent reinforcers, readily self-administered by rats, cats, dogs, rhesus monkeys, baboons, and humans under a broad range of experimental conditions regardless of the nature of the behavior being maintained (12,44,57,113,121). In fact, much of the early research exploring the relationship among the organism, its environment, and the reinforcing properties of drugs was carried out using psychomotor stimulant drugs. As has been pointed out elsewhere (71), the reinforcing properties of a drug are the result of an interaction between the drug and the environmental circumstances under which it is administered. The abuse liability of a drug is in part related to the range of conditions (e.g., route, schedule of availability) under which it can maintain behavior leading to its delivery. The defining feature of dependence potential is a measure of

the toxic consequences of that drug at doses that are readily self-administered.

The intravenous route of administration has been the most frequently tested in the self-administration paradigm, and abundant examples of the reinforcing properties of psychomotor stimulant drugs exist (e.g., refs. 58, 73). Cocaine and amphetamine have also been shown to maintain responding when delivered intramuscularly (54), intragastrically (6), and, for amphetamine, orally (23) and directly into the nucleus accumbens (63).

The efficacy of these drugs as reinforcers has most clearly been demonstrated by the range of schedules of availability under which they can maintain behavior. These include ratio, interval, concurrent and discrete trial, as well as second-order schedules (71). These studies have shown that, as with other nondrug reinforcers, the characteristics of responding are largely determined by the characteristics of the schedule of delivery and not the drug. Related to their reinforcing properties, administration of some psychomotor stimulant drugs appears to potentiate the effects of conditioned reinforcers (114). If true, this enhancement of the reinforcing properties of other stimuli provides insight into our understanding of the behavioral mechanisms of action of these drugs.

Central Nervous System Effects of Stimulant Self-Administration

It is well known that psychomotor stimulant drugs enhance the effects of catecholamines in a number of ways, including blocking their reuptake, retarding their breakdown, and potentiating their release (30). Studies by Yokel and Wise (149) and de Wit and Wise (35) have implicated the role of dopamine in the mediation of the reinforcing properties of these drugs. Using pimozide as a dopaminergic blocker and manipulating dose and time of pretreatment, they showed that dopaminergic blockade antagonized the reinforcing properties of both amphetamine and cocaine and led to extinction of the self-administration behavior. In addition, other dopaminergic agonists are self-administered (113,142,145), but both α- and β-adrenergic agents are not, and both α- and β-adrenergic blocking agents do not have specific effects on cocaine or amphetamine self-administration (35,113). These data suggest that it is the dopaminergic activity shared by both cocaine and the amphetamines that is critical to their reinforcing properties. However, changes in responding caused by CNS lesions or antagonist administration could also be related to modification of the general effects of the drug rather than only its reinforcing property.

Drug Discrimination

A traditional approach to the classification of abused drugs has been the evaluation of their subjective effects in human volunteers (40). Obviously, since humans have unique verbal abilities, this approach has not been possible in the animal laboratory. However, the development of methods for establishing drugs as discriminative stimuli has made possible comparable procedures in nonhuman research subjects (120). When the psychomotor stimulant drugs have been studied, either amphetamine or cocaine has generally functioned as the training drug, and it has been shown that these drugs are capable of controlling differential responding in a variety of species including pigeons (31), rats (27), cats (79), gerbils (66), squirrel monkeys (147), rhesus monkeys (7), and humans (24). The discriminative stimulus properties of these two drugs are similar, supporting the report that experienced users do not accurately differentiate them (48), and, in general, amphetamine appears to be more potent than cocaine (28,65), although several studies (e.g., ref. 31) suggest that these two drugs may be equal in potency.

As with their reinforcing properties, it has been demonstrated that the discriminative stimulus properties of the psychomotor stimulant drugs are mediated by dopaminergic mechanisms. Dopaminergic blocking agents such as haloperidol, pimozide, and spiperone (28,29,64,98) antagonize the ability of these drugs to act as discriminative stimuli. Less clearly, the direct-acting dopaminergic agonists such as apomorphine, piribidel, bromocriptine, and amantadine (143) only partially substitute for amphetamine or cocaine. It is also possible that norepinephrine may play a role in the discriminative stimulus properties of amphetamine, since the norepinephrine blocker nisoxetine substitutes for amphetamine (143). As with their reinforcing properties, the discriminative stimulus properties of cocaine and amphetamine are not affected by α- and β-noradrenergic receptor blockers (64). Thus, the evidence suggests that dopamine is largely responsible for mediating the discriminative stimulus properties of cocaine and amphetamine. To the extent that the behaviors observed with this procedure reflect mechanisms similar to those measured by verbal report information collected in humans, the data provide interesting insights into the subjective effects of drugs in humans.

Toxicity

Abuse liability and dependence potential are defined by both the reinforcing properties of a drug and its toxicity at readily self-administered doses. There would be little public concern if the use of these drugs did not lead to toxic consequences.

Unlimited Access to Drug

Despite the importance of such studies, there are few that have evaluated the effects of unlimited access to psychomotor stimulants in the animal laboratory. Rhesus monkeys given unlimited access to amphetamine or cocaine self-administer substantial amounts of the drug and do so in a somewhat cyclic pattern, alternating days of high intake with days of low intake (34,72). The behavioral changes seen include restlessness, stereotypic movements, tremors, mydriasis, piloerection, and ataxia. Animals allowed access to 0.2 mg/kg/infusion cocaine died in less than 5 days, whereas all animals given access to 0.05 mg/kg/infusion d-amphetamine or 0.025 mg/kg/infusion d-

methamphetamine also died but tended to survive longer than animals exposed to cocaine (72). Food intake decreased during the initial days of stimulant self-administration but returned to near base-line levels within 7 days in those animals who survived. The behavioral changes seen are comparable to those reported for monkeys maintained on large doses of methamphetamine (42) and for rats given unlimited access to d- or l-amphetamine or d- or l-methamphetamine (148) or cocaine (16). The toxicity of these drugs is substantial, with animals self-administering highly debilitating amounts within a few days of their availability. In fact, in a comparison of the effects of unlimited access to 1 mg/kg/infusion cocaine or 100 μg/kg/infusion heroin in rats (16), it was found that the mortality rate over 30 days was 36% for heroin and 90% for those self-administering cocaine. As with laboratory animals, human cocaine users who appear for treatment report control over their initial stimulant use, but as use continues and availability increases, binges continue in a more and more uncontrolled fashion (51).

The extreme toxicity of cocaine is further evidenced by its potency as a reinforcer. It has been found that rhesus monkeys given a choice between 0.3mg/kg/infusion or five 1-g food pellets/delivery almost exclusively chose the drug reinforcer, a pattern of behavior that led to weight loss and marked behavioral toxicity (4). Rhesus monkeys will also self-administer cocaine when the choice is between drug and the opportunity to have social access to another monkey (W. L. Woolverton, *personal communication*). The loss of control and compulsion to take cocaine described for the human cocaine abuser has thus been clearly mirrored in the animal laboratory.

Behavioral Disruption

Another aspect of the toxicity of a drug is reflected in its ability to disrupt ongoing behavior and/or interfere with the acquisition of new behavior patterns. Although the effects of psychomotor stimulant drugs on schedule-controlled behavior are multiply determined, the principle of rate dependency accounts for many of the effects observed with this class of drugs, indicating that base-line rate of responding, systematically and inversely correlated with response rate after drug administration, is an important determinant of the effects of cocaine and the amphetamines (116,133). Thus, whether responding is maintained under ratio, interval, or multiple schedules or is not a schedule-controlled operant, in rats, pigeons, or monkeys, this principle has utility in the prediction of the disruptive effects of psychomotor stimulant drugs on behavior.

The nature of the reinforcing event can frequently play an important role in determining the effects of amphetamine and cocaine on schedule-controlled behavior. It has been suggested (14) that amphetamine often has differential effects on responding maintained under fixed-ratio schedules of food presentation and stimulus–shock termination, whereas behaviors maintained under fixed-interval schedules are largely independent of the event maintaining behavior. Other determinants of the effects of cocaine and amphetamine on schedule-controlled behavior include environmental events (93) and prior behavioral history of the organism (13). Few studies have been carried out investigating these manipulations, and further studies are needed to determine the contextual variables, relevant behavioral histories, and existing behaviors that influence the effects of psychomotor stimulant drugs.

Using a repeated acquisition of behavioral chains, Thompson and Moerschbaecher (132) have developed a procedure in which animals are required to learn a chain of four responses on three keys. Under conditions in which the sequence of four responses changes from session to session, the animals quickly develop a steady state of acquisition behavior against which the effects of specific drugs can be measured. Under these conditions, 2 mg/kg d-amphetamine in the dog, 1 mg/kg d-amphetamine and 10 mg/kg cocaine in the rat, increased within-session errors, interfering with acquisition of the response chain. This was true whether behavior was maintained by food delivery or an avoidance contingency. Increasing dose produced increases in error rate and decreases in response rates. The overall rate-increasing effects of these drugs were only seen when the avoidance contingency was in effect despite the fact that such rate increases resulted in an increase in frequency of shocks. This is a characteristic effect of these drugs on free operant avoidance (60).

Amphetamine also has disruptive effects on social behavior (13,29). Not only does this drug differentially affect the rate of occurrence of aggressive and affiliative behaviors in group-living rhesus monkeys, but it affects patterns of social relationships within the group. For example, in those animals given d-amphetamine, aggression toward nonadult monkeys increased, more towards kin-related than non-kin-related, whereas aggression directed at adult monkeys decreased. One of the determinants of the effect of amphetamine in squirrel monkeys is the social status of the animal; dominant animals totally reverse their characteristic patterns of interaction (95). Clearly, disruptions in social interactions can be important toxic manifestations of a drug's effect and deserve more laboratory attention.

REPEATED LONG-TERM USE

Tolerance and Sensitization

A major contribution of behavioral pharmacology has been the investigation of the behavioral actions of drugs given repeatedly, since this is the usual manner in which these drugs are taken or prescribed for therapeutic purposes. It has generally been found that prior dose experience is likely to modify the subsequent action of psychomotor stimulant drugs. Most commonly, prior experience with a drug tends to decrease responsivity to its effects, a process called tolerance. Under other conditions, multiple administrations of a psychomotor stimulant can result in an increased effect of a specific dose, a process referred to as sensitization.

Sensitization

Sensitization to the effects of psychomotor stimulants has been described for a number of dependent variables: activity, stereotypy, startle response, seizures, and brain stimulation (80). In general, increased sensitivity to the effects of psychomotor stimulant drugs occurs after intermittent repetitive administration (107), although Kilbey and Sannerud (80) have suggested that the injection regimen may not be the critical variable. In fact, when the effects of administering amphetamine once or three times daily to rats were investigated (88), regardless of the regimen, repeated amphetamine administration resulted in an enhancement of the stereotyped behavior and locomotor stimulant effects of the drug. However, Nelson and Ellison (96) showed that although rats receiving once-daily injections of amphetamine for 7 or 30 days showed greater levels of amphetamine-induced stereotypy than controls, those with subcutaneous pellet implants, and thus constant drug levels, did not show this augmented effect. The compulsive repetitive patterns characteristic of stereotyped behavior have been reported for humans as well as nonhumans (59). These perseverative behaviors generally occur during the first 8 hr after injection, while the positive mood-enhancing effects of the drug are present, and thus are associated with those aspects of the drug.

The sensitization to increases in locomotor activity elicited by one psychomotor stimulant drug generalizes to others in that class (106) and persists for long periods of time after administration is terminated.

Leith and Kuczenski (88) suggested that the process involved in the development of sensitization may reflect the increased susceptibility to psychoses elicited by psychomotor stimulant drugs with repeated use. Ellinwood and Kilbey (37) have reported that once an individual develops an amphetamine psychosis, it is easy to reinitiate that psychosis with a moderate dose of drug. This was illustrated by Bell (15), who precipitated a psychotic reaction in an abstinent amphetamine user after administering 120 mg i.v. amphetamine, and it was recently reported (117) that the psychotic episode precipitated by repeated methamphetamine intake is longer in duration and induced after considerably less drug subsequent to the initial episode.

A "kindling" model has been developed by Post (104), who compared the repetitive administration of psychomotor stimulant drugs to the increased widespread afterdischarges often leading to major seizures seen after daily electrical stimulation of the amygdala. It is not currently clear whether kindling and the sensitization produced by repeated doses of amphetamine and cocaine occur by similar mechanisms.

In an excellent review of the available literature, Demellweek and Goudie (33) concluded that the "causes and mechanisms of sensitization remain an enigma." The most reasonable suggestion to date of the mechanisms underlying sensitization is that increased sensitivity to a drug may be the primary pharmacological effect of repeated administration (121). This effect, however, can be modified when compensatory mechanisms are activated by, for example, reinforcement loss.

Tolerance

The most commonly reported change produced by prior experience with a drug is a decrease in responsiveness to its effects. Tolerance develops differentially to specific behavioral effects of drugs, and variables such as reinforcement loss and degree of stimulus control have been found to be important.

It has been hypothesized that the consequences of the drug-induced behavioral disruption are a major determinant of the development of tolerance to the psychomotor stimulant drugs (119). Thus, tolerance develops when drug administration results in a decrease in reinforcement density but does not when reinforcement density is increased or remains the same. Studies investigating the development of tolerance to the anorectic effects of amphetamine and cocaine have supported this hypothesis (121,146). Interestingly, and in contrast to rats receiving cocaine prior to their milk-drinking sessions, rats receiving cocaine after their milk-drinking session not only showed no tolerance but showed sensitization to the anorectic effects of cocaine (146). Both cross tolerance and cross sensitization between cocaine and amphetamine were seen. In addition, despite a suggestion that the attenuation of anorexia after repeated amphetamine administration was related to weight loss (89), Demellweek and Goudie (32) showed that tolerance developed in rats given supplemental feeding, which prevented weight loss during the amphetamine maintenance regimen. They also eliminated the possibility that the contingent tolerance effect is an artifact of the development of a conditioned taste aversion.

The contingent tolerance hypothesis has been well supported by studies investigating the development of tolerance to the effects of amphetamine and cocaine on schedule-controlled behavior (e.g., 33,119,130). There are, however, exceptions to this (e.g., ref. 134). These findings are compatible with a modified reinforcement density hypothesis in which the change in the total behavioral "economy" (or cost of responding) of the organism, rather than the reinforcement loss per se, is the stimulus for tolerance development (33). In that way, tolerant subjects minimize the energy expenditure required to obtain a reinforcer.

Other behavioral variables are relevant in the development of tolerance to the disruptive effects of amphetamine and cocaine. Behavior under strong exteroceptive stimulus control shows tolerance to repeated drug administration more rapidly than does behavior under weak stimulus control (33). Balster (11) presented data from rats working under a multiple fixed-consecutive-number schedule of food delivery. In one condition, responding was under strong stimulus control, and repeated administration of amphetamine produced decrements in performance, which rapidly dissipated. In contrast, behavior under weaker stimulus control showed the initial decrement, which was followed by little or no recovery with repeated amphetamine treatment.

Not all tolerance to the behavioral effects of psychomotor stimulant drugs is a behavioral adaptation. Rhesus monkeys working under a food-reinforced operant schedule developed tolerance to doses of methamphetamine well above those found to be lethal in the nontolerant monkey (42). Monkeys not in contact with the reinforcement contingencies during a similar drug regimen showed comparable tolerance to those that were (39). Animals on such drug regimens showed irreversible depletion of brain dopamine after methamphetamine cessation (123), and it is possible that neurochemical mechanisms contributed to this tolerance.

There is an acute tolerance development to the cardiovascular and subjective effects of cocaine in humans (46). This occurs when an intravenous dose of 16, 32, or 48 mg is administered 1 hr after a single intranasal dose of 96 mg. In addition, when constant cocaine blood levels are maintained in human volunteers for a period of 4.5 hr (124), tolerance to the subjective effects of the drug rapidly appear, but the effect on heart rate and blood pressure is more variable. This tolerance development to the effects of intravenous cocaine is also seen when volunteer research subjects are allowed to self-administer the drug repeatedly within a 1-hr session (44). Under these conditions, despite continuously rising cocaine blood levels above 1,200 ng/ml, heart rate, blood pressure, and most of the verbal report measures of the effects of cocaine return toward base-line levels. Thus, although there is clearly no tolerance development to the reinforcing properties of cocaine, its positive mood-enhancing properties appear to decrease with repeated dosing. This has also been reported for the amphetamines (59) and for users binging on cocaine, who describe a pattern of steadily increasing doses during a binge despite an inability to attain the level of positive subjective effects achieved earlier in that drug-taking occasion (52).

With few exceptions (92) there does not seem to be any tolerance development to effects of the psychomotor stimulants as positive reinforcers (118). In contrast, the development of tolerance to the positive mood or "euphorigenic" effects of cocaine and amphetamine (44,46,124) brings into question the hypothesis that the ability of a drug to produce "euphoria" is an index of its reinforcing effectiveness and abuse potential (e.g., ref. 94). Further, tolerance may, in fact, occur to some of the aversive properties of drugs (e.g., the nausea-producing effects of i.v. cocaine), thus making it possible for the reinforcing effects to be unmasked (21). The interaction of tolerance development with psychomotor stimulant use is a complex issue and requires further investigation before treatment interventions can be designed based on these data.

Toxic Effects

There is both clinical and experimental evidence suggesting that irreversible morphological and behavioral toxicity may result from repeated high-dose use of cocaine and the amphetamines (25,38,82,115,126). An initial report that a necrotizing angiitis was frequently found in methamphetamine users (25) was followed by a laboratory study in which 1.5 mg/kg methamphetamine was intravenously administered to rhesus monkeys every other day for 2 weeks (115). Extensive neurological effects including petechial hemmorhages and cerebral edema resulted. A subsequent study (125) did not replicate these results, however, nor were morphological changes found in rhesus monkeys maintained on high doses of methamphetamine for 3 to 6 months (123). The brains of monkeys in this latter study, however, showed an apparently irreversible reduction of up to 70% in caudate dopamine levels. Evidence of morphological toxicity after long-term psychomotor stimulant use therefore still remains questionable.

Although a cocaine toxic psychosis has not been experimentally induced, administration of amphetamine to normal volunteers with no histories of psychosis (56) resulted in a clear-cut paranoid psychosis in five of the six subjects who received *d*-amphetamine for 1 to 5 days (120–700 mg). These symptoms, as well as malnutrition, anorexia, and complications dependent on route of administration, have also been reported for uncontrolled cocaine users (128). Route-related toxic effects are common in the uncontrolled cocaine user. Cocaine free-base smoking has been linked to impaired pulmonary gas exchange (140). Inhalation of cocaine hydrochloride leads to chronic rhinitis or sinusitus and, rarely, to necrosis and perforation of the nasal septum (137). Intravenous users suffer the complications of other i.v. drug users such as hepatitis, septicemia, endocarditis, and acquired immunodeficiency disorder. Clinical descriptions of the toxic consequences of repeated cocaine use report the existence of a withdrawal syndrome including depression, craving, tremor, muscle pain, EEG changes, and sleep and eating disturbances (52,77). Although a syndrome has not been documented in the laboratory, the possible existence of this pattern of abstinence effects is of great importance in consideration of treatment issues.

The amphetamine psychosis caused by increasing doses of *d*-amphetamine represents a reasonably accurate model of schizophrenia (10), including symptoms of persecution, hyperactivity and excitation, visual and auditory hallucinations, and changes in body image. These symptoms have been reported in uncontrolled users requiring treatment for cocaine abuse (52) and disappear when the drug is discontinued. It has further been suggested that there is sensitization to the development of a stimulant psychosis: once an individual has experienced this toxic effect, it is readily reinitiated, even following long drug-free periods (36,84).

HUMAN BEHAVIORAL PHARMACOLOGY

Self-Administration

Cocaine is self-administered via a number of different routes including oral, intranasal, intravenous, and by smoking. Coca leaves have been harvested and chewed for more than 3,000 years by the Indians living in the Andes Mountains in South America (22). When chewed with the addition of an alkaline substance, dose-related blood levels of up to 95 ng/ml peaked shortly after cessation of chewing (100). Despite elevated plasma levels, little "high" was reported in these chewers (19). The absorption of the drug probably occurred through the mucous membrane of the mouth as well as through the lower gastrointestinal tract, since saliva containing the coca juice was swallowed as chewing continued. This absorption from the gastrointestinal tract was documented by Van Dyke et al. (136), who administered cocaine-filled gelatin capsules to volunteers and found that plasma concentrations peaked at approximately 65 min after ingestion and dissipated about as rapidly as after intravenous administration (141).

The most common nonmedical route of cocaine self-administration is "snorting" or inhaling the drug as a white powder. The user experiences 20 to 40 min of stimulation with no initial "rush." Peak plasma levels after intranasal crystalline cocaine occur at 30 to 40 minutes subsequent to inhalation (67,141), with 96 mg resulting in peak levels of 150 to 200 ng/ml. Cocaine via this route has a half-life of about 40 min (68).

The intravenous route of administration is popular with "serious" and perhaps more experienced drug users, since the drug goes rapidly to the brain, and subjective effects, including an intense "rush," are reported within 1 or 2 min (67,111). Estimates of dose made by laboratory subjects suggest that the average dose of cocaine injected intravenously by users in a recreational setting is approximately 16 mg/injection, comparable to 10 mg *d*-amphetamine (48). Cocaine plasma levels are correlated with dose of intravenous cocaine (14,68), and plasma levels of approximately 300 ng/ml have been recorded after single 32-mg doses (67). The elimination half-life of cocaine by this route may be dose-related at very high doses but has generally been estimated to be approximately 40 min (68).

The smoking of coca paste has been reported to be widespread in Peru, Ecuador, Colombia, and Bolivia (69), and plasma levels as high as 975 ng/ml have been reported after smoking 0.5 g of paste (101). A more efficient method of smoking cocaine has emerged in recent years. Cocaine "free base," volatile at temperatures above 90°, provides an active drug for smoking (41,126). Although no pharmacokinetic or blood level studies have been published, chronic cocaine free base smokers have shown plasma levels of 800 to 900 ng/ml 3 hr after smoking (126).

Cocaine is readily self-administered in the laboratory by volunteer subjects with histories of cocaine use (44). Subjects given a choice between injections of intravenous cocaine or saline approximately once every 6 min for 1 hr consistently chose cocaine (16 or 32 mg). As with laboratory animals, drug injections were fairly regularly spaced, with plasma levels of approximately 1,200 ng/ml after 224 mg cocaine. Subjects indicated that they felt high, stimulated, "weird," and anorexic for 2 to 3 hr after these sessions; several subjects indicated that they had difficulty sleeping 8 to 14 hr later. A similarly designed choice procedure was carried out in which volunteers were allowed to choose between a 5-mg capsule of *d*-amphetamine and placebo (74). Drug was reliably chosen over placebo, and reports of significant changes in mood were most evident 3 hr after drug ingestion. Both of these drugs, therefore, have been shown to serve as positive reinforcers in humans and can maintain drug-taking behavior under limited access conditions over a period of several weeks.

Subjective Effects

Experienced drug users, given a variety of stimulant drugs, often cannot differentiate among cocaine, amphetamine, methamphetamine, and methylphenidate (48,91), all of which appear to have similar profiles of action. Cocaine and amphetamine produce changes on a number of scales of the Profile of Mood States, including vigor, elation, friendliness, arousal, and positive mood (45,47,74,131). The similarities are impressive, given the fact that neither route of administration nor dose was controlled.

Scores on the Addiction Research Center Inventory reflect the fact that both amphetamine and cocaine are psychomotor stimulant drugs. Administration of either of these drugs intravenously causes increases in scores on the amphetamine, benzedrine general, morphine–benzedrine-general, and LSD scales and decreases on the pentobarbital-chlorpromazine–alcohol general scale (48,91). When cocaine is smoked as the base, 37 mg of smoked base and 20 mg of i.v. cocaine have approximately comparable effects (103). Similar reports of cocaine's effects were obtained after intranasal administration, but the effect was less intense, slower in onset, and without an initial "rush" (111). Doses as high as 96 mg had no effect on scores on the Profile of Mood States. Cocaine given as a capsule containing 2 mg/kg produced an increase in ratings of "high," which peaked at 75 min after ingestion (136).

Cocaine, when compared with the synthetic local anesthetics, appears to share at least some stimulus properties with procaine. Like cocaine, procaine maintains responding in laboratory animals leading to its delivery (74), and these drugs seem to share discriminative stimulus properties in both nonhuman (144) and human (47) research subjects. This does not seem generally to be the case for lidocaine (45,144).

A biphasic response to the effects of cocaine has been reported (111), beginning with stimulant effects and followed 30 to 60 min after drug by a "crashing" effect "characterized by feelings of anxiety, depression, fatigue, and wanting more cocaine." Although described by "street" users, this effect has generally not been documented in laboratory studies. Gunne (59) reported that the combination of an initial stage of euphoria after amphetamine administration followed by dysphoria and depression is difficult to demonstrate after low doses but is easily recognized when large parenteral doses have been employed. For example, a 200-mg intravenous dose of dl-amphetamine given to experienced amphetamine users was followed by a 10- to 12-hr euphoric response and then a period of dysphoria that persisted for 48 hr. The inability to document a "crash" in the laboratory after cocaine may simply be related to dose or level of tolerance.

The self-reported euphoric effect of 200 mg amphetamine was reduced by 50% by administration of 2 g α-methyl-p-tyrosine (AMPT) and virtually eliminated by 4 g of that drug (59). Daily administration of 4 g AMPT rendered volunteers insensitive to the subjective effects of amphetamine, and enhancement of the amphetamine effects followed withdrawal of that compound. Other blockers of the subjective effects of amphetamine, such as chlorpromazine and pimozide, were less effective. Clinical reports of treatment for cocaine abuse with methylphenidate and pimozide are based on the hypothesis that these drugs will serve as substitute maintenance drugs, much as methadone does for opiate users. In an open trial of these drugs (51), methylphenidate, in fact, appeared to serve as a stimulus cue for cocaine taking. Lithium, which was not found to block the positive subjective effects of either amphetamine or cocaine (8,111), also did not appear to be generally useful in treating cocaine abusers (49).

Learning and Performance

A procedure adapted from Thompson and Moersch-baecher (132) to measure repeatedly acquisition of behavior in individual research subjects was used to compare the effects of cocaine and amphetamine. It was found that at sufficient doses (32 mg i.v.), cocaine, but not amphetamine, interferes with the acquisition of new behavior patterns, increasing error rate without affecting response rate (41). This differential effect may reflect the fact that only one amphetamine dose was tested, although dose–response functions were obtained for both intravenous and intranasal cocaine.

Cocaine users frequently report that the drug enhances performance, but with few exceptions this effect has never been investigated experimentally. Neither 10 nor 25 mg intravenous or intranasal cocaine has an effect on hand-grip strength (113), nor does inhalation of 96 mg cocaine affect performance of a reaction time task in rested subjects (43). However, when subjects were deprived of sleep for 24 to 48 hr, which resulted in a fatigue-induced decrement in performance, inhalation of 96 mg cocaine reversed (after 24 hr) or partially reversed (after 48 hr) the decrement. Although no other research has been carried out investigating the effects of cocaine on performance in humans, substantial data do exist indicating that, in general, the amphetamines have minimal effects on performance in the non-sleep-deprived subject (86,138,139) but are generally successful in returning to its predeprivation level performance that has deteriorated as a result of fatigue. Laties and Weiss (86) have argued persuasively that the small changes in performance induced by amphetamines can result in the 1 to 2% improvement that can make the difference in a close athletic competition. Although the facilitation in performance after amphetamine does not appear to be substantial, it is sufficient to "spell the difference between a gold medal and a sixth place." Animal laboratory data reporting dose-dependent decreases in reaction times after methamphetamine (62) lend support to this hypothesis of the facilitatory effects of amphetamine. Such data are not available for cocaine; anecdotal evidence suggests that it does not have similar properties (86), and its short duration of action argues against the usefulness of such an effect. The recent flirtation of athletes with this drug, however, suggests that it has not gone untested.

SUMMARY

Animal laboratory research has clearly provided us with the data to predict the uncontrolled psychomotor stimulant use and concomitant toxicity that have appeared in cycles for both amphetamine and cocaine. The amphetamine epidemic of the 1950s and 1960s gave way to the cocaine epidemic of the 1970s and 1980s, although reports from Japan suggest a recurrence of the amphetamine problem. A difference in these two drugs, which in low doses do not necessarily make the user dysfunctional, may be that although initial low-dose use of the amphetamines was daily, it was generally by prescription and therefore at least partially controlled. Even low-dose cocaine use depends on illicit suppliers and therefore has the potential for unlimited availability. The unlimited-access variable obviously carries with it severe potential for toxicity and may therefore make it more difficult to initiate effective prevention programs for cocaine abuse. Current programs, as indicated by epidemiologic data, have not had sufficient impact, and treatment interventions (discussed by J. Jaffe, *this volume*) are still in the early stages of development.

The seductiveness of the psychomotor stimulant drugs lies, at least in part, in their ability to elevate mood and give the user a sense of behavioral enhancement. The general facilitation of energy, alertness, and perhaps of the reinforcing properties of other stimuli, the increases in low rates of responding seen in schedule-controlled responding, the slight "edge" in performance seen in professional athletes, and the restoration of performance that has deteriorated as a result of boredom or fatigue, all provide important data for understanding why humans use cocaine. Such behavioral facilitation, although perhaps dose or situation specific and certainly transitory, is clearly powerful in maintaining subsequent psychomotor stimulant use.

ACKNOWLEDGMENT

Preparation of this manuscript was supported by PHS Grants DA-03818, DA-03476, and DA-02588.

REFERENCES

1. Abelson, H., and Fishburne, P. (1976): *National Survey—Main Findings 1976: Nonmedical Use of Psychoactive Substances.* National Technical Information Service, Springfield, VA.
2. Abelson, H. I., and Miller, J. D. (1985): In: *Cocaine Use in America: Epidemiologic and Clinical Perspectives,* edited by N. J. Kozel and E. H. Adams, pp. 35–49. NIDA Research Monograph 61, U.S. Government Printing Office, Washington.
3. Adams, E. H., and Durrell, J. (1984): In: *Cocaine: Pharmacology, Effects and Treatment of Abuse,* edited by J. Grabowski, pp. 9–14. NIDA Research Monograph 50, U.S. Government Printing Office, Washington.
4. Aigner, T. G., and Balster, R. L. (1978): *Science,* 201:534–535.
5. Alles, G. (1933): *J. Pharmacol. Exp. Ther.,* 47:339–354.
6. Altshuler, H., Weaver, S., and Phillips, P. (1975): *Life Sci.,* 17: 883–890.
7. Ando, K., and Yanagita, T. (1978): In: *Stimulus Properties of Drugs: Ten Years of Progress,* edited by F. C. Colpaert and J. A. Rosecrans, pp. 125–136. Elsevier/North-Holland Biomedical Press, Amsterdam.
8. Angrist, B., and Gershon, S. (1979): *Am. J. Psychiatry,* 136:806–810.
9. Angrist, B., and Sudilovsky, A. (1978): In: *Handbook of Psychopharmacology, Vol. 11,* edited by L. I. Iverson, S. D. Iverson, and S. H. Snyder, pp. 99–165. Plenum Press, New York.
10. Angrist, B., and Van Kammen, D. P. (1984): *Trends Neurosci.,* 7:388–390.
11. Balster, R. L. (1985): In: *Behavioral Pharmacology: The Current Status,* edited by L. S. Seiden and R. L. Balster, pp. 403–418. Alan R. Liss, New York.
12. Balster, R. L., Kilbey, M. M., and Ellinwood, E. H. (1976): *Psychopharmacology,* 46:229–233.
13. Barrett, J. E. (1977): *Science,* 198:67–69.
14. Barrett, J. E., and Katz, J. L. (1981): In: *Advances in Behavioral Pharmacology,* edited by T. Thompson, P. B. Dews, and W. A. McKim, pp. 119–168. Academic Press, New York.
15. Bell, D. S. (1973): *Arch. Gen. Psychiatry,* 29:35–40.
16. Bozarth, M. A., and Wise, R. A. (1985): *J.A.M.A.,* 254:81–83.
17. Brill, H., and Hirose, T. (1969): *Semin. Psychiatry,* 1:179–194.
18. Byck, R. (1974): *Cocaine Papers.* Stonehill, New York.
19. Byck, R., Van Dyke, C., Jatlow, P., and Barash, P. (1980): In: *Cocaine, 1980,* edited by F. R. Jeri, pp. 250–256. Pacific Press, Lima.
20. Caldwell, J. (1980): In: *Amphetamines and Related Stimulants: Chemical, Biological, Clinical, and Sociological Aspects,* edited by J. Caldwell, pp. 1–12. CRC Press, Boca Raton, FL.
21. Cappell, H., and LeBlanc, A. E. (1981): In: *Research Advances in Alcohol and Drug Dependence,* edited by Y. Israel, F. B. Gaser, H. Kalant, R. E. Popham, W. Schmidt, et al., pp. 159–196. Plenum Press, New York.
22. Carroll, E. (1977): In: *Cocaine: 1977,* edited by R. Petersen, and R. Stillman, pp. 35–46. NIDA Research Monograph 13, U.S. Supt. of Documents, Washington.
23. Carroll, M. E., and Stotz, D. C. (1983): *J. Pharmacol. Exp. Ther.,* 227:28–34.
24. Chait, L. D., Uhlenhuth, E. H., and Johanson, C. E. (1985): *Psychopharmacology,* 86:307–312.
25. Citron, B. P., Halpern, M., McCarron, M., Lundberg, G. D., McCormick, R., et al. (1970): *N. Engl. J. Med.,* 283:1003–1011.
26. Clayton, R. R. (1985): In: *Cocaine Use in America: Epidemiologic and Clinical Perspectives,* edited by N. J. Kozel and E. H. Adams, pp. 8–34. NIDA Research Monograph 61, U.S. Government Printing Office, Washington.
27. Colpaert, F. C., Niemeegers, C. J. E., and Janssen, P. A. J. (1976): *Psychopharmacologia,* 46:169–177.
28. Colpaert, F. C., Niemeegers, C. J. E., and Janssen, P. A. J. (1978): *Neuropharmacology,* 17:937–942.
29. Colpaert, F. C., Niemeegers, C. J. E., and Janssen, P. A. J. (1979): *Pharmacol. Biochem. Behav.,* 10:535–546.
30. Costa, E., and Garattini, S., eds. (1970): *Amphetamines and Related Compounds.* Raven Press, New York.
31. de la Garza, R., and Johanson, C. E. (1985): *Psychopharmacology,* 85:23–30.
32. Demellweek, C., and Goudie, A. J. (1983a): *Psychopharmacology,* 79:58–66.
33. Demellweek, C., and Goudie, A. J. (1983b): *Psychopharmacology,* 80:287–307.
34. Deneau, G., Yanagita, T., and Seevers, M. H. (1969): *Psychopharmacologia,* 16:30–48.
35. de Wit, H., and Wise, R. A. (1977): *Can. J. Psychol.,* 31:195–203.
36. Ellinwood, E. H. (1979): In: *Handbook on Drug Abuse,* edited by R. L. Dupont, A. Goldstein, and J. O'Donnell, pp. 221–231. U.S. Government Printing Office, Washington.
37. Ellinwood, E., and Kilbey, M. M. (1977): In: *Predicting Dependence Liability of Stimulant and Depressant Drugs,* edited by T. Thompson and K. Unna, pp. 81–123. University Park Press, Baltimore.
38. Escalante, O. D., and Ellinwood, E. H. (1972): In: *Current Concepts on Amphetamine Abuse,* edited by P. G. Bourne, pp. 97–106. Department of Health, Education, and Welfare Publication No. 72-9085, U.S. Government Printing Office, Washington.
39. Finnegan, K. T., Recaurte, G., Seiden, L. S., and Schuster, C. R. (1982): *Psychopharmacology,* 77:43–52.
40. Fischman, M. W. (1977): In: *Predicting Dependence Liability of Stimulant and Depressant Drugs,* edited by T. Thompson and K. Unna, pp. 261–284. University Park Press, Baltimore.
41. Fischman, M. W. (1984): In: *Cocaine: Pharmacology, Effects and Treatment of Abuse,* edited by J. Grabowski, pp. 72–91. NIDA Research Monograph 50, U.S. Government Printing Office, Washington.
42. Fischman, M. W., and Schuster, C. R. (1977): *J. Pharmacol. Exp. Ther.,* 201:593–605.
43. Fischman, M. W., and Schuster, C. R. (1980): *Psychopharmacology,* 72:1–8.
44. Fischman, M. W., and Schuster, C. R. (1982): *Fed. Proc.,* 41: 241–246.
45. Fischman, M. W., Schuster, C. R., and Hatano, Y. (1983): *Pharmacol. Biochem. Behav.,* 18:123–127.
46. Fischman, M. W., Schuster, C. R., Javaid, J. I., Hatano, Y., and Davis, J. (1986): *J. Pharmacol. Exp. Ther.,* 235: 677–682.
47. Fischman, M. W., Schuster, C. R., and Rajfer, S. (1983): *Pharmacol. Biochem. Behav.,* 18:711–716.
48. Fischman, M. W., Schuster, C. R., Resnekov, L., Shick, J. F. E., Krasnegor, N. A., et al. (1976): *Arch. Gen. Psychiatry,* 33:983–989.
49. Gawin, F. H., and Kleber, H. D. (1984): *Arch. Gen. Psychiatry,* 41:903–909.
50. Gawin, F. H., and Kleber, H. D. (1985): In: *Cocaine Use in America: Epidemiologic and Clinical Perspectives,* edited by N. J. Kozel, and E. H. Adams, pp. 182–192. NIDA Research Monograph 61, U.S. Government Printing Office, Washington.

51. Gawin, F. H., Riordan, C., and Kleber, H. D. (1985): *Am. J. Drug Alcohol Abuse*, 11:193–197.
52. Gawin, F. H., and Kleber, H. D. (1986): *Arch. Gen. Psychiatry*, 43:107–113.
53. Gold, M. S., Washton, A. M., and Dackis, C. A. (1985): In: *Cocaine Use in America: Epidemiologic and Clinical Perspectives*, edited by N. J. Kozel, and E. H. Adams, pp. 130–150. NIDA Research Monograph 61, U.S. Government Printing Office, Washington.
54. Goldberg, S. R., Morse, W. H., and Goldberg, D. M. (1976): *J. Pharmacol. Exp. Ther.*, 199:278–286.
55. Grabowski, J., ed. (1984): *Cocaine: Pharmacology, Effects, and Treatment of Abuse*. NIDA Research Monograph 50, U.S. Government Printing Office, Washington.
56. Griffith, J. D., Cavanaugh, J. H., Held, J., and Oates, J. A. (1970): In: *Amphetamines and Related Compounds*, edited by E. Costa and S. Garattini, pp. 897–904. Raven Press, New York.
57. Griffiths, R. R., Bigelow, G. E., and Henningfield, J. E. (1980): In: *Advances in Substance Abuse: Behavioral and Biological Research*, edited by N. K. Mello, pp. 1–90. Jai Press, Greenwich, CT.
58. Griffiths, R. R., Winger, G., Brady, J. V., and Snell, J. D. (1976): *Psychopharmacology*, 50:251–258.
59. Gunne, I. M. (1977): In: *Drug Addiction II: Amphetamine, Psychotogen, and Marihuana Dependence*, edited by W. R. Martin, pp. 247–275. Springer-Verlag, Berlin.
60. Heise, G. A., and Boff, E. (1962): *Psychopharmacologia*, 3:264–282.
61. Herning, R. I., Jones, R. T., Hooker, W. D., Mendelson, J., and Blackwell, L. (1985): *Electroencephalogr. Clin. Neurophysiol.*, 60:470–477.
62. Hienz, R. D., Lukas, S. E., and Brady, J. V. (1985): *Psychopharmacology*, 85:476–482.
63. Hoebel, B. G., Monaco, A. P., Hernandez, E. F., Aulisi, B. G., and Stanley, L. L. (1983): *Psychopharmacology*, 81:158–163.
64. Jarbe, T. U. C. (1978): *Psychopharmacology*, 59:183–187.
65. Jarbe, T. U. C. (1982): *Pharmacol. Biochem. Behav.*, 17:671–675.
66. Jarbe, T. U. C., and Kroon, E. R. (1980): *Gen. Pharmacol.*, 11:153–156.
67. Javaid, J. I., Dekirmenjian, H., Davis, J. M., and Schuster, C. R. (1978): *J. Chromatogr.*, 152:105–113.
68. Javaid, J. I., Musa, M. N., Fischman, M. W., Schuster, C. R., and Davis, J. M. (1983): *Biopharmacol. Drug Dispos.*, 4:9–18.
69. Jeri, F. R., Sanchez, C. C., del Pozo, T., Fernandez, M., and Carbajal, C. (1980): In: *Cocaine 1980*, edited by F. R. Jeri, pp. 76–85. Pacific Press, Lima.
70. Johanson, C. E. (1980): *Psychopharmacology*, 67:189–194.
71. Johanson, C. E. (1984): In: *Cocaine: Pharmacology, Effects & Treatment of Abuse*, edited by J. Grabowski, pp. 54–71. NIDA Research Monograph 50, U.S. Government Printing Office, Washington.
72. Johanson, C. E., Balster, R. L., and Bonese, K. (1976): *Pharmacol. Biochem. Behav.*, 4:45–51.
73. Johanson, C. E., and Schuster, C. R. (1975): *J. Pharmacol. Exp. Ther.*, 193:676–688.
74. Johanson, C. E., and Uhlenhuth, E. H. (1980): *Psychopharmacology*, 71:275–279.
75. Johnston, L. D. (1985): *Drugs Drug Abuse Educ. Newslett.*, 16:91–98.
76. Johnston, L. D., O'Malley, P. M., and Bachman, J. G. (1984): *Highlights from Drugs and American High School Students: 1975–1983*. NIDA, U.S. Government Printing Office, Washington.
77. Jones, R. T. (1984): In: *Cocaine: Pharmacology, Effects & Treatment of Abuse*, edited by J. Grabowski, pp. 34–53. NIDA Research Monograph 50, U.S. Government Printing Office, Washington.
78. Kandel, D. B., Murphy, D., and Karus, D. (1985): In: *Cocaine Use in America: Epidemiologic & Clinical Perspectives*, edited by N. J. Kozel, and E. H. Adams, pp. 76–110. NIDA Research Monograph 61, U.S. Government Printing Office, Washington.
79. Kilbey, M. M., and Ellinwood, E. H. (1979): *Psychopharmacology*, 63:151–153.
80. Kilbey, M. M., and Sannerud, C. A. (1985): In: *Behavioral Pharmacology: The Current Status*, edited by L. S. Seiden and R. L. Balster, pp. 295–322. Alan R. Liss, New York.
81. Klein, D. F., and Davis, J. M. (1969): *Diagnosis and Drug Treatment of Psychiatric Disorders*. Williams & Wilkins, Baltimore.
82. Kloss, M. W., Rosen, G. M., and Rauckman, E. J. (1984): *Biochem. Pharmacol.*, 33:169–173.
83. Kozel, N. J., and Adams, E. H., eds. (1985): *Cocaine Use in America: Epidemiologic and Clinical Perspectives*, NIDA Research Monograph 61, U.S. Government Printing Office, Washington.
84. Kramer, J. C., Fischman, V. S., and Littlefield, D. C. (1967): *J.A.M.A.*, 201:89–93(305–309).
85. Lasagna, L. (1980): In: *Obesity*, edited by A. Stunkard, pp. 292–299. W. B. Saunders, Philadelphia.
86. Laties, V. G., and Weiss, B. (1981): *Fed. Proc.*, 40:2689–2692.
87. Leake, C. D. (1958): *The Amphetamines, Their Actions and Uses*. Charles C. Thomas, Springfield, IL.
88. Leith, N. J., and Kuczenski, R. (1981): *Pharmacol. Biochem. Behav.*, 15:399–404.
89. Levitsky, D. A., Strupp, B., and Lupoli, J. (1981): *Pharmacol. Biochem. Behav.*, 14:661–667.
90. Lewander, T. (1977): In: *Drug Addiction II: Amphetamine, Psychotogen, and Marihuana Dependence*, edited by W. R. Martin, pp. 247–275. Springer-Verlag, Berlin.
91. Martin, W. R., Sloan, J. W., Sapira, J. D., and Jasinski, D. R. (1971): *Clin. Pharmacol. Ther.*, 12:245–258.
92. McCown, T. J., and Barrett, R. J. (1980): *Pharmacol. Biochem. Behav.*, 12:137–141.
93. McKearney, J. W., and Barrett, J. E. (1975): *Psychopharmacology*, 41:23–26.
94. Mello, N. K. (1977): In: *Predicting Dependence Liability of Stimulant and Depressant Drugs*, edited by T. Thompson and K. R. Unna, pp. 243–260. University Park Press, Baltimore.
95. Miczek, K. A., and Gold, L. H. (1983): *Psychopharmacology*, 81:183–190.
96. Nelson, L. R., and Ellison, G. (1978): *Neuropharmacology*, 17:1081–1084.
97. Newmeyer, J. A. (1978): In: *Amphetamine Use, Misuse & Abuse*, edited by D. E. Smith, D. R. Wesson, M. E. Buxton, R. B. Seymour, J. T. Ungerleider, et al. pp. 55–72. J. K. Hall, Boston.
98. Nielson, E. B., and Jepsen, S. A. (1985): *Eur. J. Pharmacol.*, 111:167–176.
99. O'Malley, P. M., Johnston, L. D., and Bachman, J. G. (1985): In: *Cocaine Use in America: Epidemiologic and Clinical Perspectives*, edited by N. J. Kozel, and E. H. Adams, pp. 50–75. NIDA Research Monograph 61, U.S. Government Printing Office, Washington.
100. Paly, D., Jatlow, P., Van Dyke, C., Cabieses, F., and Byck, R. (1980): In: *Cocaine 1980*, edited by F. R. Jeri, pp. 86–89. Pacific Press, Lima.
101. Paly, D., Van Dyke, C., Jatlow, P., Jeri, F. R., and Byck, R. (1980): In: *Cocaine 1980*, edited by F. R. Jeri, pp. 106–110. Pacific Press, Lima.
102. Parkes, J. D., Tarsy, D., Marsden, C. D., Bovill, K. T., Phipps, J. A., et al. (1975): *J. Neurol. Neurosurg. Psychiatry*, 38:232–237.
103. Perez-Reyes, M., Di Guiseppi, S., Ondrusek, G., Jeffcoat, A. R., and Cook, C. E. (1982): *Clin. Pharmacol. Ther.*, 32:459–465.
104. Post, R. M. (1977): In: *Cocaine and Other Stimulants*, edited by E. H. Ellinwood and M. M. Kilbey, pp. 353–372. Plenum Press, New York.
105. Post, R. M. (1980): *Life Sci.*, 26:1275–1282.
106. Post, R. M. (1981): In: *Research Advances in Alcohol and Drug Problems*, edited by Y. Israel, F. B. Glaser, H. Kalant, R. E. Popham, W. Schmidt, et al. pp. 1–65. Plenum Press, New York.
107. Post, R. M., and Contel, N. R. (1983): In: *Stimulants: Neurochemical, Behavioral, and Clinical Perspectives*, edited by I. Creese, pp. 169–203. Raven Press, New York.
108. Post, R. M., Gillin, J. C., Wyatt, R. J., and Goodwin, F. K. (1974): *Psychopharmacologia*, 37:59–66.
109. Post, R. M., Kotin, J., and Goodwin, F. K. (1974): *Am. J. Psychiatry*, 131:511–517.
110. Rechtschaffen, A., and Maron, L. (1964): *Electroencephalogr. Clin. Neurophysiol.*, 16:438–445.
111. Resnick, R. B., Kestenbaum, R. S., and Schwartz, L. K. (1977): *Science*, 195:696–699.

112. Resnick, R. B., Kestenbaum, R. S., and Schwartz, L. K. (1980): In: *Cocaine 1980*, edited by F. R. Jeri, pp. 17–20. Pacific Press, Lima.
113. Risner, M. C., and Jones, B. E. (1976): *Biol. Psychiatry*, 11:625–634.
114. Robbins, T. W., Watson, B. A., Gaskin, M., and Ennis, C. (1983): *Psychopharmacology*, 80:113–119.
115. Rumbaugh, C. L., Bergeron, R. T., Scanlan, R. L., Teal, J. S., Segall, H. D., et al. (1971): *Radiology*, 101:345–351.
116. Sanger, D. J., and Blackman, D. E. (1976): *Pharmacol. Biochem. Behav.*, 4:73–83.
117. Sato, M. (1985): Paper presented at the Annual Meeting of the American College of Neuropsychopharmacology.
118. Schuster, C. R. (1978): In: *Behavioral Tolerance: Research and Treatment Implications*, edited by N. Krasnegor, pp. 4–17. NIDA Research Monograph 18, U.S. Government Printing Office, Washington.
119. Schuster, C. R., Dockens, W., and Woods, J. (1966): *Psychopharmacologia*, 9:170–182.
120. Schuster, C. R., Fischman, M. W., and Johanson, C. E. (1981): In: *Behavioral Pharmacology of Human Drug Dependence*, edited by C. E. Johanson, and T. Thompson, pp. 116–129. NIDA Research Monograph 37, U.S. Government Printing Office, Washington.
121. Schuster, C. R., and Johanson, C. E. (1981): In: *Anorectic Agents: Mechanisms of Action and Tolerance*, edited by S. Garratini and R. Samanin, pp. 63–77. Raven Press, New York.
122. Seiden, L. S., and Balster, R. L., eds. (1985): *Behavioral Pharmacology: The Current Status*. Alan R. Liss, New York.
123. Seiden, L. S., Fischman, M. W., and Schuster, C. R. (1975): *Drug Alcohol Depend.*, 1:215–219.
124. Sherer, M., Kumar, K., Thompson, L., Cone, E., and Jaffe, J. (1985): Paper presented at the Annual Meeting of the American College of Neuropsychopharmacology.
125. Shybut, G. T., Richter, W. R., and Schuster, C. R. (1976): *Res. Commun. Chem. Pathol. Pharmacol.*, 15:53–73.
126. Siegel, R. K. (1982): *J. Psychoact. Drugs*, 14:271–359.
127. Siegel, R. K. (1984): In: *Cocaine: Pharmacology, Effects and Treatment of Abuse*, edited by J. Grabowski, pp. 92–110. NIDA Research Monograph 50, U.S. Government Printing Office, Washington.
128. Siegel, R. K. (1985): In: *Cocaine Use in America: Epidemiologic and Clinical Perspectives*, edited by N. J. Kozel, and E. H. Adams, pp. 204–220. NIDA Research Monograph 61, U.S. Government Printing Office, Washington.
129. Smith, E. O., and Byrd, L. D. (1985): *Pharmacol. Biochem. Behav.*, 22:135–139.
130. Smith, J. B., and McKearney, J. W. (1977): *Psychopharmacology*, 53:151–157.
131. Tewes, P. A., and Fischman, M. W. (1982): *J. Pharmacol. Exp. Ther.*, 221:373–383.
132. Thompson, D. M., and Moerschbaecher, J. M. (1979): In: *Advances in Behavioral Pharmacology*, edited by T. Thompson and P. B. Dews, pp. 229–260. Academic Press, New York.
133. Thompson, T., Dews, P. B., and McKim, W. (1981): *Advances in Behavioral Pharmacology*. Academic Press, New York.
134. Tilson, H. A., and Sparber, S. B. (1973): *J. Pharmacol. Exp. Ther.*, 187:372–379.
135. Van Dyke, C., Barash, P. G., Jatlow, P., and Byck, R. (1976): *Science*, 191:859–861.
136. Van Dyke, C., Jatlow, P., Ungerer, J., Barash, P. G., and Byck, R. (1978): *Science*, 200:211–213.
137. Villensky, W. (1982): *J. Forens. Sci.*, 27:958–962.
138. Weiss, B. (1968): In: *Abuse of Central Stimulants*, edited by F. Sjoquist and M. Tottie, pp. 31–66. Raven Press, New York.
139. Weiss, B., and Laties, V. G. (1962): *Pharmacol. Rev.*, 14:1–36.
140. Weiss, R. D., Goldenheim, P. D., and Mirin, S. M. (1981): *Am. J. Psychiatry*, 138:1110–1112.
141. Wilkinson, P., Van Dyke, C., Jatlow, P., Barash, P., and Byck, R. (1980): *Clin. Pharmacol. Ther.*, 27:386–394.
142. Wise, R. A. (1984): In: *Cocaine: Pharmacology, Effects and Treatment of Abuse*, edited by J. Grabowski, pp. 15–33. NIDA Research Monograph 50, U.S. Government Printing Office, Washington.
143. Woolverton, W. L. (1984): *Pharmacologist*, 26:1621.
144. Woolverton, W. L., and Balster, R. L. (1982): *Pharmacol. Biochem. Behav.*, 16:491–500.
145. Woolverton, W. L., de la Garza, R., and Johanson, C. E. (1986): In: *Problems of Drug Dependence, 1985*, edited by L. Harris, p. 504. NIDA Research Monograph Series, U.S. Government Printing Office, Washington.
146. Woolverton, W. L., Kandel, D., and Schuster, C. R. (1978): *J. Pharmacol. Exp. Ther.*, 205:525–535.
147. Woolverton, W. L., and Trost, R. C. (1978): *Pharmacol. Biochem. Behav.*, 8:627–630.
148. Yokel, R. A., and Pickens, R. (1973): *J. Pharmacol. Exp. Ther.*, 187:27–33.
149. Yokel, R. A., and Wise, R. A. (1976): *Psychopharmacology*, 48:311–318.

Psychopharmacology:
The Third Generation of Progress,
edited by Herbert Y. Meltzer.
Raven Press, New York © 1987.

CHAPTER **167**

Opioids, Receptors, and Abuse Liability

James H. Woods and Gail Winger

Medical records indicate that opium was used for the treatment of pain in the first century A.D. and perhaps earlier. Abuse of opium has a considerably shorter history, becoming a problem in China in the 17th century after the technique of pipe smoking had become popular. Since that time, however, the use of opioid drugs has been closely entwined with abuse of these compounds. This class of drugs today remains our most effective treatment for severe pain and the source of one of our more serious drug abuse problems. These two facets of opioid drugs form a basis for the need to continue to develop new opioid compounds with novel spectra of action.

The objective of discovering a strong analgesic without some liability for abuse has not yet been achieved. Until this goal is met, there will be continuing concern that the physician, in providing relief from pain, may, under some circumstances, contribute to the genesis of abuse. Even when the goal of developing a dependence-free opioid analgesic is met, abuse of heroin will most likely continue to be a serious problem throughout many regions of the world. The same opioid drug development programs that are searching for dependence-free opioid analgesics offer the best hope for the discovery of agents that will be therapeutically effective for treatment of heroin abuse.

The research and theory described in this chapter deal primarily with the efforts that have been made towards discovering abuse-free opioid analgesics. There are three very relevant, more thorough reviews of past work in this area that should be consulted (38,39,71). Our treatment, although more current, is by necessity of space limitations far more selective.

In the course of the search for abuse-free analgesics, a theoretical concept developed that became a major modern framework for the study of opioid analgesics. This was the concept of multiple opioid receptors, a concept that blends and incorporates current notions on how opioids influence the behaviors most intimately involved with their abuse. The two opioid receptors that are discussed in this chapter are the μ and κ receptors, since it is with these classes of the opioid receptor that the most progress has been made toward achieving the stated objective. The discussion takes advantage of the major findings of the last three decades and attempts to put these findings into a perspective that will allow a more rapid analysis and more rational classification of new drugs as they are discovered in the future. Progress toward understanding current opioid analgesics and developing new ones has been considerable, and it is reasonable to suggest that even greater strides will be made in the future if the past serves as our guide.

HISTORY

With the benefit of hindsight, it is clear that the discovery of the actions of nalorphine in various pharmacological preparations represented a critical turning point both in the basic understanding of the actions of opioids and in the search for dependence-free analgesics. Discovery of its major pharmacological and behavioral properties was to lead to revolutions in drug discovery programs throughout the world. Nalorphine provided the first clue that the effects of opioids could specifically be antagonized when it was found to reverse the acute effects of morphine (13,58). This provided important evidence for the theory that opioid effects were mediated through occupation of specific receptors; these effects could be antagonized by prior or subsequent occupation of opioid receptors by a drug with affinity but less efficacy at those receptors (e.g., ref. 38). The further finding that nalorphine could precipitate morphine withdrawal signs in morphine-dependent humans, signs that differed from those of morphine deprivation only in their onset and duration (66), gave credence to the idea that it was the removal of morphine from these opioid receptors that resulted in withdrawal.

Nalorphine had effects in addition to its antagonist properties, however, and these effects included analgesia in man (19,26,30). Nalorphine analgesia in animals was difficult to demonstrate in some morphine-sensitive assays (67), although analgesic effects were observed in animals using phenylquinone stretching tests (47). Enthusiasm about the possibility that nalorphine-like agents might be the group from which a dependence-free analgesic would come was tempered by the fact that nalorphine produced a dysphoric reaction in man that was often less acceptable than the pain for which it had been given (30). This dysphoric effect was one of the first clues that the acute effects of nalorphine and morphine, apart from their mutual ability to produce analgesia, were quite different. In postdependent addicts, the subjective effects of nalorphine and morphine were different as well. For example, morphine produced dose-related reports of "itchy skin" and "coasting," whereas nalorphine produced dose-related reports of "drunken" and "sleepy" (36).

Chronic administration of nalorphine to postaddicts also produced dysphoric reactions that prevented escalation in dose (20). When the dose was increased more slowly, tolerance appeared to develop to these dysphoric effects, and the patients became rather indifferent to the acute effects of the drug (37). When nalorphine administration was abruptly discontinued, withdrawal signs such as scratching and yawning developed that were obviously different from those seen with morphine withdrawal (37).

Chronic administration of nalorphine to monkeys (69) also resulted in withdrawal signs that were qualitatively different from those observed with morphine but quite similar to those observed in humans withdrawn from chronically administered nalorphine.

The different subjective effects of nalorphine and morphine in man as well as their distinctive type of physiological dependence provided early indications that (a) morphine-like subjective effects of opioid analgesics could be eliminated without removing the analgesic action, and (b) the development of an opioid analgesic without morphine dependence-producing potential was feasible. This set the stage for attempts to develop, through chemical variations, an opioid analgesic with reduced likelihood of either physiological or psychological dependence potential. It also set the stage for important developments in the theory of opioid analgesic action. With an extensive review of the literature and a novel theoretical approach, Martin (38) argued that nalorphine and morphine produced analgesia by different mechanisms (receptor dualism) and that the different subjective effects were also mediated by different receptors. All involved receptors were opioid receptors, since effects of both compounds could be reversed by the newly discovered "pure antagonist" naloxone.

These findings and this theory were widely incorporated into subsequent opioid research, and the possibilities for drug development using mixed opioid agonist–antagonists were widely discussed. A next important theoretical devel-

opment was the discovery of a novel compound, ketazocine, and shortly thereafter the slightly more potent ethylketazocine (42). These drugs were very close in structure to cyclazocine, a nalorphine-like drug, but, as shown on smooth muscle preparations (28) and in the whole animal (42,56), they had little, if any, antagonist action. They neither precipitated nor suppressed abstinence in morphine-dependent monkeys (56), raising the question of whether they produced a dependence of a type different from morphine or whether they produced no dependence at all.

The ketazocines were poor analgesics in rat tail-flick assays but were potent analgesics in stretching assays in the mouse (42). The agonist effects of these drugs, both as analgesics in the rodent and as inhibitors of the twitch of smooth muscle preparations, were four to five times more difficult to antagonize with naloxone than were the effects of morphine, although the antagonism that developed was competitive (28). Thus, their analgesic effects may reflect activity at different receptors.

In the chronic spinal dog preparation, Martin and his colleagues did evaluations of the effects of ketazocine and ethylketazocine in normal, in morphine-dependent, and in cyclazocine-dependent preparations. The acute effects of both of the ketazocine drugs were quite different from those of morphine. Ethylketazocine did not suppress or precipitate abstinence in morphine-dependent dogs, and ketazocine's ability to precipitate morphine abstinence was marginal at best. Both ketazocine and ethylketazocine suppressed cyclazocine withdrawal. When chronic administration of ketazocine replaced that of cyclazocine, the ketazocine withdrawal syndrome was similar to cyclazocine withdrawal signs. The effects of ethylketazocine and ketazocine were not identical to those of cyclazocine, however; cyclazocine had the capacity to elicit morphine withdrawal signs and also had some agonist actions that differed from those of the ketazocines (9). These observations led Martin and colleagues to conclude that ketazocine was a prototypic agonist on the opioid receptor previously defined by nalorphine as distinct from the morphine (μ) receptor, a receptor they labeled as the κ receptor. Cyclazocine had actions at this receptor as well as acting as an antagonist at the μ receptor and having additional actions independent of these (9).

Shortly therafter, it was shown that neither ketazocine nor ethylketazocine would maintain self-injection responding in rhesus monkeys (69). At the time, it was known that all opioids with abuse liability were reinforcers of self-injection behavior but that nalorphine was not. Thus, in animals, these κ agonists showed, in common with nalorphine, a lack of reinforcing effect; it was not yet clear, however, that the lack of reinforcing property was part of a common action at the κ receptor.

Subsequent to the development of ketazocine and ethylketazocine, a number of κ agonists of note have been developed. Bremazocine is a benzomorphan, close in structure to earlier drugs such as cyclazocine. It was considerably more potent as a κ agonist than ethylketazocine when assessed in either *in vivo* or *in vitro* assay systems (49). It retained a potent μ antagonist action as well (65), making it similar to nalorphine and cyclazocine. Because bremazocine became available in a tritiated form, it has been very useful with *in vitro* assays, and this drug has received considerable attention.

Tifluadom, a member of a chemical class associated with antianxiety agents, was also shown to have many of the biochemical and behavioral properties of a κ agonist (51). Tifluadom did not, however, have biochemical or behavioral properties of an antianxiety agent and also did not have μ antagonist effects. This drug was strikingly selective at the κ receptor site *in vitro,* and this aspect, in conjunction with its novel chemical structure, has made it of continuing interest.

There is also widespread interest in a drug labeled U-50,488, a compound with an interesting and novel chemical structure from a class of compounds not known for having opioid activity (25,64). *In vitro,* it appeared to have a 1,300-fold selectivity at κ relative to μ opioid receptor binding sites (21). This represents the greatest κ selectivity demonstrated thus far.

There has been a considerable neuroscientific interest whetted by the finding that dynorphin and related endogenous peptides shared *in vitro* pharmacological actions with κ opioid agonists (2), thus establishing them as potential endogenous ligands at the κ receptor. This study and many related studies have led to a variety of interesting avenues of basic research far beyond the scope of this chapter. This discovery has not, on the other hand, led as yet to peptide-related compounds with novel analgesic profiles, but it has enhanced our understanding of the potential sites and mechanisms of action of these drugs and could lead to interesting progress in drug development in the future.

μ AND κ OPIATE RECEPTOR AGONISTS

The assessment of abuse liability of opioids depends critically on a balanced view of their acute and chronic actions in relation to the desired effect, i.e., analgesia. In the following section on the actions of opioids that act on μ and κ receptor sites, the behavioral effects in the rhesus monkey are emphasized; in addition, comparisons are made to man and other animal species where they appear especially important or relevant. The discussion does not include actions of substances at other receptors, opioid or nonopioid. Apart from a question of unduly wide scope, there is little information on *in vivo* behavioral effects in primates of drugs active at other putative opioid receptors [e.g., δ receptors (34)].

The most thoroughly described behavioral actions of μ and κ opioids may be classified into direct effects (those in which the drug does not serve as a stimulus in a behavioral conditioning procedure), dependence-producing effects (those observed only when the agent is removed or antagonist administration produces effects equivalent to drug removal), discriminative effects (wherein a drug is used to signal an appropriate response), and reinforcing effects (when a drug is used to maintain an operant response). Each of these effects is discussed in turn, and its ability to differentiate μ and κ opioid agonists is described.

Direct Effects

Analgesia

The analgesic effects of morphine and similar compounds have been assessed by a variety of techniques. As an example, morphine in doses of 0.3 to 10 mg/kg reduced the speed with which rhesus monkeys withdrew their tails from hot water (5). A variety of κ agonists have been shown to be active in the rhesus monkey in the same assay procedure (6). It is difficult to demonstrate κ-agonist-induced thermal analgesia in rodents (e.g., refs. 57,59); the lack of analgesia to thermal stimuli and the corresponding presence of analgesia to chemical stimuli in rodents may be a distinguishing feature of κ agonists. Since these drugs have not been evaluated as analgesics in man, it is not known whether κ agonists will produce analgesia to thermal stimuli or other stimuli in this species.

Recently, the opioid antagonist quadazocine (WIN 44441-3) has been used to reverse the analgesic actions of morphine and of the κ agonists bremazocine, ethylketazocine, and U-50,488. The affinity of antagonists for receptor sites may be estimated *in vivo* by examining a measure called the pA_2. It is expressed as the negative logarithm of the dose of antagonist necessary to administer in order to achieve the same effect when the dose of the agonist is doubled. Thus, the larger the pA_2 value, the higher is the affinity of the antagonist for a given receptor site. Apparent pA_2 values for the κ agonists were similar (6.1–6.4) but markedly different from that of morphine (8.5). In addition, β-funaltrexamine, a μ-selective antagonist, was effective in preventing the analgesic action of morphine but left unchanged the analgesia produced by ethylketazocine (7). These data suggest that κ agonists produce analgesia that can be differentiated from that of morphine by antagonists selective for opioid receptor type, and they support the theory of receptor dualism of Martin (38) described above.

Fluid Balance

The κ agonists induced a marked diuresis in a variety of animal species (e.g., ref. 31). Morphine, on the other hand, failed to change or suppressed urine output in many species. In the rat, the κ-agonist-induced effect may result in large part from the reduction of vasopressin (53). κ agonists, in doses below those that induce thermal analgesia, produced a large increase in urine output in rhesus monkeys. The analgesic and diuretic potencies of the κ agonists in the monkey have the same rank order potency, i.e., bremazocine > ethylketazocine > tifluadom = U-50,488 (6). In keeping with the broad generality of this effect, ketazocine also increased urine output in humans (K. M. Kumor and D. R. Jasinski, *personal communication*).

Discriminative Effects

One can learn important characteristics of the internal stimulus effects of a drug by teaching an organism to report when it has received that drug. This can be accomplished in a procedure in which two responses are possible. One of two responses results in reinforcement following administration of the training drug; the other response is reinforced when the vehicle is administered. Once subjects have learned the appropriate discrimination, they make the response associated with drug administration following administration of other drugs that have stimulus properties in common with the training drug and make the nondrug response following administration of drugs that do not have stimulus properties in common with the drug on which they were trained.

It is currently thought that the discriminative effects of drugs may predict the type of subjective effect obtained in human subjects. μ and κ agonists produced different discriminative effects in a variety of species (e.g., ref. 18). Ketazocine produced a pattern of subjective effects quite different from morphine in postaddict human subjects (28a), with ketazocine having a greater similarity to the more extensively studied κ mixed agonist–antagonists, nalorphine and cyclazocine, than to morphine or other μ agonists. This was entirely concordant with studies in rhesus monkeys. Rhesus monkeys trained to discriminate ethylketazocine from saline made drug-appropriate responses when given a wide variety of other κ agonists (see Table 1) but not when given morphine or a wide variety of other μ agonists (e.g., codeine, etorphine) or nonopioids

(e.g., apomorphine, pentobarbital) (14). The discriminative properties clearly reside in the κ agonist action rather than the μ antagonist action of these drugs, since not all of these compounds have antagonist properties. Conversely, rhesus monkeys trained to discriminate the μ agonist etorphine from saline made drug-appropriate responses following administration of other μ agonists but not when given κ agonists (e.g., see ref. 16). Quaternary nalorphine failed to produce ethylketazocine-appropriate responses at much higher doses than those necessary for the tertiary form (14). Also, morphine was much more potent when given directly into the ventricles of the brain (33), and morphine's effects, though readily blocked by naltrexone, were not blocked by the quaternary form of naltrexone (60). Thus, both the κ- and μ-type discriminative effects appeared to be centrally mediated.

There are stereoactive κ or μ forms of opioids that produce the appropriate type of discriminative effect (14,16), indicating the stereoselective nature of the effects. The discriminative effects of κ and μ agonists could be selectively antagonized; quadazocine was a surmountable antagonist of the discriminative effects of μ or κ agonists. Its pA_2, however, was much higher for μ than κ agonists (1,7). The pA_2 for the effects of quadazocine against the discriminative effects of μ and κ agonists was comparable to those found for the analgesic effects of these opioids, as noted above. β-Funaltrexamine (β-FNA) failed to antagonize ethylketazo-

TABLE 1. *Behavioral potencies of κ agonist/antagonists in rhesus monkeys*

Compound	Potency relative to ethylketazocine training dose	Capacity to precipitate morphine abstinence[a]	References[b]	
			Disc. effects	Abstinence
Bremazocine	3.0	+	6	11
Mr 2033[c]	1.0	−	16	69
UM 715[d]	1.0	+	25	25
UM 928[e]	0.7	+	25	25
Ketazocine	0.5	−	25	69
Cyclazocine	0.3	+	16	60
Levallorphan	0.1	+	16	UO
U-69,593[f]	0.1	NT	UO	—
Tifluadom	0.1	NT	6	—
N-Allylnormetazocine	0.03	+	16	UO
Oxilorphan	0.03	+	73	UO
U-50,488[g]	0.03	−	6	UO
Nalorphine	0.03	+	16	60
Mr 1268[h]	0.01	−	16	69
Nalmefene	0.01	+	UO	UO
β-FNA[i]	0.001	+	7	10

[a] NT, not tested.
[b] UO, unpublished observations.
[c] (±)-(1R/S,5R/S,9R/S,-2″R/S)-5,9-Dimethyl-2′-hydroxy-2-tetrahydrofurfuryl-6,7-benzomorphan.
[d] N-Cyclopropylmethyl-7-(2-hydroxy-5-methyl-2-hexyl)-6,14-*endo*-ethenotetrahydronororipavine.
[e] N-Cyclopropylmethyl-7-(2-hydroxy-2-pentyl)-6,14-*endo*-ethenotetrahydronororipavine.
[f] (5α,7α,8β)-(+)-N-Methyl-N-[7-(1-pyrrolidinyl)-1-oxaspiro(4,5)dec-8-yl]benzeneacetamide.
[g] *trans*-3,4-Dichloro-N-methyl-N[2-(1-pyrrolidinyl)cyclohexyl]benzeneacetamide.
[h] 2-(2-Methyl-3-furylmethyl)-2′-hydroxy-5,9α-dimethyl-6,7-benzomorphan.
[i] β-Funaltrexamine.

cine under conditions in which it clearly prevented the actions of μ agonists (7).

These data on antagonism of μ and κ agonists provide strong support for the involvement of these receptors in the discriminative effects generated by opioid drugs. A drug development objective should be to synthesize an analgesic shorn of significant subjective effect. The behavioral assays described above are sufficient to evaluate this. It may be that previously developed compounds may offer leads in this respect, although none of the currently popular pharmacological prototypes offers significant hope. That such selectivity of action may be obtained is shown by the accomplishments with selective opioid antidiarrheal agents (e.g., ref. 62).

Reinforcing Effects

If a μ agonist has a rapid onset of action, it is likely to maintain self-injection responding. This generalization has been established firmly with a variety of compounds from different chemical families (e.g., ref. 72). It is equally clear that under the same conditions, κ agonists fail to maintain reinforced responding. Table 2 lists a set of κ compounds that have been evaluated for their reinforcing effects. Each of these compounds has been classified as a κ agonist by one or more *in vitro* or *in vivo* assays for direct effect, e.g., diuresis. None of these drugs maintained rates of responding above those maintained by saline. In fact, in the rhesus monkey, U-50,488 (69a), nalorphine, cyclazocine, ketazocine, and ethylketazocine (69) rates of responding can be below those maintained by saline. U-50,488 also failed to maintain self-injection responding in rats (29). These findings suggested that κ agonists may have aversive effects, a possibility that is currently under study.

Dependence

Both μ and κ agonists induce a state of physiological dependence. As noted above, dependence associated with nalorphine-like agents has been thought for a long time to be different from morphine dependence. With the discovery of much more selective agonists, this has been borne out in primates (10), although it is not clear in rodents as yet. Chronic administration of U-50,488 to rhesus monkeys produced a dependence that was identified either by termination of U-50,488 administration or by administration of naltrexone or quadazocine. The distinctive signs of withdrawal in rhesus monkeys following establishment of U-50,488 or morphine dependence are shown in Table 3. Withdrawal from U-50,488 had signs in common with bremazocine, Mr 2033, nalorphine, and cyclazocine withdrawal and could be elicited selectively. That is, β-funaltrexamine precipitated morphine withdrawal but not U-50,488 withdrawal. The signs were also selectively suppressed by appropriate agonists; only κ agonists suppressed U-50,488 withdrawal, and only μ agonists suppressed morphine withdrawal (11).

There were strong correlations between the potencies of μ agonists in tests of various behavioral effects described above. Thus, morphine-like agents that were relatively potent in maintaining self-injection responding were also relatively potent in suppressing morphine abstinence (72). Likewise, the potencies of μ agonists as reinforcing stimuli were highly correlated with their potencies as morphine-like discriminative stimuli (*unpublished observations*).

With κ agonists, the number of compounds that have been assessed in these tests is too small to allow the same generalization. Nevertheless, the following potency order has been established for the analgesic, discriminative, diuretic, and sedative properties of κ agonists in the rhesus monkey: bremazocine > ethyketazocine = Mr 2033 > tifluadom > U-50,488 (6).

This brief survey of the properties of μ and κ agonist actions should serve at least two purposes. It gives behavioral clarification to the differential effects of drugs that act on these receptors. In addition, it serves as a guide for evaluating the actions of mixed agonist–antagonists and other drugs whose effects are not clearly of one type or another. With the benefit of clear understanding of the nature of κ and μ

TABLE 2. *κ agonists that fail to maintain self-injection responding in primates*

Compound	Doses tested (μg/kg/inj)	Schedule conditions[a]	Dose/drug used to establish/maintain behavior	Reference[b]
EKC (UM 975)	0.1–10	FR 30	0.32 mg/kg/inj codeine	69
Ketazocine (UM 974)	0.1–30	FR 30	0.32 mg/kg/inj codeine	69
Mr 2033 (UM 1072)[c]	0.01–40	FR 30	0.32 mg/kg/inj codeine	69
Mr 1353 (UM 911)[d]	1.0–1,000	FR 30	0.32 mg/kg/inj codeine	69
Mr 2184 (UM 1070)[e]	0.1–10	FR 30	0.32 mg/kg/inj codeine	69
Mr 1268 (UM 909)[f]	3.0–1,000	FR 30	0.32 mg/kg/inj codeine	69
Bremazocine	0.018–0.10	FR 1	0.10 mg/kg/inj morphine	51
U-50,488[g]	0.32–100	FR 30	0.32 mg/kg/inj codeine	UO

[a] FR, fixed ratio.
[b] UO, unpublished observations.
[c] (±)-(1R/S,5R/S,2″R/S)-5,9-Dimethyl-2′-hydroxy-2-tetrahydrofurfuryl-6,7-benzomorphan.
[d] α-5,9-Dimethyl-2-(furylmethyl)-2′-hydroxy-6,7-benzomorphan.
[e] (±)-5,9β-Dimethyl-2′-hydroxy-2-tetrahydrofurfuryl-6,7-benzomorphan.
[f] α-5,9-Dimethyl-2-(furylmethyl)-2′-hydroxy-6,7-benzomorphan.
[g] trans-3,4-Dichloro-methyl-N[2-(1-pyrrolidinyl)cyclohexyl]benzeneacetamide.

TABLE 3. *Signs produced by antagonist administration or agonist deprivation in rhesus monkeys*

Morphine withdrawal	U-50,488 withdrawal
Abdominal defense reaction	General hyperactivity
Apprehension/aggression towards handlers[a]	Unusual tongue movements[c]
Coughing, retching, or vomiting	Yawning
Miosis	Excessive scratching
Apprehension towards other monkeys[b]	Excessive grooming of other monkeys
Grimacing during handling	Picking of fingers and toes
Excessive vocalization	

[a] Monkey is hesitant or refuses to come out of cage and is resistant to handling.
[b] Monkeys are avoiding each other, grimacing, vocalizing, or fighting.
[c] Monkey's tongue is turned and positioned towards the side of the mouth.
Adapted from Gmerek et al. (11), with permission.

agonist actions, for example, true partial agonists can be defined with respect to certain specific functions [e.g., diuretic actions (31)]. Some of the complex effects of drugs of this type are described in the section below.

MIXED AGONISTS AND MIXED AGONIST–ANTAGONISTS

μ Opiate-like

Butorphanol

Butorphanol is an opioid that has been marketed as an analgesic for humans and as an antitussive for dogs. It was similar to the κ agonists in that it was active in rodent analgesia tests using phenylquininone but less active in analgesia measures using thermal stimuli (45). It also increased urine output, which would be a κ rather than a μ action, except that this effect was not blocked by naloxone (43). Other agonist actions of butorphanol were quite similar to those of μ opioid agonists. When substituted for codeine in tests of the reinforcing effects with intravenous delivery, it maintained rates well above those maintained by saline, although these rates were considerably lower than those maintained by the optimal dose of codeine (73). Rhesus monkeys trained to discriminate administration of the μ agonist etorphine and rats trained to discriminate morphine responded completely on the drug-appropriate lever following administration of butorphanol (18,73). Squirrel monkeys trained to discriminate morphine, however, showed only partial generalization to butorphanol, even when quite high doses were given (18). Rhesus monkeys trained to discriminate ethylketazocine showed no generalization to butorphanol (73).

Administration of butorphanol to morphine-dependent rhesus monkeys produced no signs of withdrawal. When morphine-dependent monkeys were deprived of morphine for 14 hr, however, butorphanol produced mild exacerbation rather than reduction of the morphine withdrawal signs

(68). Despite this tendency to exacerbate rather than attenuate withdrawal in the monkey, butorphanol was effective in reducing the jumping response to morphine deprivation in morphine-dependent mice (52). Chronic administration of butorphanol to rhesus monkeys followed by drug deprivation produced mild withdrawal signs much like those that developed following withdrawal of κ agonists and distinct from μ-agonist withdrawal signs. Administration of naloxone produced much more severe signs, however, and naloxone-precipitated withdrawal in monkeys given chronic butorphanol was indistinguishable from morphine withdrawal (68).

In summary, although butorphanol is frequently referred to as a κ agonist in the literature (e.g., refs. 44, 46, 55), data obtained in rhesus monkeys as well as in some other species indicated that it also had marked actions at the μ receptor. These were primarily agonist actions in the nondependent monkey, but slight antagonist actions were observed in the morphine-dependent, morphine-withdrawn monkey. The κ agonist signs were revealed only when butorphanol was withdrawn by natural withdrawal following chronic administration. Thus, butorphanol can be described as a compound with mixed-agonist actions and with only slight antagonist actions. Studies in methadone-maintained clients indicated that butorphanol had antagonist actions similar to those of naloxone (G. E. Bigelow and K. L. Preston, *personal communication*); thus, the antagonist actions of butorphanol may be more obvious in man than in the monkey.

Nalbuphine

Nalbuphine is an opioid analgesic with a spectrum of action that is similar in many ways to that of butorphanol. Like butorphanol, nalbuphine had clear reinforcing effects in rhesus monkeys but did not maintain rates of responding as high as those maintained by codeine (73). Also like butorphanol, nalbuphine produced drug-appropriate responding in monkeys trained to discriminate etorphine but not in monkeys trained to discriminate ethylketazocine (73). Nalbuphine also resembled butorphanol in its ability to produce exacerbation of withdrawal signs in morphine-deprived, morphine-dependent rhesus monkeys. It differed from butorphanol in that it produced withdrawal signs in both withdrawn and nonwithdrawn morphine-dependent rhesus monkeys (68). Nalbuphine also produced morphine-like withdrawal reactions in morphine-dependent mice (52).

Following chronic administration of nalbuphine, monkeys became tolerant to the ability of the drug to produce stupor and muscle relaxation; on drug deprivation, mild to moderate withdrawal signs developed that were like morphine withdrawal signs. Morphine withdrawal signs of greater severity were observed following naloxone precipitation of nalbuphine withdrawal. Nalorphine was unable to precipitate withdrawal signs in nalbuphine-dependent monkeys (68). In mice, chronic nalbuphine administration appeared to produce a very mild dependence; drug deprivation did not result in jumping in the mice, and very large doses of naloxone were required to precipitate the jumping response (52).

Nalbuphine had clear μ-like agonist activity in nondependent monkeys and opioid antagonist activity in morphine-dependent monkeys. It appeared to have more antagonist actions than did butorphanol, and, in contrast to butorphanol, it did not appear to have any κ agonist actions. It thus appears appropriate to classify nalbuphine as a μ-like mixed agonist–antagonist in the monkey.

Acute administration of nalbuphine to human postaddicts produced morphine-like subjective effects that did not increase above a certain dose. At higher doses, subjective reports were more like those found with nalorphine and cyclazocine. Subjects reported liking the low doses of nalbuphine. Nalbuphine precipitated abstinence in subjects maintained on morphine. As in the monkey, chronic administration of nalbuphine produced dependence that could be revealed by naloxone but not by nalorphine administration. The abstinence syndrome was similar to that observed following morphine withdrawal (24).

Buprenorphine

Buprenorphine is an opioid analgesic with an unusual and interesting profile of action. It also has a very long duration of action, an attribute that could be advantageous in an analgesic compound or in one with potential usefulness in treating opioid abuse. Buprenorphine has promise for both of these applications. The analgesic action of buprenorphine was apparent in both phenylquinone stretching tests and thermal tests in rodents. Its potency in the chemical tests was more than 100 times greater than in the thermal tests (57); the considerably lower potency in tests using heat stimuli suggests analgesia mediated through κ receptors, at least in the rodent. The promise of buprenorphine's usefulness in treating opioid abuse was shown by demonstrations of the drug's capacity to reduce heroin self-administration in human heroin users under experimental conditions (41).

The drug produced a full etorphine-like cue in monkeys trained to discriminate etorphine and no ethylketazocine-like cue in monkeys trained to discriminate ethylketazocine

(73). Nondependent human opioid abusers also indicated that the subjective effects of buprenorphine were similar to those of morphine (23), and human subjects indicated that they liked the effects of buprenorphine. Studies in monkeys showed that buprenorphine maintained self-administration (40,71,73), but at rates of responding that were lower than those maintained by the base-line opioid. Buprenorphine was not as efficacious as morphine, butorphanol, or nalbuphine in maintaining self-administration in the baboon (35).

Low doses of buprenorphine did not suppress morphine withdrawal signs in morphine-withdrawn, morphine-dependent rhesus monkeys, and higher doses exacerbated the signs of withdrawal in these monkeys. Buprenorphine also precipitated withdrawal in nonwithdrawn monkeys in a dose-related manner. Thus, buprenorphine has a profile of action similar to nalbuphine in the morphine-dependent monkey. The ability of morphine to reverse withdrawal precipitated by buprenorphine was attenuated in these monkeys (12), suggesting that buprenorphine's long duration of action may be related to a demonstrated, relatively strong attachment of this drug to the μ receptor (48). Administration of buprenorphine to opioid-dependent humans resulted in a fairly mild withdrawal syndrome in one group of methadone-maintained patients (22) and a considerably more severe withdrawal in another group of methadone-stabilized patients (32).

Chronic administration of buprenorphine to rhesus monkeys resulted in tolerance to the sedative effects of this drug. Withdrawal reactions could not be elicited by drug deprivation or by nalorphine or naloxone administration. Slight increases in restlessness and irritability were observed following administration of naloxone or following drug deprivation. These were quite mild, however, and did not warrant an indication of drug withdrawal (12). Morphine-like physiological dependence to buprenorphine has been reported in man, although it was mild and did not develop until about 14 days following cessation of chronic administration (23).

These observations combine to give a profile of a very interesting opioid compound. A drug with clear opioid actions on acute administration but with little ability to produce dependence warrants considerable attention. Many of the unusual aspects of buprenorphine are likely related to its long duration of action, which is, in turn, likely to result from its strong attachment to the μ receptor. The fact that withdrawal reactions are slight under either drug deprivation or antagonist-induced conditions may be because buprenorphine is very slowly removed from this receptor and because it is difficult to displace buprenorphine from this receptor by administration of an antagonist. Thus, buprenorphine may very well be capable of producing dependence; the difficulty is in demonstrating withdrawal signs, which is the only way of defining the state of dependence. With some clever and different methodology, Dum et al. (4) have shown greater acute dependence on morphine in rats that had been given buprenorphine prior to the administration of morphine. The fact that buprenorphine may produce dependence that is hidden by the kinetics of the drug–receptor interaction is, at some levels of discussion, irrelevant. It is these very kinetics that make the drug of special interest and of great potential usefulness as an analgesic and in the treatment of opioid addiction. Buprenorphine's actions can be summarized as mixed agonist–antagonist with the additional characterization of a long duration of action and little potential for producing withdrawal.

κ Opiate-like

Nalorphine

The history of opioid analgesics described above points out the critical role of nalorphine in the development of novel and interesting compounds. In the late 1950s through the 1960s, nalorphine was shown to have both acute effects and dependence properties that differed markedly from those of morphine, in addition to the fact that it was a morphine antagonist. More recent work in the rhesus monkey demonstrated the similarities between the agonist properties of nalorphine and those of κ agonists. Nalorphine did not support self-administration behavior (3); rates of intravenous nalorphine-maintained responding were less than rates maintained by saline and very similar to the low rates maintained by intravenous ketazocine and ethylketazocine (69). Studies of the discriminative effects of nalorphine demonstrated that in the monkey this drug had stimulus effects in common with ethyketazocine (14).

In the rat, nalorphine and other κ drugs appeared to retain a partial μ agonist effect (17). Its most appropriate characterization in the monkey, however, seemed to be that of a μ antagonist and a κ agonist. The μ antagonist effects of nalorphine were evident not only in the early descriptions of its ability to antagonize the analgesic effects of morphine and to precipitate morphine withdrawal in morphine-dependent monkeys but also in its more recently described ability to antagonize the discriminative effects of acute administration of codeine (66a). In doses that shifted the codeine dose–effect curve to the right in these studies, nalorphine either had no effect on discrimination of ethylketazocine or shifted the ethylketazocine discrimination dose–effect curve to the left. Nalorphine was not entirely without κ antagonist effects in primates. In monkeys made dependent on U-50,488, nalorphine administration resulted in withdrawal signs typical of deprivation-induced κ agonist withdrawal (11). Nalorphine may bear a relationship to κ agonists that resembles the relationship of nalbuphine or buprenorphine to μ agonists, i.e., it is a κ agonist in nondependent monkeys, but retains some κ antagonist properties in monkeys dependent on a κ agonist.

Cyclazocine

Cyclazocine was one of the first drugs synthesized to take advantage of the interesting properties of nalorphine (36). The antagonist properties of cyclazocine were similar to those of nalorphine, and the drug also produced analgesia in man (27). Although it did not appear to produce as much dysphoria as nalorphine in man (8,27), there was

cross tolerance between these compounds (36). Chronic administration of cyclazocine to postaddict prisoners resulted in dependence that was very similar to that found with nalorphine. The addicts had been disinterested in the drug during chronic administration, responding with "don't care" when asked if they would like to take the drug every day. They maintained similar states of equanimity during cyclazocine withdrawal, not requesting further drug injections although recognizing the mild withdrawal state (36). The withdrawal signs were qualitatively different from those produced by morphine, and cyclazocine did not substitute for morphine in morphine-dependent individuals. Like nalorphine, it produced abstinence in these addicts.

More recent studies in monkeys demonstrate that cyclazocine had κ agonist actions in that it produced drug-appropriate responding in monkeys trained to discriminate ethylketazocine (16); it was not self-administered by rhesus monkeys (69).

Like nalorphine, cyclazocine produced withdrawal reactions in morphine-dependent rhesus monkeys (63). It also reversed the discriminative effects of codeine in monkeys trained to report the enteroceptive effects of this drug but did not reverse the discriminative stimulus effects of ethylketazocine (66a). The primary difference between cyclazocine and nalorphine lay in additional properties of cyclazocine that were lacking in nalorphine: cyclazocine had some effects in common with phencyclidine. The nature of these effects depended on the species tested and the isomer of cyclazocine that was used (16). The stimulus properties of d-cyclazocine were similar to those of ketamine, whereas the stimulus properties of l-cyclazocine were similar to those of ethylketazocine (54). In the monkey, therefore, the levo isomer of cyclazocine was quite similar to nalorphine in its agonistic and antagonistic effects, whereas the dextro isomer was not an opioid.

Bremazocine

The spectrum of action of bremazocine is similar to that of nalorphine and l-cyclazocine in the monkey but with an apparently larger ratio of κ agonist to μ antagonist effects. In the rhesus monkey, bremazocine produced generalization to ethylketazocine (6), was not self-administered intravenously (51), and attenuated withdrawal from U-50,488 (10). Intravenous administration of bremazocine every 4 hr produced dependence on this drug in monkeys as demonstrated by κ-like withdrawal signs of yawning and scratching on deprivation-induced withdrawal (51). These were all effects to be expected from a κ agonist. Bremazocine was different from nalorphine and l-cyclazocine in that it did not antagonize the discriminative effects of codeine, indicating that it did not have μ antagonist effects in the nondependent monkey (66a). In morphine-dependent monkeys, however, bremazocine was capable of inducing withdrawal, suggesting a weak μ antagonist property of this compound that can be revealed in monkeys sensitive to this property. Bremazocine thus can be classified as a mixed κ agonist–antagonist, although its antagonist properties are not as marked as those of nalorphine or cyclazocine.

CONCLUSION

The concept of multiple opioid receptors represents a significant economy of explanation of the wide spectrum of action of the opioid class of drugs. Behavioral pharmacological procedures have been instrumental both in describing the broad range of effects opioids can have and in identifying the behavioral actions that are associated with two of the currently recognized opioid receptors. We therefore know that whereas both μ and κ agonists produce analgesia and have antagonist-reversible behavioral effects, only μ agonists support self-administration behavior. Likewise, μ and κ agonists are completely separable on the basis of their discriminative effects and the types of physiological dependence that they produce.

With a good behavioral pharmacological description of the effects of prototypic μ and κ receptor agonists, it has been possible to sort out the complicated information presented by opioids with so-called mixed agonist, partial agonist, and agonist–antagonist actions. Opioid drugs with additional nonopioid actions have also been characterized. Since it currently seems likely that novel analgesics with reduced abuse potential will be drugs with multiple actions rather than drugs with relatively "pure" actions on one opioid receptor, it is especially important that we have the tools necessary to identify and characterize these drugs. It seems clear that the discipline of behavioral pharmacology has contributed to the tools and concepts to make the appropriate identification and clarification.

ACKNOWLEDGMENTS

Original research reported herein and the writing of this chapter were supported by USPHS Grants DA 00154 and DA 00254 and the Committee on Problems of Drug Dependence. The secretarial assistance of R. McLaughlin and the editorial assistance of Drs. Griffiths and Mello are greatly appreciated.

REFERENCES

1. Bertalmio, A. J., Winger, G., and Woods, J. H. (1984): *Fed. Proc.*, 43:966.
2. Chavkin, C., and Goldstein, A. (1981): *Nature*, 291:591–593.
3. Deneau, G. A., Yanagita, T., and Seevers, M. H. (1969): *Psychopharmacologia*, 16:30–48.
4. Dum, J., Blasig, J., and Herz, A. (1981): *Eur. J. Pharmacol.*, 70:293–300.
5. Dykstra, L. A., and Woods, J. H. (1986): *J. Pharmacol. Methods*, 15:263–269.
6. Dykstra, L. A., Gmerek, D. E., Winger, G., and Woods, J. H. (1987): *J. Pharmacol. Exp. Ther.* (in press).
7. Dykstra, L. A., Gmerek, D. E., Winger, G., and Woods, J. H. (1987): *J. Pharmacol. Exp. Ther.* (in press).
8. Fraser, H. F., and Rosenberg, D. E. (1966): *Int. J. Addict.*, 1:86–98.
9. Gilbert, P. E., and Martin, W. R. (1976): *J. Pharmacol. Exp. Ther.*, 198:66–82.
10. Gmerek, D. E., and Woods, J. H. (1986): *Life Sci.*, 39:987–992.
11. Gmerek, D. E., Dykstra, L. A., and Woods, J. H. (1987): *J. Pharmacol. Exp. Ther.* (in press).
12. Gmerek, D. E., and Woods, J. H. (1985): *J. Pharmacol. Exp. Ther.*, 235:296–301.
13. Hart, E. R., and McCawley, E. L. (1944): *J. Pharmacol. Exp. Ther.*, 82:339–348.
14. Hein, D. W., Young, A. M., Herling, S., and Woods, J. H. (1981): *J. Pharmacol. Exp. Ther.*, 218:286–291.
15. Herling, S., Coale, E. H., Jr., Hein, D. W., Winger, G., and Woods, J. H. (1981): *Psychopharmacology*, 73:286–291.
16. Herling, S., and Woods, J. H. (1981): *Life Sci.*, 28:1571–1584.
17. Holtzman, S. G. (1983): In: *Theory in Psychopharmacology, Vol. 2.*, edited by S. J. Cooper, pp. 1–45. Academic Press, New York.
18. Holtzman, S. G. (1985): *Drug Alcohol Depend.*, 14:263–282.
19. Houde, R. W., and Wallenstein, S. L. (1956): *Fed. Proc.*, 15:440–441.
20. Isbell, H. (1956): *Fed. Proc.*, 15:442.
21. James, I. F., and Goldstein, A. (1984): *Mol. Pharmacol.*, 25:337–342.
22. Jasinski, D. R., Henningfield, J. E., Hickey, J. E., and Johnson, R. E. (1982): *NIDA Res. Monogr.*, 43:92–98.
23. Jasinski, D. R., Pevnick, J. S., and Griffith, J. D. (1978): *Arch. Gen. Psychiatry*, 35:501–516.
24. Jasinski, D. R., and Mansky, P. A. (1972): *Clin. Pharmacol. Ther.*, 13:78–90.
25. Katz, J. L., Woods, J. H., Winger, G., and Jacobson, A. E. (1982): *Life Sci.*, 31:2375–2378.
26. Keats, A. S., and Telford, J. (1956): *J. Pharmacol. Exp. Ther.*, 117:190–196.
27. Keats, A. S., and Telford, J. (1964): *J. Pharmacol. Exp. Ther.*, 143:157–164.
28. Kosterlitz, H. W., Waterfield, A. A., and Berthoud, V. (1973): In: *Problems of Drug Dependence*, pp. 131–151. NIDA Research Monograph Series, U.S. Government Printing Office, Washington.
28a. Kumor, K. M., Haertzon, C. A., Johnson, R. E., Kocher, T., and Jasinski, D. (1986): *J. Pharmacol. Exp. Ther.*, 238:960–968.
29. Lahti, R. A., and Collins, R. J. (1982): *Pharmacol. Biochem. Behav.*, 17:107–109.
30. Lasagna, L., and Beecher, H. K. (1954): *J. Pharmacol. Exp. Ther.*, 112:356–363.
31. Leander, D. J. (1985): In: *Neurology and Neurobiology, Vol. 13: Behavioral Pharmacology: The Current Status*, edited by L. S. Seiden and R. L. Balster, pp. 93–110. Alan R. Liss, New York.
32. Lewis, J. W. (1985): *Drug Alcohol Depend.*, 14:363–372.
33. Locke, K. W., and Holtzman, S. G. (1985): *Psychopharmacology*, 87:1–6.
34. Lord, J. A. H., Waterfield, A. A., Hughes, J., and Kosterlitz, H. W. (1977): *Nature*, 267:495–499.
35. Lukas, S. E., Griffiths, R. R., and Brady, J. V. (1983): In: *Problems of Drug Dependence, 1982*, edited by L. S. Harris, pp. 178–183. NIDA Research Monograph Series No. 43, U.S. Government Printing Office, Washington.
36. Martin, W. R., Fraser, H. F., Gorodetzky, C. W., and Rosenberg, D. E. (1965): *J. Pharmacol. Exp. Ther.*, 150:426–436.
37. Martin, W. R., and Gorodetzky, C. W. (1965): *J. Pharmacol. Exp. Ther.*, 150:437–442.
38. Martin, W. R. (1967): *Pharmacol. Rev.*, 19:463–521.
39. Martin, W. R. (1983): *Pharmacol. Rev.*, 35:283–323.
40. Mello, N. K., Bree, M. P., and Mendelson, J. H. (1981): *Pharmacol. Biochem. Behav.*, 154:215–225.
41. Mello, N. K., Mendelson, J. H., and Kuehnle, J. C. (1982): *J. Pharmacol. Exp. Ther.*, 223:30–39.
42. Michne, W. F., Pierson, A. K., and Albertson, N. F. (1974): In: *Problems of Drug Dependence*, pp. 524–526. NIDA Research Monograph Series, U.S. Government Printing Office, Washington.
43. Miller, M. (1975): *Neuroendocrinology*, 19:241–251.
44. Morley, J. E., Levine, A. S., Kneip, J., Grace, M., Zeugner, H., et al. (1985): *Eur. J. Pharmacol.*, 112:17–25.
45. Pachter, I. J., and Evens, R. P. (1985): *Drug Alcohol Depend.*, 14:325–338.
46. Pallasch, T. J., and Gill, C. J. (1985): *Oral Surg. Oral Med. Oral Pathol.*, 59:15–20.
47. Pearl J., Stander, H., and McKean, D. B. (1969): *J. Pharmacol. Exp. Ther.*, 167:9–13.
48. Rance, M. J. (1979): *Br. J. Clin. Pharmacol.*, 7:281s–286s.
49. Romer, D., Buscher, H., Hill, R. C., Maurer, R., Petcher, T. J., et al. (1980): *Life Sci.*, 27:971–978.

50. Romer, D., Buscher, H. H., Hill, R. C., Maurer, R., Petcher, J. J., et al. (1982): *Nature,* 298:759–760.
51. Romer, D., Hill, R. C., and Maurer, R. (1982): In: *Learning and Memory Drugs as Reinforcers,* edited by S. Saito and T. Yanagita, pp. 286–293. Excerpta Medica, Amsterdam.
52. Schmidt, W. K., Tam, S. W., Shotzberger, G. S., Smith, D. H., Clark, R., et al. (1985): *Drug Alcohol Depend.,* 14:339–363.
53. Slizgi, G. R., and Ludens, J. H. (1982): *J. Pharmacol. Exp. Ther.,* 220:585–591.
54. Solomon, R. E., Herling, S., and Woods, J. H. (1981): In: *Advances in Endogenous and Exogenous Opioids, Proceedings of the International Opioid Research Conference, Kyoto, Japan,* pp. 484–486. Kodansha, Tokyo.
55. Su, T. P. (1985): *J. Pharmacol. Exp. Ther.,* 232:144–148.
56. Swain, H. H., and Seevers, M. H. (1974): In: *Problems of Drug Dependence,* pp. 1168–1195. NIDA Research Monograph Series, U.S. Government Printing Office, Washington.
57. Tyers, M. B. (1982): *Life Sci.,* 31:1233–1236.
58. Unna, K. (1943): *J. Pharmacol. Exp. Ther.,* 79:27–31.
59. Upton, N., Sewell, R. O. E., and Spencer, P. S. S. (1982): *Eur. J. Pharmacol.,* 78:421–429.
60. Valentino, R. J., Herling, S., Woods, J. H., Medzihradsky, F., and Merz, H. (1981): *J. Pharmacol. Exp. Ther.,* 217:652–659.
61. Valentino, R. J., Katz, J. I., Medzihradsky, F., and Woods, J. H. (1983): *Life Sci.,* 32:2887–2896.
62. Van Bever, W., and Lal, H. (1976): *Modern Pharmacology-Toxicology, Vol. 7.* Marcel Dekker, New York.
63. Villarreal, J. E., and Karbowski, M. G. (1973): *Adv. Biochem. Psychopharmacol.,* 8:703–789.
64. Von Voigtlander, P. F., Lahti, R. A., and Ludens, J. H. (1983): *J. Pharmacol. Exp. Ther.,* 224:7–12.
65. Von Voigtlander, P. F., and Lewis, R. A. (1982): *Prog. Neuropsychopharmacol. Biol. Psychiatry,* 6:467–470.
66. Wikler, A. R., Carter, L., Fraser, H. F., and Isbell, H. (1952): *Fed. Proc.,* 11:402.
66a. Winger, G., Dykstra, L., Gmerek, D. E., and Woods, J. H. (1987): *Fed. Proc.,* 46:382.
67. Winter, C. A., Orahovats, P. A., and Lehman, E. G. (1957): *Arch. Intern. Pharmacodyn. Ther.,* 110:186–207.
68. Woods, J. H., and Gmerek, D. E. (1985): *Drug Alcohol Depend.,* 14:233–248.
69. Woods, J. H., Smith, C. B., Medzihradsky, F., and Swain, H. (1979): In: *Mechanisms of Pain and Analgesic Drugs,* edited by R. F. Beers, Jr., and E. G. Bassett, pp. 429–445. Raven Press, New York.
69a. Woods, J. H., and Winger, G. (1987): *Drug Alcohol Depend. (in press).*
70. Woolverton, W. L., and Schuster, C. R. (1983): *Pharmacol. Rev.,* 35:33–52.
71. Yanagita, T., Katch, S., Wakase, Y., and Dinuma, N. (1982): In: *Problems of Drug Dependence, 1981,* edited by L. Harris, pp. 208–214. NIDA Research Monograph Series No. 41, U.S. Government Printing Office, Washington.
72. Young, A. M., Swain, H. H., and Woods, J. H. (1981): *Psychopharmacology,* 74:329–335.
73. Young, A. M., Stephens, K. R., Hein, D. W., and Woods, J. H. (1984): *J. Pharmacol. Exp. Ther.,* 229:118–126.

Psychopharmacology:
The Third Generation of Progress,
edited by Herbert Y. Meltzer.
Raven Press, New York © 1987.

CHAPTER **168**

Marijuana

Jack H. Mendelson

Marijuana smoking is the most frequent form of illicit drug use in America. Although there is evidence that a gradual decline has occurred in marijuana usage by young adults in the United States from 1975 through 1984 (53), it is estimated that at least one in every 20 high school seniors smokes marijuana on a daily basis. The health benefits associated with a decline in the age of onset of marijuana smoking (100) may be offset by an increase in the potency of marijuana available in many locations in the United States (109,113). The importance of marijuana use in the causation of derangements in health, psychological status, and social function remains a subject of controversy. In this chapter we review and attempt to evaluate some pertinent biomedical and psychosocial factors associated with marijuana abuse and dependence. Because of space limitations, this review is necessarily selective. However, a number of extensive and excellent critical reviews on the effects of marijuana on biologic and behavioral function are currently available for readers who wish to obtain more detailed information (29,78,113).

CHEMISTRY AND PHARMACOLOGY

An extensive review of the chemistry, pharmacology, and toxicology of cannabis compounds was described by Harris in *Psychopharmacology: A Generation of Progress* published in 1978. Over 400 compounds in addition to the psychoactive agent Δ^9-tetrahydrocannabinol (THC) have been identified in marijuana cigarettes. The usual marijuana cigarette, prepared from the leaves and flowering tops of the plant *Cannabis sativa,* contains 0.5 to 1 g of plant material. The THC concentration in typical marijuana cigarettes may range between 5 and 20 mg, but concentrations as high as 100 mg per cigarette have been detected. Hashish is prepared from concentrated resin of *Cannabis sativa* and contains a THC concentration between 8 and 12% by weight. "Hash oil," a lipid-soluble plant extract, may contain a THC concentration as high as 25 to 60%. "Hash oil" has been added to marijuana cigarettes in order to increase the concentration of THC. During pyrolysis of a marijuana cigarette, over 150 compounds in addition to the THC are present in smoke and fumes.

Following marijuana cigarette smoking, THC is quickly absorbed from the lungs and is then sequestered rapidly from blood into body tissues. The THC is metabolized chiefly in the liver, where it is converted to 11-hydroxy-THC, a psychoactive compound, and more than 20 other metabolites. The THC metabolites are excreted via the feces at relatively slow rates.

Although many investigations of the effects of marijuana smoking on behavior (including determinations of levels of intoxication and the subjective "high") have been reported, it has been difficult to establish good correlations between clinical effects and plasma THC levels (8,34,110–112,118). In general, peak levels of intoxication occur later and persist longer than peak levels of THC in plasma. Undoubtedly, one problem in establishing covariance between behavioral effects and plasma THC levels is the complex pharmacokinetic profile of THC in humans (46). However, recent data indicate that more sophisticated analysis of pharmacologic responses and plasma THC levels with compartmental models and phase plots may yield significant correlations (17). Chiang and Barnett (17) have reported that the effect compartment for psychologic high is directly coupled to the central (plasma) compartment. These investigators concluded that "the effect is directly proportional to mean THC levels from approximately 1 to 4 hr after the start of smoking a marijuana cigarette." When data obtained in previous studies (112) were reanalyzed with the model proposed by Chiang and Barnett, good correlations were obtained between rapid behavioral and physiologic effects after marijuana smoking and plasma THC levels (17).

Delayed physiologic and pathophysiologic effects of marijuana smoking may be caused by accumulation of critical plasma levels of a major metabolite, 11-nor-COOH-THC (9-carboxy-THC) (135). Good correlations have been reported between radioimmunoassay analysis and gas chromatograph–mass spectroscopy analysis of THC and 9-carboxy-THC in plasma obtained from men and women following marijuana smoking (112), and no differences between men and women have been observed with respect to conversion of THC to 9-carboxy-THC (135).

Hunt and Jones have noted that if THC in biological fluids were confined only to blood, 99% of an intravenous dose (and presumably a similar dose administered via inhalation) would be metabolized in less than 30 min (46). However, the swift decline of THC in plasma is associated with a very rapid intake of the drug into tissue compartments. It has been calculated that approximately 70% of the THC in plasma following an i.v. dose rapidly enters the tissue compartment, and 30% is converted to metabolites. Hunt and Jones (46) state that "after approximately 6 hr the rate-limiting step for elimination of unchanged THC is not metabolism as implied by Lemberger et al. (71) but rather is a slow return to plasma of THC sequestered in tissues."

EFFECTS ON BEHAVIOR: SENSORY PROCESSES AND PERCEPTION

Since automobile accidents are a major cause of death and disability in America, marijuana effects on perceptual and sensory functions that are essential for driving are of considerable importance. Early studies (47) showed that heavy marijuana smokers often experienced distortions in the sizes of objects and also had impaired distance perception of objects and their rate of approach. Marijuana smoking reduces accurate detection of peripheral light stimuli as a consequence of impaired ocular motor control (103). Decrements in visual reaction time (104), ocular motor tracking function (4), and color discrimination have also been reported (4). Impairment in auditory function such as auditory reaction time and auditory signal detection occurs after marijuana smoking (102).

A number of investigators have reported a unique marijuana-related aberration of perceptual processes: distortion of time sense (15,36,47,132,137). Impairment of time sense perception following marijuana smoking may not only increase risk for automobile accidents but also contribute to disturbance of ideational states under nondriving conditions (83,98).

There is a strong positive correlation between the dose of marijuana used and degree of driving impairment (60,70,123). The duration of marijuana effects on driving function may persist for over 2 hr (117). Since marijuana smoking impairs driving ability, it is not surprising that the drug also adversely affects a pilot's performance during simulated instrument flying (13,49,50). Moreover, pilot performance has been shown to be impaired as a consequence of marijuana hangover effects. Recent studies have shown that significant impairment in a pilot's function may persist for as long as 24 hr following acute marijuana smoking (141).

COGNITIVE FUNCTION

Marijuana effects on cognitive function are dependent on the dose of marijuana used, the route of administration, plus the demand characteristics of the task such as difficulty, complexity, and familiarity or practice. A significant correlation between dose effects and task difficulty and complexity has been established by a number of investigators (14,115,116,140). Complex cognitive tasks are especially sensitive to marijuana effects (14,116). The acquisition of new information that requires systematic study and learning is also compromised by marijuana use (1,119,126,134). It has also been reported that marijuana use may impair short-term memory function (10,21,22,69,82,121).

MOTIVATION

Perhaps one of the most controversial purported adverse effects of marijuana use is the "amotivational syndrome" (81). Although some investigators have concluded that amotivation and loss of interest in conventional social goals is an indirect concomitant of marijuana use (107), others believe that marijuana directly impairs motivation and achievement (25,27,52,77). A major problem inherent in evaluation of clinical reports of "amotivation" is the reliability and validity of procedures employed to measure motivation.

Several studies have attempted to assess effects of marijuana smoking on motivation to obtain socially desirable goals such as money reinforcement (84,85,88,90,91). These studies indicated that marijuana smoking (including heavy marijuana smoking) did not significantly suppress operant acquisition of either marijuana cigarettes or money. However, the operant task employed in these studies, as well as those utilized by other investigators (99), was relatively easy to perform. Adverse effects of marijuana on personal achievement cannot, at present, be explained by a specific and unique drug effect on motivation.

PSYCHIATRIC DISORDERS

Marijuana-induced intoxication is similar to intoxication caused by ethanol. Marijuana users usually report enhanced mood states following smoking, but there are also reports of anxiety, depersonalization, and dissociation after marijuana smoking (19,47,58,83,107,127). Popular folklore has argued that marijuana use facilitates aggressive behavior, but objective clinical observations have not supported this notion. Some experts have suggested that poor impulse control and enhanced aggressive behavior may occur in a minority of individuals either during active use (2,54) or during drug withdrawal (29).

Although marijuana smoking does not induce *de novo* psychiatric disorders, there is considerable evidence that marijuana smoking may aggravate preexisting illness. Paranoid symptoms as well as affective disorders may be exacerbated during marijuana use (18,37,106,127). Anxiety and panic reactions have also been reported following marijuana use in susceptible individuals (98,109,138).

TOLERANCE AND PHYSICAL DEPENDENCE

Significant tolerance develops to marijuana effects during chronic use. This process is associated with the tendency to increase dose and/or frequency of marijuana use through time (84,85,88,90,91). As tolerance progresses, psychological dependence may occur (32,113). Evidence of overt physical dependence in males has been reported by Jones et al. (57,59). The marijuana abstinence syndrome consists of anorexia, anxiety, agitation, depression, restlessness, irritability, tremor, as well as severe insomnia (56). There have also been recent reports of physical dependence on marijuana by women who were studied under controlled research ward conditions. Abrupt cessation of marijuana use following 21 days of heavy smoking caused an abstinence syndrome consisting of sweating, exaggerated deep tendon reflexes, lateral gaze nystagmus, tremulousness of the tongue and extremities, anxiety, dysphoria, insomnia, and anorexia. Onset of withdrawal signs and symptoms occurred 10 hr following cessation of marijuana smoking, and symptom intensity was greatest 48 hr after smoking. The dose of THC sufficient to induce dependence was 3.2 mg/kg body weight per day for 3 consecutive weeks (94).

PHYSIOLOGIC EFFECTS

Respiratory System

Because the most common route of self-administration of marijuana is through inhalation of pyrolyzed material, it is not surprising that respiratory disorders are common in chronic marijuana smokers. Clinical reports have implicated marijuana smoking in the causation of persistent rhinitis, dyspnea, and decreased exercise tolerance (40). Marijuana smokers are also at increased risk for developing chronic cough and bronchitis (3,129). Pulmonary function studies have shown that marijuana may produce a significant impairment in vital capacity and ventilatory function (40,86,105,128). Recent studies of pulmonary function in women who smoke marijuana revealed a striking reduction in gas diffusion across the surface of lung cell membranes (131). Women who smoked marijuana plus tobacco cigarettes had even greater impairment of lung function than

those women who smoked marijuana only. Since there is evidence that women are increasing both cigarette smoking and marijuana smoking, it is reasonable to anticipate that the prevalence of pulmonary disease in women smokers will increase in future years.

Cardiovascular System

One of the most consistent effects observed in humans following marijuana smoking is tachycardia (5,9,20,35, 51,55). Electrocardiographic studies have shown that elevations of the S–T segment, increase in amplitude of the P wave, and inversion or flattening of the T wave occur following marijuana smoking (9,24,62,120,139). High doses of marijuana can induce premature ventricular contractions (62).

Blood pressure changes following marijuana smoking are variable. Increased and decreased pressure responses as well as marijuana-induced postural hypotension have been reported (11,12,55,114,136). Although no cardiovascular-related deaths directly attributable to marijuana use have been reported, it is probable that chronic marijuana smoking may exacerbate cardiac problems in individuals with preexisting cardiovascular disease (78).

Central Nervous System

Marijuana is used primarily to induce changes in mood states and behavior, but the neural mechanisms underlying this process remain to be determined. Marijuana smoking produces changes in the electrical activity (EEG) of the brain, principally a reduction in peak power of the α rhythm, a decrease in β rhythm activity, and an increase in the amplitude of the contingent negative variation (30,31,43,56,61,65,75,76). The relationship between marijuana-induced changes in the EEG and neurophysiologic impairment is unknown. Marijuana-induced structural damage to the central nervous system has not been observed in postmortem studies. Previous impressions that gross structural changes occur in the intact brains of heavy marijuana smokers have not been confirmed by studies utilizing CAT scan procedures (23,68).

Reproductive System

Marijuana-induced decrements in plasma testosterone levels observed in one laboratory (24,63,64) have not been confirmed by a number of other studies (28,38,87,89,92,122). However, marijuana smoking has been reported to cause a decrease in sperm cell count and motility (39). Marijuana-induced abnormalities in sperm cell morphology have also been reported (39,48,101).

Experimental animal studies have consistently shown that relatively small doses of THC may have adverse effects on reproductive hormones in females (6,7,16,45,66,67,79, 108,124,125). Marijuana smoking affects reproductive hormones in women differently at different phases of the menstrual cycle (95–97). Paradoxically, marijuana stimulates the luteinizing hormone (LH) surge during the periovulatory phase of the menstrual cycle and thus may increase probability of ovulation (96). But marijuana smoking during the luteal phase of the menstrual cycle suppresses LH (96) and enhances risk for a shortened luteal phase and compromises optimal conditions for maintenance of pregnancy. If pregnancy is sustained, adverse effects of marijuana on LH and uterine function may increase the probability for occurrence of fetal abnormalities. Taken together, these data suggest that acute marijuana smoking may stimulate ovulation but that maintenance of pregnancy may be compromised and, if pregnancy is sustained, there is increased risk for damage to the fetus. Marijuana-induced changes in reproductive hormones may be one important factor that contributes to congenital malformation and behavior disorders that have been reported to occur in newborns whose mothers were chronic marijuana smokers (74).

Acute marijuana smoking suppresses prolactin levels in women (97), a finding that is consistent with data reported in studies with female rodents and monkeys (7,16,44,45,66, 67,133). Marijuana-related suppression of plasma prolactin levels appears unique for women, since marijuana has not been found to suppress prolactin levels in men (64,72,93). Although it remains to be determined if marijuana-induced suppression of prolactin occurs in lactating as well as nonlactating females, inhibition of prolactin secretion during lactation could impede adequate nurturance of newborns who are maintained on schedules of breast-feeding. It is also possible that marijuana-induced prolactin suppression in women could have therapeutic applications for the management of neoplastic disease associated with prolactin hyperstimulation. More precise delineation of the sites of marijuana action on neuroendocrine function should be carried out with provocative tests that have been shown to be efficacious in clinical medicine for identifying hypothalamic and pituitary dysfunction (80).

There have been a number of reports of adverse effects of marijuana smoking on fetal growth and development. A high frequency of low-birth-weight children has been reported for women who chronically use marijuana during pregnancy (130). Prospective studies with large population groups revealed that there was a significant inverse relationship between number of marijuana cigarettes smoked by pregnant women and birth weight of their children. The lowest birth weight of newborns occurred in women who were the heaviest marijuana smokers. Longitudinal studies also revealed that a number of prominent features of the fetal alcohol syndrome were also commonly observed in the offspring of heavy marijuana users (42). Behavioral evaluation of newborns whose mothers smoked marijuana heavily showed that these infants had a higher frequency of tremor and startle responses in comparison to offspring of women who never smoked marijuana (33,74).

POTENTIAL THERAPEUTIC USES FOR MARIJUANA

Because marijuana is classified as a drug that has no applications for medical use (FDA schedule 1), few investigations have been carried out to assess any possible therapeutic uses. In 1976, Cohen and Stillman edited a volume that highlighted a number of possibilities for therapeutic potentials of marijuana (26). Unfortunately, few effective therapeutic uses for marijuana have been discovered and confirmed in controlled clinical trials. One exception is the development of synthetic cannabis compounds that appear to be efficacious for reduction of nausea and vomiting associated with chemotherapy for neoplastic disease (41,73).

SUMMARY

Although recreational use of marijuana by young adults in the United States is decreasing, millions of persons consistently abuse the drug. Since inhalation of pyrolyzed marijuana leaf remains the most common route of administration, marijuana-induced pulmonary disease is likely to become a major public health problem. At present, considerable evidence for marijuana-related impairment of pulmonary function has been well documented in clinical studies. Many specialists in pulmonary medicine believe that marijuana smoking, similar to cigarette smoking, enhances risk for development of lung cancer. Persons who appear to be at greatest risk are women who smoke both marijuana and tobacco cigarettes.

Initial reports that marijuana suppresses testosterone levels in males have not been confirmed, but marijuana use does reduce sperm cell motility and function. The significance of these effects on male fertility have not yet been determined.

Marijuana smoking produces significant changes in female reproductive hormone function. In addition, low-birth-weight children and fetal abnormalities have been reported in the offspring of mothers who regularly smoke marijuana during pregnancy.

Persons who constantly use marijuana in high dosage often have concomitant social, occupational, and interpersonal problems. These individuals are also at greater risk for developing polydrug abuse disorders. However, the specific and unique antecedent biologic, psychologic, and social factors that enhance risk for marijuana or other drug abuse disorders have not been discovered.

Although much has been learned about the chemistry and pharmacology of marijuana and other cannabis compounds, their mechanism of action in the central nervous system is not well understood. Similar to other self-administered intoxicating agents (e.g., alcohol), tolerance and dependence (psychologic and physiologic) on marijuana may occur in men and women.

ACKNOWLEDGMENT

Preparation of this chapter was supported, in part, by grants DA 00064 and DA 02905 from the National Institute on Drug Abuse.

REFERENCES

1. Abel, E. L. (1975): *Int. Rev. Neurobiol.*, 18:329–356.
2. Abel, E. L. (1977): *Psychol. Bull.*, 84:193–211.

3. Abramson, H. A. (1974): *J. Asthma Res.*, 11(3):97.
4. Adams, A. J., Brown, B., Flom, M. C., Jones, R. T., and Jampolsky, A. (1975): *Am. J. Optom. Physiol. Opt.*, 52:729–735.
5. Aronow, W. W., and Cassidy, J. (1974): *N. Engl. J. Med.*, 291:65–67.
6. Asch, R. H., Fernandez, E. O., Smith, C. G., and Pauerstein, C. J. (1979): *Fertil. Steril.*, 31:331.
7. Asch, R. H., Smith, C. G., Siler-Khodr, T. M., and Pauerstein, C. J. (1979): *Fertil. Steril.*, 32:571–575.
8. Barnett, G., Chiang, C. N., Perez-Reyes, M., and Owens, S. M. (1982): *J. Pharmacokinet. Biopharmacol.*, 10:495–506.
9. Beaconsfield, P., Ginsburg, J., and Rainsbury, R. (1972): *N. Engl. J. Med.*, 2878:209–212.
10. Belmore, S. M., and Miller, L. L. (1980): *Pharmacol. Biochem. Behav.*, 13(2):199–203.
11. Benowitz, N. L., and Jones, R. T. (1975): *Clin. Pharmacol. Ther.*, 18:287–297.
12. Benowitz, N. L., and Jones, R. T. (1977): *Clin. Pharmacol. Ther.*, 21:336–342.
13. Blaine, J. D., Meacham, M. P., Janowsky, D. S., Schoor, M., and Bozzetti, L. P. (1976): In: *Pharmacology of Marijuana, Vol. 1*, edited by M. C. Braude and S. Szara, pp. 445–447. Raven Press, New York.
14. Butler, J. L., Gaines, L. S., and Lenox, J. R. (1976): *Percept. Mot. Skills*, 42(3):1059–1065.
15. Cappell, H., and Pliner, P. (1974): In: *Marijuana: Effects on Human Behavior*, edited by L. L. Miller, pp. 233–264. Academic Press, New York.
16. Chakravarty, I., Shah, P. G., Sheth, A. R., and Ghosh, J. J. (1975): *Fertil. Steril.*, 26:947–948.
17. Chiang, C.-W., and Barnett, G. (1984): *Clin. Pharmacol. Ther.*, 36:234–238.
18. Chopra, G. S. (1973): *Int. J. Addict.*, 8:1015–1026.
19. Chopra, G. S., and Smith, J. W. (1974): *Arch. Gen. Psychiatry*, 30:24–27.
20. Clark, S. C., Greene, C., Karr, G. W., MacConnell, U. L., and Milstein, S. L. (1974): *Can. J. Physiol. Pharmacol.*, 52:706–719.
21. Clark, W. C., Goetz, R. R., McCarethy, R. H., Bemporad, B., and Zeidenberg, P. (1979): In: *Marijuana: Biological Effects-Analysis, Metabolism, Cellular Responses, Reproduction and Brain*, edited by G. G. Nahas and W. D. M. Paton, pp. 665–680. Pergamon Press, New York.
22. Clopton, P. L., Janowsky, D. S., Clopton, J. M., Judd, L. L., and Huey, L. (1979): *Psychopharmacology*, 61:203–206.
23. Co, B. T., Goodwin, D. W., Gado, M., Mikhael, M., and Hill, S. Y. (1977): *JAMA*, 237:1229–1230.
24. Cohen, S. (1976): *Ann. N.Y. Acad. Sci.*, 282:217–218.
25. Cohen, S. (1982): In: *Marijuana and Youth: Clinical Observations on Motivation and Learning*, pp. 2–11. U.S. Government Printing Office, Washington.
26. Cohen, S., and Stillman, R. C., eds. (1976): *The Therapeutic Potential of Marihuana*. Plenum Press, New York.
27. Creason, C. R., and Goldman, M. (1981): *Psychol. Rep.*, 48:447–454.
28. Cushman, P. (1975): *Am. J. Drug Alcohol Abuse*, 2:269–276.
29. Fehr, K. O., and Kalant, H., eds. (1983): *Cannabis and Health Hazards*. Addiction Research Foundation, Toronto.
30. Fink, M. (1978): In: *Psychopharmacology: A Generation of Progress*, edited by M. A. Lipton, A. DiMascio, and K. F. Killam, pp. 691–698. Raven Press, New York.
31. Fink, M., Volavka, J., Panayiotopoulos, C. P., and Stefanis, C. (1976): In: *Pharmacology of Marijuana, Vol. 1*, edited by M. C. Braude and S. Szara, pp. 383–391. Raven Press, New York.
32. Finnell, W. S. (1973): *Dissert. Abstr.*, 33A:4875–4876.
33. Fried, P. A. (1980): *Drug Alcohol Depend.*, 6:415–424.
34. Galanter, M., Wyatt, R. J., Lemberger, L., Weingartner, H., Vaughan, T. B., et al. (1972): *Science*, 176:934–936.
35. Galanter, M., Weingartner, H., Vaughan, T. B., Roth, W. T., and Wyatt, R. J. (1973): *Arch. Gen. Psychiatry*, 28:278–281.
36. Greenberg, I., Mendelson, J. H., Kuehnle, J. C., Mello, N. K., and Babor, T. F. (1976): *Ann. N.Y. Acad. Sci.*, 282:72–84.
37. Harmatz, J. S., Shader, R. I., and Salzman, C. (1972): *Arch. Gen. Psychiatry*, 26:108–112.
38. Hembree, W. C., Nahas, G. G., Zeidenberg, P., and Dyrenfurth, I. (1976): *Clin. Res.*, 24(3):272A.
39. Hembree, W. C., Nahas, G. G., Zeidenberg, P., and Huang, H. F. S. (1979): In: *Marihuana: Biological Effects—Analysis, Metabolism, Cellular Responses, Reproduction, and Brain*, edited by G. G. Nahas and W. D. M. Paton, pp. 429–439. Pergamon Press, New York.
40. Henderson, R. L., Tennant, F. S., and Guerry, R. (1972): *Arch. Otolaryngol.* 92:248–251.
41. Herman, T. S., Jones, S. E., Dean, J., Leigh, S., Dorr, R., et al. (1977): *Biomedicine*, 27:331–334.
42. Hingson, R., Alpert, J. J., Day, N., Dooling, E., Kayne, H., et al. (1982): *J. Safety Res.*, 13:33–38.
43. Hollister, L., Sherwood, S., and Cavasino, A. (1970): *Pharmacol. Res. Commun.*, 2:305–308.
44. Hughes, C. L., Jr., Everett, J. E., and Tyrey, L. (1981): *Endocrinology*, 109:876–880.
45. Hughes, C. L., Jr., and Tyrey, L. (1982): *Endocrinol. Res. Commun.* 9:25–36.
46. Hunt, C. A., and Jones, R. T. (1980): *J. Pharmacol. Exp. Ther.*, 215:35–44.
47. Isbell, H., Gorodetzky, C. W., Jasinski, D. R., Claussen, U., von Spulak, F., et al. (1967): *Psychopharmacologia*, 11:184–188.
48. Issidorides, M. R. (1979): In: *Marijuana: Biological Effects—Analysis, Metabolism, Cellular Responses, Reproduction, and Brain*, edited by G. G. Nahas and W. D. M. Paton, pp. 377–388. Pergamon Press, New York.
49. Janowsky, D. S., Meacham, M. P., Blaine, J. D., Schorr, M., and Bozzetti, L. P. (1976): *Am. J. Psychiatry*, 133:383–388.
50. Janowsky, D. S., Meacham, M. P., Blaine, J. D., Schorr, M., and Bozzetti, L. P. (1976): *Aviat. Spac. Environ. Med.*, 47:124–128.
51. Johnson, S., and Domino, E. F. (1971): *Clin. Pharmacol. Ther.*, 12:762–768.
52. Johnston, L. D., Bachman, J. G., and O'Malley, P. (1980): *Highlights from Student Drug Use in America, 1975–1980*. National Institute on Drug Abuse, DHHS Publ. No. (ADM) 81-1066, U.S. Government Printing Office, Washington.
53. Johnston, L. D., O'Malley, P. M., and Bachman, J. G. (1985): *Use of Licit and Illicit Drugs by America's High School Students 1975–1984*. National Institute on Drug Abuse, DHHS Publ. No. (ADM)85-1394, U.S. Government Printing Office, Washington.
54. Jones, R. T. (1975): In: *Marijuana and Health Hazards: Methodological Issues in Current Research*, edited by J. R. Tinklenberg, pp. 115–120. Academic Press, New York.
55. Jones, R. T. (1977): In: *Marihuana Research Findings: 1976*, edited by R. C. Petersen, pp. 128–178. U.S. Government Printing Office, Washington.
56. Jones, R. T., and Benowitz, N. (1976): In: *Pharmacology of Marijuana, Vol. 2*, edited by M. C. Braude and S. Szara, pp. 627–642. Raven Press, New York.
57. Jones, R. T., Benowitz, N., and Bachman, J. (1976): *Ann. N.Y. Acad. Sci.*, 282:221–239.
58. Jones, R. T., and Stone, G. (1970): *Psychopharmacologia*, 18:108–117.
59. Jones, R. T., Benowitz, N. L., and Herning, R. I. (1981): *J. Clin. Pharmacol.*, 21:143S–152S.
60. Klonoff, H. (1974): *Science*, 186:317–324.
61. Klonoff, H., and Low, M. D. (1974): In: *Marijuana: Effects on Human Behavior*, edited by L. L. Miller, pp. 121–155. Academic Press, New York.
62. Kochar, M. S., and Hosko, M. J. (1973): *JAMA*, 225:25–27.
63. Kolodny, R. C. (1975): In: *Marihuana and Health Hazards: Methodological Issues in Current Research*, edited by J. R. Tinklenberg, pp. 71–81. Academic Press, New York.
64. Kolodny, R. C., Masters, W. H., Kolodner, R. M., and Gelson, T. (1974): *N. Engl. J. Med.*, 290:872–874.
65. Kopell, B. S., Tinklenberg, J. R., and Hollister, L. E. (1972): *Arch. Gen. Psychiatry*, 27:809–811.
66. Kramer, J., and Ben-David, M. (1974): *Proc. Soc. Exp. Biol. Med.*, 147:484.
67. Kramer, J., and Ben-David, M. (1978): *Endocrinology*, 103:452–457.
68. Kuehnle, J. C., Mendelson, J. H., Davis, K. R., and New, P. F. J. (1977): *JAMA*, 237:1231–1232.
69. Lantner, I. L. (1982): In: *Marijuana and Youth: Clinical Observations on Motivation and Learning*, pp. 84–92. U.S. Government Printing Office, Washington.

70. LeDain, G., Campbell, I. L., Lehmann, H., Stein, J. P., and Bertrand, M. A. (1972): *A Report to the Commission of Inquiry into the Non-medical Use of Drugs: Cannabis.* Information Canada, Ottawa.

71. Lemberger, L., Axelrod, J., and Kopin, I. J. (1971): *Ann. N.Y. Acad. Sci.,* 191:142–152.

72. Lemberger, L., Crabtree, R., Rowe, H., and Clemens, J. (1973): *Life Sci.,* 16:1339–1343.

73. Lemberger, L., and Rowe, H. (1975): *Clin. Pharmacol. Exp. Ther.,* 18:720–725.

74. Linn, S., Shoenbaum, S., Monson, R. R., Rosner, R., Stubblefield, P. C., and Ryan, K. J. (1983): *Am. J. Publ. Health,* 73(10):1161–1164.

75. Linton, P. H., Kuechenmeister, C. A., White, H. B., and Travis, R. P. (1975): *Res. Commun. Chem. Pathol. Pharmacol.,* 10:201–219.

76. Low, M. D., Klonoff, H., and Marcus, A. (1973): *Can. Med. Assoc. J.,* 108:157–164.

77. Manno, J. E., Manno, B. R., Kiplinger, G. F., and Forney, R. B. (1974): In: *Marijuana: Effects on Human Behavior,* edited by L. L. Miller, pp. 46–72. Academic Press, New York.

78. *Marijuana and Health, Fourth Annual Report to the U.S. Congress from the Secretary of Health, Education and Welfare* (1974): U.S. Government Printing Office, Washington.

79. Marks, B. H. (1973): In: *Progress in Brain Research, Drug Effects on Neuroendocrine Regulation, Vol. 10,* edited by E. Zimmerman, W. H. Gispen, B. H. Marks, and D. DeWied, pp. 331–338. Elsevier, Amsterdam.

80. Martin, J. B., Reichlin, S., and Brown, G. M., eds. (1977): *Clinical Neuroendocrinology.* F. A. Davis, Philadelphia.

81. McGlothlin, W. H., and West, L. J. (1968): *Am. J. Psychiatry,* 125:370–378.

82. Melges, F. T., Tinklenberg, J. R., Hollister, L. E., and Gillespie, H. K. (1970): *Science,* 168:1118–1120.

83. Melges, F. T., Tinklenberg, J. R., Hollister, L. E., and Gillespie, H. K. (1970): *Arch. Gen. Psychiatry,* 23:204–210.

84. Mello, N. K. (1987): In: *Methods of Assessing the Reinforcing Properties of Abused Drugs,* edited by M. A. Bozarth (*in press*).

85. Mello, N. K., and Mendelson, J. H. (1985): *J. Pharmacol. Exp. Ther.,* 235(1):162–171.

86. Mendelson, J. H., Meyer, R. E., Rossi, A. M., Bernstein, J. G., Patch, V. D., et al. (1972): In: *Marihuana: A Signal of Misunderstanding, Vol. I,* pp. 68–246. U.S. Government Printing Office, Washington.

87. Mendelson, J. H., Kuehnle, J. C., Greenberg, I., and Mello, N. K. (1974): *N. Engl. J. Med.,* 291:1051–1055.

88. Mendelson, J. H., Rossi, A. M., and Meyer, R. E., eds. (1974): *The Use of Marihuana: A Psychological and Physiological Inquiry.* Plenum Press, New York.

89. Mendelson, J. H., Kuehnle, J. C., Ellingboe, J., and Babor, T. F. (1975): In: *Marihuana and Health Hazards: Methodological Issues in Current Research,* edited by J. R. Tinklenberg, pp. 83–93. Academic Press, New York.

90. Mendelson, J. H., Babor, T. F., Kuehnle, J. C., Rossi, A. M., Bernstein, J. G., et al. (1976): *Ann. N.Y. Acad. Sci.,* 282:186–210.

91. Mendelson, J. H., Kuehnle, J. C., Greenberg, I., and Mello, N. K. (1976): In: *Pharmacology of Marijuana, Vol. 2,* edited by M. C. Braude and S. Szara, pp. 643–653. Raven Press, New York.

92. Mendelson, J. H., Ellingboe, J., Kuehnle, J. C., and Mello, N. K. (1978): *J. Pharmacol. Exp. Ther.,* 207:611–617.

93. Mendelson, J. H., Ellingboe, J., and Mello, N. K. (1984): *Pharmacol. Biochem. Behav.,* 20:103–106.

94. Mendelson, J. H., Mello, N. K., and Lex, B. W. (1984): *Am. J. Psychiatry,* 141:1289–1290.

95. Mendelson, J. H., Cristofaro, P., Ellingboe, J., Benedikt, R. A., and Mello, N. K. (1985): *Pharmacol. Biochem. Behav.,* 23:765–768.

96. Mendelson, J. H., Mello, N. K., Cristofaro, P., Ellingboe, J., and Benedikt, R. A. (1985): In: *Problems of Drug Dependence 1984,* edited by L. S. Harris, pp. 24–31. U.S. Government Printing Office, Washington.

97. Mendelson, J. H., Mello, N. K., and Ellingboe, J. (1985): *J. Pharmacol. Exp. Ther.,* 232:220–222.

98. Meyer, R. E. (1975): In: *Marijuana and Health Hazards: Methodological Issues in Current Research,* edited by J. Tinklenberg, pp. 133–152. Academic Press, New York.

99. Miles, C. G., Congreve, G. R. S., Gibbins, R. J., Marshman, J., Devenyi, P., et al. (1974): *Acta Pharmacol. Toxicol.,* 34:1–44.

100. Miller, L. D., and Cisin, I. H. (1983): *Highlights from the National Survey on Drug Abuse 1982.* National Institute on Drug Abuse, Rockville, MD.

101. Morishima, A. (1984): In: *Marijuana Effects on the Endocrine and Reproductive Systems,* edited by M. C. Braude and J. P. Ludford, pp. 25–45. U.S. Government Printing Office, Washington.

102. Moskowitz, H., and McGlothlin, W. (1974): *Psychopharmacologia,* 40:137–145.

103. Moskowitz, H., Sharma, S., and McGlothlin, W. (1972): *Percept. Mot. Skills,* 35:876–882.

104. Moskowitz, H. (1976): In: *Research Advances in Alcohol and Drug Problems,* edited by R. J. Gibbons, Y. Israel, H. Kalant, R. E. Popham, W. Schmidt, et al., pp. 283–399. John Wiley & Sons, New York.

105. Moss, I. R., and Friedman, E. (1976): *Life Sci.,* 19:99–104.

106. Naditch, M. P. (1974): *J. Abnorm. Psychol.,* 83:394–403.

107. Negrete, J. C. (1973): *Can. Med. Assoc. J.,* 108:195–196.

108. Nir, I., Ayalon, D., Tsafriri, A., Cordova, T., and Lindner, H. R. (1973): *Nature,* 243:470–471.

109. Novak, W. (1980): *High Culture.* Alfred A. Knopf, New York.

110. Ohlsson, A., Lindgren, J.-E., Wahlen, A., Agurell, S., Hollister, L. E., et al. (1980): *Clin. Pharmacol. Ther.,* 28:409–416.

111. Ohlsson, A., Lindgren, J.-E., Wahlen, A., Agurell, S., Hollister, L. E., et al. (1982): *Biomed. Mass. Spectrom.,* 9:6–120.

112. Perez-Reyes, M., DiGuiseppi, S., Davis, K. H., Schindler, V. H., and Cook, C. E. (1982): *Clin. Pharmacol. Ther.,* 31:617–624.

113. Petersen, R. C., ed. (1980): *Marijuana Research Findings: 1980.* U.S. Government Printing Office, Washington.

114. Prakash, R., Aronow, W. S., Warren, M., Laverty, W., and Gottschalk, L. A. (1975): *Clin. Pharmacol. Ther.,* 18:90–95.

115. Rao, A. V., Chinnian, R. R., Pradeep, D., and Rajagopal, P. (1975): *Int. J. Psychiatry,* 17:233–237.

116. Ray, R., Prabhu, G. G., Mohan, D., Nath, L. M., and Neki, J. S. (1978): *Drug Alcohol Depend.,* 3:365–368.

117. Reeve, V. C. (1980): Presented at the American Academy of Forensic Sciences 32nd Annual Meeting, New Orleans.

118. Reeve, V. C., Grant, J. D., Robertson, W., Gillespie, H. K., and Hollister, L. E. (1983): *Drug Alcohol Depend.,* 11:167–175.

119. Rickles, W. H., Cohen, M. J., Whitaker, C. A., and McIntyre, K. E. (1973): *Psychopharmacologia,* 30:349–354.

120. Roth, W. T., Tinklenberg, J. R., Kopell, B. S., and Hollister, L. E. (1973): *Clin. Pharmacol. Ther.,* 14:533–540.

121. Roth, W. T., Tinklenberg, J. R., and Kopell, B. S. (1977): *Electroencephalogr. Clin. Neurophysiol.,* 42:381–388.

122. Schaefer, C. F., Gunn, C. G., and Dubowski, K. M. (1975): *N. Engl. J. Med.,* 22:867–868.

123. Sharma, S., and Moskowitz, H. (1972): *Percept. Mot. Skills,* 35:891–894.

124. Smith, C. G., Besch, N. F., Smith, R. G., and Besch, P. K. (1979): *Fertil. Steril.,* 31:335–339.

125. Smith, C. G., Smith, M. T., Besch, N. F., Smith, R. G., and Asch, R. H. (1979): In: *Advances in the Biosciences, Vol. 22–23, Marihuana: Biological Effects,* edited by G. G. Nahas and W. D. M. Paton, pp. 449–467. Pergamon Press, Oxford.

126. Smith, D. E., and Seymour, R. B. (1982): In: *Marijuana and Youth: Clinical Observations on Motivation and Learning,* pp. 61–72. U.S. Government Printing Office, Washington.

127. Tart, C. T. (1970): *Nature,* 226:701–704.

128. Tashkin, D. P., Shapiro, B. J., Lee, Y. E., and Harper, C. E. (1976): *N. Engl. J. Med.,* 294:125–129.

129. Tennant, F. S. (1980): In: *Problems of Drug Dependence 1979,* edited by L. S. Harris, pp. 309–315. U.S. Government Printing Office, Washington.

130. Tennes, K. (1984): In: *Marijuana Effects on the Endocrine and Reproductive Systems,* edited by M. C. Braude and J. P. Ludford, pp. 115–123. U.S. Government Printing Office, Washington.

131. Tilles, D., Goldenheim, P., Johnson, D. C., Mendelson, J. H., Mello, N. K. et al. (1986): *Am. J. Med.,* 80:601–606.

132. Tinklenberg, J. R., Kopell, B. S., Melges, F. T., and Hollister, L. E. (1972): *Arch. Gen. Psychiatry,* 27:812–815.

133. Tyrey, L., and Hughes, C. L., Jr. (1983): In: *The Cannabinoids: Chemical, Pharmacologic and Therapeutic Aspects,* edited by S. Agurell, W. L. Dewey, and R. E. Willette, pp. 487–495. Academic Press, New York.

134. Voth, H. M. (1980): *How to Get Your Child Off Marihuana.* Patient Care Publications Inc. for Citizens for Informed Choices on Marihuana, Inc., Stamford, CT.

135. Wall, M. E., Sadler, B. M., Brine, D., Taylor, H., and Perez-Reyes, M. (1983): *Clin. Pharmacol. Ther.,* 34:352–363.

136. Warren, R., Simpson, H., Hilchie, J., Cimbura, G., Lucas, D., et al. (1981): In: *Alcohol, Drugs and Traffic Safety,* edited by L. Goldberg, pp. 203–217. Almqvist and Wiksell, Stockholm.

137. Waskow, I. E., Olsson, J. E., Salzman, C., and Katz, M. M. (1970): *Arch. Gen. Psychiatry,* 22:97–107.

138. Weil, A. T., Zinberg, N. E., and Nelson, J. M. (1968): *Science,* 162:1234–1242.

139. Wendkos, M. H. (1973): *JAMA,* 226:78.

140. Wig, N. N., and Varma, V. K. (1977): *Drug Alcohol Depend.,* 2:211–219.

141. Yesavage, J. A., Leirer, V. O., Denari, M., and Hollister, L. E. (1985): *Am. J. Psychiatry,* 142(11):1325–1329.

Psychopharmacology:
The Third Generation of Progress,
edited by Herbert Y. Meltzer.
Raven Press, New York © 1987.

CHAPTER **169**

The Behavioral Pharmacology of Phencyclidine

Robert L. Balster

Phencyclidine was synthesized in 1956 at the Parke-Davis Company. The circumstances surrounding its initial synthesis and subsequent pharmacological development have been described by Maddox (93), Chen (41), and McCarthy (96). Phencyclidine is 1(1-phenylcyclohexyl)-piperidine, and in the initial full publication on its pharmacology (43), it was abbreviated PCP, with the initials representing the three rings in its structure. It is interesting that some of the earliest street names for phencyclidine were PCP and PeaCe Pill (26); apparently the abuse community reads the scientific literature. The PCP abbreviation has stuck, and now, like LSD, the drug may best be known by its initials.

Parke-Davis' interest in PCP was as an injectable anesthetic, and indeed PCP has a unique and potentially useful profile as an anesthetic (51,67,79). It produced a "dissociated" state in which patients were generally unresponsive and analgesic. They were amnesic for the surgery, and the anesthesia was not accompanied by normal signs of CNS depression. Cardiovascular signs were, if anything, increased, with pressor effects and tachycardia. Phencyclidine was given the trade name Sernyl®. Unfortunately, occasionally unpredictable anesthetic effects and relatively frequent prolonged and bizarre emergence precluded its general introduction as an anesthetic for humans. Ketamine, which is chemically and pharmacologically similar to PCP (97), was introduced and remains in use at present. Phencyclidine was used for some time as a veterinary anesthetic, particularly for nonhuman primates, under the name Sernylan®, but it is no longer marketed in the United States. The early published literature on PCP often refers to it only as Sernyl® or Sernylan® (13).

The initial published report of PCP abuse was in 1969 (88), and an epidemic of abuse was well under way in the early 1970s with a number of descriptions of PCP abuse appearing in the mid-1970s (25,26,46,56,57,113). These papers describe typical patterns and methods of PCP use and clinical problems encountered in treating both PCP overdosage and chronic use. An extensive ethnographic study of PCP users has also been conducted (59).

The first compilation of scientific papers on PCP appeared in 1976 as Volume 9, Issue 4, of *Clinical Toxicology,* and a bibliography of biomedical research on PCP prior to 1978 is available (13). The National Institute on Drug Abuse (NIDA) sponsored a workshop in 1978 on PCP, the proceedings of which were published (114). The NIDA recently sponsored another workshop whose proceedings will also be published (45). The *Journal of Psychedelic Drugs* devoted an entire issue (Volume 12, Numbers 3–4, 1980) to epidemiological and clinical papers on PCP. In addition, E. F. Domino organized a published workshop on PCP for the 1979 ACNP meeting (52), and he coorganized a joint U.S.–French seminar in 1982 (81).

HUMAN PSYCHOPHARMACOLOGY

Information on the effects of PCP in humans can be obtained from a variety of studies. The effects of acute high doses have been studied in the course of PCP's evaluation as an anesthetic (47,67,79). These effects are very similar to those that are seen in PCP overdosage in abusers (3,25).

Because of the bizarre behaviors occasionally occurring during emergence from PCP anesthesia, some studies were carried out to characterize these lower-dose effects in human subjects. The most extensive report is by Pollard et al. (117). They administered PCP to normal subjects in a laboratory situation and tape recorded their verbal behavior and made other observations. Luby and colleagues (89,90,120) also studied the effects of subanesthetic doses of PCP in humans. They reported that PCP seemed to produce a dissociation from the environment that had features in common with the effects of sensory deprivation. They also advanced the notion that PCP intoxication had some similarities to psychiatric disease and that PCP effects could be used as a model for schizophrenia (53,54). This relationship is supported by other similar studies (50) and by evidence that PCP exacerbates schizophrenia in patients (73) and that some PCP abusers develop schizophreniform behaviors after chronic use (2,91,112,133). This possible relationship between PCP and schizophrenia has served as a rationale for studying the dopaminergic effects of PCP (75,100).

Subsequent to these studies in the 1950s and early 1960s there have been few laboratory studies of PCP effects in humans (49,99). The only other information on the effects of PCP comes from observations and interviews of PCP users. Because human subject concerns have undoubtedly limited laboratory studies with PCP in humans, most of the recent knowledge we have on the behavioral pharmacology of PCP comes from animal research.

AMPHETAMINE-LIKE EFFECTS

The pharmacological classification of PCP proved troublesome and has varied. It was initially classified as an anesthetic, but PCP anesthesia is quite dissimilar to that produced by typical general anesthetics (51). In the early years of its abuse, PCP was often classified as a hallucinogen; however, clinical experience and research have found more differences than similarities in the effects of PCP and classical hallucinogens such as LSD. However, PCP has a broad spectrum of pharmacological and behavioral actions, some of which are shared by other drugs of abuse. Other effects are unique to PCP and PCP-like drugs.

Graham Chen, who pioneered the pharmacology of PCP, often characterized PCP as a "sympathomimetic anesthetic" (40), and the reference drug to which it was initially compared was methamphetamine (39). Phencyclidine has many behavioral actions characteristic of dopaminergic agonists (75,100). Among these effects are the production of stereotyped behavior (35,141), ipsilateral rotation in substantia-nigra-lesioned rats (82), increased motor activity (43,74,77,139), decreased food consumption (160), enhancement of the effects of amphetamine (11), and suppression of plasma prolactin levels (123). These amphetamine-like actions are often blocked by antipsychotic drugs (35,60,94,100,106,140,150), although in the case of motor activity increases, it appears that the less-specific antipsychotics such as chlorpromazine are sometimes more effective antagonists than pure dopamine-receptor blockers such as haloperidol (61,62). Also, there is some evidence that PCP-induced rotation cannot solely be accounted for by dopaminergic actions (65,78,134). The lack of cross sensitization

between PCP and d-amphetamine for the production of increased locomotion also suggests that different mechanisms may be involved (66). In addition, Nabeshima and his associates (109,110) have also found evidence for a serotonergic component to the stereotyped behavior produced by PCP.

The effects of PCP on schedule-controlled behavior are also often similar to those of amphetamine, with large increases in rates of responding and rate-dependent effects (7,10,21,115,152); however, PCP's effects on operant behavior are less consistently blocked by antipsychotics (9,84,151). Although amphetamine-like effects on operant behavior have been seen in mice, pigeons, and monkeys, the amphetamine-like stereotyped behavior and hyperactivity are particularly prominent in rodents. The most prominent observable effect of PCP in pigeons is catalepsy (39,84). Monkeys exhibit decreased responsivity, motor incoordination, changes in visual attention, and, at high doses, a characteristic anesthesia (10). These species differences in overt behavioral effects of PCP lead to the speculation that dopaminergic actions are less prominent in primate species, possibly including humans.

The effects of PCP also differ in other important ways from those of amphetamines. The well-known aggregate toxicity seen with amphetamine does not occur with PCP (85), and chlorpromazine does not prevent PCP lethality in mice (86). Phencyclidine and amphetamine intoxication in humans also differs considerably. Consistent with this, PCP and amphetamine do not share discriminative stimulus properties in animals, nor are PCP's discriminative effects blocked by antipsychotics (116,124,157).

Nonetheless, the amphetamine-like dopaminergic actions of PCP are of considerable interest because of the aforementioned connection between PCP and schizophrenia. The biochemical bases for PCP's amphetamine-like behavioral effects have been studied extensively, implicating indirect dopaminergic actions (75,100; K. M. Johnson, Jr., *this volume*). Phencyclidine's dopaminergic effects may be responsible for its schizophreniform manifestations in humans. Like amphetamines, PCP would be expected to exacerbate schizophrenia, and users with this or related disorders or with latent psychiatric diseases may be at considerable risk from taking PCP.

BARBITURATE-LIKE EFFECTS

Although the anesthesia produced by PCP and typical CNS depressants differs considerably (51), PCP has a number of behavioral and pharmacological effects similar to those of depressants such as the barbiturates (14). Phencyclidine has profound motor effects as evidenced by effects on rotorod performance and similar measures (4,80). Like barbiturates, PCP also has anticonvulsant effects in various animal models (43,64,68,122). There is also some evidence that PCP has anxiolytic-like effects in animal models (17,38,153). Perhaps most clinical significance, PCP very markedly enhances the sedative effects of classical depressant drugs, including barbiturates and ethanol. This interaction has been shown in pigeons, rodents, and primates using a number of different behavioral measures, and quantitatively the interaction can be as large as the interaction among CNS depressants (37,145,146,155,159).

DISCRIMINATIVE STIMULUS EFFECTS

The discriminative stimulus effects of PCP differ qualitatively from those of other drugs (115,124). Animals trained to discriminate PCP from nondrug do not generalize stimulus control by PCP to other drugs of abuse including stimulants, depressants, and hallucinogens, nor do animals trained to discriminate representatives of other drug classes generalize to PCP (115,124). Thus, these data are consistent with the ability of PCP to produce a unique type of intoxication in humans and with its separate classification as representative of a distinct class of psychoactive drugs. It has also recently been shown that the same discriminative stimulus effects of PCP are produced in rats whether the drug is injected or inhaled (156), the typical route for human use. Because of the pharmacological specificity of the discriminative stimulus effects of PCP, they have been extensively studied in animals as a model of PCP intoxication in humans.

Although the discriminative stimulus effects of PCP are not shared by other major classes of psychoactive drugs, they are not unique to PCP. Many arylcyclohexylamine analogs of PCP, including ketamine, have PCP-like discriminative effects, and the structural requirements for these effects are being established (18,48,124,127,128, 135,136). The good correspondence between the results of these structure–activity studies and the results of binding studies is among the strongest evidence in support of the hypothesis that the binding site is a physiologically relevant "PCP receptor" and that this receptor mediates the discriminative stimulus effects of these PCP-like drugs (163; K. M. Johnson, Jr., *this volume*).

More recently, drugs from other chemical classes have been shown to have PCP-like discriminative effects as well. Dexoxadrol and etoxadrol, which are 1,3-substituted dioxolanes, are generalized in PCP-trained pigeons, rats, and monkeys (22,79,127). This class of PCP-like drugs is of particular interest because, unlike arylcyclohexylamines, they demonstrate considerable stereospecificity (70,127,131). Stereospecific PCP-like discriminative stimulus effects have also been obtained with 2-methyl-3,3-diphenyl-3-propanolamine (143), a representative of another distinct chemical class. This evidence for stereospecificity provides additional support for the hypothesis that the discriminative stimulus properties of PCP and related drugs are receptor mediated. Phencyclidine-like discriminative effects have also been obtained with benz[f]isoquinoline derivatives (162). These nonarylcyclohexylamine PCP-like drugs are important research tools for investigating cellular mechanisms of action.

σ-AGONIST EFFECTS

Perhaps the most important nonarylcyclohexylamine drugs that share discriminative stimulus effects with PCP are the psychotomimetic opioids. Shannon (124) found that rats trained to discriminate PCP from vehicle generalized to N-allylnormetazocine (NANM); NANM (also referred to as SKF-10,047) is the model agonist for the σ-opioid receptor described by Martin and his colleagues (95). N-Allylnormetazocine and other opioids such as cyclazocine with σ-agonist effects in animals produce disturbing "psychotomimetic" effects in humans; thus, it is possible that there is a PCP-like component to these effects. This possibility was given further support when binding studies found that NANM (165) and other σ-agonist opioids (163) displace ^{3}H-PCP from its recognition sites in brain. This has led to many studies, both biochemical and behavioral, further exploring the relationships among PCP and σ agonists.

Many opioids, including cyclazocine and other N-substituted 6,7-benzomorphans and dextrorphan, have been found to have PCP- and/or ketamine-like discriminative stimulus effects in a variety of animal species (19,69–72,125). There is a lack of stereospecificity of these opioids for PCP-like effects, but there is an important stereoselectivity favoring the *dextro* isomers. This is the reverse of the well-established selectivity for classical opiate actions produced by the *levo* isomers. For example, in the case of NANM, binding studies generally show that the *d* isomer is somewhat more potent for displacing ^{3}H-PCP, although both isomers have affinity for this site (101,107,142,164). In drug discrimination studies too, the *d* isomer is either more potent than the *l* isomer for producing PCP-like effects (126), or, in some studies, only the *d* isomer produces PCP-like effects (8,20). Studies with the *l* isomer of NANM show that it has far greater affinity for classical opiate binding sites than for PCP sites (164) and has potent opioid agonist/antagonist effects *in vivo* (1). Thus, *l*-NANM is a more potent opiate agonist/antagonist than it is a PCP-like drug, and these opiate actions can mask the *in vivo* PCP-like effects of this isomer and/or the racemate under certain conditions. This would account for the inconsistency and lack of complete overlap in the effects of PCP and *l*-NANM and *d,l*-NANM. On the other hand, *d*-NANM appears to be a relatively specific PCP-like drug devoid of classical opiate actions (1). In addition to sharing discriminative stimulus effects with PCP, *d*-NANM also has effects on schedule-controlled behavior similar to PCP (83), shows cross tolerance and cross dependence to PCP (138), produces anticonvulsant effects similar to PCP (67), and functions as a reinforcer (130). Thus, PCP and *d*-NANM appear to have a nearly complete overlap in their behavioral and pharmacological effects.

EFFECTS ON LEARNING AND MEMORY

Relatively little is known about the effects of PCP on learning and memory. Thompson and Moerschbaecher have used a procedure that is often referred to as repeated acquisition to study the effects of PCP and other drugs of abuse. In this procedure, subjects learn a new response sequence every day. The effects of drugs on this acquisition of new behavior are compared to the effects on performance of the same response sequence every day. Phencyclidine has consistently been found to disrupt acquisition at lower doses than those that disrupt a well-learned performance, an effect also produced by *d*-amphetamine and pentobarbital (103,105,145,147). Using another procedure in which conditional discriminations are acquired at each test session, they again found that learning was more sensitive to disruption by PCP than performance (102). Although these error-increasing effects of PCP were often accompanied by changes in overall rates of responding, there were occasions when response rate decreases were not observed with increases in error rates (105,148). In this respect, PCP seemed to have a more selective effect on learning than did heroin or methadone (105).

Interestingly, this selective effect of PCP on learning was shared by the σ agonists NANM (104) and cyclazocine (105). Similar effects of PCP and σ agonists on acquisition were also reported by Tang and Franklin (144). In rats, the σ agonists cyclazocine and NANM impaired the acquisition of a brightness discrimination under conditions in which morphine, nalorphine, pentazocine, chlorpromazine, and scopolamine did not. In the only study of specific effects on memory, McMillan (98) found that PCP decreased matching accuracy in a delayed matching-to-sample procedure in pigeons. A similar effect was found for pentobarbital but not for morphine, *d*-amphetamine, or tetrahydrocannabinol. Thus, a number of studies show PCP to have relatively selective effects on learning and memory. In some cases PCP produces these effects under conditions in which some other drugs of abuse do not, suggesting that PCP may be among the more disruptive drugs for these processes.

EFFECTS ON AGGRESSIVE BEHAVIOR

Phencyclidine has often been associated with violent behavior on the part of users (58,129). This has led to a number of laboratory studies of the effects of PCP on animal aggression. Although a few studies resulted in modest increases in aggressive behavior by the animal receiving PCP at a single dose and/or under limited conditions (24,55,108,118), the bulk of the evidence indicates that PCP decreases aggression at most doses under most conditions (44,55,108,118,121,149). Indeed, in studies of intraspecies aggression, it has been found that there were increases in aggression by the nontreated animal towards the animal receiving PCP (121,150). We have given PCP on many occasions to normally aggressive laboratory monkeys. Rather than making these animals more difficult to handle, PCP nearly always has a taming effect. Thus, there is little evidence from animal research that the clinical association of PCP abuse and violence is caused by a profound direct effect of PCP on aggressive behaviors; it is more likely a complex interaction of the propensity of the individuals attracted to PCP use with the conditions of its use.

TOLERANCE AND DEPENDENCE

Repeated PCP administration can be shown to produce both tolerance and dependence in animals (6,16). Studies of tolerance have most commonly utilized changes in effects on operant behavior. The magnitude of tolerance is usually relatively small, with two- to fourfold shifts in dose–effect curves commonly obtained (16,23,36,154). Most of the tolerance appears to be accountable for by pharmacological mechanisms, including some evidence for biodispositional changes (63,76,111,150,158), although in one study (158) there was some evidence that behavioral factors played a role in the rate of loss of tolerance.

In a study of unlimited-access self-administration of PCP in which monkeys took very large daily doses of PCP resulting in blood levels of 100 to 300 ng/ml for periods of over a month, we (15) observed quite dramatic withdrawal signs when PCP access was terminated. Signs included vocalizations, bruxism, oculomotor hyperactivity, diarrhea, piloerection, difficulty remaining awake, tremors, and in one case convulsions. These signs appeared within 8 hr of abstinence and were most severe at about 24 hr, corresponding to the rapid decline in plasma PCP levels. A withdrawal syndrome has also been reported to occur in rats after high-dose (45–72 mg/kg/day) repeated PCP administration (137,138). The syndrome in rats also included signs of CNS hyperexcitability such as twitches, hyperresponsivity, and increased susceptibility to audiogenic seizures.

We (132) have some evidence that more modest regimens of PCP administration can produce dependence. The operant behavior of rhesus monkeys infused i.v. with 1.2 mg/kg/day for 10 days was markedly disrupted during withdrawal. Grossly observable signs of withdrawal were not remarkable, but the animals ceased responding for food 8 hr after terminating PCP infusion, and responding often did not recover completely for 7 to 9 days. These behavioral effects of withdrawal could be reversed immediately by PCP administration. These behavioral changes during withdrawal are evidence for a more subtle behavioral dependence, which may be produced by PCP and which may contribute to its repeated use (5).

SELF-ADMINISTRATION OF PCP

Data showing that PCP was readily self-administered intravenously by rhesus monkeys (12) were among the first evidence that PCP had behavioral effects that differed considerably from those of classical hallucinogens, which typically are not easily established as reinforcers in animals. The reinforcing properties of PCP in animals have subsequently been demonstrated under a number of conditions in rhesus monkeys (15,22,33,130,161), baboons (92), dogs (119), and rats (32). These studies have also found that many analogs of PCP sharing discriminative stimulus properties with PCP also function as reinforcers. Taken together, these results suggest that many PCP analogs may have PCP-like abuse potential and may well appear in the near future as "designer drugs."

Although early studies of PCP self-administration by laboratory animals used the i.v. route, Carroll and her colleagues have been very successful in getting animals to drink PCP solutions (27–29,33). Even extended sequences of behavior leading to PCP availability can be established using second-order schedules (30,31). One of the interesting findings using this model has been the demonstration that food deprivation reliably and markedly increases rates of PCP self-administration (31–33). This food-deprivation effect occurs with other drug reinforcers such as cocaine, *d*-amphetamine, ethanol, and the potent opioid etonitazine (34) and suggests that general motivational state may play an important role in the propensity to use PCP and other drugs.

SUMMARY AND CONCLUSIONS

Although originally developed as an anesthetic, PCP has received recent scientific attention primarily because of its abuse. Its effects have also been proposed as a model of schizophrenia. Phencyclidine has a unique spectrum of behavioral effects. The most specific behavioral effects are its discriminative stimulus effects. These effects are only produced by PCP, chemical analogs of PCP, a few chemically unrelated drugs with other PCP-like effects, and σ-agonist opioids. There is good evidence that these discriminative stimulus effects of PCP and its biologs are mediated by a specific receptor mechanism. It is not clear how many other of the effects of PCP can be attributed to this mechanism.

Other important effects of PCP include its amphetamine-like actions, which have been attributed to PCP's dopaminergic biochemical effects. These effects are of particular interest to those studying PCP as a psychotomimetic. Phencyclidine also has some classical CNS depressant effects including what may be a clinically significant interaction with CNS depressant drugs. Phencyclidine has been shown to produce tolerance and, at high doses in animals, physical dependence. More subtle behavioral signs of withdrawal at more modest doses can also be shown. Phencyclidine is also readily self-administered using animal models, consistent with its high abuse potential.

Research interest in PCP remains high, partly because PCP continues to be abused at a fairly high rate but also because it has proven to have such interesting neurobehavioral effects. Evidence that PCP may produce its discriminative stimulus effects via a specific receptor mechanism raises the question of what endogenous chemicals normally interact with that receptor. Further study of the behavioral neuropharmacology of PCP will provide important insights into possible functions for this receptor system.

ACKNOWLEDGMENTS

A large part of the research reviewed in this chapter has been supported by the National Institute on Drug Abuse, including research from my laboratory, which has been supported since 1976 by NIDA Grant DA-01442. I also wish to acknowledge my trainees and colleagues who appear as coauthors with me on the papers cited here. They have contributed considerably to the ideas and research results reviewed here.

REFERENCES

1. Aceto, M. D., and May, E. L. (1983): *Eur. J. Pharmacol.,* 91: 267–272.
2. Allen, M. R., and Young, S. J. (1978): *Am. J. Psychiatry,* 135: 1081–1084.
3. Aronow, R., and Done, A. K. (1978): *J. Am. Coll. Emerg. Physicians,* 7:56–59.
4. Balster, R. L. (1980): *Pharmacology,* 20:46–51.
5. Balster, R. L. (1985): In: *Behavioral Pharmacology: The Current Status,* edited by L. S. Seiden and R. L. Balster, pp. 403–418. Alan R. Liss, New York.
6. Balster, R. L. (1986): In: *Phencyclidine,* edited by D. H. Clouet, pp. 148–162. National Institute on Drug Abuse Research Monograph 64, DHHS Pub. No. (ADM) 86–1443. U.S. Government Printing Office, Washington.
7. Balster, R. L., and Baird, J. B. (1979): *Pharmacol. Biochem. Behav.,* 11:617–623.
8. Balster, R. L., and Brady, K. T. (1982): In: *Drug Discrimination: Applications in CNS Pharmacology,* edited by F. C. Colpaert and J. L. Slangen, pp. 99–108. Elsevier Biomedical Press, Amsterdam.
9. Balster, R. L., and Chait, L. D. (1976): *Clin. Toxicol.,* 9:513–528.
10. Balster, R. L., and Chait, L. D. (1978): In: *Phencyclidine (PCP) Abuse: An Appraisal,* edited by R. C. Petersen and R. C. Stillman, pp. 53–65. National Institute on Drug Abuse Research Monograph 21, DHEW Pub. No. (ADM) 78–728, U.S. Government Printing Office, Washington.
11. Balster, R. L., and Chait, L. D. (1978): *Eur. J. Pharmacol.,* 48: 445–450.
12. Balster, R. L., Johanson, C. E., Harris, R. T., and Schuster, C. R. (1973): *Pharmacol. Biochem. Behav.,* 1:167–172.
13. Balster, R. L., and Pross, R. S. (1978): *J. Psychedel. Drugs,* 10: 1–15.
14. Balster, R. L., and Wessinger, W. L. (1983): In: *Phencyclidine and Related Arylcyclohexylamines: Present and Future Applications,* edited by J.-M. Kamenka, E. F. Domino, and P. Geneste, pp. 291–309. NPP Books, Ann Arbor.
15. Balster, R. L., and Woolverton, W. L. (1980): *Psychopharmacology,* 70:5–10.
16. Balster, R. L., and Woolverton, W. L. (1981): In: *PCP (Phencyclidine): Historical and Current Perspectives,* edited by E. F. Domino, pp. 293–306. NPP Books, Ann Arbor.
17. Bandao, M. L., Fontes, J. C. S., and Graeff, F. G. (1980): *Pharmacol. Biochem. Behav.,* 13:1–4.
18. Brady, K. T., and Balster, R. L. (1981): *Pharmacol. Biochem. Behav.,* 14:213–218.
19. Brady, K. T., and Balster, R. L. (1982): *Life Sci.,* 31:541–549.
20. Brady, K. T., Balster, R. L., and May, E. L. (1982): *Science,* 212: 178–180.
21. Brady, K. T., Balster, R. L., Meltzer, L. T., and Schwertz, D. (1980): *Pharmacol. Biochem. Behav.,* 12:67–71.
22. Brady, K. T., Woolverton, W. L., and Balster, R. L. (1982): *J. Pharmacol. Exp. Ther.,* 220:56–62.
23. Brocco, M. J., Rastogi, S. K., and McMillan, D. E. (1983): *J. Pharmacol. Exp. Ther.,* 226:449–454.
24. Burkhalter, J. E., and Balster, R. L. (1979): *Psychol. Rep.,* 45: 571–576.
25. Burns, R. S., and Lerner, S. E. (1976): *Clin. Toxicol.,* 9:477–501.
26. Burns, R. S., Lerner, S. E., Corrado, R., James, S. H., and Schnoll, S. H. (1975): *West. J. Med.,* 123:345–349.
27. Carroll, M. E. (1982): *Psychopharmacology,* 78:116–120.
28. Carroll, M. E. (1982): *Drug Alcohol Depend.,* 9:213–214.
29. Carroll, M. E. (1982): *Pharmacol. Biochem. Behav.,* 17:341–346.
30. Carroll, M. E. (1984): *Pharmacol. Biochem. Behav.,* 20:779–787.
31. Carroll, M. E. (1985): *J. Pharmacol. Exp. Ther.,* 232:351–359.
32. Carroll, M. E., France, C. P., and Meisch, R. A. (1981): *J. Pharmacol. Exp. Ther.,* 217:241–247.
33. Carroll, M. E., and Meisch, R. A. (1980): *J. Pharmacol. Exp. Ther.,* 214:339–346.
34. Carroll, M. E., and Meisch, R. A. (1984): In: *Advances in Behavioral Pharmacology, Vol. 4,* edited by T. Thompson, P. B. Dews, and J. E. Barrett, pp. 47–88. Academic Press, New York.
35. Castellani, S., and Adams, P. M. (1981): *Neuropharmacology,* 20:371–374.
36. Chait, L. D., and Balster, R. L. (1978): *J. Pharmacol. Exp. Ther.,* 204:77–87.
37. Chait, L. D., and Balster, R. L. (1978): *Commun. Psychopharmacol.,* 2:351–356.

38. Chait, L. D., Wenger, G. R., and McMillan, D. E. (1981): *Pharmacol. Biochem. Behav.,* 15:145–148.
39. Chen, G. (1965): *Arch. Int. Pharmacodyn. Ther.,* 157:193–201.
40. Chen, G. (1973): *Can. Anaesth. Soc. J.,* 20:180–185.
41. Chen, G. (1981): In: *PCP (Phencyclidine): Historical and Current Perspectives,* edited by E. F. Domino, pp. 9–16. NPP Books, Ann Arbor.
42. Chen, G., Ensor, C. R., and Bohner, B. (1965): *J. Pharmacol. Exp. Ther.,* 149:71–78.
43. Chen, G., Ensor, C. R., Russell, D., and Bohner, B. (1959): *J. Pharmacol. Exp. Ther.,* 127:241–250.
44. Cleary, J., Herakovic, J., and Poling, A. (1981): *Pharmacol. Biochem. Behav.,* 15:813–818.
45. Clouet, D. H., ed. (1986): *Phencyclidine.* National Institute on Drug Abuse Monograph 64, DHHS Pub. No. (ADM) 86–1443, U.S. Government Printing Office, Washington.
46. Cohen, S. (1977): *J.A.M.A.,* 238:515–516.
47. Collins, V. J., Gorospe, C. A., and Rovenstine, E. A. (1960): *Anesth. Analg.,* 39:302–306.
48. Cone, E. J., McQuinn, R. L., and Shannon, H. E. (1984): *J. Pharmacol. Exp. Ther.,* 228:147–153.
49. Cook, C. E., Brine, D. R., Jeffcoat, A. R., Hill, J. M., Wall, M. E., et al. (1982): *Clin. Pharmacol. Ther.,* 31:625–634.
50. Davies, B. M., and Beach, H. R. (1960): *J. Ment. Sci.,* 106:912–924.
51. Domino, E. F. (1964): *Int. Rev. Neurobiol.,* 6:303–347.
52. Domino, E. F., ed. (1981): *PCP (Phencyclidine): Historical and Current Perspectives.* NPP Books, Ann Arbor.
53. Domino, E. F., and Luby, E. D. (1973): In: *Psychopathology and Psychopharmacology,* edited by J. O. Cole, A. M. Freedman, and A. J. Friedhoff, pp. 37–50. Johns Hopkins University Press, Baltimore.
54. Domino, E. F., and Luby, E. D. (1981): In: *PCP (Phencyclidine): Historical and Current Perspectives,* pp. 401–418. NPP Books, Ann Arbor.
55. Emly, G. S., and Hutchinson, R. R. (1983): *Pharmacol. Biochem. Behav.,* 18:163–166.
56. Fauman, B., Aldinger, G., Fauman, M., and Rosen, P. (1976): *Clin. Toxicol.,* 9:529–538.
57. Fauman, B., Baker, F., Coppleston, L. W., Rosen, P., and Segal, M. B. (1975): *J. Am. Coll. Emerg. Physicians,* 4:223–225.
58. Fauman, M. A., and Fauman, B. J. (1979): *Am. J. Psychiatry,* 136:1584–1586.
59. Feldman, H. W., Agar, M. H., and Bescher, G. M. (1979): *Angel Dust, An Ethnographic Study of PCP Users.* D. C. Heath, Lexington, MA.
60. Finnegan, K. T., Kanner, M. I., and Meltzer, H. Y. (1976): *Pharmacol. Biochem. Behav.,* 5:650–651.
61. Freed, W. J., Bing, L. A., and Wyatt, R. J. (1984): *Neuropharmacology,* 23:175–181.
62. Freed, W. J., Weinberger, D. R., Bing, L. A., and Wyatt, R. J. (1980): *Psychopharmacology,* 71:291–297.
63. Freeman, A. S., Martin, B. R., and Balster, R. L. (1984): *Pharmacol. Biochem. Behav.,* 20:373–377.
64. Geller, E. B., Adler, L. H., Wonjo, C., and Adler, M. W. (1981): *Psychopharmacology,* 74:97–98.
65. Glick, S. D., Meibach, R. C., Cox, R. D., and Maayani, S. (1980): *Brain Res.,* 196:99–107.
66. Greenberg, B. D., and Segal, D. S. (1985): *Pharmacol. Biochem. Behav.,* 23:99–105.
67. Greifenstein, F. E., DeVault, M., Yoshitake, J., and Gajewski, J. E. (1958): *Anesth. Analg.,* 37:238–294.
68. Hayes, B. A., and Balster, R. L. (1985): *Eur. J. Pharmacol.,* 117:121–125.
69. Herling, S., Coale, E. H., Hein, D. W., Winger, G., and Woods, J. H. (1981): *Psychopharmacology,* 73:286–291.
70. Herling, S., and Woods, J. H. (1981): *Life Sciences,* 28:1571–1584.
71. Holtzman, S. G. (1980): *J. Pharmacol. Exp. Ther.,* 214:614–619.
72. Holtzman, S. G. (1982): *Psychopharmacology,* 77:295–300.
73. Itil, T., Keskiner, A., Kiremitici, N., and Holden, J. M. C. (1967): *Can. Psychiatr. Assoc. J.,* 12:209–212.
74. Iwamoto, E. T. (1984): *Psychopharmacology,* 84:374–382.
75. Johnson, K. M. (1982): *Fed. Proc.,* 42:2579–2583.

76. Johnson, K. M., and Balster, R. L. (1981): *Subst. Alcohol Actions Misuse,* 2:131–142.
77. Johnson, K. M., Gorgon, M. B., and Ziegler, M. G. (1978): *Pharmacol. Biochem. Behav.,* 9:563–565.
78. Johnson, K. M., and Snell, L. D. (1985): *Pharmacol. Biochem. Behav.,* 22:731–735.
79. Johnstone, M., Evans, V., and Baigel, S. (1959): *Br. J. Anesth.,* 31:433–439.
80. Kalir, A., Edery, H., Pelah, Z., Balderman, D., and Porath, G. (1969): *J. Med. Chem.,* 12:473–477.
81. Kamenka, J.-M., Domino, E. F., and Geneste, P., eds. (1983): *Phencyclidine and Related Arylcyclohexylamines: Present and Future Applications.* NPP Books, Ann Arbor.
82. Kanner, M., Finnegan, K., and Meltzer, H. Y. (1975): *Psychopharmacol. Commun.,* 1:393–401.
83. Katz, J. L., Spealman, R. D., and Clark, R. D. (1985): *J. Pharmacol. Exp. Ther.,* 232:452–461.
84. Koek, W., Woods, J. H., Rice, K. C., Jacobson, A. E., Hugenin, P. N., et al. (1985): *Eur. J. Pharmacol.,* 106:635–638.
85. Landauer, M. L., and Balster, R. L. (1982): *Toxicol. Lett.,* 12:171–176.
86. Landauer, M. L., Woolverton, W. L., and Balster, R. L. (1982): *Res. Commun. Subst. Abuse,* 3:287–295.
87. Leander, J. D. (1982): *Subst. Alcohol Actions Misuse,* 2:197–203.
88. Lindgren, J. E., Hammer, C. G., Hessling, R., and Holmstedt, B. (1969): *Am. J. Psychiatry,* 141:86–90.
89. Luby, E. D., Cohen, B. D., Rosenbaum, G., Gottlieb, J. S., and Kelly, R. (1959): *Arch. Neurol. Psychiatry,* 81:363–369.
90. Luby, E. D., Gottlieb, J. S., Cohen, B. D., Rosenbaum, G., and Domino, E. F. (1962): *Am. J. Psychiatry,* 119:61–67.
91. Luisada, P. V., and Brown, B. I. (1976): *Clin. Toxicol.,* 9:539–545.
92. Lukas, S. E., Griffiths, R. R., Brady, J. V., and Wurster, R. M. (1984): *Psychopharmacology,* 83:316–320.
93. Maddox, V. H. (1981): In: *PCP (Phencyclidine): Historical and Current Perspectives,* edited by E. F. Domino, pp. 1–8. NPP Books, Ann Arbor.
94. Martin, J. R., Berman, M. H., Krewsun, I., and Small, S. F. (1979): *Life Sci.,* 24:1699–1704.
95. Martin, W. R., Eades, C. G., Thompson, J. A., Huppler, R. E., and Gilbert, P. E. (1967): *J. Pharmacol. Exp. Ther.,* 197:517–532.
96. McCarthy, D. A. (1981): In: *PCP (Phencyclidine): Historical and Current Perspectives,* edited by E. F. Domino, pp. 17–23. NPP Books, Ann Arbor.
97. McCarthy, D. A., Chen, G., Kaump, D. H., and Ensor, C. (1965): *J. New Drugs,* 5:21–33.
98. McMillan, D. E. (1981): *Neurotoxicology,* 2:485–498.
99. Meltzer, H. Y., Holtzman, P. S., Hassan, S. Z., and Guschwan, A. (1972): *Psychopharmacologia,* 26:44–53.
100. Meltzer, H. Y., Sturgeon, R. D., Simonovic, M., and Fessler, R. G. (1981): In: *PCP (Phencyclidine): Historical and Current Perspectives,* edited by E. F. Domino, pp. 207–242. NPP Books, Ann Arbor.
101. Mendelsohn, L. G., Karla, V., Johnson, B. G., and Kerchner, G. A. (1985): *J. Pharmacol. Exp. Ther.,* 233:597–602.
102. Moerschbaecher, J. M., and Thompson, D. M. (1980): *Pharmacol. Biochem. Behav.,* 13:887–894.
103. Moerschbaecher, J. M., and Thompson, D. M. (1980): *J. Exp. Anal. Behav.,* 33:369–381.
104. Moerschbaecher, J. M., and Thompson, D. M. (1983): *J. Pharmacol. Exp. Ther.,* 226:738–748.
105. Moerschbaecher, J. M., Thompson, D. M., and Winsauer, P. J. (1985): *Pharmacol. Biochem. Behav.,* 22:1061–1069.
106. Murray, T. F., and Horita, A. (1979): *Life Sci.,* 24:2217–2226.
107. Murray, T. F., and Leid, M. E. (1984): *Life Sci.,* 34:1899–1911.
108. Musty, R. E., and Consroe, P. F. (1982): *Life Sci.,* 30:1733–1738.
109. Nabeshima, T., Yamada, K., Yamaguchi, K., Hiramatsu, M., Furukawa, H., et al. (1983): *Eur. J. Pharmacol.,* 91:455–462.
110. Nabeshima, T., Yamaguchi, K., Hiramatsu, M., Amano, H., Furukawa, H., et al. (1985): *Pharmacol. Biochem. Behav.,* 21:401–408.

111. Nabeshima, T., Sivam, S. P., Tai, C. Y., and Ho, I. K. (1982): *J. Pharmacol. Methods,* 7:239–253.
112. Pearlson, G. D. (1981): *Johns Hopkins Med. J.,* 148:25–33.
113. Perry, D. C. (1976): *Clin. Toxicol.,* 9:339–348.
114. Petersen, R. C., and Stillman, R. C., eds. (1978): *Phencyclidine (PCP) Abuse: An Appraisal.* National Institute on Drug Abuse Research Monograph 21, DHEW Pub. No. (ADM) 78-728, U.S. Government Printing Office, Washington.
115. Poling, A. D., Cleary, J., Jackson, K., and Wallace, S. (1981): *Pharmacol. Biochem. Behav.,* 15:357–361.
116. Poling, A. D., White, F. J., and Appel, J. B. (1979): *Neuropharmacology,* 18:459–463.
117. Pollard, J. C., Uhr, L., and Stern, E. (1965): *Drugs and Phantasy: The Effects of LSD, Psilocybin and Sernyl on College Students.* Little, Brown, Boston.
118. Rewerski, W., Kostowski, W., Piechocki, T., and Rylski, M. (1971): *Pharmacology,* 5:314–320.
119. Risner, M. E. (1982): *J. Pharmacol. Exp. Ther.,* 221:627–644.
120. Rosenbaum, G., Cohen, B. D., Luby, E. D., Gottlieb, J. S., and Yelen, D. (1959): *Arch. Gen. Psychiatry,* 1:651–656.
121. Russell, J. W., Greenberg, B. D., and Segal, D. S. (1984): *Biol. Psychiatry,* 19:195–202.
122. Sagratella, S., Passarelli, F., and de Carolis, A. S. (1983): *Arch. Int. Pharmacodyn. Ther.,* 266:294–307.
123. Saller, C. F., Zerbe, R. L., Bayorh, M. A., Lozovsky, D., and Kopin, I. J. (1982): *Eur. J. Pharmacol.,* 83:309–312.
124. Shannon, H. E. (1981): *J. Pharmacol. Exp. Ther.,* 216:543–551.
125. Shannon, H. E. (1982): *J. Pharmacol. Exp. Ther.,* 222:146–151.
126. Shannon, H. E. (1982): *Eur. J. Pharmacol.,* 84:225–228.
127. Shannon, H. E. (1983): In: *Phencyclidine and Related Arylcyclohexylamines: Present and Future Applications,* edited by J.-M. Kamenka, E. F. Domino, and P. Geneste, pp. 311–335. NPP Books, Ann Arbor.
128. Shannon, H. E., McQuinn, R. L., Vaupel, D. B., and Cone, E. J. (1983): *J. Pharmacol. Exp. Ther.,* 224:327–333.
129. Siegel, R. K. (1978): In: *Phencyclidine (PCP) Abuse: An Appraisal,* edited by R. C. Petersen and R. C. Stillman, pp. 272–288. National Institute on Drug Abuse Research Monograph 21, DHEW Pub. No. (ADM) 78-728, U.S. Government Printing Office, Washington.
130. Slifer, B. L., and Balster, R. L. (1983): *J. Pharmacol. Exp. Ther.,* 225:522–528.
131. Slifer, B. L., and Balster, R. L. (1985): *Subst. Alcohol Actions Misuse,* 5:273–280.
132. Slifer, B. L., Balster, R. L., and Woolverton, W. L. (1984): *J. Pharmacol. Exp. Ther.,* 230:399–406.
133. Smith, D. E., and Wesson, D. R. (1980): *J. Psychedel. Drugs,* 12:293–299.
134. Snell, L. D., and Johnson, K. M. (1985): *J. Pharmacol. Exp. Ther.,* 235:50–57.
135. Solomon, R. E., Herling, S., Domino, E. F., and Woods, J. H. (1982): *Neuropharmacology,* 21:1329–1336.
136. Solomon, R. E., Herling, S., and Woods, J. H. (1982): *Eur. J. Pharmacol.,* 82:233–237.
137. Spain, J. W., and Klingman, G. I. (1985): *J. Pharmacol. Exp. Ther.,* 234:415–424.
138. Stafford, I., Tomie, A., and Wagner, G. C. (1983): *Drug Alcohol Depend.,* 12:151–156.
139. Stavchansky, S., Riffee, W., and Geary, R. (1985): *Res. Commun. Chem. Pathol. Pharmacol.,* 48:189–202.
140. Sturgeon, R. D., Fessler, R. G., London, S. F., and Meltzer, H. Y. (1981): *Eur. J. Pharmacol.,* 76:37–53.
141. Sturgeon, R. D., Fessler, R. G., and Meltzer, H. Y. (1979): *Eur. J. Pharmacol.,* 59:169–179.
142. Tam, S. W. (1983): *Proc. Natl. Acad. Sci. U.S.A.,* 80:6703–6707.
143. Tang, A. H., Cangelosi, A. A., Code, R. A., and Franklin, S. R. (1984): *Pharmacol. Biochem. Behav.,* 20:209–213.
144. Tang, A. H., and Franklin, S. R. (1983): *Pharmacol. Biochem. Behav.,* 18:873–877.
145. Thompson, D. M., and Moerschbaecher, J. M. (1982): *Pharmacol. Biochem. Behav.,* 16:159–165.
146. Thompson, D. M., and Moerschbaecher, J. M. (1982): *Pharmacol. Biochem. Behav.,* 17:353–357.
147. Thompson, D. M., and Moerschbaecher, J. M. (1984): *Pharmacol. Biochem. Behav.,* 21:453–457.
148. Thompson, D. M., Moerschbaecher, J. M., and Winsauer, P. J. (1983): *J. Exp. Anal. Behav.,* 39:175–184.
149. Tyler, C. B., and Miczek, K. A. (1982): *Pharmacol. Biochem. Behav.,* 17:503–510.
150. Wagner, G. C., Franko, C. M., and Tomie, A. (1984): *Pharmacol. Biochem. Behav.,* 20:379–382.
151. Wagner, G. C., Masters, D. B., and Tomie, A. (1984): *Psychopharmacology,* 84:32–38.
152. Wenger, G. R. (1976): *J. Pharmacol. Exp. Ther.,* 196:172–179.
153. Wenger, G. R. (1980): *Pharmacol. Biochem. Behav.,* 12:865–870.
154. Wenger, G. R. (1983): *J. Pharmacol. Exp. Ther.,* 225:646–652.
155. Wessinger, W. D., Balster, R. L., and Hayes, B. A. (1982): *Fed. Proc.,* 41:1541.
156. Wessinger, W. D., Martin, B. R., and Balster, R. L. (1985): *Pharmacol. Biochem. Behav.,* 23:607–612.
157. Woods, J. H. (1983): In: *Phencyclidine and Related Arylcyclohexylamines: Present and Future Applications,* edited by J.-M. Kamenka, E. F. Domino, and P. Geneste, pp. 337–345. NPP Books, Ann Arbor.
158. Woolverton, W. L., and Balster, R. L. (1979): *Psychopharmacology,* 64:19–24.
159. Woolverton, W. L., and Balster, R. L. (1981): *J. Pharmacol. Exp. Ther.,* 217:611–618.
160. Woolverton, W. L., Martin, B. R., and Balster, R. L. (1980): *Pharmacol. Biochem. Behav.,* 12:761–766.
161. Young, A. M., and Woods, J. H. (1981): *J. Pharmacol. Exp. Ther.,* 218:720–727.
162. Zimmerman, D. M., Woods, J. H., Hynes, M. D., Cantrell, B. E., Reamer, M., et al. (1983): In: *Phencyclidine and Related Arylcyclohexylamines: Present and Future Applications,* edited by J.-M. Kamenka, E. F. Domino, and P. Geneste, pp. 59–69. NPP Books, Ann Arbor.
163. Zukin, R. S., and Zukin, S. R. (1983): In: *Phencyclidine and Related Arylcyclohexylamines: Present and Future Applications,* edited by J.-M. Kamenka, E. F. Domino, and P. Geneste, pp. 107–124. NPP Books, Ann Arbor.
164. Zukin, S. R., Brady, K. T., Slifer, B. L., and Balster, R. L. (1984): *Brain Res.,* 294:174–177.
165. Zukin, S. R., and Zukin, R. S. (1979): *Proc. Natl. Acad. Sci. U.S.A.,* 76:5372–5376.

Psychopharmacology:
The Third Generation of Progress,
edited by Herbert Y. Meltzer.
Raven Press, New York © 1987.

CHAPTER **170**

Neurochemistry and Neurophysiology of Phencyclidine

Kenneth M. Johnson, Jr.

Our knowledge of the mechanisms underlying the behavioral effects of PCP has been advanced dramatically since 1979 by the investigation of structure–activity relationships (SAR) in studies of the PCP/σ receptor site and of the discriminative stimulus properties of PCP. There is an excellent correlation between the rank-order potencies of those drugs that share subjective discriminative properties with PCP and those that are able to displace ^{3}H-PCP from its binding site in brain membranes. These data have prompted the formulation of the hypothesis that the discriminative properties of PCP are mediated by action at a brain receptor specific for PCP-like substances. The SAR studies also suggest that the discriminative properties of PCP-like drugs are similar across species, including primates. If neurochemical or physiological mechanisms underlying the behavioral effects of PCP can be delineated in enough detail, it should then be possible to design appropriate chemotherapeutic interventions for the toxic effects of PCP (i.e., the development of a PCP antagonist). Perhaps even more important is that the discovery of PCP/σ receptors in brain tissue from several species, including man (99), implies that PCP-like drugs are capable of mimicking an unknown endogenous substance. Since PCP produces psychotomimetic behavioral effects, this hypothesized endogenous substance may play a unique role in brain function and possibly in the etiology of schizophrenia and affective disorders in man.

Also significant to our understanding of PCP actions are the effects of PCP that may appear to be nonspecific or unrelated to the PCP receptor. These effects may occur subsequent to a receptor-mediated event, but because they are secondary or tertiary in nature, their SAR profile may not strictly coincide with that of a primary event. In addition, it is entirely conceivable that important effects of PCP are the consequence of biological mechanisms completely independent of the PCP receptor.

The extensive pharmacologic literature on PCP-like drugs precludes an exhaustive review. This chapter primarily examines biochemical and electrophysiological studies of PCP that have used central nervous system (CNS) tissue from mammals. Some neurophysiological research on PCP is not covered, including electroencephalography (EEG), cardiovascular pharmacology, and the *in vitro* electrophysiology of muscle tissue. Muscle electrophysiology, EEG, and other areas of PCP research from leading laboratories around the world are included in the proceedings of two workshops organized by Domino (28,52) and in two monographs edited by the National Institute on Drug Abuse staff (22,84).

EVIDENCE FOR A PCP/σ RECEPTOR

A saturable, proteinaceous, high-capacity site that binds ^{3}H-PCP with modest affinity ($K_D = 200$ nM) was found in rat brain membranes by two independent groups in 1979 (122,131). This site was somewhat unusual in that it was subject to competitive inhibition by monovalent cations and to noncompetitive inhibition by divalent cations in the physiological concentration range (120). The significance of this finding is still unclear, but some investigators feel that the PCP binding site may be associated with one or more ionic conductance channels (3,59). The pharmacologic specificity of this site was originally found to be unique in that only drugs from the arylcycloalkylamine and psychotomimetic benzomorphan classes were able to displace ^{3}H-PCP from its binding site (122,131). The apparent affinities of these drugs were highly correlated with their ability to inhibit rotarod performance, suggesting that this binding site might be a physiologically relevant receptor (122,131).

The list of drugs with moderately high affinity for the ³H-PCP binding site now has been expanded to include some substituted dioxolane dissociative anesthetics (35), benz[f]isoquinolines (78), dihydropyridine calcium channel antagonists (89), noncompetitive antagonists of the nicotinic-receptor-associated sodium channel (54), and the potassium channel antagonist 4-aminopyridine (56). The behavioral effects of the first three classes above have been studied extensively in animals trained to discriminate between the interoceptive cues produced by PCP and saline. These and the arylcycloalkylamine class share discriminative stimulus properties with PCP (38,95,97,126). Moreover, the SAR of the discriminative stimulus properties of these drugs is parallel to the SAR determined using displacement of ³H-PCP from brain membranes (127,132). This correlation and the pharmacologic specificity of the discriminative stimulus properties of PCP have convinced most investigators in this area that the ³H-PCP binding site is the recognition site of an important receptor, referred to most commonly as the PCP/σ receptor.

The use of the term σ derives from the observation that N-allylnormetazocine (NANM) or SKF 10,047, originally described as the prototypic agonist for σ opiate receptors (70), is one of the benzomorphans with PCP-like discriminative stimulus properties (38,95). Inasmuch as the original observations on most of the naloxone-reversible actions of NANM have been refuted (115) and opiate antagonists have little or no effect on PCP-induced behavioral patterns (18,115), it is likely that the behavioral effects shared by PCP and σ opiates such as NANM are mediated through nonopiate receptors. Thus, the term PCP/σ receptor is somewhat unfortunate in that it implies a nonexistent opiate connection (see G. Pasternak, *this volume,* for a review of opiate receptors).

This matter has become more complicated recently because of the discovery of a naloxone-insensitive site with a high affinity for the (+) isomers of several benzomorphans, including both σ and κ opiates (40,57,68,111). A similar but not identical site has also been described using either ³H-NANM or ³H-ethylketocyclazocine in the presence of opiate blocking agents (108,110). Both sites have been referred to as the σ site. These sites have a high affinity for some dopamine agonists and antagonists, such as (+)3-(3-hydroxyphenyl)-N-(1-propyl)piperidine (3-PPP) and haloperidol, and a moderate affinity for PCP and substituted dioxolanes (40,68,110,111).

The (+)benzomorphan site has several characteristics that have prompted investigators to propose its involvement in the psychotomimetic effects of benzomorphans and PCP. First, there is evidence that various (+)benzomorphans are more selective than the corresponding (−) isomers for PCP-like discriminative effects (17,100) and for reinforcing effects (100). Additionally, pentazocine, which is known to produce psychotomimetic symptomatology in humans (41), has a high affinity for this site but little or no affinity for the PCP site (111).

Regardless of these similarities, two facts are very clear: the PCP-like discriminative stimulus properties of the benzomorphans are not correlated with the (+)benzomorphan

site (38,97,108,111), and these sites can easily be discriminated on both pharmacologic and biochemical grounds. For example, the (+)benzomorphan site has a high stereoselectivity in favor of the (+) isomers of both σ and κ agonists (40,108,111), whereas the PCP/σ receptor has only a slight and inconsistent stereoselectivity for σ agonists and has almost no affinity at all for κ agonists (127,128). These sites also differ greatly with regard to density, localization, and sensitivity to cations (57,88,120,129,131).

Other complications arise from the fact that some of the σ agonist racemates and (−) isomers of the benzomorphan series that have prominent PCP-like behavioral effects also have a high affinity ($K_d \sim 10$ nM) for μ, δ, and κ opiate receptors (85,111,127; G. Pasternak, *this volume*). Also adding to the confusion is that under certain conditions the low-affinity binding sites of both ³H-cyclazocine and ³H-NANM represent binding to the PCP/σ receptor (45,129,133).

In summary, the binding data are quite complex. Nevertheless, the pharmacological specificity of the two sites labeled by ³H-PCP or ³H(+)benzomorphans is distinctive. The physiologic and behavioral relevance of what has been referred to here as the PCP/σ receptor appears to be well established. However, the significance of the "σ" site [here referred to as the (+)benzomorphan site] remains to be established. The important questions remaining concern the identification of the endogenous ligand(s) for these sites and the function of these substances. Some progress has been made on the first concern, with three laboratories recently presenting preliminary evidence for a peptide with appropriate activity in binding and/or biological assays (88,109,130). The second concern is one of the primary focus points of the remainder of this chapter. The possible function of the unknown endogenous substances is addressed by reviewing the effects of PCP and other PCP-like drugs on various neurotransmitter systems, paying particular attention to structure–activity relationships where possible. The transmitter substances discussed here include the excitatory amino acids, norepinephrine, dopamine, acetylcholine, and serotonin.

EXCITATORY AMINO ACIDS

Of the several endogenous amino acids that depolarize various neuronal membranes, glutamate and aspartate are generally considered the most likely candidates to mediate excitatory transmission (123). The effects of glutamate and aspartate are thought to be mediated by three or four receptor subtypes, which were classified primarily on the susceptibility of several depolarizing agonists to a variety of structurally related antagonists. Depolarization induced by agonists such as N-methyl-D-aspartate (NMDA), quisqualate, and kainate varies in time of onset and recovery as well as in alterations of membrane conductance involving Na^+, K^+, and Ca^{2+} (25,74,94,105). In spinal motoneurons it appears that one type of receptor is preferentially activated by NMDA and antagonized by 2-amino-5-phosphonovalerate (APV), and a second is activated by quisqualate and antagonized by glutamate diethylester. The third receptor type is activated by kainate but not blocked by either of the above antagonists. In the spinal cord, Lodge and co-workers found that the PCP analog ketamine was a stereoselective antagonist of the excitatory response evoked by NMDA, whereas little or no effect was observed on responses to quisqualate or kainate (64). Antagonism of NMDA-induced excitation of either cat or rat spinal neurons was later found for PCP (5) and several other agents that possessed PCP-like behavioral properties, including etoxadrol and dexoxadrol (10), cyclazocine (6), N-allylnormetazocine (11), and dextrophan (21). Less or no effect was found for drugs such as levoxadrol, pentazocine, ethylketocyclazocine, and levorphanol, which have little PCP-like behavioral activity.

Excitatory amino acids are thought to evoke ^{3}H-ACh release from rat striatal slices labeled with ^{3}H-choline by activating NMDA receptors (60). It has recently been demonstrated that submicromolar concentrations of PCP-like representatives from three distinct chemical classes, including the arylcycloalkylamines, substituted dioxolanes, and σ-agonist benzomorphans, inhibit NMDA-stimulated striatal ^{3}H-ACh release with potencies that are highly correlated with their potencies as inhibitors of ^{3}H-PCP binding (102,103). This response was stereoselectively antagonized by cyclazocine and dioxadrol, drugs with PCP-like behavioral properties (103). Phencyclidine had no effect on ^{3}H-ACh release stimulated by quisqualate or kainate. Similar selectivity for NMDA was observed in the nucleus accumbens and hippocampus using either transmitter release or CA$_1$ pyramidal cell depolarization as the dependent variables, respectively (30,51). However, blockade of quisqualate- and kainate-stimulated ^{3}H-DA release from the striatum has been reported, suggesting that PCP may not be entirely selective for the NMDA receptor subtype (102,103).

These data suggest the possibility that activation of the PCP/σ receptor and the NMDA receptor have opposing effects on the Na$^+$ and/or K$^+$ conductance, which probably underlies the excitatory effects of NMDA. Data from my laboratory indicate that PCP probably does not inhibit the NMDA receptor competitively, in that PCP shifted the NMDA concentration–response curve to the right in a nonparallel fashion when either striatal ACh or DA release was measured (103). This nonparallel shift to the right has also been observed when measuring NMDA-evoked release of either ACh from the cortex (65) or norepinephrine (NE) from the hippocampus (S. M. Jones and K. M. Johnson, Jr., *unpublished observations*).

The agreement between SAR studies of the NMDA receptor and the discriminative stimulus properties of PCP suggests that this receptor may be very important to the actions of PCP-like drugs. Additionally, NMDA antagonists (and PCP) have been shown to be anticonvulsant (20,24) and to block long-term potentiation in the hippocampus (23,106), a phenomenon many feel is related to memory. Thus, there appears to be considerable circumstantial evidence that some of the behavioral properties of PCP are related to the ability of these drugs to antagonize the NMDA-preferring excitatory amino acid receptor.

In summary, PCP-like drugs potently and selectively antagonize a variety of responses to excitatory amino acids, probably by acting in a noncompetitive manner at NMDA-preferring receptors. The precise mechanism of inhibition is not understood, but it has been speculated that the action of ketamine at the NMDA receptor–ionophore complex may be analogous to the action of the noncompetitive GABA antagonist picrotoxin in decreasing the rate of flow of ions through the Cl$^-$ channel without directly binding to the GABA recognition site or altering the individual channel conductance (36).

NOREPINEPHRINE

Based on observations of locomotor stimulant and anticonvulsant properties of PCP, Chen and co-workers (20) proposed a central adrenergic mechanism for PCP. More recently it has been shown that performance in an avoidance–escape task that was dependent on brightness discrimination was impaired by PCP, ketamine, and dexoxadrol but not levoxadrol (112). The effects of PCP on brightness discrimination (and locomotor activity between trials) were blocked by specific α$_1$ antagonists and by an α$_2$ agonist. Although PCP has no effect on the binding of ^{3}H-dihydroalprenolol to β receptors (121), it is not known whether the apparent α effect discussed above could be directly mediated at the α-adrenergic receptor.

The effect of PCP on brain norepinephrine (NE) synthesis and metabolism is still unclear. Levels of NE have been reported to be unchanged by PCP in mouse forebrain (48) and guinea pig forebrain and brainstem (46) but to be decreased both in rat whole brain (61) and in individual rat brain nuclei known to play a role in cardiovascular function (9). Phencyclidine has been demonstrated to decrease the apparent synthesis of NE at the level of tyrosine hydroxylase (37), an effect thought to be consistent with the observation that PCP decreased the firing rate of noradrenergic cell bodies in the locus coeruleus (90). Both of these effects may well be secondary, compensatory responses to the ability of PCP to block NE reuptake competitively and to enhance its release (34,101,113).

At the electrophysiological level, PCP has been shown to produce effects in the cerebellum and hippocampus that are consistent with its ability to enhance the synaptic concentration of NE. Pressure injection of PCP, ketamine, and the 3-methylpiperidine derivative of PCP (PCMP) depressed the spontaneous firing rate of cerebellar Purkinje cells (71–73). This effect was stereoselective (72), reversed by neuroleptics and lithium (73), and was absent in rats whose noradrenergic input had been destroyed by 6-hydroxydopamine (73). Similar effects have been observed with hippocampal CA$_1$ pyramidal cells (12,93). However, another group that measured the effect of i.v. PCP administration on synaptically activated CA$_1$ pyramidal cell discharges found no evidence for the involvement of NE in PCP's depressant effect (107). Moreover, these workers found that both spontaneous activity and glutamate-evoked activity were depressed by either i.v. or iontophoretic application of PCP or behaviorally active analogs (91). Thus, although there is not a consensus, there seems to be sufficient evidence to suggest that PCP alters NE function in a physiologically relevant manner.

DOPAMINE

There is considerable evidence that PCP has amphetamine-like behavioral properties, particularly in rodents. Because PCP induces in some people a psychosis that resembles paranoid schizophrenia, the effects of PCP on dopamine (DA) biochemistry and DA-mediated behaviors have received much attention. These areas have recently been reviewed by Meltzer (77) and Johnson (43) and are discussed in the chapter by R. L. Balster (*this volume*).

Phencyclidine is known to inhibit competitively the uptake of ^{3}H-DA into rat striatal slices (116) and synaptosomes (34,101). At somewhat higher concentrations, PCP is also able to enhance the spontaneous efflux of preloaded ^{3}H-DA from synaptosomes (8,26) and slices (7,118). Whether the ability of PCP to release DA is mechanistically related to its ability to inhibit reuptake is uncertain, with seemingly solid evidence on both sides (7,16,117,118). Phencyclidine is approximately equipotent with amphetamine as an uptake blocker (16) but is about 10 times less potent as a releasing agent (7,16,118).

Similarities between PCP and nonamphetamine stimulants have been noted by investigators who showed that although PCP alone had no effect on striatal DA turnover, it augmented the enhanced utilization of DA produced by haloperidol (26,48). This effect was blocked by γ-butyrolactone or baclofen, suggesting that it is dependent on nigrostriatal impulse flow. This effect of PCP is also characteristic of methylphenidate, pemoline, and amfonelic acid but not amphetamine (33,75,98).

In contrast to the studies cited above in which PCP alone had no effect on DA turnover, there is other evidence suggesting that PCP does alter DA metabolism *in vivo*. With different techniques used to estimate striatal DA synthesis, it has been shown that PCP inhibits tyrosine hydroxylase activity *in vivo* (26,37). This action of PCP may well be a transsynaptically mediated compensatory response of the nigrostriatal DA pathway to the DA release and blockade of DA reuptake by PCP (26). Evidence supporting the hypothesis of transsynaptic down-regulation of tyrosine hydroxylase is indirect. First, in striatal synaptosomes PCP stimulates rather than inhibits tyrosine hydroxylase activity [probably as a result of decreasing end-product feedback inhibition subsequent to DA release (117)]. However, in striatal slices, PCP decreased the enhanced tyrosine hydroxylase activity associated with neuronal depolarization. Second, *in vivo* voltammetry shows that PCP enhances and then decreases striatal extracellular DA (S. Howard-Butcher, *personal communication*). At higher doses, only the decrease in DA release is observed (39). Finally, the decrease in striatal DA metabolite levels observed after a high PCP dose (26) could be accounted for by a decrease in either tyrosine hydroxylase activity or DA reuptake following an increased release of DA.

Electrophysiologic studies of the DA system also support the hypothesis that PCP releases DA *in vivo*. The spontaneous activity of single neurons in the caudate that was inhibited by local application of DA was also inhibited by local application of PCP (50). Inhibition by PCP was antagonized by neuroleptics and reduced in rats pretreated with either reserpine or 6-hydroxydopamine, suggesting

that the effect of PCP was presynaptic (50). The effects of PCP have also been studied on the DA cell bodies of the nigrostriatal pathway (A_9) and the mesolimbic pathway (A_{10}). A biphasic effect on A_9 and A_{10} cells was observed, with low (i.v.) doses increasing firing rate and higher doses decreasing firing rate (31). Only the high-dose effect was blocked by haloperidol. Both enantiomers of the σ benzomorphan NANM increased firing rate in A_9 and A_{10} neurons, with no rate-decreasing effect at higher doses observed. Iontophoretic application of PCP to DA-sensitive A_9 and A_{10} cells resulted in little or no effect on firing rate, suggesting that the effects of PCP were transsynaptically mediated (31). It is interesting to note that the common effect of PCP and NANM was the nondopaminergic rate-increasing effect.

Evidence from nonstriatal systems implicating DA in PCP's mechanism of action is rather sparse, but it is supportive of the hypothesis. For example, PCP inhibits prolactin secretion (66) and retards the α-methyl-*p*-tyrosine-induced increase in prolactin secretion (76). Both effects are undoubtedly related to the ability of PCP to release DA and increase its concentration in the pituitary stalk (76). Tolerance develops to this effect of PCP after chronic administration (66). This tolerance may be related to a decrease in the density of DA receptors labeled with ^{3}H-spiroperidol (66,92). In addition to the similar effects that PCP produces on A_9 and A_{10} neurons, there are data that support the involvement of brain areas that receive A_{10} projections in the mechanism of PCP. For example, PCP increases the concentration of DA metabolites in the frontal cortex (15) and enhances DA release from slices of the nucleus accumbens (S. M. Jones and K. M. Johnson, Jr., *unpublished observations*). Also, PCP-induced locomotor activity in rats can be dramatically reduced by bilateral 6-hydroxydopamine lesions of the nucleus accumbens (32).

In spite of the evidence implying a role for DA in the behavioral properties of PCP, very few studies have addressed this issue using the SAR approach. Two studies examined the effects of the enantiomers of PCMP and found that the behaviorally active (+) isomer was more potent than the (−) isomer in inhibiting prolactin release (66) and in inhibiting the firing of caudate neurons (50). Structure–function relationships in the inhibition of synaptosomal DA uptake by PCP-like drugs have been examined in two studies. In the first, PCP and eight arylcycloalkylamine analogs were tested, and their IC_{50} values were found to be highly correlated ($r = 0.93$) with their IC_{50} values for inhibition of ^{3}H-PCP binding (119). In the second, this correlation for arylcycloalkylamines was verified but was found not to extend to either the substituted dioxolanes or psychotomimetic σ benzomorphans with PCP-like behavioral activity (49). Thus, it seems likely that the PCP/σ receptor and the DA uptake site are not associated with each other. In a similar series of experiments conducted in my laboratory, it was shown that neither striatal DA release *in vitro* nor haloperidol-induced DA metabolism *in vivo* by 13 PCP-like drugs was correlated with their affinity for the ^{3}H-PCP binding site (104).

In summary, PCP inhibits striatal DA reuptake, facilitates its release, and subsequently affects DA synthesis and metabolism in the rodent. These effects are correlated with electrophysiological effects in the caudate and are probably related to behavioral effects such as enhanced locomotor activity and stereotypy (77). However, behavioral effects of PCP, such as its discriminative stimulus effects, which are shared by drugs from the psychotomimetic benzomorphan class and the dissociative anesthetic dioxolane class, are probably not mediated by these dopaminergic mechanisms. In addition, the effects of PCP itself on striatal dopaminergic neurotransmission likely do not involve the PCP/σ receptor. However, recent evidence showing a dramatic decrease in the binding of ^{3}H-PCP in the nucleus accumbens following 6-hydroxydopamine-induced lesions of the ventral tegmental area suggests that PCP/σ receptors may modulate dopaminergic neurotransmission in the mesolimbic pathway (32).

ACETYLCHOLINE

Pharmacologic manipulation of PCP-induced locomotor activity (1), stereotypy (80), and turning behavior (53) suggested that PCP also has anticholinergic properties in addition to its indirect dopaminergic properties. Interestingly, behavioral studies have also shown that mice rendered tolerant to PCP showed cross tolerance with physostigmine and oxotremorine, a muscarinic agonist (86). Physostigmine has also been shown both to potentiate the effects of a low dose of PCP and to block partially the effects of a higher dose of PCP on operant behavior in monkeys (19). The mechanisms that underlie these apparent cholinergic and anticholinergic effects of PCP are unclear but could be related to the observation that ACh and PCP have very similar electrostatic charge distributions, particularly when considered in the vicinity of the muscarinic receptor (67,124).

As might be predicted from such an observation, PCP has been shown to be a weak inhibitor of acetylcholinesterase (47,67) and of binding to the muscarinic ACh receptor (55). Comparison of these activities of PCP to those of two PCP metabolites and the enantiomers of NANM suggested that neither of these activities was correlated with either rotorod activity or the discriminative stimulus properties of PCP (47). It has also been argued that the antimuscarinic property of PCP is too weak to elicit an anticholinergic response following a pharmacologically effective dose (42).

Phencyclidine has also been shown to interact with the nicotinic receptor in various muscle and electric organ membrane preparations. For example, in frog sartorius muscle, PCP potentiated neuromuscular transmission by inhibiting delayed rectification and prolonging the action potential, suggesting that PCP blocks potassium conductance (114). Phencyclidine does not bind to the ACh recognition site of the nicotinic receptor but does bind to the ionic channel associated with it in the electric organ of *Torpedo ocellate* (4). Structure–activity relationships among the benzomorphans suggest that this action is not behaviorally relevant to mammals (54). On the other hand, the ability of PCP to block potassium conductance in muscle may be relevant to its action in CNS tissue (2). Phencyclidine has been shown to block potassium conductance in rat brain synaptosomes, as estimated by measuring potassium-stim-

ulated ^{86}Rb efflux (14). Only the flux through the voltage-regulated, noninactivating potassium channel is inhibited by PCP-like drugs in a manner consistent with the behavioral properties of these drugs (13). The relevance of this mechanism is unknown inasmuch as it predicts that PCP would increase transmitter release as a result of blocking repolarization and prolonging the action potential duration. Although PCP increases dopamine release at concentrations similar to those required for potassium conductance inhibition, the release is unaffected by tetrodotoxin, which suggests that an action potential is not required (118). However, this particular conductance mechanism may not exist on dopamine terminals and may be more important on as yet untested transmitter substances.

The release of ACh itself is affected by PCP as mentioned above in connection with excitatory amino acids. At somewhat higher concentrations, PCP inhibits potassium-stimulated striatal ACh release (62). The ability of haloperidol to antagonize this effect of PCP suggested that this might be the indirect result of the release of the inhibitory neurotransmitter DA onto cholinergic interneurons in the striatum. However, this hypothesis was not borne out by SAR studies of ACh and DA release (63,104). Inasmuch as K$^+$-stimulated release was inhibited by PCP, (+)NANM, and ethylketocyclazocine in a haloperidol-reversible manner, it is conceivable that this phenomenon may be related to activation of the "σ" or (+)benzomorphan site (*vide supra*). If this effect observed *in vitro* is relevant, one could predict that PCP would decrease striatal ACh turnover *in vivo*. However, no effect of PCP was observed on either striatal or hippocampal ACh turnover, although ACh turnover in the whole brain, frontal cortex, and parietal cortex was enhanced by PCP (29,79). The discrepancy between the *in vivo* and *in vitro* effects of PCP may arise from activation of compensatory mechanisms *in vivo* that rely on nonstriatal mechanisms not extant in the slice preparation. Thus, in summary, the effects that PCP exerts on cholinergic neurotransmission are complex, and their behavioral significance has not been identified.

SEROTONIN

Phencyclidine and ketamine have several pharmacological effects that potentially could be mediated by serotonin (5-HT), including analgesia, hallucinations, stereotypy, sedation, and anesthesia. Whether these effects are actually mediated by direct alterations of serotonergic neurotransmission is unknown. Although there has been little work done at an electrophysiological level in serotonergic systems, PCP and ketamine have been demonstrated to inhibit selectively a dorsal root potential in the lower spinal cord evoked by stimulation of brainstem serotonergic cell bodies (58). Comparative studies with the isomers of ketamine and LSD suggested that this effect was not related to the hallucinogenic properties of PCP. However, the depression of this root potential was correlated in time and dose with the sedative–anesthetic effects in cats (58). A similar selectivity of depression has also been shown in which inhibitory bulbar pathways were more sensitive to PCP than facilitatory ones (27). The cell bodies of the descending serotonergic system have not been studied directly, but PCP was shown to have no effect on the firing rate of cells in an adjacent ascending serotonergic nucleus (90).

In spite of the paucity of electrophysiological data, several biochemical studies have implicated 5-HT in the actions of PCP. The most clear-cut effect of PCP and ketamine is that they are potent inhibitors of 5-HT uptake into synaptosomes from rat cortex (101). Both drugs also reduce the turnover of 5-HT (44,69,125), perhaps as a compensatory response to reduced 5-HT reuptake. Acute but not chronic administration of PCP increased cortical 5-HT levels in mouse brain (81). Similarly, the decrease in 5-HT turnover observed in rat forebrain following acute PCP administration was not observed following 14 daily administrations (44). This apparent tolerance may be related to the finding that chronic, but not acute, PCP administration resulted in significant reduction in the density of 5-HT$_2$ binding sites in rat cortex (82). Additional studies of the interactions between PCP-like drugs and the serotonergic system appear to be warranted by these interesting findings.

SUMMARY AND CONCLUSIONS

Understanding how PCP works at physiological, biochemical, and molecular levels is an important scientific goal not only because of PCP's illicit use but because its effects may mimic the actions of an endogenous substance which may play an important role in brain function and may contribute to disordered behaviors such as schizophrenia. Research in the last decade, particularly since 1979, has had considerable impact on this goal. We now know a great deal about the effects of PCP on various neurotransmitter systems in mammalian brain, particularly those that utilize catecholamines, acetylcholine, and excitatory amino acids. We also know some of the anatomical, biochemical, and pharmacological characteristics of the PCP/σ receptor, and we are beginning to understand some of the physiological and behavioral consequences of activating this receptor. What is primarily needed in the future is research with the following objectives: (a) identification of the structure of the endogenous ligand(s) that act(s) at the PCP/σ receptor, (b) identification of the mechanisms by which this ligand is synthesized, stored, released, and metabolized, (c) identification of functional bioassays of the effects of this substance and PCP-like drugs, (d) identification of drugs that are capable of antagonizing PCP-like substances, and finally, (e) determination of the biochemical and physiological mechanisms underlying the diverse behavioral effects of these drugs.

ACKNOWLEDGMENTS

Much of the research reviewed here has been supported by the National Institute on Drug Abuse, including research from my laboratory, which has been supported since 1979 by NIDA grant DA-02073.

REFERENCES

1. Adams, P. M. (1980): *Neuropharmacology,* 19:151–153.
2. Aguayo, S. G., Weinstein, H., Maayani, S., Glick, S. D., Warnick, J. E., et al. (1984): *J. Pharmacol. Exp. Ther.,* 288:80–87.
3. Albuquerque, E. X., Aguayo, L. G., Warnick, J. E., Weinstein, H., Glick, S. D., et al. (1981): *Proc. Natl. Acad. Sci. U.S.A.,* 78:7792–7796.
4. Albuquerque, E. X., Tsai, M.-C., Aronstam, R. S., Eldefrawi, A. T., and Eldefrawi, M. E. (1980): *Mol. Pharmacol.,* 18:167–178.
5. Anis, N. A., Berry, S. C., Burton, N. R., and Lodge, D. (1983): *Br. J. Pharmacol.,* 79:565–575.
6. Anis, N. A., Berry, S. C., Burton, N. R., and Lodge, D. (1983): *J. Physiol. (Lond.),* 338:37–38P.
7. Ary, T. E., and Komiskey, H. L. (1982): *Neuropharmacology,* 21:639–645.
8. Bagchi, S. P. (1981): *Neuropharmacology,* 20:845–851.
9. Bayorh, M. A., Zukowska-Grojec, Z., Palkovits, M., and Kopin, I. J. (1984): *Brain Res.,* 321:315–318.
10. Berry, S. C., Anis, N. A., and Lodge, D. (1984): *Brain Res.,* 307:85–90.
11. Berry, S. C., Dawkins, S. L., and Lodge, D. (1984): *Br. J. Pharmacology,* 83:179–185.
12. Bickford, P. C., Palmer, M. R., Rice, K. C., Hoffer, B. J., and Freedman, R. (1981): *Neuropharmacology,* 20:733–742.
13. Blaustein, M. P., Bartschat, D. K., and Sorensen, R. G. (1986): In: *Phencyclidine,* edited by D. H. Clouet, National Institute on Drug Abuse Monograph DHHS Publication. U.S. Govt. Printing Office, Washington, D.C.
14. Blaustein, M. P., and Ickowicz, R. K. (1983): *Proc. Natl. Acad. Sci. U.S.A.,* 80:3855–3859.
15. Bowers, M. B., Jr., and Hoffman, F. J., Jr. (1984): *Psychopharmacology,* 84:136–137.
16. Bowyer, J. F., Spuhler, K. P., and Weiner, N. (1984): *J. Pharmacol. Exp. Ther.,* 229:671–680.
17. Brady, K. T., Balster, R. L., and May, E. L. (1982): *Science,* 212:178–180.
18. Browne, R. G., Welch, W. M., Kozlowski, M. R., and Duthu, G. (1983): *Phencyclidine and Related Arylcyclohexylamines: Present and Future Applications,* edited by J.-M. Kamenka, E. F. Domino, and P. Geneste, pp. 639–666. NPP Books, Ann Arbor.
19. Chait, L. D., and Balster, R. L. (1979): *Pharmacol. Biochem. Behav.,* 11:37–42.
20. Chen, G., Ensor, C. R., Russell, D., and Bohner, B. (1959): *J. Pharmacol. Exp. Ther.,* 127:241–250.
21. Church, J., Lodge, D., and Berry, S. C. (1985): *Eur. J. Pharmacol.,* 111:185–190.
22. Clouet, D. H., ed. (1986): *Phencyclidine: An update.* National Institute on Drug Abuse Monograph, 64, DHHS Pub. No. (ADM) 86-1443. U.S. Government Printing Office, Washington, D.C.
23. Collinridge, G. L., Kehl, S. J., and McLennan, H. (1982): *J. Physiol. (Lond.),* 322:53P.
24. Czuczwar, S. J., Frey, H. H., and Loscher, W. (1985): *Eur. J. Pharmacol.,* 108:273–280.
25. Dingledine, R. (1983): *Fed. Proc.,* 42:2881–2885.
26. Doherty, J. D., Simonovic, M., So, R., and Meltzer, H. Y. (1980): *Eur. J. Pharmacol.,* 65:139–149.
27. Domino, E. F. (1964): *Int. Rev. Neurobiol.,* 6:303–347.
28. Domino, E. F., ed. (1981): *PCP (Phencyclidine): Historical and Current Perspectives.* NPP Books, Ann Arbor.
29. Domino, E. F., and Wilson, A. E. (1972): *Psychopharmacologia,* 25:291–298.
30. Duchen, M. R., Burton, N. R., and Biscoe, T. J. (1985): *Brain Res.,* 342:149–153.
31. Freeman, A. S., and Bunney, B. S. (1984): *Eur. J. Pharmacol.,* 104:287–293.
32. French, E. D., Pilapil, C., and Quirion, R. (1985): *Eur. J. Pharmacol.,* 116:1–9.
33. Fuller, R. W., Perry, K. W., Bymaster, F. P., and Wong, D. T. (1978): *J. Pharm. Pharmacol.,* 30:197–198.
34. Garey, R. E., and Heath, R. G. (1976): *Life Sci.,* 18:1105–1110.
35. Hampton, R. Y., Medzihradsky, F., Woods, J. H., and Dahlstrom, P. J. (1982): *Life Sci.,* 30:2147–2154.
36. Harrison, N. L., and Simmonds, M. A. (1985): *Br. J. Pharmacol.,* 84:381–391.
37. Hitzemann, R. J., Loh, H. H., and Domino, E. F. (1973): *Arch. Int. Pharmacodyn.,* 202:252–258.
38. Holtzman, S. G. (1980): *J. Pharmacol. Exp. Ther.,* 214:614–619.
39. Howard-Butcher, S., Blaha, C. D., and Lane, R. F. (1984): *Brain Res. Bull.,* 13:497–501.

40. Itzhak, Y., Hiller, J. M., and Simon, E. J. (1984): *Mol. Pharmacol.,* 27:46–52.
41. Jasinski, D. R. (1977): In: *Handbook of Experimental Pharmacology, Vol. 45,* edited by W. R. Martin, pp. 197–245. Springer-Verlag, New York.
42. Johnson, K. M. (1982): *Pharmacol. Biochem. Behav.,* 17:53–57.
43. Johnson, K. M. (1982): *Fed. Proc.,* 42:2579–2583.
44. Johnson, K. M. (1982): *J. Neurol. Transm.,* 53:179–186.
45. Johnson, K. M. (1983): *Res. Commun. Subst. Abuse,* 4:33–47.
46. Johnson, K. M., Gordon, M. B., and Ziegler, M. G. (1978): *Pharmacol. Biochem. Behav.,* 9:563–565.
47. Johnson, K. M., and Hillman, G. R. (1982): *J. Pharm. Pharmacol.,* 34:462–464.
48. Johnson, K. M., and Oeffinger, K. C. (1981): *Life Sci.,* 28:361–369.
49. Johnson, K. M., and Snell, L. D. (1985): *Pharmacol. Biochem. Behav.,* 22:731–735.
50. Johnson, S. W., Haroldsen, P. E., Hoffer, B. J., and Freedman, R. (1984): *J. Pharmacol. Exp. Ther.,* 229:322–332.
51. Jones, S. M., Snell, L. D., and Johnson, K. M. (1985): *Soc. Neurosci. Abstr.,* 11:342.
52. Kamenka, J.-M., Domino, E. F., and Geneste, P., eds. (1983): *Phencyclidine and Related Arylcyclohexylamines: Present and Future Applications.* NPP Books, Ann Arbor.
53. Kanner, M., Finnegan, K., and Meltzer, H. Y. (1975): *Psychopharmacol. Commun.,* 1:393–401.
54. King, C. T., Jr., and Aronstam, R. S. (1983): *Eur. J. Pharmacol.,* 90:419–422.
55. Kloog, Y., Rehavi, M., Maayani, S., and Sokolovsky, M. (1977): *Eur. J. Pharmacol.,* 45:221–227.
56. Lai, W. S., and El-Fakahany, E. E. (1985): *Soc. Neurosci. Abstr.,* 11:597.
57. Largent, B. L., Gundlach, A. L., and Snyder, S. H. (1984): *Proc. Natl. Acad. Sci. U.S.A.,* 81:4983–4987.
58. Larson, A. A. (1984): *Neuropharmacology,* 23:785–791.
59. Lazdunski, M., Bidard, J.-N., Romey, G., Tourneur, Y., Vignon, J., et al. (1983): In: *Phencyclidine and Related Arylcyclohexylamines: Present and Future Applications,* edited by J.-M. Kamenka, E. F. Domino, and P. Geneste, pp. 83–106. NPP Books, Ann Arbor.
60. Lehmann, J., and Scatton, B. (1982): *Brain Res.,* 252:77–89.
61. Leonard, B. E., and Tonge, S. R. (1969): *Life Sci.,* 8(Part 1):815–825.
62. Leventer, S. M., and Johnson, K. M. (1983): *J. Pharmacol. Exp. Ther.,* 225:332–337.
63. Leventer, S. M., and Johnson, K. M. (1984): *Life Sci.,* 34:793–801.
64. Lodge, D., Anis, N. A., and Burton, N. R. (1982): *Neurosci. Lett.,* 29:282–286.
65. Lodge, D., and Johnston, G. A. R. (1985): *Neurosci. Lett.,* 56:371–375.
66. Lozovsky, D., Saller, C. F., Bayorh, M. A., Chiueh, C. C., Rice, K. C., et al. (1983): *Life Sci.,* 32:2725–2731.
67. Maayani, S., Weinstein, H., Ben-Zvi, N., Cohen, S., and Sokolovsky, M. (1974): *Biochem. Pharmacol.,* 23:1263–1281.
68. Martin, B. R., Katzen, J. S., Woods, J. A., Tripathi, H. L., Harris, L. S., et al. (1984): *J. Pharmacol. Exp. Ther.,* 231:539–544.
69. Martin, L. L., and Smith, D. J. (1982): *Neuropharmacology,* 21:119–125.
70. Martin, W. R., Eades, C. G., Thompson, J. A., Huppler, R. E., and Gilbert, P. E. (1976): *J. Pharmacol. Exp. Ther.,* 197:517–532.
71. Marwaha, J., Palmer, M., Hoffer, B., and Freedman, R. (1980): *Life Sci.,* 26:1509–1515.
72. Marwaha, J., Palmer, M., Hoffer, B., Freedman, R., Rice, K. C., et al. (1981): *Naunyn Schmiedebergs Arch. Pharmacol.,* 315:203–209.
73. Marwaha, J., Palmer, M. R., Woodward, D. J., Hoffer, B. J., and Freedman, R. (1980): *J. Pharmacol. Exp. Ther.,* 215:606–613.
74. Mayer, M. L., Westbrook, G. L., and Guthrie, P. B. (1984): *Nature,* 309:261–263.
75. McMillen, B. A., and Shore, P. A. (1978): *J. Pharm. Pharmacol.,* 30:464–466.
76. Meltzer, H. Y., Simonovic, M., and Gudelsky, G. (1985): *Eur. J. Pharmacol.,* 110:143–146.
77. Meltzer, H. Y., Sturgeon, R. D., Simonovic, M., and Fessler, R. G. (1981): In: *PCP (Phencyclidine): Historical and Current Perspectives,* edited by E. F. Domino, pp. 207–242. NPP Books, Ann Arbor.
78. Mendelsohn, L. G., Kerchner, G. A., Kalra, K., Zimmerman, D. M., and Leander, J. D. (1984): *Biochem. Pharmacol.,* 33:2525–2529.
79. Murray, T. F., and Cheney, D. L. (1981): *J. Pharmacol. Exp. Ther.,* 217:733–737.
80. Murray, T. F., and Horita, A. (1979): *Life Sci.,* 24:2217–2226.
81. Nabeshima, T., Hiramatsu, M., Furukawa, M., and Kameyama, T. (1985): *Life Sci.,* 36:939–946.
82. Nabeshima, T., Noda, Y., Yamaguchi, K., Ishikawa, K., Furukawa, H., et al. (1985): *Eur. J. Pharmacol.,* 109:129–130.
83. Nabeshima, T., Sivam, S. P., Norris, J. C., and Ho, I. K. (1981): *Res. Commun. Subst. Abuse,* 2:343–354.
84. Petersen, R. C., and Stillman, R. C., eds. (1978): *Phencyclidine (PCP) Abuse: An Appraisal.* National Institute on Drug Abuse Research Monograph 21, DHEW Pub No. (ADM) 78-728, U.S. Govt. Printing Office, Washington.
85. Pfeiffer, A., and Herz, A. (1982): *Mol. Pharmacol.,* 21:266–271.
86. Pinchasi, I., Maayani, S., and Sokolovsky, M. (1978): *Psychopharmacology,* 56:37–40.
87. Quirion, R., DiMaggio, D. A., French, E. D., Contreras, P. C., Shiloach, J., et al. (1984): *Peptides,* 5:967–973.
88. Quirion, R., Hammer, R. P., Jr., Herkenham, M., and Pert, C. B. (1981): *Proc. Natl. Acad. Sci. U.S.A.,* 78:5558–5881.
89. Quirion, R., and Pert, C. B. (1982): *Eur. J. Pharmacol.,* 83:155–156.
90. Raja, S. A. N., and Guyenet, P. G. (1980): *Eur. J. Pharmacol.,* 63:229–233.
91. Raja, S. A. N., and Guyenet, P. G. (1982): *Brain Res.,* 236:289–304.
92. Robertson, H. A. (1983): *Brain Res.,* 267:179–182.
93. Rose, G., Pang, K., Palmer, M., and Freedman, R. (1984): *Neurosci. Lett.,* 45:141–146.
94. Segal, M. (1981): In: *Advances in Biochemical Psychopharmacology,* edited by G. Dichara and G. L. Gessa, pp. 271–275. Raven Press, New York.
95. Shannon, H. E. (1981): *J. Pharmacol. Exp. Ther.,* 216:543–551.
96. Shannon, H. E. (1982): *Eur. J. Pharmacol.,* 84:225–228.
97. Shannon, H. E. (1983): *J. Pharmacol. Exp. Ther.,* 225:144–151.
98. Shore, P. A. (1976): *J. Pharm. Pharmacol.,* 28:855–858.
99. Sircar, R., and Zukin, S. R. (1983): *Life Sci.,* 33(Sup. 1):259–262.
100. Slifer, B. L., and Balster, R. L. (1983): *J. Pharmacol. Exp. Ther.,* 225:522–528.
101. Smith, R. C., Meltzer, H. Y., Arora, R. C., and Davis, J. M. (1977): *Biochem. Pharmacol.,* 26:1436–1439.
102. Snell, L. D., and Johnson, K. M. (1985): *J. Pharmacol. Exp. Ther.,* 235:50–57.
103. Snell, L. D., and Johnson, K. M. (1986): *J. Pharmacol. Exp. Ther.,* 238:938–946.
104. Snell, L. D., Mueller, Z. M., Gannon, R. L., Silverman, P. B., and Johnson, K. M. (1984): *J. Pharmacol. Exp. Ther.,* 231:261–269.
105. Sonnhof, U., and Buhrle, C. (1981): In: *Advances in Biochemical Psychopharmacology,* edited by G. Dichara and G. L. Gessa, pp. 195–204. Raven Press, New York.
106. Stringer, J. L., Greenfield, L. J., Hackett, J. T., and Guyenet, P. G. (1983): *Brain Res.,* 280:127–138.
107. Stringer, J. L., and Guyenet, P. G. (1982): *Brain Res.,* 252:343–352.
108. Su, T.-P. (1981): *Eur. J. Pharmacol.,* 75:81–82.
109. Su, T.-P., and Weissman, A. D. (1985): *Soc. Neurosci. Abstr.,* 11:309.
110. Tam, S. W. (1983): *Proc. Natl. Acad. Sci. U.S.A.,* 80:6703–6707.
111. Tam, S. W. (1985): *Eur. J. Pharmacol.,* 109:33–41.
112. Tang, A. H., and Franklin, S. R. (1983): *J. Pharmacol. Exp. Ther.,* 225:503–508.
113. Taub, H. D., Montel, H., Hau, G., and Starke, K. (1975): *Naunyn Schmiedebergs Arch. Pharmacol.,* 291:47–54.
114. Tsai, M.-C., Albuquerque, E. X., Aronstam, R. S., Eldefrawi, A. T., Eldefrawi, M. E., et al. (1980): *Mol. Pharmacol.,* 18:159–166.
115. Vaupel, D. B. (1983): In: *Phencyclidine and Related Arylcycloh-*

exylamines: Present and Future Applications, edited by J.-M. Kamenka, E. F. Domino, and P. Geneste, pp. 347–368. NPP Books, Ann Arbor.

116. Vickroy, T. W., and Johnson, K. M. (1980): *Subst. Alcohol Actions Misuse*, 1:351–354.

117. Vickroy, T. W., and Johnson, K. M. (1981): *Eur. J. Pharmacol.*, 71:463–473.

118. Vickroy, T. W., and Johnson, K. M. (1982): *J. Pharmacol. Exp. Ther.*, 223:669–674.

119. Vignon, J., and Lazdunski, M. (1984): *Biochem. Pharmacol.*, 33:700–702.

120. Vignon, J., Vincent, J. P., Bidard, J. N., Kamenka, J. M., Geneste, P., et al. (1982): *Eur. J. Pharmacol.*, 81:531–542.

121. Vincent, J. P., Cavey, D., Kamenka, J. M., Geneste, P., and Lazdunski, M. (1978): *Brain Res.*, 152:176–182.

122. Vincent, J. P., Kartalovski, B., Geneste, P., Kamenka, J., and Lazdunski, M. (1979): *Proc. Natl. Acad. Sci. U.S.A.*, 76:5372–5376.

123. Watkins, J. C., and Evans, R. H. (1981): *Annu. Rev. Pharmacol. Toxicol.*, 21:165–204.

124. Weinstein, H., Maayani, S., Cohen, S., and Sokolovsky, M. (1973): *Mol. Pharmacol.*, 9:820–834.

125. Ylitalo, P., Saarnivaara, L., and Ahtee, L. (1976): *Acta Anesth. Scand.*, 20:216–220.

126. Zimmerman, D. M., Woods, J. H., and Hynes, M. D. (1983): In: *Phencyclidine and Related Arylcyclohexylamines: Present and Future Applications*, edited by J.-M. Kamenka, E. F. Domino, and P. Geneste, pp. 107–124. NPP Books, Ann Arbor.

127. Zukin, S. R., Brady, K. T., Slifer, B. L., and Balster, R. L. (1984): *Brain Res.*, 294:174–177.

128. Zukin, S. R., Fitz-Syage, M. L., Nichtenhauser, R., and Zukin, R. S. (1983): *Brain Res.*, 258:277–284.

129. Zukin, S. R., Tempel, A., Gardnen, E. L., and Zukin, R. S. (1986): *J. Neurochem.*, 46:1032–1041.

130. Zukin, S. R., Zukin, R. S., Vale, W., Rivier, J., Nichtenhauser, R., Smell, L. D., and Johnson, K. M. (1987): *Brain Res. (in press)*.

131. Zukin, S. R., and Zukin, R. S. (1979): *Proc. Natl. Acad. Sci. U.S.A.*, 76:5372–5376.

132. Zukin, S. R., and Zukin, R. S. (1981): In: *PCP (Phencyclidine): Historical and Current Perspectives*, edited by E. F. Domino, pp. 105–130. NPP Books, Ann Arbor.

133. Zukin, R. S., and Zukin, S. R. (1981): *Mol. Pharmacol.*, 20:246–254.

Psychopharmacology:
The Third Generation of Progress,
edited by Herbert Y. Meltzer.
Raven Press, New York © 1987.

CHAPTER 171

Tobacco Dependence

Reese T. Jones

In 1982 in the United States, 623 billion cigarettes (or about 6.2 trillion doses of nicotine) were sold to 55 million tobacco users who smoke mainly to experience tobacco's psychoactive effects. Most smokers would like to quit but find they cannot stop smoking (25,49,55,64). They behave as if they are addicted. Finally, a consensus has developed (among researchers of tobacco psychopharmacology, at least) that "nicotine is a prototypic drug of abuse" (39,76). As happens in science, what was obvious and proven to a few gradually has become accepted by the majority. Over the past 10 years, discussions of the tobacco smoking "habit" have, with increasing frequency, included the terms dependence or addiction to characterize that behavior (26,39,49).

Information relevant to the psychopharmacology of tobacco has grown enormously in the last 10 years. The handful of researchers publishing data suggesting "cigarette smoking is probably the most addictive and dependence-producing form of object-specific, self-administered gratification known to man" (64) has grown to dozens of major research programs on tobacco psychopharmacology and an enormous, exponentially expanding literature.

This chapter cites only a portion of the literature relevant to tobacco dependence, selecting topics that are important because of uncertainties resolved or because new findings set the stage for further research. Fortunately, recent books, reviews, and conference proceedings cover the whole of tobacco psychopharmacology and provide a more balanced and complete review of progress (1,5,7,13,16,18,20, 21,26,28,38,49,56,58,60,64,76). The periodic Surgeon General's reports to Congress on Smoking and Health and the National Institute on Drug Abuse Research Monograph series (see ref. 26 for a 10-year listing) offer comprehensive reviews of selected topics.

ECONOMICS OF TOBACCO DEPENDENCE

Tobacco use and its consequences have economic import far greater than other psychoactive drugs. Economics must be considered when trying to understand tobacco dependence and to understand seemingly inconsistent public policy. The tobacco industry ranks in the top five U.S. industries (24). Tobacco users spent almost $25 billion on tobacco products in 1982, accounting for 1% of personal disposable income and 6% of nondurable goods expenditures. Tobacco use contributes about $60 billion to the United States economy or 2.5% of the gross national product (24).

Tobacco use results in enormous economic burdens as well. Cigarette smoking is the principal cause of preventable morbidity and premature mortality (24,25). Excess mortality from cigarette smoking exceeds 350,000 deaths each year in the United States. Total direct health care costs associated with tobacco smoking exceed $16 billion annually in the United States. Indirect costs from lost productivity and earnings add $37 billion (24).

IS COMPULSIVE TOBACCO USE A MATTER OF PERSONAL CHOICE, JUST A HABIT, OR DEPENDENCE?

As judged by most surveys, more than 90% of all people and 60 to 80% of all tobacco smokers believe smoking to be harmful to health (25,49,55,64,65). When asked, 50 to 97% of tobacco smokers say they would stop smoking if they could. At least 60% have attempted to stop smoking before returning to tobacco use (64). Tobacco industry spokesmen maintain the position that cigarette smoking is merely a matter of "personal choice" and "a freely chosen adult custom." Nevertheless, tobacco dependence is now included as a diagnosis in the third revision of the American Psychiatric Association's *Diagnostic and Statistical Manual* (DSM-III). The package insert for prescribed nicotine warns about nicotine dependence. Comprehensive reviews of tobacco psychopharmacology generally conclude that tobacco smoking has all the attributes of drug use considered to be addicting (21,26,28,36,38–40,49,64,76).

When cigarette smoking is suddenly stopped, irritability, restlessness, difficulty concentrating, hunger, depression, craving, and other subjective, behavioral, and physiologic changes rapidly appear (22,26,38,43,49,64,70,75). Smokers with a high preabstinence nicotine intake, as measured by biochemical markers of smoke intake (plasma nicotine levels, expired air carbon monoxide), experience the most intense symptoms (75). Daily cigarette consumption does not predict withdrawal syndrome intensity, supporting the belief that inhaled dose is not measured by simply counting number of cigarettes smoked per day. Partial replacement of nicotine lost during abstinence by oral, transdermal, or intravenous nicotine reduces withdrawal discomfort (26,34,39,46,63,68,70). Smokers who stop using tobacco generally gain body weight rapidly and typically are 8 to 10 lb heavier 6 months or a year after stopping (35). Greater weight gain is associated with more cigarettes smoked per day and a past history of higher body weight. The use of nicotine gum does not always prevent weight gain during tobacco abstinence (35,68).

THE IMPORTANCE OF NICOTINE IN TOBACCO PRODUCTS

If tobacco contained no nicotine, it is unlikely that people would smoke, chew, or snuff as persistently as they do. If smokers did not develop tolerance to nicotine, most tobacco-induced problems would diminish because less tobacco would be used less often. People smoke tobacco for many reasons—psychological, social, cultural—but pharmacological effects, mainly produced by nicotine, provide the basis for continued smoking and other tobacco use even though most users are quite unaware of most of them (26,36,40,53,56,64,69,75).

Nicotine, in doses taken by tobacco smokers, is a remarkably versatile and potent psychoactive drug with diverse effects. Depending on dose, history of nicotine exposure, and the specific biological system under study, nicotine produces a complex array of stimulant and depressant effects involving central and peripheral nervous (6,7,21,43,60), cardiovascular (16), endocrine (57,58), gastrointestinal, and skeletal motor (20,21,56) systems. Nicotine can stimulate or relax (6,7,21,43,60) and enhance learning and attention (7,21,74) under drug administration conditions that allow practiced smokers to regulate dose delivered to brain precisely (5,44). Older studies of nicotine phar-

macology often used doses much higher than commonly consumed in tobacco smoking. Thus, pharmacology textbook descriptions of nicotine as mainly a stimulant of autonomic ganglia and nicotinic muscarinic receptors are describing high-concentration effects for the most part. For a typical tobacco smoker, nicotine's actions are more complex, depending on dose, presmoking autonomic tone, tobacco exposure, and other drug history (6,7,21,22,40,56,60,65).

WHY DO PEOPLE START SMOKING?

The pharmacology of nicotine or tobacco does not explain why someone first begins to smoke. Tobacco effects are initially aversive. A person must learn to smoke (49). A typical 13-year-old beginner smokes more for social, psychological, and cultural reasons rather than to experience the stimulant effects of nicotine or because of an abstinence syndrome associated with nicotine dependence. Only after a smoker learns to inhale and to manipulate dose and establishes a regular smoking pattern do pharmacological considerations become primary in maintaining nicotine dependence (38,64,65). The transition from experimentation and usually intermittent smoking to nicotine dependence associated with regular, intensive tobacco use takes less than 2 or 3 years and perhaps for some smokers only months or even weeks (5,7,28,49).

As the smoking pattern evolves and becomes well practiced, stimuli such as tobacco flavor, aroma, and a host of other associated elements of the complex smoking ritual interact with social and psychological considerations (40,49,56). A $2.65 billion per year tobacco use education activity (sometimes called advertising and promotion) (24) enhances secondary associations among psychological, physiological, pharmacological, and social aspects of tobacco dependence (28,49,56,64). It may be the secondary associations and ancillary stimuli that make nicotine the powerful reinforcer that it is for humans (21,38,61,62).

NEURAL MECHANISMS

What seem to be a variety of nicotinic receptors in brain (and elsewhere) offer a range of very-high-, high-, and low-affinity variations (2–4,45,51). Much remains to be learned about mechanisms of nicotine actions in the central nervous system. It is unclear whether all nicotinic receptors are cholinergic, what the function of these receptors is, or how they are involved in tolerance, dependence, antianxiety, muscle relaxant, and memory-enhancing effects of nicotine (4). *In vivo* nicotine, at doses producing EEG arousal, releases acetylcholine as it does in *in vitro* preparations (20). Thus, presynaptic nicotinic receptors may enhance release of acetylcholine. At higher nicotine concentrations, presynaptic muscarinic receptors inhibit acetylcholine release from cholinergic neurons (60). Stimulation of peripheral afferents and subsequent release of catecholamines, other neurotransmitters, and neuromodulators (serotonin, dopamine, histamine, endorphins) may enhance the direct central effects of nicotine (20,57,58). Nicotine or tobacco smoking markedly decreases phasic stretch reflexes (for example, patellar reflex) by central and peripheral mechanisms, depending on dose. Magnitude of effect varies among individual skeletal muscles. The combination of psychic and physiologic arousal concurrent with skeletal muscle relaxation may be one element in the appeal of nicotine to a tobacco user (20,60).

DOSE CONSIDERATIONS: THE WELL-ENGINEERED CIGARETTE

In understanding the psychopharmacology of tobacco, a fundamental consideration is measuring or specifying dose consumed. One of the important advances during the past 10 years is a better appreciation of the complexity of characterizing nicotine or smoked tobacco dose (11,15,18,23,36).

The modern cigarette is a carefully engineered, efficient device for getting the maximum amount of nicotine to the brain in concentrated form. During the past 20 years, the average nicotine yield of cigarettes smoked in the United States has decreased from 2.3 mg to 1.2 mg, and the average tar yield from 38 mg to less than 12 mg per cigarette (25,48). Brands delivering as little as 0.1 mg of nicotine per cigarette have a significant share of the market (25). It is important to understand that low-yield cigarettes do not contain any less nicotine and in some instances contain more nicotine than so-called high-yield cigarettes (11).

Specifying yields of cigarettes does not necessarily specify nicotine dose actually absorbed (11,14,44,48). Low yield is mainly a result of removing tar and nicotine by filtration systems or cigarette design allowing for dilution of mainstream smoke with air during smoking. For some cigarette brands, nicotine dose per puff depends on whether filter ventilation holes are covered by the smoker's finger or lips (48,50). Measures of nicotine and other tobacco combustion products in plasma show that, except perhaps in the case of extremely low-tar, low-nicotine delivery cigarettes, actual drug intake is relatively independent of dose implied by nicotine or tar delivery figures as measured by smoking machines (16,38,48,67,69).

CIGARETTE SMOKING IS A COMPLEX BEHAVIOR

Smoking is a complex, highly practiced, overlearned, relatively automatic behavior (18,27). Without awareness, smokers adjust dose on a puff-by-puff basis (5,48,50,72,73). Estimates of cigarettes smoked per day usually used in studies of smoking and health-related consequences do not adequately characterize individual daily doses of nicotine and the other substances in burning tobacco (11,14–16,67,69). Some smokers change puff number and rate as the nicotine content of the cigarette or the amount of nicotine delivered in the smoke of the cigarette varies (8,18,27,36). Other smokers or, to a degree, all smokers alter puff volume, inhalation volume, and rate and thus vary the nicotine dose and combustion products actually absorbed (8,11,14,29,41,42,44,48,54,59,77).

A typical puff contains 30 to 40 ml of mainstream smoke (29,41). A typical inhalation contains from 0.5 to 1 liter or more of the mixture of mainstream smoke in the puff and ambient room air, thus diluting smoke actually delivered to lung alveoli, where most cigarette smoke absorption occurs (42,44). Nicotine is steam distilled just ahead of the burning phase of the tobacco rod and is inhaled as a fine aerosol of 0.2- to 0.5-μm particles. The kinetics of aerosol transport from inhaled air to blood are complex and in the case of nicotine not well studied. Measuring carboxyhemoglobin changes as an index of nicotine absorption is only partially predictive (14,44,54), possibly because of differences in absorption of aerosols and gases in the lung and because the kinetics of nicotine and carbon monoxide are so different (13,16).

WHAT A DIFFERENCE A PUFF MAKES

Each puff during the 10 min or so that a typical cigarette is smoked should be considered as a single dose. As a cigarette is smoked, the concentration of nicotine and carbon monoxide in each successive individual puff increases. The last puff of 10 contains much more nicotine than the first because of progressive filtering and nicotine accumulation in the tobacco rod (47). Thus, one or two additional puffs can markedly change total dose absorbed from a cigarette no matter what its machine-determined yield.

The actual nicotine content of tobacco products is a limiting factor in self-dose regulation. By tradition, the nicotine content of cigarettes or other tobacco products is not listed or even considered in such classifications as the Federal Trade Commission rankings of nicotine and tar yields. Tobacco varieties range from 0.2 to almost 5% in nicotine content. Thus, by agricultural and genetic manipulations and blending, it is possible to vary nicotine content over a wide range if a low-nicotine cigarette was merely the goal. However, on average, almost all present-day cigarettes sold in the United States contain 8 to 9 mg of nicotine with little variation among most popular brands (11). Perhaps smokers as a group will not settle for much less.

PHARMACOKINETICS AND METABOLISM OF NICOTINE

It should not be surprising that nicotine has pharmacokinetic characteristics that make it an ideal psychoactive drug for self-administration (16). The regular use of nicotine by a billion smokers throughout the world suggests that nicotine is a very special drug.

Absorption

Nicotine is a weak base with a pK_a of 7.9. At the pH of blood (7.4), nicotine is about 69% ionized and 31% unionized. Its water or lipid solubility and ability to cross membranes depend on pH. In acidic environments, for example in cigarette smoke (pH 5.5), little buccal or upper airway absorption occurs. In contrast, nicotine in the alkaline (pH 8.5) smoke of air-cured pipe, cigar, and occasionally cigarette tobacco is significantly absorbed in the mouth. When tobacco smoke reaches the 70 m² membranes of the capillary vessel network of lung alveoli and small airways, 80 to 90% of the nicotine is rapidly absorbed independent of smoke pH. A typical smoker of leading North American brand cigarettes absorbs about 1 mg of nicotine per cigarette (15,16,23,67).

Distribution in the Body

Smoking is the most efficient way of delivering a drug to the brain short of carotid artery or direct intracerebral injections. Entry to brain via the lung is more rapid and offers less opportunity for drug metabolism, binding, and distribution than does injection into the systemic venous circulation or oral routes (16). Nicotine reaches the brain within 7 sec after inhalation while smoking a cigarette. Brain levels rise rapidly and then decline as rapidly as nicotine is subsequently distributed to skeletal muscle and other body tissues (16). Nicotine has high affinity for skeletal muscle (occupying, for example, 40 to 50% of the body weight in the monkey), though there is marked accumulation of nicotine in brain as well (16,20). The time course of central nervous system effects while smoking a cigarette is more determined by distribution half-life (8 min) than elimination half-life of nicotine (2 hr) (16,23).

Modern cigarettes are formulated and engineered to produce smoke suitably flavored and nonirritating enough to be inhaled deeply into lung alveoli. Nicotine concentrations and rate of change in concentration in the blood reaching the brain after each puff are greater than would be possible to produce with intravenous injection of a similar dose into an arm vein. Arterial and brain levels of nicotine are higher than what is measured in peripheral venous blood during or immediately after smoking. The smoking process allows for relatively precise puff-by-puff dose regulation that would be difficult to mimic even with repeated intravenous administration. The rapid brain uptake and consequences of a concentrated bolus of nicotine may account for the highly reinforcing nature of cigarette smoking as compared to tobacco chewing or snuffing.

Animal self-administration experiments with nicotine must consider the special nature of nicotine delivery to brain by lung if the data are to be most relevant to understanding cigarette smoking. Unfortunately, it is difficult to get most animals to smoke tobacco as readily as humans dependent on nicotine do, though clearly animals will both smoke and self-inject nicotine if "ancillary" variables are adequately considered (7,21,38,61,62).

Elimination

Nicotine is extensively metabolized in the liver and, to a lesser extent, kidney and lung (16). Renal excretion accounts for 10 to 35% of total elimination but is dependent on urinary pH and flow. At highly acid pHs, renal clearance is 208% greater than at usual levels and is associated with a compensatory increase in nicotine intake during smoking

(16,17). Nicotine terminal half-life averages 2 hr but varies greatly (range 1 to 4 hr) (9,23). Nicotine's major metabolites, cotinine and nicotine-N-oxide, have been reported to be without biological activity in most (12) but not all studies (61). Because of its 17-hr half-life, cotinine is a useful marker of nicotine intake and provides an approximate index of daily nicotine consumption (12,13,15,30).

NICOTINE LEVELS DURING A TYPICAL DAY OF SMOKING

Typically, approximately 10 puffs are taken from a cigarette over 10 min, though number and duration vary greatly (44). Thus, a one- to two-pack-a-day smoker can be considered as taking 200 to 400 doses of nicotine each 24 hr (23,64,65). The first few puffs and inhalations deliver less nicotine in each milliliter of puff volume than do the last few puffs of each cigarette (47). Rapid tolerance develops to many effects of nicotine (9,46) so that the effects from each microgram of nicotine in the first few puffs are greater than the effects of the last few puffs even on a single first cigarette of the day. There is considerable peak-to-trough oscillation in plasma nicotine levels between cigarettes (10,15,64,65). Nicotine accumulates over the 16 hr of regular smoking during a typical day and diminishes overnight, but measurable levels remain in the morning (10,15,44). Thus, tobacco smoking results in continual exposure to nicotine and other components of tobacco smoke 24 hr a day. Late afternoon plasma nicotine levels range from 10 to 50 ng/ml (10). The increment in plasma nicotine levels while smoking each single cigarette ranges from 5 to 30 ng/ml, depending on just how the cigarette is smoked (15,23,44).

Nicotine content of tobacco snuffed or chewed is similar to that of cigarette tobacco. Nicotine is well absorbed from nasal or oral mucosa. Although absorbed more slowly, nicotine and cotinine levels in plasma of tobacco snuffers or chewers are similar to those of tobacco smokers (52,66,68,71).

EXPERIMENTS ON NICOTINE DOSE REGULATION

Studies manipulating nicotine dose leave little doubt that nicotine is a very important, if not the most important, variable in controlling tobacco smoking (38,39,53,64). Tobacco smokers will not happily smoke material containing no nicotine. Smokers adjust, albeit not perfectly, smoking behavior to regulate what appears to be an individually determined range of nicotine levels in their body. Varying tobacco smoke concentration (36), manipulating body levels of nicotine by deprivation or by oral or intravenous preloading (63), or varying nicotine delivery (18,29) results in smoking behavior changes and other effects consistent with that notion. When smoking a cigarette delivering smaller amounts of nicotine per puff than regular smokers are used to, smoking behavior changes so as to increase dose (41). After manipulations that deliver more nicotine per puff, smoking behavior tends to change in ways that should decrease dose of nicotine absorbed (73). Smokers will self-administer intravenous nicotine (37,39).

However, it is also clear that besides the contribution of the nicotine, many psychosocial, environmental, and biological factors influence tobacco use, as with any other psychoactive drug use. A weakness in much research on the importance of nicotine seeking as an explanation for smoking behavior is that individual experiments tend to emphasize either biological or psychological–sociological or environmental influences on tobacco smoking and often do not consider all factors concurrently.

A proper model for characterizing smoking behavior must consider both biological and psychosocial factors. For example, Kozlowski (40,48) describes a model of tobacco use that assumes that the biological regulation of tobacco intake (nicotine) is governed by upper and lower regulatory regions or boundary areas rather than a precise plasma or other tissue level of nicotine implied by some so-called nicotine titration models (38,53). The upper and lower boundary region limits are determined by individual constitutional (genetic, receptor, or other) differences and history of tobacco use. The upper boundary defines a region characterized by increasing overdose or toxic effects of nicotine, and the lower boundary a region defined by insufficient nicotine intake that, when entered, results in the smoker experiencing a progressively severe abstinence syndrome.

Between the pharmacologic and biologically determined upper and lower boundaries (regions) is a zone that varies in size for individuals where the precise nicotine dose (or tissue level) is less important in determining smoking behavior than are a host of concurrent psychosocial factors. A partial list of psychosocial factors includes the level of motivation to smoke or not, intensity of concern about health, the setting, experiencing learned cues for lighting up a cigarette, environmental influences and social pressures to smoke or not to smoke, constraints against smoking in the workplace, friends, work associates, or family encouraging smoking or not smoking, and availability of alternatives that satisfy need to smoke. Thus, within an acceptable range of tissue levels of nicotine, whose upper and lower limits vary among smokers for a host of biological reasons, operate a complex mix of psychosocial factors. This mix of factors, rather than simply nicotine dose or tissue level, determines when a cigarette is lit and how it is smoked. For example, a smoker whose nicotine levels are at the upper boundary would respond differently to a decrease in a cigarette's nicotine delivery than would a smoker of the same number of cigarettes per day whose nicotine levels are in the area of the lower boundary. The upper-boundary smoker might not change smoking behavior at all, whereas the lower-boundary smoker would more likely increase number of cigarettes smoked or otherwise increase delivered nicotine dose (40,48).

SOME USEFUL NICOTINE EFFECTS

Nicotine gives pleasure. It stimulates, relaxes, relieves boredom, and improves performance (56). Nicotine has effects similar to other cholinergic agonists in improving information-processing task performance (7,21,38,74). Performance decrements during sustained vigilance tasks are less after nicotine. Speed and accuracy on rapid experimenter-paced visual information-processing tasks are increased. When nicotine is given prior to training, acquisition and storage of new information are facilitated. When given after learning, retention of learned material is facilitated. Nicotine's effects can be state dependent. Dose–effect functions are not monotonic; higher doses produce decrements in information processing. Nicotine-induced reversal of performance decrements associated with tobacco abstinence could explain enhanced performance in dependent individuals tested when abstinent for some hours. However, nondependent animals and humans show a similar pattern of enhanced information processing after nicotine.

TREATMENT OF TOBACCO DEPENDENCE

An estimated 95% of ex-tobacco smokers quit tobacco use without any formal help (25,55). As with other drugs, those users who seek treatment when trying to stop are a distinct minority of all users. Unfortunately, most of the data on the treatment of tobacco dependence comes from intensive study of a minority of tobacco users. Whether on their own or after formal treatment programs, the 2 to 3% of smokers who quit each year and remain abstinent are characterized by distinctive motivations, good self-management skills for quitting, and good social supports (25,31,33,55). The greater the number of reasons for quitting, the greater is the likelihood it will be successful. Less dependence on nicotine (22) and lower nicotine intake (32,55) may be associated with greater success.

Even minimal interventions such as physician advice to quit produce 10 to 60% 1-year quit rates among high-risk patients (25,55). Intensive smoking dependence treatment programs typically produce 15 to 25% 1-year quitting rates; exceptional programs produce 40 to 50% (25,34,55). The more successful programs combine multicomponent behavioral and psychological interventions with some variations on rapid or aversive smoking exercises (31,33–35). Biochemical markers of smoking status (breath or blood carbon monoxide levels, blood or saliva cotinine or thiocyanate) allow for objective verification of outcome and are now expected in any well-designed treatment research (13,30,32,55). Research has increasingly focused on reducing high relapse rates of even the more successful treatments (31,35,55) or providing treatment in special settings (19,55).

Pharmacologic Approaches to Treatment

Pharmacologic intervention is an old notion (26). Lobeline, an alkaloid with similar effects, has been used as a nicotine substitute. But lobeline's effects are weak. It does not substitute for nicotine in animal self-administration studies. Possibly because of the subtle, almost concurrent, stimulant and depressant actions of nicotine, substitution of other CNS stimulants has not been therapeutically useful. A problem when substituting other, nonsmoked drugs for nicotine is that dose regulation can be so flexible with inhaled nicotine. Also, nicotine kinetics are quite different from those of amphetamine and most other stimulants. Substitution of other psychostimulants without consideration of the very special attributes of nicotine smoking is unlikely to be effective.

Receptor blockade at the nicotine receptor level or subsequent to the initial sites of action has been tried. In principle, a drug blocking the rewarding effects of nicotine could serve as a useful therapeutic agent. Propranolol and other β-adrenergic blockers diminish peripheral cardiovascular effects of smoking but have no effect on mood and other psychoactive effects. Clonidine, an α_2 agonist, diminishes craving for tobacco, at least for relatively short periods of time. The central or peripheral mechanisms warrant further examination. Mecamylamine blocks many subjective effects of nicotine, leading to increased smoking, possibly to overcome the receptor blockade (38). However, mecamylamine has unpleasant side effects at doses producing full blockade. Incomplete blockade does not provide an adequate test of the extinction model.

As in treating opiate dependence, blockade and behavior extinction strategies have been unsatisfactory. An extinction model of treatment may not be appropriate or at least practical for humans considering the multitude of continued pressures for an ex-smoker to resume. Pharmacologic aversion therapies, for example, with emetine or apomorphine have not been effective, perhaps for similar reasons.

Considering the alternatives, nicotine substitution remains the most useful pharmacologic adjunct. Nicotine as a substitute for tobacco smoking has been given by almost every conceivable route. Bioavailability, safety, and social acceptability constrain route of administration. Oral nicotine absorption is relatively slow, but about 30% of the drug reaches systemic circulation (16,70). Well-conceived therapeutic trials have not been done using that route. Safety considerations suggest other routes or dose forms. Nicotine rectal suppositories would partially substitute but probably would be unacceptable to the consumer. Nicotine injections would need to be frequent and present logistical problems. Transdermal delivery offers adequate bioavailability and sustained delivery. Enough nicotine is absorbed from a small patch on the skin to decrease craving and preference for smoke containing high nicotine levels (63).

In principle, nicotine aerosols with suitable particle size and consistency should provide alveolar absorption similar to the nicotine aerosol produced during tobacco smoking. However, no completely satisfactory nonsmoking aerosol delivery systems have been developed for nicotine. Dose regulation problems and irritation to throat and upper airways have limited long-term aerosol use (26).

Nasal sprays of nicotine reproduce blood nicotine concentrations produced by tobacco snuff. The nicotine is absorbed relatively rapidly and efficiently. Nicotine-containing tablets or lozenges for sublingual administration have been marketed to help manage smoking dependence but have not had adequate clinical trials (26).

The current popular pharmacologic adjunct is a nicotine-containing chewing gum developed in the early 1970s (34,38,68). Besides providing a controlled, relatively slow delivery of nicotine, the gum was thought to be a substitute for oral activity important to some smokers. The gum contains 2- or 4-mg doses of nicotine in a resin complex with release dependent on rate and vigor of chewing. About 90% of the nicotine is released during 30 min of moderate chewing. The gum is buffered to maintain an oral pH of about 8.5, allowing optimal absorption of nicotine through buccal mucosa. Rate of absorption is slow. Peak plasma concentrations occur 15 to 30 min after chewing is begun. A piece of gum containing 4 mg of nicotine chewed each hour will, after a period of 3 hr, produce plasma nicotine concentrations similar to those measured in frequent cigarette smokers, though with less marked peaks and troughs. The gum produces cardiovascular effects similar to nicotine, has modest inhibitory effects on concurrent smoking behavior, and, most important for treatment, decreases intensity and duration of withdrawal symptoms.

ACKNOWLEDGMENTS

Preparation of this review supported in part by Grants DA01696 and DA00053 from the National Institute on Drug Abuse.

REFERENCES

1. Abel, E. L. (1980): *Hum. Biol.,* 52:593–625.
2. Abood, L. G., Grassi, S., and Noggle, H. D. (1985): *Neurochem. Res.,* 10:259–267.
3. Abood, L. G., Lowy, K., Tometsko, A., and Booth, H. (1978): *J. Neurosci. Res.,* 3:327–333.
4. Aceto, M. D., Martin, B. R., and May, E. L. (1984): In: *CRC Handbook of Stereoisomers: Drugs in Psychopharmacology,* edited by D. F. Smith, pp. 67–78. CRC Press, Boca Raton, FL.
5. Adams, P. I. (1978): In: *Smoking Behaviour—Physiological and Psychological Influences,* edited by R. E. Thornton, pp. 349–360. Churchill-Livingstone, London.
6. Ashton, H., Marsh, V. R., Millman, J. E., Rawlins, M. D., Telford, R., et al. (1980): *Br. J. Clin. Pharmacol.,* 10:579–589.
7. Battig, K., ed. (1978): *Behavioral Effects of Nicotine.* S. Karger, Basel.
8. Battig, L., Buzzi, R., and Nil, R. (1982): *Psychopharmacology,* 76: 139–148.
9. Benowitz, N. L., Jacob, P., III, Jones, R. T., and Rosenberg, J. (1982): *J. Pharmacol. Exp. Ther.,* 221:368–372.
10. Benowitz, N. L., Kuyt, F., and Jacob, P., III (1982): *Clin. Pharmacol. Ther.,* 32:758–764.
11. Benowitz, N. L., Hall, S. M., Herning, R. I., Jacob, P., III, Jones, R. T., et al. (1983): *N. Engl. J. Med.,* 309:139–142.
12. Benowitz, N. L., Kuyt, F., Jacob, P., Jones, R. T., and Osman, A.-L. (1983): *Clin. Pharmacol. Ther.,* 309:139–142.
13. Benowitz, N. L. (1984): In: *Measurement in the Analysis and Treatment of Smoking Behavior,* NIDA Research Monograph No. 48, edited by J. Grabowski and C. S. Bell, pp. 6–26. U.S. Government Printing Office, Washington.
14. Benowitz, N. L., and Jacob, P., III (1984): *Clin. Pharmacol. Ther.,* 36:265–270.
15. Benowitz, N. L., and Jacob, P., III (1984): *Clin. Pharmacol. Ther.,* 35:499–504.
16. Benowitz, N. L. (1986): In: *Research Advances in Alcohol and Drug Problems, Vol. 9,* edited by H. Cappell et al., pp. 1–52. Plenum Press, New York.
17. Benowitz, N. L., and Jacob, P., III (1985): *J. Pharmacol. Exp. Ther.,* 234:153–155.
18. Creighton, D. E., and Lewis, P. H. (1978): In: *Smoking Behaviour: Physiological and Psychological Influences,* edited by R. E. Thornton, pp. 289–298. Churchill-Livingstone, London.
19. Danaher, B. G. (1980): *Public Health Rep.,* 95:149–157.
20. Domino, E. F. (1979): In: *Electrophysiological Effects of Nicotine,*

edited by A. Remond and C. Izard, pp. 133–146. Elsevier/North-Holland Biomedical Press, Amsterdam.

21. Emley, G. S., and Hutchinson, R. R. (1984): In: *Advances in Behavioral Pharmacology, Vol. 4,* edited by T. Thompson, P. B. Dews, and J. E. Barrett, pp. 105–129. Academic Press, New York.

22. Fagerstrom, K. (1978): *Addictive Behav., 3:*235–241.

23. Feyerabend, C., Ings, R. M. J., and Russell, M. A. H. (1985): *Br. J. Clin. Pharmacol., 19:*239–247.

24. Fielding, J. E. (1985): *N. Engl. J. Med., 313:*491–498.

25. Fielding, J. E. (1985): *N. Engl. J. Med., 313:*555–561.

26. Grabowski, J., and Hall, S. M., eds. (1985): *Pharmacological Adjuncts in Smoking Cessation,* NIDA Research Monograph No. 53, U.S. Government Printing Office, Washington.

27. Griffiths, R. R., Henningfield, J. E., and Bigelow, G. E. (1981): *J. Pharmacol. Exp. Ther., 230:*256–263.

28. Gritz, E. R. (1980): In: *Advances in Substance Abuse, Vol. 1,* edited by N. Mello, pp. 91–158. JAI Press, Greenwich, CT.

29. Gust, S. W., and Pickens, R. W. (1982): *Clin. Pharmacol. Ther., 36:*418–422.

30. Haley, N. J., Axelrod, C. M., and Tilton, K. A. (1983): *Am. J. Public Health, 73:*1204–1207.

31. Hall, R. G., Sachs, D. P. L., Hall, S. M., and Benowitz, N. L. (1984): *J. Consult. Clin. Psychol., 52:*574–581.

32. Hall, S. M., Herning, R. I., Jones, R. T., Benowitz, N. L., and Jacob, P. (1984): *Clin. Pharmacol. Ther., 35:*810–814.

33. Hall, S. M., Rugg, D., Tunstall, C., and Jones, R. T. (1984): *J. Consult. Clin. Psychol., 52:*372–382.

34. Hall, S. M., Tunstall, C., Rugg, D., Jones, R. T., and Benowitz, N. (1985): *J. Consult. Clin. Psychol., 53:*256–258.

35. Hall, S. M., Ginsberg, D., and Jones, R. T. (1986): *J. Consult. Clin. Psychol., 54:*342–346.

36. Henningfield, J. E. (1983): In: *Measurement in the Analysis and Treatment of Smoking Behavior,* National Institute on Drug Abuse Research Monograph No. 48, edited by J. Grabowski and C. Bell, pp. 27–38. U.S. Government Printing Office, Washington.

37. Henningfield, J. E., Miyasato, K., and Jasinski, D. R. (1983): *Pharmacol. Biochem. Behav., 19:*887–890.

38. Henningfield, J. E. (1984): In: *Advances in Behavioral Pharmacology, Vol. 4,* edited by T. Thompson, P. B. Dews, and J. E. Barrett, pp. 131–210. Academic Press, New York.

39. Henningfield, J. E., Miyasato, K., and Jasinski, D. R. (1985): *J. Pharmacol. Exp. Ther., 234:*1–12.

40. Herman, C. P., and Kozlowski, L. T. (1979): *J. Drug Issues, 9:*185–196.

41. Herning, R. I., Jones, R. T., Bachman, J., and Mines, A. H. (1981): *Br. Med. J., 283:*187–193.

42. Herning, R. I., Hunt, J. S., and Jones, R. T. (1983): *Behav. Res. Methods Instrum., 15:*561–568.

43. Herning, R. I., Jones, R. T., and Bachman, J. (1983): *Psychophysiology, 20:*507–512.

44. Herning, R. I., Jones, R. T., Benowitz, N. L., and Mines, A. H. (1983): *Clin. Pharmacol. Ther., 33:*84–90.

45. Ikushima, S., Muramatsu, I., Sakakibara, Y., Yokotani, K., and Fujiwara, M. (1982): *J. Pharmacol. Exp. Ther., 222:*463–470.

46. Jones, R. T., Farrell, T. R., and Herning, R. I. (1978): In: *Self-Administration of Abused Substances,* National Institute on Drug Abuse Research Monograph Series No. 18, edited by N. A. Krasnegor, pp. 202–208. U.S. Government Printing Office, Washington.

47. Kiefer, J. E. (1972): In: *The Chemistry of Tobacco and Tobacco Smoke,* edited by I. Schmeltz, pp. 167–176. Plenum Press, New York.

48. Kozlowski, L. T., and Herman, C. P. (1984): *J. Appl. Soc. Psychol., 14:*244–256.

49. Krasnegor, N. A., ed. (1979): *Cigarette Smoking as a Dependence Process.* National Institute on Drug Abuse Research Monograph Series No. 23, U.S. Government Printing Office, Washington.

50. Lombardo, T., Davis, C. J. U., and Prue, D. M. (1983): *Addict. Behav., 8:*67–69.

51. Martin, B. R., Tripathi, H. L., Aceto, M. D., and May, E. L. (1983): *J. Pharmacol. Exp. Ther., 226:*157–163.

52. McCusker, K., McNabb, E., and Bone, R. (1982): *J.A.M.A., 248:*577–578.

53. McMorrow, M. J., and Foxx, R. M. (1983): *Psychol. Bull., 93:*302–327.

54. Nemeth-Coslett, R., and Griffiths, R. R. (1985): *Drug Alcohol Depend., 15:*1–13.

55. Orleans, C. T. (1985): In: *Annual Review of Medicine,* edited by W. P. Creger, pp. 51–61. Annual Reviews, Palo Alto.

56. Pomerleau, O. F. (1980): In: *Behavioral Medicine: Changing Health Lifestyles,* edited by P. Davidson, pp. 94–115. Brunner/Mazel, New York.

57. Pomerleau, O. F., Fertig, J. B., Seyler, L. E., and Jaffe, J. (1983): *Psychopharmacology, 81:*61–67.

58. Pomerleau, O. F., and Pomerleau, C. S. (1984): *Neurosci. Biobehav. Rev., 8:*503–513.

59. Rawbone, R. G., Murphy, K., Tate, M. E., and Kane, S. F. (1978): In: *Smoking Behaviour: Physiological and Psychological Influences,* edited by R. E. Thornton, pp. 171–179. Churchill-Livingstone, Edinburgh.

60. Remond, A., and Izard, C., eds. (1979): *Electrophysiological Effects of Nicotine.* Elsevier, Amsterdam.

61. Risner, M. E., and Goldberg, S. R. (1983): *J. Pharmacol. Exp. Ther., 224:*319–326.

62. Risner, M. E., Goldberg, S. R., Prada, J. A., and Cone, E. J. (1985): *J. Pharmacol. Exp. Ther., 234:*113–119.

63. Rose, J. E., Herskovic, J. E., Trilling, Y., and Jarvik, M. E. (1975): *Clin. Pharmacol. Ther., 38:*450–456.

64. Russell, M. A. H. (1976): In: *Research Advances in Alcohol and Drug Problems, Vol. 3,* edited by R. J. Gibbins, Y. Israel, H. Kalant, R. E. Popham, W. Schmidt, and R. G. Smart, pp. 1–48. John Wiley & Sons, New York.

65. Russell, M. A. H., and Feyerabend, C. (1978): *Drug Metab. Rev., 8:*29–57.

66. Russell, M. A. H., Jarvis, M. J., and Feyerabend, C. (1980): *Lancet.* 1:474–475.

67. Russell, M. A. H., Jarvis, M., Iyer, R., and Feyerabend, C. (1980): *Br. Med. J., 280:*972–976.

68. Russell, M. A. H., Raw, M., and Jarvis, M. J. (1980): *Br. Med. J., 280:*1599–1602.

69. Russell, M. A. H., Sutton, S. R., Iyer, R., Feyerabend, C., and Vesey, C. J. (1982): *Br. J. Addict., 77:*145–158.

70. Shiffman, S. M., Gritz, E. R., Maltese, J., Lee, M. A., Schneider, N. G., et al. (1983): *Clin. Pharmacol. Ther., 33:*800–805.

71. Squires, W. G., Branton, T. A., Zinkgraf, S., Bonds, D., Hartung, G. H., et al. (1984): *Prev. Med., 13:*195–206.

72. Stepney, R. (1982): *J. Epidemiol. Commun. Health, 36:*109–112.

73. Tobin, M. J., and Sackner, M. A. (1982): *Am. Rev. Respir. Dis., 126:*258–264.

74. Warburton, D. M., and Wesnes, K. (1984): *Neuropsychobiology, 11:*121–132.

75. West, R. J., and Russell, M. A. H. (1985): *Psychopharmacology, 87:*334–336.

76. Wyngaarten, J. B., and Smith, L. H., Jr. (1985): *Cecil Textbook of Medicine,* 17th edition. W. B. Saunders, Philadelphia.

77. Zacny, J. P., and Stitzer, M. L. (1985): *Clin. Pharmacol. Ther., 38:*109–115.

Psychopharmacology:
The Third Generation of Progress,
edited by Herbert Y. Meltzer.
Raven Press, New York © 1987.

CHAPTER 172

Multiple Drug Abuse Patterns and Medical Consequences

Mary Jeanne Kreek

In this brief discussion of multiple drug abuse patterns and medical consequences, only a few substances can be mentioned. Greatest attention is given to those substances that, when abused alone or in combination, are the most likely to cause serious and costly early medical complications or significant behavorial and social problems and that thus have the greatest potential for negative impact on the individual. These substances, alone and in combination, are the most costly drugs of abuse for society. We therefore focus primarily on heroin addiction and cocaine abuse alone, in combination with each other or with alcohol abuse, and, to a much lesser extent, on heroin and cocaine abuse in combination with marijuana and other drugs. Some attention is also given to multiple drug abuse patterns that have been observed in patients receiving chronic pharmacological treatment for heroin addiction either with the opioid agonist methadone or with the opioid antagonist naltrexone.

MULTIPLE DRUG ABUSE PATTERNS

Alcohol, cigarettes, and marijuana are the top three drugs "used nonmedically" according to the most recently published National Institute on Drug Abuse (NIDA) statistics (34,36,38). The percentage of persons in the United States who reported having "ever used" these agents were 86% for alcohol, 75% for cigarettes (tobacco), and 31% for marijuana and hashish; the percentage of persons reporting "current user" status defined as use within the last month before the survey were 55%, 33%, and 11%, respectively (34–36,38–40).

In the National Survey on Drug Abuse of 1982, a NIDA-sponsored household population survey, it was found that 64% of the 18- to 25-year-old age group had used marijuana at least one time and that 27% of this age group had used marijuana within the last month (34). Of these, almost all reported use of alcohol during the same time period (34). In this same survey, 12% of the 18- to 25-year-old age group reported use on at least one occasion during the preceding month of cocaine, heroin, or a hallucinogen or nonmedical use of a psychotherapeutic drug. Essentially all of these young adults also reported use of alcohol during the same time period, with concomitant use of alcohol and another drug or drugs as a common pattern of use (34). Thus, purposeful simultaneous use of alcohol with another drug is very common.

Despite the fact that cigarettes and marijuana are two of the three top drugs used "nonmedically," the negative immediate impact for the individual and for society is much greater when heroin and cocaine are used. The number of heroin abusers reported is very large indeed: in a 1982 NIDA survey, 1.88 million persons in the United States were reported to have used heroin at some time (34,36,38). In 1985, 258,000 persons in New York State alone were reported to be current regular heroin abusers, and it is estimated that there are over one-half million untreated heroin addicts nationwide (42). Most heroin abusers initially, or after a brief period of transnasal administration, use heroin by the parenteral route (subcutaneous or intravenous self-administration), and a substantial proportion become heroin addicts with multiple heroin injections required each day to maintain the narcotic-tolerant and -dependent state. Secondly, the numbers of cocaine abusers are increasing rapidly. In a 1982 survey, 21.57 million persons in the United States were reported to have used cocaine at some time, and 4.12 million persons had used cocaine at least once in the month prior to the survey (34,36,38,41). Most abusers initiate cocaine use with sporadic intermittent transnasal self-administration of cocaine in the salt form, but some progress to regular frequent self-administration of the more bioavailable free-base form of cocaine administered transnasally, and others turn to parenteral use of cocaine to achieve greater desired effects (34,36,38,41,42).

The fact that these two agents, heroin and cocaine, are often used in combination with alcohol (which is the most widely used drug or chemical, with 157.75 million persons in the United States reporting some alcohol use in the 1982 survey), in combination with other drugs, or with each other has added to the prevalence and severity of immediate toxic complications from each drug when used alone as well as to the multitude of direct and indirect medical complications that may result from heroin and cocaine abuse, especially when used by a parenteral route of administration (34–36,38–43).

Persistent nonnarcotic drug abuse, especially alcohol and cocaine abuse, is unfortunately common during outpatient "drug-free" treatment of narcotic addiction and during pharmacological treatment of narcotic addiction either with the long-acting opioid agonist methadone (and with *l*-alphaacetylmethadol, LAAM, an experimental drug with a more prolonged duration of action than methadone) or with the opioid antagonist naltrexone. Such alcohol, cocaine, and other drug abuse during chronic pharmacological treatment of narcotic addiction may complicate treatment by direct toxic consequences, problems resulting from drug interactions, or by introduction of other medical complications (11,18–20,43). It has been determined that 25 to 50% of street heroin addicts and 25 to 50% of methadone-maintained patients abuse alcohol (11,19,20). Cocaine abuse, including both intermittent, infrequent use and regular extensive use, has been found in up to 50% of youthful methadone-maintained former heroin addicts and is also common in naltrexone-treated patients (3,14,25). The precise prevalence of alcohol abuse, cocaine abuse, and other drug abuse in other populations of methadone-maintained, LAAM-treated, and naltrexone-treated as well as in "drug-free" patients in outpatient treatment needs to be determined more carefully. Such determinations should be made on a regular basis, since alcohol, cocaine, and other drug abuse patterns are in a constant state of flux, depending on many diverse factors.

According to the 1982 NIDA-sponsored Drug Abuse Warning Network (DAWN) survey of emergency rooms in the United States, three of the top five drugs of abuse mentioned as causing problems necessitating acute medical care were (a) alcohol used in combination with other drugs, most frequently cited, accounting for 24.4% of all drug-related episodes (excluding those episodes related to alcohol use alone, for which data were not collected); (b) in third place, heroin, cited as need for emergency room care in 10.4% of cases; and (c) in fifth place, cocaine, which was responsible for 5.2% of emergency room episodes. Benzodiazepine drugs, especially diazepam (Valium®), and aspirin were the second and fourth most frequently cited drugs (36). According to the same DAWN reports of emergency room visits in 1982 for drug-related problems, heroin was reported to be used in combination with alcohol and/or

one or more other drugs in 41% of the heroin abuse cases reported, and cocaine was reported as used in combination with alcohol and/or one or more other drugs in 71% of the cocaine abuse cases (34).

In New York State during the period of 1982 to 1985, heroin continued to be the leading drug implicated in drug-induced or drug-related emergency room episodes, with 3,199 cases of heroin-related problems seen in emergency rooms in New York in 1984 (42). Cocaine was the second leading drug identified as causing drug-induced emergency room episodes in New York State, with 2,610 cases reported in 1984 (41). The same three drugs, i.e., alcohol used in combination with other drugs, heroin, and cocaine, were among the top eight drugs most frequently cited by medical examiners in the United States in postmortem examination reports as causes of death or related to death in drug-related cases. Two other narcotics, codeine and *d*-propoxyphene, were two additional drugs among the eight most frequently cited as causes of, or related to, deaths. Alcohol used in combination with other drugs was cited in 31.6% of medical-examiner-reported drug-related cases, heroin in 27.4% of cases (codeine and *d*-propoxyphene in an additional 20.6% of cases), and cocaine in 6.7%. In all sets of data, it should be emphasized that alcohol in combination with other drugs was the most frequently cited cause for drug-related emergency room visits and also drug-related causes of death in medical examiner cases. A very large proportion, possibly the majority, of all drug-related emergency room visits and deaths were caused by drugs used in combination with alcohol and/or in combination with one or more other drugs.

In New York State, actual drug-dependent mortality has been assessed, as contrasted with assessment of "mentions" by all medical examiners of drugs present at time of postmortem examination, as reported in the national surveys (34,36,38,41,42). In New York State, the numbers of deaths caused primarily by chronic or acute intraveneous heroin use were 582 in 1983 and 427 in 1984 (42). In 1984 there were 91 deaths attributed to cocaine abuse, whereas in 1983 there were only seven deaths reported to be caused by cocaine (41). In a separate survey of deaths of all causes among narcotic abusers in New York State in 1984, only 32% of deaths were from narcotic drugs per se, 9% were from alcohol abuse, and 59% of deaths in this group were from other causes including AIDS (26%), pneumonia (15%), and other causes (18%) (42).

To address questions concerning the extent of use and abuse of psychoactive prescription drugs in the New York State household population, a household survey was conducted by the New York State Division of Substance Abuse Services (DSAS) in 1981 (39). It was determined that of 14.3 million household residents in New York State, 3.5 million had used prescription drugs "medically" (under medical supervision) during the year prior to the survey, 1.0 million household residents had used prescription drugs "nonmedically" (beyond the dose prescribed or use of prescriptions obtained from a nonmedical source), and 389,000 had used prescription drugs both "medically and nonmedically" during the year (39). Stimulants, tranquilizers, and sedatives were the prescription drugs most frequently used nonmedically, although the prescription drugs that attracted the largest number of new "nonmedical" users in 1981 were stimulants (271,000 household residents) and analgesics or cough medicines with codeine (168,000 household residents) (39). In the household survey, 765,000 persons were using both prescription drugs nonmedically and also illicit drugs; of these, 439,000 household residents were using illicit drugs other than marijuana (39). Therefore, use of combinations of drugs including both licit and illicit drugs was the rule, not the exception.

More extensive data about the prevalence of specific combinations of drugs abused, with or without concomitant use of alcohol, would be of interest, along with more precise data on deaths directly and also indirectly attributed to drug and alcohol abuse used alone or in specific defined combinations. It is of interest that the most commonly prescribed drugs in 1983 requiring use of the triplicate prescription procedure of New York State were three narcotic analgesic drugs: oxycodone (Percodan®), meperidine (Demerol®), and hydromorphone (Dilaudid®), accounting for over 257,000 prescriptions written in 1 year. These were followed by barbiturates with over 77,000 prescriptions written in that year. These drugs thus would have been those most often misused or used with alcohol in combination with illegally obtained or illicit drugs.

A new major combined drug abuse problem has been emerging over the last few years. According to street sources, there appears to be an increase in demand for heroin as a direct consequence of cocaine abuse (42). Persons who use cocaine frequently and/or in large amounts, especially those who use the free-base form of cocaine or use cocaine by the intravenous route of administration, experience a highly anxious and nervous state or "overstimulation" along with rebound dysphoria (so-called "crash") following cocaine use. Self-medication of this state has included use of alcohol as well as various sedative–hypnotics and tranquilizers. Increasing numbers of regular cocaine users have now found that these undesired aftereffects of cocaine use are apparently alleviated by use of heroin (42). Therefore, many of these cocaine abusers have now become regular abusers of heroin; many have become heroin addicts by the definition of the development of tolerance, physical dependence, and drug-seeking (heroin) behavior on a regular multiple-dose-per-day basis. Cocaine abuser heroin addicts are now being identified as they enter drug treatment programs.

The better-known long-standing pattern of combined use of cocaine and heroin, "speedballing," the simultaneous intravenous administration of both cocaine and heroin to obtain certain desired effects conferred by these drugs when used in combination, remains common also, and according to street observers, this practice may be increasing because of the relative increase in purity of heroin available at this time, thus enhancing the interactive effects with cocaine (42).

It has been reported that street heroin addicts wishing to withdraw or detoxify themselves from heroin will self-administer gradually decreasing amounts of heroin along with gradually increasing amounts of cocaine (12). Addicts following this procedure have reported that cocaine provides relief from the physiological withdrawal symptoms that usually accompany the cessation of heroin use in a tolerant and dependent person (12). Several workers have suggested, based on findings from animal studies and clinical obser-

vations, that cocaine may potentiate several narcotic effects including general depressant effects on the brain as well as the specific respiratory depressant effect when high doses of cocaine are used simultaneously with heroin (3,12). Workers have also reported that greater amounts of an opioid antagonist such as naltrexone are required to block narcotic actions when cocaine has been administered (3). It has been suggested by some that cocaine may cause the production and/or release of endogenous opioids, thereby augmenting opioid-like action. Thus, it is apparent that combined cocaine and heroin use, either simultaneously or sequentially, is increasing and, on one hand, may cause more severe and unique adverse reactions to the drugs per se (following simultaneous administration of both drugs) yet may, in fact, protect against some of the adverse effects of each drug when used alone (sequential use) (42). It is well recognized that drug dealers who once sold only heroin or cocaine now sell both drugs (42).

A recent report of the effects of cocaine use in pregnant women included an assessment of the effects of the use of cocaine by opioid-free women and use of cocaine in former heroin addicts in methadone maintenance treatment for narcotic addiction as contrasted with women who were not abusing cocaine, including otherwise drug-free methadone-maintained former heroin addicts and control women receiving no medications and with no history of drug abuse (4,52). It was noted that women using cocaine had a significantly higher prevalence of spontaneous abortion, as well as abruptio placenta, both in the opiate-free and methadone-maintained cocaine abusers (4,52). Several other adverse reactions were found in pregnant women abusing cocaine but who were not in methadone maintenance treatment, suggesting to the authors that methadone maintenance treatment may have prevented some of the adverse effects of cocaine abuse in this pregnant population (4).

Parenteral use of cocaine, an increasingly common practice, exposes the user to all of the medical complications that are inherent to parenteral drug abuse of any type and that have been most commonly identified in the past in heroin addicts. Direct drug effects, adverse drug effects related to interactions between drugs or alcohol, and medical complications related to parenteral drug abuse are discussed.

In 1982, a NIDA-sponsored National Drug and Alcoholism Treatment Utilization Survey (NDATUS) report stated that 173,479 patients were enrolled in some kind of drug treatment program in the United States, with an overall utilization of 88% of available treatment places (35). At that time, it was estimated that 72,000 former heroin addicts were in methadone maintenance treatment programs in the United States, with 97% utilization of the available methadone maintenance treatment places. Heroin addiction is still the most prevalent drug abuse problem in persons seeking public (federal or state) supported programs. In the years 1982, 1983, and 1984, 62 to 72% of patients admitted to drug treatment programs in New York State (3,500 to 4,300 patients admitted each year) had heroin addiction as a primary drug abuse problem. Concomitant alcohol, cocaine, and other drug abuse problems were common.

With all New York State drug treatment programs filled to greater than 100% of capacity, along with increased voluntary retention in treatment and longer durations of treatment, the apparent recent decline in percentages of heroin addicts entering treatment (primarily entering methadone maintenance treatment programs) is misleading (43). The waiting list for entry into treatment programs for heroin addiction, particularly for entry into the methadone maintenance treatment programs, has grown steadily, and in many locations the waiting period for admission to treatment is up to 1 year. Potential patients have found it frustrating to attempt to enter a drug treatment program at this time because of the greater than 100% utilization of treatment resources and the resultant long waiting lists. Many heroin addicts may have given up attempts to enter treatment at this time despite the ongoing AIDS epidemic. In this setting, the number of admissions of heroin addicts into the detoxification programs of the New York State Corrections Department has increased again in 1985. This fact, along with other indirect indicators, suggests that heroin addiction remains the most serious drug abuse problem in New York State. The second most serious drug abuse problem in New York State is cocaine abuse. In 1984, cocaine was the primary drug of abuse in 3,159 patients entering New York State drug treatment programs. At this time there are still very limited resources for treatment of cocaine abuse.

MEDICAL CONSEQUENCES

Medical Consequences of Direct Drug Effects and Drug Interactions

Toxic effects of intrinsic toxicity of a drug or a drug metabolite, adverse clinical reaction resulting from pharmacodynamic and/or pharmacokinetic drug interactions, and drug interactions resulting in increased or accelerated production of toxic metabolites of drugs all contribute to the medical consequences of direct drug effects, especially in the setting of multiple drug abuse. Since many patients in pharmacological treatment of narcotic addiction may continue to abuse alcohol, cocaine, and other drugs, it is of considerable importance to consider whether any drug interactions may occur that cause or enhance the intrinsic toxicity of the treatment drug, contribute to a direct drug-related adverse reaction, or alter treatment efficacy. As in the previous section, abuse of three agents, alcohol in combination with other drugs, heroin, and cocaine, is considered, along with use of two orally effective agents used in treatment of narcotic addiction, the long-acting opioid agonist methadone and the opioid antagonist naltrexone. More research is needed to determine the extent and clinical impact of drug interactions between drugs of abuse and use in humans, with emphasis on delineating dispositional interactions, the underlying mechanisms of these interactions, and their impact on neuroendocrine, neurological, immunological, and metabolic functioning as well as on behavior (19–21).

The intrinsic toxicities of alcohol for many organs and physiological systems are the best known and studied of all drug-induced toxicities (29). It is known that alcohol is a dose-dependent hepatotoxin; that is, continued use of large amounts of alcohol will predictably cause hepatocellular damage ranging from the mild lesion of hepatic steatosis to the more severe hepatic diseases of alcoholic hepatitis and alcoholic cirrhosis (29). It is known that regular use of small, apparently nonhepatotoxic amounts of alcohol (less than 3 oz equivalent of whiskey or 8 oz of wine per day) as well as much larger amounts may cause alterations in functions of the liver, including enhancement of the hepatic mixed-function oxidase microsomal P-450-dependent drug- and steroid-metabolizing enzyme activities, thereby accelerating the metabolism of a variety of drugs and steroids (29). Conversely, large amounts of alcohol, such as may be used in an abuse setting, may inhibit or retard the metabolism of drugs by the hepatic microsomal P-450-dependent enzymes by direct inhibition when alcohol is present in high concentrations (19,20). Consequences of opiate–alcohol interactions have been reviewed in detail recently (19,20).

Alcohol is also a dose-dependent neurotoxin, causing adverse effects on both the central and peripheral nervous systems. As in the case of alcohol-induced liver disease, brain and neurological damage caused by alcohol may or may not be completely reversible following alcohol withdrawal. Alcohol is also a direct toxin to the heart, causing myocardopathy, and to the gastrointestinal tract, causing gastritis, altered intestinal function, and pancreatic disease. Alcohol may also alter neuroendocrine and peripheral endocrine function through direct effects on the brain, hypothalamus, pituitary, adrenal gland, and gonads and by indirect effects caused by liver damage (29). Since use of large amounts of alcohol may cause central nervous system depression, concomitant use of other drugs with central nervous system depressant action may lead to adverse medical consequences because of the additive effects of the two agents.

Cocaine and/or one or more of its metabolites may be directly toxic to some organs or organ systems, and cocaine itself may also be indirectly toxic to various organs by way of its local anesthetic and peripheral sympathomimetic effects as well as its stimulatory and depressant effects on the central nervous system. Although acute tolerance may develop to the positive chronotropic effects of cocaine, use of large amounts of cocaine can cause tachycardia, increased cardiac irritability with resultant arrhythmias, and hypertension (5,9,28,51). Angina pectoris and myocardial infarction associated with cocaine abuse have been reported recently (51). Since one action of cocaine is prevention of norepinephrine and epinephrine reuptake at adrenergic nerve terminals, resulting in an increase of norepinephrine levels, action of adrenergic neurotransmitters may be potentiated at peripheral sites, causing a variety of effects including vasoconstriction, which may lead to hyperthermia. Combined use or abuse of any drug with similar effects such as adrenergic agents can add to the toxicity of cocaine.

More unusual complications directly resulting from cocaine abuse have been identified recently (10,55). Renal infarction, followed in turn by hypertension, has been documented in one patient who used cocaine intravenously. It is postulated that increased adrenergic stimulation with resultant hypertension increased heart rate, and increased cardiac output caused by the intravenous cocaine use in association with a preexisting arterial thrombus led to end-organ (renal) infarction (55). Cocaine-induced colitis, a new syndrome, has been described as a pseudomembranous colitis with an ischemic component in cocaine-abusing patients with no other identifiable cause for this type of colitis (10). This syndrome is felt to be caused by elevated levels and activity of catecholamines causing mucosal ischemia. Diarrhea, one of the symptoms in cocaine-induced colitis, is a relatively common problem among cocaine abusers. Again, combined use of drugs with similar enhancement of catecholamine activity in sympathetically innervated organs could lead to increased occurrence of these newly recognized unusual consequences of cocaine abuse.

Cocaine is not known to alter the disposition or metabolism of any other drug. However, the metabolism of cocaine may be altered by agents that either enhance hepatic microsomal mixed-function oxidase P-450-dependent enzyme activities or inhibit esterase activities. Clinical observations have suggested that cocaine is hepatotoxic. Careful studies using animal models have shown that the hepatotoxin is one or more metabolites resulting from oxidative metabolism of cocaine. In these studies, it was shown that pretreatment with an agent such as phenobarbital, which enhances microsomal P-450-dependent enzymes, sensitizes animals to develop cocaine-induced hepatotoxicity and also increases latent cocaine-induced lethality. Inhibition of hepatic and serum esterase activities also results in hepatocellular damage and necrosis of the liver. Both enhancement of the microsomal P-450-dependent enzyme systems and inhibition of esterase enzymes increased the biotransformation of cocaine by oxidative pathways to form the major N-demethylated metabolite norcocaine and norcocaine metabolites. It has been shown that norcocaine and its metabolites are the primary hepatotoxic agents derived from cocaine. Several animal studies have shown that ethanol enhances hepatic microsomal mixed-function oxidase P-450-dependent drug-metabolizing enzyme systems. It recently has been directly shown that ethanol pretreatment potentiates cocaine-induced liver disease (centrolobular hepatic necrosis) as well as cocaine-induced lethality. Similar interactions between ethanol and cocaine may well occur in man and explain the various anecdotal reports of hepatotoxicity of cocaine, especially when combined with alcohol use.

It has been suggested that enhanced oxidative biotransformation of cocaine, which has been documented to lead to hepatic necrosis, may also explain in part the central nervous system toxicity of cocaine, since enzymatic activities essential for such oxidative biotransformation of cocaine have been identified in brain tissue. If this is the case, then combined use of alcohol, barbiturates, or any other agents that enhance microsomal P-450 drug-metabolizing enzyme activities may increase the central nervous system toxicity as well as the hepatotoxicity of cocaine. Such a hypothesis, if correct, could explain the very high prevalence of combined use of cocaine and alcohol in those cocaine-related cases requiring acute emergency medical care or leading to death and examination by medical examiners. As discussed above, the simultaneous intravenous administration of cocaine plus heroin can result in sudden death thought to be primarily from respiratory depression, representing one

type of addictive or, more likely, synergistic effect of these two agents on the central nervous system. More research is needed to find the mechanisms of cocaine-induced hepatotoxicity and neurotoxicity. Clinical studies are needed to determine the prevalence of cocaine-induced hepatotoxicity in cocaine use alone and in combination with alcohol and also to determine the potential effects of cocaine injury superimposed on preexistent viral or alcohol injury to the liver.

Heroin, the illicit drug of narcotic addiction, along with most other narcotics used both illicitly and licitly for relief of pain, such as morphine, meperidine (Demerol®), oxycodone (Percodan®), and hydromorphone (Dilaudid®), are all short-acting narcotics with durations of action from 3 to 8 hr in humans. Heroin and morphine require parenteral administration for maximum effect. Methadone, which when used on a chronic basis in steady doses, has been documented to be the most effective treatment to date for narcotic addicts (60–80% voluntary retention in treatment for 2 years or more with less than 5% with illicit narcotic use) is an orally effective, long-acting narcotic with a duration of action of 24 to 36 hr in humans (37). Methadone has been shown by rigorous long-term prospective studies not to have any intrinsic toxicity for any organ or organ system (8,17,22,25,37,52). Although rigorous prospective studies have not been performed, apparently neither heroin nor morphine has any intrinsic toxicity either. Chronic use of any of these narcotic drugs for any purpose, licit or illicit, will lead to the development of tolerance and physical dependence and in many individuals to drug-seeking behavior.

The short-acting narcotics, such as heroin, whether used acutely or on a chronic basis, cause profound disruptions of several endocrine and neuroendocrine systems (17,27,28). Following narcotic administration, when drug levels are high, suppression of levels of ACTH, cortisol, and probably β-endorphin, all part of the hypothalamic–pituitary–adrenal axis, will occur along with suppression of levels of LH and the peripheral gonadal steroids, most notably testosterone, of the hypothalamic–pituitary–gonadal axis. Tolerance does not develop to these effects during chronic short-acting narcotic use, probably because of the intermittant narcotic effects followed by effects of relative withdrawal several times each day during each dosing interval.

Although methadone may cause similar effects during acute or short-term administration with ascending doses given, during chronic steady-dose methadone treatment, a steady state of drug levels is achieved, and normalization of neuroendocrine–endocrine function occurs with normal levels and circadian rhythms of levels of ACTH, β-endorphin, and cortisol and of FSH, LH, and testosterone (17,18,24,27,28). During chronic methadone treatment, responses to the provocative tests of neuroendocrine function, the metyrapone test of hypothalamic–pituitary reserve and the dexamethasone suppression test, become normal, whereas both of these tests are abnormal during cycles of heroin addiction (26–28). The normalization of neuroendocrine function occurs around the time of normalization of functional status and behavior (24,26–28). Prolactin levels are increased following administration of either short- or long-acting narcotics (18,24). This effect does not disappear during chronic methadone treatment, suggesting that the endogenous opioids may play an important role in prolactin release, probably by countering the inhibition of prolactin release by dopamine (41,42).

Alcohol, when used in large amounts on a chronic basis, has a biphasic effect on methadone metabolism, first inhibiting the metabolism of methadone by competition for the microsomal P-450-dependent enzymes when alcohol is present in large amounts, and then by accelerating methadone metabolism after alcohol has been cleared from the body because of the enhancement of hepatic microsomal enzyme activities in response to chronic alcohol use (19,20). Studies of the effects of use of alcohol on neuroendocrine function in methadone-maintained patients have been initiated. Concomitant use of certain other drugs such as barbiturates, the antituberculosis drug rifampin, and the anticonvulsant drug phenytoin (Dilantin®) also accelerates methadone metabolism by enhancing hepatic P-450-dependent enzymes and results in a lowering of plasma levels of methadone, thereby causing the appearance of narcotic withdrawal signs and symptoms prior to the end of the 24-hr dosing interval. The relative narcotic abstinence syndrome that appears may lead to drug-seeking behavior, which is usually prevented by chronic methadone treatment (21).

Naltrexone, an orally effective opioid antagonist, has been shown to be useful in the treatment of only 15 to 20% of "street" heroin addicts and up to 50% or more of small special groups such as health care professionals. Naltrexone does not seem to be intrinsically toxic to any organ or organ system except for the liver. Naltrexone does not seem to be hepatotoxic in most patients when recommended treatment doses (an average of 50 mg/day) are used. Naltrexone has been found to be a dose-dependent hepatotoxin (30,33). Significant abnormalities in liver function, specifically three- to sixfold elevations of serum transaminases (SGOT, SGPT) reflecting hepatocellular damage, have been observed in around 20% of subjects receiving 100 mg or 300 mg per day of naltrexone in attempts to manage obesity or senile dementia (2,30,33). A lower percentage of patients receiving standard treatment doses of naltrexone averaging 50 mg/day (given as 50-, 100-, 150-, or 200-mg doses) in attempts to manage obesity, irritable bowel syndrome, or narcotic addiction have been documented to sustain less dramatic elevations of serum transaminase levels. In those patients who have been followed, the abnormalities observed return to base-line levels within weeks following cessation of naltrexone administration.

Over 60% of former heroin addicts have chronic liver disease of viral and/or alcoholic origin with persistent liver test abnormalities, making it difficult to detect early or mild additional hepatic injury (1,17,18,22,32,44,57). Therefore, careful monitoring of liver function is essential during naltrexone treatment of narcotic addicts. Combined use or abuse of drugs, especially alcohol, could prove to be of great importance with respect to naltrexone effects on the liver. Unfortunately, it is not yet known whether naltrexone itself is the hepatotoxin or, as in the case of cocaine (discussed above), whether one or more of the naltrexone metabolites formed by oxidative metabolism by hepatic microsomal P-450-dependent enzyme systems may be the hepatotoxin(s). The precise hepatotoxin needs to be determined by use of appropriate animal models accompanied by careful observational studies of humans receiving the drug.

Naltrexone has essentially the opposite effects on neuroendocrine function as heroin. Naltrexone causes elevations in levels of ACTH, β-endorphin, cortisol, LH, and testosterone; moderate elevations of some of these hormone levels persist in patients during chronic naltrexone treatment (14–16,31,32,53). The possible effects of abuse of alcohol or drugs during naltrexone treatment on endocrine function have not yet been determined.

Medical Consequences of Parenteral Use of Drugs

An enormous variety of both common and very unusual disease entities have been observed as a result of parenteral drug abuse because of (a) infectious agents introduced by use of dirty needles and syringes contaminated with the blood of previous users as well as materials used to extend or "cut" the drugs or introduced during preparation of the drug for injection or (b) by chemicals or other substances used to extend (or "cut") or prepare the drug for self-administration. The types of medical consequences to have occurred as a result of parenteral drug abuse include localized cellulitis and abscesses, necrotizing fasciitis, bacteremia or septic arthritis, osteomyelitis with multiple bone abscesses, chronic bronchitis, lung abscesses, pneumonia, tuberculosis, transverse myelitis, brachial and lumbosacral plexitus, mononeuropathy, symmetrical polyneuropathy similar to Guillain–Barré syndrome, acute rhabdomyolysis, tetanus, botulism, malaria, and glomerulonephritis as well as other disorders. The three most commonly encountered severe diseases resulting from parenteral drug abuse, whether heroin or cocaine abuse, are bacterial or fungal endocarditis involving a number of unusual as well as usual organisms, viral hepatitis of several types including hepatitis B virus infection (markers showing prior or ongoing infection in 90% of heroin addicts), non-A, non-B hepatitis virus infection (markers not yet available for study), and δ agent hepatitis (markers showing prior or acute infection in over 10% of heroin addicts), and acquired immunodeficiency syndrome (AIDS) (1,6,7,17,18,22,25,32,37,44–47,50,57).

Parenteral drug abuse is the second most prevalent risk factor for development of AIDS, accounting for over 17% of cases as a single risk factor and contributing to 25 to 33% of cases if considered in combination with the most common risk factor, homosexuality. Most cases of AIDS in women and in infants are related directly or indirectly to parenteral drug abuse by direct exposure, heterosexual transmission, or *in utero* or perinatal transmission (6,7,47,50). Whether or not parenteral drug abuse, by way of introducing multiple potential antigenic stimuli or by direct drug effects not only on endocrine function but possibly also on immunological status, may enhance the risk of AIDS virus infection or development of the full-blown AIDS syndrome is not yet known. The possible role of combined use of alcohol and one or more drugs in the development of AIDS infection is not known, although it is appreciated that alcohol abuse may alter endocrine and immunological function significantly.

In New York City over 60% of parenteral abusers (heroin or cocaine) have been shown to be positive for the HTLV-III/LAV antibody as a marker of AIDS in 1984–85 (6,7,47,50). In other regions of the United States and in Europe, from fewer than 5% to over 80% of parenteral drug abusers have been found to be positive for the HTLV-III/LAV antibody, with sharp increases in local prevalence between 1983 and 1985 (47).

We have shown that early intervention with effective treatment for narcotic addiction has had a dramatic impact on the prevention of AIDS virus infection; fewer than 10% of former heroin addicts admitted to methadone treatment programs prior to 1978 had positive tests for the HTLV-III/LAV antibody (6,47,50). Despite the fact that up to 50% of these patients may have sporadic or intermittent parenteral drug abuse, primarily cocaine, this occasional parenteral drug abuse in no way compares with the frequency of parenteral drug abuse of the untreated heroin addict. Effective treatment of narcotic addiction, primarily methadone maintenance treatment, which is effective in 60 to 80% of typical heroin addicts, needs to be made generally available as soon as possible to prevent AIDS infection in those not yet infected and to prevent further spread of AIDS by those already showing evidence of this viral infection (47).

ACKNOWLEDGMENTS

This work was supported in part by a contract from The New York State Division of Substance Abuse Services. Dr. Kreek is a recipient of an ADAMHA-NIDA Research Scientist Award, DA00049.

REFERENCES

1. Alter, M. J. (1985): *Morbid. Mortal. Weekly Rep.*, 34:1SS–10SS.
2. Atkinson, R. L., Berke, L. K., Drake, C. R., Bibbs, M. L., Williams, F. L., et al. (1985): *Clin. Pharmacol. Ther.*, 38:419–422.
3. Blumberg, H., and Ikeda, C. (1978): *J. Pharmacol. Exp. Ther.*, 206:303–310.
4. Chasnoff, I. J., Burns, W. J., Schnoll, S. H., and Burns, K. A. (1985): *N. Engl. J. Med.*, 313:666–669.
5. Chow, M. J., Abbre, J. J., Ruo, T. I., Atkinson, A. J., Bowsher, D. J., et al. (1985): *Clin. Pharmacol. Ther.*, 38:318–324.
6. Des Jarlais, D. C., Marmor, M., Cohen, H., Yancovitz, S., Garber, J., et al., and Centers for Disease Control (1984): *Morbid. Mortal. Weekly Rep.*, 33:377–379.
7. Des Jarlais, D. C., Friedman, S. R., and Hopkins, W. (1985): *Ann. Intern. Med.*, 103:755–759.
8. Dipalma, J. R. (1981): *Am. Fam. Physician*, 24:236–238.
9. Fishbain, D. A., and Wetli, C. V. (1981): *Ann. Emerg. Med.*, 10:531–532.
10. Fishel, R., Hamamoto, G., Barbul, A., Jiji, V., and Efron, G. (1985): *Dis. Colon Rectum*, 28:264–266.
11. Hartman, N., Kreek, M. J., Ross, A., Khuri, E., Millman, R. B., et al. (1983): *Alcoholism Clin. Exp. Res.*, 7:316–320.
12. Hunt, D. E., Lipton, D. S., Goldsmith, D., and Strug, D. (1984): *Drug Alcohol Depend.*, 13:375–387.
13. Kloss, M. W., Rosen, G. M., and Rauckman, E. J. (1984): *Biochem. Pharmacol.*, 33:169–173.
14. Kosten, T. R., Kreek, M. J., Raghunath, J., and Kleber, D. (1986): In: *Proceedings of the 47th Annual Scientific Meeting of the Committee on Problems of Drug Dependence*, Vol. 67, edited by L. S. Harris, pp. 362–365. NIDA Research Monograph Series, Rockville, MD.
15. Kosten, T. R., Kreek, M. J., Raghunath, J., and Kleber, H. D. (1986): *Biol. Psychol.*, 21:217–220.
16. Kosten, T. R., Kreek, M. J., Raghunath, J., and Kleber, H. D. (1986): *Life Sci.*, 39:55–59.
17. Kreek, M. J. (1973): *J.A.M.A.*, 223:665–668.
18. Kreek, M. J. (1978): *Ann. N.Y. Acad. Sci.*, 311:110–134.
19. Kreek, M. J. (1981): *Ann. N.Y. Acad. Sci.*, 362:36–49.
20. Kreek, M. J. (1984): *Adv. Alcohol Subst. Abuse*, 3:35–46.
21. Kreek, M. J. (1986): In: *Strategies for Research on the Interactions of Drugs of Abuse*, Vol. 68, edited by M. C. Braude & H. M. Ginzburg, pp. 193–225. NIDA Research Monograph Series, Rockville, MD.
22. Kreek, M. J., Dodes, L., Kane, S., Knobler, J., and Martin, R. (1972): *Ann. Intern. Med.*, 77:598–602.
23. Kreek, M. J., Gutjahr, C. L., Garfield, J. W., Bowen, D. V., and Field, F. H. (1976): *Ann. N.Y. Acad. Sci.*, 281:350–370.
24. Kreek, M. J., and Hartman, N. (1982): *Ann. N.Y. Acad. Sci.*, 398:151–172.
25. Kreek, M. J., Khuri, E., Fahey, L., Miescher, A., Arns, P., et al. (1986): In: *Proceedings of the 47th Annual Scientific Meeting of the Committee on Problems of Drug Dependence*, Vol. 67, edited by L. S. Harris, pp. 307–309. NIDA Research Monograph Series, Rockville, MD.
26. Kreek, M. J., Raghunath, J., Plevy, S., Hamer, D., Schneider, B., et al. (1984): *Neuropeptides*, 5:277–278.
27. Kreek, M. J., Wardlaw, S. J., Friedman, J., Schneider, B., and Frantz, A. G. (1981): In: *Advances in Endogenous and Exogenous Opioids*, edited by E. Simon and H. Takagi, pp. 364–366. Kodansha Ltd. Publishers, Tokyo, Japan.
28. Kreek, M. J., Wardlaw, S. L., Hartman, N., Raghunath, J., Friedman, J., et al. (1983): *Life Sci.*, 33:409–411.
29. Lieber, C. S. (1977): *Metabolic Aspects of Alcoholism*. University Park Press, Baltimore.
30. *Medical Letter* (1985): *Med. Lett.*, 22:11–12.
31. Mendelson, J. H., Ellingboe, J., Kuehnle, J. C., and Mello, N. K. (1980): *J. Pharmacol. Exp. Ther.*, 214:503–506.
32. Miller, D. J., Kleber, H., and Bloomer, J. R. (1979): *Yale J. Biol. Med.*, 52:135–140.
33. Mitchell, J., Knopman, D., Levine, A. S., and Morley, J. E. (1985): *Gastroenterology*, 88:1646.
34. National Institute on Drug Abuse (1983): *Highlights from the National Survey in Drug Abuse: 1982 U.S. Department HHS-DHS-ADAMHA (DHHS Publication (ADM) 83-1277)*. U.S. Government Printing Office, Washington.
35. National Institute on Drug Abuse (1983): *National Drug and Alcoholism Treatment Utilization Survey (NDATUS) Series F No. 10, U.S. Department HHS-PHS-ADAMHA DHS Publication (ADM) 83-1284*. U.S. Government Printing Office, Washington.
36. National Institute on Drug Abuse (1983): *Statistical Series: Annual Data 1982; Data from Drug Abuse Warning Network (DAWN) Series 1, Number 2, U.S. Department HHS-PHS-ADAMHA (DHHS Publication No. (ADM) 83-1283)*. U.S. Government Printing Office, Washington.
37. National Institute on Drug Abuse (1983): *Treatment of Narcotic Addiction: State of the Art*, edited by J. Cooper, NIDA Research Monograph Series (DHSS Publication No. (ADM) 83-1281). NIDA, Rockville, MD.
38. National Institute on Drug Abuse (1984): *Capsules—1984 U.S. Department HHS-PHS-ADAMHA*. U.S. Government Printing Office, Washington.
39. New York State Division of Substance Abuse Services (1982): *Use of Psychoactive Prescription Drugs Among New York States' Household Population*. DSAS, Albany.
40. New York State Division of Substance Abuse Services (1984): *Recent Drug Abuse Statistics*. DSAS, Albany.
41. New York State Division of Substance Abuse Services (1985): *Cocaine Update for New York State*. DSAS, Albany.

42. New York State Division of Substance Abuse Services (1985): *Heroin Update for New York State.* DSAS, Albany.

43. New York State Division of Substance Abuse Services (1985): *State-Wide Comprehensive Five Year Plan 1984–88; Second Annual Update.* DSAS, Albany.

44. Novick, D. M., Enlow, R. W., Gelb, A. M., Stenger, R. J., Fotino, M., et al. (1985): *Gut,* 26:8–13.

45. Novick, D. M., Farci, P., Karayiannis, P., Gelb, A. M., Stenger, R. J., et al. (1985): *J. Med. Virol.,* 15:351–356.

46. Novick, D. M., Gelb, A. M., Stenger, R. J., Yancovitz, S. R., Adelsberg, B., et al. (1981): *Am. J. Gastroenterol.,* 75:111–115.

47. Novick, D. M., Khan, I., and Kreek, M. J. (1986): *United Nations Bulletin on Narcotics,* 38:15–25.

48. Novick, D. M., Kreek, M. J., Fanizza, A. M., Yancovitz, S. R., Gelb, A. M., et al. (1981): *Clin. Pharmacol. Ther.,* 30:333–336.

49. Novick, D. M., Kreek, M. J., Arns, P. A., Lau, L. L., Yancovitz, S. R., et al. (1985): *Alcoholism Clin. Exp. Res.,* 9:349–354.

50. Novick, D., Kreek, M. J., Des Jarlais, D., Spira, T. J., Khuri, E. T., et al. (1986): In: *Proceedings of the 47th Annual Scientific Meeting of The Committee on Problems of Drug Dependence,* Vol. 67, edited by L. S. Harris, pp. 318–320. NIDA Research Monograph Series, Rockville, MD.

51. Pasternack, P. F., Colvin, S. B., and Baumann, F. G. (1985): *Am. J. Cardiol.,* 55:847.

52. Pond, S. M., Kreek, M. J., Tong, T. G., Raghunath, J., and Benowitz, N. L. (1985): *J. Pharmacol. Exp. Ther.,* 234:1–6.

53. Ragavan, V. V., Wardlaw, S. L., Kreek, M. J., and Frantz, A. G. (1983): *Neuroendocrinology,* 37:266–288.

54. Rutgi, U. K., McGuire, M., Wise, T. N., and Cooper, J. N. (1985): *Gastroenterology,* 88:1563.

55. Sharff, J. A. (1984): *Ann. Emerg. Med.,* 13:1145–1147.

56. Smith, A. C., Freeman, R. W., and Harbison, R. D. (1981): *Biochem. Pharmacol.,* 30:453–458.

57. Stimmel, B., Vernace, S., and Schaffner, F. (1975): *J.A.M.A.,* 234:1135–1138.

58. Washton, A. M., Gold, M. S., and Pottash, A. C. (1984): *Adv. Alcohol Subst. Abuse,* 4:51–57.

Psychopharmacology:
The Third Generation of Progress,
edited by Herbert Y. Meltzer.
Raven Press, New York © 1987.

CHAPTER **173**

Pharmacological Agents in Treatment of Drug Dependence

Jerome H. Jaffe

This chapter focuses on the work of the last decade aimed at developing and evaluating pharmacological agents to ameliorate withdrawal syndromes, modify drug-seeking behavior, or treat psychiatric disorders among drug-dependent individuals. The vast new literature on mechanisms of action of drugs of abuse and on the clinical implications of the psychopathology now recognized to be present among drug-dependent patients is left to other chapters. Despite these exclusions, space limitations make it necessary, in many instances, to cite recent literature reviews rather than the original or definitive studies.

MANAGEMENT OF THE OPIOID WITHDRAWAL SYNDROME

Substitution of methadone (by mouth) for other opioids, such as heroin, is still viewed as the standard method against which other withdrawal techniques are measured. Among hospitalized patients, reductions of about 20% per day (usually 5 to 10 mg) from the initial stabilization doses permit the process to be completed in a week or two, but low-level withdrawal symptoms, including sleep and mood disturbance, typically persist for several weeks after the last dose, and relapse soon after discharge is common, especially among those patients who have been active heroin users prior to admission.

For ambulatory heroin addicts who have recently been stabilized on methadone, total withdrawal from methadone is difficult and is not routinely successful. Extending the period of gradual dose reduction from about 3 weeks to 6 weeks does not appear to increase significantly the likelihood of successful abstinence, nor does permitting patients to self-regulate the rate of reduction over this period, nor does the use of opioids, such as L-α-acetylmethadol (L-AAM), which has a longer duration of action than methadone (89). Indeed, abrupt withdrawal of L-AAM is associated with greater likelihood of successful detoxification than gradual reduction over 13 weeks (44). Even for patients who have been stabilized on methadone for several months, complete withdrawal is difficult. There have been some studies suggesting that a very gradual dose reduction (for example, 10% of dose per week, then 3% per week when the dose is below 20 mg) produces less mood disturbance and better long-term outcome (86). Expected new FDA regulations should permit such extended detoxification schedules.

Other Detoxification Agents

Clonidine (Catapres®), an α_2 agonist drug now marketed as an antihypertensive, has been used in both inpatient and outpatient settings to facilitate withdrawal from opioids (7,98). Many of the autonomic components of the opioid withdrawal syndrome are reduced by clonidine (1 to 2 mg/day), but many of the more subjective components of withdrawal, such as craving, lethargy, insomnia, and restlessness, are not well suppressed (5,7,45). Inpatients stabilized on 30 mg of methadone or less per day can be switched abruptly to clonidine. Although dosages up to 2.5 mg/day have been used, 1.25 to 1.5 mg is more typical. Even at these lower doses, episodes of severe hypotension have not been uncommon. Sedation is another major side effect seen with clonidine. Although the dropout rate appears to be somewhat higher with clonidine, the overall outcome of inpatient detoxification appears to be comparable to that achieved with reduction of methadone over 10 days (5,7).

Clonidine detoxification has been used to facilitate the initiation of naltrexone use in heroin addicts (6,98).

In a double-blind study of outpatient detoxification, patients maintained on 20 mg/day or less of methadone who had developed a relationship with the staff were about as successful after abrupt substitution of clonidine as after reduction of methadone by 1 mg/day. Approximately 40% of both groups were successfully detoxified as measured by a naloxone test or by no opioid use for 10 days after the last dose of methadone. In both groups the majority of those who were successful initially were again using illicit opioids 3 months later. The relatively low rates of successful detoxification in this outpatient study are consistent with other outpatient studies and contrast with success rates of more than 80% reported for inpatient studies using clonidine. Higher doses of clonidine and the supportive inpatient environment are likely explanations (46).

Clonidine is less useful for detoxifying addicts directly "off the street." Other α_2-adrenergic agonists such as lofexidine and guanfacine may also ameliorate aspects of the opioid withdrawal syndrome, but they have not yet been subjected to careful controlled studies (78,98). Clonidine has not yet been approved by the FDA for use in treating opioid dependence, although it is available as an antihypertensive agent.

Opioid Antagonists

The use of opioid antagonists to treat opioid dependence was originally based on the hypothesis that classically and operantly reinforced drug-seeking behavior contributes to high relapse rates following detoxification. It was postulated that blocking the reinforcing effects of opioids would lead to extinction of the drug-seeking behavior and of those opioid withdrawal symptoms that had become conditioned to environmental stimuli. Several different opioid antagonists have been tried clinically in double-blind studies, but results have not been dramatic. For the most part, opioid addicts at public clinics do not continue to take the drugs long enough or consistently enough to achieve the postulated extinction (23,74).

After almost 12 years as an investigational drug, in 1984, naltrexone (Trexan®) became the first opioid antagonist approved by the FDA for clinical use in treating opioid users. It is a long-acting, orally effective agent that, given daily in 50 mg/day dosage or three times weekly on a schedule of 100 mg on weekdays and 150 mg on weekends, produces substantial blockade of the effects of large doses of injected opioid drugs (such as 25 mg of heroin i.v.) (74). In a large, double-blind, multiclinic study, the dropout rate was so high that it was not possible to demonstrate significant clinical benefits attributable to naltrexone. The average time in treatment for clinic patients appears to be about 6 weeks (23). Although two double-blind studies have found that some individuals given naltrexone experience mild dysphoria, which is distinct from withdrawal (9,34), it does not appear that the high rate of dropout from treatment is directly related to such effects.

Although low levels of compliance have been observed in double-blind studies with opioid addicts having minimal occupational skills and social supports, experienced clinicians have found that naltrexone is beneficial for patients who are well motivated, have strong family support, and are actively engaged in legitimate careers (such as addicted physicians and other professionals). Such patients are much more likely to continue to take the drug for several months (53,99). Those who do so are also far more likely to be opioid abstinent at the 1-year follow-up period, and rates as high as 70% among such individuals have been reported (99). Those public programs combining naltrexone with high levels of rehabilitative support services have higher compliance and retention rates than are observed in double-blind studies, and patients in these programs who take the drug for more than 2 months are less likely to be opioid dependent at follow-up (74,99).

Patients maintained on naltrexone who were asked to "cook up" and self-inject saline under double-blind conditions as part of an effort to extinguish conditioned stimuli that elicit craving found the procedure very aversive, complained of severe withdrawal and craving, and discontinued the experiment. In a subsequent study utilizing less powerful stimuli and more psychological supports, gradual reduction of conditioned craving occurred in a substantial percentage of subjects following repeated cue exposure (60). In clinical trials with heroin addicts, toxicity was generally low. However, some nonaddict obese subjects given doses of 300 mg of naltrexone per day developed elevated transaminase values (SGPT values three to 19 times higher than base line), suggesting that such doses can produce hepatocellular injury. The use of naltrexone is, therefore, contraindicated in acute hepatitis or liver failure.

Opioid Maintenance

The use of methadone as a maintenance agent in treating opioid dependence was initiated by Dole and Nyswander in 1964. It is now established as one of the major treatment approaches in the United States and several other countries. However, as the number of programs utilizing methadone grew, and more disturbed and less motivated patients were admitted to treatment, the positive results were often less dramatic than those observed by Dole and Nyswander. Nevertheless, recent reviews support the position that the benefits to patients are substantial and outweigh the associated problems and costs. Most methadone programs continue to find that, on average, patients engage in less criminal activity, reduce illicit opioid and nonopioid drug use, and show decreased psychological symptoms such as depression (29,61,88).

Currently, treatment programs utilizing methadone maintenance vary with respect to the average dose of methadone prescribed, tolerance of continued antisocial behavior, and long-term goals of treatment. Many early programs used doses of methadone (80 to 120 mg/day) high enough to suppress the postulated "drug hunger" and block the effects of illicit opioids. Patients were encouraged to remain on methadone indefinitely, since it was assumed that opioid drug hunger would return following detoxification and lead to relapse. The need for methadone was seen as being comparable to a diabetic's need for insulin.

Many later programs found that lower doses of methadone (30 to 60 mg/day) were adequate to suppress most drug-seeking behavior despite inadequate cross tolerance to large doses of heroin. Some programs now see methadone as a transitional stage to eventual detoxification, emphasize behavioral change, are less tolerant of continued use of illicit drugs, and may encourage efforts at gradual withdrawal.

Retention rates during the first year vary from under 50% to 85%. Programs viewing methadone as a transitional treatment on the way to total abstinence, those using only low doses (20 to 40 mg), and those using confrontational techniques tend to have lower retention rates than programs favoring indefinite treatment, those using high or flexible doses of methadone, or those using supportive techniques (4,29). There is evidence that lower doses (29,59) or lower plasma levels despite prescribed high doses (35) are associated with increased illicit use of opioids and nonopioids, but the issue remains controversial.

Long-Term Effects of Methadone Maintenance

Although the relative safety of methadone is well established, it is now clear that tolerance to many of its opioid agonist actions is incomplete, and continuing pharmacological effects are seen in some patients. These effects include constipation (which can sometimes be severe enough to cause fecal impaction and intestinal obstruction), excessive sweating, and complaints of decreased libido and sexual dysfunction. Opioids reduce plasma levels of testosterone and follicle-stimulating hormone (FSH), for which tolerance is often incomplete. However, the abnormally low plasma levels of hormones and sexual dysfunction are not highly correlated. Other abnormalities, such as sweating, constipation, decreased sensitivity of CNS receptors to hypoxia, and decreased testosterone levels, are sometimes seen even after a year of treatment (49). Sleep abnormalities, including insomnia, nightmares, and altered EEG sleep patterns, frequently occur during the first months of treatment. The EEG sleep patterns appear to return to base line, but complaints of sleep abnormalities may persist (49). Not all patients develop tolerance to the mood-elevating effects of methadone; patients in double-blind studies report feeling an increased sense of well-being a few hours after ingesting their daily dose (57).

Detoxification from Methadone and Long-Term Outcome

The likelihood of remaining abstinent over the short term is uncertain even for those patients who successfully detoxify after a period of maintenance. Long-term abstinence once withdrawal is completed is not predicted by the same factors that predict retention and positive outcome in treatment. The percentage of patients who remain abstinent for 1 to 3 years after detoxification ranges from 12 to 28% for unselected samples of patients, some of whom were detoxified for violation of clinic rules, to 83% when analysis is restricted to those patients who elect to be withdrawn with both staff and patient concurring that treatment is complete (29,91). A multiclinic follow-up study found that 40% of former methadone patients interviewed were abstinent from all illicit opioids and did not have any other significant drug problems 6 years after completing their initial treatment (88).

Heroin Versus Methadone

A random assignment study comparing legally prescribed i.v. heroin to methadone was conducted at a London clinic. Subjects assigned to treatment with legally prescribed heroin continued to inject heroin and continued to be involved with the drug culture. Some of the subjects assigned to oral methadone maintenance refused to participate and left treatment immediately. One year later, 29% of patients assigned to oral methadone were still in treatment; 40% had left the clinic but were no longer using opioids regularly. Over the year between initial random assignment and follow-up, fewer patients assigned to oral methadone than to heroin had been admitted to hospitals for drug-related problems or had died. The impact of each treatment on crime is difficult to evaluate because of differences in baseline rates of criminality (30).

Other Opioid Maintenance Drugs

L-α-Acetylmethadole (L-AAM, methadylacetate), currently an investigational drug, is pharmacologically more complex than methadone but similar in its actions. Because it is converted into active metabolites that have very long biological half-lives, L-AAM can be given as infrequently as three times per week. Because different patients form and metabolize the various active metabolites at different rates, its use demands more clinical skill than methadone does (51).

Both double-blind and large-scale multicenter open studies have found L-AAM to be equivalent to methadone in suppressing illicit opioid use and facilitating productive activity. However, more patients drop out of treatment with L-AAM than with methadone used at dosages of 80 to 100 mg/day (51). Some patients complain of side effects such as nervousness and stimulation not commonly seen with methadone, although in one study, patients who had taken both L-AAM and methadone rated L-AAM to be preferable in most respects (96). Its major advantage seems to be the reduction of drug diversion and of negative interactions with clinic personnel about medication take-home privileges. After more than 17 years from its first use in opioid addicts, it remains an investigational new drug.

Buprenorphine (Temgesic®), available as an analgesic in

Europe and Australia, has been proposed as an alternative to methadone in opioid maintenance programs, but it has not yet been tried in outpatient settings for this purpose. It is considered a partial μ-receptor agonist, producing morphine-like effects at low doses but exhibiting a ceiling effect so that the intensity of its actions does not seem to exceed that achieved with 30 to 60 mg of morphine. This ceiling may limit risk of overdose. Given chronically, buprenorphine blocks the subjective effects of parenterally administered morphine or heroin (41). In experimental settings, chronic heroin users maintained on subcutaneous buprenorphine while being given access to i.v. heroin sharply reduced their heroin intake (63). It is not clear whether the blocking action results from cross tolerance or from antagonist-like actions. Given to subjects on high doses of opioids, buprenorphine precipitates abstinence; in subjects on low doses, it suppresses withdrawal (54). The drug binds quite firmly to receptors. Doses of naloxone up to 4 mg do not precipitate withdrawal, although higher doses may do so.

Drugs Used to Treat Psychiatric Disorders in Opioid Users

Up to 87% of opioid addicts seeking treatment meet RDC criteria for a psychiatric diagnosis other than drug addiction in their lifetime. The most common of these are affective disorders (74%), antisocial personality (27%), alcoholism (35%), and anxiety disorders (16%) (76). Opioid users with frank schizophrenic or manic–depressive features have responded well to antipsychotic agents and lithium, respectively. However, despite the high prevalence of depressive symptoms, the role of antidepressants is not firmly established. Although in one study doxepin appeared to speed the reduction of depressive symptoms beyond that seen with placebo, in other work with newly admitted addicts, improvement with placebo or without specific pharmacotherapy was rapid and significant, making it difficult to demonstrate efficacy of antidepressants such as imipramine (47).

The prescription of benzodiazepine anxiolytics for those opioid addicts with anxiety syndromes is controversial because some patients use such drugs (whether prescribed or obtained by other means) to the point of obvious oversedation, ataxia, and dysarthria. For those opioid addicts meeting diagnostic criteria for alcoholism or alcohol abuse, making treatment with methadone contingent on use of disulfiram produces a clear reduction in alcohol use (92). However, in a randomized double-blind study with methadone-maintained patients, both disulfiram and placebo produced equal degrees of improvement (52). The two drugs do not appear to produce adverse interactions. A study in which methadone patients with alcohol problems were randomly assigned to intensive Alcoholics Anonymous-type programs, behavioral modification, or no special intervention also revealed no significant differences in outcome measures despite enthusiastic participation in interventions by patients and staff (90).

In general, since those addicts with the greatest severity of psychiatric symptoms respond least well to any of the standard treatments for opioid dependence (62), we can expect increased attention to the problems of treating associated psychopathology by means of psychotherapy.

COCAINE: CRAVING AND WITHDRAWAL

The course of the cocaine abstinence syndrome appears to be more complex than an acute "crash" lasting several days followed by a general and gradual recovery over a period of weeks. Instead, it has been described as a three-phase syndrome. In the first phase, lasting up to about 4 days, the early agitation, anorexia, and high craving for cocaine are succeeded by a loss of craving associated with fatigue, exhaustion, depression, desire for sleep (or hypersomnia), and hyperphagia. This is followed by a second phase lasting 1 to 10 weeks. During the early part of this phase, mood improves, and sleep normalizes; but later, high levels of cocaine craving return, especially when stimuli associated with cocaine use are presented. It is during this later stage of the second phase, when craving returns, that the patient is most likely to relapse. This pattern may underlie the repeated cycles ("binges") typical of cocaine dependence, which resemble the "runs" or sprees of amphetamine abusers (20). It is postulated that some aspects of craving become conditioned so that even if the patient successfully reaches the third phase, where mood and hedonic responses are generally normal for patients without additional psychiatric diagnoses, environmental stimuli may still trigger craving for cocaine even months after last use (10,20).

Since the acute "crash" phase of withdrawal is neither life threatening nor of long duration, there have been few efforts to develop pharmacological agents to reduce acute withdrawal symptoms other than the "craving" for cocaine. To date, most efforts to treat cocaine craving or use have been based on one of three hypotheses. The first is that the craving represents a dysregulation of neurotransmission in the catecholaminergic reward systems, including the dopaminergic system (19,20), or a dopaminergic deficiency primarily (10). The second hypothesis is that cocaine is used, at least in part, to ameliorate some additional psychiatric syndrome (e.g., cyclothymic or attention deficit disorder) (20); and the third is that cocaine craving can be a conditioned response to stimuli previously associated with cocaine use (10,20).

Several pilot studies of pharmacological treatment of cocaine craving based on a catecholamine dysregulation or dopamine depletion hypothesis have been reported. Bromocriptine, given orally, appeared to reduce self-rated craving more than did placebo in two female patients. It has also been suggested that administration of tyrosine may be helpful (10), but additional data on the use of tyrosine following the first early reports have not emerged. In an open study using desipramine in doses of 25 to 100 mg, cocaine craving appeared to be reduced and abstinence facilitated (93). Similar benefits were found in patients with various depressive syndromes as well as in those without additional diagnoses in another open study when doses of desipramine up to 200 mg/day were used (19). To date, only one double-blind placebo-controlled study with a total N of 22 has been reported. This study used doses of desipramine up to 150 mg/day; 45% of both groups dropped out within the first week. Because of the small N, results are difficult to interpret, but the placebo group did about as well on all measures as the group receiving desipramine (94).

There are several case studies suggesting that methylphenidate may reduce craving in cocaine users with clearly established attention deficit disorder, residual type (45).

Lithium has been reported to attenuate cocaine-induced psychoactive effects (8) and to be helpful for some cocaine users (8,19,20), but no long-term or controlled studies have been reported. In an open study, lithium was helpful in cocaine users with cyclothymic disorders, but the investigators were not impressed with the effects of lithium in those patients without additional diagnoses (however, only 10 patients were treated with lithium). The benefits of lithium did not appear to be related to any significant reduction in the euphorigenic effects of cocaine (19).

In all of the studies describing treatments using pharmacological agents, the authors emphasize the importance of combining the agents with psychological support groups that reinforce the need for total abstinence. It is conceivable that chronic blockade of dopaminergic receptors could alter craving in the same way that naltrexone can alter craving in heroin users. In heroin users, the cognitive recognition that the presence of the blocker will minimize the reinforcing effects of heroin actually reduced craving (67). However, unlike naltrexone, which has only modest subjective effects, current dopaminergic blockers such as haloperidol may have distinctly dysphoric effects at usual doses. Some investigators have found that acute administration of drugs such as thioridazine to recently withdrawn cocaine users results in increased reports of craving (10). Whether dopaminergic blockers can help extinguish conditioned cocaine craving and, if so, whether this therapeutic possibility outweighs the risk of tardive dyskinesia is not known at this time. It has been postulated that by interfering with the mechanism of action of cocaine, tricyclic antidepressants might also act to reduce its euphorigenic effects in addition to any actions they might exert in reversing cocaine-induced changes in dopaminergic systems (19).

AMPHETAMINE DEPENDENCE

Although the subjective effects of amphetamines are quite similar to those of cocaine, there appear to be important differences in their mechanisms of action. It is not entirely clear why the cocaine epidemic beginning in the late 1970s should have stimulated so many more attempts at psychopharmacological intervention than did the amphetamine ("speed") epidemic that occurred only a decade previously. Whatever the reason, there is remarkably little that can be stated with certainty about pharmacological treatment of amphetamine dependence or its complications.

Dopaminergic blockers, such as haloperidol, have been widely accepted as the agents of choice for treating those amphetamine-induced paranoid and psychotic states that do not subside spontaneously within a few days. In the late 1960s, studies of the effects of depletion of catecholamines by α-methyl-para-tyrosine (aMT) on amphetamine-induced

euphoria in amphetamine addicts showed that self-rated euphoria was reduced to 50% by administration of 2 g aMT and almost eliminated by 4 g daily. It was suggested that long-term amphetamine blockade could be maintained by giving aMT at 2-day intervals. Dopaminergic blockers, such as chlorpromazine and pimozide, produced blockade equivalent to 2 g aMT, but additional blockade could not be achieved by increasing the dose (26). Animal studies suggest that in contrast to its efficacy in reducing the actions of amphetamine, aMT is unable to block the effects of methylphenidate, nomifensine, or cocaine (13).

Case reports of amphetamine abusers and one controlled trial in patients with affective disorders (97) showed that lithium tended to blunt or block the euphorigenic effects of amphetamine. However, in an open but controlled study of substance abusers in which an amphetamine challenge was given before and after 6 days of lithium stabilization, the degree of attenuation of induced euphoria was variable, with two of eight subjects reporting blockade and three of eight reporting no change (1). In a crossover study of lithium, of eight patients with affective disorder or alcoholism, lithium did attenuate some of the activating effects of i.v. methylphenidate (36).

There have been both animal and clinical pilot trials of the use of dopaminergic blockers to block euphorigenic effects in a manner analogous to the use of naloxone and cyclazocine in blocking the euphoric effects of opioids. These approaches never gained clinical acceptance.

The use of tricyclic antidepressants has been recommended to reduce postamphetamine depression and drug craving (13), an approach that seems to be gaining favor in treatment of cocaine dependence (see above). However, some investigators report having no success with the use of tricyclics, even in those cases in which they believed depression was a significant factor motivating the use of amphetamine (101).

DRUGS USED IN THE TREATMENT OF ALCOHOLISM

The use of drugs in the treatment of alcoholism and alcohol intoxication has been reviewed recently (21,39,83) and was the central focus of a recently published book (12).

Despite active research, there are as yet no drugs that specifically can antagonize the acute effects of alcohol. Naloxone was reported to have some beneficial effects in reversing alcohol-induced coma, but it now seems likely that beneficial effects when observed are related to actions on endogenous opioids that were aggravating the basic pathology causing the coma (11). Despite the traditional use of coffee as a sobering agent, caffeine has little demonstrable antidotal effect (71).

Zemelidine, an antidepressant that appears to be a specific serotonin uptake inhibitor, has been reported to reduce the memory-impairing effects of acute ethanol administration (100) and to alter alcohol intake in nonalcoholic heavy drinkers (70). In subsequent experiments, however, zemelidine appeared to aggravate the performance-impairing effects of ethanol and its effect on mood (69). Further exploration of these findings was inhibited by the withdrawal from clinical use of zemelidine by the manufacturer.

The Alcohol Withdrawal Syndrome

The alcohol withdrawal syndrome varies greatly in severity. Although severity of withdrawal is generally proportional to the level and duration of alcohol intake, many other factors, such as previous episodes of dependence and concurrent medical illness, also influence syndrome severity. Most episodes of withdrawal are mild and require neither hospitalization nor pharmacological intervention (103). Although some clinicians avoid use of any sedative agents in managing withdrawal on an ambulatory basis, others emphasize the value of the same drugs demonstrated to be useful in hospitalized alcoholics (39). In addition to the use of drugs directed specifically at the treatment of the alcohol withdrawal syndrome (see below), good nursing care, the routine use of nutritional supplements, and prompt attention to complicating illnesses are all responsible for the present low rate of delirium tremens and mortality from alcohol withdrawal.

More than 100 different drugs and drug combinations have been described for the treatment of alcohol withdrawal. There is evidence that the benzodiazepines, paraldehyde, chloral hydrate, barbiturates, and clomethiazole (chlormethiazole, Heminevrin®) are all effective in suppressing the alcohol withdrawal syndrome, as is alcohol itself. The benzodiazepines are superior to the phenothiazines in preventing seizures and when given in adequate dosage are probably as effective as the older sedative agents (21,39,83,87).

Available benzodiazepines vary greatly in complexity of metabolic transformation, duration of action of the parent compound, and in the number and activity of metabolites formed. In using the benzodiazepines to treat alcohol withdrawal, the basic principle is rapid substitution of a sufficient amount to suppress withdrawal, followed by a gradual tapering of drug levels over several days. Recent experiments demonstrated that in many cases, those drugs with long-acting metabolites such as chlordiazepoxide and diazepam are, for practical purposes, self-tapering. After administration of loading doses sufficient to suppress withdrawal (for example, 20 mg of diazepam orally with an additional 20 mg every 2 hr if needed), little additional medication was needed (85). Since the very rapidly metabolized entities will require more attention to the process of dose reduction, longer-acting drugs are better choices.

Parenteral administration must be considered when patients cannot take drugs by mouth. Lorazepam is promptly and reliably absorbed from intramuscular sites in contrast to chlordiazepoxide and diazepam, which are slowly and inconsistently absorbed. If suppression of withdrawal is delayed and hallucinosis develops, dopaminergic blockers such as haloperidol may be required in addition to benzodiazepines (21,83).

Barbiturates are still preferred for treating alcohol withdrawal in some European countries. Chloral hydrate has no significant advantages over the benzodiazepines, and paraldehyde, because of its toxicity, should be considered

obsolete. Clomethiazole (chlormethiazole, Heminevrin®) is a sedative–hypnotic that is commonly used in Great Britain and Europe; it is not available in the United States. It has a rapid onset of action but a shorter duration of action than benzodiazepines such as diazepam. As with other sedatives, abuse and overdosage have been reported (21,83,87).

Phenytoin (diphenylhydantoin) is sometimes used as part of the treatment of alcohol withdrawal, but there is no good evidence that it ought to be used routinely except in those patients who have a history of seizures unrelated to alcohol withdrawal. If phenytoin maintenance has been used prior to admission and has been stopped for several days, a loading dose followed by daily maintenance is indicated. Unlike phenytoin, valproic acid does suppress alcohol withdrawal seizures in animals; it has been used with good results in Europe and Australia in treating alcohol withdrawal (21,83,87). Lithium has been tried but has no practical place in the withdrawal phase of treatment.

Drugs Used in the Postwithdrawal Phase of Treatment of Alcoholism

Drugs to Deter Alcohol Consumption

Pharmacological agents can deter alcohol consumption by making the ingestion of alcohol aversive (sensitizing drugs) or by producing unpleasant effects that are deliberately linked to the ingestion of alcohol to create a conditioned aversion to alcohol (conditioning agents).

Although many drugs alter the body's response to alcohol and make its ingestion unpleasant (see below), only two, disulfiram and carbimide, have been widely used in the treatment of alcoholism. Both of these agents inhibit the enzyme aldehyde oxidoreductase (ALDH, aldehyde dehydrogenase), which metabolizes acetaldehyde to acetic acid. When this enzyme is inhibited, ingestion of alcohol causes a rise in acetaldehyde and brings on an unpleasant syndrome characterized by facial flushing, tachycardia, pounding in the chest, decreased blood pressure, nausea, vomiting, shortness of breath, sweating, dizziness, and confusion. In severe syndromes, there may be myocardial infarction, cerebrovascular hemorrhage, cardiovascular collapse, congestive failure, and seizures (84). In volunteers in whom the disulfiram–alcohol reaction (DER) was deliberately induced, the drug 4-methylpyrazol, which inhibits the metabolism of alcohol to acetaldehyde, produced a prompt fall in blood acetaldehyde levels and a decrease in symptoms (50). Disulfiram inhibits ALDH (as well as a number of other enzymes) irreversibly, and renewed enzyme activity is a function of protein synthesis; the effects are, therefore, long-lasting. Carbimide is much shorter acting. Disulfiram is associated with numerous side effects unrelated to the DER. These include drowsiness, lethargy, and peripheral neuropathy. Presumably because it inhibits dopamine β-hydroxylase, resulting in increased brain levels of dopamine, its use has been associated with exacerbation of schizophrenia.

Although disulfiram has been used for more than 35 years, it has been difficult to design an experiment that would demonstrate its clinical value. In the few controlled studies that have been done, differences between subjects on placebo and those on disulfiram were few. In the most carefully designed study to date, equally motivated patients were randomly assigned to 1 mg of disulfiram, 250 mg of disulfiram, or placebo; the latter group knew they were receiving a vitamin and not disulfiram. Using a life table analysis, the investigators concluded that the two groups receiving disulfiram did better in terms of complete abstinence than the placebo control, especially in the early months of treatment. However, there were no clinically important differences among the three groups in terms of days worked or days drinking or family stability (17). Since the study was restricted to male subjects who were not living alone and who volunteered to participate (and who tend to have a better prognosis in general), it is conceivable that the use of disulfiram could have had a greater influence on the course of alcoholism in the very patients who were less willing to participate and who had fewer social supports. A multicenter study using essentially the same design and involving a much larger number of alcoholic patients made essentially similar findings. There were no important differences among groups in terms of continuous abstinence, but among drinking men, there appeared to be a reduction in extent of alcohol use. In all three groups, including those who knew they were taking a vitamin rather than disulfiram, there was a very close relationship between compliance and continuous abstinence (18).

Disulfiram has been implanted subcutaneously, but blood levels from such implants are probably too low to produce sensitizing effects over periods long enough to justify the procedure, and any benefits are thought to have resulted from psychological factors (3,18). Disulfiram has been administered surreptitiously in some countries and has been made mandatory in some court-related programs (39), but in view of its toxicity, serious ethical questions are raised by these procedures.

Clinicians differ on the criteria used to decide if disulfiram use is contraindicated. Most include as contraindications myocardial disease, severe pulmonary insufficiency, liver dysfunction, renal failure, organic mental disturbances, neuropathy, psychosis, difficulty in impulse control, and suicidal ideation. The need for certain medication, such as vasodilators, β-adrenergic antagonists, MAO inhibitors, or antipsychotic agents, may also be considered a contraindication. Some clinicians recommend extensive initial mental, physical, and laboratory examinations followed by monthly or quarterly repetitions of selected tests (84); other clinicians believe that such criteria and repeated examination requirements would largely preclude the use of disulfiram in most alcoholics.

Calcium carbimide (citrated calcium carbimide, calcium cyanamide, Temposil®) produces a reversible inhibition of ALDH; its duration of action is shorter than that of disulfiram (less than 1 day), and it does not inhibit the same wide range of enzyme systems inhibited by disulfiram or cause as many adverse drug interactions and side effects (84). However, the evidence for its efficacy in reducing relapse is no more solid than that of disulfiram.

Other natural materials and clinically useful drugs causing altered sensitivity and adverse responses to ethanol including MAO inhibitors, certain antibiotics, some oral hypoglycemic agents, hydrogen sulfide, tetraethyl lead, pyrogallol, 4-bromopyrazole, and coprine, the active ingredient in the inky-cap mushroom (55,84). None of these agents has been used in controlled trials to treat alcoholism. Metronidazole (Flagyl®) also sensitizes some individuals but did not prove useful in treatment of alcoholism.

Drugs Used to Create Conditioned Aversion to Alcohol

Emetine-induced nausea coupled with the ingestion of alcohol has been used for more than 40 years to induce aversion to alcohol. But it is only in the last decade that controlled studies have demonstrated that conditioned aversion to alcohol can, in fact, be established and that such conditioning contributes to a positive clinical outcome. The use of lithium as an emetic can also produce clinically relevant aversion (36% abstinence for experimental subjects versus 12% for controls at 6 months). Efforts to demonstrate useful alcohol aversions with electrical shocks have not been successful (60). Apomorphine, which can produce emesis, has also been used as a conditioning agent, but it has been used for its other pharmacological actions as well (see below).

Drugs Used for Postwithdrawal Anxiety and Affective Disturbance

At the beginning of withdrawal, the majority of alcoholics report symptoms typical of depression. Most improve fairly quickly, but 15% to 30% continue to report high levels of depression and anxiety on self-rating instruments such as the Beck Depression Inventory, the SCL-90, or the Zung. There is some controversy about the clinical significance of these elevated scores and whether intervention apart from efforts to prevent relapse is indicated (39,80,81). However, it is clear that, using DSM-III criteria, the majority of alcoholics who seek treatment have diagnosable lifetime disorders in addition to alcoholism (33). Among the more common are major and minor depression, bipolar depression, depressive personality, antisocial personality, drug dependence, borderline personality, agoraphobia with panic episodes, and attention deficit disorder, residual type (33,39). When the manifestations of these disorders do not reach diagnosable levels prior to onset of alcoholism, some clinicians consider these additional diagnoses as secondary and unlikely to affect importantly the course of the primary alcoholism (80). However, most of these diagnoses do produce affective disturbances even in the absence of alcoholism. How these affective states are related to post-alcohol-withdrawal disturbances is not clear, since excessive alcohol probably induces a variety of organic affective states, and the insomnia and anxiety of withdrawal probably persist for many weeks. A number of drugs have been used or proposed for treatment of postwithdrawal anxiety and depressive states, including tricyclic antidepressants, MAO inhibitors, benzodiazepines, propranolol, lithium, dopaminergic agonists, and phenothiazines and other dopaminergic blockers.

The tricyclic antidepressants are frequently prescribed for alcoholics, but there is little firm evidence for their efficacy, even in "primary depressives" with alcoholism. Controlled studies of these agents have generally been conducted in heterogeneous groups of alcoholics. Although reviewers are generally negative in their assessments of the value of tricyclics (81), nonefficacy has not been proven. Failure to control for subtypes of depression, to measure plasma levels to assure adequate dosage and compliance, or to measure mood changes as well as patterns of alcohol use are among the methodological problems complicating interpretation of existing data. In addition, most studies were initiated soon after withdrawal, when rapid spontaneous improvement would obscure drug-related improvement. It is now clear that alcoholics metabolize imipramine more rapidly than controls, and in all probability most studies did not prescribe what would today be considered adequate dosage (39). Despite all of these biases against positive findings, one study of doxepin and one study of amitriptyline in selected alcoholics showed some positive effects on mood (39). Tricyclics have not yet been studied systematically in alcoholics as antianxiety or anti-panic-disorder agents. Concerns about liver toxicity and the need for careful compliance with dietary restrictions appear to have limited trials with MAO inhibitors in alcoholism. But for these concerns, MAO inhibitors would appear to be logical candidates for study in this group, many of whom have panic episodes and depressive symptoms more like those seen in atypical depression than in primary affective disorder.

Although the benzodiazepines have largely replaced other sedative agents in the treatment of postwithdrawal anxiety and sleep disturbance, many physicians and most nonmedical personnel involved in the treatment of alcoholism hold a strong bias against the use of any drug that can induce any variety of dependence. Although there may be some alcoholics who could benefit from these drugs and not abuse them, the preponderant tendency is to avoid their use in order to avoid a combined dependence. There is some suggestion that a combined alcohol and anxiolytic dependence may increase the incidence of depressive symptoms (79). In reducing tension in recently detoxified alcoholics, propranolol, a β-adrenergic blocker, is reported to be superior to placebo in one study and superior to diazepam in another. Low doses of thioridazine were superior to placebo in reducing tension and insomnia, but the placebo group did better in terms of work and activity. As with studies of tricyclics, studies of dopaminergic blockers were probably biased against positive findings. Since many dopaminergic blockers are somewhat dysphoric in their actions, there is probably little urgency in subjecting patients to additional clinical trials in treatment of depression and dysphoric states. Buspirone, an antianxiety agent that appears to be efficacious in neurotic outpatients, did not produce accentuated effects when combined with alcohol in normal volunteers and had little or no euphorigenic effect in drug abusers (39).

Apomorphine, a dopaminergic agonist, has been used as an aversive conditioning agent and as treatment for tension and craving. Clinicians who have used it for the latter effects over many years are enthusiastic about its capacity

to reduce relapse (16). No controlled studies have been reported.

In two early double-blind studies, patients assigned to lithium spent fewer days drinking and had fewer days of incapacitating drinking. In one, but not the other, only those categorized as depressed seemed to benefit (48,66,76). In a more recent random-assignment study of 84 volunteers, of whom 87% were considered depressed by SADS interview at the start of treatment, compliance with medication and serum lithium levels greater than 4 mEq/liter predicted a better outcome (15). Another study of 47 patients randomly assigned to lithium and placebo used a 3-month crossover design, which revealed no drug/placebo differences in terms of drinking or measures of depression, but the authors retrospectively concluded that the crossover design might have been inappropriate for testing the hypothesis (73). In double-blind placebo-controlled studies in normals and recently detoxified alcoholics, lithium blunts the sense of intoxication produced by alcohol; in the alcoholics, it also reduces the self-rated desire to continue drinking (43a). Among the drugs potentially available for treating alcoholics, lithium has the major advantage of agreed-on therapeutic levels and readily available methods for monitoring these levels. Its disadvantages are its many side effects and relatively narrow safety range.

PHARMACOLOGICAL APPROACHES TO TREATMENT OF TOBACCO DEPENDENCE

When relatively heavy smokers abruptly stop smoking, the following signs and symptoms (the tobacco withdrawal syndrome) typically emerge: craving for nicotine, irritability, impatience, hostility, restlessness, anxiety, depression, difficulty concentrating, confusion, trouble sleeping, increased appetite and caloric intake, weight gain, decreased heart rate, and increased slow waves in the EEG. There is some variability in the syndrome, depending in part on whether smokers stop in their natural environment or under laboratory conditions (37,38,77).

As is the case with alcohol and opioids, pharmacological treatments for tobacco dependence can be divided into three broad groups: (a) agents intended to produce some of the effects produced by nicotine (e.g., stimulation, relaxation, appetite suppression, or suppression of the nicotine withdrawal syndrome); (b) alternative means of delivering nicotine itself, but with reduced toxicity; and (c) agents intended to block the reinforcing effects of smoking or to make smoking aversive.

As a broad generalization, drugs that attempt to produce alerting, stimulation, or appetite suppression (e.g., amphetamines) are not of demonstrable value in helping smokers stop smoking. Indeed, under double-blind conditions, amphetamines increase the rate of smoking, as do alcohol and heroin (25,31,64). Nor has it been shown that sedatives or tranquilizers or propranolol can be of substantial aid in smoking cessation.

Lobeline, an alkaloid obtained from *Lobelia inflata,* has been proposed as a treatment for tobacco dependence and withdrawal on the basis of its structural similarity to nicotine and the observation that cross tolerance to nicotine develops in some systems. Although it continues to be marketed as an over-the-counter preparation, it has been exceedingly difficult to find consistent evidence that it is superior to nonspecific (placebo) agents in helping smokers stop smoking. In laboratory experiments, smokers not trying to reduce their intake showed no change in number of cigarettes smoked or weight of butts when given lobeline at the dosage recommended by the manufacturer (82).

Mecamylamine has been shown to block the subjective and reinforcing effects of nicotine at doses that produce no significant adverse effects (32). Smokers seeking treatment for their tobacco use have voluntarily ingested mecamylamine on an outpatient basis, and some of those found it helpful (95). Neither long-term follow-up of this group nor data from controlled studies are available.

In contrast to these negative or only tentative results, there is ample evidence that nicotine in the form of nicotine chewing gum can suppress important components of the tobacco withdrawal syndrome and can be of practical value in helping smokers achieve long-term success in quitting.

On the basis of several independent studies (38,40,77,102), it is now clear that compared to placebo, nicotine gum can suppress some of the elements of the tobacco withdrawal syndrome, thus demonstrating a relationship of these symptoms to nicotine withdrawal and not merely to the interruption of repeatedly reinforced behavior. The symptoms most consistently relieved by chewing nicotine gum containing 2 mg nicotine are irritability and impatience. Some studies also find reduction in difficulty in concentrating, restlessness, anxiety, hunger, insomnia, and changes in heart rate. Nicotine at this dose level was not usually effective in reducing the increased craving for cigarettes. However, whenever a total score of symptoms is constructed, nicotine produces greater reductions than does placebo. In two early studies, nicotine gum had no effect on withdrawal, but measures of the gum effect were confounded by continued smoking of cigarettes (77).

It is not clear whether failure to relieve all symptoms of withdrawal is related to dose or to route of administration or to other factors. Because nicotine gum in dosage forms currently available does not substantially alleviate craving, the use of the gum as an adjunct to smoking cessation must be combined with careful instruction on its use and on what can reasonably be expected.

When nicotine gum is used to treat patients seeking to end their smoking and is combined with intensive behavioral modification techniques, the combination produces some of the highest 1-year abstinence rates reported (40–50%) (28). Even when combined with lesser degrees of instruction, nicotine gum produces significant increases in the percentage of smokers who remain abstinent at 6 months and at 1 year. However, if smokers are not given specific instructions in how to chew the gum, what they can reasonably expect to experience, and what contribution they must make in the effort to quit, the prescription of the nicotine gum is not associated with higher abstinence rates than placebo gum (77). Nevertheless, even in minimal-intervention dispensary studies, those subjects who used more than one box of the gum had far higher success rates than those who were given only advice about smoking cessation and than those who were given the gum but did not use it. It does

seem that, as a minimum, patients must be given instruction on proper initial use of the gum and encouragement to continue to use it over at least several weeks.

Smokers vary in their nicotine intake and also in the severity of the nicotine abstinence syndromes they experience. In two early studies of psychological intervention, levels of serum cotinine (a principal and longer-lasting metabolite of nicotine) were predictive of withdrawal symptoms and success in cessation (27,104). On the assumption that those smokers most physically dependent on nicotine would be more likely to benefit from treatment with nicotine gum, several groups have examined the relationship between measures of nicotine dependence and/or pretreatment measures of nicotine intake and the response to the treatment. The results with biochemical indices of intake have not been entirely consistent. In two similar but independent studies using 2-mg nicotine gum, one found no significant relationship between pretreatment plasma levels of cotinine and the likelihood that patients would do better on nicotine gum than on placebo. In the other, those patients whose cotinine levels were above the median did poorly without nicotine gum (28). However, clinical estimates of nicotine tolerance and dependence do appear to predict which smokers will be helped more by nicotine gum than by nonpharmacological approaches (14). Nicotine-containing gum–resin complex has been available for research purposes for more than a decade and was available on a prescription basis in Scandinavia, England, and Canada for several years before its approval by the U.S. Food and Drug Administration in the spring of 1984. Only the 2-mg dosage form is currently available in the United States, but 2- and 4-mg size pieces of gum are available elsewhere.

In addition to nicotine gum, other means to deliver nicotine have been developed. These include nicotine nasal sprays and skin patches (75). Some of these have been studied by academic researchers. One device that, to the best of this reviewer's knowledge, has been marketed but not studied is a hollow plastic tube virtually identical in appearance to a filter cigarette and containing at the distal end a filter-like material that delivers nicotine vapor when the user inhales through the tube. The legal status of these devices, each of which is said to deliver the nicotine equivalent of three cigarettes, is uncertain. They are sold over the counter in cigarette-like packets containing five devices.

Many former smokers have adopted the use of oral tobacco in the form of snuff or chewing tobacco. Although this practice reduces the hazards associated with tobacco smoke inhalation, it is not clear whether the use of smokeless tobacco qualifies as a pharmacologic treatment of tobacco dependence.

In a single double-blind 24-hr crossover study, clonidine in doses tolerated by ambulatory subjects more effectively reduced craving for tobacco (as experienced at about 12 to 24 hr of abstinence) than did placebo or alprazolam (24).

BARBITURATES AND SEDATIVE–HYPNOTIC DEPENDENCE

The barbiturate withdrawal syndrome is generally managed by stabilizing patients on amounts of a short-acting barbiturate, such as pentobarbital, sufficient to suppress withdrawal symptoms and then slowly reducing the dosage. Substitution of phenobarbital, which has a much longer duration of action, allows for smooth and gradual reduction in dosage (56).

Benzodiazepine withdrawal is generally managed by gradual withdrawal of the specific drug on which dependence has developed. Since all benzodiazepines seem to occupy the same receptors, substitution of longer-acting metabolites for shorter-acting congeners, such as diazepam for triazolam, seems rational.

There are no specific pharmacological treatments available or proposed for treating the postwithdrawal phase of barbiturate or sedative–hypnotic dependence.

CANNABIS DEPENDENCE

Some individuals use cannabis on a daily or almost daily basis. Many experience serious impairment of their capacity to function normally. A withdrawal syndrome (not life threatening and resembling mild sedative withdrawal) has been reported in experimental situations (43,65), but its relationship to marijuana-seeking behavior remains unclear. A request for help (treatment) in breaking the cannabis-using patterns is no longer uncommon. At present, there are no therapeutic agents that are specific for either cannabis withdrawal or dependence.

PHENCYCLIDINE AND RELATED COMPOUNDS

To date, no drugs have been put forward as pharmacological treatments for PCP dependence, although, in one open study, desipramine was reported helpful. Withdrawal phenomena have been described in monkeys (2), suggesting that physical dependence can develop; there is no clear evidence that physical dependence plays an important role in chronic self-administration of PCP in man. The pharmacological treatment of PCP intoxication is built on a somewhat firmer empirical base. The removal of PCP, which is sequestered in acidic gastric fluids, can be aided by judicious use of gastric drainage, but acidification of urine, which also accelerates excretion, is no longer routinely used. Dopaminergic blockers such as haloperidol appear to be of value in the treatment of the PCP acute psychotic states (58), and there has been a report suggesting that opioids such as meperidine and morphine may be of equal value (22). The use of drug-specific antibody fragments (antigen-binding fragments of IgG) has been shown to reverse digoxin toxicity in both animals and man and is now being evaluated in PCP intoxication in animals (72).

SUMMARY

Pharmacological agents now play a significant role in medical treatment of a variety of drug dependence syndromes. Over the past decade, the advent of α_2 agonists such as clonidine has introduced new flexibility into the management of opioid withdrawal. Naltrexone, finally

available, has a limited but useful role in treating selected opioid-dependent individuals. Opioid maintenance with methadone is still being refined, and new agents with some advantages (such as buprenorphine, L-AAM) are under development. Nicotine has now been demonstrated to suppress components of the tobacco withdrawal syndrome, and nicotine gum represents a significant advance in treatment of tobacco dependence. Although there are no agents of demonstrable value for treating cocaine dependence, several are under investigation. The benzodiazepines are now established as the agents of choice in managing alcohol withdrawal, and the evidence that lithium could play some role in the postwithdrawal phase of treatment is at least as strong as the evidence supporting the use of disulfiram and antidepressants.

The development of a criteria-based diagnostic system has led to the rediscovery of the psychopathology that commonly accompanies various forms of drug dependence. This rediscovery has led, in turn, to renewed interest in understanding the role of psychopathology in drug dependence and developing more effective treatments of those pathologies. Recent research on the genetics of alcoholism and sociopathy supports the notion of a genetically transmitted vulnerability to alcoholism and has generated intense interest in exploring the biology of this vulnerability. It is likely that the interest in psychopathology related to addictions and in the genetics of vulnerability will overlap and generate new therapeutic agents in the future. Such new agents could conceivably alter the current bleak prognosis for some of the personality disorders characterized by aggression, impulsivity, and affective instability.

REFERENCES

1. Angrist, B., and Gershon, S. (1979): *Am. J. Psychiatry,* 136:806–810.
2. Balster, R. L. (1986): In: *Phencyclidine: An Update,* edited by D. H. Clouet, pp. 148–162. NIDA Res. Monograph 64, DHHS Publ. No. (ADM)86-1443, U.S. Government Printing Office, Washington.
3. Bergstrom, B., Ohlin, H., Lindblom, P. E., and Wadstein, J. (1982): *Lancet,* I:49–50.
4. Brown, B. S., Waters, J. K., Iglehart, A. S., and Akins, C. (1983): *Am. J. Drug Alcohol Abuse,* 9:129–140.
5. Cami, J., de Torres, S., San, L., Sole, A., Guerra, D., et al. (1985): *Clin. Pharmacol. Ther.,* 38:336–341.
6. Charney, D. S., Riordan, C. E., Kleber, H. D., Murburg, M., Braverman, P., et al. (1982): *Arch. Gen. Psychiatry,* 39:1327–1333.
7. Charney, D. S., Sternberg, D. E., Kleber, H. D., Heninger, G. R., and Redmond, D. E., Jr. (1981): *Arch. Gen. Psychiatry,* 38:1273–1277.
8. Cronson, A. J., and Flemenbaum, A. (1978): *Am. J. Psychiatry,* 135:856–857.
9. Crowley, T. J., Wagner, J. E., Zerbe, G., and MacDonald, M. (1985): *Am. J. Psychiatry,* 142:1081–1084.
10. Dackis, C. A., and Gold, M. S. (1985): *J. Subst. Abuse Treat.,* 2:139–145.
11. Dole, V. P., Fishman, J., Goldfrank, L., Khanna, J., and McGivern, R. F. (1982): *Alcoholism: Clin. Exp. Res.,* 6:275–279.
12. Edwards, G., and Littleton, J., eds. (1984): *Pharmacological Treatments for Alcoholism.* Methuen, New York.
13. Ellinwood, E. H. (1979): In: *Handbook on Drug Abuse,* edited by R. I. Dupont, A. Goldstein, and J. O'Donnell, pp. 221–231. U.S. Government Printing Office, Washington.
14. Fagerstrom, K. O., and Mellin, B. (1985): In: *Pharmacological*

Adjuncts in Smoking Cessation, edited by J. Grabowski and S. M. Hall, pp. 102–109. NIDA Res. Monograph 53, DHHS Publ. No. (ADM)85-1333, U.S. Government Printing Office, Washington.

15. Fawcett, J., Clark, D. C., Gibbons, R. D., Aagesen, C. A., Pisani, V. D., et al. (1984): *J. Clin. Psychiatry,* 45:494–499.

16. Feldmann, H. (1983): *Psychiatr. J. Univ. Ottawa,* 8:30–37.

17. Fuller, R. K., and Williford, W. O. (1980): *Alcoholism Clin. Exp. Res.,* 4:298–301.

18. Fuller, R. K., Branchey, L., Brightwell, D. R., Derman, R. M., and Emrick, C. D. (1986): *J.A.M.A.* (*in press*).

19. Gawin, F. H., and Kleber, H. D. (1984): *Arch. Gen. Psychiatry,* 41:903–909.

20. Gawin, F. H., and Kleber, H. D. (1986): *Arch. Gen. Psychiatry,* 43:107–113.

21. Gessner, P. K. (1979): In: *The Biochemistry and Pharmacology of Ethanol,* edited by E. Majchrowicz and E. Noble, pp. 375–434. Plenum Press, New York.

22. Giannini, A. J., Loiselle, R. H., Price, W. A., and Giannini, J. D. (1985): *J. Clin. Psychiatry,* 46:52–54.

23. Ginzburg, H. M. (1986): In: *Advances in Alcohol & Substance Abuse,* edited by B. Stimmel, pp. 83–101. The Haworth Press, New York.

24. Glassman, A. H., Jackson, W. K., Walsh, B. T., and Roose, S. P. (1984): *Science,* 226:864–866.

25. Griffiths, R. R., Bigelow, G. E., and Liebson, I. (1976): *J. Exp. Anal. Behav.,* 25:279–292.

26. Gunne, L. M. (1977): In: *Drug Addiction II,* edited by W. R. Martin, pp. 247–275. Springer-Verlag, Berlin.

27. Hall, S. M., Herning, R. I., Jones, R. T., Benowitz, N. L., and Jacob, P., III (1984): *Clin. Pharmacol. Ther.,* 35:810–814.

28. Hall, S. M., and Killen, J. D. (1985): In: *Pharmacological Adjuncts in Smoking Cessation,* edited by J. Grabowski and S. M. Hall, pp. 131–143. NIDA Res. Monograph 53, DHHS Publ. No. (ADM)85-1333, U.S. Government Printing Office, Washington.

29. Hargreaves, W. A. (1983): In: *Research on the Treatment of Narcotic Addiction,* edited by J. R. Cooper, F. Altman, B. Brown, and D. Czechowicz, pp. 19–79. NIDA Treatment Res. Monograph Series, DHHS Publ. No. (ADM)83-1281, U.S. Government Printing Office, Washington.

30. Hartnoll, R. L., Mitcheson, M. D., Battersby, A., Brown, G., Ellis, M., et al. (1980): *Arch. Gen. Psychiatry,* 37:877–884.

31. Henningfield, J. E., and Griffiths, R. R. (1981): *Clin. Pharmacol. Ther.,* 30:497–505.

32. Henningfield, J. E., Miyasato, K., Johnson, R. E., and Jasinski, D. R. (1983): In: *Problems of Drug Dependence 1982,* edited by L. S. Harris, pp. 259–265. NIDA Res. Monograph 43, DHHS Publ. No. (ADM)83-1264, U.S. Government Printing Office, Washington.

33. Hesselbrock, M. N., Reyer, R. E., and Keener, J. J. (1985): *Arch. Gen. Psychiatry,* 42:1050–1055.

34. Hollister, L. E., Johnson, K., Boukhabza, D., and Gillespie, H. K. (1981): *Drug Alcohol Depend.,* 8:37–41.

35. Holmstrand, J., Anggard, E., and Gunne, L.-M. (1978): *Clin. Pharmacol. Ther.,* 23:175–180.

36. Huey, L. Y., Janowsky, D. S., Judd, L. L., Abrams, A., Parker, D., et al. (1981): *Psychopharmacology,* 73:161–164.

37. Hughes, J. R., and Hatsukami, D. K. (1986): *Arch. Gen. Psychiatry,* 43:289–294.

38. Hughes, J. R., Hatsukami, D. K., Pickens, R. W., Krahn, D., Malin, S., et al. (1984): *Psychopharmacology,* 83:82–87.

39. Jaffe, J. H., and Ciraulo, D. (1985): In: *The Diagnosis and Treatment of Alcoholism,* edited by J. H. Mendelson and N. K. Mello, pp. 355–389. McGraw-Hill, New York.

40. Jarvis, M. J., Raw, M., Russell, M. A. H., and Feyerabend, C. (1982): *Br. Med. J.,* 285:537–540.

41. Jasinski, D. R., Pevnick, J. S., and Griffith, J. D. (1978): *Arch. Gen. Psychiatry,* 35:501–516.

42. Jasinski, D. R., Johnson, R. E., and Kocher, T. R. (1985): *Arch. Gen. Psychiatry,* 42:1063–1066.

43. Jones, R. T. (1983): In: *Cannabis and Health Hazards,* edited by K. O. Fehr and H. Kalant, pp. 617–689. Addiction Research Foundation, Toronto.

43a. Judd, L. L., and Huey, L. Y. (1984): *Am. J. Psychiatry,* 141:1517–1520.

44. Judson, B. A., Goldstein, A., and Inturrisi, C. E. (1983): *Arch. Gen. Psychiatry,* 40:834–840.

45. Khantzian, E. J., Gawin, F. H., Riordan, C., and Kleber, H. D. (1984): *J. Subst. Abuse Treat.,* 1:107–112.

46. Kleber, H. D., Riordan, C. E., Rounsaville, B., Kosten, T., Charney, D., et al. (1985): *Arch. Gen. Psychiatry,* 42:391–394.

47. Kleber, H. D., Weissman, M. M., Rounsaville, B. J., Wilber, C. H., Prusoff, B. A., et al. (1983): *Arch. Gen. Psychiatry,* 40:643–649.

48. Kline, N. S., Wren, J. C., Cooper, T. B., Varga, E., and Canal, O. (1974): *Am. J. Med. Sci.,* 268:15–22.

49. Kreek, M. J. (1983): In: *Research on the Treatment of Narcotic Addiction,* edited by J. R. Cooper, F. Altman, B. S. Brown, and D. Czechowicz, pp. 456–482. NIDA Treatment Res. Monograph Series. DHHS Publ. No. (ADM)83-1281, U.S. Government Printing Office, Washington.

50. Lindros, K. O., Stowall, A., Pikkarainen, P., and Salaspuro, M. (1981): *Alcoholism Clin. Exp. Res.,* 5:528–530.

51. Ling, W., Dorus, W., Hargreaves, W. A., Resnick, R., Senay, E., et al. (1984): *Arch. Gen. Psychiatry,* 41:193–199.

52. Ling, W., Weiss, D. G., Charuvastra, V. C., and O'Brien, C. P. (1983): *Arch. Gen. Psychiatry,* 40:851–854.

53. Ling, W., and Wesson, D. R. (1984): *J. Clin. Psychiatry,* 45:46–48.

54. Lukas, S. E., Jasinski, D. R., and Johnson, R. E. (1984): *Clin. Pharmacol. Ther.,* 36:127–132.

55. Marchner, H. (1984): In: *Pharmacological Treatments for Alcoholism,* edited by G. Edwards and J. Littleton, pp. 491–530. Methuen, New York.

56. Martin, P. R., Kapur, B. M., Whiteside, E. A., and Sellers, E. M. (1979): *Clin. Pharmacol. Ther.,* 26:256–264.

57. McCaul, M. E., Bigelow, G. E., Stitzer, M. S., and Liebson, I. (1982): *Clin. Pharmacol. Ther.,* 31:753–761.

58. McCarron, M. M. (1986): In: *Phencyclidine: An Update,* edited by D. H. Clouet, pp. 209–217. NIDA Res. Monograph 64, DHHS Publ. No. (ADM)86-1443, U.S. Government Printing Office, Washington.

59. McGlothlin, W. H., and Anglin, M. D. (1981): *Arch. Gen. Psychiatry,* 38:1055–1063.

60. McLellan, A. T., and Childress, A. R. (1985): *J. Subst. Abuse Treat.,* 2:187–191.

61. McLellan, A. T., Luborsky, L., O'Brien, C. P., et al. (1982): *J.A.M.A.,* 247:1423–1427.

62. McLellan, A. T., Luborsky, L., Woody, G. E., O'Brien, C. P., and Druley, K. A. (1983): *Arch. Gen. Psychiatry,* 40:620–625.

63. Mello, N. K., and Mendelson, J. H. (1980): *Science,* 207:657–659.

64. Mello, N. K., Mendelson, J. H., Sellers, M. L., and Kuehnle, J. C. (1980): *Psychopharmacology,* 67:45–52.

65. Mendelson, J. H., Mello, N. K., Lex, B. W., and Bavli, S. (1984): *Am. J. Psychiatry,* 141:1289–1290.

66. Merry, J., Reynolds, C. M., Bailey, J., and Coppen, A. (1976): *Lancet,* 2:481–482.

67. Meyer, R. E., and Mirin, S. M. (1979): *The Heroin Stimulus.* Plenum Press, New York.

68. Morland, J., Johnsen, J., Bache-Wiig, J. E., Ripel, A., Stensrud, T., et al. (1984): In: *Pharmacological Treatments for Alcoholism,* edited by G. Edwards and J. Littleton, pp. 573–578. Methuen, New York.

69. Naranjo, C. A., Sellers, E. M., Kaplan, H. L., Hamilton, C., and Khouw, V. (1984): *Clin. Pharmacol. Ther.,* 36:654–660.

70. Naranjo, C. A., Sellers, E. M., Roach, C. A., Woodley, D. V., Sanchez-Craig, M., et al. (1984): *Clin. Pharmacol. Ther.,* 35:374–381.

71. Nuotto, E., Mattila, M. J., Seppala, T., and Konno, K. (1982): *Clin. Pharmacol. Ther.,* 31:68–76.

72. Owens, S., and Mayersohn, M. (1986): In: *Phencyclidine: An Update,* edited by D. H. Clouet, pp. 112–126. NIDA Research Monograph 64, DHHS Publ. No. (ADM)86-1443, U.S. Government Printing Office, Washington.

73. Pond, S. M., Becker, C. E., Vandervoort, R., Phillips, M., Bowler, R. M., et al. (1981): *Alcoholism: Clin. Exp. Res.,* 5:247–251.

74. Resnick, R. B., Schuyten-Resnick, E., and Washton, A. M. (1980): *Annu. Rev. Pharmacol. Toxicol.,* 20:463–474.

75. Rose, J. E., Herskovic, J. E., Trilling, Y., and Jarvik, M. E. (1985): *Clin. Pharmacol. Ther.,* 38:450–456.

76. Rounsaville, B. J., Weissman, M. M., Kleber, H., and Wilber, C. (1982): *Arch. Gen. Psychiatry,* 39:161–166.

77. Schneider, N. G., and Jarvik, M. E. (1985): In: *Pharmacological Adjuncts in Smoking Cessation,* edited by J. Grabowski and S. M. Hall, pp. 83–101. NIDA Research Monograph 53, DHHS Publ No. (ADM)85-1333, U.S. Government Printing Office, Washington.

78. Schubert, H., Fleischhacker, W. W., Meise, U., and Theohar, C. (1984): *Am. J. Psychiatry,* 141:1271–1273.

79. Schuckit, M. A. (1983): *Am. J. Psychiatry,* 140:711–714.

80. Schuckit, M. A. (1985): *Arch. Gen. Psychiatry,* 42:1043–1049.

81. Schuckit, M. A. (1986): *Am. J. Psychiatry,* 143:140–141.

82. Schuster, C. R., Lucchesi, B. R., and Emley, G. S. (1979): In: *Cigarette Smoking as a Dependence Process,* edited by N. A. Krasnegor, pp. 91–99. NIDA Res. Monograph 23, DHHS Publ. No. (ADM)82-800, U.S. Government Printing Office, Washington.

83. Sellers, E. M., and Kalant, H. (1982): In: *Encyclopedic Handbook of Alcoholism,* edited by E. Kaufman and E. M. Pattison, pp. 141–166. Gardner Press, New York.

84. Sellers, E. M., Naranjo, C. A., and Peachey, J. E. (1981): *N. Engl. J. Med.,* 305:1255–1262.

85. Sellers, E. M., Naranjo, C. A., Harrison, M., Devenyi, P., Roach, C., et al. (1983): *Clin. Pharmacol. Ther.,* 34:822–826.

86. Senay, E. C., Dorus, D. W., Goldberg, F., and Thornton, W. (1977): *Arch. Gen. Psychiatry,* 34:361–367.

87. Shaw, G. K. (1982): *Br. Med. Bull.,* 38:99–102.

88. Simpson, D. D., Joe, G. W., and Bracy, S. A. (1982): *Arch. Gen. Psychiatry,* 39:1318–1326.

89. Sorensen, J. L., Hargreaves, W. A., and Weinberg, J. A. (1982): *Arch. Gen. Psychiatry,* 39:167–171.

90. Stimmel, B., Cohen, M., Sturiano, V., Hanbury, R., Korts, D., et al. (1983): *Am. J. Psychiatry,* 140:862–866.

91. Stimmel, B., Goldberg, J., Kotkopf, E., and Cohen, M. (1977): *J.A.M.A.,* 237:1216–1220.

92. Stitzer, M. L., Bigelow, G. E., Liebson, I. A., and McCaul, M. E. (1984): In: *Behavioral Intervention Techniques in Drug Abuse Treatment,* NIDA Res. Monograph 46, edited by J. Grabowski, M. L. Stitzer, and J. E. Henningfield, pp. 84–103. DHHS Publ. No. (ADM)84-1282, U.S. Government Printing Office, Washington.

93. Tennant, F. S., Rawson, R. A., and McCann, M. A. (1981): *Am. J. Psychiatry,* 138:845–847.

94. Tennant, F. S., and Tarver, A. L. (1985): In: *Problems of Drug Dependence 1984,* edited by L. S. Harris, pp. 159–163. NIDA Res. Monograph 55, DHHS Publ. No. (ADM)85-1393, U.S. Government Printing Office, Washington.

95. Tennant, F. S., and Tarver, A. L. (1985): In: *Problems of Drug Dependence 1984,* edited by L. S. Harris, pp. 291–297. NIDA Res. Monograph 55, DHHS Publ. No. (ADM)85-1393, U.S. Government Printing Office, Washington.

96. Trueblood, B., Judson, B. A., and Goldstein, A. (1978): *Drug Alcohol Depend.,* 3:125–132.

97. van Kammen, D. P., and Murphy, D. L. (1975): *Psychopharmacologia,* 44:215–224.

98. Washton, A. M., and Resnick, R. G. (1981): *Pharmacotherapy,* 1:140–146.

99. Washton, A. M., Gold, M. S., and Pottash, A. C. (1985): In: *Problems of Drug Dependence 1984,* edited by L. S. Harris, pp. 185–190. NIDA Res. Monograph 55, DHHS Publ. No. (ADM)85-1393, U.S. Government Printing Office, Washington.

100. Weingartner, H., Buchsbaum, M. S., and Linnoila, M. (1983): *Life Sci.,* 33:2159–2163.

101. Wesson, D. R., and Smith, D. E. (1978): In: *Amphetamine Use, Misuse, and Abuse,* edited by D. E. Smith, pp. 260–274. G. K. Hall, Boston.

102. West, R. J., Jarvis, M. J., Russell, M. A. H., Carruthers, M. E., and Feyerabend, C. (1984): *Br. J. Addict.,* 79:215–219.

103. Whitfield, C. (1980): In: *Phenomenology and Treatment of Alcoholism,* edited by W. E. Frann, I. Karacan, A. D. Pokorny, and R. Williams, pp. 305–320. Spectrum Publications, New York.

104. Zeidenberg, P., Jaffe, J. H., Kanzler, M., Levitt, M. D., Langone, J. L., et al. (1977): *Compr. Psychiatry,* 18:93–101.

Psychopharmacology:
The Third Generation of Progress,
edited by Herbert Y. Meltzer.
Raven Press, New York © 1987.

CHAPTER **174**

Evaluating Laboratory Models of Drug Dependence

Chris-Ellyn Johanson, William L. Woolverton, and Charles R. Schuster

As the chapters in this section amply demonstrate, research on the behavioral effects of psychoactive drugs has made great strides in the last 10 years in increasing our understanding of their abuse. One of the most important achievements, begun in the 1920s, is the development of models of drug dependence using both humans and other animal species in experimental laboratory investigations. These models have enabled researchers to develop new psychoactive drugs with low dependence potential, to develop successful treatment strategies, and to increase the understanding of environmental as well as biological factors that influence the likelihood that humans will abuse a drug. There is little doubt that the trend of increasing knowledge that can be seen in the preceding chapters will continue and that within the next decade our ability to decrease the prevalence and incidence of drug abuse will improve dramatically.

Despite this deserved optimism, it is still important to evaluate critically the strategies that are currently being employed in this research in an attempt to accelerate the progress. Therefore, the purpose of this chapter is to evaluate the validity and usefulness of human and animal laboratory models of drug dependence that have been developed to assess the dependence potential of psychoactive drugs, to design treatment interventions, and to understand the pharmacological and behavioral mechanisms underlying drug dependence. Although researchers within the field are confident that the research strategies used in studies of drug dependence will result in continued progress in this field, the strengths and weaknesses of the models have not been critically examined. For instance, despite an extensive literature demonstrating the reliability, generality, and va-

lidity of many laboratory methods used in studying drug dependence (e.g., refs. 49, 65), the criteria used to judge these attributes, the definition of key concepts, and the intent of the model are seldom made explicit. By making such an evaluation, it is possible to see how the models can be improved and expanded to cover more aspects of drug dependence.

The present chapter is divided into three parts. In the first part, a review of the types of research approaches and specific procedures that are considered integral features of models of drug dependence is presented. Since other chapters in this volume have reviewed individual procedures and strategies extensively, this description is brief but puts forth some fundamental concepts essential for subsequent discussions. The second part contains a general discussion of the criteria used to evaluate reliability, generality, and validity of different methods. The principal intent of this section is to provide a framework for judging the usefulness of any laboratory model of drug dependence. In the final section, the adequacy of models of drug dependence that use drug self-administration procedures is evaluated.

The importance of judging the status of the laboratory models of drug dependence that presently exist lies not only in assuring their continued productivity but also in the impact they have on the development of prevention and treatment strategies for drug abuse. Obviously, demonstrating that research findings are reliable and valid is a general concern of all science. These considerations become a major issue, however, when researchers assert that they have a model of a human behavioral disorder, such as drug dependence, that can be used to understand its etiology and treatment. Moreover, in the area of prevention, laboratory models are also used to evaluate the dependence potential of new drugs for regulatory purposes, and this evaluation has far-reaching therapeutic and economic consequences.

LABORATORY METHODS USED IN MODELS OF DRUG DEPENDENCE

Drug Self-Administration Methods

The World Health Organization's definition of drug dependence includes as the salient feature of this disorder the "compulsion to take the drug" (68). For models of drug dependence this has been translated into objective measures of drug-seeking behavior. Therefore, drug self-administration procedures that measure the reinforcing effects of drugs are considered an integral and perhaps the primary component of laboratory models of drug dependence. The basic premise of drug self-administration studies is that psychoactive drugs, like many other stimulus events, can control behavior by functioning as positive reinforcers. There are numerous reviews, including many in the present volume, that have described self-administration procedures designed to assess the reinforcing properties of drugs in both animals and humans as well as the central position of these measures in models of drug dependence (5,26,35,42,45,51).

In order to evaluate critically models of drug dependence that include the assessment of reinforcing properties, it is essential to describe their goals. There are at least three purposes of models of drug dependence that use drug self-administration methods. The first purpose is to evaluate the dependence potential[1] of drugs in order to prevent new drugs of abuse from entering the market and to provide a rational basis for regulating the availability of therapeutically necessary drugs that have dependence potential. A second purpose of drug dependence models is to determine what types of pharmacological and environmental manipulations decrease drug-taking behavior in order to develop new treatment approaches (60). A third is to serve as a means of investigating the pharmacological and behavioral mechanisms underlying drug dependence. This includes studies designed to determine the factors besides the drug itself that are important in controlling the initiation and persistence of drug-seeking and drug-taking behaviors and to determine the neurochemical and neuroanatomical substrates mediating drug reinforcement (e.g., ref. 6).

---

[1] There are several excellent reviews of the methods that are used in the evaluation of the dependence potential of drugs (e.g., 7,69) and the reader should refer to these documents for a thorough description of procedures. In addition, there are also outstanding documents that review the terminology used in these evaluations (e.g., 7,68). For instance, terms such as dependence potential, dependence liability, and abuse liability are often used interchangeably by different investigators. For some this has been a distressing situation which they have attempted to resolve by suggesting a common set of terms. Since it was not the purpose of this chapter to argue terminology or the importance of having a single set of terms, we have chosen to use only the term dependence potential. While this choice is to some extent arbitrary, it is consistent with our past writings. In addition, it is the term adopted by WHO (68).

Other Methods

As previously stated, the most important method in models of drug dependence involves the assessment of the reinforcing properties of drugs in humans and other animals. As a result of this central position, the emphasis in this chapter is on evaluating models of drug dependence that include self-administration studies. However, there are other methods available that are useful, particularly for predicting dependence potential. Although space limitations prevent a thorough evaluation of their reliability, generality, and validity, a brief discussion is warranted.

Physical Dependence

Historically, early research on drug dependence involved the investigation of opiate analgesics and included studies in both humans and animals. One of the most salient characteristics of this class of drugs is the ability to produce physical dependence, which is defined by the occurrence of a withdrawal syndrome following the cessation of repeated drug administration. The demonstration that an opiate analgesic could produce physical dependence was considered the best indication that the drug would be abused, i.e., that the drug had dependence potential. Regardless of the causes of the original use of drugs, such as morphine or heroin, it was believed that the production of the aversive state of withdrawal had motivational properties that led humans to continue drug use. Therefore, if this property of a drug could be eliminated or minimized, the abuse of such drugs would not occur. With this assumption, the emphasis of early studies designed to evaluate experimentally the dependence potential of drugs was on the development of methodologies in both humans and monkeys for assessing the ability of drugs to produce physical dependence (see refs. 17, 50). Although the analysis of the ability of drugs to produce physical dependence has led to important discoveries about underlying biological substrates of the actions of drugs, this property does not necessarily covary with drug-seeking behavior and is now believed to be a limited indicator of a drug's dependence potential (e.g., ref. 8). Physical dependence does have relevance, however, as a variable that can potentiate the reinforcing properties of certain types of drugs.

Physiological and Subjective Effects

A variety of procedures have been developed at the Addiction Research Center (ARC) that are considered integral to models of drug dependence designed to assess dependence potential. The approach is to measure a wide range of effects for prototypic drugs such as morphine and to compare this profile to the profile of effects of an unknown drug. To the extent that the two profiles are similar, i.e., that the effects of the two compounds are the same across a wide range of measures, it is possible to predict that the dependence potential of the new compound will be similar to that of the prototypic agent. The types of effects that are included in these profiles are to some extent drug class specific (e.g., changes in pupil diameter for opiates, changes in catecholamine levels for stimulants) but include both physiological and subjective effects.

Although the importance of the subjective effects of drugs had begun to be appreciated by others (e.g., ref. 4), in large measure the development of quantitative methods for assessing subjective effects of drugs in humans was accomplished at the ARC. In the late 1940s, Isbell recognized that the effects of morphine-like drugs in postdependent subjects could be used to classify other compounds and attempted to define and assess the subjective changes produced by morphine and related drugs that were felt to contribute to their dependence potential. As Isbell (32) said: "Since most persons begin the use of drugs and become addicted because the drugs produce effects which they regard as pleasurable, the detection of euphoria is a very important procedure in evaluating addiction liability." At first the methods used were observational, but the research of Beecher (4), which quantitatively assessed the analgesic effects of drugs using subjective responses, led to the development of the single-dose opiate questionnaire (20). Since the single-dose questionnaire was only relevant to opiate analgesics, the Addiction Research Center Inventory (ARCI) was introduced to distinguish between drugs of different classes (30).

Other measures of subjective effects that have been found to be useful in the study of drugs include the Profile of Mood States (e.g., ref. 44), assessments of monetary street value (29), and questions on liking (e.g., ref. 39). Although a wide range of subjective effects are measured and reported, many investigators emphasize those subjective effects that are considered measures of euphoria such as the MBG scale of the ARCI, positive mood of the POMS, or measures of liking. It is these measures, either because the production of euphoria by a drug is believed to be the reason for its subsequent abuse (see previous Isbell quotation) or because euphoria is considered an indirect measure of reinforcing effects (33), that are integral to models of drug dependence. Additionally, however, the entire profile of subjective effects added to the profile of physiological effects can be used to compare the dependence potential of a new drug to a known drug of abuse.

Discriminative Stimulus Properties

This same reasoning provides the rationale for including measures of the discriminative stimulus effects of drugs in laboratory models of drug dependence. Beginning in the 1960s, studies were conducted that demonstrated that experimental organisms could be trained to make one type of response when they were administered drug and another type of response when they were administered saline. The emergence of differential responding was taken as an indication that the animals were discriminating the presence or absence of the drug or, by implication, a drug-induced interoceptive state. Furthermore, if these trained animals were given drugs pharmacologically similar to the training drug, they responded as if they had received the training drug. On the other hand, when drugs from other pharmacological classes were administered, the animals responded

as if they had received saline; i.e., there was pharmacological specificity. As a result, it is possible to use this type of procedure to classify drugs in terms of their interoceptive properties. Many investigators believe this procedure to be analogous to studying the subjective effects of drugs in humans (see ref. 61). To the extent that they correspond, drug discrimination studies can also be viewed as integral to models of drug dependence either as an indirect measure of reinforcing properties or as part of the profile of effects of a compound that will be compared to the profile of effects of prototypic drugs of abuse.

Consequences of Drug Dependence

In addition to compulsive drug use, the World Health Organization's definition of drug abuse includes the criterion of the production of deleterious consequences to society or the individual (68). Drug self-administration studies can and should include measures of the physiological and behavioral toxicity produced at doses of the drug that are self-administered (e.g. refs. 3, 7, 38, 53). Unfortunately, few studies of this type have been done. Studies on the consequences of drug taking are also relevant when it can be demonstrated that they affect the reinforcing properties of drugs and therefore contribute directly to their continued use. For instance, prolonged use of cocaine may, through depletion of central monoamines, lead to a state of depression that the user may try to treat by increasing cocaine use. Finally, special attention should be paid to behavioral changes not usually assessed as part of toxicological analyses. One of the behavioral changes often noted with drugs of abuse is the control they assume over the entire behavioral repertoire of the organism because of their strong reinforcing properties. Although a drug may not have any other toxic effect when it is self-administered, if organisms become completely involved in taking the drug to the exclusion of other alternatives, this is an important consequence to assess (e.g., ref. 1). Although little research has been done in this area, methods are available for this purpose and should be utilized (7).

EVALUATING MODELS OF DRUG DEPENDENCE

The behavioral disorder of drug dependence is exceedingly complex. As with other types of excessive behaviors, factors relevant to its etiology and maintenance may differ from drug to drug, from individual to individual, and even from time to time. Many clinicians, in emphasizing this complexity, express doubt that models such as those described to study the phenomenon experimentally are valid or useful for the problem as it exists in the real world. Models of drug dependence cannot be simply "scaled-down" versions of the human disorder. Such a model would not be useful, since the result would be as difficult to analyze as the situation being modeled. The advantage of models, and in fact their main purpose, is to identify the salient features of a complex disorder so that important variables can be studied, at least at first, in isolation of others. As more controlling variables are understood, complexity can be gradually introduced by systematically studying how these variables interact.

Models of drug dependence are evaluated by the same standards that are used to evaluate any body of scientific data. The first consideration is the reliability of the results. Experiments can be repeated with the same subjects (intrasubject reliability) or with new subjects (intersubject reliability). In fact, any experiment that uses more than one subject is determining intersubject reliability. Within experiments, intrasubject reliability is determined by returning animals to standard conditions between manipulations. Across experiments, reliability is assured by using positive and negative controls. For instance, when Johanson and Schuster (43) assessed the reinforcing properties of cathinone, they included d-amphetamine as a positive control. If the results with d-amphetamine did not correspond to previous studies, the reliability of the results with cathinone would be suspect.

Reliability also involves the assessment of the generality of the results across species or across different experimental contexts (systematic replication: 63). For instance, if the ability of an opiate antagonist to decrease the self-administration of an agonist can be demonstrated using different experimental procedures (e.g., ref. 31 versus ref. 48), different species (56), as well as different agonist drugs (morphine versus heroin), the belief in the generality of the result that opiate antagonists block the reinforcing effects of opiate agonists is strengthened. Furthermore, if a single independent variable can be shown to have large effects in a variety of situations, its importance or robustness as a relevant variable is also increased.

In most research in the area of drug dependence, meticulous attention is paid to assessing reliability. Review articles devote much attention to proving the consistency of a functional relationship by discussing the reliability of experimental results. In the area of drug self-administration, there are many excellent reviews of this type (e.g., refs. 26, 28). An explicit example of the concern with generality or systematic replication can be found in Johanson and Balster (37). By summarizing results provided by investigators from many laboratories, these authors demonstrated that despite wide variations in experimental procedures and design, the assessments of the reinforcing properties of narcotic analgesics, nonnarcotic analgesics, sedatives, psychomotor stimulants, plus a broad range of other CNS drugs were the same. Demonstrating the importance of a single independent variable is also an example of generality. For instance, Meisch and Thompson (52) originally demonstrated that lowering the body weight of rats increased the rate of self-administration of ethanol. Since ethanol has caloric value, the significance of this finding was not clear. However, it has now been shown that deprivation conditions including both weight reduction and acute food restriction affect the self-administration of drugs from many pharmacological classes under a variety of experimental conditions and in several species (9). As a result, the importance of food access conditions as an independent variable is now well accepted as a result of demonstrating the generality of its influence.

One of the difficulties in evaluating whether a body of experimental evidence, in this case models of drug dependence, has generality is that there are no acceptable criteria for judging when an adequate range of conditions has been tested. Furthermore, some types of systematic replication are more persuasive than others for accepting the importance of a particular variable. For instance, demonstrating that the results of an experiment using primates as subjects can also be replicated with humans has more influence than a replication with rats. Sidman (63) eloquently stated that a great deal of inductive judgment is involved in assessing generality, and by its very nature this judgment is not always quantitative or logical.

Although reliability is of fundamental importance (a necessary condition) in evaluating the results generated in laboratory models of drug dependence, more concern has been focused on validity. There are many types of validity. For example, predictive validity refers to whether the experimental results are useful for predicitng what they purport to measure. Construct validity implies that the constructs of the experimental situation allow a parsimonious interpretation of the experimental findings within a theoretical framework. If a manipulation such as providing an alternative reinforcer in a drug self-administration paradigm decreases drug intake in an experimental situation, this can be viewed as compatible with epidemiological findings that abuse is more likely to occur in populations with limited resources, and clinical evidence that treatment is often more successful if patients acquire new skills, new jobs, or new recreational interests. Models that can be shown to have such construct validity can provide clues concerning underlying mechanisms that are causal of the phenomenon under study.

One problem with evaluating validity, as with assessments of generality, is that there is no metric for determining what degree of correlation (or how to calculate it) is required to conclude that the results generated by a particular method have predictive validity. An indirect way of evaluating the validity of one procedure is to determine the concordance of its predictions with the results from other methods purporting to measure the same phenomenon. If all the methods result in similar predictions, belief in the validity of each is strengthened.

In the area of assessing dependence potential, validity is often evaluated by determining the correspondence of results across different methods. For instance, Griffiths and Balster (25) demonstrated that for opioids, the same drugs that are self-administered in laboratory studies are those that produce a morphine-like profile of subjective effects. As they conclude: "This good concordance between the human and animal results further validates each procedure and suggests the possibility that both the human and animal procedures are measuring a common underlying pharmacological property, which relates to abuse potential of drugs."

De Wit et al. (15) have also shown that individual differences in self-administration of amphetamine in humans are correlated with differences in reported subjective effects in the same individuals. Woolverton and Schuster (67) reported on the concordance between human subjective effects and laboratory animal drug discrimination results for opioids. However, it is important to point out that the status of drug discrimination methods as valid indicators of dependence potential is still unknown. Although many believe that the discriminative stimulus properties of drugs in animals and the subjective effects of drugs in humans are evaluating similar properties, this relationship has not been unequivocally established. One approach to determining the nature of the relationship is to study both of these properties simultaneously in humans. For instance, Chait et al. (10) trained normal human volunteers to discriminate between 10 mg *d*-amphetamine and placebo and simultaneously measured subjective effects using the Profile of Mood States (POMS), the Addiction Research Center Inventory (ARCI), and visual analog scales. The strategy then was to measure the ability of other drugs both to substitute for *d*-amphetamine as a discriminative stimulus and to produce a similar profile of subjective effects in order to determine the concordance of the two measures. In subsequent studies, Chait et al. (11,12) showed that although drugs like phenmetrazine substituted for *d*-amphetamine and produced similar subjective effects, other drugs like mazindol substituted for *d*-amphetamine but produced a different profile of subjective effects. Although further research is required to evaluate the role of discriminative stimulus properties as indicators of dependence potential, the general point is that one way of judging validity is to determine the correspondence of results across different measures.

EVALUATION OF THE USEFULNESS OF DRUG SELF-ADMINISTRATION PROCEDURES IN MODELS OF DRUG DEPENDENCE

As previously noted, because of their central importance, the emphasis of this chapter is on drug self-administration methods within the model of drug dependence. Therefore, in this section, the usefulness of only this method is evaluated. Also previously stated was the idea that the evaluation of any method could only be done if the intent of the model was specified. In the following sections, self-administration studies are reviewed according to their purpose. These purposes include predicting dependence potential, developing treatment interventions, and determining the pharmacological and environmental mechanisms underlying drug dependence.

Dependence Potential

One of the most important goals of models of drug dependence is to assess the dependence potential of drugs. It is important to distinguish between dependence potential and actual drug abuse. The models under review are concerned with measuring dependence potential as an approximation of the expected extent of abuse that will occur in the natural environment. There are several reasons why it is unrealistic to expect a 100% correlation between predictions of dependence potential and extent of abuse,

most of which do not reflect on the adequacy of the experimental models. First, the measures of actual incidence and prevalence of drug abuse are not adequate (26). Even compared to some other complex behavioral disorders, there is great disagreement about what constitutes drug abuse, and even where there is agreement, the methods for measuring it lack the precision that is found in the laboratory models. Second, there are a variety of variables that determine whether the dependence potential of a drug is actualized to its maximum. For instance, if a synthetic drug found to have high dependence potential is extremely difficult to manufacture, abuse may be minimal because of its availability and/or price relative to other drugs. There are vagaries of the street distribution system and fads, which may, at least for short periods of time, be a major influence on which drugs are actually abused. If a famous person or star becomes involved in the abuse of a particular drug, certain types of people or people of certain ages are likely to abuse this drug as a way of emulation. In summary, there are a variety of reasons why the extent of abuse may not be in accord with the substance's dependence potential. In evaluating the adequacy of the models, the reasons for these discrepancies should be pursued before the methods are considered inadequate.

Despite these problems, the concordance between drugs that can serve as positive reinforcers in laboratory studies and those that are commonly abused by humans is remarkable (26,37). However, there are some important exceptions. For instance, hallucinogens are not self-administered under laboratory conditions yet are considered drugs of abuse (28). Likewise, local anesthetics such as procaine are self-administered by both rhesus monkeys (19) and humans (M. W. Fischman and C. R. Schuster, *unpublished data*) but do not appear to be abused by humans in the natural environment. In the latter case, there are good explanations for the discrepancy that do not indicate problems with the model (see ref. 19). Even with these exceptions, it appears that drug self-administration procedures are reasonably valid predictors of whether a drug has significant dependence potential. The difficulty lies, however, in estimating the relative dependence potential of drugs. This is a particularly important issue in drug development, where it may be unrealistic to expect that a drug will have no dependence potential but may very well have less than those drugs currently available for medical use (e.g., nalbuphine versus morphine).

For the sake of this review, the dependence potential of a drug can be viewed as varying along three dimensions, each of which is assessed with a different strategy. The first dimension is that of the inherent reinforcing properties of a drug molecule. It is assumed that drugs vary in their relative reinforcing efficacy as a function of differences in their pharmacological actions in the central nervous system. Studies attempting to place specific drugs on this dimension compare the reinforcing actions of a wide variety of drugs under standard conditions to determine their relative efficacy. The most useful procedures to begin the evaluation of a drug's reinforcing properties are substitution procedures (e.g., ref. 37). These procedures allow the determination of whether a drug will serve as a positive reinforcer under conditions in which it has previously been shown that a variety of drugs of abuse are self-administered. Substitution procedures do not, however, give an accurate estimate of a drug's relative reinforcing efficacy because of the use of rate of self-administration as the operational definition of reinforcing properties. With this definition, if responding maintained by one drug is greater than responding maintained by a second drug, the first drug could be assumed to have greater reinforcing properties. However, under many conditions there are alternative explanations for differences in rate of responding maintained by drugs (see ref. 35 for a discussion of this issue).

For the purpose of evaluating relative reinforcing properties, other procedures such as choice procedures (e.g., ref. 40) and progressive-ratio schedules (e.g., ref. 27) are used. In choice procedures, subjects are given an opportunity to choose between two mutually exclusive drug conditions. The number of trials during which one option rather than the other is selected is used as a rate-free measure of reinforcing efficacy. This method appears to be a direct means of comparing the relative reinforcing efficacy of drugs. It has been shown, for example, that both procaine and cocaine serve as positive reinforcers in substitution procedures. When, however, rhesus monkeys are given a choice between the two drugs, cocaine is chosen exclusively (36). Similar results have been obtained in laboratory investigations of the reinforcing actions of cocaine and procaine in humans (M. W. Fischman and C. R. Schuster, *unpublished data*). By a series of comparisons with known drugs of abuse, it would be possible to create a preference ranking of drugs that could be compared to epidemiological estimates of their prevalence of dependence. At the present time, however, not enough systematically obtained preference data are available to assess adequately the validity of the choice procedure for predicting the relative dependence potential of drugs. The data that have been collected suggest that the method may be useful particularly if choice procedures can be modified to make them less time consuming.

Progressive-ratio methods also have been used as predictors of relative dependence potential. The amount of effort or work an organism is willing to emit is an intuitively appealing metric for assessing the value of a drug reinforcer. In the progressive-ratio method, the number of responses required for each drug delivery is sytematically increased until responding declines to below some criterion rate. The ratio value that leads to this criterion reduction is called the breaking point. By comparing the greatest effort different drug reinforcers maintain, it should be possible to create a ranking of predicted dependence potential. For example, Griffiths et al. (27) compared the progressive-ratio performance maintained by three different psychomotor stimulants in baboons and found that the breaking point for cocaine was higher than the breaking point of any dose of diethylpropion, which confirmed findings of Johanson and Schuster (41) showing the same ranking in a choice paradigm. This correspondence in results despite differences in species and procedures indicated that these methods have promise in predicting relative dependence potential. Unfortunately, however, little research of this type has been attempted, most likely because of its time-consuming nature.

A second dimension along which the dependence potential of a drug may vary involves the range of conditions under which it can function as a reinforcer (62). In studies of this type, a single drug is evaluated extensively with the assumption that a drug that can control behavior under a broad range of experimental conditions has greater dependence potential than a drug that is a positive reinforcer only under a limited range of conditions. Stated in another way, the generality of a drug's reinforcing properties increases the likelihood that the drug will be used under conditions favoring its abuse.

The assessment of a drug's reinforcing properties under a wide variety of conditions is an example of systematic replication (63). There have been dozens of experiments, for example, in which the positive reinforcing properties of cocaine have been demonstrated. These experiments have used different species (e.g., rats, 57; dogs, 58; squirrel monkeys, 21; rhesus monkeys, 66; baboons, 27; humans, 18) and different schedules of reinforcement (e.g., fixed ratio, 66: fixed interval, 2; second-order, 21). This systematic replication establishes the reliability of the observation that cocaine serves as a reinforcer in any one experiment and as well establishes the generality of the finding. These results with cocaine can be contrasted to studies investigating the reinforcing effects of nalorphine. In most studies nalorphine has been shown to have aversive properties. That is, animals can be trained to make a response that avoids or escapes its infusion. However, there are conditions under which it is self-administered (22). It is important to note that under the limited conditions in which nalorphine serves as a positive reinforcer, it may be highly efficacious. This illustrates the manner in which dimensions one and two may be independent.

The failure to appreciate that drugs may differ in their ranking along these two dimensions can give rise to confusion and controversy. For example, clinicians who observe a serious case of dependence on a drug often conclude that it is a serious public health problem, whereas epidemiologists reach a different conclusion because the prevalence of abuse of the drug is low. In this case, the clinician may have had contact with an individual who was exposed to esoteric conditions under which a drug like nalorphine would have efficacious reinforcing properties. In contrast, because of the limited population exposed to the esoteric conditions necessary for this drug to serve as a reinforcer, a low prevalence of dependence would be found by the epidemiologist.

Although this second dimension, i.e., range of conditions, has been recognized for some time as important (e.g., ref. 62), it has received little systematic exploration. This is at least in part because of the failure to develop acceptable criteria for determining the various situations in which a drug's reinforcing effects should be tested to determine generality. Currently, such variations are largely a function of idiosyncratic approaches used by different laboratories that happen to be investigating the reinforcing properties of the same drug. This results in a great deal of systematic replication of results with drugs of current interest (e.g., cocaine) but relatively little with other less-well-known ones (e.g., chlorphentermine). Clearly, a more systematic approach must be developed if it is to be determined whether ranking along the second dimension will be a valid predictor of a drug's dependence potential.

The third dimension on which drugs may vary in their dependence potential is sensitivity to variables that potentiate their reinforcing action. It has recently been demonstrated that food deprivation enhances the reinforcing actions of many drugs (9), but the extent of this effect with different classes of drugs needs to be investigated in order to determine whether drugs differ in their sensitivity to potentiation. Another example is that the reinforcing properties of opiates are potentiated when a physically dependent organism is deprived of the drug or withdrawal is precipitated by the administration of an opiate antagonist (64). Again, whether comparable potentiation of the reinforcing properties occurs with other classes of drugs that produce physical dependence is not established (8). This third dimension becomes particularly important to assess when potentiation of the reinforcing effects of a drug leads to its intake at toxic levels.

In summary, the first purpose of models of drug self-administration procedures is to evaluate dependence potential. This property of drugs is determined by measuring their reinforcing properties, which, as described above, may vary along three dimensions. At present, it is impossible to determine the relative importance of each of these three dimensions, nor can they be regarded as equally validated. Nevertheless, it seems likely that drugs with the highest dependence potential are those with the greatest inherent reinforcing properties that are manifest under the broadest range of conditions and that are most sensitive to variables that further potentiate their reinforcing actions. In order to validate more adequately the predictiveness of these three dimensions, additional systematic research is necessary.

Treatment Interventions

The second general use of drug self-administration procedures is in the development of treatment interventions. This area has recently been extensively reviewed (60) and therefore is only highlighted here. Drug self-administration procedures have been found to be useful in the evaluation of the therapeutic potential of pharmacological approaches to the treatment of drug dependence. Validiation of these procedures has consisted of demonstrating that interventions such as treatment with methadone or narcotic antagonists decrease the reinforcing properties of opiates in the laboratory as they do in the clinic (14,46–48). Further, the laboratory demonstration that narcotic antagonists are aversive (16) would lead to the prediction that patient compliance with antagonist therapy would be poor, which in fact is the clinical reality. More recently, these same procedures have been used to investigate the effects of the mixed agonist–antagonist buprenorphine on opiate self-administration (54,55). The results of these experiments suggest that buprenorphine would make an excellent maintenance drug in the treatment of opiate dependence. The finding that buprenorphine has reinforcing properties in monkeys (70), is identified as an opiate in drug discrim-

ination studies (13), and produces subjective effects in postdependent addicts that indicate liking (34) would lead to the prediction that its acceptance by patients in treatment for heroin dependence would be excellent.

In summary, these studies indicate that laboratory models of drug dependence can be used to make valid predictions of the therapeutic potential of new pharmacological agents for the treatment of opiate dependence. However, the demonstration of the validity of these models is limited by the absence of research on pharmacotherapies for dependence on other classes of abused drugs. In addition, relatively little effort has been made to investigate the usefulness of laboratory models of drug dependence for the determination of the efficacy of behavioral therapies. Since it is likely that drug self-administration procedures will be used for the development of pharmacotherapy for dependence on other classes of drugs as well as behavioral therapies, the model will be further validated if these efforts are successful.

Mechanisms of Drug Dependence

The most important purpose of laboratory models of drug dependence is to investigate the biological and behavioral mechanisms underlying drug dependence as well as the variables that modulate this phenomenon. Although this purpose may be the most important, the generality and validity of such studies are the most difficult to demonstrate. For biological studies, the difficulty lies in the relative inability to replicate findings in humans. Therefore, generality and validity must be demonstrated indirectly. For behavioral studies, particularly those purporting to demonstrate the relevance of a process, the difficulty lies in verifying its role in the natural environment. To demonstrate whether a functional relationship between an independent and a dependent variable is relevant for understanding drug dependence, the finding must generate a theoretical framework that predicts the results of other independent studies, all of which ultimately lead to the successful development of prevention and treatment approaches.

A recent study demonstrating that there are separate brain sites mediating physical dependence and reinforcing effects of opiates illustrates the difficulty in generalizing from animals to humans (6). Although the results of such experiments are intrinsically important, most researchers hope that their results are applicable to humans. Since such studies use procedures that, for ethical or practical reasons, cannot be carried out using humans, validation of their findings must be indirect. Systematic replication in other infrahuman species can increase confidence in the applicability of the findings to humans. Further indirect support that reinforcing properties and the ability of a drug to produce physical dependence are separate phenomena comes from observations in both rhesus monkeys and humans that opiates can serve as reinforcers under conditions in which physical dependence cannot be demonstrated (59,66). The best indirect support for this finding will be the discovery of drugs that differentially affect the ability of opiates to serve as reinforcers and produce physical dependence. Thus, through systematic replication, evidence can be gathered that increases the confidence in the validity of results from animals as a predictor of the sites of action of opiates in humans.

Verifying the role of environmental variables affecting drug dependence in the natural environment is extremely difficult. For instance, experimental studies have shown that certain kinds of manipulations will affect the initiation of drug use. It has been very difficult to demonstrate that infrahumans will ingest alcohol for its pharmacological actions. In many instances, procedures involving food or water deprivation are used, which confound alcohol's caloric and thirst-satisfying properties with any possible reinforcement based on its psychoactive properties. It has recently been found that nondeprived rats will drink alcohol in order to be able to drink a saccharin solution. After alcohol ingestion was well established, access to the saccharin solution was omitted, and the rats continued to ingest alcohol at intoxicating doses (24). Similar results were obtained in a systematic replication of this study in rhesus monkeys (23). Although the ability to replicate this study in two species increases the belief in the reliability of the findings, it is not clear if they are relevant to the initiation of alcohol use in humans. To determine relevance, it is necessary to go beyond the specific operations to specify the general processes involved, i.e., that initiation of drug use is related to contingencies in the environment that are only satisfied by drug-taking behaviors. It is obvious that this parallels the experience of many young drug users who begin using drugs in order to obtain social reinforcers from drug-using peers. Drug use may then continue because the drug acquires conditioned reinforcing properties by virtue of its association with social reinforcers. It may also be the case that repeated exposure allows the development of tolerance to a drug's aversive effects so that its positive reinforcing properties may then emerge. Implications of experiments such as these (e.g. 23,24) are often unrecognized because researchers fail to go beyond a description of the operations involved in their experiments to the general processes they are studying. It is no wonder, therefore, that clinicians reading experimental literature may fail to see the relevance of such work to the clinical situation.

CONCLUSIONS

The present chapter has been an attempt to place the research reviewed in the preceding chapters into a critical perspective concerning its reliability and validity. The contribution of experimental laboratory investigations with both humans and other animals to our understanding of the etiology and maintenance of drug dependence has been outstanding, and the avenues of research that have been opened, particularly in the last 10 years, productive. As with any developing approach, there is a recurrent need to evaluate its progress not only in terms of the data gathered but also in terms of the adequacy of the strategies employed. The present chapter has attempted to evaluate the latter primarily to emphasize that models of drug dependence have made important and sound advances in our knowledge of drug dependence and, more importantly, are likely to

continue to do so in the future. This review has also pointed out that the validity of these models has not been completely explored, and in addition there are areas (e.g., behavioral treatment modalities) that have been ignored where additional research is of vital importance. However, since the progress to date has been excellent, it seems clear that researchers are capable of filling these important gaps in our knowledge.

ACKNOWLEDGMENT

The preparation of this manuscript was supported by PHS grant DA00250.

REFERENCES

1. Aigner, T. G., and Balster, R. L. (1978): *Science*, 201:534–535.
2. Balster, R. L., and Schuster, C. R. (1973): *J. Exp. Anal. Behav.*, 20:119–129.
3. Balster, R. L., and Woolverton, W. L. (1980): *Psychopharmacology*, 70:5–10.
4. Beecher, H. K. (1959): *Measurement of Subjective Responses.* Oxford University Press, New York.
5. Bigelow, G., Griffiths, R., and Liebson, I. (1976): *Pharmacol. Rev.*, 27:523–531.
6. Bozarth, M. A., and Wise, R. A. (1984): *Science*, 224:516–517.
7. Brady, J., and Lukas, S. (1984): *Testing Drugs for Physical Dependence Potential and Abuse Liability.* Department of Health and Human Services, Washington.
8. Cappell, H., and LeBlanc, A. E. (1981): In: *Research Advances in Alcohol and Drug Problems, Vol. 6,* edited by Y. Israel, F. Glaser, H. Kalant, R. Popham, W. Schmidt, et al., pp. 159–196. Plenum Press, New York.
9. Carroll, M. E., and Meisch, R. A. (1984): In: *Advances in Behavioral Pharmacology, Vol. IV,* edited by T. Thompson and P. B. Dews, pp. 47–88. Academic Press, New York.
10. Chait, L. D., Uhlenhuth, E. H., and Johanson, C. E. (1985): *Psychopharmacology*, 86:307–312.
11. Chait, L. D., Uhlenhuth, E. H., and Johanson, C. E. (1986): *Psychopharmacology*, 89:301–306.
12. Chait, L. D., Uhlenhuth, E. H., and Johanson, C. E. (1986): *Pharmacol. Biochem. Behav.*, 24:1665–1672.
13. Colpaert, F. C. (1978): *Pharmacol. Biochem. Behav.*, 9:863–887.
14. Cooper, J., Altman, F., Brown, B., and Czechowicz, D., eds. (1983): *Research on the Treatment of Narcotic Addiction: State of the Art.* (DHEW Publication No. ADM 83-1281. NIDA Research Monograph Series). U.S. Government Printing Office, Washington.
15. deWit, H., Uhlenhuth, E. H., and Johanson, C. E. (1986): *Drug Alcohol Depend.*, 16:341–360.
16. Downs, D. A., and Woods, J. H. (1975): *J. Exp. Anal. Behav.*, 23:415–427.
17. Eddy, N. B. (1973): *The National Research Council Involvement in the Opiate Problem.* The National Academy of Sciences, Washington.
18. Fischman, M. W., and Schuster, C. R. (1983): *Psychopharmacol. Bull.*, 19:772–773.
19. Ford, R. D., and Balster, R. L. (1977): *Pharmacol. Biochem. Behav.*, 6:289–296.
20. Fraser, H. F., Van Horn, G. D., Martin, W. R., Wolbach, A. B., and Isbell, H. (1961): *J. Pharmacol. Exp. Ther.*, 133:371–387.
21. Goldberg, S. R. (1973): *J. Pharmacol. Exp. Ther.*, 186:18–30.
22. Goldberg, S. R., Hoffmeister, F., Schlichting, U., and Wuttke, W. (1971): *J. Pharmacol. Exp. Ther.*, 179:268–276.
23. Grant, K., Johanson, C. E., and Schuster, C. R. (1985): *Alcoholism: Clin. Exp. Res.*, 9:205.
24. Grant, K. A., and Samson, H. H. (1985): *Psychopharmacology*, 86:475–479.
25. Griffiths, R. R., and Balster, R. L. (1979): *Clin. Pharmacol. Ther.*, 25:611–617.

26. Griffiths, R. R., Bigelow, G. E., and Henningfield, J. E. (1980): In: *Advances in Substance Abuse,* edited by N. K. Mello, pp. 1–90. JAI Press, Greenwich, CT.
27. Griffiths, R. R., Brady, J. V., and Snell, J. D. (1978): *Psychopharmacology,* 56:5–13.
28. Griffiths, R. R., Brady, J. V., and Bradford, L. D. (1979): In: *Advances in Behavioral Pharmacology, Vol. II,* edited by T. Thompson and P. B. Dews, pp. 163–208. Academic Press, New York.
29. Griffiths, R. R., McLeod, D. R., Bigelow, G. E., Liebson, I. A., Roache, J. D., et al. (1984): *J. Pharmacol. Exp. Ther.,* 229:501–508.
30. Haertzen, C. A. (1966): *Psychol. Rep.,* 18:163–194.
31. Harrigan, S. E., and Downs, D. A. (1978): *J. Pharmacol. Exp. Ther.,* 204:481–486.
32. Isbell, H. (1948): *Ann. N.Y. Acad. Sci.,* 51:108–122.
33. Jasinski, D. R. (1977): In: *Handbook of Experimental Pharmacology: Drug Addiction I,* edited by W. R. Martin, pp. 197–258. Springer-Verlag, New York.
34. Jasinski, D. R., Pevnick, J. S., and Griffith, J. D. (1978): *Arch. Gen. Psychiatry,* 35:501–516.
35. Johanson, C. E. (1978): In: *Contemporary Research in Behavioral Pharmacology,* edited by D. E. Blackman and D. J. Sanger, pp. 325–390. Plenum Press, New York.
36. Johanson, C. E., and Aigner, T. (1980): *Pharmacol. Biochem. Behav.,* 15:49–53.
37. Johanson, C. E., and Balster, R. L. (1978): *Bull. Narc.,* 30:43–54.
38. Johanson, C. E., Balster, R. L., and Bonese, K. (1976): *Pharmacol. Biochem. Behav.,* 4:45–51.
39. Johanson, C. E., Kilgore, K., and Uhlenhuth, E. H. (1983): *Psychopharmacology,* 81:144–149.
40. Johanson, C. E., and Schuster, C. R. (1975): *J. Pharmacol. Exp. Ther.,* 193:676–688.
41. Johanson, C. E., and Schuster, C. R. (1977): In: *Cocaine and Other Stimulants,* edited by E. Ellinwood and M. Kilbey, pp. 545–570. Plenum Press, New York.
42. Johanson, C. E., and Schuster, C. R. (1981): In: *Advances in Substance Abuse: Behavioral and Biological Research,* edited by N. K. Mello, pp. 219–297. JAI Press, Greenwich, CT.
43. Johanson, C. E., and Schuster, C. R. (1981): *J. Pharmacol. Exp. Ther.,* 219:355–362.
44. Johanson, C. E., and Uhlenhuth, E. H. (1980): *Psychopharmacology,* 71:275–279.
45. Johanson, C. E., and Uhlenhuth, E. H. (1982): *Fed. Proc.,* 41:228–233.
46. Jones, B. E., and Prada, J. A. (1975): *Psychopharmacologia (Berl.),* 41:7–10.
47. Jones, B. E., and Prada, J. A. (1977): *Psychopharmacologia (Berl.),* 54:109–112.
48. Killian, A. K., Bonese, K. N., and Schuster, C. R. (1978): *Drug Alcohol Depend.,* 3:245–251.
49. Martin, W. R., ed. (1977): *Handbook of Experimental Pharmacology: Drug Addiction I,* Springer-Verlag, New York.
50. Martin, W. R., and Jasinski, D. R. (1977): In: *Handbook of Experimental Pharmacology: Drug Addiction I,* edited by W. R. Martin, pp. 159–196. Springer-Verlag, New York.
51. Meisch, R. A. (1977): In: *Advances in Behavioral Pharmacology, Vol. 1,* edited by T. Thompson and P. Dews, pp. 35–84. Academic Press, New York.
52. Meisch, R. A., and Thompson, T. (1974): *Pharmacol. Biochem. Behav.,* 2:589–596.
53. Mello, N. K., Bree, M. P., Mendelson, J. H., Ellingboe, J., King, N. W., et al. (1983): *Science,* 221:677–679.
54. Mello, N. K., Bree, M. P., and Mendelson, J. H. (1983): *J. Pharmacol. Exp. Ther.,* 223:378–386.
55. Mello, N. K., Mendelson, J. H., and Kuehnle, J. C. (1982): *J. Pharmacol. Exp. Ther.,* 225:30–39.
56. Meyer, R. E., and Mirin, S. M., eds. (1979): *The Heroin Stimulus: Implications for a Theory of Addiction.* Plenum Press, New York.
57. Pickens, R., and Thompson, T. (1968): *J. Pharmacol. Exp. Ther.,* 161:122–129.
58. Risner, M. E., and Jones, B. E. (1980): *Psychopharmacology,* 71:83–89.
59. Robins, L. N., Helzer, J. E., Hessebrock, M., and Wish, E. (1980): In: *Yearbook of Substance Use and Abuse,* pp. 222–240. Human Services Press, New York.
60. Schuster, C. R. (1986): In: *Behavioral Analysis of Drug Dependence,* edited by S. Goldberg and I. Stolerman, pp. 357–385. Academic Press, New York.
61. Schuster, C. R., Fischman, M. W., and Johanson, C. E. (1981): In: *Behavioral Pharmacology of Human Drug Dependence,* edited by T. Thompson and C. E. Johanson, pp. 116–129. National Institute on Drug Abuse Research Monograph Series #37, NIDA, Washington.
62. Schuster, C. R., and Thompson, T. (1969): *Annu. Rev. Pharmacol.,* 9:483–502.
63. Sidman, M. (1960): *Tactics of Scientific Research.* Basic Books, New York.
64. Thompson, T., and Schuster, C. R. (1964): *Psychopharmacologia (Berl.),* 5:87–94.
65. Thompson, T., and Unna, K. R., eds. (1977): *Predicting Dependence Liability of Stimulant and Depressant Drugs.* University Park Press, Baltimore.
66. Woods, J. H., and Schuster, C. R. (1968): *Int. J. Addict.,* 3:231–236.
67. Woolverton, W. L., and Schuster, C. R. (1983): *Pharmacol. Rev.,* 35:33–52.
68. World Health Organization. (1969): *WHO Tech. Rep. Ser.,* 407:1–21.
69. World Health Organization. (1981): *Bull. WHO,* 59:225–242.
70. Young, A. M., Stephens, K. P., Hein, D. W., and Woods, J. H. (1984): *J. Pharmacol. Exp. Ther.,* 229:118–126.

Psychopharmacology:
The Third Generation of Progress,
edited by Herbert Y. Meltzer.
Raven Press, New York © 1987.

CHAPTER 175

Psychoactive Phenylisopropylamines

Richard A. Glennon

From a chemical standpoint, phenylisopropylamine (i.e., 1-phenyl-2-aminopropane) is a relatively simple structural unit that forms the general backbone of a wide variety of pharmacologically active substances. Phenylisopropylamine itself, known more commonly as amphetamine, is a central stimulant; however, minor structural modification of phenylisopropylamine results in agents that can produce a broad spectrum of effects. Representative examples include norephedrine (decongestant), fenfluramine (anorexic), tranylcypromine (monoamine oxidase inhibitor), 1-(2,5-dimethoxy-4-methylphenyl)-2-aminopropane (DOM) (hallucinogen), and bupropion (antidepressant) (see Fig. 1 for structures). The purpose of this present chapter is to

assemble some of the available information on the effect that structural modification of the phenylisopropylamine (PIA) skeleton can have on central activity. Emphasis is placed on psychoactive agents that possess abuse potential (as central stimulants or hallucinogenic agents) and, in particular, on several agents that have recently attracted widespread attention.

The term "amphetamine" refers to a particular phenylisopropylamine (i.e., phenylisopropylamine itself); substituted phenylisopropylamines should probably not (with several exceptions) be referred to as substituted amphetamines. As discussed by Shulgin (48), the term "amphetamine" bears with it the connotation of amphetamine-like pharmacological activity as well as suggestions of legal constraints that are typically associated with amphetamine-like stimulants. However, not all PIA-containing agents necessarily produce "amphetamine-like" effects. For example, the phenylisopropylamine DOM, often called 2,5-dimethoxy-4-methylamphetamine, produces effects in animal (including human) subjects that are quite distinct from those produced by amphetamine. There probably are a few cases in which the application of amphetamine-type nomenclature is justified, e.g., N-monomethylamphetamine (methamphetamine). Nevertheless, the indiscriminate use of this type of nomenclature should be discouraged.

PHENYLISOPROPYLAMINE DERIVATIVES: STRUCTURE–ACTIVITY CONSIDERATIONS

Few agents have received as much attention or are as readily recognized (by health professionals and the lay public alike) as amphetamine; thus, it is not uncommon to feel, intuitively, that agents with an amphetamine-type structure should probably possess amphetamine-like character. As just mentioned, this is not necessarily the case. Amphetamine, despite its simple structure, produces a

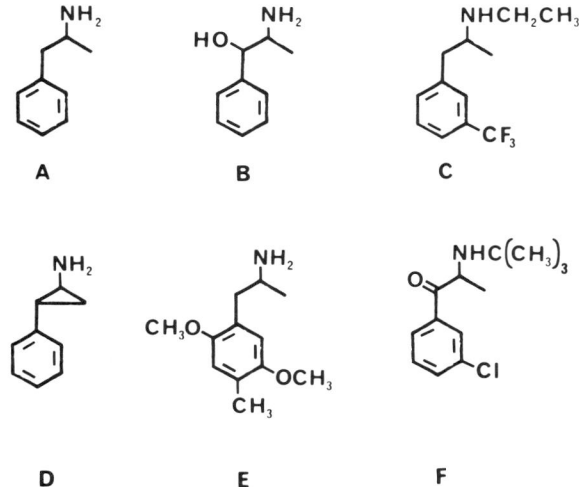

FIG. 1. Chemical structures of some common phenylisopropylamines: amphetamine (**A**), norephedrine (**B**), fenfluramine (**C**), tranylcypromine (**D**), DOM (**E**), and bupropion (**F**). Stereochemistry is not indicated.

variety of effects; most notable are its central stimulant, anorexic, and vasoconstrictor properties. About 10 years ago, Biel and Bopp (6) thoroughly reviewed the structure–activity relationships (SAR) of amphetamine with respect to central stimulant, anorexic, and psychotomimetic activity, monoamine oxidase inhibition, and neurotransmitter uptake. Structural modification of amphetamine can result in the enhancement of one of these effects at the expense of another or can result in an entirely new spectrum of action. With respect to the behavioral properties discussed herein, the simple PIAs are divided into two general groups: central (CNS) stimulants and hallucinogenic agents. Furthermore, for the sake of discussion, the phenylisopropylamine molecule can be arbitrarily divided into three major structural components: (a) the aromatic nucleus, (b) the terminal amine, and (c) the isopropyl side chain. The effects of structural modification of each of these components are discussed. An aromatic ring separated from a terminal amine by a two-carbon spacer appears to be necessary for both types of activity; however, further associated with each of these activities is a fairly distinct SAR.

Central Stimulants

The central stimulant properties and mechanism of action of amphetamine have been well studied (e.g., see refs. 3, 11, 29, 53 for reviews); however, much less is known about substituted PIAs as a group. Although a number of such agents have been evaluated, the great variety of techniques that have been used makes it somewhat difficult to formulate a comprehensive SAR. In an early study by van der Schoot et al. (54), the effects of a large number of PIA derivatives on spontaneous locomotor activity of mice were examined in such a fashion as to allow comparisons to be made. Unfortunately, it is unclear whether this study employed optically active materials or racemic mixtures. Nevertheless, this study still constitutes an important contribution to our understanding of the SAR of PIA derivatives. Subsequent studies have been conducted by other groups of investigators, but the effects of large numbers of agents have rarely been compared in the same study. Another technique that has seen considerable application for the evaluation of PIA derivatives is the drug discrimination paradigm; the use of this method has provided extensive information on which types of structures produce amphetamine-like stimulus effects in animals. The discriminative stimulus properties of amphetamine and related PIA derivatives have been recently reviewed by Young and Glennon (58). In general, there is a fairly good qualitative agreement, from an SAR standpoint, between the results of locomotor stimulation and drug discrimination studies (where comparisons are possible), and the present discussion draws heavily on the findings of such studies. Human data, where available, are also discussed; Shulgin (48) has reviewed the literature with regard to the effect of PIA derivatives on human subjects.

Aromatic Nucleus

In general, substitution on the aromatic nucleus of PIA results in agents that are less potent than amphetamine or that are inactive as CNS stimulants. Substitution by electron-withdrawing groups (e.g., Cl, Br), particularly at the 4 position, affords agents that are potent depleters of serotonin (13). Several such agents have been investigated as potential antidepressants (48). With respect to alkyl derivatives, human data are available only on several methyl-substituted compounds. There are three monomethyl derivatives of PIA; these agents are, at best, only weakly active as central stimulants in humans (48). Hydroxylated derivatives appear to be too polar to penetrate the blood–brain barrier and usually display minimal (if any) central activity. For example, 3-hydroxy- and 4-hydroxy-PIA were inactive as locomotor stimulants (54), and the 4-hydroxy analog failed to serve as a training drug in tests of stimulus control of behavior (33). The 4-hydroxy derivative (Paredrine®) also lacks any significant central effect in humans (48). There are three possible monomethoxy derivatives; these are the 2-, 3-, and 4-methoxy analogs OMA, MMA, and PMA, respectively. Of these, OMA and MMA have not been evaluated in humans; PMA has been reported to produce a "psychotomimetic syndrome" at total doses of 60 to 80 mg but possesses a very low therapeutic index. Shulgin (48) has commented that PMA is a treacherous agent to study in human subjects. All three monomethoxy analogs are weak central stimulants; for example, each produces locomotor stimulation in rodents, but none is more potent than amphetamine (38,53). In one study in which all three agents were compared with amphetamine as locomotor stimulants in rats, the order of potency was (+)-amphetamine > PMA > MMA > OMA (38). In tests of discriminative control of behavior using (+)-amphetamine as the training drug, the amphetamine stimulus generalized to all three monomethoxy derivatives (24,28), but again, all were less potent than amphetamine (Table 1); potency decreased

TABLE 1. *Potencies of selected phenylisopropylamines in stimulus generalization studies employing (+)-amphetamine-trained rats[a]*

Agent	ED50 (mg/kg)	Agent	ED50 (mg/kg)
Amphetamine	0.6	Cathinone	0.7
(+)-Amphetamine	0.4	(+)-Cathinone	4.4
(−)-Amphetamine	1.2	(−)-Cathinone	0.3
OMA	7.8	3,4-MDA	2.3
MMA	3.5	(+)-MDA	0.9
PMA	1.9	(−)-MDA	NSG[c]
Phenethylamine	NSG[b]	MDMA	1.6
(+)-Methamphetamine	0.4	2,3-MDA	NSG[c]

[a] Rats were trained to discriminate 1.0 mg/kg of (+)-amphetamine sulfate from saline; data are from Glennon et al. (19,20,23,24). NSG, stimulus generalization (i.e., >80% amphetamine-appropriate responding) did not occur. Data are for racemates unless otherwise stated.

[b] Phenethylamine produced saline-appropriate responding at 5.75 mg/kg and disruption of behavior at higher doses.

[c] R(−)-3,4-MDA and 2,3-MDA produced saline-appropriate responding at 2.0 and 2.75 mg/kg, respectively, and disruption of behavior at slightly higher doses. Note: none of the agents in Table 2 showed complete generalization in (+)-amphetamine-trained rats.

in the order (+)-amphetamine > PMA > MMA > OMA (24). PMA has recently been used as a training drug in tests of discriminative control of behavior in rats (56).

There are six possible dimethoxy analogs (DMAs) and six different trimethoxy analogs (TMAs) of PIA. Relatively little work has been done with these agents as a group. The 3,4-dimethoxy analog (3,4-DMA), perhaps because of its structural similarity to dopamine, has been examined in several different studies: 3,4-DMA seems to be inactive as a locomotor stimulant (53), does not result in (+)-amphetamine stimulus generalization (58), and is essentially inactive (or only weakly active) in humans (48). Both the 2,4- and 2,5-dimethoxy analogs (2,4-DMA and 2,5-DMA, respectively) are hallucinogenic in man, but both possess a considerable component of amphetamine-like stimulation (48). The remaining DMAs, 2,3-DMA, 2,6-DMA, and 3,5-DMA, have not been evaluated in humans. Of the TMAs, two (2,3,4-TMA and 2,3,5-TMA) appear to be inactive at the 50- to 100-mg (oral) dose range, whereas too little human data are available on 2,3,6-TMA to draw any conclusions (48). The remaining three positional isomers (3,4,5-TMA, 2,4,5-TMA, and 2,4,6-TMA) are hallucinogenic and are discussed in the following section. The stimulus effects of 11 of the 12 DMAs and TMAs (the exception being 2,3,6-TMA) have been examined using animals trained to discriminate (+)-amphetamine from saline; although none of these agents resulted in amphetamine stimulus generalization, 2,4-DMA, 2,5-DMA, 2,4,5-TMA, 2,4,6-TMA, and 3,4,5-TMA produced partial generalization (i.e., circa 50% amphetamine-appropriate responding) (24). These results suggest that certain of these hallucinogenic DMAs and TMAs may produce some amphetamine-like effects.

Terminal Amine

Very little has been done in the way of a detailed examination of terminal amine substituents. Amphetamine possesses a primary amine function, and N-monomethylation affords methamphetamine; methamphetamine produces amphetamine-like effects in animals trained to discriminate amphetamine from saline (Table 1) and is at least as potent as amphetamine as a central stimulant in humans (3,11). Methamphetamine is about 60 to 70% more potent than amphetamine as a locomotor stimulant; further extension of this alkyl function to ethyl and n-propyl results in retention of activity but in a gradual decrease in potency (53). The four-carbon (n-butyl), five-carbon (amyl), and benzyl derivatives are much less potent or are inactive (53). Introduction of N-ethyl or N-propyl groups to less potent stimulants such as OMA, PMA, and 3,4-DMA affords compounds that are inactive as locomotor stimulants, and addition of a second methyl group to methamphetamine (i.e., N,N-dimethylamphetamine) reduces its potency by an order of magnitude (53).

Side Chain

The most important feature of the side chain of amphetamine is an asymmetric carbon atom, and its presence gives rise to two optical isomers. The S(+) isomer (i.e., the

d isomer) is called dextroamphetamine, whereas the R(−) isomer (i.e., the l isomer) is known as levoamphetamine (Fig. 2). With respect to peripheral effects, the isomers of amphetamine are equipotent; however, centrally, S(+)-amphetamine is about three times (2–10 times) (39,54) more potent than its R(−) enantiomer. This has been found to be the case in drug discrimination studies involving amphetamine-trained animals (Table 1) (58), in human studies (11), and in various other pharmacological studies. Likewise, S(+)-methamphetamine and S(+)-3,4-DMA are three times more potent than their R(−) isomers in producing amphetamine-like effects in rats (4,44,54).

The aromatic nucleus of amphetamine is separated from its terminal amine by a two-carbon chain; this chain is branched such that the asymmetric carbon atom bears a methyl group (i.e., the α-methyl group). This α-methyl group is another important feature of the side chain. Removal of this group from amphetamine affords phenethylamine; phenethylamine is a very weak locomotor stimulant, presumably because of its rapid metabolism in vivo. Likewise, α-demethylation of other PIAs with central activity generally reduces their potency or abolishes activity altogether (53). Homologation of the methyl group of amphetamine to an ethyl group reduces potency (as a locomotor stimulant) by approximately 85%; addition of a second methyl group (i.e., gem-dimethyl) reduces potency by 50% (53). If an additional methylene group is inserted into the side chain of amphetamine (to afford 1-phenyl-3-amino-butane), the resultant compound is inactive as a locomotor stimulant; similarly, the "extended" derivatives of 3,4-DMA, 2,4,5-TMA, and 2,4,6-TMA are also inactive (9). Hydroxylation of the benzylic carbon of amphetamine and various other PIAs serves (a) to introduce a new asymmetric carbon atom (and hence the possibility of diastereoisomers) and (b) to reduce potency as a central stimulant. Certain of these agents, for example, ephedrine, behave as locomotor stimulants (53) and produce amphetamine-like stimulus effects (28) but are less potent than amphetamine.

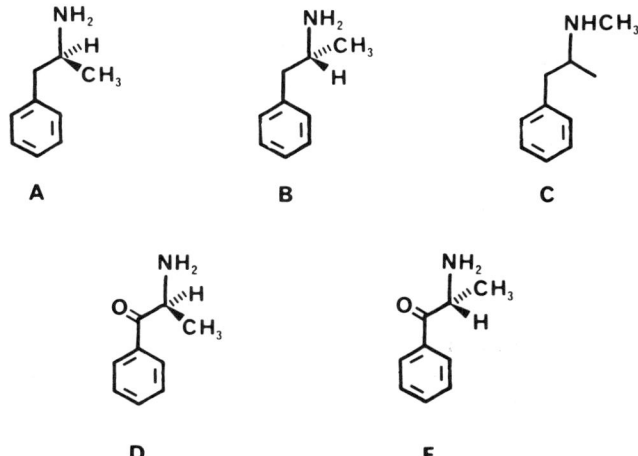

FIG. 2. Structures of S(+)-amphetamine (**A**), R(−)-amphetamine (**B**), racemic methamphetamine (**C**), S(−)-cathinone (**D**), and R(+)-cathinone (**E**). Note the structural similarity, optical rotation, and absolute configuration of S(+)-amphetamine and S(−)-cathinone.

Up to this point, mention has been made of only one structural change of the amphetamine molecule that does not result in a decrease in central stimulant potency (i.e., *N*-monomethylation). There is one additional example; oxidation of the benzylic hydroxy group of norephedrine gives rise to cathinone, a central stimulant that produces amphetamine-like effects. Cathinone, a naturally occurring compound, has been isolated from the fresh leaves of *Catha edulis* (khat). The term "cathinone" was originally used to designate only the *S*(−) isomer (i.e., the naturally occurring isomer). Through common usage, the term now applies to the racemic mixture, and the optical isomers are designated as *S*(−)-cathinone and *R*(+)-cathinone (Fig. 2). (Note: some authors still refer to the naturally occurring material as cathinone.) Khat chewing has become a major drug abuse problem in certain countries; the isolation and identification of *S*(−)-cathinone in 1979 and the finding that this agent may be the active constituent responsible for the stimulant effects of khat have prompted considerable research in this area. Several review articles describing the chemistry, pharmacology, and botany of khat are now available (34–36,52). With respect to activity as a locomotor stimulant, *S*(−)-cathinone is more potent than either its racemate or *R*(+) enantiomer and is one-fourth to one-sixth as potent as (+)-amphetamine [for a review, see Kalix and Braenden (35)]. Johanson and Schuster (32) have found that *S*(−)-cathinone is one-half to one-fourth as potent as (+)-amphetamine and equipotent with racemic cathinone in decreasing operant responding in monkeys. In animals trained to discriminate (+)-amphetamine from saline, *S*(−)-cathinone was essentially equipotent with the training drug (Table 1) and 10 times more potent than *R*(+)-cathinone (24). Racemic cathinone has also been used as a training drug in drug discrimination studies; in cathinone-trained animals, *S*(−)-cathinone was equipotent with racemic cathinone and (+)-amphetamine, three times more potent than *R*(+)-cathinone, and about 10 times more potent than its naturally occurring reduced counterpart (+)-norpseudoephedrine (22,46). The cathinone stimulus, like the amphetamine stimulus, generalizes to methamphetamine and cocaine (45).

Although khat has been used/abused for many centuries, there are essentially no human data available on cathinone. On the other hand, there is a considerable amount of information available on khat. The variety of effects produced in humans by khat are quite reminiscent of those produced by amphetamine (34,35). There have also been reports of khat-induced psychoses with symptomatology resembling that of amphetamine psychoses (2,26,35).

Hallucinogens

Prior to a discussion of these agents, it should be noted that there still exists a lack of consensus as to exactly what constitutes a hallucinogenic agent, whether or not all hallucinogenic agents produce similar effects (involving a similar mechanism), and, indeed, whether all hallucinogenic agents produce true hallucinations. Nevertheless, where human data are discussed, the term "hallucinogenic agent" is used in its broadest sense (for a further discussion of this topic, see ref. 31). Reviews are available on the general SAR of hallucinogenic phenylisopropylamines (based on the results of human and animal studies) (42,48) and on their mechanism of action (15,30). The discriminative stimulus properties of these agents have also been reviewed (21).

Aromatic Nucleus

Those PIA derivatives that produce a hallucinogenic effect (excluding amphetamine psychoses) in humans invariably possess an aromatic ring bearing alkoxy (e.g., methoxy) substituents. For example, 2,4-DMA and 2,5-DMA, as mentioned above, are hallucinogenic; these agents appear to be effective at the 50- to 60-mg (oral) dose range (48). Recently, Cassels and Gomez-Jeria (10) have claimed that the active dose commonly reported for 2,5-DMA is low and, based on their studies, should be revised upwards by a factor of about two. Addition of a third methoxy group can either increase or decrease potency depending on its location. Table 2 lists these TMAs as well as some additional analogs; 2,3,4-TMA is inactive at oral doses of up to 100 mg, and 2,3,5-TMA and 2,3,6-TMA are in need of further evaluation (48). One of the more potent TMAs as a hallucinogenic agent is 2,4,5-TMA (Table 2). Replacement of the 4-position methoxy group of 2,4,5-TMA by certain alkyl and other substituents gives rise to some of the most potent of the PIA hallucinogens. For example, the methyl, ethyl, and propyl derivatives of 2,5-DMA (i.e., DOM, DOET, and DOPR, respectively) are active at total oral doses of 1 to 5 mg (48); likewise, the 4-bromo and iodo analogs (i.e., DOB and DOI) are also very potent (Table 2). Where they have been evaluated, the *R*(−) isomers are about two to 10 times more potent than their *S*(+) enantiomers. The chloro (DOC) and fluoro (DOF) counterparts are active in animals but have not been studied in humans.

Two hallucinogenic PIA derivatives have been employed as training drugs in drug discrimination studies: DOM (21,49) and DOI (16). In general, the DOM stimulus generalizes to those PIAs that have been reported to be hallucinogenic in humans, and a significant correlation exists between human hallucinogenic potencies and discrimination-derived ED50 values (21). Some selected data are shown in Table 2. With the exception of 3,4-MDA (which is discussed separately below), the DOM stimulus did not generalize to any of the PIA derivatives to which the amphetamine stimulus generalized, and the amphetamine stimulus did not generalize to any of the PIA derivatives to which the DOM stimulus generalized.

Terminal Amine

Although there are very few examples of this phenomenon, *N*-monomethylation reduces the human hallucinogenic potency of PIAs (1). The *N*-methyl derivative of DOM (i.e., *N*-Me-DOM) is approximately $\frac{1}{10}$ as potent as DOM (48). Similar results were obtained in tests of stimulus generalization using DOM-trained animals (Table 2). The DOM

TABLE 2. *Potencies of selected methoxy-substituted phenylisopropylamines*

Agent	R_2	R_3	R_4	R_5	R_6	R'	Approx. human hallucinogenic dose (mg)[a]	Generalization ED50 (mg/kg)[b]
2,3-DMA	OMe	OMe	H	H	H	H	ND	NSG
2,4-DMA	OMe	H	OMe	H	H	H	60	4.9
2,5-DMA	OMe	H	H	OMe	H	H	50–100	5.5
2,6-DMA	OMe	H	H	H	OMe	H	ND	NSG
3,4-DMA	H	OMe	OMe	H	H	H	300–400(?)	NSG
3,5-DMA	H	OMe	H	OMe	H	H	ND	NSG
2,3,4-TMA	OMe	OMe	OMe	H	H	H	ND	7.8
2,3,5-TMA	OMe	OMe	H	OMe	H	H	ND	16.5
2,3,6-TMA	OMe	OMe	H	H	OMe	H	ND	ND
2,4,5,-TMA	OMe	H	OMe	OMe	H	H	20	3.6
2,4,6-TMA	OMe	H	OMe	H	OMe	H	30	3.7
3,4,5-TMA	H	OMe	OMe	OMe	H	H	160–200	6.3
DOM	OMe	H	Me	OMe	H	H	2–5	0.4
R(−)-DOM	OMe	H	Me	OMe	H	H	1–3	0.2
N-Me-DOM	OMe	H	Me	OMe	H	Me	20–50	4.0
DOET	OMe	H	Et	OMe	H	H	1–4	0.2
R(−)-DOET	OMe	H	Et	OMe	H	H	2	0.1
S(+)-DOET	OMe	H	Et	OMe	H	H	8	0.9
DOPR	OMe	H	n-Pr	OMe	H	H	1–2	0.2
DOBU	OMe	H	n-Bu	OMe	H	H	10	0.9
DON	OMe	H	NO_2	OMe	H	H	—	0.8
DOB	OMe	H	Br	OMe	H	H	1–2	0.2
R(−)-DOB	OMe	H	Br	OMe	H	H	0.5	0.1
S(+)-DOB	OMe	H	Br	OMe	H	H	5	0.8
DOI	OMe	H	I	OMe	H	H	1–2	0.4

[a] Human hallucinogenic potency represents total oral dose; doses are approximate. Most data are from Shulgin (48); see text for further discussion and references. ND, agent not tested or human potency not yet determined.

[b] Results of stimulus generalization studies employing rats trained to discriminate 1.0 mg/kg of DOM from saline as reviewed by Glennon et al. (21). NSG, stimulus generalization (i.e., >80% DOM-appropriate responding) did not occur.

stimulus also generalized to the *N*-propyl and *N,N*-dimethyl analogs of DOM, but both agents were less potent than DOM itself (21,25).

Side Chain

In contrast to what is usually found for amphetamine and related stimulants, the *R*(−) isomers of hallucinogenic PIAs are more potent than their *S*(+) enantiomers and/or racemates. This effect has been demonstrated both in human and in animal studies. The stereochemical aspects of hallucinogenic PIAs have been reviewed (14).

Removal of the α-methyl group of hallucinogenic PIAs usually results in retention of activity but in a decrease in potency. For example, α-demethylation of 3,4,5-TMA affords mescaline, which is orally active in humans at a dose of 300 to 500 mg (48). Similarly, the α-demethyl analogs

of DOM and DOB are active at doses of between 10 and 15 mg (48). Comparable results have been obtained in drug discrimination studies (21). The results of studies in humans reveal that homologation of the α-methyl group of hallucinogenic PIAs appears to abolish or alter activity. Only one such example has been examined in drug discrimination studies using DOM-trained rats. The DOM stimulus generalized to the α-ethyl homolog of DOM; although it was about 10 times less potent than DOM, the *R*(−) isomer was still more potent than its *S*(+) enantiomer (21).

Stimulant Hallucinogens

Certain agents seem to possess both stimulant and hallucinogenic character; generally, one activity predominates. For example, 2,4-DMA and 2,5-DMA are generally classified as hallucinogens or as psychotomimetics but are reported to produce some amphetamine-like stimulation (48). One agent that presents a particular problem when it comes to classification is the 3,4-methylenedioxy analog of amphetamine (i.e., 3,4-methylenedioxyphenylisopropylamine, 3,4-MDA, MDA); for a lack of a better term, it will be classified here as a stimulant hallucinogen. Prior to discussing this agent, it is appropriate to describe the nomenclature of MDA and MDA-related drugs. There are two positional isomers of MDA: 2,3-MDA and 3,4-MDA (Fig. 3). The older of the two isomers is 3,4-MDA, and as a consequence it is commonly referred to simply as MDA; this agent, often called the "love drug," is discussed below in greater detail. The other, 2,3-MDA, was first synthesized and characterized by Soine et al. (50) in 1983; its behavioral properties appear to be distinct from those of either amphetamine or DOM (23).

Introduction of a methoxy group to 3,4-MDA results in a series of analogs that are named on the basis of the position of the methoxy group. The *meta*-methoxy analog (i.e., 3-methoxy-4,5-methylenedioxyphenylisopropylamine) is known as MMDA. Two *ortho*-methoxy analogs are possible, MMDA-2 (i.e., 2-methoxy-4,5-methylenedioxyphenylisopropylamine) and MMDA-3a (i.e., 2-methoxy-3,4-methylenedioxyphenylisopropylamine). Each of these three agents is psychoactive (48), and MMDA has been explored by Naranjo as an adjunct to psychotherapy (40). There are also three positional isomers of methoxy-2,3-MDA; the *ortho, meta,* and *para* isomers are called MMDA-5, MMDA-4, and MMDA-3b, respectively. Of these, MMDA-4 has not been evaluated in humans, and only scant data are available on the other two isomers (48). Several dimethoxy and trimethoxy analogs of 2,3-MDA and 3,4-MDA can also be formulated, but most have not yet been synthesized or evaluated.

In humans, 3,4-MDA produces effects that are somewhat similar to, yet distinct from, those produced by LSD and other hallucinogenic agents (41). At the same time, 3,4-MDA produces certain effects that are characteristic of central stimulants; Shulgin (48) suggests that these latter effects might be attributable to the $S(+)$ isomer. Much of the human data on racemic MDA are of an anecdotal nature (e.g., ref. 55); however, $R(-)$-MDA is more potent than either its racemate or $S(+)$ isomer (48), and the $R(-)$ isomer has been evaluated in several clinical studies (12,51,57).

In animals, MDA produces effects that are both LSD- or hallucinogen-like and amphetamine-like (e.g., ref. 43). The LSD-like effects are associated with the $R(-)$ isomer, whereas the $S(+)$ isomer produces amphetamine-like effects. Mar-

quardt et al. (37) have provided evidence suggesting that the metabolites of 3,4-MDA may be responsible for at least some of the pharmacological and toxicological effects observed after administration of 3,4-MDA. In drug discrimination studies using amphetamine-trained rats, Shannon has reported that racemic MDA produces saline-like effects at low doses and disruption of behavior at higher doses (47). Glennon and Young subsequently reported that amphetamine stimulus generalization occurs with racemic MDA and $S(+)$-MDA but not with $R(-)$-MDA (17–19). W. L. Woolverton (*personal communication*) has found that MDA does not produce amphetamine-like effects with rats as subjects but does result in stimulus generalization in five of six amphetamine-trained rhesus monkeys. These studies employed different training and testing procedures, different species of animals, and/or different training doses of amphetamine; thus, it is difficult to draw any conclusions at this time. Interestingly, racemic MDA and $R(-)$-MDA but not $S(+)$-MDA produce stimulus generalization in DOM-trained animals (20). These results support the contention that each optical isomer of MDA may be primarily responsible for producing a different effect.

When 3,4-MDA has been employed as a training drug in drug discrimination studies (18), the MDA stimulus generalized with PIA stimulants (e.g., amphetamine) and PIA hallucinogens (e.g., DOM); generalization also occurred with cocaine (to which an amphetamine stimulus but not a DOM stimulus generalizes) and LSD (to which a DOM stimulus but not an amphetamine stimulus generalizes) (17–19). The 3,4-MDA stimulus also generalized to 2,3-MDA (an agent to which neither an amphetamine or a DOM stimulus generalized) (23); as such, this might be an interesting candidate for further evaluation.

There are only two structural modifications of 3,4-MDA that have received any attention: α-demethylation and N-alkylation. The α-demethyl or phenethylamine counterpart of 3,4-MDA (i.e., homopiperonylamine, HPA) appears to be inactive in humans (48) and in rats trained to discriminate DOM from saline (20). N-Alkylation results in a series of agents that has recently attracted some attention. The N-monomethyl analog of 3,4-MDA (i.e., N-monomethyl-3,4-methylenedioxyphenylisopropylamine, MDMA, "XTC," "ecstasy," "Adam") is perhaps the most noteworthy. In humans, the potency of MDMA (effective oral dose 100–160 mg) is similar to that of 3,4-MDA; however, unlike 3,4-MDA, the $S(+)$ isomer of MDMA (effective dose 80–120 mg) is more potent than its $R(-)$ enantiomer (effective dose estimated to be in the vicinity of 300 mg) (1). Qualitatively, most of the effects produced by the racemate are similar to those observed with the $S(+)$ isomer (1). In animals, stimulus generalization was obtained with MDMA in amphetamine-trained rats (19) but not in DOM-trained rats (20); furthermore, the DOM stimulus did not generalize to either isomer of MDMA. Stimulus generalization did occur in 3,4-MDA-trained animals (19). W. L. Woolverton (*personal communication*) has found that MDMA results in partial generalization in amphetamine-trained rats but in complete generalization (regardless of route of administration) in amphetamine-trained rhesus monkeys. MDMA has now been demonstrated to serve as an effective training drug (at 1 mg/kg; ED50 = 0.5 mg/kg)

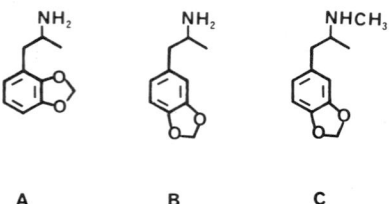

FIG. 3. Structures of 2,3-MDA (**A**), 3,4-MDA ("MDA") (**B**), and MDMA (**C**).

in discriminative control of behavior in rats (R. A. Glennon and M. Tocarz, *unpublished data*). Several other *N*-mono-alkyl and *N,N*-dialkyl derivatives of 3,4-MDA have been reported. The *N*-monoethyl analog (i.e., MDEA; "Eve") is slightly less potent than MDMA in humans (7); the *N-n*-propyl, *N*-isopropyl, and several related agents, were less potent (or were inactive) relative to MDEA (7,8); 3,4-MDA produces locomotor stimulation in mice (8,27); MDMA is severalfold more potent than 3,4-MDA; and MDEA is approximately equiactive with MDMA (7,8).

Summary of SAR

Derivatives of phenylisopropylamine can produce predominantly central stimulant or hallucinogenic effects depending on the presence and location of certain substituent groups; that is, each effect is associated with a distinct SAR. Unsubstituted phenylisopropylamine (i.e., amphetamine) is a central stimulant, and the introduction of substituents to the aromatic nucleus tends to decrease its potency. Removal or extention (i.e., homologation) of the side chain α-methyl group decreases or abolishes central stimulant activity. Introduction of a benzylic hydroxyl function reduces potency, but oxidation of this hydroxyl group to a keto (i.e., carbonyl) group essentially restores activity/potency. The *N*-monomethyl derivative of amphetamine is at least as potent as, if not more potent than, amphetamine as a central stimulant. For those PIAs with central stimulant activity, the *S* isomer is severalfold more potent than the *R* enantiomer. With respect to hallucinogenic/psychotomimetic activity, the presence of two or three aromatic alkoxy groups is important. Within the 2,5-dimethoxy series, potency increases dramatically when the 4 position is additionally substituted by a small alkyl group such as methyl, ethyl, or *n*-propyl or by halogen. From the information available to date, it appears that the side chain can not be altered without an ensuing decrease in potency. *N*-Alkylation of the terminal amine group of hallucinogenic PIAs decreases potency or abolishes activity. In contrast to what is found for the stimulant PIAs, the *R* isomers are more potent than the racemates and/or *S* isomers as hallucinogenic agents.

The drug 3,4-MDA is unique from several standpoints. First, it seems to possess both stimulant and hallucinogenic character and may produce effects that result from a combination of these properties; alternatively, it may produce an effect that is distinct from these properties (with the stimulant and hallucinogenic effects being "side effects"). Second, because 3,4-DMA is only a weakly active agent, it might not have been anticipated that 3,4-MDA would be as active as it is; however, it might not be justifiable to extrapolate from alkoxy to methylenedioxy. Thus, 3,4-MDA is unique in that it possesses a methylenedioxy group. From here, the SAR seem to follow what is expected. Being substituted in the aromatic ring, 3,4-MDA would be anticipated to be less potent than amphetamine as a stimulant; also, the *S* isomer, as with amphetamine, should be more potent than the *R* isomer in this regard. The *R* isomer should be the more potent as a hallucinogenic agent; this appears to be the case. *N*-Monomethylation, to afford MDMA, would be expected to increase (or at least not decrease) stimulant activity but would be expected to decrease hallucinogenic activity/potency. As a consequence of enhancing the amphetamine-like aspects of this agent, the *S*(+) isomer should be more potent than its enantiomer; this, too, seems to be the case. The question still remains whether MDA (and, for that matter, MDMA) produces a unique effect. Only additional clinical evaluation can answer this question.

DESIGNER DRUGS

"Designed drugs" and "designer drugs" differ primarily with respect to who is doing the designing. Armed with a variety of information, including the available structure–activity relationships for a series of compounds, medicinal chemists routinely strive to modify the molecular structures of given agents so as to (a) enhance potency, (b) alter pharmacodynamic properties (e.g., stability, solubility), and/or (c) highlight a specific activity (i.e., to remove structural features that might be responsible for undesirable side effects). Other factors (e.g., economic) may also be important considerations. This process is referred to as drug design. Within the context of PIAs, anorexic agents might serve as a retrospective example. In the search for an amphetamine-like anorexic agent with diminished stimulant properties, structures that might be considered are those that incorporate structural features known to have an adverse effect on central stimulation. These features, as discussed above, include substitution on the aromatic nucleus, substitution on the α position of the side chain with long alkyl groups or *gem*-dialkyl groups, and substitution on the terminal amine with large alkyl or *N,N*-dialkyl groups. Indeed, many of the commonly used PIA anorexic agents bear these features.

The term "designer drug" is a colloquialism that has been applied to the end product of drug design as performed in clandestine laboratories. That is, structure–activity relationships can be applied to design analogs of an abused substance that is in short supply or to design new derivatives of a known agent such that they will not be covered under the Controlled Substances Act; MDMA, for example, has been termed (although perhaps not rightfully so) a designer drug. With the looming possibility that other novel designer drugs may appear on the illegitimate market (5), it is prudent to continue efforts to understand the generalities surrounding these agents prior to their appearance. One way in which this can be done is to have a thorough grounding in, and an appreciation for, the concept of structure–activity relationships.

REFERENCES

1. Anderson, G. M., Braun, G., Braun, U., Nichols, D. E., and Shulgin, A. T. (1978): *NIDA Res. Monogr. Ser.*, 22:8–15.
2. Angrist, B. (1983): In: *Stimulants: Neurochemical, Behavioral, and Clinical Perspectives,* edited by I. Creese, pp. 1–30. Raven Press, New York.
3. Angrist, B., and Sudilovsky, A. (1978): In: *Handbook of Psychopharmacology, Vol. 11: Stimulants,* edited by L. L. Iversen, S. D. Iversen, and S. H. Snyder, pp. 99–166. Plenum Press, New York.

4. Barfknecht, C. F., and Nichols, D. E. (1972): *J. Med. Chem.*, 15: 109–110.
5. Baum, R. M. (1985): *Chem. Eng. News*, 9:7–16.
6. Biel, J. H., and Bopp, B. A. (1978): In: *Handbook of Psychopharmacology, Vol. 11: Stimulants*, edited by L. L. Iversen, S. D. Iversen, and S. H. Snyder, pp. 1–39. Plenum Press, New York.
7. Braun, U., Shulgin, A. T., and Braun, G. (1980): *J. Pharm. Sci.*, 69:192–195.
8. Braun, U., Shulgin, A. T., and Braun, G. (1980): *Arzneim. Forsch.*, 30:825–830.
9. Buxton, D. A. (1972): *Prog. Brain Res.*, 36:171–181.
10. Cassels, B. K., and Gomez-Jeria, J. S. (1985): *J. Psychoact. Drugs*, 17:129–130.
11. Creese, I., ed. (1983): *Stimulants: Neurochemical, Behavioral, and Clinical Perspectives.* Raven Press, New York.
12. Di Leo, F. B. (1981): *J. Psychoact. Drugs*, 13:319–324.
13. Fuller, R. W., Baker, J. C., Perry, K. W., and Molloy, B. B. (1975): *Neuropharmacology*, 14:739–746.
14. Glennon, R. A. (1984): In: *Handbook of Stereoisomers: Drugs in Psychopharmacology*, edited by D. F. Smith, pp. 327–368. CRC Press, Boca Raton, FL.
15. Glennon, R. A. (1985): In: *Pharmacology of Serotonin*, edited by A. R. Green, pp. 253–280. Oxford University Press, Oxford.
16. Glennon, R. A., and McKenney, J. D. (1985): *Pharmacologist*, 27:194.
17. Glennon, R. A., and Young, R. (1984): *Eur. J. Pharmacol.*, 99: 249–250.
18. Glennon, R. A., and Young, R. (1984): *Life Sci.*, 34:379–383.
19. Glennon, R. A., and Young, R. (1984): *Pharmacol. Biochem. Behav.*, 20:501–505.
20. Glennon, R. A., Young, R., Rosecrans, J. A., and Anderson, G. M. (1982): *Biol. Psychiatry*, 17:807–814.
21. Glennon, R. A., Rosecrans, J. A., and Young, R. (1983): *Med. Res. Rev.*, 3:289–340.
22. Glennon, R. A., Schechter, M. D., and Rosecrans, J. A. (1984): *Pharmacol. Biochem. Behav.*, 21:1–3.
23. Glennon, R. A., Young, R., and Soine, W. (1984): *Gen. Pharmacol.*, 15:361–362.
24. Glennon, R. A., Young, R., and Hauck, A. E. (1985): *Pharmacol. Biochem. Behav.*, 22:723–729.
25. Glennon, R. A., McKenney, J. D., Titeler, M., and Lyon, R. A. (1986): *J. Med. Chem.*, 29:914–921.
26. Gough, S. P., and Cookson, I. B. (1984): *Lancet*, 1:455.
27. Gunn, J. A., Gurd, M. R., and Sachs, I. (1939): *J. Physiol. (Lond.)*, 95:485–500.
28. Huang, J.-T., and Ho, B. T. (1974): *Pharmacol. Biochem. Behav.*, 2:669–673.
29. Iversen, L. L., Iversen, S. D., Snyder, S. H., eds. (1978): *Handbook of Psychopharmacology, Vol. 11, Stimulants.* Plenum Press, New York.
30. Jacobs, B. L. (1982): In: *Psychopharmacology 1. Part 1. Preclinical Psychopharmacology*, edited by D. G. Grahame-Smith and D. J. Cowen, pp. 344–376. Elsevier Science Publishing Co., New York.
31. Jacobs, B. L., ed. (1984): *Hallucinogens: Neurochemical, Behavioral, and Clinical Perspectives.* Raven Press, New York.
32. Johanson, C. E., and Schuster, C. R. (1981): *J. Pharmacol. Exp. Ther.*, 219:355–362.
33. Jones, C. N., Hill, H. F., and Harris, R. T. (1974): *Psychopharmacologia*, 36:347–356.
34. Kalix, P. (1984): *Gen. Pharmacol.*, 15:179–187.
35. Kalix, P., and Braenden, O. (1985): *Pharmacol. Rev.*, 37:149–164.
36. Kennedy, J. G., Teague, J., and Fairbanks, L. (1980): *Cult. Med. Psychiatry*, 4:311–344.
37. Marquardt, G. M., DiStefano, V., and Ling, L. L. (1978): In: *Psychopharmacology of Hallucinogens*, edited by R. C. Stillman and R. E. Willette, pp. 84–104. Pergamon Press, New York.
38. Menon, M. K., Tseng, L.-F., and Loh, H. H. (1976): *J. Pharmacol. Exp. Ther.*, 197:272–279.
39. Moore, K. E. (1978): In: *Handbook of Psychopharmacology, Vol. 11: Stimulants*, edited by L. L. Iversen, S. D. Iversen, and S. H. Snyder, pp. 41–98. Plenum Press, New York.
40. Naranjo, C. (1973): *The Healing Journey.* Pantheon, New York.
41. Naranjo, C., Shulgin, A. T., and Sargent, T. (1967): *Med. Pharmacol. Exp.*, 17:359–364.
42. Nichols, D. E., and Glennon, R. A. (1984): In: *Hallucinogens: Neurochemical, Behavioral, and Clinical Perspectives*, edited by B. L. Jacobs, pp. 95–142. Raven Press, New York.
43. Nozaki, M., Vaupel, D. B., and Martin, W. R. (1977): *Eur. J. Pharmacol.*, 46:339–349.
44. Roth, L. W., Richards, R. K., Shemano, I., and Morphis, B. B. (1954): *Arch. Int. Pharmacodyn. Ther.*, 98:362–368.
45. Schechter, M. D., and Glennon, R. A. (1985): *Pharmacol. Biochem. Behav.*, 22:913–916.
46. Schechter, M. D., Rosecrans, J. A., and Glennon, R. A. (1984): *Pharmacol. Biochem. Behav.*, 20:181–184.
47. Shannon, H. (1980): *Psychopharmacology*, 67:311–312.
48. Shulgin, A. T. (1978): In: *Handbook of Psychopharmacology, Vol. 11: Stimulants*, edited by L. L. Iversen, S. D. Iversen, and S. H. Snyder, pp. 243–333. Plenum Press, New York.
49. Silverman, P. B., and Ho, B. T. (1980): *Psychopharmacology*, 68: 209–215.
50. Soine, W. H., Shark, R. E., and Agee, D. T. (1983): *J. Forens. Sci.*, 28:386–390.
51. Turek, I. S., Soskin, R. A., and Kurland, A. A. (1974): *J. Psychedel. Drugs*, 6:7–14.
52. United Nations (1980): *Bull. Narc.*, 32(3):1–99.
53. Van der Schoot, J. B., Ariens, E. J., van Rossum, J. A., and Hurkmans, J. A. T. M. (1962): *Arzneim. Forsch.*, 12:902–907.
54. Van Kammen, D. P., Ninan, P. T., and Hommer, D. (1984): In: *Handbook of Stereoisomers: Drugs in Psychopharmacology*, edited by D. F. Smith, pp. 297–315. CRC Press, Boca Raton, FL.
55. Weil, A. T. (1976): *J. Psychedel. Drugs*, 8:336–337.
56. Winter, J. (1984): *Pharmacol. Biochem. Behav.*, 20:201–203.
57. Yensen, R., Di Leo, F. B., Rhead, J. C., Richards, W. A., Soskin, R. A., et al. (1976): *J. Nerv. Ment. Dis.*, 163:233–245.
58. Young, R., and Glennon, R. A. (1986): *Med. Res. Rev.*, 6:99–130.

Psychopharmacology:
The Third Generation of Progress,
edited by Herbert Y. Meltzer.
Raven Press, New York © 1987.

CHAPTER **176**

Introduction: Development of New Drugs

M. Goldberg and B. Dubnick

"How do CNS drugs get onto the market." One objective for this section is to describe drug discovery and development for those relatively new in the field. Such a chapter has not been part of the previous two volumes of this series. What idea produces a chemical which then becomes a drug? Can that progression be made comprehensible? We have described the process in five parts from conception to therapeutic acceptance: from synthesis by the medicinal chemist, to testing by preclinical pharmacologists, then by the clinician for human efficacy trials, followed by regulatory approval and postmarketing surveillance.

A typical simplified scheme, then, can be represented as follows:

1. OBJECTIVE

(e.g., To find an anxiolytic without concomitant sedation, ataxia, amnesia, withdrawal convulsions, potentiation of alcohol and barbiturates)

2. LEAD COMPOUND

Medicinal chemist ← feedback → Pharmacologist

Select approach(es) for choosing test compounds

Evaluate test results ↕

Synthesize new compounds for test

Screen and evaluate
Tests for efficacy
in vivo:
    behavioral (conflict);
    anticonvulsant
    (metrazol)
in vitro:
    diazepam receptor
    binding
Tests for side effects
in vivo:
    acute toxicity-
    observational battery
    (LD_{50}, preliminary
    profile);
    rod walking
    (coordination,
    sedation);
       feedback
inclined screen
(muscle relaxation);

convulsant-anticonvulsant profile;
alcohol or barbiturates interactions (sleep)
memory test

3. PRECLINICAL DEVELOPMENT (begin Good Laboratory Practice in accordance with government regulations)

Pharmaceutical (e.g., dosage forms)   Chemical (e.g., bulk chemical)   Safety Evaluation (toxicology, pharmacokinetics and biotransformation)

Broad Pharmacological Evaluation (autonomic, cardiovascular-renal respiratory, etc.)

4. CLINICAL CANDIDATE (IND package to FDA for approval of new drug investigation

Clinical Monitor (in house)   Support (e.g., statistics, regulatory affairs)   Clinical Center

5. CLINICAL INVESTIGATION (Phases I–III leading to New Drug Application

6. REGULATORY APPROVAL of NDA

7. POSTMARKETING SURVEILLANCE (Phase IV)

However, the process of drug development is conceptual as well as methodological, attended by difficulties particularly associated with the study of psychiatric disorders in animals. In the absence of authentic disease models and a deficient basic understanding of CNS diseases, procedures used in screening for new drugs have been based on clinical findings. The current array of antipsychotics, antidepressives/antimanics, and anxiolytics (the principal therapeutic categories that we address) had to be based on clinical discoveries. Reserpine, from folk medicine, and chlorpromazine (an antihistamine by design), originally selected to potentiate anesthesia and lower body temperature based on its animal pharmacology, were recognized as having useful psychological effects in patients; "neuroleptic" properties, including effects on avoidance behavior, were then defined in animals. The antidepressant properties of imipramine, noted in the clinic, were surprising in view of its chemical and pharmacological similarity to the tricyclic neuroleptics; special animal tests for antidepressants (based, for example, on reversal of the reserpine syndrome) were devised only after the fortuitous and separate clinical observations with imipramine and with iproniazid. In the latter case, the probable mechanism (monoamine oxidase inhibition) was known as a property of the antitubercular hydrazide before either the clinical observation or the animal pharmacology. The use of alcohol to reduce "anxiety" is ancient and traditional; but the modern era of anxiolytics started with meprobamate, originally conceived as a centrally acting muscle relaxant and found to produce clinical antianxiety effects with advantages over barbiturates. Thus procedures used in pharmaceutical laboratories as screening tests for new drugs depended first on the discovery of clinical efficacy but then on the interplay of empiricism and conceptual approaches derived from current and basic findings in our science, in many cases contributed by the pharmaceutical laboratories themselves.

The first volume of this series, *Psychopharmacology: A Review of Progress, 1957–1967*, covering the decade since neuropsychopharmacology emerged as a discipline, broadly speaking defined the subject, dealing with neurotransmitters, drugs, and behavior and several specific therapeutic classes of drugs (antineurotics, addictive agents, antidepressants, antipsychotics, and psychotomimetics). The clinical effects of chlorpromazine, reserpine, imipramine, iproniazid, and LSD had already been observed and reported before 1957, as were the presence in the CNS and assay of 5-HT, "sympathin," and the first hints of dopamine. The reviews in that first volume dealt with the classical neurotransmitters (acetylcholine, 5-HT, norepinephrine, dopamine): regulation of biosynthesis and release, histochemical and subcellular localization, uptake and storage, and neuronal function and specificity. The clinical papers dealt largely with developing ethics, and quantitative methods for measuring the phenomena produced by the same drug across species, including humans. During this period, pharmaceutical laboratories contributed new behavioral methods and phenomenology. Their scientists used current quantitative biochemical measurements as well as specially devised procedures to characterize extant and new drugs and to conceptualize therapeutic improvements. As methods were developed to measure dynamic qualities (neurotransmitter turnover, regulation, adaptive responses), often with new drug substances as tools, these methods or their implications became part of the drug development process. The second volume, *Psychopharmacology: A Generation of Progress*, continued the general focus on neurotransmitters, drugs, and behavior and the specific therapeutic areas: schizophrenia, depression, anxiety, neurological disorders, and the special concerns involved in pediatics, geriatrics, and drug abuse. Chapters in that volume reviewed the histochemical mapping of monoaminergic pathways, elucidating their function; neuroendocrine connections; amino acids and peptides as prospective neurotransmitters and receptors as entities that can be measured. Receptor methodology, of course, became standard in applied pharmaceutical

research. Both the "receptors" and original ligands have often been a contribution from a pharmaceutical laboratory.

In Chapter 177 Hesp and Resch present a systematic view particular to CNS drugs from the vantage of medicinal chemists. Instances where the biological methods are standard and the endpoint well defined are discussed as well as the difficult circumstance (such as Alzheimer's disease) where little is known about the disease or its treatment. Since the medicinal chemist must work closely with a biologist, Chapter 178 by Weissman and Koe offers the pharmacologist's view, introspective and personal, with examples showing what may be perceived on the periphery of standard methods. Spilker, in Chapter 179, has taken a pragmatic approach in describing the clinician's concerns in developing drugs with CNS indications. Informed consent, carryover to humans from *deficient* animal models, and practical considerations relating to the design and conduct of studies at single and multiple centers are among his ethical and practical issues. Finally, Fisher (Chapter 180) and Leber (Chapter 181) deal with regulatory aspects. Fisher reviews the history and problems of postmarketing surveillance for adverse reaction and side effects. After a discussion of the current FDA requirements, he suggests a future direction. Leber's review provides a historical and current (evolving) view of the responsibility of the FDA for the IND process under the Federal Food, Drug, and Cosmetic Act.

Pharmaceutical companies will continue to be the source of new and improved CNS drugs; the process by which they are developed will continue to be both rational and intuitive, and overall an interactive one. The institution itself *requires* its various applied scientists (medicinal chemists, pharmacologists, pharmacists, clinicians, molecular biologists, computer and library specialists, etc.) to work together toward a common goal. The scientists with pharmaceutical affiliations will themselves continue to be participants and contributors to the development and dissemination of basic information in our science. More formal industry/academic interactions in very basic areas such as molecular biology have been encouraged by the current economic climate. Obviously, the question is not whether there will be an impact of new technology on the (applied) drug discovery process, but how soon and what. The application of new, noninvasive, imaging techniques (computerized axial tomography, positron emission tomography, nuclear magnetic resonance) in the clinic will influence how data in animals are obtained and presented to support early human pharmacology. As knowledge develops to clarify reactions that occur after receptor activation, such as the dynamics of receptor participation in subsequent events and the signals that mediate adaptive regulation, then drugs will be sought to modify those reactions. Neuropeptides are bound to provide one direction for our search, and molecular biology will be a strong influence: natural products, such as neurotropic factors, and modified natural products; how function is related to structure; possibly a better understanding of the genetic basis of certain CNS diseases and how to treat them. Perhaps the methods of molecular biology will provide a better basis for understanding behavioral pharmacology and the adaptive responses to training and environment, as well as to drug treatments. A preview of the next decade of drug discovery.

Psychopharmacology:
The Third Generation of Progress,
edited by Herbert Y. Meltzer.
Raven Press, New York © 1987.

CHAPTER **177**

The Medicinal Chemist's Approach to CNS Drug Discovery

Barrie Hesp and James F. Resch

Discussions of drug-hunting for CNS disorders usually begin by dividing known agents into classes according to their therapeutic utility. Thus we might speak separately of antidepressants, anxiolytics, antipsychotics, and so on. This would be an entirely pharmacological distinction. Only rarely would a medicinal chemist doing CNS research classify himself as he would the drugs themselves, and terms such as "anxiolytic chemist" or "antidepressant chemist" seem quite artificial to those in the field. Any medicinal chemist is first of all an organic chemist, skilled in the assembly of novel chemical structures, and his expertise in this area is easily transferred from one project to another. This much is widely recognized. Moreover, the basic tools of medicinal chemistry, particularly as they have become specialized for use in CNS research, are quite generally applicable to research on diverse disease types. But how are these tools employed in the search for a novel CNS drug? What will the CNS chemist use as his starting point in designing a new chemical series? How will he optimize activity once it is discovered?

The answers to these questions will differ markedly, depending on the type of drug-hunting program in which the medicinal chemist finds himself. Some projects will depend on pragmatic whole-animal models of the disease state, whereas others will originate from precisely defined goals at the molecular level. Between these extremes lies a continuum of possible environments for the medicinal chemist. Our discussion of the medicinal chemist's role in drug discovery will be simplified if we first consider three representative types of drug-hunting programs, which we will label the disease-model approach, the mechanism-based approach, and the systems approach. We will then show that a unified approach, which blends aspects of these three prototypical programs, can broaden the chemist's

understanding of the targeted disorder and so increase the likelihood of success in drug discovery. The importance of the clinic cannot be overlooked, especially when considering CNS drug therapy, and accordingly we will describe the types of clinical feedback that can generate new leads for the medicinal chemist. Finally, we will consider the difficulties inherent in beginning work on a disease for which no effective treatment exists, and thereby explore the contributions a medicinal chemist can make in planning a new integrated research program.

THE DISEASE-MODEL APPROACH

Many of today's psychotropic drugs originated in skillful exploitation of a shrewd clinical observation with a drug originally intended for a quite different indication. For example, the prototype phenothiazine neuroleptic chlorpromazine (Structure 1) was synthesized in an attempt to increase the sedative component first observed in the pharmacology of the related structure promethazine (Structure 2), a drug under clinical investigation at the time as a potent antihistamine. The remarkable activity of chlorpromazine stimulated the search for animal models that could be used to characterize chlorpromazine pharmacologically and as screens in the search for additional novel agents with similar, if not identical, profiles. These tests were used to evaluate large numbers of compounds in which various structural features in the prototype molecules were varied systematically, limited only by the chemists' imagination and versatility. Their objective was to provide an entree for their companies into this particular marketplace.

Such efforts based on novel chemistry, with compounds evaluated in largely empirical behavioral models of the disease, may be termed the "disease-model" approach. In the absence of an understanding of the mechanistic basis of a test, the medicinal chemist may be forced to view the biological system as a "black box" providing little or no explanation for the activity elicited by his compounds. Despite these constraints, an impressive list of achievements has stemmed from this form of chemical evolution, which in some respects resembles the Darwinian version. Thus, most structural changes confer no benefit and the products make little or no sustained impact under the pressures of the world of medicine; others, seemingly trivial (at the time), result in an improved profile and commercial success, such as in thioridazine (Structure 3), a neuroleptic with less propensity to induce extrapyramidal side effects, a property now known to be subserved by the enhanced anticholinergic activity introduced through the structural modifications.

Not infrequently the change in pharmacology induced by a series of small stepwise structural alterations results in a qualitative change in profile and a new class of drug. In such fashion the phenothiazine neuroleptics were the forerunners of the first tricyclic antidepressant, imipramine (Structure 4), with amitriptyline (Structure 5) and doxepin (Structure 6) as just two of the numerous analogs subsequently synthesized.

Although some medicinal chemists have criticized the disease-model approach as unimaginative, it has not only led to remarkable advances in therapies, but has also contributed much to our present-day concept of "bioisosterism" (25), the ability of one functional group to mimic another in its recognition by biological systems. Bioisosteric replacements in the above-mentioned tricyclic antidepressant structures are the substitution of the methylene and nitrogen group in Structure 4 by a carbon-carbon double bond in Structure 5, and the subsequent substitution of a methylene group in the seven-membered ring of Structure 5 by an oxygen atom in Structure 6.

The law of diminishing returns usually applies as a particular series is increasingly worked over and several thousand analogs have been synthesized, as is often the case. Arguably the greatest scope for creativity in the disease-model approach lies in the selection of a novel target structure for subsequent manipulation. The choice of the potent analgesic meperidine (Structure 7) as the starting point for a broad disease-model approach to CNS

drug discovery by Janssen et al. led directly to the second major class of neuroleptics, the butyrophenones, typified by haloperidol (Structure 8). A third class, the benzamides, originated in chemical modification of the antiarrhythmic drug procainamide (Structure 9). Interestingly, there are major national differences in psychotropic drug usage, a fact not without influence on the "local" medicinal chemist. Though not approved for use in the United States, sulpiride (Structure 10), a member of the benzamide class, is the most frequently used neuroleptic in France and Japan and in these countries far outsells drugs familiar to the U.S. physician. Not surprisingly, therefore, the benzamide class remains a very active research topic for the chemist in parts of Europe and in Japan.

One final example, the benzodiazepine anxiolytics, will serve to demonstrate the continuing usefulness of the disease-model approach. This series, typified by diazepam (Structure 11), itself the product of the disease-model approach, has captured the attention of many medicinal chemists and has spawned numerous "lookalikes" which together have served to delineate the structure-activity relationships (SAR) in the general series. By the mid-1970s one would have thought there was little further scope for chemical modification in this series, but yet one more surprise was in store. Incorporation of an amino-alkyltriazole moiety, as in adinazolam (Structure 12), resulted in compounds with antidepressant activity (9) in addition to the usual anxiolytic activity, again as measured in disease-model screens. The cooccurrence of anxiety with depression is common in the clinical situation and compounds with this profile may be of value.

Undoubtedly the disease-model approach has been highly successful as the path to most of today's psychotropic drugs. In the case of the neuroleptics, it has also provided a rich diversity of chemical structures with similar pharmacological and clinical profile. This perhaps is the approach's greatest weakness: we can be reasonably confident that new drugs identified on the basis of these same models will be active in the target disease in humans. Rather, the issue is whether they will be significantly different from what has gone before. In this context the medicinal chemist would question the clinician as to whether the major chemical classes of neuroleptics differ in their positive attributes or solely on the basis of their side effect profiles. In the next section we shall see how important the answer to this question is as we discuss the potential value of detailed neurochemical profiles of these superficially similar drugs.

THE MECHANISM-BASED APPROACH

The "dopamine hypothesis," and the recognition that all neuroleptics are antagonists of dopamine at postsynaptic receptors, facilitated a more mechanism-based approach to the design of drugs for the treatment of schizophrenia. For the chemist, the challenge from these findings was to understand the details of the interaction between dopamine and its receptors, or to be more specific, to identify the conformation (i.e., three-dimensional shape) of dopamine in the bound form. With such information he would attempt to design alternative structures with similar affinity for the receptor but lacking key structural features essential for activating the receptor. Central to this hypothesis is the assumption that receptor binding involves only discrete regions of the ligand structure, the remaining structural framework serving to fix these key regions in the appropriate spatial relationships. Alternative frameworks may be considered, leading to novel structures for synthesis and evaluation.

In contrast to many enzymes, no receptors have been crystallized and subjected to structural scrutiny. Neither are there direct analytical methods for determining the conformation of ligands at their receptors, and the chemist must conceptualize from a knowledge of the structures of the agonists and antagonists that bind to the receptor of interest. From an analysis of the structures of semirigid analogs of dopamine, the latter is thought to bind to at least one class of dopamine receptor in the conformation depicted in Structure 13. In the solid state, as determined by X-ray crystallography, the aminopropyl chain in chlorpromazine is oriented toward the ring containing the chlorine substituent, as drawn in Structure 1. On the basis of this finding, chemists have suggested that the receptor "recognizes" elements of the dopamine structure in chlorpromazine, as depicted in the composite Structure 14. It will be apparent from a consideration of the hypothetical conformation depicted for sulpiride in Structure 10 that similar reasoning could be applied to other neuroleptic drugs. The reader is referred to the original literature (12) for a sophisticated analysis of the structure of one such drug, butaclamol.

In some respects such analyses have been simplified with the finding that there are heterogeneous populations of dopamine receptors. Since dopamine may possibly bind in different conformations to D_1 and D_2 receptors, data that could not be accommodated on the single receptor model may be interpretable in terms of two binding modes. There is currently great interest in the ramifications of dopamine receptor heterogeneity in the context of drugs to treat schizophrenia. Today's most frequently used drugs are much more selective for D_2 than for D_1 receptors, and it is an open question whether drugs with a different balance of D_1/D_2 receptor antagonism would have improved profiles with respect to side effects such as the tardive dyskinesias, or even whether selective D_1 receptor antagonists would be effective antipsychotic agents in their own right. SCH 23390 (Structure 15) and sulpiride (Structure 10) are among the most selective antagonists available at present (23) for D_1 and D_2 receptors, respectively, and as such encode important structural information for the medicinal chemist.

The availability of receptor binding assays has made it a relatively simple procedure to profile a particular drug against a battery of such assays. Such studies can be particularly informative when they are used to compare different structural types within a single therapeutic class. For example, differences within the various chemical classes of neuroleptic drugs are readily evident, though they share the common property of high affinity for the dopamine receptor. Snyder (7) has noted that the diphenylbutyl-piperidine subset of neuroleptic drugs, such as pimozide (Structure 16), also bind to receptors for calcium channel antagonists of the nitrendipine type. This property may subserve a potentially important clinical difference between this class and other neuroleptics, namely, their effectiveness in ameliorating some of the negative symptoms of schizophrenia. Though extremely speculative, this is precisely the type of clue the chemist needs, since it provides the basis for a new chemical approach to drugs that may be qualitatively different from those currently available to the clinician.

The search for more selective and faster-acting antidepressant drugs has likewise benefited from a mechanism-based approach. Most tricyclic antidepressants potentiate noradrenergic neurotransmission, and this property probably underlies their therapeutic activity. In terms of neurochemistry, these drugs prevent reuptake of norepinephrine and serotonin into the presynaptic terminal. They are also antagonists at central muscarinic receptors. With this knowledge, chemists have produced a variety of structures lacking the anticholinergic component of the pharmacology, and/or selective for norepinephrine or serotonin with respect to reuptake blockade, the objective being to eliminate troublesome side effects and to delineate the mechanism of action of antidepressants at the level of the synapse. Maprotiline (Structure 17), a close structural analog of imipramine (Structure 4), is a selective antagonist of norepinephrine reuptake. Viloxazine (Structure 18) is also a selective antagonist of norepinephrine reuptake but lacks significant anticholinergic activity. Minor structural changes can result in remarkable changes in pharmacology, as is evident with nisoxetine (Structure 19) and fluoxetine (Structure 20), selective antagonists of norepinephrine and serotonin, respectively. The consensus is that selective

13

14

15

16

nists of norepinephrine and serotonin uptake are each effective antidepressants. Indeed, evidence is accumulating for a functional interaction between noradrenergic and serotonergic systems in certain brain areas (22).

17   18   19   20

Alternative mechanisms for potentiating noradrenergic transmission may result in drugs with superior efficacy to the tricyclics and fewer, or at least different, side effect profiles. One such mechanism under investigation in several companies involves modulation of the inhibitory feedback loop with a presynaptic α_2-adrenergic antagonist. In considering what to synthesize when assigned such a project, the chemist will typically survey the known structures with α_2-receptor agonist or antagonist activity. Most chemists would recognize three structural types as worthy of serious consideration. The centrally acting antihypertensive agent clonidine (Structure 21) is a potent selective α_2-agonist. Piperoxan (Structure 22) is a potent α-receptor antagonist but is essentially nonselective between α_1- and α_2-receptors. Yohimbine (Structure 23), a member of the rauwolfia alkaloid family, is a potent α_2-antagonist but has several other, undesirable pharmacological actions. As might be expected, the creative process leads different chemists down different tracks. Workers at Reckitt and Colman (3) in Great Britain hybridized the clonidine (Structure 21) and piperoxan (Structure 22) structures to give idazoxan (Structure 24), whereas Merck chemists (11) in the United States elected to start with the complex yohimbine structure and produced the simpler analog L-654,284 (Structure 25). Both idazoxan and L-654,284 are potent and selective α_2-antagonists, and it will be most interesting to chart their progress.

21   22   23   24   25   26

The latency of onset of clinical improvement with the tricyclic antidepressants has long puzzled bi20scientists and chemists alike, since these drugs typically were discovered on the basis of acute effects in animal models. Recently, it has been suggested that the neurochemical correlate of antidepressant activity is a time-dependent adaptive change in central β-receptors. This has stimulated the search for novel agents that would down-regulate central β-receptors more rapidly than existing antidepressants. Studies with combinations of α_2-antagonists, such as yohimbine, and norepinephrine-uptake blockers, such as imipramine, have demonstrated that this desensitization of β-receptors occurs more rapidly with the combination than with either agent alone (18). This finding has spurred medicinal chemists to attempt to incorporate both properties into a single molecule, but in practice this has been a difficult task. Most drugs have more than a single component to their pharmacology, but this has rarely been by design. We do not know the reasoning that led to the synthesis of FCE-20124 (Structure 26), but as drawn it has a striking structural resemblance to viloxazine, nisoxetine, and fluoxetine. FCE-20124 is a potential antidepressant currently in clinical trials, and has this particular combination of properties (13). As such it should provide a test of this mechanistic hypothesis.

THE SYSTEMS APPROACH

In the mechanism-based approach, a specific disease target has already been chosen, and the initial challenge for the researcher is to select an appropriate mechanism as a template for drug design. The systems approach goes one step further, in that an enzyme or receptor system may be chosen as a target for drug intervention, even in the absence of a clear link between the system and any known disease state. To be sure, there will always be conjecture about possible therapeutic applications for any drug derived from this systems approach, and pragmatists will pressure the researcher to justify his work in terms of postulated mechanisms for specific disorders. In the end, however, only clinical evaluation can determine which, if any, disease state will respond to such treatment. Here the aim of preclinical pharmacology will be to demonstrate that the selected neurotransmitter system has been manipulated in the desired manner *in vivo*. Following the necessary assurances from animal toxicology, the drug can be screened in the clinic to assess its actual value in the treatment of diseased patients. Such clinical screening will be broadly based, and of course expensive, but it offers the researcher the opportunity of finding the rare breakthrough in CNS drug therapy.

Historically speaking, prevailing attitudes about CNS drug research have been too conservative to permit a widespread application of the systems approach. Today there is a growing belief among medicinal chemists, pharmacologists, and clinicians alike that at least some speculative programs must be implemented in order to provide truly novel drugs in the future. Perhaps the best candidates for a systems approach to CNS drug design are to be found in the plethora of neuropeptides that have been discovered in the last decade. Their number is continually increasing, far in advance of any useful information on their function in CNS disorders. The first challenge, and perhaps the greatest gamble, lies in knowing which of these to choose as the basis for such a program.

One neuropeptide that warrants consideration is neurotensin (Structure 27), which will serve to illustrate many of the challenges posed by such peptides. The role of neurotensin in the mammalian CNS is poorly understood, but it is known to be concentrated in areas of the brain thought to be involved in behavioral homeostasis, including the nucleus accumbens and the locus ceruleus. Central administration of neurotensin in rats produces a significant hypothermia and prolongs the sedation induced by phenobarbital. It is also a potent antinociceptive agent. As such the neurotensin system promises to exert profound effects in the mammalian CNS (15), and based on available evidence it appears a likely candidate for the systems approach.

pyro Glu – Leu – Tyr – Glu – Asn – Lys – Pro – Arg – Arg – Pro – Tyr – Ile – Leu – OH

<u>27</u>

In formulating a drug-hunting strategy for the neurotensin system, the first step is to decide whether to potentiate the effects of this peptide in the CNS or to antagonize its actions. Ideally, we would wish to investigate the therapeutic potential of both agonists and antagonists, but for the sake of argument we will limit discussion to the former. One approach could be to administer neurotensin itself, but like most similarly sized peptides, it is not expected to be absorbed into the bloodstream following oral dosing, owing to rapid degradation in the digestive tract. Once in circulation, such a peptide would be vulnerable to protease attack, and probably would not cross the blood-brain barrier. Alternatively, we could attempt to increase the brain's own native supply of this peptide, perhaps by stimulating production of those enzymes involved in its synthesis, or by inhibiting those which degrade it. Unfortunately, the former is not currently feasible, whereas the latter depends on a more extensive knowledge of neurotensin-specific peptidases than is now available. One strategy would be to design an agonist of neurotensin that overcomes the natural peptide's pharmacokinetic liabilities. Since the receptor for neurotensin has not been characterized, the medicinal chemist's sole lead is the structure of neurotensin itself.

By conventional standards, the size and complexity of neurotensin are intimidating. Mere combinatorial arguments can be staggering; there are 20^{13} possible tridecapeptide analogs that could be synthesized, limiting ourselves only to the 20 naturally occurring amino acids. This is of course no place to start. Our first attempt would be to simplify the target; perhaps smaller fragments of the neurotensin structure will retain the parent molecule's activity. Barring this happy circumstance, we must attempt to visualize neurotensin in a way that mimics the receptor itself. What is the most likely shape of this very large and conformationally flexible molecule? At which points on this three-dimensional surface are there concentrations of charge suitable for ionic or hydrogen-bonding interactions? What is the placement of hydrophobic sidechains that could

indicate complementary binding regions at the receptor? Established techniques such as nuclear magnetic resonance (NMR) spectroscopy and X-ray crystallography may provide some insight into the solution and solid state conformations of the peptide.

In future drug-hunting programs, molecular modeling programs that feature high-speed computational techniques will become increasingly important as medicinal chemists target molecules as complex as neurotensin. Using such packages, the medicinal chemist will be able to generate a set of minimum energy conformations for neurotensin, and then calculate any of various types of electronic surfaces for the molecule. Graphics terminals that provide an illusion of three-dimensionality will allow visualization of the results of these calculations, giving a glimpse of the molecule that mimics the perspective of the receptor itself. Even in the absence of information about the structure of the neurotensin receptor, an imaginative chemist could construct a reasonable model complementary to the neuropeptide's structure. Ideally, he would make use of molecular modeling as an initial "screen" before committing himself to the perhaps lengthy synthesis of a proposed drug candidate.

Having obtained all this valuable information, where is the chemist likely to begin a synthetic program? At first, he would probably prepare peptides that bear considerable analogy to neurotensin. The first encouraging finding might well be activity in an appropriate *in vitro* test, such as a receptor binding assay. This would permit him to test and modify his original hypotheses. Rapid increases in potency and selectivity may develop in response to repeated iterations of synthesis and *in vitro* testing. All of this improvement, however, might well come at the expense of unexplored pharmacokinetic parameters. Thus it is unlikely that any of the "optimized" structures will possess the structural characteristics necessary for oral absorption, adequate half-life in circulation, or ability to penetrate the blood-brain barrier.

The incorporation of these properties into peptides and peptide analogs, once thought a nearly impossible task, has become an active area of research in medicinal chemistry (19). Much excitement has been generated by the discovery of isosteric replacements for the amide bond that links amino acid residues within a peptide. Thus it has become possible in many instances to preserve the desired activity while conferring resistance to metabolic attack. For instance, ketomethylene, alkylidene, retro-, and N-methyl amide linkages are all reasonable substitutes for the peptide bond, and are all poor substrates for most proteases. Additional metabolic stability may be achieved by substituting unnatural D-amino acids where sterically permissible. Workers at Sandoz (17) in search of a synthetic enkephalin agonist have produced a pentapeptide, FK 33-824 (Structure 28), in which three of the five amino acid residues have been modified to limit metabolic attack. The resulting peptide produced analgesic activity even after oral administration, and was 30,000 times more potent than natural Met-enkephalin (Structure 29) when given intracerebroventricularly.

By no means does the list of possible structural modifications end here. The incorporation of bridges between proximal residues in a large three-dimensional structure will lend metabolic stability by increasing conformational

Tyr – D – Ala – Gly – (N – Me)Phe – Met – (S →O) – ol   Tyr – Gly – Gly – Phe – Met – OH

28   **29**

Ala – Gly – Cys – Lys – Asn – Phe – Phe – Trp   (N – Me)Ala – Thr – D – Trp
| | | |
Cys – Ser – Thr – Phe – Thr – Lys   Phe – Val – Lys

30   **31**

rigidity, and may increase affinity for the target receptor in the bargain. In what may be the most elegant example of neuropeptide conformational analysis to date, Veber and his co-workers at Merck (27) have deduced the bioactive conformation of the hormone somatostatin (Structure 30) from its NMR properties and those of synthetic analogs. This information, coupled with molecular modeling, has led to synthesis of the cyclic hexapeptide L-363,586 (Structure 31), which is 50 to 100 times more potent than the endogenous substance in some assays, and is far more stable to metabolic cleavage.

Over time, the medicinal chemist may attempt to replace the entire peptidic backbone with an alternative molecular scaffolding that presents the peripheral functional groups to the receptor in an appropriate three-dimensional array (5). Although we know of no examples where this has yet been accomplished, the task is by no means hopeless. The chemist in search of inspiration needs only consider the opiate alkaloids as a naturally occurring example of stable, orally active, nonpeptidic structures that efficiently enter the brain and compete for neuropeptide binding sites.

Once the preclinical goal of a systems approach has been met, in the present example by an orally active agonist of neurotensin, clinical testing will determine the fate of the program. Failure to indicate therapeutic potential in humans for such an agent would of course put an end to the speculation on which this systems approach was based. On the other hand, clinical success would indicate a new mechanism of treatment for some CNS disorder and in so doing would likely spawn numerous mechanism-based approaches to its therapy. There is an immense scientific and commercial advantage awaiting the adventurous industrial researcher who undertakes the systems approach and in so doing discovers a novel CNS agent. This is perhaps an appropriate reward given the risks inherent in the systems approach; in it one can be confident of the mechanistic novelty of a new drug without having any assurance whatsoever of its utility in humans.

THE UNIFIED APPROACH

We have seen that the decisions reached by a medicinal chemist in planning new chemical series depend critically on the broader drug-hunting environment in which he is placed. Varying degrees of dependency on *in vitro* as opposed to *in vivo* screens will alter dramatically his choice of tools in optimizing activity. Ideally, he would prefer to

work in an environment that combines aspects of all three previously described approaches. In such a unified approach, he would expect to encounter *in vivo* behavioral screens with a clear logical connection to the target disease. This would be complemented by neurochemical screens that would confirm the desired mechanism of action for his drug candidate, guard against false positives in the behavioral paradigms, and identify the occasional serendipitous new lead. Ideally, the targeted profile and mechanism of action would be sufficiently different from established therapies that the novelty of the chemist's efforts would be guaranteed. It is into these unified approaches that drug-hunting programs logically develop as they mature and confidence is gained in the basic understanding of the targeted disorder.

Soon after the introduction of the first benzodiazepines for anxiety in the early 1960s, effective animal models became available to help the researcher identify novel anxiolytic structures. Under this disease-model approach, it obviously made a great deal of sense for the chemist to begin with the active benzodiazepine structure, and untold thousands of benzodiazepine analogs were prepared for screening. Although an assortment of new anxiolytics was added to the marketplace, the basic benzodiazepine structure (and the underlying animal pharmacology) remained essentially unchanged.

The mechanism of action of these drugs remained a mystery until 1977, when Squires and Braestrup (20) announced the discovery of high-affinity binding sites for benzodiazepines in brain tissue. The discovery of this new receptor spurred the search for endogenous ligands, leading to the isolation from urine of a potent displacer of radio-labeled benzodiazepines, ethyl β-carboline 3-carboxylate (β-CCE) (Structure 32) in 1980. Although the formation of β-CCE was later dismissed as an artifact of the isolation procedure, its discovery provided medicinal chemists with a new, nonbenzodiazepine structural lead. By this time it had become obvious to medicinal chemists worldwide that such receptor binding studies could be a powerful tool for identifying structurally diverse anxiolytics. There followed the discovery of such compounds as zopiclone (Structure 33), CGS 9896 (Structure 34), PK 8165 (Structure 35), and a multitude of β-carbolines related to β-CCE, none of which bears any obvious relationship to the benzodiazepine structure (28).

32   **33**

34   **35**

Many of these newer compounds were remarkably active not only in benzodiazepine receptor binding assays but also in the classical behavioral screens for anxiolytics, and as such could have been discovered a decade earlier under the simple disease-model approach. There are undoubtedly several reasons for this embarrassing delay. The phenomenal success of chlordiazepoxide and diazepam pressured companies to enter the anxiolytic market as rapidly as possible during the 1960s and 1970s, and relatively minor variations on the benzodiazepine structure sufficed to meet the demands of chemical novelty in patent law. However, with the proliferation of new patent claims, it became increasingly difficult to find latitude for continued work on the benzodiazepine nucleus. Moreover, clinical feedback indicated that, despite minor differences, all of the benzodiazepine anxiolytics suffered to some extent from undesirable side effects, namely sedation, propensity to potentiate the CNS depressant effects of alcohol, and liability for dependence.

It was into this climate that benzodiazepine receptor binding assays were introduced. Medicinal chemists, now more keenly interested in nonbenzodiazepine structures, could interpret flickers of activity in behavioral models in conjunction with receptor affinity studies. Weakly active compounds once lightly dismissed as "false positives" became interesting leads whenever good *in vitro* activity was discovered. As such they could be further modified and improved in cycles of synthesis and testing. An example from our own laboratories shows that even in the absence of *in vivo* activity, weak *in vitro* activity can initiate work on a successful chemical series. Accelerated decomposition studies on the nonbenzodiazepine anxiolytic tracazolate (Structure 36) generated traces of desbutyltracazolate (Structure 37). Unlike tracazolate, desbutyltracazolate was found to displace radiolabeled benzodiazepines, albeit very weakly. No behavioral activity could be demonstrated for desbutyltracazolate following oral administration. However, chemical modification of this lead produced the orally active pyrazolopyridine ICI 174,329 (Structure 38), which was two orders of magnitude more potent than desbutyltracazolate *in vitro,* and equipotent with diazepam in several animal models of anxiety.

cases, receptor binding assays may fail to discriminate between molecules with agonist and antagonist properties. One relatively new approach the medicinal chemist can explore in such circumstances is Quantitative Structure-Activity Relationship (QSAR) analysis. This technique seeks to express mathematically the observed biological activity as a function of free energy terms contributed by the drug's substituents. Although most published QSAR studies have been retrospective in nature, an immense potential exists for predictive value when QSAR is employed during the development of a new chemical series.

So it was that the development of receptor binding assays transformed the disease-model-based search for anxiolytics into a more unified approach. The chemists' efforts soon rendered the situation more complex, as subtypes of the benzodiazepine receptor, and ligands selective for them, were reported (10) beginning in 1979. Studies with one ligand selective for the type I receptor subtype, CL 218,872 (Structure 39), suggested that the adverse sedative and muscle relaxant components of the benzodiazepines' pharmacological profile might be attributable to the latter's indiscriminate affinity for type II binding sites. As such it was widely held that type-I-selective agents would deliver the desired "anxioselective" profile in humans.

This receptor selectivity theory was not without its detractors. Shortly thereafter there arose an alternative hypothesis that held that the anxiolytic/anticonvulsant/sedative profile common to most benzodiazepines could be traced to their full agonist activity at the receptor. It was argued that partial agonists might retain anxiolytic activity but lack the sedative effects of full agonists. At least two chemical series have emerged that demonstrate that very small structural changes can alter the agonist character of the molecule. Workers at Ciba-Geigy (30) have shown that CGS 9896 (Structure 34) shares some, but not all properties of benzodiazepine full agonists, whereas CGS 8216 (Structure 40) behaves as nearly a pure antagonist and CGS 9895 (Structure 41) appears intermediate in profile. In a series of β-carbolines related to β-CCE, Schering AG (21) have produced a spectrum of profiles including full agonists such as ZK 93423 (Structure 42), partial agonists typified by ZK 91296 (Structure 43), and antagonists represented by ZK 93426 (Structure 44). Inverse agonists have also been prepared; these induce anxiety, increase muscle tone, and are proconvulsant. Although inverse agonists are not likely to become useful in therapy, there exists the possibility that partial inverse agonists would act as CNS stimulants, enhancing vigilance and cognition processes; FG 7142 (Structure 45) appears to belong in this interesting category (21).

Within any unified approach, inconsistencies can arise whenever good *in vitro* activity does not translate into *in vivo* potency. This may be due to variations in pharmacokinetic parameters that depend on such physical properties of the drug molecule as lipophilicity and solubility. In other

42   43   44   45

48

It is apparent that a unified approach to anxiolytic drug discovery has given the medicinal chemist the most information, and with it, the greatest freedom to design and test novel drug structures. From this unified approach have arisen a number of challenging (and conflicting) hypotheses regarding anxiolytic drug action that could never have been suggested within the confines of earlier approaches. We must await the imminent clinical evaluation of a whole generation of promising new anxiolytics before passing judgment on the validity of these proposals.

THE CLINICAL DIMENSION

In contrast to several other therapeutic areas, for example, hypertension, the CNS chemist must admit that there have been relatively few breakthroughs following the introduction of the first antidepressants, neuroleptics, and anxiolytics a quarter of a century ago. It is perhaps ironic that at the very time when preclinical research on benzodiazepine-like agents holds such promise for new anxioselective drugs, the wheel has turned full circle and an unexpected advance has come, once again, from the clinic.

Buspirone (Structure 46) is a novel anxiolytic agent (24) introduced recently in Europe and whose approval in the United States appears imminent. Preclinically this compound, which originated in a classical disease-model approach to neuroleptic drugs, profiled as a dopamine antagonist, and as such was selected for clinical trial in schizophrenia. The results in schizophrenia were disappointing, but subsequent clinical research suggested that buspirone was effective in anxiety neurosis and this finding was confirmed in several controlled studies. In practice buspirone and diazepam are equally efficacious in anxiety, but the former is anxioselective. These clinical findings were clearly a breakthrough and offered great potential for the medicinal chemist, though it was far from obvious how to proceed.

46   R^1,R^2 = (CH$_2$)$_4$
47   R^1 = R^2 = Me

Buspirone was soon found to be an ineffective ligand for the benzodiazepine binding site and hence differed from diazepam mechanistically. There followed a flurry of activity aimed at further characterizing buspirone in the laboratory. Activity in several behavioral models of anxiety eventually resulted but the underlying mechanism remained to be clarified. The medicinal chemist can work with a disease model if that is all that is available, but as we have seen in earlier sections, he prefers a mechanism-based, or ideally, a unified approach. It was particularly important to determine whether the anxiolytic properties were independent of dopaminergic mechanisms since, at least theoretically, dopaminergic mechanisms offer the potential for undesirable side effects.

A tentative answer to this question has emerged very recently with the finding that two close structural analogs, gepirone (Structure 47) (4) and TVX Q 7821 (Structure 48) (26), are equieffective with buspirone in certain laboratory models of anxiety but are essentially inactive as dopamine antagonists. The value of a battery of receptor binding assays in profiling drugs within a single therapeutic class was highlighted in The Mechanism-Based Approach and in the present context is clearly evident from Table 1. Both buspirone and TVX Q 7821 are highly effective ligands for the 5-HT$_{1A}$ subtype of serotonin receptor labeled by tritiated 2-dipropylamino-8-hydroxytetralin (DPAT). Though not examined in this particular study, gepirone is also selective for the 5-HT$_{1A}$ receptor (29). The complete story has not yet unfolded and awaits clinical experience with these drugs, but the evidence implicates an involvement of 5-HT$_{1A}$ neuronal systems in buspirone's mechanism of action.

In the space of just a few years, laboratory research with buspirone and analogs has moved through several distinct phases, from a disease model for neuroleptics, through a disease model for anxiolytics, to a mechanism-based, and even a unified approach. The key point is that all the preclinical precedents directed buspirone toward clinical evaluation in schizophrenia. Shrewd clinical investigation uncovered buspirone's anxiolytic profile and paved the way for a new class of anxioselective drugs that promises to be a significant therapeutic advance over the benzodiazepines.

In comparison with the present, it was easier to progress a speculative compound to the clinic twenty-five or so years ago, and certainly very much less expensive and on a much shorter timescale. The value of the clinic as an extension of the laboratory, with timely feedback to the chemist, cannot be overemphasized. In the most difficult areas, such as depression, the clinician's finding may well be the key stimulus for the chemist in the search for truly novel therapies. Seemingly, there is an endless stream of potential antidepressants headed for the clinic and it will be the clinician who provides the data to single out the breakthrough from the majority that are typically reported as "about as efficacious as imipramine."

TABLE 1. *Interaction of buspirone and TVX Q 7821 with neuronal membrane binding sites[a]*

Radioligand	Receptor	IC$_{50}$ (nM)	
		Buspirone	TXV Q 7821
[³H]DPAT	5-HT$_{1A}$	24 ± 4	9.5 ± 2
[³H]Spiperone	Dopamine (D$_2$)	380 ± 70	3,000 ± 300
[³H]WB 4101	α$_1$-Adrenergic	1,400 ± 500	58 ± 10
[³H]Spiperone	5-HT$_2$	2,100 ± 600	10,000 ± 7,000
[³H]Pyrilamine	Histamine (H$_1$)	4,700 ± 1,000	4,700 ± 600
[³H]Yohimbine	α$_2$-Adrenergic	7,100 ± 8,000	2,200 ± 200
[³H]5-HT	5-HT$_{1B}$	26,000 ± 7,000	26,000 ± 7,000
[³H]Nitrendipine	Calcium channel	65,000 ± 3,000	100,000
[³H]QNB	Muscarinic cholinergic	76,000 ± 10,000	97,000 ± 10,000
[³H]Flunitrazepam	Benzodiazepine	>100,000	>100,000

[a] Adapted from ref. 16.

CHOOSING AN APPROACH TO A NEW TARGET

In previous sections we have discussed historical, current, and possible new approaches to CNS disorders for which there are already well-tried and useful drugs. Perhaps the greatest challenge for the chemist is to be assigned to a target disease area for which there are either no useful drugs or, at best, only drugs steeped in controversy. How does he proceed in such circumstances?

Millions of dollars are currently being spent annually in the pharmaceuticals industry in the search for drugs to treat senile dementia, and Alzheimer's disease in particular. The diagnosis of Alzheimer's disease has reached almost epidemic proportions with the increase in the population aged 65 and over, and it is the fourth leading cause of death in the United States. Up to 10% of the population over 65 years old suffers from Alzheimer's disease, and this proportion rises to 20% or more beyond age 80. Considering that the population in the United States over 85 is expected to more than double to 5.1 million by the end of the century, the statistics speak for themselves.

Once again there are large cultural and territorial differences in attitudes toward treatments for cognitive disorders, including Alzheimer's disease. In the United States the prevailing opinion is that there are no useful drugs for cognitive disorders, though one drug combination, the ergoloid mesylates (Hydergine, Structure 49) has been approved for dementia. Elsewhere, particularly on the European mainland and in Japan, Hydergine, and to a lesser extent piracetam (Structure 50) are widely used. To put this in perspective, world sales of Hydergine are not far behind diazepam, though it is difficult to estimate the extent to which Hydergine is used for cognitive disorders since prescription data show broad usage, with both general ischemic cerebrovascular disease and essential benign hypertension as the main diagnoses.

Piracetam (Structure 50) is the first member of the nootropic class of drugs. The term nootropic was coined in Europe to indicate drugs, acting at the level of the cerebral cortex, that improve integrative brain mechanisms associated with mental performance (6). Briefly, piracetam

was first prepared as an analog of γ-aminobutyric acid (GABA) in a mechanism-based approach to novel hypnotic drugs. In practice it was neither a GABAergic agent, nor a hypnotic, but ultimately it was shown to improve overall mental efficiency in humans, particularly in the learning situation. Subsequently several animal models of learning situations were developed in which piracetam's learning-enhancement properties were clearly evident. Such "disease models" have been the basis for the development of several more potent analogs including pramiracetam (Structure 51) and aniracetam (Structure 52).

Clearly, the chemist could find many additional active analogs of the "racetams" and one would expect a steady progression of structural changes leading ultimately to new compounds structurally distinct from the early members of the series. For the chemist Hydergine is an enigma. As a mixture of complex structures, with a diversity of neurochemical properties, it is extremely difficult to select a structural feature to elaborate. However, to return to the central theme for this section, there remains little, if any, convincing evidence that Hydergine or the nootropics are of value in treating Alzheimer's disease, and if this is the exclusive target then the chemist had best look elsewhere for a lead.

There are several candidates for a mechanism-based approach. The brains of Alzheimer patients consistently show degeneration of cholinergic neurons, especially in the nucleus basalis of Meynert. Marker enzymes of cholinergic activity, such as choline acetyltransferase and acetyl cholinesterase, are also below the level observed in the appropriate controls. There is an obvious analogy with the dopaminergic deficit in Parkinson's disease. Several animal models have been developed in which learning deficits are induced by lesions in the cholinergic system, for example by the neurotoxin AF64A (8), which is structurally similar to choline. A variety of cholinergic agents, such as the cholinesterase inhibitor physostigmine (Structure 53) and the muscarinic agonist bethanechol (Structure 54), are effective in several animal models in which the cholinergic system has been compromised, and even in behavioral models that are less clearly dependent on a cholinergic deficit.

There have been many clinical trials in which attempts have been made to potentiate central cholinergic neurotransmission by a variety of methods, including the above, but despite flickers of activity the trials have been uniformly disappointing, certainly in comparison with the L-dopa analogy in Parkinsonism. Nevertheless, we believe there remains scope for further work in this area. A postsynaptic muscarinic agonist, selective for the CNS, and therefore free from unpleasant and potentially dangerous peripheral side effects, would appear to be the best candidate for a definitive test of the cholinergic hypothesis. (Agents acting presynaptically might be severely limited if there has been substantial degeneration of cholinergic neurons.) The requirement for selectivity for the CNS almost certainly requires a "prodrug" approach in which the active entity is delivered to the brain packaged as an inert substance which is subsequently metabolized *in situ* to the active species. This is a demanding requirement, but there is precedent in a method developed recently by Bodor (1), which is exemplified here for dopamine but is likely to be of general applicability. In Bodor's method dopamine is first protected as the dipivalyl ester, then "packaged" as an amide (Structure 55) of a dihydropyridine that readily penetrates the brain. Once inside the brain, the dihydropyridine is oxidized to the quaternary derivative (Structure 56), which is unable to cross the blood-brain barrier in the reverse direction and slowly releases the dopamine component through hydrolytic cleavage.

The progressive loss of cholinergic neurons is but one of several deficits in Alzheimer's disease. Recently it has been suggested (14) that the destruction of somatostatin-containing neurons may be of critical importance in the etiology of the disease, in which case somatostatin replacement therapy, for example with a somatostatin agonist, would be a logical approach. The challenge posed to the chemist by neuropeptides has been discussed in detail in The Systems Approach, and reference was made to the potent somatostatin agonist L-363,586 (Structure 31). An early report (2) of a trial with this compound in Alzheimer patients is not encouraging, but there is much scope for further work, particularly with delivery to the CNS in mind.

Several pituitary peptides, and fragments or analogs thereof, are active in learning paradigms in animals. Again, the clinical results are disappointing with all compounds of this type tested to date in Alzheimer's disease. Since deficits in pituitary peptides are not considered to be primary markers for Alzheimer's disease, chemistry based on such systems is intrinsically risky.

There is no shortage of yet more speculative mechanism-based approaches to the target. To give just one final example: Very recent studies have shown significant decreases in RNA and protein synthesis in the brains of Alzheimer patients, giving rise to speculation that a decrease in protein synthesis may underlie the progressive loss of neurons typically found in the disease. The deficit in brain RNA is, in turn, subserved by a deficit in an endogenous inhibitor of alkaline ribonuclease. It is argued that this process could be prevented or reversed by administration of an exogenous inhibitor of alkaline ribonuclease.

In summary, the task of finding useful therapies in a new disease area such as Alzheimer's disease is one of the toughest challenges facing the medicinal chemist. Although there exist several animal models based on learning and memory deficits, none of the compounds active in these screens is convincingly active in Alzheimer's disease in humans. There is considerable risk in basing a drug-hunting program on disease models that have not been validated with a clinically effective drug. There is no lack of biochemical speculation on the etiology of the disease, including the well-known cholinergic deficit hypothesis. More recently there has been an increased awareness of the possible involvement of somatostatin. Though results from the clinic have been far from encouraging, there remains considerable scope for further chemistry with both cholinergic and somatostatin agonists, particularly with targeted delivery to the CNS in mind. From our standpoint the several other mechanism-based approaches are too speculative for the chemist to take seriously unless he is tempted by extremely long odds.

PERSPECTIVE

With the benefit of hindsight, some would suggest that the major CNS drug classes were discovered through a combination of opportunity and good fortune. Such a view would belittle the efforts of the chemists who produced today's invaluable drugs given the knowledge base of their time. Following their lead, today's medicinal chemists have become adept at modifying and optimizing activity through application of the disease-model approach. Although the probability of clinical success with such an approach is reasonably high, true advances in therapy have emerged only rarely, and then almost always by accident. The mechanism-based approach, which has been greatly facilitated by the explosive growth of neurochemistry in the past decade, provides the chemist with an opportunity to develop structurally diverse drug molecules that may offer an advantage over existing therapies. This approach, in turn, is limited by preexisting concepts of the disease mechanism. In the majority of cases, our understanding of CNS disorders lags far behind the basic neuroscience, and here the systems approach may provide the most effective route to truly novel therapeutic agents. Within any strategy, the more informed the medicinal chemist can become about the target disorder, the more likely he is to succeed in developing a useful drug. As such, he is most comfortable with established animal models of the disease that can be correlated with neurochemical tests for mechanistic validity. Such unified approaches are now becoming possible in many areas of CNS research, and are expected to offer key improvements in drug therapy for the major affective disorders.

Clinical trials provide the ultimate test of the medicinal chemist's ideas, and seminal contributions from the clinician can still provide the chemist with the lead he needs to begin work on tomorrow's drugs. It is most distressing to the medicinal chemist that today's economic and regulatory pressures have made it more difficult to justify evaluation of a new compound in humans and have extended the timescale for feedback of clinical information.

The immense social and commercial urgency associated with a CNS disorder such as Alzheimer's disease presents special difficulties for the preclinical researcher. In the absence of an established etiology or therapy for a disease state, the medicinal chemist finds himself at the mercy of conflicting biological hypotheses and with no good structural leads. Under such circumstances, medicinal chemists and pharmacologists together must judge which of these approaches is most likely to succeed. If the chemists' initial efforts do not provide useful therapies for such diseases, it is anticipated that they will at least provide further mechanistic insight into the disease process.

REFERENCES

1. Bodor, N., and Brewster, M. E. (1983): *Pharmacol. Ther.,* 19:337–386.
2. Cutler, N. R., Haxby, J. V., Narang, P. K., May, C., Burg, C., and Reines, S. A. (1985): *N. Engl. J. Med.,* 312:725.
3. Doxey, J. C., Roach, A. G., and Smith, C. F. C. (1983): *Br. J. Pharmacol.,* 78:489–505.
4. Eison, M. S., Yevich, J. P., and Farney, R. F. (1985): *Drugs Fut.,* 10:456–457.
5. Farmer, P. S. (1980): In: *Drug Design, Vol. 10,* edited by E. J. Ariëns, pp. 119–143. Academic Press, New York.
6. Giurgea, C. E. (1982): *Drug Dev. Res.,* 2:441–446.
7. Gould, R. J., Murphy, K. M. M., Reynolds, I. J., and Snyder, S. H. (1983): *Proc. Natl. Acad. Sci. USA,* 80:5122–5125.
8. Hanin, I., DeGroat, W. C., Mantione, C. R., Coyle, J. T., and Fisher, A. (1983): In: *Conference on Biological Aspects of Alzheimer's Disease,* edited by R. Katzman, p. 243. Cold Spring Harbor Laboratory, Cold Spring Harbor, NY.
9. Hester, J. B., Rudzik, A. D., and VonVoigtlander, P. F. (1980): *J. Med. Chem.,* 23:392–402.
10. Hirsch, J. D., Garrett, K. M., and Beer, B. (1985): *Pharmacol. Biochem. Behav.,* 23:681–685.
11. Huff, J. R., Anderson, P. S., Baldwin, J. J., Clineschmidt, B. V., Guare, J. P., Lotti, V. J., Pettibone, D. J., Randall, W. C., and Vacca, J. P. (1985): *Pharmacologist,* 27:153.
12. Humber, L. G., Philipp, A. H., Bruderlein, F. T., Götz, M., and Voith, K. (1979): In: *Computer-Assisted Drug Design,* edited by E. C. Olson and R. E. Christoffersen, pp. 227–241. American Chemical Society, Washington, DC.
13. Melloni, P., Carniel, G., Torre, A. D., Lazzari, E., Bonsignori, A., Ricciardi, S., and Rossi, A. C. (1982): *Abstracts North Am. Med. Chem. Symp.,* Toronto (20–24 June), abstr. 45.
14. Morrison, J. H., Rogers, J., Scherr, S., Benoit, R., and Bloom, F. E. (1985): *Nature,* 314:90–92.
15. Nemeroff, C. B. (1980): *Biol. Psychiatry,* 15:283–302.
16. Peroutka, S. J. (1985): *Biol. Psychiatry,* 20:971–979.
17. Roemer, D., Buescher, H. H., Hill, R. C., Pless, J., Bauer, W., Cardinaux, F., Closse, A., Hauser, D., and Huguenin, R. (1977): *Nature,* 268:547–549.
18. Scott, J. A., and Crews, F. T. (1983): *J. Pharmacol. Exp. Ther.,* 224:640–646.
19. Spatola, A. F. (1983): In: *Chemistry and Biochemistry of Amino Acids, Peptides, and Proteins,* edited by B. Weinstein, pp. 267–357. Marcel Dekker, New York.
20. Squires, R. F., and Braestrup, C. (1977): *Nature,* 266:732–734.
21. Stephens, D. N., Kehr, W., Schneider, H. H., and Schmiechen, R. (1984): *Neurosci. Lett.,* 47:333–338.
22. Stockmeier, C. A., Martino, A. M., and Kellar, K. J. (1985): *Science,* 230:323–325.
23. Stoof, J. C., and Kebabian, J. W. (1984): *Life Sci.,* 35:2281–2296.
24. Taylor, D. P., Eison, M. S., Riblet, L. A., and VanderMaelen, C. P. (1985): *Pharmacol. Biochem. Behav.,* 23:687–694.
25. Thornber, C. W. (1979): *Chem. Soc. Rev.,* 8:563–580.
26. Traber, J., Davies, M. A., Dompert, W. U., Glaser, T., Schuurman, T., and Seidel, P.-R. (1984): *Brain Res. Bull.,* 12:741–744.
27. Veber, D. F., Saperstein, R., Nutt, R. F., Freidinger, R. M., Brady, S. F., Curley, P., Perlow, D. S., Paleveda, W. J., Colton, C. D., Zacchei, A. G., Tocco, D. J., Hoff, D. R., Vandlen, R. L., Gerich, J. E., Hall, L., Mandarino, L., Cordes, E. H., Anderson, P. S., and Hirschmann, R. (1984): *Life Sci.,* 34:1371–1378.
28. Williams, M. (1983): *J. Med. Chem.,* 26:619–628.
29. Yocca, F. D., and Maayani, S. (1985), *Pharmacologist,* 27:195.
30. Yokoyama, N., Ritter, B., and Neubert, A. D. (1982): *J. Med. Chem.,* 25:337–339.

Psychopharmacology:
The Third Generation of Progress,
edited by Herbert Y. Meltzer.
Raven Press, New York © 1987.

CHAPTER **178**

Contributions of Industrial Research to Basic Neuropsychopharmacology: Preclinical Screening and Discovery

Albert Weissman and B. Kenneth Koe

We take our world of receptors, enzymes, neurotransmitters, and selective neurophysiological pathways so much for granted that we sometimes forget that modern psychopharmacology began as a series of clinical accidents superimposed on mostly folkloric medicines. The discovery histories of three early epochal drugs, chlorpromazine, iproniazid, and imipramine, need no recounting. But few of us consider the extent to which agents that came subsequently, that constitute our therapies and scientific tools, that shaped the development of our field, and that derive almost exclusively from industrial research, also evolved unpredictably. Molecular pursuits in neuropsychopharmacology, as described in most preclinical sections of these volumes, have analyzed or exploited discoveries frequently made serendipitously with whole animal and inductive methods now often ignored or taken for granted. This is often the relationship between invention and science.

SOURCES OF NEW DRUG DISCOVERY

The impact made by drugs discovered or promulgated outside the industry must be acknowledged. Dopa therapy of Parkinson's disease and lithium therapy for mania, as two examples, each impacting on laboratory research, owe debts to individuals outside the drug industry, although industrial developmental roles have not been trivial. The dopa example constitutes an excellent example of rational drug discovery. Following studies showing Parkinson's disease to be a "striatal dopamine deficiency syndrome" (31), the logical step of administering dopa (subsequently levodopa) to replenish dopamine was rewarded with success (11). Lithium therapy, on the other hand, originated from the fortuitous observation that lithium carbonate, administered to animals to improve the solubility of urates, produced lethargy (8,66).

Such instances notwithstanding, most modern drug therapies and tools derive directly not from unaffiliated individuals, not from foundations, not from academe, not from public institutions, but rather from private pharmaceutical industry research. The contribution to basic neurobiology deriving from industry is too easily overlooked in favor of the therapeutic and economic fallout of drug discoveries. It is ironic to hear companies depicted as feeding on basic discoveries made in academic and institutional laboratories. In the neurosciences, at least, the converse is more truthful: Neuropsychopharmacology in its most basic sense has been built almost entirely on the study of drugs discovered in industrial laboratories and that serve as independent experimental variables.

DRUGS AS TOOLS

The most important contribution of industry-discovered drugs is more subtle than their therapeutic utility and economic impact, or than their use in the countless experiments whose results in sum constitute modern neuropsychopharmacology. Centrally acting drugs and their actions cement chemical, psychological, biological, and clinical disciplines in such a way as to establish a molecular basis for behavior and psychiatric illness. The evident nature of this truth provides the impetus for societal support for our efforts, and has swept away many vestiges of mentalism that would otherwise have continued into the last decades of this millennium.

Less globally, industry-discovered drug tools have penetrated into every crevice of neurobiology. The explosive development of the field of neurotransmitter receptors and binding sites well illustrates the impact of industry-discovered drugs on basic neuroscience. This line of research may be said to have begun in the early 1960s, when discoveries were made pertaining to neuronal membrane pumps for norepinephrine (2,34). Requisite drug tools for such studies were available in the form of tricyclic antidepressants, following on the accident of imipramine's clinical discovery. Analogous studies were conducted on uptake systems for dopamine, using benztropine (12,30), and on uptake systems for serotonin, using tricyclic antidepressants (37,68) or chlorpheniramine (51), which eventually evolved into the serotonin uptake blocking drug, zimelidine.

For the moment, let us sketch the relevance of these reuptake explorations to subsequent developments in the field of depression. One avenue of research yielded drugs incorporating tailored uptake blocking properties, such as nomifensine (dopamine and norepinephrine), clovoxamine (norepinephrine and serotonin), and zimelidine, fluoxetine, and sertraline (serotonin). Following the widespread introduction of membrane receptor binding methodology, another avenue led to the characterization of drug binding sites in brain membranes and platelets. Continuing efforts were made to identify binding sites for [^{3}H]imipramine (14), which could serve as biochemical markers of depression, illustrating the use of drug tools in nosology. Studies of uptake blocking drugs enabled conjectures that binding of [^{3}H]imipramine (45,46), [^{3}H]desipramine (61), and [^{3}H]cocaine, [^{3}H]mazindol, or [^{3}H]nomifensine (65) may label sites associated with transport of serotonin, norepinephrine, and dopamine, respectively. New mechanisms of depression were advanced based, for instance, on [^{3}H]imipramine binding studies, i.e., that repeated administration of imipramine down-regulates a binding site for an endogenous imipramine-like ligand, causing enhanced reuptake of serotonin. The decreased serotonergic activity disinhibits noradrenergic neurons, yielding antidepressant activity (3). That enhanced noradrenergic activity might be induced by repeated administration of serotonin uptake blockers, was concluded from a different viewpoint (43). A laboratory correlate of delayed antidepressant drug onset is the finding that subacute administration of clinically active antidepressants down-regulates β-receptors and desensitizes norepinephrine-sensitive adenylate cyclase in limbic forebrain or frontal cortex regions (41,75). Down-regulation has been determined by use of β-adrenergic antagonist ligands, such as [^{3}H]dihydroalprenolol or [^{125}I]iodopindolol. Through the application of selective β_1- and β_2-antagonists, regional localization of both subtypes of β-receptors was established in rat brain (60). The β-receptor down-regulated

by long-term antidepressant drug or electroconvulsive shock (ECS) treatment is the β_1-subtype (39,53).

But depression-related research comprises only one facet of broader and more momentous sequelae to the early reuptake findings. Using the simple methodology of synaptosomal uptake studies, e.g., incubation of radioactive ligands with brain membrane preparations and centrifugation or, more conveniently, rapid filtration to recover membrane-ligand complexes (30), investigators discovered opiate binding sites in brain, initially by the demonstration of stereospecific binding of [^{3}H]dihydromorphine, [^{3}H]naloxone, and [^{3}H]etorphine to crude membrane preparations (57,71,77). The correlation of binding affinities with pharmacological potencies in vitro and in vivo provided evidence that these binding sites have functional significance (13,87). After the pioneering experiments with opiates, membrane binding systems were described for the amine neurotransmitters, excitatory amino acids, adenosine, various neuropeptides, and diverse exogenous CNS active drugs, such as drugs associated with the γ-aminobutyric acid (GABA)-benzodiazepine-barbiturate/picrotoxin complex (86,88). Drugs emanating from pharmaceutical companies were and continue to be indispensable to this burgeoning area of neuroscience. Not only have they contributed primordial agents from which most radioactive ligands derive, but they provide a vast assortment of selective synthetic agonists and antagonists essential to the characterization of binding site subtypes. The rapid proliferation of identified receptor or binding site subtypes has often outpaced the discovery of correlated physiological or behavioral functions, making understanding of the significance of some binding sites a continuing challenge.

For studies of receptors and binding sites, appropriately derivatized drugs can be used for affinity labeling, photoaffinity probes, and preparation of affinity resins for the isolation and purification of receptor proteins (78). There are many methodological extensions of the study of receptors and binding sites, such as the localization of such sites in various brain regions through the application of autoradiography (25,44). Quantitative autoradiography enables determination of binding parameters much as in homogenate binding, but affords detailed regional localization of receptors not possible by the latter method (6,60,65). Localization of receptors in human brain using suitably labeled drug ligands has also been carried out with the positron emission tomography (PET scan) technique (16).

One representative example of the role played by industrially discovered drugs in the development of this area of neuropsychopharmacology is that afforded by the benzodiazepines. Early pharmacological characterization of chlordiazepoxide and diazepam was undertaken in ignorance of the existence of highly specific binding sites in the brain for these synthetic compounds. The analogy with the well-known opiate receptor story is striking, except that morphine derives from a natural product. Using [^{3}H]diazepam, several groups discovered benzodiazepine binding sites in brain, and found excellent correlation of pharmacological activity with binding potency for a large number of industry-discovered benzodiazepines (48,54,73). It had been known that diazepam facilitates electrophysiological effects of

GABA. Exploration of membrane receptor binding enabled the formulation of a molecular model for the modulation of GABA transmission via the chloride channel by diazepam and similarly acting benzodiazepines (7). The "GABA receptor-benzodiazepine receptor-picrotoxin/barbituate binding site complex" is now believed to be the site of action for GABA agonists and antagonists, benzodiazepine agonists, receptor antagonists (e.g., Ro 15-1788), partial agonists and "inverse agonists" (agents exhibiting actions opposite to those of diazepam), and anticonvulsant and convulsant drugs. The catalog is still growing (38,58). The possibility of receptor subtypes (15,26) has fueled efforts to synthesize more selective agents. In addition, peripheral benzodiazepine binding sites have been investigated with the ligands, Ro 5-4864 and PK 11195 (47,55). Facile binding experiments have enabled a broadening of structural types known to exhibit the various actions of the classical benzodiazepine cluster. Basic nondrug discoveries have followed the identification of benzodiazepine binding sites, for example, characterization of brain polypeptides such as GABA modulin and DBI, the latter a supposed endogenous diazepam binding inhibitor, that may play a role in normal physiological modulation of the chloride channel (49).

Comparable discussions to those just presented for the receptor binding subdiscipline of neurobiology could as easily be written for neuroanatomical mapping, stimulus control of behavior, experimental social psychology, neuroenzymology, neuronal cell culture, and scores of others. Industry-discovered drugs have been indispensable to the development of modern neurobiology.

Conversely, there are examples illustrating how the lack of selective drugs may hamper development of an area of neuroscience. Consider the question of the functional role of epinephrine-containing neurons in brain. Neuroanatomical mapping methods have enabled localization of phenylethanolamine N-methyltransferase (PNMT) in brain medullary regions and in axons projecting to hypothalamus and spinal cord (28). Although localization of PNMT neurons implies that epinephrine may be involved in synaptic transmission, it is difficult to know for sure. The lack of drugs that selectively affect epinephrine metabolism, release, reuptake, and receptor interactions leaves the manipulation of synthesis via PNMT inhibition as the primary means of affecting epinephrine concentrations in brain. Efforts of the drug industry in the 1970s provided several effective PNMT inhibitors (20); however, some PNMT inhibitors are also antagonists of α_2-adrenergic receptors (56,79), a property that can confuse the interpretation of experiments. Evidence indicating a functional role for epinephrine in the CNS remains sketchy, with the possible exception of neuroendocrine regulation (69).

FORTUITOUS DISCOVERY

Drug companies did not presciently seek from the outset of modern neurobiology to discover drugs oriented towards a future receptor-oriented technology, nor have their ambitions often been successfully directed towards purely mechanistic targets in the central nervous system, defined in advance. On the contrary, many of the most valuable drug tools, whether or not used therapeutically, derive from what retrospectively might be considered mundane phenomenology. There was once a time, for example, when industrial pharmacologists feverishly sought *any* demonstrable laboratory effect from imipramine, *in vivo* or *in vitro,* that would distinguish that newly identified clinically active antidepressant from moderately potent phenothiazine neuroleptics. *In vivo* effects quite remote from any perceived biochemical rationales have often been the key findings in discovering new CNS drugs and, much as the term accident is used, it understates the actual contribution of fortuitous findings and *ad hoc* inspiration. The situation is similar in biological and medical sciences in general (9). One reason for this understatement is that published accounts of industrial discoveries, like the memoirs of generals, naturally reinterpret events to make them appear more logical than was actually the case. Seldom have industrial researchers or their managements cared to acknowledge openly the many variants whereby important findings have derived from seemingly chance events.

Here is a rare, candid exception, describing the moment of discovery within a large pharmaceutical company of a commercially and scientifically important substance that works at peripheral taste receptors. This account derives from an affidavit by a chemical research assistant, Mr. J. M. Schlatter, as cited by Mazur (50):

In December, 1965, I was working with Dr. Mazur on the synthesis of the C-terminal tetrapeptide of gastrin [in a project intended to find drugs acting in the gastrointestinal system]. We were making intermediates and trying to purify them. In particular . . . I was recrystalizing aspartylphenylalanyl methyl ester (aspartame) which had been prepared by the hydrogenolysis of the protected dipeptide ester prepared and given to me by Dr. Mazur. I was heating the aspartame in a flask with methanol when the mixture bumped onto the outside of the flask. As a result, some of the powder got onto my fingers. At a slightly later stage, when licking my finger to pick up a piece of paper, I noticed a very strong, sweet taste. Initially I thought that I must have still had some sugar on my hands from earlier in the day. However, I quickly realized this could not be so, since I had washed my hands in the meantime. I therefore traced the powder on my hands back to the container into which I had placed the crystallized aspartylphenylalanine methyl ester. I felt that this peptide ester was not likely to be toxic and I therefore tasted a little of it and found that it was the substance which I had previously tasted on my finger.

Mazur (50) notes that the sweetness of aspartame could not have been predicted from the tastes of aspartic acid, phenylalanine, or deesterified aspartylphenylalanine.

The above account must represent an extremely rare kind of fortuity, although it is reminiscent of Hofmann's famous notebook description (e.g., 27) of his discovery of LSD's action in 1943. Far more common, although seldom disclosed, must be drug discovery scenarios similar to many the present authors can recollect from their own careers. Our citing such experiences is not intended to exaggerate unduly the importance of our own work. Rather, for the reason cited above, we are hesitant in accepting published accounts of the discovery experiences of others.

In the late 1950s, in a synthesis/screening search for amphetamine-like anorectics, one of us unexpectedly observed that *p*-and *m*-trifluoromethylamphetamine were nonstimulant anorectics in rats (29,84). Reports of this finding led scientists at a French company (5) to synthesize the *N*-ethyl derivative of the latter (fenfluramine), leading to the availability of that substance as a tool, especially for studying serotonin pathways (32). Fenfluramine, in turn, served as an intellectual precursor to other contemporary drug tools for studying serotonin receptors and function, such as *m*-trifluoromethylphenylpiperazine (21,70) and 1-(*p*-aminophenylethyl)-4-trifluoromethylphenylpiperazine (1).

A routine screen in our laboratories in the early 1960s was the determination of catecholamine and serotonin levels in rat brain, as an adjunct to simple drug interaction tests. Following reports from competitor companies that *p*-chloroamphetamine lowered concentrations of serotonin in rat brain, we decided to test likely metabolic precursors to *p*-chlorophenethylamine derivatives, among them, PCPA. Fortuitously, biochemical endpoints were examined at both 1 and 24 hr after treatment. Later careful studies showed that marked depletion of serotonin levels could *only* have been detected after approximately 24 hr. Publication of our studies (42) rapidly attracted the interest of pharmacologists, neuroscientists, behaviorists, and clinicians.

In 1965, shortly after the disclosure that α-methyltyrosine (AMT) inhibits tyrosine hydroxylase (72,80), we discovered that our company had coincidentally synthesized an ample supply of a one-step chemical precursor to AMT for a different purpose, enabling us rapidly to conduct *in vivo* pilot experiments. It was predicted by one of us that AMT-elicited blockade of catecholamine synthesis would *increase* a rat's sensitivity to the behavioral effects of amphetamine, then widely believed to act in the central nervous system directly at postsynaptic sites. Presumably, AMT would potentiate the stimulant effects of amphetamine by what was then termed denervation supersensitivity. The experiments conducted (82,83) yielded exactly opposite effects to those expected, with important continuing implications for our present understanding of the mechanism of action of amphetamine.

In the middle 1970s, as part of an antipsychotic research approach seeking inhibitors of the enzyme indole *N*-methyltransferase (INMT), we routinely checked for possible "miscellaneous antipsychotic activities" of certain indole-like structures that modestly inhibited INMT. We unexpectedly found neuroleptic activity and, in collaboration with medicinal chemists, synthesized and identified flutroline and structural analogs as extraordinarily potent neuroleptics, with structural implications for dopamine receptors (22,23,85).

In the late 1960s, synthesis of 1-aminotetralins was initiated at our company, based on neuroleptic properties of 2-chloro-*cis*-doxepin. Possible active conformations of these dibenzoxepines led to the idea that the active moiety might correspond to a rigid 1-aminotetralin structure. The resulting compound, lometraline, did not exhibit the expected neuroleptic effects but unexpectedly reversed tetrabenazine depression and trifluoperazine catalepsy on the one hand, and exerted anticonflict activity on the other

(64). Following introduction of a 4-phenyl substituent to improve brain penetration and pharmacokinetic properties, the prototype compound (tametraline) unexpectedly blocked the uptake of norepinephrine (63) and dopamine (40). Subsequently, the introduction of chlorine substituents into the pendant phenyl ring unexpectedly enhanced serotonin and catecholamine uptake blocking activity. Separation of the isomeric mixture yielded the pure (*cis*) 1*S*,4*S*-3,4-dichloro derivative, sertraline, which, again unexpectedly, potently and highly selectively inhibited serotonin uptake (43).

The examples cited above describe important biological findings that were not predicted or sought in advance of the studies conducted, and in some cases the findings were precisely opposite to those expected. We could also provide anecdotes depicting more improbable drug discoveries emanating from occurrences such as the testing by error of incorrectly numbered samples, or the conduct of experiments suggested by citations from remote disciplines and encountered seemingly by chance. Although many "rational" projects were also undertaken during our years of conducting industrial screening, and with findings of note, the relative importance of our fortuitous discoveries seems remarkable.

The sympathetic reader, even if agreeing with our emphasis on the role of fortuity, may want to know something of the laboratory backdrop against which it has occurred. We now proceed to discuss screening tests in general, and then the dilemmas for new discovery as posed by the existing state of our science, the burgeoning of molecular rationales, and what we perceive to be the disparity between the reality of past fortuity and the voguish supposition that we enjoy precognitive abilities to predict what modifications of which unexplored molecular mechanisms will alter human behavior in new and useful ways.

SCREENING PROCEDURES

All scientific experiments can be formalized as consisting of three components: (a) a testing system; (b) independent variables delivered to that system; and (c) selected measures, termed dependent variables, on which the effects of the independent variables are ascertained. In the instance of contemporary pharmaceutical screening, the independent variables are still typically relatively pure, low-molecular-weight chemical compounds with relatively unknown activities. We have not yet reached the point where high-molecular-weight proteins and polypeptides are available for screening, and although natural products testing is enjoying a renaissance, largely because modern analytical tools and techniques of molecular biology enable isolation, identification, and synthesis of actives faster than heretofore, such samples still comprise an infinitesimal fraction of all samples examined. The bases for selecting compounds as deserving of biological testing may range from extremely empirical, even intentionally random methods, through highly rational medicinal chemical bases, as described in the preceding chapter.

Industrial pharmacologists have usually been eclectic in their choice of testing systems and dependent variables, using neurobiological systems that seemed to work, and seldom dwelling seriously on how well screens fulfill the accepted requirements for "good tests" in the formal, statistical sense: reliability and validity. Practicality, volume, simplicity, and speed of testing methods are all-important considerations when large-scale compound exposure is desired.

Let us enumerate the more common types of screening tests used in industrial screening, even though such listing trivializes their variety and evolution. Discerning readers will understand that efforts to itemize procedures comprehensively are foredoomed, nor would such efforts be very purposeful, since several books and monographs attempt such cataloging (e.g., 17–19,62). Model data from an industrial laboratory noted for the volume, quality, and discovery history of its screening output may also be consulted (e.g., 35,36).

A naive observer, familiar with the organization of university departments, the National Institute of Mental Health (NIMH), or many neurobiology textbooks, or having read industrial placement advertisements, might assume that screening tests would be classifiable within traditional disciplines such as "experimental psychology," "biochemistry," "autonomic pharmacology," "neurophysiology," etc. Although that is in part true, it tends to obscure the generic importance of one very large family of tests that has most commonly been exploited in industrial screening for centrally acting drugs: *in vivo* neurological examinations of intact, unanesthetized animals, usually rodents, often in conjunction with drug interaction protocols.

Because this family of tests is poorly identified within the rubric of academic disciplines, its vast contribution to discovery is seldom identified, but more agents acting on the central nervous system have been sought and found using these techniques than by using any others. In addition to the well-known Irwin (33) type of symptomatology screen in mice, there are diverse means to efficiently screen blockers or potentiators of dopamine agonists, amine releasers, convulsants, cholinergics, drugs presumed to cause pain, and an enormous variety of other challenge agents that rapidly elicit readily observed symptoms or death. In many instances the discovery within the drug industry of just these challenge agents, e.g., oxotremorine, or of the simple and reproducible signs they produce, e.g., "writhing" after 2-phenyl-1,4-benzoquinone, has itself impacted neurobiology in far-reaching ways. If one adds the many comparable techniques enabling facile determination of *in vivo* interactions with nonpharmacological challenges, then electroconvulsant antagonism tests, analgetic tests such as hot plate and tail flick tests, various psychomotor tests, simple motor function tests, swimming tests, and even observational tests using social stimuli, would also have to be included.

There is no well-accepted distinguishing label for this plethora of technically simple observational tests taken collectively. Are they "behavioral," "pharmacological," or "neurological"? In any case, their stand-alone output as simple, high-capacity screening methods for drugs has been enormous. For many years they have also been a reliable source of *in vivo* functional data with which receptor, enzymologic, or other biochemical screening data could be correlated. The scope of their use would be apparent to any inexperienced reader who perused methods sections of journals such as the *Journal of Medicinal Chemistry, Arzneimittelforschung,* or *Drug Development Research.*

Among biochemical techniques most frequently used are receptor binding techniques, *in vivo* and *ex vivo,* with all their ligand and methodogical diversity. An important corollary of drug action at receptors is receptor adaptation, resulting in secondary tests such as down-regulation of β-adrenergic receptors and preclinical markers of antidepressant activity. Other screens are based on the modulation of synaptic activity, such as tests for blockade of reuptake, facilitation of release, or inhibition of degradative enzymes of neurotransmitters, cotransmitters, or neuromodulators. The converse, interference with synthetic pathways of these brain constituents, also serves as the basis of screening tests. Levels of neurotransmitters, of their metabolites, or of turnover are frequently measured. Ratios from diverse screening data are examined for presumed "selectivity" of interesting compounds. Component parts of second messenger or effector systems (cyclic AMP, cyclic GMP, phosphoinositide cleavage products) may serve as screening substrates, e.g., activity of various phosphodiesterases or adenylate cyclases, accumulation of cyclic nucleotides, accumulation of inositol phosphates.

Turning to screening for behavioral effects in conditioned subjects, those systems used most frequently are almost all instrumental, rather than respondent conditioning procedures. The first of these to achieve wide acceptance was discrete-trial conditioned avoidance behavior (10), used primarily to detect neuroleptics. Conflict testing, conditioned emotional response (CER) testing, and similar tests using punishment-suppressed behavior are well-known tests (cf. 67) used primarily for seeking behaviorally disinhibiting agents such as diazepam, widely, but very imprecisely, also termed anxiolytics. (The distinction between characterizing diazepam-like compounds as "behaviorally disinhibiting agents" and as "anxiolytics" is not trivial. There are certain older drugs, such as thioridazine and doxepin, that have yielded good evidence of therapeutic activity in some patients characterized clinically as "anxious," but these drugs are generally inactive in laboratory tests for behavioral disinhibition. Furthermore, one can readily conjure hypotheses for possible useful behavioral actions of benzodiazepine antagonists only by using the former terminology. The common usage, "anxiolytic tests," for animal screening procedures is in any case flagrantly anthropomorphic.) Drug discrimination techniques have been used for determining "subjective" effects of many drug classes, and self-administration procedures have sought to identify agents with reinforcing properties, possibly reflecting abuse potential. In these last two cited procedural classes, drugs may be construed less as independent variables than as elicitors of unique internal states. A noteworthy trend during the last 25 years has been the steady diminution of any impact on industrial drug discovery of steady-state, free operant behavior maintained by traditional reinforcement schedules.

Animal neurophysiological techniques continue to be far less used in screening than methods mentioned above, because the preparative time and skills required to build up sample sizes appropriate for the variability and the relatively short viability of many preparations are not often compatible with the needs of high-throughput testing. Practitioners, if they can neglect these considerations, most often study spinal reflexes, subcortical evoked potentials, and after discharges, electroencephalograms (EEGs), sleep patterns, and spontaneous neuronal firing. There is a recent increase in *in vitro* neurophysiological screening using cell culture and tissue slice techniques, and of single-cell recording from intact animals.

RELIABILITY AND VALIDITY

Insuring test reliability in the above domains is seldom a theoretical problem, although, in practice, a decision on which of several chemical synthetic paths to pursue is too often based solely on initial small-sample data. A frequent source of error arises when screening data are expressed as ratios between dependent variables, since there is a tendency to underestimate the impact of multiplicative error factors on the reliability of the ratios. There are no substitutes for soundly designed followup assays (e.g., employing randomized latin squares with concurrently tested positive and negative standards, and investigators blinded as to the identity of all samples) using the screening protocol, to avoid needless blind alleys.

In vitro receptor binding tests provide the best example of biological systems with highly replicable results, provided that assay conditions are held reasonably constant. But most methodologically simpler *in vivo* tests tend also to be highly replicable. One example is afforded by convulsant challenge testing, which has proven so important not only in identifying antiepileptic drugs, but in the early discovery and classification of benzodiazepine. More complex *in vivo* tests tend to have greater reliability problems, but achieve adequate reliability when experimenters carefully attend to spurious environmental or subject variation, or to matters of design, particularly sample size. It must be conceded that there are examples of important drugs for which data obtained on critical endpoints in different laboratories are in direct conflict. This is illustrated by the behavioral testing literature on the new, supposed anxiolytic drug, buspirone. Although there is widespread agreement that this compound lacks the typical central nervous system properties of benzodiazepines such as diazepam, its behavioral–disinhibiting properties in rats and monkeys trained on conflict or similar testing procedures are in dispute. Sometimes these effects are depicted as at least comparable to those of diazepam (24,76), sometimes as present, but quantitatively less than those of benzodiazepines (59,81), and sometimes as entirely absent (74). Adding to the confusion is the mixed pharmacological profile of buspirone, which includes weak dopamine antagonist activity (52) and serotonin (5-HT_{1A}) agonist or partial agonist activity (76).

The validation of screening tests designed to uncover new therapeutic entities, i.e., the demonstration that results, even if reliable, predict the desired efficacy in humans, is extraordinarily difficult in almost all instances. As noted at the outset, the main therapeutic action of the earliest modern drugs in psychopharmacology, e.g., chlorpromazine, were discovered in humans. That such drugs enjoyed hitherto unsuspected therapeutic activity enabled *post hoc* laboratory analysis. In the case of chlorpromazine, such analysis led retrospectively to the development of tests for blockade of amphetamine and apomorphine stereotypy, and tests for the selective blockade of conditioned avoidance behavior. Many test systems that once seemed sensible, such as efforts to assay the ability of chlorpromazine-like drugs to block actions of LSD in animals, were discarded. Dopamine-oriented biochemical tests came only later. Empirical validation of all these tests depended at first on clinical results from only a single agent (chlorpromazine), but human testing then became available from a group of close analogs (e.g., other phenothiazines and closely related tricyclics), and still later from structurally dissimilar compounds (e.g., butyrophenones, diphenylbutylpiperidines, molindone, benzamides) with more-or-less similar biology. Unfortunately, logical attempts to assess test validation can be undone by the use of such shibboleths as "atypical" or "paradoxical" neuroleptics.

But how are screening protocols for discovery of entirely new types of drugs to be validated? The escalating and often legally mandated costs and controls imposed on both preclinical and clinical developmental research by governmental agencies appreciably decrease the likelihood that serendipitous findings, as were once possible, can be repeated. The same factors have made rapid clinical evaluation of exploratory laboratory actives far more difficult than it once was. Society as a whole, as well as pharmaceutical industry managements, now attempts energetically to rationalize all prospective discovery research to focus costly resources, to minimize risk, and to satisfy a widespread belief that the science of pharmacology has advanced sufficiently to enable all new drugs to be discovered by deductive logic. These understandable efforts exact the severe, though difficult-to-measure, price of undermining those very sorts of serendipitous, *ad hoc* discoveries that historically have provided the foundations of our science.

Returning to the validation of screens, some may be validated empirically on the basis of correlating quantitative differences in laboratory effects with relatively small clinical shadings among known entities, particularly on side effect profiles, usually resulting at best in the possibility of theoretically minor advances. In practice, though, there are rarely, if ever, direct clinical data in support of screening for novel mechanisms, and highly speculative theory has to be relied upon for presumptions of "face validity." In some cases these presumptions are proven wrong even before attempts at drug-based clinical validation can occur. One example is the search for presumed antipsychotic agents that block the enzyme indole N-methyltransferase. Projects toward this end were undertaken by several pharmaceutical companies, in the belief that methylated indoles such as bufotenin and N,N-dimethyltryptamine play a role in idiopathic psychosis. That theory has since come into disrepute. In other cases, discovery of target compounds to test a speculative theory proves intractable. The search for agents that block the "receptor" binding of phencyclidine or its behavioral effects in the belief that there is a natural receptor for an endogenous phencyclidine-like psychotogen may provide a suitable example. And there are cases in which newly discovered drugs have been claimed to satisfy theoretical demands for a mechanistically novel therapeutic entity, only to fail on clinical testing.

The appeal to logic as a means of validating novel screening programs can be tedious and tenuous, and the data supporting the logic may be only marginally reliable. When clinical claims take on commercial interest, as of "rapid-acting antidepressants," of "neuroleptics lacking extrapyramidal effects," or of "nonsedating anxiolytics," disproportionate effort can be expended in pursuit of ephemeral screening results and small selectivity differences. In just this fashion, superficially rational projects supporting the clamor for discovery based on a "new biology" have become dominant in what may be still predominantly phenomenological areas of neuropsychopharmacology, and have been treated as if they constitute validated approaches.

Some readers will no doubt misconstrue our emphasis on fortuitous discovery as being grossly anachronistic in the current scientific milieu, when neurobiology laboratories are expected to emphasize molecular biological mechanisms. The necessity for highly rational approaches in some areas of neurobiology, as biology in general, cannot be denied, yet inappropriate reductionism, overdependence on nonvalidated theoretical rationales, or denigration of the "chemical approach" (cf., e.g., 4) in domains that are still phenomenological can be counterproductive when imposed on scientific talent.

DILEMMAS

The current emphasis on rational planning in screening, contrasted with historic evidence that fortuitous discovery has been focal in shaping modern neuropsychopharmacology, brings us to the consideration of selected dilemmas of conducting biological discovery research within the pharmaceutical industry. The issues to be cited touch on nonscientific matters, as they would if the research were conducted under any auspices. For clarity, the dilemmas will be posed as if they were all-or-none, although circumstances are never so simple.

Therapeutic Versus Mechanistic Rationales

Should screening emphasize therapeutic goals, as reflected by face-valid functional tests, or should it emphasize mechanistic goals to the exclusion of function? Many biochemical systems are more tentatively related to diseases than the literature might indicate. Substance P, as one example, is known for its distribution in spinal areas, suggesting a role in pain sensation, and it has been implicated in psychic depression. One should recall that no pharmaceutically feasible antagonist of its action or inhibitor of its synthesis has been discovered, hindering simple probes of its functional role. In mounting resources for screening, should a company define the mission of its researchers as finding a substance P antagonist and, only after appreciable success, ascertaining the activity of such an antagonist in functional tests? Or should it rapidly be ascertained whether or not even weakly acting lead antagonists exert analgetic, antidepressant, or other action? The former approach insures

sustained mechanistic research, but may lead to a long cul-de-sac. The alternative may put an onerous testing burden on investigators armed with the skill to perform basic biochemical research on substance P, diluting their output. The premature assignment of criterion status to functional testing tends to subvert basic mechanistic research.

Molar Versus Molecular Rationales

Scientific reductionism to the level of enzyme biochemistry and receptor analysis is common in neuropsychopharmacology. Reductionism provides "explanatory" verbiage in science, although lower-level mechanisms are not the only mechanisms, and are themselves susceptible to further reduction. Most observers would agree that it is evidently premature for human social sciences to be explained in terms of biochemical reactions, even if few would doubt that social interactions do, in fact, depend on biochemical underpinnings in the brains of many individuals. A biochemical level of discovery is nevertheless being forced onto the discovery component of neuropsychopharmacology, even when no adequate foundation justifies this. There remain no widely accepted biochemical data correlated with, let alone causative of, core phenomenological functional data, such as human verbal behavior, animal schedule-controlled behavior, or a host of functions elaborated in the *Diagnostic and Statistical Manual of Mental Disorders,* 3rd edition (DSM-III) as essential to delineating diagnostic categories.

Novel Versus Derivative Rationales

Should discovery teams attempt to create novel approaches to therapy, or should they be content with incremental derivative approaches, taking advantage of knowledge of the properties of clinically active drugs? Novel approaches are difficult to synthesize without understanding the causes of the disorders for which one seeks new psychotherapeutic agents. Not only is there little chance of finding an active or useful drug, but a certain amount of "free experimentation" is needed to establish the new rationale proposed or to develop even the rudiments of the basic science involved.

The Paradox of Serendipity

There are those who would deny that serendipity may be fostered, and who cite the seeming paradox in believing that favorable accidents can be "arranged." There is no necessary conflict between serendipity and planning. Although it may be useful, administratively, to subordinate youthful scientific talent to team approaches, and to require some amount of justification in their selection of experiments, individual intellectual curiosity at its apogee must still be allowed to flourish. Although all approaches require some amount of deductive reasoning, the need for rationales should not be so doctrinaire as to prevent individuals from delving into ancillary empirical matter that kindles their interest. Scientific, as well as commercial, implications of prospective or completed experimentation are relevant in pharmaceutical research. Pharmacology managements must be careful to enable human organisms to pass through the "jurisdictional membranes" separating disciplines, objectives, and laboratories if growth is to be nourished and information exchanged. The close restriction of internal communications or of scientific publications in the interests of security must not be allowed to withhold information unnecessarily from just those junior, slightly off-center, or unknown outside scientists whose interests may be aroused, and who may provide needed fresh outlooks. The restriction of *ad hoc* experimentation on compounds subject to regulatory review, lest difficult-to-explain findings arise, can serve as well to preclude unexpected serendipitous results. On the training and hiring side, there is as much need for acculturated opportunists in sprawling disciplines such as neuropsychopharmacology as there is for highly specialized technologists.

SUMMARY

Tests correlating with therapeutic targets have not been tabulated cookbook style, for any attempt to have done so would have been impossible and antithetical to our belief that important new drugs are rarely discovered by formula. We began by emphasizing that important modern drugs emanate predominantly from industrial laboratories, and that their discoveries are often fortuitous. That fortuity has been fundamental in providing every subdiscipline within our science with its basic tools. Test systems using the simplest of phenomenological endpoints have contributed heavily to new drug discovery. Such techniques, frequently divorced from the mainstream of our increasingly molecular science, often provide its bedrock. Principles of sound testing apply fully to screening. Tests must be both reliable and valid. Errors in the former domain may usually be corrected by sound experimental design. Inadequate validation is less easily, if at all, corrected, and we express concern at the extent to which the validation of prolonged research efforts is provided by molecular rationales lacking convincing data. A sensible balance between functional, phenomenological screening on the one hand, and theoretical, molecular approaches, on the other, is a hard one to reach, but like other dilemmas in organizing screening efforts, it must be carefully and objectively considered. The future of molecular biology in the discovery of new central nervous system drugs enthralls us, but successes from the recent past have much to teach.

ACKNOWLEDGMENT

We gratefully acknowledge the technical assistance provided by Mrs. Marylouise Stachon in preparing the manuscript.

REFERENCES

1. Asarch, K. B., Ransom, R. W., and Shih, J. C. (1985): *Life Sci.*, 36:1265–1273.
2. Axelrod, J., Whiteby, L. G., and Hertting, G. (1961): *Science*, 133:383–384.
3. Barbaccia, M. L., Brunello, N., Chuang, D. M., and Costa, E. (1983): *Neuropharmacology*, 22:373–383.
4. Bartholini, G. (1983): In: *Decision Making in Drug Research*, edited by F. Gross, pp. 123–139. Raven Press, New York.
5. Beregi, L. G., Hugon, P., LeDouarec, J. C., Laubie, M., and Duhault, J. (1978): In: *International Symposium on Amphetamine and Related Compounds*, edited by E. Costa and S. Garattini, pp. 21–61. Raven Press, New York.
6. Biegon, A., and Rainbow, T. C. (1982): *Eur. J. Pharmacol.*, 82:245–246.
7. Biggio, G., and Costa, E., eds. (1983): *Benzodiazepine Recognition Site Ligands: Biochemistry and Pharmacology.* Raven Press, New York.
8. Cade, J. F. J. (1949): *Med. J. Aust.*, 2:349–352.
9. Comroe, J. H., Jr. (1977): *Am. Rev. Respir. Dis.*, 115:853–860, 1035–1044.
10. Cook, L., and Weidley, E. (1957): *Ann. NY Acad. Sci. USA*, 66:740–752.
11. Cotzias, G. C., Van Woert, M. H., and Schiffer, L. M. (1967): *N. Engl. J. Med.*, 276:374–379.
12. Coyle, J. T., and Snyder, S. H. (1969): *Science*, 166:899–901.
13. Creese, I., and Snyder, S. H. (1975): *J. Pharmacol. Exp. Ther.*, 194:205–219.
14. Davis, A. (1984): *Experientia*, 40:782–794.
15. Dubnick, B., Lippa, A. S., Klepner, C. A., Coupet, J., Greenblatt, E. N., and Beer, B. (1983): *Pharmacol. Biochem. Behav.*, 18:311–318.
16. Farde, L., Hall, H., Ehrin, E., and Sedvall, G. (1986): *Science*, 231:258–261.
17. Fielding, S., and Lal, H., eds. (1974): *Neuroleptics (Industrial Pharmacology, Vol. 1).* Futura Publishing Co., Mount Kisco, NY.
18. Fielding, S., and Lal, H., eds. (1975): *Antidepressants (Industrial Pharmacology, Vol. 2).* Futura Publishing Co., Mount Kisco, NY.
19. Fielding, S., and Lal, H., eds. (1977): *Anxiolytics (Industrial Pharmacology, Vol. 3).* Futura Publishing Co., Mount Kisco, NY.
20. Fuller, R. W. (1982): *Annu. Rev. Pharmacol. Toxicol.*, 22:31–55.
21. Fuller, R. W., Snoddy, H. D., Mason, N. R., and Molloy, B. B. (1978): *Eur. J. Pharmacol.*, 52:11–16.
22. Harbert, C. A., Plattner, J. J., Welch, W. M., Weissman, A., and Koe, B. K. (1980): *Mol. Pharmacol.*, 17:38–42.
23. Harbert, C. A., Plattner, J. J., Welch, W. M., Weissman, A., and Koe, B. K. (1980): *J. Med. Chem.*, 23:635–643.
24. Hartmann, R. J., and Geller, I. (1981): *Proc. West. Pharmacol. Soc.*, 24:179–181.
25. Herkenham, M. (1984): In: *Brain Receptor Methodologies, Part A: General Methods and Concepts. Amines and Acetylcholine*, edited by P. J. Marangos, I. C. Campbell, and R. M. Cohen, pp. 127–152. Academic Press, Orlando, FL.
26. Hirsch, J. D., Garrett, K. M., and Beer, B. (1985): *Pharmacol. Biochem. Behav.*, 23:681–685.
27. Hofmann, A. (1968): In: *Drugs Affecting the Central Nervous System, Vol. 2*, edited by A. Burger, pp. 169–235. Marcel Dekker, New York.
28. Hokfelt, T., Johansson, O., and Goldstein, M. (1984): In: *Classical Transmitters in the CNS, Part I*, edited by A. Bjorklund and T. Hokfelt, pp. 157–276. Elsevier Science Publishers, Amsterdam.
29. Holland, G. F., Buck, C. J., and Weissman, A. (1963): *J. Med. Chem.*, 6:519–524.
30. Horn, A. S., Coyle, J. T., and Snyder, S. H. (1971): *Mol. Pharmacol.*, 7:66–80.
31. Hornykiewicz, O. (1973): *Fed. Proc.*, 32:183–190.
32. Invernizzi, R., Berettera, C., Garattini, S., and Samanin, R. (1986): *Eur. J. Pharmacol.*, 120:9–15.
33. Irwin, S. (1968): *Psychopharmacologia*, 13:222–226.
34. Iversen, L. L. (1967): *The Uptake and Storage of Noradrenaline in Sympathetic Nerves.* Cambridge University Press, London.
35. Janssen, P. A. J., Neimegeers, C. J. E., and Schellekens, K. H. L. (1965): *Arzneimittelforsch.*, 15:104.
36. Janssen, P. A. J., Neimegeers, C. J. E., Schellekens, K. H. L., Lenaerts, F. M., Verbruggen, F. J., VanNeuten, J. M., and Schaper, W. K. A. (1970): *Eur. J. Pharmacol.*, 11:139–154.
37. Kannengiesser, M. H., Hunt, P., and Raynaud, J. P. (1973): *Biochem. Pharmacol.*, 22:73–84.

38. Karobath, M., and Supavilai, P. (1985): *Pharmacol. Biochem. Behav.,* 23:671–674.
39. Kellar, K. J., Stockmeier, C. A., Rainbow, T. C., and Wolfe, B. B. (1985): *Soc. Neurosci. Abstr.,* 11:812.
40. Koe, B. K. (1976): *J. Pharmacol. Exp. Ther.,* 199:649–661.
41. Koe, B. K., and Vinick, F. J. (1984): *Annu. Rep. Med. Chem.,* 19: 41–50.
42. Koe, B. K., and Weissman, A. (1966): *J. Pharmacol. Exp. Ther.,* 154:499–516.
43. Koe, B. K., Weissman, A., Welch, W. M., and Browne, R. G. (1983): *J. Pharmacol. Exp. Ther.,* 226:686–700.
44. Kuhar, M. J. (1985): In: *Neurotransmitter Receptor Binding,* edited by H. I. Yamamura, S. J. Enna, and M. J. Kuhar, pp. 153–176. Raven Press, New York.
45. Langer, S. Z., Moret, C., Raisman, R., Dubocovich, M. L., and Briley, M. (1980): *Science,* 210:1133–1135.
46. Langer, S. Z., and Raisman, R. (1983): *Neuropharmacology,* 22: 407–413.
47. LeFur, G., Guilloux, F., Rufat, P., Benavides, J., Uzan, A., Renault, C., Dubroeucq, M. C., and Gueremy, C. (1983): *Life Sci.,* 32:1849–1856.
48. Mackerer, C. R., Kochman, R. L., Bierschenk, B. A., and Bremner, S. S. (1978): *J. Pharmacol. Exp. Ther.,* 206:405–413.
49. Massotti, M., Guidotti, A., and Costa, E. (1981): *J. Neurosci.,* 1: 409–418.
50. Mazur, R. H. (1984): In: *Aspartame: Advances in Physiology and Biochemistry,* edited by L. D. Stegink and L. J. Filer, Jr., pp. 3–9. Marcel Dekker, New York.
51. Meek, J. L., Fuxe, K., and Carlsson, A. (1971): *Biochem. Pharmacol.,* 20:707–709.
52. Meltzer, H. Y., Simonovic, M., Fang, V. S., and Gudelsky, G. A. (1982): *Psychopharmacology,* 78:49–53.
53. Minneman, K. P., Dibner, M. D., Wolfe, B. B., and Molinoff, P. B. (1979): *Science,* 204:866–868.
54. Mohler, H., and Okada, T. (1977): *Science,* 198:849–851.
55. Pellow, S., and File, S. E. (1984): *Neurosci. Behav. Rev.,* 8:405–413.
56. Pendleton, R. G., and Hieble, J. P. (1981): *Res. Commun. Chem. Pathol. Pharmacol.,* 34:399–408.
57. Pert, C. B., and Snyder, S. H. (1973): *Science,* 179:1011–1014.
58. Polc, P., Bonnetti, E. P., Schaffner, R., and Haefely, W. (1982): *Naunyn Schmiedebergs Arch. Pharmacol.,* 321:260–264.
59. Porter, J. H., Johnson, D. N., and Jackson, J. Y. (1985): *Soc. Neurosci. Abstr.,* 11:426.
60. Rainbow, T. C., Parsons, B., and Wolfe, B. B. (1984): *Proc. Natl. Acad. Sci. USA,* 81:1585–1589.
61. Raisman, R., Sette, M., Pimoule, C., Briley, M., and Langer, S. Z. (1982): *Eur. J. Pharmacol.,* 78:345–351.
62. Rubin, A. A., ed. (1978): *New Drugs: Discovery and Development.* Marcel Dekker, New York.
63. Sarges, R., Koe, B. K., and Weissman, A. (1974): *J. Pharmacol. Exp. Ther.,* 191:393–402.
64. Sarges, R., Tretter, J. R., Tenen, S. S., and Weissman, A. (1973): *J. Med. Chem.,* 16:1003–1011.
65. Scatton, B., Dubois, A., Dubocovich, M. L., Zahniser, N. R., and Fage, D. (1985): *Life Sci.,* 36:815–822.
66. Schou, M. (1959): *Psychopharmacologia,* 1:65–78.
67. Sepinwall, J., and Cook, L. (1978): In: *Handbook of Psychopharmacology, Vol. 13,* edited by L. L. Iversen, S. D. Iversen, and S. S. Snyder, pp. 345–393. Plenum Press, New York.
68. Shaskan, E. G., and Snyder, S. H. (1970): *J. Pharmacol. Exp. Ther.,* 175:404–418.
69. Sheaves, R., Laynes, R., and Mackinnon, P. C. B. (1985): *Endocrinology,* 116:542–546.
70. Sills, M. A., Wolfe, B. B., and Frazer, A. (1984): *J. Pharmacol. Exp. Ther.,* 231:480–487.
71. Simon, E. J., Hiller, J. M., and Edelman, I. (1973): *Proc. Natl. Acad. Sci. USA,* 70:1947–1949.
72. Spector, S., Sjoerdsma, A., and Udenfriend, S. (1965): *J. Pharmacol.,* 147:86–95.
73. Squires, R. F., and Braestrup, C. (1977): *Nature,* 266:32–34.
74. Sullivan, J. W., Keim, K. L., and Sepinwall, J. (1983): *Soc. Neurosci. Abstr.,* 9:434.
75. Sulser, F., Janowsky, A. J., Okado, F., Manier, D. H., and Mobley, P. L. (1983): *Neuropharmacology,* 22:425–431.
76. Taylor, D. P., Eison, M. S., Riblet, L. A., and Vandermaelen, C. P. (1985): *Pharmacol. Biochem. Behav.,* 23:687–694.
77. Terenius, L. (1973): *Acta Pharmacol. Toxicol.,* 32:317–320.
78. Thomas, J. W., and Tallman, J. F. (1984): In: *Brain Receptor Methodologies, Part A: General Methods and Concepts. Amines and Acetylcholine,* edited by P. J. Marangos, I. C. Campbell, and R. M. Cohen, pp. 95–113. Academic Press, Orlando, FL.
79. Toomey, R. E., Horng, J. S., Hemrick-Luecke, S. K., and Fuller, R. W. (1981): *Life Sci.,* 29:2467–2472.
80. Udenfriend, S., Zaltman-Nirenberg, P., and Nagatsu, T. (1965): *Biochem. Pharmacol.,* 14:837–845.
81. Weissman, B. A., Barrett, J. E., Brady, L. S., Witkin, J. M., Mendelsohn, W. B., Paul, S. M., and Skolnick, P. (1984): *Drug Dev. Res.,* 4:83–93.
82. Weissman, A., and Koe, B. K. (1965): *Life Sci.,* 4:1037–1048.
83. Weissman, A., Koe, B. K., and Tenen, S. S. (1966): *J. Pharmacol. Exp. Ther.,* 151:339–352.
84. Weissman, A., and Schneider, J. A. (1960): *Pharmacologist,* 2:71.
85. Welch, W. M., Ewing, F. E., Harbert, C. A., Weissman, A., and Koe, B. K. (1980): *J. Med. Chem.,* 23:949–952.
86. Williams, M., and U'Pritchard, D. C. (1984): *Annu. Rep. Med. Chem.,* 19:283–292.
87. Wilson, R. S., Rogers, M. E., Pert, C. B., and Snyder, S. H. (1975): *J. Med. Chem.,* 18:240–242.
88. Yamamura, H. I., Enna, S. J., and Kuhar, M. J., eds. (1985): *Neurotransmitter Receptor Binding.* Raven Press, New York.

Psychopharmacology:
The Third Generation of Progress,
edited by Herbert Y. Meltzer.
Raven Press, New York © 1987.

CHAPTER **179**

Practical Considerations in the Clinical Development of CNS Drugs

Bert Spilker

This chapter describes some practical guidelines on study design and conduct to assist individuals planning or conducting studies. A broad approach would be to discuss issues that relate to almost all clinical studies. This approach has previously been followed (14,15). A more specific approach would be to discuss practical considerations relating to each individual CNS disease, syndrome, and disorder. That type of approach has been attempted in numerous texts.

The approach chosen for this chapter emphasizes practical considerations that are relevant for most clinical studies conducted with drugs used to treat CNS diseases. Overlap with both the general and the specific approaches is unavoidable. Considerations of CNS effects resulting from drugs intended for non-CNS diseases will not be specifically addressed.

Two major sections of this chapter briefly discuss current issues in developing drugs with CNS indications and considerations relating to study design and conduct. The four current issues are (a) the ability of patients to give an informed consent; (b) the problem of inadequate animal models for identifying compounds to develop in humans; (c) the number and types of efficacy parameters and raters to use in clinical studies; and (d) proper control populations to use in CNS drug studies. Considerations relating to study design and conduct are presented in a series of tables. Separate tables present information suitable for different phases of study and for specific factors, such as placebo, compliance, and adverse reactions.

The clinical monitor who is responsible for developing and implementing the clinical evaluation of a potential new drug usually receives a large quantity of information to assist in planning activities. These reports include data on preclinical studies conducted in pharmacology, biochemistry, toxicology, metabolism, and other scientific disciplines. Reports and/or publications of any clinical studies that have been previously conducted are also included. Establishing a clinical plan, preparing a protocol for the initial study, and developing an investigator's brochure are usually the first steps conducted.

CURRENT ISSUES FOR DEVELOPING DRUGS FOR CNS INDICATIONS

Ability of Patients to Give an Informed Consent

There must be adequate safeguards to protect patients who are not mentally competent to understand their rights and provide an informed consent. This may be done through family members, professional staff, legal guardians, and/or Investigational Review Boards (IRBs). This issue is especially pertinent in studies with drugs that treat CNS diseases or problems, since patients may be mentally retarded, brain damaged, senile, psychotic, severely depressed, or otherwise handicapped. It may be relevant to give patients a simple "test" to determine if they have the minimum level of understanding required to give their informed consent. The particular criteria chosen to allow patients to sign an informed consent must be acceptable to the IRB that approved the study.

At present there is no accepted "test" to verify that a patient is mentally qualified to provide informed consent. Consent forms describe various aspects of a study and detail the rights of patients, but many patients cannot adequately comprehend this material. Having a patient read and sign a form does not insure the patient's understanding of the contents.

It is often possible to enhance patients' understanding of the contents of an informed consent by (a) requiring a written or verbal test of the patient, (b) having discussion sessions with groups of patients and family members, and/or (c) repeating the warnings contained in the informed consent several times during the study. There are several reasons why it is not advisable to follow these methods. The basis of evaluating an informed consent is that it contains information required by law and is written in a manner that is understandable.

A potential problem is that these methods may improve patients' understanding at the price of instilling fear and misunderstanding, and thus may be counterproductive. Patients or volunteers who enter studies are generally unable to fully evaluate the medical information presented. Thus, the use of these techniques may cause patients to be less likely, rather than more likely, to do what is in their best medical interest.

A different approach that may reassure the investigator and IRB that patients enrolled have a general comprehension of the contents of the informed consent is achieved by asking patients three questions and discussing their responses prior to signing the informed consent. These questions which are not intended to meet any specific legal standards, are intended as a rough gauge of the patient's capacity to consent to participate in research. It is preferable for the questions to be discussed rather than just answered with a yes or no.

1. Do you understand that by signing this informed consent document you are agreeing to participate in a clinical study for up to _____ (days, weeks, months) and to cooperate in following these general requirements: _____ ?
2. Do you understand that the following alternative treatments exist (if any), plus the alternative not to participate, and you can withdraw from the study at any time without jeopardizing the care and concern of the health care providers?
3. Do you understand that you would be participating in research and you may risk possibly harmful adverse effects from this treatment and (if applicable) some potential benefits from this treatment?

Although these questions are covered in most informed consent forms and may be discussed in some instances, adopting a formal discussion procedure as part of obtaining informed consent assures that critical issues will be discussed beyond a simple reading of the form.

How Does One Deal with the Problem of Inadequate Animal Models in Choosing Compounds to Develop in Humans?

In some areas of medicine (e.g., infectious diseases), the predictability of data from animal models for human outcomes is excellent, whereas in other areas the predict-ability is poor. Animal models of CNS diseases are a varied group, but in general are near the poor end of the predictability spectrum. There are numerous neurological diseases where animal models either are not present or are inadequate for generating adequate information of drug activity. A few such diseases include Alzheimer's, multiple sclerosis, and Parkinson's disease. There are no suitable animal models for most psychiatric diseases such as schizophrenia or panic disorder. There are some CNS diseases, however, where reasonable animal models do exist; these include (a) inborn errors in metabolism, (b) antidepressants, and (c) anticonvulsants. Animal models in psychopathology are described by Bond (1). The process of extrapolating from animal models to human testing is described by Spilker (15).

There is no simple solution to the problem of inadequate animal models. The best approach is to (a) use state-of-the-art methods; (b) evaluate standard drugs as well as test compounds in the models; (c) utilize a battery of both *in vitro* and *in vivo* models; (d) evaluate and compare dose-response relationships of several drugs obtained in several models, species, and conditions; (e) consult eminent authorities in the field; and (f) use models that evaluate biochemical as well as physiological mechanisms. Factors to consider in extrapolating data from animal models to humans are listed in Table 1.

How Many Efficacy Parameters and Independent Raters Should Be Used in Clinical Studies?

It is important to use objective, validated efficacy measures whenever possible in a study and to develop such methods

TABLE 1. *Factors to consider in extrapolating results from animal models of CNS diseases to humans*

1. There are no animal models that accurately mimic schizophrenia, endogenous depression, or senile dementia. Therefore, neuropharmacological dysfunctions of the brain that are believed to be present in these diseases are created in animals and then used as models. It is essential to carefully evaluate data obtained with standard drugs.
2. Extrapolating results obtained in these models to humans assumes that the target human disease is associated with the dysfunction(s) created. Another major assumption is that the organization and function of the animal brain is similar to the human brain insofar as the target disease is concerned.
3. Animal models exist at multiple levels of organization (e.g., subcellular, cellular, tissue, organ, organism) and utilize techniques from a wide range of scientific disciplines (e.g., biochemistry, pharmacology) to obtain data.[a]
4. Drugs presumed to act on the nervous system solely, either centrally or peripherally, may have other actions as well. These additional effects should be searched for and evaluated by various techniques (e.g., autoradiographic distribution, pithed animals, pharmacological research tools, comparing the time course of various effects, establishing dose-response relationships).

[a] See Table 1 in ref. 4.

when they do not exist. When only subjective or quasiobjective measures (e.g., questionnaires, clinical global impressions) are available to evaluate drug efficacy, many studies include multiple efficacy parameters. The number of parameters and statistical tests conducted, however, must be limited, or else there will be a high probability of having significant effects occurring by chance alone. This creates a difficulty in that there is an uncertainty in knowing whether positive results are clinically important and whether the treatment is effective.

Several approaches to this issue are to (a) include fewer tests and/or parameters in the study; (b) use only the most appropriate scales or tests for a particular situation; (c) prioritize all of the possible efficacy measures prior to the test, so that a statistically significant result observed in a minor test is not later used to claim drug efficacy; (d) define *a priori* the magnitude of effect for each of the primary parameters that would be clinically important; and/or (e) combine various tests and/or parameters to obtain either a single overall index value or a smaller number of parameters to evaluate. If this last approach is adopted, it should be followed in all appropriate clinical studies conducted on the investigational drug, not just those in which it is convenient (and beneficial) to use the index. There should be a scientific rationale for choosing the tests and parameters that are combined into an index score, as well as for any weighting of individual parameters or scores. The index should be validated with data from standard drugs (if standard drugs exist) before it is used with investigational drugs. The validation may be done with historical data, if necessary.

Another related issue is whether a scale is being used appropriately (i.e., in the correct patients and in the correct manner). For instance, the Hamilton Anxiety Scale was designed to measure the severity of anxiety in patients with a diagnosis of anxiety disorder, but is sometimes used to measure effects in depressed patients, even though the assumptions of the test are not necessarily relevant. The practice of using this test in patients with other diagnoses has been questioned (7).

When objective criteria and data are used to evaluate drug efficacy, it is unnecessary to use multiple raters. But when a drug's activity is judged using subjective data, especially if they are elicited in an interview, it is often valuable to have two independent raters.

Using two raters who each rate the same patient throughout a study usually improves a study, whereas multiple raters for different patients usually adds variability and may seriously affect the outcome. Raters whose evaluations differ from their colleagues will adversely affect a study.

There are many reasons why a single rater may obtain incorrect or misleading data. Using a second rater will help control for possible sources of error. The sources of error include those related to the (a) investigator (e.g., training, experience, attitudes and biases toward the study and patient, ability to obtain relevant and sufficient information from the patient, inadequate duration of evaluations because of time constraints); (b) therapist (when the therapist is not the rater of the patient); (c) patient (e.g., degree of cooperativeness, attitude toward the study, attitude toward each investigator or rater); (d) study design and conduct (e.g.,

too few evaluations, use of too many subjective parameters); and (e) study instruments (e.g., excessively long scales may be completed too rapidly because of time constraints or completed improperly because of patient frustration).

The major difficulties of using a second rater include (a) expense; (b) problems of training; (c) difficulties of analyzing additional data; (d) difficulties in interpreting results, which may be biased if patients behave differently toward different raters; and (e) necessity of evaluating interrater differences prior to incorporating the concept in a protocol.

Derogatis et al. (3) reported that when two independent raters were used with the Inpatient Multidimensional Psychiatric Scale there was an increase in power of statistical tests used, and the sample size required to achieve a given power was reduced by about 16%.

It was reported (2) that interrater reliability for the Hamilton and Raskin Depression Rating Scales was greater at the end of the study when fewer symptoms were present than during patient randomization. They also reported that interrater reliability was greater for factor or total scores than for individual items in the scales.

What Control Populations Should Be Included in CNS Drug Studies?

Variations in patient responses to CNS drugs are generally greater than in other therapeutic areas. The primary reasons for this situation may relate to the imprecision in diagnosis, heterogeneity of disease characteristics, and increased number of subjective, emotional, and psychological factors that are part of many CNS diseases. Control of these factors will tend to decrease both intra- and interpatient variability.

The issue of identifying the best control group(s) arises in many studies of CNS drugs. Multiple control populations and treatments are often required but are rarely included in studies. For example, in studies on autistic children, control groups are often matched with patients based on mental and chronological ages. Matching controls are based on intellectual development, since autistic children have disturbances of speech, language, and nonverbal communication. Tsai and Beisler (17) reported that two commonly used tests of language comprehension (the Peabody Picture Vocabulary Test and the Test for Auditory Comprehension of Language) do not yield similar results for choosing language-matched controls. This raises the additional problem of identifying the best means to choose control patients once the nature of the control group is established.

In the field of schizophrenia there is a lack of agreement on whether subtypes exist and if they do, how they should be defined. Subtypes have been described in numerous categories, including paranoid-nonparanoid, acute-chronic, process-reactive, and good-poor premorbid. Lewine (8) has noted that making comparisons between subtypes and control groups unrelated for subtype characteristics makes it impossible to determine if "subtype differences are: (a) specific to schizophrenia, (b) characteristic of severe psychiatric disorder, (c) characteristic of severe disorder in general, or (d) normal variations in personality." He characterizes many research studies as either omitting nonschizophrenic control groups or assuming that their control

TABLE 2. *Considerations for phase I evaluations of CNS drugs*

1. Patients, in lieu of or in addition to normal volunteers, should be enrolled in phase I studies whenever possible.
2. Patients with certain diseases (e.g., epilepsy) who have induced hepatic microsomal enzymes from concomitant drugs may metabolize drugs differently than normal volunteers.
3. Tests should be included to probe for CNS-related adverse reactions (e.g., behavioral, performance, and psychological tests).
4. Tests such as those that assess mood or feelings are often helpful in obtaining subclinical information on potential CNS areas where adverse reactions may occur with higher doses or with repeated doses.
5. Phase I studies present an opportunity to evaluate the effects of a drug on behavioral rating scales, psychometric tests, and performance tests in normal volunteers. These tests include measurement of perceptual skills, mental acumen, motor skills and accuracy, coordination, judgment, and social skills.
6. Effects of drugs on electroencephalograms of normal volunteers and/or abnormal patients may be assessed.
7. Phase I studies may be conducted with patients as well as normals to obtain data on (a) how the drug is absorbed, metabolized, and eliminated, and (b) how the drug is tolerated on a subchronic basis (e.g., 2 or 4 weeks).
8. It is difficult to obtain efficacy data during phase I, because characteristics of safety and dosage regimen are unknown. In some situations, however, changes in laboratory or other parameters may provide indications about efficacy.
9. Effects of drugs on the CNS may be affected by the type and level of activities and noise in the study environment, as well as by the amount and type of movies, television programs, and physical activities permitted.

group is homogeneous. He suggests multiple control groups to evaluate paranoid schizophrenics including (a) normals, (b) medical patients, and (c) nonschizophrenic psychiatric patients who have paranoid attributes.

The use of control groups was evaluated in a review of 478 articles published between 1970 and 1979 for studies involving schizophrenic patients. Because schizophrenics are not always psychotic, it is important to control for psychosis in studies with schizophrenic patients. Controls for psychosis were present in only 11% of the articles reviewed. Most studies included nonpsychiatric controls (primarily normals), and a smaller number of studies included nonpsychotic psychiatric controls (10). Of the 478 studies, only 13 (2.7%) were comprehensively controlled.

The size of the control (and treatment) groups is an important, related issue. The size of the patient population to be enrolled in a study should be established using statistical techniques prior to the study. When an excessive number of patients is entered in a study, the power may be adequate to detect very small differences between groups. These statistically significant differences often are not clinically important. On the other hand, when an inadequate number of patients is enrolled, the power of the study is too small. In either situation an article may be published that may inadvertently mislead the medical community.

CONSIDERATIONS RELATING TO STUDY DESIGN AND CONDUCT

Numerous considerations relating to various aspects of study design and conduct are presented in Tables 2 to 14. These tables are divided into two broad categories:

1. Phases of drug studies—Tables 2 to 5
2. Factors relating to study design (e.g., placebo, compliance, adverse reactions)—Tables 6 to 14.

TABLE 3. *Considerations for phase II evaluations of CNS drugs*

A. Factors relating to study design
1. Use of single-patient experiments with CNS drugs is justified under certain circumstances, especially when multiple treatments within the same patient may be randomized on a daily (or weekly) basis.[a]
2. Pilot studies to evaluate efficacy do not provide adequate demonstrations of a drug's efficacy but hopefully indicate the dosage regimen to be used in controlled studies.
3. All pilot studies should be well designed and well controlled. This includes using double-blind techniques whenever possible to minimize the possibility of obtaining false positive data.[b]
4. Concomitant use of psychotherapy during a study must be controlled. Terminating psychotherapy just prior to a study may cause a carryover effect.
5. An adequate washout period must be allowed after previous drug and/or nondrug treatment is discontinued.
6. Length of study must be sufficient to convince both regulatory agencies (when appropriate) and the prescribing physician that the drug has activity under appropriate clinical conditions to adequately treat the illness.
7. The use of placebo is highly controversial in some studies but justifiable in most studies. Ethical issues should be discussed with the IRB.
8. An initial single-blind placebo period for all patients may be used to eliminate the placebo responders from a study prior to randomization for certain CNS diseases (e.g., Parkinson's disease).
9. Followup evaluations of patients after completion of drug treatment may provide important data on the reemergence of disease symptoms, potential carryover benefits of treatment, and possible withdrawal effects of the drug.
10. Most studies evaluating CNS-active drugs do not use a crossover design, primarily because of the instability of chronic CNS diseases. Under certain conditions it is possible to conduct crossover studies in epilepsy.
11. Clinical Global Impression Scale (CGI) is an important measure of efficacy, especially when used in double-blind controlled study designs. The CGI may be general and unstructured, or it may focus on one or a few specific symptoms or criteria.

TABLE 3. (*Continued*)

12. It is often worthwhile for the CGI to be completed by nurses and/or family of the patient as well as by investigators. The form used must be carefully worded to obtain information on the (a) presence of symptoms, (b) intensity of symptoms, (c) degree to which symptoms (if present) appear to be bothersome, and (d) change from baseline.
13. Since psychopathology may markedly affect the patient's perception of his or her own status and change, a CGI should be completed by patients when it is believed that they can provide meaningful self-ratings. In addition, their desire to please or displease the investigator will also affect their responses on the CGI.

B. Factors relating to patients enrolled in a study
1. Patient diagnoses should be established with *Diagnostic and Statistical Manual of Mental Disorders,* 3rd edition (*DSM-III*) and/or other standard criteria established by professional societies or other groups.
2. When a study is evaluating patients whose diagnoses are not clearly established (e.g., schizophrenia), it may be valuable to have patients diagnosed by two independent raters.
3. Psychiatric patients who refuse to participate in studies may differ significantly from those who do.[c] One group[d] reported that patients who refused to participate were more hostile on initial approach by the interviewer and were more likely to abuse alcohol and drugs.
4. Depressed and schizophrenic patients who are excluded from an inpatient study may differ in age, sex, legal status, and other factors from patients admitted to studies.[e]
5. Establish previous response to medical therapy whenever possible, to confirm that patients have the ability to respond to treatment (i.e., eliminate known nonresponders from a study before it starts).
6. Patients who have an imminently high risk of being suicidal should almost always be eliminated from studies, especially if there is a chance that they may receive placebo or if the efficacy of the study drug has not yet been demonstrated.
7. It is usually preferable to enroll a homogeneous population of patients in pivotal phase II studies; however, assuring patient uniformity is often difficult.
8. Study specific disease subtype(s) whenever possible, in lieu of mixed patient populations (e.g., in epilepsy, schizophrenia).
9. Patients with potentially confounding diseases should be excluded (e.g., alcoholics, demented) unless the study is designed to utilize such patients as the target population.
10. Patients with two concomitant diseases (e.g., depression and anxiety) may be identified as a target population.
11. Studies should either randomize patients by sex or analyze data by sex to determine if there is any possible influence on the results.[f]
12. Patients sometimes use old drugs or trade drugs with other patients. Urine may be monitored for presence of other drugs.

C. Other factors relating to phase II studies
1. Design and layout of psychiatric wards may have a significant effect on interpatient socialization, which may affect responses to drugs in inpatient studies.[g]
2. The milieu of the ward is well known to have an influence on patient outcome in a drug treatment protocol.
3. Restricting or fostering interpatient contact and socialization may affect the outcome of a drug study.
4. Investigators and/or staff should be trained to conduct comparable patient interviews.[h]
5. Agreement between two (or more) raters for certain psychiatric tests should be evaluated both prior to and during a study to validate data obtained by different investigators. Interrater reliability has been reported to be both poor[i] and excellent[j] for physicians who judged the severity of depression.
6. Staff to patient ratios may vary widely between sites and could affect treatment outcome.
7. Since the diagnosis of anxiety raises a possibility of psychosis, a standard test(s) to evaluate psychosis should be considered for studies evaluating antianxiety drugs.
8. Have relevant evaluations (e.g., work performance, social skills) completed by the patient's family when possible.
9. Studies on orphan drugs may require multicenter studies or novel study designs.[k]
10. Having the study pay for bed costs in inpatient studies may accelerate rate of patient entry; however, the study could become too expensive to conduct.
11. Evaluate whether pharmacokinetic parameters are the same in patients as in normal volunteers.

[a] Ref. 20.
[b] See Chapter 32 in ref. 15.
[c] Ref. 12.
[d] Ref. 5.
[e] Ref. 9.
[f] Wahl (18) reported that of 131 studies of schizophrenia (published in three journals, 1974–1976) 29 studies reported using patients of only one sex, and of the remainder (102 studies) only 11 studies mentioned analysis of the data for each sex. He also reported that 44 of 131 studies failed to mention the sex of their patients.
[g] Ref. 19.
[h] Russell et al. (11) describe 34 simulated patient characteristics used in a training session for staff.
[i] Refs. 6 and 2.
[j] Ref. 7.
[k] Ref. 16.

TABLE 4. *Considerations for phase III evaluations of CNS drugs*

1. Drug interaction studies are important to conduct with alcohol, commonly used drugs (e.g., diazepam), and standard treatments.
2. Various types of control groups may be considered, including patients who receive psychotherapy at an intense level, those who receive it at a minimal level, and those who receive usual care (see Issue number 5 in text).
3. Tests for physical dependence and abuse potential of a new drug may be assessed in populations of drug abusers, addicts, and/or patients with the disease being treated, but the first two populations are preferable.[a]
4. It may be relevant to assess evaluations of tolerance to both efficacy and adverse reactions.
5. After drug treatment is stopped it may be relevant to assess the onset of signs and symptoms in patients. These may result from either drug withdrawal or reemergence of the disease.
6. Special studies may be conducted to evaluate psychomotor performance, motor performance, or behavior (e.g., disability scales, vigilance tests, reaction times).
7. Evaluate whether plasma levels correlate with clinical effects and toxicity, as for certain antiepileptic and tricyclic antidepressant drugs.
8. Periodic evaluations of physical and mental growth and development should be included in long-term pediatric studies.
9. If too many investigators participate in a multicenter study each will generally provide only a few patients and introduce great variability.

[a] There is no means to know with certainty whether regulatory authorities will schedule a drug, and if so, in what class. Data that may be used to address this issue are important to obtain.

TABLE 5. *Considerations for phase IV evaluations of CNS drugs*

1. Many over-the-counter drugs are associated with CNS adverse reactions (e.g., sedation, dizziness) and may confound data collected with prescription drugs.[a]
2. Data sources must be carefully chosen since uses and responses to CNS drugs differ markedly between (a) in- and outpatients; (b) community and academic hospitals; (c) primary, secondary, and tertiary care facilities; and (d) indigent patients and those in the upper middle class.

[a] A list of examples is given by Shader and Greenblatt (13).

Although only a few selected study factors are discussed in this chapter, they illustrate that careful attention to detail with existing methodologies usually provides meaningful data. The opposite conclusion is also true: Lack of attention to details in study design and conduct makes it difficult for meaningful data to be obtained.

TABLE 6. *Situations when use of placebo in a study of CNS drugs is ethically justifiable[a]*

1. There is no alternative treatment available.
2. It can be shown that placebo-treated patients did as well in previous studies as patients on active drug.
3. Patients may be rapidly discontinued from the study on showing initial signs of deterioration or lack of improvement.
4. Some patients do well without receiving any treatment.

[a] When ethical standards do not permit the use of placebo drugs, other forms of controls are often necessary. A number of alternatives to placebo control groups are described in ref. 14. These include dose-response relationships, active drug controls, and in selected cases historical controls.

TABLE 7. *Location of populations used to study CNS drugs*

1. Inpatients in hospital wards or psychiatric wards
2. Outpatients at a hospital clinic
3. Nursing home residents
4. Daycare residents (e.g., for evaluating conduct disorders in children)
5. Emergency rooms in psychiatric hospitals
6. Family practice clinics

TABLE 8. *CNS problems of patients that may compromise compliance*

1. Diagnosis of dementia or other organic CNS problem
2. Diagnosis of schizophrenia or mania
3. Lack of motivation to cooperate in the study
4. Overenthusiastic patients who have difficulty adhering to requirements of the study
5. Confusion created by a complex dosing regimen for either one or multiple medications
6. Anger or upset reactions created by unpleasant, onerous, boring, or excessive demands of the study
7. Occurrence of behavioral, psychological, or other CNS adverse reactions

TABLE 9. *Possible approaches toward improving compliance*

1. Evaluate the degree of each patient's compliance and identify any reason(s) for decrease.
2. Evaluate patient's mental and physical status to assure that the requirements of the study do not surpass the patient's abilities.
3. Determine what factors would increase the patient's motivation (e.g., providing meals and/or transportation, providing a stipend).
4. Simplify the patient's dosage regimen as much as possible within limits set by the protocol.
5. Decrease the drug dosage to reduce or eliminate adverse reactions.
6. Minimize demands of the study that bother patients.
7. Provide counseling to the patient.
8. Assess whether there is a previous history of noncompliance prior to the study. Exclude patients if it is considered that there is a high likelihood of its recurring.

TABLE 10. *CNS problems of patients that may lead to adverse reactions, and possible approaches toward a solution*

A. Problems that may lead to adverse reactions
   1. Not taking the drug as prescribed (e.g., taking too many, too few, or an irregular amount of drug). This could be deliberate or forgetful.
   2. Symptoms of a concurrent illness that may be partly or entirely responsible for the adverse reactions.
   3. Adverse reactions from concomitant medications confounding results with the study drug.
   4. "Contact effects" of certain adverse reactions may occur when multiple patients are housed in one room. This leads to a falsely elevated incidence of the particular problem (e.g., nausea, malaise, fatigue, ataxia, or an even more serious problem).
B. Possible approaches toward a solution
   1. Evaluate all adverse reactions and carefully assess the reason(s) for their occurrence.
   2. Follow the course of the adverse reaction and any concurrent illness to determine if any association is present.
   3. Modify the drug dosage and evaluate changes in adverse reactions.
   4. Perform psychological tests to identify possible clues that may lead toward patient improvement.
   5. Conduct a psychiatric evaluation to probe for hidden motivations.
   6. Conduct a physical examination to probe for organic explanations.
   7. Place patients in separate rooms or in rooms with only one (or two) roommates.

TABLE 11. *Factors to consider in evaluating efficacy of CNS drugs*

1. Some efficacy scales are not linear throughout the range tested (e.g., a difference on the Hamilton Depression Scale of 5 points is quite different for scores changing from 10 to 5 and from 25 to 20).
2. Some drugs (e.g., nomifensine) appear to have documented efficacy in outpatient studies, but not in inpatient studies.
3. Enrolling drug-naive patients usually reduces the number of nonresponders in a study of many CNS drugs; however, drug-sophisticated patients generally respond "better" to certain drugs (e.g., cannabinoids). In addition, it is usually difficult to locate and enroll drug-naive patients.
4. Use performance, behavioral, and physical disability tests when appropriate.
5. Use additional tests/parameters to evaluate efficacy (e.g., compare rate of patient dropout for groups on test drug, active control drug, and placebo; compare number of days in a hospital over a year or other period).[a]

[a] See ref. 15 for list of numerous other efficacy parameters that may be measured.

TABLE 12. *Factors to consider in measuring quality of life in studies with CNS drugs*

1. Degree of physical abilities and disabilities
2. Degree of psychological abilities and disabilities
3. Ability of patients to function on their own versus depending on others
4. Number of days a patient is able to work
5. Number of episodes of disease or medical problems in a given period
6. Ability of patients to cope with their problems
7. Degree to which unpleasant adverse reactions are avoided
8. Degree to which patient is productive and feels positive about himself/herself

TABLE 13. *Specific factors to control in studies of CNS drugs both intrasite and intersite*

1. Use of concomitant drugs and/or concomitant nondrug treatments
2. Differences in ward procedures between different sites of a multicenter study, relating to drug dispensing and study conduct that may influence patient reactions
3. Housing too many patients in a single room, since this may lead to "contact" reactions
4. Ward design may influence patient contact and socialization[a]
5. Artificially separating inpatients from normal social contact will eventually create adverse reactions
6. Attitude and behavior of the investigator toward the patient usually has a major influence on the rate and degree of improvement on treatment in psychiatric studies
7. Degree of adherence to the protocol

[a] Ref. 19.

TABLE 14. *Advantages of inpatient studies*

1. Potential sources of external stress (e.g., family, employer) are reduced.
2. Conditions for all patients are more comparable than for outpatients.
3. The same staff usually treat and evaluate all patients.[a]
4. More complex study designs may be used.

[a] This often applies to outpatient studies too.

ACKNOWLEDGMENTS

The author appreciates reviews of the manuscript by Drs. J. Davidson, C. Gorodetsky, and J. Schoenfelder.

REFERENCES

1. Bond, N. W., ed. (1984): *Animal Models in Psychopathology.* Academic Press, New York.
2. Cicchetti, D. V., and Prusoff, B. A. (1983): *Arch. Gen. Psychiatry,* 40:987–990.
3. Derogatis, L. R., Bonato, R. R., and Yang, K. C. (1968): *Arch. Gen. Psychiatry,* 19:689–699.

4. Drews, J. (1983): In: *Decision Making in Drug Research,* edited by F. Gross, pp. 44–55. Raven Press, New York.
5. Edlund, M. J., Craig, T. J., and Richardson, M. A. (1985): *Am. J. Psychiatry,* 142:624–627.
6. Fisch, H.-U., Hammond, K. R., Joyce, C. R. B., and O'Reilly, M. (1981): *Br. J. Psychiatry,* 138:100–109.
7. Gjerris, A., Bech, P., Bojholm, S., et al. (1983): *J. Affective Disord.,* 5:163–170.
8. Lewine, R. R. J. (1978): *Schizophr. Bull.,* 4:244–247.
9. Miller, R. D., Strickland, R., Davidson, J., and Parrott, R. (1983): *Am. J. Psychiatry,* 140:1205–1207.
10. Ritzler, B. A., and Rinehart, K. (1981): *Schizophr. Bull.,* 7:729–735.
11. Russell, M. L., Ghee, K. L., Probstfield, J. L., and Insull, W., Jr. (1983): *Controlled Clin. Trials,* 4:197–208.
12. Schubert, D. S. P., Patterson, M. B., Miller, F. T., and Brocco, K. J. (1984): *Psychiatry Res.,* 12:313–320.
13. Shader, R. I., and Greenblatt, D. J. (1982): *J. Clin. Psychiatry,* 43:8–18.
14. Spilker, B. (1984): *Guide to Clinical Studies and Developing Protocols.* Raven Press, New York.
15. Spilker, B. (1986): *Guide to Clinical Interpretation of Data.* Raven Press, New York.
16. Spilker, B. (1986): In: *Orphan Diseases and Orphan Drugs,* edited by I. H. Scheinberg and S. Walshe, pp. 119–134. Manchester University Press, Manchester, UK.
17. Tsai, L. Y., and Beisler, J. M. (1984): *J. Am. Acad. Child Psychiatry,* 23:700–703.
18. Wahl, O. F. (1977): *J. Abnorm. Psychol.,* 86:195–198.
19. Whitehead, C. C., Polsky, R. H., Crookshank, C., and Fik, E. (1984): *Am. J. Psychiatry,* 141:639–644.
20. Wolfrum, C., Klieser, E., and Lehmann, E. (1984): *Neuropsychobiology,* 12:152–157.

Psychopharmacology:
The Third Generation of Progress,
edited by Herbert Y. Meltzer.
Raven Press, New York © 1987.

CHAPTER 180

Postmarketing Surveillance of Adverse Drug Reactions

Seymour Fisher

On May 13, 1959, a New Drug Application (NDA) was approved by the Food and Drug Administration (FDA) for imipramine (Tofranil). Since February 1960 more than six labeling changes have been made to reflect new information on adverse drug reactions, including stroke and other cardiovascular warnings, alcohol potentiation, inappropriate antidiuretic hormone secretion syndrome, and interaction with cimetidine. By March 1967 enough information was available for the manufacturer to request a labeling change to reflect a new beneficial effect (i.e., for treating childhood enuresis), although final FDA approval for the labeling change was not granted until April 1973.

Trazodone (Desyrel) was first marketed in the United States on March 17, 1982. According to Scher et al. (43), the first case of priapism in a patient taking trazodone was reported to the manufacturer in July 1982, and although Scher's case report was not published until October 1983, the trazodone package insert was voluntarily changed by the manufacturer in March 1983.

And as this chapter is being written in January 1986, nomifensine (Merital)—first marketed in Europe in 1976 and in the U.S. in July 1985—has just been voluntarily withdrawn by the manufacturer from the worldwide market after accumulating reports of hemolytic anemias.

Here, then, are three examples of postmarketing surveillance in action. The issues to be discussed in this chapter concern the strengths and weaknesses of existing systems; in addition, a description of a new complementary approach will be briefly presented.

A well-functioning postmarketing surveillance system should be capable of providing answers to two primary questions:

1. How can we best detect a new adverse reaction or beneficial effects (including new therapeutic indications) from a recently FDA-approved drug? The detection function for adverse reactions comprises both an alerting mechanism for suspected side effects and a confirming or verification mechanism for definitively attributing a suspected adverse reaction to the drug.

2. When we detect an unexpected side effect of a drug (i.e., confirm its attribution), how can we best estimate its actual population incidence?

KEY DEFINITIONS

Adverse Clinical Event

All inferences about drug-induced reactions must first begin with accurate identification and description of the reactions themselves. An adverse clinical event (ACE) is simply any undesirable, unwanted reaction, either sign or symptom, either expected or unexpected, that may or may not be caused by a particular drug. If an ACE's onset clearly follows the initiation of drug treatment, it has passed the first test for being a valid ACE and can be considered as a possible adverse drug reaction.

Adverse Drug Reaction

An adverse drug reaction (ADR) is any valid ACE for which reasonably conclusive evidence exists attributing the reaction to a particular drug. All ADRs must be valid ACEs, but all ACEs are definitely not ADRs; in fact, the likelihood of any ACE turning out to be an ADR is inversely related to the number of factors other than the target drug that are capable of producing the ACE. A "new" ADR could be an ACE that previously had never been thought to be caused by the drug (i.e., the expected ADR incidence was assumed to be zero) or a previously identified ADR with a greater true incidence than expected. Some people use the term "side effect" synonomously with ADR; others tend to refer to common and expected ADRs as "side effects," reserving "ADRs" for more rare and serious drug-induced ACEs (e.g., amitriptyline-related dry mouth as a "side effect," amitriptyline-induced cardiac arrhythmia as an "ADR"). A "side effect" may also turn out to be a therapeutic effect for some other indication.

Spontaneous Reporting System

This term broadly covers all voluntary spontaneous reporting by physicians to manufacturers, journals, and governmental agencies (e.g., FDA, WHO). At the heart of this general system is the FDA's Drug Experience Report (form 1639), on which all suspected adverse reactions from marketed drugs are required to be reported to the FDA by the drug manufacturer. Jones (25) states that the FDA receives 85% of its reports from manufacturers and 15% directly from physicians. Published anecdotal reports and other monitoring studies reported in the medical literature are also part of the "spontaneous reporting" concept, since it depends on the initiative of practicing physicians and investigators to make their observations public. Voluntary reporting systems theoretically seem best suited for the alerting function of postmarketing surveillance, but can rarely confirm an ACE to be an ADR; they also have little capability for estimating ADR incidences (24).

Formal Surveillance Systems

Over the years a number of attempts have been made to establish more systematic approaches to monitoring new drugs. Some were initiated by independent "pharmacoepidemiologists," whereas others were initiated by manufacturers. The term "phase IV studies" has been applied to formal investigations, often performed by the manufacturer after NDA approval, that take place under conditions of usual clinical use of the drug; these studies commonly include no control or comparison groups. Theoretically, phase IV studies would be best capable of accurate ADR incidence estimates whenever new ADRs are successfully detected.

HISTORY OF POSTMARKETING SURVEILLANCE SYSTEMS

As a supplement to their textbooks and journals, physicians have always had an "invisible college" (i.e., word-of-mouth from colleagues) to educate them about possible adverse effects of the drugs they use. The current United States postmarketing surveillance system has evolved into a somewhat haphazard network of resources that, like the federal government itself, somehow manages to do a rea-

sonably creditable job of fulfilling its function. Since 1960 the FDA has maintained its spontaneous adverse reaction reporting system, which was supplemented in the late 1960s by other data bases from collaborating sources. Following a 1980 report by the Joint Commission on Prescription Drug Use (23), originally created by Senator Edward Kennedy in 1976, the FDA joined with the Department of Commerce's Experimental Technology Incentives Program, resulting in three publications providing an overview of existing postmarketing activities (26). Since then, the FDA has actively continued its efforts to improve existing resources and to develop new approaches to meet postmarketing needs. The FDA funds several different registries that collect ADR data, and has the authority to mandate phase IV studies as part of an NDA approval (this was done for L-dopa some years ago). In 1980 there were nine manufacturer-initiated postmarketing studies in progress, and several new psychopharmacologic agents currently under review will also require phase IV monitoring. Summaries of the FDA's current surveillance programs were recently presented at an American Public Health Association annual meeting (1,10).

In the United Kingdom, the thalidomide tragedy led W. H. W. Inman and the Committee on Safety of Medicines to establish in 1964 a "Yellow Card" alerting system for physician use (18). Subsequently, in an attempt to improve on the voluntary reporting system, Inman (19) in 1981 initiated his Prescription-Event Monitoring (PEM) program, which links prescription information with physician reports and hospital records. Many other British investigators (e.g., 3, 6, 9, 28, 35, 44) are actively pursuing improvements in existing postmarketing surveillance systems.

A 1981 NATO conference report (49) is an excellent source for a general overview of monitoring methods used in other foreign countries.

PROBLEMS IN POSTMARKETING SURVEILLANCE SYSTEMS

With recent U.S. expediting of the FDA's procedures for NDA reviews, the need for increased postmarketing surveillance of new psychotropic drugs is greater than ever. It is essential to be able to observe and correctly interpret the real-life performance of newly approved therapeutic agents in the course of usual medical practice, where patient characteristics and other factors often differ widely from those that prevailed in the premarketing clinical trials. The need is particularly compelling for drugs being used by ambulatory patients, where continual patient monitoring is considerably more difficult than with hospitalized patients.

Sources of ACE Information

Although a Medicine in the Public Interest conference report (39) concluded that the voluntary physician reporting system was "the single most important source of suspected ADRs" and further characterized the published case reports and letters-to-the-editor system as its "most valuable" form, this spontaneous reporting system suffers from serious underdetection (7,20,38,42,48). The FDA's early warning monitoring system was found by Rossi and Knapp (41) to be somewhat inferior to physician reports published in the medical literature; clearly, these "systems" each contribute to a general alerting mechanism for suspected ADRs. But there is widespread agreement that sole reliance on systems of voluntary reporting by physicians to manufacturers, journals, and government agencies (e.g., FDA, WHO) is clearly unsatisfactory (46,47)—especially for psychiatric outpatients, many of whom cannot be followed adequately after initiating treatment with a newly approved drug.

Most attempts by manufacturers and other investigators to set up formal surveillance systems in the United States have been notably unsuccessful (16,32,42). In the United Kingdom, although Venning (45) noted that the practolol disaster (drug-induced oculomucocutaneous syndrome) was not detected by the Yellow Card system in the mid-1970s, Inman (17) defends the system—in combination with his PEM program, which also allows for incidence estimates—as fulfilling its intended functions.

A number of different approaches to formal systems have been explored in the United States. Most depend on physician judgments in one form or another, including record-linkage methods such as utilization of Medicaid drug-event data (25) or data relating pharmacy prescriptions to hospital record information (15,20–22). Direct consumer contact via survey methods has been used by Mellinger (37). The Upjohn Company has reported a phase IV study based on staff-initiated direct contacts with patients by mail and telephone (2,34). It is noteworthy that there has always been a general mistrust of any voluntary *patient-initiated* formal reporting system, although most suspected ADRs in ambulatory populations stem initially from patients' spontaneous reports of ACEs. One such system—to be described below in more detail—has been recently developed by Fisher et al. (12,13) and is soon expected to be tested for its sensitivity and overall utility in detecting ADRs with newly approved antidepressants and anxiolytics.

Problems in Identifying Valid ACEs

If an ACE is to be considered a possible ADR, the foremost requirement is to ensure that the ACE was not already present before treatment with the target drug was started. This is so obvious, yet with an ambulatory patient who may be questioned up to 2 or 3 weeks after the prescription was written, the patient has to rely on memory not only as to when s/he actually began to take the medication but also for its temporal relation to the onset of the symptom(s). In one of our recent studies, we found that when patients were interviewed approximately 2 weeks after picking up a new prescription, even when told we only wanted to know about "new or unusual changes that could be possible side effects," about 25% of the ACEs first elicited were later revealed, upon close questioning, to have been present prior to starting the drug (32.4% for 1,119 patients taking tricyclic antidepressants and 21.8% for 2,062 antibiotic patients).

A second problem has to do with determining independent ACEs. Deaths following the initiation of psychopharmacologic treatment can be unambiguously counted as individual adverse events. Hospital admissions are also easy to count, but it may not always be clear whether a readmission 1 week after discharge should be meaningfully counted as a second ACE. Counting becomes fuzzier when a patient reports multiple symptoms, especially when one may be a restatement of another in slightly different words. Should "nervous" be counted as a separate symptom from "butterflies in my stomach"? Are "tired" and "sleepy" one or two ACEs? When are "tingling" and "numbness" to be considered as two ACEs rather than one?

For a related issue, consider the following: A patient states that she has been urinating frequently since starting her medication; later she mentions her mouth has been dry, and in the course of the interview also notes that she has been drinking a great deal of water. Similarly, a patient may report ACEs and also mention that the presence and severity of these ACEs kept him from getting out of bed on occasion—should "inability to get out of bed" be identified as a separate adverse clinical event?

A careful and thorough description of the onset and pattern of each ACE can sometimes help to resolve these problems rationally (e.g., if urinary frequency preceded the dry mouth the two are probably independent), but when all ACEs have occurred nearly simultaneously or in a temporal sequence consistent with a causally linked chain (e.g., pain began at 10 p.m., followed by sleep disturbance that night), specific guidelines are required for appropriate quantification. In our ongoing studies, we have arbitrarily decided that if a patient explicitly and spontaneously links two or more ACEs causally, then the dependent symptoms are considered invalid and only the "causative" symptom is a valid ACE. We are undoubtedly missing some genuine valid ACEs by using the patient's awareness of a causal link to invalidate some ACEs, but the alternative of counting each symptom as an independent valid ACE seems even more prone to false positive errors in detecting primary ADRs.

Determining Drug Causality

As noted earlier, ACEs may or may not turn out to be true ADRs, depending upon additional information that permits inferences about causality; but all ADRs must first be valid ACEs. The basic problem, of course, is that in the absence of a controlled randomized study, an observed ACE may always be caused by factors other than the target drug:

1. Other medications, foods, or substances taken concomitantly with the target drug
2. The natural course of the primary illness for which the target drug was prescribed
3. One or more complications secondary to the primary illness
4. The unexpected onset of a new illness
5. Any one of many physical, psychological, or environmental factors capable of producing the ACE
6. Placebo effects associated with starting the target drug

Much has been written about the difficulties of inferring drug causality from uncontrolled observations of ACEs (5,6,27,30,31,38,46). But history fortunately shows that in many instances we *are* able to avoid logical pitfalls and reach the right conclusions—even when ethical and practical considerations preclude withholding treatment as part of a controlled trial or by stopping and starting the drug repeatedly (i.e., instituting dechallenge and rechallenge tests) in individual patients. Nevertheless, especially in postmarketing surveillance studies where random assignment is virtually impossible, the desirability of some kind of concurrent control groups is so obvious that a method of "approximate controls" should be routinely included in every monitoring study: When a new drug is marketed there is generally a transition period of some months (possibly years) while the drug is being used increasingly in practice. In most instances physicians will have been using one or more "standard" drugs for the same indication, so that ACEs obtained from these patients can be compared with ACEs from patients being given the new drug. During the early postmarketing phases, the "control" observations may well constitute 80 to 90% of the total sample, but as the new drug gains acceptance the sample sizes will begin to balance out. Even if one questions the basic assumption that patients being given the older "standard" drug are no different from those patients for whom the new drug is being prescribed, ACEs identified with significantly greater frequency in the New Drug group are indeed most likely to be true ADRs that have different incidences from the standard drug. Similarly, *less* frequently identified ACEs in the New Drug group would be indicative of the new drug's advantages. A method similar to this is being used by Inman (19) in his Prescription Event Monitoring program, and seems to represent the best possible attempt to control for such biases as possible differences in therapeutic indications along with numerous other nondrug confounding variables including regional and seasonal factors. It is important to bear in mind, however, that if the incidence of a particular ACE in the New Drug group does not differ from the ACE incidence in the Standard Drug group, this does not imply that the ACE is not a genuine drug-induced adverse reaction; it only means that, relative to the Standard Drug selected for comparison, it cannot be considered a new ADR since the ACE could be an ADR common to both drugs.

Frequency and Severity of ACEs

Most surveillance systems are especially targeted for early warnings about unsuspected toxicity. However, the need for monitoring "nonserious" as well as "serious" adverse events, strongly adovocated by Jones (25), was highlighted in a discussion of Jones's paper when Finney (25, p. 216) wondered whether thalidomide-induced peripheral neuropathy would probably not have been detected by the FDA's voluntary reporting system since physicians tend to complete and submit a form 1639 only for the more blatent ACEs (39). A comprehensive system must be capable of detecting true incidence differences in less noxious ADRs as well as those that are of great societal concern. The more pernicious ACEs, because they have relatively few nondrug causal factors, are rarely seen. And although this is fortunate for the public, it is not so fortunate for monitoring systems. The FDA is properly concerned with alerting the medical community to extremely serious ADRs. But other less serious ADRs also play a major role in medical practice. The FDA also requires in official package inserts a list of numerous ACEs for which there are varying degrees of evidence supporting their status as true ADRs. And here we have the paradox that, although existing reporting systems suffer from underreporting of true ADRs, they tend to overreport ACEs that are most likely not true ADRs. One recent methodologically oriented study found when patients were interviewed about possible side effects 2 weeks after beginning antibiotic therapy that, in contrast to spontaneously reported symptoms, ACEs elicited by a detailed review of symptom areas actually impaired the accurate detection of some well-known, common antibiotic ADRs (12,13). With increasing patient demand for information about side effects (14,36), it is more important than ever that the FDA be able to better discriminate ADRs from ACEs so that the official labeling will include primarily those adverse clinical events with a high probability of being true adverse drug reactions.

FUTURE DIRECTIONS

Klein et al. (29) attempted to summarize the known ADRs from tricyclic antidepressants along with their estimated incidences. Although some of the studies on which the summary was based came from premarketing controlled trials, many were postmarketing reports. The authors note that "the data on side effects are often confusing and show great variation from study to study."

Similar comments could be made about most psychotropic drugs currently in use. In large part, this ignorance reflects the primitive state of our postmarketing methodologies when applied to adverse drug reactions. It has taken medicine in general, and psychiatry in particular, many decades to reach an appreciation of the need for assessing therapeutic effects using standardized instruments and methods.

The practitioner's judgment of "I think s/he's (mildly, moderately, or greatly) improved" is simply inadequate—although not to be discarded. Yet, with only a few notable exceptions, standardized documentation of possible ADRs is woefully lacking. Most practitioners and researchers seeking to identify and measure ADRs use some form of clinical interview as their starting point. The ACEs may have been elicited during "interviews" ranging from a casual inquiry about how the patient has been feeling since starting the drug to a detailed review of organ systems (e.g., 35,37,40,46). Even in controlled clinical trials, it is usually impossible to tell from the published paper how adverse effects were elicited and measured. In a thorough review of the antidepressant properties of trazodone, Bryant and Ereshefsky (4) were able to create a table describing in detail each of 14 different studies, specifying the rating scales and other assessment measures used to evaluate *therapeutic* improvement; but no evaluations of adverse effects could be included in the table, reflecting the authors' inability to determine that information from the primary published sources. Recent development of standardized interviews like the National Institute of Mental Health's "Systematic Assessment for Treatment Emergent Events" (33) may help to increase the level of sophistication in eliciting and reporting adverse clinical events.

There is little doubt that the 1980 report of the Joint Commission on Prescription Drug Use spurred much interest and activity in the postmarketing surveillance area. The commission explicitly commended the FDA for its progress, and then recommended that postmarketing surveillance should be a priority program of the FDA. (The report also recommended the establishment of a private, nonprofit "Center for Drug Surveillance" to provide a single systematic and comprehensive system of postmarketing surveillance; this recommendation has not been implemented to date.)

It is clear that a meaningful systematic approach demands the development and application of multiple complementary methods. Physician-initiated and record linkage systems are essential monitoring components, but there is considerable room for innovative supplements. One particular promising direction, mentioned earlier, is in the development of a pharmacy-based, patient-initiated monitoring system for ambulatory populations. A cohort of patients filling a prescription for a newly approved drug is recruited as consenting, active "participants," while a comparable "control" group filling new prescriptions for a standard drug is concurrently recruited. The information given to the patient at the time of recruitment (and repeated on the written consent form) states that important information is being collected about how often side effects of medicines can occur; that the prescribed medicine(s) have been proved to be safe and effective; that there is no reason to believe that the medicine(s) should cause any special problem, although all prescription medicines may occasionally cause unwanted side effects in some patients; and that the patient is being asked to use a toll-free telephone to report any "new or unusual symptoms," other adverse health events (including hospitalizations), or any unexpected health benefits. The patient is given a full explanation of what else is expected during the defined monitoring period (which could be as short as 2 weeks after starting the medication to possibly 1 year or longer). Consenting patients are given removable stickers with a toll-free number along with a summary of details about how and when to report any new ACEs; it is suggested that the stickers be placed on their bathroom mirror or elsewhere as a general reminder. Patients who do not call should be periodically sent letters reminding them that when they are not heard from, it is assumed that they have not experienced any unusual health events (these letters almost always produce additional calls). A brief questionnaire should be included with each reminder letter, not only for related information, but particularly to know that contact with the patient is being maintained. The basic ACE reports, then, are obtained from these patient-generated telephone calls to carefully trained staff who conduct a standardized computer-assisted interview each time. Computer-directed interviews have the special advantage that, after the patient's presenting complaints have been recorded verbatim, the necessary followup questions appearing on the interviewer's video screen are almost completely determined by the patient's prior response; an additional advantage lies in the fact that most of the patient's responses are entered directly into the database at the time of the interview (8).

Telephone reports must be supplemented, when necessary, by individual case investigations searching for unreported hospitalizations and deaths in patients with whom contact has been lost.

At any one time the system will be accumulating ACEs simultaneously from the New Drug and Standard Drug cohorts. A statewide or nationwide network of collaborating pharmacies could readily recruit many thousands of New Drug exposures annually without difficulty. A computer can be easily programmed to continuously scan each new ACE and compare its relative frequency in the two cohorts. The ACEs can be coded for combinations of ACEs and diagnoses as well as individual signs and symptoms. As telephone reports are received from patients, whenever a difference in relative frequencies is detected between the two groups, the computer can signal an alert. The threshold level for defining a "difference" could depend, in part, upon the nature of the ACE: *any* rare or potentially serious adverse event identified in the New Drug group (e.g., vomiting of blood, seizures, unexplained episodes of loss of consciousness, yellowing of eyes or skin, sudden numbness, or hospitalization for an unexpected illness) should be immediately flagged for comparison with the Standard Drug group. For less noxious ACEs, whenever four or more reports of a single symptom or combination of symptoms (syndrome) accumulate in any drug group, the alert could be sequentially signaled if the incidence estimates are different at, say, less than the .20 probability level. Once a New Drug ACE has been signaled as being different from the Standard Drug (remembering that an ACE may be signaled because its relative frequency is greater in the Standard Drug group), changes in significance levels could be followed continuously over the entire monitoring period.

This kind of patient-initiated reporting system has several attractive features:

1. The system is simple. Direct staff-initiated patient contact is minimal, so that for every 10,000 patients recruited into the study only a small percentage will result in a full interview. And under appropriate conditions, patient-initiated reports of ACEs can be highly reliable.

2. The system is highly cost effective. The cost of having physicians or other staff systematically conduct interviews (repeated several times at various intervals) with an entire cohort of patients is exorbitant compared to the funding required to support an efficient patient-initiated system.

3. The system is efficient in obtaining results even while one particular study is ongoing. Phase IV studies generally do not (i.e., read "can not") analyze their data until the patient monitoring period has been completed and all data have been collected. With a patient-initiated system the data analyses are sequential and continuous.

4. The system contains ADR verification potential as opposed to the mere reporting of ACEs associated with target drug use. The computer-generated alert for new ACEs with a larger New Drug incidence compared to the

Standard Drug goes a long way toward identifying a "semiconfirmed" ADR, thereby reducing the number of false positives.

5. The system has the potential for more accurate incidence estimates of newly detected ADRs, since accurate information is available for the denominator of such rates (the actual number of patients who started taking the target drug).

6. The system permits the identification of potential drug advantages by detecting reduced incidences of expected ADRs.

7. The system need not be limited to adverse drug reactions. By including in the patient instructions a request for reports of any unexpected benefits as well as adverse health events, the system may uncover unsuspected therapeutic indications for the target drug.

However, there are some obvious intrinsic limitations to a voluntary, spontaneous patient-initiated reporting system that should be recognized:

1. The system may be most applicable only with patients who clearly understand what is required of them and agree to participate actively, thereby introducing a possible bias in interpreting and generalizing the results.

2. Incidence estimates based on the system are still likely to be underestimated for various reasons:

(a) The system by itself is unlikely to detect drug-induced mortality and must be supplemented by death registry searches.

(b) The system may underdetect drug-induced hospital admissions that will go unreported by telephone because of inconvenience to the patient.

(c) Long-delayed insidious ADRs (e.g., interstitial nephritis, endometrial cancer) may never be detected within the system, nor will any ADRs that are only first detectable by a clinical laboratory procedure (e.g., low sperm count or leukocytosis).

(d) Some patients may be hesitant in reporting certain kinds of ACEs (e.g., genital-urinary) to lay interviewers (although it may be easier to discuss them by telephone than in a face-to-face situation).

(e) From our previous research it appears that patient motivation to report *new* ACEs by telephone may decrease over time, especially if use of the target medication has been terminated before the required reporting period has ended. To even approach the quintessential level of patient-initiated appropriate actions, the system not only must select well-motivated patients initially but probably has to be supplemented by staff-initiated periodic mailings of "Reminder" letters to participating patients.

Despite these limitations, the system is substantially simpler and more cost effective than any other direct patient-contact approach currently being used in phase IV and other formal surveillance systems. The development and validation of such a system is currently being supported by the National Institute of Mental Health (12,13). By complementing voluntary physician-initiated systems with valid and sensitive patient-initiated reporting systems, we may be closer to achieving the ultimate goal of having a more comprehensive system of postmarketing surveillance.

ACKNOWLEDGMENTS

I am indebted to my colleagues Stephen G. Bryant, Pharm.D., Bruce Mansbridge, Ph.D., and Brenda L. Solovitz, Dr. P.H., who have worked so closely with me on our current postmarketing surveillance project. The study is supported in part by a research grant (MH-39661) from the National Institute of Mental Health.

REFERENCES

1. Anello, C., and O'Neill, R. T. (1985): Presented at the American Public Health Association meeting, November 17–21, 1985, Washington, DC.
2. Borden, E. K., and Lee, J. G. (1982): *J. Chronic Dis.*, 35:803–816.
3. Bridgman, K. M., Carr, M., and Tattersall, A. B. (1984): *J. Int. Med. Res.*, 12:40–45.
4. Bryant, S. G., and Ereshefsky, L. (1982): *Clin. Pharmacy*, 1:406–417.
5. Castle, W. M., and Lewis, J. A. (1984): *Br. Med. J.*, 288:1458–1459.
6. Castle, W. M., Nicholls, J. T., and Downie, C. C. (1983): *Br. J. Clin. Pharmacol.*, 16:581–585.
7. Cluff, L. E., Thornton, G. F., and Seidl, L. G. (1964): *JAMA*, 188:976–983.
8. Crawley, J. A., Houchard, R. A., and Krieger, K. S. (1983): *Clin. Res. Pract. Drug Reg. Affairs*, 1:303–311.
9. Crombie, I. K., Brown, S. V., and Hamley, J. G. (1984): *J. Epidemiol. Community Health*, 38:226–231.
10. Faich, G. A. (1985): Presented at the American Public Health Association meeting, November 17–21, 1985, Washington, DC.
11. Finney, D. J. (1984): In: *Detection and Prevention of Adverse Drug Reactions*, edited by H. Bostrom and N. Ljungstedt, p. 216. Almqvist & Wiksell International, Stockholm.
12. Fisher, S., Bryant, S. G., and Kluge, R. M. (1986): *Psychopharmacol. Bull.*, 22:272–277.
13. Fisher, S., Bryant, S. G., and Kluge, R. M. (1986): *Psychopharmacology*, 90:347–350.
14. Fisher, S., Mansbridge, B., and Lankford, A. (1982): *Arch. Gen. Psychiatry*, 39:707–711.
15. Gardner, P., and Watson, L. J. (1970): *Clin. Pharmacol. Ther.*, 11:802–807.
16. Hollister, L. E., and Overall, J. E. (1984): *J. Clin. Pharmacol.*, 24:3–5.
17. Inman, W. H. W. (1983): *Br. Med. J.*, 286:719–720.
18. Inman, W. H. W. (1983): *Practitioner*, 227:1443–1449.
19. Inman, W. H. W. (1984): *Acta Med. Scand. (Suppl.)*, 683:119–126.
20. Jick, H. (1977): *N. Engl. J. Med.*, 296:481–485.
21. Jick, H. (1985): *Pharmacotherapy*, 5:280–284.
22. Jick, H., Walker, A. M., and Spriet-Pourra, C. (1979): *JAMA*, 242:2310–2314.
23. Joint Commission on Prescription Drug Use (1980): *Report of the Commission.* Rockville, MD.
24. Jones, J. K. (1982): *Drug Inf. J.*, 16:87–92.
25. Jones, J. K. (1984): In: *Detection and Prevention of Adverse Drug Reactions*, edited by H. Bostrom and N. Ljungstedt, pp. 203–214. Almqvist & Wiksell International, Stockholm.
26. Jones, J. K. (1985): In: *Clinical and Social Pharmacology Postmarketing Period*, edited by J. L. Alloza, pp. 14–24. Editio Cantor, Aulendorf, FR Germany.
27. Karch, F. E., and Lasagna, L. (1977): *Clin. Pharmacol. Ther.*, 21:247–254.
28. Kay, C. R. (1983): *J. R. Coll. Gen. Pract.*, 33:438–441.
29. Klein, D. F., Gittelman, R., Quitkin, F., and Rifkin, A. (1980):

Diagnosis and Drug Treatment of Psychiatric Disorders: Adults and Children. Williams and Wilkins, Baltimore.

30. Knapp, D. E., Zax, B. B., Rossi, A. C., and O'Neill, R. T. (1980): *Drug Intell. Clin. Pharmacy,* 14:23–27.

31. Kramer, M. S., Leventhal, J. M., Hutchinson, T. A., and Feinstein, A. R. (1979): *JAMA,* 242:623–632.

32. Lasagna, L. (1983): *JAMA,* 249:2224–2225.

33. Levine, J., and Schooler, N. (1984): *Clin. Neuropharmacol. (Suppl.),* 7:856–857.

34. Luscombe, F. A. (1984): Presented at the Drug Information Association Workshop, October 19, 1984, Bethesda, MD.

35. Maclay, W. P., Crowder, D., Spiro, S., and Turner, P. (1984): *Br. Med. J.,* 288:911–914.

36. Mansbridge, B., and Fisher, S. (1984): *Psychopharmacology,* 82:225–228.

37. Mellinger, G. D. (1984): Presented at the American College of Neuropsychopharmacology meeting, December 10–14, 1984, San Juan, PR.

38. MIPI (1975): *Adverse Drug Reactions in the United States.* Medicine in the Public Interest, Washington, DC.

39. MIPI (1977): *Postmarketing Surveillance of Drugs.* Medicine in the Public Interest, Washington, DC.

40. Rauch, E. F. (1979): *Drug Inf. J.,* 13:75–83.

41. Rossi, A. C., and Knapp, D. E. (1984): *JAMA,* 252:1030–1033.

42. Rossi, A. C., Knapp, D. E., Anello, C., O'Neill, R. T., Graham, C. F., Mendelis, P. S., and Standley, G. R. (1983): *JAMA,* 249:2226–2228.

43. Scher, M., Krieger, J. N., and Juergens, S. (1983): *Am. J. Psychiatry,* 140:1362–1363.

44. Venning, G. F. (1982): *Br. Med. J.,* 284:249–252.

45. Venning, G. F. (1983): *Br. Med. J.,* 286:199–202.

46. Venulet, J., Berneker, G., and Ciucci, A. G., eds. (1982): *Assessing Causes of Adverse Drug Reactions.* Academic Press, New York.

47. Wardell, W. M., Tsianco, M. D., Anavekar, S. N., and Davis, H. T. (1979): *J. Clin. Pharmacol.,* 19:85–94.

48. Wardell, W. M., Tsianco, M. D., Anavekar, S. N., and Davis, H. T. (1979): *J. Clin. Pharmacol.,* 19:169–184.

49. Wardell, W. M., Velo, G., and Jarocha, N. M., eds. (1981): *Drug Development, Regulatory Assessment, and Postmarketing Surveillance.* Plenum Press, New York.

Psychopharmacology:
The Third Generation of Progress,
edited by Herbert Y. Meltzer.
Raven Press, New York © 1987.

CHAPTER 181

FDA: The Federal Regulation of Drug Development

Paul Leber

The Food and Drug Administration (FDA) is the agency within the Department of Health and Human Services that is responsible for the administration and enforcement of the federal Food, Drug, and Cosmetic Act. The act gives the FDA sweeping authority over the development, clinical testing, and marketing of drug products.

Under the act, a new drug may not be commercially marketed, that is, introduced into interstate commerce, until its sponsor (i.e., its vendor) has submitted, and the Food and Drug Administration has approved, a New Drug Application (NDA) for the product.

Under the act, a sponsor and/or investigator may not carry out clinical studies with a new drug unless the FDA has determined that it is reasonably safe to do so.

This chapter describes how major provisions of the act apply to the development of new drugs.

HISTORICAL BACKGROUND

Federal regulation of drug development and marketing did not come about precipitously. Current requirements of the federal Food, Drug, and Cosmetic Act are reflections of more than 80 years of congressional responses to societal concerns about unacceptable free market conditions. As this section on the history of the development of our domestic drug laws illustrates, major regulatory legislation has often been enacted in the wake of publicity surrounding some especially egregious or tragic event, but, by and large, the legislation enacted has been carefully considered, balancing societal interests with the rights of those regulated.

Although the first federal law governing the quality of drug products was enacted in 1848 (it concerned the importation of products failing to meet pharmacopeial standards), authorities on the history of drug regulation agree that the first significant congressional attempt to control the distribution and marketing of drugs did not occur until the turn of the century.

In the period following our Civil War, the urbanization of what had been a largely rural society generated the need for an entirely new industry to distribute foodstuffs from the producer to the consumer (6,7). Unfortunately, many in the ranks of the rapidly expanding food packing and processing business were unscrupulous. Agricultural products were commonly adulterated and/or stored, processed, and packaged in the midst of filth and pestilence (7,8). Toxic chemicals were sometimes used as adulterants or preservatives. As the facts about the industry became known, public pressure for reform and corrective regulation grew. In particular, the public's concern was stimulated by a series of exposés and a "muckraking" press (4). In fact, Dr. Harvey Wiley, a physician who was to be the first head of the FDA's institutional antecedent, the Bureau of Chemistry of the Department of Agriculture, played an important role in exposing the toxicity of various food additives and adulterants by feeding them to a group of "volunteers" in the Department of Agriculture. Dr. Wiley was evidently quite willing to report the results of his studies with his "Poison Squad" to the press (7).

It was, therefore, in a climate of public indignation about unwholesome conditions in the food processing industry that Congress, in 1906, passed the Pure Food and Drugs Act. The act made the interstate shipment of adulterated or misbranded foods and drugs illegal.

It is worth noting that the Pure Food and Drugs Act of 1906 sought only to ensure that drug products were truthfully labeled as to their chemical contents. Preventing false claims of safety and efficacy, at least as we would understand the concept today, was *not* a goal of the act at least insofar as the courts were concerned.

For example, when the government sought to prevent a sponsor from making a claim that his product cured cancer on the grounds that the claim was false and that the product was, therefore, "misbranded," the Court (the opinion was given by the famous physician and jurist Oliver Wendell Holmes) ruled it could not (United States vs Johnson, 1911; cited in ref. 5, pp. 303–304). Holmes argued that whether or not a drug product contained what its label claimed it contained was clearly an issue that Bureau of Chemistry staff were competent to evaluate. On the other hand, he could not believe that Congress ever intended to ask the staff to assess matters of truth about "medical effects."

Actually, Holmes' speculation about Congress' probable intent was evidently incorrect. Within a year (1911), Congress amended the act (the Sherley Amendment) to make a fraudulent claim for a therapeutic effect an illegal act. The Sherley Amendment is, therefore, a sort of legal progenitor of the efficacy requirement of our current domestic drug regulatory law, the federal Food, Drug, and Cosmetic Act.

This historical vignette emphasizes an important point. Holmes' decision illustrates the conservative manner in which courts often interpret regulatory powers and explains, in part, why regulations promulgated by agencies must not expand an agency's authority beyond the intended goals of Congress. The regulations construed under an act of Congress must keep faith with both the literal letter of the law and the existing socio-political-scientific Zeitgeist. In 1906 the concept of efficacy, certainly as we understand it today, would have been difficult for most to comprehend. Whether or not a treatment was efficacious was seen as a matter of professional opinion and judgment and not as a matter that could be proven right or wrong (7).

Clearly, society's collective understanding of a problem, be it impure foods, unsafe drugs, ineffective remedies, or environmental hazards, and a regulatory agency's ability to enforce a law enacted to deal with the problem, are inexorably linked to one another as well as to the state of scientific knowledge and belief. The rules, standards, and policies enforced by the agency in 1938, let alone those in place in 1985, could not possibly have been applied in 1906; the scientific groundwork for such regulation simply did not exist.

Although a lack of scientific knowledge and understanding may automatically impose limits on the extent of regulation, public awareness of scientific advances may have an opposite effect. Increasing scientific knowledge is linked, often unrealistically, to increasing expectations for successful and immediate control of newly recognized risks. Of course, every societal expectation is not immediately converted into some expanded regulatory requirement. Rather, as most experts in the history of drug regulation have noted, societal expectations accumulate unfulfilled until some dramatic event occurs that focuses public and congressional attention on the entire area. This point is well illustrated by the circumstances that led to revision of the 1906 Pure Food and Drugs Act.

A major push for comprehensive reform of the 1906 act began in earnest under the New Deal. In 1933, Rex Tugwell, a New Dealer and Assistant Secretary of Agriculture, got a major new drug bill to the Senate floor. It got no further, however, as many in Congress were wary of central federal authority, in general, and the New Deal, in particular. A major theme espoused by those who opposed the reform bill was that it lacked sufficient procedural safeguards to protect those regulated from the exercise of bureaucratic caprice (2). This concern is worth noting, as the procedural safeguards incorporated in current law reflect in large measure the concerns voiced in Congress more than 50 years ago. Thus, Tugwell's bill floundered for several years. In 1937, however, a tragedy changed the political landscape dramatically.

A large ethical drug manufacturer developed and marketed a new sulfonilamide drug product. Because the sulfonilamide was sparingly soluble in water, the company's chemists had elected to dissolve it in diethylene glycol. Prior to shipment, the product was tested for appearance, palatability, and fragrance, but not for toxicity. The product proved to be a deadly poison and more than a hundred individuals died as a direct result of its administration. A major irony of the entire tragic episode was the fact that the agency was able to seize the product not because it was unsafe, but because it was misbranded. The firm had called their product an Elixir; under law this constituted misbranding, as the term Elixir refers exclusively to alcohol-solubilized products and the firm's product contained only diethylene glycol.

In the aftermath of the tragedy, Congress passed the federal Food, Drug, and Cosmetic Act of 1938. The act prohibited the marketing of a new drug without prior agency approval of a New Drug Application. The sponsor was to submit the application and the FDA was to allow it to become "effective" unless it failed to provide full reports of tests showing the safety of the drug product. The 1938 act did not mention efficacy but did require that the drug product's labeling not be "false or misleading" in any particular. (This was an important change because the Sherley Amendment banning fraudulent therapeutic claims had been exceedingly difficult to enforce. Sponsors charged with making fraudulent claims escaped conviction by foreswearing any purposeful intent to deceive. A fraudulent act, it seems, must involve willful intent.)

The 1938 act was a marked improvement on its 1906 antecedent; however, it was far from a perfect regulatory instrument. In particular, because a submitted application automatically became effective 60 days after its receipt, the agency could be placed under inordinate and unfair pressure to act on an application without adequate review and consideration. Admittedly, the agency did have a right, provided the sponsor was notified within 60 days, to postpone the effective date of an application for a period of up to 180 days. However, the administrative burden of postponement, especially in the face of a large volume of submissions, was always a potential problem. Furthermore, the passive approval/active disapproval stance of the 1938 act did not provide "fail-safe" protection. Specifically, such a procedure creates the possibility, probably remote, that a totally unreviewed drug might, through administrative or clerical error, become marketed. There is, however, no record of this having occurred; when the 1938 act failed, it did so in an entirely unexpected way.

The 1938 act also had other major deficiencies. It did not require a sponsor to show that a drug was effective for the uses claimed in its labeling. False or misleading claims, of course, could *not* be made for a drug, but proof of a plausible claim was not required. Why a demonstration of efficacy was not required is a matter of speculation.

Assuredly, most physicians have always understood that an ineffective drug is potentially harmful if its administration delays access to definitive effective therapy. This, however, is unlikely to have been a major concern when the number of curative remedies in medicine was vanishingly small. Prior to the mid-1940s, most products were palliative in nature, and if one product did not work one could switch to another without much being lost. It is difficult to chronicle, but the postwar growth of scientific knowledge and the appearance of antibiotics as curative remedies may have altered public and medical attitudes about the efficacy question (7).

Indeed, forces favoring an efficacy requirement were gathering as early as 1951. The legislative history of the 1951 Humphrey-Durham Amendment clarifying the agency's authority to assign a drug to prescription status clearly indicates that Congress believed that the safety of drugs would be considered in the context of their efficacy. Specifically, the house version of the amendment contained a clause, eventually stricken from the bill enacted, that stated that a determination of prescription status should rest on whether or not experts believed a drug was "safe and *efficacious* for use only after professional diagnosis" (7).

In any event, by the time the next major tragedy involving drug development occurred, the scientific medical community had become very much concerned about the question of drug efficacy.

The sociopolitical climate was evolving as well. Advocates of consumer protection were increasingly active during the later part of President Eisenhower's administration. In late 1959, Senator Estes Kefauver began hearings on the question of excess profits in the drug industry. Kefauver's concern about the disadvantaged position of consumers in the purchase of drugs is evident in a quotation cited by Temin: "He who orders does not buy, he who buys does not order" (7).

It was in this evolving climate favoring reform that the thalidomide tragedy occurred. Thalidomide, an effective hypnotic drug, was undergoing clinical testing in the United States when, in late 1961, its teratogenic potential was discovered as a result of an epidemic of limb reduction defects (phocomelia) that occurred in children born following its marketing in Europe and England. A New Drug Application for thalidomide had been submitted to the FDA in 1960, but had not been permitted to become effective because the FDA's clinical reviewer, Dr. Frances Kelsey, had determined that the application lacked adequate tests to show the drug to be safe. Nonetheless, although the application had been rejected in the United States, more than two and a half million tablets of the hypnotic had been distributed domestically to more than 1,200 physicians for testing (7).

To be clear, this extensive exposure of the public, which caused a small but definite cluster of nine or so cases of phocomelia, was not illegal. Although commonly unappreciated, the 1938 act made provision for the investigational use of experimental drugs by qualified experts. The regulations construed under this provision of the 1938 act [Sec 505 (i)], however, only required that investigational drugs be labeled as such and that the investigator maintain records on any investigations conducted; there was no restriction on the extent of investigational use. Had there been, the harm caused by the domestic study of thalidomide might have been substantially limited, perhaps entirely avoided.

It is commonly held that the Kefauver-Harris Amendments to the Food, Drug, and Cosmetic Act were passed in 1962 as a consequence of public response to the thalidomide tragedy. Although this may be a bit of an oversimplification, it does illustrate, as did the sulfonilamide tragedy a quarter of a century earlier, the importance of specific events as catalysts to congressional action.

The 1962 amendments altered the act in two major ways:

First, the method and requirements for the approval of NDAs were changed. The demonstration of efficacy, based on "substantial" evidence derived from adequate and well-controlled clinical investigations, was made a *sine qua non* of drug approval and the passive approval/active disapproval system that allowed applications to become effective was replaced by a system requiring the agency to approve each application affirmatively.

Second, and perhaps of greater importance to those involved in clinical research, the clinical investigation of new drugs was placed under much closer regulatory supervision.

The 1962 amendments authorize the Secretary of Health and Human Services to place conditions and limitations upon any exemption granting permission for the investigational use of new drugs. Prior to the initiation of any proposed clinical investigation, the secretary has the right to require submission of the results of investigations "or preclinical tests (including tests on animals) of such drugs to justify the proposed clinical testing." The amendments also empower the secretary to (a) control the extent of and fix responsibility for the distribution and clinical use of experimental drugs, and (b) set requirements for both record keeping and periodic reporting of the results of clinical investigations.

The 1962 amendments have profoundly altered drug development in the United States and in the world. Whatever one's personal view of the value of these amendments and the added burdens they impose, it is clear that they have served as a major force driving the development of techniques and methods to assess drug safety and efficacy.

In the remainder of this chapter, the application of law, regulations, and policy to the FDA's supervision of clinical drug research is described. It must be noted that this chapter is written at a time when a major revision of the regulations governing drug research (i.e., the "IND Rewrite") is awaiting final clearance in the Office of Management and Budget. Although the proposed version of the new regulation has been published (1), the final form and content of the regulations are not yet known. The IND Rewrite is primarily intended to clarify IND procedures and to restrict and/or remove regulatory requirements that may needlessly interfere with the conduct of research. By and large, the changes implemented do not reflect any major shift in regulatory policy or philosophy. The changes, however, should promote the efficiency of IND regulation. Where important, possible changes and/or effects of the Rewrite are described.

Incidentally, in recent years, two new acts have been passed that affect drug development and marketing. In 1983 the Orphan Drug Act was passed to encourage and support the development of drugs under conditions that offer commercial sponsors little chance for profit. In 1984 the Drug Price Competition and Patent Term Restoration Act was passed to permit generic copies of approved drugs to be marketed under circumstances that do not undercut the motivation of sponsors to develop new drug products.

THE REQUIREMENTS OF THE FEDERAL FOOD, DRUG, AND COSMETIC ACT

Clinical Investigations

Under existing federal regulations, the investigation of a new drug in human volunteers or patients may only take place if authorized by the FDA. The formal instrument used by drug sponsors to obtain authorization, the IND, is officially known as a Notice of Claimed Investigational Exemption for a New Drug. It owes its peculiar-sounding official name to the way in which the Federal Food, Drug, and Cosmetic Act is written.

Under the provisions of the act, a new drug may *not* move in interstate commerce unless it is the subject of an approved NDA. Further, the sponsor or vendor of the new drug, even a drug with an approved NDA, may only ship the drug in interstate commerce for the purposes of use described in the product's approved labeling. Consequently, a sponsor or vendor would violate the new drug provisions of the act if he knowingly shipped any drug in interstate commerce for any experimental or investigational use. Therefore, to allow clinical investigation of new drugs, Congress included a provision in the act allowing exemptions from the ban on interstate shipment of unapproved new drugs for drugs intended solely for investigational use by experts qualified by training and experience to conduct clinical investigations. As noted earlier, the conditions for obtaining this exemption were modified significantly by the 1962 amendments.

The mechanism of granting an exemption has been promulgated in regulations (21 CFR 312) that permit a sponsor (either a firm or an individual investigator) to apply for an exemption, obtain supplies of the drug, and proceed with a planned experiment *unless,* within a period of 30 days of the agency's receipt of this notice, the agency objects to the proposal. An agency objection is expressed as a request that the applicant withhold and/or restrict the scope of the proposed research. (The request is commonly known as a "hold" and is discussed in greater detail in the next section.)

The strategy employed places the agency in a passive approval/active disapproval role, one quite similar to its position in regard to NDA evaluation during the period between 1938 and 1962. As noted earlier, the passive approval/active disapproval approach is not a "fail–safe" method. However, agency procedures assure that an active and complete review of virtually every IND occurs within a 30-day interval. Furthermore, the risk to the public health posed by inadvertent initiation of an unsafe investigation is far less than that which could accompany unintended marketing of a dangerous drug. Consequently, the passive approval/active disapproval approach to the assessment of INDs seems more than adequate.

The Philosophical Basis of IND Policy

The agency's primary obligation in its administration of INDs is to ensure that subjects who participate in clinical trials will not be exposed to any unnecessary risk. It is important to emphasize that the obligation is envisioned as a need to prevent unnecessary risk, not as a mandate to ensure absolute safety. The risks of human experimentation can be minimized, but cannot be totally removed.

In this context, provided that there is adequate informed consent, agency policy holds that the safe investigation of new drugs should be permitted to proceed without undue hindrance. Indeed, as noted earlier, the IND procedures themselves are designed to permit research to proceed almost automatically upon the filing of a relatively simple notice.

For the IND process to work efficiently, however, the sponsor of an IND must understand the obligations of the process and must cooperate as fully and completely as possible. If the agency is to fulfill its obligation to assess the risks of a research proposal, it must have adequate information at its disposal to do so. Each IND must contain all the relevant evidence that would allow a responsible expert to reach a reliable conclusion that the proposed experimental use is reasonably safe. Further, the information must be organized in a manner that permits efficient review. The 30 calendar days allotted for review do not allow much leeway. Consequently, the IND should be well organized, contain the required information, and provide a cogent presentation of the case for allowing the research to proceed.

Not surprisingly, many who submit INDs miss this point and a significant proportion of holds occur because the applicant has failed to provide information the agency's professional staff must have to complete its assessment of the application rather than because the staff has reached an affirmative conclusion that the project involves "unreasonable and significant risk."

THE IND PROCESS IN OPERATION

The Usual IND: Approval Through Silence (Occasionally Broken by a Muted Comment or Two)

If the agency does not object within 30 days of its receipt of the notice, the sponsor may proceed with the experiment(s) proposed.

Because the date of receipt is initially known only to the agency, the agency issues a letter acknowledging the submission of the notice. In addition, the letter provides the sponsor with the official number assigned to the IND, a number to be used in any and all correspondence with the agency. This should not be confused with permission to initiate clinical testing; a sponsor must still wait until the required 30 days have elapsed to initiate clinical testing.

On many occasions, agency staff may offer comments about a proposed investigation that are intended solely as helpful advice. These comments are just that: advice offered in a cooperative spirit. There is no regulatory requirement that the investigator or sponsor adhere to the advice. Of course, if the advice is sensible and applies to the design of studies that are intended to serve as sources of evidence of drug efficacy, it does seem prudent for a sponsor to consider it seriously.

On still other occasions, the staff may identify some readily repairable, but nevertheless serious, defect in a proposed study. In such cases an attempt is made to inform the sponsor of the problem before the 30-day interval elapses. If the sponsor agrees to repair the defect, the study is allowed to proceed without any delay. Indeed, this approach is used to deal with the vast majority of INDs that have serious but readily correctable defects.

Incidentally, once an IND is underway, a sponsor may wish to modify his research proposal (e.g., to add additional protocols, new investigators, etc.). To do this, he amends the IND by submitting a new protocol *before* proceeding with it. There is, however, no additional 30-day pause before he can proceed. Again, the passive approval/active disapproval mode of the IND requires that agency procedures assure timely review of new protocol amendments.

The Clinical Hold: An Explicit Demand to Withhold Initiation of Clinical Testing or to Suspend Testing Already Initiated

There are circumstances, however, where the defects in an IND are so numerous or so serious that the agency finds either that it cannot permit initial clinical testing to begin, or that it must suspend testing already underway. Current regulations, however, provide only general guidance about the nature of such circumstances. Thus, a major feature of the proposed new IND regulations is the specification of the circumstances that the agency considers to justify the imposition of a hold.

The Rewrite proposes to limit holds for initial clinical testing to four situations. A hold may be implemented if (a) there is an "unreasonable and significant risk" to subjects; (b) the clinical investigators who intend to conduct the research are unqualified; (c) the "investigator brochure" (a compilation of information about the drug—a sort of provisional drug labeling) is false, inaccurate, or incomplete; or (d) the IND application does not provide sufficient information to permit its proper assessment.

However, in later phases of a drug's development, where exposure in a given trial is much more extensive, a hold may be imposed if "the plan or protocol for the investigation is clearly deficient in design to meet its stated objectives."

An important distinction about the timing of holds is worth noting. If the agency wishes to prevent clinical testing from being *initiated,* it must notify the sponsor of its decision to hold the investigation within 30 days of the agency's receipt of the IND. However, the agency is free to hold an IND at any time. Once an investigation has begun it may ordinarily continue according to plan, but if information is obtained showing that ongoing research, either a particular new protocol or the entire effort, is *not* reasonably safe, the agency has the obligation and the absolute authority to require immediate suspension of some or all clinical testing.

Usually, if a hold on initial testing is imposed, the applicant learns of the decision by phone. The call is typically made by a Consumer Safety Officer (CSO), who is generally only able to provide a rough outline of the reasons for the agency's action. Within as short an interval as possible following the call, however, the agency issues a letter providing a detailed explanation for its action and enumerates the deficiencies.

What to Do About an IND Placed on Hold

The sponsor is expected to repair the deficiencies enumerated by the agency. If the applicant fails to understand the nature of the deficiencies cited, or encounters some other sort of specific problem, the CSOs in each drug review division are available to offer advice.

In some instances, the sponsor is not able to accomplish the repair of a cited deficiency without the help of an outside party. For example, a sponsor-investigator often depends on access to confidential information held in an IND belonging to a commercial sponsor. Another common example, affecting commercial firms and independent sponsor-investigators alike, involves confidential Drug Master Files (DMFs) that contain vital information about the manufacture or stability of a drug product. If the information contained in a particular DMF is inadequate, the IND must be placed on hold until the holder (owner) of the DMF supplies the necessary information.

There will be instances, however, in which an applicant believes the hold is unfair or unjustified or the proposed remedy unreasonable. The applicant should feel entirely free to argue the case. The agency's professional staff always review each applicant's response to a deficiency or hold letter and are prepared to discuss it with the applicant. Of course, understanding an applicant's argument is not equivalent to agreeing with it. Therefore, if, after learning of the basis for a division's decision, an applicant continues to believe that the decision is wrong, he is free and is encouraged to pursue an appeal at a higher organizational level within the agency.

It is appropriate, however, to close this section on a more sanguine note. The vast majority of INDs submitted are *never* placed on hold. Further, most of the small number that are held, provided that they are not abandoned by the sponsor, are eventually allowed to proceed. Indeed, in many cases, initial holds are lifted within days. Of course, there are holds that remain for months, even years. It is rare, however, that any hold is imposed with the expectation that research with the drug will never be allowed. In fact, it is usually the sponsor, not the agency, who decides to abandon further clinical testing of a drug.

The IND: What It Allows and What It Doesn't

Permission to initiate clinical testing (whether inferred from FDAs silence at 30 days or gained explicity from an agency communication lifting a hold) is *not* an unlimited license to use the experimental drug, but is a permission that carries many caveats, conditions, and obligations. These are detailed in the official forms that are used by sponsors and investigators to apply for an IND (a 1571, and, depending on the stage of proposed investigation, either a 1572 or 1573 or both). Space does not permit a full discussion of all IND requirements. It is important, however, to emphasize that the permission granted is limited to the use of the drug for the purposes and under the conditions specified in the initial IND application or subsequent amendments to it. The purpose for which the vast majority of INDs are granted is bona fide research; that is, research that has, by design, a reasonable potential to generate scientifically valid data to evaluate a drug's safety, efficacy, or directions for use.

An IND is not intended to be a means to allow individuals to use an unapproved new drug without restriction in their private or institutional practice of medicine. An IND is not a means to sell and/or distribute an unapproved new drug to others, regardless of one's professed motivations. In short, an IND is a limited license to permit legitimate research. A notable exception are INDs issued for the treatment of single patients or groups of patients who suffer from a disease or condition for which effective alternative treatment is not available. Current policy permits review divisions to grant INDs for treatment; under the Rewrite, a "treatment" IND will be recognized formally in regulations.

The IND: A Device to Meter the Rate of Human Exposure to a New Drug

As reviewed earlier, the 1962 amendments that created the authority for INDs were passed in the aftermath of the thalidomide tragedy. Especially shocking at the time was the notion that an unapproved and, as it turned out, very dangerous drug could be widely used in human experiments without adequate safeguards. The IND authority thus reflects Congress' intent that the investigation of new drugs be carried out under carefully controlled conditions that minimize the risk of injury to the general public.

In light of this mandate, the regulatory assessment of each new drug, especially new chemical entities (NCEs), is undertaken with considerable caution. Sanguine assumptions advanced by sponsors about the potential value of a new drug, even those supported by current theories and beliefs, are put aside. The evaluation of each new drug begins with the recognition that it may be dangerous and/or ineffective, a sort of regulatory "null hypothesis." It is the sponsor's burden to conduct experiments and provide evidence to reject the hypothesis.

Because of the potential risk to subjects, the process of gathering evidence to reject the regulatory null hypothesis must be carried out in a series of measured steps. The steps are commonly identified as the phases (I, II, and III) of new drug development. Agency regulations outline the aims of these phases relatively clearly.

The first phase of drug development that falls under agency regulation is the introduction of a new chemical entity into a human for the first time. Initial studies are short-term and limited to a few patients. Gradually, the duration, dose, and numbers of patients exposed are increased.

It should be appreciated that the agency's authority applies only to drug development by domestic companies. A drug extensively investigated in humans elsewhere in the world will usually enter the domestic drug evaluation process at a later phase than would be allowed in the absence of prior experience.

However, it is critical to bear in mind that the value of foreign experience is a function of its quality, not its extensiveness. In particular, essential information regarding a product's clinical pharmacology (pharmacokinetics, dose-response, effect on organ system performance, etc.) may not be available although the product may have been used at some dose under uncontrolled conditions in thousands of foreign patients. Consequently, before full-scale (i.e., late phase II/phase III) domestic study of such a drug would be permitted, remedial phase I experiments might have to be carried out to provide the information needed to assess the drug's risks by American standards. This is not chauvinism. Foreign governments are free to permit drug testing under any set of circumstances they choose; their standards, however, are not ours and cannot substitute for ours.

This caveat given, consider the typical case of a new chemical entity proposed for initial clinical testing within the United States. Before clinical testing can proceed, a *minimum* amount of information about the drug product's composition and its effects on biological systems and animals must be obtained, the amount depending on the specific human studies proposed.

The so-called chemistry requirements are intended to ensure that the planned investigations employ the product nominally identified and that the product is reasonably pure. Thus, a sponsor must provide documentation that the drug product is (a) chemically (i.e., in regard to structure, physical state, etc.) what it is claimed to be; (b) reasonably free of unwanted materials (starting reagents, intermediate products, by-products, pyrogens, etc.); and (c) manufactured, packed, and stored within containers according to currently accepted standards.

The chemistry requirements that must be met before initial clinical testing may begin are intentionally set at a less demanding level than those required for large-scale clinical testing or marketing. This flexible approach to setting requirements bears emphasis because it applies not only to chemistry requirements but to those involving preclinical and clinical investigations as well (*vide infra*).

The linkage between the phase of drug development and preclinical testing illustrates the tie between the extent of testing required and the extent of potential human exposure. For example, before a typical new drug may be marketed, a sponsor will have to have (a) conducted 1-year toxicity testing in two species; (b) performed carcinogenicity testing in two species (usually an 18- to 24-month mouse and a 24-month rat study); and (c) evaluated the product's teratogenicity, its capacity to affect reproductive performance, and its ability to cause neonatal injury. In contrast, for initial phase I clinical studies (i.e., those limited to single doses or repeated doses for only a few days *in toto*), it is usually only necessary to carry out (a) acute toxicity testing in three or four species (at least one a nonrodent) by the route to be employed clinically; and (b) subacute toxicity tests in two species (one a nonrodent) for 2 weeks at three dosage levels. Similarly, if a drug is intended for single-dose parenteral use, its animal testing requirements will be reduced below those for the typical oral drug product intended for extended use. In short, the requirements for animal testing are carefully linked to the stage of drug development and the extent and duration of potential human exposure.

Space, again, does not permit a discussion of the details of these requirements. They, of course, may be modified or adjusted to some extent if circumstances warrant. Indeed, as noted above, if there is extensive human experience outside the United States, the early toxicity testing requirements, which are intended to support early human exposure, may be modified by the agency on an *ad hoc* basis. There is, however, no routine or automatic waiver of toxicity testing requirements based on nondomestic clinical experience. Indeed, teratogenicity and carcinogenicity testing are invariably required regardless of prior nondomestic human experience because these risks are exceedingly difficult to assess in clinical trials or from postmarketing data. The point emphasized is that the agency's requirements for clinical trials are linked in a logical way to the stage of a drug's development. Some requirements are relaxed with increasing clinical experience; others are implemented anew as the size of the population at potential risk for injury grows.

Exceptions to Policy Involving Sequential Drug Development

Obviously, the uniform implementation of a strategy of sequential drug development occasionally leads to situations where a sponsor believes it is appropriate to conduct a study at a time before the usual prerequisite animal or clinical testing has been completed. The prudent sponsor

who is aware of the policy will include a justification for any proposed exception along with the proposal for the study. A classic example is a request that Women of Childbearing Potential (WCBP) be permitted to enroll in a clinical investigation before the usual requirements [completion of the female part of segment I (fertility/general reproductive performance), segment II (teratogenicity), and documentation of preliminary clinical evidence of therapeutic effectiveness] have been met. Sometimes the request may be honored because the circumstances clearly warrant the exception. For example, the division would certainly waive the requirement for complete preclinical teratogenicity testing under the following set of conditions: (a) The disease for which the treatment is proposed is fatal, progressive, or very serious; (b) no effective alternative treatments exist; and (c) there is a modicum of evidence from controlled experiments suggesting efficacy. Often, however, the rationale offered is inadequate to justify an exception. As noted previously, regulation of drug development does place restrictions on the freedom of individual sponsors and investigators. The agency is always willing to consider a request for an exemption to policy, but, as with any other matter, disagreements may not be resolved in a manner satisfactory to the sponsor.

The IND as a Device to Ensure the Quality of Research

As noted repeatedly, the primary goal of government regulation of clinical drug research is the protection of subjects from needless risk and injury. Does the agency have any obligation or authority to influence the quality of clinical research? Indirectly, of course, NDA approval requirements are generally agreed to have a salutary effect on clinical research designs and conduct. Certainly, a sensible and prudent sponsor will not waste money supporting research that he knows the agency will reject as inadequate. The question, however, is more focused. Can the agency *directly* prevent clinical research on the grounds that it is grossly inadequate because of some aspect of its design?

The proposed Rewrite of the IND regulations makes the agency's authority to control the quality of research clear. After the completion of early clinical testing (i.e., beyond phase I), the Rewrite makes explicit FDA's authority to hold a proposed clinical investigation if "the plan or protocol for the investigation is clearly deficient in design to meet its stated objectives."

The agency recognizes, however, that authority to place limitations on the conduct of research for reasons other than safety must be used with great care. Many a major advance in science has occurred because someone had the wisdom to recognize that the seemingly irrational or impossible wasn't "crazy." Thus, the agency will *not* use its authority to suppress legitimate scientific inquiry. The agency is also well aware that a good part of drug research is only remotely intended to lead to the development of new drug products. The agency recognizes the legitimacy of research in which drugs are used to evaluate normal physiology and the pathophysiology of disease. As long as there is adequate protection of subjects and full informed consent, the agency does not interfere with fundamental pharmacological and biological research.

The agency's commitment to avoid unnecessary interference in the conduct of research should not be taken as evidence of a lack of interest in the quality of research. The agency makes a substantial effort to ensure the quality of clinical studies carried out to provide evidence of drug safety and efficacy. The FDA cooperates with national medical and scientific organizations in diverse efforts to improve and/or refine methodologies for the design, performance, and analysis of clinical trials, and working with such groups has developed more than 25 clinical guidelines. In addition, agency staff review and offer constructive commentary on the vast majority of commercial drug development programs and clinical trial protocols, both at formal meetings (end of phase II or pre-NDA meetings) and during less formal contacts.

Space does not permit a discussion of the considerations the agency applies to the design and execution of clinical studies carried out in support of NDAs for psychopharmacologic drug products. The interested reader may gain some insight into current agency views on design issues by referring to a recent review by the author (3).

Ongoing Obligations Under the IND: Reporting Requirements

While the IND allows a sponsor to conduct clinical studies, the extent of the activity permitted varies with the extent of information extant about the drug's risks and benefits. As emphasized earlier, permission to initiate clinical testing is not permission to weigh anchor and proceed unfettered on some uncharted course to an unknown destination.

The IND process requires continuing interaction between the agency and the sponsor. Some of the interaction is formally mandated by regulations. Other contacts are voluntary, spurred by a mutual interest in ensuring the safe and efficient development of new drugs. It is expected that the sponsor (and investigators involved) will continuously inform the agency of progress and setbacks, successes and, most critically, disasters or near disasters. Routine findings may be reported periodically, but any unexpected and serious event must be communicated to the agency immediately. The need to inform the agency rapidly about serious risks is, beyond a legal obligation of the IND holder, an ethical one. Unknown to the sponsor, especially if he is an independent sponsor-investigator, other patients may be exposed to the drug or a closely related one. Early receipt of information about a previously unappreciated risk may save others needless injury.

Commercial Versus Single-Investigator INDs: Some Important Contrasts

This chapter's focus on the regulation of the clinical investigation of drugs precludes any major discussion of the NDA approval process. It would be remiss, however, not to emphasize the important role the commercial IND plays in the development of drugs intended for marketing. In contrast to the typical IND submitted by an academic

sponsor-investigator, the commercial IND is the vehicle through which sponsors and agency staff jointly work out the specific requirements for the approval of the NDA. Before its completion, the typical commercial drug development program will lead to the exposure of between one and two thousand human volunteers and patients. To gain permission to conduct programs of this magnitude, commercial sponsors must mount truly comprehensive support programs. These include the full panoply of animal studies as well as the special clinical investigations needed to characterize the drug's pharmacodynamics, its effects on special populations, and its biopharmacokinetic parameters. The breadth of the commercial IND license is proportional to the supporting data provided by the sponsor.

In contrast, the academic sponsor-investigator who applies to use a new chemical entity typically provides very little information about the drug, unless, of course, he is able to reference information in a commercial IND. Clearly, without access to the data in a commercial IND, the sponsor-investigator cannot provide the extensive supporting information required to allow large-scale human exposure. Nevertheless, in part because the agency believes that Congress never intended to preclude academic investigation, the agency permits small-scale experiments to be carried out by qualified clinical investigators on the basis of information that would not be considered adequate to support commercial development of a drug. There is, however, a *quid pro quo* involved. The investigator must be very explicit about what he intends to do and must provide sufficient detail about any proposed study to allow agency staff to reach a conclusion, independently, that the proposal is reasonably safe and well monitored.

The IND as a Vehicle for Treatment

As noted earlier, the IND authority is clearly intended to permit the legitimate investigation of drugs. Congress probably did not anticipate that the testing and evaluation of drugs would take as long as it does. In any case, drugs are often identified as potentially useful in the treatment of disease in advance of their approval for marketing. Clearly, this creates a legitimate interest by physicians and informed patients in gaining access to many unapproved new drugs, particularly where the new agent is thought to have unique features. Unfortunately, open access of everyone to all drugs effectively bypasses the requirements of the Food, Drug, and Cosmetic Act. Furthermore, many allegedly effective drugs are not only ineffective, but unsafe.

In an attempt to deal with this problem, the agency has long had a policy of permitting drugs for which there is some evidence of safety and efficacy, but not sufficient to allow approval, to be used in the treatment of selected patients. As noted earlier, such "treatment" INDs will become recognized in regulations under the proposed Rewrite. At present, however, two approaches are used.

In the more common, a physician is granted permission to use an unapproved new drug to treat a single patient (occasionally two, or even three) who suffers from an illness for which no treatment is available. This option is also used in circumstances where effective marketed treatments are available, but the patient has responded poorly or not at all or cannot tolerate the treatment.

In such circumstances, the IND is said to be granted on "compassionate" grounds. The physician who applies for an IND on a compassionate basis must make a compelling case justifying the exception if alternative treatments for the condition exist. On the other hand, when a very rare and dangerous condition for which no recognized treatment exists is the aim of treatment, evidence justifying the diagnosis is more than adequate documentation provided there is some basis to believe the drug is effective and reasonably safe.

Commercial sponsors may also seek permission to treat groups of patients with an unapproved new drug at a relatively late stage (i.e., after the completion of phase II) in the commercial drug development process. In such circumstances, evidence of efficacy and safety is often available, but an NDA has either not been submitted or has not yet been approved. The sponsor, principally as a public service, submits a "treatment" protocol under its commercial IND and makes the private physician for each patient to whom it agrees to supply drug one of its clinical investigators.

This process should be distinguished from what are called "extension" protocols. Often, in the course of the commercial development of an investigational agent, patients who participate in controlled trials do unexpectedly well. Clinicians, understandably, are reluctant to withdraw such patients from treatment. Of course, improvement may always be due to chance or regression to the mean, so even in such circumstances, the agency tends to wait until fairly persuasive evidence of safety and efficacy is available before permitting the more or less routine admission of patients completing controlled trials into "extension" protocols.

Incidentally, an IND is not required to use an approved drug for an unapproved indication in the practice of medicine.

CLOSING COMMENTS

The supervision and monitoring of clinical drug research conducted under INDs is but one aspect of FDA regulatory activity involving drugs. Indeed, some might say it is a relatively minor activity considering the importance of the NDA approval process, the Generic Drug Program, the Post-Marketing Surveillance Programs, and FDA's compliance activities that are carried out throughout the land.

However, the IND process is far more important than its relative budget and manpower allotments might suggest. The regulation of INDs is probably the single most important medium for the mutual exchange of ideas and scientific information between agency scientists and their counterparts in the academic and commercial world. By the time an NDA is evaluated, issues have hardened and decisions are made on the basis of what already has or has not been done. In contrast, the IND review process allows all the division's regulatory disciplines to interact in an innovative and constructive manner with those regulated, be they commercial developers, clinical investigators, or wet-bench molecular biologists. In a way, the IND is both a training ground and a proving ground. Used wisely, the agency's supervision of drug research is a tool for the advancement of clinical pharmacology and therapeutics as well as a regulatory device to protect the public from undue risk.

REFERENCES

1. FDA (1983): *Proposed New Drug, Antibiotic, and Biologic Drug Product Regulation,* FR 48:26720–26749, No. 12, June 9.
2. Hoffman, J. E. (1984): In: *Seventy-Fifth Anniversary Commemorative Volume of Food and Drug Law,* Chapter 1, pp. 1–26. Food and Drug Law Institute Series. Food and Drug Law Institute, Washington, DC.
3. Leber, P. (1986): *Psychopharmacol. Bull.,* 22, 23:30–32.
4. Levine, A. S., Laboza, T. B., and Morhey, J. E. (1985): *N. Engl. J. Med.,* 312:628–634.
5. Merrill, R. A., and Hutt, P. B. (1980): *Food and Drug Law, Cases and Materials.* Foundation Press, Mineola, NY.
6. Pfeifer, E. M. (1984): In: *Seventy-Fifth Anniversary Commemorative Volume of Food and Drug Law,* Chapter 3, pp. 72–113. Food and Drug Law Institute Series. Food and Drug Law Institute, Washington, DC.
7. Temin, P. (1980): *Taking Your Medicine: Drug Regulation in the United States.* Harvard University Press, Cambridge.
8. Ziporyn, T. (1985): *JAMA,* 254:2037–2046.

Psychopharmacology:
The Third Generation of Progress,
edited by Herbert Y. Meltzer.
Raven Press, New York © 1987.

CHAPTER 182

Future Directions and Goals in Basic Psychopharmacology and Neurobiology

Floyd E. Bloom

The intellectual exchange between fundamental neurobiology and neuropsychopharmacology has traditionally emphasized neurotransmitters, their biochemistry, physiology, and anatomy, and the macromolecular changes in these indices produced by mental illnesses or the drugs or procedures currently available to diagnose or treat them. What has been far less amenable to the College's interests are the numerous other waves of progress currently driving the general area of neuroscience. Such areas of active ferment not yet linked to psychopharmacology include the characterization of intermediate filaments by which neuronal and glial structure is maintained, the sharing of cell surface markers with cells of the immune system and with certain neurotropic viruses, and the early isolation of the growth-regulating factors of neurons and glia that operate at least during brain organogenesis, and which may also operate to adjust circuitry in the adult brain. As we try to peer into the next generation's efforts to draw from neurobiology the ideas and methods that can advance our understanding of human mental illness, it seems likely that we can count on the neurotransmitters continuing to be in the center of the stage.

Given this traditional focus, it seems clear that we must change our expectations of how drugs are designed and how new diagnostic procedures and treatments are to be derived from the interplay between basic and clinical neurosciences. My best guesses of where future directions are likely to be gained still focus on the interface between cellular and molecular neurobiology. This is the frontier at which the most extensive progress has been made over the past decade: the discovery of multiple new neuronally made substances satisfying many of the criteria of neurotransmitters, as I broadly define them (2); the recognition of new anatomic connections linking neurons in circuits; and the recognition that the newly recognized chemicals in the newly recognized circuits can produce effects on the transmission process that transcend classical views of how transmitters act, and how disease and drugs may alter transmitter actions.

The next generation should clarify the standards by which the effects of transmitter substances can be classified and compared, to look beyond "factors" assessed *in vitro* for biochemical regulatory actions, and characterize how and where physiological regulators operate within the context of their circuit anatomy and receptors. Formerly the nervous system was thought of as a rather dry place in which the transmitters were narrowly restricted to excitatory or inhibitory roles. In less than a decade this picture has changed to one of a very juicy, flexible nervous system in which transmitters act on many different receptor transduction mechanisms and provide a very enriched repertoire of signaling capabilities across widely differing spatial domains and widely variant durations of action. Here is where the major conceptual changes should be expected to be further refined: no longer need "real" transmitters be viewed strictly as primary communicators. They can also furnish more complex signals that can modify the response of the intended target cells to the other classical transmitter signals they are receiving simultaneously. These added signaling capabilities will not only give new meaning to the fundamentals of neuronal communication and the regulation of behavior, but will also provide new avenues to examine for pathophysiological mechanisms and drug actions.

MONOAMINES: CONTINUING EXEMPLARS

Monoamines were among the first chemically defined transmitters to meet the more rigorous tests as central transmitters and to gain prominence in psychopharmacology. This was due to two specific advantages: the broader armamentarium of drugs available to manipulate the central monoaminergic systems, and the detailed structural information on these systems that grew from sensitive methods for their cytochemical localization. However, their unique cellular morphology—with a highly divergent axonal arborization connecting pontine nuclei with cortical regions by routes never visualized by the empirical methods of the metal impregnation era—and their unique electrophysiological actions—altering membrane potential without increased ionic conductance and relying on second messenger systems for amplification and intermediation (see 5, 9 for recent reviews) helped force the initial expansion of the concepts of neurotransmitters. There has clearly been an enormous profusion of new neural circuitry as revealed by transmitter or ligand markers, and that thrust is likely to continue unabated for some time to come.

By comparison with more classical hierarchical neurons, or more numerous local circuit neurons, the single-source, divergent circuitry of most monoaminergic and some peptidergic neurons operates over much larger spatial domains with much less constrained connectivities. Confidently, we may predict that the work of the next generation will be largely to assemble and integrate these chemically denoted, functionally diverse circuits with behavior.

Given the exemplary role played by studies of monoamine anatomy, physiology, and pharmacology in formulating of normal brain operations and in conceptualizing principles of human psychopharmacology, future progress is destined to reveal the errors of oversimplification based on the fact that virtually all these data have come from studies of rodent brains. Monoamine systems in primate neocortex and subcortical regions show considerably greater regional and laminar specificity (and presumably in their cellular connectivity) than was previously deducible from the extensive prior neuroanatomic studies of rodent brain. These findings strongly suggest that the concept of "diffuse nonspecificity" for monoamine systems, as is widely conjectured, is incorrect.

In our view, an effective evaluation of the catecholamine/indoleamine/monoamine hypotheses of affective disorders or the dopamine-oriented concept of schizophrenia requires a more accurate determination of the structure and function, at the cellular and systems level, of the monoamine neural circuits in the human brain. In the absence of methods and specimens that will permit effective studies of these systems at any time soon, the only viable alternative for future studies is to concentrate on the primate nervous system.

These observations suggest that coincident with the extensive phylogenetic development and functional differentiation of neocortex in the primate there has been a parallel elaboration and differentiation of the ascending noradrenergic, dopaminergic, and serotonergic projections. However, the possible changes in this complementary regional and laminar innervation will require exploration in the generation ahead. Even for the normal human cerebral cortex, the brain region we must presume to be crucial to diseases of cognitive processes and higher cerebral function, we remain woefully ignorant of the detailed internal circuitry. Moreover, the transmitters that operate there, and the way in which these transmitters interact to perform the phenomena we refer to operationally as perceiving, learning, and remembering, are unsolved fields of intense activity. Thus, examining the possible pathological mechanisms that could arise in such systems should provide new ways of conceptualizing the catecholamine hypotheses, and of devising testable methods of determining where the pertinent functional changes occur.

TRANSMITTER INTERACTIONS

The work of the past decade has emphasized transmitter-drug-behavior effects largely in isolation, as though single transmitter systems were monologists acting in a covertly admitted multiple character ensemble. Recent evidence of transmitter coexistence and synergistic interactions between transmitters influencing a single target cell suggests there is much to be learned here about physiology, pathophysiology, and drug design.

One example is the ability of vasoactive intestinal polypeptide (VIP) and norepinephrine to act synergistically on cortical neurons, an effect observed both biochemically and electrophysiologically. Our electrophysiological indications of a VIP-norepinephrine interaction at the cellular level in rodent neocortex may arise from their common ability to stimulate cyclic AMP generation *in vitro*. The reported enhancement by norepinephrine of synaptic and other transmitter responses (including inhibitory ones) may depend on such shared biochemical mechanisms (see 1, 5). Two modes of indirect amplification of postsynaptic target cell mechanisms may be involved in these interactions, namely a cyclic AMP-mediated activation of protein kinases (as with β-adrenergic and other responses) and a calcium activation of protein kinases (as with α_1-adrenergic and other transmitter or hormone responses (see 8). However, it is not yet clear how these metabolic and electrophysiologic events actually interact, and such events will require linkage for more complete understanding.

Other important interactive transmitter regulations are becoming recognized. For example, consider the oligopeptide somatostatin. Although discovered and named for its ability to impair the release of growth hormone from somatotropes, the same peptide is ubiquitous throughout the central, peripheral, and diffuse gastrointestinal nervous systems and the endocrine pancreas. Among the nonendocrine regions of the rat and primate central nervous system where this peptide has been localized to large numbers of neurons are the hippocampus and cerebral cortex. In rat hippocampus, direct tests of somatostatin alone on neurons *in vitro* and *in vivo* suggest that the peptide shows many of the qualities of action of so-called "classical" inhibitory messenger molecules, depressing spontaneous discharge rate, hyperpolarizing the postsynaptic membrane, and increasing membrane conductance. However, at doses that had little or no direct effect on spontaneous discharge rate, somatostatin showed interesting selective effects enhancing responses of hippocampal pyramidal neurons to acetylcholine (6,7). The most notable effect was an increased responsiveness of the test neuron to acetylcholine; under these test conditions neurons showed more potent and somewhat longer-lasting effects of acetylcholine-induced (but not glutamate-induced) firing, with a more rapid onset and offset than the "direct" depressant effects of somatostatin. The ability of intoxicating doses of ethanol to enhance somatostatin actions, and thereby enhance acetylcholine effects, suggests the likely importance of these transmitter interactions to the further analysis of CNS drug effects.

ARE NEUROPEPTIDES THE NEW EXEMPLARS?

Although we routinely speak of peptide-containing neurons as though they were peptidergic, there are, in fact, no instances yet of which I am aware in which all or any of the effects of a peptide-containing system in the mammalian CNS have been identified as being peptidergic. Moreover, given the existing anatomic data, there are few places other than the hypothalamic paraventricular nucleus (4) where such stimulation paradigms might be effectively attempted. Nevertheless, as a field of scientific investigation, neuropeptides offer both the fundamental and the clinical pharmacologist enormous opportunities.

Two obvious future developments seem likely to become reality in the near term. The first involves the *biosynthetic process* of prohormone peptide synthesis by perikaryal ribosomes and raises the exciting prospects of genetic expression and its regulation, as well as alternative routes for peptide precursor processing. Each of these regulated steps suggests innumerable testable hypotheses of neurological and psychiatric disorder when a currently inexplicable disease can be reconceived in terms of the production of messenger peptides in abnormal amounts or in abnormal molecular forms. Second, we can readily accept the importance of *diverse receptor mechanisms* ranging from direct regulation of ion permeability to more complex synergistic regulation of intracellular metabolism. These and other mechanisms will provide a wide dynamic range of actions attributable to neuropeptides.

Ultimately, the concerns of the College will be whether there are any special properties of peptides as intercellular signals that either transcend or follow from their obvious chemical differences from amino acid or monoamine transmitters. More specifically, we might ask whether peptides have special properties as cell regulators that suggest they serve in different roles than conventional amino acid, monoamine, or ionic signals.

Potentially useful frames of reference for future work here will center on (a) the relatively modest amounts of peptides relative to other recognized transmitter substances; (b) their diverse molecular structures that allow for groupings according to amino acid sequence homologies, and may suggest evolutionary functional relationships; (c) their frequent coexistence with amine or amino acid transmitters; and (d) their ability to influence the response of target cells to other chemical signals.

Although these facets of peptides will undoubtedly be polished by more work, their reflections of future basic operating principles are still murky. Such studies will hopefully clarify the meaning of the relatively poor correlation between peptide cellular distributions (as revealed by detailed cytochemistry or microdissection sample assay) and presumptive peptide receptor distributions (indicated by ligand binding of synthetic analogs or drugs that show receptor correlations). At face value, peptides may be recognized by binding sites that are at considerable distances from their sites of release. Does this mean peptides act by diffusing to distant receptors to regulate local activity with little constraint by moment-to-moment neural events? Or does it mean that more data are needed to detect the subsets of "all possible binding sites" that are routinely utilized to respond normally to endogenously released peptides? A grand campaign for the next generation will be to answer this question: Is the brain more properly regarded as a precisely wired, chemically transmitted switchboard, or as a collection of loosely bounded chemical ponds acting on shifting cellular shores?

TRANSMITTER PEPTIDES AND BRAIN DISORDERS

Even without wistful looks into the future, a considerable body of recent basic neuropeptide knowledge still awaits direct clinical assessment. Thus, the recognition of countless new anatomical circuits in the brain, plus the opportunity to assign to these circuits one of the rapidly increasing numbers of peptides and other transmitters, offers the beginnings of a vast new world of selective neuropathology which has for the most part yet to be applied comprehensively to the human brain.

NEUROPEPTIDES: HOW MANY MORE?

Recently two new strategies have been plumbed to discover new peptides that may greatly lengthen the list emerging from the era of the hypophysiotrophic factors. In one approach, a directed search was made for medium-sized peptides whose C-terminal amino acids are amidated (a feature shared by many of the gut and CNS peptides). In the other, recombinant DNA sequencing methods were directed at the determination of the precursor forms of brain, pituitary, and gut peptides whose structures were already known. The unexpected discovery, which has now occurred in sufficient repetitions to make this seem almost a principle of peptide biology: precursors of neuropeptides contain the makings of more possible final products than just the one originally recognized. Whether cosynthesized peptides may represent occasionally required, alternative messengers or critical embellishments of routine intercellular signaling is just one of the questions most easily envisioned already. Furthermore, a general method for elucidating the neuron-specific genes for peptide messengers could be viewed as a great untapped resource for the discovery of the next generations of neurotransmitters, as well as an elegant way to derive the sequence of transmitter-related proteins, such as receptors, and the ion channels they may regulate. Such endpoints, once considered hopeless pipe dreams to solve in molecular terms, are now becoming routine end-products of the molecular neurobiology era.

There are enormous difficulties to be solved in extending this approach to genotypic segments whose biochemistry and physiology cannot now be predicted. However, a comprehensive search strategy (10, see also 3) to reveal all the segments of the gene library coding for specific neuronal secretory products could yield invaluable information. Every new neurotransmitter discovered is an important preclinical opportunity, providing a means to reveal new structural relationships, to define new regulatory commands within the chemical vocabulary of neurons, and to promote new tests by which to reveal pathology and to devise therapies.

Based on the premier example of Parkinson's disease, the emerging discipline of neurochemical pathology has primarily focused on loss of a neurotransmitter system as the indication of disease, and at the replacement of that missing transmitter as the primary means of therapy. Although L-dopa therapy has been a notable success for the nigrostriatal degeneration of the dopaminergic pathway, no subsequent comparable successes have yet been documented for the other major neurologic or psychiatric disorders.

It now seems clear that other neurodegenerative disorders, such as Alzheimer's dementia, are unlikely to be explainable in terms of such unidimensional transmitter deficiencies. In fact, for Alzheimer's disease it would appear that several monoamine systems as well as peptide systems are involved, in terms of their selective loss in postmortem specimens. However, none of these losses *per se* are able to explain the dementing symptoms or provide for means to treat or prevent the disorder, let alone to explain the cellular mechanisms underlying the pathology.

If the conditional postsynaptic effects of adrenergic, cholinergic, and certain peptidergic systems we have observed in rats were also to apply to human cortical processes, it is clear that the combined chemical pathologies already documented could severely incapacitate the cortex. The multiple transmitter systems involved in the senile dementia of the Alzheimer's type (SDAT) pathologic process suggest that no single transmitter can provide a therapeutic strategy, and that the nature of the primary pathologic insult remains the primary question to be answered. New modes of understanding this and other brain-wasting dementing disorders, including untreatable chronic schizophrenia, will surely require more than one more generation.

NEUROPEPTIDES AND TREATMENT

The recent history of peptide research has provided a cardinal lesson pertinent for future therapeutic expectations even if pathologic correlations were to establish the cells that make or respond to them as likely etiologic factors:

peptide messengers isolated originally from gut or brain for specific actions in those systems are almost always later found to be far more widely distributed and to act on targets far more pervasive than was anticipated from the bioassay by which they were discovered. The multiorgan occurrences pose important issues for the clinical pharmacologist interested in developing synthetic agonists or antagonists of these peptides. The existence of multiple sites of specific regulatory actions for almost every messenger substance implies that there may also be multiple sites at which unwanted side effects may be evoked. Thus, pharmacological expectations for specific agonists and antagonists to peptides must be tempered by our ignorance as to what effects such drugs might be expected to produce on the whole organism.

At the same time as one recognizes these potential disadvantages of peptides for novel conventional drugs, peptides also present several new faces that may in fact make them more amenable to drug interventions, aside from their several additional enzymes required for prohormone processing and postresponse catabolism. The aura of molecular biological tricks to come holds that gene expression may be amenable to manipulation, given neurotropic viruses as carriers that can target to specific neurons, and once there reprogram missing or hyperactive genes back into a reasonable physiological status. The ability to incorporate antisense strand RNA into a cell is an alternative means of inactivating a potentially harmful gene product within the cell that makes it, rather than inactivating the receptors on target cells that may be more generally distributed.

There is a widely held view that mental activity ultimately rests on molecular and cellular biological phenomena, and that brain activity *per se* drives gene expression to account for cellular and behavioral plasticity. Given that premise, there is at least some reason to predict that when the genetic explanations for brain disorders are recognized more completely, behavioral therapies alone may be able to evoke the desired biological responses.

UNEXPECTED MOLECULAR DIVIDENDS

Recent findings on the molecular properties shared by some neuropeptides deserve close attention for the development of therapeutic ligands. Thus, analysis of secondary structural features within unrelated linear amino acid sequences has revealed a novel homology in zones that may exhibit helical structures when interacting with their receptors. The distribution of hydrophilic and hydrophobic residues within these potential helices yields patches or faces of hydrophilicity and hydrophobicity. Thus, at least two possible lessons emerge: (a) linear sequence substitutions may have unexpected effects on ligand-receptor binding that would depend on these second-order structural features; and (b) a critical aspect of a "good" peptide messenger may depend on such secondary internal helical domains, perhaps induced in part by properties of the receptor proteins themselves.

A second recent study of the physical properties of protein-protein interaction also merits close attention. This study used synthetic peptide fragments to raise polyclonal antisera against different domains of large proteins whose X-ray crystallographic structures were resolved. Antipeptide antibodies against regions with high atomic mobility produced much stronger immune interactions with the native proteins then did antisera against well-ordered and stable regions. This suggests that ligand-receptor interactions we may regard as homologous to interactions between neuropeptides and their receptors may not match the traditional "lock and key" construct. If these ligand-antibody interactions are validly extended to peptide-receptor interactions, attention to atomic mobility features may provide conformational flexibility that will clarify receptor activation processes and facilitate development of peptide drugs with appropriate atomic features.

CONCLUSIONS: WHITHER OR WITHER?

There is, however, a notable gap between recognition of a possible molecular pathology, however that may be determined, and the construction of a functional conceptual model of a CNS disorder. How does that molecular process lead to effects on the operations of cell systems, and how do those interconnected ensembles generate behaviors, as the organism senses, anticipates, or reacts to events in its internal and external environments? Put more simply, we do not yet have insight into how molecular events are translated through regulation of neuroal biology into the integrative actions we attribute to the behaving brain and which may be at fault in the unresolved CNS disorders.

There is likely to be continued progress in the detailed anatomy, physiology, and behavioral correlates of specific transmitter systems in both vertebrates and invertebrates that will help to reveal those specific molecular events in those defined cellular sites that underlie not only simple elements of memory and learning, but the more complex forms that are achievable with more complex neuronal circuitry. In fact, there is a great possibility that in the decade ahead, we can anticipate that human mental activities will become far more thoroughly explainable in these terms, although obviously not with the direct confirmations possible for simpler behavioral events in animals.

Noninvasive methods for the assessment of neuroendocrine or electrophysiological indices of brain pathophysiology in normal or psychotic humans will likely gain much from the development of improved methods for determining the origin of electroencephalographic (EEG) phenomena. Such progress will include those EEG events summed with a computer into event-related potentials for better temporal correlations of mental phenomena and electrophysiology, and those analyzed with magnetic probes for greater spatial resolution of sites far below the cortex. An important aspect of these studies is the attempt to draw from these human indices possible clues as to the pathophysiology of the brain and incorporate them into animal models of brain disorder in animals.

Perhaps the only future-directed conclusion worth drawing is that the fields of fundamental neurobiology and psychopharmacology are actively engaged in an era of discovery, and about the only certain discovery we will face is that we don't really know what to expect.

ACKNOWLEDGMENTS

The author's work is supported by grants AA 06420, NS 22347 and the Whittier Foundation.

REFERENCES

1. Bloom, F. E. (1984): *Am. J. Physiol.,* 246:C184–C194.
2. Bloom, F. E. (1986): In: *Neuropeptides in Neurologic and Psychiatric Disease,* edited by J. B. Martin and J. Barchas, pp. 335–349. Raven Press, New York.
3. Bloom, F. E., Battenberg, E., Milner, R. J., and Sutcliffe, G. (1986): In: *Neurohistochemistry: Modern Methods and Applications,* edited by P. Panula, H. Päivärinta, and S. Soinila, pp. 3–19. Allan R. Liss, New York.
4. Buijs, R. M., and Van Heerikhuize, J. J. (1982): *Brain Res.,* 252: 71–76.
5. Foote, S. L., Bloom, F. E., and Aston-Jones, G. (1983): *Physiol. Rev.,* 63:844–914.
6. Mancillas, J. R., Siggins, G. R., and Bloom, F. E. (1986): *Science,* 231:161–163.
7. Mancillas, J. R., Siggins, G. R., and Bloom, F. E. (1986): *Proc. Natl. Acad. Sci. USA,* 83:7518–7521.
8. Nestler, E. J., and Greengard, P. (1984): *Protein Phosphorylation in the Nervous System.* John Wiley and Sons, New York.
9. Siggins, G. R., and Gruol, D. L. (1986): In: *Handbook of Physiology, Vol. IV: Intrinsic Regulatory Systems of the Brain,* edited by F. E. Bloom, Vol. IV, pp. 1–114. American Physiological Society, Bethesda, MD.
10. Sutcliffe, J. G., Milner, R. J., Shinnick, T. M., and Bloom, F. E. (1983): *Cell,* 33:671–682.

Psychopharmacology:
The Third Generation of Progress,
edited by Herbert Y. Meltzer.
Raven Press, New York © 1987.

CHAPTER **183**

Future Directions in Biological Psychiatry

Frederick K. Goodwin and Peter P. Roy-Byrne

In preparing a chapter describing the future of any medical discipline, authors have traditionally catalogued all the exciting developments on the horizon, often emphasizing that the availability of new technologies will provide the understanding necessary to control and/or eradicate human disease. Although the advent of new and exciting tools to explore brain function will no doubt enlarge the scope and yield of subsequent investigations in clinical psychiatry, future research goals must not be based primarily on these new technologies, but must derive from consideration of the strengths and limitations of the various paradigms we have used in the past to understand and interpret our data. That is, as we continue to gather new knowledge, we must simultaneously rethink our current knowledge along new lines.

This discussion about concepts and hypotheses should also remind us that the term "biological psychiatry" in the title of this chapter may be misunderstood as denoting a "type" of, or subspecialty area in, psychiatry. As E. O. Wilson has written in his discussion of the development of scientific disciplines (42), new disciplines are created out of the hierarchy of existing disciplines (i.e., physics-chemistry-biology-psychology-social science) when the lower-order macrodiscipline is reformulated according to the laws of the higher-order microdiscipline. Hence, physics changed chemistry into physical chemistry, chemistry changed biology into molecular biology, and now biology is changing psychiatry into biological psychiatry. This implies that eventually there will be no other kind of psychiatry: not that psychiatry will be reduced to the study of the mechanisms involved in brain function, but rather that this new knowledge will inform, change, and potentially rearrange psychological constructs so that they are more consistent with what we are learning about the biology of human thought, mood, and behavior. The clinical implications of

this for the practice of psychoanalysis have been recently addressed (8).

In this chapter, we will begin by highlighting some problems with existing approaches to psychiatric illness and brain-behavior relationships before moving on to the possibilities and promises of the current technological revolution. We will then conclude with a discussion of how the combination of new technologies and new conceptual approaches will guide future attempts at understanding how biology shapes the genesis, occurrence, and outcome of various psychiatric disorders.

CURRENT PROBLEMS

The State of Our Scholarship

The wealth of information presented in previous chapters reflects the exponential increase in data that has occurred in our field over the past few years. As new technologies continue to proliferate, providing new and more accurate ways to measure various aspects of brain function, there needs to be an equally vigorous effort to keep pace conceptually with this "data explosion" by seeking new ways of understanding observed relationships between brain and behavior. Powerful computer techniques that permit the high-speed analysis of multivariate data have radically changed the conduct of scientific investigation. In the past researchers often would have to wait for their data to emerge; thus, there was ample time to carefully consider and reevaluate hypotheses, meticulously review the literature, and develop research strategies and goals for the future. Now, because of the increased technological ability to generate data, the enhanced speed of data analysis, and the academic pressure to "publish or perish," time constraints can limit the breadth and depth of literature reviews, as well as the ability to keep pace conceptually with the hypotheses and findings of others. Thus, we face a potential paradox: diminished understanding in the face of (and perhaps because of) increasing amounts of data.

There are other problems related to the design of experiments. The use of linear statistical models that reduce the variance in groups in order to facilitate the analysis of group differences also promotes the assumption that clinical phenomena are homogeneous and encourages investigators to view intra- and interindividual differences in a given parameter as "noise." The large numbers of "negative" psychiatric studies with small n values highlight the problem of type II or "beta" statistical error (i.e., the high likelihood that a true difference has not been detected), which makes such negative findings uninterpretable (10). The plethora of such studies may be, in part, the result of a pressure to publish results prematurely.

Another problem derives from the increasing availability of powerful new assay methods that can now measure previously unmeasurable substances. This development has caused investigators discouraged by the current lack of a general theory of cerebral and mental functioning to believe the problem is that they just haven't found or focused on the right neurotransmitter or neuromodulator. Assay availability, then, determines research direction with investigators repeating the mistakes of the past, measuring the new substance in two groups, and demonstrating or not demonstrating group mean differences. As noted above, negative findings are often uninterpretable because of small sample sizes, and even "positive" ones may be too quickly accepted, with investigators moving on to the next substance rather than pausing to figure out what their positive findings mean. Thus, by letting our tools and our statistics do our thinking for us and hoping that something new will clarify the old confusion, we avoid the obvious: if little is gained from using approach "A" on neurotransmitters X, Y, and Z, the problem may be in the approach rather than in the neurotransmitters that we select to study.

Although some of the methodological problems previously mentioned might be easily addressed (i.e., calculation of beta errors and use of larger sample sizes), others might require more forethought. For example, the solution to the practice of using powerful multivariate statistics to fit psychiatric phenomena to a linear model might involve an attempt to focus on and better characterize the variance obtained in samples of patients. It has recently been appreciated by a number of investigators looking at the noradrenergic system in depression that abnormalities in this system appear to be better characterized by the term "dysregulation" than by an absolute increase or decrease at a given period in time (36). Mandell et al. (23) have described a number of ways to find order, regularity, and pattern in the variance of enzyme kinetic phenomena, and these tools may also be applicable to more complex biological systems (see later section entitled "Conceptual and Technologic Leads for the Future"). Above all, it must be emphasized that no statistical technique, no matter how powerful, can substitute for a clear hypothesis, capable of being disproven, and for *replication*.

The decline in scholarship may require solutions directed at changing the values and reward systems of the scientists involved in the funding and conduct of clinical research. For example, the current peer review system controlling the allocation of grants with the requirement for specific detailed proposals may discourage innovative thinking and "scientific revolutions." More than a few distinguished scientists have suggested it might be preferable to fund *people* rather than *projects* (44). In a similar vein, grants might be made available for the performance of scholarly reviews in a given area rather than for generation of data in that area, or to allow individual investigators to serve as journal reviewers rather than requiring a free contribution of time which often compromises the ability to perform careful, scholarly reviews. Since scholarship is not synonymous with statistics or methodology, in addition to recent attempts to standardize the methodology of clinical research (20), there also needs to be standardization in the various psychiatric research journals for the *quality* of scholarship. Since the attempt to standardize clinical methodology grew out of a specific conference that addressed this specific issue as one of its concerns, it might be possible to tackle this more ambiguous issue by a similar method.

The "Medical Model" and Research Design

Although the term "medical model," as it is used in psychiatry, generally denotes a view of psychiatric dysfunction as disease or illness, there are more specific implications of the term with regard to research in biological psychiatry. Our notions of medical illness initially grew out of the infectious disease or "inborn errors of metabolism" models, which assumed that a single agent or deficiency was responsible for the illness and demonstrated that their respective removal or correction was curative. This approach was mirrored in "pharmacologic bridge" strategies that explored the neurochemical mechanisms of therapeutically effective drugs in animals and attempted to reason backwards, inferring an opposite "cause" in psychiatrically ill humans. In addition to other limitations of this paradigm (15,34), its focus on a single "cause" was doubtless a conceptual liability. In schizophrenia, for example, a recent review of the contradictory evidence for neurochemical abnormalities in the illness (9) notes that few studies have simultaneously considered more than a single variable.

Even the exploration of multiple variables, however, can be tied to a view that disease is caused by too much or too little of some specific thing. In affective illness, multiple neurotransmitter, endocrine, and peptide "abnormalities" (too much or too little) have been identified (31), and one is left with the problem of determining how all these specific abnormalities fit together and how specific they are to the illness. When taken with the fact that lithium carbonate, a highly specific drug for bipolar affective illness, also has widespread effects that are not at all specific (i.e., interaction with cyclic AMP-mediated processes in multiple tissues), one wonders if there might be a more generalized abnormality contributing to the illness (i.e., membrane defect) and giving rise to numerous epiphenomena. Although membrane hypotheses have certainly been considered, these and other hypotheses of a generalized abnormality have not received the attention given to specific transmitter systems, possibly because they don't lend themselves to the linear approach so popular at present.

An additional legacy of the medical model is the danger of focusing only on the biological cause when the mainstream of medicine has itself moved to a more systems-oriented view that emphasizes the importance of host factors for infectious disease and health habits for a variety of other illnesses. In our eagerness to free ourselves from the limitations of earlier psychosocial paradigms, there is a danger of ignoring relevant psychosocial variables. For example, studies of social groups of monkeys have shown that response to serotonin agonists is dependent on the animal's position in the dominance hierarchy, such that a change in position from alpha to lower-order male can result in dramatic and categorically different behavioral responses (33). The role of context has also been emphasized in pharmacologic studies of both tolerance and sensitization phenomena. For example, theories of opiate craving in abstinent heroin addicts suggest that the development of tolerance may be associated with neurochemical changes in an opposite or compensatory direction from changes induced by opiates, and that such changes can be triggered on a conditioned basis when the abstinent addict enters an old context or setting where he had previously used heroin, neurochemically setting off a kind of "withdrawal" state (35). Sensitization in rats to the psychomotor effects of repeated doses of cocaine can also be greatly amplified if the cocaine challenge occurs in the same cage or test environment in which the original cocaine doses had been administered (32). Both these phenomena suggest that neurochemical changes, originally the result of pharmacologic stimuli, can be conditioned and reelicited by certain contextual "cues." These considerations may become vitally important as we continue our exploration of the biology of formerly labeled "neuroses" (i.e., anxiety, minor depression, somatoform disorders) and certain "personality disorders," since similar kinds of conditioning may play an important role in these disorders' seeming plasticity in the face of environmental change, a plasticity formerly thought to indicate that such disorders are fundamentally "nonbiological" in nature.

Finally, emphasis on how the mind and social context can affect body and brain should be supplemented by newer ways of viewing the effects of "body" on mind. An exclusive focus on the brain as the organ of interest could obscure recent discoveries that suggest a renewed focus on the periphery and how it affects the brain [i.e., peptides secreted by blood cells that might affect brain functioning (37) and provide a model for parts of the body other than brain mediating mood and behavior]. No doubt, this "new psychosomatic medicine" will provide additional details of how peripheral peptides involved in peripheral organ pathology might themselves mediate some of the behavioral effects traditionally associated with these illnesses (depression in carcinoma of the pancreas or other paraneoplastic syndromes). Communication between the immune system and the brain may serve as a model for the discovery of other peripheral-central lines of communication and could provide a new view of the James-Lang theory of emotion where the brain's interpretation of signals from the periphery is not solely a "cognitive" event, but depends on the biological nature of the peripheral message. That is, the neuroanatomical site of action of such a messenger, along with its known biological characteristics, may help enlarge and further clarify our notions of "cognitive" psychology. Do the peripherally secreted peptides in question bind to areas of the brain more involved with planning and the anticipation of action (prefrontal cortex), to areas of the brain more involved with the primary expression of emotions (septum, amygdala), or to areas primarily involved in the short-term consolidation of memory (hippocampus)? Are such peripherally secreted peptides known on the basis of their action in the brain to be modulators of other neurotransmitters with their own particular cognitive, mood, and behavioral effects?

Specificity of Biological Findings

Although our modern diagnostic entities have greater reliability and predictive validity than ever before, biological findings related to them have poor specificity, with abnormalities crossing diagnostic lines more often than not (i.e., the overlap between affective, eating, and anxiety disorders in neuroendocrine function and treatment response) (15). Methodologically, this is partially due to the fact that most studies are diagnostically, rather than biologically, based (i.e., observable symptom complexes are used as the dependent variable). When biological variance is then found within a given disorder or group of disorders, it is virtually impossible to determine whether it is due to some global aspect of the syndrome or to specific symptoms, behaviors, or personality traits associated with them.

There are several solutions to the problem. Foremost would be to develop a new system of biological typologies by beginning with the biological variable and attempting to specify the clinical variables that are most strongly associated with it, regardless of diagnosis. Although some studies have employed this strategy, it has often been within the confines of a given diagnostic category (e.g., depression), which has limited its utility since certain biological abnormalities might underlie behavior that crosses diagnoses (e.g., a decreased serotonin metabolite level in association with aggression). This approach might uncover new relationships between syndromes not previously thought to be strongly related (e.g., the role of endorphins in the modulation of both affect and pain). More importantly, however, many behavioral abnormalities may lie on a continuum with normal personality "traits," and hence there is a need to understand the normal cerebral mechanism mediating fluctuations in cognition, mood, and behavior before attempting to understand abnormalities or deviations from these mechanisms. Although this implies that the biology of such traits (i.e., depression, aggression) must be explored in normal individuals, it has been more difficult to study individuals without psychiatric illness or individuals with psychiatric illness in remission, partly because of a long-standing debate about the public health value versus the knowledge generation value of research funded with government dollars. Concerned individuals without scientific backgrounds often want to target research dollars exclusively toward the study of ill patients, despite the fact that in working with this population certain flaws in experimental design are difficult to avoid (e.g., confounding effects of medication, which may exist even if a washout period of several weeks is utilized, since it is not clear what kind of long-standing changes in brain chemistry, or in the presumed abnormality in brain chemistry responsible for an illness, are induced).

A more complete implementation of the "biological typology" approach would require enlargement of the usual clinical descriptions beyond simple cataloguing of symptoms to include dimensional rather than categorical measures of personality, life stress, social role, etc. Ethological approaches that have abandoned self-report and even traditional observer rating scales to emphasize instead an atheoretical approach to behavioral description might also be employed (30). The 1982 Dahlem Conference on the origins of depression made a series of recommendations specifying the kinds of clinical variables that might be involved in biological studies in psychiatry (20). Adherence to these recommendations should facilitate metaanalytic approaches that can compensate for small sample sizes by pooling the results of many studies. Although metaanalysis has been recently employed in examining psychotherapy efficacy, it has probably been underutilized in biological studies.

Another approach to the question of specificity involves the study of biological correlates of individual symptoms (e.g., insomnia) as they occur across different syndromes (e.g., primary insomnia, depression, anxiety disorder). Optimally such an approach should be combined with epidemiologic methods (18). After selecting populations with an extremely high or low incidence of a given disease and also searching for large pedigrees with the disease in question, large-scale studies might try to identify etiologic agents, indicators, or risk factors associated with specific *components* of these diseases (e.g., deficits in attention, cognition, and mood in schizophrenia). The clustering of specific phenomena on a geographical, seasonal, or other spatiotemporal basis might provide valuable clues as to which factors are relevant for a given illness. Because a given phenomenon might appear descriptively similar across individuals, but still be the final common pathway for disparate biologic abnormalities, the use of clustering and other epidemiologic techniques may help clarify biological variations found within certain individual factors.

CONCEPTUAL AND TECHNOLOGIC LEADS FOR THE FUTURE

Frame of Reference for Observations

One of the more productive conceptual shifts occurring in recent times has been the move to consider not just cross-sectional aspects of affective disorder, but temporal ones as well. Kraepelin's initial emphasis on the longitudinal *course* of manic-depression was somehow lost in this country as subsequent writers focused on the present state of the patient and proximate (precipitating?) life events. Only recently has there been a renewed focus on the temporal aspects of the illness (16,45), fueled especially by the development of maintenance pharmacological treatments. We highlight this shift to note that it has given rise to two novel and important theories about affective disorder. First, consideration of the intermittent and repetitive nature of affective illness spurred Robert Post and colleagues at the National Institute of Mental Health to ask whether the process underlying this pattern might resemble the processes

responsible for electrical kindling and behavioral sensitization—two phenomena where responsivity to the same stimulus applied intermittently over time, progressively increases. They noted that the probability of recurrent affective episodes also seemed to increase over time in some patients. From this came the notion that carbamazepine, which retards electrical kindling in animals, might be particularly effective in various forms of rapidly cycling affective illness—a rare occurrence in psychiatry, where a theory of pathophysiology suggested a particular clinical application for an existing drug treatment. A second example occurred when focus on the cyclic aspects of illness that occur within a given day (i.e., early morning wakening, diurnal variation of mood, early morning switches of mood state) led Wehr, Goodwin, and colleagues at NIMH to become interested in circadian rhythms and how they might be related to phenomena common to both the cross-sectional state and longitudinal fluctuations of the illness. This has already proven helpful in understanding the antidepressant effect of sleep deprivation (39), and suggesting a modification of the technique to partial (second half of the night) sleep deprivations that could be repetitively administered (unlike total sleep deprivation), and hence provide more long-lasting effects. It also provided a new understanding of the possible mode of action of antidepressant drugs which were found in animal studies to lengthen the periodicity of strong circadian oscillators, theoretically realigning them with weak oscillators and correcting out-of-phase phenomena that are present in many patients (phase advance of many rhythms) (43). This shift in perspective has also spurred interest in seasonal variations in affective disorder and the possible roles of light and melatonin in the etiology and treatment of affective disorder.

Further consideration of other aspects of course of illness is particularly relevant to issues raised earlier regarding the clinical specificity of biological findings. For example, some biological abnormalities observed in the depressed state may be partially dependent on variations in the prior course of the illness (i.e., number of prior episodes, length of longest remission, duration of most recent episode). This possibility might be important in schizophrenia research, where a major confounding factor has been the large number of chronically ill patients studied and the paucity of studies examining acute, first-time patients.

A more complex example of this shift from static to dynamic paradigms is encompassed in Mandell's use of nonlinear mathematical models to understand the behavior of living systems (22). Although these approaches initially arose as a result of some unexpected nonlinear responses in experiments in enzyme kinetics (24), they have been useful in the hands of other investigators to describe the structure of apparently random rat behavior in response to stimulants (14) and the structure of the heart rate variation observed in psychiatric patients before and after psychotropic drug treatment (4). Because the concepts underlying such approaches are primarily mathematical, it is difficult to articulate them without the benefit of mathematical equations. Briefly, however, Mandell found that enzyme activity in the living brain occurs at substrate and cofactor concentrations below the saturation conditions assumed to exist in linear enzyme kinetic models. While examining enzyme activity *in vitro* as a function of small increments in substrate and cofactor concentrations similar to that found *in vivo,* Mandell showed that the relation between enzyme activity and substrate concentration deviated radically from that described by ideal enzyme kinetics (i.e., with successive small changes, enzyme activity changed in a variable manner that seemed, however, to follow a certain pattern). By using time series analysis, Mandell was able to examine this variation in terms of its frequency or periodicity, as well as its amplitude. He observed that there were only a few, rather than an infinite variety, of patterns of variation (23). In the study alluded to above (4), the periodicity of heart rate variation in psychiatric patients was described by time series analysis and found to be decreased after successful drug treatment of psychosis, suggesting that a reduction in a system's variance was a sign of enhanced functioning in the system.

Essentially what Mandell has done is to bring to psychiatric research techniques from other fields that reveal the degree of order, regularity, and predictability existing in variation previously described as random. Implicitly, this model might allow psychiatric investigators to more elegantly and precisely explore and describe the "dysregulation" that they are now postulating to occur in various neurotransmitter systems. That is, this notion suggests that dysregulation is not equivalent to chaos, disorder, and a lack of equilibrium, but merely represents a different kind of equilibrium that can be described with the benefit of these new models. Mandell further suggests that each living larger system is composed of a multitude of smaller fluctuating systems that act in some kind of harmony. Thus, apparently variable, dysregulated, or chaotic behavior in smaller systems may produce more regular patterns of behavior in larger systems. The clinical correlate of this may be the regular periodicity of episodes observed in certain forms of manic-depressive illness, a regularity in the larger (behavioral) system arising out of some presumed derangement in the smaller (neurochemical) systems controlling mood and behavior. It is possible that these approaches may be applied to find new ways of analyzing both psychometric data involving self and observer ratings of patients' mood and behavior, and the fluctuations in neurochemicals and neurotransmitters obtained from various bodily fluids.

The New Neurology of Psychiatric Disease

More recently, advances in the neurosciences have provided psychiatric investigators with an increased ability to image the brain. The precursor to these advances was the advent of computed tomographic (CT) brain scanning, which resulted in a series of studies of brain and ventricular size, focused particularly on the schizophrenic population. More recently, however, investigators have recognized that ventricular enlargement also occurs in a substantial proportion of patients with major affective disorder and that such patients also show an incidence of soft neurologic signs similar to that previously noted in the schizophrenic population (19). Other investigators have focused on related neurologic abnormalities in patients with borderline personality disorder (1). Thus, it is likely that neurological

approaches need not be confined to the more traditionally severe or psychotic psychiatric disorder, but may yield useful information about a wide array of behavioral abnormalities.

These initial CT scan studies carefully examined only structural changes, with no attempt to simultaneously look at neurochemical changes in the same population. More recently, however, studies have begun to link neurochemical changes to structural atrophy in the brain in an attempt to bridge the gap between biochemical and neuroanatomical approaches. However, since both technologies (CT scanning and the analysis of chemical changes in bodily fluids) are unable to detect changes in specific brain areas, they are of somewhat limited value. This limitation, however, has now been overcome by the development of magnetic resonance imaging (MRI) which will allow more refined imaging of brain *structure,* such that it more closely approximates that obtained by direct autopsy. Thus, the size and configuration of various nuclei and subcortical areas may be visualized and a study similar to the recently reported analysis of hippocampal/temporal lobe tissue densities in autopsied schizophrenic brains (5) might be done on living patients. This could be of immeasurable help in exploring, for example, congenital, degenerative, or viral etiologic theories of the schizophrenias. In addition, investigators might combine *in vivo* imaging with postmortem studies, employing, among other techniques, autoradiography to map systems of neurotransmitters and neuromodulators in discrete brain areas. This new technology might also allow investigators to take advantage of naturally occurring medical models of psychiatric illness. For example, the precise location of plaques in multiple sclerosis (MS) patients with mood disorders might be compared with those seen in MS patients without mood disorders to gain new knowledge about the neuroanatomy of mood. At present, in addition to problems with resolution, the long time in which a subject is required to remain motionless makes the study of certain behavioral conditions difficult. However, developments will likely shorten the required time and thus increase the number *and* type of patient (e.g., more severely ill) able to be studied.

Even more important than the ability to examine brain *structure* is the possibility of more closely examining brain *function.* Because human behavior is a dynamic series of changing states, it follows that abnormalities in behavior (i.e., psychiatric disorder) can only be understood by exploring how brain physiology changes across different behavioral states and conditions. Using this strategy, Weinberger et al. (40) have recently applied cerebral blood flow techniques to the study of schizophrenic patients under a series of behavioral (cognitive) conditions and found specific abnormalities in prefrontal cortical blood flow only when patients were performing a task previously found in primate studies (11,25) to depend specifically on intact prefrontal cortical functioning. This exciting finding also points out the utility of studying individuals in other than basal conditions (no blood flow differences were found between patients and controls at rest), as well as the importance of drawing on work in primate neuropsychology in designing research protocols. With regard to schizophrenia, information processing models of this illness (6) may yield additional behavioral paradigms that could be tested with this method.

Other studies by this same group have examined blood flow changes in normal subjects under simulated emotional states. Once abnormalities in discrete parts of the brain are found to be associated with behavioral changes, investigators might combine this with a biochemical/pharmacological approach by administering drugs that affect a discrete neurotransmitter system known to be important in the given brain region with abnormal blood flow and see if it can independently affect both blood flow and the behavioral change.

The above strategy is likely to be made more useful because of the development of the positron emission tomography (PET) scan. The PET scan is now providing psychiatric investigators with the exciting possibility of having direct access to the local biochemistry of the living human brain (29). Previously, investigators only had the ability to make inferences about biochemical processes in the brain by combining global biochemical measures derived from *in vivo* study of body fluids (e.g., cerebrospinal fluid, blood, urine) with more specific information about local biochemistry gleaned from animal studies. These methods had the inherent limitations of animal models, which may only approximate some aspects of human brain physiology. With this new tool, however, it is possible to measure the localization of a specific type of isotope that has been attached to a given compound and administered intravenously to a living patient. PET techniques will also allow investigators to move beyond the identification of a given structural lesion to specification of the functional results of this lesion (i.e., what connections running through this involved area are disturbed, where do they go, and hence what other brain areas are also dysfunctional?) (29). This will permit better understanding of how the brain works.

However, although the theoretical implications of this are great (i.e., various neurotransmitter, hormone, and peptide analogs can theoretically be labeled with positron-emitting nucleotides and their distribution in the brain over time can be traced so that both presynaptic events and the activity of receptor systems thought to be involved in various human behaviors can be examined), there are numerous technical and scientific problems (7). To begin with, investigators must select an isotope and a compound to be tagged with it. This alone generates numerous problems: How is the isotopically labeled compound metabolized? What are the specific chemical forms of isotope in various metabolic compartments and how do they vary over time? What does the "localization" obtained mean? In addition, certain anatomic regions are small compared with the resolution capacity of the scanner, so the size of any area of interest is confounded with the quantitative measure of isotopic activity. Other technical sources of variance include artifact induced by subtle subject movement (e.g., eye blink) and large (20–25%) coefficients of variation obtained among normal subjects when measuring the same area.

Even more important and relevant to this chapter are certain scientific limitations. Consistent with earlier-noted caveats regarding the importance of studying patients without psychiatric illness, the future of PET scanning in the short run should probably involve the careful study of normal brain functioning so that the role of particular neurochemicals and anatomic pathways in mediating rela-

tionships between brain and behavior in normal subjects can be described carefully before attempting to understand the deviations in these relationships that may be responsible for psychopathology. Currently, this is not being pursued with the same vigor as studies of patient populations. Additional problems include the need to specify response sets and behavioral conditions, as done in the blood flow studies of Weinberger et al., so that the range of values of other confounding variables will be somewhat restricted, increasing the chances of differentiating "abnormal" from "normal." Finally, there is the usual dilemma of determining the meaning of any "abnormal" finding (e.g., decreased activity in a given anatomic region in schizophrenia). Is this the real "cause" of the disease, is it an epiphenomenon or result, or are both the disease and the abnormality epiphenomena of some third as yet unidentified factor? Other problematic aspects involved in the interpretation of brain-behavior data have been dealt with elsewhere (34).

These limitations suggest that there is a long way to go and much more needed besides the development of new ligands before PET scanning can be used to explore, for example, dopamine systems in schizophrenia, benzodiazepine systems in anxiety disorders, cholinergic systems in the dementias, and the noradrenergic system in both mood and anxiety disorders. It should be noted that, analogous to the PET scan, it may be possible to give paramagnetic substances tagged to different drugs or neurotransmitters and utilize MRI scanning in the same way as PET.

Another newly developed tool that gives a cross-sectional computer-derived image of both structure and function is electroencephalographic (EEG) topographic mapping, which uses computer techniques to determine the distribution of electrical activity over the cortical surface. This is particularly useful when employed to measure a subject's response under a variety of different behavioral conditions (e.g., pain, cognitive task) or in the presence of a given drug. It might also be useful, however, in examining cortical function in patients suffering "toxic" psychoses.

Molecular Genetics

Over the past decade, the development of molecular genetic techniques has advanced our understanding of certain human genetic diseases. These techniques now hold the promise not only of clarifying the genetic components of major psychiatric disorders through gene-mapping strategies, but of discovering previously unknown peptides and other gene products that might mediate behavioral disturbances using brain-specific mRNA and subtraction hybridization techniques (3).

The combination of powerful recombinant DNA techniques with the traditional methods of genetic linkage analyses has recently led to the discovery of a DNA marker linked to Huntington's disease (17). DNA sequence variations are detected using enzymes (restriction endonucleases) that specifically digest DNA and yield variously sized fragments (restriction fragment length polymorphisms or RFLPs), depending on the type of base sequence present at the site of enzyme action. These sequence variations (RFLPs) display mendelian inheritance and can be used as genetic markers in linkage studies. Thus, one can look for a gene without knowing anything about it. However, in order to apply this technique, investigators must first identify large pedigrees in which the gene is segregating in order to obtain a statistically significant incidence of coinheritance of marker and disease. This is further complicated by the fact that psychiatric illnesses demonstrate complex inheritance (i.e., variable penetrance), making the method of case identification of paramount importance. Ethological approaches to psychiatry have emphasized that behavior is naturally selected just as certain physical characteristics are and that this selection depends on its *adaptive value* for the population in question (30). Thus, genetic strategies may need to add *functional* criteria to the symptom criteria that are used to make certain diagnoses. Such a modification in diagnostic criteria has recently been employed (13) and found to decrease the reported incidence of major depression in family members of individuals without the illness, further strengthening proband-normal control differences in the incidence of familial affective disorder.

It is important to emphasize that the above gene-mapping strategies should not be expected to pinpoint the specific gene or genes involved in the illness in question (and by implication the peptide, neurotransmitter, or receptor abnormalities). However, DNA hybridization techniques can now be used to search for unique brain-specific mRNAs in postmortem brain tissue of psychiatric patients, with the advantage that recombinant molecules carrying sequences derived from polyadenylated mRNA will represent only those genes being transcribed in the tissue from which the mRNA was obtained. Such a strategy was recently employed to identify a unique mRNA whose expression is increased in both scrapie-infected brains of mice and senile plaques in human brain from patients with Alzheimer's disease (41). The usefulness of such a strategy for psychiatric illness probably will depend on searching for unique mRNAs in brain regions already suspected of being important in the pathophysiology of the illness (e.g., the nucleus basalis and areas receiving cholinergic projections or areas of greatest plaque and tangle density in Alzheimer's disease) and using subtraction techniques and data from normals to factor out normal mRNAs. After this, it might be possible to translate the unique mRNA and synthesize the protein it codes for.

Recombinant DNA technology can also be used to discover new peptides and other protein substances that seem structurally similar to already known proteins. These can then be localized to certain brain areas using radioactive DNA probes or peptide analogs synthesized and applied iontophoretically to the same brain regions in order to test for their biological activity. Although this strategy may help clarify and enlarge our understanding of normal brain function, it is possible that numerous newly discovered peptides could merely represent "evolutionary debris" and have no meaningful function in humans (26).

Endogenous Ligands

The discovery of saturable, high-affinity, and stereospecific recognition sites for opiate drugs in brain soon led to the isolation and identification of endogenous opiate-like sub-stances that were thought to interact with these receptors under normal physiological conditions (27,28). However, the variety of substances discovered (i.e., various enkephalins, endorphins, dynorphins) suggests that it is an oversimplification to speak of *an* endogenous ligand for *the* opiate receptor. Furthermore, endogenous substances relevant to the function of a given system may function as *modulators* rather than actual transmitters. For example, the discovery of the benzodiazepine receptor (38) has led to a search for endogenous anxiolytic or anxiogenic substances that might normally occupy these sites and regulate the γ-aminobutyric acid (GABA) receptor-coupled chloride ion channel. Recently, Costa and colleagues (12) have isolated and purified from rat and human brain a neuropeptide that displaces diazepam from benzodiazepine receptors and seems to have proconflict action similar to that of certain anxiogenic β-carbolines. In addition to this work, Paul's group has discovered an endogenous steroid that modulates the GABA receptor-coupled chloride ion channel in the GABA-ben-zodiazepine receptor complex and may serve as an "endogenous barbiturate-like" compound without actually being a direct ligand for the receptor (21). These results will no doubt spur additional searches for other endogenous ligands or modulators that might well serve as more appropriate models for understanding pathophysiology and for developing new treatment strategies. Currently, work at NIMH has focused on identifying and characterizing endogenous inhibitors of imipramine binding and serotonin uptake (2). Future investigators might search for naturally occurring amphetamine, neuroleptic, or phencyclidine (PCP)-like compounds that might point the way toward understanding psychosis and appetite dysregulation in certain disorders. As this work proceeds, the use of bioassays as opposed to static receptor binding assays takes on greater importance, since modulators can only be discovered when the biological function of the system is examined.

CLINICAL ISSUES

As the excitement of technological and conceptual advances seizes hold of investigators, there is often a temptation to draw premature closure on the potential clinical implications of a given finding. Perhaps the best example of this in recent years is the initial enthusiasm for the dexamethasone suppression test as a specific diagnostic laboratory test for depression, followed by more sober recognition of its many limitations and a realization that the transition from the research to the clinical setting had been made too quickly. Unfortunately, the media fuel this tendency because journalists are always eager for a story and may oversimplify in an attempt to "package" scientific information for the public. The upshot of such developments is that they widen the credibility gap between researchers and clinicians and undermine clinicians' faith in research and its potential applications for clinical practice. Since the cooperation and participation of clinicians in research are obviously crucial for recruitment of patients, it is important they perceive researchers as careful, cautious, and responsible.

Clinicians may also be important for the conduct of research by helping to inform researchers about subtleties of clinical phenomena that might shape future research directions. There is a need to provide channels for better communication from the clinician to the researcher. For example, in the field of drug development research, one wishes there could be developed a type of "reverse detail man" who could not only bring drug industry information to the clinician, but might also carry back observations and concerns from the clinician to the researcher in industry.

A word should also be said about underdeveloped areas that will require vigorous attention. Although advances in the pathophysiology and treatment of affective and anxiety disorders have occurred over the last decade, this has not been the case for the schizophrenic disorders. This is especially tragic in light of the major disability caused by this illness. No doubt newer brain imaging techniques may contribute to advances in schizophrenia, but it may be that novel conceptual approaches are more sorely needed. The importance of conducting biological studies under various behavioral conditions has already been highlighted in the previously cited work of Weinberger et al. (40). This shift in experimental paradigm may prove to be analogous to paradigmatic shifts involving temporal approaches that have yielded new developments in affective disorders.

Finally, as we contemplate the excitement of neuroscience advances and the potential of new investigative tools, we should not lose sight of the fundamental importance of careful clinical observation. In this regard, the recent emergence of reliable criteria for diagnosis is double-edged. On the one hand, the criteria can help by serving as a frame of reference for new observations, but on the other hand, they can lock us into the present by encouraging a false sense of closure. The great European tradition of descriptive psychiatry virtually died out early in this century—consumed on the continent by two world wars and in the United States diverted by efforts to extend psychoanalytic models to the major disorders. Descriptive psychiatry must now be reinvigorated if we are to realize the clinical potential of the brain sciences.

REFERENCES

1. Andrulonis, P. A., Glueck, B. C., Stroebel, C. F., Vogel, N. G., Shapiro, A. L., and Aldridge, D. M. (1981): *Psychiatr. Clin. North Am.,* 4:47–66.
2. Angel, I., Goldman, M. E., Skolnick, P., Pisano, J. J., and Paul, S. M. (1985): In: *Endocoids,* edited by H. Lal, F. LaBella, and J. Lane, pp. 457–464. Alan R. Liss, New York.
3. Barnstable, C., Jessell, T., Sanes, J., Stevens, C., and Robertson, M. (1983): *Nature,* 306:14–16.
4. Blackburn, M. R. (1982): *Psychopharmacol. Bull.,* 18:51–55.
5. Brown, R., Colter, N., Corsellis, J. A. N., Crow, T. J., Firth, C. D., Jague, R., Johnstone, E. C., and Marsh, L. (1986): *Arch. Gen. Psychiatry,* 43:36–42.
6. Callaway, E., and Naghdi, S. (1982): *Arch. Gen. Psychiatry,* 39:339–350.
7. Cohen, R. M., Semple, W. E., and Gross, M. (1986): *Psychiatr. Clin. North Am.,* 9:63–79.
8. Copper, A. M. (1985): *Am. J. Psychiatry,* 142:1395–1402.
9. DeLisi, L. E., and Wyatt, R. J. (1985): In: *Handbook of Neurochemistry, Vol. 10,* edited by A. Lajtha, pp. 553–587. Plenum Publishing, New York.
10. Edlund, M. J., Overall, J. E., and Rhoades, H. M. (1985): *J. Psychiatr. Res.,* 19:563–567.
11. Evarts, E. V., Shinoda, Y., and Wise, S. P. (1984): In: *Neurophysiological Approaches to Higher Brain Function,* pp. 65–89. John Wiley and Sons, New York.
12. Ferrero, P., Guidotti, A., Conti-Tronconi, B., and Costa, E. (1984): *Neuropharmacology,* 23:1359–1362.
13. Gershon, E. S., Weissman, M. M., Guroff, J. J., Prusoff, B. A., and Leckman, J. F. (1986): *J. Affective Disord.,* 11:125–131.
14. Geyer, M. A. (1982): *Psychopharmacol. Bull.,* 18:48–51.
15. Goodwin, F. K. (1984): In: *Frontiers in Biochemical and Pharmacological Research in Depression,* edited by E. Usdin, pp. 11–26. Raven Press, New York.
16. Goodwin, F. K., and Jamison, K. R. (1988): In: *Manic-Depressive Illness,* Oxford University Press, New York (*in press*).
17. Gusella, J. F., Tanzi, R. E., Anderson, M. A., Hobes, W., Gibbons, K., Raschtchian, R., Gilliam, T. C., Wallace, M. R., Wexler, N. S., and Conneally, P. M. (1984): *Science,* 225:1320–1326.
18. Jablensky, A. (1984): *J. Psychiatric Res.,* 18:541–554.
19. Jeste, D. V., and Goodwin, F. K. (1987): *Am. J. Psychiatry* (*in press*).
20. Kupfer, D. J., and Rush, A. J. (1983): *Arch. Gen. Psychiatry,* 40:1031.
21. Majewska, M. D., Harrison, N. L., Schwartz, R. D., Barker, J. L., and Paul, S. M. (1986): *Science,* 232:1004–1007.
22. Mandell, A. J. (1982): *Psychopharmacol. Bull.,* 18:59–63.
23. Mandell, A. J., Knapp, S., Ehlers, C., and Russo, P. V. (1984): In: *Neurobiology of Mood Disorders,* edited by R. M. Post and J. C. Ballenger, pp. 744–776. Williams and Wilkins, Baltimore.
24. Mandell, A. J., and Russo, P. V. (1981): *J. Neurosci.,* 1:380–389.
25. Milner, B. (1964): In: *The Frontal Granular Cortex and Behavior,* edited by J. M. Warren and K. Akert, pp. 313–334. McGraw-Hill, New York.
26. Newmark, P. (1983): *Nature,* 303:665.
27. Pert, C. B., Pert, A., Chang, J.-K., and Fong, B. T. W. (1976): *Science,* 194:330–332.
28. Pert, C. B., and Snyder, S. H. (1973): *Science,* 179:1011–1014.
29. Phelps, M. E., and Mazziotta, J. C. (1985): *Science,* 228:799–809.
30. Polsky, R., and McGuire, M. T. (1979): *J. Nerv. Ment. Dis.,* 167:56–65.
31. Post, R. M., and Ballenger, J. C. (1984): In: *Neurobiology of Mood Disorders,* edited by R. M. Post and J. C. Ballenger, pp. vii–viii. Williams and Wilkins, Baltimore.
32. Post, R. M., Rubinow, D. R., and Ballenger, J. C. (1984): In: *Neurobiology of Mood Disorders,* edited by R. M. Post and J. C. Ballenger, pp. 432–466. Williams and Wilkins, Baltimore.
33. Raleigh, M. J., McGuire, M. T., Brammer, G. L., and Yuwiler, A. (1984): *Arch. Gen. Psychiatry,* 41:405–410.
34. Rose, S. P. R. (1984): *J. Psychiatry Res.,* 18:351–360.
35. Siegel, S. (1979): In: *Psychopathology in Animals: Research and Clinical Applications,* edited by J. D. Keehn, pp. 143–165. Academic Press, New York.
36. Siever, L. J., and Davis, K. L. (1985): *Am. J. Psychiatry,* 142:1017–1031.
37. Smith, E. M., and Blalock, J. E. (1981): *Proc. Natl. Acad. Sci. USA,* 78:7530–7534.
38. Squires, R. F., and Braestrup, C. (1977): *Nature,* 266:732–734.
39. Wehr, T. A., Wirz-Justice, A., Goodwin, F. K., Duncan, W., and Gillin, J. C. (1979): *Science,* 206:710–713.
40. Weinberger, D. R., Berman, K. F., and Zec, R. F. (1986): *Arch. Gen. Psychiatry,* 43:114–125.
41. Wietgrefe, S., Zupancic, M., Haase, A., Chesebro, B., Race, R., Frey, W., Rustan, T., and Freidman, R. L. (1985): *Science,* 230:1177–1179.
42. Wilson, E. O. (1978): *On Human Nature.* Harvard University Press, Cambridge.
43. Wirz-Justice, A., Wehr, T. A., Goodwin, F. K., Kafka, M. S., Naber, D., Marangos, P. J., and Campbell, I. C. (1980): *Psychopharmacol. Bull.,* 16:45–52.
44. Yalow, R. S. (1986): *Biol. Psychiatry,* 21:1–2.
45. Zis, A. P., and Goodwin, F. K. (1979): *Arch. Gen. Psychiatry,* 36:835–839.

Psychopharmacology:
The Third Generation of Progress,
edited by Herbert Y. Meltzer.
Raven Press, New York © 1987.

CHAPTER **184**

Future Prospects for Clinical Psychopharmacology

Gerald L. Klerman

In this chapter I attempt an assessment of the future prospects of clinical psychopharmacology, especially in the next decade.

Any assessment of the future of human endeavor is influenced by the assessment of the current situation. In psychopharmacology, currently, there is a mixture of optimism and pessimism. Compared to 25 years ago, at the founding of the American College of Neuropsychopharmacology, progress has been considerable. Although the pace of introduction of new therapeutic compounds has slowed considerably (Chapter 3), advances in neuroscience, molecular biology, genetics, and brain imaging are rapid and exciting. Researchers in psychopharmacology are optimistic. Researchers are confident that given enough time and resources—especially space, funding, and access to patients—research will yield new knowledge. Moreover, they are confident that the rational development of new therapeutic interventions will derive from basic knowledge of neuroscience.

However, the practitioners of clinical psychiatry (especially the psychotherapists, but also biological psychiatrists and psychopharmacologists) are less optimistic. There is a sense of malaise: In fact, many are pessimistic. The limitations of existing treatments are too readily apparent, and economic regulations weigh heavily on practitioners and hospital and academic administrators as national efforts to control the federal deficit and rising health care costs restrict clinical practice and research. Among researchers, especially

young researchers, there is apprehension that future funding will be limited.

Much of this malaise derives from outside psychopharmacology, mostly from the state of political and national economic forces. However, other aspects of our malaise derive from limitations inherent in our current treatment technologies. Our treatments have serious adverse effects for some patients: tardive dyskinesia with the neuroleptics, hypertensive crises with monoamine oxidase inhibitors. Among depressives there is a growing group of patients resistant to electroconvulsive therapy and other forms of treatment.

Given this situation, how can we approach an assessment of the next decades? To the extent that the past is a valid guide to the future, the future of clinical psychopharmacology, at least as far as the development of new therapeutic agents is concerned, is predictably unpredictable. Most of the major therapeutic advances in our field have come from serendipity rather than from the rational development of new drugs. What serendipitous discoveries lie ahead cannot be clearly stated. However, from the perspective of a clinical psychopharmacologist one can identify what the needs are and indicate not only what is hoped for, but, perhaps also, in what direction future knowledge may lie.

In my attempt to assess the future, I will first outline my views of the ideal paradigm of medical research and therapeutics, then discuss the state of clinical psychopharmacology in general; following which I will focus on one disorder, schizophrenia, and predict how the future may achieve this ideal.

THE IDEAL PARADIGM: RATIONAL DEVELOPMENT OF THERAPEUTIC AGENTS FOR PSYCHIATRIC DISORDERS

Since the late eighteenth century, Western medicine has been dominated by a view of the ideal development of therapeutics. In this ideal, treatments (pharmacologic, surgical, or even psychotherapeutic) are developed from an understanding of the etiology and pathophysiology of the disease to be treated. Understanding of diseases best derives from scientific investigation of biological processes.

This complex of ideas constitutes what Thomas Kuhn, the historian of science, calls a "paradigm." A scientific problem is shared by a group of investigators who form a community. In Kuhn's view, scientific change occurs with the emergence of new paradigms to solve difficult problems. The history of a science is the chronicle of the emergence, victory, and downfall of paradigms. Scientific fields are the areas for competition among paradigms attempting to understand some aspect of natural or human functioning.

Today we take this paradigm for granted. We should remember that in the eighteenth century the medical paradigm for mental illness competed with paradigms of demonic possession and witchcraft, astrological influence, and religious retribution for sin and transgression.

Competing Paradigms in Psychiatric Illness: Continuum or Discrete Psychiatric Disorders

It is important to note that this modern paradigm presupposes a nosologic concept of multiple disease: Each disease will have its specific etiology and, hopefully, specific treatment. This concept of separate disorders derives from the writings of Sydenham and was applied to psychiatric disorders in the mid to late nineteenth century by French and German psychiatrists, culminating in the monumental work of Kraepelin and Bleuler.

The appropriateness of this approach to mental illness has frequently been the subject of controversy. After World War II the dominant paradigm in psychiatry was that there were no discrete mental illnesses, but rather a continuum from mental health, with psychosis being the most severe form of mental illness.

The dramatic clinical effects of new psychopharmacologic agents introduced in the early 1950s contributed to the downfall of the continuum of this paradigm. It became apparent that the clinical actions of the new drugs corresponded to the classical categories in psychiatry, i.e., an-

tianxiety, antidepressant, antimanic. When there was only one valued treatment, psychotherapy, as there was in the 1940s and 1950s, it did not matter what disorder the patient might have; but with the advent of treatments with selective and differential effects, the need for selection of patients for specific treatments, i.e., diagnosis, became evident.

American psychiatry underwent a major paradigm shift in the 1960s. Diagnostic categories were employed and the role of manifest symptoms and descriptive psychopathology in diagnosis became important [Klerman in *Diagnostic and Statistical Manual of Mental Disorders*, 3rd edition, International Volume (DSM-III)].

Specificity of Treatment

The greatest specificity occurs when treatments impact on some etiologic agent. Treatments other than those of this nature are considered less than ideal and are often called "nonspecific." The goal of therapeutic research has been to develop drugs with greater and greater specificity.

This goal has been best achieved for infectious diseases, for nutritional deficiencies, and for endocrinopathies. Such disorders were considered serious psychiatric problems which have largely disappeared because of the success of preventive and therapeutic agents. Consequently, today, psychiatrists see less frequently the delirium associated with fevers due to infection. Significantly, general paresis due to central nervous system syphilis is now almost nonexistent. It is to be noted that CNS syphilis made up about 15% of admissions to public mental hospitals. Pellagra, due to vitamin B_6 deficiency, also previously of high prevalence, is no longer found in the United States due to vitamin-supplemental dietary foods, particularly bread.

Thus, what we now treat are not disorders for which we know the etiology, but various syndromal disorders: depressions, psychoses, dementias, etc. Does this mean that the treatments we have are *just* symptomatic treatments?

Psychopharmacology and Treatments of the Middle Ground

In the classic view of therapeutics there are two types of specific treatments, such as antibiotics and vitamins, and other interventions that are relegated to the category of care and management. In the absence of specific treatments (i.e., those directed at etiology), the role of the clinician is one of healer: to provide humane care and management, to reduce symptomatic distress, and to minimize social disability. In my opinion it is necessary to modify this view of therapeutics to take note of new classes of treatments

TABLE 1. *Older view of treatment goals*

Type of treatment	Treatment target	Role of the doctor	Examples from medicine	Examples from psychiatry
Specific treatment	Causal agent	Scientific medicine	Antibiotics	Penicillin for CNS syphilis
Nonspecific	Symptoms	Care and management	Analgesics for pain	Barbiturates for insomnia

TABLE 2. *Revised view of treatment*

	Level of clinical intervention		Examples of medical diseases	Examples of psychiatric disorders
Specific treatments	Etiologic agent	Bacterial agents	Antibiotics	CNS Syphilis
Treatments of middle ground	Pathophysiology of syndrome	Reverse pathological process	Diuretics/hypertension	Antidepressants
Care and management	Symptom formation	Relieve distress of particular symptoms	Aspirin/fever	Barbiturates/insomnia

whose action is specific, however, not at the level of etiology, i.e., agents, but at the level of syndrome. I call these interventions "treatments of the middle ground."

Many of the important treatments developed since World War II in medicine as well as in psychiatry have been of this intermediate nature. Drugs such as steroids for asthma and other allergic disorders, diuretics for hypertension, and insulin for diabetes reverse abnormal homeostatic mechanisms and alter the pathophysiologic basis for the clinical syndrome. They seldom attack the specific etiologic process.

Treatments of the middle ground have a number of features in common. The syndromes that they treat are often chronic or recurrent. Left untreated, the pathophysiologic process produces progressive disability and often premature death. When treatments of the middle ground are successful, the rate of deterioration is slowed and at times even stopped, and the degree of symptomatic distress and social disability markedly reduced. Because these treatments are seldom etiologic, they often require long-term application.

The etiology of most of these syndromes is unknown. One possibility is that they may be heterogeneous as to etiology, and thus, there may be multiple diseases that present a common clinical syndrome. The other view is that of multifactorial causation. Thus, we do not know the etiology of hypertension or of arteriosclerosis. In this respect, our colleagues in internal medicine have a similar situation to psychiatry. As in schizophrenia and bipolar disease, it is uncertain whether we are dealing with heterogeneous clinical conditions or, as is often suggested, a multifactorial model, in which genetic, social status, and life style factors play a role. However, our colleagues in internal medicine know more about the pathophysiology of the conditions and are better able to identify and test the nature of the disturbances. Nevertheless, from the point of view of treatment, we are in similar situations. The treatments we have in psychiatry are of this nature; they are treatments of the middle ground.

The Developing Therapies Aimed at Etiology

The success in psychopharmacology has been to make available treatments of the middle ground for psychiatric disorders: for syndromes such as psychoses, depression, mania, and panic anxiety. Previously, syndromal treatments were not available for the majority of patients under psychiatric care, particularly for the "functional" psychoses. Not only did these new drugs significantly revolutionize the pattern of psychiatric care, they contributed to a significant paradigm shift in psychiatry. It soon developed that the best conceptual basis for understanding these drugs' clinical action was to reevaluate the classic syndromes described in nineteenth-century psychiatry. The actions of the new drugs corresponded roughly to the categories of syndromes described by the generation of Kraepelin, Bleuler, and the other French, German, and English observers of the nineteenth century. This had a profound impact on the intellectual trends in psychiatry and resulted in a reawakening.

In my view, psychopharmacology is now eagerly poised to move from treatments of the middle ground, aimed at reversing the pathophysiology of syndromes, to the rational development of treatment aimed at etiologic agents. In this process, not only will important knowledge be required from basic sciences, such as neuroscience and molecular biology, but the current role of the clinical investigator will require modification.

THE CURRENT STATE OF KNOWLEDGE IN SCHIZOPHRENIA

Rather than survey the future range of clinical applications of psychopharmacology, I have chosen to focus on one disorder, schizophrenia, and review the current situation in some depth with the intent of identifying future prospects.

The field of schizophrenia illustrates many of the points I have described in my general view of therapeutic paradigms. Significantly, schizophrenia also illustrates some important aspects of the interplay among scientific research, clinical practice, and public policy and politics.

Schizophrenia, because of its high rate of chronicity and the extensive social disability it engenders in patients, contributes heavily to the public costs of mental illness. Government agencies assume responsibility for the care of schizophrenics whether in institutions or deinstitutionalized. For many centuries, this aspect of psychiatry has been the focus of public attention and often of friction and misunderstanding among the public at large, government officials, and psychiatric physicians.

Background

The first two effective antipsychotic drugs, chlorpromazine, the prototypic phenothiazine, and reserpine, the prototypic rauwolfia derivative, were discovered to be clinically effective by serendipity.

Chlorpromazine was synthesized and developed at the Rhone-Poulenc Laboratories in France in their search for a more effective antihistamine agent. Clinical observations by Laborit, a surgeon who was investigating treatments of shock, and by anesthesiologists led Delay and Denniker to use the compound between 1950 and 1952 to treat acutely excited psychotics, mainly manics and schizophrenics. H. Lehmann replicated their observations in Montreal, Canada, and by 1954 the new age of psychopharmacology had begun.

At the same time, researchers at CIBA had isolated reserpine as one of the active ingredients of rauwolfia serpentine, "the snake root," used in India. Clinicians found it reduced blood pressure. Although reserpine was primarily developed for its antihypertensive action, it was soon observed by Kline to have antipsychotic actions. Were reserpine to be the only antipsychotic compound available, it would be considered highly desirable. However, it was soon shown to be less clinically effective than the phenothiazines. Research on rauwolfia contributed to the knowledge in neuropharmacology, particularly the observations of its depletion of biogenic amines, including dopamine, norepinephrine, and serotonin.

The concept of "neuroleptic" was proposed by the French clinicians in the mid-1950s to emphasize the apparent unity of antipsychotic efficacy with extrapyramidal effects. It was almost a decade later that basic research in neuropharmacology showed dopamine to be the neurotransmitter involved in the extrapyramidal actions. During the 1960s and 1970s, the anatomy of dopamine neurons and their terminals, its synthesis and metabolism were extensively studied. In these neuropharmacologic discoveries, the Swedish investigators were preeminent.

The hypothesis linking the clinical effects of neuroleptic to the actions of dopamine, has provided the basis for scientific understanding of neuroleptic actions in relationship to schizophrenia. The neurotransmitter approach to understanding the pathophysiology of schizophrenia was paralleled in the affective disorders by the intellectual excitement generated in the mid-1960s by the catecholamine theory. In the 1970s, rethinking of the nature of anxiety was provided by the discovery of the benzodiazepine receptor and its relationship to the neurotransmitter γ-aminobutyric acid (GABA).

The Past Decade: Loss of Momentum in Research on Schizophrenia

We must acknowledge that the past decade has not been one of great optimism and triumph in the field of schizophrenia and the field has not flourished. This has recently become the matter of concern in Congress and in the federal agencies as well as among scientists, clinicians, and even the families of patients with this disorder.

As has been noted by Hollister and others, we have not had any dramatically new drugs for schizophrenia. The drugs we have seem replicas of the classic neuroleptics, the phenothiazines and the butyrophenones, with their variable ability to block dopamine at postsynaptic receptors. Tragi-

cally, at the same time the growing frequency of tardive dyskinesia has set serious limits on therapeutic optimism and contributed to significant public policy debate.

These frustrations converge to emphasize a crucial therapeutic test of the dopamine hypothesis of schizophrenia. The hope was to develop a dopamine blocking agent with actions on the ONS urstate for cognitive and psychological efficacy of schizophrenia, but devoid of effects on extrapyramidal centers producing dyskinesia.

Neuroleptics, Tardive Dyskinesia, and Reinstitutionalization: The Limitations of Halfway Technologies

The current status of neuroleptic treatment of schizophrenia highlights problems of treatments of the middle ground. Lewis Thomas considers these treatments "halfway technologies." The neuroleptics have made our patients "better but not well." They have reduced psychotic symptoms and have contributed to shortened duration of hospital stay, thus reducing the hospital population. These effects are advantageous to patients and should be of benefit to society. However, translated into the public policy of deinstitutionalization, the results have had adverse consequences.

It is interesting to note that the beginning of psychopharmacology in the early 1950s coincided with the introduction of streptomycin and other drugs for the treatment of tuberculosis. We hoped that the patterns in psychiatry would follow those in tuberculosis. Like mental illness, tuberculosis had high prevalence and was a chronic disorder. It required major public responsibility. Most states had one or more sanitariums and there were statutes for compulsory treatment and involuntary hospitalization. Almost all the public TB hospitals have been closed or converted into chronic disease hospitals. Although the patient census of public mental hospitals has dropped dramatically from a peak of 600,000 in 1955 to below 150,000 in 1985, few of the mental hospitals have closed. In fact, there are more state mental hospitals today than in 1955. One of the important differences between drugs for TB and those for mental disorders is that drugs for TB cured the disease. Streptomycin was an antibiotic with specific action on the etiologic agent, the tubercular bacillus.

We do not know the agent for schizophrenia, or even whether there is one agent. In the 1950s, a number of agents were hypothesized, including schizophrenogenic mothers, social class, and urban poverty. These hypothesized agents were not substantiated by further research, and treatments derived from psychological and social theories proved to be inadequate.

The neuroleptic drugs, however, are treatments of the middle ground. The patients are sufficiently improved, but not well enough to be socially independent. The combination of limited technology plus social policy has contributed to large numbers of patients becoming discharged but remaining socially disabled and living in urban centers where there are inadequate community facilities for residential care or rehabilitation.

Deinstitutionalization as a public policy was the result of a curious alliance of civil libertarians (often with a romantic view of schizophrenia derived from the writings of Szasz and Laing) and fiscal conservatives interested mainly in reducing the expenditures of state budgets. The hope was that patients released into the community would lose their psychotic symptoms when embraced by a loving community. That hope proved ill-founded. The "locked door" has given way to the "revolving door," and with a growing housing shortage in major cities, the ranks of the homeless have increased. Approximately 50% of the homeless are mentally ill and have high rates of physical illness and are subject to molestation, rape, and robbery by urban predators. Interestingly, there is no call for reinstitutionalization, and when queried about their wishes, former mental patients rarely express the wish to return to the hospital. In this situation the profession of psychiatry has fared poorly. Psychiatrists on the one hand are attacked by civil libertarians and on the other hand blamed by families for the ravages of tardive dyskinesia.

I believe research and therapeutic efforts on schizophrenia have lost considerable momentum in the past decade. The excitement in psychopharmacology has been in the other fields, such as in depression, with the better understanding of the newer antidepressants and the development of highly specific serotonin-blocking agents. In the field of anxiety, the clinical separation of panic anxiety from generalized anxiety has generated new research on the pathophysiology of anxiety and the use of the lactate infusion as an experimental model for panic anxiety, contributing not only to validity of diagnosis, but also to a testing of hypotheses as to the pathophysiology of this form of anxiety.

Interest in schizophrenia research seemed to decrease. Many psychiatrists withdrew from public hospitals. In keeping with the conservatism of the time, the interest in public psychiatry in community mental health has gradually decreased, and the number of psychiatrists serving as commissioners of mental health in the various states, or as superintendents of mental hospitals, has greatly decreased. In part, this is a defensive response to the public criticism of psychiatry, but also, it is an awareness of the frustrations inherent in current treatments.

FUTURE PROSPECTS FOR SCHIZOPHRENIA

There are encouraging signs that this situation is about to be altered. Influential members of Congress, particularly the Senate, have expressed their interest in seeking ways to intensify efforts in schizophrenia and chronic mental illness. The National Institute of Mental Health (NIMH) in its recent reorganization has created a schizophrenia research branch and developed strategies for increased activity in this area.

We are, thus, in a position to expect that the next decade will offer more hope. Among the urgent priorities are some immediate treatment needs, as well as long-term strategies to develop interventions aimed at etiologic agents and processes, as is currently the case, rather than treatments of the middle ground.

Immediate Treatment Needs

First: to develop effective treatments for tardive dyskinesia.

Second: to perfect a neuroleptic drug with minimum or no effects on extrapyramidal systems.

In both of these efforts, the hope is that recent knowledge of neuropharmacology of the dopamine system will enhance the ability of medicinal chemists to target compounds.

We know a great deal about the dopamine receptors system, particularly the role of D1 and D2, and the changes that are likely to have occurred in tardive dyskinesia. The concept that supersensitivity of the dopamine receptor is the mechanism for tardive dyskinesia has been widely accepted but is now being challenged by some respected authorities. Hopefully, it will be possible to develop antipsychotic compounds that will not produce tardive dyskinesia and permit a resolution of its symptoms in those that already experience its ravages. Clozapine may be such a compound but it produces a high rate of granulocytopenia.

Similarly, knowledge of the dopaminergic system gives hope of the development of a new safer clozapine-like compound. The excitement generated by clozapine was based on its clinical efficacy combined with its almost complete absence of extrapyramidal side effects. This clinical pattern was paralleled by neuropharmacologic findings that indicated high affinity for dopamine receptors in projections to the frontal cortex and minimal effects on projections to the basal ganglia.

Testing the Dopamine Cortex Theory

One reason the dopamine theory of schizophrenia has lost some of its momentum in the 1970s is the lack of suitable methods for demonstrating abnormalities in patients *in vivo,* particularly to demonstrate the hypothesized changes in dopamine metabolism postulated by the dopamine hypothesis at specific anatomical sites.

We know most about the dopaminergic projections to the hypothalmus which are related functionally to the control of hormonal secretion by the anterior pituitary, particularly prolactin. This is related to the clinical use of prolactin measures as an indicator of neuroleptic effect.

Similarly, we know a great deal about the role of the dopamine system in the regulation of the functioning of the extrapyramidal motor system. This knowledge formed the basis of our understanding of the adverse extrapyramidal effects, as well as the successful dopa treatment of Parkinson's disease.

Recent knowledge indicates that there is more than one dopamine receptor, and the multiplicity of dopamine receptors offers the hope that the different receptors will be related to different biological functions.

At this point we should recall that the frontal cortex has been for many decades implicated in the pathogenesis of schizophrenia. Prefrontal lobotomy, one of the most controversial treatments in the history of psychiatry, was developed serendipitously by E. Moniz, a Portuguese neurosurgeon, who observed changes in the thinking behavior of a patient following a traumatic injury to the frontal area of the patient's brain.

However, abnormalities in frontal cortex in schizophrenics have not been demonstrated by conventional neuropathologic techniques, and autopsy studies have been inconclusive.

For the past few years, it appears that brain imaging techniques are beginning to prove fruitful. Earlier findings using computerized axial tomography (CAT) scan imaging demonstrated enlarged cerebral ventricles in schizophrenia and contributed to a renewed search for abnormalities in the frontal lobe. Earlier reports of frontal asymmetry were difficult to confirm. However, the recent research conducted by the NIMH group (11), using positron emission tomography (PET) scan, and the Iowa group (1,9), using nuclear magnetic resonance (NMR), indicates the increasing evidence for structural abnormalities in the frontal systems in schizophrenia. Convergence of findings from these two methodologies gives greater validity to the findings. Thus, three aspects of schizophrenia have been unified:

1. Structural abnormalities in the frontal lobe
2. Changes in attention and cognition, particularly manifested by negative systems
3. Dopamine action in CNS

Movement from Syndromal to Etiologic Focus

It can be argued, however, that these changes in dopamine metabolism are more indicative of the syndrome of psychosis than specific to the etiology of schizophrenia. It is to be noted that dopamine abnormalities have also been implicated in the effects of cocaine, and the cocaine psychosis in many respects is a far better model of psychosis for schizophrenia than LSD and other hallucinogens.

The dopamine hypothesis appears to be an increasingly convincing explanation of the pathophysiology of psychotic states. Neuroleptic treatment is a treatment of the middle ground. How to move from an understanding of the pathophysiology to etiology is a challenge. There are two lines of investigation that seem to offer promise: the frontal lobe structures lesion and the genetic hypothesis.

A possible viral agent has received far less attention and empirical support than the genetic hypothesis. Torrey and others have pointed out that schizophrenia was not described in the clinical literature before the late eighteenth and early nineteenth centuries. Although there were many descriptions of visual hallucinations and other psychotic states throughout the ancient, medieval, and Renaissance periods, there are no convincing descriptions of schizophrenia in the ancient literature commensurate with the excellent clinical descriptions of mania, depression, and dementia. Partial support for a viral hypothesis came from the Moscow investigators who claimed changes in immune responses in schizophrenics. However, their results have only partially been substantiated by the multinational World Health Organization (WHO) study. The recent techniques of immunology have only begun to be applied to possible abnormalities in schizophrenia. However, viral factors have been implicated in two other disorders with similarities in clinical history to schizophrenia. The demonstration of a latent virus in Kuru has given greater credence to the role of viruses in CNS diseases. More interesting is the relation-

ship between coxsackievirus and human lymphocyte antigen (HLA) antibodies in diabetes. It is now fairly well established that the juvenile form of diabetes is associated with a genetically determined abnormality in HLA antibodies and that children with this genetic vulnerability, when exposed to an infection with the coxsackievirus, develop damage to the pancreas. Thus, a genetic predisposition becomes clinically manifest only when exposed to a specific environmental stimulus.

A *genetic abnormality* in schizophrenia, or at least in some subtypes, has gained increasing acceptance, particularly from the data derived from twin studies and from the Scandinavian adoption studies. Translating these findings of population genetics into laboratory genetics is only now beginning. A number of informative families are being gathered by investigators, such as Rettenberg in Sweden and Kendler. This is a promising area and the techniques are just being applied to schizophrenia.

Further progress in elucidating possible genetic contributions in schizophrenia is dependent on important developments in clinical research, particularly genetic epidemiology. Numerous observers have pointed out the great potential of the techniques of molecular biology and their potential application to psychiatry. The example of Huntington's disease is informative. The breakthrough with this disease came with the identification of informative families in Venezuela willing to identify the chromosome on which the Huntington gene is likely to reside.

Similar to the advances in the understanding of Huntington's disease are advances in muscular dystrophy.

CONCLUSIONS: THE ROLE OF THE CLINICAL INVESTIGATOR

It is useful to conclude with a reassessment of the role of clinical investigators. In clinical psychopharmacology, the major role of the clinical investigator has been to design, conduct, and analyze data from clinical trials to test the efficacy of therapeutic agents. Clearly, one of the main contributions of psychopharmacology to clinical research has been the stimulus provided for the improvement of methodology: The techniques of the randomized trial have had profound impact on all clinical research.

Techniques of sampling, rating scale development, and use of multivariant statistics were perfected in the 1960s in the attempt to demonstrate the efficacy of the new drugs against the many skeptics and critics. Recently, new techniques have been developed for the assessment of diagnostic classes. Structured interviews, such as the SADS-RDC, the DIS, the PSE, and SCID, have evolved to insure comprehensive and systematic assessment of current and past psychopathology. These interview techniques have been linked to operational criteria embodied in the RDC, the DSM-III, and, hopefully, the ICD-10. Thus, there has been a reciprocal and iterative process whereby problems in clinical research have contributed to basic psychopharmacology.

Given these developments, the skills required of clinical investigators will increasingly be quantitative: knowledge of advanced techniques in statistical method plus development of mathematical models appropriate to testing hypotheses, be they genetic, neurochemical, or viral.

The art of prophecy is far from being a science. The history of clinical psychopharmacology, as has often been noted, is mainly that of a serendipitous discovery of new compounds. The hope of movement from serendipity to rational development of therapies remains a goal of psychopharmacology. The application of recent knowledge to schizophrenia indicates the directions in which progress is likely to occur. Hopefully, the next decade will be more fruitful and productive than the recent decade has been.

REFERENCES

1. Andreasen, N., Nasrallah, H. A., Dunn, V., Olson, S. C., Grove, W. M., Ehrardt, J. C., Coffman, J. A., and Crossett, J. H. W. (1986): *Arch. Gen. Psychiatry,* 43:136–144.
2. Berman, K. F., Zec, R. F., and Weinberger, D. R. (1986): *Arch. Gen. Psychiatry,* 43:126–135.
3. Black, J. L., and Richelson, J. W. (1985): *Mayo Clin. Proc.,* 60:777–789.
4. Dakis, C. A., and Gold, M. S. (1985): *Neurosci. Biobehav. Rev.,* 9:469–477.
5. DeLisi, L. E., Goldin, L. R., Hamovit, J. R., Maxwell, M. E., Kurtz, D., and Gershon, E. S. (1986): *Arch. Gen. Psychiatry,* 43:148–153.
6. Leff, J. (1985): In: *Recent Advances in Clinical Psychiatry, Vol 5,* edited by K. Granville-Grossman. Churchill Livingston, London.
7. Linn, S. C., Olson, K. C., Okazaki, H., and Richelson, E. (1986): *J. Neurochem.,* 46:274–279.
8. McGlashon, T. H. (1986): *Arch. Gen. Psychiatry,* 43:167–176.
9. Nasrallah, H. A., Olson, S. C., McCalley-Whitters, M., Chapman, S., and Jacoby, C. G. (1986): *Arch. Gen. Psychiatry,* 43:157–159.
10. Stahl, S. M., Thiemann, S., Faull, K. F., Barchus, J. D., and Berger, P. A. (1986): *Arch. Gen. Psychiatry,* 43:161–164.
11. Weinberger, D. R., Berman, K. F., and Zec, R. F. (1986): *Arch. Gen. Psychiatry,* 43:114–124.

Subject Index

urinary MHPG affected by, and attention deficit disorder with hyperactivity, 841

Desmethylchlordiazepoxide, formation of, in elderly, 1145

Desmethylclobazam, lipid solubility of, 1378

Desmethyldiazepam
lipid solubility of, 1378
and onset of action, 1379
pharmacokinetics of, hepatic dysfunction affecting, 1399,1400
plasma levels of, treatment response correlated with, 1333
plasma protein binding of, 1378–1379

N-Desmethyldiazepam
metabolism of, cigarette smoking affecting, 1400–1401
plasma levels of, and clearance concepts, 1326–1327

Desmethylflunitrazepam, lipid solubility of, 1378

Desmethylimipramine
antiarrhythmic effect of, 1440
binding, MAO inhibitors affecting, 548
cognition and memory affected by, 1468–1469
cortisol secretion affected by, and correlation between adult and childhood affective disorders, 854
maternal behavior affected by, 1480
for obsessive-compulsive disorder, in children, 1213
orthostatic hypotension caused by, 1438

Developmental disorders
axis II, pediatric psychopharmacology and diagnostic validity of, 1213–1214
pervasive. See Autism; Pervasive developmental disorders

Dexamethasone
carbamazepine affecting, 573
pharmacology of, dexamethasone suppression test outcome affected by, 609
receptors for, in brain, 596–597
suppression test. See Dexamethasone suppression test

Dexamethasone suppression test, 609–615
in elderly, as predictor of antidepressant treatment response, 1152
in psychiatry, 609–615
general approach to studies of, 610
as predictor of treatment response, 612–613,1033,1074,1152,1251
response to
in affective disorders, 610–611
age affecting, 595
in autism, 831
in childhood affective disorders, 853
circadian rhythm disturbances affecting, 598
correlation with other suicide markers, 662
drugs affecting, 592
in eating disorders, 1263
and β-endorphin activity, 640–641
factors influencing, 609–610
in major depressive disorder in children and adolescents, as predictor of imipramine response, 1251
in melancholia, 660–661
in obsessive-compulsive disorder, 1206
plasma tryptophan/amino acid ratio as predictor of, 516
as predictor of antidepressant treatment response, 612–613,1033,1152
as predictor of electroconvulsive therapy response, 578,1074
as predictor for suicide, 665–666

serotonergic mechanisms affecting, 518
somatostatin affecting, 624–625
specificity of, for depression, 611–612
in suicide attempters, 660–661
technique affecting, 609–610

Dexetimide, binding affinities of, 243

Dextroamphetamine
in attention deficit disorder with hyperactivity, noradrenergic effects of, 841
cortisol responses to, in depressed patients, 499
for depression in elderly, 1154–1155
growth hormone response to, in depressed patients, 498
for hyperactivity in children, and psychotherapy, 1220
for narcolepsy, 1309
for obesity, 1282
from side chain substitution of phenylisopropylamine, 1629

Dextrophan
competition of nalaxone binding by, 282
and PCP discriminative stimulus effects, 1575

DFP. See Anticholinesterase diisopropylfluorophosphate; Diisopropyl fluorophosphate

DHE. See Dihydroergocriptine

DHEA. See Dehydroepiandrosterone

DHLA. See Dihomo-γ-linoleic acid

Diabetes, α_2-adrenoceptor antagonists for, 153

Diacylglycerol
calcium release regulated by, 454
in PI cycle, 18
as second messenger, 96
as second messenger product, 322–323
tyrosine hydroxylase activity affected by, 75–76

1,2-Diacylglycerol
and α_1-adrenoceptors, 250–251
and H_1 receptors, 275–276

Diagnostic interview schedule, for diagnosis of anxiety, 1184–1185

Diagonal band of Broca, cholinergic neurons in, 212

Diagonal band-septum complex, galanin-positive cells in, 408

Diamino puridines, cholinergic function affected by, 225

Diazepam
abuse of, emergency treatment needed for, 1598
adenosine-mediated systems affecting, 295
aggressive behavior affected by, 700
for agitation in the elderly, 1174
for alcohol withdrawal syndrome, 1610
in alcoholics, use of, 1612
amnestic effects of, 221
as an antipsychotic, 32
for anxiety, 1195–1197
and behavioral effects of locus ceruleus stimulation, 969
and benzodiazepine recognition sites, 266–268
binding
in Alzheimer's disease, 892
electroconvulsive therapy affecting, 584
and impact of industry-discovered drugs on basic neuroscience, 1650–1651
inhibitor for, 429–434. See also Diazepam binding inhibitor
and cognitive impairment
age affecting, 1451–1452
alcohol affecting, 1452
caffeine affecting, 1452

dose-response relationships and, 1450–1451
disease-model approach to discovery of, 1638
drug effect offset curves for, 1363,1459
and drug interaction and cross tolerance, pharmacodynamic mechanisms affected by, 1464
extent of nonmedical use of, 1536–1537
frequency of use, 1378
and $GABA_A$ receptor function, 267
high-dosage, for acute schizophrenia, 1098–1099
hysteresis curves and, 1461
intravenous administration of, 1288
learning affected by, 1449
lipid solubility of, 1378
locus ceruleus neurons affected by, 167,968
memory affected by, 1449–1450
mesoprefrontal dopamine neurons affected by, 89
metabolism of
cigarette smoking affecting, 1400–1401
ethanol affecting, 1402
metabolites of, clinical importance of, 1383–1384
in neuroleptic malignant syndrome treatment, 1428
and onset of action, 1379
for panic disorder, 1200
performance affected by, 1450
pharmacokinetic and pharmacodynamic half-lives of, 1462
and pharmacokinetic-pharmacodynamic relationship, 1460–1464
pharmacokinetics of, 1381
in elderly, 1145
hepatic dysfunction affecting, 1399,1400
physical dependence following high daily doses, and withdrawal signs and symptoms, 1539
physical dependence following therapeutic doses, 1539–1540
plasma binding of, concentration at site of action affected by, 1328
plasma levels of
and clearance concepts, 1326–1327
clinical effects correlated with, 1460–1464
treatment response correlated with, 1333
plasma protein binding of, 1378–1379
reinforcing effects of, 1537–1538
serotonergic neurons affected by, 162
tic behaviors affected by, 1242–1243
withdrawal responses to, 1197
yohimbine-induced anxiety affected by, 987–988

Diazepam binding inhibitor, 428–434
biochemistry of, 429
brain distribution of, 430–432
dynamic equilibrium of, mRNA hybridization to study, 432–433
as endogenous anxiogenic substance, 982
as endogenous benzodiazepine receptor ligand, 267
GABA transmission modulated by, 433
histochemical studies of, 430–432
in human brain and cerebrospinal fluid, 434
pharmacology of, 429–430
physiological relevance of, 430–433
as precursor, 433
rat versus human, 434
release of, 432

Dichotomizing, in psychopharmacologic research, 1009

Extrapyramidal motor dysfunction, animal
   models of
   adrenal medulla grafts in, 474–475
   brain tissue transplantation in, 471–479
   and dissociated cells in brain tissue
     transplantation, 473
   functional effects of brain grafts in,
     472–473
   for Huntington's chorea, 477
   and immunology of brain tissue
     transplantation, 467
   intraocular grafting studies in, 471–472
   and limits of neurite growth in brain tissue
     transplantation, 467
   mechanisms of action of brain tissue
     transplantation in, 475–476
   and other behavioral effects of brain tissue
     transplantation, 473–474
   pheochromocytoma cell grafts in, 475
   and substantia nigra graft maturation,
     471–472
Extrapyramidal side effects, from
   neuroleptics, 1096–1097
   antiparkinson drugs for, 1097
Extrapyramidal syndrome, neuroleptic acute
   differential diagnosis of, 1412–1413
   as tardive dyskinesia risk factor, 1414

F

FAB/MS. *See* Fast atom bombardment mass
   spectrometry
Facial motor nucleus, 5-HT$_2$ receptors in, 146
Fallopian tubes, GABA in, 176
False transmitters
   acetylcholine synthesis affected by,
     234–235
   AF64A as, 344
   choline analogs as, 234–235
   cholinergic transmission affected by,
     234–235
   and experimental model of
     hypocholinergic state, 236
   and MAO inhibitors, 550
False-transmitter concept, 43
Family psychoeducation, in schizophrenia,
   1117
Family studies
   of alcoholism, 1527–1528,1529–1532
   of Alzheimer's disease, 930–931
   of autism, 827–828
   of childhood affective disorders, 845–847
   of chronic anxiety disorders, 961–962
   of major affective disorders, 482–483
   of panic and generalized anxiety disorders,
     1178,1180
   of panic disorder and agoraphobia, 1181
   of personality traits, 960–961
   of posttraumatic stress disorder, 1185
   of related disorders in relatives of affective
     patients, 483
   of schizophrenia, and viral etiology
     hypothesis, 766
   of simple phobias, 1182
   of somatization, 962–963
     Briquet's syndrome, 962–963
     diversiform somatization, 963
   of tic disorders, 1240–1241
Family therapy, in schizophrenia, 1115–1117
   behavioral, 1116–1117
   expressed emotion affecting, 1116
   and psychoeducation, 1117
   and variation of drug treatment,
     1115–1116
FAS. *See* Fetal alcohol syndrome
Fast atom bombardment mass spectrometry
   (FAB/MS), in search for neuropeptides,
   440–441

Fatty acids, in schizophrenia
   as prostaglandin precursors, 762–763
   supplementation of, in treatment for,
     763–764
Feedback pathways, A9 dopamine cells
   regulated by, 117–118
Feeding. *See* Eating
   sham. *See* Sham feeding
Femoxetine
   for depression, 34
   as developmental antidepressant, 1046
Fenfluramine
   antidepressant effects of, 519
   and 5-HT levels, autistic symptoms
     affected by, 831
   for infantile autism, 1227–1229
     biochemical abnormalities as rationale
      for treatment with, 1227
     indications for, 1226
   as modification of phenylisopropylamine,
     1627
   neurotoxic effect of, 363
   for obesity, 1282
   prolactin response in depressed patients
     affected by, 518
   receptor sensitivity to, clinical evaluation
     of, in depressed patients, 540
   REM sleep affected by, 514
   in schizophrenia, 754
   sexual behavior affected by, 1478
   structure of, 1627
   urinary MHPG affected by, and attention
     deficit disorder with hyperactivity, 841
Fengabine
   for depression, 189–190
   GABA$_B$ binding affected by, 190
Fenoldopam, as D$_1$ dopamine receptor
   agonist, 259
Fetal alcohol syndrome (FAS), 1518–1519
FG 7142 (methyl-β-carboline-3-
   carboxamide)
   dopamine metabolism affected by, 90
   unified approach to discovery of, 1643
Fisher statistic, for combining results from
   multiple independent trials, 1014
FK 33-824
   for affective disorder treatment, 642
   antipsychotic effects of, 735,1137
   and systems approach to CNS drug design,
     1641
Flagyl. *See* Metronidazole
Flame ionization detector, for gas
   chromatography measurement of
   plasma drug concentrations, 1324
Flunitrazepam
   and benzodiazepine recognition sites,
     266–268
   binding, in Alzheimer's disease, 892
   and colocalization of GABA and
     benzodiazepine binding sites, 427
   and GABA$_A$ receptor function, 267
   lipid solubility of, 1378
   pharmacokinetics of, 1381
   plasma protein binding of, 1378–1379
Fluorescence polarization, to study
   pharmacology of alcohol, 1521
5-Fluorotryptamine, phosphoinositide
   hydrolysis affected by, 96–98
Fluoxetine
   β-adrenoceptors affected by, 537
   antiobsessional properties of, 1209
   clinical effects of, 1043
   for depression, 34
   in elderly, efficacy of, 1150
   GABA$_B$ binding affected by, 190
   and 5-HT uptake blockade, 519–520
   interactions with, 1043
   major characteristics of, 1047

mania during treatment with, 521
   mechanism of action of, 519–520
   mechanism-based approach to discovery
     of, 1639
   overdosage of, 1043
   side effects of, 1043
   structure, pharmacology, development,
     and pharmacokinetics of, 1043
   uptake studies of, and impact of industry-
     discovered drugs on basic
     neuroscience, 1650
Flupentixol
   and D$_1$ and D$_2$ receptor binding, 258
   as D$_1$ dopamine receptor antagonist, 259
   and D$_1$ dopamine receptor labeling, 258
cis-Flupentixol
   dopamine dose-response curves affected
     by, 121–122
   receptor affinity profile of, 1130
Fluperlapine
   action of, 1134
   antipsychotic effect of, 1134
   receptor affinity profile of, 1130
Fluphenazine
   animal behavior affected by, 1469
   as D$_1$ dopamine receptor antagonist, 259
   depot injection of, 1288
   in elderly
     for agitation, 1170
     for depression, 1155
     efficacy of, 1150
   hepatotoxicity of, 1435
   in neuroleptic malignant syndrome, 1421
   plasma levels of
     clinical response correlated with,
      1334,1347–1348
     radioimmunoassay for, 1325
     radioreceptor assay for,
      1325–1326,1342–1343
   in schizophrenia
     dosage of, in long-term treatment,
      1106–1107
     and family therapy, 1115–1116
     high-dose, 1099
     and psychosocial treatment and
      compliance, 1112
   somatostatin affected by, 624
   therapeutic window for, 1347–1348
   tics suppressed by, 1241
Flurazepam
   blood levels of, in elderly, 1145
   and cognitive impairment, age affecting,
     1451–1452
   frequency of use, 1378
   lipid solubility of, 1378
   and onset of action, 1379
   performance affected by, 1450
   pharmacokinetics of, 1381
   physical dependence following therapeutic
     doses, 1539–1540
   for sleep disorders in elderly, 1162
Flurazepam aldehyde, lipid solubility of, 1378
Flurothyl, for seizure induction in affective
   disorders, 1073
Fluvoxamine
   cognition and memory affected by, 1468
   for depression, 34
   as developmental antidepressant, 1046
FMRF-NH$_2$, antibodies to, across species,
   442
Food, Drug, and Cosmetic Act,
   requirements of, 1678–1679
   and clinical investigations, 1678
   philosophical basis of, 1678–1679
Food and Drug Administration (FDA)
   and regulation of development of new
     drugs, 1675–1683
     historical background, 1675–1678

THIP for, 178
γ-vinyl GABA for, 179
HV interval, tricyclic antidepressants affecting, 1439
HVA. *See* Homovanillic acid
HW 165, as autoreceptor-selective agonist, 87
Hybridization, *in situ,* in search for neuropeptides, 443
Hydergine
  discovery of, for Alzheimer's disease, 1645
  and tardive dyskinesia treatment, 1417
Hydrazinopropionic acid, sexual behavior affected by, 1480
Hydrogen sulfide, for alcoholism treatment, 1611
Hydromorphone
  toxicity of, 1601
  use or abuse of, with alcohol, 1599
Hydroxyamitriptyline, plasma binding of, concentration at site of action affected by, 1238
γ-Hydroxybutyrate, for schizophrenia, 722,756
17-Hydroxycorticosteroids (17-OCHS), excretion of, in affective disorders, 599
Hydroxydesipramine
  elimination of, and renal function, 1359
  plasma levels of
    and clearance concepts, 1326–1327
    liquid chromatography measurement of, 1324
2-Hydroxydesipramine, increased steady-state concentrations of, in elderly, 1152–1153
8-Hydroxy-2-(di-*N*-propylamine)tetralin (8-OH-DPAT)
  appetite affected by, 514
  and 5-HT behavioral syndrome, 308
  and 5-HT receptors
    autoreceptors, 307
    classification of, 304
    5-HT₁ receptors, 305
    and 5-HT₁ₐ receptor selectivity, 145
  and MAO inhibitors, 548–549
  phosphoinositide hydrolysis affected by, 96–98
6-Hydroxydopa, as aminergic neurotoxin, 353
5-Hydroxydopamine, and localization of catecholamines, 49–59
6-Hydroxydopamine
  and β-adrenoceptor supersensitivity, lithium affecting, 560
  aggressive behavior affected by, 700–701
  as aminergic neurotoxin, 352–353
    mechanism of, 353
  carbamazepine affected by, 569
  and dopamine receptor supersensitivity, lithium affecting, 559
  drinking modulated by, 1269–1270
  maternal behavior affected by, 1480
  and methamphetamine-induced dopamine neurotoxicity, 361–362
  resistance to, by TIDA neurons, 130
  sexual behavior affected by, 1479
Hydroxyethyl flurazepam, lipid solubility of, 1378
Hydroxyimipramine, plasma levels of, liquid chromatography measurement of, 1324
2-Hydroxyimipramine, antiarrhythmic effect of, 1440
5-Hydroxyindoleacetic acid (5-HIAA)
  AF64A affecting, 344
  in affective disorders
    in CSF, 692
    as vulnerability marker, 487,488
  and aggressive behavior, CSF levels, 700
  in Alzheimer's disease, in CSF, 898,899
  in anorexia nervosa, in CSF, 1264

in anxiety, in CSF, 959
in bulimia, 1264
carbamazepine affecting, 569
CSF levels of
  and habituation, 665
  height, sex, and environmental factors affecting, 515
  personality traits and, 664
  tryptophan loading affecting, 515
CSF levels in depression, 515–516
  antidepressants affecting, 516
  correlation with brain 5-HIAA, 515
  depressive symptomatology and, 516
  electroconvulsive therapy affecting, 516
CSF levels and suicide, 516
  correlation with other suicide markers, 662
  low levels as vulnerability marker, 661–662
  as predictor of suicide, 661,665
  in suicide attempters, 657–658,659
in Down's syndrome, in CSF, 900
electroconvulsive therapy affecting, 578–579
lithium affecting, 555
MAO inhibitors affecting, 550,1299
methamphetamine affecting, 362–363
MPTP affecting, 354
in obsessive-compulsive disorder, 1208–1209
in postmortem brains of suicide victims, 656
as predictor of antidepressant response, 1033–1034
in premenstrual syndrome, 682
in prepubertal major depressive disorder, suicidal behavior and, 852
in schizophrenia
  in brain studies, 753–754
  in CSF, 754
  with lateral ventricular enlargement, 775
in Tourette's syndrome, in CSF, 1242
and violent behavior, CSF levels in, 663
Hydroxylation, of tricyclic antidepressants, 1353–1354
6-Hydroxymelatonin, studies of, in depressed patients, 501
1-Hydroxymethyl midazolam, lipid solubility of, 1378
p-Hydroxy-methylphenidate
  gas chromatography for measurement of, 1390
  in pharmacology of methylphenidate, 1389
4-Hydroxymidazolam, lipid solubility of, 1378
3-Hydroxy-*N*-allylmorphinan, competition of nalaxone binding by, 282
6-Hydroxynorepinephrine, as aminergic neurotoxin, 353
Hydroxynortriptyline
  elimination of, and renal function, 1359
  plasma binding of, concentration at site of action affected by, 1328
  plasma levels of, treatment response correlated with, 1330
10-Hydroxynortriptyline
  increased steady-state concentrations of, in elderly, 1152–1153
  plasma concentrations of, 34
5-Hydroxytryptamine
  action of, in facial motor nucleus, 146
  adenosine modulating release of, 292
  and adenylate cyclase/cyclic AMP signal cascade, 100–101
  AF64A affecting, 344
  in affective disorders, and learned helplessness studies, 693
  aggressive behavior affected by, 46,699

in Alzheimer's disease
  binding, 892
  presynaptic cortical transmitter activities of, 889,890
in autism, biochemical markers for, 1227
behavioral hyperactivity and, 308
carbamazepine affecting, 569
carbohydrate intake affected by, 1269
in central appetite regulation, 1268
coexistence with neuropeptides, 405
in cortex, laminar distribution of, 69–70
CRH/ACTH release affected by, 593
and cyclic AMP production, 101
  high-affinity system for, 101
depletion of, by methamphetamine, 362–363
in depression, 513–526
  animal models for, 515
  appetite affected by, 514
  body temperature affected by, 514
  circadian rhythms affected by, 514
  and electroconvulsive therapy, 521
  fenfluramine affecting, 519
  and 5-hydroxyindoleacetic acid levels in CSF, 515–516
  5-hydroxytryptophan affecting, 518–519
  lithium affecting, 556
  lithium potentiation of antidepressants and, 520–521
  and manic reactions following treatment, 521
  mood affected by, 514
  neuroendocrine studies of, 517–518
  and neurotransmission affected by antidepressants, 521
  and noradrenergic, dopaminergic, and GABAergic interaction, 522
  and organic brain diseases, 522
  pain sensitivity affected by, 514
  and plasma tryptophan levels, 516–517
  precursors affecting, 518–519
  sexual function affected by, 514
  sleep affected by, 514
  somatic functions affected by, 513–515
  tryptophan affecting, 518
  uptake and imipramine binding in platelets in, 517
  uptake blockers affecting, 519–520
and detection of satiety, 1261–1262
discovery of, 39
drinking modulated by, 1269–1270
electroconvulsive therapy affecting, 578–579
  in human studies, 583
  in rodents, 583
in ethanol-seeking behavior, 45
facial motoneurons affected by, 146
fluoxetine affecting, 1043
functions and pathophysiologic significance of, 45
high-affinity labeling of, 155–156
and 5-HT receptor labeling, 303
  5-HT₁c site, 305
  5-HT₂ site, 305–306
light-dark cycle affecting, 160–161
lithium affecting, 555–556
  animal studies of, 555–556
  clinical studies of, 556
locus ceruleus neurons affected by, 968
maternal behavior affected by, 1479
in mental functions, 39
in midbrain, physiology of, 141–149. *See also* Midbrain serotonin system
and monoamine oxidase
  inhibitors affecting, 1298,1299
  subtypes, 1299
motor and sensory processing and, 66
MPTP affecting, 354

5-Hydroxytryptamine *(contd.)*
  neuronal uptake of, presynpatic receptors
      modulating, 155–156
  neurophysiologic effects of, 307–308
  neurophysiologic sensitivity to,
      antidepressant treatment affecting,
      538
  in obsessive-compulsive disorder,
      1208–1209
  peptide coexistence affecting function of,
      411
  phencyclidine and, 1585–1586
  and phosphoinositide hydrolysis,
      activation of, 96–98
  precursors of, in depression, 518–519
  in premenstrual syndrome, 682
  receptors for. *See* 5-Hydroxytryptamine
      receptors
  release of
      5-HT autoreceptors modulating, 154
      and receptor-mediated changes, 101–102
  reuptake of
      clomipramine affecting, 1208–1209
      studies of, and impact of industry-
          discovered drugs on basic
          neuroscience, 1650–1651
  in schizophrenia
      brain studies in, 753–754
      evidence for, 754
      whole blood and platelet studies, 754
  and serotonin receptor classification, 304
  sexual behavior affected by, 1478
  sleep-wake cycle modulating, 161
  somatostatin affecting, 623
  and stress-induced changes in TIDA
      neurons, 137
  and suicide
      cortisol response in attempters, 658
      metabolites of, in attempters,
          657–658,659
      in postmortem brain, 654–657
      in prepubertal major depressive
          disorder, 852
      trazadone affecting, 1045
      in violent individuals, 663
5-Hydroxytryptamine autoreceptors, 307
  antagonists for, use in depression, 154
  appetite affected by, 514
  5-HT agonists and antagonists affecting,
      307
  5-HT$_{1A}$ subtype of, in dorsal raphe, 145
  presynaptic
      MAO inhibitors affecting, 1298
      and serotonin release, 154
5-Hydroxytryptamine motor syndrome, 146
5-Hydroxytryptamine receptors
  abnormalities in, in Alzheimer's disease,
      892
  activation of
      and adenylate cyclase/cyclic AMP signal
          cascade, 100–101
      and changes in 5-HT release, 101–102
      and hydrolysis of membrane
          phosphoinositides, 95–100
      neurochemical consequences of, 95–103
  and adenylate cyclase activity, 100
  and adenylate cyclase in hippocampus, 101
  antagonists, in schizophrenia, 1136
  antibody to, hyperserotonemia in autism
      caused by, 832
  antidepressant treatment affecting, 537,541
  binding studies of, 303–306
      and differentiation of receptor subtypes,
          304
      preliminary, 303–304
  classification of, 304
  clozapine affecting, 1133–1134
  in depression, 517

  and differentiation of receptor subtypes,
      future strategies for, 309
  down-regulation of, and monoamine
      oxidase inhibitors, 1298
  electroconvulsive therapy affecting, 579
  fluperlapine affecting, 1134
  lithium affecting, 561
  MAO inhibitors affecting, 548
  mianserin affecting, 1044
  on NCB-20 cells, 101
  and phosphoinositide hydrolysis, 96–100
      antagonists affecting, 98
  physiologic models of, 306–309
      autoreceptors and, 307
      behavioral studies and, 308
      neurophysiologic effects of 5-HT and,
          307–308
      phosphoinositide turnover and, 307
      serotonin-sensitive adenylate cyclase
          and, 306–307
  sensitivity of, clinical evaluation of, in
      depressed patients, 540
  subtypes, 95,304–306
      classification of, 144
      drugs selective for, 95
      functional correlates of, 306
      5-HT$_1$, 144–146,304. *See also* 5-HT$_1$
          receptors
      5-HT$_2$, 146–148. *See also* 5-HT$_2$
          receptors
      in mediation of behavior, 308
      physiologic correlates of, 144–148
  trazadone affecting, 1045
5-Hydroxytryptamine uptake blockers
  as antidepressants, 519–520
  behavioral effects of long-term treatment
      with, 538
  and monoamine oxidase inhibitor
      coadministration, 1038
  monoaminergic receptor sensitivity
      affected by, 536
  in social interaction studies of anxiety, 693
5-Hydroxytryptamine-immunoreactive
      (5-HT-IR) cells
  anatomic distribution of, 61–73
  in brainstem of *M. fascicularis,* 63,64
  cell bodies of, 61–66
      caudal brainstem group of, 64–66
      rostral brainstem group of, 62–64
  cellular organization of, 65–66
  in hypothalamus, 63–64,65
  in nucleus centralis superior, 62
  in nucleus prosupralemniscus, 62–63
  in nucleus raphe dorsalis, 62
  in nucleus raphe magnus, 64–65
  in nucleus raphe obscurus, 64
  in nucleus raphe pontis, 62
  in nucleus raphe ventricularis, 65
  in nucleus reticularis-paragigantocellularis
      lateralis, 65
  pathways of, 66–70
      ascending projections to forebrain,
          68–70
      in brainstem, 66
      descending projection to spinal cord
          and brainstem, 66–68
      dorsal raphe cortical tract, 68
      in hippocampus, 70
      medial forebrain bundle, 68
      raphe magnus spinal tract, 67
      raphe obscurus spinal tract, 66
      in spinal cord, 66–67
      subcortical distribution of, 69
      in substantia gelatinosa, 66–67
  in raphe pallidus, 64
5-Hydroxytryptophan (5-HTP)
  aggressive behavior affected by, 699
  antidepressant effect of, 518–519

  behavioral hyperactivity and, 308
  cortisol response to
      in affective disorders, 517
      correlation with other suicide markers,
          662
  mania or hypomania following treatment
      with, 521
  peptide coexistence affecting function of,
      411
  for preventive treatment of bipolar
      disorder, 1055
  prophylactic use of, 519
  receptor sensitivity to, clinical evaluation
      of, in depressed patients, 540
  in schizophrenics with lateral ventricular
      enlargement, 775
  and tardive dyskinesia treatment, 1416
D,L-5-Hydroxytryptophan (D,L-5-HTP),
      cortisol response to, in affective
      disorders, 517
L-5-Hydroxytryptophan
  antidepressant effect of, 518–519
  coadministration of, in depression,
      518–519
  hypomania during treatment with, 521
Hydroxyzine, as antianxiety agent, 1197
Hyperactivity, in children. *See also*
      Attention deficit disorder with
      hyperactivity
  bupropion for, 1223
  caffeine for, 1222
  clonidine for, 1223
  EEG event-related potentials in, 797
  failed treatments for, 1223
  magnesium pemoline for, 1222
  monoamine oxidase inhibitors for,
      1222–1223
  and pharmacotherapy and psychotherapy
      combined, 1219–1221
  pharmacotherapy of, 1215–1224
  psychostimulants for, 1215–1222
  and risk for alcoholism, 1531
Hyperammonemia, inborn metabolic
      disorder associated with, 862
Hypercortisolemia, agitated dysphoria
      associated with, 960
Hypercortisolism, in psychiatric disorders,
      620–622
Hyperdynamic β-adrenergic circulatory
      state, 986
Hyperglycinemia, idiopathic, inborn
      metabolic disorder associated with, 862
Hyperhidrosis, iontophoresis for, 1290
Hyperinsulinism, in violent individuals, 663
Hyperkinesia, initial, differential diagnosis
      of, 1412–1413
Hyperkinesis. *See* Attention deficit disorder
      with hyperactivity
Hyperlysinemia, inborn metabolic disorder
      associated with, 862
Hyperolinemia, inborn metabolic disorder
      associated with, 862
Hyperparathyroidism, and neuroleptic
      malignant syndrome, differential
      diagnosis of, 1423
Hyperphagia. *See* Eating disorders; Anorexia
      nervosa; Bulimia; Obesity
Hyperphenylalaninemia, 863–865. *See also*
      Phenylketonuria
Hyperpolarization, of dopamine neurons,
      intracellular recording of, 121
Hyperserotonemia, in autistic and mentally
      retarded patients, 830–831
  autoimmune processes in, 832
Hypertension
  α_1-adrenoceptor antagonists for, 152–153
  α_2-adrenoceptor agonists for, 153

DATE DUE